PRINCIPLES AND PRACTICE OF

Ophthalmic Plastic and Reconstructive Surgery

alibris

EXLIBOOKS
10600 DUTCHESS WAY
WOODSTOCK, MD 21163
UNITED STATES

To: ALIBRIS APEX DC 76906305-27
APEX
800 AVONDALE AVE.
GRANDVIEW HEIGHTS, OH 43212-3473

Shipping Instructions for EXLIBOOK

Print this Packing Slip and enclose inside the front cover of the book.

Please ship this item no later than Wed Sep 23, 2026.

Ship to:

ALIBRIS APEX DC 76906305-27
APEX
800 AVONDALE AVE.
GRANDVIEW HEIGHTS, OH 43212-3473
UNITED STATES

PN #	Item ID	Alibris ID	Media Type	Title / Author	Seller List Price	Order Date
76906305-27	FAL-533	B084287035	BOOK	Principles and Practice of Ophthalmic Plastic and Reconstructive Surgery Bosniak, Stephen, MD, Facs	$129.00	Sep, 11 2026

76906305-27

VOLUME I

PRINCIPLES AND PRACTICE OF

Ophthalmic Plastic and Reconstructive Surgery

Stephen Bosniak, M.D.
Associate Clinical Professor, State University of New York at Stony Brook;
Director, Ophthalmic Plastic and Reconstructive Surgery, Nassau County Hospital and Kings County Hospital;
and Associate Attending Surgeon, Manhattan Eye, Ear, and Throat Hospital and
New York Eye and Ear Infirmary, New York, New York

Section Editors

Giulio Bonavolontà, M.D.
Professor and Chairman of Ophthalmology (Eye Institute),
University of "Federica II" School of Medicine,
University of Naples,
Naples, Italy

Stephen Bosniak, M.D.
Associate Clinical Professor,
State University of New York at Stony Brook;
Director, Ophthalmic Plastic and Reconstructive Surgery,
Nassau County Hospital and Kings County Hospital;
and Associate Attending Surgeon, Manhattan Eye, Ear, and Throat Hospital
and New York Eye and Ear Infirmary,
New York, New York

Robert Alan Goldberg, M.D.
Associate Professor of Ophthalmology,
University of California, Los Angeles, School of Medicine;
and Chief, Orbital and Ophthalmic Plastic Surgery,
Jules Stein Eye Institute,
Los Angeles, California

Russell S. Gonnering, M.D.
Associate Professor of Ophthalmology,
University of Wisconsin School of Medicine;
and Active Staff, St. Luke's Medical Center,
Milwaukee, Wisconsin

James W. Karesh, M.D.
Assistant Professor, Johns Hopkins University School of Medicine, Wilmer Ophthalmologic Institute
and the University of Maryland School of Medicine;
Director, Ophthalmic Plastic and Reconstructive Surgery,
Krieger Eye Institute, Sinai Hospital of Baltimore,
Baltimore, Maryland

Don Liu, M.D.
Associate Professor, Department of Ophthalmology,
University of Southern California School of Medicine,
Los Angeles, California

Jeffrey A. Nerad, M.D.
Professor of Ophthalmology,
University of Iowa College of Medicine;
and Director, Oculoplastic, Orbital, and Oncology Service,
University of Iowa Hospitals and Clinics,
Iowa City, Iowa

Robert A. Weiss, M.D.
Clinical Associate Professor of Ophthalmology,
Oculoplastic and Reconstructive Surgery
and Ophthalmic Oncology, University of Illinois at Chicago,
and the Chicago Eye Institute, Chicago, Illinois

Ralph E. Wesley, M.D.
Director, Ophthalmic Plastic and Orbital Surgery, and
Clinical Professor of Ophthalmology,
Vanderbilt University Medical Center;
Chief of Ophthalmology, Baptist Medical Center,
Nashville, Tennessee

Ted H. Wojno, M.D.
Associate Professor of Ophthalmology,
Emory University School of Medicine;
and Director, Oculoplastic and Orbital Surgery,
Emory Clinic, Atlanta, Georgia

W.B. SAUNDERS COMPANY
A Division of Harcourt Brace & Company
Philadelphia London Toronto Montreal Sydney Tokyo

W.B. SAUNDERS COMPANY
A Division of Harcourt Brace & Company

The Curtis Center
Independence Square West
Philadelphia, Pennsylvania 19106

Library of Congress Cataloging-in-Publication Data

Principles and practice of ophthalmic plastic and reconstructive surgery / [edited by] Stephen Bosniak. — 1st ed.

p. cm.

ISBN 0-7216-3559-8

1. Ophthalmic plastic surgery. I. Bosniak, Stephen
[DNLM: 1. Eye—surgery. 2. Surgery, Plastic. WW 168 P957 1996]
RE87.P75 1996 617.7′1—dc20
DNLM/DLC 95-12616

Principles and Practice of Ophthalmic Plastic and Reconstructive Surgery
Volume 1 ISBN 0-7216-6033-9
Volume 2 ISBN 0-7216-6034-7
Two-Volume Set ISBN 0-7216-3559-8

Printed in the United States of America

Last digit is the print number: 9 8 7 6 5 4 3 2 1

Dedication

For **Marian,** *who changed my life.*

S.B.

Contributors

Ronald G. Amedee, M.D.
Associate Professor of Otolaryngology, Department of Otolaryngology, Tulane University Medical School; Chief of Surgical Services, Eye, Ear, Nose, and Throat Hospital, New Orleans, Louisiana.
Ophthalmic Manifestations of Mucoceles

Catherine Atzen, P.M.A., CIDESCO Diplomat
Catherine Atzen Laboratories; Vice-President, Aesthetics International Association, Campbell, California.
The Role of the Aesthetician Before and After Surgery

John C. Baer, M.D.
Assistant Professor, Department of Ophthalmology, University of Maryland School of Medicine; Staff, Veterans Affairs Medical Center, Baltimore, Maryland.
Ocular Manifestations of Systemic Immune Disease

George B. Bartley, M.D.
Chair, Department of Ophthalmology, Mayo Clinic and Mayo Foundation; Associate Professor of Ophthalmology, Mayo Medical School, Rochester, Minnesota.
The Eyelids in Graves' Ophthalmopathy; Secondary Acquired Lacrimal Drainage Obstruction

Henry I. Baylis, M.D.
Clinical Professor of Ophthalmology, University of California, Los Angeles, School of Medicine; Founding Chief, Orbital and Ophthalmic Plastic Surgery, Jules Stein Eye Institute, University of California, Los Angeles, Los Angeles, California.
Transconjunctival Lower Blepharoplasty

Fred S. Bodker, M.D.
Private Practice, Kansas City Eye Clinic, Overland Park, Kansas.
Harvesting and Use of Biological Tissue Grafts

Giulio Bonavolontà, M.D.
Professor and Chairman of Ophthalmology (Eye Institute), University "Federico II" School of Medicine, University of Naples, Naples, Italy.
Surgical Approaches to the Orbit; Anterior, Medial, Lateral, and Combined Surgical Approaches for Orbital Tumor Resection

Stephen Bosniak, M.D.
Associate Clinical Professor, State University of New York at Stony Brook; Director, Ophthalmic Plastic and Reconstructive Surgery, Nassau County Hospital and Kings County Hospital; and Associate Attending Surgeon, Manhattan Eye, Ear, and Throat Hospital and New York Eye and Ear Infirmary, New York, New York.
Alternative Techniques of Fat Removal

Jeffrey Bruce, M.D.
Assistant Professor of Clinical Neurosurgery (in Pathology), Columbia University; Assistant Attending Physician in Neurological Surgery, Columbia Presbyterian Medical Center, New York, New York.
Neurogenic Tumors

Cora Buggea
Electrolysis Instructor, Gina's School of Aesthetics and Electrology, Toronto, Ontario, Canada.
Electrology and Eyebrow Contouring

Richard C. Cape, M.D.
Private Practice; Staff, Methodist Hospital, Dyersburg, Tennessee.
Surgical Intervention in Conjunction with Medical Treatment of Cicatricial Pemphigoid

Keith D. Carter, M.D.
Associate Professor of Ophthalmology, Oculoplastics, Orbital and Oncology Services, Associate Professor, University of Iowa Hospitals and Clinics, Iowa City, Iowa.
Primary Acquired Nasolacrimal Duct Obstruction

Phillip Casson, M.D.
Associate Professor of Surgery (Plastic), New York University School of Medicine; Assistant Attending Surgeon, Tisch Hospital, Bellevue Hospital, New York Eye and Ear Infirmary, and Veterans Affairs Medical Center, New York, New York.
Autologen: Autologous, Injectable Dermal Collagen

William P. Chen, M.D.
Assistant Clinical Professor of Ophthalmology, Jules Stein Eye Institute, University of California, Los Angeles, School of Medicine; Associate Clinical Professor of Ophthalmology, University of California, Irvine, College of Medicine; Senior Attending Surgeon, Ophthalmic Plastic Surgery Service, Harbor-UCLA Medical Center, Torrance, California.
Tarsoconjunctival Polishing with Mucous Membrane Grafting for Cicatricial Entropion and Trichiasis; Enucleation and Evisceration

David B. Christie, M.D.
Instructor in Ophthalmology, Tufts University School of Medicine, Boston, Massachusetts.
Basic Surgical Techniques, Technology, and Wound Repair

Jonathan Christenbury, M.D.
Attending Physician, Presbyterian Hospital, Carolinas Medical Center, Charlotte, North Carolina.
Aponeurotic Ptosis

Chieh Chung, M.D.
Assistant Professor of Ear, Nose, and Throat Medicine, Yang Ming Medical School, Taipei, Taiwan.
Auricular Acupuncture in the Treatment of Blepharospasm

Michael Clarke, M.A., M.B., B.Chir., D.O., F.R.C.S., F.R.C.Ophth.
Acting Head, Department of Ophthalmology, Medical School, University of Newcastle; Consultant Paediatric Ophthalmologist, Royal Victoria Infirmary, Newcastle Upon Tyne, England.
Mesenchymal and Fibro-osseous Tumors

Marc S. Cohen, M.D.
Assistant Professor, Thomas Jefferson University School of Medicine; Assistant Surgeon, Wills Eye Hospital, Philadelphia, Pennsylvania.
Lower Eyelid Retraction and Cicatricial Ectropion; Optic Nerve Sheath Decompression

Harvey P. Cole III, M.D.
Clinical Instructor of Ophthalmology, Emory University School of Medicine; Staff, Southeastern Oculoplastic Center, Piedmont Hospital, Atlanta, Georgia.
Conjunctiva: Structure and Function; Basic Techniques of Conjunctival Surgery; Treatment of Squamous Papillomas of the Conjunctiva

M. Ronan Conlon, M.D., F.R.C.S.C.
Assistant Clinical Professor of Ophthalmology, University of Saskatchewan; Staff, Saskatoon City Hospital, Saskatoon, Saskatchewan, Canada.
Pigmented Conjunctival Neoplasms; Benign Eyelid Tumors

Philip L. Custer, M.D.
Associate Professor of Ophthalmology, Washington University School of Medicine; Director, Orbital Center, Barnes Hospital, St. Louis, Missouri.
Lower Eyelid Blepharoplasty

Roger A. Dailey, M.D.
Assistant Professor of Ophthalmology, Casey Eye Institute, Oregon Health Sciences University; Active Staff, Oregon Health Sciences University, Veterans Affairs Medical Center, Good Samaritan Hospital, St. Vincent Hospital, and Emanuel Hospital, Portland, Oregon.
Medial Canthal Reconstruction

Carlo de Conciliis, M.D.
Staff, Ophthalmic Plastic Reconstructive and Orbital Surgery, Department of Ophthalmology and Visual Science, Scientific Institute H. S. Raffaele, Milan, Italy.
Epidemiology of Orbital Pathology

Robert D. Deitch Jr., M.D.
Assistant Clinical Professor, Department of Ophthalmology, Indiana University School of Medicine, Indianapolis, Indiana.
Management of Pterygia

Dale P. DeVore, Ph.D.
Chief Scientific Officer, Autogenesis Tech, Inc., Acton; Managing Director, Organogenesis, Inc., Canton, Massachusetts.
Autologen: Autologous, Injectable Dermal Collagen

Marcos T. Doxanas, M.D.
Staff, Department of Ophthalmology, Greater Baltimore Medical Center, Baltimore, Maryland.
Malignant Epithelial Eyelid Tumors

Steven C. Dresner, M.D.
Associate Clinical Professor of Ophthalmology, Jules Stein Eye Institute, University of California, Los Angeles, Los Angeles, California.
Reconstruction of the Lower Eyelid and Lateral Canthus

Nancy Dugan, B.A.
Paramedical Camouflage Consultant
Principles of Camouflage Make-up and the Postoperative Patient

Jonathan J. Dutton, M.D., Ph.D.
Professor, Duke University Eye Center, Durham, North Carolina.
Replacement of Conjunctival Mucous Membrane

Steven Fagien, M.D., F.A.C.S.
Boca Raton Center for Ophthalmic Plastic and Reconstructive Surgery; Director, Boca Raton Center for Ophthalmic Plastic and Reconstructive Surgery, Boca Raton, Florida.
Autologen: Autologous, Injectable Dermal Collagen

James C. Fleming, M.D.
Assistant Professor, Department of Ophthalmology, University of Tennessee Center for the Health Sciences, University of Tennessee, Memphis, Tennessee.
Surgical Intervention in Conjunction with Medical Treatment of Cicatricial Pemphigoid

Jill A. Foster, M.D.
Director of Oculoplastic and Orbital Surgery Service, Division of Ophthalmology, Cleveland Clinic Foundation, Cleveland, Ohio.
Congenital Eyelid Anomalies

Tamara R. Fountain, M.D.
Clinical Instructor and Clinical Fellow, Department of Ophthalmic Plastic and Reconstructive Surgery, Doheny Eye Institute, University of Southern California, Los Angeles, California.
Considerations for Oculoplastic Surgery in the African American Patient

Craig D. Friedman, M.D.
Staff, Department of Otolaryngology, Yale University Medical Center, New Haven, Connecticut.
Harvesting and Use of Biological Tissue Grafts

Constance L. Fry, M.D.
Clinical Professor of Oculoplastics and Orbital Disease, Tulane University; Staff, Oculoplastics and Orbital Surgery Service, Ochsner Clinic, and Eye, Ear, Nose, and Throat Hospital, New Orleans, Louisiana.
Eyelid Infections and Inflammations

Steven L. Galetta, M.D.
Associate Professor and Director, Neuro-ophthalmology Service, Department of Neurology and Ophthalmology, University of Pennsylvania School of Medicine, Philadelphia, Pennsylvania.
Facial Paralysis: Diagnosis and Management

Linda Garofallou, B.S.
Director of Training, Dr. Hauschka Skin Care, USA; Authorized International Trainer, WALA Heilmittel, GmbH, Germany.
Lymphatic Drainage Massage

Steven M. Gilbard, M.D.
Consultant, Ophthalmic Plastic Surgery, St. Joseph's Hospital and Medical Center and Barrow Neurological Institute, Phoenix, Arizona.
Involutional and Paralytic Ectropion

Gregory G. Gion, B.A., B.S., C.M.I.
Adjunct Faculty, Department of Biomedical Communications, Graduate School of Biomedical Sciences, University of Texas Southwestern Medical Center, Dallas, Texas.
Orbital Prostheses

Robert Alan Goldberg, M.D.
Associate Professor of Ophthalmology, University of California, Los Angeles, School of Medicine; Chief, Orbital and Ophthalmic Plastic Surgery, Jules Stein Eye Institute, University of California, Los Angeles, Los Angeles, California.
Entropion; Transconjunctival Lower Blepharoplasty

Stacia H. Goldey, M.D.
Attending Surgeon, Florida Hospital, Eustis; and Leesburg Regional Medical Center, Leesburg, Florida.
Transconjunctival Lower Blepharoplasty

Russell S. Gonnering, M.D.
Associate Clinical Professor, University of Wisconsin School of Medicine; Active Staff, St. Luke's Medical Center, Milwaukee, Wisconsin.
Eyelid Trauma

Holly Gore, M.D.
Clinical Instructor, Department of Ophthalmology, Tulane University School of Medicine, New Orleans; Corneal Specialist, North Lake Eye Center, Slidell, Louisiana.
Vascular Tumors of the Orbit

Diana Habrich
Staff, Sunnyside Medical Office, Kaiser Permanente, Clackamas, Oregon.
Medial Canthal Reconstruction

Barrett G. Haik, M.D.
Professor and Chairman, Department of Ophthalmology, University of Tennessee School of Medicine, Memphis, Tennessee.
Vascular Tumors of the Orbit; Ophthalmic Manifestations of Mucoceles

Lawrence F. Handler, M.D.
Clinical Instructor, Scheie Eye Institute, University of Pennsylvania School of Medicine, Philadelphia, Pennsylvania.
Facial Paralysis: Diagnosis and Management

Annette Hanson, B.A.
President, Atelier Esthétique, Inc., New York, New York.
Principles of Camouflage Make-up and the Postoperative Patient

Will Harms, M.D.
Former Office Medical Director, Anchor Norridge Medical Office, Norridge, Illinois.
Pseudotumors

Ramzi K. Hemady, M.D.
Assistant Professor, Department of Ophthalmology, University of Maryland School of Medicine; Chief, Ophthalmology Section, Baltimore Veterans Affairs Medical Center, Baltimore, Maryland.
Ocular Manifestations of Systemic Immune Disease

John B. Holds, M.D., F.A.C.S.
Associate Professor of Ophthalmology and Otolaryngology, St. Louis University Health Sciences Center, Anheuser-Busch Eye Institute, St. Louis, Missouri.
Essential Blepharospasm and Hemifacial Spasm; The Role of Paranasal Sinus Disease in Orbital Cellulitis

Anne R. Horan, M.D.
Instructor in Ophthalmology, Vanderbilt University Department of Ophthalmology and Visual Sciences, Vanderbilt University Medical Center, and Nashville Veterans Affairs Medical Center, Nashville, Tennessee.
Conjunctival and Limbal Neoplasia: Diagnosis and Management

Wen Ming Hsu, M.D.
Associate Professor, Department of Ophthalmology, Yang Ming-University School of Medicine; Director, Oculoplastic Section, Department of Ophthalmology, Veterans General Hospital–Taipei, Taipei, Taiwan.
Auricular Acupuncture in the Treatment of Blepharospasm

William D. James, M.D.
Chief, Dermatology Service, Walter Reed Army Medical Center, Washington, D.C.
Cutaneous and Multisystemic Processes Affecting the Ocular Adnexa

Walter J. Johnson
Board-Certified Ocularist, Fellow, American Society of Ocularists, Denver Optic Company, Englewood, Colorado.
The Perfect Socket: The Ocularist's View

Kelly Jones, M.D.
Staff, Department of Ophthalmology, University of Maryland School of Medicine, Baltimore, Maryland.
Neoplastic and Related Conditions of the Orbital and Adnexal Structures

David R. Jordan, M.D., F.A.C.S., F.R.C.S.(C)
Associate Professor, University of Ottawa Eye Institute, Ottawa, Ontario, Canada.
Reconstruction of the Upper Eyelid; Evaluation of the Tearing Patient

Sara A. Kaltreider, M.D.
Associate Professor of Ophthalmology, University of Virginia School of Medicine, Charlottesville, Virginia.
Orbital Fractures

Leonard P. Kapcala, M.D., F.A.C.P.
Associate Professor of Medicine and Physiology, University of Maryland School of Medicine; Attending Physician, Endocrinology Division, University of Maryland Hospital, Baltimore, Maryland.
Diagnosis and Management of Thyrotoxicosis; Diagnosis and Management of Hyperparathyroidism

James W. Karesh, M.D.
Assistant Professor, Johns Hopkins University School of Medicine, Wilmer Ophthalmologic Institute and the University of Maryland School of Medicine; Director, Ophthalmic Plastic and Reconstructive Surgery, Krieger Eye Institute, Sinai Hospital of Baltimore, Baltimore, Maryland.
Neoplastic and Related Conditions of the Orbital and Adnexal Structures; The Ocular Manifestations of Non–Thyroid-Related Endocrine Disease

James A. Katowitz, M.D.
Associate Professor of Ophthalmology (Children's Hospital), University of Pennsylvania School of Medicine; Attending Physician, Hospital of the University of Pennsylvania, Philadelphia, Pennsylvania.
Congenital Eyelid Anomalies

Jonathan Kay, M.D.
Staff, Department of Anesthesiology, St. Luke's Medical Center, Milwaukee, Wisconsin.
Anesthetic Considerations for Oculoplastic Surgery: An Update for the 1990s

Michael Kazim, M.D.
Assistant Professor of Clinical Ophthalmology and Clinical Surgery, Columbia University College of Physicians and Surgeons and Columbia-Presbyterian Medical Center, New York, New York.
Neurogenic Tumors

Charles D. Kelman, M.D.
Clinical Professor, New York Medical College, Valhalla; Attending Surgeon, New York Eye and Ear Infirmary, New York, New York.
Autologen: Autologous, Injectable Dermal Collagen

Robert C. Kersten, M.D.
Assistant Professor of Ophthalmology, Department of Ophthalmology, University of Cincinnati College of Medicine, Cincinnati, Ohio.
Congenital Lacrimal Abnormalities

Don O. Kikkawa, M.D.
Assistant Professor and Director of Orbital and Oculoplastics Service, Department of Ophthalmology, University of California, San Diego, LaJolla; Attending Staff, Surgical Service, Veterans Affairs Medical Center, San Diego, California.
Orbital Anatomy and Embryology

Jan W. Kronish, M.D.
Clinical Assistant Professor, Department of Ophthalmology, Bascom Palmer Eye Institute, University of Miami School of Medicine, Miami; Delray Eye Associates, Delray Beach, Florida.
Eyelid and Orbital Considerations in AIDS; Metastatic Tumors

Kurt Laedrach, M.D., D.M.D.
Assistant Professor, University Hospital of Bern, Bern, Switzerland.
Craniofacial Congenital Anomalies: The Subcranial Approach

Brian Leatherbarrow, B.Sc., M.B.Ch.B., F.R.C.S., F.R.C.Ophth.
Honorary Lecturer, University of Manchester; Consultant Ophthalmic, Oculoplastic, and Orbital Surgeon, Manchester Royal Eye Hospital, Manchester, United Kingdom.
Benign Eyelid Tumors

Bradley N. Lemke, M.D.
Clinical Professor, Department of Ophthalmology and Visual Sciences, University of Wisconsin, Madison; Staff, Davis Duehr Dean Clinic, Madison, Wisconsin.
Clinical Eyelid Anatomy; Orbital Anatomy and Embryology

Peter S. Levin, M.D.
Director, Ophthalmic Plastic and Orbital Surgery, Stanford University School of Medicine, Stanford, California.
Orbital Exenteration

Richard D. Lisman, M.D., F.A.C.S.
Clinical Associate Professor of Ophthalmology, New York University School of Medicine; Clinic Chief, Division of Ophthalmic Plastic Surgery, Manhattan Eye and Ear Hospital, New York, New York.
Diagnosis and Management of Sebaceous Gland Carcinoma

Don Liu, M.D.
Associate Professor, Department of Ophthalmology, University of Southern California School of Medicine; Head of Oculoplastics, Doheny Eye Institute, Los Angeles, California.
An Overview: Cultural Background and Anatomic Considerations in the Asian Patient; Asian Blepharoplasty; Eyelid Tumors in Chinese

John A. Long, M.D.
Clinical Assistant Professor, University of Alabama, Birmingham, Alabama.
Entropion

Mahmood F. Mafee, M.D.
Professor of Radiology, University of Illinois at Chicago Medical Center; Director, MRI Center, and Director, Radiology Section, Eye and Ear Infirmary, University of Illinois at Chicago, Chicago, Illinois.
Neuroradiologic Imaging of the Orbit and Globe

Hector M. Marines, M.D.
Assistant Professor of Ophthalmic Plastic and Orbital Surgery, and Ocular Pathology, Department of Ophthalmology, Hospital San Jose, Instituto Tecnologico y de Estudios Superiores de Monterrey; Associate Member, Instituto de Oftalmologia, S.C., Monterrey, N.L. Mexico.
Male Blepharoplasty

Alice Y. Matoba, M.D.
Associate Professor, Baylor College of Medicine; Chief, Ophthalmology Service, Houston Veterans Affairs Medical Center, Houston, Texas.
Conjunctival Procedures for Corneal Disease

Joseph F. Mazza, Jr., M.D.
Private Practice, Ft. Myers, Florida.
Blepharopigmentation: Techniques, Indications, and Comparison of Modalities

Steven A. McCormick, M.D., F.C.A.P.
Associate Professor of Pathology, Ophthalmology and Otolaryngology/Head and Neck Surgery, New York Medical College, Valhalla; Director of Pathology and Laboratory Medicine, New York Eye and Ear Infirmary, New York, New York.
Idiopathic Orbital Inflammation and Lymphoid Tumors of the Orbit

Timothy F. McDevitt, M.D.
Staff Ophthalmologist, Faulkner Institute, Honolulu, Hawaii.
Alternative Techniques of Fat Removal

Michael E. Migliori, M.D., F.A.C.S.
Clinical Assistant Professor of Ophthalmology, Brown University; Director of Ophthalmic Plastic and Reconstructive Surgery, Rhode Island Hospital, Providence, Rhode Island.
Evaluation and Management of the Anophthalmic Socket

James P. Milite, M.D.
Associate Adjunct Attending Ophthalmologist and Fellow in Ophthalmic Pathology, New York Eye and Ear Infirmary, New York, New York.
Idiopathic Orbital Inflammation and Lymphoid Tumors of the Orbit

Neil R. Miller, M.D.
Professor of Neuro-ophthalmology, Johns Hopkins Medical Institutions, Baltimore, Maryland.
Disorders of Eyelid Function Caused by Systemic Disease

Ronald L. Moy, M.D.
Assistant Professer, University of California, Los Angeles, School of Medicine; Director of Dermatologic Surgery, Veterans Affairs Medical Center—West Los Angeles, Los Angeles, California.
Mohs' Surgery for Periorbital Malignancies

Howard Murad, M.D.
Assistant Clinical Professor of Dermatology, University of California, Los Angeles, California.
Chemical Peels

Brent A. Murphy, M.D.
Assistant Professor of Ophthalmology and Director of Ophthalmic Plastic and Orbital Surgery, University of South Alabama College of Medicine, Mobile, Alabama.
Management of Conjunctival Amyloidosis; Kaposi's Sarcoma of the Conjunctiva; Lymphoid Tumors of the Conjunctiva

Marjorie Murphy, M.D.
Former Resident, Wills Eye Hospital, Philadelphia, Pennsylvania.
Lower Eyelid Retraction and Cicatricial Ectropion

Jeffrey A. Nerad, M.D.
Professor of Ophthalmology, University of Iowa College of Medicine; Director, Oculoplastic, Orbital, and Oncology Service, University of Iowa Hospitals and Clinics, Iowa City, Iowa.
Benign Eyelid Tumors; Eyelid Causes of Tearing; Primary Acquired Nasolacrimal Duct Obstruction; Osseointegration for the Exenterated Orbit

Russell W. Neuhaus, M.D.
Clinical Professor of Ophthalmology, University of Texas Health Science Center at San Antonio, San Antonio, Texas.
Eyelid Infections and Inflammations

Nelson Lee Novick, M.D., F.A.C.P., F.A.A.D.
Associate Clinical Professor of Dermatology, Mount Sinai School of Medicine; Associate Attending Physician, Mount Sinai Medical Center, New York, New York.
Total Facial Rejuvenation

Thaddeus S. Nowinski, M.D.
Clinical Associate Professor, Jefferson Medical College; Associate Surgeon, Oculoplastics Service, Wills Eye Hospital, Philadelphia, Pennsylvania.
Anatomy and Physiology of the Lacrimal System

William R. Nunery, M.D., F.A.C.S.
Clinical Associate Professor of Ophthalmology, Indiana University School of Medicine; Staff, Methodist Hospital, Indiana University Hospital, Wishard Hospital, and Meridian Plastic Surgery Center, Indianapolis, Indiana.
Enucleation and Evisceration

Denis M. O'Day, M.D.
Chairman and George Weeks Hale Professor, Vanderbilt University Department of Ophthalmology and Visual Sciences; Professor of Ophthalmology, Vanderbilt University Medical Center, Nashville Veterans Affairs Medical Center, Nashville, Tennessee.
Conjunctival and Limbal Neoplasia: Diagnosis and Management

Brian Patrick O'Donnel, M.D.
Private Practice, Portland, Maine.
Cutaneous and Multisystemic Processes Affecting the Ocular Adnexa

Nita Patel, M.D.
Affiliated Dermatology, Inc., Los Angeles, California.
Chemical Peels

James R. Patrinely, M.D.
Associate Professor of Ophthalmology and Plastic Surgery, Baylor College of Medicine; Clinical Assistant Surgeon of Ophthalmology and Clinical Assistant Professor in the Division of Surgery, Department of Head and Neck Surgery, University of Texas, M.D. Anderson Cancer Center, Houston, Texas.
Male Blepharoplasty

Jay M. Pensler, M.D.
Associate Professor, Northwestern University Medical School; Attending Plastic Surgeon, Children's Memorial Hospital, Evanston Hospital, and Northwestern Memorial Hospital, Chicago, Illinois.
Diagnostic and Presurgical Evaluation of Congenital Craniofacial Anomalies

Roswell R. Pfister, M.D.
Clinical Professor, University of Alabama School of Medicine; Director of Eye Research, Brookwood Medical Center, Birmingham, Alabama.
Chemical and Thermal Injuries of the Cornea and Conjunctiva

Phillip F. Pierce, M.D.
Associate Professor of Medicine and Microbiology, Georgetown University School of Medicine, Washington, D.C.
Infections of the Orbit and Orbital Structures

Holla'e Ploof, B.A.
Director, Training Clinical Electropigmentation, The Holla'e Methode Inc., Tucson, Arizona.
Electropigmentation and the Cosmetic Surgery Patient

Jeffrey C. Popp, M.D., F.A.C.S.
Assistant Clinical Professor and Director, Oculoplastic Orbital Oncology Service, University of Nebraska School of Medicine, Omaha, Nebraska.
Facial Paralysis: Diagnosis and Management

Jeffrey C. Posnick, D.M.D., M.D.
Associate Professor, Division of Plastic Surgery; Department of Periodontics; and Department of Ear, Nose, and Throat, Georgetown University Medical Center, Washington, D.C.
Orbital Deformities: Anterior Cranial Base Approach

David A. B. Price, B.A.
Medical Photographer, David Price Photography, New York, New York.
Photography of the Ophthalmic Plastic Surgery Patient

Peter T. Pugliese, M.D.
Chairman and Chief Scientific Officer, Milmar Research, Inc., Bernville, Pennsylvania.
Lymphatic Drainage Massage

Cynthia Rager, C.P.M.E.
Adjunct Staff, Edison Community College, Ft. Myers, Florida.
Blepharopigmentation: Techniques, Indications, and Comparison of Modalities

Sankaran Rajagopalan, M.D.
Staff, Department of Ophthalmology, University of Maryland School of Medicine, Baltimore, Maryland.
Neoplastic and Related Conditions of the Orbital and Adnexal Structures

Joram Raveh, M.D., D.M.D.
Head and Professor, University Hospital of Bern, Bern, Switzerland.
Craniofacial Congenital Anomalies: The Subcranial Approach

David M. Reifler, M.D., F.A.C.S.
Clinical Associate Professor of Surgery/Ophthalmology, Michigan State University College of Human Medicine (GRAMEC); Attending Physician, Butterworth Hospital and Blodgett Memorial Medical Center, Grand Rapids, Michigan.
Upper Eyelid Blepharoplasty

Daniel Rivlin, M.D.
Chief, Mohs' Surgery Unit, Mt. Sinai Medical Center, Miami Beach, Florida.
Mohs' Surgery for Periorbital Malignancies

Wallace A. Roberts, A.S.E.E.
Electrology Instructor, Newbury College, Brookline, Aquinas College, Milton, and Roberts Institute, Brookline, Massachusetts.
Electrology and Eyebrow Contouring

Merlyn M. Rodrigues, M.D., Ph.D.
Professor, University of Maryland Medical School, Baltimore, Maryland.
Neoplastic and Related Conditions of the Orbital and Adnexal Structures

Geoffrey E. Rose, B.S., M.B.B.S., M.S., M.R.C.P., F.R.C.S., F.R.C.Ophth.
Honorary Lecturer in Ophthalmology, Institute of Ophthalmology, University of London; Consultant Ophthalmic Surgeon, Moorfields Eye Hospital, London; Honorary Consultant Ophthalmic Surgeon, Hospital for Sick Children, London, United Kingdom, and Royal Victoria Hospital, Belfast, Northern Ireland.
Clinical Examination in Orbital Disease; Lacrimal Gland Neoplasia

Marian Rubenfeld, M.D.,Ph.D.
Clinical Associate Professor, Department of Ophthalmology, University of Minnesota School of Medicine; Subsection Chief, Minneapolis Veterans Affairs Medical Center, Minneapolis, Minnesota.
Neuro-ophthalmic Considerations in Orbital Disease

Peter A.D. Rubin, M.D.
Assistant Professor, Department of Ophthalmology, Harvard Medical School; Director, Eye Plastics and Orbital Surgery, Massachusetts Eye and Ear Infirmary, Boston, Massachusetts.
Pigmented Conjunctival Neoplasms

Steven J. Rubin, M.D.
Assistant Professor, Department of Radiation and Cellular Oncology, University of Chicago School of Medicine; Instructor, University of Illinois at Chicago, Chicago, Illinois.
Radiation Therapy in Orbital Disease

Evan H. Sacks, M.D.
Assistant Attending Physician, Manhattan Eye, Ear and Throat Hospital and Beth Israel Medical Center, New York, New York.
Diagnosis and Management of Sebaceous Gland Carcinoma

Curt P. Samlaska, M.D.
Assistant Professor of Medicine, University of Hawaii; Chief, Dermatology Service, Tripler Army Medical Center, Honolulu, Hawaii.
Cutaneous and Multisystemic Processes Affecting the Ocular Adnexa

Jeffrey Schiller, M.D.
Professor of Ophthalmology, Chairman of Ophthalmology University "Federico II" of Naples School of Medicine, Institute of Ophthalmology, Naples, Italy.
Translator for *Surgical Approaches to the Orbit; Anterior, Medial, Lateral, and Combined Surgical Approaches for Orbital Tumor Resection*

Norman Shorr, M.D., F.A.C.S.
Clinical Professor of Ophthalmology and Director, Fellowship in Orbital and Ophthalmic Plastic and Reconstructive Surgery, Jules Stein Eye Institute, University of California, Los Angeles, Los Angeles, California.
Suborbital Augmentation

Joseph P. Shovlin, M.D.
Associate in Ophthalmology; Director, Division of Ophthalmic Plastic and Reconstructive Surgery, Geisinger Medical Center, Danville, Pennsylvania.
Clinical Eyelid Anatomy; Amyloidosis and Idiopathic Orbital Conditions

David I. Silbert, M.D.
Active Staff, Lancaster General Hospital, Lancaster; and Courtesy Staff, Wills Eye Hospital, Philadelphia; Lancaster General Hospital, Lancaster; and Wills Eye Hospital, Philadelphia, Pennsylvania.
Malignant Eyelid and Orbital Tumors

Mary A. Stefanyszyn, M.D.
Assistant Professor, University of Pennsylvania Hospital; Clinical Instructor, Thomas Jefferson University; Associate Surgeon, Wills Eye Hospital, Lankenau Hospital, and Thomas Jefferson University Hospital, Philadelphia; Associate Surgeon, Lankenau Hospital, Wynnewood, Pennsylvania.
Malignant Eyelid and Orbital Tumors

Kenneth D. Steinsapir, M.D.
Visiting Assistant Professor of Ophthalmology, Jules Stein Eye Institute, University of California, Los Angeles, School of Medicine, Los Angeles, California.
Suborbital Augmentation

Darlene P. Story, B.A.
President, Lasting Impression I, Inc., Englewood, New Jersey.
Micropigmentation and the Patient with Facial Burn and Facial Reconstruction

Richard W. Story, B.A.
Lasting Impression I, Inc., Englewood, New Jersey.
Micropigmentation and the Patient with Facial Burn and Facial Reconstruction

Gerald G. Striph, M.D.
Clinical Assistant Professor, Medical College of Ohio, Toledo, Ohio.
Disorders of Eyelid Function Caused by Systemic Disease

Nancy C. Swartz, M.D.
Instructor, Wills Eye Hospital, Philadelphia, Pennsylvania.
Lower Eyelid Retraction and Cicatricial Ectropion

Myron Tanenbaum, M.D., F.A.C.S.
Assistant Clinical Professor, Department of Ophthalmology, Bascom Palmer Eye Institute, University of Miami School of Medicine, Miami, Florida.
Orbital Decompression for Graves' Orbitopathy

Thierry Vuillemin, M.D., D.M.D.
Assistant Professor, University Hospital of Bern, Bern, Switzerland.
Craniofacial Congenital Anomalies: The Subcranial Approach

Susanne S. Warfield, B.S.
President, Paramedical Consultants, Inc., Ridgewood, New Jersey.
The Practical Application of Aestheticians in the Plastic and Reconstructive Surgeon's Office

Robert A. Weiss, M.D.
Clinical Associate Professor of Ophthalmology, Oculoplastic and Reconstructive Surgery and Ophthalmic Oncology, University of Illinois at Chicago and the Chicago Eye Institute, Chicago, Illinois.
Brow Ptosis; Harvesting and Use of Biological Tissue Grafts

Ralph E. Wesley, M.D.
Director, Ophthalmic Plastic and Orbital Surgery and Clinical Professor of Ophthalmology, Vanderbilt University Medical Center; Chief of Ophthalmology, Baptist Medical Center, Nashville, Tennessee.
Conjunctiva: Structure and Function; Basic Techniques of Conjunctival Surgery; Management of Conjunctival Amyloidosis; Kaposi's Sarcoma of the Conjunctiva; Lymphoid Tumors of the Conjunctiva; Treatment of Squamous Papillomas of the Conjunctiva; Management of Conjunctival Prolapse; Conjunctival Dermolipoma Surgery

William White, M.D.
Clinical Instructor of Ophthalmology, Children's Mercy Hospital, University of Missouri; Staff, Baptist Medical Center, Kansas City, Missouri.
Disorders of the Canaliculus and Punctum

Fred M. Wilson II, M.D.
Professor of Ophthalmology, Department of Ophthalmology, Indiana University School of Medicine, Indianapolis, Indiana.
Management of Pterygia

Jonathan D. Wirtschafter, M.D.
Professor, Departments of Ophthalmology, Neurology, and Neurosurgery; Director, Neuro-ophthalmology, Orbit, and Oculoplastics Service, University of Minnesota, Minneapolis, Minnesota.
Neuro-ophthalmic Considerations in Orbital Disease

Ted H. Wojno, M.D.
Associate Professor of Ophthalmology, Emory University School of Medicine; Director of Oculoplastic and Orbital Surgery, Emory Clinic, Atlanta, Georgia.
Preoperative Evaluation; Alternative Techniques of Fat Removal; Management of Blepharoplasty Complications; Indications for Orbital Surgery; Operative Principles and Instrumentation

John J. Woog, M.D.
Clinical Associate Professor, Tufts University School of Medicine; Clinical Instructor, Harvard Medical School; Co-Director, Eye Plastics and Orbit Service, New England Eye Center; Staff, Ophthalmic Consultants of Boston, Boston, Massachusetts.
Basic Surgical Techniques, Technology, and Wound Repair; Disorders of the Canaliculus and Punctum

Allan E. Wulc, M.D., F.A.C.S.
Assistant Professor and Director, Oculoplastic Orbital Service, Scheie Eye Institute, University of Pennsylvania School of Medicine, Philadelphia, Pennsylvania.
Facial Paralysis: Diagnosis and Management

Nai Jiang Xu, M.D.
Professor, Division of Ophthalmic Plastic and Reconstructive Surgery, Ninth People's Hospital, Shanghai, China.
Eyelid Tumors in Chinese

Guang-Xi Zhao, M.D.
Professor of Ophthalmology, Beijing Medical University; Vice Chief Editor, Chinese Language Edition of *Archives of Ophthalmology*; Editor, *Chinese Journal of Ophthalmology*, Beijing, China.
Eyelid Tumors in Chinese

Foreword

It has become obvious that the borders of our oculoplastic surgery discipline have now been expanded further with this magnum opus by Stephen Bosniak. Not too long ago an authoritative text on ophthalmic plastic surgery would be considered complete if it contained the requisite number of chapters dealing with the standard periorbital problems of ectropion, entropion, ptosis, and lid reconstruction. *Principles and Practice of Ophthalmic Plastic and Reconstructive Surgery*'s 112 chapters force us to realize that from now on much more will be expected of an oculoplastic textbook and an oculoplastic surgeon than previously.

The first section teaches us that, above all, we oculoplastic surgeons are physicians and thus must be diagnostically alert to the periorbital manifestations of systemic disease. Conjunctiva, the "Rodney Dangerfield" of the orbit because it "gets no respect," is handsomely treated in the second section with 100 pages of text, starting with an elegantly written chapter on anatomy. The third and fourth sections, which discuss the eyelids, are textbooks within themselves, especially the relevant sections on cosmetic procedures. In this decade of declining remuneration by third party insurers, cosmetic oculoplastic surgery, a "fee-for-service business," is becoming more a part of everyone's practice—patients also desire this kind of surgery more now then ever before. As such, the chapters on preoperative and postoperative aesthetics will be somewhat of a surprise to most ophthalmologists, but they should be read. Section 5 is a well-written, fascinating glimpse into the Eastern mind and culture with respect to eyelid surgery and, together with other chapters in this section, makes us realize that our practice will be more internationally based in future years.

The closing sections on lacrimal surgery, orbital disease and fractures, and the ophthalmic socket are updated and germane to modern oculoplastic surgery. The final small section of craniofacial disorders is excellent, but proportional in length to its relevance in our specialty.

It is often said that a multidiscipline-author book suffers from uneven writing, inconsistent illustration material, and the inability to mesh different styles of writing, not to mention the archenemy of all textbooks—repetition. Dr. Bosniak's book has none of this. On the other hand, obvious advantages of a multiauthor text show in that different cross sections of oculoplastic surgery practice are presented in one source—how else can you find a chapter written by authors in private practice who see the "regular" patients of an unskewed population and thus provide insight to those who work "in the trenches?" At the same time, institutional studies have great merit in that by analyzing referred series of patients they bring together the experience of professors combined.

To become an oculoplastic surgeon of the 1990s, we can no longer be content that we know several versions of operations for entropion or a handful of classic techniques for ptosis correction. We must have more than a passing knowledge of the use of endoscopic surgery, and we certainly must know of the indications for

diagnostic procedures like flow cytometry in tumor analysis. With the influx of immigrants we must be aware of the social and cultural differences of our patients, and we must be ready to diagnose the systemic diseases that many of the immigrants bring with them. It also can be said that if we wish to survive in the era of managed care, we all must become more familiar with cosmetic eyelid surgery, which does not just mean "how to do a blepharoplasty," but the indications for brow lifting and the different ways to do it, cosmetology consultation, and even the method for performing a skin peel.

Principles and Practice of Ophthalmic Plastic and Reconstructive Surgery will never be an obsolete book. The wealth of information contained herein is encyclopedic and well referenced. With its multitude of illustrations it presents a systematized approach to oculoplastic surgery, and many of us will spend the better part of our remaining careers attempting to read and retain all the facts contained herein.

Dr. Bosniak and all the section editors have truly left what Longfellow penned as "footprints in the sands of time."

MICHAEL A. CALLAHAN, M.D.

Preface

Writing books and sharing information with physicians and surgeons who have interests in common with me have been driving forces in my life. W.B. Saunders Company has provided me with the opportunity to present a magnum opus. With this book, I have had the luxury and pleasure of working with Giulio Bonavolontà, Robert Goldberg, Russell Gonnering, James Karesh, Don Liu, Jeffrey Nerad, Robert Weiss, Ralph Wesley, and Ted Wojno— a new generation of creative minds.

During the years spent organizing and compiling this project, dramatic advances in technology have become available to the ophthalmologist. Ophthalmic plastic and reconstructive surgeons have sought the most effective and appropriate applications of this technology. In this book we have strived to incorporate these latest advances and to describe the indications for their use.

In *Principles and Practice of Ophthalmic Plastic and Reconstructive Surgery,* we have emphasized an approach to the patient as a whole. We have allotted a complete section to systemic diseases and a discussion of systemic perioperative preparation of the surgical patient, including postoperative treatment to enhance and accelerate wound healing. Current and historical surgical advances in eyelid reconstruction, ptosis correction, and entropion and ectropion repair are thoroughly presented and documented. A separate section on conjunctival diseases and surgery has been included to highlight their importance and the necessity for alternative techniques in handling conjunctival tissue. The orbital section is voluminous to accommodate the current advanced status of diagnosing and documenting orbital pathology. The anatomic and physiologic distinctions of ethnic ophthalmic patients are also represented in a separate section. In addition, the significance of a multidisciplinary approach to the orbit in selected cases is clearly established. The state-of-the-art techniques of socket reconstruction are also presented in a separate section.

Ophthalmic plastic surgeons are endeavoring to competitively enter into the arena of aesthetic surgery. The section on cosmetic surgery not only provides the surgical principles but also introduces adjunctive techniques essential to a cosmetic surgical practice: topical home care products, in-office peeling agents, camouflage make-up, and lymphatic drainage massage. New surgical modalities have been introduced: radiosurgery and ultra-pulse laser surgery.

I am joined with the section editors in the commitment to a totally new presentation of the state-of-the-art ophthalmic plastic surgery. Not only is the content updated but the presentation is revitalized. The two-volume presentation of the text lends itself to easy accessibility and logical organization of material.

STEPHEN BOSNIAK

Acknowledgments

This book would not have been possible without the diligence of the section editors and authors. Our editors at W.B. Saunders, Nellie McGrew and Kim Kist, have facilitated and coordinated this complex project. Drs. Marian Cantisano Zilkha, Charles Crane, and Ferdinand Tan have been of invaluable assistance in the preparation, editing, and proofreading of the manuscripts. I also would like to thank my office staff, Barbara Bozzone, Sharon Murphy, June Hummel, and Rene Harris, for their secretarial support.

S.B.

Contents

VOLUME 1

SECTION I

Orbital and Periorbital Manifestations of Systemic Diseases . . . 1

James W. Karesh

Introduction . . . 1

James W. Karesh

CHAPTER 1

Cutaneous and Multisystemic Processes Affecting the Ocular Adnexa . . . 3

Curt P. Samlaska, Brian Patrick O'Donnel, and William D. James

CHAPTER 2

Neoplastic and Related Conditions of the Orbital and Adnexal Structures . . . 53

Merlyn M. Rodrigues, Sankaran Rajagopalan, Kelly Jones, and James W. Karesh

CHAPTER 3

Disorders of Eyelid Function Caused by Systemic Disease . . . 72

Gerald G. Striph and Neil R. Miller

CHAPTER 4

Ocular Manifestations of Systemic Immune Disease . . . 94

John C. Baer and Ramzi K. Hemady

Ocular Manifestations of Systemic Endocrine Diseases . . . 121

CHAPTER 5

Diagnosis and Management of Thyrotoxicosis . . . 121

Leonard P. Kapcala

CHAPTER 6

Diagnosis and Management of Hyperparathyroidism . . . 132

Leonard P. Kapcala

CHAPTER 7

The Ocular Manifestations of Non–Thyroid-Related Endocrine Disease . . . 137

James W. Karesh

CHAPTER 8

Infections of the Orbit and Orbital Structures . . . 146

Phillip F. Pierce

SECTION II

Conjunctiva . . . 157

Ralph E. Wesley

Introduction . . . 157

Ralph E. Wesley

CHAPTER 9

Conjunctiva: Structure and Function . . . 159

Harvey P. Cole III and Ralph E. Wesley

CHAPTER 10

Basic Techniques of Conjunctival Surgery . . . 163

Harvey P. Cole III and Ralph E. Wesley

CHAPTER 11

Replacement of Conjunctival Mucous Membrane . . . 170

Jonathan J. Dutton

CHAPTER 12

Pigmented Conjunctival Neoplasms . . . 178

M. Ronan Conlon and Peter A. D. Rubin

CHAPTER 13

Diagnosis and Management of Sebaceous Gland Carcinoma . . . 190

Evan H. Sacks and Richard D. Lisman

CHAPTER 14

Surgical Intervention in Conjunction with Medical Treatment of Cicatricial Pemphigoid . . . 196

James C. Fleming and Richard C. Cape

CHAPTER 15

Tarsoconjunctival Polishing with Mucous Membrane Grafting for Cicatricial Entropion and Trichiasis . . . 203

William P. Chen

CHAPTER 16
Management of Pterygia 208
Robert D. Deitch, Jr., and Fred M. Wilson II

CHAPTER 17
Chemical and Thermal Injuries of the Cornea and Conjunctiva 222
Roswell R. Pfister

CHAPTER 18
Conjunctival and Limbal Neoplasia: Diagnosis and Management . . . 231
Anne R. Horan and Denis M. O'Day

CHAPTER 19
Management of Conjunctival Amyloidosis 238
Brent A. Murphy and Ralph E. Wesley

CHAPTER 20
Kaposi's Sarcoma of the Conjunctiva 242
Brent A. Murphy and Ralph E. Wesley

CHAPTER 21
Lymphoid Tumors of the Conjunctiva 244
Brent A. Murphy and Ralph E. Wesley

CHAPTER 22
Conjunctival Procedures for Corneal Disease 248
Alice Y. Matoba

CHAPTER 23
Treatment of Squamous Papillomas of the Conjunctiva 251
Ralph E. Wesley and Harvey P. Cole III

CHAPTER 24
Management of Conjunctival Prolapse 253
Ralph E. Wesley

CHAPTER 25
Conjunctival Dermolipoma Surgery 255
Ralph E. Wesley

SECTION III
Eyelids 259
Robert Alan Goldberg and Russell S. Gonnering
Introduction 259
Robert Alan Goldberg and Russell S. Gonnering
Basic Sciences 261

CHAPTER 26
Clinical Eyelid Anatomy 261
Joseph P. Shovlin and Bradley N. Lemke

CHAPTER 27
Basic Surgical Techniques, Technology, and Wound Repair 281
David B. Christie and John J. Woog

CHAPTER 28
Anesthetic Considerations for Oculoplastic Surgery: An Update for the 1990s 294
Jonathan Kay

CHAPTER 29
Malignant Eyelid and Orbital Tumors 300
Mary A. Stefanyszyn and David I. Silbert

Clinical Sciences 307

CHAPTER 30
Eyelid Infections and Inflammations 307
Constance L. Fry and Russell W. Neuhaus

CHAPTER 31
Benign Eyelid Tumors 323
M. Ronan Conlon, Brian Leatherbarrow, and Jeffrey A. Nerad

CHAPTER 32
Malignant Epithelial Eyelid Tumors 342
Marcos T. Doxanas

CHAPTER 33
Mohs' Surgery for Periorbital Malignancies 352
Daniel Rivlin and Ronald L. Moy

CHAPTER 34
Reconstruction of the Upper Eyelid 356
David R. Jordan

CHAPTER 35
Medial Canthal Reconstruction 387
Roger A. Dailey and Diana Habrich

CHAPTER 36
Reconstruction of the Lower Eyelid and Lateral Canthus 400
Steven C. Dresner

CHAPTER 37
Congenital Eyelid Anomalies 407
Jill A. Foster and James A. Katowitz

CHAPTER 38
Entropion 413
John A. Long and Robert Alan Goldberg

CHAPTER 39
Involutional and Paralytic Ectropion 422
Steven M. Gilbard

CHAPTER 40
Lower Eyelid Retraction and Cicatricial Ectropion 438
Nancy C. Swartz, Marjorie Murphy, and Marc S. Cohen

CHAPTER 41
Aponeurotic Ptosis 447
Jonathan Christenbury

CHAPTER 42
Eyelid Trauma 452
Russell S. Gonnering

CHAPTER 43
Facial Paralysis: Diagnosis and Management 465
Lawrence F. Handler, Steven L. Galetta, Allan E. Wulc, and Jeffrey C. Popp

CHAPTER 44
Suborbital Augmentation 484
Kenneth D. Steinsapir and Norman Shorr

CHAPTER 45
Essential Blepharospasm and Hemifacial Spasm 504
John B. Holds

CHAPTER 46
The Eyelids in Graves' Ophthalmopathy 514
George B. Bartley

CHAPTER 47
Eyelid and Orbital Considerations in AIDS 525
Jan W. Kronish

CHAPTER 48
Micropigmentation and the Patient with Facial Burn and Facial Reconstruction 535
Richard W. Story and Darlene P. Story

SECTION IV
Cosmetic Surgery 543
Ted H. Wojno and Stephen Bosniak
Introduction 543
Stephen Bosniak

CHAPTER 49
Preoperative Evaluation 545
Ted H. Wojno

CHAPTER 50
Photography of the Ophthalmic Plastic Surgery Patient 551
David A. B. Price

CHAPTER 51
Total Facial Rejuvenation 560
Nelson Lee Novick

CHAPTER 52
The Practical Application of Aestheticians in the Plastic and Reconstructive Surgeon's Office 573
Susanne S. Warfield

CHAPTER 53
The Role of the Aesthetician Before and After Surgery 576
Catherine Atzen

CHAPTER 54
Brow Ptosis 578
Robert A. Weiss

CHAPTER 55
Electrology and Eyebrow Contouring 589
Wallace A. Roberts and Cora Buggea

CHAPTER 56
Upper Eyelid Blepharoplasty 596
David M. Reifler

CHAPTER 57
Lower Eyelid Blepharoplasty 617
Philip L. Custer

CHAPTER 58
Transconjunctival Lower Blepharoplasty 626
Robert Alan Goldberg, Henry I. Baylis, and Stacia H. Goldey

CHAPTER 59
Male Blepharoplasty 632
Hector M. Marines and James R. Patrinely

CHAPTER 60
Alternative Techniques of Fat Removal 638
Stephen Bosniak, Timothy F. McDevitt, and Ted H. Wojno

CHAPTER 61
Management of Blepharoplasty Complications 643
Ted H. Wojno

CHAPTER 62
Lymphatic Drainage Massage 651
Peter T. Pugliese and Linda Garofallou

CHAPTER 63
Principles of Camouflage Make-up and the Postoperative Patient . . 657
Annette Hanson and Nancy Dugan

CHAPTER 64
Chemical Peels 662
Howard Murad and Nita Patel

CHAPTER 65
Autologen: Autologous, Injectable Dermal Collagen 670
Dale P. DeVore, Charles D. Kelman, Steven Fagien, and Phillip Casson

CHAPTER 66
Electropigmentation and the Cosmetic Surgery Patient 676
Holla'e Ploof

CHAPTER 67
Blepharopigmentation: Techniques, Indications, and Comparison of Modalities 682
Joseph F. Mazza, Jr., and Cynthia Rager

VOLUME 2

SECTION V
Ethnic Ophthalmic Plastic Surgery 689
Don Liu
Introduction 689
Don Liu

CHAPTER 68
An Overview: Cultural Background and Anatomic Considerations in the Asian Patient 691
Don Liu

CHAPTER 69
Asian Blepharoplasty 702
Don Liu

CHAPTER 70
Considerations for Oculoplastic Surgery in the African American Patient 715
Tamara R. Fountain

CHAPTER 71
Auricular Acupuncture in the Treatment of Blepharospasm 718
Chieh Chung and Wen Ming Hsu

CHAPTER 72
Eyelid Tumors 721
Don Liu, Guang-Xi Zhao, and Nai Jiang Xu

SECTION VI
Lacrimal Surgery 729
Jeffrey A. Nerad
Introduction 729
Jeffrey A. Nerad

CHAPTER 73
Anatomy and Physiology of the Lacrimal System 731
Thaddeus S. Nowinski

CHAPTER 74
Evaluation of the Tearing Patient 748
David R. Jordan

CHAPTER 75
Eyelid Causes of Tearing 762
Jeffrey A. Nerad

CHAPTER 76
Congenital Lacrimal Abnormalities 777
Robert C. Kersten

CHAPTER 77
Primary Acquired Nasolacrimal Duct Obstruction 784
Keith D. Carter and Jeffrey A. Nerad

CHAPTER 78
Secondary Acquired Lacrimal Drainage Obstruction 797
George B. Bartley

CHAPTER 79
Disorders of the Canaliculus and Punctum 821
William White and John J. Woog

SECTION VII
The Orbit 835
Robert A. Weiss and Giulio Bonavolontà
Introduction 835
Robert A. Weiss and Giulio Bonavolontà

CHAPTER 80
Orbital Anatomy and Embryology 837
Don O. Kikkawa and Bradley N. Lemke

CHAPTER 81
Epidemiology of Orbital Pathology 853
Carlo de Conciliis

CHAPTER 82
Clinical Examination in Orbital Disease 860
Geoffrey E. Rose

CHAPTER 83
Neuro-ophthalmic Considerations in Orbital Disease 874
Marian Rubenfeld and Jonathan D. Wirtschafter

CHAPTER 84
Neuroradiologic Imaging of the Orbit and Globe 885
Mahmood F. Mafee

CHAPTER 85
Vascular Tumors of the Orbit 913
Barrett G. Haik and Holly Gore

Orbital Inflammatory Disorders 935

CHAPTER 86
The Role of Paranasal Sinus Disease in Orbital Cellulitis 935
John B. Holds

CHAPTER 87
Amyloidosis and Idiopathic Orbital Conditions 944
Joseph P. Shovlin

CHAPTER 88
Idiopathic Orbital Inflammation and Lymphoid Tumors of the Orbit 952
James P. Milite and Steven A. McCormick

CHAPTER 89
Pseudotumors 964
Will Harms

CHAPTER 90
Orbital Decompression for Graves' Orbitopathy 967
Myron Tanenbaum

Orbital and Periorbital Neoplasia. 983

CHAPTER 91
Neurogenic Tumors. 983
Michael Kazim and Jeffrey Bruce

CHAPTER 92
Mesenchymal and Fibro-osseous Tumors 994
Michael Clarke

CHAPTER 93
Lacrimal Gland Neoplasia 999
Geoffrey E. Rose

CHAPTER 94
Metastatic Tumors 1007
Jan W. Kronish

CHAPTER 95
Ophthalmic Manifestations of Mucoceles 1015
Barrett G. Haik and Ronald G. Amedee

CHAPTER 96
Radiation Therapy in Orbital Disease 1023
Steven J. Rubin

Orbital Surgery 1035

CHAPTER 97
Enucleation and Evisceration. 1035
William R. Nunery and William P. Chen

CHAPTER 98
Indications for Orbital Surgery 1046
Ted H. Wojno

CHAPTER 99
Operative Principles and Instrumentation. 1048
Ted H. Wojno

CHAPTER 100
Surgical Approaches to the Orbit 1050
Giulio Bonavolontà

CHAPTER 101
Optic Nerve Sheath Decompression 1056
Marc S. Cohen

CHAPTER 102
Anterior, Medial, Lateral, and Combined Surgical Approaches for Orbital Tumor Resection 1060
Giulio Bonavolontà

CHAPTER 103
Orbital Exenteration 1070
Peter S. Levin

CHAPTER 104
Harvesting and Use of Biological Tissue Grafts. 1077
Craig D. Friedman, Fred S. Bodker, and Robert A. Weiss

Orbital Trauma 1085

CHAPTER 105
Orbital Fractures 1085
Sara A. Kaltreider

SECTION VIII
Anophthalmic Socket 1103
Robert A. Weiss and Stephen Bosniak

CHAPTER 106
Evaluation and Management of the Anophthalmic Socket. 1105
Michael E. Migliori

CHAPTER 107
The Perfect Socket: The Ocularist's View. 1127
Walter J. Johnson

CHAPTER 108
Orbital Prostheses 1134
Gregory G. Gion

CHAPTER 109
Osseointegration for the Exenterated Orbit 1150
Jeffrey A. Nerad

SECTION IX
Craniofacial Deformities 1161
Robert A. Weiss

CHAPTER 110
Craniofacial Congenital Anomalies: The Subcranial Approach 1163
Joram Raveh, Kurt Laedrach, and Thierry Vuillemin

CHAPTER 111
Diagnostic and Presurgical Evaluation of Congenital Craniofacial Anomalies. 1178
Jay M. Pensler

CHAPTER 112
Orbital Deformities: Anterior Cranial Base Approach 1187
Jeffrey C. Posnick

Index i

SECTION I

Orbital and Periorbital Manifestations of Systemic Diseases

SECTION EDITOR

James W. Karesh

Introduction

James W. Karesh

When considering the ocular manifestations of systemic disease, the conditions that most commonly come to mind include diseases such as diabetes mellitus, hypertension, and hyperthyroidism. However, a myriad of diseases, both common and rare, can involve the eye and the structures surrounding it. The following chapters are devoted to a discussion of systemic diseases as they affect the periorbital and orbital structures. Some of these diseases may also involve the globe and its contents, but a consideration of these manifestations is beyond the limits of the discussion presented in this section. The interested reader is directed elsewhere for information regarding these subject areas.

Section I has six separate chapters. Each chapter covers a distinct type of systemic disease affecting the periorbita or orbit. The first and longest of these is concerned with cutaneous diseases. This is probably the most diverse group, because it includes descriptions of collagen vascular diseases, systemic and metabolic diseases, vesicobullous diseases, dermatoses, and hypersensitivity disorders. The chapter on neoplastic disorders describes a variety of conditions including malignant lymphoproliferative disorders, metastatic tumors, paraneoplastic syndromes, systemic inflammatory conditions such as Wegener's granulomatosis, amyloidosis and sarcoidosis, neoplastic cutaneous disorders, and periorbital neoplasia. The description of systemic neurologic conditions has been limited to those entities affecting the eyelids manifesting themselves as either blepharoptosis or eyelid retraction. Facial nerve palsies and the syndromes of benign essential blepharospasm are covered in other sections, and diseases affecting the other cranial nerves are beyond the limits of the discussion presented here. Systemic immune disease is another diverse area and includes bullous diseases, idiopathic inflammatory conditions, and systemic vasculitic conditions. The discussion of endocrine disease has been divided into three parts. The most important of these is related to the diagnosis and management of thyrotoxicosis. There is also a short section on hyperparathyroidism and other non–thyroid-related diseases such as diabetes and the various polyendocrine diseases. The final chapter in this section is devoted to a discussion of the various infectious processes that can involve the orbit and periorbital structures.

The intent of each of the authors of the chapters included in this section is to be current and, to the greatest extent possible, comprehensive. However, this has led to some duplication of coverage between the chapters. For example, sarcoidosis, thyroid disease, and paraneoplastic disorders are discussed in more than one chapter. Even though this redundancy can be criticized, it was believed that the overall content of this section would be strengthened by descriptions of similar entities from different points of view. In contrast, there is no section devoted to a discussion of either genetic or dysmorphic syndromes. Some of these are addressed in the various chapters in this section, for example, the phakomatoses, whereas others are addressed elsewhere in the sections devoted to craniofacial and congenital anomalies. Those readers who are interested in a more comprehensive discussion of these entities are referred to the excellent text by Gorlin and associates listed in the following general references. The editor realizes that, as with most multiauthored texts, there is some variability of style between the various chapters. No attempt was made to constrain the authors in this regard. The authors for each chapter were chosen because of their expertise in a particular area and, in many instances, because as nonophthalmologists they would have a more comprehensive understanding of the systemic nature of the disease processes they were describing. It is hoped that this will heighten the usefulness and quality of this section's content. Finally, a short list of texts describing the ocular manifestations of systemic diseases is provided here. It is hoped that the interested reader will refer to these for further information.

GENERAL REFERENCES

Cogan DG: Ophthalmic Manifestations of Systemic Vascular Disease. Philadelphia, WB Saunders, 1974.

Dinning WJ: Systemic Inflammatory Disease and the Eye. Bristol, England, Wright, 1987.

Gold DH, Weingeist TA: The Eye in Systemic Disease. Philadelphia, JB Lippincott, 1990.

Gordon DM: The eye in systemic disease. Int Ophthalmol Clin 7(3):1967.

Gorlin RJ, Cohen MM Jr, Levin LS: Syndromes of the Head and Neck, 3rd ed. New York, Oxford University Press, 1990.

Griffith DG, Salasche SJ, Clemons DE: Cutaneous Abnormalities of the Eyelid and Face. New York, McGraw-Hill, 1987.

Kanski JJ, Thomas D: The Eye in Systemic Disease, 2nd ed. Boston, Butterworths-Heinemann, 1990.

Korting GW: The Skin and Eye. Philadelphia, WB Saunders, 1973.

Kritzinger EE, Wright BE: A Colour Atlas of the Eye and Systemic Disease. London, Wolfe Medical Publications, 1984.

Mausolf FA: The Eye and Systemic Disease, 2nd ed. St. Louis, CV Mosby, 1980.

Miller NR: Walsh and Hoyt's Clinical Neuro-ophthalmology, 4th ed. Baltimore, Williams & Wilkins, 1991.

Ryan SJ, Smith RE: Selected Topics on the Eye in Systemic Disease. New York, Grune & Stratton, 1974.

Spencer WH: Ophthalmic Pathology: An Atlas and Textbook, 3rd ed. Philadelphia, WB Saunders, 1986.

CHAPTER 1

Cutaneous and Multisystemic Processes Affecting the Ocular Adnexa

Curt P. Samlaska, Brian Patrick O'Donnel, and William D. James

A vast number of cutaneous and systemic disorders can affect the ocular adnexa. Indeed, in many instances the eyelid findings are quite specific for disorders such as discoid lupus erythematosus (DLE), dermatomyositis, amyloidosis, lipoid proteinosis, ulerythema ophryogenes, granuloma annulare, alopecia areata, acanthosis nigricans, and multiple mucosal neuroma syndrome. These ocular adnexal findings in combination with other cutaneous and systemic abnormalities frequently result in establishing the correct diagnosis. To review such a large topic, the disorders are grouped into collagen vascular diseases, systemic and metabolic disorders, vesicobullous diseases, and dermatoses and hypersensitivity disorders. This chapter concentrates on those noninfectious cutaneous and systemic diseases involving the eyelids, orbit, lacrimal system, and sinuses. A critical review of systemic diseases involving the globe and intraocular structures is beyond the scope of this chapter. Some intraocular findings associated with ocular adnexal disease are mentioned for completeness, with emphasis on clinical presentation in relation to other cutaneous and systemic findings.

COLLAGEN VASCULAR DISEASES

A wide range of seemingly dissimilar disorders are classified as collagen vascular diseases, also referred to as *connective tissue diseases*. This group encompasses disorders such as lupus erythematosus, rheumatoid arthritis, rheumatic fever, polyarteritis nodosa, scleroderma, dermatomyositis, and mixed connective tissue diseases. Collectively, they exhibit an autoimmune process resulting in faulty T cell function that allows unchecked B cells to produce gamma globulins. The resulting dysproteinemias (cryoglobulinemia and hypergammaglobulinemia), autoimmune antibodies, and antigen-antibody immune complexes are capable of inducing vasculitis and small vessel obstruction.

The tremendous variability in clinical and laboratory findings has promoted establishing criteria to define many of these conditions. Several distinct diseases may be seen in the same patient, resulting in overlap syndromes. Others may have evidence of several of the conditions; however, they do not fulfill the criteria for any one collagen vascular disease and are thus classified as undifferentiated connective tissue diseases. Although all of these conditions have cutaneous lesions, only those with involvement of the eyelids and ocular adnexa are discussed. Sjögren's syndrome with keratoconjunctivitis sicca can be found in any collagen vascular disease.

Lupus Erythematosus

Lupus erythematosus (Fig. 1 – 1) is a chronic autoimmune disease with a wide spectrum of clinical forms. The polar expression of disease ranges from the purely cutaneous DLE at one end to systemic lupus erythematosus (SLE) with its protean manifestations of multisystem involvement at the other. Intermediate disorders that may or may not have associated SLE include disseminated DLE, subacute cutaneous lupus erythematosus (SCLE), mixed connective tissue disorders with lupus erythematosus features, and antiphospholipid antibody syndromes, including lupus anticoagulant and anticardiolipin antibody syndrome.

The reported prevalence of SLE in the continental United States ranges between 14.6 and 50.8 cases per 100,000 persons, and estimated incidence rates range between 1.8 to 7.6 cases per 100,000 persons per year.[1] The diagnosis of SLE requires 4 of 11 criteria established by the American Rheumatism Association (Table 1 – 1).[2] Cutaneous involvement is observed in 75% to 88% of all patients with SLE and is second only to joint disease in frequency of occurrence.[3] Cutaneous disease is the presenting manifestation of SLE in 25% of patients.[3] Cutaneous lesions account for 4 of the 11 criteria shown in Table 1 – 1 and are often key clinical findings in establishing the diagnosis.

Cutaneous manifestations of lupus erythematosus

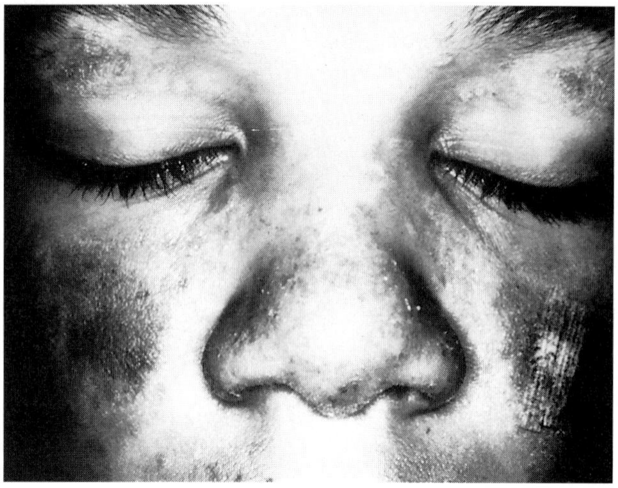

Figure 1–1. Lupus erythematosus.

may be divided into those that have classic histologic features on biopsy specimens for lupus erythematosus (lupus erythematosus–specific) and those that do not (lupus erythematosus–nonspecific).[4, 5] Lupus erythematosus–specific lesions can further be divided into chronic cutaneous lupus erythematosus (CCLE), SCLE, and acute cutaneous lupus erythematosus (ACLE), as shown in Table 1–2. The hallmark of ACLE is the "butterfly rash," a photosensitive process that begins as an erythematous patch that progresses into confluent symmetric involvement of the cheeks and lower eyelids with a connecting bridge over the dorsum of the nose. The patches can evolve into edematous plaques. The clinical appearance may simulate a drug-induced photosensitive eruption, polymorphous light eruption, dermatomyositis, seborrheic dermatitis, or acne rosacea.[3, 5]

TABLE 1–1

1982 Revised Criteria for Systemic Lupus Erythematosus[2,*]

1. Malar rash
2. Discoid rash
3. Photosensitivity
4. Oral ulcers
5. Nonerosive arthritis
6. Serositis
    - Pleuritis
    - Pericarditis
7. Renal disease
    - Proteinuria >0.5 g/d
    - Cellular casts
8. Neurologic disorders
    - Psychosis
    - Seizures
9. Hematologic disorders
    - Hemolytic anemia
    - Leukopenia
    - Lymphopenia
    - Thrombocytopenia
10. Immunologic disorders
    - Positive LE cell preparation
    - Anti-DNA antibody to native DNA
    - Anti-Sm
    - False-positive serologic test for syphilis
11. Positive antinuclear antibody results

*Diagnosis of systemic lupus erythematosus requires at least 4 of 11 criteria.
LE, lupus erythematosus; DNA, deoxyribonucleic acid.
Adapted from Tan EM, Cohen AS, Fries JR, et al: The 1982 revised criteria for the classification of systemic lupus erythematosus. Arthritis Rheum 25:1271–1277, 1982.

TABLE 1–2

Classification of Mucocutaneous Lesions of Lupus Erythematosus

Lupus Erythematosus–Specific Histologic Pattern (LE specific)
- Acute cutaneous lupus erythematosus (ACLE)
    - Malar erythema
    - Photosensitivity
    - Generalized erythema
    - Bullous lupus erythematosus
- Subacute cutaneous lupus erythematosus (SCLE)
    - Annular
    - Papulosquamous
    - Neonatal lupus erythematosus
    - C_2-deficient lupus erythematosus–like syndrome
    - Drug-induced SCLE[6]
        - Hydrochlorothiazide
        - Procainamide
        - Oxprenolol
        - Penicillamine
        - Sulfonylurea
        - Griseofulvin[7]
- Chronic cutaneous lupus erythematosus (CCLE)
    - Discoid lupus erythematosus (widespread and localized)
    - Hypertrophic and verrucous lupus erythematosus
    - Palmar and plantar lupus erythematosus
    - Oral discoid lupus erythematosus
    - Lupus panniculitis (lupus profundus)

Lupus Erythematosus–Nonspecific Mucocutaneous Lesions (LE nonspecific)
- Urticarial lesions
- Vascular lesions[3]
    - Vasculitis
    - Raynaud's phenomenon
    - Periungal erythema
    - Palmar erythema
    - Livedo reticularis
    - Thrombophlebitis
    - Chronic ulcers
    - Peripheral gangrene
    - Lupus pernio
    - Degos-like dermal infarcts or atrophy blanche
- Oral erosions
- Nonscarring alopecia
- Periungal erythema[3]
- Telangiectasias[3]
- Chilblain lupus[3]
- Rheumatoid-like nodules[3]
- Soft tissue calcification[3]
- Associated mucocutaneous disorders and findings
    - Dermal mucinosis
    - Porphyrias
    - Lichen planus
    - Psoriasis
    - Sjögren's syndrome
    - Squamous cell carcinoma

Adapted from Callen JP: Treatment of cutaneous lesions in patients with lupus erythematosus. Dermatol Clin North Am 8:355–365, 1990.

The most frequent ocular abnormalities (Table 1–3) are flame-shaped retinal hemorrhages and cotton-wool spots.[14, 22] These findings are not specific for SLE and may be seen in a variety of disorders. In the series by Frith and associates,[9] the most significant external ocular findings in SLE were episcleritis, blepharitis, and sicca syn-

TABLE 1-3

Ocular Complications of Systemic Lupus Erythematosus Disease and Therapy[8]

Adnexal
Cutaneous lid involvement[9]
Periorbital edema
Proptosis
Myopathy
Neuro-ophthalmologic
Cranial neuropathy[10]
Bilateral internuclear ophthalmoplegia[11,12]
Migraine-like syndrome[13]
Intracerebral vasculitis[14]
Optic neuritis[15]
Anterior Segment
Keratoconjunctivitis sicca
Subconjunctival hemorrhage
Uveitis[16]
Scleritis (episcleritis)[17]
Posterior Segment
Retinal vasculitis[18]
Pseudotumor cerebri[19-21]
Central retinal vein occlusion
Cotton-wool spots
Choroidopathy[22]
Drug-Induced Visual Loss
Corticosteroids[23]
Antimalarial agents[24]
Ibuprofen[25]
Indomethacin[26]

Adapted from Rubin BR, De Horatius RJ: Acute visual loss in systemic lupus erythematosus. J Am Osteopath Assoc 89:73–77, 1989.

drome. Acute visual loss has been reported with retinal vasculitis, central retinal vein occlusion, intracerebral vasculitis, uveitis,[19] scleritis,[20] and optic neuritis.[8,21] As previously noted, keratoconjunctivitis sicca may be seen in all of the collagen vascular diseases. The patient complains of a dry, gritty sensation in both eyes. On examination there is decreased tearing (as measured by the Shirmer's test), corneal staining, and epithelial debris in the tear film. Additional ocular complications of SLE are listed in Table 1–3.

Medications used to treat patients with SLE may result in gradual or rapid ocular complications (see Table 1–3). Systemic and topical steroids have been associated with increased intraocular pressure and glaucoma.[8,23] Visual loss can also occur through the development of posterior subcapsular cataract formation in patients on long-term corticosteroid therapy. Rapid tapering of systemic steroids has been reported to precipitate pseudotumor cerebri.[8] The antimalarials chloroquine and hydroxychloroquine can produce visual disturbances such as poor vision and halos around lights.[24] The most significant ocular complication of the antimalarials is irreversible retinal toxicity leading to blindness.

It has long been known that certain drugs, particularly procainamide, hydralazine, and isoniazid, may be associated with a lupus-like syndrome called *drug-related lupus*, *drug lupus*, and *hydralazine lupus* (Table 1–4).[27-29] Drug-related lupus is classified separately from SLE owing to a lower incidence of cutaneous, renal, and central nervous system findings. Much emphasis has been placed on the detection of antihistone antibodies, which approaches 100% of patients with symptoms, compared with 25% of patients with idiopathic SLE.[28] However, the detection of antihistone antibodies alone does not mean that the patient has drug-related lupus, because 50% to 100% of patients on procainamide will test positive after one year of therapy.[28] Symptoms include polyarthralgias, myalgias, pericarditis, fever, and weight loss. Pleuropulmonary disease resulting in effusions, pulmonary infiltrates, and pleuritis is common. Although patients with drug-related lupus usually have milder symptoms than do patients with idiopathic SLE, occasionally more severe forms are reported.[29] This is also true for ocular disease where procainamide use has been shown to be associated with scleritis and severe retinal vaso-occlusive disease[28,30]

The concept of SCLE was introduced to the medical community by Gilliam in 1977.[3,6] Although approximately 50% of these patients fulfill the criteria for SLE, SCLE represents only 5% to 10% of all patients with lupus erythematosus in the United States. In general, systemic manifestations are mild and cutaneous features are prominent. Two morphologic patterns have been identified (annular-polycyclic and papulosquamous-psoriasiform) involving the face, the upper trunk, and the dorsal surface of the arms and hands in a clear photosensitive pattern. Ocular findings in patients with SCLE without SLE are usually cutaneous lesions involving the eyelids. Photosensitivity occurs in 70% to 100% of reported cases and is a key clinical finding.[6] SCLE may be distinguished from DLE by the absence of dermal atrophy (scarring) and lack of follicular plugging. Although SCLE lesions heal without scarring, central lesion dyspigmentation may be observed. Antibodies to Ro/SSA have been sug-

TABLE 1-4

Drugs Related to Lupus Erythematosus[27,28]

Proved	*Possible*
Procainamide	Acetazolamide
Hydralazine	Captopril
Isoniazid	Chlorthalidone
Probable	Cimetidine
Acetylprocainamide	Gold salts
Allopurinol	Griseofulvin
Chlorpromazine	Methysergide
Ethosuximide	Oral contraceptives
Lithium carbonate	Other beta-blockers
Mephenytoin	Penicillin
Methyldopa	Phenylbutazone
Methylthiouracil	Streptomycin
Nitrofurantoin	Sulfonamides
Penicillamine	Tetracycline
Practolol	
Propylthiouracil	
Quinidine	
Reserpine	
Trimethadione	

gested as a serologic marker for SCLE. Of the 331 patients reported to have been tested for anti-Ro/SSA, 56% were positive compared with 25% anti-Ro/SSA for SLE.[6] Further evidence for the significance of anti-Ro/SSA antibodies in the development of SCLE comes from the detection of these antibodies in patients who develop drug-induced SCLE (see Table 1-2).[6, 7] The anti-Ro antibody response appears to be directed against the anti-Ro/SSA epitopes. The histologic features of SCLE are similar to those found in lupus erythematosus, and immunofluorescence studies are positive 50% of the time for immunoglobulin or complement deposition at the dermoepidermal junction.[3]

The most common form of CCLE is DLE, which is considered the clinical hallmark for this group of patients (see Table 1-2). The term *DLE* refers to a specific type of cutaneous lesion and does not refer to a subset of patients.[5] In fact, DLE lesions are observed in 20% to 30% of SLE patients, and 15% to 20% of all SCLE patients throughout the course of their disease.[30] Conversely, only 5% to 10% of all CCLE patients will develop systemic disease. Characteristic features of DLE lesions include a discrete erythematous plaque with thick adherent scale, follicular dilation with keratin plugging, peripheral hyperpigmentation with central atrophy and central hypopigmentation, and telangiectasias.[3, 5, 30] It occurs most commonly in women in their third to fifth decades of life. Although DLE may be seen on both light-exposed and light-protected surfaces, there is a strong correlation to ultraviolet exposure, with lesions predominating in the sun-exposed areas of the face, ears, arms, and V of the neck and chest.[5] Traditionally, DLE is divided into two subsets: localized and widespread disease. Although there is no serologic marker for DLE and the incidence of developing SLE is quite low, patients with widespread DLE are at a higher risk of developing systemic features than are patients with localized disease.[5, 30] The histology is characteristic for lupus erythematosus, and immunofluorescent studies demonstrate immunoglobulin deposits at the dermoepidermal junction in 80% of cases.[3]

The eyelids are not considered to be a strong site of predilection for DLE, but lesions nonetheless often occur there and are frequently a diagnostic challenge.[31-34] DLE of the eyelid may be misdiagnosed as chronic blepharitis, eczema, psoriasis, and even fungal dermatitis. The diagnosis is easy to make if the characteristic discoid lesions are identified and biopsy is performed. Blepharoconjunctivitis, in addition to DLE, can be caused by staphylococci (most common), atopic dermatitis, medications, other bacterial infections, viral infections, pediculosis, and sebaceous cell carcinoma.[33] Biopsies performed for histologic and immunofluorescent studies will establish the diagnosis. Identification of discoid lesions elsewhere on the face or other sites of the body supports the diagnosis of DLE. Stromal keratitis associated with DLE has also been described.[35] Loss of lashes and exacerbation with sun exposure are additional historical clues. Surgical manipulation of untreated DLE involving the eyelid may result in wound dehiscence and poor wound healing.[34] Treatment with topical steroids alone or in combination with hydroxychloroquine has been reported to be effective.

Lupus panniculitis, also known as *lupus profundus*, is an inflammatory subcutaneous process resulting in hyaline fat necrosis and eventual atrophic scarring.[3, 5] Sites of predilection include the face, shoulders, upper arms, and buttocks. The lesions begin as tender, erythematous, firm, subcutaneous nodules. Multiple sites may be involved, and the overlying skin may be normal in appearance, erythematous, or dyspigmented or show features of DLE. Histologic features include hyaline fat necrosis with a patchy or nodular lymphohistiocytic infiltrate, hyalinization of blood vessels, and endothelial swelling. The epidermis and overlying dermis may exhibit typical features of lupus erythematosus but may also be normal. Immunofluorescence studies are positive 70% of the time, showing granular immunoglobulin and complement deposition at the dermoepidermal junction. Nowinski and colleagues[36] reported three cases of lupus panniculitis involving the eye that resulted in lid edema and proptosis. Use of antimalarials such as chloroquine was effective in controlling the disease.

Confirming the diagnosis of SLE is difficult owing to the marked variation in clinical presentations. Astute interpretation of clinical findings and laboratory results is often required. The most important laboratory studies advocated historically are the lupus band test, the fluorescent antinuclear antibody (ANA) test, and the detection of antinative deoxyribonucleic acid (n-DNA) antibodies. ANA results are extremely sensitive for the detection of SLE but are not very specific. Of the serum autoantibodies, the most specific for SLE is the n-DNA or double-strand DNA (ds-DNA) antibody.[2, 37] Detection of antibodies to Sm and the lupus erythematosus cell preparation are fairly specific indicators of SLE. If the clinical findings suggest the possibility of a hypercoagulable state, laboratory evaluations should include studies to rule out antiphospholipid antibodies. Laboratory tests for lupus anticoagulant and anticardiolipin antibodies both should be ordered because the two disorders do not always overlap.[38]

Skin biopsies of cutaneous lesions frequently demonstrate histologic features of lupus erythematosus. Major features include hyperkeratosis, follicular plugging, atrophic stratum malpighii, vacuolar alteration of the epidermal basal cell layer, and thickening of the basement membrane. Dermal changes consist of a thickened basement membrane, perivascular and periadnexal mononuclear infiltrates, fibrin deposition between collagen bundles, edema, vascular ectasia, extravasated erythrocytes, and increased dermal acid mucopolysaccharides.

Prednisone remains the drug of choice for SLE, with the aim of improving clinical symptoms and normalizing n-DNA titers, serum complement, and urinary sediment. Management of cutaneous lesions includes education, liberal use of sunscreens, topical steroids, selected intralesional therapy, and antimalarial agents.[5] When standard treatment regimens fail to control cutaneous disease, additional treatment modalities may be required, such as azathioprine, cyclophosphamide, methotrexate, cyclosporine, retinoids, dapsone, auranofin, thalidomide, and lasers.[5]

Dermatomyositis

Dermatomyositis is an idiopathic inflammatory disease of muscle with far-ranging systemic complications. The disorder is one of the idiopathic inflammatory myopathies in which the cutaneous findings are characteristic, involving the fingers and eyelids. There are two peak incidence rates: one in childhood and another in the fifth decade.[39] It affects women more than men by two to one and appears to be less common in African American patients.[39,40]

Clinical criteria used to establish the diagnosis are listed in Table 1-5. Although there are fewer cutaneous lesions in dermatomyositis than in SLE, they are highly characteristic. A violaceous suffusion of the eyelids and upper cheeks is called a *heliotrope.* Patients develop a photosensitive edematous-erythematous eruption similar to that seen in SLE and SCLE. Gottron's papules are also highly characteristic of dermatomyositis. Features include flat-topped, violaceous, lichenoid papules distributed over the dorsal distal interphalangeal and proximal interphalangeal joint spaces. Additional cutaneous findings, such as periungual telangiectasias, cuticular hypertrophy with punctate infarcts, poikiloderma, and calcinosis cutis, may be observed.[42] Calcinosis cutis is a prominent feature in childhood dermatomyositis.[41] Approximately 11% of patients develop amyopathic dermatomyositis and exhibit the classic cutaneous lesions for as long as 8 years before developing myopathy.[43]

Extracutaneous manifestations of dermatomyositis are broad in scope. Proximal muscle weakness involving the upper extremities and neck is often the first symptom noted, and these sites are often the most severely involved. Arthralgias and dysphagia, particularly in childhood dermatomyositis, are common symptoms. Pulmonary disease manifested as interstitial fibrosis, hypoxemia, localized atelectasis, and nonproductive cough can be life threatening.[39,42] Cardiovascular involvement includes cardiomyopathy, cor pulmonale, tachyarrhythmias, conduction abnormalities, pericarditis, and heart failure. Gastrointestinal and renal disease (glomerulonephritis) have also been observed.

TABLE 1-5

Diagnostic Criteria for Dermatomyositis*[41,42]

1. Symmetric proximal muscle weakness†
2. Elevation of serum muscle enzyme levels
3. Electromyographic evidence of myopathy
4. Muscle biopsy with features of an inflammatory myopathy
5. Typical cutaneous eruptions of dermatomyositis
   - Heliotrope rash involving eyelids and facial regions
   - Gottron's papules over knuckles and joint spaces

* *Definitive* diagnosis: three or four criteria plus rash; *probable* diagnosis: two criteria plus rash; *possible* diagnosis: one criterion plus rash.

† With or without dysphagia and respiratory muscle weakness.

In addition to the heliotrope, periocular diseases such as conjunctivitis, episcleritis, and Sjögren's syndrome have been reported.[44-47] Paralysis of the external ocular muscles and proptosis may develop.[46] Intraocular disorders include severe retinal vasculitis with hemorrhages, cotton-wool exudates, retinal edema, iritis, glaucoma, and vascular tortuosity.[44-47] Retinitis appears to be the most frequently reported intraocular finding and is seen mostly in childhood dermatomyositis.

Although childhood dermatomyositis is not associated with malignancy, the adult forms may be. Malignancy-associated dermatomyositis is a controversial area, with some authors describing a higher association in patients with more acute and potentially more devastating variants.[39,42,48] Most patients found to have occult malignancy have abnormalities on history, physical examination, or laboratory studies. Basic evaluation of adult patients with dermatomyositis should include a complete history and physical examination (including rectal, stool guaiac, pelvic, and breast), routine laboratory tests (complete white blood cell count, serum electrolytes, stool guaiac on three separate occasions, and urinalysis), chest roentgenogram, and mammography in women.[42]

Although the diagnosis of dermatomyositis is established by a combination of characteristic skin lesions, muscle biopsy, electromyographic changes, and muscle enzyme studies, a variety of environmental agents have been implicated in inducing chronic myopathies. More than 20 drugs have been reported, some of which may cause cutaneous findings consistent with dermatomyositis. Marie and coworkers[49] reported a case of a lichenoid drug eruption that simulated cutaneous features of dermatomyositis, including facial erythema with eyelid edema, due to chronic hydroxyurea therapy. Skin biopsies should be performed whenever the diagnosis is in question.

Systemic corticosteroids are the mainstay of treatment. In amyopathic dermatomyositis, hydroxychloroquine alone or in combination with prednisone has been proved effective.[43] Additional agents include azathioprine, methotrexate, cyclophosphamide, and chlorambucil alone or in combination with prednisone.[39]

Scleroderma

Scleroderma (Fig. 1-2) is the result of a process of cutaneous thickening and induration due to excessive tissue deposition of collagen and other matrix proteins. Tradi-

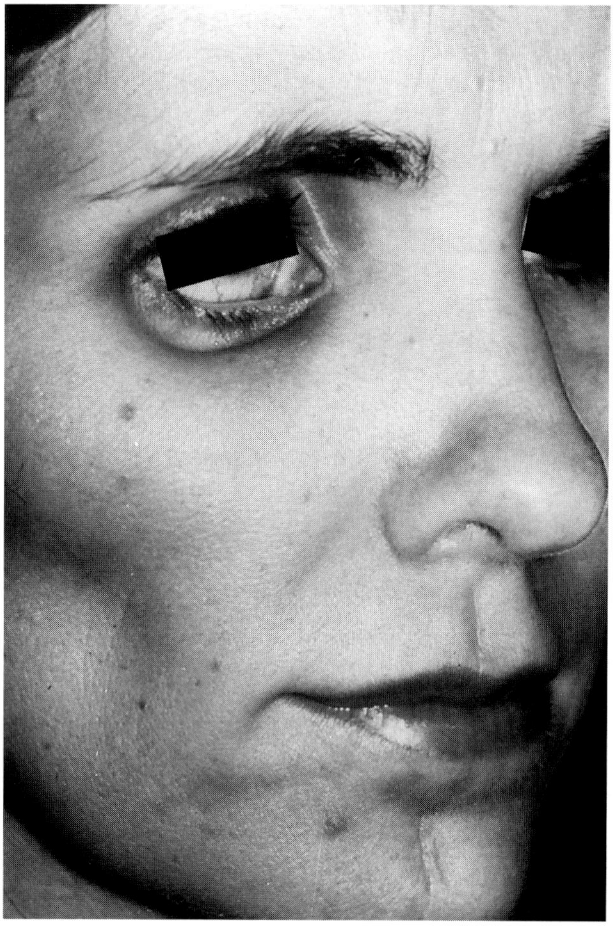

Figure 1 – 2. Linear scleroderma.

tional classification divides the various disorders into localized cutaneous forms, associated with little or no systemic disease, and systemic forms that manifest more symmetric generalized cutaneous involvement. Localized scleroderma can be divided into morphea, generalized morphea, and linear scleroderma.[50] More recent classification schemes include scleroderma variants, such as scleredema, eosinophilic fasciitis, and scleromyxedema.[50] There are also overlap syndromes with features of other rheumatologic disorders. In addition, a variety of conditions may manifest sclerodermoid features, including genetic disorders (progeria, Werner's syndrome), environmental causes (polyvinylchloride exposure, silicosis, rapeseed oil), metabolic disorders (porphyria, amyloidosis, POEMS syndrome, thyroiditis, childhood diabetes), chemical exposure (bleomycin, isoniazid, valproate sodium), malignancy (carcinoid syndrome, metastatic melanoma, bronchoalveolar carcinoma), postinfectious states (acrodermatitis chronica atrophicans, lipodystrophy) and neurologic disorders (dermal fibrosis in spinal injury, limb immobilization).[50] The following discussion is confined to localized scleroderma, systemic sclerosis, and CREST syndrome.

Localized scleroderma, or morphea, may be seen anywhere on the body and has several different clinical forms. The most common is the plaque variety in which circumscribed, edematous plaques in the skin become sclerotic, ivory-colored, smooth, devoid of hair, and slightly depressed. This form is most frequently observed on the trunk.[51] When the lesions are active and enlarging, a lilac or erythematous color to the advancing margin may appear. Multiple small plaques are referred to as *guttate*; when numerous, they evolve into the more debilitating generalized form of morphea. There is not a high association with visceral abnormalities. Another form is called *linear morphea.* Linear morphea involving the extremities may extend to deeper structures resulting in contractures and ankylosis of the involved joints.

A facial form of linear morphea resembles the healed wound from a saber cut, thus the Gallic description "en coup de sabre." The typical location is in the distribution of the supraorbital nerve in a linear fashion extending across the frontoparietal regions and may involve the eye.[52–54] Characteristically, this form of scleroderma involves one half of the face.[54] Patients may present to the ophthalmologist with symptoms long before the diagnosis has been established.[54] Early symptoms include pain, redness, eyelid edema, hypopigmentation, hyperpigmentation, and ptosis.[52–54] After the initial inflammatory phase, a sclerotic depression of the forehead develops, often extending through the eyelid with loss of the eyebrows and eyelashes in the involved sites. Additional ocular manifestations are listed in Table 1 – 6. Extension of the process can result in the facial hemiatrophy of

TABLE 1 – 6

Ocular Manifestations of Facial Linear Scleroderma[52–54]

Adnexal
Eyelid edema
Eyelid redness
Eyelid hyperpigmentation or hypopigmentation
Loss of eyelashes
Narrowed palpebral fissure
Extropion and ectropion
Ptosis
Excessive lacrimation
Retro-orbital inflammation with proptosis
Eyeball deeply set in orbit
Ocular muscle atrophy and paresis
Neuro-ophthalmologic
Ipsilateral neurocytoma of optic nerve
Anterior Segment
Iritis
Heterochromia
Uveitis
Sector iris atrophy
Corneal epithelial opacity
Decreased corneal sensitivity
Cataract
Glaucoma
Phthisis bulbi
Posterior Segment
Retinal hemorrhage
Central vein occlusion
Phthisis bulbi

Parry-Romberg syndrome.[51] The eyelids may occasionally be involved with plaque-type morphea, and bilateral eyelid disease has been described.[55]

The classification of systemic scleroderma into systemic sclerosis and CREST syndrome is based on mode of onset, patterns of cutaneous involvement, severity, and prognosis.[56] Overall, the average age of onset is between 40 to 50 years, with a female-to-male ratio of three to one.[57] Women are at their highest risk during the childbearing years between ages 30 to 39, and fewer than 10% will develop disease before the age of 20.[57]

Newer classification schemes attempt to define high-risk patients based on the site of onset and progression of sclerosis, such as acrosclerosis and diffuse scleroderma. CREST syndrome is the prototypical form of acrosclerosis. The acronym CREST stands for *c*alcinosis cutis, *R*aynaud's phenomenon, *e*sophageal dysfunction, *s*clerodactyly, and *t*elangiectasias.[58] Raynaud's phenomenon, edema of the hands, and arthralgias are frequently the first signs of disease. The edema gradually subsides, revealing sclerosis and atrophy of the distal extremities. The sclerotic phase slowly progresses into the typical features of sclerodactyly, namely, tapered fingers, tight hidebound skin, and a claw-like deformity secondary to muscle atrophy and joint contractures. Calcinosis cutis is often marked in the fingertips, resulting in transepithelial elimination and the subsequent development of ulcerations. Patients are also more prone to traumatic and vasospastic digital ulcers. The process slowly progresses in a distal-to-proximal direction on the extremities and, with time, may involve the chest, the face, and the scalp. Telangiectasias are prominent, particularly on the face, including the eyelids, and the distal extremities.[57, 58] The degree of telangiectasis often separates CREST syndrome from systemic sclerosis.[57] The morphology and distribution of the telangiectasia are similar to those seen in hereditary hemorrhagic telangiectasia, also known as *Osler-Weber-Rendu disease*.

Systemic sclerosis may begin much like CREST syndrome; however, it progresses more quickly and becomes more generalized. Initial onset of sclerosis on the trunk is a particularly poor prognostic sign.[57] Edema involving the upper chest is rapidly replaced by fibrosis, which subsequently spreads to the upper extremities and head and neck regions. The rate of progression may occur so quickly that sclerodactyly does not have time to develop. Additional cutaneous findings include diffuse hyperpigmentation resembling Addison's disease, postinflammatory hypopigmentation, calcinosis cutis, Raynaud's phenomenon, and telangiectasias. The facial features of systemic sclerosis are characteristic: The face is immobile and bound-down, with a youthful wrinkle-free appearance. The nose is small with a pinched look. The mouth is small with thin lips retracted into a permanent grimace. Sclerosis may also involve the eyelids, leading to blepharophimosis and lagophthalmos. Additional ocular findings include keratoconjunctivitis sicca, Sjögren's syndrome, cataracts, and retinal cotton-wool exudates.[59, 60]

Systemic scleroderma can involve all organs but has a predilection for the skin, gastrointestinal tract, lungs, heart, and kidneys. Gastrointestinal disturbances are seen in as many as 80% of patients, resulting in dysphagia, regurgitation, malabsorption, and constipation.[50] Myocardial disease is found in 80% of autopsy patients and is a frequently overlooked complication. Heart disease includes myocardial fibrosis, pericarditis, contraction band necrosis, conduction system fibrosis, and coronary artery disease.[57] Pulmonary fibrosis may result in lung cancer and pulmonary hypertension.[50] In patients with CREST syndrome, pulmonary hypertension is one of the leading causes of death. Acute fulminant malignant hypertension is a leading cause of death in systemic sclerosis. The presence of renal disease in scleroderma is still regarded as a poor prognostic sign. Arthralgias and myalgias occur during the inflammatory stages of the disease and may be confused with rheumatoid arthritis.[50]

The cause of scleroderma is still unknown. There is much evidence suggesting that the disorders are autoimmune in nature, resulting in activation of fibroblasts and altered collagen synthesis. A detailed discussion of these processes can be found in the review by Krieg and Meurer.[56] Many patients have positive ANA tests with a speckled or nucleolar pattern. Anticentromere antibodies are positive in CREST disease 49% to 96% of the time compared with positive 3% to 12% in systemic sclerosis.[57] Anti-Scl-70 is very specific for systemic sclerosis and is detected in as many as 60% of cases. Detection of anti-Scl-70 and anticentromere antibodies in the same patient is extremely rare.[57]

Treatment is supportive with close observation for the development of hypertension, heart disease, and respiratory complaints. Vasoactive agents such as nicotinic acid, dipyridamole, prazosin, calcium channel blockers, and beta-blocking agents may aid in controlling Raynaud's phenomenon and digital ulcers. Anti-inflammatory agents help control symptoms of arthralgia and myalgia. Systemic steroids have also been employed to control inflammatory periods. Vasoactive agents such as nifedipine, captopril, and minoxidil have proved effective in the control of malignant hypertension. The immunosuppressive agents azathioprine, cyclophosphamide, and cyclosporine yield variable results. D-Penicillamine and isotretinoin have been used with some success in halting the rate of progression; however, use of these agents must be considered with respect to possible drug-induced complications.[50]

Wegener's Granulomatosis

The respiratory vasculitides comprise Wegener's granulomatosis, Churg-Strauss syndrome, and lymphomatoid granulomatosis. Granulomatous inflammation of medium- and small-sized blood vessels and a predilec-

TABLE 1-7

1990 Criteria for Classification of Wegener's Granulomatosis*

1. Nasal or oral inflammation
   - Painful or painless oral ulcers
   - Purulent or bloody nasal discharge
2. Abnormal chest roentgenograms
   - Nodules, infiltrates, or cavities
3. Abnormal urinary sediment
   - Microhematuria (>5 red blood cells per high-power field)
   - Casts in urine sediment
4. Granulomatous inflammation on biopsy
   - Within vessel wall
   - Perivascular or extravascular areas

*Presence of two or more of the four criteria yields a sensitivity of 88.2% and a specificity of 92.0%.

Adapted from Leavitt RY, Fauci AS, Bloch DA, et al: The American College of Rheumatology 1990 criteria for the classification of Wegener's granulomatosis. Arthritis Rheum 33:1101–1107, 1990.

tion for pulmonary involvement are common features. Although these three disorders may have a similar clinical presentation, they are different disease processes that may require different treatment modalities. For these reasons it is important to be able to differentiate between them.

Wegener's granulomatosis is a multifocal necrotizing vasculitis that, in its classic form, involves the lungs, upper respiratory tract, and kidneys.[60–64] Another type of Wegener's granulomatosis is the limited form that fails to develop renal disease and has a better overall prognosis.[60] Classic Wegener's granulomatosis has a peak incidence during the fourth and fifth decades but may occur at any age. There is no sex or racial predilection for the classic form; however, the limited form affects women more frequently than men.[60–64] Criteria established by the American College of Rheumatology for the diagnosis of Wegener's granulomatosis are listed in Table 1–7.[65]

Clinically, these patients may present with a productive cough, hemoptysis, pneumonia, sinusitis, serous otitis media, or renal failure. Chest roentgenograms demonstrate waxing and waning pulmonary infiltrates, cavitary and noncavitary nodules, or frank consolidation. The pulmonary findings are bilateral, and rarely, pleural effusions, atelectasis, or mediastinal lymphadenopathy may occur. Glomerulonephritis is a late manifestation, and fewer than 10% of patients will present with renal disease.[60] Inflammation of medium- and small-sized vessels may involve any organ system, resulting in fibrinoid degeneration, aneurysmal dilation, thrombosis, and hemorrhage. In the series by Bullen and associates,[64] 48% developed hemorrhagic cutaneous lesions, 29% developed endocarditis, and 24% developed polyneuritis. Additional cutaneous findings include urticarial lesions, papules, vesicles, erythema, petechiae, purpura, ulcerative lesions, and pyoderma gangrenosum.[66] Chondritis of the nose results in a typical saddle deformity of the nose.

The same incidence rates of ocular disease exist for classic and limited forms. Eye involvement ranges between 28% and 58% and may be focal or contiguous.[60, 61] Focal ocular disease most commonly involves the sclera and episclera (20% to 38%), uveal tract (10% to 20%), peripheral cornea (14% to 38%), and retinal vasculature (7% to 18%).[60, 64] Orbital inflammation is observed in contiguous ocular disease, which occurs in 18% to 22% of patients.[67] Contiguous ocular involvement is the result of direct spread from paranasal sinuses. Cutaneous lesions involving the eyelids may occur. Additional sites of ocular involvement for Wegener's granulomatosis are listed in Table 1–8. Wegener's granulomatosis may present initially with eye findings and visual impairment progressing to blindness and possible enucleation.[60, 68]

TABLE 1-8

Ocular Abnormalities of the Respiratory Vasculitides[61,62]

Features	Wegener's Granulomatosis	Churg-Strauss Syndrome	Lymphomatoid Granulomatosis
Incidence	28–58%	Uncommon	Uncommon
Adnexa	Dacryoadenitis Nasolacrimal duct obstruction Eyelid granulomas	Eyelid granulomas	Eyelid granulomas
Orbit	Bilateral proptosis	Unaffected	Unaffected
Neuro-ophthalmologic	Ischemic papillopathy Papilledema Cranial nerve palsies	Ischemic papillopathy Amaurosis fugax	Cranial nerve palsies
Anterior Segment	Conjunctivitis Conjunctival hemorrhage Scleritis Episcleritis Limbal changes Keratitis Uveitis Marginal corneal furrows	Conjunctival nodules Episcleritis Marginal corneal furrows	Conjunctival infiltrates
Posterior Segment	Retinal vasculitis Retinitis Choroidal and retinal detachments	Posterior uveitis	Retinal panvasculitis

Although a number of mechanisms have been proposed, such as atopy, defective cell-mediated immunity, and other immune-mediated defects, the cause remains unknown. The differential diagnosis includes other forms of respiratory vasculitis such as microvascular polyarteritis, infectious diseases (tuberculosis, syphilis, histoplasmosis, blastomycosis, and coccidioidomycosis), and noninfectious granulomatous diseases (sarcoidosis, berylliosis, and midline lethal granuloma).[60, 61] Differentiation between these various disorders may be difficult because the diagnosis is based on clinical presentation, histology, and cultures. Skin biopsies in patients with Wegener's granulomatosis demonstrate necrotizing granulomas with a polymorphous infiltrate of neutrophils, plasma cells, and histiocytes.[69] The diagnosis of Wegener's granulomatosis has recently been facilitated by the identification of specific circulating autoantibodies to neutrophil cytoplasmic determinants.[61, 70] Two such antineutrophil cytoplasmic autoantibodies (ANCAs) have been shown to be helpful in classifying vascular disorders: cytoplasmic ANCA (directed against a 29-kD protease) is specific for Wegener's granulomatosis, and perinuclear ANCA (directed against myeloperoxidase) is specific for microvascular polyarteritis.[61]

Treatment of Wegener's granulomatosis, including ocular disease, requires systemic therapy. Local ocular treatment fails to arrest disease progression.[60] Current therapeutic recommendations include systemic corticosteroids in combination with cytotoxic agents such as cyclophosphamide. Pulsed intravenous corticosteroids and cyclophosphamide, and plasma exchange have also been used successfully during the acute phase of disease.[60–64] Some success has recently been reported with the use of trimethoprim-sulfamethoxazole alone or in combination with steroids in patients with slowly progressive localized disease, and this approach may prove to be an additional adjunct to combination therapy for systemic disease.[66]

Churg-Strauss Syndrome

Allergic granulomatosis and angiitis was first described by Churg and Strauss[71] in 1951. The syndrome is characterized by asthma, eosinophilia, fever, and systemic vasculitis.[60, 65, 71, 72] Earlier clinical series reported a fulminant course and high morbidity. There is no gender predilection, and age of onset ranges between 20 and 40 years.[69] The American College of Rheumatology has proposed a new classification scheme, as shown in Table 1–9.

The onset of asthma usually, but not always, precedes the onset of systemic vasculitis by many years. Presenting symptoms include fever, weight loss, and generalized malaise. Abdominal pain with gastrointestinal vasculitis and hesitancy with prostatic disease has been reported. Upper respiratory tract involvement and abnormal chest roentgenograms demonstrating transient patchy, nodular, or cavitary infiltrates are indistinguishable from Wegener's granulomatosis.[60] Lymphadenopathy is commonly observed. The cutaneous manifestations in the series by Masi and colleagues[72] included palpable purpura (40%), maculopapular eruptions (40%), and subcutaneous nodules (20%). Other reported findings are erythema multiforme–like lesions and hemorrhagic dermatitis.[60] The usual distribution is the scalp and extremities. Eyelid involvement is rare, but nodular granulomatous lesions of the eyelids and conjunctiva have been reported.[60] Associated ocular abnormalities are shown in Table 1–8.

TABLE 1–9

1990 Criteria for the Classification of Churg-Strauss Syndrome*

1. Asthma
2. Eosinophilia
3. Mononeuropathy or polyneuropathy
4. Paranasal sinus abnormalities
History of acute or chronic paranasal sinus pain
Sinus tenderness on physical examination
Opacification of the paranasal sinuses on roentgenograms
6. Eosinophils on biopsy
Biopsy of artery, arteriole, or venule with eosinophils in extravascular areas

*Presence of four or more of the six criteria yields a sensitivity of 85% and a specificity of 99.7%.

Adapted from Masi AT, Hunder GG, Lie JT, et al: The American College of Rheumatology 1990 criteria for the classification of Churg-Strauss syndrome (allergic granulomatosis and angiitis). Arthritis Rheum 33:1094–1100, 1990.

Biopsy specimens for Churg-Strauss syndrome demonstrate necrosis of small arteries and venules, fibrinoid collagen degeneration, granuloma formation with accumulation of epithelioid and giant cells in a perivascular location, and eosinophils.[60, 65, 68, 72] The necrotizing vasculitis observed in Churg-Strauss syndrome is not pathognomonic for this disorder and has been observed in other disease processes, such as polyarteritis nodosa and hypersensitivity angiitis.[72] In addition to eosinophilia, elevation of serum immunoglobulin E (IgE) has been described.[60]

Unlike in Wegener's granulomatosis, which responds poorly to monotherapy with systemic steroids, in Churg-Strauss syndrome the patients usually experience a good response. In those patients who do not remit with systemic steroids alone, the addition of azathioprine or cyclophosphamide is recommended.[60, 72]

Lymphomatoid Granulomatosis

In 1972 Liebow and coworkers[73] described 40 patients with an "angiocentric and angiodestructive lymphoreticular proliferative and granulomatous disease involving predominantly the lungs." Since then more than 300 cases of *lymphomatoid granulomatosis* have been described.[74] The most commonly involved organ systems include the lungs, skin, and central nervous system.[60, 69, 74–77] Men are affected more often than women, with peak incidence rates in the third to sixth decades.[74]

Patients present with fever, cough, chest pain, malaise, weight loss, and dyspnea.[74-77] Arthralgias and myalgias are infrequent complaints.[60,76] Pulmonary lesions develop in all patients throughout the course of their disease. There is a high mortality rate (65% to 90%) related to respiratory failure.[74] Approximately 13% to 18% of patients with lymphomatoid granulomatosis experience an evolution into classic malignant lymphoma. Indeed, numerous authors now believe that many cases of lymphomatoid granulomatosis are malignant lymphomas from the onset. Chest roentgenograms reveal bilateral nodular infiltrates in the lower lung fields. Skin is the extrapulmonary organ most commonly involved, with reports ranging between 40% and 60%.[69,74] Cutaneous lesions can be the presenting sign in 20% of cases, many of which (as many as 75%) do not have evidence of pulmonary disease.[74] Skin lesions frequently are transient, polymorphous, and asymptomatic.[76] The primary lesions are dermal nodules and plaques that may evolve into annular plaques. Additional descriptions include macules, macular erythema, papules, tumors, ulcerations, vesicles, ichthyosis, alopecia, and necrobiosis lipoidica-like lesions.[74,76] The differential diagnosis of these findings includes granuloma annulare, sarcoidosis, lymphoma cutis, leukemia cutis, lymphomatoid papulosis, and Hansen's disease.[77] About one third of patients develop neurologic symptoms manifested as peripheral neuropathy, mental confusion, ataxia, hemiparesis, seizures, and cranial nerve palsies.[60,69] Other organ systems (hepatic, cardiac, renal, adrenal, and splenic) can be involved but are not important clinically and are detected on autopsy.[76]

The most frequent ocular manifestations are due to cranial nerve palsies.[60] Findings include facial nerve palsies, ptosis, diplopia, and transient blindness. Infiltration of the eyelid with granulomatous lesions and cutaneous lymphoma can occur.[60,76] Additional ocular abnormalities associated with lymphomatoid granulomatosis are listed in Table 1-8.

The cause of lymphomatoid granulomatosis is unknown. Cutaneous and open lung biopsies are paramount to confirmation of the diagnosis. Skin biopsy findings demonstrate a destructive granulomatous perivascular infiltrate in the dermis comprising atypical lymphoid cells and plasma cells. There can be extensive necrosis and infiltration of small- and medium-sized arteries and veins. More than 50% atypical lymphoreticular cells indicates a poor prognosis.[69] A paucity of eosinophils and polymorphonuclear leukocytes differentiates lymphomatoid granulomatosis from Wegener's granulomatosis and Churg-Strauss syndrome. Immunohistochemical studies have demonstrated mostly T cells, and many authors believe that this disorder is a variant of peripheral T cell lymphoma.[69,74]

Fauci and associates[75] have been successful in inducing long-term remission in lymphomatoid granulomatosis with the use of combined prednisone and cyclophosphamide. Once the disease has progressed to frank malignant lymphoma, however, the chance of successful medical management even with more aggressive multiple chemotherapeutic regimens is small.

SYSTEMIC AND METABOLIC DISEASES

This section reviews inborn and acquired metabolic abnormalities and systemic disorders that do not fit into more specific categories. Admittedly, inclusion into this group is somewhat arbitrary owing to the limited knowledge of etiology. Every attempt was made to discuss the various diseases based on shared clinical and systemic findings. For example, scleredema and scleromyxedema are reviewed in this section instead of the section on collagen vascular diseases owing to similar clinical and histologic findings in comparison with thyroid disease states. In many instances the eyelid or ocular abnormalities may be incidental and in others constitute the earliest manifestations of the underlying systemic disease process.

Hyperthyroidism

Graves' disease is the most common form of hyperthyroidism (Fig. 1-3) and afflicts mostly women between the ages of 10 and 45 years.[78-80] Patients with thyrotoxicosis present with fatigue, irritability, heat intolerance, weight loss, palpitations, and fine tremors. Classic Graves' disease consists of the triad of hyperthyroidism with a diffuse goiter, ophthalmopathy, and infiltrative dermopathy manifested as pretibial myxedema. Cutaneous manifestations include smooth, warm skin and puffy thickening of the eyelids, sometimes associated with hyperpigmentation. The appearance may be indistinguishable from myxedema.[81] Without treatment, the disease usually burns itself out within 1 to 3 years.

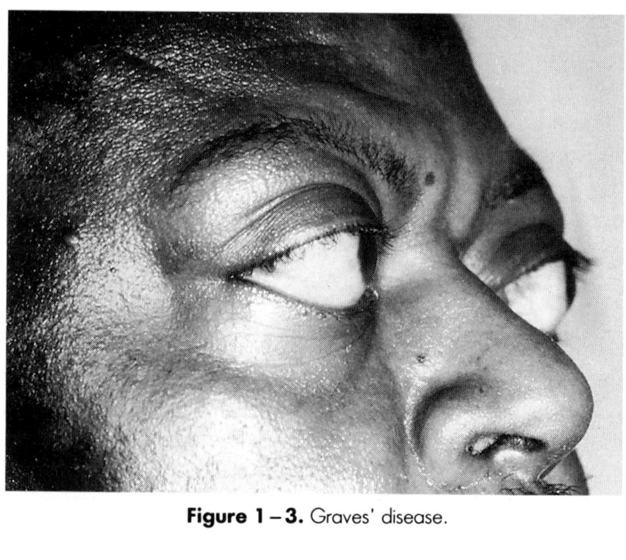

Figure 1-3. Graves' disease.

Ocular manifestations of thyroid dysfunction are referred to as *Graves' ophthalmopathy, dysthyroid ophthalmopathy, dysthyroid orbitopathy, endocrine exophthalmos, Graves' orbitopathy, infiltrative ophthalmopathy, thyroid eye disease,* and *malignant exophthalmos.*[79] The most common manifestations of Graves' ophthalmopathy are upper and lower eyelid retraction, lagophthalmos, conjunctival chemosis, restricted eye movement manifesting as diplopia, eyelid edema, and axial exophthalmos.[79, 80, 82] Edema and thickening of the eyelids can also be found in hypothyroidism (myxedema), scleromyxedema, trichinosis, dermatomyositis, amyloidosis, hypersensitivity reactions, and Melkersson-Rosenthal syndrome. Severe orbital disease can result in loss of vision from exposure keratitis or optic nerve compression.

The most common form of unilateral or bilateral exophthalmos in adults is dysthyroid ophthalmopathy, and more than 80% who develop severe eye findings do so within 18 months of detection of thyroid disease.[79, 80] However, many systemic disease processes can result in exophthalmos, and as many as 25% of patients referred to an ophthalmologist for consideration of dysthyroid ophthalmopathy have other causes, including metastatic disease and pseudotumors.[80] Table 1–10 lists some of the systemic diseases that are associated with exophthalmos.

The pathogenesis of dysthyroid ophthalmopathy remains obscure. The diagnosis of Graves' ophthalmopathy is not difficult, and a variety of eye signs on physical examination aid in the diagnosis.[80] Laboratory evaluations should include free thyroxine (T_4) index, thyroid-

TABLE 1–10

Systemic Diseases Associated with Exophthalmos

Endocrine Disorders
- Graves' ophthalmopathy
- Hypothyroidism
- Acromegaly
- Cushing's syndrome
- Hyperparathyroidism

Lymphoid and Hematologic Disorders
- Malignant lymphoma
- Multiple myeloma
- Leukemia
- Myelodysplastic syndrome[85]

Histiocytic and Macrophage Disorders
- Histiocytosis X
  - Hand-Schüller-Christian disease
  - Letterer-Siwe disease
  - Eosinophilic granuloma
- Juvenile xanthogranuloma
- Sinus histiocytosis with massive lymphadenopathy
- Systemic xanthogranulomatosis (Erdheim-Chester disease)
- Necrobiotic xanthogranuloma

Noninfectious Orbital Inflammation
- Sarcoidosis
- Multifocal fibrosclerosis
- Lupus erythematosus
- Dermatomyositis
- Scleroderma[52]
- Giant cell polymyositis
- Wegener's granulomatosis
- Polyarteritis nodosa
- Cogan's syndrome (atypical form)
- Lethal midline granuloma
- Angiolymphoid hyperplasia with eosinophilia (Kimura's disease)
- Amyloidosis

Infectious Orbital Inflammation
- Pyemic cellulitis
- Tuberculosis
- Syphilis
- Mucormycosis
- Aspergillosis
- Echinococcosis (hydatid cyst)
- Trichinosis
- Amebiasis
- Lyme disease

Fibro-osseous Lesions
- Fibrous dysplasia and Albright's syndrome
- Brown tumor in hyperparathyroidism
- Orbital osteomas in Gardner's syndrome
- Multiple enchondromatosis (Ollier's disease)
- Infantile cortical hyperostosis (Caffey's disease)
- Hereditary diaphyseal dysplasia (Engelmann's disease)
- Osteopetrosis (Albers-Schonberg disease)

Phakomatoses and Vascular Syndromes
- Neurofibromatosis
- Wyburn-Mason syndrome
- Osler-Weber-Rendu syndrome
- Klippel-Trenaunay-Weber syndrome
- Sturge-Weber syndrome

Benign Intracranial Disorders
- Orbital encephaloceles[86]
- Leptomeningeal cysts[87]

Metastatic Tumors to the Orbits
- In children
  - Neuroblastoma
  - Ewing's sarcoma
  - Wilms' tumor
  - Medulloblastoma
  - Sarcoma
  - Other cancers
- In adults
  - Breast adenocarcinoma
  - Lung cancer[88]
  - Prostate cancer
  - Gastrointestinal tract cancer
  - Renal cell carcinoma
  - Thyroid cancer
  - Melanoma
  - Carcinoid
  - Other cancers

Congenital Craniofacial Deformities
- Crouzon's disease
- Apert's syndrome
- Pfeiffer's syndrome
- Kleeblattschadel anomaly
- Lowry's syndrome
- Hermann-Opitz syndrome
- Sakati-Nyhan-Tisdale syndrome
- Other craniofacial disorders

Reprinted with permission from Int Ophthalmol Clin 31:143–162, 1991.

stimulating hormone (TSH), thyrotropin receptor antibodies, serum antimicrosomal antibodies, and serum antithyroglobulin antibodies.[80-83] Good control of the hyperthyroid state is recommended; however, the ophthalmopathy does not necessarily parallel the thyroid state.[79] Results of surgical correction of exophthalmos and eyelid retraction are variable and should be considered when there is a potential for developing progressive chemosis and exposure keratitis.[79, 80, 84]

Myxedema

Myxedematous states consist of a group of disorders ranging from localized to systemic disease. On skin biopsy they all have characteristic histologic features, namely, mucin deposition within the dermis. Hypothyroidism is the classic systemic disorder associated with myxedema. Clinical presentation is often slow and progressive with complaints of mental obtundation, sluggishness, weight gain, asthenia, anemia, cold temperature intolerance, hypohidrosis, constipation, and voice changes.[89-93] The skin is dry, wax-like, translucent, and indurated and frequently has fine scaling consistent with xerosis.

Mucopolysaccharide accumulation in the skin results in nonpitting edema particularly involving the pretibial regions and the eyelids. Facial features include puffy eyes and cheeks (Fig. 1–4); dull and expressionless facies; a broad, thick nose; and fat lips. Diffuse scalp alopecia and loss of the outer portions of the eyebrows along with generalized sparse, dry, and thin hair may occur (Fig. 1–5). Intraocular associations are rare in hypothyroidism; however, an increased incidence of glaucoma and cataracts in myxedematous patients has been reported.[93, 94] Eyelid myxedema may be an early finding in these patients, resulting in presentation to a plastic surgeon for cosmetic correction.[93]

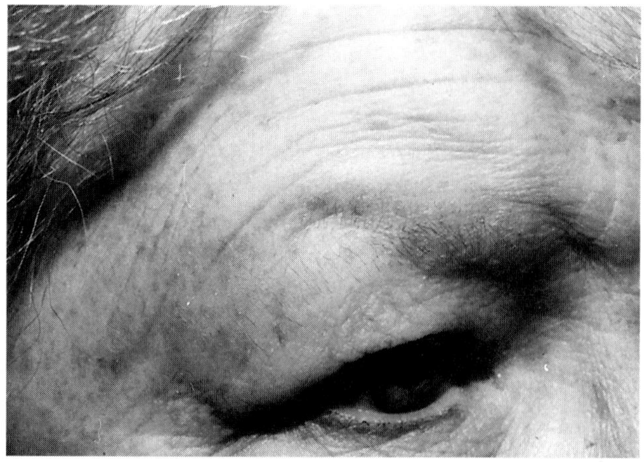

Figure 1–5. Hypothyroidism, with loss of lateral eyelashes.

Cretinism is the result of untreated congenital hypothyroidism. Clinical features include dwarfism; wide-set eyes; thick lips; macroglossia; and pale, edematous skin. Frequently, the child develops a hoarse cry and a "pot belly." Mental retardation is severe.[95]

Screening laboratory examination for hypothyroidism should include a free T_4 index and TSH levels. Treatment with desiccated thyroid, L-thyroxine (Synthroid), L-triiodothyronine (Cytomel), or liotrix (Euthroid) results in improvement of myxedema caused by hypothyroidism.[95]

Scleromyxedema

Scleromyxedema (Fig. 1–6) is a rare fibromucinous disorder affecting adults between 28 and 76 years of age with clinical features similar to systemic sclerosis.[96-100] Scleromyxedema is considered to be a variant of lichen myxedematosus or papular mucinosis.[100] Characteristic

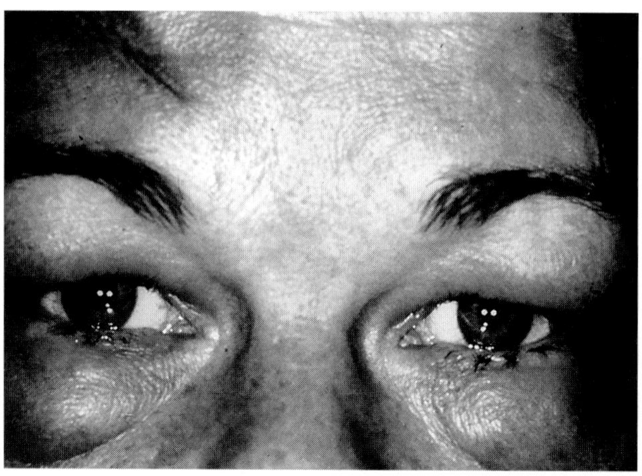

Figure 1–4. Myxedema.

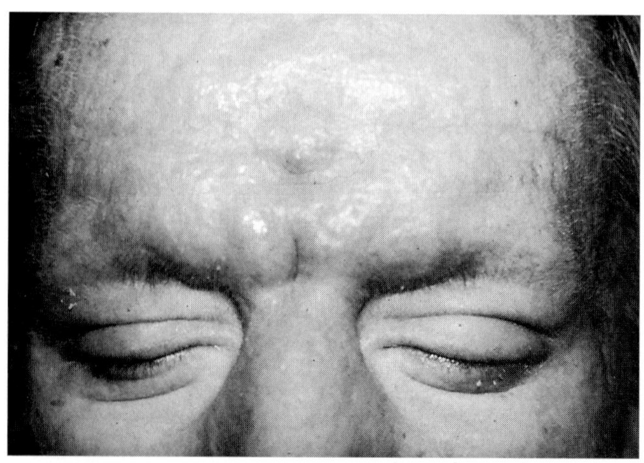

Figure 1–6. Scleromyxedema. (Courtesy of Dr. Neil Fenske.)

clinical features include onset of a cutaneous eruption composed of flesh-colored waxy papules progressing to marked sclerosis and induration of the skin involving the hands, arms, and face. The trunk and lower extremities may also be involved but to a lesser extent. Although the degree of sclerosis may result in restricted range of motion, the skin lacks the bound-down quality seen in scleroderma.[97] Acrosclerosis, stiff hands, and flexion contractures can develop in scleromyxedema. However, other findings of systemic sclerosis, such as Raynaud's phenomenon, calcinosis cutis, telangiectases, decreased carbon monoxide diffusion, and digital ulcers, rarely occur.[96, 97] As the disease progresses, the forehead and glabellar regions may become deeply furrowed, resulting in a leonine facies. Facial expressions are blunted owing to restricted range of motion.

Many cases are associated with paraproteinemia, most notably monoclonal gammopathy of the IgG and, to a lesser extent, the IgA class. Numerous systemic manifestations have been associated with scleromyxedema, including neurologic symptoms, renal insufficiency, cardiovascular disorders, amyloidosis, connective tissue disorders, Waldenström's macroglobulinemia, and non-Hodgkin's lymphoma.[96-98] Necrotizing myositis, dermatomyositis, and esophageal aperistalsis have also been described.[96-99] Acute psychosis is the most common neurologic manifestation. Depression, paresthesia, paralysis, encephalopathy, coma, transient ischemic attacks, meningioma, and carpal tunnel syndrome are additional neurologic complications.[97]

The eyelids can be involved, showing thickening and induration.[101] Impairment of eyelid closure usually does not occur. Mucinous infiltration into skin results in loss of eyebrows and eyelashes.[97] Corneal deposits of hyaluronic acid and amyloid P component in Bowman's membrane manifest as blurred vision.[101, 102]

The differential diagnosis includes thyroid-induced myxedema, systemic sclerosis, systemic amyloidosis, multiple myeloma, and Hansen's disease. Skin biopsies demonstrate mucinous infiltration of the papillary dermis that is distinctly different from the marked sclerosis and destruction of adnexal structures observed in scleroderma.[96] The mucopolysaccharide consists of hyaluronic acid and is indistinguishable from that seen in the skin of pretibial myxedema. Thyroid studies are normal.

Treatment of scleromyxedema has been ineffective and frequently results in complications. Corticosteroids, alkylating agents, mechlorethamine hydrochloride, urethane, methotrexate, melphalan, cyclophosphamide, plasmapheresis, etretinate, psoralen plus ultraviolet A (PUVA), dermabrasion, and electron beam and radiation therapies have been used with variable results.[96-100] Good responses with isotretinoin have recently been reported, with fewer potential side effects than some of the other treatment options.[97, 98]

Scleredema

Scleredema, also known as *scleredema adultorum of Buschke*, is a rare condition of unknown etiology and is characterized by excess deposition of acid mucopolysaccharides in the dermis.[103-106] Initially, this was considered to be a benign self-limited disease that often occurred following influenza or streptococcal infections in children.[104] More recent literature, however, suggests that this may be a more progressive disorder, particularly when found in adults.

Scleredema is characterized by the development of nonpitting, symmetric cutaneous induration with a peculiar wooden-like consistency.[107] The brawny induration begins on the nape of the neck and subsequently progresses to involve the upper torso, arms, face, and eyelids.[103-106] Reported additional sites of involvement include the abdomen, tongue, pharynx, skeletal muscle, joints, pericardium, and pleura.[105] Early eyelid involvement is observed more in pediatric patients and must be differentiated from Melkersson-Rosenthal syndrome and angioneurotic edema. In addition to induration of the eyelids, conjunctival and corneal changes have been observed.[104] In the pediatric age group the disorder is usually self-limited, resolving in 1 to 2 years.[104, 108] In adults the disease is frequently associated with adult-onset insulin-resistant diabetes mellitus. Associations with paraproteinemia and primary hyperparathyroidism have also been reported.[105, 106]

Histologic examination reveals an expanded dermis with swollen collagen bundles. The collagen is separated by fenestrations containing deposits of mucopolysaccharides that stain positively with Alcian blue. There is no effective treatment for the cutaneous changes, although strict control of diabetes, if present, is recommended.

Melkersson-Rosenthal Syndrome

Melkersson-Rosenthal syndrome is a bizarre entity consisting of the triad of orofacial swelling of the lips, intermittent facial nerve palsy, and fissuring of the tongue called lingua plicata.[109-113] Miescher's cheilitis granulomatosa is considered by some investigators to be a monosymptomatic form involving only the lips.[109] Melkersson-Rosenthal syndrome afflicts mostly young adults, with a peak incidence rate in the second decade of life. Caucasian, Japanese, and Middle Eastern patients have been reported, with approximately equal distribution between the sexes.[109, 110]

Patients present with a history of intermittent orofacial swelling and transient facial nerve palsies. The clinical signs do not necessarily appear simultaneously, and disease-free intervals may range from months to years.[109] In the series of 58 patients reported by Alexander and James,[113] 86% developed orofacial swelling, 90% developed facial paralysis, and 77% had a fissured tongue. Oral swelling can involve the gingiva, palate, and tongue. Swelling of the cheek, forehead, and eyelids is not uncommon. The swelling is often asymmetric, nonerythematous, painless, and nonpruritic. Additional ocular manifestations include retrobulbar neuritis, lagophthalmos, exposure keratitis, corneal opacity, epiphora, and keratoconjunctivitis sicca.[109, 112] In addition to facial nerve palsies, migraine headaches, hyperhidrosis, hypogeusia, acroparesthesia, and hyperacusis have been reported.[109]

Potential systemic disease associations with Melkersson-Rosenthal syndrome include atopic dermatitis, leukemia, and rheumatoid arthritis.[109, 113, 114] Crohn's disease and sarcoidosis may have similar clinical and histologic findings; however, most authors believe that Melkersson-Rosenthal syndrome is a separate entity. The differential diagnosis of cheilitis granulomatosis includes all three of these disorders.[110, 115]

The cause of Melkersson-Rosenthal syndrome is unknown. The differential diagnosis includes sarcoidosis, Crohn's disease, lymphatic obstruction, Ascher's syndrome (facial swelling with cutaneous atrophy), recurrent erysipelas, hereditary angioedema, contact dermatitis, and facial edema with eosinophilia.[109-113] Biopsy specimens demonstrate dermal edema and noncaseating granulomas with Langhans' giant cells.[109] Numerous treatment modalities have been used with only temporary improvement, including intralesional steroids, danazol, clofazimine, salazosulfapyridine, radiation therapy, and surgical reduction cheiloplasty.[109-113] Surgical procedures performed without postoperative intralesional or systemic corticosteroids may result in an exaggerated recurrence.[109]

Sarcoidosis

Sarcoidosis (Fig. 1-7) is a multisystemic disorder that can affect any organ of the body. The most characteristic features are hilar lymphadenopathy, pulmonary infiltration, and ocular or cutaneous disease.[116, 117] The diagnosis is confirmed on identification of typical clinicoradiographic findings in conjunction with histologic evidence of widespread epithelioid granulomas in more than one system.[116] Peak age of onset is in the second to fourth decades, and there is no sex predilection.[117] In Europe it is most prevalent in the Scandinavian countries, particularly Sweden. In the United States it affects mostly African Americans, although Asian Americans and Caucasians may also be afflicted.[117]

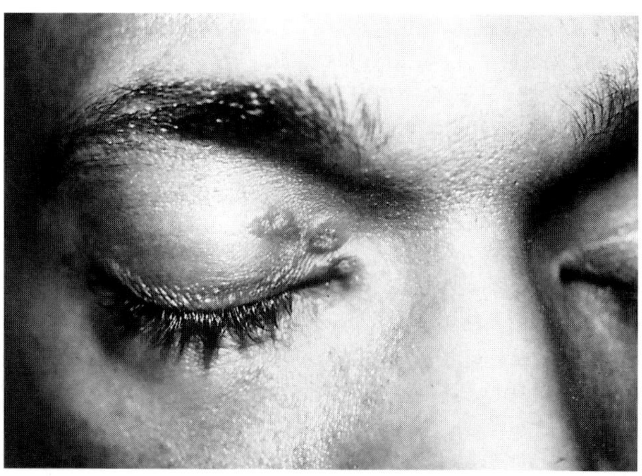

Figure 1-7. Sarcoidosis.

Chest roentgenograms are abnormal in more than 90% of patients with sarcoidosis.[118] The lungs and mediastinal lymph nodes are the most frequently involved organ systems. Indeed, in view of normal chest roentgenogram findings, the diagnosis of sarcoidosis is questionable considering the vast number of disorders that may present with infiltrating granulomas. Lymphadenopathy is common. Additional organ systems involved, in order of frequency, are ocular (7% to 33%), cutaneous (30%), hepatic (20%), and nervous (10%) systems.[117, 119, 120] Cutaneous manifestations are diverse and offer an easy site for biopsy confirmation. One of the most common cutaneous manifestations is tender nodular lesions of the lower extremities known as *erythema nodosum*. Erythema nodosum is a reactionary process (biopsy results do not show sarcoidal granulomas) and is one component of Lofgren's syndrome.[121] Features of Lofgren's syndrome are fever, polyarthralgias, uveitis, bilateral hilar adenopathy, fatigue, and erythema nodosum.[117, 121] Papular sarcoid, also known as *miliary sarcoid*, demonstrates numerous indurated small papules located over the face, eyelids, neck, and shoulders. Additional cutaneous types include hypopigmented, lupus pernio, psoriasiform, verrucose, ulcerative, subcutaneous, Hutchinson's plaque, erythrodermic, ichthyosiform, and mucosal forms.[117] Although only 20% of patients develop clinical evidence of hepatic disease, blind liver biopsy results are positive in 60% of patients.[117] Facial nerve palsies are the most common neurologic manifestation of sarcoidosis.[120] Patients with Heerfordt's syndrome develop uveitis, parotitis, and facial or other cranial nerve palsies.[121]

In the series by Obenauf and colleagues,[118] the most common manifestation of ocular sarcoidosis was uveitis (52%), lacrimal gland disease (16%), acute iritis (15%), iris nodules (11%), chorioretinitis (11%), and periphlebitis (10%). The most frequent ocular findings in the series by Karma and coworkers[122] were conjunctival granulomas (47%) and lacrimal gland disease (46%). Conjunctival nodules are frequently asymptomatic and occur mainly during active stages.[119, 122] Retinal periphlebitis producing the "candle-wax drippings" observed on ophthalmoscopic examination is a rarely observed hallmark of ocular sarcoid.[118] Vitreous opacities may produce grayish-white bodies in chains referred to as a "string of pearls."[118] Optic nerve disease is frequently associated with intracranial involvement and may produce papil-

TABLE 1-11

Ocular Manifestations of Sarcoidosis[118-120,122]

Adnexal
Lacrimal gland enlargement
Dacryoadenitis
Papular lesions involving the eyelids
Eyelid edema
Orbital granulomas
Orbital tumors
Exophthalmos[69]
Abnormal ocular motility
Neuro-ophthalmologic
Cranial nerve palsies
Papilledema
Papillitis
Optic disk granulomas
Optic neuritis
Anterior Segment
Acute and chronic uveitis
Iris nodules
Acute iritis
Episcleritis
Cataracts
Glaucoma
Keratoconjunctivitis sicca
Conjunctival granulomas
Symblepharon
Band keratitis
Interstitial keratitis
Staphyloma[123]
Posterior Segment
Chorioretinitis
Periphlebitis
Chorioretinal nodules
Vitreous opacities
Vitreous hemorrhage
Retinal neovascularization
Acute posterior multifocal placoid pigment epitheliopathy[124]

ledema, papillitis, optic neuritis, and granulomas infiltrating the optic disk.[118] Additional ocular findings are listed in Table 1-11.

Although the cause of sarcoidosis is unknown, it is considered a lymphoproliferative disorder resulting in depression of delayed-type hypersensitivity, an imbalance of helper and suppressor T lymphocyte subsets, and hyperactive B cell lymphocytes resulting in an increase in circulating immune complexes.[116, 117] The differential diagnosis is quite large based on clinical and histologic features. Detection of granulomas on tissue samples must be interpreted carefully because more than 70 different infectious and noninfectious disorders may have similar histologic findings.[125] This is particularly important for infectious disorders such as syphilis, tuberculosis, cat-scratch disease, lymphogranuloma, and deep fungal infections, which may have ocular and systemic features suggestive of sarcoidosis.[125, 126] Biopsy specimens demonstrate sarcoidal granulomas consisting of well-demarcated, avascular, eosinophilic epithelioid cells, which may fuse to form epithelioid multinucleated Langhans' giant cells.[117, 121] The giant cells and epithelioid cells may contain various inclusions called Schaumann's bodies and asteroid bodies.[117, 126] Random bilateral conjunctival biopsies have been shown to be positive for sarcoidal granulomas in 71% of proven and 29% of suspected sarcoid patients.[127]

Markers of disease activity include an elevation in serum angiotensin-converting enzyme levels, elevated serum calcium values, a positive Kveim-Siltzbach skin test, intrathoracic uptake of radioactive gallium, and abnormal fluorescein angiography.[116] In patients with uveitis suspected to be caused by sarcoid, serum angiotensin-converting enzyme values greater than 50 U/L yielded a sensitivity of 84%, a specificity of 95%, and a predictive value of 47% for the diagnosis of sarcoidosis.[128] Many patients are anergic on skin testing.

Systemic corticosteroids are the mainstay for treating systemic disease. Antimalarials and isotretinoin have been used with variable success for treatment of cutaneous manifestations.[117] Acute anterior uveitis responds well to local corticosteroids and mydriatics.[119, 121, 122] Sarcoidosis involving the posterior segment is best treated with systemic corticosteroids.[121, 122] Vitreous hemorrhages may absorb spontaneously within 12 months. If visual impairment exists after this time, a vitrectomy may result in significant improvement.[119] Acute optic nerve disease should be treated with systemic corticosteroids at the time of presentation.[119]

Amyloidosis

Amyloidosis (Fig. 1-8) is a group of disease entities that result in deposition of amyloid material in tissue, producing considerable organ dysfunction.[129] On light microscopy using hematoxylin-eosin stain, amyloid deposits consists of amorphous homogenous eosinophilic material. Regardless of the cause, amyloid is composed of 7.5- to 10-nm rigid, linear, nonbranching, aggregated, paired, hollow fibrils of indefinite length.[129] It is an end-stage glycoprotein that the body cannot metabolize.

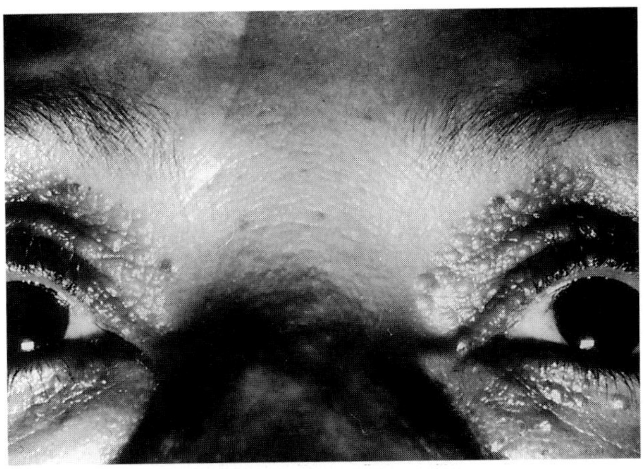

Figure 1-8. Amyloidosis.

TABLE 1–12

Classification Schema for Amyloidosis[129–131]

Clinical Types of Amyloidosis	Amyloid Fibril Protein*
Systemic	
Primary	AL
Myeloma associated	AL
Secondary	AA
Hemodialysis associated	β_2-Microglobulin
Heredofamilial	
Familial Mediterranean fever	AA
Muckle-Wells syndrome	AA
Familial amyloid polyneuropathy (FAP)	
FAP type 1 (Portuguese, Japanese)[130]	Prealbumin
FAP type 2 (Indiana, Maryland)[130]	Prealbumin
Swedish type [129,130]	Prealbumin
Organ Limited	
Nodular	AL
Primary localized cutaneous	
Nodular	AL
Macular amyloidosis	? Altered keratin
Lichen amyloidosis	? Altered keratin
Ocular[129,130]	
Vitreous	? Prealbumin
Endocrine	
Pancreatic	? Proinsulin
Thyroid	? Precalcitonin
Senile	
Senile cardiac	ASc1
Senile cerebral/Alzheimer's associated	APCP
Heredofamilial	
Hereditary cerebral	Cystatin C

*AA, amyloid A; AL, amyloid L; APCP, amyloid plaque core protein; ASc1, amyloid senile cardiac protein-1.

Amyloid fibril proteins are derived from different precursor substances, reflecting the underlying disease process. The two most common amyloid fibril proteins are amyloid L and amyloid A, which are derived from immunoglobulin light chains and serum amyloid A protein, respectively. Protein amyloid A is derived from an acute-phase reactant called *serum amyloid A,* an apolipoprotein of high density (HDL_3) found in normal people. Some cutaneous forms are the result of altered keratin filaments (Table 1–12). The type of amyloid fibril protein is helpful in the classification of amyloidosis.[129]

Table 1–12 lists a classification schema for the many forms of amyloidosis. This scheme is based on a number of principles. Systemic disease involves many organs of the body, whereas organ-limited disease is confined to a single organ system. Systemic amyloidosis may be divided further into primary systemic disease, which is the result of an occult plasma cell dyscrasia, multiple myeloma, and a secondary type associated with a variety of chronic illnesses. Disorders causing secondary systemic amyloidosis include chronic infection, rheumatoid arthritis, inflammatory bowel disease, Hodgkin's lymphoma, solid nonlymphoid tumors, venous ulcerations, psoriatic disease, lepromatous leprosy, hidradenitis suppurativa, chronically infected burns, chronic skin infection in drug addicts, ulcerated basal cell carcinoma, epidermolysis bullosa acquisita, and X-linked anhidrotic ectodermal dysplasia.[129] The remainder of the organ-limited disorders are classified based on the organ system involved and the type of amyloid fibril protein. Solitary plasmacytomas found in the respiratory or urinary tracts and around the eye are classified as nodular organ–limited amyloidosis. Some authors classify vitreous amyloid as nodular organ–limited disease.[129] Ocular organ–limited disease has been added to the classification schema (see Table 1–12) because more than 30 cases of sporadic vitreous amyloid have been reported.[130, 132, 133] In addition, Gorevic and associates[130] have shown that vitreous amyloid deposition in some sporadic amyloid cases is due to prealbumin (not amyloid L).

In primary and myeloma-associated systemic amyloidosis, the amyloid L deposits can involve the tongue, heart, gastrointestinal tract, skeletal and smooth muscle, carpal ligaments, nerves, and skin. The organ systems involved in secondary systemic amyloidosis are the liver, spleen, kidneys, and adrenal glands.[129] Patients with primary systemic and myeloma-associated disease present with symptoms of fatigue, weight loss, paresthesias, hoarseness, edema, dyspnea, and lightheadedness or syncope. Carpal tunnel syndrome, macroglossia, mucocutaneous lesions, hepatomegaly, and edema are frequent physical findings. Cutaneous lesions include petechiae, purpura, and ecchymoses; waxy, translucent, or purpuric papules; nodules; plaques; tumefactive lesions; pigmentary changes; scleroderma-like infiltration; bullous lesions; alopecia; cord-like blood vessel thickening; and nail dystrophy.[129] Purpuric lesions are pronounced on flexural regions such as the eyelid, nasolabial fold, neck, axillary, umbilical, and anogenital regions. Eyelid purpura may be induced by coughing, Valsalva maneuver, vomiting, forced expiration during spirometric testing, proctoscopy (postproctoscopic palpebral purpura), and pinching (pinch purpura).[129] Papulonodular amber and xanthelasma-like papules characteristically involve the eyelids (amyloidosis palpebrarum).[134] Tumefactive lesions on the face can produce a leonine appearance. Scleroderma-like diffuse infiltration may affect the face, the hands, and the feet.[129] A myxedematous appearance may develop, manifesting with rigidity of facial expression; thick, drooping eyelids; pendulous lips; and projecting ears.[129]

As previously noted, ocular disease may be localized or part of systemic amyloidosis. Localized ocular forms can manifest as flat, pink, well-vascularized conjunctival lesions, ptosis, vitreous opacities, and painless induration or tumefaction of the eyelids or conjunctiva.[130, 135, 136] Bilateral corneal amyloid in a patient with retrolental fibroplasia has also been reported.[137] The most frequent intraocular finding in patients with systemic amyloidosis is vitreous opacification.[130, 138] Visible corneal nerves have been reported. There are two forms of familial lattice corneal dystrophy, and a familial corneal and conjunctival subepithelial form of amyloidosis known as *primary gelatinous drop-like dystrophy.*[129, 139] Corneal opacities are not observed in familial amyloid polyneuropathy types 1 or 2, and lattice corneal dystrophy does not react to prealbumin on immunohistologic studies.[130] Proptosis has also been reported for systemic disease.[79] Multiple myeloma associated with amyloidosis may also present with primary ocular findings. Maisel and coworkers[140] reported a case of painful unilateral ocular inflammation and acute blindness associated with multiple myeloma. Additional ocular adnexal manifestations of multiple myeloma include proptosis, cranial nerve compression, conjunctival crystal deposition, and sludging blood column in conjunctival vessels.[140]

The differential diagnosis of amyloidosis is quite large and dependent on the clinical presentation. Cutaneous disease must be distinguished from other infiltrative processes such as scleroderma, scleromyxedema, thyroid-induced myxedema, necrobiotic xanthogranuloma, other xanthomatous lesions, bullous disorders, ligneous conjunctivitis, lipoid proteinosis, and infectious disorders such as Hansen's disease. Histologic, immunohistochemical, and electron microscopic examination of biopsy tissue is the key to diagnosis. Results of fine-needle biopsy of abdominal subcutaneous fat from clinically normal skin are positive for amyloid in 95% of primary systemic, 66% of secondary systemic, and 86% of heredofamilial disease.[129] Secondary amyloidosis lacks cutaneous findings. Biopsies of cutaneous lesions in primary systemic, myeloma-associated, and heredofamilial disease invariably yield positive histologic findings for amyloid. Biopsies of conjunctival lesions and vitreous sampling are also high-yield procedures.[136, 138] Cresyl violet, Congo red, and thioflavine T special stains aid in identification of amyloid deposits in tissue.[129] Serum prealbumin levels in affected patients with familial amyloid polyneuropathy 1 and 2 can be decreased and may have diagnostic value.[130] Laboratory studies to rule out the possibility of multiple myeloma should be performed in those patients with systemic features.

There is no effective treatment for primary or secondary systemic disease. Management of secondary systemic disease is directed at treatment of the underlying cause. For patients with localized disease, there are more therapeutic options available and these are reviewed in the article by Breathnach.[129] Treatment for vitreous amyloidosis is pars plana vitrectomy.[141]

Necrobiotic Xanthogranuloma

In 1980 Kossard and Winkelmann[142] described eight patients with multiple xanthomatous plaques and subcutaneous nodules associated with paraproteinemia. Histologic examination revealed xanthogranulomatosis and necrobiosis, resulting in the proposed name *necrobiotic xanthogranuloma with paraproteinemia.* Review of the literature by these authors resulted in the identification of a number of similar case reports labeled as atypical multicentric reticulohistiocytosis with paraproteinemia, particularly involving the trunk and eyelids.[143] More than 48 cases of this newly described disease have been reported. The age of onset ranges between 17 and 85 years (average 54 years), and there is no sex predilection.[143]

All patients develop cutaneous lesions described as indurated papules, nodules, or plaques. The coloration varies from violaceous to red-orange, but yellow is most often noted, particularly in the periorbital region. Some lesions may become atrophic and develop telangiectases.[143] The cutaneous sites slowly evolve into infiltrating plaques ranging from 0.3 to 25 cm in diameter. Central clearing or ulceration may be observed. Although most lesions are asymptomatic, tenderness, pain, pruritus, and a "burning" sensation may be reported.[143] The most frequent site of involvement is the periorbital region (81% of reported cases), followed by the trunk, face, arms, thighs, and distal lower extremities.[143]

Necrobiotic xanthogranuloma is a systemic disease, and many patients have hepatosplenomegaly on physical examination. Multiple myeloma has been reported in three patients.[143, 144] A variety of seemingly unrelated illnesses have been documented to include hypertension, chronic obstructive pulmonary disease, pulmonary fibrosis, cardiomyopathy, pituitary adenoma, lung carcinoma, Graves' disease, primary biliary cirrhosis, carpal tunnel syndrome, epilepsy, peripheral neuropathy, colonic carcinoma, and lymphatic leukemia.[143] Future studies are required to determine if these findings are indeed associated with necrobiotic xanthogranuloma. In the patients followed at the Mayo Clinic, more than half have died from malignancies.[143]

About half of the patients develop ophthalmic complaints, including burning, pruritus, blurred vision, painful eyes, diplopia, dry eyes, periorbital swelling, and acute transient loss of vision.[143, 145] Eyelid lesions often resemble xanthelasma; however, on palpation, there is deep induration not observed in xanthelasma.[145] Additional ocular findings include orbital masses, conjunctivitis, keratitis, scleritis, episcleritis, iritis, anterior uveitis, cataracts, glaucoma, ptosis, and ectropion.[143, 145]

The cause of necrobiotic xanthogranuloma with paraproteinemia is unknown. The differential diagnosis includes necrobiosis lipoidica diabeticorum, amyloidosis, xanthelasma, sarcoidosis, chalazion, generalized normolipemic plane xanthoma, xanthoma disseminatum, and juvenile xanthogranuloma.[143] Laboratory findings are significant for the detection of an IgG paraproteinemia in more than 80% of patients.[143] Biopsy specimens are remarkable for palisading xanthogranulomas associated with necrobiosis. Touton giant cells, foreign body granulomas, and cholesterol clefts can also be observed. Histiocytes and lymphoid aggregates are the predominant cell types.[143] Similar histologic features have been demonstrated in the spleen, heart, kidneys, and ovaries on autopsy.[143]

Treatment for necrobiotic xanthogranuloma has resulted in some success, particularly with the use of chlorambucil. Radiation therapy for periorbital lesions has also been effective.[146] Additional treatment options are melphalan, hydroxychloroquine, and plasmapheresis.[143] According to Robertson and Winkelmann,[145] excision followed by intralesional corticosteroids has been unsuccessful for localized cutaneous disease. Methotrexate is ineffective in these patients.[143]

Ligneous Conjunctivitis

Ligneous conjunctivitis is a rare form of chronic pseudomembranous conjunctivitis first reported by Borel[147] in 1933. *Ligneous* means "woody hard" and refers to the wood-like pseudomembranous lesions of the tarsal conjunctiva that are often refractory to therapy.[148] The disease usually affects children, particularly after recurrent infections, but may occur at any age. It is a chronic, progressive systemic disorder involving mucous membranes and frequently results in visual loss and ocular destruction.[149]

Patients may present with symptoms of stringy eye mucus, discharge, conjunctival masses, injection, decreased vision, and inflammation.[147–150] Upper eyelid masses have also been reported.[148] Pseudomembranes may extend to the cornea, resulting in vascularization.[150] Other mucous membranes and organ systems may be involved, such as the larynx, vocal cords, trachea, nasopharynx, vagina, gingiva, middle ear, and tympanic membrane.[149] A familial predisposition has also been reported for ligneous conjunctivitis and hydrocephalus, anophthalmos, and recurrent respiratory infections.[149] Hidayat and Riddle[150] believe there are two phases to ligneous conjunctivitis: (1) an acute phase, which occurs in association with systemic signs and symptoms such as fever, upper respiratory tract and urinary tract infections, otitis media, sinusitis, vulvovaginitis, and cervicitis; and (2) the chronic phase, which may present without systemic features and result in progressive ocular disease.

The cause of ligneous conjunctivitis remains poorly understood. Vasculopathy, hypersensitivity reaction, defective glycosaminoglycan metabolism, exaggerated inflammatory response, viral infection, trauma, and disturbed wound healing all have been proposed, based mostly on immunohistochemical and electron microscopic studies.[149,150] The differential diagnosis of ligneous conjunctivitis includes all forms of chronic membranous conjunctivitis, pyogenic granuloma, lipoid proteinosis, and amyloidosis.[150] The predominant histologic findings are subepithelial deposits of eosinophilic, amorphous material that greatly resembles amyloid on histologic studies. Indeed, Congo red stain for amyloid may actually be positive; however, on electron microscopy these deposits lack amyloid fibrils.[148,150] Examination with special stains and immunohistochemical studies has resulted in the identification of mucopolysaccharides, albumin, fibrin, and immunoglobulin.[149,150] A mixed acute and chronic inflammatory infiltrate is frequently observed.[148]

Treatment of this rare disorder has been based on the various substances deposited in tissues.[149] Antibiotics, topical steroids, cromolyn sodium, hyaluronidase, chymotrypsin, azathioprine, and cyclosporine have been used with variable success.[149,150] In most chronic forms, these treatment regimens have been unsuccessful.

Lipoid Proteinosis

Lipoid proteinosis, also known as *Urbach-Wiethe disease, lipoproteinosis, lipoglycoproteinosis, lipidosis cutis et mucosae, hyalinosis cutis et mucosae,* and *nevus ichthyosiformis,* is a rare autosomal recessive inherited condition characterized by the deposition of a hyalin glycoprotein in the skin and mucous membranes of the eyelids, mouth, larynx, and pharynx. About 300 cases have been described, mostly in people of European and South African descent.[151] Patients lacking severe laryngeal obstruction have a normal life expectancy.[151]

The earliest clue to the diagnosis is hoarseness, due to hyalin infiltration of the vocal cords, which may be present at birth.[151–154] Cutaneous lesions, most often involving the face and extremities, develop about the time the child begins to walk. These initial lesions are vesiculopustular and may be mistaken for impetigo.[151] Healing results in depressed acneiform scars. Subsequent deposition of hyaline material in the dermis produces yellow nodules and diffuse cutaneous thickening.[151–154] Nodular lesions 1 to 3 mm in diameter affect the face, neck, and lid margins. The eyelid lesions are small yellowish, translucent pearly papules located around the eyelashes and along the lid margin. At least two thirds of the cases develop these characteristic eyelid lesions referred to as *moniliform blepharosis,* and their detection is a useful diagnostic clue.[152] Nodular lesions have also been reported to involve the scrotum, vulva, perineum, and perianal areas.[151] Verrucous plaques may develop over the hands, elbows, knees, and other sites exposed to trauma and irritation. Additional cutaneous findings include generalized waxy cutaneous thickening, pigmentary changes (particularly in non-Caucasian patients), patchy hair loss, and nail dystrophies.[151–154] Mucous membrane disease can result in a hoarse voice; diffuse, irregular thickening of the lips; macroglossia with geographic furrowing of the tongue and epiglottitis; and lesions involving the buccal mucosa, tonsils, vaginal vestibules, or rectum.[151–154] Laryngeal or pharyngeal obstruction may necessitate performance of a tracheostomy. Patients have been reported to have psychomotor seizures (due to bilateral calcifications near the dorsum sellae, a pathognomonic roentgenographic sign), impaired hearing, and mental retardation.[151,152] Visceral involvement has been described in virtually every organ system but with much less hyaline deposition than the skin and upper airways.[154] Diabetes mellitus, hyperlipoproteinemia, hypogonadism, congenital insensitivity to pain, and carpal tunnel syndrome have been documented in some patients with lipoid proteinosis.[151, 152]

In addition to moniliform blepharosis, a number of ocular complications may occur. Glaucoma, drusen of Bruch's lamina vitrea, corneal opacities, and retinal degeneration are later manifestations.[151-153] Corectopia developed shortly after birth in a case reported by Johnson and Hepler.[155] Another patient developed pseudomembranous conjunctivitis that failed to respond to surgical management at 4 months of age and had histologic findings consistent with lipoid proteinosis on conjunctival biopsy.[152]

The differential diagnosis of lipoid proteinosis includes amyloidosis, xanthomatoses, ligneous conjunctivitis, and erythropoietic protoporphyria.[151, 152] The differential diagnosis of moniliform blepharosis is amyloidosis, syringomas, Darier's disease, and multiple mucosa neuroma syndrome. Histologic examination of cutaneous lesions establishes the diagnosis. Amorphous eosinophilic material is demonstrated around blood vessels, and larger hyalin deposits with cleft formation are found in the upper dermis.[151] The substance surrounds sweat glands, hair follicles, and errector pili muscles while sparing eccrine ducts and apocrine sweat glands. The hyaline material is strongly periodic acid–Schiff (PAS) positive, fat stain (Sudan black) positive, and Congo red negative (stain for amyloid).

There is no definitive therapy for lipoid proteinosis. The challenge is mostly a cosmetic one, because few patients develop life-threatening complications. Cosmetic improvement has been achieved with dermabrasion. Surgical removal of vocal cord nodules results in improved function. Wong and Lin[156] reported a dramatic improvement in one case treated with oral dimethyl sulfoxide. Dimethyl sulfoxide works by dissolving the hyalin deposits and has also been used successfully in patients with localized cutaneous amyloid.

Darier's Disease

Keratosis follicularis, or Darier's disease, is an autosomal dominant inherited condition with cutaneous and mucosal involvement. Cutaneous lesions described as reddish keratotic follicular papules involving the scalp, face, central chest, and intertriginous zones are initial manifestations.[157] As the disease progresses, the lesions develop a dirty, warty character and coalesce into symmetric, malodorous, vegetative plaques.[157] The cutaneous lesions may become generalized. Occasionally, the skin lesions are hemorrhagic or bullous, and exacerbations with systemic steroids and lithium have been reported.[158-161] The nails develop characteristic subungual hyperkeratosis, fragility, splintering, and triangular nicking of the free edges.[157] Mucous membrane involvement results in a "cobblestone" appearance of the hard palate, tongue, larynx, esophagus, and anorectal mucosa.[157, 158] The disorder is worse during the summer months because of photosensitivity.

Large scaling, keratotic crusts at the base of the eyelashes are more extensive than those found in patients with seborrheic dermatitis. Staphylococcal blepharitis is a frequent complication, particularly in patients treated with retinoids.[158, 162] The most common ocular abnormalities are irregular peripheral intraepithelial corneal deposits and linear, thread-like or verticillate whorls in the more central cornea.[158] Additional ocular features include dense yellowish peripheral pannus, corneal stromal opacities, endothelial cystic focal lesions, trichiasis, red-green defect, amblyopia, and aphakia.[158] Abnormal dark adaptation has also been reported.[163]

The differential diagnosis of keratosis follicularis includes acanthosis nigricans, ichthyosis vulgaris, keratosis pilaris, and seborrheic dermatitis.[158] Most of these conditions can be excluded on clinical grounds; however, skin biopsies should be performed whenever the diagnosis is in question. Keratosis follicularis demonstrates characteristic histologic features, including acanthosis, formation of suprabasal lacunae, upward proliferation of villi into the lacunae, acantholytic dyskeratotic cells, corps ronds, and grains. Acantholysis is responsible for the formation of clefts called *lacunae.* Corps rond cells demonstrate basophilic nuclear staining surrounded by a slight halo. Grains are small dark cells with a pyknotic nucleus.[157] Ocular findings are most likely to be confused with lipoid proteinosis or seborrheic blepharitis. Verticillate whorls in the corneal epithelium have also been reported in Fabry's disease, chloroquine and amiodarone therapy, and map-dot-fingerprint dystrophy of the cornea.[158]

Treatment with systemic retinoids, such as 13-*cis*-retinoic acid, has resulted in dramatic improvement in most patients with keratosis follicularis. Systemic retinoid therapy may result in staphylococcal blepharitis that responds well to topical antibiotics. Local therapy may also be effective and includes topical corticosteroids, moisturizing ointments, salicylic acid, tar, and tretinoin (Retin-A). Intralesional triamcinolone is effective for temporary relief of localized disease. For more hypertrophic or recalcitrant disease, dermabrasion, laser vaporization, and excision and grafting have been successful in selected cases.[157, 164]

Multiple Mucosal Neuroma Syndrome

Multiple mucosal neuroma syndrome, also known as *multiple endocrine neoplasia III* (MEN 3) and *multiple endocrine neoplasia type 2b*, is a rare disorder characterized by mucosal neuromas associated with medullary thyroid carcinoma, pheochromocytoma, marfanoid habitus, medullated corneal nerves, and gastrointestinal ganglioneuromatosis.[165,166] More than 50 cases have been reported in the world literature; half of these are inherited in an autosomal dominant fashion, and the remaining are sporadic. It is distinguished from multiple endocrine neoplasia type I (Werner's syndrome), which has hyperplasia and tumors of the pituitary, parathyroids, and pancreatic islets as characteristic features. Patients with multiple endocrine neoplasia type II (Sipple's syndrome) develop medullary thyroid carcinoma, pheochromocytoma, and hyperparathyroidism.

The earliest clinical manifestations are small neuromas involving the tongue, which may be evident within a few years after birth.[167] All patients develop cutaneous and mucosal neuromas, and the most frequently involved sites are the lips, oral cavity, and eyelids (by the end of the first decade).[165,166] Lip involvement results in a characteristic "blubbery," "bumpy," "negroid," or diffusely thickened appearance. The papular neuromas range between 2 and 6 mm in diameter and are particularly prominent over the anterior portion of the tongue.[165] Acanthosis nigricans can give a similar appearance of tongue and lip involvement. Neuromas have also been reported to involve the conjunctiva, corneas, other cutaneous sites, and the laryngeal, pharyngeal, and nasal mucosa.[165,166] There is a characteristic facial appearance, similar to that observed in patients with acromegaly.[166] Although patients with multiple mucosal neuroma syndrome may have a marfanoid habitus, they do not develop ocular, enzymatic, or cardiovascular abnormalities associated with Marfan's syndrome.[165] Additional physical findings include café-au-lait macules (22%), fibromas, and neurofibromas.[166] Gastrointestinal ganglioneuromatosis most commonly involves the intestine, although esophageal and gastric disease have also been reported.[165,166] Gastrointestinal disease manifests with difficulties swallowing, megacolon, and constipation. A subnormal wheal-and-flare response to histamine has been documented for many patients and may be of some diagnostic value.[166]

More than 90% of patients with multiple mucosal neuroma syndrome develop medullary thyroid carcinoma in their teens.[166] The earliest detected case was at 6 months of age.[165] The malignancy remains confined to the head and neck region for long periods before metastatic disease develops. Early manifestations of medullary thyroid carcinoma include a thyroid nodule and diarrhea, although most patients are asymptomatic.[165,166] At least 65% of patients develop bilateral and multifocal pheochromocytomas later in life (the second decade). Although these associated pheochromocytomas are usually benign, malignant cases have been reported.[165]

Ocular abnormalities may be the first clinical sign of disease in many patients with multiple mucosal neuroma syndrome, and the ophthalmologist can make the diagnosis before any of the associated malignancies have become metastatic.[167,168] The most frequent ocular findings are prominent corneal nerves on slit-lamp examination.[167-170] The incidence of many ocular findings is difficult to estimate owing to the lack of thorough ophthalmoscopic examinations on earlier reported cases. In a series by Robertson and associates,[170] all patients examined for corneal nerve enlargement were positive. Estimates on other ocular findings include conjunctival neuromas (87%), eyelid neuromas (80%), dry eyes (67%), and prominent perilimbal conjunctival blood vessels (40%).[170] Khairi and colleagues[166] reported a series of kindred with medullated corneal nerves and mucosal neuromas as isolated findings without subsequent development of endocrine neoplasia. Visible corneal nerves have also been reported in neurofibromatosis, keratoconus, Refsum's syndrome, primary amyloidosis, and "collodion skin" syndrome.[168] The nerves in these conditions, however, are much smaller and less visible than in multiple mucosal neuroma syndrome. Eyelid neuromas are pinkish sessile papules along the lid margins that displace the lashes rostrally. Palpebral-conjunctival tumors range between 0.6 and 3 mm in diameter.[167,168] Neural involvement of the tarsal plate results in symmetric thickening of the eyelids. Additional ocular findings are listed in Table 1-13.

The differential diagnosis of multiple mucosal neuroma syndrome includes other multiple endocrine neoplasia disorders, von Recklinghausen's disease (neurofibromatosis), tuberous sclerosis, and von Hippel-Lindau syndrome.[165] Indeed, there has been much discussion in the literature as to overlap of these disorders due to shared clinical features.[165-169] When the disease is fully expressed, there is little question that it is a separate disorder, and the challenge remains in early detection of the potentially life-threatening complications. The differential diagnosis of eyelid neuromas includes neurofibromatosis, lipoid proteinosis, and amyloidosis. The number of palpebral lesions noted in multiple mucosal neuroma syndrome is usually less than that observed in lipoid proteinosis. Many of the reported patients had single to

TABLE 1-13

Ocular Manifestations of Multiple Mucosal Neuroma Syndrome[166-170]

Adnexal
Diffuse or nodular thickening of eyelids
Eyelid papules
Rostral displacement of eyelashes
Eversion of eyelids
Subconjunctival neuromas
Thickened conjunctival nerves
Nasal displacement of lacrimal puncta
Decreased tear formation
Anterior Segment
Prominent corneal nerves in clear stroma
Impaired pupillary dilation
Increased intraocular pressure
Thickened nerves in iris

several lesions involving the eyelids. Biopsy is helpful in establishing the diagnosis. Histologically, the papules are unencapsulated masses of convoluted nerve fibers surrounded by a thickened perineurium.[165] These findings are consistent with plexiform neurofibromas. Some authors note a lack of increased connective tissue stroma, in contrast with neurofibromas.[166] The neuromas found in patients with multiple mucosal neuroma syndrome do not undergo malignant transformation.[165, 166] Examination of corneal nerves on electron microscopy has shown that they consist of numerous closely packed axons and Schwann cells.[168, 169]

Early screening and surgical intervention result in a greatly increased survival of these patients and a normal life span. Some authors have suggested prophylactic total thyroidectomy and prophylactic bilateral adrenalectomy.[165] Currently, this is not considered the treatment of choice.[165] Excision of mucosal and cutaneous neuromas may be performed for cosmetic and functional reasons.

Acanthosis Nigricans

Acanthosis nigricans (Fig. 1–9) is a common cutaneous finding that is associated with many different disorders. The diagnosis in most patients can be made on clinical grounds. The cutaneous findings are characterized by symmetric, velvety to verrucous, hyperkeratotic and hyperpigmented plaques with a predilection for the axilla, the nape of the neck, and other flexural surfaces.[171] More generalized forms may occur involving the extremities, central chest, central back, and facial regions.[171–174] The severity and extent of cutaneous involvement do not necessarily correlate with a type of systemic disease, such as internal malignancy.[175, 176]

Table 1–14 lists those disorders that have been reported to be associated with acanthosis nigricans. The most common association is obesity and insulin resistance. Stuart and coworkers[177] examined 1412 school children and detected acanthosis nigricans in 7.1%. The findings were equally distributed between both sexes. There was an ethnic predilection, with 13% of African Americans, 6% of Hispanics, and 0.5% of Caucasians being affected. Diabetes mellitus, polycystic ovarian disease, and thyroid disease states are the most frequently associated endocrinopathies.[175] Crouzon's disease has a predilection for involvement of the eyelids with acanthosis nigricans.[179] Other congenital disorders may have additional ocular associations, such as pigmented retinopathy in patients with Alström's syndrome and conjunctival telangiectasis in ataxia-telangiectasia.[178, 183] Genetic studies have shown an autosomal dominant form of non-neoplastic type of acanthosis nigricans that may resemble ichthyosis hystrix.[176, 188] Drug-induced acanthosis nigricans, particularly caused by niacin, is not uncommon and usually resolves with discontinuation of the medication.[189]

Malignant acanthosis nigricans is a cutaneous marker of internal and external cancer. The degree of skin findings associated with malignancy is not necessarily the most severe or generalized. As a rule, most of these patients are older than 40 years of age when they present

TABLE 1–14
Disorders Associated with Acanthosis Nigricans[171,172,176]

Disorders
Non-neoplastic
Insulin-resistant disorders
Obesity[177]
Endocrinopathies[171,176]
Diabetes mellitus (types A, B, and C)
Polycystic ovary disease (Stein-Leventhal syndrome)
Ovarian hyperthecosis
Acromegaly
Cushing's disease
Addison's disease
Lipodystrophy
Hyperthyroidism
Hypothyroidism
Pinealoma or pineal hyperplasia[178]
Congenital syndromes[171,176]
Crouzon's syndrome[179,180]
Bloom's syndrome[181]
Rud's syndrome[182]
Prader-Willi syndrome[180]
Ataxia-telangiectasia[183]
Cutis gyratum, acanthosis nigricans, and other abnormalities[184]
Alström syndrome[185]
Rabson's syndrome[186]
Leprechaunism[171]
Capozucca's syndrome[182]
Syndrome of acral hypertrophy and muscle cramps[187]
Autosomal dominant inherited
Ichthyosis hystrix type[188]
Drug-induced disorders
Nicotinic acid (niacin)[189,190]
Diethylstilbestrol[191]
Glucocorticoids[192]
Oral contraceptives[179]
Miscellaneous[171]
Lupoid hepatitis
Pemphigus vulgaris
Pemphigus foliaceus[193]
Osteoectasia (juvenile Paget disease of bone)
Neoplastic[172]
Gastric adenocarcinoma
Hepatocellular
Uterine and cervical cancers
Hodgkin's and non-Hodgkin's lymphoma
Mycosis fungoides[194]
Breast carcinoma
Lung adenocarcinoma and alveolar cell and squamous cell carcinomas
Pancreatic tumors
Colorectal malignancies
Ovarian neoplasms
Esophageal tumors
Gallbladder adenocarcinoma
Prostatic carcinoma
Osteogenic sarcoma
Thyroid adenocarcinoma
Lymphosarcoma
Renal cell carcinoma
Testicular cancer
Lip cancers
Pharyngeal cancers
Laryngeal cancers
Fibrosarcoma
Unknown primary cancer

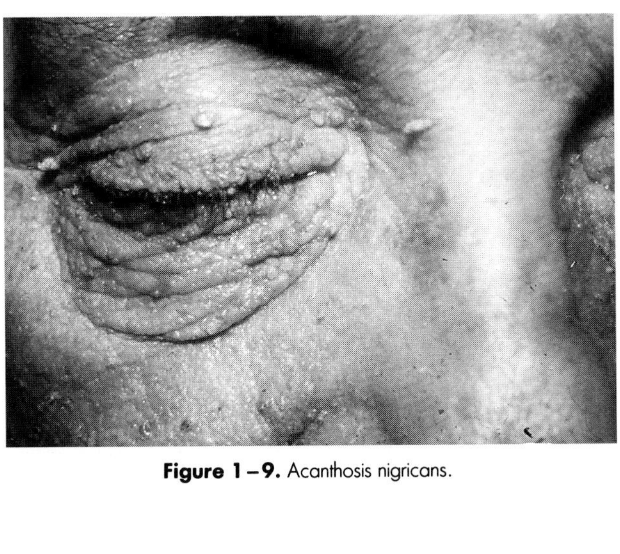

Figure 1–9. Acanthosis nigricans.

with acanthosis nigricans that frequently pursues an aggressive course.[172] Pruritus is an important symptom, and 30% to 40% of patients develop oral manifestations. Oral lesions are not always pigmented and are described as papillomatous growths on the tongue and lips.[172, 176] The oral findings may be difficult to distinguish clinically from multiple mucosal neuroma syndrome and lipoid proteinosis.[151, 176] Malignant acanthosis nigricans can precede, accompany, or follow the onset of malignancy. More than half of all cases reported were caused by gastric adenocarcinoma.[172] Most cases resolve after the tumor is removed or treated.

Characteristic velvety, hyperkeratotic plaques may involve the eyelids and progress to verrucoid papules. The conjunctiva as well as other mucosal membranes such as the vagina, the esophagus, and the pharynx may also be involved.[176] Surgical procedures performed on involved eyelid skin result in prominent scarring, and incisions should be avoided if possible.[179]

The cause of acanthosis nigricans is poorly understood. Androgenic steroids, urogastrone, corticotropin, alpha-melanocyte-stimulating hormone–like protein, human growth hormone, TSH, and amine precursor uptake and decarboxylation cell secretion have been implicated as causative agents.[172] The differential diagnosis is quite large and reflects additional physical and laboratory features of the associated disease process. Addison's disease, arsenic poisoning, hemochromatosis, and ichthyosis hystrix should be considered with generalized acanthosis nigicans.[176] In those patients with oral, ocular, and other sites of facial involvement, there may be confusion with amyloidosis, keratosis follicularis, multiple mucosal neuroma syndrome, lipoid proteinosis, Cowden's disease, bromoderma, and condyloma acuminatum.[176] Histologic features include hyperkeratosis, papillomatosis, acanthosis alternating with atrophic regions, and normal to increased amounts of melanin in the basal epidermis.[171, 176] Laboratory abnormalities reflect the underlying cause. Treatment is directed at controlling the primary disease.

Neurofibromatosis

Neurofibromatosis (Fig. 1–10), also known as *von Recklinghausen's disease*, is a conglomeration of neurocutaneous disorders with overlapping features and systemic complications.[195] There is no racial, ethnic, or geographic predilection. It is a common autosomal dominant trait affecting 1 in 3500 births.[196,197] More than half of the cases represent new mutations, and it has been stated that neurofibromatosis has one of the highest reported mutation rates in humans.[198] Although there is virtually 100% penetrance, marked variation in expression ranges from diffuse disfiguring tumors to a few café-au-lait macules without cutaneous neurofibromas. Because of this heterogeneity, Riccardi[199, 200] has proposed classification into eight types based on clinical features. For the clinician, however, it is best to divide the neurofibromatoses into three groups[197]: (1) neurofibromatosis 1, the classic form characterized by café-au-lait spots, multiple neurofibromas, and Lisch nodules; (2) neurofibromatosis 2, defined by bilateral acoustic neuromas, posterior subcapsular lenticular opacities, and cranial as well as paraspinal meningiomas; more specific classification criteria are listed in Table 1–15; and (3) the remaining six types, classified together as "incomplete forms," which include a segmental variant Riccardi classified as type 5. The following discussion is restricted to the three forms currently known to have ocular findings (types 1 and 2 and segmental neurofibromatosis).

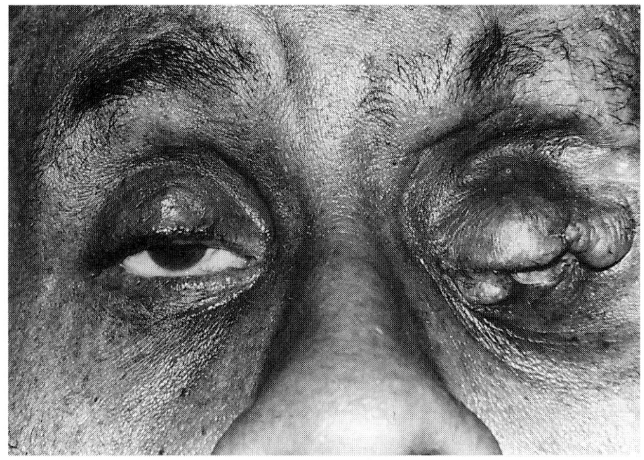

Figure 1–10. Neurofibromatosis.

TABLE 1–15

1988 Diagnostic Criteria for the Neurofibromatoses

Neurofibromatosis 1 (requires two or more of the following)

1. Six or more café-au-lait macules
   >5 mm in greatest diameter in prepubertal persons
   >15 mm in greatest diameter in postpubertal persons
2. Two or more neurofibromas of any type, or one plexiform neurofibroma
3. Freckling of the axillary or inguinal regions
4. Optic glioma
5. Two or more Lisch nodules
6. Osseous lesions such as sphenoid dysplasia and thinning of long bone (with or without pseudoarthrosis)
7. First-degree relative (parent, sibling, or offspring) with neurofibromatosis 1 (diagnosis established by the above criteria)

Neurofibromatosis 2 (requires either of the following)

1. Bilateral eighth nerve masses (computed tomography or magnetic resonance imaging)
2. First-degree relative with neurofibromatosis 2 and either unilateral eighth nerve mass or two of the following:
   Neurofibroma
   Meningioma
   Glioma
   Schwannoma
   Juvenile posterior subcapsular lenticular opacity

Adapted from Neurofibromatosis Conference Statement: National Institutes of Health Consensus Development Conference. Arch Neurol 45:575–578, 1988.

Cutaneous manifestations of neurofibromatosis 1 are some of the earliest features detected.[197] Café-au-lait spots are brown, flat, oval macules and patches with sharp borders that may be present at birth.[196, 197] People with other congenital disorders and those who are normal can have café-au-lait spots. Thus, the size and number are important in establishing the diagnosis, as shown in Table 1–15. Freckling in the axillary or inguinal region is also a helpful diagnostic clue. Neurofibromas arise from small nerves and may be found anywhere on the body. Initially, they are violaceous, minimally elevated papules that evolve into soft fleshy papules of varying size.[196, 197] A characteristic finding is invagination with gentle pressure through a defect in the dermis, called "buttonholing."[197] Large plexiform neurofibromas consist of tortuous coils or rope-like masses that feel like a "bag of worms" on palpation.[197] Plexiform neurofibromas are cosmetically disfiguring, particularly in the craniofacial regions, resulting in hypertrophy known as *elephantiasis neuromatosa.* Lisch nodules are clear to yellowish brown, dome-shaped, hamartomatous projections from the iris believed to be pathognomonic for neurofibromatosis.[196, 197] Additional abnormalities and symptoms include skeletal (scoliosis, pseudarthrosis, hemihypertrophy), neurologic (mental deficiencies, seizures, headaches, learning disabilities), and vascular abnormalities (occlusion, stenosis such as renal artery or vein); pruritus; macrocephaly; short stature; congenital heart disease; lung disease (pulmonary fibrosis, mediastinal neurofibromas); gastrointestinal disease (visceral neurofibromas and ganglioneuromas resulting in pain, bleeding, perforation, anemia, constipation); urologic disease; and endocrinopathies (hypoparathyroidism).[196, 197]

Patients with neurofibromatosis 1 have a propensity for the development of malignancies. Neurofibrosarcomas and malignant schwannomas are common.[196] Fewer than than 1% will develop pheochromocytomas.[196] Additional associated malignancies include Wilms' tumor, rhabdomyosarcomas, granulocytic leukemia (associated with xanthogranulomas), astrocytomas, meningiomas, neurilemmomas, gliomas, neuroblastomas, medullary-thyroid carcinoma, and possibly cutaneous and choroidal malignant melanoma.[196, 197, 201–203]

Neurofibromatosis 2 is an autosomal dominant disorder with a lower rate of mutation than neurofibromatosis 1 and a prevalence rate of 0.1 per 100,000 persons.[197] Bilateral acoustic neuromas (schwannomas) are the hallmark of this type of neurofibromatosis; however, the diagnosis can be made in some patients with unilateral acoustic neuromas (see Table 1–15).[204] Patients usually present with hearing loss, ataxia, and headache in the second to third decades of life. Only half have the characteristic café-au-lait spots, and rarely are more than six spots found on clinical examination. Approximately 20% have typical neurofibromas.[197] Lisch nodules are also notably absent in these patients; however, 50% develop presenile lens opacities and cataracts.[205] About 20% develop other central nervous system tumors such as meningiomas, other schwannomas, and spinal cord ependymomas.[197,204] Optic gliomas, astrocytomas, and hamartomas do not appear to be associated with neurofibromatosis 2.[204]

Segmental neurofibromatosis is defined by limitation of café-au-lait spots and neurofibromas to a given region of the body.[206] Riccardi believes that a postzygotic somatic mutation in neural crest cells is the most likely mechanism resulting in unilateral and noninherited forms of disease.[207] Roth and associates[206a] have identified the following four subtypes of segmental neurofibromatosis reported in the literature:

1. The noninherited true segmental form (the most frequently identified), for example, involvement of a single limb
2. Segmental neurofibromatosis with deep involvement — Biemer and Muhlbauer[206a] reported a case of segmental neurofibromatosis involving the face, soft tissue, and bone
3. A hereditary form of segmental disease — Rubenstein and colleagues[208] reported two families with inherited segmental disease, noting right flank neurofibromas in the father and plexiform neurofibroma of the left side of the face in the daughter in one family. In the second family, the father had right flank neurofibromas and a single café-au-lait spot and his son had neurofibromatosis 1
4. Bilateral segmental disease that can present with interesting findings such as café-au-lait spots on one side and neurofibromas in the same distribution on the other side[206]

Ocular features of the neurofibromatoses are shown in Table 1–16. In a series on neurofibromatosis 1 by Riccardi and Lewis,[200] the most frequent findings were Lisch nodules (92%), eyelid neurofibromas and café-au-lait spots (25%), and corneal disease (25%) manifesting as prominent nerves and posterior embryotoxon. In the series by Huson and coworkers,[209] Lisch nodules were found in 96%, choroidal hamartomas in 35%, and eyelid neurofibromas in 16% of cases. Bilateral Lisch nodules are a common and pathognomonic sign for neurofibromatosis 1.[211] Although rare, unilateral Lisch nodules have been reported in as many as 9% of patients in one series.[204] In another series by Lubs and associates,[211] there was no association between the detection of Lisch nodules and the severity of neurofibromatosis 1. All patients older than 20 years of age were found to have Lisch nodules compared with fewer than 5% for children younger than 3 years of age.[211] Patients with neurofibromatosis 2 lack Lisch nodules and are much more likely to develop presenile cataracts, particularly involving the posterior capsule. Cutaneous neurofibromas and café-au-lait spots are found much less frequently in neurofi-

TABLE 1-16

Ocular Manifestations of the Neurofibromatoses[200,204,209-211]

Features	Neurofibromatosis 1	Neurofibromatosis 2	Periorbital Segmental
Adnexal	Eyelid neurofibromas and plexiform neurofibromas Eyelid café-au-lait spots Sphenoid wing dysplasia Orbital neurofibromas	None	Eyelid neurofibromas Plexiform neurofibromas Café-au-lait spots[206-208] ?*
Neuro-ophthalmologic	Optic nerve glioma (proptosis)[212,213] Strabismus Ocular motor apraxia[214]	Intracranial tumors (meningiomas)	?*
Anterior Segment	Lisch nodules Choroidal nevi and hamartomas Choroidal melanomas Prominent corneal nerves Conjunctival neurofibromas and nerve enlargement Conjunctival melanomas[210] Posterior embryotoxon Neurofibromas[216] Congenital glaucoma	Presenile lens opacities and cataracts[205]	Lisch nodules (unilateral)[215] ?*
Posterior Segment	Optic disk drusen Sectoral chorioretinal scar Myelinated nerve fibers Peripheral retinoschisis Congenital hypertrophy, retinal pigment epithelium Neurofibromas[216] Neurilemmoma[216] Retinal astrocytomas[204]	None	?*

*Indicates that in segmental disease, particularly the localized deep type, any of the ocular findings noted for neurofibromatosis 1 are theoretically possible.

bromatosis 2 than in neurofibromatosis 1. Although eyelid findings are yet to be reported, it is possible that cutaneous eyelid involvement may occur. Visual loss in patients with neurofibromatosis 2 is most frequently related to anterior-placed tumors of the central nervous system.[204] Weleber and Zonana[215] reported a case of segmental neurofibromatosis with Lisch nodules, numerous right-sided café-au-lait spots (including the face), and right shoulder freckling. Because patients with segmental disease, particularly of the deep type, have developed many findings seen in neurofibromatosis 1 within the involved segment, it is possible that patients with periocular segmental neurofibromatosis may develop ocular findings similar to those found in more classic forms.

The heterogeneity of this group of neurocutaneous disorders is further exemplified by genetic linkage analysis. The abnormal gene for neurofibromatosis 1 has been identified on chromosome 17, whereas the gene for neurofibromatosis 2 has been identified on chromosome 22.[204,210] The differential diagnosis depends on the clinical presentation and the sites of involvement. Histologic examination of neurofibromas reveals compact cords of fusiform cells surrounded by abundant matrix that stains positively for mucopolysaccharides.[197] Lymphocytes and mast cells are often found. Treatment is supportive, and close observation is recommended for early detection of potential malignant disease and compromised organ function. Genetic counseling should be provided for inherited forms of neurofibromatosis.

Tuberous Sclerosis

Tuberous sclerosis, also known as *Bourneville's disease*, is an autosomal dominant inherited disorder that comprises the classic triad of epilepsy, mental retardation, and adenoma sebaceum.[157,217,218] As in neurofibromatosis, there is a high spontaneous mutation rate, reaching as high as 80% in some series.[217] Both sexes are equally affected, and incidence rates range between 1 in 20,000 to 300,000 births.[217]

A wide spectrum of cutaneous and systemic abnormalities has resulted in the proposed diagnostic criteria by Gomez shown in Table 1-17.[219] The earliest signs of tuberous sclerosis are ash leaf spots.[218] They may appear at birth and are well-circumscribed macules or patches with partial pigment loss. Frequently, the areas are white leaf-shaped macules (ash leaf spots), and the number identified per patient can vary from 1 to 100.[157,218] Approximately 1% of normal newborns have congenital hypopigmented macules (nevus depigmentosus) that are clinically indistinguishable from ash leaf macules.[218]

TABLE 1-17

Diagnostic Criteria for Tuberous Sclerosis

Primary Criteria (requires one or more of the following for diagnosis)
Angiofibromas (adenoma sebaceum)
Subungual fibromas (Koenen's tumor)
Fibrous plaque involving the forehead or scalp
Retinal hamartomas
Cortical tubers
Subependymal glial nodules
Renal hamartomas (angiomyolipomas)
Secondary Criteria (requires two or more of the following for presumptive diagnosis)
Ash leaf macules (hypopigmented macules and patches)
Shagreen patch
Gingival fibromas
Single peripapillary retinal hamartoma
Seizures (including infantile spasms)
Subcortical or cortical calcification
Multiple subcortical hypomyelinated lesions
Cardiac rhabdomyoma
Pulmonary lymphangiomyomatosis
First-degree relative with tuberous sclerosis

Adapted from Gomez MR (ed): Criteria for diagnosis. *In* Tuberous Sclerosis, 2nd ed. New York, Raven Press, 1988, pp. 9–19.

Central facial angiofibroma, called *adenoma sebaceum*, occurs in 46% to 90% of patients and is characterized by yellowish red, translucent, discrete, waxy papules.[157, 218] Biopsy-confirmed angiofibromas involving the face are believed to be pathognomonic for tuberous sclerosis.[157] *Shagreen patches* are connective tissue nevi that appear as "knobby" flesh-toned plaques with the appearance of "pigskin," "gooseflesh," or "shark skin." This lesion is observed in 28% to 83% of patients and most frequently involves the trunk. *Koenen's tumors* (subungual fibromas) are asymptomatic digitate angiofibromas protruding from the base of the nail, affecting 19% to 52% of patients. Subungual fibromas are frequently found in women after puberty, most often involve the toes, and are associated with renal hamartomas.[218] Similar angiofibromas may be found in the mouth, scalp, neck, and axilla.[218]

The most common systemic complications are intracranial subependymal nodules and hamartomas called *cortical tubers*.[218] Seizures are the most frequent symptom, which is often related to cortical tubers and cerebral calcifications. Additional systemic features include mental retardation, rhabdomyomas of the heart, renal hamartomas, pulmonary lymphangiomyomas, and bony abnormalities such as cysts and sclerosis.[157, 218]

The term *phakoma* is derived from the Greek word *phakos*, which means "mother spot."[217] Phakomata are the white lesions involving the posterior pole; these are angiogliomatous hamartomas on histologic examination. Three types exist[217]: (1) the flat, smooth, translucent form, which has the same color as the background or is light grayish yellow; (2) the classic "mulberry" or "salmon egg" form, which may have lesions as large as two optic disk diameters; and (3) the intermediate one between the first two forms. The differential diagnosis of phakomata includes retinoblastoma, choroiditis, optic disk drusen, and Coats' disease.[217] Angiofibromas, shagreen patches, and ash-leaf macules may involve the eyelids. Additional ocular findings are listed in Table 1–18. Visual disturbances are rare; however, vitreous hemorrhage resulting in impaired vision has been reported. Phakoma can result in ocular pain and blindness due to retinal detachment and secondary glaucoma.

In those patients suspected of having tuberous sclerosis, a systematic evaluation is recommended. Wood's light examination will accentuate ash leaf macules on the skin. Skin biopsies of angiofibromas, shagreen patches, and ash leaf macules are helpful. Skull roentgenograms reveal cerebral calcification. Computed tomographic and magnetic resonance imaging scans should be considered in patients with a seizure history. In selected patients, evaluation of the heart (echocardiogram), distal extremities (roentgenograms for cysts), and kidneys (ultrasonography) should be performed.[157, 217–219]

Treatment is supportive. Facial angiofibromas can be disfiguring, and the best cosmetic results have been obtained with dermabrasion and laser therapy.[157] Genetic counseling is recommended.

Porphyria Cutanea Tarda

The porphyrias are enzymatic disorders of heme biosynthesis in which excessive formation of porphyrins pro-

TABLE 1-18

Ocular Manifestations of Tuberous Sclerosis

Adnexal
Eyelid angiofibromas
Eyelid shagreen patches
Eyelid ash leaf macules
Subconjunctival nodules
Poliosis of eyelashes
Neuro-ophthalmologic
Strabismus
External ophthalmoplegia
Papilledema
Optic atrophy
Anterior Segment
Depigmented sectors of iris
Coloboma of the iris, lens, and choroid
Megalocornea
Posterior embryotoxon
Glaucoma
Posterior Segment
Angiogliomatous hamartomas (phakomata)
Peripheral punched-out depigmented areas (ash leaf patch)
Retinitis pigmentosa
Vitreous hemorrhage
Hemorrhagic retinopathy

Adapted from Williams R, Taylor D: Tuberous sclerosis. Surv Ophthalmol 30(3):143–154, 1985.

duces photosensitization and liver disease.[220, 221] Seven clinical forms exist ranging from acute intermittent porphyria (AIP), which lacks significant cutaneous disease, to congenital erythropoietic protoporphyria, which results in severe photosensitivity and progressive scarring. Although AIP has been associated with intraocular disease (ischemia, transient visual loss, retinal infarcts with cotton-wool exudates, hemorrhage, disk edema, and optic atrophy), there is no involvement of the ocular adnexa, except muscle palsies.[222] Only those forms resulting in significant involvement of the ocular adnexa are reviewed.

Porphyria cutanea tarda (PCT) is the most common form of porphyria.[220] A deficiency in the enzyme uroporphyrinogen decarboxylase is the basic defect found in all four types of the disease, namely, sporadic (type 1), familial autosomal dominant (type 2), familial disease localized to liver involvement (type 3), and toxic (type 4).[220] The most common are the sporadic and familial forms (type 2), which are also similar clinically, producing hepatic and cutaneous disease. Acquired toxic forms (type 4) have been reported with exposure to hexachlorobenzene, 2,3,7,8-tetrachlorodibenzo-*para*-dioxin, and 2,4,5-trichlorophenol.[220, 221] In addition, a variety of drugs may induce PCT, including ethyl alcohol, estrogens, chloroquine, tetracyclines, furosemide, nalidixic acid, dapsone, pyridoxine, and naproxen.[221] Indeed, there is a high association with alcohol intake and estrogen use in many patients with PCT. Development of clinically overt PCT requires inactivation of hepatic uroporphyrinogen decarboxylase activity to below 50% of normal.[220]

The most notable clinical manifestation is photosensitivity resulting in bullae, superficial erosions due to cutaneous fragility, milia, onycholysis, scarring, and hyperpigmentation. Hypertrichosis may develop on the face. A pink violaceous hue involving the face, the neck, and the periorbital regions may be observed. Sclerodermatous changes have also been reported, particularly involving the cheeks, back of the neck, preauricular areas, ears, thorax, fingers, and scalp (resulting in alopecia). Although many of these effects are the result of sun exposure, acute photosensitivity is uncommon.[220]

Despite elevated transaminases, liver disease as a direct result of PCT is unusual.[220] Systemic associations include nonalcoholic liver disease, cirrhosis (20%), hepatocellular carcinoma, hemochromatosis, SLE, non–insulin-dependent diabetes mellitus, reticuloendotheliosis, and Hodgkin's lymphoma.[220, 221] A similar bullous dermatitis associated with elevated porphyrins has been reported in patients on chronic hemodialysis, referred to as *therapy-induced porphyria* or *pseudoporphyria*.[221] Hemodialysis-associated disease does not result in hypertrichosis, hyperpigmentation, or the sclerodermatous changes observed in PCT.

Periocular disease may develop. Hypertrichosis of the eyebrows and lateral canthal regions occurs in males, whereas a more diffuse form of hypertrichosis occurs in females. There may be scarring of the eyelids without bullae formation.[223] Additional ocular findings include conjunctival hyperemia, conjunctival erosions progressing to conjunctival-scleral adhesions, senile-type hyaline plaques, blepharospasm, corneal scarring, corneal vascularization, cataracts, glaucoma, and descemetocele.[223] Photophobia is the most common ocular complaint.

Porphyrins absorb ultraviolet radiation in the Soret band (400-nm range) with emission of light in the 619- to 634-nm range.[221] This results in the production of singlet O from O_2 and eventual damage to lysosomes and cellular membranes. The cellular injury and inflammation promote bullae formation. The differential diagnosis of PCT includes other photosensitizing porphyrias, polymorphous light eruption, drug-induced photosensitization, and other vesicobullous diseases, such as pemphigus vulgaris and bullous pemphigoid (BP). Histologic examination reveals noninflammatory bullae with sharp undulations along the free-floating epidermis called *festooning*.[221] The capillary walls are thickened owing to deposition of a PAS-positive hyalin-like material. The diagnosis is confirmed on porphyrin analysis of plasma, urine, and feces.

Patients with PCT should avoid hepatic toxins such as alcohol. Sun avoidance and sun protection measures, such as use of sunscreens, are recommended. Phlebotomy of 500 mL at 2-week intervals is effective in reducing cutaneous sensitivity. Chloroquine therapy has also been used successfully. Additional treatment options include small-volume plasmapheresis and desferrioxamine.[120,121] Genetic counseling should be provided to patients with inherited forms of PCT.

Variegate Porphyria

Variegate porphyria is an autosomal dominant inherited disease characterized by cutaneous lesions, abdominal crises, gastrointestinal symptoms, and neurologic manifestations.[220,221] Protoporphyrinogen oxidase is the deficient enzyme. Clinical features of variegate porphyria are mixed, having cutaneous findings similar to PCT and systemic features, such as abdominal colic and psychiatric disturbances, suggestive of AIP. Symptoms rarely develop before puberty and relatives may have silent disease.[220, 221] Approximately 25% of patients with variegate porphyria also have concomitant PCT.[224] Clinical evaluation, laboratory studies, and treatment of coexistent disease are the same as those described for PCT. Plasma in patients with variegate porphyria contains a unique and diagnostic porphyrin complex with fluorescence emission peaks at 624 to 626 nm. In those patients with acute disease, such as abdominal crisis and acute psychosis, use of the same therapeutic agents used for AIP may be considered. Oral or intravenous glucose loading, opiates, hematin infusions, and high-dose propranolol have resulted in clinical improvement.[225]

Erythropoietic Protoporphyria

Erythropoietic protoporphyria (EEP) is an autosomal dominant inherited deficiency of ferrochelatase (heme synthetase) activity and is the second most common porphyria.[220, 221] Patients present in early childhood with acute photosensitivity characterized by intense pricking, pruritus, and burning sensations within 5 to 30 minutes of sunlight exposure. At times the symptoms may be delayed as much as 7 hours. Additional acute cutaneous features include erythema, edema, crust formation, small vesicles, petechiae, and photo-onycholysis. With repeated exposure the skin may become thickened, waxy, and pitted. Linear and circular scars have also been reported.[220] Chronic cutaneous changes frequently involve the knuckles and face, particularly the bridge of the nose, the perioral regions, and the eyelids.

Although uncommon, fulminant hepatic disease may occur in these patients. Hepatic cirrhosis, gallstones, portal hypertension, and esophageal varices have been reported.[226] Some patients may develop a mild hypochromic microcytic anemia.[220]

Other porphyrias must be distinguished from EEP. The diagnosis is confirmed on identification of typical cutaneous lesions, raised erythrocyte protoporphyrin content, fluorescent erythrocytes (634 nm), and the absence of porphyrinuria.[220, 221, 226] Treatment is supportive and directed at protecting against ultraviolet exposure. Sun avoidance, sunscreens, and beta-carotene are recommended treatment options that have been used with some success.

Congenital Erythropoietic Porphyria

Congenital erythropoietic porphyria (CEP), also known as *Günther's disease*, is an autosomal recessive–inherited deficiency of uroporphyrinogen III cosynthetase with onset in infancy or early childhood.[220, 221] Severe photosensitivity with bullae formation is the hallmark of this disease. Another characteristic feature is the development of reddish brown teeth that fluoresce on exposure to Wood's light. Bullous lesions heal with scarring and progressive photomutilation, especially on the face. Hypertrichosis is severe resulting in hair growth on the cheeks and temporal regions, profuse eyebrows, and long eyelashes. In the past many of these unfortunate people have been referred to as "monkey face" and "werewolf."[221] Additional cutaneous features include cicatricial alopecia, skin fragility, and irregular hyperpigmentation and hypopigmentation.[221] A chronic hemolytic anemia, often accompanied by splenomegaly, is a constant feature. Recently, another form has been described that starts after the second decade of life, is much more common than the 100 reported cases of classic Günther's disease, is much less severe than the infantile form, and may be mistaken for PCT.[227, 228]

In addition to scarring of the eyelids, other ocular complications may be found. The most frequent eye complaint is photophobia. Ectropion, symblepharon, and keratoconjunctivitis are common findings.[221]

The diagnosis is confirmed on identification of the typical clinical features and porphyrins in erythrocytes, urine, and feces.[221] Treatment is supportive and directed at decreasing ultraviolet exposure. A splenectomy may result in decreased hemolysis and less cutaneous disease. Chelation therapy with deferoxamine mesylate, oral charcoal therapy, and frequent blood transfusions have also had some treatment success.[221]

VESICOBULLOUS DISEASES

Vesicobullous disease encompasses a diverse group of blistering disorders that involve the epithelium of the skin or mucous membranes. Some of these conditions may involve the ocular adnexa. Because of their large number, only those disorders with prominent or critically focal ocular manifestations are reviewed.

Some basic principles apply to all blistering disorders. Blisters smaller than 5 mm are referred to as *vesicles* and larger lesions are called *bullae.* The site of cleavage also helps define characteristics of the blisters. Intraepidemal blisters are flaccid, break easily, and tend to heal without scarring. Many disease processes can result in intraepidermal lesions, such as bacterial infections (staphylococcal scalded skin syndrome), viral infections (herpes simplex and varicella), and autoimmune disorders (pemphigus vulgaris). Cleavage below the level of the basement membrane produces a tense blister that is resistant to rupture and extension with applied pressure (Nikolsky's sign). Because the basal layer is frequently lost at the site of blister formation, scarring is much more prominent. Dystrophic forms of epidermolysis bullosa (EB), cicatricial pemphigoid (CP), erythema multiforme (EM), and toxic epidermal necrolysis (TEN) are examples of subepidermal bullous disorders that may develop significant ocular disease. Distinguishing the site of blister formation within the dermis or epidermis requires specialized studies, such as immunofluorescence, electron microscopy, and immunoelectron microscopy.

A number of vesicobullous disorders may develop mild ocular features; however, they are minimal findings compared with other sites of involvement and are unlikely to aid in the diagnosis or become clinically significant. These conditions include epidermolytic hyperkeratosis, acrodermatitis enteropathica, bullous disease of childhood, bullous diabeticorum, Hailey-Hailey disease, herpes gestationis, and subcorneal pustular dermatosis.

Epidermolysis Bullosa

EB, also referred to as *mechanobullous diseases,* comprises some 30 different inherited and acquired disorders that are phenotypically different.[229, 230] Common features include cutaneous fragility and the formation of blisters, erosions, and in some patients, progressive scarring. The clinical spectrum ranges from mild nonscarring peeling of the palms and soles to life-threatening and destructive disease. The most useful classification is based on the level at which blister formation occurs.[230] Separation within the epidermis results in minimal if any scarring and is referred to as the *epidermolytic subgroup.* Bullae formation within the lamina lucida of the basement membrane is referred to as a *lamina lucidolytic* or *junctional subgroup.* Many authors prefer the term *junctional EB* because the exact site of separation between the epidermis and dermis is debatable and is not considered to be at the level of the lamina lucida.[230] The third and last subtype of EB is the *dystrophic* or *dermolytic* form with blister formation below the basal lamina. An acquired form of EB, referred to as *epidermolysis bullosa acquisita,* has the same level of bullae formation and similar clinical features reported for dominant dystrophic EB.[231] Only the forms of EB known to have ocular involvement are reviewed.

Epidermolytic EB comprises 17 different inherited forms.[230] In epidermolysis bullosa simplex, blisters and erosions may be present at birth or develop as late as several weeks of age. The lesions occur most commonly on the acral areas (distal extremities) and flexural surfaces. Warm weather aggravates the disease, as does increased sweating (hyperhydrosis).[229, 230] Hyperkeratosis of the palms and soles is a common feature but is usually mild. Secondary bacterial infections may also occur. Most patients, particularly females, improve at puberty. In Weber-Cockayne epidermolysis bullosa, trauma-induced blistering is mild and involves the hands and the feet. Symptoms are often delayed in onset and develop later in childhood. Epidermolysis bullosa herpetiformis, also known as *Dowling-Meara disease,* commonly results in acral blistering; however, more generalized variants have been reported.[230, 232] Although the healed lesions may appear atrophic and have milia, true scarring rarely occurs. Dystrophic nails, hyperkeratosis of the palms and soles, oral blistering, dental abnormalities, esophageal casts, and flexion contractures are potential complications of Dowling-Meara disease. Ocular manifestations in the epidermolytic forms of EB are mild and include chronic blepharitis and blistering of the eyelids, as shown in Table 1–19.

Of the six forms of junctional EB, four types may result in significant ocular disease (see Table 1–19). Epidermolysis bullosa letalis, or Herlitz variant, is the most common form. Generalized erosions and blisters are present at birth, particularly over the distal extremities.[230, 235] The lesions heal slowly with scarring and atrophy. Vegetative plaques may involve the perioral regions. Nails are frequently lost or absent. Multiple organ systems may be involved to include the mucous membranes (oral, nasal, pharyngeal, esophageal, anal, and vaginal), small intestine, gallbladder, urethra, kidneys, pylorus, and teeth.[229,230] Ocular features may be severe and result in significant visual loss. Although most patients die within a few weeks, a few have been reported to survive into adolescence.[230] Epidermolysis bullosa mitis is also present at birth and is very similar to epidermolysis bullosa letalis. Scarring in this form tends to result in more atrophy than does Herlitz disease. In the EB localized form the blistering and scarring occur over the hands, feet, and some-

TABLE 1–19

Ocular Manifestations of Inherited Epidermolysis Bullosa (EB)[230,232–237]

Subgroups and Types	Inheritance	Ocular Manifestations
Epidermolytic		
EB simplex[233]	AD	Corneal erosions
EB, Weber-Cockayne[232]	AD	Blepharitis
EB herpetiformis[232] (Dowling-Meara)	AD	Blepharitis, eyelid blistering
Junctional		
EB Herlitz (letalis)[232–235]	AR	Eyelid blistering; blepharitis; cicatricial ectropion; congenital strabismus; foveal hypoplasia; corneal scarring; retinal disease; edema of the lens, optic nerve, ciliary body, iris, and trabecular network
EB mitis[232,236] (generalized atrophic benign)	AR	Corneal scarring, absent lashes, broadening of the limbus
EB, localized[236]	AR	Conjunctival tethering, broadening of the limbus, corneal scarring
EB, inverse[236]	AR	Conjunctival tethering, corneal scarring
Dermolytic[230,232,233,237]		
EB, dominant dystrophic	AD	Eyelid scarring, cicatricial conjunctivitis, keratitis, corneal erosions
EB, recessive dystrophic	AR	Loss of eyelashes, eyelid blistering and scarring, cicatricial ectropion, exposure keratitis, keratoconjunctivitis, limbal broadening, corneal erosions and ulcers, corneal opacities, cicatrical band formation, symblepharon

AD, autosomal dominant; AR, autosomal recessive.

times the pretibial areas (onset at birth). Additional sites of involvement include the nails, eyes, nasal and oral mucosa, and teeth.[230, 235] EB inverse is characterized by neonatal erosions and blisters involving the axilla and groin. At times acral involvement may occur. The lesions heal with mild atrophy, and the nails may also be involved. Additional organ involvement includes the eyes, oral and anal mucosa, and esophagus.

The dermolytic subgroup is divided into two types based on inheritance: (1) four autosomal dominant (EB dominant dystrophic) forms; and (2) two autosomal recessive (EB recessive dystrophic) forms.[230] In general, the autosomal dominant forms, characterized by the Cockayne-Touraine variant, are less severe than the recessive inherited forms, and this also applies to ocular disease (see Table 1-19). Patients with dominant dystrophic disease develop acral and generalized blistering, to varying degrees, at birth or during infancy. Ocular disease may also be significant. Additional sites of involvement include the nails, oral mucosa, esophagus, and teeth. An increased risk of developing squamous cell carcinomas has been reported.[230] The prototypical form of EB recessive dystrophic is the Hallopeau-Siemens variant.[229] These patients develop severe progressive blistering and scarring. Onset is at birth or shortly thereafter. Progressive scarring results in a mitten deformity of the hands and syndactyly of the toes. As many as 82% of patients with recessive dystrophic EB develop eye involvement.[237] Keratitis and corneal erosions are the most common ocular complications (see Table 1-19).[230, 232] Additional systems involved include the oral, esophageal, anal, and vaginal mucosa; bladder; urethra; kidneys; and teeth. Anemia is common, and these patients are also susceptible to the development of cutaneous squamous cell carcinomas.[230] Growth and development are retarded. Life expectancy is shortened, particularly in the more severe forms.

More than 60 cases of epidermolysis bullosa acquisita have been reported.[231] There is no racial or sex preference, and the disease may develop at any time from childhood to the ninth decade (mean is fifth decade).[231] Clinically, there are two forms of cutaneous expression. In the classic presentation, there is noninflammatory bullous disease involving the acral regions and marked cutaneous fragility, similar to that observed in dystrophic EB. The sites heal with scarring and milia. Alopecia and nail dystrophies have also been reported. The second form results in more widespread tense vesicobullous lesions similar to those seen in patients with BP.[231] This type is characterized by pruritus, minimal skin fragility, and healing without scarring. About 30% to 50% of patients develop oral erosions and blistering reminiscent of CP.[231] Ocular disease has been reported and includes symblepharon, increased lacrimation, scarring of the lacrimal points, scarring of the conjunctiva tarsi, dry eyes, and corneal vesicles.[238-240] Association between Crohn's disease and SLE has been conclusively shown.[231, 241] Other potential disease associations include rheumatoid arthritis, chronic thyroiditis, idiopathic pulmonary fibrosis, chronic lymphocytic leukemia, cryoglobulinemia, and diabetes mellitus.[231]

The cause of EB in many types is unknown. In some instances it appears to be related to the formation of antibodies (epidermolysis bullosa acquisita) to or inherited deficiencies of normal constituents of the basal cell layer, basement membrane, or anchoring fibrils.[229-231] In patients with recessive dystrophic EB, there are excessive amounts of dermal collagenases.[229] Morphologic defects include rudimentary or absent hemidesmosomes in junctional EB, reduction or absence of anchoring fibrils in patients with dominant and recessive forms of dystrophic EB, and clumped tonofilaments within basilar keratinocytes in the Dowling-Meara variant.[229] The differential diagnosis of facial vesicobullous disorders includes pemphigus vulgaris, BP, benign mucous membrane pemphigoid, ocular pemphigoid, dermatitis herpetiformis, linear IgA dermatosis, PCT, congenital syphilis, EM, TEN, and acute dermatophytosis.[238] The histologic findings in the inherited forms are reviewed by Pearson.[230] The histologic picture for epidermolysis bullosa acquisita is similar to PCT.[231]

Treatment for most forms is supportive. For junctional EB, use of intensive systemic steroids and epidermal autografts to facial regions has been successful in some patients.[157] Phenytoin has shown promise in treating recessive dystrophic EB.[157] Surgical intervention may be required to prevent exposure keratitis and improve ocular function.[237]

Cicatricial Pemphigoid

CP (Fig. 1-11) is an autoimmune subepidermal blistering disorder that involves the mucous membranes and skin.[242, 243] Although a disease predominantly of the elderly (mean age 70 years), it has been reported in children.[244] There is no racial or geographic predilection, and

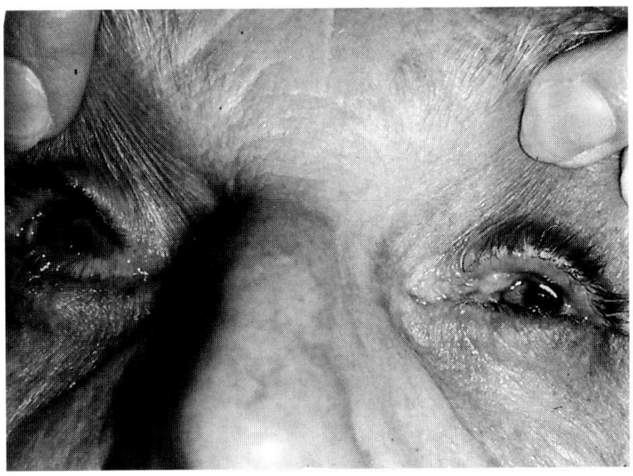

Figure 1-11. Cicatricial pemphigoid.

it affects women more often than men, with ratios varying from 1.6:1 to 1.8:1.[243] Of patients treated in an ophthalmology clinic, it is estimated that 1 in 15,000 to 40,000 may have CP.[242] There are many forms of CP, ranging from localized cutaneous to disseminated disease.[242]

The onset of CP is usually insidious. Common features are vesicles, bullae, or erosions involving the mucous membranes and skin. The most frequently involved mucous membranes are the oral cavity (85%) and eyes (65%).[242] Additional sites include the nose, pharynx, larynx, trachea, esophagus, anus, and genitalia. Ocular disease usually begins with unilateral chronic conjunctivitis with symptoms of burning, irritation, and excess tearing that progresses to bilateral disease within 2 years.[242, 243] Some patients may be asymptomatic. Mucous threads, vascular dilation, and patches of ocular surface epitheliopathy have also been reported.[242] Ocular CP may be slowly or rapidly progressive, leading to conjunctival cicatrization and blindness.[245] Subepithelial scarring with gradual obliteration of Meibomian gland orifices and lacrimal gland ducts results in xerosis. Points on the bulbar and palpebral conjunctivae fuse resulting in symblepharon. A band of symblepharon stretching like a clothesline across the medial aspect of the lower cul-de-sac is an early feature of CP. Eyelid malposition, symblepharon formation, and trichiasis promote keratopathy and eventual visual loss. Additional eye complications include eyelid scarring, shrinkage of the conjunctiva, conjunctival vesicles and bullae, entropion, glaucoma, and corneal neovascularization. More than 25% of CP patients develop cutaneous disease. Erythematous plaques progressing to recurrent blisters that heal with atrophic scarring may develop on the scalp, neck, and face. CP may develop nonscarring vesicobullous lesions on the trunk that are similar to BP. About 20% of CP patients develop genital lesions. Nasopharyngeal, laryngeal, esophageal, and anal disease often result in severe symptoms and significant sequelae.[242]

There are numerous clinical forms of CP, such as childhood, Brunsting-Perry, localized oral, localized ocular, disseminated, and drug-induced varieties.[242] A number of topical medications have been reported to induce ocular CP, including idoxuridine, echothiophate iodide, pilocarpine, demecarium, timolol, epinephrine, Phospholine iodide, and dipivefrin.[243] In addition, systemic use of D-penicillamine and practolol has been associated with CP.[242, 243]

The cause of CP is unknown. Many authors believe that an initial triggering event results in the conversion of normal CP or BP precursor proteins into a form that is antigenic.[242] Stevens-Johnson syndrome and EM have recently been shown to be disorders that may progress to CP.[243, 246] The differential diagnosis is large and dependent on the clinical presentation. Although BP and CP are histologically and immunopathologically identical, there are some important differences.[242] Rare shrinkage of conjunctival membranes has been reported for BP; however, cutaneous disease is the major clinical finding. Skin lesions for BP are large, tense vesicles and bullae involving the arms, legs, and trunk.[242] In contrast with CP, BP lesions heal without scarring and mucous membrane involvement is uncommon. Conjunctival scarring may be caused by chemical burns (especially alkali), scleral buckles, and conjunctival carcinoma (usually unilateral).[243] Trachoma also promotes conjunctival scarring. Symblepharons have been reported with Sjögren's syndrome, atopic keratoconjunctivitis, and sarcoidosis.[243] Infectious causes of conjunctival scarring include adenovirus, herpes simplex, diphtheria, and beta-hemolytic streptococci. Conjunctival shrinkage may be associated with drug-induced CP as previously described. Other inflammatory and bullous disorders, such as pemphigus, EM major, linear IgA disease, and Stevens-Johnson syndrome, may be confused with CP.[242, 243] Histologic examination frequently aids in excluding other bullous disorders; however, immunofluorescence studies may be required in some patients.

On histologic examination there is a subepidermal bulla without acantholysis. A mixed inflammatory infiltrate in the dermis is frequently observed. Immunofluorescent studies demonstrate deposition of complement and immunoglobulins along the basement membrane zone 80% to 97% of the time.[242] The deposits are linear, smooth, homogeneous or ribbon-like and are comprised most often of the IgG class of immunoglobulin. Circulating IgG antibasement membrane antibodies are detected (by indirect immunofluorescence) in 20% to 30% of patients with CP.[242] Indirect immunofluorescence using salt-split skin is a diagnostic technique for the detection of circulating antibasement membrane antibodies. In a recent series by Sarret and colleagues,[247] 55% had circulating IgA compared with 18% circulating IgG.

Treatment includes local and systemic regimens. Local care includes artificial tears, antibiotics (topical or systemic), correction of entropion and trichiasis, local débridement, intralesional steroids, and therapeutic soft contact lenses.[242, 243] Topical corticosteroid therapy is ineffective in ocular CP. Surgical intervention must be considered early in the course of disease because stimulation of acute inflammation with rapid conjunctival shrinkage has been associated with later stages.[243] A large number of systemic agents has been used in patients with CP, including cyclophosphamide, prednisone, azathioprine, diaminodiphenylsulfone (dapsone), and cyclosporine.[242, 243, 245] Treatment success with systemic agents is also more likely in earlier stages of the disease.[245] In a recent series by Neumann and coworkers,[245] of 104 patients treated with systemic therapy and followed over a 4-year period, 22% experienced relapse of their disease.

Pemphigus

Pemphigus is another autoimmune disorder of the skin and mucous membranes. There are six different variants (including drug-induced pemphigus) based on clinical features, histologic findings, and epidemiology.[248] In the group of pemphigus disorders, there is intraepidermal blister formation and acantholysis as a result of antibody production against cellular constituents. It is a rare disease, with an incidence rate of 0.5 to 3.2 cases per 100,000 persons per year. Although it is a disease mostly of middle age, reported cases have ranged from 3 to 89 years.[248] It is a disease afflicting all racial and ethnic groups, but the incidence is increased in the Jewish population.

The most common variant of pemphigus is pemphigus vulgaris. Patients present with oral blisters and erosions 50% to 70% of the time. Cutaneous lesions may take several months to develop after the onset of mucosal involvement. The entire oral cavity may be involved. Mucous membrane disease can involve the pharynx, larynx, esophagus, conjunctiva, urethra, cervix, and anal mucosa.[248, 249] Skin lesions are flaccid blisters that break easily, leaving denuded areas of skin. Lateral pressure applied to the edge of the blister or normal skin results in epidermal separation (Nikolsky's sign). Nikolsky's sign may also be positive in patients with TEN, BP, and some types of EB.[248] The most common sites of involvement are the scalp, face, axilla, and oral cavity, although more generalized lesions may occur.[248, 249]

Pemphigus foliaceus is also known as *superficial pemphigus*.[248] Patients develop recurrent, superficial, shallow erosions; erythema; scaling; and crust formation. Because of their superficial nature and easy fragility, intact blisters are flaccid, infrequently observed, and small in size. The lesions occur most commonly in a seborrheic distribution, involving the face, scalp, upper chest, and back. In severe cases, there is generalized cutaneous disease. Mucous membrane involvement in this form of pemphigus is rare.[248] Fogo selvagem, also known as *endemic pemphigus foliaceus*, is another type that is endemic in rural areas of South America, particularly Brazil. Fogo selvagem is histologically and immunopathologically indistinguishable from pemphigus foliaceus; however, it is different on epidemiologic and clinical grounds (ocular disease). It is endemic in rural jungle areas, and epidemics occur when forest is cleared for urbanization. Fogo selvagem afflicts children and young adults in contrast with pemphigus foliaceus, which affects middle-aged adults.[250, 251] The epidemiology of this disease suggests the possibility of an infectious agent. Patients with fogo selvagem may develop significant ocular disease. Facial blistering and crust formation can be severe and result in progressive eyelid scarring and loss of eyebrows.[252] Additional ocular features are described later.

Pemphigus vegetans results in hypertrophic granulation tissue and pustules close to the sites of bullae formation. The most common sites of involvement are the axilla, groin, flexural surfaces, and oral cavity.[248] Vegetative lesions in pemphigus vegetans are particularly resistant to treatment. Rarely, there may be cutaneous involvement of the mouth, midface, and eyelids.[253]

Pemphigus erythematosus, also called *Senear-Usher syndrome*, is characterized by erythematous, scaling, hyperkeratotic plaques distributed in a butterfly pattern over the nose and malar surfaces.[248] The upper chest, back, scalp, and buttocks are also frequently involved. Like pemphigus foliaceus, mucosal findings are rare. There have been reports of pemphigus erythematosus being associated with lupus erythematosus.[248]

A variety of drugs may induce pemphigus. The most commonly reported forms of drug-induced pemphigus are pemphigus erythematosus and pemphigus foliaceus.[248] Penicillamine is the most frequent offending agent. Additional reported medications include captopril, rifampin, thiopronine (mercaptopropionylglycine), phenobarbital, and piroxicam.[248]

Pemphigus has been associated with an increased incidence of myasthenia gravis and thymoma.[254] In addition, there are 16 patients reported to have developed all three diseases. Lymphoreticular malignancies, particularly Kaposi's sarcoma, are also associated with pemphigus. Lymphoreticular malignancies were documented in 37 of 60 pemphigus patients (61%) reported to have developed malignancies.[254]

Little has been reported on ocular disease developing in pemphigus patients. The most significant abnormalities are associated with fogo selvagem. Amendola[252] reported a large series of patients with ocular disease in 1949 (clinical observations were made in 1944). Although these observations were reported before immunohistochemical studies were available, the clinical picture of fogo selvagem is distinct. Some 240 patients underwent cutaneous, slit lamp, and corneal microscopic examination over a 1-year period. Progressive eyelid disease resulted in erythema, edema, fibrosis, ectropion, lagophthalmos, entropion, tylosis, trichiasis, madarosis, and blepharophimosis. Patients with eyelash deviation upward experienced repetitive trauma to the cornea, producing superficial infiltrations, pannus formation, vascularization, and keratitis. Muscular palpebral atrophy was observed and confirmed on biopsy. Conjunctival disease included hyperemia, conjunctival contraction, and catarrhal secretion. The author believed that catarrhal secretion and scleroconjunctival hyperemia was a result of microbial disease and not directly related to fogo selvagem. Additional corneal disease included blisters, infiltration, corneal pannus, and synechiae. Corneal vesicles were positive for Nikolsky's sign. Twelve of the 240 patients developed cataracts.

Cutaneous involvement of the eyelids can occur in any form of pemphigus. Patients with pemphigus vulgaris may develop eye complaints such as irritation, excessive watering of the eyes, and a foreign body sensation.[255] Clinical findings include conjunctival hyperemia, conjunctivitis, erosions, symblepharon, ciliary infections, mucoid discharge, and, rarely, synechiae.[255,256] In a series of 11 patients reported by Hodak and associates,[255] in which all had ocular symptoms, only 3 were shown on blind conjunctival biopsies (none of the patients had conjunctival vesicles or bullae) to have histologic and direct immunofluorescence studies confirming the diagnosis of pemphigus vulgaris. Although Kaposi's sarcoma rarely involves the conjunctiva, there is an increased association of Kaposi's sarcoma and pemphigus.[254] Jaimovich and colleagues[257] reported a case of pemphigus erythematosus treated with systemic steroids with the subsequent development of conjunctival and generalized cutaneous Kaposi's sarcoma.

The exact cause of pemphigus is under investigation, and much has been learned. The evidence suggests that circulating antibodies are pathogenic; however, the underlying events inducing the production of these autoantibodies are still unknown.[248] Many of the epidermal cellular antigens have been identified and are reviewed by Korman.[248] The differential diagnosis includes BP, CP, dermatitis herpetiformis, EB, EM, bullous impetigo, and drug eruptions. On biopsy pemphigus vulgaris demonstrates characteristic findings, such as suprabasal intraepidermal blister formation with loss of cellular cohesion (acantholysis). The basal epidermal layer of cells usually is intact and resembles a row of tombstones at the bottom of the blister. In pemphigus foliaceus, fogo selvagem, and pemphigus erythematosus, separation and acantholysis occur within the granular layer of cells in the epidermis, resulting in subcorneal blisters. Patients with pemphigus vegetans develop suprabasilar acantholysis within a thickened epidermis (epidermal hyperplasia) and abscesses composed of eosinophils. Direct immunofluorescence studies tested against keratinocyte cell surfaces are positive in 100% of patients with pemphigus for IgG, 50% for C_3, and 30% for IgM or IgA.[248] Indirect immunofluorescence testing is positive in 80% to 90% of patients.[248]

Glucocorticoids are the mainstay of treatment for all forms of pemphigus. Immunosuppressive agents have also been used with success, including methotrexate, cyclophosphamide, and azathioprine. Combinations of prednisone and an immunosuppressive agent in patients with severe disease are used together for their steroid-sparing effects. Parenteral gold is another adjuvant form of therapy. Additional therapeutic options include dapsone, cyclosporine, and plasmapheresis.[248] Local wound care should not be forgotten. Silver sulfadiazine (Silvadene) and topical antibiotics should be used to treat cutaneous lesions. Oral lesions may require antiseptic mouthwashes and use of viscous lidocaine before meals.

Erythema Multiforme

EM is an acute inflammatory cutaneous disorder. There are three clinical forms: (1) EM minor involves only skin and is generally self-limited; (2) EM major, also known as *Stevens-Johnson syndrome*, is characterized by severe mucosal involvement, marked cutaneous disease, toxemia, and ocular manifestations (Fig. 1 – 12)[243, 246]; and (3) TEN, also known as *Lyell's syndrome* (Fig. 1 – 13). Patients with TEN develop massive desquamation of the epidermis.[243, 258] Some authors believe that the clinical presentation of TEN is distinct, whereas others believe that it is simply a more severe form of Stevens-Johnson syndrome.[259] In a recent population-based study involving three institutions, the overall incidence rate of Stevens-Johnson syndrome resulting in hospitalization was 6.1 in 1 million persons per year.[260] For TEN it was less than 1 in 1 million hospitalized patients per year.[260] These values are much lower than previously believed and suggest that the risk of severe forms of drug-induced EM is quite low.

Patients with EM have prodromal symptoms and may present with malaise, fever, upper respiratory tract symptoms, prostration, and headache.[243, 258] There are many different cutaneous varieties of EM minor, such as macular, papular, nodose, vesicular, or bullous disease. The most common presentation is that of annular, circinate, iris-shaped, or target lesions (bull's eye) involving the distal extremities. The onset is rapid, occurring over 12 to 24 hours. The most frequent sites of involvement include the face, neck, forearms, legs, and dorsal surfaces of the hands and feet.[258] The most frequent cause of EM minor is herpes infections.[243, 258]

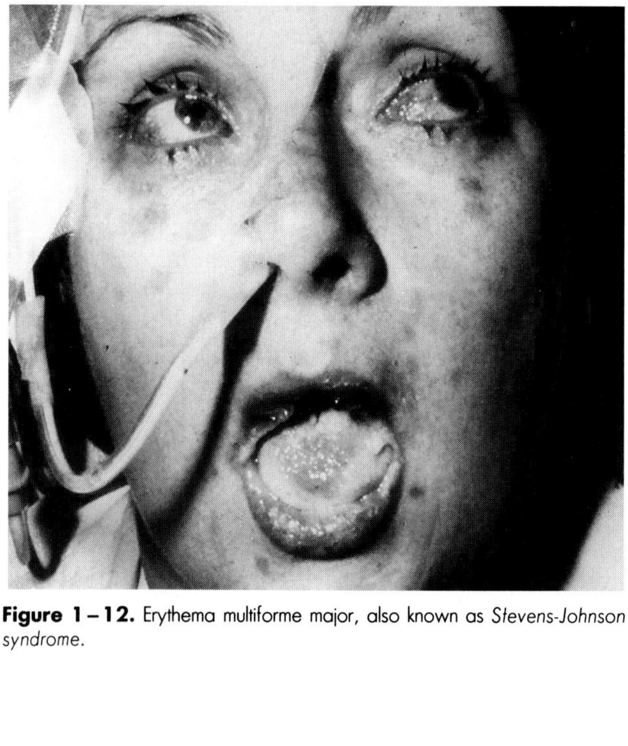

Figure 1 – 12. Erythema multiforme major, also known as *Stevens-Johnson syndrome*.

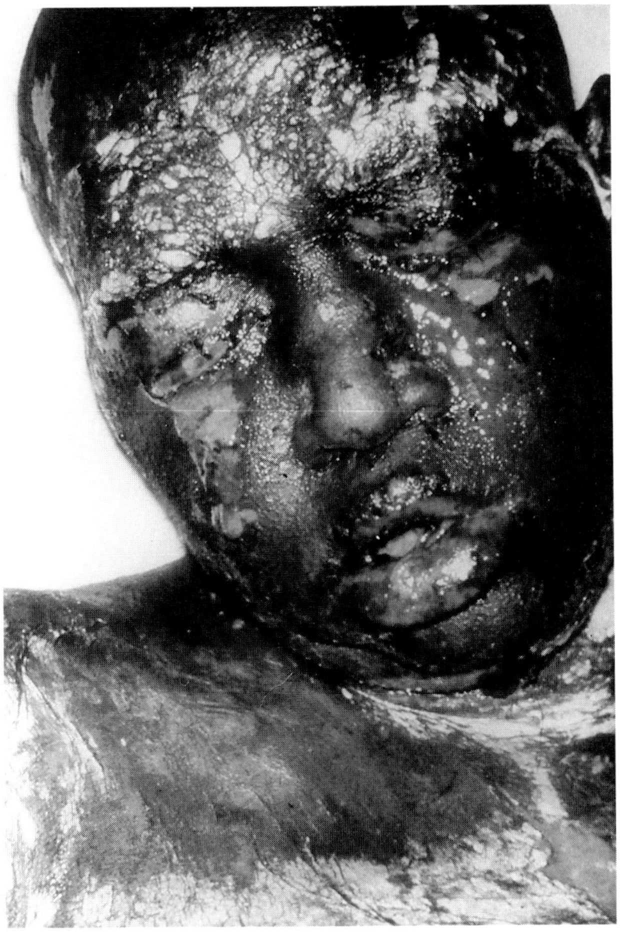

Figure 1–13. Toxic epidermal necrolysis, also known as *Lyell's syndrome.*

Patients with Stevens-Johnson syndrome experience an abrupt onset of fever, headache, malaise, and soreness of the throat and mouth. Constitutional symptoms soon develop to include a rapid weak pulse, tachypnea, prostration, and joint pains. Stomatitis is an early finding that begins with vesicles on the lips, tongue, and buccal mucosa.[258] Oral findings may rapidly progress to pseudomembranous exudation, salivation, and ulcerations. Other mucosal membranes may be involved, resulting in conjunctivitis, corneal ulcers, rhinitis with epistaxis, erosive vulvovaginitis, anal erosions, and balanitis. Cutaneous lesions initially are the same as those described for EM minor; however, they often become more generalized and severe. Complications of the disease include gastrointestinal disturbances, bronchial pneumonia, arthritis, convulsions, coma, cardiac arrhythmias, pericarditis, myositis, hepatitis, septicemia, and death.[258] Stevens-Johnson syndrome afflicts mostly children and young men. Males outnumber females by two to one, and there is an increased incidence during the winter and spring months.[258]

The controversy over the separation of TEN and Stevens-Johnson syndrome is complicated by one of definition and cause. Some cases of classic Stevens-Johnson syndrome may progress and result in large areas of cutaneous desquamation suggestive of TEN. However, although herpes and *Mycoplasma pneumoniae* infections are well-known causes of Stevens-Johnson syndrome, they are not implicated in causing TEN, suggesting that they are different disease processes.[259] In addition, graft-versus-host disease may result in TEN but has not been implicated in causing Stevens-Johnson syndrome.[259] Roujeau and coworkers[259] define Stevens-Johnson syndrome as the combination of severe mucosal erosions, discrete target-like macules, and occasional cutaneous blistering involving less than 10% of the body's surface area. The diagnosis of TEN is made when sheet-like desquamation of the epidermis involves more than 10% of the body surface area.[259] In an attempt to better define these disorders, Ruiz-Maldonado has proposed the term *acute disseminated epidermal necrosis* (ADEN) types 1, 2, and 3.[261] Type 1 ADEN corresponds to "classic" Stevens-Johnson syndrome, type 2 to classic TEN, and type 3 to transitional forms. Roujeau and associates[259] have not noted any difference in pathology, etiology, complications, or prognosis between ADEN type 2 and ADEN type 3 disease.

Drugs are the most frequent cause of TEN.[27, 259] It begins with fever, malaise, diarrhea, angina, or vomiting, followed by cutaneous features of erythema and tenderness. The sites of erythema may rapidly progress to form large flaccid bullae. Within hours the skin begins to peel off in large sheets, exposing raw dermis.[27] This presentation is similar to that observed in staphylococcal scalded skin syndrome in children. Staphylococcal scalded skin syndrome is a superficial blistering disorder caused by the production of a staphylococcal exotoxin.[27] In both conditions there is a positive Nikolsky's sign. The disorders may be differentiated on biopsy because staphylococcal scalded skin syndrome results in vesicobullous disease high in the epidermis, whereas in TEN the separation is below the basal cell layer. Less frequently, a generalized scarlatiniform erythema has been observed.[259] In a recent review of TEN by Roujeau and colleagues,[259] the authors stated that mucosal involvement occurs in 85% to 95% of patients. In our experience mucosal involvement in classic TEN is less common than that reported for Stevens-Johnson syndrome but may result in pronounced ocular complications, particularly in the severest forms. Stevens-Johnson syndrome can last for weeks and result in considerable scarring. Approximately 20% to 30% of patients die from their disease, and sepsis is the most frequent underlying cause.[259] A poor prognosis is associated with age, extensive necrolysis, and elevation of serum urea.[27, 259]

Ocular disease is most commonly associated with Stevens-Johnson syndrome.[243, 262–264] The acute phase of ocular disease lasts between 2 and 3 weeks. Swelling and crusting of the eyelids and a membranous conjunctivitis are frequent findings. A purulent conjunctivitis may develop secondary to bacterial infections.[243] Anterior uveitis has also been reported.[263] Chronic ocular complications include symblepharon, conjunctival shrinkage, ankyloblepharon, entropion, trichiasis, lagophthalmos, exposure keratitis, obliteration of the lacrimal puncta, epiphora, dry eyes, punctate corneal erosions, corneal pannus, corneal ulcers, and corneal opacification. Most corneal ulcers are secondary to bacterial infections.[243] In severe forms of classic TEN, patients may develop conjunctivitis, conjunctival scarring, synechiae, exposure keratitis, ectropion, and madarosis.[27, 259, 265]

Table 1–20 lists some of the infectious and drug-related causes of EM. The most commonly implicated causative agents of EM minor and Stevens-Johnson syndrome are herpes and *Mycoplasma pneumoniae* infections. However, many other infectious disorders may cause EM, as shown in Table 1–20. Drugs are also frequent offenders, particularly the aminopenicillins.[259]

The differential diagnosis of EM minor and Stevens-Johnson syndrome includes other vesicobullous diseases, collagen vascular diseases, and infectious dermatoses. For TEN the differential diagnosis includes staphylococcal scalded skin syndrome, toxic shock syndrome, Kawasaki disease, second-degree burns, other forms of drug eruptions, and disseminated pustular disor-

TABLE 1–20

Suspected Causes of Erythema Multiforme[*,243, 258–260, 263, 264]

Infectious Agents
- Viral
  - Herpes
  - Asian flu
  - Lymphogranuloma venereum
  - Infectious mononucleosis
  - Measles
  - Milker's nodules
  - Mumps
  - Coxsackie viruses
  - Echoviruses
  - Poliomyelitis
- Bacterial
  - *Mycoplasma pneumoniae*
  - Brucellosis
  - Diphtheria
  - Erysipeloid
  - Glanders
  - *Yersinia*
  - Psittacosis
  - Tuberculosis
  - Tularemia
  - Lepromatous leprosy
  - Typhoid fever
- Protozoan
  - Malaria
  - Trichomoniasis

Drugs
- Allopurinol
- Antipyrine
- Arsenic
- Barbiturates
- Bromides
- Carbamazepine (TEN)
- Chloramphenicol (TEN)
- Cyclines (TEN)
- Dapsone
- Digitalis
- Disulfiram (TEN)
- Erythromycin (TEN)
- Ethambutol (TEN)
- Fenbufen (TEN)
- Gold salts
- Griseofulvin (TEN)
- Hydralazine
- Iodides
- Isoniazid (TEN)
- Isoxicam (TEN)
- Mercurials
- Naproxen (TEN)
- Penicillamine
- Penicillins
- Phenylbutazone
- Phenytoin (Dilantin)
- Piroxicam (TEN)
- Pyrazolones (TEN)
- Quinolones (TEN)
- Rifampicin (TEN)
- Salicylates
- Sulfonamides
- Sulindac (TEN)
- Tetracycline
- Tolbutamide
- Trimethoprim-sulfamethoxazole
- Vancomycin (TEN)

Allergenic Skin Contactants
- Bromofluorine
- Fire sponge (*Tedania egnis*)
- *Toxicodendron* (3-pentadecylcatechol)

Vaccines
- Bacille Calmette-Guérin
- Smallpox
- Hepatitis B
- Measles-mumps-rubella
- Diphtheria-tetanus
- Poliomyelitis

Collagen Vascular Diseases
- Systemic lupus erythematosus
- Chronic discoid lupus erythematosus

Neoplasia
- Carcinoma
- Hodgkin's disease
- Lymphoma
- Myeloma
- Leukemia
- Polycythemia

Miscellaneous
- Graft-versus-host disease (TEN)
- Hormonal changes (pregnancy and menstruation)
- Loeffler's syndrome

*Erythema multiforme includes erythema multiforme minor, Stevens-Johnson syndrome, and toxic epidermal necrolysis (TEN).

ders such as acute pustular psoriasis.[259] On histologic examination there is frequently papillary edema and separation or bullae formation below the basal layer of epidermal cells. In more severe forms there is epidermal necrosis manifesting as eosinophilic-appearing necrotic keratinocytes.[258] Mononuclear cells are found in a perivascular distribution. Direct immunofluorescence studies frequently demonstrate immunoglobulins C_3 and C_4 within blood vessels.[243, 263] Conjunctival and skin biopsy results are similar.

Treatment is supportive. Although systemic steroids have been recommended by authors in the past, there has never been a controlled study. In patients with TEN involving more than 20% total surface area, steroids are presently believed to be contraindicated owing to an associated increase in secondary infections.[27] Many authors continue to recommend systemic corticosteroids (60 to 80 mg of prednisone daily) early in the course of disease for patients with less severe forms.[243] Local wound care includes wet dressings, local débridement, baths, hydration, analgesics, saline mouthwashes, topical anesthetics, and topical corticosteroids.[243, 259] Systemic antibiotics should be administered only if there is evidence of infection. In extensive cutaneous disease patients should be considered for care in a burn center. Local treatment for ophthalmic complications appears to have little influence.[243] The most important treatable acute complication is infection. Frequent cultures should be performed followed by initiation of topical antibiotics when ocular infections are suspected. Early lysis of symblepharon, although rarely effective, should be attempted. Once the acute inflammation has subsided, patients may require artificial tears, destruction of aberrant lashes, soft contact lenses to protect the cornea, and topical antibiotics to manage superinfection.[243] The lacrimal puncta may be scarred and require surgical intervention. If the patient has dry eyes, the lacrimal ducts should be closed.[266] Topical retinoids have been shown to be ineffective in reversing conjunctival keritinization.[267] Chronic corneal ulceration may require tarsorrhaphy.[243] Mucous membrane grafts have been used to reconstruct the fornices. Localized conjunctival epidermization may be treated by tarsal polishing followed by full-thickness buccal mucous membrane grafting.[243] Kerito-epithelioplasty has also been used successfully in patients with Stevens-Johnson syndrome.[268] A keratoprosthesis should be considered for those patients with severe symblepharon, ankyloblepharon, and keratinization of the ocular surface epithelium.[243]

DERMATOSES AND HYPERSENSITIVITY DISORDERS

A number of dermatoses and hypersensitivity disorders may involve the ocular adnexa. Papulosquamous diseases include seborrheic dermatitis, pityriasis rubra pilaris, psoriasis, lichen planus, lichen simplex chronicus, atopic dermatitis, and exfoliative dermatitis. Additional epidermal processes include the ichthyoses and hypersensitivity disorders. Dermal inflammatory diseases include acne rosacea, urticaria, granuloma annulare, and granuloma faciale. There are two disorders that may involve hair structures: alopecia mucinosa and alopecia areata. Most of these conditions are restricted to the skin; however, some may develop systemic features or result in significant ocular disease, or both. Clinical presentation and cutaneous biopsies are frequently all that are needed to establish the correct diagnosis. The histology for many of these disorders is complex and beyond the scope of this chapter.

Seborrheic Dermatitis

Seborrheic dermatitis (Fig. 1–14) is a common chronic, superficial inflammatory skin disease of unclear etiology. The onset usually occurs between puberty and middle age, often involving the scalp first. The sites of predilection are areas of high sebaceous gland density, with the course paralleling active sebaceous gland size and function.[269–273]

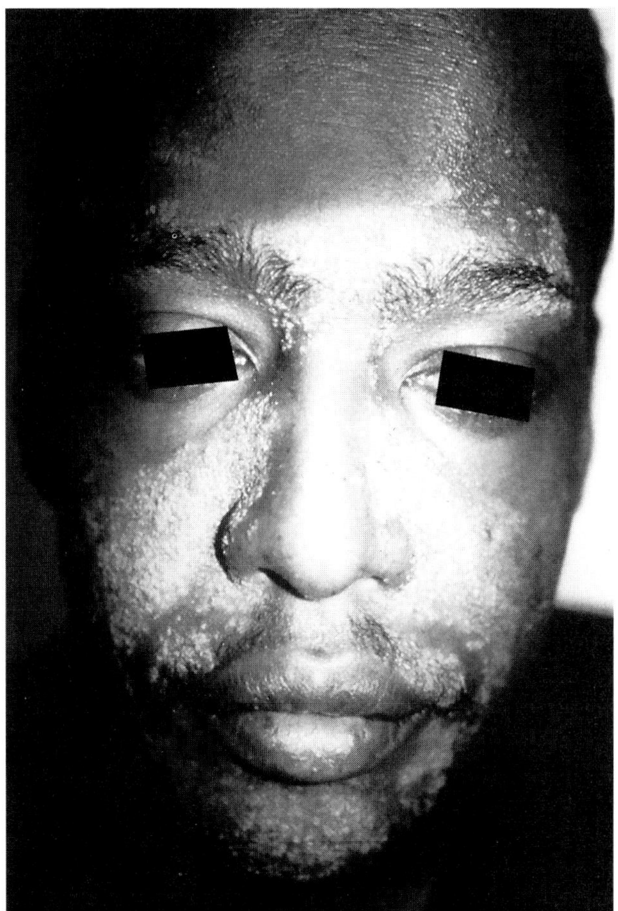

Figure 1–14. Seborrheic dermatitis in a patient with human immunodeficiency virus infection.

A seborrheic dermatitis-like eruption has a reported incidence of 40% to 83% in human immunodeficiency virus (HIV) disease and may be the presenting manifestation.[274] It is an unusually severe dermatitis, and exacerbations often correlate with the clinical deterioration of the patient and decreasing helper-to-suppressor T cell ratio. The dermatitis is characterized by loose, superficial, greasy, scaly patches with indistinct borders. Periods of exacerbation and remission are common. The typical distribution includes the scalp, eyebrows, eyelids, nasolabial folds, and retroauricular and sternal areas.

The eyebrows may have typical skin lesions with no associated alopecia. Inflammation is found along the anterior ciliary portion of the eyelids with variable extension onto the margin (marginal blepharitis). Collarettes of debris around the lashes may lead to misdirection or loss of eyelashes. Associated staphylococcal superinfection is common and will increase the inflammatory appearance and formation of external or internal hordeolum. Meibomian glands may become inflamed (meibomianitis). Increased inflammation raises the likelihood of associated conjunctivitis or keratitis. Hypersensitivity to staphylococcal exotoxin can lead to marginal corneal ulceration.[275] Approximately one third of patients with seborrheic blepharoconjunctivitis have associated keratoconjunctivitis sicca owing to tear film abnormalities.

Although the pathogenesis may involve sebaceous gland dysfunction, recent studies have implicated, although not proved, an etiologic role for the lipophilic, pleomorphic fungus *Malassezia ovalis* (*Pityrosporum ovale*).[273] The differential diagnosis includes psoriasis, contact dermatitis, pityriasis rosea, dermatophytosis, and Hailey-Hailey disease.

Treatment of the eyebrow area with low-potency corticosteroid creams or lotions is often effective. Scalp seborrhea can usually be controlled with 1% selenium sulfide shampoo. Ketoconazole cream and shampoo are also proven therapeutic options. In patients with severe, treatment-resistant disease, coexistent HIV disease should be suspected.

Rosacea

Acne rosacea (Fig. 1-15) is a common, chronic, inflammatory disorder with a predilection for middle-aged females. Although the onset usually occurs between the ages of 25 and 50 years, the disorder has been reported in children.[276-281] Skin lesions occur on the eyelids, brow, and midface, often consisting of variable combinations of patchy erythema, telangiectases, small papules, pustules, and hypertrophic sebaceous glands. Rhinophyma is the result of collagen deposition in the dermal and subcutaneous tissues of the nose. Although ocular involvement is found in as many as 60% of patients, it is often underdiagnosed. To address this problem, Browning and Proia[282] have devised a point system that emphasizes the skin findings of rosacea over the often nonspecific ocular findings. Relatively mild skin changes can be accompanied by severe ocular involvement.

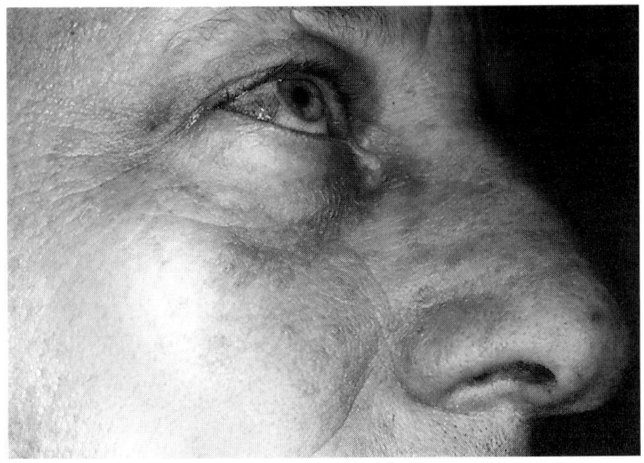

Figure 1-15. Rosacea of the face and conjunctiva.

Lid manifestations include relentless blepharitis, meibomianitis, and recurrent chalazia. Ocular involvement is usually characterized by conjunctival hyperemia. Approximately 5% of patients demonstrate infiltrates of the inferior cornea leading to vascularization and ulceration; this often results in thinning of the cornea, scarring, and occasional perforation. A coexisting tear deficiency occurs in more than 30% of patients.[283, 284] *Staphylococcus aureus*, although not considered an underlying cause of rosacea, is often cultured from the lids of most patients with blepharitis. Those with recurrent chalazia are often found to have rosacea.[285, 286]

Lupus miliaris disseminatus faciei (Fig. 1-16) is an asymptomatic papular eruption previously thought to be a tuberculid. Most authors believe that it is a variant of acne rosacea.[287] The primary lesions are reddish-brown aggregated papules with a predilection for the central face. The eyelid is the most common site of involvement.

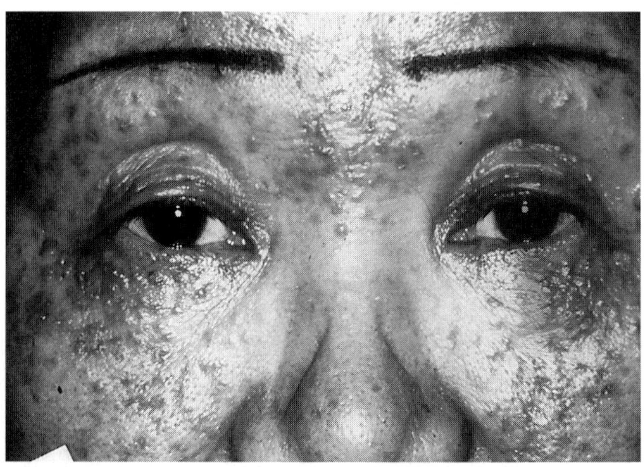

Figure 1-16. Lupus miliaris disseminatus faciei.

Over a 1- to 3-year period, the disorder often resolves spontaneously, leaving pock-like scars.

A number of factors have been implicated in the pathogenesis of acne rosacea. Vasomotor lability, psychogenic stimuli, endocrine factors, ultraviolet light exposure, heat, *Demodex folliculorum,* and topical fluorinated steroid usage have been proposed as etiologic factors. The clinical features result from attendant inflammation, capillary proliferation, and collagen depostion.[276-281] The differential diagnosis includes acne vulgaris, seborrhea, lupus erythematosus, syphilis, cutaneous tuberculosis, and sarcoidosis. Other generalized telangiectatic processes may also simulate rosacea. The diagnosis is based on clinical findings, which can be corroborated with biopsies if necessary. Schirmer's testing for adequacy of tear production should be performed.

Treatment consists of tetracycline 250 mg four times a day. This dosage is tapered to 250 mg daily or every other day as the disease process comes under control. Lupus miliaris disseminatus faciei responds slowly to tetracycline, in 2 to 4 months. Topical metronidazole and isotretinoin have been successful in difficult cases, but relapses have been observed.[288] Although steroids offer temporary relief of ocular symptoms, their use in patients with corneal involvement may contribute to corneal "melting" and perforation. Artificial tears often afford considerable symptomatic relief, even in those cases with apparently normal amounts of tear formation, suggesting that there may be qualitative tear alterations as well. Tear supplementation may also result in objective improvement in corneal manifestations.

Pityriasis Rubra Pilaris

Pityriasis rubra pilaris is a rare condition affecting both sexes equally. Familial and acquired forms of the disease have been described. The age of onset has a bimodal distribution, with peaks in the first and sixth decades.

Five types of pityriasis rubra pilaris are recognized. The adult types are generally characterized by relatively rapid caudal spread of follicular hyperkeratosis and erythema. Characteristic small islands of normal skin are found within the involved areas. An exfoliative erythroderma may result. There is facial and palmar-plantar hyperkeratosis with a typical orange hue. The juvenile types may have an associated family history, often being less generalized in extent.[289, 290]

The eyelids may have follicular papules at the cilia, and confluent lesions frequently result in ectropion. Other abnormalities rarely observed are papules of the bulbar conjunctiva, generalized thickening of the entire conjunctiva, corneal epithelial erosions, generalized corneal epithelial thickening with pannus formation, interstitial keratitis, iridocyclitis, and chorioretinitis.[291, 292]

Clinical and histologic features suggest that a vitamin impairment, particularly vitamin A, may be involved in the pathogenesis. The differential diagnosis includes psoriasis, drug eruption, ichthyosis, and lichen planopilaris. The combination of classic clinical features with a supportive biopsy establishes the diagnosis.

Isotretinoin is the treatment of choice for systemic therapy in adult patients. Etretinate is equally effective; however, the long elimination half-life limits its use in women of child-bearing age. Both retinoids are highly teratogenic.[293]

Psoriasis Vulgaris

Psoriasis vulgaris (Fig. 1 – 17) is a genetic multifactorial disease of controversial pathogenesis affecting 1% to 2% of the population. The onset usually occurs between 15 and 30 years of age but may develop as early as infancy. Accelerated epidermal cell proliferation and accompanying polymorphonuclear inflammation are important features.[294-296]

Classic psoriasis is characterized by well-demarcated erythematous plaques covered with a thick, micaceous scale. Pinpoint bleeding occurs (Auspitz's sign) on forcible removal of this scale. Involvement is usually symmetric, with a predilection for the scalp, nails, extensor aspects of the extremities, and sacral region. Typical lesions may appear at sites of trauma (Koebner isomorphic response). The extent of involvement is variable, ranging from isolated scaling papules to exfoliative erythroderma (Fig. 1 – 18). Pustular variants also occur. Arthritis is seen in 6% of patients, characteristically affecting the terminal interphalangeal joints.

Ocular signs occur in 10% of psoriatic patients, with a 2:1 predilection for males. Lid involvement presents as a scaling process, often affecting the base of the lashes. It may lead to inflammatory ectropion with trichiasis or madarosis, often accompanied by conjunctivitis, iritis, nodular episcleritis, keratoconjunctivitis sicca, posterior subcapsular cataracts (zonular, shield shaped), and cor-

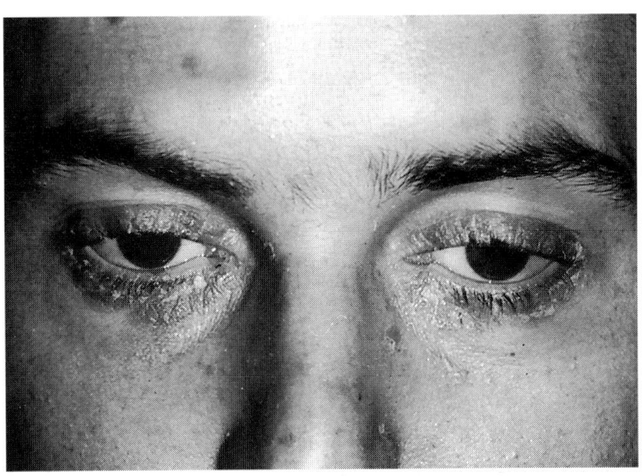

Figure 1 – 17. Psoriasis vulgaris.

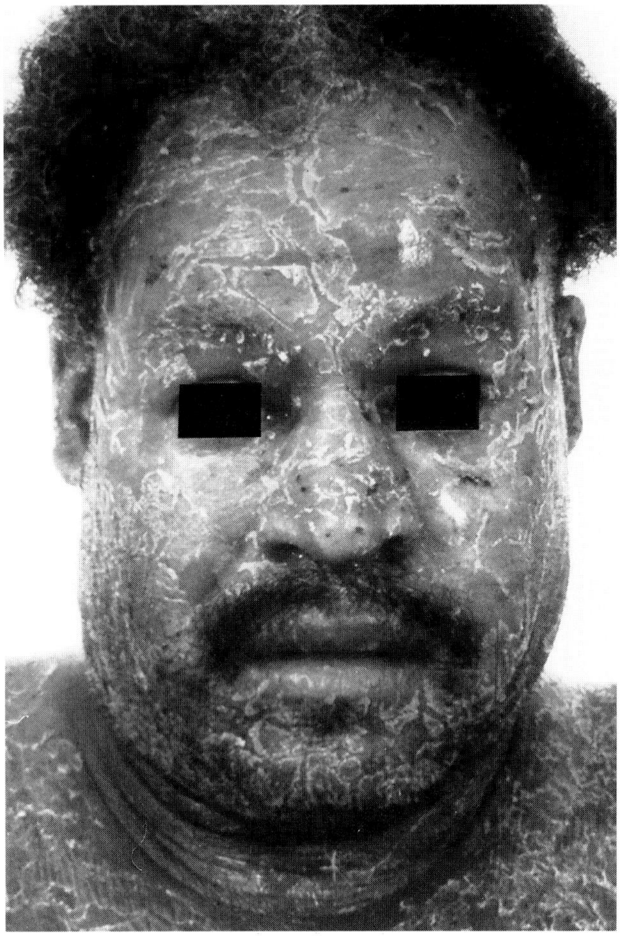

Figure 1 – 18. Erythrodermic psoriasis.

neal disease (erosions, opacities, vascularization, or ulcers).[297,298]

Although there is a genetic tendency for the development of psoriasis, this is not always the case, and the exact cause remains unknown. The differential diagnosis includes seborrheic dermatitis, pityriasis rosea, lichen planus, eczema, and pityriasis rubra pilaris. Clinical characteristics are usually sufficient to differentiate these diseases; however, biopsy findings will corroborate the diagnosis, if necessary.

Treatment options include topical corticosteroids in creams and lotions, intralesional steroid injections, tar preparations, ultraviolet light, aromatic retinoids, and systemic antimetabolites. Although there is often a good response to these treatment options, the disease process is chronic and usually lifelong.

Urticaria and Angioedema

Approximately 0.1% of the population will have urticaria on physical examination, and the cumulative prevalence rates are between 15% and 25%.[299] Urticaria and angioedema (Fig. 1 – 19) are classified into three categories: immunologic, nonimmunologic, and idiopathic. Immunologic urticaria is either IgE dependent or complement mediated, whereas the nonimmunologic forms are caused by drugs, dyes, and radiopaque media. The clinical finding of an erythematous, evanescent, elevated swelling associated with pruritus reflects increased vascular permeability and extravasated proteins and fluids into the extracellular space. Mast cell degranulation, with the release of its mediators, is involved in the vascular aberration.[300]

Eyelid swelling due to urticaria occurs when the edema is in the dermal tissue, and angioedematous swelling reflects a deeper subcutaneous reaction. Reactive conjunctival vascular dilation can also lead to a boggy and sometimes massive conjunctival edema (chemosis).

Determining the underlying cause is the central concern in urticaria and angioedema. The goal is to eliminate the inciting factor. Often, the cause cannot be determined, in which case oral antihistamines are the drugs of choice to attenuate the secondary reactions. Alternative therapy includes tricyclic antidepressants, beta-adrenergic agents, and, occasionally, corticosteroids.[301]

Lichen Planus

Lichen planus is a common pruritic, inflammatory dermatitis. Disease occurrence is predominantly between the ages of 30 and 60 years, with both sexes affected equally. Contact allergens, systemic drugs, and graft-versus-host reactions may induce lesions similar to lichen planus. Genetic influence may also play a role, as familial cases are seen, and HLA-A3 and HLA-B5 have been reported with increased frequency.[302–314]

Characteristic skin lesions are 2- to 4-mm flat-topped violaceous papules, frequently exhibiting fine whitish lines on the surface called *Wickham's striae.* Cutaneous injury may stimulate the formation of white, reticular lesions that may ulcerate. Nail changes are reported in 10%

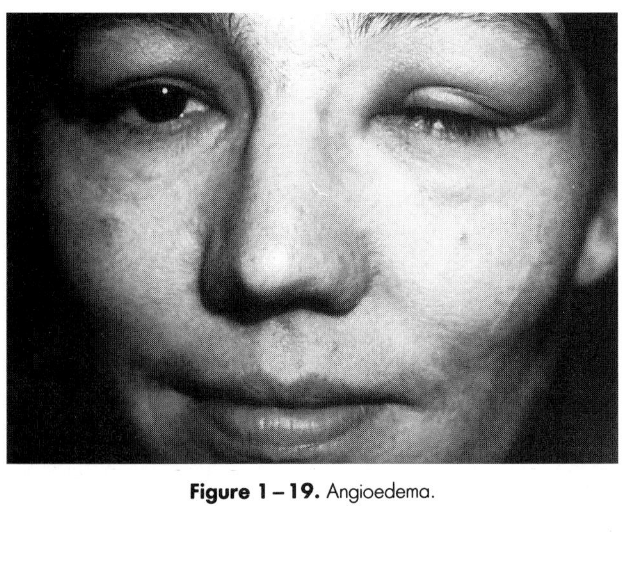

Figure 1 – 19. Angioedema.

of patients. Several variants of lichen planus have been identified. The onset may be acute and can lead to a generalized eruption, or it may be chronic and demonstrate only localized lesions. The morphologic changes can vary from papules, plaques, bullae, erosions, and atrophy. The configuration may be linear, annular, or grouped. At times lichen planus involves only the hair follicles (lichen planopilaris), leading to scarring alopecia. Isolated mucous membrane involvement is often present.[304, 305]

Eyelid and facial involvement in this condition are uncommon but not unreported. Typical violaceous papules and plaques have been documented to involve the eyelids. The conjunctiva may show white, reticular, lace-like involvement, similar to that observed in oral lichen planus. Additional ocular findings include blepharitis, conjunctivitis, keratitis, punctate corneal opacities, iridocyclitis, and chorioretinitis.[306, 307]

The cause of lichen planus is unknown, although current theories implicate an autoimmune cell-mediated process. Although the classic papules are clinically distinct, the differential diagnosis can be wide ranging, depending on lesion morphology and configuration. Biopsy for routine microscopy should be diagnostic in all forms.

Therapy is usually topical, intralesional, or systemic corticosteroids. Oral lesions respond to topical or oral vitamin A derivatives. Acute generalized lichen planus usually resolves in 6 to 18 months, but the oral, hypertrophic, and follicular variants tend to be chronic. Squamous cell carcinoma may complicate the hypertrophic, ulcerative, or chronic oral variety.[304]

Lichen Simplex Chronicus

Lichen simplex chronicus is a common pruritic disorder with an increased frequency of occurrence in Asian Americans and a slight female preponderance. The age of onset varies, although the disease seldom afflicts children.[308–311] Repeated scratching or rubbing of the skin results in oval, well-circumscribed, scaling, lichenized plaques. There is often associated hyperpigmentation. Usual sites of involvement include the back, sides of the neck, scalp, perineal and perianal regions, wrists, and ankles. Most patients have only a single site affected. Facial lesions may be seen, and eyelid thickening, accompanied by scale and hyperpigmentation, is present when this area is involved. The upper lid is most commonly affected.

Lichen simplex chronicus is also referred to as *neurodermatitis circumscripta*, in reference to the belief that this disorder is directly related to stress and anxiety. The differential diagnosis includes psoriasis, atopic dermatitis, stasis dermatitis, contact dermatitis, and lichen amyloidosis. The disease should be suspected on identification of an extremely pruritic, persistent, lichenized plaque in a patient with no known underlying cause. Biopsies are also helpful in establishing the diagnosis.

Treatment consists of prevention of scratching. Patient education combined with topical or intralesional steroids may be effective. Using the steroids under occlusion has the advantage of reminding the patient not to scratch.

Exfoliative Erythroderma

Exfoliative erythroderma is a severe cutaneous reaction to an underlying systemic or cutaneous disease process.[312] Although the clinical presentation is similar in most patients, the causes are protean. In as many as 40% of patients, the cause is idiopathic. Nearly one half of reported cases result from exacerbation of a preexisting skin disease, with psoriasis, eczema, and seborrheic dermatitis being most frequent. Drug reactions to either topical or systemic agents account for another 10% to 15% of reported cases, and lymphomas or leukemias are present in another 10%.[313] Diffuse scaling erythroderma has also been reported in late stages of HIV disease.[314]

When a drug reaction, underlying reticulosis, contact allergy, or infection is present, the onset is usually acute, whereas gradual progression is the rule if an exacerbation of a cutaneous disease is the cause. Nail dystrophy and alopecia often accompany confluent erythema and scaling. The eyelids are often involved in the exfoliation, and ectropion may result. Corneal anesthesia and ulcerations have also been reported. Additional ocular features include keratitis, bullous keratopathy, symblepharon, and keratomalacia.[315, 316]

The most frequent drugs implicated in causing exfoliative erythroderma include allopurinol, sulfa drugs, gold, phenytoin, phenobarbital, isoniazid, and iodine. The differential diagnosis is related to the underlying cause of the reactive skin state and includes those diseases previously described. A thorough history, physical examination, and skin biopsies identify the cause in most patients.

Treatment is directed toward the underlying disease state. The prognosis is further improved if complications such as high-output cardiac failure, septicemia, and pneumonia can be avoided.

Atopic Dermatitis

Atopic dermatitis (Fig. 1–20) is often associated with a family history of atopy, asthma, or hay fever and occurs in approximately 2% of the population. Clinical signs of disease appear in 75% of patients between 3 and 6 months of age and vary with the age of the patient.[317,318] Facial erythema and crusting with lichenification over the extensor surfaces of the extremities are infantile manifestations. After 2 years of age, lichenification, ero-

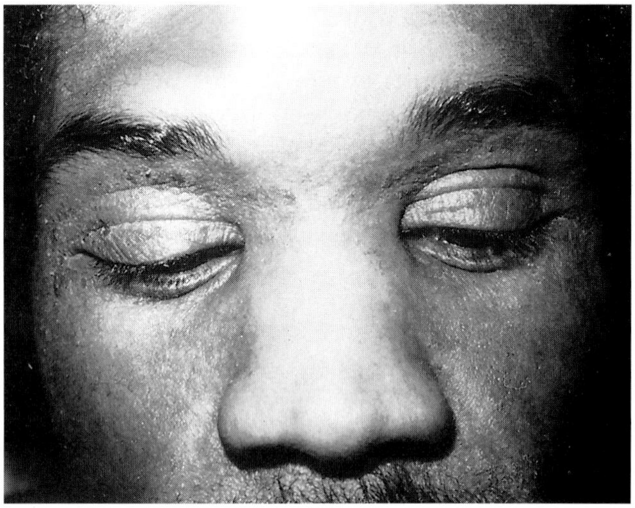

Figure 1–20. Atopic dermatitis.

sions, and hyperpigmentation and hypopigmentation develop over the extensor surfaces of the extremities. Other diseases may be associated with atopic dermatitis, including ichthyosis vulgaris, keratosis pilaris, and pityriasis alba. Secondary viral, bacterial, and fungal infections are frequent complications.

Eyelid changes are common and consist of thickening, induration, lichenification, and weeping eczematous lesions. Nonulcerative blepharitis with secondary staphylococcal infections can progress to frank periocular cellulitis. Eversion or stenosis of the lacrimal puncta may also occur. An infraorbital lid crease, called a *Dennie-Morgan fold,* is present in 25% of patients.[319] Darkening of the periorbital skin and absence of the lateral eyebrow (de Hertoghe's sign) are additional signs of atopic dermatitis. Conjunctivitis is often associated with pruritus and a conjunctival papillary reaction. The papillae are usually less than 1 mm in diameter and diffusely arranged on the palpebral conjunctiva. Chronic atopic conjunctivitis can eventuate into progressive cicatrization. Keratoconjunctivitis with infiltration and neovascularization of the corneal circumference is uncommon but quite characteristic for the disease. Anterior cortical shield-like cataracts and posterior subcapsular cataracts are frequently found. Retinal detachments have been reported at a higher rate in patients with atopic dermatitis. Keratoconus is another infrequent ocular complication.[320–325]

The pathogenesis of atopic dermatitis is unknown. Some authors believe it is an immunologic aberration resulting in increased IgE levels and depressed cell-mediated immunity, whereas others believe it is a disorder of dysfunctional beta-adrenergic receptors. The differential diagnosis includes lichen simplex chronicus, allergic contact dermatitis, nummular eczema, and seborrheic dermatitis.

Treatment includes intensive patient education, avoidance of known exacerbating factors, topical corticosteroid preparations, antibiotics, and antihistamines. Surgical intervention for the ocular complications of cataracts and keratoconus may be necessary and is associated with an increased incidence of perioperative complications. The prognosis in young children is excellent for spontaneous resolution; however, in adolescent and adult patients a chronic course characterized by intermittent exacerbations and remissions is expected.

Contact Dermatitis

Irritant and allergic contact dermatitis (Fig. 1–21) are the most common eruptions involving the eyelid. Airborne pollen, dust, volatile agents (alcohol and isoparaffins), and other chemicals (propylene glycol and soap emulsifiers) may produce an irritant contact dermatitis.[326] Allergic (type 4) contact dermatitis involves the activation of a T cell via the presentation of a foreign antigen by Langerhans' cells or macrophages.[327] Eruptions of this type are most commonly related to hair cosmetics, creams, or nail polish that inadvertently contact the eyelids. Medications or cosmetics resulting in an allergic contact dermatitis are also applied directly to the periocular regions.[328–336]

Clinical findings are related to the severity and chronicity of the reaction. Erythema, edema, papules, and vesicles accompany acute dermatitis, whereas a chronic process demonstrates scaling, lichenification, and hyperpigmentation. Infraorbital folds, usually seen in atopic patients, may be present if the lower lid is involved with chronic eczematous dermatitis. Conjunctivitis has also been reported.

The differential diagnosis of contact dermatitis of the eyelids includes atopic dermatitis, psoriasis, seborrheic dermatitis, and lichen simplex chronicus. Evaluations for a suspected contact dermatitis should include a thorough history, a trial test of the suspected agent on flexural forearm skin, and formal open or closed patch testing. There is no diagnostic test for contact dermatitis caused by primary irritants.

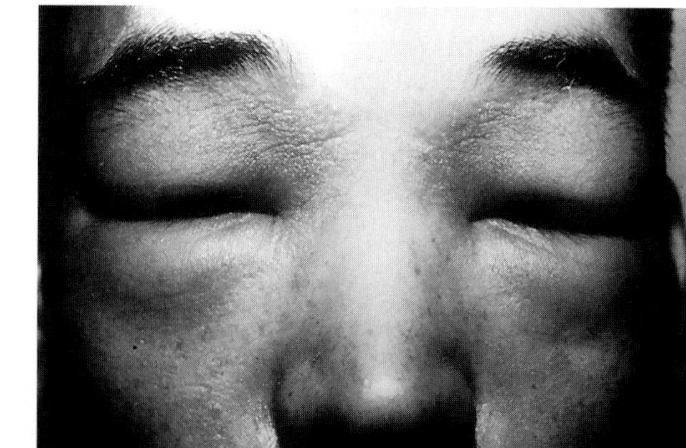

Figure 1–21. Allergic contact dermatitis (poison ivy).

Treatment involves avoidance of the suspected agent and topical corticosteroids. Systemic steroids may be indicated in severe allergic contact dermatitis.

Granuloma Annulare

Granuloma annulare (Fig. 1–22) is an uncommon condition with a 2:1 predilection for women over men. In two thirds of reported patients with localized granuloma annulare, the onset is prior to 30 years of age compared with 30 to 70 years of age for patients with generalized disease.[336–339]

Cutaneous lesions are characterized by skin-colored to reddish-brown, firm dermal papules arranged in an annular configuration. The most common site of involvement is the distal extremities. Variations in clinical patterns include generalized or disseminated, and subcutaneous types (pseudorheumatoid nodules). Periorbital involvement has been rarely reported.[340–343] The lateral aspects of the upper lids and the lateral canthal regions may be involved with both papular and nodular lesions.

The cause of granuloma annulare is unknown. The differential diagnosis includes sarcoidosis, syringomas, lipoid proteinosis, alopecia mucinosis, basal cell carcinoma, molluscum contagiosum, epidermal inclusion cysts (nodular type), and neurofibromas (nodular type). Biopsy is often necessary, and the histologic features of granuloma annulare are diagnostic.

Intralesional steroid injections for localized disease are successful 70% of the time. A variety of other therapeutic options have been employed to include systemic steroids, intramuscular triamcinolone acetonide, dapsone, isotretinoin, niacinamide, and potassium iodide.[340] Therapeutic intervention should be tempered with the knowledge that granuloma annulare is a benign, self-limited disease that spontaneously resolves within 2 years in more than 50% of patients.

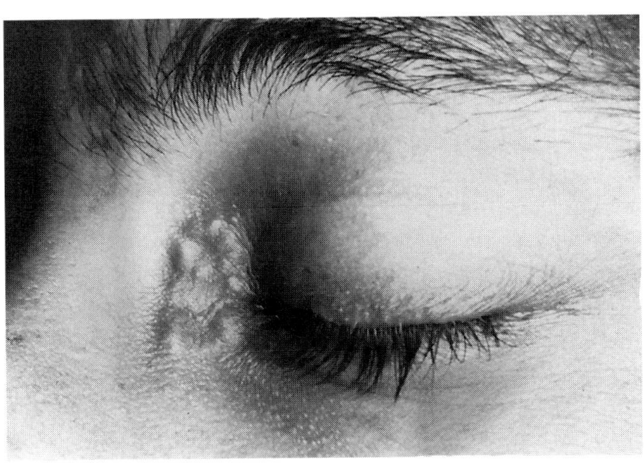

Figure 1–22. Granuloma annulare.

Granuloma Faciale

Granuloma faciale is a rare inflammatory disease that is more often seen in men between the ages of 40 to 60 years.[344–346] Typical lesions are characterized by multiple, purple-red to dull brown nodules primarily involving the face. Additional sites include the periorbital regions, trunk, and extremities. The lesion surface is often smooth, and telangiectasias or dilated follicular orifices, or both, may be observed.

Although actinic damage and altered local immunologic reactivity have been suggested as possible inciting factors, the cause of granuloma faciale remains unknown. The differential diagnosis includes sarcoidosis, lymphoma, pseudolymphoma, DLE, mycosis fungoides, insect bite reactions, and lymphocytoma cutis. Biopsy findings are essential in establishing the diagnosis.

Granuloma faciale is often a therapeutic challenge. Intralesional steroids have generally been the most successful. Additional treatment options include surgical excision, cryotherapy, electrosurgery, dermabrasion, antimalarial agents, dapsone, and argon or carbon dioxide lasers.[347–349]

Mastocytoma and Mastocytosis

A mastocytoma is a localized, dermal accumulation of mast cells that forms a characteristic reddish-brown nodule in infants. Spitz nevus (spindle and epithelioid nevus) and juvenile xanthogranuloma have similar clinical appearances. Darier's sign is pathognomonic and is elicited by stroking the tumor, producing urtication (erythema and edema) and occasional blistering at the site. Mastocytomas usually involve the trunk and extremities; however, they may occur on the face and occasionally around the eyes.[350]

The mastocytoma is only one expression of a larger group of mast cell disease known collectively as *urticaria pigmentosa*.[351–353] Additional presentations include single or multiple brownish macules and papules, generalized doughy infiltration of the skin, and numerous hyperpigmented, telangiectatic, pruritic macules. In some patients, excessive histamine and other vasoactive amines lead to flushing, pruritus, diarrhea, palpitations, and even histamine shock. Visceral involvement, especially bone, may occur. There are no known ocular manifestations of these other forms of urticaria pigmentosa.

Ulerythema Ophryogenes

Ulerythema ophryogenes is a rare clinical syndrome characterized by childhood onset of inflammatory keratotic papules arising in the lateral third of the eyebrows, alopecia involving the eyebrows, and atrophy of the contiguous skin.[354] A similar process on the cheeks eventuates in a pattern of reticulated follicular pits resembling a honeycomb (atrophoderma vermicularis). Keratosis pilaris is an associated condition with lesions occurring on the extensor aspect of the upper extremities, thighs, and buttocks. An autosomal dominant transmission has been suggested but remains unproved. Ulerythema may be associated with atopic dermatitis, mental retardation, and Noonan's syndrome.[355, 356] There is no definitive treatment available. Keratolytic agents, topical steroids, and emollients may offer temporary symptomatic improvement.

Alopecia Mucinosa

Alopecia mucinosa (Fig. 1–23) is classified into three categories and usually begins between the ages of 10 and 40 years. The first form is benign and self-limited; it afflicts younger patients, and lesions are limited to the head and neck. The second form is characterized by onset in an older age group and widespread lesions. Patients with the third form are older patients with mycosis fungoides who develop widespread alopecia mucinosa.[357–361]

The primary cutaneous lesions are grouped follicular papules with varying degrees of inflammation and induration. Coalescing papules fuse to form plaques that may subsequently become scaly, erythematous, indurated, and boggy. Alopecia is present within the lesions. Any of the various types of lesions may develop in the periorbital region, but it is the early-onset form that is typically localized to the head and neck area.

The cause of alopecia mucinosa is unknown. The differential diagnosis includes psoriasis, tinea corporis, sarcoidosis, and granuloma faciale. Biopsy findings are diagnostic.

The benign form of alopecia mucinosa may respond to topical or intralesional steroids. Additional treatment options include dapsone, PUVA, and fractional radiation therapy. Treatment of an underlying lymphoma, if present, should be considered the highest priority. Spontaneous resolution over 2 to 3 years is the rule for the benign type of alopecia mucinosa.

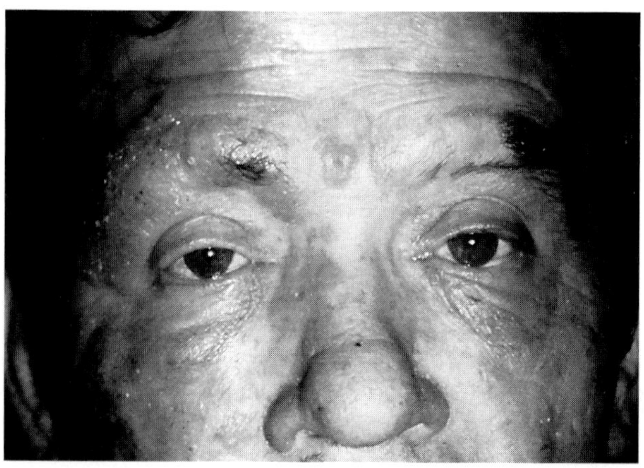

Figure 1–23. Alopecia mucinosa secondary to mycosis fungoides.

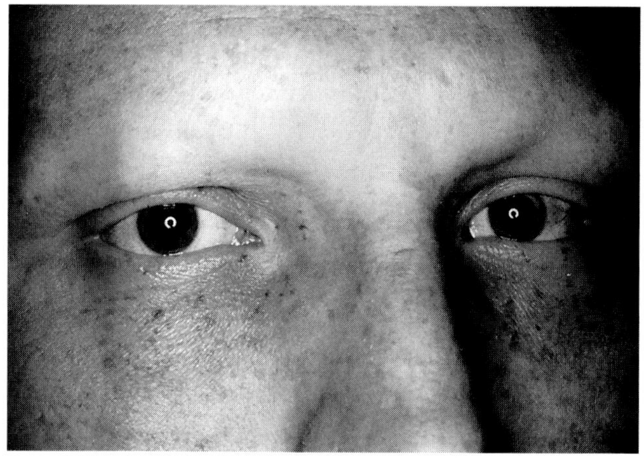

Figure 1–24. Alopecia universalis.

Alopecia Areata

Alopecia areata (Fig. 1–24) is a common disorder characterized by the sudden onset of patchy, well-circumscribed, nonscarring hair loss. The peak incidence is between the third and sixth decades. Approximately 25% of patients have a positive family history. Classification schemes are based on clinical features, prognosis, and associated diseases. Recognition of the heterogeneous nature of alopecia areata is more significant than the specifics of any system of categorization.[362–365]

The most common clinical presentation is complete loss of hair (alopecia) in round or oval patches involving a single locus. Multiple sites may occur, and with progressive increase in size the sites can fuse into large irregular patches. In the most severe forms there can be complete alopecia involving the scalp (alopecia totalis) or the entire cutaneous surface (alopecia universalis). At the periphery of the patches of alopecia are loose broken-off hairs called "exclamation point" hairs, which have a characteristic tapered hair shaft when plucked and examined. Exclamation point hairs are believed to be pathognomonic for alopecia areata. Pitting of the nails occurs in 10% to 20% of patients. The eyelids are involved in approximately 10% of cases, and loss of eyelashes portends a poorer prognosis for spontaneous recovery.[365] Additional ocular findings include lens opacities and retinal pigmentary alterations.

The pathogenesis of alopecia areata remains unknown. Numerous case reports of abnormalities of cell-mediated immunity suggest an immunologic cause. The clinical features are usually diagnostic; however, tinea capitis, early lupus erythematosus, congenital triangular alopecia, alopecia neoplastica, and trichotillomania should be considered in the differential diagnosis.

Intralesional steroid injections are the mainstay of therapy for the eyebrows. Generally, this area responds to treatment even when it is ineffective elsewhere; however, repeated injections are needed to sustain growth. Additional therapeutic modalities include topical irritants such as anthralin, topical immunotherapy with selected contact allergens (dinitrochlorobenzene or squaric acid dibutyl ester), photochemotherapy using 8-methoxypsoralen, ultraviolet light, topical minoxidil, and immunomodulation with inosiplex.[362, 363] The prognosis for regrowth is variable, being worse with more generalized disease.

Ichthyosis

The ichthyoses (Fig. 1–25) are a heterogeneous group of disorders of keratinization, and a number of them may be associated with ocular disease.[366–369] Ichthyosis vulgaris is a common autosomal dominant inherited disease with onset during the first year of life (not present at birth). Generalized fine light scales with flexural sparing are present and may involve the eyelids and eyelashes. Corneal changes include gray stromal opacities, punctate epithelial erosions, gray elevated nodules, and band-shaped keratopathy. These corneal lesion may be associated with photophobia, lacrimation, and eye discomfort.

X-linked ichthyosis occurs in 1 in 6000 male births, with onset within the first year of life. Large dark scales are typical with involvement of the flexural surfaces. Corneal opacities may occur in the region of Descemet's membrane by the second or third decade of life. Even though these opacities involve the cornea diffusely, they do not lead to decreased visual acuity. Similar opacities have been seen in female carriers. Additional associations include an increased incidence of testicular cancer, cryptorchidism, and delayed or failed parturition.

Autosomal recessive ichthyoses include lamellar ichthyosis and congenital ichthyosiform erythroderma. Lamellar ichthyosis is a rare condition that is present at birth. There are large thick, uniform scales in a generalized distribution. Eyelid and eyelash scaling is frequently present. There may be keratinization and papillary formation of the conjunctiva. In addition, ectropion occurs in more than half of the cases. Exposure keratitis with secondary corneal scarring and vascularization may result.[370] Congenital ichthyosiform erythroderma is an autosomal recessive ichthyosis recently distinguished from lamellar ichthyosis. Salient clinical findings include prominent erythema, mild ectropion, fine white scales, and a variable course.

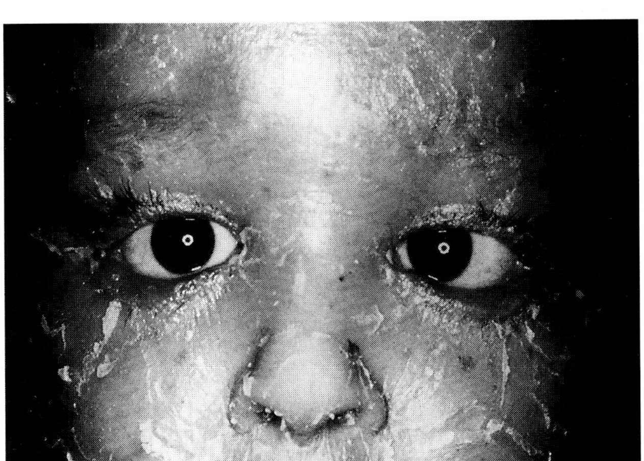

Figure 1–25. Congenital bullous ichthyosiform erythroderma.

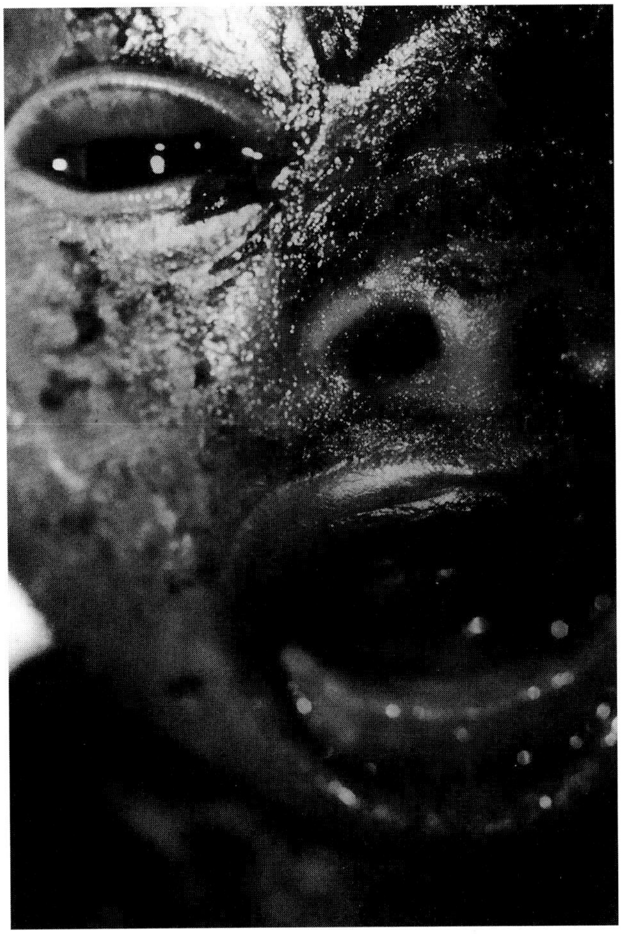

Figure 1–26. Harlequin fetus.

Epidermolytic hyperkeratosis is a rare autosomal dominant inherited disorder that presents at birth with red moist skin and blisters. Thick verrucous scales form within several days. The entire cutaneous surface is affected; however, facial involvement is usually mild.

Several unusual syndromes have ichthyosiform skin changes and associated findings. The harlequin fetus (Fig. 1–26) is a rare recessively inherited disease that presents at birth with massive hyperkeratosis, eclabium, ectropion, and absent pinnae. Death usually ensues in the first few weeks of life. The collodion baby is a phenotypic expression of several genotypes. The infant is encased in a shiny, parchment-like membrane that sheds by 6 months of age. The underlying skin may be normal, may develop lamellar ichthyosis, or may manifest one of the rare ichthyoses (such as Refsum's disease and

Sjögren-Larsson syndrome). Approximately 33% have bilateral ectropion.[371]

Refsum's disease is an autosomal recessive metabolic deficiency of alpha-phytanic acid alpha-hydroxylase resulting in the accumulation and storage of phytanic acid. The skin changes are mild, showing only small white scales. Progressive neural degeneration is the cause of death in most patients. Night blindness occurs in childhood secondary to a pigmentary retinopathy. Treatment involves restriction of dietary phytanic acid.

Sjögren-Larsson syndrome is another rare autosomal recessive disorder presenting during the first few months of life with an ichthyosiform erythroderma. Additional features include spastic paralysis, mental retardation, and oligophrenia. Visual impairment from chorioretinitis with macular and perimacular pigmentary degeneration is seen in 20% to 30% of patients. A defect in long-chain fatty acid metabolism has been suggested as the cause, and fatty alcohol oxidoreductase deficiency may serve as a diagnostic marker.

The chondrodysplasia punctata syndromes are an ill-defined group of disorders characterized by epiphyseal dysplasia in association with abnormal facies, cataracts, and an unusual patterned ichthyosis. The syndromes have been classified into a severe autosomal recessive type of rhizomelic dwarfism and the more variable dominantly inherited Conradi-Hünermann syndrome. The radiographic finding of stippled epiphyses in the cartilaginous skeleton of an affected infant is characteristic. This manifestation usually resolves after infancy. Skin changes occur in 25% of cases and consist of thick scales in a whorl-like pattern on a background of erythema. Bilateral cataracts, with or without optic atrophy, may be present at birth.

The KID syndrome is a disease characterized by a vascularizing *k*eratitis, *i*chthyosiform skin changes, and neurosensory *d*eafness. Blindness results from progressive keratitis in 75% of patients. The keratitis generally begins in infancy, although the onset may be as late as the second decade of life.[372]

Trichothiodystrophy, or sulfur-deficient brittle hair, serves as a marker for a neuroectodermal symptom complex characterized by mental and growth retardation, lamellar ichthyosis, decreased fertility, dental caries, pili torti, and trichoschisis (transverse fracturing of the hair shaft). Small punctate cataracts have been reported to occur in this syndrome.[373]

Hydration techniques, keratolytic agents, and retinoids have been of use in the treatment of most forms of ichthyosis.[374] Ectropion may require surgical intervention.[375]

REFERENCES

1. Hochberg MC: Systemic lupus erythematosus. Rheum Dis Clin North Am 16:617–639, 1990.
2. Tan EM, Cohen AS, Fries JR, et al: The 1982 revised criteria for the classification of systemic lupus erythematosus. Arthritis Rheum 25:1271–1277, 1982.
3. Watson R: Cutaneous lesions in systemic lupus erythematosus. Med Clin North Am 73:1091–1111, 1989.
4. Gilliam JN: The cutaneous signs of lupus erythematosus. Contin Educ Fam Physician 6:34–40, 1977.
5. Callen JP: Treatment of cutaneous lesions in patients with lupus erythematosus. Dermatol Clin North Am 8:355–365, 1990.
6. Sontheimer RD: Subacute cutaneous lupus erythematosus: A decade's perspective. Med Clin North Am 73:1073–1089, 1989.
7. Miyagawa S, Okuchi T, Shiomi Y, Sakamoto K: Subacute cutaneous lupus erythematosus lesions precipitated by griseofulvin. J Am Acad Dermatol 21:343–346, 1989.
8. Rubin BR, De Horatius RJ: Acute visual loss in systemic lupus erythematosus. J Am Osteopath Assoc 89:73–77, 1989.
9. Frith P, Burge SM, Millard PR, Wojnarowska F: External ocular findings in lupus erythematosus: A clinical and immunopathological study. Br J Ophthalmol 74:163–167, 1990.
10. Macrae D, O'Reilly S: On some neuro-oto-ophthalmological manifestations of systemic lupus erythematosus and periarteritis nodosa. Eye Ear Nose Throat 36:721–726, 1957.
11. Jackson G, Miller M, Littlejohn G, et al: Bilateral internuclear ophthalmoplegia in systemic lupus erythematosus. J Rheumatol 13:1161–1162, 1986.
12. Cogen MS, Kline LB, Duvall ER: Bilateral internuclear ophthalmoplegia in systemic lupus erythematosus. J Clin Neuro Ophthalmol 7:69–73, 1987.
13. Brandt KD, Lessel S: Migrainous phenomena in systemic lupus erythematosus. Arthritis Rheum 21:7–16, 1978.
14. Lessell S: The neuro-ophthalmology of systemic lupus erythematosus. Doc Ophthalmol 47:13–42, 1979.
15. Deutsch TA, Corwin HL: Lupus optic neuritis with negative serology. Ann Ophthalmol 20:383–384, 1988.
16. Gold DH, Morris DA, Henkind P: Ocular findings in systemic lupus erythematosus. Br J Ophthalmol 56:800–804, 1972.
17. Watson P, Hayreh SS: Scleritis and episcleritis. Br J Ophthalmol 60:163–191, 1976.
18. Jabs DA, Fine SL, Hochberg ME, et al: Severe retinal vaso-occlusive disease in systemic lupus erythematosus. Arch Ophthalmol 104:558–563, 1986.
19. Parnass SM, Goodwin JA, Patel DV, et al: Dural sinus thrombosis: A mechanism for pseudotumor cerebri in systemic lupus erythematosus. J Rheumatol 14:152–155, 1987.
20. Li EK, Ho PCP: Pseudotumor cerebri in systemic lupus erythematosus. J Rheumatol 16:113–116, 1989.
21. Li EK, Chan MSY: Is pseudotumor cerebri in SLE a thrombotic event [letter]? J Rheumatol 17:983–984, 1990.
22. Jabs DA, Hanneken AM, Schachat AP, Fine SL: Choroidopathy in systemic lupus erythematosus. Arch Ophthalmol 106:230–234, 1988.
23. David DS: Adrenal glucocorticoids after 20 years: A review of their clinically relevant consequences. J Chronic Dis 22:637–711, 1970.
24. Rynes RI, Krohel G, Falbo A, et al: Ophthalmologic safety of long-term hydroxychloroquine treatment. Arthritis Rheum 22:832–836, 1979.
25. Collum LMT, Bowen DI: Ocular side effects of ibuprofen. Br J Ophthalmol 55:472–477, 1971.
26. Rhymer AP, Gengos DC: Indomethacin. Clin Rheum Dis 5:541–552, 1979.
27. Arnold HL Jr, Odom RB, James WD (eds): Contact dermatitis: Drug eruptions. *In* Andrews' Diseases of the Skin, 8th edition. Philadelphia, WB Saunders, 1990, pp. 89–130.
28. Turgeon PW, Slamovits TL: Scleritis as the presenting manifestation of procainamide-induced lupus. Ophthalmology 96:68–71, 1989.
29. Hess E: Drug-related lupus. N Engl J Med 318:1460–1462, 1988.
30. Hymes SR, Jordon RE: Chronic cutaneous lupus erythematosus. Med Clin North Am 73:1055–1071, 1989.
31. Cyran S, Douglass MC, Silverstein JL: Chronic cutaneous lupus erythematosus presenting as periorbital edema and erythema. J Am Acad Dermatol 26:334–338, 1992.
32. Huey C, Jakobiec FA, Iwamoto T, et al: Discoid lupus erythematosus of the eyelids. Ophthalmology 90:1389–1398, 1983.
33. Anderson LL, Grimwood RE: Discoid lupus erythematosus

manifesting as chronic blepharitis. J Assoc Military Dermatol 15:12–15, 1989.
34. Meiusi RS, Cameron JD, Holland EJ, Summers CG: Discoid lupus erythematosus of the eyelid complicated by wound dehiscence. Am J Ophthalmol 111:108–109, 1991.
35. Raizman MB, Baum J: Discoid lupus keratitis. Arch Ophthalmol 107:545–547, 1989.
36. Nowinski T, Bernardino V, Naidoff M, Parrish R: Ocular involvement in lupus erythematosus profundus (panniculitis). Ophthalmology 89:1149–1154, 1982.
37. Provost TT, Reichlin M: Antinuclear antibody-negative systemic lupus erythematosus. J Am Acad Dermatol 4:84–89, 1981.
38. Samlaska CP, James WD: Superficial thrombophlebitis. Part I: Primary hypercoagulable states. J Am Acad Dermatol 22:975–989, 1990.
39. Plotz PH, Dalakas M, Leff RL, et al: Current concepts in the idiopathic inflammatory myopathies: Polymyositis, dermatomyositis, and related disorders. Ann Intern Med 111:143–157, 1989.
40. Norins AL: Juvenile dermatomyositis. Med Clin North Am 73:1193–1209, 1989.
41. Caro I: Dermatomyositis as a systemic disease. Med Clin North Am 73:1181–1192, 1989.
42. Richardson JB, Callen JP: Dermatomyositis and malignancy. Med Clin North Am 73:1211–1220, 1989.
43. Euwer RL, Sontheimer RD: Amyopathic dermatomyositis (dermatomyositis sine myositis). J Am Acad Dermatol 24:959–966, 1991.
44. DeVries S: Retinopathy in dermatomyositis. Arch Ophthalmol 46:432–435, 1951.
45. Liebman S, Cook C, Donaldson DD: Retinopathy with dermatomyositis. Arch Ophthalmol 74:704–705, 1965.
46. Harrison SM, Frenkel M, Grossman BJ, Matalon R: Retinopathy in childhood dermatomyositis. Am J Ophthalmol 76:786–790, 1973.
47. Fong LP, Yeung J: Spontaneous regression of retinal neovascularization in juvenile dermatomyositis. Aust N Z J Ophthalmol 18:107–108, 1990.
48. Cox NH, Lawrence CM, Langtry JA, Ive FA: Dermatomyositis: Disease associations and an evaluation of screening investigations for malignancy. Arch Dermatol 126:61–65, 1990.
49. Marie R, Truchetet F, Friedel J, et al: Skin lesions simulating chronic dermatomyositis during long-term hydroxyurea therapy. J Am Acad Dermatol 21:797–798, 1989.
50. Tuffanelli DL: Systemic scleroderma. Med Clin North Am 73:1167–1180, 1989.
51. Falanga V: Localized scleroderma. Med Clin North Am 73:1143–1156, 1989.
52. David J, Wilson J, Woo P: Scleroderma "en coup de sabre." Ann Rheumatol Dis 50:260–262, 1991.
53. Goldenstein-Schainberg C, Rereira RMR, Gusukuma MC, et al: Childhood linear scleroderma "en coup de sabre" with uveitis. J Pediatr 117:581–584, 1990.
54. Suttorp-Schulten MSA, Koornneef L: Linear scleroderma associated with ptosis and motility disorders. Br J Ophthalmol 74:694–695, 1990.
55. El Baba F, Frangieh GT, Iliff WJ, et al: Morphea of the eyelids. Ocular Pathol Clinicians 89:1285–1288, 1982.
56. Krieg T, Meurer M: Systemic scleroderma. J Am Acad Dermatol 18:457–481, 1988.
57. Velagos EE, Masi AT, Stevens MB, Shulman LE: The CREST syndrome: Comparison with systemic sclerosis (scleroderma). Arch Intern Med 139:1240–1244, 1979.
58. Pollack IP, Becker B: Cytoid bodies of the retina. Arch Ophthalmol 54:655–660, 1962.
59. Manschot WA: Generalized scleroderma with ocular symptoms. Ophthalmologica 149:131–137, 1965.
60. Robin JB, Schanzlin J, Meisler VP, et al: Ocular involvement in the respiratory vasculitides. Surv Ophthalmol 30:127–140, 1985.
61. Charles SJ, Meyer PAR, Watson PG: Diagnosis and management of systemic Wegener's granulomatosis presenting with anterior ocular inflammatory disease. Br J Ophthalmol 75:201–207, 1991.
62. Koyama T, Matsuo N, Watanabe Y, et al: Wegner's granulomatosis with destructive ocular manifestations. Am J Ophthalmol 98:736–740, 1984.
63. Fauci AS, Haynes BF, Katz P, et al: Wegener's granulomatosis: Prospective clinical and therapeutic experience in 85 patients for 21 years. Ann Intern Med 98:76–85, 1983.
64. Bullen CL, Liesegang TJ, McDonald TJ, DeRemme RA: Ocular complications of Wegener's granulomatosis. Ophthalmology 90:279–290, 1983.
65. Leavitt RY, Fauci AS, Bloch DA, et al: The American College of Rheumatology 1990 criteria for the classification of Wegener's granulomatosis. Arthritis Rheum 33:1101–1107, 1990.
66. Specks U, DeRemme RA: Granulomatous vasculitis; Wegener's granulomatosis and Churg-Strauss syndrome. Rheum Dis Clin North Am 16:377–397, 1990.
67. Haynes BF, Fishamn ML, Fauci AS, Wolff SM: The ocular manifestations of Wegener's granulomatosis: fifteen years' experience and review of the literature. Am J Med 63:131–141, 1977.
68. Pavelka K, Dostal C, Rossman P, et al: Wegener's granulomatosis with bilateral necrotizing scleritis, polyarthritis, and renal failure efficiently treated with immunosuppressive therapy. Clin Rheumatol 5:112–117, 1986.
69. Yevich I: Necrotizing vasculitis with granulomatosis. Int J Dermatol 27:540–560, 1988.
70. Pulido JS, Goeken JA, Nerad JA, et al: Ocular manifestations of patients with circulating antineutrophil cytoplasmic antibodies. Arch Ophthalmol 108:845–850, 1990.
71. Churg J, Strauss L: Allergic granulomatosis, allergic angiitis, and periarteritis nodosa. Am J Pathol 27:277–301, 1951.
72. Masi AT, Hunder GG, Lie JT, et al: The American College of Rheumatology 1990 criteria for the classification of Churg-Strauss syndrome (allergic granulomatosis and angiitis). Arthritis Rheum 33:1094–1100, 1990.
73. Liebow AA, Carrington CRB, Friedman PJ: Lymphomatoid granulomatosis. Hum Pathol 3:457–558, 1972.
74. Camisa C: Lymphomatoid granulomatosis: Two cases with skin involvement. J Am Acad Dermatol 20:571–578, 1989.
75. Fauci AS, Haynes BJ, Costa J, et al: Lymphomatoid granulomatosis. N Engl J Med 306:69–74, 1982.
76. James WD, Odom RB, Katzenstein ALA: Cutaneous manifestations of lymphomatoid granulomatosis. Arch Dermatol 117:196–202, 1981.
77. Jambrosic J, From L, Assad DA, et al: Lymphomatoid granulomatosis. J Am Acad Dermatol 17:621–631, 1987.
78. Hamburger JI: Ophthalmopathy and thyroid disorders. N Engl J Med 296:1002–1003, 1977.
79. Marines HM, Patrinely JR: Systemic associations of exophthalmos. Int Ophthalmol Clin 31:143–162, 1991.
80. Char DH: The ophthalmopathy of Graves' disease. Med Clin North Am 75:97–119, 1991.
81. Lynch P, Maize J, Sisson J: Pretibial myxedema and nonthyrotoxic thyroid disease. Arch Dermatol 107:107–111, 1973.
82. Hamilton HE, Schultz RO, DeGowin EL: Endocrine eye lesion in hyperthyroidism. Arch Intern Med 105:675–685, 1960.
83. McDougall IR: Graves' disease current concepts. Med Clin North Am 75:79–95, 1991.
84. Pearl RM, Vistnes L, Troxel S: Treatment of exophthalmos. Plast Reconstr Surg 87:236–244, 1991.
85. Yamagami S, Ando K, Akahoshi T, Yamashita H: Exophthalmos in myelodysplastic syndrome. Acta Ophthalmol (Copenh) 69:261–265, 1991.
86. Cataltepe O, Ozcan OE: Bilateral orbital encephaloceles: An unusual cause of exophthalmos. J Clin Neuro Ophthalmol 10:131–134, 1990.
87. Abernethy LJ, Whittle IR, Sellar RJ: Leptomeningeal cyst of the orbit presenting with pulsatile exophthalmos. Clin Radiol 40:531–532, 1989.
88. Spaide RF, Granger E, Hammer BD, et al: Rapidly expanding exophthalmos: An unusual presentation of small cell lung cancer. Br J Ophthalmol 73:461–462, 1989.
89. Caron GA: Pretibial myxedema and LATS. Arch Dermatol 98:310, 1968.
90. Watanakunakorn C, Hodges R, Evans T: Myxedema: A study of 400 cases. Arch Intern Med 116:183–190, 1965.
91. Christianson H: Cutaneous manifestations of hypothyroidism including purpura and ecchymoses. Cutis 17:45–52, 1976.
92. Jakubovic HR, Salama SS, Rosenthal D: Multiple cutaneous focal mucinoses with hypothyroidism. Ann Intern Med 96:56–58, 1982.

93. Gilmore J, Mellon D: The rare presentation to the cosmetic and plastic surgeon of a patient with myxedema. Ann Plast Surg 25:484–486, 1990.
94. Block R, Henkind P: Ocular manifestations of endocrine and metabolic diseases. *In* Duane TD, Jaeger EA (eds): Duane's Clinical Ophthalmology, vol 5. Philadelphia, JB Lippincott, 1987, pp. 1–26.
95. Arnold HL Jr, Odom RB, James WD (eds): Mucinoses. *In* Andrews' Diseases of the Skin, 8th edition. Philadelphia, WB Saunders, 1990, pp. 186–188.
96. Gabriel SE, Perry HO, Oleson GB, Bowles CA: Scleromyxedema: A scleroderma-like disorder with systemic manifestations. Medicine 67:58–64, 1988.
97. Milam CP, Cohen LE, Fenske NA, Ling NS: Sceromyxedema: Therapeutic response to isotretinoin in three patients. J Am Acad Dermatol 19:469–477, 1988.
98. Hisler BM, Savoy LB, Hashimoto K: Improvement of scleromyxedema associated with isotretinoin therapy. J Am Acad Dermatol 24:854–857, 1991.
99. Rothe MJ, Rivas R, Gould E, Kerdel FA: Scleromyxedema and severe myositis. Int J Dermatol 28:657–660, 1989.
100. Harris AO, Altman AR, Tschen JA, Wolf JE: Scleromyxedema. Int J Dermatol 28:661–667, 1989.
101. Goldin HM, Axelrod AJ, Bronson DM, et al: Scleromyxedema with corneal deposits. Ophthalmology 94:1334–1338, 1987.
102. Pusateri TJ, Margo CE, Groden LR: Corneal manifestations of scleromyxedema. Ophthalmology 94:510–513, 1987.
103. Fleischmajer R, Lara JV: Scleredema: A histochemical and biochemical study. Arch Dermatol 92:643–652, 1965.
104. Bradford WD, Cook CD, Vawter GF, et al: Scleredema of childhood: Report of five cases. J Pediatr 68:391–399, 1966.
105. Curtis AC, Shulak BM: Scleredema adultorum: Not always a benign self-limited disease. Arch Dermatol 92:526–541, 1965.
106. Parker SC, Fenton DA, Black MM: Scleredema. J Exp Dermatol 14:385–386, 1989.
107. Berk MA, Lorincz AL: Scleredema adultorum of Buschke and primary hyperparathyroidism. Int J Dermatol 27:647–649, 1988.
108. Hurwitz S: Unclassified disorders. *In* Clinical Pediatric Dermatology. Philadelphia, WB Saunders, 1981, pp. 435–455.
109. Greene RM, Rogers RS: Melkersson-Rosenthal syndrome: A review of 36 patients. J Am Acad Dermatol 21:1263–1270, 1989.
110. Williams PM, Greenberg MS: Management of cheilitis granulomatosa. Oral Surg Oral Med Oral Pathol 72:436–439, 1989.
111. Pryce DW, King CM: Orofacial granulomatosis associated with delayed hypersensitivity to cobalt. Clin Exp Dermatol 15:384–386, 1990.
112. Minor MW, Fox RW, Bukantz SC, Lockey RF: Melkersson-Rosenthal syndrome. J Allergy Clin Immunol 80:64–67, 1987.
113. Alexander RW, James RB: Melkersson-Rosenthal syndrome. J Oral Surg 30:599–604, 1972.
114. Eggelmeijer F, Kijkmans BAC: Melkersson-Rosenthal syndrome and arthritis [letter]. J Am Acad Dermatol 23:1186, 1990.
115. Kano Y, Shiohara T, Yagita A, Nagashima M: Granulomatous cheilitis and Crohn's disease. Br J Dermatol 123:409–412, 1990.
116. James DG: Definition and classification of granulomatous disorders. Semin Respir Med 8:1–9, 1986.
117. Arnold HL Jr, Odom RB, James WD (eds): Macrophage/monocytic and lymphocytic infiltrates. *In* Andrews' Diseases of the Skin, 8th edition. Philadelphia, WB Saunders, 1990, pp. 831–853.
118. Obenauf CD, Shaw HE, Sydnor CF, Klintworth GK: Sarcoidosis and its ophthalmic manifestations. Am J Ophthalmol 86:648–655, 1978.
119. Graham E: Ocular involvement in sarcoidosis. Semin Respir Med 8:59–64, 1986.
120. Sharma OP, Sharma AM: Sarcoidosis of the nervous system. Arch Intern Med 151:1317–1321, 1991.
121. Mayers M: Ocular sarcoidosis. Int Ophthalmol Clin 30:257–263, 1990.
122. Karma A, Huhti E, Poukkula A: Course and outcome of ocular sarcoidosis. Am J Ophthalmol 106:467–472, 1988.
123. Zeiter JH, Bhavsar A, McDermott ML, Siegel MJ: Ocular sarcoidosis manifesting as an anterior staphyloma. Am J Ophthamol 112:345–347, 1991.
124. Dick DJ, Newman PK, Richardson J, et al: Acute posterior multifocal placoid pigment epitheliopathy and sarcoidosis. Br J Ophthalmol 72:74–77, 1988.
125. Klech H: Sarcoidosis: Differential diagnosis. Semin Respir Med 8:72–94, 1986.
126. Gibbs AR, Williams WJ: The pathology of sarcoidosis. Semin Respir Med 8:10–16, 1986.
127. Karcioglu ZA, Brear R: Conjunctival biopsy in sarcoidosis. Am J Ophthalmol 99:68–73, 1985.
128. Baarsma GS, Hey EL, de Vries GJ, Kijlstra A: The predictive value of serum angiotensin-converting enzyme and lysozyme levels in the diagnosis of ocular sarcoidosis. Am J Ophthalmol 104:211–217, 1987.
129. Breathnach SM: Amyloid and amyloidosis. J Am Acad Dermatol 18:1–16, 1988.
130. Gorevic PD, Rodrigues MM, Spencer WH, et al: Prealbumin: A major constituent of vitreous amyloid. Ophthalmology 94:792–798, 1987.
131. Falls HF, Jackson J, Carey JH, et al: Ocular manifestations of hereditary primary systemic amyloidosis. Arch Ophthalmol 54:660–664, 1955.
132. Schwartz MF, Green WR, Michels RG, et al: An unusual case of ocular involvement in primary systemic nonfamilial amyloidosis. Ophthalmology 89:394–401, 1982.
133. Lieberman TW, Ferry AP: Bilateral amyloidosis of the vitreous body without systemic involvement. Trans Am Ophthalmol Soc 73:302–328, 1974.
134. Natelson EA, Duncan WC, Macossay CR, Fred HL: Amyloidosis palpebrarum. Arch Intern Med 125:304–307, 1970.
135. Smith ME, Zimmerman LE: Amyloidosis of the eyelid and conjunctiva. Arch Ophthalmol 75:42–50, 1966.
136. Rosenblatt M, Spitz GF, Friedman AH, Kazam ES: Localized conjunctival amyloidosis: Case reports and review of literature. Ophthalmologica 192:238–245, 1986.
137. Stafford WR, Fine BS: Amyloidosis of the cornea. Arch Ophthalmol 75:53–56, 1966.
138. Bene C, Kranias G: Ocular amyloidosis: Clinical points learned from one case. Ann Ophthalmol 22:101–102, 1990.
139. Stock EL, Feder RS, O'Grady RB, et al: Lattice corneal dystrophy type IIIA: Clinical and histopathologic correlations. Arch Ophthalmol 109:354–358, 1991.
140. Maisel JM, Miller F, Sibony PA, Maisel LM: Multiple myeloma presenting with ocular inflammation. Ann Ophthalmol 19:170–174, 1987.
141. Doft BH, Machemer R, Skinner M, et al: Pars plana vitrectomy for vitreous amyloidosis. Ophthalmology 94:607–611, 1987.
142. Kossard S, Winkelmann RK: Necrobiotic xanthogranuloma. Australas J Dermatol 21:85–88, 1980.
143. Mehregan DA, Winkelmann RK: Necrobiotic xanthogranuloma. Arch Dermatol 128:94–100, 1992.
144. Venencie PY, Puissant A, Verola O, et al: Necrobiotic xanthogranuloma with myeloma: A case report. Cancer 59:588–592, 1987.
145. Robertson DM, Winkelmann RK: Ophthalmic features of necrobiotic xanthogranuloma with paraproteinemia. Am J Ophthalmol 97:173–183, 1984.
146. Char DH, LeBoit PE, Ljung B-ME, Wara W: Radiation therapy for ocular necrobiotic xanthogranuloma. Arch Ophthalmol 105:174–175, 1987.
147. Borel G: Un nouveau syndrome palpebral. Bul Soc Franc Ophthalmol 46:168–180, 1933.
148. Newcomer V, Klein A: Ligneous conjunctivitis. Arch Dermatol 113:511–512, 1977.
149. Marcus DM, Walton D, Donshik P, et al: Ligneous conjunctivitis with ear involvement. Arch Ophthalmol 108:514–519, 1990.
150. Hidayat AA, Riddle PJ: Ligneous conjunctivitis: A clinicopathologic study of 17 cases. Ophthalmology 94:949–959, 1987.
151. Aubin F, Blanc D, Badet JM, Choubaut JC: Lipoid proteinosis: Case report. Pediatr Dermatol 6:109–113, 1989.
152. Barthelemy H, Mauduit G, Kanitakis J, et al: Lipoid proteinosis with pseudomembranous conjunctivitis. J Am Acad Dermatol 14:367–371, 1986.
153. Jensen AD, Khodadoust AA, Emery JM: Lipoid proteinosis: Report of a case with electron microscopic findings. Arch Ophthalmol 88:273–277, 1972.
154. Caplan RM: Visceral involvement in lipoid proteinosis. Arch Dermatol 95:149–155, 1967.

155. Johnson LN, Hepler RS: Corectopia and lipoid proteinosis. Br J Ophthalmol 73:394-396, 1989.
156. Wong CK, Lin CS: Remarkable response of lipoid proteinosis to oral dimethyl sulfoxide. Br J Dermatol 119:541-544, 1988.
157. Arnold HL Jr, Odom RB, James WD (eds): Some genodermatoses. *In* Andrews' Diseases of the Skin, 8th edition. Philadelphia, WB Saunders, 1990, pp. 637-681.
158. Blackman HJ, Rodrigues MM, Peck GL: Corneal epithelial lesions in keratosis follicularis (Darier's disease). Ophthalmology 87:931-943, 1980.
159. Jones W, Nix T, Clark W: Hemorrhagic Darier's disease. Arch Dermatol 89:523-527, 1968.
160. Hori Y, Tsuru N, Niimura M: Bullous Darier's disease. Arch Dermatol 118:278-279, 1982.
161. Milton GP, Peck GL, Fu JJL, et al: Exacerbation of Darier's disease by lithium carbonate. J Am Acad Dermatol 23:926-928, 1990.
162. Blackman HJ, Peck GL, Olsen TG, Bergsma DR: Blepharoconjunctivitis: A side effect of 13-*cis*-retinoic acid therapy for dermatologic diseases. Opthalmology 86:753-758, 1979.
163. Elliott S, Buxman M, Weleber R: Abnormal dark adaptation in Darier's disease [abstract]. J Invest Dermatol 72:207, 1979.
164. McElroy JA, Mehregan DA, Roenigk RK: Carbon dioxide laser vaporization of recalcitrant symptomatic plaques of Hailey-Hailey and Darier's disease. J Am Acad Dermatol 23:893-897, 1990.
165. Kirk JF, Flowers FP, Ramos-Caro FA, Browder JF: Multiple endocrine neoplasia type III: Case report and review. Pediatr Dermatol 8:124-128, 1991.
166. Khairi MRA, Dexter RN, Burzynski NJ, Johnston CC: Mucosal neuroma, pheochromocytoma and medullary thyroid carcinoma: Multiple endocrine neoplasia type 3. Medicine 54:89-112, 1975.
167. Spector B, Klintworth GK, Wells SA: Histologic study of the ocular lesions in multiple endocrine neoplasia syndrome type IIb. Am J Ophthalmol 91:204-215, 1981.
168. Baum JL, Adler ME: Pheochromocytoma, medullary thyroid carcinoma, multiple mucosal neuroma. Arch Ophthalmol 87:574-584, 1972.
169. Riley FC, Robertson DM: Ocular histopathology in multiple endocrine neoplasia type 2b. Am J Ophthalmol 91:57-64, 1981.
170. Robertson DM, Sizemore GW, Gordon H: Thickened corneal nerves as a manifestation of multiple endocrine neoplasia. Trans Am Acad Ophthalmol Otolaryngol 79:772-787, 1975.
171. Rendon MI, Cruz PD, Sontheimer RD, Bergstresser PR: Acanthosis nigricans: A cutaneous marker of tissue resistance to insulin. J Am Acad Dermatol 21:461-469, 1989.
172. Schmidt KT, Massa MC, Welykyj SE: Acanthosis nigricans and a rectal carcinoid. J Am Acad Dermatol 25:361-365, 1991.
173. Hisler BM, Savoy LB: Acanthosis nigricans of the forehead and fingers associated with hyperinsulinemia [letter]. Arch Dermatol 123:1441-1442, 1987.
174. Matsuoka LY, Wortsman J, Gavin JR, et al: Acanthosis nigricans, hypothyroidism, and insulin resistance. Am J Med 81:58-62, 1986.
175. Matsuoka LY, Wortsman J, Gavin JR, et al: Spectrum of endocrine abnormalities associated with acanthosis nigricans. Am J Med 83:719-725, 1987.
176. Sedano HO, Gorlin RJ: Acanthosis nigricans. Oral Surg Oral Med Oral Pathol 63:462-467, 1987.
177. Stuart CA, Pates CJ, Peters EJ: Prevalence of acanthosis nigricans in an unselected population. Am J Med 87:269-272, 1989.
178. Brown J, Winkelmann RK: Acanthosis nigricans: Study of 90 cases. Medicine 47:33-51, 1968.
179. Breitbart AS, Eaton C, McCarthy JG: Crouzon's syndrome associated with acanthosis nigricans: Ramifications for the craniofacial surgeon. Ann Plast Surg 22:310-315, 1989.
180. Reed WB, Ragsdale W, Curtis RC, et al: Acanthosis nigricans in association with various genodermatoses. Acta Derm Venereol (Stockh) 48:465-473, 1968.
181. Curth HO: Bloom's syndrome. Arch Dermatol 90:349-350, 1986.
182. Safai B, Grant J, Kurtz R, et al: Cutaneous manifestation of internal malignancies. Part I: Acanthosis nigricans. Int J Dermatol 17:312-315, 1978.
183. Grunfield C: Insulin resistance: Pathophysiology, diagnosis, and therapeutic implications. Spec Top Endocrinol Metab 6:193-240, 1984.
184. Stevenson RE, Ferlauto GJ, Taylor HA: Cutis gyratum and acanthosis nigricans associated with other anomalies: A distinctive syndrome. J Pediatr 92:950-952, 1978.
185. Connolly MB, Jan JE, Couch RM, et al: Hepatic dysfunction in Alstrom disease. Am J Med Genet 40:421-424, 1991.
186. Perez-Corral F, de la Vina S, Carbo M, et al: Rabson's syndrome: Model of insulin resistance of decreased number and affinity of insulin receptors in erythrocytes. Diabetologia 19:306-319, 1980.
187. Flier JS, Young JB, Landsberg L: Familiar insulin resistance with acanthosis nigricans: Acral hypertrophy and muscle cramps. N Engl J Med 303:970-973, 1980.
188. Tasjian D, Jarrat M: Familial acanthosis nigricans. Arch Dermatol 120:1351-1354, 1984.
189. Elgart ML: Acanthosis nigricans and nicotinic acid. J Am Acad Dermatol 5:709-710, 1981.
190. Appeltauer LC: Megavitamin and megamineral therapy in childhood [letter]. Can Med Assoc J 145:104-105, 1991.
191. Fishbein HA: Acanthosis nigricans following prolonged use of stilbestrol. Arch Dermatol 81:153-154, 1960.
192. Randle HW, Winkelmann RK: Steroid-induced acanthosis nigricans in dermatomyositis. Arch Dermatol 115:587-588, 1979.
193. Muramatsu T, Matsumoto H, Yamashina Y, et al: Pemphigus foliaceus associated with acanthosis nigricans-like lesions and hepatocellular carcinoma. Int J Dermatol 28:462-463, 1989.
194. Schweitzer WJ, Coldin HM, Bronson DM, Brody PE: Acanthosis nigricans associated with mycosis fungoides. J Am Acad Dermatol 19:951-953, 1988.
195. Riccardi VM: Neurofibromatosis: The importance of localized or otherwise atypical forms. Arch Dermatol 123:882-883, 1987.
196. Riccardi VM: Von Recklinghausen neurofibromatosis. N Engl J Med 305:1617-1627, 1981.
197. Dunn DW: Neurofibromatosis in childhood. Curr Probl Pediatr 8:450-497, 1987.
198. Sergeyev AS: On the mutation rate of neurofibromatosis. Hum Genet 28:129-138, 1975.
199. Riccardi VM: Neurofibromatosis: Clinical heterogeneity. Curr Probl Cancer 7:1-34, 1982.
200. Riccardi VM, Lewis RA: Von Recklinghausen neurofibromatosis. Ophthalmology 88:348-354, 1981.
201. Neurofibromatosis Conference Statement: National Institutes of Health Consensus Development Conference. Arch Neurol 45:575-578, 1988.
202. Morier P, Merot Y, Paccaud D, et al: Juvenile chronic granulocytic leukemia, juvenile xanthogranulomas, and neurofibromatosis. J Am Acad Dermatol 22:962-965, 1990.
203. To KW, Rabinowitz SM, Friedman AH, et al: Neurofibromatosis and neural crest neoplasms: Primary acquired melanosis and malignant melanoma of the conjunctiva. Surv Ophthalmol 33:373-379, 1989.
204. Mulvihill JJ, Parry DM, Sherman JL, et al: Neurofibromatosis 1 (Recklinghausen disease) and neurofibromatosis 2 (bilateral acoustic neurofibromatosis). Ann Intern Med 113:39-52, 1990.
205. Pearson-Webb MA, Kaiser-Kupfer MI, Eldridge R: Eye findings in bilateral acoustic (central) neurofibromatosis: Association with presenile lens opacities and cataracts but absence of Lisch nodules [letter]. N Engl J Med 315:1553-1554, 1986.
206. Roth RR, Martines R, James WD: Segmental neurofibromatosis. Arch Dermatol 123:917-920, 1987.
206a. Biemer E, Muhlbauer WD: Ein Fall einer lokalisierten Neurofibromatosis der rechten Gesichtshalfte. *In* Hohler H (ed): Plastische und Wiederherstellungs-Chirurgie. Stuttgart, Schattauer, 1975, pp. 357-361.
207. Riccardi VM: Neurofibromatosis heterogeneity. J Am Acad Dermatol 10:518-519, 1984.
208. Rubenstein AE, Bader JL, Aron AA, Wallace S: Familial transmission of segmental neurofibromatosis. Neurology 33[Suppl]: 76, 1983.
209. Huson S, Jones D, Beck L: Opthalmic manifestations of neurofibromatosis. Br J Ophthalmol 71:235-238, 1987.
210. To KW, Rabinowitz SM, Friedman AH, et al: Neurofibromatosis and neural crest neoplasms: Primary acquired melanosis and malignant melanoma of the conjunctiva. Surv Ophthalmol 33:373-379, 1989.

211. Lubs MLE, Bauer MS, Formas ME, Djokic B: Lisch nodules in neurofibromatosis type 1. N Engl J Med 324:1264–1266, 1991.
212. Listernick R, Charrow J, Greenwald MJ, Esterly NB: Optic gliomas in children with neurofibromatosis type 1. J Pediatr 114:788–792, 1989.
213. de Keizer RJW, de Wolff-Rouendaal D, Bots GTAM, et al: Optic glioma with intraocular tumor and seeding in a child with neurofibromatosis. Am J Ophthalmol 108:717–725, 1989.
214. Glover AT, Powe L: Ocular motor apraxia and neurofibromatosis [letter]. Arch Ophthalmol 103:763, 1985.
215. Weleber RG, Zonana J: Iris hamartomas (Lisch nodules) in a case of segmental neurofibromatosis. Am J Ophthalmol 96:740–743, 1983.
216. Freedman SF, Elner VM, Donev E, et al: Intraocular neurilemmoma arising from the posterior ciliary nerve in neurofibromatosis. Ophthalmology 95:1559–1564, 1988.
217. Williams R, Taylor D: Tuberous sclerosis. Surv Ophthalmol 30:143–154, 1985.
218. Pinto FJ: Disorders of hypopigmentation in children. Pediatr Clin North Am 38:991–1017, 1991.
219. Gomez MR (ed): Criteria for diagnosis. *In* Tuberous Sclerosis, 2nd ed. New York, Raven Press, 1988, pp. 9–19.
220. Elder GH: The cutaneous porphyrias. Semin Dermatol 9:63–69, 1990.
221. Arnold HL Jr, Odom RB, James WD (eds): Errors of metabolism. *In* Andrews' Diseases of the Skin, 8th edition. Philadelphia, WB Saunders, 1990, pp. 599–636.
222. Wolter JR, Clark RL: Ocular involvement in acute intermittent porphyria. Am J Ophthalmol 74:666–674, 1972.
223. Sevel D, Burger D: Ocular involvement in cutaneous porphyria: A clinical and histologic report. Arch Ophthalmol 85:580–585, 1971.
224. Day RS, Eales L, Meissner D: Coexistent variegate porphyria and porphyria cutanea tarda. N Engl J Med 307:36–41, 1982.
225. Corey TJ, DeLeo VA, Christianson H, Poh-Fitzpatrick MB: Variegate porphyria: Clinical and laboratory features. J Am Acad Dermatol 2:36–43, 1980.
226. Romslo I, Gadeholt HG, Hovding G: Erythropoietic protoporphyria terminating in liver failure. Arch Dermatol 118:668–671, 1982.
227. Nordmann Y, Deybach JC: Congenital erythropoietic porphyria. Semin Dermatol 5:106–114, 1986.
228. Horiguchi Y, Horio T, Yamamato M, et al: Late-onset erythropoietic porphyria. Br J Dermatol 121:255–262, 1989.
229. Fine JD, Johnson LB, Wright JT: Inherited blistering diseases of the skin. Pediatrician 18:175–187, 1991.
230. Pearson RW: Clinicopathologic types of epidermolysis bullosa and their nondermatological complications. Arch Dermatol 124:718–725, 1988.
231. Woodley DT, Briggaman RA, Gammon WT: Review and update of epidermolysis bullosa acquisita. Semin Dermatol 7:111–122, 1988.
232. Gans LA: Eye lesions of epidermolysis bullosa: Clinical features, management, and prognosis. Arch Dermatol 124:762–764, 1988.
233. Granek H, Baden HP: Corneal involvement in epidermolysis bullosa simplex. Arch Ophthalmol 98:469–472, 1980.
234. Aurora AL, Madhavan M, Rao S: Ocular changes in epidermolysis bullosa letalis. Am J Ophthalmol 79:464–470, 1975.
235. Holbrook KA: Extracutaneous epithelial involvement in inherited epidermolysis bullosa. Arch Dermatol 124:726–731, 1988.
236. McDonnell PJ, Schofield OM, Spalton DJ, Eady RAJ: Eye involvement in junctional epidermolysis bullosa. Arch Ophthalmol 125:1635–1637, 1989.
237. Iwamoto M, Haik BG, Iwamoto T, et al: The ultrastructural defect in conjunctiva from a case of recessive dystrophic epidermolysis bullosa. Arch Ophthalmol 109:1382–1386, 1991.
238. Zierhut M, Thiel HJ, Weidle EG, et al: Ocular involvement in epidermolysis bullosa acquisita. Arch Ophthalmol 107:398–401, 1989.
239. Richter BJ, McNutt S: The spectrum of epidermolysis bullosa acquisita. Arch Dermatol 115:1325–1328, 1979.
240. Gammon WR, Briggaman MD, Woodley DT, et al: Epidermolysis bullosa acquisita: A pemphigoid-like disease. J Am Acad Dermatol 11:820–832, 1984.
241. Boh E, Roberts LJ, Lieu TS, et al: Epidermolysis bullosa acquisita preceding the development of systemic lupus erythematosus. J Am Acad Dermatol 22:587–593, 1990.
242. Ahmed AR, Kurgis BS, Rogers RS: Cicatricial pemphigoid. J Am Acad Dermatol 24:987–1001, 1991.
243. Mondino BJ: Cicatricial pemphigoid and erythema multiforme. Ophthalmology 97:939–952, 1990.
244. Oranje AP, van Joost T. Pemphigoid in children. Pediatr Dermatol 6:267–274, 1989.
245. Neumann R, Tauber J, Foster CS: Remission and recurrence after withdrawal of therapy for ocular cicatricial pemphigoid. Ophthalmology 98:858–862, 1991.
246. Chan LS, Kaz Soong H, Foster S, et al: Ocular cicatricial pemphigoid occurring as a sequela of Stevens-Johnson syndrome. JAMA 266:1543–1546, 1991.
247. Sarret Y, Hall R, Cobo M, et al: Salt-split human skin substrate for the immunofluorescent screening of serum from patients with cicatricial pemphigoid and a new method of immunoprecipitation with IgA antibodies. J Am Acad Dermatol 24:952–958, 1991.
248. Korman NJ: Pemphigus. Dermatol Clin North Am 8:689–700, 1990.
249. Lever WF: Pemphigus. Medicine 32:1–123, 1953.
250. Diaz LA, Sampaio SA, Rivitti EA, et al: Endemic pemphigus foliaceus (fogo selvagem). Part II: Current and historic epidemiologic studies. J Invest Dermatol 92:4–12, 1989.
251. Diaz LA, Sampaio SA, Rivitti EA, et al: Endemic pemphigus foliaceus (fogo selvagem). Part I: Clinical features and immunopathology. J Am Acad Dermatol 20:657–669, 1989.
252. Francisco A: Ocular manifestations of pemphigus foliaceus. Am J Ophthalmol 32:35–44, 1949.
253. Winkelmann RK, Su WPD: Pemphigus vegetans. Arch Dermatol 115:446–448, 1979.
254. Younus J, Ahmed AR: The relationship of pemphigus to neoplasia. J Am Acad Dermatol 23:498–502, 1990.
255. Hodak E, Kremer I, David M, et al: Conjunctival involvement in pemphigus vulgaris: A clinical, histopathological, and immunofluorescence study. Br J Dermatol 123:615–620, 1990.
256. Bean SF, Holubar K, Gillet RB: Pemphigus involving the eyes. Arch Dermatol 111:1484–1486, 1975.
257. Jaimovich L, Calb I, Kaminsky A: Kaposi's sarcoma of the conjunctiva. J Am Acad Dermatol 14:589–592, 1986.
258. Arnold HL Jr, Odom RB, James WD (eds): Erythema and urticaria. *In* Andrews' Diseases of the Skin, 8th edition. Philadelphia, WB Saunders, 1990, pp. 131–158.
259. Roujeau JC, Chosidow O, Saiag P, Guillaume JC: Toxic epidermal necrolysis (Lyell syndrome). J Am Acad Dermatol 23:1039–1058, 1990.
260. Strom BL, Carson JL, Halpern AC, et al: A population-based study of Stevens-Johnson syndrome: Incidence and antecedent drug exposures. Arch Dermatol 127:831–838, 1991.
261. Ruiz-Maldonado R: Acute disseminated epidermal necrosis types 1, 2, and 3: Study of sixty cases. J Am Acad Dermatol 13:623–635, 1985.
262. Foster CS, Fong LP, Azar D, Kenyon KR: Episodic conjunctival inflammation after Stevens-Johnson syndrome. Ophthalmology 95:453–462, 1988.
263. Tilden ME, Rosenbaum JT, Fraunfelder FT: Systemic sulfonamides as a cause of bilateral, anterior uveitis. Arch Ophthalmol 109:67–69, 1991.
264. Genvert GI, Cohen EJ, Donnenfeld ED, Blecher MH: Erythema multiforme after use of topical sulfacetamide. Am J Ophthalmol 99:465–468, 1985.
265. Bennett TO, Sugar J, Sahgal S: Ocular manifestations of toxic epidermal necrolysis associated with allopurinol use. Arch Ophthalmol 95:1362–1364, 1977.
266. Tuberille AW, Frederick WR, Wood TO: Punctal occlusion in tear deficiency syndromes. Ophthalmology 89:1170–1172, 1982.
267. Soong HK, Martin NF, Wagoner MD, et al: Topical retinoid therapy for squamous metaplasia of various ocular surface disorders: A multicenter, placebo-controlled double-masked study. Ophthalmology 95:1442–1446, 1988.
268. Turgeon PW, Nauheim RC, Roat MI, et al: Indications for keratoepithelioplasty. Arch Ophthalmol 108:233–236, 1990.
269. McCulley J, Dougherty J, Deneau D: Classification of chronic blepharitis. Ophthalmology 89:1173–1180, 1982.
270. McCulley J: Blepharoconjunctivitis. Int Ophthalmol Clin 24:65–77, 1984.

271. Arnold HL Jr, Odom R, James WD (eds): Seborrheic dermatitis, psoriasis, recalcitrant palmoplantar eruptions, and erythroderma. *In* Andrews' Diseases of the Skin, 8th edition. Philadelphia, WB Saunders, 1990, pp. 194–214.
272. Plewig G: Seborrheic dermatitis. *In* Fitzpatrick T, Eisen A, Wolff K, et al (eds): Dermatology in General Medicine, 3rd edition. New York, McGraw-Hill, 1987, pp. 978–981.
273. Heng M, Henderson C, Barker D, Haberfeld G: Correlation of *Pityrosporum ovale* density with clinical severity of seborrheic dermatitis as assessed by a simplified technique. J Am Acad Dermatol 23:82–86, 1990.
274. Sadick N, McNutt N, Kaplan M: Papulosquamous dermatoses of AIDS. J Am Acad Dermatol 22:1270–1277, 1990.
275. Wright J, Merger G: Allergic keratoconjunctivitis secondary to seborrheic dermatitis. Am J Ophthalmol 53:686–687, 1962.
276. Jenkins M, Brown S, Lempert S, et al: Ocular rosacea. Am J Ophthalmol 88:618–622, 1979.
277. Brown S, Shahimian I: Diagnosis and treatment of rosacea. Tran Am Acad Ophthalmol 85:779–786, 1978.
278. Rebora A: Rosacea. J Invest Dermatol 88[Suppl]:56–60, 1987.
279. Martin D, Turner M, Williams C: Recent onset of smooth, shiny, erythematous papules on the face: Steroid rosacea secondary to topical fluorinated steroid therapy. Arch Dermatol 125:828–831, 1989.
280. Stevens G, Lemp M: Acne rosacea. *In* Gold D, Weingeist T (eds): The Eye in Systemic Disease. Philadelphia, JB Lippincott, 1990, pp. 604–606.
281. Arnold HL Jr, Odom R, James WD (eds): Acne. *In* Andrews' Diseases of the Skin, 8th edition. Philadelphia, WB Saunders, 1990, pp. 250–267.
282. Browning D, Proia A: Ocular rosacea. Surv Ophthalmol 31:145–158, 1986.
283. Lemp MA, Mahmood MA, Weiler HH: Rosacea and keratoconjunctivitis sicca. Arch Ophthalmol 102:556–557, 1984.
284. Browning D: Tear studies in ocular rosacea. Am J Ophthalmol 99:530–533, 1985.
285. Lempert S, Jenkins M, Brown S: Chalazia and rosacea. Arch Ophthalmol 97:1652–1653, 1979.
286. Coskey R, Liioi J, Robbins T: Diagnosis and treatment of chalazia. J Am Acad Dermatol 15:345–347, 1986.
287. Anderson L, McCollough M, Grabski W: Lupus miliaris disseminatus faciei. J Assoc Military Dermatol 15:8–11, 1989.
288. Bleicher P, Charles J, Sober A: Topical metronidazole therapy for rosacea. Arch Dermatol 123:609–614, 1987.
289. Baden H: Pityriasis rubra pilaris. *In* Fitzpatrick T, Eisen A, Wolff K, et al (eds): Dermatology in General Medicine, 3rd edition. New York, McGraw-Hill, 1987, pp. 517–519.
290. Cohen P, Prystowsky J: Pityriasis rubra pilaris: A review of diagnosis and treatment. J Am Acad Dermatol 20:801–807, 1989.
291. Duke-Elder S (ed): System of Ophthalmology, vol 7. St. Louis, CV Mosby, 1965, p. 560.
292. Pearlman MD: A Catalogue of Eye Signs in Systemic Disorders. Springfield, IL: Charles C Thomas, 1965, pp. 119–120.
293. Borok M, Lowe N: Pityriasis rubra pilaris: Further observations of systemic retinoid therapy. J Am Acad Dermatol 22:792–795, 1990.
294. Zelickson BD, Muller SA: Generalized pustular psoriasis: A review of 63 cases. Arch Dermatol 127:1339–1345, 1991.
295. Baadsgaard O, Fisher G, Voorhees J, et al: The role of the immune system in the pathogenesis of psoriasis. J Invest Dermatol 95[Suppl]:32–34, 1990.
296. Whitmore P: Skin and mucous membrane disorders. *In* Tasman W, Jaeger E (eds): Duane's Clinical Ophthalmology, vol 5. Philadelphia, JB Lippincott, 1980, pp. 12–13.
297. Kaldeck R: Ocular psoriasis. Arch Dermatol 68:44–49, 1953.
298. Lambert J, Wright V: Eye inflammation in psoriatic arthritis. Ann Rheum Dis 35:354–356, 1976.
299. Cooper K: Urticaria and angioedema: Diagnosis and evaluation. J Am Acad Dermatol 25:166–176, 1991.
300. Soter N: Acute and chronic urticaria and angioedema. J Am Acad Dermatol 25:146–154, 1991.
301. Kennard C, Ellis C: Pharmacologic therapy for urticaria. J Am Acad Dermatol 25:176–189, 1991.
302. Fox B, Odom R: Papulosquamous diseases: A review. J Am Acad Dermatol 12:597–624, 1985.
303. Arndt K: Lichen planus. *In* Fitzpatrick T, Eisen A, Wolff K, et al (eds): Dermatology in General Medicine, 3rd edition. New York, McGraw-Hill, 1987, pp. 967–973.
304. Boyd A, Nelder K: Lichen planus. J Am Acad Dermatol 25:593–619, 1991.
305. Soper D, Patterson J, Hurt W, et al: Lichen planus of the vulva. Obstet Gynecol 72:74–76, 1988.
306. Goldsmith J: Deep keratitis associated with atypical lichen planus. Arch Ophthalmol 40:138–146, 1948.
307. Vogel P, James WD: Lichen planus of the eyelids. J Am Acad Dermatol 27:638–639, 1992.
308. Cleveland D: Lichen simplex chronicus: 170 consecutive cases encountered in private practice. Arch Dermatol Syph 33:316–326, 1936.
309. Shaffer B, Beerman H: Lichen simplex chronicus and its variants. Arch Dermatol 64:340–351, 1951.
310. Arnold HL Jr, Odom R, James WD (eds): Pruritus and neurocutaneous dermatoses. *In* Andrews' Diseases of the Skin, 8th edition. Philadelphia, WB Saunders, 1990, pp. 51–67.
311. White J: Eczematous reaction patterns. *In* Sams W Jr, Lynch P (eds): Principles and Practice of Dermatology. New York, Churchill Livingstone, 1990, pp. 381–383.
312. Thestrup-Pedersen K, Halkier-Sorensen L, Sogaard H, Zachariae H: The red man syndrome. J Am Acad Dermatol 18:1307–1312, 1988.
313. Hasan I, Jansen C: Erythroderma: A follow-up of fifty cases. J Am Acad Dermatol 8:836–840, 1983.
314. Kaplan M, Sadick N, McNutt N, et al: Dermatologic findings and manifestations of acquired immunodeficiency syndrome (AIDS). J Am Acad Dermatol 16:485–506, 1987.
315. Pearlman M: A Catalogue of Eye Signs in Systemic Disease. Springfield, IL, Charles C Thomas, 1965, pp. 54.
316. Duke-Elder S: System of Ophthalmology, vol 8. St. Louis, CV Mosby, 1965, p. 548.
317. Hanifin J, Lobitz W Jr: Newer concepts of atopic dermatitis. Arch Dermatol 113:663–669, 1977.
318. Arnold HL Jr, Odom R, James WD (eds): Atopic dermatitis, eczema, noninfectious immunodeficiency disorders. *In* Andrews' Diseases of the Skin, 8th edition. Philadelphia, WB Saunders, 1990, pp. 68–74.
319. Uehara M: Infraorbital fold in atopic dermatitis. Arch Dermatol 117:627–629, 1981.
320. Ingram R: Retinal detachment associated with atopic dermatitis and cataract. Br J Ophthalmol 49:96–97, 1965.
321. Longmore L: Atopic dermatitis cataract and keratoconus. Australas J Dermatol 11:139–141, 1970.
322. Rich L, Hanifin J: Ocular complications of atopic dermatitis and other eczemas. Int Ophthalmol Clin 25:61–76, 1985.
323. Garrity J, Liesegang T: Ocular complications of atopic dermatitis. Can J Ophthalmol 19:21–24, 1984.
324. Rapoza P, Chandler J: Atopic dermatitis. *In* Gold D, Weingeist T (eds): The Eye in Systemic Disease. Philadelphia, JB Lippincott, 1990, pp. 606–609.
325. Brunsting L, Reed W, Bair H: Occurrence of cataracts and keratoconus with atopic dermatitis. Arch Dermatol 72:237–241, 1955.
326. Dooms-Goosens A, Debusschere K, Gevers D, et al: Contact dermatitis caused by airborne agents. J Am Acad Dermatol 15:1–10, 1986.
327. Bergstresser P: Immune mechanism in contact dermatitis. Dermatol Clin 8:3–11, 1990.
328. Fisher A: Cosmetic dermatitis of the eyelids. Cutis 34:216–221, 1984.
329. Maibach HI, Engasser PG: Dermatitis due to cosmetics. *In* Fisher A (ed): Contact dermatitis, 3rd edition. Philadelphia, Lea & Febiger, 1986, pp. 368–393.
330. Nethercott J, Nield G, Holness L: A review of 79 cases of eyelid dermatitis. J Am Acad Dermatol 21:223–230, 1989.
331. Bloomfield S: Clinical allergy and immunology of external eye. *In* Tasman W, Jaeger E (eds): Duane's Clinical Ophthalmology, vol 9. Philadelphia, JB Lippincott, 1986, pp. 1–25.
332. Wilhelm K, Maibach H: Factors predisposing to cutaneous irritation. Dermatol Clin North Am 8:17–22, 1990.
333. Sher M: Contact dermatitis of the eyelids. S Afr Med J 55:511–513, 1979.
334. Svensson A, Moller H: Eyelid dermatitis: The role of atopy and contact allergy. Contact Dermatitis 15:178–182, 1986.

335. Burkhart C: Looking at the eyelid lesions—a clinical roundup. Geriatrics 36:91–95, 1981.
336. Muhlbauer J: Granuloma annulare. J Am Acad Dermatol 3:217–230, 1980.
337. Ghadially R, Sibbald R, Walter J, Haberman H: Granuloma annulare in patients with human immunodeficiency virus infections. J Am Acad Dermatol 20:232–235, 1989.
338. Dabski K, Winkelmann R: Generalized granuloma annulare: Clinical and laboratory findings in 100 patients. J Am Acad Dermatol 20:39–47, 1980.
339. Samlaska CP, Sandberg GD, Maggio KL, LA Sakas: Generalized perforating granuloma annulare. J Am Acad Dermatol 27:319–322, 1992.
340. Lawton AW, Karesh JW: Periocular granuloma annulare. Surv Ophthalmol 31:285–290, 1987.
341. Rao N, Font R: Pseudorheumatoid nodules of the ocular adnexa. Am J Ophthalmol 79:471–478, 1975.
342. Coskey R: Facial granuloma annulare. Arch Dermatol 155:866–868, 1979.
343. McFarland J, Kauh Y, Luscombe H: Periorbital granuloma annulare. Arch Dermatol 118:190–191, 1982.
344. Pedace G, Perry H: Granuloma faciale. Arch Dermatol 94:387–395, 1966.
345. Apfelberg D, Druker D, Maser M, et al: Granuloma faciale: Treatment with argon laser. Arch Dermatol 119:573–576, 1983.
346. Burgdorf W, Goltz R: Granuloma faciale. *In* Fitzpatrick T, Eisen A, Wolff K, et al (eds): Dermatology in General Medicine, 3rd edition. New York, McGraw-Hill, 1987, pp. 1317–1319.
347. Sears J, Gitter D, Stone M: Extrafacial granuloma faciale. Arch Dermatol 5:742–743, 1991.
348. Dinehart S, Gross D, Davis C, Herzberg A: Granuloma faciale: Comparison of different treatment modalities. Arch Otolaryngol Head Neck Surg 116:849–851, 1990.
349. Guill M, Aton J: Facial granuloma responsive to dapsone therapy. Arch Dermatol 118:332–335, 1982.
350. Scheck O, Horny H, Ruck P, et al: Solitary mastocytoma of the eyelid: A case report with special reference to the immunocytology of human tissue mast cells, and a review of the literature. Virchows Arch A Pathol Anat Histopathol 412:31–36, 1987.
351. Soter N: The skin in mastocytosis. J Invest Dermatol 96[Suppl]:32–39, 1991.
352. Metcalfe D: The treatment of mastocytosis: An overview. J Invest Dermatol 96[Suppl]:55–56, 1991.
353. Metcalfe D: Classification and diagnosis of mastocytosis: Current status. J Invest Dermatol 96[Suppl]:2–3, 1991.
354. Davenport D: Ulerythema ophryogenes. Arch Dermatol 89:74–80, 1964.
355. Pierini D, Pierini A: Keratosis pilaris atrophicans faciei (ulerythema ophryogenes): A cutaneous marker in the Noonan syndrome. Br J Dermatol 100:409–416, 1979.
356. Bennett J, Schwartz M, Berberian B: Ulerythema ophryogenes with multiple congenital anomalies. J Am Acad Dermatol 18:437–440, 1988.
357. Emmerson R: Follicular mucinosis: A study of 47 patients. Br J Dermatol 81:395–413, 1969.
358. Coskey R, Mehregan A: Alopecia mucinosa: A follow-up study. Arch Dermatol 102:193–194, 1970.
359. Truhan A, Roenigk H: The cutaneous mucinoses. J Am Acad Dermatol 14:1–18, 1986.
360. Gibson L, Muller S, Leiferman K, Peters M: Follicular mucinosis: Clinical and histopathologic study. J Am Acad Dermatol 20:441–446, 1989.
361. Arnold HL Jr, Odom R, James WD (eds): Mucinoses. *In* Andrews' Diseases of the Skin, 8th edition. Philadelphia, WB Saunders, 1990, pp. 190–191.
362. Perret C, Steijlen P, Happle R: Alopecia areata: Pathogenesis and topical immunotherapy. Int J Dermatol 29:83–88, 1990.
363. Mitchel A, Krull E: Alopecia areata: Pathogenesis and treatment. J Am Acad Dermatol 11:763–775, 1984.
364. Mitchell A, Balle M: Alopecia areata. Dermatol Clin North Am 5:553–564, 1987.
365. Giovinazzo V, Rodriguez-Sains R: Ophthalmologic oncology: Alopecia of the eyelids. J Dermatol Surg Oncol 10:182–185, 1984.
366. Williams M, Elias P: Genetically transmitted, generalized disorders of cornification. Dermatol Clin 5:155–178, 1987.
367. Shwayder T, Ott F: All about ichthyosis. Pediatr Clin North Am 38:835–857, 1991.
368. Cherubini T: Entropion and ectropion of the eyelids. Clin Plast Surg 5:583–591, 1978.
369. Sever R, Frost P, Weinstein G: Eye changes in ichthyoses. JAMA 206:2283–2286, 1968.
370. Rose H: Lid changes in nonbullous ichthyosiform erythroderma. Br J Ophthalmol 55:750–752, 1971.
371. Orth D, Fretzin D, Abramson V: Collodion baby with transient bilateral upper lid ectropion. Arch Ophthalmol 91:206–207, 1974.
372. Langer K, Konrad K, Wolff K: Keratitis, ichthyosis, and deafness (KID) syndrome: Report of three cases and a review of the literature. Br J Dermatol 122:689–697, 1990.
373. Price V, Odom R, Ward W, Jones R: Trichothiodystrophy. Arch Dermatol 116:1375–1384, 1980.
374. Baden H, Buxman M, Weinstein G, et al: Treatment of ichthyosis with isotretinoin. J Am Acad Dermatol 6:716–720, 1982.
375. Peled I, Bar-Lev A, Wexler M: Surgical correction of ectropion in lamellar ichthyosis. Ann Plast Surg 8:429–431, 1982.

CHAPTER 2

Neoplastic and Related Conditions of the Orbital and Adnexal Structures

Merlyn M. Rodrigues, Sankaran Rajagopalan, Kelly Jones, and James W. Karesh

This chapter describes systemic malignant neoplasms and lesions simulating malignancy and their relationships to the orbital and adnexal structures. The diagnosis of metastatic orbital lesions is usually associated with a poor prognosis; thus, accurate clinical and histologic diagnosis and prompt management are of paramount importance.[1] Newer clinical diagnostic techniques have greatly facilitated prompt recognition of orbital lesions.[1] Computed tomographic scans and magnetic resonance imaging have been particularly invaluable diagnostic tools to alert the clinician to the existence of these lesions. These techniques have also facilitated diagnosis of these lesions through either a surgical or guided radiologic approach.[2,3]

The chapter considers the following topics: (1) metastatic tumors to the orbital and adnexal structures; (2) carcinoid tumors; (3) malignant melanoma; (4) paraneoplastic syndromes; (5) lymphoma and related diseases; (6) histiocytosis X; (7) multiple myeloma and plasmacytoma; (8) sarcoidosis; (9) amyloidosis; (10) idiopathic midline destructive disease (IMDD) and Wegener's granulomatosis; (11) xeroderma pigmentosum; (12) pseudorheumatoid nodules; (13) rare pigmentary lesions (basal cell nevus and dysplastic syndromes and squamous papilloma); and (14) extension into the orbital and adnexal tissues from primary tumors, for example, adenoid cystic carcinoma.

DIAGNOSIS

Procedures such as fine-needle aspiration biopsy[4] and open biopsy are important diagnostic techniques that along with other selected histologic techniques can determine the origin of poorly differentiated tumors and may be helpful in determining specific hormonal therapy. There have been exciting advances in laboratory techniques that provide insight into the diagnosis, prognosis, and treatment of tumors. Important markers of tumor prognosis include the following:

1. Proliferation indicators: These include Ki-67, proliferating cell nuclear antigen, deoxyribonucleic acid (DNA) synthetic cell analysis, mitosis counting (s phase), and thymidine labeling index.
2. Hormone-growth receptor analyses: These consist of receptors for estrogen, progesterone, androgen, insulin, and growth factors.[5]
3. Ploidy analysis using flow cytometry.
4. Cytogenetic analysis: This is used to detect consistent chromosomal deletions, translocations (as in chronic myeloid leukemia), and double-minute chromosomes or C-bandless chromosomes.
5. Oncogene analysis: Changes in cancer cells represent exaggerations or distortions of normal cell physiology, usually resulting from a gene mutation that produces an abnormal protein.[6] Oncogene analysis includes testing for *myc* genes (amplification), *ras* genes (mutations), and HER 2/*neu* (amplification-overexpression).
6. Predictors of invasion and metastasis: These include the detection of enzymes and tissue inhibitors of metalloproteinases (metastasis suppressor proteins),[7] *ras* mutations, adhesion molecules, and loss of basement membrane components.
7. Tumor-suppressor gene analysis: This is used for detection of the retinoblastoma gene and p53.[6]
8. Multidrug-resistant (MDR) genes: Oncogenes, tumor-suppressor genes, and MDR genes represent the major areas of new investigations and are important in assessing tumor prognosis.[6] In addition, the wide range of therapeutic options currently available in the modern treatment armamentarium has dramatically altered the outlook for many patients with cancer.

Ophthalmologists can play an important role in the diagnosis of metastatic ocular and orbital cancer. Orbital metastatic cancer appears to have increased in frequency during the past 2 decades.[1] The prevalence of orbital metastasis in relation to all orbital diseases has been estimated to be 1.5% to 3.3%[1]; however, Henderson and Farrow[8] described a 10% prevalence of orbital metastases among all orbital neoplasms. Breast, lung, and prostate carcinomas and melanoma are the most common primary sites (Figs. 2-1 to 2-3), but it is not unusual that

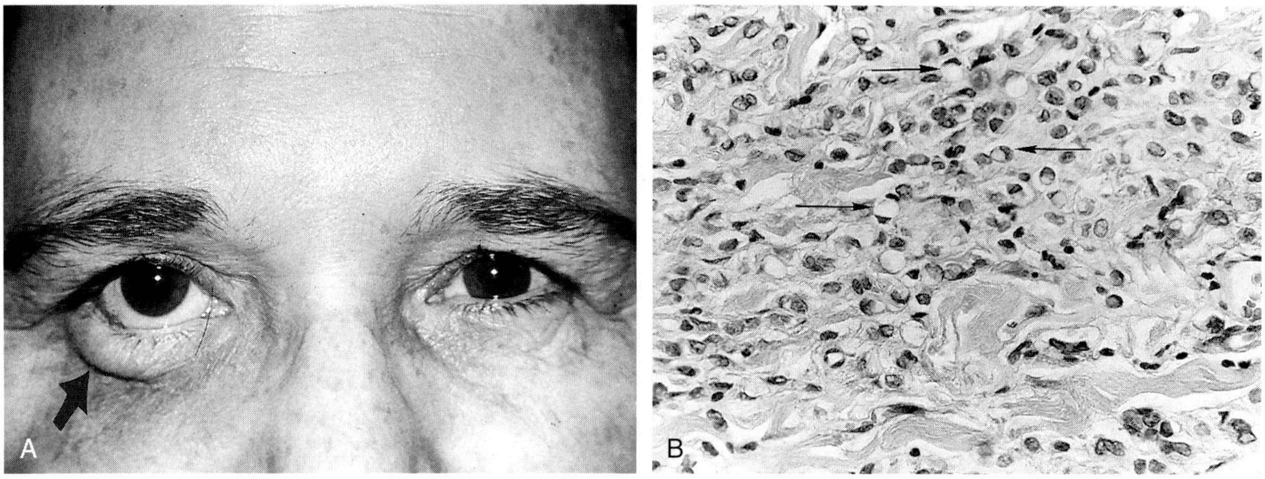

Figure 2–1. *A*, Metastatic tumor to the lower eyelid presenting as an initial manifestation of breast cancer. *B*, Metastatic adenocarcinoma cells are arranged in lobular and single-file fashion. The tumor cells display mucin secretion with large intracytoplasmic vacuoles *(arrows)*. ×640.

the primary site cannot be definitely established.[9–14] More unusual orbital metastases have also been observed (Figs. 2–4 to 2–6).[15–18] Some reports have indicated that orbital metastatic tumors have a tendency to lateralize, suggesting that metastases occur preferentially in the left orbit.[9–13] However, other studies have disputed this view, and recent reports have indicated that the right orbit is more frequently involved than the left.[1] Although some have suggested that the superior and medial orbits are the most common sites of predilection of orbital tumors, Goldberg and associates reported that the lateral orbit may be the most common quadrant affected.[1]

There has been an increasing tendency to diagnose the primary tumor before the orbital metastasis appears. However, in approximately 25% of patients with systemic metastatic cancer, orbital involvement may be the initial clinical manifestation, thus providing an important diagnostic challenge to the ophthalmologist.[14]

Metastatic tumors to the orbit and eyelids are uncommon compared with metastatic ocular tumors. Goldberg and associates[1] reported that the incidence of orbital metastases of systemic cancer appears to have been increasing in frequency during the past 2 decades. However, with current advances in chemotherapy and other treatment modalities, patients generally have increased longevity. Improved methods of diagnosis have enabled the ophthalmologist to institute appropriate treatment earlier than in the past, often resulting in an improved prognosis. Among metastatic tumors, there appears to be a difference in the type of lesion in children and adults.[1,12] In adults the most common metastatic tumors are carcinoma of the lung, breast (in women), and prostate and

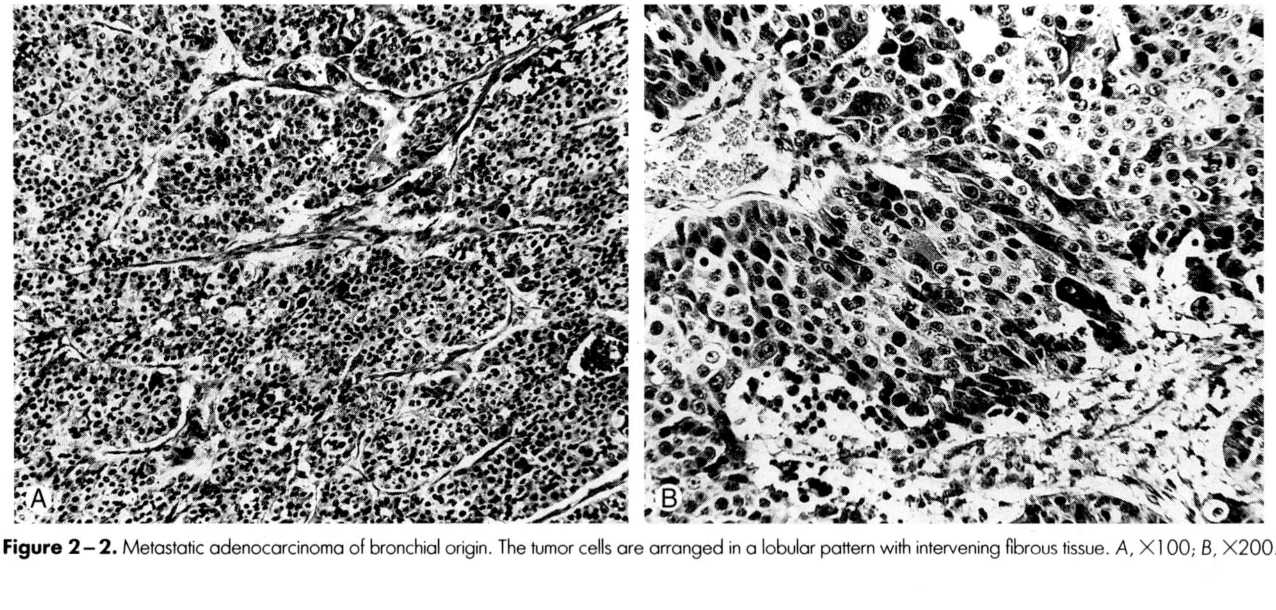

Figure 2–2. Metastatic adenocarcinoma of bronchial origin. The tumor cells are arranged in a lobular pattern with intervening fibrous tissue. *A*, ×100; *B*, ×200.

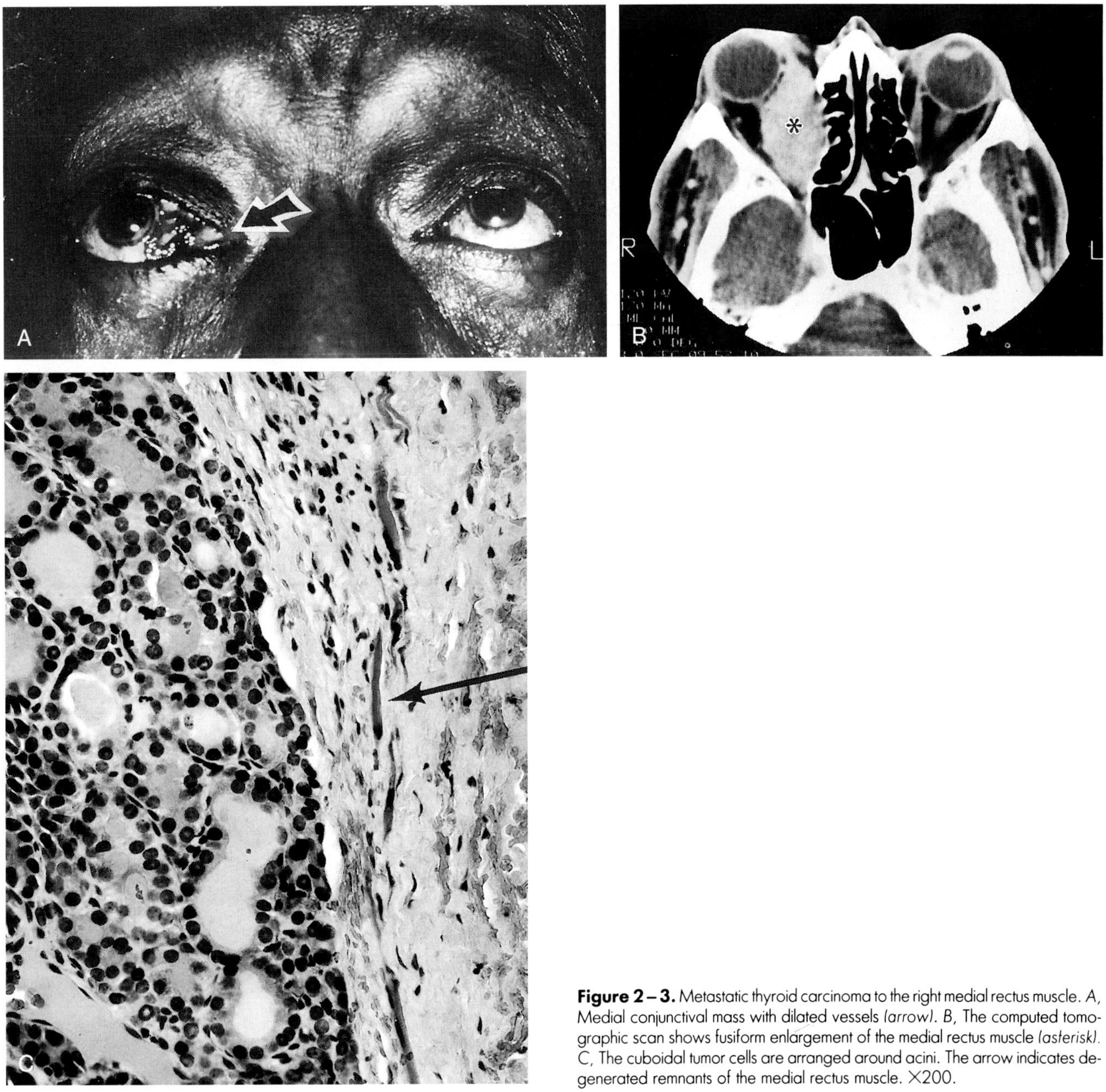

Figure 2–3. Metastatic thyroid carcinoma to the right medial rectus muscle. *A*, Medial conjunctival mass with dilated vessels *(arrow)*. *B*, The computed tomographic scan shows fusiform enlargement of the medial rectus muscle *(asterisk)*. *C*, The cuboidal tumor cells are arranged around acini. The arrow indicates degenerated remnants of the medial rectus muscle. ×200.

testicle (in men) in addition to tumors of unknown origin and lymphomas.[1] In children the most common primary types are neuroblastoma, embryonal sarcoma, medulloblastoma, and Wilms' tumor. In adults, metastatic carcinomas occur in the orbit about 10% less frequently than metastases to the eye. These tumors usually occur in the 6th and 7th decades. The metastases are generally unilateral and are characterized clinically by pain, periorbital swelling, and a disturbance of extraocular motility. In metastatic breast cancer, a considerable delay can occur between the diagnosis of the primary lesion and the development of ocular or orbital metastases[1]; latency periods of 20 to 30 years have been reported. Patients with breast, lung, kidney, prostate, and other cancers can present with their orbital lesions before the primary tumor has been detected.[1] Thus, incisional biopsy of the lesion is important to determine the primary site. The histopathology of various types of primary tumors displays a considerable degree of variation. In primary breast cancers the individual tumor cells can exhibit a lobular appearance, or a single column, Indian-file infiltrating pattern. Mucinous differentiation can be confirmed with

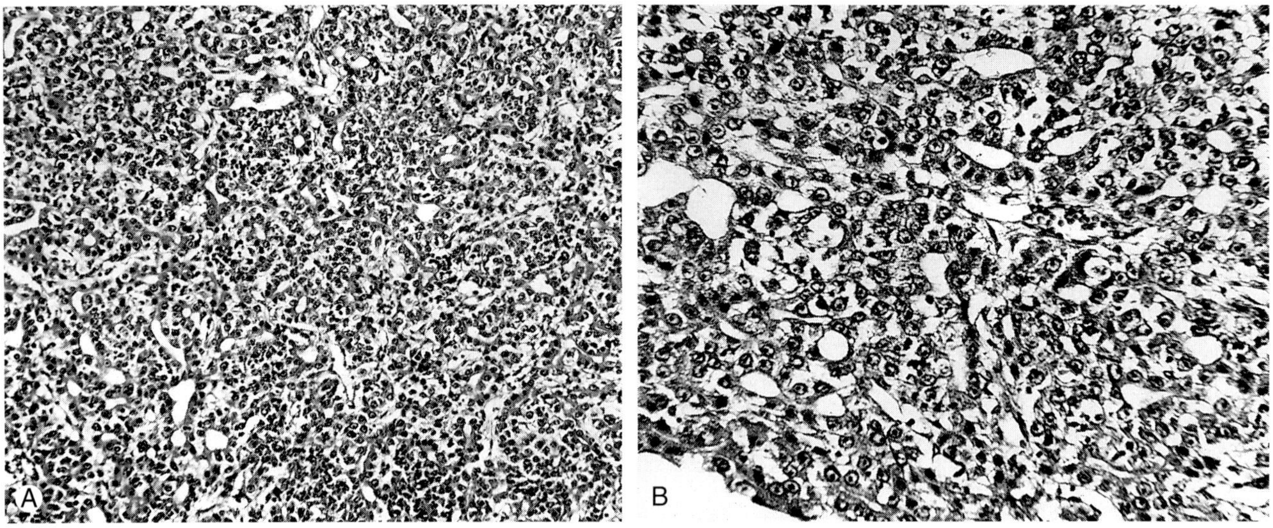

Figure 2–4. Metastatic hepatoblastoma to the orbit. The tumor cells exhibit an array of poorly differentiated cells arranged in an alveolar pattern. *A*, ×100; *B*, ×200.

special stains such as Alcian blue and mucicarmine.[14] Mucin production can also occur in lung or gastrointestinal primary tumors.

In lung cancer, the most common metastasis is the oat cell type where small anaplastic tumor cells are arranged in infiltrating sheets or trabeculae as well as larger sheet-like aggregates. In prostate cancer, the detection of acid phosphatase in the cytoplasm of tumor cells is helpful in establishing the diagnosis. Most carcinomas also display immunoreactivity for keratin protein.

Eyelid metastases are relatively rare. Among the most common primary sites are breast, cutaneous melanoma, lungs, and gastrointestinal tract carcinoma. These lesions may manifest as rapidly enlarging eyelid lesions that are sometimes mistaken for a chalazion or a meibomian gland carcinoma. Histochemical stains are particularly useful in distinguishing primary tumor sites. Thyroid carcinoma may have a protracted course with a relatively long interval between the diagnosis of primary thyroid cancer and the appearance of orbital metastasis. Thyroid cancer involves the posterior portion of the orbit; more rarely, isolated metastases to an extraocular muscle can occur.[15,16] Multiple endocrine neoplasia (MEN) types 2A and 2B are associated with medullary thyroid carcinoma and high levels of plasma calcitonin.[19] MEN type 2A has an increased incidence of prominent corneal nerves[20]

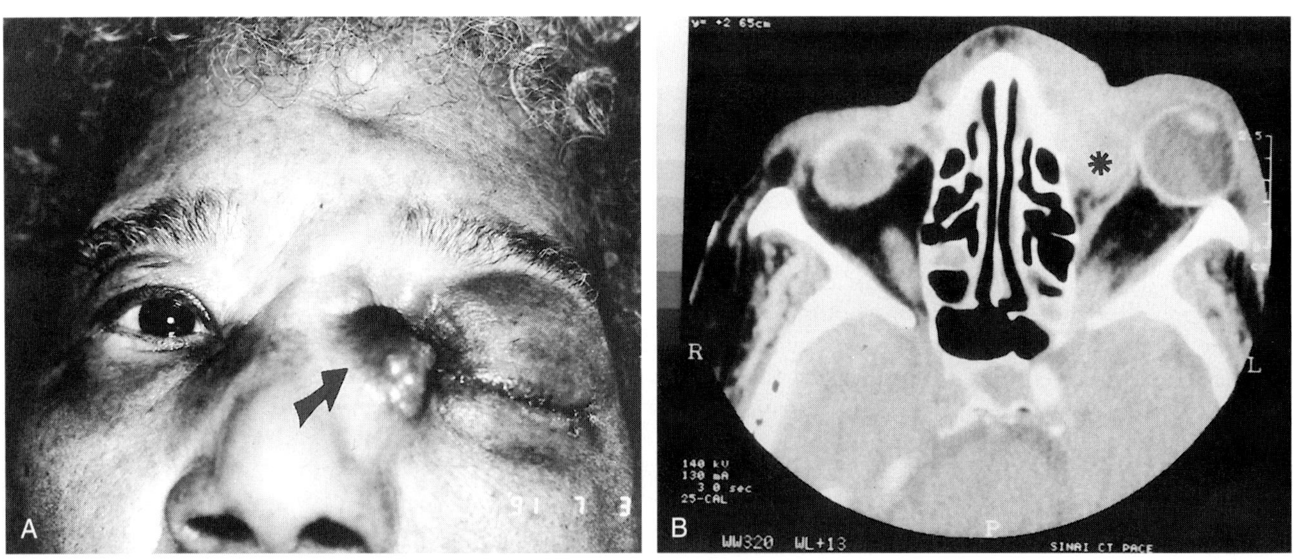

Figure 2–5. Metastatic squamous cell carcinoma. *A*, Fungating necrotic medial mass (*arrow*). *B*, The computed tomographic scan shows diffuse soft tissue involvement (*asterisk*) with lateral displacement of the medial rectus muscle.

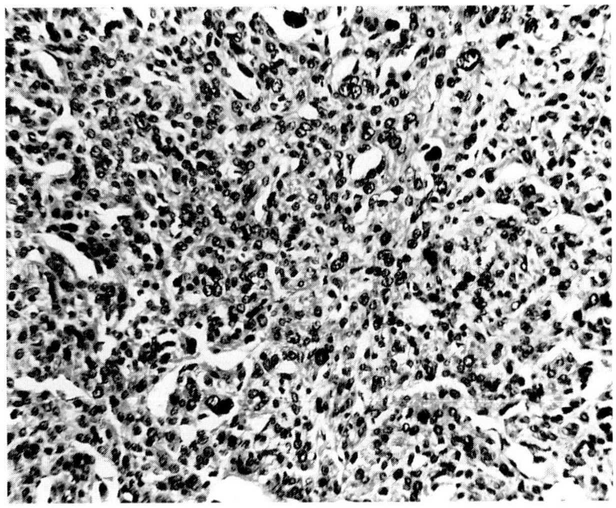

Figure 2–6. Metastatic leiomyosarcoma to the orbit. Microscopic examination shows atypical spindle cell proliferation of smooth muscle cells. ×200.

and MEN type 2B is associated with a marfanoid habitus and thickened eyelids and lips. In orbital metastatic cutaneous malignant melanoma, a latent period of several years to as long as 40 years has been observed. However, following occurrence of metastasis, the progress of the disease becomes much more rapid. Immunocytochemical markers such as HMB-45 can be helpful in the diagnosis of metastatic melanoma, although other tumors also express this protein.[21–23]

Among orbital metastases, the most common presenting symptoms and signs are proptosis and disturbances of ocular motility. A decrease in vision and proptosis may also be noted.

TREATMENT

The treatment of orbital metastatic tumors is usually palliative. The principal therapeutic modalities include radiotherapy, chemotherapy, hormonal therapy, surgery, and monoclonal antibodies in selected patients.[24] Radiotherapy is typically administered in divided doses for 1 or 2 weeks, with a total dosage of 3000 to 4000 rads (30 to 40 Gy). This regimen may be followed by dramatic improvement, particularly in patients with lymphomas. Precautions should be taken with field placement, dosimetry, and shielding of the globe to minimize complications of radiotherapy. Hormonal therapy is useful in certain cancers derived from organs with cell surface hormone receptors, particularly metastatic breast and prostate carcinoma. The presence of surface hormone receptors in these tumors can be measured with adequate fresh tissue specimens. McGuire[5] reported that 55% to 60% of metastatic breast carcinomas with positive estrogen receptor respond to endocrine ablative treatment.

Chemotherapy is particularly effective in small cell carcinoma of the lung and in neuroblastoma. Surgery is usually not indicated unless the tumor is small, circumscribed, and easily accessible, as in metastatic carcinoid tumor, or if there is marked proptosis and severe pain for which radiotherapy and chemotherapy have been unsuccessful.

LABORATORY TESTS

Laboratory tests are useful in the differential diagnosis of an orbital mass. For example, primary prostate cancers secrete prostatic acid phosphatase, and human chorionic gonadotropin is expressed in seminoma cells. Carcinoid tumors may secrete 5-hydroxyindoleacetic acid into the urine, particularly in the presence of carcinoid syndrome. The immunocytochemistry for keratin is also useful in establishing the diagnosis of cancer. Melanomas can be detected by Fontana's stain or by the presence of melanin by electron microscopy. Immunohistochemical stains, particularly HMB-45, are useful in the diagnosis of melanoma, including conjunctival melanoma.[23] However, this protein is also present in adenocarcinoma[22] and in sweat gland tumors.[21]

SPECIFIC TUMOR TYPES

Carcinoid Tumors

Carcinoid tumors metastatic to the orbit are uncommon. Riddle and associates[25] and Shetlar and colleagues[26] reported a total of seven cases of orbital carcinoid tumors documented by histochemistry and electron microscopy. Most carcinoid tumors metastatic to the orbit arise from primary ileal carcinoids, whereas most reported metastatic uveal carcinoids have originated from primary bronchial tumors. Carcinoid orbital metastases show a granular content of the tumor cells, and electron microscopy shows dense cytoplasmic granules (Fig. 2–7).

Immunocytochemical markers such as chromogranin A, synaptophysin, and serotonin are useful in diagnosis. In addition, DNA flow cytometry can be of prognostic value; DNA aneuploidy has been correlated with an unfavorable clinical outcome.[26] The management of carcinoid tumor is by surgical excision or radiotherapy and chemotherapy.

Malignant Melanoma

Melanomas involving the orbit are infrequent and generally result from a choroidal or conjunctival melanoma spreading into the orbit by continuity or from a metastatic cutaneous melanoma.[18] Rarely, melanomas of the lacrimal sac and sinuses may also invade the orbit. Primary malignant melanomas are characterized histologi-

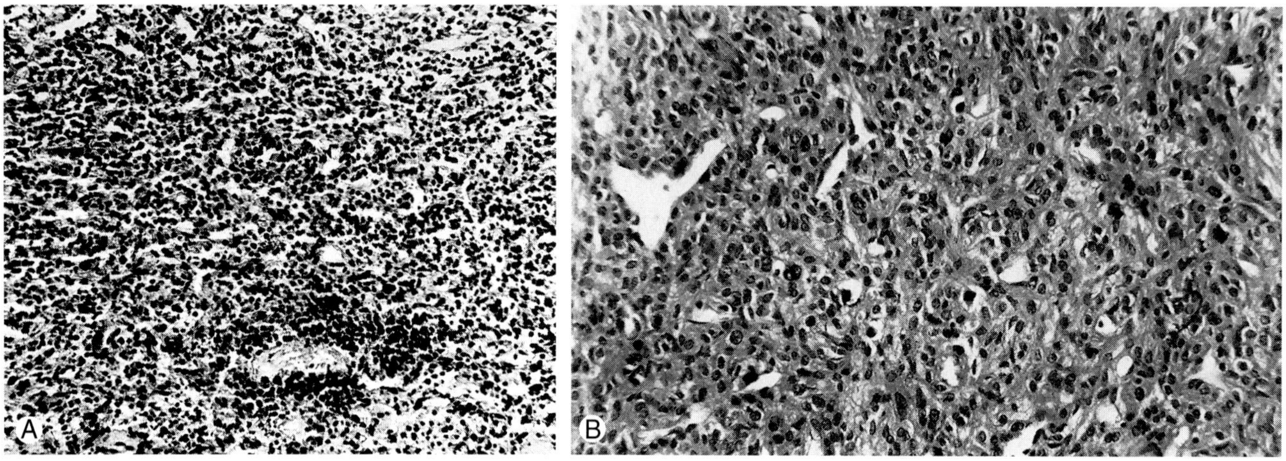

Figure 2–7. Metastatic carcinoid tumor from a primary lung lesion. The tumor cells are arranged in a lobular pattern. *A*, ×200; *B*, ×400.

cally by variable pigmented cells with a spindle cell proliferation or a mixture of spindle and epithelioid cells (Fig. 2–8). In amelanotic lesions, special stains and electron microscopy are useful diagnostic techniques. Clinically, patients should be examined for periocular cutaneous pigmentation or pigmentation in the distribution of the trigeminal nerve or for the existence of pigmented lesions elsewhere on the skin. Exenteration is the preferred treatment for primary orbital melanoma.

Paraneoplastic Syndromes

Paraneoplastic syndromes are the symptom complexes that result from remote, nonmetastatic effects of tumors. These syndromes are presumably caused by autoimmune mechanisms or by mediators (hormones and growth factors) produced by tumor cells. Ocular remote effects include cancer-associated retinopathy, autoimmune retinal degeneration, uveal melanocytic tumors often associated with uveitis, and eye movement disorders.[27] Recently, paraneoplastic pemphigus, cicatricial conjunctivitis, and acanthosis nigricans were observed in a patient with bronchogenic squamous cell carcinoma.[28]

Lymphoma and Related Disease

Lymphoid tumors constitute an important group of orbital neoplasms that includes malignant lymphoma, reactive lymphoid hyperplasia, multiple myeloma, and lymphoplasmacytoid tumors. The orbital systemic lymphomas include non-Hodgkin's lymphoma, lymphosarcoma, Burkitt's tumor, Hodgkin's disease, mycosis fungoides, and reticulum cell sarcoma. Because the orbit does not normally contain lymph vessels, any orbital lymphoid mass is abnormal. On the other hand, there are lymphoid aggregates in the conjunctiva that may become hyperplastic and form focal lymphoid hyperplasia or that may be part of a systemic disease (Fig. 2–9). Lymphoid

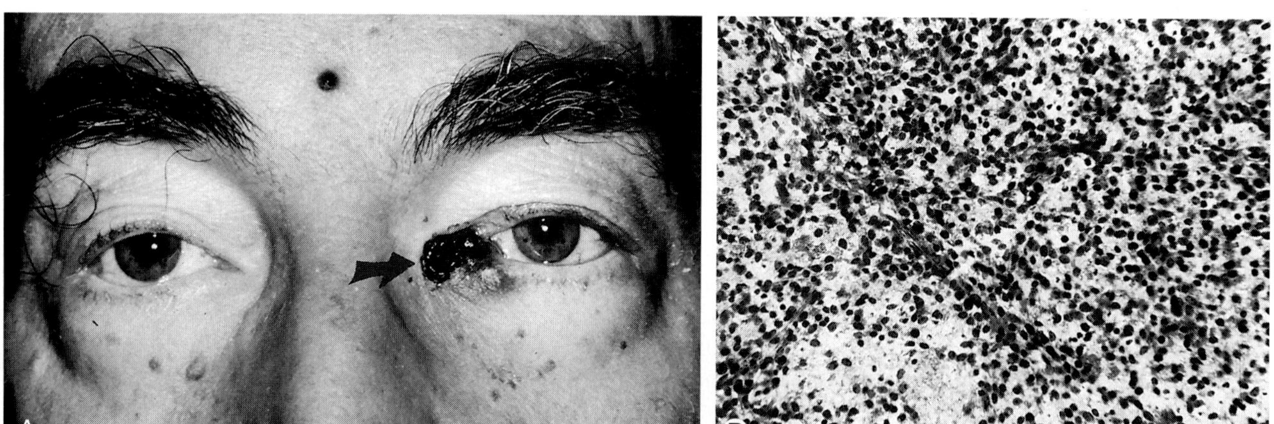

Figure 2–8. Poorly differentiated malignant melanoma. *A*, Darkly pigmented fungating necrotic tumor in the medial canthus *(arrow)*. *B*, From a different patient, poorly differentiated tumor cells with scant pigment. ×200.

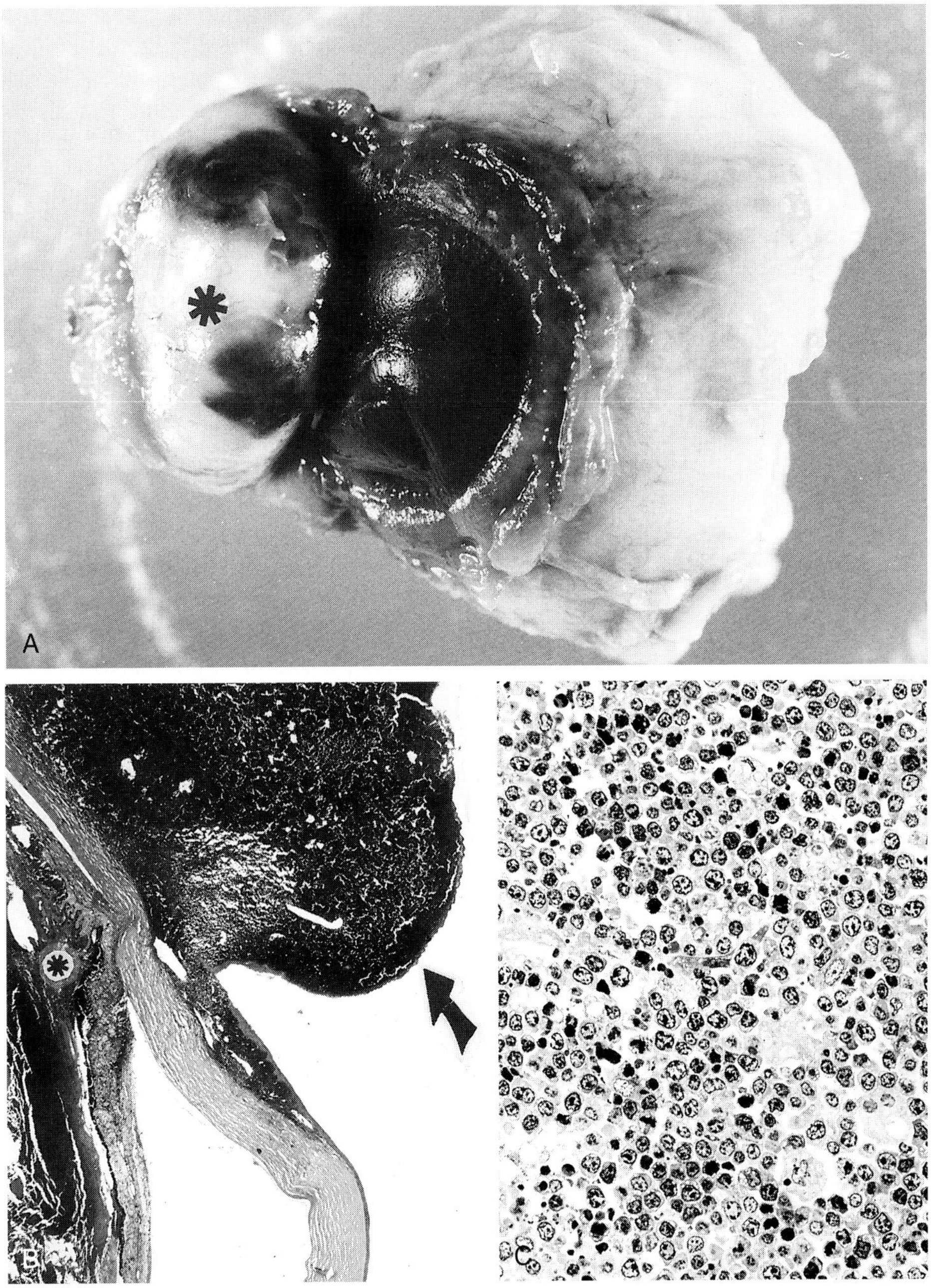

Figure 2–9. *A*, Extraocular nodular limbal lesion *(asterisk)* in a patient with B cell lymphoma and leukemia. *B*, Corneoscleral invasion with intraocular *(asterisk)* and epibulbar *(arrow)* involvement. ×15. *C*, The tumor cells display large hyperchromatic nuclei with prominent nucleoli. Immunoperoxidase staining was positive for L-26 antigen. ×500.

lesions of the conjunctiva usually present clinically as fleshy pink salmon-colored masses that are generally movable over the epibulbar surface because they involve the substantia propria and do not cause proptosis or problems with extraocular motility. On the other hand, orbital lesions are associated with proptosis and can cause motility disturbances as well as displacement of the eye. Tumors located within the skin of the eyelid or extended to the lid from a deeper orbital involvement have a prognosis similar to orbital lymphomas.

Newer histologic techniques have permitted a more accurate assessment of the type of lymphoid tumor and are valuable indicators of the prognosis. Markers for B and T cell lesions are useful to determine the cellular constituents of the lymphoid tumor.[29–31] Finfer and Jakobiec[32] showed that extranodal noncutaneous lymphomas represent a progressive spectrum of B cell neoplasia up to and including malignant lymphoma. More recently, Jakobiec and Knowles[31] applied molecular genetic studies for the analysis of adnexal lymphoid tumors. The most favorable prognosis was noted in conjunctival lymphomas; orbital lymphoma had an intermediate prognosis; and lid lesions had the worst prognosis. In an overview of ocular adnexal tumors, Knowles and colleagues[33] reported that the single most important and statistically significant prognostic factor was the extent of disease at the time of presentation with the ocular adnexal lesion. B cells produce surface immunoglobulins, particularly L26, that can be detected in paraffin sections. Both the light chains (kappa or lambda), and the heavy chains (M, G, A, D, or E) of the immunoglobulins can be stained by immunoperoxidase or immunofluorescence techniques. T cells that are responsible for cell-mediated immunity have cell subsets, including helper, suppressor, and natural killer cells, that are better demonstrated in frozen unfixed tissue but can also be detected in paraffin sections using antibodies against T cell surface antigens such as UCHL-1. The results of light and electron microscopy and immunohistochemical staining should be correlated with a careful clinical history, physical evaluation, and followup to accurately determine prognostic implications.

Well-differentiated monoclonal B cell tumors have approximately a 10% possibility of being part of a systemic disease process, whereas poorly differentiated B cell neoplasms have a higher than 50% likelihood. Polyclonal lesions have been associated with a more benign, yet fully understood, prognosis.

Van der Gaag[34] reviewed immunologic responses in the eyelid and the orbit: A local response dependent on the presence of lymphoid tissues is present in the conjunctival tissue and in the lacrimal gland but not in the orbit. A local immune response is also present in the palpebral conjunctiva. In addition to lymphocyte cell markers studies used in the histologic assessment of lymphoid lesions, other useful techniques are imprint smears as well as cell sorter analysis by flow cytometry. The term *polyclonal* indicates that there is an admixture of B and T lymphocytes, with different immunoglobulins characterizing the B cells. In most benign pseudolymphomatous orbital hyperplasia there is a predominance of T cells that can be further identified by the sheep erythrocyte rosetting formation or by alpha-naphthyl acetate esterase (ANAE) reactions. The evaluation of the nuclear outlines is helpful histologically because neoplastic T lymphocytes often display hyperchromatic nuclei, whereas reactive non-neoplastic T lymphocytes are generally rounded in configuration.

Lymphoid lesions of the orbit tend to present initially without inflammatory clinical signs. Patients are generally in their 5th and 6th decades, and these tumors are relatively rare in childhood, when leukemia tends to be more common. The lesions tend to occur most frequently in the superior orbit and can be suspected in the computed tomographic scan. In contrast with idiopathic inflammatory pseudotumors, lymphoid lesions are usually localized masses, although they can invade the optic nerve.[35] In the orbit most lymphomas are of the non-Hodgkin's variety because Hodgkin's disease rarely involves the lacrimal gland or orbital soft tissue and then only in advanced stages of the disease. Hodgkin's disease shows the typical binucleated Reed-Sternberg cells. The Epstein-Barr virus has been detected in paraffin-embedded tissues of Hodgkin's disease using in situ hybridization and polymerase chain reaction.[36] The T cell lymphoma as exemplified by mycosis fungoides is rare in the eyelid and conjunctiva and is extremely rare in the orbit.[37] According to the Rappaport classification of non-Hodgkin's lymphoma, there are four recognized categories, as follows:

1. Low grade, consisting of well-differentiated small lymphocytic or follicular type
2. Intermediate grade, with larger follicles and a diffuse histiocytic type
3. High grade, with immunoblastic plasmacytoid type and Burkitt's lymphoma
4. A miscellaneous group including hairy cell leukemia, mycosis fungoides, and malignant histiocytosis

Some examples of non-Hodgkin's lymphoma are illustrated as follows: (1) multiple myeloma, (2) plasmacytoid tumor, and (3) benign plasmacytomas of the orbit. Multiple myeloma is related in a sense to malignant lymphomas because the plasma cell is derived from a highly differentiated type of the B lymphocyte.

Leukemias

Leukemias are diseases that originate in the bone marrow and then involve the blood stream and multifocal organ and soft tissue sites. The most common orbital leukemic involvement is granulocytic disease such as acute lymphocytic leukemia in children and chronic lymphocytic leukemia in adults. Granulocytic differentiation is characterized by the presence of esterase and lysosomal cytoplasmic enzymes. These can be demonstrated by the Leder stain; histiomonocytic cells show reactivity with esterase and ANAE. It has been found that proptosis associated with leukemia is relatively rare, particularly with the use of systemic chemotherapy. Because the orbit has fenestrated blood vessels, chemotherapeutic agents can have access to the extravascular spaces that harbor tumor cells. In certain advanced cases, unilateral or bilateral proptosis can develop in rapidly growing tumors. The electron microscopy of acute monocytic leukemia is characterized by distinctive cytoplasmic organelles with a tubular complex composed of cylindrical aggregates of rough endoplasmic reticulum around a central dilated cisterna. Leukemic cells usually display vesicular nuclei without the coarse heterochromatin of lymphoma cells.

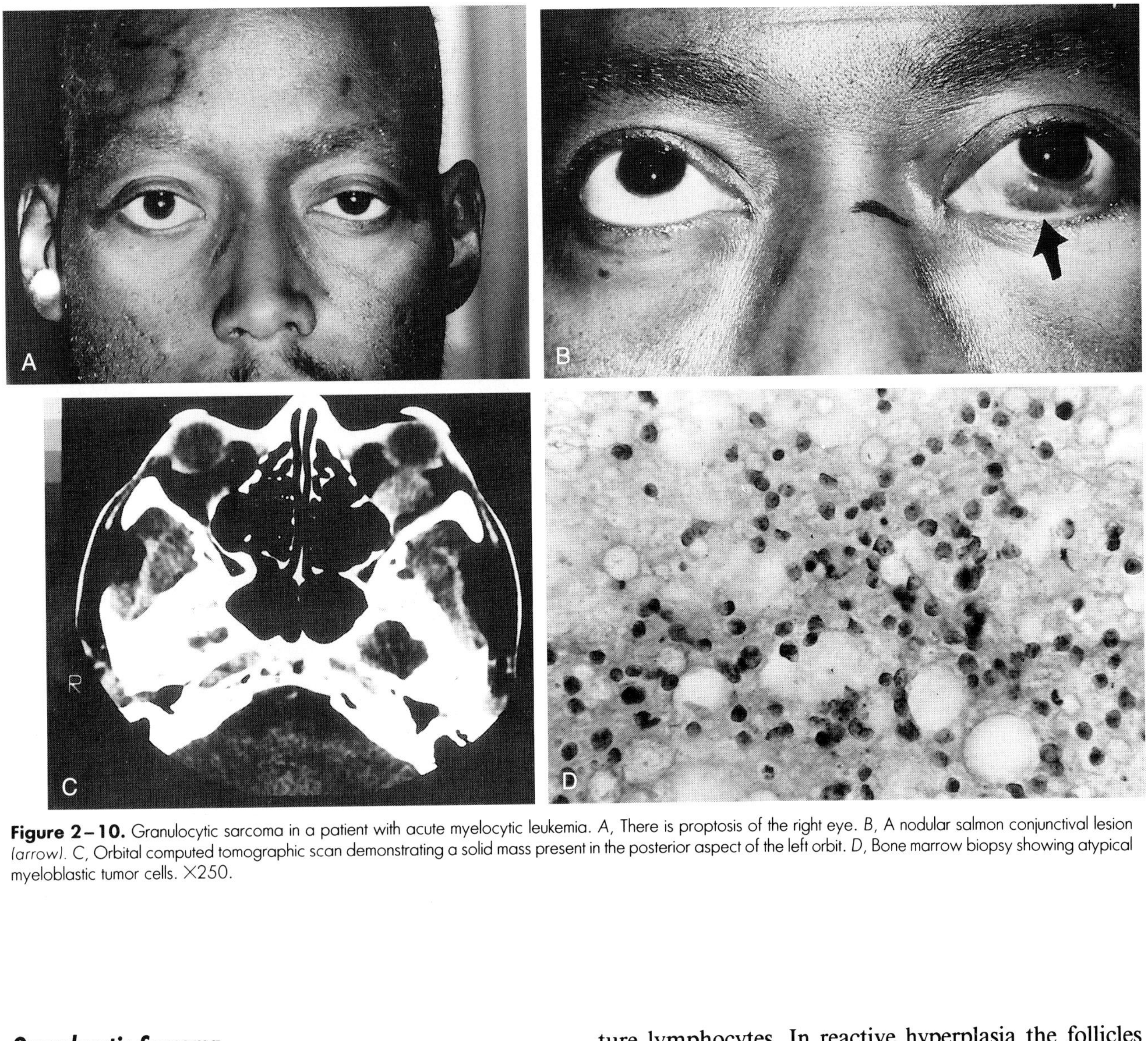

Figure 2–10. Granulocytic sarcoma in a patient with acute myelocytic leukemia. *A*, There is proptosis of the right eye. *B*, A nodular salmon conjunctival lesion (arrow). *C*, Orbital computed tomographic scan demonstrating a solid mass present in the posterior aspect of the left orbit. *D*, Bone marrow biopsy showing atypical myeloblastic tumor cells. ×250.

Granulocytic Sarcoma

The tumor known as *granulocytic sarcoma* has been referred to as a *chloroma* in the past because of the greenish hue observed clinically as a result of myeloperoxidase activity (Fig. 2–10). Histologically, the diagnosis is made by observing large, undifferentiated round tumor cells. The Leder stain for esterase or immunohistochemical stains for lysosomes such as muramidase and ANAE can establish cytoplasmic differentiation and lysosomal inclusions. Early diagnosis is extremely important so that the appropriate chemotherapy can be started before peripheral blood involvement occurs.

Benign Reactive Lymphoid Hyperplasia

Benign reactive lymphoid hyperplasia is characterized by having prominent germinal centers with a mixture of central large blastic cells and a peripheral mantle of mature lymphocytes. In reactive hyperplasia the follicles tend to be irregularly shaped, and there is a peripheral admixture of plasma cells, histiocytes, or eosinophils with a polymorphic pattern. There is also considerable capillary endothelial proliferation.

In atypical lymphoid hyperplasia there is a borderline lesion characterized by a monomorphous sheet or diffusely proliferating lymphoid cells that may be somewhat larger than the mature lymphocytes. There are abortive follicles, and in many lesions, mitotic activity may be sparse or absent. Some of these lesions cannot be conclusively diagnosed; they are in a so-called "gray zone" and require further followup. In a malignant lymphoma the lesions are generally diffuse proliferations with only 10% showing a follicular pattern. The tumors are composed of poorly differentiated or sometimes less well-differentiated cells. Mitotic activity is not as marked in the germinal centers as in reactive benign lymphoid hyperplasia. Endothelial cell proliferation is also not prominent.

However, even orbital lesions diagnosed as benign reactive lymphoid hyperplasia have a 15% to 25% possibility of systemic disease. Lesions diagnosed as atypical lymphoid hyperplasia have approximately a 40% chance of extraorbital disease after 5 years. In contrast, lesions diagnosed as malignant lymphoma have a higher than 60% likelihood of being associated with systemic disease after 5 years. A 10-year mortality rate for atypical lymphoid hyperplasia ranges from 19% to 34%, but reactive lymphoid hyperplasia stays constant at 6%.[33]

Mycosis Fungoides

Mycosis fungoides is a type of cutaneous lymphoma that has three stages clinically: erythematous, placoid, and tumor.[38] In patients with biopsy-proved mycosis fungoides, those with lid involvement usually have multiple lid tumors, including conjunctival involvement. In the microscopic examination of the erythematous stage, there are nonspecific changes similar to those in other inflammatory dermatoses. In the placoid stage the histologic changes consist of a polymorphic cellular infiltrate composed of histiocytes, eosinophils, plasma cells, lymphoid cells, and lymphoid reticulum cells known as *mycosis cells.* The latter display hyperchromatic nuclei and scant cytoplasm. The small mycosis cell (Lutzner's cell) shows a lobulated nuclear membrane that is quite characteristic. Epidermal involvement by the atypical cell infiltrate shows mycosis cells arranged singularly or in small clusters known as *Pautrier's microabscesses.* In the tumor stage the infiltrate is composed of large atypical anaplastic cells with a monomorphic appearance that may closely resemble other malignant lymphomas of the skin.

Sinus Histiocytosis with Lymphadenopathy

In sinus histiocytosis there is generally bilateral proptosis. Usually, children are affected, but involvement can also occur in adults (Fig. 2–11).[39] There is generally marked generalized lymphadenopathy with sparing of the viscera and the skin. Histologically, there are sheets of histiocytic cells with vesicular nuclei and abundant cytoplasm. There may be phagocytosis of lymphocytes and erythrocytes, and the histiocytic sheets are separated sometimes by mature lymphoid tissue. Occasionally, a follicular appearance is present. In the orbit the histiocytes and lymphocytes may be randomly dispersed in the orbital soft tissues. The disease is self-limited and does not respond well to radiotherapy or chemotherapy. The overall prognosis is good.

Plasma Cell Tumors

Multiple myeloma is associated with multifocal lesions involving the bone marrow and affects the orbit and lymph nodes, producing punched-out lesions in the skull. In this condition the plasma cells are recognized by the eccentrically placed nucleus with a cartwheel pattern and may be associated with amyloid deposits.[40] Lymphoplasmacytoid tumors are composed of cells that resemble both lymphocytes and plasma cells and secrete immunoglobulins (Fig. 2–12). An example of this entity is Waldenström's macroglobulinemia, which is associated with the production of immunoglobulin M. Serum and urine electrophoresis can establish some of the immunoglobulin abnormalities involved.

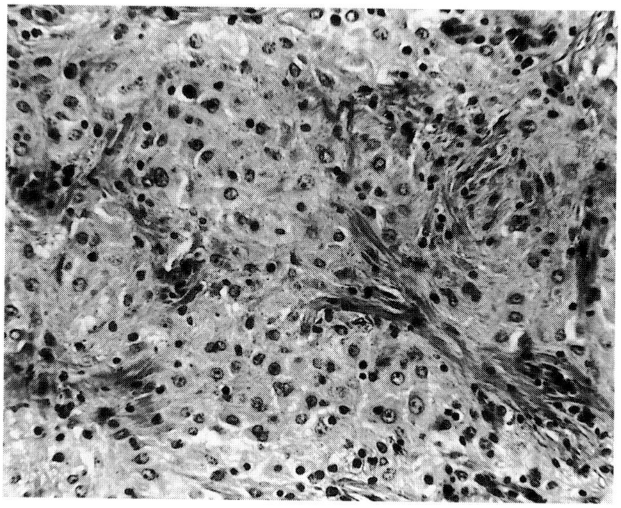

Figure 2–11. Sinus histiocytosis. The tumor cells display a follicular pattern consisting of pale histiocytic cells and a proliferation of lymphocytes. ×200.

Histiocytic Disorders

The orbit can be involved in a variety of disorders, including (1) eosinophilic granuloma (Fig. 2–13); (2) sinus histiocytosis with massive lymphadenopathy[39]; (3) juvenile xanthogranuloma; (4) Erdheim-Chester disease; and (5) pseudorheumatoid nodule. Eosinophilic granuloma and other entities have been referred to in the past as *histiocytosis X.* However, it is now recognized that there is no histopathologic difference between the localized and disseminated forms of this disease in which there is an involvement of histiocytes and other inflammatory cells. This entity is also sometimes referred to as *Langerhans' cell histiocytosis.* This condition generally affects younger people within the 1st decade of life with involvement of the orbit, visceral organs, lymph nodes, and cutaneous lesions. In older children, the triad of lytic skull defects, proptosis, and diabetes insipidus is known as *Hand-Schüller-Christian disease.* In eosinophilic granuloma there is a predilection for the superior temporal bone at the orbital rim with irregular lytic skull lesions. Light microscopic examination shows large, pale histiocytic cells with folded nuclei and occasional giant cells as well as considerable infiltrates of eosinophils, lympho-

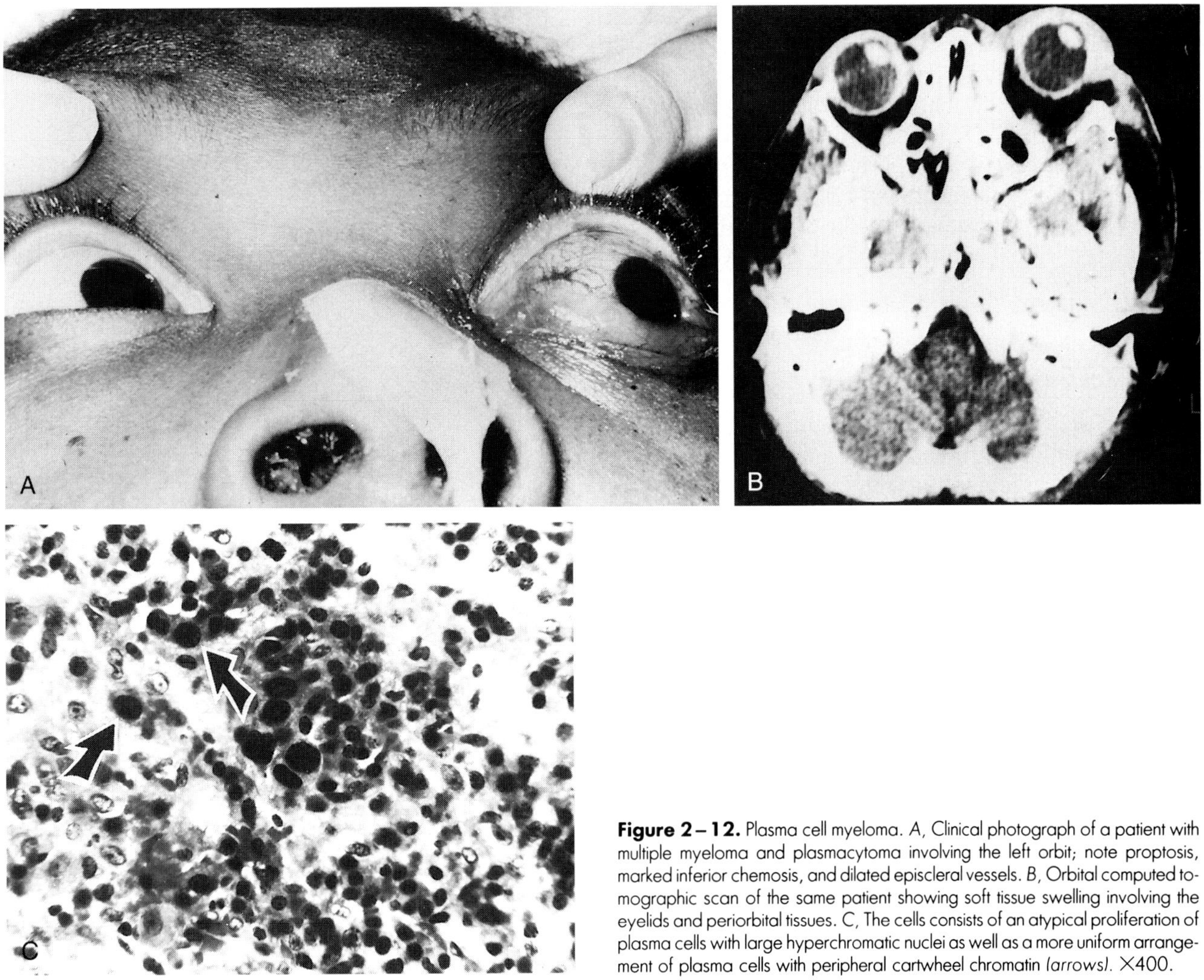

Figure 2–12. Plasma cell myeloma. *A*, Clinical photograph of a patient with multiple myeloma and plasmacytoma involving the left orbit; note proptosis, marked inferior chemosis, and dilated episcleral vessels. *B*, Orbital computed tomographic scan of the same patient showing soft tissue swelling involving the eyelids and periorbital tissues. C, The cells consists of an atypical proliferation of plasma cells with large hyperchromatic nuclei as well as a more uniform arrangement of plasma cells with peripheral cartwheel chromatin *(arrows)*. ×400.

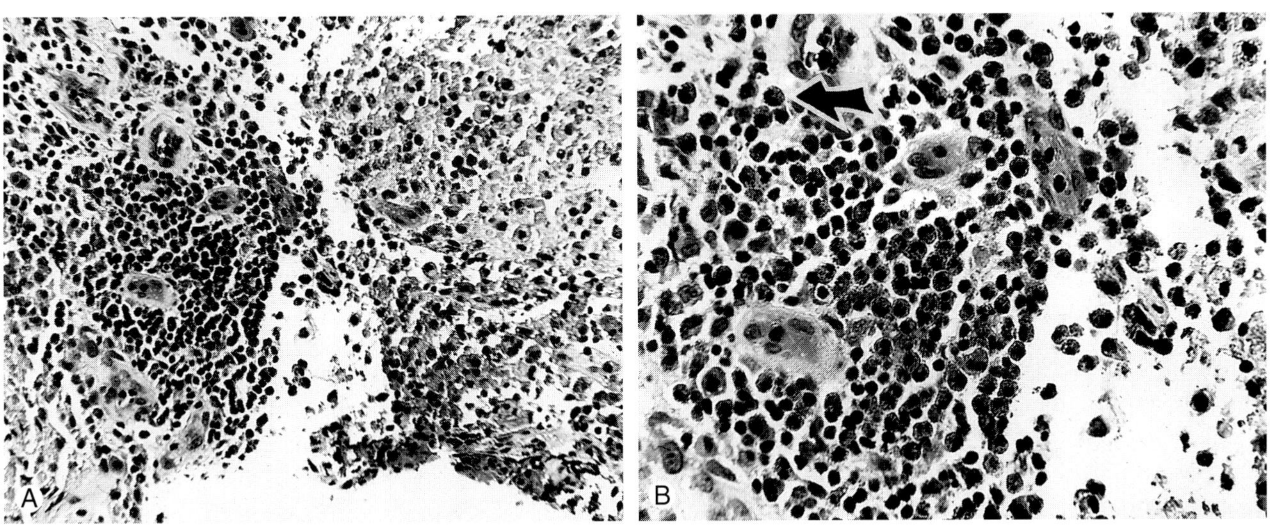

Figure 2–13. Eosinophilic granuloma (*A* and *B*). The cells are composed of an accumulation of eosinophils with bilobed nuclei and granular cytoplasm (*arrow* in *B*). *A*, ×200; *B*, ×400.

cytes, and plasma cells. The lesion is often associated with hemorrhage because of the rich vascularity and lipidization that can occur in some cells. There are also scattered Langerhans' cells that are macrophages characterized by cytoplasmic rod-like inclusions known as *Birbeck granules* that have a typical appearance when viewed by electron microscopy. Langerhans' cells are a type of macrophage that stains positive with the S-100 protein and with the monoclonal antibody OKT-6 and are normally present in the conjunctiva.[41]

Juvenile Xanthogranuloma

Juvenile xanthogranuloma is a condition that characteristically involves the eyelid and skin with modular yellow lesions. It is frequently accompanied by iris involvement that often results in hyphema. The histologic appearance is characterized by the Touton giant cell, a multinucleated cell with a paracentral ring-like accumulation of nuclei and peripheral vacuolated cytoplasm containing lipid material. There are adjacent aggregates of lymphocytes and plasma cells. These lesions respond to systemic steroids and low dosages of radiation.

Erdheim-Chester Disease

Orbital involvement by Erdheim-Chester disease is rare and is characterized by orbital lesions causing retinal stria, optic atrophy, ophthalmoplegia, and xanthelasma-like lid lesions. Histologically, the lesions are composed of histiocytic cells with occasional Touton giant cells and scattered lymphocytes and plasma cells (Fig. 2–14). The histiocytic cells have abundant pale cytoplasm containing lipid material and small, centrally placed nuclei. The

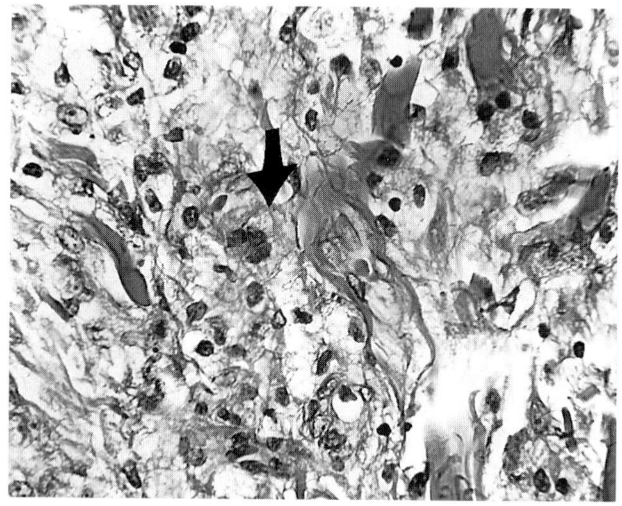

Figure 2–14. Erdheim-Chester disease. The cell infiltrate consists of Touton giant cells *(arrow)* with peripheral foamy cytoplasm and vacuolated histiocytes. ×200.

condition can be confused with inflammatory pseudotumors and should be suspected in patients with bilateral proptosis and xanthelasma-like lesions. Treatment with systemic corticosteroids can result in some improvement of the proptosis.

Sarcoidosis

Sarcoidosis is a systemic disease that affects the visceral organs, lymph nodes, skin, salivary glands, lacrimal glands, sinuses, central nervous system, and lungs. Intraocular involvement also occurs. However, not all cases of orbital sarcoidosis are associated with systemic disease: in some older people the involvement may be unilateral and localized to the orbit (Fig. 2–15). In the orbit, the lac-

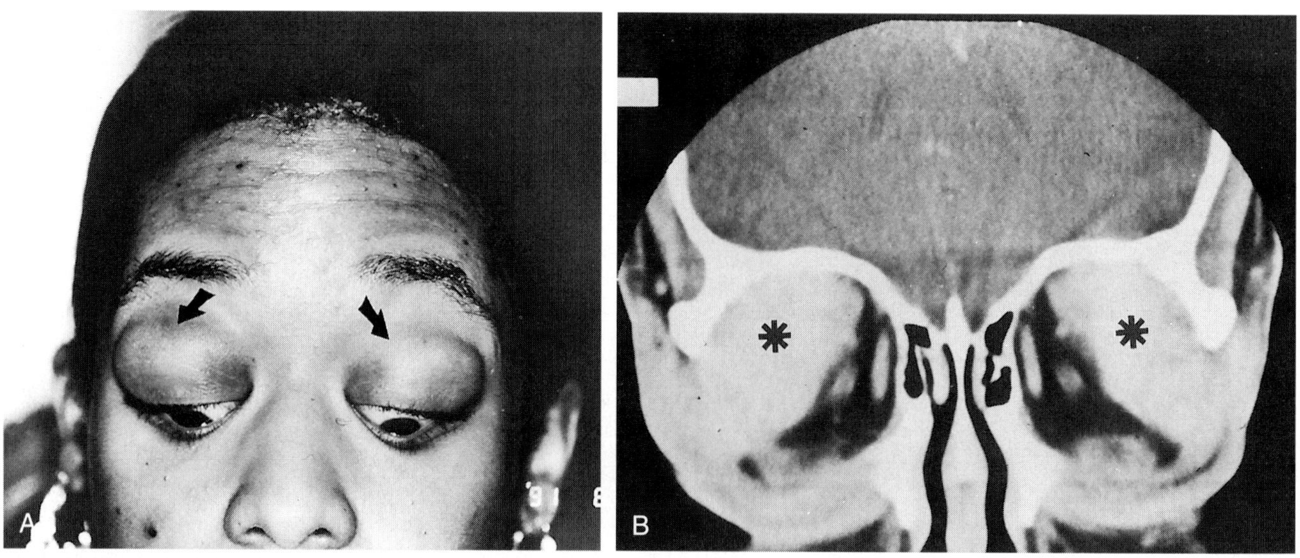

Figure 2–15. Orbital sarcoidosis. *A*, Sarcoidosis showing bilateral superior orbital nodular involvement *(arrows)*. *B*, Computed tomographic scan showing an orbital lesion with massive bilateral lacrimal gland involvement *(asterisks)*.

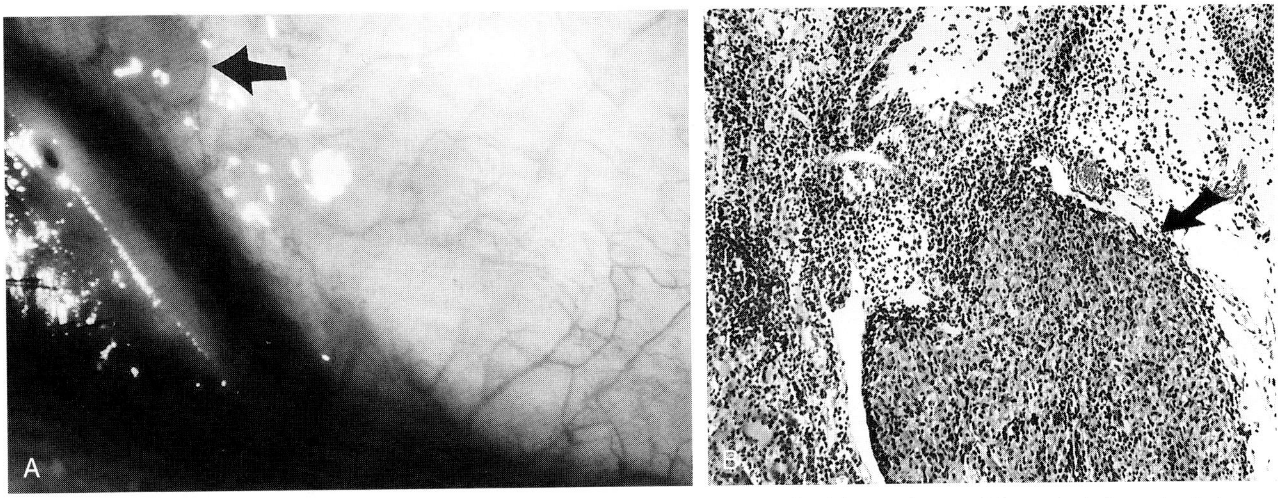

Figure 2–16. *A*, Conjunctival sarcoid with a nodular lesion in the inferior fornix *(arrow)*. *B*, Areas of nodular granulomatous inflammation in the conjunctival stroma *(arrow)*. ×100.

rimal gland is most frequently involved. Gallium scanning is useful in the detection of this involvement. Enlargement of the hilar lymph nodes can be detected by chest radiographs, which can also demonstrate the presence of pulmonary infiltrates. Blood studies for angiotensin-converting enzyme and hypercalcemia may be useful. The Kveim test (cutaneous injection of sarcoid antigen) is also used as a diagnostic test. Random conjunctival biopsies of patients with suspected sarcoidosis may be positive in approximately 25% of subjects, who can thus be spared higher-risk invasive techniques such as transbronchial biopsy and mediastinoscopy.[42] Conjunctival involvement manifests as visible yellowish-gray nodules in the fornices, and a biopsy can readily establish the diagnosis (Fig. 2–16). A biopsy of the lacrimal gland can be performed through the lid, and a biopsy of the deeper orbital lobe rather than the superficial palpebral lobe can be done.[43] Histopathologically, the lesions are composed of noncaseating aggregates of histiocytes with scattered multinucleated giant cells and lymphocytes at the periphery. There are also cytoplasmic inclusions known as *asteroid bodies* and *Schaumann's bodies.* In the immunohistochemical characterization of sarcoid, T lymphocytic helper cells appear to be localized in the central areas, whereas at the periphery there are usually T suppressor cytotoxic cells. Sarcoidosis can be managed with high dosages of prednisone for several months followed by a tapering of these dosages.

Amyloidosis

The eyelids and conjunctivae as well as the orbit may be involved in primary systemic amyloidosis. However, the eyelid skin is the primary site of predilection for this disease. Secondary localized amyloidosis is characterized by accumulation of amyloid in the conjunctiva and orbit (Fig. 2–17). Histologically, the amyloid deposits are

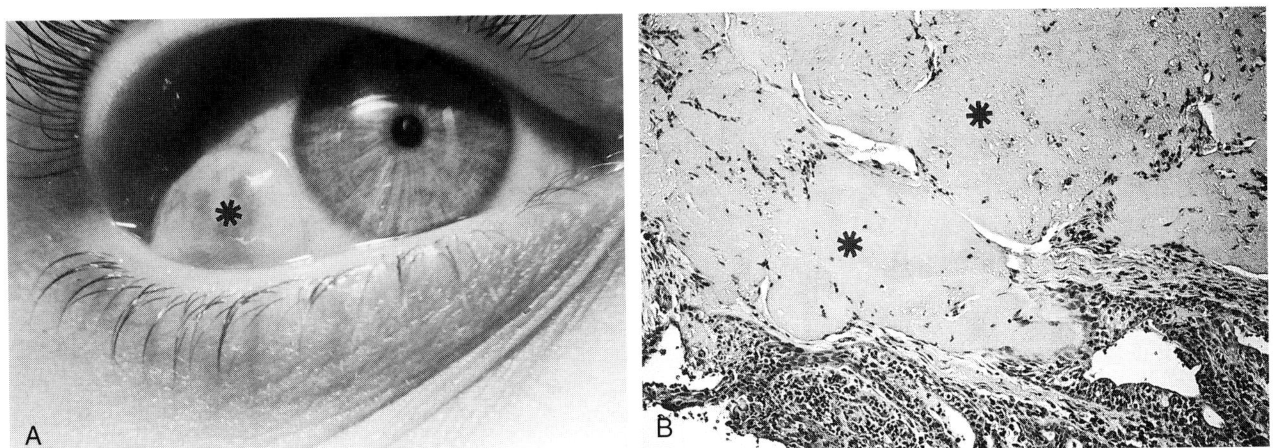

Figure 2–17. Conjunctival amyloid. *A*, Nodular conjunctival lesion *(asterisk)*. *B*, Subepithelial accumulation of amorphous material that stained positive with Congo red and was birefringent with polarized light *(asterisks)*. ×250.

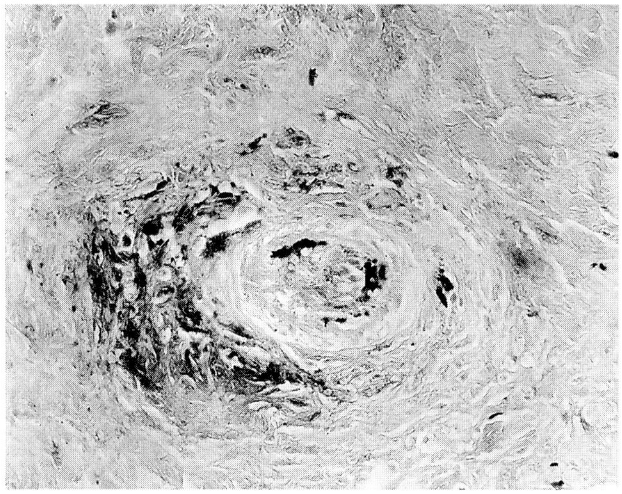

Figure 2–18. Idiopathic midline granuloma. The lesion shows peripheral palisading of histiocytic infiltrates and marked necrosis of the soft tissues. ×80.

characterized by accumulation of amyloid proteins that stain with Congo red and show dichroism with polarized light. Electron microscopy displays the typical 9- to 10-nm–diameter randomly oriented filaments.

Idiopathic Midline Destructive Disease

IMDD is one of a rare number of disorders once designated as the *midline granuloma syndrome* (Fig. 2–18).[44] These conditions, which include Wegener's granulomatosis, malignant reticulosis, nasal carcinoma, and lymphoma, manifest as a variable degree of upper airway obstruction. Orbital and ocular involvement occur due to obstruction of the nasolacrimal ducts and the proximity of the orbits to the nasopharynx with extension of the disease into the orbits. These lesions can also involve the eyelids and brow, as reported by Chu and associates.[44] Microscopic examination shows areas of sclerosis, loss of cellularity, and nodular zones of fibrinoid necrosis adjacent to blood vessels. The results of examination with special stains for fungi and bacteria are usually negative. There appears to be a gray zone between lesions that are considered IMDD and Wegener's granulomatosis: IMDD is a disease of the midline face and upper airways, whereas Wegener's granulomatosis is a systemic lesion involving the kidneys and lower respiratory tract in addition to the face. The skin of the nose is usually disrupted in IMDD but is preserved in Wegener's granulomatosis. The two entities must be distinguished because localized radiotherapy is the treatment of choice in IMDD, whereas cyclophosphamide and corticosteroids are used for the treatment of Wegener's granulomatosis. Thus, IMDD appears to be a rare, chronic inflammatory disorder mainly resulting in necrosis of the midline face and upper airways.

Wegener's Granulomatosis. Orbital involvement is among the most common ophthalmic lesions in the classic or limited forms of Wegener's granulomatosis (Fig. 2–19).[45] Accurate histologic interpretation is essential for diagnosis and treatment. The classic triad of histopathologic features in Wegener's granulomatosis including vasculitis, tissue necrosis, and granulomatous inflammation is seen in 54% of patients with this disorder. Clinical correlation with the antinuclear cytoplasmic antigen test and histopathology are essential for diagnosis.

Xeroderma Pigmentosum

Xeroderma pigmentosum is a rare autosomal recessive systemic disorder. Cutaneous manifestations of the affected patients are sun sensitivity, xerosis, pigmentary anomalies including both depigmentation and hyperpig-

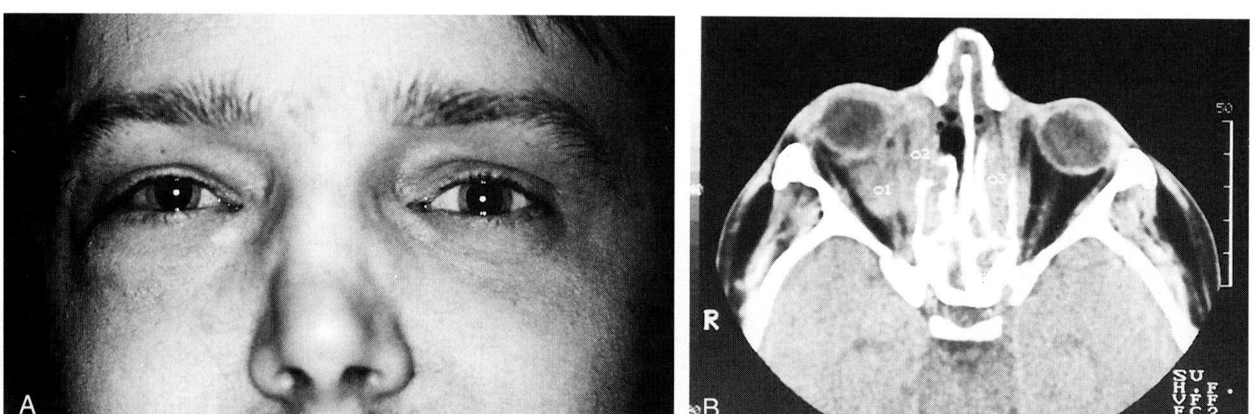

Figure 2–19. *A*, A 24-year-old patient with Wegener's granulomatosis involving the right orbit and sinuses; note the nasal deformity and right globe dystopia. *B*, Computed tomographic image of the same patient showing bony destruction of the sinus walls, the nasal cavity, and the vomer; note the soft tissue involvement of the sinuses, the right orbit, the lacrimal system, and the nasal cavity.

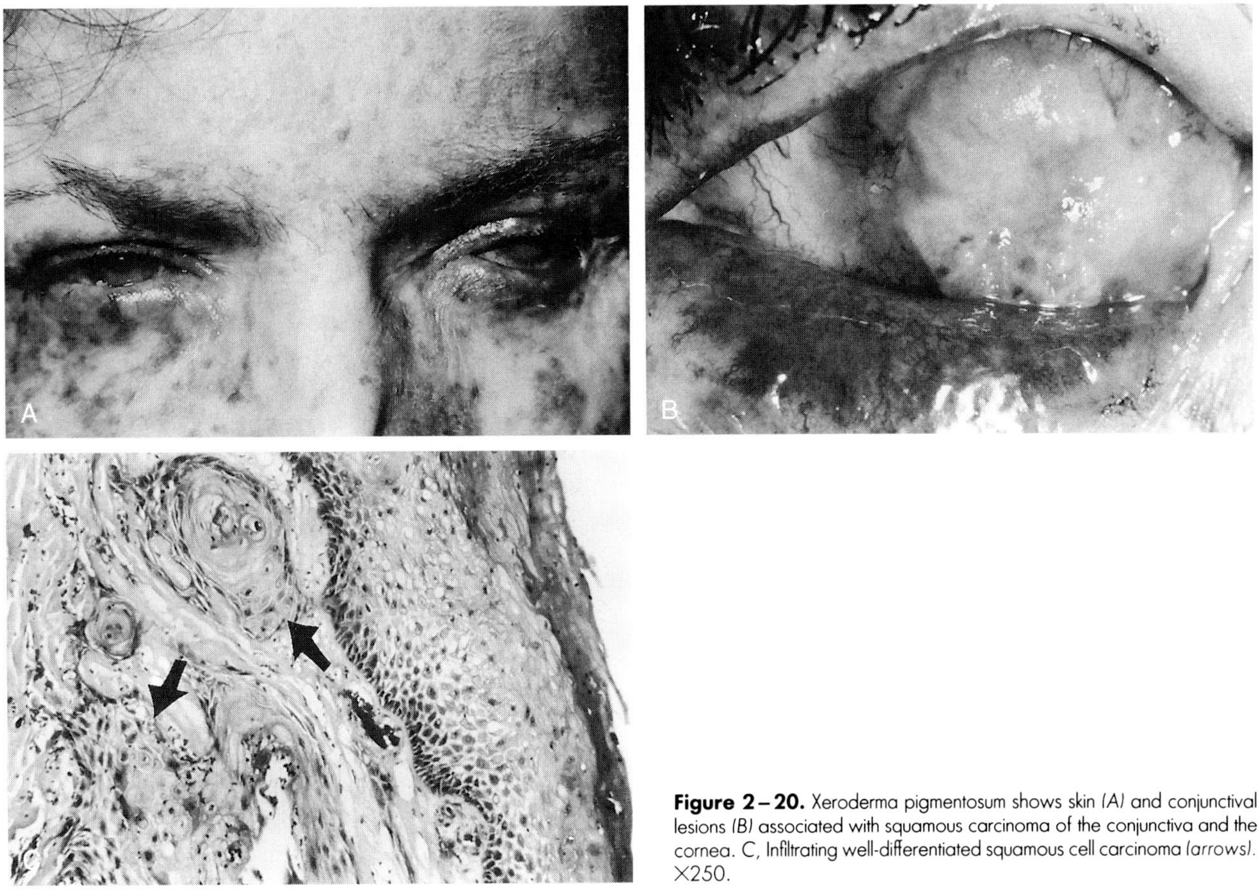

Figure 2–20. Xeroderma pigmentosum shows skin *(A)* and conjunctival lesions *(B)* associated with squamous carcinoma of the conjunctiva and the cornea. C, Infiltrating well-differentiated squamous cell carcinoma *(arrows)*. ×250.

mentation, and benign and malignant tumor formation of sun-exposed areas. Malignancies of the eyelids and conjunctivae occur in most of the patients and are considered a major manifestation of the disease. Patients with xeroderma pigmentosum have defective repair of DNA after ultraviolet light–induced damage associated with sun sensitivity and the development of multiple cutaneous tumors. Conjunctival tissues are involved in the DNA repair defect. The eyelids, conjunctiva, and cornea are involved in this disease (Fig. 2–20).[46] The lid lesions include basal cell carcinoma, squamous cell carcinoma, and malignant melanoma. In some instances, squamous cell carcinoma from the conjunctiva can infiltrate the cornea, as reported by Gaasterland and associates.[46]

Pseudorheumatoid Nodules

Pseudorheumatoid nodules generally occur in otherwise healthy children without evidence of systemic rheumatic disease. Reports of epibulbar and orbital disease have shown necrobiotic granulomas of areas of palisading fibroblasts and epithelioid cells. There is no evidence of fibrinoid necrosis.

Rare Skin and Mucous Membrane Lesions

Basal Cell Nevus Syndrome

Basal cell nevus syndrome is an autosomal dominant disease with variable penetrance characterized by multiple basal cell carcinomas involving the eyelids, lips, nose, and ears (Fig. 2–21). Other features of this entity include palmar and plantar pits, mandibular cysts, frontal bossing, ectopic cranial calcification, and, occasionally, medulloblastoma. Treatment includes surgical excision of skin lesions. Isotretinoin may be effective in preventing the development of basal cell carcinoma in basal cell nevus syndrome.[47]

Dysplastic Nevus Syndrome

Dysplastic nevi are an important indicator of risk of cutaneous and ocular malignant melanoma (Fig. 2–22). Since the original description of dysplastic nevi in 1978,[48] attempts have been made to characterize the clinical and histologic features of this entity. The major histologic

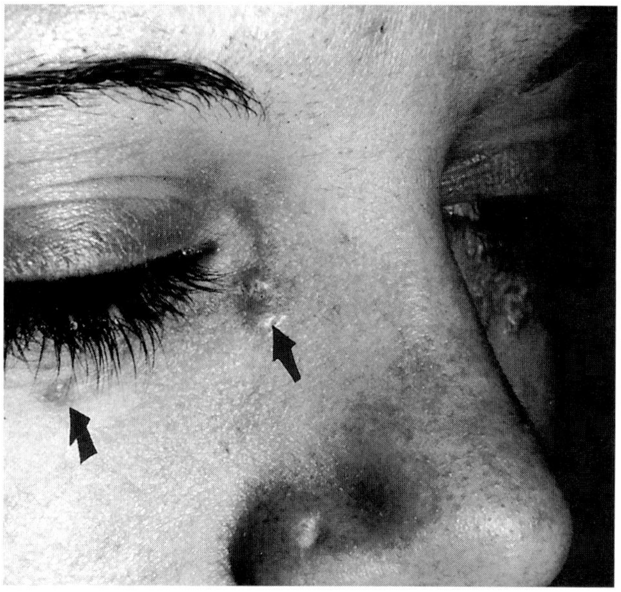

Figure 2–21. Basal cell nevus syndrome. Nodular lesions of the medial canthus and the lower lid are shown *(arrows)*.

criteria established by the World Health Organization Melanoma Program are as follows:

1. Basilar proliferation of atypical nevomelanocytes (extending at least three rete ridges or "pegs" beyond any dermal nevocellular component)
2. Organization of this proliferation in a lentiginous or epithelioid cell pattern

Ackerman[49] disputed the original concept of dysplastic nevi as precursors of melanoma and suggested that most lesions diagnosed as dysplastic nevi are in fact melanoma in situ, thus accounting for the progression of dysplastic nevi to melanoma.[49–51] This controversy is not yet entirely resolved.[51]

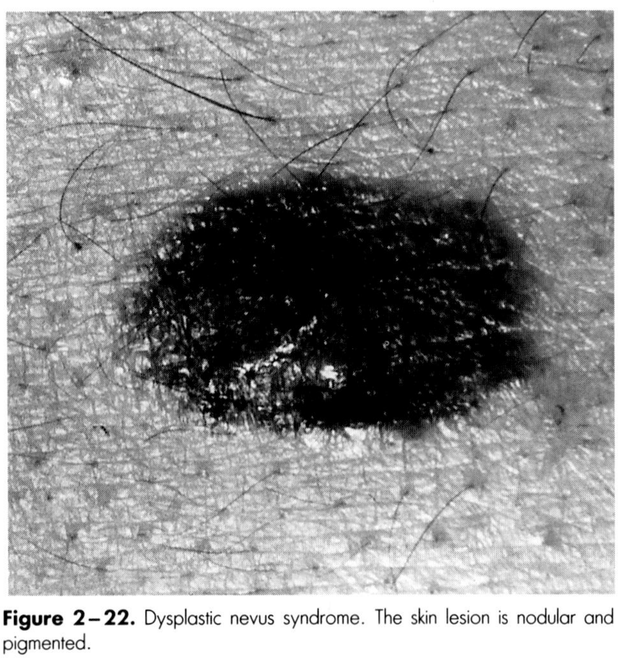

Figure 2–22. Dysplastic nevus syndrome. The skin lesion is nodular and pigmented.

Squamous Papilloma

Orbital involvement can occasionally be secondary to a schneiderian (inverted) papilloma of the paranasal sinuses.[52] Recurrent sessile conjunctival papilloma can be associated with several dysplasias (Fig. 2–23) and can cause nasolacrimal duct obstruction.[52] Conjunctival papillomas are frequently associated with human papillomavirus types 2 and 6, demonstrated by polymerase chain reaction and in situ hybridization.[53] The role of human papillomavirus in conjunctival dysplasias and malignant transformation is unclear.[54]

Secondary Tumors

Secondary tumors are neoplasms that are derived from ocular lesions or from the sinuses, conjunctivae, or lids with secondary orbital invasion. The most common site of a carcinoma invading the orbit is from an adjacent sinus, with the antrum the most frequent site of origin followed by the ethmoid and frontal sinuses. Histopathologically, most of these lesions are squamous cell carcinoma, moderately or poorly differentiated, with solid lobules of epithelial-like cells. The second most common source of secondary epithelial invasion of the orbit is from basal cell and squamous cell carcinoma from these sites and also from malignant melanoma.

Mucoepidermoid Carcinoma

Mucoepidermoid carcinoma of the lacrimal gland is a tumor containing both squamous (epidermoid) and mucin-secreting cells (Fig. 2–24).[55] This tumor is relatively rare in the lacrimal gland and the conjunctiva.[56]

Adenoid Cystic Carcinoma

Adenoid cystic carcinoma of the lacrimal gland is a highly malignant epithelial tumor associated with perineural infiltration of orbital tissue (Fig. 2–25), including the extraocular muscles.[38] Bone changes occur in about 80% of the patients, and tumor invasion of the superior orbital tissue and temporal fossa have been observed. Histologically, the neoplastic cells can appear deceptively bland with a basaloid or cribriform pattern surrounded by fibrosis and basement membrane material. A worse prognosis was reported with basaloid tumor growth in one study[38] but was not confirmed by others.[57] Mortality is due to intracranial spread resulting from perineural in-

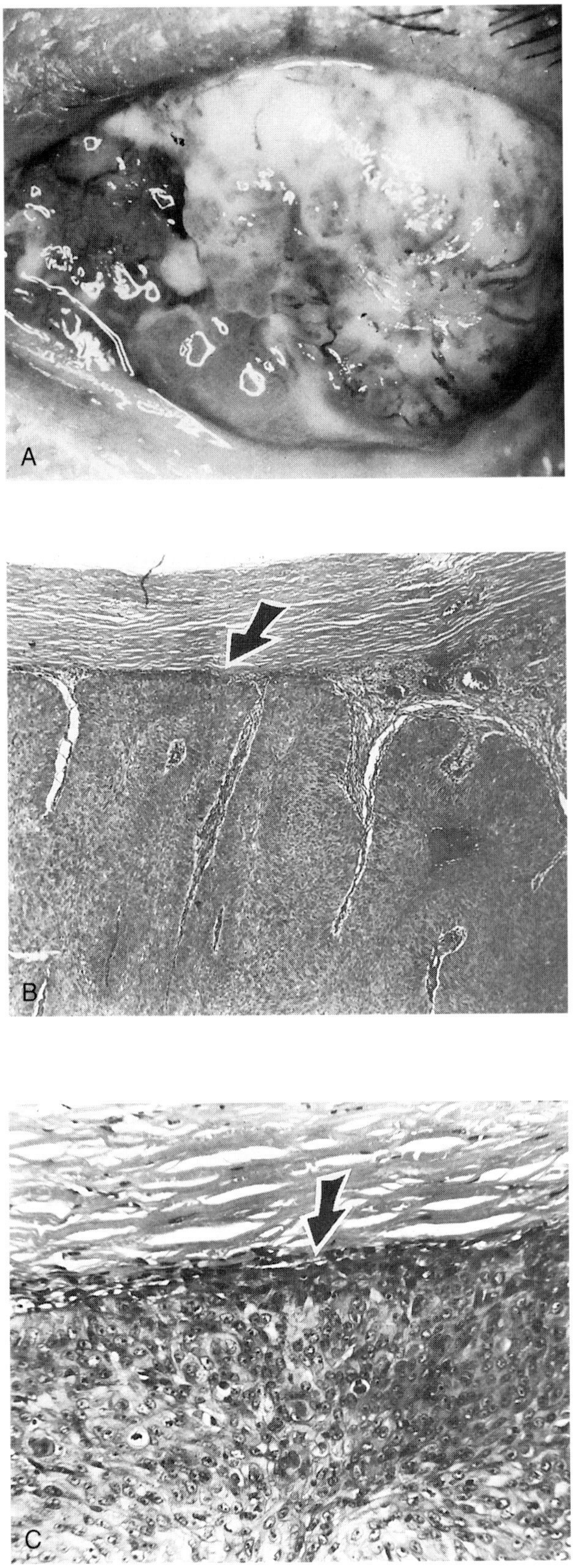

Figure 2–23. Recurrent conjunctival squamous papilloma. *A*, Clinical appearance shows a large fungating epibulbar lesion. (*A* courtesy of Dr. Richard Smith.) *B* and *C*, Histologic appearance of atypical extensions of dysplastic squamous epithelium (*arrows*). *B*, ×40; *C*, ×200.

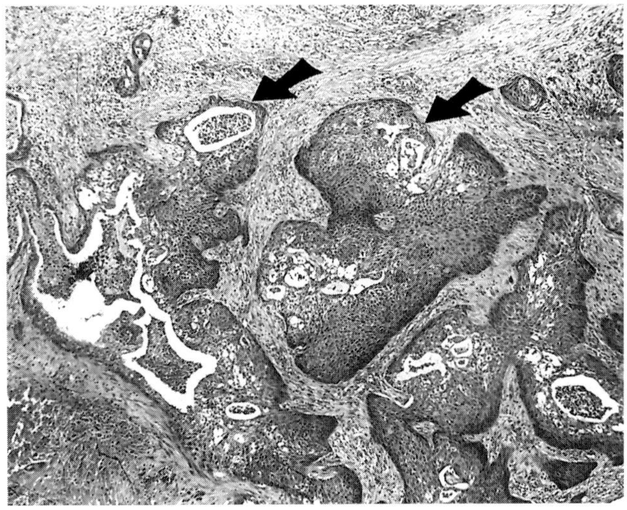

Figure 2–24. Mucoepidermoid carcinoma invading the nasal ethmoid sinus. The tumor is composed of infiltrating lobules of squamous epithelium with scattered mucin-secreting cystic and intracytoplasmic areas (*arrows*). ×40.

vasion through the superior orbital tissue into the middle cranial fossa. Because of the poor results with exenteration alone, some surgeons have used a single en bloc excision, whereas others have recommended exenteration with orbitectomy. Adjunctive postoperative radiotherapy has also been advocated. Considerable controversy exists regarding management of this tumor.

Limbal Tumors

Limbal tumors include melanocytic lesions, benign and malignant squamous cell lesions, lymphoid tumors, and solid dermoids. Garner[58] reported that more than 50% of the lesions in a series of 636 limbal lesions from

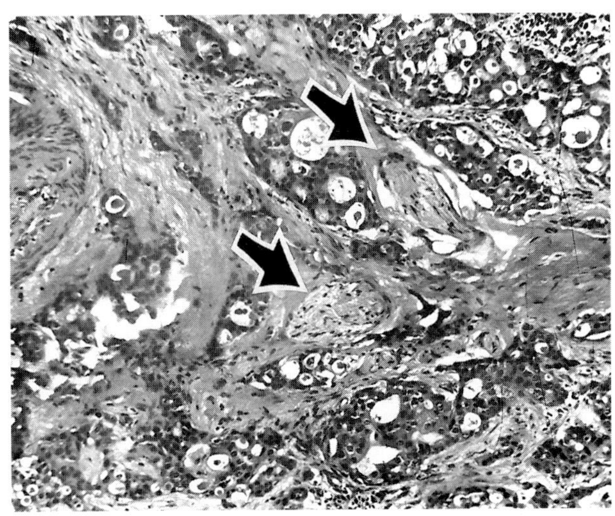

Figure 2–25. Adenoid cystic carcinoma of the lacrimal gland showing perineural invasion (*arrows*). ×100.

the Institute of Ophthalmology involved melanocytes. Approximately 20% of the tumors were of squamous origin, mainly squamous carcinoma (73 patients) and rare papillomas. Solid dermoids constituted 10% of all limbal tumors.[58]

SUMMARY

Orbital and adnexal tumors are a heterogenous group of neoplasms in which clinicopathologic correlation and ancillary radiologic studies, laboratory tests, and histologic studies are of paramount importance in establishing an accurate diagnosis. Improved diagnostic techniques, including immunohistochemistry and the polymerase chain reaction, are extremely valuable tools that can facilitate this process.

REFERENCES

1. Goldberg RA, Rootman J, Cline RA: Tumors metastatic to the orbit: A changing picture. Surv Ophthalmol 35:1–24, 1990.
2. Taveras JL, Haik BG: Magnetic resonance imaging in ophthalmology. *In* Masters BR (ed): Noninvasive Diagnostic Techniques in Ophthalmology. New York, Springer-Verlag, 1990, pp 32–46.
3. Peyster RG, Shapiro MD, Haik BG: Orbital metastasis: Role of magnetic resonance imaging and computed tomography. Radiol Clin North Am 25:647–662, 1987.
4. Dresner SC, Kennerdell JS, Dekker A: Fine-needle aspiration biopsy of metastatic orbital tumors. Surv Ophthalmol 27:397–398, 1983.
5. McGuire WL: Current status of estrogen receptors in human breast carcinoma. Cancer 36:638–644, 1975.
6. Fenoglio-Preiser CM, Willman CL: Molecular Diagnostics in Pathology. Baltimore, Williams & Wilkins, 1990, p 167.
7. Liotta LA: Cancer cell invasion and metastasis. Sci Am 266:54–63, 1992.
8. Henderson JW, Farrow GM: Metastatic carcinoma. *In* Henderson JW (ed): Orbital Tumors, 2nd ed. New York, Brian C Decker, 1980, pp 451–471.
9. Ferry AP, Font RL: Carcinoma metastatic to the eye and orbit: Clinical pathologic study of 227 cases. Arch Ophthalmol 92:276–286, 1974.
10. Jenson OA: Metastatic tumors of the eye and orbit: A histopathological analysis of a Danish series. Acta Pathol Microbiol Scand (Suppl) 212:201–214, 1970.
11. Freedman MI, Folk JC: Metastatic tumors to the eye and orbit: Patient survival and clinical characteristics. Arch Ophthalmol 105:1215–1220, 1987.
12. Shields CL, Shields JA, Peggs M: Tumors metastatic to the orbit. Ophthalmol Plast Reconstr Surg 4:73–80, 1988.
13. Reese AB: Expanding lesions of the orbit [Bowman Lecture]. Trans Ophthalmol Soc UK 91:85–104, 1971.
14. Rodrigues MM, Font RL, Shannon G: Metastatic mucous-secreting mammary carcinoma of the eyelid. Br J Ophthalmol 58:877–882, 1974.
15. Friedman J, Karesh J, Rodrigues M, Sun C-C: Thyroid carcinoma metastatic to the medial rectus muscle. Ophthalmol Plast Reconstr Surg 6:122–128, 1990.
16. Capone A Jr, Slamovits TL: Discrete metastasis of solid tumors to extraocular muscles. Arch Ophthalmol 108:237–243, 1990.
17. Lubin JR, Grove AS Jr, Zakov ZN, et al: Hepatoma metastatic to the orbit. Am J Ophthalmol 89:268–273, 1980.
18. Bond JB, Wesley RE, Reynolds VH, et al: Orbital metastasis from cutaneous melanoma. South Med J 79:1439–1442, 1986.
19. Spector B, Klintworth GK, Wells SA Jr: Histologic study of the ocular lesions in multiple endocrine neoplasia syndrome type IIb. Am J Ophthalmol 91:204–210, 1981.
20. Kinoshita S, Tanaka F, Ohashi Y, et al: Incidence of prominent corneal nerves in multiple endocrine neoplasia type IIA. Am J Ophthalmol 111:307–311, 1991.
21. Kanitakis J, Hermier C, Chouvet B, Thivolet J: Reactivity of HMB-45 monoclonal antibody with sweat gland tumors of the skin. Acta Derm Venereol 71:426–428, 1991.
22. Hancock C, Allen BC, Herrera GA: HMB-45 detection in adenocarcinoma. Arch Pathol Lab Med 115:886–890, 1991.
23. McDonnell JM, Sun YY, Wagner D: HMB-45: Immunohistochemical staining of conjunctival melanocytic lesions. Ophthalmology 98:453–458, 1991.
24. Waldman TA: Monoclonal antibodies in diagnosis and therapy. Science 252:1657–1662, 1992.
25. Riddle PJ, Font RL, Zimmerman LE: Carcinoid tumors of the eye and orbit: A clinicopathologic study with histochemical and electron microscopic observations. Arch Ophthalmol 13:459–469, 1982.
26. Shetlar DJ, Font RL, Ordonez N, et al: A clinicopathologic study of three carcinoid tumors metastatic to the orbit. Ophthalmology 97:257–264, 1990.
27. Alexander KR, Fishman GA, Peachey NS, et al: "On" response defect in paraneoplastic night blindness with cutaneous malignant melanoma. Invest Ophthalmol Vis Sci 33:477–483, 1992.
28. Sugar A: Paraneoplastic pemphigus and ophthalmology. Ophthalmology 99:5–6, 1992.
29. Knowles DM, Halper JP, Jakobiec FA: The immunologic characterization of 40 extranodal lymphoid infiltrates: Usefulness in distinguishing between benign pseudolymphoma and malignant lymphoma. Cancer 49:2321–2335, 1982.
30. Jakobiec FA, Neri A, Knowles DM II: Genotypic monoclonality in immunophenotypically polyclonal orbit lymphoid tumors: A model of tumor progression in the lymphoid system. Ophthalmology 94:980–994, 1987.
31. Jakobiec FA, Knowles DM: An overview of ocular adnexal lymphoid tumors. Trans Am Ophthalmol Soc 87:420–442, 1990.
32. Finfer M, Jakobiec FA: Extranodal noncutaneous lymphoid hyperplasias represent a continuous spectrum of B-cell neoplasia: Demonstration by molecular genetic analysis. Blood 73:1635–1645, 1989.
33. Knowles DM, Jakobiec FA, McNally L, Burke JS: Lymphoid hyperplasia and malignant lymphoma occurring in the ocular adnexa (orbit, conjunctiva and eyelids): A prospective multiparametric analysis of 108 cases during 1977 to 1987. Hum Pathol 21:959–973, 1990.
34. Van der Gaag R: Immunological responses in the eyelid and orbit. Eye 2:158–163, 1988.
35. Christmas N, Mead MD, Richardson EP, Albert DM: Secondary optic nerve tumors. Surv Ophthalmol 36:196–206, 1991.
36. Weiss LM, Chen Y-Y, Liu X-F, Shibata D: Epstein-Barr virus and Hodgkin's disease: A correlative in situ hybridization and polymerase chain reaction study. Am J Pathol 139:1259–1265, 1991.
37. Lauer SA, Fischer J, Jones J, et al: Orbital T-cell lymphoma in human T-cell leukemia virus-1 infection. Ophthalmology 95:110–114, 1988.
38. Jakobiec FA, Font RL: Orbit. *In* Spencer WH, Font RL, Green WR, et al (eds): Ophthalmic Pathology: An Atlas and Textbook, 3rd ed, vol 3. Philadelphia, WB Saunders, 1986, pp 2459–2860.
39. Friendly DS, Font RL, Rao NA: Orbital involvement in sinus histiocytosis. Arch Ophthalmol 95:2006–2011, 1977.
40. Rodman HI, Font RL: Orbital involvement in multiple myeloma: Review of the literature and report of three cases. Arch Ophthalmol 87:30–35, 1972.
41. Rodrigues MM, Rowden G, Hackett J, Bakos I: Langerhans' cells in the normal conjunctiva and peripheral cornea of selected species. Invest Ophthalmol Vis Sci 21:759–762, 1981.
42. Karcioglu ZA, Brear R: Conjunctival biopsy in sarcoidosis. Am J Ophthalmol 99:68–73, 1985.
43. Weinreb RN: Diagnosing sarcoidosis by transconjunctival biopsy of the lacrimal gland. Am J Ophthalmol 97:573–576, 1984.
44. Chu FC, Rodrigues M, Cogan DG, Fauci AS: The pathology of idiopathic midline destructive diseases in the eyelid. Ophthalmology 90:1385–1390, 1984.
45. Kalina PH, Qie JT, Campbell RJ, Garrity JA: Diagnostic value and limitations of orbital biopsy in Wegener's granulomatosis. Ophthalmology 99:120–124, 1992.
46. Gaasterland D, Rodrigues M, Moshell A: Ocular changes in xeroderma pigmentosum. Ophthalmology 89:980–986, 1982.

47. Goldberg LH, Hsu SH, Alcalay J: Effectiveness of isotretinoin in preventing the appearance of basal cell carcinomas in basal cell nevus syndrome. J Am Acad Dermatol 21:144–145, 1989.
48. Clark WH Jr, Reimer RR, Green MH, et al: Origin of familial malignant melanomas from heritable melanocytic lesions: The B-K mole. Arch Dermatol 114:732–738, 1978.
49. Ackerman AB: What nevus is dysplastic, a syndrome, and the commonest precursor of malignant melanoma? A riddle and an answer. Histopathology 13:241–256, 1988.
50. Vink J, Crijns MB, Mooy CM, et al: Ocular melanoma in families with dysplastic nevus syndrome. J Am Acad Dermatol 23:858–862, 1990.
51. Cook MG, Fallowfield ME: Dysplastic naevi—an alternative view. Histopathology 16:29–35, 1990.
52. Migliori ME, Putterman AM: Recurrent conjunctival papilloma causing nasolacrimal duct obstruction. Am J Ophthalmol 110:17–22, 1990.
53. McDonnell JM, McDonnell PJ, Sun YY: Human papillomavirus DNA in tissues and ocular surface swabs of patient with conjunctival epithelial neoplasia. Invest Ophthalmol Vis Sci 33:184–189, 1992.
54. McDonnell JM, Wagner D, Ng ST, et al: Human papillomavirus type 16 DNA in ocular and cervical swabs of women with genital tract condylomata. Am J Ophthalmol 112:61–66, 1991.
55. Levin LA, Popham J, To K, et al: Mucoepidermoid carcinoma of the lacrimal gland: Report of a case with oncocytic features arising in a patient with chronic dacryops. Ophthalmology 98:1551–1555, 1991.
56. Margo CE, Groden LR: Intraepithelial neoplasia of the conjunctiva with mucoepidermoid differentiation. Am J Ophthalmol 108:600–601, 1989.
57. Lee DA, Campbell RJ, Waller RR, Ilstrup DM: A clinicopathologic study of primary adenoid cystic carcinoma of the lacrimal gland. Ophthalmology 92:128–134, 1985.
58. Garner A: The pathology of tumors at the limbus. Eye 3:210–217, 1989.

CHAPTER 3

Disorders of Eyelid Function Caused by Systemic Disease

Gerald G. Striph and Neil R. Miller

A variety of systemic and neurologic diseases produce disorders of eyelid function, particularly eyelid retraction and ptosis. It is important to recognize these disorders to separate them from the more common local conditions such as levator dehiscence and dysthyroid orbitopathy so that affected patients can be managed appropriately. In this chapter, we discuss the common systemic and neurologic conditions that may affect eyelid position and movement.

EYELID RETRACTION

Neuropathic

Supranuclear: The Dorsal Mesencephalic Syndrome

Supranuclear lesions may cause both true and simulated eyelid retraction. True supranuclear neuropathic eyelid retraction is most often caused by a lesion near the posterior commissure in the dorsal mesencephalon and is usually part of a more extensive neurologic disturbance called the *dorsal midbrain syndrome* (DMS). This condition, which is also called Parinaud's syndrome, the sylvian aqueduct syndrome, or the dorsal mesencephalic syndrome, most often results from extrinsic pressure on the structures of the dorsal mesencephalon in patients with congenital or acquired hydrocephalus or masses in the region of the pineal gland, such as pinealomas, astrocytomas, and germ cell tumors. Numerous other extrinsic and intrinsic tumors in this region can produce the same clinical picture, however, such as multiple sclerosis, closed-head trauma, bulbar poliomyelitis, Landry-Guillain-Barré syndrome, Fisher's syndrome, epidemic encephalitis, and mesencephalic infarction. The clinical history, other symptoms and signs, as well as neuroimaging findings will differentiate among these distinct causes.

The presenting complaint in patients with DMS is variable. Frequently, patients experience difficulty in rapid upward gaze that they notice while at work, playing sports, or after reading. On examination, upward slow eye movements (pursuit movements) may seem normal in both velocity and range, but upward fast eye movements (saccades) are slow, limited, and often accompanied by convergence and retraction of the globes into the orbit (convergence-retraction nystagmus). In severe cases, both upward pursuit and saccades are abnormal. The abnormality of upward eye movements seen in DMS is almost always associated with bilateral eyelid retraction (*Collier's sign*[1]) (Fig. 3–1), but it occasionally may seem to be unassociated with any abnormality of eye movement. Other neurologic disturbances associated with DMS are pupils that may be anisocoric and often have a reduced or absent reaction to light stimulation but a normal or near-normal reaction to near stimuli. Downward gaze deficiencies are a late finding in DMS, and third and fourth nerve palsies may eventually cause diplopia. Since eyelid retraction may be the first overt finding in a patient with DMS, a careful neurologic examination is warranted in addition to the usual screening for thyroid disease (the most common cause of eyelid retraction).

The eyelid retraction that occurs in DMS can easily be differentiated from that which occurs in dysthyroid orbitopathy. It is maintained in upward gaze as well as in primary position; and, unlike the eyelid retraction of dysthyroid orbitopathy, there is no lid lag when the patient looks downward (Figs. 3–2 and 3–3). As the eye moves downward, levator tonus is smoothly decreased and the lid follows the eye down normally. Proptosis is also not present in DMS but is a frequent finding in thyroid disease. The difficulties with upward gaze that occur in patients with DMS can best be detected by inducing *voluntary* upward saccades. The use of an optokinetic drum or tape rotating or moving downward to produce upward saccades is quite useful in bringing out not only the difficulties with upward gaze but also the convergence-retraction nystagmus that may accompany them.

Supranuclear eyelid retraction is occasionally seen in conditions other than DMS. Episodic supranuclear eyelid retraction has been described in a boy with "chorea"[2] and in a patient with impending tentorial herniation.[3] Vertical movements by oculocephalic testing (doll's eye maneuver) were preserved in this child, thus confirming

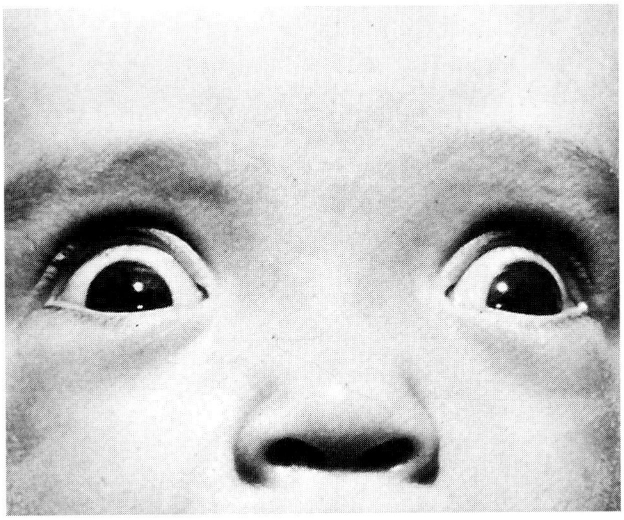

Figure 3–1. Collier's sign. Bilateral eyelid retraction in an infant with communicating hydrocephalus. Upward movements of the eyes were also limited. (From Miller NR: Walsh and Hoyt's Clinical Neuro-ophthalmology, 4th ed, vol 2. Baltimore, Williams & Wilkins, 1985, p 946.)

the supranuclear location. Clonic lid retraction can also occur during attacks of myoclonic or petit mal seizures. Clonic bilateral lid retraction in association with spastic downward deviation of the eyes has been reported in infants. These findings disappear after several weeks.[4]

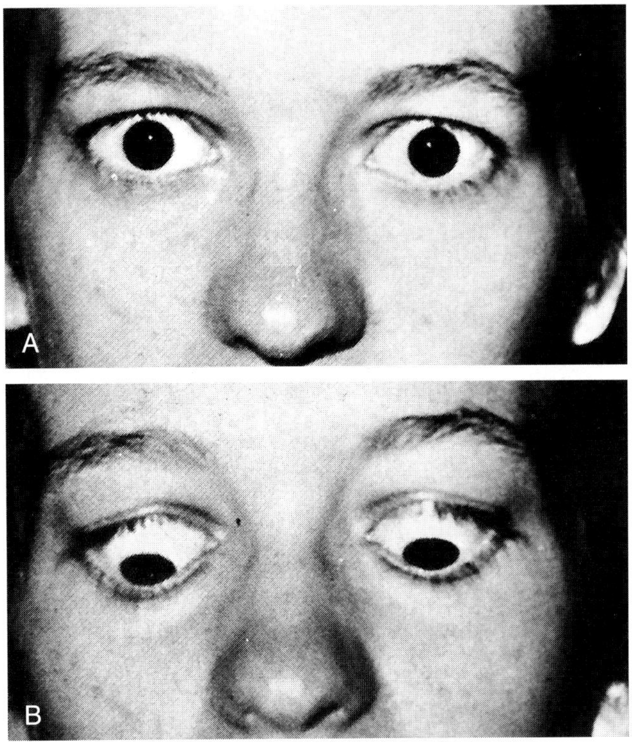

Figure 3–3. Bilateral eyelid retraction (*A*) and lid lag on downward gaze (*B*) in a patient with dysthyroid orbitopathy. (From Miller NR: Walsh and Hoyt's Clinical Neuro-ophthalmology, 4th ed, vol 2. Baltimore, Williams & Wilkins, 1985, p 953.)

Nuclear and Infranuclear Lesions

In 1883, Robert Marcus Gunn[5] described a patient whose eyelid retracted during opening of the mouth and certain movements of the jaw. Since this report, many patients have been described in whom congenital unilateral or bilateral eyelid retraction is associated with various actions of the facial muscles (Fig. 3–4). These represent abnormal congenital interconnections between the trigeminal nerve nuclei or nerve branches and the oculomotor subnucleus or nerve branches subserving the levator muscle. In the resting state, affected patients usually have unilateral or bilateral ptosis. The eyelid elevates in response to movement of the internal or, more commonly, the external pterygoid (trigemino-oculomotor synkinesis). Occasionally, synkineses with other cranial nerves may result in unusual movements of the eyelid during other activities, such as tongue protrusion.

Acquired jaw-winking and related abnormal movements can occur from aberrant regeneration of damaged peripheral cranial nerve axons. The injury that causes such a phenomenon is usually a crushing blow to the orbit.

Eyelid retraction can occur during horizontal eye movements. Like the eyelid retraction that occurs during facial movements, this condition may be congenital or acquired. There is, in most normal persons, some physiologic synkinesis between the portion of the oculomotor

Figure 3–2. Collier's sign in a young man with a dorsal mesencephalic syndrome. *A*, The patient has mild bilateral eyelid retraction when looking straight ahead. *B*, On attempted upward gaze, the eyes do not elevate, but the eyelids elevate normally, producing marked eyelid retraction and stare. *C*, On attempted downward gaze, the eyelids move normally with the eyes. There is no retraction or lag. (From Miller NR: Walsh and Hoyt's Clinical Neuro-ophthalmology, 4th ed, vol 2. Baltimore, Williams & Wilkins, 1985, p 946.)

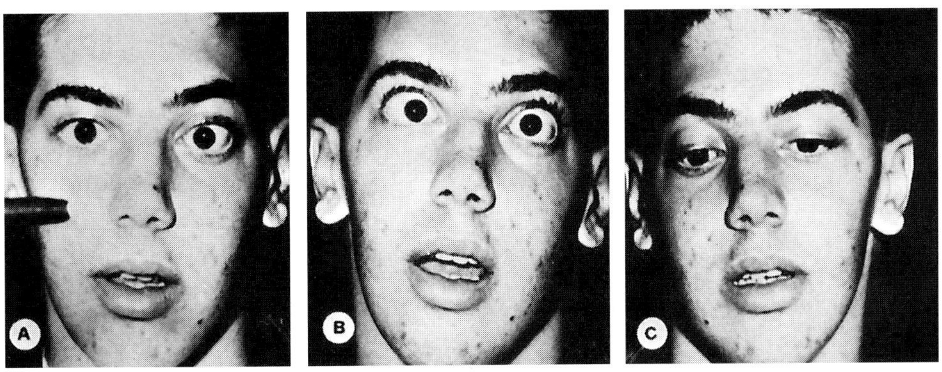

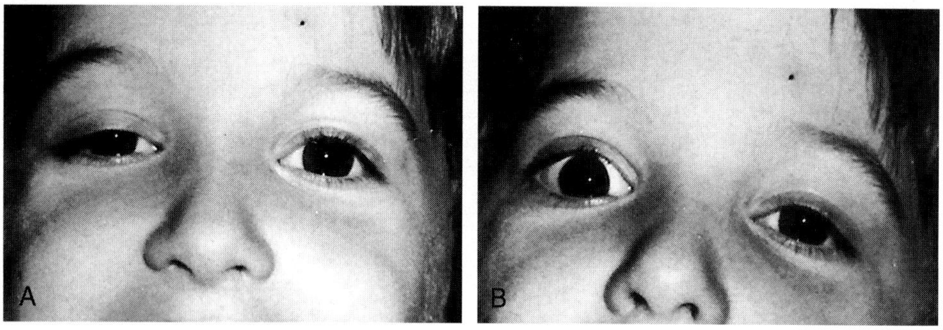

Figure 3–4. The Marcus Gunn jaw-winking phenomenon. *A*, The patient has a congenital right ptosis. *B*, When the patient moves her mouth to the left side, the right upper eyelid elevates, and the ptosis disappears. (Courtesy of Dr. Nicholas Iliff.)

nerve system that innervates the levator palpebrae superioris and the abducens nerve system. This synkinesis probably occurs in the brain stem. The result of this synkinesis is that there is a slight degree of retraction of the eyelids during attempted horizontal gaze (Fig. 3–5). This retraction may increase significantly on the side of an abducens nerve paresis when the patient attempts to look toward that side (Fig. 3–6). Marked retraction of the eyelids during horizontal gaze may also occur in patients with certain congenital syndromes associated with oculomotor synkineses, such as Duane's retraction syndrome,[6] and in both congenital and acquired cases of misdirected regeneration of the oculomotor nerve. In the latter, the levator often contracts during attempted adduction or depression of the eye, producing mild to marked eyelid retraction (pseudo-Graefe's sign) (Fig. 3–7).

Unilateral eyelid retraction can occur on the side opposite a ptotic lid as a consequence of Hering's law of equal innervation (Fig. 3–8). This contralateral eyelid retraction results from increased stimulation of the levator palpebrae superioris in an attempt to correct the ptosis. The same innervation is sent to the contralateral levator muscle, and the eyelid thus retracts. This type of eyelid retraction usually resolves when the ptotic eyelid is manually raised or the affected eye is covered, since the excess innervation is no longer necessary.

Occasionally, in the setting of a facial nerve palsy, the reduced tone in the orbicularis oculi will result in mild lid retraction. In most of these cases, however, it is lower eyelid retraction rather than upper eyelid retraction that is most prominent.

Neuromuscular

A variety of conditions may be associated with eyelid retraction on the basis of stimulation of the neuromuscular junction. Topical medications such as phenylephrine drops used for routine eye dilation may cause eyelid retraction by directly stimulating Müller's muscle. A similar mechanism may be responsible for the eyelid retraction that is produced by apraclonidine, a topical, antiglaucoma medication that is an alpha-adrenergic agonist. Anticholinesterase inhibitors may produce elevation of the eyelids in patients with myasthenia gravis by allowing accumulation of acetylcholine in the neuromuscular junction, although transient eyelid retraction may also occur in patients with myasthenia gravis for other reasons. Eyelid retraction in patients with myasthenia gravis may occur in three other settings[7]: (1) transiently, after prolonged elevation probably due to post-tetanic facilitation of the levator[8]; (2) transiently, after prolonged downward gaze (Cogan's lid twitch—see later); and (3) with contralateral ptosis—the result of a relatively normal levator palpebrae superioris responding to an increased neural signal attempting to elevate the ptotic eyelid (see Fig. 3–8). Depolarizing drugs, such as succinylcholine, can also produce eyelid retraction by causing an initial release of acetylcholine.

Myopathic

The most common myopathic cause of eyelid retraction is dysthyroid ophthalmopathy and is discussed else-

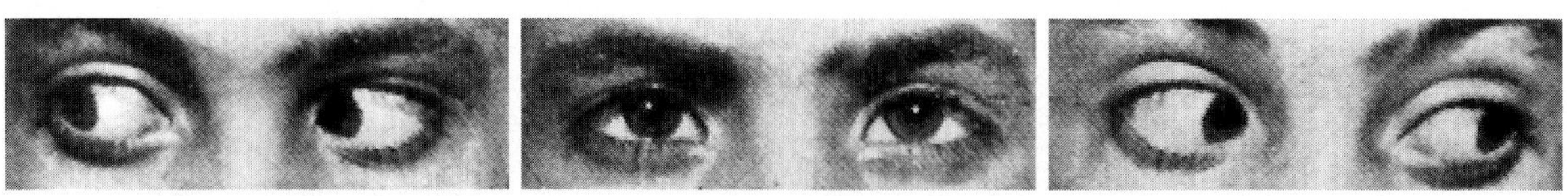

Figure 3–5. Physiologic synkinesis between normal horizontal eye movement and the eyelids. The patient has normal ocular motility but develops bilateral upper eyelid retraction during extreme rightward and leftward gaze. (From Ticho U: Synkinesis of upper lid elevation occurring in horizontal eye movements. Acta Ophthalmol 49:232–238, 1971.)

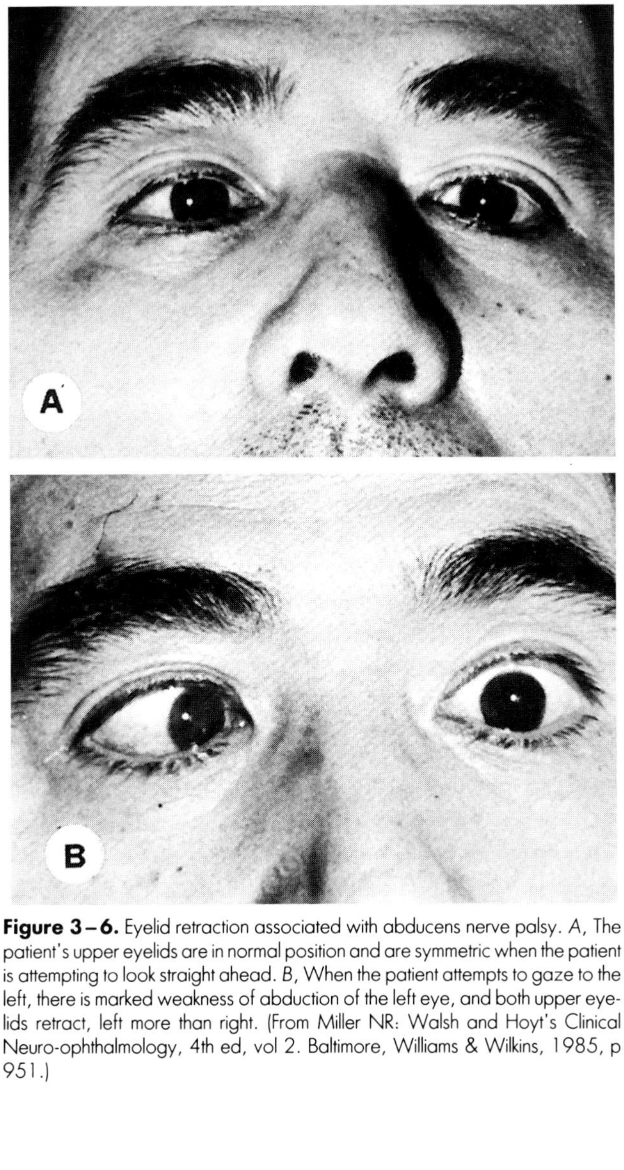

Figure 3–6. Eyelid retraction associated with abducens nerve palsy. *A*, The patient's upper eyelids are in normal position and are symmetric when the patient is attempting to look straight ahead. *B*, When the patient attempts to gaze to the left, there is marked weakness of abduction of the left eye, and both upper eyelids retract, left more than right. (From Miller NR: Walsh and Hoyt's Clinical Neuro-ophthalmology, 4th ed, vol 2. Baltimore, Williams & Wilkins, 1985, p 951.)

where in this text. Nevertheless, there are a few other myopathic causes of eyelid retraction. Patients with hepatic cirrhosis, for instance, may exhibit lid retraction (Fig. 3–9).[9, 10] The mechanism by which eyelid retraction occurs in this setting is unknown.

PTOSIS

Neuropathic

Supranuclear

Most cases of neuropathic ptosis are caused by congenital or acquired damage to the portion of the oculomotor nerve nucleus, fascicle, or peripheral nerve that supplies the levator palpebrae superioris (see later). Nevertheless, supranuclear causes of ptosis exist. They are rare but may be early presenting signs of significant central nervous system disease.

Ptosis resulting from a supranuclear lesion in the cerebral cortex is usually unilateral and contralateral to the side of the lesion. Cogan[11] described a patient with unilateral ptosis that appeared to have resulted from damage to the contralateral angular gyrus. Walsh and Hoyt[3] reported the case of an epileptic woman with a left temporal lobe seizure focus, right-sided ptosis, and no evidence of oculomotor or oculosympathetic disease (Fig. 3–10). Caplan[12] reported a series of 13 patients with ptosis from strokes caused by emboli in the distribution of the middle cerebral artery. Eight of these patients had unilateral ptosis. In six of these eight patients, the ptosis was contralateral to the side of the lesion. It was suggested by Caplan[12] that the two patients with apparent unilateral ptosis ipsilateral to the side of the lesion may have had bilateral findings masked by facial paralysis. Lowenstein and colleagues[13] reported two patients with chronic, acquired, unilateral ptosis from contralateral hemispheric arteriovenous malformations that improved with surgical removal of the vascular lesion. Afifi and associates[14] described two patients with seizure-associated miosis and ptosis with temporal lobe abnormalities that were seen using magnetic resonance imaging. One of these patients had ptosis that was contralateral to the temporal lobe defects; the other, however, had ptosis on the ipsilateral side. Afifi and associates[14] hypothesized that the contralateral ptosis and miosis were caused by the irritative effects of the temporal lobe disease and that the ipsilateral eye findings in the second patient were the result of a decrease in impulse production from the ipsilateral side, al-

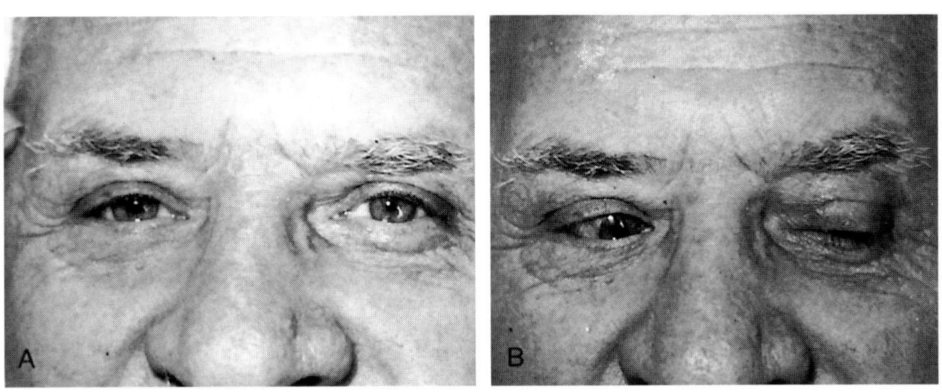

Figure 3–7. Eyelid retraction in a patient with aberrant regeneration (misregeneration) of the oculomotor nerve. *A*, In the primary position, there is a mild right ptosis. *B*, When the patient looks down and to the left, the upper eyelid retracts (pseudo-Graefe's sign). (From Miller NR: Walsh and Hoyt's Clinical Neuro-ophthalmology, 4th ed, vol 2. Baltimore, Williams & Wilkins, 1985, p 681.)

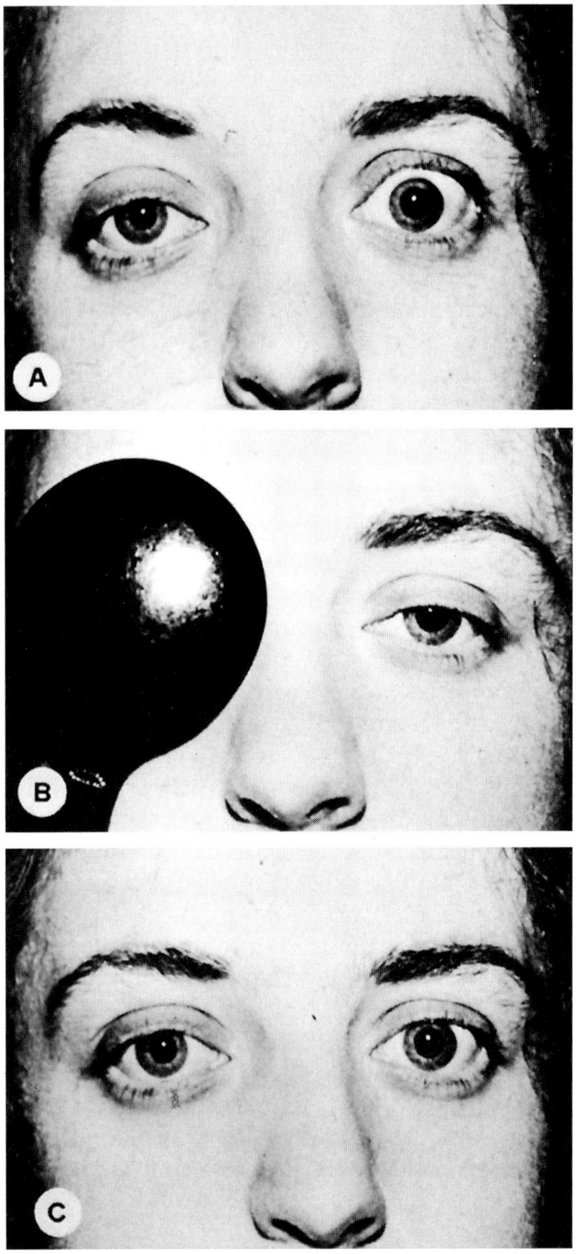

Figure 3–8. Eyelid retraction secondary to Hering's law of equal innervation in a patient with myasthenia gravis and contralateral ptosis. *A*, The patient has moderate right ptosis and left eyelid retraction. *B*, When the right eye is occluded, the left eyelid retraction disappears, and the patient actually develops left ptosis. *C*, After administration of edrophonium chloride (Tensilon), the right ptosis improves, as does the left eyelid retraction. (From Miller NR: Walsh and Hoyt's Clinical Neuro-ophthalmology, 4th ed, vol 2. Baltimore, Williams & Wilkins, 1985, p 952.)

lowing impulses from the normal, contralateral side to predominate.

Rarely, cerebral ptosis may be bilateral despite single hemisphere involvement (Fig. 3–11). As noted earlier, Caplan[12] reported a series of 13 patients with ptosis caused by emboli in the territory of the middle cerebral artery. Five of these patients had obvious bilateral ptosis, and two patients with apparent ptosis ipsilateral to the hemisphere disease were thought to have had bilateral

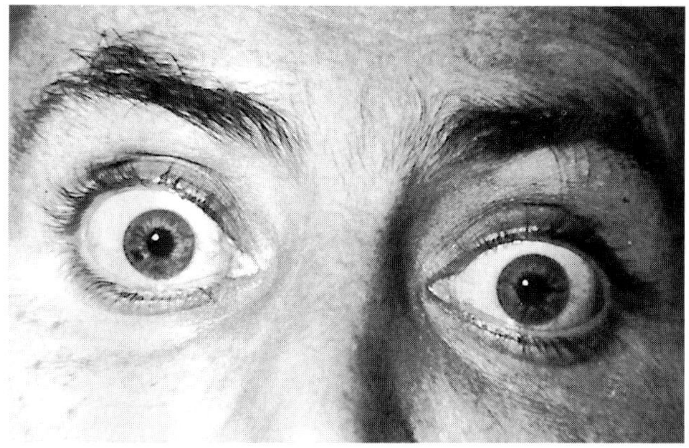

Figure 3–9. Summerskill's sign: bilateral eyelid retraction in a patient with severe hepatic disease. (From Miller NR: Walsh and Hoyt's Clinical Neuro-ophthalmology, 4th ed, vol 2. Baltimore, Williams & Wilkins, 1985, p 952.)

ptosis with masking of the ptosis on the contralateral side by an associated facial paralysis. Similar cases of bilateral neuropathic ptosis caused by damage to one or both cerebral hemispheres have been reported by others.[15, 16] Lepore[17] described a series of 13 patients with bilateral ptosis after acute right frontotemporoparietal lesions. The ptosis lasted about 5 days in five of the patients and persisted in the others. All patients had right-sided deviation of conjugate gaze, and many had associated facial weakness. Lepore[17] suggested that the transient nature of the ptosis was the result of the intact hemisphere gradually assuming control of levator function.

Not all supranuclear ptosis is caused by damage to the cerebral hemispheres. Buttner-Ennever and associates[18] reported a patient with a midbrain glioma that caused bilateral ptosis and a supranuclear downward gaze paralysis. These authors suggested that their case supports other experimental animal evidence of an eyelid control area in the region dorsal to the third nerve nucleus. Ptosis may also be a part of the "locked-in" syndrome, a condition that is characterized by complete absence of all voluntary

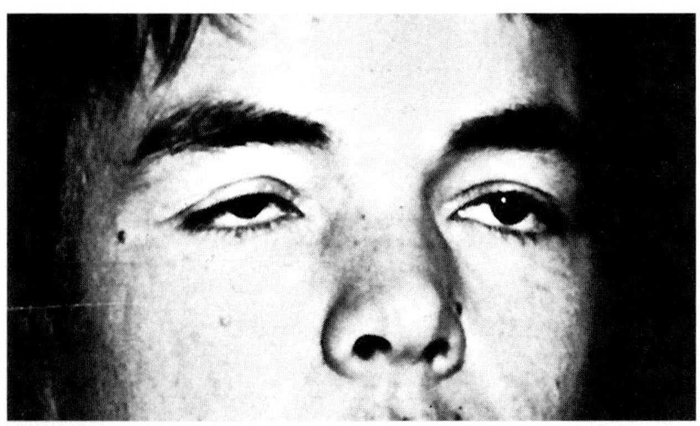

Figure 3–10. Unilateral supranuclear ptosis. The patient had seizures with an electroencephalographic focus in the left temporal lobe. The patient had no evidence of sympathetic or oculomotor nerve dysfunction. (From Miller NR: Walsh and Hoyt's Clinical Neuro-ophthalmology, 4th ed, vol 2. Baltimore, Williams & Wilkins, 1985, p 937.)

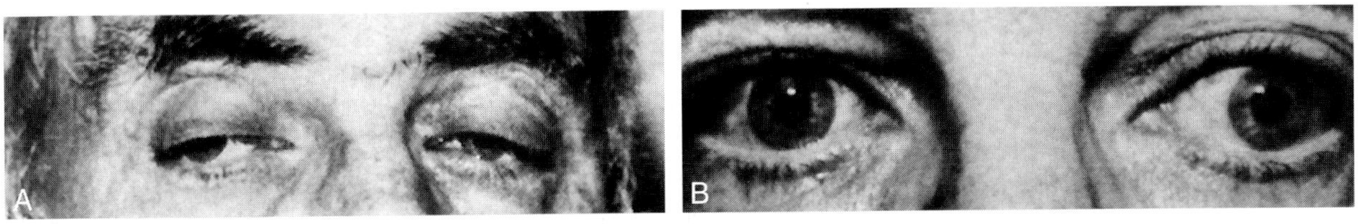

Figure 3–11. Bilateral supranuclear ptosis and recovery. *A*, The patient has bilateral severe ptosis. Computed tomographic scan showed changes consistent with bilateral frontal lobe infarctions. *B*, The ptosis has completely resolved 2 months later. (From Krohel GB, Griffen JF: Cortical blepharoptosis. Am J Ophthalmol 85:632–634, 1978. Published with permission from The American Journal of Ophthalmology. Copyright by The Ophthalmic Publishing Company.)

motor function except for eye movements and movements of the eyelids.[19, 20] This condition is usually caused by severe brain stem disease, usually an infarction of the midbrain or pons.

Nuclear

Both levator palpebrae superioris muscles are innervated by a single, caudal, midline subnucleus in the oculomotor nuclear complex. Thus, ptosis caused by lesions of the oculomotor nucleus is always symmetric and bilateral (Fig. 3–12). Mesencephalic ptosis can be produced by a variety of causes, including ischemic, inflammatory, infiltrative, compressive, and toxic lesions. The ptosis may be isolated or in conjunction with other neurologic deficits.[21–25]

Infranuclear

Damage to the oculomotor fascicle or nerve is the most common cause of neuropathic ptosis. It is always unilateral unless both oculomotor nerves are affected, as in trauma or herniation. Generally, ptosis caused by oculomotor nerve damage is associated with other evidence of third nerve dysfunction, such as strabismus, a dilated and poorly reactive pupil, or both (Fig. 3–13), but occasionally it will be the presenting finding. Good[26] reported a patient with a posterior communicating artery aneurysm in whom ptosis was the only sign of oculomotor dysfunction, and we have seen similar cases in patients with intracranial aneurysms and cavernous sinus meningiomas. In one series of pituitary tumors, third nerve palsies occurred in 14% and several of these patients presented with ptosis.[27] Small and Buckley[28] described a patient with recurrent ptosis as the sole sign of oculomotor nerve paresis in the setting of a pituitary adenoma. Similarly, Yen and colleagues[29] reported a small series of patients with pituitary tumors that presented with ptosis and then later developed other signs of third nerve paresis. We have seen one patient in whom ptosis was the primary sign of a pituitary adenoma. Careful examination revealed that the patient actually had a superior division third nerve paresis, but involvement of the superior rectus was so mild that he did not complain of vertical diplopia. We believe it is possible that other patients with "isolated" ptosis caused by third nerve paresis may, in fact, have mild superior division pareses of the third nerve. Wand[30] reported a patient with unilateral ptosis as the presenting sign of meningitis and postulated that it was caused by irritation of the oculomotor nerve in the subarachnoid space.

Ptosis caused by damage to the oculomotor nerve has the same large differential diagnosis of all oculomotor nerve pareses. Compressive lesions of the third nerve from the midbrain to the orbit must always be considered, particularly aneurysms and tumors. Other causes include trauma, ischemia, inflammation, infiltrative processes, and toxins.

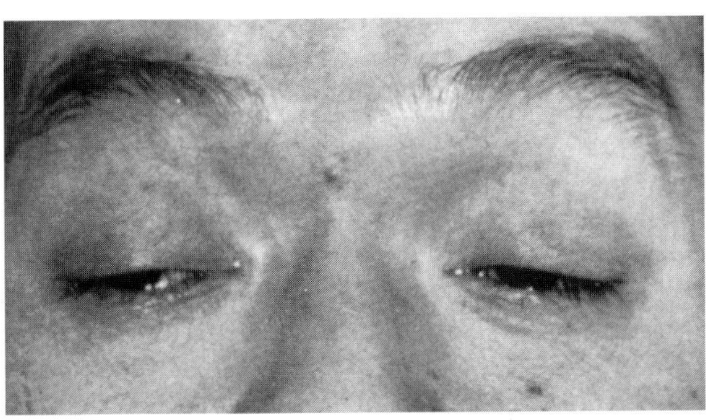

Figure 3–12. Midbrain ptosis. The patient had brain stem encephalitis and a discrete inflammatory focus in the caudal mesencephalon. Note that the ptosis is bilateral and symmetric. It was unassociated with any limitation of eye movement. (From Conway VH, Rozdilsky B, Schneider RJ, Sundaram M: Isolated bilateral complete ptosis. Can J Ophthalmol 18:37–40, 1983.)

Sympathetic

An interruption in the oculosympathetic pathway anywhere from the hypothalamus to the orbit results in a unilateral ptosis and ipsilateral miosis (Horner's syndrome). In some cases, Horner's syndrome is associated with other neurologic deficits, but it is often an isolated finding. The ptosis is typically mild (1 to 2 mm), and there is a corresponding elevation ("upside-down ptosis") of the lower eyelid (Fig. 3–14). Other findings may include ipsilateral facial anhidrosis, relative ocular hypotony, changes in iris pigmentation (generally in congenital lesions), and increased accommodative amplitude.

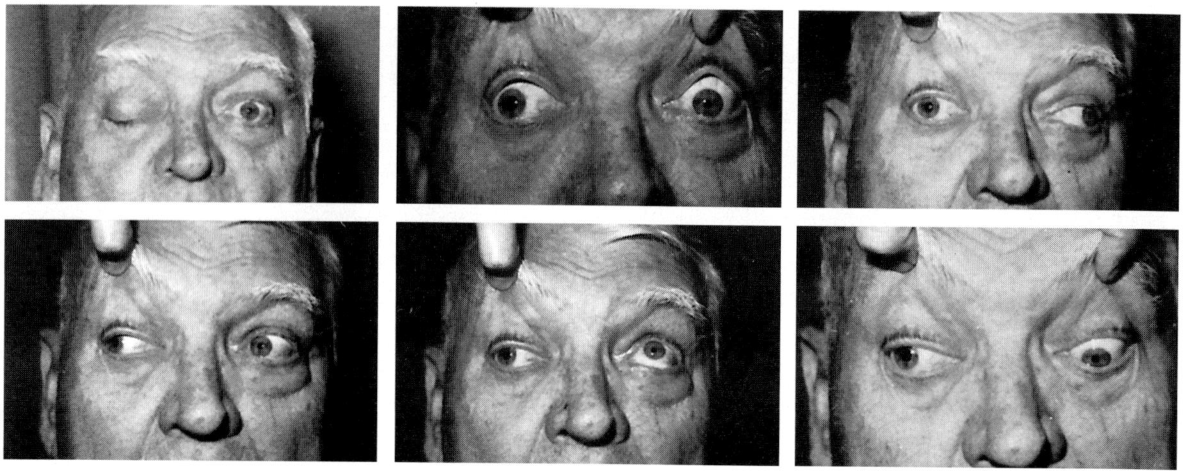

Figure 3–13. Unilateral ptosis associated with a complete oculomotor (third) nerve palsy. The patient had a right-sided intracranial aneurysm at the junction of the internal carotid and posterior communicating arteries. Note other signs of oculomotor nerve palsy, including a dilated right pupil and limitation of adduction, elevation, and depression of the right eye. ((From Miller NR: Walsh and Hoyt's Clinical Neuro-ophthalmology, 4th ed, vol 2. Baltimore, Williams & Wilkins, 1985, p 666.)

The upper eyelid ptosis of Horner's syndrome is caused by paresis of the sympathetically innervated Müller's muscle (a smooth muscle). Paresis of a similar muscle in the lower eyelid produces the lower lid elevation, and the resultant narrowing of the lid fissure can simulate enophthalmos.

The anisocoria that occurs in Horner's syndrome is caused by a paresis of the dilator muscle of the iris. Because the condition only affects the sympathetic pathway to the eye and not the parasympathetic innervation of the iris constrictor muscle, pupillary inequality is most apparent in dim light and may be minimal in bright light. Constriction of the pupil not only is normal but, in fact, is faster than normal because of the loss of sympathetic tone.

Sympathetic innervation to the eye consists of a three-neuron chain. The first or central neuron runs from the hypothalamus to the lower cervical–upper thoracic cord to synapse in the ciliospinal center of Budge and Waller. The second, or preganglionic, neuron begins in this center and travels over the apex of the lung and upward to synapse in the superior cervical ganglion. The third, or postganglionic, neuron leaves the ganglion and accompanies the internal carotid artery through the foramen lacerum into the carotid canal and then into the cavernous sinus. Within the cavernous sinus, the fibers destined for the eyelids and iris dilator muscle join briefly with the abducens nerve and then leave it to join with the ophthalmic division of the trigeminal nerve. These fibers enter the orbit through the superior orbital fissure with the nasociliary branch of the trigeminal nerve and then separate from it, becoming the long posterior ciliary nerves.

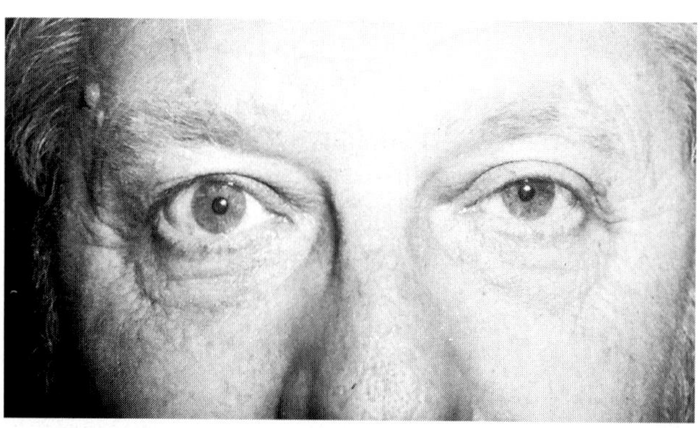

Figure 3–14. Left Horner's syndrome in a patient with episodic headaches. Note the ptosis of the left upper eyelid, the slight inverse ptosis of the left lower eyelid, and anisocoria, with the left pupil slightly smaller than the right.

Horner's syndrome can occur from damage to any portion of the three-neuron oculosympathetic pathway. The frequency with which central, preganglionic, or postganglionic Horner's syndrome occurs varies with the patient population studied. Maloney and colleagues[31] reported the Mayo Clinic experience of 450 patients, some of whom were hospitalized and some of whom were seen as outpatients. They were able to determine the etiology in 270 (60%) of these and found that 13% were central in origin, 44% were preganglionic, and 43% were postganglionic.

It is important to determine whether a Horner's syndrome is central, preganglionic, or postganglionic because the nature and potential severity of the causative lesion varies considerably with the location. The lesions that cause completely isolated postganglionic Horner's syndromes are usually benign, whereas there is a high incidence of neoplasms and other serious diseases with isolated central and preganglionic Horner's syndromes.[31, 32]

The first part of the evaluation of a patient with Horner's syndrome is a careful examination looking for other signs of neurologic dysfunction. Horner's syndromes caused by disease in the brain stem or cavernous sinus, for example, are often associated with enough other findings to determine the site of the lesion. When the location cannot be determined with certainty by the history or clinical examination, the location of the lesion

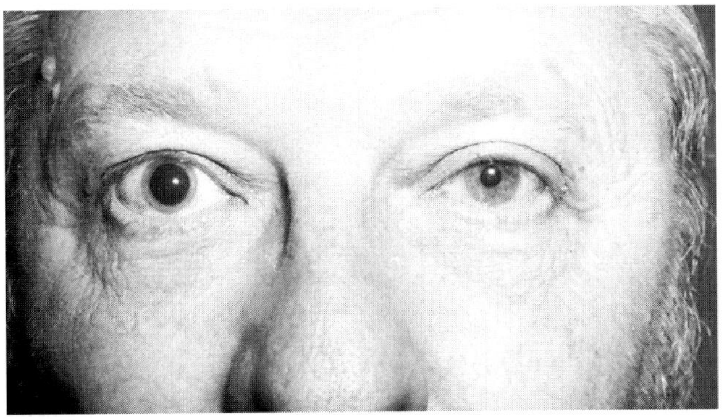

Figure 3–15. Cocaine test for Horner's syndrome. Two drops of 10% cocaine were instilled into the lower cul-de-sac of both eyes of the patient seen in Figure 3–14. Forty-five minutes later, the right pupil is widely dilated, but the left pupil has dilated only a slight amount. This test is thus positive for left Horner's syndrome.

can be at least partially determined by pharmacologic testing.

The second part of the evaluation of a patient with Horner's syndrome is pharmacologic diagnosis and localization. This usually requires a two-step approach. In the first step, 2 drops of a solution of 10% cocaine are placed in the lower cul-de-sac of both eyes (the normal eye acts as a control) on two occasions 5 minutes apart. The eyes are then examined every 15 minutes for the next 45 minutes (patients with particularly dark irides may require additional dosing and waiting time). Cocaine blocks norepinephrine reuptake by the nerve endings within the iris. Normal pupils thus dilate because of the persistent release and gradual accumulation of the neurotransmitter. Patients with a lesion of the sympathetic pathway in *any of the three* neurons show minimal or no pupillary dilation, since the amount of norepinephrine being released at the neuromuscular junctions of the iris is too small to produce dilation (Fig. 3–15).

Once the presence of Horner's syndrome is confirmed by cocaine testing, it is then necessary to determine if the causative lesion is affecting the postganglionic neuron (third order) or is in the preganglionic or central portion of the system. On a separate day (so that the effects of the cocaine are gone), 1% hydroxyamphetamine hydrobromide solution (Paredrine) is applied to both eyes in the same manner as the cocaine. This drug directly causes the release of norepinephrine from the postganglionic nerve terminals. It will result in the dilation of normal pupils and most miotic pupils from central and preganglionic lesions, since the intact postganglionic neuron has stores of norepinephrine for release. However, lesions of the postganglionic sympathetic neuron result in eventual disappearance of the neurotransmitter, and no dilation will occur during this test. A solution of 5% tyramine hydrochloride (which must be custom-made) can be substituted for Paredrine with similar results.

In both the cocaine and Paredrine tests, we recommend placing the topical solution first in the cul-de-sac of the eye with the suspected lesion and then in the cul-de-sac of the normal eye. Cocaine, in particular, stings considerably and elicits a reflex blepharospasm. Placing it in the presumably affected eye first ensures adequate delivery of the drug; dilation in the normal eye serves as a control. Nothing should disrupt the corneal epithelium before these tests are performed to help ensure equal corneal penetration. It thus is best to defer corneal sensation testing and applanation tonometry if possible. The pupils should be examined in dim light to maximize the anisocoria. Many authors recommend documentation with photographs for a permanent record. However, in most cases the anisocoria is of sufficient magnitude that precise photographic measurements are not required for diagnosis.

Neuromuscular

Persons with diseases of the neuromuscular junction usually present with multiple cranial nerve motor deficits but may present with ptosis either first or most overtly. The most common disease affecting the neuromuscular junction in the eyelids is *myasthenia gravis*, although other conditions that damage the neuromuscular junction can also produce ptosis.

Myasthenia Gravis

In myasthenia gravis, the function of acetylcholine at the postsynaptic neuromuscular junction is impaired by antibody-mediated damage. These antibodies, found in about 90% of myasthenic patients, are believed to interrupt acetylcholine's normal neurotransmitter function by various mechanisms, including blocking the receptors, damaging the postsynaptic membrane that houses the receptors, increasing the rate of receptor degradation, and decreasing the rate of receptor synthesis.[33–36] Antibody levels do not always correlate with clinical severity of disease and may be difficult to detect in patients with only ocular findings. There is evidence to suggest that thymic dysfunction and both the T-cell and B-cell lymphocyte system are involved with the disease process.

Myasthenia gravis occurs in persons of all races and ages. The prevalence has been estimated at 1 in 10,000 to 50,000. The mean age at onset is 26 years in women and 31 years in men, and the disease is at least twice as likely to occur in women (although this may reverse late in life). About 65% of these patients have a "hyperplastic" thymus, and an additional 10% to 15% have thymomas; in this latter group, 60% are male.[37, 38]

Myasthenia gravis is characterized by fluctuating weakness of voluntary muscles, with a general progression of weakness with repeated or maintained activities and as the day goes on. The levator palpebrae superioris and the extraocular muscles are the first voluntary muscle to be affected in about 70% of patients with myasthe-

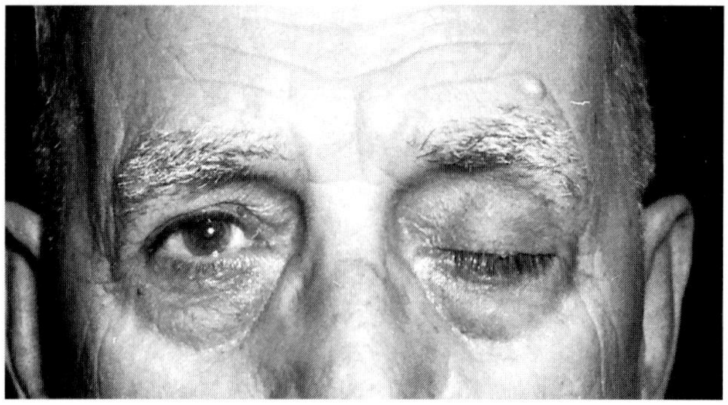

Figure 3–16. Unilateral ptosis in myasthenia gravis. Note the virtually complete ptosis on the left. The right upper eyelid is in a reasonably normal position.

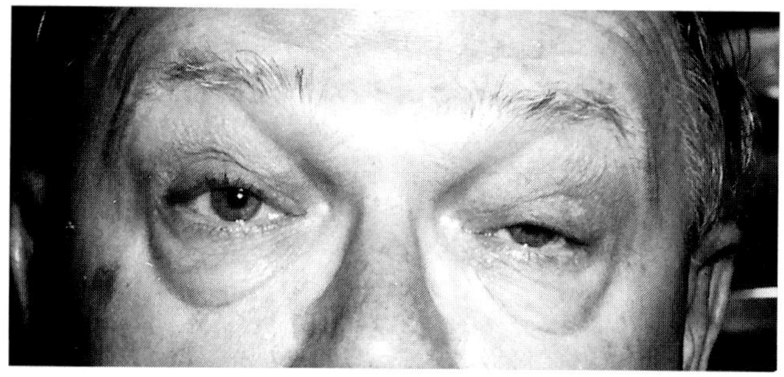

Figure 3–17. Bilateral asymmetric ptosis in myasthenia gravis. Note the relative positions of both upper eyelids. The patient is attempting to overcome the ptosis by using his frontalis muscle.

nia gravis and ultimately become affected in 90% of myasthenics.[39–43] Adults with myasthenia have been classified in several ways, based on their presentation and response to therapy.[41, 44] Group I consists of patients with purely ocular findings. Typically, if no other skeletal muscle groups become involved within 2 years, the symptoms remain confined to the eyes. Group II consists of patients with mild to moderate generalized disease with gradual onset and spread and reasonable response to treatment. Group III consists of patients with acute, fulminant disease with bulbar and skeletal muscle weakness. The respiratory musculature is frequently involved. Response to treatment may be poor and mortality may be high. Group IV consists of patients from the first two groups who progress to severe symptoms after at least 2 years of stability; they typically do not respond well to therapy at this point. The incidence of thymomas is highest in these last two groups.

The ptosis of myasthenia gravis may be unilateral or bilateral (Figs. 3–16 through 3–18). When bilateral, it may be symmetric or asymmetric. Severe, symmetric ptosis is usually accompanied by ophthalmoplegia. Cogan[45] described a *lid twitch* response that is commonly seen in myasthenics. The patient is instructed to look down for about 20 seconds and is then asked to rapidly refixate in the primary position. The eyelids will characteristically overshoot upward and slowly droop or quiver before settling into position. Gorlick and associates[46] described the "enhanced ptosis" of patients with myasthenia gravis and ptosis. When one eyelid is manually elevated, the opposite eyelid becomes ptotic or preexisting ptosis worsens (Fig. 3–19). This phenomenon seems to be a result of Hering's law of equal innervation. When one eyelid is manually elevated, it requires less of an impulse to raise it. Consequently, the contralateral levator palpebrae superioris is sent fewer neural impulses.

The ophthalmoparesis of myasthenia gravis mimics virtually every other cause of limitation of eye movements except for a pupil-involved third nerve palsy, since patients with myasthenia gravis never have clinically evident involvement of the pupils. Patients with myasthenia gravis may have unilateral or bilateral disorders of ocular motility. They may appear to have a pupil-sparing third nerve paresis, a superior division third nerve paresis, a fourth nerve paresis, a sixth nerve paresis, a horizontal or vertical gaze paresis, an internuclear ophthalmoplegia, a one-and-a-half syndrome, or any combination of these.

Children with acquired myasthenia gravis typically

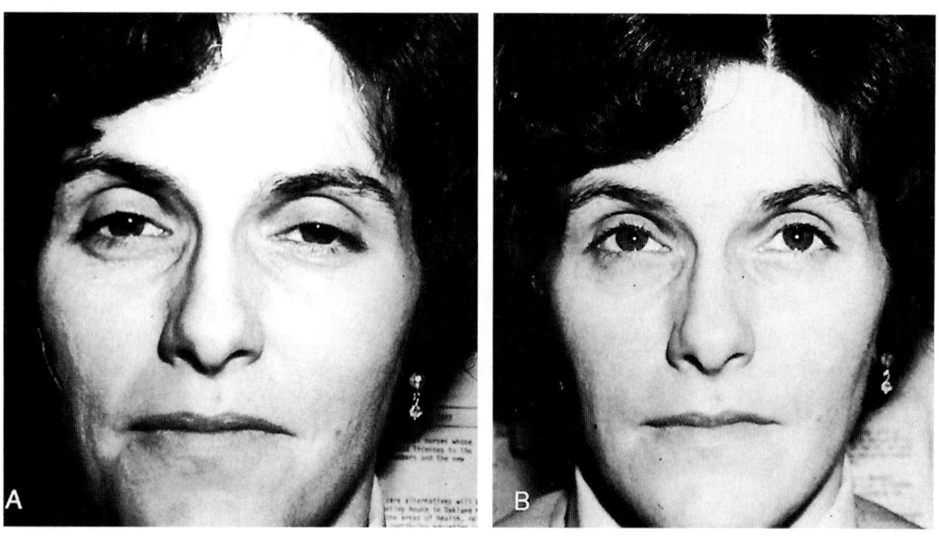

Figure 3–18. Bilateral symmetric ptosis in a patient with myasthenia gravis, with resolution after an intravenous injection of edrophonium chloride (Tensilon). *A*, The patient has bilateral symmetric ptosis. Note a slight symmetric weakness of the face. *B*, After injection of Tensilon, the ptosis has resolved, and the patient's facial expression is more pronounced. (From Miller NR: Walsh and Hoyt's Clinical Neuro-ophthalmology, 4th ed, vol 2. Baltimore, Williams & Wilkins, 1985, p 851.)

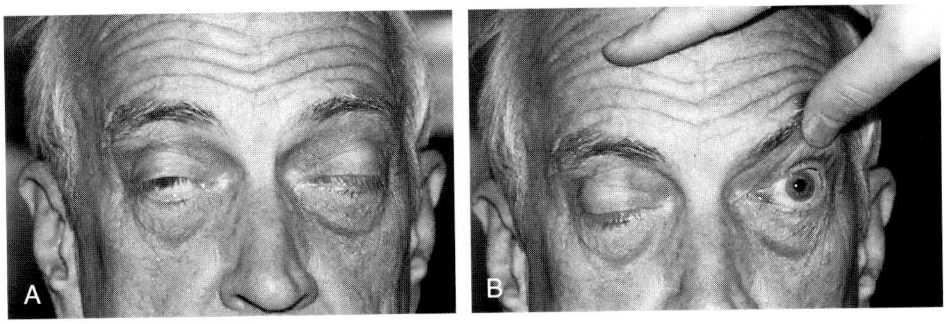

Figure 3–19. Enhancement of ptosis in myasthenia gravis. *A*, The patient has bilateral ptosis; the left is greater than the right. *B*, When the left upper eyelid is manually elevated, the right eyelid becomes more ptotic.

follow the same pattern as adults. However, newborns presenting with myasthenia gravis can follow several different patterns.[47] The most common is transient myasthenia gravis immediately after birth from a myasthenic mother. It is the result of circulating maternal anti–acetylcholine receptor antibodies and clears within 12 weeks as the infant clears the offending antibodies. Not all children of myasthenic mothers have symptoms, however, and the severity of the presentation does not correlate with the status of the mother's myasthenia control. Other congenital forms of myasthenia gravis are quite rare and are caused by a variety of immunologic abnormalities other than autoantibodies to acetylcholine receptors. Such patients may or may not have a mother with myasthenia gravis.

The ptosis and ophthalmoparesis of patients with myasthenia gravis or one of the myasthenic syndromes can simulate the manifestations of a variety of other conditions. It thus is important to consider myasthenia gravis in the differential diagnosis of all patients with ptosis with or without ophthalmoparesis because the approach to their care is markedly different. The diagnosis is usually based on the constellation of results of history, clinical examination, pharmacologic tests, electrophysiologic studies, blood and serologic assays, and muscle biopsy with receptor assays.

Pharmacologic testing is the most common screening examination for myasthenia performed in the ophthalmologist's office. The patient is given an anticholinesterase agent and then observed for a reversal of the muscular weakness. Atropine needs to be given or be available in the event of marked cholinergic side effects (e.g., nausea, bradycardia). There are two common test medications: edrophonium hydrochloride (Tensilon) and neostigmine methylsulfate (Prostigmin). One or both may be used in a given patient.

The Tensilon test is ideal for the adult with obvious ptosis, with or without ophthalmoparesis. Tensilon is administered intravenously. Its effects on the levator and the extraocular muscles are rapid, and side effects are minimal and resolve quickly. A variety of techniques have been described for this test.[48, 49] The position of the eyelids is measured and, if appropriate, documented photographically. Ten milligrams (1 mL) of Tensilon is drawn up in a 3-mL syringe. Slowly, 2 to 3 mg (0.2 to 0.3 mL) of Tensilon is injected intravenously, and the patient is observed for any change in the position of the eyelids (see Fig. 3–18). If no improvement is noted in several minutes, the remainder of the Tensilon is injected, either as a bolus or in two divided doses about 3 minutes apart.

There are three possible results: (1) a negative test—no change in eye findings; (2) a positive test—the ptosis resolves or improves for several minutes, eventually returning as the effects of the drug wear off; and (3) a "paradoxic" result— the eye findings get worse or perhaps reverse (the ptotic eyelid retracts and the previously normal eyelid droops) with the medication.

A negative Tensilon test is better termed *nondiagnostic*. It does not eliminate myasthenia gravis as the cause of the patient's symptoms and signs. Indeed, we have seen patients who had several negative Tensilon tests before one was positive, and we have also seen several patients with negative Tensilon tests but positive Prostigmin tests. Patients with symptoms and signs that strongly suggest myasthenia gravis but who have a negative Tensilon test should undergo repeat testing with Tensilon, and if this test is also negative, such patients should undergo a Prostigmin test as well as nonpharmacologic testing by a neurologist or a specialist in neuromuscular disease.

A positive Tensilon test usually indicates myasthenia (especially when a placebo is used with the Tensilon), but there are anecdotal reports of false-positive responses in patients with intracranial tumors and other lesions of the ocular motor nerves.[50] We thus recommend that any patient with purely uniocular signs (i.e., unilateral ptosis, ophthalmoparesis, or both) and a positive Tensilon test nevertheless undergo magnetic resonance imaging of the brain as part of the subsequent evaluation.

The significance of a paradoxic response during the Tensilon test is controversial. It is best to consider such a response as negative. If a strong clinical suspicion exists, repeat testing, further testing, or both is warranted. Occasionally, patients with paradoxic responses during a standard Tensilon test give a clearly positive response when Tensilon is given slowly in 0.1- to 0.2-mL increments.

The advantages of Tensilon are that it is fast acting and that the side effects pass quickly. The disadvantages are that intravenous access is required (including all of the risks of an intravenous injection and rapid dosing of a cardioactive substance) and that in some patients re-

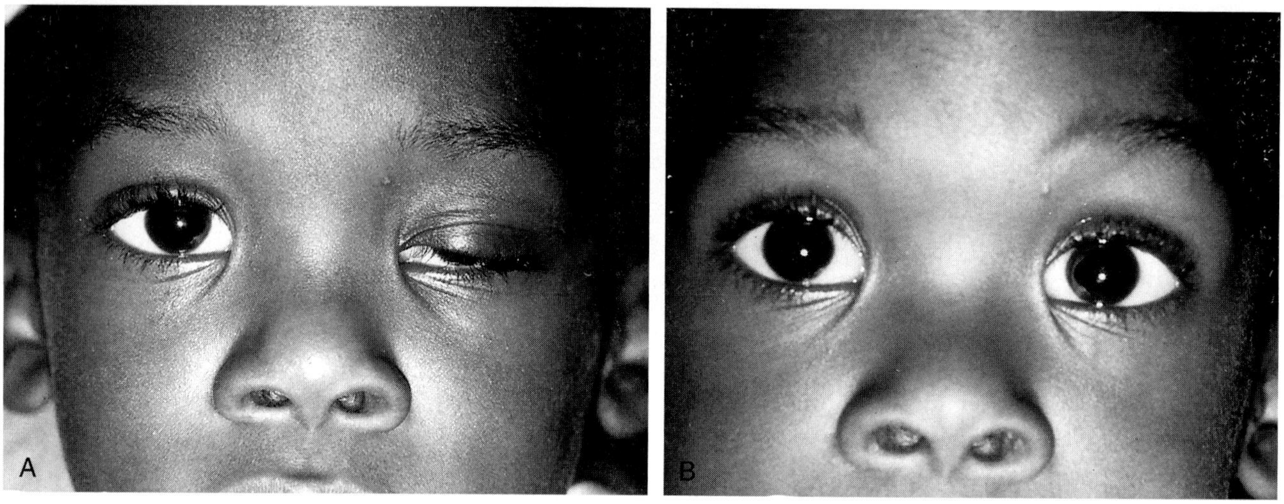

Figure 3–20. Positive Prostigmin test in myasthenia gravis. The patient is a 4-year-old boy with unilateral ptosis. *A*, The patient has an almost complete left ptosis. *B*, Thirty minutes after receiving an intramuscular injection of atropine sulfate combined with neostigmine bromide, the patient's ptosis has completely disappeared.

sponses are difficult to measure in a relatively brief period. These characteristics are reversed with Prostigmin.

The Prostigmin test is ideal for children, particularly when they have variable or no ptosis but measurable strabismus. The test is performed as follows. The positions of the eyelids are measured and documented by photography if appropriate. The ocular alignment and range of movement of the eyes are measured. Atropine sulfate (0.4 to 0.6 mg) is mixed with Prostigmin (0.02 mg/kg for adults and 0.04 mg/kg for children—not to exceed 1.5 mg) in a 3-mL syringe and given intramuscularly. The patient is observed for a response after 30 to 45 minutes. The results are interpreted in the same manner as the Tensilon test, but there is about a 30-minute window to observe and remeasure the positions of the eyelids (Fig. 3–20).

There are a few useful nonpharmacologic tests in diagnosing myasthenia gravis that may be performed by the ophthalmologist. Sethi and coworkers[51] reported using an "ice pack" test in patients with suspected ocular myasthenia who had negative pharmacologic testing. This test exploits the tendency of cold temperature to improve neuromuscular function. Ice packs are applied to the ptotic eyelids, and the effects of the packs are determined over several minutes. In the cases reported by Sethi and coworkers,[51] ptosis improved in 8 of 10 patients with myasthenia gravis but in none of 7 control subjects. Other authors have reported similar findings.[52]

Another test that is safe and useful in elderly patients with heart disease in whom one suspects myasthenia gravis but does not want to risk pharmacologic testing is the "sleep test."[53] This test is based on the tendency for the strength of muscles affected by myasthenia gravis to improve with rest. Such muscles are often strongest when the patient awakens after a night's sleep, for example. In this test, the positions of the eyelids are determined photographically (Fig. 3–21*A*). The patient is then led to a quiet area where there is a bed or couch. The patient sleeps for 30 to 40 minutes, following which he or she is awakened and the positions of the eyelids are reassessed photographically (see Fig. 3–21*B*). Improvement in ptosis on awakening from sleep may be considered highly suggestive, if not diagnostic, of myasthenia gravis.

In addition to tests that are often performed by the ophthalmologist, other tests for myasthenia gravis that are usually performed by a neurologist or specialist in

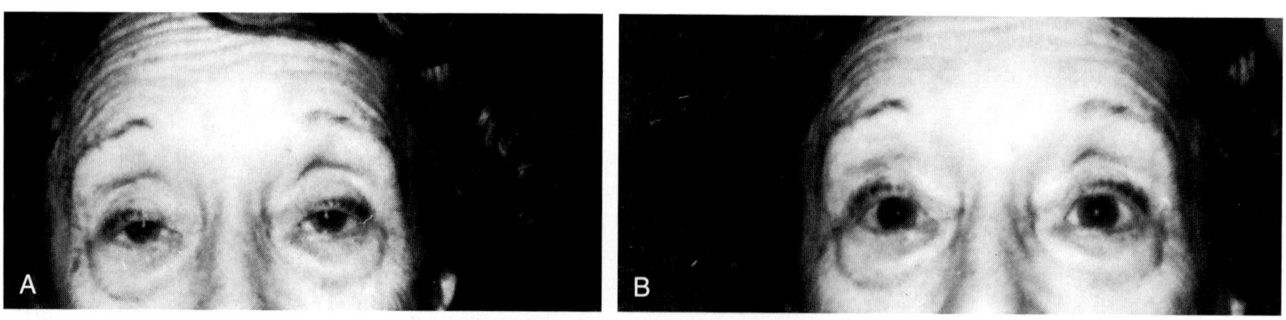

Figure 3–21. The sleep test for myasthenia gravis. The patient is an 80-year-old woman with recent onset of bilateral ptosis and generalized fatigue. She has severe cardiac disease. *A*, Before the test, the patient has moderate bilateral ptosis. She is using her frontalis muscle to elevate the eyelids. *B*, The patient has just been awakened after sleeping for 60 minutes. Note the improvement in ptosis.

neuromuscular diseases include evaluation of the amplitude of the miniature end-plate potential amplitudes in various skeletal muscles (reduced in myasthenia), evaluation of the electromyographic response to repetitive stimulation (decremental in myasthenia), and evaluation of a single motor fiber electromyogram recording for "jitter" (a measure of the variability of muscular response to nerve stimulation that is increased in myasthenics). These techniques have reasonable sensitivity in patients with generalized myasthenia but may be less reliable in purely ocular myasthenia gravis. Blood can be screened for anti-acetylcholine receptor antibodies, and muscle biopsy specimens can similarly be assayed for acetylcholine receptors.[54] There are frequently other immunologic abnormalities such as circulating antinuclear antibodies and anti-skeletal muscle antibodies.[55] A combination of pharmacologic, electrophysiologic, serologic, and pathologic tests yields an extremely high sensitivity and specificity in diagnosis.[56]

A number of other autoimmune disorders have been noted to be more frequent in the myasthenic population than in the normal population. Thyroid disorders, including hypothyroidism and hyperthyroidism, thyroid carcinoma, and Hashimoto's thyroiditis, occur in 5% to 10% of myasthenic patients. Arthropathies similar to rheumatoid arthritis or ankylosing spondylitis are not uncommon. Aplastic anemia, pernicious anemia, systemic lupus erythematosus, pemphigus vulgaris, ulcerative colitis, sarcoidosis, Sjögren's syndrome, diabetes mellitus, hepatitis, Kaposi's sarcoma, and orbital lymphoid tumors have all been reported in association with myasthenia gravis.

Myasthenic Syndromes

Conditions that mimic myasthenia gravis and that affect the neuromuscular junction in much the same way as myasthenia gravis are termed *myasthenic syndromes.* The best known of these is the Eaton-Lambert syndrome of muscle weakness in association with a malignancy (usually oat cell carcinoma of the lung).[57] In some of these cases, the diagnosis of cancer has already been made at the time ptosis and ophthalmoparesis become evident, whereas in others, these signs precede detection of the malignancy. Myasthenic syndromes may also occur in association with a variety of autoimmune diseases, such as pernicious anemia,[58] thyroid disease,[59] and Sjögren's syndrome[60] or even myasthenia gravis itself.[61-63] Some patients with Eaton-Lambert syndrome have elevated titers of serum antibodies to voltage-gated calcium channels; this test shows promise in aiding to make the diagnosis as well as in elucidating the underlying pathophysiology of this syndrome.[64]

Patients with the myasthenic syndrome usually present with generalized muscle weakness. Ocular involvement is less common than in myasthenia gravis, but ptosis and strabismus occur and may be severe.[65] The pathophysiologic basis for the syndrome is impaired acetylcholine release; the small amount released has a normal effect for its size on the receptor. Unlike myasthenia gravis, there is no impairment of the acetylcholine receptor. This defect results in the phenomenon of *facilitation.* Muscle action potentials (and, for example, in the eyes, saccadic velocity) increase with rapid stimulation because of the ultimate accumulation of small amounts of neurotransmitter. Calcium and guanidine augment the release of acetylcholine, and the former is the treatment of choice for patients with myasthenic syndrome.

Neuromuscular Toxins

Certain drugs and toxins can cause ptosis from their effects on the neuromuscular junctions of the levator palpebrae superioris. Botulism is the result of poisoning with a toxin produced by the organism *Clostridium botulinum.* The toxin blocks acetylcholine release at the nerve terminal. The disease has three methods of transmission: food-borne, wound, and infantile. In food-related disease, incompletely cooked food containing the toxin is ingested. Symptoms begin in 8 to 36 hours and consist of nausea, pooling of secretions, and diffuse muscle weakness. Ptosis, ophthalmoparesis, and dilated pupils that are nonreactive or poorly reactive are commonly present. Wound botulism results from contaminated injuries that allow toxin to be produced and absorbed systemically (Fig. 3-22). In infantile botulism, the gastrointestinal tract in populated with toxin-producing bacteria. In addition to its peripheral effects, botulinum toxin can produce central nervous system abnormalities presumably through its effects on central cholinergic synapses. A related toxin produced by *Clostridium tetani* has more pronounced central nervous system effects (tetanus) and may produce similar ocular findings as well. The therapeutic use of botulinum toxin (Botox, available from Allergan Pharmaceuticals, Irvine, CA) in the treatment of benign essential blepharospasm, hemifacial spasm, and Meige's syndrome has been associated with both ptosis (16% incidence) and vertical muscle imbalance (17% incidence).

Certain arthropods and reptiles produce venom that can block neuromuscular transmission. In most cases, the toxicity is severe and widespread, with the eye findings not being significant in the overall disease process. Arthropods whose stings can produce neuromuscular damage that includes ptosis include the black widow spider, certain ticks, scorpions, and wasps. Reptiles such as the sea snakes of the South Pacific Ocean and certain land snakes on the continent of Australia can also produce similar findings.

A long list of drugs may disrupt neuromuscular transmission. Many seem to cause a worsening of symptoms and signs in patients with preexisting myasthenia gravis, whereas others produce new disease that mimics myasthenia. Drugs that can exacerbate myasthenia gravis or

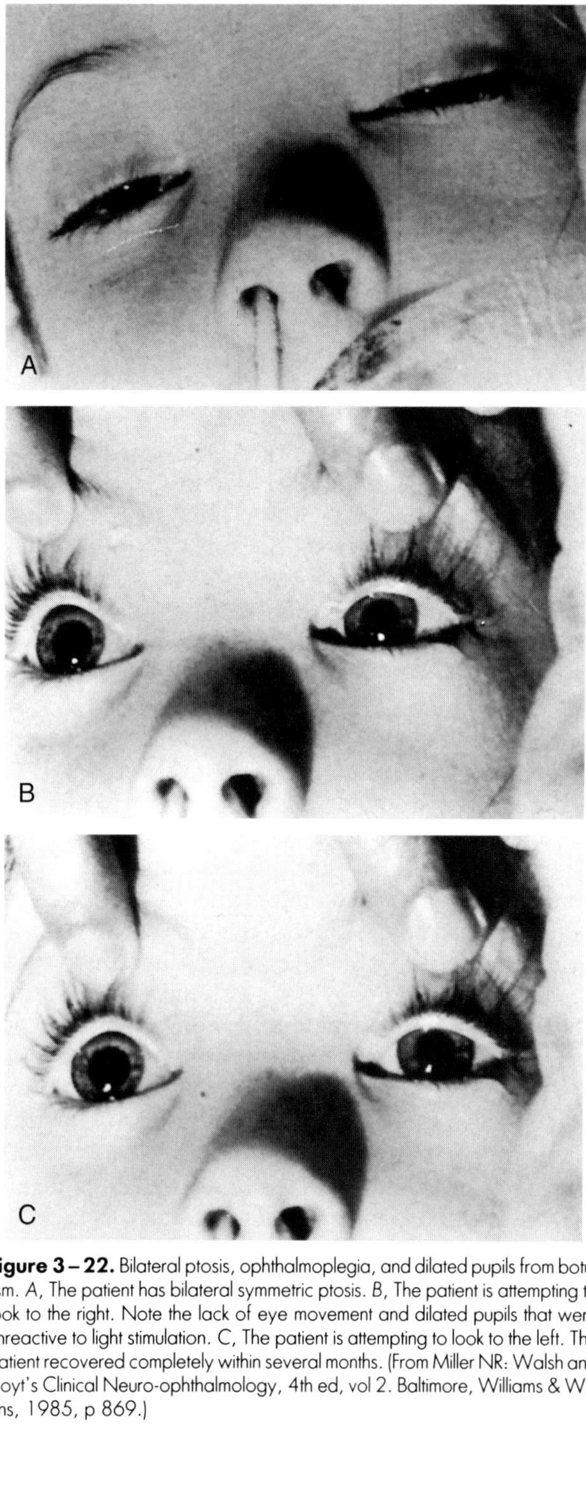

Figure 3–22. Bilateral ptosis, ophthalmoplegia, and dilated pupils from botulism. *A*, The patient has bilateral symmetric ptosis. *B*, The patient is attempting to look to the right. Note the lack of eye movement and dilated pupils that were unreactive to light stimulation. *C*, The patient is attempting to look to the left. The patient recovered completely within several months. (From Miller NR: Walsh and Hoyt's Clinical Neuro-ophthalmology, 4th ed, vol 2. Baltimore, Williams & Wilkins, 1985, p 869.)

produce a myasthenic syndrome include D-penicillamine, phenothiazines, tetracyclines, procainamide, quinidine, polymyxins, aminoglycosides, phenytoin, certain beta-blockers, chloroquine, cisplatin, magnesium, and lithium. Berstein and Henkind[66] reported ptosis after topical timolol therapy for glaucoma and speculated that it was caused by neuromuscular blockade. Poisoning with commercial anticholinesterase agents (primarily in pesticides) frequently begins with diplopia and ptosis but rapidly progresses to a cholinergic crisis.

Myopathic

Structural Myopathies

Generalized diseases of muscles can produce ptosis and diplopia. In most of these conditions, the systemic problems far overshadow the ophthalmic signs. However, a few conditions are characterized primarily by ocular involvement.

There are several structurally defined congenital myopathies that may, in their course of affecting all muscles, cause ptosis and diplopia. Their common bond is morphologic abnormalities present within the muscle itself. Their clinical course is usually nonprogressive. *Central core myopathy* was first described in 1956 by Shy and Magee.[67] Muscle biopsies revealed a central azurophilic central core with trichrome staining. Clinically, muscle weakness appears in early childhood and is worse in the lower extremities. Nevertheless, the facial and extraocular muscles may be affected. A different morphologic pattern (numerous granules or rods within the muscle fibers) is present in *nemaline myopathy* (also called rod myopathy). Clinically, the disease is similar to central core myopathy, although no patients with eye involvement have been reported. *Centronuclear (myotubular) myopathy* describes a heterogeneous group of conditions in which muscle fibers show an area without enzymatic activity around the centrally located nucleus. The clinical presentation is similar to other congenital myopathies, and ocular involvement is more common with patients who have symptoms present at a younger age (Fig. 3–23). *Multicore* disease is distinguished pathologically by many areas of involvement in the muscle fibers rather than one specific region in the cell. Clinical disease is similar to the others. Isolated bilateral ptosis has been reported.[68] Other entities that are poorly defined seem to result in the same early-onset generalized muscle weakness and may affect the extraocular muscles as well. The difficulty in exactly characterizing these conditions probably reflects our lack of knowledge of their underlying genetic and biochemical defects.

Muscular Dystrophy

Muscular dystrophy encompasses a group of genetically determined diseases that cause progressive wasting and weakness of the skeletal muscles by directly affecting the muscle cells (unlike the congenital structural myopathies). The different types are separated by their inheritance pattern, age at onset, and clinical features. Only the *Fukuyama type* of congenital muscular dystrophy has ocular involvement consisting of optic nerve hypoplasia and atrophy, myopia, cataracts, and orbicularis muscle weakness. This condition is devastating and usually results in death by age 10.[69, 70]

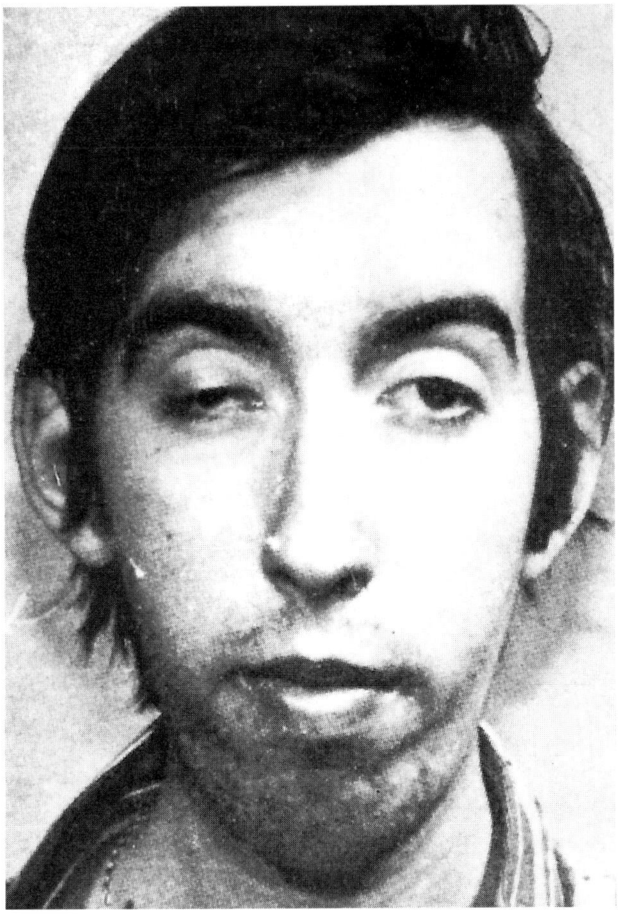

Figure 3–23. Bilateral asymmetric ptosis in a patient with a congenital systemic disorder known as *centronuclear myopathy*. He also had generalized muscle weakness, a high-arched palate, moderate scoliosis, and winged scapulae. (From Jadro-Santel D, Grčevic N, Dogan S, et al: Centronuclear myopathy with type I fibre hypotrophy and "fingerprint" inclusions associated with Marfan's syndrome. J Neurol Sci 45:43–56, 1980.)

Myotonia and Myotonic Disorders

Myotonia refers to persistent muscle contraction after a strong stimulus or continuous muscle fiber activity when it should be relaxed. It is believed to be a disorder of the muscle cell membrane.[71] Myotonia can occur congenitally. Ptosis and ophthalmoplegia rarely occur in the congenital form, although blepharospasm is common.

Myotonic dystrophy is the most common myotonia and is distinguished from the others by involvement of other tissues and organs.[72, 73] Patients become symptomatic in early adulthood with myotonia and muscle atrophy. Frequent early signs include the inability to release from a handshake and inability to open the eyelids after a forced closure. Systemic involvement may consist of mental retardation; cardiac hypertrophy; weakness of respiratory and pharyngeal muscles; skeletal malformations and thickening of the calvaria; atrophy of the tongue; weakness of the smooth muscles leading to constipation, incontinence, and prolonged labor; high-frequency hearing loss; and testicular atrophy. Ptosis is a frequent finding (Fig. 3–24), and many patients also demonstrate generalized weakness of the orbicularis oculi that results in infrequent blinking and deficient lid closure. Paradoxically, once the lids are closed, the myotonia may hamper their reopening. Other eye findings include slowed saccades and strabismus, iridescent cataracts, sluggish pupillary responses, iris blood vessel malformations that lead to hyphemas with minimal trauma, hypopigmented and shortened ciliary processes that can lead to hypotony, and a nonspecific chorioretinopathy (Fig. 3–25). Electroretinographic abnormalities are useful in detecting asymptomatic carriers of the disease.[74]

Myotonic dystrophy is an autosomal dominant disease that is caused by a specific molecular defect on chromosome 19q13.3.[75] Biopsies of affected striated muscle (including affected extraocular muscles) may be normal initially but ultimately demonstrate increased nuclei arranged in long rows centrally. As the disease advances, the muscle fibers are replaced with connective and adipose tissue. Other tissues demonstrate variable atrophy.

Familial periodic paralysis encompasses a group of hereditary myotonic disorders in which patients experience

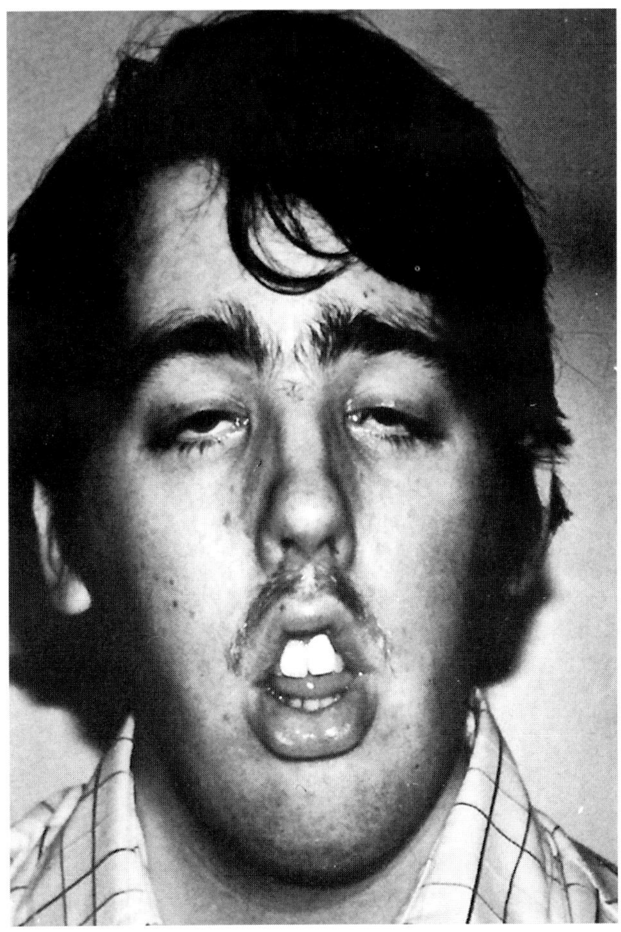

Figure 3–24. Bilateral severe ptosis in a patient with myotonic dystrophy. The patient also has mental retardation and cataracts. Note the myopathic facies. (From Miller NR: Walsh and Hoyt's Clinical Neuro-ophthalmology, 4th ed, vol 2. Baltimore, Williams & Wilkins, 1985, p 797.)

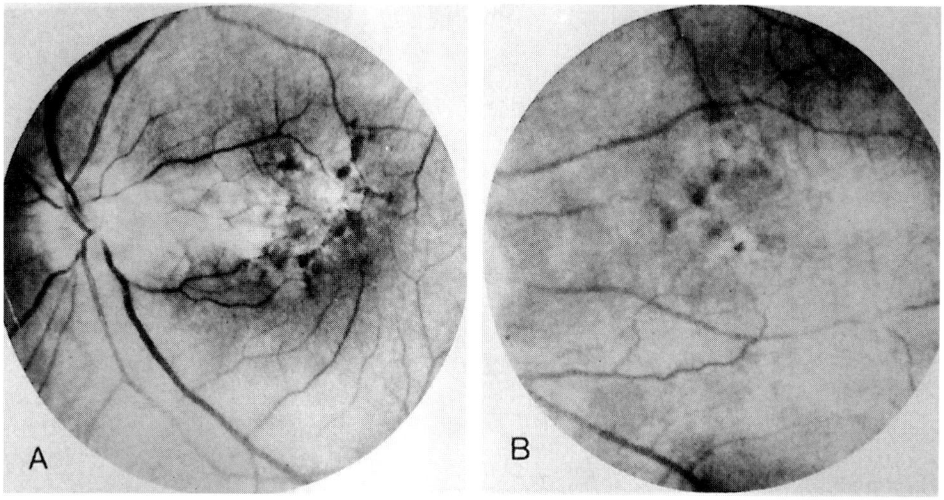

Figure 3–25. Pigmentary retinopathy in myotonic dystrophy. Note the clumping of pigment in the posterior pole in a 50-year-old man (*A*) and in a 36-year-old woman (*B*). (From Burian HM, Burns CA: Ocular changes in myotonic dystrophy. Am J Ophthalmol 63:22–34, 1967. Published with permission from The American Journal of Ophthalmology. Copyright by The Ophthalmic Publishing Company.)

repeated attacks of flaccid muscle paralysis. Eye findings during attacks may include ptosis, lid lag, or lid retraction, but they are often overshadowed by the more widespread and dramatic systemic muscle findings (Fig. 3–26). Different subgroups of patients exist in whom the serum potassium level is elevated, decreased, or, very rarely, normal during the episodes. The treatment generally consists of altering the potassium level in the correct direction with medication (oral potassium or glucose with insulin). All forms seem to share the same muscle biopsy morphology: a vacuolization centrally within the muscle fibers.

Oculopharyngeal dystrophy was first described in two generations of French Canadians[76] but has since been reported in other pedigrees and with various modes of genetic inheritance. Onset of symptoms is usually around age 40 and consists of dysphagia followed by ptosis. The ptosis is usually symmetric, severe, and occasionally accompanied by weakness of the extraocular muscles.[77] Muscle biopsy specimens have shown variable abnormalities.

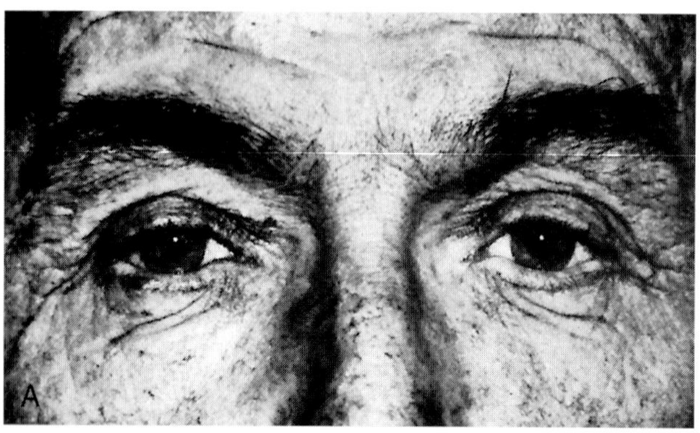

Figure 3–26. Ptosis and eyelid retraction in a patient with hyperkalemic familial periodic paralysis. *A*, There is mild bilateral symmetric ptosis when the patient looks straight ahead. *B*, When the patient looks downward, there is marked lid retraction and lid lag that disappear within 1 minute. (From McArdle B: Adynamia episodica hereditaria and its treatment. Brain 85:121–148, 1962. By permission of Oxford University Press.)

Chronic Progressive External Ophthalmoplegia

Certain disorders characterized by primary muscle dysfunction are caused by defective mitochondria. The most common of these disorders produces ptosis and ophthalmoparesis without involvement of the pupils and is called *chronic progressive external ophthalmoplegia* (CPEO).[78] Muscle biopsy specimens of patients with CPEO show typical morphologic changes in a small portion of the muscle fibers scattered throughout the field as well as muscle size variability and atrophy. Abnormal fibers have an irregular outline and stain darkly with Gomori's trichrome stain. Called *ragged-red fibers*, these abnormal muscle fibers have an appearance that is caused by mitochondrial accumulations beneath the plasma membrane and between the myofibrils.[79–81] Under the electron microscope, the mitochondria can be seen to be irregularly sized and shaped as well as increased in number. Mitsumoto and colleagues[82] demonstrated that mitochondrial function was decreased in CPEO muscle specimens, and Johnson and associates[83] found a partial deficiency in cytochrome-*c* oxidase function, but the genetic and biochemical defects are not defined. Clinical and pathologic abnormalities in patients with CPEO may not be confined to muscles. Many patients have abnormalities in the retina, heart, endocrine system, and central nervous system. Such patients are frequently said to have CPEO-plus.

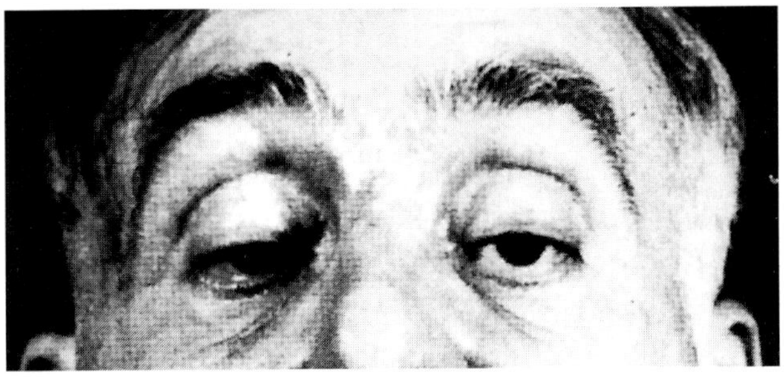

Figure 3-27. Myopathic facies in a patient with the mitochondriopathy known as *chronic progressive external ophthalmoplegia*. Note the flat, expressionless facial features associated with continuous wrinkling of the frontalis muscle and a posterior head tilt to compensate for bilateral ptosis. (Courtesy of Dr. I. Lewis.)

Ptosis is usually the first sign of ocular involvement in CPEO. It is usually bilateral and symmetric, and it may appear at any age. Ultimately, head tilt and frontalis use are required to clear the visual axis (Fig. 3-27). There is a symmetric reduction in ocular movements so *patients are not usually aware of any diplopia or gaze limitation* (Fig. 3-28). In advanced disease, the patients must manually elevate their eyelids and turn their head in the direction of interest to see.

It is important to evaluate patients with ptosis and external ophthalmoplegia for other systemic findings (ophthalmoplegia plus). For example, Kearns and Sayre[84] reported two patients with CPEO, pigmentary retinopathy simulating retinitis pigmentosa, and complete heart block. The recognition of this Kearns-Sayre syndrome at an early stage is important if one is to prevent the systemic consequences of the cardiac disease. Other authors have described gastrointestinal disturbances associated with progressive external ophthalmoplegia.[85, 86] Such patients often present with severe malabsorption that is misdiagnosed if the eye findings, which are usually asymptomatic, are ignored. The hereditary pattern of the mitochondrial cytopathies is maternal.

As noted earlier, some patients with CPEO develop a pigmentary retinopathy that superficially resembles retinitis pigmentosa. There is a "salt and pepper" pattern of pigment deposition and retinal pigment epithelium depigmentation that is heaviest in the peripapillary region (Fig. 3-29). Peripheral bone spicule formation is rare. Night blindness is mild and not consistently present. The blood vessel attenuation and waxy optic disc pallor that is usually seen in typical retinitis pigmentosa does not occur, and visual loss is much less severe in this condition than in retinitis pigmentosa. Histologically, atrophy of the retinal pigment epithelium with destruction of the

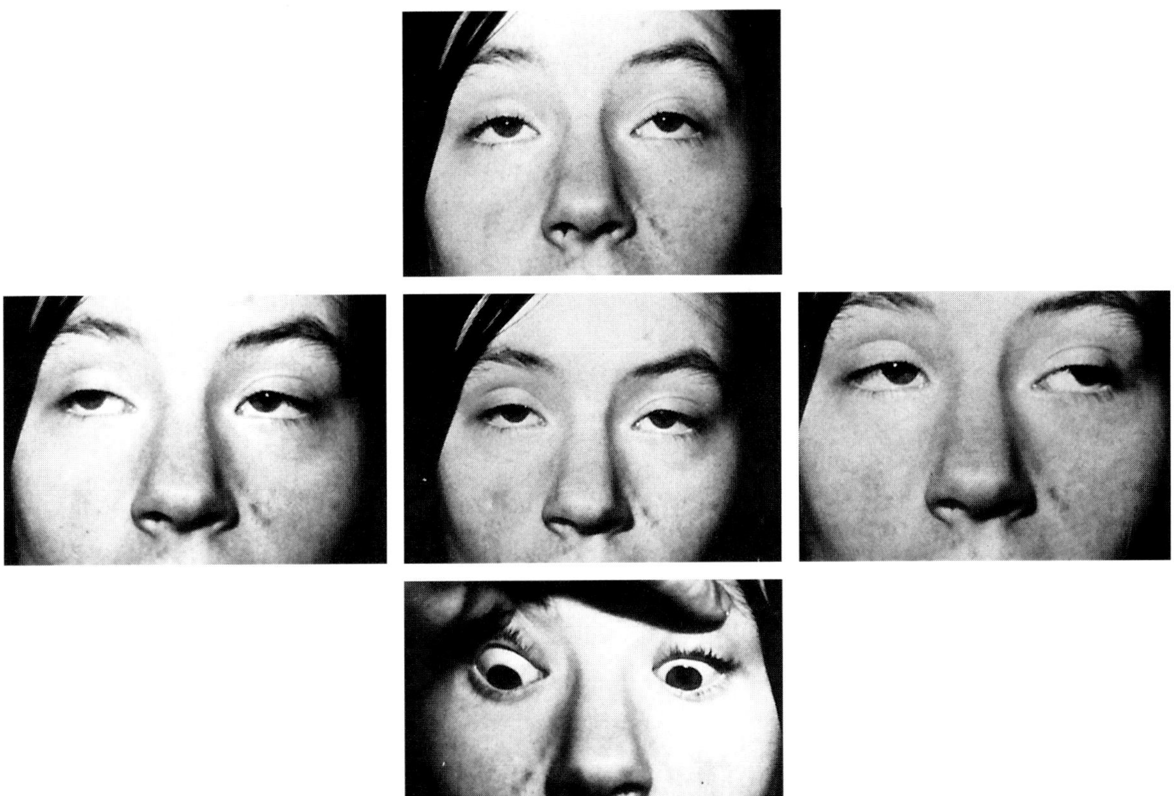

Figure 3-28. Bilateral symmetric ptosis and ophthalmoplegia with normal pupils in a patient with the mitochondriopathy known as *chronic progressive external ophthalmoplegia*. The patient also has mild pigmentary retinopathy. (From Miller NR: Walsh and Hoyt's Clinical Neuro-ophthalmology, 4th ed, vol 2. Baltimore, Williams & Wilkins, 1985, p 817.)

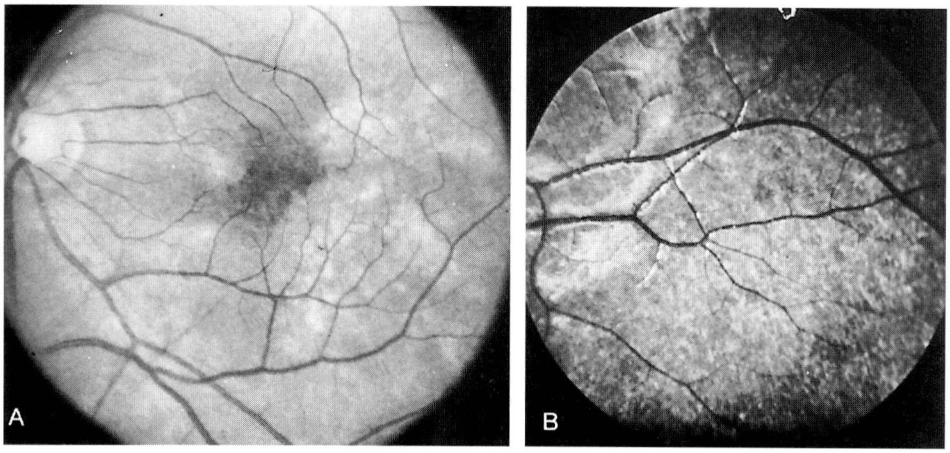

Figure 3–29. Pigmentary retinopathy in patients with Kearns-Sayre syndrome. *A*, Posterior pole of a 17-year-old man shows a mild pigmentary disturbance with pigment clumping overlying white streaks. Note the resemblance to the appearance of the fundus in myotonic dystrophy (see Fig. 3–25). *B*, Stippled (salt-and-pepper) pigmentary disturbance in a 35-year-old woman. (From Miller NR: Walsh and Hoyt's Clinical Neuro-ophthalmology, 4th ed, vol 2. Baltimore, Williams & Wilkins, 1985, p 818.)

overlying retinal cells was most pronounced posteriorly and abnormal mitochondria were spread about the choroid, retinal pigment epithelium, and sensory retina.[87–89]

Cardiac conduction disturbances, severe enough to result in sudden death, are common in patients with CPEO and may worsen in parallel with the course of the ptosis and ophthalmoparesis. In addition to heart block, other cardiac abnormalities such as valve disease have been reported. All patients with CPEO should have periodic cardiac evaluations.

Somatic muscles other than the levator palpebrae superioris and the extraocular muscles may eventually become affected in patients with CPEO, especially in the head and neck region. This may exacerbate the ptosis because the patient is unable to use the frontalis muscle to elevate the eyelids.

Patients with CPEO may develop significant neurologic deficits, including cerebellar ataxia, nystagmus, hearing loss, vestibular dysfunction, and decreased intellectual function. Cerebrospinal fluid protein levels may be elevated. Coulter and Allen[90] documented spongy vacuolization of the brain stem, and it is possible that some of the cases of sudden death that have occurred in patients with CPEO were caused not by cardiac disease but by acute neurologic deterioration. Brain stem auditory evoked response studies have been advocated as a screening tool, although it is unclear how the patients so identified would be treated.

Endocrine abnormalities including short stature and hypoparathyroidism[91, 92] and other biochemical abnormalities have inconsistently been reported in patients with CPEO.

Inflammatory and Infiltrative Myopathies

Inflammatory and infiltrative myopathies can produce ptosis, although their effect on the other extraocular muscles is usually more striking. Snead and colleagues[93] reported ptosis from sarcoidosis of the levator palpebrae superioris, and we have seen several patients who developed ptosis with idiopathic inflammatory orbital pseudotumor. Most of these patients have also had some degree of proptosis and ophthalmoparesis. We have also seen a patient in whom an orbital lymphoma initially produced ptosis from infiltration of the levator muscle without significant involvement of the superior rectus or other extraocular muscles. Susac and coworkers[94] described a woman with ptosis and other signs of external ophthalmoplegia along with extremity weakness as a presentation of dermatomyositis, but this is a most unusual presentation. Primary or secondary amyloidosis may infiltrate muscles in the orbit. Orbital involvement is much more common in the primary form, and ptosis may rarely be the presenting sign of this condition.[95]

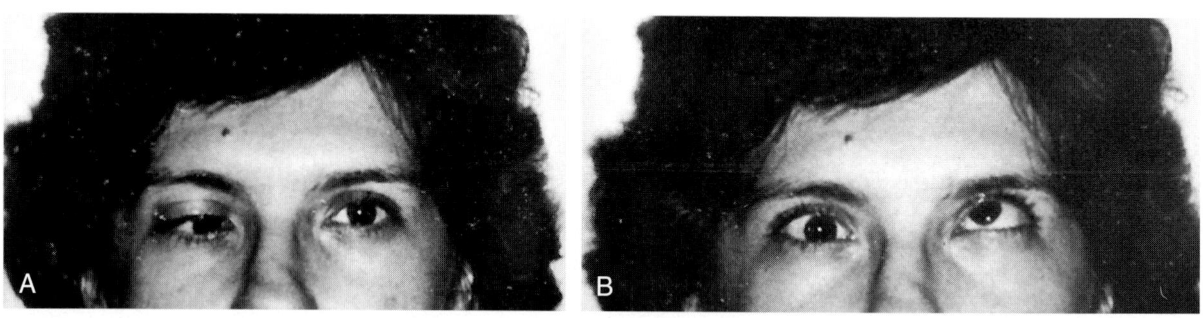

Figure 3–30. Pseudoptosis associated with vertical strabismus. *A*, The patient has a marked right hypotropia and esotropia and is fixating with the left eye. The right upper eyelid seems to be ptotic, but, in fact, it is at the appropriate level for the position of the eye. *B*, When the patient fixates with the left eye, the apparent ptosis disappears, because the right eye is now in normal position. (Courtesy of J. E. Morris, C.O.)

PSEUDOPTOSIS AND EYELID RETRACTION

A number of systemic and local ocular conditions can produce changes in the upper eyelid that mimic ptosis or eyelid retraction. Patients with vertical strabismus, for example, may appear to have ptosis or eyelid retraction depending on the eye being used to fixate (Fig. 3–30). If a normally hypertropic eye fixates, the contralateral eye will be hypotropic, and the eyelid on that side will appear ptotic relative to the opposite side. If the patient attempts to fixate with the hypotropic eye, the opposite eye will now be hypertropic, and the eyelid on that side may appear retracted. Alternatively, when a patient with mechanical restriction of upward gaze (e.g., a patient with a fracture of the orbital floor or involvement of the inferior rectus muscle in dysthyroid orbitopathy) attempts to fixate with the hypotropic eye, the eyelid on that side, which is not mechanically restricted and which receives the same innervation as the superior rectus, will markedly elevate, producing secondary eyelid retraction. Similarly, patients with downward gaze paralysis may preserve eyelid function. When they attempt to look down, the lids depress but the eyes remain in primary position.[96]

Orbital tumors and inflammatory conditions may simulate ptosis by infiltrating the eyelid and displacing the globe or normal eyelid structures.

Blepharospasm may result from a variety of causes, including ocular irritation (e.g., iritis, keratoconjunctivitis sicca) and stroke, but it most often occurs as an idiopathic syndrome that is called *essential blepharospasm.* Essential blepharospasm is characterized by bilateral, spasmodic eyelid closure (Fig. 3–31). When accompanied by face, cheek, mouth, and tongue movements it is called *Meige's syndrome.* It is more common in women and usually appears in patients older than the age of 50.[97] In the early stages of the disease, the patient may complain of difficulty keeping the eyes open, and this may be interpreted as ptosis (Fig. 3–32). Such patients are often

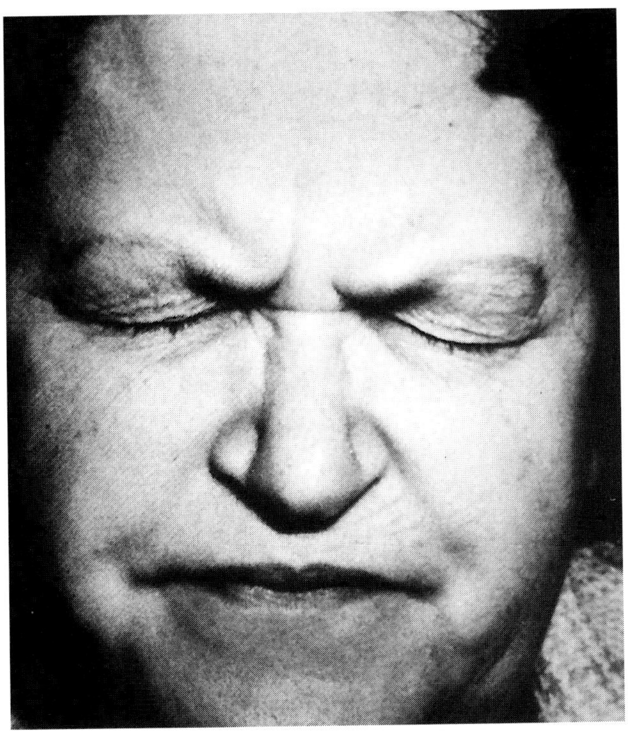

Figure 3–31. Essential blepharospasm. The patient has severe blepharospasm causing both eyelids to close involuntarily. Such patients are often suspected of having myasthenia gravis because of their complaints that they cannot keep their eyes opened during the day. (From Miller NR: Walsh and Hoyt's Clinical Neuro-ophthalmology, 4th ed, vol 2. Baltimore, Williams & Wilkins, 1985, p 977.)

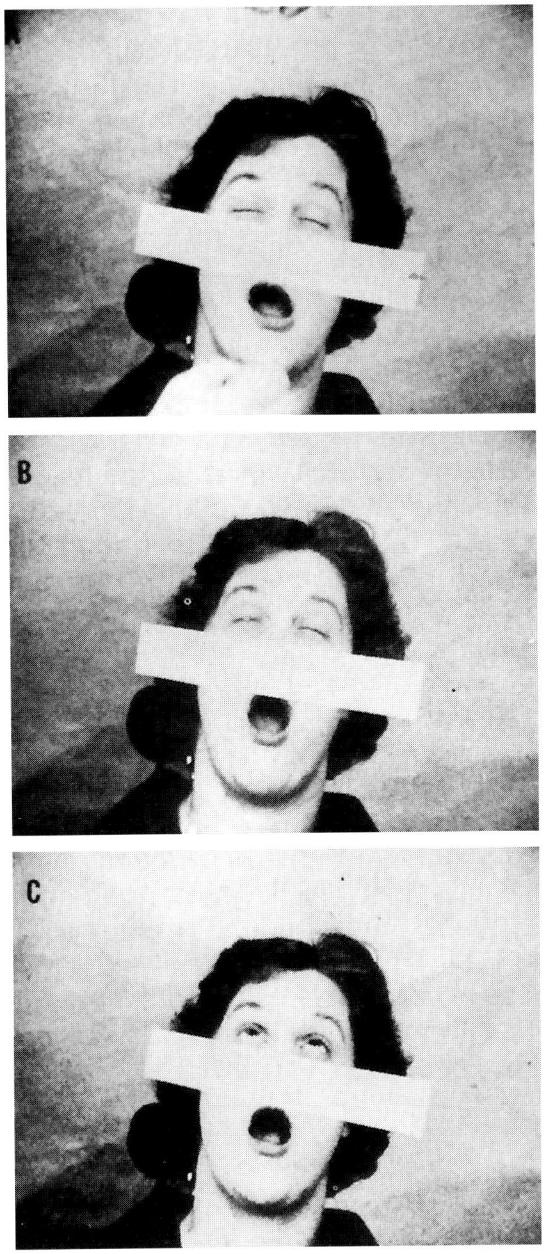

Figure 3–32. Apraxia of eyelid opening, producing an appearance of ptosis. *A,* The patient is attempting to open her eyes on command. Her eyes remain closed, but her mouth opens and her frontalis muscle contracts. *B,* The patient begins to thrust her head backward, and her eyes begin to open slightly. *C,* The patient's neck remains hyperextended, and her eyelids elevate to a normal position, showing the eyes themselves to be elevated. (The photographs were reproduced from a motion picture.) (From Goldstein JE, Cogan DG: Apraxia of lid opening. Arch Ophthalmol 73:155–159, 1965. Copyright 1965, American Medical Association.)

evaluated for possible myasthenia gravis until the spasmodic nature of the eyelid closure becomes evident.

Hemifacial spasm resembles Meige's syndrome except that it is unilateral rather than bilateral (Fig. 3–33). Patients with this condition experience paroxysmal bursts of involuntary muscle activity that initially affect only the orbicularis oculi and simulate intermittent ptosis. With time, however, the spasms spread to affect the entire side of the face. The spasms usually continue during sleep (unlike blepharospasm), and between spasms, facial strength is normal or slightly weak. Most patients with chronic hemifacial spasm have both clinical and electromyographic evidence of aberrant regeneration of the facial nerve.[98] The cause of hemifacial spasm is thought to be compression of the facial nerve root as it exits the brain stem. It is thus important for all patients with this condition to undergo a complete neurologic examination and magnetic resonance imaging of this region of the brain stem to eliminate the possibility of a mass lesion such as a tumor or aneurysm compressing the facial nerve.

The management of blepharospasm, Meige's syndrome, and idiopathic hemifacial spasm has been greatly advanced through the use of botulinum toxin type A (Botox). Although in the past extensive myectomies or extirpation of several branches of the facial nerve were all that was available for controlling these debilitating conditions, intramuscular or subcutaneous injections of botulinum toxin have provided relief of symptoms in over 90% of patients. The symptom-free interval can last anywhere from 2 to 6 months, after which additional injections are required. This interval usually does not decrease with repeated injections. In general, the periocular dose ranges from 1.25 to 5.0 units per injection site, with the maximum cumulative dose in a 30-day period being 200 units. Complications of this treatment have included ptosis, vertical muscle deviations, facial palsy, corneal exposure, dry eye symptoms, and ocular irritation.

Another condition that simulates ptosis is *apraxia of eyelid opening*, also called atypical blepharospasm. This disorder, which occurs most frequently in patients with Parkinson's disease or Huntington's chorea, is associated with intermittent flaccid closure of both eyelids. It is caused primarily by supranuclear inhibition of the innervation of the levator muscles,[99] but, like blepharospasm, there is some spasmodic orbicularis contraction. Patients often attempt to overcome this supranuclear inhibition of eyelid opening by a backward thrusting of the head; the movement interrupts the levator muscle inhibition (see Fig. 3–32). Other patients simply open their eyelids

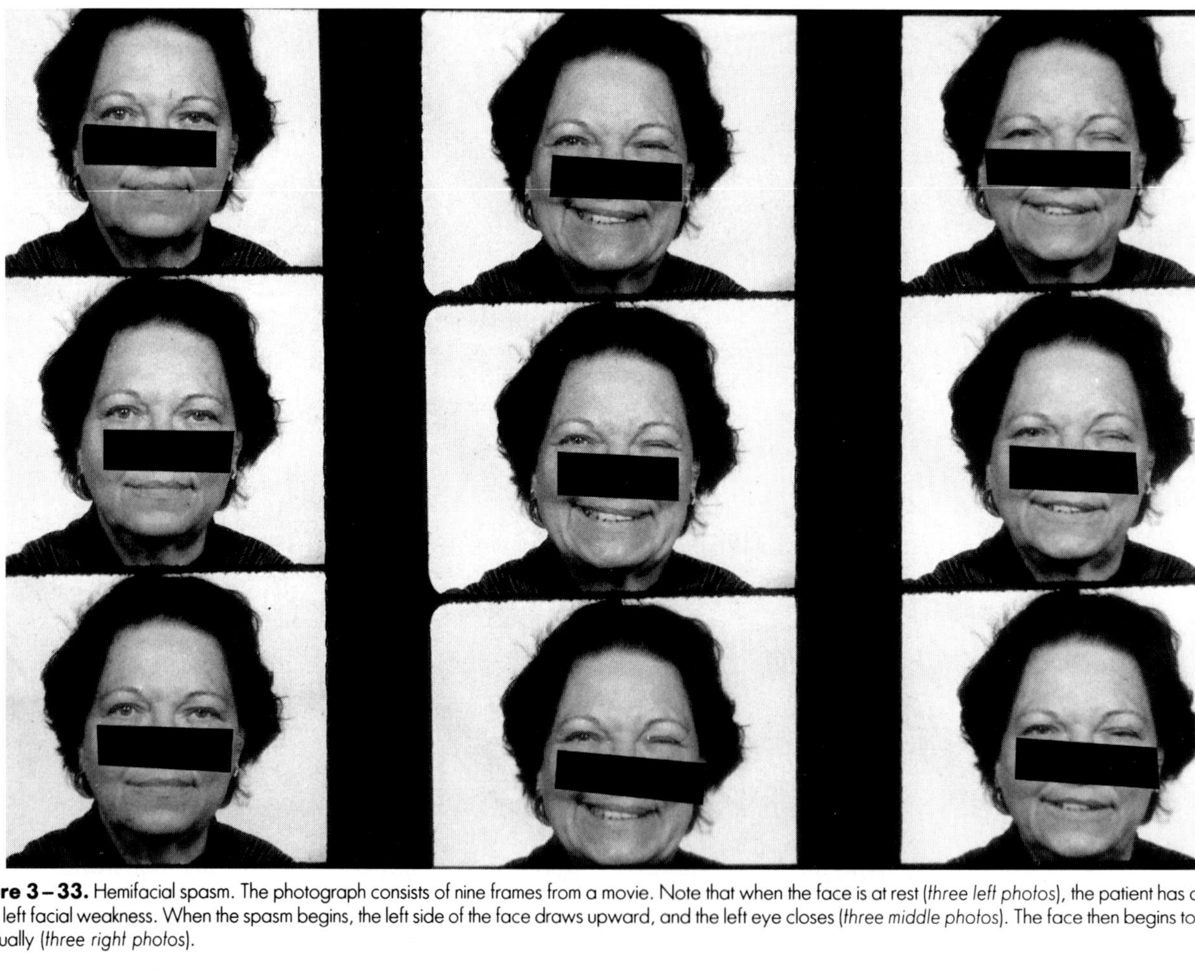

Figure 3–33. Hemifacial spasm. The photograph consists of nine frames from a movie. Note that when the face is at rest (*three left photos*), the patient has a very slight left facial weakness. When the spasm begins, the left side of the face draws upward, and the left eye closes (*three middle photos*). The face then begins to relax gradually (*three right photos*).

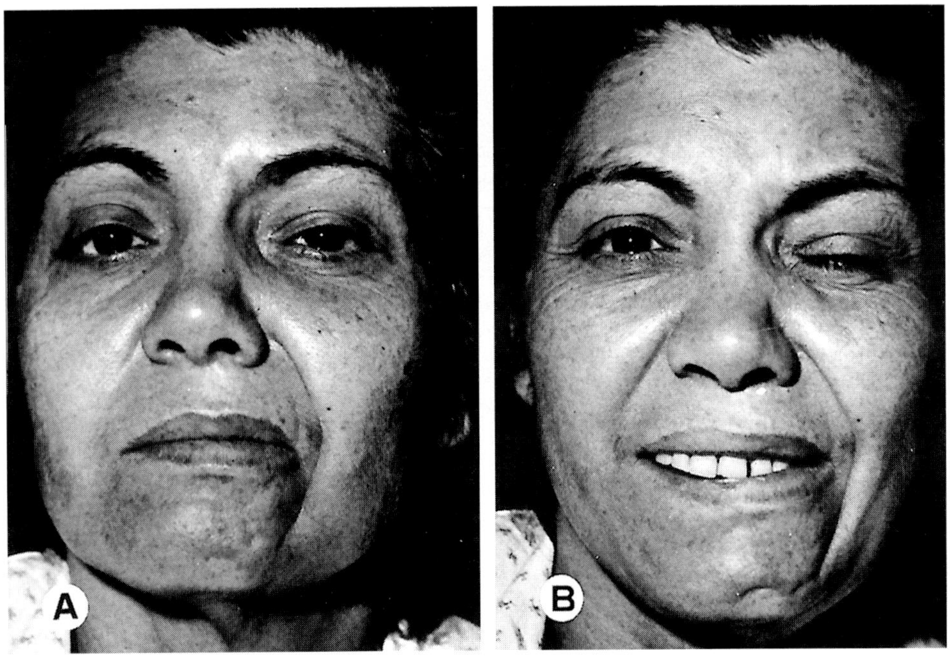

Figure 3–34. Apparent ptosis from aberrant regeneration (misregeneration) of the facial (seventh) nerve following Bell's palsy. *A*, The patient has a slightly narrowed lid fissure and a deep-ended nasolabial fold on the left. *B*, Movement of the corner of the left side of the mouth (such as when the patient is asked to smile) produces left eyelid closure. (From Miller NR: Walsh and Hoyt's Clinical Neuro-ophthalmology, 4th ed, vol 2. Baltimore, Williams & Wilkins, 1985, p 975.)

manually. Some patients are unable to separate their eyelids after blinking.[100] Patients with apraxia of eyelid opening have no ptosis between attacks. Botox may also be helpful in treating this condition.

Patients with *aberrant regeneration of the facial nerve* after Bell's palsy may develop such severe eyelid closure during movements of the mouth and lower face that they are thought to have ptosis (Fig. 3–34). The true nature of the condition can be determined by noting the normal eyelid position when the other facial muscles are inactive.

REFERENCES

1. Collier J: Nuclear ophthalmoplegia: With especial reference to retraction of lids and ptosis and to lesions of posterior commissure. Brain 50:488–498, 1927.
2. Posey WC: Unusual choreiform alterations in the width of the palpebral fissure of both eyes, occasioned by spasm of the levator palpebrae muscles. J Nerv Ment Dis 29:419–421, 1902.
3. Walsh FB, Hoyt WF: Clinical Neuro-ophthalmology, 3rd ed, vol 1. Baltimore, Williams & Wilkins, 1969, p 305.
4. Hoyt CS, Mousel DK, Weber AA: Transient supranuclear disturbances of gaze in healthy neonates. Am J Ophthalmol 89:708–713, 1980.
5. Gunn RM: Congenital ptosis with peculiar associated movements of the affected lid. Trans Ophthalmol Soc UK 3:283–287, 1883.
6. Ticho U: Synkinesis of upper lid elevation occurring in horizontal eye movements. Acta Ophthalmol 49:232–238, 1971.
7. Kansu T, Subutay N: Lid retraction in myasthenia gravis. J Clin Neuro Ophthalmol 7:145–150, 1987.
8. Puklin JE, Sacks JG, Boshes B: Transient eyelid retraction in myasthenia gravis. J Neurol Neurosurg Psychiatry 39:44–47, 1976.
9. Miller NR: Hepatic cirrhosis as a cause of eyelid retraction. Am J Ophthalmol 112:760–761, 1991.
10. Summerskill WHJ, Molnar GD: Eye signs in hepatic cirrhosis. N Engl J Med 266:1244–1248, 1962.
11. Cogan DG: Neurology of the Ocular Muscles, 2nd ed. Springfield, IL, Charles C Thomas, 1956, pp 139–148.
12. Caplan LR: Ptosis. J Neurol Neurosurg Psychiatry 34:1–7, 1974.
13. Lowenstein DH, Kock TK, Edwards MS: Cerebral ptosis with contralateral arteriovenous malformation: A report of two cases. Ann Neurol 21:404–407, 1987.
14. Afifi AK, Corbett JJ, Thompson HS, Wells KK: Seizure-induced miosis and ptosis: Association with temporal lobe magnetic resonance imaging abnormalities. J Child Neurol 5:142–146, 1990.
15. Nutt JG: Lid abnormalities secondary to cerebral hemisphere lesions. Ann Neurol 1:149–151, 1977.
16. Krohel GB, Griffin JF: Cortical blepharoptosis. Am J Ophthalmol 85:632–634, 1978.
17. Lepore FE: Bilateral cerebral ptosis. Neurology 37:1043–1046, 1987.
18. Buttner-Ennever JA, Acheson JF, et al: Ptosis and supranuclear downgaze paralysis. Neurology 39:385–389, 1989.
19. Plum F, Posner JB: The Diagnosis of Stupor and Coma, 3rd ed. Philadelphia, FA Davis, 1980.
20. Dehaene I, Dom R, Marchau M, Geens K: Locked-in syndrome with bilateral ptosis: Combination of bilateral horizontal pontine paralysis and nuclear oculomotor nerve paralysis. J Neurol 232:366–367, 1985.
21. Stevenson GC, Hoyt WF: Metastasis to midbrain from mammary carcinoma: Cause of bilateral ptosis and ophthalmoplegia. JAMA 186:514–516, 1963.
22. Growden JH, Winkler GF, Wray SH: Midbrain ptosis: A case with clinicopathologic correlation. Arch Neurol 30:179–181, 1974.
23. Meienberg O, Mumenthaler M, Karbowski K: Quadriparesis and nuclear oculomotor palsy with total bilateral ptosis mimicking coma: A mesencephalic "locked-in syndrome"? Arch Neurol 36:708–710, 1979.
24. Conway VH, Rozdilsky B, Schneider RJ, Sundaram M: Isolated bilateral complete ptosis. Can J Ophthalmol 18:37–40, 1983.
25. Fleet WS, Rapcsak SZ, Huntley WW, Watson RT: Pupil-sparing oculomotor palsy from midbrain hemorrhage. Ann Ophthalmol 20:345–346, 1988.
26. Good EF: Ptosis as the sole manifestation of compression of the oculomotor nerve by an aneurysm of the posterior communicating artery. J Clin Neuro-Ophthalmol 10:59–61, 1990.
27. Robert CM Jr, Feigenbaum JA, Stern WE: Ocular palsy occurring with pituitary tumors. J Neurosurg 38:17–19, 1973.
28. Small KW, Buckley EG: Recurrent blepharoptosis secondary to a pituitary tumor. Am J Ophthalmol 106:760–761, 1988.
29. Yen MY, Liu JH, Jaw SJ: Ptosis as the early manifestation of pituitary tumour. Br J Ophthalmol 74:188–191, 1990.

30. Wand O: Ptosis associated with aseptic meningitis. Arch Ophthalmol 88:334–335, 1972.
31. Maloney WF, Younge BR, Moyer NJ: Evaluation of the causes and accuracy of pharmacologic localization in Horner's syndrome. Am J Ophthalmol 90:394–402, 1980.
32. Miller NR: Walsh and Hoyt's Clinical Neuro-ophthalmology, 4th ed, vol 2. Baltimore, Williams & Wilkins, 1985, pp 504–507.
33. Elias SB, Appel SH: Current concepts of pathogenesis and treatment of myasthenia gravis. Med Clin North Am 63:745–757, 1979.
34. Drachman DA, Adams RN, Stanley EF, Pestronk A: Mechanisms of acetylcholine receptor loss in myasthenia gravis. J Neurol Neurosurg Psychiatry 43:601–610, 1980.
35. Lindstrom JM, Seybold ME, Lennon VA, et al: Antibody to acetylcholine receptor in myasthenia gravis: Prevalence, clinical correlates, and diagnostic value. Neurology 26:1054–1059, 1976.
36. Lindstrom JM: Experimental autoimmune myasthenia gravis. *In* Aguayo A, Karpati G (eds): Current Topics in Nerve and Muscle Research. Amsterdam, Excerpta Medica, 1979, p 104.
37. Simpson JA: An evaluation of thymectomy in myasthenia gravis. Brain 81:112–144, 1958.
38. Schwab RS, Leland CC: Sex and age in myasthenia gravis as critical factors in incidence and remissions. JAMA 153:1270–1273, 1953.
39. Mattis RD: Ocular manifestations of myasthenia gravis. Arch Ophthalmol 26:969–982, 1941.
40. Osserman KE: Ocular myasthenia gravis. Invest Ophthalmol 6:277–287, 1967.
41. Daroff RB: Ocular myasthenia: Diagnosis and therapy. *In* Glaser JS (ed): Neuro-Ophthalmology, vol. 10. St. Louis, CV Mosby, 1980, pp 62–71.
42. Simpson JA: Myasthenia gravis and myasthenic syndromes. *In* Walton J (ed): Disorders of Voluntary Muscle, 4th ed. Edinburgh, Churchill Livingstone, 1981, pp 585–624.
43. Oosterhuis HJGH: The ocular signs and symptoms of myasthenia gravis. Doc Ophthalmol 52:363–378, 1982.
44. Osserman KE: Myasthenia Gravis. New York, Grune & Stratton, 1958.
45. Cogan DB: Myasthenia gravis: A review of the disease and a description of lid twitch as a characteristic sign. Arch Ophthalmol 74:217–221, 1965.
46. Gorlick PB, Rosenberg M, Pagano RJ: Enhanced ptosis in myasthenia gravis. Arch Neurol 38:531, 1981.
47. Patten BM: Myasthenia gravis: Review of diagnosis and management. Muscle Nerve 1:190–205, 1978.
48. Burde RM, Savino PJ, Trobe JD: Clinical Decisions in Neuro-ophthalmology. St. Louis, CV Mosby, 1985, pp 175–177.
49. Bartley GB, Bullock JD: The Tensilon test using a three-way stopcock and double syringe. Ophthal Plast Reconstr Surg 2:95–96, 1986.
50. Moorthy G, Behrens MM, Drachman DB, et al: Ocular pseudomyasthenia or ocular myasthenia "plus": A warning to clinicians. Neurology 39:1150–1154, 1989.
51. Sethi KD, Riuner MH, Swift TR: Ice pack test for myasthenia gravis. Neurology 37:1383–1385, 1987.
52. Ertas M, Arac N, Kumral K, Tuchay T: Ice test as a simple diagnostic aid for myasthenia gravis. Acta Neurol Scand 89:227–229, 1994.
53. Odel JG, Winterkorn JM, Behrens MM: The sleep test for myasthenia gravis. A safe alternative to Tensilon. J Clin Neuro-ophthalmol 11:288–292, 1991.
54. Pestronk A, Drachman DB, Josifek LF: Measurement of junctional ACh receptors in myasthenia gravis: Diagnostic value and clinical correleates. Neurology 31:83, 1981.
55. Feltkamp TEW, van den Berg-Loonen PM, Nijenhuis LE, et al: Myasthenia gravis, autoantibodies and HL-A antigens. Br Med J 1:131–133, 1974.
56. Kelly JJ Jr, Daube JR, Lennon VA, et al: The laboratory diagnosis of mild myasthenia gravis. Ann Neurol 12:238–242, 1982.
57. Lambert EH, Rooke ED, Eaton LM, Hodgson CH: Myasthenic syndrome occasionally associated with bronchial neoplasm: Neurophysiologic studies. *In* Viets HR (ed): Myasthenia Gravis: The 2nd International Symposium Proceedings. Springfield, IL, Charles C Thomas, 1961, pp 362–410.
58. Gutmann L, Crosby TW, Takamori M, Martin JD: The Eaton-Lambert syndrome and autoimmune disorders. Am J Med 53:354–356, 1972.
59. Norris FH Jr: Neuromuscular transmission in thyroid disease. Ann Intern Med 64:81–86, 1966.
60. Brown JW, Nelson JR, Herrmann C Jr: Sjögren's syndrome with myopathic and myasthenic features. Bull Los Angeles Neurol Soc 33:9–20, 1968.
61. Brown JC, Johns RJ: Clinical and physiological studies of the effect of guanidine on patients with myasthenia gravis. Johns Hopkins Med J 124:1–8, 1969.
62. Takamori M, Gutmann L: Intermittent defect of acetylcholine release in myasthenia gravis. Neurology 21:47–54, 1971.
63. Schwartz MS, Stalberg E: Myasthenia gravis with features of the myasthenic syndrome. Neurology 25:80–84, 1975.
64. Leys K, Lang B, Johnston I, Newsom-Davis J: Calcium channel autoantibodies in the Lambert-Eaton myasthenic syndrome. Ann Neurol 29:307–314, 1991.
65. Cruciger MP, Brown B, Denys EH, et al: Clinical and subclinical oculomotor findings in the Eaton-Lambert syndrome. J Clin Neuro-Ophthalmol 3:19–22, 1983.
66. Berstein LP, Henkind P: Additional information on adverse reactions to timolol. Am J Ophthalmol 92:295–296, 1981.
67. Shy GM, Magee KR: A new congenital nonprogressive myopathy. Brain 79:610–622, 1956.
68. Engel AG, Gomez MR, Groover RV: Multicore disease: A recently recognized congenital myopathy associated with multifocal degeneration of muscle fibres. Mayo Clin Proc 46:666–681, 1971.
69. Fukuyama Y, Kawazura M, Haruna H: A peculiar form of congenital progressive muscular dystrophy: Report of 15 cases. Paediatr Univ Tokyo 4:5, 1960.
70. Tsutsumi A, Uchida Y, Osawa M, Fukuyama Y: Ocular findings in Fukuyama type congenital muscular dystrophy. Brain Dev 11:413–419, 1989.
71. Aström KE, Adams RD: Myotonic disorders. *In* Mastaglia FL, Walton J (eds): Skeletal Muscle Pathology. Edinburgh, Churchill Livingstone, 1982, pp 266–286.
72. Kuhn E, Fiehn W: Adult form of myotonic dystrophy. *In* Huber A, Klein D (eds): Neurogenetics and Neuro-ophthalmology. Amsterdam, Elsevier/North-Holland, 1981, pp 31–49.
73. Babel J: Ophthalmological aspects of myotonic dystrophy. *In* Huber A, Klein D (eds): Neurogenetics and Neuro-ophthalmology. Amsterdam, Elsevier/North-Holland, 1981, pp 19–30.
74. Creel DJ, Crandall AS, Ziter FA: Identification of minimal expression of myotonic dystrophy using electroretinography. Electroencephalogr Clin Neurophysiol 61:229–235, 1985.
75. Achiron A, Magal N, Shem-Tor N, et al: Myotonic dystrophy gene analysis in affected Israeli families. Isr J Med Sci 30:622–625, 1994.
76. Taylor EW: Progressive vagus-glossopharyngeal paralysis with ptosis: Contribution to group of family disease. J Nerv Ment Dis 42:129–139, 1915.
77. Johnson CC, Kuwabara T: Oculopharyngeal muscular dystrophy. Am J Ophthalmol 77:872–879, 1974.
78. Harding AE, Sanders MD, Petty RKH, Morgan-Hughes JA: The neuro-ophthalmological features of mitochondrial myopathy. Presented at the Fifth Meeting of the International Neuro-ophthalmology Society. Antwerp, Belgium, May 14–18, 1984.
79. Engel WK: Muscle biopsies in neuromuscular diseases. Pediatr Clin North Am 14:963–995, 1967.
80. Engel WK, Cunningham GG: Rapid examination of muscle tissue: An improved trichrome method for rapid diagnosis of muscle biopsy fresh-frozen section. Neurology 13:919–923, 1963.
81. Olson W, Engel WK, Walsh GO, Einaugler R: Oculocraniosomatic neuromuscular disease with "ragged-red" fibers: Histochemical and ultrastructural changes in limb muscles of a group of patients with idiopathic progressive external ophthalmoplegia. Arch Neurol 26:193–211, 1972.
82. Mitsumoto H, Aprille JR, Wray SH, et al: Chronic progressive external ophthalmoplegia (CPEO): Clinical, morphologic, and biochemical studies. Neurology 33:452–461, 1983.
83. Johnson MA, Turnbull DM, Dick DJ, Sherratt HSA: A partial deficiency of cytochrome-*c* oxidase in chronic progressive external ophthalmoplegia. J Neurol Sci 60:31–53, 1983.
84. Kearns TP, Sayre GP: Retinitis pigmentosa, external ophthalmo-

plegia, and complete heart block. Arch Ophthalmol 60:280–289, 1958.
85. Bardosi A, Creutzfeldt W, Di Mauro S, et al: Myo-, neuro-, gastrointestinal encephalopathy (MNGIE syndrome) due to partial deficiency of cytochrome-*c*-oxidase. A new mitochondrial multisystem disorder. Acta Neuropathol (Berl) 74:248–258, 1987.
86. Threlkeld AB, Miller NR, Golnik KC, et al: Ophthalmic involvement in myo-neuro-gastrointestinal encephalopathy syndrome. Am J Ophthalmol 114:322–328, 1992.
87. Newell FW, Polascik MA: Mitochondrial disease and retinal pigmentary degeneration. Council Ophthalmol 1:615–617, 1979.
88. Eagle RC Jr, Hedges TR, Yanoff M: The atypical pigmentary retinopathy of Kearns-Sayre syndrome: A light and electron microscopic study. Ophthalmology 89:1433–1440, 1982.
89. Eagle RC Jr, Hedges TR, Yanoff M: The Kearns-Sayre syndrome: A light and electron microscopic study. Trans Am Ophthalmol Soc 80:218–234, 1982.
90. Coulter DI, Allen RJ: Abrupt neurological deterioration in children with Kearns-Sayre syndrome. Arch Neurol 38:247–250, 1981.
91. Marks H, Headington J, Allen RJ: Hypoparathyroidism associated with oculocraniosomatic syndrome [abstract]. Presented before the Fifth National Meeting of the Child Neurology Society, 1976.
92. Toppet M, Telerman-Toppet N, Szliwowski HB, et al: Oculocraniosomatic neuromuscular disease with hypoparathyroidism. Am J Dis Child 131:437–441, 1977.
93. Snead JW, Seidenstein L, Knific RJ, et al: Isolated orbital sarcoidosis as a cause for blepharoptosis. Am J Ophthalmol 112:739, 1991.
94. Susac JO, Garcia-Mullin R, Glaser JS: Ophthalmoplegia in dermatomyositis. Neurology 23:305–310, 1973.
95. Gonnering RS, Sonneland PR: Ptosis and dermatochalasis as presenting signs in a case of occult primary systemic amyloidosis. Ophthalmic Surg 18:495–497, 1987.
96. LoBue TD, Feldon SE: Reverse Collier's sign: Pseudoblepharoptosis associated with downgaze paralysis. Am J Ophthalmol 95:120–121, 1983.
97. Frueh BR, Callahan A, Dortzbach RK, et al: A profile of patients with intractable blepharospasm. Trans Am Acad Ophthalmol Otolaryngol 81:591–594, 1976.
98. Kim P, Fukushima T: Observations on synkinesis in patients with hemifacial spasm: Effect of microvascular decompression and etiological considerations. J Neurosurg 60:821–827, 1984.
99. Schilder P: Neuer Beitrag zur Pathologie der Lidbewegungen, kipfmitbewegungen aphatiker beim öffnen und Schlissen der Augen. Dtsch Z Nervenheilkd 98:161–168, 1927.
100. Goldstein JE, Cogan DG: Apraxia of lid opening. Arch Ophthalmol 73:155–159, 1965.

CHAPTER 4

Ocular Manifestations of Systemic Immune Disease

John C. Baer and Ramzi K. Hemady

This chapter addresses systemic inflammatory diseases that affect the lids, the adnexa, or the orbit and are of autoimmune, or presumed autoimmune, etiology. Three broad classes of diseases are considered: bullous diseases, sarcoidosis, and vasculitic diseases. Although the chapter is oriented toward the orbital and adnexal signs and symptoms of these diseases, the full range of ocular manifestations is presented. Inflammatory diseases whose manifestations are restricted to the globe, sparing the orbit and the adnexa, are not included. A brief review of general immunologic concepts is included to serve as a foundation for the sections describing the specific disease entities.

THE IMMUNE SYSTEM

A basic understanding of the cell types involved in immune reactions, the role of complement and immunoglobulins, the classification of immune reactions, and the basis of laboratory techniques is important to the ophthalmologist in establishing a clinical diagnosis and treatment regimen for autoimmune diseases. A review of these principles is presented. The reader is referred to standard immunology texts for a more detailed description of these topics.

Cells of the Immune System

Macrophages

Macrophages and monocytes are phagocytic cells of bone marrow origin. In addition to their direct phagocytic role, macrophages play two other important roles in promoting immune responses. Macrophages act as antigen-presenting cells that ingest antigen, process it intracellularly, and present it to T lymphocytes (see later discussion) in an acceptable form to result in T cell activation and cell-mediated and humoral immune responses. In addition, macrophages secrete a wide array of biologically active substances that stimulate or attract other leukocytes, affect blood vessel permeability and smooth muscle tone, modify the extracellular matrix, and affect wound healing.

Lymphocytes

Lymphocytes are found throughout the body tissues, with especially high concentrations in the spleen, lymph nodes, and thymus. Lymphocyte traffic between organs occurs via the blood and the lymphatics.

Lymphocytes are derived from bone marrow stem cells but are divided into two subpopulations called *B cells* and *T cells,* based on their site of maturation and cell characteristics. T cells have been processed in the thymus, whereas B cells, which mature in the bursa of Fabricius in birds, mature in the bursa equivalent in humans and other mammals without a bursa. This bursa-equivalent site is probably the bone marrow in humans.

Subpopulations of T lymphocytes participate in a wide range of immunologic reactions. They cooperate with other lymphocytes in inducing immune reactions (e.g., helper T cells with B lymphocytes for antibody production). T cells also down-regulate immune reactions (suppressor T cells), and participate in direct killing of target cells (cytotoxic T cells). These T cell subpopulations can be differentiated by using monoclonal antibodies (see later discussion) to markers on the cell surface. The CD4 marker is present on human T helper/inducer cells. Monoclonal antibodies for this marker are OKT4 and Leu-3a. T suppressor and T cytotoxic lymphocytes are CD8 positive (OKT8 and Leu-2a antibodies). The CD3 marker (OKT3 and Leu-4 antibodies) is present on all mature T cells.

As described, T cells play a wide variety of important roles in immune reactions. Conceptually, they are most often associated with the arm of immune response termed *cell-mediated immunity.*

B lymphocytes, on the other hand, are conceptually associated with humoral immune responses mediated by antibodies. After interaction with T helper cells and under proper conditions, B cells become antibody-producing plasma cells. Although in some instances antibody production can occur without T cell help, for example, in the presence of pneumococcal cell walls, lipopolysaccharide, and some mitogens, most clinically important antibody production requires T cell help. Most B cells have immunoglobulins on their surface that can be used as cell markers.

Null cells are lymphocytes that lack the surface markers specific for either T or B cells. Included in this heterogeneous group are natural killer (NK) cells and killer (K) cells. NK cells are cytotoxic cells that do not require prior sensitization to kill target cells. They are probably important in surveillance for tumors and in transplantation rejection. K cells act against antibody-coated targets in a reaction termed *antibody-dependent cell-mediated cytotoxicity.*

Granulocytes

Neutrophils respond to inflammatory sites by margination within blood vessels, adhesion to the blood vessel endothelium, and emigration through the vessel wall into the perivascular tissues. They play an important role in the inflammatory process by phagocytosis and by release of lysosomal enzymes, which are cytotoxic and aid in degradation of extracellular components and cellular debris.

Basophils and mast cells may or may not share the same stem cell origin, but they have many similarities. Basophils are derived in the bone marrow from the same stem cell as other granulocytes. The origin of mast cells is less clear. Basophils are circulating cells, whereas mast cells are identified in tissue. Both cell types have receptors on their cell surface for immunoglobulin E (IgE). When two cell-surface IgE molecules attach to the same bivalent antigen, a chain reaction is set in motion that results in mast cell or basophil degranulation and release of multiple biologically active products, including histamine, serotonin, prostaglandins, leukotrienes, and chemotactic factors for neutrophils and eosinophils. Histamine, serotonin, prostaglandins, and leukotrienes have pronounced effects (some of which are contradictory) on vascular permeability and smooth muscle contraction. Leukotriene B_4 and chemotactic factors attract neutrophils and eosinophils to the site of inflammation.

Eosinophils produce many of the same enzymes as neutrophils. They are attracted to inflammatory sites by mast cell degranulation products. One role that eosinophils may play is modulation of mast cell activation. Eosinophils are also found in high numbers at sites of parasitic infection.

Antibodies

Antibodies are the product of plasma cells. In humans, antibodies are proteins that share a common underlying structure and are referred to as *immunoglobulins.* The basic building block from which all immunoglobulins are built consists of a monomer containing four polypeptide chains: two light chains and two heavy chains. There are five classes of immunoglobulins: IgA, IgD, IgE, IgG, and IgM. The heavy chains determine the class of immunoglobulin and are named with the corresponding Greek letters: alpha, delta, epsilon, gamma, and mu. The two different light-chain polypeptides are known as kappa and lambda.

At the amino-terminal end of all four polypeptide chains of an immunoglobulin molecule is a variable region that is the antigen-binding site. The variation in the amino ends and among clones of plasma cells means that the "catalog" of antibodies can recognize a wide variety of antigens. The carboxyl end has a more constant amino acid sequence, and it is this end of the immunoglobulin molecule that binds to cell surfaces. The cell-surface receptors for the carboxyl end of immunoglobulins are referred to as *Fc receptors.*

IgM is a pentamer composed of five covalently bonded copies of the basic monomer. On first exposure to an antigen the primary antibody response is IgM. Therefore, the presence of IgM helps confirm infections of recent onset. IgM is an effective agglutinating antibody and is one of two antibody classes present on B lymphocyte cell surfaces.

IgG, a monomer, is the most abundant immunoglobulin in the serum. IgG is also produced on first exposure to an antigen, but it peaks later and persists longer than IgM. IgG and IgM are the two classes of immunoglobulins that activate the complement cascade ("fix" complement). Another important characteristic of IgG is its ability to cross the placenta.

IgE attaches to mast cell and basophil surface receptors, and, as discussed earlier, is important in mast cell degranulation. IgE is believed to be an important mediator of allergic reactions, including anaphylaxis.

IgD is found on B cell surfaces and is a receptor for antigen-specific B cell stimulation.

IgA is found at mucosal surfaces and in tears, saliva, and nasal, bronchial, and gastrointestinal secretions. At mucosal surfaces, IgA occurs as a dimer with an additional secretory piece that is synthesized by the mucosal epithelial cells. The probable role for IgA is to help protect mucosal surfaces from invasion by environmental pathogens.

The Complement System

The complement system is a cascade of nine serum proteins that is activated in the presence of membrane-bound antigen-antibody complexes to produce holes in the membrane that, in turn, promote cell lysis. An alternate pathway for complement activation exists that does not require antibody. The alternate pathway is activated directly by a variety of substances, including bacterial cell walls, bacterial endotoxins, and polysaccharide. Cleavage products of complement activation not involved in the lytic process mediate chemotaxis, smooth muscle contraction, and mast cell degranulation.

Classic Immune Reactions ("hypersensitivity reactions")

Gell and Coombs classified inflammatory reactions into four types based on their mechanism: types I, II, and III involve interaction between antibody and antigen, and type IV, also known as *delayed hypersensitivity,* is a cell-mediated process involving T cells.

Type I Hypersensitivity (anaphylactic response). Type I hypersensitivity is the reaction of antigen with the IgE bound to the mast cell surface resulting in mast cell degranulation and release of the soluble mediators, described earlier, and is the hypersensitivity reaction associated with allergic reactions and anaphylaxis. Tissue edema is one hallmark of type I hypersensitivity. A classic example is the development of skin wheal and flare after intradermal injection of an antigen.

Type II Hypersensitivity (cytotoxic response). In type II hypersensitivity, antibody binds to cell membrane–bound antigen resulting in cell killing by one of three different mechanisms: (1) activation of complement; (2) phagocytosis that is facilitated by the presence of antibody (opsonization); and (3) antibody-dependent cell-mediated cytotoxicity. A classic example of type II hypersensitivity is a transfusion reaction, in which lysis of red blood cells occurs in sensitized people who have antibodies to cell-surface antigens on the donor red blood cells. Type II hypersensitivity may play a role in cicatricial pemphigoid and other bullous diseases.

Type III Hypersensitivity (immune complex reaction). When circulating antigen-antibody complexes (immune complexes) are deposited in blood vessel walls and surrounding tissues, complement is activated and neutrophils are attracted to the site. Serum sickness is an example of this type of reaction. It occurs 1 to 2 weeks after injection of a foreign protein (e.g., tetanus antitoxin from horse serum) and results in fever, lymphadenopathy, urticarial rash, and hypocomplementemia. The histology demonstrates vasculitis.

Another example of type III hypersensitivity is the Arthus reaction. Under the right conditions, injection in the skin of soluble antigen produces vasculitis and neutrophil infiltration. The reaction is maximal after about 4 hours. In later stages, there is an increase in the number of mononuclear cells. The reaction disappears after about 12 hours. This timing contrasts with type I reactions, which are almost immediate. It has been suggested that type III mechanisms play a role in rheumatoid arthritis, lupus erythematosus, and vasculitic diseases.

Type IV Hypersensitivity (delayed reaction). Type IV hypersensitivity differs from types I to III because it is mediated by sensitized T cells (cell-mediated immunity) rather than antibody (humoral immunity). The term *delayed hypersensitivity* reflects the fact that the reaction does not reach its peak for about 1 to 3 days. In this reaction, T cell receptors, rather than the variable region of an antibody, recognize antigen. The activated T cell secretes lymphokines that attract inflammatory cells, including macrophages, lymphocytes, and granulocytes. Lymphokines may themselves be cytotoxic. An example of type IV hypersensitivity is the skin reaction 48 hours after injection of purified protein derivative tuberculin into a patient previously exposed to tuberculosis. Transplantation rejection is another important example.

Histocompatibility Antigens

The histocompatibility antigens are termed *histocompatibility leukocyte antigens* (HLA) in humans and are located on chromosome six. The HLA genes, or genes closely linked to this region, are important in immune responsiveness. Two classes of antigens have been identified: (1) class I antigens are found on nucleated cells, and the loci for these antigens have been termed *HLA-A, HLA-B,* and *HLA-C;* (2) class II antigens are produced by the HLA-D/DR loci. Class II antigens must match between a macrophage (or other antigen-presenting cells) and a T cell for successful antigen presentation to occur, and the process is said to be class II restricted. In a similar fashion, T cell interaction with B cells is class II restricted. Mismatched class I antigens are the principal target of the immune response in allograft rejection, hence matching class I HLA loci between donor and recipient enhances graft survival in many instances. In addition, class I antigens serve as recognition sites for cytotoxic T cells when they attack cells whose surface antigens have been altered by viral infection or neoplastic transformation.

Monoclonal Antibodies

In vivo, when the immune system is presented with an antigen, many clones of B cells are stimulated. The individual B cells respond to different portions of the antigen (epitopes) and produce antibodies of different affinity for the antigen. In this circumstance, the heterogeneous antibodies from a serum sample are said to be *polyclonal antibodies* to the antigen. By fusing an antibody-producing B cell with an immortalized myeloma cell line, a large number of identical B cells result, all producing antibody of the same specificity and affinity for the antigen. Therefore, large quantities of identical antibody can be produced. The availability of monoclonal antibodies has been a crucial tool in both the basic science and clinical setting in the understanding, diagnosis, and treatment of immune and other diseases.

Laboratory Testing

Proper interpretation of test results by the ophthalmologist depends on an understanding of the test methods. The techniques for the enzyme-linked immunosorbent assay (ELISA) and for immunofluorescent and immunohistochemical staining of smears and tissue sections are described.

ELISA involves fixing antigen to a surface, for example, the bottom of a plastic laboratory plate. Serum, which may contain antibody to the test antigen, is added and time allowed for antibody to combine with the antigen. The serum is washed gently away, removing any unbound antibody. A monoclonal antibody specific for immunoglobulin, which is chemically linked to an enzyme, is added to the plate. If serum antibody is bound to the antigen, the monoclonal antibody against immunoglobulin will, in turn, bind to the serum antibody. The excess monoclonal antibody is washed off. Finally, a substrate that can be cleaved by the enzyme is added. The substrate and enzyme are chosen such that cleaving the substrate results in a color change that can be measured by spectrophotometry. The degree of color change is related to the number of enzyme molecules, which, in turn, is related to the quantity of bound serum antibody.

Immunofluorescent and immunohistochemical staining use monoclonal antibodies to identify antigens in tissue sections and smears. Fixation of the tissue in formalin or strong fixatives may chemically alter antigens in such a way that they are no longer recognized. Because of this, immune staining is often performed on frozen sections. Before the tissue specimen is obtained, the ophthalmologist must discuss the preparation and handling of the specimen with the ocular pathologist to avoid unreliable results or the need to repeat the biopsy.

After the tissue has been appropriately prepared and sectioned for immunofluorescence, the slide is incubated with antibody against the desired antigen, which has been conjugated to fluorescein or rhodamine (direct immunofluorescence). After washing off the unbound antibody, the specimen is examined by fluorescent microscopy, and a qualitative assessment is made in comparison with positive and negative control slides. For greater sensitivity, the tissue can be incubated with antigen-specific monoclonal antibody without a fluorescent tag. Then, a second fluorescent monoclonal antibody specific for immunoglobulin is added. Since more than one anti-immunoglobulin antibody may bind to each of the antigen-specific monoclonal antibodies, an amplification of the fluorescence may result. If the patient's serum is substituted for the first monoclonal antibody, serum antibodies to the target tissue can be detected and a titer determined (indirect immunofluorescence).

In immunohistochemical staining, an enzymatic reaction is used to cleave a substrate, as in ELISA. The colored product is deposited in the tissue at the site of the antigen, and the specimen is examined by light microscopy. Amplification can be obtained using biotinylated antibodies. Enzyme is bound to avidin, which is capable of binding to biotin in large quantities. Therefore, more than one copy of the enzyme is present for each copy of antigen.

Pharmacology of Therapeutic Agents

Corticosteroids have been the primary treatment for ocular inflammatory diseases since the 1950s. Because of their pronounced side effects and their inability to control the most severe inflammatory and autoimmune diseases, cytotoxic agents, including the alkylating agents (chlorambucil and cyclophosphamide) and the antimetabolites (azathioprine and methotrexate), have been used in instances when steroids alone are insufficient or poorly tolerated. More recently, cyclosporine has shown promise in some instances.

Corticosteroids form a complex with a cell-surface receptor and are transported to the nucleus, where they act on deoxyribonucleic acid (DNA) transcription. Most organ systems are affected by pharmacologic doses of corticosteroids. The effect on the immune system includes movement of T helper cells out of the intravascular compartment that results in a reduced recruitment of other inflammatory cells to the active inflammatory site. Although there is an increase in neutrophil production and an increase in the leukocyte count in peripheral blood, there is a reduced ability of neutrophils to migrate out of blood vessels. Counts of circulating monocytes, eosinophils, and basophils may be reduced. In addition to changes in the cell populations in the circulation, there are profound changes in cellular function as well, including a decrease in leukocyte phagocytosis and decreased lymphokine production.

Alkylating agents act by alkylating DNA guanine residues. This can result in miscoding of the DNA, scission of the DNA chain, or cross-linking of the two DNA chains. Rapidly dividing clones of inflammatory cells are profoundly affected. Cyclophosphamide exerts its effects predominantly on leukocytes, whereas chlorambucil, at least transiently, affects red blood cell production as well.

The antimetabolites azathioprine and methotrexate alter purine and folate metabolism, respectively. Azathioprine is a pro-drug that is converted to 6-mercaptopurine. Incorporation of 6-mercaptopurine into the 5′-phosphate ribonucleotide inhibits the production of adenosine monophosphate and guanosine monophosphate and the metabolism of DNA and ribonucleic acid. Methotrexate acts by inhibiting dihydrofolate reductase, which is important in the production of tetrahydrofolate. Tetrahydrofolate is incorporated into coenzymes that are important in purine and pyrimidine synthesis.

Cyclosporine is cyclic peptide derived from fungi. It

primarily affects a T cell's ability to recruit and activate other leukocytes. Cyclosporine may act by blocking the release of interleukin-2 (IL-2) or by reducing the number of IL-2 receptors, or both.

BULLOUS DISEASE

The skin, mucous membranes, and ocular surface may be involved in bullous diseases. Bullae are intraepithelial or subepithelial collections of fluid in spaces created by the dissolution of intracellular matrices. Many bullous diseases are of presumed autoimmune etiology. Ocular involvement in many of these diseases follows a similar pattern: conjunctival inflammation followed by cicatrization, entropion, trichiasis, dry eyes, and corneal opacification and neovascularization. A discussion of the five bullous diseases that commonly affect the eyes follows.

Cicatricial Pemphigoid

Background

Cicatricial pemphigoid is a relatively rare systemic autoimmune disease affecting the skin and the mucous membranes. Several different names have been used to refer to this disease in the past, including *ocular pemphigoid, benign mucous membrane pemphigoid,* and *essential shrinkage of the conjunctiva.*[1-3] Pemphigoid was long considered a form of pemphigus but was separated from it in 1953 after the pioneering work of Lever.[4] The ocular manifestations of this disease are characterized by progressive conjunctival inflammation with loss of vision from corneal opacification.[1, 5-7]

Epidemiology

Cicatricial pemphigoid affects 1 in 15,000[8] to 1 in 46,000[9] ophthalmic patients. These data may, however, be deceptively low, since early involvement with cicatricial pemphigoid is difficult to diagnose.[1] Patients with early forms of the disease may therefore be excluded from epidemiologic estimates. The average age at onset in one large ophthalmic series was 64 years (range of 20–87 years).[1] In another ophthalmic series, the mean age at initial examination was 70 years (range of 43 to 88 years).[7] Women outnumber men[1,7,10,11]; there is no known racial or geographic predilection for the disease.[1,3,7,10]

Ocular Manifestations

Ocular involvement with cicatricial pemphigoid is second only to that of the oral mucosa in frequency and affects 60% to 75% of patients.[1, 2, 11] Ocular inflammation may be the presenting manifestation in as many as one third of patients.[1] Alternatively, ocular inflammation may begin years after the onset of inflammation elsewhere.[1, 10] Chronic and progressive conjunctival inflammation, punctuated by acute exacerbations, is typical.[1,11] Spontaneous remissions are rare. Ocular symptoms are nonspecific and include irritation, injection, burning, and itching.[1, 2, 5-7, 10, 11]

Conjunctival injection is commonly present on examination.[1, 5-7] Subepithelial fibrosis, the primary destructive process in cicatricial pemphigoid, is seen as fine white subepithelial lines on the inferior palpebral conjunctiva.[1, 5-7] If left untreated, the fornices progressively foreshorten and symblepharon form.[1, 2, 5-7, 10, 11] These may best be detected by asking the patient to look up while pulling the lower lid down. Late in the disease, the conjunctival sac may become obliterated, resulting in ankyloblepharon and a frozen globe.[1, 5-7] Corneal and conjunctival bullae are rarely seen.[1, 2, 5-7] Eyelid abnormalities that contribute to blinding keratopathy include entropion, trichiasis, lagophthalmos, and abnormal blink.[1, 2, 5-7]

Conjunctival scarring from chronic inflammation may lead to occlusion of the lacrimal gland ducts and destruction of the goblet cells, resulting in tear film instability and deficiency.[1, 5-7] This usually occurs at advanced stages of the disease.[1] The tear film in patients with cicatricial pemphigoid may also contain elevated levels of harmful inflammatory mediators.[1] The hostile environment created by the abnormal tear film, defective lid function, and trichiasis eventually leads to corneal surface breakdown, keratinization, neovascularization, scarring, and blindness.[1, 2, 5-7] Poor control of inflammation, trichiasis, topical corticosteroids, ocular surgery, and bandage contact lenses may predispose patients with cicatricial pemphigoid to secondary microbial keratitis, most commonly with gram-positive organisms.[12]

Glaucoma may be more prevalent in patients with cicatricial pemphigoid. In one ophthalmic series, 29 (26%) of 111 patients with cicatricial pemphigoid had glaucoma.[13] The reason for this relationship was unclear. Genetic susceptibility to both diseases or to conjunctival scarring secondary to topical medications, drug-induced cicatricial pemphigoid, and cicatricial pemphigoid–induced alterations to aqueous outflow all are possible mechanisms.[13]

Systemic Manifestations

Cicatricial pemphigoid is a disease of the mucosa and the skin.[1, 2] All mucosal surfaces may be involved, most commonly the oral mucosa (in 91% of patients), followed in descending order by the pharynx, the nose, the larynx, the genitalia, the anus, and the esophagus.[1, 2, 7] Oral lesions may be desquamative or vesicobullous,[1, 2, 6, 7] or both. Scarring of the vagina, the urethra, and the anus may be asymptomatic until strictures form.[1,6,14] Asphyxiation secondary to laryngeal strictures may be fatal; tracheostomies may be required.[1-3,15] Esophageal strictures usually involve the upper one third of the esophagus and may lead to dysphagia or to asphyxiation and death if food is entrapped.[1,3,16] Esophageal dilation or surgical repair of strictures may become necessary.[16]

The skin is affected less commonly than the mucosa (in 9% to 24% of patients).[1,2,5-7] Skin lesions may be vesicobullous types that are recurrent and nonscarring and involve the inguinal area and the extremities, or well-circumscribed erythematous plaques (Brunsting-Perry) with overlying vesicles and bullae that develop on the scalp and the face near affected mucous membranes and leave atrophic scars after they heal.[1,2,6]

Clinical Stages

Two clinical staging systems based on changes in the conjunctiva are commonly used for documenting and monitoring ocular disease progression. One was proposed by Mondino and Brown and consists of four stages reflecting fornix shrinkage.[6] Zero to 25%, 25% to 50%, and 50% to 75% of the fornix is lost in stages 1 to 3, respectively. In stage 4, the fornix is totally obliterated, and keratinization of the ocular surface has begun.

Another method was proposed by Foster[1] and later modified by Tauber and associates.[17] In this staging system, stage 1 consists of chronic conjunctivitis and subepithelial fibrosis; stage 2, fornix foreshortening; stage 3, symblepharon formation; and stage 4, end-stage disease with ankyloblepharon, dry eyes, and keratinization. Stages 2 and 3 are each further divided into subclasses a, b, c, and d, depending on the amount of fornix depth lost (stage 2) and the horizontal dimension of the symblepharon (stage 3).

Histopathology

Bullae, the hallmark of cicatricial pemphigoid, develop subepithelially within the lamina lucida of the basement membrane.[1-3,7] In early cicatricial pemphigoid, the conjunctiva is infiltrated with lymphocytes and plasma cells.[1,3,6,7] Histiocytes and mast cells may also be found. Mast cells in cicatricial pemphigoid are typically of the connective-tissue type; these have been implicated in the pathogenesis of several other fibrotic disorders.[18] Neutrophils invade in acute exacerbations.[1] Squamous metaplasia of the epithelium, keratinization, and fibrosis follow the acute inflammation.[1,6,7] Conjunctival goblet cells may be markedly decreased in number in late stages.[1,6,7] Findings on electron microscopic examination include increased desmosomes; prominent tonofilaments and tonofibrils in the epithelium; disorganized collagen fibrils; reduced vascular spaces; and thickening, discontinuity, and duplication of the basal lamina.[1,6,7]

Immunopathology. Immunofluorescent staining demonstrates linear deposition of all classes of immunoglobulins (especially IgG and IgA) and complement at the basement membrane in 20% to 100% of conjunctival biopsies.[1,2,7,19-22] Only one class of immunoglobulin may be deposited in as many as 25% of patients.[1] In one case report of a patient with cicatricial pemphigoid, IgA deposition at the basement membrane was granular, and electron microscopic examination was suggestive of immune complex deposition.[23] The target antigen of immunofluorescent staining is found in the lamina densa and the lamina lucida of the basement membrane.[1,2,21] During active inflammation, immunoglobulins may also bind to the epithelium.[1,6,16,19] Foster has suggested that demonstration of immune deposits along the basement membrane is a requirement for the diagnosis of cicatricial pemphigoid and that immune deposits may be found in all patients with the disease if immunostaining is properly performed.[1,24] Others have suggested that the absence of such immune deposits may not refute the diagnosis of cicatricial pemphigoid, but the presence of the deposits confirms the clinical impression.[6,7] Immunodeposition at the basement membrane has also been noted in Mooren's ulcer and *Staphylococcus*-induced keratitis.[7] These may be differentiated from those seen in cicatricial pemphigoid by their granularity.[1,6,7]

Although local immune deposits at the basement membrane were present in all patients with cicatricial pemphigoid reported by Foster, circulating anti–basement membrane and antiepithelial cell antibodies were present in only 26 (20%) of 130 patients.[1] These may be more common in acute stages of the disease.[1,25] Similar findings have been reported by others.[19,26-28]

Other immunologic phenomena associated with cicatricial pemphigoid include increased T helper cells, macrophages, and B cells in the epithelium and the substantia propria.[1,2,6,7,19] Antinuclear antibodies were present in 56 (43%) of 130 patients reported by Foster.[1] Many of the immunohistopathologic alterations described earlier may reverse after immunosuppression has been achieved.[1]

Pathogenesis

Cicatricial pemphigoid is an autoimmune disease resulting from an immunologic attack against the basal epithelial cells of the mucosa and the skin.[1-3,6,7] Two antigenic targets in the skin were recently identified by Niimi and colleagues.[29] Types II and III hypersensitivity reactions have been implicated in this process[1]; this is supported by the immunohistopathologic findings presented previously. According to one generally accepted hypothesis, antibody deposition at the lamina lucida and the lamina densa of the basement membrane is followed by activation of the complement pathway and resultant inflammation.[1,2] The conjunctiva and mucous membranes share common antigens; this may explain the ocular involvement in the autoimmune attack.[30] The association of cicatricial pemphigoid with other autoimmune diseases further supports an autoimmune etiology.[1] An association with HLA types B12, DR4, DR5,

DQw3, A2, B8, B35, and B49 has been reported, suggesting a genetic susceptibility to develop cicatricial pemphigoid.[31,32]

Differential Diagnosis

All causes of cicatricial conjunctivitis, including trauma and infections, may be included in the differential diagnosis of cicatricial pemphigoid.[1,2,6,7] In contrast with cicatricial pemphigoid, trachoma usually involves the upper fornix. Topical and systemic medications have been implicated in drug-induced pemphigoid, which may be clinically and immunohistopathologically indistinguishable from cicatricial pemphigoid.[33–38] Conjunctival cicatrization may also be found in Sjögren's syndrome and sarcoidosis.[6,7] In bullous pemphigoid, the mucous membranes and the ocular surface are rarely involved, circulating anti–basement membrane antibodies are common, and there is no sex predilection.[2,39] Conjunctival scarring and shrinkage are rare in pemphigus. Erythema multiforme occurs in younger people, rarely progresses after the acute phase, and exhibits typical skin lesions, and an inciting agent may be elicited.[5,7] Cicatrization is nonprogressive in toxic epidermal necrolysis, dermatitis herpetiformis (where mucosal involvement is uncommon), atopy, rosacea, porphyria cutanea tarda, and erythroderma ichthyosiform congenita.[1]

Treatment

Effective control of inflammation is essential for successful management of cicatricial pemphigoid, and systemic immunosuppression is key to achieving this end. Prednisone, dapsone, cyclophosphamide, and azathioprine all have been successfully used, individually or in combination, to control inflammation in cicatricial pemphigoid.[1,5–7,23,39–47] Corticosteroids are particularly effective in controlling acute exacerbations. Tauber and colleagues proposed using dapsone alone in the initial management of mild to moderately inflamed eyes and cyclophosphamide for highly active cases.[47] Azathioprine may only be useful as adjunctive and not primary therapy. The efficacy and safety of cyclosporine in controlling cicatricial pemphigoid–associated inflammation have not been adequately investigated.[2,48] Immunosuppressive drugs are potentially toxic and should be administered only by physicians trained in their use. Adverse effects of these drugs include lymphopenia, hemolytic anemia, secondary neoplasms, sterility, renal failure, and hemorrhagic cystitis.[48] If expertly used, however, immunosuppressive agents may be more effective and safer than corticosteroids in the chronic management of cicatricial pemphigoid.[1,47,48]

Local ocular therapeutic measures include aggressive lubrication, preferably with preservative-free solutions; topical retinoids if keratinization is present; aggressive treatment of meibomianitis and blepharitis; and treatment of infections as they arise.[1,5–7,49,50] The efficacy of topical corticosteroids is controversial.[1,6,7] The results of laser treatment of corneal vascularization in patients with cicatricial pemphigoid have been disappointing.[51]

All ocular and adnexal surgical procedures in patients with cicatricial pemphigoid must be deferred until inflammation is controlled. This cannot be overstressed, since the consequences of operating on actively inflamed eyes may be disastrous. Specifically, results of penetrating keratoplasty have been uniformly disappointing even in the setting of adequate preoperative control of inflammation.[1,7] Severe sicca, keratinization, and lid disease have usually set in by the time keratoplasty is required and preclude successful results. Better success may be achieved with keratoprosthesis.[1,6,7,52–54] The results of cataract extraction in adequately immunosuppressed patients are generally favorable.[55] Additional systemic corticosteroids perioperatively may be necessary for best results. Surgical correction of misdirected eyelashes, entropion, punctal occlusion, obliterated fornices, and surface keratinization may be necessary, and the outcome is frequently successful.[1,6,7,56–60]

Erythema Multiforme

Background

Erythema multiforme is an acute, usually self-limited disease of the skin and mucous membranes.[5,7,11,39,61] Erythema multiforme is commonly divided into major and minor forms.[5,7,11,61,62] The major form, also known as *Stevens-Johnson syndrome,* is a systemic disease of the skin and the mucosa. Erythema multiforme major may be life threatening; fortunately, it is uncommon. The minor form is more common and is known as *erythema multiforme minor.* Erythema multiforme minor is less severe than erythema multiforme major and primarily affects the skin; mucosal involvement in erythema multiforme minor is rare. The mortality rates in erythema multiforme minor and erythema multiforme major are approximately 1%, and 2% to 25%, respectively.[7] The differential diagnosis of erythema multiforme is similar to that of cicatricial pemphigoid.

Epidemiology

The peak incidence of erythema multiforme is in the third and fourth decades; 20% of cases occur in children and adolescents.[5,7,61] Males slightly outnumber females,[61] and no racial or geographic predilection is known.[5,7,61]

Ocular Manifestations

The eyes are involved in 60% to 80% of patients with erythema multiforme major; ocular involvement in erythema multiforme minor is far less common.[5,7,11] The prognosis of the ocular complications in erythema multiforme depends on the severity of systemic inflammation.[5, 7, 63] Corneal scarring and neovascularization may lead to visual loss in 35% of patients and blindness in 5% to 6% of patients with erythema multiforme.[5, 7, 62, 64, 65]

Acutely, varying degrees of bilateral mucopurulent conjunctivitis, papillae, and pseudomembranes are present, lasting 2 to 3 weeks.[5, 7, 11, 39, 62, 63, 65] Like cicatricial pemphigoid, corneal and conjunctival bullae are rarely seen. Chronically, the ocular findings are similar to those seen in cicatricial pemphigoid.[5, 7, 11, 39, 62, 63, 65] Unlike cicatricial pemphigoid, however, the inflammation is self-limited and scarring is not progressive. Rarely, inflammation of the conjunctiva is episodic and recurrent.[66] Conjunctival scarring, symblepharon formation, epithelial squamous metaplasia, surface keratinization, trichiasis, and entropion may develop.[5, 7, 62, 63, 65] Destruction of the conjunctival goblet cells and cicatrization of the lacrimal and accessory lacrimal gland ducts may lead to severe sicca. Breakdown of the corneal epithelial surface from trichiasis, lagophthalmos, and dry eyes may lead to corneal infections (most commonly with gram-positive cocci) and corneal perforation.[12] Tear outflow obstruction may develop secondary to scarring of the lacrimal puncta and canaliculi. Uveitis, panophthalmitis, and lacrimal gland cysts have also been described.[5, 7, 67]

Systemic Manifestations

Erythema multiforme is diagnosed clinically.[61] Findings vary from an asymptomatic papular eruption to a generalized bullous reaction with systemic toxicity, hence the name *multiforme*.[5, 7, 39, 61, 62] Commonly, a prodromal phase characterized by malaise, fever, upper respiratory tract symptoms, vomiting, diarrhea, and headache precedes the skin and mucosal eruptions by 1 to 14 days.[5, 7, 39, 61, 62] The eruptions are usually symmetric, occur in crops, and have an explosive onset. In erythema multiforme minor, these are usually limited to the skin and last 1 to 3 weeks. In erythema multiforme major, the eruptions are more generalized and may last as long as 6 weeks. Target lesions consisting of a red center surrounded by a pale area that, in turn, is surrounded by a red rim are characteristic skin findings.[5, 7, 61] Macules, papules, vesicles, and bullae may also develop and are generally painless.

All mucosal surfaces, most commonly the oral mucosa, may be involved. Tense mucosal bullae develop that may rupture, causing pain. Unlike the conjunctiva, the skin and mucosal lesions resolve without scarring but with residual hyperpigmentation. Systemic inflammation may recur in as many as 20% of patients with erythema multiforme.[5]

Immunohistopathology

Histopathologic and immunopathologic studies of ocular findings in erythema multiforme are scarce. Most such information is derived from the dermatologic literature. The classic triad of histopathologic findings in the skin includes endothelial cell swelling, mixed lymphocyte-histiocyte infiltration, and dermal edema. Subepithelial bullae are characteristic.[11, 61] The dermis overlying the bullae is frequently damaged and exhibits intercellular edema and hydropic degeneration and necrosis of the basal cells.[5, 7, 39] Acutely, mononuclear cells infiltrate the dermis and may surround vessels. Neutrophils are notably rare.[5, 7] Mucosal lesions are histopathologically similar to those seen in the skin. Unlike the skin, however, neutrophils are prominent in the mucosa.[5, 7] Pseudomembranes, and in severe cases, true membranes, may form. Except in patients with recurrent conjunctival inflammation, true vasculitis is uncommon.[5, 7, 39, 66] Chronically, squamous metaplasia, surface keratinization, and diminished numbers of goblet cells may be found.[5, 7, 39, 64]

Circulating immune complexes may be found in the sera of patients with erythema multiforme.[68–70] Complement, immunoglobulins, and fibrin have been found in dermal blood vessels and at the dermoepidermal junction by direct immunofluorescent staining.[7, 66, 68]

Cytotoxic/suppressor T lymphocytes outnumber helper/inducer T lymphocytes in the epidermis; the opposite is true in the dermis.[71] Foster and colleagues reported deposition of immunoreactants in the walls of conjunctival vessels in patients with recurrent ocular inflammation.[66] This was in contrast with findings in primary erythema multiforme where true vasculitis was not seen.[7, 66] In contrast with cicatricial pemphigoid, deposition of immunoreactants at the basement membrane and circulating anti–basement membrane antibodies have not been described in erythema multiforme. Some of these immunohistopathologic findings may reverse after therapy.

Pathogenesis

The etiology of erythema multiforme is uncertain. Infections and drugs are the most common predisposing factors.[5, 7, 72–78] Other inciting factors include malignancies, certain foods, radiation therapy, vaccines, and collagen vascular diseases. Approximately 50% are idiopathic. Predisposing infectious agents include bacteria, viruses, fungi, and *Mycoplasma pneumoniae*. *Mycoplasma* infections may precede the onset of erythema multiforme major in 20% of patients, and epidemics of erythema multiforme have been associated with outbreaks of *Mycoplasma* infections.[5, 7] Herpes simplex virus infections have been implicated in as many as 15% of patients with erythema multiforme minor, and recurrences of erythema multiforme minor may follow recurrent herpes simplex virus eruptions. Topical and systemic sulfonamides are the most commonly implicated drugs. It is often difficult to ascertain whether erythema multiforme was caused by a drug or whether the drug was given in response to the prodromal symptoms of erythema multiforme, which may resemble a flu. Cases of erythema multiforme have followed the administration of drugs given for symptoms unrelated to the flu-like prodromata of erythema multiforme, however.[7] A history of allergies or atopy may be elicited in as many as one third of patients.[78] Mondino and colleagues reported an increased prevalence of HLA-Bw44, a subtype of HLA-B12, in Caucasian patients with erythema multiforme major and ocular involvement, suggesting an immunogenetic susceptibility to develop the disease.[79]

Erythema multiforme may be secondary to a type III hypersensitivity reaction. This is supported by the presence of circulating and vessel wall immune complexes in patients with erythema multiforme.[5,7,66,68–70] In patients with recurrent conjunctival inflammation, circulating immune complexes may deposit in previously damaged predisposed vessels, leading to vasculitis.[66]

Treatment

Treatment of erythema multiforme is nonspecific and primarily supportive. Possible precipitating factors should be eliminated. Extensive skin bullae are treated as burns, with wet dressings, lubricants, baths, hydration, analgesics, and maintenance of electrolyte balance and nutritional requirements.[5,7,61] In severe cases, treatment in burn centers may improve the chance for survival.[80] Mouth care includes mouthwashes, local anesthetics, and steroids. Systemic antibiotics are given for infections. The therapeutic usefulness of systemic corticosteroids and immunosuppressive drugs is controversial. In one report, hospitalization was prolonged and complications were increased in patients treated with systemic corticosteroids.[81]

Local ocular treatment has little influence on the severity of the ophthalmic complications of erythema multiforme.[63] Early and frequent lysis of symblepharon with a glass rod and stripping of membranes have been recommended by some authors.[5,7,39] Manipulation of the conjunctiva may lead to increased conjunctival scarring, however, and is not favored by others.[11,61] Placement of a scleral shell to limit symblepharon formation and irrigation of the exudates may be preferable.[39] The efficacy of topical ocular antibiotics and corticosteroids in patients with erythema multiforme has yet to be properly evaluated. Secondary infections are treated with antibiotics as needed.[12] Blepharitis and dry eyes should be aggressively managed.[7] Topical retinoids may help reverse keratinization of the ocular surface.[49,82] Because of the nonprogressive nature of the inflammation in erythema multiforme, surgical correction of eyelid deformities, conjunctival scarring, and trichiasis may yield results superior to those achieved in patients with cicatricial pemphigoid.[65]

Pemphigus

Background

Pemphigus is a term used to describe a collection of autoimmune diseases characterized by blistering of the skin and the mucous membranes.[11,83,84] Pemphigus is generally divided into two main variants: pemphigus vulgaris and pemphigus foliaceus.[21,83] Pemphigus vulgaris is the commoner and more severe form of pemphigus[11,83,85] and is the main subject of the discussion that follows.

Epidemiology

Pemphigus affects males and females equally and is most common in the 4th and 5th decades of life.[83,84] Pemphigus vulgaris has a predilection for people of Jewish and Mediterranean descent[83,84] and is associated with HLA-DR4, especially among Jewish patients.[86,87]

Ocular Manifestations

The eyes are involved in 16% of patients with pemphigus vulgaris.[88] Common ocular symptoms include tearing and foreign body sensation.[11,89] The primary ocular lesions are usually transient and may precede other manifestations of the disease.[89] The commonest ocular findings are purulent conjunctivitis, with or without pseudomembranes, and blepharitis.[39,88] Rarely, corneal bullae, trichiasis, and symblephara develop.[90] Blindness from corneal opacification, in contrast with untreated cicatricial pemphigoid, is extremely uncommon.[11] The eyes usually improve after initiation of systemic immunosuppression. In one report of pemphigus foliaceus from Brazil, 5% of patients developed lens opacities.[11] Eyelid basal cell carcinoma in a patient with chronic pemphigus vulgaris has been reported[91]; this was possibly related to chronic immunosuppressive therapy. Ocular involvement in paraneoplastic pemphigus may be more aggressive.[92]

Systemic Manifestations

The primary lesions in pemphigus are blisters.[21,83–85] The blisters in pemphigus are large and very fragile, and they rupture easily. Ruptured blisters lead to denuded skin and secondary lesions—erosions—which are commonly the predominant clinical sign in patients with pemphigus. As in toxic epidermal necrolysis, Nikolsky's sign (separation of the epidermis from the dermis after traction) may be positive.[83,84] The oral mucosa is most commonly involved, and lesions typically affect the oral mucosa first, then become generalized over weeks, months, or years. The course of pemphigus is usually relentless, eventually involving the rest of the body. Fatalities secondary to sepsis and fluid and electrolyte loss were common in the past.[11, 39, 83, 84] Immunosuppressive therapy has markedly improved the prognosis, however, such that mortality from pemphigus vulgaris is now uncommon. The diagnosis is established by demonstrating acantholysis histopathologically, positive staining of the intercellular space by immunofluorescence, and typical clinical features.[11,39,83,84]

Immunohistopathology

Acantholysis is the histologic hallmark of pemphigus.[21,83,84] Acantholysis starts with intercellular edema in the epidermis, followed by dissolution of intercellular bridges ending in cell-to-cell detachment; this manifests clinically as blisters. In pemphigus vulgaris, these changes are mainly suprabasilar in the epidermis.[39] The basilar cells remain normal and attached to the underlying basement membrane.[39, 83, 84] Inflammation is generally absent early but may be present later.

Highly specific autoantibodies are present in 90% of patients with pemphigus. The autoantibodies are both tissue fixed and circulating and react to surface and intercellular epidermal components (pemphigus antigens).[21, 39, 83, 84] Although the IgG4 subclass of immunoglobulins predominates, IgG1 may best correlate with disease activity.[93] The tissue-fixed autoantibodies may be found in the mucous membranes, the skin, and the conjunctiva.[21, 83, 84, 88, 89] These autoantibodies are probably directed against intercellular bridges that are important for epithelial cell adhesion.[94] The "pemphigus antigen" is a normal constituent of suprabasilar epidermal cells and reacts with the circulating autoantibodies present in the sera of patients with the disease. These antigens may be directly involved in cell adhesion in the epidermis.[83]

Pathogenesis

That pemphigus is an autoimmune disease is supported by the demonstration of tissue and circulating autoantibodies in patients with the disease. Much evidence implicates these autoantibodies in the pathogenesis of pemphigus. For example, the titers of these autoantibodies usually correlate with disease activity.[95, 96] Also, transplacental transfer of IgG may lead to transient pemphigus in neonates born to mothers with pemphigus vulgaris.[97] Pemphigus vulgaris serum or immunoglobulins from pemphigus vulgaris serum can lead to acantholysis in human skin explants and epidermal cell detachment in murine epidermal cell cultures.[98-100] Injection of these immunoglobulins into mice neonatally leads to blisters with immunohistologic features identical to those seen in pemphigus vulgaris.[39]

Differential Diagnosis

Lever, in 1953, was the first to provide the clinical and histologic distinction between pemphigus and cicatricial pemphigoid.[4] Histologically, a key difference is the presence of acantholysis in the mucosa and skin of patients with pemphigus.[4, 83] In pemphigus, the split is in the epidermis; in cicatricial pemphigoid, the split is subepidermal. Circulating autoantibodies are rare in cicatricial pemphigoid and are common in pemphigus. Tissue-fixed autoantibodies are directed against the basement membrane in cicatricial pemphigoid and against the intercellular spaces of the epidermis in pemphigus vulgaris.

Treatment

Systemic immunosuppression is the therapy of choice for pemphigus.[11, 21, 39, 83, 84] The rationale for this treatment is based on the autoimmune nature of the disease. Systemic corticosteroids are the mainstay of therapy. Before the use of corticosteroids, pemphigus was almost uniformally fatal. Methotrexate, cyclophosphamide, azathioprine, gold, and dapsone have also been used successfully. Plasmapheresis may offer temporary relief.[93, 101] Autoantibody titers may be used to monitor disease activity and response to therapy.[95, 96]

Epidermolysis Bullosa

Background

Epidermolysis bullosa is a group of rare hereditary diseases of the skin and mucous membranes characterized by the development of bullae at sites of minor trauma.[21, 102] Epidermolysis bullosa is classified as epidermolytic, lamina lucidolytic or junctionolytic, or dermolytic based on the level of separation in the skin where the bullae develop.[102] The *epidermolytic class* includes the various forms of epidermolysis bullosa simplex.[102] These are generally nonscarring and dominantly inherited. The *junctionolytic class* includes junctional epidermolysis bullosa and Herlitz's disease.[102] These are uncommon, generally nonscarring, and recessively inherited and may be lethal in infancy. The *dermolytic* class includes the dominantly and recessively inherited dystrophic (scarring) forms of epidermolysis bullosa and epidermolysis bullosa acquisita.[102] The latter typically has its onset in adulthood and an absent family history of blistering diseases and is often confused with cicatricial pemphigoid.[103,104] Epidermolysis bullosa acquisita is usually the most benign and least scarring form of epidermolysis bullosa but may be associated with other systemic diseases such as multiple myeloma, diabetes mellitus, and amyloidosis.[105]

Epidemiology

Most forms of epidermolysis bullosa are dominantly inherited; a few are recessive.[102, 105, 106] Most are congenital and manifest at birth, during infancy, or early in childhood.[102, 105] No race or sex predilection is known. Epidermolysis bullosa acquisita is the only nonhereditary form of epidermolysis bullosa and is acquired in adulthood; the average age at onset of epidermolysis bullosa acquisita is 47 years.[103] An association with HLA-DR2 has been described for epidermolysis bullosa acquisita.[103]

Ocular Manifestations

Ocular involvement is possible in all forms of epidermolysis bullosa, but it is more common in the recessive dystrophic and junctional forms of the disease and is rare in epidermolysis bullosa simplex.[106–109] In one series of 11 patients with dystrophic epidermolysis bullosa, 11% had ocular involvement.[106] In contrast, in a review of 78 patients with various forms of epidermolysis bullosa, none had conjunctival scars or symblepharon.[110] Visual outcome in this series was good. In general, the severity of the ocular involvement in epidermolysis bullosa follows the severity of the systemic disease.

Ocular findings in epidermolysis bullosa are mostly confined to the ocular surface.[108] Bullae may be seen on the eyelids, the conjunctiva, and the cornea.[107, 110, 111] Corneal bullae are usually at the basal epithelial level and occur in a ring-like fashion around the periphery.[107, 111] These may lead to recurrent corneal erosions, the frequency of which diminishes with advancing age.[107, 109, 111] Corneal scars, ulcers, and perforation may also result.[112] Pannus formation and broadening of the limbus are typical corneal findings.[106, 113] Chronic and progressive conjunctivitis may lead to conjunctival scarring, pseudomembranes, and symblepharon formation.[110, 112, 113] Junctional epidermolysis bullosa and epidermolysis bullosa acquisita more commonly involve the cornea and spare the conjunctiva, whereas the dystrophic forms may involve the conjunctiva, sparing the cornea.[110, 113] Blepharitis and loss of eyelashes are common. Cataracts may form at an early age, suggesting involvement of the lens epithelium in the pathologic process.[108] Retinal involvement in epidermolysis bullosa is rare.[114]

Systemic Manifestations

Epidermolysis bullosa is diagnosed by a combination of typical history, inheritance, and immunohistopathology.[115] All epithelial skin and mucosal surfaces may be involved.[108] The manifestations, severity, and prognosis of epidermolysis bullosa depend on the subtype and are worst in patients with junctional epidermolysis bullosa and the recessive dystrophic forms.[102, 116] Patients with junctional epidermolysis bullosa may die shortly after birth, whereas patients with milder forms such as epidermolysis bullosa simplex may have minimal findings and lead normal and healthy lives.

Bullous formation after minor trauma is the hallmark of the different forms of epidermolysis bullosa.[21, 102, 115, 116] Bullae may be generalized or localized. Nail deformities and hair loss are common.[102] Scarring may be severe, leading to syndactyly, skin atrophy, and hypopigmentation.[102] The number and shape of teeth may be abnormal, with discoloration and increased caries.[102, 108] The oral mucosa is the most commonly involved mucosal surface.[102] Strictures may form in the esophagus, the vagina, and the anus.[102, 108] Respiratory system involvement may extend from the nares to the tertiary or segmental bronchi and lead to respiratory difficulties.[108] Stunted growth and malnutrition are common. Milia are prominent in epidermolysis bullosa acquisita at the sites of healed blisters.[103] Extensive blistering may lead to septicemia. Epidermolysis bullosa acquisita is often confused with bullous or cicatricial pemphigoid[103, 117, 118]; Gammon and Woodley and colleagues estimated that 10% to 15% of patients previously diagnosed with bullous pemphigoid may actually have epidermolysis bullosa acquisita.[103, 118]

Immunohistopathology

Immunohistopathologic descriptions of ocular involvement in epidermolysis bullosa are scarce. Most such information is derived from the dermatologic literature. Epidermolysis bullosa is a disease of the dermoepidermal junction. A brief description of the layers of the basement membrane helps elucidate the histopathologic findings in epidermolysis bullosa. The normal basement membrane consists of four layers: (1) the basal cell plasma membrane; (2) an electron-lucent lamina lucida; (3) an electron-dense lamina densa (often called the *basal lamina*); and (4) lamina lucida fibrous components.[119, 120] In the epidermolytic class of epidermolysis bullosa, the separation (or bullae formation) is within the epidermal layer such that the lamina densa forms the roof of the bullae.[102] In the lamina lucidolytic or junctionolytic class, the separation is in the plane of the lamina lucida of the basement membrane. In the dermolytic class, the separation is beneath the basal lamina.[102] In comparison, the split in cicatricial pemphigoid is such that the basal epidermal cells form the roof of bullae and the lamina lucida forms the base. Anchoring fibrils and hemidesmosomes are diminished or absent in epidermolysis bullosa.[121]

Immunopathology has been best studied in epidermolysis bullosa acquisita.[21, 103, 122–126] Linear deposits of IgG, C3, and fibrinogen have been detected in the skin and oral mucosa. Deposits of IgG, IgM, and complement have been noted in the conjunctiva of patients with epidermolysis bullosa. Circulating anti–basement membrane antibodies have also been reported. In epidermolysis bullosa acquisita, deposits of IgG and electron-dense homogeneous material have been noted below and at the lamina densa. In 1984, Woodley and coworkers isolated a circulating basement membrane antigen in patients with epidermolysis bullosa acquisita and termed it the *epidermolysis bullosa acquisita antigen.*[103, 125] This antigen is located at the lamina densa and consists of a glycoprotein representing the globular carboxyl terminus of type VII procollagen. Fine later reported a similar circulating antigen in other hereditary forms of epidermolysis bullosa.[120]

Treatment

General supportive measures, including antibiotics, soft diets, skin lubricants, and proper hygiene, are recommended in all patients with epidermolysis bullosa.[103] A 4- to 6-week trial of systemic corticosteroids, with or without azathioprine or dapsone, has been recommended by some authors; however, the results of such treatment have often been disappointing.[103] Systemic cyclosporine has shown promise in patients with epidermolysis bullosa recalcitrant to other modes of treatment.[127, 128] Local ocular measures include lubrication, antibiotics to prevent infections, cycloplegics for comfort, and therapeutic contact lenses.[110] Eyelid taping should be avoided, since this may lead to blistering of the skin.[110] Surgical correction of eyelid deformities may become necessary, although the success of such surgical procedures is uncertain.

Toxic Epidermal Necrolysis

Background

Toxic epidermal necrolysis, or Lyell's disease, is a rare, rapidly progressive, often life-threatening disease of unknown etiology affecting the skin and mucous membranes.[129–131] It is the most severe skin disease attributed to a drug reaction and is one of the few true dermatologic emergencies. Objective diagnostic criteria and a universal definition for toxic epidermal necrolysis are still lacking.[131] In 1987, Goldstein and colleagues proposed the following working definition: explosive and widespread onset of blisters and skin tenderness involving at least 10% of total body surface, absence of target lesions, and full-thickness epidermal confluent keratinocytic necrosis with minimal infiltration of the dermis.[131]

Epidemiology

Toxic epidermal necrolysis is a rare disease, with an estimated incidence of 10 in 1 million per year.[132] One of the largest single series of patients with toxic epidermal necrolysis was recently reported by a group from Creteil, France.[130] In this series, a slight predilection for females was noted. The mean age was 45.8 ± 22.7 years, with a range of 2 to 90 years. No racial or geographic predilection was described.

Ocular Manifestations

Ocular involvement in toxic epidermal necrolysis is common. In one large series of patients, the eyes were involved in 68 (78%) of 87 patients.[130] This was second only to oral mucosal involvement. Although the eyes were rarely involved alone in this series of patients, ocular lesions were the most common disabling sequelae of toxic epidermal necrolysis, occurring in 15 (17%) of 87 patients. Severe loss of vision may result; this is usually secondary to corneal opacification. Generally, the ocular findings are similar to those seen in erythema multiforme and include dry eyes, trichiasis, entropion, punctate keratopathy, and corneal scarring and neovascularization.[130, 133–135] These usually develop a few weeks after the acute process.

Systemic Manifestations

Toxic epidermal necrolysis is a life-threatening disease; the mortality rate may be as high as 60%.[130, 136] The main causes of death are infections, most commonly with *Staphylococcus aureus* and *Pseudomonas aeruginosa,* and hypovolemia.[129, 135, 136] Prognosis is inversely related to age, area of necrolysis, and serum urea level.[130] Fever, malaise, and pharyngitis may precede the cutaneous and mucosal eruptions. Mucosal erosions in toxic epidermal necrolysis are similar to those seen in erythema multiforme.[130] The oral mucosa is most commonly involved, followed by ocular and genital mucosa.[137, 138] Mucosal lesions usually antedate skin involvement. Skin and mucosal lesions may be maximal by 24 hours, or they may continue to spread and develop for as long as 15 days. Once cutaneous involvement is complete, moderate traction on the skin may lead to separation of the epidermis from the dermis (Nikolsky's sign).[130, 134] The skin heals rapidly in the absence of infections; residual pigmentary changes are common, but mucous membrane erosions usually last longer. Involvement of the viscera heralds a poor prognosis.

Immunohistopathology

The epidermis in toxic epidermal necrolysis is typically necrotic, with mild mononuclear cell infiltration.[134, 138] Intercellular edema is usually most marked near the epidermal basal cells. The dermis is relatively normal and characteristically free of inflammation.[136] Similar histopathologic findings may be seen in some patients with graft-versus-host disease.[139] Bullae form within the epidermis or subepidermally.[136, 137]

Immunoglobulin and complement deposition may be

found intercellularly in the basal cell layer of the epidermis, suggesting that the basal cells may be the target of an immune attack.[140] One report of a patient with drug-induced toxic epidermal necrolysis described drug-dependent binding of circulating antibodies to the epidermis.[141]

Pathogenesis

Toxic epidermal necrolysis is a disease of presumed autoimmune etiology; T cells and lymphokines have been implicated in its pathogenesis.[131, 136] A role for circulating toxins and toxic drug metabolites has also been suggested.[141] A genetic association with HLA-B12 has been described—this is the same HLA type that has been linked to erythema multiforme, a closely related disease.[142] Predisposing factors for toxic epidermal necrolysis include drugs and infections.[129, 134, 136–138, 143] In one large series of patients with toxic epidermal necrolysis, 77% of cases were clearly ascribed to drugs.[144] Sulfonamides (especially sulfamethoxazole and trimethoprim), anticonvulsants, and nonsteroidal anti-inflammatory agents are the most commonly implicated drugs.

Differential Diagnosis

In view of the marked differences in treatment and prognosis of scalded-skin syndrome and toxic epidermal necrolysis, differentiation of these often similar diseases is important.[129, 137] The scalded-skin syndrome is predominantly a pediatric disease with excellent prognosis; toxic epidermal necrolysis may occur in any age group and may have a poor prognosis.[129, 136] The scalded-skin syndrome is caused by *S. aureus* toxins; toxic epidermal necrolysis is usually secondary to drugs. Mucosal involvement is absent in scalded-skin syndrome and common in toxic epidermal necrolysis. Bacteriology is usually not helpful, since the skin in scalded-skin syndrome may be sterile, whereas colonization of the skin with *S. aureus* in toxic epidermal necrolysis is common. Definitive differentiation is made histopathologically.[137, 145] Bullae form superficially in the epidermal granular layer without necrolysis or inflammation in the scalded-skin syndrome and intraepidermally and subepidermally with epidermal necrosis in toxic epidermal necrolysis.

Differentiation of toxic epidermal necrolysis from erythema multiforme is more difficult because similarities in the mucosal and skin lesions abound.[141] They are believed by some authors to be part of a spectrum of one disease. In fact, Ruiz-Maldonado proposed the term *acute disseminated epidermal necrosis* to encompass both toxic epidermal necrolysis and erythema multiforme.[138] Generally, toxic epidermal necrolysis is a more severe disease with a worse prognosis, involving at least 10% of the total body surface without target lesions.

Treatment

Improvements in measures to control infections and fluid imbalance during the past 20 years have led to increased survival of patients with toxic epidermal necrolysis.[136, 137, 146, 147] Fluid replacement is calculated as in burn patients: 5 to 7 L may be required in the first 24 hours. Intravenous lines should be discontinued as soon as possible owing to the danger of colonization and infection. Control of infection is of paramount importance, since half of all deaths are secondary to infections. Bacterial colonization of the skin is rapid and massive. Blood, skin, and mucous membranes are cultured daily. Intravenous lines and catheters are cultured and replaced every 3 days. Broad-spectrum antibiotics are given on admission or are withheld until early sepsis develops. Sulfonamides are to be avoided because they are often implicated in the pathogenesis of the disease. Local application of an antiseptic and bathing are encouraged. Necrotic epidermis, especially after it has become folded over, should be peeled off. Epidermis may regrow, or grafting of biologic or hydrocolloidal dressings may be required. Some authors recommend systemic corticosteroids; however, the efficacy of this practice has not been proved. In fact, many contemporary investigators discourage their use.[136,138] In view of the proposed role of T lymphocytes in the pathogenesis of toxic epidermal necrolysis, cyclosporine may be a reasonable therapeutic alternative.[148]

Local therapeutic ocular measures include topical antibiotics with or without corticosteroids.[134] Synechiae may be broken as they form.

SARCOIDOSIS

Background

Sarcoidosis is a multisystem granulomatous disorder of unknown etiology characterized by the presence of noncaseating granulomas in affected tissues. Sarcoidosis most commonly affects the lungs, the eyes, and the skin. The overall prognosis is usually favorable, with a mortality rate of 1% to 5%; many patients recover with little or no residual effects. The term *sarcoid* was first introduced by Boeck because of the resemblance between the histologic appearances of the skin lesions in sarcoid and sarcoma.[149]

Epidemiology

Epidemiologic studies of sarcoidosis are hampered by the lack of a standardized case definition. Sarcoidosis is more common in young adults 20 to 40 years of age[149–151]; it is unusual before 16 and after 70 years of age but may be more severe in older patients. Pediatric sarcoidosis is relatively rare and is divided into two subsets based on the age of onset.[152] Females are involved two or three times more frequently than males.[149-151] Familial associations have been reported.[153-155] African Americans are more likely to develop sarcoidosis than are Caucasians and more commonly develop ocular disease.[149-151, 156, 157] In the United States, sarcoidosis is more prevalent in residents of the South Atlantic and South Central states.[149-151] Worldwide, sarcoidosis is more common in rural areas.[149-151] An association with HLA-B8 and HLA-A1 has been reported.[158, 159]

Ocular Manifestations

Twenty-five percent to 50% of patients with sarcoidosis develop ocular manifestations, and 3% to 7% of patients with uveitis may have systemic sarcoidosis.[156, 160] Ocular findings may be the presenting manifestation of sarcoidosis.[160] As many as 12.5% of patients with ocular sarcoidosis may lose their vision from secondary glaucoma, cataract, retinal destruction, fundal neovascularization, optic nerve damage, and corneal band keratopathy; another 12.5% become visually handicapped.[156, 160-163]

Bilateral, recurrent anterior granulomatous uveitis is the commonest ocular manifestation of sarcoidosis.[157, 160, 161, 163, 164] The onset is typically insidious and painless; less commonly, it is acute and symptomatic. Granulomas in the eyelids, lacrimal glands, and conjunctiva may be easily accessible for diagnostic biopsies.[156,157,161,163-165] Granulomas may also be found in the iris, the retina, and the choroid. [156, 157, 161, 163-166] Choroidal granulomas may occur in the absence of other signs of ocular inflammation.[167]

Posterior-segment inflammation occurs in as many as 25% of patients with ocular sarcoidosis.[162] Vitreous inflammation ("snow banking" and "string of pearls"), retinal hemorrhages, perivascular infiltrates ("candle wax drippings"), macular edema, and retinal and choroidal granulomas may be seen.[157, 161, 162, 164-166] Retinal, subretinal, and disc neovascularization may develop and herald a worse visual prognosis.[162, 166, 168] Optic nerve involvement, in the form of optic neuritis, papillitis, disc swelling, or true papilledema, may develop secondary to severe uveitis or direct optic nerve inflammation and often accompanies neurosarcoidosis.[157, 161-163, 165, 166, 169, 170]

Orbit involvement typically consists of painless bilateral enlargement of the lacrimal glands.[171] This condition may lead to granulomatous dacryoadenitis in 7% to 26% of patients and may accompany parotid gland enlargement (Mikulicz's syndrome).[163] Granulomatous inflammation of the orbit is rare and may lead to proptosis.[172] Granulomatous inflammation of the extraocular muscles is similarly rare but may lead to diplopia, which may be the presenting sign of systemic sarcoidosis.

Systemic Manifestations

Granulomatous inflammation may develop in any organ but has a predilection to affect the lungs and thoracic lymph nodes.[149-151] The onset may be insidious or acute and may be subclinical. The prognosis is generally more favorable in patients with an acute onset of the condition. The lungs are involved in 90% of patients with sarcoidosis.[149] Lung involvement is divided into three stages based on radiologic criteria.[150] Most commonly, hilar lymphadenopathy or interstitial infiltrates, or both, are noted. Symptoms of lung involvement include cough, wheezing, and hemoptysis.[149] Dyspnea is usually a late symptom and heralds a worse prognosis. Lymphatic involvement includes hilar adenopathy and hepatosplenomegaly. Skin involvement in the form of erythema nodosum (a subcutaneous hypersensitivity reaction that is tender and self-limited) or nontender granulomatous nodules is common.[150] Acute arthritis may develop, mimicking rheumatoid arthritis; chronic arthritis is less common.[173] Other organ involvement includes the kidneys, skeletal muscles, bones, and central and peripheral nervous systems.[149, 150] Neurosarcoidosis consisting of facial nerve palsies, disc edema, peripheral neuropathy, myopathy, or meningitis may develop.

Immunohistopathology

Sarcoidosis is characterized by the presence of noncaseating granulomas in involved organs. These granulomas are not specific for sarcoidosis, however, and may be seen in other granulomatous diseases such as certain infections and neoplastic diseases; immunologic diseases such as systemic lupus erythematosus and Wegener's disease; and reactions to irritants such as beryllium.[151,174] Granulomas may be also be found in organs free of active disease.[151] The granulomas found in sarcoidosis consist of focal collections of mononuclear cells (epithelioid cells, macrophages, and multinucleated giant cells) surrounded by activated T lymphocytes, mostly of the helper subset.[151] Granuloma formation may be triggered by unknown antigens, infectious agents, or immune complexes.[149]

The immune system in a patient with sarcoidosis may best be characterized as that of heightened cellular immune processes at sites of disease contrasted with generalized anergy.[149, 151, 174] Systemic humoral immunity may be nonspecifically exaggerated with increased production of all classes of immunoglobulins, including autoantibodies. Conversely, systemic T helper levels and functions may be suppressed. Circulating immune complexes have also been described.[149, 151] T lymphocytes from lung tissue may secrete a chemotactic factor for monocytes and IL-2.[173, 175] The findings discussed earlier support an immune etiology for sarcoidois.[149, 151, 163, 173]

In the eye, Gass and Olson reported epithelioid and giant cells in the vitreous, retina, and retinal pigment epithelium in a patient with sarcoidosis.[170] The choroid was notably free of epithelioid cells, however. The optic nerve head was invaded by granulomas, and localized areas of optic nerve tissue destruction were noted. Chan and associates described T helper cells in and around granulomas.[176] Within the granulomas, macrophages, T cells, and epithelioid cells showed IL-2 receptors and were capable of releasing interferon-gamma. Class II HLA antigens were diffusely distributed. In contrast, the choroid was mostly spared from inflammation. Barth and colleagues isolated an acid-fast organism from the aqueous humor of a patient with ocular sarcoidosis.[177]

Diagnosis

A clinical impression of sarcoidosis should prompt an appropriate workup, including laboratory and radiologic tests, and histopathologic confirmation.[171, 174] Unfortunately, absolute diagnostic criteria for sarcoidosis are lacking.[149] Many investigators rely on the demonstration of typical noncaseating granulomas in affected tissues for definitive diagnosis.[163, 171, 173, 174] One should consider the most accessible tissues, such as skin, lymph nodes, conjunctiva, and lacrimal gland, as potential biopsy sites.[174] Transbronchial or open lung biopsies may be attempted, if necessary. The yield of conjunctival and lacrimal gland biopsies increases significantly in the presence of detectable conjunctival or eyelid nodules or granulomas and enlarged lacrimal glands, especially if guided by a positive gallium 67 scan, and in patients with proven sarcoidosis.[178-182]

Chest radiographs are the most widely used diagnostic tests for sarcoidosis and may show bilateral hilar adenopathy with or without parenchymal involvement.[149, 151, 174] A gallium 67 scan of the lung and head is especially helpful when chest radiographic findings are negative, but it is not specific for sarcoid.[174] Pulmonary function tests are useful for characterizing disease activity and the extent of lung involvement and may be abnormal before the onset of radiologic changes.[174] Ancillary evidence includes elevated serum angiotensin-converting enzyme (ACE) levels. The sources of ACE in sarcoidosis are epithelioid cells and monocytes.[149, 171, 174] Although not a specific sign in this instance, ACE levels may be elevated in 60% to 90% of patients with active sarcoidosis and may be useful in evaluating response to therapy and monitoring recurrences, since ACE serum levels reflect the total body mass of ACE-producing granulomas. It may be difficult to interpret ACE levels in children due to the normally high levels of the enzyme in the pediatric age group.[152] Anergic responses to common antigens by skin testing are typical in sarcoidosis and reflect the generalized state of cellular unresponsiveness.[151, 171, 173] Elevated levels of serum and urine calcium may be present secondary to increased sensitivity to or increased levels of vitamin D. Elevated lysozyme levels may also be found.[171, 174] Autoantibodies such as rheumatoid factor and antinuclear antibody levels as well as circulating immune complexes may be present.[149, 151, 171, 173] Negative results of these tests do not exclude a diagnosis of sarcoidosis.

The Kveim test is now rarely used, since the testing agent is not commercially available; it has to be prepared from tissue obtained from a patient with sarcoidosis.[149, 161] Furthermore, 6 weeks are required to interpret the test, and transmission of infectious agents may be possible.

Differential Diagnosis

The differential diagnosis of sarcoidosis depends on the organ system involved and generally includes other granulomatous diseases such as infections, including tuberculosis, histoplasmosis, and coccidioidomycosis; connective tissue diseases such as Wegener's granulomatosis; and exposure to irritants such as beryllium and talc.[151, 173] The anterior-segment and posterior-segment manifestations of sarcoidosis must be differentiated from other causes of granulomatous uveitis, vasculitis, and pars planitis such as tuberculosis and syphilis.[164, 166] Fundal neovascularization may resemble proliferative diabetic retinopathy. Lacrimal gland enlargement may occur in neoplastic diseases such as lymphomas, immune-mediated diseases such as Sjögren's syndrome, and inflammatory diseases such as pseudotumor. These conditions can be excluded and a diagnosis of sarcoidosis established by following the diagnostic procedures suggested in the previous section.

Treatment

The prognosis of systemic sarcoidosis is generally favorable; many patients may not require systemic therapy.[149-151] Corticosteroids are the mainstay of treatment in sarcoidosis.[149-151, 161, 173, 183] Chloroquine and hydroxychloroquine have also been used to treat chronic lung disease.[161] Published case reports suggest a possible role for cyclosporine in the treatment of pulmonary and central nervous system sarcoidosis.[173, 184] Topical corticosteroids and cycloplegics may be sufficient to treat anterior uveitis.[157, 164-166] Posterior-segment inflammation and inflammation of the orbit, lacrimal glands, and extraocular muscles usually respond to systemic corticosteroids. Surgical intervention may be attempted in patients with visually significant cataracts and uncontrolled glaucoma.[166] Increased ocular inflammation is common postoperatively. Retinal and disc new vessels may respond to corticosteroids; however, subretinal new vessels may require laser therapy.[166]

diseases such as syphilis, tuberculosis, and fungi may present as granulomatous orbital disease without primary vasculitis. Culture and special stains of biopsy material in conjunction with careful systemic history, physical examination, and laboratory workup eliminate these possibilities. Sarcoidosis may involve the orbit but is not accompanied by a primary vasculitis and may be distinguished by its other accompanying systemic manifestations. Lethal midline granuloma is not a single disease but is attributable to any of a number of midfacial destructive entities, including those in the differential diagnosis.[206]

Polyarteritis Nodosa

Background

Polyarteritis nodosa is a vasculitic disease of medium and small blood vessels whose description is attributed to von Rokitansky[207] and Kussmaul and Maier.[208] The blood vessels of the kidney, bowel, skin, muscle, heart, nervous system, and eye may be involved, but unlike Wegener's granulomatosis and lymphomatoid granulomatosis, the pulmonary vessels are usually spared.

Epidemiology

Because polyarteritis is uncommon, epidemiologic characteristics can be based only on retrospective reviews and summary data. Mean age of onset of symptoms is estimated to occur at 45 years,[209] but the range in age is broad.[210] There is a male predominance of between 2:1 and 4:1.[199,209,210]

Systemic Manifestations

Systemic involvement in polyarteritis nodosa is protean.[209] Constitutional symptoms include weakness, malaise, weight loss, and fever. Seventy percent to 80% of patients have renal vascular involvement.[209,210] Although it does not usually have early symptoms,[209,210] it can be severe, leading to malignant hypertension, renal failure, and death, if untreated. Arthralgias, myalgias, and arthritis occur in 64% of patients and are probably due to vascular involvement in the muscles and to immune complex-mediated joint disease.[209] Gastrointestinal symptoms include nausea, vomiting, and abdominal pain. All segments of the alimentary canal as well as the gallbladder and the pancreas can be involved. Bowel ischemia and vasculitis may result in life-threatening gastrointestinal hemorrhage or bowel perforation.[209] Both peripheral and central nervous systems can be involved. Multiple peripheral nerves, both motor and sensory, may be involved simultaneously.[210] Stroke, altered mental state, and seizures are the most common central signs.[209,210] Subarachnoid hemorrhage has been reported. Ischemia and infarction of skin may present as nodules, ulcers, gangrene, urticaria, or a characteristic reticular pattern (livedo reticularis).[211] Testicular involvement is manifested by pain or tenderness.[212] Liver and cardiac involvement are commonly found at autopsy.[209] Unlike in Wegener's granulomatosis, the lungs are rarely involved.

Ocular Manifestations

Ocular blood vessel may be primarily affected by vasculitis or may demonstrate the secondary effects of severe hypertension that accompanies renal involvement. The choroidal, posterior ciliary, and retinal vessels are most frequently affected.[213] As in other organs, retinal vasculitis results in vascular occlusion or aneurysm. Choroiditis, scleritis, peripheral ulcerative keratitis, conjunctival vasculitis, and uveitis also occur.[201,214-218] Orbital involvement can present as exophthalmos[219] and may be the initial sign of polyarteritis nodosa.[220] The extraocular muscles and optic nerves may be involved.[199,221] It has been suggested that the orbital inflammation may be contiguous with adjacent sinusitis.[222] The presence of bilateral orbital pseudotumor suggests a systemic disease, and polyarteritis nodosa must be considered.

Laboratory Findings

The diagnosis of polyarteritis nodosa is based on the presence of typical signs and symptoms in addition to laboratory evaluation. A formal system of criteria has been proposed.[212] Using this system, rheumatoid arthritis, systemic lupus erythematosus, and Wegener's granulomatosis should first be considered, and one of these diagnoses confirmed, if appropriate, based on clinical and laboratory findings. If the criteria for these diagnoses are not met, it is suggested that evaluation of 10 variables, any three of which need to be positive, yields a diagnosis of polyarteritis nodosa with a sensitivity and specificity higher than 80%. The criteria include weight loss, livedo reticularis, testicular pain, muscle pain or weakness, mononeuropathy or polyneuropathy, increased diastolic blood pressure, elevated blood urea nitrogen or creatinine levels, or antibody or antigen to hepatitis B.

The remaining two criteria are angiographic and biopsy findings from an affected organ system. Angiography demonstrates aneurysms or occlusions of vessels. Muscle, nerve, testicle, liver, kidney, and skin tissues may be obtained by biopsy and examined for granulocytic and mononuclear involvement of the wall of small-sized and medium-sized muscular arteries.[209,211,223,224]

Because lesions are segmental and may scar as they become chronic, orbital biopsy may not demonstrate classic lesions of polyarteritis nodosa with full-thickness involvement of the small-sized and medium-sized arteries, fibrinoid necrosis, and edema. Nonetheless, perivascular inflammation without inflammation elsewhere on the biopsy specimen and the presence of eosinophils are suggestive findings. Granulomatous changes and the presence of giant cells are not characteristic and should raise the possibility of alternate diagnoses.[213]

Pathogenesis

Polyarteritis nodosa appears to be the result of deposition of antigen-antibody complexes and complement in vessel walls with inflammatory changes involving the full thickness of the vessel. In some instances, the antigen-antibody complexes have been composed of hepatitis B surface antigen and complement-fixing antibody against this antigen. Association with other infectious agents has also been suggested.[209]

Differential Diagnosis

The differential diagnosis for polyarteritis includes other vasculitic disease: Wegener's granulomatosis, giant cell arteritis, Takayasu's arteritis, and allergic granulomatous angiitis. Of these diseases, Wegener's granulomatosis most commonly involves the orbit and should be considered in a patient who presents with pseudotumor. Giant cell arteritis may involve the posterior ciliary vessels but can usually be distinguished by its clinical presentation. Takayasu's arteritis and allergic granulomatous angiitis rarely, if ever, present with orbital signs and symptoms.

Treatment

If untreated, polyarteritis nodosa is almost uniformly fatal. Corticosteroids may induce partial remission in some patients. Systemic chemotherapy with a cytotoxic agent such as cyclophosphamide is considered the treatment of choice.[217] Plasma exchange may have a role in the treatment of polyarteritis, especially in those who show evidence of hepatitis B infection.[224]

Temporal Arteritis

Temporal arteritis is well known to ophthalmologists because of its dramatic ocular presentation. It is a systemic disease that affects medium and large muscular arteries, primarily in the head,[225] hence the alternate name *cranial arteritis.* The term *giant cell arteritis* is used by some authors to describe temporal arteritis, but Takayasu's arteritis, which occurs in young women and affects primarily the aortic arch, also is an arteritis with giant cells on histologic examination and may properly be considered one of the giant cell arteritides.[225] Takayasu's arteritis presents with transient, position-dependent visual loss and retinal changes that are caused by ischemia, but orbital disease is not a characteristic finding.

The incidence of temporal arteritis increases with age, with a dramatic increase in the very elderly.[226] Even though more than 95% of cases occur in patients 50 years of age and older, age alone is not sufficient to rule out this diagnosis.[225] Average age of onset of first symptoms is 70 years.[225] There is a female predominance of 3:1.[227]

The systemic symptoms of temporal arteritis include headache or head tenderness, malaise, fatigue, fever, jaw claudication, and polymyalgia rheumatica, characterized by proximal muscle weakness or pain and arthralgias. Loss of the temporal artery pulse, tenderness over the artery, or abnormality detected by palpation of the artery may occur, but the diagnosis should be considered even in the absence of these signs. Because many of the systemic symptoms are nonspecific, this diagnosis is often not considered until ocular symptoms are reported.

Vision loss is the most prominent ocular symptom and is associated with ischemic optic neuropathy or occlusion of any of the ophthalmic central retinal or branch retinal arteries. Signs of anterior ischemia, including uveitis, low intraocular pressure, rubeosis, corneal edema, episcleritis, scleritis, and cataract, may occur.[227] Of relevance to the ophthalmic plastic surgeon, diplopia, ptosis, and periorbital pain may also occur.[198] Ophthalmoplegia may also occur in a few patients because of ischemia of the extraocular muscles.[228] Orbital involvement usually does not present as proptosis.

Laboratory findings include a dramatically elevated erythrocyte sedimentation rate. Mild anemia and elevated liver enzyme levels may be present.[225] The diagnosis is confirmed by the results of biopsy, most often of the temporal artery, which show segmental involvement of the media with a predominantly mononuclear infiltrate with multinucleated giant cells and disruption of the internal elastic lamina.[213,225,229] Orbital biopsy may demonstrate involvement of the long or short posterior ciliary arteries[199, 225, 229] and ischemic lesions of the extraocular muscles.[228, 230] Because the temporal artery lesions may be segmentally involved (so-called skip lesions or skip areas),[223, 231] harvesting of an adequate biopsy specimen and careful histologic examination along the entire length of the specimen increase the diagnostic yield. Some authors believe that bilateral biopsy may be indicated in some circumstances to firmly establish the diagnosis, given the significant complications of high-dose, long-term corticosteroid therapy.

The treatment for temporal arteritis is high-dose corticosteroids. Because the second eye may become involved within days to weeks, and the active inflammatory findings do not revert immediately, treatment should be begun immediately, even if the biopsy must be delayed. Efficacy of treatment is guided by relief of symptoms and normalization of the sedimentation rate.

Other vasculitic diseases, for example, polyarteritis nodosa, should be considered if the biopsy specimen demonstrates vasculitis without giant cells.[225]

Allergic Granulomatous Angiitis

Background

Allergic granulomatous angiitis is an entity that is often considered to be part of the polyarteritis nodosa family of diseases. The unique feature of allergic granulomatous angiitis is asthma that is followed, sometimes years later, by multisystem vasculitis.[232]

Epidemiology

The mean age of onset of systemic symptoms in allergic granulomatous angiitis is 44 years, and with a male to female ratio of 1.3:1.[209]

Systemic Manifestations

Systemic symptoms of allergic granulomatous angiitis include pulmonary signs and symptoms in almost all patients. The pulmonary symptoms are often the presenting sign. In addition to asthmatic symptoms, nodular or patchy infiltrates or diffuse interstitial disease may be present on chest radiograph. Involvement of other organ systems occurs a mean of 2 years after pulmonary symptoms (range of 0 to 30 years).[209] Skin nodules and purpura occur as in classic polyarteritis nodosa. Livedo reticularis is less common. Inflammatory bowel lesions with bleeding occur in 40% of patients. Peripheral neuropathies, central nervous system involvement, coronary vasculitis, and renal involvement also occur, although renal involvement is less common than in classic polyarteritis nodosa.

Ocular Manifestations

Vasculitic lesions of allergic granulomatous angiitis often involve vessels of the eye itself and manifest as uveitis. The iris, ciliary body, retina, choroid, and sclera may be involved.[232-234] Granulomata of the eyelids and conjunctiva have been observed, sometimes in an apparently limited form of the disease.[235-237]

Laboratory Findings

Laboratory findings are similar to those in polyarteritis nodosa. However, in allergic granulomatous angiitis, peripheral eosinophil counts higher than 1000/mm^3 occur sometime during the course of the disease in 85% of patients. As mentioned earlier, most patients have abnormal chest radiographs, and transient infiltrates are common.

Segmental lesions of small-sized and intermediate-sized arteries are identical to those of classic polyarteritis nodosa. Veins, venules, and arterioles may also be affected. In addition, eosinophilic infiltrates and granulomata are seen and are a common histopathologic feature of skin lesions even in the absence of vasculitis.

Differential Diagnosis

Diagnosis of allergic granulomatous angiitis is established by biopsy of a symptomatic organ system. Lung, muscle, and skin are potential sites. The differential diagnosis includes classic polyarteritis nodosa, Wegener's granulomatosis, sarcoidosis, and aspergillosis. Unlike classic polyarteritis nodosa, there is frequent involvement of the pulmonary vessels with eosinophilic tissue infiltrates. The clinical findings of severe asthma and peripheral blood eosinophilia also help distinguish the two entities.

Pathogenesis

The lesions of allergic angiitis are immune complex mediated (type III hypersensitivity), and allergens have been implicated as triggering the disease.

Treatment

When allergic granulomatous angiitis is untreated, the 5-year survival rate is 4%.[238] Pulmonary, cardiac, and renal lesions are common causes of death. With corticosteroid treatment, 5-year survival rate improves to 50% to 60%. As in classic polyarteritis nodosa, chemotherapeutic agents can induce remission and have prevented relapse over a 10-year period.[224]

Lymphomatoid Granulomatosis and Polymorphic Reticulosis

Background

Lymphomatoid granulomatosis was first described by Liebow and associates[239] as a vasculitic disorder predominantly involving the lung and has been grouped with Wegener's granulomatosis and allergic granulomatous angiitis as one of the respiratory vasculitic diseases.[240] Because it has been so widely described in earlier literature as a true vasculitis, it is included in this chapter. It is now regarded as a lymphoproliferative disorder, as described in the following sections.

Epidemiology

The first symptoms commonly appear in the 5th or 6th decade,[241, 242] although the condition has been reported in children.[241, 243] There is a slight male predominance.[241, 242, 244, 245] The disease is uncommon, with fewer than 200 cases reported in the literature by 1980.[241, 245] However, it is increasingly being recognized in patients with acquired immunodeficiency syndrome[246-248] or other immunosuppressive disorders.[249]

Systemic Manifestations

The clinical presentation is characterized by respiratory symptoms, including cough and dyspnea, and constitutional symptoms, including fever, malaise, and weight loss. Of the extrapulmonary manifestations, skin and neurologic involvement are most common. Cutaneous involvement occurs in approximately 40% of patients[241, 245, 251] and most commonly consists of scattered nodules or ulcers on the face or extremities.[251] As many as 30% of patients have neurologic involvement, including central nervous system signs and symptoms, cranial nerve palsies, and peripheral neuropathy. Visceral involvement is also reported.

Polymorphic reticulosis, which has been described as a destructive process of the midface,[252, 253] is now regarded as the part of the same pathologic process as lymphomatoid granulomatosis.[206, 254, 255] Lymphomatoid granulomatosis involving the upper respiratory tract continues to be referred to as *polymorphic reticulosis* by some authors. The nose, sinuses, pharynx, and palate may be affected.

Ocular Manifestations

Intraocular involvement in lymphomatoid granulomatosis is uncommon. Uveitis,[246] retinal vasculitis and vitritis,[257] choroiditis,[243] and scleritis[190] have been reported. Patients with cranial nerve palsies can have ocular manifestations, including strabismus and ptosis. Periocular involvement by midfacial disease can present with periorbital edema,[258] proptosis, involvement of the skin of the lid and brow,[259] orbital infiltrate, ophthalmoplegia, vascular occlusion, and sudden blindness.[256]

Laboratory Findings

The diagnosis is made by biopsy of an affected organ. The histology has been characterized as angiocentric and angiodestructive with a triad of features: (1) a polymorphic infiltrate of lymphoid and plasma cells; (2) location of the infiltrate around arteries and veins with transmural involvement of the vessel walls by lymphocytes; and (3) necrosis in the center of the lymphoid nodules.[239] The presence of necrosis and the polymorphic nature of the infiltrate can make histologic diagnosis difficult. Immunocytochemical staining and studies of gene rearrangement by Southern blot are necessary to determine the cell lineage of the lymphoid infiltrates.

Other laboratory testing is based on the organ system involved. Because lung involvement is common, a chest radiograph should be obtained. The typical finding includes bilateral nodular densities in the lower lung fields. Pleural effusion, cavitation, or infiltration may also be present.[241]

Pathogenesis

Lymphomatoid granulomatosis is widely accepted as a lymphoproliferative disease and is believed to be a type of malignant lymphoma.[242] Most cases have been of T cell origin and fall in the category of extranodal peripheral T cell lymphomas.[242] Some cases have been classified as B cell in origin,[249, 260] but controversy persists.[261] It is clear that several different types of lymphomas affect the midface.[262] The possibility of a role for Epstein-Barr virus in the pathogenesis of lymphomatoid granulomatosis has been raised.[249, 263]

Differential Diagnosis

The differential diagnosis for lymphomatoid granulomatosis includes other lymphomas, Wegener's granulomatosis, and the wide variety of disorders that present clinically as lethal midline granuloma.

Treatment

Untreated, the prognosis for lymphomatoid granulomatosis is poor. Treatment strategies have included radiation therapy, chemotherapy, and corticosteroids. Evaluation of the various regimens is difficult because of the diagnostic difficulties and heterogeneity of patients treated.[262] Currently, 5-year survival with a variety of treatment regimens appears to be approximately 50%.

Lethal Midline Granuloma

The term *lethal midline granuloma* has been used to describe a clinical condition that is characterized by progressive destruction of midfacial tissues, with inflammation and necrosis.[264, 265] Older literature tends to regard this as a specific diagnostic entity, whereas more recently the term has been reserved to describe a clinical condition of midfacial destruction that can result from a number of disease entities.[265, 266] The differential diagnosis includes lymphomas (including polymorphic reticulosis), carcinomas (basal cell, squamous cell, adenocystic, and nasopharyngeal), infectious diseases (syphilis, tuberculosis, leprosy, and fungal infection), Wegener's granulomatosis, sarcoidosis, cocaine abuse, and other entities.[206, 267] Even this differential diagnosis has been the subject of controversy.[268, 269]

To confuse the picture further, the term *midline malignant reticulosis* also appears in the literature. Some authors have considered this to be synonymous with polymorphic reticulosis, whereas others use it as a synonym for lethal midline granuloma.[258] The term *idiopathic midline destructive disease* should probably be reserved for use as a diagnosis of exclusion.[268, 269]

REFERENCES

1. Foster CS: Cicatricial pemphigoid. Trans Am Ophthalmol Soc 84:527–663, 1986.
2. Fine JD: Cicatricial and localized pemphigoid. *In* Jordan RE (ed): Immunologic Diseases of the Skin. Norwalk/San Mateo, CA, Appleton & Lange, 1991, pp 303–313.
3. Person JR, Rogers RS: Bullous and cicatricial pemphigoid: Clinical, histopathologic, and immunopathologic correlates. Mayo Clin Proc 52:54–66, 1977.
4. Lever WF: Pemphigus. Medicine 32:1–123, 1953.
5. Mondino BJ: Cicatricial pemphigoid and erythema multiforme. Int Ophthalmol Clin 23:63–79, 1981.
6. Mondino BJ, Brown, SI: Ocular cicatricial pemphigoid. Ophthalmology 88:95–100, 1981.
7. Mondino BJ: Cicatricial pemphigoid and erythema multiforme. Ophthalmology 97:939–952, 1990.
8. Bettelheim H, Kraft D, Zehetbauer G: Uber den sogenanneten augenpemphigus (pemphigus ocularis, pemphigus conjunctivae). Klin Auggenheilkd 160:65–75, 1972.
9. Smith RC, Myers EA, Lamb HD: Ocular and oral pemphigus: Report of case with anatomic findings in eyeball. Arch Ophthalmol 11:635–640, 1934.
10. Mitchell RD, Smith NHH: Cicatricial pemphigoid: A review of eleven cases. Aust Dental J 24:260–265, 1979.
11. Unis ME: The skin and the eye. Dermatol Clin North Am 8:297–311, 1990.
12. Ormerod LD, Fong LP, Foster CS: Corneal infection in mucosal scarring disorders and Sjögren's syndrome. Am J Ophthalmol 105:512–518, 1988.
13. Tauber J, Melamed S, Foster CS: Glaucoma in patients with ocular cicatricial pemphigoid. Ophthalmology 96:33–37, 1989.
14. Frith P, Charnock M, Wojnarowska F: Cicatricial pemphigoid diagnosed from ocular features in recurrent severe vulval scarring: Two case reports. Br J Obstet Gynaecol 98:482–484, 1991.
15. Mills RP, O'Connor MJ, Shun-Shin GA: Mucous membrane pemphigoid—a preventable cause of laryngeal stenosis. J Laryngol Otol 97:761–765, 1983.
16. Lekas MD, Thayer WR: Dysphagia from benign mucocutaneous pemphigoid. Ear Nose Throat J 67:113–116, 1988.
17. Tauber J, Jabbur N, Foster CS: Improved detection of disease progression in ocular cicatricial pemphigoid. Cornea 11:446–451, 1992.
18. Hoang-Xuan T, Foster CS, Raizman MB, Greenwood B: Mast cells in conjunctiva affected by cicatricial pemphigoid. Ophthalmology 96:1110–1114, 1989.
19. Mondino BJ, Ross AN, Rabin BS, Brown SI: Autoimmune phenomena in ocular cicatricial pemphigoid. Am J Ophthalmol 83:443–450, 1977.
20. Leonard JN, Hobday CM, Haffenden GP, et al: Immunofluorescent studies in ocular cicatricial pemphigoid. Br J Dermatol 118:209–217, 1988.
21. Helm K, Peters MS: Immunodermatology update: The immunologically mediated vesiculobullous diseases. Mayo Clin Proc 66:187–202, 1991.
22. Rogers RS, Perry HO, Bean SF, Jordan RE: Immunopathology of cicatricial pemphigoid: Studies of complement deposition. J Invest Dermatol 68:39–43, 1977.
23. Proia AD, Foulks GN, Sanfilippo FP: Ocular cicatricial pemphigoid with granular IgA and complement deposition. Arch Ophthalmol 103:1669–1672, 1985.
24. Ahmed AR, Khan KNA, Wells P, et al: Preliminary serological studies comparing immunofluorescence assay with radioimmunoassay. Curr Eye Res 8:1011–1019, 1989.
25. Franklin RM, Fitzmorris CT: Antibodies against conjunctival basement membrane zone: Occurrence in cicatricial pemphigoid. Arch Ophthalmol 101:1611–1613, 1983.
26. Dantzig P: Circulating antibodies in cicatricial pemphigoid. Arch Dermatol 108:264–266, 1973.
27. Wright P: Enigma of ocular cicatricial pemphigoid: A comparative study of clinical and immunological findings. Trans Ophthalmol Soc UK 99:141–145, 1979.
28. Kelly SE, Wojnarowska F: The use of chemically split tissue in the detection of circulating anti-basement membrane zone antibodies in bullous pemphigoid and cicatricial pemphigoid. Br J Dermatol 118:31–40, 1988.
29. Niimi Y, Zhu XJ, Bystryn JC: Identification of cicatricial pemphigoid antigens. Arch Dermatol 128:54–57, 1992.
30. Anhalt GJ, Wicha MX, Sugar A, et al: Distribution of pemphigus and pemphigoid antigens, laminin, and type VI collagen in corneal epithelium. Invest Ophthalmol Vis Sci 21:879–882, 1981.
31. Mondino BJ, Brown SI, Rabin BS: HLA antigens in ocular cicatricial pemphigoid. Arch Ophthalmol 97:479, 1979.
32. Zaltas MM, Ahmed R, Foster CS: Association of HLA-DR4 with ocular cicatricial pemphigoid. Curr Eye Res 8:189–193, 1989.
33. Patten JT, Cavanagh HD, Allansmith MR: Induced ocular pseudopemphigoid. Am J Ophthalmol 82:272–276, 1976.
34. Lass JH, Thoft RA, Dohlman CH: Idoxuridine-induced conjunctival cicatrization. Arch Ophthalmol 101:747–750, 1983.
35. Pouliquen Y, Patey A, Foster CS, et al: Drug-induced cicatricial pemphigoid affecting the conjunctiva. Ophthalmology 93:775–783, 1986.
36. Fiore PM, Jacobs IH, Goldberg DB: Drug-induced pemphigoid. Arch Ophthalmol 105:1660–1663, 1987.
37. Fiore PM: Drug-induced ocular cicatrization. Int Ophthalmol Clin 29:147–150, 1989.
38. Kremer I, Rozenbaum D, Aviel E: Immunofluorescence findings in pseudopemphigoid induced by short-term idoxuridine administration. Am J Ophthalmol 111:375–377, 1991.
39. Anhalt GJ, Bahn CF, Diaz LA: Bullous diseases. Int Ophthalmol Clin 25:37–59, 1985.
40. Brody HJ, Pirozzi DJ: Benign mucous membrane pemphigoid: Response to therapy with cyclophosphamide. Arch Dermatol 113:1598–1599, 1977.
41. Person JR, Rogers RS: Bullous pemphigoid responding to sulfapyridine and the sulfones. Arch Dermatol 113:610–615, 1977.
42. Lang PG: Sulfones and sulfonamides in dermatology today. J Am Acad Dermatol 1:479–492, 1979.
43. Foster CS: Immunosuppressive therapy for external ocular inflammatory disease. Ophthalmology 87:140–150, 1980.
44. Foster CS, Wilson LA, Ekins MB: Immunosuppressive therapy for progressive ocular cicatricial pemphigoid. Ophthalmology 89:340–353, 1982.
45. Rogers RS, Seehafer JR, Perry HO: Treatment of cicatricial (benign mucous membrane) pemphigoid with dapsone. J Am Acad Dermatol 6:215–223, 1982.
46. Mondino BJ, Brown SI: Immunosuppressive therapy in ocular cicatricial pemphigoid. Am J Ophthalmol 96:453–459, 1983.
47. Tauber J, Sainz de la Maza M, Foster CS: Systemic chemotherapy for ocular cicatricial pemphigoid. Cornea 10:185–195, 1991.
48. Hemady R, Tauber J, Foster CS: Immunosuppressive drugs in immune and inflammatory ocular disease. Surv Ophthalmol 35:369–385, 1991.
49. Tseng SCG, Maumenee AE, Stark WJ, et al: Topical retinoid treatment for various dry-eye disorders. Ophthalmology 92:717–727, 1985.
50. Herbort CP, Matter M, Uffer S: Topical retinoic acid treatment of drug-induced pseudopemphigoid. Ophthalmologica 193:27–33, 1986.
51. Baer JC, Foster CS: Corneal laser photocoagulation for treatment of neovascularization. Ophthalmology 99:173–179, 1992.
52. Girard LJ, Hawkins RS, Nieves R, Borodofsky T, Grant C: Keratoprosthesis: A 12-year follow-up. Trans Am Acad Ophthalmol Otolaryngol 83:252–267, 1977.
53. Cardona H, DeVoe AG: Prosthokeratoplasty. Trans Am Acad Ophthalmol Otolaryngol 83:271–280, 1977.
54. Kozarsky AM, Knight SH, Waring GO: Clinical results with a ceramic keratoprosthesis placed through the eyelid. Ophthalmology 94:904–911, 1987.
55. Sainz de la Maza M, Tauber J, Foster CS: Cataract surgery in ocular cicatricial pemphigoid. Ophthalmology 95:481–486, 1988.
56. Beyer CK: The management of special problems associated with Stevens-Johnson syndrome and ocular pemphigoid. Trans Am Acad Ophthalmol Otolaryngol 83:701–707, 1977.

57. McCord CD, Chen WP: Tarsal polishing and mucous membrane grafting for cicatricial entropion, trichiasis, and epidermalization. Ophthalmic Surg 14:1021–1025, 1983.
58. Millman AL, Katzen LB, Putterman AM: Cicatricial entropion: An analysis of its treatment with transverse blepharotomy and marginal rotation. Ophthalmic Surg 20:575–579, 1989.
59. Naumann GOH, Lang GK, Rummelt V, Wigand ME: Autologous nasal mucosa transplantation in severe bilateral conjunctival mucus deficiency syndrome. Ophthalmology 97:1011–1017, 1990.
60. Shore JW, Foster CS, Westfall CT, Rubin PAD: Results of buccal mucosal grafting for patients with medically controlled ocular cicatricial pemphigoid. Ophthalmology 99:383–395, 1992.
61. Huff JC: Erythema multiforme. *In* Jordan RE (ed): Immunologic Diseases of the Skin. Norwalk/San Mateo, CA, Appleton & Lange, 1991, pp 463–470.
62. Howard GM: The Stevens-Johnson syndrome: Ocular prognosis and treatment. Am J Ophthalmol 55:893–900, 1963.
63. Arstikaitis MJ: Ocular aftermath of Stevens-Johnson syndrome. Arch Ophthalmol 90:376–379, 1973.
64. Magli A, Sammartino A, Loffredo A, et al: Stevens-Johnson syndrome: A clinical and histological study. Ophthalmologica 183:122–127, 1981.
65. Wright P, Collin JRO: The ocular complications of erythema multiforme (Stevens-Johnson syndrome) and their management. Trans Ophthalmol Soc UK 103:338–341, 1983.
66. Foster CS, Fong LP, Azar D, Kenyon KR: Episodic conjunctival inflammation after Stevens-Johnson syndrome. Ophthalmology 95:453–462, 1988.
67. Harris GJ: Marsupialization of a lacrimal gland cyst. Ophthalmic Surg 14:75–78, 1983.
68. Imamura S, Yanase K, Taniguchi S, et al: Erythema multiforme: Demonstration of immune complexes in the sera and skin lesions. Br J Dermatol 102:161–166, 1980.
69. Wuepper KD, Watson PA, Kazmierowski JA: Immune complexes in erythema multiforme and the Stevens-Johnson syndrome. J Invest Dermatol 74:368–371, 1980.
70. Bushkell LL, Mackel SE, Jordan RE: Erythema multiforme: Direct immunofluorescence studies and detection of circulating immune complexes. J Invest Dermatol 74:372–374, 1980.
71. Margolis RJ, Tonnesen MG, Harrist TJ, et al: Lymphocyte subsets and Langerhans' cells/indeterminate cells in erythema multiforme. J Invest Dermatol 81:403–406, 1983.
72. Rubin Z: Ophthalmic sulfonamide-induced Stevens-Johnson syndrome. Arch Dermatol 113:235–236, 1977.
73. Ward B, McCulley JP, Segal RJ: Dermatologic reaction in Stevens-Johnson syndrome after ophthalmic anesthesia with proparacaine hydrochloride. Am J Ophthalmol 86:133–135, 1978.
74. Yetiv JZ, Bianchine JR, Owen JA: Etiologic factors of the Stevens-Johnson syndrome. South Med J 73:599–602, 1980.
75. Kiernan JP, Schanzlin DJ, Leveille AS: Stevens-Johnson syndrome associated with adenovirus conjunctivitis. Am J Ophthalmol 92:543–545, 1981.
76. Howland WW, Golitz LE, Weston WL, Huff JC: Erythema multiforme: Clinical, histopathologic, and immunologic study. J Am Acad Dermatol 10:438–446, 1984.
77. Genvert GI, Cohen EJ, Donnenfeld ED, Blecher MH: Erythema multiforme after use of topical sulfacetamide. Am J Ophthalmol 99:465–468, 1985.
78. Sherertz EF, Reed JW, Zanolli MD, Goldsmith SM: Severe allergic conjunctivitis and erythema multiforme after a routine eye examination: Discerning the cause. Ann Ophthalmol 23:173–176, 1991.
79. Mondino BJ, Brown SI, Biglan AW: HLA antigens in Stevens-Johnson syndrome with ocular involvement. Arch Ophthalmol 100:1453–1454, 1982.
80. Marvin JA, Heimbach DM, Engrav LH, Harnar TJ: Improved treatment of the Stevens-Johnson syndrome. Arch Surg 119:601–605, 1984.
81. Rasmussen JE: Erythema multiforme in children: Response to treatment with systemic corticosteroids. Br J Dermatol 95:181–186, 1976.
82. Singer L, Brook U, Romem M, Fried D: Vitamin A in Stevens-Johnson syndrome. Ann Ophthalmol 21:209–210, 1989.
83. Dugan EM, Anhalt GJ, Diaz LA: Pemphigus. *In* Jordan RE (ed): Immunologic Diseases of the Skin. Norwalk/San Mateo, CA, Appleton & Lange 1991, pp 279–291.
84. Korman N: Pemphigus. J Am Acad Dermatol 18:1219–1238, 1988.
85. Stanle JR: Pemphigus: Skin failure mediated by autoantibodies. JAMA 264:1714–1717, 1990.
86. Park MS, Terasaki PI, Ahmed AR, Tiwari JL: HLA-DRW4 in 91% of Jewish pemphigus vulgaris patients. Lancet 2:441–442, 1979.
87. Brautbar C, Moscovitz M, Livshits T, et al: HLA-DRW4 in pemphigus vulgaris patients in Israel. Tissue Antigens 16:238–243, 1980.
88. Bean SF, Holubar K, Gillett RB: Pemphigus involving the eyes. Arch Dermatol 111:1484–1486, 1975.
89. Hodak E, Kremet I, David M, et al: Conjunctival involvement in pemphigus vulgaris: A clinical, histopathological and immunofluorescence study. Br J Dermatol 123:615–620, 1990.
90. Carroll JM, Kuwabara T: Ocular pemphigus: An electron microscopic study of the conjunctival and corneal epithelium. Arch Ophthalmol 80:683–695, 1968.
91. Pagani WA, Rimondi AP, Chiacchiarini A, Lorenzi G: Basal cell carcinoma arising in pemphigus vulgaris of the lower eyelid. J Dermatol Surg Oncol 16:1152–1154, 1990.
92. Lam S, Seabury Stone M, Goeken JA, et al: Paraneoplastic pemphigus, cicatricial conjunctivitis, and acanthosis nigricans with pachydermatoglyphy in a patient with bronchogenic squamous cell carcinoma. Ophthalmology 99:108–113, 1992.
93. David M, Katzenelson V, Hazaz B, et al: Determination of IgG subclasses in patients with pemphigus with active disease and in remission. Arch Dermatol 125:7787–7790, 1989.
94. Wolff K, Schreiner E: Ultrastructural localization of pemphigus autoantibodies within the epidermis. Nature 229:59–61, 1971.
95. O'Loughlin S, Goldman GC, Provost TT: Fate of pemphigus antibody following successful therapy: Preliminary evaluation of pemphigus antibody determinations to regulate therapy. Arch Dermatol 114:1769–1772, 1978.
96. Fitzpatrick RE, Newcomer VD: The correlation of disease activity and antibody titers in pemphigus. Arch Dermatol 116:285–290, 1980.
97. Moncada B, Kettelsen S, Hernandez-Moctezuma JL, Ramirez F: Neonatal pemphigus vulgaris: Role of passively transferred pemphigus antibodies. Clin Res 28(2):251A, 1980.
98. Schiltz JR, Michel B: Production of epidermal acantholysis in normal human skin in vitro by the IgG fraction from pemphigus serum. J Invest Dermatol 67:254–260, 1976.
99. Frab RM, Dykes R, Lazarus GS: Anti–epidermal-cell-surface pemphigus antibody detaches viable epidermal cells from culture plates by activation of proteinase. Proc Natl Acad Sci USA 75:459–463, 1978.
100. Diaz LA, Marcelo CL: Pemphigoid and pemphigus antigens in cultured epidermal cells. Br J Dermatol 98:631–637, 1978.
101. Ruocco V, Rossi A, Argenziano G, et al: Pathogenicity of the intercellular antibodies of pemphigus and their periodic removal from the circulation by plasmapheresis. Br J Dermatol 98:237–241, 1978.
102. Pearson RW: Clinicopathologic types of epidermolysis bullosa and their nondermatological complications. Arch Dermatol 124:718–725, 1988.
103. Woodley DT, Gammon WR, Briggaman RA: Epidermolysis bullosa acquisita. *In* Jordan RE (ed): Immunologic Diseases of the Skin. Norwalk/San Mateo, CA, Appleton & Lange, 1991, pp 321–333.
104. Richter BJ, McNutt NS: The spectrum of epidermolysis bullosa acquisita. Arch Dermatol 115:1325–1328, 1979.
105. Roengik HH, Ryan JG, Bergfeld WF: Epidermolysis bullosa acquisita: Report of three cases and review of all published cases. Arch Dermatol 1971: 1–10.
106. McDonnell PJ, Spalton DJ: The ocular signs and complications of epidermolysis bullosa. J R Soc Med 81:576–578, 1988.
107. Granek H, Baden HP: Corneal involvement in epidermolysis bullosa simplex. Arch Ophthalmol 98:469–472, 1980.
108. Holbrook KA: Extracutaneous epithelial involvement in inherited epidermolysis bullosa. Arch Dermatol 124:726–731, 1988.
109. Steuhl KP, Anton-Lamprecht I, Arnold ML, Thiel HJ: Recurrent bilateral corneal erosions due to an association of epidermolysis

bullosa simplex Kobner and X-linked ichthyosis with steroid sulfatase deficiency. Graefes Arch Klin Exp Ophthalmol 226:216–223, 1988.
110. Gans LA: Eye lesions of epidermolysis bullosa. Arch Dermatol 124:762–764, 1988.
111. Zierhut M, Thiel HJ, Weidle EG, et al: Ocular involvement in epidermolysis bullosa acquisita. Arch Ophthalmol 107:398–401, 1989.
112. Lang PG, Tapert MJ: Severe ocular involvement in a patient with epidermolysis bullosa acquisita. J Am Acad Dermatol 16:439–443, 1987.
113. McDonnell PJ, Schofield OMV, Spalton DJ, Eady RAJ: Eye involvement in junctional epidermolysis bullosa. Arch Ophthalmol 107:1635–1637, 1989.
114. Aurora AL, Madhavan M, Rao S: Ocular changes in epidermolysis bullosa letalis. Am J Ophthalmol 79:464–470, 1975.
115. Craighead JE: Pathogenesis, clinical features, and management of the non-dermatological complications of epidermolysis bullosa. Arch Dermatol 124:705, 1988.
116. Kaluza C, Kennedy BJ, Harman L: Head and neck complications of epidermolysis bullosa. Laryngoscope 95:599–600, 1985.
117. Dahl MGC: Epidermolysis bullosa acquisita—a sign of cicatricial pemphigoid? Br J Dermatol 101:475–483, 1979.
118. Gammon WR, Briggaman RA, Woodley DT, et al: Epidermolysis bullosa acquisita—a pemphigoid-like disease. J Am Acad Dermatol 11:820–832, 1984.
119. Eady RAJ: The basement membrane—interface between the epithelium and the dermis: Structural features. Arch Dermatol 124:709–712, 1988.
120. Fine JD: Antigenic features and structural correlates of basement membranes: Relationship to epidermolysis bullosa. Arch Dermatol 124:713–717, 1988.
121. Hashimoto I, Gedde-Dahl T, Schnyder UW, Anton-Lamprecht I: Ultrastructural studies in epidermolysis bullosa hereditaria. Part IV: Recessive dystrophic types with junctional blistering (infantile or Herlitz-Pearson and adult type). Arch Dermatol Res 257:17–32, 1976.
122. Kushniruk W: The immunopathology of epidermolysis bullosa acquisita. Can Med Assoc J 108:1143–1146, 1973.
123. Gibbs RB, Minus HR: Epidermolysis bullosa acquisita with electron microscopical studies. Arch Dermatol 111:215–220, 1975.
124. Nieboer C, Boorsma DM, Woerdemna MJ, Kalsbeek GL: Epidermolysis bullosa acquisita: Immunofluorescence, electron microscopic, and immunoelectron microscopic studies in four patients. Br J Dermatol 102:383–392, 1980.
125. Woodley DT, Briggaman RA, O'Keefe EJ, et al: Identification of the skin-basement membrane autoantigen in epidermolysis bullosa acquisita. N Engl J Med 310:1007–1013, 1984.
126. Mooney E, Falk RJ, Gammon WR: Studies on complement deposits in epidermolysis bullosa acquisita and bullous pemphigoid. Arch Dermatol 128:58–60, 1992.
127. Crow LL, Finkle JP, Gammon WR, Woodley DT: Clearing of epidermolysis bullosa with cyclosporine. J Am Acad Dermatol 19:937–942, 1988.
128. Layton AM: Clearing of epidermolysis bullosa acquisita with cyclosporine. J Am Acad Dermatol 22:535, 1990.
129. Lyell A: Toxic epidermal necrolysis (the scalded-skin syndrome): A reappraisal. Br J Dermatol 100:69–86, 1979.
130. Revuz J, Penso D, Roujeau JC, et al: Toxic epidermal necrolysis: Clinical findings and prognosis in 87 patients. Arch Dermatol 123:1160–1165, 1987.
131. Goldstein SM, Wintroub BW, Elias PM: Toxic epidermal necrolysis: Unmuddying the waters. Arch Dermatol 123:1153–1155, 1987.
132. Bottiger LE, Strandberg I, Westerholm B: Drug-induced febrile mucocutaneous syndrome. Acta Med Scand 198:229–233, 1975.
133. Björnberg P, Björnberg K, Gisslen H: Toxic epidermal necrolysis with ophthalmologic complications. Acta Ophthalmol 42:1084–1095, 1964.
134. Bennett TO, Sugar J, Sahgal S: Ocular manifestations of toxic epidermal necrolysis associated with allopurinol use. Arch Ophthalmol 95:1362–1364, 1977.
135. Belfort R, de Smet M, Whitcup SM, et al: Ocular complications of Stevens-Johnson syndrome and toxic epidermal necrolysis in patients with AIDS. Cornea 10:536–538, 1991.
136. Rasmussen J: Toxic epidermal necrolysis. Med Clin North Am 64:901–920, 1980.
137. Kint A, Geerts ML, de Weert J: Le syndrome de Lyell. Dermatologica 163:433–454, 1981.
138. Ruiz-Maldonado R: Acute disseminated epidermal necrolysis types 1, 2, and 3: Study of sixty cases. J Am Acad Dermatol 13:623–635, 1985.
139. Peck G, Herzig GP, Elias PM: Toxic epidermal necrolysis in a patient with graft-versus-host reaction. Arch Dermatol 105:561–569, 1972.
140. Stein KM, Schlappner OLA, Heaton CL, Decherd JW: Demonstration of basal cell immunofluorescence in drug-induced toxic epidermal necrosis. Br J Dermatol 86:246–252, 1972.
141. Hensen EJ, Claas FHJ, Veermer BJ: Drug-dependent binding of circulating antibodies in drug-induced toxic epidermal necrolysis. Lancet 2:151–152, 1981.
142. Roujeau JC, Huynh TN, Bracq C, et al: Genetic susceptibility to toxic epidermal necrolysis. Arch Dermatol 123:1171–1173, 1987.
143. Ellman MH, Fretzin DF, Olson W: Toxic epidermal necrolysis associated with allopurinol administration. Arch Dermatol 111:986–990, 1975.
144. Guillaume JC, Roujeau JC, Revuz J, et al: The culprit drugs in 87 cases of toxic epidermal necrolysis (Lyell's syndrome). Arch Dermatol 123:1166–1170, 1987.
145. Amon RB, Dimond RL: Toxic epidermal necrolysis: Rapid differentiation between staphylococcal and drug-induced disease. Arch Dermatol 111:1433–1437, 1975.
146. Halebian PH, Corder VJ, Madden MR, et al: Improved burn center survival of patients with toxic epidermal necrolysis managed without corticosteroids. Ann Surg 204:503–512, 1986.
147. Revuz J, Roujeau JC, Guillaume JC, et al: Treatment of toxic epidermal necrolysis: Creteil's experience. Arch Dermatol 123:1156–1158, 1987.
148. Biren CA, Barr RJ: Dermatologic applications of cyclosporine. Arch Dermatol 122:1028–1032, 1986.
149. Bresnitz EA, Strom BL: Epidemiology of sarcoidosis. Epidemiol Rev 5:124–156, 1983.
150. Siltzbach LE, James DG, Neville E, et al: Course and prognosis of sarcoidosis around the world. Am J Med 57:847–852, 1974.
151. Thomas PD, Hunninghake GW: Current concepts of the pathogenesis of sarcoidosis. Am Rev Respir Dis 135:747–760, 1987.
152. Hoover DL, Khan JA, Giangiacomo J: Pediatric ocular sarcoidosis. Surv Ophthalmol 30:215–228, 1986.
153. Headings VE, Weston D, Young RC, Hackney RL: Familial sarcoidosis with multiple occurrences in eleven families: A possible mechanism of inheritance. Ann NY Acad Sci 278:377–385, 1976.
154. Sharma OP, Neville E, Walker AN, James DG: Familial sarcoidosis: A possible genetic influence. Ann NY Acad Sci 278:386–400, 1976.
155. British Thoracic and Tuberculosis Association: Familial associations in sarcoidosis. Tubercle 54:87–98, 1973.
156. Jabs DA, Johns CJ: Ocular involvement in chronic sarcoidosis. Am J Ophthalmol 10:297–301, 1986.
157. Obenauf CD, Shaw HE, Sydnor CF, Klintworth GK: Sarcoidosis and its ophthalmic manifestations. Am J Ophthalmol 86:648–655, 1978.
158. Brewerton DA, Cockburn C, James DCO, James DG: HLA antigens in sarcoidosis. Clin Exp Immunol 27:227–229, 1977.
159. Olenchock SA, Heise ER, Marx JJ, et al: HLA-B8 in sarcoidosis. Ann Allergy 47:151–153, 1981.
160. Foster CS: Ocular manifestations of sarcoidosis preceding systemic manifestations. *In* Grassi C, Rizzato G, Pozzi E (eds): Sarcoidosis and Other Granulomatous Diseases. New York, Elsevier, 1988, pp 177–181.
161. James DG, Neville E, Langley DA: Ocular sarcoidosis. Trans Ophthalmol Soc UK 96:133–139, 1976.
162. Spalton DJ, Sanders MD: Fundus changes in histologically confirmed sarcoidosis. Br J Ophthalmol 65:348–358, 1981.
163. Klintworth GK: Sarcoidosis. *In* Gold DH, Weingeist TA (eds): The Eye in Systemic Diseases. Philadelphia, JB Lippincott, 1990, pp 289–293.
164. Smith RE, Nozik RA: Sarcoidosis. *In* Smith RE, Nozik RA (eds):

Uveitis: A Clinical Approach to Diagnosis and Management. Baltimore, Williams & Wilkins, 1983, pp 161–163.
165. O'Connor GR: Endogenous uveitis: Sarcoidosis. *In* Kraus-Mackiw E, O'Connor GR (eds): Uveitis: Pathophysiology and Therapy. New York, Thieme, 1986, pp 93–97.
166. Nussenblatt RB, Palestine AG: Sarcoidosis. *In* Nussenblatt RB, Palestine AG (eds): Uveitis: Fundamentals and Clinical Practice. Chicago, Year Book, 1989, pp 198–211.
167. Campo R, Aaberg TM: Choroidal granuloma in sarcoidosis. Am J Ophthalmol 97:419–427, 1984.
168. Gragoudas ES, Regan CDJ: Peripapillary subretinal neovascularization in presumed sarcoidosis. Arch Ophthalmol 99:1194–1197, 1981.
169. Beardsley TL, Brown SVL, Sydnor CF, et al: Eleven cases of sarcoidosis of the optic nerve. Am J Ophthalmol 97:62–77, 1984.
170. Gass JDM, Olson CL: Sarcoidosis with optic nerve and retinal involvement. Arch Ophthalmol 94:945–950, 1976.
171. Lamkin JC, Raizman MB: Update on laboratory tests for diagnosis of orbital disease. Int Ophthalmol Clin 32:27–44, 1992.
172. Collison JMT, Miller NR, Green WR: Involvement of orbital tissues by sarcoid. Am J Ophthalmol 102:302–307, 1986.
173. Spillberg I: Sarcoidosis. *In* Schumacher HR, Klippel JH, Robinson DR (eds): Primer on the Rheumatic Diseases. Atlanta, Arthritis Foundation, 1988, pp 190–192.
174. Weinreb RN, Tessler H: Laboratory diagnosis of ophthalmic sarcoidosis. Surv Ophthalmol 28:653–664, 1984.
175. Hunninghake GW, Bedell GN, Zavala DC, et al: Role of interleukin-2 release by lung T-cells in active pulmonary sarcoidosis. Am Rev Respir Dis 128:634–638, 1983.
176. Chan CC, Wetzig RP, Palestine AG, et al: Immunohistopathology of ocular sarcoidosis: Report of a case and discussion of immunopathogenesis. Arch Ophthalmol 105:1398–1402, 1987.
177. Barth CL, Judge MS, Mattman LH, Hessburg PC: Isolation of an acid-fast organism from the aqueous humor in a case of sarcoidosis. Henry Ford Hosp Med J 27:127–133, 1979.
178. Nichols CW, Eagle RC, Yanoff M, Menocal NG: Conjunctival biopsy as an aid in the evaluation of the patient with suspected sarcoidosis. Ophthalmology 87:287–291, 1980.
179. Merritt JC, Lipper SL, Peiffer RL, Hale LM: Conjunctival biopsy in sarcoidosis. J Natl Med Assoc 72:347–349, 1980.
180. Merritt JC, Ross G, Avery A: Conjunctival biopsy in sarcoidosis: Four-year NCMH experience. N C Med J 44:636–637, 1983.
181. Weinreb RN: Diagnosing sarcoidosis by transconjunctival biopsy of the lacrimal gland. Am J Ophthalmol 97:573–576, 1984.
182. Karcioglu ZA, Brear R: Conjunctival biopsy in sarcoidosis. Am J Ophthalmol 99:68–73, 1985.
183. Baughman RP, Ploysongsang Y, Roberts RD, Srivastava L: Effects of sarcoid and steroids on angiotensin-converting enzyme. Am Rev Respir Dis 128:631–633, 1983.
184. Kavanaugh AF, Andrew SL, Cooper B, et al: Cyclosporine therapy of central nervous system sarcoidosis. Am J Med 82:387, 1987.
185. Straatsma BR: Ocular manifestations of Wegener's granulomatosis. Am J Ophthalmol 44:789–799, 1957.
186. Haynes BF, Fishman ML, Fauci AS, Wolff SM: The ocular manifestations of Wegener's granulomatosis: Fifteen years' experience and review of the literature. Am J Med 63:131–141, 1977.
187. Bullen CL, Liesegang TJ, McDonald TJ, DeRemee RA: Ocular complications of Wegener's granulomatosis. Ophthalmology 90:279–290, 1983.
188. Soukiasian SH, Foster CS, Niles JL, Raizman MB: Diagnostic value of antineutrophil cytoplasmic antibodies in scleritis associated with Wegener's granulomatosis. Ophthalmology 99:125–132, 1983.
189. Spalton DJ, Graham EM, Page NGR, Sanders MD: Ocular changes in limited forms of Wegener's granulomatosis. Br J Ophthalmol 65:553–563, 1981.
190. Fauci AS, Haynes BF, Costa J, et al: Lymphomatoid granulomatosis: Prospective clinical and therapeutic experience over 10 years. N Engl J Med 306:68–74, 1982.
191. Cupps TR, Fauci AS: Wegener's granulomatosis. *In* Smith LH (ed): Major Problems in Internal Medicine, vol 11. Philadelphia, WB Saunders, 1981, pp 72–87.
192. Kalina PH, Garrity JA, Herman DC, et al: Role of testing for anticytoplasmic autoantibodies in the differential diagnosis of scleritis and orbital pseudotumor. Mayo Clin Proc 65:1110–1117, 1990.
193. Allen JC, France TD: Pseudotumor as the presenting sign of Wegener's granulomatosis in a child. J Pediatr Ophthalmol 14:158–159, 1977.
194. Liliequist B, Link H: Wegener's granulomatosis: Report of a case. Angiology 19:215–224, 1968.
195. Fauci AS, Wolff SM: Wegener's granulomatosis: Studies in eighteen patients and a review of the literature. Medicine 52:535–561, 1973.
196. Cassan SM, Divertie MV, Hollenhorst RW, Harrison EG: Pseudotumor of the orbit and limited Wegener's granulomatosis. Ann Intern Med 72:687–693, 1970.
197. Kay CM, McCrary JA: Multiple cranial nerve palsies in late metastasis of midline malignant reticulosis. Am J Ophthalmol 88:1087–1090, 1979.
198. Jakobiec FA, Jones IS: Orbital inflammations. *In* Tasman W, Jaeger EA (eds): Duane's Clinical Ophthalmology. Philadelphia, JB Lippincott, 1989, pp 1–75.
199. Jakobiec FA, Font RL: Noninfectious orbital inflammations. *In* Spencer WH (ed): Ophthalmic Pathology: An Atlas and Textbook, 3rd ed. Philadelphia, WB Saunders, 1985, pp 2765–2812.
200. Hardwig PW, Bartley GB, Garrity JA: Surgical management of nasolacrimal duct obstruction in patients with Wegener's granulomatosis. Ophthalmology 99:133–139, 1992.
201. Cogan DG: Corneoscleral lesions in periarteritis nodosa and Wegener's granulomatosis. Trans Am Ophthalmol Soc 53:321–344, 1965.
202. Brubaker R, Font RL, Shepherd EM: Granulomatous sclerouveitis: Regression of ocular lesions with cyclophosphamide and prednisone. Arch Ophthalmol 86:517–524, 1971.
203. Kalina PH, Lie JT, Campbell RJ, Garrity JA: Diagnostic value and limitations of orbital biopsy in Wegener's granulomatosis. Ophthalmology 99:120–124, 1992.
204. Specks U, Wheatlye CL, McDonald TJ, et al: Anticytoplasmic autoantibodies in the diagnosis and follow-up of Wegener's granulomatosis. Mayo Clin Proc 64:28–36, 1989.
205. Leavitt RY, Fauci AS: Wegener's granulomatosis and other systemic granulomatous conditions. Curr Opin Rheumatol 2:55–59, 1990.
206. Seidman JD: Case 2: 1990 [letter; comment]. N Engl J Med 324:1371, 1991.
207. Von Rokitansky C: Ueger einige der wichtigsten Krankheitin der Arterien. Denkscher d k Akad D Wissensch 4:49, 1852.
208. Kussmaul A, Maier K: Uber eine bisher nicht beschriebene eigenthumliche Arterienerkrankung (periarteritis nodosa), die mit Morbus Brightii un rapid fortschreitender allgemeiner Muskellahmung einhergeht. Dtsch Arch Klin Med 1:484–517, 1866.
209. Cupps TR, Fauci AS: Systemic necrotizing vasculitis of the polyarteritis nodosa group. *In* Smith LH (ed): Major Problems in Internal Medicine, vol 11. Philadelphia, WB Saunders, 1981, pp 26–49.
210. Frohnert PP, Sheps SG: Long-term follow-up study of periarteritis nodosa. Am J Med 43:8–14, 1967.
211. Moreland LW, Ball Gene V: Cutaneous polyarteritis nodosa. Am J Med 88:426–430, 1990.
212. Lightfoot RW, Michel BA, Block DA, et al: The American College of Rheumatology 1990 criteria for the classification of polyarteritis nodosa. Arthritis Rheum 33:1088–1093, 1990.
213. Jakobiec FA, Jones IS: Orbital inflammations. *In* Duane TD (ed): Clinical Ophthalmology. Philadelphia, Harper & Row, 1981, pp 30–35.
214. Goldsmith J: Periarteritis nodosa with involvement of the choroidal and retinal arteries. Am J Ophthalmol 29:435–446, 1946.
215. Moore JG, Sevel D: Corneoscleral ulceration in polyarteritis nodosa. Br J Ophthalmol 50:651–655, 1966.
216. Harbert F, McPherson SD: Scleral necrosis in polyarteritis nodosa. Am J Ophthalmol 30:727–732, 1947.
217. Foster CS: Basic ocular immunology. *In* Kaufman HE, Barron BA, McDonald MB, Waltman SR (eds): The Cornea. New York, Churchill Livingstone, 1988, pp 85–122.
218. Purcell JJ, Birkenkamp R, Tsai CC: Conjunctival lesions in periarteritis nodosa: A clinical and immunopathologic study. Arch Ophthalmol 102:736–738, 1984.
219. Van Wien S, Merz EH: Exophthalmos secondary to periarteritis nodosa. Am J Ophthalmol 56:204–208, 1963.

220. Hope-Robertson WJ: Pseudo-tumour of the orbit as a presenting sign in periarteritis nodosa. Trans Ophthalmol Soc N Z 8:56–66, 1956.
221. Solomon SM, Solomon JH: Bilateral central retinal artery occlusions in polyarteritis nodosa. Ann Ophthalmol 10:567–569, 1978.
222. Walton EW: Pseudo-tumour of the orbit and polyarteritis nodosa. J Clin Pathol 12:419–426, 1959.
223. Albert DA, Rimon D, Silverstein MD: The diagnosis of polyarteritis nodosa. Part I: A literature-based decision analysis approach. Arthritis Rheum 31:1117–1127, 1988.
224. Guillevin L, Jarrousse B, Lok C, et al: Long-term follow-up after treatment of polyarteritis nodosa and Churg-Strauss angiitis with comparison of steroids, plasma exchange, and cyclophosphamide to steroids and plasma exchange: A prospective, randomized trial of 71 patients. J Rheumatol 18:567–574, 1991.
225. Cupps TR, Fauci AS: Giant cell arteritides. *In* Smith LH (ed): Major Problems in Internal Medicine, vol 11. Philadelphia, WB Saunders, 1981, pp 99–115.
226. Hauser WA, Ferguson RH, Holley KE, Kurland LT: Temporal arteritis in Rochester, Minnesota, 1951 to 1967. Mayo Clin Proc 46:597–602, 1971.
227. Glaser JS: Topical diagnosis: Prechiasmal visual pathways. *In* Duane TD (ed): Clinical Ophthalmology. Philadelphia, Harper & Row, 1989, pp 1–85.
228. Glaser JS: Infranuclear disorder of eye movement. *In* Duane TD (ed): Clinical Ophthalmology. Philadelphia, Harper & Row, 1988, pp 1–85.
229. Gold DH: Ocular manifestations of connective tissue (collagen) disease. *In* Duane TD (ed): Clinical Ophthalmology. Philadelphia, Harper & Row, 1980, pp 1–30.
230. Barricks ME, Traviesa DB, Glaser JS, Levy IS: Ophthalmoplegia in cranial arteritis. Brain 100:209–221, 1977.
231. Klein RG, Campbell RJ, Hunder GG, Carney JA: Skip lesions in temporal arteritis. Mayo Clin Proc 51:504–510, 1976.
232. Churg J, Strauss L: Allergic granulomatosis, allergic angiitis, and periarteritis nodosa. Am J Pathol 27:277–301, 1951.
233. Cury D, Breakey AS, Payne F: Allergic granulomatous angiitis associated with uveoscleritis and papilledema. Arch Ophthalmol 55:261–266, 1966.
234. Chumbley LC, Harrison EG Jr, DeRemee RA: Allergic granulomatosis and angiitis Churg-Strauss syndrome: Report and analysis of 30 cases. Mayo Clin Proc 52:477–484, 1977.
235. Ashton N, Cook C: Allergic granulomatous nodules of the eyelid and conjunctiva. The XXXV Edward Jackson Memorial Lecture. Am J Ophthalmol 87:1–28, 1979.
236. Meisler DM, Stock EL, Wertz RD, et al: Conjunctival inflammation and amyloidosis in allergic granulomatosis and angiitis (Churg-Strauss syndrome). Am J Ophthalmol 91:216–219, 1981.
237. Nissim F, Von der Balde J, Czenobilksy B: A limited form of Churg-Strauss syndrome: Ocular and cutaneous manifestations. Arch Pathol Lab Med 106:305–307, 1982.
238. Rose GA, Spencer H: Polyarteritis nodosa. Q J Med 26:43–48, 1957.
239. Liebow AA, Carrington CRB, Friedman PJ: Lymphomatoid granulomatosis. Hum Pathol 3:457, 1972.
240. DeRemee RA, Weiland LH, McDonald TJ: Respiratory vasculitis. Mayo Clin Proc 55:492–498, 1980.
241. Cupps TR, Fauci AS: Lymphomatoid granulomatosis. *In* Smith LH (ed): Major Problems in Internal Medicine, vol 11. Philadelphia, WB Saunders, 1981, pp 88–98.
242. Myers JL: Lymphomatoid granulomatosis: Past, present, future? Mayo Clin Proc 65:274–278, 1990.
243. Pearson ADJ, Craft AW, Howe JM: Choroidal involvement in lymphomatoid granulomatosis. Br J Ophthalmol 75:688–689, 1991.
244. Pisani RJ, DeRemee RA: Clinical implications of the histopathologic diagnosis of pulmonary lymphomatoid granulomatosis. Mayo Clin Proc 65:151–163, 1990.
245. Katzenstein AL, Carrington CB, Liebow AA: Lymphomatoid granulomatosis: A clinicopathologic study of 152 cases. Cancer 43:360–373, 1979.
246. Colby TV: Central nervous system lymphomatoid granulomatosis in AIDS? Hum Pathol 20:361–369, 1989.
247. Anders KH, Latta H, Chang BS, et al: Lymphomatoid granulomatosis and malignant lymphoma of the central nervous system in the acquired immunodeficiency syndrome. Hum Pathol 20:326–334, 1989.
248. Mittal K, Neri A, Feiner H, et al: Lymphomatoid granulomatosis in the acquired immunodeficiency syndrome. Cancer 65:1343–1349, 1990.
249. Najjar T, Gadol C, Khan MY: Immune deficiency with polymorphic reticulosis. Oral Surg Oral Med Oral Pathol 67:322–326, 1989.
250. Fauci AS, Haynes BF, Katz P, Wolf SM: Wegener's granulomatosis: Prospective clinical and therapeutic experience with 85 patients for 21 years. Ann Intern Med 98:76–85, 1983.
251. Carlson KC, Gibson LE: Cutaneous signs of lymphomatoid granulomatosis. Arch Dermatol 127:1693–1698, 1991.
252. Eichel BS, Harrison EG, Devine KD, et al: Primary lymphoma of the nose including a relationship to lethal mid-line granuloma. Am J Surg 112:597–605, 1966.
253. McDonald TJ, DeRemee RA, Harrison EG Jr, et al: The protean clinical features of polymorphic reticulosis (lethal midline granuloma). Laryngoscope 86:936–945, 1976.
254. DeRemee RA, Weiland LH, McDonald TJ: Polymorphic reticulosis, lymphomatoid granulomatosis: Two diseases or one? Mayo Clin Proc 53:634–640, 1978.
255. Gaulard P, Henni T, Marolleau J, et al: Lethal midline granuloma (polymorphic reticulosis) and lymphomatoid granulomatosis. Cancer 62:705–710, 1988.
256. McKay D, Ell J, Williams R, Taylor F: Lymphomatoid granulomatosis presenting as sudden blindness. Aust N Z J Ophthalmol 182:215–219, 1990.
257. Robin JB, Schanzlin DJ, Meisler DM, et al: Ocular involvement in the respiratory vasculitides. Surv Ophthalmol 30:127–140, 1985.
258. Whittaker S, Foroni L, Luzzatto L, et al: Lymphomatoid granulomatosis—evidence of a clonal T-cell origin and an association with lethal midline granuloma. Q J Med 68:645–655, 1988.
259. Font RL, Rosenbaum PS, Smith JL: Lymphomatoid granulomatosis of eyelid and brow with progression to lymphoma. J Am Acad Dermatol 23:334–337, 1990.
260. Lin-Greenberg A, Villacin A, Moussa G: Lymphomatoid granulomatosis presenting as ulcerodestructive gastrointestinal tract lesions in patients with human immunodeficiency virus infection. Arch Intern Med 150:2581–2583, 1990.
261. Gold JE, Castella A: Polymorphic reticulosis: T- or B-cell malignancy. Laryngoscope 99:989–990, 1989.
262. Ratech H, Burke JS, Blayney DW, et al: A clinicopathologic study of malignant lymphomas of the nose, paranasal sinuses, hard palate, including cases of lethal midline granuloma. Cancer 64:2525–2531, 1989.
263. Harabuchi Y, Yamanaka N, Kataura A, et al: Epstein-Barr virus in nasal T-cell lymphomas in patients with lethal midline granuloma. Lancet 335:128–130, 1990.
264. Stewart JP: Progressive lethal granulomatous ulceration of the nose. J Laryngol Otol 48:657–701, 1933.
265. Spear GS, Walker WG Jr: Lethal midline granuloma (granuloma gangraenescens) at autopsy. Bull Johns Hopkins Hosp 99:313–332, 1956.
266. Salman SD, Graeme-Cook F: Case records of the Massachusetts General Hospital (case 2-1990). N Engl J Med 322:116–123, 1990.
267. Daggett RB, Haghighi P, Terkeltaub RA: Nasal cocaine abuse causing an aggressive midline intranasal and pharyngeal destructive process mimicking midline reticulosis and limited Wegener's granulomatosis. J Rheumatol 17:838–840, 1990.
268. Pickens JP, Modica L: Current concepts of the lethal midline granuloma syndrome. Otolaryngol Head Neck Surg 100:623–630, 1989.
269. Kornblut AD: Current concepts of the lethal midline granuloma syndrome. Otolaryngol Head Neck Surg 102:201–202, 1990.

Ocular Manifestations of Systemic Endocrine Diseases

CHAPTER 5

Diagnosis and Management of Thyrotoxicosis

Leonard P. Kapcala

Graves' disease is the most common and important cause of thyrotoxicosis. Infiltrative ophthalmopathy is one of three abnormalities that can constitute the diagnosis of Graves' disease. Other abnormalities include hyperthyroidism with diffuse goiter due to thyroid-stimulating immunoglobulins and also pretibial myxedema. Consequently, one can make the diagnosis of Graves' disease based on one or any combination of these abnormalities. Considering that hyperthyroidism is the most common abnormality associated with Graves' disease, the focus in this chapter is on the diagnosis and management of thyrotoxicosis. Special related conditions such as euthyroid hyperthyroxinemia, hyperthyroidism and pregnancy, thyroid storm, and euthyroid Graves' disease are also reviewed. Because ophthalmopathy per se is dealt with in other chapters, it is not discussed in depth in this chapter.

THYROID-ASSOCIATED OPHTHALMOPATHY

Autoimmune-mediated inflammation of the extraocular muscles and periorbital connective tissue results in ophthalmopathy termed *thyroid-associated ophthalmopathy* (TAO) because it is associated with autoimmune thyroid disease. Whereas the overwhelming majority of patients (approximately 85%) with TAO have Graves' hyperthyroidism, a small group (approximately 15%) have Hashimoto's thyroiditis, subclinical thyroiditis, or thyroid immunologic abnormalities without Hashimoto's thyroiditis or Graves' hyperthyroidism. This last group of patients are considered as having *euthyroid Graves' disease.*[1, 2] Conversely, it has been estimated that approximately half of those persons with Graves' hyperthyroidism and 5% of those with Hashimoto's thyroiditis exhibit ophthalmopathy.[1] Despite the fact that one typically thinks of Graves' hyperthyroidism when dealing with ophthalmopathy, these observations illustrate that this infiltrative and inflammatory ophthalmopathy is not specifically related to Graves' disease or Graves' hyperthyroidism but is specifically related to autoimmune thyroid disease. Furthermore, only a small minority (approximately 10%) of patients exhibit severe orbitopathy requiring aggressive therapy. Most people with mild to moderate disease can be managed conservatively. Frequently, ophthalmopathy settles down and becomes relatively quiescent once the thyroid disorder has been treated.

In some cases, patients may present with bilateral or unilateral ophthalmopathy and will be euthyroid clinically as well as on the basis of biochemical testing.[1] Such patients may be diagnosed as having Graves' disease, with ophthalmopathy being their sole presenting feature. Other causes of proptosis should be excluded, especially with computed tomography (CT) of the orbits. Although these patients are clinically euthyroid and show normal peripheral thyroid hormone levels, including serum-free thyroxine (T_4) and triiodothyronine (T_3), they may also exhibit other more subtle biochemical abnormalities and a goiter. These potential abnormalities[3] consist of antithyroid antibodies (particularly antimicrosomal antibodies), and other more sophisticated research immunologic markers, suppressed serum thyroid-stimulating hormone (TSH) levels, and either blunted or exaggerated serum TSH responses to thyrotropin-releasing hormone (TRH).[3] Occasionally antithyroid antibodies may be so high as to suggest the presence of Hashimoto's thyroiditis. In short, patients with euthyroid ophthalmopathy can often show subtle and subclinical evidence of autoimmune thyroid disease. Nevertheless, regardless of the subclinical abnormality, treatment need not be directed at the thyroid gland but rather should be directed toward the ophthalmopathy if any treatment is required.

Although the precise pathophysiology of TAO remains to be elucidated, a significant body of evidence has provided insight into this problem.[1] The pathology shows infiltration of inflammatory cells and fluid in and around extraocular muscle cells as well as an increase in connective tissue elements, including fibroblasts, collagen, and different ground substances termed *glycosaminoglycans*. Typically, TAO is bilateral. However, not infrequently asymmetric disease occurs and, rarely, unilateral disease can also present and be diagnosed as TAO.

It is believed that the autoimmune reaction to extraocular muscle is the main site of the pathophysiologic disturbance.[1] A leading hypothesis holds that cytotoxic antibodies and sensitized T lymphocytes, or both react against antigens common to thyroid and extraocular muscle cells. Although circulating antibodies to TSH receptor, thyroglobulin, or thyroid microsomes may be present in TAO, they do not play a role in the pathogenesis of this orbitopathy. Other less attractive hypotheses propose that thyroid dysfunction alters the immune system, leading to a loss of tolerance to orbital antigens, and that autoimmune thyroid disorders and ophthalmopathy are genetically linked. Presently, immunologic testing is not routinely performed in nonacademic research settings to identify TAO. Nevertheless, sophisticated research testing utilizing the antibody-dependent cell-mediated cytotoxicity assay or measurement of eye-muscle antibodies by sodium dodecyl sulfate–polyacrylamide gel electrophoresis or Western blotting methods are relatively sensitive and specific methods for illustrating immunologic abnormalities in the majority of patients with TAO.[1]

Major clinical features of TAO include symptoms of dry, gritty, or watery eyes, pain, diplopia, or reduced vision. Signs include proptosis, extraocular muscle paresis or palsy, lid retraction or ptosis, lid and conjunctival swelling, and corneal ulceration. Orbital CT or ultrasonography typically illustrates orbital pathology. Although CT should not necessarily be performed routinely, ultrasonography can be considered as a more routine baseline test in the newly diagnosed patient with TAO. Intraocular pressure on upward gaze is also abnormally increased in many patients with moderately advanced disease. Furthermore, measurement of exophthalmos or proptosis can be monitored on clinical visits. It is optimal that patients with TAO be managed jointly by endocrinologists and ophthalmologists. Although various reports have correlated changes in ophthalmopathy with changes in thyroid function or treatment of the thyroid, it is not clear nor likely that changes in thyroid hormone levels play a causal role.[4, 5]

Conservative management consisting of close follow-up and attention to mechanical abnormalities (e.g., taping lids at night or artificial tears) is used in the vast majority of cases with TAO. More severe cases may require anti-inflammatory (e.g., glucocorticoid) or immunosuppressive drugs, plasmapheresis, radiotherapy, or surgery. Presently, it is not possible to predict the course of TAO in various patients. However, it is hoped that prospective studies of patients with Graves' hyperthyroidism will reveal temporal relationships between immunologic markers and eye findings that will facilitate a means for identifying patients at greater risk for developing ophthalmologic complications and, correspondingly, for treating such patients prophylactically before these complications develop or become significant.

PHYSIOLOGIC REGULATION OF HYPOTHALAMIC-PITUITARY-THYROID AXIS

To understand the diagnosis and management of thyroid dysfunction such as thyrotoxicosis or hypothyroidism it is imperative to have a basic understanding of the physiology[6] of thyroid hormone secretion, which is regulated by the hypothalamic-pituitary-thyroid axis[7] (Fig. 5–1). TRH is synthesized in neurons of the paraventricular nucleus of the hypothalamus. After axonal transport of TRH to the median eminence, it is released into the hypothalamic-pituitary portal capillaries and transported to the anterior pituitary, where it stimulates synthesis and release of TSH. Major hypothalamic regulators exerting inhibitory effects on TSH secretion include dopamine and somatostatin. Circulating TSH acts at multiple levels in the thyroid cell and increases iodide uptake, thyroglobulin synthesis, production of T_3 and T_4, thyroglobulin proteolysis, and secretion of T_4 and T_3. Twenty to 25% of circulating T_3 is normally derived from thyroid secretion. The rest of T_3 is derived from peripheral conversion (especially in liver and kidney) of T_4 to T_3. Both T_4 and T_3 circulate bound (>99%) to proteins. T_4 is bound to thyroxine-binding globulin (TBG), prealbumin, and albumin. T_3 is bound to TBG and albumin. The free level of thyroid hormone determines the physiologic effects through stimulation of nuclear T_3 receptors

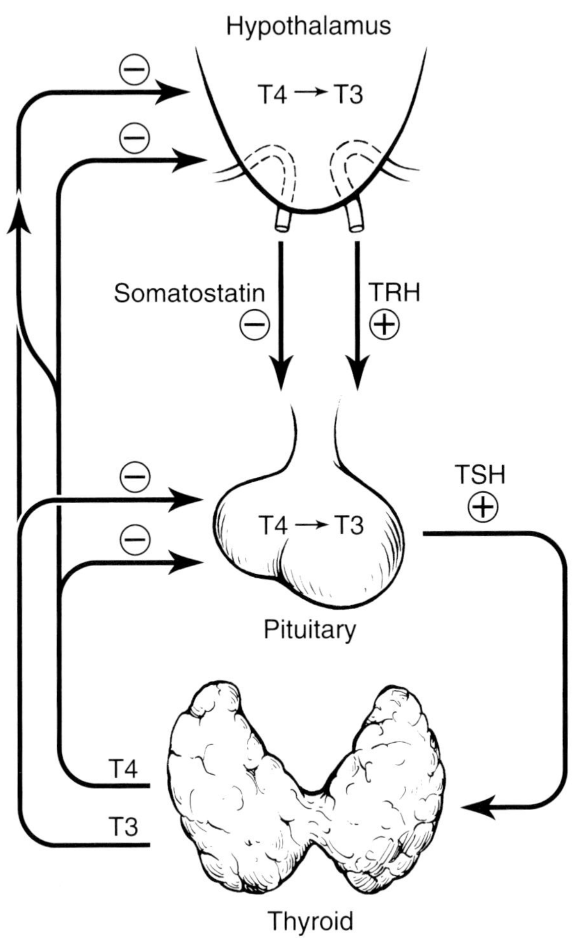

Figure 5–1. Diagram of regulation of the hypothalamic-pituitary-thyroid axis. T_4, thyroxine; T_3, triiodothyronine; TRH, thyrotropin-releasing hormone; TSH, thyroid-stimulating hormone. (From Reichlin S: Hypothalamus and pituitary neuroendocrinology. *In* Wilson JD, Foster DN [eds]: Williams Textbook of Endocrinology, 8th ed. Philadelphia, WB Saunders, 1992, p 169.)

that interact with genomic DNA sites in different tissues. Evidence has suggested that T_3 is the major physiologic thyroid hormone and that T_4 is predominantly a prohormone that serves as a source of T_3. Thyroid hormones exert a regulatory effect on the axis by acting at both hypothalamic and pituitary levels. Clearly, they exert a potent negative feedback effect on TRH-mediated TSH secretion at the pituitary level. Evidence has also suggested a negative feedback effect on TRH gene expression. Cortisol or other glucocorticoids and growth hormone can also exert inhibitory effects on TSH release from the pituitary, and estrogen can enhance TSH release.

THYROTOXICOSIS VERSUS HYPERTHYROIDISM

Before reviewing various considerations related to hyperthyroidism, it is important to define *hyperthyroidism* and distinguish this entity from *thyrotoxicosis*.[8] These terms are often used synonymously but inaccurately. Thyrotoxicosis is a clinical condition resulting from increased circulating free thyroid hormones (T_4, T_3) that exert biologic effects. In contrast, hyperthyroidism is a clinical condition resulting from increased circulating levels of free T_4 or T_3 that exert biologic effects and are related to hyperfunction of the thyroid gland. For example, patients with clinical manifestations related to excessive free T_4 or T_3 levels derived from ingestion of excessive amounts of thyroid hormone or increased dysregulated release of preformed T_4 or T_3 due to thyroid inflammation (thyroiditis) would be thyrotoxic but not hyperthyroid. Patients with clinical manifestations of excessive free T_4 or T_3 due to increased function of the thyroid (e.g., diffuse thyroid hyperfunction—Graves' disease or nodular hyperfunction) would exhibit hyperthyroidism. Thus, all patients who exhibit hyperthyroidism are also thyrotoxic, but all patients with thyrotoxicosis do not necessarily exhibit hyperthyroidism.

THYROTOXICOSIS

Clinical Manifestations

The clinical presentation of thyrotoxicosis is extremely variable.[9, 10] It may present as a single complaint or in association with few or many clinical features consisting of a variety of symptoms and signs (Table 5–1). As a general rule, the number and severity of clinical manifestations correlate with the magnitude of the biochemical abnormalities. However, in some instances, the presentation may be subtle and may not consist of many symptoms or signs related to hyperadrenergic function (e.g., nervousness, sweating, palpations or tachycardia, shakiness or tremor). Such patients are characterized as ex-

TABLE 5–1

Symptoms and Signs Associated with Thyrotoxicosis

Symptoms	Signs
Nervousness/anxiety	Tachycardia/atrial fibrillation
Diaphoresis	Goiter (diffuse)
Heat intolerance/sensitivity	Solitary or multiple thyroid nodules
Palpitation	Skin changes
Fatigue/weakness	Tremor
Weight loss	Muscle weakness (proximal > distal)
Dyspnea	Thyroid bruit/thrill
Muscle weakness	Gynecomastia
Hyperphagia	Galactorrhea
Eye complaints	Splenomegaly
Leg swelling	Lymphadenopathy
Hyperdefecation/diarrhea	Onycholysis
	Digital acropachy
	Eye signs:
	Lid lag
	Stare
	Exophthalmos/proptosis
	Extraocular muscle paresis/palsy
	Chemosis

hibiting "apathetic" thyrotoxicosis, often presenting with fatigue or weight loss or both. This presentation is much more prevalent in elderly patients. In other instances, thyrotoxicosis may present solely as new onset of atrial fibrillation. However, frequently when such patients or others with few major complaints are questioned and examined closely, other subtle abnormalities can be noted. Occasionally some patients diagnosed with thyrotoxicosis seem essentially asymptomatic, but mildly abnormal signs or symptoms are usually present when they are closely sought.

Biochemical Diagnosis

When signs or symptoms consistent with thyrotoxicosis are present, the diagnosis should be established or excluded by biochemical testing.[11] Initially, a screening approach with minimal testing is recommended. The test or tests selected in screening for thyrotoxicosis may vary according to the style of the practitioner. In recent years, many clinicians have opted for screening with a "sensitive" serum TSH determination. Because thyroid hormones exert a potent negative feedback effect on the pituitary-thyroidal axis directly at the level of the pituitary by inhibiting TSH release, thyrotoxicosis is typically associated with a decreased serum TSH value. Initially, first-generation TSH assays were not able to distinguish decreased from normal TSH levels but second-generation, more sensitive TSH assays provided a lower limit of normal and therefore illustrated decreased TSH values in thyrotoxic patients. More recently, extremely sensitive third-generation TSH assays,[12] using chemoluminescent techniques, have illustrated serum TSH values as low as 0.005 μU/mL and allow specific discrimination of normal from suppressed TSH concentrations. In these assays, thyrotoxicosis is typically associated with serum TSH levels of less than 0.05 μU/mL. In contrast, most patients with other causes of decreased TSH, such as subclinical thyrotoxicosis, severe nonthyroidal illness or euthyroid sick syndrome, or drugs (dopamine or glucocorticoids) inhibiting TSH secretion, show diminished TSH levels and usually normal free T_4 levels, but their TSH levels (> 0.01 but < 0.1 μU/mL) are much higher than those of overtly thyrotoxic patients. Consequently, screening for thyrotoxicosis with a "sensitive" TSH assay is a good approach that is reasonably cost-effective. The most sensitive TSH assays provide more specificity with regard to diagnosing overt thyrotoxicosis. The only potential problem with using a serum TSH test to screen for thyrotoxicosis is that one could miss diagnosing patients with the rare syndrome of thyrotoxicosis due to inappropriate TSH secretion (e.g., TSH-secreting pituitary adenomas or selective pituitary resistance to thyroid hormone).[13]

When a decreased serum TSH level, consistent with thyrotoxicosis, is obtained, one should assess the level of peripheral thyroid hormones. Normally, most thyrotoxic patients exhibit an increased serum free T_4 value. Older tests such as serum T_4 (measuring total T_4) and T_3 resin uptake (test inversely illustrating available binding sites for thyroid hormones) when multiplied provide a serum free T_4 index (FTI) that generally shows a good correlation with the actual serum free T_4 level. Potential exceptions to this principle are the coincidental presence of nonthyroidal illness or euthyroid sick syndrome[14, 15] or severe disturbances in thyroid hormone binding proteins. Because thyroid hormones (T_4 and T_3) are predominantly protein bound, marked increments in thyroid hormone–binding proteins can result in an increased FTI and can potentially be misleading. Another important test for diagnosing thyrotoxicosis is the serum T_3 (measuring total T_3). The serum T_3 concentration is typically elevated in most cases of thyrotoxicosis regardless of etiology, and this test is especially helpful in the relatively rare syndrome of T_3 toxicosis (increased serum total and free T_3 but normal serum total and free T_4).[11]

One can also screen for thyrotoxicosis with a serum free T_4 or, if this is not available, with a serum FTI. Most patients with thyrotoxicosis will exhibit an elevated serum free T_4 or FTI. This approach will also identify those with inappropriate TSH secretion producing hyperthyroidism but will not identify those with the relatively uncommon (but still much more common syndrome than that of TSH-induced hyperthyroidism) syndrome of T_3 toxicosis. If an elevated serum free T_4 level or FTI is obtained, one should confirm thyrotoxicosis with a sensitive TSH determination that in the overwhelming majority of cases will be suppressed. As outlined, one can screen for thyrotoxicosis with a serum TSH test, free T_4 assay, or FTI. In most cases of thyrotoxicosis, the clinician will detect abnormal results with any of these approaches, but it is important to be aware of the potential pitfalls using a specific screening strategy in which patients with specific etiologies of thyrotoxicosis could be missed. Whenever a screening test result is abnormal and consistent with thyrotoxicosis, it is important to perform a battery of tests that will provide a more comprehensive picture and delineate the severity of the biochemical dysfunction. This test battery should consist of serum TSH ("sensitive"), free T_4 (or at least FTI if free T_4 is not available), and T_3 determinations. Previously, TRH stimulation tests were performed in difficult cases exhibiting equivocal peripheral thyroid hormone values. With this test, TRH (200–500 μg) was usually administered intravenously and blood was sampled at various intervals (TSH at 0, 20, 30, 60 minutes; T_3 at 0, 90, 120, 150 minutes). A normal response consisted of a peak TSH increment ranging between 2 and 25 μU/mL at 20 to 30 minutes and a T_3 increment ($\geq$30% above the basal value). Patients with thyrotoxicosis show a blunted TSH response. More precisely, TSH responses measured by sensitive assays are typically absent in thyrotoxic patients. Similarly, elevated T_3 values in these patients do not change in response to TRH. However, with the advent of sensitive TSH assays, the TRH test has essentially become outdated and is rarely used or indicated.

Determination of Etiology

After thyrotoxicosis has been diagnosed, attention should be directed toward determining the cause (Table 5–2).[11] Specific tests potentially useful for this purpose include 24-hour radioactive iodine uptake (RAIU), thyroid scan, antithyroid antibody (especially antimicrosomal antibody) tests, and determination of serum thyroglobulin, serum human chorionic gonadotropin, and urinary iodide concentrations. As alluded to earlier in discussing the distinction between thyrotoxicosis and hyperthyroidism, an elevated 24-hour RAIU will usually demonstrate that one is dealing with hyperthyroidism and, if combined with a diffuse goiter or diffuse uptake on a scan, will support the likely diagnosis of Graves' hyperthyroidism. Specific patterns of various tests (Table 5–3) will usually delineate the specific cause of the thyrotoxicosis.

Management

After diagnosis of thyrotoxicosis, management[16, 17] generally consists of one or a combination of treatment options, including medical therapy,[17, 18] radioactive iodine (RAI),[17, 19] and surgery.[17, 20] Medical management can be subdivided into using drugs that decrease thyroid hormone production, secretion, or both and drugs that diminish the biologic effects of excessive thyroid hormones. Thiourea drugs such as propylthiouracil (PTU) or methimazole act at multiple levels within the thyroid cell and diminish the production of thyroid hormones and therefore ultimately diminish their release. PTU is typically begun using 300 to 450 mg daily in divided doses (three times a day). In contrast, methimazole is usually started using 30 to 40 mg daily as a single dose because it has a longer half-life than PTU. Although PTU also has the theoretic advantage of inhibiting peripheral conversion of T_4 to T_3, a process that usually accounts for approximately 80% of T_3 production, the actual practical benefit of this theoretic advantage is not clear. Multiple side effects, including among others fever, rash, and agranulocytosis, have been reported with either drug. The most serious reaction is agranulocytosis, which appears to be idiosyncratic. One cannot necessarily predict in whom it may occur or when, but a sore throat is often associated as a presenting manifestation of this abnormality. Therefore, whenever a patient who takes one of these drugs develops a significant sore throat, a white blood cell count should be obtained. Despite a slight decrease of white blood cell count after initiation of PTU or methimazole, the diagnosis of agranulocytosis is an absolute contraindication and requires discontinuation of the drug. Rash is a relatively common side effect of either drug and may resolve despite continued usage. There is also a certain degree (≤20%) of cross-reactions between both drugs. After medical treatment is begun, the patient is seen in follow-up in 4 to 8 weeks. Because the maximal effect of inhibiting thyroid hormone production requires several weeks, this interval allows one to determine the efficacy of the initial medical treatment. At this visit, levels of peripheral thyroid hormones (T_3 and free T_4) are obtained, and depending on clinical responses of thyroid hormone levels, PTU or methimazole is continued at the same dose or at a lower dose. In many instances, either drug is often decreased to approximately 50% of the initial dosage for chronic management. Because approximately one third of patients with Graves' hyperthyroidism may experience a spontaneous clinical and biochemical remission within 1 year of medical therapy, this modality is often used to allow such patients this opportunity. A lesser probability of experiencing a spontaneous remission is correlated with the presence of a large goiter or a prolonged history of Graves' hyperthyroidism especially with active hyperthyroidism.

Beta-adrenergic antagonists such as propranolol (nonselective) or atenolol or metoprolol (beta$_1$-selective) are also an important group of drugs used to diminish the biologic effects of excessive thyroid hormones. Because thyrotoxicosis increases beta-adrenergic receptors that facilitate enhanced beta-adrenergic tone, the use of beta-adrenergic antagonists is important for diminishing clinical manifestations (tachycardia, tremor, diaphoresis, nervousness) resulting from this phenomenon. A major advantage of these agents is their rapid onset of efficacy and the potential for making patients feel much better in a short period. These benefits allow one to use a beta-

TABLE 5–2
Causes of Thyrotoxicosis

Increased Thyroidal Radioactive Iodine Uptake
Graves' disease
Toxic multinodular goiter
Solitary toxic nodule
Trophoblastic disorders
Hydatidiform mole
Choriocarcinoma
Hashitoxicosis
Selective pituitary thyroid hormone resistance
TSH-producing pituitary adenoma
Decreased Thyroidal Radioactive Iodine Uptake
Subacute thyroiditis
Silent/painless thyroiditis
Postpartum thyroiditis
Exogenous thyroid hormone ingestion
Ingestion of thyroid tissue
Graves' disease after iodine exposure
Jod-Basedow disease (after iodine exposure)
Struma ovarii
Metastatic functioning thyroid carcinoma

TSH, thyroid-stimulating hormone.

TABLE 5-3

Characteristic Test Results in Various Etiologies of Thyrotoxicosis

Etiology	Serum T_4	Serum T_3	Serum Free T_4	Serum FTI	Serum TSH	Serum Antithyroid Antibodies*	Serum TSI	Serum Thyroglobulin	Serum hCG	24-Hour RAIU	Thyroid Scan	Miscellaneous
Graves' disease	↑	↑	↑	↑	↓	+	+	↑	–	↑	Diffuse goiter homogeneous uptake	
Toxic multinodular goiter	↑	↑	↑	↑	↓	–	–	↑	–	↑	Multiple nodules of uptake	
Solitary toxic nodule	↑	↑	↑	↑	↓	–	–	↑	–	↑	Single nodule of uptake (rest of thyroid suppressed)	
Trophoblastic disorders	↑	↑	↑	↑	↓	–	–	↑	↑	↑	Diffuse goiter homogeneous uptake	Pelvic ultrasonography shows lesion
Hashitoxicosis	↑	↑	↑	↑	↓	++	+	↑	–	↑	Diffuse goiter inhomogeneous uptake	Previous history of Hashimoto's thyroiditis
Selective pituitary thyroid hormone resistance	↑	↑	↑	↑	↑/nl	–	–	↑	–	↑	Diffuse goiter homogeneous uptake	Normal serum α-subunit; increased TSH response to TRH; no discrete pituitary adenoma on CT or MRI
TSH-producing pituitary adenoma	↑	↑	↑	↑	↑/nl	–	–	↑	–	↑	Diffuse goiter homogeneous uptake	Increased serum α-subunit; no TSH response to TRH; pituitary adenoma or CT or MRI

Subacute thyroiditis	↑	↑	↑	↑	↓	±	–	↑	–	↓	Decreased inhomogeneous uptake	Leukocytosis, increased sedimentation rate, needle biopsy shows granulomatosis and inflammation
Silent/painless or postpartum thyroiditis	↑	↑	↑	↑	↓	+	–	↑	–	↓	Decreased inhomogeneous uptake	Biopsy shows lymphocytic thyroiditis
Ingestion of exogenous thyroid hormone or tissue	↑	↑	↑	↑	↓	–	–	↓	–	↓	Decreased homogeneous uptake	
Graves' disease after iodine exposure	↑	↑	↑	↑	↓	+	+	↑	–	↓	Decreased homogeneous uptake	Increased serum and/or urinary iodine
Jod-Basedow disease	↑	↑	↑	↑	↓	–	–	↑	–	↓	Decreased homogeneous uptake	Increased serum and/or urinary iodine
Struma ovarii	↑	↑	↑	↑	↓	–	–	↑	–	↓	Decreased homogeneous uptake	Pelvic mass shown by ultrasonography, CT, or MRI takes up ^{131}I
Metastatic functioning thyroid carcinoma	↑	↑	↑	↑	↓	–	–	↑/nl	–	↓	Decreased uptake in thyroid bed	Whole-body ^{131}I scanning shows functioning metastases

*Antithyroid antibodies = antimicrosomal and/or antithyroglobulin.

T_4, thyroxine; T_3, triiodothyronine; FTI, free thyroxine index; TSH, thyroid-stimulating hormone; TSI, thyroid-stimulating immunoglobulins; hCG, human chorionic gonadotropin; RAIU, radiolabeled iodine uptake; TRH, thyrotropin-releasing hormone; CT, computed tomography; MRI, magnetic resonance imaging.

adrenergic blocker as sole therapy before and after radioactive iodine therapy, particularly in younger patients with mild to moderate biochemical thyrotoxicosis. These drugs are also the agents of choice for treating symptomatic patients with transient thyrotoxicosis owing to subacute thyroiditis or silent thyroiditis rather than thiourea drugs, which are contraindicated because hyperthyroidism is not present in these disorders.

Other drugs play a limited role in the medical management of thyrotoxicosis but mainly in special circumstances. These include iodide (Lugol's solution or supersaturated potassium iodide—SSKI, sodium iodide), lithium, glucocorticoids, and iodine-containing dyes (iopanoic acid or sodium iopodate). Iodides can inhibit thyroid hormone release directly and demonstrate a rapid (within hours) onset of action. Lithium can also inhibit thyroid hormone release. Glucocorticoids in pharmacologic doses inhibit peripheral conversion of T_4 to T_3 and may also decrease thyroid hormone release. Iodide-containing radiographic contrast agents that inhibit peripheral T_4 to T_3 conversion can also inhibit thyroid hormone production.

Radioactive iodine (^{131}I) therapy[17, 19] is typically used as definitive treatment for Graves' or nodular hyperthyroidism. It is often considered the treatment of choice in most older ($\geq$40 years old) patients because it is relatively inexpensive and safe. Despite the inclination of concern by the lay public about radioactive exposure and risk of cancer with ^{131}I usage, after many years (approximately 50) of ^{131}I usage there is no evidence of a higher risk of cancer in treated versus untreated patients. Medical therapy with antithyroid drugs is often used before administration of ^{131}I in patients with severe biochemical thyrotoxicosis or in elderly patients in whom grave consequences could result from exacerbation of their thyrotoxicosis by a radiation-induced thyroiditis and increased release of preformed thyroid hormones. However, in such cases, the thiourea drugs are held for approximately 4 days before and after ^{131}I administration to facilitate maximum uptake of ^{131}I. Because of many anecdotal experiences relating instances of discovering pregnancy immediately before or just after RAI treatment, one cannot rely on a patient's history of regular monthly menses or denial of sexual relations for many months or years. Unless the patient has entered menopause or has had a hysterectomy, it is a wise, safe, and imperative practice to perform a pregnancy test in all patients of child-bearing age before RAI treatment regardless of the patient's menstrual or sexual history. Determination of a suitable dose of ^{131}I for Graves' disease is directly related to thyroid size and inversely related to the 24-hour RAIU. Estimation of the ^{131}I dose is made using the formula

$$^{131}\text{I required} = \text{estimated thyroid size (g)} \times 100\ \mu\text{Ci/g thyroid/24-hour RAIU}$$

Frequently, Graves' disease is treated with 5 to 15 mCi of ^{131}I. In contrast, solitary nodular thyrotoxicosis or multiple nodular thyrotoxicosis is relatively more resistant to ^{131}I therapy and requires greater quantities (e.g., 15 to 30 mCi ^{131}I). One should be aware of the potential but rare development of radiation-induced thyroiditis and consequent release of residual thyroid hormones that can result in exacerbation of thyrotoxicosis if ^{131}I treatment has not been preceded by adequate antithyroid medical therapy. Depending on specific clinical circumstances, patients are usually seen in followup at 6 to 12 weeks after therapy. A maximum effect of ^{131}I is usually seen between 2 and 4 months but no later than 6 months after therapy. If the patient has not become euthyroid or hypothyroid in 4 to 6 months, repeat treatment with ^{131}I is required.

The main side effect of ^{131}I treatment is permanent hypothyroidism. The incidence during the first year varies between 5% and 20% and generally correlates with the dose of ^{131}I. In subsequent years, the incidence of the development of hypothyroidism approximates 2% to 3% per year. Consequently, most patients are expected to demonstrate hypothyroidism after a prolonged interval (e.g., >20 years) after RAI treatment. In some instances, immediately after ^{131}I therapy, hypothyroidism may be transient. Because it is not possible to distinguish whether the onset of hypothyroidism is permanent or transient, most clinicians usually assume it is permanent and treat patients with thyroid hormone. The only way to determine if it is transient is to taper thyroid hormone replacement at a later date and see if thyroid hormone levels decrease significantly or remain essentially normal. If hypothyroidism develops, thyroid hormone replacement with L-thyroxine is begun using full replacement doses (0.1–0.15 mg/d) based on approximately 1.6 μg/kg in younger ($\leq$40 years old) individuals without cardiovascular disease. Older patients (>than 40 years old) or those with cardiovascular disease are commonly begun on low doses of thyroxine (e.g., 0.025 mg or 25 μg) and the dose is gradually increased by this amount every 3 to 4 weeks until full replacement is determined on the basis of a normalization of serum TSH. One should also be aware of the possibility that the prolonged duration of previous thyrotoxicosis may result in prolonged suppression of TSH secretion, which may persist when the free T_4 level decreases below normal and clinical hypothyroidism ensues. Usually TSH begins to rise within 2 to 3 months of the onset of untreated hypothyroidism.

Subtotal thyroidectomy is also a potential therapeutic option,[17, 20] which is rarely used at this time except in special circumstances. Such instances include patients who are children, patients who want definitive therapy but who do not want ^{131}I, and pregnant patients (during second trimester) whose disease cannot be managed medically. In most cases, postoperative patients go into a remission and are "cured." Rarely do such patients experience relapse because of stimulation of residual thyroid tissue by thyroid-stimulating immunoglobulins. Surgically treated patients can also develop hypothyroidism at a delayed interval after surgery, but this is much less common than after RAI treatment. Surgery is also associated with a distinct but low morbidity (hypoparathyroidism and recurrent laryngeal nerve dysfunction) and mortality in the hands of an experienced thyroid surgeon and is also significantly more costly in the short term than the other treatment modalities.

EUTHYROID HYPERTHYROXINEMIA

Euthyroid hyperthyroxinemia[21] manifested by an increased serum T_4 (total T_4) value can be related to several diverse causes (Table 5–4). This hyperthyroxinemia can potentially be misleading and makes one consider whether the patient may be thyrotoxic. However, it can be distinguished from thyrotoxicosis by demonstrating a normal serum free T_4, FTI, or "sensitive" TSH. Furthermore, these laboratory findings are associated with a euthyroid state on clinical grounds. Consequently, caution should be exercised and determination of thyroid status should be evaluated by these other important tests and supported on a clinical basis by the absence of symptoms and signs of thyrotoxicosis.

HYPERTHYROIDISM IN PREGNANCY

Hyperthyroidism usually due to Graves' disease can occur during pregnancy.[22, 23] If it occurs during pregnancy, it is most typical during the first trimester and may improve or remit during subsequent trimesters because of the relative immunosuppression that develops at these times. Because pregnancy is often associated with many signs and symptoms (e.g., tachycardia, palpitations, diaphoresis, fatigue, heat intolerance) also associated with thyrotoxicosis, mild thyrotoxicosis can be masked during pregnancy and may not be clinically obvious. To compound the situation further, pregnant patients tolerate symptoms of mild thyrotoxicosis relatively well and may not complain about them. Somewhat unique biochemical test results are found in thyrotoxic, pregnant patients. Increased estrogen levels found during pregnancy increase the serum TBG concentration, and this alteration results in increased serum T_4 and T_3 levels and decreased T_3 resin uptake, but serum free T_4, FTI, and TSH values remain normal. Considering that thyrotoxicosis produces increased serum T_4, T_3, free T_4, and FTI values, and the effects of both thyrotoxicosis and pregnancy appear to be additive on thyroid function tests, thyrotoxic pregnant patients typically show a relatively high serum T_4 and T_3 and normal T_3 resin uptake but still exhibit the characteristic increased serum free T_4 or FTI and decreased TSH found in thyrotoxic patients without pregnancy.

Special considerations need to be raised during the management of thyrotoxic, pregnant patients. RAI (^{131}I) treatment is an absolute contraindication in pregnant patients because of concern about radiation-induced teratogenicity even if the pregnancy has progressed beyond the normal period of organogenesis occurring mainly in the first trimester. The rationale for this principle in the latter stages of pregnancy appears more likely related to medicolegal considerations and potential psychological guilt if the infant exhibits any abnormalities even if they are not likely related to radioactive exposure. Radioactive diagnostic tests are also not performed during pregnancy for the same reasons.

Management of thyrotoxicosis during pregnancy is limited to medical therapy at any time or surgery during the second trimester.[22, 23] Under special circumstances in which thyrotoxicosis is very mild and the patient does not want to take drugs, the patient can be observed. Although risks of maternal thyrotoxicosis or hypothyroidism to the fetus have not unequivocally been established, there are studies suggesting potentially deleterious effects of maternal thyrotoxicosis or hypothyroidism on fetal development or childhood development.[23] There is no significant transplacental transfer of thyroid hormones. Nevertheless, the rationale follows the approach that it is theoretically better for the fetus to develop in a euthyroid mother than in one with thyrotoxicosis or hypothyroidism. When medical therapy is selected, the antithyroid drug PTU is the drug of choice. Methimazole is not usually used because of concern about the potentially rare development of aplasia cutis in the fetus. PTU is usually begun in a dose such as 100 mg given three times a day and adjusted to maintain the free serum free T_4 value at an upper normal or slightly elevated level and to control symptoms of thyrotoxicosis reasonably. Because PTU can cross the placenta and result in fetal goiter, which can complicate delivery on a mechanical basis, the lowest dose of PTU that allows one to achieve the desired clinical response and level of serum free T_4 is used. Beta-

TABLE 5–4

Causes of Euthyroid Hyperthyroxinemia
Increased thyroxine-binding globulin
Hereditary
Acute hepatitis
Chronic liver disease
Hyperestrogenemia
Porphyria
Drugs (e.g., perphenazine, methadone)
Familial dysalbuminemia
Euthyroid sick syndrome/nonthyroidal illness
Acute psychiatric decompensation
Hyperemesis gravidarum
Thyroxine antibodies causing assay artifact
Thyroid hormone resistance/generalized

blockers are not used because of a concern of potentially detrimental effects on fetal development. If medical therapy cannot be used or must be discontinued because of side effects and if thyrotoxicosis is clinically significant, surgery is optimally performed in the second trimester. One should also be prepared for the possible development of transient hyperthyroidism or hypothyroidism in the newborn due to placental transfer of thyroid-stimulating or thyrotropin-blocking antibodies, respectively. Clinical circumstances will dictate whether the newborn requires transient therapy until the antibodies have cleared the circulation.

THYROID STORM

Although patients with thyroid storm usually exhibit severe thyrotoxicosis, the presence of severe thyrotoxicosis is not equivalent to nor synonymous with thyroid storm. Thyroid storm is a clinical diagnosis and cannot necessarily be established by any single thyroid function test or combination of tests.[24] Major clinical features suggesting thyroid storm include fever, severe cardiovascular (tachycardia, arrhythmias, hypotension, high output, heart failure), central nervous system (altered mental status, seizures), and gastrointestinal (diarrhea, nausea/vomiting, abdominal pain) symptoms. The diagnosis or consideration of the diagnosis of thyroid storm constitutes a medical emergency. It can be precipitated in thyrotoxic patients by stress, trauma, infections, surgery, and iodine-containing contrast dyes or by discontinuation of antithyroid medical therapy.

When thyroid storm is considered, the history is reviewed and a physical examination and tests are performed to establish the diagnosis of thyrotoxicosis. If the diagnosis of thyroid storm is seriously entertained, then treatment is a medical emergency because of the high mortality associated with it. Treatment should be initiated before the return of results of thyroid function tests. Major goals include reducing the levels of thyroid hormones, antagonizing their effects, and providing supportive measures. Large doses of thiourea drugs (300–400 mg PTU or 30–40 methimazole q8h PO) that inhibit synthesis of thyroid hormones are used. PTU is preferable because of its theoretic advantage of also inhibiting T_3 production by inhibiting peripheral conversion of T_4 to T_3. If the patient cannot take these drugs orally, they can be given by means of a nasogastric tube but cannot be given parenterally. They block organification and synthesis of thyroid hormones and ultimately result in their decreased release. Iodide orally (10–20 drops of Lugol's solution or 5 drops of SSKI every 8 hours) or intravenously (0.5–1.0 g sodium iodide) inhibit release of thyroid hormones rapidly but should not be given until at least 1 hour after antithyroid drugs to prevent the iodide from being rapidly incorporated into newly synthesized thyroid hormone. Lithium (600 mg orally initially and then 400 mg every 6 hours) can also be used to inhibit thyroid hormone release rapidly and to complement the effects of iodide. However, lithium is not always needed nor necessarily used and caution should be exercised relative to the narrow range between therapeutic and toxic levels of lithium. If lithium is used, serum levels should be monitored closely and maintained at less than 1.5 mEq/mL. Contraindications for the use of lithium include cardiac arrhythmias, heart failure, and significant azotemia.

Inhibition of peripheral conversion of T_4 to T_3 can also be achieved by high doses of beta-blockers (e.g., propranolol 40–120 mg PO q4–8h or 1 mg/min IV up to 2–10 mg q4h IV) and glucocorticoids (e.g., dexamethasone 2 mg q6h IV). It is also possible to achieve a similar effect with contrast medium–containing dyes (iopanoic acid [Telepaque] or sodium ipodate [Oragrafin], 1 g/d PO), but the conventional agents discussed previously are typically used. Aggressive use of beta-blockers antagonizes the effects of the increased sympathomimetic tone resulting from excessive thyroid hormones.

Treatment of thyroid storm with supportive measures is also important and includes suppression of high fever with acetaminophen. Salicylates should not be used because high doses of these drugs displace bound T_4 and can increase free T_4 levels. High doses of glucocorticoids also suppress fever and prevent the possible development of adrenal insufficiency for any reason. Careful attention should also be given to the type and volume of appropriate fluids required.

Acknowledgments

The author thanks John Wilber, M.D., for reviewing this chapter and making helpful comments and Theresa O'Brocki and Connie Ball for secretarial help.

REFERENCES

1. Wall JR: Pathogenesis and management of thyroid associated ophthalmopathy: An update. Thyroid Today 14(1):1, 1991.
2. Feldon SE: Diagnosis levels and clinical techniques in the evaluation of Graves' ophthalmopathy. *In* Wall JR, How JS (eds): Pathogenesis and Management of Graves' Ophthalmopathy. Oxford, Blackwell Scientific, 1990, p 79.
3. Salvi M, Zhang ZO, Ilaegert D, et al: Patients with endocrine ophthalmopathy not associated with overt thyroid disease have multiple thyroid immunological abnormalities. J Clin Endocrinol Metab 70:87, 1990.
4. Gorman CA: Temporal relationship between onset of Graves' ophthalmopathy and diagnosis of thyrotoxicosis. Mayo Clin Proc 58:515, 1983.
5. Tamai H, Nakagawa T, Onsako N: Changes in thyroid function in patients with euthyroid Graves' disease. J Clin Endocrinol Metab 50:108, 1980.
6. Stockigt JR: Serum thyrotropin and thyroid hormone measurements and assessments of thyroid hormone transport. *In* Braverman LE, Utiger RD (eds): Werner and Ingbar's The Thyroid. Philadelphia, JB Lippincott, 1991, p 463.
7. Reichlin S: Hypothalamus and pituitary neuroendocrinology. *In* Wilson JD, Foster DN (eds): Williams Textbook of Endocrinology. Philadelphia, WB Saunders, 1992, p 135.
8. Braverman LE, Utiger RD: Introduction to thyrotoxicosis. *In* Bra-

verman LE, Utiger RD (eds): Werner and Ingbar's The Thyroid. Philadelphia, JB Lippincott, 1991, p 645.

9. Nordyke RA, Gilbert FI Jr, Harada ASM: Graves' disease: Influence of age on clinical findings. Arch Intern Med 148:626, 1988.
10. Trzepacz FT, Klien I, Robert M, et al: Graves' disease: An analysis of thyroid hormone levels and hyperthyroid signs and symptoms. Am J Med 87:558, 1989.
11. Ladenson PW: Diagnosis of thyrotoxicosis. *In* Braverman LE, Utiger RD (eds): Werner and Ingbar's The Thyroid. Philadelphia, JB Lippincott, 1991, p 880.
12. Spencer CA, LoPresti JS, Patel A: Applications of a new chemiluminometric thyrotropin assay to subnormal measurement. J Clin Endocrinol Metab 70:453, 1990.
13. Gesundheit N: Thyrotropin-induced hyperthyroidism. *In* Braverman LE, Utiger RD (eds): Werner and Ingbar's The Thyroid. Philadelphia, JB Lippincott, 1991, p 682.
14. Wartofsky L, Burman KD: Alterations in thyroid function in patients with systemic illness: The "euthyroid sick syndrome." Endocr Rev 3:164, 1982.
15. Tibaldi JM, Surks MI: Effects of nonthyroidal illness on thyroid function. Med Clin North Am 69:899, 1985.
16. Solomon B, Glinoer D, Lagasse R, Wartofsky L: Current trends in the management of Graves' disease. J Clin Endocrinol Metab 70:1518, 1990.
17. Cooper DS: Treatment of thyrotoxicosis. *In* Braverman LE, Utiger RD (eds): Werner and Ingbar's The Thyroid. Philadelphia, JB Lippincott, 1991, p 887.
18. Cooper DS: Antithyroid drugs. N Engl J Med 311:1353, 1984.
19. Graham GD, Burman KD: Radioiodine treatment of Graves' disease. Ann Intern Med 105:900, 1986.
20. Hedley AJ, Bewsher PD, Jones SJ: Late-onset hypothyroidism after subtotal thyroidectomy for hyperthyroidism: Implications for long-term follow-up. Br J Surg 70:740, 1983.
21. Borst GC, Eil C, Burman KD: Euthyroid hyperthroxinemia. Ann Intern Med 89:366, 1983.
22. Burrow GN: Thyroid function and hyperfunction in the pregnant woman. Adv Exp Med Biol 299:157, 1991.
23. Emerson CH: Thyroid disease during and after pregnancy. *In* Braverman LE, Utiger RD (eds): Werner and Ingbar's The Thyroid. Philadelphia, JB Lippincott, 1991, p 1263.
24. Gavin LA: Thyroid crises. Med Clin North Am 75:179, 1991.

CHAPTER 6

Diagnosis and Management of Hyperparathyroidism

Leonard P. Kapcala

In rare instances, hyperparathyroidism is associated with orbital pathology. Primary or secondary hyperparathyroidism producing bone disease may result in a bone cyst or brown tumor of the orbit. Considering this presentation, the diagnosis and management of primary hyperparathyroidism are briefly reviewed.

REGULATION OF CALCIUM METABOLISM

Normal total serum calcium (Ca^{2+}) levels (8.5 – 10.5 mg/dL) are maintained by hormonal regulation of Ca^{2+} in bone, the gastrointestinal tract, and kidneys.[1] Bone serves as the body's main reservoir of Ca^{2+}, which enters the extracellular fluid depending on the net regulation of bone resorption and mineralization of osteoid. Parathyroid hormone (PTH) is a major regulator of Ca^{2+} metabolism. PTH increases the serum Ca^{2+} level by stimulating bone resorption, indirectly enhancing intestinal Ca^{2+} absorption by stimulation of an active vitamin D metabolite (1,25-dihydroxycholecalciferol), and increasing renal tubular reabsorption of Ca^{2+}. The active metabolite of vitamin D facilitates PTH-induced bone resorption and enhances renal tubular Ca^{2+} reabsorption. Calcitonin, derived from parafollicular cells of the thyroid, inhibits bone resorption. However, the physiologic importance of calcitonin's action is not clear. Free serum Ca^{2+}, which is approximately half of the total serum Ca^{2+}, is physiologically important for regulating many cellular processes. The other half of total serum Ca^{2+} is predominantly bound to proteins (particularly albumin). Thus, a significant change in a Ca^{2+}-binding protein as albumin can alter total serum Ca^{2+} but does not alter serum ionized Ca^{2+} and therefore does not have physiologic relevance. A small proportion of bound Ca^{2+} is also bound to organic complexes. Free ionized serum Ca^{2+} regulates secretion of PTH insofar as lower levels stimulate PTH release and higher levels inhibit it. Reduction of ionized Ca^{2+} stimulates renal 1α-hydroxylase, which is critical for producing the most potent vitamin D metabolite.

DIAGNOSTIC CONSIDERATIONS

There are many causes of hypercalcemia (Table 6 – 1).[2] However, primary hyperparathyroidism or a malignancy account for more than 90% of patients with hypercalcemia. Unless there are extenuating circumstances, the general approach is to consider primary hyperparathyroidism or a malignancy initially. The history and setting in which hypercalcemia presents is important in suggesting the probability of these two main considerations. Whereas hospitalized patients exhibiting hypercalcemia are often diagnosed with a malignant etiology, subjects exhibiting hypercalcemia in an outpatient setting, often during biochemical screening, are usually diagnosed with primary hyperparathyroidism. A prolonged history (>6 months) of asymptomatic hypercalcemia strongly suggests primary hyperparathyroidism, particularly when subsequent investigations show that it was demonstrated years earlier but ignored or not recognized.

The most important biochemical test in the evaluation of hypercalcemia is measurement of serum PTH. In the overwhelming majority of patients with primary hyperparathyroidism, the serum PTH level, measured by the double antibody technique that detects the intact PTH molecule, is elevated.[3-5] Patients with malignancy or other causes of hypercalcemia show decreased or low-normal serum intact PTH levels. If the clinical presentation or serum intact PTH level does not suggest primary hyperparathyroidism, an evaluation should proceed to exclude a malignancy unless another benign cause is suggested on clinical grounds. If such is the case, specific tests can be ordered in a prioritized approach to establish or exclude specific suspected etiologies. In addition, measurement of parathyroid-related protein (which is elevated in many malignancies) has become available.[6] Although this peptide shows only minor amino acid homology with PTH at the amino-terminal end, it exhibits similar biologic effects as PTH and is believed to stimulate the PTH receptor.

Particular attention needs to be given to the specific methodology measuring PTH. Before the development of the double antibody technique, many radioimmunoassays measuring PTH were directed toward the midpor-

TABLE 6-1

Causes of Hypercalcemia

Causes of Hypercalcemia
Primary Hyperparathyroidism
Cancer
Carcinomas (squamous cell of lung or head and neck, renal, esophageal) secrete parathyroid-related protein
Lymphoma
Leukemia
Breast
Endocrine Disorders (Nonparathyroid)
Thyrotoxicosis
Adrenal insufficiency
Pheochromocytoma
Granulomatous Diseases (1,25-Dihydroxyvitamin D_3 Hypersecretion)
Sarcoid
Tuberculosis
Fungal (histoplasmosis, coccidioidomycosis)
Berylliosis
Drugs
Thiazides
Lithium
Sex steroids (during cancer treatment)
Vitamin Intoxication
Vitamin A
Vitamin D
Miscellaneous Etiologies
Milk-alkali syndrome
Familial hypocalciuric hypercalcemia
Immobilization (especially in growing children and adolescents or people with Paget's disease)
Acute renal failure due to rhabdomyolysis
Severe or critical illness

tion or carboxy-terminal portion of a circulating fragment of PTH that does not exert biologic activity.[3, 5] Because this fragment is cleared primarily by the kidney, even minor or subclinical impairment of renal function can result in elevated PTH levels without any relationship to the hypercalcemia. Clinicians unaware of this information can misdiagnose patients as having primary hyperparathyroidism. Older methodologic testing using assays with mid- or carboxy-terminal–directed PTH antisera, however, could be helpful in suggesting primary hyperparathyroidism when they reveal an elevated serum PTH level associated with clearly normal renal function. Older testing methodology measuring an increased amino-terminal PTH fragment, which exerts biologic activity and which is not significantly affected by impaired renal function, can also point to the diagnosis of primary hyperparathyroidism. In summary, knowledge about the type of PTH assay obtained can have important clinical implications.

CLINICAL MANIFESTATIONS

Primary hyperparathyroidism may present as an "asymptomatic" disorder, diagnosed as a result of biochemical screening or may be diagnosed after clinical manifestations related to one or several organ systems.[4, 7, 8] "Stones" (renal), "bones" (bone and skeletal), "groans" (gastrointestinal), and "moans" (central nervous system) refer to the different organ systems that may be affected and exhibit clinical symptoms or signs leading to the diagnosis of primary hyperparathyroidism. During the past 2 decades, most patients with this disorder have taken on a different presentation, with the overwhelming majority exhibiting relatively mild disease of the aforementioned organ systems, nonspecific symptoms, particularly fatigue and weakness, or no clear symptoms. Previously, many patients diagnosed with primary hyperparathyroidism exhibited renal stones and nephrocalcinosis or significant bone disease consisting of the classic finding of osteitis fibrosa cystica or both. Despite this change in presentation, the frequency of diagnosis has increased substantially in recent years. The age-adjusted (average) incidence of primary hyperparathyroidism has been estimated as approximately 28 per 100,000 (with a heavy skewing toward older patients, especially women older than 60 years old).[7]

The reason for discussing hyperparathyroidism in this chapter relates to the occasional, albeit rare, presentation of hyperparathyroid bone disease as orbital disease. Bony enlargement of the orbit may be secondary to a true bone cyst or to a brown tumor (also known as an osteoclastoma). True bone cysts are fluid-filled cysts that remain indefinitely after successful parathyroid surgery.[9] In contrast, brown tumors are cysts composed of highly vascularized fibrous tissue with hemorrhagic zones containing accumulated blood pigment and of osteoclasts intermixed with poorly mineralized woven bone.[9] Patients with primary or secondary hyperparathyroidism (resulting from chronic renal disease) may develop hyperparathyroid-related bone disease, and brown tumors and true bone cysts can also occur in secondary hyperparathyroidism. Brown tumors resolve after surgical cure of hyperparathyroidism[9] and the skeleton undergoes remineralization.[10] Examples of a brown tumor of the orbit are shown in Figures 6–1 through 6–6. Such lesions can also be delineated by bone scanning.[11] Because both types of cysts have a similar radiologic appearance, they can be distinguished only by the postoperative course or by surgical biopsy.

Other presentations of bone disease of hyperparathyroidism include (1) "salt and pepper" appearance of the skull, (2) subperiosteal resorption in specific locations such as the radial portion of the second and third phalanges and distal clavicles, (3) loss of the lamina dura around the roots of the teeth, and (4) diffuse osteoporosis. These findings are more commonly seen now than osteitis fibrosis cystica, which is associated with severe bone involvement. Enhanced bone turnover due to increased resorption by osteoclasts leads to bone disease. Generally, it has been believed that cortical bone is primarily affected. However, more recently, a serious question

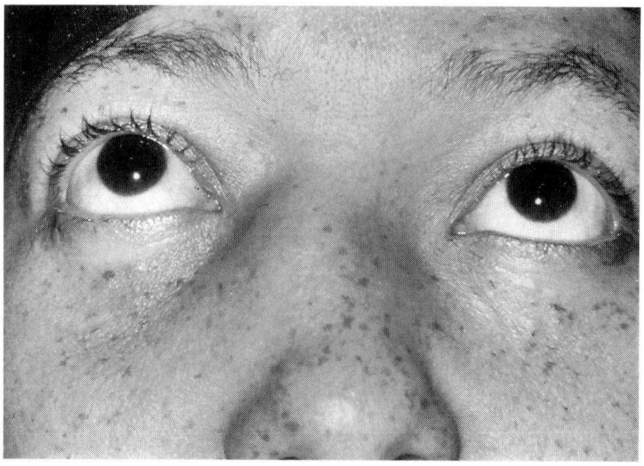

Figure 6–1. Mild right proptosis and a mass involving the nasal bridge. (From Karesh J, Lawton A: Case report. Ophthalmic Pract 9:285, 1991.)

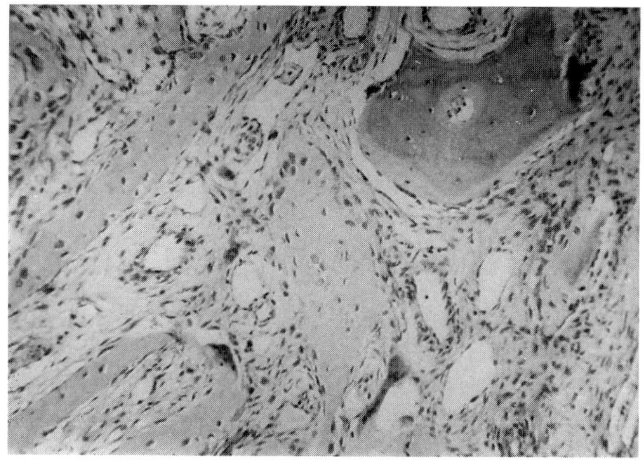

Figure 6–3. Light micrograph of a tumor demonstrating fibrous stroma with new bone formation. H & E, ×32. (From Karesh J, Lawton A: Case report. Ophthalmic Pract 9:285, 1991.)

about involvement of trabecular bone has been raised.[9] Osteoclastic activity is normally coupled to osteoblastic activity in bone modeling units, and this coupling is often maintained in mild hyperparathyroidism. Nevertheless, more sensitive diagnostic procedures such as bone scanning[11] or quantitative techniques for measuring bone density[12] (single- or dual-photon absorptiometry, dual energy x-ray absorptiometry, quantitative computed to-

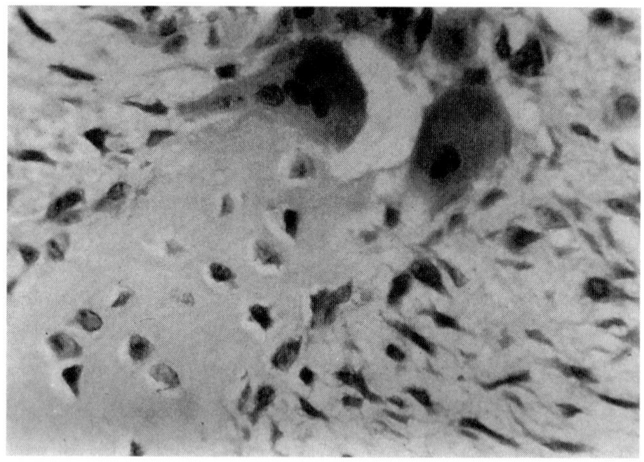

Figure 6–4. High-powered view of osteoclastic activity in association with new bone formation. H & E, ×128. (From Karesh J, Lawton A: Case report. Ophthalmic Pract 9:285, 1991.)

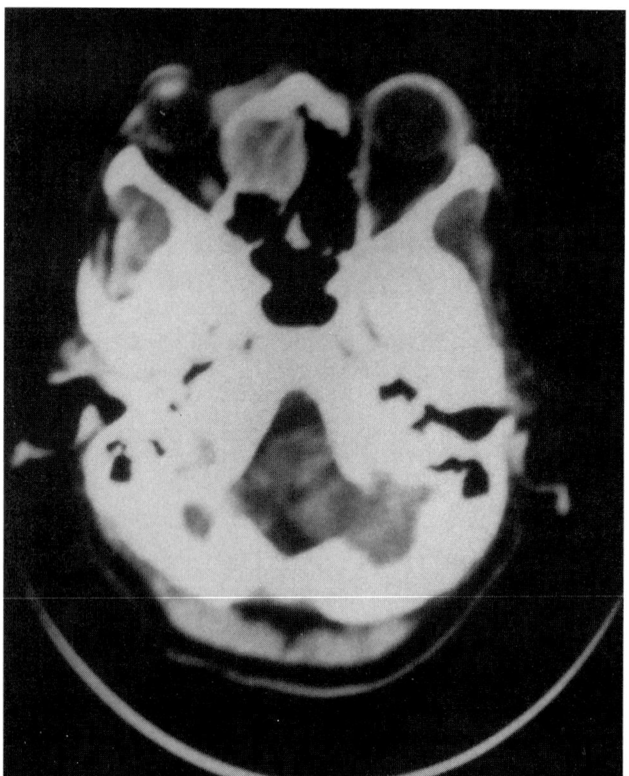

Figure 6–2. Computed tomographic image of a right-sided intraosseous orbital and nasal tumor with a thin calcified rim and internal calcifications. (From Karesh J, Lawton A: Case report. Ophthalmic Pract 9:285, 1991.)

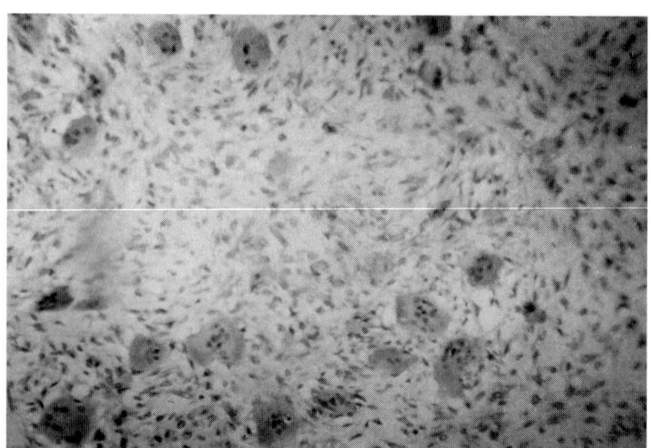

Figure 6–5. Brown tumor stoma demonstrating scattered osteoclasts. H & E, ×32. (From Karesh J, Lawton A: Case report. Ophthalmic Pract 9:285, 1991.)

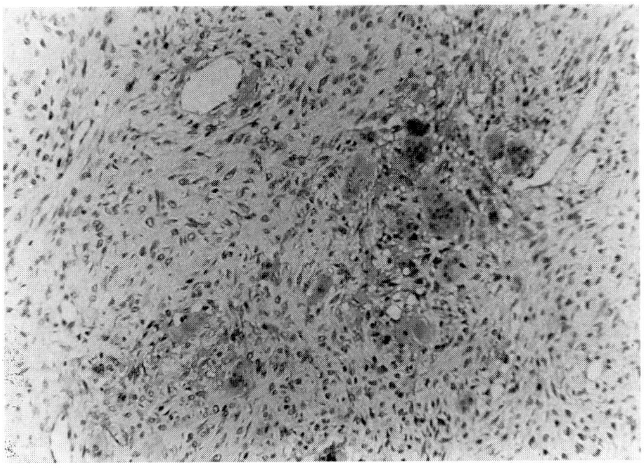

Figure 6-6. Light micrograph of tumor demonstrating numerous multinucleated giant cells (osteoclasts) in a cluster within dense fibrous stroma. H & E, ×32.

mography) may reflect dysfunctional coupling of osteoclast and osteoblast with predominant primary activity of the former. These more sensitive methods for detecting osteoporosis facilitate the diagnosis of the abnormality even in the presence of normally appearing bones on radiography.[11-13]

Many other clinical manifestations are also found with hyperparathyroidism. Renal manifestations can include mild to moderate azotemia, which may be functional and reversible owing to a decrease of glomerular filtration by hypercalcemia or irreversible because of complications of nephrocalcinosis, renal calculi, or both. Gastrointestinal complications can include nausea, vomiting, abdominal discomfort, and constipation. Central nervous system and other neurologic dysfunction consisting of mild dementia or difficulty in concentration, unusual behavior due to exacerbation of underlying psychiatric disease, anorexia leading to weight loss, muscle weakness, and diminished deep tendon reflexes are also reported and are common in patients with hyperparathyroidism. Furthermore, the majority of patients with clinical evidence of disease complain of nonspecific symptoms of fatigue and generalized weakness.

MANAGEMENT

Management of hypercalcemia can be viewed from an acute and chronic perspective. Although severe hypercalcemia has been defined as a serum Ca^{2+} of greater than 14 mg/dL associated with a normal serum albumin value, it is reasonable and wise to treat hypercalcemia of more than 12.5 mg/dL aggressively regardless of symptoms. Acute treatment initially includes aggressive use of intravenous fluid such as normal saline (aggressiveness varies directly with the severity of fluid depletion).[2] Elderly patients or those with cardiac disease particularly require close observation of cardiovascular status during fluid treatment and may require specific adjustments in the normally aggressive rehydration approach. Once fluids have been initiated and intravascular volume is replete, concomitant diuresis is begun with a potent diuretic such as furosemide (e.g., 20 mg IV q1-2h initially and in lesser doses at more prolonged intervals once a significant effect has been obtained) in conjunction with close monitoring of vital signs and urinary responses. Rehydration increases glomerular filtration, which enhances urinary Ca^{2+} excretion, and furosemide also enhances urinary Ca^{2+} excretion. These measures are critical initially but are only relatively temporary therapeutic measures. It is also important to initiate specific drugs that produce more prolonged effects to inhibit the increased bone resorption and thereby control the hypercalcemia over a longer period. Such drugs include a bisphosphonate (e.g., etidronate or pamidronate), gallium, and calcitonin. Although glucocorticoids may be especially beneficial in specific causes of hypercalcemia, they do not play any significant role in the management of hyperparathyroidism.

In considering the best approach for managing hyperparathyroidism, consideration of the natural history of the disorder is important. Despite numerous attempts to define this natural history, it is clear that some patients experience little or no symptoms over a prolonged period, others develop complications after a prolonged period, and others present with complications.[4, 7, 14-16] Unfortunately, for those presenting with essentially asymptomatic disease, it is not possible to predict its course. Because of the lack of efficacy of any oral drugs for chronic medical management of hyperparathyroidism, the main approach consists of parathyroid exploration and surgical resection of a parathyroid adenoma (which is found in approximately 90% or more patients who undergo surgical exploration by an experienced parathyroid surgeon) or close followup and observation. The remainder of patients exhibit parathyroid hyperplasia (four gland) or, rarely, parathyroid carcinoma. Of those with hyperplasia, this disorder may be sporadic or familial and associated with other endocrine tumors (e.g., multiple endocrine neoplasia type I or II).[17] The chronic management and decision about who should undergo surgical exploration has been the subject of controversy for many years. A National Institutes of Health (NIH) consensus conference[15] has suggested guidelines for surgical intervention (Table 6-2).

Operative complications[18] of parathyroid exploration include laryngeal nerve damage, transient or permanent hypoparathyroidism, and "hungry bone syndrome" in which the patient experiences hypocalcemia typically for a short time in the postoperative period but which can be extended over weeks. Before surgery there is no clear benefit of any imaging procedure, and it is not necessary to perform PTH sampling to try to localize the probable parathyroid adenoma unless a previous surgical exploration has been negative.

If there is no clear reason for surgery, prolonged sur-

TABLE 6-2

Guidelines for Parathyroid Surgical Exploration
Typical parathyroid-related symptoms involving skeletal, renal, or gastrointestinal systems
Sustained increase in serum calcium level >12 mg/dL (3 mmol/L)
Significant decline in renal function
Nephrolithiasis or worsening calciuria
Significant decline in bone mass
Significant neuromuscular or select psychological symptoms without another obvious cause
Inability or unwillingness to continue under medical observation

veillance is a reasonable approach as long as careful followup at periodic intervals is performed along with reassessment of the benefits of surgery versus continued followup. Consideration can also be given to the fact that patients with borderline contraindications for surgery are likely to develop clear-cut contraindications as they age if they continue to be observed. The surgery is well tolerated by young and relatively healthy patients, and thus a surgical cure prevents the possible development of complications or difficulties that can increase the risk of surgery.

Acknowledgments

The author wishes to thank Drs. Thomas Connor and Luis Martin for helpful comments in the review of this chapter and Theresa O'Brocki for secretarial assistance.

REFERENCES

1. Mallette LE: Regulation of blood calcium in humans. Endocrinol Metab Clin North Am 18:601-610, 1989.
2. Bilezikian JP: Management of acute hypercalcemia. N Engl J Med 326:1196-1203, 1992.
3. Blind E, Schmidt-Gayk H, Scharla S, et al: Two-site assay of intact parathyroid hormone in the investigation of primary hyperparathyroidism and other disorders of calcium metabolism compared with a midregion assay. J Clin Endocrinol Metab 67:353-360, 1988.
4. Potts JT Jr: Management of asymptomatic hyperparathyroidism. J Clin Endocrinol Metab 70:1489-1493, 1990.
5. Ashby JP, Thakkar H: Diagnostic limitations of region-specific parathyroid hormone assays in the investigation of hypercalcemia. Ann Clin Biochem 25:275-279, 1988.
6. Insogna K: Humoral hypercalcemia of malignancy: The role of parathyroid-related protein. Med Clin North Am 18:779, 1989.
7. Heath DA: Primary hyperparathyroidism. Endocrinol Metab Clin North Am 18:631-646, 1983.
8. Chu BC, Gillott AR, Beck J: Primary hyperparathyroidism: Ten-year experience. Contemp Surg 35:72-77, 1989.
9. Parisien M, Silverberg SJ, Shane E, et al: Bone disease in primary hyperparathyroidism. Metab Bone Dis 19:19-34, 1990.
10. Abugassa S, Nordenstrom J, Eriksson S, et al: Skeletal remineralization after surgery for primary and secondary hyperparathyroidism. Surgery 107:128-133, 1990.
11. Clarke SE, Fogelman I: Bone scanning in metabolic and endocrine bone disease. Endocrinol Metab Clin North Am 18:977-994, 1989.
12. Wahner HW: Measurements of bone mass and bone density. Endocrinol Metab Clin North Am 18:995-1012, 1989.
13. Cooper KL: Radiology of metabolic bone disease. Endocrinol Metab Clin North Am 18:955-976, 1989.
14. Lafferty FW, Hubay CA: Primary hyperparathyroidism: A review of the long-term surgical and nonsurgical morbidities as a basis for a rational approach to treatment. Arch Intern Med 149:789-796, 1989.
15. Diagnosis and management of asymptomatic primary hyperparathyroidism. National Institutes of Health Consensus Development Conference Statement. October 29-31, 1990. 8:1-18, 1990.
16. Rao DS, Wilson RJ, Kleerekoper M, Parfitt AM: Lack of biochemical progression or continuation of accelerated bone loss in mild asymptomatic primary hyperparathyroidism: Evidence for biphasic disease course. J Clin Endocrinol Metab 67:1294-1298, 1988.
17. Fitzpatrick LA: Hypercalcemia in the multiple endocrine neoplasia syndromes. Endocrinol Metab Clin North Am 18:741-752, 1989.
18. Niederle B, Woloszczuk W, Klaushofer K, et al: Successful parathyroidectomy in primary hyperparathyroidism: A clinical follow-up study of 212 consecutive patients. Surgery 102:903-909, 1987.

CHAPTER 7

The Ocular Manifestations of Non–Thyroid-Related Endocrine Disease

James W. Karesh

Although thyroid disease is the most common endocrine abnormality associated with extraocular ophthalmologic findings, a number of other endocrinopathies can also involve the orbital and periocular structures. Both thyroid and parathyroid pathology have already been discussed elsewhere in this section. In this chapter a brief description is provided of some of the other associations between endocrinopathies and the extraocular structures.

DIABETES MELLITUS

Diabetes mellitus is well known for its ocular complications, in particular, diabetic retinopathy, which is a leading cause of blindness in the industrialized world. However, there are a number of extraocular manifestations of this disease. In general, these are related to orbital infections and neuro-ophthalmic complications, although there are a number of associated cutaneous processes. The causes of the various extraocular complications of diabetes mellitus are not entirely understood. Metabolic abnormalities related to activation of aldose reductase and the polyol pathway may result in metabolic and cellular alterations. These may cause the microvascular abnormalities, such as capillary basement membrane thickening, pericyte loss, decreased oxygen diffusion, and changes in blood flow, that are hypothesized to cause monocranial neuropathies.[1, 2] These same microvascular abnormalities may also be the underlying mechanism for the increased incidence of infection associated with diabetes.[3] The cutaneous manifestations of diabetes may be related to either microvascular disease or abnormalities of collagen cross-linking associated with protein glycosylization.[4, 5] The extraocular complications of diabetes mellitus are listed in Table 7–1.

Orbital Infection

Phycomycosis of the orbit and sinus represents one of the most devastating infections occurring in the diabetic patient. This class of nonseptate fungi, Phycomycetes, contains several orders, including Mucorales of which the family Mucoraceae is but one family. The three genera of this family, *Absidia, Mucor*, and *Rhizopus*, are all human pathogens. These fungi are ubiquitous, occurring in soil, air, and bread molds. Transmission to humans is through inhalation. In general, individuals with normal immune systems are able to mount an adequate immune response to eradicate these organisms. This is not the case in patients who have inadequate immune systems, in particular, diabetics in ketoacidosis. Other conditions that predispose to infection with these organisms include leukemia, lymphoma, multiple myeloma, tuberculosis, malnutrition, renal disease, and chronic antibiotic or corticosteroid therapy.[6–9]

Fungal infection with the phycomycetes begins with the inhalation of spores and a mild pharyngitis and sinusitis. This is followed by invasion of the walls of contiguous arteries and occlusion of the lumen of these vessels, leading to tissue ischemia and necrosis.[8, 9] Large vessels, such as the carotid artery and the cavernous sinus as well as the ophthalmic artery, are not infrequently involved in the infectious process. Although the nasopharynx, sinuses, and orbit are the most common sites of infection, since inhalation is the means by which spores enter the body, pulmonary, disseminated, gastrointestinal, and cutaneous infections can also occur.[9]

Symptoms suggestive of phycomycosis include multiple cranial nerve palsies and disturbance of globe motility; proptosis; unilateral orbital or facial pain; acute periorbital and orbital inflammatory symptoms such as erythema, edema, ptosis, and chemosis; headache; and acute loss of vision. Nasal discharge, sinusitis, pharyngitis, eschar formation in areas of tissue necrosis, and facial paresthesias have also been reported.[9] These symptoms are particularly suggestive of phycomycosis when a patient also has diabetes and metabolic acidosis or of any of the previously mentioned conditions associated with immunosuppression.

Evaluation by computed tomography or magnetic resonance imaging is helpful in delineating the extent of the disease process.[10, 11] Involvement of bone is unusual.[11] A tissue biopsy or fungus culture is important for confirmation of the diagnosis. Early diagnosis is essential to

TABLE 7-1

Extraocular Associations of Diabetes Mellitus

Location	Manifestation
Orbit	Cellulitis, phycomycosis, rhinoscleroma
Cranial nerves	Motor nerve pareses (mononeuropathies of cranial nerves III, IV, V, and VII)
	Idiopathic optic disc edema/anterior ischemic optic neuropathy (cranial nerve II mononeuropathy)
	Corneal hypesthesia (cranial nerve V mononeuropathy)
	Malignant external otitis (associated with cranial nerve VII mononeuropathy)
	Kearns-Sayre syndrome (chronic progressive ophthalmoplegia, ptosis, heart conduction defect, pigmentary retinopathy, diabetes mellitus, other endocrinopathies)
	Wolfram syndrome (optic atrophy, diabetes mellitus, urinary atony, diabetes insipidus, neurosensory deafness)
Skin and eyelids	Necrobiosis lipoidica diabeticorum
	Granuloma annulare
	Acanthosis nigricans
	Vitiligo
	Eruptive xanthomas
	Skin tags
	Cutaneous infections (*Candida albicans, Corynebacterium minutissimum*)
	Carotenemia
	Hemochromatosis
	Bullous pemphigoid
	Werner's syndrome (premature aging, atrophic skin, cataracts, osteoporosis, papillary thyroid carcinoma, gonadal atrophy)
	Ataxia-telangiectasia (ataxia, oculocutaneous telangiectasia, ocular motor defects, immunologic deficiencies, adrenal cortical hypoplasia, gonadal dysgenesis)
	Fanconi's syndrome (short stature, bone marrow hypoplasia, skin pigmentation, radius malformations, panhypopituitarism, adrenal atrophy, gonadal atrophy)
Periocular	Myotonic dystrophy (muscular dystrophy, ptosis, ocular motility impairment, facial weakness, cataracts, baldness, cardiac disease, gonadotropin and growth hormone abnormalities, hypothyroidism, primary gonadal failure)

achieving a successful outcome because phycomycosis is associated with a high incidence of mortality, especially when intracranial invasion occurs.

Therapy for phycomycosis is based around systemic and local antifungal agents, aggressive surgical debridement, and control of the underlying disease process. Amphotericin B remains the antifungal agent of choice.[9, 12–14] Newer antifungal agents such as flucytosine, clotrimazole, and miconazole have not been shown to be of value in the treatment of this disease.[9, 14] An aggressive surgical approach involves multiple debridements of necrotic tissue and, in some cases, orbital and sinus cavity exenteration. Packing the sinus and exenteration cavities with amphotericin B–soaked packing may also be helpful since extensive areas of ischemia may prevent adequate delivery of systemic amphotericin B. The use of hyperbaric oxygen has been recommended as adjunctive therapy, although as yet no definitive study supporting this therapy has been published.[15]

Rhinoscleroma is an unusual chronic inflammatory condition involving the respiratory tract. It is endemic to Central America and Africa. *Klebsiella rhinoscleromatis* is the underlying causative organism.[16] Patients usually present with complaints of nasal congestion, although orbital apex syndrome has been reported.[17, 18] Diabetes has been reported in conjunction with this disease process.[18] On examination of the nasal cavity, patients frequently demonstrate crusted erythematous granular or nodular swellings. Proptosis has also been noted in several cases.[19] Computed tomography shows evidence of soft tissue swelling of the nasal cavity and sinuses. Definitive diagnosis is made by tissue biopsy and immunoperoxidase staining. Nodules of plasma cells with Russell bodies or vacuolated histiocytes (Mikulicz's cells) are characteristically observed in addition to vasculitis and acute inflammation, ulceration, submucosal keratin cysts, and pseudoepitheliomatous hyperplasia.[17, 20] The management of this disorder is difficult, since it is not unusual for the disease course to be protracted with multiple exacerbations and recurrences.[19] Rifampicin as well as many other antibiotics have been used with varying success in its treatment.[21]

Malignant external otitis is an invasive infection caused by *Pseudomonas aeruginosa*. It usually occurs in elderly diabetics.[22, 23] Symptomatology includes severe ear pain and tenderness of the mastoid and periaural tissues. Persistent drainage from the external ear canal as well as the occurrence of granulation tissue at the junction of the osseous and cartilaginous portions of the external ear are characteristic.[24] The infection spreads to the mastoid and temporal bones and is frequently associated with facial nerve palsy.[24] Osteomyelitic extension to the petrous bone is associated with multiple cranial nerve palsies, and all cranial nerves except the first and the fourth have been involved.[25] Although modern antibiotic therapy has improved the prognosis of this disease, a mortality rate of 60% to 80% has been reported.[25] Treatment includes aminoglycosides and anti-*Pseudomonas* penicillins, such as ticarcillin, as well as the newer fluoroquinolones.[22, 23] Hyperbaric oxygen has been used as adjunctive therapy.[26]

Cranial Nerve Palsies

Idiopathic optic disc edema is occasionally encountered in both adult-onset and juvenile-onset diabetes.[27–29] One study has reported an incidence of 0.4% in all diabetic patients.[29] Unlike the significant decrease in vision often seen in anterior ischemic optic neuropathy, in this condition vision is usually normal or only slightly decreased. There is no associated pain, diplopia, or other cranial nerve palsies. Fundus examination reveals either unilateral or bilateral optic disc swelling with occasional dilatation of radial peripapillary vessels. Telangiectatic vessels may be present over the disc.[30] The disc edema may be segmental.[31] Occasionally there is an associated proliferative retinopathy requiring laser photocoagulation. More often the disc edema is an isolated ocular finding that resolves spontaneously without therapeutic intervention. Rarely there may be residual segmental or diffuse atrophy.[31] Visual field examination in these patients usually shows only an enlarged blind spot. However, arcuate, nerve fiber bundle defects have been described.[29, 30] Fluorescein angiography may reveal diabetic retinopathy but disc swelling does not by itself suggest that retinopathy will occur or worsen. It appears that the etiology of these findings is related to a reversible and self-limited microvasculopathy and may represent a limited form of anterior ischemic optic neuropathy.[27, 30, 32]

Cranial nerve mononeuropathies and polyneuropathies are not uncommonly associated with diabetes mellitus. All the motor nerves to the eye and periocular structures including the oculomotor, trochlear, abducens, and facial nerves have been reported to be involved either alone or in combination.[31, 33, 34] Paralysis of the third and sixth cranial nerves has been most commonly reported. The underlying mechanism for these neuropathies appears to be an ischemic infarction of the nerve,[34] although others suggest that it is due to microinfarctions within the brain stem with fascicular disruption.[31] In general, these neuropathies are of short duration, usually lasting 2 to 6 months before spontaneously resolving. In addition, these mononeuropathies may be the initial presenting sign of diabetes mellitus. For this reason, it is not unreasonable to perform a screening fasting blood glucose test on patients presenting with isolated cranial nerve palsies who do not have a history of diabetes mellitus. However, it must be remembered that the fasting blood glucose value may be normal in the presence of a mildly abnormal glucose tolerance test.[34]

Classically, diabetes-related third nerve paresis is painless and sudden in onset, only incompletely involves the extraocular muscles, and does not affect any pupillomotor fibers. However, these clinical findings are not absolute. In 60% to 80% of cases there may be some mild periorbital pain.[34, 35] In 20% of cases the pupil may be either slightly dilated or may show a light-near dissociation.[36, 37] This contrasts to oculomotor nerve palsies secondary to aneurysms in which pupillary findings are present in almost all cases. In general, the pupillary abnormality is not nearly as significant as that seen in a third nerve palsy caused by an aneurysm of the posterior communicating artery. In some cases, however, it may be necessary to perform a diagnostic imaging study such as computed tomography, magnetic resonance imaging, or angiography to exclude the existence of an aneurysm. Although usually a unilateral condition, rarely oculomotor paresis may be bilateral.[38]

Sixth nerve palsies occur only slightly less commonly than third nerve palsies in patients with diabetes.[33, 39] However, it should be kept in mind that intracranial neoplasia is also a significant cause of this problem. For this reason, diabetic patients with sixth nerve palsies who present with additional neurologic symptoms or worsening of their paresis should undergo imaging studies to rule out intracranial neoplasia.

Other cranial neuropathies also occur in association with diabetes mellitus; for example, it is responsible for about 5% of all fourth nerve palsies.[39] Decreased corneal sensation has also been demonstrated in these patients.[40] Diabetes mellitus has also been reported to be present in a significant number of patients with seventh nerve palsies.[41] Bell's palsy may precede the occurrence of ophthalmoplegia by several years.[31] Multiple cranial nerve palsies and complete ophthalmoplegia with and without optic nerve involvement mimicking an orbital apex syndrome can also occur in association with diabetes mellitus.[42, 43] This must be differentiated from mucormycosis and other inflammatory, infectious, and neoplastic causes of this condition. Finally, although not a mononeuropathy or polyneuropathy, the chronic progressive external ophthalmoplegia, ptosis, pigmentary retinopathy, and cardiac conduction defects that make up the Kearns-Sayre syndrome have been associated with multiple endocrinopathies, including diabetes mellitus, hypogonadism, hypoparathyroidism, growth hormone deficiency, and adrenal dysfunction.[44, 45] Kearns-Sayre syndrome, despite its rarity, should be considered in the differential diagnosis of the diabetic patient who presents with ophthalmoplegia.

Optic atrophy, diabetes mellitus, diabetes insipidus, neurosensory deafness, and atony of the urinary tract is an association of findings known as Wolfram or DIDMOAD syndrome.[46–49] This is an autosomal recessive disorder whose underlying pathology includes atrophy of the hypothalamic nuclei as well as degeneration of the optic nerves, chiasm, and tracts.[48] The cause of the diabetes mellitus is not understood. However, all patients have insulin-dependent diabetes mellitus. Optic atrophy occurs late and progresses at a variable rate.

Skin Disorders[4, 50]

Necrobiosis lipoidica diabeticorum[51] is a rare skin disorder that only occasionally involves the eyelids.[52, 53] It occurs in about 0.3% of patients with diabetes mellitus. It is more common in women, especially those in the 30- to 40-year age groups. It exclusively occurs in Caucasians. Characteristically an irregular, orange-red plaque with well-defined margins is seen. The shins are the most common site of occurrence. The lesion slowly enlarges, becoming centrally erythematous then yellow or sclerotic, finally resembling porcelain. It is covered with telangiectases. Often the lesion will ulcerate spontaneously or after minor trauma. Histopathologically, both granulomatous and necrobiotic reactions are seen. The latter shows large ill-defined areas of amorphous collagen in the dermis with a mixed inflammatory cell response and collagen degeneration. The pathogenesis is unknown. Treatment consists of topical and intralesional steroids and occlusive dressings. Aspirin and dipyridamole have also been used to treat this condition. Results of treatment are generally disappointing.

Granuloma annulare is a benign, self-limited, and usually symptomless disorder consisting of multiple annular papules.[54] These lesions may appear anywhere on the body, including the eyelids and face.[54–57] There is a 2 : 1 predilection for females, and in over two thirds of patients lesions will occur before the age of 30. Characteristically, the lesions are skin colored to reddish brown and measure 1 to 5 mm. They may slowly enlarge and most commonly involve the extremities. There are localized, generalized, perforating, and deep subcutaneous (pseudorheumatoid nodules) forms of the disease.[54, 57] Histopathologically, there is a granulomatous, inflammatory process involving the mid to upper dermis with focal collagen degeneration and mucopolysaccharide deposition. Mucin surrounded by palisades of lymphocytes, histiocytes, and fibroblasts may also be seen.[54] Although most cases resolve spontaneously, successful treatment of these lesions has been carried out with intralesional and topical corticosteroids.

Acanthosis nigricans is a hyperpigmented, hyperkeratotic, papillomatous dermatosis most often involving areas such as the groin, axilla, dorsa of the fingers, and neck. It is strongly associated with insulin resistance and obesity as well as a variety of endocrinopathies, including diabetes mellitus, gonadal disease, and thyroid disease.[58, 59] In addition, it has been associated with a number of neoplastic conditions, most particularly, adenocarcinoma of the gastrointestinal tract, as well as Crouzon's syndrome.[60, 61] There is also an autosomal dominant type that begins in childhood.[62] The involved areas of skin generally have a velvety and flaky appearance owing to the presence of the desquamating hyperkeratosis. The papillomatous changes often look like small multiple warts. Although the autosomal dominant type tends to progress over time, the type related to endocrine disease will regress with weight loss or treatment of the endocrine disorder. The paraneoplastic form may improve with treatment of the underlying malignancy. Histopathologic evaluation of skin biopsy specimens from patients with any type of acanthosis nigricans reveals hyperkeratosis and papillomatosis as well as thinning of the suprapapillary epidermis and widening of the dermal rete ridges. Despite the apparent increased pigmentation seen clinically, histopathologically there is no increase in basal melanin.

Vitiligo is an acquired disease characterized by patchy or diffuse well-demarcated areas of hypopigmentation or depigmentation due to a loss of cutaneous melanocytes. Generally the disease process begins in the second or third decades of life and affects females more than males.[63–65] There is a 25% to 30% familial incidence.[66] Although the exact cause of vitiligo is unknown, there is a significant association with a variety of autoimmune diseases, including diabetes mellitus (1% to 7%), thyroid disease (40%), pernicious anemia (1%), Vogt-Koyanagi-Harada syndrome, and sympathetic ophthalmia.[67–72] For this reason it is hypothesized that vitiligo also has an autoimmune etiology.[73, 74] In addition, cutaneous melanoma has also been associated with hypopigmentation of the skin. Therefore, it is important to screen patients with vitiligo for thyroid disease, diabetes mellitus, and other autoimmune diseases, as well as for evidence of cutaneous melanoma.[75, 76]

Skin involvement in vitiligo can have a variety of distributional patterns. These have been variously characterized as generalized, acrofacial, localized, and segmental. The first of these consists of a random distribution of symmetric macules of depigmentation. The acrofacial variety involves the extremities and face (particularly the eyelids) and may also be associated with poliosis, depigmentation of the choroid and retinal pigment epithelium, and Vogt-Koyanagi-Harada syndrome.[64, 77–79] Segmental vitiligo follows a dermatomal pattern and most often occurs along the distribution of the trigeminal nerve.[80] Localized vitiligo consists of one to several patches of depigmentation in a particular body area. Histopathologically, all types of vitiligo show a decrease in the number of melanocytes and melanin at the dermoepidermal junction. Antimelanocyte antibodies have been demonstrated in these patients. Perivascular inflammatory cell infiltration has been seen in up to 90% of biopsy specimens.[81] Treatment of vitiligo is for cosmetic purposes. However, because of the psychologic distress associated with this disease, counseling is an important adjunct to other treatments. Cosmetic camouflage with water-insoluble cosmetics is very effective in the management of localized depigmentation.[82] Therapy with psoralens and UVA light (PUVA) will repigment many patients.[82, 83] Other repigmentation regimens with corticosteroids, 5-fluorouracil, cyclophosphamide, and tattooing have also been used.[84, 85] Some patients with large areas of depigmentation may prefer total depigmentation with monobenzyl ether of hydroquinone.[82]

Eruptive xanthomas represent deposition of lipid in the dermis of patients with abnormal plasma lipid levels.[86] Unlike xanthelasmas, which are common, plaque-like depositions of lipid usually occurring in the medial portion of the upper or lower eyelids and which are most often unrelated to any metabolic derangement, xanthomas are always the result of defects in lipid metabolism. They are usually nodular or slightly raised, yellow or reddish yellow papules of lipid within the dermal layer of the skin. Their name comes from their tendency to appear suddenly in crops of papules measuring 1 to 4 mm in diameter. They may appear in the conjunctiva, peripheral cornea, and oral mucosa as well as in the eyelid skin and margin, buttocks, thighs, knees, and elbows.[87, 88]

Their appearance indicates the presence of significant hypertriglyceridemia due either to diabetes mellitus or to one of the autosomal dominant hyperlipoproteinemias.[86, 89, 90] In addition to lipid-laden histiocytes or "foam cells" in the dermal layer of the skin, inflammatory cells and fibrosis are also seen on histopathologic evaluation of skin biopsy specimens. Reduction in plasma lipid levels usually results in the disappearance of the xanthomas.[90, 91]

Carotenemia is usually the result of ingesting excess amounts of vitamin A or foods rich in carotene.[92] Its major manifestation is a yellowish pigmentation of the skin. In addition, there are a number of systemic diseases associated with this phenomenon, including diabetes mellitus, hypothyroidism, hypopituitarism, liver disease, anorexia nervosa, and inborn errors of metabolism.[92–94] The most common areas affected are the palms, soles, and nasolabial areas, although, the entire skin area can become involved. The cause of this condition in endocrine disease is not understood but may be the result of abnormal excretion or metabolism of carotene. The condition usually resolves with treatment of the underlying metabolic derangement.

Hemochromatosis exists in both an acquired and an inherited form.[95, 96] The former is associated with multiple blood transfusions or rarely with an excessive dietary iron intake. Idiopathic hemochromatosis is an autosomal recessive disorder characterized by abnormal iron metabolism with excessive storage of iron in the liver, pancreas, adrenals, pituitary, heart, and skeletal musculature.[97, 98] Men are more commonly affected than women because of an increased iron loss in women over the course of their lifetime. The disease frequently does not become clinically evident until the fourth decade of life, although it has been described in younger individuals.[99] About 80% of individuals with hemochromatosis develop diabetes mellitus, which in most cases is insulin dependent.[100, 101] In 50% of cases diabetes is the presenting condition suggesting the diagnosis of hemochromatosis. Hyperpigmentation of the skin is due to an increased deposition of epidermal melanin. Hemosiderin can be seen in dermal macrophages and in perivascular areas. The skin changes in hemochromatosis are often overlooked since they progress gradually. Patients may appear slightly bronzed ("bronze diabetes"), metallic gray, or brown. Color changes may be more obvious in sun-exposed areas, scars, areas of flexure, or areolae. The mucous membranes may be involved in up to 20% of cases, and hyperpigmentation of the external genitalia may also be seen. Other skin changes found in this disease process include hair loss, skin atrophy, spider angiomas, ichthyosis-like changes, palmar erythema, and nail abnormalities. A number of endocrinologic abnormalities associated with pituitary insufficiency are also found in patients with hemochromatosis, including decreased levels of prolactin, testosterone, and gonadotropin.[102] Other complications associated with hemochromatosis include liver failure, cirrhosis, cardiac dysrhythmias, and pseudopericarditis.[96] Treatment is related to removal of excess iron. Both weekly phlebotomies and deferoxamine, an iron-chelating agent, have been successfully used in the management of this disease.[96, 103, 104]

POLYENDOCRINE DISEASE AND OTHER ENDOCRINOPATHIES

Addison's disease is an uncommon disease whose major manifestation is the primary failure of the adrenal glands.[105, 106] It has multiple causes, including chronic infection, autoimmune disease, vasculitis, or neoplasia. About 80% of all cases of Addison's disease is autoimmune and may occur as part of various polyglandular autoimmune syndromes.[107, 108] Tuberculosis remains the next most common cause of this disease. The difficulty in diagnosing Addison's disease is due to the nonspecific, multisystemic nature of its clinical features. These include weight loss, asthenia, nausea, and hypoglycemia.[109] However, the first sign of Addison's disease in 20% to 40% of patients is the presence of cutaneous darkening. With time, almost every patient will have significant pigmentary changes.[110] This is due to the effect of chronic pituitary secretion of corticotropin or melanocyte-stimulating hormone. Patients may have darkening of nevi and the occurrence of lentigo-type lesions. In addition to these skin changes, vitiligo will be present in 15% of patients, especially in those with polyglandular autoimmune disease. Cortisol deficiency will also result in hypothyroidism, hyperprolactinemia, and hypercalcemia. The diagnosis of Addison's disease is based on the presence of adrenocortical insufficiency and the results of various adrenal stimulation tests. Treatment of this disease is through replacement therapy with glucocorticoids.

Polyglandular autoimmune syndromes can be divided into two types.[111, 112] In both types the principal endocrine features include adrenal insufficiency and Addison's disease, autoimmune thyroid disease, insulin-dependent diabetes mellitus, and gonadal failure.

Pernicious anemia and vitiligo may also occur. Although most cases are sporadic, a genetic basis has been suggested in those instances in which several family members are affected.[113] In type I disease, the onset is in childhood, and mucocutaneous candidiasis and acquired hypoparathyroidism are features. In addition, chronic active hepatitis, malabsorption, and alopecia may occur. In type II disease, insulin-dependent diabetes and autoimmune thyroid disease are more frequent than in type I disease and onset tends to occur later in life.[113] In both types there are low levels of circulating hormones as well as antibodies to one or more endocrine glands.

Pheochromocytomas are tumors of the chromaffin cells in the medulla of the adrenal gland.[114, 115] This portion of the gland is responsible for producing the catecholamines epinephrine and norepinephrine. Rarely these tumors may have an extramedullary origin in the segmental ganglia of the sympathetic chain. Clinically, these tumors are well encapsulated with fibrous tissue or compressed adrenal cortex.[114] They appear lobular owing to the presence of fibrous septa and are gray or light brown with areas of hemorrhage and necrosis. Although they usually occur in adults between 30 and 50 years of age, pheochromocytomas may also occur in children. There is no difference between males and females in the frequency of occurrence. About 9% of these tumors are bilateral or multiple. Usually in these cases the tumor occurs as part of either a phakomatosis or multiple endocrine neoplasia. Pheochromocytomas have been reported to occur in about 1% of patients with neurofibromatosis and up to 25% of patients with von Hippel-Lindau disease.[116–118] They are also a characteristic finding in multiple endocrine neoplasia type II (MEN IIa) and III (MEN IIb).[116, 119] The clinical presentation of pheochromocytoma includes headaches, uncontrolled hypertension, dyspnea, angina, tachycardia, and transient or permanent ischemic events.[120] Patients will often experience periods of extreme nervousness and apprehension. A high index of suspicion is required to diagnose these tumors. Diagnosis is based on the demonstration of increased levels of urinary or plasma catecholamines or their metabolites.[121, 122] Treatment consists of surgical removal of the tumor.[123, 124] Although most of these tumors are benign, about 5% are malignant and unresponsive to either chemotherapy or radiation.[124, 125] The 5-year survival rate for these patients is about 45%.

MEN syndromes comprise three well-delineated disease complexes.[116, 126–128] These all have an autosomal dominant pattern of inheritance. Type I (MEN I; Wermer's syndrome) is characterized by hyperplasia of the parathyroids, pancreatic islet cells, and the pituitary gland.[129, 130] Two thirds of patients present with adenomas of two or more endocrine systems, and about 20% develop adenomas of three or more systems. The major clinical findings in these patients include peptic ulcer; hypoglycemia; hypercalcemia and renal calculi; symptoms of pituitary dysfunction including headaches, visual field loss, and secondary amenorrhea; and multiple lipomas and leiomyomas of the skin. In addition, up to 10% of patients will have acromegaly, Cushing's syndrome, nonfunctional thyroid adenomas, hyperthyroidism, hepatomegaly, or the carcinoid syndrome. MEN II (MEN IIa; Sipple's syndrome) consists of pheochromocytoma, medullary thyroid carcinoma, and parathyroid hyperplasia.[129] Patients will present with symptoms of catecholamine excess, including headache, palpitations, diaphoresis, and hypertension. The medullary thyroid carcinoma is often multifocal. The only effective treatment for this carcinoma is the total removal of the thyroid. Measurement of serum calcitonin levels can be utilized to assess the completeness of the surgical removal. Chemotherapy and radiation therapy have been of only limited value in the management of this disease. MEN III (MEN IIb; multiple mucosal neuroma syndrome) like MEN II is characterized by medullary thyroid carcinoma and pheochromocytoma.[131, 132] However, in addition, patients with MEN III demonstrate multiple neuromas of the conjunctival, nasal, labial, and buccal mucosa, tongue, and other portions of the gastrointestinal tract. Multiple mucosal neuromas can also occasionally occur as a sporadic syndrome. Patients with MEN III also have an asthenic habitus, kyphosis, lordosis, muscular hypotonia, joint laxity, café-au-lait spots or diffuse freckling, enlarged corneal nerves, large bulbous lips, pseudoprognathism, pes cavus, and genu valgum. An absent flare response to intradermal histamine is characteristic of this syndrome. Treatment of this condition, like that of MEN II, revolves around surgical excision of the thyroid neoplasm and pheochromocytoma.

Acromegaly is the result of an excessive secretion of growth hormone, usually due to the presence of a pituitary adenoma.[133, 134] Very rarely, pituitary hyperplasia will occur in the presence of a carcinoid that produces growth hormone–releasing hormone.[135, 136] Excessive growth hormone secretion results in hypertrophy of periosteal bone and cartilage. This causes frontal bossing; prognathism; widely spaced teeth; large ears, hands, and feet; and gigantism.[137] Growth hormone produces an increase in dermal collagen with deposition of glycosaminoglycans, including chondroitin sulfate, hyaluronic acid, and dermatan sulfate. This is manifested clinically by furrowing and accentuation of skin folds in the nasolabial area, forehead, and scalp. In addition, there is thickening of the eyelids, lips, and nose.[137] Dermal and epidermal hyperplasia results in enlarged skin pores, skin tags, and thickened nails. There is increased eccrine, apocrine, and sebaceous glandular activity. About 40% of patients will have hyperpigmentation of sun-exposed skin, skin folds, and genitalia.[138] Body hair may become coarse, or in severe cases there may be loss of body hair and thinning of the scalp hair. Glucose intolerance, diabetes mellitus, and hypertension are also common in these patients.[137] Peripheral neuropathies and polyostotic fibrous dysplasia have also been reported in association with acromegaly.[138–140] About one third of patients with acromegaly have adenomas producing both growth hormone and prolactin with symptoms of hyperprolactinemia including amenorrhea, gynecomastia, galactorrhea, sexual dysfunction, and infertility.[138] Hypersecreting pituitary adenomas often do not produce compressive symptoms involving the optic nerve, chiasm, and tracts. However, masses 10 mm or larger frequently result in visual symptomatology and clinical findings including visual field loss, loss of vision, color vision deficits, an afferent pupillary defect, papilledema, and optic atrophy.[140, 141] Cranial nerve palsies can occur with extension of the tumor into the cavernous sinus.[141] Although treatment of acromegaly is based on the surgical removal of the pituitary tumor producing growth hormone or the tumor producing ectopic growth hormone-releasing hormone, adjunctive radiation therapy and chemotherapy are useful in those cases in which complete surgical ablation is not possible.[142, 143] Bromocriptine, a dopamine agonist, and octreotide, a long-acting somatostatin analogue given subcutaneously, are used in the medical management of acromegaly.[144, 145]

Polyostotic fibrous dysplasia is a bone disorder characterized by patchy areas of rarefaction associated with a pseudocystic appearance.[146] The lesions can be found throughout the skeleton but are most common in the lower limbs. They are less frequent in the upper limbs and uncommon in the skull.[147, 148] When the skull is involved there is dense sclerotic overgrowth of bone including the jaw, facial bones, and skull. The bony lesions in the long bones are associated with pathologic fractures and limb deformity.[149, 150] Biopsy of the skeletal lesions shows poorly differentiated fibrous tissue with interspersed fibrous bone trabeculae and, occasionally, islands of cartilage. Although not invariably present, skin lesions and endocrine abnormalities are common in this condition.[146] The skin lesions consist of brown elevated pigmented patches with irregular borders. They may overlie areas of abnormal bone and can be segmental or unilateral. Endocrine abnormalities associated with this disease include sexual precocity, Cushing's syndrome, acromegaly, hyperparathyroidism, hyperprolactinemia, nodular toxic goiter, hyperphosphatemia, and pheochromocytoma.[146, 150-152] Treatment of polyostotic fibrous dysplasia is directed toward management of the multiple endocrine abnormalities associated with it and surgical treatment of the skeletal deformities, including craniofacial reconstruction.[153, 154]

REFERENCES

1. Stribling D, Armstrong FM, Perkins CM, Smith JC: Aldose reductase in the etiology of diabetic complications: III. Neuropathy. J Diabetic Complications 3:139-148, 1989.
2. Marano CW, Matschinsky FM: Biochemical manifestations of diabetes mellitus in microscopic layers of the cornea and retina. Diabetes Metab Rev 5:1-15, 1989.
3. Shami SK, Chittenden SJ: Microangiopathy in diabetes mellitus: II. Features, complications and investigation. Diabetes Res 17:157-168, 1991.
4. Huntley AC: Cutaneous manifestations of diabetes mellitus. Dermatol Clin 7:531-546, 1989.
5. Edidin DV: Cutaneous manifestations of diabetes mellitus in children. Pediatr Dermatol 2:161-179, 1985.
6. Maniglia AJ, Mintz DH, Novak S: Cephalic phycomycosis: A report of eight cases. Laryngoscope 92:755-760, 1982.
7. Forteza G, Burgeno M, Martorell V, Sierra I: Rhinocerebral mucormycosis: Presentation of two cases and review of the literature. J Craniomaxillofac Surg 16:80-84, 1988.
8. Schwartz JN, Donnelly EH, Klintworth GK: Ocular and orbital phycomycosis. Surv Ophthalmol 22:3-28, 1977.
9. Ferry AP, Abedi S: Diagnosis and management of rhino-orbitocerebral mucormycosis (phycomycosis): A report of 16 personally observed cases. Ophthalmology 90:1096-1104, 1983.
10. Yousem DM, Galetta SL, Gusnard DA, Goldberg HI: MR findings in rhinocerebral mucormycosis. J Comput Assist Tomogr 13:878-882, 1989.
11. Gamba JL, Woodruff WW, Djang WT, Yeates AE: Craniofacial mucormycosis: Assessment with CT. Radiology 160:207-212, 1986.
12. Parfrey NA: Improved diagnosis and prognosis of mucormycosis: A clinicopathologic study of 33 cases. Medicine 65:113-123, 1986.
13. Bhattacharyya AK, Deshpande AR, Nayak SR, et al: Rhinocerebral mucormycosis: An unusual case presentation. J Laryngol Otol 106:48-49, 1992.
14. Sugar AM: Mucormycosis. Clin Infect Dis 14(Suppl 1):S126-S129, 1992.
15. De la Paz MA, Patrinely JR, Marines HM, Appling WD: Adjunctive hyperbaric oxygen in the treatment of bilateral cerebro-rhino-orbital mucormycosis. Am J Ophthalmol 114:208-211, 1992.
16. Batsakis JG, el-Naggar AK: Rhinoscleroma and rhinosporidiosis. Ann Otol Rhinol Laryngol 101:879-882, 1992.
17. Stiernberg CM, Clark WD: Rhinoscleroma: A diagnostic challenge. Laryngoscope 93:866-870, 1983.
18. Nayar RC, Mathur RP, Gulati A, Mann SB: Orbital apex syndrome due to rhinoscleroma: A case report. J Laryngol Otol 99:597-599, 1985.
19. Lubin JR, Jallow SE, Wilson WR, et al: Rhinoscleroma with exophthalmos: A case report. Br J Ophthalmol 65:14-17, 1981.
20. Meyer PR, Shum TK, Becker TS, Taylor CR: Scleroma (rhinoscleroma): A histologic immunohistochemical study with bacteriologic correlates. Arch Pathol Lab Med 107:377-383, 1983.
21. Gamea AM: Local rifampicin in treatment of rhinoscleroma. J Laryngol Otol 102:319-321, 1988.
22. Salit IE, McNeely DJ, Chait G: Invasive external otitis: Review of 12 cases. Can Med Assoc J 132:381-384, 1985.
23. Rubin J, Stoehr G, Yu VL, et al: Efficacy of oral ciprofloxacin plus rifampin for treatment of malignant external otitis (see comments). Arch Otolaryngol Head Neck Surg 115:1063-1069, 1989.
24. Babiatzki A, Sade J: Malignant external otitis. J Laryngol Otol 101:205-210, 1987.
25. Damiani JM, Damiani KK, Kinney SE: Malignant external otitis with multiple cranial nerve involvement. Am J Otol 1:115-120, 1979.
26. Mader JT, Love JT: Malignant external otitis: Cure with adjunctive hyperbaric oxygen therapy. Arch Otolaryngol 108:38-40, 1982.
27. Pavan PR, Aiello LM, Wafai MZ, et al: Optic disc edema in juvenile-onset diabetes. Arch Ophthalmol 98:2193-2195, 1980.
28. Katz B: Disc swelling in an adult diabetic patient. Surv Ophthalmol 35:158-163, 1990.
29. Barr CC, Glaser JS, Blankenship G: Acute disc swelling in juvenile diabetes: Clinical profile and natural history of 12 cases. Arch Ophthalmol 98:2185-2192, 1980.
30. Hayreh SS, Zahoruk RM: Anterior ischemic optic neuropathy: VI. In juvenile diabetics. Ophthalmologica 182:13-28, 1981.
31. Burde RM: Neuro-ophthalmic associations and complications of diabetes mellitus. Am J Ophthalmol 114:498-501, 1992.
32. Schwartz JS, Pavan PR: Optic disc edema. Int Ophthalmol Clin 24:83-91, 1984.
33. Watanabe K, Hagura R, Akanuma Y, et al: Characteristics of cranial nerve palsies in diabetic patients. Diabetes Res Clin Pract 10:19-27, 1990.
34. Rush JA: Extraocular muscle palsies in diabetes mellitus. Int Ophthalmol Clin 24:155-159, 1984.
35. Tuescher AU, Meienberg O: Ischaemic oculomotor nerve palsy: Clinical features and vascular risk factors in 23 patients. J Neurol 232:144-149, 1985.
36. Gilmore PC, Carlow TJ: Diabetic oculomotor paresis with pupil fixed to light. Neurology 30:1229-1230, 1980.
37. Naghmi R, Subuhi R: Diabetic oculomotor mononeuropathy: Involvement of pupillomotor fibers with slow resolution. Horm Metab Res 22:38-40, 1990.
38. Sergott RC, Glaser JS, Berger LJ: Simultaneous bilateral diabetic ophthalmoplegia: Report of two cases and discussion of differential diagnosis. Ophthalmology 91:18-22, 1984.
39. Rush JA, Younge BR: Paralysis of cranial nerves III, IV, and VI: Cause and prognosis in 1,000 cases. Arch Ophthalmol 99:76-79, 1981.

40. Schwartz DE: Corneal sensitivity in diabetics. Arch Ophthalmol 91:174–178, 1974.
41. Pecket P, Schattner A: Concurrent Bell's palsy and diabetes mellitus: A diabetic mononeuropathy? J Neurol Neurosurg Psychiatry 45:652–655, 1982.
42. Jabs DA, Miller NR, Green WR: Ischaemic optic neuropathy with painful ophthalmoplegia in diabetes mellitus. Br J Ophthalmol 65:673–678, 1981.
43. Luco CF, Valenzuela RF: Diabetic complete external ophthalmoplegia. J Clin Neuro Ophthalmol 10:206–209, 1990.
44. Tanabe Y, Miyamoto S, Kinoshita Y, et al: Diabetes mellitus in Kearns-Sayre syndrome. Eur Neurol 28:34–38, 1988.
45. Bastiaensen LA, Frenken CW, Ter Laak HJ, et al: Kearns syndrome: A heterogeneous group of disorders with CPEO, or a nosological entity? Doc Ophthalmol 52:207–225, 1982.
46. Najjar SS, Saikaly MG, Zaytoun GM, Abdelnoor A: Association of diabetes insipidus, diabetes mellitus, optic atrophy, and deafness: The Wolfram or DIDMOAD syndrome. Arch Dis Child 60:823–828, 1985.
47. Dreyer M, Rudiger HW, Bujara K, et al: The syndrome of diabetes insipidus, diabetes mellitus, optic atrophy, deafness, and other abnormalities (DIDMOAD syndrome): Two affected sibs and a short review of the literature (98 cases). Klin Wochenschr 60:471–475, 1982.
48. Carson MJ, Slager UT, Steinberg RM: Simultaneous occurrence of diabetes mellitus, diabetes insipidus, and optic atrophy in a brother and sister. Am J Dis Child 131:1382–1385, 1977.
49. Cremers CW, Wijdeveld PG, Pinckers AJ: Juvenile diabetes mellitus, optic atrophy, hearing loss, diabetes insipidus, atonia of the urinary tract and bladder, and other abnormalities (Wolfram syndrome): A review of 88 cases from the literature with personal observations on 3 new patients. Acta Paediatr Scand Suppl 264:1–16, 1977.
50. Huntley AC: Diabetes and the skin. J Am Acad Dermatol 7:427–455, 1982.
51. Muller SA, Winklemann RK: Necrobiosis lipoidica diabeticorum: A clinical and pathological investigation of 171 cases. Arch Dermatol 93:272–281, 1966.
52. Küta A, Sobkovä M: Diabetes mellitus, necrobiosis lipoidica and xanthelasma palpebrarum. Cesk Dermatol 42:95–99, 1967.
53. Schwartz ME: Necrobiosis lipoidica and granuloma annulare: Simultaneous occurrence in a patient. Arch Dermatol 118:192–193, 1982.
54. Muhlbauer JE: Granuloma annulare. J Am Acad Dermatol 3:217–230, 1980.
55. Coskey RJ: Facial granuloma annulare. Arch Dermatol 115: 866–868, 1979.
56. McFarland JP, Kauh YC, Luscombe HA: Periorbital granuloma annulare. Arch Dermatol 118:190–191, 1982.
57. Rao NA, Font RL: Pseudorheumatoid nodules of the ocular adnexa. Am J Ophthalmol 79:471–478, 1975.
58. Rendon MI, Cruz PJ, Sontheimer RD, Bergstresser PR: Acanthosis nigricans: A cutaneous marker of tissue resistance to insulin. J Am Acad Dermatol 21:461–469, 1989.
59. Matsuoka LY, Wortsman J, Gavin JR, Goldman J: Spectrum of endocrine abnormalities associated with acanthosis nigricans. Am J Med 83:719–725, 1987.
60. Breitbart AS, Eaton C, McCarthy JG: Crouzon's syndrome associated with acanthosis nigricans: Ramifications for the craniofacial surgeon. Ann Plast Surg 22:310–315, 1989.
61. Rogers DL: Acanthosis nigricans. Semin Dermatol 10:160–163, 1991.
62. Brown J, Winkelmann RK: Acanthosis nigricans: A study of 90 cases. Medicine 47:33–51, 1968.
63. Jaisankar TJ, Baruah MC, Garg BR: Vitiligo in children. Int J Dermatol 31:621–623, 1992.
64. Cowan CJ, Halder RM, Grimes PE, et al. Ocular disturbances in vitiligo. J Am Acad Dermatol 15:17–24, 1986.
65. Barsky S, Knapp DP, Levine M, Schuller GS: Vitiligo in a black population. Arch Dermatol 115:225, 1979.
66. Das SK, Majumder PP, Chakraborty R, et al: Studies on vitiligo: I. Epidemiological profile in Calcutta, India. Genet Epidemiol 2:71–78, 1985.
67. Macaron C, Winter RJ, Traisman HS, et al: Vitiligo and juvenile diabetes mellitus. Arch Dermatol 113:1515–1517, 1977.
68. Gould IM, Gray RS, Urbaniak SJ, et al: Vitiligo in diabetes mellitus. Br J Dermatol 113:153–155, 1985.
69. Bloch MH, Sowers JR: Vitiligo and polyglandular autoimmune endocrinopathy. Cutis 36:417–419, 1985.
70. Betterle C, Caretto A, De Zio A, et al: Incidence and significance of organ-specific autoimmune disorders (clinical, latent or only autoantibodies) in patients with vitiligo. Dermatologica 171: 419–423, 1985.
71. Grunnet I, Howitz J, Reymann F, Schwartz M: Vitiligo and pernicious anemia. Arch Dermatol 101:82–85, 1970.
72. Barnes L: Vitiligo and the Vogt-Koyanagi-Harada syndrome. Dermatol Clin 6:229–239, 1988.
73. Goudie RB, Spence JC, MacKie R: Vitiligo patterns simulating autoimmune and rheumatic diseases. Lancet 2:393–395, 1979.
74. Bystryn JC: Immune mechanisms in vitiligo. Immunol Ser 46:447–473, 1989.
75. Albert DM, Sober AJ, Fitzpatrick TB: Iritis in patients with cutaneous melanoma and vitiligo. Arch Ophthalmol 96:2081–2084, 1978.
76. Schallreuter KU, Levenig C, Berger J: Vitiligo and cutaneous melanoma: A case study. Dermatologica 183:239–245, 1991.
77. Albert DM, Nordlund JJ, Lerner AB: Ocular abnormalities occurring with vitiligo. Ophthalmology 86:1145–1160, 1979.
78. Wagoner MD, Albert DM, Lerner AB, et al: New observations on vitiligo and ocular disease. Am J Ophthalmol 96:16–26, 1983.
79. Albert DM, Wagoner MD, Pruett RC, et al: Vitiligo and disorders of the retinal pigment epithelium. Br J Ophthalmol 67:153–156, 1983.
80. Flint S, Scully C: Isolated trigeminal sensory neuropathy: A heterogeneous group of disorders. Oral Surg Oral Med Oral Pathol 69:153–156, 1990.
81. Morohashi M, Hashimoto K, Goodman TF Jr, et al: Ultrastructural studies of vitiligo, Vogt-Koyanagi syndrome, and incontinentia pigmenti achromians. Arch Dermatol 113:755–766, 1977.
82. Antoniou C, Katsambas A: Guidelines for the treatment of vitiligo. Drugs 43:490–498, 1992.
83. Prystowsky JH, Keen MS, Rabinowitz AD, et al: Present status of eyelid phototherapy: Clinical efficacy and transmittance of ultraviolet and visible radiation through human eyelids. J Am Acad Dermatol 26:607–613, 1992.
84. Goldstein E, Haberman HF, Menon IA, Pawlowski D: Non-psoralen treatment of vitiligo: I. Cosmetics, systemic coloring agents, and corticosteroids. Int J Dermatol 31:229–236, 1992.
85. Goldstein E, Haberman HF, Menon IA, Pawlowski D: Non-psoralen treatment of vitiligo: II. Less commonly used and experimental therapies. Int J Dermatol 31:314–319, 1992.
86. Parker F: Xanthomas and hyperlipidemias. J Am Acad Dermatol 13:1–30, 1985.
87. Alexander LJ: Ocular signs and symptoms of altered blood lipids. J Am Optom Assoc 54:123–126, 1983.
88. Winder AF, Dodson PM, Galton DJ: Ophthalmological complications of the hypertriglyceridaemias. Trans Ophthalmol Soc UK 100:119–122, 1980.
89. Winder AF: Factors influencing the variable expression of xanthelasmata and corneal arcus in familial hypercholesterolaemia. Birth Defects 18:449–462, 1982.
90. Vermeer BJ, Poland MK: A case of xanthomatosis and hyperlipoproteinemia type V probably induced by overdosage of insulin. Dermatologica 151:43–50, 1975.
91. Matsuzawa Y, Yamashita S, Funahashi T, et al: Selective reduction of cholesterol in HDL2 fraction by probucol in familial hypercholesterolemia and hyperHDL2 cholesterolemia with abnormal cholesteryl ester transfer. Am J Cardiol 62:66B–72B, 1988.
92. Lascari AD: Carotenemia: A review. Clin Pediatr 20:25–29, 1981.
93. Hoerer E, Dreyfuss F, Herzberg M: Carotenemic, skin colour and diabetes mellitus. Acta Diabetol Lat 12:202–207, 1975.
94. Stawiski MA, Voorhees JJ: Cutaneous signs of diabetes mellitus. Cutis 18:415–421, 1976.
95. Holland HK, Spivak JL: Hemochromatosis. Med Clin North Am 73:831–845, 1989.
96. McLaren GD, Muir WA, Kellermeyer RW: Iron overload disorders: Natural history, pathogenesis, diagnosis, and therapy. Crit Rev Clin Lab Sci 19:205–266, 1983.

97. Milder MS, Cook JD, Stray S, Finch CA: Idiopathic hemochromatosis, an interim report. Medicine 59:34–49, 1980.
98. Nichols GM, Bacon BR: Hereditary hemochromatosis: Pathogenesis and clinical features of a common disease. Am J Gastroenterol 84:851–862, 1989.
99. Lamon JM, Marynick SP, Roseblatt R, Donnelly S: Idiopathic hemochromatosis in a young female: A case study and review of the syndrome in young people. Gastroenterology 76:178–183, 1979.
100. Phelps G, Chapman I, Hall P, et al: Prevalence of genetic haemochromatosis among diabetic patients. Lancet 2:233–234, 1989.
101. Singh BM, Grunewald RA, Press M, et al: Prevalence of haemochromatosis amongst patients with diabetes mellitus. Diabet Med 9:730–731, 1992.
102. Walton C, Kelly WF, Laing I, Bullock DE: Endocrine abnormalities in idiopathic haemochromatosis. Q J Med 52:99–110, 1983.
103. Niederau C, Fischer R, Sonnenberg A, et al: Survival and causes of death in cirrhotic and in noncirrhotic patients with primary hemochromatosis. N Engl J Med 313:1256–1262, 1985.
104. Hershko C, Pinson A, Link G: Iron chelation. Blood Rev 4:1–8, 1990.
105. Davenport J, Kellerman C, Reiss D, Harrison L: Addison's disease. Am Fam Physician 43:1338–1342, 1991.
106. Kannan CR: Diseases of the adrenal cortex. Dis Mon 34:601–674, 1988.
107. Muir A, Maclaren NK: Autoimmune diseases of the adrenal glands, parathyroid glands, gonads, and hypothalamic-pituitary axis. Endocrinol Metab Clin North Am 20:619–644, 1991.
108. Bigazzi PE: Autoimmunity in diabetes mellitus and polyendocrine syndromes: Current concepts of pathogenesis and etiology. Immunol Ser 52:295–322, 1990.
109. Burke CW: Adrenocortical insufficiency. Clin Endocrinol Metab 14:947–976, 1985.
110. Feingold KR, Elias PM: Endocrine-skin interactions: Cutaneous manifestations of adrenal disease, pheochromocytomas, carcinoid syndrome, sex hormone excess and deficiency, polyglandular autoimmune syndromes, multiple endocrine neoplasia syndromes, and other miscellaneous disorders. J Am Acad Dermatol 19:1–20, 1988.
111. Leshin M: Polyglandular autoimmune syndromes. Am J Med Sci 290:77–88, 1985.
112. Neufeld M, Maclaren NK, Blizzard RM: Two types of autoimmune Addison's disease associated with different polyglandular autoimmune (PGA) syndromes. Medicine 60:355–362, 1981.
113. Butler MG, Hodes ME, Conneally PM, et al: Linkage analysis in a large kindred with autosomal dominant transmission of polyglandular autoimmune disease type II (Schmidt syndrome). Am J Med Genet 18:61–65, 1984.
114. Medeiros LJ, Wolf BC, Balogh K, Federman M: Adrenal pheochromocytoma: A clinicopathologic review of 60 cases. Hum Pathol 16:580–589, 1985.
115. Ram CV: Pheochromocytoma. Cardiol Clin 6:517–535, 1988.
116. Schimke RN: Multiple endocrine neoplasia: How many syndromes? Am J Med Genet 37:375–383, 1990.
117. Riccardi VM: Neurofibromatosis update. Neurofibromatosis 2:284–291, 1989.
118. Martz CH: Von Hippel-Lindau disease: A genetically transmitted multisystem neoplastic disorder. Semin Oncol Nurs 8:281–287, 1992.
119. Sheps SG, Jiang NS, Klee GG, van Heerden JA: Recent developments in the diagnosis and treatment of pheochromocytoma. Mayo Clin Proc 65:88–95, 1990.
120. Cryer PE: Phaeochromocytoma. Clin Endocrinol Metab 14:203–220, 1985.
121. Rosano TG, Swift TA, Hayes LW: Advances in catecholamine and metabolite measurements for diagnosis of pheochromocytoma. Clin Chem 37:1854–1867, 1991.
122. Eckfeldt JH, Engelman K: Diagnosis of pheochromocytoma. Clin Lab Med 4:703–716, 1984.
123. Levine SN, McDonald JC: The evaluation and management of pheochromocytomas. Adv Surg 17:281–313, 1984.
124. Shapiro B, Gross MD: Endocrine crises: Pheochromocytoma. Crit Care Clin 7:1–21, 1991.
125. Dow CJ, Palmer MK, O'Sullivan JP, Kirkham JS: Malignant phaeochromocytoma: Report of a case and a critical review. Br J Surg 69:338–340, 1982.
126. Caruso DR, O'Dorisio TM, Mazzaferri EL: Multiple endocrine neoplasia. Curr Opin Oncol 2:108–116, 1990.
127. Caruso DR, O'Dorisio TM, Mazzaferri EL: Multiple endocrine neoplasia. Curr Opin Oncol 3:103–108, 1991.
128. Schimke RN: Genetic aspects of multiple endocrine neoplasia. Annu Rev Med 35:25–31, 1984.
129. Schimke RN: Multiple endocrine adenomatosis syndromes. Adv Intern Med 21:249–265, 1976.
130. Brandi ML: Multiple endocrine neoplasia type I: General features and new insights into etiology. J Endocrinol Invest 14:61–72, 1991.
131. Gorlin RJ, Vickers RA: Multiple mucosal neuromas, pheochromocytoma, medullary carcinoma of the thyroid and marfanoid body build with muscle wasting: Reexamination of a syndrome of neural crest malmigration. Birth Defects 7:69–72, 1971.
132. Carney JA, Sizemore GW, Hayles AB: Multiple endocrine neoplasia, type 2b. Pathobiol Annu 8:105–153, 1978.
133. Chang DB, Jackson IM: Diagnosis and endocrine testing in acromegaly. Endocrinol Metab Clin North Am 21:649–668, 1992.
134. Melmed S: Etiology of pituitary acromegaly. Endocrinol Metab Clin North Am 21:539–551, 1992.
135. Faglia G, Arosio M, Bazzoni N: Ectopic acromegaly. Endocrinol Metab Clin North Am 21:575–595, 1992.
136. Melmed S: Extrapituitary acromegaly. Endocrinol Metab Clin North Am 20:507–518, 1991.
137. Molitch ME: Clinical manifestations of acromegaly. Endocrinol Metab Clin North Am 21:597–614, 1992.
138. Nabarro JD: Acromegaly. Clin Endocrinol 26:481–512, 1987.
139. Kupcha PC, Guille JT, Tassanawipas A, Bowen JR: Polyostotic fibrous dysplasia and acromegaly. J Pediatr Orthop 11:95–99, 1991.
140. Woo CC: Neurological features of acromegaly: A review and report of two cases. J Manipulative Physiol Ther 11:314–321, 1988.
141. Baumann G: Acromegaly. Endocrinol Metab Clin North Am 16:685–703, 1987.
142. Fahlbusch R, Honegger J, Buchfelder M: Surgical management of acromegaly. Endocrinol Metab Clin North Am 21:669–692, 1992.
143. Barkan AL: Acromegaly: Diagnosis and therapy. Endocrinol Metab Clin North Am 18:277–310, 1989.
144. Sassolas G: The role of Sandostatin in acromegaly. Metabolism 4:39–43, 1992.
145. Sachdev Y, Gopal K, Garg VK: Bromocriptine therapy in acromegaly: A long-term review of 35 cases. Postgrad Med J 57:210–216, 1981.
146. Mauras N, Blizzard RM: The McCune-Albright syndrome. Acta Endocrinol Suppl 279:207–217, 1986.
147. Johns WD, Gupta SM, Kayani N: Scintigraphic evaluation of polyostotic fibrous dysplasia. Clin Nucl Med 12:627–631, 1987.
148. Machida K, Makita K, Nishikawa J, et al: Scintigraphic manifestation of fibrous dysplasia. Clin Nucl Med 11:426–429, 1986.
149. Hjelmstedt A, Ljunghall S: A case of Albright's syndrome treated with calcitonin. Acta Orthop Scand 50:251–253, 1979.
150. Lee PA, Van DC, Migeon CJ: McCune-Albright syndrome: Long-term follow-up. JAMA 256:2980–2984, 1986.
151. Harris RI: Polyostotic fibrous dysplasia with acromegaly. Am J Med 78:539–542, 1985.
152. Lipson A, Hsu TH: The Albright syndrome associated with acromegaly: Report of a case and review of the literature. Johns Hopkins Med J 149:10–14, 1981.
153. Dohler JR, Hughes SP: Fibrous dysplasia of bone and the Weil-Albright syndrome: A study of thirteen cases with special reference to the orthopaedic treatment. Int Orthop 10:53–62, 1986.
154. Moore AT, Buncic JR, Munro IR: Fibrous dysplasia of the orbit in childhood: Clinical features and management. Ophthalmology 92:12–20, 1985.

CHAPTER 8

Infections of the Orbit and Orbital Structures

Phillip F. Pierce

This chapter reviews infections of the orbit and orbital structures, with emphasis on the epidemiologic, diagnostic, and therapeutic differentiation of orbital from periorbital cellulitis. Posterior globe infections often imitate orbital tumors. The recent literature of hydatid disease, cysticercosis, and tuberculosis is detailed. Neurologic complications of systemic infections such as polio and tetanus are compared in their manifestations of ocular muscle palsies. The complications of varicella zoster are specified. Additionally, miscellaneous structural abnormalities such as periorbital edema are detailed, and causes of infectious dacryoadenitis are reviewed. In the final section, trachoma, the major cause of blindness in the world, is analyzed.

PERIORBITAL AND ORBITAL CELLULITIS

Spreading inflammatory processes involving the eyelids and deeper orbital structures can be broadly divided into periorbital (preseptal) and orbital (postseptal) cellulitis. The anatomic basis of this distinction can be seen in Figure 8 – 1. The orbital septum is fascia that acts as an anatomic barrier between the soft tissues of the lids and the orbital contents. Infections involving the preseptal region result in lid edema but no impairment of visual acuity or gaze restriction. The latter are present when orbital structures are involved; chemosis and proptosis are additional findings of postseptal orbital cellulitis. Predisposing factors, bacteriology, and treatment all differ for these conditions. A classification of orbital inflammation by Smith and Spencer,[1] subsequently modified by Chandler,[2] clarifies this complex area (Table 8 – 1).

Periorbital inflammation may arise from local trauma or secondary to localized infection. *Staphylococcus aureus* or group A streptococci is the major pathogen in this setting. Patients with this condition do not have proptosis, pain on eye movement, or external ophthalmoplegia. Specific systemic diseases, such as trichinosis and mononucleosis, have been associated with periorbital edema rather than inflammation.

Orbital cellulitis (group II) most commonly occurs in the setting of sinusitis or trauma. In Jackson and associates' 1986 series,[3] sinusitis was the predisposing factor in 64% of patients; 89% of these patients had maxillary sinus involvement. In addition to direct trauma, dental extraction is a frequent predisposing factor.

The signs and symptoms of inflammation due to orbital cellulitis, based on Jackson and associates' experience with 39 patients, are displayed in Table 8 – 2. Figure 8 – 2 demonstrates the typical appearance of a child with preseptal cellulitis, whereas Figure 8 – 3 shows chemosis and proptosis in postseptal cellulitis. Clinically, abscesses manifest with similar but more severe symptoms, such as exophthalmos, chemosis, and decreased visual acuity, than does orbital cellulitis.

Bacteriology

Bacterial causes of orbital cellulitis are similar to those bacterial causes of sinusitis: *S. aureus, Streptococcus pneumoniae,* hemolytic streptococcus, and *Haemophilus influenzae.* Because of the deep structures involved, isolates are frequently not obtained until after broad-spectrum antibiotic therapy has been initiated.

Periorbital and orbital cellulitis in children have several distinct features compared with those in adults. Periorbital cellulitis occurred 10-fold more frequently than orbital cellulitis in Israele and Nelson's[4] review of 10 years of hospital admissions. Periorbital cellulitis was related to an upper respiratory tract infection (20%), otitis media (18%), and skin infections or trauma (24%). It was related to sinusitis in only 13%. Orbital cellulitis in the pediatric group was similar to that in adults in that 75% were secondary to sinusitis. Periorbital cellulitis in pediatric patients is most often caused by *H. influenzae,* whereas, like in adults, *Staphylococcus* and *Streptococcus* are the predominant pathogens (80%) in orbital cellulitis. *Haemophilus* rates may decline with the advent of *H. influenzae* vaccine as they have for pediatric meningitis. *Haemophilus* is rarely a pathogen after age 5.

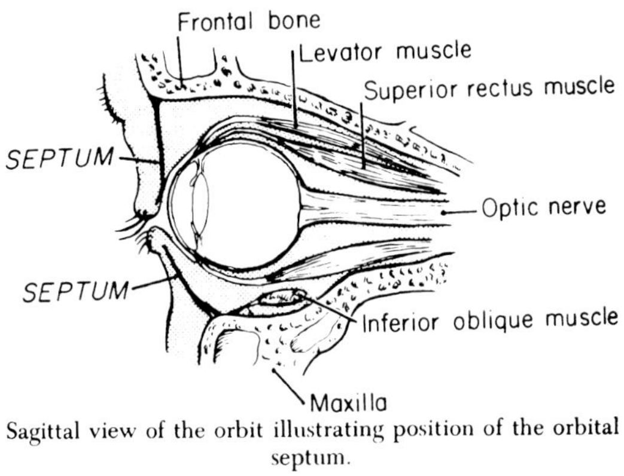

Figure 8–1. Anatomy of the orbit. (Reproduced by Permission of *PEDIATRICS*, Vol 62, Page 1006, Copyright 1978.)

TABLE 8–2

Presenting Signs and Symptoms of Orbital Cellulitis

Signs and Symptoms	Prevalence No.	Prevalence Percentage
Periorbital swelling	37/39	95
Periorbital edema	37/39	95
Proptosis	33/37	89
Orbital pain	30/35	85
Limitation of globe movement	27/37	73
Chemosis	24/37	65
Leukocytosis (>10,000/mm^3)	23/36	64
Radiographs suggestive of sinusitis	22/36	61
Visual disturbance	17/30	56
Nasal discharge	13/39	33
Abnormal retina	8/32	25
Eye discharge	9/39	23
Fever (100.5°F or greater)	9/38	23
Abnormal pupil	9/38	23
Decreased visual acuity	7/34	20

From Jackson K, Baker SR: Clinical implications of orbital cellulitis. Laryngoscope 96:568–574, 1986.

Hematogenous dissemination of bacteria to the orbit from distant body sites represents a small percentage of cases but is an important consideration in the pathogenesis of orbital cellulitis. Uncommon causes, such as fungi and protozoa, are reviewed at the end of this chapter.

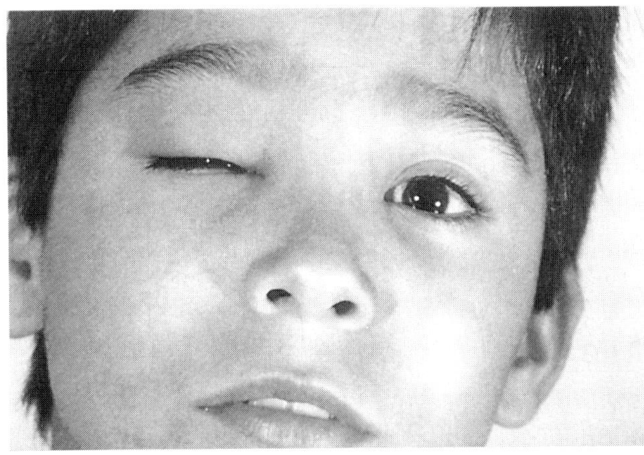

Figure 8–2. Preseptal cellulitis. (From Infectious Disease News, May 1992, p 10.)

Radiographic Diagnosis

Computed tomographic (CT) scanning has truly advanced the diagnostic and therapeutic evaluation of orbital inflammation. Not only are contiguous structures clearly visualized but the more advanced stages of inflammation, particularly orbital abscess, are detectable.

All patients with orbital cellulitis should have a sinus radiograph performed to evaluate the sinuses as the potential source of the cellulitis. Although the sphenoid sinus is the least common sinus to be involved as the site of origin of orbital cellulitis, it may be undetected in 15% of patients.[5]

Although medical therapy is often adequate for group II orbital inflammation (orbital cellulitis), subperiosteal abscess and orbital abscesses require surgical drainage. Because the signs and symptoms most consistent with an abscess—proptosis, chemosis, and visual loss—overlap between these entities, CT scanning has become a routine part of the evaluation. Contrast enhancement assists the differentiation between orbital cellulitis and abscess.[6]

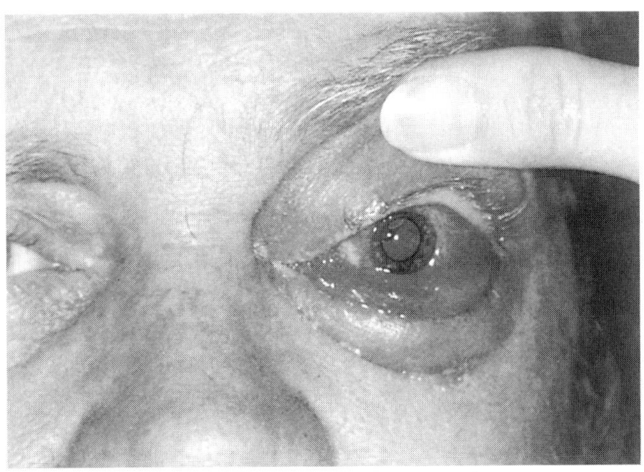

Figure 8–3. Postseptal cellulitis. (From Sinnot JT, IV, Rodnite JA, Ruland RT: What is it? Is this orbital or periorbital cellulitis? Postgrad Med 85:267–269, 1989.)

TABLE 8–1

Orbital Inflammation

Group	Characteristics
I	Inflammatory edema
II	Orbital cellulitis
III	Subperiosteal abscess
IV	Orbital abscess
V	Cavernous sinus thrombosis

In orbital cellulitis the normal fat shadows are lost. Abscess can be demonstrated as discrete lesions that enhance. Not all authors have advocated the use of intravenous contrast medium for this purpose.[7]

The adequacy of CT scanning to guide therapeutic decisions has also been questioned.[8, 9] The diagnostic yield can be improved by adding coronal sections to axial views, particularly in patients with subperiosteal abscess.[10] Surgical intervention is recommended for groups III, IV, and V orbital infections as well as for those patients with orbital infection who do not improve within 48 hours after the institution of appropriate antibiotics.

Orbital abscess and cellulitis should be viewed as a continuum in a spectrum of organization of inflammation: Orbital cellulitis occurs relatively early and is analogous to a phlegmon in a closed space, whereas an abscess has discrete borders. Serial CT scanning assists the clinician in observing this evolution and in timing surgical intervention such as the drainage of an orbital abscess. Surgical intervention is also indicated for the absence of improvement after 48 hours of intense antibiotic therapy.

Representative CT scans are shown in Figures 8–4 and 8–5.

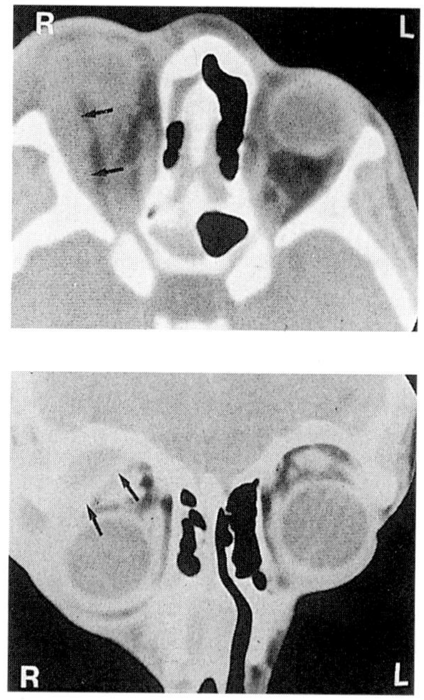

Figure 8–5. Computed tomographic image of a subperiosteal abscess in a child with ethmoiditis. Coronal section *(bottom)* demonstrates abscess more clearly. (From Langham-Brown JJ, Rhys-Williams S: Computed tomography of acute orbital infection: The importance of coronal sections. Clin Radiol 40:472, 1989.)

Medical Management

Antibiotic therapy is directed at the four major pathogens: *S. aureus,* group A streptococci, *S. pneumoniae,* and *Haemophilus.* Empirical therapy to encompass these pathogens includes (1) a second-generation cephalosporin or ticarcillin disodium combined with clavulanate potassium (Timentin) monotherapy or (2) combination therapy of vancomycin for gram-positive cocci and a second- or third-generation cephalosporin for *Haemophilus.* Blood culture studies should be obtained before therapy is instituted. Abscesses should be drained surgically, and Gram's stain and culture should be performed on the drainage material. Sinus drainage should be considered in those patients in whom extension from the maxillary or ethmoid sinuses was the primary site of infection.

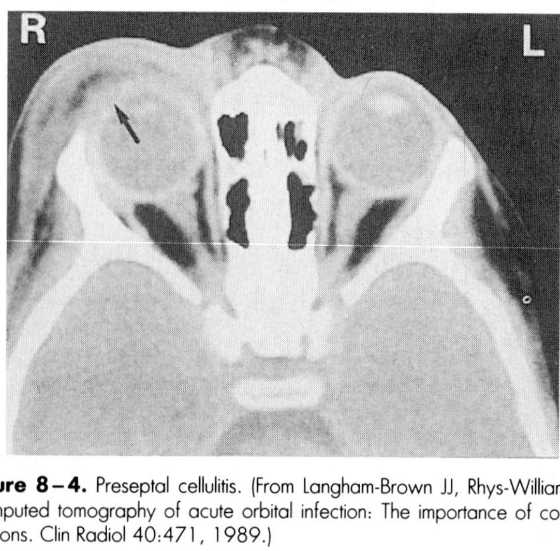

Figure 8–4. Preseptal cellulitis. (From Langham-Brown JJ, Rhys-Williams S: Computed tomography of acute orbital infection: The importance of coronal sections. Clin Radiol 40:471, 1989.)

Complications

Serious complications may accompany orbital inflammation. Because venous drainage of the orbit is to the cavernous sinus, extension of infection into this venous channel may result in cavernous sinus thrombosis. Meningitis and brain abscess have been reported to occur not infrequently. Eye complications include decreased vision, optic atrophy, and keratitis. Blindness occurred in 20% of patients with postseptal inflammation before antibiotic therapy.[11] Patt and Manning[11] reported an incidence of 10.5% in 1991; none of the patients had a discrete abscess on CT scan. Visual loss may be related to pressure ischemia of the central retinal artery, ischemia secondary to thrombophlebitis, or optic neuritis.

Orbital apex syndrome is characterized by ptosis, proptosis, complete internal and external ophthalmoplegia, neuralgia of the ophthalmic division of the trigeminal nerve, and visual loss. Anatomically, this syndrome involves the cone of the orbit where the optic nerve and the retinal artery as well as the orbital muscles can be insulted simultaneously. Orbital cellulitis with abscess, mucormycosis, *Aspergillus* infections, and syphilis are the infectious conditions causing orbital apex syndrome.

Presently, the case fatality rate of orbital cellulitis is 2%, and the rate for periorbital cellulitis is 0.2%.

OCULOGLANDULAR DISEASE

Localized conjunctival inflammation associated with regional lymph nodes, such as the preauricular nodes, is termed *oculoglandular disease.* The two most common conditions causing oculoglandular disease in the United States are cat-scratch disease and tularemia. Rare additional causes are tuberculosis, syphilis, and lymphogranuloma venereum.

Cat-Scratch Disease

Oculoglandular involvement attributed to the cat-scratch bacillus was originally described in 1889. The condition has been termed *Parinaud's syndrome,* or *oculoglandular syndrome of Parinaud,* after the author of the original article. Subsequent reports, particularly that of Carithers,[12] have provided clarification of the frequency and presenting manifestations of this entity. In Carithers' series of 585 patients with cat-scratch disease, 14 had oculoglandular disease.[12] All the patients in Carithers' series were children or adolescents who had contact with cats or kittens. Rather than direct inoculation, such as with a scratch, indirect inoculation of the palpebral conjunctiva by the hands of the patient following cat contact is the proposed mode of transmission. Moriarty and Margileth reported the conjunctiva as the primary inoculation site in 7% of patients in their series.[13] A maculopapular lesion, generally smaller than 1 cm in diameter, develops on the conjunctiva 1 week after inoculation, and regional adenopathy develops 5 to 10 days later. Suppuration occurs in 15% of the conjunctival papules; lymphadenopathy developing over weeks to months is typical. Conjunctival discharge, either mucoid or purulent, is atypical. Generally, patients are not systemically ill.

Criteria for the diagnosis in the past have been (1) lymphadenopathy, (2) intimate cat exposure, (3) the presence of an inoculation site on an eye structure, and (4) a positive skin test to cat-scratch antigen of known potency.[12] Recent developments have modified the diagnostic approach. The skin test antigen has never been generally available. Although no instances of adverse reactions have been reported, concerns of possible transmission of blood-borne pathogens have particularly limited wider distribution. A gram-negative bacillus has been identified in tissue section in lymph nodes[14] and in conjunctival biopsy specimens[15] using Warthin-Starry silver impregnation stain. Although biopsies are not indicated in typical cases, the stain should be applied to all material that is ultimately pathologically examined. Suggestive histology has features of lymphoid hyperplasia, granulomas, and microabscesses.

Intense investigation into identifying the specific bacterial origin of cat-scratch disease has followed the histopathologic description of a bacteria in tissue. Using polymerase chain reaction studies and serologic responses, a *Rochalimaea* sp. has been implicated as the causative organism.[16] *Rochalimaea* sp. is a rickettsial-like organism that has also been recently linked to bacillary angiomatosis and peliosis hepatis. Alternative bacterial agents have also been proposed.[17] Antibiotic therapy has been attempted, especially since a bacterial cause has been confirmed, but has not been consistently successful.

Cat-scratch disease has been infrequently associated with nonorbital ophthalmologic signs, including optic neuritis and neuroretinitis.[18]

Tularemia

The oculoglandular form of tularemia differs dramatically from that described earlier for cat-scratch disease. Tularemia is caused by *Francisella tularensis,* a gram-negative coccobacillus. It is an arthropod-borne disease principally affecting rodents. Cases are reported throughout the United States but principally in the East and southwest central states.

Human cases may result from direct inoculation of tularemia by a tick or through aerosolization or direct contact with an infected mammal. Rabbits are the most common animal associated with tissue transmission to humans, although 100 different mammals have been found to be infected with tularemia. Eye involvement results from inoculation of the conjunctiva during the process of wild mammal skinning or evisceration.

Clinically, patients have unilateral purulent conjunctivitis associated with preauricular or cervical adenopathy. The conjunctivitis is painful. Initially, small nodular lesions are present at the site of inoculation in the palpebral conjunctiva; these lesions subsequently ulcerate.

Generally, the diagnosis is made clinically with the history of animal exposure and the findings described earlier. Isolation on routine bacteriologic media is not possible, but the organism does grow on specialized media, such as chocolate agar supplemented with cystine or cysteine. A microagglutination serology test that becomes positive during the second or third week of symptoms is available.

Oculoglandular tularemia represents only 1% or 2% of all cases of tularemia in the United States. Treatment is with intramuscular streptomycin. Alternative therapeutic choices include gentamicin, tetracycline, and chloramphenicol.

INFECTIOUS CAUSES OF NODULAR ERUPTIONS OF THE LIDS AND SURROUNDING STRUCTURES

A wide variety of infectious organisms may involve the lids or adjacent structures. Although these organisms have no predilection for the eye, infection may be limited to these areas. These infections generally present as small nodules, although they may be plaques. The infections considered in this section are sporotrichosis and leishmaniasis and those due to *Nocardia* and atypical mycobacteria (*Mycobacterium kansasii* and *Mycobacterium marinum*).

The patient's exposure history is important in differentiating these entities. Sporotrichosis occurs most typically after contact with thorny plants such as roses, and sphagnum moss. Facial involvement occurs most often in children. The initial lesion, a red, painless papule, appears at the site of inoculation after an incubation period of 1 to 12 weeks. Ulceration may occur. Frequently, new lesions develop along the lymphatics, giving rise to lymphocutaneous sporotrichosis. The organism may be isolated from the exudate, but biopsy with culture and histology is most often necessary. Figure 8–6 illustrates sporotrichosis involving the upper lid.

Leishmaniasis is rarely acquired in the United States; cases have been reported from Texas. Endemic geographic areas are Central and South America and the Middle East. A small erythematous papule appears 2 to 8 weeks following the bite of the vector, the sandfly. This papule may ulcerate, leaving a raised border with a granulating base. The organism can be seen on biopsy and, in experienced hands, cultivated. Pentavalent antimonials are the treatment of choice.

When facial involvement occurs, the conjunctiva is often affected and presents as a granular or papilliform conjunctivitis. As the facial lesions (including those involving the eyelids) become more chronic, they may evolve into papular, verrucous, or ulcerative lesions. Multiple lesions of the face are common. Leishmanial infections are usually self-limited after 6 months to 1 year. A depressed scar, termed the *Oriental sore*, is a manifestation of previous infection.

Diffuse cutaneous leishmaniasis (DCL) (Fig. 8–7) is a chronic form of leishmanial infection that develops in patients with inadequate cell-mediated immune response to the organism. DCL is recognized by the redundant nodules that progressively spread across the face and the extremities. Eyelid involvement is common.

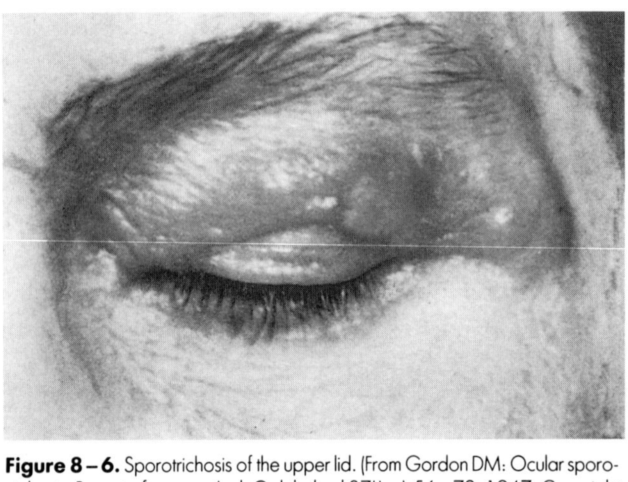

Figure 8–6. Sporotrichosis of the upper lid. (From Gordon DM: Ocular sporotrichosis: Report of a case. Arch Ophthalmol 37(Jan):56–72, 1947; Copyright 1947, American Medical Association.)

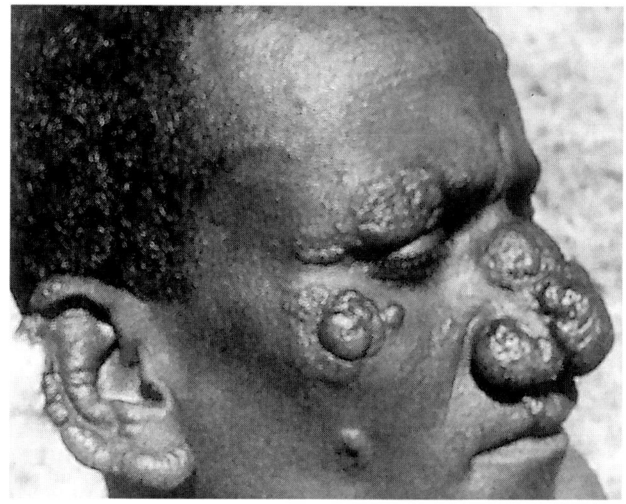

Figure 8–7. Diffuse cutaneous leishmaniasis. Note the eyelid and ear involvement. (From Manson-Bahr PEC, Bell DR: Manson's Tropical Diseases, 19th ed. London, Baillière Tindall, 1987, p 733.)

Cutaneous nocardial infection is an exceptional presentation of this respiratory tract pathogen. Because the organism is a soil saprophyte, direct inoculation is the probable pathogenicity.

Atypical mycobacteria may involve the skin. *M. marinum* typically involves the upper extremities as a result of inoculation during fish tank cleaning. The lesions are lymphocutaneous nodules. *M. kansasii* likewise can form similar sporotrichoid nodules.

MISCELLANEOUS CAUSES OF ORBITAL CELLULITIS, EXOPHTHALMOS, AND LID EDEMA

Atypical organisms may cause orbital cellulitis. These cases often arise in immunocompromised patients (*Mucor* infection, aspergillosis) or in people from areas of the world with endemic exotic diseases (hydatid cyst, cysticercosis).

Mucormycosis

Rhinocerebral mucormycosis occurs most typically in diabetic patients (80%) but complicates the course of immunosuppressed patients and those with burns. It occurs rarely in normal hosts. This infection is caused by fungi in the class Phycomycetes. The principal genera causing infection in humans are *Rhizopus, Mucor,* and *Absidia.* Orbital infection occurs by direct extension from the sinuses. Eye involvement is often dramatic, with rapid evolution from proptosis to visual loss. This is related to the rapid growth of this fungi and its propensity to invade blood vessels. Schwarz and colleagues[19] reported visual loss in 50% of patients with mucormycosis, but only 10% had ocular invasion. Optic nerve ischemia may account for visual loss.

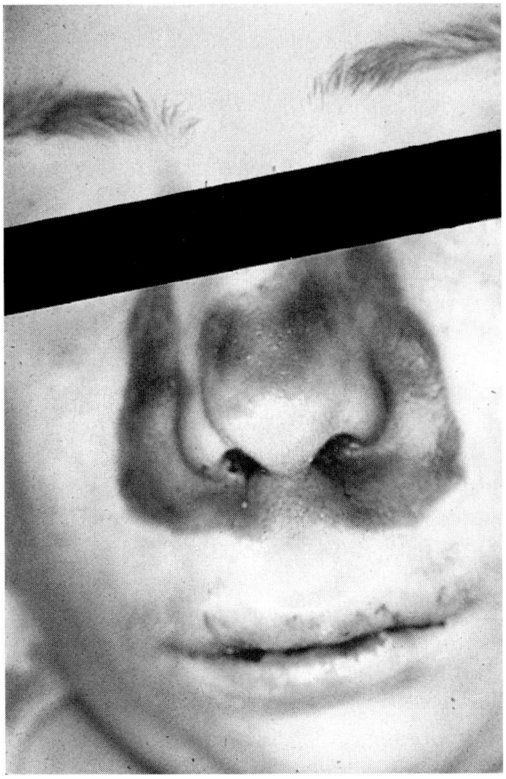

Figure 8–8. Rhinocerebral mucormycosis in a leukemic child.

Periocular disease occasionally is the dominant feature.[20] Generally, symptoms begin as sinusitis or rhinitis and progress to headache and facial pain. Tissue infarction by invasion of blood vessels occurs early and rapidly progresses, distinguishing this entity from other infections. Nasal involvement is manifested by necrotic turbinates; palatal ulcers that perforate are seen in the mouth (Fig. 8–8). Sinus involvement presents with pain and edema.

Proptosis and ophthalmoplegia are the cardinal ophthalmologic findings.[21]

Ocular invasion implies advanced disease. Aggressive therapy including surgery and amphotericin has improved the overall survival rate to 50%; however, rare survivors of ocular invasion have been recorded.[22]

Hydatid Cyst

Hydatid cysts are caused by *Echinococcus,* a tapeworm whose natural host is the dog. Humans are incidental hosts following ingestion of eggs that subsequently form oncospheres and penetrate the gut, ultimately encysting throughout the body. The liver and lung are the principal organs involved with echinococcal cysts, which present as mass lesions with compression of surrounding tissues. The orbit is involved in 1% of all patients and presents as unilateral exophthalmos that must be differentiated from an orbital tumor. In Morales'[23] series of 35 patients from Argentina, the median age was 16 years. The young age at presentation was related to the closed space of the orbit compared with the liver and lungs, where cystic growth of 1 cm per year may be unappreciated for many years—symptoms evolve over months to years. Visual acuity was reduced in most patients, and impairment of extraocular muscles was common.

Ultrasonographic or CT scan demonstrates a cystic lesion. Operative intervention generally results in substantial decrease in proptosis and improvement in visual acuity.

Cysticercosis

Cysticercosis, a disease caused by the larva of the pork tapeworm, is well recognized for its capacity to establish itself at body sites distant from the intestine. Oncospheres penetrate the gut wall following the ingestion of *Taenia solium* eggs and encyst throughout the body, principally in muscle. Central nervous system involvement is common, with seizures as the typical clinical manifestation.

Ophthalmic complications most commonly involve the globe. Orbital cysticercosis is relatively rare and typically presents as proptosis and extraocular muscle palsy. Symptoms generally evolve over 4 to 8 weeks. Cyst-like lesions can be defined by using ultrasonographic or imaging techniques other than plain radiography.[24] This appearance is helpful in differentiating cysticercosis from an orbital pseudotumor. Surgical excision is the appropriate therapeutic approach. Cysticercosis is particularly endemic in India and Central America.

PERIORBITAL EDEMA

Infectious causes of periorbital edema include mononucleosis, mumps, and trichinosis. Unilateral periorbital edema is seen in Chagas' disease following transmission by the reduviid bug. There is generally little difficulty distinguishing between these entities. Mononucleosis is manifested by generalized lymphadenopathy and exudative pharyngitis. Atypical lymphocytes are found in the peripheral smear and serologic tests (heterophil or Epstein-Barr viral titers) are positive. Although 50% of patient with mononucleosis may have periorbital edema, periorbital edema may occasionally be present before any other symptoms develop.[25]

Trichinella spiralis, a tissue nematode that encysts in muscles, causes bilateral periorbital edema during the acute phase. Eye movement is painful, probably as a result of ocular muscle involvement. Generalized muscle tenderness and splinter hemorrhages are present, and creatine phosphokinase levels are elevated. Eosinophilia is typically present. A history of ingestion of undercooked pork or bear meat is helpful. Supportive care is sufficient therapy, although corticosteroids may be useful in patients with severe infection.

The unilateral periorbital edema of Chagas' disease, termed *Romaña's sign,* results from invasion of the protozoa *Trypanosoma cruzi* into the skin adjacent to the eye or through the conjunctiva. *T. cruzi* is transported by the reduviid bug, which passes this parasite in its feces. The periorbital edema is the initial manifestation of an illness characterized by fever, malaise, and occasional generalized lymphadenopathy and hepatosplenomegaly. The endemic area for Chagas' disease is Central and South America. Fewer than five acute cases have been recognized in the United States.[26]

PARESIS INVOLVING THE ORBITAL NERVES

Infectious diseases occasionally result in neurologic sequelae. Paresis of cranial nerves is commonly seen in botulism, polio, and rabies.

Botulism, caused by the toxins of *Clostridium botulinum,* generally occurs following ingestion of home-canned foods. Neurologic symptoms dominate the presentation, and the cranial nerves are usually involved first. Diplopia, blurred vision, and photophobia are commonly the presenting neurologic complaints. Symmetric cranial nerve abnormalities, including dilated, unreactive pupils, postural hypotension, dry mucous membranes, and descending paralysis, are cardinal manifestations. Patients are afebrile.

Polio contrasts with botulism by the typical presence of fever before the onset of paralysis. Meningeal signs such as frequent headache and neck stiffness accompany the fever. Flaccid paralysis results from spinal cord involvement, and cranial nerves are not involved. Pure bulbar poliomyelitis accounts for 10% of all patients with paralysis; mixed bulbospinal involvement is more common. The most common cranial nerves involved are cranial nerves IX and X. Ocular palsies and pupillary disturbances are present in 11% of patients.

In rabies, ocular involvement is minimal, and ocular palsies are rare. Sympathetic stimulation results in mydriasis.

Tetanus, caused by a neurotoxin elaborated by *Clostridium tetani,* generally presents with trismus and subsequently increasing muscle rigidity that becomes generalized. Lacerations of the lid complicated by infection with *C. tetani* can result in cephalic tetanus. In this setting, ophthalmoplegia or spasm of the extraocular muscles occurs.

VARICELLA ZOSTER

Varicella (herpes) zoster is a double-stranded deoxyribonucleic acid virus, a member of the herpes family that has multiple manifestations within the orbit and orbital structures. Varicella is endemic in temperate climates worldwide, with a 90% attack rate before adulthood. Tropical zones are less affected, and adults leaving tropical areas frequently present with varicella during travel to temperate zones.

Primary varicella infection is manifested by the cutaneous vesicular eruption commonly termed *chickenpox.* This neurotropic virus achieves latency in nerve ganglion, including the trigeminal and spinal ganglia. Reactivation results typically in dermatomal involvement along the affected nerve root, that is, herpes zoster. Immunosuppression is one factor that may result in reactivation, although most people with herpes zoster do not have a recognized immunodeficiency. Disseminated zoster—extension beyond a dermatome—is associated with immunosuppression and typically occurs in the setting of chemotherapy, leukemia, or human immunodeficiency virus infection. Postherpetic neuralgia occurs in approximately 25% to 50% of elderly people with herpes zoster.

The most common manifestation of varicella in the orbit and orbital structures is herpes zoster ophthalmicus. This results from reactivation of varicella zoster in the ophthalmic branch of the trigeminal nerve. Vesicle formation often preceded by pain erupts along the distribution of the branch, including the lids. Ocular muscle paresis has been reported in 31% of patients with herpes zoster ophthalmicus.[27]

Nonorbital, that is, globe, complications are common, particularly anterior uveitis and stromal keratopathy. Occasionally, encephalitis occurs during acute herpes zoster ophthalmicus; this most likely is related to a cerebral vasculitis.

Treatment of dermatomal zoster in an immunocompetent patient is generally supportive. Analgesics and topical dressings are generally sufficient. Localized zoster in immunosuppressed patients should be treated with oral acyclovir. Involvement of the ophthalmic branch of the trigeminal nerve should be treated with acyclovir, regardless of the immune status of the patient. The intravenous formulation has been recommended for ophthalmic involvement; however, studies of oral acyclovir have demonstrated decreased intraocular complications especially in those receiving 800 mg of acyclovir five times per day within 72 hours of the onset of symptoms.[28]

TUBERCULOSIS

Tuberculosis involving the eye is rarely seen in the late twentieth century. In the prechemotherapy era the incidence of ocular involvement was found to be 1.4% in an analysis of 10,000 patients in a sanatorium.[29] The uveal tract was most commonly involved. Keratitis, conjunctivitis, and corneal ulcers represented 25% of patients in this series.

Tuberculosis was among the causes of chronic

dacryoadenitis until the advent of specific chemotherapy. Few cases have been cited since 1960, even in the developing world.[30] Tuberculosis dacryoadenitis typically presents as painless, progressive swelling of the lateral aspect of the upper lid. Histologically, caseation or sclerosis may be seen, but identification of acid-fast organisms is unusual.

Tuberculosis involving the orbit is rare. When it does occur, it generally presents as progressive, painless proptosis. Active disease may be present elsewhere, such as in a contiguous sinus or pericardium.[29] Drainage is not necessary because medical therapy reduces the inflammatory response adequately. Spread may be by direct extension or hematogenesis. Sinus involvement with extension into the orbit typically demonstrates bony erosion and occasionally cutaneous fistulas.[31]

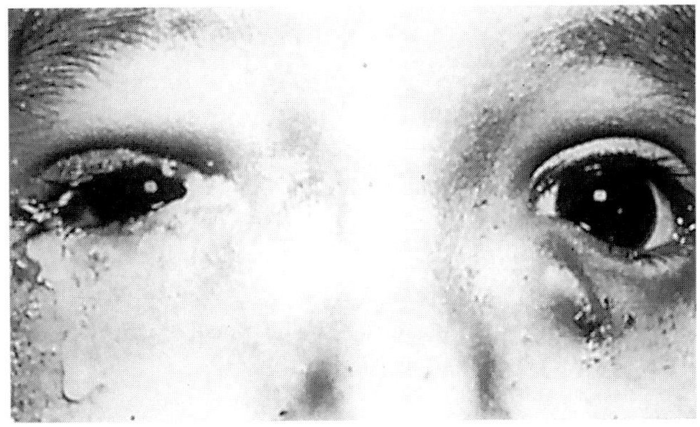

Figure 8–9. Dacryocystitis. (From Boruchoff SA, Boruchoff SE: Infections of the lacrimal system. Infect Dis Clin North Am 6:925–932, 1992.)

SYPHILIS

Syphilitic involvement of the eye may occur at any stage of the infection. Primary syphilis results from direct inoculation and may cause a chancre on the lid or conjunctiva. Involvement of the lacrimal gland is rare. Secondary syphilis produces macules or papules diffusely, and the lids may be affected. Lesions are nonpruritic. A plasma cell infiltrate is seen on biopsy. The spirochete can be visualized using a Warthin-Starry stain. In tertiary syphilis gummas cause ulcerations and bony destruction. Periostitis in the orbital apex may result in ocular palsies. Periostitis of the paranasal sinuses is manifested by proptosis, ophthalmoplegia, or trigeminal neuralgia.

DACRYOADENITIS ASSOCIATED WITH SYSTEMIC INFECTION

The lacrimal system occasionally is coincidentally infected during generalized infection or incidentally involved with regional infection. Acute bacterial dacryoadenitis is most commonly caused by *S. aureus. Streptococcus, Chlamydia,* and *Neisseria gonorrhea* are typical pathogens. Acute dacryoadenitis is manifested by painful swelling of the lateral aspect of the lid. The patient may exhibit systemic signs of fever and malaise; regional adenopathy occurs.

Chronic dacryoadenitis is associated with a systemic infection, particularly a viral type. Mumps generally causes bilateral involvement and occurs simultaneously with parotid gland involvement. Measles, Epstein-Barr virus, cytomegalovirus, and enteroviruses also result in dacryoadenitis.

Chronic dacryoadenitis is associated with systemic granulomatous processes, such as tuberculosis, syphilis, and leprosy. These must be listed as rare complications. Sarcoid and Sjögren's syndrome should be strongly considered in the differential diagnosis.

Herpes simplex virus may reside in the lacrimal gland following ocular herpes and is a potential reservoir for recurrent infection. Canalicular stenosis has been associated with antecedent ocular herpes. Actinomycosis is a common pathogen causing canaliculitis. It is associated with the expression of sulfur granule concretions from the puncta and can be seen on Gram's stain and recovered in culture. Treatment of canaliculitis is with local therapy—expression, curettage, and topical antibiotics—directed at the recovered organism.

Acute infectious dacryocystitis presents as painful swelling beneath the medial aspect of the lower lid (Fig. 8–9). Bacterial pathogens similar to dacryoadenitis are the most common organisms and can often be recovered by applying pressure over the lacrimal sac and simultaneously culturing purulence from the punctum. Gram-negative bacilli and fungi are associated with chronic infection. Systemic antibiotic therapy rather than topical agents should be used.

LEPROSY

Leprosy, caused by *Mycobacterium leprae,* frequently has extraocular and intraocular manifestations. Keratitis may result from nerve involvement that impedes lid closure. An avascular punctate keratitis may occur. This condition, scleritis, iridocyclitis, and uveitis are not considered further in this section.

Leprosy affects the orbital structures by involvement of the cranial nerves and skin infiltration. In the tuberculoid form of leprosy, neurologic signs and symptoms are more common. Skin lesions are discrete macules or plaques, hypopigmented and anesthetic. Peripheral nerve involvement is common secondary to Schwann cell proliferation and caseation in the nerves. Cranial nerve VII involvement results in lower lid ectropion and lagophthalmos. Cranial nerve V involvement complicates this inefficient lid closure, further predisposing the patient to exposure keratitis. Finally, infiltration of the upper lid and levator muscle dysfunction results in a wide-open stare.

Lepromatous leprosy, the opposite "pole" of tuberculoid leprosy, has more skin and fewer neurologic features. *M. leprae* bacilli are much more abundant in tissue, and the inflammatory response is diminished. Intraocular involvement is more common. The principal orbital manifestation of lepromatous leprosy is the loss of eyebrows (madarosis). The outer third of the brow is usually affected first; this occurs as an early manifestation of disease. Eyelash loss is also common.

Several surgical procedures have been designed to treat lagophthalmos, including the temporalis sling operation and the Kuhnt operation. The systemic infection of leprosy has traditionally been treated with dapsone, a sulfa drug. Resistance appears to be increasing, and combination therapy is now recommended by the World Health Organization (WHO).

TRACHOMA

Chlamydia trachomatis is the major cause of blindness worldwide. *Chlamydia* affects the eye through a chronic process of reinfection that results in scarring of the palpebral conjunctiva, which, in turn, damages the cornea. An acute chlamydial conjunctivitis that occurs in neonates is acquired during passage through the birth canal. This infection, similar in pathogenesis to neonatal gonococcal conjunctivitis, is not considered further and is unrelated to trachoma.

Epidemiology

The WHO has estimated that 2 million people worldwide are blind as a result of trachoma and that 400 million are infected. Trachoma is clustered geographically and socioeconomically. Endemic infections occur principally in the Middle East, northern Africa, and northern India. Within these countries, the low-income population groups are principally infected because conditions of poor sanitation and poor personal hygiene are necessary to maintain the cycle of fomite contact and person-to-person spread of secretions containing *C. trachomatis.* The disease is three times more prevalent among women than among men, probably related to more frequent exposure that women experience during child care.

Bacteriology

C. trachomatis is a bacteria of the order Chlamydiales that is unique in its development. It has two distinct forms: the elementary body and the reticulate body. Elementary bodies are the extracellular form and are metabolically inactive. This form is the transmittable agent, principally by insect vectors, such as flies, or by person-to-person spread. The elementary body attaches to host cells and undergoes phagocytosis. Following phagocytosis, fission begins within the vacuole, forming reticulate bodies. This appears microscopically as a glycogen, or inclusion, body. These ultimately will become elementary bodies, completing the life cycle.

Pathogenesis

Trachoma initially involves the palpebral and bulbar conjunctivae resulting in submucosal follicles. With repeated infection, scarring of the conjunctiva develops, resulting in trichiasis and entropion. Secondary bacterial conjunctivitis is common. Infection of the bulbar conjunctiva results in neovascularization of the cornea, that is, pannus formation. Blindness is a result of pannus and additional scarring from entropion and trichiasis.

Trachoma is a chronic inflammatory condition requiring prolonged infection or multiple reexposures. The chronic infection of the conjunctiva proceeds through a recognized evolution from conjunctivitis to a papillary response, a follicular response, scarring, and pannus formation. There are overlapping stages, complicated by reinfection. The initial infection resembles other bacterial or viral conjunctivitis. Subsequently, papillae, congested capillary tufts, appear in the upper tarsus, upper fornix, and lower lid. These are small, erythematous papules. Follicles, elevated avascular lesions 0.2 to 3 mm in diameter, occur throughout the conjunctiva. Earlier in the disease, smaller lesions are typical; they are composed of lymphocytes and macrophages. Follicles may rupture, and Herbert's pits form in the limbus at the site of rupture. Limbal follicles are smaller than those involving the palpebral conjunctiva. Conjunctival scarring and peritarsal fibrosis progress to lid deformity and result in trichiasis and entropion.

Corneal involvement results from direct inflammation from *Chlamydia* but is complicated by the recurrent injury from the trichiasis and entropion. Epithelial and subepithelial punctate keratitis are characteristic; the former require slit-lamp examination. Pannus, superficial vascularization of the cornea, appears typically over the upper half of the cornea. Different patterns, including circum-

TABLE 8-3

MacCallan's Four-Level Staging System for Trachoma

Stage	Characteristics
I	Trachoma at onset: immature follicles with early corneal changes
II	Established or florid trachoma: mature follicles (necrotic, rupturing under light pressure) with papillary hypertrophy and limbal follicles or Herbert's pits
III	Cicatrizing trachoma: conjunctival scarring together with some of the conjunctival signs of stage I or II
IV	Cicatrized or healed trachoma: conjunctival scarring without signs of active trachoma

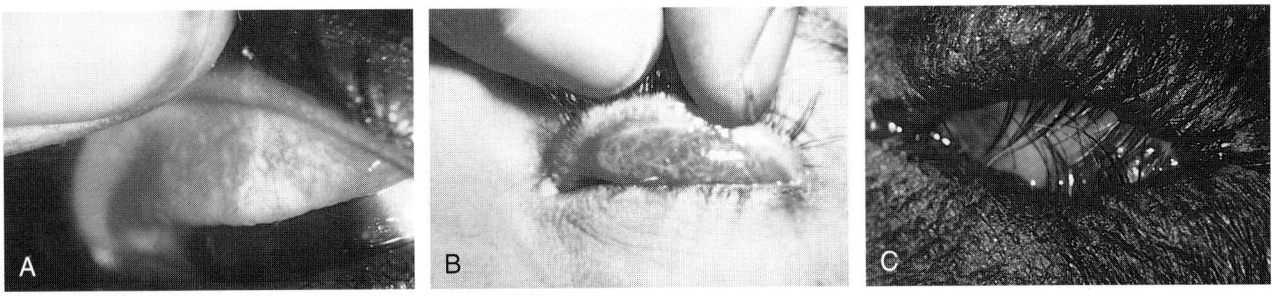

Figure 8–10. Stages of trachoma. *A*, Follicles; *B*, Pannus; and *C*, Trichiasis. (*A* to *C* courtesy of Dan Connor, MD, Armed Forces Institute of Pathology.)

corneal pannus, and papillary covering occur. Corneal scarring is a late manifestation.

MacCallan[1] developed a four-level staging system for trachoma in 1936 (Table 8–3). Subsequently, modifications have been recommended to include a scoring system of papillae and follicles.[32]

Clinical Presentation

Clinical findings in trachoma are dependent on the stage of pathology at the time of examination. Early infection is similar to other types of purulent acute bacterial conjunctivitis. Conjunctival follicles are the hallmark of the intermediate stage of the disease; these are 0.5 to 1 mm in diameter and erythematous. Patients note a foreign body sensation, photophobia, and mucopurulent discharge. With progressive scarring, entropion and trichiasis ensue. Pannus develops simultaneously with the palpebral conjunctival findings. Pannus is infrequent before the late adolescent years or early 20s (Fig. 8–10).

Diagnosis

Confirmation of diagnosis is made by direct immunofluorescence in which a conjunctival scraping is smeared onto a slide impregnated with *Chlamydia* antibody and counterstained with another immunofluorescent-tagged antibody. A Giemsa stain of a conjunctival smear demonstrates the inclusion body. Culture for *Chlamydia* is less readily available and requires a cell culture system. Tear antibody detection is an alternative sensitive methodology.

Clinical Treatment

Systemic antibiotic therapy is the indicated medical treatment for trachoma. Topical therapy has not resulted in acceptable outcome. Tetracycline 500 mg four times daily for 3 weeks is the drug of choice for adults or doxycycline 100 mg twice daily for 3 weeks. Duration of therapy has been prolonged to 40 days in more chronic cases. In children, erythromycin is the drug of choice.

REFERENCES

1. Smith AT, Spencer JT: Orbital complications resulting from lesions of the sinuses. Ann Otol Rhinol Laryngol 57:5, 1948.
2. Chandler JR, Langenbrunner DJ, Stevens ER: Pathogenesis of orbital complications in acute sinusitis. Laryngoscope 80:1414–1428, 1970.
3. Jackson K, Baker SR, Arbor A: Clinical implications of orbital cellulitis. Laryngoscope 96:568–573, 1986.
4. Israele V, Nelson J: Periorbital and orbital cellulitis. Pediatr Infect Dis J 6:404–410, 1987.
5. Wyllie JW, Kern EB, Djalilian M: Isolated sphenoid sinus lesions. Laryngoscope 83:1252–1265, 1973.
6. Leo JS, Halpern J, Sacher JP: Computed tomography in the evaluation of orbital infections. Comput Tomogr 4:133, 1980.
7. Towbin R, Han BK, Kaufman RA: Postseptal cellulitis: CT in diagnosis and management. Radiology 158:735–737, 1986.
8. El-Simily O, Stearns MP: Orbital infection and sinusitis [correspondence]. J Roy Soc Med 80:660, 1987.
9. Niyadurupola T: Orbital infection [correspondence]. J R Soc Med 80:194, 1987.
10. Langham-Brown JJ, Rhys-Williams S: Computed tomography of acute orbital infection: The importance of coronal sections. Clin Radiol 40:471–474, 1989.
11. Patt BS, Manning SC: Blindness resulting from orbital complications of sinusitis. Otolaryngol Head Neck Surg 104:789–795, 1991.
12. Carithers HA: Oculoglandular disease of Parinaud. Am J Dis Child 132:1195–1200, 1978.
13. Moriarty RA, Margileth AM: Cat-scratch disease. Infect Dis Clin North Am 1:575–590, 1987.
14. Wear DJ, Margileth AM, Hadfield TL, et al: Cat-scratch disease: A bacterial infection. Science 221:1403–1405, 1983.
15. Wear DJ, Malaty RH, Zimmerman LE, et al: Cat-scratch disease bacilli in the conjunctiva of patients with Parinaud's oculoglandular syndrome. Ophthalmology 92:1282–1287, 1985.
16. Regenery RL, Olson JG, Perkins BA, Bibb W: Serologic response to *Rochalimaea henselae* antigen in suspected cat-scratch disease. Lancet 339:1443–1445, 1992.
17. Brenner DJ, Hollis DG, Moss CW, et al: Proposal of *Afipia* gen. nov., with *Afipia felis* sp. nov. (formerly the cat-scratch disease bacillus), *Afipia clevelandensis* sp. nov. (formerly the Cleveland Clinic Foundation strain), *Afipia broomeae* sp. nov., and three unnamed genospecies. J Clin Microbiol 29:2450–2460, 1991.
18. Chousos GA, Drach AV, Young M, et al: Neuroretinitis in cat-scratch disease. J Clin Neuropathol 10:92–94, 1990.
19. Schwarz JN, Donnelly EH, Klintworth GK: Ocular and orbital phycomycosis. Surv Ophthalmol 22:3–28, 1977.
20. Best M, Obstbaum SA, Friedman B, et al: Survival in orbital phycomycosis. Am J Ophthamol 71:1078–1080, 1971.
21. Mohan RCC, Gupta VP, Sarada P, et al: Ophthalmic complications most commonly involve the globe. Indian J Ophthalmol 28:69–72, 1980.
22. Dr. James Karesh, personal communication.
23. Morales AG, Croxatto JO, Crovetto L, Ebner R: Hydatid cysts of the orbit: A review of 35 cases. Ophthalmology 95:1027–1032, 1988.

24. Murthy H, Kumar A, Verma L: Orbital cysticercosis—an ultrasonic diagnosis. Acta Ophthalmol 68:612–614, 1990.
25. Decker GR, Berberian BJ, Sulica VI: Periorbital and eyelid edema: The initial manifestation of acute infectious mononucleosis. Cutis 47:323–324, 1991.
26. Schiffler RJ, Mansur GP, Navin TR: Indigenous Chagas' disease (American trypanosomiasis) in California. JAMA 251:2983–2984, 1984.
27. March RJ, Dulley B, Kelley V: External ocular motor palsies in ophthalmic zoster: A review. Br J Ophthalmol 61:677–682, 1977.
28. Cobo LM, Foulks GN, Liesegung T, et al: Oral acyclovir in the therapy of acute herpes zoster ophthalmicus. Ophthalmology 92:1574–1583, 1985.
29. Donahue HC: Ophthalmic experience in a tuberculosis sanitorium. Am J Ophthamol 64:742–748, 1967.
30. Baghdassarian SA, Zakharia H, Asdourian KK: Report of a case of bilateral caseous tuberculosis dacryoadenitis. Am J Ophthamol 74:744–746, 1972.
31. Spoor TC, Harding SA: Orbital tuberculosis. Am J Ophthalmol 91:644–647, 1981.
32. Schacter J, Moncada J, Dawson CR, et al: Nonculture methods for diagnosing chlamydial infection in patients with trachoma: A clue to the pathogenesis of the disease? J Infect Dis 158:1347–1352, 1988.

SECTION II

Conjunctiva

SECTION EDITOR

Ralph E. Wesley

Introduction

Ralph E. Wesley

Conjunctival diseases represent the most treacherous part of ophthalmic plastic surgery. Malignant neoplasms such as sebaceous gland carcinoma and melanoma are potentially deadly lesions in which the clinical presentation may be subtle, the interpretation of pathologic specimens difficult, and the surgical treatment confusing. Inflammatory disorders such as pemphigoid may follow a course resulting in blindness if they are not properly monitored and treated. Chemical and thermal burns of the conjunctiva present another group of problems that requires understanding of the clinical and pathologic stages to preserve ocular function. In brief, most conjunctival disorders beyond simple lesions tend to require a complex system of management.

Surgery on the conjunctiva tends to be fraught with difficulty because of the tendency of conjunctival or mucous membrane grafts to contract in the presence of inflammation. Elegant geometric patterns of flaps that work well with skin lesions tend to contract and thicken with conjunctival lesions such that restriction of the globe may become a problem. In general, the less conjunctival surgery the better. Even so, the chapters in this section provide what appear to be the most predictable techniques for treating disorders of the conjunctiva.

The following chapters are formulated to provide exposure of the ophthalmic plastic surgeon or the general ophthalmologist to the major conjunctival disorders and to present strategies and techniques for treating the condition, with a bibliography for quick reference to the basic sources in each area. The areas selected represent the conjunctival diseases encountered during the past 15 years on the Ophthalmic Plastic and Reconstructive Surgery Service at Vanderbilt University Medical Center that I found most often required research and consultation in the field of oculoplastic surgery.

CHAPTER 9

Conjunctiva: Structure and Function

Harvey P. Cole III and Ralph E. Wesley

The conjunctiva is a thin, transparent, vascularized mucous membrane that covers the pericorneal surface of the globe and the posterior surface of the upper and lower eyelids. The conjunctiva, like all mucous membranes, consists of the epithelium and the substantia propria. This intact epithelium serves as a barrier to foreign particles and inhibits the invasion of exogenous bacteria. The conjunctival secretions allow a smooth palpebral surface for eyelid closure without damage to the cornea. This surface is important in corneal nourishment and the transportation of secretions to the nasal lacrimal outflow system.

The conjunctiva is encountered by all ophthalmic surgeons. This tissue is intimately involved in glaucoma filtration surgery, both fornical and limbal strabismus approaches, cataract extraction, orbital approaches, and transconjunctival eyelid surgery and serves as a marker of many systemic diseases.

EMBRYOLOGY

The conjunctiva is a continuous membrane that shares a common origin from ectodermal and mesodermal tissues with the cornea and eyelids. The earliest embryonic development is observed at 6 weeks (10- to 15-mm stage), when surface ectoderm bulges outward, forming the buds that will become the eyelid folds.[1] At 10 weeks (40- to 45-mm stage), the conjunctival epithelium differentiates from the eyelid skin and cornea when goblet cells and glandular ducts become visible. By 12 weeks (50- to 55-mm stage), caruncular development from the nasal aspect of the lower lid fold and further epithelial invaginations to form the accessory glands of Krause and Wolfring are seen. A soft, moveable fold (plica semilunaris) is also seen between the caruncle and the globe at this stage. The semilunar fold corresponds to the nictitating membrane (third lid) that may be actively moved in certain mammals.

MACROSCOPIC ANATOMY

The conjunctiva is arbitrarily subdivided into the bulbar, palpebral, fornical (fornix conjunctivae), plica semilunaris, and caruncular areas for clinical convenience.

The *bulbar conjunctiva* is translucent and loosely adherent to the underlying Tenon's capsule and white sclera. The bulbar conjunctiva becomes firmly attached approximately 3 mm from the limbus, where it becomes continuous with the corneal epithelium. This relationship is important during dissection of limbal-based flaps. The bulbar conjunctiva is further attached to the rectus muscles via their envelope of Tenon's capsule and then becomes continuous with the loose and redundant fornical conjunctiva.

Unlike the bulbar conjunctiva, the *palpebral conjunctiva* is firmly adherent to the tarsal plate. This portion extends from the mucocutaneous junction posterior to the cilia of the eyelid margin and lines the inferior portion of the upper and lower eyelids to become continuous with the fornical conjunctiva. The marked adherence to the tarsal plate allows clinical signs of reactive follicular and papillary formation that may be helpful in identifying viral, bacterial, and allergic conditions. However, this same firm adherence is the basis for tarsoconjunctival flaps transferring as a composite unit.

The *fornical conjunctiva* swells easily, being thrown into multiple folds because of loose adherence to the orbital septum. The fornix is a transitional zone uniting the bulbar and palpebral conjunctivae. The superotemporal fornical conjunctiva contains ducts of the lacrimal gland and extends just behind the equator of the globe. The medial portion loses the fornix to become continuous with the plica semilunaris and the caruncle.[2] This change is paramount in the relationship of the punctum to the lacrimal lake to allow maximal lacrimal pump outflow efficiency.

The bulbar and fornical conjunctivae unite at the medial canthus to become continuous with the *plica semilunaris* and the *caruncle.* The semilunar fold is a vertical crescent of modified conjunctiva believed to be a vestigial remnant of the nictitating membrane in lower animals. This soft, moveable fold is important to preserve in conjunctival surgery because it may cause marked restriction and symblepharon formation if inadvertently sutured during conjunctival closure. The caruncle is essentially modified skin and may normally contain lanugo hairs, sebaceous and sweat glands, striated muscle (Horner's), and lobules of lacrimal gland.[1] The caruncle and the trochlea are the only two places in the orbital region where cartilage is normally encountered.

MICROSCOPIC ANATOMY

Epithelium

The conjunctival epithelium is predominantly stratified columnar epithelium that becomes stratified squamous epithelium at the limbal and palpebral margins. This two- to five-layer–thick epithelium rests on a loose connective tissue layer termed *substantia propria* (Fig. 9–1). The basal cells are cuboidal and evolve into flat polyhedral surface cells. The epithelium is always nonkeratinized in healthy people but may assume the characteristics of keratinized skin with chronic exposure and drying. The nonkeratinized mucosal epithelium has a relatively abrupt transition to keratinized stratified squamous epithelium at the mucocutaneous junction of the lid margin. A more gradual transition from nonkeratinized stratified columnar epithelium of conjunctiva to the nonkeratinized stratified squamous epithelium occurs at the corneal limbus. Melanocytes are universally found in the basal epithelial layer and manifest ethnic variations in proportion to skin pigmentation.

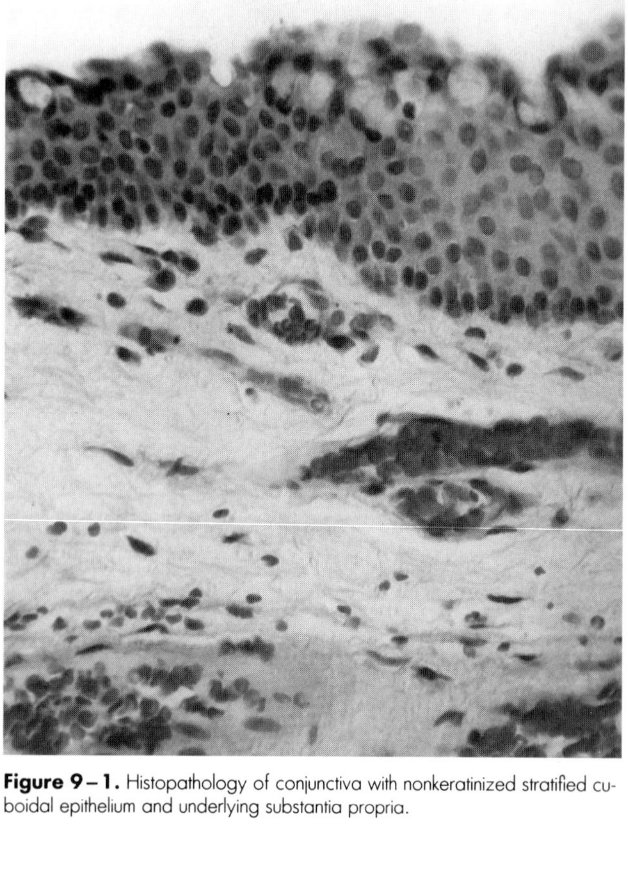

Figure 9–1. Histopathology of conjunctiva with nonkeratinized stratified cuboidal epithelium and underlying substantia propria.

Stroma

The conjunctival stroma is a richly vascularized connective tissue separated from the epithelium by a basement membrane. This substantia propria varies in density and thickness depending on its location. The palpebral conjunctiva contains thin, compact stroma with firm connections between the epithelium and the tarsal plate. This relationship accounts for the frequent clinical sign of upper palpebral papillae. The bulbar and fornical conjunctivae contain thick, loose stroma, the classic site for large quantities of transudate called *chemosis.*

The conjunctival stroma is further subdivided into a superficial lymphoid layer and a deeper fibrous layer. The lymphoid or adenoid layer is most predominant in the bulbar and fornical conjunctivae. This lymphoid tissue does not develop until 2 to 3 months postnatally, which explains why a neonate is unable to produce a follicular reaction. The deeper fibrous layer is tightly adherent to the inner margins of the tarsal plate and is continuous with the vascular network and the smooth palpebral muscle of Müller.

Glands

The conjunctiva contains many glandular structures that are responsible for maintaining moisture and precorneal tear film stability. These glands may be classified as either mucous glands or accessory lacrimal glands.

The mucous glands are unicellular goblet cells located within the epithelium that secrete a wetting agent and tear film–stabilizing agent termed *mucin.* These apocrine glands are not found in the corneal epithelium and are therefore essential to maintaining the overall integrity of the precorneal tear film, principally by lowering the surface tension. The goblet cells are most numerous in the inferonasal conjunctiva and most dense in children and young adults.[3] Therefore, the inferonasal conjunctiva is a favored site of diagnostic biopsy.

These mucin secretors may be decreased with destructive disorders like cicatricial pemphigoid and acute alkali burns or increased in density with long-standing inflammation such as with a poorly fitting ocular prosthesis with resultant increased mucous discharge.[4] There are additional mucin secretors along the tarsal conjunctiva called *crypts of Henle* and in a perilimbal ring termed *glands of Manz*; however, these are considered of minor importance in humans.

The accessory lacrimal glands of the conjunctiva are

located in the substantia propria. The glands of Krause are found predominantly in the fornices (42 upper and 6 to 8 lower) and have a similar histologic composition as the main lacrimal gland.[1] The upper border of the tarsus contains other accessory lacrimal glands called *glands of Wolfring*. The location of these accessory lacrimal glands is critical in planning procedures that involve the superior tarsus, as with the Fasanella-Servat procedure for blepharoptosis. The inadvertent excision of these accessory lacrimal glands may cause or enhance a dry eye condition.

Blood Supply

The conjunctiva has a rich vascular supply derived from the ophthalmic artery, which is derived from the internal carotid artery. The palpebral conjunctiva is nourished from the peripheral and marginal arterial arcades of the eyelid. The bulbar conjunctiva is supplied by the anterior ciliary artery. The fornical conjunctiva is nourished by an anastomosis of the blood supply from the palpebral and bulbar regions. The superficial location of the conjunctival vessels is important diagnostically because these vessels constrict with topical instillation of 1:1000 epinephrine. These vessels also appear bright red and move with a cotton-tipped applicator as compared with the purplish color and lack of movement with the deeper episcleral vessels. The venous supply for the palpebral conjunctiva communicates with the orbital veins and the pterygoid plexus. The bulbar conjunctiva has a venous network continuous with the intrascleral and episcleral venous plexus.

Nerve Supply

The sensory nerve supply of the conjunctiva may be found in the substantia propria and is derived entirely from the first and second division of the trigeminal nerve. There are sympathetic nerves that accompany the blood vessels and also innervate Müller's muscle.

Lymphatic Supply

The lymphatic drainage of the conjunctiva may be found in all portions of the substantia propria. The lymphatic channels from the medial bulbar and palpebral conjunctivae drain into the submandibular nodes, whereas the lateral conjunctiva drains to the preauricular nodes. These collecting lymphatic channels may be visible with the biomicroscope in certain conditions.

PHYSIOLOGY

The conjunctiva plays a major role in ocular inflammation and secondary wound healing. The principal features to consider in conjunctival inflammation are the type of discharge, the characteristics of the reaction, and the presence or absence of lymphadenopathy. The conjunctival epithelial cells are important in wound healing and have been shown to be responsible for repair of peripheral corneal abrasions.[5] This property of conjunctival epithelial cells is used clinically by the popular trend toward incisions further away from the surgical limbus in cataract surgery and in other conjunctival approaches in ocular surgery.

TISSUE HANDLING

The relationship between the ophthalmic surgeon and the pathologist is critical when the surgeon is handling conjunctival tissue. The removal of conjunctival tissue should be done in a gentle fashion, so that clinically normal tissue is removed along with the pathologically involved area. The evolving edge may offer more diagnostic information about the entire disease process.

The conjunctival specimen should be gently spread out flat on an adherent surface such as the paper wrapping from gloves, specific filter paper, or paper available from the inside of a suture package. Some institutions use specific adherence vehicles like dehydrated cucumber, dehydrated slices of squash, and even a business card containing information about the surgeon. Pinning the tissue may cause crush artifact or possible rust deposition that may be confused with melanin. The tissue is spread evenly and then allowed to dry for approximately 30 seconds. This minimal amount of time prevents the tissue from curling, which would make investigation and orientation difficult. The tissue on this adherent surface is then placed face up in 10% neutral buffered formalin, unless a specific fixative is needed for special studies, as in the case of specimens submitted in Michel's solution for basement membrane fluorescent studies in pemphigoid. The specimen information should include whether the conjunctival specimen is bulbar, fornical, or palpebral in origin.

Special studies may be indicated based on preoperative consultation with the ophthalmic pathologist. A "touch prep" can be done immediately to provide cytologic detail with suspected lymphoid lesions. The tissue is sent to the pathologist unfixed but lightly moistened in a saline-soaked gauze. The pathologist can then touch the fresh tissue to several glass slides before fixating the specimen in alcohol and staining. Immunopathologic analysis to differentiate neoplastic from reactive lymphoid lesions can be performed on fresh conjunctival tissue, usually taking a few additional days for a result.

Preserving some tissue in glutaraldehyde provides an opportunity for electron microscopy at a later date should a question arise as to the origin of the tumor cells. Electron microscopy requires approximately 4 or 5 days for processing and interpretation.

REFERENCES

1. Spencer WH, Zimmerman LE: Conjunctiva. *In* Spencer WH (ed): Ophthalmic Pathology, 3rd ed. Philadelphia, WB Saunders, 1985, pp 109–117.
2. Srinivasan BD, Jakobiec FA, Iwamoto T: Ocular Anatomy, Embryology, and Tetralogy. Philadelphia, Harper & Row, 1982.
3. Kessing SV: Mucous gland system of the conjunctiva. Acta Ophthalmol Suppl 95:1–9, 1968.
4. Ralph RA: Conjunctival goblet cell density in normal subjects and in dry eye syndromes. Invest Ophthalmol Vis Sci 14:299–302, 1975.
5. Mann I: A study of epithelial regeneration in the living eye. Am J Ophthalmol 28:26–40, 1944.

CHAPTER 10

Basic Techniques of Conjunctival Surgery

Harvey P. Cole III and Ralph E. Wesley

Conjunctiva is a translucent mucous membrane that covers the anterior segment of the sclera and lines the posterior surface of the eyelids. This tissue is essential for the integrity of the tear film and serves as a barrier to exogenous organisms.

The conjunctiva is normally abundant and elastic, allowing repair by simply undermining and direct closure in many minor injuries or removal of lesions. However, with more extensive tissue loss, shrinkage, or chemical injury, a restorative procedure may be necessary. Specialized techniques of conjunctival surgery may be required for pterygium, chalazion, symblepharon, corneal exposure, keratomycosis, chemical and herpetic keratitis, socket contracture, neurotrophic ulceration, and chronic prolapsing conjunctival chemosis.

The novice surgeon can be easily misled by texts and articles showing elegant geometric flaps to reconstruct conjunctival defects. The greatest limitation on conjunctival surgery comes from subsequent inflammation and contraction that affect the ultimate outcome of a procedure. Knowledge of the possible ultimate biologic response to the surgery is as important as the ability to perform procedures such as a Z-plasty or V-Y plasty, simple lysis, excision and direct closure, a free conjunctival graft, or a mucous membrane graft. This chapter describes basic techniques of conjunctival surgery for the surgeon to determine which procedure is applicable to the specific ocular condition. Additional special techniques are described in detail in subsequent chapters.

CONJUNCTIVAL FLAPS

The need for full conjunctival flaps has decreased because of the advent of soft contact lenses, collagen shields, and improved keratoplasty techniques. However, conjunctival flap surgery is a procedure of necessity with localized conjunctival defects such as symblepharon and traumatic avulsion and when chronic sterile corneal ulcers fail to respond to traditional medical treatment. The main types of conjunctival flaps are the transpositional (Z-plasty) conjunctival flap, the partial (bridge) sliding flaps, and the complete (Gundersen) sliding flaps.

Transpositional Conjunctival Flap

The Z-plasty is the classic transpositional flap used to relieve tension and redirect scar bands and is a core procedure in conjunctival oculoplastic surgery. Variations include transpositional flaps such as V-plasty to Y-plasty, Y-plasty to V-plasty, O-plasty to Z-plasty, and W-plasty.

In the classic Z-plasty, two triangular flaps of conjunctiva are formed by three incisions of equal length cut at 60 degrees to the conjunctival scar (Fig. 10–1*A*). A central limb is made directly over the length of the scar; the side arms are then fashioned at 60 degrees from the central limb. After the conjunctival flaps are undermined, they are transposed and then sutured into position with 6-0 fast-absorbing plain catgut (Fig. 10–1*B*). The advantage of this transpositional procedure is to elongate the conjunctival scar and disperse and realign the tension direction. Long-term results are not usually as good as those shown in diagrams because of the tendency for conjunctiva to contract, which counteracts the theoretic geometry of the flap.

Partial Conjunctival Flap

A partial conjunctival flap is particularly beneficial in the treatment of localized corneal disease such as sectorial corneal edema and peripheral nonhealing ulcers. The bridge flap is based on surgical principles similar to those of the complete conjunctival flap but has the advantage of preserving the visual axis, thereby maintaining or improving preoperative vision.

Figure 10–2 shows a technique to swing a flap of conjunctiva from the fornix onto a localized defect after removal of a lesion. This type of flap should be used when allowing the defect to heal by spontaneous closure would contract and restrict the globe. The flap will undergo thickening and contraction in the weeks after the procedure. This type of flap can be helpful when covering a thin part of the sclera is important to maintain the structural integrity of the globe.

Figure 10–3*A* demonstrates a technique to recess contracted conjunctiva off the globe. The edge of the recessed

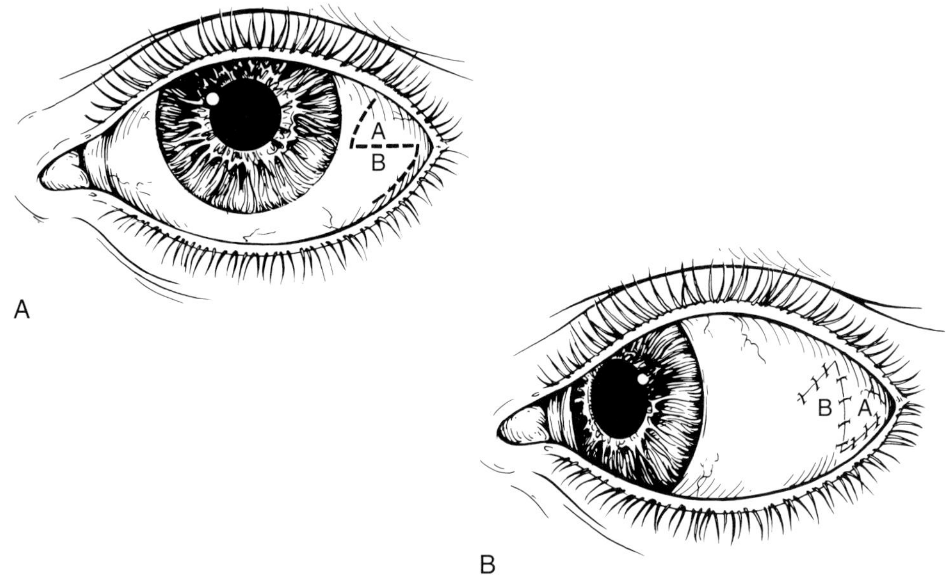

Figure 10–1. *A*, Z-plasty drawn to release a medial restriction of the conjunctiva. Traction will be released along the long horizontal portion of the marked Z. *B*, Standard limbs of Z-plasty transposed to lengthen the conjunctiva horizontally to relieve traction.

flap is fixated with 8-0 Vicryl sutures to the episclera or Tenon's layer to prevent localized contraction (Fig. 10–3*B*). The bare area on the globe should be treated with topical steroid drops until spontaneous secondary epithelialization occurs. This works best for patients with localized disease rather than with a generalized cicatricial process such as pemphigoid, in which the procedure would nearly always fail.

Flaps over the rounded convex surface of the globe heal most favorably; however, flaps over the globe are least often needed. Flaps and grafts in the medial fornix have perhaps the worst prognosis for smooth, uncontracted healing. On the other hand, defects in this area more often need replacement of conjunctival tissue compared with other areas. The lateral fornix is more plentiful and less likely to cause restriction than the medial fornix. The upper and lower fornices can tolerate some shortening as long as lagophthalmos or entropion is not produced. Larger defects of the upper and lower fornices require reconstruction, which is usually best carried out with conjunctival replacement rather than geometric flaps.

Complete Conjunctival Flap

In 1958, Gundersen[1] described a conjunctival flap that has since been termed simply the *Gundersen flap.* This type of flap provides a vascular supply and serves as a protective barrier to nonhealing corneal conditions.

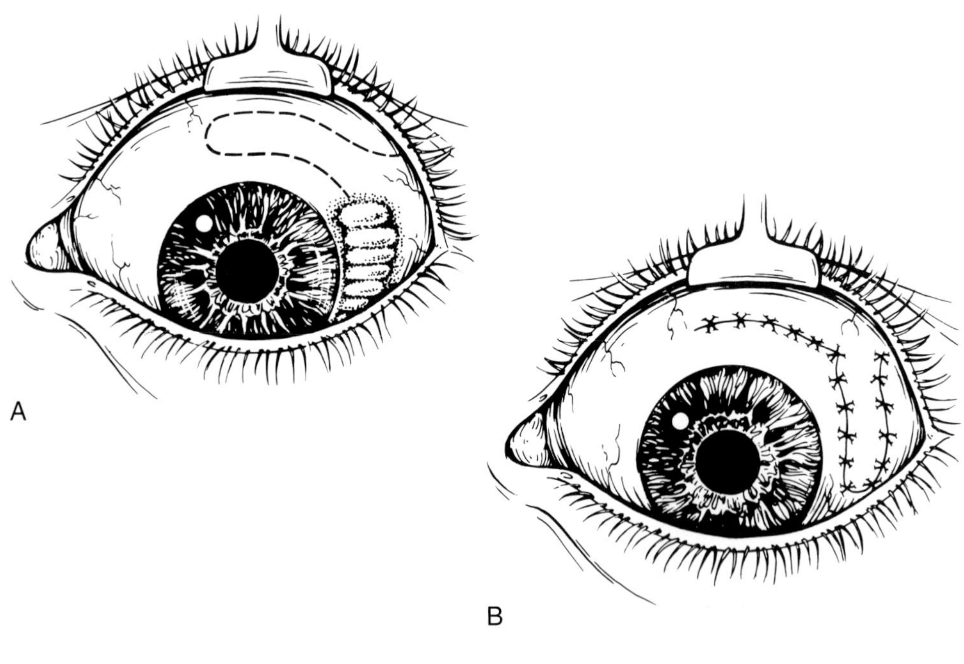

Figure 10–2. *A*, Flap drawn to cover a conjunctival lesion. *B*, Lesion is excised and covered with a transpositional flap. This technique should be used on fresh surgical defects rather than scars or contractures to avoid a thickened, cicatricial flap.

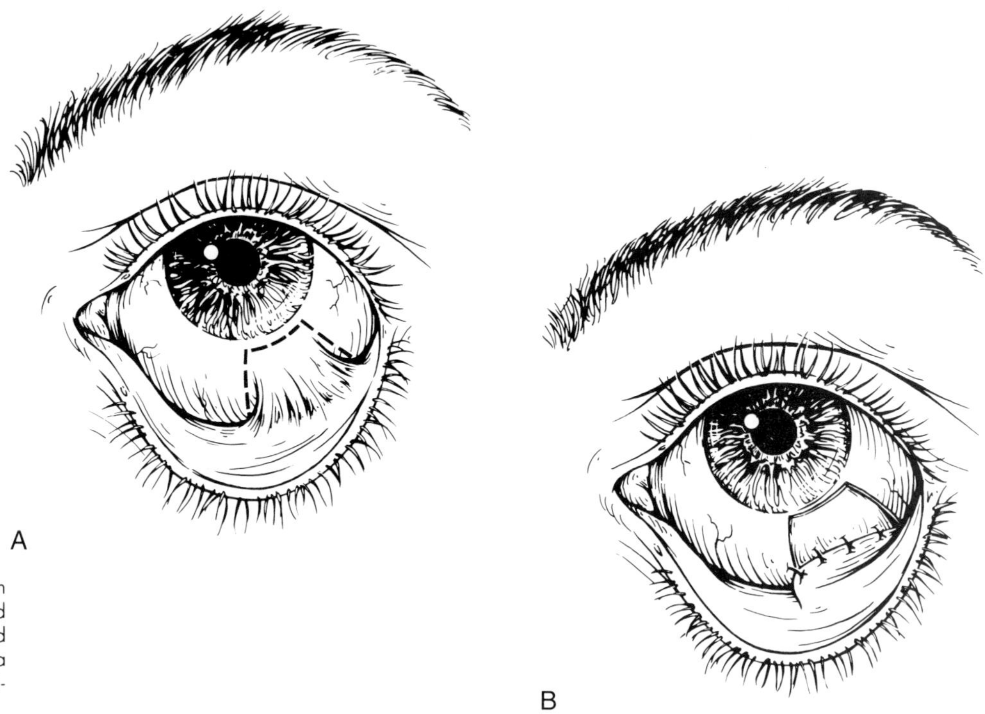

Figure 10–3. *A*, Localized adhesion of conjunctiva in the lower fornix marked for recession. *B*, Scar and flap recessed to the inferior fornix, allowing bare sclera to heal with epithelialization by secondary intention.

The main principles to bear in mind with the Gundersen flap are that the corneal epithelium must be completely removed, the flap must be conjunctiva only and not include Tenon's fascia, and the flap should be typically left in place for 1 year to allow stability of the underlying disease process. A detailed description of the surgical technique is presented by Matoba in Chapter 22.

The principal disadvantages of a complete conjunctival flap are decreased vision potential for the patient, impairment of intraocular pressure assessment, decreased absorption of drugs administered intraocularly, and difficulty in the assessment of possible progression of corneal ulceration or melting. The postoperative complication rate is low but may include retraction of the flap, cyst formation, corneal perforation, vascularization and opacification of the flap, and, rarely, ptosis.

A partial conjunctival flap to cover the inferior cornea can be helpful in cases of persistent inferior corneal exposure encountered in some patients after ptosis surgery and in patients with facial palsy and symptomatic neurogenic lagophthalmos. The ideal patient is one in whom closure cannot be reasonably obtained with other procedures and who has chronic, symptomatic inferior-exposure keratitis. Patients with stable, long-standing inferior-exposure keratitis without symptoms do not require surgical intervention.

Figure 10–4*A* shows inferior corneal exposure with secondary inferior corneal vascularization. A flap of inferior conjunctiva can be advanced onto the cornea after removal of the epithelium. The inferior conjunctiva is prepared by undermining inferiorly, but avoiding the insertion of, the inferior rectus muscle. The flap is sewed to the cornea with superficial bites using the operating microscope to secure the flap with a running 10-0 nylon suture (Fig. 10–4*B*). The patient should be maintained on antibiotic eyedrops postoperatively until the suture is removed 10 to 14 days later; the inferior cornea at that time is covered with a thicker layer of epithelium from the conjunctiva (Fig. 10–4*C* and *D*) that is more resistant to exposure. The flap always retracts after the sutures are removed. The lower, most exposed portion of the cornea receives a thicker flap than the thinner portion closer to the optical axis.

CONJUNCTIVAL GRAFTS

Free Conjunctival Graft

The ophthalmic surgeon should always choose like tissue to replace like tissue, if available. A free conjunctival graft may be harvested from the opposite fornix of the same eye or from the fornix of the fellow eye. Techniques for conjunctival transplant are described by Deitch and Wilson, Pfister, and Matoba in Chapters 16, 17, and 22, respectively.

The desired amount of conjunctival tissue needed for the defect is estimated recognizing that the free graft should be 10% to 15% larger than the recipient site. The upper eyelid, if chosen, may be everted over a Desmarres retractor to maximally expose the fornix conjunctiva. The donor site is infiltrated subconjunctivally with 2% lidocaine with 1:100,000 epinephrine and allowed to balloon away from the underlying Tenon's fascia and possibly Müller's muscle. The graft is then carefully harvested

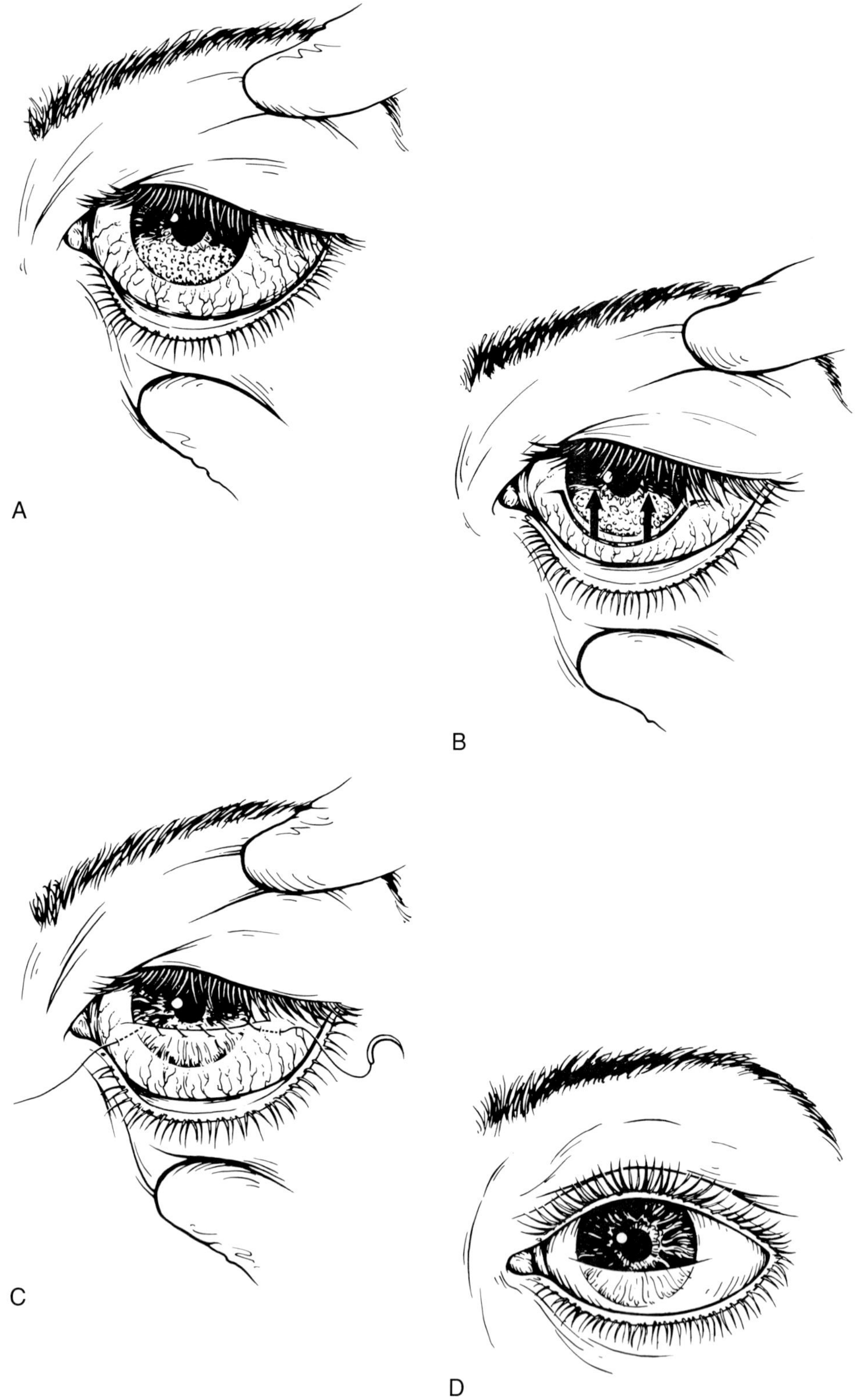

Figure 10–4. *A*, Inferior corneal vascularization from chronic inferior corneal exposure and keratitis. *B*, Inferior conjunctival flap sutured to de-epithelialized inferior cornea using 10-0 nylon running suture. *C*, Appearance of the cornea after the conjunctival flap has healed onto the outer portion of the inferior cornea and the suture has been removed. *D*, A thin conjunctival flap is more resistant to exposure than is corneal epithelium.

with 0.12-mm forceps and blunt-tipped spring-action scissors. Special care is needed to keep the donor tissue from curling and causing difficulty in determining which surface is raw or lined with mucous membrane. If the surgeon becomes uncertain, 2% fluorescein may be applied to the graft, which will show uptake to the raw surface only. The donor site may be gently undermined and closed primarily with 6-0 fast-absorbing catgut sutures or allowed to reepithelialize secondarily. The free graft is sutured with adjacent conjunctiva at the recipient site with 6-0 fast-absorbing plain catgut. Sterile ointment is then applied to the conjunctival surfaces, and the eye is patched. An optional symblepharon conformer or fornix suture may be used to maintain the furrow between bulbar and tarsal conjunctivae.

Mucous Membrane Grafts

Split-thickness Mucous Membrane Graft

In many instances a free conjunctival graft is inadequate to cover larger mucous membrane defects. When tarsal support remains, the ideal mucous membrane material for socket and fornix reconstruction is buccal mucosa. A split-thickness buccal mucosa graft is ideal for large bulbar conjunctival defects with better thickness and color match than full-thickness buccal grafts.

Usually under general anesthesia, towel clamps are applied at the corner of one side of the mouth to pull the cheek away from the teeth and possibly the endotracheal tube. A local anesthetic of 2% lidocaine with 1:100,000 epinephrine and hyaluronidase is infiltrated submucosally to allow the mucosal surface to balloon out and become taut and flattened to facilitate graft uniformity when harvesting. A Castroviejo mucotome at a 0.3-mm–thickness setting is then applied at a 45-degree angle in an anteroposterior direction, with the assistant putting firm and constant inward pressure on the external cheek to maintain this flat surface. Care is taken to stay inferior to the parotid (Stensen's) duct located adjacent to the second upper molar. As the surgeon advances the mucotome, the assistant grasps the mucous membrane graft with a forceps and maintains gentle but firm pressure to prevent reengagement of the graft by the oscillating cutting blades. Once the desired graft length is obtained, the mucotome is stopped and the graft is excised from the donor site with Westcott scissors or a scalpel. The size of the donor graft should be 25% to 30% larger than the recipient site to allow for shrinkage. The harvested graft is then oriented on a tongue blade, rinsed with gentamicin solution, and kept moistened until sutured at the recipient site. A portion of Gelfoam soaked with topical thrombin is applied to the donor site. The donor site should not be cauterized to reduce postoperative pain. The oral mucosal surface will resurface in 2 or 3 days. Because this donor site heals without scarring, it may be used again.

The split-thickness buccal mucosal graft is then handled in a similar fashion described earlier for free conjunctival grafts. It is sutured into position with 6-0 fast-absorbing plain catgut, a symblepharon conformer placed, sterile ointment applied, and the eye patched. The symblepharon ring is important to maintain the fornix configuration and to discourage graft shrinkage. The conformer may be sutured to the orbital rim periosteum, or the suture (5-0 chromic catgut) may be passed through the full thickness of the eyelid. Regardless of the technique used, the integrity of the cornea should be monitored closely.

Full-thickness Mucous Membrane Graft

The increased glandularity, persistent pinkish color, and bulkiness of a full-thickness buccal mucosal graft is the principal reason that a full-thickness mucous membrane graft is not preferred for large bulbar conjunctival defects. However, the full-thickness "free-handed" buccal graft is an excellent graft for complex socket and fornix reconstruction.

Under general anesthesia, towel clamps are placed at the ends of the lower lip, which is everted over an assistant's finger or a rolled gauze pad for counterpressure. The desired graft size is then demarcated with a methylene blue marking pen, recalling that this donor graft should be approximately 25% to 30% larger than the desired recipient site to allow for shrinkage. Care is taken not to include the mucocutaneous junction at the vermilion or to make the graft wide enough to alter the gum line. We prefer the lower lip buccal mucosa for a full-thickness mucous membrane graft because of the excellent exposure obtained for dissection. The upper lip and cheek regions may similarly be used, but they are technically more difficult. The mucosal region previously outlined is then ballooned up with the local anesthetic. A no. 15 surgical blade is used to make the entire full-thickness incision. The graft is then harvested with blunt scissors dissection, being careful not to include the underlying submucosal fat and buccinator muscle. The graft may be further thinned by placing the mucosal surface tautly over a gloved finger and trimming the irregular areas. The care of the donor site and use of the mucous membrane graft are the same as described earlier for the split-thickness buccal mucosal graft.

Split-thickness Skin Graft: Anophthalmic Sockets

The split-thickness skin graft is the preferred graft material with severe socket contracture and very large conjunctival defects. We have found that this type of graft is the most resistant to postoperative shrinkage and gives the best postoperative result, where indicated. A full-thickness skin graft involves epidermal and dermal elements versus a split-thickness skin graft that contains epidermal elements only. This thinness of a split-thickness skin graft enables it to require less vascular supply. Split-thickness grafts are more pliable than full-thickness grafts; the donor site of split-thickness skin grafts requires a dressing but does not involve the closure required with full-thickness grafts.

The preferred donor skin site is the upper outer thigh. This area is first injected with 2% lidocaine with 1:100,000 epinephrine, then is shaved, cleansed with povidone-iodine, marked with a methylene blue pen, and covered with a thin film of mineral oil. Our preferred instrument is the Padgett electric dermatome set at a harvest thickness of 0.015 inch. This instrument is applied at a 30-degree angle with firm, even pressure while the assistant maintains tautness of the skin with a tongue blade approximately 1 cm in front of the advancing dermatome. The harvested graft bunches at the oscillating blade site if left unattended and should therefore be held on stretch by the assistant while the dermatome is advanced. The donor site should have fine oozing only from the dermal papilla if the correct depth is obtained. Brisk bleeding is encountered if the graft is harvested too thick. Once the desired length is obtained, the dermatome is released and slowly backed up approximately 1 cm to allow the surgeon to separate the graft with scissors from the donor site. This graft is then rinsed with gentamicin solution and soaked in cool saline until it is placed at the recipient site.

The graft bed should have excellent hemostasis and be on stretch to allow the maximal surface area exposure for the best survival of the graft. The harvested graft is removed from the saline solution, and the epidermis is placed face up. The epidermal side may be distinguished from the raw surface because it contains the previously marked methylene blue, and the epithelial side tends to roll in toward the raw surface at the edges. The graft is then draped into the fornix, allowing for the necessary redundancy in this region. The tissue is sutured, like all grafts, from the loose graft to the fixed recipient tissue. We prefer 6-0 fast-absorbing plain catgut (or 6-0 chromic catgut) for graft fixation. The graft is held in position at the fornix region by placement of full-thickness sutures of double-armed 5-0 chromic catgut with the knot tied externally at the skin surface. A symblepharon ring or similar conformer is then placed into the fornix, antibiotic steroid ointment is applied, and the eye is either patched or sutured closed temporarily.

The donor site has a moistened gauze with 1:100,000 epinephrine and topical thrombin in firm contact during the operative procedure once the graft is harvested. At the conclusion of the procedure, an occlusive dressing (Op-Site or Tegaderm) is applied, and the epidermis is allowed to heal by secondary intention over the next couple of weeks. No further care is indicated at the donor site postoperatively.

Split-thickness skin grafts are used only when severe contractures or large defects exist in the anophthalmic socket. The resistance to contraction provides an advantage, but the requirement to clean the socket of desquamated epithelial keratin daily is the major disadvantage.

MISCELLANEOUS TECHNIQUES

Chalazion Surgery

A chalazion arises from obstruction of meibomian glands, inciting a chronic inflammatory lipogranuloma in the tarsus of the eyelid. If the chalazion is acute, it may often be adequately treated with warm compresses, systemic antibiotics, and, possibly, an injection of noncrystalloid steroids deep to the orbicularis. If medical treatment fails or the lesion becomes large enough to cause ptosis, corneal stigmatism, or a cosmetic blemish, then surgical excision is indicated. The important differential diagnosis of sebaceous gland carcinoma should always be considered with recurrent lesions and atypical-appearing lid masses. We recommend that all excised lesions be submitted for histopathologic evaluation regardless of size, frequency, or developmental history. If sebaceous gland carcinoma is suspected, the excised lesion should be submitted fresh or in saline in anticipation of specialized lipid stains. These specialized stains are not usually required by pathologists experienced in eyelid lesions.

After two drops of proparacaine 0.5% are instilled into the eye, the area surrounding the chalazion is injected with 2% lidocaine and 1:100,000 epinephrine. It is important to infiltrate enough anesthetic along the lid margin to anesthetize the area where the chalazion clamp will be placed. The clamp is placed, and the eyelid is everted. A vertical incision parallel to the meibomian gland is performed to protect the integrity of the adjacent meibomian glands. Westcott scissors are then used to cut through the septate trabeculations to allow removal of the caseous material. It is typically necessary to use a curette to "scoop out" the fibrous debris from the loculated compartments. The pseudocapsule should be removed if possible. We prefer to inject noncrystalloid steroids before releasing the chalazion clamp to decrease any possibility of central retinal artery embolization. The clamp is then slowly loosened while a disposable hand-held cautery or pressure is used to obtain hemostasis. No sutures are required at the conclusion. Antibiotic steroid ointment and a patch are applied. Patients are instructed to remove the patch when they arrive home and to apply a covered ice cube to the operative site for approximately 4 hours.

Conjunctival Lacerations

The most significant clinical issue with conjunctival lacerations involves the question of whether ocular or periocular injury has occurred. Simple conjunctival lacerations can be closed with 6-0 plain interrupted sutures, which will dissolve and not require tedious removal; these 6-0 plain gut sutures are unlikely to irritate the cornea or the undersurface of the eyelid.

The posterior conjunctival surface of a full-thickness eyelid laceration does not require closure when the lid has been properly aligned because the conjunctival edge resurfaces without sutures. When traumatic loss of conjunctiva threatens late contracture and motility restriction, immediate replacement with flap or free graft should be performed as part of the primary repair.

The greatest complication in conjunctival trauma is an unrecognized corneoscleral penetrating intraocular injury or laceration of the extraocular muscles or the tear drainage system.

REFERENCE

1. Gundersen T: Conjunctival flaps in the treatment of corneal disease with reference to a new technique of application. Arch Ophthalmol 60:880, 1958.

CHAPTER 11

Replacement of Conjunctival Mucous Membrane

Jonathan J. Dutton

Conjunctival epithelium is a specialized mucous membrane that covers the posterior surface of the eyelid and overlies the anterior surface of the globe, except for the cornea. It serves to protect the underlying tissues from trauma, desiccation, and infection. The conjunctiva contains numerous mucin-producing goblet cells that contribute to ocular surface lubrication. Epithelium continues over the corneal surface, but this differs histologically from that of the conjunctiva in being thicker, more tightly packed, having more desmosomes and hemidesmosomes, and lacking goblet cells. It also differs biochemically in having a more sluggish tricarboxylic acid cycle and a higher level of hexose monophosphate shunt activity.[1] When conjunctival epithelium grows over denuded corneal stroma, it is capable of transforming both biochemically and morphologically into corneal epithelium.[2]

Loss of conjunctiva may be seen following a wide variety of circumstances. In congenital microphthalmos or anophthalmos the socket is generally smaller than normal, the palpebral fissure is horizontally shortened, and the conjunctival surface is often severely reduced. Enucleation during childhood may lead to failure of the socket to grow normally and insufficient conjunctiva to allow wearing of a prosthesis. Trauma commonly results in some loss of tissue, either primarily or as a result of excision of devitalized or severely disorganized mucosa. Poor reconstructive technique can also lead to loss of surface epithelium. Chemical injury with acid or alkali typically results in marked contraction and symblepharon formation. Infectious processes, such as severe blepharitis, meibomianitis, and trachoma, can also cause conjunctival contraction with tarsal deformity.[3] Inflammatory disorders, such as Stevens-Johnson syndrome and cicatricial ocular pemphigoid (Fig. 11–1), usually lead to contraction of the epithelial surface. Surgical injury, for example following excision of malignant tumors, may also leave the patient with significant loss of conjunctiva. Irradiation may cause severe contraction coupled with impaired vascular supply. Resurfacing of the tarsus or eyelid may also be used in the management of inflammatory diseases such as vernal conjunctivitis.[4]

The physiologic consequences of conjunctival loss may vary from mild to severe. Small symblepharon may have little effect on eyelid function, but when large, they may prevent normal eyelid motility. Ptosis may result in loss of visual field and even functional blindness. Eyelid retraction and lagophthalmos are common sequelae that can cause corneal desiccation and ulceration. Reduction in goblet cell function may reduce ocular surface lubrication, resulting in epithelialization of the conjunctiva, corneal abrasions, vascularization, and opacification. Cicatrization of the conjunctiva leads to foreshortening of the posterior eyelid lamella, with blunting or loss of the fornices, entropion, and secondary trichiasis.

Repair of the conjunctival surface may be achieved by a number of reconstructive techniques. For minor degrees of contraction, scarring, or symblepharon formation, excision of scar bands accompanied by simple closure or minor tissue rearrangement usually gives adequate results. Small areas of bare episclera can even be left to epithelize spontaneously from the surrounding conjunctiva. However, where larger areas are involved, or when a fibrotic subconjunctival bed is present, more extensive surgery will be needed for a successful outcome. It is important to excise all vestiges of fibrosis to minimize subsequent contraction. Replacement mucous membrane with various types of grafts can then be positioned into a prepared bed. Skin grafts in the orbit are to be condemned, and the results are uniformly unacceptable, including not only a thick, inflexible lining but also desquamation and an unhygienic, foul-smelling discharge. When a more rigid material is needed for replacement of both mucosa and tarsus, compound grafts are more appropriate.

SPONTANEOUS GRANULATION

Small areas of denuded conjunctiva reepithelialize spontaneously without difficulty. Such beds are frequently left following excision of pingueculae, pterygia, neoplastic lesions, or symblepharon. Whenever possible, it is best to leave the underlying subconjunctival layer

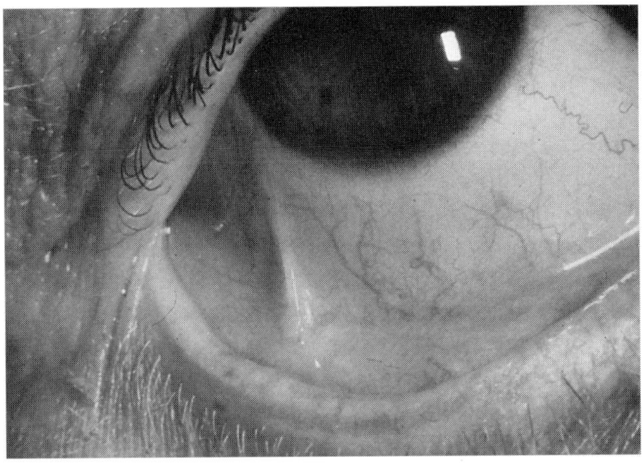

Figure 11–1. Early cicatricial ocular pemphigoid with blunted conjunctival fornix and symblepharon formation.

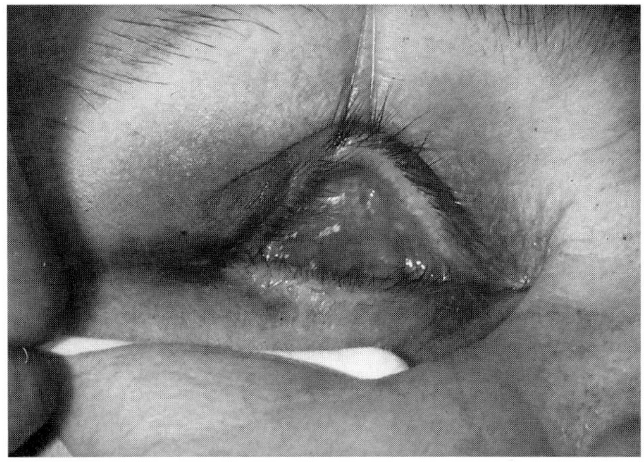

Figure 11–2. Anophthalmic socket with mild contraction of the superior fornix.

and Tenon's capsule, although resurfacing will occur directly over bare sclera. To prevent adhesions between the eyelid and globe, it is important that only one surface be denuded. The defect should not extend into the apex of the fornix.

ALLOPLASTIC GRAFTING AND SPONTANEOUS EPITHELIALIZATION

When larger areas of conjunctiva are lost, it is possible to encourage granulation, but contraction may be significant. Tight splinting of the defect allows resurfacing while it minimizes surface contraction. Kaufman and Thomas[5] emphasized the value of alloplastic grafting and noted the large size of a defect that can be resurfaced without the need for mucosal grafts. It is important, however, that opposing denuded surfaces be separated to prevent adhesions. Many materials have been used in the past to separate these surfaces, including methyl methacrylate conformers, plastic wrap, silicone sheeting, and rubber gloves.[6–10]

Polytetrafluoroethylene (polytef) has been used as a pericardial, vascular, and abdominal patch graft material for years.[11, 12] The material is an extruded Teflon that is biologically inert, nonantigenic, easily cut and molded, and resistant to infection.[13, 14] This material is available as a 0.1-mm nonporous, thin surgical membrane. We have used this material as an alloplastic exograft for a variety of eyelid and socket reconstructive procedures. It is pliable enough to allow molding into the contours of the socket and soft enough to use along the eyelid margins and adjacent to the corneal limbus with minimal discomfort (Figs. 11–2 and 11–3).[15] The smooth surface acts as a surface splint and as an ideal temporary separator that allows conjunctival epithelium to slide beneath the graft to resurface large areas of the globe or eyelid within 2 to 3 weeks (Figs. 11–4 and 11–5).

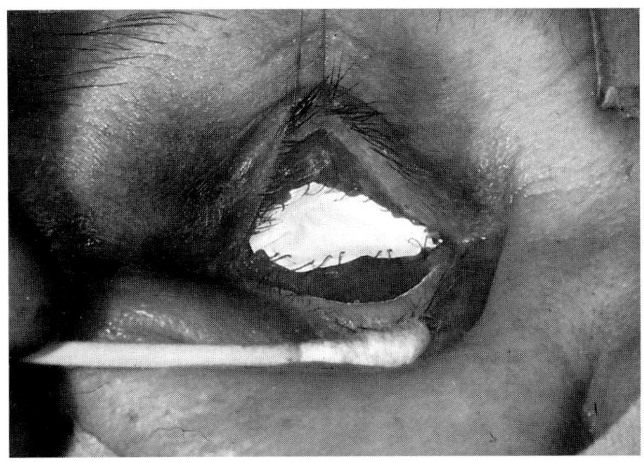

Figure 11–3. Same patient as in Figure 11–2 following dissection of the superior fornix and placement of a polytetrafluoroethylene alloplastic graft.

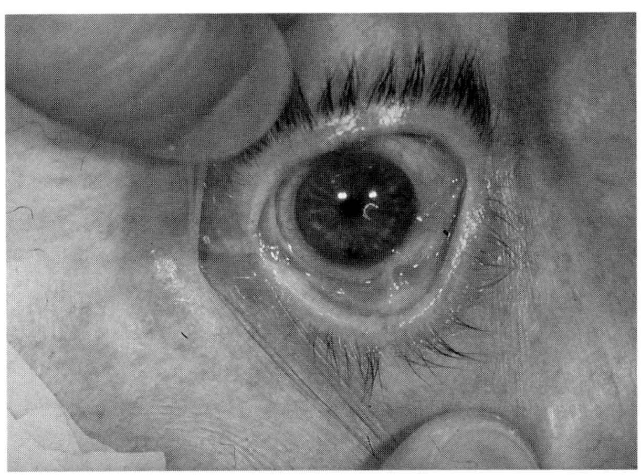

Figure 11–4. Cicatricial ocular pemphigoid with contraction of the inferior fornix.

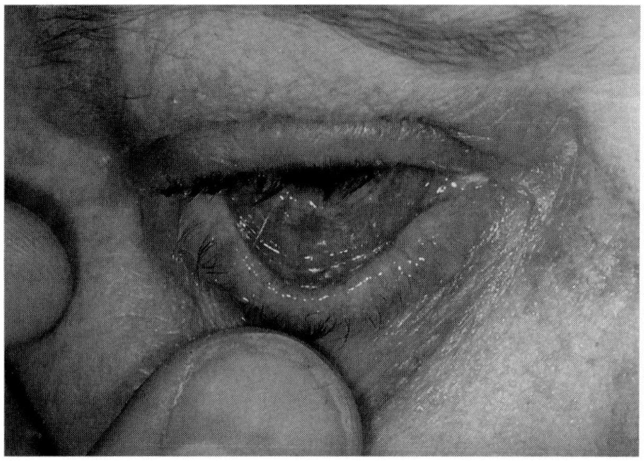

Figure 11–5. Same patient as in Figure 11–4 after removal of a polytetrafluoroethylene alloplastic graft. The conjunctiva has completely resurfaced the dissection bed.

The host surgical bed is prepared as for standard mucosal grafting. In the presence of socket contraction, the fornices are reconstructed by dissecting in a plane posterior to the capsulopalpebral fascia in the lower eyelid or to Müller's sympathetic muscle in the upper eyelid. The dissection is carried to the level of the orbital rims. In cicatricial diseases, such as ocular pemphigoid, the bulbar and palpebral surfaces are first separated, and the fornices are reestablished. As for mucous membrane grafts, the host bed must be free of submucosal fibrosis to prevent subsequent recurrent contracture. The technique works best when cicatrization is minimal. Hemostasis is ensured with bipolar cautery. If loss of conjunctiva resulted from resection of a neoplastic lesion, no further preparation is needed.

The polytef alloplastic graft is cut from a sheet. The graft should be slightly larger than is required to cover the host defect to allow the graft to overlap the mucosal edges by about 1 to 2 mm. It is positioned over the eyelid or globe and sutured into position with interrupted or running sutures of 6-0 polyglactin 910 (Vicryl). To help fixate the graft when it extends into the deep fornices, several double-armed 4-0 chromic Quickert-Rathbun–type sutures may be passed through the eyelid from the graft to the skin, as for fornix reconstruction. In an anophthalmic socket a conformer or a symblepharon ring may be used to hold the graft into the fornix, and a temporary tarsorrhaphy keeps the graft flat. If the bulbar conjunctiva is being replaced, the graft can be sutured directly to the pericorneal limbus with a running 7-0 stitch. When epithelium is missing from the eyelid margin, the graft is folded over the eyelid and sutured directly to the skin surface. The Vicryl sutures usually dissolve in about 2 to 3 weeks; by then the defect is resurfaced with conjunctival epithelium. If necessary, any remaining sutures are cut and removed. If any bare areas are noted, especially in the deep fornices, the graft can be left in position for an additional week.

Polytef has proved to be superior to more rigid materials used as a separator, such as methylmethacrylate and silicone. Its nonporous surface prevents adhesions, resists infection, and does not incite an inflammatory reaction. It is well tolerated by patients, even when sutured along the corneal limbus and over the eyelid margins. The new mucosal surface clinically resembles normal conjunctiva and, in our experience, gives good long-term results. However, in many cicatricial diseases, contraction of persistent submucosal fibrosis is common with this material as with mucous membrane grafts. Polytef has several additional advantages: large areas can be covered without the need for harvesting mucosa from many sites in the mouth, and no special instrumentation is needed. Use of this material in carefully selected cases may obviate the need for mucosal grafting when that process may be difficult because of concurrent oral mucosal disease or when repeat surgery is anticipated.

CONJUNCTIVAL TRANSPLANTATION

For small areas of bulbar or palpebral mucosal defects, transplantation of conjunctiva from the ipsilateral eye provides an excellent source of graft material. Unless previously injured, this material is normal conjunctiva, with goblet cells and characteristic conjunctival physiology. In patients for whom the corneal epithelium is also lacking, such grafts can be overlapped onto the corneal stroma where they undergo transformation into corneal epithelium.[16]

The size of the conjunctival transplant is limited and usually should not exceed 1.5 × 2 cm. The graft is taken from the superior quadrants, because these areas allow larger grafts and are more completely covered by the upper eyelid. Mucosa should be harvested from the bulbar surface only. At least 4 mm of conjunctiva should be left around the corneal limbus and over the insertion of the superior rectus muscle.[17] The donor site can be closed primarily but can be allowed to granulate spontaneously. As with all grafts, the recipient bed must have an adequate vascular supply. The graft is sutured edge to edge into the defect with 7-0 Vicryl or chromic suture, and, if necessary, it is splinted with a symblepharon ring to hold it flat.

ORAL MUCOUS MEMBRANE GRAFTS

For mucosal defects larger than 2 to 3 cm in diameter, nonconjunctival mucous membrane grafts are necessary. Numerous donor sites have been proposed, such as maxillary sinus mucosa,[18] but these may require special surgical skills not readily available from the ophthalmologist. Oral mucosa has proved to be the most useful material for eyelid and socket reconstruction. It is easily harvested as a full-thickness graft by direct dissection or in partial thickness using a mucotome. Grafts as large as 2 × 4 cm can be harvested from the lower lip, and additional grafts may be taken from the buccal surfaces so that an entire contracted socket may be repaired as a single procedure.

Although oral mucosal grafts can be harvested under local anesthesia, it is preferable to use a general anesthetic. For lower lip grafts, it is important that the graft not extend to within 2 mm of the vermilion border or the frenulum. The lip is everted using towel clips to expose the posterior surface. The mucosa is hydraulically elevated with local anesthetic containing hyaluronidase and 1:200,000 dilution of epinephrine for hemostasis. For partial-thickness grafts, a Castroviejo mucotome is used (Fig. 11–6). A very taut mucosal surface facilitates cutting without injury to deeper layers. For replacement of palpebral conjunctiva, a graft of 0.4 to 0.5 mm thickness is obtained. However, for grafting onto the bulbar surface a thinner graft of about 0.3 mm should be used to prevent an irregular surface and possible dellen formation. Although split-thickness grafts take extremely well, they typically undergo some degree of shrinkage, so a graft that is at least 25% to 30% larger than needed should be used. The patient is instructed to gargle with antiseptic solution for 5 to 7 days after surgery. Healing is rapid and remarkably painless.

When postoperative contraction is a concern, as in chemical burns, in a previously irradiated socket, or in the presence of excessive fibrosis, a full-thickness graft is preferred. In this instance, the donor area is marked and incised with a scalpel blade.[19] A thin sheet of epithelium is carefully dissected, leaving behind as much submucosal tissue as possible. If additional mucosa is needed, the cheek is everted, and a full-thickness graft is harvested from one or both sides. The graft should not exceed about 1.5 cm horizontally by 3 cm vertically and must avoid the opening of Stensen's duct located opposite the upper second molar tooth. The donor sites are packed with a sponge moistened with thrombin. Excessive cautery should be avoided. Buccal donor beds are closed with a running stitch of 5-0 Vicryl suture, but the lower lip bed is left to granulate. The patient is placed on a bland diet for several days after surgery, and the donor site is kept moist with bacitracin ointment. Healing takes place over several weeks.

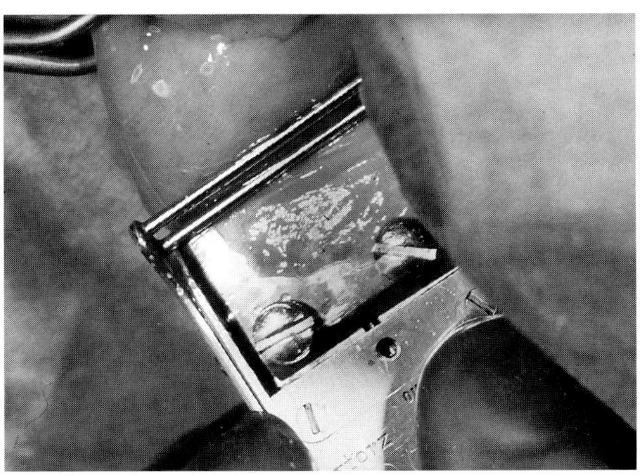

Figure 11–6. Harvesting of partial-thickness oral mucous membrane with a Castroviejo mucotome.

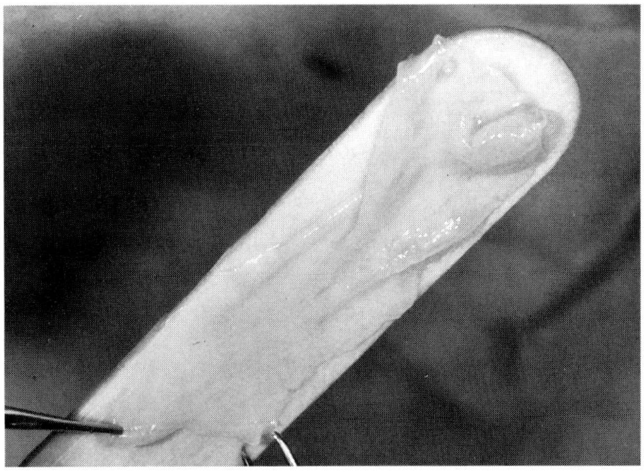

Figure 11–7. The graft is stored until use, mucosal side up, and soaked in gentamicin solution. Note that the edges of the graft roll away from the epithelial surface.

Complications at the donor site are unusual. Scarring and contraction may be seen, along with symblepharon formation.[20] If the contracting zone is symptomatic and functionally limiting, steroids can be injected into the area, or the scar bands can be excised and repaired with one or multiple tandem Z-plasties.

The mucosal graft should be stored on a flat surface with the mucosal surface upward (Fig. 11–7). The surfaces can usually be identified because the graft edges will characteristically roll away from the epithelial side owing to contraction of elastic fibers in the subconjunctival layer. The graft is covered with gentamicin solution until it is used.

Before placement of any mucosal graft, all scarred and fibrotic tissue must be excised from the recipient bed. When the tarsal surface is epidermalized and irregular, epithelium is removed using a diamond bur.[21] If entropion and trichiasis are present, the anterior skin–muscle lamella should be elevated and recessed about 2 mm away from the lid margin. If deeper fornices are required, conjunctiva is dissected from the orbital socket, and a pocket is formed immediately behind the capsulopalpebral fascia and Müller's muscle in the lower eyelid (Fig. 11–8) and the levator aponeurosis and Müller's muscle in the upper eyelid. Meticulous hemostasis must be ensured. The mucosal graft is sutured into the recipient bed with a running stitch of 6-0 Vicryl or chromic sutures (Fig. 11–9). Large folds and dog-ears are avoided, because these will not be in contact with the vascular bed. If necessary, large folds should be excised and the defects repaired. For trichiasis or tarsal deformity, the graft is folded over the lid margin and sutured to the recessed

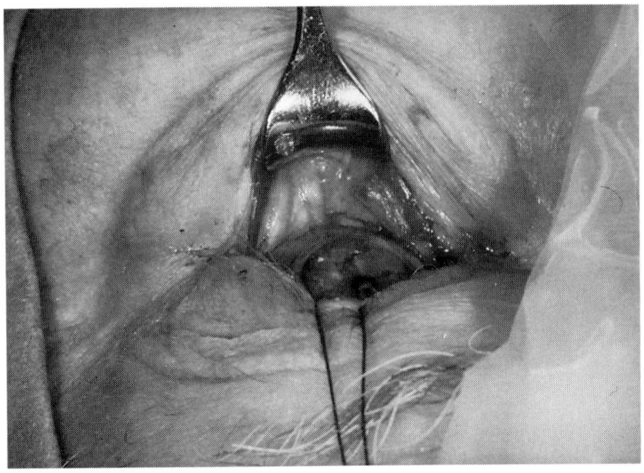

Figure 11–8. Preparation of the recipient bed with dissection of a pocket for reconstruction of the inferior fornix.

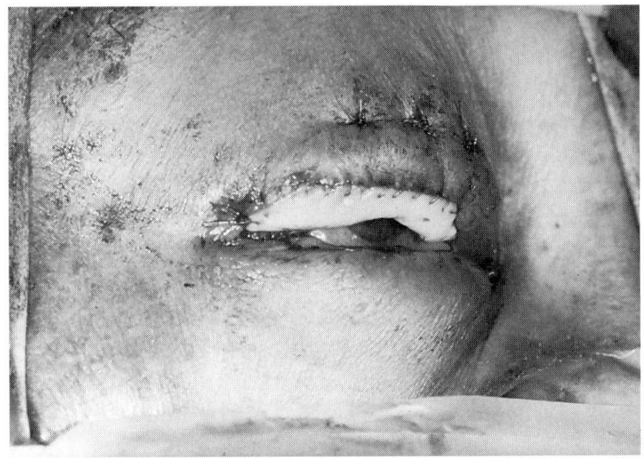

Figure 11–10. The graft is folded over the eyelid margin and sutured to the recessed skin–muscle lamella.

skin–muscle lamella (Fig. 11–10). Following placement of the graft an adequate splint is positioned. In the presence of a seeing eye, a symblepharon ring with a very large central opening can be placed to hold the mucosa into the fornices (Figs. 11–11 and 11–12).[22] Alternatively, a 2.5-cm length of 10 French catheter tubing can be placed into the fornices and secured with double-armed 4-0 sutures passed through the catheter and fornix and out onto the skin surface. A temporary-suture tarsorrhaphy is placed for 7 to 10 days to help keep the graft flat. For repair of a previously totally contracted socket, a specially designed thick conformer can be wrapped with mucosa, epithelial side in, and fixed to small holes drilled into the superior and inferior orbital rims.[23] However, the success rate in such cases is not high, and further contraction is common.

Complications at the recipient site are few. Graft failure is unusual and is related to a poorly vascular bed or large folds in the graft. Granulomas at the junctions of the graft with normal mucosa may occur and should be excised to prevent mechanical ectropion or difficulty in

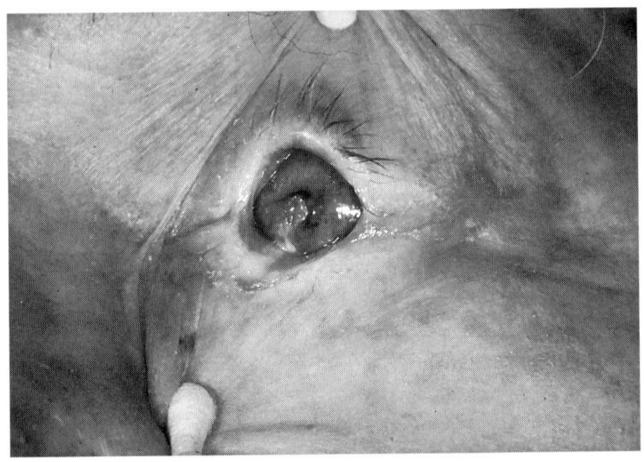

Figure 11–11. Severe cicatricial ocular pemphigoid with near total loss of conjunctiva.

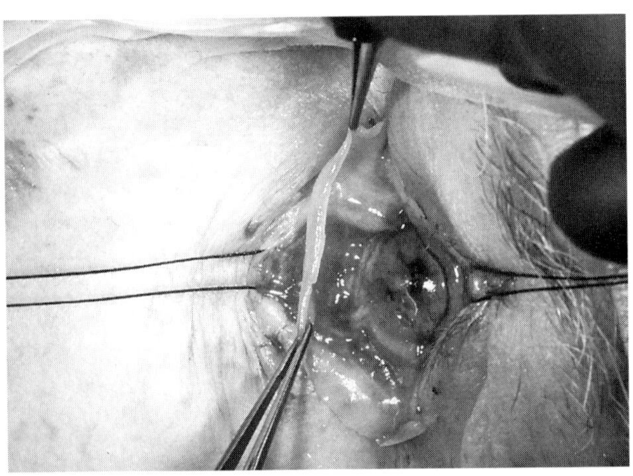

Figure 11–9. The mucous membrane graft is sutured to the edges of the remaining conjunctiva in the prepared recipient bed.

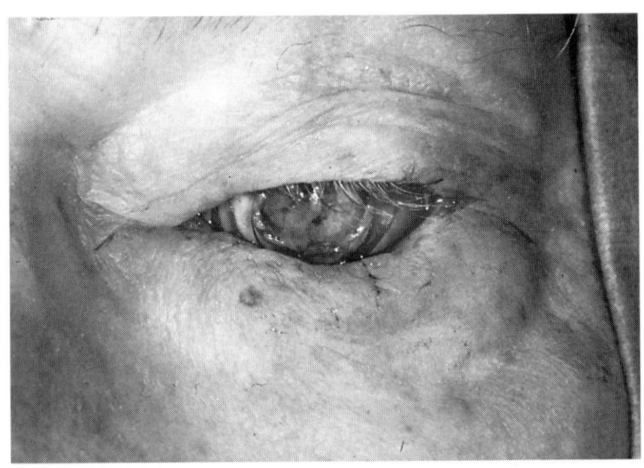

Figure 11–12. Same patient as in Figure 11–11 after placement of a mucous membrane graft. The graft is stented with a symblepharon ring.

wearing a prosthesis.[24] Infraorbital anesthesia is rare and results from too aggressive dissection of the inferior fornix with injury to branches of the infraorbital nerve. Ankyloblepharon with secondary blepharophimosis may result from fusion of adjacent raw surfaces when both eyelid margins are grafted. These are easily divided with repair of the margins, if needed. Minor infections are seen infrequently and generally are managed with oral and topical antibiotics. We do not routinely place our patients on prophylactic antibiotics. Ptosis of the upper eyelid results from injury to the levator aponeurosis during dissection of the superior fornix. Care must be taken to remain behind Müller's muscle to the level of Whitnall's ligament. Levinson and associates[25] described a patient who developed a perilimbic mass within a graft. This was composed of Fordyce's nodules of mature sebaceous glands located in the buccal mucosa. Contraction of the graft postoperatively is more related to the recipient bed than to the graft itself.[26] In previously contracted or irradiated sockets, all fibrotic tissue must be excised prior to graft placement. If repeat surgery is needed, this should be delayed for at least 1 year until the cicatricial stage has stabilized.

In patients with eyelid marginal deformity and secondary trichiasis, it may be desirable to rotate the lash-bearing skin lamella forward without resurfacing the palpebral conjunctiva. In this instance, a thicker graft with greater stability is needed. Hard palate mucous membrane is ideal for this purpose; it is harvested from the lateral hard palate as a strip measuring 2 to 2.5 cm in length by 5 mm in width. The defect is left to granulate. The lid margin is split along the gray line, and the graft is interposed between the two lamellae.[27]

FREE TARSOCONJUNCTIVAL GRAFTS

In many patients both conjunctiva and tarsus are contracted, and the tarsal plate is deformed, resulting in marginal entropion (Fig. 11–13). Also, following trauma or excision of malignant or benign lesions, segments of full-thickness eyelid may be missing. In all such patients both elements of the posterior lamella—conjunctiva and a tarsal substitute—will have to be replaced. Although numerous materials have been used, certainly the most appropriate is similar eyelid tissue. Free tarsoconjunctival grafts taken from the ipsilateral or contralateral upper eyelid are easily harvested and rarely, if ever, fail to take if properly supported by a vascular flap. The donor upper eyelid is everted over a Desmarres retractor with the use of the marginal traction suture. A rectangular block of tarsus and conjunctiva measuring approximately 20 mm long and 6 mm wide is cut with a scalpel blade, leaving 3 to 4 mm of tarsus along the eyelid margin for structural support (Fig. 11–14). The tarsus is carefully dissected from the underlying levator aponeurosis and excised along its upper border. If the block extends to the superior border of the tarsal plate, it must be separated from Müller's muscle. The donor site is not closed, because this may result in eyelid retraction.

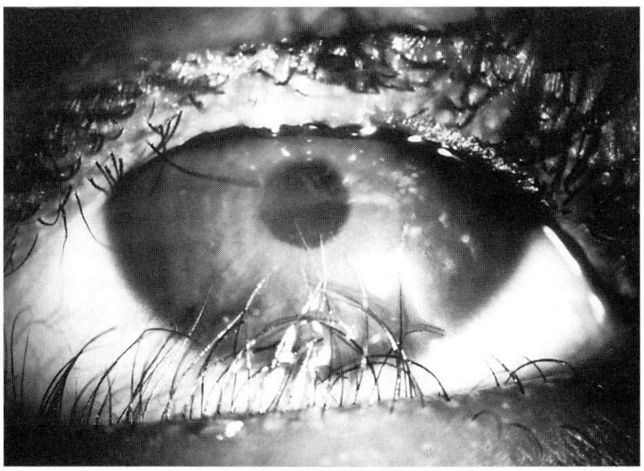

Figure 11–13. A young patient with Stevens-Johnson syndrome, cicatricial entropion of the lower eyelid, and secondary trichiasis.

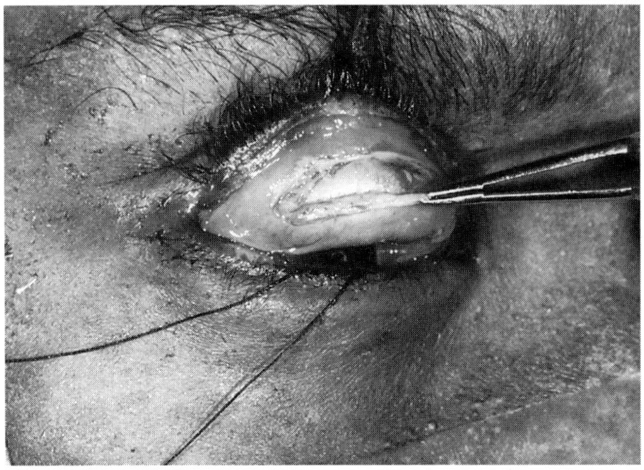

Figure 11–14. Same patient as in Figure 11–13. A free tarsoconjunctival graft is harvested from the ipsilateral upper eyelid and carefully dissected from the levator aponeurosis.

For entropion repair, the recipient bed is prepared by making a horizontal incision through the contracted conjunctiva and tarsus, and the marginal segment is separated from the underlying orbicularis (Fig. 11–15). The graft is placed into the bed, mucosal side facing the globe, and sutured with buried stitches to the edges of the defect (Fig. 11–16). For eyelid reconstruction the graft is positioned into the posterior lamellar defect and sutured to the remaining tarsus on either side or to the tarsus and stump of the canthal tendon. The graft should be oriented with the cut surfaces of the meibomian glands directed toward the new eyelid margin. The capsulopalpebral fascia is sutured to the graft along its inferior edge with a running stitch of 6-0 Vicryl suture. A skin–muscle advancement, rotational, or transpositional flap is placed over the graft for vascular support. It is important to recess the skin 1 mm below the graft margin to avoid epidermidalization of the new lid margin.

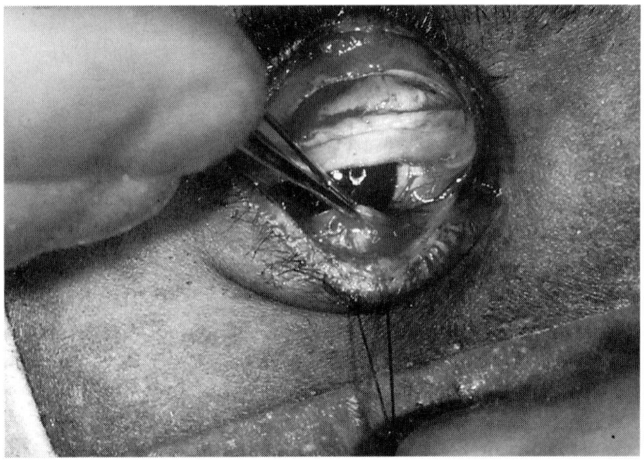

Figure 11–15. Same patient as in Figure 11–13. A horizontal incision is made in the contracted posterior lamella of the lower eyelid.

CARTILAGE-MUCOSAL COMPOUND GRAFTS

Another source for posterior lamellar replacement is the cartilage-mucosal compound graft.[28] This can be obtained directly from the nasal septum, or it can be prepared from ear cartilage. In the case of nasal septum the nose is packed with cotton sponges soaked in 4% cocaine. The base of the nasal ala is injected with 2% lidocaine containing epinephrine. A 4-0 silk suture is passed through the ala for traction, and an incision is made along its base to separate it from the face. Retraction of the ala exposes the nasal septum. A graft up to 1 × 1.5 cm is outlined parallel to the direction of the turbinates, and an incision is made through mucosa and cartilage only, leaving the mucosa on the opposite side intact. The graft is dissected off with fine scissors. The ala is resutured to the facial skin with 5-0 silk sutures, and the nose is packed with antibiotic ointment and a pressure stent inside the finger of a latex glove. The cartilage usually must be thinned prior to use in the eyelid.

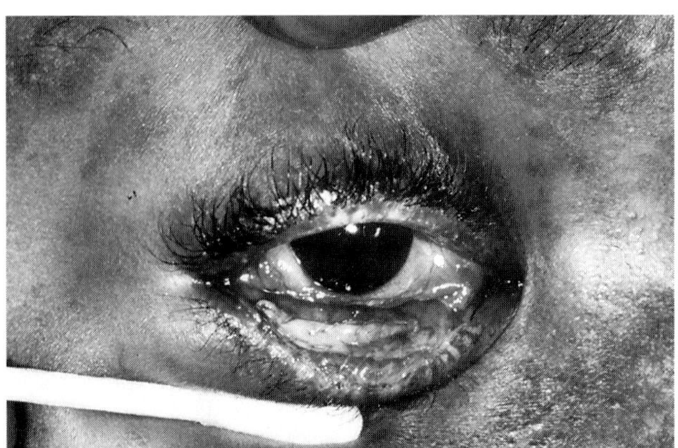

Figure 11–16. Same patient as in Figure 11–13. The free tarsoconjunctival graft is placed into the recipient defect and sutured with buried 6-0 Vicryl sutures.

When a larger graft is needed, auricular cartilage is harvested from the pinna through a posterior skin incision. If the graft is excessively curved, partial-thickness incisions can be made in the convex surface parallel to the curvature axis to flatten it. A submucosal pocket is prepared in the cheek, and the cartilage graft is inserted. The defect is repaired with a running stitch of 6-0 chromic suture. After 2 to 3 weeks the graft is vascularized and the composite mucosal graft can be harvested.

REFERENCES

1. Kinishita JH, Masurat T, Helfant M: Pathways of glucose metabolism in the corneal epithelium. Science 122:72, 1955.
2. Thoft RA, Friend J: Biochemical transformation of regenerating ocular surface epithelium. Invest Ophthalmol Vis Sci 16:14–20, 1977.
3. Hosni FA: Repair of trachomatous cicatricial entropion using mucous membrane graft. Arch Ophthalmol 91:49–51, 1974.
4. Tse DT, Mandelbaum S, Epstein E, et al: Mucous membrane grafting for severe palpebral vernal conjunctivitis. Arch Ophthalmol 101:1879–1883, 1983.
5. Kaufman HE, Thomas EL: Prevention and treatment of symblepharon. Am J Ophthalmol 88:419–423, 1988.
6. Guibor P, Smith B: Symblepharon shield. Trans Am Acad Ophthalmol Otol 77:484–485, 1977.
7. Zagora E: Eye Injuries. Springfield, IL, Charles C Thomas, 1970, pp 409–412.
8. Choy AE, Asbell RL, Taterka HB: Symblepharon repair using a silicone sheet implant. Ann Ophthalmol 9:197–204, 1977.
9. Stallard HB: Eye Surgery. Baltimore, Williams & Wilkins, 1973, pp 779–782.
10. Clark G: Use of silicone in eye surgery. Bull Dow Corning Cent Aid Med Res 5:3, 1963.
11. Hammer-Hodges DW, Scott NB: Replacement of an abdominal wall defect using expanded PTFE sheet (Gore-Tex). J R Coll Surg Edinb 30:65–67, 1985.
12. Savrin RA, Record GT, McDowell DE: Axillofemoral bypass. Arch Surg 121:1016–1020, 1986.
13. Hanel KC, McCabe C, Abbott WM, et al: Current PTFE grafts: A biochemical, scanning electron, and light microscopic evaluation. Ann Surg 195:456–463, 1982.
14. Sugarman B: In vitro adherence of bacteria to prosthesis vascular grafts. Infection 10:9–12, 1982.
15. Levin PS, Dutton JJ: Polytef (polytetrafluoroethylene) alloplastic grafting as a substitute for mucous membrane. Arch Ophthalmol 108:282–285, 1990.
16. Thoft RA: Conjunctival transplantation as an alternative to keratoplasty. Ophthalmology 86:1084–1091, 1979.
17. Vastine DW, Stewart WB, Schwab IR: Reconstruction of the periocular mucous membrane by autologous conjunctival transplantation. Ophthalmology 89:1072–1081, 1982.
18. Fry TL, Woods CI: Readily available full-thickness mucous membrane graft. Arch Otolaryngol Head Neck Surg 113:770–771, 1987.
19. Weiss RA, McCord CD, Ellsworth RM: Reconstruction of the anophthalmic socket: Lower eyelid malposition and canthal tendon laxity. Adv Ophthalmic Plast Reconstr Surg 8:192–198, 1990.
20. Neuhaus RW, Baylis HI, Shorr N: Complications of mucous membrane donor sites. Am J Ophthalmol 93:643–646, 1982.
21. McCord CD, Chen WP: Tarsal polishing and mucous membrane grafting for cicatricial entropion, trichiasis, and epidermalization. Ophthalmic Surg 14:1021–1025, 1983.
22. Karesh JW, Putterman AM: Reconstruction of the partially contracted ocular socket or fornix. Arch Ophthalmol 106:552–556, 1988.
23. Putterman AM, Karesh JW: A surgical technique for the successful and stable reconstruction of the totally contracted ocular socket. Ophthalmic Surg 19:194–201, 1988.

24. Mathur SP: Cicatricial entropion of the upper eyelid: A modification of the operation. Ophthalmologica 152:207–211, 1966.
25. Levinson AW, Jakobiec FA, Reifler DM, Hornblass A: Ectopic epibulbar Fordyce nodules in a buccal mucous membrane graft. Am J Ophthalmol 100:724–727, 1985.
26. Vistnes LM: Management of the contracted socket. *In* Hornblass A (ed): Oculoplastic, Orbital, and Reconstructive Surgery, vol 2. Baltimore, Williams & Wilkins, 1990, pp 1313–1319.
27. Silver B: The use of mucous membrane from the hard palate in the treatment of trichiasis and cicatricial entropion. Ophthalmic Plast Reconstr Surg 2:129–131, 1986.
28. McCord CD, Tannenbaum M: Oculoplastic Surgery, 2nd ed. New York, Raven Press, 1987, pp 17–19.

CHAPTER 12

Pigmented Conjunctival Neoplasms

M. Ronan Conlon and Peter A. D. Rubin

Pigmented neoplasms encompass a wide spectrum of disease ranging from benign complexion-associated melanosis (racial melanosis) to malignant conjunctival melanoma. In no area of ophthalmology has the terminology applied to a group of conditions changed so often and, in doing so, generated so much confusion in the interpretation of these lesions. The optimal management of a patient requires close communication between the ophthalmic surgeon and a pathologist who is familiar with the conjunctiva. Although conjunctival pigmentation is not an uncommon observation in ophthalmic practice, the occurrence of conjunctival melanoma is relatively rare, thus diminishing general ophthalmologists' familiarity with this condition. Conjunctival melanoma is estimated to be 1/30 to 1/40 as common as choroidal melanoma, of which 1500 new cases are diagnosed yearly in the United States,[1] so it is assumed that approximately 40 new cases of conjunctival melanoma are diagnosed annually in the United States.

It is particularly important for the ophthalmologist to be able to distinguish between benign conjunctival pigmentations and conjunctival melanoma, for the latter is associated with a mortality rate of 25%.[2] The difficulty in the management of these neoplasms is complicated by the importance of the conjunctiva to the maintenance of the functional integrity of the globe. Thus, one is not at the same liberty to excise these lesions, as one would be if dealing with a cutaneous melanoma. The management of pigmented neoplasms of the conjunctiva has moved in a more conservative direction over the last decade, with the ultimate goals of preserving the patient's life and yet maintaining useful vision.

The effective management of these tumors is founded on early clinical recognition, appropriate histopathologic interpretation, and institution of adequate treatment. Toward furthering these goals, this chapter places particular emphasis on the clinical manifestations, assessment, and management of these tumors.

ANATOMY

The conjunctiva is a mucous membrane composed of two to five cell layers of nonkeratinized squamous epithelium that lies on a delicate connective tissue known as the *substantia propria.* The basilar layer of epithelium is composed of 5% conjunctival melanocytes, which are normally found in a circumlimbal distribution. The normal conjunctival melanocyte has a dendriform appearance; however, on cytologic fixation it assumes a more rounded appearance with a clear cytoplasm, which allows it to be distinguished histopathologically from adjacent epithelial cells. Changes in the metabolic rate and growth of the normal conjunctival melanocytes can give rise to a number of pigmented lesions in the conjunctiva.

In contrast with the skin epithelium, the conjunctival epithelium is nonkeratinized and contains goblet cells. Although the subepithelial layers of the skin are stratified into papillary and reticular dermis, the subepithelial layer of the conjunctiva (substantia propria) lacks this division (Fig. 12–1).

For the purpose of clinical description the conjunctiva can be divided into three topographic zones: (1) the tarsal (palpebral) conjunctiva, which is densely adherent to the tarsal plate, starts at the mucocutaneous junction of the eyelid, and ends in the fornix; (2) the fornix conjunctiva, which lines the fornices, is abundant in the area, giving rise to loose folds; and (3) the bulbar conjunctiva, which lines the surface of the globe, is normally freely mobile over the surface of the eye, except at the limbus where the bulbar conjunctiva fuses with underlying connective tissue to become closely adherent to the globe. The conjunctiva also contains several glandular structures, including the accessory lacrimal glands of Krause and Wolfring, which are found in the fornix and at the upper border of the tarsus, respectively.[3–5]

TERMINOLOGY

The terminology used to describe pigmented lesions of the conjunctiva has evolved in recent years. It is important for the ophthalmologist to be aware of the terminology when interpreting biopsy results from this area. Basic definitions of current terminology are as follows:

1. *Melanosis* refers to pigmentation secondary to the production of melanin as opposed to pigmentation

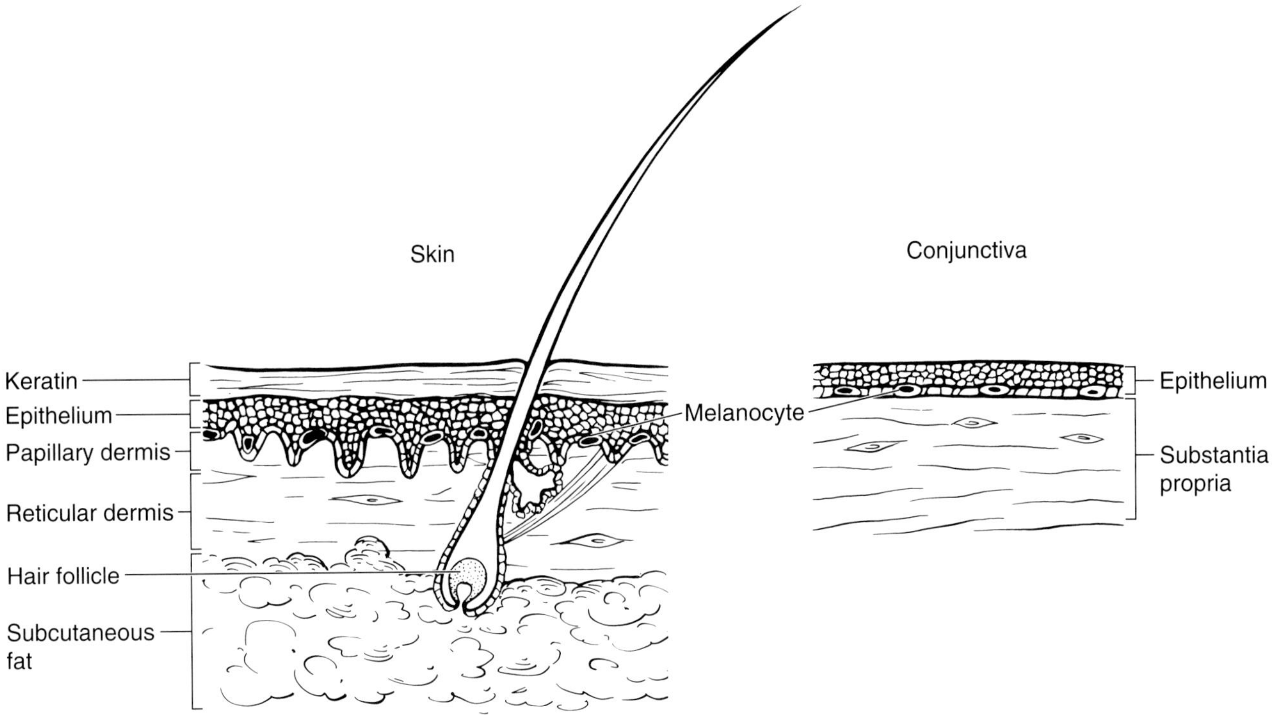

Figure 12-1. Schematic diagram comparing the histopathologic stratification of the conjunctiva and the skin.

secondary to a pharmacologic agent (such as epinephrine) or systemic disease (such as Addison's disease). It has been used in both the dermatologic and ophthalmologic literature.

2. A *nevus* is a benign proliferation of roundish cells that are believed to be derived from dendritic melanocytes.
3. *Basilar hyperplasia* is a proliferation of basilar epithelial cells with confinement of the cell to this location and no evidence of migration either downward or into the suprabasilar epithelium.
4. *Pagetoid spread* refers to a growth pattern where atypical cells are present in the suprabasilar epithelium (pagetoid cells). In primary acquired melanosis (PAM) this pattern of growth is highly predictive of lesions likely to progress to malignant melanoma.
5. *Atypia* notes the presence of polyhedral or irregularly shaped cells in which the nucleus is hyperchromatic. These cells typically lack the cohesiveness of normal epithelial cells.
6. *Lentigo maligna* (Hutchinson's freckle) is a term used in dermatology to describe variably pigmented tumors of the skin with poorly demarcated edges. Histopathologically, lentigo maligna is characterized by atypical melanocytes located along the basilar epithelium that have a tendency to spread around adnexal structures. Although this term has been applied to the description of PAM of the conjunctiva, we do not advocate its use.
7. *Lentigo maligna melanoma, superficial spreading melanoma,* and *nodular melanoma* all refer to different types of cutaneous melanoma. These terms should not be applied to the description of conjunctival melanoma (see later).

CLASSIFICATION

The classification of conjunctival tumors has changed considerably over the last decade. Furthermore, the classification of pigmented conjunctival tumors used by ophthalmopathologists is not completely analogous to that used by dermatopathologists. Because conjunctival biopsies are not interpreted exclusively by ophthalmopathologists, it is important for the ophthalmologist to have some familiarity with differences in terminology so that confusion can be avoided (Table 12-1).

The term *primary acquired melanosis,*[6] previously referred to as *precancerous melanosis,*[7] *benign acquired melanosis,*[8] *primary idiopathic melanosis,*[8] and *atypical melanocytic hyperplasia,*[9] has been adopted by ophthalmologists to describe a patchy pigmentation of the conjunctiva that is distinct from conjunctival nevi and melanoma. Although dermatopathologists have suggested that the term *carcinoma in situ* should be applied to PAM,[10-12] ophthalmologists have resisted this designation, primarily because *carcinoma in situ* suggests an inexorable progression to malignant melanoma yet does not reflect the diversity of clinical manifestations seen in patients with PAM.

TABLE 12-1

Comparison of Classifications of Conjunctival Pigmented Tumors

Ophthalmopathologists	Dermatopathologists
PAM without atypia	Conjunctival melanosis
PAM with atypia	Atypical melanocytic hyperplasia
Low risk of progression	Lentiginous
High risk of progression to	Transepithelial
Suprabasilar atypical melanocytes	
Epithelioid cells	
Malignant melanoma	Malignant melanoma
With PAM	With a radial growth phase (lentiginous)
Malignant melanoma	
Without PAM	Without a radial growth phase

PAM, primary acquired melanosis.

Adapted from Folberg R, McLean MC: Primary acquired melanosis and melanoma: Terminology, classification, and biological behavior. Hum Pathol 17:653, 1986.

For the ophthalmologist the information needed about these patients includes (1) the likelihood of clinical progression to conjunctival melanoma and (2) who needs aggressive treatment. Folberg and associates,[13] in a series from the Armed Forces Institute of Pathology (AFIP), showed that patients with PAM are a heterogeneous group separated by the absence (PAM without atypia) or presence (PAM with atypia) of atypical cells in the conjunctival epithelium. The same study showed that patients with PAM without atypia were virtually at no risk for developing malignant melanoma, whereas in patients with PAM with atypia, the risk approached 50%. Thus, the term *primary acquired melanosis* is useful for the ophthalmologist in both a clinical and histopathologic sense: (1) it identifies a patient who requires a conjunctival biopsy prior to definitive treatment, because one cannot distinguish between PAM without and with atypia on clinical grounds alone, and (2) the histopathologic subdivision into PAM without and with atypia allows one to tailor treatment accordingly.

In as many as 75% of patients with conjunctival melanoma, a component of PAM can be found histopathologically. Attempts to apply the classification of cutaneous melanoma (nodular, superficial spreading, lentigo maligna) to the PAM component of conjunctival melanoma have met with difficulty.[9, 13] One of the main problems is that the PAM component of conjunctival melanoma may have areas that resemble both superficial spreading melanoma and lentigo maligna and are thus not easily classifiable; other difficulties relate to tumor thickness. Clark and coworkers' classification of tumor thickness of cutaneous melanoma based on tumor location with the epidermis and dermis is not readily applicable to conjunctival melanoma because the substantia propria lacks the same histopathologic stratification (see Fig. 12-1).[14, 15]

CLINICAL FEATURES

Complexion-associated Melanosis

Complexion-associated melanosis is a benign condition seen more frequently in dark-skinned than in light-skinned people.[16-18] Its importance lies in being able to distinguish it from more ominous pigmented tumors of the conjunctiva. Increased metabolic activity of basilar melanocytes without a proliferation in their absolute number is the underlying pathologic change in complexion-associated melanosis. The "switched-on" melanocytes in this condition liberate melanin, which is readily incorporated into the adjacent basal epithelial cells. Clinically, the condition appears as a bilateral golden-brown patchy pigmentation of the bulbar conjunctiva that is interpalpebral and perilimbal in distribution (Fig. 12-2). Typically, the degree of pigmentation fades toward the fornices, and one does not see involvement of the tarsal conjunctiva. Although this pigmentation abuts the corneal epithelium, it does not spread centrally onto the corneal epithelium significantly. In the absence of inflammatory pannus, which may draw pigmented cells centrally onto the cornea, the presence of central corneal pigmentation should suggest diagnostic possibilities other than complexion-associated melanosis (Fig. 12-3).[19, 20]

The differential diagnosis of complexion-associated melanosis includes PAM, malignant melanoma, melanosis oculi, and argyrosis. Differentiating features of PAM and malignant melanoma are discussed later in this chapter. Melanosis oculi is a rare condition that may infrequently be confused with complexion-associated melanosis.[21-23] The underlying pathologic abnormality in this condition is an arrest in embryogenesis of the normal migration of neural crest-derived melanocytes to the uveal tract, with their sequestration within the sclera.[24] This gives rise to a blue-gray appearance of the sclera (Fig. 12-4). Caucasian patients with ocular me-

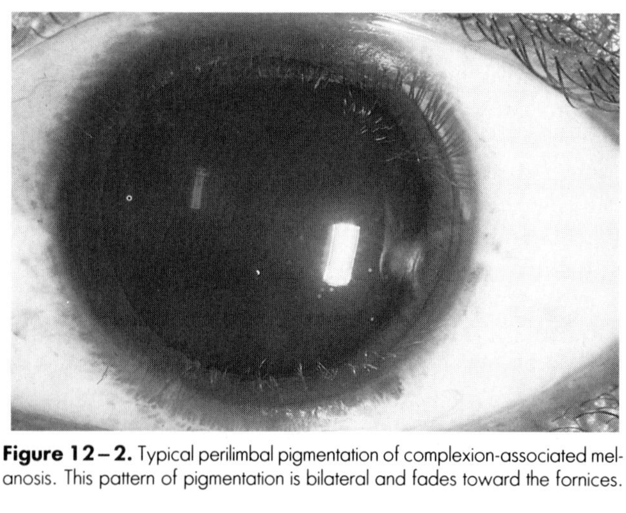

Figure 12-2. Typical perilimbal pigmentation of complexion-associated melanosis. This pattern of pigmentation is bilateral and fades toward the fornices.

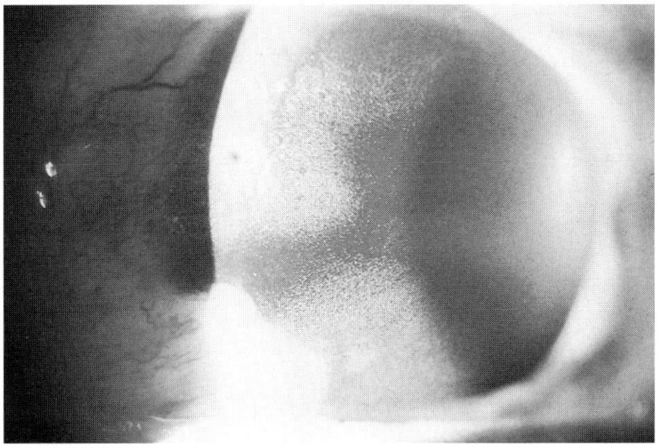

Figure 12–3. Migration of pigment on the central corneal epithelium in the absence of inflammation suggests the diagnosis of primary acquired melanosis with atypia. Involvement of the corneal epithelium generally does not extend beyond a few millimeters of the limbus in complexion-associated melanosis.

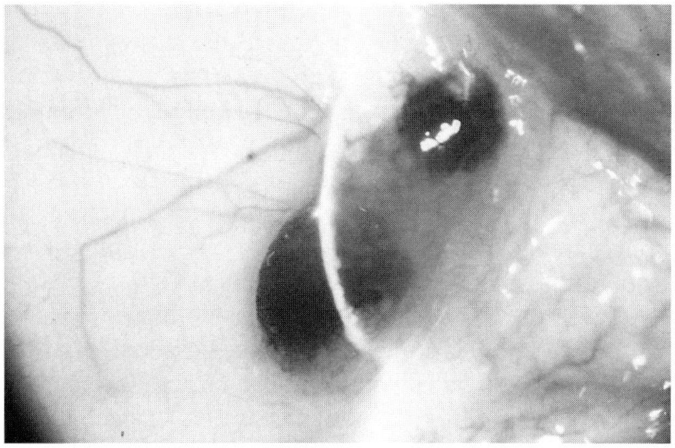

Figure 12–5. Conjunctival nevus. The nevus in the region of the plica semilunaris demonstrates the characteristic features of pseudocysts that are composed of conjunctival epithelial inclusion cysts and goblet cells.

lanocytosis are at an increased risk for developing uveal melanoma, and two studies have calculated ocular melanocytosis to be 30 to 35 times more common in patients with uveal melanoma.[25] Careful slit-lamp examination of the patient reveals that the overlying conjunctiva is not involved by the process and moves freely over the discolored sclera.

Conjunctival Nevi

Nevi of the conjunctiva usually develop during the first decade of life and appear as well-circumscribed, brownish lesions often in a juxtalimbal location (Fig. 12–5). The degree of pigmentation of a nevus may be variable, and as many as 30% may be nonpigmented (Fig. 12–6).[18,26] Nevus cells are believed to be transformed melanocytes that have assumed a more rounded appearance and have a marked tendency to adopt a nesting pattern.[5, 27] The normal maturation of nevus cells is characterized by a gradual descent from the epithelium into the underlying substantia, and this gives rise to the following histopathologic classification:

1. Junctional—nevus cells at the junction of the epithelium and subepithelial tissue
2. Compound—nevus cells in the epithelium and the substantia propria
3. Subepithelial—nevus cells within the substantia propria

The presence of epithelial inclusion cysts is a characteristic feature of a nevus and is suggestive of a benign process; however, one must remember that this is not absolute, because as many as 25% of conjunctival melanomas have histologic evidence of arising from a nevus.[2, 16]

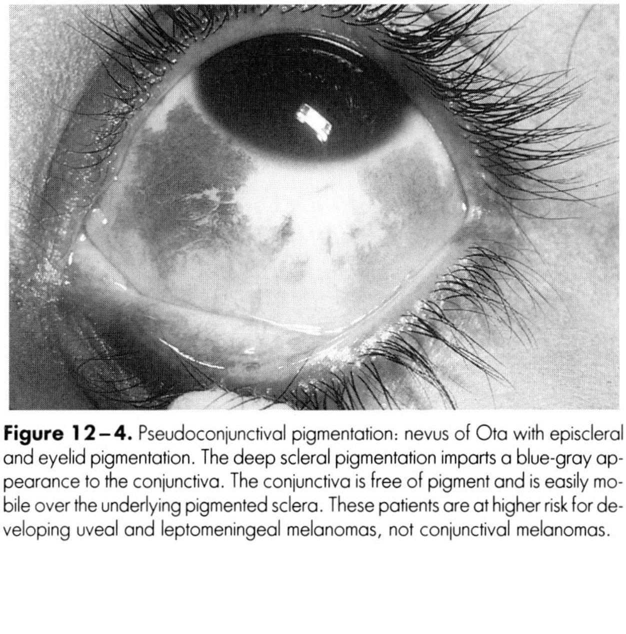

Figure 12–4. Pseudoconjunctival pigmentation: nevus of Ota with episcleral and eyelid pigmentation. The deep scleral pigmentation imparts a blue-gray appearance to the conjunctiva. The conjunctiva is free of pigment and is easily mobile over the underlying pigmented sclera. These patients are at higher risk for developing uveal and leptomeningeal melanomas, not conjunctival melanomas.

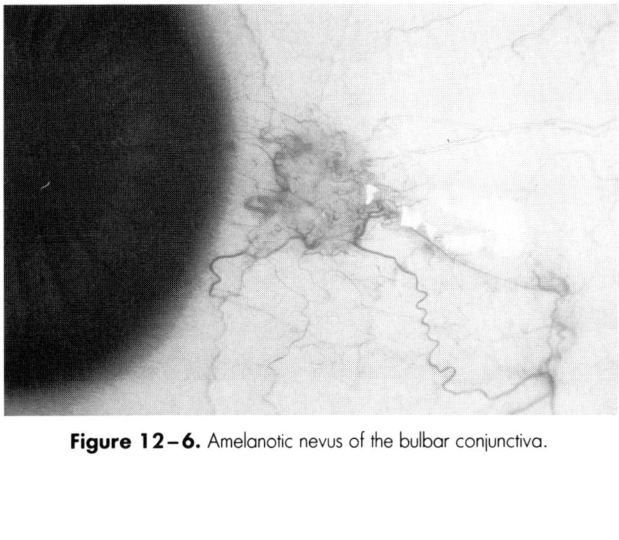

Figure 12–6. Amelanotic nevus of the bulbar conjunctiva.

Most nevi are benign, and excision is not required unless cosmesis is a concern or the patient has undue fears regarding cancerous change. These lesions may grow during childhood, change in coloration, and increase in vascularity. Although these are important points, they are not especially helpful in predicting if the lesion has undergone a malignant transformation. Inflammation, actinic damage, hormonal changes (such as in pregnancy and Addison's disease), trauma, and malignant change all may stimulate melanin production within nevus cells. Conjunctival melanoma in children is exceedingly rare, as is malignant transformation of a conjunctival nevus.

The clinical differential diagnosis of a suspected conjunctival nevus includes conjunctival melanoma, Axenfeld's nerve loop, and extrascleral extension of a uveal melanoma (Fig. 12–7). Conjunctival melanoma is frequently associated with PAM, and careful inspection of the conjunctiva should be made for this entity during examination of a suspected nevus of the conjunctiva.[2] The presence of cysts within the lesion is more suggestive of a benign nevus, as is confinement of the lesion to the conjunctiva. Extrascleral extension of a uveal melanoma can simulate a nevus; however, the adherence of the lesion to the underlying sclera should make the distinction possible on clinical examination. Other tests used to exclude extrascleral extension of a uveal melanoma include transillumination of the globe, gonioscopy, ultrasonography, and dilated fundus examination.

Primary Acquired Melanosis

PAM is a unilateral condition that typically appears as a patchy brown pigmentation of the conjunctiva in people in their early 40s. The pigment has the following specific noteworthy characteristics: (1) variability in the degree and location (often referred to as *waxing and waning*); (2) flatness; (3) golden brown in color; and (4) edges that are indistinct (Fig. 12–8).[7,13,16,28]

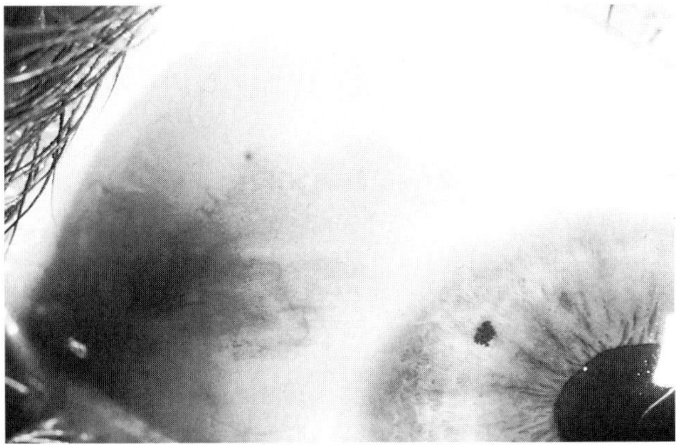

Figure 12–8. Primary acquired melanosis of the conjunctiva with fine, flat epibulbar pigmentation with feathery borders.

What is the risk of a patient with PAM developing malignant melanoma? The answer to this question is related to the histopathologic appearance of the lesion, which has been subclassified into PAM without atypia and PAM with atypia, based on the absence or presence of atypical melanocytes within the epithelium (Fig. 12–9). In a study based on material from the AFIP, PAM without atypia was found to be associated with a good prognosis.[13] Of the 13 patients with PAM without atypia, none later developed malignant melanoma. However, in patients with PAM with atypia, the risk of progression to malignant melanoma approached 50%. This risk increased to 70% if epithelioid cells were present and to 90% if a suprabasilar (pagetoid) distribution of melanocytes was present.[2] One cannot distinguish clinically between PAM without atypia and with atypia, so when the diagnosis is suspected, a biopsy is indicated. Additionally, evidence suggests that progression to conjunctival melanoma in patients with PAM with atypia is more likely in the first 6 years of diagnosis and is very unlikely thereafter.[2]

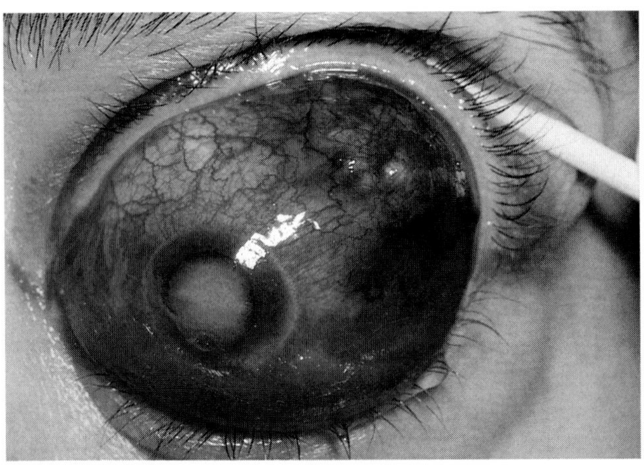

Figure 12–7. Extrascleral extension of a choroidal melanoma body simulating a primary conjunctival melanoma.

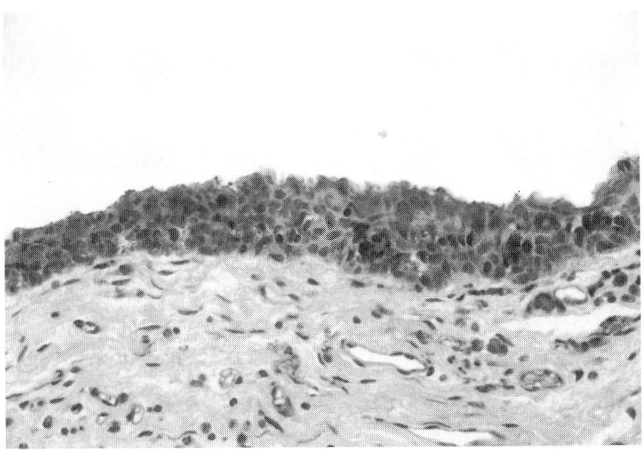

Figure 12–9. Histologic section demonstrating the appearance of primary acquired melanosis with atypia.

Malignant Melanoma

Malignant melanoma of the conjunctiva most often arises in the context of preceding PAM (75%),[2] whereas the remainder of cases occurs in association with a preexisting nevus or de novo. The average age of presentation is the early 50s, and the tumor is exceedingly rare in African American patients.[2, 29] It is important to inquire about a history of a preexisting blemish, because this is present in as many as 30% of patients.[29]

By definition, conjunctival melanoma is heralded by the invasion of melanoma cells into the substantia propria (Fig. 12–10). The development of a nodule in a previously flat area of pigmentation should alert the clinician to the possibility of invasive melanoma. Less dramatic evidence of melanoma developing in an area of PAM is localized thickening of the conjunctiva, increased vascularity, and inflammatory changes in a previously quiet area.[29] Malignant melanoma of the conjunctiva may involve any region of the conjunctiva (bulbar, fornical, palpebral), caruncle, or lid margin.[30, 31]

The overall mortality rate from metastatic spread in patients with melanoma of the conjunctiva is approximately 25%.[2] In melanoma associated with PAM, histopathologic analysis of the PAM component may provide useful information regarding the future risk of metastatic spread.[2] Features in the PAM component associated with a higher incidence of metastatic spread include the presence of atypical melanocytes, palpebral involvement, and absence of clinical pigmentation (sine pigmento) and small polyhedral cells. In Folberg and coworkers' series,[2] tumor thickness did not invariably correlate with metastatic spread; however in other studies tumors thicker than 1.5 mm were consistently associated with metastatic spread.[9, 29] In approximately 20% to 30% of conjunctival melanomas, a nevus component can be identified pathologically; however, this has not been found to be predictive of metastatic spread.[2, 29] In regard to location, Jakobiec and colleagues[29] have commented that metastatic spread is rarely seen in purely juxtalimbal conjunctival melanomas, whereas with fornical and palpebral involvement metastatic spread is more likely owing, in part, to the delay of recognition of lesions outside the palpebral zone and the greater accessibility of fornix-based lesions to the lymphatics.

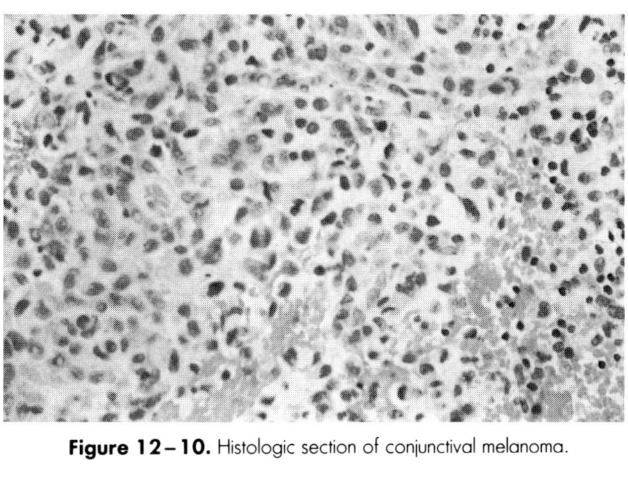

Figure 12–10. Histologic section of conjunctival melanoma.

TABLE 12–2

Evaluation of Pigmented Conjunctival Tumors

I. History
   A. Age
   B. Date first noticed
   C. Growth
   D. Change in color, vascularity
   E. Use of eye drops
   F. Trauma—foreign body
   G. Pregnancy
      1. Systemic illnesses
         a. Endocrine disorders
II. Clinical evaluation
   A. External examination
      1. Eyelid pigmentation
      2. Lid contour suggesting mass
      3. Palpation of ocular adnexa
      4. Palpation of regional lymph nodes
   B. Anterior segment examination
      1. Pigmentation—flat or elevated
      2. Mobile or nonmobile
      3. Tenderness—Axenfeld's nerve loop
      4. Location—bulbar, forniceal, or palpebral
      5. Eversion and double eversion of the eyelids
      6. Gonioscopy, echography
   C. Posterior segment examination
      1. Scleral indentation—rule out ciliary body tumor

CLINICAL EVALUATION

It is important to have a systematic approach, an algorithm, to evaluating a patient with a pigmented conjunctival lesion. The following section outlines important points to elicit during the history and features to assess on clinical examination (Table 12–2). This is not meant to be a dogmatic approach but rather a useful guideline.

History

A good history is essential to the clinician in determining the malignant potential of a given pigmented tumor of the conjunctiva. To rule out lesions simulating a conjunctival melanoma, attention should be paid to any history of previous trauma to the eye. The patient may forget an old injury, and with time a foreign body in the conjunctiva may simulate a conjunctival tumor (Fig. 12–11). Specific inquiry should be made about the use of eye drops in the past because compounds containing epinephrine and silver can give rise to adrenochrome and argyrosis, respectively, which can mimic pigmented tumors of the conjunctiva. The appearance of a newly pigmented lesion of the conjunctiva in a person 20 years of age or older should raise suspicion, and a biopsy of the lesion should be performed. In addition, lesions that are

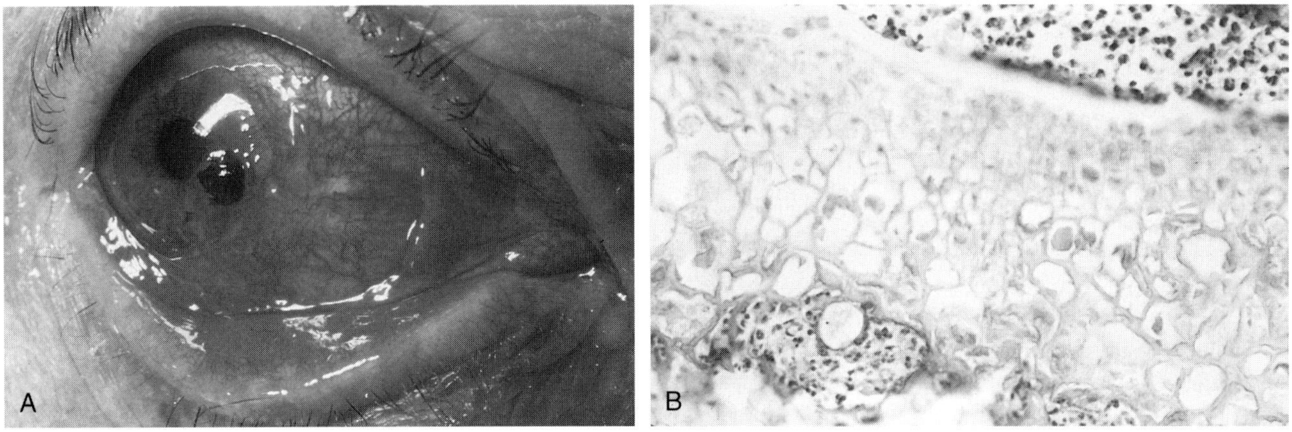

Figure 12–11. Pseudomelanocytic lesion: a wood foreign body. *A*, This pigmented lesion of the limbus and adjacent inflammation with conjunctival thickening was suggestive of an amelanotic melanoma with a pigmented component at the limbus. Removal of the limbal mass and microscopic evaluation *(B)* revealed a vegetative structure consistent with a wood foreign body.

enlarging should undergo biopsy. Benign conjunctival nevi may also increase in size, vascularity, and pigmentation with time. Systemic illness (adrenal insufficiency, ochronosis) or physiologic states (pregnancy) that can cause increased pigmentation of the conjunctiva should be pursued in the appropriate clinical context.

Examination

Careful examination of the area under slit-lamp magnification is essential in all patients with a pigmented conjunctival lesion. The use of an ultraviolet light is useful in detecting subtle areas of pigmentary spread on the conjunctiva as well as the lid margin. It is most important to assess the location of the lesion and be aware of the implications of location in terms of clinical diagnosis and prognosis. Accurate diagrams of the pigmentation location or photographic documentation should be performed at each visit so that the progression of the disease can be closely monitored.

Pigmentation in non–sunlight-exposed areas such as the palpebral and fornical conjunctivae is highly unusual, so a biopsy should be performed. The likelihood of a benign nevus arising in either of these locations is low. Double eversion of the eyelids should be performed in all patients being evaluated for pigmentation of the conjunctiva to permit maximal viewing of the conjunctival surface (Fig. 12–12). The spread of juxtalimbal pigmentation onto the central cornea or isolated central corneal pigmentation is a feature of PAM and can be a useful distinguishing feature (see Fig. 12–3). The level of conjunctival pigmentation should be determined. Conjunctival nevi and PAM are confined to the conjunctival epithelium and should move freely with the conjunctiva. The presence of deeper involvement can be assessed clinically by applying topical 1% proparacaine to the conjunctiva and then gently assessing the conjunctival mobility with a cotton-tipped applicator. Sometimes gently moving the lower eyelid up against the area of involvement and noting whether the conjunctiva moves freely are sufficient to exclude clinical involvement of the deeper tissues. Immobility of the conjunctiva suggests either invasion of the deeper tissues or the possibility of extrascleral spread of a uveal melanoma (see Fig. 12–7). The latter condition can be distinguished from the former by the use of echography, gonioscopy, transillumination, and indirect ophthalmoscopy combined with scleral depression. It is not possible to determine accurately the mobility of the conjunctiva near the limbus owing to the fusion of the conjunctiva with the underlying Tenon's fascia in this area.

Following careful slit-lamp examination the ocular adnexa and regional nodes should be carefully palpated to detect localized spread. This should be repeated on subsequent examinations in patients at risk for the development of conjunctival melanoma or who have been treated for conjunctival melanoma. Contrary to uveal

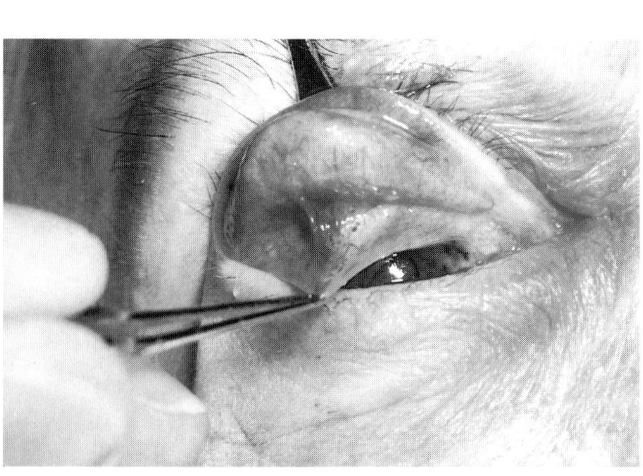

Figure 12–12. Double eversion of the upper eyelid is the best technique to visualize the fornical conjunctiva.

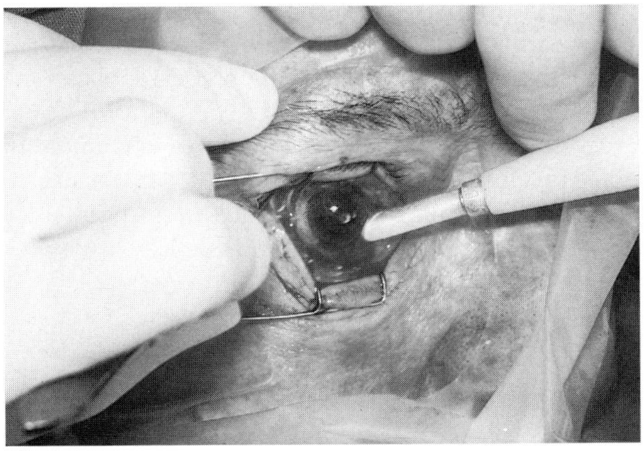

Figure 12–13. Cryotherapy application to the epibulbar surface and conjunctival edges to eliminate residual melanocytes following excision of a conjunctiva melanoma.

melanoma, which metastasizes to the liver first, conjunctival melanoma spreads initially via the lymphatics to the regional nodes in the head and neck.

MANAGEMENT

The management of pigmented conjunctival tumors has changed greatly over the last decade.[5, 32–36] Although controversies exist about the optimal management, certain points are generally accepted. Cryotherapy as an adjunctive therapy for PAM with atypia and conjunctival melanoma has proved to be a useful modality (Fig. 12–13).[5, 32–34, 36, 37] The ability of cryotherapy to selectively destroy pigmented tumor cells in the conjunctiva has made it extremely useful in treating a tumor and minimizing collateral tissue loss and damage.[38] In managing these patients, one has to balance the desire to eradicate the disease process entirely with the unsatisfactory situation of creating a nonfunctioning eye. The following section outlines the treatment regimens for different conjunctival tumors, based on the extent of the disease, the patient's age and level of comfort, and the condition of the ocular surface.

Conjunctival Nevi

The management of conjunctival nevi is simple observation, because most of these lesions remain benign. Benign nevi can grow, especially during puberty, but this is not necessarily an indication for removal. Likewise, the degree of pigmentation of the lesion may change over the course of time without its becoming malignant. Pigmented lesions of the palpebral or fornical conjunctiva should be excised regardless of their appearance, because nevi do not typically occur in these locations.

At surgery topical anesthetic is applied to the surface of the lesion and the undersurface is infiltrated with 1% lidocaine with epinephrine. We recommend that a 2-mm margin of normal-appearing conjunctiva be removed with the lesion because nonpigmented cells may extend beyond the visible surface of the lesion. It is unnecessary to remove the underlying substantia propria or apply adjunctive cryotherapy to the base of the lesion. The resultant defect can be closed with interrupted 7-0 Vicryl sutures or often is small enough not to require a suture. It is usually unnecessary to patch the eye at the time of surgery, and the application of antibiotic-steroid combination eye drops for 1 week after surgery is generally adequate.

Primary Acquired Melanosis

The absence of clear clinical signs to distinguish PAM without atypia from PAM with atypia makes it mandatory to perform a biopsy on any lesion suspected of being PAM. For a small lesion an excisional biopsy can be performed under local anesthesia. The area of involved conjunctiva is infiltrated with 1% lidocaine, and the area is excised with a 2-mm border of normal conjunctiva. The resulting defect can be closed with an absorbable suture or be left to heal spontaneously. If the pathologic diagnosis is PAM without atypia, then no further treatment is required. If the diagnosis is PAM with atypia and the lesion has been completely excised, then no additional treatment is required. In patients with inadequately excised localized PAM with atypia, reexcision or cryotherapy to the involved margin is indicated.

In patients with diffuse conjunctival pigmentation in which initial biopsy specimens demonstrate PAM with atypia, additional incisional map biopsies of the conjunctiva are indicated to identify the extent of the disease. Usually, 10 to 15 small incisional map biopsies of the conjunctiva are adequate. The technique we prefer is to infiltrate the conjunctiva with 1% lidocaine and obtain the biopsy specimens by tenting small areas of the conjunctiva with 0.12 mm toothed forceps and removing the sample with curved Westcott scissors. The specimens can be placed on a piece of filter paper and sent in individual containers of formalin to the pathology laboratory, along with a diagram illustrating the biopsy sites. The biopsy sites do not need to be sutured. Areas that show PAM with atypia require adjunctive treatment with cryotherapy using a double freeze-thaw technique.

Once the area of PAM with atypia has been identified by map biopsies, definitive destructive treatment is indicated. We usually delay cryotherapy to the conjunctiva approximately 2 weeks after conjunctival biopsies are performed to allow for healing of the conjunctiva; this facilitates the subconjunctival injection of lidocaine. The eyelids are retracted with a wire eyelid speculum and topical anesthetic is instilled. In some instances it is necessary to give an adjunctive facial nerve block. An area of involved conjunctiva, as determined by conjunctival map biopsy, is ballooned up using 1% lidocaine with epinephrine in a 30-gauge needle. Using a sealed flat-topped cryoprobe (Frigitronics), the probe is placed on the conjunctiva until an iceball begins to form; when the conjunctiva is engaged, the probe is pulled away from the globe. This maneuver allows one to give an adequate treatment to the conjunctiva without damaging the underlying tunics of the globe. The cryoprobe is applied to the conjunctiva for 20 to 30 seconds. We do not routinely use a thermocouple because this length of treatment is adequate. Saline irrigation is useful in helping to release the conjunctiva from the cryoprobe. A second application is delivered to the conjunctiva after the first in a double freeze-thaw fashion. The maximum area of conjunctiva treated in one session is two quadrants. If additional areas of conjunctiva require treatment, it is best to wait 4 to 6 weeks between treatment sessions (Fig. 12–14).

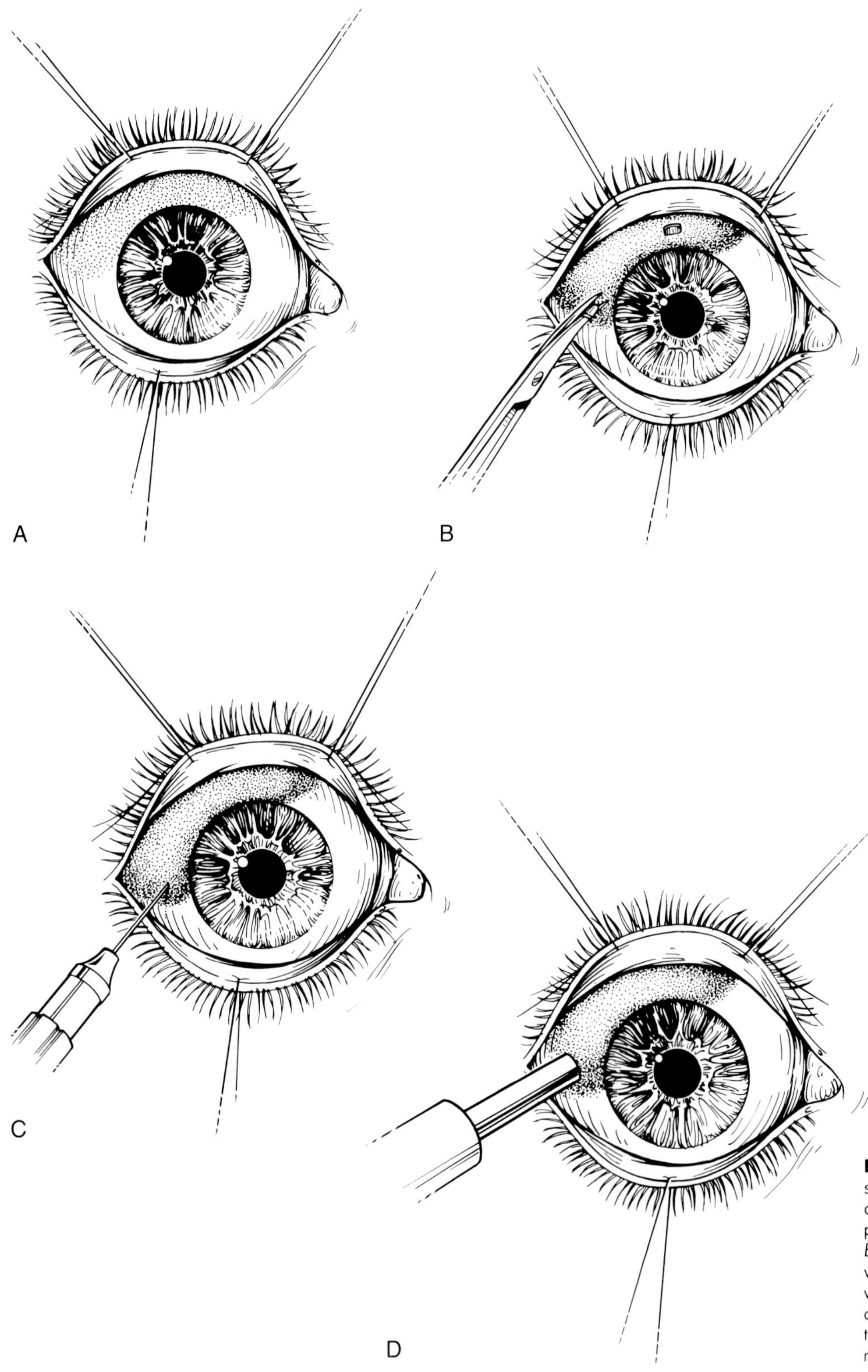

Figure 12–14. Diagrammatic representation of the treatment of primary acquired melanosis with atypia. *A*, Diffuse pigmentation of the bulbar conjunctiva. *B*, Multiple map biopsies. *C*, Two weeks later, ballooning the conjunction with local anesthetic. *D*, The application of cryotherapy to the area of conjunctiva with features of primary acquired melanosis with atypia.

In patients with corneal involvement we recommend pretreatment of the involved epithelium with 4% cocaine. Pledgets soaked in absolute alcohol should be applied briefly to the area, which should be débrided with a fine scalpel blade, with care taken not to violate Bowman's layer. The area should then be copiously irrigated with balanced salt solution. The specimen should be placed on moistened filter paper and submitted to the pathology laboratory. It is rare for Bowman's layer to be penetrated by atypical cells; however, if there is evidence of invasion, then a superficial keratectomy is recommended. If there is extensive dissection of the epibulbar, tarsal, or fornical conjunctiva, consideration should be given to fitting the patient with a ring conformer in the immediate postoperative period in an effort to minimize symblepharon formation.

After surgery, patients are placed on 60 to 80 mg of prednisone daily in addition to topical steroids and cycloplegics. The oral and topical steroids are typically tapered according to the degree of intraocular inflammatory response. Most patients are completely tapered by 4 weeks. Close followup immediately after treatment is required because cryotherapy may induce an intense inflammatory reaction. The followup of these patients is extremely important, and examination every 3 months is indicated for patients with PAM with atypia.

Malignant Melanoma

The treatment of malignant melanoma of the conjunctiva is primarily surgical, with the goal to remove the entire tumor, if possible. The type of the surgery depends on the location of the tumor, the presence or absence of associated PAM, tumor thickness, and histologic type. A solitary lesion suspicious for malignant melanoma should undergo excisional biopsy. The excisional biopsy should include a superficial sclerectomy in the area of the base of the tumor if deep tumor spread is suspected. Adjunctive cryotherapy is applied to the base and margins of the tumor. The freeze is applied directly to the tumor base and epibulbar conjunctiva for 20 seconds in a double freeze-thaw fashion. A surrounding 2-mm edge of normal-appearing conjunctiva should also be treated; this is best done by pulling the conjunctiva away from the globe once it has become adherent to the ice ball. This technique minimizes the morbidity caused by the cryotherapy.

In the case of nodular melanoma arising in an area of PAM, the nodule is completely excised, with a superficial sclerectomy performed if indicated clinically or histopathologically. The base, edges, and involved adjacent conjunctiva are treated with double freeze-thaw cryotherapy. If there is widespread involvement of the conjunctiva by flat pigmentation following excision of a nodular melanoma, map biopsies are performed and cryotherapy is directed toward the most atypical areas. Multiple treatment sessions may be required to stay ahead of the disease. Treatment of extensive conjunctival disease is usually limited to two quadrants in one treatment session. The total amount of cryotherapy has to be titrated against the age of the patient, with older patients' conjunctiva being less resilient to the complications of cryotherapy. In very extensive disease (more than two quadrants), it may not be possible to totally eradicate the disease in one setting without severe morbidity to the globe. In this setting the treatment goal may be to reduce the tumor load and decrease the chance of metastatic spread. Conjunctival adjunctive cryotherapy appears to have the greatest benefit in patients with unifocal conjunctival melanoma or extensive lesions of only PAM.[38]

Malignant melanoma involving the palpebral conjunctiva is treatment by full-thickness wedge resection of the lesion. The eyelid is allowed to heal for 6 weeks and then cryotherapy is applied to the surgical wound and any adjacent pigmentation. Cryotherapy is avoided immediately after eyelid repair because the secondary eyelid edema distorts the wound and may cause wound dehiscence.

An aggressive anti-inflammatory regimen must be used to minimize the postoperative complications (Table 12–3) following excision and cryotherapy of conjunctival melanoma. The inflammatory response is particularly marked with application of the cryotherapy to the outer tunics of the eye or to the palpebral conjunctiva. In addition to patching and local therapy consisting of anti-inflammatory and cycloplegic eye drops, the patients are placed on 60 to 80 mg of prednisone daily for a week. Oral prednisone is tapered quickly and discontinued after 14 days. An intense anterior chamber and vitreous inflammatory response, including hyphema and hypopyon, can occur after cryotherapy. Potential complications such as cataract formation, severe conjunctival scarring, transient hypotony, symblepharon formation, iritis, and ptosis can be minimized using this anti-inflammatory regimen (Table 12–4).

The management of aggressive conjunctival melanoma that has spread deeper into the eyelid tissues, fornices, globe, or orbit or is multifocal in distribution is dictated by the patient's age and general health and the goals of treatment. Exenteration has not been shown to prevent metastatic disease once orbital involvement has

TABLE 12–3

Complications of Cryotherapy

Subepithelial corneal opacification
Iritis and vitritis
Ocular hypotony
Symblepharon
Secondary diplopia
Keratoconjunctivitis sicca
Loss of eyelashes
Depigmentation
Ptosis
Pupil irregularities
Decreased accommodation

TABLE 12-4

Typical Care Following Cryotherapy of the Conjunctiva

I. Immediate postoperative period
  A. Apply an antibiotic-steroid ointment (e.g., Tobradex) and a cycloplegic agent (atropine)
  B. Patch for 24 hr
  C. Administer oral steroids (prednisone) 60–80 mg daily, and taper over 1–2 wk
  D. Provide analgesia as needed (e.g., acetaminophen with codeine)
  E. Administer atropine 1% 1 drop qid
  F. Administer antibiotic drops qid until reepithelialization occurs
  G. Patch in between eye drop application if conjunctiva is slow to reepithelialize
II. Intermediate postoperative period
  A. After removal of the patch, begin topical steroid and taper over 2 weeks according to inflammation
  B. Administer topical antibiotic coverage until conjunctiva and cornea heal
  C. Administer topical artificial tears for lubrication
III. Long-term followup to avoid complications
  A. Monitor for symblepharon formation
  B. Provide lysis of conjunctival adhesions
  C. Check for fading of pigmentation in the treatment area
  D. Perform another biopsy if there is a suspicious or inadequate response or if further disease develops
  E. Recheck the patient every 3 to 4 months

occurred, with most patients (89%) developing metastases following exenteration.[39] In the same study 15 (43%) of 35 patients without orbital involvement at the time of exenteration later developed metastatic disease. Generally, exenteration is reserved for younger patients when one is attempting to totally eradicate the tumor and when orbital involvement is not suspected. In older patients, less aggressive approaches may be taken by debulking the tumor in the belief that the patients' quality of life would be better served by a subtotal procedure and that exenteration is not likely to prolong their life span. The practice of prophylactic lymph node dissection at the time of exenteration is theoretically reasonable because conjunctival melanoma spreads via the lymphatics; however, definitive studies showing its benefit are unavailable. So, in these advanced cases, the clinician cannot offer the patient an improved prognosis even with the most aggressive intervention.

In some patients pigmentation of the conjunctiva may be accompanied by adjacent pigmentation of the eyelid margin (Fig. 12–15). In a review of 112 patients with conjunctival melanomas, Robertson and coworkers[30] found pigmentation of the eyelid margin to be present in 17 patients. Usually, the pigmentation is confined to within a few millimeters of the eyelid margin. In this study, the presence of coexistent eyelid margin pigmentation was a poor prognostic feature, with 12 (70%) of the patients in this group eventually dying of metastatic disease. In the same study the mortality rate from metastatic disease associated with conjunctival melanoma was found to be 26%. Thus, it is important to note clinically the presence or absence of eyelid pigmentation because this may alert the physician to the presence of particularly aggressive disease. The treatment of this form of disease should include complete resection of the involved eyelid margin as well as excision and cryotherapy of associated conjunctival melanoma.

CONCLUSION

An appreciation of the clinical characteristics of different forms of pigmented lesions of the conjunctiva is the first step in the successful management of this group of patients. Attention to the details of the history, the age of the patient, and the physical characteristics of the pigmentation help the clinician determine need for a biopsy. Confusion in the management of these pigmented lesions will always exist in part owing to the absence of clinical features that would distinguish benign PAM from PAM with atypia. Clearer parameters for the management of the subsequent biopsy specimen are unavailable;

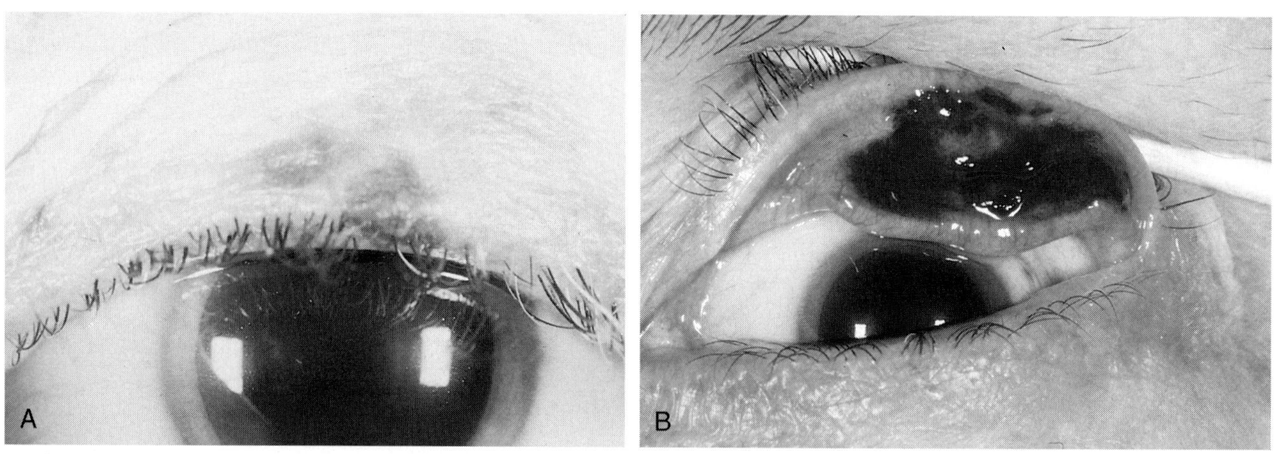

Figure 12–15. *A*, A 50-year-old woman presenting with juxtamarginal eyelid pigmentation. *B*, Eversion of the eyelid revealed a large area of melanoma involving the palpebral conjunctiva. (*A* and *B* courtesy of Jeffrey Nerad, MD.)

however, difficult questions still remain to be answered regarding the ultimate prognostic significance of a biopsy specimen demonstrating an occasional atypical cell or the risk of the patient with PAM without atypia developing atypia in the future. Answering these questions may prove difficult; however, the clinician now has a clearer set of guidelines by which to manage these patients.

REFERENCES

1. Scotto J, Fraumeni JJ, Lee J: Melanomas of the eye and other noncutaneous sites: Epidemiological aspects. J Natl Cancer Inst 56:489–491, 1976.
2. Folberg R, McLean IW, Zimmerman LE: Malignant melanoma of the conjunctiva. Hum Pathol 16:136–145, 1985.
3. Fine SB, Yanoff M: Ocular Histology, 2nd ed. Hagerstown, MD, Harper & Row, 1979.
4. Hogan MJ, Alvarado JA, Weddell JE: Histology of the Human Eye. Philadelphia, WB Saunders, 1971.
5. Jakobiec FA, Brownstein S: Cryotherapy for conjunctival melanotic neoplasms. *In* Jakobiec FA, Sigelman J: Advanced Techniques in Ocular Surgery. Philadelphia, WB Saunders, 1984.
6. Folberg R, McLean IW: Primary acquired melanosis and melanoma of the conjunctiva: Terminology, classification, and biologic behavior. Hum Pathol 17:652–654, 1986.
7. Reese A: Tumors of the Eye, 3rd ed. Hagerstown, MD, Harper & Row, 1976.
8. Zimmerman LE: Criteria for the management of melanosis. Arch Ophthalmol 76:307, 1966.
9. Silvers D, Jakobiec FA, Freeman TR, et al: Melanoma of the conjunctiva: A clinicopathological study. *In* Jakobiec FA (ed): Ocular and Adnexal Tumors. Birmingham, Aesculapius, 1978, pp 583–599.
10. Ackerman AB: Malignant melanoma in situ: The flat curable stage of malignant melanoma. Pathology 17:298–300, 1985.
11. Ackerman AB: Primary acquired melanosis [letter]. Hum Pathol 16:1077, 1985.
12. Ackerman AB, Sood R, Koenig M: Primary acquired melanosis of the conjunctiva is melanoma in situ. Mod Pathol 4:253–263, 1991.
13. Folberg R, McClean I, Zimmerman L: Primary acquired melanosis of the conjunctiva. Hum Pathol 16:129–135, 1985.
14. Clark WHJ: A classification of malignant melanoma in man correlated with histogenesis and biological behavior. *In* Montagna W, Hu F (eds): Advances in Biology of the Skin: The Pigmentary System. London, England, Pergamon Press, 1967, pp 621–647.
15. Clark WHJ, From L, Bernardino EA, Mihm MC: The histogenesis and biological behavior of primary human malignant melanomas of the skin. Cancer Res 29:705, 1969.
16. Folberg R, Jakobiec FA, Bernardino VB, Iwamoto T: Benign conjunctival melanocytic lesions: Clinicopathologic features. Ophthalmology 96:436–461, 1989.
17. Zimmerman LE: The histogenesis of conjunctival melanomas: The First Algernon B. Reese lecture. *In* Jakobiec FA (ed): Ocular and Adnexal Tumors. Birmingham, Aesculapius, 1978, pp 600–630.
18. Henkind P: Conjunctival melanocytic lesions: Natural history. *In* Jakobiec FA (ed): Ocular and Adnexal Tumors. Birmingham, Aesculapius, 1978, pp 572–582.
19. Jakobiec FA, Folberg R, Iwamoto T: Clinicopathologic characteristics of premalignant and malignant melanocytic lesions of the conjunctiva. Ophthalmology 96:147–166, 1989.
20. Jakobiec FA: Corneal tumors. *In* Kaufman H, Barron B, McDonald M, et al (eds): The Cornea. New York, Churchill Livingstone, 1988, pp 563–598.
21. Cowan TH, Balistocky M: The nevus of Ota or oculodermal melanocytosis: The ocular changes. Arch Ophthalmol 65:483–492, 1961.
22. Fitzpatrick TB, Zeller R, Kukita A, Kitamura H: Ocular and dermal melanocytes. Arch Ophthalmol 56:483–492, 1956.
23. Ota M, Tanino H: Navus fusco-caeruleus ophthalmomaxillus. Tokyo Med J 63:1243–1245, 1939.
24. Reese AB: Melanosis oculi. Am J Ophthalmol 8:865–870, 1925.
25. Wagoner MD, Beyer C, Gonder JR, Albert DM: Common presentations of sebaceous gland carcinoma of the eyelid. Ann Ophthalmol 14:159–163, 1982.
26. Jay B: Naevi and melanomata of the conjunctiva. Br J Ophthalmol 49:169–204, 1965.
27. Lever WF, Schaumburg-Lever G: Histopathology of the Skin, 6th ed. Philadelphia, JB Lippincott, 1983.
28. Reese AB: Precancerous and cancerous melanosis. Am J Ophthalmol 61:1272–1277, 1966.
29. Jakobiec FA, Rini FJ, Fraunfelder FT, Brownstein S: Cryotherapy for conjunctival primary acquired melanosis and malignant melanoma. Ophthalmology 95:1058–1070, 1988.
30. Robertson DM, Hungerford JL, McCartney A: Pigmentation of the eyelid margin accompanying conjunctival melanoma. Am J Ophthalmol 108:435–439, 1989.
31. Giblin ME, Shields JA, Shields CL, Eagle RCJ: Primary eyelid malignant melanoma associated with primary conjunctival malignant melanoma. Aust N Z J Ophthalmol 16:127–131, 1988.
32. Jakobiec FA, Brownstein S, Wilkinson RD: Combined surgery and cryotherapy for diffuse malignant melanoma of the conjunctiva. Arch Ophthalmol 98:1390–1396, 1980.
33. Brownstein S, Jakobiec FA, Wilkinson RD: Cryotherapy for precancerous melanosis (atypical melanocytic hyperplasia) of the conjunctiva. Arch Ophthalmol 99:1224–1231, 1981.
34. Jakobiec FA, Brownstein S, Wilkinson RD, Katzin HM: Adjuvant cryotherapy for focal nodular melanoma of the conjunctiva. Ophthalmology 100:115–118, 1982.
35. Jakobiec FA, Brownstein S, Albert W, et al: The role of cryotherapy in the management of conjunctival melanoma. Ophthalmology 89:502–515, 1982.
36. Codère F, Brownstein S, Garwood JL, Dresner SC: Carbon dioxide laser treatment of the conjunctiva and the cornea. Ophthalmology 95:37–45, 1988.
37. Jakobiec FA: Tumors of the lids. *In* Symposium on Diseases and Surgery of the Lids, Lacrimal Apparatus, and Orbit. St. Louis, CV Mosby, 1982, pp 288–292.
38. Jakobiec FA, Iwamoto T: Ultrastructural effects of cryotherapy for intraepithelial conjunctival melanocytic proliferations. Arch Ophthalmol 101:904–912, 1983.
39. Folberg R, McLean IW, Zimmerman LF: Conjunctival melanosis and melanoma. Ophthalmology 91:673–678, 1984.

CHAPTER 13

Diagnosis and Management of Sebaceous Gland Carcinoma

Evan H. Sacks and Richard D. Lisman

Sebaceous gland carcinoma is a relatively rare malignancy comprising between 0.2% and 0.8% of all eyelid lesions and 1% to 4.7% of all malignant eyelid lesions, as encountered in large series.[1-5] Sebaceous carcinomas are often highly malignant tumors that occur most frequently in women in their sixth to eighth decades of life.[6-9] The rare patients younger than 40 years of age usually have a history of radiation therapy.[6, 10] All racial groups are affected, with a significant number of patients from Asian populations.[6] Sebaceous carcinoma is encountered with greater frequency in China than in Western countries, where it is found to be second in frequency of all malignant eyelid lesions (32.7%).[9, 11]

Sebaceous carcinoma arises almost exclusively in the ocular adnexa.[12] The ocular adnexa contains various sebaceous glands from which carcinomas can arise. These include the meibomian glands located in the tarsus; the glands of Zeis at the lid margins; the glands in the caruncle and the eyebrow; and those associated with the fine hair follicles throughout the eyelid skin (Fig. 13–1). Most sebaceous carcinomas involve the tarsus or eyelid margin or both.[8, 13] Some tumors are multicentric in origin, arising from both the meibomian glands and glands of Zeis, although sometimes the precise site of origin cannot be determined.[8, 6, 14] Sebaceous carcinoma arises more frequently in the upper eyelid than in the lower eyelid, corresponding to the more numerous meibomian glands in the upper tarsus compared with the lower.[6, 8, 13] This differs markedly from basal cell carcinoma, which has a strong predilection for the lower eyelid and the medial canthus.[6]

CLINICAL FEATURES

Sebaceous carcinoma of the eyelids is a highly malignant tumor that can have a wide variety of clinical presentations. Most often it are evidenced as a nontender, enlarging lid mass.[8] Often, this tumor produces a chalazion as its initial misleading manifestation. Atypical or recurring chalazions showing a rubbery consistency should raise levels of suspicion. When the tumor arises in the meibomian glands, a diffuse, plaque-like thickening of the tarsus may occur (Fig. 13–2). A fungating or papillomatous growth resembling a squamous cell papilloma or carcinoma may also develop. Lash loss associated with a diffuse or nodular thickening of the eyelids is highly suspicious for sebaceous cell carcinoma, the lash loss being secondary to neoplastic involvement of the lash follicles (Fig. 13–3). These lesions often have a yellowish hue to them, related to the oily content of the tumor.[13] Lesions originating from the glands of Zeis may appear as small, yellow nodules situated at the lid margin anterior to the gray line, whereas those arising from the caruncle's sebaceous glands appear as subconjunctival multilobular yellow-gray masses covered by an intact epithelium. Small tumors may be overlooked until after they have spread into the orbit, lacrimal gland, or regional lymph nodes. The most frequent evidence of metastasis is enlarged preauricular or cervical lymph nodes.

Sebaceous carcinoma has the ability to masquerade as many other disease processes, possibly mimicking a chalazion, cutaneous horn, cicatricial pemphigoid, blepharoconjunctivitis, carcinoma in situ, or a squamous or basal cell carcinoma. Commonly misdiagnosed as a squamous or basal cell carcinoma, its deep origins and absence of significant ulceration or papillary mass on the cutaneous surface distinguish the sebaceous cell carcinoma.

The term *masquerade syndrome* refers to a distinctive clinical feature of some sebaceous carcinomas that presents as a persistent unilateral conjunctivitis, blepharitis, meibomitis, or blepharoconjunctivitis and does not respond completely to antibiotic therapy and lid hygiene. This inflammatory disease appearance in sebaceous carcinoma is caused by the invasion of sebaceous carcinoma cells into the overlying epithelium, forming single-cell and small multiple-cell nests. This pattern of tumor spread is referred to as *pagetoid invasion* (Fig. 13–4), named after the breast carcinoma it resembles; it occurs in 40% to 80% of all patients with sebaceous carcinoma.[7, 8] In addition to individual nests of cells, the sebaceous carcinoma cells may replace the epithelium in its full thickness, producing an intraepithelial carcinoma. The oily contents of these sebaceous carcinoma cells produce an inflammatory reaction as the cells spread through the epithelium. These spreading foci of intraepi-

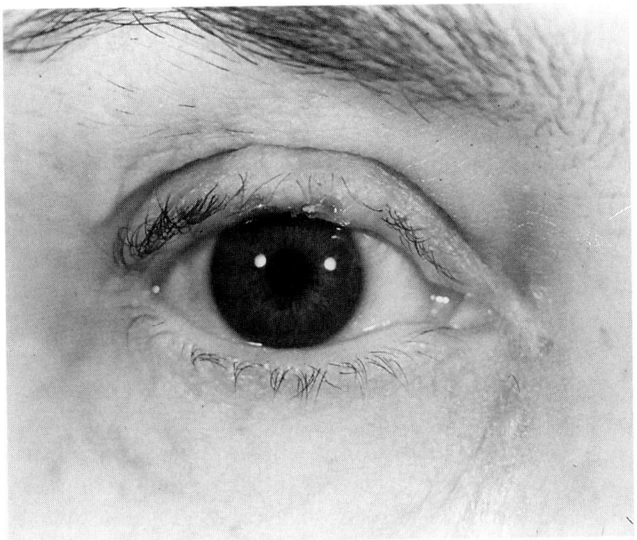

Figure 13–1. This 60-year-old woman had a long-standing blepharoconjunctivitis and palpable thickening of the right upper eyelid. Full-thickness biopsy revealed sebaceous carcinoma; later map biopsies demonstrated spread into the superior fornical and bulbar conjunctiva as intraepithelial pagetoid extension. The loss of cilia in the midposition of the eyelid is a significant clinical finding, raising suspicion of a carcinoma without an obvious mass. This patient underwent resection of the right upper eyelid after conjunctival map biopsies to determine the exact extent and spread of the lesion.

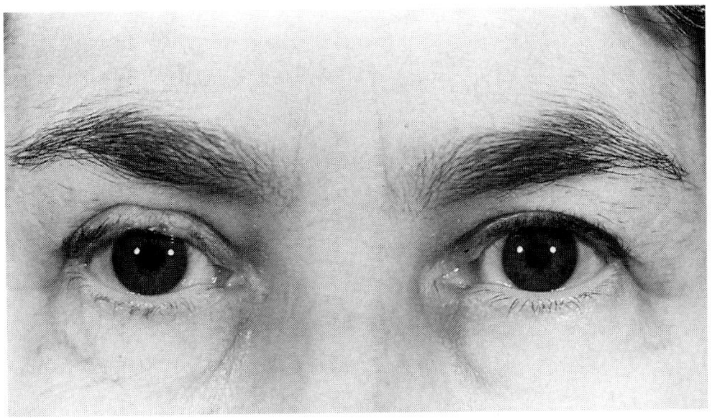

Figure 13–3. A 69-year-old patient with thickening of the right upper eyelid with loss of cilia, without palpable nodule or mass. Again, the loss of cilia and chronic blepharitis, without resolution, raised a suspicion of a sebaceous gland carcinoma of the right upper lid.

thelial malignant cells invade the lids, the conjunctiva, and even the corneal epithelium, causing a neoplastic pannus of scarring and vascularization. Patients with sebaceous carcinoma who present with diffuse blepharoconjunctivitis may remain undiagnosed for months to years. Because of the highly malignant nature of this disease and its ability to masquerade as various common ocular complaints, it is important to keep in mind the following six clinical features that should raise levels of suspicion, as pointed out by Boniuk and Zimmerman:[6]

1. Atypical or recurrent chalazions, particularly with a peculiar consistency at the time of surgery
2. Any yellowish lid margin tumor with lash loss
3. Diffuse or nodular tumors involving the upper and lower lids
4. Atypical unilateral blepharitis, meibomitis, or blepharoconjunctivitis with or without associated keratitis
5. Any orbital mass developing after removal of an unspecified or questionably interpreted lid or canalicular tumor
6. Any lid tumor seen following excessive radiation therapy to the eye, ocular adnexa, or face

In any of these situations or others when the diagnosis of sebaceous carcinoma is raised, a biopsy specimen must

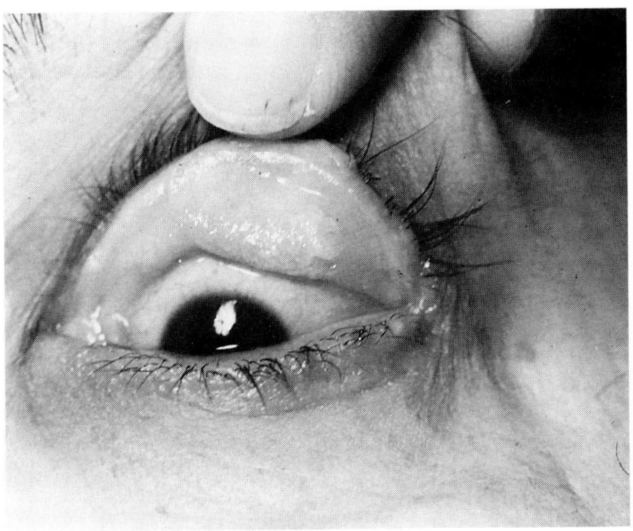

Figure 13–2. A 59-year-old patient with a chronic blepharoconjunctivitis, without an obvious palable mass of the left upper eyelid. Keratinization of the mucocutaneous junction was apparent, with loss of cilia. Eversion of the eyelid revealed this mass lesion of the palpebral conjunctiva, and map biopsies were taken to determine that intraepithelial pagetoid extension had indeed spread to the two upper quadrants of the globe. This patient was treated with adjunctive cryotherapy to the palpebral conjunctiva following resection and reconstruction of the left upper eyelid.

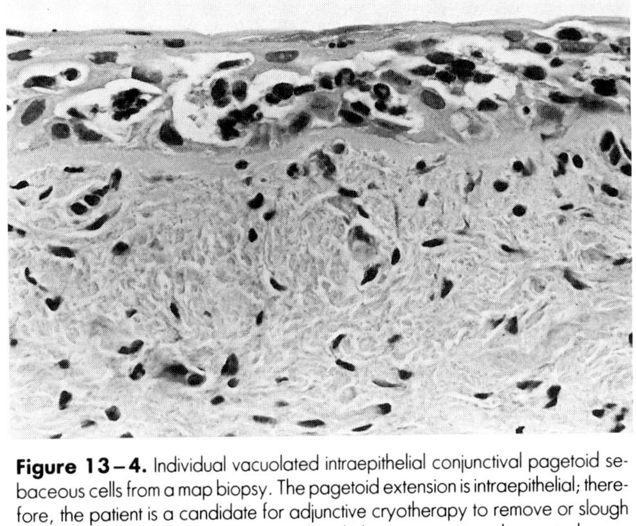

Figure 13–4. Individual vacuolated intraepithelial conjunctival pagetoid sebaceous cells from a map biopsy. The pagetoid extension is intraepithelial; therefore, the patient is a candidate for adjunctive cryotherapy to remove or slough the epithelium. The surrounding normal epithelium migrates into the treated areas to fill the gap with uninvolved conjunctival epithelium. H & E, ×280.

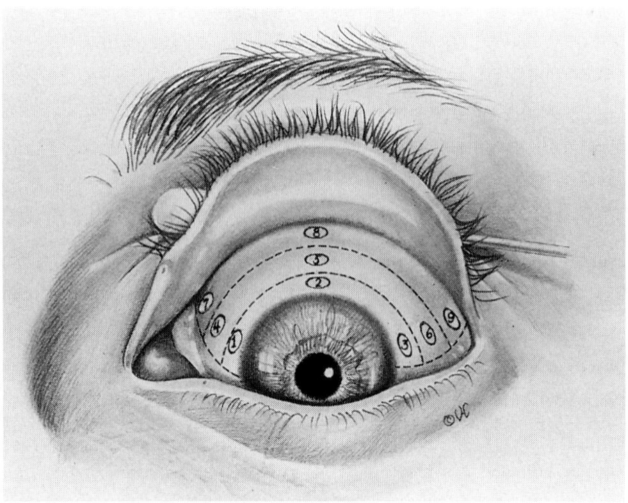

Figure 13–5. Map biopsies are performed whenever suspicion for conjunctival extension is present. Small ellipses of conjunctiva are taken from the suspected quadrants. The map includes both bulbar and palpebral conjunctivae, and each specimen is put into its own specimen bottle and sent to the laboratory for examination. A map is made of the specimens taken from the limbal area, the bulbar palpebral reflection, and an area between the two. Six to nine biopsy specimens are taken from each hemisphere, including seemingly uninvolved areas, because of pagetoid extension.

be obtained for pathologic study. In suspected lid masses, full-thickness lid tissue is usually necessary to make the diagnosis of sebaceous carcinoma; if pagetoid invasion is clinically apparent, multiple biopsy specimens of the conjunctiva are necessary for proper staging (Fig. 13–5).

PATHOLOGY

The histologic features of sebaceous carcinoma have been elaborated on in superb series.[1,6–8,13] Sebaceous carcinoma of the eyelid is occasionally misdiagnosed as squamous or basal cell carcinomas by pathologists just as by clinicians unfamiliar with the entity. Sebaceous carcinomas display lobules and cords of tumor cells with different degrees of sebaceous differentiation and infiltration into the surrounding tissue (Fig. 13–6). The lobules of sebaceous carcinoma re-create the patterns seen in normal sebaceous glands, with differentiation progressing from the periphery toward the center of the lobules and the formation of increasing amounts of cytoplasmic lipid as one approaches the center of the neoplastic lobule. The well-differentiated cells contain foamy or vacuolated basophilic cytoplasm, whereas less-differentiated cells contain more deeply basophilic cytoplasm and more miotic figures. These cells are more likely to be found in the periphery of infiltrating lobules. This pattern can simulate basal cell carcinoma. Some sebaceous carcinomas demonstrate squamous features with distinct foci of keratinization, similar to the keratinization and squamous differentiation found in the normal meibomian gland ducts near the lid margin. This pattern of growth may be confused with squamous cell carcinoma. Different histologic patterns of growth include the comedo pattern, with large lobules and central necrosis resembling ductal carcinomas of breasts; the lobular pattern, with well-demarcated lobules of variable size resembling basal cell carcinoma; and the papillary pattern, composed of papillary fronds of neoplastic cells resembling squamous cell carcinoma and having a tendency to occur in the conjunctival surface. Mixed patterns of tumor often show an admixture of the different patterns mentioned earlier.

Tumors may also be classified according to the varying patterns of infiltration. Minimally infiltrative neoplasms consist of compact lobules with only minor extensions of neoplastic cells into the adjacent stroma. Highly infiltrative tumors are composed of infiltrating cords of malignant cells, occasionally in single rows (single-file appearance), with little or no areas of lobule formation.

Sebaceous gland carcinoma demonstrates two modes of neoplastic spread into the epithelium of the conjunctiva, cornea, and skin. These epithelial changes are usually associated with moderately to highly infiltrative carcinomas. In pagetoid spread, the neoplastic cells invade the epithelium as single cells or as small clusters of cells that are devoid of intercellular bridges (Fig. 13–7). The pagetoid cell has a hyperchromatic nucleus and abundant lipid-laden vacuolated cytoplasm. It is this irritating lipid content that attracts the inflammatory component responsible for the clinically discernible masquerade syndrome.

In the second mode of intraepithelial spread, sebaceous carcinoma cells replace the full thickness of the surface epithelium. These changes resemble squamous cell carcinoma in situ. The cells seen in this form of intraepithelial spread are large pleomorphic cells with high levels of mitotic activity. The epithelium of the conjunctiva, cornea, and epidermis can display multifocal involvement with skip areas.

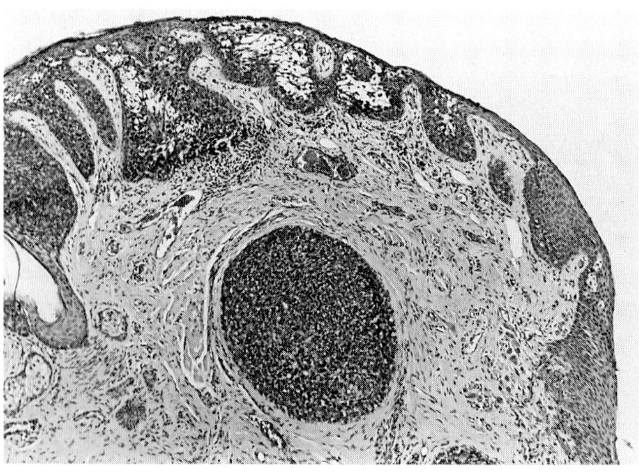

Figure 13–6. Pagetoid intraepithelial sebaceous carcinoma at the mucocutaneous junction. The lobule of infiltration sebaceous carcinoma is noted below. H & E, original magnification ×140.

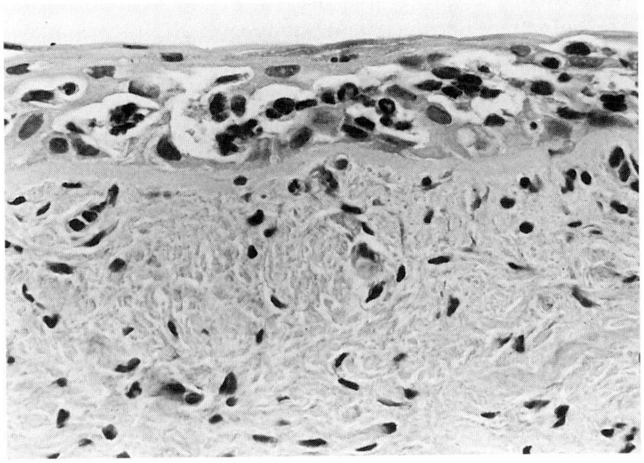

Figure 13–7. Neoplastic cells invade the epithelium as single cells, or small clusters of cells, that are devoid of intracellular bridges. This represents pagetoid extension with cells containing hyperchromatic nuclei and abundant lipid-laden vacuolated cytoplasm.

Sebaceous carcinomas can be multicentric in origin.[6] Upper and lower lid independent focal involvement has been observed in 6% to 10% of patients with sebaceous carcinoma.[6, 8, 14] In addition to intraepithelial spread and multicentric foci of disease, sebaceous carcinoma can spread by direct extension into the adjacent structures: the orbit, the paranasal sinuses, and the intracranial vault.[15] Perineural infiltration and direct spread into the lymphatics has been seen in moderately to poorly differentiated tumors.[8, 13] In one series, direct orbital invasion occurred in 19% of patients and metastases to preauricular or cervical lymph nodes or both in 23% of patients.[16] In this same series, vascular invasion with distant metastases was associated with previous or simultaneous spread to regional lymph nodes.

PROGNOSIS AND MANAGEMENT

The prognostic significance of the location, size, site of origin, duration of symptoms before surgery, histologic pattern, degree of cellular differentiation, and deoxyribonucleic acid (DNA) characteristics by DNA flow cytometry have been analyzed in various studies.[8, 16, 17] Location of the tumor in the upper eyelid, maximal diameter larger that 10 mm, meibomian gland origin, symptoms existing longer than 6 months, an infiltrative growth pattern, and poor differentiation all indicated a poor prognosis. The presence of vascular or lymphatic invasion frequently indicated a fatal outcome. Such invasion was present only in tumors with minimal to moderate degrees of sebaceous differentiation and a highly infiltrative pattern with invasion of the surrounding tissues. Such tumors usually exhibited large numbers of mitotic figures. These features were also apparent in tumors that had invaded the orbit or metastasized to the regional lymph nodes.

High mortality rates were associated with both upper and lower eyelid involvement and multicentric origin from meibomian glands and glands of Zeis. Pagetoid and carcinoma in situ changes in the epithelia were associated in one study with a 59% mortality rate, whereas those tumors without intraepithelial spread had a mortality rate of 11%.[8] DNA flow cytometric studies showed a direct correlation between aneuploidy and pagetoid spread and lesser degrees of differentiation. In most series, the patients with pagetoid spread were those who were correctly diagnosed late and treated for a long time as having primary inflammatory conditions.[8, 16]

Early, accurate diagnosis and adequate treatment can significantly affect prognosis. Incompletely excised sebaceous carcinoma has a high recurrence rate[13]; therefore, complete, wide surgical excision with frozen section control is the only treatment recommended. Radiation therapy has little, if any, beneficial effect in controlling sebaceous carcinoma and should be reserved only for palliation in patients unfit for surgery.[6, 13, 18]

Patients with suspected sebaceous carcinoma should have a biopsy of the suspected lesion or lesions before treatment is planned. Palpation of the cervical and preauricular lymph nodes is mandatory, as is biopsy of any suspicious adenopathy, before further possibly radical surgery is performed.

Full-thickness biopsies of lid lesions are less likely to yield false negative results or misreadings by pathologists, and if pagetoid spread is suspected, as evidenced by reddened or thickened conjunctiva, multiple mapping biopsies should be performed.[18, 19] These biopsies should include the obviously involved conjunctiva or lid and beyond. Skip areas and multicentricity of origin are not uncommon in sebaceous carcinoma. When the tumor is limited to one eyelid and the pagetoid extension is within two quadrants of the epibulbar surface, Lisman and associates[19] have recommended wide local resection of the eyelid with frozen section control and first-stage reconstruction at that session, as indicated by the type of resection performed. At the time of the second-stage reconstruction, or at 4 to 6 weeks after surgery if only single-stage reconstruction was indicated, cryotherapy is applied to the areas determined to be positive for intraepithelial disease on biopsy.

In the technique for cryosurgery, the conjunctiva is ballooned away from the globe with lidocaine injection (Fig. 13–8). Using a nitrous oxide cryogen, the tip is applied to the conjunctiva, which is then immediately pulled away from the sclera once adhesion occurs (Fig. 13–9). When a complete freeze is noted (in approximately 10 to 15 seconds), the iceball is allowed to thaw without irrigation. This procedure is repeated one time to each area treated. The goal in any approach to sebaceous carcinoma is the complete resection of the solid tumor and eradication by thermal destruction of any pagetoid or intraepithelial disease. Wide destruction with cryotherapy to the pagetoid spread has been tremendously suc-

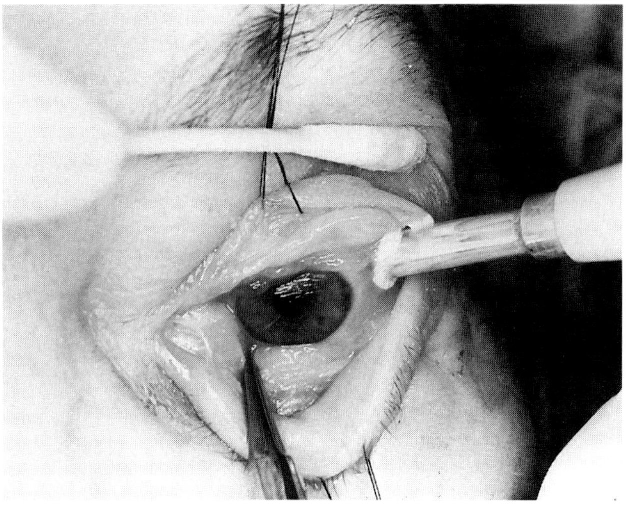

Figure 13–8. Cryotherapy with a Soll Cryomedic unit is applied to the involved conjunctiva. As soon as the cryoprobe is applied to the conjunctiva, the cyroprobe is lifted to prevent extensive thermal damage to the scleral surface. Once the iceball forms (in 4 to 8 seconds), the freeze is ended. Irrigation is not used to loosen the iceball. Each section is frozen at least two times, but it is vital to lift the probe and iceball off the scleral surface at the moment of the freeze.

cessful when the intraepithelial component has been two quadrants of the epibulbar surface or less. The major complications of this technique are the subsequent dry eye and symblepharon formation. Special symblepharon conformers help prevent adhesions from forming, and the dry eye symptoms can be medically and surgically treated.[19] Following this conservative approach to sebaceous carcinoma, mapping biopsies should be repeated every 6 months for the first 3 to 5 years (see Fig. 13–5). These biopsies should cover the previously treated area, specifically from the limbal region, the bulbar-palpebral reflection, and midway between between these two, in a distribution involving at least 50% of the globe's surface. In our series, 10 (90%) of 11 patients

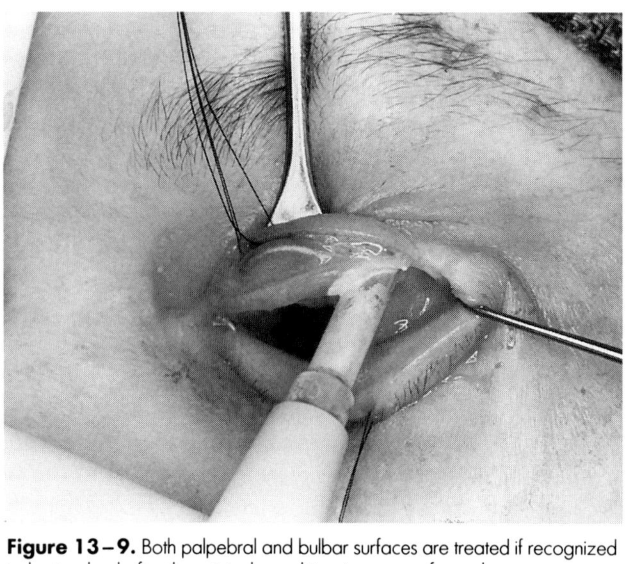

Figure 13–9. Both palpebral and bulbar surfaces are treated if recognized to be involved after the original map biopsies are performed.

treated with cryotherapy following eyelid resection have remained free of intraepithelial pagetoid involvement for longer than 48 months. In this series, one patient, who was a poor candidate for cryotherapy, went on to exenteration and mediastinal metastases. This patient initially presented with four quadrants of bulbar conjunctival epithelial involvement but refused exenteration initially. One patient with three-quadrant involvement and another with four-quadrant involvement remain tumor free at 48 months, but we recommend limiting cryotherapy to those whose conjunctival involvement has been mapped as two quadrants or less. When greater degrees of cryotherapy are applied in patients with three-quadrant and four-quadrant involvement, visual loss is notable owing to diffuse punctate keratitis, corneal ulceration, and symblepharon.

Mohs' surgery, which has been effective in reducing the incidence of recurrence in periocular basal and squamous cell carcinomas, is not recommended in sebaceous cell carcinoma because of the multicentric nature of many of these tumors and the incidence of skip areas in the intraepithelial disease.[20]

In many patients with long-standing sebaceous carcinoma who have withstood diagnosis, exenteration is the only form of effective wide excision. This includes disease with orbital extension, extensive two-lid involvement more than two quadrants of epibulbar intraepithelial spread, or lacrimal gland extension.

All patients should be followed carefully, whatever mode of treatment they have had, for local recurrence or metastasis to the ipsilateral preauricular, submandibular, or cervical nodes. If lymph node metastasis develops, then the patient should have a radical neck dissection. If, at initial presentation, enlarged preauricular or cervical lymph nodes are present, biopsy will confirm the presence of any tumor metastasis.[1] Radical neck dissection is recommended for tumor metastasis at the time of exenteration if lymph node biopsy results are positive for tumor.[1] In some patients, radiation therapy (4800 to 6600 rad) may be an effective adjunct in the management of tumors that have extended to the regional lymph nodes.[1]

In conclusion, treatment of sebaceous carcinoma is simplified by high levels of suspicion early in the clinical care of the patient, pathologic confirmation, and wide local excision with frozen section control of the surgical margins. Cryotherapy is indispensable in treating intraepithelial disease limited to two or fewer epibulbar quadrants. Tumors that are more diffuse or that extend into the orbit require exenteration. Early awareness, diagnosis, and treatment are the essential elements of improving prognosis.

REFERENCES

1.. Donazas MT, Green R: Sebaceous gland carcinoma: Review of 40 cases. Arch Ophthalmol 102:245–249, 1984.

2. Welch RB, Duke JR: Lesions of the lids: A statistical note. Am J Ophthalmol 45:415–416, 1958.
3. Kwitko ML, Boniuk M, Zimmerman LE: Eyelid tumors with reference to lesions confused with squamous cell carcinoma. Part I: Incidence and errors in diagnosis. Arch Ophthalmol 69:693–697, 1963.
4. Ginsberg J: Present status of meibomian gland carcinoma. Arch Ophthalmol 73:271–277, 1965.
5. Aurora AL, Bloodi FC: Lesions of the eyelids: A clinicopathological study. Surv Ophthalmol 15:94–104, 1970.
6. Boniuk M, Zimmerman LE: Sebaceous carcinoma of the eyelids, eyebrow, caruncle, and orbit. Trans Am Acad Ophthalmol Otolaryngol 72:619–642, 1968.
7. Wolfe JT, Yeatts RP, Wick MR, et al: Sebaceous carcinoma of the eyelid: Errors in clinical and pathologic diagnosis. Am J Surg Pathol 8:597–606, 1984.
8. Rao NA, Hidayat AA, McLean IW, Zimmerman LE: Sebaceous carcinomas of the ocular adnexa: A clinicopathologic study of 104 cases, with five-year follow-up data. Hum Pathol 13:113–122, 1982.
9. Ni C, Kuo P-K: Meibomian gland carcinoma: A clinicopathological study of 156 cases with long-period follow-up of 100 cases. Jpn J Ophthalmol 23:388–401, 1979.
10. Lemos LB, Santa-Cruz DJ, Baba N: Sebaceous carcinoma of the eyelid following radiation therapy. Am J Surg Pathol 2:305–311, 1978.
11. Ni C, Searl SS, Kuo P-K, et al: Sebaceous gland carcinoma of the ocular adnexa. Int Ophthalmol Clin 22:23–61, 1982.
12. Rulon DB, Holwog EB: Cutaneous sebaceous neoplasms. Cancer 33:82–102, 1974.
13. Spencer WH: Ophthalmic Pathology: An Atlas and Textbook, vol 3. Philadelphia, WB Saunders, 1986.
14. Cavanagh HD, Green WR, Goldberg HK: Multicentric sebaceous adenocarcinoma of the meibomian gland. Am J Ophthalmol 77:326–332, 1974.
15. Shields JA, Font RL: Meibomian gland carcinoma presenting as a lacrimal gland tumor. Arch Ophthalmol 92:304–306, 1974.
16. Rao NA, McLean IW, Zimmerman LE: Sebaceous carcinoma of the eyelid and caruncle: Correlation of clinical pathologic features with prognosis. *In* Jakobiec FA (ed): Ocular and Adnexal Tumors. Birmingham, Aesculapius, 1978, p 461.
17. Sakol PJ, Simons KB, McFadden PW, et al: DNA flow cytometry of sebaceous cell carcinomas of the ocular adnexa: Introduction to the technique in the evaluation of periocular tumors. Ophthalmic Plast Reconstr Surg 8:77–87, 1992.
18. Khan JA, Doane JF, Grove AS Jr: Sebaceous and meibomian carcinomas of the eyelid: Recognition, diagnosis, and management. Ophthalmic Plast Reconstr Surg 7:61–66, 1991.
19. Lisman RD, Jakobiec FA, Small P: Sebaceous carcinoma of the eyelids: The role of adjunctive cryotherapy in the management of conjunctival pagetoid spread. Ophthalmology 96:1021–1026, 1989.
20. Folberg R, Whitaker DC, Tse DT, Nera JA: Recurrent and residual sebaceous carcinoma after Mohs' excision of the primary lesion. Am J Ophthalmol 103:817–823, 1987.

CHAPTER 14

Surgical Intervention in Conjunction with Medical Treatment of Cicatricial Pemphigoid

James C. Fleming and Richard C. Cape

GENERAL ASPECTS OF CICATRICIAL PEMPHIGOID

Cicatricial pemphigoid is a relatively uncommon systemic disorder with devastating ocular manifestations. Its frequency has been estimated to be anywhere from 1 in 12,000 to 1 in 60,000 ophthalmic patients.[1] Cicatricial pemphigoid is believed to be an immunoregulatory dysfunction, even though this mechanism is not fully understood. It usually affects the elderly population, with mean age in the 60s and 70s, and it is almost nonexistent in people 30 years of age or younger. Women are affected more than men by a 2:1 ratio. There is no racial or geographic predilection. This disease has cutaneous, mucous membrane, and ocular manifestations.[2,3]

Cicatricial pemphigoid follows a course of gradual scarring that progresses to blindness in many patients if untreated. It has varying levels of severity, and in certain patients it becomes inactive spontaneously. During the course of their disease, many patients require surgical treatment for entropion, trichiasis, repair of significant scarring, and other ocular problems (such as cataracts). This chapter discusses the rationale and the timing for medical and surgical interventions in patients with cicatricial pemphigoid.

Cutaneous Manifestations

Fewer than 25% of patients with cicatricial pemphigoid have skin involvement. When it does occur, the face, neck, and scalp areas are most often involved. Many patients are asymptomatic, whereas others note a burning or itching sensation. The lesions are erythematous plaques with overlying blisters that ultimately leave scarring. Less frequently, the extremities, genitalia, and shoulders are involved. These vesiculobullous lesions are usually nonscarring as compared with the facial lesions.[4,5]

Nonocular Mucous Membrane Manifestations

There is great variation in ophthalmic, dermatologic, and dental studies noting the percentage of patients with cicatricial pemphigoid and mucous membrane involvement. It is probably in the range of 70% with marked variation in severity. The bullous lesions that occur may leave scarring or strictures, causing significant morbidity and even mortality in some instances. Nasopharyngeal or laryngeal involvement may cause obstructive sleep apnea and ultimately require surgery. The most devastating and only life-threatening manifestation of cicatricial pemphigoid is involvement of the esophagus: Death from asphyxiation may occur in patients with esophageal strictures.[5] Any patient with cicatricial pemphigoid who has complaints of dysphagia should be seen immediately by a gastroenterologist for evaluation with endoscopy and barium swallow.

Ocular Manifestations

The characteristic feature of cicatricial pemphigoid with ocular involvement is subepithelial bullous formation and subsequent conjunctival scarring and fibrosis. The disease is bilateral and may present in various stages of involvement. Chronic conjunctivitis is the earliest and least specific finding. In the later stages, fibrosis, symblepharon formation, entropion, aqueous and mucin deficiency, and fornix foreshortening may ultimately lead to blindness from corneal opacification. Corneal epithelial changes are secondary to the inflammatory process of the disease itself or from complications of the disease, such as entropion and tear insufficiency. Culture results from patients with cicatricial pemphigoid have been positive more than 80% of the time, with *Staphylococcus* being the most common pathogen. This blepharoconjunctivitis can exacerbate the disease process.[6,7]

Staging of Ocular Manifestations

Two different staging systems have been proposed, with both based on conjunctival scarring (Table 14–1). Mondino and Brown[8] based their staging system on the percentage of conjunctival shrinkage. Stage 0 consists of no conjunctival shrinkage, and stage 1 consists of 25% or

TABLE 14-1

Staging of Ocular Cicatricial Pemphigoid

Stage	Characteristics: Mondino and Brown[8]	Characteristics: Foster and Associates[9]
0	No conjunctival shrinkage	—
1	≤25% conjunctival shrinkage	Conjunctival injection and subepithelial fibrosis
2	25%–50% conjunctival shrinkage	Foreshortening of inferior cul-de-sac
3	75% conjunctival shrinkage	Symblepharon formation
4	End stage	End stage

TABLE 14-2

Drugs Associated with Ocular Pemphigoid

Topical
- Demecarium
- Dipivefrin
- Echothiophate iodide
- Epinephrine
- Idoxuridine
- Pilocarpine
- Timolol

Systemic
- Practolol

less shrinkage of conjunctival fornices. In stage 2 there is 25% to 50% shrinkage of the conjunctival fornices. Stage 3 consists of 75% shrinkage, and stage 4 is the end stage, characterized by absent tears, obliterated conjunctival fornices, ankyloblepharon, and a keratinized ocular surface epithelium. Mondino and Brown compared patients in different stages and found that patients in the later stages were more likely to have dry eye, corneal vessels, trichiasis, and lid and conjunctival cultures positive for pathogens. Their studies also revealed that the disease is more likely to progress in the later stages as compared with the earlier stages.[8]

Foster and associates[9] developed a staging system more descriptive of the ocular findings and progression in cicatricial pemphigoid. Stage 1 is characterized by conjunctival inflammation, mucoid discharge, small patches of rose bengal–staining epithelium, and conjunctival subepithelial fibrosis. The white striae, as seen by slit-lamp examination, are indicative of subepithelial fibrosis. In stage 2, there is foreshortening of the inferior conjunctival cul-de-sac; this is caused by the subepithelial fibrosis. In stage 3, there is symblepharon formation (Fig. 14–1) and varying degrees of keratopathy, corneal neovascularization, generalized conjunctival shrinkage, trichiasis, districhiasis, and tear insufficiency. Stage 4 is end-stage disease with severe sicca syndrome, ocular surface keratinization, and ankyloblepharon.[9] Inflammation is clinically determined by the amount of conjunctival redness and is graded from 0 to 4+. The staging and inflammatory activity do not necessarily correlate; both are important when considering the prognosis and treatment for these patients.

Drug-induced Pemphigoid

Antiviral and topical antiglaucoma medications have been implicated in causing conjunctival scarring that mimics cicatricial pemphigoid (Table 14–2). There are many similarities between cicatricial pemphigoid and drug-induced ocular scarring: Patients with drug-induced changes may have immunoglobulins bound to the basement membrane of the conjunctiva (Fig. 14–2); these patients also respond to immunosuppressive therapy. Foster[6] has found similar histopathology in patients with cicatricial pemphigoid. Topical timolol, pilocarpine, idoxuridine, epinephrine, echothiophate iodide, dipivefrin, and demecarium all have been implicated in causing unilateral scarring in an eye treated with these medications. Systemic practolol, a beta-blocker, has also

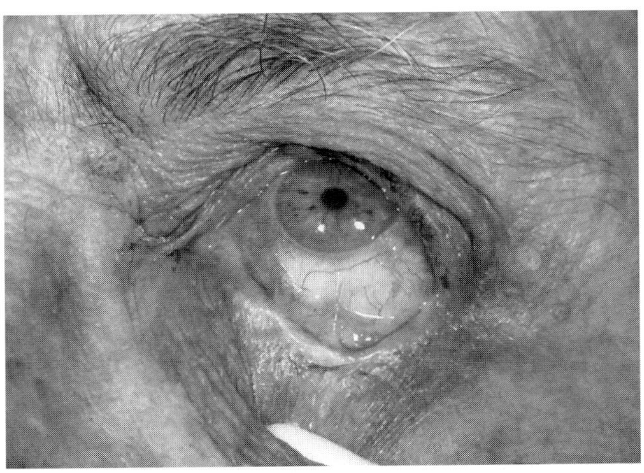

Figure 14–1. Stage 3 (Foster's classification) showing symblepharon formation.

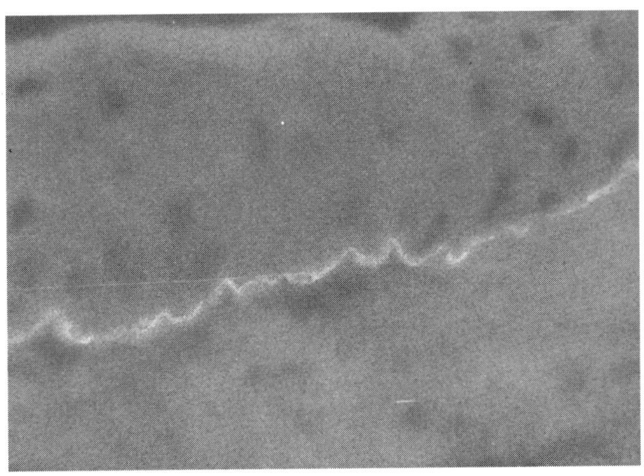

Figure 14–2. Immunofluorescent study with immunoglobulin deposit on the basement membrane.

been reported to cause ocular scarring. For patients using these medicines, it must be decided whether the agents are causing the conjunctival scarring or whether they are exacerbating the pemphigoid in the patients who ultimately would be destined to have this disease. If possible, the drug should be discontinued in patients with pemphigoid changes. For most of these patients further treatment is unnecessary. However, some of these patients have progression of the disease even when these medications are discontinued and will subsequently be given the diagnosis of cicatricial pemphigoid. In patients who need these medications, progression of conjunctival scarring should be closely monitored, and the patient may ultimately require immunosuppressive therapy to prevent further ocular damage.[5,6]

Histopathology

Pemphigoid is characterized by separation of the plasma membrane of the basal cells from the underlying basement membrane, creating a subepidermal blister as opposed to pemphigus, which has blisters that develop within the epidermis. In the early stages, there is usually a granulation tissue infiltrate of chronic inflammatory cells such as lymphocytes and plasma cells within the substantia propria. In acute phases, an active inflammation characterized by neutrophils and occasional eosinophils can be found. In the later stages, scarring within the substantia propria is more pronounced, causing foreshortening of the conjunctiva. There is derangement in the T cell helper to suppressor ratio, with more helper than suppressor T cells. This suggests an underregulation of the immunologic system.[6]

Immunopathology

One of the most striking features of cicatricial pemphigoid is the characteristic binding of immunoglobulins and complement system to the basement membrane of the skin and mucosal areas. Immunofluorescence using IgG, IgA, IgM, and C3 should be obtained. There is a great variance in the percentage of positive biopsy results, ranging from 20% to 84%. Foster[6] also tests IgE, IgD, properdin, factor B, and C4 to increase the sensitivity of the immunofluorescent studies. If the standard immunofluorescence is negative, he uses the avidin-biotin complex (ABC) immunoperoxidase technique, which is 1000 times more sensitive.[6]

The percentage of circulating antibodies to the basement membrane varies from zero to 50%, with IgA and IgG being the most common.[10] One study linked circulating antibodies to the degree of clinical activity.[5] Some patients have also been found to have circulating autoantibodies to the pancreas, thyroid, and adrenal gland. More commonly, antinuclear antibodies, fluorescent antinuclear antibodies, and rheumatoid factor have been found.[2, 6] There have been numerous studies trying to link cicatricial pemphigoid with a histocompatibility linkage antigen, but none of these studies has been conclusive.[6]

TABLE 14-3

Differential Diagnosis in Cicatricial Pemphigoid
Bullous pemphigoid
Chemical or toxic injury
Cicatricial IgA bullous dermatoses
Dermatitis herpetiformis
Drug-induced pemphigoid
Epidermolysis bullosa
Infectious diseases
Paraneoplastic pemphigus
Pemphigus vulgaris
Sarcoid
Sjögren's syndrome
Stevens-Johnson syndrome
Trauma

Differential Diagnosis

A pertinent history should rule out other disorders (Table 14–3), including previous chemical burns and trauma that have caused conjunctival scarring. Infections such as herpes, adenovirus, and trachoma must also be ruled out. Most of these do not have the chronic nature of cicatricial pemphigoid. Sarcoid and Sjögren's syndrome can rarely cause conjunctival scarring, but the scarring is usually mild and not as extensive as in cicatricial pemphigoid.

There are other bullous diseases that must be differentiated from cicatricial pemphigoid. Pemphigus vulgaris has rarely been associated with conjunctival involvement. It is an epithelial process in contrast with cicatricial pemphigoid, which is a subepithelial process. The immunoglobulin and complement bind to the epithelium in immunofluorescent studies.[4, 5] Stevens-Johnson syndrome is an acute bullous disease usually precipitated by infection or a drug reaction in younger patients. It may cause extensive conjunctival shrinkage in acute episodes but usually does not progress. There have been reports of cicatricial pemphigoid developing in patients who previously had Stevens-Johnson syndrome; the mucosal injury from this disorder may have precipitated this occurrence.[11] Bullous pemphigoid and cicatricial pemphigoid both have subepidermal involvement as well as similar immunofluorescent and histopathologic study outcomes. They can be differentiated on the different sites of involvement: Bullous pemphigoid has a predilection for the skin and usually causes nonscarring lesions; it rarely involves the conjunctiva. Cicatricial pemphigoid, on the other hand, has a predilection for mucous membranes with less frequent involvement of the skin; it usually causes scarring lesions. Circulating antibasement membrane zone antibodies are much more common in bullous pemphigoid as compared with cicatricial pemphigoid.[12–14] A newly described entity, paraneoplastic pemphigus, must also be considered in the differential diagnosis for cicatricial conjunctivitis. The disease process is a nonmetastatic effect of a distant malignancy and causes progressive scarring of the conjunctival mucosa.[15,16]

Associated Disorders

There has been an association between cicatricial pemphigoid and other autoimmune disorders.[2] Rheumatoid arthritis and systemic lupus erythematosus have been most commonly associated with cicatricial pemphigoid. Foster[6] found in a large series that 17.7% of the patients had an associated autoimmune disorder. There have also been reports of an increased incidence of systemic malignancies in patients with cicatricial pemphigoid, but the association appears coincidental. In most large studies, the incidence of malignancy has been found to be no higher for patients with cicatricial pemphigoid than for the general population.[6]

TREATMENT OF CICATRICIAL PEMPHIGOID

To decide on treatment, which may involve immunosuppression, one must have a clear clinical diagnosis. Once a diagnosis of cicatricial pemphigoid has been determined, then staging of the patient is used (see section on staging). The second aspect of evaluating the disease process is the degree of active inflammation. Because the clinical course is variable, assessment of disease activity and evidence of progression are quite helpful in determining timing for medical treatment or surgical intervention. Our experience has been that patients with evidence of scarring without evidence of inflammation tend to follow a much slower course and may even be stable. Surgical intervention in these patients, once inactivity has been confirmed, is possible and has been done without exacerbating the disease process. We have also used conjunctival biopsy, both hematoxylin and eosin stains as well as immunofluorescence, to assess the level of activity within the conjunctiva.[6]

Medical Treatment

In the earlier stages, it may be appropriate to treat patients symptomatically and watch for progression of the disease, especially if they have other underlying illnesses that would make them less tolerant of immunosuppressive therapy. All patients with positive culture results should be treated appropriately; lid scrubs and an antibiotic ointment may suffice. Patients with dry eyes should be treated with preservative-free artificial tears solution or ointment and possibly punctal occlusion. A topical retinoid may be employed in patients with cicatricial pemphigoid. If it is not found to be effective in 1 to 2 months, it should be discontinued.

Active progressive cicatricial pemphigoid poses a difficult problem for all clinicians. A number of drugs have been used with varying success. Corticosteroids have been relatively unsuccessful in protracted use and appear to serve only in an adjunctive role to control the inflammation. The advent of immunosuppression therapy has made major changes in the treatment of this disease. Azathioprine was first used in the early 1970s as an alternative treatment modality to corticosteroids.[17,18] Since then, other immunosuppressive drugs have been used. Cyclophosphamide (Cytoxan) has been the most widely used and successful of these medications. Dapsone (sulfapyridine), a drug previously used to treat leprosy, has also been shown to be efficacious in the treatment of cicatricial pemphigoid. Because of the severe potential side effects of these treatment modalities, they have been reserved only for advanced and active disease processes. There must be at least stage 3 disease according to Foster's classification or stage 2 disease by Mondino and Brown's scheme with an active inflammatory process for immunosuppressive therapy to be considered.[8,9]

Several authors favor dapsone for the less active, less progressive disease. The medication carries fewer side effects and is better tolerated by patients. Dapsone is begun at 2 $mg \cdot kg^{-1} \cdot day^{-1}$ with prednisone 1 $mg \cdot kg^{-1} \cdot day^{-1}$. The maximum dose of dapsone is 200 mg daily. Patients have been reported to show response to this regimen; however, one third of the patients who initially respond relapse within 6 months of cessation of dapsone. Even though it is usually less toxic, it still has significant side effects, including aplastic anemia, hemolytic anemia, and agranulocytosis. The dose-related hemolysis is the most common side effect. Patients with glucose-6-phosphate dehydrogenase (G6PD) deficiencies are more susceptible to this adverse side effect. A G6PD level must be determined before dapsone treatment is initiated. Dapsone is a sulfone derivative and may cause an allergic reaction in patients allergic to sulfa.[6,19]

Cyclophosphamide has been our choice in patients with active, progressive disease. The initial dosage is 1 to 2 $mg \cdot kg$. It is then modified based on clinical judgment, bone marrow tolerance, and side effects. White blood cell counts are maintained at at least 2500 cell/mm and a platelet count at at least 70,000/mm^3. Blood counts are obtained biweekly and urinalysis at least monthly. Patients who are taking cyclophosphamide are followed constantly and monitored by physicians familiar with the use of immunosuppression.[20] Other drugs such as azathioprine (Imuran) and methotrexate have also been employed in these patients. Complications from immunosuppressive therapy include hemorrhagic cystitis, dermatitis, alopecia, weight loss, gastrointestinal distress and bleeding, anemia, and severe leukopenia. Defective oogenesis or spermatogenesis has been reported in a number of patients treated with methotrexate or cyclophosphamide.[5,6,8,9]

The goal of immunosuppression is to stop progression of the disease. Patients on immunosuppression therapy are maintained on this drug level for 6 months to 1 year. If prednisone is begun for the initial inflammation, this may be gradually tapered and discontinued within a few months, depending on clinical response. Cessation of immunosuppressive therapy is based on clinical judgment and, as reported by some authors, response may also be assessed by serial biopsies for immunofluorescence.[21]

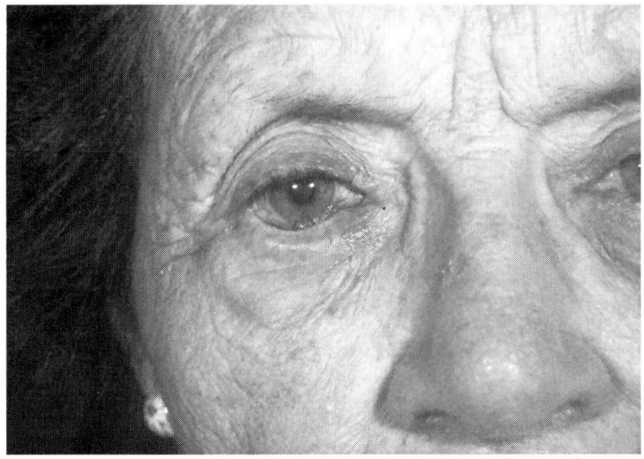

Figure 14–3. Entropion formation in a patient with cicatricial pemphigoid.

Surgical Intervention

Treatment, as noted earlier, is primarily medical; however, a number of patients with ocular pemphigus require surgical intervention at some time during the course of their disease process. It has been noted in the literature that surgical intervention in these patients has worsened or hastened conjunctival scarring and advanced the disease process.[22–25] We have performed 22 surgical procedures on patients with cicatricial pemphigoid without causing significant worsening of their disease process and obtaining improvement in the condition that was addressed surgically. This has been achieved by obtaining an adequate diagnosis, staging the disease, proceeding with appropriate medical treatment when necessary, and timing the surgical procedure with the level of activity to their disease process. By using this approach, we believe that surgical intervention can be done, minimizing the risk of causing worsening of the disease.

Surgery in Early Stages

The need for surgical treatment in stage 1 or early ocular pemphigus is quite rare. In this stage of the disease process there is primarily conjunctival inflammation, mucoid discharge, and conjunctival subepithelial fibrosis. If a patient does happen to have a preexisting ocular problem that will require surgery, it is probably best to observe him or her for a period to see if one can document progression, and, if this stage is fairly stable, then lid surgery can probably be done without pretreatment with immunosuppressive agents.

Surgery in More Advanced Stages

In surgical treatment of patients with cicatricial pemphigoid in more advanced stages it must be decided whether the inflammatory response is being caused by the disease process or if it is being caused by complications of the disease such as entropion and trichiasis. Stabilization of the disease process with the administration of immunosuppressives should be obtained prior to surgical intervention, if possible. If this is not possible because of secondary complications such as trichiasis, immunosuppression should be instituted before surgical intervention is considered.

Procedures

Entropion. Entropion repair may be either an involutional type or a cicatricial type. Both types have been noted in our series in patients with cicatricial pemphigoid. An involutional type may be coincidental or secondary to chronic rubbing and swelling, causing a dehiscence of the inferior lid retractors and stretching of the lateral canthal tendon. Cicatricial changes are expected secondary to the scarring from the disease process.

Involutional entropion can be corrected at any time and can be achieved through an external approach that does not violate the conjunctival surface or minimally incises the conjunctival surface at the lateral canthus. Cicatricial entropion (Figs. 14–3 and 14–4) poses more of a problem. Patients with this type of entropion have more advanced cicatricial pemphigoid and require either

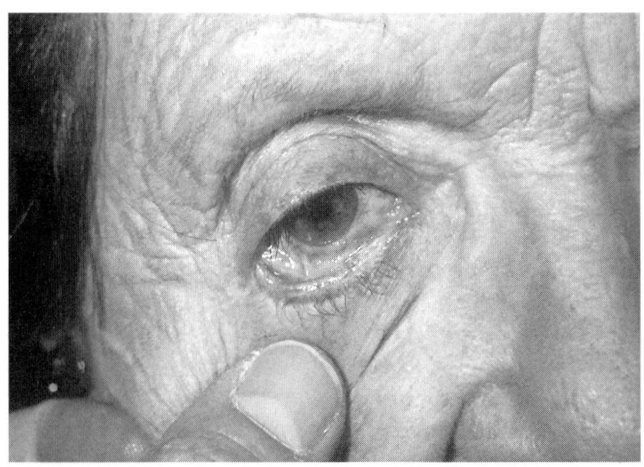

Figure 14–4. Same patient as in Figure 14–3, with eversion of the lower lid revealing symblepharon formation.

evidence that the disease is stabilized and nonprogressive or pretreatment with immunofluorescence and adequate stabilization. It is our preference, if possible, to delay correction as long as possible, but scarring that is occurring secondary to the lashes must be taken into account in deciding when to correct this.

Trichiasis and Districhiasis. Cryoablation has been helpful in the treatment of this condition; however, one should realize that cryoablation to large areas causes loss of tissue and structure within the lid, and cryoablation should be directed to the lash follicle with care taken to minimize tissue loss in the surrounding area. Cryoprobes 2 to 3 mm in length have been helpful in obtaining this. Lid-splitting procedures can be performed, but they also require stabilization of the disease process before proceeding. Conjunctival procedures involved with grafting and rearrangement pose a much higher risk to the patient with cicatricial pemphigoid.

The goal in these patients is not the creation of a deep cul-de-sac and removal of all symblepharon but stabilization of the disease process and, through surgical intervention, prevention of the trichiasis, entropion, and scarring from causing progressive vision loss. Grafting, in our series, has been directed primarily to lid margins, and surgery to the cul-de-sac has not been addressed.

Altered Tear Production. Lacrimal surgery in many patients is primarily closure of the puncta to increase tear production as performed in an office setting. Many of these patients require no punctum closure because the disease process has already achieved this. As noted in the literature, tear production may or may not be affected in the earlier stages of the disease; therefore, a percentage of these patients have required lacrimal surgery for chronic tearing once their disease process has stabilized. Dacryocystorhinostomy and conjunctivodacryocystorhinostomy have been of benefit in particular patients.

Other Ocular Surgery in Patients with Cicatricial Pemphigoid

Cataract surgery has been successful in patients with cicatricial pemphigoid when the ocular inflammation is under control. These patients can be placed on chemotherapy for 6 months after the surgery to prevent any reactivation of the disease process. Corneal transplantation, on the other hand, has not been successful in these patients, because they usually have mucosal keratinization and severely dry eyes that make them poor candidates.

Patients who present with advanced scarring and conjunctival shrinkage have a poor prognosis with all forms of therapy. Heroic surgical measures in these patients in our hands have not shown prolonged benefit. A number of authors have used keratoprosthesis with some success in these patients.

Conclusion

Because cicatricial pemphigoid is such a devastating ocular process, appropriate and timely intervention must be initiated. Immunosuppression is an important therapy in this disease, but surgical intervention must also be employed at times. This is especially true if complications are exacerbating the disease process. As the combination of medical and surgical intervention has developed, the prognosis for this disease has been greatly enhanced.

REFERENCES

1. Lever WF, Talbot JH: Pemphigus: A historical study. Arch Dermatol Syph 46:800–823, 1942.
2. Person JR, Rogers RS 3rd: Bullous and cicatricial pemphigoid: Clinical, histopathologic and immmunopathologic correlations. Mayo Clin Proc 52:54–66, 1977.
3. Fine JD: Cicatricial pemphigoid. *In* Wojnarowski F, Briggaman RA (eds): Management of Blistering Diseases. New York, Raven Press, 1992, pp 83–91.
4. Mondino BJL: Bullous diseases of the skin and mucous membranes. Duane's Clinical Ophthalmology, vol 4. Philadelphia, JB Lippincott, 1991, pp 1–19.
5. Mondino BJ: Cicatricial pemphigoid. Ophthalmology 97:939–950, 1990.
6. Foster CS: Cicatricial pemphigoid. Trans Am Ophthalmol Soc 84:527–663, 1986.
7. Mondino BJ, Brown SI: Ocular cicatricial pemphigoid. Ophthalmology 88:95–100, 1981.
8. Mondino BJ, Brown SI: Immunosuppressive therapy in ocular cicatricial pemphigoid. Am J Ophthalmol 96:453–459, 1983.
9. Foster CS, Wilson LA, Ekins MB: Immunosuppressive therapy for progressive ocular cicatricial pemphigoid. Ophthalmology 89:340–353, 1982.
10. Franklin RM, Fitzmorris CT: Antibodies against conjunctival basement membrane zone: Occurrence in cicatricial pemphigoid. Arch Ophthalmol 101:1611–1613, 1983.
11. Chan LS, Soong HK, Foster CS, et al: Ocular cicatricial pemphigoid occurring as a sequela of Stevens-Johnson syndrome. JAMA 266:1543–1546, 1991.
12. Frith PA, Venning VA, Wojnarowski F, et al: Conjunctival involvement in cicatricial and bullous pemphigoid: A clinical and immunopathological study. Br J Ophthalmol 73:52–56, 1989.
13. Laskaris G, Angelopoulos A: Cicatricial pemphigoid: Direct and indirect immunofluorescent studies. Oral Surg 51:43–54, 1981.
14. Venning VA, Frith PA, Bron AJ, et al: Mucosal involvement in bullous and cicatricial pemphigoid: A clinical and immunopathological study. Br J Dermatol 118:7–15, 1988.
15. Lam S, Stone MS, Goeken JA, et al: Paraneoplastic pemphigus, cicatricial conjunctivitis, and acanthosis nigricans with pachydermatoglyphy in a patient with bronchogenic squamous cell carcinoma. Ophthalmology 99:108–113, 1992.
16. Sugar A: Paraneoplastic pemphigus and ophthalmology [editorial]. Ophthalmology 99:5–6, 1992.
17. Dantzig PI: Immunosuppressive and cytotoxic drugs in dermatology. Arch Dermatol 110:393–406, 1974.
18. Dave VK, Vickers CFH: Azathioprine in the treatment of mucocutaneous pemphigoid. Br J Dermatol 90:183–186, 1974.
19. Rogers RS 3rd, Seehafer JR, Perry HO: Treatment of cicatricial (benign mucous membrane) pemphigoid with dapsone. J Am Acad Dermatol 6:215–223, 1982.
20. Brody HJ, Pirozzi DJ: Benign mucous membrane pemphigoid: Response to therapy with cyclophosphamide. Arch Dermatol 113:1598–1599, 1977.
21. Stevens-Johnson Syndrome (Erythema Multiforme Major), pp 221–224. Basic and Clinical Science Course. San Francisco, American Academy of Ophthalmology, 1987.

22. Sainz de la Maza M, Tauber J, Foster CS: Cataract surgery in ocular cicatricial pemphigoid. Ophthalmology 95:481–486, 1988.
23. McDonald M: Questions and answers. Arch Ophthalmol 109:785, 1991.
24. Belin MW, Hannush SB: Mucous membrane abnormalities. *In* Abbott RL (ed): Surgical Intervention in Corneal and External Diseases. Orlando, Grune & Stratton, 1987, pp 259–276.
25. Robin JB, Dugel R: Immunologic disorders of the cornea and conjunctiva. Kaufman H, et al (eds): The Cornea. New York, Churchill Livingstone, 1988, pp 523–528.

CHAPTER 15

Tarsoconjunctival Polishing with Mucous Membrane Grafting for Cicatricial Entropion and Trichiasis

William P. Chen

In patients with cicatricial entropion and trichiasis, corneal surface irritation results from chronic assault from ingrown and aberrant eyelashes, roughened lid margin scarring from epidermalization, and in severe cases, retraction and poor closure of the eyelid margins. These findings are manifested in Stevens-Johnson syndrome, ocular pemphigoid, postinflammatory processes such as trachoma, and chemical and metal burns and, rarely, after therapeutic use of antiglaucoma medications such as echothiophate iodide and pilocarpine. In Stevens-Johnson syndrome,[1, 2] one sees a cicatrization of mucosal surface, keratinization, metaplasia of the meibomian glands, and a quantitative decrease in the density of goblet cells in the conjunctiva.[3] These findings are also evident in ocular pemphigoid.

For the past 15 years, I have used the method of tarsal polishing with full-thickness buccal mucous membrane graft with satisfactory improvement in the symptoms of these patients.[4]

CLINICAL FEATURES

In patients who have had trachoma, the upper tarsus is typically scarred with evidence of Arlt's line, an inward migration of the mucocutaneous border (from contracture and epidermalization), trichiasis (as a result of tarsal margin contracture and metaplasia of the meibomian glands), and a slight degree of inward buckling and thickening of the tarsal plate.

In patients with Stevens-Johnson syndrome and ocular pemphigoid, the conjunctival surface has undergone severe autoimmune-based "membranous" conjunctivitis, creating a contracted and pale tarsoconjunctival surface with a decrease in goblet cell density in the chronic phase. Often, one sees symblepharon formation as a result of conjunctival melting. Patients with cicatricial trichiasis after chronic use of echothiophate iodide develop a "pseudo-ocular pemphigoid syndrome." Similar changes can occur following burn injuries.

The treatment consists of the following:

1. Removal of diseased and metaplastic conjunctival elements through tarsal polishing.
2. Replacement of roughened tarsal conjunctiva and lid margin with a smooth mucosal surface through grafting of full-thickness buccal mucous membrane.
3. Correction of the inwardly directed lashes (either from being pulled in by conjunctival contracture or from metaplasia of the hair follicles next to a meibomian gland) by recession of the skin–muscle layer and advancement of the tarsoconjunctival layer.

SURGICAL METHODS

Unless contraindicated, the procedure of tarsal polishing with full-thickness buccal mucous membrane graft is performed under general anesthesia for ease of surgical maneuvering and harvesting of the buccal mucous membrane graft.

The offending eyelid and the donor site on the lip are preinfiltrated with 2% lidocaine with 1:100,000 epinephrine, mixed 10 mL to 150 U of hyaluronidase. With two 4-0 silk sutures placed along the lid margin, the lid is everted (Fig. 15–1) to allow for examination of the scarred and epidermalized conjunctival surface. A 3-mm, smooth diamond polishing tip on a rotary handle (such as a Hall drill or a Stryker roto-osteotome) is used to polish away the diseased tarsal conjunctiva (Fig. 15–2). The underlying tarsus shows fine capillary oozing after adequate tarsal polishing.

For those patients with trichiasis in addition to a roughened tarsal surface and lid margin, it is important to include recession of the skin–muscle layer (or advancement of the tarsoconjunctival layer). With magnification, the surgeon uses a super-sharp blade to split the lid margin along the gray line into an anterior skin–muscle layer and a posterior tarsoconjunctival layer (Fig. 15–3). The dissection is carried out further along the anterior tarsal plane to allow for recession of the skin–

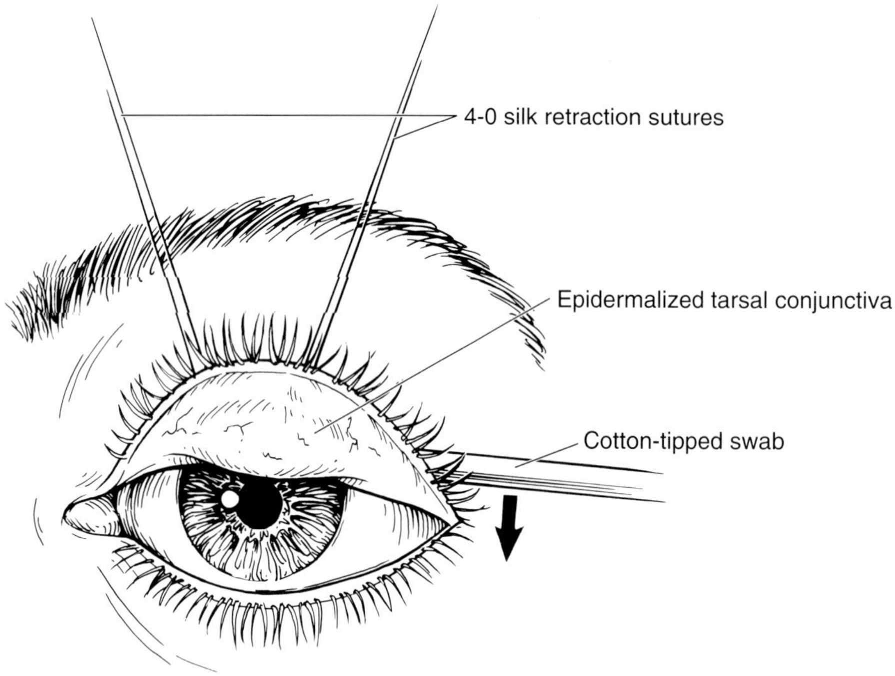

Figure 15–1. The lid margin is everted with 4-0 silk sutures. (From McCord CD Jr, Chen WP: Tarsal polishing and mucous membrane grafting for cicatricial entropion, trichiasis, and epidermalization. Ophthalmic Surg 14:1021–1025, 1983.)

muscle layer relative to the tarsoconjunctival layer. This is facilitated by a transverse Müllerotomy above the superior tarsal border of the upper lid. A 2-mm vertical relaxing incision is performed at each end of the tarsus to allow for a 1.5- to 2-mm advancement of the tarsoconjunctival layer relative to the skin–muscle layer. If any aberrant lashes are seen on the tarsoconjunctival layer under direct or microscopic visualization, they are removed. The two layers are then secured in this recessed position using three 4-0 silk sutures, placing them full thickness through the lid in the fashion described by Pang (Fig. 15–4).[5] The sutures are applied full thickness above the superior edge of the upper tarsus, while in the lower lid, they are placed directly below the inferior edge of the lower tarsus.

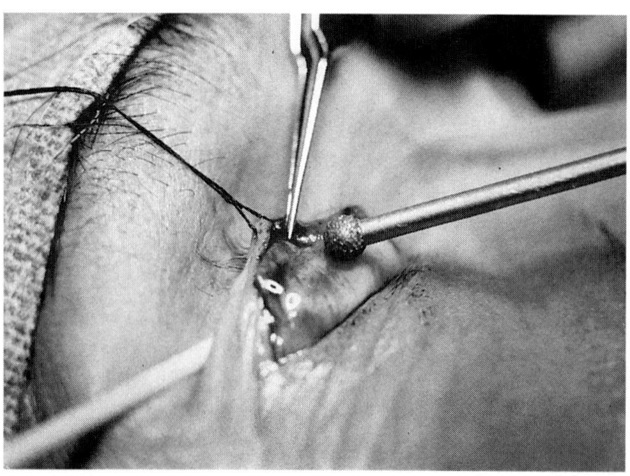

Figure 15–2. Three-millimeter diamond bur used to polish away diseased tarsal conjunctiva, providing a smooth tarsal plate for grafting.

The buccal mucous membrane graft is obtained in the following fashion: The lower lip is everted using surgical clips, and a strip of buccal mucous membrane measuring 20 × 40 mm is designed (Fig. 15–5). The graft is taken, noting that it will shrink 2 ½ to 3 times in size after the

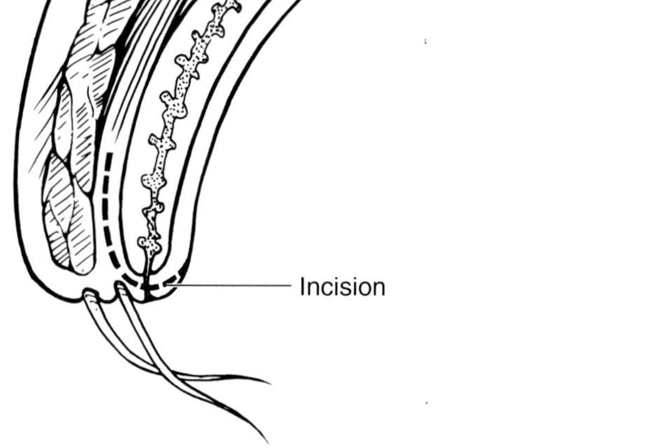

Figure 15–3. Cross-section view of upper lid showing the plane of surgical dissection along the lid margin dividing the lid into an anterior skin–orbicularis layer and a posterior tarsoconjunctival layer. Excision of Müller's muscle facilitates advancement of the tarsoconjunctival layer. (Modified from Tasman W, Jaeger E [eds]: Duane's Clinical Ophthalmology, vol 5. Philadelphia, JB Lippincott, 1985, pp 1–54.)

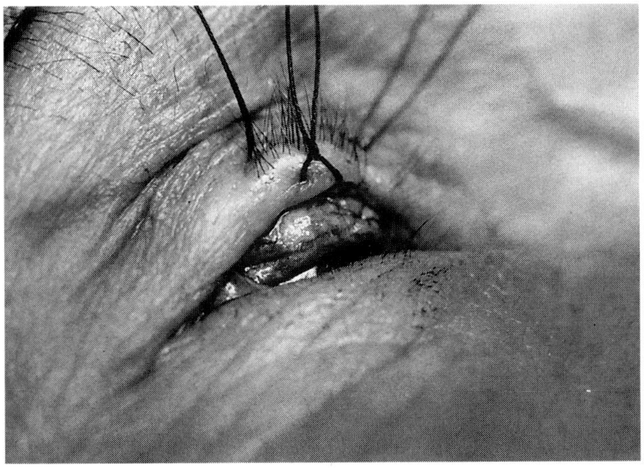

Figure 15–4. Anterior skin–muscle layer recessed 2 mm relative to the tarsal border and anchored in place using two or three 4-0 silk sutures passed full thickness through the lid just above the superior edge of the upper tarsus.

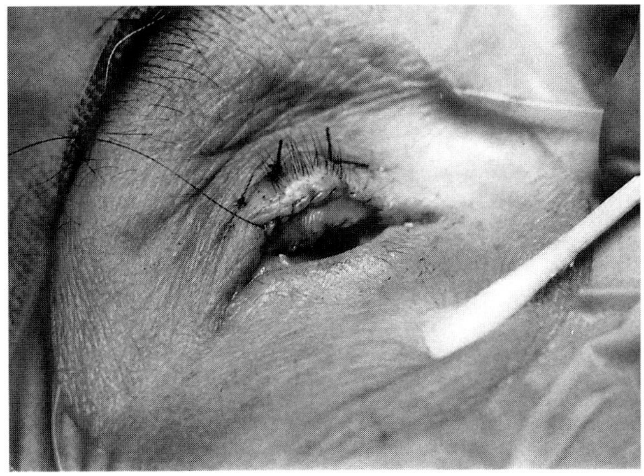

Figure 15–6. Rectangular strip of full-thickness buccal mucous membrane graft sutured onto the underside of the abnormal portion of the tarsus. The grafts curve around the tarsal edge onto the anterior, exposed surface of the advanced tarsal plate. The suture knot is exteriorized.

harvesting. It is carefully cleansed of any submucosal fatty tissue and then soaked in diluted gentamicin solution. The donor site bleeds minimally and can be easily compressed with a strip of Gelfoam.

The buccal mucous membrane is trimmed to the proper dimensions and applied over the polished tarsal surface and lid margin, especially over the exposed anterior tarsal surface if skin–muscle recession was performed. Sutures of 6-0 black nylon on a P-1 needle are then used to anchor the buccal mucous membrane graft onto the tarsus, starting laterally to medially and then again exiting laterally with the sutures tied externally (Fig. 15–6 to 15–8). In most patients, both the upper and lower eyelids undergo the mucous membrane grafting. Two or three double-armed 4-0 silk sutures are then used as an intermarginal suture to splint the buccal mucous membrane grafts at the lid margins together (Fig. 15–9). The patient is given a cephalosporin antibiotic intravenously followed by an oral regimen for 7 days postoperatively. The sutures are removed in 5 to 7 days.

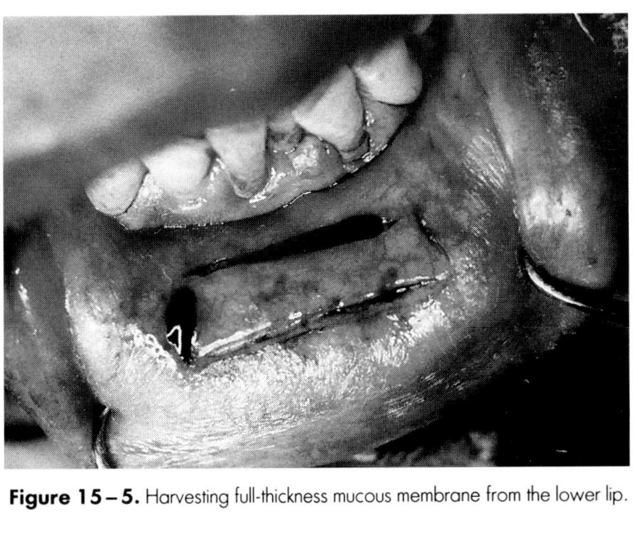

Figure 15–5. Harvesting full-thickness mucous membrane from the lower lip.

CLINICAL RESULTS

Almost all patients who have undergone the tarsal polishing with full-thickness buccal mucous membrane graft procedure report a lessening of ocular irritation and pain and a decrease in the degree of tearing. Some patients report an improvement in visual acuity, most likely from a decrease in reflex tear secretion and lessening of photophobia that is often seen in association with corneal irritation. The buccal mucous membrane graft usually takes well and appears as an erythematous lid margin for 3 to 4 months, after which the hyperemia recedes and the graft assumes a flesh color (Fig. 15–10).

Complications have included suture irritation of the cornea (which can be avoided by careful edge-to-edge placement of the nylon suture), necrosis of the graft from excessive compression of the intermarginal suture, and recurrent trichiasis when lash follicles were inadvertantly left on the tarsal border. The donor site on the lower lip usually heals within 2 to 3 weeks, and postoperative discomfort is almost always transient.

CONCLUSION

The tarsal polishing with full-thickness buccal mucous membrane graft procedure is especially effective in the surgical management of patients with cicatricial trichiasis and entropion, as a result of trachoma, Stevens-Johnson syndrome, ocular pemphigoid, or a chemical burn. All of these patients have scarring and epidermalization of the tarsal conjunctiva and secondary corneal irritation. Tarsal polishing removes the offending rough surface and, when combined with the grafting of a full-

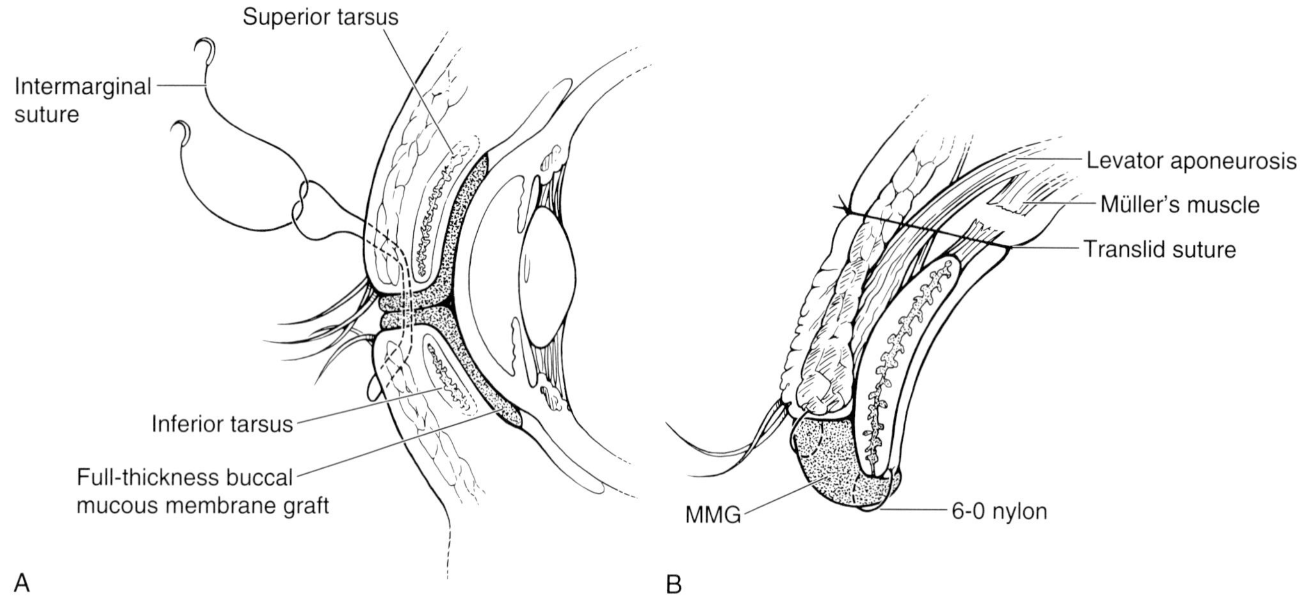

Figure 15-7. Placement of graft. *A*, The grafts are placed on the tarsal border and back surface of the tarsus when tarsal polishing but no skin-muscle recession is performed. B, The graft is placed on the back surface, the tarsal border, and the front surface of the tarsus when both tarsal polishing and skin-muscle recession are performed. (MMG, mucous membrane graft.) (*A* and *B* modified from McCord CD Jr, Chen WP: Tarsal polishing and mucous membrane grafting for cicatricial entropion, trichiasis, and epidermalization. Ophthalmic Surg 14:1021-1025, 1983.)

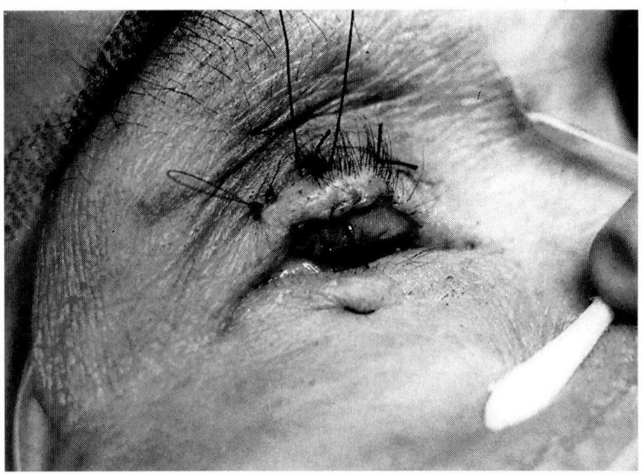

Figure 15-8. Doubled-armed 4-0 black silk suture passed from lower lid margin through mucous membrane graft on upper lid margin. (The patient had only the upper lid margin grafted.) Upper lid shown with full-thickness anchoring sutures and externalized suture knot of 6-0 nylon.

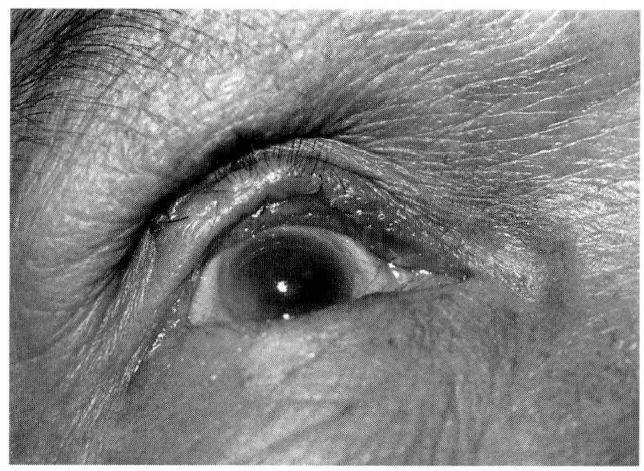

Figure 15-10. Postoperative appearance of mucous membrane graft. Abnormal tarsal surface is replaced with smooth mucosal surface.

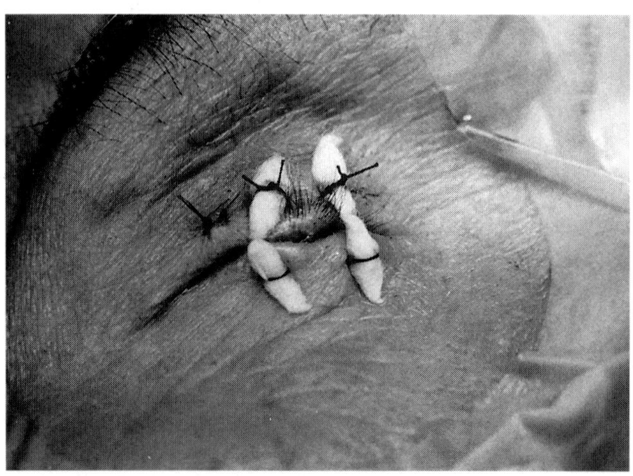

Figure 15-9. Two intermarginal sutures placed across cotton bolsters to splint the buccal mucous membrane graft.

thickness buccal mucous membrane, results in the following effects:

1. The interposition of a smooth mucosal lining between the diseased tarsus and the cornea.
2. The addition of goblet cells, which secrete mucin, to the overall mucosal surface of the eyelid fissure. The attendant mucin and increased vascular perfusion, which leads to higher ambient oxygen tension, may help improve the stability of the precorneal tear film.

REFERENCES

1. Yetiv JZ, Bianchine JR, Owen JA: Etiologic factors of the Stevens-Johnson syndrome. South Med J 73:599-602, 1980.

2. Arstikaitis MJ: Ocular aftermath of Stevens-Johnson syndrome. Arch Ophthalmol 90:376–379, 1973.
3. Ralph RA: Conjunctival goblet cell density in normal subjects and in dry eye syndromes. Invest Ophthalmol Vis Sci 14:299–302, 1975.
4. McCord CD Jr, Chen WP: Tarsal polishing and mucous membrane grafting for cicatricial entropion, trichiasis, and epidermalization. Ophthalmic Surg 14:1021–1025, 1983.
5. Pang HG: Surgical formation of upper lid fold. Arch Ophthalmol 65:783–784, 1961.

CHAPTER 16

Management of Pterygia

Robert D. Deitch, Jr., and Fred M. Wilson II

A pterygium is a horizontally oriented, fleshy, triangular tumor of the bulbar conjunctiva near the limbus that grows across the superficial cornea, toward the visual axis, in the interpalpebral fissure. The lesion insinuates itself between the corneal epithelium and Bowman's layer, disrupting the latter.

The word *pterygium* is derived from the Greek word, *pteryx*, meaning wing, which describes the characteristic shape. Pterygia have been recognized since ancient times as described by the world's first known ophthalmologist, Susruta, as early as 1000 B.C.[1-3]

Pterygia most commonly occur nasally but can occur temporally, with their bases directed toward the respective canthi. When both nasal and temporal pterygia occur in the same eye, the temporal lesion usually develops later. Approximately 25% of pterygia are bilateral. Four pterygia have been reported in the same person.[2]

The decision to remove a pterygium surgically should be made only with an understanding, and due consideration, of the anatomy, histopathology, pathogenesis, differential diagnosis, prognosis, complications, and treatment alternatives.

ANATOMY

Pterygia have been classically described as having three parts: a body, a neck, and a head. The anatomic boundaries between these parts are imprecise. The body of a pterygium arises from the bulbar conjunctiva or occasionally from the semilunar fold or conjunctival fornix (particularly in recurrent pterygia). The upper and lower borders of the body present folds under which a probe can be placed for some distance because the attachment to underlying tissue is less in extent than the apparent vertical height. The anterior portion of Tenon's capsule becomes incorporated into the body of the pterygium and contributes to its vasculature and bulk.[4] The body of the pterygium joins the neck near the limbus. The neck is horizontally oriented, as is its vasculature. This portion of the pterygium can be elevated or flat and is adherent to the underlying Bowman's layer of the cornea. The head of the pterygium is the distal 1 to 2 mm of the lesion closest to the visual axis. The head is tightly adherent to the underlying cornea. A "crown," or "cap," of grayish opacification at the level of Bowman's layer is seen around the head of the pterygium. This opacification often has a fimbriated central edge, with some areas having lost their contiguity with the crown. These more central, local, detached areas of opacification are called *islets of Fuchs.* A Stocker's line is an epithelial deposition of iron-containing pigment, similar to a Hudson-Stähli line, that can often be found in the otherwise uninvolved corneal epithelium. The Stocker's line conforms to the shape of the head of the pterygium and often denotes chronicity since rapidly growing lesions do not allow time for the iron to be deposited in the epithelium.

Anatomic differences are apparent with respect to the activity of the lesion and the stage of development. Actively growing lesions are raised and hyperemic, whereas inactive ones are flat and pale gray. The clinical significance of activity is discussed later. The anatomic boundaries separating the body, neck, and head are more indistinct with early pterygia because of their small size. These early lesions extend into the cornea 1 to 2 mm from the limbus, have minimal vasculature, and tend to progress slowly. As growth continues, the features described earlier become apparent.

HISTOPATHOLOGY

Pterygia are characterized histopathologically by abnormal subepithelial fibrovascular connective tissue. The overlying epithelium is not primarily involved in the process; it can be thickened or thinned but is usually normal.

The collagen of the conjunctival subepithelial tissue is described as having undergone "elastotic degeneration." This refers to the staining of this tissue with elastic stains but its resistance to lysis with elastase, thereby demonstrating that this tissue is not true elastin. A large component of this elastotic material has been shown to be derived from newly synthesized elastic fiber precursors and abnormally formed elastic fibers that undergo secondary degeneration.[5] Other involved components of the subepithelial tissue include ground substance, abnormal fibroblasts, and normal and abnormal true elastic tissue. As pterygia encroach on the cornea, Bowman's layer is replaced by a fibrovascular pannus. The histopathologic changes do not extend deeper than Bowman's layer.

A "recurrent pterygium" is histopathologically distinct from the primary lesion. The former is a fibrovascular scar, arising from the excision site, that is composed of exuberant fibroblasts and vasculature and that has been likened to a keloid of the skin. Therefore, the term *recurrent pterygium* may be technically inappropriate, although it is well established and, we believe, clinically useful.[6,7]

PATHOGENESIS

Pterygia are quite common, but little is known regarding their pathogenesis. Several theories have been developed to explain their occurrence. Since pterygia are believed to be degenerative responses, stimuli that possibly contribute to their occurrence include those such as ultraviolet radiation, airborne allergens, chemical irritants, wind, dust, heat, and dry climate. These ocular irritants usually cause a chronic keratoconjunctivitis that is believed to lead to the development of pterygia.[1,8–10] Men have pterygia more often than women. This male predominance may be explained by a presumably increased environmental insult.

Ultraviolet-induced damage to the conjunctiva, with or without other associated irritants, is the most popular mechanism proposed to explain the induction of pterygia. This theory is supported by studies showing that the incidence of pterygia increases with proximity to the equator. Cameron mapped the worldwide distribution of pterygia and found that the prevalence is generally highest within the 30th-latitude parallels.[1] The prevalence of pterygia is lowest north of the northern 40th parallel and south of the southern 40th parallel. Cameron also noted that the incidence of pterygium rose among the British who migrated to the more equatorial Australia.[1] The incidence is also higher for people such as fishermen and farm workers, who have increased actinic exposure as a result of employment or lifestyle.[11] A study of welders, who are exposed to greater levels of ultraviolet light, demonstrated a direct relationship between the length of employment and the incidence of pterygium.[12] In Australia the incidence of primary pterygia was found to be 15% in people who did not wear eyeglasses and 3% in those who wore eyeglasses since before the age of 15 years.[1] The predilection for the nasal aspect of the globe is thought to be secondary to increased actinic exposure in this region as a result of the reflection of ultraviolet light from the nose or from scattered and indirect ultraviolet light concentrated in this area by corneal internal reflection.[13,14] Some evidence exists that susceptibility to environmental factors that predispose to the development of pterygia may be inherited as an autosomal dominant trait with partial penetrance.[2,15,16]

Factors other than ultraviolet radiation can probably lead to pterygia. The prevalence among Punjab Indians in British Columbia who work in indoor sawmills as compared with those who work as outdoor farmers in the Indian Punjab region is strikingly high.[17] In a study of the sawmill workers, sawdust was thought to be the stimulant responsible for the presence of pterygia. Further support for other factors, in addition to actinic exposure, being able to incite pterygia is found in studies that show that pterygia are not closely linked to the chronic actinic disorder of climatic droplet keratopathy.[18]

Tear film abnormalities have been proposed as a cause for pterygia.[8,19] Elevation of the pterygium head, leading to delle formation and epithelial irregularity with subsequent inflammation, followed by vascularization, has been proposed as a mechanism stimulating advancement of the lesion. According to this theory, pterygia are initiated by delle formation adjacent to pingueculae.[8,20]

In 1892 Fuchs popularized the idea that all pterygia arise from pingueculae.[21] Even though both lesions are believed to be initiated by exposure to environmental stimuli, particularly ultraviolet radiation, pterygia do not invariably arise from pingueculae.[22]

DIFFERENTIAL DIAGNOSIS

True pterygia should be distinguished from pseudopterygia. The latter arise as a result of an inflammatory process affecting the external ocular surface, such as that initiated by chemical injury, thermal injury, other trauma (including surgical), peripheral corneal ulceration (infectious or autoimmune), and cicatrizing conjunctivitis. Pseudopterygia can cross the limbus in any axis and do not have a predilection for the interpalpebral area, as do true pterygia. One commonly described feature that helps in distinguishing pseudopterygia from true pterygia is that a probe can often be passed beneath the former at the limbus and cannot be with the latter. A true pterygium remains firmly fixed to the underlying tissue throughout most of its extent, whereas a pseudopterygium is often adherent only at its apex.

Fuchs' superficial marginal keratitis and Terrien's marginal degeneration are unusual causes of pseudopterygia that are important to recognize because of the underlying corneal thinning.[23,24] Perforations have occurred with resections of these pseudopterygia. A limbal dermoid or phlyctenular pannus may also occasionally be confused with an atypical pterygium.

Other considerations in the differential diagnosis of pterygia include conjunctival intraepithelial neoplasia and squamous cell carcinoma. These lesions usually develop from corneal stem cells at the limbus in the interpalpebral fissure. The involved epithelium is thickened, opalescent, and loosely adherent to underlying tissues. With time, papillomatous growth can occur, and there may be associated inflammation and prominent vascularity. Both conjunctival intraepithelial neoplasia and squamous cell carcinoma of the conjunctiva have been reported rarely to occur in association with a pterygium. It is surprising that this does not occur more often since chronic exposure to ultraviolet light is currently believed to be the primary pathogenic mechanism for each of these lesions. Pterygia are not otherwise precursors to epithelial dysplasia or carcinoma.

PROGNOSIS

Recurrence of a pterygium after surgical resection is common—often it is worse than the primary lesion.[1, 20] Recurrent pterygia tend to be larger, thicker, more hyperemic, and more aggressive than the initial lesion. The recurrent lesions can be associated with the formation of symblepharon and restricted ocular motility.

Factors that are related to a high risk of recurrence of pterygia after resection include the following:

1. Large size
2. Recent activity and progression
3. Previous recurrence
4. Younger patient age
5. Living nearer to the equator and other forms of increased actinic exposure or environmental insult
6. Inadequate surgery

In temperate climatic zones, relatively small and asymptomatic pterygia are best observed. Patients who have such lesions should be provided with explanations, reassurance (including the fact that pterygia are not "cancers"), and periodic observation and should actually be discouraged from having surgery. They should be informed that surgical intervention can have disappointing results.

It is sometimes suggested that small pterygia should perhaps be handled more aggressively in tropical and subtropical areas because of a greater likelihood of progression as the result of more intense actinic exposure. However, some clinicians in Israel have essentially given up excising pterygia of any size because of poor results and complications despite the careful use of excellent surgical techniques. These clinicians concluded that it is preferable to observe pterygia until they threaten the visual axis or become otherwise unacceptable and then perform corneal transplantation.[25] Such an extreme approach is not appropriate for most parts of the world, but it does emphasize the need for caution.

INDICATIONS FOR SURGERY

In temperate climates, primary pterygia rarely extend to the visual axis; many of these lesions do not progress. Most pterygia in patients who are older than 50 years of age are atrophic and inactive. Inactive pterygia are pale, thin, and membranous. An inactive lesion in a patient of any age should probably be left undisturbed, although inactive lesions are much less apt to recur following surgical excision. Aggressive and recurrent pterygia have a tendency to occur in younger patients.[26] Active pterygia grow demonstrably over time and are fleshy, vascular, usually hyperemic, and raised above the surrounding cornea. Aside from their cosmetic problems, most pterygia are asymptomatic. Surgery cannot reliably be expected to eliminate irritative symptoms, such as feelings of dryness. The following guidelines are acceptable indications for the surgical removal of pterygia (if the patient fully understands and accepts the risks of the procedure):

1. Advancement of an active pterygium to, or beyond, a point halfway between the limbus and the visual axis
2. Obvious progression of a bothersome and worrisome pterygium, even if it does not extend halfway to the visual axis
3. A need to correct complications such as symblepharon and restricted motility, keeping in mind that these problems can occasionally be corrected without attacking the pterygium itself
4. A desire to improve vision for a patient whose pterygium has caused decreased visual acuity by having invaded the visual axis (sometimes also requiring corneal transplantation, traditional superficial keratectomy, or excimer laser phototherapeutic keratectomy because of remaining corneal scarring) or by having produced astigmatism (flattening of the corneal curvature in the horizontal meridian)[27, 28]
5. A need to improve the appearance of the eye
6. Occasionally to eliminate symptoms such as foreign body sensation and mild photophobia
7. Insistence by an informed patient that surgery be done

Pterygia have also been shown to cause decreased contrast sensitivity and greater glare disability.[29] Guidelines for the use of these parameters in the decision to remove pterygia have not been established.

NONSURGICAL MANAGEMENT

There are no known nonsurgical treatments to cause regression of a pterygium. Medical management is directed toward preventing its development or slowing its growth when surgical removal is not indicated. The goal of medical therapy is to decrease or eliminate the chronic keratoconjunctivitis that is believed to stimulate the growth of a pterygium.

Certainly, the avoidance of environmental irritants is recommended. Exposure to ultraviolet radiation can be lessened by wearing protective glasses and a brimmed hat. The effects of wind can be lessened by wearing glasses with side shields. Goggles can protect the eyes from dust. Changing geographic location can also be helpful but is seldom practical.

Artificial tears are helpful in comforting the eye and in possibly allowing the ocular surface to heal. Preservatives in some artificial tears can be toxic to the ocular surface if used routinely at a frequency greater than four or five times daily, especially if the eyes are dry. Nonpreserved artificial tears should be prescribed when tears are to be used more often.

Topical corticosteroids decrease inflammation but are not recommended for chronic use because of potential complications. Topical nonsteroidal anti-inflammatory agents (flurbiprofen, diclofenac, suprofen, and ketorolac) have not been evaluated as to their efficacy for the chronic reactive keratoconjunctivitis that is believed to precede the development of pterygia. Topical vasoconstrictors help the appearance of the eye by temporarily lessening redness but are not believed to inhibit the progression of pterygia.

TREATMENT ALTERNATIVES

Many surgical techniques are described in the literature as having been used for the treatment of pterygia. The number of procedures described attests to the fact that pterygia pose difficult management problems and that an optimal procedure has not been found. Also, because all pterygia are different, varying in their size, rate of growth, and effect on the function of the eye, different procedures for their management have been developed. These procedures have included avulsion with redirection or resection of the head; the bare-sclera technique (BST); and resection with use of various conjunctival flaps, lamellar limbal transplants, free conjunctival grafts, buccal mucous membrane grafts, split-thickness skin grafts, or corneal transplantation. These techniques may be used with adjunctive therapies such as beta radiation, thiotepa, and mitomycin C.

PREOPERATIVE EVALUATION

General preoperative measures include searching for nearby possible sources of infection, such as blepharitis, canaliculitis, and dacryocystitis, that should be treated before surgery. Preoperative evaluation that pertains specifically to pterygia includes ascertaining (1) the number of previous recurrences; (2) the techniques used in any previous surgical procedures; (3) the extent of the patient's past, present, and future exposure to sunlight or other inciting factors; (4) whether the patient has had any prior treatment with beta radiation, thiotepa, or mitomycin C and, if so, how much; (5) the presence of symptomatic symblepharon or restriction of ocular movement; and (6) the presence or absence of any corneal thinning beneath the pterygium as can be associated with previous disease or surgery.

SURGICAL MANAGEMENT — HISTORIC

Numerous techniques for the management of pterygia have been devised since Susruta first described the removal of these lesions more than 3000 years ago.[3] Two popular techniques in the past were avulsion and burying the head of the pterygium.

Avulsion

Avulsion as a method of pterygium removal was devised before the development of modern microsurgical instrumentation and techniques. The advantages of avulsion are that it is simple and quick.[30] Under local anesthesia, the surgeon grasps the head of the pterygium with toothed forceps and pulls it from the underlying cornea to the limbus. The head, neck, and body are then excised with Westcott scissors. When recurrent lesions are treated with avulsion techniques, the risk of corneal perforation is high because of underlying corneal thinning from previous surgery. This technique leads to an approximately 50% long-term recurrence rate.[1]

Burying the Head

Desmarres was the first to propose redirecting the head of the pterygium away from the cornea.[19] The McReynolds operation of 1902 involves mobilizing the head of the pterygium, turning it, and burying it beneath the inferior conjunctiva.[31] Knapp developed a similar technique for the management of broad-headed pterygia: A horizontal incision divides the pterygium into equal upper and lower halves. Incisions are also made along the upper and lower borders of the lesion to about one half of its length. After the pterygium is rendered free of the cornea, each half of the head is turned toward its respective fornix and buried beneath the corresponding uninvolved bulbar conjunctiva.[32] Similar procedures have been described by others.[2, 33] These techniques have largely been replaced by more modern methods of pterygium removal.

SURGICAL MANAGEMENT — CURRENT

The foundation of all currently favored procedures for management of pterygia is the BST of excision, with or without adjunctive chemotherapy, radiation therapy, or conjunctival flaps or autografts. The operating microscope is generally useful in pterygium surgery because it allows the surgeon to perform more precise corneal dissection, thus lessening the chance of excessive removal of tissue or perforation into the anterior chamber, in addition to providing other advantages.

Anesthesia

Subconjunctival injection of a local anesthetic, such as lidocaine, in the area of planned conjunctival surgery is often used along with a topical anesthetic, such as proparacaine or cocaine, for the remaining conjunctiva and cornea. Epinephrine in the subconjunctival injection may be used to help minimize bleeding. Since surgical landmarks can become distorted by the volume of anesthetic injected into the subconjunctival space, they should be noted or marked with cautery or an agent such as methylene blue prior to injection. Less cooperative patients, or those with larger lesions requiring extensive dissection, should receive a retrobulbar or peribulbar injection with or without an eyelid block. Rarely, general anesthesia is required for uncooperative or extremely anxious patients.

Bare-Sclera Technique

The BST in 1948 supplanted the previously popular McReynolds operation.[1, 20, 25, 31, 34] The BST is widely used, but its principles are also widely misunderstood and misapplied. Despite the fact that the BST is a currently popular surgical procedure, recurrence rates run as high as 40% to 50% (and even higher for large and recently active lesions).[20, 25] The use of adjunctive beta radiation or topical thiotepa significantly reduces the rate of recurrence. Some recurrences can be prevented simply by performing the surgery correctly; others are unnecessary because surgery should not have been performed at all.

The fundamental concept of the BST is that it is designed to give the corneal epithelium a "head start" in a "race for the limbus."[25] The surgery creates denuded areas of cornea, limbus, and sclera that epithelialize secondarily. The pterygium will almost certainly recur if proliferating conjunctival tissue reaches the limbus (and crosses onto the cornea) before the corneal epithelium regrows to this landmark.

The BST involves dissecting the head and neck of the pterygium from the cornea and removing the remainder of the lesion from the underlying sclera, leaving behind an area of bare sclera. The dissection of the corneal portion of the pterygium should be performed as superficially and smoothly as possible, realizing that pterygia do not extend beneath Bowman's layer unless previous surgery has been performed. A very superficial delineating keratotomy is performed around the head of the pterygium. This is followed by a shallow lamellar keratectomy to free the tightly adherent head of the lesion from the underlying cornea (Fig. 16–1*A*). After the head has been freed, the neck of the pterygium is dissected from the cornea to the limbus. The neck is much less adherent, and less dissection is necessary to free this portion of the lesion. The neck is removed from the limbus later, after the area of bare sclera has been fashioned. The cut edges of the corneal epithelium (and conjunctiva) should be left as smooth and as regular as possible.

An area of bare sclera of adequate vertical, as well as horizontal, extent should then be created. This is done by cutting through normal conjunctiva and the underlying tissue with Westcott scissors, around the body of the pterygium. The body is then dissected free of the underlying sclera (Fig. 16–1*B*). The pterygium then remains attached only at the limbus (a limbus-based flap of the pterygium body and a limbus-based flap of the head and neck). The excision is completed by cutting the last remaining attachments at the limbus with Westcott scissors (Fig. 16–1*C*). In this manner the pterygium is removed in one piece.

The point at which the conjunctival excision reaches the limbus should be at least 1 clock-hour from where the corneal excision reaches the limbus (Fig. 16–1*B*). This gives an advantage to the corneal epithelium for resurfacing the corneal and limbal defect before the remaining conjunctiva or proliferating fibrovascular tissue reach the denuded cornea.

Excessive amounts of cautery should be avoided, especially if beta radiation is to be used, because cautery and beta radiation are believed to be synergistic in increasing the risk of late scleral melting. Excessive cautery might also result in the formation of granulation tissue, and this can increase the chance for recurrence of the pterygium.

Any remaining corneal and limbal irregularities should be polished. This may be done by holding a no. 64 Beaver blade perpendicular to the tissue and scraping repeatedly (Fig. 16–1*D*). A fine, rotating diamond bur has also been recommended for this. It is unnecessary to remove all the corneal scarring, but it is believed that reepithelialization is aided if the tissue is left as smooth and as normally contoured as possible.

If there is involvement of the semilunar fold (plica semilunaris), caruncle, or fornices, it is often not necessary to remove all the pterygium. The body of the pterygium should be removed in its entirety as far as approximately 5 mm from the limbus so as to not expose the insertion of the rectus muscle. More may be removed if the insertion of the muscle is later covered by conjunctiva. The caruncle may be excised without untoward effect, but it is usually not necessary to do so. The cut edges of conjunctiva may be sutured to the globe or to themselves with 8-0 to 10-0 nylon, silk, or Vicryl sutures (Fig. 16–1*E*). Displacement of the plica can occur but should be minimized, because postoperative cicatrization can lead to restrictive

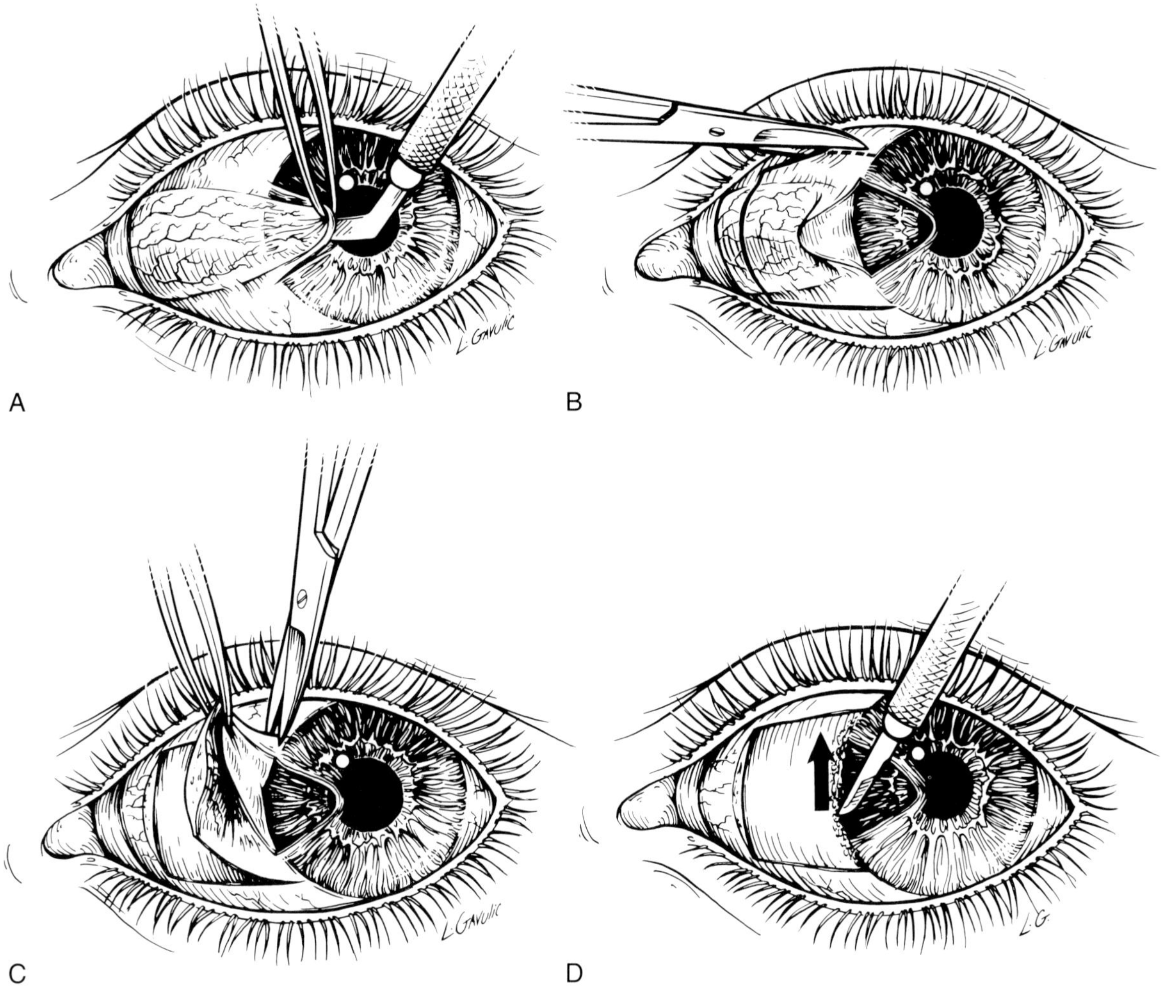

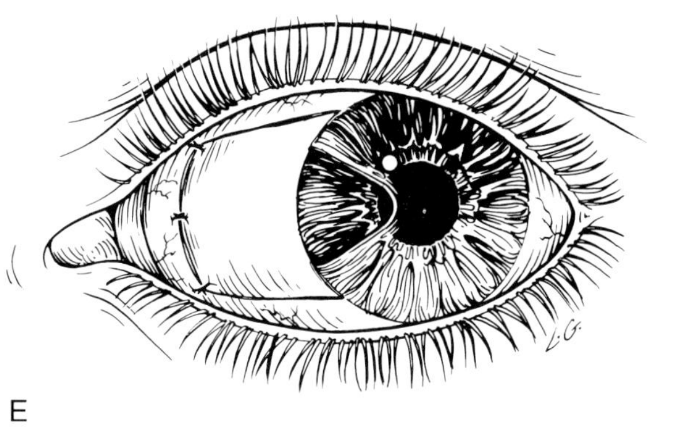

Figure 16–1. *A*, The head of the pterygium is excised superficially from the cornea. *B*, The head and neck of the pterygium are reflected to the limbus. The conjunctival incision is made such that the point at which the limbus is reached is about 1 clock-hour from the point at which the corneal incision reached this landmark. *C*, The limbus-based flap of the head and neck, and the limbus-based flap of the body, of the pterygium are excised from the limbus with Westcott scissors. *D*, The limbal area is "polished" by scraping with a no. 64 Beaver blade or a rotating bur. *E*, The cut edge of the conjunctiva is sutured to the sclera.

esotropia. Also, a displaced plica often maintains an unsightly, fleshy appearance after healing has occurred.

If insufficient conjunctiva remains to allow suturing to the sclera without obliterating the fornix, the cut edge of tissue should be sewn into the fornix to reconstruct this space. This can be accomplished by passing both arms of a double-armed suture through the conjunctival edge and the full thickness of the eyelid deep within the fornix. The two ends of the suture are tied over a pledget of foam rubber, or cotton on the skin, the suture being left in place for 5 to 7 days. This technique is useful also for revising preexisting symblepharon (as can occur after prior surgery); the adhesion is severed from the globe, and the free end is rotated and then sutured into the adjacent fornix. Symblepharon can be avoided by not leaving areas that are devoid of epithelium on opposing bulbar and palpebral conjunctival surfaces.

Care should be taken not to cut the insertion of the rectus muscle or leave it exposed. Inadvertent disinsertion of the medial rectus muscle has been reported, particularly with resection of large or recurrent pterygia.[35] Identification (and isolation with a muscle hook) of the rectus muscle tendon and insertion prior to dissection can prevent this complication. Tenon's capsule should not be left exposed because this (as well as exposure of the muscle insertion) can lead to the production of excessive granulation tissue and subsequent recurrence of the pterygium. Intravitreal migration of a scleral suture has been reported following the repair of an inadvertent scleral perforation during the resection of a recurrent pterygium.[36] Release of adhesions around the medial rectus muscle, sometimes with recession or marginal myotomy, can be necessary if cicatricial esotropia has developed.

One author recommended (in 1950) preserving the conjunctiva overlying a pterygium while removing as much of the fibrovascular component as possible.[32] Since the conjunctival epithelium is usually not involved by the pterygium, this approach has some rational basis but is technically difficult and not currently used as far as we know; the technique could also defeat the basic principle of the BST.

Lamellar Grafts

Lamellar corneal or corneoscleral grafts have long been known to impede the recurrence of pterygia. These grafts are usually circular, semicircular, or oval and are placed so as to straddle the affected limbus (Fig. 16–2). Such a graft is fashioned to fit precisely into the host bed.

One method of performing lamellar grafting in the area of resection of a pterygium involves using an 8-mm trephine to create the host bed straddling the limbus. The trephine is positioned to incorporate 3 mm of the peripheral cornea and 5 mm of the adjacent sclera. Care is taken to avoid the insertion of the rectus muscle. An approximately 0.2-mm-deep trephination is made, followed by lamellar excision of this tissue. Caution should be used near the insertion of the muscle where the sclera is only 0.3-mm thick. The donor graft is fashioned from a whole globe or a preserved cornea, using the same 8-mm trephine. This is followed by lamellar dissection, attempting to keep the graft 0.2- to 0.3-mm thick. Alternatively, a full-thickness graft may be used. The graft is sewn into the host bed with 10-0 nylon running or interrupted sutures. These sutures are left in place for 2 to 3 months. The conjunctiva may then be closed over the scleral portion of the graft, using absorbable sutures. With corneoscleral grafts, the donor limbus is placed at the position of the host's limbus to maintain the anatomy of the limbal sulcus.

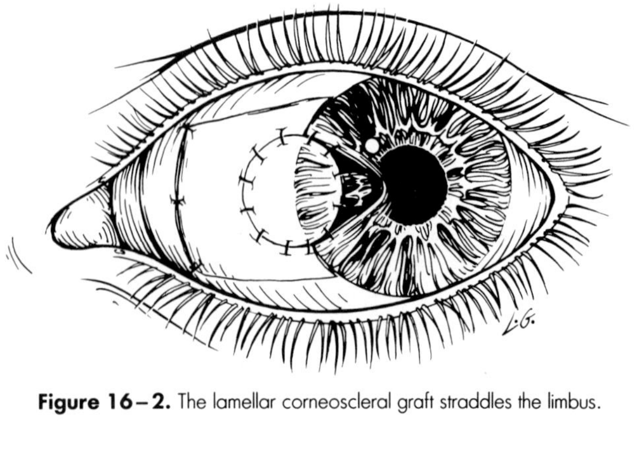

Figure 16–2. The lamellar corneoscleral graft straddles the limbus.

Grafts probably inhibit recurrence of pterygia by providing a new bed of healthy tissue that can epithelialize quickly and a fibrous barrier at the donor–host interface, across which the pterygium is less likely to grow.

Grafts are usually reserved for the most extreme situations, but their advantage of providing a fibrous barrier can also be achieved by fashioning a curvilinear groove of one-half to two-thirds scleral depth at the limbus. This simple but little-known adjunct is called *Newton's groove.*[37] The groove can be made with a no. 64 Beaver blade and can then be closed with a few interrupted sutures to speed healing and minimize any astigmatic effects. We use this to supplement the BST whenever we are especially worried about recurrence.

Conjunctival Flaps

Many types of conjunctival flaps have been created to cover the exposed sclera after resections of pterygia. Such flaps are not inconsistent with the goals of the BST because they consist of essentially normal tissue. The conjunctiva in the area from which the flap is to be created is bluntly dissected from the underlying Tenon's fascia. The free conjunctival edges are then anastomosed with 8-0 to 10-0 nylon or Vicryl sutures, which may also incorporate the underlying sclera if desired for fixation.

Occasionally, the defect resulting from excision of a pterygium may be closed primarily, particularly if radial relaxing incisions are used (Fig. 16–3*A*). In 1943 Bangerter[38] described a technique of using a conjunctival flap brought from either the superior or inferior bulbar conjunctiva into the defect (Fig. 16–3*B*). In 1967 Aratoon[39] described a pedicle conjunctival graft fashioned from a distant site (Fig. 16–3*C*). A conjunctival bridge flap that is transferred from the opposite limbus has been described by Demartini and Vastine (Fig. 16–3*D*).[40]

We seldom use conjunctival flaps, generally preferring conjunctival autografts.

Conjunctival Autograft

Conjunctival autografting is a technique that is quite useful in the management of recurrent pterygia or aggressive primary lesions and is a means of treating cases complicated by conjunctival scarring causing restriction of ocular motility or fornical foreshortening.[40–43] The recurrence rates of pterygia treated with this method generally vary between 2% and 7%.[44] One exceptional study randomized patients (who had pterygia) on a tropical is-

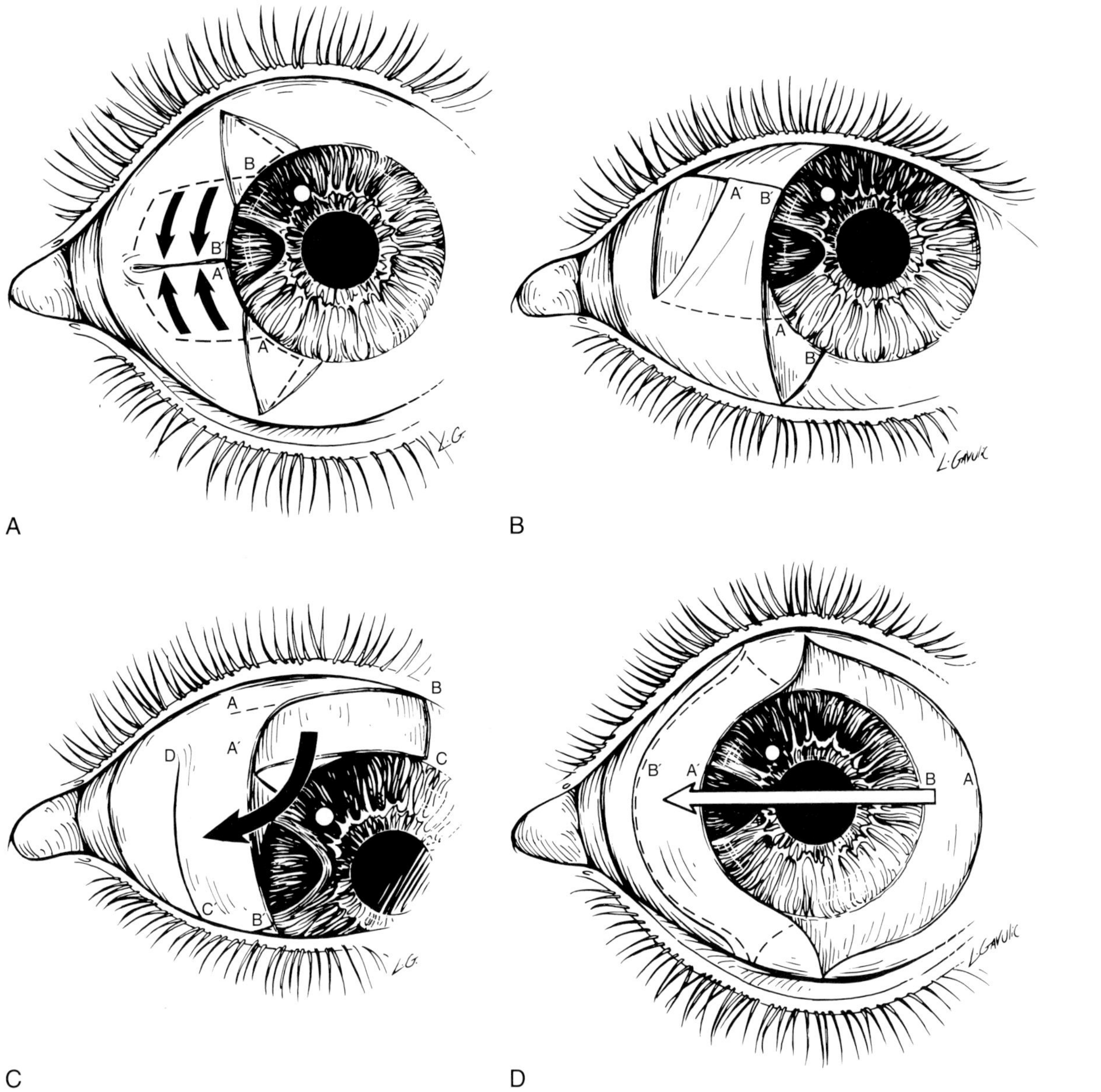

Figure 16–3. Methods of closure of the conjunctival defect with flaps include the following: radial relaxing incisions *(A)*, an inferior conjunctival flap as described by Bangerter[38] *(B)*, a pedicle conjunctival flap as described by Aratoon[39] *(C)*, and a conjunctival bridge flap transferred from the opposite limbus *(D)*.

land to bare-sclera resection alone or resection followed by conjunctival autografting. After 15 months of mean followup, the rate of recurrence in the grafted cases (4 of 19 cases [21%]) was not statistically significantly different from the recurrence rate in the bare-sclera group (6 of 16 cases [37%]).[45]

When using a conjunctival autograft, the pterygium is resected as described for the BST. A free autograft is taken from the conjunctiva of the supratemporal aspect of the ipsilateral eye, and this graft is then sutured into the resulting defect (Figs. 16–4).

The autograft is harvested by measuring with calipers the conjunctival defect resulting from resection of the pterygium. Traction sutures are placed at the limbus to infraduct the globe, thus allowing access to the supratemporal bulbar conjunctiva. The measurements of the conjunctival defect are transferred to the conjunctiva in this region, and markings are made with cautery or methylene blue (Fig. 16–4*A*). An injection of subconjunctival anesthetic helps separate the conjunctiva from underlying Tenon's capsule. This injection should not be made through the conjunctiva that is to be excised but should be made from the side so as not to buttonhole the graft. The free conjunctival autograft is fashioned by making the posterior circumferential cut with Westcott scissors. The radial cuts are then made, followed by excising the tissue from the limbus. Care must be taken to maintain orientation of the graft with respect to the epithelial surface and the limbal edge. This may be facilitated by use of a stent placed under the graft prior to excision from the limbus (Fig. 16–4*B*).

The free conjunctival graft is transferred to the site of

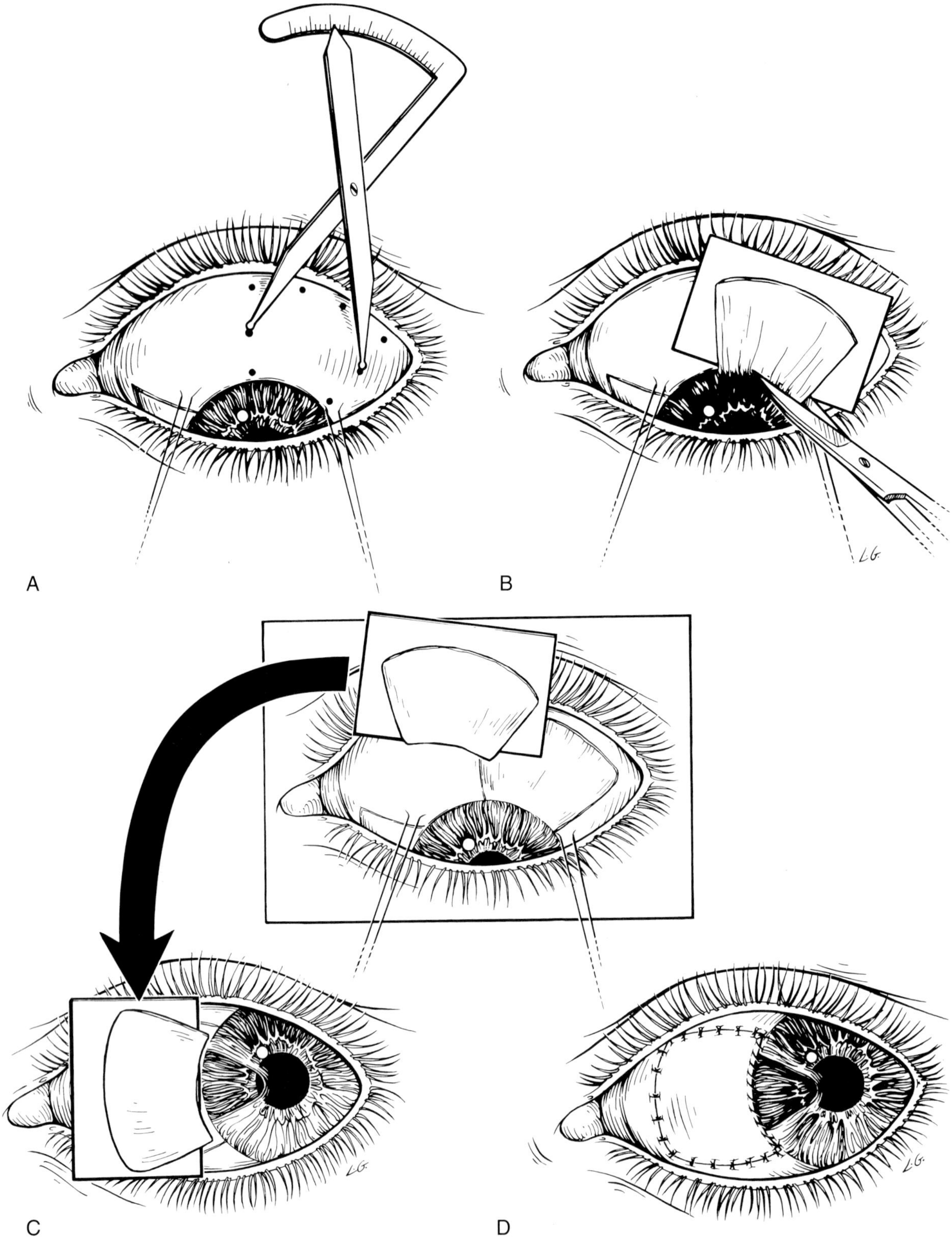

Figure 16–4. *A*, The measurement of the conjunctival defect is transferred to the superotemporal bulbar conjunctiva. *B*, After partial excision of the graft, a stent is placed beneath it to maintain orientation of the tissue before freeing it from the limbus. C, The graft is moved to the defect and oriented such that the limbal portion is placed at the limbus and the epithelial surface is external. *D*, The graft is sutured into place.

bare sclera, placing the limbal portion of the graft at the limbus (Fig. 16–4*C*). The graft is sutured into position with interrupted 10-0 nylon or 8-0 Vicryl sutures (Fig. 16–4*D*).

It is unnecessary to close the donor site since this protected area under the eyelid nearly always heals uneventfully, although a case of postoperative diplopia resulting from subconjunctival fibrosis at the harvest site has been reported.[46] Tenon's layer, when not violated, sufficiently covers the superior rectus and tendon insertion. Tissue should not be excised past the superior fornix to avoid symblepharon formation.

Several problems and complications can occur with this technique. Conjunctival graft edema, corneoscleral dellen, and epithelial cysts occur infrequently. Graft edema may occur, usually within the first 10 days, and persists for 2 to 4 weeks. Less frequently encountered problems include Tenon's granuloma, hematoma, and retraction or necrosis of the graft. These complications can be minimized by limiting surgical manipulation, excising Tenon's tissue completely from the host bed and the donor graft, orienting the tissue properly, maintaining adequate hemostasis, and harvesting a graft of adequate size.[44]

We treated a 39-year-old Hispanic man who had undergone three previous operations for pterygia (one initial and two recurrent), with the technique just described plus intraoperative beta radiation to the bare sclera before the free conjunctival graft was sutured into place. He had been without recurrence for 2 years when the photograph in Fig. 16–5 was taken.

Buccal Mucous Membrane Graft

Buccal mucosal grafts are not frequently used because they often do not achieve the same cosmetic appearance provided by conjunctival autografts. Buccal mucous membrane grafts can be harvested from the lower lip with a mucotome. These grafts should be 0.1 to 0.2 mm in thickness and can be fashioned to fit the conjunctival defect. Thicker grafts tend to remain red and thickened after healing.

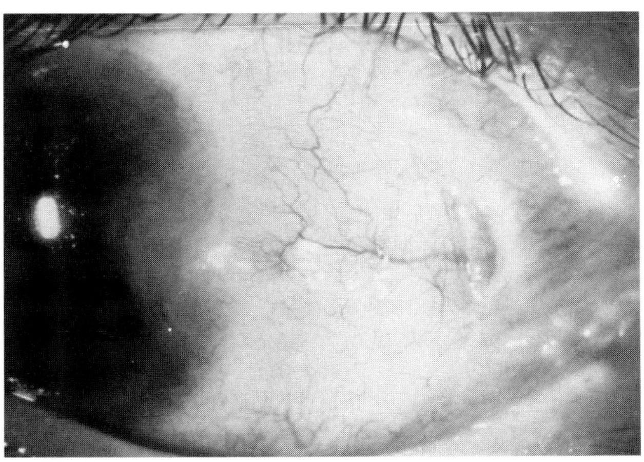

Figure 16–5. Two years after recurrent pterygium resection (the patient had three previous operations) using intraoperative beta radiation before placement of a free conjunctival autograft. There is peripheral superficial corneal scarring but no recurrence of the lesion.

A symblepharon can usually be handled simply by releasing it from the globe and suturing the free end into the conjunctival fornix as described earlier. Mucous membrane or conjunctival grafts may occasionally be required to prevent two surfaces without epithelium from being opposed, thus preventing symblepharon formation. Split-thickness skin grafts have also rarely been used.[47]

ADJUNCTIVE THERAPY

In addition to surgery, certain adjunctive measures have been used to reduce the rate of recurrence of pterygia or to improve the visual result. These include beta radiation, thiotepa, mitomycin C, argon laser, excimer laser, and corticosteroids.

Beta Radiation

Beta radiation, when used as an adjunct to surgery, significantly reduces the rate of recurrence of pterygia. Beta radiation consists of electrons emitted with great velocity during radioactive decay. Strontium 90, the beta-radiation source that is used clinically, has a half-life of 28.7 years. The older unit for strontium 90 application is the rep (roentgen equivalent physical), which equals 1.08 rad (radiation absorbed dose). One rad is equal to 1 centigray (cGy), which is the currently used International unit.

The strontium 90 contained in the end of an applicator rod is held against the bare sclera in the area from which the pterygium was excised. The length of time that the strontium 90 is applied to the surgical site determines the dose of beta radiation. The usual treatment takes seconds to minutes, depending on the dose to be given and the age of the strontium 90 source. The source is placed against the bare sclera and rotated slowly so as to distribute the radiation evenly.

Beta particles have limited ability to penetrate tissue. The dosage at the surface is reduced to approximately 50% at 1-mm tissue depth, 25% at 2-mm tissue depth, and 6% at 4-mm tissue depth.[48] Therefore, a much larger dose is applied to the relatively radioresistant sclera, and the radiosensitive lens is largely spared.

Administration of beta radiation after the BST reduces overall recurrence rates from approximately 30% to 50% to 0.5% to 33%, with most studies reporting recurrence rates of less than 5%.[32, 49] One review of 205 pterygia revealed a 54.7% recurrence rate for pterygia when surgery alone was used. Superficial radiation applied in one dose of 800 to 900 cGy at the time of surgery decreased the recurrence rate to 1.5%.[50] Even when recurrences appear, they are likely to be smaller and less active after beta radiation.[1,8,20] Recurrent pterygia, not previously irradiated, when treated with subsequent surgery using the BST followed by fractionated beta radiation, are controlled at a rate of 89% according to one study.[51] The radiation is best applied within 24 hours after surgery, although some evidence suggests that as long as 3 days is acceptable. Fractionated dosage schedules such as 1000 rep given on days 0, 7, and 14, as supported in the older literature, have largely been replaced by a single application because of convenience and similar efficacy. We usually use 1500 to 2200 cGy in a single dose, depending on our estimation of the likelihood of recurrence and whether or not beta radiation has been previously given. Adverse effects are minimized if total lifetime dosage to a given site does not exceed 5000 cGy. Reports of scleral melting, with or without secondary infection, at the site of previous beta application are found in the literature but are generally associated with the use of excessive radiation.[52,53] Visually significant cataract occurs with doses of beta radiation in the range of 8000 to 10,000 rep.[47] Peripheral lens changes can occur with doses as small as 1500 to 2500 rep.[47] Although some practitioners prefer beta radiation as a routine measure, we do not believe that it is necessary for primary excisions unless these lesions appear unusually aggressive.

Beta radiation is of value only following surgical excision of pterygia. Radiation therapy is of no value for pterygia that have not been surgically excised very recently because it acts mainly on immature and rapidly proliferating fibrovascular tissue, causing an obliterative endarteritis.[47] The effects of incomplete surgery cannot be negated by the use of this adjunct. Beta radiation is not readily available in many areas, and this fact increases the popularity of techniques using conjunctival flaps or grafts after pterygium resection.

Thiotepa

Thiotepa (triethylenethiophosphoramide) is a radiomimetic drug that has effects on the healing process similar to those of beta radiation.[54] It is a nitrogen mustard alkylating agent that presumably inhibits vascular endothelial proliferation and fibroblast proliferation.[55–57] Meacham[56] introduced the drug in 1962 as adjunctive treatment following pterygium resection by the BST. Recurrence rates of zero to 16% have been reported.[55,58–60] In a double-blind study by Harrison and associates,[61] comparing thiotepa to beta radiation, there was one recurrence in the radiation group (n = 25) and none in the thiotepa group (n = 24). The use of a 1:2000 dilution of the drug (15 mg in 30 mL of Ringer's lactate solution) has been consistently described in the literature. Thiotepa is seldom used because it is not readily available and must be given four to six times daily for 6 to 8 weeks postoperatively. It is also recommended that the medication be stored in the refrigerator.

Adverse effects are more likely with thiotepa than with beta radiation. Reported complications include conjunctival injection and irritation, conjunctival granuloma formation, allergic reactions, bacterial superinfection, and permanent eyelid depigmentation (especially in people who are darkly pigmented).[54,62,63] This last side effect is primarily responsible for the unpopularity of thiotepa. No systemic toxicity has been reported with topical use.

Mitomycin C

Mitomycin C is an antibiotic-antineoplastic agent that inhibits the synthesis of deoxyribonucleic acid, ribonucleic acid, and protein in rapidly dividing cells.[64] Its mode of action mimics that of ionizing radiation, and as with beta radiation, the complications associated with the drug seem to be related to total cumulative dose. Mitomycin C is approved for cancer therapy and is marketed by Bristol-Meyers under the trade name Mutamycin.

In 1963 the first report of using topical mitomycin C postoperatively to decrease the risk of recurrence of pterygium was made by Kunitomo and Mori.[65] They used a 0.04% concentration three times daily for 1 to 2 weeks. Additional reports regarding the use of topical mitomycin (0.02% to 0.04%) following pterygium excision by the BST are encouraging, but the optimal frequency of instillation and duration of therapy have not been determined.[66–68] Proposed regimens for mitomycin C instillation range from using a 0.02% concentration twice daily for 5 days to using a 0.04% concentration four times daily for 2 weeks.[67,68] In view of recent reports of serious complications arising from mitomycin C use, the lower dosage schedule seems prudent.[69] Some investigators recommend a single application of mitomycin C at the time of surgery.

Recurrence rates of 1.4% to 16% have been found in several published series, with most reported rates being lower than 5%.[18,64,66,67,70,71]

One study[68] addressed the issue as to whether postoperative mitomycin C instillation or conjunctival autograft transplantation is more efficacious in preventing recurrence of pterygium. Fifteen patients were treated with mitomycin C, and fifteen patients were treated with conjunctival autograft transplantation. Only one pterygium recurred overall, and this was in the conjunctival autograft transplantation group.

Mitomycin C results in remarkably avascular scleral beds, and the avascularity can persist indefinitely. In filtration surgery there is evidence that a single application of this agent can have a lifelong (local) effect on fibroblast activity and conjunctival healing.[72]

Reported complications following the use of mitomycin C include conjunctival, scleral, and corneal melting, corneal edema, corneal perforation, infection, local ischemia, glaucoma, sudden-onset cataract, uveitis, scleral calcification, and intractable pain with or without photophobia.[69] Many of these complications occurred months to years after the excision site had apparently healed. Concerns regarding mutagenicity also require further investigation. Complications can be minimized if mitomycin C is used after the area of pterygium excision is covered with a flap or graft. Mitomycin C is not recommended for patients who have keratoconjunctivitis sicca, rosacea, atopic dermatitis, ichthyosis, herpetic keratitis, or neurotrophic keratitis.[69]

Occupational Safety and Health Administration guidelines pertaining to the preparation, administration, and handling of mitomycin C must be complied with when this drug is used. If mitomycin C is dispensed to a patient, it should be prescribed in a small volume; after treatment, the unused portion should be retrieved and disposed of properly. The drop form is purple and should be refrigerated. Special precautions for the use of this agent by the patient when the drop is instilled include wearing gloves and placing the gloves and any tissues that come into contact with the agent into a plastic bag, to be returned to the physician or pharmacy.[73]

Because of the recent reports of complications associated with the use of mitomycin C,[69] conjunctival autograft transplantation is believed to be the procedure of choice, except possibly in those instances when an unusually aggressive lesion has been excised. Even in those instances, consideration should be given to using a single application of mitomycin C at the time of surgery.

Argon Laser

Use of the argon laser has been advocated for ablating neovascular twigs that are growing toward, or into, the cornea after surgery for pterygium. A 50-μ spot size is used, with a power of 0.2 to 0.3 W, and a duration of 0.1 second, to ablate immature conjunctival vessels at the limbus. The goal of the laser application is to ablate the vessels without causing thermal damage to surrounding tissue that could cause additional fibrosis and inflammation. Treatment of these vessels may begin once the eye is relatively quiet and can be repeated every 1 to 2 weeks. Questions regarding the long-term efficacy of this procedure remain, especially because thermal cautery of such vessels is generally agreed to be ineffective.

Excimer Laser

The excimer laser has been used to smooth the corneal surface in the area of pterygium resection, as well as to remove scarring in Bowman's layer. This technique has not been perfected, and high residual astigmatism has occurred.

Corticosteroids

The postoperative use of topical steroids might be of some value for reducing cicatrization, especially if symblepharon and restrictions of ocular motility are a concern. After surgery, they might also theoretically inhibit corneal edema by stabilizing vascular permeability and prevent or reduce neovascularization by inhibiting inflammation.[58] Overall, their ability to reduce the rate or severity of recurrence of pterygia is doubtful. Corticosteroids should not be used until the corneal epithelium has healed.

GENERAL CONSIDERATIONS

The lesion excised during pterygium resection should be submitted for histopathologic evaluation. Occasionally, premalignant or malignant tumors can mimic pterygia, and surgery may spread or stimulate their growth.[2]

Simultaneous pterygium and intraocular surgery may be safely performed in areas where pterygium is endemic and medical facilities inadequate. One report from Nigeria describes pterygium resection in 15 patients, 11 of whom had simultaneous cataract extraction and 4 of whom had trabeculectomy, without increased incidence of pterygium recurrence or complications with the intraocular surgery.[74] Generally, intraocular surgery may be performed safely and in routine fashion in the presence of an inactive pterygium (especially in older patients), as though the lesion were not even present. For example, it is entirely acceptable simply to cut across the pterygium when making a limbal incision in such a situation.

Penetrating keratoplasty is reserved for those situations in which the visual axis is involved by scarring not amenable to lamellar keratectomy or excimer laser phototherapeutic keratectomy. Visually significant residual irregular astigmatism can often be successfully neutralized with a hard contact lens, but keratoplasty is occasionally needed. Perforation at the time of pterygium excision can also necessitate penetrating keratoplasty. Postoperative measures for reducing the patient's exposure to sunlight and irritating environmental conditions seem to be reasonable, although no good evidence exists that such precautions are of value in the immediate postoperative period. Pterygia that recur immediately after resection are not the result of further environmental insult. Recurrences have occurred as early as 2 weeks from the time of excision. One theory to explain such early recurrence is the formation of granulation tissue that subsequently contracts, resulting in conjunctivalization of the limbus and the cornea. A recurrence is heralded by horizontally oriented blood vessels, arising from the cut edge of the conjunctiva at the limbus, making their way onto the cornea. Beta radiation, thiotepa, argon laser, or corticosteroids are treatments that may limit the progression of an early recurrence and that should be considered.

Artificial tears, patching, or soft contact lenses can be generally helpful for encouraging healing of the corneal epithelium, when necessary, perhaps thus lessening the likelihood of recurrence.

CONCLUSION

Optimal management of pterygia requires an understanding of the pathogenesis, anatomy, histopathology, prognosis, and treatment alternatives associated with these lesions. The decision to operate for pterygia can be difficult and must be tempered by the understanding that these lesions can recur. The popular BST for removal of pterygia seems to have been improved substantially by the supplemental use of conjunctival flaps or (preferably) free conjunctival autografts. These techniques are believed to rival the use of beta radiation or topical mitomycin C, in association with the BST, in efficacy for lessening the chance for recurrences and seem to be associated with fewer severe complications. Nevertheless, we continue to use both beta radiation and conjunctival grafting (with the former being applied before placement of the graft) for especially difficult cases.

Acknowledgment

This work was supported in part by grants from Research to Prevent Blindness, Inc., New York, New York, and from the Indiana Lions Eye Bank, Inc., Indianapolis, Indiana.

REFERENCES

1. Cameron ME: Pterygium Throughout the World. Springfield, IL, Charles C Thomas, 1965.
2. Duke-Elder S: Diseases of the outer eye. *In* Duke-Elder S (ed): System of Ophthalmology, vol 8. St. Louis, CV Mosby, 1965, pp 573.
3. Rosenthal JW: Chronology of pterygium therapy. Am J Ophthalmol 36:1601, 1953.
4. Townsend WM: Pterygium. *In* Kaufman HE, McDonald MB, Barron BA, et al (eds): The Cornea. New York, Churchill Livingstone, 1988, p 461.
5. Austin P, Jakobiec FA, Iwamoto T: Elastodysplasia and elastodystrophy as the pathologic bases of ocular pterygia and pingueculae. Ophthalmology 90:96, 1983.
6. Cameron ME: The treatment of beta irradiation necrosis of the sclera. Aust J Ophthalmol 6:88, 1978.
7. Spencer WH, Zimmerman LE: Conjunctiva. *In* Spencer WH (ed): Ophthalmic Pathology. Philadelphia, WB Saunders, 1985, p 174.
8. Paton D: Pterygium management based upon a theory of pathogenesis. Trans Am Acad Ophthalmol Otolaryngol 79:603, 1975.
9. Pinkerton OD, Yoshitsugi H, Shigemura BA: Immunologic basis for the pathogenesis of pterygium. Am J Ophthalmol 98:225, 1984.
10. Wong WW: A hypothesis on the pathogenesis of pterygiums. Ann Ophthalmol 810:303, 1978.
11. Taylor HR, West SK, Rosenthal FS, et al: Corneal changes associated with chronic UV irradiation. Arch Ophthalmol 107:1481, 1989.
12. Karai I, Horiguchi S: Pterygium in welders. Br J Ophthalmol 68:347, 1984.
13. Coroneo MT: Albedo concentration in the anterior eye: A phenomenon that locates some solar diseases. Ophthalmic Surg 21:60, 1990.
14. Coroneo MT, Muller-Stolzenburg NW, Ho A: Peripheral light focusing by the anterior eye and the ophthalmohelioses. Ophthalmic Surg 22:705, 1991.
15. Hecht F, Shoptaugh MG: Winglets of the eye: Dominant transmission of early adult pterygium of the conjunctiva. J Med Genet 27:392, 1990.
16. Neal AJ, Irwin C, Hope-Stone HF: The role of strontium-90 beta irradiation in the management of pterygia. Clin Oncol 3:105, 1991.
17. Detels R, Dhir SP: Pterygium: A geographical study. Arch Ophthalmol 78:485, 1967.
18. Hill JC, Maske R: Pathogenesis of pterygium. Eye 3:218, 1989.
19. Adamis AP, Starck T, Kenyon KR: The management of pterygium. Ophthalmol Clin North Am 3:611, 1990.
20. Rich LF: Pterygium and pseudopterygium. *In* Fraunfelder FT, Roy FH (eds): Current Ocular Therapy, 2nd ed. Philadelphia, WB Sanders, 1985, p 299.
21. Fuchs E: Uber das pterygium. Graefes Arch Clin Exp Ophthalmol 38:1, 1892.
22. Johnson GJ: Etiology of spheroidal degeneration of the cornea in Labrador. Br J Ophthalmol 65:270, 1981.
23. Bierly JR, Dunn JP, Dawson CR: Fuchs' superficial marginal keratitis. Am J Ophthalmol 113:541, 1992.
24. Goldman KN, Kaufman HE: Atypical pterygium: A clinical feature of Terrien's marginal degeneration. Arch Ophthalmol 96:1027, 1978.
25. Youngson RM: Recurrence of pterygium after excision. Br J Ophthalmol 56:120, 1972.
26. Zauberman H: Pterygium and its recurrence. Am J Ophthalmol 62:1780, 1967.
27. Ashaye AO: Refractive astigmatism and pterygium. Afr J Med Sci 19:225, 1990.
28. Oldenburg JB, Garbus J, McDonnell JM: Conjunctival pterygia: Mechanism of corneal topographic changes. Cornea 9:200, 1990.
29. Lin S, Reiter K, Dreher AW, et al: The effect of pterygia on contrast sensitivity and glare disability. Am J Ophthalmol 107:407, 1989.
30. Zolli CL: Experience with avulsion technique in pterygium surgery. Ann Ophthalmol 11:1569, 1979.
31. McReynolds JO: The nature and treatment of pterygia. JAMA 39:296, 1902.
32. King JH Jr: The pterygium: Brief review and evaluation of certain methods of treatment. Arch Ophthalmol 44:854, 1950.
33. Berens C: New method for transplanting pterygium. Arch Ophthalmol 21:30, 1939.
34. D'Ombrain A: Surgical treatment of pterygium. Br J Ophthalmol 32:65, 1948.
35. Raab EL, Metz HS, Ellis FD: Medial rectus injury after pterygium excision. Arch Ophthalmol 107:1428, 1989.
36. Solomon A, Rosen N, Treister G, et al: Intravitreal suture: A complication of pterygium surgery. Ophthalmic Surg 22:56, 1991.
37. Newton FH: Operation for recurrent pterygium. Am J Ophthalmol 44:258, 1957.
38. Bangerter A: Pterygium operation and covering of conjunctival defects. Ophthalmologica 106:316, 1943.
39. Aratoon V: Surgery of pterygium by conjunctival pedicle flap. Am J Ophthalmol 63:1778, 1967.
40. Demartini DR, Vastine DW: Pterygium. *In* Abbott RL (ed): Surgical Intervention in Corneal and External Diseases. Orlando, Grune & Stratton, 1988, p 141.
41. Dowlut MS, Laflamme MY: Les pterygions recidivants: Frequence et correction par autogreffe conjunctivale. Can J Ophthalmol 16:119, 1981.
42. Hartman DC: Use of free grafts in correction of recurrent pterygia, pseudopterygia, and symblepharon. Calif Med 75:279, 1951.
43. Kenyon KR, Wagoner MD, Hettinger ME: Conjunctival autograft transplantation for advanced and recurrent pterygium. Ophthalmology 92:1461, 1985.
44. Starck T, Kenyon KR, Serrano R: Conjunctival autograft for primary and recurrent pterygia: Surgical technique and problem management. Cornea 10:196, 1991.
45. Lewallen S: A randomized trial of conjunctival autografting for pterygium in the tropics. Ophthalmology 96:1612, 1989.
46. Vrabec MP, Weisenthal RW, Elsing SH: Subconjunctival fibrosis after conjunctival autograft. Cornea 12:181, 1993.
47. Jaros PA, DeLuise VP: Pingueculae and pterygia. Surv Ophthalmol 33:41, 1988.

48. Sharma SC: Strontium-90 eye application. Med Dosim 14:229, 1989.
49. Haik GM, Ellis GS, Nowell JF: The management of pterygia, with special reference to surgery combined with beta irradiation. Trans Am Acad Ophthalmol Otolaryngol 66:776, 1962.
50. Nowell JF: Management of pterygia: 20 years later. South Med J 79:1382, 1986.
51. Campbell OR, Amendola BE, Brady LW: Recurrent pterygia: Results of postoperative treatment with Sr-90 applicators. Radiology 174:565, 1990.
52. Altman AJ, Cohen EJ, Berger ST, Mondino BJ: Scleritis and *Streptococcus pneumoniae.* Cornea 10:341, 1991.
53. MacKenzie FD, Hirst LW, Kynaston B, Bain CB: Recurrence rate and complications after beta irradiation for pterygia. Ophthalmology 98:1776, 1991.
54. Kleis W, Pico G: Thiotepa therapy to prevent postoperative pterygium occurrence and neovascularization. Am J Ophthalmol 76:371, 1973.
55. Liddy BSL, Morgan JF: Triethylene thiophosphoramide (thiotepa) and pterygium. Am J Ophthalmol 61:888, 1966.
56. Meacham R: Triethylene phosphoramide in the prevention of recurrent pterygium. Am J Ophthalmol 54:751, 1962.
57. Rock RL: Inhibition of corneal vascularization by triethylene thiophosphoramide (thiotepa). Arch Ophthalmol 69:330, 1963.
58. Cassidy JR: The inhibition of pterygium recurrence by thiotepa. Am J Ophthalmol 61:886, 1966.
59. Joselson GA, Muller P: Incidence of pterygium recurrence in patients treated with thiotepa. Am J Ophthalmol 81:891, 1976.
60. Mori S: A new treatment of pterygium. Acta Soc Ophthalmol Jpn 66:990, 1962.
61. Harrison M, Kelly A, Ohlrich L: Pterygium: Thiotepa versus beta radiation, a double-blind trial. Trans Aust Coll Ophthalmol 1:64, 1969.
62. Asregadoo ER: Surgery, thiotepa, and corticosteroid in the treatment of pterygium. Am J Ophthalmol 74:960, 1972.
63. Orlander K, Haik KG, Haik G: Management of pterygia: Should thiotepa be used? Ann Ophthalmol 10:853, 1978.
64. Singh G, Wilson MR, Foster CS: Mitomycin eye drops as treatment for pterygium. Ophthalmology 95:813, 1988.
65. Kunitomo N, Mori S: Studies on the pterygium. Part IV: A treatment of the pterygium by mitomycin C instillation. Acta Soc Ophthalmol Jpn 67:601, 1963.
66. Hayasaka S, Noda S, Yamamoto Y, et al: Postoperative instillation of low-dose mitomycin C in the treatment of primary pterygium. Am J Ophthalmol 106:715, 1988.
67. Hayasaka S, Noda S, Yukari Y, Setogawa T: Postoperative instillation of mitomycin C in the treatment of recurrent pterygium. Ophthalmic Surg 20:580, 1989.
68. Singh G, Wilson RW, Foster CS: Long-term follow-up study of mitomycin eye drops as adjunctive treatment for pterygia and its comparison with conjunctival autograft transplantation. Cornea 9:331, 1990.
69. Rubinfeld RS, Pfister RR, Stein RM, et al: Serious complications of topical mitomycin C after pterygium surgery. Ophthalmology 99:1647, 1992.
70. Chayakul V: Prevention of recurrent pterygium by mitomycin C. Fortschr Ophthalmol 84:422, 1987.
71. Oka PM: Mitomycin C therapy to prevent pterygium recurrence. Trans Asia Pacific Acad Ophthalmol 6:617, 1976.
72. Palmer SS: Mitomycin as adjunct chemotherapy with trabeculectomy. Ophthalmology 98:317, 1991.
73. Spires R: Postoperative instillation of mitomycin eye drops in the treatment of primary pterygium. J Ophthalmic Nurs Technol 10:15, 1991.
74. Ibechukwu BI: Simultaneous pterygium and intraocular surgery. Br J Ophthalmol 74:265, 1990.

CHAPTER 17

Chemical and Thermal Injuries of the Cornea and Conjunctiva

Roswell R. Pfister

Chemical or thermal injury of the eye and adnexa constitutes one of the most catastrophic insults to the visual system, often resulting in partial or complete loss of sight. The spectrum of injury is broad, ranging from damage to the anterior segment of the eye alone to extensive involvement of the eye and the entire integumentary system, with pulmonary and esophageal exposure. The objective of treatment is to deliver emergency and intermediate-stage care before healing has stabilized and then to plan for subsequent definitive surgical repair. Consultation with a corneal surgeon during each of these phases can help immeasurably, with the ultimate expectation of corneal surgery.

NATURE OF THE INJURY

The character and extent of the injury have a substantial effect on the repair processes and outcome. The severity of a chemical injury is predicated on the type and concentration of the chemical and the duration of contact. Acid injuries are often relatively mild because the concentrations are low, the ions are weakly dissociated, and the resultant precipitation of protein acts as an impediment to its penetration through the tissues. When the acid concentrations are high, especially those used in the semiconductor and paper pulping industries, ocular damage can be extremely severe. Thermal burns of the eye can occur from splashes of molten metal or from direct exposure to flames or thermal elements. Liquefaction and shrinkage of collagen lead to extreme damage of the eye and adnexa that might destroy any chance for rehabilitation. Studies have concentrated on the most common severe injury: the alkali-injured eye. Since severe chemical and thermal injuries tend to follow a course similar to that of the alkali-injured eye, the following discussion centers on this disease entity.

The work for this chapter was supported by NEI grant EY04716. The skillful editorial assistance of Sarah L. Alvarez, PhD, is gratefully acknowledged.

EPIDEMIOLOGY

The most common cause of a severe alkali burn of the eye in the United States is an assault.[1] Data gathered from a large urban hospital show that young black men are at greatest risk, usually in a domestic setting where there is low-income, high-density housing and a record of alcoholism and prior assaults. In the industrial sector, approximately 10% of 52,142 cases of ocular trauma reported from 16 states were chemical burns (1.6% acid and 0.6% alkali). Safety awareness, monitors, and strict Occupational Safety and Health Administration requirements in the industrial setting have reduced the incidence of job-related eye injuries. Despite such programs, the storage and use of powerful alkalis under extreme pressure and high temperature continue to pose serious threats even to the properly attired worker wearing protective clothing and goggles. Farmers using liquid ammonia as fertilizer and homeowners using powerful cleansing agents, without wearing eye protection, are examples of people who continue to be at special risk.

Natural Clinical History

Pain, lacrimation, and blepharospasm following an alkali ocular burn result from direct stimulation of free nerve endings located in the epithelium of the cornea and conjunctival lining. With severe injuries, there is a sudden, painful, spiking increase in the intraocular pressure, lasting about 10 minutes, caused primarily by shrinkage of the collagen coat of the eye. A more prolonged increase in pressure quickly follows, secondary to prostaglandin release.[2] Strong alkali in the external eye continues to penetrate into the eye until it is flushed away. Within a minute the severe rise in aqueous humor pH causes lysis of cells lining and adjacent to the anterior chamber, destroying the blood–aqueous barrier and releasing cellular debris into the aqueous humor. This leads to a severe fibrinous inflammatory reaction in the entire anterior segment of the eye. Glaucoma may also develop from inflammatory products accumulating in the aqueous humor and especially the inferior chamber angle, promoting anterior synechial closure inferiorly. The trabeculum and the ciliary body may be injured directly by penetration of alkali through the sclera or by contact with alkaline aqueous humor percolating through the meshwork. Ocular hypertension, hypotension, or both may occur at different periods, depending on the predominance of one or more of those factors influencing aqueous humor dynamics. Chemical injury to the iris, the crystalline lens, and the ciliary body may produce mydriasis, cataract, and even phthisis bulbi, respectively.

Natural Repair

An alkali ocular burn injury frequently extends well beyond the limits of the cornea, destroying the limbal palisades of Vogt, the source of stem cells producing new corneal epithelium. If all corneal epithelial stem cells have been destroyed, the remaining conjunctival epithelial cells must first spread over damaged collagenous tissues of the episclera and then continue over corneal stroma. On the cornea this rate of spread is initially similar to epithelial recovery occurring after a simple abrasion.[3] At 84 hours epithelial movement usually stops as a result of the leading edge losing its adherence to the underlying corneal stroma and then at 96 hours subsequently peels back loosely from the stroma. The specific cause of this loss of epithelial adhesion is unknown. It may result, in large part, from loss of the corneal phenotype repopulating the cornea; accelerated degradation of fibrinogen on the stromal surface by plasminogen activator, a substance probably secreted in excessive amounts by the basal epithelial cells in the alkali-injured eye; or other unknown factors.

Healing of the corneal stroma in a timely manner is the key to avoidance of ulceration and perforation of the globe. Two events proceed simultaneously in the repair process: degradation and removal of tissue debris and replacement of portions of the collagenous matrix, glycosaminoglycans, and fixed cells.

Neutrophils play a significant role in the initial phases of repair in the chemically injured eye. The initial degradative phase is initiated by inflammatory mediators released from the alkali-injured cornea that draw polymorphonuclear neutrophil leukocytes (PMNs) into the damaged tissue, where they are stimulated to undergo a respiratory burst to fuel their phagocytic and degranulation activities. Degranulation involves the release and activation of enzymes contained in the specific and azurophilic granules of the PMNs, breaking down the corneal stroma. The influx of neutrophils thus can lead to ulceration and perforation of the eye.[3] If the injury is extremely severe, then massive invasion of PMNs rapidly converts the corneal tissue into a necrotic sequestrum. In these instances the entire cornea degrades and perforates.

After injury, repair fibroblasts invade the cornea slowly, less so, or not at all in extremely severe injuries when a large amount of necrosis is present. The best result that can be obtained in an eye after a severe alkali injury is a totally vascularized and scarred cornea that has not undergone ulceration and in which glaucoma has not developed.

CLASSIFICATION

The prognosis of a chemical burn of the eye is predicated on the extent and severity of lid and adnexal injury, corneal stromal opacification (marbleization), and perilimbal whitening.[4] To gain a more accurate prognosis it may by prudent to delay the final assessment for as long as 48 hours. A group of drawings is presented (Fig. 17–1) to simplify the classification. The legends detailing the course and prognosis of each burn are intended to provide only a general guide. Extensive lid damage causing lagophthalmos or interference with normal lid physiology and blink patterns seriously diminishes the chance for a favorable outcome from a given degree of chemical or thermal injury.

EMERGENCY CARE

Common sense demands that immediate irrigation with water at the site of the injury be performed to remove a continuing source of cauterization.[5] In the emergency department, irrigation (with lactated Ringer's or other sterile solution) is essential until the pH of the cul-de-sac is 8 or less. Irrigation of a severe injury should be performed for at least 1 to 2 hours but is not likely to be useful after 4 hours. A scleral shell (with an inflow cannula [Mediflow Lens—Morgan Lens, Torrington, WY]) attached to an intravenous infusion bottle facilitates the continuous flow of fluid over the eye.

Although there is no universal agreement on this point, paracentesis of the anterior chamber and reformation with a balanced salt solution may be advantageous, if performed less than 2 hours after the injury. This recommendation is based on the finding that the pH of aqueous humor 100 minutes after injury of the rabbit eye is still higher than 10, even when copious lavage is begun 7 minutes after the injury.[5] Animal studies by Bennett have confirmed the advantage of early paracentesis.[6] In contrast, Grant's studies of alkali-burned rabbit eyes showed aqueous humor pH levels no higher than 10 and no clinical improvement of the eyes after ocular lavage.[7] In my opinion, although there is immediate damage inflicted by the chemical, continuing cauterization by the alkaline aqueous humor demands its removal if the patient is seen within 2 hours from the time of the injury.

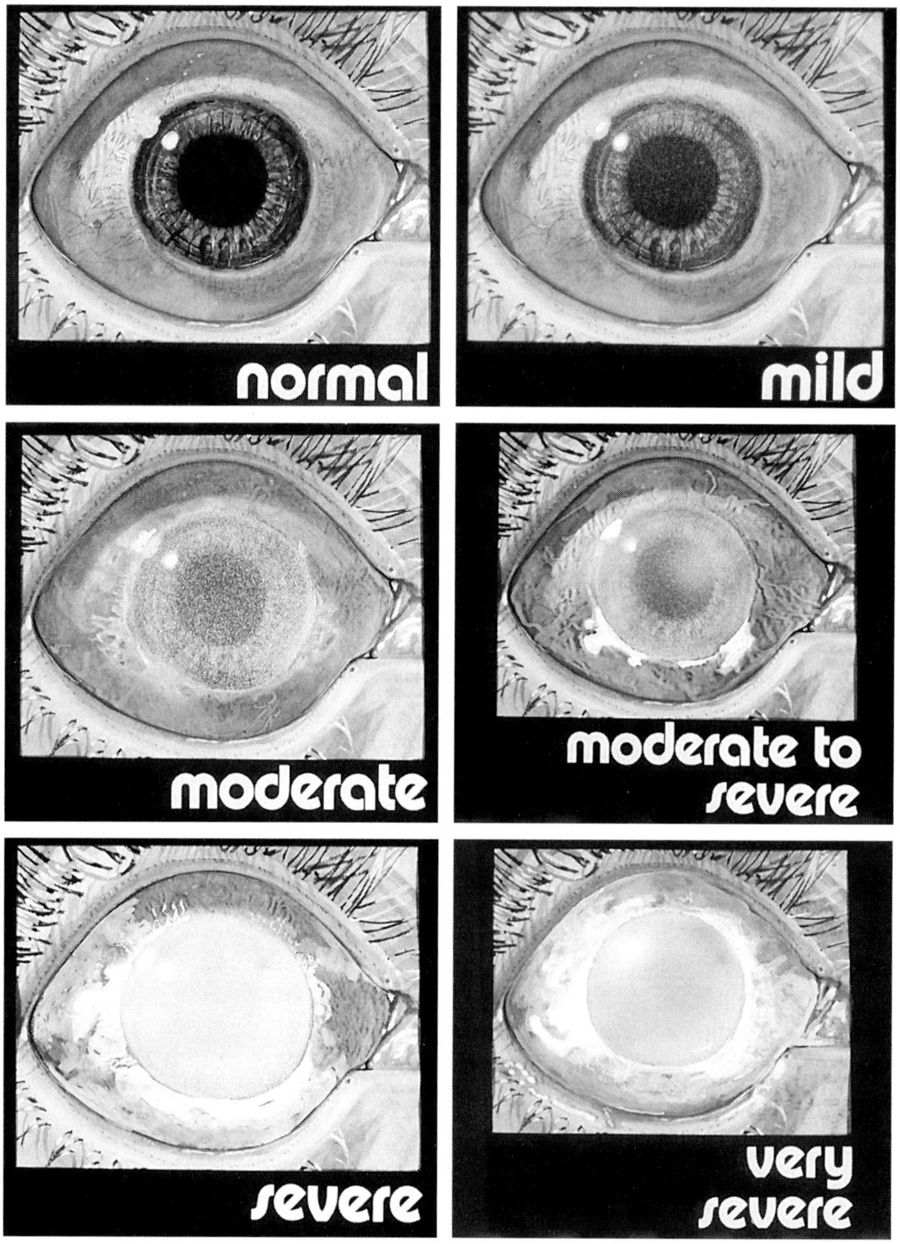

Figure 17–1. Classification of alkali-burned eyes. *Normal* eye, First drawing. *Mild*, Corneal epithelial erosion, faint anterior stromal haziness, and no ischemic necrosis of perilimbal conjunctiva and sclera. Prognosis: Healing with little or no corneal scarring; visual loss usually no greater than one or two lines. *Moderate*, Moderate corneal opacity and little or no significant ischemic necrosis of perilimbal conjunctiva. Prognosis: Slow healing of epithelium with moderate scarring, peripheral corneal vascularization, and visual loss of two to seven lines. *Moderate to severe*, Corneal opacity blurring iris details and ischemic necrosis of conjunctiva limited to less than one third of perilimbal conjunctiva. Prognosis: Prolonged corneal healing with significant corneal vascularization and scarring; vision usually limited to 20/200 or less. *Severe*, Blurring of pupillary outline, ischemia or approximately one to two thirds of perilimbal conjunctiva, and cornea that is often marbleized. Prognosis: Greatly prolonged corneal healing with inflammation and high incidence of corneal ulceration and perforation. In the best cases, severe corneal vascularization and scarring with counting-fingers vision. *Very severe*, Pupil not visible, greater than two-thirds ischemia of perilimbal conjunctiva, and completely marbleized cornea. Prognosis: Healing greatly prolonged, with frequent conversion of corneal stroma into necrotic sequestrum; ulceration and perforation frequent; and very severe corneal vascularization and scarring. Phthisis bulbi may occur with or without ulceration or perforation. (Reprinted by permission from the SOUTHERN MEDICAL JOURNAL [75:418, 1982].)

Paracentesis may be performed under topical anesthesia in the emergency department or clinician's office by making a nonperforating, slanting stab incision at the limbus with a no. 11 Bard-Parker blade, a razor blade, or a supersharp knife to create a tract facilitating the entry of a 27-gauge needle into the anterior chamber. After withdrawal of an aliquot of aqueous humor, balanced salt solution can be used to re-form the anterior chamber. Mydriasis and cycloplegia should be induced by 1% atropine drops twice daily. A broad-spectrum topical antibiotic, such as ciprofloxacin or ofloxacin, are administered four times daily as long as an epithelial defect persists. Acute secondary glaucoma is treated with carbonic anhydrase inhibitors, beta-adrenergic blockers, or both. During the first few days, it is occasionally necessary to treat severe increases in intraocular pressure by paracentesis; this helps remove the necrotic debris and fibrin that accumulate in the anterior chamber and obstruct the outflow channels. Over the subsequent few days, depression of the posterior lip of the paracentesis incision at the slit-lamp releases aqueous humor to control the intraocular pressure repeatedly, if necessary, during the transient pressure increase.

Recent studies show that alkali-injured ocular tissues generate inflammatory mediators that attract and activate PMNs. Although not yet proven to be clinically relevant, débridement of necrotic tissues tenuously attached to the surface of the eye appears to be a reasonable way to diminish PMN activation.

INTERMEDIATE CARE

Loss of conjunctival epithelium and damage to subconjunctival tissues and blood vessels results in an outpouring of plasma proteins with the result that fibrinous adhesions form between surfaces denuded of epithelium. To reduce the chances of symblepharon, remove—rather than lyse—these strands with a cotton-tipped applicator once or twice a day under topical anesthesia. The use of plastic food wrap sutured to line the cul-de-sacs has been advocated to prevent adhesions from forming during the acute stage. Methyl methacrylate rings have also been inserted to prevent synechial adhesions and cicatricial conjunctival contraction in the subacute phase. Although acceptable, it is not clear that such approaches offer any additional advantage in the early phases of treatment. If extensive conjunctival shrinkage and ankyloblepharon do develop later, conjunctivoplasty with incision of the cul-de-sacs, excision of scar tissue, and insertion of a symblepharon ring allow reconstruction when the acute inflammatory phase has subsided. Placement of medial and lateral tarsorrhaphies prevents shell extrusion and offers hope of improved mobility of the eyeball and lid. The tarsorrhaphies can be opened after 3 or 4 months and the shell removed with less danger of conjunctival shrinkage.

Corneal exposure resulting from lid retraction, incomplete blinking, or unconsciousness must be quickly and aggressively treated. Artificial tears and ointment may be satisfactory for the milder problem. If the adjacent facial skin is not burned, a commercially available plastic bubble will form a tight seal with adhesive to the skin. When the facial and lid skin is severely burned, a moist chamber may be temporarily created over the eye with the use of thin plastic food wrap stretched over the external lids and held in place with ointment. Later, skin grafts and lid surgery can be performed.

Persistence of an epithelial defect after an alkali burn is common and often one of the most serious problems encountered because it increases the risk of corneal ulceration. It is important to observe and follow the closure of an epithelial defect with the aid of fluorescein and intervene if epithelial movement does not continue. Patching is only occasionally helpful but may be done even when there are extensive facial burns by using a plastic wrap around the head. A therapeutic or disposable soft contact lens, fitted with 1 to 2 mm of movement, may encourage and maintain corneal reepithelialization by acting as a bandage against the shearing force of the lids. Soft contact lenses should not be used when there is extensive lagophthalmos since they will dry on the surface of the cornea and peel off the epithelium when removal is attempted. The use of nonpreserved artificial drops hourly helps maintain hydration and lens mobility. In very severe burns, epithelial movement from the palpebral conjunctiva may not reach the cornea for weeks or months, growing in only when deep and superficial vessels have penetrated the corneal stroma.

Corneal ulcers are more likely to develop in eyes sustaining corneal *and* perilimbal burns with alkali or strong acids. One approach to treatment has been to inhibit the enzyme collagenase released into the cornea, which in turn destroys the corneal collagen. Although controversy still exists, acetylcysteine (Mucomyst), L-cysteine, and ethylenediaminetetra-acetic acid (EDTA) all appear to inhibit mammalian collagenase in vitro and significantly reduce the incidence of ulceration in animal corneas after alkali burns. More recent studies in extreme alkali-injured rabbit eyes showed no favorable effect of acetylcysteine when compared with control eyes (81% versus 75%).[8] When L-cysteine (0.2 M solution) was begun on the 7th day after a total alkali burn in 33 eyes, only one perforated.[9] A similar study in 28 human eyes substantiated the favorable effect of L-cysteine in preventing acute-stage perforation in total alkali-injured eyes, in aiding ulcer healing, and improving corneal transplantation outcome. In 35 patient eyes with corneal ulceration (diseases unspecified) treated with 0.2 M of EDTA, 30 (86%) healed or remained unchanged compared with 12 (46%) of the 26 control eyes.[10] Cysteine and acetylcysteine are both effective inhibitors of collagenase, but the latter has the advantage of greater stability and availability. Although it is suspected that acetylcysteine (Mucomyst 10%) has a favorable effect in some human alkali-injured corneas, this has not been proved by a clinical trial.

The use of topical steroids after chemical burns is controversial. If the steroid is used four times a day for the first 7 days after injury, it may possibly decrease the inflammatory reaction of the entire anterior segment, possibly reducing some of the late side effects, such as glaucoma. If used longer than 7 days, topical steroids interfere with the repair process and may result in corneal ulceration and perforation. It seems reasonable to avoid topical steroids if possible, but especially later than 7 to 10 days after the injury.

THE CONJUNCTIVA AND TEAR FRAME

Eyelid dysfunction must not be overlooked as a cause, or contributing cause, of corneal epithelial defects, infiltration of inflammatory cells, or ulceration. Chemical or thermal injuries can shorten the eyelid, necrose the eyelid margin, and induce partial blinking, resulting in extreme forms of exposure keratitis. In the presence of a brief or self-limited ocular exposure, ointment, temporary closure of the eyelid with a patch, or tape applied directly to the eyelid may prevent further damage to the corneal stroma. When the periorbital skin is damaged or the lids are unable to close, a temporary moist chamber can be created by having the patient wear swim goggles or by covering the orbital opening with plastic wrap adhered to the orbital rim with an ointment. Temporary or permanent tarsorrhaphy soon after the injury is rarely indicated since this tends to encourage symblepharon formation in the early course of the disease. However, tarsorrhaphy might be desirable later when corneal exposure leads to epithelial disturbances and defects.

After ocular scarring has completed its course, the tear frame and conjunctiva must be reevaluated. Minimal and mild conjunctival symblepharon should be left untouched if they do not interfere with eyelid function. More severe adhesions between the lid and globe interfering with function must be revised. Moderate symblepharon can often be incised directly and a symblepharon ring inserted to reduce the chance of reattachment. In the more substantial adhesions, a two-pillar tarsorrhaphy placed after the conjunctival surgery is required to decrease the likelihood of ring expulsion. When the cul-de-sacs are absent, mucosal grafts from the mouth are often necessary to reline the palpebral and bulbar surfaces of the eye. This procedure may be combined with, or be performed shortly before, perilimbal conjunctival transplantation from the other eye or as a homograph. It is imperative that buccal mucosa not be left as the final resurfacing epithelial cells of the cornea because it lacks stem cells with a corneal phenotype, ultimately leading to corneal epithelial defects, neovascularization, and scarring.

Scarring of the eyelid resulting in lagophthalmos usually responds to a pinch graft to lengthen the lid. Trichiasis must be eliminated by cryoablation, electrolysis, or, in the case of entropion, marginal eyelid rotation. If most of the intricate anatomy and physiology of the eye are not restored before corneal transplantation, then the chance for graft failure increases appreciably.

THE TEAR FILM

The quantity and quality of the tear film layer are also critically important to the health and integrity of the corneal epithelium. After alkaline injuries of the conjunctiva, the excretory tear ducts are scarred, reducing the aqueous component of the tear film. The aqueous phase constitutes the bulk of the thickness of the precorneal tear film (about 7 μm) lying between the superficial lipid layer and the deeper mucin on the epithelial cells. Between blinks the aqueous component thins from evaporation and from flow into the nasolacrimal passages. As the aqueous portion thins, the superficial lipid layer approaches the deepest mucin layer. If the aqueous component of the tear film is not replenished by blinking or is inadequate in volume, lipid then contaminates the underlying mucin coacervate adjacent to the surface cells, creating a localized hydrophobic epithelium. If such a dry area persists, partial-thickness or full-thickness epithelial breakdown may occur.

The importance of the superficial lipid layer rests largely on its ability to retard the evaporation of tears (by a factor of 10). Lipid deficiencies occur when there is destruction of the meibomian glands. This destruction can occur in lid resections, after alkali injuries, after diseases producing scarring, with isotretinoin (Accutane) therapy, and in severe and recalcitrant blepharitis.[11]

Mucin is the spreading agent of the tears produced from conjunctival goblet cells. It is spread out on the surface of the eye by blinking and becomes adsorbed to the plasma membrane of surface epithelial cells. Goblet cell density, and hence mucin production, decreases significantly after alkaline injuries, thereby interfering with the spreading of the aqueous component of the tears. Dry eye is a common and serious sequela of chemical eye injuries.

Treatment of dry eye after alkali injury is similar to that of most other dry eye syndromes. Mild cases of dry eye are successfully treated with artificial tears used every hour and ointment at bedtime. Nonpreserved preparations are preferable, especially if epithelial disturbances already exist. Preparations with higher viscosity are preferred by patients with the driest eyes. If three consecutive Schirmer's I tests on different days give values of 3 to 5 mm of wetting, permanent occlusion of the lower lacrimal punctae is indicated. If testing shows 0 to 2 mm of wetting, then closure of upper and lower punctae is reasonable. Eyeglasses with side panels that create higher-humidity atmospheres around the eyes are useful for patients with the most severe form of dry eye syndrome.

Filamentary keratitis, almost always associated with dry eye syndrome, usually responds to mechanical removal of the filament at its base by severing cleanly with a jeweler's forceps and restitution of tears. Some patients may require a soft contact lens to prevent re-formation of the filaments.

INFLUENCE OF PERILIMBAL EPITHELIAL LOSS

The size and specific areas of epithelial loss after alkali injury influence the course and the permanence of corneal epithelial recovery. In the absence of substantial basement membrane or stromal injury, epithelial defects that do not exceed the limits of the cornea usually heal

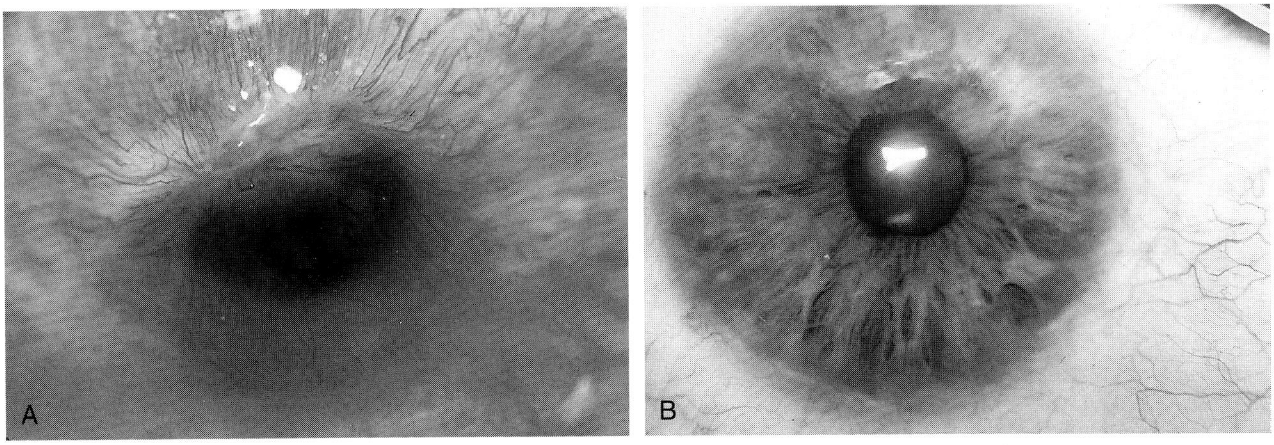

Figure 17–2. *A*, Moderate alkali injury resulted in total corneal pannus. Clear cornea is seen below the surface. *B*, Incisions were made to allow retraction of the pannus to 2 mm behind the limbus. Five years later, a small pannus from above and central epithelial irregularity prompted pannus excision. The resulting persistent epithelial defect did not heal until a limbal conjunctival transplant restored the previous 20/25 acuity. (Reprinted by permission from the SOUTHERN MEDICAL JOURNAL [75:418, 1982].)

without incident. When epithelial damage is more extensive and includes most of the perilimbal palisades of Vogt, epithelial regrowth occurs. The conjunctival epithelium transdifferentiates on the corneal surface but never develops a corneal phenotype. In this circumstance healing is slow and incomplete, resulting in epithelial defects, inflammation, neovascularization, and scarring.

When corneal scarring is relatively superficial or a pannus is present, a simple keratectomy may be all that is required to regain corneal clarity (Fig. 17–2*A*). If healthy bulbar conjunctiva is transplanted from the healthy eye to the limbus of the alkali-injured eye, the vision improves and the ocular surface stabilizes (Fig. 17–2*B*).[12] In the first study of bulbar conjunctival transplantation in alkali-injured eyes, 7 of 10 eyes had improved sight, and all eyes showed an improved and more stable ocular surface. Subsequent immunohistochemical studies have revealed the presence of a discrete group of pluripotential cells (stem cells), 1.5-mm wide, located in the depths of a narrow zone straddling the perilimbal conjunctiva and peripheral cornea. There is indirect evidence that these cells are progenitors of corneal epithelium. The specific 64 kD keratin marker for corneal epithelial cells stains all of the corneal cells but not the deep cells at the limbus. They also react to a specific monoclonal antibody believed to be specific for corneal stem cells.[13] These cells show an enhanced growth curve compared with corneal or conjunctival epithelium. Furthermore, clinical observations confirm that excision of all limbal epithelium from a normal eye leads to poor corneal epithelialization and extensive corneal vascularization, a sign that a critical element has been removed from the generative source of corneal epithelial cells. These basic experimental data and clinical experience give strong support to the current recommendation of limbal conjunctival autograft from the uninjured eye to the injured eye for those patients who have sustained extensive unilateral stem cell injury.[14] This approach works well in conditions such as unilateral chemical injury but poses difficult problems in bilateral chemical injuries.

The surgical technique requires lamellar excision of the epithelium and scar from the cornea, retracting the conjunctiva about 3 mm beyond the limbus. Each limbal transplant containing stem cells (about 3 mm on a side) is obtained from the healthy eye by delineating the conjunctiva to be excised with wet field cautery, incising it, and carrying the dissection to the limbus. Two or three tissue grafts can be disinserted from the donor eye by careful incision of the limbal area with scissors or a small piece of cornea removed with it using a Graefe knife. The graft is then sutured into its anatomically corresponding position in the recipient eye. If the full thickness of cornea is scarred, then a limbal stem cell transplant can be followed by corneal transplantation about 4 months later.

VISUAL REHABILITATION

If corneal surgery is delayed 18 months to 2 years after a chemical burn, it is more likely to be successful, especially if there has been no preexisting ulceration, perforation, or glaucoma.[15] Preparatory procedures to lyse symblepharon, expand cul-de-sacs, or eliminate lagophthalmos are often required to reestablish normal lid physiology and anatomy. If all limbal stem cells have been lost, limbal transplants from the other eye are required to ensure the corneal phenotype required to maintain an intact epithelial surface. Secondary glaucoma must also be controlled with medications, cyclocryotherapy, or filtration surgery. Corneal surgery is indicated for the worst eye in bilateral burns when

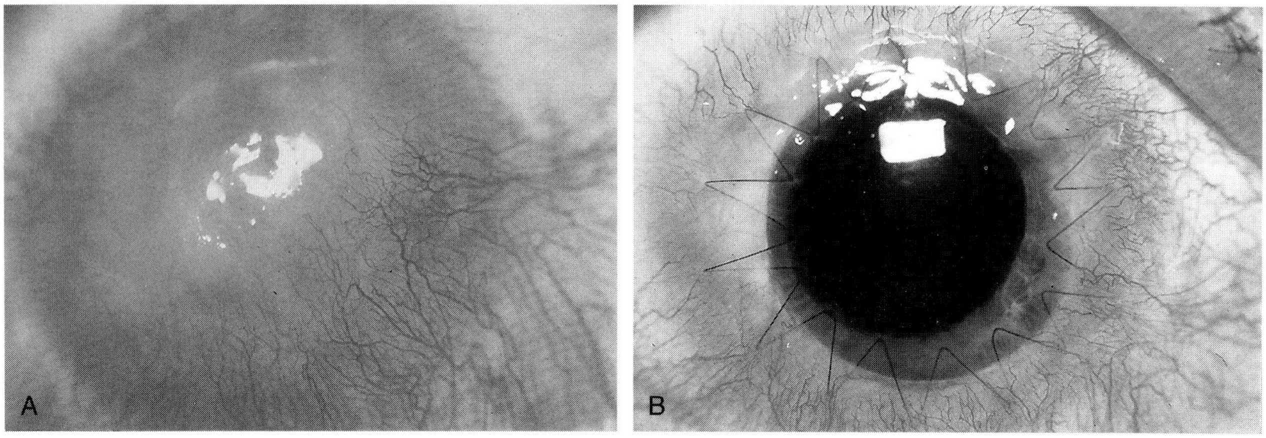

Figure 17–3. *A*, A severe alkali injury caused severe scarring and vascularization of the cornea. *B*, Firmer corneal tissues allowed placement of a continuous 10-0 nylon suture. The 20/30 result has been stable. (Reprinted by permission from the SOUTHERN MEDICAL JOURNAL [75:418, 1982].)

serviceable vision is not available. Corneal transplantation should not be encouraged in patients with severe monocular injuries if a definite need for binocularity does not exist. It is reasonable, however, to give the patient the right of choice, understanding that the procedure is fraught with numerous potential complications.

The chance for visual improvement in chemically burned eyes has been enhanced appreciably from earlier reports (Fig. 17–3). It is important to maintain meticulous attention to the details of surgery, including a fresh, intact epithelium on the donor, punched from the posterior, 0.5 mm larger than the recipient bed; simultaneous removal of cataract, if present; and implantation of an intraocular lens and closure with 10-0 nylon suture. Interrupted sutures are preferred for the more extensively vascularized corneas because of the tendency for sutures to cut through the vascularized recipient bed. Sutures that become loose and break through the epithelium should be removed immediately. If an epithelial defect will not heal, then a soft contact lens is fitted for continuous wear.

When the severity of the injury defies oculoplastic reconstruction of the external eye or when repeated corneal transplantation has failed, then visual rehabilitation can be achieved only with implantation of a keratoprosthesis. The operation is advisable only in those bilateral severe injuries when serviceable vision is not present in either eye. If there is considerable conjunctiva left, the stem of the keratoprosthesis is brought out between the lids (Fig. 17–4). If the conjunctiva is virtually gone, then it is surfaced through the upper lid. The devices are investigational; they are complex to implant and sometimes are associated with serious and untreatable complications.

If vision return is not of primary concern, as in a unilateral injury, the eye can be prepared for a cosmetic shell. This may require a reconstitution of the cul-de-sacs prior to cosmetic shell fitting.

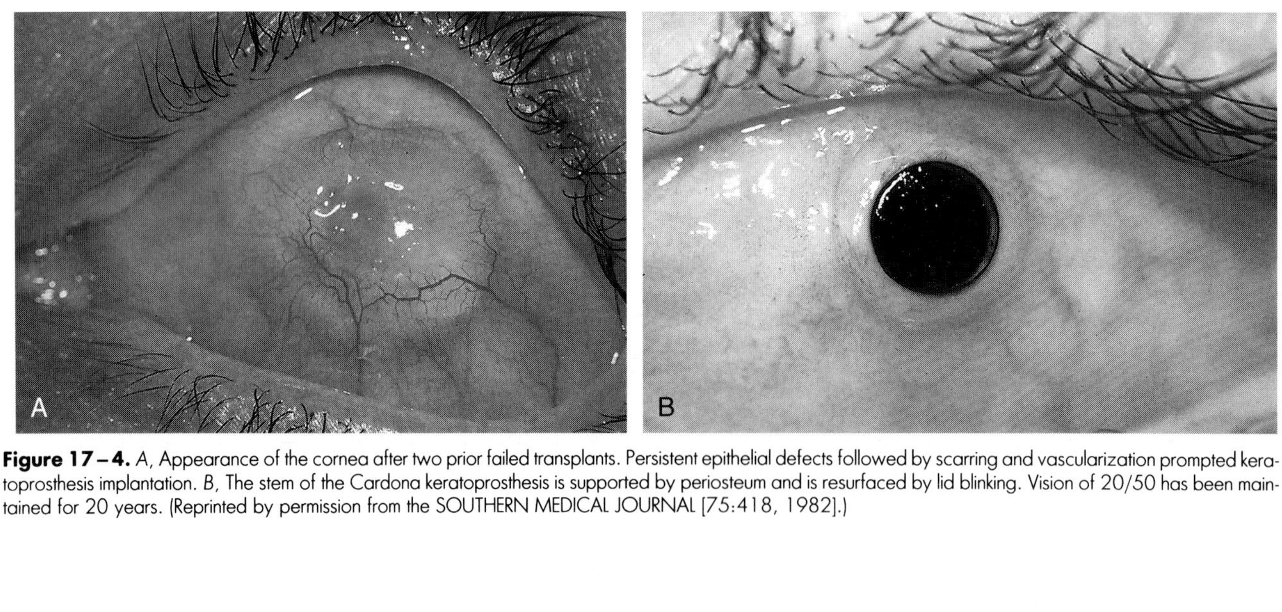

Figure 17–4. *A*, Appearance of the cornea after two prior failed transplants. Persistent epithelial defects followed by scarring and vascularization prompted keratoprosthesis implantation. *B*, The stem of the Cardona keratoprosthesis is supported by periosteum and is resurfaced by lid blinking. Vision of 20/50 has been maintained for 20 years. (Reprinted by permission from the SOUTHERN MEDICAL JOURNAL [75:418, 1982].)

NEW RESEARCH FINDINGS

Newer studies have focused on the basic biochemical, physiologic, and anatomic changes in the anterior segment of the eye after severe injury. This effort has encouraged new thinking in developing the concept of orthomolecular approaches to treatment. To obtain the greatest possible success in treating alkali injuries of the eye, it may be necessary to employ all of the traditional approaches to treatment coupled with the newest molecular therapy.

Ascorbate

In animal experiments, ascorbic acid in the aqueous humor was depressed to one third of normal after severe alkali injuries of the eye. Topical or subcutaneously administered ascorbate (10%) significantly decreased the incidence of corneal ulcerations and perforations if the aqueous humor ascorbate level could be elevated to 15 mg/dL.[16] Light and electron microscopy and radioactive tracer experiments showed that the mechanism of action is replenishment of ascorbic acid to the scorbutic fibroblasts of the cornea. Ascorbic acid is a powerful reducing agent required by fibroblasts to synthesize collagen, thereby promoting healing of damaged corneal tissues.[17]

Citrate

A new idea is the inhibition of PMNs in situ with topical citrate. Sodium citrate prevents the accumulation, phagocytosis, and subsequent release of degradative enzymes and free oxygen radicals from PMNs. Animal and laboratory studies with citrate have shown sodium citrate to be a chelator of extracellular calcium. Calcium is probably necessary for the activation of the PMNs, acting as an important intracellular second messenger in the neutrophil. Inhibition of the PMNs through calcium depletion may be caused by interference with calcium–calmodulin-modulated microfilament or microtubule interfaces in the plasma membrane.[18] Hence, topical treatment with citrate brings the entire set of PMN activities to a halt. Citrate has been shown to be extremely effective in decreasing the incidence of corneal ulceration after alkali injury of the animal eye. Citrate inhibits the efferent part of the inflammatory response by interfering with the adherence of PMNs to vascular endothelium, decreasing the migration of PMNs into damaged cornea, and diminishing the discharge of hydrolytic enzymes, and probably superoxide radicals, into the corneal stroma. My colleagues and I believe that citrate chelation of extracellular calcium creates a plasma membrane and cellular deficiency of this important intracellular second messenger. Interference with the production of activated calcium-binding proteins (in particular, calmodulin) inhibits many intracellular processes, notably receptor movement and the function of microfilaments.

Ascorbate and citrate reduce the incidence of corneal ulceration in alkali-injured eyes by different mechanisms.[19, 20] This accounts for the substantial further reduction in corneal ulceration in alkali-injured animals from an untreated rate of corneal ulceration of 80% to a transitory 4.6% when citrate and ascorbate eye drops are concurrently alternated throughout the day.[21]

A national randomized clinical trial of ascorbate or citrate in the treatment of alkali injuries of the human eye is still in progress. Criteria for entry include moderately severe or worse burns occurring less than 29 days previous and without ulceration (see the section on classification). Study medications provided to the patient are either ascorbate, citrate, or a placebo given as hourly eye drops and capsules every 6 hours. Patients may be entered into the trial by their own physician, a local corneal specialist, or a participating ophthalmologist in that area. To discuss entering an alkali-injured patient, call the clinical coordinator at (205) 877-1747 or Dr. Pfister at (205) 877-2837.

The use of tetracycline, subconjunctival progesterone, intramuscular nortestosterone, or thiol dipeptides all have shown favorable effects in animal models of alkali injuries. However, a clinical trial must be performed before any of these approaches can be considered for routine human use.

OTHER POSSIBLE CHEMICAL TREATMENTS

Fibronectin has been implicated as a key element in wound healing for its involvement in cell-to-cell and cell-to-matrix adhesion and cell spreading. Eye trauma causes exudation of large proteins such as fibrinogen from conjunctival blood vessels, reaching the bare basement membrane, where polymerization and deposition take place. Epithelial defects occurring in herpetic keratitis and trophic corneal ulcers and after cataract surgery have responded to fibronectin drops when used in an open-labeled study. An alternative explanation for this favorable effect is suggested by an animal study showing that albumin eye drops were as effective as fibronectin in the treatment of persistent epithelial defects after alkali injuries in rabbits.[22] This finding suggests a nonspecific response. The determination of the value of fibronectin in persistent epithelial defects can be gleaned only from a prospective, randomized clinical trial.

Epidermal growth factor (EGF) enhances the rate of healing and induces hyperplasia in corneal epithelium.[23, 24] EGF stimulated complete epithelial healing after alkali injury in two studies, but in each instance recurrent erosions reestablished the defect.[25, 26] Epithelial proliferation is clearly stimulated by EGF, but its usefulness in corneal diseases is unknown. Its use may be limited to certain types of persistent epithelial defects in which adhesion problems are least significant. Growth factors may find a more favored place in the acceleration of wound strength by the mechanism of enhancement of macromolecular synthesis.

REFERENCES

1. Klein R, Lobes LA Jr: Ocular alkali burns in a large urban area. Ann Ophthalmol 8:1185–1189, 1976.
2. Paterson CA, Pfister RR: Intraocular pressure changes after alkali burns. Arch Ophthalmol 91:211–218, 1974.
3. Pfister RR, Burstein N: The alkali-burned cornea. Part I: Epithelial and stromal repair. Exp Eye Res 23:519–535, 1976.
4. Pfister RR: Chemical injuries of the eye. Ophthalmology 90:1246–1253, 1983.
5. Paterson CA, Pfister RR: Aqueous humor pH changes after experimental alkali burns. Am J Ophthalmol 79:414–419, 1975.
6. Bennett TO, Peyman GA, Rutgard J: Intracameral phosphate buffer in alkali burns. Can J Ophthalmol 13:93–95, 1978.
7. Grant WM: Experimental investigation of paracentesis in the treatment of ocular ammonia burns. Arch Ophthalmol 44:399–404, 1950.
8. Pfister RR, Nicolaro ML, Paterson CA: Sodium citrate reduces the incidence of corneal ulcerations and perforations in extreme alkali-burned eyes—acetylcysteine and ascorbate have no favorable effect. Invest Ophthalmol Vis Sci 21:486–490, 1980.
9. Brown SI, Akiya S, Weller CA: Prevention of the ulcers of the alkali-burned cornea: Preliminary studies with collagenase inhibitors. Arch Ophthalmol 82:95–97, 1969.
10. Slansky HH, Dohlman CH, Berman MB: Prevention of corneal ulcers. Trans Am Acad Ophthalmol Otolaryngol 75:1208–1211, 1971.
11. Mathers WD, Shields BS, Sachdev MS, et al: Meibomian gland dysfunction in chronic blepharitis. Cornea 10:277–285, 1991.
12. Thoft RA: Conjunctival transplantation as an alternative to keratoplasty. Ophthalmology 86:1084–1092, 1979.
13. Zieske JD, Bukusoglu H: Numbers of limbal basal cells expressing a 50-kD antigen increase after wounding. Invest Ophthalmol Vis Sci 31[Suppl]:538, 1990.
14. Kenyon KR, Tseng SC: Limbal autograft transplantation for ocular surface disorders. Ophthalmology 96:709, 1989.
15. Kramer S: Late numerical grading of alkali burns to determine keratoplasty prognosis. Trans Am Ophthalmol Soc 81:97–106, 1983.
16. Pfister RR, Paterson CA: Additional clinical and morphological observations on the favorable effect of ascorbate in experimental ocular alkali burns. Invest Ophthalmol Vis Sci 16:478–487, 1977.
17. Pfister RR, Paterson CA: Ascorbic acid in the treatment of alkali burns of the eye. Ophthalmology 87:1050–1057, 1980.
18. Pfister RR, Haddox J, Dodson R: Polymorphonuclear leukocytic inhibition by citrate, other metal chelators, and trifluoperazine: Evidence to support calcium-binding protein involvement. Invest Ophthalmol Vis Sci 25:955–970, 1984.
19. Pfister RR, Paterson CA, Hayes SA: The efficacy of sodium citrate in the treatment of severe alkali burns of the eye is influenced by the route of administration. Cornea 1:205–211, 1982.
20. Pfister RR, Paterson CA, Hayes SA: Topical ascorbate decreases the incidence of corneal ulceration after experimental alkali burns. Invest Ophthalmol Vis Sci 17:1019–1024, 1978.
21. Pfister RR, Haddox JL, Barr D: The combined effect of citrate/ascorbate treatment in alkali-injured rabbit eyes. Cornea 10:100–104, 1991.
22. Boisjoly H, Beaulieu A, Giasson M, Menard C: The effect of fibronectin compared to albumin on rabbit epithelial wound healing. Invest Ophthalmol Vis Sci 28[Suppl]:52, 1987.
23. Cohen S: Isolation of a mouse submaxillary gland protein accelerating incisor eruption and eyelid opening in the newborn animal. Am J Ophthalmol 98:411, 1984.
24. Ho PC, Davis WH, Elliott JH, Cohen SP: Kinetics of corneal epithelial regeneration and epidermal growth factor. Invest Ophthalmol Vis Sci 13:804, 1974.
25. Eiferman R, Schultz GS: Treatment of alkali burns in rabbits with epidermal growth factor. Invest Ophthalmol Vis Sci 28[Suppl]:52, 1987.
26. Singh G, Foster CS: Epidermal growth factor in alkali-burned corneal epithelial wound healing. Am J Ophthalmol 103:802–807, 1987.

CHAPTER 18

Conjunctival and Limbal Neoplasia: Diagnosis and Management

Anne R. Horan and Denis M. O'Day

Conjunctival malignancies are relatively rare. As such, the oculoplastic surgeon may be much less familiar with the diagnosis and management of these neoplasms than with those of the eyelid and orbit. Squamous cell carcinoma is the most frequently encountered conjunctival malignancy. Melanoma of the conjunctiva, which constitutes approximately 2% of all ocular malignancies, is less common, followed by lymphoid tumors and Kaposi's sarcoma.[1]

One of the more prevalent eyelid malignancies, sebaceous cell carcinoma, often spreads to involve the conjunctiva. It has been suggested that sebaceous cell carcinoma may develop directly from the conjunctival epithelium as well as from the lid structures; however, this has not been well documented.[2]

Unlike the eyelid, where basal cell carcinoma is the most common malignancy, basal cell carcinoma of the conjunctiva is exceedingly rare. It is estimated that the ratio of conjunctival squamous cell carcinoma to basal cell carcinoma ranges from 10:1 to 20:1.[1,3]

SQUAMOUS CELL CARCINOMA

Myriad terms have been used in the past to identify epithelial neoplasia of the conjunctiva. Fortunately, much of the resultant confusion has now been eliminated with the adoption of an ordered terminology that defines the neoplasia in stages. Conjunctival intraepithelial neoplasia (CIN) indicates that the neoplastic process has not crossed the basement membrane of the conjunctival epithelium. The degree of epithelial dysplasia is classified as either mild or severe, depending on whether the dysplastic cells constitute less than or greater than 50% of the epithelial thickness. The term *squamous cell carcinoma* is used when there is penetration of the basement membrane. The neoplasm is classified as microinvasive if only the substantia propria is involved. When structures such as the cornea, sclera, iris, or orbit are affected by tumor spread, the tumor is identified as invasive squamous cell carcinoma.[4] Mucoepidermoid carcinoma is a rare but particularly aggressive version of squamous cell carcinoma. It is prone to recurrence after excision and is much more likely than squamous cell carcinoma to invade the globe or orbit.[5]

Approximately 75% of all patients with CIN or squamous cell carcinoma are elderly men.[1] Although the precise etiology of these tumors is unknown, the predilection for the exposed limbal regions in the interpalpebral fissure would argue for ultraviolet exposure as a possible risk factor.[6]

Odrich and associates[7] recently presented two cases of bilateral squamous dysplasia of the conjunctiva, with CIN in one eye and invasive squamous cell carcinoma in the other. Molecular hybridization analysis determined that the lesions in both patients harbored human papillomavirus (HPV)-16 deoxyribonucleic acid sequences, raising the possibility that this viral agent may have a role in epithelial neoplasia of the conjunctiva.[7]

CIN is frequently described as a gray, intraepithelial plaque-like lesion located in the palpebral fissure and involving the limbal region (Fig. 18–1). Squamous cell carcinomas tend to have a mulberry appearance due to the presence of superficial vessels coursing through the gelatinous-looking tumor (Fig. 18–2). Less frequently, and not unlike CIN, squamous cell carcinoma may appear leukoplakic or papillomatous.

In the setting of an elderly patient presenting with chronic, refractory, unilateral "conjunctivitis," the diagnosis of diffuse involvement of bulbar and palpebral conjunctivae with squamous cell carcinoma should always be considered. Scraping of the conjunctiva for exfoliative cytology may exhibit malignant cells with large nuclei.[8]

The diagnosis of epithelial neoplasia is made by excisional biopsy. In CIN, there is proliferation of the basal epithelial cells with prominent nuclei and mitotic figures, disruption of the normal horizontal polarization of the squamous epithelial cells, and an intact basement membrane. The findings are similar in squamous cell carcinoma, with the exception that tumor cells are found to have involved the substantia propria deep to the basement membrane as well (Fig. 18–3).[9]

Squamous cell carcinoma infrequently invades the underlying sclera or adjacent cornea.[10] Intraocular extension is even less common and is quite difficult to

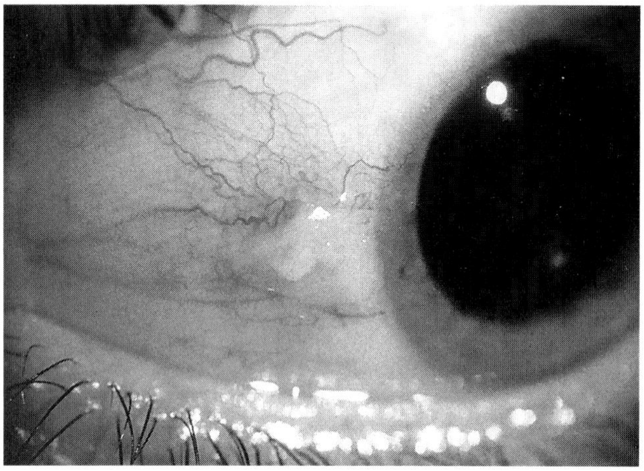

Figure 18–1. This limbal lesion, located in the palpebral fissure, has the typical gray, plaque-like appearance of a conjunctival neoplasm.

diagnose.[11-14] Anterior chamber inflammation may be the only clue to intraocular tumor spread. If intraocular extension is suspected, paracentesis to obtain specimens for cytology is indicated.[11,13]

Squamous cell carcinoma of the conjunctiva rarely metastasizes. Only three deaths attributed to squamous cell carcinoma of the conjunctiva have been reported in this country. Of these, only one has been substantiated with an autopsy.[12,15,16]

The rates of recurrence for CIN and squamous cell carcinoma treated with simple excision are high (ranging from 20% to 40% in most series).[17,18] This has prompted the trial of alternative treatment modalities. Currently, excision combined with cryotherapy appears to be the treatment of choice.

The long-term results of treatment by excision combined with cryotherapy have been studied by Peksayar and coworkers[17] in a series of 22 eyes of 20 patients—10 with CIN and 12 with squamous cell carcinoma—followed for 5 to 12 years. All patients underwent excision of the conjunctival lesion with 2 mm of apparently healthy surrounding conjunctiva. Nitrous oxide cryotherapy was then applied to all of the conjunctival margins, the limbus, and the sclera at the base of the lesion. After primary closure of the conjunctiva, the limbus and the conjunctiva were retreated with additional cryotherapy. The recurrence rate for this series was 9% (2 eyes), with both recurrences presenting within 2 years of initial treatment.[17] Fraunfelder and Wingfield followed 36 patients for more than 3 years and reported an 8% recurrence rate after treatment with excision and liquid nitrogen cryotherapy.[19]

Char[1] indicated that the rate of recurrence can be as low as 5% when excision is guided by frozen-section examination, providing a thorough resection. The "tumor-free" conjunctival margins, limbus, and bare sclera are then treated with double freeze-thaw cryotherapy. Finally, the conjunctiva is either closed primarily, or, in the case of a particularly large defect, grafted with autologous conjunctiva or buccal mucous membrane.[1] Recurrent lesions typically develop at the limbus and spread onto the cornea. They have been successfully treated in much the same manner: either with excision and cryotherapy or cryotherapy alone.[17]

In some instances of invasion beyond the substantia propria, excision may need to include a full-thickness sclerokeratectomy.[10,19] The excision needed to fully encompass the lesion may encroach significantly onto the cornea if routine trephination is employed. This may be avoided by free-hand tailoring of the excision and replacement graft. We prefer to use donor corneal tissue, but some surgeons use sclera or a corneoscleral graft. In time, the clear corneal graft usually opacifies (Fig. 18–4).

Orbital involvement is usually confined to the anterior orbit; therefore, total exenteration is rarely indicated. Advanced intraocular extension or orbital spread can be managed by anterior exenteration in most patients.[1]

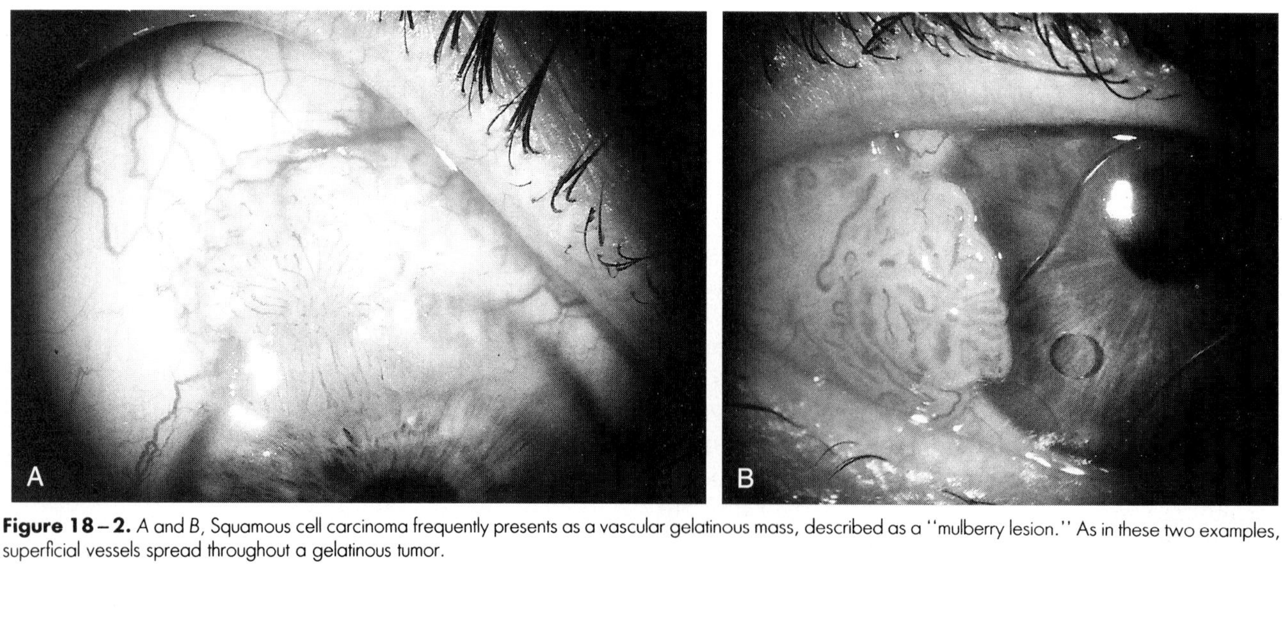

Figure 18–2. *A* and *B*, Squamous cell carcinoma frequently presents as a vascular gelatinous mass, described as a "mulberry lesion." As in these two examples, superficial vessels spread throughout a gelatinous tumor.

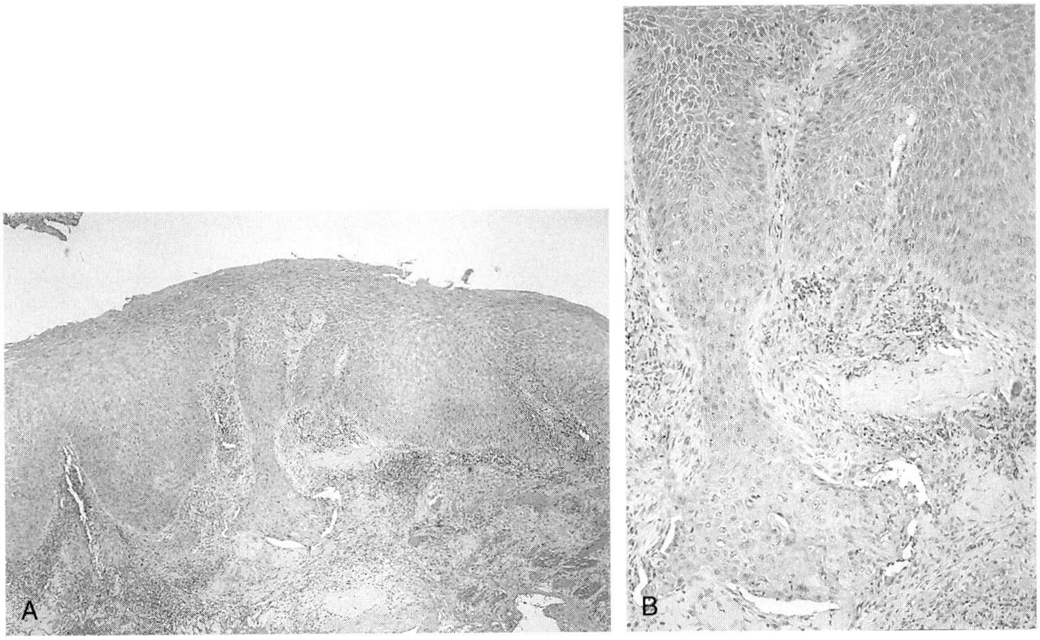

Figure 18–3. Photomicrographs at ×20 *(A)* and ×40 *(B)* magnification illustrate squamous cell carcinoma that has invaded beyond the basement membrane to involve the substantia propria of the conjunctiva.

MALIGNANT MELANOMA

Although primary malignant melanoma is the second most frequently occurring conjunctival malignancy, it accounts for only 2% of all ocular melanomas.[20] Much attention has been directed toward elucidation of the pathogenesis and prognostic indicators of this potentially fatal neoplasm.[20–28] Malignant melanoma of the conjunctiva has been shown to arise from preexisting nevi, primary acquired melanosis (PAM), as well as de novo. The association of PAM with subsequent development of melanoma is seen in approximately 60% to 75% of patients. Approximately 20% of all patients with conjunctival melanoma either have a history of conjunctival nevus or are found to have histologic evidence of a preexisting nevus.[22,23,25,29]

Malignant melanoma of the conjunctiva is rare in children. Including three young adults, there are only nine reported cases in the literature.[26] Conjunctival melanoma is most commonly seen in middle age, with an average age at presentation of 50 to 55 years.[20,23] Women are more frequently affected than men.[20,29,30]

Conjunctival melanoma must be differentiated from benign simulating lesions. Ocular melanocytosis and oculodermal melanocytosis involve not only the conjunctiva but also the episclera and superficial sclera. Ma-

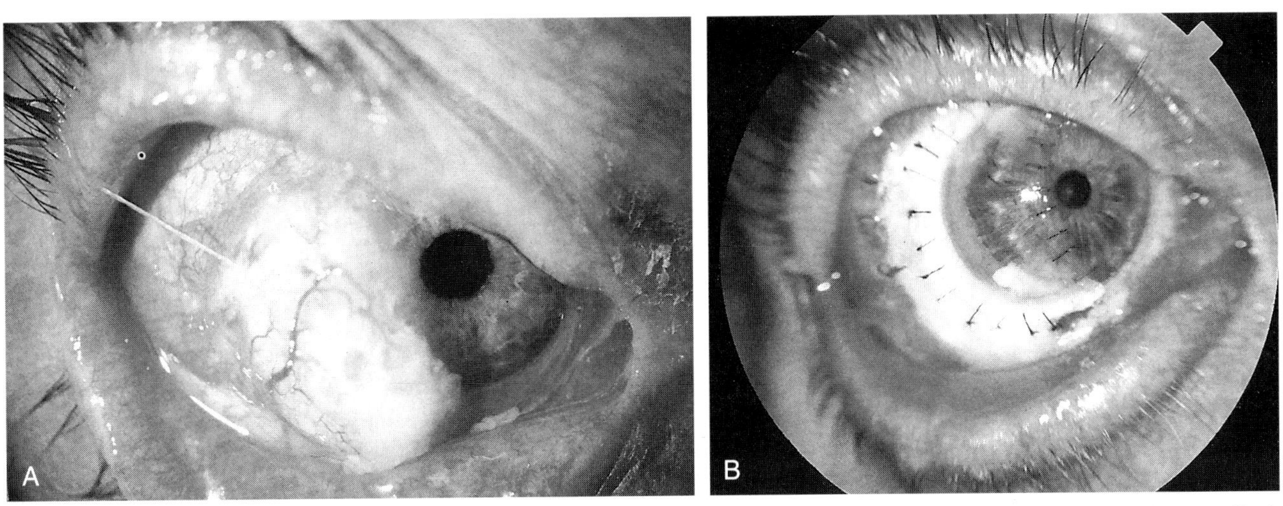

Figure 18–4. Removal of a large lesion *(A)* such as this one involves both sclera and cornea in addition to conjunctiva and may require free-hand tailoring *(B)* of both the excision site and the graft.

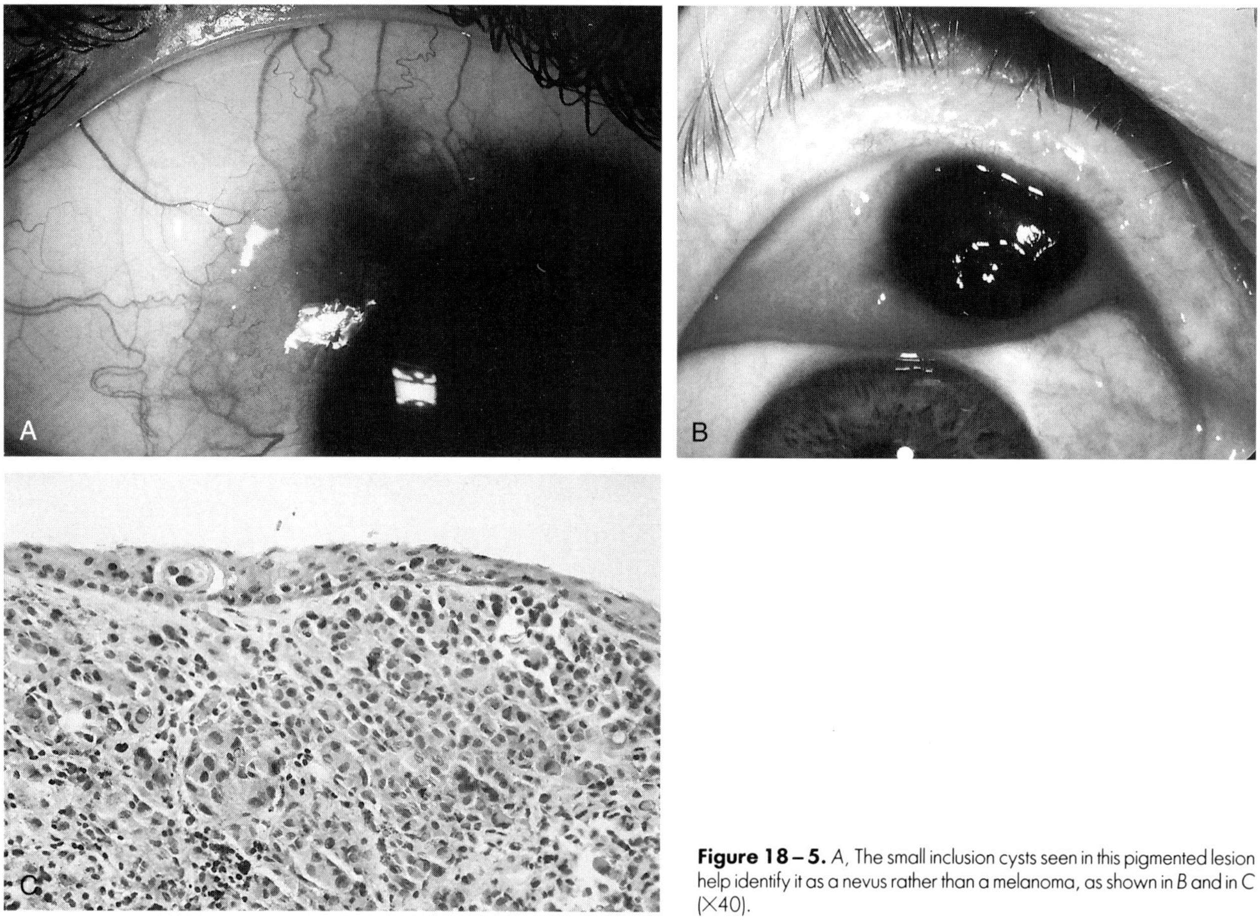

Figure 18–5. *A*, The small inclusion cysts seen in this pigmented lesion help identify it as a nevus rather than a melanoma, as shown in *B* and in *C* (×40).

lignant transformation is extremely rare.[31] Nevi of the conjunctiva frequently contain inclusion cysts, a useful finding when attempting to differentiate between nevi and melanomas on clinical examination (Fig. 18–5). Nevi rarely undergo malignant transformation.[31] Acquired racial melanosis is a benign bilateral perilimbal pigmentation occurring predominantly in patients whose skin is heavily pigmented.

Clinically, PAM of the conjunctiva is manifested as unilateral patches of golden brown to chocolate-colored flat conjunctival pigmentation.[25] Histologically, it is possible to identify two distinct types of PAM: without atypia and with atypia. PAM without atypia is characterized by the presence of either hyperplasia of melanocytes without evidence of cytologic atypia or increased pigmentation within the melanocytes due to increased production of melanin; PAM without atypia is unlikely to undergo malignant transformation.[25] PAM with atypia is a known precursor of melanoma, with nearly 50% progressing to melanoma development.[22] The presence of epithelioid cells or a pattern of intraepithelial pagetoid extension increases to 75% or greater the chance of undergoing melanomatous change. Since the distinction between PAM with and without atypia cannot be made clinically, a biopsy is useful in determining which lesions can be safely observed over time and which should be excised.[22] Increasing nodularity, thickening, vascularity, or inflammation of an area of PAM may signal progression to melanoma and mandates excision.[1]

Folberg and coworkers[23] have shown that the more favorable prognosis for patients with cutaneous melanoma in association with an acquired nevus does not hold true for conjunctival melanomas. Other attempts to apply cutaneous melanoma classification systems to the conjunctival neoplasms have been similarly unfruitful. Jakobiec's[32] conclusion that tumor thickness is the "sovereign prognostic factor" in conjunctival melanomas appears to be quite accurate. Tumor thickness of 0.8 mm or more is associated with a higher risk of metastases than that of thinner melanomas. Tumor thickness of 0.8 to 1.5 mm was shown by Folberg and coworkers[23] to be responsible for a 29% mortality rate. Lommatzsch and colleagues[20] have reported a 31.4% metastasis rate for conjunctival melanomas that are thicker than 2 mm or involve the fornix, palpebral conjunctiva, caruncle, or cornea. However, the unpredictable nature of conjunctival melanoma should be reinforced by the recognition that some patients in this series had distant metastases with very thin tumors, and others developed no metastatic disease after exenteration for very thick lesions.

Unlike uveal melanomas, small conjunctival melanomas should not be observed for evidence of growth—they should be thoroughly excised upon identification.[33] Delay in excision may permit metastatic spread to regional lymph nodes (preauricular, submandibular, and cervical) as well as distant metastases. Jakobiec and associates[25] recommended cryotherapy to the base of the excision as well as "the surrounding conjunctiva for the eradication of any accompanying PAM." Histologic evidence of tumor at the margin of the specimen indicates the need for wide reexcision or treatment of the surgical site with cryotherapy.

Exenteration may be a surgical option in the management of diffuse fornical involvement, intraocular invasion, or orbital extension; however, it has not been shown to alter the long-term prognosis.[22, 29] A complete metastatic workup should precede the decision to perform exenteration. Robertson and colleagues[34] suggested that an eyelid-sparing exenteration may not be appropriate in patients identified as having ipsilateral eyelid margin pigmentation in association with conjunctival melanoma. Even in the absence of eyelid malignancy, this proved to be an ominous sign. A comparison of deaths due to metastatic disease in patients with and without eyelid pigmentation is impressive: 70% in the former group and 26% in the latter.[34]

Any patient who has been treated for conjunctival melanoma should have serial examinations every several months. In addition to a complete ophthalmologic assessment, palpation to detect possible preauricular, submandibular, or cervical adenopathy should be performed with each visit.[25] Complaints of even minor symptoms that are referable to the nasal cavity or paranasal sinuses should elicit prompt consultation for examination of these structures. Robertson and associates[35] reported four patients in whom epistaxis or symptoms of nasal obstruction were associated with melanoma in the nasal cavity and paranasal sinuses. Each of these patients had been treated months to years earlier for conjunctival melanoma. Subsequent management may be influenced by the presence of nasal cavity or paranasal sinus melanoma, since the prognosis is much poorer than for conjunctival melanoma.

LYMPHOID TUMORS

Conjunctival lymphoid tumors are rare, comprising less than 1% of all ocular tumors.[36] Lymphoid lesions of the conjunctiva typically present as "salmon patches": elevated masses with a smooth surface and fleshy appearance (Fig. 18–6).

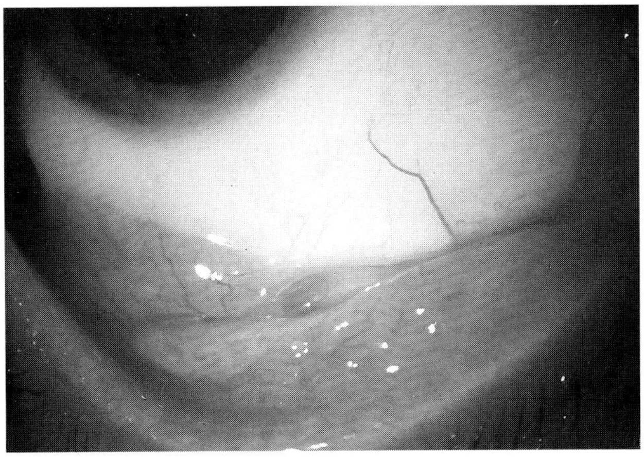

Figure 18–6. The "salmon patch" lymphoid tumor is an orange-pink, elevated, fleshy mass with a smooth surface.

Localization of lymphoid infiltrates to the conjunctiva appears to be associated with a lower incidence of extraocular lymphoma (20%) than involvement of the orbit (35%) or lid (67%).[37] There is little else about the clinical appearance that would indicate whether a particular infiltrate is benign or malignant in nature. Histopathology, and possibly immunophenotypic analysis, can provide useful prognostic information.

In Jakobiec and Knowles' series[37, 38] of 108 patients with 117 lymphoid tumors of the ocular adnexa, 30 (28%) had tumors involving the conjunctiva; 3 (10%) of these patients had concurrent systemic lymphoma. None of the patients with conjunctival lymphoid neoplasia had a prior history of nonocular lymphoma.

Small lymphocytic and intermediate lymphocytic lymphomas of the conjunctiva were associated with systemic lymphoma less frequently than those with the higher grade cell types such as immunoblastic large cell and follicular center cleaved cell.[38] Medeiros and Harris[39] reported that one third of the cases they reviewed were histologically indeterminate and malignancy could only be determined by immunohistologic studies. In contrast with this finding, Jakobiec and Knowles[38] indicated that elaborate immunophenotypic analysis of adnexal lymphoid tumors offers no advantage in predicting the association of systemic disease than does a careful histopathologic examination. Highly sensitive molecular genetic analyses may ultimately prove to be more accurate indicators of malignancy. However, their diagnostic value has not been fully evaluated.

It is sobering to note that nonocular disease has been shown to occur with approximately the same frequency in association with "benign" lymphoid hyperplasia as with well-differentiated lymphocytic lymphoma.[38] In light of this, all patients with biopsy-proven lymphoid infiltrates of the conjunctiva should undergo a thorough evaluation for systemic lymphoma.

The prognosis for ocular adnexal lymphoid tumors is excellent: 67% of these tumors are not associated with nonocular disease when followed for 4 years. However, systemic disease may be more frequently seen with longer followup.[38] The extent of lymphoid proliferation at the time of presentation with the conjunctival mass is the most significant prognostic factor with respect to development of systemic lymphoma.[37] When there is no evidence of nonocular disease at the time of presentation, the tumor is considered to be stage IE.[38] Over a 3-year period of followup, as many as 86% of patients with stage IE disease will remain free of extraocular lymphomatous disease. Stage IE patients with bilateral conjunctival tumors fared no worse than those with unilateral lesions.[37]

Surgical management of conjunctival lymphoid tumors is limited to excisional biopsy to provide adequate tissue for specific diagnosis (Fig. 18–7). Stage IE lymphoid tumors respond well to radiation therapy of the conjunctiva.[36] In the presence of nonocular disease, systemic chemotherapy also effectively treats the conjunctival mass. If the response of the conjunctival lesion is less than complete, chemotherapy can later be supplemented with local radiation therapy. Radiation therapy and chemotherapy may be employed simultaneously in patients with particularly large conjunctival tumors.[38]

KAPOSI'S SARCOMA

Prior to the advent of the acquired immunodeficiency syndrome (AIDS) epidemic, Kaposi's sarcoma was rarely seen in this country. This multifocal hemorrhagic sarcoma typically presented as violaceous macular lesions in elderly men of "Central European, Jewish, or Mediterranean extraction."[40] In most patients, the sarcomas were successfully treated with excision or local irradiation.

A more aggressive form of Kaposi's sarcoma that is less amenable to treatment has been identified in immunosuppressed patients, particularly those with AIDS.[41,42] In these patients, erythematous or violaceous lesions develop on the skin or mucous membranes.[42]

Ocular Kaposi's lesions involve the lids and the conjunctiva. Conjunctival Kaposi's sarcoma has been shown in several studies to occur in 5% to 10% of AIDS patients, and it may be their first manifestation of Kaposi's sarcoma.[41–44] The reddish-blue vascular subconjunctival masses may be misdiagnosed as subconjunctival hemorrhages, pyogenic granulomas, or cavernous hemangiomas, particularly when the patient has yet to be identified as immunodeficient.[42,44]

Because ophthalmic Kaposi's sarcoma tends to progress slowly, without invasive behavior, treatment is generally reserved for symptomatic lesions that produce discomfort or obstruct vision.[41] Owing to minimal adherence to the surrounding tissues, surgical resection of these lesions is relatively simple. Despite their highly vascular nature, excision can be performed without significant bleeding.[42] Histopathologic examination of surgical specimens has shown fascicles of "spindle-shaped cells with elongated oval nuclei," with tumor cells forming "irregular clefts, round lumina, and mantles around medium-sized vessels."[45] Deep within the lesions, there is "widespread extravasation of erythrocytes and deposition of hemosiderin."[40]

Kaposi's sarcoma has been shown to be quite sensitive to radiation therapy.[41, 45, 46] In the setting of AIDS, Kaposi's sarcoma is multifocal. Excision alone, even of a presumed isolated lesion, is unlikely to provide a cure. Systemic chemotherapy may produce regression of ocu-

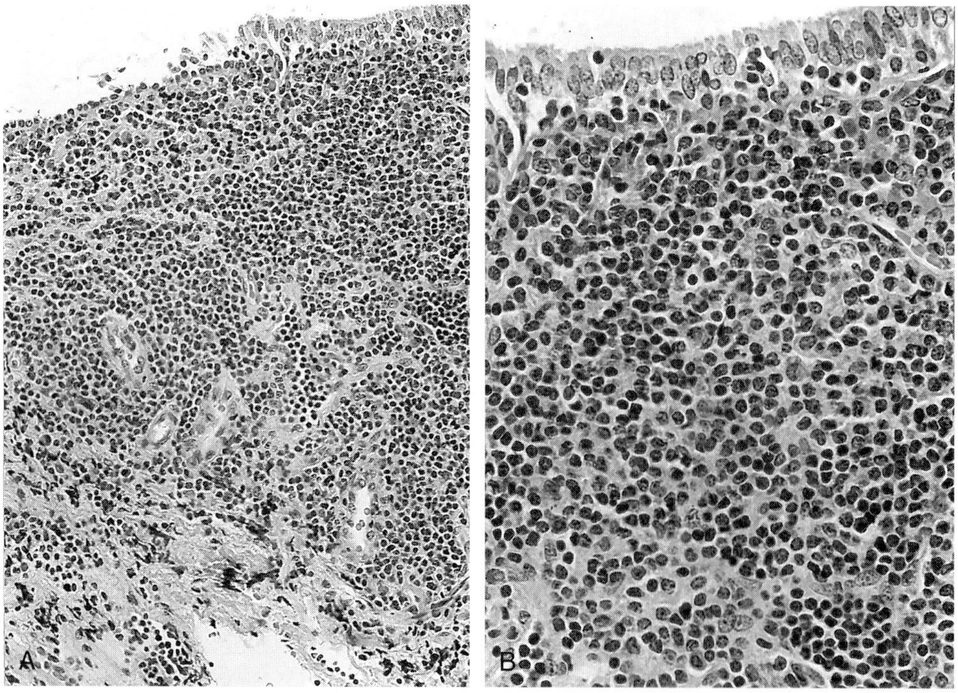

Figure 18–7. Biopsy specimen from a B cell lymphoma shown at ×20 *(A)* and ×40 *(B)* magnification.

lar lesions. If the response of ocular lesions is suboptimal, or if the disease is believed to involve solely the lid or conjunctiva, or both, local radiation therapy is recommended.[41]

REFERENCES

1. Char DH: Clinical Ocular Oncology. New York, Churchill Livingstone, 1989, pp 63–87.
2. Margo CE, Lessner A, Stern GA: Intraepithelial sebaceous carcinoma of the conjunctiva and skin of the eyelid. Ophthalmology 99:227–231, 1992.
3. Reese AB: Tumors of the Eye, 3rd ed. Hagerstown, MD, Harper & Row, 1976, p 53.
4. Cameron JD, Folberg R, Kincaid MC, et al: Ophthalmology Basic and Clinical Science Course. Section 11 Ophthalmic Pathology. San Francisco, CA, American Academy of Ophthalmology, 1990, p 146.
5. Margo CE, Groden LR: Intraepithelial neoplasia of the conjunctiva with mucoepidermoid differentiation. Am J Ophthalmol 108:600–601, 1989.
6. Erie JC, Campbell RJ, Liesegang TJ: Conjunctival and corneal intraepithelial and invasive neoplasia. Ophthalmology 93:176–183, 1986.
7. Odrich MG, Jakobiec FA, Lancaster WD, et al: A spectrum of bilateral squamous conjunctival tumors associated with human papillomavirus type 16. Ophthalmology 98:628–635, 1991.
8. Spinak M, Friedman AH: Squamous cell carcinoma of the conjunctiva: Value of exfoliative cytology in diagnosis. Surv Ophthalmol 21:351–355, 1977.
9. Apple DJ, Rabb MF: Ocular Pathology: Clinical Applications and Self-Assessment, 3rd ed. St. Louis, CV Mosby, 1985, pp 459–460.
10. Freedman J, Rohm G: Surgical management and histopathology of invasive tumours of the cornea. Br J Ophthalmol 63:632–635, 1979.
11. Nicholson DH, Herschler J: Intraocular extension of squamous cell carcinoma of the conjunctiva. Arch Ophthalmol 95:843–846, 1977.
12. Iliff WJ, Marback R, Green WR: Invasive squamous cell carcinoma of the conjunctiva. Arch Ophthalmol 93:119–122, 1975.
13. Li WW, Pettit TH, Zakka KA: Intraocular invasion by papillary squamous cell carcinoma of the conjunctiva. Am J Ophthalmol 90:697–701, 1980.
14. Wexler SA, Wallow IHL: Squamous cell carcinoma of the conjunctiva presenting with intraocular extension. Arch Ophthalmol 103:1175–1177, 1985.
15. Carroll JM, Kuwabara T: A classification of limbal epitheliomas. Arch Ophthalmol 73:545–551, 1965.
16. Ash JE, Wilder HC: Epithelial tumors of the limbus. Am J Ophthalmol 33:1203–1219, 1950.
17. Peksayar G, Soyturk MK, Demiryont M: Long-term results of cryotherapy on malignant epithelial tumors of the conjunctiva. Am J Ophthalmol 107:337–340, 1989.
18. Elkon D, Constable WC: The use of strontium-90 in the treatment of carcinoma in situ of the conjunctiva. Am J Ophthalmol 87:84–86, 1979.
19. Fraunfelder FT, Wingfield D: Management of intraepithelial conjunctival tumors and squamous cell carcinomas. Am J Ophthalmol 95:359–363, 1983.
20. Lommatzsch PK, Lommatzsch RE, Kirsch I, Fuhrman P: Therapeutic outcome of patients suffering from malignant melanomas of the conjunctiva. Br J Ophthalmol 74:615–619, 1990.
21. Zimmerman LE: Melanocytic tumors of interest to the ophthalmologist. Ophthalmology 87:497–502, 1980.
22. Folberg R, McLean IW, Zimmerman LE: Conjunctival melanosis and melanoma. Ophthalmology 91:673–678, 1984.
23. Folberg R, McLean IW, Zimmerman LE: Malignant melanoma of the conjunctiva. Hum Pathol 16:136–143, 1985.
24. Folberg R, McLean IW: Primary acquired melanosis and melanoma of the conjunctiva. Hum Pathol 17:652–654, 1986.
25. Jakobiec FA, Folberg R, Iwamoto T: Clinicopathologic characteristics of premalignant and malignant melanocytic lesions of the conjunctiva. Ophthalmology 96:147–166, 1989.
26. McDonnell JM, Carpenter JD, Jacobs P, et al: Conjunctival melanocytic lesions in children. Ophthalmology 96:986–993, 1989.
27. Hayton S, Lafreniere R, Jerry LM, et al: Ocular melanoma in Alberta: A 38-year review pointing to the importance of tumor size and tumor histology as predictors of survival. J Surg Oncol 42:215–218, 1989.
28. Fuchs U, Kivela T, Liesto K, Tarkkanen A: Prognosis of conjunctival melanomas in relation to histopathological features. Br J Cancer 59:261–267, 1989.
29. Jakobiec FA, Rini FJ, Fraunfelder FT, Brownstein S: Cryotherapy for conjunctival acquired melanosis and malignant melanoma. Ophthalmology 95:1058–1070, 1988.
30. Jakobiec FA, Brownstein S, Albert W, et al: The role of cryotherapy in the management of conjunctival melanoma. Ophthalmology 89:502–515, 1982.
31. Folberg R, Jakobiec FA, Bernardino VB, Iwamoto T: Benign conjunctival melanocytic lesions: Clinicopathologic features. Ophthalmology 96:436–461, 1989.
32. Jakobiec FA: Conjunctival melanoma: Unfinished business. Arch Ophthalmol 98:1378–1384, 1980.
33. Jakobiec FA, Brownstein S, Wilkinson RD, Katzin HM: Adjuvant cryotherapy for focal nodular melanoma of the conjunctiva. Arch Ophthalmol 100:115–118, 1982.
34. Robertson DM, Hungerford JL, McCartney A: Pigmentation of the eyelid margin accompanying conjunctival melanoma. Am J Ophthalmol 108:435–439, 1989.
35. Robertson DM, Hungerford JL, McCartney A: Malignant melanomas of the conjunctiva, nasal cavity, and paranasal sinuses. Am J Ophthalmol 108:440–442, 1989.
36. Dunbar SF, Lingood RM, Doppke KP, et al: Conjunctival lymphoma: Results and treatment with a single anterior electron field—a lens-sparing technique. Int J Radiat Oncol Biol Phys 19:249–257, 1990.
37. Knowles DM, Jakobiec FA, McNally L, Burke JS: Lymphoid hyperplasia and malignant lymphoma occurring in the ocular adnexa (orbit, conjunctiva, and eyelids): A prospective multiparametric analysis of 108 cases during 1977 to 1987. Hum Pathol 21:959–973, 1990.
38. Jakobiec FA, Knowles DM: An overview of ocular adnexal lymphoid tumors. Trans Am Ophthalmol Soc 87:420–444, 1989.
39. Medeiros LJ, Harris NL: Lymphoid infiltrates of the orbit and conjunctiva: A morphologic and immunophenotypic study of 99 cases. Am J Surg Pathol 13:459–471, 1989.
40. Weiter JJ, Jakobiec FA, Iwamoto T: The clinical and morphologic characteristics of Kaposi's sarcoma of the conjunctiva. Am J Ophthalmol 89:546–552, 1980.
41. Shuler JD, Holland GN, Miles SA, et al: Kaposi's sarcoma of the conjunctiva and eyelids associated with acquired immunodeficiency syndrome. Arch Ophthalmol 107:858–862, 1989.
42. Macher AM, Palestine A, Masur H, et al: Multicentric Kaposi's sarcoma of the conjunctiva in a male homosexual with the acquired immunodeficiency syndrome. Ophthalmology 90:879–884, 1983.
43. Holland GN, Pepose JS, Pettit TH, et al: Acquired immune deficiency syndrome: Ocular manifestations. Ophthalmology 90:859–873, 1983.
44. Palestine AG, Rodrigues MM, Macher AM, et al: Ophthalmic involvement in acquired immunodeficiency syndrome. Ophthalmology 91:1092–1099, 1984.
45. Howard GM, Jakobiec FA, DeVoe AG: Kaposi's sarcoma of the conjunctiva. Am J Ophthalmol 79:420–423, 1975.
46. Cooper JS, Fried PR: Treatment of aggressive epidemic Kaposi's sarcoma of the conjunctiva by radiotherapy. Arch Ophthalmol 106:20–21, 1988.

CHAPTER 19

Management of Conjunctival Amyloidosis

Brent A. Murphy and Ralph E. Wesley

Amyloidosis encompasses a group of disorders of unclear etiology with extracellular deposition of amyloid—an amorphous, heterogeneous, proteinaceous material that has distinctive ultrastructural, x-ray diffraction, and biochemical properties. Although amyloid is deposited in all body tissue as part of the normal aging process,[1] amyloidosis occurs based on distinct patterns and abnormal quantities.

Amyloid, meaning starch-like, is the term adopted by Virchow in 1854 to name the deposits in sectional organs resembling starch when stained with iodine and treated with dilute sulfuric acid.[2] Ultrastructurally, amyloid is composed of a protein component and a P component that form fine, nonbranching filaments that occur in a beta B-pleated sheet[2, 3] that renders amyloid resistant to phagocytosis. Amyloid demonstrates Congo red–induced green birefringence (change in refractive index when the plane of polarized light is varied), dichroism (change in color as polarized light is rotated through the tissue), and metachromasia with crystal violet.[4] The P component, an alpha-glycoprotein, comprises 5% to 10% of amyloid. The protein composition of amyloid varies with the specific type of amyloidosis.[5,6]

Three major amyloid protein groups are known: (1) the amyloid light chain (AL) protein, derived from plasma cells, which shows homology to immunoglobulin light chains and is found in the primary forms of amyloidosis; (2) amyloid A (AA) (believed to be derived from serum amyloid–associated protein), which has a homology with C-reactive protein[2, 3, 7] and is found in the secondary types of amyloidosis; and (3) amyloid F (AF), which occurs in several heredofamilial forms of amyloidosis (prealbumin makes up the protein component).

Clinically, amyloidosis is classified into six broad categories based on the presence or absence of underlying disease, family predisposition, and whether the disease is localized or systemic (Table 19–1). Primary and secondary systemic amyloidosis are by far the most common of these entities. However, conjunctival involvement is rare in primary systemic amyloidosis and to our knowledge is unknown in secondary systemic amyloidosis.[8–12]

When conjunctival involvement is present in primary systemic amyloidosis, additional ocular and extraocular manifestations of the disease are usually present (see Table 19–1). The most commonly involved site in primary systemic amyloidosis is the eyelid skin, virtually a pathognomonic sign of systemic disease.[5, 12] The conjunctival involvement may consist of characteristic amyloid nodules or may be diffuse and clinically inapparent.

No laboratory study is specific for amyloidosis. Elevated sedimentation rate and blood urea nitrogen and creatinine levels and proteinuria may occur.[13] Serum protein electrophoresis may be useful. Definitive diagnosis requires histopathologic study of biopsy material.

The prognosis for patients with primary systemic disease is poor, with an average survival of 1 to 4 years.[7] There is no proven effective therapy for this or any other form of amyloidosis, although colchicine may be helpful in slowing progression of the disease.[7] The most common cause of death is renal failure.

Secondary systemic amyloidosis is associated with multiple infectious and inflammatory disease states, as noted in Table 19–1. Conjunctival involvement is not seen in this form of the disease. Likewise, conjunctival involvement in amyloidosis occurring with multiple myeloma is not seen.[5,12]

Although certain heredofamilial forms of amyloidosis demonstrate ocular involvement (deposition of amyloid in the vitreous and cornea, adjacent to retinal vessels, and in ciliary nerves), conjunctival involvement has not been found (see Table 19–1).[1,5,12]

Localized forms of amyloidosis, as with systemic disease, may be primary or secondary. Localized amyloidosis, however, is significantly less common and involves only one organ. Primary localized amyloidosis is known to occur in a variety of sites (see Table 19–1), including the conjunctiva, and occurs in the absence of other predisposing diseases. Once believed to represent a forme fruste of systemic amyloidosis, it is known now that primary localized amyloidosis rarely, if ever, progresses to systemic disease.[12,14]

Primary localized conjunctival amyloidosis usually occurs in the fourth and fifth decades of life and affects men and women equally. Often asymptomatic for years,

TABLE 19-1
Classification of Amyloidosis

Amyloidosis Classification	Associated Diseases	Amyloid Type	Locations	Eye Involvement
Primary systemic	None	AL	Skin, heart, tongue, gastrointestinal tract, nerves, kidney	Rare: vitreous, extraocular muscles, trigeminal nerve branches, lacrimal gland, conjunctiva
Secondary systemic	Rheumatoid arthritis, tuberculosis, leprosy, Crohn's disease, ulcerative colitis, osteomyelitis, Hodgkin's disease, renal cell carcinoma	AA	Spleen, kidney, adrenal glands, liver	Rare
Multiple myeloma	Multiple myeloma	AL	Kidney, heart, joints, tongue,nerves, gastrointestinal tract	Cornea
Primary localized associated	None	AL*	Skin, uterus, heart, larynx, gastrointestinal system, tracheobronchial tree	Conjunctiva and lids, cornea, orbit, levator muscle
Secondary localized	Trachoma, tumor, sarcoid, chronic conjunctivitis, interstitial keratitis, psoriasis	AA	Skin	Conjunctiva
Heredofamilial	None	AF	Variable	Vitreous, cornea, retina

*One case reported with IgD heavy chain determinant.[16]
AL, amyloid light chain; AA, amyloid A; AF, prealbumin or protein A.
Adapted from Rosenblatt M, Spitz GF, Friedman AH, Kazam ES: Localized conjunctival amyloidosis: Case reports and review of the literature. Ophthalmologica 192:238-245, 1986; with permission of S. Karger, Basel.

its most common presentation is a swollen or ptotic eyelid.[5, 12] Ocular irritation and recurrent subconjunctival hemorrhage are less frequently presenting complaints.[8,12]

Amyloid commonly appears in the superior fornical or palpebral subconjunctival space as a discrete, yellow, waxy tumefaction, but any conjunctival location may be involved (Figs. 19-1 and 19-2). Ptosis can occur as shown in Figure 19-3 from mechanical factors or involvement of the levator aponeurosis.[12,15] Histopathologically, the lesions show irregular accumulations of amorphous, eosinophilic, hyaline substance with a variable degree of chronic inflammation.[1, 5] Diagnosis may be confirmed by biopsy tissue demonstrating green birefringence with Congo red stain.

Treatment of primary localized conjunctival amyloidosis should be undertaken in patients who manifest significant symptoms, bearing in mind that treatment is

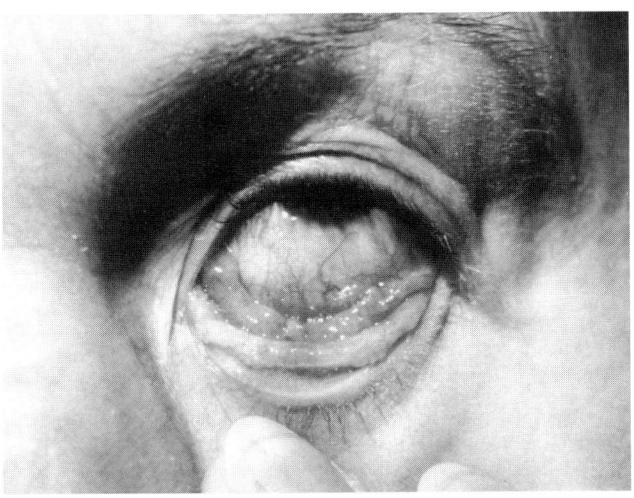

Figure 19-1. Amyloid in inferior fornix beneath the conjunctiva seen in at least two ridges.

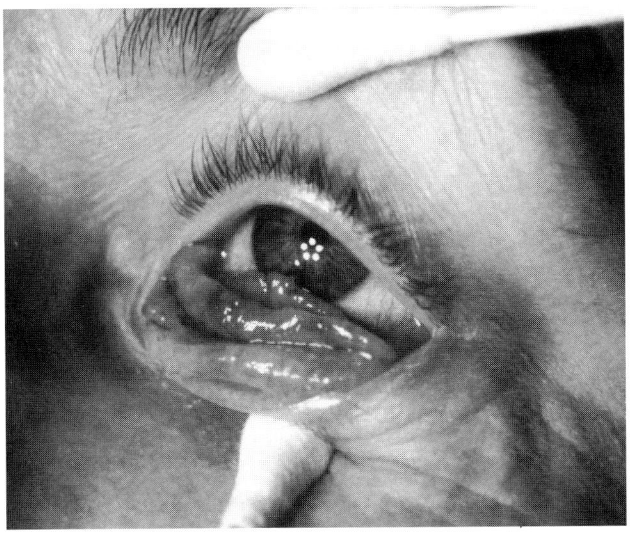

Figure 19-2. Massive amyloid creating irregular ridges in the inferior fornix. The irregular surface of the inferior conjunctival fornix makes salvaging conjunctiva difficult during surgery. Aggressive removal tends to cause loss of conjunctival lining of the inferior fornix.

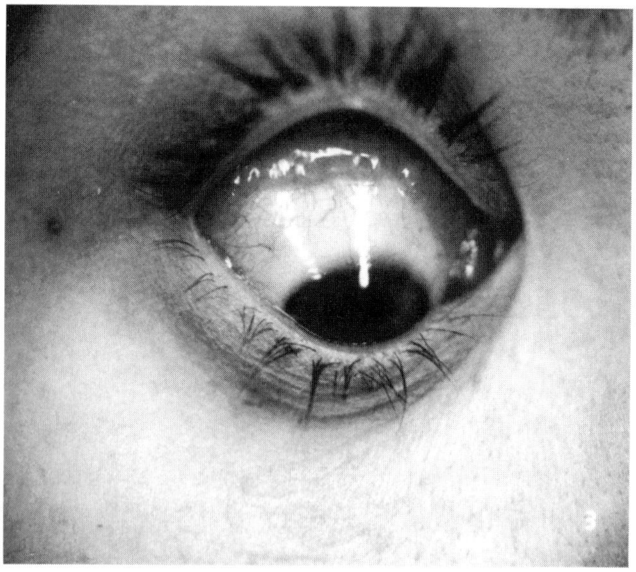

Figure 19–3. Patient with ptosis from amyloid, which can be seen under the superior bulbar conjunctiva.

palliative and recurrence highly likely. Pecora and associates[13] treated one case of localized conjunctival amyloidosis with external beam radiation. The total dose given was 3900 rads. This therapy produced partial regression of the disease, but surgical debulking was required 3 months after completion of the radiation therapy. Patrinely and Koch[15] reported two cases of advanced conjunctival and eyelid amyloidosis that were treated with meticulous debulking of the amyloid deposits while normal anatomic planes were respected. Both patients had good surgical results, but reaccumulation of amyloid occurred 6 months and 2 years postoperatively in these patients. Meticulous removal of amyloid deposits in primary conjunctival amyloidosis would appear preferable to other modalities of treatment, including radiation and en bloc excision in patients seeking palliation of symptoms. Orbital computed tomographic or magnetic resonance scanning may help delineate the extent of disease prior to surgical intervention.

The surgeon should remove just enough amyloid to provide satisfactory relief from the bulk effect of the amyloid. Aggressive removal may result in shortening the conjunctiva such that an ocular restrictive syndrome can be produced. One should assume that further accumulation and deposition of the amyloid will occur. The eyelids may be displaced away from the globe owing to massive accumulation of the material. The fornices are frequently shortened after the most conservative and careful surgical removal.

Ptosis is a common complication that must be treated in longstanding cases. Repeated repairs and removal of the amyloid can provide improvement for considerable periods, but the amyloid and ptosis relentlessly recur.

Secondary localized conjunctival amyloidosis can occur in the setting of chronic inflammatory disease (see Table 19–1). These include, but are not limited to, basal cell carcinoma, conjunctival sarcoid, chronic bacterial conjunctivitis, interstitial keratitis, and most commonly in trachoma.[12] The amyloid deposits found in secondary localized disease are usually diffuse and are not evident clinically; however, they may be detected histopathologically. Treatment in these cases is aimed at the underlying ocular disease.

SUMMARY

Amyloidosis is a heterogeneous group of diseases with unclear etiology and no proven effective treatment. The pathogenesis of amyloid formation is related to both the overproduction of precursor proteins and their defective degradation in either a localized or systemic fashion.[2] Conjunctival involvement may occur in primary systemic amyloidosis and necessarily occurs in primary and secondary localized conjunctival amyloidosis. This conjunctival involvement may bring the patient to the ophthalmologist in the nodular form as seen in primary localized conjunctival amyloidosis and in primary systemic amyloidosis.

Localized conjunctival amyloidosis is a benign, local process, whereas conjunctival disease plus amyloid deposits in eyelid skin heralds systemic disease.

The diagnosis of amyloidosis must be made histopathologically. Once made, consultation with an internist is advisable to clearly establish whether the disease is localized or systemic. Once the appropriate workup is complete, consideration may be given to surgical intervention related to conjunctival and ocular adnexal disease.

REFERENCES

1. Knowles PM, Jakobiec FA, Rosen M, Howard G: Amyloidosis of the orbit and adnexal. Surv Ophthalmol 19:367–384, 1975.
2. Robbins SL, Cotran RS, Kumar V: Pathologic Basis of Disease, 3rd ed. Philadelphia, WB Saunders, 1984, pp 195–205.
3. Schrier SL: Amyloidosis. *In* Rubenstein E, Federman DD (eds): Scientific American Medicine. New York, Scientific American, 1988, Section 5-IX, pp 8–10.
4. Yanoff M, Fine BS: Ocular Pathology: A Text and Atlas, 2nd ed. Philadelphia, Harper & Row, 1982, pp 287–288.
5. Rosenblatt M, Spitz GF, Friedman AH, Kazam ES: Localized conjunctival amyloidosis: Case reports and review of the literature. Ophthalmologica 192:238–245, 1986.
6. Borodic GE, Beyer-Machule CK, Millin J, et al: Immunoglobulin deposition in localized conjunctival amyloidosis. Am J Ophthalmol 98:617–622, 1984.
7. Cohen AS: Amyloidosis. *In* Petersdorf RG, Adams RD (eds): Harrison's Principles of Internal Medicine, 10th ed. New York, McGraw-Hill, 1983, pp 368–371.
8. Iijima S: Primary systemic amyloidosis: A unique case complaining of diffuse eyelid swelling and conjunctival involvement. J Dermatol 19:113–118, 1992.

9. Bene C, Kranias G: Ocular amyloidosis: Clinical points learned from one case. Ann Ophthalmol 22:101–102, 1990.
10. Purcell JJ Jr, Birkenkamp R, Tsai CC, Riner RN: Conjunctival involvement in primary systemic nonfamilial amyloidosis. Am J Ophthalmol 95:845–847, 1983.
11. Stansburg JR: Conjunctival amyloidosis in association with systemic amyloid disease. Am J Ophthalmol 59:24–29, 1965.
12. Brownstein MH, Elliott R, Helwig EB: Ophthalmologic aspects of amyloidosis. Am J Ophthalmol 69:423–430, 1970.
13. Pecora JL, Sambursky JS, Vargha Z: Radiation therapy in amyloidosis of the eyelid and conjunctiva: A case report. Ann Ophthalmol 14:194–196, 1982.
14. Schwartz MF, Green WR, Michels RG, et al: An unusual case of ocular involvement in primary systemic non-familial amyloidosis. Ophthalmology 89:394, 1982.
15. Patrinely JR, Koch DD: Surgical management of advanced ocular adnexal amyloidosis. Arch Ophthalmol 110:882–885, 1992.
16. Schaldernbrand JD, Keren DF: IgD amyloid in IgD-lambda monoclonal conjunctival amyloidosis. Arch Pathol Lab Med 107:626, 1983.

CHAPTER 20

Kaposi's Sarcoma of the Conjunctiva

Brent A. Murphy and Ralph E. Wesley

Kaposi's sarcoma was a rare endemic disease of equatorial Africa before the onset of acquired immunodeficiency syndrome (AIDS) from infection with human immunodeficiency virus.[1-4] Kaposi's sarcoma now occurs in approximately 37% of patients with AIDS; 20% have ophthalmic involvement.[5,6] This entity of multiple idiopathic hemorrhagic vascular sarcomas of skin, mucosal surfaces, lymph nodes, and viscera was first described by Moricz Kaposi in 1872.[7]

Conjunctival lesions occur most often in the inferior fornix as deep red or violaceous macules, plaques, or nodules (Fig. 20–1) that may be mistaken for a subconjunctival hemorrhage.[8] These lesions may be the slow-growing, asymptomatic presentation of AIDS. Some lesions enlarge to cause ectropion, ptosis, or direct visual obstruction.

Histopathologically, the tumors have spindle-shaped cells with nuclear pleomorphism, dilated vascular clefts with prominent endothelial cells with well-formed capillaries, and a perivascular and diffuse chronic inflammatory infiltrate. The conjunctiva may demonstrate squamous metaplasia. There may be extravasation of erythrocytes from the vascular channels with hemosiderin deposition.[9,10]

Vasoformative mesenchymal cells, specifically endothelial cells and pericytes, are believed to be the progenitors of this tumor. Factor VIII–related antigen on immunoperoxidase staining and Weibel-Palade bodies with electron microscopy[11,12] are markers characteristic of vascular endothelium found in Kaposi's sarcoma.[13]

TREATMENT

Treatment of conjunctival Kaposi's sarcoma in patients with AIDS is predominantly palliative since excision is rarely curative. Multifocal lesions and widespread cutaneous and visceral involvement are common. Treatment is indicated for lesions causing visual obstruction, ocular irritation, and surface problems and sometimes for cosmetic reasons. Treatment is not necessary for all diagnosed cases of conjunctival Kaposi's sarcoma. Before the advent of AIDS, local excision of isolated lesions was frequently curative,[8,9] but Kaposi's sarcoma in patients with AIDS is more fulminant than in patients without AIDS.[14-16]

Treatment modalities for patients with conjunctival Kaposi's sarcoma include cryotherapy, radiation therapy, and excision.[7,17,18] Chemotherapy and immunotherapy are available for systemic disease. Radiation therapy has been used with good results and minimal ocular toxicity using 3000 rads delivered in 10 fractions of 300 rads over 2 weeks.[17] Despite treatment by excision, radiation therapy, or cryotherapy, the lesions frequently recur within the first year.

Systemic disease may be treated with chemotherapy. Ocular lesions unresponsive to systemic therapy usually respond to focal irradiation.

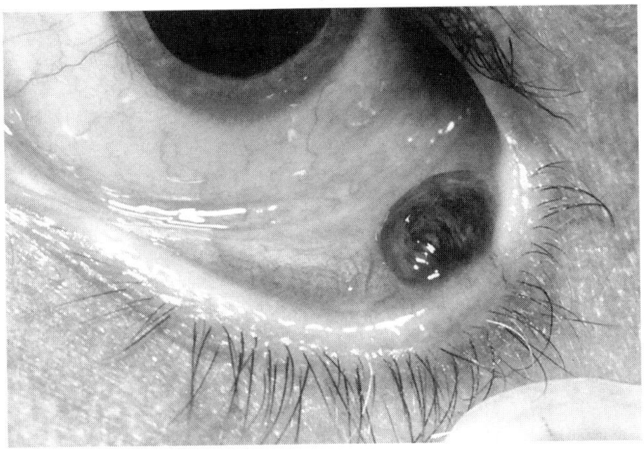

Figure 20–1. Conjunctival Kaposi's sarcoma.

REFERENCES

1. Laor Y, Schwartz RA: Epidemiologic aspects of American Kaposi's sarcoma. J Surg Oncol 12:299–303, 1979.
2. Rothman S: Remarks on the sex, age, and racial distribution of Kaposi's sarcoma and on possible pathogenetic factors. Acta Un Int Cancr 18:326–329, 1962.
3. Oettle AG: Geographical and racial differences in the frequency of Kaposi's sarcoma as evidence of environmental or genetic causes. Acta Un Int Cancr 18:330–363, 1962.
4. Safai B, Good RA: Kaposi's sarcoma: A review and recent developments. CA 31:2–12, 1981.
5. Centers for Disease Control: Update: Acquired immunodeficiency syndrome—United States. MMWR 35:17–21, 1986.
6. Shuler JD, Holland GN, Miles SA, et al: Kaposi sarcoma of the conjunctiva and eyelids associated with the acquired immunodeficiency syndrome. Arch Ophthalmol. 107:858–862, 1989.
7. Kaposi M: Idiopathesches multiples Pigments, Sarcom de Haut. Arch Derm Syph (Wein) 4:256, 1872.
8. Shuler JD, Engstrom RE Jr, Holland GN: External ocular disease and anterior segment disorders associated with AIDS. Int Ophthalmol Clin 29:98–104, 1989.
9. Weiter JJ, Jakobiec FA, Iwanoto T: The clinical and morphologic characteristics of Kaposi's sarcoma of the conjunctiva.
10. Howard GM, Jakobiec FA, Devoe AG: Kaposi's sarcoma of the conjunctiva. Am J Ophthalmol 79:420–423, 1975.
11. Gokel JM, Kurzi R, Hubner G: Fine structure and origin of Kaposi's sarcoma. Pathol Eur 11:45–47, 1976.
12. Nadji M, Morales AR, Ziegles-Weissman J, et al: Kaposi's sarcoma: Immunohistologic evidence for an endothelial origin. Arch Pathol Lab Med 105:274–275, 1981.
13. Thorgeirsson G, Robertson AL Jr: The vascular endothelium: Pathobiologic significance. Am J Pathol 93:803–848, 1978.
14. Hymes KB, Cheung T, Greene JB, et al: Kaposi's sarcoma in homosexual men—a report of eight cases. Lancet 2:598–600, 1981.
15. Macher AM, Palestine A, Masur H, et al: Multicentric Kaposi's sarcoma of the conjunctiva in a male homosexual with the acquired immunodeficiency syndrome. Ophthalmology 90:879–884, 1983.
16. Holland GN, Pepose JS, Pettit TH, et al: Acquired immune deficiency syndrome: Ocular manifestations. Ophthalmology 90:859–873, 1983.
17. Cooper JS, Fried PR: Treatment of aggressive epidemic Kaposi's sarcoma of the conjunctiva by radiotherapy. Arch Ophthalmol 106:20–21, 1988.
18. Cooper JS, Fried PR: Defining the role of radiation therapy in the management of epidemic Kaposi's sarcoma. Int J Radiat Oncol Biol Phys 13:35–39, 1987.

C H A P T E R 2 1

Lymphoid Tumors of the Conjunctiva

Brent A. Murphy and Ralph E. Wesley

Benign and malignant lymphoid tumors of the conjunctiva are often difficult to differentiate based on clinical and histopathologic analysis alone.[1-4] Immunophenotypic studies in conjunction with improved histopathologic classification have aided in accurate diagnosis of these tumors but have added little to the ability to predict the subsequent development of extraocular lymphoma.[5,6] Most published studies investigating ocular adnexal lymphoid neoplasms have extrapolated data from a relatively small number of patients with conjunctival tumors.

HISTOLOGY

The conjunctiva contains lymphoid tissue with lymphocytes and plasma cells found in the substantia propria of the conjunctiva, with greatest density in the fornices.[7,8] Scattered lymphocytes are also found in conjunctival epithelium. Conjunctival lymphatics drain to the preauricular, submental, and cervical lymph nodes. This population of lymphocytes gives rise to primary conjunctival neoplasms.

CLASSIFICATION AND CLINICAL FEATURES

Lymphoid neoplasms of the ocular adnexa account for 10% to 15% of all orbital tumor masses.[9] Although reports vary, conjunctival lymphoid tumors account for just less than half of all orbital tumors.[10] Lymphoid neoplasms of the conjunctiva (and orbit) may be classified by histopathologic and immunophenotypic methods as reactive lymphoid hyperplasia, as atypical lymphoid hyperplasia, as indeterminate, or as malignant non-Hodgkin's lymphoma. Lymphoid hyperplasias are subclassified as diffuse or follicular type. Malignant lymphomas are subclassified according to the Working Formulation for Non-Hodgkin's Lymphoma based on cytomorphologic features.[11] Virtually all ocular adnexal lymphomas are B cell lymphomas, with small cell lymphocytic lymphoma being by far the most common. To our knowledge only one report of an ocular adnexal tumor composed predominantly of T lymphocytes exists in the literature.[12]

Clinically, these tumors are often indistinguishable, presenting as freely movable salmon-colored patches (Fig. 21 – 1) commonly in the fornices or on the epibulbar conjunctiva. Ellis and coworkers[13] have correlated multinodular, minimally elevated lesions with a greater likelihood of benignity and larger, smooth lesions with a greater likelihood of malignancy. Diagnosis depends on the biopsy results of suspicious lesions.

HISTOPATHOLOGIC ANALYSIS

Histopathologically, benign lesions include diffuse and follicular lymphoid hyperplasia. The diffuse variant displays a monomorphous infiltrate of small, mature lymphocytes, whereas the follicular variant demonstrates these lymphocytes with activated germinal centers. Both lesions are richly vascularized and often have prominent endothelial cells.[4] The histogenesis of these tumors is not well understood but is believed to represent a reaction to an exogenous or endogenous stimulus. Atypical lymphoid hyperplasia appears as a nodular or diffuse infiltrate containing mature lymphocytes, plasma cells, and atypical lymphoid cells with larger, hyperchromatic nuclei.

Malignant lesions are composed of dense, homogeneous small lymphocytes with significant cellular atypia. Similar-appearing infiltrates that demonstrate minimal cellular atypia are considered indeterminate lesions.

IMMUNOPHENOTYPIC ANALYSIS

Immunophenotypic analysis is used to identify the presence or absence of B and T lymphocytes and the clonality of the B cells present, performed on either cell suspensions or frozen sections. This technique presumably allows for better characterization of the benign (polyclonal immunoglobulin expression) or malignant

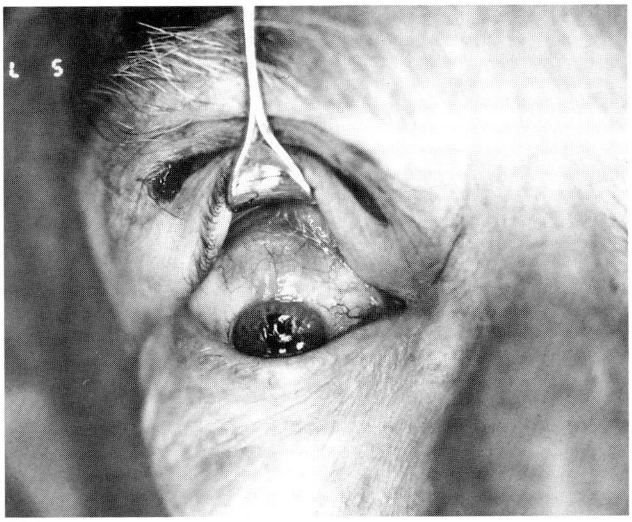

Figure 21 – 1. Subconjunctival lymphoma in the superior fornix.

(monoclonal immunoglobulin expression) nature of lymphoid tumors not otherwise discernible by histopathologic study. This technology has shown that polyclonal lesions generally have a predominance of T lymphocytes (3:2 T to B), whereas monoclonal lesions often have less than 40% T cells.[7] Although this technology is of diagnostic aid, studies have demonstrated that as many as 30% of patients with polyclonal tumors have or develop subsequent extraocular monoclonal lymphoma.[7, 13] Therefore, classifying lesions as histopathologically and immunophenotypically benign or malignant is not useful in predicting the occurrence of extraocular lymphoma.

MOLECULAR GENETIC ANALYSIS

Molecular genetic analysis of deoxyribonucleic acid extracted from cells of biopsy specimens can be used to identify unique gene rearrangement patterns indicative of malignancy in lymphoid cell populations.[14] With this technology, clonal B cell populations can be detected at a level otherwise undetectable by morphologic and immunophenotypic analysis. Tumors from patients with bilateral ocular adnexal lymphoid neoplasms were studied and demonstrated that these bilateral lesions were essentially identical proliferations in both benign and malignant diseases. Greater availability and application of molecular genetic analysis of ocular adnexal lymphoid neoplasms promise to provide better diagnostic and treatment approaches.

DEMOGRAPHICS

Conjunctival lymphoid neoplasia is predominantly a disease of the elderly. Median ages reported in most series fall in the early 60s and do not differ for lymphoid hyperplasia and malignant lymphoma.[1, 6, 13, 15] Women are affected somewhat more often than men. Bilateral conjunctival disease is not common and ranges anywhere from 0% to 50% depending on the study reviewed.[13, 14] Conflicting data exist regarding unilateral versus bilateral disease and the incidence of malignancy in each. Some studies indicate that unilateral and bilateral disease do not differ in rates of malignancy and extraocular lymphoma,[6] whereas others demonstrate that bilaterality is often indicative of malignancy.[13, 14] Sufficient numbers of patients are lacking to draw firm conclusions. Malignant lesions outnumber benign lesions 3:1. Primary ocular adnexal lymphomas are estimated to account for 5% to 14% of all extranodal non-Hodgkin's lymphomas.[16, 17] Approximately half of these occur in the conjunctiva.[10] Small cell lymphocytic lymphoma is by far the most common type encountered. Between 25% and 30% of patients diagnosed with lymphoid hyperplasia have concurrent extraocular malignant lymphoma or develop extraocular disease subsequent to their diagnosis.[7, 13] A similar number of patients with diffuse small or intermediate lymphocytic lymphoma have or develop extraocular disease. For this reason these two groups of patients receive similar treatment and share similar prognoses. In contradistinction, nearly half of patients with all other types of malignant lymphoma present with or develop systemic disease.[6]

Prognosis, therefore, relates primarily to histopathologic diagnosis and the disease stage at presentation. Five-year actuarial survival rates for patients with high- and low-grade lymphoma are 59% and 80%, respectively.[18] Those diagnosed with indeterminate lesions had an 88% 5-year survival. At 10 years the survival rates drop to 25%, 63%, and 68%, respectively. The survival curve for those patients with low-grade and indeterminate lesions parallels that of the general population. In addition, more than half of the patients in one study died of intercurrent illness unrelated to lymphoma. Other studies have corroborated these data and suggest that patients with lymphoid hyperplasia and low-grade lymphoma share similar clinical courses.

PATIENT EVALUATION

The workup of patients with conjunctival lymphoid lesions does not differ for patients with lymphoid hyperplasia or malignant lymphoma. All lesions should undergo biopsy. Once a working diagnosis is established, every patient should have a systemic evaluation by a hematologist or oncologist. This evaluation typically includes a complete history and physical examination, complete blood cell count, serum protein electrophoresis, chest radiography, abdominal computed tomography, and bone marrow biopsy. Computed tomography of the orbits and brain is not indicated in the absence of orbital or central nervous system signs or symptoms.[10] Extraocular lymphoma is found at the initial systemic workup or within 6 months of presentation in most patients.[6] Systemic reevaluation is recommended every 6 months thereafter for 5 years since some patients will develop systemic disease beyond the initial 6-month period. The stage of the disease will determine the appropriate therapy and does carry with it useful prognostic information. In their study of ocular adnexal lymphoid hyperplasia and malignant lymphoma, Knowles and colleagues[6] found a statistically significant difference in survival rates for patients with stage 1E disease (reactive lymphoid hyperplasia and malignant lymphoma) as compared with patients with systemic lymphoma.

TREATMENT

Treatment issues for conjunctival lymphoid hyperplasia and lymphoma are complex. In general, radiation therapy is the treatment of choice for all ocular adnexal lesions whether they are associated with systemic disease or not. Surgery alone, as well as systemic therapy with corticosteroids or chemotherapeutic agents, is ineffective for treating ocular disease.[19] The goal of therapy is complete regression of the ocular lesion while minimizing ocular morbidity. A total dose of 1500 to 2000 rads, delivered to the entire conjunctiva, has been recommended for localized unilateral or bilateral ocular adnexal lymphoid hyperplasia and small and intermediate lymphocytic lymphomas. Total doses of 2000 to 3000 rads are advocated for higher-grade lymphomas.[6, 10, 19] The doses are generally fractionated into 200 rads per day for 5 days per week or 250 rads per day for 4 days per week.

Regression rates of ocular adnexal disease after radiation therapy are high. Dunbar and associates[20] have described the use of anterior electron beam therapy in the treatment of conjunctival lymphoma with good results and low morbidity. Chemotherapy is indicated, in addition to the radiation therapy, if there is systemic lymphoma and often in younger patients with isolated ocular adnexal disease.

Ocular morbidity associated with local radiation therapy, despite shielding techniques, includes cataract formation, radiation keratitis, keratitis sicca, radiation retinopathy, ptosis, madarosis, and orbital fat atrophy.[13] With advances in delivery and shielding techniques, these complications have been greatly reduced. The lens is the most radiosensitive structure in the orbit, and cataract formation is the primary concern with modern therapy.[10] Posterior subcapsular cataracts form due to irradiation of the germinative zone of the anterior lens epithelium that resides in the lens periphery.[21] The cataract latent period after exposure is 6 months to 30 years and is inversely related to the total dose of radiation. The goal during therapy is to limit lens exposure to less than 600 rads, and this is frequently possible using a contact lens with a central lead shield.[10, 21]

SUMMARY

Lymphoid tumors of the conjunctiva are tumors seen in the elderly population and are not uncommon. Despite this fact, little is known about their pathogenesis and the relationship between reactive lymphoid hyperplasia and malignant lymphoma. Clinically, it is not possible to distinguish benign lymphoid proliferations from malignant lymphoma. Through histopathologic, immunophenotypic, and molecular genetic analysis, classifications of benign, indeterminate, and malignant disease are possible, yet benign and indeterminate disease may later give rise to malignant lymphoma or exist concurrently with systemic malignant lymphoma. The benign, indeterminate, and low-grade malignant lesions share similar prognosis and treatment. Higher-grade malignant lesions carry a more guarded prognosis.

Critical to the diagnostic and treatment process of these patients is the multidisciplinary approach involving the ophthalmologist, oncologist, and radiation oncologist. Radiation therapy for conjunctival lymphoid neoplasms is often rewarding, with complete regression of the tumor; however, these patients must be followed for a long period for evidence of recurrence. Recurrent ocular adnexal disease in a patient previously diagnosed with reactive lymphoid hyperplasia requires repeat biopsy testing to rule out malignant lymphoma.

REFERENCES

1. Knowles DM, Jakobiec FA: Ocular adnexal lymphoid neoplasms: Clinical, histopathologic, electron microscopic, and immunologic characteristics. Hum Pathol 13:148–162, 1982.
2. Knowles, DM, Jakobiec FA: Cell marker analysis of extranodal lymphoid infiltrates: To what extent does the determination of mono- or polyclonality resolve the diagnostic dilemma of malignant lymphoma vs. pseudolymphoma in an extranodal site? Semin Diagn Pathol 2:163–168, 1985.
3. Jakobiec FA, McLean I, Font R: Clinicopathologic characteristics of orbital lymphoid hyperplasia. Ophthalmology 86:948–966, 1979.
4. Knowles DM, Jakobiec FA: Orbital lymphoid neoplasms: A clinicopathologic study of 60 patients. Cancer 46:576–589, 1980.
5. Khalil HA, de Keizer RJW, Kevin PM, et al: Clinical course and pathologic features of conjunctival non-Hodgkin's lymphoma. Graefes Arch Clin Exp Ophthalmol 228:246–251, 1990.
6. Knowles DM, Jakobiec FA, McNally L, Burke JS: Lymphoid hyperplasia and malignant lymphoma occurring in the ocular adnexa (orbit, conjunctiva and eyelids): A prospective, multiparametric analysis of 108 cases during 1977 to 1987. Hum Pathol 21:959–973, 1990.
7. Jakobiec FA, Lefkowitch J, Knowles DML: B and T lymphocytes in ocular disease. Ophthalmology 91:635–654, 1984.
8. Jakobiec FA, Iwamoto T: Ocular adnexa: Introduction to lids, conjunctiva and orbit. *In* Jakobiec FA (ed): Ocular Anatomy, Embryology, and Teratology. Philadelphia, Harper & Row, 1982, pp 677–731.
9. Reese AB: Expanding lesions of the orbit. Trans Ophthalmol Soc UK 91:85, 1971.
10. Jereb B: Radiation therapy of the neoplasms of the eye and orbit. *In*

Hornblass A (ed): Oculoplastic, Orbital, and Reconstructive Surgery, Vol 2, Orbit and Lacrimal System. Baltimore, Williams & Wilkins, 1990, pp 1089-1101.

11. The non-Hodgkin's lymphoma pathologic classification project. National Cancer Institute-sponsored study of classification of non-Hodgkin's lymphoma: Summary and description of a working formulation for clinical usage. Cancer 49:2112-2135, 1982.
12. Laroche L, Pavlakis E, Saraux H: Immunological characterization of an ocular adnexal lymphoid T tumor by monoclonal antibodies. Ophthalmologica 187:43-49, 1983.
13. Ellis JH, Banks PM, Campbell RJ, Liesegang TJ: Lymphoid tumors of the ocular adnexa: Clinical correlation with the working formulation classification and immunoperoxidase staining of paraffin sections. Ophthalmology 92:1311-1324, 1985.
14. McNally L, Jakobiec FA, Knowles DM: Clinical morphologic, immunophenotypic, and molecular genetic analysis of bilateral ocular adnexal lymphoid neoplasms in 17 patients. Am J Ophthalmol 103:555-568, 1987.
15. Medeiros LJ, Harris NL: Lymphoid infiltration of the orbit and conjunctiva: A morphologic and immunophenotypic study of 99 cases. Am J Surg Pathol 13:459-471, 1989.
16. Horwich A, Peckham MJ: "Bad risk" non-Hodgkin's lymphomas. Semin Haematol 20:35-56, 1983.
17. Timothy AR, Lister TA, Katz D, Jones AE: Localized non-Hodgkin's lymphoma. Eur J Cancer 16:799-807, 1980.
18. Bessell EM, Henk JM, Wright JE, Whitelocke RAF: Orbital and conjunctival lymphoma treatment and prognosis. Radiother Oncol 13:237-244, 1988.
19. Jereb B, Lee H, Jakobiec FA, Kutcher J: Radiation therapy of conjunctival and orbital lymphoid tumors. Int J Radiat Oncol Biol Phys 10:1013-1019, 1984.
20. Dunbar SF, Lingood RM, Doppke KP, et al: Conjunctival lymphoma: Results and treatment with a single anterior electron field —a lens-sparing approach. Int J Radiat Oncol Biol Phys 19:249-257, 1990.
21. Bessell EM, Henk JM, Whitelocke RAF, Wright JE: Ocular morbidity after radiotherapy of orbital and conjunctival lymphoma. Eye 1:90-96, 1987.

CHAPTER 22

Conjunctival Procedures for Corneal Disease

Alice Y. Matoba

GUNDERSEN CONJUNCTIVAL FLAP TECHNIQUE

Indications

The primary indications for a conjunctival flap are poor visual potential of the eye in conjunction with chronic ocular surface disease compromising the integrity of the corneal epithelium, debilitating chronic pain, and significant risk of infection. In patients with good visual potential, alternative therapy is dictated by the nature of the underlying problem.

Contraindications to placement of a conjunctival flap include active microbial or viral corneal infection, poor structural integrity (presence of a descemetocele or corneal perforation), and necessity for visualization of the anterior chamber. In patients with marked conjunctival scarring or chronic inflammatory conditions such as cicatricial pemphigoid, the conjunctiva is usually not suitable for the creation of a conjunctival flap.

Surgical Technique (Gundersen Type)

A 360-degree peritomy is created at the limbus and the conjunctiva is dissected for several millimeters with blunt scissors. A traction suture can be placed through the superficial sclera near the limbus at the 12 o'clock position to facilitate downward rotation of the globe. The eye is rotated inferiorly, and a horizontal incision is placed through the upper conjunctiva after the reflection of the bulbar conjunctiva on the superior tarsal fold. The incision should be approximately 3 cm, extending from canthus to canthus. The conjunctiva is dissected down to the limbus with blunt scissors (Fig. 22–1). The tip of the scissors should be continuously visualized through the conjunctival flap to prevent inadvertent perforation. If some visualization of the anterior chamber is desired, the flap should be dissected thinly. Once the dissection has been completed and is continuous with the peritomy, the dissection should be extended laterally and medially. Relaxing incisions should be made along the superior incision as necessary to ensure that there is no traction on the conjunctival flap when it is placed over the cornea.

Corneal and perilimbal epithelia are removed completely with a no. 64 Beaver blade. The flap is then placed over the cornea and secured just below the limbus at the 5 and 7 o'clock positions with 7-0 Vicryl mattress sutures. A running suture is used to close the inferior conjunctiva (Fig. 22–2). Three to four interrupted sutures are placed through the superficial sclera to secure the upper border of the flap. If inadvertent perforation has occurred, 10-0 nylon sutures can be used to seal the perforation. Partial thickness bites are passed with the knots exposed so that the nylon suture is not in direct contact with the surface of the cornea. Factors important to the success of a conjunctival flap include complete removal of corneal and limbal epithelium, adequate dissection of the graft to avoid tension, and avoidance of perforation, particularly in the area that directly covers the cornea.

Postoperative Management

Bacitracin-polymyxin or erythromycin ophthalmic ointment may be used three to four times a day until the sclera is epithelialized. Perforation, retraction, or erosion of the flap from traction or exposure is most likely during the first 3 weeks postoperatively.

CONJUNCTIVAL RESECTION FOR SUPERIOR LIMBIC KERATOCONJUNCTIVITIS

Indications

Conjunctival resection can be considered in a patient with superior limbic keratoconjunctivitis, which is characterized by the presence of redundant, slightly chemotic superior bulbar conjunctiva. Other clinical features of superior limbic keratoconjunctivitis include hyperemia of the superior bulbar conjunctiva, staining of the superior bulbar conjunctival epithelium with rose bengal, fine papillary reaction of the superior tarsal conjunctiva, filament formation on the superior cornea, and symptoms of foreign-body sensation.

Alternative therapy providing short-term relief of

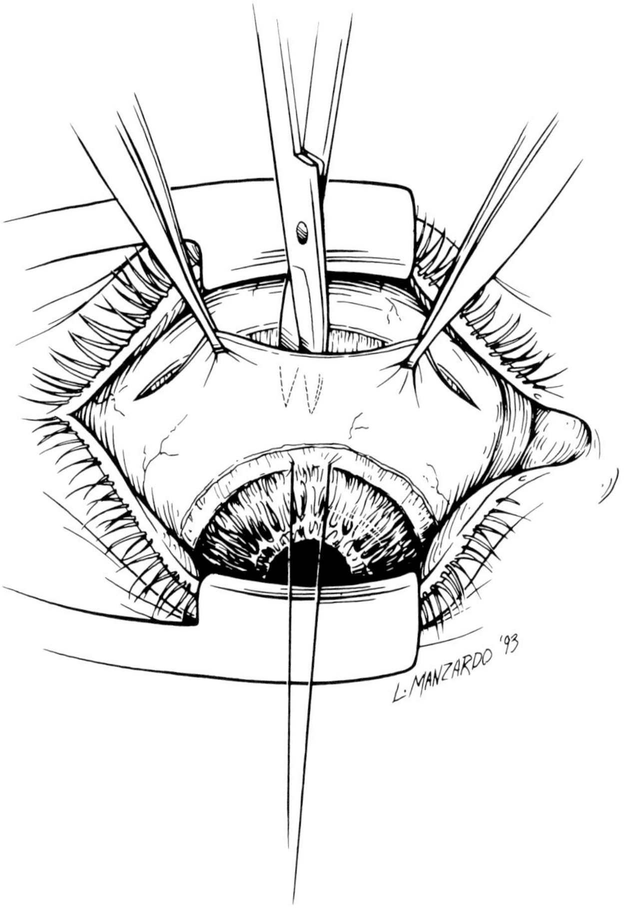

Figure 22–1. Gundersen flap technique: the conjunctiva is dissected down to the limbus, with the tip of the blunt scissors continuously visualized through the conjunctival flap to prevent inadvertent perforation.

symptoms includes treatment with 0.5% silver nitrate and placement of a therapeutic soft contact lens. In view of the association of therapeutic soft contact lenses with increased risk for development of microbial keratitis, the use of a therapeutic contact lens should be considered an adjunctive or temporary therapeutic modality. Cauterization of the superior bulbar conjunctiva may also be effective by producing conjunctival shrinkage.

Surgical Technique

Rose bengal 1% is applied to the superior bulbar conjunctiva to delineate the area of epithelial abnormality, which usually coincides with the area of greatest bulbar conjunctival redundancy. After instillation of topical anesthetic and with observation with the slit lamp biomicroscope, the physician should gently press the superior bulbar conjunctiva with an applicator stick to delineate the area of most pronounced conjunctival redundancy. If necessary, the conjunctiva can be marked with gentian violet. After insertion of the lid speculum, the superior bulbar conjunctiva should be excised 0.5 mm from the superior limbus up to 7 mm from the limbus, between the 10 and 2 o'clock positions. Care should be made to avoid the area of insertion of the superior rectus muscle. The perilimbal epithelium should not be removed so as to spare the putative corneal epithelial stem cells.

The eye should be patched after instillation of topical antibiotic and corticosteroid ointment. Thereafter, bacitracin-polymyxin or erythromycin ointment is administered three to four times per day until the epithelium is intact. Topical corticosteroid is added if significant inflammation develops.

CONJUNCTIVAL AUTOGRAFT TO REPOPULATE THE CORNEAL EPITHELIUM

Indication

The major indication for conjunctival autografts to treat ocular surface epithelial deficiency is chronic, unilateral, diffuse corneal epithelial deficiency, characterized by recurrent epithelial erosion, superficial vascularization, or both. This condition is usually due to chemical injury. The pathogenesis is believed to be a deficiency of the limbal epithelial stem cells. Alternative therapy includes keratoepithelioplasty and limbal stem cell transplantation from the fellow eye. If the limbal epithelium is intact in the fellow eye, limbal stem cell trans-

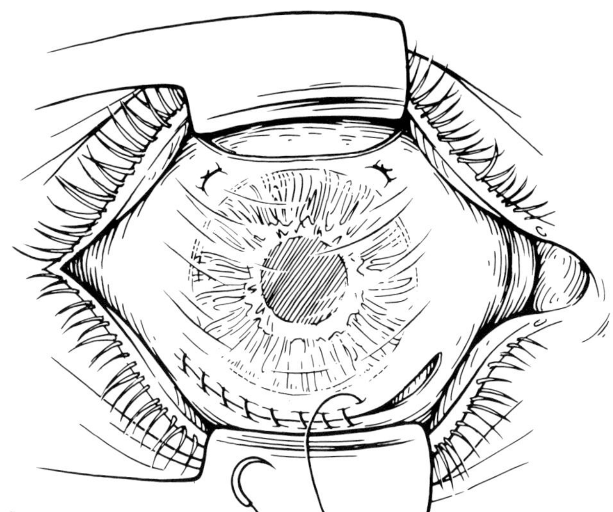

Figure 22–2. Gundersen flap closed inferiorly with 10-0 nylon running suture. Three or four interrupted sutures are placed through the superficial sclera to secure the upper border of the flap. Inadvertent perforations can be sealed with 10-0 nylon sutures.

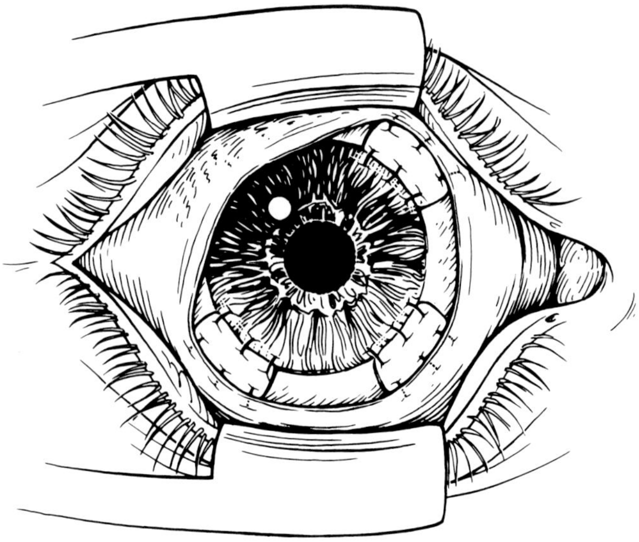

Figure 22–3. Conjunctival grafts are placed at the limbus of the injured eye, with the edge of the graft just bridging the limbus.

plantation is preferable because it is associated with less vascularization of the recipient cornea.

Surgical Technique

The corneal epithelium and superficial pannus is removed with a no. 64 Beaver blade or other suitable instrument. The perilimbal conjunctiva and corneal pannus are excised in all heavily vascularized quadrants. The donor conjunctival grafts, which are approximately 3 × 4 mm, are harvested from the superior bulbar conjunctiva of the fellow eye. Up to four conjunctival grafts are placed at the limbus of the injured eye, with the edge of the graft just bridging the limbus (Fig. 22–3). Epithelium is not transplanted to quadrants with minimal pannus and healthy-appearing limbal tissue. The grafts are secured with 10-0 nylon with the knots buried. A large-diameter extended-wear soft contact lens is applied. Broad-spectrum antibiotic solution is used two to four times per day until the epithelium is intact.

CHAPTER 23

Treatment of Squamous Papillomas of the Conjunctiva

Ralph E. Wesley and Harvey P. Cole III

Squamous papillomas of the conjunctiva tend to occur in younger patients as a fleshy nuisance arising primarily from the medial portion of the conjunctiva near the caruncle, the upper and lower fornices, and the bulbar area (Fig. 23–1). Although most of these lesions respond to excision or cryotherapy, as many as 20% of patients have multiple recurrences that are difficult to eradicate.[1]

Conjunctival papillomas may occur in elderly patients, but most of the recurrences have been in young children, who require general anesthesia to excise lesions or treat recurrences.

Some smaller lesions may be asymptomatic with little elevation above the conjunctival surface. Most lesions are usually unilateral, multifocal lesions that may create some redness to the affected area and are accentuated with a mucous discharge as the mass and number of lesions increase. The fleshy red to grayish lesions can become so prominent between the eyelids to partially obliterate and fissure and cover the cornea (Figs. 23–2 and 23–3). Even in older patients we have not encountered any malignancies, but type 11 human papillomavirus involves laryngeal, conjunctival, and cervical mucosal surfaces associated with cervical dysplasia, carcinoma in situ, and even invasive carcinoma of the cervix.[2–4]

We treat lesions at once when conjunctiva papillomas have been detected. Early, aggressive treatment may prevent local spread of a lesion of viral origin. The eyelids should be everted to inspect the upper and lower fornices. We tend to treat the lesions with cryotherapy and then excise them; other surgeons prefer to debulk the lesion and treat the surrounding base with cryotherapy. Either method seems to work as well as the other.

Cautious excision of the papilloma does not seem to lead to conjunctival shortage or constriction. The cryotherapy can affect the lesions by killing the virus or stimulating inflammatory response in the surrounding tissue that may lead to necrosis of the papilloma.

Most patients will respond to treatment and not experience recurrence. The group that has return of lesions frequently will experience this rather rapidly, often in the first 4 to 6 weeks after treatment. The treatments for recurrent papilloma of the conjunctiva include surgical excision, cryotherapy, immunotherapy, and laser therapy.

Bosniak and associates[1] have provided the best documentation regarding treatment of difficult cases of squamous papillomas of the conjunctiva with multiple recurrences. With followup exceeding 1 year, none of seven cases recurred after treatment with carbon dioxide laser vaporization. Immunotherapy for recalcitrant cases includes dinitrochlorobenzene[5,6] or interferon.[7,8]

Our approach has been to treat initial recurrences with other surgery and cryotherapy since most patients respond to that regimen. With a second recurrence we tend to use the carbon dioxide laser for vaporization. Although cryotherapy and surgical excision tend to be simple, inexpensive techniques, the carbon dioxide laser offers the theoretical advantage that vaporization should not spread the virus, whereas mechanical surgical excision may allow other portions of the conjunctiva to become infected.

TREATMENT TECHNIQUE

We inject local anesthesia containing epinephrine to aid hemostasis regardless of whether the procedure is being done with the use of local or general anesthesia. Smaller lesions, especially single isolated lesions, are clinically excised using microforceps and Westcott scissors. Removing papillomas rarely requires special closure or flaps since the bases of the lesions are small. Lesions of the caruncle are treated with complete excision, trying to avoid removing the substance of the caruncle.

With larger lesions, the cryoprobe is first placed on the lesion with a quick-freeze, slow-thaw cycle carried out for two applications. The bulbar conjunctival lesions can usually be lifted off the globe to prevent freezing of the cornea or sclera. Once the lesion has fully thawed, the papilloma is excised. Minimal cautery is applied. Hemostasis can usually be achieved by placing a cotton-tipped applicator with epinephrine or thrombin against the treated area. An important aspect of surgery is the careful inspection to identify all areas of conjunctival pathology.

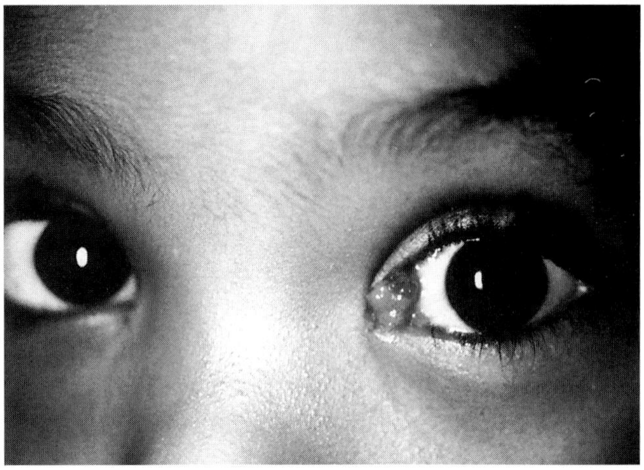

Figure 23–1. Squamous papillomas at the left medial canthus.

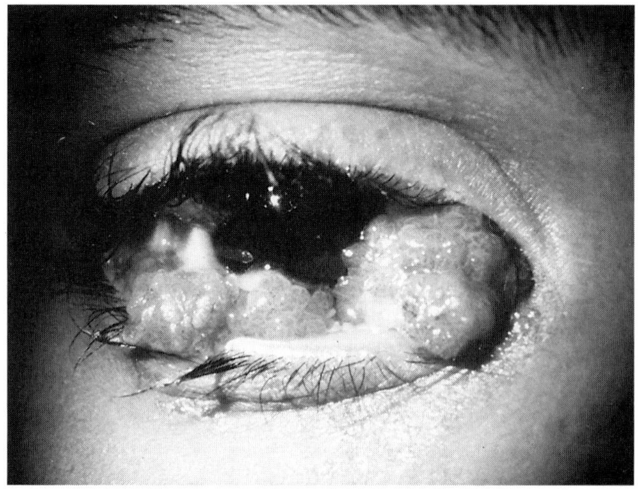

Figure 23–3. The papilloma has reached such size as to occlude vision.

Postoperatively, the patient is treated with an antibiotic ointment or eye drop primarily for the soothing value.

When treating lesions with the carbon dioxide laser, we use a large spot size that is first tested on the palpebral conjunctiva rather than starting directly on bulbar lesions. The cornea should be protected, but frequently the normal corneal protectors will not allow adequate access to the conjunctiva. A small piece of moistened gelatin sponge helps prevent injury to the cornea. By using a 2-mm spot size, the conjunctiva can be treated with good control as to the depth of the burn. Charred tissue can be carefully swabbed away between treatments. We prefer to use a hand-held applicator rather than the microscope for better ease in reaching the different portions of the conjunctiva. The carbon dioxide laser maintains good hemostasis while vaporizing the intracellular water of the treated tissue.

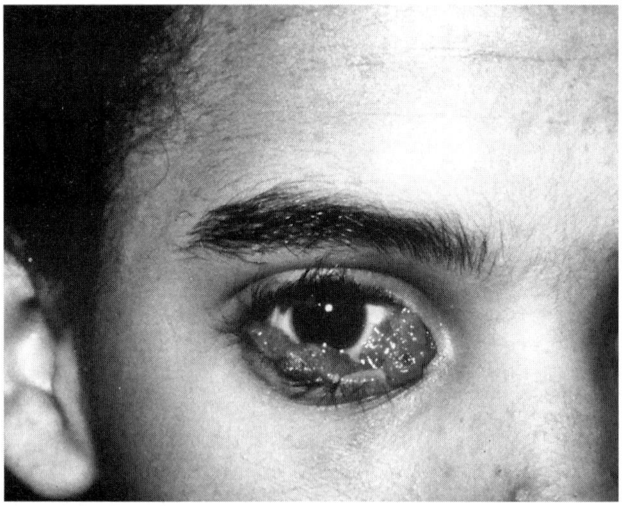

Figure 23–2. Extensive papillomas at the right lower and medial fornices.

For lesions that recur despite early, aggressive surgery, some type of immunotherapy such as interferon can be considered. Immunotherapy has only been used in small numbers of patients with uncontrolled trials. We predict the most effective treatments in the future will come from chemotherapy or immunotherapy rather than from surgical ablation.

REFERENCES

1. Bosniak SL, Novick NL, Sachs ME: Treatment of recurrent squamous papillomata of the conjunctiva by carbon dioxide laser vaporization. Ophthalmology 98:1078–1082, 1986.
2. Bissmann L, Wolnik L, Ikenberg H: Human papillomavirus types 6 and 11 DNA sequences in genital and laryngeal papillomas and some cervical cancers. Proc Natl Acad Sci USA 80:560–563, 1983.
3. Lancaster WD, Kurman RJ, Sanz LE: Human papillomavirus: Detection of viral DNA sequences and evidence for molecular heterogeneity in metaplasias and dysplasias of the uterine cervix. Intervirology 20:202–212, 1983.
4. Lass JH, Grove AS, Papale JJ: Detection of human papillomavirus DNA sequences in conjunctival papilloma. Am J Ophthalmol 96:670–674, 1983.
5. Petrelli R, Cotlier E, Robins S, Stoessel K: Dinitrochlorobenzene immunotherapy of recurrent squamous papilloma of the conjunctiva. Ophthalmology 88:1221–1225, 1981.
6. Ferry AP, Meltzer MA, Taub RN: Immunotherapy with dinitrochlorobenzene (DNCB) for recurrent squamous cell tumor of conjunctiva. Trans Am Ophthalmol Soc 74:154–171, 1976.
7. Lass JH, Foster CS, Grove AS, et al: Interferon-alpha therapy of recurrent conjunctival papillomas. Am J Ophthalmol 103:294–301, 1987.
8. Chiemchaisri Y, Dongosintr N, Wasi C, et al: The regression of recurrent conjunctival papillomas by lymphoblastoid interferon treatment. J Med Assoc Thai 73:406–413, 1990.

CHAPTER 24

Management of Conjunctival Prolapse

Ralph E. Wesley

Conjunctival prolapse can present as a minor nuisance of exaggerated conjunctival edema that slowly resolves without treatment. On the other end of the spectrum lies conjunctiva that is prolapsed to such a degree that a cycle of drying and the mass effect of subconjunctival edema prevent resolution without intervention.

Prolapse of conjunctiva should be treated according to the specific cause when possible. When the superior conjunctiva prolapses and fails to resolve after levator resection in blepharoptosis surgery, temporary sutures may be required to reattach the conjunctiva to the suspensory attachments of the superior fornix that were disturbed during surgery. Prolapse from massive traumatic or spontaneous orbital hemorrhage usually resolves spontaneously as the primary hemorrhage resorbs. Prolapse from an orbital tumor such as a rapidly expanding lymphoma ceases once the tumor is treated with chemotherapy or irradiation. Conjunctival prolapse from xerophthalmia or from arteriovenous fistulas responds to correction of the underlying cause.

In other instances, prolapse may occur after surgical procedures such as retinal procedures or even blepharoplasty. Interruption of the lymphatics of the lower conjunctiva due to electrocautery during lower lid blepharoplasty can cause persistent edema with conjunctival prolapse that may last for months. In some situations, massive edema may disrupt the normal suspensory attachments between the fornix and the base of the conjunctiva.

Treatment with artificial tears during the day and lubricating, nonpreserved ointment at night hastens the resolution. Occasionally, a mild corticosteroid eye drop reduces the edema and shortens the healing process. Taping the eyes shut at night, using petrolatum and plastic wrap or occlusive moisture bubbles, combined with elevating the head can hasten healing in cases involving more than moderate severity.

However, there are instances in which conjunctival edema with prolapse does not resolve satisfactorily and intervention is warranted. Caution should be exercised to delay procedures in more moderate cases. Sometimes an annoyed patient presses the surgeon to act when patience and medical therapy would suffice with least risk of complication.

Patching the eye usually reduces the conjunctival edema, providing the lids are closed over the cornea. If the conjunctiva protrudes through the lids when patched shut, edema may be trapped in the subconjunctival space. An injection into the conjunctiva of local anesthetic and corticosteroid can speed the resolution of the edema, although self-limited subconjunctival hemorrhage may occur right after the injection. A mixture of 0.5 mL of 1% lidocaine with 1:100,000 epinephrine and 0.5 mL of triamcinolone acetate (20 mg/mL) injected into the subconjunctival space followed by 24 hours of a light pressure dressing will sometimes cause resolution of the edematous, prolapsed conjunctiva.[1]

Next to be considered is placing fornix mattress sutures that hold the conjunctiva down into the fornix.[2] These can be used in the upper or lower fornix. I prefer to use a moderately short-acting suture such as 5-0 chromic that will persist for nearly 10 days.

With the conjunctiva anesthetized, the double-armed 5-0 chromic suture is passed into the lower fornix and out through the skin or in a similar manner in the upper fornix. The most important part of the technique is to avoid penetration of the globe with the needle. The sutures dissolve and rarely leave any residual scar on the skin surface. These sutures may possibly re-form suspensory attachments of the fornix and the conjunctiva. If the eye is not proptotic, the upper and lower lids can be sewn together with lamellar 5-0 chromic sutures. With proptosis, sewing the lids shut to reduce conjunctival swelling risks neurovascular occlusion.

In the most severe instances in which previous techniques have failed or will not apply and further delay cannot be tolerated, a small portion of the conjunctiva can be resected and the suture line closed.[3] This should be used only in extreme situations for fear of producing conjunctival shortage. Excising a small amount of severely distended conjunctiva seems to involve little risk of creating shortage of mucous membrane in the fornix.

Most problems of conjunctival prolapse resolve with more conservative methods. Even when the conjunctiva is severely desiccated, permanent change does not occur as happens with an exposed cornea. In some instances, massive swollen conjunctiva can provide coverage and protection for the cornea.

REFERENCES

1. Witherspoon CD, Cogen MS, Kuhn F: Chemotic prolapse of the conjunctiva. Ophthalmic Surg 22:241–242, 1991.
2. Levine MR, Buckman G: Conjunctival prolapse. Arch Ophthalmol 109:1614, 1991.
3. Malone TJ, Tse DT: Surgical treatment of chemotic conjunctival prolapse following vitreoretinal surgery. Arch Ophthalmol 108:890–891, 1990.

CHAPTER 25

Conjunctival Dermolipoma Surgery

Ralph E. Wesley

Just as the *Titanic* approached the iceberg without fear of the impending disaster, surgeons and patients may approach subconjunctival dermolipomas without an understanding for the disastrous, uncorrectable complications that can occur after removal of such innocuous-appearing lesions.

Dermolipomas, or lipodermoids, are usually found in the superior temporal quadrant of the orbit in a subconjunctival location that extends nearly to the limbus (Fig. 25-1). Part of the treachery of these lesions comes from the poorly defined borders of the tumor that may permeate the levator aponeurosis, the lacrimal gland, the lateral rectus muscle, and the peripheral cornea. The tumor may be inseparably fused with a portion of the lateral conjunctiva. Even carefully following the tumor borders can lead the surgeon into structures that can cause permanent blepharoptosis from injury to levator apparatus, dry eye from destruction of lacrimal secretory ductules, or strabismus from injury to the lateral rectus muscle. A restriction of ocular motility can occur from removal of even small amounts of the thickened lateral conjunctiva.

Dermolipomas arise from first branchial cleft defects, resulting in the inclusion of surface ectoderm and mesoderm in the closure of the cleft. Many tumors are only partially visible on external examination, appearing as a fold of conjunctiva in the lateral fissure. Most are discovered during infancy or childhood. Few have symptoms, although irritation of the eye for some other reason may bring the patient for ophthalmic examination. The lesions may enlarge slightly over time, but rapid growth would be unusual. A much more benign lesion is the prolapse of normal fat that occurs in the superior temporal conjunctival area seen more frequently in the elderly, as shown in Figure 25-2.

Dermolipomas are composed of adipose tissue underneath a thickened conjunctiva that may be keratinized near the lateral fornix. Other adnexal structures such as hair, sweat and sebaceous glands, hair follicles, or lacrimal secretory glands may be found in parts of the tumors. Dermolipomas are solid tumors as opposed to the well-demarcated dermoid cyst. The tumor is a true choristoma since fatty tissue does not normally occur anterior to the orbital septum. The lipodermoid may present as part of oculoauriculovertebral dysplasia (Goldenhar's syndrome), most often diagnosed by the associated preauricular skin tags.

I have found that most ophthalmologists and even specialists in ophthalmic plastic and orbital surgery are not familiar with the literature regarding complications from removal of dermolipomas. Several papers spell out in no uncertain terms the classic complications.[1-4] Beard[3] has emphasized that every surgeon who contemplates removal of a lipodermoid tumor from the orbital region should be aware of "the horrors that may occur following lipodermoid surgery."

COMPLICATIONS

Complications arise from removal of conjunctiva or from following the tumor into other vital structures. During surgery there is a desire to provide a pleasing cosmetic result. The firm adherence or fusing of the tumor to the conjunctiva may convince the surgeon to remove some of the abnormal, thickened, keratinized conjunctiva. Removal of virtually any conjunctiva can result in a shortening of the lateral fornix, which will prevent the globe from rotating medially or even deviate the globe into exotropia. Subsequent mucous membrane or free conjunctival grafts or flaps may not correct the deformity.

Trying to follow the tumor to the posterior extent can lead to damage of other vital structures. The patient may not have ptosis preoperatively even though the lesion extends upward into the upper eyelid through the levator aponeurosis. Once the tumor is removed, the patient may develop a ptosis that defies correction. The ptosis can arise from either damage to the retractors or scar contracture of the conjunctiva.

In some instances the levator aponeurosis can be repaired—usually with less severe cases of ptosis. Well documented in the literature are cases of ptosis that could not be repaired in which the patient had a permanent deformity that was unsuspected before surgery. When am-

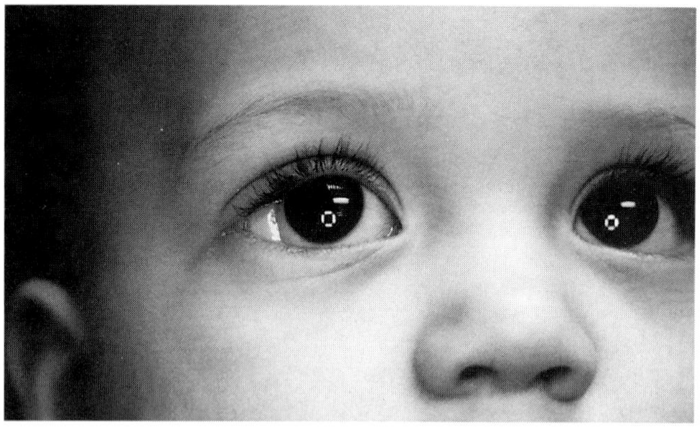

Figure 25–1. Subconjunctival lipodermoid seems innocuous in the right temporal area between the limbus and the lateral canthus. Its removal can involve uncorrectable complications.

blyopia occurs, treatment may not be possible because of the ptosis. A secondary esotropia may occur with the amblyopia—all from the removal of an innocuous lesion.

Direct damage to the lateral rectus and sometimes superior rectus muscle can also cause strabismus. Damage of the lacrimal ductules may leave the patient with a lifelong unilateral dry eye condition with severe keratitis.

EXCISION OF DERMALIPOMAS

Clearly, the surgeon and the patient should be aware of the complications from dermolipomas. Informed consent includes providing the patient and family with an analysis of the risks and benefits. The most important issue is for the patient and family to realize that (1) severe complications can occur that would never be expected by the innocent appearance of the lesion, (2) that failing to remove the lesion is unlikely to cause harm, and (3) that complications may not be correctable.

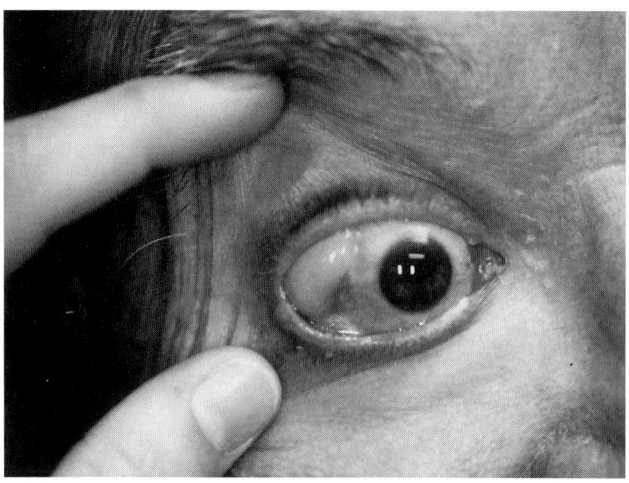

Figure 25–2. Prolapsed fatty tissue frequently seen in the superior temporal area of the conjunctiva represents the prolapse of normal fat.

I have removed numerous lipodermoids after discussing these issues with the patient and family. I do not ordinarily schedule the surgery during the first consultation, preferring to allow some time in which the patient or family can further consider this surgery and contemplate further questions.

With appreciation for the treacherous nature of these lesions, I have removed several dozen without major complications using a conservative approach in which the bargain I have with the patient is that I strongly prefer him or her to return postoperatively dissatisfied that not enough lipodermoid was removed rather than suffering the complications from trying to remove as much tumor as possible.

I routinely use the operating microscope for best visualization. I try to remove no conjunctival surface, although at times that means leaving thickened, keratinized conjunctiva. A traction stitch is placed to identify the lateral rectus muscle during surgery.

With the globe rotated inferomedially, I use blunt-tipped Westcott scissors to make a circumferential incision in the superior temporal quadrant of the conjunctiva over the tumor at the most anterior edge. The most treacherous dissection is from the conjunctiva. The portion next to the globe usually comes out easily. Some gentle pressure on the globe helps the fatty tumor to come into view, but the technique is to remove the anterior portion without following the tumor upward toward the lid and lacrimal area or toward the lateral rectus muscle. Once the anterior portion of the lipodermoid has been removed, the conjunctiva will usually heal flat against the globe without further herniation of the more posterior lipodermoid. Beard[4] has recommended deep suturing of the conjunctiva to the sclera during the conjunctival closure approximately 10 mm from the limbus to make a barrier to reappearance of the tumor. The lateral conjunctival will still be somewhat thickened at the conclusion of the resection, which is far preferable to replacement with mucous membrane grafts.

Although many patients decline surgery once they are informed of the considerations mentioned previously, I have found those submitting to surgery have been pleased and satisfied even when a greater resection might have been advantageous cosmetically.

TREATMENT OF COMPLICATIONS

When lacrimal ductules are destroyed or the lacrimal gland is removed, the tear secretory function cannot be restored. Artificial tears and ointments are usually required. Closure of the lacrimal puncta on the involved side may help with a severe dry eye condition. With cases intractable to medical treatments, a small lateral tarsorrhaphy may be helpful at the price of some cosmetic disfigurement.

Strabismus can sometimes be corrected or reduced. These cases are extremely difficult and require that the first operation be done by the most experienced strabismus surgeon available. When the deviation comes from a restrictive conjunctival syndrome, replacement with buccal mucous membrane or free conjunctiva can be helpful in less severe cases. The grafts need to be treated vigorously postoperatively with corticosteroids to reduce the inevitable contraction of the graft.

Ptosis should be treated with replacement grafting of mucous membrane if it results from a restrictive syndrome. When ptosis appears to come from a defect in the retractors, a direct repair should be attempted through an external lid incision. Mucous membrane grafts can be placed on the conjunctival surface at the same operating setting. Those patients requiring a frontalis suspension have generally had poor results.

REFERENCES

1. Sullivan GL: Caveat chirurgicus. Trans Am Ophthalmol Soc 70:328–336, 1972.
2. Paris GL, Beard C: Blepharoptosis following dermolipoma surgery. Ann Ophthalmol 5:697–699, 1973.
3. Beard C: *In* Ptosis, 2nd ed. St. Louis, CV Mosby, 1976, p 66.
4. Beard C: Dermolipoma surgery, or, "An ounce of prevention is worth a pound of cure." Ophthalmic Plast Reconstr Surg 6:153–157, 1990.

SECTION III

Eyelids

SECTION EDITORS

Robert Alan Goldberg
Russell S. Gonnering

Introduction

Robert Alan Goldberg and Russell S. Gonnering

"See one, do one, teach one."

This simple dictum is the summation of one approach to the teaching of surgery. Although it could be argued as an appropriate emphasis for the sequence of maneuvers necessary to complete a surgical procedure, this approach is fundamentally flawed. If it were taken literally, surgery would become a static profession, since no new surgical approaches would be possible.

Such an approach also minimizes the cognitive function of the surgeon by reducing surgery to a technical exercise. Although surgery is indeed technical, it is, or should be, much more. Surgery in general, and surgery of the eyelids in particular, is an art and a science. With the skillful application of technical expertise, disease or deformity is eradicated or improved. Operative techniques are only some of the tools the surgeon uses to solve a particular problem. Although the events in the operating room are important to the success of the treatment, the *why* and *when* of surgery are every bit as important as the *how*.

The most difficult aspect of surgical skill to teach is that of surgical judgment: the *why* and *when*. Ptosis surgery, in particular, demands rapid integration of complex variables, including preoperative measurements of anatomy and physiology, intraoperative anatomic variability, influence of pharmacologic agents on intraoperative levator function, and so on. A mechanistic "cookbook" approach to eyelid surgery will produce significant and uncomfortable postoperative surprises for both the patient and the surgeon!

This presents an inherent difficulty. How does one acquire surgical judgment? Experience may be one way, providing the surgeon has the capacity to learn from both successes and failures. Knowledge is another, providing the surgeon has the ability to discern what is valid from what is not.

The skilled surgeon is, first and foremost, a trained observer. To solve a problem, it must first be identified as such. Only with a firm grounding in anatomy and pathophysiology can these problems be accurately identified and the proper diagnosis made. It makes no difference that the ptosis procedure was expertly performed if the lymphoma causing the drooping eyelid was not diagnosed because it was not looked for. Likewise, if a patient's tearing problem was caused by subtle ectropion, a masterful dacryocystorhinostomy done in record time will not produce satisfying results.

The skilled surgeon is also a careful listener. Not all anatomic abnormalities require repair. Asymptomatic malignancies or other significant disease must of course be found and brought to the attention of the patient, but subtle variations in eyelid position or other inconsequential findings that are not perceived to be problems by the patient are best left alone. *Primum non nocere* holds true for eyelid surgery.

The skilled surgeon is always questioning and "pushing the envelope." Although anatomy does not change, our understanding of it does. Witness the evolution of our understanding of the medial canthal "tendons" and "ligaments." Likewise, our understanding of the pathophysiology of disease processes becomes more sophisticated with each scientific paper presented in the literature. Surgeons who fail to continue their education throughout their practice will never reach their full potential.

Disease is likewise dynamic. The influx of refugees into the United States has brought the need for an awareness of diseases not encountered in surgical training of but a few years ago. New diseases, such as the acquired immunodeficiency syndrome, must be confronted even by the eyelid surgeon.

If disease is dynamic, so is technology. New instrumentation, new drugs, and new treatment modalities all continue to be described in the ophthalmic literature. Many more changes with great potential for eyelid surgery are described in the nonophthalmic literature. The skilled surgeon must pick which of these new ideas to learn and apply.

Finally, eyelid surgery will not be immune from the significant socioeconomic crisis medicine in general will face in the next decade. Our medical abilities are rapidly outstripping our financial resources. Hard choices must be faced by society at large, by physicians in general, and by surgeons in particular. New practice dynamics are already operative in the way surgeons are accessed by patients. Whereas in the past the practice of medicine was driven into increasing specialization by the flood of knowledge, this may be reversed by global budgets, capitation, and provider networks. The skillful surgeon will most likely need to become somewhat of a statistician and advocate, by first defining outcomes of various treatment modalities, measuring those outcomes, balancing the cost–benefit equation for the individual patient and society, and communicating his or her recommendations to the person who makes the decision regarding care. Yes, skilled surgeons will surely need to be adaptable in the future.

Introductions such as this offer medical authors a singular opportunity to wax philosophically. We need not adhere to the strict guidelines of medical writing but can explain why we undertook this work and state what it is we hope the reader will gain through its reading. In this section, the reader has the opportunity to learn the approach of various skilled surgeons to problems of the eyelid. They are by no means the only approaches. It is hoped that they will not prove to be even the best approaches, because if they are, surgery of the eyelid will not advance.

Instead of "see one, do one, teach one," "identify the problems, weigh the potential solutions, learn from your actions."

Basic Sciences

CHAPTER 26

Clinical Eyelid Anatomy

Joseph P. Shovlin and Bradley N. Lemke

The eyelids are specialized structures composed of thin skin, superficial muscle, connective tissue, secretory glands, and mucous membrane that function to protect the eye and lubricate the corneal surface while maintaining an aperture for unobstructed vision. Abnormalities of these supporting structures result in malpositions, restrictions, or deformities that may interfere with the eyelids' ability to perform these functions. An appreciation of the anatomy and function of the eyelids will help to avoid mishap when performing surgery in this region.

A thorough understanding of the superficial anatomy of the eyelids enables the recognition of eyelid malpositions and the physiologic consequences of these malpositions (Fig. 26–1). The opening between the upper and lower lids comprises the palpebral fissure. The fissure measures 10 to 12 mm vertically in the adult. The upper eyelid rests at the upper corneoscleral limbus in the child and 1.5 to 2.0 mm below it in the adult. The lower lid reaches the level of the inferior corneoscleral limbus with the eye in primary position. The upper eyelid forms a gentle curve with the highest point located just nasal to the pupil. The lowest point of the lower lid is just temporal to this. The contour of the closed eyelids is similar to that of the open lower lid. The angles created by the fusion of the upper and lower lids form the medial and lateral canthi with the points of union known as the commissures. The lateral commissure rests upon the globe, while the caruncle and plica semilunaris separate the medial commissure from the globe. The horizontal palpebral fissure, the distance between the medial and lateral commissures, measures 28 to 30 mm in the adult and is decreased in traumatic telecanthus and the blepharophimosis syndrome.

The eyelid creases represent the superficial insertions of the levator aponeurosis and the lower lid retractors. The prominent upper lid crease of the Occidental, located approximately 10 mm from the lid margin in the female and 8 mm from the lid margin in the male, represents the primary insertion of the levator aponeurosis into the pretarsal orbicularis (Fig. 26–2).[1] In patients undergoing levator surgery the upper lid crease should be re-formed by anchoring the pretarsal orbicularis to the upper border of the tarsus or to the levator aponeurosis. Migration of the lid crease upward may indicate levator disinsertion, dehiscence, or attenuation found in involutional ptosis.

The lower eyelid crease begins lateral to the medial canthus 4 to 5 mm below the eyelid margin and angles inferotemporally. A malar crease may also be present that represents the junction of the orbicularis and the malar fat pad. This crease forms the lower border seen in eyelid edema and accentuates with contraction of the facial musculature during a smile.

Horizontal skin folds (laugh lines) radiating from the lateral commissure represent folding of the skin due to vertical shortening of the lateral orbicularis oculi muscle (Fig. 26–3). The laugh lines follow the relaxed skin tension lines that run perpendicular to the underlying muscle fibers. The lateralmost orbicularis fibers run vertically and are tangential to the elliptical orbital orbicularis. Excessive skin and underlying orbicularis present in infants form epicanthal and epiblepharon folds. Epiblepharon folds located in the lower lid may mechanically push the lashes against the globe, causing chronic conjunctivitis.[2] Epicanthal folds when asymmetric simulate esotropia with no ocular misalignment present. These folds become less prominent and disappear in the Occidental

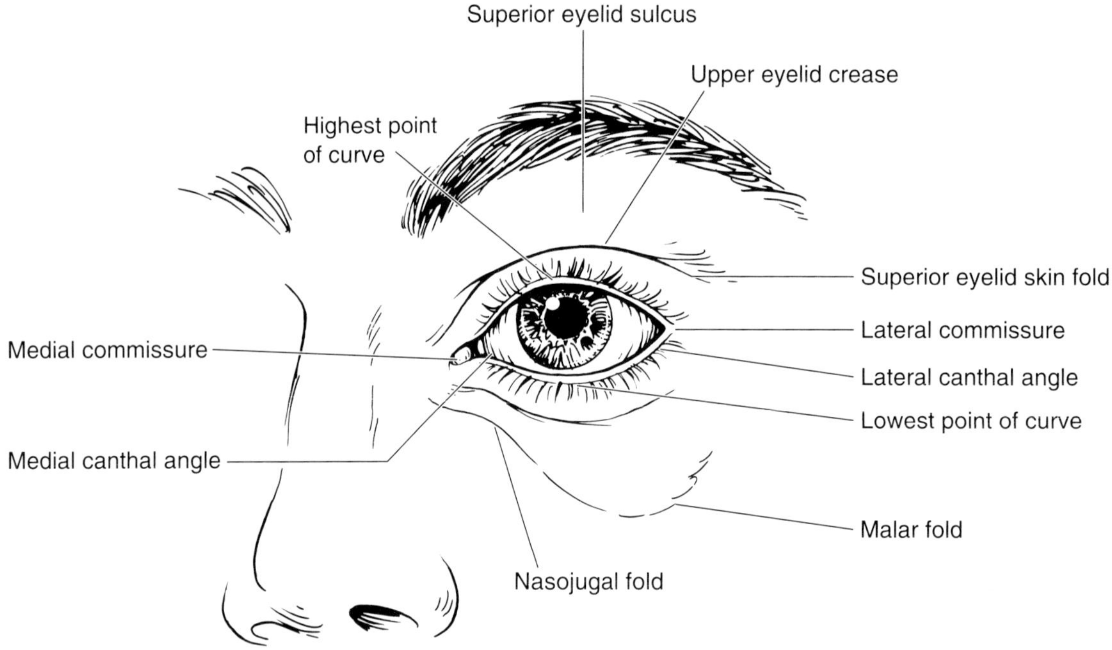

Figure 26–1. Topographic anatomy of the eyelid. (From Lemke BN: Anatomy of the ocular adnexa and orbit. *In* Smith BC, Della Rocca RC, Lisman RD, Nesi FA [eds]: Ophthalmic Plastic and Reconstructive Surgery. St. Louis, CV Mosby, 1987.)

with growth of the orbital bones and facial skeleton. Occasionally, epiblepharon requires removal of the excess skin and orbicularis for treatment of chronic conjunctivitis.

The thin skin of the eyelids undergoes abrupt transition into the thicker skin of the brow and malar regions. The skin attaches less firmly to the areas above and below the tarsi and possesses great elasticity, allowing for collection of edema fluid. Microscopically, the eyelid skin consists of a keratinized squamous epithelium with a poorly defined papillary dermis.[3] The reticular dermis also contains scant connective tissue with an abundance of elastic tissue. The dermis does not contain subcutaneous fat. The loose attachment and stretching of the skin above the tarsus in the upper lid with age allows for the redundancy of the skin seen in elderly individuals known as dermatochalasis.

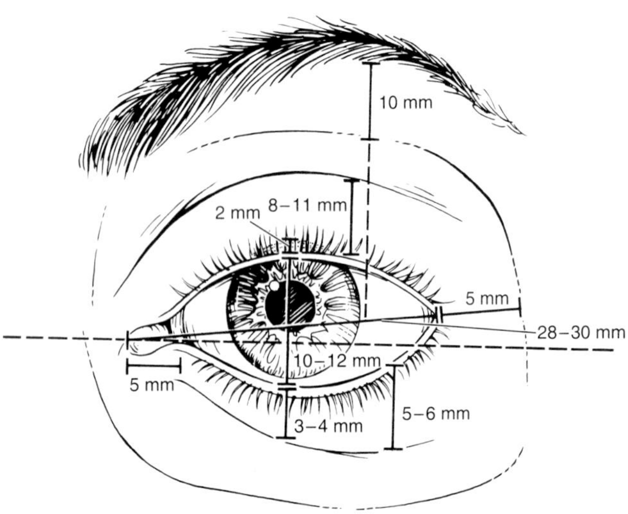

Figure 26–2. Average measurements of the superficial anatomy of the eyelids in the Occidental. The female brow is arched with the highest point at the lateral limbus. The male brow is horizontal and somewhat lower. The male lid crease and lateral canthus also tend to be lower than in the female.

The area between the upper eyelid crease and the superior orbital margin known as the superior orbital sulcus becomes more prominent with loss of orbital volume. Fat atrophy, increased orbital volume from fractures, and loss of volume from enucleation deepen the superior orbital sulcus. Bulges within the superior sulcus most commonly represent herniation of orbital fat through an attenuated orbital septum; laterally they may be due to a prolapsed lacrimal gland.

EYEBROW

The eyebrow, a specialized structure composed of pilosebaceous units, muscle, and fat, protects the eye from light and sweat and is an important component of facial expression. The orbital orbicularis oculi, frontalis, procerus, and corrugator supraciliaris muscles interdigitate in the region of the eyebrow (Fig. 26–4). The eyebrow rests on a fat pad, which improves motility and provides a cushion over the supraorbital rim. Contraction of the frontalis elevates the brow, while forced contraction of the orbital orbicularis depresses it. The corrugator supraciliaris depresses and pulls the brow toward the midline. The corrugator arises from the superomedial margin of the orbit on the frontal bone medial to the supraorbital

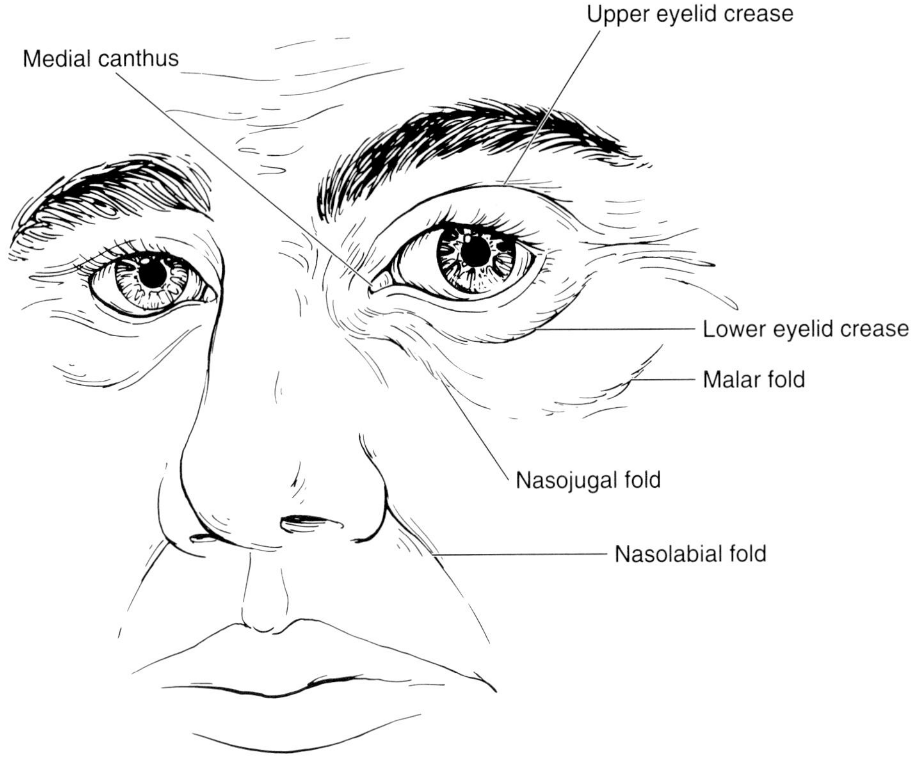

Figure 26–3. The adult wrinkled face demonstrating the relaxed skin tension lines running perpendicular to the underlying orbicularis. (From Lemke BN: Anatomy of the ocular adnexa and orbit. *In* Smith BC, Della Rocca RC, Lisman RD, Nesi FA [eds]: Ophthalmic Plastic and Reconstructive Surgery. St. Louis, CV Mosby, 1987.)

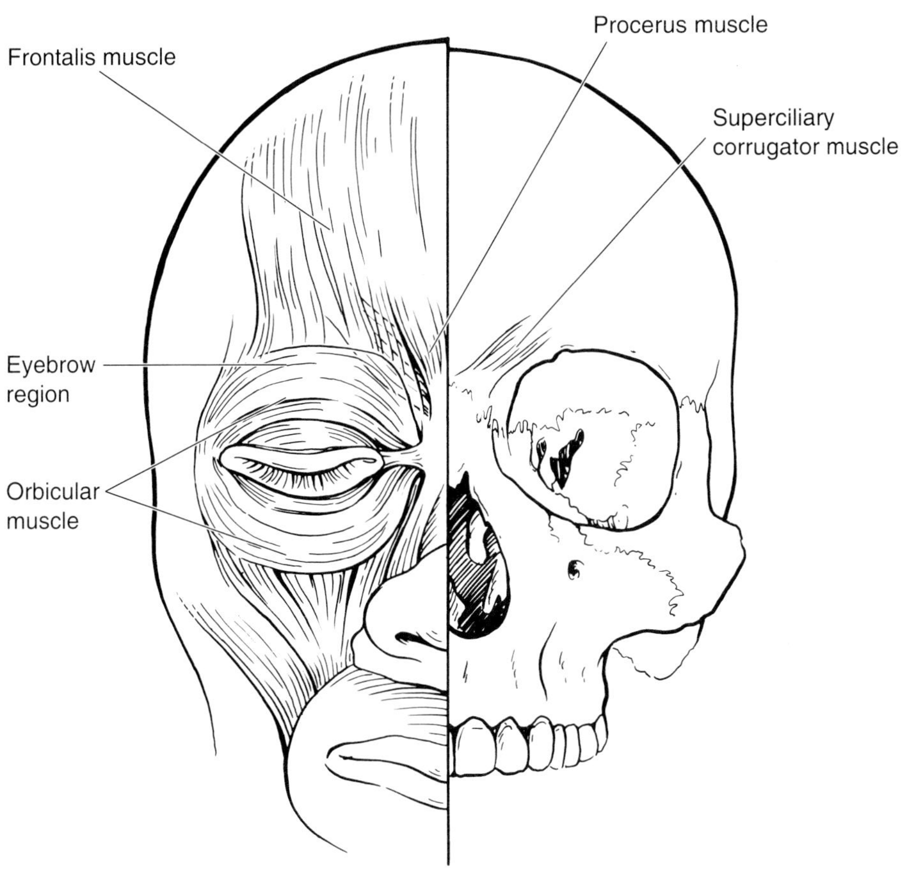

Figure 26–4. Superficial muscle plane of the face showing the interrelationships of the muscles of facial expression.

notch and runs superiorly and laterally for 2 to 3 cm to insert superficially into the medial half of the eyebrow. The corrugator originates deep to the orbicularis and procerus, blends with the overlying orbicularis, and inserts into the overlying skin surrounding the hair follicles. The procerus muscle superficially appears as a medial extension of the frontalis muscle, which inserts on the nasal bone. The procerus represents a separate muscle innervated by a separate branch of the facial nerve[4]; it contracts with the orbicularis and corrugator to depress the brow.

The frontalis has no bony attachments; rather, it arises and inserts within the galea aponeurotica. The galea splits at the origin of the frontalis to provide the frontalis with a fascial investment—the superficial and deep galea. The deep galea bifurcates again, encircling the brow fat pad with anterior and posterior deep galea. The posterior deep galea joins with the periorbita and the orbital septum at the arcus marginalis[5] The anterior deep galea continues on as the posterior orbicularis fascia.[6] This frontalis origination within the galea represents the anterior belly of the occipitofrontalis. It glides over the periosteum of the frontal bone, inserts in the skin of the eyebrow around the hair follicles, and interdigitates with the orbicularis muscle. The loose adhesion between the galea and the periosteum of the cranium provides a plane of dissection down to the superior orbital rim where these tissues are firmly adherent. This plane is below the vascular and nerve supply to the area, thus facilitating dissection. The temporal branch of the superficial facial nerve innervates the frontalis. The eyebrow attaches to the deeper osseous supraorbital ridge through dense attachments on the underside of the brow fat pad.[7] The supraorbital ridge traverses only the medial one half to two thirds of the orbit, and deep brow support is lost temporally. The frontalis muscle belly also terminates temporally; these two factors cause brow ptosis to begin laterally.

The direction of eyebrow hair is constant in the adult. Embryologically, forehead hair flows downward to meet an upward flow from the glabella (Fig. 26–5). These two streams meet, and a whorl develops as the hair direction diverts laterally. In the adult, the follicles angulate horizontally between 30 and 40 degrees, being slightly less laterally (Fig. 26–6). When the surgeon is performing vertical incisions through the eyebrow, the scalpel should be angulated 40 degrees in the medial brow and 30 degrees in the lateral brow.[8] The vertical angulation of the follicles is upward in the lower brow and downward in the upper brow with an abrupt transition at the vertical midpoint of the brow. The superior margin follicles point downward between 15 and 20 degrees. An incision along the superior brow border with an angulation of 25 to 30 degrees will minimize damage to the follicles. The inferior border follicles point upward approximately 30 degrees in the medial brow and decrease to 7 degrees laterally. An incision along the inferior border of the brow should be angulated upward 40 degrees over the medial half and 20 degrees upward over the lateral half of the brow. Minimizing damage to the follicles will preserve the camouflaging effects of the brow lashes.

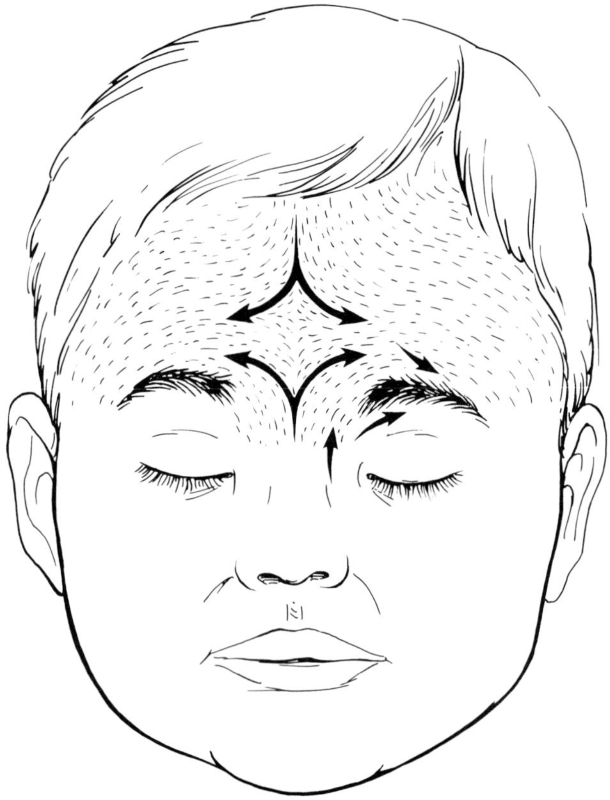

Figure 26–5. Drawing of a newborn showing the direction of frontal hair growth. This symmetric pattern occurs only 25% of the time, yet direction of eyebrow hair is remarkably constant in the adult. (From Lemke BN, Stasior OG: Eyebrow incision making. Adv Ophthalmol Plast Reconstruct Surg 2:19–23, 1983.)

EYELID PROTRACTORS

The orbicularis oculi is divided into orbital, preseptal, and pretarsal portions based on the anatomic structures that lie beneath (Fig. 26–7). On gross examination the orbicularis is continuous, but the functions of these portions differ. The orbital portion depresses the brow and assists in forced eyelid closure. The preseptal portion also aids in forced eyelid closure as well as contributes to the lacrimal pump. The pretarsal orbicularis is responsible for the involuntary eyelid blink and contributes to the central portion of the deep medial and lateral orbicularis insertions.

The orbital and preseptal orbicularis share many similarities and may be considered together. These loosely associated fibers travel in an arc encompassing the orbital and preseptal regions. In some dissections there may be vertical fibers of the orbital orbicularis laterally that are

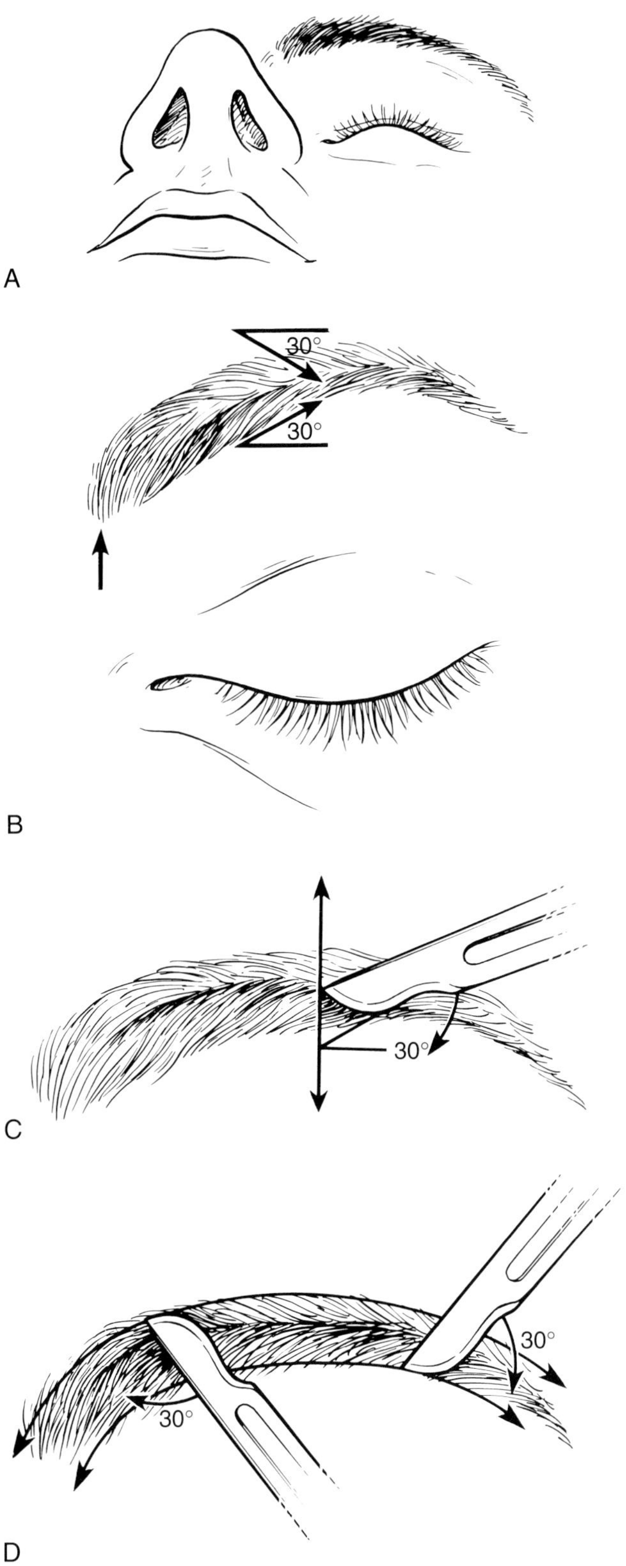

Figure 26–6. Hair direction in the adult eyebrow. *A*, Hair angulation is about 30 degrees downward from vertical in the upper eyebrow and about 30 degrees upward in the lower brow with an abrupt transition at the center of the eyebrow. This reversal does not occur at the medial end of the eyebrow, where hair sweeps upward uninterrupted from below. *B*, Hair also angles laterally at least 30 degrees from the vertical. *C* and *D*, Horizontal and vertical eyebrow hair angulations coincident to about 30 degrees serve as useful guides when making incisions in this area. (From Lemke BN: Anatomy of the ocular adnexa and orbit. *In* Smith BC, Della Rocca RC, Lisman RD, Nesi FA [eds]: Ophthalmic Plastic and Reconstructive Surgery. St. Louis, CV Mosby, 1987.)

oriented tangential to the inner curves.[9] The orbital and preseptal orbicularis loosely associate with the underlying tissues except where they are attached to bone at the lateral palpebral raphe, the supraorbital ridge, the naso-orbital valley, and the malar crease. Grossly, the orbital and preseptal orbicularis appear to terminate along the lateral palpebral raphe; however, microscopically, the fibers travel through uninterrupted. Medially, the superficial heads terminate above and below the superficial head of the medial canthal ligament in the adult. In infants and young children, skin and orbicularis pass superficial to the medial canthal ligament and may form epicanthal folds. Deep preseptal fibers insert above and below the deep pretarsal fibers on the lacrimal fascia to complete Horner's lacrimal muscle.

The pretarsal fibers of the orbicularis firmly adhere to the tarsus and may be separated only by sharp dissection. The fibers travel an elliptical path around the palpebral fissure. Laterally, these fibers form superficial and deep heads. The deep head inserts 3 to 4 mm posterior to the lateral palpebral raphe at the lateral orbital tubercle of Whitnall behind the lateral canthal ligament (Fig. 26–8). As noted earlier, the superficial head contributes to the lateral palpebral raphe. Medially, the pretarsal orbicularis splits into superficial and deep heads. The superficial head inserts with the orbital and preseptal orbicularis above and below the medial canthal ligament while the deep head dives posterior to the lacrimal sac to gain access to the posterior lacrimal crest (Fig. 26–9). These deep preseptal and pretarsal heads, known collectively as Horner's muscle, pull the lid posteriorly to follow the contour of the globe. Horner's muscle is predominantly an upper eyelid structure corresponding to the greater height of the superior tarsus when compared with the inferior tarsus.[10] The insertion of Horner's muscle on the lacrimal bone of the posterior lacrimal crest extends to the lacrimal-ethmoidal suture. Laxity or anterior displacement of this structure may contribute to medial ectropion.

The anterior limb of the medial canthal ligament inserts on the anterior lacrimal crest formed by the frontal process of the maxilla (Fig. 26–10). The anterior limb arises from the frontal process of the maxilla as a triangular band extending from the anterior lacrimal crest toward the nasomaxillary suture.[11] The anterior limb passes laterally as a fibrous band anterior to the lacrimal sac. Average measurements of the anterior limb of the medial canthal ligament are 11.7 mm in length, 2 to 4 mm in width, and 4.9 mm in thickness.[12, 13] This portion of the ligament is involved in naso-orbital fractures that produce traumatic telecanthus, which may require transnasal wiring or miniplate fixation. The less substantial posterior limb of the medial canthal ligament passes across the lacrimal fascia and diaphragm to insert to the posterior lacrimal crest just posterior to the lacrimal fascia. The posterior limb forms the anterior fascia of Horner's muscle.

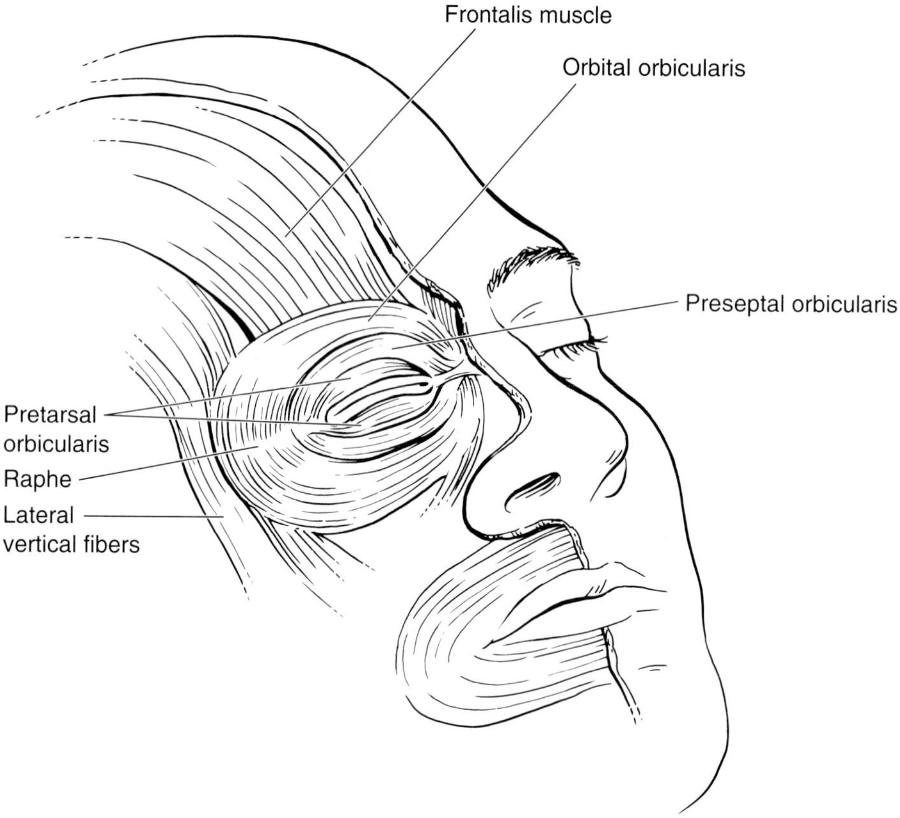

Figure 26–7. Superficial relations of the orbicularis oculi muscle.

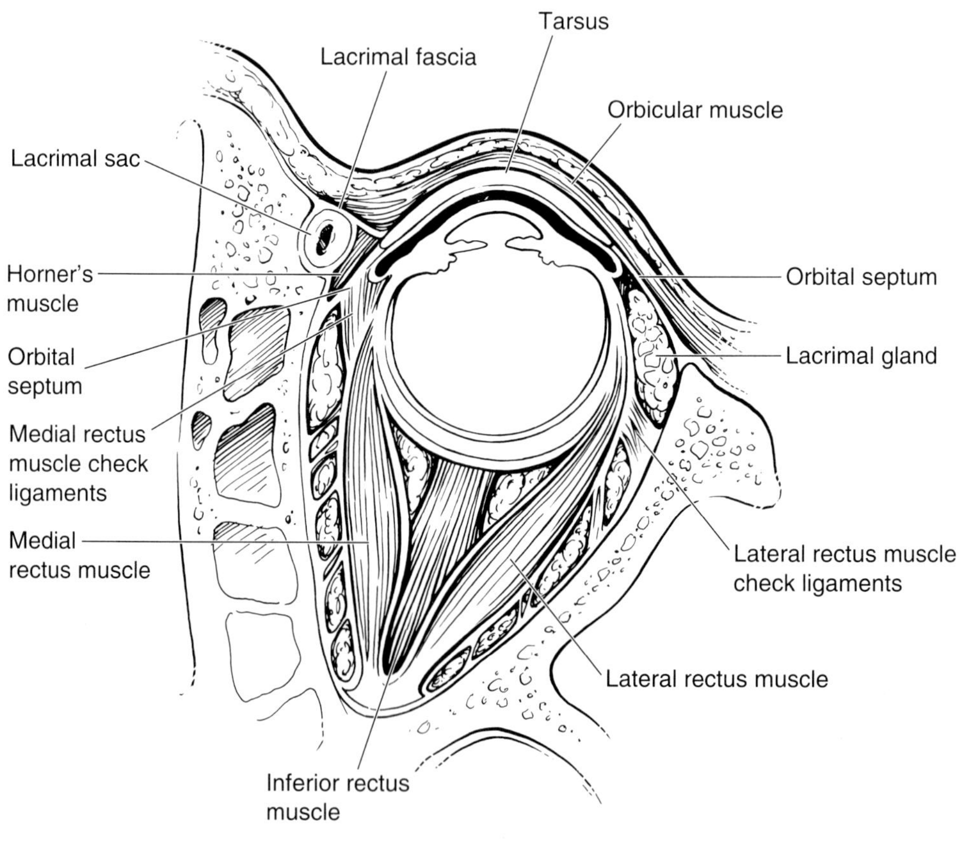

Figure 26–8. Horizontal section through the upper lid near the palpebral margin. Posterior fibers in Horner's muscle arise from pretarsal orbicularis muscle, while the more anterior fibers inserting on the lacrimal fascia originate in the preseptal orbicularis. Horner's muscle lines the posterior surface of the posterior crux of the medial canthal ligament.

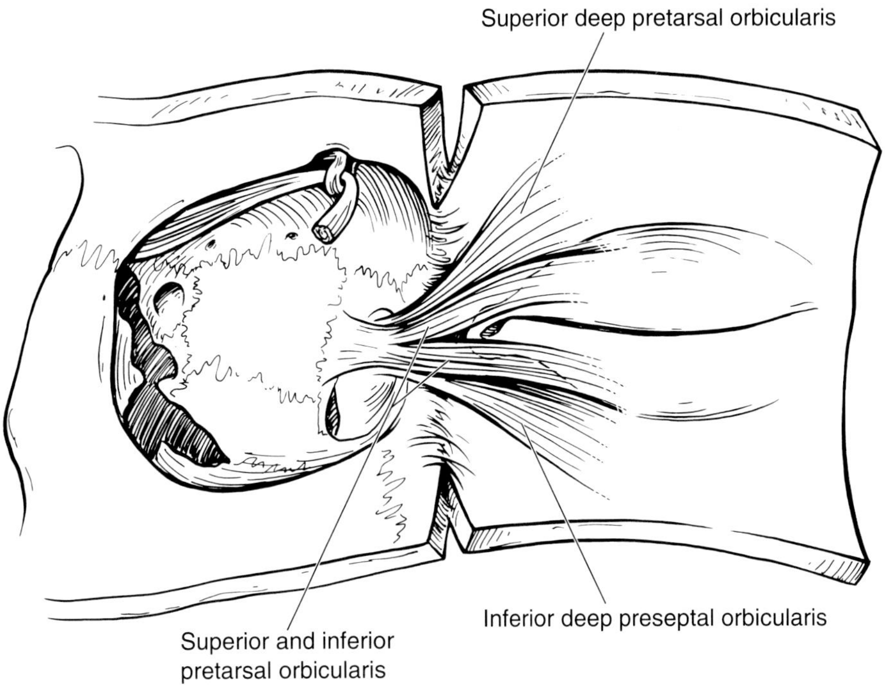

Figure 26–9. The eyelid skin and muscle are reflected medially. Note the superior and inferior deep pretarsal orbicularis joining to form Horner's muscle and inserting on the posterior lacrimal crest. The inferior and superior deep preseptal orbicularis join to insert on the lacrimal fascia.

sure within the canaliculus.[12] The deep heads of the pretarsal and preseptal orbicularis that insert on the lacrimal fascia and posterior lacrimal crest pull on the lacrimal sac, possibly creating a negative pressure within the sac.[14] Lid laxity and seventh nerve palsies disrupt the pump mechanism, resulting in epiphora even with proper punctal position and a patent lacrimal excretory system.

Small mounds of soft tissue on the medial lid margin

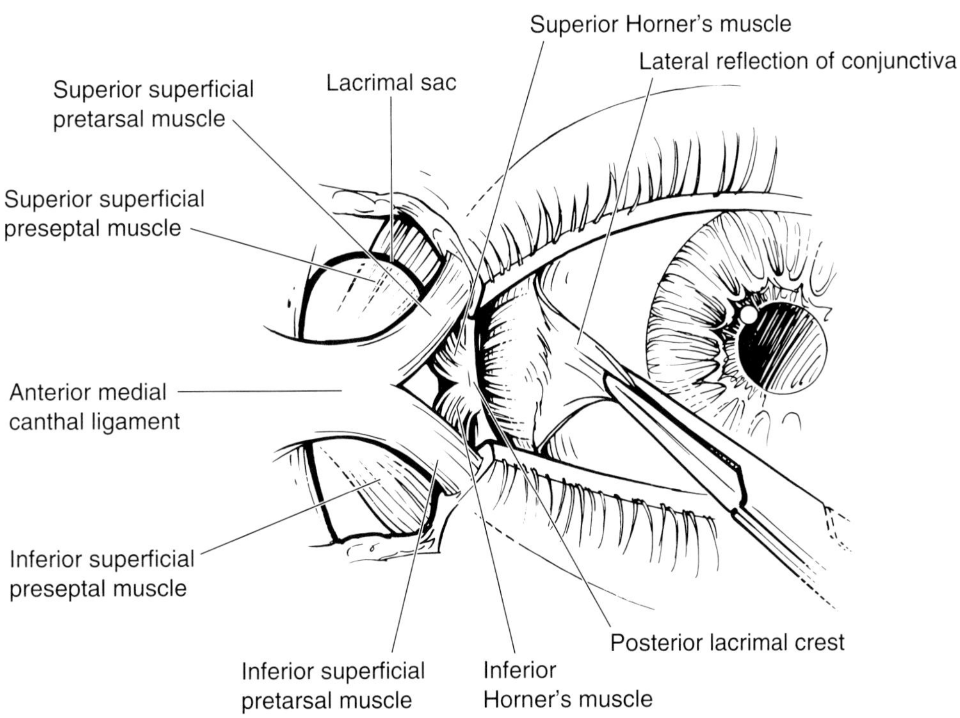

Figure 26–10. Diagram illustrating the insertion of the anterior crux of the medial canthal ligament on the frontal process of the maxilla. The medial canthal ligament is a fibrous structure that attaches the tarsal plate to the maxillary and lacrimal bones. (From Ahl NC, Hill JC: Horner's muscle and the lacrimal system. Arch Ophthalmol 100:448–493, 1982. Copyright 1982, American Medical Association.)

form the superior and inferior puncta. The upper papilla rests against the globe approximately 6.0 mm from the medial canthal angle, with the lower papilla found 6.5 mm from the medial canthus at the termination of the gray line. Medial to the puncta the lid margin assumes a rounded contour with cilia and meibomian glands no longer present. These relationships and a change in lid contour aid in the identification of imperforate or stenotic puncta. The puncta appear pale in comparison to the remainder of the lid margin owing to their high connective tissue content and their lack of vasculature. A dense ring of connective tissue surrounds a lumen that measures 0.2 to 0.3 mm wide. With the eyes in primary position the puncta lie in the marginal tear strip in a groove between the plica semilunaris and the bulbar conjunctiva. The punctal aperture is round or oval in childhood but often collapses into a fishmouth or slit configuration with age.[15] The puncta lead to ducts lined with nonkeratinized stratified squamous epithelium known as the canaliculi. The canaliculi pass vertically for 2 mm before dilating to form an ampulla (Fig. 26–11). The canaliculi then turn 90 degrees to run medially parallel to the lid margin. Pretarsal orbicularis fibers surround the ampulla and canaliculi to compress and shorten them with each blink. At the medial canthal angle the canaliculi travel behind the medial canthal ligament, joining in 90% of the cases to form a common canaliculus before entering the lacrimal sac.[4] The common canaliculus enters the lacrimal sac superior and posterior to the middle of the lateral wall, 2 to 3 mm behind the medial canthal ligament. The canalicular portion of the eyelid contains less connective tissue than the ciliary portion lateral to it, thus making the canalicular portion particularly vulnerable to avulsion by lateral tractional forces.[16]

The eyelash follicles at the lid margin separate a portion of the pretarsal orbicularis from the remainder. This portion, known as the muscle of Riolan, forms the clinical landmark, the gray line.[17] This landmark allows accurate reapproximation of the lid margin after lid lacerations or full-thickness lid procedures or may be used to split the lid into anterior and posterior lamellae. The gray line is more visible in younger individuals. Medial to the puncta the gray line is no longer present because the muscle of Riolan joins with the rest of the pretarsal orbicularis head to contribute to the lacrimal muscle of Horner.

The orbital septum constitutes the posterior limit of the superficial muscle plane, more recently designated the superficial musculoaponeurotic system (SMAS), and defines the anterior extent of the orbit. Elastic and fibrous connective tissue organized in lamellae compose the orbital septum, serving to preclude the spread of infection or hemorrhage posteriorly to the orbit.[5] The septum of the upper lid arises at the arcus marginalis with a fusion of the periorbita and deep posterior galea. At the supraorbital notch the septum traverses the notch on a periosteal bridge and then passes in front of the trochlea.[18] The septum then descends along the medial orbital rim to gain access to the posterior lacrimal crest just posterior to Horner's muscle. It passes anteriorly as a posterior boundary of the pars lacrimalis muscle to gain access to the anterior lacrimal crest. The septum follows the inferior orbital rim fused with the orbital periosteum. In the upper lid the septum passes down from the arcus margin-

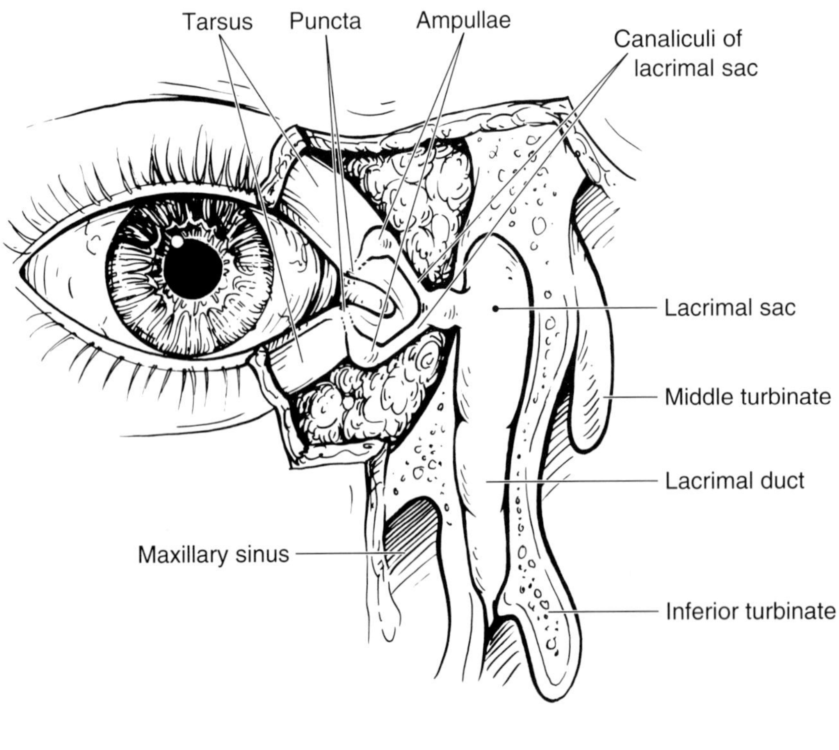

Figure 26–11. Approximate positions of the nasolacrimal excretory system. In the adult the length of the system is about 35 mm; in the newborn the system measures about 25 mm.

alis anterior to the preaponeurotic fat pad. It then joins the aponeurotic fibers of the levator just superior to the levator's primary insertion into the pretarsal orbicularis muscle.[1] Adipose tissue is frequently noted anterior to the orbital septum that is separate and distinct from the preaponeurotic fat.[5] In the lower lid, the septum passes from the orbital margin superiorly, anterior to the orbital fat, to combine with the lower lid retractors 4 to 5 mm below their collective insertion around the lower border of the tarsus.[19]

The septum tends to becomes attenuated with age, and regional differences in the thickness of the septum account for the location of fat prolapse seen in some elderly patients. The septum is thickest superolaterally where it stretches from the arcus marginalis to the lateral palpebral raphe, which it reinforces.[18] It is thin in the lower lid and most delicate superomedially in the upper lid. Attenuation of the septum with age permits prolapse of orbital fat in the lower lid and of the preaponeurotic nasal fat in the upper lid.

A thin connective tissue capsule surrounds the preaponeurotic fat located just posterior to the orbital septum in the upper lid. Fine wispy connective tissue septa extend from the capsule of the preaponeurotic fat anteriorly to the orbital septum and posteriorly to the levator aponeurosis. Connective tissue septa also divide the preaponeurotic fat into lobules. In the upper eyelid the fascial extensions from the trochlea divide the preaponeurotic pockets into nasal fat pads (Fig. 26–12). Clinically, the preaponeurotic fat tends to be more yellow compared with the relatively white nasal fat pads. Anatomically, the nasal fat pad is continuous with the deeper orbital fat. The levator aponeurosis and Whitnall's ligament define the posterior extent of the preaponeurotic fat. The orbital lobe of the lacrimal gland lies temporal to the preaponeurotic fat and must be avoided during blepharoplasty.

Although three distinct fat pads in the lower lid have not been demonstrated anatomically,[20] clinically the inferior oblique muscle and the arcuate expansion of this muscle divide the fat in the lower lid into three segments. The medial fat pad is separated from the middle fat pad by the inferior oblique as the muscle travels from its anterior origin on the maxilla posterolaterally into the orbit. The arcuate expansion of the inferior oblique, also known as the anterior expansion of Lockwood's ligament, divides the middle and the lateral fat pads.

The lacrimal sac resides outside the confines of the orbit located anterior to the septum. When dacryocystitis results in fistula formation, the fistula usually drains anteriorly to the skin beneath the medial canthal ligament rather than posteriorly to the orbit.

EYELID RETRACTORS

The lower lid retractors form a complex structure analogous to the levator aponeurosis and Müller's muscle of the upper lid. The lower lid retractors represent the capsulopalpebral head of the inferior rectus muscle. This capsulopalpebral head has multiple attachments to the terminal inferior rectus muscle and tendon that vary in strength. A small portion of the capsulopalpebral head travels anteriorly and inferiorly through the orbital fat to insert by means of a fine network in the orbital fat and to the periosteum of the orbital floor (Fig. 26–13).[19] The bulk of the capsulopalpebral head of the inferior rectus passes anteriorly, dividing to encircle the inferior

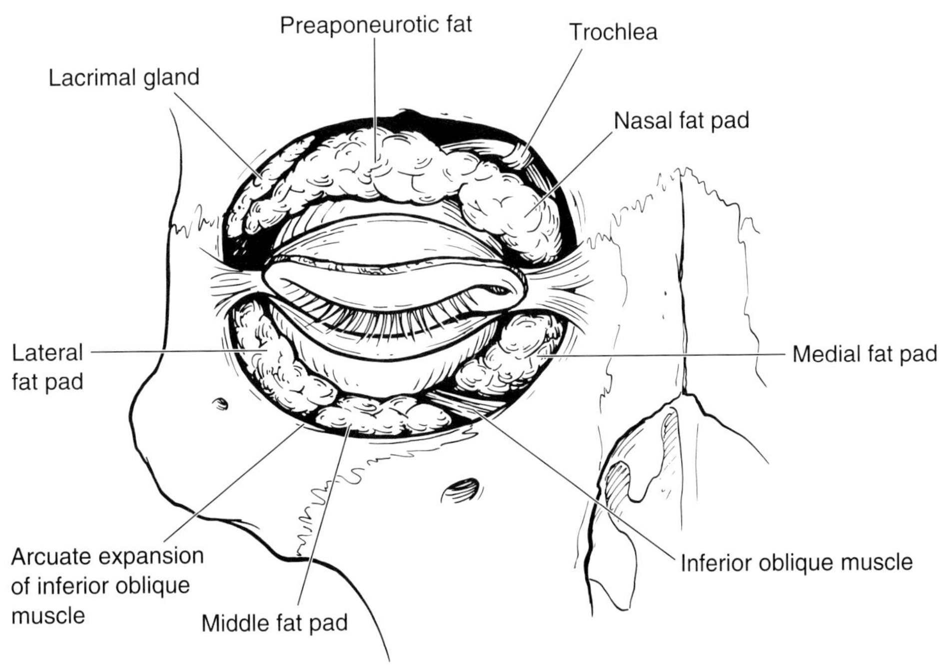

Figure 26–12. Anterior orbital fat seen after removal of the orbital septum. Deeper dissection of orbital fat pads shows fascial extensions of the trochlea dividing fat pads in the upper lid. The inferior oblique and the anterior expansion of Lockwood's ligament (arcuate expansion of the inferior oblique) divide the fat pads of the lower lid into medial, middle, and lateral.

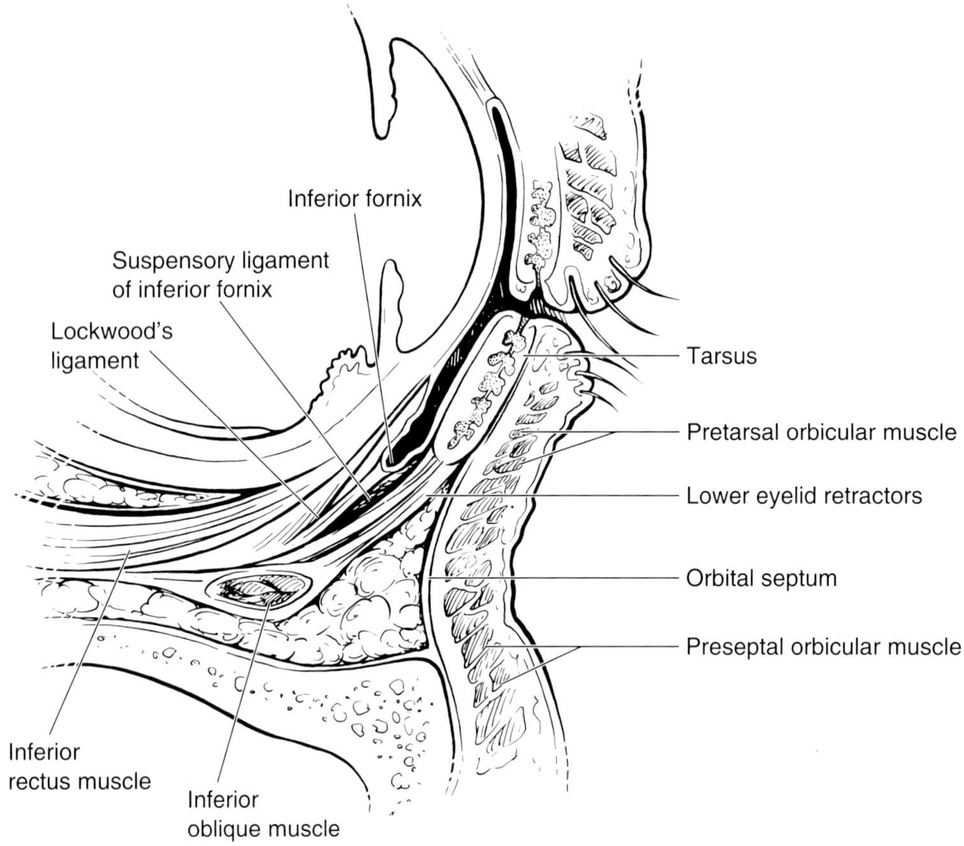

Figure 26–13. Anatomy of the lower eyelid retractors. Note the orbital septum joins the capsulopalpebral fascia before jointly inserting around the inferior border of the tarsus. Also note the fine connective tissue strands that pass through the orbital fat to insert on the periorbita of the orbital floor. (From Hawes MJ, Dortzbach RK: The microscopic anatomy of the lower lid retractors. Arch Ophthalmol 100:1313–1318, 1982. Copyright 1982, American Medical Association.)

oblique. The smooth muscle of the inferior tarsal muscle begins within the fibroelastic capsulopalpebral head anterior to the inferior rectus. The inferior tarsal muscle passes anteriorly with the capsulopalpebral fascia to fuse with the orbital septum. The septum joins the capsulopalpebral fascia 4 to 5 mm beneath the inferior tarsal border before the fascia inserts around the lower border of the tarsus. The smooth muscle fibers of the inferior tarsal muscle taper gradually and terminate approximately 2.5 mm from the inferior edge of the tarsus. Thinning and dehiscence of the lower lid retractors has been implicated as a contributing factor in involutional entropion[21, 22] and ectropion.[23] Relaxation of the inferior tarsal muscle results in the slight apparent enophthalmos seen in Horner's syndrome.

The retractor system of the upper lid parallels that of the lower lid but is much more developed. It provides for continued protection of the globe in downward gaze as well as unobstructed vision in primary and upward gaze. The 15 mm of upper lid excursion versus the 2 to 3 mm excursion of the lower lid results from a well-developed capsulopalpebral head of the superior rectus—the levator superioris. The levator arises outside the annulus of Zinn above the superior rectus on the lesser wing of the sphenoid. The levator proceeds anteriorly separated from the periorbita of the orbital roof by a thin layer of fat, the supraorbital artery, the frontal nerve, and the supratrochlear nerve. The levator and superior rectus may be easily separated from one another, except along the medial border where they are attached by a fascial sheath (Fig. 26–14). These attachments become stronger anteriorly as Whitnall's ligament is approached. The superior division of the oculomotor nerve supplies the superior rectus and the levator entering on the inferior aspects of the muscles approximately 12 mm from the orbital apex. The nerve gains access to the levator by traveling around the medial border of the superior rectus.

The muscle sheath of the levator is thin except medially, where it fuses with the sheath of the superior rectus. Behind the superior orbital rim the levator begins to fan out and become more tendinous. At this point, a fibrous condensation known as Whitnall's ligament attaches to the superior aspect of the levator. The attachments of Whitnall's ligament to the levator vary in strength, being more firm medially and laterally.[24] Medially, Whitnall's ligament terminates in the fascia that surrounds the trochlea, more posteriorly to the frontal bone beneath the superior oblique muscle and anteriorly blending with the fascia, closing the supraorbital notch (Fig. 26–15). Laterally, this ligament joins the capsule of the lacrimal gland and the periosteum of the frontal bone. The superior transverse ligament of Whitnall

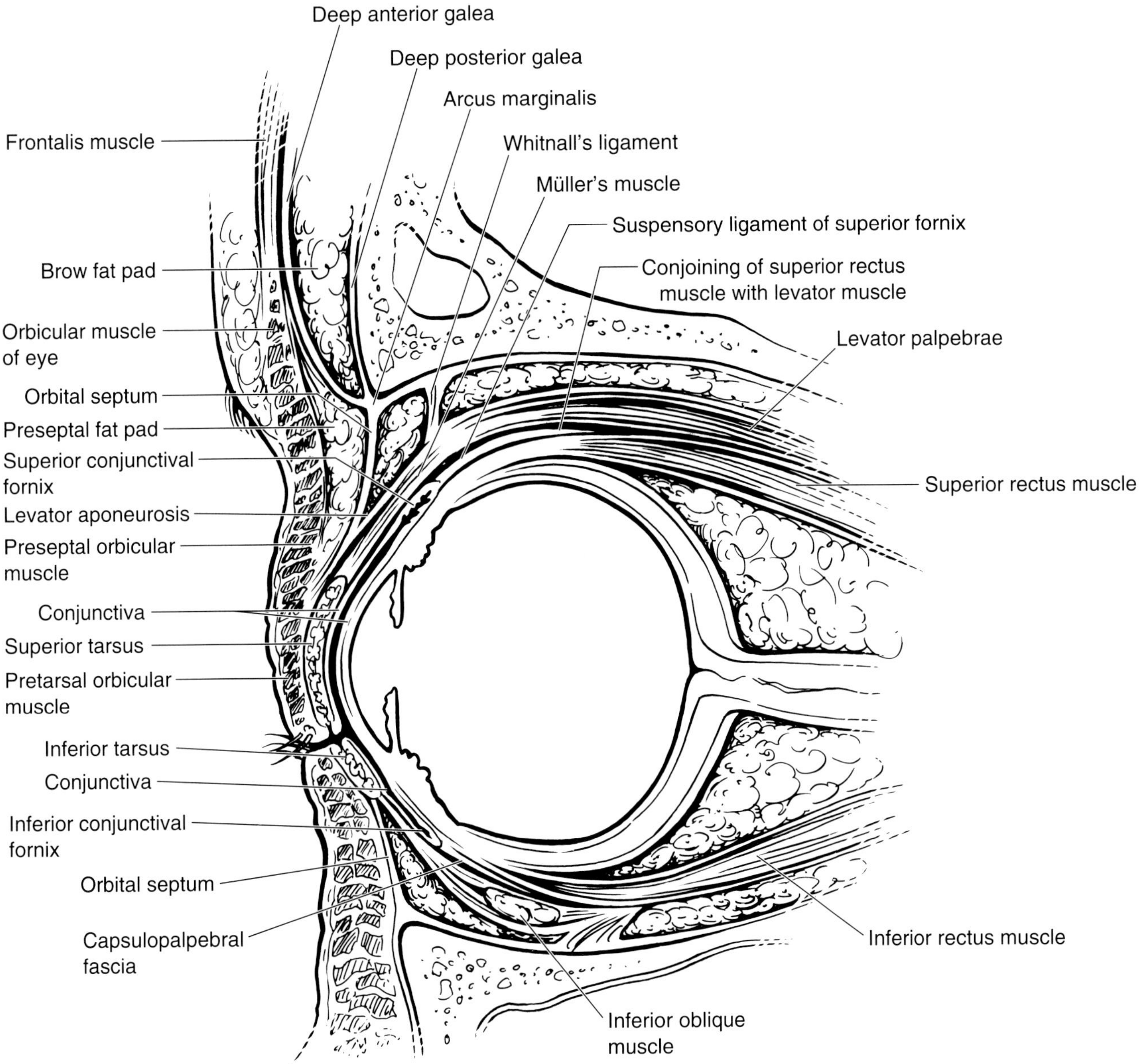

Figure 26–14. Parasagittal section of anterior orbital structures.

limits the movement of the levator longitudinally and in children may provide some vertical support for it. Dynamic high-resolution magnetic resonance imaging may demonstrate tenting of the levator superiorly by Whitnall's ligament in downward gaze, which suggests a vector-changing force supplied by Whitnall's ligament.[25] The globe supplies the principal vertical support to the upper lid[26] and after enucleation there is an immediate increase in the space between the levator and the orbital roof.[27] A thin fibrous sheet passes from the superior transverse ligament to the superior orbital rim, serving as the posterior border for the preaponeurotic fat.

The length of the levator from its origin to Whitnall's ligament averages 36 mm. The width of the levator is 4 mm at its origin and 8 mm at its midpoint and then fans out to 18 mm at the superior transverse ligament and becomes aponeurotic. The aponeurotic portion measures 14 to 20 mm, advancing to insert primarily in the orbicularis oculi with a secondary insertion on the anterior lower third of the tarsus. The levator inserts into the pretarsal orbicularis by means of a complex network of elastic fibers that forms the lid crease in the overlying skin.[1] The lid crease may be found higher than normal in patients with involutional ptosis. The levator sends projections medially and laterally known as the horns, which blend with the medial and lateral retinacula. The lateral horn of the levator is much stronger than the medial horn and incompletely splits the lacrimal gland into orbital and palpebral lobes before it joins with the lateral retinaculum to send fibers to the lateral orbital tubercle.[24] The medial horn is a delicate structure passing inferiorly to attach with the posterior limb of the medial canthal liga-

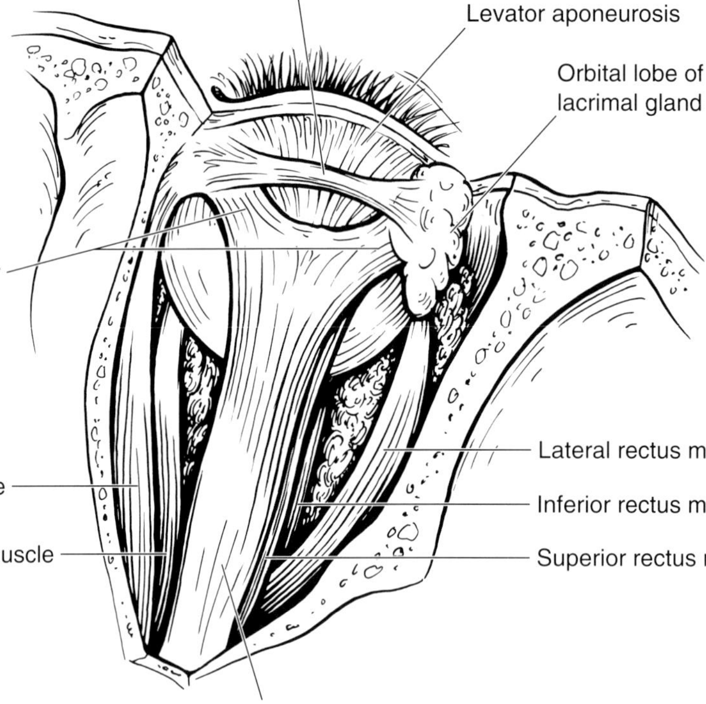

Figure 26–15. Superior view of the levator palpebrae superioris muscle and its relations. Note Whitnall's ligament attaching medially to the trochlear fascia and laterally to the fascia investing the lacrimal gland. The levator is bound on its medial side to the superior rectus and is innervated by the superior division of the oculomotor nerve.

ment on the posterior lacrimal crest and the medial orbital wall.[28]

There exists a dense condensation of fascia between the anterior aspects of the levator and the superior rectus. This fascia binds these muscles firmly together, although some play exists owing to several millimeters of fascial membrane length. The suspensory ligament of the superior fornix arises from this fascial condensation closer to the levator. The suspensory ligament originates 25 mm above the superior tarsal border and inserts into the conjunctiva of the superior fornix.

The sympathetic muscle of Müller begins from the undersurface of the levator just anterior to the intermuscular fascia. This smooth muscle proceeds anteriorly 12 to 15 mm to insert through a tendon on the superior border of the tarsus. The tendinous insertion contains numerous tightly arranged elastic fibers.[1] Müller's muscle adheres firmly to the levator only at its origin and can be easily separated from the underside of the aponeurosis anterior to this, forming a potential postaponeurotic space.[29] Müller's muscle is firmly adherent to the underlying conjunctiva just above the superior tarsal border. Dissection between Müller's muscle and the conjunctiva may be performed more easily near the origin of Müller's muscle.

Sympathetics that travel from the carotid plexus enter the orbit between the third and sixth nerves to innervate Müller's muscle. The orbital course of the sympathetics has not been completely described. Interruption of these sympathetics results in the 2 mm of blepharoptosis characteristic of Horner's syndrome. Müller's muscle may also become fibrotic as a result of the orbital inflammation of Graves' disease, often causing retraction of the upper lid.

EYELID MARGIN

Dense fibrous connective tissue forms the tarsal plates providing support and structural integrity to the eyelids. Two principal factors as described by Mustarde[30] provide for this support. The first is the lamination factor produced by the joining of the anterior and posterior lamellae. Through this lamination the strength of the lid is greater than the sum of the strength of the components. The second factor strengthening the lid margin is the phalange effect produced as the dense connective tissue of the tarsal plates intermingle and support the bulk of the cilia at the lid margin. The interdigitation of the tarsus and the lashes forms a ciliary mass that provides the bulk of the support to the lid margin. This effect is more pronounced in the upper lid and is analogous to the rigidity achieved by bending the edge of a sheet material over at a right angle, such as with an angle iron. These two factors provide the lid with its semirigid structure.

The average height of the tarsal plates is 10 mm in the upper lid and 4 to 5 mm in the lower lid.[31] These heights are in proportion to the amount of globe covered by the

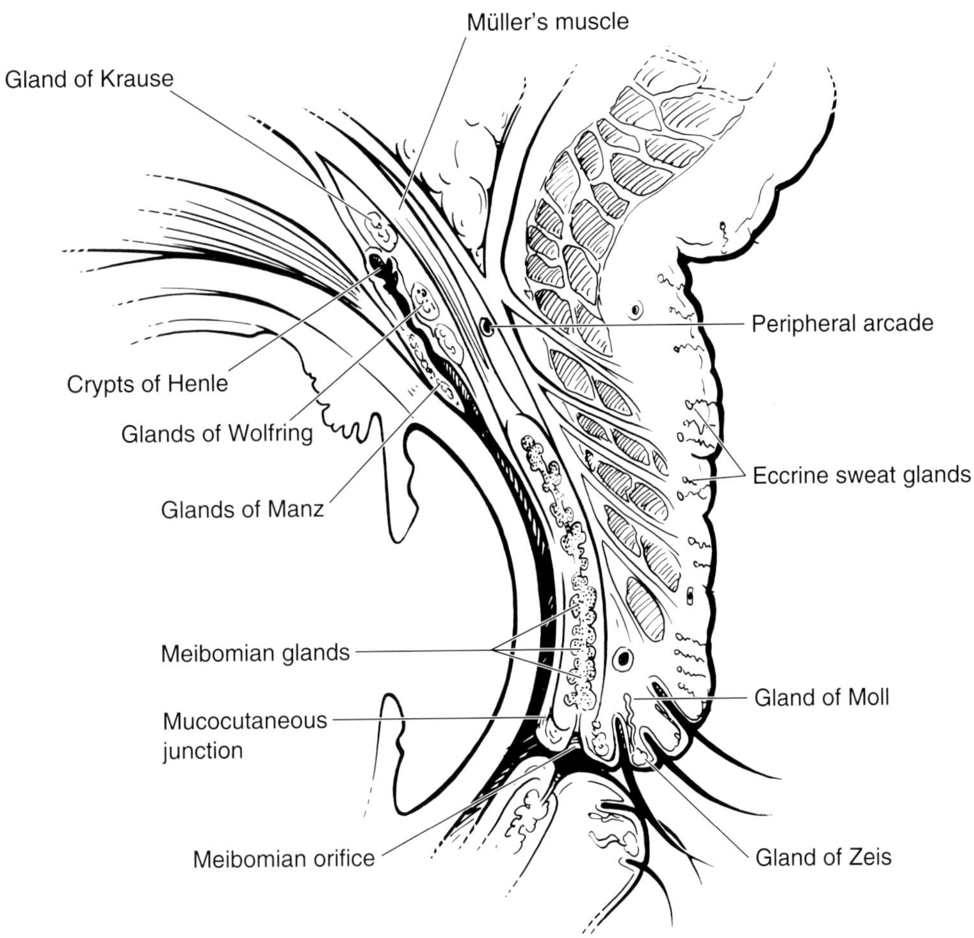

Figure 26–16. Accessory lacrimal glands of Krause and Wolfring. Mucous glands of Manz and Henle. Sebaceous glands of Zeis and Meibom. Apocrine gland of Moll and eccrine sweat glands.

respective lid. The tarsal plates support the meibomian glands and orifices, numbering 25 to 35 in the upper lid and 15 to 25 in the lower lid.[32] These branched acinal glands extend nearly the vertical height of the tarsus and through holocrine secretion produce the oil layer of the tear film. The meibomian gland orifices are located just posterior to the gray line and anterior to the mucocutaneous junction (Fig. 26–16). Keratinized squamous epithelium lines the ducts. The hydrophobic substance produced by holocrine secretion composes the outermost layer of the tear film, which retards evaporation of the tear film as well as limits the flow of tears over the lid margin. The meibomian glands may develop hair follicles congenitally or after chronic inflammation. Rarely, these glands may undergo malignant change, producing sebaceous cell carcinoma.

The eyelashes (cilia) line the eyelid margin with their bulbs resting on the tarsal plate and the lashes projecting anterior to the gray line. The cilia number slightly more than 100 in the upper lid and 50 in the lower. The lash follicle separates a portion of the pretarsal orbicularis, forming the muscle of Riolan. This bundle of pretarsal orbicularis located just anterior to the mucocutaneous junction forms the anatomic landmark known as the gray line. Sebaceous glands of Zeis and apocrine glands of Moll empty their secretions into the lumen of the follicle. The eyelashes most likely represent a sensory organ, and their bulbs are richly innervated with sensory nerve endings. In chronic inflammatory states the eyelashes may become misdirected, resulting in trichiasis. Sweat glands are also located at the lid margin. These eccrine glands have tortuous ducts that open onto the skin superior to the lashes. They are present throughout the eyelid up to the brow and play a role in temperature regulation. The apocrine and eccrine glands may form sudiferous cysts filled with clear fluid that transilluminate.

ARTERIAL SUPPLY

Both the internal and external carotid systems supply arterial blood to the eyelids. The arterial supply possesses many anastomoses, making the eyelids highly vascular structures. The external carotid system supplies the eye-

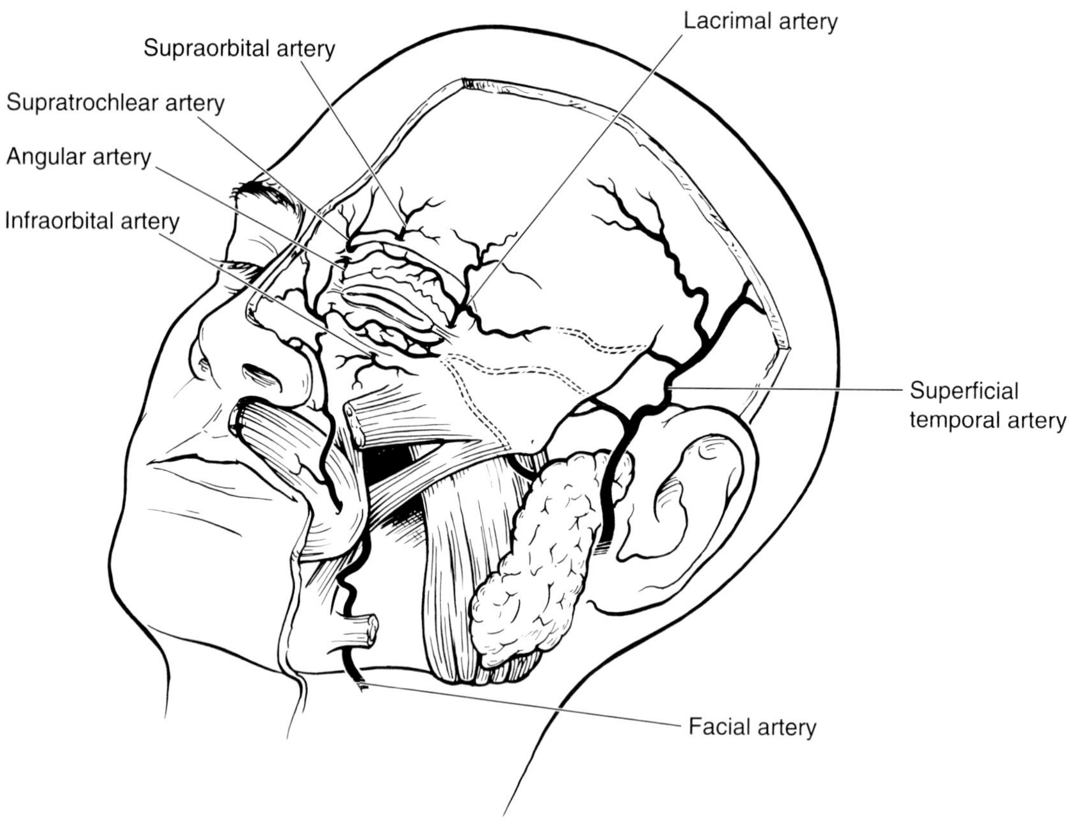

Figure 26–17. Superficial arteries of the ocular region.

lid through the facial and superficial temporal arteries (Fig. 26–17). The facial artery branches from the external carotid, crossing the mandible anterior to the masseter muscle and traveling toward the nasolabial fold. It rises alongside the nose beneath the levators of the lips and then becomes more superficial between the levator labii superioris and levator alae nasi muscles. The facial artery terminates as the angular artery, which lies beneath the orbicularis muscle 6 to 8 mm medial to the inner canthus. It travels along the line of the nasojugal skin fold and passes superficial to the medial canthal ligament. In this location the angular artery may cause profuse bleeding if severed during dacryocystorhinostomy. The artery then perforates the orbital septum to anastomose with branches of the ophthalmic artery in the superomedial orbit.

The external carotid artery terminates as the superficial temporal artery, which travels up behind the jaw and surfaces anterior to the ear, resting above the temporal fascia. The artery runs a sinuous course superiorly, giving off three branches to the eyelid: the frontal, zygomaticofacial, and transverse facial. The frontal branch passes upward and medially to supply the frontalis and orbicularis oculi, anastomosing with the supraorbital and lacrimal branches of the ophthalmic artery. The zygomaticofacial branch passes along the upper border of the zygoma, supplying the lateral aspects of the lids. The transverse facial artery runs forward below the zygoma, anastomosing with the infraorbital and lacrimal arteries at the lateral border of the lower lid.

Two branches of the ophthalmic artery, the lacrimal and the dorsonasal artery, anastomose to form the marginal and peripheral arcades of the upper eyelid (Fig. 26–18). The medial vessels arise from the terminal branch of the ophthalmic artery, usually before perforating the orbital septum. The marginal arcade traverses the anterior surface of the tarsus 2 to 3 mm from the lid margin and should be avoided during reconstructive tarsal-sharing techniques. The peripheral arcade rests above the upper border of the tarsus beneath the levator and above Müller's muscle in the postaponeurotic space. Both the marginal and peripheral vascular arcades contribute to the blood supply of the conjunctiva. Perforating conjunctival branches form a posterior tarsal plexus that affords a rich blood supply to the tarsal conjunctiva. The peripheral arcade also gives rise to the posterior conjunctival artery, which supplies the superior fornix and anastomoses with the anterior ciliary branches near the limbus. The lower lid contains a marginal arcade that arises medially from a branch of the nasal artery and joins the lacrimal and zygomaticotemporal arteries. The peripheral arcade in the lower lid is poorly developed and does not supply the conjunctiva.

The venous system also possesses anastomoses be-

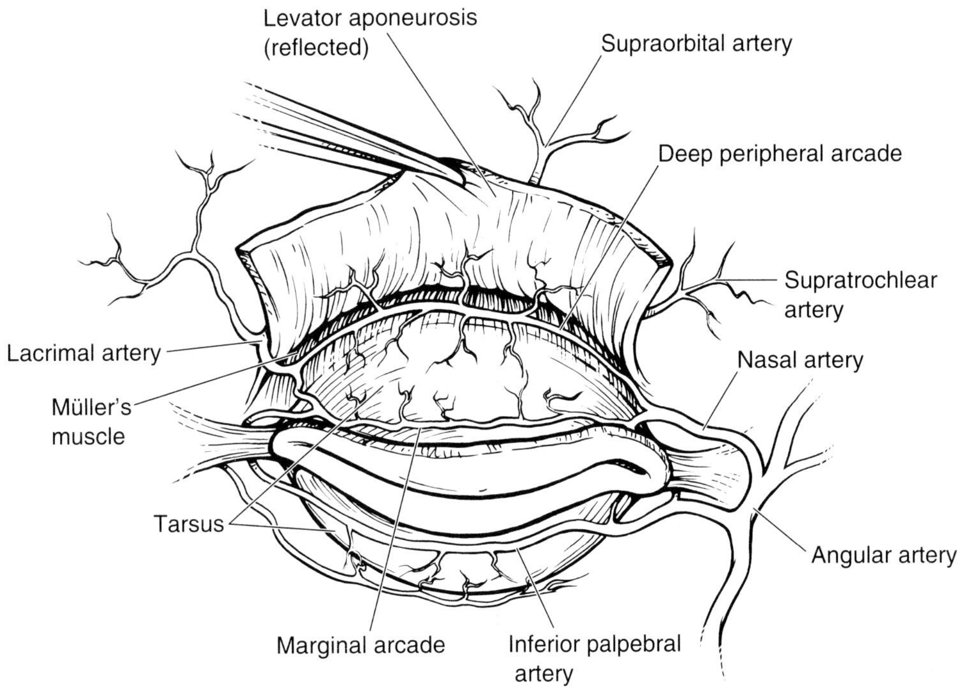

Figure 26–18. Tarsal arterial arcades. Marginal artery is larger than peripheral artery and is located 2 to 3 mm from the tarsal margin. The peripheral arcade in the upper lid is located between Müller's muscle and the levator aponeurosis above the tarsus. The angular artery and the superficial temporal artery are branches from the external carotid artery, while the supraorbital and lacrimal arteries originate from the internal carotid system.

tween the superficial veins of the face draining into the jugular and the deep veins of the orbit, which drain into the cavernous sinus. The frontal and supraorbital veins join at the medial eyebrow to form the angular vein (Fig. 26–19). The angular vein rests superficially 6 to 8 mm medial to the inner canthus, medial to the artery where it may be visualized, and should be avoided during dacryocystorhinostomy. The angular vein becomes the facial vein, which travels just lateral to the facial artery. The supraorbital vein travels horizontally beneath the orbicularis parallel to the superior orbital margin joining the frontal and superior ophthalmic veins. Lateral to the lateral canthus the supraorbital vein forms a preauricular plexus before draining posterior to the ear by way of the superficial temporal vein. The frontal veins run down the forehead vertically just below the skin along with the supraorbital artery and nerve.

Superficial infections of the face may spread to the cavernous and dural sinuses through anastomoses between the facial veins and the cavernous sinus. The angular vein joins the superior ophthalmic vein, which drains into the cavernous sinus. The facial vein communicates with the internal maxillary vein before it drains into the pterygoid plexus, which reaches the cavernous sinus through the inferior ophthalmic vein. These veins do not possess a well-developed system of valves and may allow the spread of superficial infections of the face to the dural sinuses.

LYMPHATICS

The lymphatic drainage of the eyelids may be divided into a small medial and larger lateral groups (Fig. 26–20). The medial group drains the medial half of the lower lid, the medial commissure, the medial end of the upper lid, the conjunctiva of the medial two thirds of the lower lid, and the caruncle. The lymphatic vessels travel with the facial vein down the face to reach the submandibular lymph nodes. The lateral group drains the majority of the upper and the lateral half of the lower lid. The lymphatics drain to the preauricular nodes located just anterior to the external auditory meatus. Sebaceous carcinomas most commonly spread by means of the lymphatics to the preauricular nodes from the upper lid.

INNERVATION

The eyelids receive motor innervation from the facial nerve and the oculomotor nerve. Sympathetics originating in the superior cervical ganglion supply Müller's muscle, the inferior tarsal muscle, and the sweat glands of the face. The ophthalmic and the maxillary divisions of the trigeminal nerve provide for sensation to the periorbital region.

The facial nerve originates in the facial nucleus within the pons. The facial nucleus receives supranuclear input from the motor cortex of the contralateral precentral gyrus. Supranuclear input to the lower face is completely contralateral, while the upper face receives bilateral input. Presence of upper facial involvement characteristic of peripheral facial nerve palsies differentiates peripheral from central facial nerve palsies. In the pons the fibers of the facial nerve pass over the abducens nerve nucleus as the genu of the facial nerve to exit the brain stem at the pontomedullary junction. The facial nerve

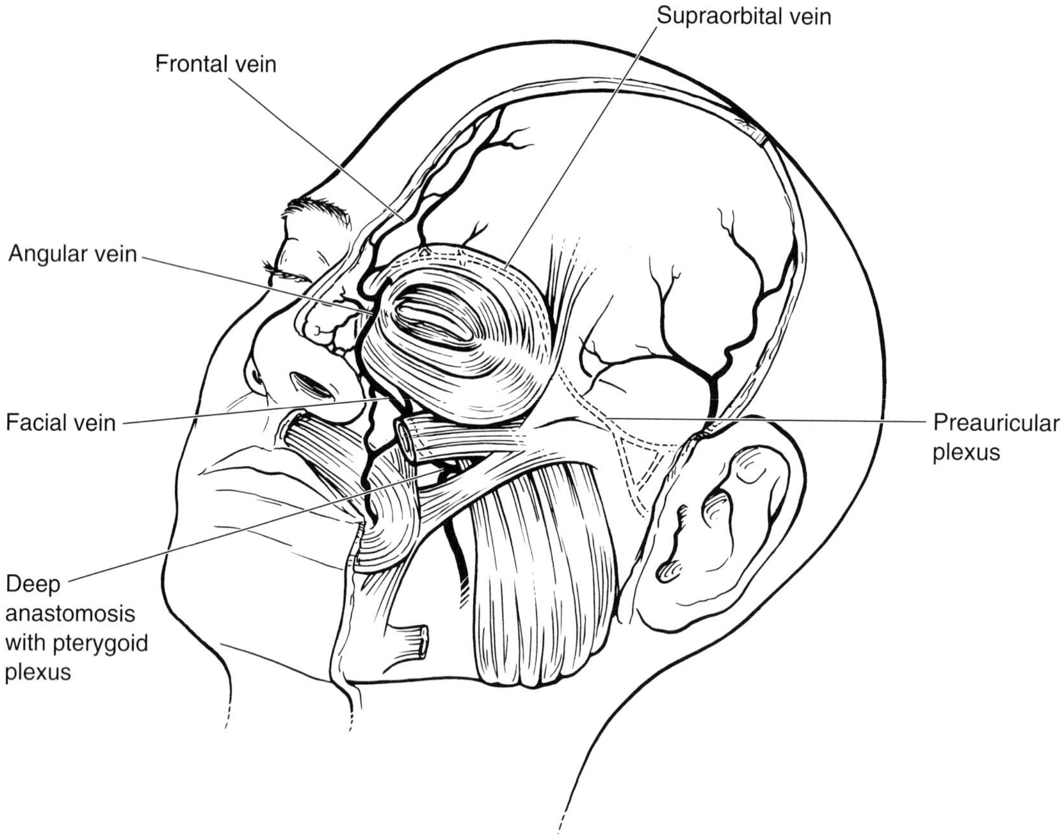

Figure 26–19. Superficial veins of the ocular region. The angular vein lies 6 to 8 mm medial to the inner commissure; it communicates superficially with the frontal and facial veins, joins the horizontal supraorbital vein beneath the orbicularis, and becomes the superior ophthalmic vein after piercing the orbital septum. (From Lemke BN: Anatomy of the ocular adnexa and orbit. *In* Smith BC, Della Rocca RC, Lisman RD, Nesi FA [eds]: Ophthalmic Plastic and Reconstructive Surgery. St. Louis, CV Mosby, 1987.)

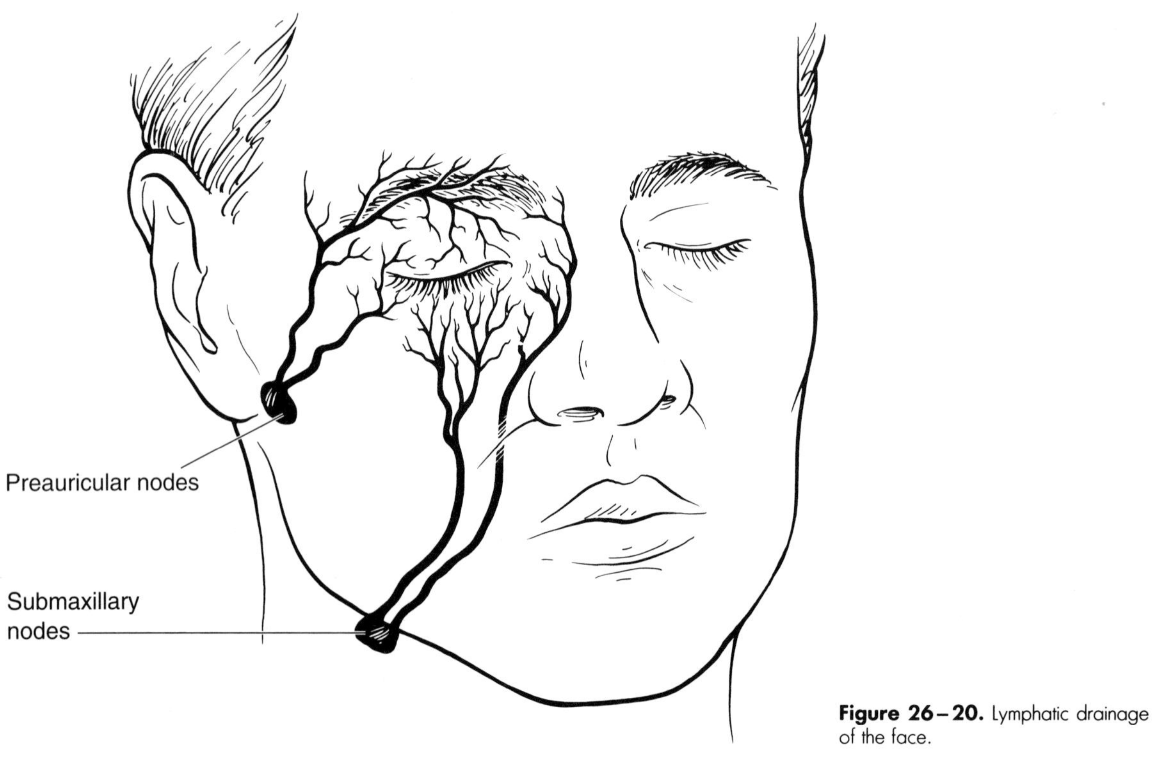

Figure 26–20. Lymphatic drainage of the face.

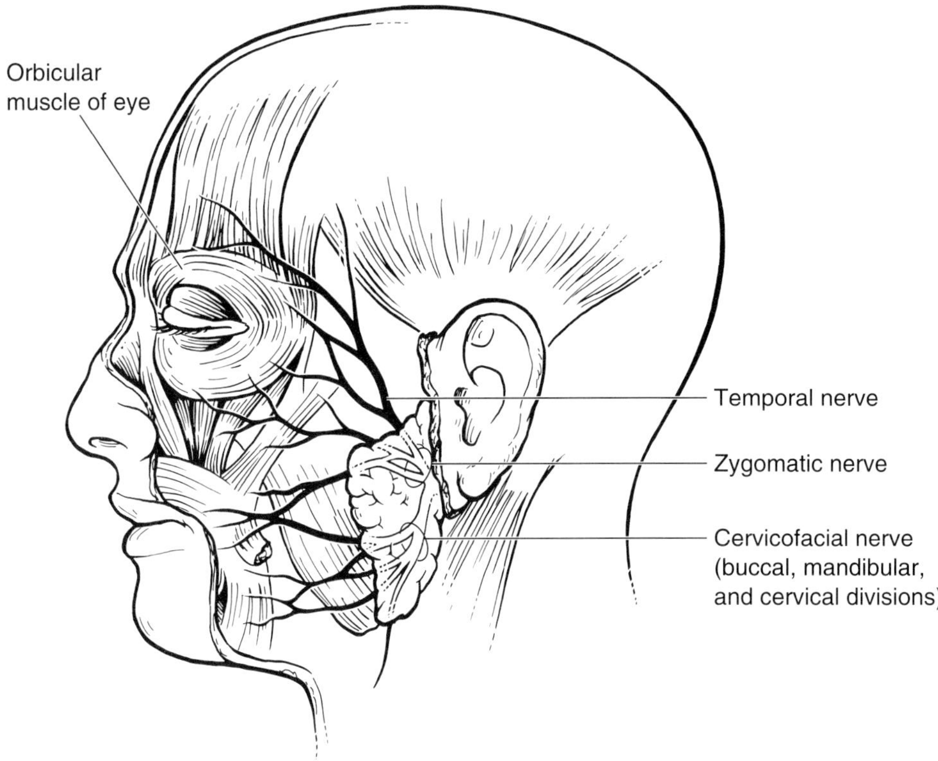

Figure 26–21. Superficial cranial nerve VII.

enters the internal acoustic meatus associated with the nervus intermedius and the acoustic nerve. The facial nerve gives off a branch to supply the stapedius muscle and then exits the auditory canal behind the styloid process by way of the stylomastoid foramen. The facial nerve then travels anteriorly and superiorly to reach the parotid gland. Within the gland the nerve divides, with the temporal, zygomatic, and buccal branches traveling superomedially to innervate the orbicularis on its undersurface (Fig. 26–21). Extensive arborization of the motor nerve fibers can be demonstrated before reaching the edge of the orbicularis oculi muscle. The facial nerve fibers are oriented horizontally at the lateral border of the orbicularis and supply the muscle through its undersurface. Perineural fusion between some large branches of the facial and trigeminal nerves exists that electrophysiologic data suggest may be unimportant.[4] Innervation to the procerus passes inferior to the orbit while the nerve to the corrugator supraciliaris may travel inferiorly or superiorly.

The oculomotor nerve divides into a superior and inferior division within the cavernous sinus or at the apex of the orbit after passing through the superior orbital fissure. The superior division innervates the levator superioris and superior rectus through its undersurface. Innervation to the levator from the oculomotor nerve nuclei is bilateral, and lesions of the oculomotor nerve nucleus may produce bilateral ptosis with involvement of the contralateral superior rectus. The inferior branch of the oculomotor nerve innervates the inferior rectus, medial rectus, and inferior oblique and supplies parasympathetics to the pupillary sphincter.

Two of the three branches of the trigeminal nerve originating in the gasserian ganglion pass through the orbit to provide sensory input from the periorbital region (Fig. 26–22). The first branch, the ophthalmic nerve, passes along the lateral wall of the cavernous sinus to enter the orbit through the superior orbital fissure. This ophthalmic branch divides into three branches: the nasociliary, frontal, and lacrimal. The frontal and lacrimal branches pass outside the muscle cone in the superior orbit, with the frontal branch further dividing into the supraorbital and supratrochlear nerves before piercing the septum. These branches provide sensation for the medial portion of the upper lid and conjunctiva, forehead, scalp, frontal sinuses, and side of the nose. The lacrimal division supplies the skin and conjunctiva surrounding the lacrimal gland, supplies the lateral third of the eyelid, and carries postganglionic parasympathetic fibers for reflex lacrimation. The nasociliary nerve passes through the muscle cone, giving rise to the long and short posterior ciliary nerves, which provide sensory fibers to the cornea, bulbar conjunctiva, and the globe. Branches of the nasociliary nerve travel with the anterior and posterior ethmoidal arteries to gain access to the anterior and posterior ethmoidal foramina. These branches provide sensory input from the medial canthus, lacrimal sac, middle and inferior turbinates, lateral nasal wall, and tip of the nose. In the upper lid, sensory fibers from branches of the supraorbital and supratrochlear nerves travel vertically in

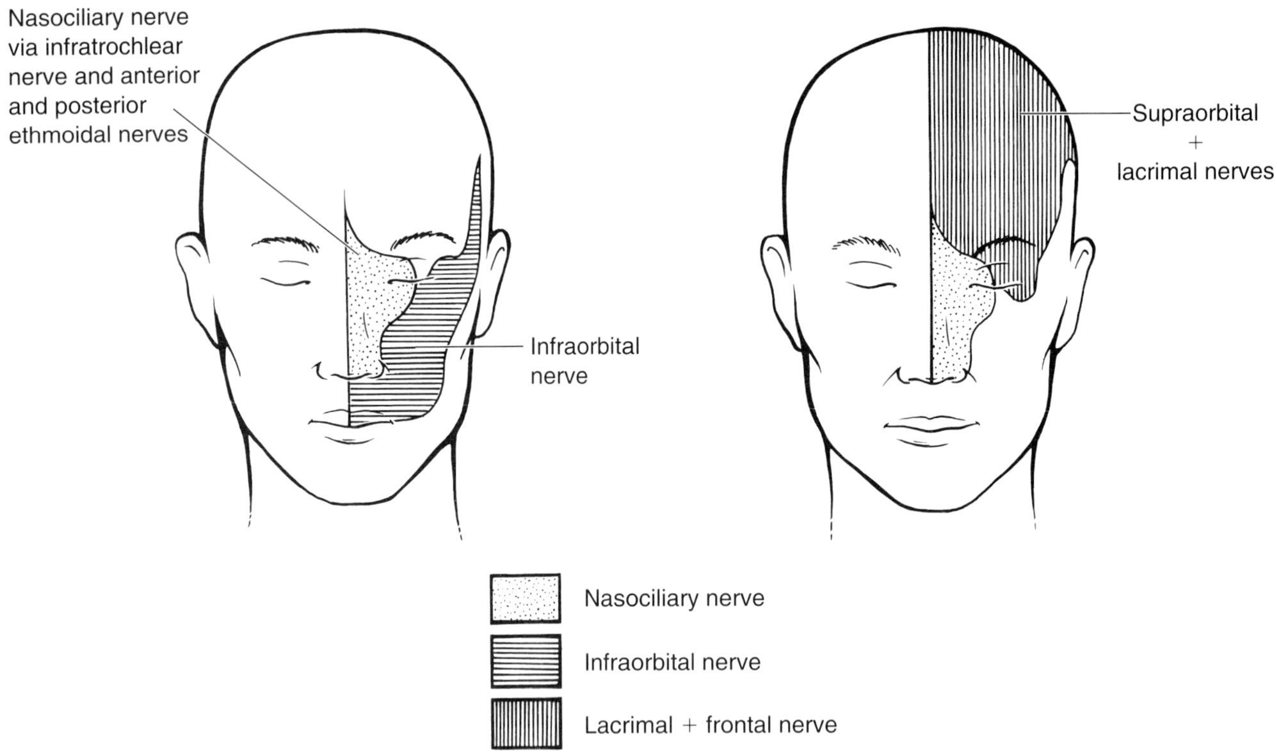

Figure 26–22. Cutaneous distribution of cranial nerve V.

the suborbicularis fascial plane, in the preorbicular plane, and within the orbicularis muscle itself.[33]

The maxillary division of the trigeminal nerve leaves the gasserian ganglion and travels through the foramen rotundum to gain access to the pterygopalatine fossa. This branch then enters the orbit through the inferior orbital fissure, passing through the infraorbital canal as the infraorbital nerve. After exiting at the infraorbital foramen the nerve divides into an inferior palpebral branch, a superior labial branch, and a nasal branch. These branches innervate the lower lid, upper lip, and side of the nose, respectively. Branches from the maxillary division also provide for sensation from the teeth, maxillary sinus, roof of the mouth, and soft palate.

REGIONAL ANESTHESIA

Anesthesia for lid surgery can be obtained either by local infiltration of the tissues or by regional nerve blocks. Local infiltration provides the advantage of improved hemostasis and longer duration of action when epinephrine is added to the anesthetic mixture. Regional nerve blocks require less volume of anesthetic and do not distort the tissues in the operative field.

Regional blocks of the motor branches of the facial nerve prevent lid closure during intraocular surgery and protect ruptured globes from increased pressure due to orbicularis spasm. Approaches to the facial nerve include sites at the stylomastoid foramen as described by Nadbath,[34] as it crosses the parotid gland as described by O'Brien,[35] and lateral to the orbital rim as described by Van Lint.[36] Blocks at the stylomastoid foramen produce a hemifacial palsy, while O'Brien and Van Lint blocks result in akinesia of the orbicularis oculi, frontalis, procerus, and corregator supraciliaris.

Anesthesia in the brow and lid region can be obtained through use of frontal, nasociliary, infraorbital, or zygomaticofacial blocks alone or more frequently in combination. The frontal block provides anesthesia for the medial two thirds of the upper lid, the eyebrow, and the forehead. After palpation of the supraorbital notch a needle is inserted just temporal to this, going back 5 to 10 mm posterior to the superior orbital rim; 1 mL of anesthetic is injected. A nasociliary block provides anesthesia for the inner canthus, lacrimal sac, skin, and mucosa of the nose. The nerve is blocked at the anterior and posterior ethmoidal foramina. The trochlea is palpated, and a needle is inserted just inferior to the trochlea and advanced 20 mm posteriorly with 1 mL of anesthetic injected. The needle is advanced 20 mm farther posterior, and an additional 1 mL is injected. This block allows dacryocystorhinostomy to be performed under local anesthesia. Possible complications include profuse bleeding from the anterior and posterior ethmoidal vessels. The infraorbital nerve may be blocked as it exits the infraorbital foramen, providing anesthesia for the lower lid, conjunctiva, and a portion of the medial canthus and lacrimal sac. The infraorbital foramen is located at the medial third of an imaginary line drawn between the ala nasi and the lateral orbital rim. The infraorbital nerve may also be blocked in the infraorbital canal by advancing a needle along the orbital floor and injecting 1 mL of anesthetic. The zygomaticofacial nerve exits the zygomaticofacial foramen located 10 mm below the lateral canthus. It may be blocked here, providing anesthesia for the lateral canthal area and the outer portion of the lower lid.

REFERENCES

1. Stasior GO, Lemke BN, Wallow IH, Dortzbach RK: Levator aponeurosis elastic fiber network. Ophthal Plast Reconstr Surg 9:1–10, 1993.
2. Lemke BN, Stasior OG: Epiblepharon. Clin Pediatr 20:661–662, 1981.
3. Srinivasan BD, Jakobiec FA, Iwamoto T: Conjunctiva. *In* Jakobiec FA (ed): Ocular Anatomy, Embryology, and Teratology. New York, Harper & Row, 1982, pp 733–760.
4. Lemke BN: Anatomy of the ocular adnexa and orbit. *In* Smith BC, Della Rocca RC, Lisman RD, Nesi FA (eds): Ophthalmic Plastic and Reconstructive Surgery. St. Louis, CV Mosby, 1987.
5. Meyer DR, Linberg JV, Wobig JL, McCormick SA: Anatomy of the orbital septum and associated eyelid connective tissues. Ophthalmic Plast Reconstr Surg 7:104–113, 1991.
6. Putterman AM, Urist MJ: Surgical anatomy of the orbital septum. Ann Ophthalmol 6:290–294, 1974.
7. Lemke BN, Stasior OG: The anatomy of eyebrow ptosis. Arch Ophthalmol 100:981–986, 1982.
8. Lemke BN, Stasior OG: Eyebrow incision making. Adv Ophthalmic Plast Reconstr Surg 2:19–23, 1983.
9. Lemke BN: Applied anatomy of the eyelids, lacrimal system and the orbit. Curr Opin Ophthalmol 1:501–505, 1990.
10. Elner VM, Lemke BN, Dortzbach RK: The histologic anatomy of the medial canthal ligament and surrounding structures. Presented to the American Society of Ophthalmic Plastic and Reconstructive Surgery, November, 1988.
11. Sullivan TJ, Welham RAN, Collin JRO: Centurion syndrome: Idiopathic anterior displacement of the medial canthus. Ophthalmology 100:328–333, 1993.
12. Ahl NC, Hill JC: Horner's muscle and the lacrimal system. Arch Ophthalmol 100:488–493, 1982.
13. Robinson TJ, Stranc MF: The anatomy of the medial canthal ligament. Br J Plast Surg 11:1–9, 1983.
14. Jones LT: An anatomic approach to problems of the eyelid and lacrimal apparatus. Arch Ophthalmol 66:111, 1961.
15. Linberg JV: Surgical anatomy of the lacrimal system. *In* Contemporary Issues in Ophthalmology, Vol 5, Lacrimal Surgery. New York, Churchill Livingstone, 1988.
16. Wulc AE, Arterberry JF: The pathogenesis of canalicular laceration. Ophthalmology 98:1243–1249, 1991.
17. Wulc AE, Dryden RM, Khatchaturian T: Where is the grey line? Arch Ophthalmol 105:1092–1098, 1987.
18. Whitnall ES: The Anatomy of the Human Orbit and the Accessory Organs of Vision. Huntington, NY, Robert E. Krieger, 1979 [facsimile of 1932 edition].
19. Hawes MJ, Dortzbach RK: The microscopic anatomy of the lower lid retractors. Arch Ophthalmol 100:1313–1318, 1982.
20. Hugo NE, Stone E: Anatomy for a blepharoplasty. Plast Reconstr Surg 53:381, 1974.
21. Dryden RM, Leibsohn J, Wobig J: Senile entropion pathogenesis and treatment. Ophthalmology 96:1883–1885, 1978.
22. Hill JC: Treatment of epiphora owing to flaccid eyelids. Arch Ophthalmol 97:323–327, 1979.
23. Putterman AM: Ectropion of the eyelid secondary to Müller's muscle–capsulopalpebral fascia detachment. Am J Ophthalmol 85:813–817, 1978.
24. Lemke BM, Stasior OG, Rosenberg PN: The surgical relations of the levator palpebrae superioris muscle. Ophthal Plast Reconstr Surg 4:25–30, 1988.
25. Goldberg RA, Wu JC, Jesmanowicz A, Hyde JS: Eyelid anatomy revisited: Dynamic high resolution magnetic resonance images of Whitnall's ligament and upper eyelid structures with use of a surface coil. Arch Ophthalmol 110:1598–1600, 1992.
26. Vistnes IM: Mechanism of upper lid ptosis in the anophthalmic orbit. Plast Reconstr Surg 58:539–545, 1976.
27. Soll DB: Evolution and current concepts in surgical treatment of the anophthalmic orbit. Ophthal Plast Reconstr Surg 2:163–171, 1986.
28. Anderson RL, Beard C: The levator aponeurosis: Attachments and their clinical significance. Arch Ophthalmol 95:1437–1441, 1977.
29. Jones LT: The anatomy of the upper eyelid and its relation to ptosis surgery. Am J Ophthalmol 73:1189–1197, 1964.
30. Mustarde JC: Repair and Reconstruction in the Orbital Region, 3rd ed. New York, Churchill Livingstone, 1988.
31. Wesley RE, McCord CD: Height of the tarsus of the lower eyelid. Am J Ophthalmol 90:102, 1980.
32. Mansour AM: Meibomian gland secretion. Orbit 7:201–209, 1988.
33. Scott KR, Tse DT, Kronish JW: Vertically oriented upper eyelid nerve fibers: A clinical, anatomic and immunohistochemical study. Ophthalmology 99:222–226, 1992.
34. Nadbath RP, Rehman I: Facial nerve block. Am J Ophthalmol 55:143–146, 1963.
35. O'Brien CS: Local anesthesia in ophthalmic surgery. JAMA 90:8, 1928.
36. Van Lint A: Paralysie palpebrae temporaire par l'operation de la cataracte. Ann Ocul 151:420, 1914.

BIBLIOGRAPHY

Atkinson WS: Anesthesia in ophthalmology. Publication #251, American Lecture Series. Springfield, IL, Charles C Thomas, 1955.

Baylis HI, Long JA, Groth MJ: Transconjunctival lower lid blepharoplasty: Techniques and complications. Ophthalmology 96:1027–1032, 1989.

Bergen MP: Some histological aspects of the connective tissue system and its relationships with the blood vessels of the human orbit. Acta Morphol Neerl Scand 20:293–308, 1982.

Beyer CK, Fabian RL, Smith B: Naso-orbital fractures, complications and treatment. Ophthalmology 5:456–463, 1982.

Biglan AW, Chang A, Hiles DA: Prolapse of conjunctiva following external levator resection. Ophthalmic Surg 11:581–583, 1982.

Buckman G, Levine MR: Treatment of prolapsed conjunctiva. Ophthal Plast Reconstr Surg 2:33–39, 1986.

Collin JR, Rathbun JE: Involutional entropion. Arch Ophthalmol 96:1058–1064, 1978.

Dresner SC: Further modifications of the Müller's muscle conjunctival resection procedure for blepharoptosis. Ophthal Plast Reconstr Surg 7:114–122, 1991.

Fink WH: An anatomic study of the check mechanism of the vertical muscles of the eyes. Am J Ophthalmol 44:800–809, 1957.

Gioia VM, Linberg JV, McCormick SA: The anatomy of the lateral canthal tendon. Arch Ophthalmol 105:529–533, 1987.

Goldberg RA, Lessner AM, Shorr N, Baylis HI: The transconjunctival approach to the orbital floor and orbital fat: A prospective study. Ophthal Plast Reconstr Surg 6:241–246, 1990.

Harvey JT, Anderson RL: The aponeurotic approach to eyelid retraction. Ophthalmology 88:513–524, 1981.

Hill JC: Treatment of epiphora owing to flaccid eyelids. Arch Ophthalmol 97:323–324, 1979.

Jones LT: A new concept of the orbital fascia and rectus muscle sheaths and its surgical implications. Trans Am Acad Ophthalmol Otolaryngol 72:755–764, 1968.

Jones LT: Epiphora. Am J Ophthalmol 43:203–212, 1957.

Klatsky S, Manson PN: Numbness after blepharoplasty: The relation of the upper orbital fat to the sensory nerves. Plast Reconstr Surg 67:20–22, 1981.

Koornneef L: Eyelid and orbital fascial attachments and their clinical significance. Eye 2:130–134, 1988.

Koornneef L: New insights in the human orbital connective tissue. Arch Ophthalmol 95:1269–1273, 1977.

Koornneef L: Orbital septa: Anatomy and function. Ophthalmology 86:876–880, 1979.

Lemke BN: Anatomic considerations in upper eyelid retraction. Ophthal Plast Reconstr Surg 7:158–166, 1991.

Lockwood CB: The anatomy of the muscles, ligaments, and fascia of the orbit, including an account of the capsule of Tenon, the check ligaments of the recti, and of the suspensory ligament of the eye. J Anat Physiol 20:1–25, 1886.

Manson PN, Clifford CM, Su CT, et al: Mechanisms of global support and post-traumatic enophthalmos: I. The anatomy of the ligament sling and its relation to intramuscular cone orbital fat. Plast Reconstr Surg 77:193–202, 1986.

Newhaus RW, Hawes MJ: Inadequate inferior cul-de-sac in the anophthalmic socket. Ophthalmology 99:153–157, 1992.

Schwab IR, Linberg JV, Gioia VM, et al: Foreshortening of the inferior conjunctival fornix associated with chronic glaucoma medications. Ophthalmology 99:197–202, 1992.

Shore JW, McCord CD: Anatomic changes in involutional ptosis. Am J Ophthalmol 98:21–27, 1984.

Silkiss RZ, Carroll RP: Transconjunctival surgery. Ophthalmic Surg 23:288–291, 1992.

Sutton JE: The fascia of the human orbit. Anat Rec 18:141–157, 1920.

Warwick R: Eugene Wolff's Anatomy of the Eye and Orbit. Philadelphia, WB Saunders, 1976, pp 205–226.

Werb A: Ptosis. Aust J Ophthalmol 18:286–287, 1976.

Westfall CT, Shore JW, Nunery WR, et al: Operative complications of the transconjunctival inferior fornix approach. Ophthalmology 98:1525–1528, 1991.

Zide BM, Jelks GW: Surgical anatomy of the orbit. Plast Reconstr Surg 74:301–305, 1984.

CHAPTER 27

Basic Surgical Techniques, Technology, and Wound Repair

David B. Christie and John J. Woog

WOUND HEALING

Healing of skin and underlying connective tissues can be divided into two general categories. Primary wound healing (healing by primary intention) occurs when the skin edges are opposed. Reapproximation of the wound is usually accomplished with sutures, although skin staples or sterile adhesive strips are used in certain situations. Secondary wound healing (healing by secondary intention) occurs in an untreated wound, with or without tissue loss. In each process, the histologic events leading to wound closure and scar formation are essentially the same, with some important exceptions described in this chapter. Although we separate the process into phases of healing, wound repair is a dynamic process and represents a continuum starting at the time of initial injury and continuing probably for years with remodeling of scar tissue.[1-3]

Primary Wound Repair

The Inflammatory Phase

Immediately after wounding, a cascade of events occurs that leads first to the formation of a barrier to the outside environment. After injury, there is release of cellular enzymes, including amines, lymphokines, and other chemotactic factors. In concert with this, initial vasoconstriction soon gives way to vasodilation and changes in capillary permeability, which assists in recruitment of macrophages, lymphocytes, and other cellular and noncellular components. This establishes the inflammatory environment needed for the intricate process of wound healing. This phase starts at the time of injury and continues for 4 to 7 days.

EPITHELIALIZATION

Initially, in a well-sutured wound, a fibrin–platelet clot bridges the cut surfaces. Migration and proliferation of epithelial cells starts in a downward orientation toward the base of the wound until an epithelial "bridge" is formed and can be complete in 12 to 24 hours. Epithelial hyperplasia is aided by capillary bud formation, which provides a framework for cellular proliferation. Reorganization and alignment of the new epithelium is seen during days 10 to 15. Starting around the 25th day after injury, the new layer starts to thin, a process that may continue for months or years thereafter.

Fibroblastic Phase

Production of collagen by fibroblasts begins around day 6 after injury. Collagen is then synthesized rapidly for the next 10 days. After day 17, there is a sharp decline in the total collagen content of the wound. By 4 weeks, no net increase in collagen is observed. Tensile strength of the wound also increases rapidly during this time; the most important process that imparts strength to the wound is collagen remodeling.

GROUND SUBSTANCE

Essential for providing a nutrient-rich environment for fibroblast proliferation and collagen synthesis is the acellular "gel" called *ground substance.* It is rich in hyaluronic acid, chondritin sulfate, and other mucopolysaccharides.

Maturation Phase

Alignment and restructuring of collagen fibers into a lattice network starts around 4 weeks after wounding and may continue for a year or more. During this phase, collagen synthesis is balanced by collagenolysis and no net increase in collagen is observed. Wound tensile strength reaches a maximum in 10 to 12 weeks; and although remodeling continues, little strength is added thereafter. It should also be noted that even years after injury, overall wound strength never quite reaches that of uninjured skin.

Secondary Wound Healing

The events leading to healing of an untreated wound occur when skin edges are left unopposed, usually after full-thickness tissue loss. Examples include avulsions, chemical injuries, and thermal or other radiation burns. Secondary healing also occurs when no tissue is lost and is occasionally utilized clinically in the management of certain infected wounds.

This type of healing is similar to that of primary wound healing and includes all three phases described earlier. In contrast to primary wound healing, wound contraction plays the predominant role. The degree of contraction in an open wound can be extensive. After clot and scab formation, epithelial migration and proliferation advance centrally. It was initially thought that epithelialization occurs beneath the scab or eschar and pushes up from below. It now appears that proteolytic enzymes are released along the advancing edge of the epithelium that uses the fibrin clot as a scaffold. The multicellular epithelial edge soon becomes a monolayer as it moves centrally. This is probably due to the relatively inhospitable environment of granulation tissue composed of capillary buds, fibroblasts, collagen, reticulin, and elastin fibers together with its ground substance matrix. As collagen synthesis proceeds, specialized fibroblasts called myofibroblasts containing the contractile proteins actin and myosin provide the forces for the central movement of the wound edges. Contraction can proceed at a rapid rate and may result in a rate of closure of 0.6 to 0.75 mm/d for 12 to 15 days after injury.[3] Contraction slows after this time but may continue for several months, depending on the extent of the wound, after which remodeling may continue for several years. The extent of wound contraction is dependent on a number of factors such as shape of the defect, connections to underlying tissues, and mobility of surrounding anatomic structures. Closure of a contracting wound may thus not always proceed at the same rate in all directions. Contraction of a full-thickness defect of the lower eyelid skin, for example, tends to result in ectropion secondary to vertical contraction of the wound, which is unopposed by the freely mobile eyelid margin.

In ophthalmic plastic surgery, healing by secondary intention has limited use and is reserved for certain cases of infection and burns and in selected cases for the management of defects after resection of cutaneous tumors particularly of the medial or lateral canthal areas.

Table 27–1 summarizes the time course of wound healing.

TABLE 27–1

Approximate Times for Phases of Wound Repair After Injury

Phase	Time
Epithelialization	12–24 hours
Inflammatory phase	4–7 days
Fibroblastic phase	6–17 days; rapid collagen production usually complete by 4 weeks
Maturation phase	4 weeks to several years
Time to maximum wound strength	10–12 weeks

HEMOSTASIS

Creating a dry surgical field is a "double-edged sword." The surgeon must maintain adequate exposure and visibility of tissue planes, while at the same time causing the least amount of tissue destruction. Considerations such as time, type of tissue, the availability and cost of each modality, and surgeon's preference all play a role in deciding the type of application necessary. General considerations such as patient use of aspirin, nonsteroidal anti-inflammatory drugs, and anticoagulants need to be specifically addressed before any surgery. Preoperative discontinuation of aspirin and anticoagulants should be discussed and coordinated with the patient's internist or other prescribing physician and the relative risk assessed. In general, aspirin and nonsteroidal agents should be stopped 10 days before surgery.[4, 5] Since warfarin activity is more dependent on individual metabolism, one or more preoperative checks of prothrombin time may be necessary. Should the risk of stopping anticoagulant therapy be too great (i.e., certain heart valves), then admission to the hospital and conversion to heparin may be needed. Heparin is stopped 4 to 6 hours before surgery and then restarted postoperatively.

Pressure Tamponade

Pressure tamponade is the simplest way to achieve hemostasis and is useful primarily in certain low flow states (e.g., capillary oozing). This technique causes little or no tissue damage. An important use in ophthalmic surgery is after transection of the optic nerve and its vessels during enucleation. Two major disadvantages to this technique are time to produce adequate hemostasis and a fragile clot. Control of bleeding may take 2 to 10 or more minutes, thereby increasing the time of the procedure and drying of the open tissues. In addition, subsequent manipulation in the area may dislodge a weak clot and cause further bleeding. This is particularly important when working behind the orbital septum with the threat of orbital hemorrhage and possible compromise of the optic nerve. Similarly, even a small subcutaneous hematoma postoperatively can be of great concern to both patient and surgeon.

Thermal Cautery and Electrocautery

Two types of thermal cautery are generally available and are provided as sterile, disposable battery-operated units. A low-temperature version (1350°F) is useful for conjunctival and other fine tissue cautery. A high-temperature model (2200°F) is adequate for many minor procedures when electrocautery is unavailable or impractical. The latter may also be very useful for surgical dissection. These instruments are small and compact and offer excellent control.

Cautery and hemostasis may also be achieved with the use of certain laser sources. These lasers include pulsed argon and holmium:yttrium-aluminum-garnet (YAG) as well as continuous-wave neodymium: YAG and CO_2 lasers.

The two types of electrocautery used most frequently are the bipolar and monopolar units. With electrocautery instrumentation, coagulation and cellular destruction are produced by generated heat from an electrical arc. A fine-tipped jeweler's type bipolar unit is excellent for most ophthalmic plastic procedures. The electrical arc is produced by close approximation of the tips with intervening tissue. The monopolar unit with a needle tip is also useful and offers both coagulation and cutting modes. The electrical current flows between the monopolar hand piece electrode to a grounding pad electrode placed on the patient. Coagulation and cutting modes differ with respect to how the electrical pulse is delivered. The coagulation mode generates a more effective electrical arc, whereas the cutting mode (and less coagulation) proceeds better with a less intense arc.

Electrosurgical instruments are available that convert electrical current into radiowave frequency. Cellular disintegration is produced by intracellular heat generated by the resistance of the tissue to the passage of high-frequency current. These units also offer cutting and coagulation modes and can accommodate a variety of different handpiece electrodes, including straight cutting and loop tips, needle tips, as well as bipolar capability. Radiosurgical devices may have the advantage of less tissue destruction and scar formation.

Two important points need to be raised here. The first concerns the use of thermal and electrocautery in the presence of oxygen. Supplemental oxygen is often used during operative procedures and is administered by mask or nasal cannula. Precautions should be taken during cautery use to limit the chance of combustion or explosion. Second, caution should be taken with the use of monopolar and radiofrequency cautery in the presence of a cardiac pacemaker. Shielded pacemakers implanted after the mid 1970s are probably safe from interference due to electrocautery use; however, if the use of these types of cautery is planned, consultation with the patient's cardiologist should be included in the preoperative evaluation.

Pharmacologic Agents

Thrombin is a proteinase that converts fibrinogen into fibrin, facilitating the clotting process. It is produced from bovine sources and available in 1000- and 5000-unit doses. Typically, 5000 units of lyophilized thrombin is reconstituted in 50 ml of saline and soaked in Gelfoam for use topically.

Epinephrine is used in conjunction with local anesthetics generally at a concentration of 1:100,000 or 1:200,000. Small volumes of more concentrated epinephrine solutions may be applied topically by means of packing materials to facilitate hemostasis during surgery, including the nasal cavity and paranasal sinuses. Being a sympathomimetic, it produces local vasoconstriction at the site of injection, decreasing capillary bleeding and delaying absorption of the anesthetic agent.

Phenylephrine and oxymetazoline are also vasoconstrictors and are used primarily for decongestion of the nasal mucosa during lacrimal surgery. Alternatively, a 4% to 10% cocaine solution can be used.

Use of the sympathomimetics during surgery needs to be tailored to the patient's overall medical condition and closely monitored by anesthesia personnel. Complications including cardiac arrest, tachycardia, arrhythmias, hypertension, and cerebral vascular events can occur rapidly, especially in susceptible individuals. Careful preoperative evaluation and judicious use of these agents during surgery will limit the possibility of serious side effects of these drugs.

Desmopressin (DDAVP) is a synthetically produced analogue of antidiuretic hormone. Although it lacks the vasoconstrictive effects of antidiuretic hormone, its mechanism of action when given intravenously or intranasally is to temporarily raise circulating levels of factor VIII and von Willebrand factor. Increases in these clotting factors may facilitate coagulation in selected individuals with hemophilia A and von Willebrand disease. Similarly, DDAVP may be useful for patients with uremia, cirrhosis of the liver, and perhaps even aspirin-induced prolongation of bleeding time.[6, 7] As noted earlier, the procoagulant effect of DDAVP is temporary and recurrent hemorrhage may be noted in treated patients.

Topically Applied Chemical Agents

Gelfoam is produced from animal skin gelatin. Although it has no hemostatic capability per se, it may serve as a tamponade material. In addition, it may be used as a sponge-like carrier for topical thrombin. It is particularly useful in the control of mucosal oozing, as is often encountered in lacrimal surgery.

Surgicel and Oxycel are forms of oxidized cellulose, are applied dry, and produce a local reaction with blood, leading to formation of an artificial clot. Care should be taken when using these agents in lacrimal and orbital surgery. There are anecdotal reports of significant swelling postoperatively, with secondary compression of vital orbital structures apparently caused by the osmotic effects of this material.[8]

Avitene is also effective in creating local hemostasis, although it is fairly expensive. It is a microcrystalline form of collagen and is sprinkled dry on areas of continued oozing. Avitene also has intrinsic hemostatic ability and provides a structure for clot formation.

Bone wax is a combination of sterile bees' wax and a softening agent and is helpful for hemostasis of cut surfaces of bone as well as subperiosteal bleeding from small perforating vessels.

All these materials are nontoxic, are relatively nonirritating, and are removed by local phagocytosis and liquefaction.

SUTURE MATERIAL

Choice of suture material for wound closure is dependent on a variety of factors, including type and location of tissue, wound tension, potential for infection (wound contamination), potential patient cooperation for suture removal, and suture handling characteristics. In general, sutures are classified as either absorbable (e.g., gut, polyglycolic acid, polydioxanone) or nonabsorbable (e.g., silk, Dacron, Polydek) and as either monofilament or braided. In general, absorbable sutures lose their tensile strength within 60 days.[9, 10] Nonabsorbable sutures retain the majority of their strength beyond this time.[11]

Absorbable Sutures

Fast absorbing gut suture is produced primarily from braided ribbons of sheep intestinal mucosa. This suture loses 50% of its tensile strength in 3 to 5 days and should be utilized only for closure of wounds under minimal or no tension (e.g., upper eyelid crease incisions).

Plain gut suture is obtained from the same source and will lose half of its strength in 7 to 10 days.

Chromic gut is made in the same manner with additional treatment in a chromic oxide solution, which prolongs the process of hydrolysis by soft tissue. It loses 50% of its tensile strength in 10 to 14 days.

Polyglycolic acid/polyglactin (e.g., Vicryl, Dexon) are synthetic braided sutures that are much less reactive than gut. Time for 50% reduction in tensile strength is around 14 days. These sutures may be easier to tie than gut but may catch when drawn through tissues.

Polydioxanone is a monofilament synthetic absorbable suture that loses half its tensile strength in 28 to 35 days.

Table 27-2 summarizes the absorption times of these sutures.

TABLE 27-2

Approximate Absorption Times for Selected Sutures

Suture Material	Time (days) for 50% Loss Tensile Strength	Time (days) for Total Absorption
Fast absorbing gut	2-3	21-42
Plain gut	7-10	50-70
Chromic gut	10-14	60-90
Polyglactin 910	14	56-70
Polydioxanone	28-35	180

Modified from Woog JJ: Penetrating eyelid trauma. *In* Shingleton BJ, et al (eds): Eye Trauma. St. Louis, CV Mosby, 1991, p 328.

Nonabsorbable Sutures

Silk is a braided suture made of naturally occurring fibers. It may be more accurately described as slowly absorbing, losing 100% of its tensile strength by 2 years. Silk causes significantly more tissue inflammation than other synthetic varieties.

Dacron (e.g., Mersilene) is made of synthetic braided fibers and is much less reactive than silk. It maintains 95% of its tensile strength at 2 years.

Teflon-coated Dacron (e.g., Polydek, Tevdek) may cause more tissue inflammation than plain Dacron, possibly from fragmentation of the Teflon. It maintains 85% to 100% of its tensile strength at 2 years.

Nylon is a monofilament synthetic suture. This suture is minimally reactive and is excellent in this regard for skin closure. Nylon and polypropylene possess significant memory and therefore may be somewhat more cumbersome to handle than other sutures. Nylon loses approximately 30% of its tensile strength at 2 years.

Polypropylene (Prolene) is another monofilament synthetic suture with tissue reactivity comparable to nylon. It maintains nearly 100% of its tensile strength at 2 years.

Stainless steel wire is used occasionally in ophthalmic plastic surgery in procedures such as transnasal wiring for telecanthus and fixation of bony fragments. It is relatively difficult to work with and causes little tissue reactivity.

Skin staples are also used occasionally for skin closure and are formed from stainless steel wire. They are provided in single use, disposable staple guns. Their use in ophthalmic plastic surgery is limited to skin closure in areas that are not cosmetically conspicuous, primarily behind the hair line.

SUTURE NEEDLES

The various types of needles and their cutting surfaces are shown in Figure 27-1. For skin closure and general purpose use, conventional cutting needles of a ⅜-circle radius come in various diameters depending on the type of tissue sutured. Reverse cutting needles can also be used for this purpose. Small ½-circle needles (see Fig. 27-1*E*) are excellent for suturing in confined spaces as in mucosal flap anastomosis during dacryocystorhinostomy and reattachment of a tarsal strip to the periosteum of the lateral orbital wall during eyelid-shortening procedures. Taper needles have no cutting surfaces other than at the tip and are particularly useful for extraocular muscle traction sutures, whereas cutting needles may cause hemorrhages in this highly vascular tissue. Spatula needles are side cutting and are very helpful in placement of partial-thickness sutures through the tarsal plate, as in ptosis surgery, or in reattachment of rectus muscles to the sclera in strabismus or orbital surgery. Most sutures are available

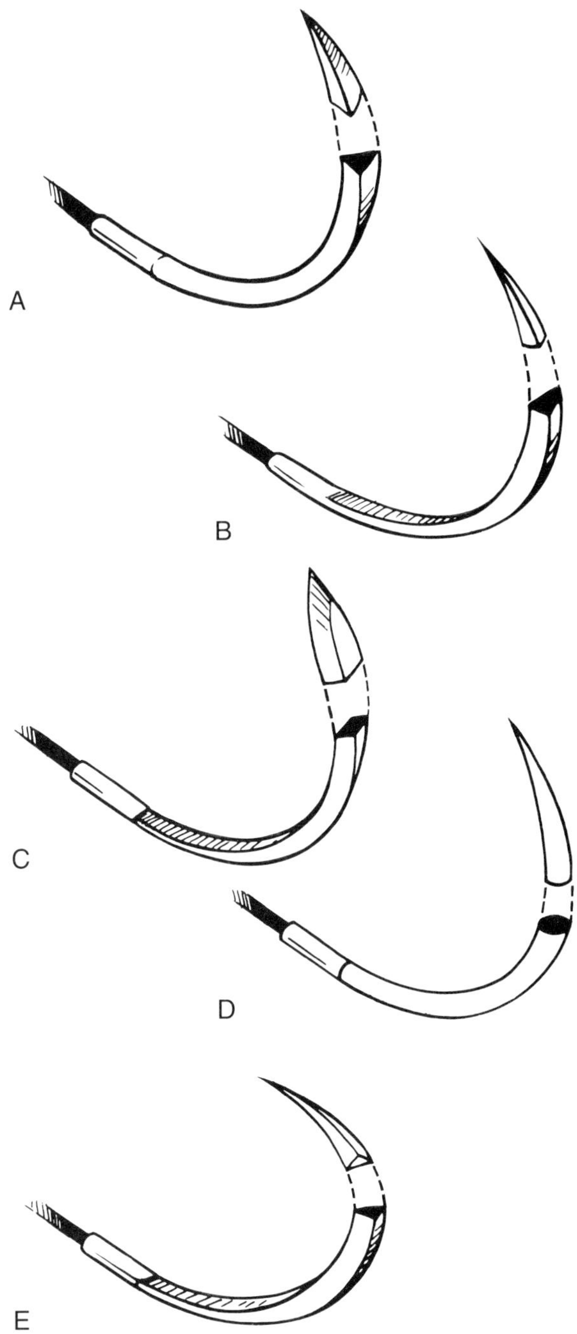

Figure 27–1. Suture needles used in ophthalmic plastic surgery. *A*, Conventional cutting. *B*, Reverse cutting. *C*, Spatula. *D*, Taper. *E*, Half-circle cutting.

swedge-locked to the base of the needle, although free needles are occasionally useful as well.

BASIC SUTURING TECHNIQUES

Suturing technique is perhaps more important than actual choice of suture material. To set up the wound for the best possible healing and least conspicuous scar formation, a number of general principles need to be considered. First it is generally preferable, when possible, to place the skin incision along relaxed skin tension lines (Fig. 27–2). A number of techniques have been utilized to determine the proper orientation of these lines, especially those of the head and neck. Some controversy exists concerning the anatomic relationship of these lines to the structures underlying the skin. In many cases, relaxed skin tension lines develop perpendicular to the action of the underlying muscle. Because of the complexity of the facial muscles, this may at times be difficult to assess. Relaxed skin tension lines may or may not have a relationship to wrinkle lines that naturally develop, further confusing the issue. According to Borges, orientation of these lines can be easily demonstrated by pinching the skin and observing the resulting furrows. By noting the characteristics of these furrows, relaxed skin tension lines can be accurately identified.[12] Incisions made parallel to these lines tend to heal with less scarring and be less noticeable than ones oriented tangentially. Second, it is generally preferable to make the initial incision perpendicular to the skin surface. Beveled wounds retard healing and are more difficult to reapproximate properly. Beveled incisions are often utilized, however, directly above the eyebrow to minimize transection of brow follicles.

During wound closure, efforts are made to minimize

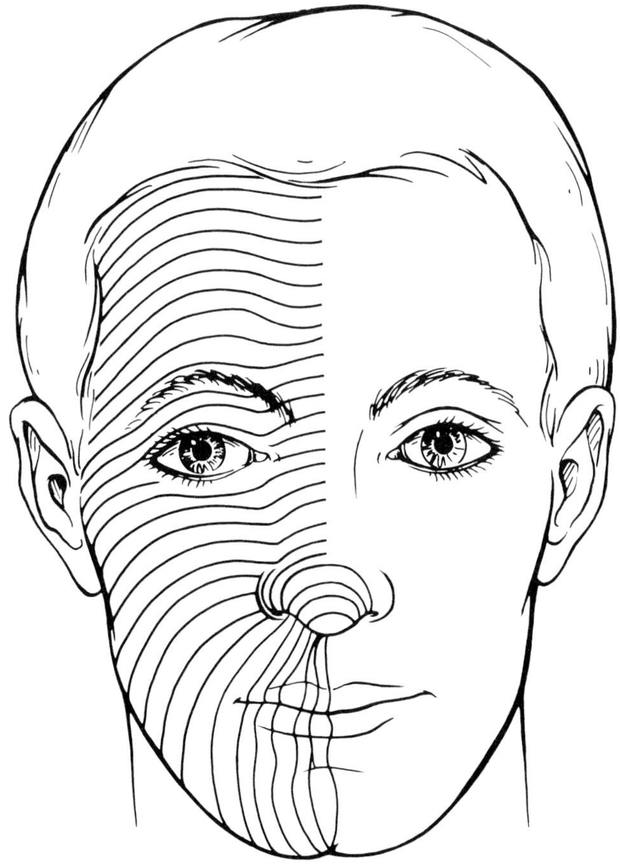

Figure 27–2. Drawing showing relaxed skin tension lines of the face.

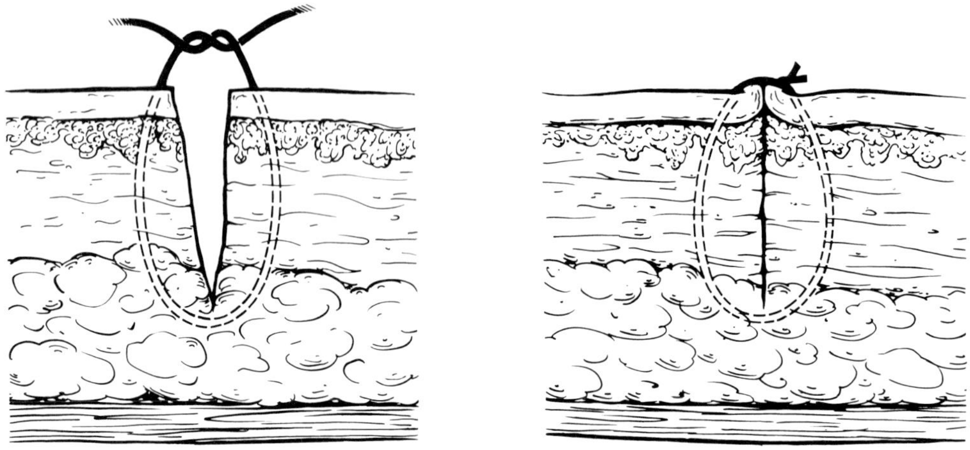

Figure 27–3. Simple interrupted percutaneous suture.

tissue drying. Evaporation from an open wound can be significant, and drying can distort tissue planes, retard healing, and make closure more difficult.

Relieving tension against the wound edges with properly placed deep sutures will help facilitate compact scar formation and adds adequate strength to the wound during the second and third phases of repair. As noted earlier, although epithelialization of a well-sutured wound may be complete in 12 to 24 hours, this adds little tensile strength to the wound. Adequate tensile strength (strength per unit area of the wound) and burst strength (strength of the entire wound) require weeks to develop, much longer than most superficial skin sutures may be left in.

Tissue handling is also important and can influence wound healing. Minimal skin edge manipulation with an appropriate fine-toothed forceps generally causes the least trauma. Crush injury from forceps should be avoided, and, where appropriate, skin edges may be grasped by dermis, further reducing epithelial disruption.

Finally, the surgeon should strive for slight eversion of the skin edges at the time of closure (Fig. 27–3). During the healing process, wound edges tend to invert along the line of the incision. This becomes particularly important in lid margin closure where even slight inversion can cause a very noticeable "notch."

Simple interruped percutaneous sutures (see Fig. 27–3) are useful for smaller wounds. These sutures produce slight eversion of the wound edges.

Running percutaneous sutures (Fig. 27–4) are helpful for longer incisions and may be used alone in areas of minimal skin tension.

Deep interrupted sutures (Fig. 27–5) are used in closing "dead" space or other tissue planes such as muscle. An exception to this is dead space involving adipose tissue. In this instance, deep sutures add little, if any, strength to the wound, increase tissue inflammation, and should be avoided.

Buried subcutaneous sutures (Fig. 27–6) are used extensively to relieve tension and add strength to the wound. The knot is tied deep in the tissue and protects against knot extrusion or noticeable "bumps" along the suture line, particularly in thin skin. This type of closure is usually supplemented with percutaneous interrupted or running sutures, or in certain instances sterile adhesive strips (Steri-Strips) may be used for proper skin edge realignment.

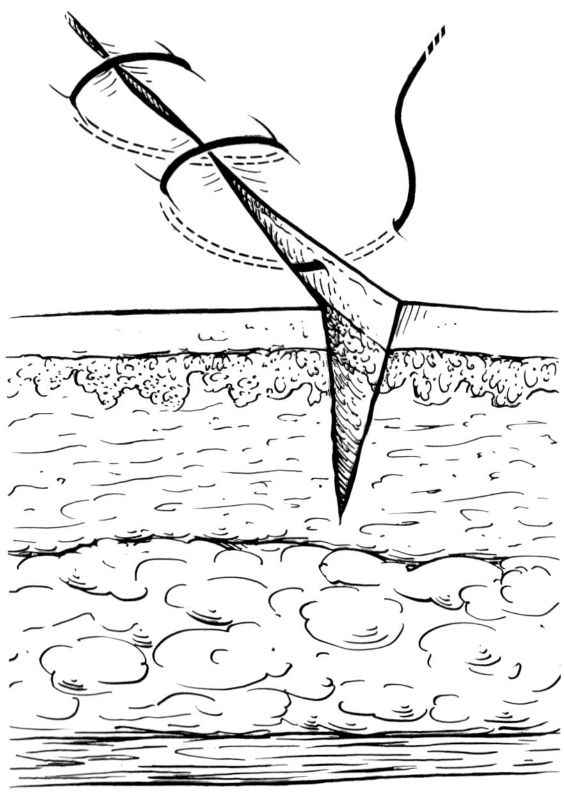

Figure 27–4. Running percutaneous suture.

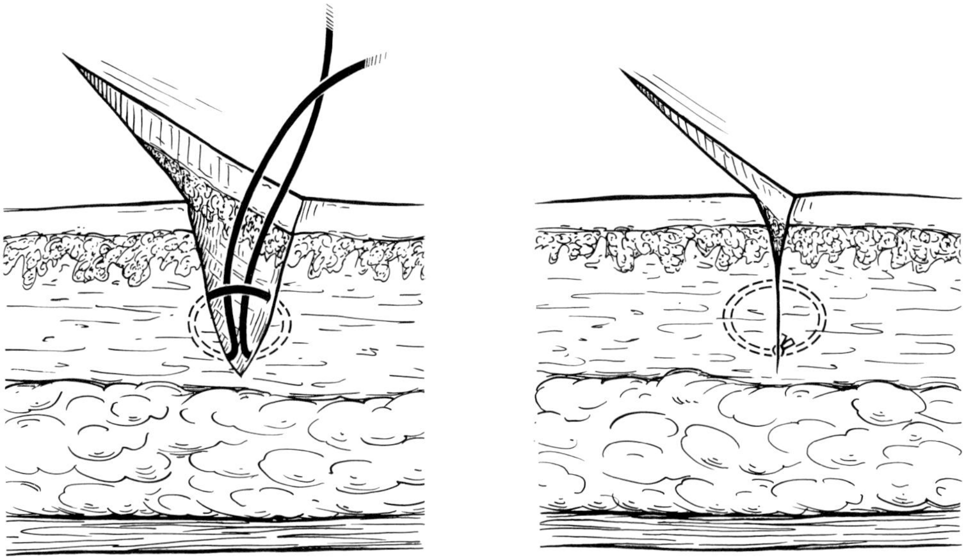

Figure 27–5. Deep interrupted suture.

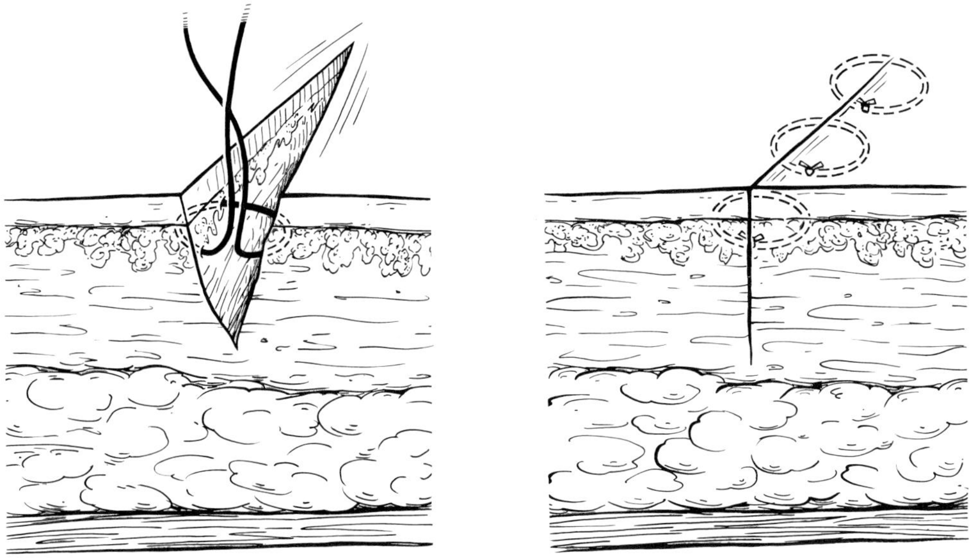

Figure 27–6. Buried subcutaneous suture.

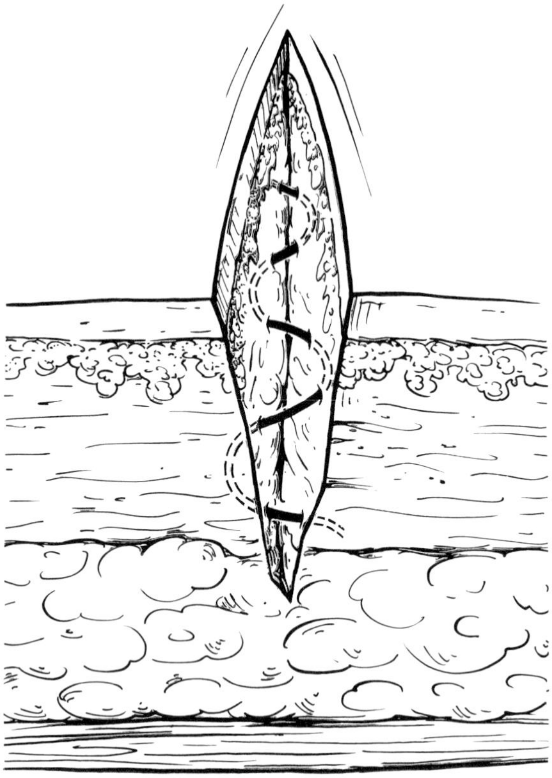

Figure 27–7. Running subcuticular suture.

Running subcuticular sutures (Fig. 27–7) are useful in closing long incisions with minimal tension. This usually requires skin with an appropriately thick dermis layer and can be totally buried using an absorbable suture (Vicryl, PDS) or a removable suture (nylon, Prolene), the ends of which are tied percutaneously.

Horizontal mattress sutures (Fig. 27–8) can be used for skin closure, but these tend to strangulate tissue more than other techniques. Buried horizontal mattress sutures may be helpful in minimizing tension on wound edges.

Half-buried horizontal mattress sutures (Fig. 27–9) are very helpful in areas of moderate wound tension and in comples closures involving flaps, as in Y-V plasty, Z plasty, and rhomboid flap closure.

Vertical mattress sutures (Fig. 27–10) combine the advantages of deep closure to eliminate tension with pronounced skin edge eversion. They can be used either as single interrupted sutures or in a running fashion.

OPHTHALMIC PLASTIC INSTRUMENTS

In general, instruments used in ophthalmic plastic surgery tend to be small and delicate. Many of the instruments utilized for ocular surgery are also used. Figure 27–11 shows a basic instrument set. Individual pieces are identified by the legend. Figures 27–12 and 27–13 include accessory kits useful in lacrimal and orbital surgery. Many types of bone saws and drills are available such as the one shown in Figure 27–14, which are occasionally needed for orbital surgery. A number of miniplating and microplating sets (Fig. 27–15) may be useful for orbital and zygomatic fracture repair. Finally, endoscopic sinus surgery instrumentation (Fig. 27–16) is helpful in facilitating conjunctival surgery and intranasal dacryocystorhinostomy.

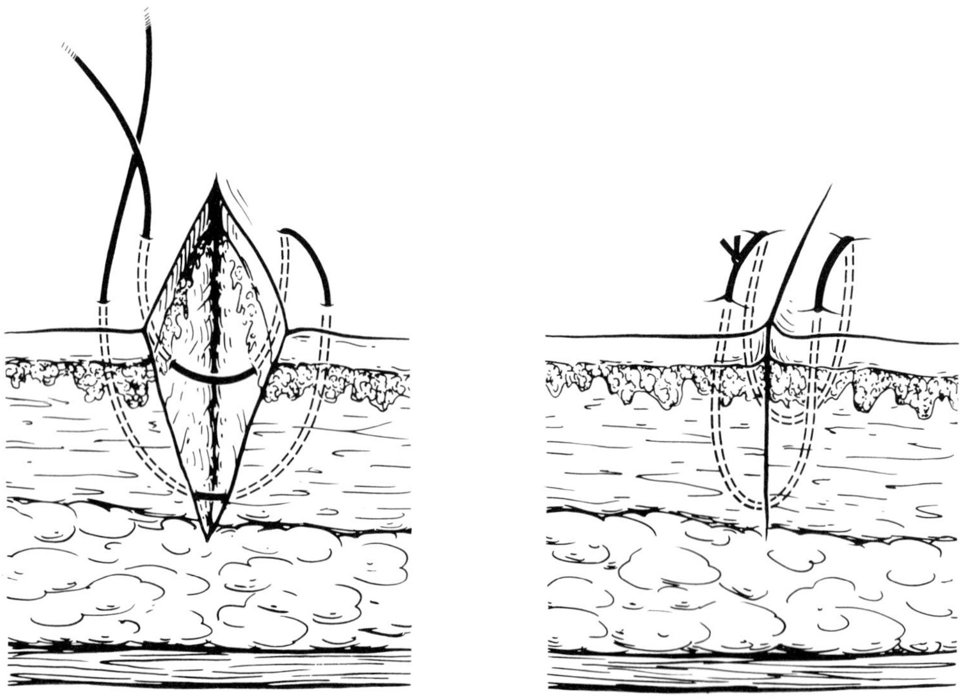

Figure 27–8. Horizontal mattress suture.

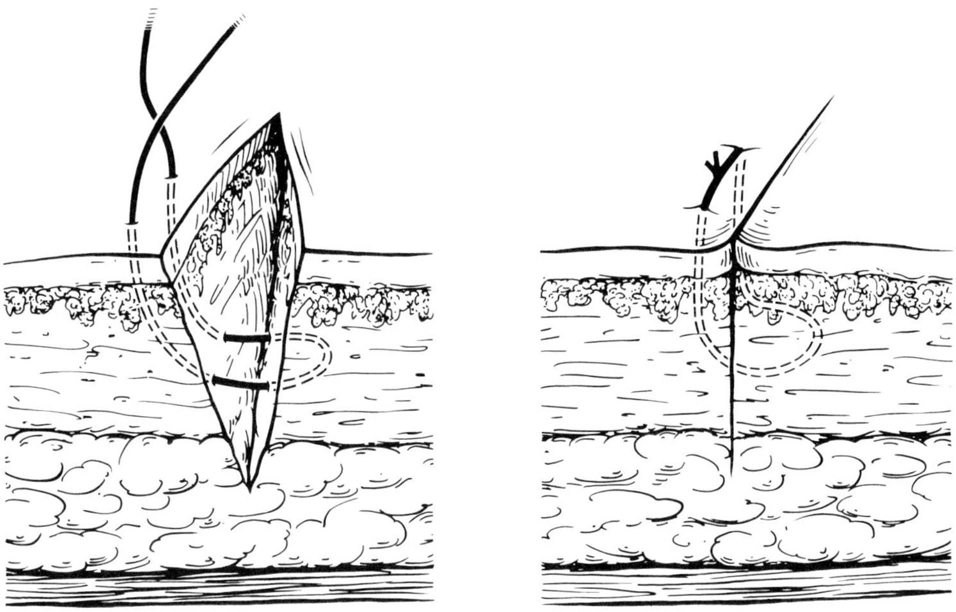

Figure 27–9. Half-buried horizontal mattress suture.

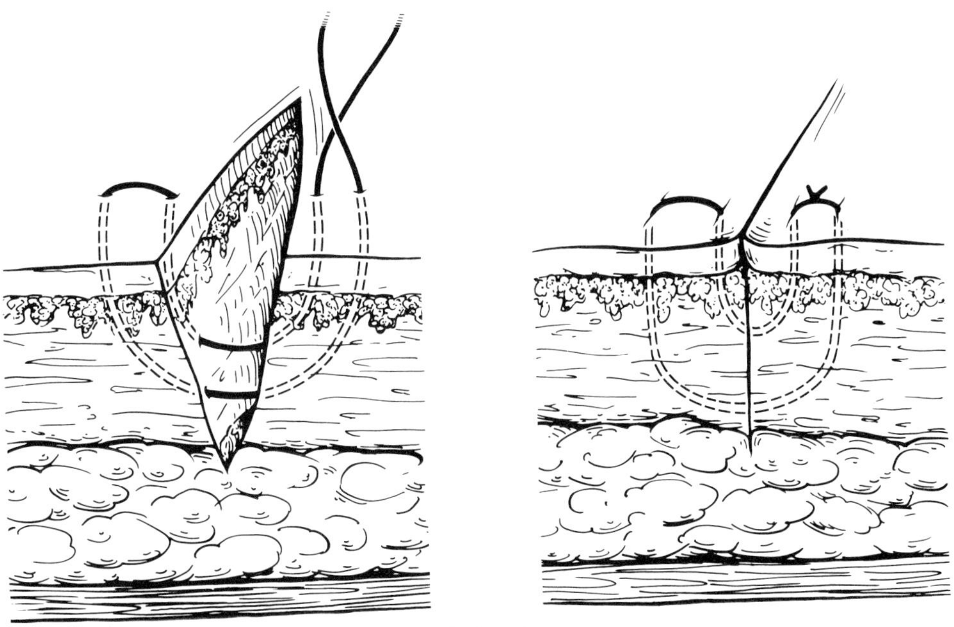

Figure 27–10. Vertical mattress suture.

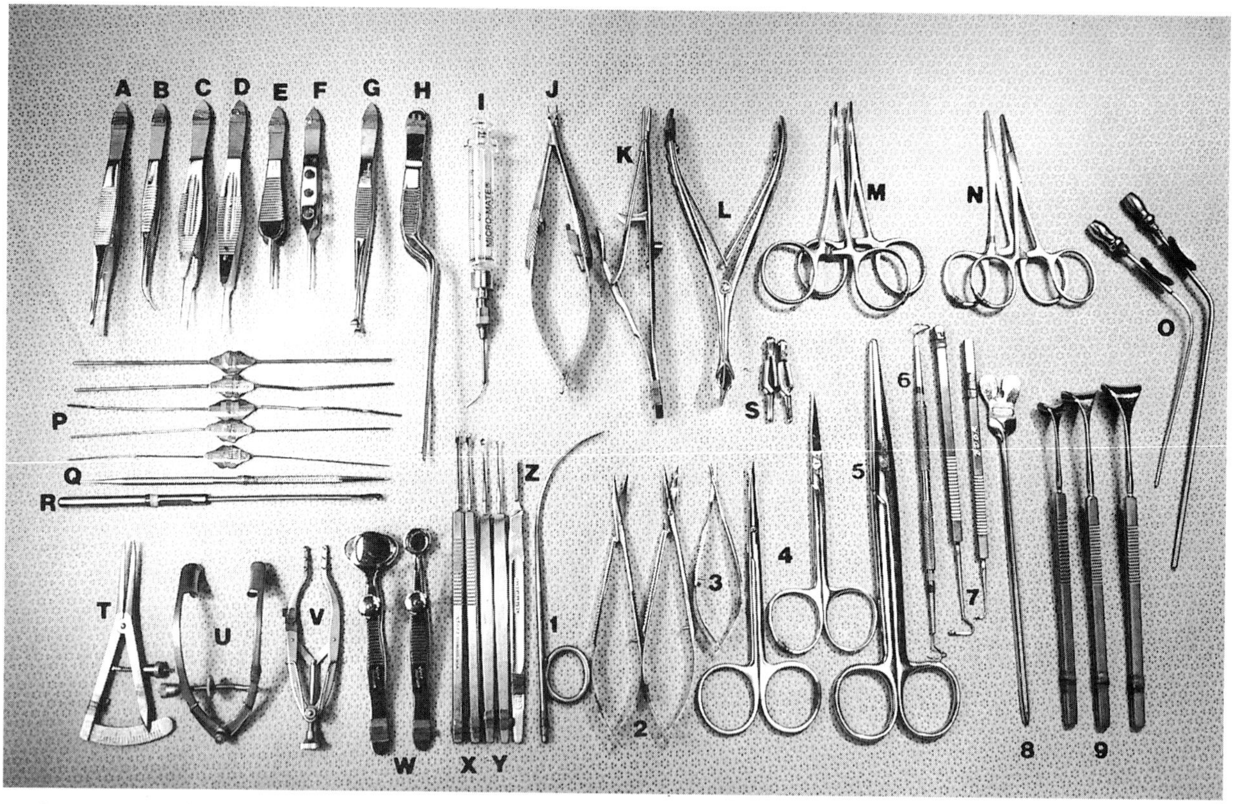

Figure 27–11. Basic ophthalmic plastic surgery kit. **A**, Utility forceps. **B**, Curved dressing forceps. **C** and **D**, Castroviejo 0.3-mm and 0.5-mm toothed forceps. **E**, Paufique toothed forceps. **F**, Bishop-Harmon toothed forceps. **G**, Graefe fixation forceps. **H**, Kennerdell bayonet forceps. **I**, Glass syringe with 23-g lacrimal irrigating cannula. **J**, Catalano needle holder. **K**, Kalt needle holder. **L**, Nasal speculum. **M** and **N**, Curved and straight hemostats. **O**, Baron suction tips. **P**, Bowman lacrimal probes. **Q**, Castroviejo double-ended lacrimal dilator. **R**, Lacrimal probe retrieval hook. **S**, Serrefine clamps. **T**, Castroviejo calipers. **U**, Lancaster lid speculum. **V**, Stevenson lacrimal sac speculum. **W**, Desmarres chalazion forceps. **X**, Double-fixation hook. **Y**, Meyeroefer chalazion curettes. **Z**, Bard-Parker scalpel handle. **1**, Wright fascia needle. **2**, Blunt and sharp Wescott scissors. **3**, Vannas scissors. **4**, Curved and straight iris scissors. **5**, Heavy dressing scissors. **6**, Worst pigtail probe. **7**, Jameson muscle hook and Stevens tenotomy hook. **8**, Quickert grooved director. **9**, Desmarres lid retractors.

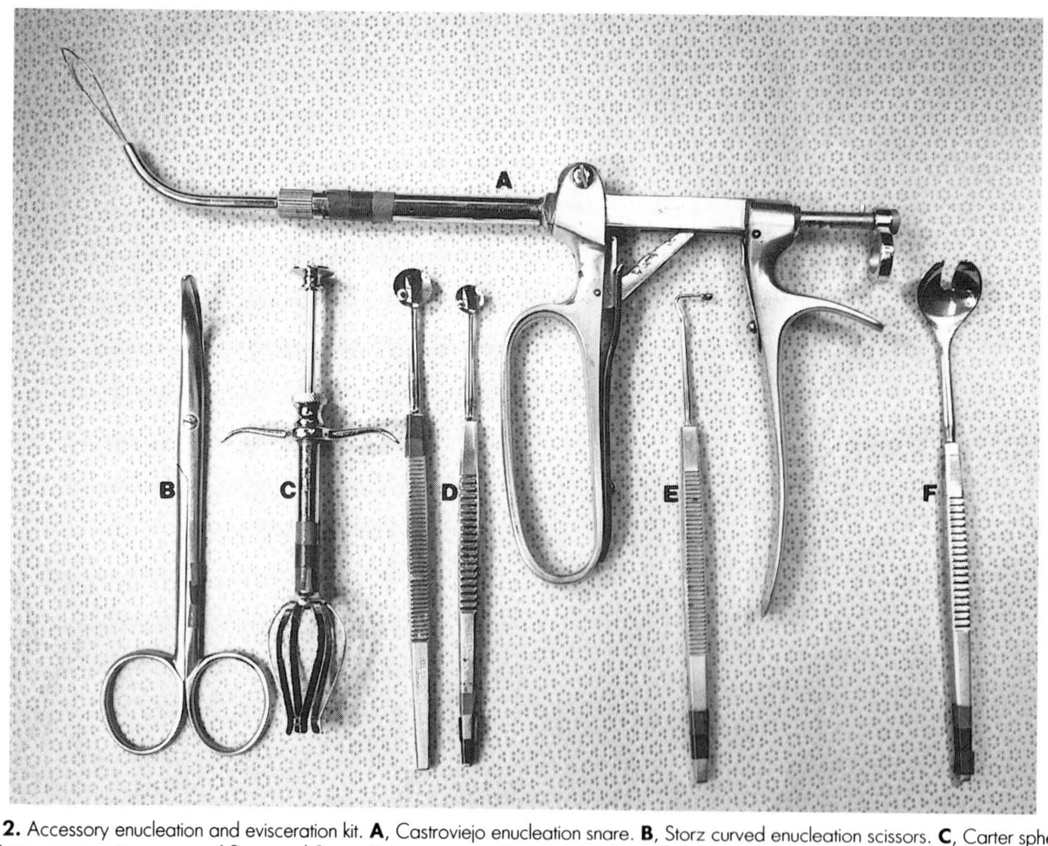

Figure 27–12. Accessory enucleation and evisceration kit. **A**, Castroviejo enucleation snare. **B**, Storz curved enucleation scissors. **C**, Carter sphere holder and introducer. **D**, Bunge evisceration spoons, 12 mm and 8 mm. **E**, Jameson muscle hook. **F**, Wells enucleation spoon.

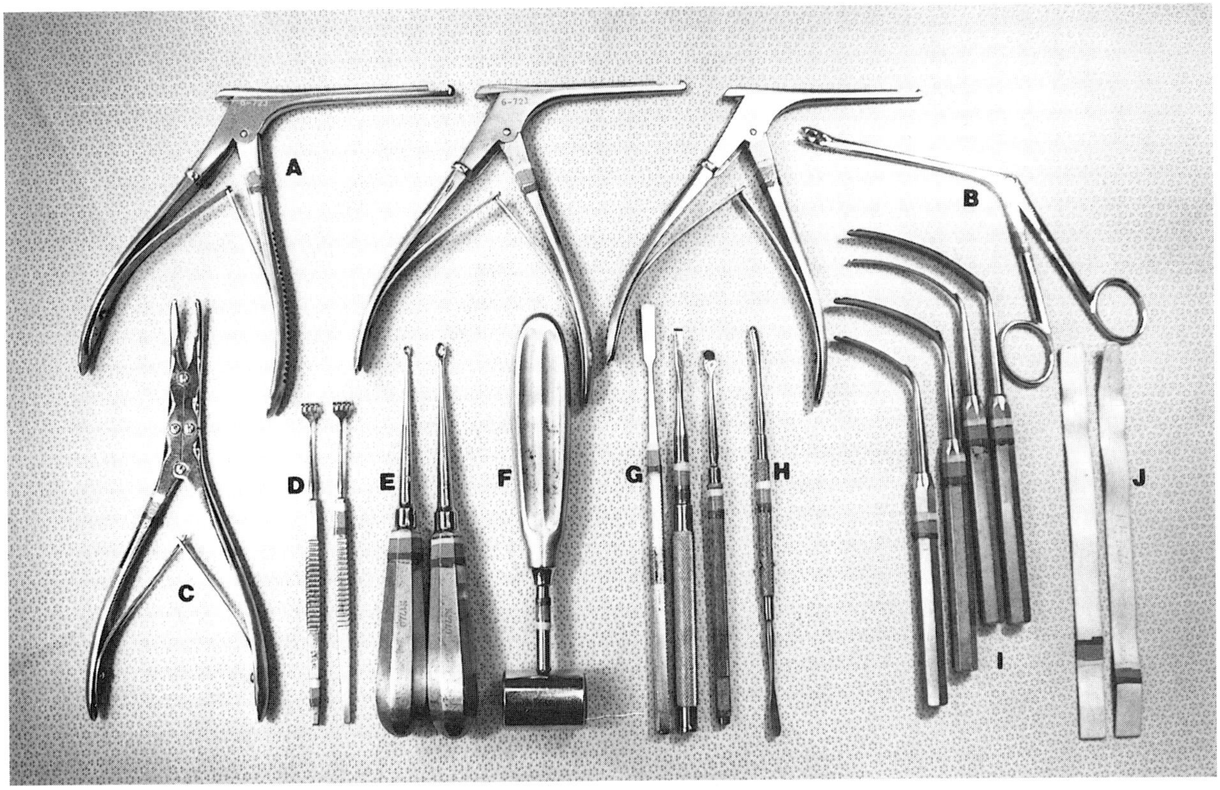

Figure 27–13. Accessory orbital and lacrimal kit. **A**, Kerrison rongeur no.1, no.2, no.3. **B**, Wilde rongeur. **C**, Zaufal-Jansen rongeur. **D**, Knapp lacrimal sac retractors. **E**, Spratt bone curettes. **F**, Lead-filled mallot. **G**, Osteotomes and West lacrimal sac chisel. **H**, Freer periosteal elevator. **I**, Sewall orbital retractors. **J**, Malleable retractors.

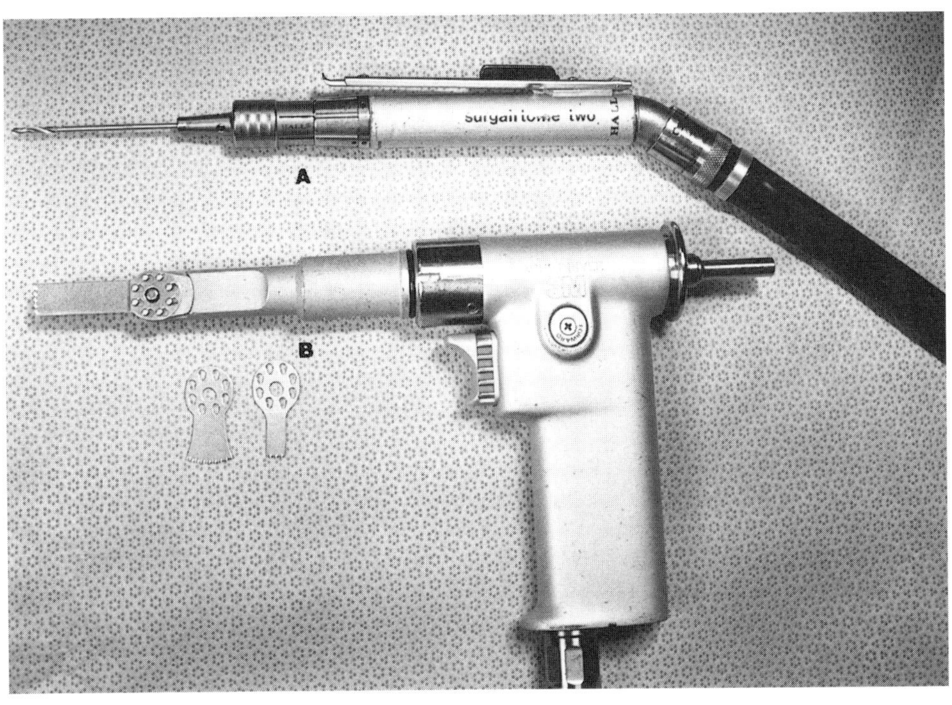

Figure 27–14. A, Hall pneumatic drill. **B**, 3M mini-driver.

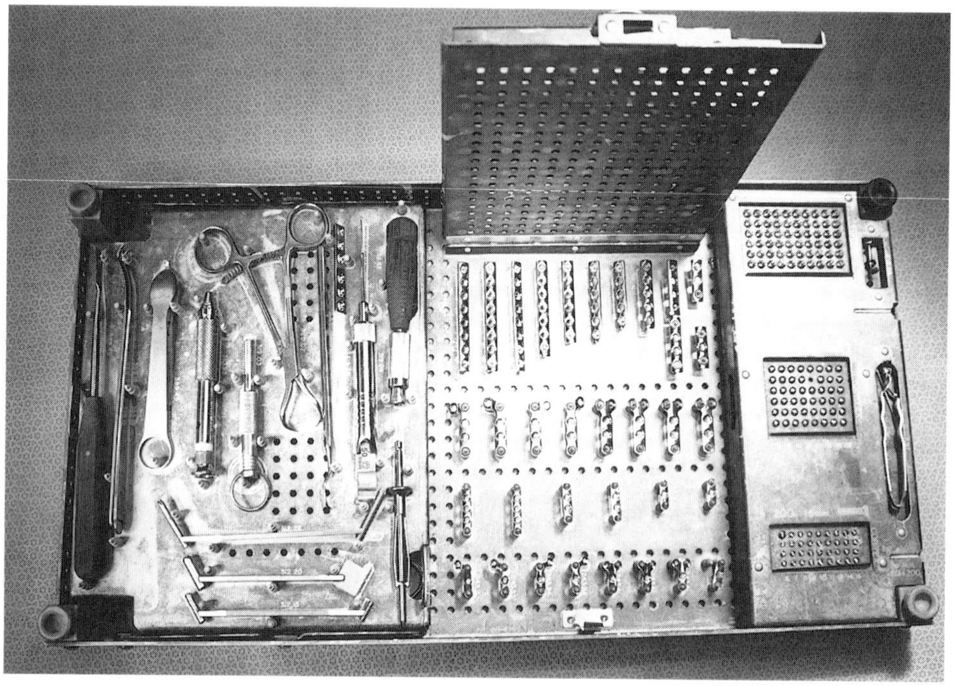

Figure 27–15. Synthes mini and microplating kit.

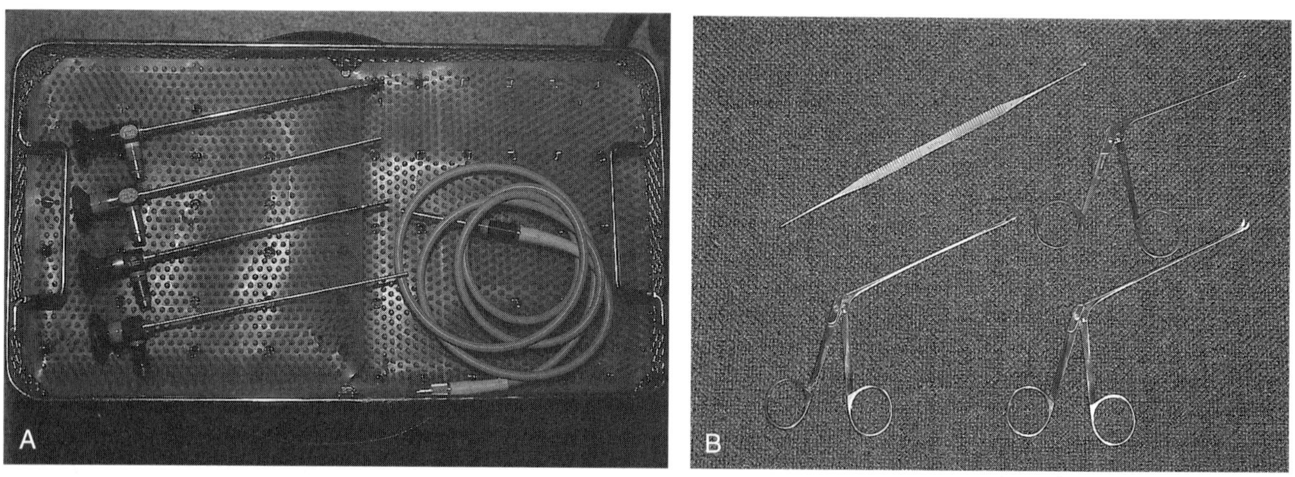

Figure 27–16. *A* and *B*, Endoscopic sinus surgery kit.

REFERENCES

1. Peacock EE Jr, Van Winkle W: Wound Repair, 2nd ed. Philadelphia, WB Saunders, 1976, pp 1–21, 61.
2. Montandon D, D'Andiran G, Gabbianig G: The mechanism of wound contraction and epithelialization. Clin Plast Surg 4:325–346, 1977.
3. Wilkins RB, Kulwin DR: Wound healing. Ophthalmology 86:507–510, 1979.
4. Amrien PC, Ellman L, Harris WH: Aspirin-induced prolongation of bleeding time and perioperative blood loss. JAMA 245:1825–1828, 1981.
5. Fiore LD, Brophy MT, Lopez A, et al: The bleeding time response to aspirin: Identifying the hyperresponder. Am J Clin Pathol 94:292–296, 1990.
6. Mannucci PM: Desmopressin: A nontransfusional hemostatic agent. Annu Rev Med 41:55–64, 1990.
7. Horrow JC: Desmopressin and antifibrinolytics. Int Anesthesiol Clin 28:230–236, 1990.
8. Johnson LP, Parkin JL: Blindness and total ophthalmoplegia: A complication of transantral ligation of the internal maxillary artery for epistaxis. Arch Otolaryngol 102:501–504, 1976.
9. Edlich RF: Physical and chemical configuration of sutures in the development of surgical infection. Ann Surg 177:679–687, 1973.
10. Ray JA, Doddi N, Regula D, et al: Polydioxanone (PDS), a novel monofilament synthetic absorbable suture. Surg Gynecol Obstet 153:497–507, 1981.
11. Postlethwait RW: Long-term comparative study of nonabsorbable sutures. Ann Surg 171:892–897, 1971.
12. Borges AF: Relaxed skin tension lines (RSTL) versus other skin lines. Plast Reconstr Surg 73:144–150, 1984.

CHAPTER 28

Anesthetic Considerations for Oculoplastic Surgery: An Update for the 1990s

Jonathan Kay

This chapter is designed to acquaint the oculoplastic surgeon with current practice in anesthesia. The pressure to do elective cases with minimum contact with the patient until the day of surgery, with minimum laboratory evaluation, and with as rapid operating room turnover as possible has impacted on the practice of anesthesia. In this chapter the focus is on current concepts in preoperative evaluation, premedication, monitoring, commonly used anesthetic agents, and some special considerations for the pediatric patient undergoing oculoplastic surgery.

PREOPERATIVE EVALUATIONS AND SCREENING TESTS: WHAT IS REALLY NEEDED AND WHY

The pressure to perform surgery on outpatients with little time to prepare them and with less and less information about their past medical history has intensified in this cost-conscious era. A cancellation under these circumstances disrupts the operating room schedule, disrupts the surgeon's schedule, and deprives the patient of the operation. Furthermore, such cancellations may be avoidable by careful planning and coordination with the anesthesiologist involved. Automated interactive questionnaires are a cost-effective way to expedite the preoperative evaluation. Such questionnaires help identify what laboratory testing is indicated based on the patient's history.[1]

Current recommendations for laboratory screening include a hemoglobin determination for all patients before major surgery and an electrocardiogram if older than age 50. Patients older than age 70 should also have a Sequential Multiple Analyzer 6 and a chest radiograph.[1, 2]

These recommendations are undergoing intense scrutiny to determine what impact laboratory results have on specific anesthetic decisions and outcome. Local mythology occasionally prevails. Thus, the following discussion serves only as a guideline.

Potassium abnormalities have been a chronic source of concern particularly for patients on diuretics or digoxin. Although somewhat controversial, good evidence suggests that in asymptomatic patients (no congestive heart failure, no digoxin therapy, and no ischemic symptoms) elective surgery may proceed if potassium values are greater than 2.8 or less than 5.9 mEq/L. Acutely elevating the potassium level by intravenous administration on the day of surgery is painful, is hazardous, and does not replete the intracellular deficit.[1, 3-5]

Another common problem is the discovery of an abnormality on the chest radiograph that is suggestive of carcinoma but does not impair the patient's respiratory status nor in turn impact on the type of anesthesia administered. The risks and benefits of delaying the exact diagnosis of the chest lesion versus delaying the desired elective eye surgery should be discussed with the patient, his or her family, and the patient's personal physician.

Marked elevations of blood glucose (greater than 350 mg/dL) or the discovery of new onset of diabetes mellitus should cause a delay in elective eye surgery. The prognosis for neurologic compromise is worse if cardiac arrest or low perfusion states are allowed to coexist with significant hyperglycemia.[6, 7]

Electrocardiographic abnormalities should be carefully evaluated despite the relatively "stress-free" nature of oculoplastic surgery. The most stable patient may quickly become hypertensive, hypotensive, tachycardic, or bradycardic in response to stimuli (such as a vasovagal reaction or claustrophobia). These hemodynamic perturbations may in turn cause a downward spiral of ischemia-induced problems. The key question in elective situations (especially medicolegally) is whether the patient is in optimal medical condition. Common abnormalities that pose problems on the electrocardiogram include "new" onset of atrial fibrillation, ST-T segment changes of ischemia, "new" myocardial infarction, and premature ventricular contractions.

New atrial fibrillation may be benign or may indicate significant ischemic disease, including myocardial in-

The drug dosages included in this chapter are meant as guides only—every effort has been made to ensure their accuracy, but the author strongly suggests checking them with local authorities and verifying them. Doses may change as a result of new information obtained after the completion of this chapter.

farction. Chronic lung disease, pulmonary emboli, or congestive heart failure can also cause new-onset atrial fibrillation. Appropriate consultation and medical workup is required when there is a finding of "new" atrial fibrillation. An old electrocardiogram demonstrating that the patient has been in long-standing atrial fibrillation indicates that a new insult (to cause the atrial fibrillation) is unlikely.

ST-T segment changes on the electrocardiogram suggestive of ischemia should similarly prompt comparison with old electrocardiograms. Stable changes in an asymptomatic patient are less troublesome than new changes in a patient with episodic chest discomfort. Similarly, the exact age of a myocardial infarction is important. The incidence of reinfarction decreases to a stable risk of about 5% by 6 months after the original myocardial infarction. Frequently, the patient's electrocardiographic abnormality is seen "in vacuo" without access to an old electrocardiogram (at 6 A.M. on the morning of surgery). Preoperative screening clinics tend to avoid such embarrassment on the day of surgery.[8, 9]

Although more than five premature ventricular contractions per minute is associated with an increased perioperative morbidity, premature ventricular contractions must be considered in the context of the patient's history. Are potassium and magnesium levels normal? Are there symptoms or signs of ischemia (e.g., cardiomegaly on the chest radiograph)? Premature ventricular contractions can occur with the abuse of caffeine, alcohol, or cocaine. Considerable judgment must be used in the decision to proceed in such situations with elective oculoplastic surgery.[10]

MANAGEMENT OF CONCURRENT MEDICATIONS

Questions frequently arise regarding which chronic medications should be taken the day of surgery and which should be held the day of surgery. We offer the following general guidelines, although it must be recognized that individual practice may vary from locality to locality.

Antihypertensive medications should be continued until the time of surgery to avoid "rebound" hypertensive crises and to avoid the risk of end-organ damage associated with uncontrolled hypertension (myocardial ischemia is of greatest concern). Medications of particular importance in this category include clonidine (both transcutaneous and oral), beta-blockers, and angiotensin-converting enzyme inhibitors. These medications can be taken with a sip of water the day of surgery despite the NPO status of the patient.[11]

Digoxin can be held if the patient is bradycardic and the intended anesthetic technique and surgical procedure are likely to worsen the bradycardia. For example, a patient for strabismus surgery who has a resting heart rate of 45 beats per minute should not take digoxin the morning of surgery. However, another patient who is receiving digoxin to control the ventricular response to atrial fibrillation should receive the normal dose of digoxin the morning of surgery if the resting heart rate is over 70 beats per minute. Note, however, that it is generally easier for the anesthesiologist to slow an underdigitalized patient's heart rate with additional doses of digoxin intravenously than it is to speed the heart rate of a patient who is digoxin intoxicated. The latter patient may require a temporary transvenous pacemaker because of the failure of medical therapy to speed the rate.

Routine anticonvulsant medications should be administered at the usual time for the patient with sips of water, since stress and particularly general anesthesia can provoke seizures in susceptible persons.[12]

The patient who has taken corticosteroids for more than 1 month within the previous 6 months before surgery traditionally is "covered" with the equivalent of 300 mg/d of hydrocortisone perioperatively. At the start of the case, 100 mg is given intravenously, an additional 100 mg is given at the end of the procedure, and the last 100 mg is given 6 hours after the procedure. Other authors suggest lower doses for procedures associated with minimal physiologic stress—in the range of 25 to 30 mg of hydrocortisone intravenously in the first 24 hours perioperatively.[13]

The automated glucose measuring devices now available to patients have made the perioperative management of diabetes more precise. For short procedures, "no insulin, no glucose" works very well, with close perioperative monitoring of the blood glucose level. In addition, during the procedure intravenous solutions without dextrose (lactated Ringer's or saline) are given. After the procedure, the patient receives a portion of the usual insulin dose (usually one half or two thirds of the usual dose) after demonstrating successful oral caloric intake. For longer procedures, insulin should be given as an infusion of at least 4 units per hour of regular insulin with monitoring of blood glucose level every 30 minutes. Alternatively, for longer cases or for the patient who tends to run higher blood glucose levels, one fourth to one half of the patient's usual daily long-acting insulin is administered at the beginning of the case and the glucose level is monitored every 30 minutes. If the glucose value goes above 200 mg/dL, an insulin drip is added.[13]

Obviously, a primary care physician may be involved to help manage the blood glucose level after the patient leaves the recovery room.

Oral hypoglycemic medications should generally be held the day of surgery because of their relatively long duration of action, which could lead to hypoglycemia late in the day if the patient's oral caloric intake has been inadequate.

Although thyroid medications have a very long half-life, they should be given on the day of surgery.[17]

Medications to Omit the Day of Surgery

Diuretics should be omitted the day of surgery. The patient having a local procedure may become uncomfortable from the full bladder caused by taking a dose of diuretic before coming to the operating room. The patient on chronic diuretic therapy may tend to become hypotensive with a general anesthetic because of chronic intravascular volume depletion.

Drugs that interfere with platelet function such as aspirin or the nonsteroidal anti-inflammatory agents (ibuprofen, indomethacin, naproxen, sulindac) should be discontinued for the duration of one platelet life span, at least 7 days. Similarly, warfarin should be discontinued until the prothrombin time has returned to normal, unless the patient has an artificial heart valve. In the case of an artificial valve (especially a mitral valve), warfarin is discontinued until the prothrombin time is around 15 seconds. Heparin may then be started and infused to appropriate anticoagulation endpoint until 2 hours before the procedure. Heparin is then restarted after the procedure (usually 12 to 24 hours postoperatively). An internist, cardiologist, or primary care provider should be involved in the management of patients with such complex problems.[14]

Nicotinic acid should not be administered before surgery done with the patient under general anesthesia because it can cause an exaggerated hypotensive response.[15] Monoamine oxidase inhibitors (although currently not commonly used) should be stopped 2 to 3 weeks before anticipated elective surgery. These drugs are associated with an exaggerated hypertensive response to indirect-acting systemically released vasopressors during general anesthesia.[16]

WHAT THE OPHTHALMOLOGIST SHOULD KNOW ABOUT COMMONLY USED ANESTHETIC AGENTS

This section is not intended as a cookbook for how to do anesthesia but rather as a guide for the oculoplastic surgeon to some of the techniques and agents currently used. The first section is on agents used for monitored anesthesia care—a popular form of sedation and monitoring for outpatients undergoing oculoplastic procedures. The next section covers general anesthetic agents and techniques. Please note that the doses are strictly intended as guidelines based on a 70-kg healthy patient and that every attempt to avoid errors in dosage or overdosage must be made. Furthermore, the agents and techniques are not inherently safe or dangerous but rather how the agents are used makes them safe or dangerous.

Monitored Anesthesia Care

The use of relatively short-acting anxiolytics, hypnotics, and narcotics for the safe sedation of patients is common. First, these agents are used either singly or in combination to blunt the pain of local infiltration or regional anesthesia blockade. They are also useful to provide comfort and anxiolysis during the procedure. Titration to effect is an art mastered by patience and experience. Remember that more drug can always be given, but that once given it is hard to get the drug back and the reversal of drug effect may be hazardous.

Anxiolytics

Midazolam (Versed). This potent amnestic/anxiolytic is given either intramuscularly 30 to 60 minutes before the procedure or intravenously 2 to 3 minutes before a stimulus (e.g., retrobulbar block). The dose intramuscularly is 2 to 4 mg, and intravenously it is 0.5 to 1 mg at a time to effect depending on the age and vigor of the patient. A cardinal sign of successful anxiolysis (and amnesia) with this class of agents is the patient's constant repetition of the same questions—the patient keeps forgetting the answer.

Diazepam (Valium). This agent is being used less because of the more rapid offset of midazolam. Dosing is almost identical to that of midazolam, but the elimination half-life of diazepam is 20 to 40 hours compared with 2 to 4 hours for midazolam. Intramuscular dosing with diazepam is notoriously unreliable because of variable absorption. Midazolam absorption through the intramuscular route is far more reliable.

Narcotics

Small amounts of short-acting narcotics may be titrated with anxiolytics to produce an excellent balance of sedation, analgesia, and amnesia.

Alfentanil (Alfenta) has its peak effect in 1.5 to 2 minutes and a duration of action of 10 to 20 minutes. It is given in titrated doses of 100 to 500 μg intravenously in the setting of monitored anesthesia care.

Fentanyl (Sublimaze) has a peak effect in 3 to 5 minutes and lasts about 30 minutes. It is given in titrated doses of 25 to 50 μg for ophthalmic monitored anesthesia care.

One hazard with rapid doses of a large amount of narcotic is that of the rigid chest. The patient turns blue, and ventilation is impossible without the addition of neuromuscular blocking agents. Another problem with narcotics is relative narcotic overdose.

Narcotics can of course be reversed with the specific antagonist naloxone. The reversal can be accomplished with titrated doses in 10- to 20-μg increments given intravenously. The duration of action of naloxone is less than 1 hour. The patient remains in jeopardy from narcotic overdose after the naloxone has worn off if sufficient narcotic effect remains.

Barbiturates

Thiopental sodium (Pentothal) in 25-mg increments every 30 seconds can be used to ensure amnesia and hypnosis for regional anesthesia or local infiltration. Such titration is tricky business especially in the elderly, in frail patients, or in those with end-organ disease or with a tendency to "lose the airway" as they become unconscious. There is a fine line between "conscious sedation" and a "punch-drunk fighter." Too rapid a dose or too large a dose may depress hemodynamics and respiration. Methohexital (Brevital) can be similarly used in increments of 10 mg titrated intravenously every 20 to 30 seconds with the same precautions that apply to Pentothal. Sneezing, coughing, and jerky movements can be associated with the administration of barbiturates, which can be disruptive to the administration of local or regional anesthesia.

Propofol (Diprivan) is a drug with unique properties of rapid hypnosis, tendency to produce bradycardia, and rapid clearance with very little "hang over" or dysphoria. It must be given through a large-bore vein or it will burn considerably. It has been associated with infectious complications if allowed to sit overnight because the intralipid vehicle promotes bacterial and yeast growth. Increments of 10 to 20 mg are used every 20 to 30 seconds to produce sedation, amnesia, or hypnosis.

Common Agents for General Anesthesia in Adults

After intravenous induction with thiopental sodium, methohexital, or propofol, anesthesia is maintained with either inhalational agents or with continuous administration of propofol (or short-acting narcotics) with nitrous oxide. The use of propofol is associated with a lower incidence of nausea and vomiting compared with "traditional anesthesia" with the inhalational agents.[18]

Newer, very fast onset and offset inhalational agents are being introduced (e.g., sevoflurane, desflurane), and their place in the anesthetic armamentarium is being defined. "Balanced anesthesia" refers to the common practice of using a multiplicity of agents in relatively low doses to avoid the toxicity and morbidity from higher doses of any one agent. The ability to use the more rapidly metabolized neuromuscular blocking agents such as atracurium (Tracrium) and mivacurium (Mivacron) as continuous infusions with user-friendly intravenous infusion pumps has allowed for the fine-tuning of neuromuscular blockade. In oculoplastic surgery, a smooth emergence without coughing on the endotracheal tube may be of importance. Airway reflexes and thus the cough mechanism may be inhibited by the use of intravenous lidocaine.

ADVANTAGES AND DISADVANTAGES OF LOCAL ANESTHETIC OR MONITORED ANESTHESIA CARE APPROACH TO OCULOPLASTIC PROCEDURES

Advantages of regional anesthesia compared with general anesthesia for oculoplastic procedures include a reduction in operating room turnover time, a lower incidence of nausea and vomiting, and less sedation and hence earlier discharge. Safety has not been shown to be greater with a regional technique (at least for cataract surgery).[19, 20]

No studies comparing regional anesthesia to general anesthesia with use of balanced anesthesia or some of the newer, faster-acting agents discussed in the previous section have been done for oculoplastic surgery.

Some patients are not candidates for local or regional anesthetic techniques. These include pediatric patients, patients with a perforated globe, patients with uncontrollable tremor or cough, patients with a bleeding diathesis, patients with language difficulties that would make communication impossible, and patients with severe claustrophobia.

True allergic reactions are extremely rare, constituting less than 1% of local anesthetic toxicity.[21, 22]

A careful history is critical in discerning true allergy from other more common problems with the administration of infiltrative anesthesia. These include the intravascular injection of epinephrine containing local anesthetic mixtures, a vasovagal attack, or even a panic attack. Sweating, tachycardia ("my heart was beating like a sledge hammer"), and headache (from the epinephrine-induced hypertension) suggest the intravascular injection of epinephrine. An overdose of local anesthetic or direct venous bolus of a large enough mass of drug produces tinnitus, a bad taste in the mouth, confusion, circumoral numbness, and slurred speech, followed by tonic clonic convulsions and cardiopulmonary arrest.

The hallmarks of a true allergic reaction to a local anestheic include wheezing, urticaria, and respiratory distress. True allergic reactions are more likely with the ester derivatives (procaine, tetracaine, chloroprocaine, and benzocaine).[23] Confounding the question of allergy to local anesthesia is the allergic response to the preservative paraben, which is widely used in multidose vials of local anesthetics and is also found in cosmetics, in food, and as a preservative for other medications.[24]

Skin testing in advance of the day of a prospective operation by appropriate personnel with adequate monitoring and resuscitation equipment nearby is desirable in patients suspected of an allergy to local anesthetics.[22] If the patient demonstrates an ester allergy, an amide may be used as an alternate anesthetic agent. Amides include mepivacaine, prilocaine, lidocaine, ropivacaine, bupivacaine, and etidocaine.

The duration of infiltrative local anesthetic action is

prolonged by the combination with epinephrine (optimal concentration 1:200,000), and the onset of action of lidocaine and bupivacaine may be hastened by adding bicarbonate (1 mL of standard bicarbonate solution for every 10 mL of lidocaine, and 0.1 mL for every 10 mL of bupivacaine).[25]

The recommended maximal dose of lidocaine for a 70-kg patient is 300 mg (500 mg if given with epinephrine), and the maximum for bupivacaine is 175 mg (225 mg if given with epinephrine).[26]

MONITORING

Monitoring of pulse oximetry and capnography have been repeatedly shown to reduce the incidence of preventable anesthetic mishaps in closed claims studies.[27] Pulse oximetry can be performed so noninvasively and expeditiously that there is no excuse for its absence. In cases in which the patient may be fidgety, a pulse oximeter that is incorporated into an adhesive strip is useful. Alternate sites include the toe, ear, and the bridge of the nose, all of which may prove useful if the patient has poor limb perfusion, absence of a limb, or had a pulse oximeter fall off while the extremity is tucked and therefore inaccessible. Low saturation values must always be believed until proven otherwise. The continuous breath-by-breath evaluation of respiration is easily provided by a precordial stethoscope and may be confirmed by observation of the chest.

Multiple systems for monitoring capnography in awake or sedated, but nonventilated patients are available. One type is incorporated into the nasal cannula. These systems are especially suited for use in oculoplastic procedures. Again, the use of a precordial stethoscope to ensure adequacy of ventilation is strongly encouraged.

Additional and customary monitoring includes electrocardiogram, blood pressure, and, where appropriate, mental status. The latter can be tricky if talking to the patient during conscious sedation results in the patient moving. One useful technique is to set up hand signals with the patient in advance—to ask the patient to squeeze the anesthesiologist's hand if all is well. (Two squeezes indicate the patient needs to communicate with the surgical team.)

INTRAOPERATIVE PROBLEMS

Bradycardia with manipulation of extraocular muscles can occur in up to 90% of patients and is more dramatic with abrupt sustained traction on the muscle. Vagal escape and fatigue of the reflex over time will occur. The reflex can occur with any of the structures innervated by the ophthalmic branch of the trigeminal nerve. Although the use of vagolytics (atropine and glycopyrrolate) has been advocated, arrhythmias from the vagolytic agents themselves are common. An alternative is to blunt the reflex by infiltrating the muscles or structure involved with local anesthetic. Note that hypercarbia augments the reflex bradycardia, which implies that controlled ventilation may be superior to spontaneous ventilation.[28-34] Other causes of bradycardia include vasovagal reactions, overdose of narcotic, and preexisting beta-blockade.

The "startle reaction" as the patient wakes up from sedation used for the infiltration or the regional block may be disruptive. Good communication between patient, anesthesiologist, and surgeon minimizes this risk. After the local agent has been given, carefully titrated reversal with naloxone or flumazenil may avoid the startle reaction. Alternatively, waiting until the sedative has worn off will facilitate patient cooperation and avoid startling. Educating the patient in advance to expect to wake up in the operating room with the drapes on, music in the background, and people talking is useful. Additionally, the patient should be coached preoperatively so that, if necessary, he or she can communicate by squeezing the anesthesiologist's hand. I have found that this "human touch" monitor goes a long way to reassure the patient in the operating room environment. Depth of sedation can also be precisely assessed with this technique.

Restlessness and fidgetiness are nonspecific signs that may represent anything from the need to void to hypoglycemia. Pain and immobility are common causes of fidgeting. Pain from the surgical field or from an arthritic joint or back can be alleviated by administering additional local anesthetic or carefully titrated doses of narcotics or by allowing the patient a stretch period when he or she can move the lower extremities. Patients should be screened in advance for claustrophobia, which can have a devastating impact on a sterile oculoplastic field when the patient decides to abruptly leave the operating room halfway through a blepharoplasty. Communication with the patient will help decide the course of action. We routinely permit the patient to wear a hearing aid and dentures for cases employing monitored anesthesia care.

PEDIATRIC PATIENTS

Blood work in the child younger than 7 years old, especially if done on the day of surgery, makes any further medical interaction more difficult. There is no evidence that abnormalities of a complete blood cell count impact the choice of anesthesia or its management in asymptomatic children.[35]

A family history of sickle trait or sickle cell disease on the other hand should lead to the performance of a Sickle-dex since this entity does affect the conduct of the anesthetic. Other laboratory work such as bleeding time or routine urinalysis is unnecessary in the healthy child and only serves to traumatize the child.[35]

Last minute cancellations in pediatric patients scheduled for elective oculoplastic surgery may be avoidable. When to perform a procedure on a child with an upper respiratory tract infection is a case in point. One must distinguish between the healthy child with allergic rhinitis who "always looks like this" (according to the parents) from the child with a fever over 38°C (100.4°F), sore throat, malaise, and anorexia. Making the parents aware of the dangers of proceeding with a general anesthetic in a child with an upper respiratory tract infection is usually sufficient to temper their disappointment at having to delay the elective procedure. Furthermore, the presence of an infectious nasal discharge may endanger the results of the surgery should the operative site become infected. I suggest that part of the preoperative teaching of the parents should include discussion of the symptoms of an upper respiratory tract infection and that a phone call be made 24 hours in advance of surgery to confirm the child's status.

REFERENCES

1. White PF: Preoperative evaluation and premedication of ambulatory surgery patients. Refresher Courses Anesthesiol 19:217–232, 1991.
2. MacPherson DS: Preoperative laboratory testing: Should any tests be "routine" before surgery? Med Clin North Am 77:289–308, 1993.
3. Vitez TS, Soperle LE, Wong KC: Chronic hypokalemia and introperative dysrhythmias. Anesthesiology 63:130, 1985.
4. Hirsh IA, Thomlinson DL, Slogoff S: The overstated risk of preoperative hypokalemia. Anesth Analg 67:131, 1988.
5. Wong KC, Schafer PG, Schultz JR: Hypokalemia and anesthetic implications. Anesth Analg 77:1238, 1993.
6. Pulsinelli WA: Increased damage after ischemic stroke in patients with hyperglycemia with or without established diabetes mellitus. Am J Med 74:540, 1983.
7. Longstreth WE, Inui TS: High blood glucose level on hospital admission and poor neurological recovery after cardiac arrest. Ann Neurol 15:59, 1984.
8. Tarhan S, Moffitt CA, Taylor WF, Guilani E: Myocardial infarction after general anesthesia. JAMA 220:1451, 1972.
9. Steers PA, Tinker JH, Tarhan S: Myocardial reinfarction after anesthesia and surgery. JAMA 239:2566, 1978.
10. Ross AF, Tinker JH: Cardiovascular disease. *In* Brown D (ed): Risk and Outcome in Anesthesia. Philadelphia: JB Lippincott, 1992, p 39.
11. Stoelting RK: NPO and aspiration pneumonitis: Changing perspectives. Refresher Courses Anesthesiol 21:41, 1993.
12. Stoelting RK, Dierdorf SF, McCammon RL: Diseases of the nervous system. *In* Stoelting RK: Anesthesia and Coexisting Disease, 2nd ed. New York: Churchill Livingstone, 1987, p 335.
13. Kay J: Endocrine disorders. *In* Cheng EY, Kay J (eds): Anesthesia and the Medically Compromised Patient. Philadelphia: JB Lippincott, 1990, p 362.
14. Florete OG, Gallagher TJ: Cardiac disease: Congestive heart failure, coronary disease, and valvular disease. *In* Cheng EY, Kay J (eds): Anesthesia and the Medically Compromised Patient. Philadelphia, JB Lippincott, 1990, p 2.
15. Roizen MG: Anesthetic implications of concurrent disease. *In* Miller RD (ed): Anesthesia, 3rd ed. New York: Churchill Livingstone, 1990, p 874.
16. El Ganzouri AR, Ivankovich AD, Braverman B, McCarthy R: Monoamine oxidase inhibitors: Should they be discontinued preoperatively? Anesth Analg 64:592, 1985.
17. Roizen MF: Disease of the endocrine system. *In* Katz J, Benumof JL, Kadis LB (eds): Anesthesia and Uncommon Diseases. Philadelphia: WB Saunders, 1990, p 260.
18. Hemelrijck JH, Gonzales JM, White PF: Pharmacology of intravenous anesthetic agents. *In* Rogers MC, Tinker JH, Covino BG, Longnecker DE (eds): Principles and Practice of Anesthesiology. St. Louis, CV Mosby, 1993, p 1140.
19. Lynch S, Wolf GL, Berlin I: General anesthesia for cataract surgery: A comparative review of 2217 consecutive cases. Anesth Analg 53:909, 1974.
20. Snow JC, Sensel S: Cataract extraction under local and general anesthesia. Anesth Analg 45:742, 1966.
21. Sobol WM, McCrary JA: Ocular anesthetic properties and adverse reactions. Int Ophthalmol Clin 29:195, 1989.
22. Aurora S, Aldrete JA: Investigation of possible allergy to local anesthetic drugs. Anesthesiology Rev 13:1976.
23. Aldrete JA, Johnson DA: Evaluation of intracutaneous testing for investigation of allergy to local anesthetic agents. Anesth Analg 49:173, 1970.
24. McLeskey CH: Allergic reaction to an amide local anesthetic. Br J Anesth 53:1105, 1981.
25. Covino BG: Pharmacology of local anesthetic agents. *In* Rodgers MC, Tinker JH, Covino BG, Longnecker DE (eds.) Principles and Practice of Anesthesiology. St. Louis: CV Mosby 1993, p 1235.
26. Covino BG: Clinical pharmacology of local anesthetic agents. *In* Cousins MJ, Bridenbaugh PH (eds): Neural Blockade in Clinical Anesthesia and Management of Pain. Philadelphia: JB Lippincott, 1988, p 111.
27. Tinker JH, Dull DL, Caplan RA: Role of monitoring devices in prevention of anesthetic mishaps: A closed claims analysis. Anesthesiology 71:541, 1989.
28. Alexander JP: Reflex disturbance of cardiac rhythm during ophthalmic surgery. Br J Ophthalmol 59:518, 1975.
29. Apt L, Isenberg S, Gaffney WL: The oculocardiac reflex in strabismus surgery. Am J Ophthalmol 76:533, 1973.
30. Berler DK: The oculocardiac reflex. Am J Ophthalmol 56:954, 1963.
31. Blanc VF, Hardy JF, Milot J: The oculocardiac reflex: A graphic and statistical analysis in infants and children. Can Anaesth Soc J 30:360, 1983.
32. Doyle DJ, Mark PWS: Reflex bradycardia during surgery, Can J Anaesth 37:219, 1990.
33. Moonie GT, Reel DL, Elton D: The oculocardiac reflex during strabismus surgery. Can Anaesth Soc J 11:621, 1964.
34. Smith RB, Douglas H, Peruscak J: The oculo-cardiac reflex and sino-atrial arrest. Can Anaesth Soc J 19:138, 1972.
35. Mulroy JJ, Lynn AM: The medical evaluation of pediatric patients. Semin Anesth 11:200, 1992.

CHAPTER 29

Malignant Eyelid and Orbital Tumors

Mary A. Stefanyszyn and David I. Silbert

The treatment of ophthalmic disease rarely involves life-threatening disorders; however, there are certain eyelid and orbital tumors that have the propensity for aggressive growth or life-threatening metastases. Early diagnosis and aggressive treatment are important in achieving cure. The most common malignant eyelid tumors include basal cell carcinoma, squamous cell carcinoma, and sebaceous adenocarcinoma. Orbital malignancies most commonly include rhabdomyosarcoma in children and lacrimal gland tumors and lymphomas in adults. Metastatic orbital tumors, malignant fibrous histiocytoma, hemangiopericytoma, liposarcoma, melanoma, alveolar soft part sarcoma, osteogenic sarcoma, and other rare tumors complete the spectrum of malignant orbital disease. Tumors of the nasolacrimal system can be very aggressive and have the potential for metastasis, necessitating aggressive management.

The approach to the management of the common malignant eyelid, orbital, and nasolacrimal sac tumors is outlined in this chapter. Excluded from this discussion are ocular malignancies such as retinoblastoma and melanoma, rare orbital tumors, metastatic disease, and nasal and sinus carcinomas that can secondarily invade the orbit.

Basal cell carcinoma is the most frequently occurring skin cancer in the United States and accounts for more than 90% of eyelid tumors.[1] Excisional surgery with frozen sections or Mohs' surgery with careful monitoring of the margins is the treatment of choice. If the margins are clear of tumor, the cure rate has been reported as 93% to 100%.[1-3] Radiation therapy or cryotherapy can be used as an alternative for small, noninfiltrating lesions in elderly patients; however, re-examinations are imperative. Fraunfelder and associates[4] reported a 94% and 97% cure rate at 5 years, respectively, for infiltrative and nodular basal cell carcinoma smaller than 10 mm in diameter treated with cryotherapy. The presence of deep morphea-sclerosing or multicentric tumors is ominous, and aggressive surgical excision is indicated. Howard and coworkers[5] reported that 8 of 11 exenterations for basal cell carcinoma were of the morphea-sclerosing type. A medial canthal location is also more likely to have a grim prognosis (Fig. 29-1). Radiation therapy is particularly ineffective in the medial canthal area, and wide primary surgical excision is important.[6] Recurrent basal cell carcinoma is difficult to eradicate since it is often embedded in scar tissue and has less distinct margins; this often necessitates aggressive surgery in spite of deformity.[7] Orbital involvement is heralded by the onset of incomitant strabismus and can be accompanied by pain, ptosis, progressive eyelid and orbital swelling, and loss of vision.[8] The average duration between the onset of a cutaneous lesion and orbital invasion was 9.8 years for basal cell carcinoma and 1 year for squamous cell carcinoma in a series reported by Howard and coworkers.[5] A life-threatening neoplasm that has extended into the orbit requires aggressive surgery, including exenteration.[9, 10] The tumor can spread to the sinuses and brain, and a team approach of oculoplastic surgeons, plastic surgeons, otolaryngologists, and neurosurgeons may best succeed in en bloc surgical excision and reconstruction.[10] Preoperative planning and postoperative followup is greatly aided by neuroimaging, including computed tomographic (CT) scanning and magnetic resonance imaging (MRI). Local and systemic chemotherapy with cisplatin, doxorubicin, or both has been described as an alternative measure or an adjunct to surgical treatment.[11, 12] The use of iridium wire implants is still lacking long-term followup, but initial results are hopeful, with cure rates of 94% for recurrent lesions and 97.4% for new lesions.[13]

Squamous cell carcinoma is responsible for 9.2% of all eyelid malignancies.[14] The invasive and malignant potential of squamous cell tumors is dependent on tumor size, degree of differentiation, etiology, and depth of dermal invasion. Tumors that arise in areas of actinic keratoses are less aggressive than those that arise de novo. Squamous cell carcinoma arising in irradiated areas, burn scars, and inflamed areas and in immunosuppressed patients tend to be more invasive. Metastases to the preauricular or submandibular nodes occur late in the disease. Orbital invasion by squamous cell carcinoma ranges from 2.5% to 8.2%.[5, 15] In contrast with basal cell carcinoma, which invades the orbit many years after original presentation, intraorbital spread occurs within 1 to 3 years from diagnosis of the primary lesion. Most difficult to diagnose and frustrating to treat is the perineural infil-

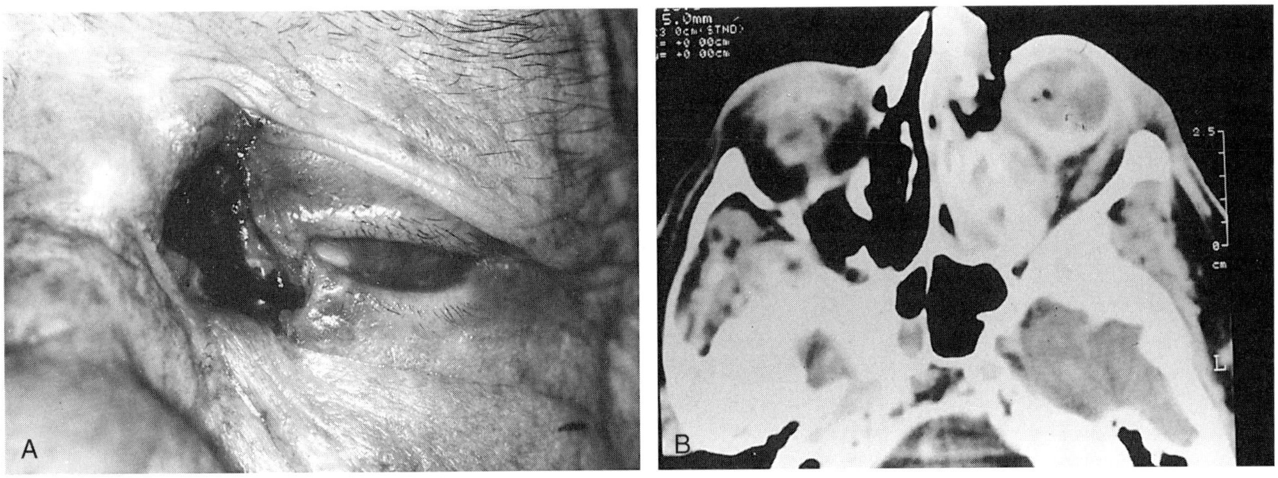

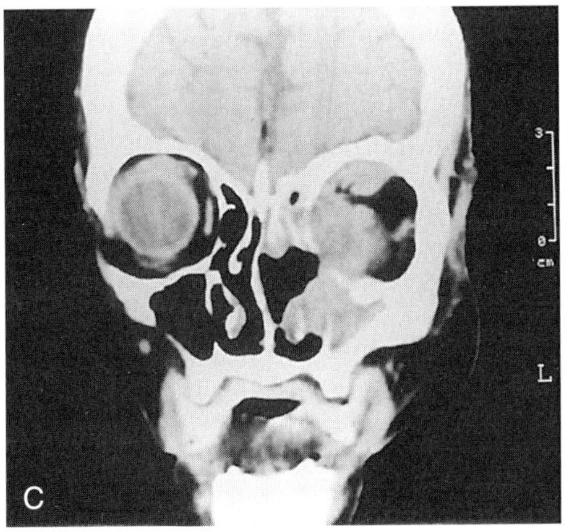

Figure 29–1. *A,* Recurrent basal cell carcinoma eroding into the orbit, nose, and sinuses. The tumor had been excised five times previously, and the area had also been treated with radiation therapy. *B,* Axial computed tomographic (CT) scan demonstrating tumor invading the left posterior orbit and ethmoidal sinus. *C,* Coronal CT scan demonstrating tumor in the maxillary sinus and left orbit.

tration of squamous cell carcinoma that results in growth into the orbit, intracranial cavity, and periorbital structures along the trigeminal nerves, extraocular nerves, and the facial nerve (Fig. 29–2). This can result in complete ptosis, ophthalmoplegia, and severe pain not responsive to chemotherapy or irradiation. Early diagnosis followed by wide excision with histopathologic control is the treatment of choice. In large lesions, preoperative and postoperative CT scan or MRI scans are helpful in delineating the extent of the disease. Unlike basal cell carcinoma, squamous cell carcinoma is relatively radioresistant, necessitating higher doses, more than 5000 rad, to achieve tumor control.[14] The lack of histologic control of tumor edges and the radiation damage to the surrounding periocular tissues limit the use of radiation therapy to patients unable or unwilling to undergo surgery. The use of cryotherapy for eyelid squamous cell carcinoma is questionable in view of its invasive and malignant potential.

Sebaceous carcinoma is a rare malignancy of the eyelids that is often misdiagnosed and has the ability to spread widely and to metastasize. Delays in clinical diagnosis, errors in pathologic diagnosis, and delays in treatment contribute to high mortality. The cases in Doxanas and Green's series[16] before 1970 were associated with a 24% mortality, whereas the cases after 1970 were associated with no mortality owing to better pathologic and clinical diagnosis. Sebaceous carcinoma can present as a chronic chalazion or blepharoconjunctivitis (Fig. 29–3). Doxanas and Green[16] correlated the blepharoconjunctivitis to intraepithelial pagetoid spread of sebaceous carcinoma cells. Rao and colleagues[17] reported a 59% mortality in cases with pagetoid involvement, as compared with 11% mortality in cases without. Poorly differentiated tumors had a 60% mortality, whereas well-differentiated tumors had a 9% mortality. Tumors of the upper eyelid had a 28% mortality, whereas tumors of the lower eyelid had 0% mortality. Tumors of both upper and lower eyelids had an 83% mortality. Tumor size was important, with tumors smaller than 6 mm in diameter having 0% mortality, whereas tumors 6 to 10 mm, 11 to 20 mm, and larger than 20 mm had mortality rates of 18%, 50%, and 60%, respectively. Patients whose duration of symptoms was less than 6 months had a mortality rate of 14%, and those with symptoms for more than 6 months had a 38% mortality. The study may not reflect present mortality rates, owing to the referral patterns of the Armed Forces Institute of Pathology and to greater awareness and earlier diagnosis of sebaceous carcinoma by the ophthalmologist.

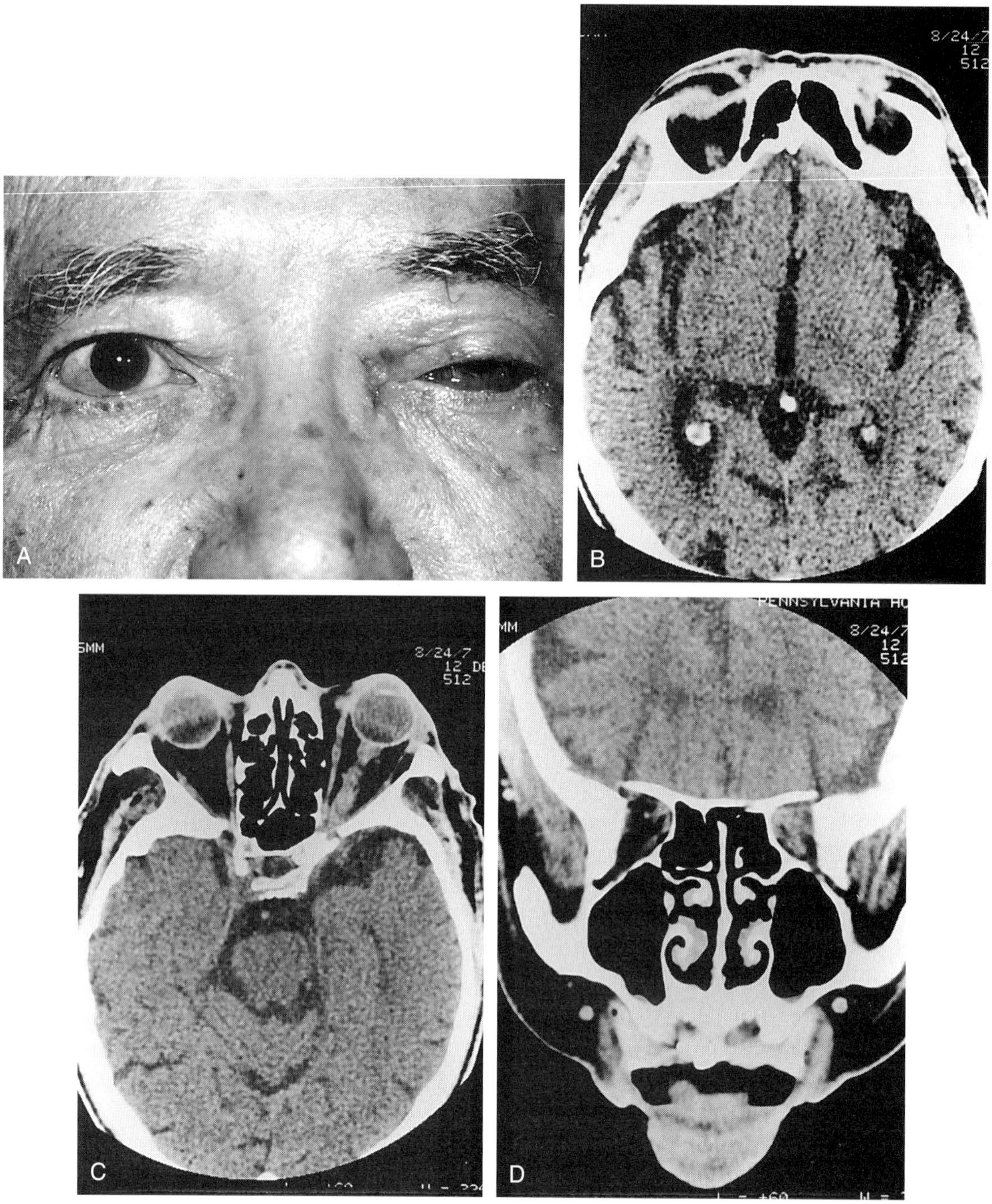

Figure 29–2. *A*, Perineural spread of squamous cell carcinoma from the forehead along the trigeminal nerves into the left orbit. The supratrochlear nerve was surrounded by tumor that grew posteriorly into the orbit. The patient complained of pain in the left temple, numbness of the left forehead, and double vision. On examination, ptosis, chemosis, restricted motility, and decreased vision were present. *B*, Axial computed tomographic (CT) scan with a soft tissue mass in the left supratrochlear area. *C*, Axial CT scan demonstrating tumor surrounding the left optic nerve. *D*, Coronal CT scan with a diffuse soft tissue mass in the left orbital apex.

A full-thickness biopsy of the eyelid is sometimes necessary to make the diagnosis of sebaceous carcinoma. Excision can be performed with frozen section control, but it is hard to determine margins if there is intraepithelial pagetoid spread of the tumor. Additional samples of the palpebral and bulbar conjunctiva should be obtained and sent for permanent sections.[18] With diffuse pagetoid involvement of the conjunctiva, Doxanas and Green[16] advocate that the bulk of the tumor be excised and the involved conjunctiva followed closely. Rebiopsy of the involved area can be performed and cryotherapy or wider excision performed at a later date. Kass and Hornblass[19] suggest wide excision of the invasive carcinoma under frozen section control with cryotherapy to the intraepithelial neoplasia. The efficacy of radiation therapy for sebaceous carcinoma has not been established. It has been

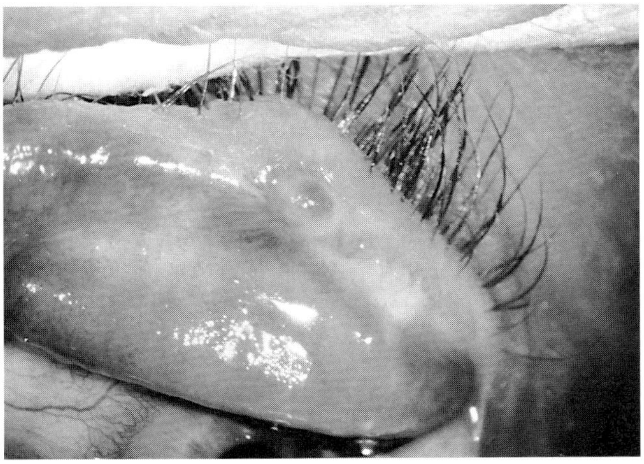

Figure 29–3. Sebaceous carcinoma can present as a chalazion or as unilateral blepharoconjunctivitis.

reserved for patients too ill for surgery and those who have refused to undergo adequate local radical surgery. Radiation therapy is also useful as a palliative modality. Pardo and associates[20] reported on 30 patients treated with radiation therapy as definitive or postoperative therapy. Local control of 90% was achieved in their cases, and they contend that the impression that sebaceous cell carcinoma is radioresistant is erroneous and that it has a place in the management of sebaceous cell carcinoma of the eyelid.

Orbital rhabdomyosarcoma is the most common malignant primary orbital tumor of childhood. Until the 1960s exenteration was the treatment of choice, with a cure rate of about 25%.[21] The current treatment combines surgery, radiation therapy, and adjuvant chemotherapy. Exenteration is reserved for the rare patient with a local recurrence. Recurrence usually occurs in the first 3 years, but a case of recurrence after 6 years has been reported.[22] The Intergroup Rhabdomyosarcoma Study of 127 orbital cases conclusively showed the efficacy of the combined regimen, reporting a local control rate of higher than 90%.[23,24] This group recommended chemotherapy for 1 year consisting of dactinomycin and vincristine. Concurrent radiation therapy is started 2 weeks after the onset of chemotherapy and consists of daily treatments of 180 rad to a total of 4140 rad for children younger than age 6 and 4500 rad for children older than age 6. Local control of the disease was attributed to radiation therapy, and distant metastatic control was attributed to chemotherapy. Late complications of radiation therapy include cataract formation, retinopathy, keratoconjunctivitis, enophthalmos, and phthisis. Facial asymmetry with bony hypoplasia of the orbit was more marked in the younger children (Fig. 29–4). Growth retardation of 20% or more was noted in 61% of patients and was believed to be secondary to the unavoidable inclusion of the pituitary in the field of radiation treatment.[24] The systemic side effects of cytotoxic drugs include epistaxis, neutropenia, abdominal pain, stomatitis, and neuropathy.[25] The extent of the late morbidity of both the chemotherapy and the irradiation is not yet fully evaluated.

Lacrimal gland neoplasms present a challenge in diagnosis and treatment. Even the benign mixed tumors can recur and undergo malignant change. In a series by Wright and associates,[26] 76% of malignant neoplasms were adenoid cystic carcinoma, 12% were adenocarcinomas, and 12% were carcinomas arising within a benign mixed tumor. Although adenoid cystic carcinoma most commonly presents in the fourth decade, two other peaks are present: the second and sixth decades.[27] Misdiagnosis is most common in the pediatric age group, in whom malignancy is least suspected.[28] Adenoid cystic carcinoma can be subdivided into five patterns: cribriform, sclerosing, basaloid, comedocarcinomatous, and tubular. The basaloid type appears to have the worst prognosis.[26,29,30] The course of the disease can be variable with long periods of remission followed by recurrent disease locally or metastases to the lungs.[31–33] Wide resection of the tumor followed by radiation therapy offered no advantage over exenteration followed by radiation therapy. At 5, 10, and 15 years, survival rates of 45%, 23%, and 14%, respectively, were noted.[31] Ten-year survival in Wright's series for adenoid cystic carcinoma with various modes of treatment was 35%. Pain was a common symptom (39%, 30%) of adenoid cystic carcinoma in the Font and Gamel series[31] and the Wright series,[26] respectively. Pain may be indicative of perineural invasion and more aggressive disease. The relentless nature of adenoid cystic carcinoma in spite of long disease-free intervals necessitates long-term followup and aggressive treatment (Fig. 29–5). Treatment and prognosis of adenocarcinoma and malignant mixed tumors is difficult to assess because of their rarity. Early diagnosis and aggressive surgical treatment combined with radiation therapy may improve survival.

Lymphomatous orbital infiltrations can be an intimidating topic to address. Advances in the field of immunohistochemistry have helped in the classification and diagnosis of lymphoproliferative disorders; however, it is hard to interpret the historical literature in which various

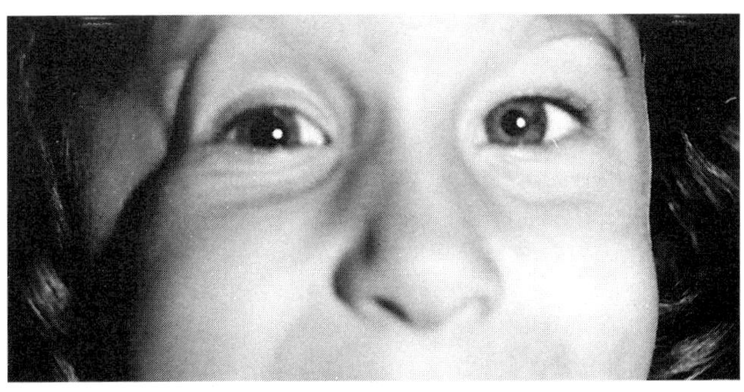

Figure 29–4. Facial asymmetry and bony hypoplasia after radiation therapy are often marked in younger children.

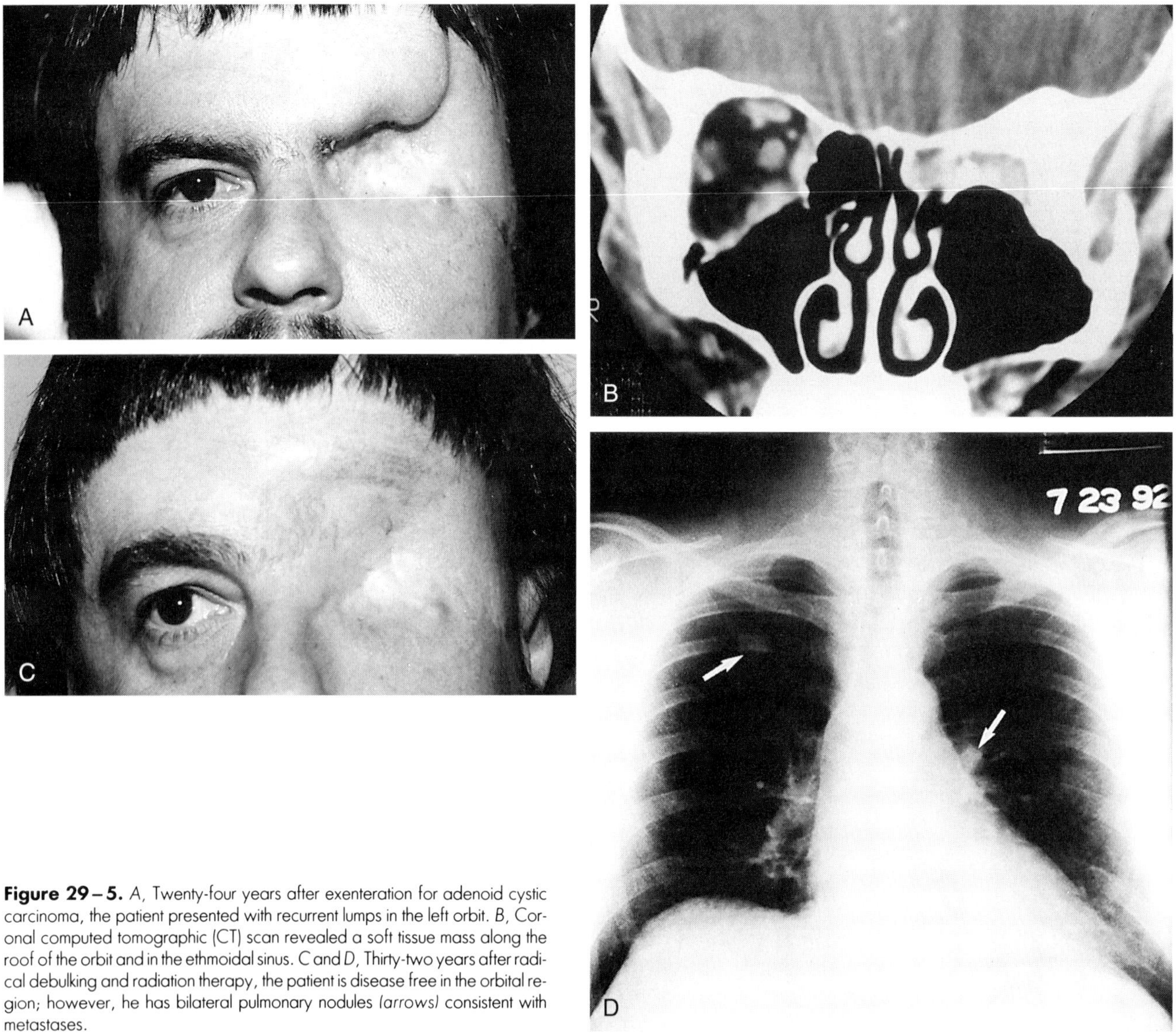

Figure 29–5. *A*, Twenty-four years after exenteration for adenoid cystic carcinoma, the patient presented with recurrent lumps in the left orbit. *B*, Coronal computed tomographic (CT) scan revealed a soft tissue mass along the roof of the orbit and in the ethmoidal sinus. *C* and *D*, Thirty-two years after radical debulking and radiation therapy, the patient is disease free in the orbital region; however, he has bilateral pulmonary nodules *(arrows)* consistent with metastases.

entities such as orbital pseudotumor, benign reactive lymphoid hyperplasia, and lymphomas were grouped together and sometimes misclassified. The benign reactive lesions are characterized by lymphoid follicles, polyclonal and polymorphous populations of lymphocytes, plasma cells, and histiocytes. These lesions respond to corticosteroids and low-dose radiation therapy. These patients can have multisystemic involvement and their tumors occasionally progress to malignant transformation.[34] The spectrum of lymphoproliferative disorders extends to the atypical lymphoid hyperplasias and lymphomas. Patients with atypical lymphoid disease vary little from those with low-grade orbital lymphomas. Lymphomas typically present in the sixth and seventh decades with orbital masses of insidious and chronic nature. Treatment of these patients varies, depending on histopathologic diagnosis, age, and systemic extent of the disease. In Rootman and associates' series of 37 lymphomas,[34] all monoclonal B cell proliferations, 60% presented as localized lesions and 40% had involvement of other sites. About 15% of patients with localized disease developed dissemination. A multidisciplinary approach to treatment is necessary with cooperation among the pathologist, ophthalmologist, radiotherapist, and oncologist.[35] Localized well-differentiated orbital lesions are treated by radiation therapy or observation. Lack of treatment does not influence later treatment once the disease becomes progressive. The less well-differentiated tumors are treated with systemic chemotherapy, low-dose irradiation (1500 to 2500 rad), or both. Local control of the disease after radiation therapy is usually excellent with low-dose radiation, and if a higher dose is needed it can be done at a later time.

Lacrimal sac tumors are rare; however, they can be life threatening, and early diagnosis and treatment are necessary. In a review of 115 lacrimal sac tumors, 50% were

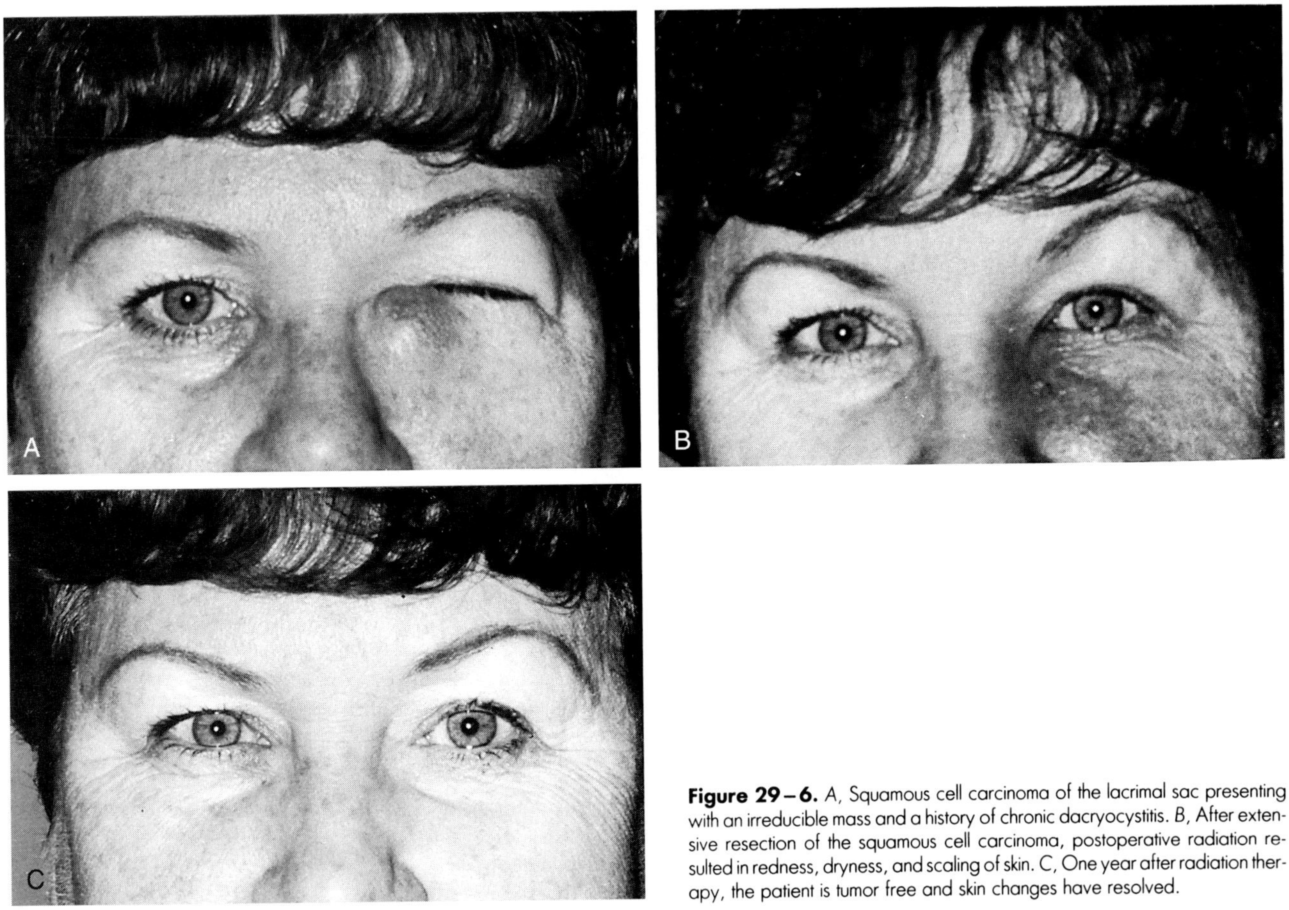

Figure 29–6. *A*, Squamous cell carcinoma of the lacrimal sac presenting with an irreducible mass and a history of chronic dacryocystitis. *B*, After extensive resection of the squamous cell carcinoma, postoperative radiation resulted in redness, dryness, and scaling of skin. *C*, One year after radiation therapy, the patient is tumor free and skin changes have resolved.

malignant lesions.[36] Of 82 epithelial tumors, 44 were malignant. Additionally, malignant lymphomas and melanomas can present as primary tumors of the lacrimal sac. Malignant epithelial lacrimal sac tumors need to be treated with wide surgical excision, including a lateral rhinostomy, and followed with high-dose radiation therapy (Fig. 29–6). In a review of the literature the recurrence rate for invasive squamous and transitional cell carcinoma was shown to be 50%, with 50% being fatal.[36] Lymphoid lesions generally respond well to radiation therapy with minimal complications. The most dismal prognosis is that of malignant melanoma, which is often fatal despite aggressive treatment. A high index of suspicion on the part of the clinician is essential in the early diagnosis of lacrimal sac tumors. Since these lesions tend to present with symptoms of dacryostenosis, dacryocystitis, or both, they are often misdiagnosed early on in the disease. Any recurrent bouts of dacryocystitis combined with a mass in the area of the lacrimal sac, bleeding from the puncta, epistaxis, ulceration, and involvement of the preauricular, submandibular, and cervical nodes are signs of neoplastic disease.

In conclusion, it is rare for the ophthalmologist or oculoplastic surgeon to deal with malignant life-threatening disease. As headway is made in the fields of histopathology and immunohistochemistry the surgeon must communicate with the pathologist to ensure the proper handling of tissues. Accurate pathologic diagnosis may require special studies, including electron microscopy and immunohistochemistry. Tissues for routine histologic examination are fixed in paraformaldehyde solution. Electron microscopy requires fixation of tissues in glutaraldehyde, and immunohistochemistry studies are best done on fresh tissue or tissue briefly fixed in acetone, Bouin's solution, or Carnoy's solution. The pathologist needs to be available for frozen section evaluation or to do cell impressions for cytology if indicated.

Once the pathologic diagnosis is available, management decisions need to be made, taking into consideration the age of the patient, the aggressiveness of the tumor, and the various modes of treatment and their side effects. A young patient with a basal cell carcinoma that is morpheaform and in the medial canthus needs a wide excision and careful followup for many years. Squamous cell and sebaceous cell carcinoma even in elderly patients should be treated with wide excision since other modes of treatment such as cryotherapy and radiation therapy are not effective. Once biopsy results are obtained the treatment of orbital malignancies such as rhabdomyosarcoma and lymphomas falls primarily into the hands of the radiotherapists and oncologists. Primary lacrimal gland and lacrimal sac malignancies are best treated with aggressive surgery followed by radiation therapy. The gravity and complexity of treating malignant orbital disease often requires the cooperation of the ophthalmologist or oculoplastic surgeon with the pathologist, oncologist, radiotherapist, otolaryngologist, neurosurgeon, and other specialists.

REFERENCES

1. Leib ML, Johnson DA, Eliezri YD: Mohs' histographic surgery and ophthalmic plastic reconstruction. Ophthal Plast Reconstr Surg 8:262–270, 1992.
2. Frank HJ: Frozen section control of excision of eyelid basal cell carcinomas: 8½ years' experience. Br J Ophthalmol 73:328–332, 1989.
3. Glatt HJ, Olson JJ, Putterman AM: Conventional frozen sections in periocular basal cell carcinoma: A review of 236 cases. Ophthalmic Surg 23:6–9, 1992.
4. Fraunfelder FT, Zacarian SA, Wingfield DL, Limmer BL: Results of cryotherapy for eyelid malignancies. Am J Ophthalmol 97:184–188, 1984.
5. Howard GR, Nerad JA, Carter KD, Whitaker DC: Clinical characteristics associated with orbital invasion of cutaneous basal cell and squamous cell tumors of the eyelid. Am J Ophthalmol 113:123–133, 1992.
6. Rodriguez-Sains RS, Robbins P, Smith B, Bosniak S: Radiotherapy of periocular basal cell carcinomas: Recurrence rates and treatment with special attention to the medial canthus. Br J Ophthalmol 72:134–138, 1988.
7. Sakura CY, Calamel PM: Comparison of treatment modalities for recurrent basal cell carcinoma. Plast Reconstr Surg 63:492–496, 1979.
8. Amoaku WMK, Bagegni A, Logan WC, Archer DB: Orbital infiltration by eyelid skin carcinoma. Int Ophthalmol 14:285–294, 1990.
9. Rathbun JE, Beard C, Quickert MH: Evaluation of 48 cases of orbital exenteration. Am J Ophthalmol 72:191–199, 1971.
10. Hornblass A, Roen JL: A combined facial, orbital, and intracranial resection of extensive basal cell carcinoma arising in the eyelid. Ophthalmic Surg 16:769–773, 1985.
11. Luxenberg LN, Guthrie TH: Chemotherapy of basal cell and squamous cell carcinoma of the eyelids and periorbital tissues. Ophthalmology 93:504–510, 1986.
12. Morley M, Finger PT, Perlin M, et al: Cisplatinum chemotherapy for ocular basal cell carcinoma. Br J Ophthalmol 75:407–410, 1991.
13. Daly NJ, DeLafontan B, Combes PF: Results of the treatment of 165 lid carcinomas by iridium wire implants. Int J Radiat Oncol Biol Phys 10:455–459, 1984.
14. Reifler MD, Hornblass A: Squamous cell carcinoma of the eyelid. Surv Ophthalmol 30:349–365, 1986.
15. Henderson J, Farrow GM: The tumor survey. *In* Orbital Tumors, 2nd ed. New York, Thieme Stratton, 1980, pp 67–74.
16. Doxanas MT, Green RW: Sebaceous gland carcinoma: Review of 40 cases. Arch Ophthalmol 102:245–249, 1984.
17. Rao NA, Hidayat AA, McLean IW, Zimmerman LE: Sebaceous carcinoma of the ocular adnexa: A clinicopathologic study of 40 cases with followup data. Hum Pathol 13:113–122, 1982.
18. Folberg R, Whitaker DC, Tse DT, Nerad JA: Recurrent and residual sebaceous carcinoma after Mohs' excision of the primary lesion. Am J Ophthalmol 103:817–823, 1987.
19. Kass LG, Hornblass A: Sebaceous carcinoma of the ocular adnexa. Surv Ophthalmol 33:477–490, 1989.
20. Pardo FS, Wang CC, Albert D, Stracher MA: Sebaceous carcinoma of the ocular adnexa: Radiotherapeutic management. Int J Radiat Oncol Biol Phys 17:643–647, 1989.
21. Porterfield JF, Zimmerman LE. Rhabdomyosarcoma of the orbit: A clinicopathologic study of 55 cases. Virchows Arch [A] 355:329–344, 1962.
22. Chestler RJ, Dortzbach RK, Kronish JW: Late recurrence in primary orbital rhabdomyosarcoma. Am J Ophthalmol 106:92–93, 1988.
23. Wharam M, Beltangady M, Hays D, et al: Localized rhabdomyosarcoma: An interim report of the Intergroup Rhabdomyosarcoma Study Committee. Ophthalmology 94:251–254, 1987.
24. Heyn R, Ragab A, Raney B, et al: Late effects of therapy in orbital rhabdomyosarcoma in children: A report from the Intergroup Rhabdomyosarcoma Study. Cancer 57:1738–1743, 1986.
25. Ghafoor SY, Dudgeon J: Orbital rhabdomyosarcoma: Improved survival with combined pulsed chemotherapy and irradiation. Br J Ophthalmol 69:557–561, 1985.
26. Wright JE: Primary malignant neoplasms of the lacrimal gland. Br J Ophthalmol 76:401–407, 1992.
27. Wright JE: Factors affecting the survival of patients with lacrimal gland tumors. Can J Ophthalmol 17:3–9, 1982.
28. Dagher G, Anderson RL, Ossoinig KC, Baker JD: Adenoid cystic carcinoma of the lacrimal gland in a child. Arch Ophthalmol 98:1098–1100, 1980.
29. Moringa S, Nakajima T, Shimosato Y, et al: Histologic factors influencing prognosis of adenoid cystic carcinoma of the head and neck. Jpn J Clin Oncol 16:29–40, 1986.
30. Hickman RE, Cawson RA, Duffy SW: The prognosis of specific types of salivary gland tumors. Cancer 54:1620–1624, 1986.
31. Font RL, Gamel JW: Epithelial tumors of the lacrimal gland: An analysis of 265 cases. *In* Jakobiec FA (ed): Ocular and Adnexal Tumors. Birmingham, AL, Aesculapius, 1978, pp 787–805.
32. Font RL, Gamel JW: Adenoid cystic carcinoma of the lacrimal gland: A clinicopathologic study of 79 cases. *In* Nicholson DH (ed): Ocular Pathology Update. New York, Masson Publishing USA, 1980, pp 277–283.
33. Lee DA, Campbell JR, Waller RR, Ilstrup DM: A clinicopathologic study of primary adenoid cystic carcinoma of the lacrimal gland. Ophthalmology 92:128–134, 1985.
34. Rootman J, Robertson W, Lapointe JS, White V: Lymphoproliferative and leukemic lesions. *In* Rootman J (ed): Diseases of the Orbit. Philadelphia, JB Lippincott, 1988, pp 205–240.
35. Rosenberg SA: Current concepts in cancer: Non-Hodgkin's lymphoma: Selection of treatment on the basis of histologic type. N Engl J Med 301:924–928, 1979.
36. Stefanyszyn MA, Hidayat AA, Pe'er JJ, Flanagan JC: Lacrimal sac tumors. Ophthal Plast Reconstr Surg 10:169–180, 1994.

CHAPTER 30

Eyelid Infections and Inflammations

Constance L. Fry and Russell W. Neuhaus

Eyelid inflammation is caused by various organisms, including bacteria, viruses, parasites, and fungi. Certain inflammatory conditions have characteristic findings, but often overlap exists between disease states. Therefore, a careful history that focuses on the onset of the inflammation, concomitant disease, travel history, and prior therapy is helpful.

Eyelid inflammation may present as a localized erythematous region, diffuse or subconjunctival involvement, ulcerative papules, painless masses, malpositioned eyelids or eyelashes, necrotic lesions, or eyelid edema (Tables 30-1 through 30-6). At times, associated lymphadenopathy or pain is present. Periorbital inflammation may also extend into the orbit.

Inflammatory conditions of the eyelid may be primary infections or may be secondary to other infections of the head and neck, or to hematogenous or lymphatic spread. Involvement of single organ systems, such as the respiratory tract, or multiple systems, as in septicemia, may give valuable clues as to the cause of the illness.

The cause of inflammatory lesions of the eyelids is often evident. However, when inflammation is either atypical or recurrent, biopsy, smears, and cultures may aid in the diagnosis of occult carcinomas or unusual bacterial, viral, parasitic, and fungal diseases. A systemic evaluation may also be valuable for particularly aggressive lesions and diseases caused by fungi and parasites.

INFLAMMATION OF THE SEBACEOUS GLANDS OF THE EYELID

Sebaceous glands of the eyelid include Moll's glands, glands of Zeis, and meibomian glands. An acute infection of Moll's glands and glands of Zeis is termed *external hordeolum*, or *stye*, and is usually caused by staphylococcal infection. In these cases, a pointed erythematous eyelid lesion with edema is present on the skin surface (Fig. 30-1). Meibomian gland inflammation may result from acute or chronic infections that are localized or generalized or secondary to occult carcinoma. Acute meibomitis, or hordeolum internum, results from staphylococcal infections. Inflammation diffusely involves the entire eyelid and bulbar conjunctiva, but localized tenderness usually reveals the involved gland. An internal hordeolum is often larger than a stye, and it points toward the conjunctival surface, where a draining abscess usually develops. It also may drain through the skin or the meibomian gland orifice.[1] Occasionally, the infectious component resolves and is replaced by a nodule of granulomatous inflammation, a chalazion (Fig. 30-2).[1] Hordeola are rarely complicated by cellulitis.

Chronic meibomitis includes meibomian seborrhea, chronic meibomitis with conjunctivitis, and chronic suppurative meibomitis. Meibomian seborrhea consists of excessive meibomian gland secretions without inflammation. Chronic meibomitis is characterized by dilated, inflamed meibomian gland ductules with a thickened tarsus (Fig. 30-3). Chronic meibomitis is probably not primarily a result of bacterial infections, but secondary bacterial growth may alter meibomian gland secretions, leading to stasis of gland secretions. Suppurative meibomitis is rare. The tarsus is thickened and purulent fluid is present in chronic suppurative meibomitis, which is rarely associated with tuberculosis or actinomyces or fungal infections.[2]

Treatment of external and internal hordeola consists of administration of warm compresses and topical antibiotics and eyelid hygiene. If the hordeolum does not spontaneously drain, incision and drainage are appropriate. Treatment of meibomian seborrhea consists of daily eyelid massage to express retained secretions, eyelid hy-

TABLE 30-1

Diseases and Organisms that Cause Painless Eyelid Masses

Candida species
Chagas' disease
Chalazion
Cysticercosis
Dirofilaria
Dracunculus medinensis
Echinococcus granulosus
Onchocerciasis
Papilloma viruses
Rhinoscleroma
Sparganosis
Syphilis
Tuberculosis
Tularemia

TABLE 30-2

Diseases and Organisms Associated with Periorbital Edema

Ancylostoma duodenale
Ascaris lumbricoides
Brugia malayi
Brugia timori
Chagas' disease
Dengue viruses or fever
Enterobius vermicularis
Gnathostoma spinigerum
Lymphogranuloma venereum
Necator americanus
Rhinosporidiosis
Schistosomiasis
Trichinosis
Wuchereria bancrofti

TABLE 30-3

Causes of Necrotic Eyelid Lesions

Anthrax
Cryptococcus neoformans
Diphtheria
Ecthyma gangrenosum
Entamoeba histolytica (amebiasis)
Gas gangrene
Glanders
Necrotizing fasciitis
Progressive synergistic gangrene
Rickettsia
Smallpox
Spider bites
Streptococcal myonecrosis

TABLE 30-4

Infections with Subconjunctival Involvement

Cysticercosis species
Dirofilaria species
Loa loa

TABLE 30-5

Infections that Cause Trichiasis, Madarosis, or Ectropion

Blastomycosis
Herpes zoster
Leishmaniasis
Paracoccidioidomycosis
Smallpox
Trachoma

TABLE 30-6

Causes of Ulcerative Eyelid Lesions

Actinomycosis
Aspergillosis
Atypical mycobacteria
Bartonellosis
Blastomycosis
Chancroid
Coccidioidomycosis
Cowpox
Cryptococcus neoformans
Entamoeba histolytica
Granuloma inguinale
Herpes simplex
Leishmaniasis
Molluscum contagiosum
Paracoccidioidomycosis
Pinta
Orf
Sporotricosis
Syphilis
Vaccinia
Varicella zoster
Yaws

giene, and occasionally warm compresses. Treatment of chronic meibomitis with conjunctivitis requires daily eyelid hygiene, warm compresses, and possibly topical antibiotics. A 1-month course of low-dose (250 mg/day) systemic tetracycline may be warranted for chronic meibomitis. The tetracycline inhibits bacterial growth and bacterial enzymes, stabilizes lipid secretions, and decreases the free fatty acid concentration of sebum.[1, 3] However, in recalcitrant infections, cultures and sensitivities should direct the choice of antibiotics.

A chalazion is classically a chronic lipogranulomatous inflammation of a meibomian gland. Occasionally, lipogranulomatous inflammation occurs in the glands of Zeis and is referred to as a *marginal chalazion.* Chalazia may develop de novo, occur secondary to hordeola, or be associated with seborrheic blepharitis, chronic meibomitis, or acne rosacea.[1, 2, 4] Chalazia are postulated to develop from blockage of the orifices of the meibomian glands and stagnation of the glands' secretions.[5] A pseudocapsule develops around the inflammation. When the inflammation subsides a firm, painless nodule remains in the eyelid with occasional erythema of the overlying skin. Chalazia are often multiple, particularly in children, and occur more commonly in the upper eyelid than in the lower. A large chalazion may induce corneal astigmatism, which is reversed by chalazion drainage.[6] The inflammatory reaction may cause posterior eyelid distortion, leading to trichiasis. Cultures of chalazia are characteristically negative.[7] Rarely, chalazia may become secondarily infected, resulting in cellulitis.[5]

Several approaches are used to treat chalazia. Conservative treatment consisting of the application of warm compresses with or without eyelid hygiene is effective in 25% to 80% of cases.[7–9] If conservative treatment fails, surgical drainage with the excision of the fibrous capsule may be performed. Either local anesthesia or general an-

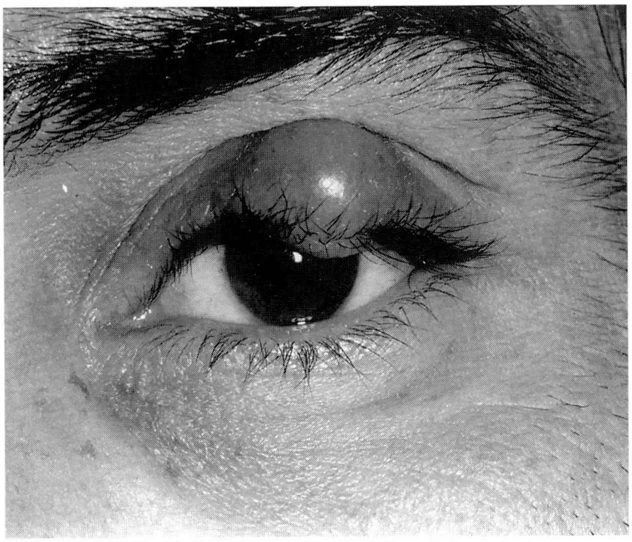

Figure 30–1. External hordeolum.

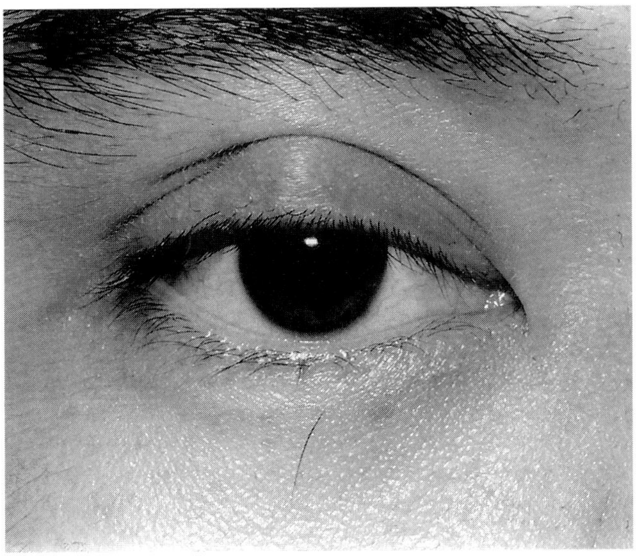

Figure 30–2. Chalazion.

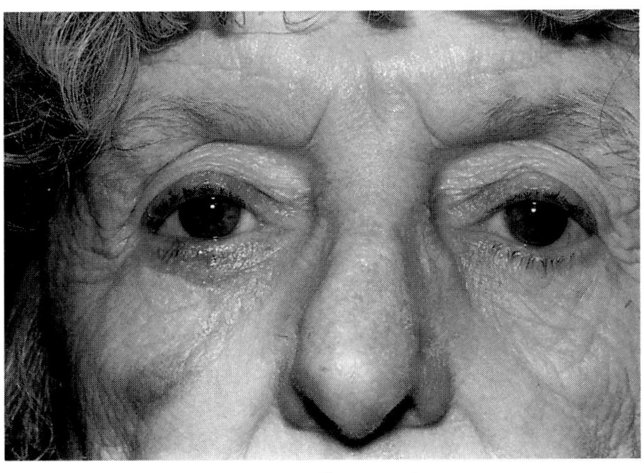

Figure 30–3. Chronic meibomitis.

esthesia for young or uncooperative patients may be employed.

Local infiltrative anesthesia consisting of 2% lidocaine (Xylocaine) with epinephrine (1:100,000) and hyaluronidase is used to ensure vasoconstriction and dispersion of the anesthetic solution. A minimum of 15 minutes should be allowed for maximal vasoconstriction and anesthesia. Administration of incremental injections of 0.5 mL of anesthetic solution at 2- to 3-minute intervals minimizes injection discomfort and maximizes the effects of anesthesia. A total of 1.5 mL of anesthetic solution is usually adequate.

A posterior conjunctival approach is preferred to allow adequate drainage and excision of necrotic material from the meibomian glands. After the chalazion clamp is in place and the eyelid is everted, a cruciate incision is made in the conjunctiva overlying the chalazion. The four flaps consisting of conjunctiva and atrophic tarsal plate are then excised. Additional mechanical expression of the adjacent meibomian gland contents should be performed. The fibrous capsule is meticulously excised with a curette or with sharp dissection. Approximately 3 mm of undisturbed tarsal plate should be preserved between the excision site and the eyelid margin to prevent eyelid margin distortion and contour abnormalities. Once the chalazion clamp is removed, excessive bleeding is managed by cauterization. After the antibiotic ointment is applied, the eye is patched for 24 hours. The resected tissue should be sent for pathologic examination if the chalazion is recurrent or has an abnormal appearance.

Other techniques for chalazion excision have been described in the literature and include excision of the chalazion through an upper eyelid crease, tarsus trephination, cutting of several vertical slits on the conjunctival surface, and use of the carbon dioxide laser.[10–12]

The use of injectable corticosteroids in the adjacent eyelid soft tissues is optional. Steroid injections may be given alone or in combination with surgical excision. In the literature, the results of steroid therapy for chalazia have varied, with larger amounts of steroid often being more effective. The commonest steroid preparations used are triamcinolone acetate or acetonide.[13–22]

Serious complications in chalazion surgery are rare; however, recurrences are common. Other complications of simple excision include secondary infection, fistula formation, eyelid notching, delayed hemorrhage, and corneal abrasion.[5, 23] Administration of intralesional steroids has resulted in incomplete cure, recurrence, hypopigmentation, and presumed retinal and choroidal vascular emboli with occlusion.[13, 14, 24]

Tumors of the eyelid may masquerade as chalazia.[25, 26] Either the tumor itself resembles a chalazion or it blocks a meibomian gland, causing a secondary chalazion. Of 168 Ontario ophthalmologists surveyed, 9% had a case diagnosed preoperatively as a chalazion that was actually a tumor.[23] This finding underscores the importance of performing histologic examination on all atypical or recurrent chalazia. The commonest tumor misdiagnosed as a chalazion is sebaceous cell carcinoma.[27–31] Other tumors that mimic chalazia include basal cell carcinoma, Merkel's cell tumors, metastatic tumors, squamous cell carcinoma, desmoplastic malignant melanoma, rhabdomyosarcoma, hemangioma, histiocytosis X, and granuloma annulare.[23, 32–35]

PRESEPTAL CELLULITIS

Two types of cellulitis affect the periorbita: preseptal and orbital cellulitis. The physician must be able to distinguish between these entities. Preseptal cellulitis often presents with marked diffuse eyelid swelling with involvement of regional lymph nodes. With progression, preseptal cellulitis may result in local abscess formation (Fig. 30–4), skin sloughing, necrotizing fasciitis, toxic shock syndrome, or orbital cellulitis.[2, 36] Orbital cellulitis usually presents with proptosis and venous congestion. Ophthalmoplegia, pain with eye movement, visual impairment, and an afferent pupillary defect may also occur. Causes of preseptal cellulitis include primary skin infections, spread from other sites, post-traumatic infections, and postoperative infections. Young children deserve special consideration when intravenous antibiotics are selected because of potential hematogenous spread from the upper respiratory tract or from otitis media caused by *Haemophilus influenzae* or *Streptococcus pneumoniae*.[2, 37]

Neonates and children younger than 6 years of age often require antibiotics that cover a different spectrum of organisms compared with those drugs used for healthy adults. In neonates (i.e., aged 1 to 30 days), gram-positive organisms are commoner when preseptal cellulitis complicates maternal mastitis, conjunctivitis, or ruptured dacryocystocele.[38, 39] In preseptal cellulitis secondary to mastitis, the initial infection begins in the gums, and the onset is characterized by unilateral facial edema and erythema. Draining fistulas may develop in the skin of the eyelids and nose and over the maxilla.[39] *Staphylococcus aureus* is almost always responsible for neonatal preseptal cellulitis. However, gram-negative bacilli have also been reported to occur in neonates.[40] Computed tomography, lumbar puncture, and blood cultures are often recommended to diagnose patients in this group.[39] In children younger than 6 years of age, preseptal cellulitis usually results from hematogenous spread from otitis media or upper respiratory tract infections. The causative organism is most commonly *H. influenzae* or *S. pneumoniae*. A violaceous hue suggests the presence of *H. influenzae*, which is a serious pathogen in young children because of the risk it carries of sepsis and meningitis. For this reason, blood cultures and lumbar puncture are often indicated in young children.[41, 42] Children 6 years of age and older may be treated as adults.

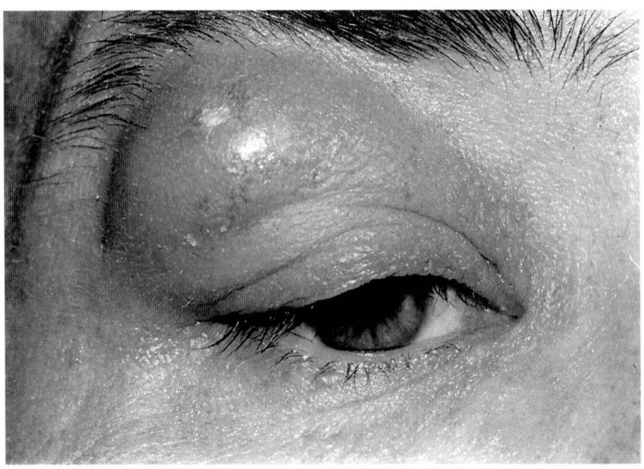

Figure 30–4. Preseptal cellulitis with abscess formation.

Primary skin infections that cause preseptal cellulitis usually result from staphylococcal and streptococcal species, including impetigo and erysipelas. Streptococcal infections are commoner in the tropics, whereas in temperate regions, mixed or staphylococcal infections predominate.[2] Impetigo, which is commoner in children than in adults, is caused by *S. aureus* or *Streptococcus pyogenes*. This infection develops as spreading erythematous macules that progress to vesicles that rupture and form a yellow crust. Satellite lesions result from secondary autoinfection. Regional lymphadenopathy is characteristic of impetigo.[2, 43–45] Impetigo may complicate pre-existing herpetic lesions or eczema.[43] Streptococcal impetigo can result in conjunctivitis, corneal ulcers, and cicatricial ankyloblepharon.[2] Erysipelas caused by *S. pyogenes* is commonest in children, the elderly, or adults with diabetes mellitus, alcoholism, and nephrotic syndrome.[45] It is characterized by a well-demarcated, rapidly spreading zone of red, indurated skin with minute vesicles at the leading edge.[2, 46] Eyelid involvement occurs as a result of lymphatic spread. Significant orbital congestion with chemosis, incomplete ophthalmoplegia, and mild proptosis may occur. This presentation of erysipelas may represent diffusion of toxins into the orbit rather than true orbital cellulitis, but neuroimaging is still warranted.[43] Erysipelas characteristically is accompanied by a high fever and it is usually self-limited if appropriate antibiotics are administered. However, in infants, the elderly, and persons with alcoholism or chronic debilitated states, it may be fatal.[2]

Another important cause of preseptal cellulitis is spread from adjacent structures. Infections of the paranasal sinuses, nasolacrimal sac, conjunctiva, and hordeola may cause secondary preseptal cellulitis.[41, 42, 47] Sinus infections result in preseptal or orbital cellulitis by direct extension or hematogenous spread.

Diabetics and other immunocompromised patients may become infected by multiple or unusual organisms, including fungi and algae.[2, 45, 48, 49] These patients should be evaluated for sepsis and bacteria-induced tissue necrosis as is discussed later.[48, 50]

Both blunt and penetrating trauma may be complicated by cellulitis. The primary causative organisms for this manifestation of cellulitis are *S. aureus* and *S. pyogenes*, although anaerobic infections may also occur.[47] Because all orbital wall fractures provide a direct communication between potentially infected sinuses and the orbital soft tissue, an increased risk of orbital or preseptal infections exits. One method of determining the likelihood of secondary infection has been proposed by Westfall and Shore,[51] who classified fractures according to wound types to determine the need for antibiotics.

Post-traumatic cellulitis resulting from human and animal bites deserves special consideration. Anaerobic bacteria, such as *Peptococcus, Peptostreptococcus, Eikenella, Fusobacterium,* and *Bacteroides*, are associated with bites.[47, 48] *Pasteurella multocida* is a serious pathogen that is associated with dog and cat bites as well as cat scratches.[52]

Rapidly spreading cellulitis that occurs after injury associated with salt or fresh water exposure may be caused by unusual organisms. Typically, salt water exposure is associated with *Vibrio vulnificus* infections and fresh water, with *Aeromonas* sp., and *Chromobacterium violaceum.* Only *C. violaceum* has been documented in preseptal cellulitis. These organisms are not susceptible to the standard antibiotics and may rapidly cause death if infection with them is not treated with the appropriate antibiotic.[53–56]

Preseptal cellulitis may also occur after ocular or periorbital surgery. Few cases are reported in the literature, but hospital-acquired organisms should be considered as the cause of this inflammation.[57]

Treatment

The treatment for cellulitis can be classified by site of origin, history of trauma, and patient age. Additionally, immunocompromised patients or a history of water exposure requires different antibiotic coverage.

In neonates with cellulitis of the face resulting from maternal mastitis, computed tomography and lumbar puncture should be obtained. If a subcutaneous abscess is present, incision and drainage are indicated, as are cultures and Gram's stain to determine the causative organism.[39] Although a penicillinase-resistant synthetic penicillin (PRSP) alone treats the commonest organism, the addition of an antipseudomonal aminoglycosidic antibiotic (APAG) to the regimen is prudent until cultures have been completed. In children younger than 6 years of age with preseptal cellulitis, cultures of the conjunctiva and blood should be obtained and a lumbar puncture should be considered. Treatment regimens in infants and children younger than 6 years of age include the administration of a PRSP plus cefuroxime or a third-generation cephalosporin.[47, 48, 58] The administration of a PRSP plus chloramphenicol is also effective. However, because of concern over chloramphenicol-induced aplastic anemia, this antibiotic is not commonly used in the United States.

Mild cellulitis secondary to skin infections is effectively treated by the administration of oral antibiotics. Severe infections should be treated by intravenous antibiotics. In both instances, a 10-day course of a PRSP or first-generation cephalosporin is effective. The addition of topical antibiotics may be effective. For patients with serious penicillin allergy, either vancomycin or penicillin skin testing is indicated. An exception to this protocol for cellulitis resulting from skin infections is erysipelas. When erysipelas manifests as severe periorbital swelling, computed tomography should be performed, and blood cultures should be obtained. Classically, the treatment included a 48- to 72-hour course of intravenous penicillin until improvement was demonstrated, and then oral therapy was instituted for a total of 10 days. However, a PRSP or first-generation cephalosporin is now the treatment of choice for the elimination of staphylococcal organisms.[43, 48] Needle aspiration of erysipelas near the orbit is contraindicated because this treatment may spread the infection beyond the orbital septum.

Atraumatic preseptal cellulitis in the absence of a primary skin infection is usually related to sinusitis, otitis, or respiratory infection. This type of cellulitis may be effectively treated by administration of oral amoxicillin-clavulanate or intravenous ampicillin-sulbactam, depending on the severity of the infection. Cefuroxime and trimethoprim-sulfamethoxazole are alternative treatments.[48]

In diabetics with cellulitis, cultures should be obtained, and bacteria-induced necrosis should be considered. A PRSP may be used to treat uncomplicated infections. If the patient appears septic, a penicillinase-resistant penicillin, given with either an antipseudomonal aminoglycoside or aztreonam, and clindamycin should be used.[48, 49] Alternatively, imipenem cilastatin may be used alone.[48]

In patients with post-traumatic suppurative cellulitis, the wound should be cultured, debrided, and vigorously irrigated. A Gram stain also should be performed. Computed tomography should be performed if an orbital cellulitis or abscess or occult orbital trauma is suspected. The treatment for uncomplicated cases is the same as for cellulitis related to skin infections (administration of a PRSP or first-generation cephalosporin). If anaerobic infections are suspected, penicillin, clindamycin, chloramphenicol, or cefuroxime should be added to the regimen. Alternatively, ampicillin-clavulanate may be used alone, particularly if the patient has human or animal bites. In addition, postexposure prophylaxis against tetanus and rabies should be given when indicated.[47] For post-traumatic injuries occurring with exposure to salt water, administration of doxycycline and an aminoglycoside is the treatment of choice against *V. vulnificus.*[54] Surgical drainage may also be necessary.[54] For fresh water injuries, administration of trimethoprim-sulfamethoxazole is the treatment of choice for *Aeromonas* sp.[59] Reported cases of *C. violaceum* have been sensitive to an APAG, tetracycline, trimethoprim-sulfamethoxazole, and chloramphenicol.[55, 56]

Other entities may be misdiagnosed as preseptal cellulitis. Two cases of subperiosteal abscesses associated with acute ethmoid sinusitis in children presented only with preseptal cellulitis.[60] In addition, a patient with acute myeloblastic leukemia presented with diffuse bilateral periorbital swelling resulting from leukemic infiltration of the skin.[61] Angiosarcoma, a malignant tumor of the elderly, may mimic chronic facial cellulitis in appearance.[62]

EYELID NECROSIS

Several causes of eyelid necrosis exist. Bacteria cause necrotizing fasciitis, streptococcal myonecrosis, progressive synergistic gangrene, gas gangrene, ecthyma gangrenosum, and nonspecific gangrene. The excellent blood supply of the eyelid margin often spares this area from necrosis.[63–65] Eyelid necrosis most commonly is caused by beta-hemolytic streptococcus. Other causative organisms or diseases described in the literature include *Clostridium hastiforme, Proteus mirabilis, Pseudomonas aeruginosa, Pseudomonas mallei,* anthrax, diphtheria, and rickettsia. Eyelid necrosis usually occurs after trauma, and most affected patients are immunocompromised (Fig. 30–5).[63, 66–72] Necrosis may also occur as a result of smallpox, cryptococcus, and spider bites (see Table 31–3).

Necrotizing fasciitis is characterized by a serosanguineous exudative necrosis of superficial fascia with extensive undermining of surrounding tissues. The involved skin is pale red with bullae and indistinct borders. The skin color progresses to purple. A cellulitis and crepitus are often present.[73] Sixteen bacterial cases of necrotizing fasciitis involving the eyelid have been described in the literature; three quarters of these patients had antecedent trauma, and almost half had either alcoholism or diabetes. Streptococcus was isolated in all but one patient and staphylococci were also cultured in almost half of the cases.[74] A case of necrotizing fasciitis of the eyelids has also been reported in which only *Cryptococcus neoformans* was found on the surgical specimen. The patient was otherwise healthy.[75] Assessment of necrotizing fasciitis consists of Gram's stain and culture, and treatment consists of immediate surgical debridement, in addition to administration of broad-spectrum antibiotics.[74] Ampicillin given in combination with an APAG and clindamycin is appropriate empiric therapy until culture results are available.[74]

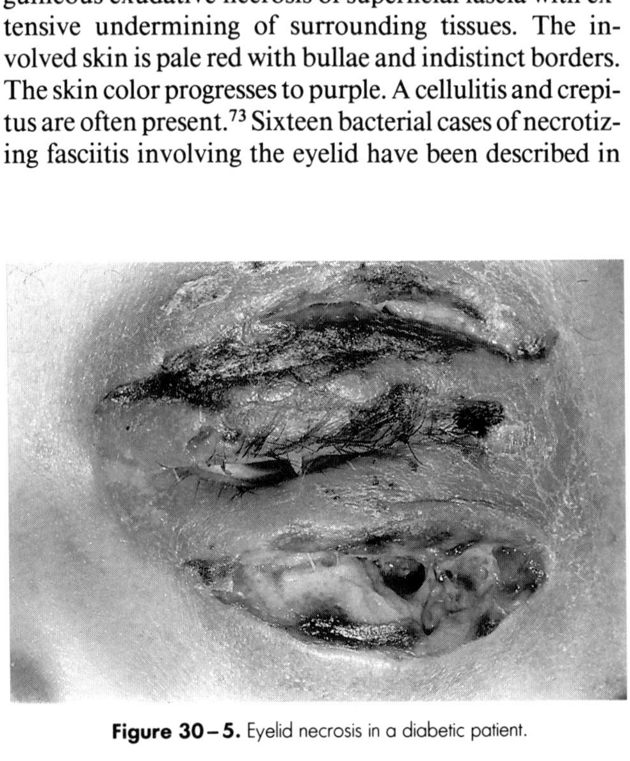

Figure 30–5. Eyelid necrosis in a diabetic patient.

Streptococcal myonecrosis is a type of gas gangrene caused by facultative or obligate anaerobic streptococci, and possibly *S. aureus.* It is characterized by pain, purulent discharge, and an infected muscle that changes from erythematous to gangrenous in appearance.[73] Several cases in the literature diagnosed as streptococcal gangrene of the eyelids appear to be streptococcal myonecrosis.[66, 71] Treatment consists of debridement and penicillin. Administration of a PRSP is appropriate when staphylococcal infections are present.[45, 76]

Progressive synergistic gangrene usually occurs postoperatively or after an abrasion. The typical lesion is painful and has a necrotic center, surrounded by concentric areas of gangrene and erythematous skin. This lesion is characterized by polymicrobial infection; cultures from the outer regions grow microaerophilic and anaerobic streptococcus, whereas those from the center grow *S. aureus* and occasionally gram-negative rods.[73] Several cases of eyelid necrosis appear in the literature that probably represent progressive synergistic eyelid necrosis.[64, 68] This type of gangrene may be effectively treated with the combination of systemic penicillin, PRSP, and APAG, or ampicillin-sulbactam or imipenem with surgical debridement of necrotic soft tissue. Hyperbaric oxygen may be useful in selected severe cases.[45, 74, 76]

Gas gangrene (clostridial myonecrosis) is a rapidly spreading myonecrosis with gas formation resulting from infection with *Clostridium* species. This infection is suggested by foul-smelling drainage, crepitus, and severe pain.[73] Bullae, bronzed skin discoloration, and areas of necrosis are also characteristic.[76] The inflammatory response is minimal.[77] One case of gas gangrene of the eyelids, resulting from infection with *Clostridium* sp., has been described.[63] Clostridia may also cause a cellulitis characterized by more crepitus but less pain, less foul odor, and no muscle involvement when compared with gas gangrene.[78] Treatment for gangrene consists of administration of penicillin G and APAG as well as aggressive surgical debridement.[76] The role of hyperbaric oxygen is debatable.

Ecthyma gangrenosum is a necrotic skin lesion caused by *Pseudomonas* species. The classic lesion is an indurated ulcer with central necrosis and minimal pain. Several cases of necrotic eyelid lesions attributed to *Pseudomonas* infection have been described.[69, 70, 72, 79]

P. mallei causes an infection in equine animals called glanders that may occasionally affect humans. This disease occurs in Asia, Africa, and South America. In glanders, vesicular lesions that become gangrenous occur in the eyelid and erode it.[2] The diagnosis is made by microscopic evaluation of scrapings of the lesion. Treatment consists of administration of streptomycin and tetracycline.[59, 80]

Anthrax, which is caused by infection with *Bacillus anthracis*, is another cause of necrotic eschars of the eyelids. This disease affects wool sorters and people who handle animal hides. It occurs sporadically in southern Europe, Africa, Asia, South America, and the United States. Three forms of anthrax exist: cutaneous, pulmonary, and intestinal. The cutaneous form is the commonest. In cutaneous anthrax, the lesion begins as a raised red papule surrounded by edema. Lymphadenopathy may be present.[81] A painless central vesicle appears and progresses to a black eschar, the malignant pustule.[82, 83] Less commonly, anthrax eyelid edema may occur. Vesicles and eschar formation may accompany the edematous form.[2] The treatment of choice is administration of penicillin G, and alternative treatments include administration of tetracycline or erythromycin.[59] Incision and debridement may increase the likelihood of bacteremia and should therefore be avoided.[45] If anthrax is left untreated, bacteremia, toxemia, and death may occur.[84] Immunization should be given to those at risk.

Diphtheria, which is caused by infection with *Corynebacterium diphtheriae*, occurs in unimmunized persons who live in the tropics; it occurs rarely in the United States. Diphtheria spreads to the eyelids from other skin or conjunctival infections. The cutaneous form develops after contamination of a wound or as a primary infection.[45] Primary cutaneous diphtheria begins as a vesicular lesion on an erythematous base. Significant pain, swelling, induration, and regional lymphadenopathy are common manifestations of the disease. In some patients, diphtheria may resemble a cellulitis.[85] Over time in all patients, a chronic ulcer with the classic overlying gray or yellow membrane develops. Gangrene of the eyelids may result from either type.[2] Cicatricial changes include symblepharon, entropion, and trichiasis. Cranial nerve palsies and Guillain-Barré syndrome have been reported in patients with cutaneous diphtheria.[45] The diagnosis is obtained from scrapings stained with methylene blue and culture on Löffler's or tellurite agar.[45] The treatment of choice is administration of erythromycin and antitoxin.[45, 48, 49, 59, 85]

Rickettsial disease, including scrub typhus and Q fever, may also cause necrotic eyelid lesions.[2] The treatment of choice for rickettsia is administration of tetracycline.[59] Smallpox has also caused gangrenous lesions of the eyelids in the past.[2]

Eyelid necrosis has also been attributed to the *Loxosceles* species of spiders, whose commonest member is the brown recluse. The venom of the spiders contains cytotoxic agents that induce dermonecrosis.[65, 86, 87] Systemic involvement includes fever arthralgias, hemolysis, thrombocytopenia, renal failure, and death.[88] Administration of systemic steroids and topical antibiotics may be helpful.

OTHER BACTERIAL INFECTIONS

The commonest manifestation of bacterial infection in the eyelid is cellulitis. Other, less common, findings include mycobacterial infiltration; tularemia, treponemal, and chancroid infections; granuloma inguinale; plague; bartonellosis; actinomyces infection; rhinoscleroma; and chlamydia infection.

Mycobacterial infections of the eyelids occur in leprosy, tuberculosis, and other uncommon mycobacteria. Leprosy, or Hansen's disease, is probably caused by *Mycobacterium leprae*. It is found throughout most of the world, including India, Asia, Australia, Africa, the Middle East, southern Europe, Central and South America, and the United States. The incidence of leprosy in the United States is increasing, possibly because of immigration from Mexico and Indochina.[89] In leprosy, madarosis, thickening of supraciliary ridges, ptosis, ectropion, entropion, and lagophthalmos may occur.[90, 91] Madarosis, supraciliary ridge thickening, and ptosis are the result of eyelid infiltration. Ptosis may also less commonly result from involvement of the third cranial nerve.[92] Entropion often occurs in areas where trachoma is endemic. Therefore, it is unclear whether the entropion is a manifestation of leprosy or of trachoma. Lagophthalmos, which results from involvement of the facial nerve, is also common.[92] The diagnosis is based on clinical findings, results of the lepromin skin test, and demonstration of acid-fast bacilli on biopsy specimens. The mainstay of medical treatment is administration of dapsone and rifampin. In some types of leprosy, clofazimine is added to the treatment regimen. Surgical correction of eyelid abnormalities may be necessary.

Eyelid involvement due to tuberculosis includes primary tuberculosis (chancre), secondary tubercle formation (lupus vulgaris), secondary extension from underlying structures (scrofuloderma), and secondary hematogenous spread (tuberculous gummata). All of these conditions are exceedingly rare.[2] Atypical mycobacteria caused a chronic eyelid abscess in two cases reported in the literature. Both patients had nasolacrimal apparatus abnormalities.[93, 94] Treatment consists of appropriate antituberculous therapy.

Tularemia, caused by the gram-negative bacillus *Francisella tularensis*, occurs in the United States, Canada, Mexico, Japan, and Russia. Ticks and deerflies are important vectors.[95] Six different types of this febrile illness exist: ulceroglandular, glandular, typhoidal, oculoglandular, oropharyngeal, and pulmonary. The organism may invade the tarsus and cause a chalazion-like swelling.[2] The diagnosis is confirmed by serologic testing. The treatment of choice is administration of streptomycin or gentamicin.[59, 95]

Spirochetal infection may rarely involve the eyelids. Primary syphilitic chancres are accompanied by regional lymphadenopathy.[2, 96] Ulcerative blepharitis, edema, and reversible alopecia of the eyebrows and scalp may occur in secondary syphilis. Gummata of the eyelids as well as tarsitis occur uncommonly with tertiary syphilis.[2]

Yaws is a nonvenereal treponemal infection. The causative organism is *Treponema pertenue*, and the disease occurs in the rural, humid tropics of Australia, Asia, Latin America, and West Africa.[97] Yaws affects the skin, cartilage, and bone. The primary lesion is an ulcerative papule. Lymphadenopathy may also be present. Secondary lesions are either macular or papillomatous. Late yaws is characterized by granulomas and gummata.[98]

Pinta, another nonvenereal treponematosis, is caused by *Treponema carateum.* It occurs in rural, semiarid tropical regions of the Americas. Unlike yaws, it affects only the skin. It is also less contagious and invasive than yaws. Pinta is characterized by the presence of chancres, skin plaques, and hyperpigmented macules, called pintids. In late disease, superficial scars and widespread depigmentation are characteristic.[97]

The diagnosis and treatment of syphilis, yaws, and pinta are similar. The diagnosis is based on clinical grounds, history of exposure to endemic locations, darkfield examination of exudate, and serologic testing including nontreponemal tests (Venereal Disease Research Laboratory, rapid plasma reagin) and treponemal tests (microhemagglutination – *Treponema pallidum*, fluorescent treponemal antibody absorption). The treatment for syphilis, yaws, and pinta is administration of penicillin.[2]

Chancroid, which is caused by *Haemophilus ducreyi* infection, is a venereal infection common in Asia, Africa, and South America. It causes painful ulceration and regional lymphadenopathy that may rarely affect the eyelid by autoinoculation. The organism may be cultured from skin lesions on special media. Accepted treatments include administration of erythromycin, ceftriaxone, or fluoroquinolones.[2, 48, 59]

Granuloma inguinale is a venereal disease caused by *Calymmatobacterium granulomatis.* It is endemic in tropical regions, but it is uncommon elsewhere, including the United States.[46] It results in painless ulcers of the skin and mucous membranes. The eyelids may become involved from autoinoculation. Smears of the lesions reveal characteristic gram-negative Donovan's bodies inside macrophages. The treatment of choice is doxycycline administration. Gentamicin or chloramphenicol therapy is reserved for resistant cases.[48, 85]

Plague is caused by the bacterium *Yersinia pestis*, the natural reservoirs of which are rodents. Transmission is by flea bites. Plague is endemic to several Asian, African, and American countries. Between 1980 and 1986, the United States was one of nine countries to report more than 100 cases. The typical findings of this febrile illness include lymphadenopathy, lymph node swellings (buboes), vessel thrombosis, and skin lesions ranging from pustules to cellulitis to abscesses. Significant bacteremia or pneumonia may be present. One case of an infraciliary abscess with periorbital swelling has been reported.[99] The diagnosis is made on the basis of the classic findings described in a patient in an endemic area with positive smears and cultures of the buboes. The treatment of choice is administration of streptomycin.[48, 59, 99]

Bartonellosis is another bacterial disease whose skin manifestations may affect the periorbita. Bartonellosis is caused by *Bartonella bacilliformis* and is confined to the valleys of the Andes mountains in South America. Bartonellosis is a febrile illness, also called Oroya fever, that is characterized by an acute hemolytic phase. A verrucous phase may develop subsequently or de novo.[46] The skin lesions range from miliary or nodular lesions to large, ulcerative tumors called *mular.* A case of a mular lesion located on the lower eyelid has been reported.[100] The diagnosis can be ascertained by blood smears and cultures during Oroya fever and skin biopsies during the verrucous phase. Effective therapy includes administration of penicillin, tetracycline, streptomycin, or chloramphenicol for the acute febrile illness.[46] However, antibiotics are not effective for verrucous lesions.[46]

Actinomycosis is a granulomatous bacterial infection caused by *Actinomyces* species. The organism has worldwide distribution and is part of normal oropharyngeal flora. Dental extraction or caries often precede overt infections. The cervicofacial form is commonest.[101] A subcutaneous nodule migrates to the skin surface. Purulent discharge with yellow "sulfur granules" containing the organism is characteristic. The face, eyelids, and orbit may become infected.[2] The diagnosis is made by examination of the sulfur granules for organisms. Administration of penicillin G or ampicillin is the treatment of choice.[48, 59, 101]

Another granulomatous disease that may affect the eyelids is rhinoscleroma, which is caused by *Klebsiella rhinoscleromatis* infection. It is commonest in the West Indies, southern Europe, Africa, and Asia.[46] Initially, subcutaneous plaques form that ultimately involve the skin. Nodules then develop, along with scarring. The disease usually begins in the nares and upper lip and may spread to the eyelids, canthus, lacrimal drainage apparatus, and conjunctiva.[2] The diagnosis is made by characteristic clinical and histologic findings. Tetracycline and streptomycin are often effective treatments, but antibiotic sensitivity should be determined.[46, 102]

Trachoma, which is caused by infection with *Chlamydia trachomatis* serotypes A, B, Ba, or C, results in a chronic follicular conjunctivitis, which causes scarring. The MacCallan classification consists of four stages. Stage I is characterized by immature follicles. In stage II, the inflammation exhibits marked follicular and papillary hypertrophy. In stage III, the cicatricial changes begin; the destruction and scar formation may result from cell-mediated immune response. In stage IV, the healing begins. At this point, cicatricial entropion and secondary trichiasis occur. Other manifestations include eyelid retraction and secondary blepharospasm.[103] The eyelid retraction occurs from primary scarring with vertical shortening of the posterior lamellae. This scarring and retraction results in lagophthalmos and secondary corneal exposure with corneal irritation and further exposure keratitis. Mild upper eyelid cicatricial entropion can be corrected with posterior tarsal surgery. In more severe cases with extensive trichiasis, posterior lamellar (tarsal) scarring, and irregular eyelid margins, mucous membrane grafts and/or composite mucoperichondrial grafts may be needed to stabilize the upper eyelid. Lower eyelid tarsotomies may not be ideal because of the shorter vertical height of the tarsal plate. Thus, inferior blepharotomies or the modified Weis procedure have been used.[103] In chronic trachoma, doxycycline therapy may be effective. However, improving health standards may have a greater effect.[104]

Lymphogranuloma venereum is caused by infection with *C. trachomatis* serotypes L1, L2, or L3. The distribution is worldwide but endemic to parts of Africa. The typical findings are a painless genital papule followed by development of bilateral inguinal lymphadenopathy.[105] The periorbital manifestations include eyelid edema, conjunctivitis, and preauricular lymphadenopathy (Parinaud's oculoglandular syndrome). The diagnosis is made from clinical findings associated with positive cultures or serologic testing. The treatment of choice is doxyycycline administration.[48]

VIRAL INFECTIONS

Virus-induced eyelid inflammation most commonly results from herpetic infections; other viruses that rarely affect the eyelids include pox, dengue, and papilloma viruses. (see Tables 30-1, 30-3, 30-5, and 30-6).

Herpetic eyelid involvement occurs with both herpes simplex and varicella zoster (herpes zoster) in primary and recurrent infections.[106] In each type of infection, a secondary bacterial cellulitis or intraocular involvement may occur.

The classic lesion of primary herpes simplex is a unilateral ulcerative blepharitis with minimal pain (Fig. 30-6). This lesion may also develop with recurrences, but such events are uncommon.[107] In addition to the typical vesicular lesion of the eyelid, herpes simplex may also cause eschar formation or isolated eyelid edema. The vesicles of herpes simplex may also occur along the distribution of the fifth cranial nerve and may mimic zoster, a condition called *zosteriform herpes*.[108] In the eyelid, herpes

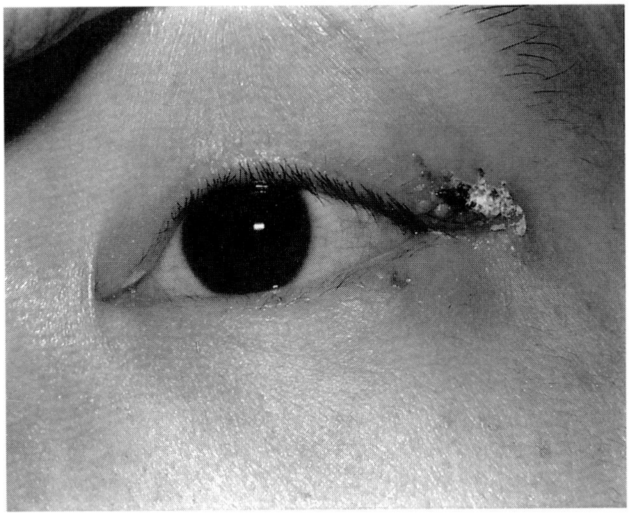

Figure 30-6. Herpes simplex eyelid infection.

simplex type 1 is commoner than type 2, although both occur.

Herpes zoster may involve either or both eyelids, depending on the involvement of the ophthalmic and maxillary divisions of the fifth cranial nerve. The vesicles are usually associated with significant pain. Eyelid involvement may result in scarring, cicatricial ectropion, eyelid retraction with lagophthalmos, trichiasis, or damage to the meibomian glands.[109]

Disseminated herpes zoster occurs mainly in immunocompromised patients. In patients with this condition, further medical evaluation for human immunodeficiency virus infection, occult lymphoma, or leukemia is indicated.[110]

The diagnosis of herpes simplex or zoster is usually on clinical grounds. When the diagnosis is not evident, such as in zosteriform herpes simplex, viral cultures, serologic testing, antigen detection, and colloidal gold immunoelectron microscopy may be used.[109]

Treatment of herpes simplex of the eyelid is primarily supportive and consists of preventing secondary bacterial infection by hygiene and possibly topical antibiotics. Application of topical 5-iodo-2′-deoxyuridine (IDU) may shorten the duration of the skin lesions. Both IDU and vidarabine ointment are recommended for the prevention of secondary keratitis when the eyelid margin is involved. The maximum duration of treatment should be 2 to 3 weeks to avoid medicamentosa.[85] Oral acyclovir therapy may be necessary for severe infections.

Acyclovir is the mainstay of treatment for herpes zoster. Ideally, it is started within 72 hours of the appearance of vesicles. In the absence of disseminated disease or in immunocompromised states, oral acyclovir may be given for 10 days. If intraocular involvement occurs, topical corticosteroid therapy is indicated. Topical antiviral agents may hasten healing. The role of systemic cortico-

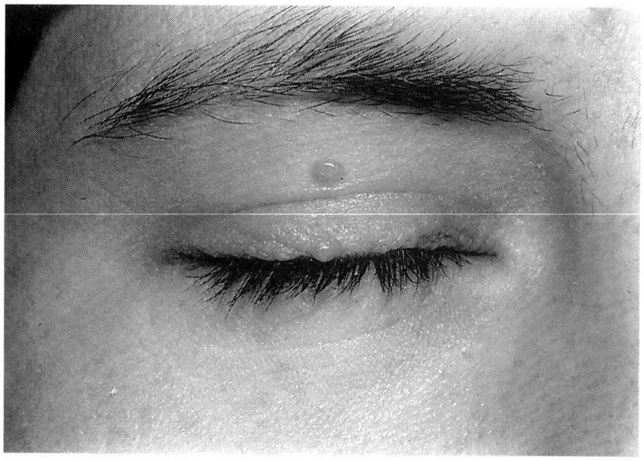

Figure 30–7. Molluscum contagiosum.

steroids and prophylaxis regimens against postherpetic neuralgia remains controversial.[109, 110]

Members of the *Poxviridae* family that rarely affect the ocular adnexa include molluscum contagiosum, smallpox, smallpox vaccine, cowpox, and orf. Molluscum contagiosum causes umbilicated lesions that affect the skin (Fig. 30–7). When the lesions occur at the eyelid margin, viral particles are shed into the conjunctival cul de sac and cause a follicular conjunctivitis and keratitis. Modes of transmission include sexual contact, direct contact, and possibly contact with fomites. The diagnosis is confirmed by histologic section.[85] Excision of the lesion or cryotherapy is curative.

Both smallpox and the vaccine against it have eyelid manifestations. Smallpox, or variola, causes a rash that may affect the eyelids. Secondary infection may cause gangrene. Involvement of the eyelid margins has been reported to cause trichiasis, madarosis, and ectropion.[2] Ocular vaccinia occurs after administration of the smallpox vaccine; it causes severe eyelid swelling with vesicles, scarring, and madarosis, as well as conjunctival ulceration and corneal involvement.[111, 112] Cowpox and orf (contagious ecthyma, or contagious pustular dermatitis) cause a painless ulcerated lesion associated with regional lymphadenopathy and a follicular conjunctivitis.[113, 114] Patients with orf usually have a history of exposure to farm animals, particularly sheep. Cultures and scrapings may be diagnostic for vaccinia and cowpox. Orf is difficult to diagnose and may require assessment by electron microscopy. Idoxuridine may be of benefit in orf and vaccinia.[112, 115] Its use has not been evaluated in ocular cowpox.

Papillomaviruses cause warts, which may be present on the eyelid and the conjunctiva. Transmission is probably by contact with fomites, direct contact, or autoinoculation. There is a worldwide distribution of papillomaviruses, but they are less common in the tropics.[113] Often, these lesions are self-limited; therefore, observation is usually the preferred method of management. Surgical excision or cryotherapy may be implemented for cosmesis or to ameliorate associated keratitis or conjunctivitis.[85]

Dengue viruses are transmitted by mosquitos in Asia, Africa, India, and Latin America. Dengue fever is a febrile illness characterized by a macular rash, gastrointestinal complaints, myalgias, and dengue facies. Dengue facies consists of edematous eyelids, suffusion of conjunctival capillaries, and flushing of the face. A retroorbital headache and pain on eye movement may also occur,[116] as may a dengue hemorrhagic fever. The diagnosis is mainly based on clinical findings. Acute and convalescent titers may be obtained.[46] The treatment is supportive.

PARASITIC INFECTIONS

Parasitic infections uncommonly involve the eyelid; however, infections with protozoans, helminths, and insect larvae have been reported.

Protozoan infections of the periorbita include leishmaniasis, trypanosomiasis, and cutaneous amebiasis. These infections may be associated with painless eyelid masses, edema, ectropion, or necrotic lesions (see Tables 30–1 through 30–3, 30–6). Leishmaniasis occurs in central Asia, Africa, the Middle East, and Central and South America. It is transmitted by a sandfly. Both a cutaneous and a visceral form of leishmaniasis exist. Several species of *Leishmania* are generally limited to the Americas (American leishmaniasis) or Asia and Africa (Old World leishmaniasis). The typical lesion, called the oriental sore in Old World leishmaniasis, is a painless papule that lacks lymphadenopathy. It is often present on the face and occasionally involves the eyelid.[117–119] The lesion evolves into a central ulcer with surrounding satellite subcutaneous nodules.[120, 121] After several months, a depressed scar forms, which may cause ectropion. A similar lesion occurs in American leishmaniasis.[122] Skin smears from the nonulcerated portion of the lesion demonstrate the organism. The diagnosis may be ascertained by tissue culture, biopsy, or the Montenegro intradermal test.[122] Cutaneous leishmaniasis occurring in the absence of mucosal disease often resolves spontaneously and is therefore not treated. However, when the eyelid is involved, treatment may prevent cicatricial changes. The mainstay of treatment is pentavalent antimony administered intravenously or intramuscularly.[123]

Trypanosoma cruzi, which causes Chagas' disease, is another protozoan that may affect the eyelid. This disease is found primarily in Central and South America and is transmitted by the kissing, or reduviid, bug. The primary lesion of Chagas' disease is an erythematous nodule, the inoculation chagoma. It often occurs in the face, including the eyelids, and is accompanied by eyelid swelling and regional lymphadenopathy. Romaña's sign, a rare but diagnostic sign, is characterized by painless edema of the periorbita. It is the classic sign of acute Chagas' disease and occurs when the infection begins in the conjunctiva.[124] Conjunctivitis, fever, and rash may occur. Blood smears and cultures may be positive. The treatment of choice is administration of nifurtimox or benzonidazole.[85, 124]

The causative organism of cutaneous amebiasis is *Entamoeba histolytica*. This protozoan infection is highly endemic in Central and South America, India, and West and South Africa. Amebiasis is contracted through fecal-to-oral contamination. Manifestations of the syndrome range from asymptomatic cyst carrier to colitis. Abscesses of the lung and liver may also be present,[125] and eyelid ulceration and necrosis may occur.[126] The diagnosis is made by histologic wet smears of tissue from the ulcer's edge that demonstrate mobile amebae.[122] Treatment strategies depend on involvement of other organ systems.[48]

Helminthic infections also involve the eyelid. They may present as migratory cystic or painless masses, subconjunctival involvement, or eyelid edema (see Tables 30-1, 30-2, and 30-4). Nematodes, cestodes, and trematodes have all been reported.

Nematodes affecting the periorbita include *Loa loa, Onchocerca volvulus, Wuchereria bancrofti, Brugia malayi, Brugia timori, Trichinella spiralis, Dirofilaria* sp., and *Dracunculus medinensis.*

L. loa, the eye worm, occurs in rain forests in central and West Africa. The vector is a tabanid fly, of the genus *Chrysops*.[127] Classically, the adult worm travels through subcutaneous tissues, eventually migrating subconjunctivally.[128] Another manifestation is a hypersensitivity reaction in persons with microfilaremia. Areas of nonpitting edema and erythema referred to as *calabar swellings* develop.[129, 130] Pruritus is characteristic. Diagnosis can be made by biopsy of the calabar swelling, the presence of peripheral eosinophilia, and positive blood smear for microfilaria. The worm should be removed from the conjunctiva. Systemic therapy includes diethylcarbamazine administration.[131]

O. volvulus, the cause of "river blindness," is predominantly seen in West Africa as well as in isolated regions of the Arabian peninsula and Central and South America. It is a leading cause of blindness.[132] It is transmitted by the blackfly, which requires rapid running water for breeding. The characteristic findings include lymphadenitis, dermatitis, subcutaneous nodules, called *onchocercomata*, and intraocular involvement.[133] The ocular manifestations include chorioretinitis as well as optic nerve involvement, iritis, glaucoma, and keratitis. The microfilaria spread subcutaneously from the site of inoculation at the insect bite.

Onchocercomata develop and may be found in the eyelid.[85] The causative organism may be recovered from a biopsy of the subcutaneous nodules. Treatment includes ivermectin administration and nodule excision. Diethylcarbamazine and suramin are alternative therapies.[48, 85, 131]

Other nematodes, *W. bancrofti, B. malayi*, and *B. timori*, are transmitted by mosquitos and are typically found in the tropics and subtropics. The classic lesion is chronic edema and elephantiasis of the lower extremities that results from lymphatic obstruction associated with a recurrent fever.[131] These organisms uncommonly cause significant eyelid edema secondary to destruction of facial lymphatics.[85] The diagnosis can be made on clinical grounds, thick blood smears, or lymph node biopsy.[122] The treatment of choice for these nematodes is ivermectin administration.[48]

T. spiralis infects humans as an incidental host when raw or incompletely cooked pork is ingested. It occurs in most parts of the world. Trichinosis has caused periorbital edema in 57% to 100% of reported cases.[134, 135] Other clinical findings include abdominal discomfort, fever, myalgias, subconjunctival hemorrhages, and headaches.[134] The diagnosis can be confirmed by antibody testing or deltoid muscle biopsy.[122] Treatment of the acute disease is thiabendazole administration.[48, 122, 134]

Dirofilaria species, a parasite of dogs and cats, classically causes either pulmonary or subcutaneous lesions in humans. These parasites may be found in Asia, Europe, and the United States. Dirofilariasis may present as a subcutaneous or subconjunctival eyelid mass with local swelling, pain, and irritation.[136, 137] The diagnosis is made by surgical excision of the cyst and worm.

A cystic mass mimicking a periorbital dermoid cyst may also occur with *D. medinensis*, the guinea worm.[138] This nematode proliferates in stagnant water, particularly in Africa, India, and the Middle East. Classically, the worm extrudes out of a lower extremity and must be removed by winding it on a stick. The cutaneous lesion is a blister with intense inflammation and a sinus tract. The diagnosis is made on clinical grounds. Treatment consists of cyst resection and worm removal.[138] Metronidazole or thiabendazole therapy decreases the inflammation related to *Dracunculus* infection and facilitates removal.[131]

Other roundworms that have been implicated in eyelid swelling include *Ascaris lumbricoides, Enterobius vermicularis, Ancylostoma duodenale, Necator americanus*, and *Gnathostoma spinigerum*.[85, 139] The treatment of choice for these roundworms is either mebendazole or pyrantel pamoate therapy, and surgical removal is indicated for *G. spinigerum*.[48, 140, 141]

Cestodes isolated from the eyelid include *Taenia solium, Diphyllobothrium* species, and *Echinococcus granulosus*. Cysticercosis is the cyst stage of *T. solium*. It is transmitted in pig feces, and humans are accidental hosts. It is common in Mexico, Latin America, India, Asia, Africa, and Europe[122] and is uncommon in the United States. Ocular cysticercosis occurs in about 20% of neurocysticercosis cases.[142] In 134 cases of ocular and periocular cysticercosis, more than 100 cases had extraocular, primarily subconjunctival, involvement.[143] The eyelid and orbit are uncommonly involved.[143, 144] Intraocular involvement is most often subretinal or in the vitreous. The painless cystic lesions of cysticercosis may be confused with noninfectious cysts, such as dermoids, unless the diagnosis is suspected and followed by cyst removal and pathologic examination.[122, 145–147] If the cyst cannot be surgically removed, praziquantel may be used. However, this agent should not be used in patients with intraocular involvement without corticosteroids to suppress the inflammatory response related to the worms' death.[142]

Sparganum mansoni is the second stage larva of *Diphyllobothrium* sp. and is found the United States and Asia.[142] Sparganosis affects humans after exposure to contaminated water or poultices of frog skin.[85] Classically, the larvae migrate subcutaneously, where they become encapsulated nodules that form abscesses.[148] A nodule firmly adherent to the eyelid skin may occur, but orbital involvement is commoner.[2] Surgical excision is the treatment of choice,[48, 85, 142] but niclosamide or praziquantel may be used.[140]

E. granulosa, the dog tapeworm, is common in Australia, New Zealand, South America, Africa, and the Middle East. Sheep and cattle act as intermediate hosts. The typical lesion is a cystic mass, which rarely occurs in the eyelid. Orbital involvement may also occur. Unlike cysticercosis, if echinococcal cysts rupture, additional cysts will form; therefore, careful excision is imperative. Cyst injection with formalin or absolute ethanol may prevent spread if cyst rupture occurs.[85] For recurrent disease, albendazole administration may be indicated.[85, 149]

Schistosomiasis of the eyelid is rare. Five species of *Schistosoma* exist, each with a specific geographic distribution, including Africa, Asia, South America, and the Middle East.[150] The infection is acquired from freshwater snails. The typical lesion is a dermatitis in the acute stage. In chronic stages, intestinal, urinary tract, and hepatic involvement predominate.[150] Schistosomiasis may cause eyelid edema and dacryoadenitis.[2, 85] Praziquantel is the recommended treatment.[48, 140, 150]

Inflammation of the eyelid may also result from parasitic arthropods, such as fly larvae and ticks.[151–156] Uncommon in the United States, ophthalmomyiasis is caused by fly larvae. Three forms of this disease exists: external, internal, and orbital. The external form presents like a cellulitis in the eyelid and conjunctiva, with localized erythema and swelling.[151–155] A draining sinus may also develop.[155] Patients with gonococcal conjunctivitis or ulcerative skin carcinomas are predisposed to this form.[134, 151] Treatment of external ophthalmomyiasis consists of removal of the organisms.

FUNGAL INFECTIONS

Fungal infections of the eyelid usually involve the lash margin; other areas of the periorbita are affected less commonly. The spectrum of disorders and organisms causing eyelid involvement includes superficial mycotic infections, *Cryptococcus*, infections secondary to hematogenous spread, and local extension from adjacent structures.

Superficial mycotic infections affecting the eyelid include *Candida* sp. and dermatophytes. *Candida albicans* infections of the face may cause eyelid granulomas.[157] Candidal infections usually occur in children and in debilitated adults. The diagnosis is confirmed by culture. Topical antifungal agents may be effective for isolated lesions. Dermatophyte infections, or ringworm fungi, present as vesicular eruptions and pustules on an erythematous base and spread as plaques affecting the eyelids or lashes. The infection may be self-limited.[158] The type of topical antifungal agent used is dictated by the type of primary infection present.[48]

C. neoformans has worldwide distribution. A cutaneous lesion of this origin may either be an isolated primary infection or part of the disseminated disease.[120] Disseminated cryptococcal infection typically occurs in an immunocompromised host. The classic lesions are papules, pustules, ulcers, subcutaneous abscesses, or nodules. A central area of ulceration may also be present, but regional lymphadenopathy is absent. Approximately 10% to 15% of cases have cutaneous involvement.[120]

Several fungal infections with primary pulmonary involvement including blastomycosis, paracoccidioidomycosis, and coccidioidomycosis, may affect the eyelids by hematogenous spread. Blastomycosis, which is caused by infection with *Blastomyces dermatitidis*, is a pulmonary infection of farmers in the southeastern United States. It is also found in Africa.[159] Eyelid involvement occurs in up to 25% of patients.[160] Two types of skin lesions exist: verrucous and ulcerative. In the verrucous type, a small papule develops a verrucous mass, which exhibits central healing. In the ulcerative type, a pustule may form that rapidly becomes ulcerative. Both types have serpiginous elevated borders.[160] Multiple black dots, representing extravasation of red cells into the dermis, may be seen at the borders.[161] Severe cicatricial ectropion requiring surgical repair may result.[157, 162–164]

Paracoccidioidomycosis is the more aggressive South American version of blastomycosis. It is a mutilating disease that primarily affects the lungs and is associated with prolonged exposure to soil. Of 44 reported cases, 35 affected the eyelid.[165] The lesion begins as a papule, which may mimic ulcerative blepharitis or a hordeolum, that progresses to central ulceration. Ultimately, an eyelid coloboma and madarosis may result.[165, 166] Uveitis may also occur.[165]

Unlike both blastomycosis and paracoccidioidomycosis, coccidioidomycosis rarely affects the eye. Coccidioidomycosis, which results from infection with *Coccidioides immitis*, primarily occurs in the deserts of the southwestern United States and South America.[159] Ocular involvement includes conjunctivitis, scleritis, and uveitis. Two manifestations of this disease occur in the eyelid, a granulomatous tubercular lesion with central ulceration and local tissue destruction and eyelid edema.

Regional lymphadenopathy is characteristic of the disease.[167, 168]

The diagnosis for blastomycosis, paracoccidioidomycosis, and coccidioidomycosis is based on the combination of clinical findings, including lung involvement, and cultures and smears of characteristic lesions. Serologic studies are also helpful for diagnosing coccidioidomycosis. The treatment for these diseases is usually ketoconazole or amphotericin B administration.[48, 140]

Sporotrichosis is caused by *Sporotrichum schenkii.* It typically occurs in people who handle dirt and plant products, especially mine workers and rosebush enthusiasts. The organism exists throughout most of the world.[159] The commonest type is a cutaneous form characterized by a painless papule with ulceration that develops along a chain of lymphatics. Plaque-like lesions then develop. Sporotrichosis rarely affects the eyelids and may invade the orbit secondarily.[2, 157, 169] It may be misdiagnosed as a chalazion.[169] The diagnosis is made by the classic cutaneous manifestations. Serologic testing and cultures are helpful in difficult cases.[170] Therapy of the cutaneous manifestations consists of potassium iodide and heat.[171, 172]

Fungal infections of the eyelid may also occur as isolated disease or from direct extension from the paranasal sinuses. A case report was published of isolated ulcerative granulomas of the eyelid due to aspergillosis.[173] The diagnosis was obtained through culture and histologic examination of scrapings. The lesion resolved with injection of amphotericin B directly into the granuloma.[173]

Rhinosporidiosis, which is caused by infection with *Rhinosporidium seeberi*, is classically a friable polypoid mass of the nose or conjunctiva. It is prevalent in India and Sri Lanka, but several cases have been reported in the United States.[174] A case report of rhinosporidiosis causing massive lower eyelid swelling was published in the literature. The diagnosis was made by observation of sporangia in the biopsy specimen. The treatment is surgical excision.[85, 174, 175]

SUMMARY

Inflammatory lesions of the eyelid may be both infectious and noninfectious. Common entities include meibomitis, chalazia, cellulitis, and herpetic disease. Less common entities include bacteria-induced necrosis of the eyelid, other viruses, and parasitic and fungal diseases. For atypical or recurrent lesions, culture and biopsy should be performed. A history of foreign travel might suggest alternate diagnoses, including unusual fungal or parasitic infections.

REFERENCES

1. McCulley JP: Meibomitis. *In* Kaufman HE, Barron BA, McDonald MB, Waltman SR (eds): The Cornea. New York, Churchill Livingstone, 1988.
2. Duke-Elder S, MacFaul PA: The ocular adnexa. *In* Duke-Elder S (ed): System of Ophthalmology, Volume XIII, Part I, Deep Inflammations of the Lids. St. Louis, CV Mosby, 1974, pp 241–250.
3. Freinkel RK, Strauss JS, Yip SY, Pochi PE: Effect of tetracycline on the composition of sebum in acne vulgaris. N Engl J Med 273:850–854, 1965.
4. Lempert SL, Jenkins MS. Brown SI: Chalazia and rosacea. Arch Ophthalmol 97:1652–1653, 1979.
5. Epstein GA: Chalazia and hordeola. *In* Lindberg JV (ed): Oculoplastic and Orbital Emergencies. Norwalk, CT, Appleton & Lange, 1990, pp 67–75.
6. Ormond AW: Notes on three cases of acquired astigmatism associated with meibomian cysts. Br J Ophthalmol 5:117–118, 1921.
7. Bohigian GM: Chalazion: A clinical evaluation. Ann Ophthalmol 11:1397–1398, 1979.
8. Perry HD, Serniuk RA: Conservative treatment of chalazia. Ophthalmology 87:218–221, 1980.
9. Cottrell DG, Bosanquet RC, Fawcett IM: Chalazions: The frequency of spontaneous resolution. BMJ 287:1595, 1983.
10. Goldberg RA, Shorr N: "Vertical slat" chalazion excision. Ophthalmic Surg 23:120–122, 1992.
11. Reifler DM, Leder DR: Eyelid crease approach for chalazion excision. Ophthal Plast Reconstr Surg 5:63–67, 1989.
12. Korn EL: Laser chalazion removal. Ophthalmic Surg 19:428–431, 1988.
13. Epstein GA, Putterman AM: Combined excision and drainage with intralesional corticosteroid injection in the treatment of chronic chalazia. Arch Ophthalmol 106:514–516, 1988.
14. Pizzarello LD, Jakobiec FA, Hofeldt AJ, et al: Intralesional corticosteroid therapy of chalazia. Am J Ophthalmol 85:818–821, 1978.
15. Garrett GW, Gillespie ME, Mannix BC: Adrenocorticosteroid injection vs. conservative therapy in the treatment of chalazia. Ann Ophthalmol 20:196–198, 1988.
16. Mohan K, Dhir SP, Munjal VP, Jain IS: The use of intralesional steroids in the treatment of chalazion. Ann Ophthalmol 18: 158–160, 1986.
17. Sloas HA, Starling J, Galentine PG, Hargett NA: Treatment of chalazia with injectable triamcinolone. Ann Ophthalmol 15:78–80, 1983.
18. King RA, Ellis PP: Treatment of chalazia with corticosteroid injections. Ophthalmic Surg 17:351–353, 1986.
19. Watson AP, Austin DJ: Treatment of chalazions with injection of a steroid suspension. Br J Ophthalmol 68:833–835, 1984.
20. Jacobs PM, Thaller VT, Wong D: Intralesional corticosteroid therapy of chalazia: A comparison with incision and curettage. Br J Ophthalmol 68:836–837, 1984.
21. Palva J, Pohjanpelto PEJ: Intralesional corticosteroid injection for the treatment of chalazia. Acta Ophthalmol (Copenh) 61:933–937, 1983.
22. Castren J, Stenborg T: Corticosteroid injection of chalazia. Acta Ophthalmol (Copenh) 61:938–942, 1983.
23. Smythe D, Hurwitz JJ, Tayfour F: The management of chalazion: A survey of Ontario ophthalmologists. Can J Ophthalmol 25: 252–255, 1990.
24. Thomas EL, Laborde RP: Retinal and choroidal vascular occlusion following intralesional corticosteroid injection of a chalazion. Ophthalmology 93:405–407, 1986.
25. Boniuk M, Zimmerman LE: Sebaceous carcinoma of the eyelid, eyebrow, caruncle and orbit. Trans Am Acad Ophthalmol Otolaryngol 72:619–642, 1968.
26. Doxanas MT, Green WR: Sebaceous gland carcinoma: Review of 40 cases. Arch Ophthalmol 102:245–249, 1984.
27. Sweebe EC, Cogan DG: Adenocarcinoma of the meibomian gland. Arch Ophthalmol 61:282–290, 1959.
28. Harvey JT, Anderson RL: The management of meibomian gland carcinoma. Ophthalmic Surg 13:56–61, 1982.
29. Kluka E, David SK, Lyons GD: Meibomian gland adenocarcinoma of the eyelid metastasizing to parotid lymph nodes. Ear Nose Throat 70:502–504, 1991.
30. Khan JA, Grove AS, Joseph MP, Goodman M: Sebaceous carcinoma: Diuretic use, lacrimal system spread, and surgical margins. Ophthal Plast Reconstr Surg 5:227–234, 1989.
31. Cavanagh HD, Green WR, Goldberg HK: Multicentric sebaceous adenocarcinoma of the meibomian gland. Am J Ophthalmol 77:326–332, 1974.

32. Mamalis N, Medlock RD, Holds JB, et al: Merkel cell tumor of the eyelid: A review and report of an unusual case. Ophthalmic Surg 20:410–414, 1989.
33. Mansour AM, Hidayat AA: Metastatic eyelid disease. Ophthalmology 94:667–670, 1987.
34. de Keizer RJW, Scheffer E: Masquerade of eyelid tumours. Doc Ophthalmol 72:309–321, 1989.
35. Roper JP, Jones T, Common JDA: Desmoplastic malignant melanoma masquerading as chalazion. Br J Ophthalmol 70:907–910, 1986.
36. Brower MF, Levine RA, Boyer KM: Preseptal cellulitis complicated by toxic shock syndrome. Arch Ophthalmol 105:1631–1632, 1987.
37. Gonnering RS, Harris GJ: Infections of the orbit. *In* Tabbara KF, Hyndiuk RA (eds): Infections of the Eye. Boston, Little, Brown & Company, 1986, pp 517–541.
38. Molarte AB, Isenberg SJ: Periorbital cellulitis in infancy. J Pediatr Ophthalmol Strabismus 26:232–234, 1989.
39. Jones DB, Steinkuller PG: Microbial preseptal and orbital cellulitis. *In* Tasman W, Jaeger EA (eds): Duane's Clinical Ophthalmology, Vol 4. Philadelphia, JB Lippincott, 1991, pp 1–24.
40. Marcy SM, Klein JO: Focal bacterial infections. *In* Remington JS, Klein JO (eds): Infectious Diseases of the Fetus and Newborn Infant. Philadelphia, WB Saunders, 1990, pp 801–809.
41. Baker RC, Bausher JC: Meningitis complicating acute bacteremic facial cellulitis. Pediatr Infect Dis J 5:421–423, 1986.
42. Siegel JD: Diagnosis and management of acute sinusitis in children. Pediatr Infect Dis J 6:95–99, 1987.
43. Jones DB, Steinkuller PG: Strategies for the initial management of acute preseptal and orbital cellulitis. Trans Am Ophthalmol Soc 86:94–112, 1988.
44. Blumer JL, Lemon E, O'Horo J, Snodgrass DJ: Changing therapy for skin and soft tissue infections in children: Have we come full circle? Pediatr Infect Dis J 6:117–122, 1987.
45. Swartz MN: Cellulitis and superficial infectons. *In* Mandell GL, Douglas RG, Bennett JE (eds): Principles and Practice of Infectious Diseases, 3rd ed. New York, Churchill Livingstone, 1990, pp 796–807.
46. Roberts SOB, Highet AS: Bacterial infections. *In* Rook A, Wilkinson DS, Ebling FJG, et al (eds): Textbook of Dermatology. Boston, Blackwell Scientific Publications, 1986, pp 725–790.
47. Jones DB, Robinson NM: Anaerobic ocular infections. Trans Am Acad Ophthalmol Otolaryngol 83:309–331, 1977.
48. Sanford JP: Guide to Antimicrobial Therapy. West Bethesda, MD, 1991.
49. Schlossberg D: Cellulitis and soft tissue infection. *In* Kass EH, Platt R (eds): Current Therapy in Infectious Disease, 3rd ed. Philadelphia, BC Decker, 1990, pp 229–231.
50. Bullock JD: Orbital infections in the immunocompromised patient. Ophthal Plast Reconst Surg 2:189–196, 1986.
51. Westfall CT, Shore JW: Isolated fractures of the orbital floor: Risk of infection and the role of antibiotic prophylaxis. Ophthalmic Surg 22:409–411, 1991.
52. Weber DJ, Wolfson JS, Swartz MN, Hooper DC: *Pasteurella multocida* infections. Medicine 63:133–154, 1984.
53. McGowan JE, del Rio C: Other gram-negative bacilli. *In* Mandell GL, Douglas RG, Bennett JE (eds): Principles and Practice of Infectious Diseases, 3rd ed. New York, Churchill Livingstone, 1990.
54. Carpenter CCJ: Other pathogenic vibrios. *In* Mandell GL, Douglas, RG, Bennett JE (eds): Principles and Practice of Infectious Diseases, 3rd ed. New York, Churchill Livingstone, 1990, pp 1646–1648.
55. Feldman RB, Stern GA, Hood I: *Chromobacterium violaceum* infection of the eye. Arch Ophthalmol 102:711–713, 1984.
56. Simo F, Reuman PD, Martinez FJ, Ayoub EM: *Chromobacterium violaceum* as a cause of periorbital cellulitis. Pediatr Infect Dis J 3:561–563, 1984.
57. Moscona R, Ullmann Y, Peled I: Necrotizing periorbital cellulitis following septorhinoplasty. Aesthetic Plast Surg 15:187–190, 1991.
58. Weiss A, Friendly D, Eglin K, et al: Bacterial periorbital and orbital cellulitis in childhood. Ophthalmology 90:195–203, 1983.
59. The choice of antibacterial drugs. Med Lett Drugs Ther 34(871): 49–56, 1992.
60. Rubin SE, Slavin ML, Rubin LG: Eyelid swelling and erythema as the only signs of subperiosteal abscess. Br J Ophthalmol 73:576–578, 1989.
61. Grossniklaus HE, Wojno TH: Leukemic infiltrate appearing as periorbital cellulitis. Arch Ophthalmol 108:484, 1990.
62. Jones WE: Some special skin tumours in the elderly. Br J Dermatol 122:71–75, 1990.
63. Lyon DB, Lemke BN: Eyelid gas gangrene. Ophthal Plast Reconstr Surg 5:212–215, 1989.
64. Mortada A: Post-operative gangrene of eyelid. Br J Ophthalmol 48:114–117, 1964.
65. Edwards JJ, Anderson RL, Wood JR: Loxoscelism of the eyelids. Arch Ophthalmol 98:1997–2000, 1980.
66. Ross J, Kohlhepp PA: Gangrene of the eyelids. Ann Ophthalmol 5:84–88, 1973.
67. Rosenthal WN, Gore HL, Insler MS: Periorbital necrotizing fasciitis. Ann Ophthalmol 19:426–427, 1987.
68. Parunovic A: *Proteus mirabilis* causing necrotic inflammation of the eyelid. Am J Ophthalmol 76:543–544, 1973.
69. Prendiville KJ, Bath PE: Lateral cantholysis and eyelid necrosis secondary to *Pseudomonas aeruginosa*. Ann Ophthalmol 20: 193–195, 1988.
70. Woog JJ, Lemke BN, Dortzbach RK: Eyelid necrosis in an anophthalmic patient. Ophthalmic Surg 17:499–501, 1986.
71. Einarsson OJ, Pers M: Streptococcal gangrene of the eyelids. Scand J Plast Reconstr Surg 20:331–335, 1986.
72. Steinkogler FJ, Huber-Spitzy V: Necrotizing destruction of the ocular adnexa by *Pseudomonas aeruginosa*. J Craniomaxillofac Surg 16:28–30, 1988.
73. Cohn I, Bornside GH: Infections. *In* Schwartz SI (ed): Principles of Surgery. New York, McGraw-Hill, 1983, pp 165–198.
74. Kronish JW, McLeish WM: Eyelid necrosis and periorbital necrotizing fasciitis. Ophthalmology 98:92–98, 1990.
75. Doorenbos-bot ACC, Hooymans JMM, Blanksma LJ: Periorbital necrotising fasciitis due to *Cryptococcus neoformans* in a healthy young man. Doc Ophthalmol 75:315–320, 1990.
76. Simmons RL, Ahrenholtz DH: Infections of the skin and soft tissues. *In* Howard RJ, Simmons RL (eds): Surgical Infectious Diseases, Norwalk, CT, Appleton & Lange, 1988, pp 377–442.
77. Dellinger EP: Crepitus and gangrene. *In* Kass EH, Platt R (eds): Current Therapy in Infectious Disease, 3rd ed. Philadelphia, BC Decker, 1990, pp 232–235.
78. Swartz MN: Subcutaneous tissue infections and abscesses. *In* Mandell GL, Douglas RG, Bennett JE (eds): Principles and Practice of Infectious Diseases, 3rd ed. New York, Churchill Livingstone, 1990, pp 808–812.
79. Treister G, Frankl O, Cohen S, Stein R: Metastatic gangrene of the lid in *Pseudomonas* septicemia. Ann Ophthalmol 7:639–641, 1975.
80. Sanford JP: *Pseudomonas* infections: Glanders and melioidosis. *In* Strickland GT (ed): Hunter's Tropical Medicine, 7th ed. Philadelphia, WB Saunders, 1991, pp 450–451.
81. Brachman PS: Anthrax. *In* Warren KS, Mahmoud AAF (eds): Tropical and Geographical Medicine. New York, McGraw-Hill Information Services Company, 1990, pp 877–880.
82. Barnshaw HD, Lovett JC: Anthrax of the eye. Am J Ophthalmol 32:106–110, 1949.
83. Barnard NAS. Anthrax of the eyelid. Ophthalmic Physiol Opt 10:300–301, 1990.
84. Velimirovic B: Anthrax. *In* Kass EH, Platt R (eds): Current Therapy in Infectious Disease, 3rd ed. Philadelphia: BC Decker, 1990, pp 318–321.
85. Starr MB. Infections and hypersensitivity of the eyelids. *In* Della Rocca RC, Nesi FA, Lisman RD (eds): Ophthalmic Plastic and Reconstructive Surgery. St. Louis, CV Mosby, 1987.
86. Zeligowski AA, Peled IJ, Wexler MR: Eyelid necrosis after spider bite. Am J Ophthalmol 101:254–255, 1986.
87. Burnett JW, Calton GH, Morgan RJ: Brown recluse spider. Cutis 36:197–198, 1985.
88. Rossignol PA, Feinsod FM: Arthropods directly causing human injury. *In* Warren KS, Mahmoud AAF (eds): Tropical and Geographical Medicine. New York, McGraw-Hill Information Services Company, 1990, pp 519–532.
89. West BC: Leprosy. *In* Kass EH, Platt R (eds): Current Therapy in Infectious Disease, 3rd ed. Philadelphia, BC Decker, 1990, pp 322–325.

90. Shields JA, Waring GO, Monte LG: Ocular findings in leprosy. Am J Ophthalmol 77:880–890, 1974.
91. Choyce DP: Diagnosis and management of ocular leprosy. Br J Ophthalmol 53:217–223, 1969.
92. Schwab IR: Ocular leprosy. *In* Tabbara KF, Hyndiuk RA (eds): Infections of the Eye. Boston, Little, Brown & Company, 1986, pp 613–624.
93. Katowitz JA, Kropp TM: *Mycobacterium fortuitum* as a cause for nasolacrimal obstruction and granulomatous eyelid disease. Ophthalmic Surg 18:97–99, 1987.
94. Kevitch R, Guyuron B: Mycobacterial infection following blepharoplasty. Aesthetic Plast Surg 15:229–232, 1991.
95. Sandford JP: Tularemia. *In* Strickland GT (ed): Hunter's Tropical Medicine. Philadelphia, WB Saunders, 1991, pp 416–417.
96. Jeyakumar W, Chithra A, Shanmugasundararaj A: Primary syphilis of the eyelid: Case report. Genitourin Med 65:192–193, 1989.
97. Hopkins DR: Nonvenereal treponematoses. *In* Kass EH, Platt R, (eds): Current Therapy in Infectious Disease, 3rd ed. Philadelphia, BC Decker, 1990, pp 376–377.
98. Hopkins DR, Perine PL: Yaws, nonvenereal treponematoses. *In* Warren KS, Mahmoud AAF (eds): Tropical and Geographical Medicine. New York, McGraw-Hill Information Services Company, 1990, pp 910–913.
99. Butler T: Plague. *In* Strickland GT (ed): Hunter's Tropical Medicine. Philadelphia, WB Saunders, 1991, pp 408–416.
100. Wignall FS: Bartonellosis. *In* Strickland GT (ed): Hunter's Tropical Medicine. Philadelphia, WB Saunders, 1991, pp 426–429.
101. Mackenzie DWR, Hay RJ: Actinomycosis. *In* Strickland GT (ed): Hunter's Tropical Medicine. Philadelphia, WB Saunders, 1991, pp 457–458.
102. Kerdel-Vegas F: Rhinoscleroma. *In* Rook A, Wilkinson DS, Ebling FJG, et al (eds): Textbook of Dermatology. Boston, Blackwell Scientific Publications, 1986, pp 766–769.
103. Nasr AM: Eyelid complications in trachoma. Acta Ophthalmol (Copenh) 69:200–204, 1991.
104. Bowie WR, Holmes KK: *Chlamydia trachomatis* (trachoma, perinatal infections, lymphogranuloma venereum and other genital infections). *In* Mandell GL, Douglas RG, Bennett JE, (eds): Principles and Practice of Infectious Diseases, 3rd ed. New York, Churchill Livingstone, 1990, pp 1426–1439.
105. Kuo C, Grayston JR: Chlamydia. *In* Warren KS, Mahmoud AAF (eds): Tropical and Geographical Medicine. New York, McGraw-Hill Information Services Company, 1990, pp 644–660.
106. Dawson CR, Togni B: Herpes simplex eye infections: Clinical manifestations, pathogenesis and management. Survey Ophthalmol 21:121–135, 1976.
107. Hyndiuk RA, Glasser DB: Herpes simplex keratitis. *In* Tabbara KF, Hyndiuk RA (eds): Infections of the Eye. Boston, Little, Brown & Company, 1986, pp 517–541.
108. Nauheim JS, Sussman W: Herpes simplex of the lids and adjacent areas. Trans Am Acad Ophthalmol Otolaryngol 75:1236–1241, 1971.
109. Liesegang TJ: Diagnosis and therapy of herpes zoster. Ophthalmology 98:1216–1229, 1991.
110. Dolin R, Reichman RC, Mazur MH, Whitley RJ: Herpes zoster-varicella infections in immunosuppressed patients. Ann Intern Med 89:375–388, 1978.
111. Ruben FL, Lane JM: Ocular vaccinia. Arch Ophthalmol 84:45–48, 1970.
112. Rennie AGR, Cant JS, Foulds WS: Ocular vaccinia. Lancet ii:273–275, 1974.
113. Nagington J, Rook A, Highet AS: Virus and related infections. *In* Rook A, Wilkinson DS, Ebling FJG, et al (eds): Textbook of Dermatology. Boston, Blackwell Scientific Publications, 1986, pp 668–697.
114. Freeman G, Bron AJ, Juel-Jensen B: Ocular infection with orf virus. Am J Ophthalmol 97:601–604, 1984.
115. Hall CJ, Stevens JD: Ocular cowpox. Lancet i:111, 1987.
116. Halstead SB: Dengue. *In* Warren KS, Mahmoud AAF (eds): Tropical and Geographical Medicine. New York, McGraw-Hill Information Services Company, 1990, pp 675–684.
117. O'Neill DPO, Deutsch J, Carmichael AJ, Taylor R: Eyelid leishmaniasis in a patient with neurogenic ptosis. Br J Ophthalmol 75:506–507, 1991.
118. Ferry AP: Cutaneous leishmaniasis (oriental sore) of the eyelid. Am J Ophthalmol 84:349–354, 1977.
119. Chu FC, Rodrigues MM, Cogan DG, Neva FA: Leishmaniasis affecting the eyelids. Arch Ophthalmol 101:84–91, 1983.
120. Font RL: Eyelids and lacrimal drainage system. *In* Spencer WH (ed): Ophthalmic Pathology: An Atlas and Textbook, 3rd ed. Philadelphia, WB Saunders, 1986, pp 2141–2312.
121. Neva F, Sacks D: Leishmaniasis. *In* Warren KS, Mahmoud AAF (eds): Tropical and Geographical Medicine. New York, McGraw-Hill Information Services Company, 1990, pp 296–308.
122. Harman RRM: Parasitic worms and protozoa. *In* Rook A, Wilkinson DS, Ebling FJG, et al (eds): Texbook of Dermatology. Boston, Blackwell Scientific Publications, 1986, pp 987–1029.
123. Pearson RD, de Queiroz Sousa A: *Leishmania* species: Visceral (kala-azar), cutaneous, and mucosal leishmaniasis. *In* Mandell GL, Douglas RG, Bennett JE (eds): Principles and Practice of Infectious Diseases, 3rd. ed. New York, Churchill Livingstone, 1990, pp 2066–2076.
124. Kirchhoff LV: *Trypanosoma* species (American trypanosomiasis, Chagas disease): Biology of trypanosomes. *In* Mandell GL, Douglas RG, Bennett JE (eds): Principles and Practice of Infectious Diseases, 3rd ed. New York, Churchill Livingstone, 1990, pp 2077–2084.
125. Ravdin JI: Amebiasis and giardiasis. *In* Kass EH, Platt R, (eds): Current Therapy in Infectious Disease, 3rd ed. Philadelphia, BC Decker, 1990, pp 366–370.
126. Beaver PC, Villegas AL, Cuello C, D'Alessandro A: Cutaneous amebiasis of the eyelid with extension into the orbit. Am J Trop Med Hyg 27:1133–1136, 1978.
127. Duke BOL: Loiasis. *In* Strickland GT (ed): Hunter's Tropical Medicine. Philadelphia, WB Saunders, 1991, pp 727–729.
128. Hubler WR Jr, Gregory JF, Knox JM, Falls H: Loaiasis. A case report and review of the literature. Arch Dermatol 108:835–836, 1973.
129. Ottesen EA: The filariases and tropical eosinophilia. *In* Warren KS, Mahmoud AAF (eds): Tropical and Geographical Medicine. New York, McGraw-Hill Information Services Company, 1990, pp 407–428.
130. Sacks HN, Williams DN, Eifrig DE: Loiasis. Arch Intern Med 136:914–915, 1976.
131. Grove DI: Tissue nematodes (trichinosis, dracunculiasis, filariasis). *In* Mandell GL, Douglas RG, Bennett JE (eds): Principles and Practice of Infectious Diseases, 3rd ed. New York, Churchill Livingstone, 1990, pp 2140–2144.
132. Duke BOL, Taylor HR: Onchocerciasis. *In* Stickland GT (ed): Hunter's Tropical Medicine. Philadelphia, WB Saunders, 1991, pp 729–743.
133. Greene BM: Onchocerciasis. *In* Warren KS, Mahmoud AAF (eds): Tropical and Geographical Medicine. New York, McGraw-Hill Information Services Company, 1990, pp 429–438.
134. Kazura JW: Trichinosis. *In* Warren KS, Mahmoud AAF (eds): Tropical and Geographical Medicine. New York, McGraw-Hill Information Services Company, 1990, pp 442–445.
135. Mauriello JA, Flanagan JC: Tumors and inflammations of the lids. *In* Maurillo JA, Flanagan JC (eds): Management of Orbital and Ocular Adnexal Tumors and Inflammations. New York, Field & Wood, 1990, p 245.
136. Christie RW: *Dirofilaria tenuis* in Vermont. N Engl J Med 297:706–707, 1977.
137. Jariya P, Sucharit S: *Dirofilaria repens* from the eyelid of a woman in Thailand. Am J Trop Med Hyg 32:1456–1457, 1983.
138. Burnier M, Hidayat AA, Neafie R: Dracunculiasis of the orbit and eyelid. Ophthalmology 98:919–924, 1991.
139. Bunnag T: Gnathostomiasis. *In* Strickland GT (ed): Hunter's Tropical Medicine. Philadelphia, WB Saunders, 1991, pp 764–767.
140. Drugs for parasitic infections. Med Lett Drugs Ther 32(814): 23–32, 1990.
141. Mahmoud AAF: Intestinal nematodes (roundworms). *In* Mandell GL, Douglas RG, Bennett JE (eds): Principles and Practice of Infectious Diseases, 3rd ed. New York, Churchill Livingstone, 1990, pp 2135–2139.
142. Pawlowski ZS: Cestodiases: Taeniasis, cysticercosis, diphyllobothriasis, hymenolepiasis, and others. *In* Warren KS, Mahmoud AAF (eds): Tropical and Geographical Medicine. New York,

McGraw-Hill Information Services Company, 1990, pp 490–504.
143. Sen DK, Mohan H: Ocular cysticercosis in India. J Pediatr Ophthalmol Strabismus 15:96–102, 1978.
144. Jampol LM, Caldwell JBH, Albert DM: *Cysticercus cellulosae* in the eyelid. Arch Ophthalmol 89:319–320, 1973.
145. Singh G, Jaswinder K: Cysticercosis of the eyelid. Ann Ophthalmol 14:947–950, 1982.
146. Sen DK: *Cysticercus cellulosae* in the lacrimal gland, orbit, and eye lid. Acta Ophthalmol (Copenh) 58:144–147, 1980.
147. Perry HD, Font RL: Cysticercosis of the eyelid. Arch Ophthalmol 96:1255–1257, 1978.
148. McGreevy PB, Nelson GS: Larval cestode infections. *In* Strickland GT (ed): Hunter's Tropical Medicine. Philadelphia, WB Saunders, 1991, pp 831–839.
149. Jones TC: Cestodes (tapeworms). *In* Mandell GL, Douglas RG, Bennett JE (eds): Principles and Practice of Infectious Diseases, 3rd ed. New York, Churchill Livingstone, 1990, pp 2151–2156.
150. Mahmoud AAF: Trematodes (schistosomiasis) and other flukes. *In* Mandell GL, Douglas RG, Bennett JE (eds): Principles and Practice of Infectious Diseases, 3rd ed. New York, Churchill Livingstone, 1990, pp 2145–2150.
151. Bosniak SL, Schiller JR: Ophthalmomyiasis in an eyelid reconstruction. Am J Ophthalmol 109:101–102, 1990.
152. Cogen MS, Hays SJ, Dixon JM: Cutaneous myiasis of the eyelid due to *Cuterebra* larva. JAMA 258:1795–1796, 1987.
153. Savino DF, Margo CE, McCoy ED, Friedl FE: Dermal myiasis of the eyelid. Ophthalmology 93:1225–1227, 1986.
154. Wilhelmus KR: Myiasis palpebrarum. Am J Ophthalmol 101:496–498, 1986.
155. Rodrigues MM, Weiss CB, Muncy DW: Ophthalmomyiasis of the eyelid caused by *Cuterebra* larva. Am J Ophthalmol 78:1024–1026, 1974.
156. Terry JE, Williams RE: *Dermacentor variabilis*: Uncomplicated eyelid involvement. Arch Ophthalmol 98:514–515, 1980.
157. Bulmer C: The ocular mycoses. Contrib Microbiol Immunol 4:56–63, 1977.
158. Ostler HB, Okumoto M, Halde C: Dermatophytosis affecting the periorbital region. Am J Ophthalmol 72:934–938, 1971.
159. Roberts SOB, Mackenzie DWR: Mycology. *In* Rook A, Wilkinson DS, Ebling FJG, et al (eds): Textbook of Dermatology. Boston, Blackwell Scientific Publications, 1986, pp 885–986.
160. Witorsch P, Utz JP: North American blastomycosis: A study of 40 patients. Medicine 47:169–200, 1968.
161. Bongiorno FJ, Leavell UW, Wirtschafter JD: The black dot sign and North American cutaneous blastomycosis. Am J Ophthalmol 78:145–147, 1974.
162. Blodi FC, Huffman WC: Cicatricial ectropion caused by cutaneous blastomycosis. Arch Ophthalmol 59:459–462, 1958.
163. Barr CC, Gamel JW: Blastomycosis of the eyelid. Arch Ophthalmol 104:96–97, 1986.
164. Wilder WH: Blastomycosis of the eyelid. JAMA 43:2026–2030, 1904.
165. de Moraes Silva MRB, Mendes RP, Lastoria JC, et al: Paracoccidioidomycosis: Study of six cases with ocular involvement. Mycopathologia 102:87–96, 1988.
166. Belfort R, Fischman O, de Camargo ZP, Almada A: Paracoccidioidomycosis with palpebral and conjunctival involvement. Mycopathologia 56:21–24, 1975.
167. Irvine AR: Coccidioidal granuloma of lid. Trans Am Acad Ophthalmol Otolaryngol 72:751–754, 1968.
168. Wood TR: Ocular coccidioidomycosis. Am J Ophthalmol 64:587–591, 1967.
169. Hill HF: *Sporothrix* infection of the eye and adnexa. Trans Am Acad Ophthalmol Otolaryngol 35:128–139, 1930.
170. Mackenzie DWR: Subcutaneous mycoses. *In* Strickland GT (ed): Hunter's Tropical Medicine. Philadelphia, WB Saunders, 1991, pp 510–514.
171. Drugs for treatment of fungal infections. Med Lett Drugs Ther 34(864):15–16, 1992.
172. Bennett JE: *Sporothrix schenckii. In* Mandell GL, Douglas RG, Bennett JE (eds): Principles and Practice of Infectious Diseases, 3rd ed. New York, Churchill Livingstone, 1990, pp 1972–1974.
173. Harrell ER, Wolter JR, Gutow RF: Localized aspergilloma of the eyelid. Arch Ophthalmol 76:322–324, 1966.
174. Bennett JE: Miscellaneous fungi. *In* Mandell, GL, Douglas RG, Bennett JE (eds): Principles and Practice of Infectous Diseases, 3rd ed. New York, Churchill Livingstone, 1990, pp 2031–2034.
175. Gupta OP: Unusual extranasal manifestations of rhinosporidiosis. Laryngoscope 76:1842–1849, 1966.

CHAPTER 31

Benign Eyelid Tumors

M. Ronan Conlon, Brian Leatherbarrow, and Jeffrey A. Nerad

This chapter is devoted to the multitude of benign tumors and related noninfectious, noninflammatory lesions that arise from the structures comprising the eyelids. The lesions are classified according to the eyelid structures from which they arise, namely the epidermis, dermis, and eyelid adnexa, whereas lesions arising from pigment cells are classified separately. Most of these benign eyelid lesions are common cutaneous lesions that occur elsewhere in the body but that are different in their character, appearance, and behavior from lesions of other locations because of the unique characteristics of the eyelid skin. A small proportion of the lesions that are described are eyelid manifestations of systemic disorders.

The purpose of this chapter is to facilitate the diagnosis and management of these benign eyelid lesions by means of a comprehensive clinical description of each, supported by clinical photographs, a histopathologic description in selected cases, and a brief discussion of the treatment options.

HISTOLOGY OF THE SKIN

The skin of the eyelids is the thinnest in the body and continues to thin with advancing age. This characteristic of the eyelids usually extends a short distance beyond the orbital rim. The eyelid skin consists of a keratinized epidermis overlying a poorly defined papillary dermis without rete ridges. A very thin areolar subcutaneous layer separates the skin from the underlying orbicularis oculi muscle.

The epidermis is composed of two cell types: keratinocytes and dendritic cells. The keratinocytes are arranged in four layers, listed here from deep to superficial: basal cell layer, squamous cell layer, granular cell layer, and horny layer. The basal keratinocytes form a single row of cells, which are columnar in shape and lie on a basement membrane firmly attached to the dermis. The basal cell layer contains variable amounts of melanin pigment derived from adjacent dendritic melanocytes. The color of the skin varies with the amount of melanin present. The squamous cell layer consists of polygonal keratinocytes that form a mosaic of cells that is usually five to ten layers thick. The cells become flattened towards the surface. The granular cell layer consists of a row of elongated, flattened cells whose cytoplasm is filled with basophilic keratohyaline granules. The horny layer consists of flat, anuclear, keratinized cells.

The undifferentiated basal cells reproduce and either remain in the proliferative pool or begin to differentiate. Differentiation in the epidermis results in the production of keratin. The developing cells migrate up the layers. By the time they reach the surface to form the horny layer, the cells have died, are anuclear, and have become filled with keratin and flattened.

Three types of dendritic cells are present in the epidermis: clear cell melanocytes, Langerhans cells, and undetermined dendritic cells. The latter two cells can be identified with certainty only by histochemical studies and electron microscopy.

The eyelid epidermal adnexa consists of the pilosebaceous unit and the eccrine and apocrine sweat glands. The sebaceous glands are holocrine. Their acini possess no lumina and extrude their secretory products by decomposition of their cells. They are composed of several lobules leading into a common secretory duct that opens into the pilosebaceous follicle. The sebaceous glands of the lashes (glands of Zeis) discharge their secretions into the follicles of the eyelid cilia. The meibomian glands are specialized sebaceous glands located within the tarsus. The sebaceous material, discharged through the meibomian gland orifices posterior to the gray line, contributes to the lipid component of the tear film.

Eccrine and apocrine glands are the two distinct types of sweat glands found in humans. Eccrine sweat glands, which are independent of the hair follicle apparatus, are found everywhere in the skin except in the vermillion border of the lip, the glans penis, and the nail bed. The glands hypersecrete mainly in response to thermal stimuli, thereby aiding in thermoregulation. The glands of the axilla, palms, and soles hypersecrete in response to emotional stimuli. The secretory cells of the glands lie coiled in the dermis with the intradermal and intraepidermal ductal segment that delivers sweat to the skin surface. A wide variety of tumors arise from the pluripotential cells destined to develop into one of the components of the eccrine sweat gland unit.

Apocrine sweat glands serve as scent glands and are active only between puberty and the climacteric. In the eyelid, these glands are referred to as *Moll's glands* and open into the eyelash follicle. They have secretory and ductal components like the eccrine sweat glands. The sweat from these glands is formed by an extrusion process of the secretory cell cytoplasm into the glandular lumen in response to emotional stimuli mediated through the sympathetic nervous system. Lesions of the apocrine sweat gland apparatus of the eyelids are common. Histopathologic examination is frequently required for the differentiation of the many different benign tumors that emanate from the sweat gland apparatus.

The eyelashes represent terminal hair follicles. The rest of the eyelid is covered with small vellus hairs associated with tiny sebaceous glands.

The dermis of the eyelid is loose and delicate. It contains bundles of collagen and variable amounts of elastic and reticulin fibers, as well as ground substance containing mucopolysaccharides. Nerve fibers, blood vessels, and lymphatics are also present.

APPROACH TO DIAGNOSIS AND MANAGEMENT

Many of the benign lesions of the eyelids may be readily diagnosed on the basis of their typical clinical appearance and behavior. Some lesions, however, cannot be easily and reliably differentiated from malignant eyelid lesions and require biopsy. For large lesions, an incisional biopsy is usually undertaken for diagnostic purposes, whereas for small lesions, an excisional biopsy fulfills two goals: diagnosis and treatment. Biopsies should include adjacent normal tissue and the base of the lesion. In cases in which the lid margin is involved and must be included in the biopsy, a pentagonal wedge resection of the eyelid is performed. Shave biopsies should be used only for lesions in which characteristic histologic changes are expected to be present in the epidermis or upper dermis, such as seborrheic keratosis. Shave biopsies are inadequate for differentiating between keratoacanthoma and squamous cell carcinoma and are contraindicated for pigmented lesions.

Most of the benign eyelid lesions are best managed by simple observation or surgical excision, but alternative treatments are discussed for individual lesions.

BENIGN LESIONS OF THE EPIDERMIS

Although most epidermal lesions exhibit benign behavior, some have clinical features that suggest malignant degeneration, ulceration, bleeding, and irregular, rapid growth. Accurate diagnosis in these cases depends on histologic examination of biopsy material.

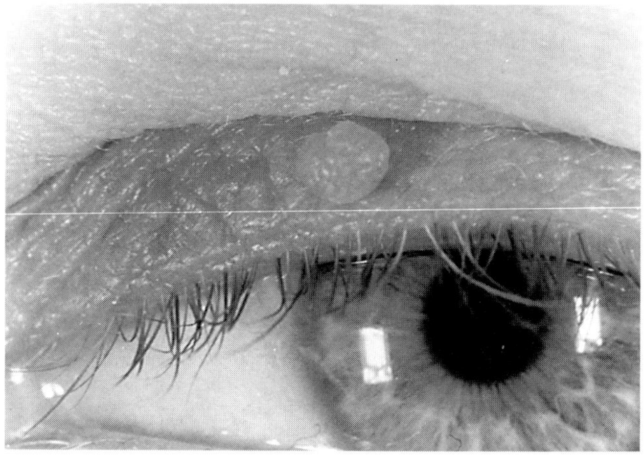

Figure 31 – 1. Typical appearance of an acrochordon (skin tag). Note that the lesion has a similar color to that of the surrounding skin and a papillomatous configuration.

Acrochordon (Skin Tag)

Skin tags (Fig. 31 – 1) are common eyelid lesions that are small, flesh-colored growths attached to the lid skin at the lid margin by a thin pedicle.[1] These lesions are frequently referred to as *papillomata*, an overused term that is merely descriptive and not diagnostic. It is a term used to describe many tumors and cutaneous lesions of numerous histopathologic diagnoses. Acrochordons may be multiple, and they may occur as larger pedunculated lesions.

Treatment consists of simple surgical transection of the lesion at its base, which can usually be performed by use of scissors and no sutures.

Milia

Milia are small, asymptomatic, raised, round, white, sharply circumscribed, superficial keratin cysts that are frequently seen on the eyelids.[2] They are particularly common in newborn infants (Fig. 31 – 2). They may arise spontaneously, follow trauma, or appear during the healing phase of bullous diseases.

Treatment consists of incision of the overlying skin

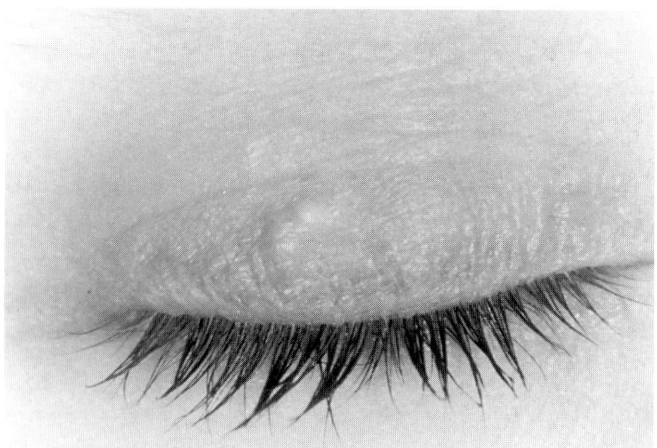

Figure 31 – 2. Milia of the lower eyelid demonstrating the typical well-circumscribed whitish appearance.

with a sharp blade or needle and expression of the contents of the cyst.

Seborrheic Keratosis

Seborrheic keratoses are common acquired eyelid lesions in middle-aged and elderly individuals and may be single or multiple. The clinical appearances vary considerably, depending on the size and degree of pigmentation of the lesions, and they are often confused with nevi, pigmented basal cell carcinomas, and melanomas (Fig. 31–3).[3] They are hyperkeratotic and usually hyperpigmented. On facial skin, they have a smooth, greasy appearance. The borders of the lesions are elevated and well demarcated with a "stuck-on" appearance. On the eyelids, the lesions may appear lobulated, papillary, or pedunculated. The surface of the lesions typically has friable, cerebriform excrescences.

The lesions are divided into three major histologic types according to their predominant histologic features: hyperkeratotic, acanthotic, and adenoid. Lesions of all three types tend to show variable degrees of hyperkeratosis, acanthosis, and papillomatosis of the epidermis. The acanthotic epidermis often contains keratin-filled cystic inclusions, referred to as *horn cysts* when they are formed within the mass and *pseudohorn cysts* when they represent invaginations of surface keratin. The dermis is uninvolved except in the case of irritated seborrheic keratoses, in which the dermis is often infiltrated by chronic inflammatory cells.

Treatment consists of shaving the lesions from the skin surface with a sharp scalpel blade. This leaves a flat surface that rapidly reepithelializes.[4] Although these lesions may be large in some cases, the superficial growth pattern excludes the need for deep scalpel excisions.

Keratoacanthoma

Keratoacanthoma has long been regarded as a benign, self-limiting lesion that mimics squamous cell carcinoma. Many pathologists, however, now regard the tumor as a low-grade squamous cell carcinoma. Its cause remains unknown, although trauma and exposure to sunlight have been implicated. It typically occurs in middle-aged to elderly patients who exhibit features of actinic damage. It may also be seen in immunosuppressed patients. Keratoacanthoma is usually a solitary lesion, although multiple variants have been described. The clinical appearances and courses are frequently very distinctive. Classically, the lesion begins as a small, flesh-colored papule, most frequently on the lower lid, which develops very rapidly over the course of a few weeks into a dome-shaped nodule with a central keratin-filled crater and elevated, rolled margins (Fig. 31–4). The lesion then gradually resolves spontaneously over the course of approximately 3 to 6 months with few visible sequelae.

Histologically, the lesion typically has a cup-shaped

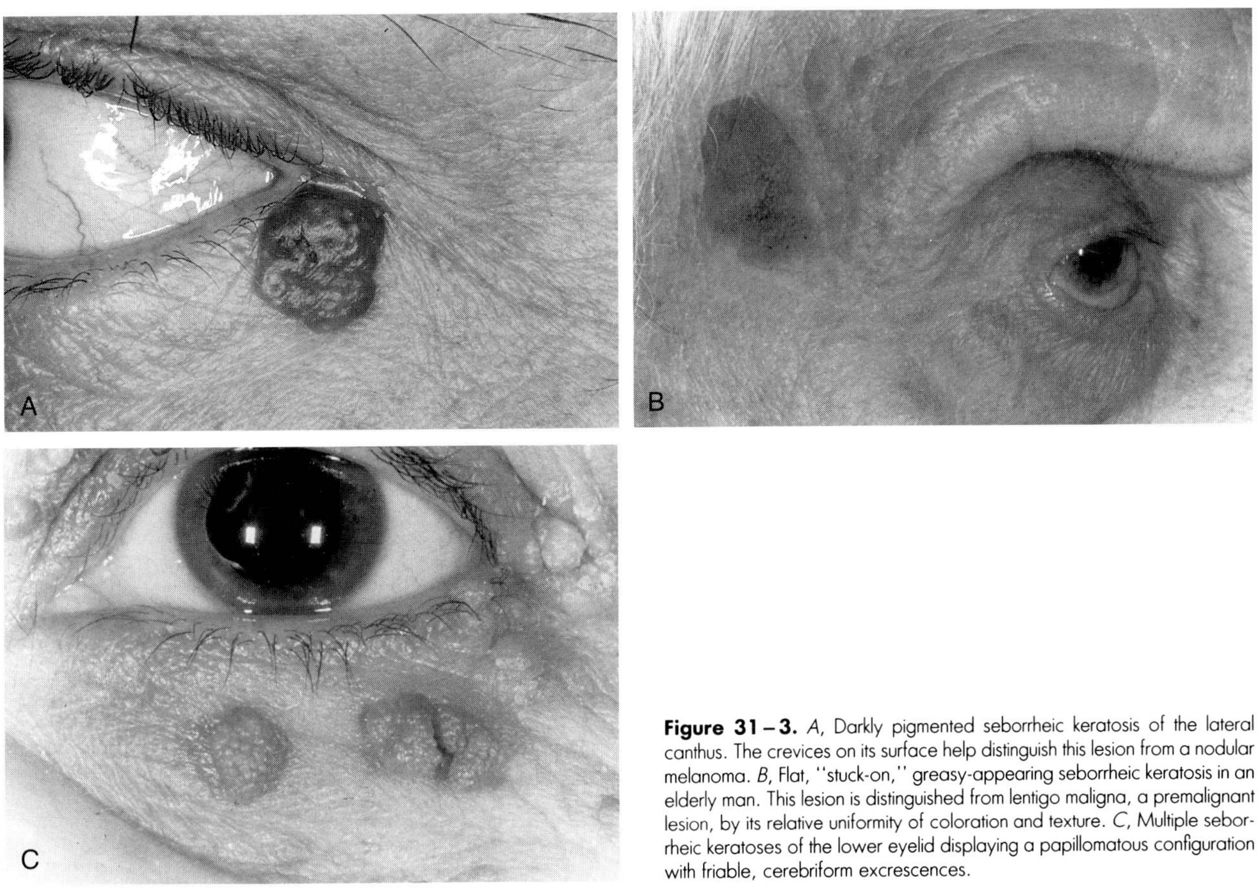

Figure 31–3. *A*, Darkly pigmented seborrheic keratosis of the lateral canthus. The crevices on its surface help distinguish this lesion from a nodular melanoma. *B*, Flat, "stuck-on," greasy-appearing seborrheic keratosis in an elderly man. This lesion is distinguished from lentigo maligna, a premalignant lesion, by its relative uniformity of coloration and texture. *C*, Multiple seborrheic keratoses of the lower eyelid displaying a papillomatous configuration with friable, cerebriform excrescences.

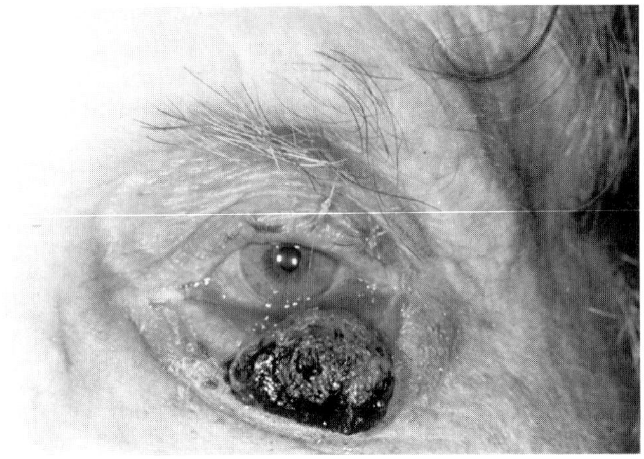

Figure 31 – 4. Large keratoacanthoma demonstrating central ulceration.

nodular elevation with thickening of the epidermis, which contains islands of well-differentiated squamous epithelium surrounding a central mass of keratin. Microabscesses may be present with the islands of squamous epithelium. The dermis often shows a polymorphous inflammatory infiltrate.

A conservative approach to treatment has been adopted in the past because the lesion is self-limiting. Few patients or physicians choose this option, however, because the healing course is prolonged, and mistakes may be made in diagnosis that delay the treatment of a potentially malignant lesion. The lesion may be surgically excised, or it can be treated with cryotherapy after a diagnostic incisional biopsy has been performed.[5] Radiotherapy for aggressive and destructive keratoacanthomas has been described,[6] but should be avoided if possible. The use of topical or intralesional 5-fluorouracil has also been described.[7-9]

Inverted Follicular Keratosis

Inverted follicular keratosis, which is usually solitary, may vary in clinical presentation and have a nodular, papillomatous, verrucous, or cystic appearance (Fig. 31 – 5). Hyperpigmentation is rare. It may also present as a cutaneous horn. The cause is unknown, but the lesion is generally considered to be a form of irritated seborrheic keratosis. Although inverted follicular keratosis has variable clinical appearances, the term was adopted to describe its distinctive histologic features.[10]

Histologically, the epithelium shows lobular acanthosis with overlying hyperkeratosis and occasional central keratin-filled, cup-shaped invagination. Proliferation of uniform basaloid cells is present, with an abrupt transition to concentrically arranged squamoid cells. The dermis is uninvolved.

Cutaneous Horn

Cutaneous horn (Fig. 31 – 6) is another clinically descriptive term and is not a diagnosis. This lesion may be associated with a benign or malignant lesion, such as seborrheic keratosis, verruca vulgaris, and squamous or basal cell carcinoma.

Treatment is directed at the underlying cutaneous lesion. Biopsy of the base of the cutaneous horn is required for diagnosis to be established.

Epidermal Inclusion Cyst

The epidermal inclusion cyst, which arises from the infundibulum of the hair follicle, may occur spontaneously or as a result of surgical or traumatic implantation of epidermis into the dermis.[11] Multiple facial inclusion cysts may be seen in patients with Gardner's syndrome, which is characterized by intestinal polyps, multiple osteomas of facial bones, fibromas and epithelial inclusion cysts of the skin, and fibromatosis (desmoid tumors) of the abdominal wall, mesentery, and breasts. The lesion is slow growing, elevated, round, smooth, and firm, and it rarely exceeds 1 cm in diameter (Fig. 31 – 7). It is freely movable and is often attached to the overlying thinned skin by the remaining pilar duct, which may appear as a pore. The lesion may rupture, causing a foreign body reaction, or

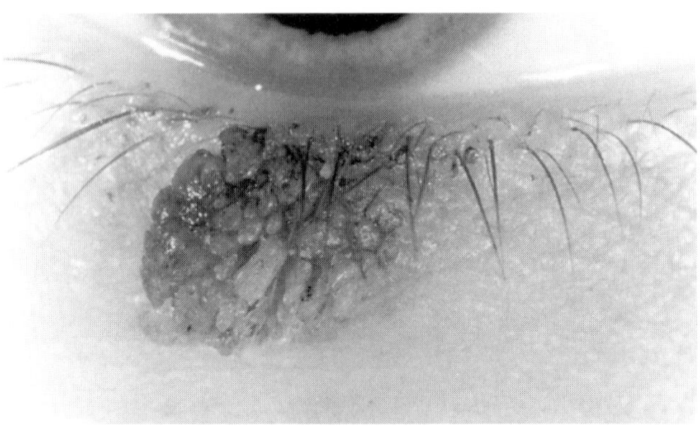

Figure 31 – 5. Solitary inverted follicular keratosis of the lower eyelid. This particular lesion has a verrucous morphology; however, other lesions may appear papillomatous or cystic.

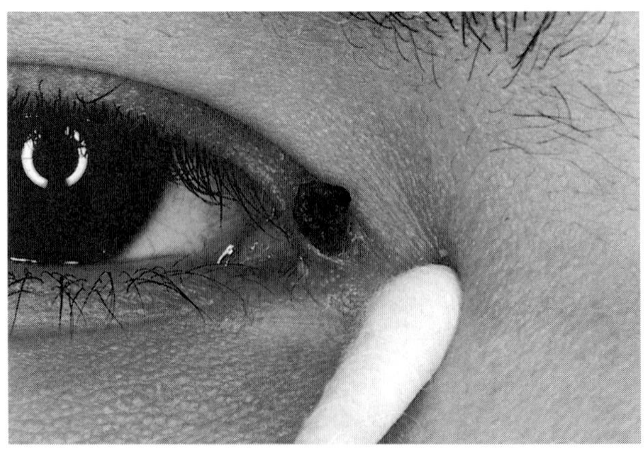

Figure 31 – 6. Cutaneous horn arising from the medial canthal area in a darkly pigmented person.

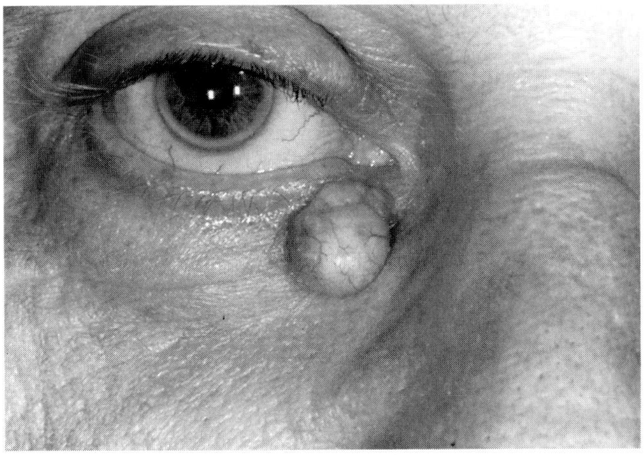

Figure 31 – 7. Epidermal inclusion cyst of the right lower eyelid. Cysts of this type are filled with desquamative keratin material produced by their epithelial cell lining.

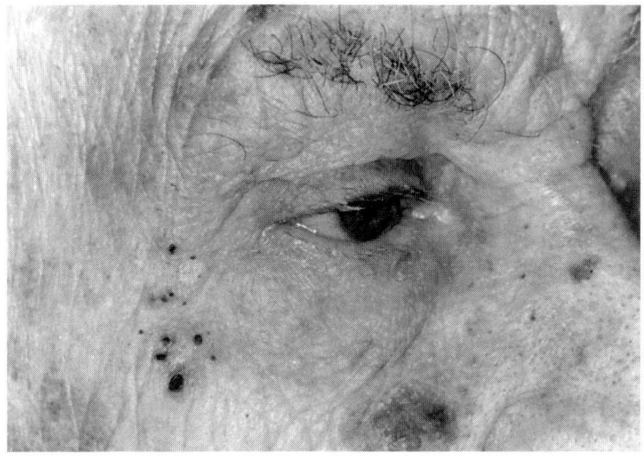

Figure 31 – 8. Multiple comedones interspersed with yellow nodules (nodular elastosis) in an elderly person with a significant history of sun exposure. Note the senile lentigo adjacent to the lesions, which also indicates solar damage.

may become secondarily infected. Malignant degeneration is extremely rare.

Treatment is by excision or by marsupialization of the cyst.

Linear Epidermal Nevus

Linear epidermal nevus may be either localized, in which only one linear lesion is present, or systematized, in which many linear lesions are present. The lesion consists of multiple, closely set, papillomatous, hyperkeratotic papules. The color of the lesions varies with the amount of hyperkeratosis and pigmentation. The lesions are occasionally associated with skeletal deformities and central nervous system disorders.[12]

Treatment is by surgical excision, which is usually curative. Alternative therapies include cryotherapy, electrodessication, application of topical retinoic acid, and dermabrasion.[13]

Nodular Elastosis with Cysts and Comedones (Favre-Racouchot Syndrome)

Nodular elastosis with cysts and comedones occurs in the solar-damaged skin of older, fair-skinned whites. It consists of multiple comedones (Fig. 31 – 8) as well as yellowish nodules containing a central comedo that mainly occurs around the lateral canthus and extends to the malar eminence and temple. The eyelid and facial skin usually show other signs of actinic damage. A variant of this condition is the actinic comedonal plaque, which is found as a solitary plaque with small nodules, dilated follicles, and numerous underlying comedones.[14]

Treatment is effected with topical application of retinoic acid and mechanical removal of the cysts and comedones.

Dermoid Cyst

Dermoid cysts are choristomas that result from the sequestration of skin along lines of embryonic closure. They contain elements of epidermis and epidermal appendages. Secretion by contained sebaceous and sweat glands causes a gradual increase in size of the cysts, which also contain hairs. They are present at birth but may not become evident until later in life. They frequently have an orbital extension. Rupture of the cyst releases highly irritating secretions that can cause a severe inflammatory reaction.[15]

Most frequently, dermoid cysts present in infants and young children (Fig. 31 – 9) and occur near the frontozygomatic suture, but dermoids may also occur medially, where they must be differentiated from a meningocele or meningoencephalocele. Dermoid cysts can be sufficiently large to compress the globe or to cause a mechanical ptosis and induce astigmatic or occlusion amblyopia. Occasionally, these cysts can become quite large and can extend into the cranium.

Histologically, the cyst is lined by stratified squamous epithelium, and the wall typically possesses adnexal structures (sebaceous and eccrine sweat glands and hair follicles) that discharge their contents directly into the

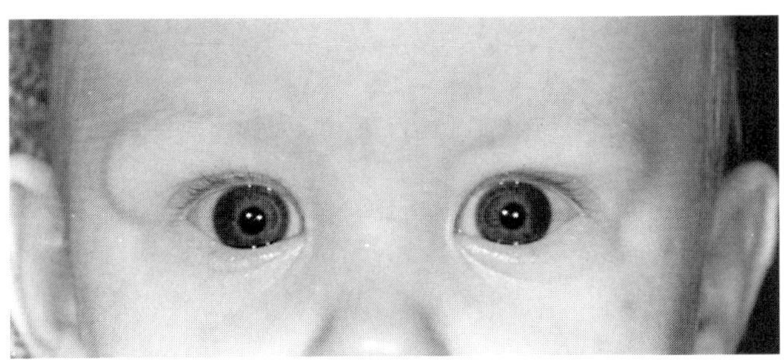

Figure 31 – 9. Typical appearance of a dermoid cyst arising over the right brow of an infant.

lumen of the cyst. Frequently, the cyst wall contains hairs that project into the cyst lumen.[16]

Treatment consists of surgical excision, which may be delayed in infants unless the cyst is large enough to cause problems or has leaked. Excision should be complete and should not cause rupture of the cyst and spillage of the irritant contents whenever possible. Occult extension deep into the orbit should be anticipated if the entire outline of the cyst is not palpable or if proptosis is present. Magnetic resonance imaging or computed tomography should be obtained preoperatively if significant orbital or intracranial involvement is suspected.

Oncocytoma

The term *oncocytoma* refers to a rare tumor composed of large eosinophilic cells (oncocytes) growing in an adenomatous pattern. Oncocytes are thought to be epithelial cells that undergo transformation with aging. Most oncocytomas arise from the caruncle, but they may also arise from the mucocutaneous border of the eyelid, the lacrimal sac, or the conjunctiva. The lesion is rare in patients under the age of 60 years. It is a slow-growing, benign tumor that rarely exceeds 15 mm in diameter. Its color varies from red to yellow, and it may have a smooth or lobulated surface.[17, 18]

Treatment is by surgical excision.

Phakomatous Choristoma

This rare lesion is believed to be a congenital neoplasm of lenticular anlage.[19–21] It always appears to be confined to the anteroinferior aspect of the lower eyelid medially (Fig. 31 – 10). It has been postulated that this lesion results from surface ectodermal cells, which are induced to form the lens plate and lens vesicle in the embryo, remaining external to the optic vesicle as the embryonic fissure closes. These cells then multiply and form the phakomatous choristoma after undergoing rudimentary differentiation. The eye is usually free from developmental defects. Its constant inferonasal position might also be explained by the ventronasal location of the embryonic choroidal fissure of the optic vesicle.

Treatment is by surgical excision.

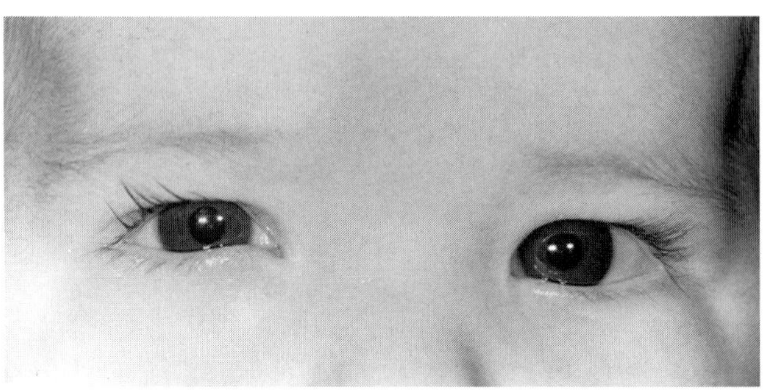

Figure 31 – 10. Phakomatous choristoma of the left lower eyelid. This rare tumor is composed of lens material that is believed to become sequestered in the eyelid during development. The eye is usually normal in these patients.

BENIGN TUMORS OF THE DERMIS

The eyelid dermis is loose and delicate and acts as a complex supporting structure for the epidermis. Its major components are collagen, elastic tissue, and ground substance. In addition, the dermis contains numerous other structures, including nerves, blood vessels, smooth muscle, and bone marrow–derived monocyte-histiocyte-macrophages, all of which can give rise to benign dermal lesions. These tumors are classified and discussed according to their dermal cellular origin.

Tumors Derived from Nervous Tissue

Neurofibroma

Neurofibromas may occur as solitary cutaneous lesions with no other associated abnormalities, or they may occur as part of neurofibromatosis (von Recklinghausen's disease). Whereas solitary neurofibromas generally arise in adulthood, the multiple cutaneous tumors of neurofibromatosis tend to appear in late childhood or adolescence and gradually increase in size and number (Fig. 31 – 11).

Neurofibromas consist of a proliferation of Schwann cells and endoneurial fibroblasts embedded in a considerable amount of endoneurial collagen. They are soft, are usually flesh colored, and tend to be pedunculated. They may be clinically indistinguishable from dermatofibromas and intradermal nevi. The diagnosis of neurofibromatosis should be excluded.

Histologically, the tumor appears to be poorly circumscribed and composed of spindle-shaped cells embedded in a loose myxoid stroma. A diffuse arrangement of fibroblasts, lymphocytes, and mast cells is found among the spindle-shaped cells.

Treatment involves excision of solitary lesions for cosmetic reasons or for the exclusion of other pathology. Surgical debulking of extensive plexiform neurofibromas may be required in cases in which a mechanical ptosis interferes with vision or visual development. The tumors are highly infiltrative, and complete excision is generally not possible without considerable sacrifice to adjacent structures. These tumors usually recur.

Neurilemoma (Schwannoma)

Neurilemomas are derived from Schwann cells of the nerve sheath. They occur along the course of peripheral nerves and are rare in the eyelid. They may be associated with neurofibromatosis. They are isolated, firm, pearly

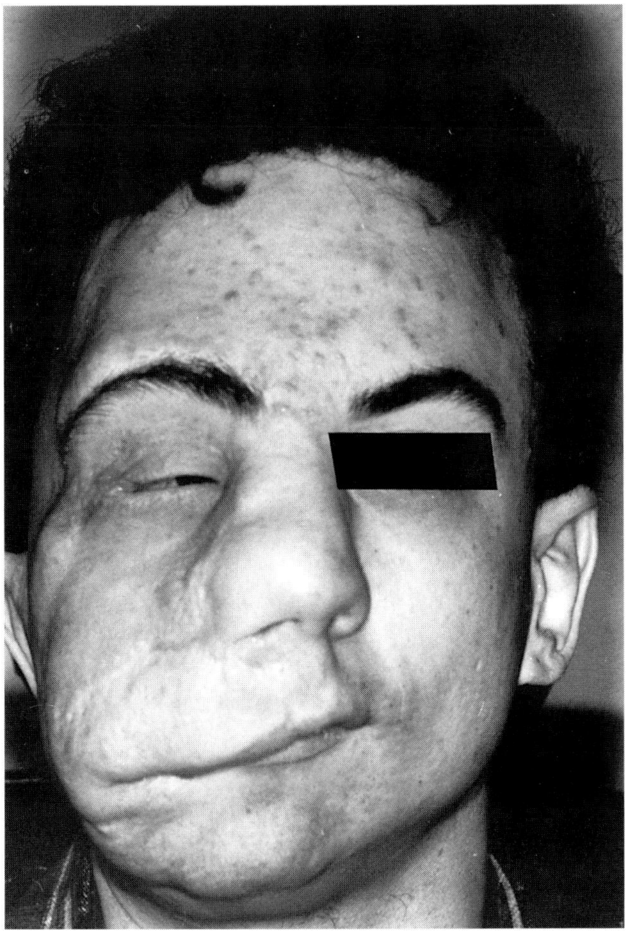

Figure 31 – 11. A 30-year-old man with hemihypertrophy of the right side of the face secondary to diffuse involvement of the dermis by neurofibromatosis.

white or yellowish subcutaneous nodules that are slow growing and benign. Malignant degeneration is extremely rare.

Histologically, the tumor appears to be well circumscribed and composed of bundles of elongated cells with thin, attenuated nuclei. These cells tend to align themselves into compact parallel rows, with intervening dense anucleate zones.

Treatment involves excisional biopsy to establish the histopathologic diagnosis.[22]

Neuroma

Neuromas are proliferations of nerve fascicles. They occur rarely in the eyelid, but when they do, they are usually part of the multiple endocrine neoplasia syndrome, in which large numbers of these small nodular lesions occur on the skin of the face, on and around the nose, and on the eyelids. They are also seen as small nodules on the mucosa of the lips, tongue, and mouth.

Treatment is by surgical excision.

Granular Cell Tumor

This rare benign tumor is thought to arise from Schwann cells of neural crest origin. It appears as a smooth, firm, well-circumscribed, subcutaneous nodule that is usually yellowish. It cannot be differentiated clinically from other nodular subcutaneous eyelid tumors.[23]

Treatment consists of surgical excision.

Tumors Derived from Smooth Muscle

Leiomyoma

Leiomyomas are benign tumors that arise from smooth muscle. They are extremely rare in the eyelids, arising from the arrector pili muscles and the smooth muscle of blood vessels. Their color varies from pink to brown. They may be single or multiple and may be painful. They cannot be differentiated clinically from other nodular subcutaneous eyelid tumors.

Treatment is by surgical excision.

Tumors Derived from Vascular Tissue

Nevus Flammeus (Port Wine Stain)

This congenital lesion is composed of capillaries that are dilated as a result of a congenital weakness of the capillary walls. It is a telangiectasia with no endothelial proliferations and is therefore not a true angioma, unlike the capillary or cavernous hemangioma with which it is frequently confused. It is characterized by one or several dull red or bluish-red patches of irregular outline that are not elevated (Fig. 31 – 12). The lesion may fade with age, but it does not undergo spontaneous regression or involution. When a facial nevus flammeus is associated with leptomeningeal angiomatosis or ocular vascular hamartomas, it is a manifestation of the Sturge-Weber syn-

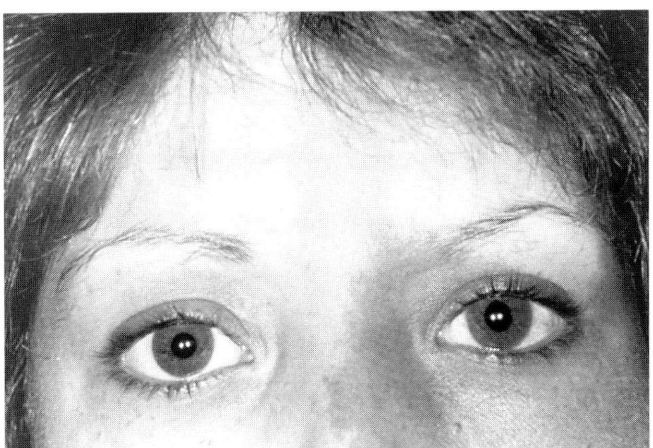

Figure 31 – 12. Nevus flammeus (port-wine stain) involving the left periocular area. This lesion is characteristically present at birth and blanches with pressure. These two features help differentiate this lesion from a capillary hemangioma.

drome. Leptomeningeal angiomatosis may cause epilepsy or hemiparesis. Ocular involvement may result in congenital or late-onset glaucoma resulting from elevated episcleral venous pressure. Histologically, dilated, mature, small capillaries with flattened endothelial lining are present in the papillary dermis.

These lesions have been treated with superficial carbon dioxide or argon laser in the past, but scarring has resulted.[24] Treatment with a pulsed-dye laser is more successful. Steroid treatment is without benefit. Alternatively, the lesions may be successfully camouflaged with cosmetics.

Capillary Hemangioma (Strawberry Nevus)

The capillary hemangioma is the commonest benign periocular tumor of infancy. It may involve the conjunctiva and orbit in addition to the eyelid. It is widely held to be a vascular hamartoma derived from endothelial cell rests. It is usually not present at birth, and approximately 95% are evident before the patient is 6 months of age. The tumor tends to grow rapidly during the first few months of life before undergoing spontaneous regression. Approximately 75% regress by the time the patient is 7 years of age, and regression may continue even up to the age of 18 years.

The clinical appearance of the capillary hemangioma varies with the depth of the lesion. When it is close to the skin surface, the tumor has a bright red or purple color (Fig. 31 – 13). It is usually elevated, it is lobulated with a spongy consistency, and it blanches with pressure. When it is deeper in the subcutaneous tissue, the lesion adopts a blue color. The eyelids may also be involved by tumor extending from the orbit. An important clinical appearance that is indicative of resolution is the appearance in a previously vascular strawberry-like lesion of fine stellate areas of pale scarring.[25]

Although entirely benign, the capillary hemangioma is associated with a high incidence of serious ocular sequelae involving occlusion or astigmatic amblyopia.[26] A rare association is the Kasabach-Merritt syndrome, in which thrombocytopenia and bleeding diathesis may be caused by entrapment of platelets within a large capillary hemangioma.

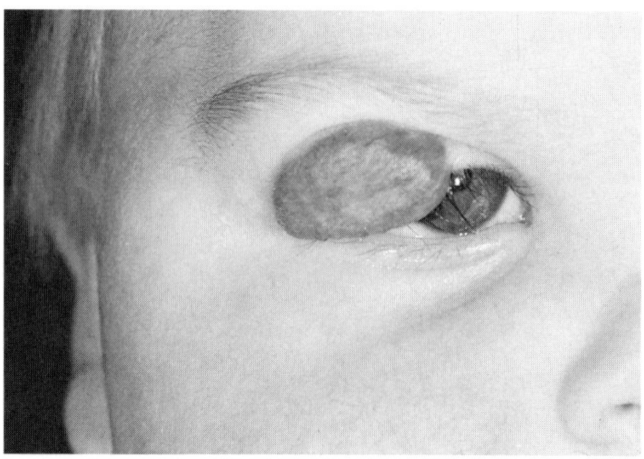

Figure 31 – 13. Capillary hemangioma involving the entire upper eyelid in a 6-month-old infant. This lesion responded well to an intralesional injection of corticosteroids.

Histologically, the dermis shows well-circumscribed collections of well-formed, small, thin-walled capillaries with a flattened endothelial cell lining and occasional buds of endothelial cells. Usually, a minimal associated inflammatory cell infiltrate is present.

Treatment is unnecessary in small tumors that do not threaten visual development. In larger tumors, especially when they are growing, orbital imaging may be indicated to assess the extent of orbital involvement. Lesions that cause or threaten to cause amblyopia should be treated with intralesional steroids.[27, 28] Failure to respond to intralesional steroids may necessitate the use of systemic steroids in selected cases, but this treatment is best avoided if possible because of the potential adverse effects associated with the high doses required. Residual tumor or tumor that is unresponsive to steroids may be managed surgically.

Cavernous Hemangioma

Cavernous hemangioma is the commonest benign primary orbital tumor of adults, but it is rarely encountered in the eyelid. Most often, capillary hemangiomas containing dilated channels that occur in infants are classified by some investigators as combined capillary-cavernous hemangiomas, but histologically they do not show the smooth muscle fibers seen in true cavernous hemangiomas. In addition, these hemangiomas behave clinically like capillary hemangiomas. In the eyelid, a true cavernous hemangioma occurs in adults and consists of one, or more commonly, multiple deep dermal and subcutaneous nodules that are often compressible.[29]

Histologically, endothelium-lined, dilated, blood-filled vascular spaces are present in the dermis and are surrounded by a thick, fibromuscular coat; capillary proliferation or endothelial buds are not present. Thrombosis or foci of calcification may be seen.

Treatment is by surgical excision, if necessary.

Varix

A varix consists of a thin-walled, dilated venule that appears as an isolated, slightly elevated, dark blue cystic lesion in elderly patients, usually no larger than 2 to 5 mm in diameter. A varix is easily compressible and is of little significance clinically.

Histologic examination shows a thickened vein wall with adventitial fibrosis. The lumen contains erythrocytes as well as fibrin deposits and scattered mononuclear cells. The lumen may be partially obliterated by an organizing thrombus, with concentric deposition of collagen,

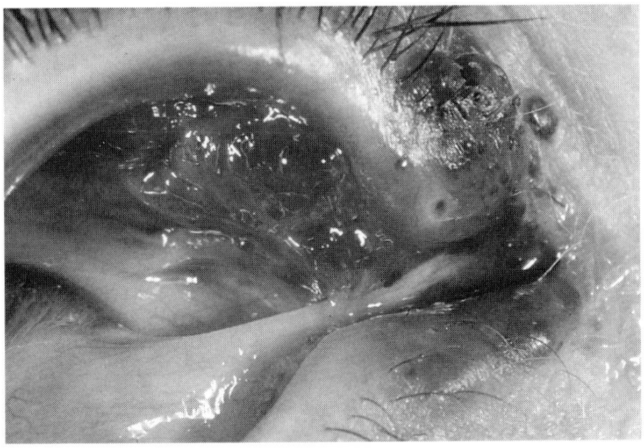

Figure 31 – 14. Lymphangioma of the right upper eyelid surrounds the punctum. This lesion demonstrates the typical features of clear cysts admixed with blood-filled cysts.

hemosiderin deposits, and foci of dystrophic calcification.

Treatment is by surgical excision, if necessary.

Lymphangioma

Three types of lymphangioma of the eyelid exist: localized lymphangioma circumscriptum, lymphangioma circumscriptum, and cavernous lymphangioma.[30] Localized lymphangioma circumscriptum consists of a single area of thick-walled vesicles that may be filled with clear lymph fluid or with an admixture of lymph and blood, giving the lesion a purplish color (Fig. 31 – 14).

In the classic lymphangioma circumscriptum, several large patches of vesicles are present, and the condition can be quite extensive. Often, a mild degree of diffuse swelling of the subcutaneous tissue lies beneath the vesicular lesions. When translucent, the vesicles may resemble a herpes simplex process. The lesions may break down and exude a serous transudate or become secondarily infected.

The cavernous lymphangioma is also referred to as a *cystic hygroma* when it is located in the neck. It appears as a soft or cystic, circumscribed or diffuse subcutaneous swelling. The lesion may be small or large and multifocal.

The presence of blood within the interstices may cause the mass to simulate a cavernous hemangioma. There may be an association with orbital and facial lymphangiomas. Large lesions may cause thickening and distortion of the eyelid, and extensive involvement may simulate the plexiform neurofibromas seen in neurofibromatosis.[31]

Histologically, large, dilated, thin-walled vascular channels are present in the dermis, with flattened endothelial cells filled with lymph fluid or occasionally red blood cells.

Treatment consists of surgery, if necessary for functional or cosmetic reasons. These lesions are unfortunately poorly responsive to steroid therapy. The infiltrative nature of these lesions limits the success of surgical resection.

Arteriovenous Malformation

An arteriovenous malformation consists of one or more endothelium-lined channels that directly communicate arterial with venous circulations at the site of involvement. They can occur spontaneously, as congenital defects, or after accidental or surgical trauma. They occur rarely in the eyelids, usually appearing secondary to orbital involvement.[32] Their clinical appearance may be confused with lymphangiomas and hemangiomas.

When treatment of isolated eyelid arteriovenous malformations is required, the feeder vessels are ligated after their identification by angiography. The vascular mass may also need to be excised. Embolization, a common treatment for orbital arteriovenous malformations, is not feasible for lesions confined to the eyelids.

Pyogenic Granuloma

It used to be widely assumed that this lesion was caused by pyogenic infection of a small wound. The histologic appearances, however, are those of a capillary hemangioma; therefore, a preferable term for this lesion is *eruptive hemangioma.* It is the commonest acquired vascular lesion of the eyelid. It appears clinically as a pedunculated, reddish lesion, frequently with superficial ulceration of the overlying epithelium (Fig. 31 – 15). Most pyogenic granulomas occur after minor trauma or surgery, and they tend to grow rapidly.

Histologically, the lesion consists of an exuberant mass of granulation tissue with prominent capillaries extending from the base to the surface of the lesion.

Treatment consists of surgical excision.

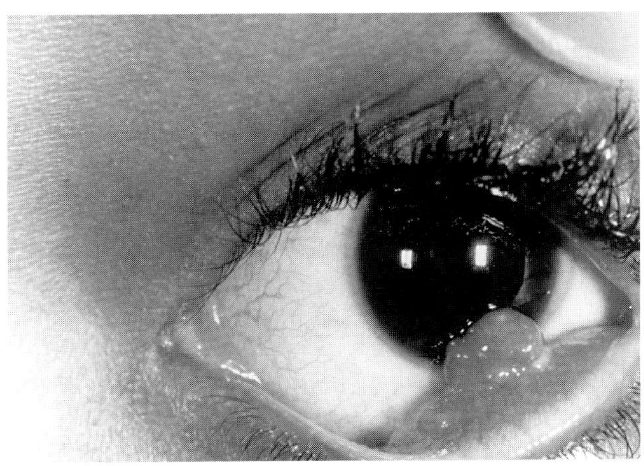

Figure 31 – 15. Pyogenic granuloma originating from the posterior aspect of the eyelid secondary to chronic inflammation caused by a chalazion.

Glomus Tumor

Two types of glomus tumor exist: the more common solitary glomus tumor and the very rare multiple variety. Both are extremely rare in the eyelid; they are more commonly found in the extremities, especially in the nail bed, where they can be very painful. In the skin, they are painful. The solitary type appears as a purplish nodule a few millimeters in diameter. Multiple tumors appear as either isolated tumors or as multiple, confluent, bluish, compressible, subcutaneous lesions varying from 5 to 20 mm in diameter.[33] This tumor may be difficult to differentiate from a lymphangioma, blue nevus, melanoma, leiomyoma, and other rare vascular tumors. Diagnosis is commonly made on biopsy.

Histologically, a well-circumscribed collection of small vascular channels is seen in the dermis, surrounded by a dense aggregate of small epithelioid cells.

Treatment is by surgical excision either for cosmetic reasons or to establish the diagnosis. The lesion may be deeply located and larger than anticipated.

Intravascular Papillary Endothelial Hyperplasia

Intravascular papillary endothelial hyperplasia is benign but is liable to be mistaken clinically and histologically for an angiosarcoma.[34] The lesion may or may not have the clinical appearance of a vascular lesion. It can vary in size from a few millimeters to 5 cm in diameter. Most of these lesions arise within a vein, but some have been found within a benign vascular lesion, such as a venous lake, hemangioma, or lymphangioma. The lesion is usually found in association with a thrombus; as a consequence, most physicians regard the lesion as an exaggerated reparative response to thrombosis within a vascular lumen. The lesion may also apparently occur spontaneously, and it may progress slowly or rapidly. It tends to affect young female adults most frequently and has a predilection for the face and extremities. Biopsy is required to establish the diagnosis.[35]

Histologically, the intraluminal mass, which is intimately attached to the vessel wall, displays collagenous cores that form papillary tufts, which are lined by a single layer of flat endothelial cells.

Treatment is by surgical excision, which, if complete, is curative.

Angiolymphoid Hyperplasia with Eosinophilia (Kimura's Disease)

In angiolymphoid hyperplasia with eosinophilia, solitary or multiple violaceous, intradermal or subcutaneous nodules occur, usually on the face and scalp, in young adult females. Significant peripheral blood eosinophilia is only occasionally encountered. The lesions histopathologically show an extensive infiltrate of lymphocytes, histiocytes, and numerous eosinophils. This lesion is

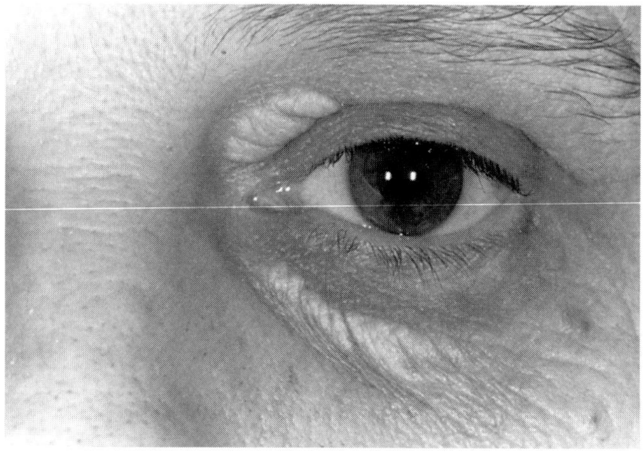

Figure 31 – 16. Typical yellow plaque-like xanthelasmas of the eyelids in a middle-aged man.

thought to be an inflammatory reactive, rather than a neoplastic, process. Biopsy is required to establish the diagnosis.

Treatment is by surgical excision, if feasible.

Tumors Derived from Histiocytes

Xanthelasma

Xanthelasmas are common dermal lesions of the medial aspects of the upper and lower eyelids that occur in middle-aged to elderly patients. Commoner in females than in males, these lesions are usually bilateral, plaque-like, yellow, flat or slightly raised deposits composed of foamy histiocytes (Fig. 31 – 16). Most patients have no underlying systemic metabolic disorder, but the lesions are occasionally found in association with diabetes and other hyperlipidemic conditions. Microscopically, the plaques consist of focal collections of foamy histiocytes distributed mainly around the vessels and adnexal structures of the dermis. There is no associated inflammation or fibrosis.

Treatment is simple surgical excision for cosmetic reasons, but recurrences are common. Surgical excision includes the full thickness of skin and sometimes the underlying orbicularis muscle. Wound closure must be accomplished without lagophthalmos or ectropion. Skin grafting is occasionally required.

Xanthoma

Xanthomas of the eyelid are more commonly associated with hyperlipidemic states than are xanthelasmas.[36] Histologically, they differ from xanthelasmas in that the lesions are situated more deeply in the dermis and show foamy histiocytes intermixed with multinucleated Touton-type giant cells as well as inflammatory cells and fibrosis.

Treatment is the same as for xanthelasmas.

Juvenile Xanthogranuloma (Nevoxanthoendothelioma)

Juvenile xanthogranuloma is a histiocytic proliferation of unknown origin that usually occurs in infants younger than 3 years of age. The lesions are nonneoplastic and self-limited. They most commonly affect the head and neck areas, but they have been reported rarely in the orbit, testes, and lung. The lesions not only affect the skin but may also affect the eye, where the conjunctiva, iris, or ciliary body may be involved.

The skin lesions, which often regress spontaneously, consist of single or multiple, elevated, orange or reddish-brown, dome-shaped nodules varying from 5 to 20 mm in diameter. Histologically, the lesions show a mixture of histiocytic foam cells, lymphocytes, histiocytes, Touton-type giant cells, and fibrosis.

Although the skin lesions carry an excellent prognosis, the intraocular lesions can cause serious problems. Spontaneous hyphema (resulting from rupture of the fragile blood vessels of the iris lesions), iritis, and secondary glaucoma may be a consequence of iris involvement. It is important to exclude juvenile xanthogranuloma as a cause of hyphema in an infant.[37] Diagnosis of juvenile xanthogranuloma may be aided by a careful skin examination for typical cutaneous lesions, which should be biopsied.

Treatment consists of administration of systemic steroids, which may expedite regression of the intraocular lesions. The cutaneous lesions resolve spontaneously in 6 to 12 months.

Tumors Derived from Fibrous Tissue

Dermatofibroma

Dermatofibromas are also known as fibrous histiocytomas, histiocytomas, and sclerosing hemangiomas. They occur in the skin as firm, indolent, single or multiple nodules, usually red to brown in color. They are usually only 2 to 3 mm in diameter but may measure 2 to 3 cm in diameter after bleeding into the tumor. In the eyelid, the lesion appears as a dome-shaped mass attached to the overlying skin. Histologic appearances vary according to the relative contribution of fibrous and cellular elements.[38, 39]

Treatment is by surgical excision.

BENIGN LESIONS OF THE ADNEXA

Tumors of Sweat Gland Origin

The eyelid eccrine and apocrine sweat glands[40] have three major components: the secretory coil lying within the dermis, the intradermal duct, and the intraepidermal duct. The eyelid eccrine glands are independent of the hair follicle apparatus, whereas the apocrine glands appear in association with the eyelashes and are referred to as Moll's glands. A wide variety of benign tumors may develop from the pluripotential cells destined to become one of the components of the eccrine sweat gland unit. With the exception of the apocrine hidrocystoma (Moll's cyst), apocrine lesions of the eyelid are relatively uncommon.

Eccrine Sweat Glands

SYRINGOMA

Syringomas are the commonest benign tumors of the eyelid adnexa. They are found most commonly in young females. Clinically, they usually appear as multiple, small, flesh-colored to yellowish, soft, waxy nodules averaging 1 to 2 mm in diameter (Fig. 31–17). The lower eyelids are predominantly affected, but the lesions may also occur on the upper lids, cheeks, and forehead. They are also occasionally found in the axillae, abdomen, and vulva. These lesions may be difficult to differentiate clinically from other benign lid lesions, and biopsy may be required for an accurate diagnosis.

Histologically, the dermis shows poorly circumscribed collections of small basaloid cells, lying in nests and strands, or individually, with many showing duct formation. The ducts contain eosinophilic keratin or amorphous material and may show a tadpole- or comma-shaped extension of small basaloid cells.

Treatment is by surgical excision, when required. Alternative treatments are electrodessication, dermabrasion, and carbon dioxide laser.[41, 42]

ECCRINE SPIRADENOMA

The eccrine spiradenoma shows differentiation toward the secretory portion of the eccrine gland. This benign tumor is an uncommon lesion that occurs as a solitary, flesh-colored nodule approximately 1 to 2 cm in diameter. Occasionally, the lesions can be multiple and larger.

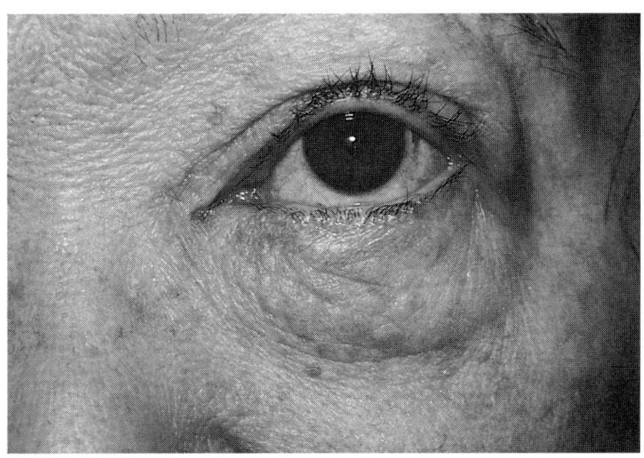

Figure 31–17. Typical periocular distribution of syringomas. The individual papules (1 to 3 mm in diameter) are firm, flesh colored, or slightly yellow in appearance.

They tend to occur in early adulthood and have no characteristic location, but the eyelid is rarely involved. The nodules can be tender and are occasionally painful.[43]

Histologically, the dermis contains well-circumscribed, deeply basophilic lobules, composed of cords and islands of two cell types: a peripherally located cell with a small, dense nucleus and a more centrally located cell with a large, pale nucleus. Eosinophilic hyaline material may surround the tumor lobules, among the cords and nests, and as hyaline droplets within the islands.

Treatment is by surgical excision.

ECCRINE ACROSPIROMA (CLEAR CELL HIDRADENOMA)

The eccrine acrospiroma shows differentiation toward both ductal and secretory portions of the eccrine gland. This tumor appears clinically as a single, nodular, solid, or cystic lesion. Rarely, several lesions may occur. The diameter of the lesions varies from 0.5 to 2 cm. The overlying skin may show ulceration, mimicking the appearance of a keratoacanthoma, but it usually is flesh-colored to reddish-blue and remains intact.[44-46]

Histologically, the dermis shows a well-circumscribed, lobular tumor mass composed of sheets and nests of large epithelioid clear cells and smaller cuboidal cells with basophilic cytoplasm. Frequently, tubular lumina occur that contain an amorphous eosinophilic material.

Treatment is by surgical excision.

ECCRINE HYDROCYSTOMA

Eccrine hydrocystomas tend to be multiple and commonly occur on the face and appear clustered around the eyelids. They tend to be small, measuring approximately 1 to 3 mm in diameter. They may simulate milia. They are regarded as ductal retention cysts, and no connection from the cyst to the overlying surface epidermis exists.[47]

Histologically, the lesions appear as large, dilated cysts, lined by a single small cuboidal or columnar cell layer and surrounded by an outer flattened myoepithelial cell layer. The cysts contain pale eosinophilic granular material.

Treatment is by surgical excision.

PLEOMORPHIC ADENOMA (MIXED TUMOR OF SKIN, CHONDROID SYRINGOMA)

The pleomorphic adenoma occurs most commonly in the head and neck regions and may involve the face and eyelids. Clinically, this lesion appears as a firm, intradermal, lobulated mass ranging from 0.5 to 3 cm in diameter (Fig. 31 – 18). Histologically, the tumor is identical to the pleomorphic adenoma of the lacrimal gland. When the lesion is located in the lateral aspect of the upper lid, it may be difficult to differentiate from a pleomorphic adenoma that arises from the palpebral lobe of the lacrimal gland.[48]

Treatment is by surgical excision.

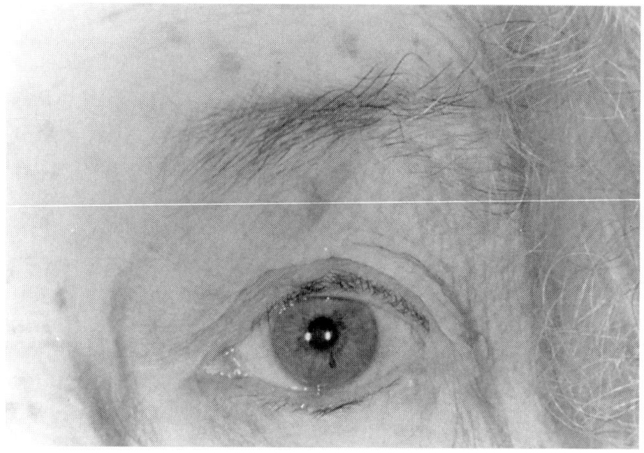

Figure 31 – 18. Chondroid syringoma (mixed eccrine tumor) presenting in a typical fashion as a firm subcutaneous nodule. This benign tumor is usually solitary and asymptomatic and most often occurs in the head and neck area.

Apocrine Sweat Glands

APOCRINE HIDROCYSTOMA (MOLL'S CYST)

The apocrine type of hidrocystoma is a true adenoma of the secretory cells of the gland rather than a retention cyst. The cells lining the cyst are not flattened, unlike in a retention cyst, and often form papillary projections into the lumen.

Most apocrine hidrocystomas occur as single lesions of the eyelids (Fig. 31 – 19). They are usually small, but they may reach a size of several centimeters. They may be skin-colored or they may have a bluish tinge. Being cystic in nature, they are compressible and tend to be translucent. The major differential diagnostic consideration is cystic basal cell carcinoma.

Treatment is by surgical excision.

CYLINDROMA

Although this tumor is known to originate generally from sweat glands, its exact origin is uncertain. It occurs

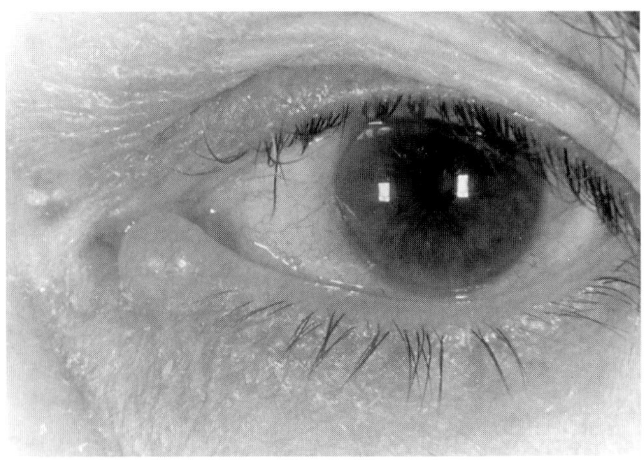

Figure 31 – 19. Typical appearance of an apocrine hidrocystoma (Moll's cyst) of the left lower eyelid.

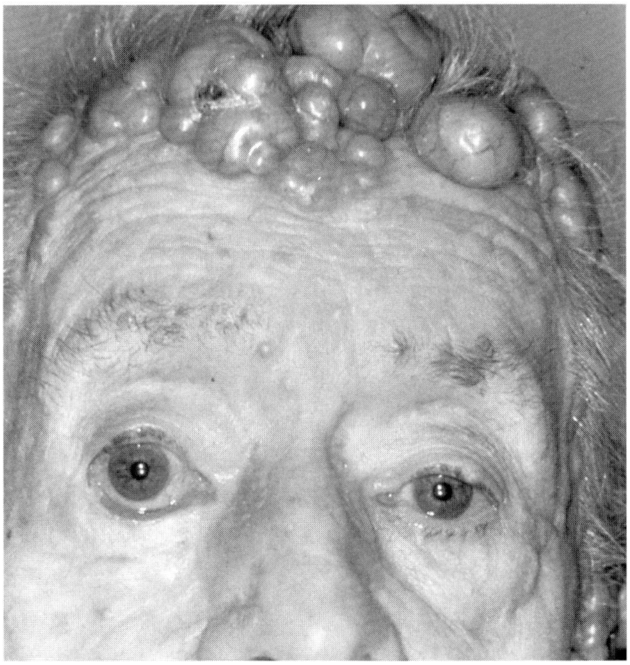

Figure 31-20. Multiple cylindromas of the scalp, the so-called turban tumor. This primitive eccrine tumor most commonly arises on the scalp and demonstrates a female preponderance (9:1). The lesion may occur in isolation or in multiple groups in a dominantly inherited variety.

as a solitary lesion or multiple lesions, and multiple lesions are dominantly inherited. Solitary lesions affect adults and appear on the face or scalp. Multiple lesions appear as dome-shaped, smooth, flesh-colored to reddish nodules of varying size on the scalp. Nodules on the scalp may be present in such large numbers that the scalp is entirely covered. Such lesions are referred to as *turban tumors* (Fig. 31-20). Multiple cylindromas may coexist with multiple trichoepitheliomas in some familial cases. Malignant degeneration of a cylindroma is a rare occurrence.

Histologically, the lesions consist of well-circumscribed islands of cells lying in a mosaic pattern and surrounded by an eosinophilic hyaline cuticle and sparse amounts of collagen. The islands contain two cell types: a large, pale-staining cell with a vesicular nucleus and a smaller, cuboidal cell with a dark-staining nucleus and less cytoplasm located at the periphery of the islands.

Treatment is by surgical excision, which may be considerably difficult when the lesions are present in large numbers.

SYRINGOCYSTADENOMA PAPILLIFERUM

Syringocystadenoma papilliferum occurs most commonly on the scalp or face, appearing at birth or during early childhood. The lesion appears clinically as a solitary papule or as multiple papules or plaques in a linear arrangement, increasing in size at puberty and becoming papillomatous.[49] The lesions may appear within a sebaceous nevus, but in the eyelid they usually arise de novo. The eyelid margin is most commonly involved in cases in which the lesion appears as a hyperkeratotic papillomatous nodule, which may mimic a basal cell carcinoma or keratoacanthoma.

Histologically, the epidermis shows cystic invagination and communication with the underlying dermal lesion. The dermis shows large cystic spaces with papillary projections in a poorly circumscribed tumor lobule. The cystic spaces are lined by two cell types: a columnar cell with an oval vesicular nucleus and abundant cytoplasm and a smaller, cuboidal cell with a round, dark nucleus and less cytoplasm. The cystic spaces are surrounded by a fibrous stroma with a dense, predominantly plasmacytic infiltrate.

Treatment is by surgical excision.

Tumors of Hair Follicle Origin[50]

TRICHOEPITHELIOMA

Trichoepithelioma occurs as both a solitary lesion and as multiple lesions inherited in an autosomal dominant manner with incomplete penetrance (epithelioma adenoides cysticum of Brooke (Fig. 31-21). The solitary lesion appears as a firm, elevated, flesh-colored nodule that may ulcerate. It tends to affect the face of older patients. Clinically, it may be difficult to differentiate from a basal cell carcinoma, intradermal nevus, neurofibroma, and other adnexal skin tumors.

In contrast, multiple trichoepitheliomas typically arise in adolescence and tend to increase in size and number. They may be present in large numbers and occur most commonly in the nasolabial fold, upper lip, eyelids, and side of the nose. They may also affect the scalp, neck, and

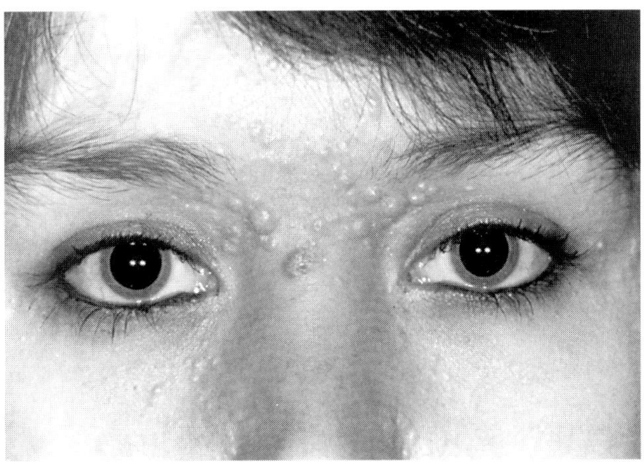

Figure 31-21. Trichoepitheliomas may be isolated or multiple and familial. Multiple flesh-colored papules are seen in a patient with familial multiple trichoepitheliomata. Histologically, this lesion is characterized by multiple squamous cell horn cysts within the epithelium representing abortive hair follicle formation.

upper trunk. The lesions should be differentiated from adenoma sebaceum, syringomas, and basal cell nevus syndrome. In contrast to basal cell nevus syndrome, ulceration is rare with multiple trichoepitheliomas. Transformation into a basal cell carcinoma has been described but is rare.

Histologically, the dermis shows a well-circumscribed nest of uniform basaloid cells surrounded by a hypercellular stroma. Often, foci of calcification and foreign body giant cells are present, as are abortive attempts at hair follicle formation.

Treatments for these tumors include simple surgical excision of individual lesions and dermabrasion or laser therapy for multiple lesions.

TRICHOFOLLICULOMA

Trichofolliculoma, which usually presents as a solitary lesion, is often confused with a sebaceous cyst. Clinically, it has characteristic features: it appears as a slightly elevated, dome-shaped, flesh-colored nodule with a diagnostic central umbilicated area that represents the opening of a keratin-filled dilated follicle. The presence of white hairs growing from the central pore is strong clinical evidence that the lesion is a trichofolliculoma. The tumor has no malignant potential.[51]

Histologically, a keratin-filled, cup-shaped invagination of the epidermis exists with numerous hair shafts. Poorly to well-differentiated secondary hair bulbs are located around the opening of the hair shafts. The dermis shows a hypercellular stroma around the secondary hair follicles.

Treatment is by simple surgical excision.

TRICHILEMMOMA

Trichilemmomas arise from the hair sheath in solitary or multiple forms. The more common solitary tumor usually occurs in older patients, in whom it appears as a flesh-colored, 3- to 8-mm verrucous or papillomatous papule on the face. It may be mistaken for a basal cell carcinoma. It most commonly appears on the nose and eyelids, where it may present as a cutaneous horn.[52]

Multiple tumors may be a cutaneous marker of Cowden's disease or multiple hamartoma syndrome, in which trichilemmomas of the nose, ear, and hands are cutaneous markers for patients with an increased risk of breast, thyroid, and gastrointestinal carcinoma.[53] In addition, retinal glioma and optic disc drusen have been reported in association with this syndrome.

Histologically, the dermis is uninvolved. The epidermis shows sheets of pale-staining to clear epithelioid cells in a lobular arrangement. The lobules show peripheral palisading and a thickened basement membrane.

Treatments include surgical excision, curettage, and electrodessication.

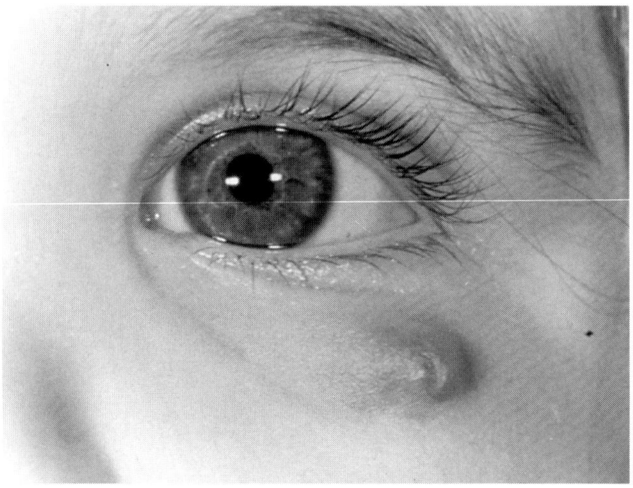

Figure 31 – 22. Pilomatrixoma (Malherbe's calcifying epithelioma) of the lower eyelid. This lesion tends to occur in adolescence as a purplish subcutaneous nodule.

PILOMATRICOMA (MALHERBE'S CALCIFYING EPITHELIOMA)

The pilomatricoma develops from hair matrix cells. The tumor, which is usually solitary, tends to occur in children. It appears as a pink to purplish, mobile, firm, irregular, subcutaneous nodule measuring 0.5 to 3 cm in diameter (Fig. 31 – 22). The face is a common site of presentation, with the eyelid and eyebrow being sites of predilection for this tumor.[54] Most of the tumors contain varying amounts of calcium. No malignant transformation has ever been reported.

Histologically, the dermis shows well-circumscribed, irregular islands of uniform, small, basophilic cells. Foci of calcification and foreign body giant cells with a variable mixed inflammatory infiltrate and fibrosis are present.

Treatment is by simple surgical excision.

Tumors of Sebaceous Gland Origin

Three subtypes of sebaceous glands are present in the eyelids: meibomian glands, glands of Zeis, and skin sebaceous glands. The meibomian glands are confined to the tarsal plates of the eyelid and contribute a surface oily layer to the tear film that retards its evaporation. The glands of Zeis are sebaceous glands associated with the eyelash follicles.

SEBACEOUS GLAND HYPERPLASIA

Hypertrophy or hyperplasia of the meibomian glands, which usually occurs in the elderly patient, appears as single or multiple small nodules in the eyelids.[55] The lids may appear thickened and may become secondarily

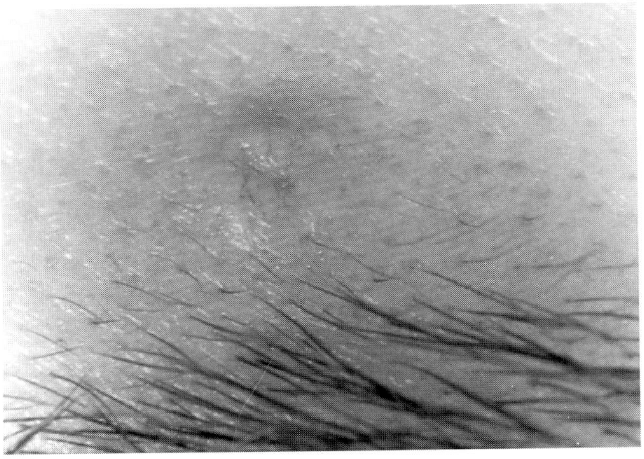

Figure 31 – 23. Sebaceous adenoma shown as a yellowish nodule above the brow in an elderly patient. This lesion may be mistaken for a basal cell carcinoma.

ectropic. Chronic blepharitis may coexist with these lesions. The differential diagnosis of sebaceous gland carcinoma must always be considered when these characteristics are present. The lesions may also mimic plexiform neuroma, amyloid, and lymphoma. A biopsy may be required to exclude these lesions.

Treatment is by surgery, if required to reposition the eyelids, and lid hygiene and administration of topical antibiotics, or steroids, or both, to treat any associated blepharitis.

SEBACEOUS ADENOMA

Sebaceous adenoma is rare and appears as a yellowish papule, usually in elderly patients (Fig. 31 – 23). It may mimic a basal cell carcinoma or a seborrheic keratosis. The lesions may affect the face, scalp, or trunk. Sebaceous adenoma may serve as a cutaneous marker for low-grade internal malignancies; this combination is known as *Torre's syndrome*.[48, 56]

Treatment is by excisional biopsy, which is usually required to establish an accurate diagnosis.

BENIGN PIGMENTARY LESIONS

Benign cutaneous pigmented tumors are derived from three sources: nevus cells, epidermal melanocytes, and dermal melanocytes. All three cells are derived embryologically from the neural crest. Nevus cells are regarded by many authorities as specialized melanocytes that show a characteristic tendency to organize into focal nests within the skin. Lesions that arise in the epidermis are derived either from nevus cells or melanocytes. In contrast, lesions arising in the dermis are believed to be derived purely from melanocytes.

Nevocellular Nevi

Considerable variation exists in the clinical appearance of nevocellular nevi. Their appearance on the eyelid skin or margin is common. They are divided in three histologic types: junctional, compound, and intradermal. Nevocellular nevi are seldom present as congenital lesions but tend to appear in childhood and increase in size and pigmentation at puberty. The histologic type may frequently be predicted on the basis of the clinical features.

Junctional nevi arise from the deeper layers of the epidermis and do not involve the underlying dermis. Most nevi affecting young children are of this type. Clinically, the lesions appear as flat, pigmented macules that are round or oval in shape. They tend to grow slowly in size, reaching up to 6 mm in diameter.

Compound nevi possess features of both junctional and intradermal nevi. Nevus cell nests may be seen in the epidermis, they may "drop off" from the epidermis into the dermis, and they may be in the dermis. Compound nevi are commoner than purely junctional nevi and affect older children and young adults. They may involve an equal portion (mirror image) of the upper and lower eyelid margins ("kissing nevi") (Fig. 31 – 24). The "kissing nevus" occurs when the developing lid folds, which contain embryonic nests of nevus cells, meet during the eighth week of gestation and remain fused until the end of the fifth month, when separation occurs.

Intradermal nevi are the commonest of the three types of nevi. They are most commonly found in adults. They usually show only very slight and occasionally no junctional activity. Melanocytes are present as discrete rests or sheets of cuboidal cells in the dermis. They appear as dome-shaped, sessile, verrucous, or even polypoid lesions, occasionally containing hairs (Fig. 31 – 25). They are often found on the eyelid margin. The degree of pigmentation is variable; the lesions may appear light brown

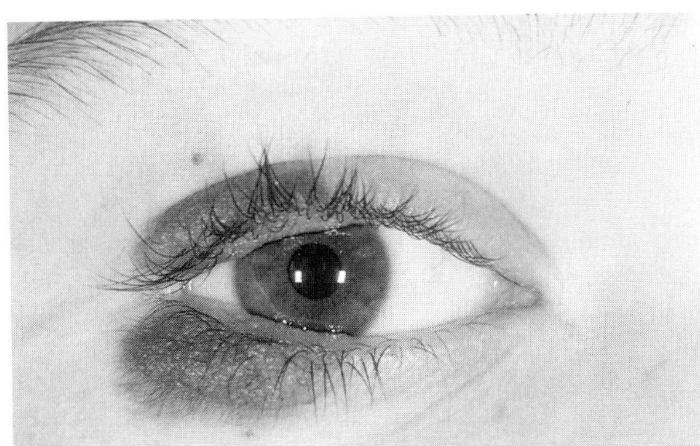

Figure 31 – 24. "Kissing nevus" secondary to the deposition of nevus cells in the eyelid fold while the lids are fused during embryogenesis.

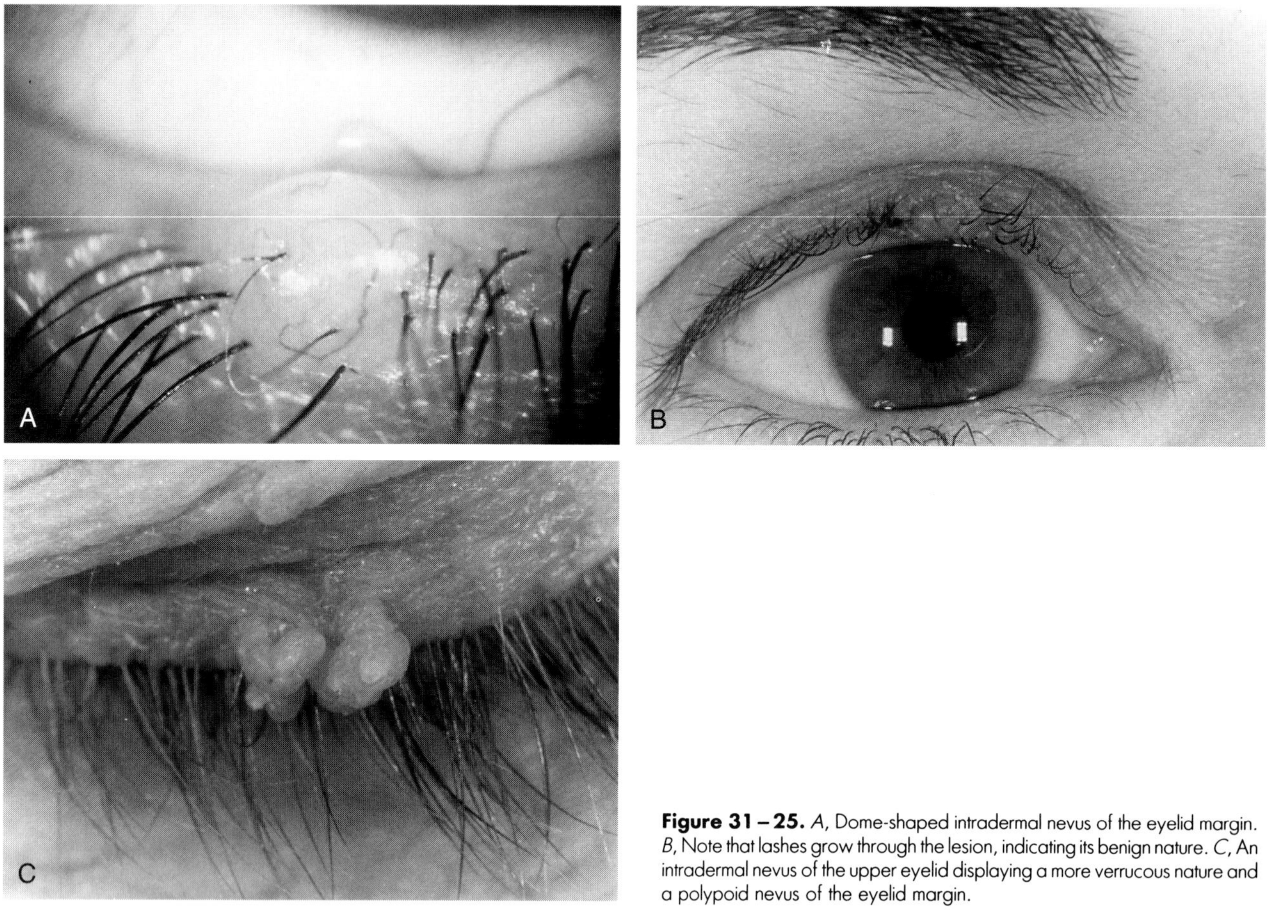

Figure 31 – 25. *A*, Dome-shaped intradermal nevus of the eyelid margin. *B*, Note that lashes grow through the lesion, indicating its benign nature. *C*, An intradermal nevus of the upper eyelid displaying a more verrucous nature and a polypoid nevus of the eyelid margin.

to flesh-colored. Junctional and compound nevi have the capacity to evolve into melanoma, although this occurrence is uncommon. Malignant change in a purely intradermal nevus is, in contrast, very rare. Signs that malignant degeneration may be occurring include a large size (>6 mm in diameter), an irregular asymmetric shape, multiple colors, and bleeding. These signs necessitate a biopsy.

Treatment consists of surgical excision for cosmetic reasons or because of concern about malignant change. A complete excision must be performed because incomplete excision may result in a recurrence, which may be difficult to differentiate clinically and histopathologically from a melanoma.

Two variants of nevocellular nevi may affect the eyelids: the balloon cell nevus and the spindle or epithelioid nevus (juvenile melanoma). The balloon cell nevus possesses no distinguishing clinical features and is very rare. Histologically, the balloon cells, which are larger than conventional nevus cells, may comprise only a small portion of an intradermal nevus, or they may appear as the major component of the nevus. Their nuclei are small and pyknotic and are located either paracentrally or eccentrically at one pole of the cell. The spindle or epithelioid nevus is a form of compound nevus that mainly affects children and young adults. The lesion appears as a dome-shaped, reddish-pink nodule. Histologically, the lesion has scattered mitotic figures and secondary inflammatory features, but despite this disturbing appearance, it usually pursues an entirely benign clinical course.

Congenital Nevus

Congenital nevi may be single or multiple and are generally larger than acquired nevi, measuring greater than 1.5 cm in diameter. Occasionally, they may be of considerable size. They are usually flat, but occasionally papules or nodules develop over time (Fig. 31 – 26). They may vary in color from dark to light brown and often contain dark coarse hairs. These nevi are of concern because of their malignant potential, which increases with lesion size. The development of melanoma is common, even in childhood.

Treatment for large nevi of the eyelids is difficult because removal would involve a potentially disfiguring procedure. Frequent observation rather than routine excision may be warranted in many cases.

Blue Nevus

The blue nevus arises from dermal melanocytes that are deeply located and have been arrested in the dermis

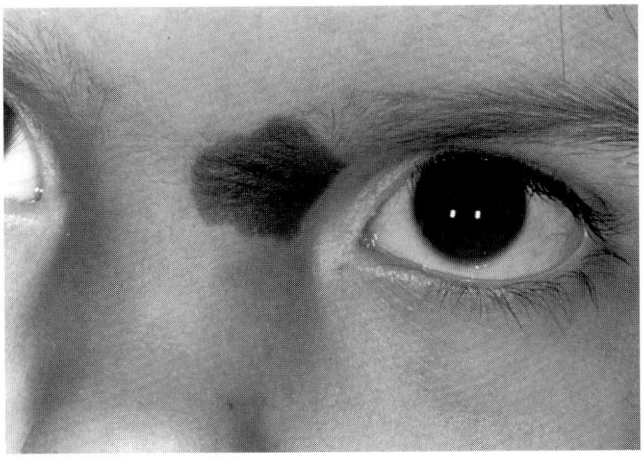

Figure 31 – 26. Fairly heavily pigmented congenital nevus in the left brow area.

before reaching the epidermis. Two types are recognized: the blue nevus and the cellular blue nevus. The blue nevus is a dome-shaped, small, blue papule or nodule that has no malignant potential. When a compound nevus is present over a conventional blue nevus histologically, the lesion is called a *combined nevus.* The cellular blue nevus consists of a bluish nodule that is usually larger than the common blue nevus. It generally measures 2 to 3 cm in diameter, but it may be larger. Malignant degeneration is recognized with lymph node metastasis, but this is a rare event.

Treatment is by surgical excision for cosmetic reasons or in cases in which the diagnosis is in doubt.

Ota's Nevus (Oculodermal Melanocytosis)

Ota's nevus is a bluish discoloration of the eyelids and periorbital skin, usually occurring unilaterally, although bilateral involvement may occur. The temple, forehead, malar region, and nose may also be involved. There is frequently a patchy bluish discoloration of the sclera of the ipsilateral eye, and occasionally also of the conjunctiva, episclera, uveal tract, and optic disc. The oral and nasal mucosa may also be involved. The lesions of Ota's nevus may be present at birth, or they may appear during the first year of life or adolescence, but they appear only rarely in childhood. They have a tendency toward gradual extension. Malignant change in the cutaneous lesions of Ota's nevus is extremely rare. The incidence of uveal melanomas is increased in patients with this condition.[57]

No specific treatment exists for Ota's nevus. Frequent follow-up with dilated fundoscopy is required to exclude the development of a uveal melanoma.

Freckle (Ephelis)

Freckles are small, well-circumscribed, red-brown macules, which appear as scattered lesions over sun-exposed areas of the skin, including the eyelids (Fig. 31 – 27). Exposure to sunlight causes darkening of the macules. The typical appearance and patient's history of darkening on sun exposure easily differentiate freckles from junctional nevi and lentigines.

Lentigo Simplex

The lesions of lentigo simplex are flat macules, brown to black in color, usually measuring 1 to 2 mm in diameter. Clinically, they are indistinguishable from junctional nevi. They are unaffected by exposure to sunlight.

Solar Lentigo

The lesions of lentigo senilis are light to dark brown, slowly expanding macules that develop in sun-exposed areas of the skin, including the eyelids. They occur in over 90% of elderly whites. They begin as small macules, 3 to 5 mm in diameter, and gradually increase in size to several centimeters in diameter (Fig. 31 – 28). Lentigo senilis must be differentiated from lentigo maligna and lentigo malignant melanoma. Lentigo maligna (Hutchinson's melanotic freckle, precancerous melanosis) is a slowly enlarging brown patch that is frequently found in the malar region in patients over the age of 50 years. Unlike lentigo senilis, a variegated brown pigmentation with irregular borders is present. After a variable period of radial extension, which may be decades, nodules of invasive melanoma develop in 30% to 50% of cases. When this occurs, the lesion is termed *lentigo maligna melanoma.* Malignant change is suggested by irregular borders, multiple colors, large size, and bleeding.

The lesions may be treated with liquid nitrogen, if the patient desires treatment.

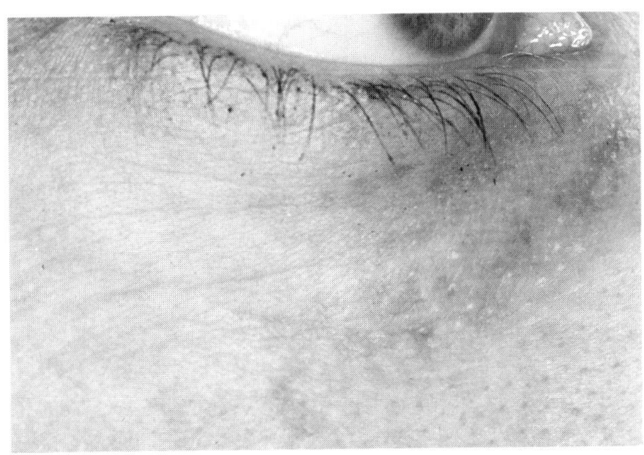

Figure 31 – 27. Freckle "ephelides" are reddish-brown macules found on sun-exposed areas of the body, including the face and the eyelids. Histologically, freckles are recognized by an increase in the distribution of pigment among basal epithelial cells without an increase in the absolute number of melanocytes.

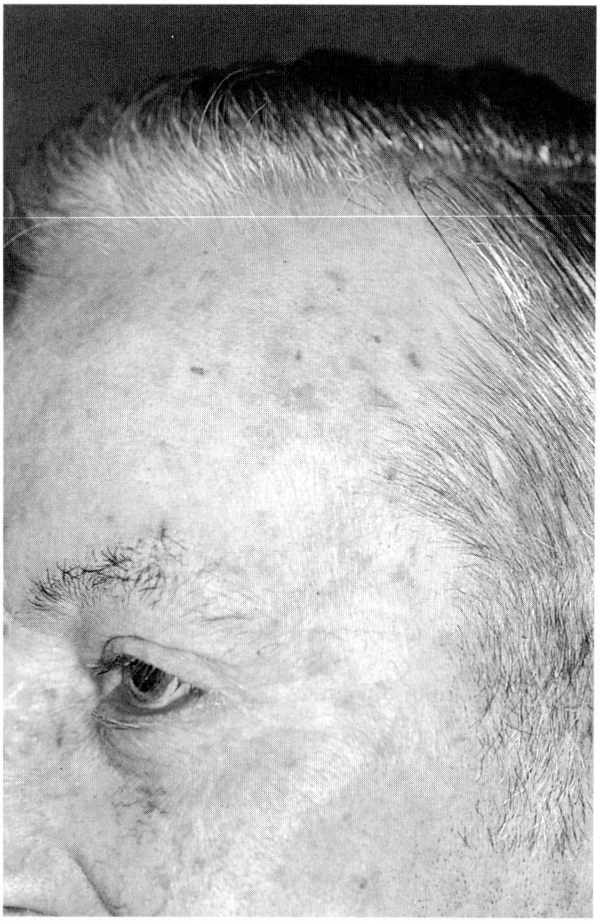

Figure 31 – 28. Solar lentigo (senile lentigo, or liver spots) are common brownish macules seen in most fair-skinned people. The pigmentation of these lesions is fairly uniform, which helps differentiate it from lentigo maligna melanoma (a precancerous condition), which is variably pigmented.

CONCLUSION

The eyelids have many components from which a multitude of benign tumors may arise. Most of these benign tumors are of cutaneous origin, arising from the structures that comprise the eyelid skin. These structures are the epidermis, the dermis, the adnexa (the pilosebaceous unit and the eccrine and apocrine sweat glands), and the associated pigment cells. Many of these cutaneous lesions arise elsewhere on the skin, but a few, such as syringomas and hydrocystomas, more commonly affect the skin of the eyelids.

The lesions may be solid or cystic, solitary or multiple. Occasionally, a diagnosis is readily made on the basis of a classic appearance and clinical behavior. In other cases, the diagnosis can be made only with the aid of a biopsy. Appropriate treatment is based on an accurate diagnosis. Importantly, because some seemingly benign eyelid lesions have malignant potential, changes in the appearance of an eyelid lesion, such as increase in size, irregular shape, or bleeding, necessitate a biopsy.

REFERENCES

1. Domonkos AN, Arnold HL, Odom RB (eds): Andrew's Diseases of the Skin. Philadelphia, WB Saunders, 1982, p 773.
2. Epstein W, Kligman AM: The pathogenesis of milia and benign tumors of the skin. J Invest Dermatol 26:1 – 11, 1956.
3. Sanderson KV: The structure of seborrheic keratosis. Br J Dermatol 80:588 – 593, 1968.
4. Scully J: Treatment of seborrheic keratosis. JAMA 213:1498, 1970.
5. Boynton JR, Searl SS, Caldwell EH: Large periocular keratoacanthoma: The case for definitive treatment. Ophthalmic Surg 17(9):565 – 569, 1986.
6. Farina AT, Leider M, Newall J, Carella R: Radiotherapy for aggressive and destructive keratoacanthomas. J Dermatol Surg Oncol 3:177 – 180, 1977.
7. Eubanks SW, Gentry RH, Patteson JW, et al: Treatment of multiple keratoacanthomas with intralesional fluorouracil. J Am Acad Dermatol 7:126 – 129, 1982.
8. Goette DK, Odom RB, Arrott JW, et al: Treatment of keratoacanthoma with topical application of fluorouracil. Arch Dermatol 118:309 – 311, 1982.
9. Odom RB, Goette DK: Treatment of keratoacanthomas with intralesional fluorouracil. Arch Dermatol 114:1779 – 1783, 1978.
10. Boniuk M, Zimmerman LE: Eyelid tumors with reference to lesions confused with squamous cell carcinoma. II: Inverted follicular keratosis. Arch Ophthalmol 69:698 – 707, 1963.
11. McGavran MH, Binnington B: Keratinous cysts of the skin. Arch Dermatol 94:499 – 508, 1966.
12. Solomon LM, Fretzin DF, Dewald RL: The epidermal nevus syndrome. Arch Dermatol 97:273 – 285, 1968.
13. Roenigk HH Jr: Dermabrasion for miscellaneous cutaneous lesions (exclusive of scarring from acne). J Dermatol Surg Oncol 3(3):322 – 328, 1977.
14. Wanjo T, Tenzel PR: Actinic comedonal plaque of the eyelid. Am J Ophthalmol 96(5):687 – 688, 1983.
15. Brownstein MH, Helwig EB: Subcutaneous dermoid cysts. Arch Dermatol 107:237 – 239, 1973.
16. Jakobiec FA, Bonanno PA, Sigelman J: Conjunctival adnexal cysts and dermoids. Arch Ophthalmol 96:1404 – 1409, 1978.
17. Rodgers IR, Jakobiec FA, Krebs, W, et al: Papillary oncocytoma of the eyelid. A previously undescribed tumor of apocrine gland origin. Ophthalmology 95(8):1071 – 1076, 1988.
18. Thaller VT, Collin JRO, McCartney ACE: Oncocytoma of the eyelid: A case report. Br J Ophthalmol 71:753 – 756, 1987.
19. Filipic M, Silva M: Phakomatous choristoma of the eyelid. Arch Ophthalmol 88:172 – 175, 1972.
20. Tripathi RC, Tripathi BJ, Ringus J: Phakomatous choristoma of the lower eyelid with psammoma body formation. Ophthalmology 88(11):1198 – 1206, 1981.
21. Zimmermann LE: Phakomatous choristoma of the eyelid, a tumor of lenticular anlage. Am J Ophthalmol 71:169 – 171, 1971.
22. Shields JA, Guibor PG: Neurilemmoma of the eyelid resembling a recurrent chalazion. Arch Ophthalmol 102:1650, 1984.
23. Friedman Z, Eden E, Neumann E: Granular cell myoblastoma of the eyelid margin. Br J Ophthalmol 57:757 – 760, 1973.
24. Noe JM, Barsky SH, Greer DE, et al: Port-wine stains and the response to argon laser therapy: Successful treatment and predictive role of color, age, and biopsy. Plast Reconstr Surg 65:130 – 136, 1980.
25. Haik BG, Jakobiec FA, Ellsworth RM: Capillary hemangioma of the lids and orbit. Ophthalmology 86:760 – 789, 1979.
26. Stigmar G, Crawford JS, Ward CM, Thomson HG: Ophthalmic sequelae of infantile hemangiomas of the eyelids and orbit. Am J Ophthalmol 85:806 – 813, 1978.
27. Glatt HJ, Putterman AM, Van Aalst JJ, et al: Adrenal suppression and growth retardation after injection of periocular capillary hemangioma with corticosteroids. Ophthalmic Surg 22(2):95 – 97, 1991.
28. Kushner B: Intralesional corticosteroid injection for infantile adnexal hemangioma. Am J Ophthalmol 93:496 – 506, 1982.
29. Jakobiec FA, Jones I: *In* Duane T (ed): Clinical Ophthalmology, vol 2. Philadelphia, Harper & Row, 37:6, 1983.
30. Pang P, Jakobiec FA, Iwamato T, Hornblass A: Small lymphangiomas of the eyelids. Ophthalmology 91(10):1278 – 1284, 1984.

31. Jones IS: Lymphangiomas of the ocular adnexa. An analysis of 62 cases. Trans Am Ophthalmol Soc 57:602–665, 1959.
32. Holt JE, Holt GR, Thornton WR: Arteriovenous malformation of the eyelid. Ophthalmic Surg 11:771–777, 1980.
33. Charles NC: Multiple glomus tumors of the face and eyelids. Arch Ophthalmol 94:1283–1285, 1976.
34. Sorenson RL, Spencer WH, Stewart WB, et al: Intravascular papillary endothelial hyperplasia of the eyelid. Arch Ophthalmol 101:1728–1730, 1983.
35. Clearkin KB, Enzinger FM: Intravascular papillary endothelial hyperplasia. Arch Pathol Lab Med 100:441–444, 1976.
36. Vinger P, Sach B: Ocular manifestations of hyperlipidemia. Am J Ophthalmol 70(4):563–573, 1970.
37. Zimmerman LE: Ocular lesions of juvenile xanthogranuloma (nevoxanthoendothelioma). Trans Am Acad Ophthalmol Otolaryngol 69:412–439, 1965.
38. John T, Yanoff M, Scheie HG: Eyelid fibrous histiocytoma. Ophthalmology 88(11):1193–1195, 1981.
39. Jordan DR, Anderson RL: Fibrous histiocytoma. An uncommon eyelid lesion. Arch Ophthalmol 107(10):1530–1531, 1989.
40. Ni C, Dryja TP, Albert DM: Sweat gland tumors in the eyelids: A clinicopathological analysis of 55 cases. Int Ophthalmol Clin 22(1):1–22, 1982.
41. Maloney ME: An easy method for removal of syringoma. J Dermatol Surg Oncol 8(11):973–975, 1982.
42. Nerad JA, Anderson RL: CO_2 laser treatment of eyelid syringomas. Ophthalmic Plast Reconstr Surg 4(2):91–94, 1988.
43. Kersting DW, Helwig EB: Eccrine spiradenoma. Arch Dermatol 73:199–227, 1956.
44. Boniuk M, Halpert B: Clear cell hidradenoma or myoepithelioma of the eyelid. Arch Ophthalmol 72:59–63, 1964.
45. Ferry AP, Hadad HM: Eccrine acrospiroma (porosyringoma) of the eyelid. Arch Ophthalmol 83:591–593, 1970.
46. Greer CH: Clear-cell hidradenoma of the eyelid. Arch Ophthalmol 80:220–222, 1968.
47. Smith JD, Chernosky ME: Hidrocytomas. Arch Dermatol 108:676–679, 1973.
48. Jakobiec FA: Sebaceous adenoma of the eyelid and visceral malignancy. Am J Ophthalmol 78(6):952–960, 1974.
49. Jakobiec FA, Streeten BW, Iwamato T, et al: Syringocystadenoma papilliferum of the eyelid. Ophthalmology 88(11):1175–1181, 1981.
50. Hashimoto K, Lever WF: Histogenesis of skin appendage tumors. Arch Dermatol 100:356–369, 1969.
51. Pinkus H, Sutton R: Trichofolliculoma. Arch Dermatol 91:46–49, 1965.
52. Hidayat AA, Font RL: Trichilemmoma of eyelid and eyebrow: A clinicopathological study of 31 cases. Arch Ophthalmol 98:844–847, 1980.
53. Brownstein MH, Mehregan AH, Bikowski JB, et al: The dermatopathology of Cowden's syndrome. Br J Dermatol 100:667–673, 1979.
54. O'Grady RB, Spoerl G: Pilomatrixoma (benign calcifying epithelioma of Malherbe). Ophthalmology 88(11):1196–1197, 1981.
55. Yanoff M, Fine BS: Ocular Pathology, 2nd ed. Philadelphia, Harper & Row, 1982, pp 34, 220, 291, 661.
56. Torre D: Multiple sebaceous tumors. Arch Dermatol 98:549–551, 1968.
57. Dutton JJ, Anderson RL, Schelper RL, et al: Orbital malignant melanoma and oculodermal melanocytosis: Report of two cases and review of the literature. Ophthalmology 91(5):497–506, 1984.
58. Hodgson C: Senile lentigo. Arch Dermatol 87:197–207, 1963.
59. Duke-Elder S: System of Ophthalmology, vol 13. St. Louis, CV Mosby, 1974, pp 470, 514.
60. Hirsch P, Helwig EB: Chondroid syringoma: Mixed tumor of the skin, salivary gland type. Arch Dermatol 84:835–847, 1961.
61. Lever WF, Schaumburg G: Histopathology of the Skin, 6th ed. Philadelphia, JB Lippincott, 1983, pp 551–553, 681–702.

CHAPTER 32

Malignant Epithelial Eyelid Tumors

Marcos T. Doxanas

Effective management of malignant epithelial eyelid tumors requires an understanding of their clinical and pathologic features. By definition, these tumors are derived from the surface epithelium or eyelid appendages and assume characteristic clinical features. Malignant epithelial tumors affecting the eyelids are generally slowly enlarging, destructive lesions that distort if not destroy eyelid anatomy. Subtle anatomic changes are evident on biomicroscopic examination with the slit lamp, allowing early evaluation and therapy. However, these lesions are diagnosed only if a high degree of clinical suspicion is applied to every eyelid tumor.

Subtle features can differentiate malignant from benign epithelial tumors. As noted, alterations in the architecture or anatomy of the eyelid margins are characteristically associated with malignant tumors. These changes vary from the loss of eyelashes to obliteration of the eyelid margin (Fig. 32–1). Inflammatory conditions of the eyelid margins such as chalazions and chronic blepharitis also occasionally result in loss of lashes but do not destroy eyelid margin architecture. Pitting or notching of the posterior lamella of the eyelid is characteristic in patients with chronic blepharitis. In benign tumors involving the eyelid margins, such as seborrheic keratosis and dermal nevi, eyelashes extend through the tumor (Fig. 32–2). In addition, the vascular pattern of these tumors is distinct from that of malignant epithelial tumors. Malignant tumors characteristically have superficial telangiectatic vessels on their surface. Benign tumors such as seborrheic keratosis have pinpoint vessels feeding each epithelial proliferation of the tumor. Biomicroscopic evaluation can highlight these various features that differentiate benign from malignant tumors.

Eyelid tumors are discussed here in order of their frequency. We reviewed eyelid tumors submitted to the eye pathology laboratory at the Wilmer Eye Institute of the Johns Hopkins Hospital over a 58-year period, which permitted a statistical tabulation of eyelid tumors (Table 32–1). Of the 5392 tumors reviewed, 749 were malignant epithelial tumors (Table 32–2).[1-3] As expected, basal cell carcinoma was the most frequently encountered type of malignant epithelial tumor. Surprisingly, sebaceous gland carcinoma was the second most frequent. Most previously reported series of malignant epithelial tumors have found squamous cell carcinoma to be the second most frequent lesion.[4-6] Review of all eyelid tumors and application of more recently described histopathologic features account for the change in the order of frequency. In addition, the aggressive behavior of the morphea pattern basal cell carcinoma and sebaceous gland carcinoma has in the past been falsely attributed to squamous cell carcinoma. Once tumors were reclassified, a unique view of malignant epithelial tumors became evident. Tumor morbidity and mortality were significantly reduced by appropriate tumor diagnosis and a systematic approach to management.[1, 2]

Clinical and histopathologic features of commonly encountered malignant epithelial tumors are discussed. Management of these tumors consists of surgical excision with monitoring of margins by frozen section controls. Specific management concerns are addressed with each tumor discussed.

BASAL CELL CARCINOMA

Basal cell carcinoma is frequently encountered on the eyelids, accounting for 12.4% (671/5392) of all eyelid tumors and 89.5% (671/749) of malignant epithelial tumors in the Wilmer Eye Institute series. Sunlight (specifically ultraviolet light) exposure is now recognized as an important etiologic factor in the development of epithelial malignancies.[7] This is particularly prevalent in fair-skinned people. The effects of sun exposure are cumulative, as reflected in the increasing incidence of the tumor with advancing age. Basal cell carcinoma may occur in younger patients, especially those with a tumor diathesis predisposing to cutaneous malignancies, such as xeroderma pigmentosa or the nevoid basal cell carcinoma syndrome.[8, 9] Basal cell carcinomas are most prominent on the lower eyelid, followed by the medial canthus. The upper lid and lateral canthus are the areas least frequently affected.

Clinically, basal cell carcinomas have a variety of presentations, as a direct reflection of the various histopathologic patterns of the tumor. The most common presen-

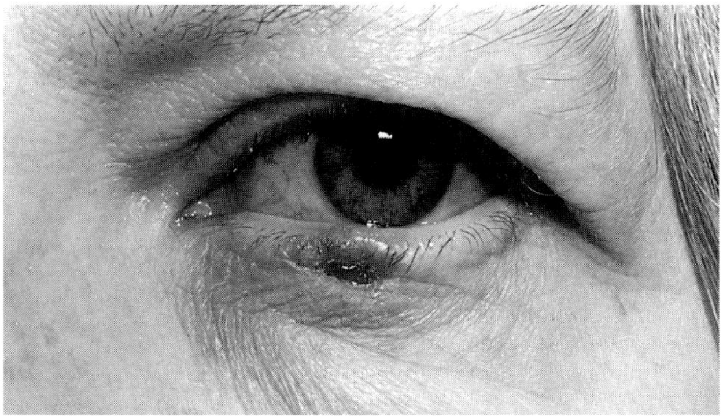

Figure 32–1. Basal cell carcinoma of the eyelid margin. Distortion of the eyelid margin architecture with loss of eyelashes is shown.

tation is a nodular pattern. The epithelial proliferation produces a solid pearly lesion contiguous with the surface epithelium. The superficial nature of telangiectatic vessels may predispose these lesions to spontaneous bleeding. With prolonged growth, central umbilication and ulceration will occur.

Nodular basal cell carcinomas may assume various clinical presentations such as papilloma (secondary to increased keratin production), a nevus (secondary to pigmentation), and a cyst (due to central tumor necrosis). The variety of clinical presentations of basal cell carcinoma accounts for the high incidence of misdiagnosis.[10, 11] However, biomiscroscopic evaluation enables the ophthalmologist to recognize the various presentations, allowing a correct diagnosis of basal cell carcinoma despite the masquerading posture of the tumor. Again, clinical awareness of the various presentations of the tumor minimizes incorrect clinical diagnoses and management.

Basal cell carcinoma may present as an infiltrative tumor, with extensive involvement of the eyelids.[12, 13] Failure to suspect and diagnose this tumor permits slow, indolent tumor progression. This pattern of basal cell carcinoma is of concern because of potential orbital extension, since actual epithelial involvement does not fully indicate the extent of the tumor.

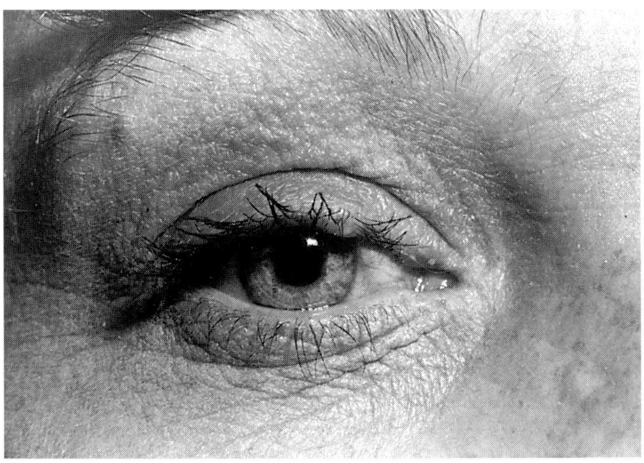

Figure 32–2. Dermal nevus of the eyelid margin. Eyelashes growing through the tumor indicate a benign tumor.

TABLE 32–1

Classificaton of Eyelid Tumors: Wilmer Eye Institute

Type of Tumor	No. Tumors
Benign surface epithelial	1995
Inflammatory	1073
Malignant epithelial	749
Mesenchymal	567
Nevocellular	513
Benign adnexal epithelial	400
Lymphocytic	37
Miscellaneous	58

The various clinical presentations of basal cell carcinoma are directly correlated with morphologic patterns of the tumor. Histologically, features of basal cell carcinoma are (1) proliferation of cells that resemble the basal layers of the epithelium, (2) peripheral palisading of the basal cells, and (3) artifactual shrinkage of the tumor from the surrounding connective tissue (Fig. 32–3). The characteristic basal cell is a small cell with an oval nucleus and scant cytoplasm. Generally, little inflammation is present in the stroma. This is in contrast with squamous cell or sebaceous gland carcinomas, in which a prominent inflammatory component may accompany stromal infiltration.

Lund[14] originally identified six morphologic patterns of basal cell carcinoma. These can be condensed to four as they pertain to the eyelids: nodular, ulcerative, morphea, and superficial spreading (multicentric). An appreciation of these patterns significantly enhances one's ability to diagnose and effectively manage these tumors.

Nodular Pattern. The nodular pattern is the most frequently encountered form of basal cell carcinoma. Clinically, these tumors present as well-demarcated epithelial lesions in which the extent of the tumor is clearly evident (Fig. 32–4*A*). The nodular pattern consists of a distinct nodular proliferation of basaloid cells with no infiltration into underlying tissues (see Fig. 32–4*B*). Compression of the surrounding connective tissue will produce a pseudocapsule, which appears to further confine or define the tumor's extension.

TABLE 32–2

Malignant Epithelial Tumors: Wilmer Eye Institute

Type of Tumor	No. Tumors
Basal cell carcinoma	671
Sebaceous gland carcinoma	40
Squamous cell carcinoma	31
Adenoacanthoma	3
Eccrine adenocarcinoma	1
Clear cell hidradenocarcinoma	1
Adnexal carcinoma	1
Transitional cell carcinoma	1

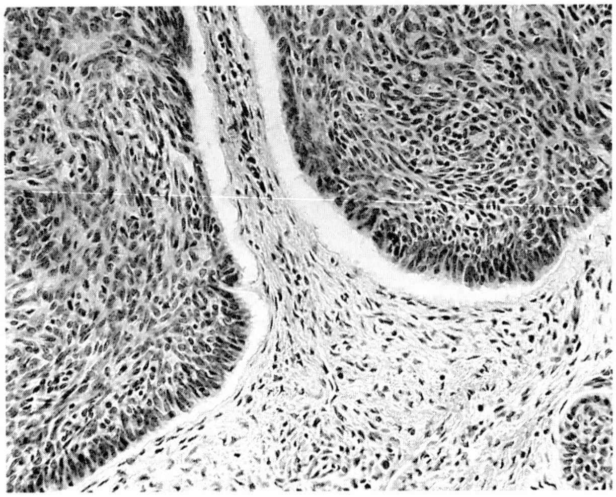

Figure 32–3. Basal cell carcinoma. Histologic features of basal cell carcinoma include basal cell proliferation, peripheral palisading of basal cells with artifactual separation of surrounding connective tissue.

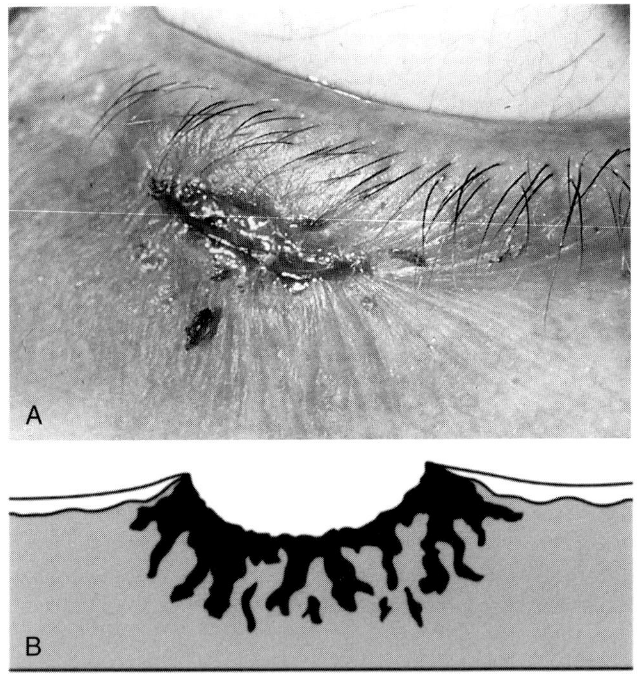

Figure 32–5. Ulcerative basal cell carcinoma. *A,* Clinical appearance. *B,* Schematic representation of ulcerative pattern, with more extensive dermal infiltration. (*B* from Doxanas MT, Green WR, Iliff CE: Factors in the successful surgical management of basal cell carcinoma of the eyelids. Am J Ophthalmol 91:726–736, 1981. Published with permission from The American Journal of Ophthalmology. Copyright by The Ophthalmic Publishing Company.)

Ulcerative Pattern. Clinically, the ulcerative pattern of basal cell carcinoma may be a direct progression of an untreated nodular pattern. Epithelial proliferation produces a raised, pearly white tumor margin that blends into the surrounding noninvolved skin (Fig. 32–5*A*). This tumor has a true central ulcerative crater devoid of surface epithelium. Spontaneous bleeding frequently occurs due to the telangiectatic vessels at or near the central crater. Histologically, the tumor extends into the dermis and potentially beyond the area of suspected clinical involvement (see Fig. 32–5*B*). This is a more aggressive pattern of basal cell carcinoma.

Morphea Pattern. The morphea pattern is an aggressive variation or form of basal cell carcinoma. Clinically, an apparent minimal involvement of the epithelium may obscure the extensive dermal infiltration of the tumor (Fig. 32–6*A*). Histopathologically, the basaloid cell proliferation is distributed in cords or islands in a dense connective tissue framework (see Fig. 32–6*B* and *C*). There may be little involvement or irregularity of adjacent surface epithelium. Complete surgical removal is difficult because of the extent of clinical involvement. Wide areas of resection are occasionally required to obtain specimens free of tumor. Monitoring of surgical margins with frozen sections is imperative in tumor management.

Superficial Spreading (Multicentric) Pattern. In the superficial spreading pattern of basal cell carcinoma, also known as the multicentric form, strands of basaloid cells extend directly from the multiple foci of the basal layer of the epithelium and superficial corium. The multiple foci of tumor involvement suggest a multicentric involvement. Involvement of the deeper layers of the corium generally does not occur, however. Clinically, the epithe-

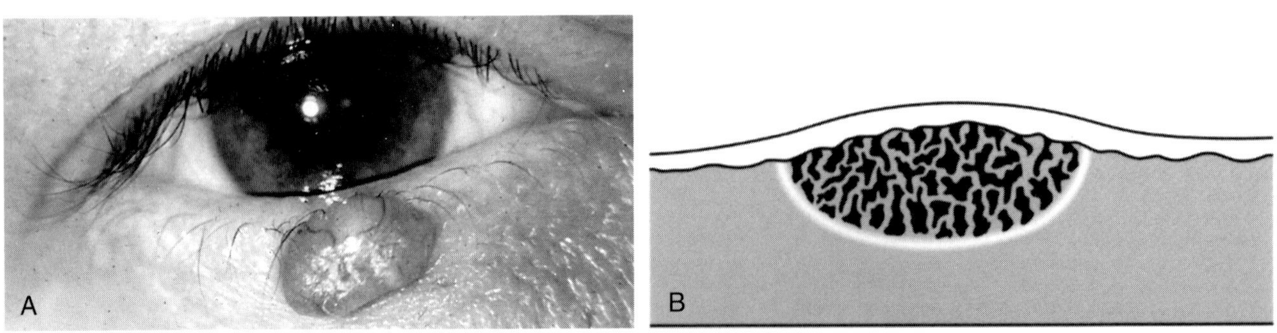

Figure 32–4. Nodular basal cell carcinoma. *A,* Clinical presentation of distinct tumor with pearly epithelial proliferation and superficial telangiectatic vessels. *B,* Schematic representation of nodular morphologic pattern that appears well circumscribed with minimal dermal infiltration. (*B,* from Doxanas M, Green WR, Iliff CE: Factors in the successful surgical management of basal cell carcinoma of the eyelids. Am J Ophthalmol 91:726–736, 1981. Published with permission from The American Journal of Ophthalmology. Copyright by The Ophthalmic Publishing Company.)

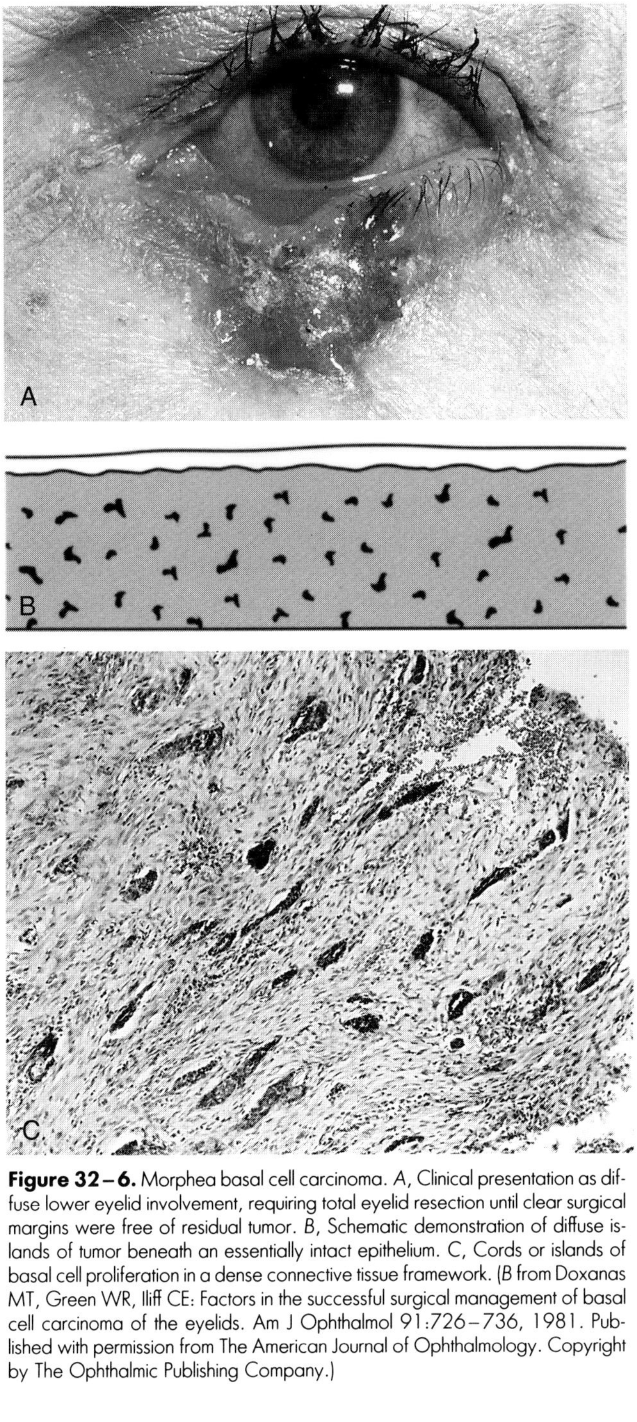

Figure 32–6. Morphea basal cell carcinoma. *A*, Clinical presentation as diffuse lower eyelid involvement, requiring total eyelid resection until clear surgical margins were free of residual tumor. *B*, Schematic demonstration of diffuse islands of tumor beneath an essentially intact epithelium. C, Cords or islands of basal cell proliferation in a dense connective tissue framework. (*B* from Doxanas MT, Green WR, Iliff CE: Factors in the successful surgical management of basal cell carcinoma of the eyelids. Am J Ophthalmol 91:726–736, 1981. Published with permission from The American Journal of Ophthalmology. Copyright by The Ophthalmic Publishing Company.)

lium assumes irregular variations and elevations reflective of underlying tumor involvement (Fig. 32–7). Again, surgical margins of excision should be monitored by frozen section controls.

A review of the tumors at the eye pathology laboratory of the Wilmer Eye Institute revealed that the most commonly encountered morphologic patterns of basal cell carcinoma were the nodular and ulcerative forms. These patterns were particularly common with primary tumors; recurrent tumors were much more likely to have a morphea pattern. All patients undergoing orbital exenteration had tumors with a morphea pattern. These features suggest that the morphea pattern is an aggressive form of basal cell carcinoma, necessitating complete tumor eradication with frozen section monitoring of surgical margins. If free margins cannot be obtained, orbital exenteration may be required. This is particularly common if the medial canthal area is involved.

Traditionally, basal cell carcinomas were thought to be relatively benign, rarely invasive tumors and were therefore casually excised. Previous studies noted an incidence of incompletely excised tumors ranging from 20% to 50%.[15–17] An earlier study at the Wilmer Eye Institute confirmed the use of frozen section controls as an effective means of minimizing recurrences, significantly reducing tumor morbidity and mortality.[1] On review of the tumors at the Wilmer Eye Institute, 15 patients were found to have extensive orbital involvement requiring exenteration. Intracranial extension resulted in induced mortality in six patients. A dedicated approach to tumor eradication is clearly essential in the management of these patients. Irradiation or cryotherapy has no role in the management of periocular basal cell carcinoma.

SEBACEOUS GLAND CARCINOMA

Considerable confusion clouds a clear appreciation of sebaceous gland carcinoma. Historically, studies report-

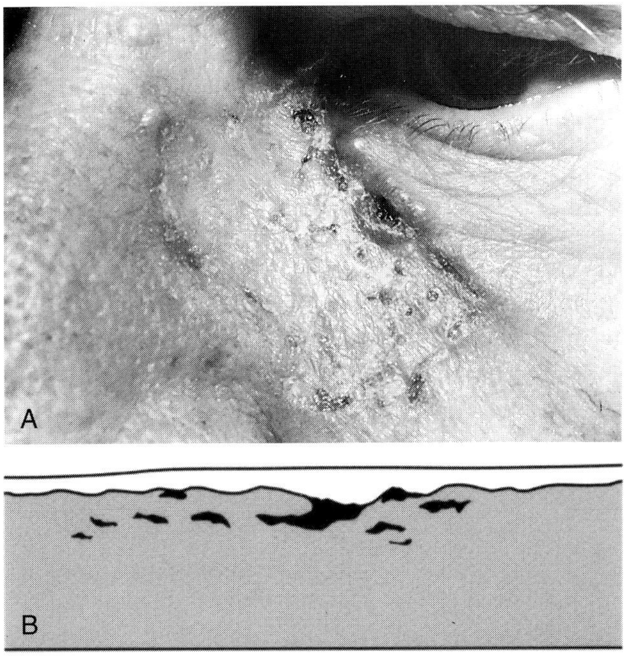

Figure 32–7. Superficial spreading basal cell carcinoma. *A*, Clinical presentation of widespread, although superficial, eyelid involvement. *B*, Schematic demonstration of multiple tumor foci from the basal layer of the epithelium. (*B* from Doxanas MT, Green WR, Iliff CE: Factors in the successful surgical management of basal cell carcinoma of the eyelids. Am J Ophthalmol 91:726–736, 1981. Published with permission from The American Journal of Ophthalmology. Copyright by The Ophthalmic Publishing Company.)

ing or tabulating eyelid tumors have failed to diagnose and report sebaceous gland carcinoma.[4–6] Straatsma's[18] study of sebaceous gland tumors in 1956 highlighted the spectrum of abnormalities from hyperplasia to carcinoma. At that time only 97 sebaceous gland carcinomas had been reported in the world literature. The unique features of sebaceous gland carcinoma of meibomian gland origin have further confused the recognition of these tumors.

Sebaceous gland carcinomas are extremely rare, with a predilection for the ocular region. Dermal pathologists rarely encounter this tumor, as is demonstrated by the space allotted to this tumor in dermal pathology textbooks. Major textbooks of dermal pathology have less than one page devoted to sebaceous gland carcinoma.[19] In addition, sebaceous gland carcinoma in the eyelids has a tendency to produce widespread metastasis, whereas such tumors occurring elsewhere on the skin rarely metastasize.[20] These unique features of the tumor on the eyelids, with its aggressive metastatic potential, account for its frequent misdiagnosis. The aggressive behavior of this tumor has traditionally led to its misdiagnosis as squamous cell carcinoma, further obscuring its understanding.

Boniuk and Zimmerman[21] extensively reviewed the clinicopathologic features of 88 patients with sebaceous gland carcinomas, highlighting some unique features of this tumor. The tumor presents not only as a solid nodule of the eyelid but also as recurrent chalazions (Fig. 32–8)[22] or chronic blepharoconjunctivitis (Fig. 32–9).[23, 24] Histopathologic features of sebaceous gland carcinoma were also highlighted, permitting consistent recognition of the tumor. Recognition of the clinicopathologic features of sebaceous gland carcinoma permits its accurate diagnosis and appropriate management. The review of eyelid tumors at the Wilmer Eye Institute showed the tumor to be the second most frequent malignant epithelial lesion.

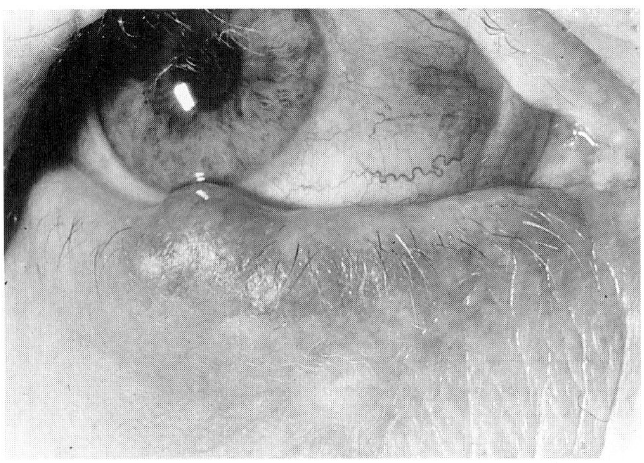

Figure 32–8. Sebaceous gland carcinoma. Clinical presentation of recurrent chalazion. Note the loss of eyelashes and distortion of the eyelid margin characteristic of malignant epithelial tumors.

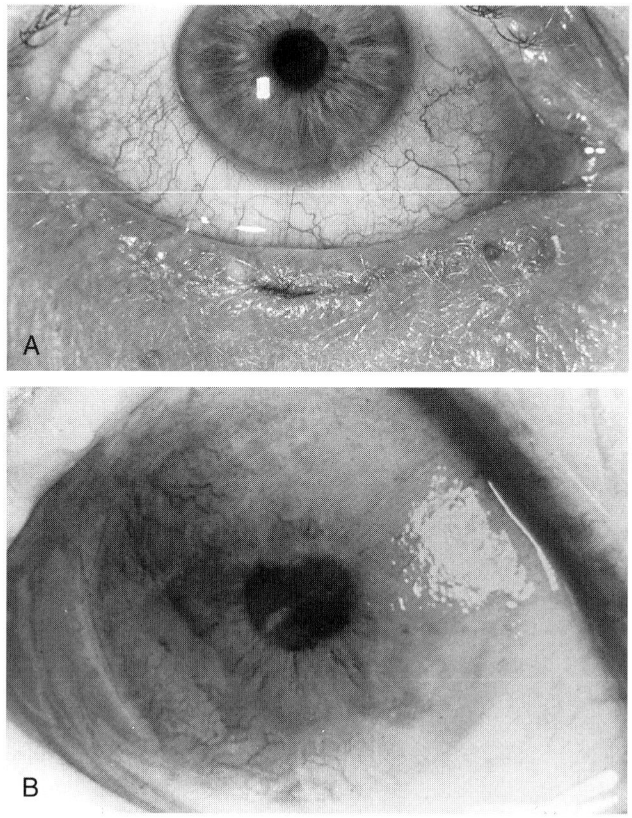

Figure 32–9. Sebaceous gland carcinoma. Clinical presentation is as chronic blepharoconjunctivitis distorting the eyelid margin architecture (*A*) or as diffuse keratoconjunctivitis (*B*).

Sebaceous gland carcinoma occurs with increasing frequency with advancing age. Patients with this type of tumor in the Wilmer Eye Institute series had a mean age of 67.9 years with a range of 39 to 88 years. The tumor has a predilection for the upper eyelid, but diffuse upper and lower eyelid involvement may occur in patients presenting with chronic blepharoconjunctivitis.

This tumor is now well recognized for its ability to masquerade as chronic blepharoconjunctivitis[23, 24] or recurrent chalazion.[22] Hagedoorn[23] first recognized the appearance of sebaceous gland carcinoma as chronic blepharoconjunctivitis. Since then, this has been recognized as a standard form of clinical presentation of the tumor, occurring in 30% to 38% of patients with sebaceous gland carcinoma. Sweebe and Cogan[22] reported the tumors presenting as recurrent chalazion. Again, since their report, recurrent chalazion or atypical solid chalazions have alerted the ophthalmologist to the possibility of underlying sebaceous gland carcinoma. This form occurs less frequently than solid tumors or blepharoconjunctivitis but accounts for 15% to 20% of sebaceous gland carcinomas. In the Wilmer Eye Institute series, recurrent chalazions had been excised as many as 8 times, with an average of 3.4 times, before appropriate histologic confirmation of the diagnosis of sebaceous gland carcinoma.

Histopathologic features of sebaceous gland carci-

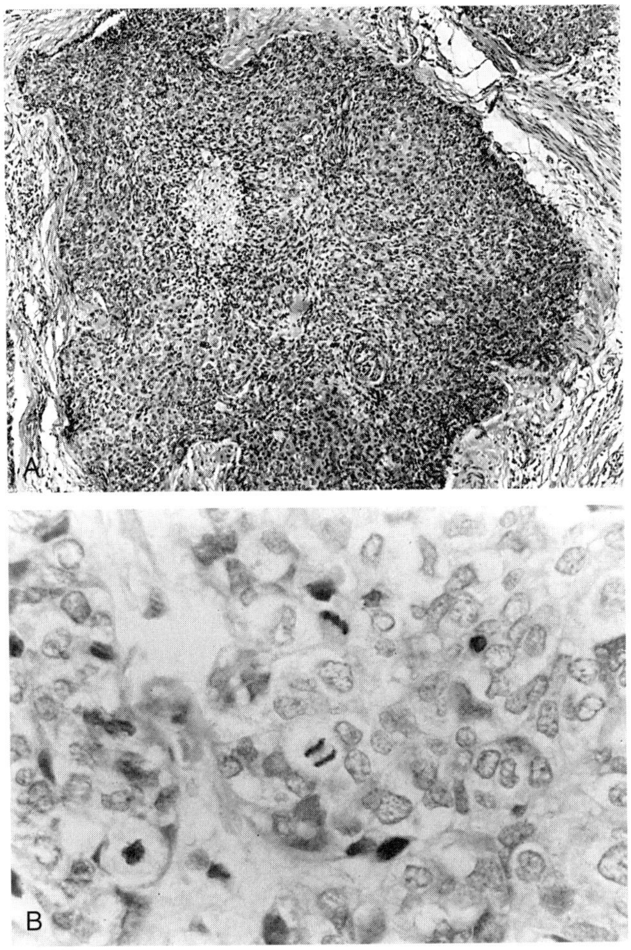

Figure 32–10. Sebaceous gland carcinoma. *A*, Histopathologic features include the loss of an orderly maturational sequence of the sebaceous gland. *B*, The sebaceous cells are replaced by large pleomorphic cells with vacuolated cytoplasm, with frequent mitotic activity.

noma are characteristic and may be confirmed by lipid stains (oil red O) on fresh tissue specimens. The normal sebaceous gland consists of a peripheral border of basaloid cells that mature to large lipid-laden cells, which undergo holocrine secretion. Sebaceous gland carcinoma is characterized by a loss of the normal maturation architecture of the gland (Fig. 32–10*A*), which is replaced by pleomorphic cells with prominent vacuolated cytoplasm (see Fig. 32–10*A*). The areas of vacuolated cytoplasm represent areas where lipid has been dissolved during the histologic processing of the tissue. Lipid can be demonstrated with oil red O staining of fresh tissues. Rao and coworkers[25] have reported a comedocarcinoma variation of the tumor in which the tumor lobules undergo central necrosis. The central necrotic area stains positively for lipid. These authors also evaluated the infiltrative features of the tumor, categorized as minimal, moderate, or highly infiltrative. Minimally infiltrative tumors are composed predominantly of lobules of varying sizes with minimal tumor extension into the surrounding stroma. Invasive tumors demonstrate diffuse infiltrating cords of cells invading the stroma with minimal areas of lobule formation. Rao and coworkers demonstrated an increased mortality correlated with greater degrees of stromal infiltration.

Cavanagh and coworkers[26] reported multicentric involvement with this type of tumor. Serial sections of their specimens revealed four distinct foci of sebaceous gland carcinoma. Multicentric sebaceous carcinoma may create problems in the management of the tumor with frozen section monitoring of surgical margins. Despite frozen section monitoring, tumor recurrence is more likely to occur than in patients with basal cell carcinoma.[27]

Clinical presentation of chronic blepharoconjunctivitis has been correlated with the pathologic features of pagetoid involvement of the surface epithelium. Paget's disease consists of intraepithelial carcinoma of the nipple and areolar skin associated with ductal carcinoma of the breast.[28] Intraepithelial carcinoma may be observed with sebaceous gland carcinoma of the eyelids and of the axillary, genital, and perianal areas. The abnormal surface epithelium contains large cells with a prominent nucleus and abundant pale-staining cytoplasm (Fig. 32–11). The cytoplasm stains positively for mucopolysaccharides with periodic acid–Schiff but does not stain positively for lipids. Pagetoid involvement of the epithelium of the axillary, genital, and perianal areas occurs without associated sebaceous gland carcinoma in 40% of instances.[29, 30] However, no cases of de novo pagetoid involvement of the eyelid and conjunctival epithelium occurred in the Wilmer Eye Institute series. Pagetoid involvement of the epithelium was noted to occur in approximately 50% of sebaceous gland carcinomas and in all of those tumors presenting as blepharoconjunctivitis.

Despite the characteristic features, the tumor is frequently misdiagnosed. Of the 40 tumors reviewed at the Wilmer Eye Institute, only 22.5 (56.2%) were initially

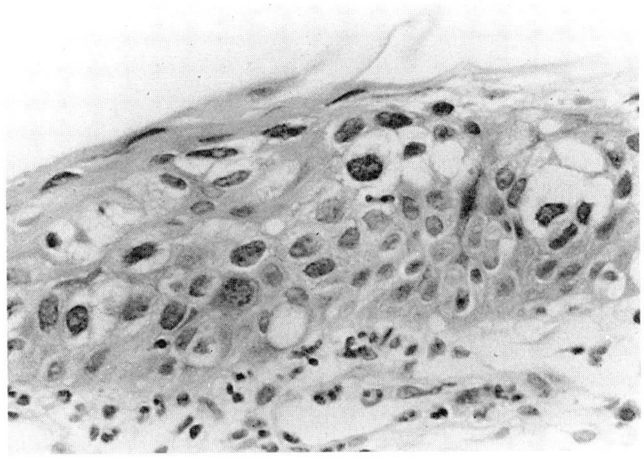

Figure 32–11. Sebaceous gland carcinoma. Pagetoid involvement of the epithelium, characterized by large cells with a prominent nucleus and pale-staining cytoplasm.

correctly diagnosed. If those patients initially evaluated by Green are excluded, the correct initial diagnostic rate decreases to 11.4%. In this series, sebaceous gland carcinoma was initially diagnosed as basal cell carcinoma (11 cases), squamous cell carcinoma (10 cases), epithelioma (1 case), or carcinoma of the lacrimal sac (1 case). The aggressive behavior and significant morbidity and mortality associated with sebaceous gland carcinomas have traditionally been attributed to the misdiagnosed tumors.

The management of sebaceous gland carcinoma consists of surgical extirpation of the tumor. With heightened appreciation of the clinical presentation of the tumor, early surgical excision significantly enhances the long-term prognosis. Rao and coworkers[25] correlated the duration of symptoms with tumor-associated mortality. Patients with symptoms of less than 6 months' duration had a tumor-associated mortality of 13%; those patients with symptoms of more than 6 months' duration had a 43% mortality rate. In the Wilmer Eye Institute study, a patient presenting with chronic blepharoconjunctivitis was actually treated with amphotericin B for suspected fungal keratitis, before a diagnosis of sebaceous gland carcinoma. In addition, numerous procedures for incision and drainage of suspected recurrent chalazions delay the appropriate diagnosis of sebaceous gland carcinoma.

Localized sebaceous gland carcinoma is managed by a biopsy to establish the diagnosis, then monitoring of surgical margins with frozen sections. A full-thickness block resection of the eyelid may be required to establish the diagnosis.[31, 32] Because of the occasional multicentric presentation of sebaceous gland carcinoma, close observation is always critical in the management of these patients to rule out recurrent disease. In patients with diffuse eyelid involvement or orbital extension, orbital exenteration is recommended.

The management of pagetoid changes of the epithelium can be challenging because of widespread involvement. The extent of pagetoid involvement can be confirmed clinically by conjunctival scrapings for a cytopathologic examination or by multiple conjunctival biopsies.[32, 33] If pagetoid changes are localized, the affected epithelium can be excised with the associated sebaceous gland carcinoma. If the pagetoid involvement is diffuse, the conjunctiva can be excised and grafted appropriately. Theoretically, removal of the underlying sebaceous gland carcinoma may permit a regression of the pagetoid changes of the epithelium.[34] Adjunctive cryotherapy in the management of pagetoid conjunctival involvement may defer orbital exenteration. Lisman and coworkers[35] advocated cryotherapy in patients who refused orbital exenteration after the primary sebaceous gland carcinoma was adequately excised. Cryotherapy was noted to result in dry eye symptoms, symblepharon, corneal erosion, and corneal vascularization. Complications were more pronounced for patients when more than two quadrants of pagetoid disease were treated.

Preauricular or anterior cervical adenopathy may be secondary to metastatic tumor or reactive hyperplasia. A biopsy of involved nodes is therefore warranted to confirm the diagnosis of metastatic disease before radical neck dissection. Two patients at the Wilmer Eye Institute had regression of cervical adenopathy after orbital exenteration, indicating a probable reactive hyperplasia of the involved nodes.

Radiation therapy has a limited role in the management of sebaceous gland carcinoma. The tumor is radiosensitive and does respond to radiation therapy, but recurrences are inevitable.[36, 37] Initially this was presumed to be due to inadequate radiation delivery, but with the total dosage increased to 5000 cGy, recurrences were still experienced. All patients treated with adjunctive radiation therapy at the Wilmer Eye Institute had recurrence of their disease. In addition, these patients had significant ocular complications such as keratitis, radiation retinopathy, and severe pain. Radiation therapy is considered a palliative procedure to reduce tumor size, but it should not be viewed as a curative modality.

The prognosis of sebaceous gland carcinoma has improved with early recognition and appropriate pathologic diagnosis of the tumor. Previous studies have documented the 5-year mortality to be in the 30% to 40% range.[21, 38] However, a review of 40 patients at the Wilmer Eye Institute revealed a 15% incidence of mortality.[2] In attempts to explain the lower mortality at the Wilmer Institute, patients were divided into those presenting before and after 1970. This date was chosen because of the arrival at the Institute in 1970 of Dr. W. Richard Green, an ophthalmic pathologist who appreciated the unique features of sebaceous gland carcinoma. For the 25 patients presenting before 1970, the mortality was 25%, whereas no tumor-associated mortality was observed in the 15 patients presenting after 1970. The dramatic reduction of tumor-associated mortality was a direct result of recognition of the clinical and histopathologic features of the tumor. In addition, guidelines for surgical management, with frozen section monitoring of surgical margins for local disease and orbital exenteration for diffuse disease, minimize tumor recurrence. The extensive study by Rao and coworkers[25] also found the duration of ocular symptoms to be one of the most significant prognostic factors. Those patients with symptoms of less than 6 months' duration had a 13% incidence of mortality, whereas those with symptoms of over 6 months' duration had a 43% incidence of mortality. The duration of symptoms, permitting tumor progression may also account for the mortality of 40% in Ni Chou's study of 146 sebaceous gland carcinomas in China.[38] It is clear that early diagnosis and appropriate therapy significantly reduce the long-term morbidity and mortality associated with this tumor.

SQUAMOUS CELL CARCINOMA

The understanding of squamous cell carcinoma is also clouded by misconceptions regarding incidence and potential morbidity and mortality. Histopathologic perception of this tumor has changed dramatically, significantly altering concepts about clinical features, morbidity, and mortality. The incidence of this tumor is now known to be significantly lower than previously recognized. Both benign and malignant tumors were previously misdiagnosed as squamous cell carcinoma. Kwitko and coworkers[5] reported a series of 115 tumors that were originally histopathologically diagnosed as squamous cell carcinoma at the Armed Forces of Institute of Pathology. Reevaluation of these tumors revealed that only 12 (10.4%) were correctly diagnosed.

Traditionally, squamous cell carcinoma was thought to be an aggressive tumor with significant tendencies toward metastasis and possible tumor-associated mortality. Close scrutiny of tumors originally evaluated at the Wilmer Eye Institute did not substantiate this impression. Tumors originally misdiagnosed as squamous cell carcinoma displayed enhanced tendencies of metastasis and tumor-induced mortality. The tumors misdiagnosed as squamous cell carcinoma included sebaceous gland carcinoma and the morphea pattern of basal cell carcinoma. If appropriate therapy is delayed in the management of these misdiagnosed tumors, significant morbidity and mortality are encountered. Squamous cell carcinoma in the eyelids is similar to that occurring elsewhere on the skin, with low metastatic potential and low tumor-induced mortality.[39-42]

Squamous cell carcinoma occurred in 31 patients in the Wilmer Eye Institute series. The incidence of squamous cell carcinoma among all eyelid tumors was 0.5% (31/5392), and among malignant epithelial tumors it was 4.13% (31/749). The tumor occurs with increasing frequency with advancing age. The range of age in the Wilmer Eye Institute study was 4 to 87 years. As with basal cell carcinomas, adolescents presenting with squamous cell carcinoma should be evaluated to rule out tumor diathesis that predisposes to malignant tumors, such as xeroderma pigmentosa and lupus vulgaris. The pediatric patient in the study did not have either of these two syndromes. There is a subtle tendency for this tumor to occur in the upper lid, although no predilection was found in the Wilmer Eye Institute experience.

Squamous cell carcinoma presents clinically as a nonspecific ulceration of the eyelid skin (Fig. 32–12). When occurring at the eyelid margin, subtle architectural features and lashes are destroyed, and occlusion of the meibomian gland orifices may produce secondary chalazions. However, squamous cell carcinomas may be derived from actinic keratoses to present as keratotic erythematous lesions. With chronicity and cicatricial changes of the skin, secondary ectropion may occur. A single patient in the current study presented with orbital extension and marked exposure keratopathy. Preoperative clinical diagnoses included basal cell carcinoma, actinic keratosis, squamous cell carcinomas, epithelioma, verruca vulgaris, chalazion, and nevus.

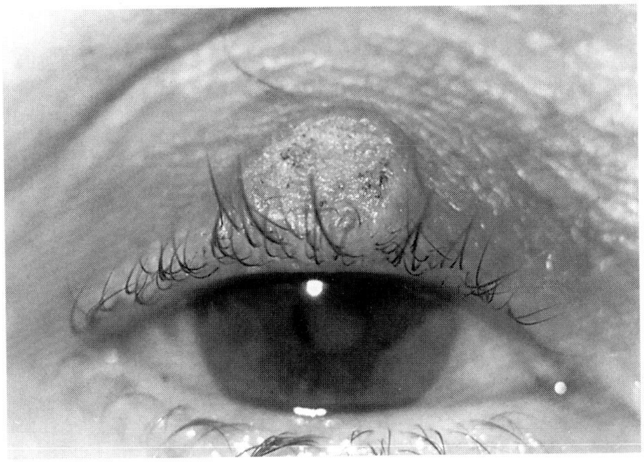

Figure 32–12. Squamous cell carcinoma. Clinical presentation of a slowly enlarging, hyperkeratotic growth of the upper eyelid is shown.

Radiation therapy is a significant etiologic factor in the production of squamous cell carcinoma. The association of radiation therapy with epithelial and soft tissue tumors does not manifest until many years after termination of therapy. Radiation therapy was used in the management of acne and chronic eczema in the 1930s and 1940s. Three patients in the Wilmer Eye Institute study developed squamous cell carcinoma after radiation therapy. A 50-year-old man who presented with a diffuse orbital tumor requiring exenteration had been treated with radiation therapy for eczema intermittently over a 30-year period. This patient had progression of the disease and died with pulmonary metastasis.

Squamous cell carcinoma is an invasive tumor derived from the surface epithelium. The clinical features of the tumor are an exaggeration of those found with actinic keratosis. Histopathologically, the progression of actinic keratosis to squamous cell carcinoma is evident.[43] These epithelial tumors are characterized by exaggerated features of a benign papilloma: acanthosis, papillomatosis, and hyperkeratosis. However, in squamous cell carcinoma, a proliferation of epidermal cells invades the dermis (Fig. 32–13*A*). The invading tumor consists of varying degrees of normal and atypical squamous cells. The greater the proportion of atypical cells, the more malignant or aggressive is the tumor. Features of atypical squamous cells include variations in their size and shape, hyperplasia and hyperchromasia of the nuclei, the absence of intracellular bridges, the keratinization of individual cells, and the presence of atypical mitotic figures (see Fig. 34–13*B*). Keratinization is variable with squamous cell carcinoma. Well-differentiated tumors exhibit

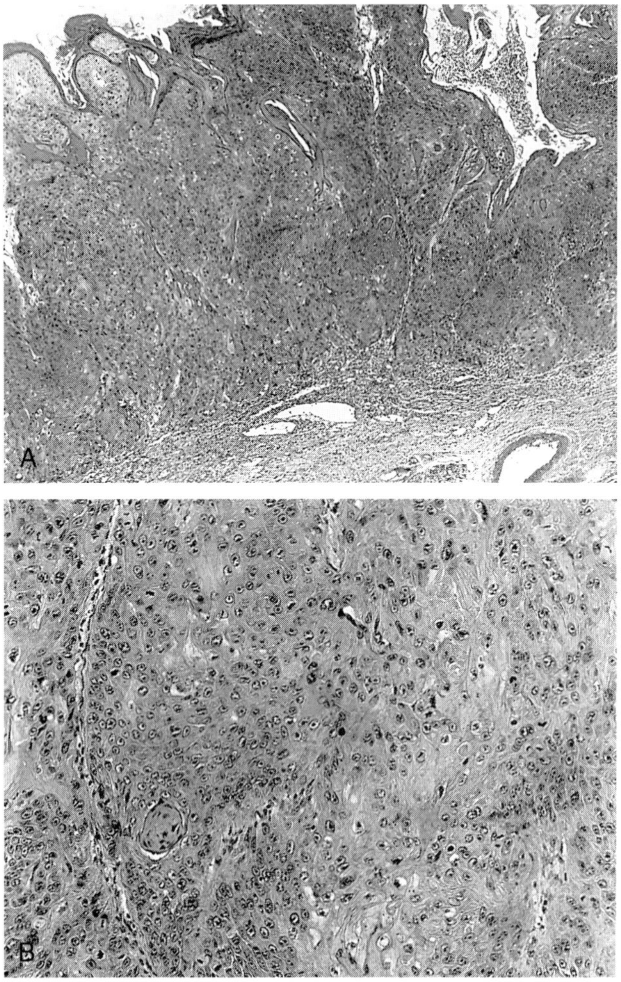

Figure 32–13. Squamous cell carcinoma. *A*, Histopathologic extension of atypical cells invading the dermis. *B*, Increased magnification of atypical squamous cells, with cellular metaplasia, hyperchromasia of nuclei, and varying degrees of keratinization.

horn pearls, which are concentric layers of squamous cells showing gradually increasing in keratinization toward their center. Dermal invasion by atypical squamous cells is the hallmark of squamous cell carcinoma.

Caya and coworkers[44] reported a variation of squamous cell carcinoma called *adenoid squamous carcinoma* (adenoacanthoma) in the periocular area. Histologically, the tumor consists of acantholysis (loss of intracellular bridges) in a pseudoglandular pattern. These tumors rarely metastasize but may locally recur. Caya and coworkers reported recurrence in 6 of the 21 patients in their series, but no widespread metastasis occurred. At the Wilmer Eye Institute, three patients had adenoacanthoma, and in none of these did local recurrence or metastasis occur.

The recognition of benign and malignant tumors that share histopathologic features with squamous cell carcinoma has led to refinement of the diagnostic criteria.[5] Benign tumors such as keratoacanthoma, inverted follicular keratosis, and pseudoepitheliomatous hyperplasia simulate features of squamous cell carcinoma. The common variable with these tumors is inflammation that stimulates epithelial proliferation. Clinically, rapid growth is characteristic of these benign lesions. Malignant tumors such as the morphea pattern of basal cell carcinoma and sebaceous gland carcinoma have also been misdiagnosed as squamous cell carcinoma. The potentially aggressive behavior of these tumors has been attributed to squamous cell carcinoma. The experience at the Wilmer Eye Institute substantiates this impression. Sebaceous gland carcinoma was misdiagnosed as squamous cell carcinoma in 10 patients, 5 of whom died with distant metastasis. The morphea pattern of basal cell carcinoma was the initial histopathologic diagnosis in four patients, and three of these required orbital exenteration; no tumor-associated deaths were noted. The aggressive behavior of these misdiagnosed tumors was inappropriately attributed to squamous cell carcinoma.

The dermatologic literature has also substantiated the changing concepts regarding the metastatic potential of squamous cell carcinoma. Cutaneous squamous cell carcinoma rarely metastasizes. Szymanski[45] and Lund[39] reported extensive series of squamous cell carcinomas, establishing a metastatic potential of 0.23% and 0.25%, respectively. However, tumors arising in areas of previous radiation therapy or osteomyelitic cutaneous fistulas had a significantly higher incidence of metastasis and mortality.[46, 47] Squamous cell carcinomas arising from previous radiation had a 20% incidence of metastasis, and those arising from osteomyelitic sinuses had a 43.6% incidence. Moller and coworkers[42] confirmed these reports of the metastatic potential of squamous cell carcinoma. The Wilmer Eye Institute series included 31 patients with squamous cell carcinoma. One patient had received radiation therapy over a 30-year period for chronic eczema and died with pulmonary metastasis, as noted earlier. No other patients at the Wilmer Eye Institute had metastasis or even local recurrence.

The management of squamous cell carcinoma consists of surgical removal of the tumor with frozen section monitoring of the excised margins.[48] If a biopsy of a suspicious tumor is done before a definitive surgical procedure, care should be taken to obtain a representative section of the tumor. Shave biopsies do not allow determination of dermal invasion by the epithelial tumor. Benign tumors such as actinic keratosis, keratoacanthoma, inverted follicular keratosis, and pseudoepitheliomatous hyperplasia can be differentiated only by evaluation of dermal extension. As such, the pathologist is frequently forced to give a diagnosis of squamous carcinoma because adequate tissue has not been submitted for review. It is not unusual for a tumor that has been reported as squamous cell carcinoma to have resolved by the time definitive surgical resection can be scheduled.

REFERENCES

1. Doxanas MT, Green WR, Iliff CE: Factors in the successful surgical management of basal cell carcinoma of the eyelids. Am J Ophthalmol 91:726–736, 1981.
2. Doxanas MT, Green WR: Sebaceous gland carcinoma: Review of 40 cases. Arch Ophthalmol 102:245–249, 1984.
3. Doxanas MT, Iliff WJ, Iliff NT, Green WR: Squamous cell carcinoma of the eyelids. Ophthalmology 94:538–544, 1987.
4. Welsh RB, Duke JR: Lesions of the lids: A statistical note. Am J Ophthalmol 45:415–416, 1958.
5. Kwitko ML, Boniuk M, Zimmerman LE: Eyelid tumors with reference to lesions confused with squamous cell carcinoma. Part I: Incidence and errors in diagnosis. Arch Ophthalmol 69:693–697, 1963.
6. Aurora AL, Blodi FC: Lesions of the eyelids: A clinicopathological study. Surv Ophthalmol 15:94–104, 1970.
7. Aubry F, MacGibbon B: Risk factors of squamous cell carcinoma of the skin. Cancer 55:907–911, 1985.
8. Milstone EB, Helwig EB: Basal cell carcinoma in children. Arch Dermatol 108:523–527, 1973.
9. Nerad JA, Whitaker DC: Periocular basal cell carcinoma in adults 35 years of age and younger. Am J Ophthalmol 106:723–729, 1988.
10. Payne JW, Duke JR, Butner R, Eifrig DE: Basal cell carcinoma of the eyelids: A long-term follow-up study. Arch Ophthalmol 81:553–558, 1969.
11. Beyer TL, Dryden RM: Basal cell carcinoma masquerading as ectropion. Arch Ophthalmol 106:170–171, 1988.
12. Glover AT, Grove AS Jr: Orbital invasion by malignant eyelid tumors. Ophthalmic Plast Reconstr Surg 5:1–12, 1989.
13. Howard GR, Nerad JA, Carter KD, Whitaker DC: Clinical characteristics associated with orbital invasion of cutaneous basal cell and squamous cell tumors of the eyelid. Am J Ophthalmol 113:123–133, 1992.
14. Lund HZ: Tumors of the skin. *In* Armed Forces Institute of Pathology, section 1, fascicle 2. Washington, DC, Armed Forces Institute of Pathology, 1957, pp 205–234.
15. Gooding CA, White G, Yatsuhashi M: Significance of marginal extension in excised basal cell carcinoma. N Engl J Med 273:923–924, 1965.
16. Einaugler RB, Henkind P: Basal cell epithelioma of the eyelid: Apparent incomplete removal. Am J Ophthalmol 67:413–417, 1969.
17. Older JJ, Quickert MM, Beard C: Surgical removal of basal cell carcinoma of the eyelids utilizing frozen section control. Trans Am Acad Ophthalmol Otolaryngol 79:658–663, 1975.
18. Straatsma BR: Meibomian gland tumors. Arch Ophthalmol 56:71–93, 1956.
19. Lever WF, Schaumburg-Lever G: Histopathology of the Skin, 5th ed. Philadelphia, JB Lippincott, 1975, p 551.
20. Rulon DB, Helwig EB: Cutaneous sebaceous neoplasms. Cancer 33:82–102, 1974.
21. Boniuk M, Zimmerman LE: Sebaceous carcinoma of the eyelid, eyebrow, caruncle and orbit. Trans Am Acad Ophthalmol Otolaryngol 72:619–642, 1968.
22. Sweebe EC, Cogan DG: Adenocarcinoma of the meibomian gland: A pseudochalazion entity. Arch Ophthalmol 61:282–290, 1959.
23. Hagedoorn A: Paget's disease of the eyelid associated with carcinoma. Br J Ophthalmol 21:234–241, 1937.
24. Foster CS, Allansmith MR: Chronic unilateral blepharoconjunctivitis caused by sebaceous carcinoma. Am J Ophthalmol 86:218–220, 1978.
25. Rao NA, McLean IW, Zimmerman LE: Sebaceous carcinoma of the eyelids and caruncle: Correlation of histopathologic features with prognosis. *In* Jakobiec F (ed): Ocular and Adnexal Tumors. Birmingham, AL, Aesculapius, 1978, pp 461–476.
26. Cavanagh HD, Green WR, Goldberg HK: Multicentric sebaceous adenocarcinoma of the meibomian gland. Am J Ophthalmol 77:326–332, 1974.
27. Folberg R, Whitaker DC, Tse DT, Nerad JA: Recurrent and residual sebaceous carcinoma after Mohs' excision of the primary lesion. Am J Ophthalmol 103:817–823, 1987.
28. Fisher ER, Beyer F Jr: Differentiation of neoplastic lesions characterized by large vacuolated intraepidermal (pagetoid) cells. Arch Pathol Lab Med 67:140–145, 1959.
29. Bowman HE, Hartman FW: Extramammary Paget's disease of the vulva. Arch Pathol Lab Med 58:304–308, 1954.
30. Kawatsu T, Miki Y: Triple extramammary Paget's disease. Arch Dermatol 104:316–319, 1971.
31. Harvey JT, Anderson RL: The management of meibomian gland carcinoma. Ophthalmic Surg 13:56–60, 1982.
32. Leibsohn J, Bullock J, Waller R: Full-thickness eyelid biopsy for presumed carcinoma in situ of the palpebral conjunctiva. Ophthalmic Surg 13:840–842, 1982.
33. Putterman AM: Conjunctival map biopsy to determine pagetoid spread. Am J Ophthalmol 102:87–90, 1986.
34. Archer CB, Louback JB, MacDonald DM: Spontaneous regression of perianal extramammary Paget's disease after partial surgical excision. Arch Dermatol 123:379–382, 1987.
35. Lisman RD, Jakobiec FA, Small P: Sebaceous carcinoma of the eyelids: The role of adjunctive cryotherapy in the management of conjunctival pagetoid spread. Ophthalmology 96:1021–1026, 1989.
36. Hendley RL, Rieser JC, Cavanagh HD, et al: Primary radiation therapy for meibomian gland carcinoma. Am J Ophthalmol 87:206–209, 1979.
37. Nunery WR, Welsh MG, McCord CD: Recurrence of sebaceous carcinoma of the eyelid after radiation therapy. Am J Ophthalmol 96:10–15, 1983.
38. Ni C, Searl SS, Kuo PK, et al: Sebaceous cell carcinoma of the ocular adnexa. *In* Ni C, Albert DM (eds): Tumors of the Eyelid and Orbit: A Chinese-American Collaborative Study, vol 22. Boston, Little, Brown & Co, 1982, pp 23–61.
39. Lund HZ: How often does squamous cell carcinoma of the skin metastasize? Arch Dermatol 92:635–637, 1965.
40. Graham JH, Helwig EB: Premalignant cutaneous and mucocutaneous disease. *In* Graham JH, Johnson WC, Helwig EB (eds): Dermal Pathology. Hagerstown, MD, Harper & Row, 1972, p 626.
41. Epstein E, Epstein NN, Bragg K, Linder G: Metastasis from squamous cell carcinoma of the skin. Arch Dermatol 97:245–251, 1968.
42. Moller R, Reymann F, Hou-Jensen K: Metastasis in dermatological patients with squamous cell carcinoma. Arch Dermatol 115:703–705, 1979.
43. Marks R, Rennie G, Selwood T: The relationship of basal cell carcinoma and squamous cell carcinoma to solar keratosis. Arch Dermatol 124:1039–1042, 1988.
44. Caya JG, Hidayat AA, Weiner JM: A clinicopathologic study of 21 cases of adenoid squamous cell carcinoma of the eyelid and periorbital region. Am J Ophthalmol 99:291–297, 1985.
45. Szymanski FJ: Keratoacanthoma. *In* Graham JH, Johnson WC, Helwig EG (eds): Dermal Pathology. Hagerstown, MD, Harper & Row, 1972, pp 625–635.
46. Martin H, Strong E, Spiro RH: Radiation induced skin cancer of the head and neck. Cancer 25:61–71, 1970.
47. Sidlin EG, Flemming JL: Epidermal carcinoma arising in chronic osteomyelitic foci. J Bone Joint Surg 45:827–837, 1963.
48. Reifler DM, Hornblass A: Surgical management of squamous cell carcinoma of the lid. Ophthalmic Plast Reconstr Surg 2:75–82, 1986.

CHAPTER 33

Mohs' Surgery for Periorbital Malignancies

Daniel Rivlin and Ronald L. Moy

Mohs' micrographic surgery has its origin in the early 1930s when Dr. Frederick Mohs discovered, serendipitously, that injection of zinc chloride into tissue caused necrosis but simultaneously fixed the tissue so that the microscopic structure was retained.[1] From this observation, Dr. Mohs realized that in situ fixation could revolutionize the way skin cancers were treated because it could allow excision with complete microscopic control. Complete microscopic control was achieved by removing tissue in layers, after application of zinc chloride paste, and sectioning the layers horizontally so that the entire undersurface of the layer was examined. The undersurface, along with the skin edge, represents the entire margin of the layer. The combination of application of zinc chloride paste to fix tissue, layered excisions, and horizontal sectioning came to be known as Mohs' chemosurgery.

During the ensuing years, Dr. Mohs had much success in treating various skin malignancies with his chemosurgical technique. However, there were several drawbacks. The most important of these was that the zinc chloride could be irritating, causing severe discomfort to the patient. This was especially true around the eyes, where the paste could cause severe conjunctivitis or keratitis.[2] Hence, in the periorbital areas, Dr. Mohs would remove the tissue unfixed and process it as a frozen section but still cut the specimen horizontally to examine 100% of the margin. This became known as the *fresh tissue technique.*[3]

In the early 1970s the fresh tissue technique was advocated by Dr. Theodore Tromovitch as the preferred technique for removal of skin cancers from all parts of the skin.[4] Studies had shown that the cure rates were as high and recurrence rates as low as that of the fixed tissue technique. In addition, frozen sections offered the advantage of allowing multiple layers to be excised on the same day if microscopic examination revealed the margins to be positive.[5] This was not the case with the fixed tissue technique because removal of a second layer required a fresh application of zinc chloride paste and a period as long as 24 hours to allow it to fix the tissue. Furthermore, the improvements in cryostats, staining techniques, and other technologic procedures resulted in frozen sections giving equal or superior clarity in terms of visualization of neoplasm as that of fixed tissue. Consequently, the fresh tissue technique is the one most commonly used today and is now renamed *Mohs' micrographic surgery.*

FRESH TISSUE TECHNIQUE

The first step in the fresh tissue technique is to assess the clinical margins of the neoplasm and mark them with a gentian violet pen. This should be done before injection of anesthesia to avoid distortion. Often, the margin may be difficult to assess. Factors that can blur the margin include inflammation, severely sun-damaged skin, the growth patterns of the neoplasm (such as morpheaform basal cell carcinoma), or the presence of scarring from a previous procedure. In such instances a reasonable guess should be made, and the margin should be marked with gentian violet.

After the margin has been marked, local anesthesia should be injected. The standard anesthetic is 1% lidocaine with 1 : 10,000 epinephrine. The anesthetic should be buffered with sodium bicarbonate because this reduces the stinging the patient feels during injection. In addition, injecting slowly decreases the discomfort. Once the lidocaine is injected, one should wait for at least 5 minutes, if possible, to allow the epinephrine to accomplish maximum vasoconstriction, which decreases the bleeding during the procedure.

For eyelid neoplasms invading the lid margin, the conjunctiva, or both, it is necessary to apply 1 or 2 drops of tetracaine solution to the eye. This allows one to administer the lidocaine injection through the lid margin or sulcus with minimum discomfort. Furthermore, if patients are psychologically uncomfortable with a needle so close to their eyes, the tetracaine will allow placement of a stainless steel contact lens that will effectively block the patient's vision.

After the area is anesthetized, the neoplasm should be debulked, especially if there is a fair amount of clinically obvious neoplasm. This can be done either by saucerization with a scalpel or with a curette. With the scalpel it is important to remove only the clinically obvious neo-

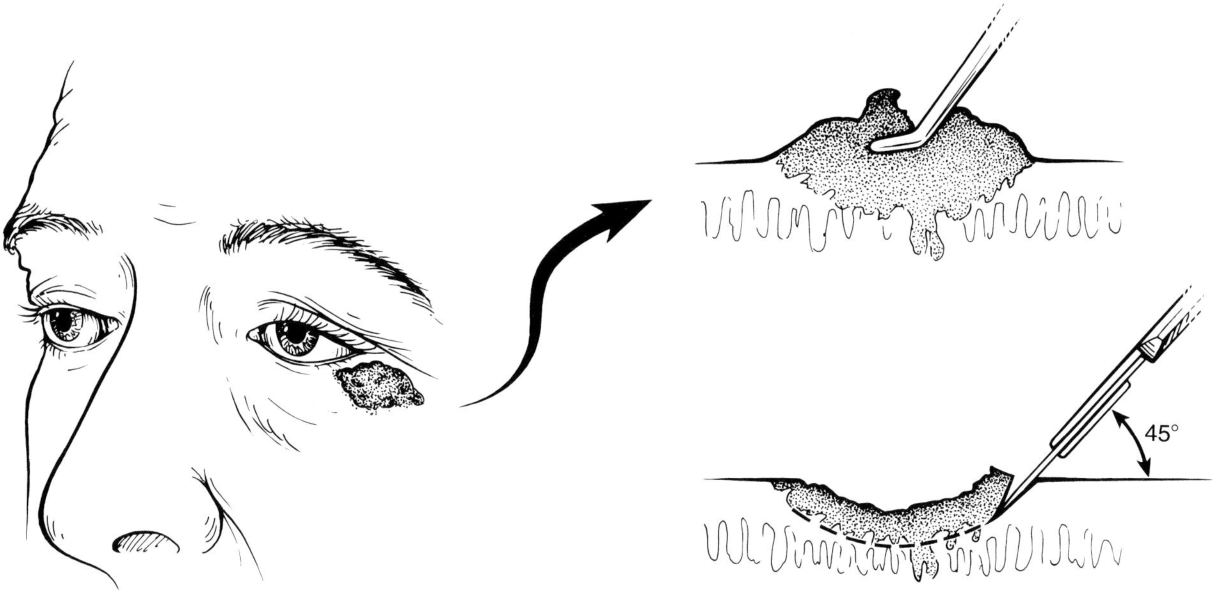

Figure 33–1. The lesion (shown on the *left*) is debulked with a curette (*right, upper*). The first stage is done with the blade at a 45-degree angle (*right, lower*).

plasm. With the curette, neoplasm will have a very soft and friable consistency. Once one encounters resistance, as with normal skin, one should stop. Curettage is also helpful in delineating clinical margins when they are difficult to visualize (Fig. 33–1*A*). Debulking saves the patient from having to have additional layers removed.

Once the neoplasm has been debulked, an initial incision should be made around the entire circumference of the lesion, placing the blade at 1 mm from the clinical margin. The incision should be made with the blade at a 45-degree angle to the skin (Fig. 33–1*B*). The depth of the incision should be approximately 1 mm because this is the ideal thickness of the layer. The incision is made in three strokes; the scalpel is held with a pencil grip by the dominant hand while the other hand is used to stretch the skin to provide tension. The strokes consist of (1) a forehand from approximately 11 o'clock to 3 o'clock; (2) a backhand from 7 o'clock to 3 o'clock; and (3) a forehand from 7 o'clock to 11 o'clock. Once the incision is made, the scalpel should be used to make small nicks at the superior, inferior, and lateral poles of the layer. The nicks should be on both sides of the initial incision, because this will be instrumental in orienting the layer. At this point, the layer is removed by continuous sweeping, side-to-side motions with the scalpel. The motion can be either forehand or backhand. With each repeated motion the angle of the blade is rotated until it is completely parallel to the plane of the skin. Once 50% of the layer is freed, the angle of the blade shifts so that it is at a negative angle to the plane of the skin. This is done so that on the last stroke, the blade exits through the initial incision.

The excised layer is than placed on a piece of gauze seated atop a pad of paper. On the pad there should be some identifying features of the patient such as name, the tumor type and location, and the date. The gauze should be premarked with an ink dot in the upper left corner so that orientation can be maintained if the gauze is turned after the tissue is placed on it. The tissue should be placed on the gauze so as to maintain anatomic orientation. This is done by coordinating the nicks on the layer with the ink dot on the gauze because the ink dot also represents the left upper corner of the patient. Next, attention is turned back to the wound, and hemostasis is achieved either chemically (with aluminum chloride or trichloroacetic acid) or electrically (with cautery or electrodesiccation). A pressure dressing is then applied, and the patient is told to wait until the tissue is processed.

The first step in processing the tissue is to draw a map of the excised layer that is as exact a replica as possible (Figs. 33–2 and 33–3). The map is essentially an outline drawing that includes the nicks to maintain orientation. The next step is to assess the size of the layer and determine whether it is small enough to fit on a glass slide (Fig. 33–4). If it is not, it must be transected into more or less equal-sized pieces that will fit on a microscope glass slide. If the tissue is transected, it must be drawn onto the map. If there is more than one piece, each piece must be numbered. The most commonly used numbering scheme is to number in a clockwise fashion. Next, each individual piece must be color coded. There are different coloring schemes, but they share a common rule, which is that each piece must have at least two different colors on two different edges so that neoplasm can be mapped precisely on each piece. The color coding is done with various permanent tissue inks.

At this point the individual pieces are ready to be frozen and cut. Each piece is positioned on a glass slide and placed into a cryostat for approximately 1 minute at

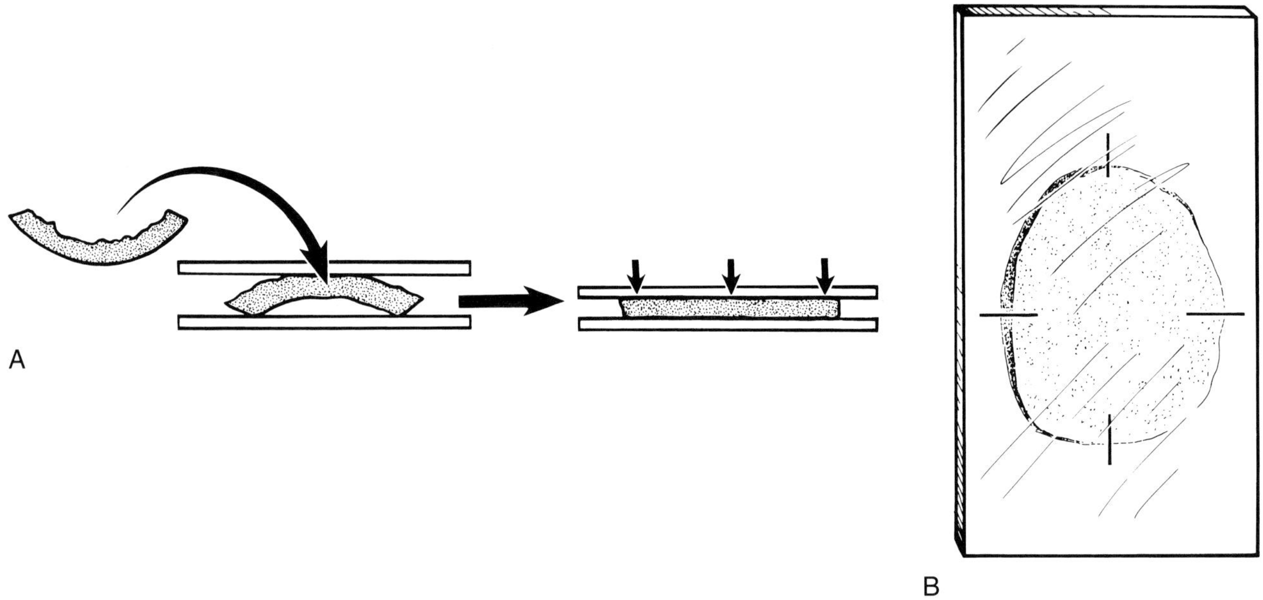

Figure 33–2. *A*, The tissue is flipped and flattened so that the entire margin is in the plane of the slide. *B*, Map sections are shown.

−24°C. The tissue at this time has a more malleable consistency so that the entire epidermal edge and bottom of the piece can be forced into the same plane that is in contact with the glass. At this point ornithine carbamoyltransferase (OCT) is applied to the piece while on the slide and placed into the cryostat until it is frozen solid. Then the OCT is placed on a chuck, and the piece is placed on the chuck with the slide still attached to the bottom so that the piece is squeezed between the chuck and the slide. This ensures that the entire margin of the piece is squeezed into a single plane. After the OCT is frozen solid, the glass slide is removed and sections are now cut with a microtome off the chuck. Of course, the sections represented the entire margin of the piece. The sections are then stained in an automatic stainer with hematoxylin and eosin.

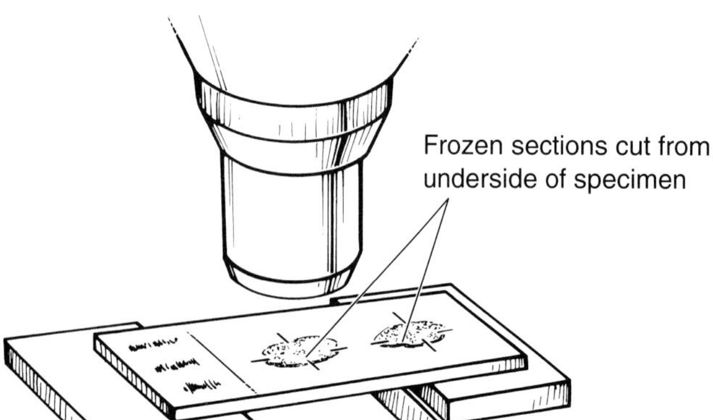

Figure 33–3. Frozen sections are cut from the underside of the specimen and are evaluated under the microscope, and areas of tumor are marked.

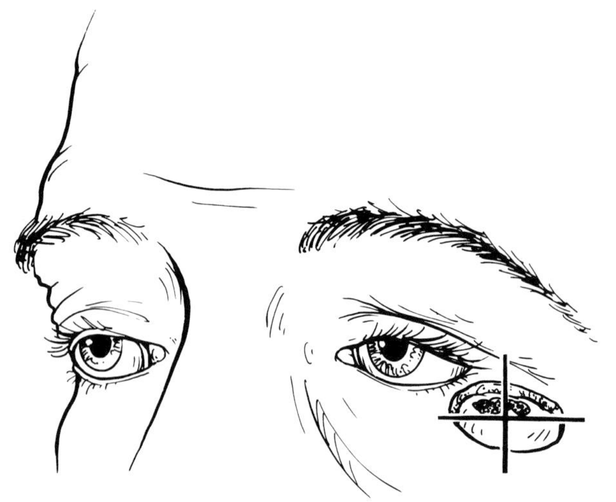

Figure 33–4. A map is made so that the location of residual tumor is pinpointed.

The microscopic sections are examined under the microscope. If neoplasm is found, it can be marked with a marking pen directly on the glass slide. The color-coded edges are also marked. The area that has been marked can then be directly marked on the map. This process is repeated for each numbered piece. Once the map is complete, a second layer can be taken just from the areas that are positive for tumor. This entire process can be repeated as many times as is necessary to clear the tumor (Figs. 33–5 and 33–6).

ADVANTAGES OF MOHS' SURGERY

As is the case with all the skin, basal cell and squamous cell carcinomas are the most common malignancies to

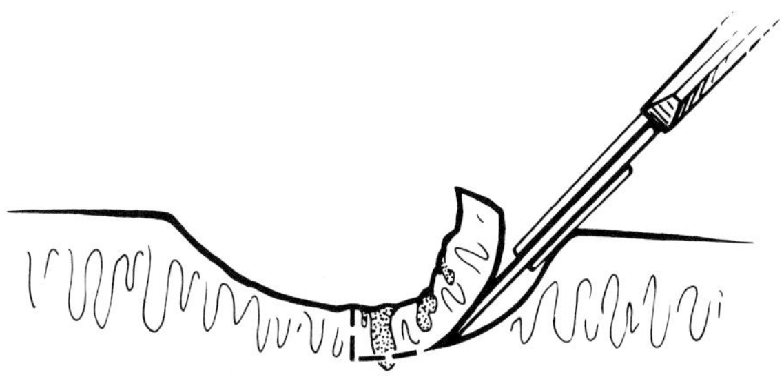

Figure 33–5. The second stage is excised with the same technique as the first.

affect the eyelid. Mohs' micrographic surgery has the highest cure rate for both of these malignancies compared with any other modality, including primary and recurrent neoplasms. The cure rate for primary basal cell carcinoma with Mohs' surgery is 98%, whereas the rates for primary surgical excision with 4-mm margins and curettage and desiccation are 93% and 90%, respectively. Radiation therapy and cryosurgery have cure rates of 91% and 92%, respectively.[6] For recurrent basal cell carcinomas, the difference between Mohs' microscopic surgery and other modalities is even more dramatic. The cure rate for Mohs' surgery is 95% whereas for surgical excision, curettage and desiccation, and radiation therapy, the cure rates are 83%, 90%, and 60%, respectively.[7]

The statistics are similar for squamous cell carcinoma, but of course the consequences of the lower cure rates are much more dire. The recurrence rates for primary squamous cell carcinoma with the various modalities are as follows: curettage and desiccation, 3.7%; surgery, 8.1%; radiation, 10%; and Mohs' surgery, 3.1%. The recurrence rate for all non-Mohs' modalities is 7.9%. For recurrent squamous cell carcinomas the recurrence rate for Mohs' surgery is 10%, whereas that for all non-Mohs' modalities is 23%.[8]

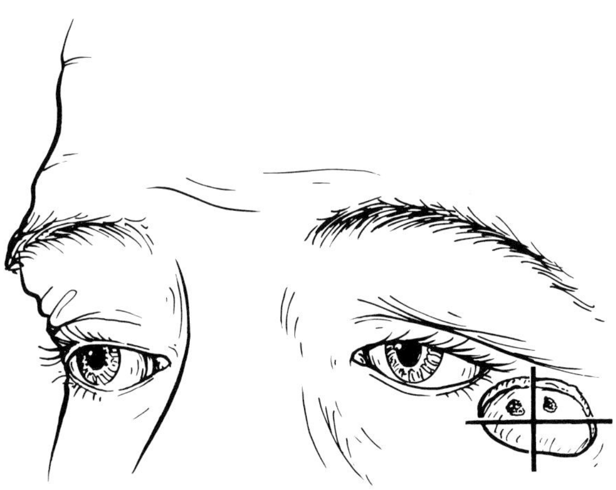

Figure 33–6. A map of residual tumor after the second stage.

The data on Mohs' surgery for other malignancies, such as sebaceous carcinoma, apocrine carcinoma, and melanoma, are less definitive because of the relative rarity of these neoplasms and the scarcity with which they have been treated with Mohs' surgery. However, the data that do exist suggest that Mohs' surgery has a higher cure rate than other modalities.

In addition to the higher cure rate, Mohs' surgery offers other advantages to patients, especially in the case of eyelid neoplasms. One critical advantage is that as much normal tissue as possible is spared with this technique. This is the consequence of the entire margin being examined microscopically, which allows extremely small surgical margins to be taken (usually 1 mm). In the case of eyelid neoplasms, this is critical because there is so little tissue to begin with that can be borrowed for a flap. Therefore, the tissue-sparing nature of Mohs' surgery helps ensure the best cosmetic result possible.

In addition to improved cosmesis, Mohs' surgery is often the most convenient modality. Most patients are "cleared" of their neoplasm with excision of just a few layers. Therefore, they know that they have been cured the day of their surgery. With standard surgical excisions, patients often wait several days for the pathology report, and when the margins are not clear, they have to undergo a second procedure. With radiation therapy, multiple visits are required, and the patients often experience radiation dermatitis during the several weeks' duration of their therapy. Curettage and desiccation always require the patient to heal by second intention, which necessitates several weeks of wound care. The same is often true of cryosurgery.

REFERENCES

1. Mohs FE, Guyer MF: Pre-excisional fixation of tissues in the treatment of cancer in rats. Cancer Res 49–51, 1941.
2. Mohs FE: Cancer of eyelids. Bull Am Coll Chemosurg 3:10–11, 1970.
3. Mohs FE: Origin and progress of Mohs' surgery. *In* Mikhail GR (ed): Mohs Micrographic Surgery. Philadelphia, WB Saunders, 1991, pp 1–10.
4. Tromovitch TA, Stegeman SJ: Microsopically controlled excision of skin tumors: Chemosurgery fresh tissue technique. Arch Dermatol 110:231–232, 1974.
5. Robins P, Henkind P, Menn H: Chemosurgery in treatment of cancers of the periorbital area. Trans Am Acad Ophthalmol Otolaryngol 70:1228–1235, 1971.
6. Rowe DE, Carroll RJ, Day CL Jr: Long-term recurrence rates in previously untreated (primary) basal cell carcinoma: Implications for patient follow-up. J Dermatol Surg Oncol 15:315–328, 1989.
7. Rowe DE, Carroll RJ, Day CL Jr: Mohs surgery is the treatment of choice for recurrent (previously treated) basal cell carcinoma. J Dermatol Surg Oncol 15:424–431, 1989.
8. Rowe DE, Carroll RJ, Day CL Jr: Prognostic factors for local recurrence, metastases, and several rates in SCC of skin, ear, and lip. J Am Acad Dermatol 26:976–990, 1991.

CHAPTER 34

Reconstruction of the Upper Eyelid

David R. Jordan

Reconstruction of the upper eyelid may be required after penetrating or avulsive traumatic injuries, for congenital anomalies, or after tumor resection. Whatever the cause of the lid defect may be, a sound knowledge of eyelid anatomy is required before consideration of lid reconstruction. The upper lid may be divided into two basic components: the anterior lamella (skin and orbicularis) and the posterior lamella (tarsus and conjunctiva). When an eyelid is being reconstructed, each of these components must be considered. For traumatic lid lacerations without tissue loss, anterior and posterior lamellae are placed together as close to a normal anatomic position as possible. For congenital defects (e.g., colobomas) and lid defects occurring after tumor resection, the surgeon must consider replacement of both the anterior and posterior lamellar components. At least one or both of these components require a blood supply. That is, during lid reconstruction either the anterior lamella should have its own blood supply and supply an underlying posterior lamellar graft or the posterior lamella should have its own blood supply and supply an overlying anterior lamellar graft. There cannot be a situation in which neither the anterior nor the posterior lamella has its own blood supply; a graft on top of a graft without a blood supply is doomed to failure.

Posterior lamella reconstructive procedures for upper (and lower) eyelids include free tarsal grafts,[1, 2] sliding tarsoconjunctival flaps,[3-5] rotating tarsal flaps,[6] and the use of various tarsal substitutes, including nasal cartilage,[7] ear cartilage,[8-10] banked sclera,[11, 12] hard palate mucosa,[13, 14] irradiated tarsus,[15, 16] irradiated aorta,[17] and composite grafts from the opposite eyelid.[18, 19] Various eyelid-sharing procedures such as the Cutler-Beard technique,[20] Hughes technique,[21, 22] and Mustardé full-thickness lid pedicle type flap have also been described.[23]

Free skin grafts, skin flaps, distal skin–muscle flaps, and myocutaneous eyelid flaps have been successfully used for anterior lamella reconstruction.[24, 25] Myocutaneous flaps are advantageous because they have their own blood supply, which is an essential requirement for a free-standing posterior lamella graft. In addition, these flaps return some mobility of the tissue since the muscle present is not totally denervated. If the myocutaneous flap is from surrounding eyelid tissue, the skin will be of a similar color and consistency, allowing a more natural appearance than if a thick flap from nonsimilar tissue is used.

The objectives of eyelid reconstruction include (1) restoration of the anatomy to allow protection of the eye, (2) motility of the reconstructed eyelid, and (3) a cosmetically acceptable result. All of the previously mentioned reconstructive techniques may satisfy the first objective (i.e., the reconstructed lids protect the globe), but the surgeon must also strive to restore motility of the lid so that the tear film is adequately exchanged and to deliver a cosmetically acceptable result. Replacing posterior lamella with tarsus and anterior lamella with skin and muscle not only provides eye protection and gives the reconstructed eyes an excellent chance of regaining motility but is also cosmetically acceptable in most cases.

RECONSTRUCTING THE TRAUMATIZED UPPER EYELID

Trauma to the upper eyelid may occur from flying missiles, motor vehicle accidents, tree branches, and dog and cat scratches or bites. The first step in the treatment of such injuries is to take a careful history to appreciate the mechanism of injury and the force and velocity with which the object approached the eye. In all eyelid trauma cases it is essential to document the visual acuity and ocular functions to rule out damage to the globe before treatment of the lid abnormality (Fig. 34–1). Penetrating eyelid trauma may involve full- or partial-thickness lacerations and may include the lid margin, canaliculus, or deeper lid structures such as the levator aponeurosis. Appropriate radiographs or computed tomographic scans are indicated when it is suspected that deeper structures such as the frontal sinus, orbital rim, and orbital wall are affected.

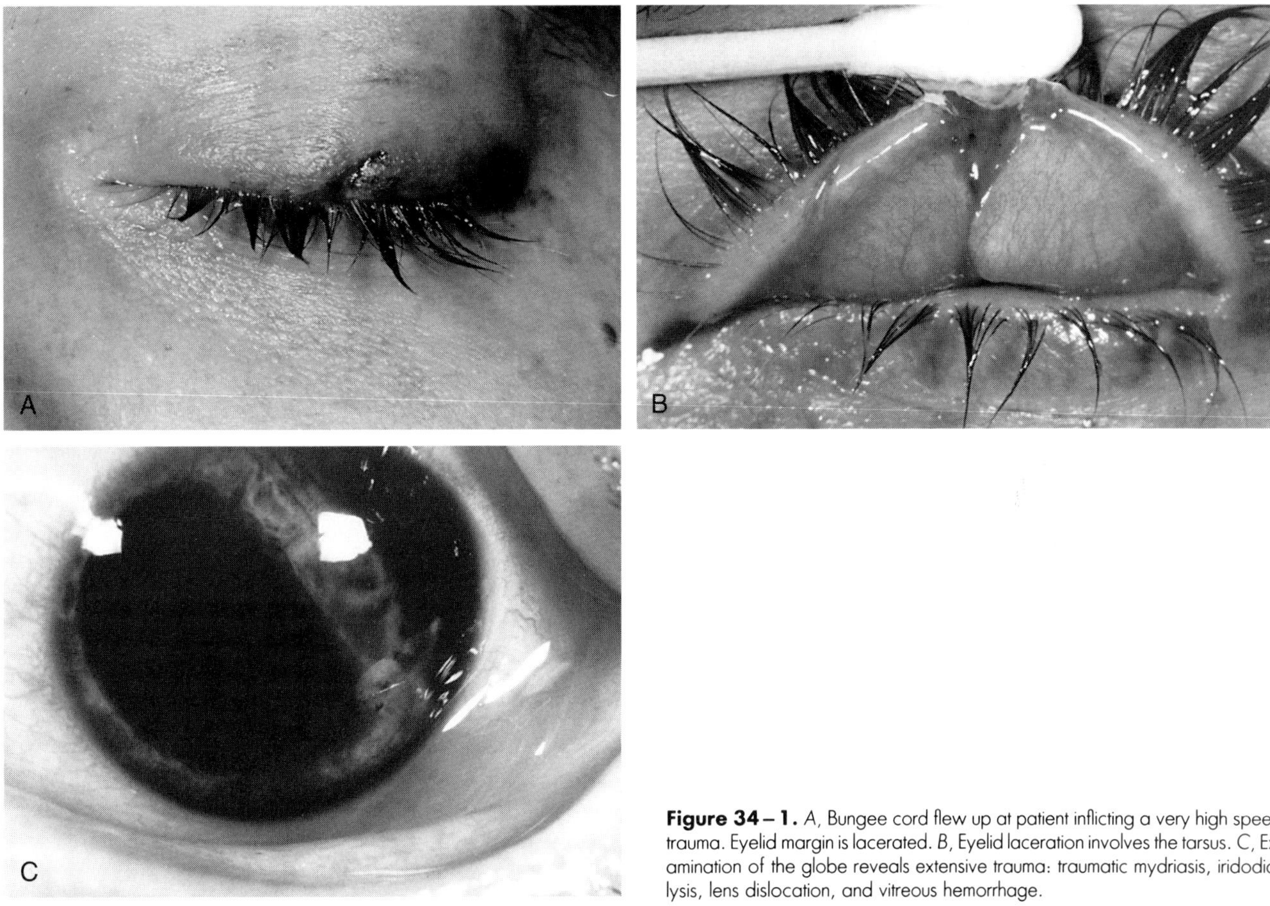

Figure 34–1. *A*, Bungee cord flew up at patient inflicting a very high speed trauma. Eyelid margin is lacerated. *B*, Eyelid laceration involves the tarsus. *C*, Examination of the globe reveals extensive trauma: traumatic mydriasis, iridodialysis, lens dislocation, and vitreous hemorrhage.

Penetrating Injuries

No Tissue Loss

For partial-thickness lid lacerations not involving the lid margin, skin closure alone is sufficient. A 6-0 silk or 6-0 or 7-0 prolene/nylon suture is best for the closure, with suture removal in 5 to 7 days. In children, a 7-0 plain or chromic suture is used so that removal is unnecessary. More extensive partial-thickness lacerations with several lacerations and shredded ends are often seen in the patient who has gone through a car windshield. Gentle cleansing of the wound is recommended, with saline irrigation and removal of foreign bodies, followed by careful reapproximation. I do not advocate routinely trimming the ends to obtain "fresh edges" as is often done during the repair of wounds on other parts of the body. Piece-by-piece approximation is preferred, using the brow line and lid crease as landmarks. The lid is extremely vascular, and tissue that often looks hopeless for survival will do well because of this rich vascularity (Fig. 34–2).

Tissue Loss

When the eyelid margin is involved, it is important to determine whether there has been tissue loss, so that lid reconstruction can be planned. Penetrating injuries due to sharp objects usually leave all the tissue present, whereas dog bite injuries often have areas of missing tissue. The lacerated lid can be dealt with in a similar fashion to the eyelid undergoing reconstruction after tumor resection. The skin and muscle represent the anterior lamella, while tarsus and conjunctiva form a posterior lamella, with both requiring reconstruction as previously mentioned.

Lid Margin Reapproximation

It is essential to reapproximate the lid margin in an accurate and meticulous fashion.[26, 27] A full-thickness lid margin laceration can be repaired either by closing the tarsus first and then the lid margin or by closing the lid margin first and then the tarsus. I prefer to close the tarsus first. The tarsal plate is closed using partial-thickness 5-0 polyglactin sutures on a spatula-type needle. The tarsal plate sutures can be temporarily tightened to check the lid margin alignment and the sutures repositioned if necessary to correct any misalignment. The lid margin is then closed. I find that the best results are obtained when the first stitch in the lid margin is placed through the meibomian gland openings using a 6-0 silk vertical mattress

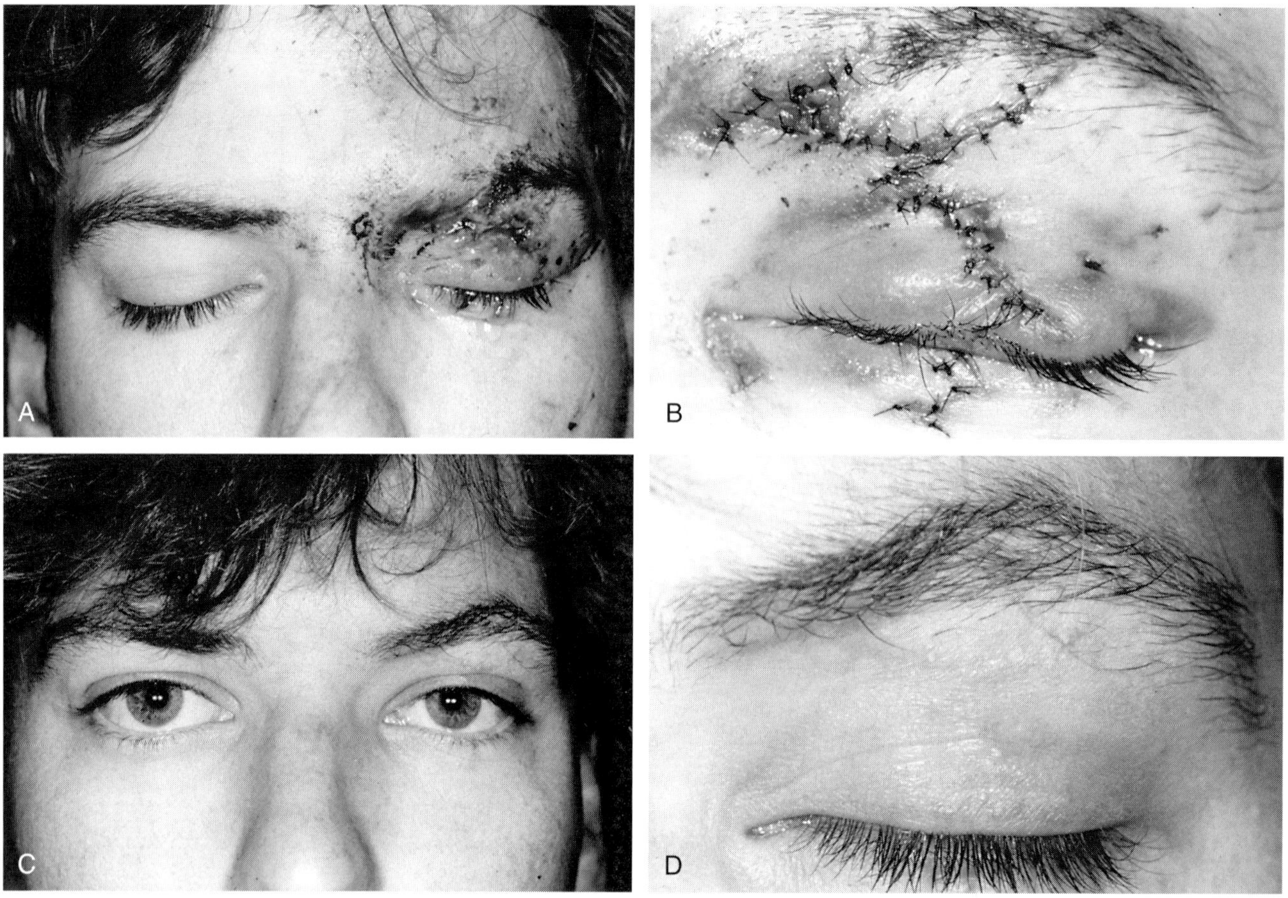

Figure 34–2. *A*, Multiple lacerations to the upper eyelid from a motor vehicle accident. *B*, Meticulous reapproximation of eyelid skin and muscle. *C*, Six months after surgery, the lid has returned to normal. *D*, Lid lacerations have healed nicely.

suture to tent up the edges. This allows a smooth lid margin to develop once the suture has been removed. Not only does this meibomian line stitch help with alignment, but the wound is also stronger when this suture is closed. A simple stitch reapproximating the lid margin is inadequate and often leads to lid notching. A second vertical mattress, and often a third, is placed through the lash line to tent up the edges. These sutures are left long and tied into skin sutures higher up on the upper lid (Fig. 34–3).

Other arthors[28, 29] have recommended that the gray line be closed first as the initial step in lid reconstruction, followed by tarsal reapproximation. Unfortunately, it is not always a visible line. In addition, it overlies the natural separation plane between anterior lamella and posterior lamella of the lid and therefore is a weak plane in the lid. Each case, however, must be assessed individually. In some instances, the gray line may be the best line to align the lid margin correctly. Once the lid margin and tarsus have been repaired, the anterior lamella is closed. The muscle does not generally need to be closed, but if it is, then additional strength is added to the wound closure. A 5-0 or 6-0 absorbable chromic or plain gut suture works well in this layer. The skin is closed with 6-0 silk or nylon or prolene in a simple stitch. The lid margin sutures are left long and tied into the simple skin sutures higher up on the lid.

If the lacerated eyelid is not reapproximated and reconstructed properly, a lid notch may occur. This disrupts the tear exchange and lubrication of the cornea. The patient is often quite uncomfortable and may have a significant cosmetic deformity (Fig. 34–4).

Extensive Injuries

With more extensive lid lacerations involving fat herniation and disruption of the levator, it is important to identify the exposed disrupted tissue, which is often in an unnatural position (Fig. 34–5). The landmark to orient oneself in the upper and lower lids is the preaponeurotic fat; the orbicularis–skin layer is anterior to this layer, while the levator aponeurosis is immediately posterior to it. The fat should be carefully repositioned. This is often aided by gentle cautery to the fat capsule, which allows it to retract into the lid. Only rarely should fat be removed. The levator is gently repositioned and sutured to either

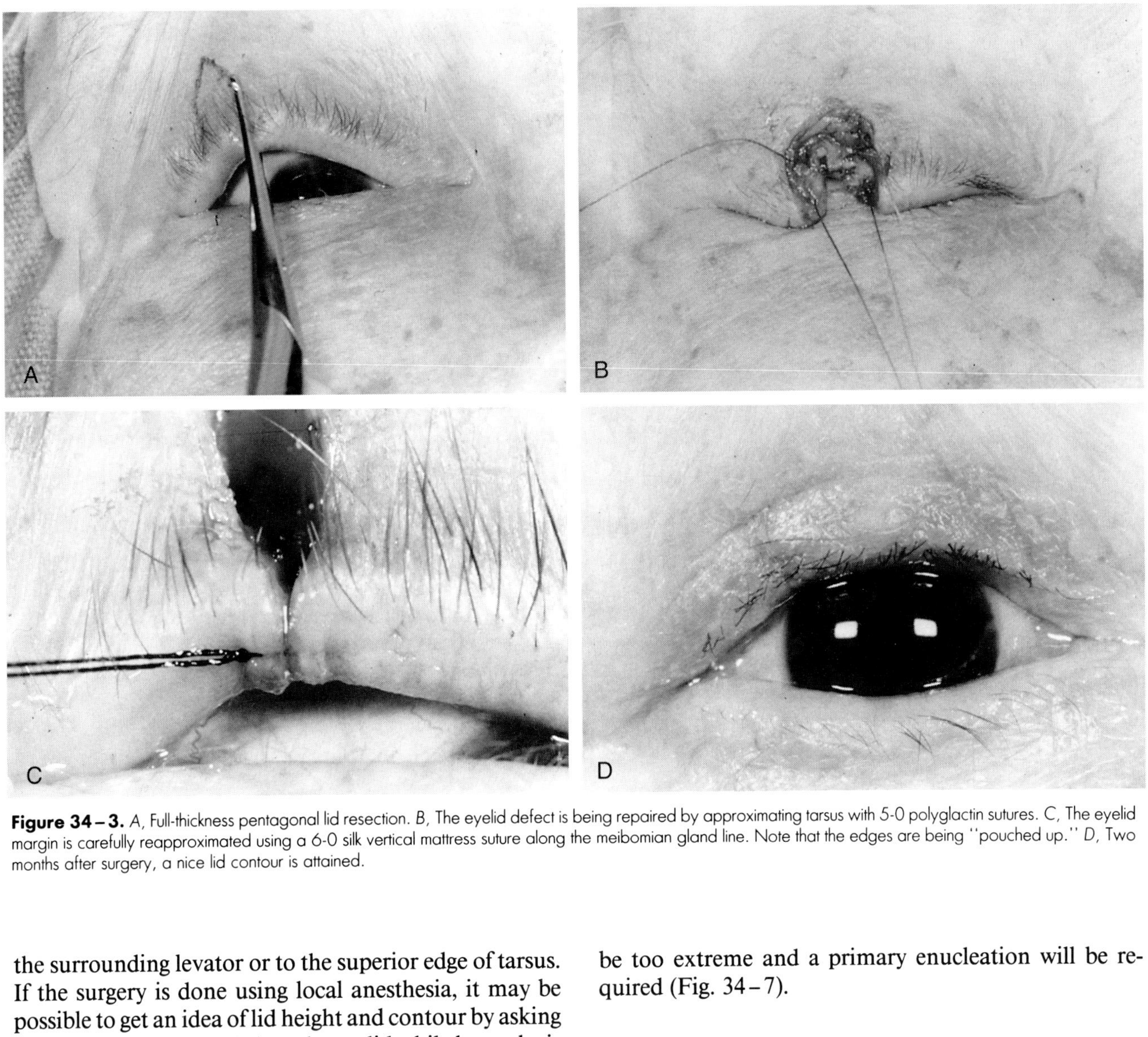

Figure 34–3. *A*, Full-thickness pentagonal lid resection. *B*, The eyelid defect is being repaired by approximating tarsus with 5-0 polyglactin sutures. *C*, The eyelid margin is carefully reapproximated using a 6-0 silk vertical mattress suture along the meibomian gland line. Note that the edges are being "pouched up." *D*, Two months after surgery, a nice lid contour is attained.

the surrounding levator or to the superior edge of tarsus. If the surgery is done using local anesthesia, it may be possible to get an idea of lid height and contour by asking the patient to open and close the eyelid while he or she is in a sitting position. An adjustment in lid height may be required at a later date. If the tarsus is involved, it is repaired as described earlier. The skin and orbicularis are closed in the usual fashion.

The lacrimal gland may occasionally prolapse into the operative field. It can be resuspended in its fossa using a double-armed 4-0 or 5-0 permanent or absorbable suture attached to the inside wall of the superior orbital rim (Fig. 34–6).

With more extensive injuries, the globe may be ruptured and should be repaired at all costs. Even if the potential for vision is almost zero, the globe should be repaired initially and then reassessed over the first 7 to 14 days to determine whether enucleation is necessary to avoid sympathetic ophthalmia.[30–32] This time allows the surgeon to assess the potential visual recovery and allows the patient time to adjust to the severity of his or her injury and to discuss the possible treatment plans, including enucleation. Occasionally, the globe disruption will be too extreme and a primary enucleation will be required (Fig. 34–7).

Canalicular Lacerations

Lacerations involving the medial upper eyelid often disrupt the medial canthal tendon, the upper or lower canaliculus, or both. There has been some controversy in the past over the role of the superior canaliculus and whether it needs repair if lacerated,[33] but several investigators have now shown its importance in tear drainage.[34–39] It must be repaired just as much as a lower canaliculus, and I hope the misconception that it does not require repair will soon be abolished.

A variety of techniques can be used to repair a canalicular laceration.[40–43] No matter which technique is chosen, two essential principles must be followed: (1) the canalicular ends should be accurately approximated (fine 7–0 or 8–0 polyglactin sutures under direct visualization may be helpful to align the canalicular ends but are not always possible to put in) and (2) a stent is required to support the canalicular walls during healing. At present,

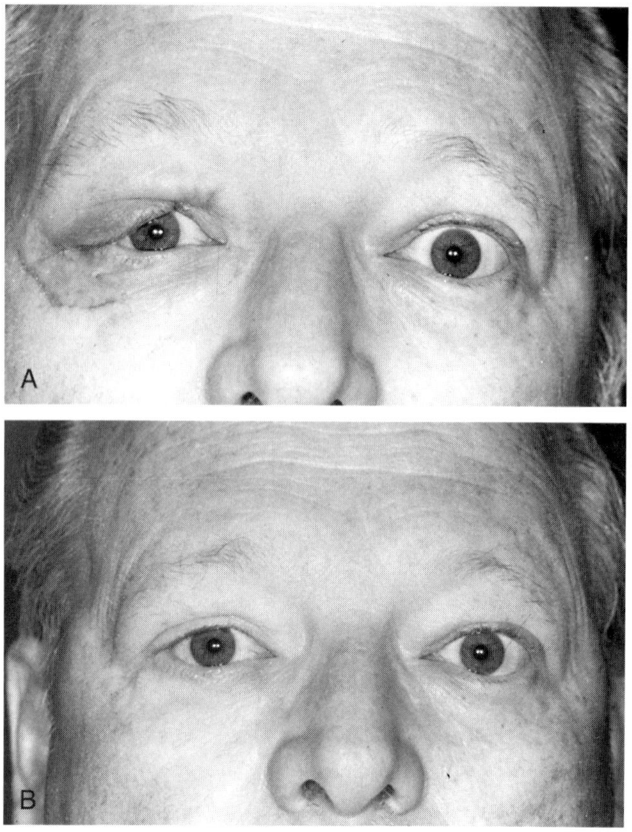

Figure 34–4. A, Upper lid laceration from a motor vehicle accident, which was improperly repaired. A large lid notch and exposure from inadequate closure and tear exchange occurred. B, Ten months after lid reconstruction the notch was excised and the tarsal plates were accurately reapproximated.

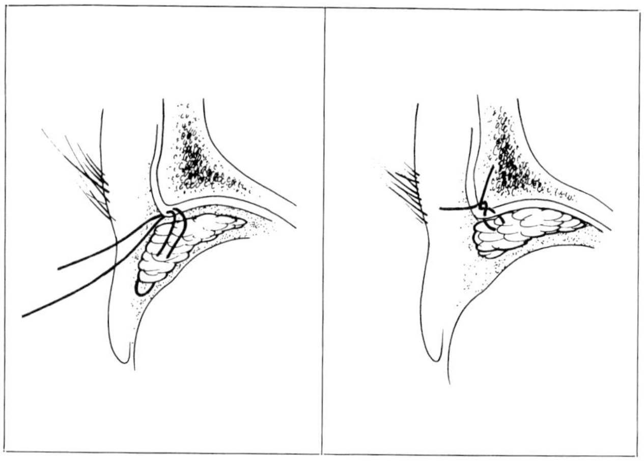

Figure 34–6. Technique to reposition lacrimal gland.

silicone tubing (0.025 inch, outside diameter, 0.012 inch, inside diameter) is the most effective stent, because it is soft, is flexible, and readily supports the canalicular walls.[44] Metal rods have been used but are difficult to keep properly positioned.[45] Placing a 3-0 or 4-0 stitch throughout the canalicular system is not effective because the canaliculus will have inadequate support.

Crawford stents[43] or similar intubation tubes may be passed through the entire nasolacrimal system, or a modified, round-tipped eyed pigtail probe may be used to place the stent (Fig. 34–8*A*).[40, 46] The Worst pigtail

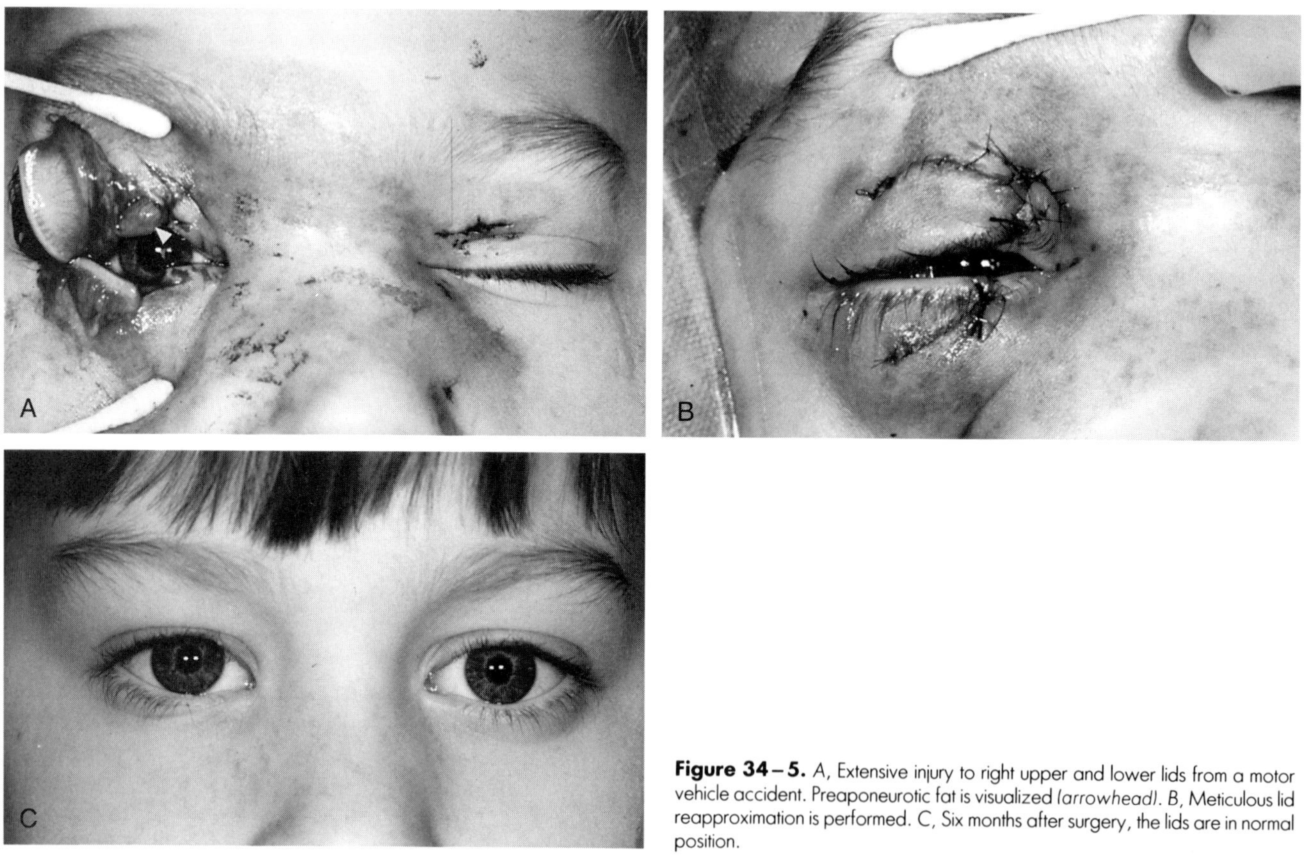

Figure 34–5. A, Extensive injury to right upper and lower lids from a motor vehicle accident. Preaponeurotic fat is visualized (arrowhead). B, Meticulous lid reapproximation is performed. C, Six months after surgery, the lids are in normal position.

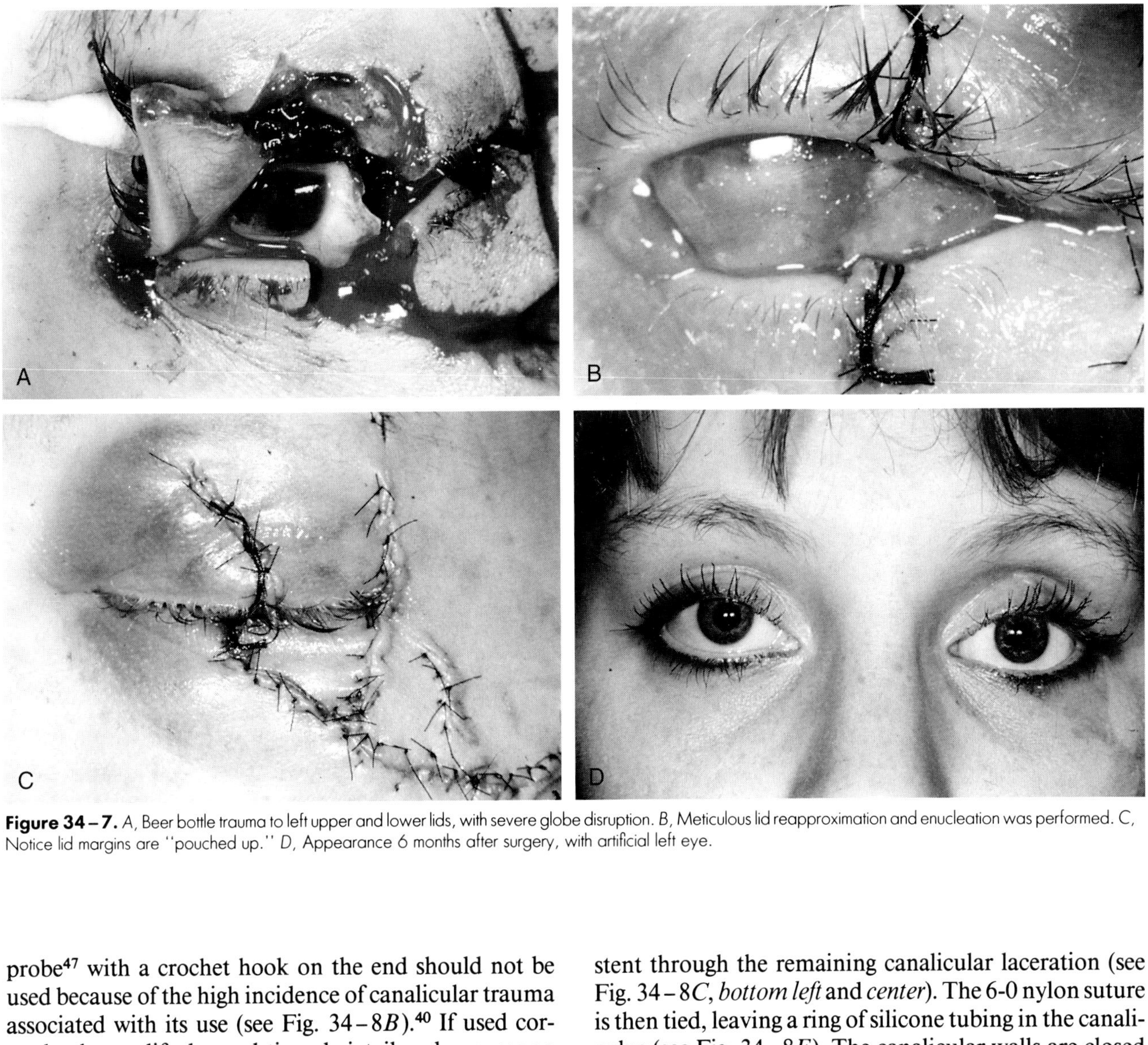

Figure 34–7. *A*, Beer bottle trauma to left upper and lower lids, with severe globe disruption. *B*, Meticulous lid reapproximation and enucleation was performed. *C*, Notice lid margins are "pouched up." *D*, Appearance 6 months after surgery, with artificial left eye.

probe[47] with a crochet hook on the end should not be used because of the high incidence of canalicular trauma associated with its use (see Fig. 34–8*B*).[40] If used correctly, the modified round-tipped pigtail probe causes no trauma and allows the surgeon to find the severed canalicular ends and reconstruct the canaliculi readily with a very high success rate.[40]

It is absolutely essential when using the round-tipped pigtail probe to rotate it with extreme care. If any pressure is applied, the risk of trauma to the canaliculus increases. Therefore, if the probe cannot be rotated smoothly, it should be abandoned for an alternative technique. The technique involves passing the probe along the uninvolved canaliculus after punctal dilation (see Fig. 34–8*C*). With careful manipulation, the probe is rotated into the lacerated canaliculus and a 6-0 nylon suture is placed through the probe eye (see Fig. 34–8*D*). The probe is then withdrawn, leaving the 6-0 nylon suture in the canaliculus. A small piece of silicone tubing, about 15 to 20 mm long, is threaded over the 6-0 nylon suture (see Fig. 34–8*E*). The silicone tubing is then compressed with forceps, and the opposite end of the nylon suture is pulled so as to rotate the stent into the damaged canaliculus. The same technique is used to pass the 6-0 nylon suture and stent through the remaining canalicular laceration (see Fig. 34–8*C*, *bottom left* and *center*). The 6-0 nylon suture is then tied, leaving a ring of silicone tubing in the canaliculus (see Fig. 34–8*F*). The canalicular walls are closed using a 7-0 or 8-0 polyglactin suture. The remaining lid is reapproximated and closed using 5-0 polyglactin suture deeply and 6-0 silk suture more superficially, as outlined for other lid lacerations.

Canthal Tendon Injuries

With more extensive medial canthal tendon injuries and avulsions, accurate realignment is required. Surgical correction must reposition the medial canthal tendon so that it is on the same horizontal plane as the tendon on the contralateral side. In addition, the tendon has to be placed posteriorly enough so that the medial eyelid hugs the globe; otherwise, a space will be left between the lid and the globe medially. It is important to reapproximate and repair the canaliculi with stents if needed. If the medial canthal tendon is avulsed, the tendon can be directly resutured to the periosteum, provided some is present. If there are multiple nasal fractures, a transnasal wire procedure may be required. Alternatively, if the bones are

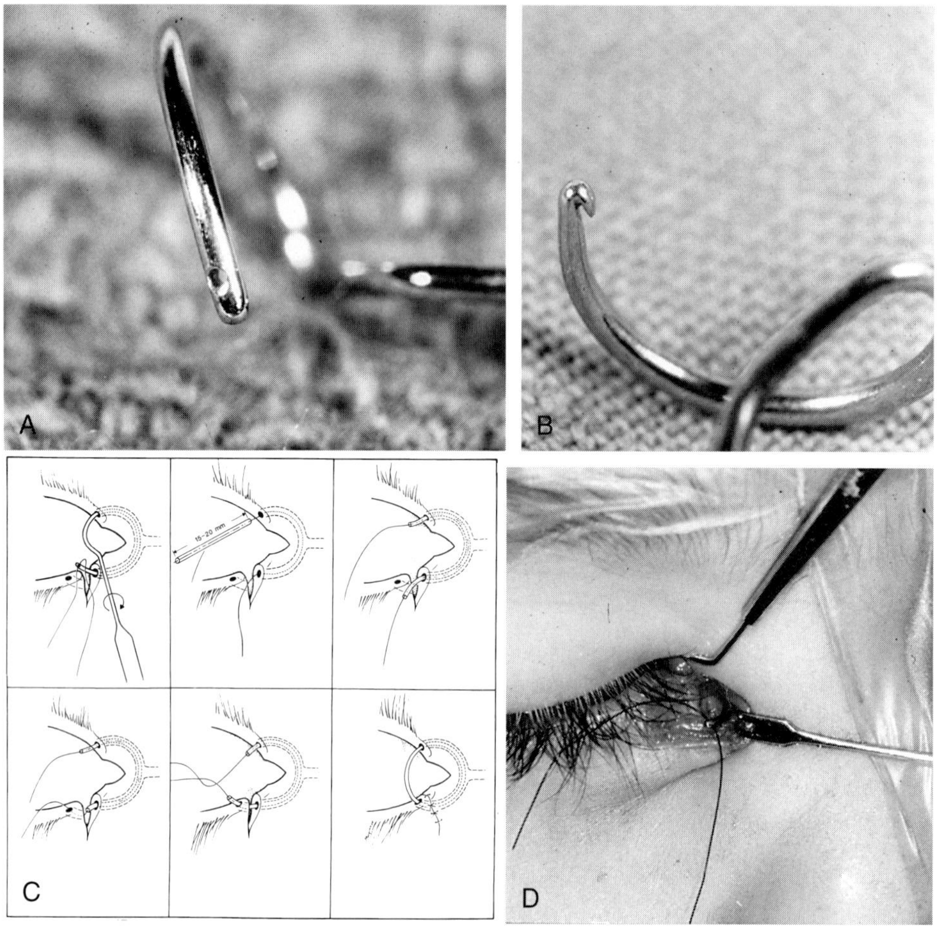

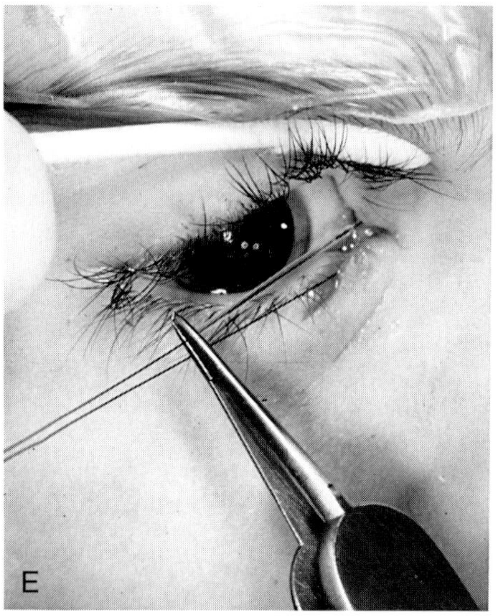

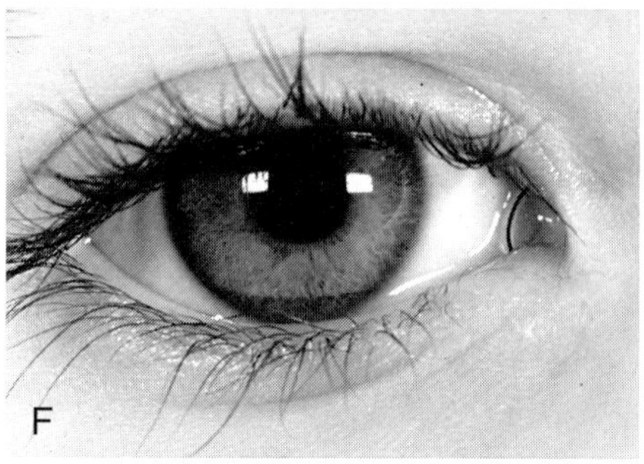

Figure 34–8. *A*, Round-tipped eyed pigtail probe. *B*, Worst-type crochet-end pigtail probe. *C*, Canalicular reconstruction technique using the pigtail probe is illustrated for a lower canaliculus. *D*, Pigtail probe has been rotated along superior canaliculus and into lacerated lower canaliculus. A 6-0 nylon suture is threaded through the probe eye. *E*, Silicone tubing is threaded onto the 6-0 nylon suture. *F*, Silicone tubing with 6-0 nylon suture in the center.

intact and stable, a Peton screw can be used to anchor the medial canthal tendon and/or lid remnants onto the frontal process of the maxilla (Fig. 34–9).[48]

Lacerations involving the lateral canthal tendon area are more straightforward because there are no canaliculi. If one or both of the lids have been lacerated laterally, it is important to reattach the canthal tendon itself or the lateral tarsus to the periosteum on the inside wall of the lateral orbital rim to achieve the proper lateral canthal approximation. If no periosteum is available, a small hole can be drilled through the lateral rim to act as an anchor site. The lateral tarsal strip procedure can be extremely useful here.[49, 50] If additional tissue is required, this can be mobilized from the lateral lid, periosteum, or temporal skin area.[6, 51, 52]

In summary, trauma to the eyelid, medial canthus, and

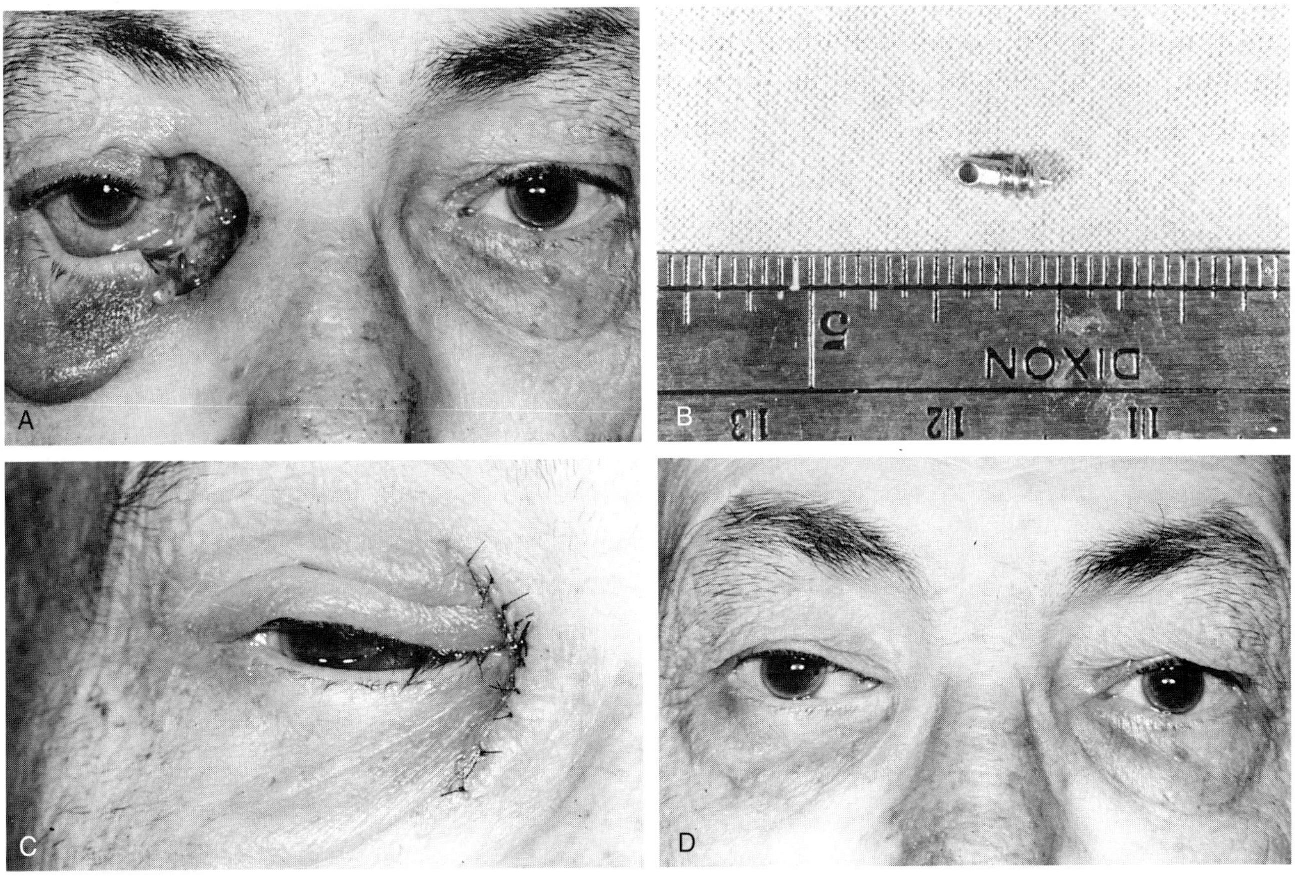

Figure 34–9. *A*, Large basal cell carcinoma removed from medial canthal area, leaving a sizable defect down to bone. *B*, Peton screw. After being secured into the frontal process of maxilla, the screw is firmly anchored. *C*, The lids are reconnected to the Peton screw. *D*, Ten months after surgery, a nice result is attained. The nasolacrimal system will be reconstructed with a Jones tube at a later date.

lateral canthus may result from blunt or penetrating injuries. Because the force and velocity of the injury can be significant, one should always be suspicious of underlying injury to the globe, orbital structures, paranasal sinuses, and bony wall. The fundamental principles involved in repairing lid and adnexal lacerations include identification of the structures involved and reapproximation of normal tissue anatomy. When tissue is lost, additional reconstructive techniques are required to replace the missing structure.

RECONSTRUCTIVE UPPER EYELID TECHNIQUES

Tarsal Substitutes

I have discovered over the past several years that posterior lamella reconstruction using such tissue as nasal cartilage or ear cartilage often gives rise to a rigid, immobile and thickened lid. Other tissue, such as sclera, provides inadequate support and may result in an unstable eyelid. These results have to be accepted at times since alternative reconstructive material may not be available. I have found that the most natural-appearing reconstructed lids have been achieved when the lost tissue is replaced with nearly identical tissue. Thus, I try to reconstruct posterior lamella with tarsus whenever possible.

Autogenous Tarsus

The patient's opposite upper lid may serve as a donor site for tarsal tissue. The technique is straightforward and easily accomplished using local anesthesia. The uninvolved upper lid is infiltrated with 2% lidocaine in combination with epinephrine. A 4-0 silk suture is placed through the lid margin, which is then everted over a lid plate. Starting 2 to 3 mm above the lid margin, a full-thickness tarsal incision is made with a no. 15 blade for the entire length of the tarsal plate. Vertical incisions are made medially and laterally. The cut edge of tarsus is elevated, and Westcott scissors are used to dissect between tarsus and overlying Müller's muscle until one reaches the superior tarsal edge. Conjunctiva is then transected at this level, and an autogenous free tarsal graft is available to use in the opposite lid requiring lid reconstruction.

Autogenous tarsus has a smooth mucosal surface to rest on the eye and is identical tissue to that lost. The donor site will heal spontaneously and is treated with an antibiotic ophthalmic ointment three or four times daily during the first week.

Sclera

Donor sclera is another alternative in posterior lamella reconstruction.[11, 12] The donor sclera is prepared according to the technique described by Flanagan[11] and rehydrated in antibiotic solution. Sclera from older donors is preferred since it tends to have increased rigidity. The sclera may be trimmed to the shape and size of the lid defect and is sutured into position with a 7-0 absorbable suture when used. Unfortunately, sclera lacks a mucosal surface and authors disagree as to whether it should be covered by conjunctiva after its placement. Sclera has been observed to undergo a variable amount of postoperative shrinkage, which represents either tissue necrosis or some degree of graft rejection. Sclera is more flexible than tarsus, and thus lid stability may not be completely satisfactory when sclera is utilized.

Auricular Cartilage

Ear cartilage may also be used as a substitute for posterior lamella.[8–10] It is relatively easy to obtain but is often thicker than tarsus, is rigid, and does not conform well to the globe. The lid may be poorly mobile with noticeable irregularities due to the cartilage. It also lacks an epithelial surface, and although it is usually reepithelialized by adjacent conjunctiva, the cornea may be extremely irritated while waiting for this to occur. It is more commonly used in the lower lid, where it can be left uncovered to be epithelialized by surrounding conjunctival tissue.

The technique for harvesting cartilage involves examining each ear to see which has the flattest portion between the helix laterally and antihelix medially. This area is known as the scaphoid fossa (Fig. 34–10). Cartilage from other areas of the ear is too curved and does not conform to the globe well. The surgeon may use an anterior or posterior approach. The posterior approach will hide the incision. The auricular skin is locally infiltrated anteriorly and posteriorly with 2% lidocaine in combination with epinephrine. The local infiltration may help dissect the perichondrium away from the cartilage itself. A towel clamp is used to grasp the helix, and the posterior aspect of the ear is exposed. A curved incision is made superiorly following the curve of the helix along the posterior surface. Sharp dissection is carried out down to cartilage, and a tissue plane is easily created between cartilage and the overlying perichondrium and skin. The desired amount of cartilage is exposed and then harvested by incising cartilage itself and then carefully dissecting skin and perichondrium away from its anterior surface. Using Westcott or Stevens scissors will aid in this dissection. Bleeding is generally minimal if epinephrine has been used. It is essential to leave a rim of cartilage superiorly, otherwise a deformed helical curve will result. No attempt is made at trying to close the cartilage defect because a severe deformity will occur. The skin is closed with a running 6-0 absorbable suture.

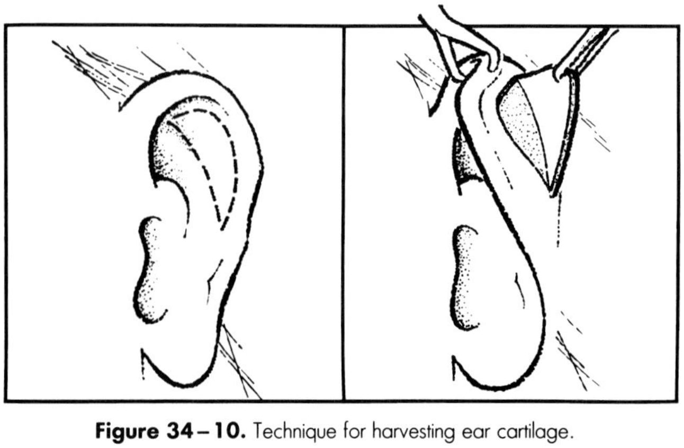

Figure 34–10. Technique for harvesting ear cartilage.

Hard Palate Mucosa

Hard palate mucosa is a useful technique for lid reconstruction.[13, 14] This material is readily available, is easy to obtain, and has rigidity similar to tarsus. Hard palate mucosa has a keratinized, stratified, squamous epithelium unlike the rest of the oral mucosa, which is nonkeratinized. In the initial postoperative period, the keratin layer may cause corneal irritation. Over time, metaplasia to nonkeratinized mucosa generally occurs and this irritation resolves. However, if it persists, the patient will be uncomfortable. Thus, it must be used cautiously in the upper lid. It is used more commonly in lower lids where there is less risk for corneal irritation.

The surgery can be performed using local anesthesia,[13] but I prefer general anesthesia because it is more comfortable for the patient and the airway is better protected if a prominent bleeding vessel should develop during harvesting. The hard palate submucosa is infiltrated with lidocaine in combination with epinephrine to obtain anesthesia as well as vasoconstriction of vessels. The graft is taken from the hard palate between the alveolar ridge and the midline, extending posteriorly to within 2 mm of soft palate. The graft is harvested laterally to the midline since mucosa is too thin centrally. It is generally 30 mm long and 10 mm wide when harvested. Two parallel incisions that are the desired length of the graft are made through the mucosa, with care being taken to avoid penetration through the underlying mucoperiosteum. The hard palate mucosa is elevated with blunt and sharp dissection using Westcott or iris scissors and a no. 15 blade. Posteriorly, care is taken to avoid damage to the palatine artery, which courses through the deep submucosal tissue at the junction of the hard and soft palate. When the graft has been removed, hemostasis is obtained with bipolar cautery and the defect is covered with a piece of absorbable gelatin sponge (Gelfoam). The adherent mucous glands and submucosa are dissected from the posterior surface of the graft. The donor site will gradually granulate in over 2 to 3 weeks. A soft diet is recommended during the first few days.

Oral Mucosa

Oral mucosa provides no tarsal support but may occasionally be required to act as a lining for a myocutaneous flap. Whenever possible, oral mucosa is harvested from the upper or lower lip. Buccal mucosa may also be used. I prefer full-thickness grafts for eyelid reconstruction because split-thickness ones tend to shrink and are not as stable after surgery.

The upper or lower lip is everted and infiltrated with 1% lidocaine in combination with epinephrine. A lip clamp may be helpful here. The approximate size of mucosal graft required is then incised and carefully dissected with sharp scissors. The plane of dissection is in the substantia propria. This can be identified by its white or yellow appearance and the presence of mulberry-shaped minor salivary glands. Deeper dissection into the muscle of the lip or cheek must be avoided. The vermilion border of the lip must be avoided. After excision, bleeding is controlled by a light application of bipolar cautery. When harvesting buccal mucosa, Stensen's duct, which is opposite the second molar, must be avoided. The lip donor site is left to close on its own, while the buccal donor site is closed with absorbable 4-0 suture.

Nasochondral Tissue

Nasochondral tissue has its own mucosa and cartilage support,[7] but unfortunately, like ear cartilage, it is extremely thick, immobile, and nonconforming to the globe. The nasochondral mucosa has numerous goblet cells and thus, when used in eyelid reconstruction, tends to have extra mucus.

The technique to harvest this tissue has been well described by Mustardé.[7] It involves packing the nose on both sides of the septum with 4% cocaine on cotton pledgets for 10 minutes. If the patient is not under general anesthesia, 2% lidocaine with epinephrine is injected beneath the mucosa on both sides of the septum, taking care not to strip the mucosa and perichondrium from the underlying cartilage on the side from which it is planned to approach it. The mucosa and perichondrium on the opposite side should be ballooned up with the local anesthesia since this will facilitate the removal of the cartilage.

In the conscious patient, a petrolatum gauze pack is placed into both nostrils as far back as possible to prevent blood running into the nasopharynx. An incision is made around the base of the ala of the nose and is carried right through so as to detach it completely. The incision for the graft should start 1 to 1.5 cm above the base of the nose in

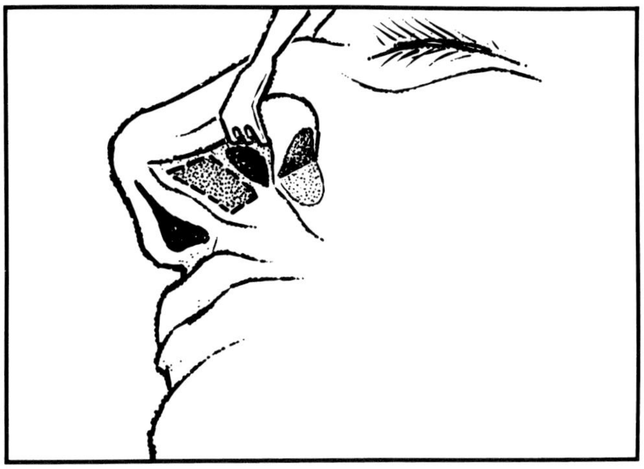

Figure 34–11. Technique for harvesting nasochondral tissue.

the groove on the outside of the nostril. This will allow sufficient exposure of the septum so as to obtain a composite septal graft up to 1.5 cm square. The required amount of mucosa is outlined and incised on the surface of the cartilage part of the septum, being careful to leave at least 0.5 cm of septal cartilage intact to form an anterior strut for the nasal bridge line. A no. 64 Beaver blade is helpful for the dissection as well as a curved no. 66 Beaver blade to facilitate making the posterior cut (Fig. 34–11).

The underlying cartilage is then incised on the same line, taking care not to perforate the contralateral perichondrium and mucosa. A flat instrument such as a Howarth septal dissector or a Freer elevator may be used to help elevate the cartilage away from the opposite perichondrium. Once enough tissue has been freed, upper and lower mucosal cuts may be made that extend down into perichondrium and cartilage, being careful not to injure perichondrium and mucosa on the opposite side. The posterior incision is then made, and the graft is removed and ready for use.

The posteriorly placed petrolatum gauze may be removed and the anterior nasal cavity packed lightly with the same petrolatum gauze.

Irradiated Tarsus and Aorta

I have been investigating the use of irradiated homologous tarsal plates[15, 16] and homologous irradicated aorta.[17] The irradiated tarsus is similar to tarsal plate without a mucosal surface. The tarsus acts as a structural framework for the host's fibroblasts to grow on. It is easy to work with, conforms to the globe, and is readily available. I have used it as the middle layer in Cutler-Beard procedures and in several lower eyelid reconstruction procedures. Because it lacks a mucosal surface, I try to bury it between two surfaces, such as in the Cutler-Beard technique. With irradiated donor aorta, I have noted similar qualities to that of irradiated tarsus and have had good results with it as the middle layer of a Cutler-Beard procedure.

Direct Closure and the Semicircular Flap Technique

The most common reconstructive procedure in the upper (and lower) eyelid is direct closure of the eyelid margin. It is applicable in cases of upper and lower eyelid defects as large as one third of the lid encountered after tumor removal, trauma, and congenital malformation (such as coloboma), when normal eyelid tissue is present on either side of the defect. These defects can generally be closed directly, even in young patients. When additional mobilization of tissue is required to close a defect, lateral canthotomy and cantholysis is suggested. In older patients with eyelid laxity, a similar closure of lid defects involving up to one half of the lid may be possible.[53]

Direct closure of an eyelid defect has many advantages. It allows the surgeon to reconstruct both the anterior (skin, muscle) and posterior (tarsus, conjunctiva) lamellae. This technique does not obstruct the visual axis and avoids multistep procedures and the use of tarsal substitutes. The eyelashes are approximated, providing a more natural-appearing reconstructed eyelid.

Direct closure can also be used in medial defects when only a remnant of medial canthal tendon or medial orbital periosteum remains. If the tissues are not elastic enough to allow direct closure, a lateral canthotomy and cantholysis will allow a large amount of additional tissue mobilization. If the superior canaliculus is involved, I recommend that a silicone stent be placed through the remaining canaliculus to maintain its patency.

For a large defect involving two thirds or more of the medial or central upper eyelid, a semicircular flap procedure is a useful technique.[54–57] This technique will allow closure of lid defects involving 50% to 70% of the central and medial lid margin. Several modifications have been suggested for this technique.[54, 57]

The procedure for a medial or central upper lid defect is straightforward. The first incision is through skin and orbicularis, directed inferiorly at the lateral canthus. The next incision heads downward and laterally in a semicircular fashion, being careful to avoid deep portions of the inferior crus of the lateral canthal tendon but beveled to include as much orbicularis as possible. The superior crus of the canthal tendon is transected, and the lid is moved medially to determine the amount of undermining that will be required at the lateral canthus. The tissue over the lateral rim area requires undermining in a submuscular plane.

Undermining laterally almost to the ear may be necessary at times to get adequate tissue mobilization. One must avoid the facial nerve in this lateral mobilization. The frontal or temporal branch of the facial nerve lies on the periosteum of the proximal one third of the zygomatic arch. This is usually 2.5 cm from the anterior border of the external auditory meatus but may vary between 0.8 and 3.5 cm from this point. The course of this nerve is oblique, running on the fascia deep to the facial muscle and passing approximately 1.5 cm to the lateral brow to enter the frontalis muscle on its undersurface not more than 2 cm above the eyebrow.[58] The dissection laterally can be done with blunt and sharp dissection just deep to the orbicularis muscle until the margin of the orbit is reached, where, owing to the increasing thickness of the skin and subcutaneous tissue, the dissection can be made more superficial to the peripheral part of the orbicularis muscle. Thus the nerve supply to the latter is present. As the dissection progresses laterally, it should not be at any deeper level than this to avoid damage to the temporal branches of the facial nerve (which runs on the fascia deep to the facial muscles). Therefore, the function of the upper part of the orbicularis and frontalis is undisturbed.[59]

Once the lid defect can be approximated, the lid margins are closed in a standard fashion.[26, 27] The skin edges at the lateral canthus are reunited and afforded deep fixation with a 4-0 polyglactin 910 suture, with a deep bite attaching underlying orbicularis to the insertion of the inferior crus of the lateral canthal tendon. The lateral canthal angle forms a natural angle, providing the reconstructed tissues are fixated to the remaining portion of lateral canthal tendon (lower crus) or posteriorly inside the orbital rim or as close to Whitnall's tubercle as possible (Fig. 34–12).

Postoperative problems are generally minor. Corneal irritation from lid margin sutures, shortage of conjunctival lining, or poor blinking may cause superficial punctate keratitis in some patients. This is readily treated with topical lubricants. In some patients, a small step off at the junction of the tarsal plate and reconstructed eyelid tissue may be noted. This notch generally smooths out with time and is not a noticeable defect. Although some degree of blepharoptosis is present early in most of these lid reconstructions, the lid usually comes up to a normal level with time. The temporal eyelid spontaneously lines itself with conjunctiva in all cases of partial lid reconstruction. The temporal conjunctiva fornix may be mildly to moderately reduced in most cases. The short temporal fornices do not seem to be a functional or cosmetic problem in any patient. Mucous membrane or tarsal grafts can be combined with this technique.

Skin Grafting and Myocutaneous Flaps

Loss of anterior lamella only (skin and muscle tissue) can, at times, be quite challenging to reconstruct. Skin grafting, utilizing skin from the opposite upper eyelid or preauricular, retroauricular, or supraclavicular regions, is a time-honored technique that can be used to fill in anterior lamellar defects. If available, the skin from the opposite upper lid is the best donor site, primarily because the grafted tissue is identical to that skin tissue lost. The eyelid crease is drawn out, and the skin is pinched up to calculate the amount available and the amount needed in a similar fashion to calculating skin removal during

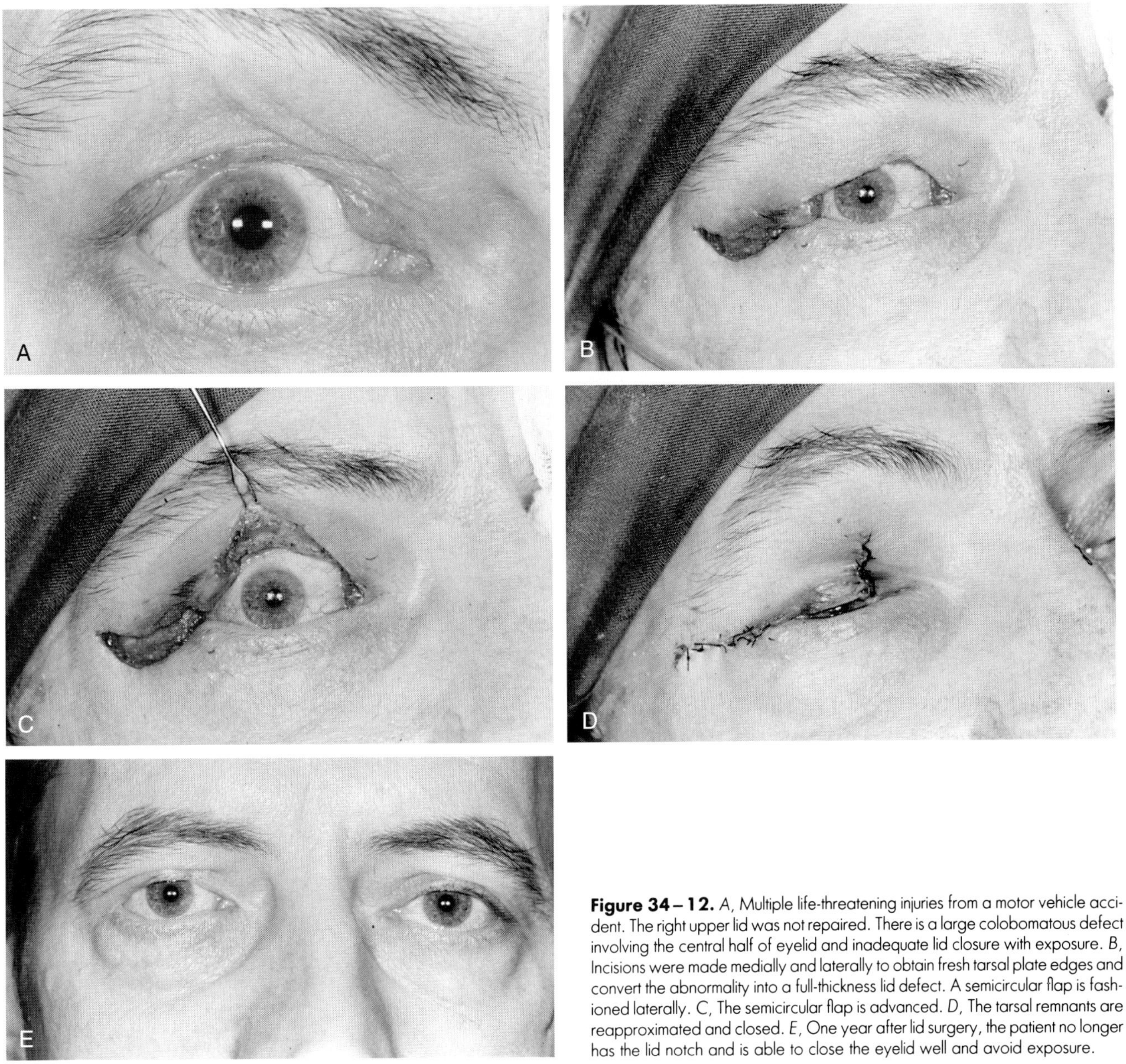

Figure 34–12. *A*, Multiple life-threatening injuries from a motor vehicle accident. The right upper lid was not repaired. There is a large colobomatous defect involving the central half of eyelid and inadequate lid closure with exposure. *B*, Incisions were made medially and laterally to obtain fresh tarsal plate edges and convert the abnormality into a full-thickness lid defect. A semicircular flap is fashioned laterally. *C*, The semicircular flap is advanced. *D*, The tarsal remnants are reapproximated and closed. *E*, One year after lid surgery, the patient no longer has the lid notch and is able to close the eyelid well and avoid exposure.

blepharoplasty. One or 2% lidocaine in combination with epinephrine is used to infiltrate the subcutaneous tissue, and the graft is incised and harvested, staying in a suborbicular plane during dissection. The bleeding vessels in the donor site are cauterized, and the skin is closed with a fine running suture. The skin graft with attached orbicularis is then put into position, trimmed to size, and sutured with multiple interrupted sutures. It is not necessary to trim off orbicularis. It is important to tie a sponge bolster over the graft for 1 week (Figs. 34–13 and 34–14).

If a full-thickness skin graft is taken from elsewhere (preauricular or retroauricular or supraclavicular), the subcutaneous tissues should be trimmed from the graft. The preauricular area in the elderly often has enough available excess skin to use as a skin graft. It is certainly much more visible to work in. It may, however, not supply enough skin and, if so, the retroauricular or supraclavicular area is used. The retroauricular skin is reasonably thin, and although its color is not identical to eyelid skin, it is a good substitute. An advantage of the retroauricular skin graft is that the donor site is hidden nicely.

The technique for harvesting retroauricular skin involves making a pattern of the defect on a glove liner. This is cut out and transferred to the retroauricular area so that it sits on the sulcus equally distributed on either side of the sulcus. Local anesthesia is injected subcutaneously to balloon off the skin from the deeper tissue. The ear is held forward with towel clamps or 4-0 silk suture. The graft is incised and then carefully dissected away.

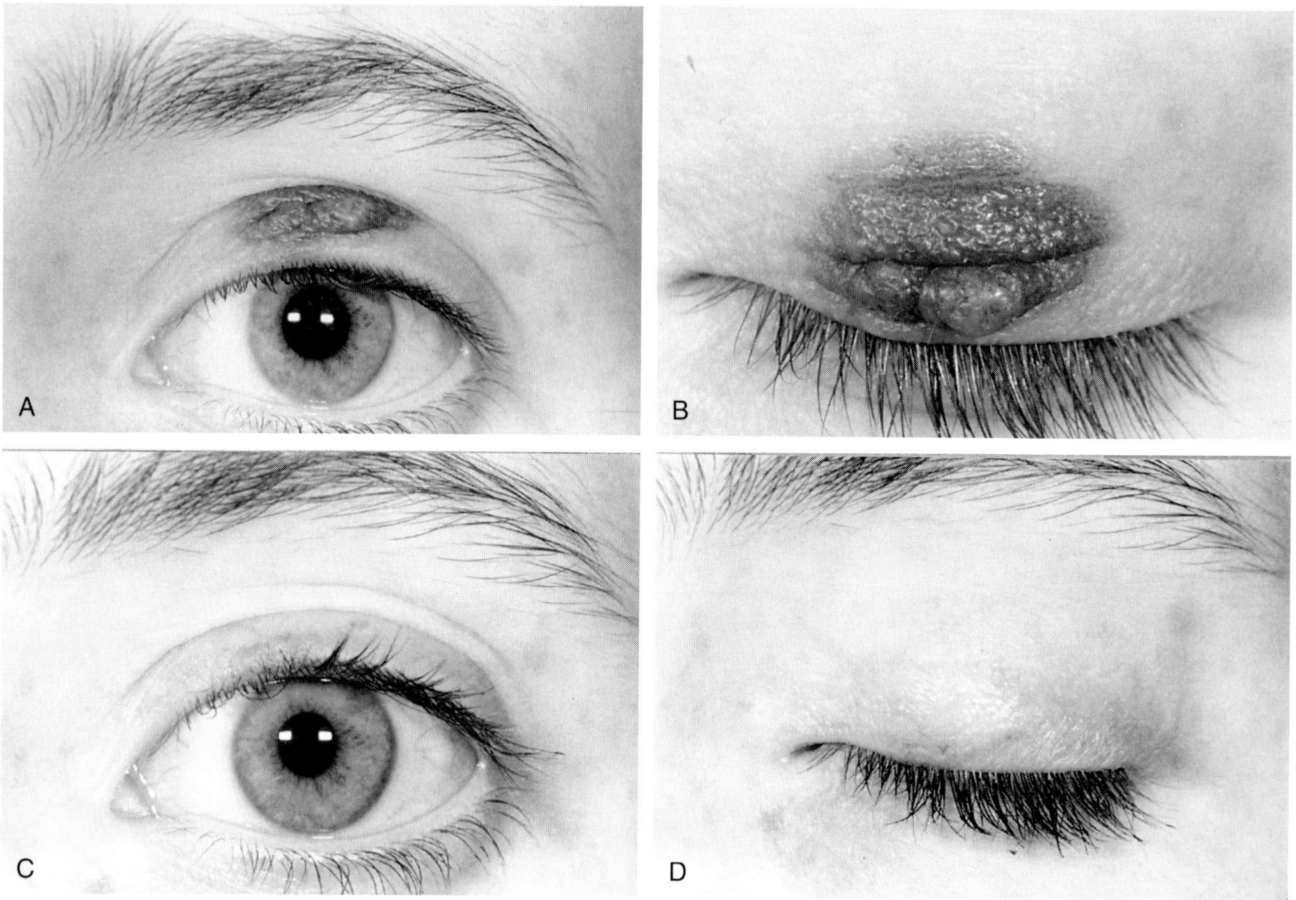

Figure 34–13. *A* and *B*, Pigmented growth illustrated on the left upper lid of a 14-year-old girl. *C* and *D*, The pigmented growth was excised and replaced with a full-thickness graft from the opposite eyelid. The graft has blended in well.

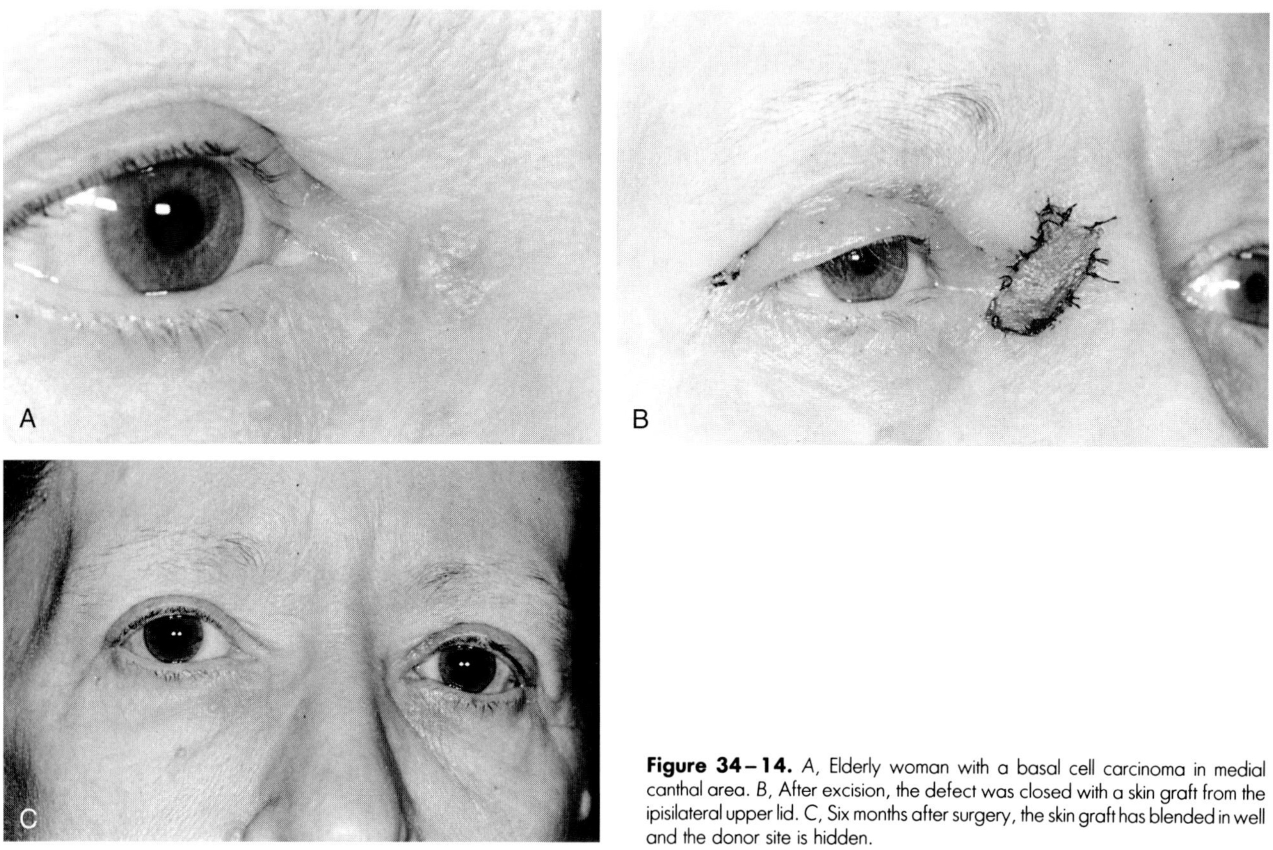

Figure 34–14. *A*, Elderly woman with a basal cell carcinoma in medial canthal area. *B*, After excision, the defect was closed with a skin graft from the ipsilateral upper lid. *C*, Six months after surgery, the skin graft has blended in well and the donor site is hidden.

After necessary cautery, closure is carried out by closing subcutaneous tissue with interrupted 4-0 chromic sutures. The skin is then closed with a running or intermittent absorbable suture. The graft should be thinned by trimming off subdermal fatty tissue. It is now ready to be used.

Split-thickness grafts are also an option but are seldom used because they tend to shrink a lot. If a split-thickness graft is considered, the assistance of a graft cutting knife or a dermatome will be required. The areas generally used for donor sites are the inner aspect of the thigh or arm, which are not too disfiguring. The skin of the upper arm has much finer hair on it except in very hirsute men.

A myocutaneous flap should always be considered when replacing anterior lamella only.[24] A myocutaneous flap formed from tissues adjacent to the defect has the advantage of replacing lost tissue with identical tissues, supported with its own blood supply. The orbicularis muscle is extremely vascular and allows more rapid healing to take place than in a standard skin graft. A valuable technique to follow in the upper eyelid involves undermining and mobilizing the skin and muscle surrounding the defect (Fig. 34–15). Dissection is started just anterior to the orbital septum to create eyelid skin–muscle flaps with orbicularis attached. A sliding flap is created with incisions that can be hidden in natural creases. The incision in the upper eyelid is placed in the eyelid crease and immediately beneath the brow. The base of the flap is fashioned wider than the distal portion, if possible. The wide flap base ensures a maximal blood supply. Care must be taken not to disinsert the levator aponeurosis while dissecting the eyelid myocutaneous flap. The extensive undermining with some of the flaps may temporarily decrease the orbicularis function and lead to a poor blink and lagophthalmos. Within a few weeks, however, the eyelid function returns, and permanent denervation is not a problem. The incision, once healed, will be hidden nicely. If the eyelid margins and posterior lamella are involved, the myocutaneous eyelid flap can be used in conjunction with other techniques for reconstruction of the posterior lamella.

The posterior lamella can be reconstructed by direct closure using tarsal advancement with or without canthotomy and cantholysis, tarsoconjunctival pedicle flaps, conjunctival flaps or grafts, free tarsal grafts, composite nasomucosal cartilage grafts, or scleral grafts. The eyelid skin muscle flap provides an excellent vascular bed for those posterior lamella grafts and flaps that cannot be obtained from skin grafts or skin flaps alone (Fig. 34–16).

Thus, the advantages of the myocutaneous flaps are (1) localized reconstruction with identical tissue, (2) one-stage reconstruction, (3) excellent blood supply, (4) vascular support for posterior lamella grafts and, (5) rapid rehabilitation with little visible scar.

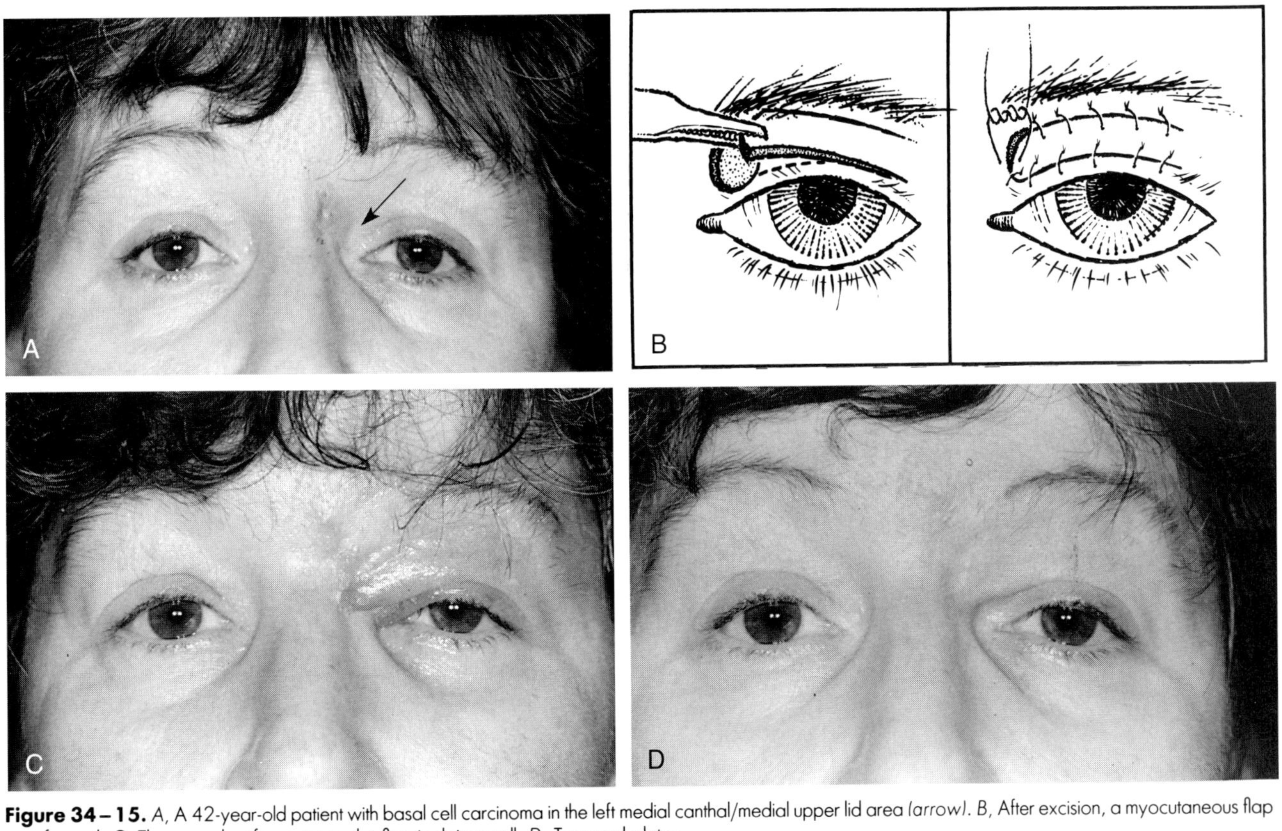

Figure 34–15. *A*, A 42-year-old patient with basal cell carcinoma in the left medial canthal/medial upper lid area *(arrow)*. *B*, After excision, a myocutaneous flap was formed. *C*, Three weeks after surgery, the flap is doing well. *D*, Ten weeks later.

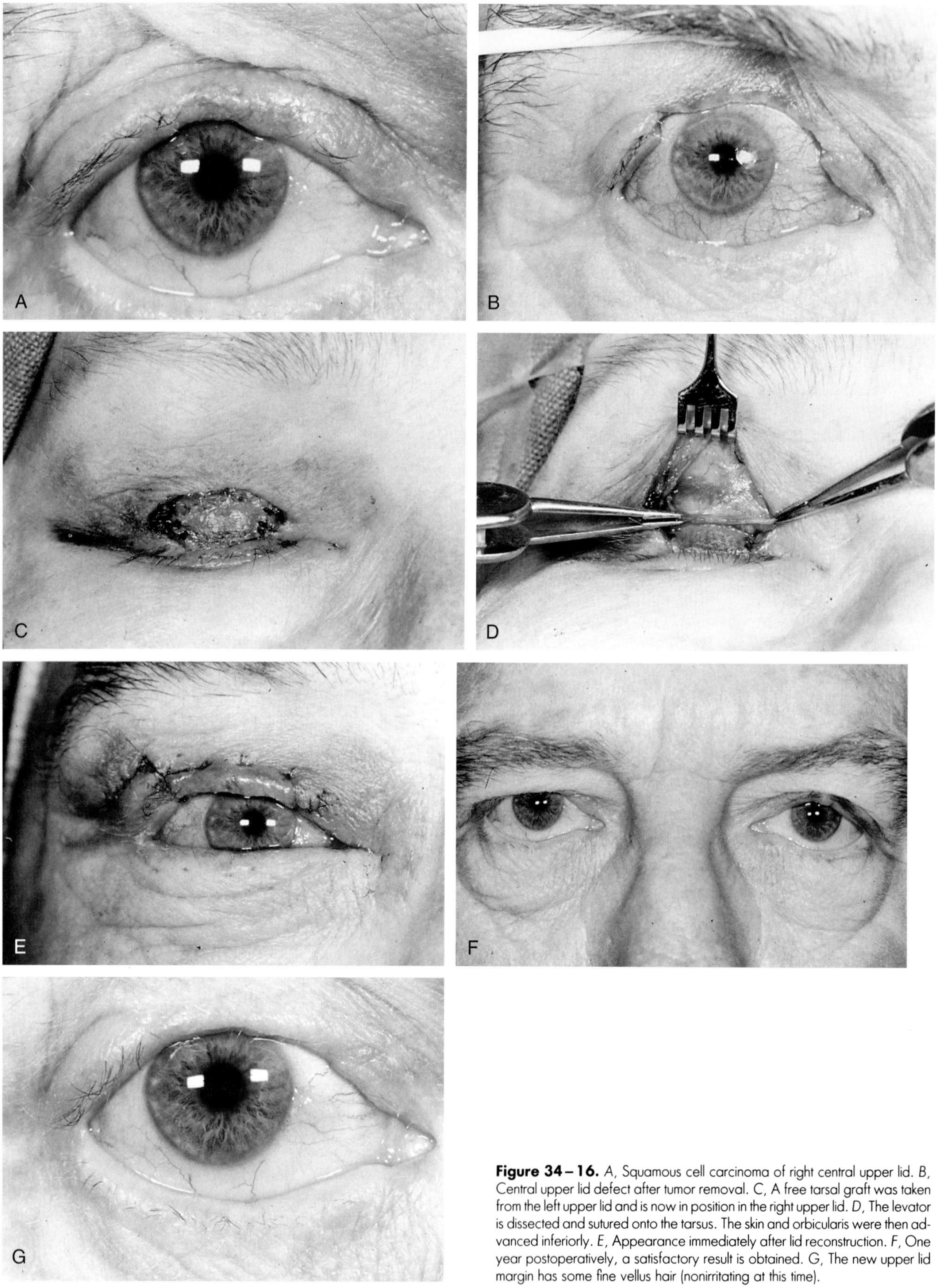

Figure 34–16. *A*, Squamous cell carcinoma of right central upper lid. *B*, Central upper lid defect after tumor removal. C, A free tarsal graft was taken from the left upper lid and is now in position in the right upper lid. *D*, The levator is dissected and sutured onto the tarsus. The skin and orbicularis were then advanced inferiorly. *E*, Appearance immediately after lid reconstruction. *F*, One year postoperatively, a satisfactory result is obtained. G, The new upper lid margin has some fine vellus hair (nonirritating at this time).

Lateral Transpositional Skin Flap

Anterior lamellar defects located laterally in the upper eyelid can also be repaired using a lateral transpositional skin flap.[60] This flap can also be used in conjunction with a posterior reconstructive technique such as the periosteal strip graft[61] or tarsal rotation flap.[62]

The technique involves marking out a vertical skin flap starting from the lateral edge of the defect and carrying it superiorly just lateral to and above the brow if necessary. The skin flap, which may be up to 1.5 cm wide, is raised and includes only subcutaneous tissue to avoid injuring branches of the facial nerve. Undermining is done on either side of the donor area to allow for easy approximation of the tissue edges once the flap is rotated into position. This flap can easily be combined with a posterior reconstructive technique, such as the periosteal strip graft (Fig. 34–17*A*). Because the transpositional flap must turn almost at a right angle, there may be some kinking in the flap. A gross amount at the time of surgery can be dealt with by excising some of the redundancy without jeopardizing the blood supply. Although the skin of the transpositional flap is not the same consistency as upper eyelid skin, it is a good substitute and has the advantage of having its own blood supply.

An alternative to the transpositional flap just described is the temporal forehead or brow flap, sometimes referred to as a Fricke flap.[63] This flap can be used for lateral upper and lower eyelid defects. The tissue being rotated into position is a much greater thickness than normal eyelid skin and should only be used if nothing else is available. In some instances, the flap has to bridge over normal tissue and thus a second stage modification is required.

The technique for harvesting the flap is straightforward. Gentian violet, methylene blue, or a similar marker is used to outline the flap above the brow. The base of the flap is temporal to the lateral orbital rim and should be as close as possible to the lateral canthus for good transposition. The flap is incised, and dissection is initiated in the subdermal fatty layer. This flap is mainly a cutaneous flap and can be quite thick. The subdermal fatty tissue may have to be trimmed to make it thinner. The tissue surrounding the pedicle may require undermining to close the donor defect. If so, dissection should be in a subcutaneous plane laterally so that facial nerve fiber in the temporal area can be avoided.

The flap is then placed into position, trimmed to size as needed, and secured to surrounding tissue. If possible, the undersurface of the flap should be secured to the lateral orbital rim periosteum in the area of Whitnall's tubercle so that a lateral canthal angle can be formed. If there is a full-thickness defect present, the flap must have a posterior lamellar lining, such as a periosteal strip graft, tarsoconjunctival flap, free tarsal graft, mucous membrane, and so on (see Fig. 34–17*B* through *G*). If the pedicle had to bridge normal tissue at the lateral canthus, a second-stage revision can be carried out in 6 to 8 weeks to trim the bridged area.

Median Forehead Flap

Anterior lamellar defects involving the medial canthal region and part of the upper lid can be repaired with the use of a median forehead flap.[63–65] The pedicle of tissue is thicker than the normal eyelid but has the advantage of bringing in its own blood supply. I find it particularly useful for large defects that involve the medial canthal area and the medial part of the upper lid.

The technique involves marking out a pedicle of tissue in the mid forehead that ideally should have a length of no more than five times its width. A longer flap may behave more as a free skin graft than as a vascular pedicle of tissue. The flap is incised and elevated, staying anterior to the frontalis muscle. Surrounding tissue is extensively undermined in the forehead area to allow the flap to rotate into the defect and allow direct closure of the donor site. As one comes down to the orbital rim area, an attempt should be made to preserve the supratrochlear vessels and supraorbital vessels.

The donor pedicle can be gently trimmed because it may be quite thick and bulky. The subcutaneous tissues are closed with 4-0 polyglactin sutures, while the skin is closed with a combination of 4-0 silk and 6-0 nylon sutures. The posterior surface of this flap may at times oppose the globe and must be lined with a posterior lamellar graft such as tarsus from the opposite eyelid, a free oral mucous membrane graft, or remnants of the conjunctiva from the lower fornices, which can be advanced upward.

The forehead flap may be attached to the levator aponeurosis with 5-0 or 6-0 polyglactin sutures to give some vertical mobility. Laterally, the flap is attached to the remaining lid with 6-0 polyglactin suture. Medially, it is important to try and tack down the flap tissue to the stump of medial canthal tendon. If the superior canaliculus has been transected, a canalicular stent is worthwhile to maintain the patency of the remaining system (Fig. 34–18).

It is not unusual to have a dog-ear of tissue over the dorsum of the nose once the median forehead flap has been rotated. This being the case, a second-stage modification can be carried out at about 8 weeks to remove the excess tissue or, in some instances, to separate the base of the flap and replace the tissue into the donor (glabellar) area to avoid narrowing the eyebrows. If the undersurface of the flap has been lined with conjunctiva from the lower lid, it can be separated in 6 weeks.

Postoperatively, some contraction of the flap will occur. Any excess bulk can be trimmed at a later date, if necessary. The eyelid will appear tight for many weeks and may not open, but, with time, it generally will open to a nice height, providing the levator was attached to it.

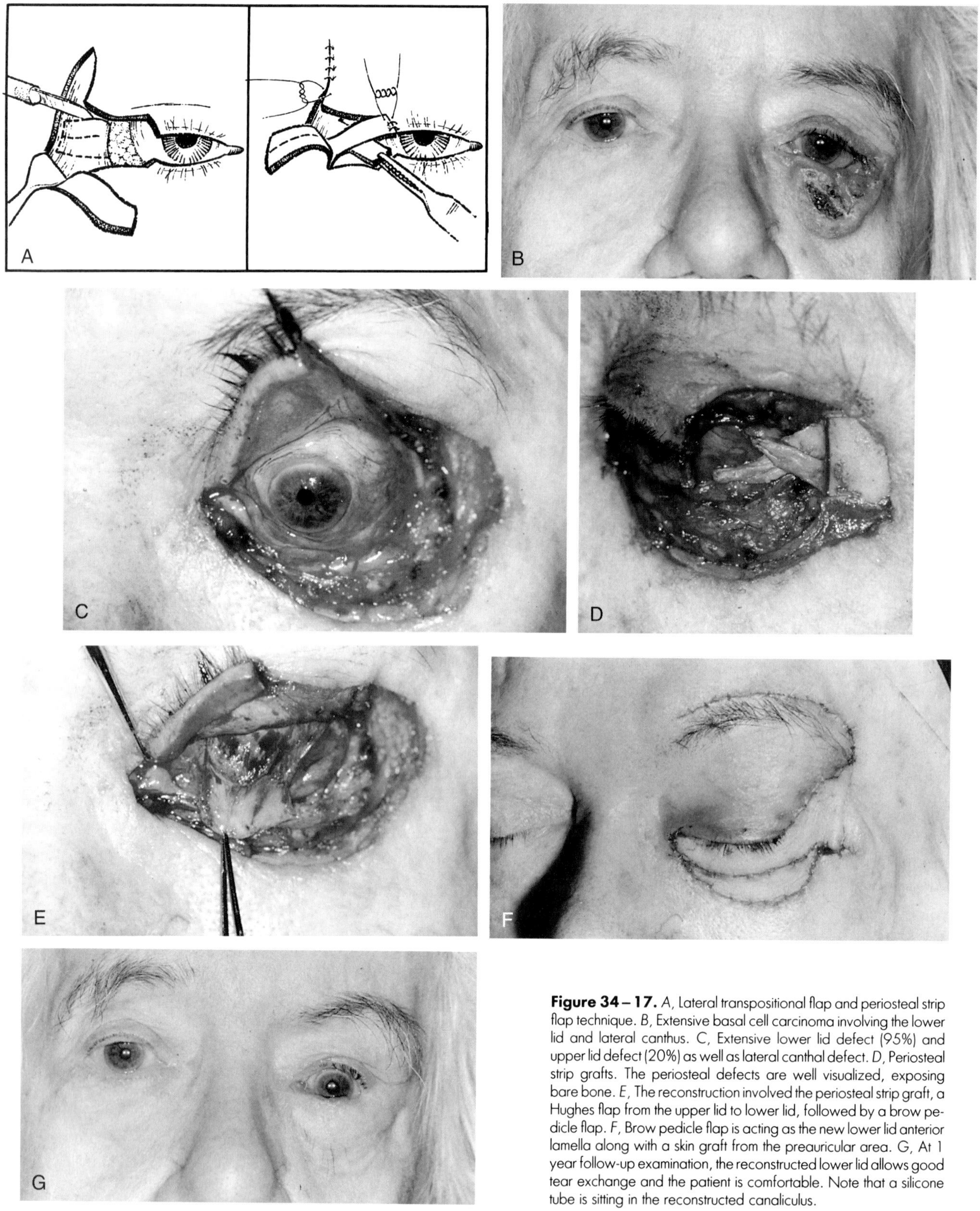

Figure 34–17. *A,* Lateral transpositional flap and periosteal strip flap technique. *B,* Extensive basal cell carcinoma involving the lower lid and lateral canthus. C, Extensive lower lid defect (95%) and upper lid defect (20%) as well as lateral canthal defect. *D,* Periosteal strip grafts. The periosteal defects are well visualized, exposing bare bone. *E,* The reconstruction involved the periosteal strip graft, a Hughes flap from the upper lid to lower lid, followed by a brow pedicle flap. *F,* Brow pedicle flap is acting as the new lower lid anterior lamella along with a skin graft from the preauricular area. G, At 1 year follow-up examination, the reconstructed lower lid allows good tear exchange and the patient is comfortable. Note that a silicone tube is sitting in the reconstructed canaliculus.

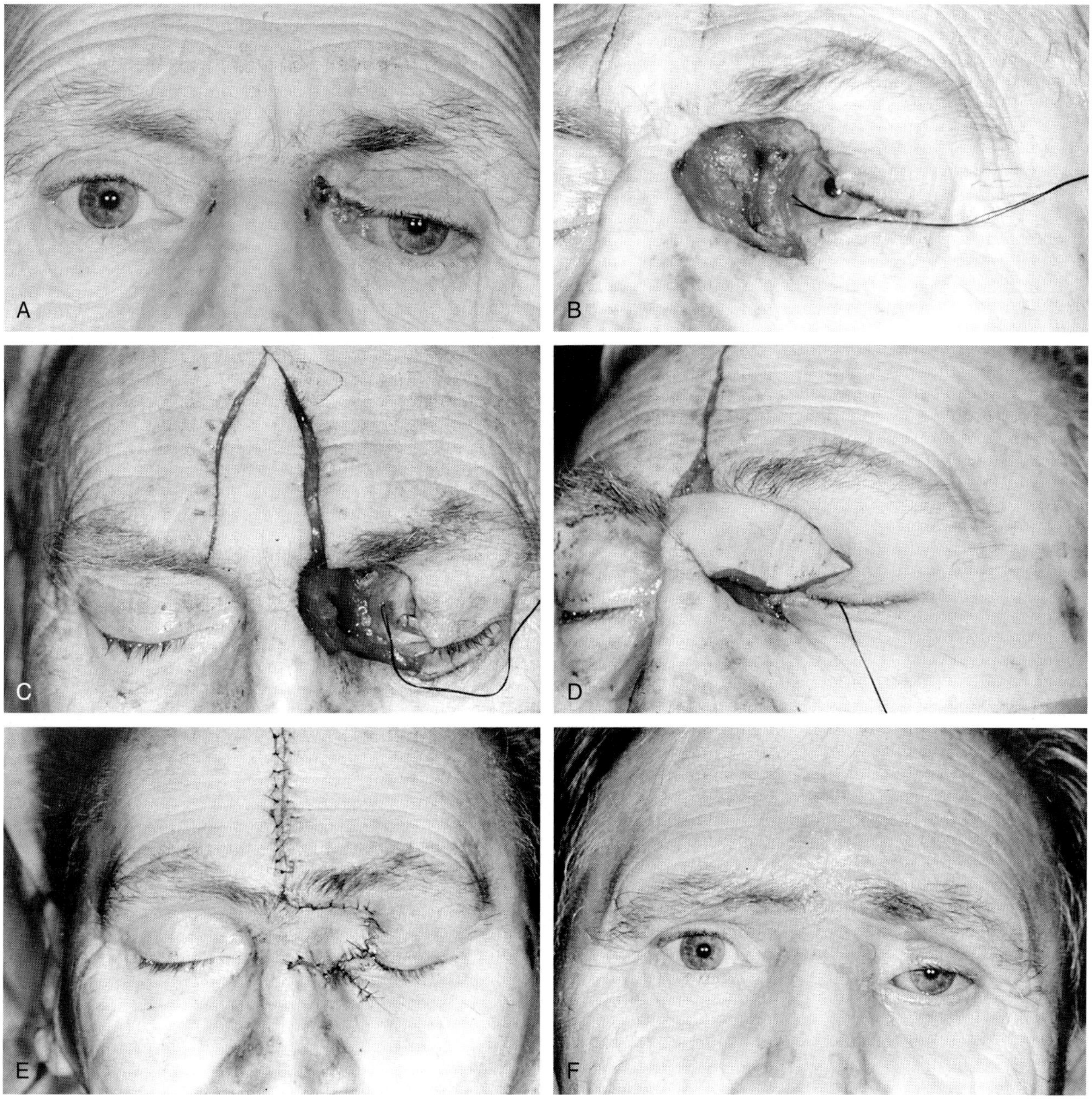

Figure 34–18. *A*, Large basal cell carcinoma is seen in the left medial canthal region. *B*, A sizeable defect involving the medial fourth of the upper and lower lids as well as the nasolacrimal system is noted. *C*, A median forehead flap is drawn out and incised. *D*, The flap is brought into position. *E*, The flap is sitting in position at the conclusion of the surgery. *F*, Six months after surgery, the result is satisfactory. Nasolacrimal reconstruction was planned, but the patient was lost to follow up.

Nasojugal Myocutaneous Flap

The orbitonasojugal or Tessier flap has been described for use in lower eyelid reconstruction in which total or subtotal loss of tissue has occurred.[66] A similar flap can be used for upper eyelid defects.[67] This technique is suited for total or subtotal upper eyelid reconstruction in cases in which a remnant of lid is present laterally (Fig. 34–19).

The transpositional flap is marked out in the orbitonasal angle and then in the nasojugal region. Its base is centered over the angular vessels and lies above the level of the medial canthal tendon. This allows the flap to reach 90-degree transposition. The flap is outlined to approximate the loss of lid tissue in the upper lid.

If posterior lamella is required, oral mucosa, conjunctiva from the inferior fornix, or a free tarsal graft from the opposite upper lid is useful. The flap once mobilized and transposed is secured to surrounding lid tissue with interrupted absorbable or nonabsorbable suture (e.g., 6-0 polyglactin suture material and 6-0 plain gut). The remnant of the levator is secured to the superior border of the graft with 5-0 polyglactin suture. The lower border of the

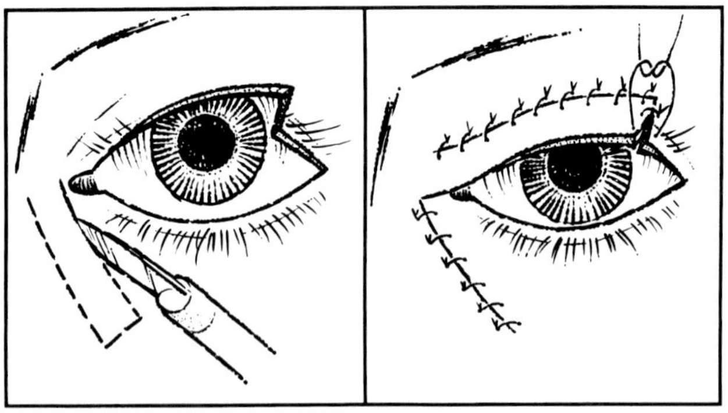

Figure 34–19. Nasojugal flap for upper lid reconstruction.

flap is sutured with a fine absorbable suture (e.g., 7-0 plain gut).

The advantage of this flap is that it can be a single-stage procedure for total or subtotal upper eyelid reconstruction. The skin of the flap is more supple and less thick than skin from the mid forehead or temporal forehead flaps. In addition, all scars are placed along normal skin folds.

The Cutler-Beard Flap

The Cutler-Beard, or lower to upper lid, bridge flap is a time-honored technique to reconstruct large full-thickness eyelid defects, including total loss of the upper lid.[68, 69] A full-thickness flap, including skin, muscle, and conjunctiva, is harvested from the lower lid and transposed into the upper lid defect. The original flap described contained little or no tarsal support.[66] A more stable upper lid is created if additional supportive tissue similar to tarsus is used between the skin and muscle and conjunctiva (e.g., sclera, ear cartilages, irradiated tarsus, irradiated aorta).[16, 17, 70]

Generally, the upper eyelid defect will contain a small remnant of tarsal plate or canthal tendon medially or laterally to use in the lid reconstruction. If there is absolutely no lid or tendon available, the Cutler-Beard flap to be harvested has to be as large as possible and additional tissue may be required to reconstruct the complete upper lid defect (e.g., a lateral periosteal strip flap in conjunction with a myocutaneous pedicle to allow additional tissues).

The technique involved in harvesting a Cutler-Beard flap involves sizing up the upper lid defect and then drawing out the flap of approximately the same size on the lower lid 4 to 5 mm below the lower lid lash line to avoid injury to the lower lid arcade vessels. A corneal protector or lid plate is placed into position. A horizontal skin muscle incision is initially made, followed by vertical skin muscle incision. The skin–muscle flap is dissected away from underlying eyelid retractors, orbital septum, and preaponeurotic fat. This dissection is carried below the level of inferior orbital rim. The lower lid retractors are next dissected carefully away from underlying conjunctiva. The conjunctiva is then incised horizontally and vertically beneath the tarsal plate and mobilized superiorly. Alternately, a full-thickness incision can be made from skin right through to conjunctiva horizontally and then vertically. Once the flap is formed, the conjunctiva can then be dissected away from the skin–muscle portion, followed by dissection and relaxation of tissue in the retractor plane. I prefer to dissect the flap in layers, as described.

The flap of conjunctiva is carefully placed under the bridge of remaining lower eyelid and sutured to the conjunctival edges of the upper lid defect with interrupted or running absorbable sutures (6-0 or 7-0 plain gut). A tarsal substitute is sutured into position medially, laterally, and to the edge of aponeurosis superiorly at this stage. Sclera and ear cartilage have been popular substitutes in the past. I find sclera to be too soft and cartilage too rigid and nonconforming. I have found irradiated homologous donor tarsus or irradiated homologous donor aorta to be excellent tarsal substitutes.[15–17] A piece of tarsal substitute is cut to the desired length and height (generally no more than 10 mm of vertical height) and then sutured into position medially, laterally, and superiorly with a 5-0 polyglactin suture. The myocutaneous flap is next passed under the bridge of the lower lid and brought into position. Additional dissection in the submuscular plane over the cheek area may be required for adequate tissue mobilization superiorly. A 6-0 or 7-0 permanent or absorbable suture is used to secure the skin edges.

Separation of the flap is carried out at no sooner than 8 weeks. After local anesthetic infiltration of the flap, the flap is incised with a blade or Stevens scissors. One to 2 mm of keratinized skin and muscle is trimmed, leaving 2 mm of extra conjunctiva to rotate anteriorly over the lid margin so that the lid margin will be composed of conjunctiva. If this is not done, corneal irritation will occur, owing to the skin surface and its fine vellus lashes rubbing on the cornea.

One must also adjust the lower lid at this stage and try to reposition the skin muscle that was sitting beneath the lower lid bridge of tissue. The lower eyelid and cheek skin muscle portion are carefully undermined so that they can be mobilized back into position. The inferior edge of the lower lid margin bridge is de-epithelialized by carefully trimming the superficial tissue. The two fresh edges are reapproximated with 6-0 or 7-0 absorbable or permanent sutures. Dog-ears are removed as needed. The conjunctival edges may be left to spontaneously unite.

The lids are then left to settle into position over the next 1 to 2 months. Further adjustments may be required, such as trimming additional skin from the upper lid, re-forming an upper lid crease, removing a lid notch, or adjusting the lower lid position, which sometimes will end up slightly ectropic after the bridge flap has been cut. The absence of normal eyelashes from the reconstructed lid is best treated with eyeshadow or artificial lashes. Although hair-bearing grafts can be attempted, they generally do not work well and have a poor appearance (Figs. 34–20 and 34–21).

Tarsoconjunctival Flap

Replacing posterior lamellar defects with the patient's own tarsus is ideal if enough tarsus remains in the ipsilateral lid to reconstruct the defect. A number of techniques have been described, including tarsal rotational flaps,[6] tarsoconjunctival advancement flaps,[4, 5] and sliding tarsal flaps.[3]

Tarsal Rotational Flap Technique

The tarsal rotational flap consists of horizontal rotation of a vertical segment of tarsus and is ideally suited for selected medial or lateral upper lid defects that have a stump of at least one third of remaining lid present. When combined with other simple techniques, such as lateral canthotomy, cantholysis, eyelid advancement,

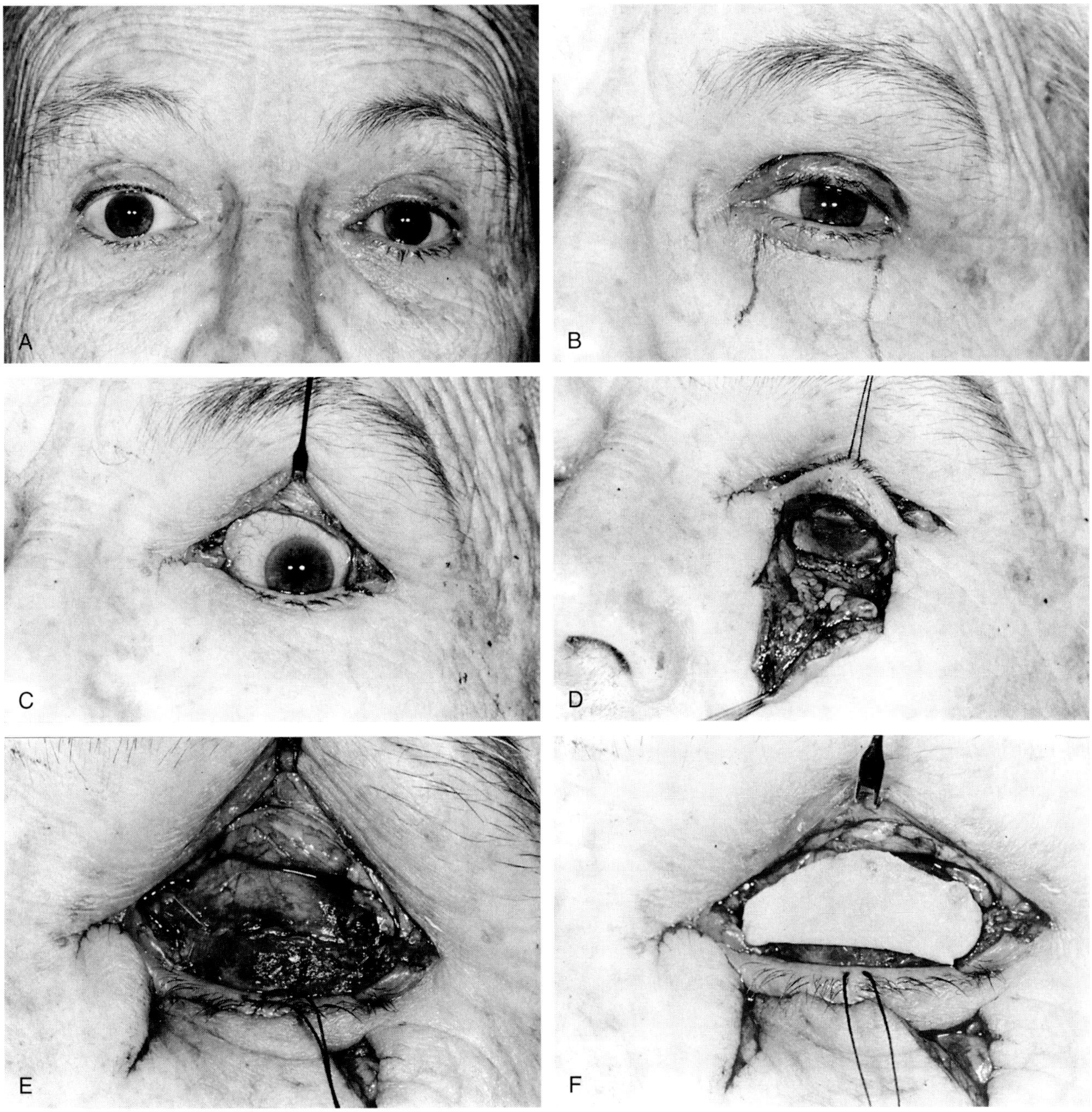

Figure 34–20. *A*, Aggressive squamous cell carcinoma of conjunctival surface of upper lid. *B*, The Cutler-Beard flap is drawn out. C, Ninety percent of the upper lid has been removed. *D*, The skin and muscle portion of the flap is dissected. *E*, Conjunctiva has been mobilized and sutured into the upper lid defect. *F*, Irradiated homologous tarsus is put into position.

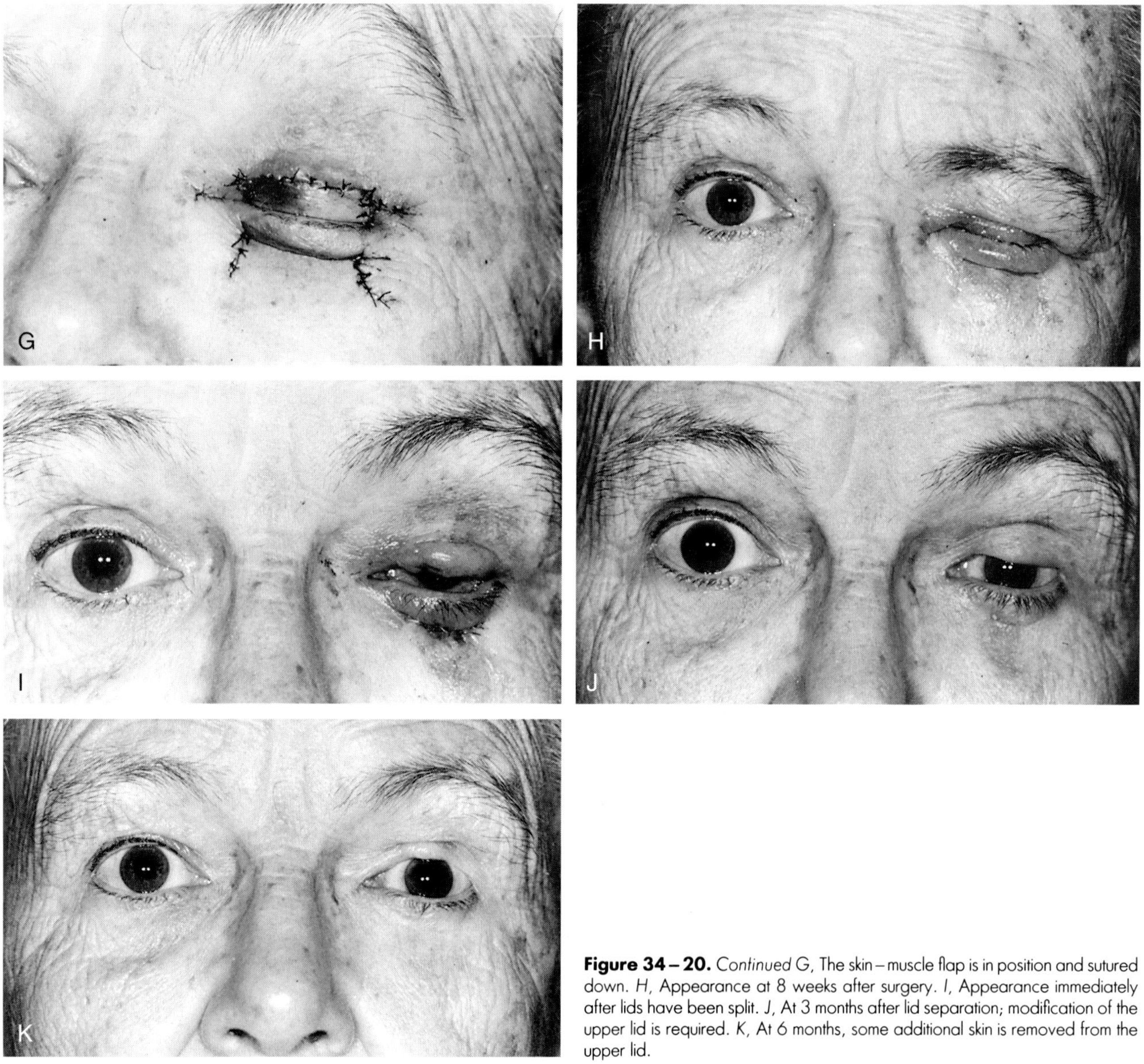

Figure 34–20. *Continued G,* The skin–muscle flap is in position and sutured down. *H,* Appearance at 8 weeks after surgery. *I,* Appearance immediately after lids have been split. *J,* At 3 months after lid separation; modification of the upper lid is required. *K,* At 6 months, some additional skin is removed from the upper lid.

and myocutaneous anterior lamellar flaps, very large medial eyelid defects can be reconstructed with excellent results.

The technique is easily carried out with topical and local anesthesia. The central upper eyelid tarsus at the edge of the lid defect is freed by sharp dissection from Müller's muscle and conjunctiva along its superior border for 3 to 4 mm. In addition, overlying levator aponeurosis and orbicularis is dissected off the anterior surface of the tarsal plate for 3 to 4 mm. Using Stevens or Westcott scissors, the surgeon creates a vertical tarsal strip 3 to 4 mm wide by making a vertical cut in the tarsus to a point 2 mm from the eyelid margin. Since the central tarsal plate is 10 to 12 mm in height, a vertical strip 7 to 10 mm long and 3 to 4 mm wide is created. This vertical strip is then rotated horizontally. The strip of tarsus is attached to the canthal tendon remnants on periosteum at the orbital rim with 4-0 polyglactin 910 or permanent sutures (Fig. 34–22*A*).

For reconstruction of large medial upper lid defects, a lateral canthotomy with superior cantholysis and skin–muscle temporal advancement flap[54] can be used to mobilize the temporal eyelid strip medially, reducing the residual medial defect requiring reconstruction. If enough conjunctiva is present in the superior fornix, the conjunctiva can be undermined, advanced, and sutured to the rotated tarsus, but I believe this is rarely required. Adequate healing has occurred in cases in which insufficient residual superior fornix conjunctiva remained to suture to the upper edge of the tarsus. Once the tarsal rotation flap is sutured into position, there is not uncommonly a small kink in the lid contour at the point where tarsus has been rotated. With time, this settles and blends in with normal lid contour.

After posterior lamellar reconstruction with this technique, the anterior lamella may be reconstructed by undermining and advancing myocutaneous flaps from adjacent areas of excess tissue. Myocutaneous flaps are ideal for this purpose (Fig. 34–23; see also Fig. 34–22*B* through *E*).

Eyelid height and contour adjustment are rarely problems with this technique since the levator aponeurosis remains attached to the remaining tarsal plate.

As a one-stage reconstructive procedure for upper lid defects, this procedure has several advantages. One is simplicity since it eliminates the need for surgery on other eyelids, nose, or ear tissue to harvest tarsal substitutes. The technique retains ipsilateral tarsus and conjunctiva as the posterior lamella, and both are more physiologic tissues than are cartilage or scleral grafts. The procedure eliminates the need to close the visual axis, which is a requirement when lower to upper eyelid sharing procedures are used, and provides normal eyelid contour and height. The procedure increases the mechanical strength of the eyelid margin by retaining the tarsus as a rotational flap rather than relying on a free graft or sliding

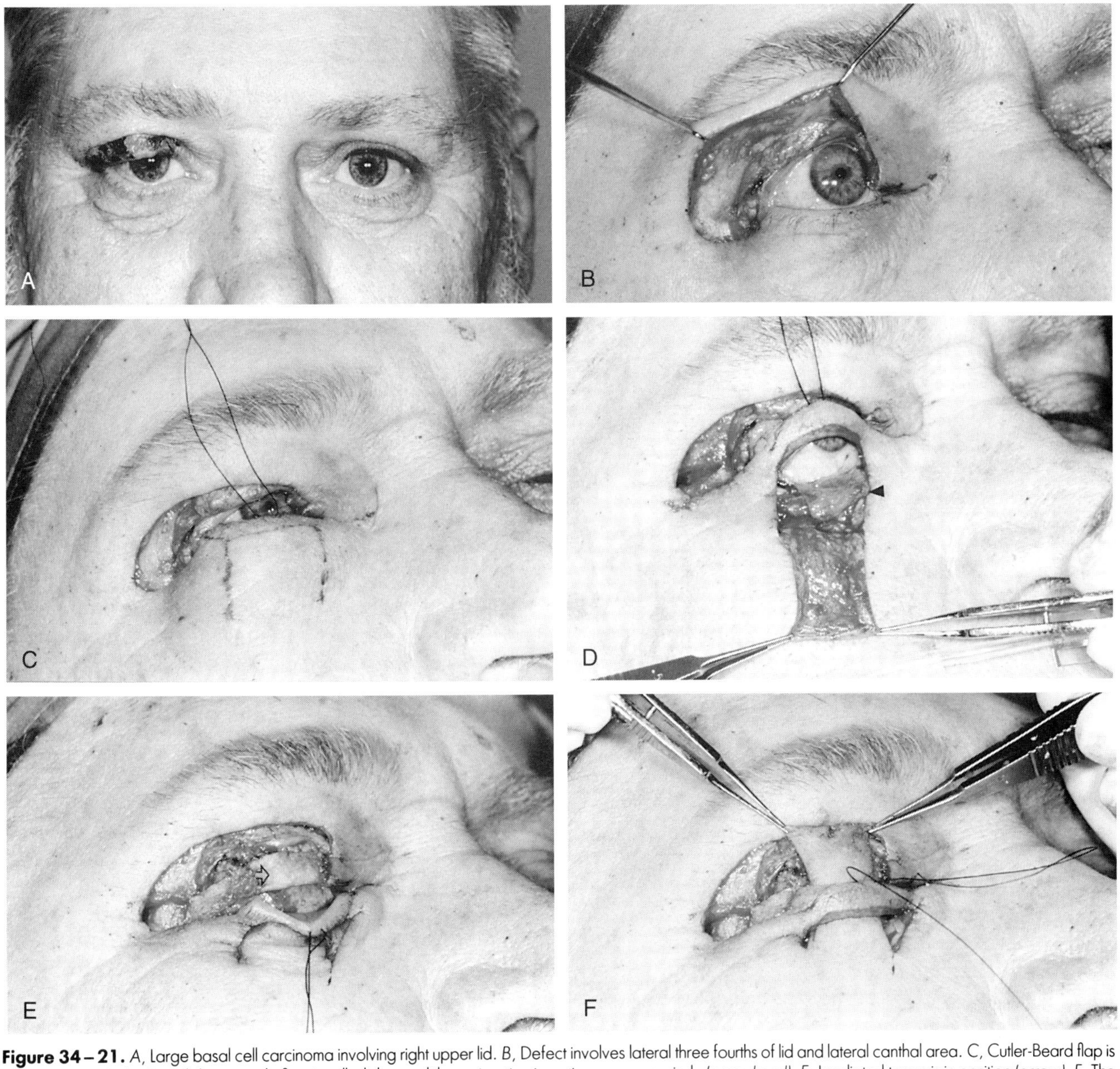

Figure 34–21. *A*, Large basal cell carcinoma involving right upper lid. *B*, Defect involves lateral three fourths of lid and lateral canthal area. *C*, Cutler-Beard flap is drawn out. *D*, Cutler-Beard skin–muscle flap is pulled down while conjunctiva is resting more superiorly (*arrowhead*). *E*, Irradiated tarsus is in position (*arrow*). *F*, The skin–muscle flap is brought into position.

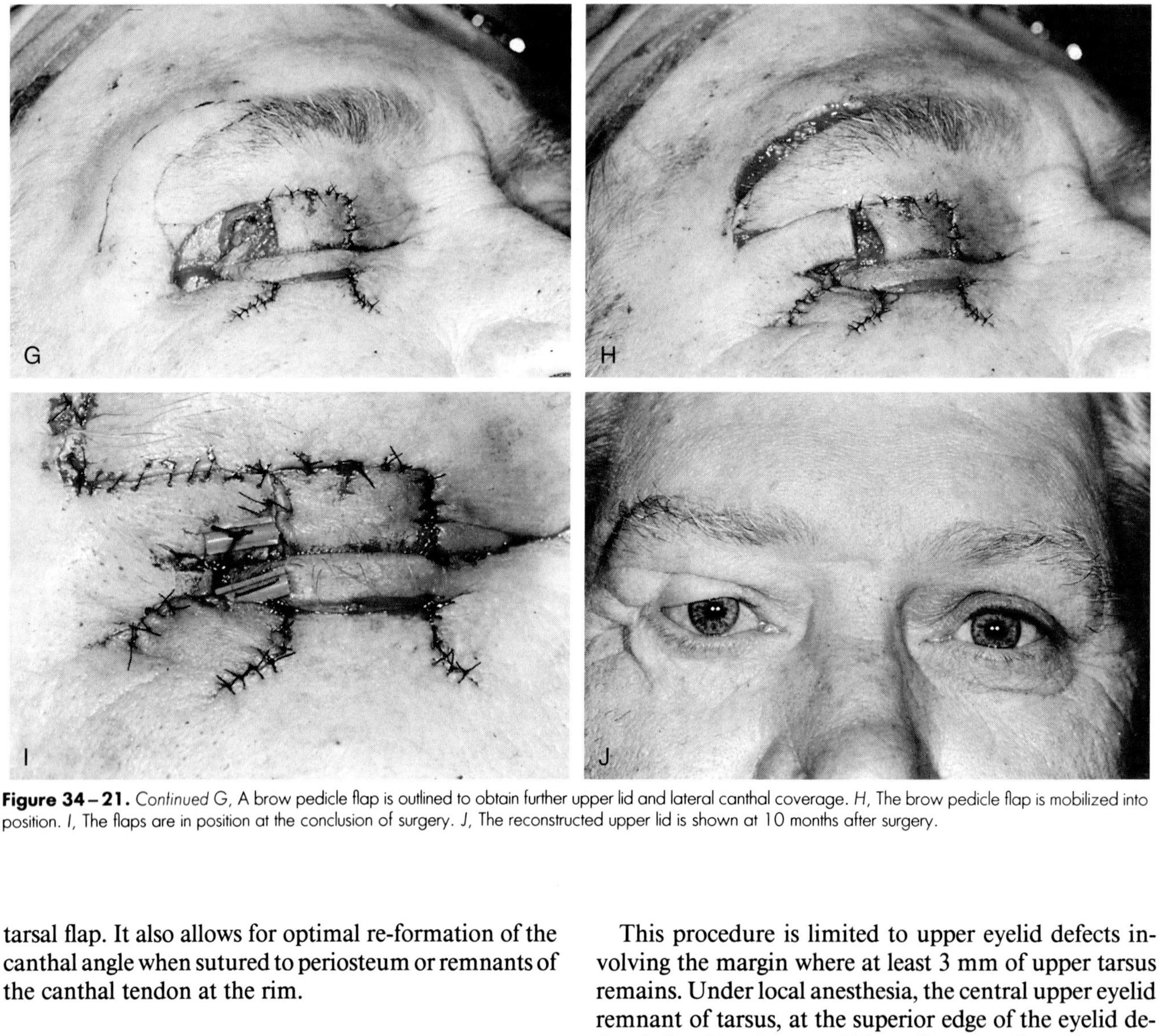

Figure 34–21. *Continued G,* A brow pedicle flap is outlined to obtain further upper lid and lateral canthal coverage. *H,* The brow pedicle flap is mobilized into position. *I,* The flaps are in position at the conclusion of surgery. *J,* The reconstructed upper lid is shown at 10 months after surgery.

tarsal flap. It also allows for optimal re-formation of the canthal angle when sutured to periosteum or remnants of the canthal tendon at the rim.

Tarsoconjunctival Flap Technique

The tarsoconjunctival flap[4] involves a technique very similar to the Hughes tarsoconjunctival flap[21, 22] commonly used in lower eyelid reconstruction yet is limited to the upper eyelid. In the Hughes flap, a tarsoconjunctival advancement flap is formed from the upper eyelid. This flap is then mobilized and secured in the lower eyelid defect, serving as the new posterior lamella. The anterior lamella is supplied by a skin graft or flap. The bridge flap is opened in 6 to 8 weeks with the use of local anesthesia.

For selected defects involving the central upper eyelid, a similar technique can be carried out. This procedure was developed to reconstruct upper eyelid defects with at least a 3-mm remnant of superior tarsal margin. The superior tarsal remnant is advanced as a tarsoconjunctival flap to re-form the deficient posterior lamella of the upper eyelid margin.

This procedure is limited to upper eyelid defects involving the margin where at least 3 mm of upper tarsus remains. Under local anesthesia, the central upper eyelid remnant of tarsus, at the superior edge of the eyelid defect, is freed by sharp and blunt dissection from the overlying tissue. A vertical incision at the medial and lateral edges of the defect is directed superiorly through the tarsus and conjunctiva to free the tarsal remnant. The levator aponeurosis is carefully dissected away from the anterior surface of the tarsal remnant and recessed superiorly. This is facilitated by infiltrating local anesthesia into the plane between the aponeurosis and Müller's muscle.

The next step involves recessing Müller's muscle from the superior tarsal border. Dissection is facilitated by infiltrating the local anesthesia in the space between Müller's muscle and conjunctiva. The levator aponeurosis and Müller's muscle should be completely freed from the conjunctiva and maximally recessed (10 to 15 mm) when only a small remnant of tarsus remains. If only a few millimeters of tarsus is missing, then less recession is required. Excessive recession of the levator and Müller's muscle is nearly impossible, since the levator has attach-

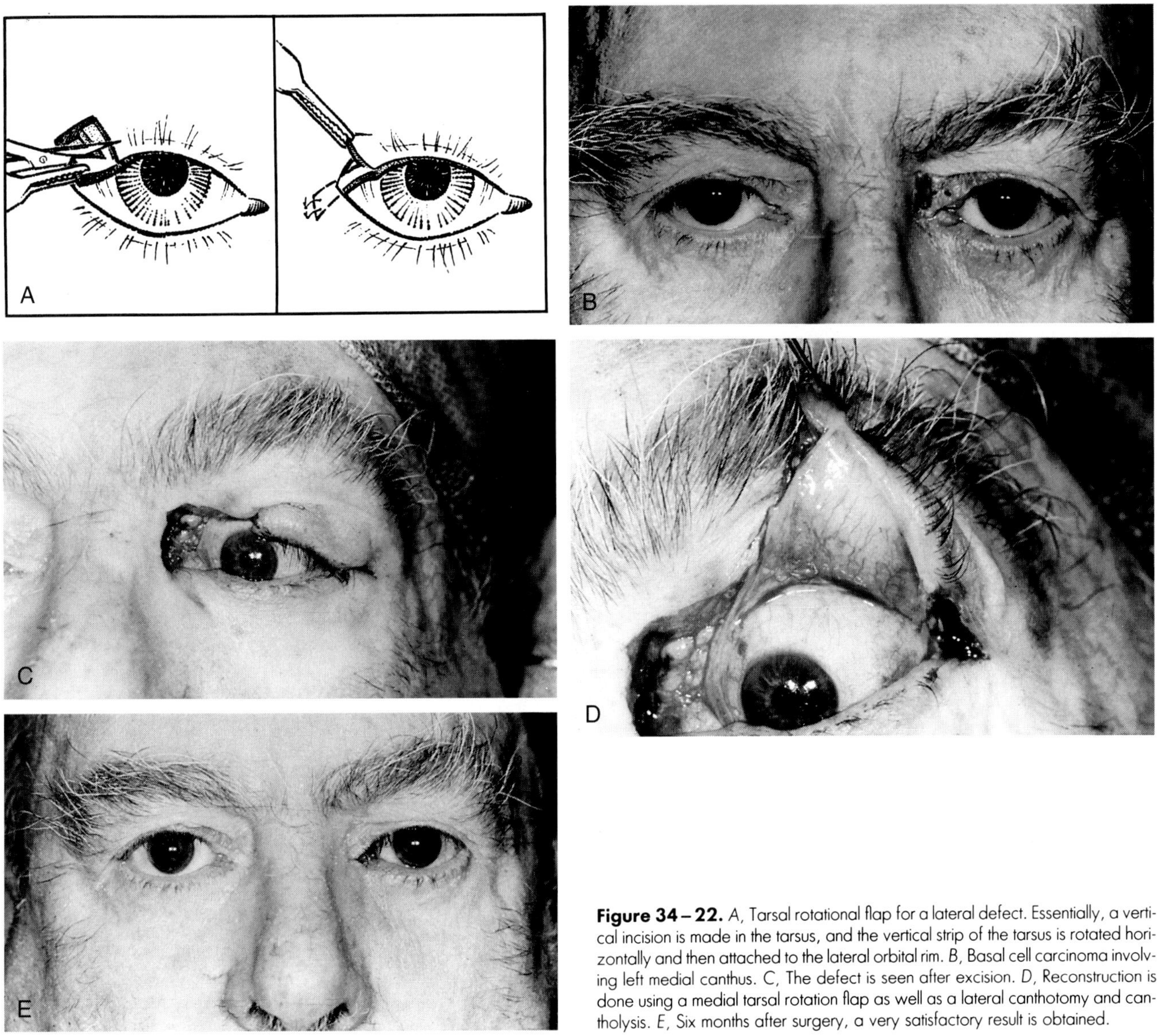

Figure 34–22. *A*, Tarsal rotational flap for a lateral defect. Essentially, a vertical incision is made in the tarsus, and the vertical strip of the tarsus is rotated horizontally and then attached to the lateral orbital rim. *B*, Basal cell carcinoma involving left medial canthus. *C*, The defect is seen after excision. *D*, Reconstruction is done using a medial tarsal rotation flap as well as a lateral canthotomy and cantholysis. *E*, Six months after surgery, a very satisfactory result is obtained.

ments to the tarsus medially and to the defect laterally. Lid retraction is a much greater concern.

The tarsal remnant is now advanced inferiorly with only its attached conjunctiva. Superior relaxing incisions in the conjunctiva (at each end of the tarsal remnant) may be required at this stage. The tarsoconjunctival advancement flap is now ready to be sutured to the remaining lid stump medially and laterally with 5-0 polyglactin sutures. Usually, the tarsoconjunctival flap is shortened slightly to correct upper eyelid laxity (if present), to reduce the portion of the reconstructed eyelid that will not have lashes, and to help avoid upper eyelid retraction in the reconstructed area. Once the posterior lamella has been reconstructed, the anterior lamella is repaired using a myocutaneous advancement flap or skin graft. If enough tissue is available above the defect, undermining in a suborbicular plane along with relaxing incisions in the skin and muscle will allow the advancement of a myocutaneous flap downward. If insufficient tissue is available, a skin graft may be used (Fig. 34–24).

Fox[71] and Leone[5] described similar procedures. However, in addition to advancing the superior remnant of tarsus and conjunctiva, Fox advocated splitting the lower lid into anterior and posterior lamellae and formed a tarsoconjunctival flap from the posterior lamella of the lower eyelid. Leone advocated incising lower lid tarsus below the lid margin and forming a tarsoconjunctival flap. In each instance, the tarsoconjunctival flap was then advanced into the upper eyelid defect to meet the tarsoconjunctival flap formed from the superior eyelid. The

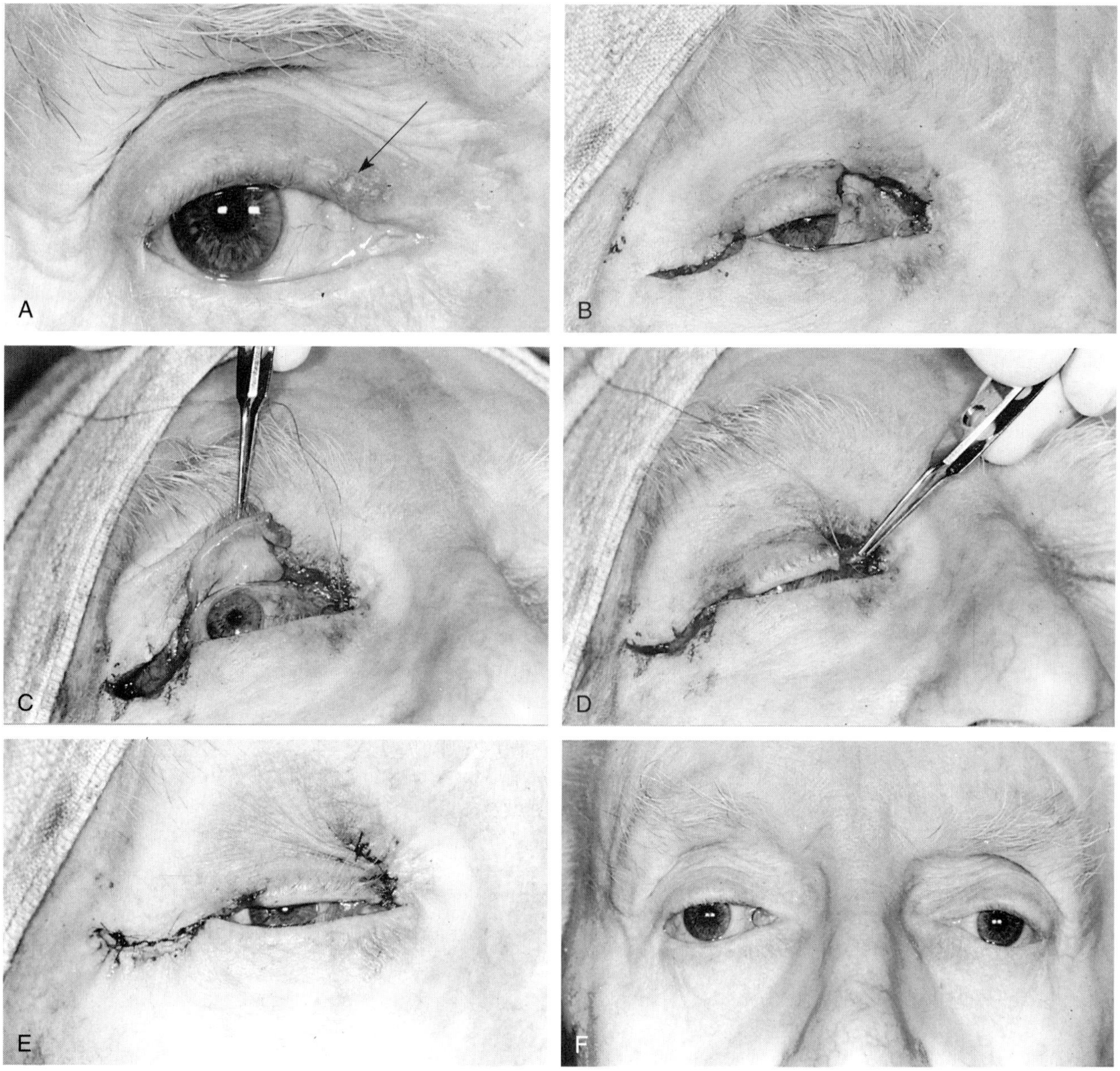

Figure 34–23. *A*, Basal cell carcinoma involving the medial upper lid *(arrow)*. *B*, The medial one third of the right upper lid was excised. A canalicular stent using a pigtail probe was required. A lateral semicircular flap has been dissected. *C*, To obtain closure of the defect, a medial tarsal rotational flap was formed on the medial upper lid. The upper lid is everted, and the tarsal rotational flap is seen medially. *D*, The tarsal rotational flap is being advanced toward the medial canthus. *E*, At the conclusion of the reconstruction, the eyelid appears tight. *F*, Ten months after surgery, the lid has a very nice appearance. The stent was removed at 12 months.

two flaps were sutured together, and the fissure was closed. The lids were then opened at a second procedure. The potential disadvantage of this latter technique include damage and instability of the lower eyelid, with possible entropion, trichiasis, lower eyelid retraction, and closing of the visual axis.

The tarsoconjunctival flap is simple and eliminates the need for additional surgery to harvest tarsal substitutes. It retains the tarsus and conjunctiva as posterior lamella; these are more physiologic tissues than are cartilage, nasolacrimal mucosa, or other tarsal substitutes. It avoids complications to normal uninvolved eyelid and does not close the visual axis.

Sliding Tarsal Flap

Isolated medial or lateral defects of the upper eyelid too large to close with direct closure may also be closed by horizontally sliding a section of tarsus from the remaining lid segment into the defect and covering the external surface with a skin graft as described by McCord and Wesley.[3]

As an example, this technique is described here for a lateral upper lid defect (Fig. 34–25). A horizontal incision is made in the remaining normal eyelid tarsal plate 4 mm above the lid margin and approximately the width of the defect. An additional relaxing incision is then made

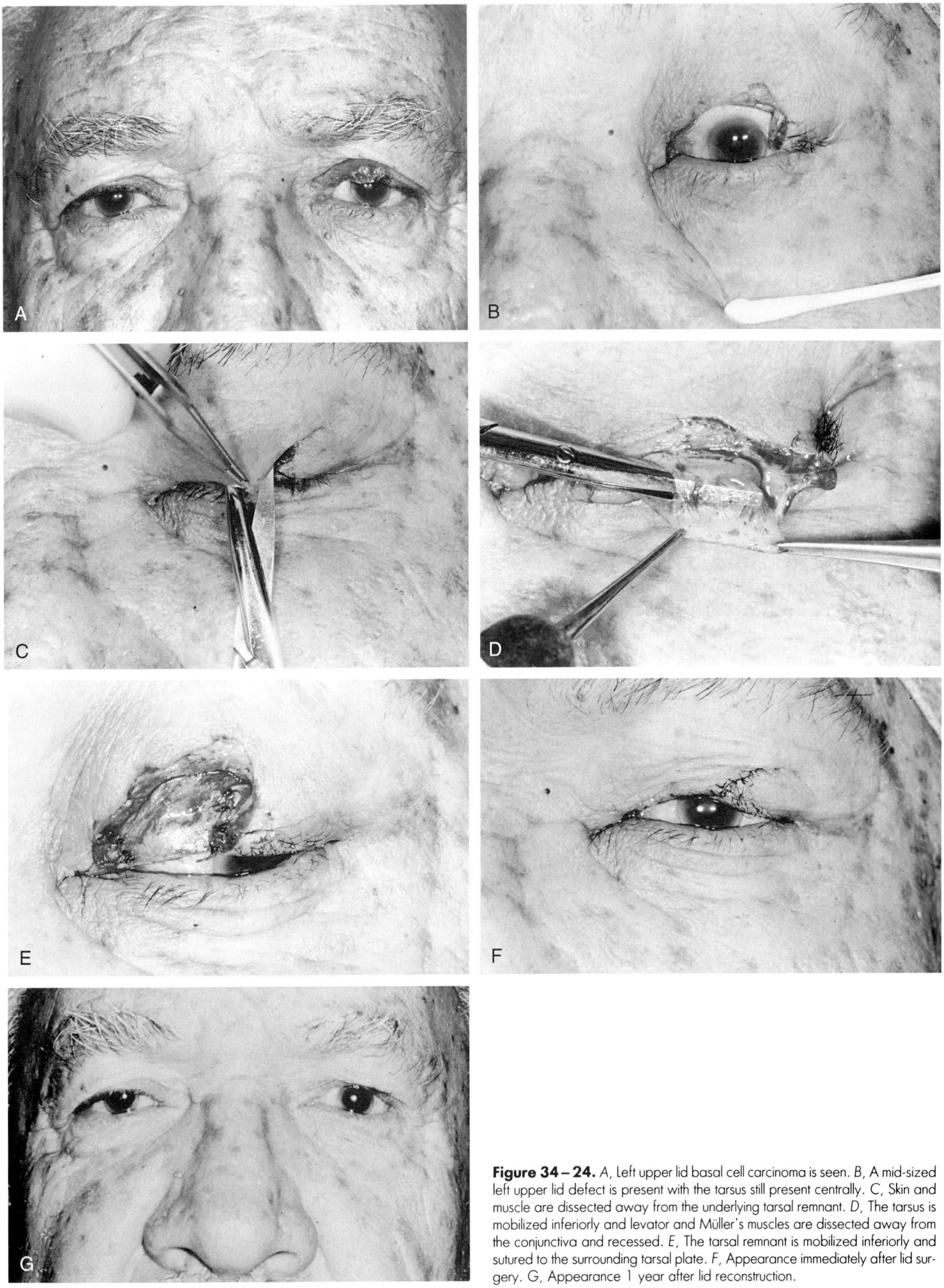

Figure 34 – 24. *A*, Left upper lid basal cell carcinoma is seen. *B*, A mid-sized left upper lid defect is present with the tarsus still present centrally. *C*, Skin and muscle are dissected away from the underlying tarsal remnant. *D*, The tarsus is mobilized inferiorly and levator and Müller's muscles are dissected away from the conjunctiva and recessed. *E*, The tarsal remnant is mobilized inferiorly and sutured to the surrounding tarsal plate. *F*, Appearance immediately after lid surgery. *G*, Appearance 1 year after lid reconstruction.

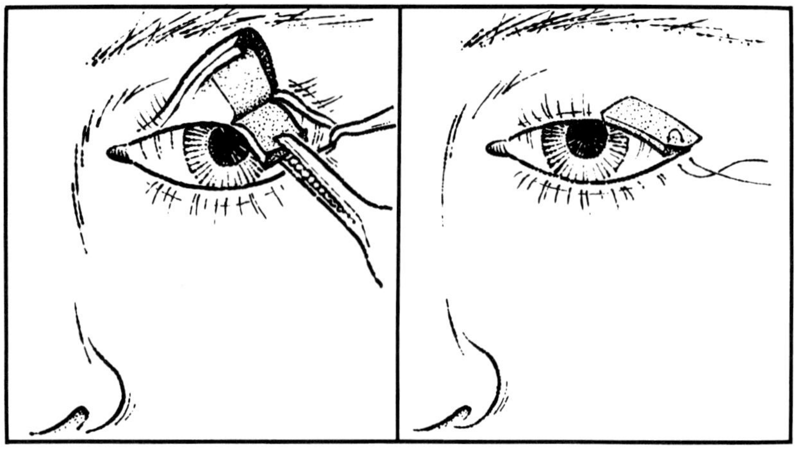

Figure 34–25. Sliding tarsoconjunctival flap.

vertically in the tarsus to the superior border of the tarsus and into the upper fornix.

The tarsoconjunctival flap is horizontally moved into the defect. The lateral edge is attached to periosteum or remnant of the lateral canthal tendon inside the orbital rim. The other edge of tarsal flap is sutured to the remaining upper lid margin with 5-0 polyglactin sutures. The cut edge of the levator may be tacked down to the superior edge of the tarsal flap. A full-thickness skin graft or myocutaneous flap is placed over the tarsoconjunctival flap and sutured into position with 6-0 or 7-0 absorbable sutures.

Defects in the upper lid occurring at the inner canthus are repaired similarly.[3, 72] The full-thickness graft or myocutaneous flap should be sutured carefully along the lid margin to avoid irritation of the cornea by keratinized epithelium.

McCord and Wesley[3] advocate an intermarginal traction suture or a Frost-type suture at the junction of the flap and eyelid margin to avoid shrinkage of the graft and notching in the area of reconstruction.

Other Techniques

The surgical technique described thus far will allow reconstruction of virtually all upper eyelid defects. There are other techniques available that are used less commonly but may be used as an alternative to those described or, in some hands, in preference to those described. These include composite grafting,[3, 9, 10, 72–75] full-thickness pedicle flaps from lower eyelid to upper eyelid,[7] and split-level eyelid grafting.[75]

Composite Grafting

Composite upper eyelid grafts are free full-thickness sections from the upper eyelids and are alternative techniques used in reconstructing surgical, traumatic, and congenital colobomatous defects of the opposite upper eyelid. They have no blood supply and must therefore rely on vascularization from the surrounding eyelid. The viability of most free grafts is from small bits of vascularized tissue that penetrate them from an overlying or underlying flap. To increase the viability of a composite graft, the full-thickness composite grafts may be divided into a skin–muscle component and a tarsoconjunctival component. After harvesting a full-thickness composite graft from the opposite upper lid, the skin and muscle are trimmed 2 mm above the lash margin. The tarsoconjunctival marginal component is sutured into the lid defect with a 5-0 or 6-0 polyglactin suture to the surrounding tarsal plate (Fig. 34–26). The lid margin is sutured using 6-0 silk vertical mattress sutures in the standard fashion.[26, 27] The donor tarsoconjunctival marginal graft may be covered with a skin–muscle flap[24] in the recipient area for maximum vascularization. Although in most cases it is not necessary, the skin–muscle flap excised from the donor graft may be used to supplement the recipient upper lid skin. Minimal cautery is important so that the tissue vascularity is not compromised. Even though the soft tissue take is excellent with good marginal restoration, in approximately 50% of persons the lashes will be lost.[3]

If direct closure of the composite graft donor site is hampered by excessive tension of the opposing eyelids, a lateral canthotomy and cantholysis can be performed to aid lid approximation in the standard fashion.[54]

Full-Thickness Pedicle Flap from Lower Lid to Upper Lid

The technique of rotating a full-thickness pedicle of lower lid onto an upper lid defect has been described by Mustardé[7] and modified by McCord and Wesley.[3] In this technique, the margin of the full-thickness lower lid pedicle is transferred to the upper lid in a two-stage procedure with placement of the pedicle into the upper lid during the first stage and separation of the pedicle and revision of the lower lid during the second stage (Fig. 34–27). It is important to outline the pedicle in the central position of the lower eyelid because it makes subsequent

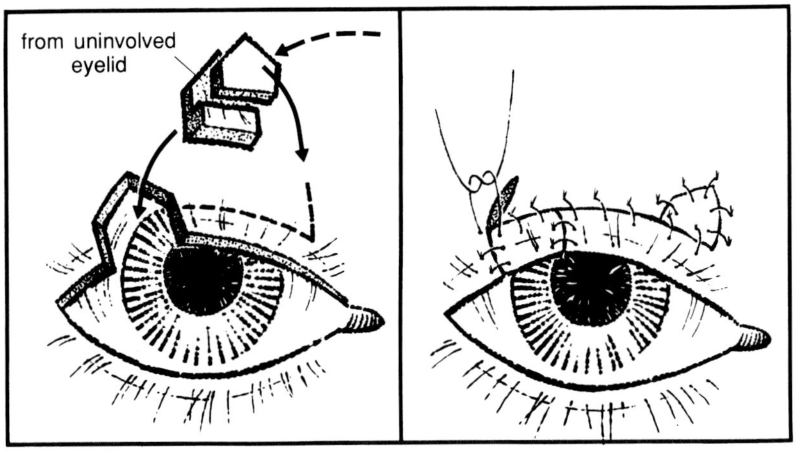

Figure 34–26. Composite grafting. A full-thickness piece of eyelid is harvested from the normal eyelid, divided into anterior and posterior lamellae, and used as grafting material in the lid to be reconstructed.

closure of the lower lid defect easier in the second stage. Care is taken after developing the pedicle to ensure that the marginal artery is included. Since vertical height of the tarsus in the lower lid averages 3.8 mm[76] and the peripheral arcade is at the base of the tarsus, a pedicle flap of at least 5 mm in height should be designed. It can be rectangular and does not have to be elliptical as in Mustardé's technique.[7] The end of the margin is rotated into position and closed, lid margin to lid margin. It is impossible to suture the flap entirely into position in the upper lid, but the end of the flap and lid edge must be approximated to establish blood supply in the upper lid. This is done with multiple fine 6-0 or 7-0 absorbable sutures. Some kinking of the rotated lid pedicle may be noted, but if the peripheral arcade from the lower lid is intact, good blood supply will ensue.

Second-stage reconstruction is generally done between 4 and 6 weeks later and involves the separation of the base of the pedicle flap from the lower lid, its rotation into the upper lid defect, and closure of the lower lid defect. Essentially, the pedicle is incised along the lower lid margin. The upper lid has to be opened so that the remaining pedicle can be mobilized into the upper lid. The pedicle edge or upper lid may be trimmed so that they fit together nicely. In the lower lid, a full-thickness incision is carried out along the previous closure junction line; and after repositioning the lower lid tarsus and trimming the lid as needed, the lid is closed. Lateral canthotomy and cantholysis may be required to close the lower lid defect if additional mobilization is needed.

This technique is an alternative to some of those already described. One advantage to it that the others are lacking is the ability to restore lashes into the lid defect. The lashes, although somewhat shorter, have a nice cosmetic appearance. This technique is not commonly used since there are other reconstructive techniques simpler to do that provide a very satisfactory result as well. The technique involved in creation of this flap is tedious (to ensure maintenance of the peripheral arcade) and involves a two-stage lid reconstruction.

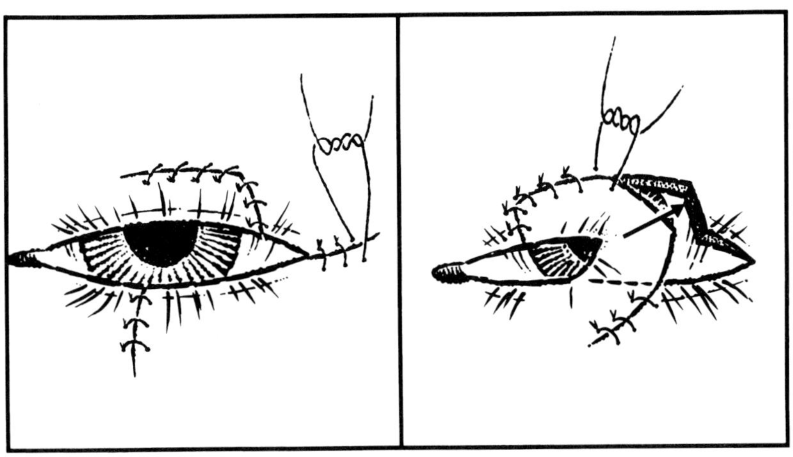

Figure 34–27. *Left,* A full-thickness pedicle flap is mobilized from the lower lid and fixated in the upper lid defect. *Right,* The appearance of the lids after secondary transection of the lower lid pedicle.

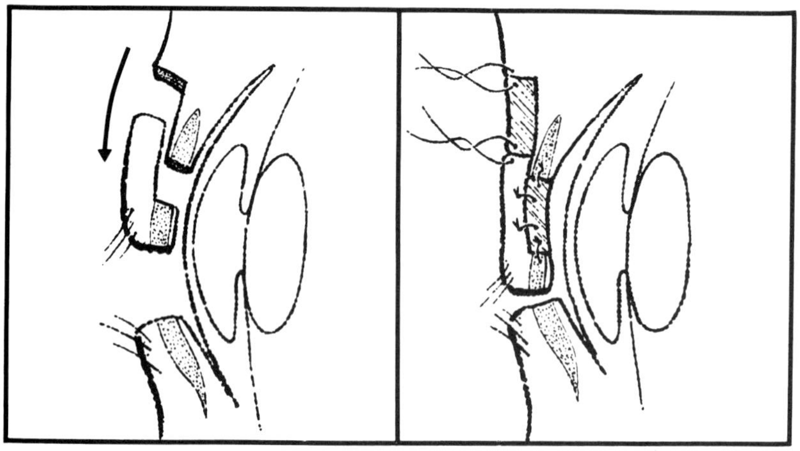

Figure 34–28. Split-level full-thickness eyelid graft technique.

Split-Level Full-Thickness Eyelid Grafts

Brown and Beard[75] described a surgical technique for correction of cicatricial eyelid retraction involving lid lengthening using eyelid grafts in the posterior and anterior lamellae at different levels. Vertically shortened upper eyelids with an intact lid margin may be caused by cicatricial changes following burns, trauma, irradiation or severe inflammation such as that seen with herpes zoster.[3] Postauricular skin is used for the anterior lamella, and oral mucous membrane is used for the posterior lamella. The upper lid is split and separated so that the two grafts are placed at different levels in the eyelid, with each graft resting on its own vascular bed (Fig. 34–28).

The technique involves placing a 4-0 silk suture through the lid margin and then everting the vertically shortened eyelid over a Desmarres retractor and making a horizontal excision through the tarsal plate 5 mm above the eyelid margin for the length of the tarsus. The retractor is removed, the lid is put on stretch, and a horizontal skin incision is made across the upper lid about 5 mm above the superior edge of the tarsus. The skin is undermined superiorly and inferiorly. All the traction bands holding the eyelid up in the retracted position are incised. The inferior undermining joins the anterior incision with the posterior incision.

With the upper lid everted over a Desmarres retractor, a full-thickness oral mucous membrane or chondral mucosal or hard palate graft is sutured into position into the posterior incision below the cut edges of the tarsus with a 6-0 or 7-0 plain gut absorbable suture. With the lid retracted downward, a preauricular or retroauricular or opposite eyelid full-thickness skin graft is placed into the anterior defect and sutured to the surrounding skin edge with multiple interrupted sutures (6-0 or 7-0 plain gut). A tie-over sponge dressing is recommended on top of the graft for 1 week to help push the graft downward onto the underlying vascular bed. I prefer to use the sponge many of the instruments are wrapped in or to cut a piece from a nondetergent scrub brush. Alternatively, Telfa and dental rolls can be used.

Marginal sutures using a 4-0 silk are recommended for 1 week to keep the lid on stretch and prevent retraction.

Eyelid Dressings

For most of the eyelid reconstruction techniques described, I prefer to apply a firm pressure dressing using two to four eye patches and occasionally 3 × 3-inch sponge rolled or folded into various dimensions to apply some pressure and relieve tension on the reconstructed tissue. A properly applied eyelid reconstruction dressing will help to stick down the various eyelid flaps and prevent edematous fluid from accumulating beneath them. In addition, it will help relax the skin tension, pulling in the opposite direction to the flap reconstruction. Dressings keep the lids at rest to allow tissue healing, and, most of all, they help protect the reconstructed eyelid from rubbing on the patient's pillow at night or from rubbing by the patient's fingers at any time.

Acknowledgment

The author wishes to thank Pat Henry for her help in preparing this chapter.

REFERENCES

1. Leone CR, Hand SI Jr: Reconstruction of the medial eyelid. Am J Ophthalmol 87:797–801, 1979.
2. Stephenson CM, Brown BZ: The use of tarsus as a free autogenous graft in eyelid surgery. Ophthal Plast Reconstr Surg 1:43–50, 1985.
3. McCord CD Jr, Wesley R: Reconstruction of the upper eyelid and medial canthus sliding tarsal flap. *In* McCord CD, Tanenbaum M (eds): Oculoplastic Surgery, 2nd ed. New York, Raven Press, 1987, pp 181–182.
4. Jordan DR, Anderson RL, Nowinski TS: Tarsoconjunctival flap for upper eyelid reconstruction. Arch Ophthalmol 107:599–603, 1989.
5. Leone CR: Tarsoconjunctival advancement flaps for upper eyelid reconstruction. Arch Ophthalmol 101:945–948, 1983.
6. Kersten RC, Anderson RL, Tse DT, Weinstein GL: Tarsal rotation flap for upper eyelid reconstruction. Arch Ophthalmol 104:918–922, 1986.

7. Mustardé JC: Repair and Reconstruction in the Orbital Region. New York, Churchill Livingstone, 1980, pp 130–151.
8. Robbins TH: Chondrodermal graft reconstruction of the lower eyelid. Br J Plast Surg 34:140–141, 1981.
9. Baylis HJ, Pernam KI, Fee DR, Sutcliffe RT: Autogenous auricular cartilage grafting for lower eyelid retraction. Ophthal Plast Reconstr Surg 1:23–27, 1985.
10. Smith B, Lisman RD: Preparation of split-thickness auricular cartilage for use in ophthalmic plastic surgery. Ophthalmic Surg 13:1018–1023, 1982.
11. Flanagan JC: Eyebank sclera in oculoplastic surgery. Ophthalmic Surg 5:45–53, 1974.
12. Wesley RE, McCord CD Jr: Transplantation of eyebank sclera in the Cutler-Beard method of upper eyelid reconstruction. Ophthalmology 87:1022–1028, 1980.
13. Kersten RC, Kulwin DR, Levartovsky S, et al: Management of lower-lid retraction with hard palate grafting. Arch Ophthalmol 108:1339–1343, 1990.
14. Bartley GB, Kay PP: Posterior lamellar eyelid reconstruction with a hard palate mucosal graft. Am J Ophthalmol 107:609–612, 1989.
15. Jordan DR, Tse DT, Anderson RL, Hansen SO: Irradiated tarsal plate banking: A new alternative in eyelid reconstruction: Technique and animal research. Ophthal Plast Reconstr Surg 6:3:158–167, 1990.
16. Jordan DR, Tse DT, Anderson RL, Hansen SO: Irradiated tarsal plate banking: A new alternative in eyelid reconstruction: II. Human data. Ophthal Plast Reconstr Surg 6:3:168–179, 1990.
17. Jordan DR, Anderson RL, McDonald H. The use of irradiated homologous aorta in eyelid reconstruction. Ophthal Plast Reconstr Surg 10:227–233, 1994.
18. Callahan A: The free composite lid grafting in eyelid reconstruction. Am J Ophthalmol 85:237–241, 1978.
19. Putterman AM: Viable composite grafting in eyelid reconstruction. Am J Ophthalmol 85:237–241, 1978.
20. Cutler NL, Beard C: A method of partial and total upper eyelid reconstruction. Am J Ophthalmol 39:1–7, 1955.
21. Hughes WL: Reconstructive Surgery of the Eyelids. St. Louis: CV Mosby, 1947, p 93.
22. Hughes WL: A new method for rebuilding a lower lid: Report of a case. Arch Ophthalmol 17:1008–1017, 1937.
23. Mustardé JC: Techniques for transfer of resurfacing materials. *In* Repair and Reconstruction in the Orbital Region, 2nd ed. New York, Churchill Livingstone, 1986, 378–381.
24. Anderson RL, Edwards JJ: Reconstruction by myocutaneous eyelid flaps. Arch Ophthalmol 97:2358–2362, 1979.
25. Anderson RL, Ceilly RI: A multispecialty approach to the excision and reconstruction of eyelid tumors. Ophthalmology 85:1150–1162, 1978.
26. Divine RD, Anderson RL: Techniques in eyelid wound closure. Ophthalmic Surg 13:283–287, 1982.
27. Jordan DR, White GL: Management of common eyelid injuries. Ophthalmic Pract 9:6:274–280, 1991.
28. Fox S: Ophthalmic Plastic Surgery. New York, Grune & Stratton, 1976, pp 121–128, 171–180, 184–193.
29. Soll DB: Management of Complications of Ophthalmic Plastic Surgery. Birmingham, AL, Aesculapius, 1976, pp 82–83.
30. Marak GE: Recent advances in sympathetic ophthalmia. Surv Ophthalmol 24:141–156, 1979.
31. Lubin JR, Albert DM, Weinstein M: Sixty-five years of sympathetic ophthalmia: A clinicopathologic review of 105 cases (1913–1978). Ophthalmology 87:109–121, 1980.
32. Brackup AB, Carter KD, Nerad JA, et al: Long-term follow-up of severely injured eyes following globe rupture. Ophthal Plast Reconstr Surg 7:194–197, 1991.
33. Anderson RL, Edwards JJ: Indications, complications and results with silicone stents. Ophthalmology 86:1474, 1979.
34. Jones LT, Marquis M, Vincent NJ: Lacrimal function. Am J Ophthalmol 73:658, 1972.
35. Lemp MA, Weller HH: How do tears exit? Invest Ophthalmol Vis Sci 24:619, 1983.
36. VanDeffer HV, Dressler J, Pabst HW: Lacrimal dacryoscintigraphy. Semin Nucl Med 14:8, 1984.
37. Lindberg JV, Moore CA: Symptoms of canalicular obstruction. Ophthalmology 95:1077, 1988.
38. Meyer DR, Antonello A, Lindberg JV: Assessment of tear drainage after canalicular obstruction using fluorescein dye disappearance. Ophthalmology 97:1371–1374, 1990.
39. Doubert J, Nik N, Chandeyssoun PA, El-Choufi L: Tear flow analysis through upper and lower systems. Ophthal Plast Reconstr Surg 6:193–196, 1990.
40. Jordan DR, Nerad JA, Tse DT: The pigtail probe revisited. Ophthalmology 97:512–519, 1990.
41. Quicker MH, Dryden RM: Probes for intubation in lacrimal drainage. Trans Am Acad Ophthalmol Otolaryngol 74:431, 1970.
42. Callahan MA: Silicone intubation for lacrimal canalicular repair. Ann Plast Surg 2:355, 1977.
43. Crawford JS: Intubation of obstructions in the lacrimal systems. Can J Ophthalmol 12:289, 1977.
44. Griffith TP: Polyethylene tubes in canalicular surgery. Br J Ophthalmol 74:203, 1963.
45. Veirs ER: Malleable rods for immediate repair of traumatically severed canaliculus. Trans Am Acad Ophthalmol Otolaryngol 66:262, 1962.
46. Pigtail probe. *In* Storz Ophthalmic Products Catalogue, #E4251-C and E4251-CB. St. Louis, Storz Instruments Company.
47. Worst JG: Method of reconstructing torn canaliculus. Am J Ophthalmol 53:520, 1962.
48. Callahan MA, Callahan A: Trauma. *In* Ophthalmic Plastic and Orbital Surgery. Birmingham, AL, Aesculapius, 1979, pp 156–182.
49. Anderson RL, Gordy DD: The tarsal strip procedure. Arch Ophthalmol 97:2192–2196, 1979.
50. Jordan DR, Anderson RL: The lateral tarsal strip revisited: The enhanced tarsal strip. Arch Ophthalmol 107:604–606, 1989.
51. Weinstein GS, Anderson RL, Tse DT: The use of periosteal strip for eyelid reconstruction. Arch Ophthalmol 103:357–359, 1985.
52. Leone CR: Lateral canthal reconstruction. Ophthalmology 94:238–241, 1987.
53. McCord CD, Wesley R: Reconstruction of the upper eyelid and medial canthus. *In* McCord CD (ed): Oculoplastic Surgery. New York, Raven Press, 1982, pp 175–188.
54. Jordan DR, Anderson RL, Holds JB: Modifications to the semicircular flap technique used in eyelid reconstruction. Can J Ophthalmol 27:129–136, 1992.
55. Tenzel RR, Stewart WB: Eyelid reconstruction by the semicircular flap technique. Ophthalmology 85:1164–1169, 1978.
56. Tenzel RR: Reconstruction of the central one-half of an eyelid. Arch Ophthalmol 93:125–126, 1975.
57. Levine MR, Buckman G: Semicircular flap revisited. Arch Ophthalmol 104:915–917, 1986.
58. Zide BM, Jelks GW: Surgical Anatomy of the Orbit. New York, Raven Press, 1985, p 16.
59. Mustardé JC: Reconstruction of the eyelid: Lower eyelids. *In* Repair and Reconstruction in the Orbital Region, 2nd ed. New York, Churchill Livingstone, 1980, pp 101–102.
60. Leone CR: Lateral canthal reconstruction. Ophthalmology 94:238–241, 1985.
61. Weinstein GS, Anderson RL, Tse DT: The use of a periosteal strip for eyelid reconstruction. Arch Ophthalmol 103:357–359, 1985.
62. Kersten RC, Anderson RL, Tse DT: Tarsal rotation flap for upper eyelid reconstruction. Arch Ophthalmol 104:918–922, 1986.
63. McCord CD, Wesley R: Reconstruction of the upper eyelid and medial canthus. *In* McCord CD, Tanenbaum M (eds): Oculoplastic Surgery. New York, Raven Press, 1987, pp. 73–91.
64. Kazanjian VH, Roopenian A: Median forehead flaps in the repair of defects of the nose and surrounding areas. Trans Am Acad Ophthalmol Otolaryngol 60:557–566, 1956.
65. Smith BC, Nesi FA: Upper lid reconstruction: A new technique for the use of mucous membrane lined pedicle flaps. Ophthalmic Surg 10:17–19, 1979.
66. Tessier P: Eyelid reconstruction or blepharopoiesis. *In* Tessier P, Hervouet F, Lekieffre M, et al (eds): Plastic Surgery of the Orbit and Eyelids. New York, Masson, 1981, pp 334–355.
67. Avram DR, Hurwitz JJ, Kratky V: Modified Tessier flap for reconstruction of the upper eyelid. Ophthalmic Surg 22:467–470, 1991.
68. Cutler N, Beard C: A method for partial and total upper lid reconstruction. Am J Ophthalmol 39:1–7, 1985.
69. Smith B, Obear MF: Bridge flap technique for reconstruction of large upper lid defects. Plast Reconstr Surg 38:45–48, 1966.

70. Wesley RE, McCord CD: Transplantation of eyebank sclera in the Cutler-Beard method of upper eyelid reconstruction. Ophthalmology 87:1022–1028, 1980.
71. Fox SA: Ophthalmic Plastic Surgery. New York, Grune & Stratton, 1976, pp 232–255.
72. Boynton JR: Subtotal reconstruction of the upper eyelid: A one-stage procedure eliminating temporary lid closure. Arch Ophthalmol 103:288–289, 1985.
73. Putterman AM: Combined viable composite graft and temporal semicircular skin flap procedure. Am J Ophthalmol 98:349–354, 1984.
74. Beyer-Machule CK, Shapiro A, Smith B: Double composite lid reconstruction: A new method of upper lid reconstruction. Ophthal Plast Reconstr Surg 1:97–102, 1985.
75. Brown BZ, Beard C: Split-level full-thickness eyelid graft. Am J Ophthalmol 87:388–392, 1979.
76. Wesley RE, McCord CD: Height of the lower tarsus of the lower eyelid. Am J Ophthalmol 90:102–105, 1980.

CHAPTER 35

Medial Canthal Reconstruction

Roger A. Dailey and Diana Habrich

Anatomic defects of the medial canthal region are most commonly a result of trauma or tumor excision. The goals of reconstruction in this area are (1) protection of the eye, (2) maintenance or reestablishment of lacrimal outflow, and (3) optimal cosmesis. In general, the options for reconstruction of the medial canthus are spontaneous granulation, a variety of flaps (using adjacent tissue), and free grafts (using remote tissue), along with fixation of the medial canthal tendon and reconstruction of the lacrimal apparatus as needed. The choice of procedure is dependent on the size and location of the defect and on the availability of appropriate tissue for reconstruction. Skin color, texture, and thickness must be considered, as well as the elasticity and abundance of excess skin in the orbital area, often a function of patient age. Functional needs to be considered are the necessity to replace mucosa, tarsus, skin, canthal tendon, and lacrimal structures. Reestablishing the directors of force in the medial canthus is extremely important in preventing anterior displacement of these structures and the accompanying medial ectropion. In addition, failure to preserve the normal intercanthal distance of approximately one half the interpupillary distance will result in telecanthus.

The pretarsal and preseptal fibers of the orbicularis separate into superficial and deep heads at the nasal border of the upper and lower tarsal plates. The superficial horizontal component of the medial canthal tendon includes the superficial heads of the preseptal muscles, attaching to the anterior surfaces of the canaliculi and the margins of the fibrous canthal tendon, as well as the superficial heads of the pretarsal muscles. The anterior aspect of the tendon fans out medially and inserts onto the anterior lacrimal crest and nasal bone. Zide and McCarthy[1] have described a vertical component of the medial canthal tendon consisting of tendinous fascia arising at the junction of the upper and lower superficial heads of the pretarsal muscles and inserting into the medial orbital rim in the region of the nasofrontal suture. Zide also describes vertical fibers of the orbicularis in the medial canthus, the depressor supercilii.[2] The deep horizontal component consists of the upper and lower preseptal fibers inserting onto the lacrimal diaphragm and posterior canaliculi and the deep heads of the upper and lower pretarsal muscles uniting to form a common insertion on the lacrimal bone behind the posterior lacrimal crest. The orbital portion of the orbicularis inserts on the anterior aspect of the orbital rim medial to the supraorbital notch and the infraorbital foramen.[1-6]

Rodriquez and Zide[6] note that the anterior horizontal component of the normal tendon is strongest, attaching most securely at the anterior lacrimal crest, followed by the vertical component of the anterior tendon and the weakest component, the posterior. They suggest that the resultant vector of these forces is best reproduced by reattaching the entire complex posterior and superior to the anterior lacrimal crest. In reconstruction, the medial end of the lid remnants must be directed toward the posterior reflection of the medial canthal tendon and fixed permanently in that position to achieve protection of the globe and facilitate function of the remaining or reconstructed lacrimal apparatus (Fig. 35–1).

SPONTANEOUS GRANULATION

Defects up to 1.5 cm that are vertically centered approximately on the medial canthal tendon and lie nasal to the canthus may be allowed to heal by second intention. Application of antibiotic ointment and daily dressing changes will allow healing of most defects within 2 to 3 weeks. Spontaneous granulation usually results in a good skin color match and maintenance of the normal depression of the medial canthal area. Equal involvement of tissue above and below this "horizontal meridian" allows equal contracture of tissues and is less likely to result in distortion and ectropion of the upper or lower lid than eccentric defects.[5, 7] The more anteriorly placed the defect lies, however, the more likely is the scar contracture to displace the medial canthus anteriorly from the globe. Spontaneous granulation may be used for residual defects in combination with any of the techniques described below.

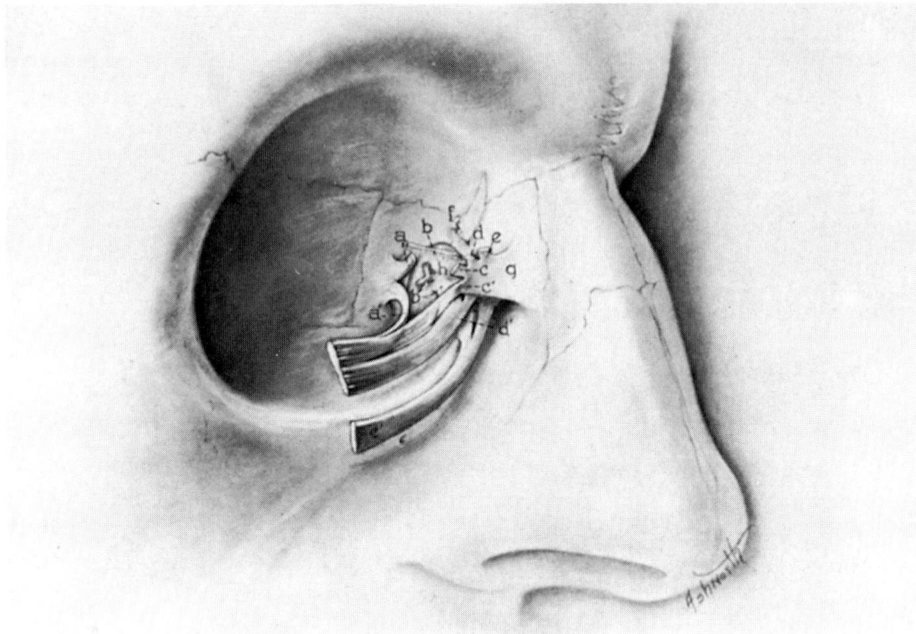

Figure 35 – 1. Insertions of pretarsal muscles in the medial canthal region. **a** and **a'**, Upper and lower deep heads of pretarsal muscles. **b** and **b'**, Upper and lower insertions of superficial heads of pretarsal muscles. **c** and **c'**, Anterior and posterior limbs of medial canthal tendon. **d**, Lower preseptal muscle. **e**, Junction of canaliculi at the lacrimal diaphragm. (From Jones LE, Wobig JL [eds]: Surgery at the Eyelid and Lacrimal System. Birmingham, AL, Aesculapius, 1976.)

DIRECT CLOSURE

Small defects may be closed directly. A narrow diamond-shaped or elliptical defect overlying or medial to the medial canthal tendon can sometimes be closed by undermining surrounding tissue, particularly in older patients with skin laxity. If less than 5 mm of medial upper or lower lid is lost, the remnant may be attached to the medial canthal tendon. Upper and lower lid remnants may be joined in a "medial tarsorrhaphy," the tarsal ends being attached to the canthal tendon with nonabsorbable suture. If the canthal tendon is absent, and less than one third of the upper and lower eyelids has been lost, the tarsal remnants may be fixed to the nasal bone or periosteum (by methods to be described later) and the remaining superficial defect allowed to heal by second intention or covered with a free graft. In most cases, defects involving significant loss of eyelid tissue or those centered above or below the medial canthal tendon are best repaired by one of the methods described below.[4-10]

MEDIAL CANTHAL TENDON FIXATION/RECONSTRUCTION

If a traumatic or postsurgical defect exists that involves the medial canthal tendon, attention must first be given to fixating the medial aspect of the remaining tarsal plate to the bony structures at the medial canthus. A tarsal strip is formed, denuded of epithelium, and attached with nonabsorbable suture to periosteum at the posterior reflection of the tendon, preventing anterior displacement of the canthus. If the canaliculus has been intubated, it is necessary to place this fixation suture posterior to the canaliculus, sometimes requiring anterior reflection of the lacrimal sac. A semicircular needle, such as the P-2 or ME-2, is helpful in placing this suture.[4, 11]

When periosteum at the desired fixation point is absent, or if the surgeon desires to create a new medial canthal tendon for fixation of eyelid remnants, a new medial canthal tendon may be created from a flap of orbital periosteum. If suitable tissue remains, a flap may be created by elevating periosteum based at the posterosuperior border of the periosteal defect. The upper and lower tarsal remnants are then sutured to this flap with nonabsorbable suture, thus giving the appropriate direction of force to prevent anterior or inferior displacement of the medial canthus (Fig. 35 – 2).[12] Moss[13] described replacement of the medial canthal tendon with local muscle flaps of orbicularis from the upper and lower lids sutured to the frontal process of the maxilla.

Unilateral transnasal wiring combined with a dacryocystorhinostomy is described by Beyer[14] and by Smith and Beyer.[15] Any remaining periosteum is stripped from the nasal and lacrimal bones to the posterior lacrimal crest, and the dacryocystorhinostomy is performed. Two holes are then drilled 1 cm apart and 3 to 4 mm from the anterior lacrimal crest. A 30-gauge stainless steel wire is then passed through these holes and out through the dacryocystorhinostomy ostium and through the medial canthal tendon remnant or its replacement (permanent suture). The wire is twisted tightly to reposition the canthal structures (Fig. 35 – 3). Wesley[16] stresses that the wire should be fixated to permanent suture (rather than directly to soft tissue) to prevent "cheesewiring" through soft tissue and migration of the canthus over time.

Yet another method of fixating a remnant of medial canthal tendon is described by Brody and Wheeler.[17]

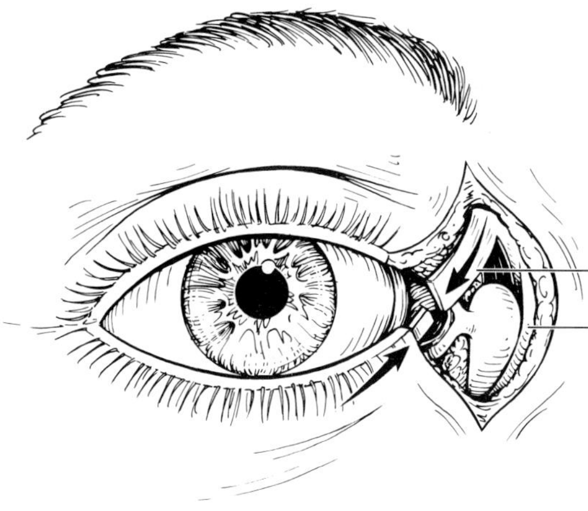

Figure 35–2. Remnant of lower tarsus advanced medially and anterior lacrimal crest. Periosteal flap is elevated and turned laterally, its base superior to the position of the medial canthal tendon and posterior to the anterior lacrimal crest.

After the tendon is identified and isolated, a bony "strut" is created approximately 2 mm in width and 4 mm in length by using a bur to create two slots in the lacrimal bone at the desired point of reattachment. A single fine drill hole is then placed 2 mm anterior to the base of the strut using a Keith or Bunnell needle as a bit. A 4-0 monofilament nylon suture is secured to the medial end of the tendon, behind the strut and through the drill hole. A slit in the remaining tendon creates a loop that encircles the strut, leaving the distal tendon intact. The suture is tied to secure the tissue in position (Fig. 35–4).

Callahan[18, 19] described a stainless steel screw set into bone with the use of a specially designed screwdriver. The screw is placed at the posterior lacrimal crest at the same horizontal level as the opposite medial canthal tendon. A "pilot" hole is made with a 1.3-mm drill bit for the first 2 to 3 mm. The (Nelson) screw comes in two lengths, 4 or 5 mm, the longer length being preferred if the bone is sufficiently thick to support its length. At the "head" of the screw is a small hole for the fixation of a permanent suture or a fascial strip (Fig. 35–5). A similar screw has been described by Mauriello and Caputo.[19a]

Shore and associates[20] describe the use of cantilevered miniplates for anterior fixation in the repair of unilateral telecanthus without adequate bony support for transnasal wiring. After exposing the nasal bone anterior to the anterior lacrimal crest, as in a dacryocystorhinostomy, periosteum is reflected posteriorly to the nasoethmoidal complex and all debris is removed. A Y-shaped miniplate is bent to conform to the bony contour, the long arm of the Y resting in the plane of the ethmoid bone inferior to the frontoethmoidal suture. While the globe is protected with a malleable retractor, a 6-mm screw is placed in a pilot hole in the inferior hole of the short arm of the Y. A 4-mm screw is placed in the superior hole, with the drill being directed slightly inferiorly to protect the cribriform plate. A 32-gauge wire is used to secure the medial canthal tendon (which may be connected with 4-0 prolene to the wire) to the appropriately positioned holes in the long arm of the miniplate. The wire is then fixated

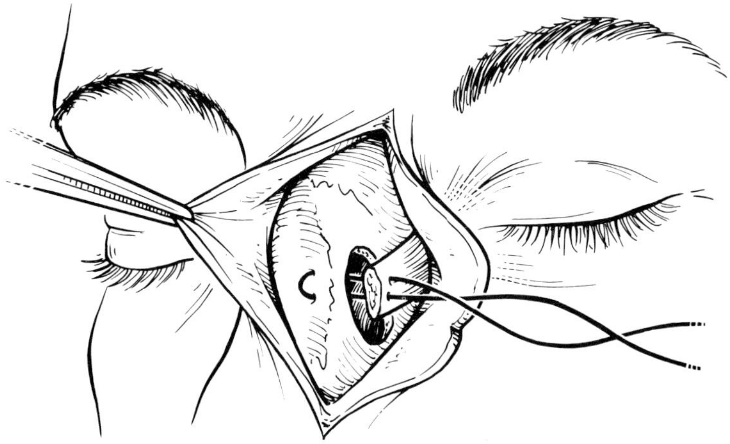

Figure 35–3. Unilateral transnasal wiring, as described by Beyer.

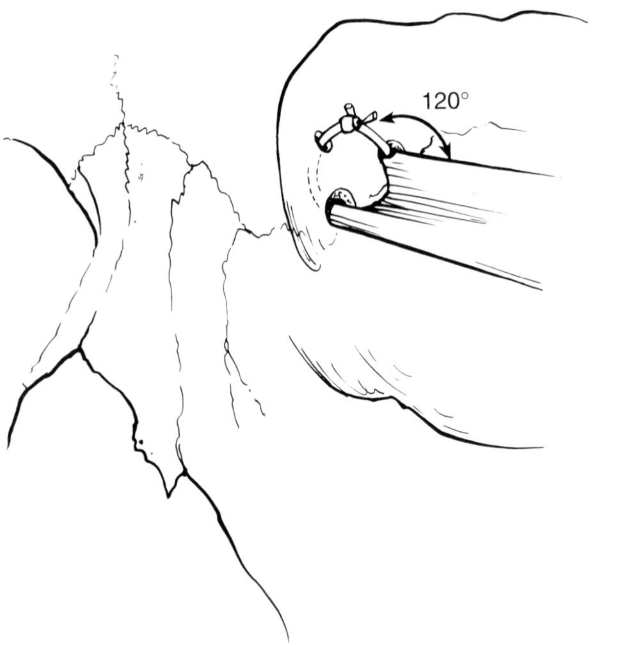

Figure 35–4. Suture fixation of medial canthal tendon with 120-degree angle between bone and tendon.

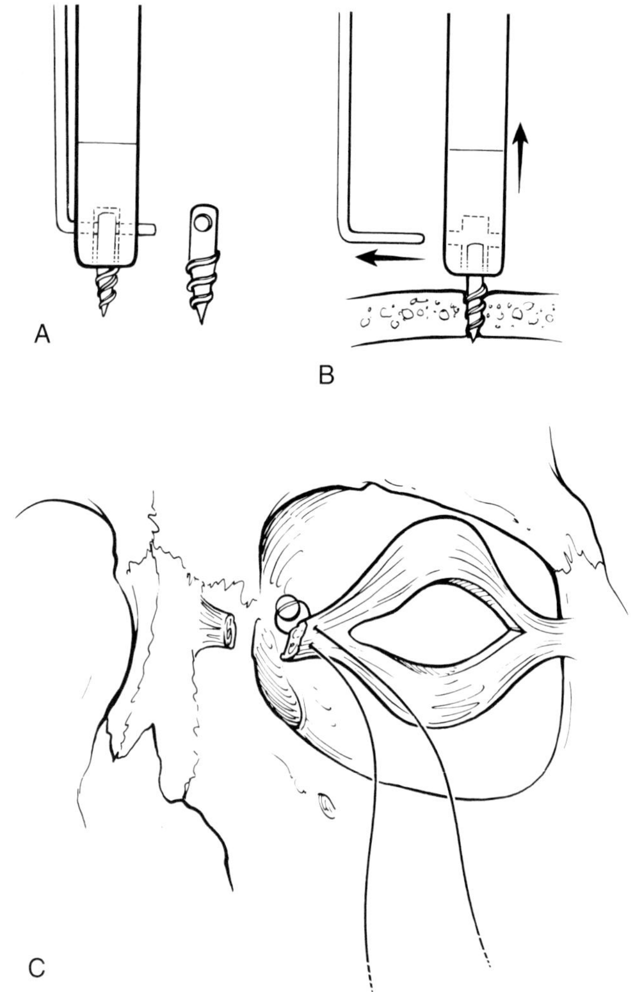

Figure 35–5. *A*, Nelson's stainless steel screw and special screwdriver. *B*, Placement of screw in bone and removal of screwdriver. *C*, Fixation screw in position with tarsi attached.

by tightening one of the anterior screws over it (Fig. 35–6).

ADVANCEMENT AND ROTATION FLAPS

In general, advancement flaps are those consisting of adjacent tissues used to fill a defect. Many modifications of such techniques exist, a few of which are described here.[5, 21–24] They may be employed over existing deep tissues (i.e., medial canthal tendon), in which case a cutaneous or myocutaneous flap is created, or they may involve the advancement of deeper tissues as well. A small circular defect in the medial canthus may be closed with a V-Y advancement flap,[25] thus avoiding a linear scar, which is more obvious and may contract.

Myocutaneous Flaps

For defects too large to close directly, a lateral canthotomy may be performed, with release of the inferior crus of the lateral canthal tendon and advancement of the full thickness of the eyelid or of a myocutaneous flap in more superficial defects (Fig. 35–7). When creating such myocutaneous flaps, the muscle and vascular bed are preserved in the advancing flap, while freeing the more lateral aspect of the flap from deeper tissues to allow its advancement.

Mustardé Technique

The Mustardé technique[24, 26] is most often employed for central or lateral eyelid defects, but it may be used to advance tissue of the malar region toward the medial canthus. The skin incision beyond the lateral canthus is directed superiorly in a gentle curve, as an extension of the curve of the lower eyelid, reaching its apex at the height of the brow. This allows for upward traction at the

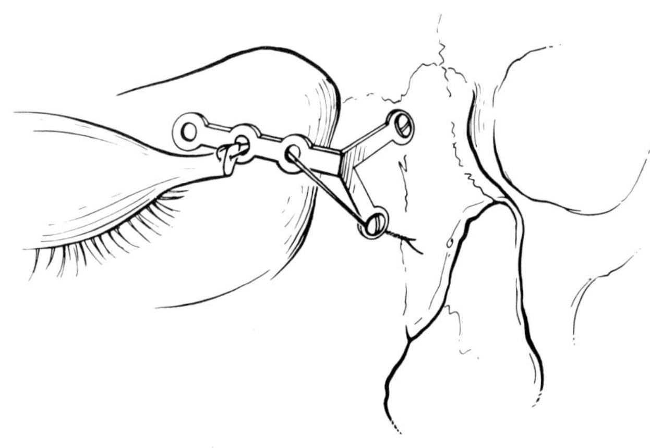

Figure 35–6. Cantilevered miniplate in position and canthal remnant attached with 32-gauge wire.

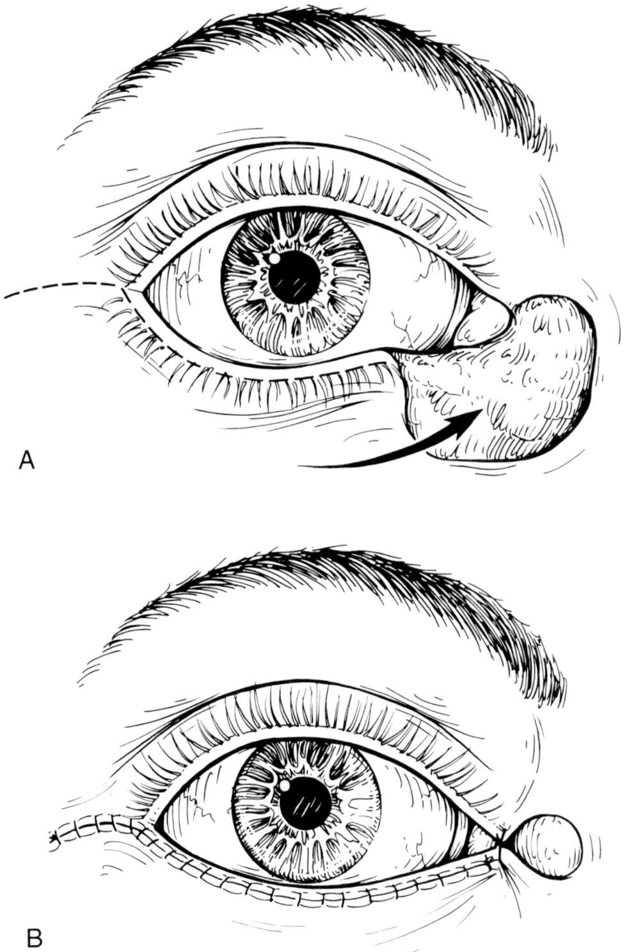

Figure 35–7. *A*, When the defect involves the eyelid as well as the medial canthus, the eyelid or a myocutaneous flap should be advanced medially after lateral canthotomy. *B*, Spontaneous granulation or a full-thickness skin graft may supplement the lower lid advancement.

new inferior crux of the lateral canthus to minimize postoperative lower eyelid contraction and ectropion. The pedicle is widely based inferolaterally to provide excellent vascular supply. The limbs of the lateral canthal tendon are severed as needed to advance the myocutaneous layer of the new eyelid. A mucous membrane graft can be used to line the posterior surface where it will contact the globe. It is extremely important to secure the tissue of the newly formed lateral canthus to the superior-temporal orbital rim periosteum to minimize inferior displacement of these tissues (Fig. 35–8).

Tenzel Flap

The Tenzel semicircular flap[27] is similar to the Mustardé technique except that it uses a smaller flap with a higher arch to close a smaller defect. The lateral extent of the flap may require a mucosal graft, but frequently sufficient conjunctiva remains so that it does not (Fig. 35–9). The most common complication of these procedures is eyelid retraction, which may require additional revision as a secondary procedure.

Sliding Tarsoconjunctival Graft

A tarsoconjunctival flap may be created by placing an incision parallel to and 4 mm from the eyelid margin, extending approximately the horizontal length of the defect. A relaxing incision is made, extending to the superior border of the tarsus into the upper fornix. The tarsoconjunctival flap is then advanced into the medial defect and fixed with a permanent suture to the periosteum or medial canthal remnant. Any identifiable remnant of levator aponeurosis may be sutured to the superior border of the advanced flap. The remaining eyelid margin is then sutured to the tarsus with sutures at partial tarsal depth. A full-thickness skin graft is placed over the flap, or tissue is advanced if available to create an anterior lamella (Fig. 35–10).[4, 5] A variation of the modified Hughes procedure (described elsewhere) may be performed medially, with the tarsoconjunctival pedicle to be divided secondarily. Small residual defects may be allowed to heal by secondary intention.[5, 27, 28]

Composite Grafts

A full-thickness defect may be covered by a flap lined with a free nasal chondromucosal or a tarsoconjunctival graft from the upper eyelid. This technique allows closure of a lower eyelid defect in the medial canthal region up to one third the horizontal length of the lid. Care must be taken in closing upper eyelid defects in this way, however, because tension may result in mechanical ptosis.

Upper Eyelid Pedicle Flap

A variety of myocutaneous flaps may be rotated from adjacent areas to fill defects in the medial canthal area. One of the easiest and most successful is the use of a flap from the upper eyelid, based medially and rotated into the defect. This is a good choice for superficial medial canthal defects because the skin color and texture match well. Although it is not truly based on a vascular pedicle, this tissue generally is well vascularized and may be placed over a minimally vascularized bed. The donor site, which lies in the usual position of an upper eyelid blepharoplasty incision, is closed primarily. A bolster is placed over the flap for 5 days, and the skin sutures are removed in 7 days (Fig. 35–11).[7]

Glabellar Flap

A V-Y flap designed from adjacent glabellar tissue provides good color and texture match for defects too large or deep to be closed with an upper eyelid flap.[4, 7] As de-

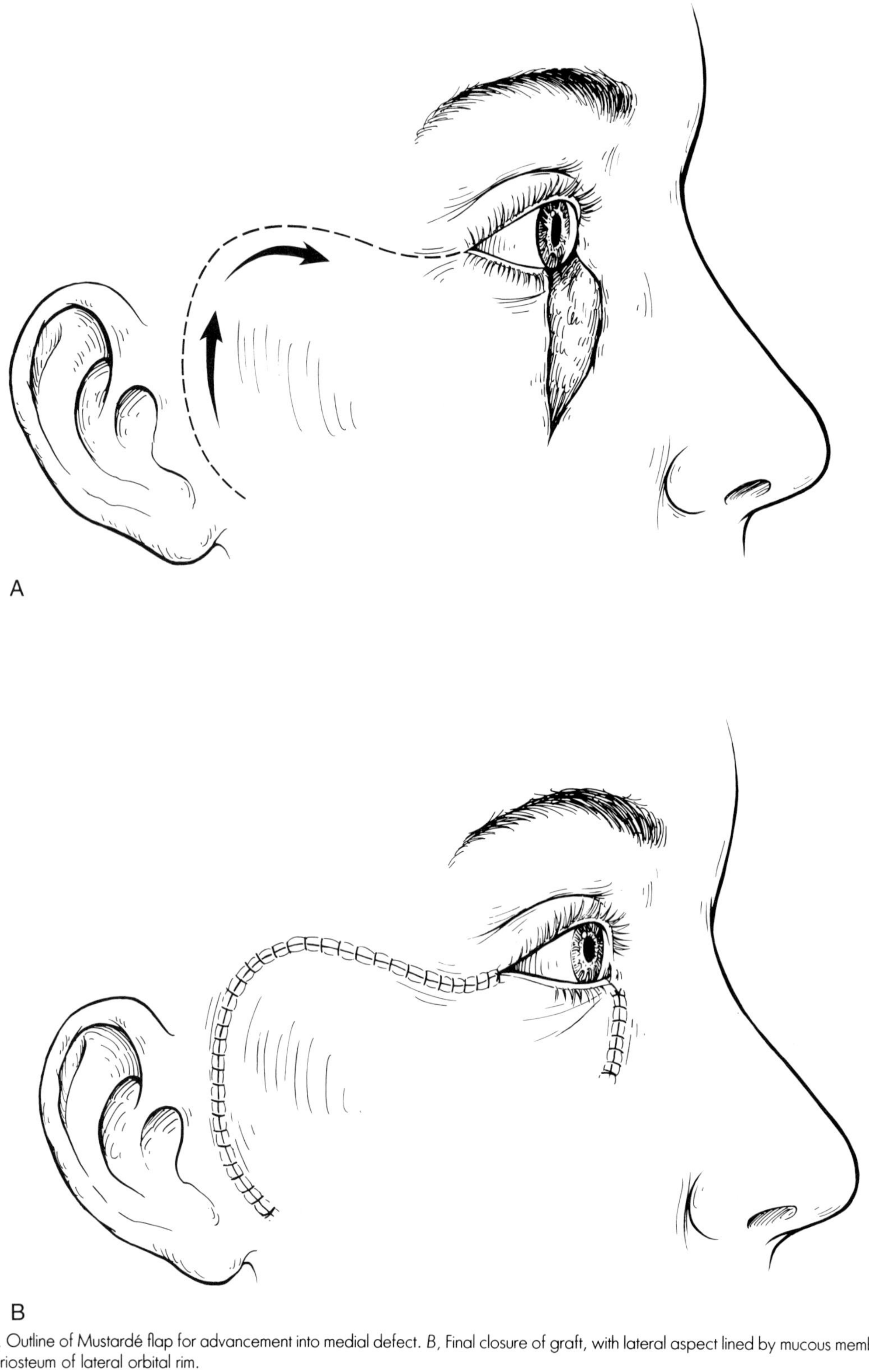

A

B

Figure 35–8. *A*, Outline of Mustardé flap for advancement into medial defect. *B*, Final closure of graft, with lateral aspect lined by mucous membrane and lateral canthus fixed to periosteum of lateral orbital rim.

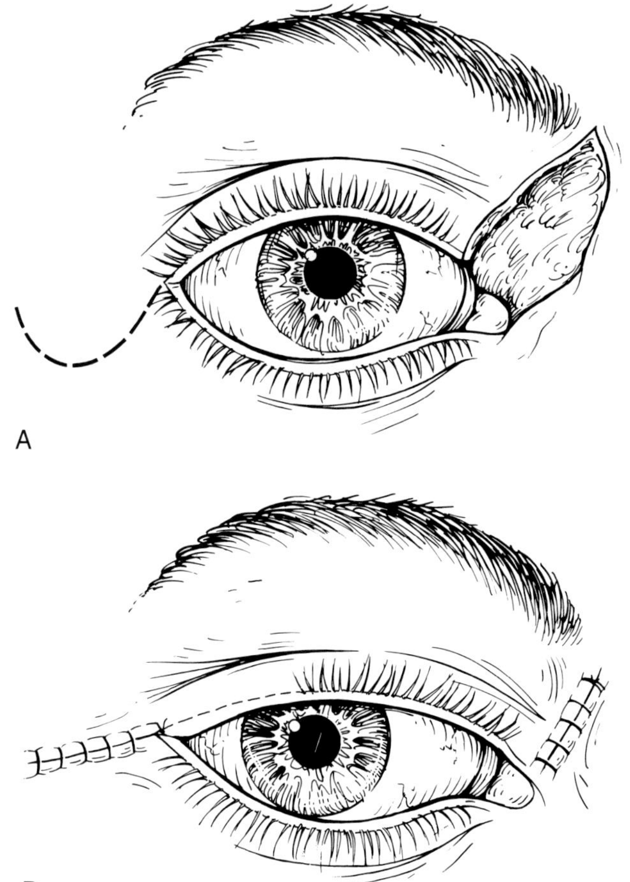

Figure 35–9. A, Tenzel flap outlined to fill a defect of upper lid and medial canthus. B, Appearance after closure.

scribed by McCord and Wesley,[4] the flap is outlined with its greatest width to cover the vertical defect in the canthus. The flap and surrounding tissue are then undermined, and the flap is rotated into the defect. The donor site is then closed in V-Y fashion, excising a small triangle at the tip of the flap if necessary for closure. The flap is secured in its position in the medial canthus with interrupted sutures, and a bolster may be applied for 5 days. The resultant donor site scar is located in Langer's lines in the glabellar area, making it relatively inconspicuous (Fig. 35–12). The excised triangle of skin may be trimmed and used to fill any residual skin defects.

MIDLINE FOREHEAD FLAP

The midline forehead flap for large, deep defects uses a flap on a subcutaneous pedicle. This flap is sometimes relatively bulky for the medial canthal area and provides a less desirable color and texture match than those previously described. The defect is measured, and the vertically oriented flap is outlined to obey the 5 : 1 rule (the length of the flap is less than five times the width).[4] The flap may be as much as 2.5 cm wide, and care must be taken to avoid extending the donor flap superiorly into hair-bearing skin. The skin is then incised, and a myocutaneous flap is elevated. Surrounding tissue at the donor site must be undermined to allow direct closure with 4-0 absorbable suture and 5-0 nylon for the skin. In a second stage after graft vascularization, redundant tissue at the base of the flap may be excised. If such a flap will directly overlie the globe, it must be lined with mucous membrane, a nasal chondromucosal graft, or conjunctiva advanced from the fornix. For large defects involving medial portions of both upper and lower eyelids, the distal segment of the flap may be bisected primarily or in a second stage to provide tissue for both upper and lower lids (Fig. 35–13).[29, 30]

Island Forehead Flap

Field[31] described a midline forehead flap based on random circulation (i.e., not designed to include an identifiable cutaneous vessel in the pedicle). This pedicle consists of subcutaneous tissue superficial to fascia and fat. The dermal-subdermal vascular plexus is left intact with a thin segment of fat-containing subcutaneous tissue. A circular myocutaneous island is outlined to fill the canthal defect, and triangular areas superior and inferior to the island are de-epithelialized. The defect thus created is closed in the midline after rotation of the pedicle. A subcutaneous tunnel allows the island pedicle to be passed from its midline donor site to the recipient bed (Fig. 35–14).

FREE SKIN GRAFTS

For superficial defects in the medial canthal region that overlie a vascular bed, full-thickness free skin grafts work well. Donor sites, in order of preference based on color and texture match, are (1) ipsilateral or contralateral upper eyelid, (2) retroauricular, (3) preauricular, (4) supraclavicular, and (5) volar aspect of upper arm. Each of these sites provides an appropriate graft of non–hair-bearing skin, and each may be closed primarily (after undermining surrounding tissues in some cases) with a minimally visible resultant scar.[4, 7, 32, 33] The defect is first carefully measured and a donor site chosen to provide adequate tissue. Paper from a suture package or other suitable substitute may be pressed against the defect, creating an imprint that is then trimmed appropriately and used as a template. The donor site is then marked, making it 20% to 30% larger than the template to allow for contracture of the graft. The skin is incised and a thin donor graft is harvested. The graft may be placed over the surgeon's gloved finger dermis up, and all subcutaneous fatty tissue is trimmed away. The graft is transferred to the recipient bed and sutured securely in

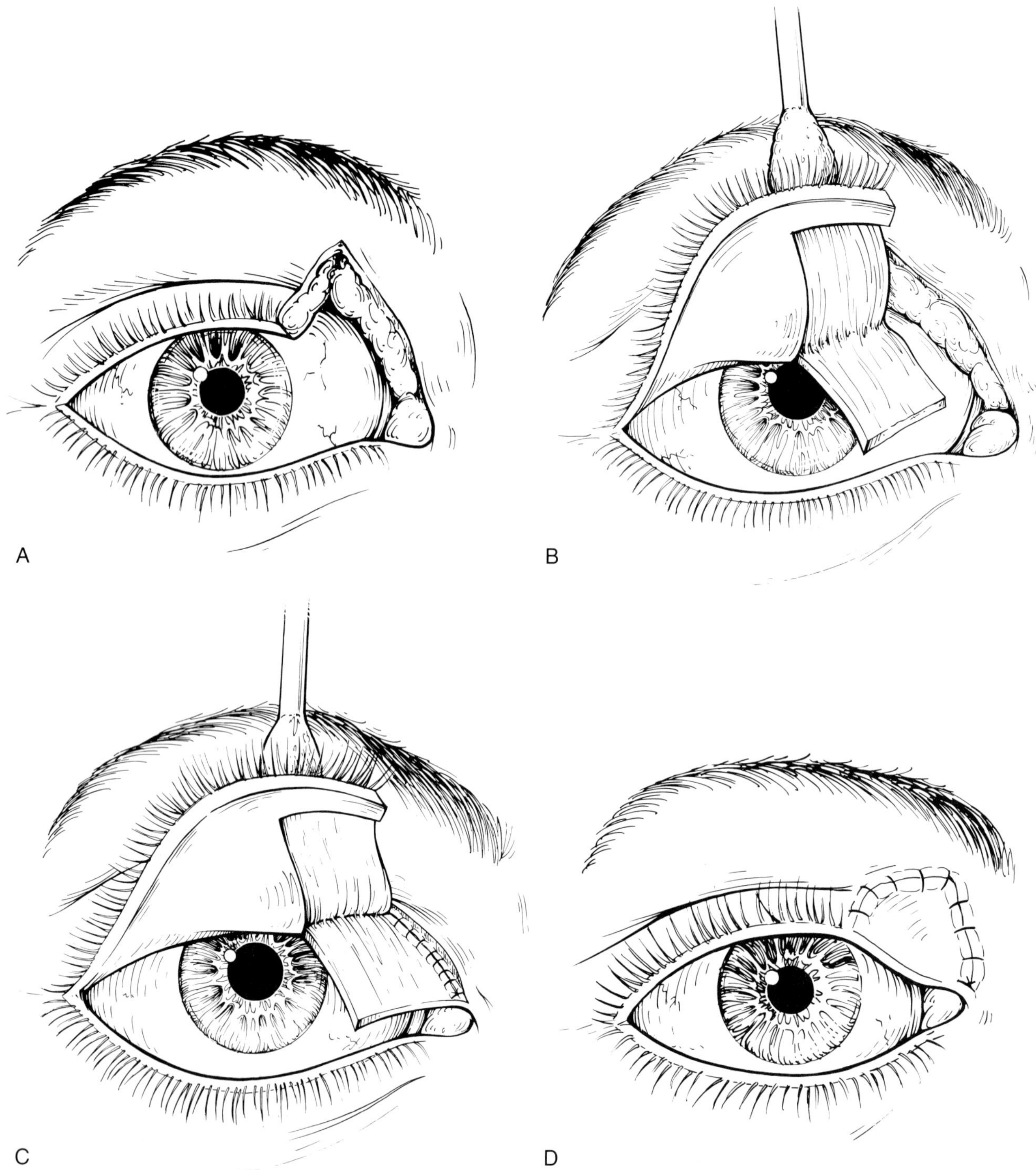
A B C D

Figure 35–10. *A*, Medial upper eyelid defect. *B*, Tarsoconjunctival flap created with eyelid everted. C, Tarsoconjunctival flap attached to periosteum or medial canthal tendon after sliding medially. *D*, Lid margin closed with sutures one-half tarsal thickness and covered with skin graft.

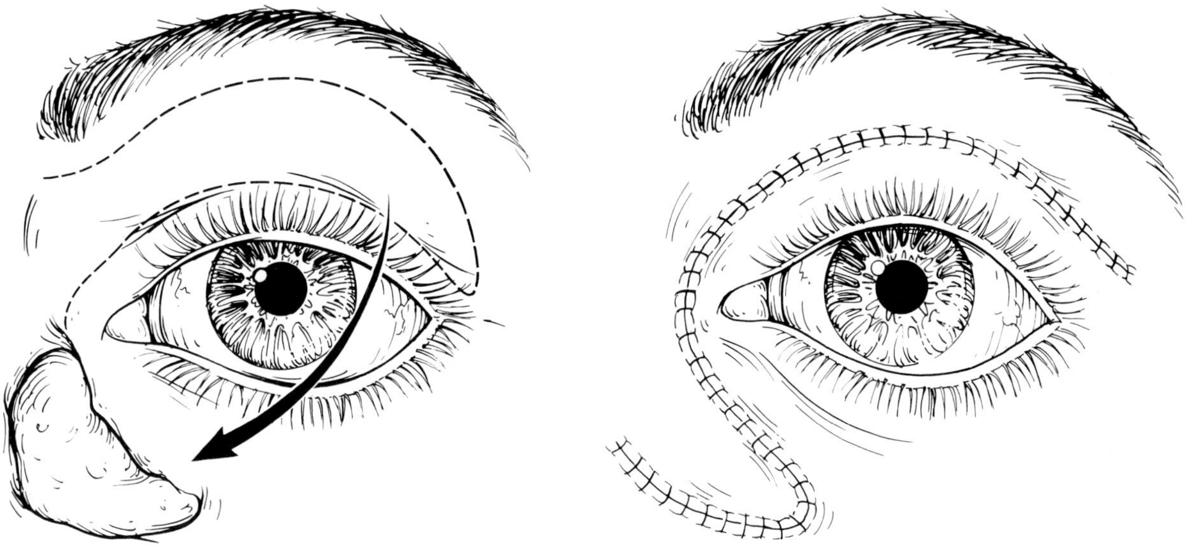

A B

Figure 35–11. Upper eyelid pedicle graft. *A*, Medial canthal defect with incision lines for pedicle from upper lid. *B*, Pedicle flap sutured into defect.

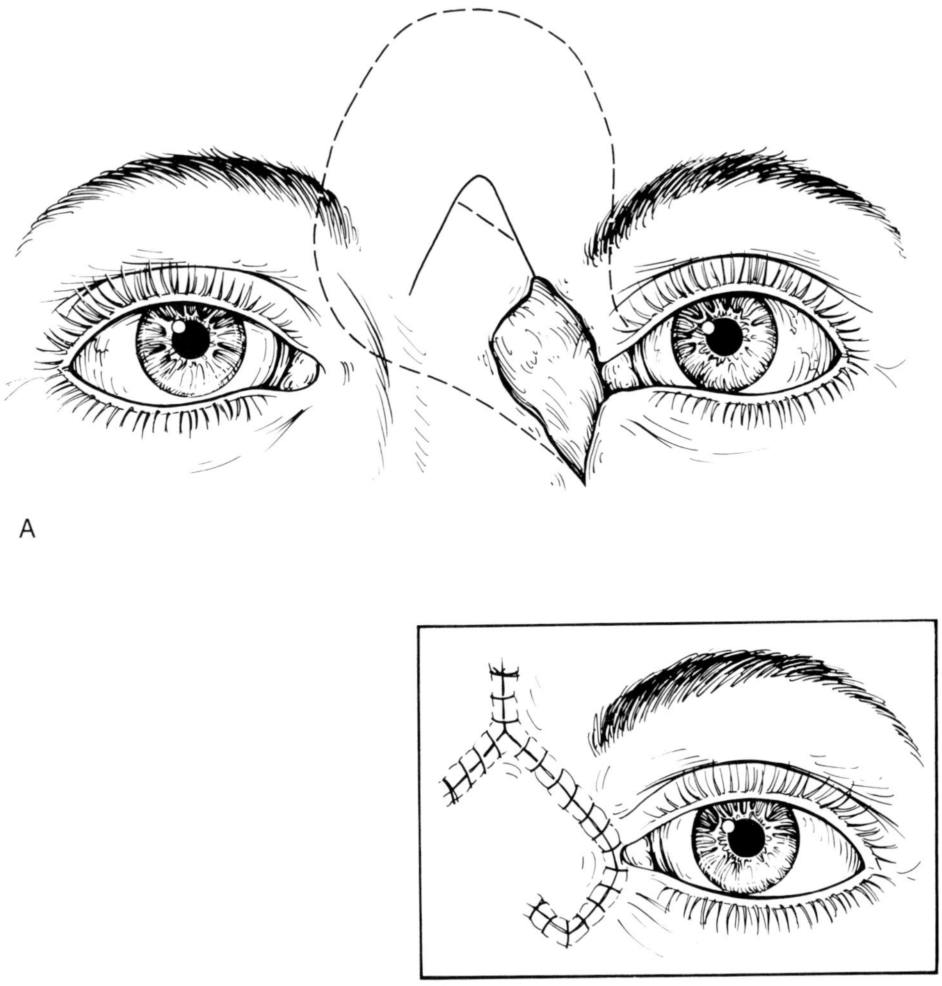

A

B

Figure 35–12. Glabellar flap. *A*, Flap outlined to cover defect. *B*, Flap sutured in place after rotation.

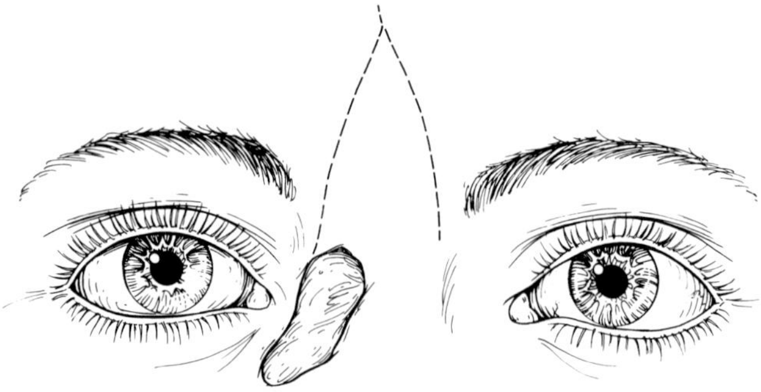

A

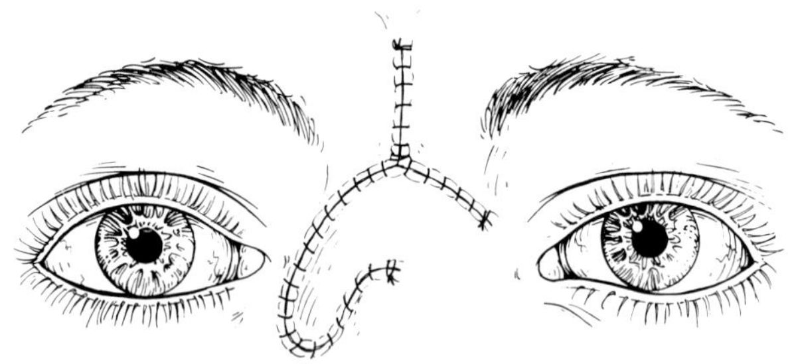

B

Figure 35–13. Midline forehead flap. *A*, Outline of proposed flap. *B*, Flap incised, undermined, rotated, and sutured.

place, first with 6-0 silk cardinal sutures, then filling in with 6-0 fast-absorbing plain gut. Although it is important to avoid excessive cautery of the graft bed, care must be taken to control any active bleeding under the graft and to evacuate all blood deep to the graft as the graft is being sutured in place. Often one or more "buttonholes" are placed in the graft to allow for drainage should any blood accumulate. Firm graft-to-vascular bed contact is important. Through-and-through sutures are placed centrally in the graft to secure it to underlying tissues. The graft is then covered with a Telfa bolster secured in place with 4-0 silk horizontal mattress sutures. This pressure dressing is left in place for 5 days. No ointments are used on grafts until after that time. Sutures are removed after 7 to 10 days (Fig. 35–15).

LACRIMAL INVOLVEMENT

Detailed discussion of lacrimal reconstruction is given elsewhere in this volume, but a few brief comments are relevant here. In many cases, particularly in older patients, the absence of a lacrimal outflow system produces few if any symptoms. Often it is best to reconstruct the medial canthal area primarily and to perform a conjunctivodacryocystorhinostomy as a secondary procedure only if epiphora is a persistent problem. When easily performed as a part of the primary repair, however, the surgeon may wish to include the lacrimal system in the reconstruction. If as little as one fourth of the canaliculus is present, the lower canaliculus can be reconstructed by the following steps (Fig. 35–16), as described by McCord and Nunery[11]:

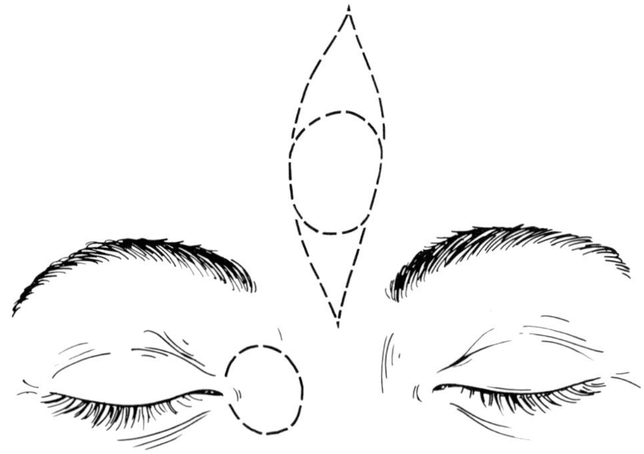

A

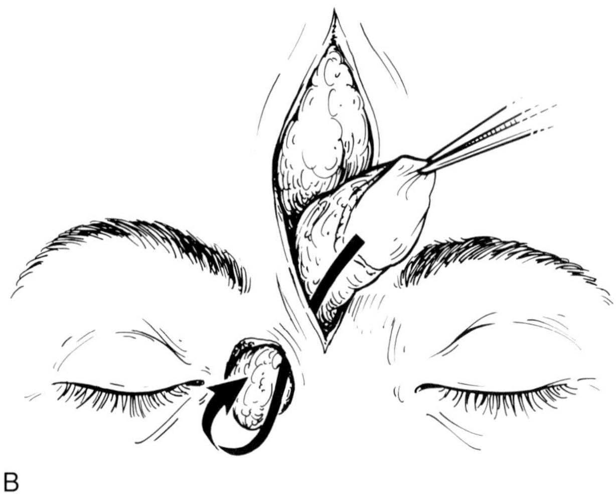

B

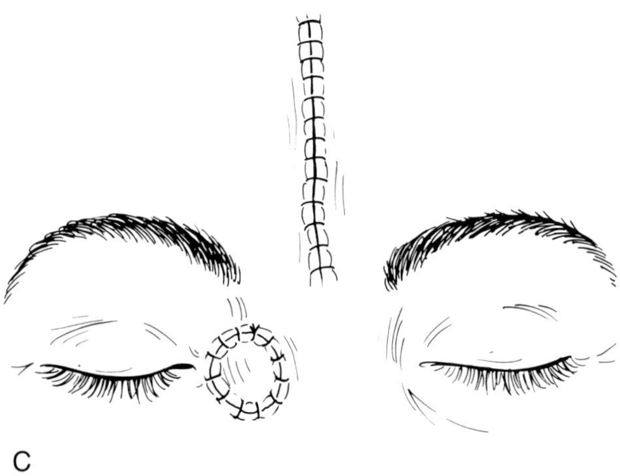

C

Figure 35–14. *A* to *C*, Island forehead flap.

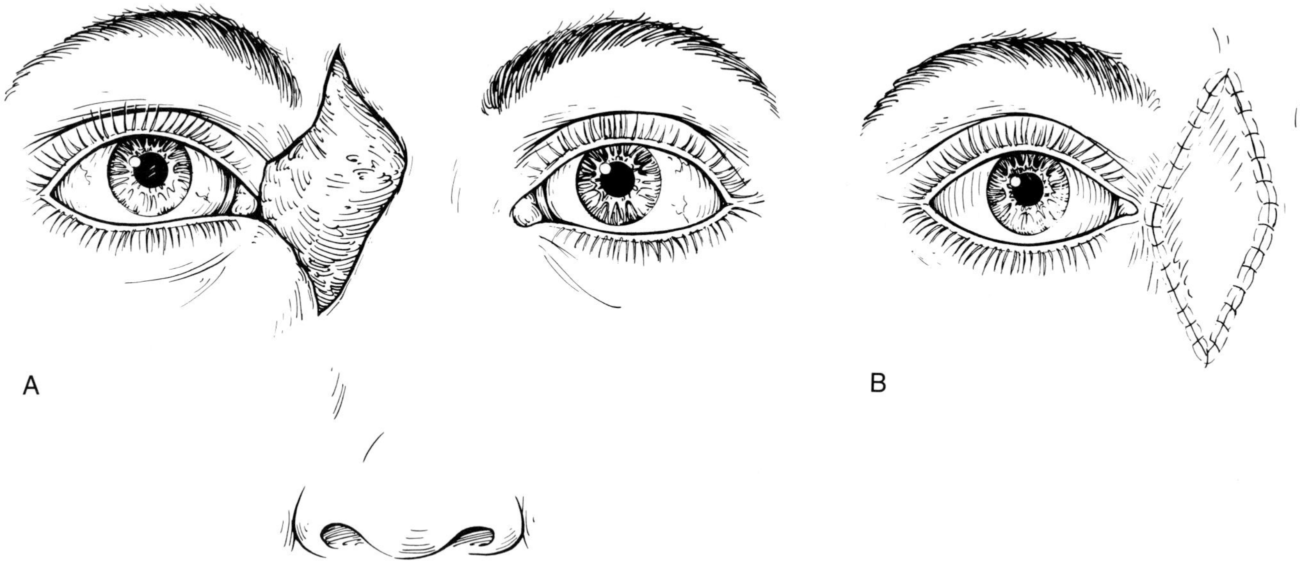

Figure 35–15. *A* and *B*, Free skin graft.

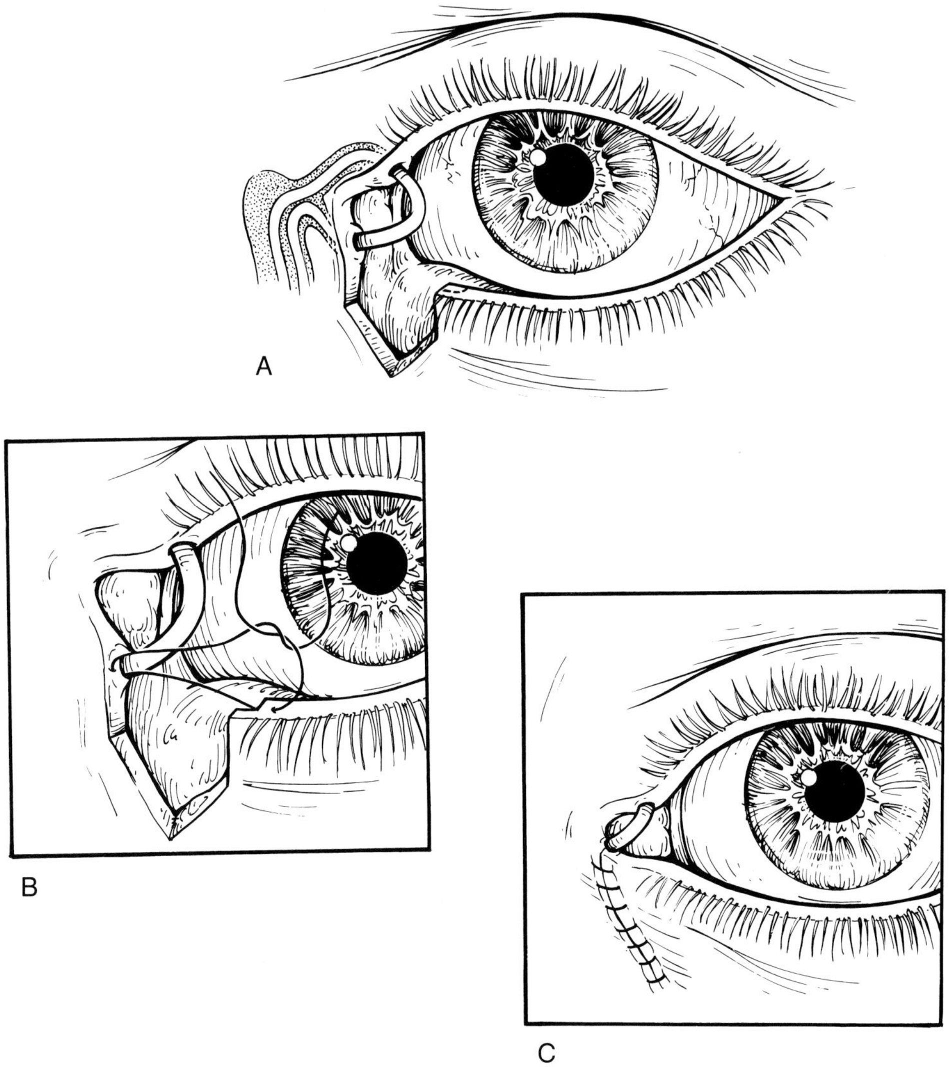

Figure 35–16. Canalicular reconstruction. *A*, Silicone intubation of remnants of canaliculus. *B*, Canaliculus sutured to posterior tarsal border. C, Skin closed with interrupted sutures.

1. Identify the distal end.
2. Undermine the tissues around the canaliculus to mobilize them.
3. Intubate the lacrimal system with Quickert-Dryden probes.
4. Reattach the medial canthal tendon posterior to the intubated canalicular remnant.
5. Create a new punctum by excising a triangle of conjunctiva and posterior tarsus at the medial end of the lid remnant.
6. Suture the canaliculus to the posterior tarsal border with 7-0 or 8-0 silk or Vicryl.
7. Tie the silicone tubing in the inferior meatus with a single square knot. It will remain in place for 6 to 8 weeks.
8. Close the skin with 7-0 silk sutures, to be removed in 5 to 7 days.

Another option is the "marsupialization" of the distal end of remaining canaliculus, as described by Older.[28] The blade of a fine iris scissors enters the canaliculus and opens that structure for 2 mm on the posterosuperior aspect. Then 7-0 chromic sutures are used to attach the cut ends to the skin and conjunctiva, leaving the canaliculus open. The lacrimal system is then intubated with silicone, which is left in place for 6 to 12 weeks.

COMPLICATIONS OF MEDIAL CANTHAL RECONSTRUCTION

As with all surgical procedures, postoperative hematoma is a complication best prevented by meticulous interoperative attention to hemostasis. A nonocclusive semipressure dressing is used postoperatively, along with ice compresses. Careful and detailed postoperative instructions must be given and a high level of suspicion maintained by the surgeon. The patient must be examined immediately if symptoms of hematoma are reported and the hematoma evacuated if necessary. In addition to the previously mentioned compromise of a skin graft by hematoma in the graft bed, one must be ever cognizant of the sight-threatening complication of orbital hematoma after reconstructive surgery.

Naso-orbital fistulas can occur if the medial orbital wall is resected with tumor or is damaged traumatically. A skin graft used to cover such a defect will have no vascular bed, increasing the likelihood of recurrence of fistula. Putterman[34] described the use of a nasolabial flap to line the deep surface of the fistula and a forehead flap to reconstruct the superficial layer.

Probably the most common postoperative complication is eyelid malposition. Ectropion of the eyelid margin may be due to the following:

1. Vertical shortage of the anterior lamella (skin). To minimize this occurrence, a full-thickness skin graft should be sized generously.[35-37] Frost or intermarginal tarsorrhaphy sutures should be used to prevent contracture, and vertical advancement flaps should be avoided.
2. Lower eyelid laxity due to excessive horizontal length. Sliding flaps (i.e., tarsoconjunctival) should be slightly undersized in comparison to the defect to provide adequate tension.
3. Lateral migration of the canthus due to inadequate fixation. Both the medial and lateral canthi must be firmly fixed to periosteum or fixation screws. As was mentioned previously, if wire is used for fixation, it should not be placed through soft tissues but should be passed through a nonabsorbable suture loop placed in the tissue.[4, 11]

REFERENCES

1. Zide BM, McCarthy JG: The medial canthus revisited: An anatomical basis for canthopexy. Ann Plast Surg 11:1, 1983.
2. Zide BM, Jelks GW: Medial canthus. *In* Surgical Anatomy of the Orbit. New York, Raven Press, 1985; pp 42–46.
3. Jones LE, Wobig JL: Anatomy of the eyelids. *In* Surgery of the Eyelid and Lacrimal System. Birmingham, AL, Aesculapius, 1976; pp 28–47.
4. McCord CD, Wesley R: Reconstruction of the upper eyelid and medial canthus. *In* McCord CD, Tannenbaum M (eds): Oculoplastic Surgery, 2nd ed. New York, Raven Press, 1987; pp 73–91.
5. Older JJ: Medial canthal reconstruction. *In* Hornblass A (ed): Oculoplastic, Orbital and Reconstructive Surgery. Baltimore, Williams & Wilkins, 1988; pp 651–658.
6. Rodriquez RL, Zide BM: Reconstruction of the medial canthus. Clin Plast Surg 15:255, 1988.
7. Becker FF: Reconstructive surgery of the medial canthal region. Ann Plast Surg 7:259, 1981.
8. Fox SA, Beard C: Spontaneous lid repair. Am J Ophthalmol 58:947, 1964.
9. Harrington JN: Reconstruction of the medial canthus by spontaneous granulation (laissez-faire): A review. Ann Ophthalmol 14:956, 1982.
10. Mehta HK: Simultaneous spontaneous and primary surgical repair of eyelid. Br J Ophthalmol 73:488, 1989.
11. McCord CD, Nunery WR: Reconstruction of the lower eyelid and outer canthus. *In* McCord CD, Tannenbaum M (eds): Oculoplastic Surgery, 2nd ed. New York, Raven Press, 1987, pp 93–115.
12. Bass CB: Medial canthal ligament reconstruction. Ann Plast Surg 3:182, 1979.
13. Moss ALH: Medial canthal tendon reconstruction. J Maxillofac Surg 12:131, 1984.
14. Beyer CK: Unilateral medial canthal wiring technique. *In* Wesley RE (ed): Techniques in Ophthalmic Plastic Surgery. New York, John Wiley & Sons, 1986, pp 436–437.
15. Smith B, Beyer CK: Medial canthaloplasty. Arch Ophthalmol 82:3448, 1969.
16. Wesley RE: Medial canthal fixation in transnasal wiring. *In* McCord CD, Tannenbaum M (eds): Oculoplastic Surgery, 2nd ed. New York, Raven Press, 1987, pp 443–444.
17. Brody GS, Wheeler ES: Medial canthal tendon reconstruction. Plast Reconstr Surg 68:789, 1981.
18. Callahan MA: Canthal fixation with a stainless steel screw: A report of ten patients. Adv Ophthalmic Plast Reconstr Surg 7:33, 1988.
19. Callahan A, Callahan MA: Fixation of the medial canthal structures: Evolution of the best method. Ann Plast Surg 11:242, 1983.

19a. Mauriello JA Jr, Caputo AR: Treatment of congenital forms of telecanthus with custom-designed titanium medial canthal tendon screws. Ophthal Plast Reconstr Surg 10:195–199, 1994.

20. Shore JW, Rubin PAD, Bilyk J: Repair of telecanthus by anterior fixation of cantilevered miniplates. Ophthalmology 99:1133–1138, 1992.

21. Avram DR, Hurwitz JJ, Kratky V: Modified Tessier flap for reconstruction of the upper eyelid. Ophthalmic Surg 22:467, 1991.
22. Iliff CE, Iliff NT: Partial and total reconstruction of the lower eyelid. Ophthalmology 87:272, 1980.
23. Matsuo K, Kiyono M, Hirose T: Lower eyelid reconstruction with orbicularis oculi musculocutaneous transposition flap and a conchal cartilage graft. Ophthalmic Plast Reconstr Surg 6:177, 1990.
24. Mustardé JC: Repair and Reconstruction of the Orbital Region: A Practical Guide. Edinburgh, Churchill Livingstone, 1980, pp 169–182.
25. Bostwick J, Vasconez LO, Jurkiewicz MJ: Basal cell carcinoma of the medial canthal area. Plast Reconstr Surg 55:667, 1975.
26. Callahan MA, Callahan A: Mustardé flap lower eyelid reconstruction after malignancy. Ophthalmology 87:279, 1980.
27. Tenzel RR, Boynton JR, Buffman FV: Technique of combined lid and medial canthus reconstruction. Ophthalmic Surg 7:25, 1976.
28. Older JJ: Canalicular reconstruction following resection of medial eyelid tumors. *In* McCord CD, Tannenbaum M (eds): Oculoplastic Surgery, 2nd ed. New York, Raven Press, 1987, pp 362–364.
29. Sakai S, Soeda S, Matsukawa A: Refinements of the island median forehead flap for reconstruction of the medial canthal area. J Dermatol Surg Oncol 15:524, 1989.
30. Sanderson RS, Rappaport I: Technique for reconstruction of carcinoma of the inner canthus. Am Surg 31:625, 1965.
31. Field LM: The midline forehead island flap. J Dermatol Surg Oncol 13:243, 1987.
32. Dryden RM, Wulc AE: The preauricular skin graft in eyelid reconstruction. Arch Ophthalmol 103:1579, 1985.
33. Hill TG: Contouring of donor skin in full-thickness skin grafts. J Dermatol Surg Oncol 13:883, 1987.
34. Putterman AM: Reconstruction of nasal fistulas of the medial canthus. Am J Ophthalmol 108:68, 1989.
35. Small RG, Sahl WJ: The use of split-thickness skin grafts for eyelid and facial reconstruction after Mohs' fresh-tissue surgery. Ophthalmic Plast Reconstr Surg 5:266, 1989.
36. Corwin TR, Klein AW, Habal MB: The aesthetics of the preauricular graft in facial reconstruction. Ann Plast Surg 9:213, 1982.
37. Bostwick J, Jurkiewicz MD: Functional anatomy of the eyelids as related to reconstruction. Am Surg 42:696, 1976.

CHAPTER 36

Reconstruction of the Lower Eyelid and Lateral Canthus

Steven C. Dresner

DIRECT CLOSURE OF DEFECTS

Small tumors or small defects from Mohs' surgery can be closed directly. The inverted pentangle design with direct end-to-end closure is useful with defects affecting up to 30% or 40% of the lower eyelid, depending on the patient's age and the elasticity of the tissues. Direct closure is the obvious choice whenever possible and gives the most cosmetically acceptable result of all lid reconstructions.

If Mohs' surgery has been performed previously, the edges must be freshened and re-excised to create perpendicular margins of tarsus. Two forceps may be used to reapproximate the margins of the defect to ensure that primary closure is possible and that no undue tension will occur. The tarsal sutures are placed primarily to ensure that the underlying architecture of the eyelid is appropriately reconstructed. Two 5-0 or 6-0 polyglactin sutures should be placed partial thickness through tarsus (Fig. 36–1).

The conjunctiva should not be included in the bite. The sutures are tied temporarily to ensure that the eyelid margin and lash line are well approximated. These sutures are untied, and the gray line is sewn with a vertical mattress suture of either 6-0 silk or 6-0 braided nylon (Nurolon). A similar suture at the lash line is also placed.

Once all these sutures are placed, the polyglactin sutures are tied permanently. The gray line and lash line sutures are tied sequentially (Fig. 36–2).

With the ends left long, the rest of the incision is then closed with interrupted sutures, bringing the ends of the lid marginal sutures into the last suture inferiorly.

LATERAL CANTHOLYSIS

If primary closure cannot be accomplished where there is undue tension on the wound, a lateral cantholysis can be performed. Traditionally, a horizontal canthal incision has been described; however, a superiorly directed incison is preferable (Fig. 36–3).

This incision can be enlarged to create a Tenzel rotation flap if necessary. The incision includes skin and orbicularis, and then the inferior crus of the lateral canthal tendon is lysed either with scissors or the electrocautery unit. Once this has been accomplished, the remnant lateral eyelid can be mobilized medially to complete the eyelid reconstruction.

TENZEL ROTATION FLAP

The Tenzel rotation flap is a semicircular myocutaneous flap originating at the lateral canthal angle. This is the most useful flap for reconstruction of central, medial, and lateral defects ranging between 40% and 70% of the lower eyelid. It yields better cosmetic results in lateral canthal defects if at least 3 to 4 mm of the lateral eyelid remains to be reapproximated to the medial eyelid remnant. It is especially useful in large, central defects by rotating the lateral cilia to a more central position, leaving the reconstructed lateral eyelid without cilia where it would be least noticeable.

The flap is designed with a marking pen beginning at the lateral canthus and extending superiorly and laterally to just below the lateral eyebrow in a curvilinear fashion (Fig. 36–4).

The incision is begun at the lateral canthus through skin and muscle. The dissection adjacent to the lateral canthus should be thicker than the flap needs to be temporally to ensure that the lateral reconstructed eyelid appears similar to the rest of the eyelid and to provide adequate orbicularis bulk to be sewn to the periorbita laterally at closure. The inferior crus of the lateral canthal tendon is lysed, and the flap is undermined from the lateral and inferior lateral orbital rim.

Precise hemostasis is necessary to ensure a dry field at completion. The flap is then rotated medially, and the lid margin remnants are closed as previously described. If desired, the remnant conjunctiva can be undermined and advanced to the new eyelid margin. Many flaps do not usually require conjunctival advancement and can be left to epithelialize.

Before closure of the temporal defect, the orbicularis adjacent to the new lateral canthus is grasped and sewn to the periorbita with 5-0 or 4-0 polyglactin suture, elevat-

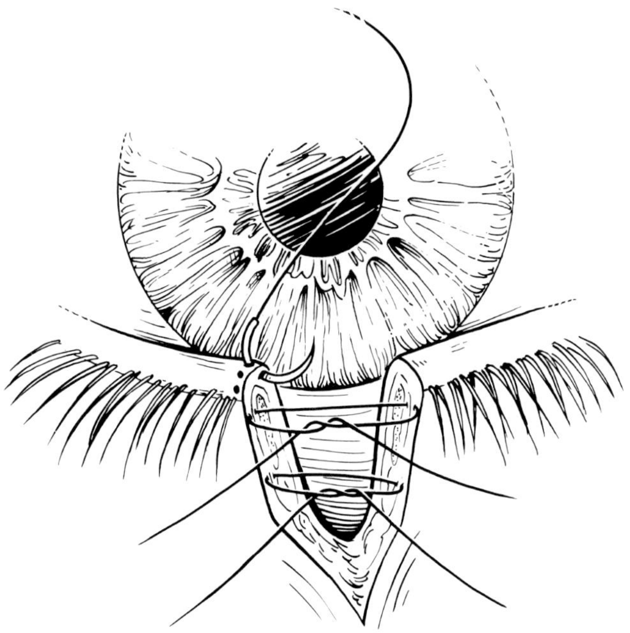

Figure 36–1. Two 5-0 or 6-0 polyglactin sutures are placed partial thickness through tarsus.

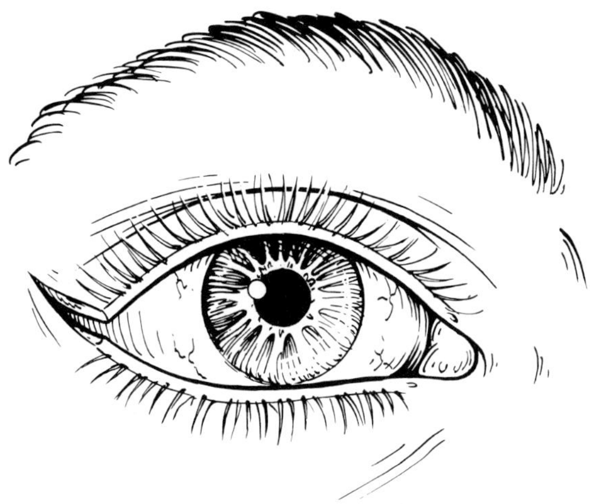

Figure 36–3. A superiorly directed canthotomy incision is made, followed by cantholysis of the inferior crus of the canthal tendon.

ing and tightening the eyelid to the appropriate tone and contour. A slight upward overcorrection is desirable, since the eyelid will usually retract or sag somewhat postoperatively. The temporal defect can be closed with a running horizontal mattress suture.

Larger flaps may require more support for the posterior lamella. A periosteal flap based at the orbital rim provides a firm support structure for the posterior lamella, which can be attached to the remnant medial eyelid. This tissue also rapidly epithelializes from the remnant conjunctiva.

After the Tenzel flap has been prepared, the lateral and superolateral orbital rim is exposed. A strip of periorbita measuring 8 to 10 mm in width is marked out, extending upward along the orbital rim (Fig. 36–5). This is incised with a no. 15 blade, undermined and rotated from its rim attachment, and sewn to the remnant tarsus with firm tension. The remnant conjunctiva can be sewn to the inferior or superior border of the periorbita. The Tenzel flap is then draped over the periosteal flap and sewn to it with 6-0 plain gut suture (Fig. 36–6).

Alternatively, the Tenzel flap can be supported by a hard palate graft or ear cartilage graft. Hard palate tissue is preferable to ear cartilage because it is more flexible and less bulky and more easily sewn. Using hard palate as a free graft can be useful in exceptionally large defects

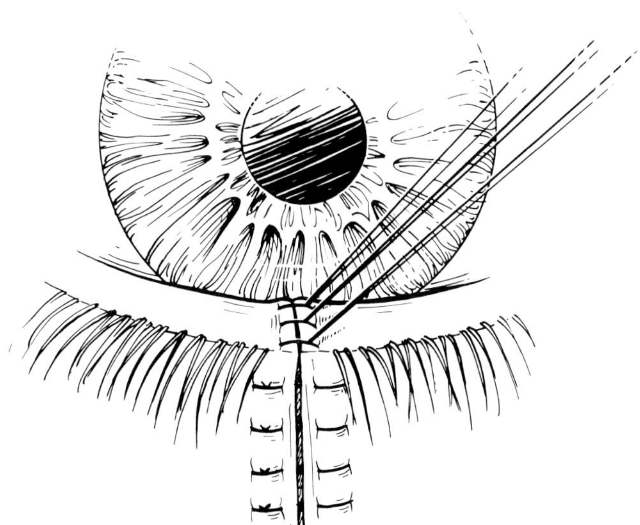

Figure 36–2. The gray line and lash line are sewn with vertical mattress sutures of 6-0 silk or 6-0 braided nylon. An additional suture between these two can also be placed.

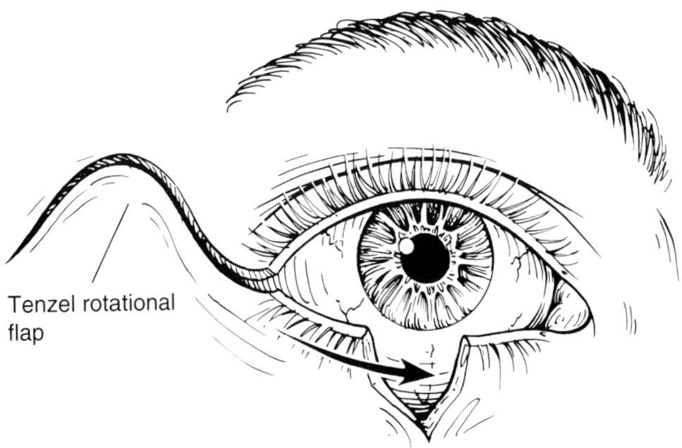

Figure 36–4. The incision can be enlarged to create a Tenzel rotation flap. (From McCord CD, Nunery WR: Reconstruction of the lower eyelid and outer canthus. *In* McCord C, Tanenbaum M [eds]: Oculoplastic Surgery, 2nd ed. New York, Raven Press, 1987, p 97.)

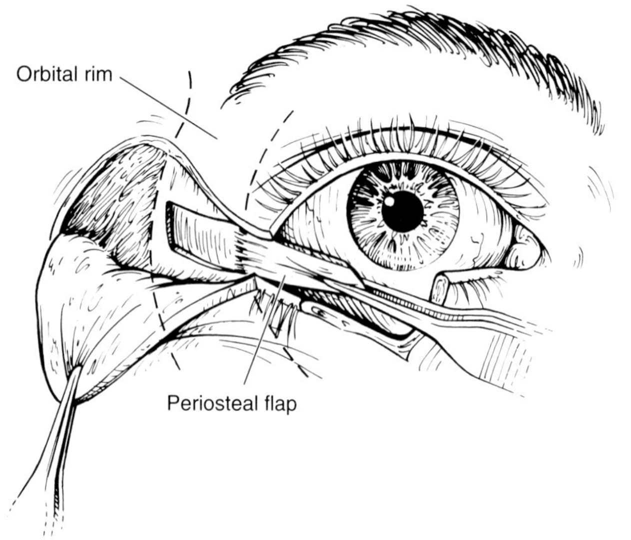

Figure 36–5. A strip of periorbita measuring 8 to 10 mm in width is incised with a no. 15 blade and reflected off the orbital rim with a periosteal elevator. (From McCord CD, Nunery WR: Reconstruction of the lower eyelid and outer canthus. *In* McCord C, Tanenbaum M [eds]: Oculoplastic Surgery, 2nd ed. New York, Raven Press, 1987, p 99.)

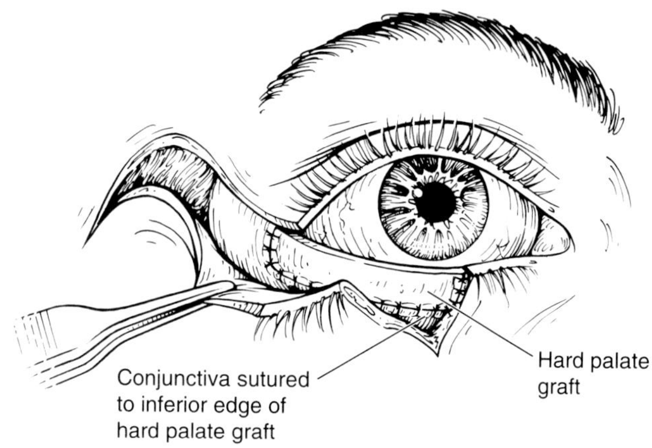

Figure 36–7. A hard palate graft is harvested and sewn between the periosteum and the remnant tarsus. (From McCord CD, Nunery WR: Reconstruction of the lower eyelid and outer canthus. *In* McCord C, Tanenbaum M [eds]: Oculoplastic Surgery, 2nd ed. New York, Raven Press, 1987, p 100.)

where there is a paucity of conjunctiva or where the patient is not a candidate for temporary lid closure as necessary with the Hughes flap.

The hard palate is harvested freehand as described previously. It is sewn to the remnant eyelid medially, the conjunctiva inferiorly, and the orbital rim laterally (Fig. 36–7). The Tenzel flap is advanced over it similar to the technique described for the periosteal flap.

HUGHES PROCEDURE

The Hughes flap is a tarsoconjunctival flap from the upper eyelid to the lower eyelid. Its best use is in defects affecting 70% or more of the lower eyelid. The lateral defects of the lower eyelid affecting 40% to 50% of the lid are also amenable to closure of the posterior lamella with a Hughes flap. Medial defects in the 40% to 50% range are better corrected with a Tenzel flap, as previously described. The disadvantage of the Hughes flap is that partial or near-complete closure of the lid fissure is required and that a second-stage procedure is needed to sever the flap. However, the flap can usually be severed at 2 to 3 weeks instead of 4 to 6 weeks as has been previously described.

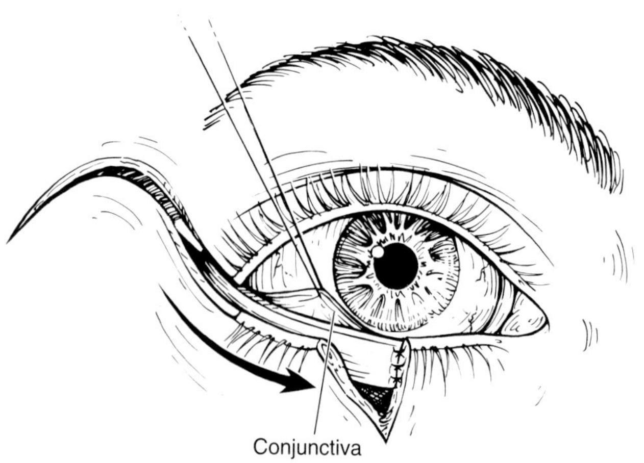

Figure 36–6. The periosteal flap is sewn to the remnant tarsus with firm tension. The remnant conjunctiva can be sewn to the periosteal flap. A Tenzel flap is then draped over the periosteal flap and sewn to it with 6-0 plain gut suture. (From McCord CD, Nunery WR: Reconstruction of the lower eyelid and outer canthus. *In* McCord C, Tanenbaum M [eds]: Oculoplastic Surgery, 2nd ed. New York, Raven Press, 1987, p 99.)

If Mohs' surgery has been performed, the edges of the defect need to be freshened and the margins of the remaining tarsus made perpendicular to the lid margin. With the remnant eyelid margin on stretch, the defect is measured in width and depth. The upper eyelid is infiltrated through the cul-de-sac with 1% lidocaine with epinephrine. The upper eyelid is everted over a Desmarres retractor. The flap is marked out with a marking pen, depending on the desired width. The horizontal incision for the flap should remain about 4 mm above the eyelid margin to avoid postoperative upper eyelid deformities and lid instability. The tarsus is incised with a no. 15 blade and dissected with scissors off the levator aponeurosis (Fig. 36–8). If a skin graft is to be used for the anterior lamella, it may be desirable to include Müller's muscle in the flap. Under most circumstances the dissection can proceed between the conjunctiva and Müller's muscle with the aid of a hand-held cautery. Eliminating Müller's muscle can help prevent postoperative upper eyelid retraction after the flap has been severed.

Once the flap has been dissected superiorly, it can be mobilized inferiorly and sewn to the remnant eyelid margins medially and laterally with 5-0 polyglactin sutures (Fig. 36–9). If no medial tarsus is remaining, the flap is sewn to the subcanalicular tissues after silicone intubation has been performed. If no lateral tarsus remains,

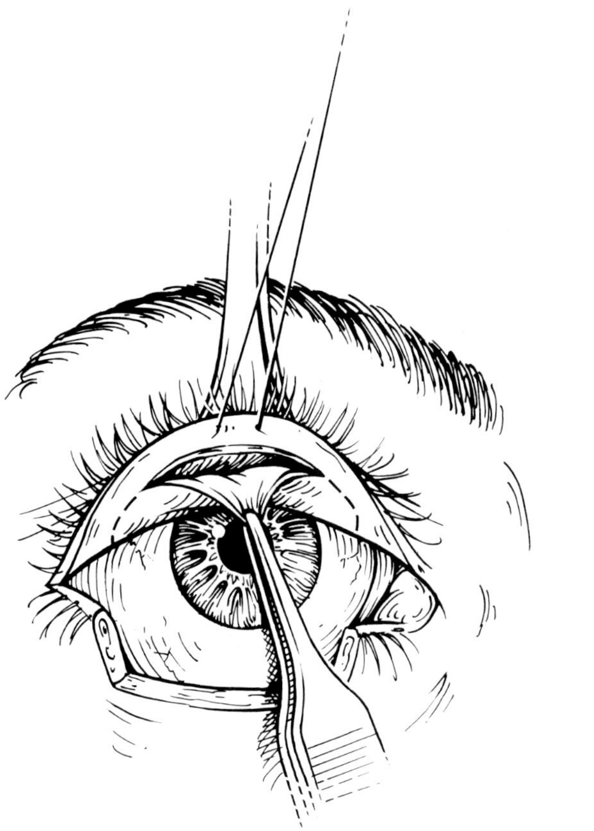

Figure 36–8. The tarsus is incised 4 mm above the lid margin with a no. 15 blade and dissected with scissors off the levator aponeurosis. (From McCord CD, Nunery WR: Reconstruction of the lower eyelid and outer canthus. *In* McCord C, Tanenbaum M [eds]: Oculoplastic Surgery, 2nd ed. New York, Raven Press, 1987, p 101.)

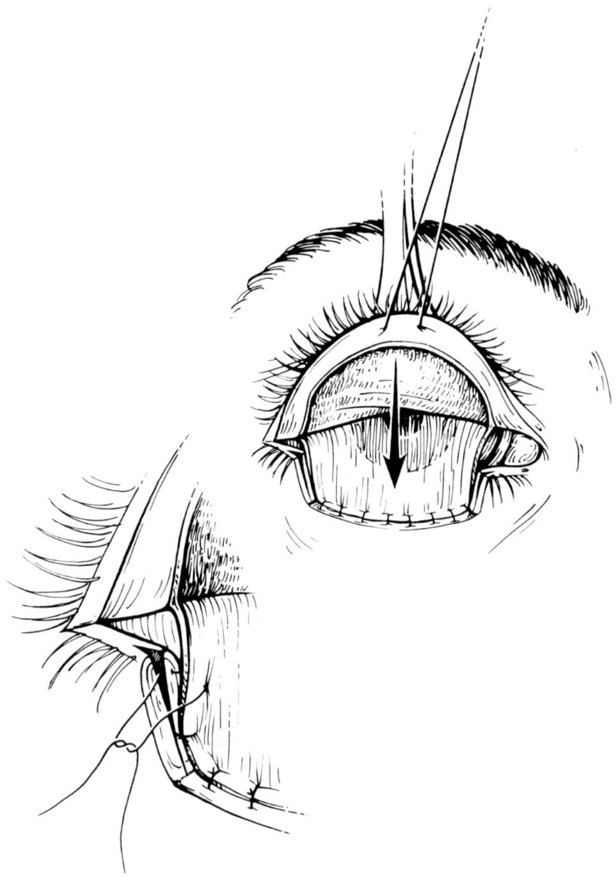

Figure 36–9. The flap is mobilized inferiorly and sewn to the remnant eyelid margins with 5-0 polyglactin sutures. (From McCord CD, Nunery WR: Reconstruction of the lower eyelid and outer canthus. *In* McCord C, Tanenbaum M [eds]: Oculoplastic Surgery, 2nd ed. New York, Raven Press, 1987, p 102.)

the flap can be sewn to the lateral periosteum or the rim with the aid of drill holes.

Once the posterior lamella has been reconstructed, the anterior lamella needs to be attended to. This can be covered by a sliding myocutaneous flap (modified Tenzel flap), a rotated myocutaneous flap (Trepier) from the upper eyelid, an advanced cheek flap, or a free skin graft.

Closure is done with a sliding myocutaneous flap, which is basically a modified Tenzel flap. The flap is designed as previously described, beginning at the lateral canthus. The tissues are undermined and advanced, trimmed appropriately, and sewn to the remnant eyelid and to the tarsoconjunctival flap.

A rotated myocutaneous flap or Trepier flap is an excellent alternative for reconstructing the anterior lamella with a lateral eyelid defect when adequate upper eyelid skin is present. A pedicle flap is marked out in the upper eyelid with its base laterally (Fig. 36–10). The flap should at least measure 8 mm in width to ensure viability. The lateral aspect of the incision should flare out for an adequate blood supply. The length of the pedicle flap should correspond to the defect.

The flap is incised with a no. 15 blade and undermined to include orbicularis. It is then rotated inferiorly, trimmed distally, and sewn to the remnant eyelid medially and inferiorly and to the tarsoconjunctival flap superiorly (Fig. 36–11). The upper eyelid defect is then closed as one would a blepharoplasty.

This type of reconstruction, like the sliding myocutaneous flap, rebuilds the lower eyelid with viable flaps from

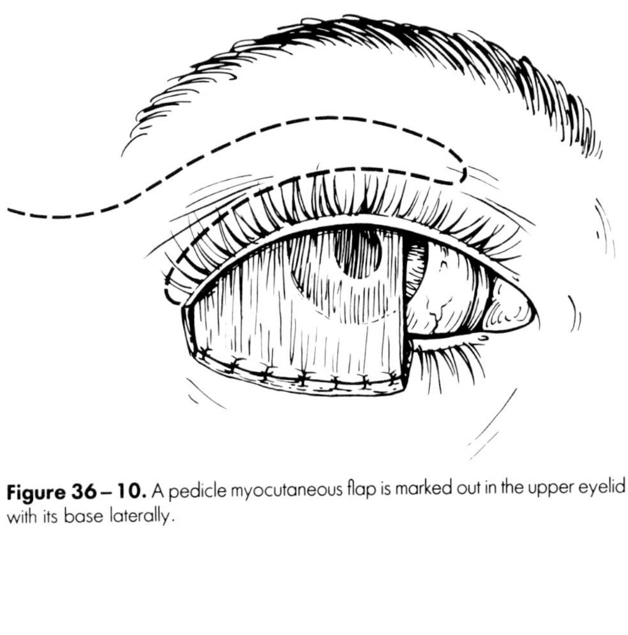

Figure 36–10. A pedicle myocutaneous flap is marked out in the upper eyelid with its base laterally.

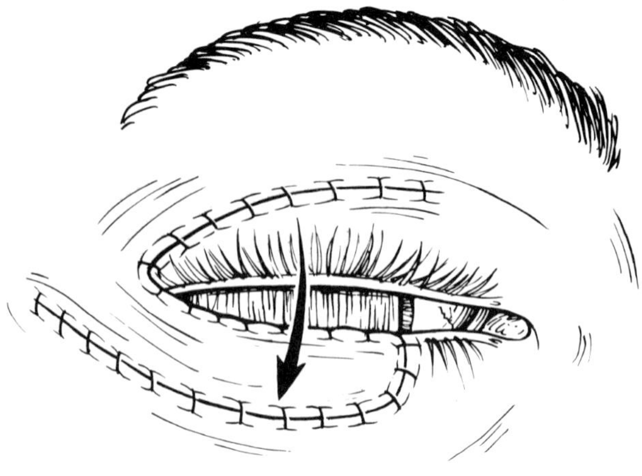

Figure 36–11. The flap is incised and undermined to include the orbicularis. It is rotated inferiorly, trimmed distally, and sewn to the remnant eyelid medially and inferiorly, and to the tarsoconjunctival flap superiorly.

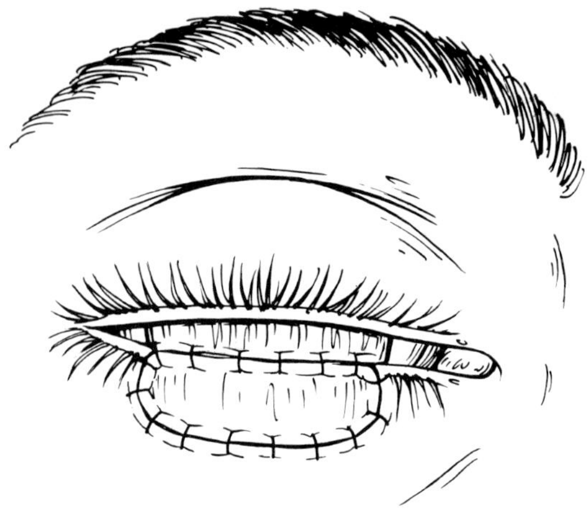

Figure 36–13. A full-thickness skin graft is harvested and sewn to the tarsoconjunctival flap and to the remnant eyelid tissues.

two separate blood supplies, giving a superb reconstructed eyelid with adequate bulk, contour, and function.

For shallow defects of the anterior lamella of the lower eyelid, the cheek skin inferiorly can be advanced superiorly and sewn to the tarsoconjunctival flap (Fig. 36–12). Small dog-ears usually need to be trimmed medially and laterally.

A free skin graft can also be placed over the tarsoconjunctival graft. If a free skin graft is desired, Müller's muscle should be included in the tarsoconjunctival graft to ensure an adequate blood supply. The graft can be taken from the upper eyelids, the postauricular or preauricular areas, or the supraclavicular area. After the graft is harvested, defatted, and trimmed, it is sewn to the tarsoconjunctival flap and remnant eyelid tissues (Fig. 36–13). A bolster can be oversewn or, alternatively, a

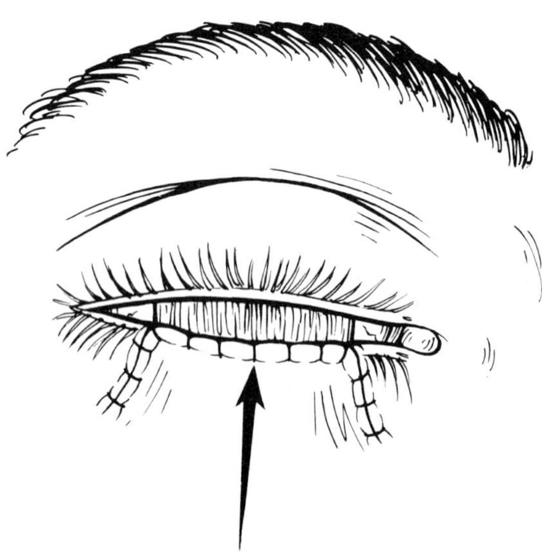

Figure 36–12. The cheek skin can be advanced superiorly and sewn to the tarsoconjunctival flap.

pressure patch applied to the orbit and left in place for 1 week.

SEVERING THE HUGHES FLAP

The Hughes flap can be separated 2 to 3 weeks after the initial surgery. This can usually be performed in an office setting with the use of local anesthesia. Topical tetracycline is placed on the tarsoconjunctival flap surface. The flap and lower eyelid are injected with 1% lidocaine with epinephrine. The tarsoconjunctival flap is elevated off the cornea, and one arm of a straight Stevens scissors is placed underneath the flap close to the under surface of the upper eyelid (Fig. 36–14). The flap is incised and allowed to retract superiorly. If there is any upper eyelid retraction, a dissection is carried out between Müller's muscle and the levator aponeurosis into the superior fornix. Usually, if a thin tarsoconjunctival flap has been previously performed without including Müller's muscle, this will be unnecessary. An incision is made along the new lower eyelid margin, and the conjunctiva is sewn to it with running 6-0 plain gut sutures (Fig. 36–15).

MUSTARDÉ FLAP

When closure of the eyelids is not desirable, large defects (greater than 80% of the lower eyelid) can be closed with a cheek rotation flap. Reconstruction of the full-thickness defect will require a graft of the posterior lamella composed either of hard palate, ear cartilage, or nasoseptal cartilage. Either of these grafts can be sewn to the remnant eyelid with 5-0 polyglactin sutures. Laterally, the graft is sewn to the periosteum. If the periosteum has been removed with the tumor, the rim can be drilled with two small holes or a small mini-plate can be placed to sew into.

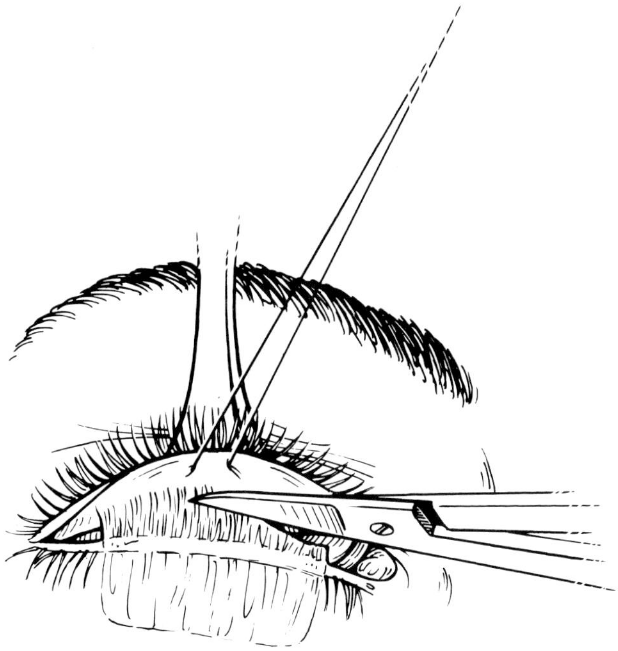

Figure 36–14. The tarsoconjunctival flap is elevated off the cornea and one arm of a straight Stevens scissors is placed underneath the flap close to the undersurface of the upper eyelid. The flap is incised and allowed to retract superiorly. (From McCord CD, Nunery WR: Reconstruction of the lower eyelid and outer canthus. *In* McCord C, Tanenbaum M [eds]: Oculoplastic Surgery, 2nd ed. New York, Raven Press, 1987, p 103.)

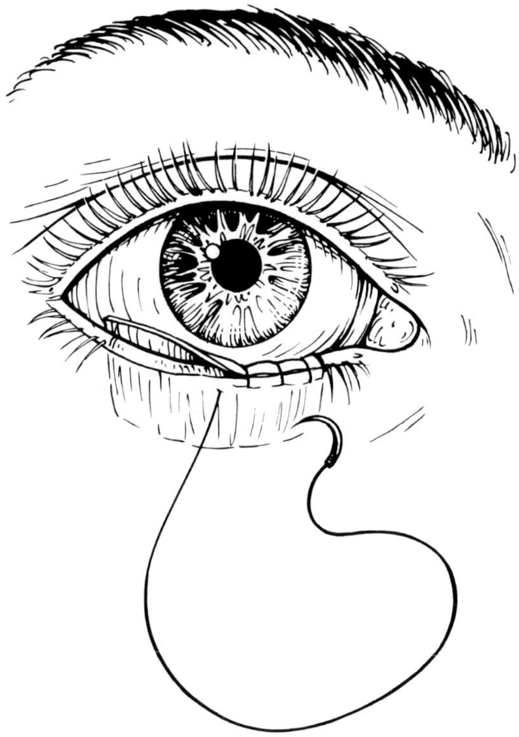

Figure 36–15. An incision is made along the new lower eyelid margin, and the conjunctiva is sewn to it with running 6-0 plain gut suture. (From McCord CD, Nunery WR: Reconstruction of the lower eyelid and outer canthus. *In* McCord C, Tanenbaum M [eds]: Oculoplastic Surgery, 2nd ed. New York, Raven Press, 1987, p 103.)

The cheek rotation flap is designed initially like a Tenzel flap, directed superiorly and laterally from the lateral canthal angle. The curve of the incision is somewhat flatter superiorly so it can continue laterally to the preauricular region. The flap is incised in a similar fashion to the Tenzel flap adjacent to the lateral canthus. A thicker skin–muscle flap is desirable in the first 2 to 2.5 cm of the incision to give the newly reconstructed eyelid more bulk and tone. Then the dissection becomes more purely subcutaneous and proceeds in a face-lift plane to the preauricular region (Fig. 36–16).

The flap is dissected as far as necessary to rotate the skin into the defect medially without tension. The flap is sewn to the remnant, eyelid, and cheek, and the lid marginal graft is sewn to the flap with 6-0 plain gut. The myocutaneous portion of the flap adjacent to the lateral canthus needs to be fixated to the orbital rim to help support the flap and the lateral canthal angle. The rest of the flap is then closed. Often a large dog-ear will remain inferiorly. This can be trimmed initially or left for any revision surgery planned thereafter.

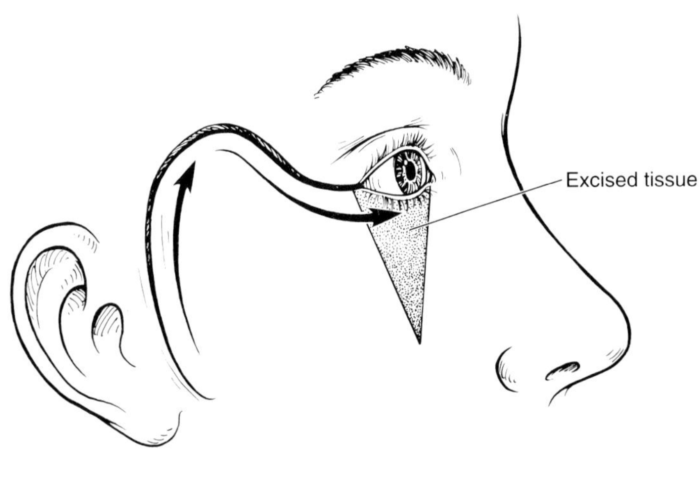

Figure 36–16. A thicker skin muscle flap is desirable in the first 2 to 2.5 cm of the incision to give the newly reconstructed eyelid more bulk and tone. Then the dissection becomes more purely subcutaneous as it proceeds in a face-lift plane to the preauricular region. (From McCord CD, Nunery WR: Reconstruction of the lower eyelid and outer canthus. *In* McCord C, Tanenbaum M [eds]: Oculoplastic Surgery, 2nd ed. New York, Raven Press, 1987, p 106.)

LOWER EYELID DEFECTS INVOLVING THE CANALICULUS

When the defect in the lower eyelid margin involves the canaliculus, reconstruction is recommended. Defects involving 100% of the upper and lower systems may be left and repaired secondarily with a Jones tube. If the distal canaliculus is obvious in the field, a stent of some type should be placed. If the distal canaliculus is not apparent, the upper puncta should be dilated and injected with 2% viscous lidocaine mixed with methylene blue. Often the distal remnant of the canaliculus will be revealed by this method. The operative microscope may be used if desired. If there is no reflux of material inferiorly, a pigtail probe may be rotated through the upper canaliculus. Lastly, sharp dissection more medially may reveal the remnant canaliculus.

Once the canaliculus has been identified, it can be intubated. A Long tube is a monocanalicular stent that can be directly placed in the canaliculus and sewn in place. A more secure stent requires bicanalicular intubation. Crawford tubes allow easy retrieval of the probes from the nose under the inferior turbinate. After retrieval the tubes are tied in a square knot and sewn to the external nasal vestibule with a 5-0 polyglactin suture and left in place for 4 to 6 weeks.

CHAPTER 37

Congenital Eyelid Anomalies

Jill A. Foster and James A. Katowitz

Because of the complexity and number of fetal growth plates in the developing face, many congenital developmental anomalies manifest in the eyes and periocular tissue. Aberrations in the orderly progression of eyelid development result in a spectrum of abnormalities.

EMBRYOLOGIC AND FETAL DEVELOPMENT OF THE EYELIDS

Eyelid folds are first identified in the seventh week of gestation.[1] During the following 2 weeks of development, the eyelid folds meet and fuse. Ectoderm on the external aspect of the lid differentiates into epithelium, while the internal pouch of ectoderm becomes conjunctiva and lacrimal secretory glands. At the junction of the lid folds, ectoderm invaginates and differentiates into meibomian glands, cilia, the glands of Zeis, and the glands of Moll. The core of mesoderm within the lid fold develops into the tarsal plate and muscles of the eyelids. The lid folds separate again in the 21st to 26th week of gestation.[2] Patterns of disruption may occur at any point along the developmental sequence.

CONGENITAL ANOMALIES

Cryptophthalmos

In cryptophthalmos, the epithelium covering the forehead passes continuously over the globe down to the cheek with complete or partial absence of the lid margin structures (Fig. 37-1). The eyebrow may be absent or temporally displaced with hair extending from the anterior hairline toward the lateral orbital margin. Although cryptophthalmos may occur as an isolated periocular finding, the condition is more often associated with other anomalies, including syndactyly, abnormal genitalia, laryngeal malformation, skeletal defects, umbilical hernia, renal agenesis, cleft lip and palate, and malformations of the nose and ears.[3, 4] The pathogenesis of cryptophthalmos is unknown, but with a predominance of bilateral cases and a familiar pattern, a genetic cause is suspect. Intrauterine infections and amniotic bands have been proposed[4] but seem less likely. Histologically, the exposed corneal tissue shows abnormal thickening of the epithelium and surface keratinization. Structures attributable to the lid folds are absent or rudimentary, suggesting that the error in development occurs during initial formation of the lid folds. Intraocular anomalies may also be present.

The surgical rehabilitation of cryptophthalmos is a challenging endeavor. With an absence of functioning lids, it is difficult to perform successful corneal transplantation even in those eyes that are otherwise normal. The prognosis for visual rehabilitation is poor, but reconstructive techniques may improve the eyelid appearance and function (see Fig. 37-1*B*). Surgical repair is done in stages beginning with separation of the lid and globe, relining the lid,[5] progressing to contouring and reconstructing the eyelid, followed by hair transplantation to the brow and lid. Mucous membrane grafts can be used to line the inner aspect of the epithelial surface, but creating a surgical space between the epithelium and the anterior chamber is often difficult. The surgeon should be prepared for corneal repair and patch grafting. Hard palate mucosa,[6] ear cartilage,[7, 8] or contralateral tarsus and conjunctiva[9] can be grafted to replace the missing tarsal elements, and hair transplantation techniques can be used to re-form the eyebrows (see Fig. 37-1*C*).

Congenital Coloboma

Coloboma can be simply defined as a "missing part in the lid." The spectrum of the congenital disorder varies from a small lid notch to almost complete absence of the lid. The defect is typically triangular, with the apex of the triangle away from the lid margin (Fig. 37-2). The most common locations are in the medial or central upper lid and the temporal lower lid.[10] In congenital coloboma there is a full-thickness absence of tissue, and the surrounding adnexal structures may be abnormal. The edges of coloboma are rounded. Colobomas may be seen in isolation or as part of Goldenhar's syndrome. Other

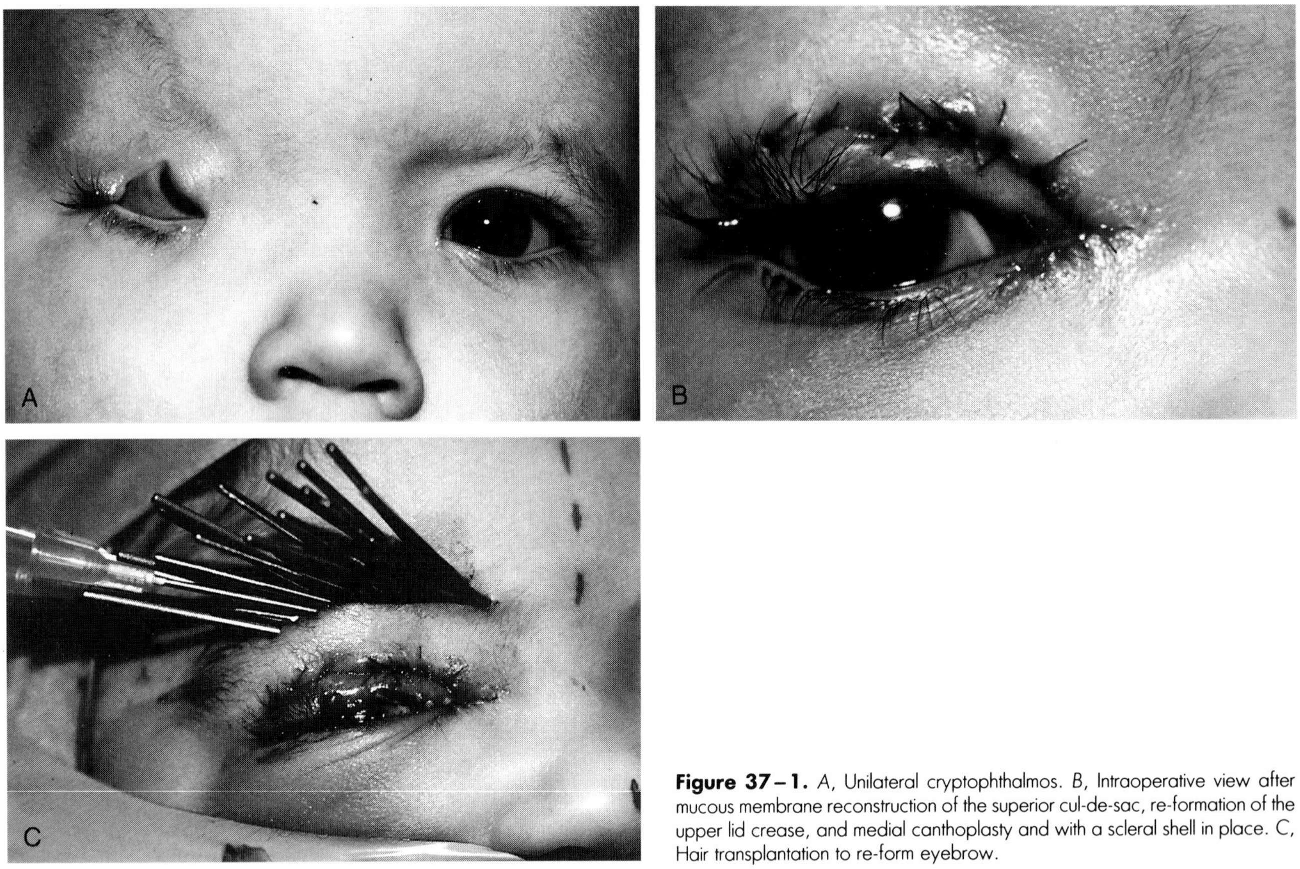

Figure 37–1. *A*, Unilateral cryptophthalmos. *B*, Intraoperative view after mucous membrane reconstruction of the superior cul-de-sac, re-formation of the upper lid crease, and medial canthoplasty and with a scleral shell in place. *C*, Hair transplantation to re-form eyebrow.

features of Goldenhar's syndrome include preauricular tags, dermatolipoma, limbal dermoid, hearing defects, and vertebral anomalies.[11]

Congenital colobomas are created by multiple mechanisms of developmental error. When seen in conjunction with digit amputations and other features of amniotic band syndrome, the coloboma is likely to result from a mechanical pressure effect of the amniotic band on the fetal eyelid. An alternative mechanism occurs when there is absence of fusion between contiguous tissue (in this

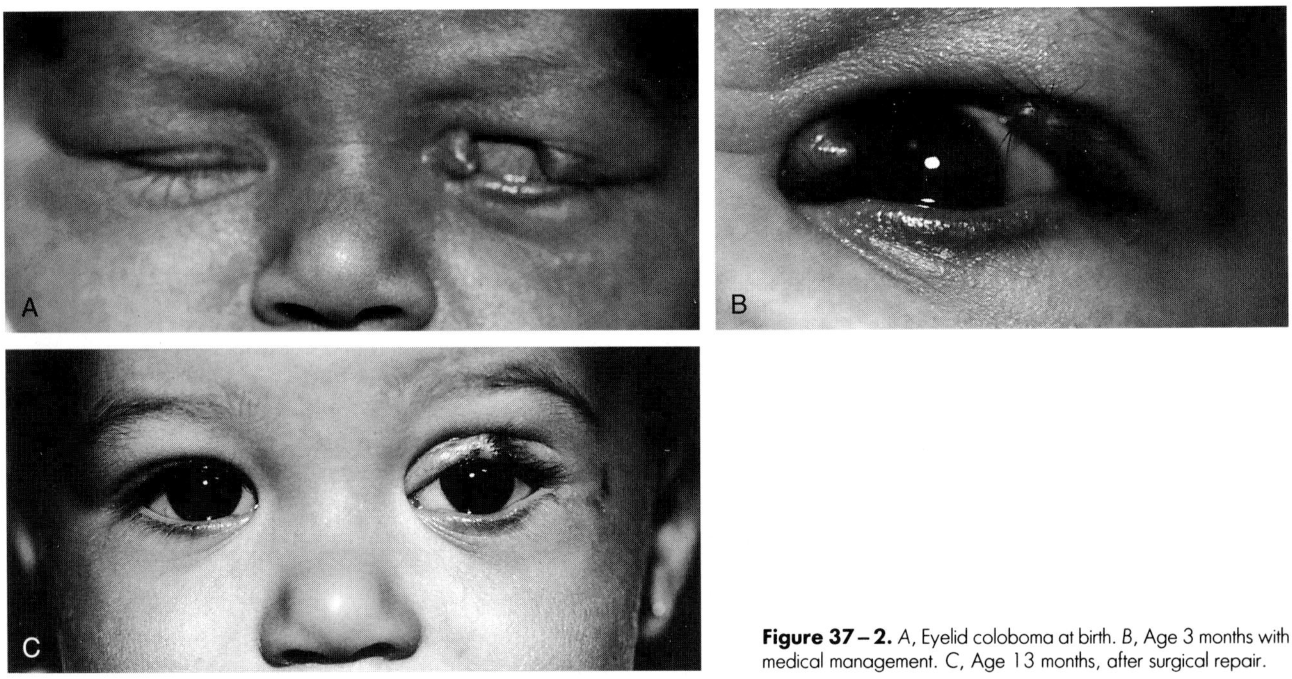

Figure 37–2. *A*, Eyelid coloboma at birth. *B*, Age 3 months with medical management. *C*, Age 13 months, after surgical repair.

case, the embryonic lid folds). In a third mechanism, mesoderm fails to advance and fill the lid fold, resulting in collapse of the intervening ectoderm.

Colobomas are initially managed with lubrication and corneal protection. If the corneal epithelium becomes irregular, or alternatively when the lids enlarge for easier flap formation (6 to 12 months of age), the coloboma is repaired. The usual techniques for eyelid margin defects are employed, but smaller percentage defects require more extensive lid modifications in children than would be necessary in adults. Small colobomas (<25% of the lid margin) may be closed primarily by creating pentagonal or triangular defects through excision of the coloboma's margins. The tarsus is closed with 7-0 Vicryl, and the lid margin is closed in a two- or three-layer fashion with 6-0 Vicryl. The 6-0 Vicryl sutures are passed from gray line to gray line, lash line to lash line, and, if possible, from mucocutaneous junction to mucocutaneous junction. The orbicularis and skin incision are also closed with 6-0 Vicryl. Larger defects (25% to 40%) may require additional horizontal laxity, which can be created with a lateral canthotomy and cantholysis or extension of the lateral canthal incision into a semicircular flap. Larger defects (>40%) may require creative flap techniques or tissue expansion.[12, 13] When possible, lid-sharing procedures are avoided in the amblyogenic age group.

When a coloboma is repaired in the upper lid, horizontal shortening may create a vertical ptosis. Advancement of the levator muscle may be necessary in conjunction with the coloboma repair.

Ankyloblepharon

In ankyloblepharon, the fused eyelid folds fail to separate. The condition may be complete, partial, or interrupted, as in ankyloblepharon filiforme. These epithelial attachments can be separated by positioning a groove director between the lid and the globe and cutting the adhesions. In cases of complete ankyloblepharon, the conjunctiva should be advanced and sutured over the lid margins to prevent reattachment of de-epithelialized surfaces.

Distichiasis

Congenital distichiasis (Fig. 37–3) occurs with an error in development along the eyelid margin; accessory cilia differentiate near and in the meibomian orifices. This results in a second and more posterior row of lashes that develops along the eyelid margin. If this more posterior row of lashes comes into contact with the cornea, epiphora, discharge, and ocular irritation may result. When corneal epithelial defects are present, the lashes may be removed with electrolysis, cryotherapy, or lid-splitting procedures.[14]

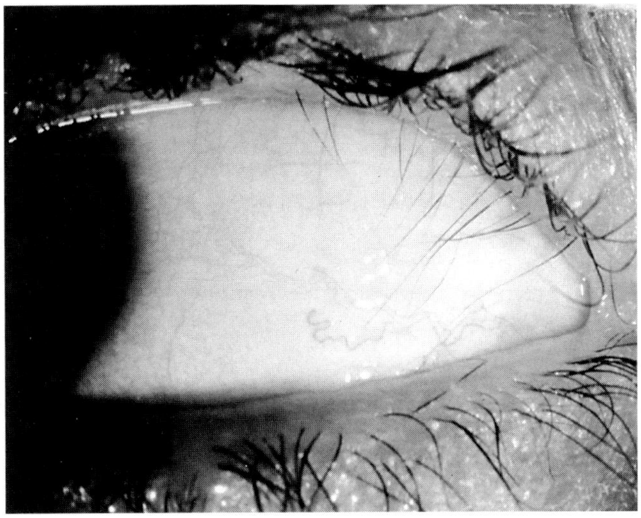

Figure 37–3. Distichiasis.

Congenital Entropion

In congenital entropion there is an inward rotation of the entire eyelid margin.[15] Entropion should be differentiated from epiblepharon, a more common condition in which there is an abnormal fold of tissue in the lower lid, sometimes pushing the lid margin toward the globe. Some of the same pathologic mechanisms associated with senile entropion are also associated with congenital entropion: defects in the lower lid retractors, hypertrophy of the preseptal orbicularis, and tarsal abnormalities.

When the lid position creates epithelial defects that are not controlled with lubrication, surgical intervention is necessary (Fig. 37–4). In milder cases, the eyelid margin can be everted by removing a base-out wedge of skin and orbicularis and by closing the wound with a suture technique that brings the lower lid retractors into attachment up with the inferior tarsal plate. Absorbable suture such as 6-0 Vicryl is used for this technique. Occasionally, tarsal modification or grafting may be necessary to evert the lid.

Epiblepharon

In congenital epiblepharon, an abnormal lid fold in the lower lid creates a mechanical force that rolls the lid margin in toward the globe. This can be mistaken for entropion. However, unlike entropion, downward force placed on the fold will return the lid margin to normal position. Epiblepharon may resolve without treatment as facial development expands the nasal bridge and midface. The pathogenesis of the abnormal fold may be a relative hypoplasia of the nasal bridge compared with the lids or an absence of the connective tissues between the capsulopalpebral fascia and the skin, allowing preseptal orbicularis to override pretarsal orbicularis. Epibleph-

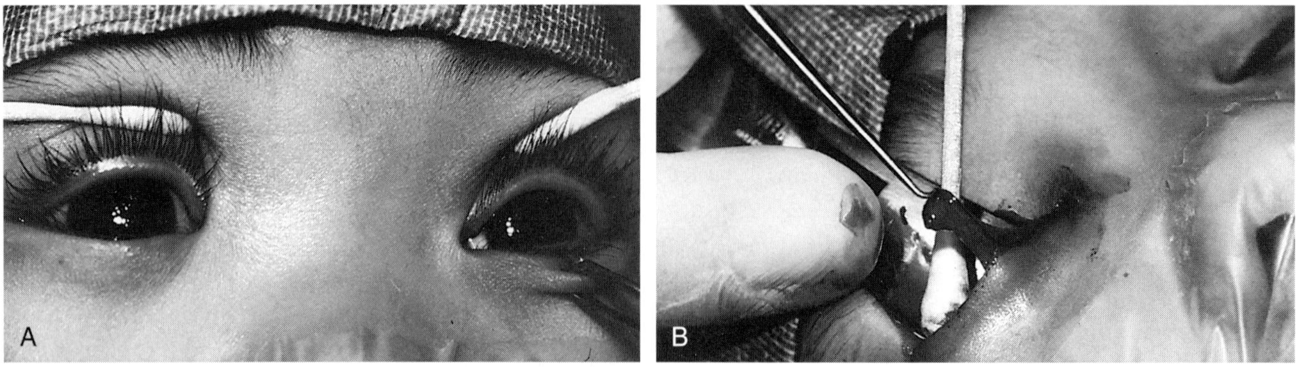

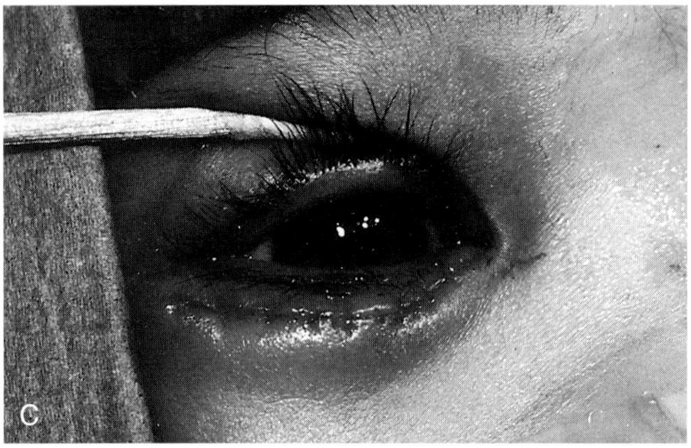

Figure 37–4. *A*, Congenital entropion. *B*, Excision of a wedge of skin and orbicularis. *C*, Postoperative appearance.

aron tends to be more prominent medially. If the epiblepharon becomes symptomatic, it is managed with the same surgical techniques used in entropion.

Congenital Ectropion

Congenital ectropion is an unusual condition in which the eyelid is rotated away from the globe (Fig. 37–5). It may occur in the upper or lower lid and is seen in association with Down syndrome and congenital eyelid syndrome. Acquired ectropion may occur on a congenital basis when tumor or congenital glaucoma has resulted in distortion of the lid.

As with entropion, the initial treatment for ectropion is lubrication. Lubrication must be monitored in the infant because unilateral visual obstruction creates a risk for amblyopia. When corneal exposure necessitates surgical repair, horizontal tightening may be performed with a lateral tarsal strip technique.[16] In children, it is usually not necessary to excise excess tissue as might commonly be the case in senile ectropion. The tarsal plate is cleared of anterior epithelium and posterior conjunctiva and may be sutured to the lateral orbital rim periosteum using 6-0 Prolene, 5-0 Mersilene, or 4-0 Vicryl.

The differential diagnosis for congenital ectropion includes acquired lid eversion due to infection or an inflammatory process. Diagnostic stains of the conjunctiva will show the infectious agent. Appropriate antibiotic therapy will reverse the process.

Epicanthal Folds

Epicanthal folds are semilunar folds that contour the lids in the medial canthal region. These folds can be seen as an isolated finding, associated with other anomalies as

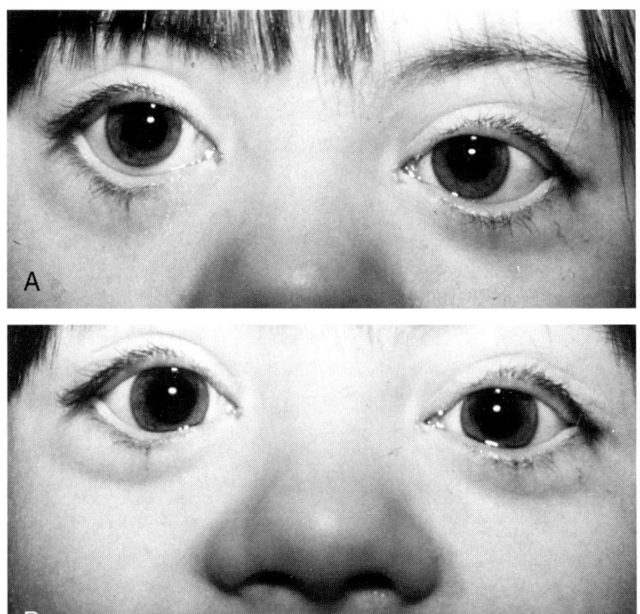

Figure 37–5. *A*, Congenital ectropion. *B*, Postoperative view after lateral tarsal strip procedure on both lower eyelids. (*A* and *B* courtesy of Michael Kazim.)

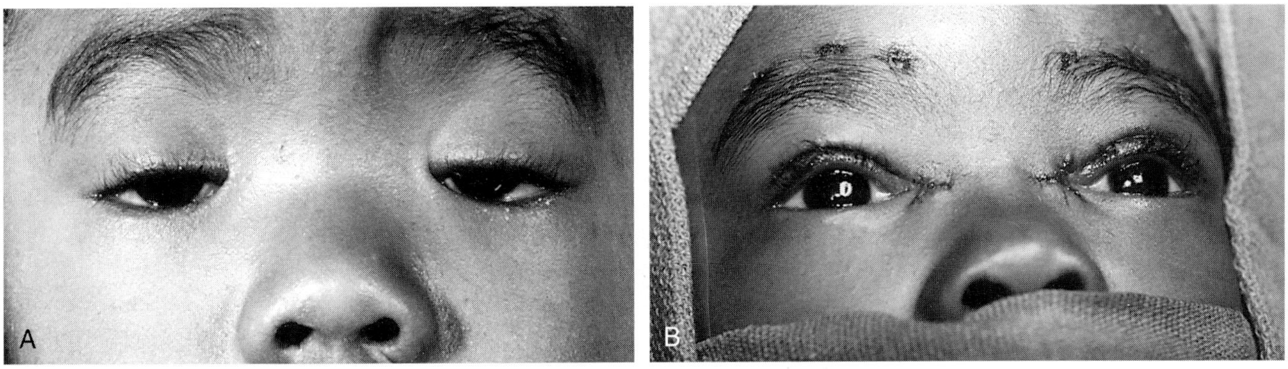

Figure 37-6. *A*, Congenital eyelid syndrome. *B*, Intraoperative appearance after frontalis suspension, medial canthoplasty, and lid crease re-formation.

part of a syndrome, as racial variation, or as part of normal development before expansion of the midface. The folds can be identified and categorized by anatomic location.[17] In epicanthus inversus the fold extends from the lower lid up through the medial canthus partially covering the inner canthal angle. This configuration is rarely a normal finding and is associated with Down syndrome and blepharophimosis syndrome. In epicanthus palpebralis, the fold extends from the tarsal region of the upper lid toward the lid margin of the lower lid. This type of fold tends to become less apparent with age as the nasal bridge enlarges relative to the rest of the face. Epicanthus tarsalis, a normal eyelid configuration in Asians, has a fold that extends from the pretarsal area of the upper lid into the medial canthal region. The fourth category of epicanthal fold is epicanthus supraciliaris. The fold comes from the eyebrow area to skin overlying the lacrimal sac.

Epicanthal folds are usually only significant to appearance, but in extreme cases they may block the horizontal visual field. When surgery is indicated for appearance or function, there are several techniques for modifying epicanthal folds.[18, 19] All variations in technique include flattening the epicanthal folds, pulling the medial canthi in toward the nose, and removing excess tissue.

Blepharophimosis Syndrome (Congenital Eyelid Syndrome)

In congenital eyelid syndrome there is a constellation of associated periocular anomalies inherited in an autosomal dominant fashion.[11, 20] Characteristics include blepharophimosis (a shortening of the eyelids in all directions), ptosis, telecanthus, and epicanthus inversus. Hypoplasia of the inferior orbital rim and lower lid ectropion may also be seen. Reconstruction of the lid anomalies may be attempted in one surgical procedure (Fig. 37-6) or may be planned in a staged fashion. This surgical reconstruction typically includes ptosis repair and modification of the telecanthus. Poor levator function is common, and frontalis suspension is often necessary for adequate ptosis repair. Various techniques may be employed in the alteration of the epicanthal folds, including V-Y plasty, Mustardé jumping-man, Roveda, and Del Campo techniques.

Congenital Lid Retraction

Upper lid retraction (Fig. 37-7) in an alert infant is not always a pathologic finding, but thyroid dysfunction and hydrocephalus should be considered in the differential diagnosis.[21] Significant corneal exposure or cosmetic defect may warrant surgical intervention. Options include internal müllerectomy, levator recession, or spacer grafts.

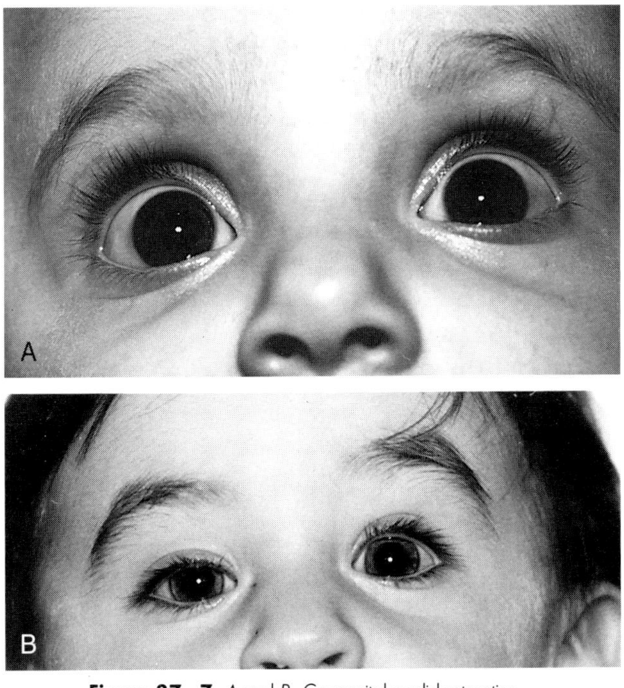

Figure 37-7. *A* and *B*, Congenital eyelid retraction.

REFERENCES

1. Arey LB: Developmental Anatomy: Textbook and Laboratory Manual of Embryology. Philadelphia, WB Saunders, 1974.
2. Duerkesen KM, Barlow WE, Stasior OG: Fused eyelids in premature infants. Abstract presented before the ASOPRS Meeting, Chicago, 1993.
3. Thomas IT, Frias JL, Felix V, et al: Isolated and syndromic cryptophthalmos. Am J Med Genet 25:85–98, 1986.
4. Duke-Elder S: System of Ophthalmology, Vol 3, Normal and Abnormal Development, Part 2, Congenital Deformities. St. Louis, CV Mosby, 1963.
5. Putterman AM, Karesh JW: A surgical technique for the successful and stable reconstruction of the totally contracted ocular socket. Ophthalmic Surg 19:193–201, 1988.
6. Kersten RC, Kulwin DR, Levartovsky S, et al: Management of lower-lid retraction with hard-palate mucosa grafting. Arch Ophthalmol 108:1339–1343, 1990.
7. Smith B, Lisman R: Preparation of full-thickness auricular cartilage for use in oculoplastic surgery. Ophthalmic Surg 13:1018–1021, 1982.
8. Markowitz GD, Wulc AE, Perman KI, Popp JC: Monopolar cautery for graft cartilage sculpting in reconstructive eyelid surgery. Ophthalmic Surg 23:489–506, 1992.
9. Stephenson CM, Brown BZ: The use of tarsus as a free autogenous graft in eyelid surgery. Ophthal Plast Reconstr Surg 1:43–50, 1985.
10. Tessier P, Hervouet F, Lekieffre M, et al: Plastic Surgery of the Orbit and Eyelids. Chicago, Year Book Medical Publishers, 1977.
11. Goodman RM, Gorlin RJ: The Malformed Infant and Child. New York, Oxford University Press, 1983.
12. Toth BA, Glafkides MC, Wandel A: The role of tissue expansion in the treatment of atypical facial clefting. Plast Reconst Surg 86:119–122, 1990.
13. Iwahira Y, Maruyama Y: Expanded preauricular full-thickness free skin graft. Plast Reconstr Surg 87:150–152, 1991.
14. Anderson RL, Harvey ST: Lid splitting and posterior lamellar cryosurgery for congenital and acquired dystichiasis. Arch Ophthalmol 99:631–634, 1991.
15. Fox SA: Primary congenital entropion. Arch Ophthalmol 56:839–842, 1956.
16. Anderson RL, Gordy DD: The tarsal strip procedure. Arch Ophthalmol 97:2192–2196, 1979.
17. Johnston CC: Epicanthus and epiblepharon. Arch Ophthalmol 96:1030–1033, 1975.
18. Callahan A: Surgical correction of blepharophimosis syndromes. Trans Am Acad Ophthalmol Otolaryngol 77:687–695, 1973.
19. Shore SW, Rubin PAD, Bilyk JR: Repair of telecanthus by anterior fixation of cantilevered miniplates. Ophthalmology 99:1133–1138, 1992.
20. Kohn R, Romano PE: Blepharoptosis, blepharophimosis, epicanthus inversus and telecanthus: A syndrome with no name. Am J Ophthalmol 72:625–632, 1971.
21. Lewis IC, MacGregor SG: Congenital hyperthyroidism. Lancet 272:14, 1957.

CHAPTER 38

Entropion

John A. Long and Robert Alan Goldberg

Entropion is the inward rotation of the eyelid margin, resulting in contact between the eyelashes and the cornea. This common malady has attracted the attention of surgeons over the centuries. Celsus, a first century surgeon, described removing a strip of skin from the lower eyelid in a logical attempt to evert the eyelid margin. Over 200 articles have been published describing the various techniques for entropion repair. In recent years, meticulous dissection of the lower eyelid and careful study of the pathophysiology of entropion have led to an anatomic basis for lower eyelid entropion and an anatomic basis for surgical repair.

Entropion of the eyelid can result from a number of diseases, but all share a fairly simple mechanical "final common pathway" related to the eyelid lamellae. The eyelids consist functionally of an anterior lamella (skin and orbicularis) and a posterior lamella (conjunctiva and tarsus) (Fig. 38–1). The first requirement for proper eyelid margin position is adequate horizontal tone. Particularly in the case of the lower eyelid, an analogy to a tennis net is appropriate: the net remains erect and straight because of its horizontal support at the net poles. If the supporting cable slackens, the net sags and is free to flop into one court or the other, depending on the wind. In the eyelid, that "wind" that determines which "court" the eyelid will flop into (entropion or ectropion) is the balance of forces between the anterior and posterior lamellae. Cicatrix of the posterior lamellae will scroll the eyelid inward, and relative shortening of the anterior lamellae will cause an outward rotation. Just as a tighter tennis net will better withstand windy conditions, a well-supported eyelid with adequate horizontal tone will be less subject to entropion or ectropion in the presence of an imbalance in the relationship of the anterior and posterior lamellae; thus, in the face of eyelid laxity, horizontal shortening is a common requirement for both entropion and ectropion surgery. Of course, severe cicatricial changes in the anterior or posterior lamellae will rotate the margin inward or outward regardless of the adequacy of horizontal support.

Assessment of eyelid tone (adequacy of horizontal support) is an important part of the evaluation of eyelid malposition. It is important to evaluate the relative contributions of eyelid laxity and mechanical changes in the anterior and posterior lamellae when designing a surgical approach to entropion in an individual patient.

Entropion may be categorized as four types: (1) congenital entropion, (2) cicatricial entropion, (3) spastic entropion, and (4) involutional entropion.

CONGENITAL ENTROPION

True congenital entropion is a very rare condition that is usually due to a dehisced lower eyelid retractor.[1] A more common variant of congenital entropion is epiblepharon. In patients with epiblepharon a fold of skin and orbicularis pushes lashes into contact with the cornea. Unlike congenital entropion, the eyelid margin remains in normal position and only the anterior lamella is found to be abnormal. This condition is most commonly seen in children of Asian ancestry and is usually asymptomatic. Epiblepharon usually spontaneously resolves with growth of the midface and nasal bridge. Occasionally, a child will experience persistent ocular irritation and epiphora caused by epiblepharon. Removing a strip of orbicularis and skin from the infraciliary region is the primary treatment. Rotation sutures that tack the orbicularis to the tarsal plate are a useful adjunct to skin and orbicularis excision.

Congenital distichiasis is another variant of congenital entropion. In this condition, abnormal lashes emerge from the meibomian gland orifices and are directed toward the cornea. The eyelid margin typically is in a normal position, and no other structural abnormalities are noted. This condition is often familial and can be treated with observation if asymptomatic. The surgical treatment of distichiasis is difficult. A variety of techniques have been described, including cryotherapy (with or without margin splitting), laser ablation of lashes, bloc excision of lashes, and tissue transplantation.[2] Each technique is moderately successful.

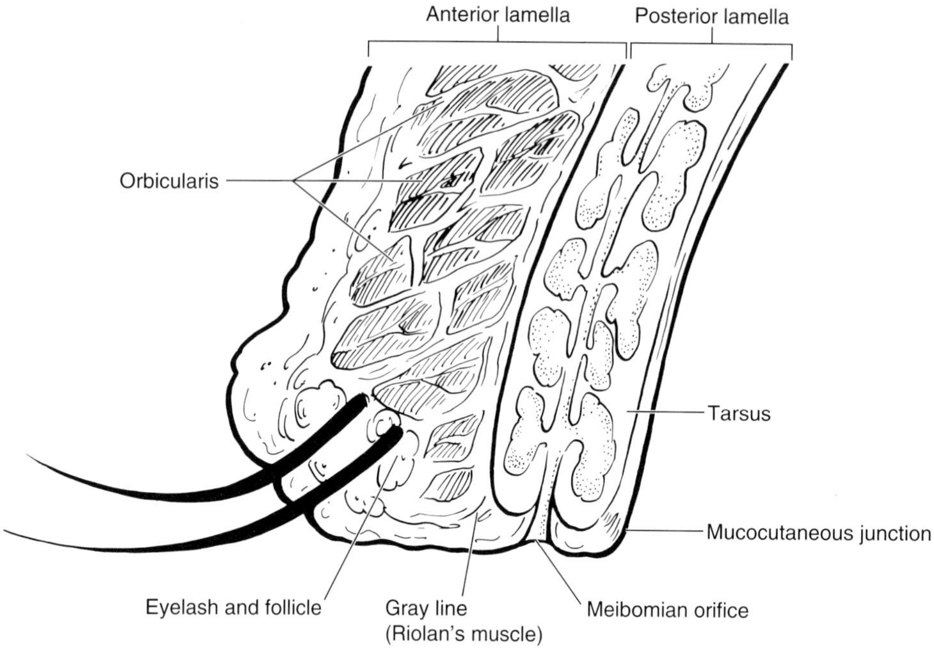

Figure 38–1. Normal eyelid anatomy: sagittal view. Anterior and posterior lamellae are in balance. Sharp, mucous membrane–covered eyelid margin functions as "windshield wiper" for corneal tear film.

CICATRICIAL ENTROPION

Cicatricial entropion is an acquired entropion caused by scarring of the inner eyelid. This condition is seen, for example, in Stevens-Johnson syndrome, ocular pemphigoid, and severe alkali burns. Mechanical shortening of the posterior lamella is the pathophysiologic basis for cicatricial entropion.

An irregularity of the position or tone of the eyelid margin may lead to imperfect spreading of the tear film and produce blurring of vision in a manner analogous to the distortion one notices when a notch forms in the windshield wiper of an automobile. Moreover, the imperfect spreading of the tear film may over time lead to embarrassment of the corneal epithelial surface, which depends on smooth spreading of the tear film for its health. More severe malpositions of the eyelid margin with inward rotation can result in posterior migration of the mucocutaneous junction with keratinized epithelium opposed to the corneal surface (Fig. 38–2). Careful examination of the eyelid margin under the slit lamp will identify the rough, nonwetting keratinized epithelium. Keratin is extremely irritating to the delicate corneal epithelium, and subtle changes in the margin that bring it into contact with the cornea can produce a severe symptomatic corneal surface abnormality, the etiology of which can elude the casual or unsophisticated observer of the eyelid margin. Most severe of all is inward rotation that brings the actual eyelashes into corneal contact. It is critical to recognize that inward rotation of the margin severe enough to cause trichiasis typically brings keratinized skin into corneal contact as well, because treatments that only remove the eyelashes will often leave the patient little better off; indeed, ablative therapies may cause additional scar tissue that will worsen posterior cicatrix and exacerbate keratin apposition. Rather, surgical therapy is directed toward lengthening the posterior lamella. Hard palate mucosal grafts have been found to be very useful as posterior lamellar eyelid extenders. The hard palate has a resilience similar to the tarsus and a surface lined with mucosa.

SPASTIC ENTROPION

Spastic entropion occurs with ocular inflammation, pain, and corneal infection. The orbicularis overrides the eyelid margin and inverts the eyelid margin, producing an entropion. Some structural instability of the lower eyelid usually exists before the development of spastic entropion. The treatment of spastic entropion is directed at removing the underlying cause.

INVOLUTIONAL ENTROPION

Involutional entropion is by far the most commonly encountered lower eyelid malposition.[3, 4] This condition is associated with increasing age and involutional eyelid changes. Four anatomic abnormalities are associated with the development of involutional entropion: (1) lower eyelid retractor disinsertion, (2) horizontal eyelid laxity, (3) overriding orbicularis, and (4) enophthalmos. With advancing age, the structural integrity of the lower eyelid begins to weaken. Any one of these underlying

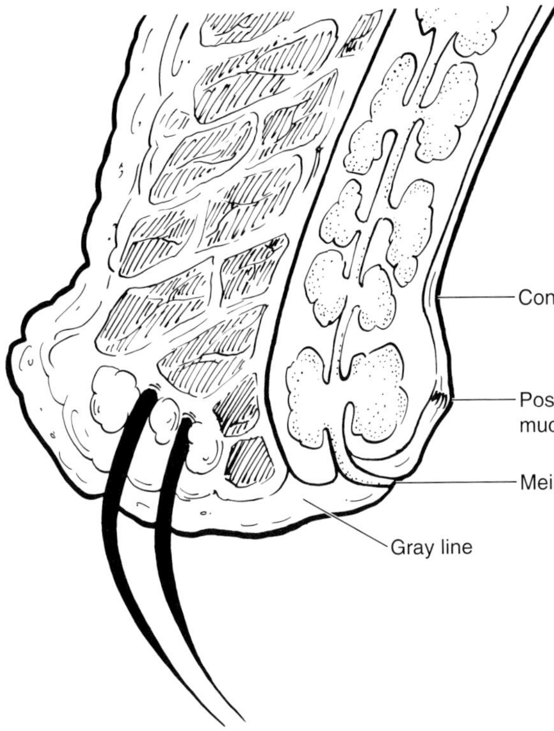

Figure 38–2. Eyelid anatomy: cicatricial entropion. Posterior lamellar contraction leads to posterior migration of the mucocutaneous junction. Keratinized epithelium comes into corneal contact. The eyelashes are rotated inward and may touch the corneal surface (trichiasis).

conditions, and, far more likely, a combination of factors, leads to involutional entropion.

Involutional entropion is an obvious clinical diagnosis, and careful examination of the eyelid will help in the understanding of the pathophysiology.

With dehiscence of the lower eyelid retractors, the attachment between the lower eyelid and inferior rectus is broken. Excursion of the lower eyelid is diminished, and a "lid lag" is noted in downward gaze. Examination of the inferior fornix may demonstrate a white band paralleling the eyelid margin. This is the edge of the dehisced lower eyelid retractor.

Horizontal eyelid laxity is demonstrated by the "snap test." The lid is distracted from the globe, and its ability to return to normal approximation of the globe is observed. With horizontal laxity of the lid, the "snap test" will demonstrate poor lid tone and an obvious slow return to its normal position.

Overriding orbicularis may be found by the "forced opening test." The upper lid is forced open while the patient actively contracts the muscle. An overriding orbicularis will force the lower eyelid margin inward.

Of the four recognized causes of involutional entropion, the correction of enophthalmos is the most problematic. With advancing age, or after orbital trauma, the connective tissue of the orbit may atrophy, leading to retroplacement of the globe. As the globe moves posteriorly away from the lower eyelid, the lid may become unstable. Replacing lost orbital volume is complicated and, in nontraumatic cases, usually not indicated.

SURGICAL APPROACH TO INVOLUTIONAL ENTROPION

With a thorough understanding of the pathophysiology of senile entropion, surgery is designed to address each of the underlying anatomic defects.[5] Combining previously described techniques into one operation allows the surgeon to reestablish the structure and function of the eyelid by correcting each of the pathophysiologic defects.

An infraciliary lid crease incision is created along the inferior border of the lower eyelid tarsus. A skin–muscle flap is directed toward the inferior orbital rim. The orbital septum is opened across the entire length of the lower eyelid, effectively separating the lid into an anterior and posterior lamella. Gentle displacement of the orbital fat will often demonstrate a dehisced lower eyelid retractor (Fig. 38–3).

Horizontal eyelid laxity is repaired with a lateral canthal tendon shortening procedure. Lower eyelid laxity is due to an elongation of the medial and lateral canthal tendons and not the tarsus itself. Lateral canthal tendon surgery avoids leaving sutures in the eyelid margin, which can be irritating and lead to lid margin notching (Fig. 38–4).

Once the lateral canthal tendon is secured to the inner aspect of the lateral orbital rim, the lower eyelid retractors are reattached to the inferior border of the tarsus (Fig. 38–5).

Overriding orbicularis is corrected by performing a

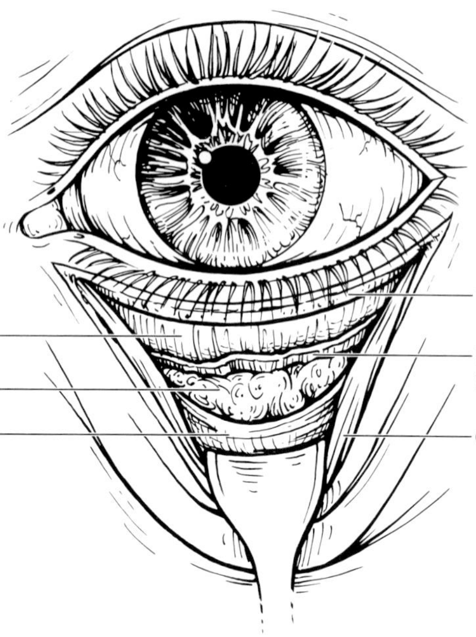

Figure 38–3. An infratarsal incision provides access to the lower eyelid retractors, which are identified as a white band closely applied to the conjunctiva. Typically in involutional entropion, a dehiscence of the lower eyelid retractors from the inferior tarsal edge can be identified.

marginal myectomy along the inferior border of the skin incision (Fig. 38–6). A strip of orbicularis is removed, which allows the lamella to form a scar adhesion to the tarsus. Once removed, the orbicularis can no longer override the eyelid margin. This procedure addresses each of the reparable causes of senile entropion.

An elegant option to a cutaneous approach is a conjunctival entropion approach described by Dresner and Karesh.[6] The surgical principles are as described earlier, but access to the lower eyelid retractors, pretarsal and preseptal orbicularis, and anterior tarsal surface is achieved through a conjunctival instead of a cutaneous incision. The conjunctival approach has the advantage of avoidance of a visible cutaneous incision and probably decreases the risk of lower eyelid retraction. Excess fat can be removed in direct transconjunctival fashion, with all of the advantages of transconjunctival lower blepharoplasty.

The combined entropion repair is extremely effective at repairing involutional entropion. Complications observed include a recurrence of the entropion, which is seen in about 1% of patients. Recurrence may be due to enophthalmos, which, as mentioned previously, is a difficult problem to treat.

Other complications include overcorrection of the entropion,[7] producing lower eyelid retraction and ectropion. In these cases, the orbital septum is usually incorporated into the lower eyelid retractor at the time of repair. The eyelid is pulled out of position by scarring and contraction of the orbital septum. Overcorrection resulting in eyelid retraction and ectropion is initially treated with gentle eyelid massage and observation. With time, the eyelid usually returns to a normal position. If conservative treatment fails, releasing the orbital septum from the surgical wound usually results in correction of the eyelid malposition.

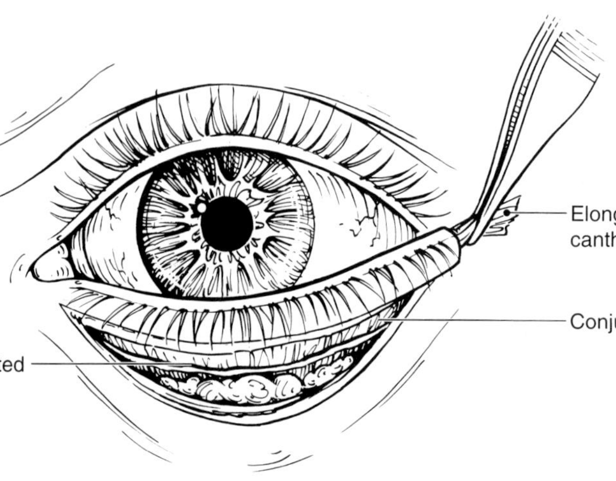

Figure 38–4. A lateral tarsal strip of 3 to 6 mm is created by disinserting the lateral canthal tendon from the lateral orbital rim and dissecting skin, eyelash-bearing margin, and conjunctiva from its stump. The tarsal strip is shortened as necessary to reestablish normal lower eyelid tone and is reattached to the internal aspect of the lateral orbital rim.

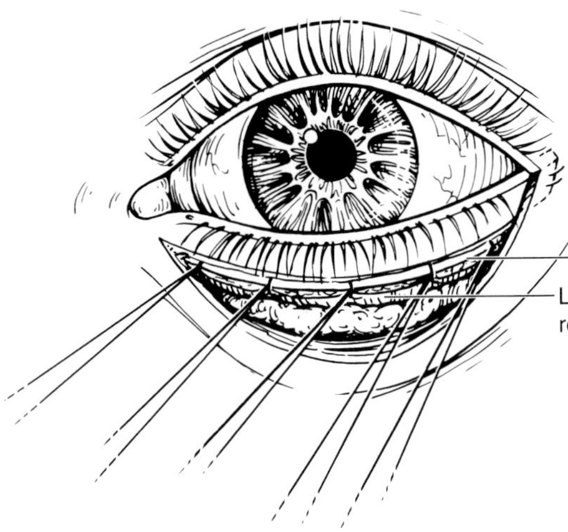

Figure 38–5. Absorbable sutures are used to advance the lower eyelid retractors onto the anterior tarsal surface; these sutures can be tied onto the tarsus or, for added rotation, brought out in mattress fashion through the skin in the region of the lower row of eyelashes to act as rotational sutures.

SURGICAL APPROACH TO CICATRICIAL ENTROPION

The primary treatment for advanced cases of cicatricial entropion with corneal epithelial damage is surgical repositioning of the eyelid margin. An important caveat relates to autoimmune progressive cicatricial disorders such as ocular cicatricial pemphigoid. There is always a danger, minimized but not eliminated by modern immunosuppressive management, that surgical intervention will "stir up" the underlying disease process, leading to worsening of the patient's overall condition.

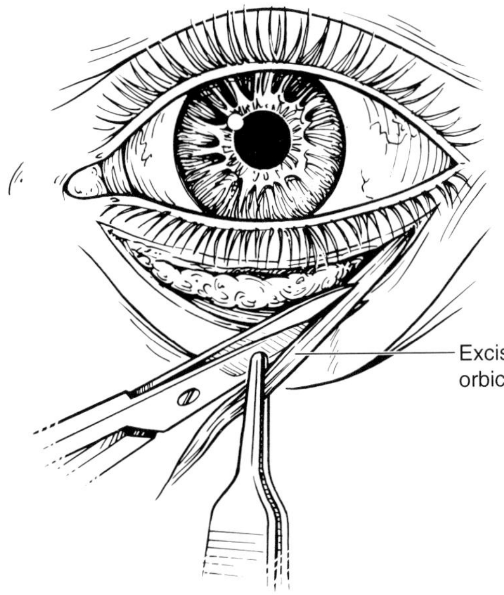

Figure 38–6. After the eyelid retractors have been reinserted and the shortened tarsal strip has been reattached to the lateral orbital rim, a strip of orbicularis is excised before closing the cutaneous wound.

In cases characterized by trichiasis without significant keratinized epithelium against the cornea, there may be a role for ablative therapies designed to destroy the hair follicles without damaging adjacent tissues. Because the hair follicles are more sensitive to freezing than the surrounding tissues, carefully applied cryotherapy to the eyelid margin can successfully ablate the aberrant eyelashes without damaging the eyelid margin.[2, 8–13] A double freeze-thaw technique with thermocouple monitoring to ensure adequate temperature (−15°C to −20°C) is recommended by most experts; a high-flow nitrous oxide probe more reliably achieves these temperatures in the eyelid than does the standard ophthalmic retinal cryoprobe. An alternative technique involves timed treatment of 45 seconds with a high-flow nitrous oxide probe instead of thermocouple monitoring.[14] Potential complications of cryotherapy[9, 14, 15] include depigmentation and scarring of the eyelid margin, in extreme cases to the point of full-thickness margin necrosis. As mentioned, cryotherapy can cause subtle worsening of posterior cicatrix, tipping a marginal case of keratinized skin entropion into corneal decompensation. Anderson and Harvey[2] observed improvement in keratinization after cryotherapy to the posterior lamella, but this has not been our experience.

Many procedures have been described over the years to rotate the margin of the eyelid away from the cornea. These various procedures can be broken down into two groups: (1) those that are characterized by "passive" rotation of the margin with tarsal fracturing, blepharotomy, rotational sutures, and other similar techniques with or without mucous membrane grafting,[16–25] and (2) those characterized by a "buttress" procedure in which some tarsal substitute is rotated, advanced, or grafted into position to reconstruct the eyelid margin.[26–30]

The passive procedures are generally easier and faster to perform but share in common a tendency for the outward rotation of the eyelid to regress over time due to second intention healing of the surgical wounds and in some cases to progression of the underlying disease. Mucous membrane grafts alone do not provide adequate reinforcement against recurrent inturning.

In our experience, "buttress" procedures in which the posterior lamella is reconstructed with a tarsal substitute have the highest likelihood of long-term success in the most severe cases.[29] A prospective study of 165 patients with trichiasis suggested that procedures that create a buttress against further rotation have an increased success rate.[31] Procedures that provide a buttress of the eyelid margin should be differentiated from procedures that lengthen the posterior lamella with a spacer but do not reconstruct the actual eyelid margin (Fig. 38–7).[20, 32–37] Posterior spacer procedures that do not reconstruct the eyelid margin may not have the same resistance to recurrent entropion, although these procedures are useful for less severe cases, particularly if keratinized epithelium is not rotated against the cornea.

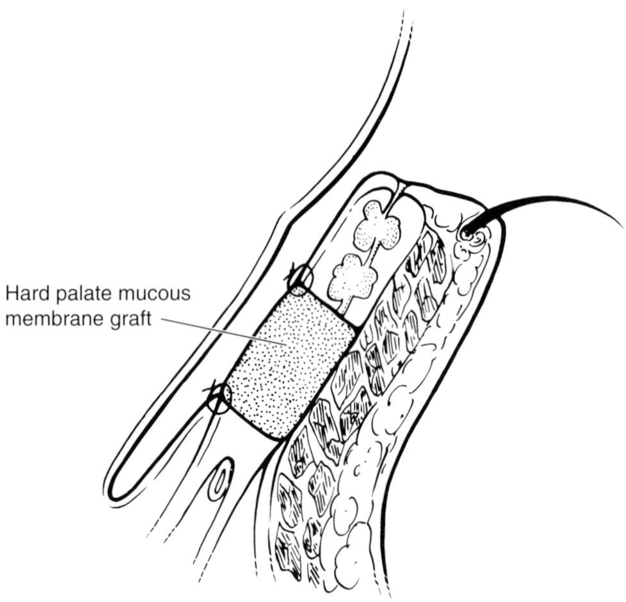

Figure 38–7. For less severe cases of cicatricial entropion, an interpositional graft of a tarsal substitute such as hard palate mucosal tissue can be used to lengthen the posterior lamella.

The primary tissue that has been used to reconstruct the eyelid margin has been tarsoconjunctiva. More recently, we have had excellent success using hard palate mucosa,[30] which has almost the same mechanical properties and resistance to shrinkage as tarsoconjunctiva and which has the additional advantages of abundant supply and the ability to harvest a piece of tissue of sufficient length to reconstruct, when necessary, the entire eyelid margin (Fig. 38–8).

Operative Technique

Local anesthesia of the eyelid is obtained with regional infiltration, and a greater palatine nerve block is performed by injecting 2 ml of 2% lidocaine with 1 : 100,000 epinephrine at the edge of the greater palatine foramen. We typically harvest the hard palate mucosal graft as a first step. Hard palate graft harvesting technique is reviewed in Chapter 40. The proposed graft is outlined with a scalpel incision in a tapered rectangular shape measuring approximately 8 by 30 mm. Less bleeding is encountered if the midline and high roof of the palate are avoided; we often take the graft 3 to 5 mm from the lateral gum line, paralleling the gum line. The graft is undermined with the scalpel or a sharp periosteal elevator and removed. It is not necessary to take a deep plane on the periosteum of the palate; in fact, a better graft is obtained with less necessity for thinning if a fairly thin plane just beneath the submucosa is observed. After the graft is removed, any frank arterial bleeding is controlled with cautery (slow oozing will spontaneously subside). The donor site is packed using Surgicel; the patient can apply some pressure with the tongue. A plastic retainer that snaps into place fixed to the upper teeth can be fashioned preoperatively by a dentist and makes an excellent stent to provide pressure for hemostasis and protect the donor site from mechanical abrasion during the first several postoperative days.

The eyelid is everted on a Desmarres retractor, and the posterior lamella is inspected. Typically the focal point of tarsoconjunctival scarring can be observed 3 to 4 mm from the gray line as a horizontal scar band. Across the entire length of involved eyelid a full-thickness tarsectomy is performed with a fresh scalpel blade in the heart of this scar band, or arbitrarily 3 mm from the gray line if a scar band is not present. The incision must pass perpendicularly through full-thickness tarsus, exposing the distal fibers of the levator aponeurosis and pretarsal orbicularis at the anterior surface of the tarsal plate.

Severe cases require a "buttress" of tarsoconjunctival substitute directly along the eyelid margin. The tarsectomy creates a distal segment of tarsus that is 2 to 3 mm in

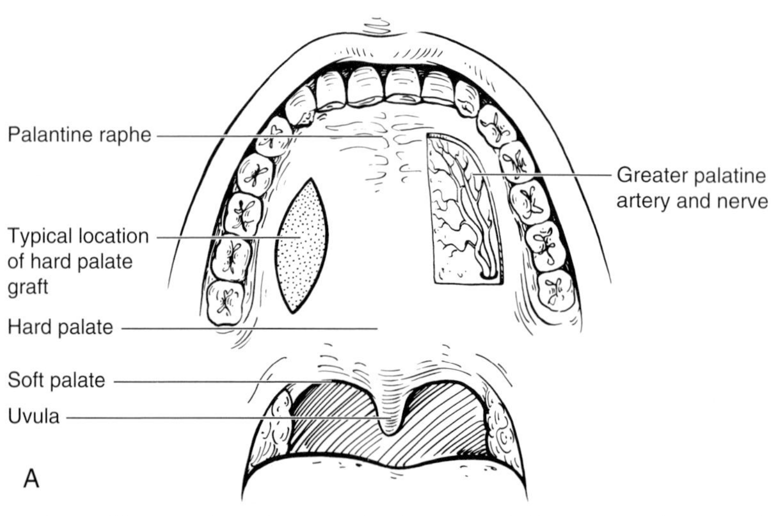

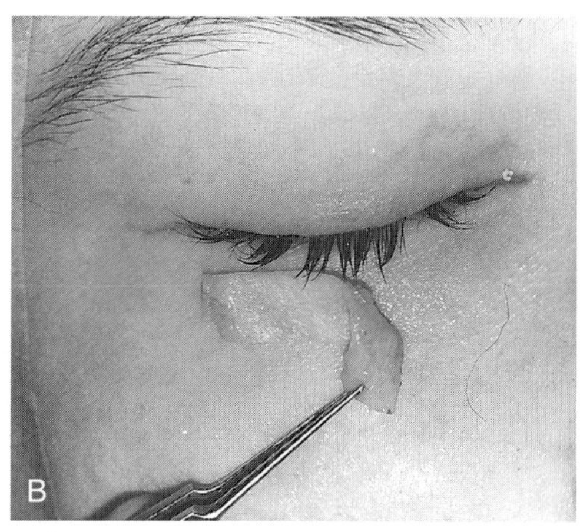

Figure 38–8. *A*, Hard palate mucosal graft donor site. *B*, The graft has thickness and pliability similar to tarsus and is covered with mucous membrane.

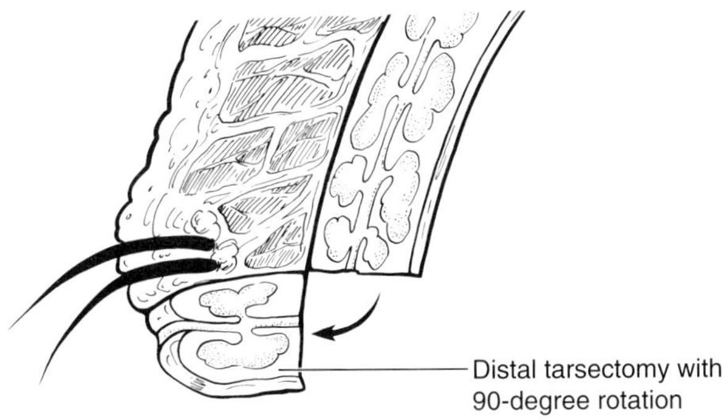

Figure 38–9. Surgical series of lower eyelid cicatricial entropion procedure. Full-thickness tarsectomy creates distal segment of tarsus approximately 3 mm in height. After limited dissection in the plane of the orbicularis, this segment is rotated externally at least 90 degrees.

height and contains the eyelash follicles (Fig. 38–9). This distal segment is further dissected from the anterior attachments until it rotates without restriction 180 degrees outward, hinged on a thin flap of skin and orbicularis. Although complete dissection of the anterior flap is critical for success, one must bear in mind that the eyelash follicles are in the anterior tarsal and pretarsal tissues of the distal segment and avoid unnecessary dissection in this area.

The hard palate mucosal graft is then sutured into position (Fig. 38–10). The proximal edge of the graft is sutured to the cut edge of normal tarsus; the suture bites should be lamellar through the tissues to minimize suture trauma to the cornea, with the knots externalized to the skin or else buried deep in the anterior tarsal tissues.

Eyelid rotation sutures are constructed from 6-0 absorbable suture on double-armed spatula needles (e.g., 6-0 Dexon on a D-1 needle), placed horizontally in lamellar fashion through the anterior graft 2 or 3 mm from the just completed anastomosis with the normal tarsal plate (Fig. 38–11). The double-armed suture ends are brought up through the distal stump of tarsus and tied in or above the lash line. The distal stump is thus rotated externally at least 90 degrees (Fig. 38–12). If the graft is 6 to 8 mm in width, there will be a significant tongue of hard palate mucosa extending beyond the eyelid margin; this is precisely the desired effect, because this 1 or 2 mm free tongue of graft at the eyelid margin will prevent early recurrence, then gradually shrink back over the first month, resulting in a smooth mucosal-lined eyelid margin. A bandage contact lens may be useful to prevent corneal irritation and abrasion from sutures and residually keratinized mucous membranes on the graft surface.

Eyelid stabilization (Frost) sutures should be placed at the end of the case, attached in horizontal mattress fashion to the cut edge of tarsus in the distal segment to enforce the outward rotation (Fig. 38–13). These sutures pass through the margin of the opposing eyelid and are fixated to the brow (for lower eyelid grafts) or thick skin of the cheek (for upper eyelid grafts).

A firm pressure dressing is applied with antibiotic steroid ointment and left untouched for 5 to 7 days to allow the graft to take. The graft edge will appear red and raw for several weeks or even months but eventually will contract, soften, and form a smooth eyelid margin (Fig. 38–14). The graft is variably keratinized when it is taken from the mouth but usually undergoes metaplasia back to a smooth mucosal surface; this process may take many months, and the graft can be irritating during this period. Lubricating ointments and bandage contact lenses can be helpful if mechanical keratitis develops; another helpful maneuver is to de-epithelialize the hard palate graft using a dermabrasion unit, allowing normal surrounding conjunctiva to reepithelialize the graft.

Finally, procedures that involve removal of the entire eyelash-bearing segment of the anterior eyelid margin have been described[38] and can be useful in recalcitrant cases of trichiasis, but only if adequate posterior lamella is present; otherwise, lower eyelid retraction and inade-

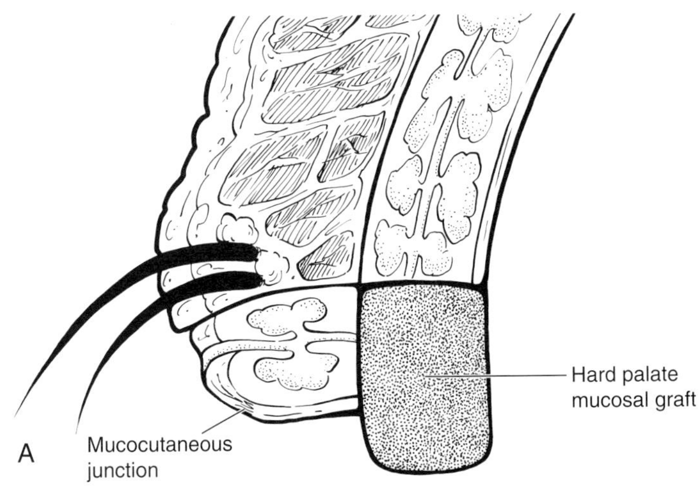

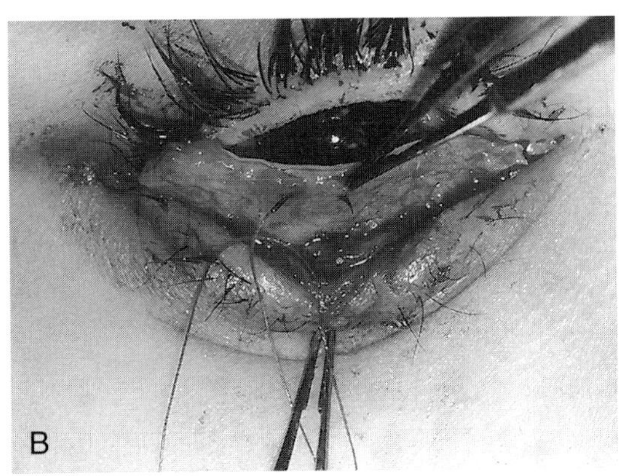

Figure 38–10. Hard palate mucosal graft *(A)* has been sutured into position edge to edge onto the proximal cut edge of tarsus. *B*, Horizontal lamellar suture is shown being placed into graft and will be brought in double-armed fashion through the tarsal stump as a rotational suture.

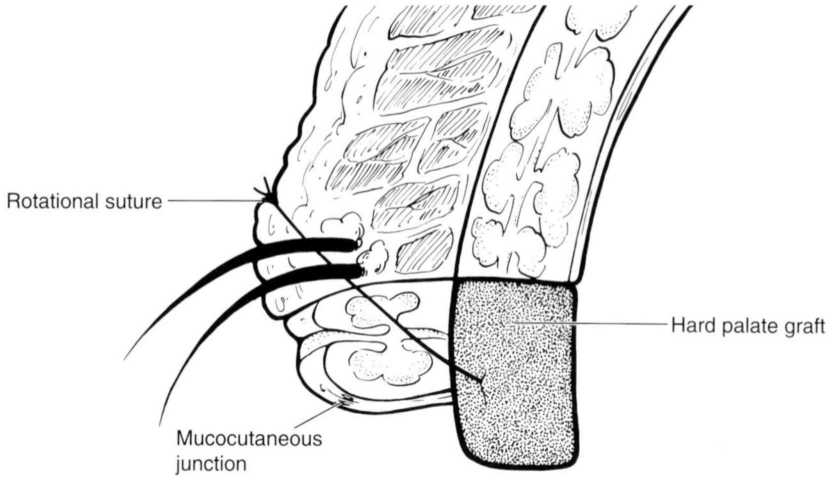

Figure 38–11. Sagittal diagram of placement of double-armed rotational suture originating in hard palate mucosal graft and tied in or just superior to the lash line.

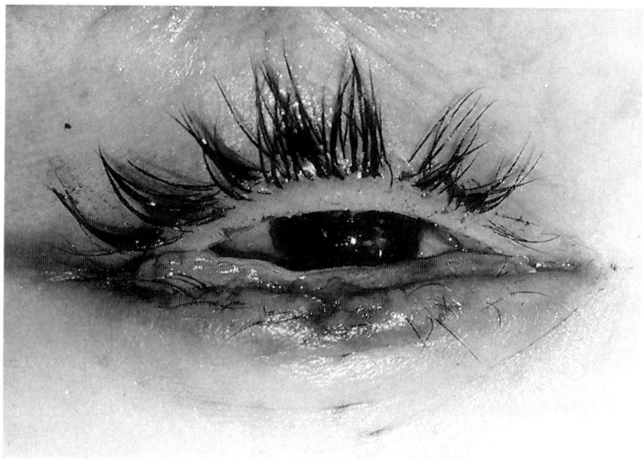

Figure 38–12. Eyelid margin after three rotational sutures have been placed across the eyelid margin. The distal stump of tarsus has been externally rotated more than 90 degrees. A 2-mm tongue of hard palate mucosa extends beyond the eyelid margin; this will shrink back over the first two postoperative months.

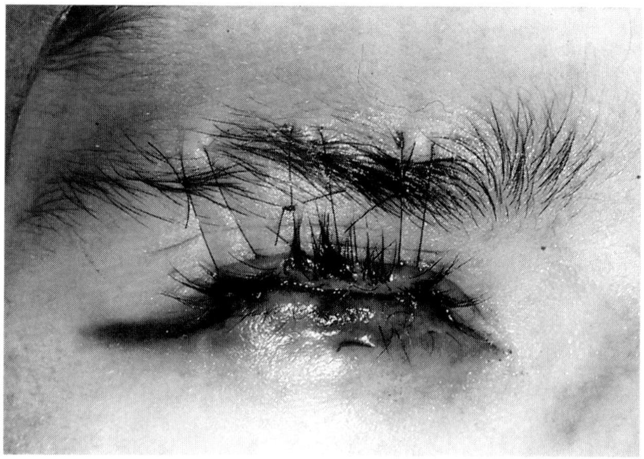

Figure 38–13. Margin fixation sutures are placed in the distal tarsal stump to further enforce external rotation and to stabilize the graft. These horizontal mattress sutures pass through the gray line of the opposing eyelid and are fixated in the eyebrow (for lower eyelid surgery) or cheek (for upper eyelid surgery).

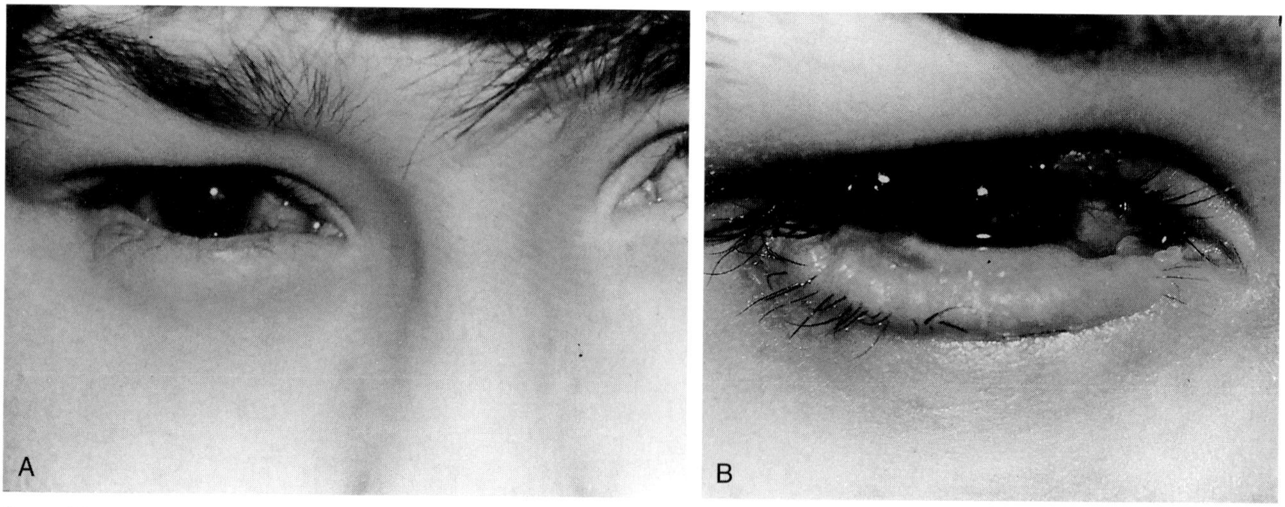

Figure 38–14. *A*, Preoperative appearance: marked lower eyelid cicatricial entropion with keratinized skin and eyelashes rubbing on corneal epithelium. *B*, Five weeks postoperative appearance: the lashes and keratinized skin have been rotated away from the corneal surface. The hard palate mucosal graft serves as a buttress to prevent recurrence and forms a mucous membrane–covered eyelid margin. There is still a tongue of graft extending beyond the eyelid margin; this will continue to contract over several months, forming a smoothly contoured eyelid margin.

quate corneal protection will result. We have used eyelid margin excision after hard palate mucosal buttress procedures with good results. The eyelash follicles reside in the deep orbicularis 2 to 3 mm from the margin, and excision must carefully include the entire row of follicles for successful elimination of the eyelashes.

REFERENCES

1. Jordan R: The lower lid retractors in congenital entropion and epiblepharon. Ophthalmic Surg 24:494–496, 1993.
2. Anderson RL, Harvey JT: Lid splitting and posterior lamella cryosurgery for congenital and acquired distichiasis. Arch Ophthalmol 99:631–634, 1981.
3. Dortzbach RK, McGetrick JJ: Involutional entropion of the lower eyelid. Adv Ophthalmic Plast Reconstr Surg 2:257–267, 1983.
4. Jones LT, Reeh MV, Wobig JL: Senile entropion: A new concept for correction. Am J Ophthalmol 72:327–329, 1972.
5. Collin RO (ed): A Manual of Systemic Eyelid Surgery, 2nd ed. New York, Churchill Livingstone, 1989; pp 7–26.
6. Dresner SC, Karesh JW: Transconjunctival entropion repair. Arch Ophthalmol 111:1144–1148, 1993.
7. Jordan DR: Ectropion following entropion: An unhappy patient and physician. Plast Reconstr Surg 8:41–46, 1992.
8. Gerkowicz K, Jedrzejewski D: Experimental studies on the effect of low temperatures on the inhibition of eyelash growth. Klin Oczńa 88:412–413, 1986.
9. Matthaus W, Matthes R: Technic and long-term results of cryogenic epilation in trichiasis and distichiasis. Klin Monatsbl Augenheilkd 196:59–61, 1990.
10. Peart DA, Hill JC: Cryosurgery for trichiasis in black patients. Br J Ophthalmol 70:712–714, 1986.
11. Sullivan JH: Cryosurgery in ophthalmic practice. Opthalmic Surg 10:37–41, 1979.
12. Sullivan JH, Beard C, Bullock JD: Cryosurgery for treatment of trichiasis. Am J Ophthalmol 82:117–121, 1976.
13. Wilkes TD, Fraunfelder FT: Principles of cryosurgery. Ophthalmic Surg 10:21–30, 1979.
14. Rice CD, Kersten RC, al-Hazzaa S: Cryotherapy for trichiasis in trachoma. Arch Ophthalmol 107:1180–1182, 1989.
15. Wood JR, Anderson RL: Complications of cryotherapy. Arch Ophthalmol 99:460–463, 1981.
16. Ballen PH: Simple procedure for relief of trichiasis and entropion of the upper eyelid. Ophthalmology 59:503–506, 1955.
17. Beyer CK, Carroll JM: Moderately severe cicatricial entropion. Arch Ophthalmol 89:33, 1973.
18. Dortzbach RK, Callahan A: Repair of cicatricial entropion of the upper eyelids. Arch Ophthalmol 85:82–89, 1971.
19. Fox SA: Cicatricial entropion of the upper eyelid. Am J Ophthalmol 57:379–382, 1964.
20. Kemp EG, Collin JR: Surgical management of upper lid entropion. Br J Ophthalmol 70:575–579, 1986.
21. Lagley ZE: Operation for entropion and trichiasis by a new method. Ann Ophthalmol 14:473–477, 1905.
22. Millman AL, Katzen LB, Putterman AM: Cicatricial entropion: An analysis of its treatment with transverse blepharotomy and marginal rotation. Ophthalmic Surg 20:575–579, 1989.
23. Teichmann KD: Correction of severe upper eyelid entropion. Int Ophthalmol 12:37–39, 1988.
24. Tenzel RR: Repair of entropion of upper lid. Arch Ophthalmol 77:675, 1967.
25. Wies FA: Spastic entropion. Trans Am Acad Ophthalmol Otolaryngol 59:503–506, 1955.
26. Baylis HI, Hamako C: Tarsal grafting for correction of cicatricial entropion. Ophthalmic Surg 10:42–48, 1979.
27. Baylis HI, Silkiss RZ: A structurally oriented approach to the repair of cicatricial entropion. Ophthal Plast Reconstr Surg 3:17–20, 1987.
28. Bosniak SL. Editorial comment: Repair of advanced cicatricial entropion: Tarsal conjunctival advancement flaps and a free mucous membrane graft. Adv Ophthalmic Plast Reconstr Surg 2:285–286, 1983.
29. Shorr N, Christenbury JD, Goldberg RA: Tarsoconjunctival grafts for upper eyelid cicatricial entropion. Ophthalmic Surg 19:316–320, 1988.
30. Silver B: The use of mucous membrane from the hard palate in the treatment of trichiasis and cicatricial entropion. Ophthal Plast Reconstr Surg 2:129–131, 1986.
31. Reacher MH, Huber MJ, Canagaratnam R, Alghassany A: A trial of surgery for trichiasis of the upper lid from trachoma. Br J Ophthalmol 74:109–113, 1990.
32. Callahan A: Correction of entropion from Stevens-Johnson syndrome. Arch Ophthalmol 94:1154–1155, 1976.
33. Carroll RP: The management of cicatricial entropion. Adv Ophthalmic Plast Reconstr Surg 2:275–284, 1983.
34. Nasr AM: Eyelid complications in trachoma: I. Cicatricial entropion. Ophthalmic Surg 20:800–807, 1989.
35. Rubenzik R, Tenzel RR, Miller GR: Repair of cicatricial entropion of the upper eyelid. Am J Ophthalmol 80:302–303, 1975.
36. Stephenson CM, Brown BZ: The use of tarsus as a free autogenous graft in eyelid surgery. Ophthal Plast Reconstr Surg 1:43–50, 1985.
37. Tenzel RR, Miller GR, Rubenzik R: Cicatricial upper lid entropion treated with banked scleral graft. Arch Ophthalmol 93:999–1000, 1975.
38. Wojno TH: Lid splitting with lash resection for cicatricial entropion and trichiasis. Ophthal Plast Reconstr Surg 8:287–289, 1992.

BIBLIOGRAPHY

Carroll RP, Allen SE: Combined procedure for repair of involutional entropion. Ophthal Plast Reconstr Surg 7:123–127, 1991.

Dresner SL, Karesh JW: Transconjunctival entropion repair. Arch Ophthalmol 111:1144–1148, 1993.

Levitt JM: Epiblepharon and congenital entropion. Am J Ophthalmol 44:112–113, 1957.

Nowinski TS: Orbicularis oculi muscle extirpation in a combined procedure for involutional entropion. Ophthalmology 98:1250–1256, 1991.

Tse DT, Anderson RL, Fratkin JD: Aponeurosis disinsertion in congenital entropion. Arch Ophthalmol 101:436–440, 1983.

Wesley RE, Collins JW: Combined procedure for senile entropion. Ophthalmic Surg 14:401–405, 1983.

CHAPTER 39

Involutional and Paralytic Ectropion

Steven M. Gilbard

Ectropion is the turning out of the eyelid margin away from the globe. In both involutional and paralytic ectropion, laxity of the eyelid tissues occurs. Because of this, some of the approaches to repair are similar. Clearly, however, both classifications require an individual approach, depending on the severity of the deformity.

INVOLUTIONAL ECTROPION

Etiology

Involutional lower lid ectropion occurs with aging changes, secondary to microinfarction and secondary atrophy, causing laxity of the eyelid tissues and resulting in turning out of the eyelid away from the globe and poor approximation of the inferior punctum to the lacrimal lake. Also included in this category are the eyelid laxity caused by the chronic pressure of an ocular prosthesis and lid–globe disparity due to marked enophthalmos. The patient experiences tearing, which causes constant wiping and further progression. Medial migration of the punctum and inefficiency of the lacrimal pump and blink mechanism also contribute to tearing. The conjunctiva becomes dry and inflamed owing to exposure, poor flow of tears, and chronic infection. This leads to keratinization of the conjunctiva, increased stretching of the eyelid tissues, and misdirection of the lashes (Fig. 39–1). With poor tear drainage, recurrent or chronic infections can occur.

The upper eyelid undergoes the same changes as the lower eyelid. Since gravity does not result in eyelid margin displacement, the upper lid usually remains in good position. However, if the lid is extremely lax and the levator muscle is advanced for the purpose of ptosis surgery, the lid may actually pull away from the globe or evert, causing significant pain and discomfort. Horizontal laxity of the upper lid may present as a disparity between upper and lower lid called floppy eyelid syndrome in which the upper lid prolapses over the lower lid margin, resulting in the lower eyelashes scrubbing the palpebral conjunctiva of the upper lid and causing chronic conjunctivitis. This disparity may increase after lower lid ectropion surgery if the upper lid laxity is not recognized and treated (Figs. 39–2 and 39–3).

Involutional ectropion is the result of a number of pathophysiologic changes. The pretarsal orbicularis that forms the medial and lateral canthal tendons serves as a dynamic hammock to suspend the lid and to keep the eyelid margin in close approximation to the globe. With laxity of the orbicularis and of the canthal tendons, the lid falls away from the globe. Predominant medial canthal laxity results in medial ectropion and punctal eversion (Fig. 39–4). Predominant lateral canthal laxity results in medial punctal migration and lateral ectropion (Fig. 39–5). Complete eversion of the entire lid margin may be the result of diffuse laxity involving both canthal tendons and the orbicularis (Fig. 39–6). Sometimes disinsertion of the lower eyelid retractor allows the tarsus to pivot more easily as the orbicularis weakens, contributing to the lower lid ectropion. Thus, repair of the lower eyelid retractors may be necessary in severe cases of ectropion.

Preoperative Evaluation

Preoperatively, the amount of horizontal eyelid laxity should be estimated. The position of the punctum should be observed by biomicroscopy and with the naked eye for possible medial migration. The normal punctal position is just lateral to the caruncle and inverted toward the lacrimal lake. The pinch test is an effective means of determining if lid laxity exists (Fig. 39–7). If the lid can be pulled more than 6 mm from the globe, then the lid is lax.[1] Grasping the lid and pinching it will also give information about canthal tendon laxity.[2] The configuration of the lateral canthal angle can be observed, and the fixation strength of the lateral canthal angle can be evaluated. If the lateral canthal tendon is not tightened before horizontal shortening of the lid, a narrowing of the horizontal palpebral aperture will result. If the punctum is displaced laterally toward the nasal limbus, medial canthal tendon laxity exists. If the lid is shortened horizontally without prior medial canthal plication, the punctum will be permanently displaced. The laxity of the upper eyelid and

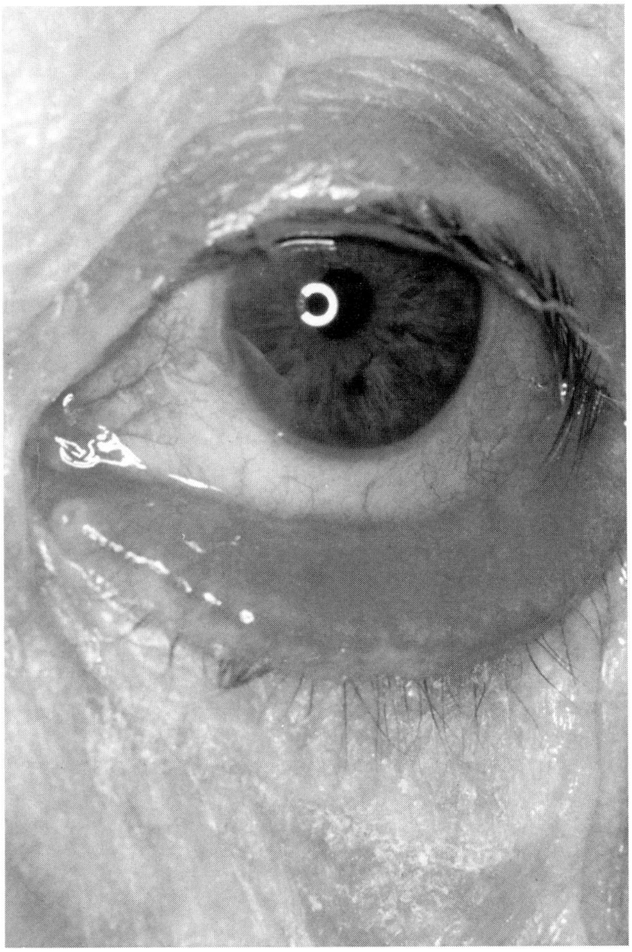

Figure 39–1. Involutional ectropion with eversion of eyelid and chronic conjunctival exposure with keratinization.

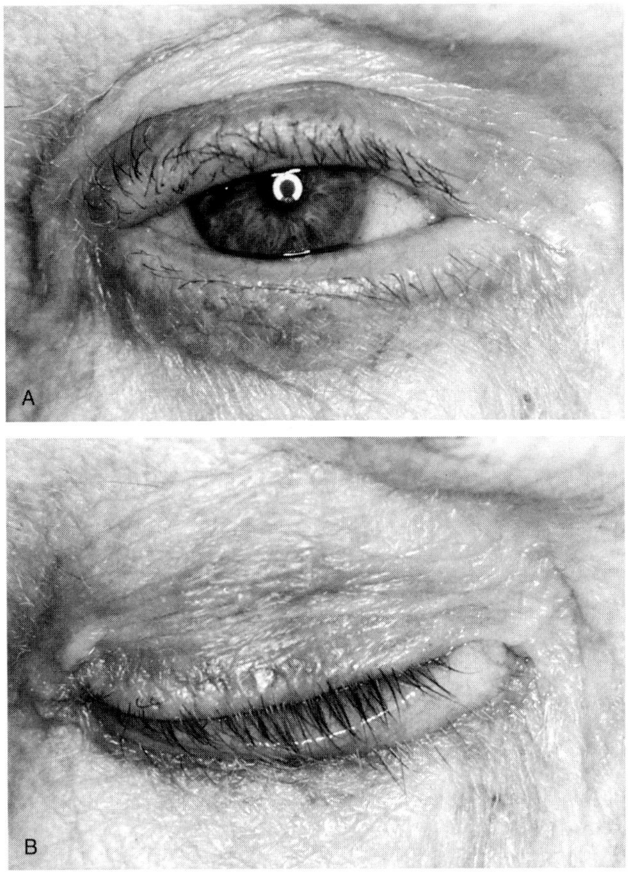

Figure 39–3. Horizontal laxity of the lower lid causing floppy eyelid syndrome. *A*, Patient opening. *B*, Patient closing.

superior limb of the medial and lateral canthal tendon should be evaluated and consideration given to shortening of the upper eyelid at the same time as lower lid repair so as not to have an upper lid grossly out of proportion to the lower eyelid with resultant floppy eyelid syndrome.

The patency of the punctum and lacrimal system should be determined. Palpebral conjunctiva that has been exposed and desiccated becomes keratinized with long-standing lower lid ectropion. If there is medial ectropion, the punctum may be obliterated. In unilateral ectropion, exacerbated by chronic wiping, tearing and nasolacrimal duct obstruction may have preceded the ectropion.

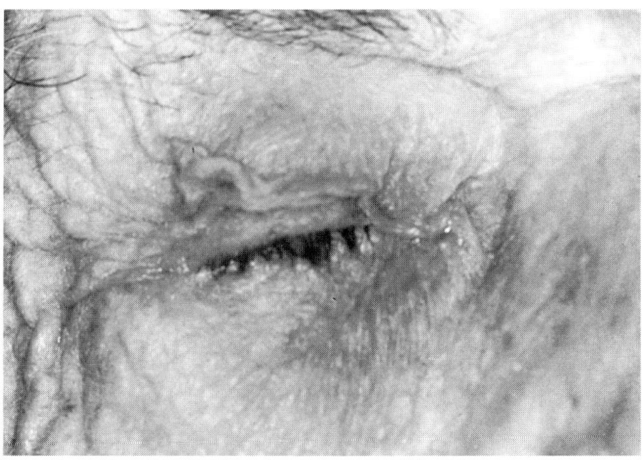

Figure 39–2. Horizontal laxity of the upper lid causing floppy eyelid syndrome.

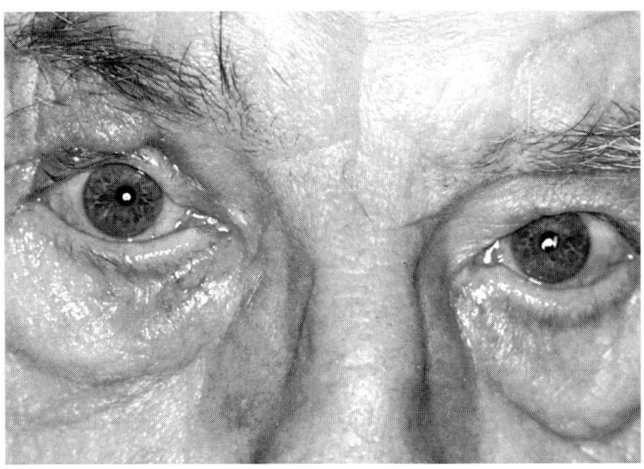

Figure 39–4. Involutional medial ectropion with punctal eversion.

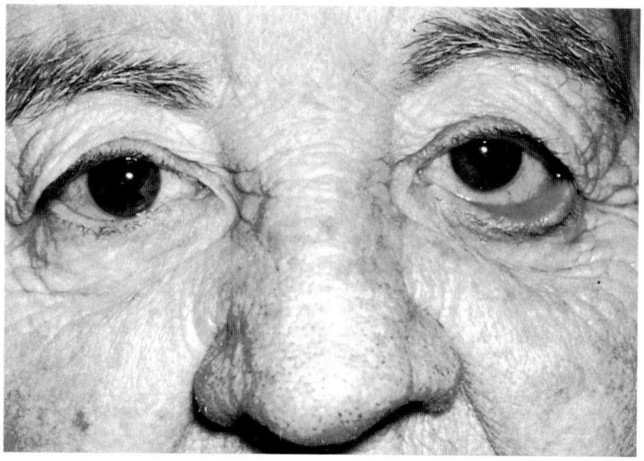

Figure 39–5. Involutional ectropion greatest laterally.

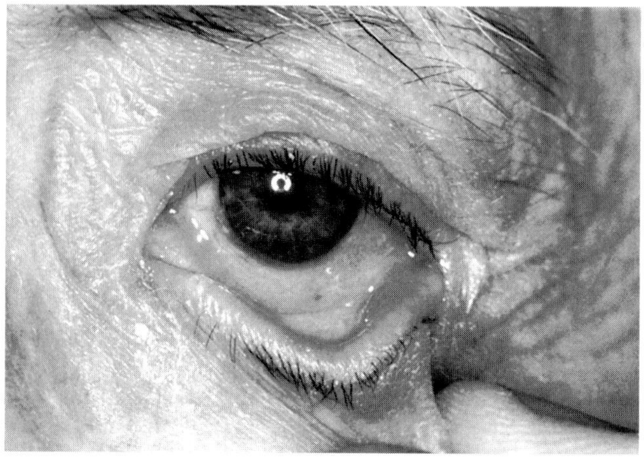

Figure 39–7. Pinch test to determine the presence of lid laxity.

The extent of skin deficiency, if present, should be noted preoperatively by grasping the lid margin and pulling it superiorly (Fig. 39–8). If it does not reach 2 mm above the inferior limbus, the lid is vertically insufficient. The anterior lamella will need to be lengthened with either a flap or a skin graft.

Lower lid retraction can accompany lower lid ectropion. This may be a function of canthal tendon laxity, shortening of the posterior lamella of the lid, proptosis, shallow orbits, or high myopia with large globes. A simple lower lid pentagonal resection may correct the ectropion but accentuate the lower lid retraction as the tightened lid rests on the convex surface of the globe inferior to the limbus. The lid must be vertically lengthened with scleral, cartilage, or fascia and supported laterally with a lateral canthoplasty, periosteal flaps, or fascial strips.

Medical Treatment

If the ectropion is of recent onset with conjunctival edema or infection, a bland or antibiotic ophthalmic ointment should be used to help protect exposed conjunctiva and corneal epithelium. This will often result in significant improvement in conjunctival engorgement, lid swelling, and lid margin position. Maximal improvement from this medical treatment is seen usually within 3 weeks. An ointment containing a corticosteroid may produce more rapid relief than a plain petrolatum ointment or an antibiotic preparation but should not be used if the corneal epithelium is not intact, if the patient is a steroid responder, or if the patient has had herpes simplex keratitis.

Surgical Treatment

Inferior Punctoplasty

In cases of mild eversion of the medial lid margin involving the punctum, a one-snip punctoplasty may relieve symptomatic tearing (Fig. 39–9). Its potential for success may be evaluated by dilating the puncta and observing a clinical response.

The technique is begun by injecting local anesthetic subconjunctivally just inferior to the punctal ampulla.

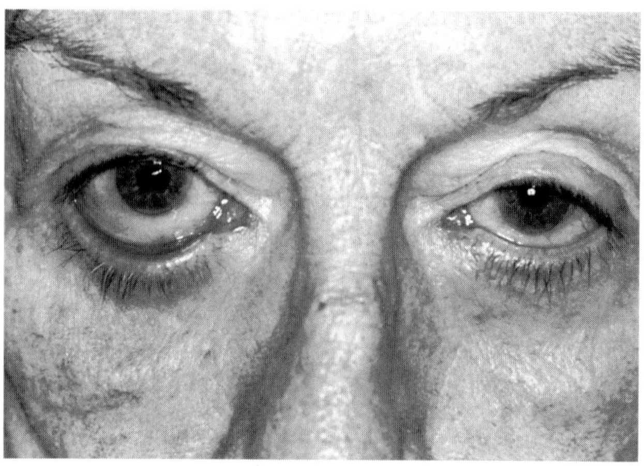

Figure 39–6. Central ectropion of the lower lid.

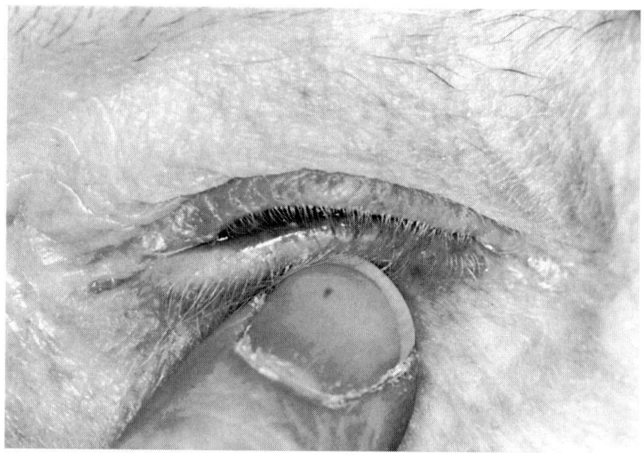

Figure 39–8. Superior displacement of lid margin to assess anterior lamenal shortening.

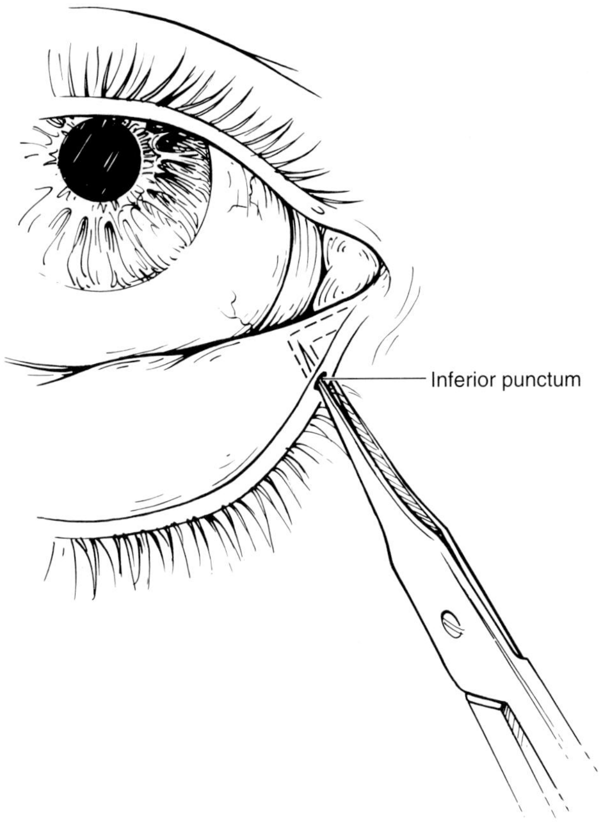

Figure 39–9. Inferior punctoplasty for mild punctal eversion.

The medial portion of the lower eyelid is then everted, and a vertical scissors cut is made in the ampulla with one blade on the conjunctival side and the other blade inside the ampulla. As this cut is made, downward pressure is exerted to prevent the tissue from sliding away. If the first snip does not gape, then a second snip is made so that a V of the ampulla is removed. To prevent scarring and closure of the punctal incisions, it is important to perform dilation at weekly intervals.

Conjunctival-Retractor Excision

In patients with more pronounced eversion of the medial lid margin involving the punctum, excision of an ellipse of conjunctiva and underlying retractors with closure is effective (Fig. 39–10).

Local anesthetic is injected subconjunctivally just inferior to the punctal ampulla. The lower canaliculus is identified by placing a lacrimal probe. An ellipse of conjunctiva and underlying retractors measuring 4 mm high and 8 mm wide is excised inferior to the punctum. The defect is then closed using three interrupted sutures of 6-0 polyglactin (Vicryl, Dexon) with buried knots. The sutures incorporate a bite of deep lid tissue in the depth of the site and the conjunctival edges to maximize the inward rotation of the punctum.

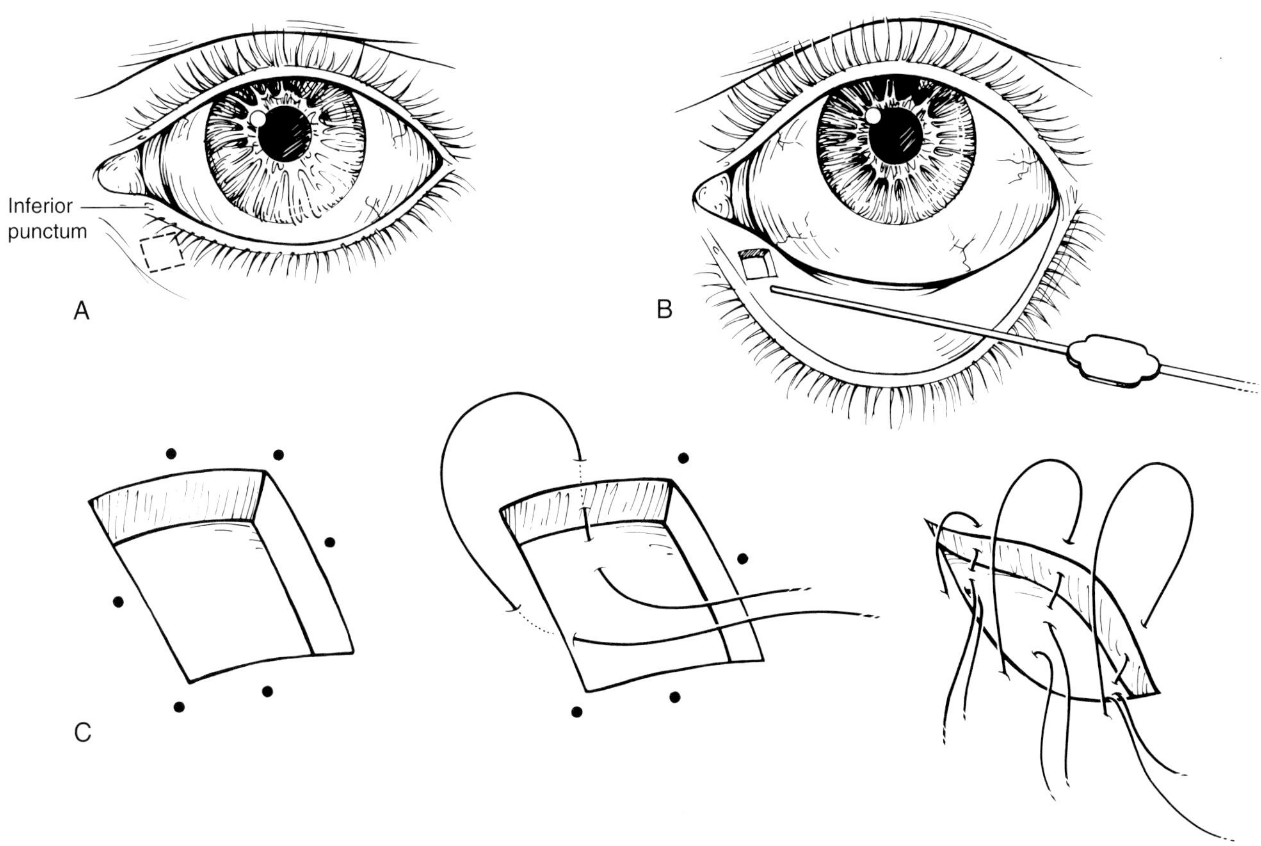

Figure 39–10. Conjunctival-retractor excision. *A*, Location of ellipse reflected onto skin plane. *B*, The ellipse of conjunctiva has been resected. *C*, Placement of 6-0 polyglactin suture.

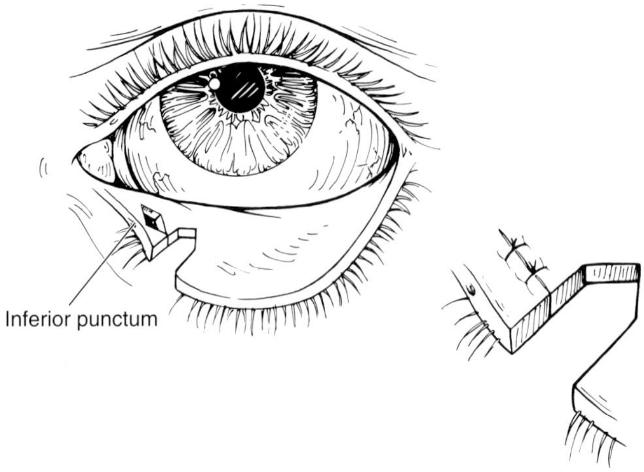

Figure 39 – 11. Smith lazy-T procedure combining conjunctival retractor excision with a pentagonal wedge resection.

Smith Lazy-T Procedure

When significant eyelid laxity is present with predominant eversion of the medial lid, and when the lateral canthal tendon is not unduly lax, the Smith lazy-T procedure is of value (Fig. 39 – 11).[3] A standard pentagonal wedge is resected 4 mm lateral to the lower punctum. The horizontal width of the pentagon is 5 to 8 mm, depending on the laxity of the lid. A conjunctival-retractor excision is then performed inferior to the punctum. This excision is made contiguous with the lid resection. The submucosa is undermined into the inferior fornix. The wound edges are overlapped, and an amount necessary to return the punctum to the lacrimal lake is resected. The conjunctiva and submucosa are closed with 6-0 plain sutures. The lid margin is closed with 6-0 black silk. The tarsus is closed with 5-0 chromic suture.

Medial Plication for Extreme Medial Canthal Laxity

If the medial attachment of the inferior tarsus is so lax that other procedures will not provide adequate tension, a medial plication should be used along with a lid-shortening procedure (Fig. 39 – 12). A lacrimal probe is placed in the lower canaliculus. A skin incision is made inferior to the canaliculus extending from just lateral to the punctum to just medial to the canthal angle. Either a nonabsorbable or a polyglactin 5-0 suture is placed to attach the medial end of the inferior tarsal plate to the anterior portion of the medial canthal tendon. The suture placement in the medial canthal tendon should be at the

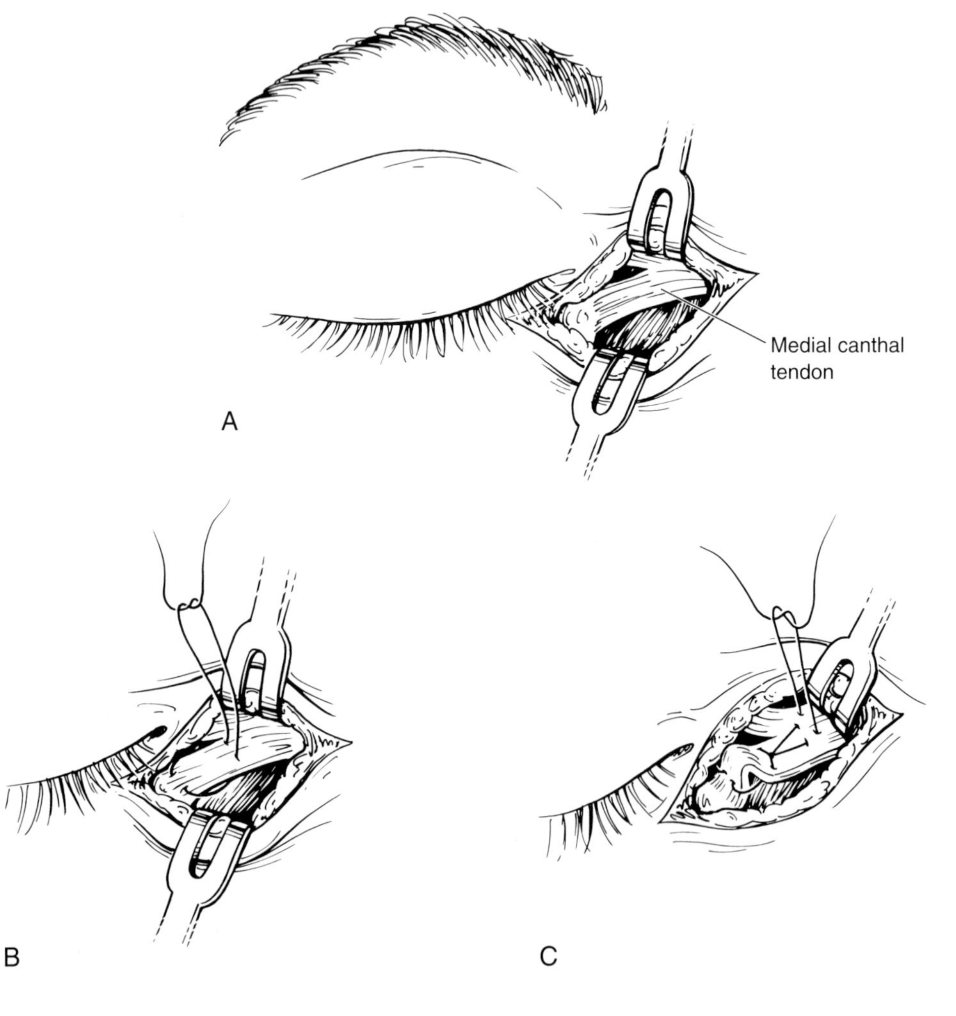

Figure 39 – 12. Medial canthal plication. *A*, Exposing the medial canthal tendon and inferior tarsus. *B* and *C*, Polyglactin 5-0 suture placement.

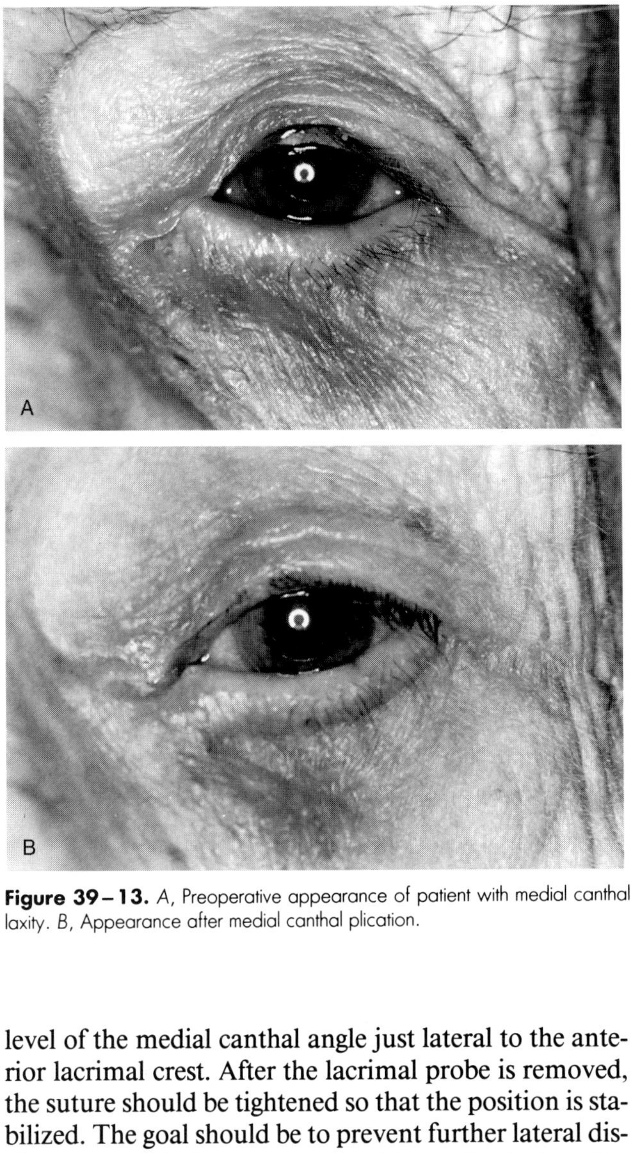

Figure 39–13. *A*, Preoperative appearance of patient with medial canthal laxity. *B*, Appearance after medial canthal plication.

level of the medial canthal angle just lateral to the anterior lacrimal crest. After the lacrimal probe is removed, the suture should be tightened so that the position is stabilized. The goal should be to prevent further lateral displacement of the lower punctum. Attempting to draw the punctum more medially may result in canalicular kinking and loss of lacrimal pump function. The skin incision is then closed (Fig. 39–13).

Horizontal Full-Thickness Eyelid Shortening

The Byron Smith modification of the Kuhnt-Szymanowski procedure combines horizontal full-thickness eyelid shortening with a blepharoplasty-type skin incision (Fig. 39–14).[4] This method is desirable when the lateral canthal tendon is stable and there is marked redundancy to lower lid skin.

Local anesthesia is injected subcutaneously. A 4-0 black silk traction suture is placed through the lid margin, and the eyelid is placed on stretch. A subciliary incision is made from the inferior punctum medially to the lateral extent of the lid. A skin flap is undermined through this wound from the cilia superiorly to the inferior orbital rim inferiorly. An inverted pentagonal wedge resection is performed at the junction of the lateral third and medial two thirds of the lid below the skin flap plane. To do this a vertical incision is first made from the lid margin to the lower border of tarsus. The wound edges are overlapped until the lid margin approximates the globe snugly. The pentagonal resection is then completed. The lid margin is reapproximated with three interrupted 6-0 black silk sutures placed first through the lash line, meibomian gland orifices, and finally the gray line. Meticulous closure is essential and depends on suture bites of equal length and depth. The reconstructed lid margin should be slightly peaked to avoid postoperative notching. The suture ends are left long so they can be anchored under the skin sutures and kept off the cornea. The tarsus and conjunctiva are closed with one or two mild 5-0 chromic sutures. The skin is closed with 6-0 nylon sutures after it has been trimmed. If there is no obvious skin redundancy, a full-thickness eyelid resection may be performed without a skin flap (Fig. 39–15).

Lateral Tarsal Strip Procedure

When there is eyelid laxity and poor lateral canthal fixation to the lateral orbital wall, re-fixation of the eyelid to the lateral orbital tubercle corrects the laxity and restores the contour of the lateral canthal angle. This concept served as the basis for the Bick procedure in which a vertical full-thickness incision in the lower eyelid is performed and the excess full-thickness eyelid tissue resected. The tarsus is then sutured to the lateral orbital rim.[5] This concept was modified and continued by fashioning a lateral tarsal strip[6–8] to shorten the lid horizontally and reestablish fixation to the area of the lateral orbital tubercle (Fig. 39–16).

The lateral tarsal strip procedure can be performed with the use of local anesthesia. A subciliary incision is made from the lateral two fifths of the eyelid extending to the lateral canthus and slightly posteriorly. The muscle is incised and spread to expose the periorbita and orbital margin. Lateral canthotomy is done, and inferior cantholysis is completed to mobilize the lateral aspect of the eyelid for its advancement superiorly and laterally. The tarsal strip is made by excising the mucosa, cilia, orbicularis, and skin at the lateral edge of the eyelid. The length of the tarsal strip and the amount, if any, of the strip to be excised is now determined, depending on the laxity of the eyelid. At least 4 to 5 mm of bare tarsal strip is left intact for attachment of the lateral orbital rim. Residual mucosa on the posterior surface of the tarsus is excised or cauterized to avoid burying epithelium when the tarsus is attached to the periorbita. A 5-0 prolene suture is passed into the periorbita 2 to 4 mm within the orbital aspect of the zygoma several millimeters above the level of the lateral commissure. The prolene suture is now passed through the stump of tarsus. After it is brought back through the tarsus, the needle is again passed into the periorbita just above the initial periorbital bite. The su-

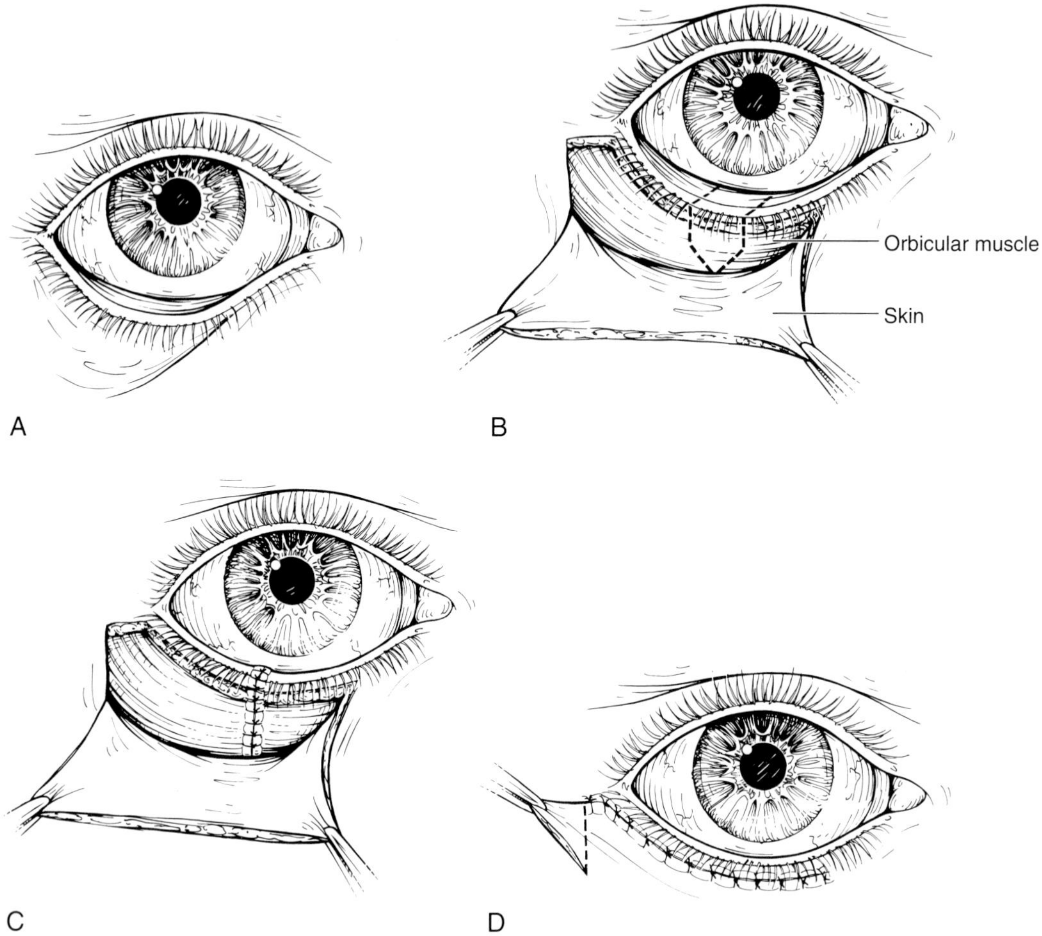

Figure 39–14. Smith modification of Kuhnt-Szymanowski. *A*, Preoperative appearance. *B*, Skin is elevated down to orbital rim, and pentagonal resection is performed. C, Closure at lid margin with 6-0 silk sutures. *D*, Skin closure.

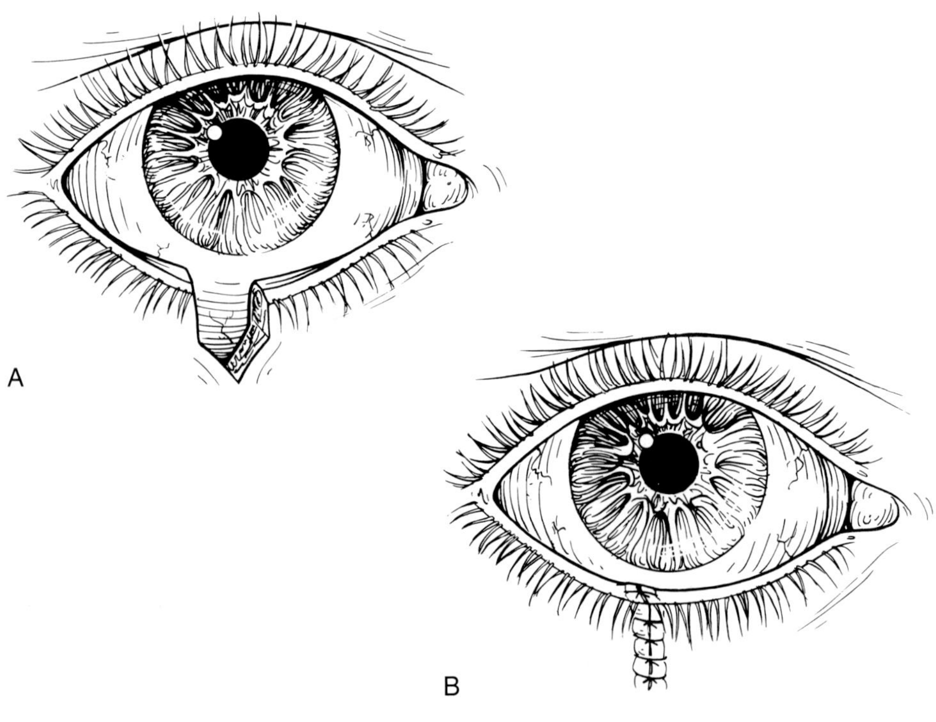

Figure 39–15. Pentagonal wedge resection. *A*, Full-thickness wedge resection. *B*, Closure with 6-0 silk sutures at lid margin, 5-0 chromic in tarsal plate, and 6-0 nylon in skin.

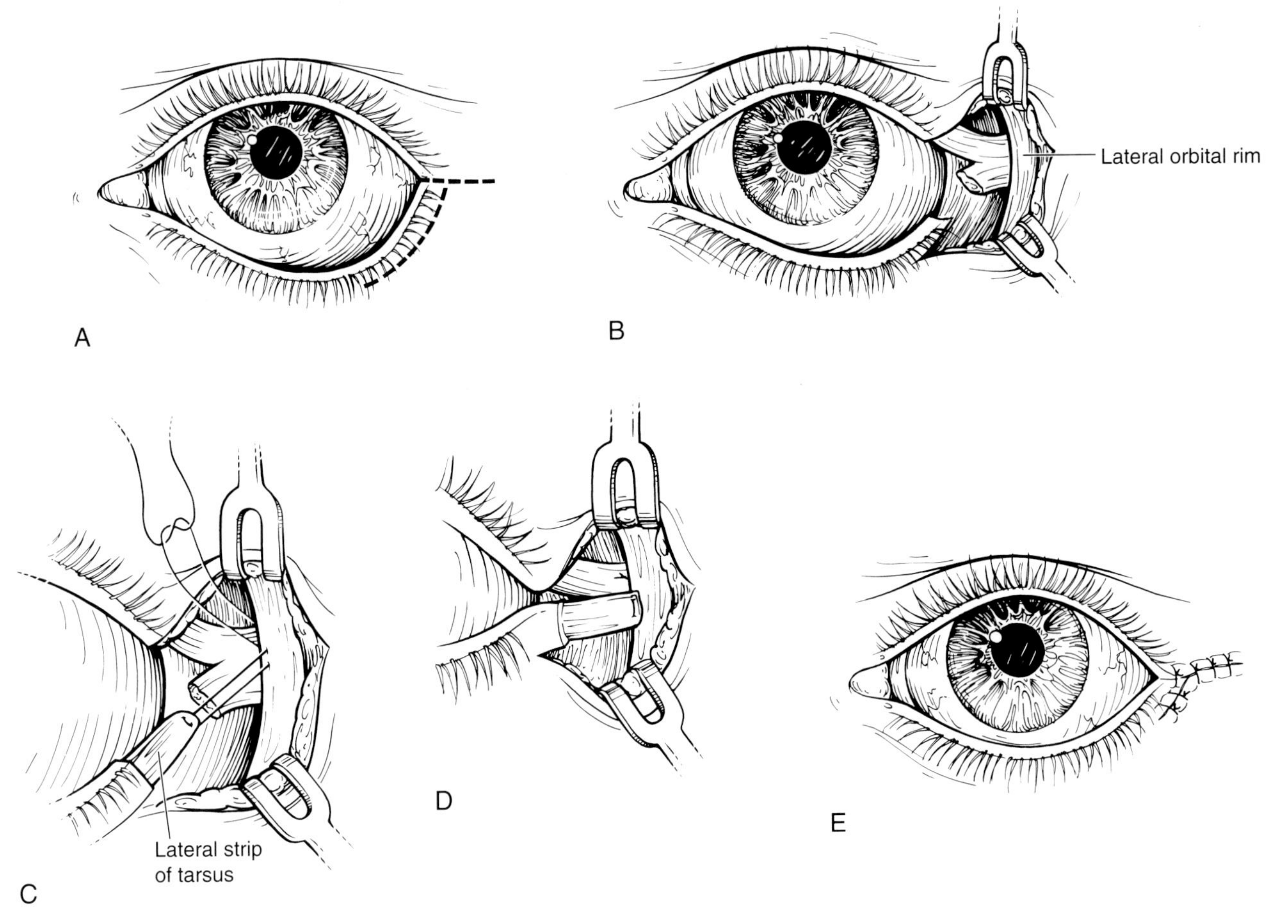

Figure 39–16. Lateral tarsal strip procedure. *A*, Subciliary incision. *B*, Cantholysis of the inferior crux of lateral canthal tendon. C, Placement of 5-0 prolene suture into periorbita and tarsal strip. *D*, Lateral tarsal strip in position. *E*, Skin closure.

ture is now tightened. The lower eyelid tarsal attachment to the periorbita can be reinforced with one or two additional 5-0 prolene sutures. The lateral commissure is redefined using 5-0 plain suture. The orbicularis plane is closed using 5-0 PDS suture. Some overcorrection at the time of surgery is desired since the lid position will drop slightly with time (Fig. 39–17).

The lateral tarsal strip procedure can be adapted for use in the upper lid for frank upper lid ectropion or to avoid significant overhang of the upper lid after lower lid ectropion surgery.

PARALYTIC ECTROPION

Etiology and Pathophysiology

Paralytic ectropion results from facial nerve paresis and secondary loss of function of the orbicularis after Bell's palsy, suppuration, trauma, tumor invasion, or resection of tumors. Over time the lower eyelid margin and the canthal tendons stretch, and the lid margin falls away from the globe secondary to the unopposed force of gravity and the lower lid retractors. These changes occur earlier and are more pronounced if there are preexisting involutional changes (Fig. 39–18).

With loss of the orbicularis contracture, voluntary and involuntary blink is lost. Tears are poorly distributed over the globe and pool over the lower lid margin. They are poorly caught because of poor punctal position, and epiphora occurs. There is failure of the lacrimal pump mechanism in which negative pressure is created in the tear sac on contracture of the attachments of the orbicularis to the walls of the tear sac. With loss of the negative tear sac pressure with blinking, tears are not sucked into the punctum and canaliculus. Chronic wiping of tears is common, which can, in turn, worsen the ectropion. Corneal exposure can occur with keratopathy. Concomitant fifth cranial nerve lesions eliminate corneal sensation, leaving the cornea even more vulnerable and subject to neuroparalytic keratopathy.

Preoperative Evaluation

Clinical history should be obtained regarding etiology and the potential for recovery determined. Facial function should be evaluated and the amount of orbicularis paresis determined. Any effect of the weight of cheek on the lower lid is observed. The House classification is a useful universal standard for facial function.[9] The amount of eyelid laxity and the integrity of the medial

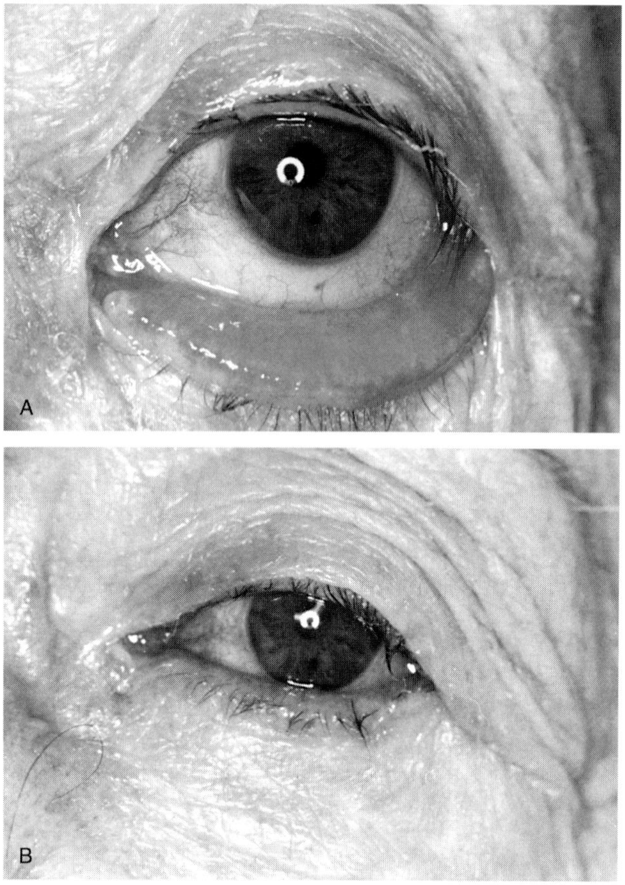

Figure 39 – 17. *A*, Preoperative appearance of patient with severe ectropion before lateral tarsal strip procedure. *B*, Postoperative appearance.

and lateral canthal tendons should be evaluated. Visual acuity is tested, and measurements are made of palpebral fissure width and inferior scleral show. The degree of voluntary and involuntary blink is assessed. Corneal sensation is tested since corneal anesthesia requires greater protection.

Medical Management

The most important part of medical management in patients with paralytic ectropion consists of artificial tears and lubricating ointments. Artificial tears allow for clear vision but may require frequent application several times every hour. Ointments provide longer lasting effects but blur vision. Frequently the use of ointment at bedtime provides lasting coverage from exposure during sleep, and the use of tears during the day allows the patient to function.

Occlusive bubble shields can be worn to reduce evaporation of natural or artificial tears. Taping the eyelids can correct irritation from ectropion. The tape should be applied across the lower eyelid, which can then be pulled upward and outward in a sweeping motion with the tape.

Surgical Treatment

Surgical Indications

Despite conservative medical management of paralytic ectropion, surgical intervention is frequently necessary. The presence of corneal deterioration is a clear indication for surgical intervention, as is marked progression of the paralytic ectropion. If the facial paralysis is expected to be permanent, then surgery is indicated. In patients with accompanying loss of the first division of the trigeminal nerve and corneal anesthesia, and in patients with accompanying dry eye, early surgical intervention is important. Lack of a good Bell phenomenon is a frequent harbinger for the need to intervene surgically. Patients with monocular vision on the paralytic side should undergo surgical correction. Finally, the noncompliant patient or the medically infirm patient who may have trouble with a regular medical regimen should have surgical correction.

Tarsorrhaphy

Tarsorrhaphy has been the classic and simplest method of providing corneal protection. A simple rapid method is the marginal adhesion tarsorrhaphy, which involves freshening opposing eyelid margin surfaces and suturing them together for 1 to 2 weeks (Fig. 39 – 19).

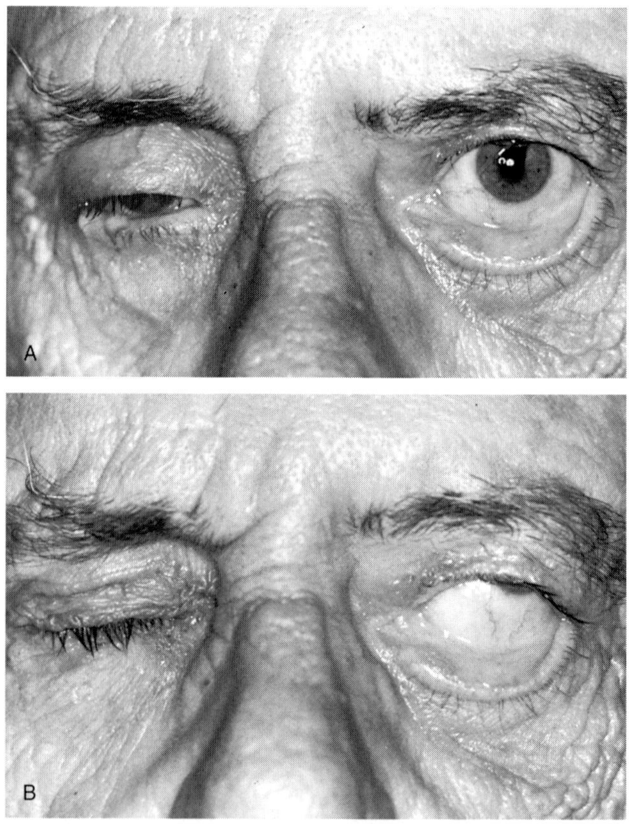

Figure 39 – 18. Longstanding paralytic lagophthalmos and ectropion. *A*, Open. *B*, Closed.

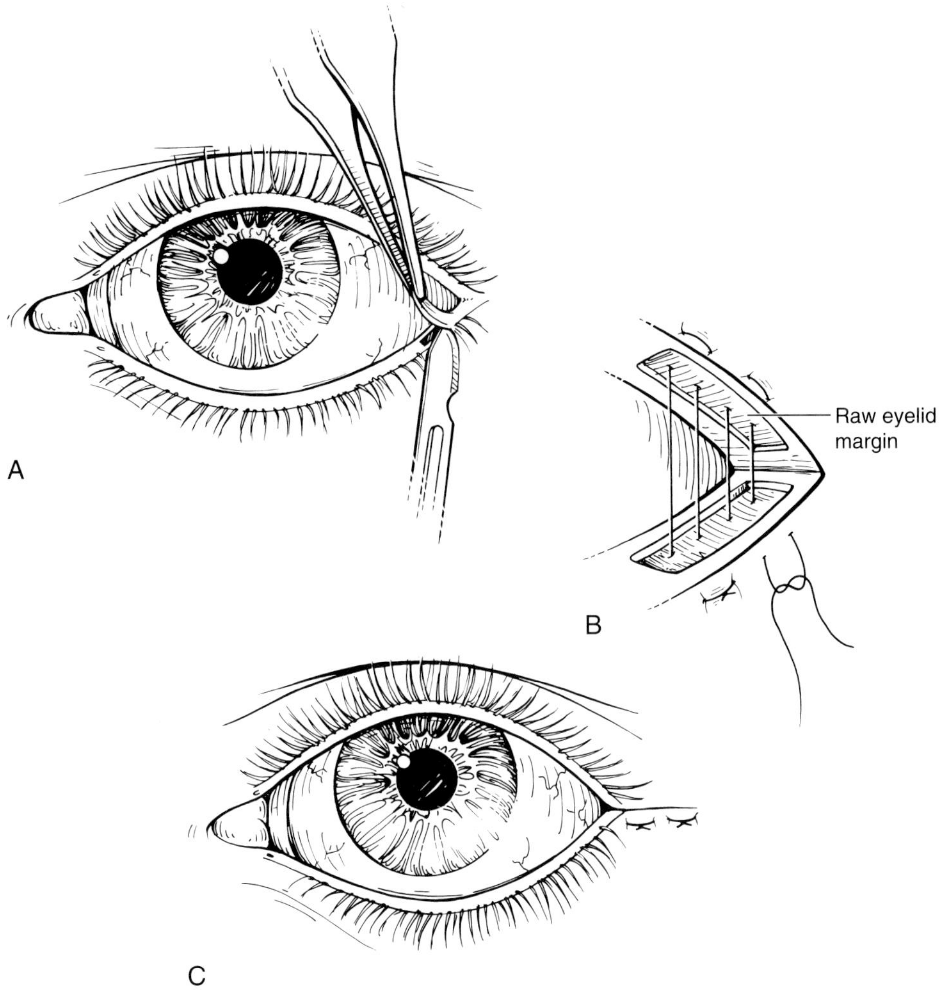

Figure 39–19. Marginal adhesion tarsorrhaphy. *A*, Roughing up opposing areas on lid margins. *B*, Placement of double-armed sutures of 4-0 chromic or silk. *C*, Tightening of the eyelid sutures.

A scalpel is used to abrade juxtaposed areas from the lateral upper and lower eyelids. Double-armed sutures enter through the center of the raw eyelid margin. The needle then enters into the opposite eyelid margin at a point corresponding within the freshened area and then exits anteriorly through the skin of the opposing eyelid. The sutures are then tied and left in place for several weeks. Opening the tarsorrhaphy is accomplished easily with a straight scissors at a future date.

If a more permanent type closure is desired, a tarsal transposition tarsorrhaphy can be performed by transposing a bridge of tarsus (Fig. 39–20). The tarsorrhaphy can be performed laterally or medially if necessary. The eyelid is divided into anterior and posterior lamellae at the tarsus–orbicularis interface with a scalpel. The depth of the division is about 5 mm, and the length of the incision is determined by the degree of eyelid closure desired. The posterior lamella is excised from the lower eyelid, and the posterior lamella from the upper eyelid is advanced into the defect thus created. The superior flap is mobilized by sharply dividing it along its medial end. Double-armed 4-0 or 5-0 chromic sutures are used to suture the flap advanced from the upper lid into the defect

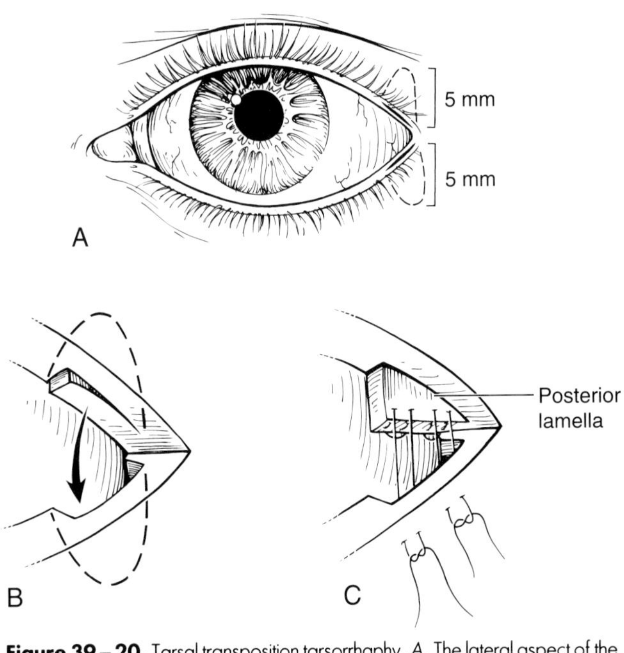

Figure 39–20. Tarsal transposition tarsorrhaphy. *A*, The lateral aspect of the eyelid margin is divided into anterior and posterior lamellae. *B*, The medial aspect of the upper eyelid posterior lamella is divided. The posterior lamella on the lower lid is excised. *C*, Double-armed 4-0 chromic sutures are placed.

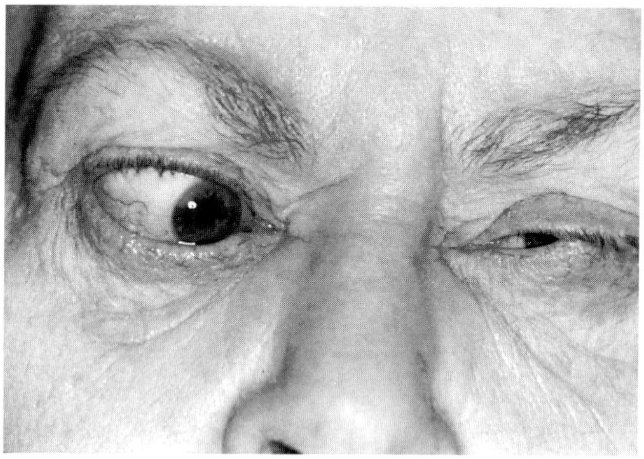

Figure 39–21. Postoperative appearance of cosmetically unacceptable tarsorrhaphy longer than 3 mm.

created in the lower lid. If a medial tarsorrhaphy is performed, the surgeon should not be concerned with reservation of the lacrimal drainage apparatus. In these cases, moisture on the ocular surface is crucial, and therefore lacrimal drainage is not desired and may be sacrificed. In addition, the lacrimal pump is usually not operating, owing to loss of orbicularis function.

By limiting the tarsorrhaphy to less than 3 mm, a somewhat acceptable cosmesis can be obtained, although many patients are less than happy with the aesthetic result (Fig. 39–21). In addition, there is limitation of peripheral vision and the cornea can still break down and scar. Sometimes lysis of the tarsorrhaphy may cause notching of the lid margin, entropion, or formation of epithelial cysts.

Lateral Canthoplasty

Lateral canthoplasties that support the lower lid from the lateral orbital rim and incorporate horizontal lid shortening are best current methods for the repair of paralytic ectropion. Edgerton and Wolfort[10] were the first to describe a technique for support of the lower eyelids in patients with orbicularis oculi palsy. Suspension of the lateral canthus is achieved with a dermal flap of adjacent eyelid skin passed through a hole in the lateral orbital rim. This procedure provides strong support for the paralyzed lid stretching the lid skin against the globe. An objection to this procedure is that it does not incorporate a horizontal lid shortening of the lower lid and thus the horizontal lid aperture remains little changed.

A lateral tarsal strip procedure as described earlier provides an excellent approach to tightening of the lower lid. In more severe cases it may be combined with recession of the lower lid retractors, which serves to weaken the antagonist of the paretic orbicularis and prevent a progressive downward movement of the eyelid (Fig. 39–22).[11]

The anesthetic used is 1% lidocaine with epinephrine. A straight hemostat is placed across the lateral canthal angle, and blunt-tipped tenotomy scissors are used to ligate the lateral canthal tendon. The scissors are then slid along the lateral orbital rim, and an inferior cantholysis is performed. A 4-0 black silk traction suture is placed through the lower lid, and the lid is everted over a Desmarres retractor. The anesthetic is infiltrated subconjunctivally. A no. 64 Beaver blade is used to incise conjunctiva at the level of the inferior tarsal border. Conjunctiva is elevated off underlying Müller's muscle plane, using a no. 64 Beaver blade and Wescott scissors. Müller's muscle and capsulopalpebral fascia are located and marked with a 4-0 black silk suture. Both muscles are dissected off overlying attachments to the orbicularis and orbital septum and from underlying attachments to conjunctiva. A spacer of either fascia lata or retroauricular muscle is used. In particularly severe cases cartilage is utilized for additional support. This is sutured to the inferior tarsal border and to the recessed lower lid retractors. The spacer is then tucked behind the orbicularis plane, and the conjunctiva is closed with a running 5-0 plain suture. A lateral tarsal procedure is then performed as described earlier. The lower eyelid is not placed on stretch (Fig. 39–23).

Eyelid Sling Procedures

The concept of forming a sling to support the lower paretic eyelid has been applied in a number of ways. It is useful especially in cases where a large bulk of atonic midfascial tissues continue to drag down the lower eyelid. Fascia lata has been used in this method for many years (Fig. 39–24). The tissue is obtained while the patient is under general anesthesia in the method described by Soll.[12] Alternatively, banked fascia lata may be utilized. Usually, a 3 × 8-mm strip is adequate. Five-millimeter horizontal linear incisions are made over the insertion of the medial and lateral canthal tendons. The fascia lata is threaded around the anterior insertion of the medial canthal tendon. It is then threaded through the entire lower lid in the pretarsal plane with a Wright needle and brought out over the insertion of the lateral canthal tendon. A bur hole is drilled in the lateral orbital rim, and the fascia lata is threaded through the hole. It is then sutured to itself around the anterior attachment of the medial canthal tendon with a buried 6-0 nylon suture. The fascia lata is then tightened to a sufficient strength to elevate the lid and sutured to itself laterally with buried 6-0 nylon. The muscle plane is closed laterally using 5-0 PDS suture, and the skin is closed using 6-0 nylon. When lower lid laxity is excessive, horizontal shortening of the eyelid may be achieved with a pentagonal resection or lateral tarsal strip, as described previously in this chapter.

The placement of fascia lata close to the eyelid margin

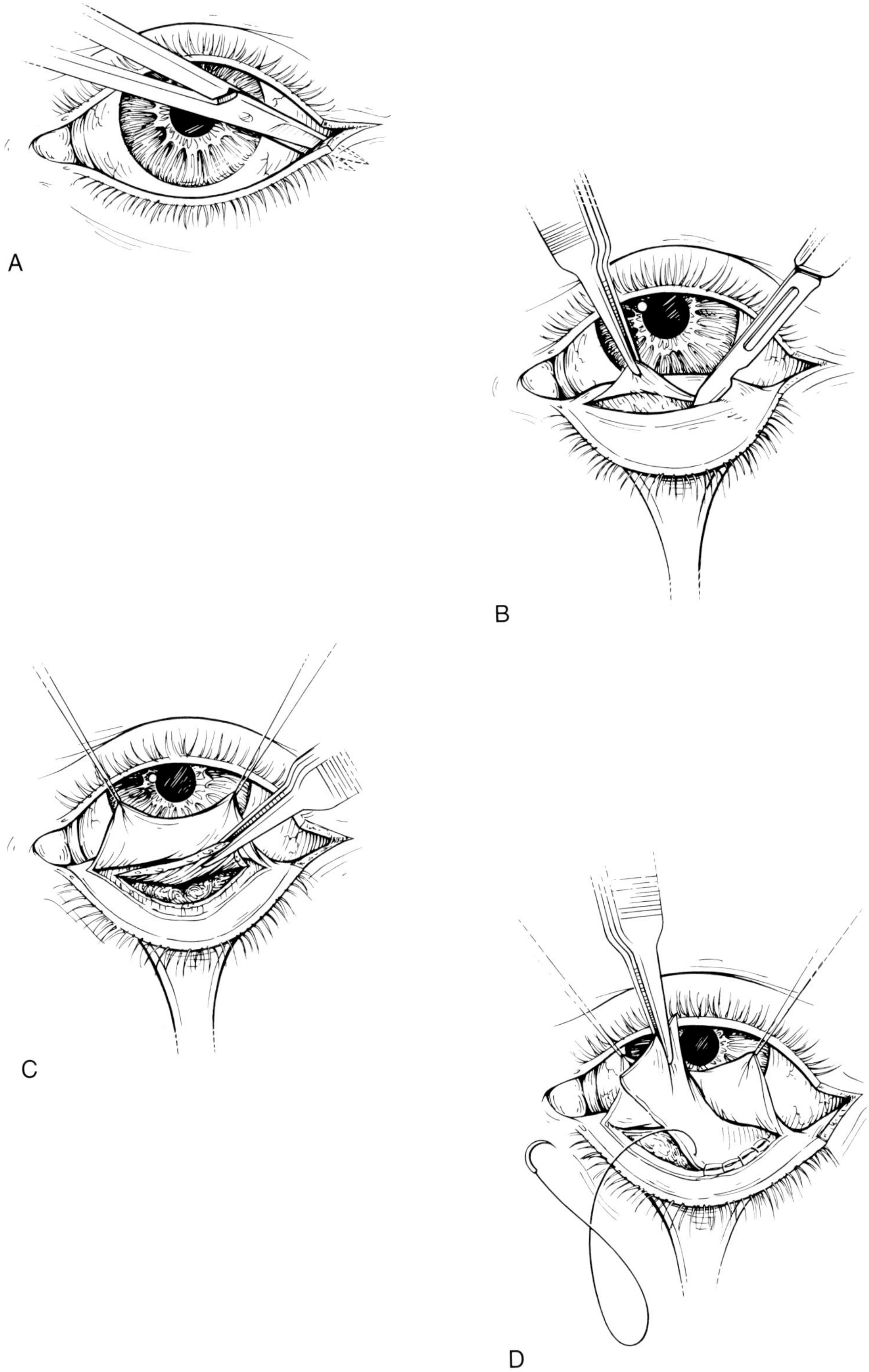

Figure 39–22. Recession of lower lid retractors and lateral tarsal strip. *A*, Lateral canthotomy and inferior cantholysis. *B*, Incising conjunctiva at level of the inferior tarsal border. *C*, Müller's muscle and capsulopalpebral fascia are dissected off overlying attachments to orbicular muscle and septum and underlying attachments to conjunctiva. *D*, Bovine fascia lata is sutured to inferior tarsal border and retractors with 5-0 Vicryl suture.

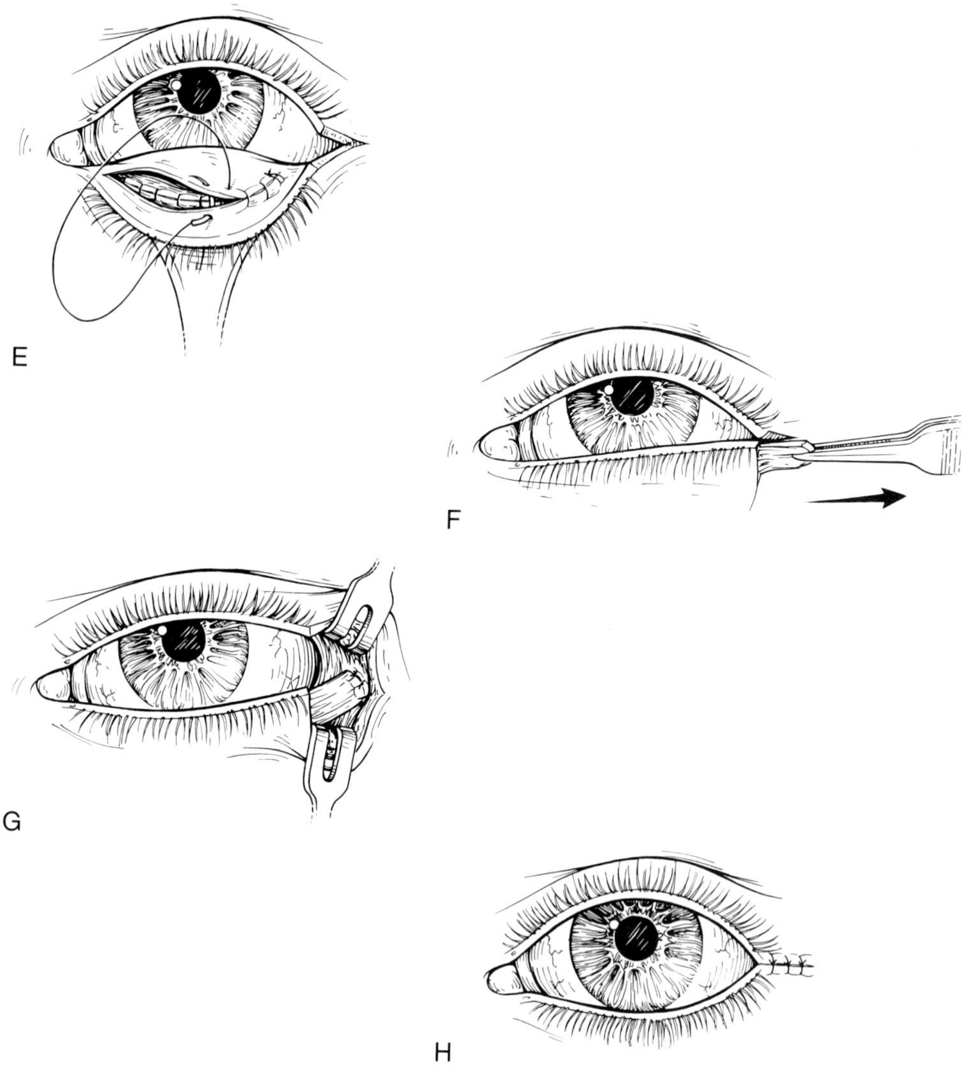

Figure 39 – 22. *Continued E*, Conjunctiva closure with running 5-0 plain suture. *F*, Lateral tarsal strip fashioned. *G*, Lateral tarsal strip sutured to lateral orbital rim with 4-0 Prolene suture. *H*, Closure with 6-0 nylon suture.

is important since placement too low will allow the lid and tarsus to rotate outward over the rigid fascia band. It is possible to see this complication late and may be due to the stretching of the fascia and medial canthal tendon. To overcome this difficulty the alloplastic material polytef (Gortex) has been recommended in place of fascia along with definitive fixation of the sling to bone using a titanium screw.[13] Polytef has a high tensile strength and little elasticity and allows for tissue integration.

Temporalis Transfer

Temporalis transfer has been effectively used to correct paralytic ectropion.[14] It is reserved for the most severe cases of paralytic ectropion that have recurred after a previous surgical procedure and when facial nerve damage is permanent. It provides a viable lower lid sling with prominent, well-supported temporal lift and functioning pretarsal muscle mass. However, it is a more complicated procedure, involving tissue not often handled by the ophthalmic surgeon. Moreover, its sling effect is most predictable laterally since the length and availability of the temporalis may limit its medial sling effect.

A lateral scalp incision overlying the midportion of the temporalis is made (Fig. 39 – 25). This dissection is made in the plane superficial to the temporalis fascia so the entire temporalis may be identified and isolated. A 10-mm strip of muscle is outlined in methylene blue, and the arc of transposition needed to reach the medial canthal tendon can be evaluated and the appropriate length determined. The epicranium, which is adherent to the temporalis fascia, is dissected free. In most cases, 1 cm of epicranium superior and distal to the superior aspect of the temporalis muscle will be essential for medial lid support. The temporalis muscle is incised and the temporalis flap elevated off the skull preserving its pedicle attachment inferiorly. It is crucial to identify and isolate the zygomatic branches of the facial nerve, which are super-

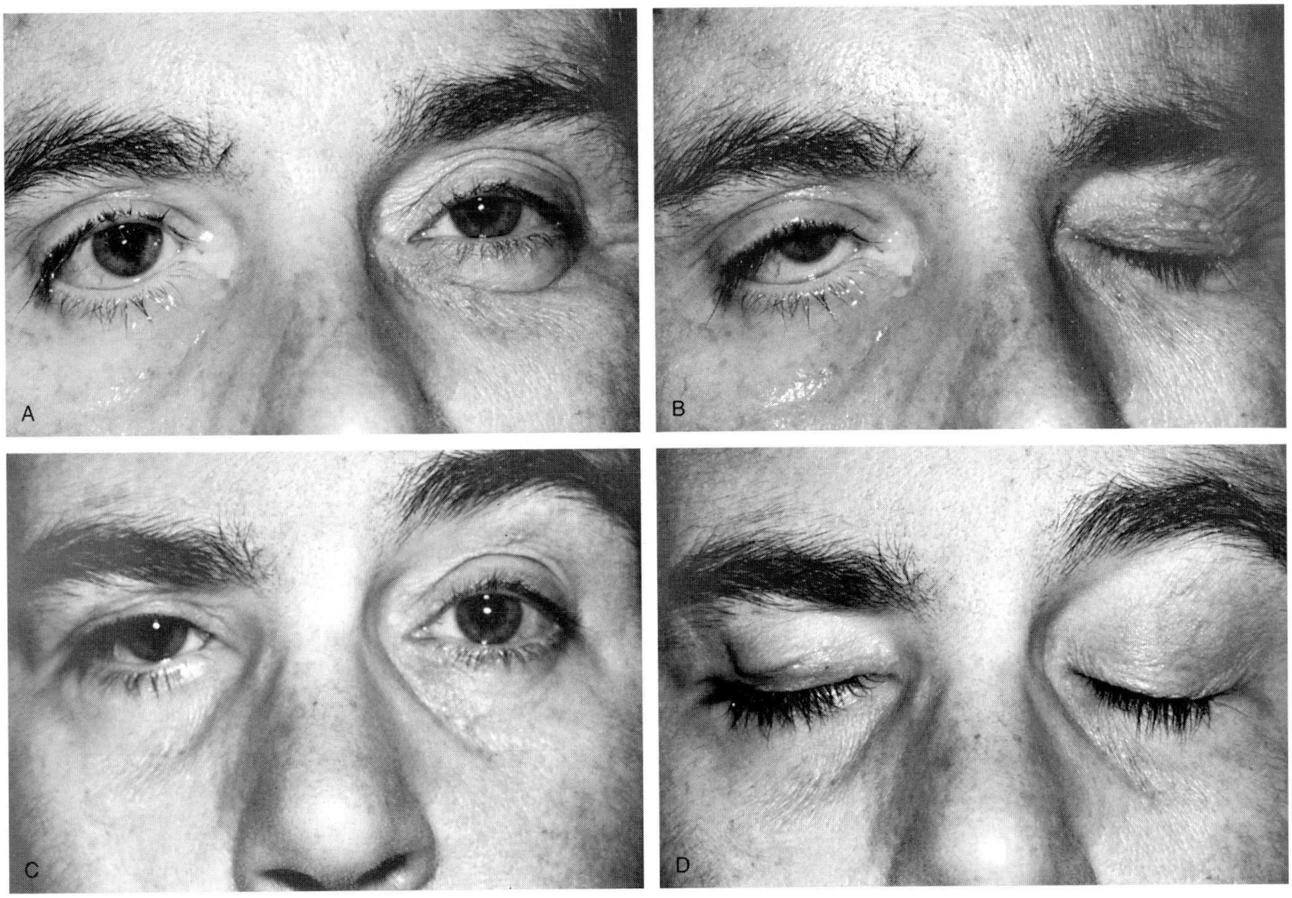

Figure 39 – 23. Preoperative and postoperative appearance of patient with total paralysis undergoing retractor recession surgery and lateral tarsal strip procedure. A gold weight has also been inserted into the upper eyelid. *A*, Preoperative appearance, open. *B*, Preoperative appearance, closed. C, Postoperative appearance, open. *D*, Postoperative appearance, closed.

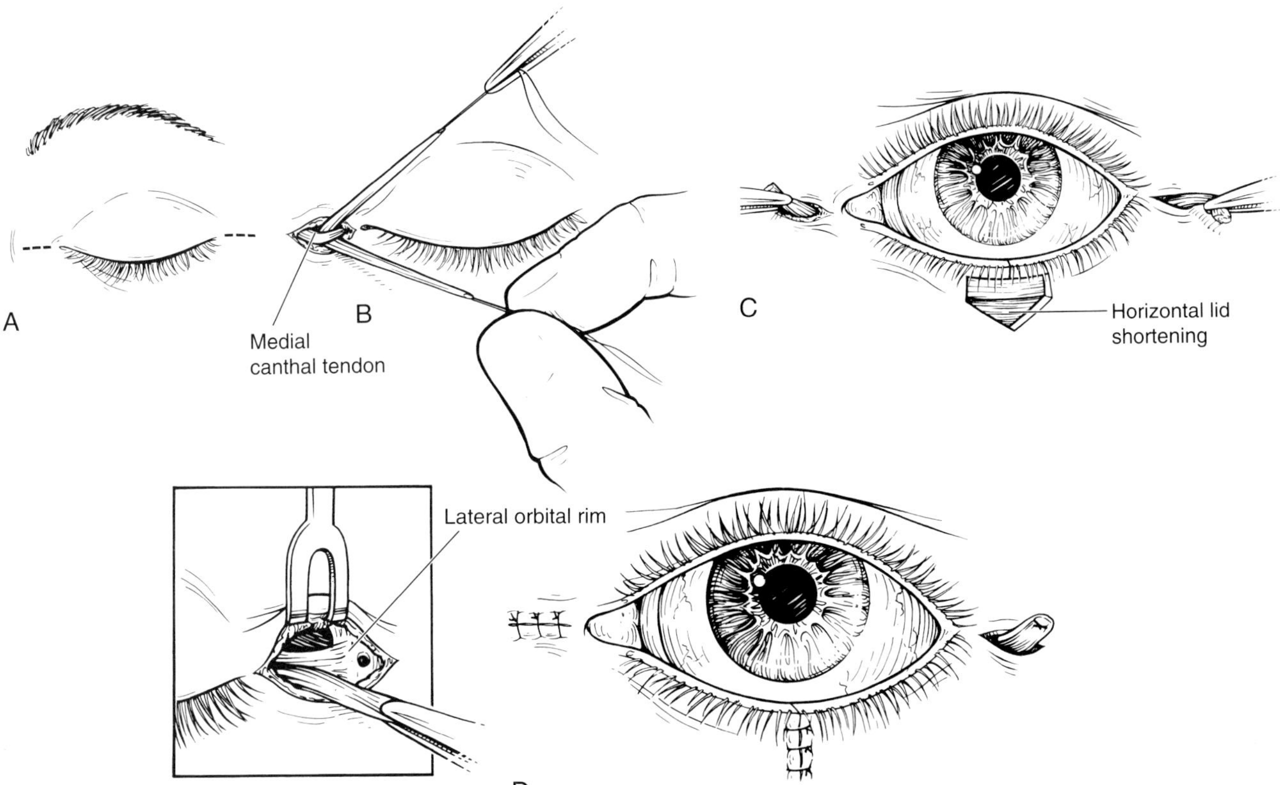

Figure 39 – 24. Repair of lower eyelid laxity using fascia lata. *A*, Five-millimeter horizontal incisions are made over the medial and lateral canthal tendons. *B*, Fascia lata is threaded around the anterior attachment of the medial canthal tendon and sutured with 6-0 nylon. C, Full-thickness pentagon of eyelid tissue has been removed centrally and fascia lata threaded through eyelid into a plane between skin and orbicularis with a Wright needle. *Inset*, Bony opening is drilled in lateral orbital wall temporal to the insertion of the lateral canthal tendon. *D*, Fascia lata has been threaded through the lower lid with the Wright needle and out through the opening in the lateral orbital wall. It is then sutured to itself with 6-0 nylon sutures.

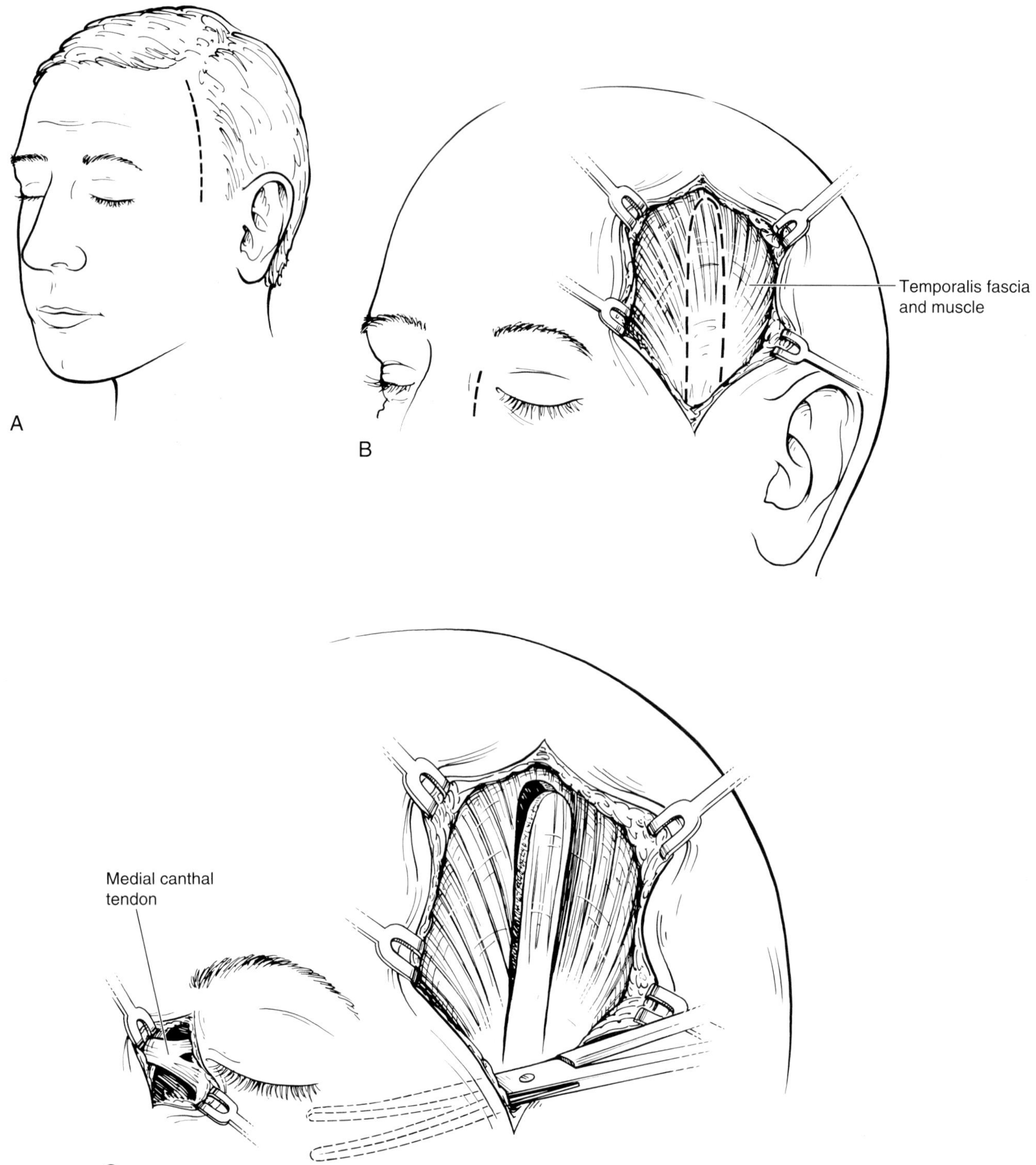

Figure 39–25. Temporalis muscle transfer. *A*, Lateral scalp incision. *B*, Temporalis muscle flap is dissected. *C*, Submuscular tunnel is created just beneath eyelashes.

ficial, overlying the zygomatic arch. A facial nerve stimulator is helpful for this portion of the technique.

A tunnel is made in a submuscular plane lateral to the lateral canthal region and extending just beneath the lashes superficial to the tarsal plate as far as the medial canthal insertion. Tunneling may be performed without a skin incision. Alternatively, if an additional wedge resection of lid is necessary, a skin–muscle flap may be prepared as in a lower lid blepharoplasty. The medial canthal tendon is then exposed. The temporalis is then transposed, passed within the pretarsal tunnel, and sutured to the medial canthal tendon with 5-0 Mersilene suture. The defect left by the transposed temporalis fascia is relatively unnoticed. A drain is placed in the area. The

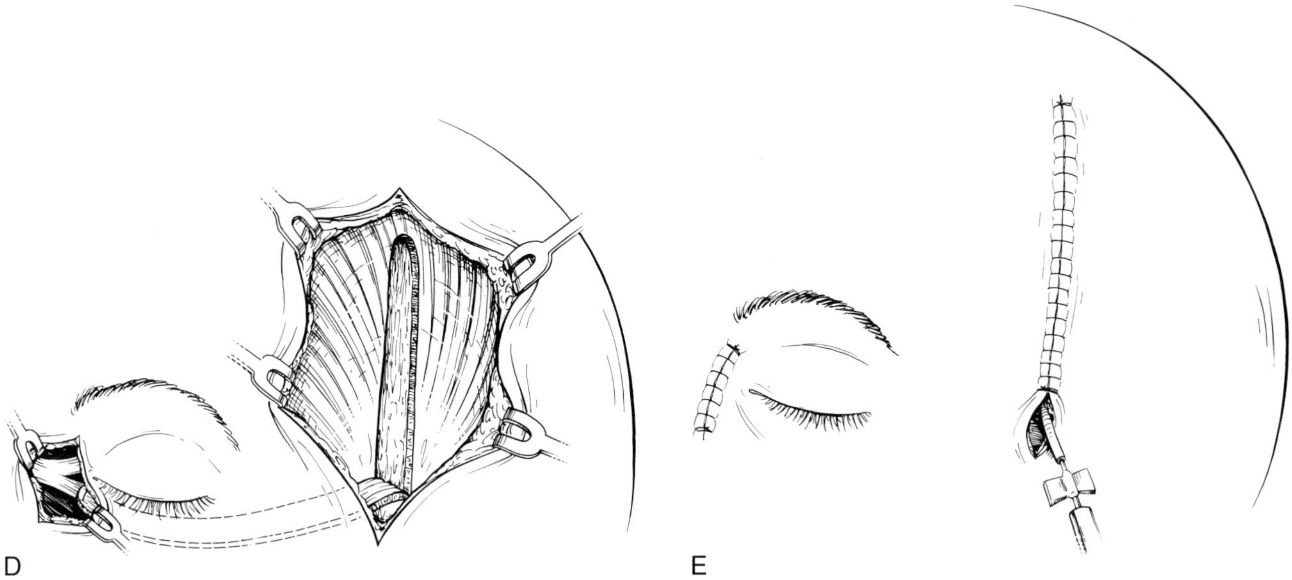

D E

Figure 39–25. *Continued D*, Temporalis muscle is transposed, and canthal tendon is sutured with 5-0 Mersilene. *E*, Closure with 4-0 chromic and 5-0 nylon sutures.

hairline incision is closed with 4-0 chromic suture deeply and 5-0 nylon suture through skin. Postoperative antibiotics are administered.

REFERENCES

1. Hill JC: Analysis of senile changes in the palpebral fissure. Trans Ophthalmol Soc UK 95:49, 1975.
2. Schaefer AJ: Lateral canthal tuck. Ophthalmology 86:1879, 1979.
3. Smith B: The "Lazy-T" correction of ectropion of the lower puctum. Arch Ophthalmol 94:1149–1150, 1976.
4. Smith B, Cherubini TD: Modification of Kuhnt-Symanowski ectopion repair. *In* Oculoplastic Surgery: A Compendium of Principles and Techniques. St. Louis, CV Mosby, 1970.
5. Bick MW: Surgical management of orbital tarsal disparity. Arch Ophthalmol 75:386, 1966.
6. Tenzel RR: Treatment of lagophthalmos of the lower lid. Arch Ophthalmol 81:366, 1969.
7. Tenzel RR, Buffam FV, Miller GR: The use of the "lateral canthal sling" in ectropion repair. Can J Ophthalmol 12:199, 1972.
8. Anderson RL, Gordy DD: The tarsal strip procedure. Arch Ophthalmol 97:2192–2196, 1979.
9. House JW, Brackmann DE: Facial nerve grading system. Otolaryngol Head Neck Surg 93:146–147, 1985.
10. Edgerton MT, Wolfort FG: The dermal-flap canthal lift for lower eyelid support. Plast Reconstr Surg 43:42, 1969.
11. Gilbard SM, Daspit CP: Reanimation of the paretic eyelid using gold weight implantation. Ophthal Plast Reconstr Surg 7:93–103, 1991.
12. Soll DB: The anophthalmic socket. *In* Soll DB (ed): Management of Complications in Ophthalmic Plastic Surgery. Birmingham, AL, Aesculapius, 1976, pp 325–327.
13. Ellis DAF, Kleiman LA: Assessment and treatment of the paralyzed lower eyelid. Arch Otolaryngol Head Neck Surg 119:1338–1344, 1993.
14. Masters FW, Robinson DW, Simonk J: Temporalis transfer for lagophthalmos due to seventh nerve palsy. Am J Surg 110:669, 1965.

CHAPTER 40

Lower Eyelid Retraction and Cicatricial Ectropion

Nancy G. Swartz, Marjorie Murphy, and Marc S. Cohen

When sclera is exposed beneath the inferior limbus in primary gaze, lower eyelid retraction is present. Many factors affect the resting position of the lower eyelid. Most commonly, eyelid retraction is caused by vertical inadequacy in one of the layers of the eyelid. Eyelid retraction can also be the result of horizontal lower eyelid laxity, malposition of the lateral canthal ligament, or proptosis.

It is essential for the surgeon to assess the anatomic cause of eyelid malposition, because this will determine the appropriate surgical plan. Problems of vertical inadequacy can occur in the anterior lamella (skin and orbicularis), the middle lamella (orbital septum and tarsus), the posterior lamella (conjunctiva and retractors), or any combination of these. In this chapter we provide a practical approach to the management of patients with lower eyelid retraction secondary to vertical inadequacy of the lower eyelid.

There are many causes of lower eyelid retraction. The most common are lower eyelid surgery, trauma, and thyroid eye disease.

Eyelid retraction is one of the most common complications of lower eyelid surgery. Anterior lamellar inadequacy occurs when excessive amounts of skin are removed during lower lid blepharoplasty. This problem is exacerbated when uncorrected lower eyelid laxity is present and when the orbicularis and septum are violated.

Middle lamellar shortening can be seen after a variety of common procedures. The septum can be shortened if it is sutured at the time of surgery. However, a more common and less recognized problem results from contracture of the scar that occurs in the plane of the septum.[1] This scar can form whenever the orbicularis and septum are violated. The scar forms a tether between the orbital rim and the tarsus; and as natural contraction of the scar occurs, it pulls the eyelid downward, causing lower eyelid retraction and a rounding and downward displacement of the lateral canthus.[2, 3] This tethering of the lower eyelid can occur whenever there is an incision that violates the septum and orbicularis. The retraction is exacerbated by resection of orbicularis and septum, but the scarring can occur even if the septum is merely incised and no tissue is removed. Patients with preoperative lower eyelid laxity are at highest risk of this postoperative retraction; however, it can occur in any patient who undergoes eyelid or orbital surgery by means of a subciliary incision.

Posterior lamellar problems can occur after inferior rectus recession, because the lower eyelid retractors are attached to the inferior rectus by the capsulopalpebral fascia. Increased retraction can also be seen after orbital decompression, since the lower eyelid retractors are often displaced from their normal anatomic position into the surgical defect in the orbital floor.

When postsurgical lower eyelid retraction is present, chemosis frequently develops, owing to conjunctival exposure and a decreased pumping action of the eyelid. This chemosis tends to weigh down the lid and further exacerbate the retraction, which sets up a vicious cycle that makes the chemosis worse.

Trauma can result in lower eyelid retraction from any of the mechanisms mentioned earlier as well as from chemical and thermal burns. Trauma often results in eyelid retraction because of defects in all layers of the eyelid.

Eyelid retraction is seen in most patients with thyroid eye disease. The lower lid retraction is frequently due to contraction of the posterior lamella and can result from multiple factors. Inflammation and fibrosis of the inferior tarsal muscle and capsulopalpebral fascia is common. Abnormal sympathetic tone in the inferior tarsal muscle can also contribute. When contracture of the superior rectus muscle is present, resultant inferior rectus hyperactivity can retract the lower lid by means of its attachment to the capsulopalpebral fascia.

Patients with lower eyelid retraction have functional and cosmetic complaints. Lower eyelid retraction can cause lagophthalmos and exposure keratopathy. This is especially true when combined with upper eyelid vertical shortening, as seen in patients after four lid blepharoplasty. Patients complain of ocular irritation and tearing due to exposure, decreased tear pump function, and punctal malposition. They are often concerned with the unnatural appearance that results from lateral canthal rounding and dystopia. This is especially true if the contour defect is asymmetric.

Treatment of eyelid retraction is directed toward the reduction of symptoms and restoration of the patient's normal appearance. Lower eyelid retraction can be addressed medically and surgically. The first goal is to lubricate and protect the eye. As a first step, the patient must be instructed to use frequent artificial tears. Next, nighttime applications of bland ointments is added. Most patients also benefit from punctal occlusion. Aggressive lubrication of the eye usually reduces the symptoms of exposure but does not affect the position of the eyelid unless there is chemosis weighing the lid down. Eyelid massage is often helpful to loosen postoperative contracture, especially if it is performed within a few weeks of surgery. Massage may also speed the resolution of chemosis.

In the early inflammatory stages of thyroid ophthalmopathy, corticosteroids may reduce orbital inflammation and cause minimal improvement in retracted lids. These agents reduce inflammation of the eyelid retractors and may also reduce pseudo-lid retraction by decreasing proptosis. Because of the significant risk of adverse side effects with corticosteroids, they are usually reserved for compressive optic neuropathy or rapidly progressive inflammation. Orbital radiation can be used in active thyroid eye disease as an alternative. Some authors advocate the use of radiation to halt the progression of inflammation.

Indications for surgical intervention of lower eyelid retraction include lagophthalmos, exposure keratopathy, and conjunctivitis that is not well controlled with medical management. Surgery is also indicated for patients who wish to obtain a more natural appearance. When evaluating the patient with eyelid retraction preoperatively, the amount of lid retraction should be measured with the patient in primary gaze. The excursion of the eyelid in upward gaze and downward gaze should be noted. Any deep fixation of the eyelid to the orbital rim should be determined by manually pulling upward on the eyelid. The surgeon should also note the presence of any horizontal lower lid laxity, lateral canthal dystopia, and proptosis.

Surgical treatment of lower lid retraction is directed at the underlying anatomic defect. Anterior lamellar defects may be corrected by skin grafts and rotational flaps. Surgery for middle lamellar shortening should be directed toward lysis of the cicatricial tissue and placement of an appropriate spacer graft. Posterior lamellar shortening is most often approached by recession of the lower eyelid retractors either alone or more often with an interpositional graft.

SURGICAL REPAIR OF ANTERIOR LAMELLAR DEFECTS

Anterior lamellar defects are most commonly corrected by replacing the vertical skin inadequacy with a skin graft. Skin grafts can be obtained from the ipsilateral or contralateral upper eyelid, the posterior auricular region, or the supraclavicular region. If excess skin is present in the upper eyelid, we prefer this approach, since this skin best matches that of the lower lid. Generally we choose the contralateral upper eyelid, because when lower eyelid retraction is present, protection of the globe is already compromised. Skin should not be removed from an upper eyelid if there is any ocular irritation due to lid retraction or lagophthalmos.

Harvesting the Graft

The upper eyelid crease is first marked with a skin marker. The predetermined ellipse of skin is then marked in a blepharoplasty-type fashion. Local anesthesia is administered subcutaneously with a mixture of lidocaine 2% with epinephrine in a 9 : 1 mixture with hyaluronidase. The injection is given 15 minutes before the first incision to allow the epinephrine to take effect. This will limit intraoperative bleeding. Hyaluronidase aids in diffusion of the anesthetic. A skin incision is made with a no. 15 Bard-Parker blade, beginning with the lid crease. The skin is then excised with either a blade or scissors, using great care not to buttonhole the tissue. The graft is then inverted over the surgeon's finger, and any excess subcutaneous tissue is removed with scissors. Thinning of the graft is essential to ensure proper vascularization of the graft. The skin at the host site is closed in standard blepharoplasty fashion. The graft tissue is kept moist in a saline-soaked gauze pad until ready for use. At the end of the case, an antibiotic corticosteroid ointment is placed on the wound.

Eyelid Surgery

Adequate local anesthesia is achieved with subcutaneous infiltration of lidocaine 2% with epinephrine in a 9 : 1 mixture with hyaluronidase. An infraciliary skin incision is made with a no. 15 Bard-Parker blade. The skin is undermined as needed. The graft is placed in position, trimmed if necessary, and sutured into position using 6-0 nylon sutures. Four interrupted cardinal sutures are placed first to position and secure the graft. The remaining skin closure can be done in an interrupted or running fashion. Three Frost-type sutures are then placed using double-armed 4-0 Prolene (Fig. 40–1). First, one arm of the suture is passed through the lower eyelid a few millimeters inferior to the margin, exiting just anterior to the margin. It is then passed through the upper eyelid, enter-

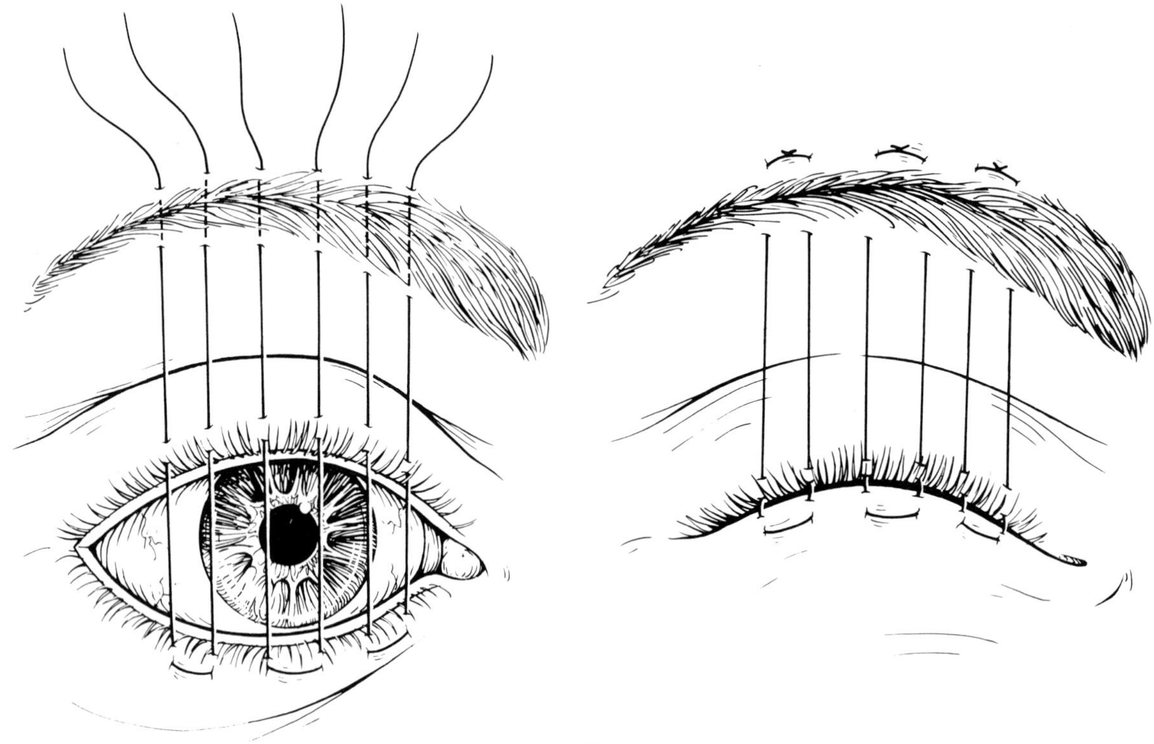

Figure 40–1. *A* and *B*, Placement of Frost-type sutures.

ing just anterior to the margin and exiting a few millimeters superior to the margin. The suture is then passed through the skin and subcutaneous tissue, entering below the brow and exiting above the brow. The second arm of the suture is placed similarly, parallel to the first. After three double-armed sutures are placed, the sutures are pulled upward, closing the eyelids, and tied. An antibiotic/corticosteroid ointment is placed on the wound edges. The graft is then covered with a Telfa dressing, which prevents the dressing from sticking to the graft and allows drainage from the site. A pressure patch is placed to immobilize the graft and is kept in place for 1 week. After 1 week the patch is removed and the Frost-type sutures are cut and removed. Prompt vascularization of the graft is enhanced by meticulous attention to hemostasis, careful suturing, proper graft thinning, and immobilization for 1 week with Frost-type sutures.

SURGICAL REPAIR OF MIDDLE AND POSTERIOR LAMELLAR DEFECTS

Tethering of the middle lamella (from the inferior tarsus to the inferior orbital rim) is the most common postoperative complication of lower eyelid blepharoplasty. Simply lysing this middle lamellar scar by an "in-glove" method, which leaves skin, orbicularis, conjunctiva, and lower eyelid retractors intact and allows healing by second intention, may result in recurrent contraction with postoperative lid retraction. Lysis of the adhesions with placement of a middle and posterior lamellar graft prevents postoperative contraction while adding to the vertical height of the retracted lid.

We recommend recession of the lower eyelid retractors with a spacer between the inferior border of the tarsus and the recessed retractors. This was first reported by Quickert and Dryden,[4] who used sclera as the interpositional graft. Others followed with modifications of this procedure. In 1985, Shorr and Fallor[3] described the "Madame Butterfly" procedure for postblepharoplasty lower lid retraction with a rounded, inferiorly displaced lateral canthus. This involved lysing the middle lamellar cicatrix, reconstructing the lateral canthus, and elevating the cheek to provide additional anterior lamellar skin. This was later modified to include the placement of a middle/posterior lamellar graft.[5]

Many different spacers have been used, including autogenous grafts (e.g., auricular cartilage, nasal septal cartilage, temporalis fascia, fascia lata, tarsus, and hard palate), homologous grafts (e.g., eye-bank sclera, banked fascia lata, and tarsus), and synthetic grafts (e.g., polytetrafluorethylene and collagen film). Although donor sclera has historically been the most popular spacer, it has numerous disadvantages. The antigenic response and associated lid erythema may persist long into the postoperative period. Variable absorption and shrinkage result in unpredictable lid height. Because no mucosal surface is present, corneal irritation may be seen in the early postoperative period. Banked fascia and tarsus have similar disadvantages. In addition, banked tarsus has a further disadvantage of limited availability.

There is much less absorption secondary to rejection with autogenous grafts. However, fascia and auricular cartilage grafts do not replace inadequate conjunctiva. Initially, ocular irritation may occur; and later contraction occurs as the conjunctiva heals. Additionally, fascia is not as stiff as tarsus and thus not optimal for maintaining eyelid contour. Auricular cartilage grafts are more stiff than tarsus and provide excellent underlying support for eyelids but result in an unnaturally firm eyelid even when crushed before placement. Host site morbidity can also occur.

Composite grafts have the distinct advantage of replacing both tarsus and conjunctiva. A tarsoconjunctival graft can be performed as a lid-sharing procedure or as a free graft. Unfortunately, adequate tissue often cannot be obtained without damaging the host lid. The use of nasal septal chondromucosa has been limited by poor access, limited tissue availability, difficulty with donor site healing, and poor graft survival. Synthetic grafts may extrude secondary to infection or erosion of tissue.

Hard palate does not have the disadvantages of the grafts previously mentioned, and we believe it is the graft material of choice in the correction of lower eyelid retraction. Hard palate is a composite graft that replaces both tarsus and conjunctiva in a single layer, thus providing a mucosal surface as well as structural support. It closely approximates the lower lid tarsus in terms of contour, thickness, and stiffness. Because it is autogenous, it is not at risk for rejection, is well tolerated when grafted into the lower lid, and undergoes only minimal shrinkage after grafting (not more than 0.5 mm). The tissue is abundant and easily obtained with minimal donor site morbidity.

Hard Palate Anatomy

The major disadvantage to the hard palate graft is the surgeon's unfamiliarity with oral surgery. Knowledge of the surgically important anatomy and histology of the palate is key to successfully harvesting a hard palate graft (Fig. 40–2). The palate is divided into two distinct regions. The anterior two thirds, the hard palate, has a bony framework consisting of the palatal processes of the maxillary and palatal bones. The posterior one third, the soft palate, has a fibromuscular basis and is supported posteriorly on each side by two arches called the fauces. The hard and soft palates can be easily distinguished from each other by color and palpation. The hard palate is firm and light pink. The soft palate is flaccid and red.

Three paired foramina open into the oral aspect of the hard palate. The incisive foramina open in the midline just behind the central incisors. They transmit the nasopalatine nerves and vessels. The greater palatine foramina are located laterally, adjacent to the distal half of the last molar or wisdom tooth. They transmit the greater palatine nerves and vessels. Just posterior to the greater palatine foramina are the lesser palatine foramina, which transmit the lesser palatine nerves and vessels. The sensory nerves supplying the palate are branches of the maxillary nerves. The nasopalatine nerve supplies the lingual gingiva and palatal mucosa anterior to the maxillary canines. The greater palatine nerve supplies the lingual mucosa and hard palate mucosa posterior to the maxillary canines. The lesser palatine nerve supplies the mucosa of the soft palate.

The oral mucosa of the hard palate can be divided into two layers: the epithelium and the lamina propria. The epithelium is composed of keratinized stratified squamous epithelium, and the lamina propria is composed mainly of collagen fibers. In the superficial lamina propria, the collagen fibers are thin and loosely arranged. Beneath this layer, the lamina has collagen arranged in thick bundles that lie parallel to one another and the surface of the mucosa. It is the dense concentration of collagen fibers in the mucosa of the hard palate that gives this tissue its stability and allows it to serve as a replacement for the tarsus.

The submucosa of the hard palate consists of loose fatty and glandular connective tissue and contains major blood vessels and nerves. The submucosa is present only in certain parts of the hard palate soft tissue. Along the medial gingival border, near the teeth, there is no defined submucosa; rather, there is a dense collagen network called the mucoperiosteum that connects the epithelium to the periosteum. A narrow zone along the midline of the palate, in the area of the palatine raphe, is also mucoperiosteum.

Hard palate grafts are harvested from the area between the gingiva and the palatine raphe. This region makes up a paired area that constitutes the majority of the roof of the mouth. In this region the submucosa is well defined and clearly separates the mucosa from the periosteum. The dissection for harvesting hard palate grafts occurs in the submucosal plane. Any fatty submucosa adherent to the graft is then excised, leaving the epithelium and firm collagenous lamina propria.

Hard Palate Surgery

This procedure is carried out using local standby anesthesia. Local block is accomplished with lidocaine 2% with epinephrine mixed with hyaluronidase in a 9:1 concentration.

The majority of the palatine mucosa and submucosa is firmly adherent to periosteum, and it is difficult to administer local infiltrative anesthesia. However, there is loose connective tissue in the regions of the incisive and greater palatine foramina. If the needle is properly placed in these regions, up to 0.5 mL of anesthetic can be easily

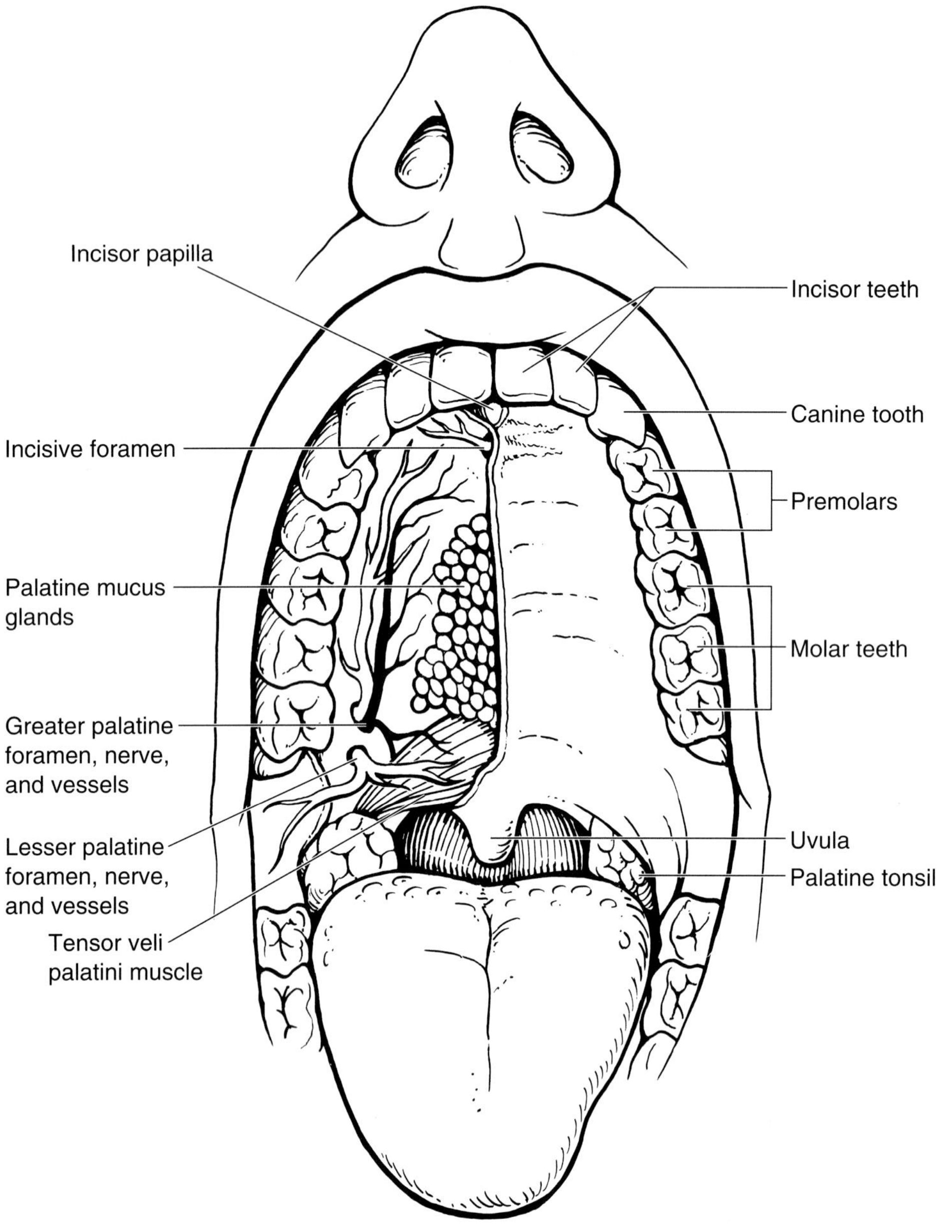

Figure 40–2. Hard palate anatomy.

administered without resistance. In addition, because the major vessels of the palate enter with the nerves, injections in the area of the foramina aid in hemostasis.

Greater Palatine Nerve Block

Due to the configuration of the mouth, the needle cannot be introduced vertically into the greater palatine foramen but must be introduced tangentially at the distal half of the last molar. The puncture is made at the apex of the curving mucosal arch between the roof of the mouth and the alveolar process (which hold the teeth). The needle is advanced superiorly, laterally, and posteriorly.

Nasopalatine Nerve Block

The mucosa in the region of the incisive foramina is elevated, forming the incisive papillae. The papillae are extremely sensitive, and thus the needle should be placed lateral to them. The direction of the needle is superior, medial, and posterior. Because of the proximity of the two nasopalatine nerves, a properly placed nasopalatine block will lead to bilateral anterior palatal anesthesia (anterior to the canines).

Harvesting the Graft

Hard palate grafts demonstrate minimal (0.5 mm) to no shrinkage, and thus the graft size need not be made ex-

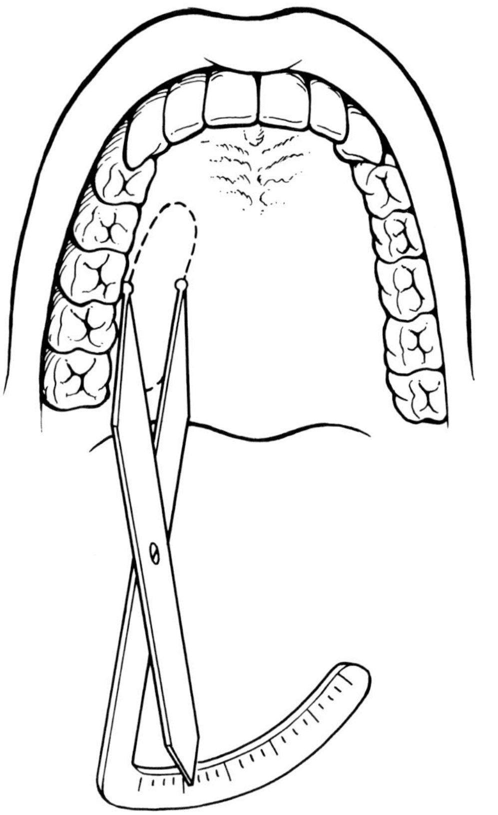

Figure 40–3. Marking the hard palate graft.

cessively large. An elliptical hard palate graft is fashioned with the vertical and horizontal dimensions closely approximating the amount of lower lid retraction. The hard palate is dried, and the predetermined size of the graft is then marked on the mucosa with a skin marker (Fig. 40–3). The mark should be made between the median raphe and the alveolar process. A no. 15 Beaver blade is then used to incise the area marked (Fig. 40–4). The edge of

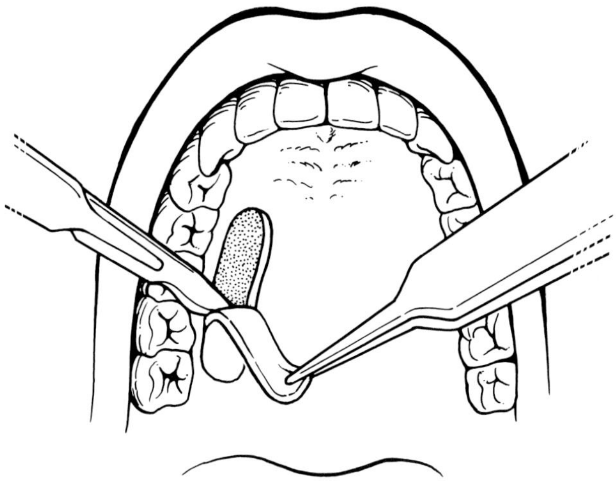

Figure 40–5. Undermining the graft.

the graft is then lifted using 0.5 Castroviejo forceps, and the dissection is carried out in the plane of the submucosa by using a Wescott scissors or a no. 15 Beaver blade (Fig. 40–5). The use of suction by the surgical assistant will control any blood that would otherwise trickle down the patient's throat. In the presence of bleeding, digital pressure is exerted through a gauze pad for a few minutes. Cautery is rarely needed. Coe-Pak (Coe Laboratories, Chicago, IL) can be placed in the defect if desired to reduce postoperative discomfort. Coe-Pak is a putty-like substance routinely used by periodontists. It can be obtained from a dental supply house. An acrylic or copolyester surgical impression plate, quickly and easily fashioned preoperatively by a dentist, can also be placed on the hard palate to aid in postoperative comfort. This is held in place by a denture adhesive (Fig. 40–6). Alternatively, a Telfa pad is placed over the wound and covered with a moistened 2 × 2-inch gauze pad. After the graft has been harvested, any adherent fatty submucosa is re-

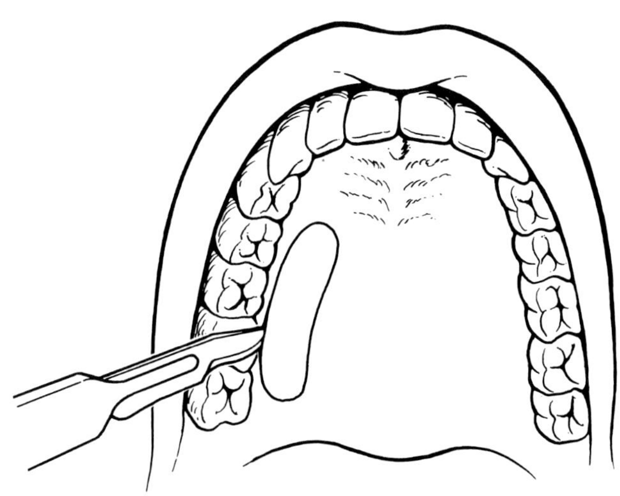

Figure 40–4. Incising the hard palate graft.

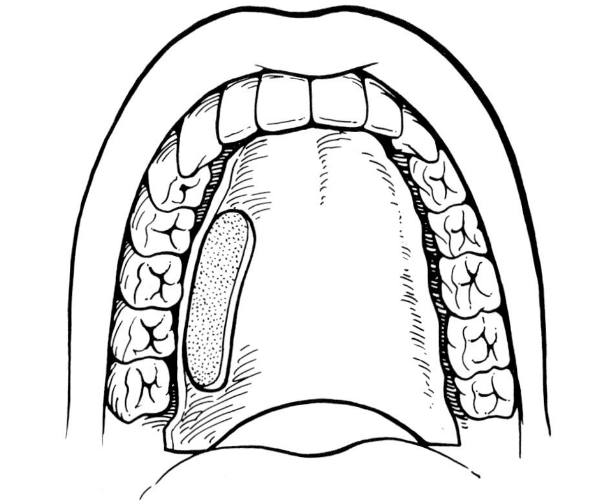

Figure 40–6. Surgical impression plate in place.

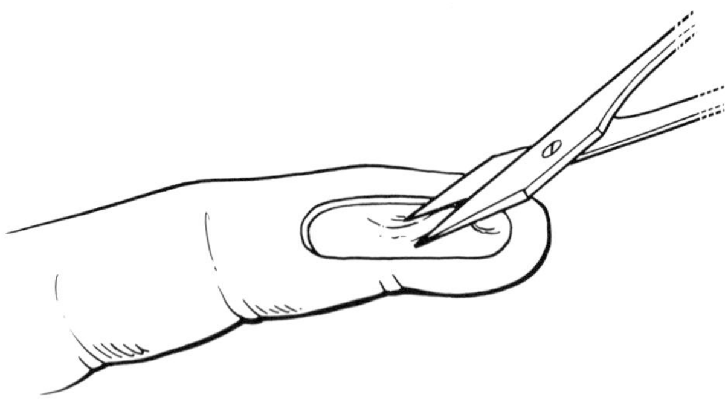

Figure 40–7. Thinning of the graft.

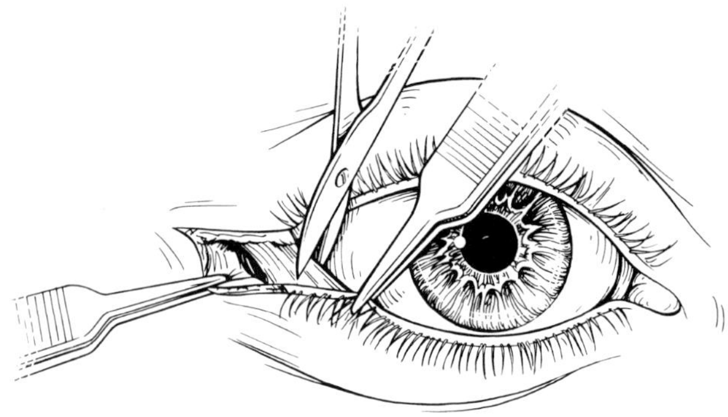

Figure 40–9. Lateral cantholysis.

moved with scissors in a manner similar to thinning a skin graft (Fig. 40–7). The graft is then wrapped in a saline-moistened gauze pad until ready for use. Although the use of Coe-Pak and a surgical impression plate reduces postoperative discomfort, these are not essential, and the wound will still heal properly even if no dressing is used.

Eyelid Surgery

The procedure is carried out using local standby anesthesia. Local infiltrative anesthesia using lidocaine 2% with epinephrine and hyaluronidase is administered subcutaneously in the lower lid and the lateral canthal region and subconjunctivally at the inferior tarsal border of the lower lid. It is also injected in the deep tissues laterally to anesthetize the periosteum of the orbital rim. A skin incision is made in the lateral canthus with a no. 15 Beaver blade (Fig. 40–8). Stevens tenotomy scissors are then used to make a lateral canthotomy and to sever the inferior limb of the lateral canthal ligament (Fig. 40–9).

A forced elevation test of the lower lid is performed to assess the resistance present (Fig. 40–10). Normal lower eyelids can be freely lifted to cover the cornea to the superior limbus. Any tethering of the middle lamella must be lysed. This can be performed by placing the Stevens tenotomy scissors through the original cathotomy incision with the blades below the inferior border of the tarsus and perpendicular to the plane of the orbital septum while the lid is held in forced elevation (Fig. 40–11). An "in-glove" dissection is performed such that all lid tissue between the orbicularis and conjunctiva is included in the incision. The surgeon will feel the cicatrix release as it is lysed. Dissection should be carried out wherever scar is present, as determined by the forced elevation test. It is not unusual for dissection to involve the entire length of the eyelid. Successful lysis is indicated by the ability to elevate the lower eyelid margin to the superior corneal limbus.

Horizontal shortening of the lower eyelid is now performed. The amount of horizontal excess is measured by draping the lower lid up into the desired position and identifying the location of the new lateral canthal angle. The eyelid margin lateral to this position is excised, taking care to remove lash follicles. A skin–muscle flap is dissected from the tarsus to the point of the new lateral canthal angle, and the underlying conjunctiva is likewise dissected free (Fig. 40–12). The periosteum of the lateral orbital rim is exposed with blunt dissection, taking care not to remove periosteum. A double-armed 5-0 Dexon horizontal mattress suture is placed through the newly fashioned tarsal tongue and periosteum but is not tied at this time (Fig. 40–13). The conjunctiva is now opened just below the inferior tarsal border.

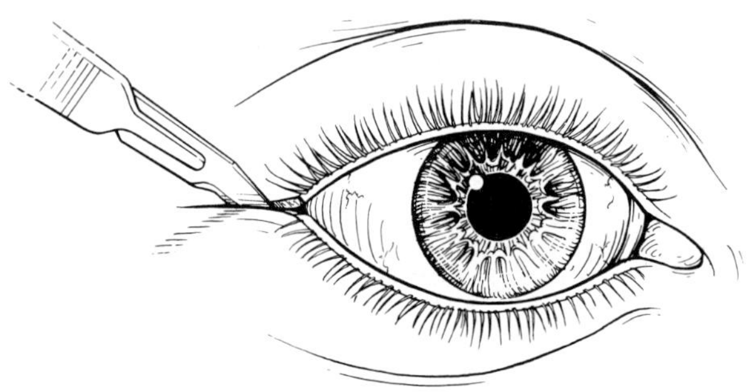

Figure 40–8. Skin incision for lateral canthotomy.

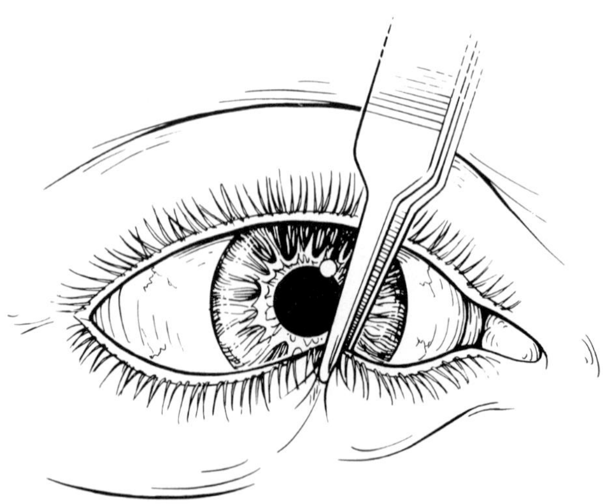

Figure 40–10. Forced elevation test of the lower lid.

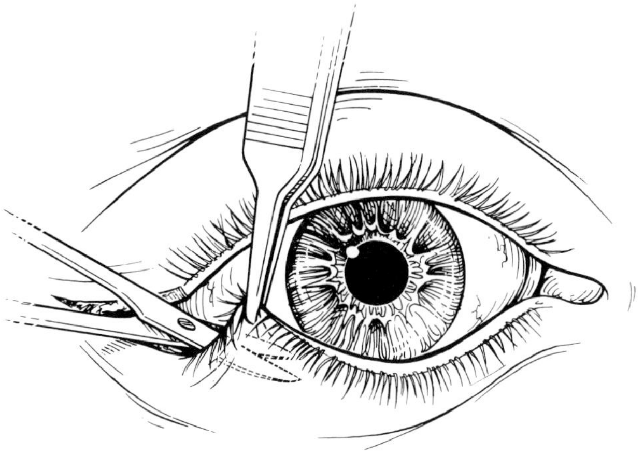

Figure 40 – 11. In-glove lysis of middle lamellar cicatrix.

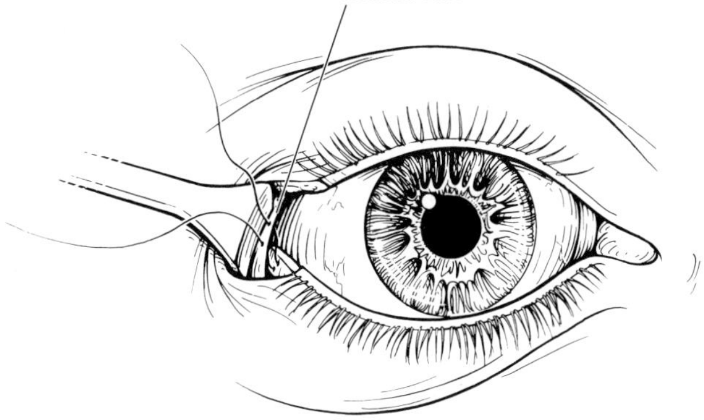

Figure 40 – 13. Suturing of the tarsal strip to the periosteum.

Attention is now turned to the hard palate graft. The graft is placed into its correct position (Fig. 40 – 14). To avoid corneal irritation, the superior edge of the graft is sutured in place with buried sutures. This is accomplished by rotating the inferior edge of the graft upward and keeping the superior edge of the graft adjacent to the superior edge of the host site. By placing partial-thickness sutures, the superior edge of the graft can be sutured in place to the tarsus with 6-0 mild chromic sutures that will become buried when the graft is returned to its proper position (Fig. 40 – 15). After suturing the superior edge and then returning the graft to its original position, the inferior edge of the graft can then be sutured to the cut edge of the conjunctiva and retractors (Fig. 40 – 16). These sutures do not cause corneal irritation because they are placed deep in the fornix. Three Frost-type sutures with brow suspension are then placed. A corticosteroid/antibiotic ointment is placed in the eye, and a pressure dressing is applied. This patch should not be removed for 1 week. The patient is advised that this patch is actually a "cast" that immobilizes the lid and graft so

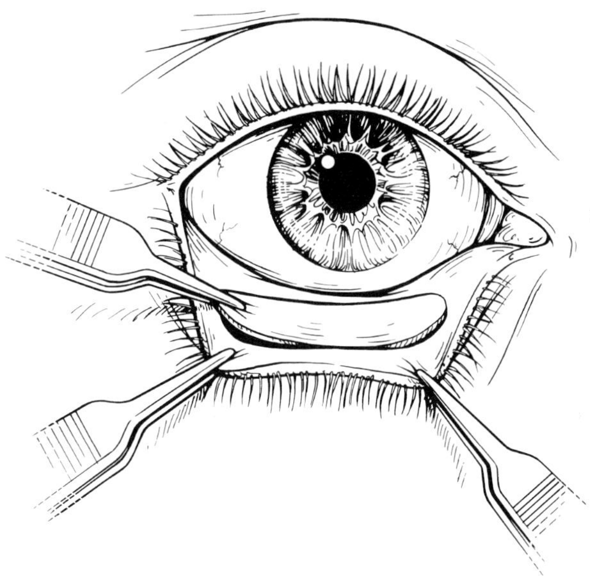

Figure 40 – 14. Placement of the graft.

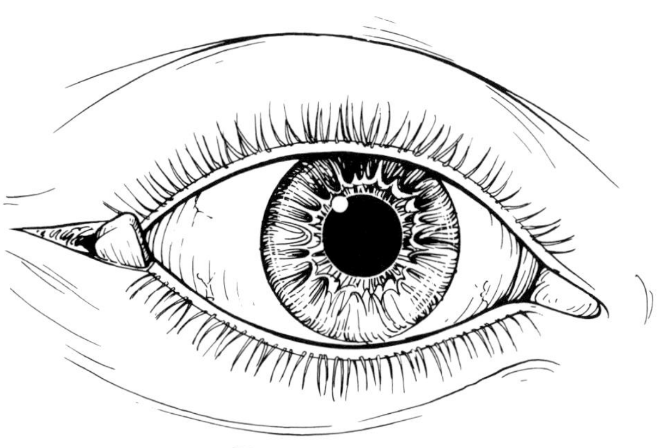

Figure 40 – 12. Creation of the lateral tarsal strip.

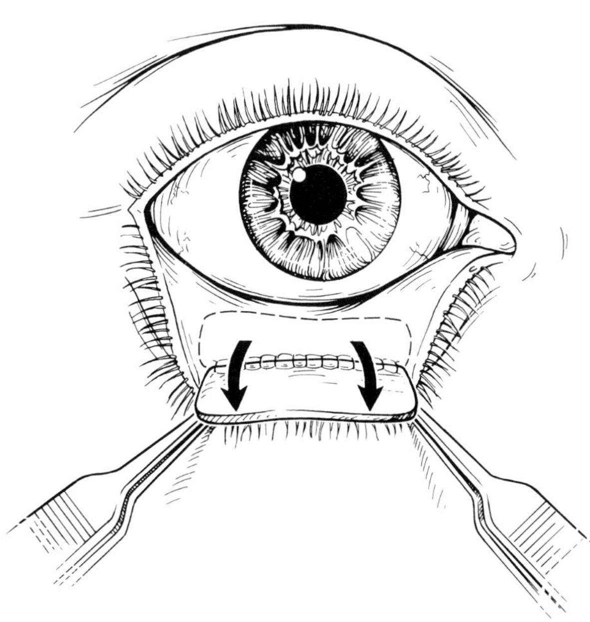

Figure 40 – 15. Placement of superior sutures with graft everted.

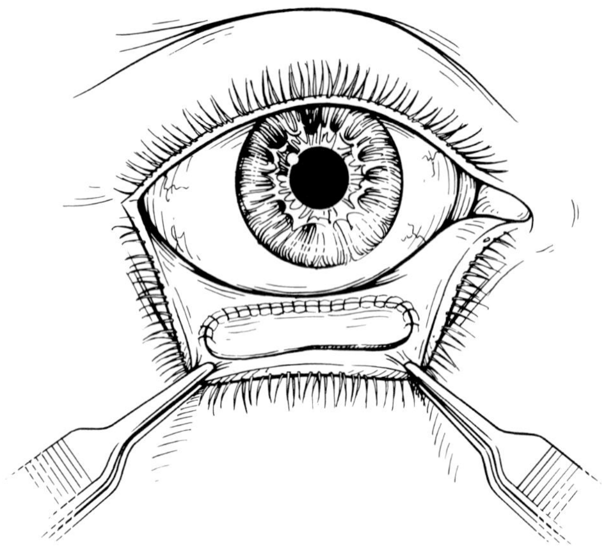

Figure 40–16. Placement of inferior sutures with graft replaced, leaving superior sutures buried.

that proper healing can occur. After 1 week the patch is removed and the Frost-type sutures are cut and removed. Prompt vascularization of the graft is enhanced by meticulous attention to hemostasis, careful suturing, proper graft thinning, and immobilization for 1 week with Frost-type sutures.

REFERENCES

1. Hamako C, Baylis HI: Lower eyelid retraction after blepharoplasty. Am J Ophthalmol 89:517–521, 1980.
2. Shore JW: Scleral show. Plast Reconstr Surg 81:812–813, 1988.
3. Shorr N, Fallor MK: "Madame Butterfly" procedure: Combined cheek and lateral canthal suspension procedure for post-blepharoplasty "round up" and lower eyelid retraction. Ophthal Plast Reconstr Surg 1:229–235, 1985.
4. Quickert MH, Dryden RM: Lower eyelid advancement. Presented at the meeting of the American Society of Ophthalmic Plastic and Reconstructive Surgery, Las Vegas, September 17, 1971.
5. Cohen MS, Shorr N: Eyelid reconstruction with hard palate mucosa grafts. Ophthal Plast Reconstr Surg 8:183–195, 1992.

CHAPTER 41

Aponeurotic Ptosis

Jonathan Christenbury

Many outstanding texts, chapters, and articles have been written describing the treatment of blepharoptosis. There are a number of sources that are constantly referred to by eyelid surgeons regarding the anatomy and physiology of the upper eyelid, as well as classic works in the treatment of blepharoptosis.[1-4] In this chapter I present my approach to the evaluation of the patient with ptosis, a philosophic rationale for choosing a particular surgical procedure, and a description of the surgical procedures, including common complications and revisions. I have developed this systematic approach to blepharoptosis after 6 years of a practice limited to ophthalmic plastic surgery. The advantages of this approach include reliability of the result; patient satisfaction; speed and efficiency of the surgery, which limits intraoperative complications; and a low rate of revision.

PATIENT EVALUATION

The patient with aponeurotic ptosis has an acquired condition,[5] resulting from a defect in transmission of the levator muscle force to the eyelid. This is caused by thinning, stretching, or disinsertion of the levator aponeurosis. The aponeurotic abnormality is most commonly an involutional change, but trauma and prior surgery are frequent causes. The patient either gives a history of a progressive ptosis that rarely varies during the day or may relate an incident after which the ptosis becomes evident, including blunt trauma or cataract or retinal surgery. A long history of daily contact lens wear may precede the development of ptosis from frequent manipulation of the eyelids. On examination, the amount of ptosis may be mild, moderate, or severe. The levator function is usually normal— 10 to 16 mm. Occasionally in a disinserted levator aponeurosis with severe ptosis the levator function is measured as low as 8 mm, owing to a very poor transmission of the levator power to the eyelid. In these cases the lid crease is often very high and the eyelid is easily everted. After ptosis correction the levator function will be measured as normal.

Measurement of the amount of ptosis is difficult. Various inaccuracies are inherent in this measurement. The simplest method involves measuring the vertical palpebral fissure, but malposition of the lower eyelid can affect this measurement. The marginal reflex distance is the measurement between the pupil light reflex and the upper eyelid margin. I dislike this measurement for three reasons: (1) it is a small number and error affects the result dramatically; (2) a bright fixation light used to create the reflex light causes many patients to squint, which alters the measurement; and (3) severe ptosis cannot be measured because the light reflex is covered. The distance between the inferior limbus and upper eyelid, I believe, is an easier measurement to make and can be compared with the fellow upper eyelid level. Also, if compensatory lid retraction is present, this can be documented with the same inferior limbus to upper eyelid measurement (normal, 9 mm). I have performed ptosis surgery many times by estimating the amount of ptosis, measuring the levator function, and taking a Polaroid photograph, without measuring the actual amount of ptosis. Since the amount of levator surgery is adjusted on the operating table and not a measured resection, the amount of ptosis is not critical to know during surgery. The lid crease should be noted, but this is more accurately measured at the time of surgery. Excess skin and fat are noted, as well as contour deformities. The patient is asked to close the eyelids tightly, and orbicularis strength and presence of Bell's phenomenon are noted simultaneously. The cornea is checked for evidence of keratitis sicca by the amount of tear film and fluorescein staining, and a baseline secretion test is done if dryness is suspected. The patient is apprised of the risks and benefits of surgery, and informed consent is obtained. All patients undergo medical clearance before surgery. Use of aspirin and nonsteroidal anti-inflammatory agents is avoided for at least 2, but preferably 4, weeks before surgery.

The upper eyelid consists of a skeleton of contoured tarsus hinged to the orbit by medial and lateral canthi. The levator muscle, an extraocular muscle, has a broad attachment to the anterior surface of the tarsus and the canthi by an aponeurotic tendon. The Müller muscle–conjunctiva complex forms a second attachment between the levator muscle and the superior border of the tarsus. The ligament of Whitnall acts as a pulley so the effective vector force of the levator muscle is changed from a horizontal to a more vertical direction, allowing eyelid elevation. Orbital fat cushions the movement of the eyelid, provides aesthetic soft tissue contours, and influences the appearance of the upper lid crease. It is an important landmark reference for identification of the levator muscle during ptosis surgery. The orbital septum extends from the superior orbital rim to the upper eyelid crease, where it fuses with the levator aponeurosis. The upper eyelid crease is the superiormost fusing of the aponeurosis with the orbicularis–skin complex.

CHOICE OF THE PROCEDURE

All of the previously mentioned structures are critical for the proper functioning and appearance of the eyelid and should be preserved if possible during surgery. Ptosis surgery should be designed to elevate the upper eyelid to a normal level and contour. Symmetry of both the eyelid margin and the lid crease should be the goal while maintaining eyelid closure. A procedure directed toward either the levator aponeurosis or Müller's muscle is usually performed, with some excision of excess skin and fat and with particular attention to re-forming the lid crease. I perform a Müller's muscle resection for 2 mm or less of ptosis that responds to phenylephrine (Neo-Synephrine) and a levator procedure for all other ptosis of an acquired condition. I rarely perform a Fasanella-Servat procedure for 2 mm or less of ptosis. The Fasanella-Servat procedure often causes a contour deformity: high lateral and low medial eyelid. Also, it is more difficult to revise both the height and the contour of an undercorrection when a tarsectomy has been performed. If a Fasanella-Servat procedure is performed, recurrent ptosis can occur months or years later and is more difficult to correct with a levator procedure. Resection of Müller's muscle can give a predictable result for minimal ptosis, provides a normal contour, avoids corneal abrasion, and is more forgiving if an overcorrection occurs.

With experience, each eyelid surgeon generally develops a fairly reliable technique to advance or resect the levator aponeurosis to a normal height. However, even the most experienced eyelid surgeon can have difficulty in providing a normal or acceptable lid contour postoperatively, especially if bilateral surgery is performed. In preoperative photographs the ptotic eyelid usually has a normal contour. It is the effect of the surgery on the structures of the eyelid that causes an abnormal contour. Understanding these effects allows a more predictable and acceptable result.

APPLIED ANATOMY

The levator aponeurosis has a broad attachment from the medial canthal area, across the tarsus, to the lateral canthal area. The thickness of the aponeurosis as well as the firmness of its attachment is stronger laterally than medially. Also, Müller's muscle attachment is weaker medially. Therefore, with any generalized shortening of advancement of the aponeurosis there will always be a tendency to elevate the lateral upper eyelid more than the medial upper eyelid, thus causing an abnormal alteration of the lid contour. This contour deformity is accentuated if the tenuous medial aponeurotic attachments are severed during ptosis surgery or if the lateral aponeurosis is overresected.

In levator resection I preserve Müller's muscle and the medial aponeurotic attachment and advance the central aponeurosis with one or more sutures. The central suture is placed and adjusted during surgery while the patient is supine and fixating straight ahead. I use nonabsorbable sutures of 6-0 prolene suture on a spatula needle. The central aponeurosis is advanced and resected, never tucked. If noticeable medial ptosis is present preoperatively or if the medial contour for some reason appears low during surgery, then the medial aponeurosis can be plicated with a horizontal mattress suture of 6-0 prolene suture. The lid crease is re-formed to the cut edge of the levator.

SURGICAL PROCEDURE

The patient is placed in the supine position in the operating room where cardiovascular monitoring and resuscitation equipment are available. An intravenous line is started and methohexital (Brevital) (25–75 mg) is given intravenously just before injection of the local anesthetic. Lidocaine (Xylocaine) 2% with 1 : 100,000 epinephrine and 0.1 mL of hyaluronidase (Wydase) per 10 mL of anesthetic is given as a subcutaneous injection with a 25-gauge ⅝-inch needle. One to 2 mL is injected just under the skin in the lid crease centrally, medially, and laterally. The skin puncture marks are helpful in identifying the upper eyelid crease after the patient is prepared and draped. The hyaluronidase allows rapid dissolution of the volume of anesthetic injected so the eyelid landmarks are easily identified.

The advantages of methohexital are that it has a rapid onset and that the patient is transiently unconscious for the injection of the local anesthetic and totally awake within 5 to 10 minutes. Apnea may occur briefly with methohexital, but respirations usually resume before the oxygen pulsimeter indicates a decline in oxygen saturation. It is imperative that a certified registered nurse anesthetist or anesthesiologist be available to manage the patient's airway. Once the surgery is underway, small amounts of midazolam (Versed) may be given if necessary to keep the patient comfortable. Too much sedation prevents patient cooperation during suture adjustment. If the patient is oversedated with midazolam, a benzodiazepine reversal agent (flumazenil [Mazicon]) is given. If the surgery is performed in the office without sedation, the local anesthetic is slowly injected using a 30-gauge needle.

The upper eyelid crease is measured and marked with a fine-tipped skin marker. The lid crease medially is 5 to 6 mm above the superior punctum, 8 to 10 mm centrally, and 6 to 8 mm superior to the lateral canthal angle. If a unilateral procedure is performed, then the fellow upper eyelid crease measurement is used. Excess skin is pinched up and marked, but care is taken to make sure the eyelid can be closed with the excess skin pinched. If the lashes evert with the skin pinch technique, caution should be used because maximal skin will be excised. The upper eyelid is placed on inferior traction. Skin and orbicularis is incised with a no. 15 blade and excised with scissors.

With scissors, blunt and sharp dissection is used to excise the skin and orbicularis off the septum. With practice, this can be a rapid maneuver and will increase the speed with which ptosis surgery or blepharoplasty can be performed. A tunnel can be made beneath the skin and muscle, which can even be dissected with unipolar cautery using a fine needle tip or with hot tip cautery.

Mild pressure is placed on the globe over the closed eyelid, the orbital septum is opened with scissors at the superior edge of the incision, and then the septum is excised. Orbital fat is swept superiorly with a Desmarres retractor, and the levator muscle and aponeurosis are identified. Rarely is dehiscence noted. The aponeurosis may be thinned or may appear normal. A hot-tipped cautery with the wire bent is used to incise over the central and lateral third of the levator aponeurosis. The medial aponeurosis is left intact. With the tarsus on inferior traction, the edge of the aponeurosis is lifted with forceps and hot-tipped cautery is used to separate the aponeurosis from its adherence to the superior border of the tarsus and underlying Müller's muscle. Dissection is carried out 10 to 12 mm superiorly. A toothed forceps is used to grasp the tarsus centrally and lift it superiorly to choose the best site for suture placement. This point of "pull" affects the lid contour. A double-armed 6-0 prolene suture with a spatula needle is placed partial thickness in the central tarsus; then each needle is passed through the advanced aponeurosis from posterior to anterior and tied in a temporary bow knot. The patient is asked to fixate at the end of a cotton-tipped applicator, and the height and contour of the eyelid margin is evaluated. The sutures are replaced through the aponeurosis until the lid margin is at, or 1 mm inferior to, the superior limbus. Excess aponeurosis is excised. If the lid contour is satisfactory, the lateral cut edge of the levator muscle is sutured where it lies on the tarsus with the eyelid gently closed.

If the medial contour is low, then a mattress 6-0 Prolene suture is placed to plicate the medial aponeurosis. Since no tarsus exists medially, the suture is passed through whatever tissue elevates the medial eyelid. Fat is excised and cauterized if it is excessive. The lid crease is re-formed with three interrupted sutures that pass from the inferior skin edge and pretarsal orbicularis, edge of levator, and superior skin edge. These sutures are located in the central, medial, and lateral eyelid. The point of crease re-formation should be confirmed with the original caliper measurement. The remaining skin wound is closed with a running suture. I prefer a 6-0 fast absorbing suture (Ethicon) for both the lid crease re-formation and the skin closure. A subcutaneous running 5-0 nylon (Ethicon) suture may also be used in younger individuals. The eye and wound are dressed with antibiotic ointment, the skin is prepared with surgical adhesive (Mastisol), and a firm dressing may be applied with two eyepads and beige paper tape. If bilateral surgery is performed, the eyes are usually not patched.

The patient is seen in the office on the first postoperative day, at which time twice-daily antibiotic ointment to the skin wound, frequent ocular lubricants of either drops or ointment, and frequent iced compresses are recommended.

COMPLICATIONS

Common complications of aponeurotic surgery are overcorrection, undercorrection, contour deformity, lid crease abnormality, soft tissue abnormality, exposure keratitis, lid lag, and lagophthalmos. I have not seen muscle imbalance, ectropion, or infection after this technique of aponeurotic surgery, but these complications have been reported. Conjunctival prolapse was a more commonly seen complication with the standard Berke levator resection when dissection was performed between Müller's muscle and conjunctiva in the superior fornix. I have not seen a case of conjunctival prolapse after aponeurotic surgery. Milia, incision tenderness, skin and cilia anesthesia, prolonged swelling, and recurrent ptosis do, however, occur with aponeurotic surgery.

OVERCORRECTION AND UNDERCORRECTION

Overcorrection is more common than undercorrection in aponeurotic surgery, while the reverse tends to be true in congenital ptosis surgery. Overcorrection occurs when the aponeurosis is overadvanced. Overadvancement is more likely to occur at the time of suture adjustment if the patient is too sedated and cannot cooperate with the surgeon during the adjustment. If the fellow eye is ptotic, and the overcorrection is 1 mm or less, surgery is performed on the fellow eye before considering revision of the first eyelid. The first eyelid may drop slightly after the second eyelid is corrected because of the innervation law of Hering. The innervation tendency works in the favor of the surgeon. This can be determined preoperatively by gently elevating the ptotic eyelid with the finger and observing whether the retracted eyelid drops to a normal level.

If the overcorrection is 1 mm or greater and both the surgeon and patient wish for revision, then a Polaroid photograph is taken and measurements are made of the amount of overcorrection. If the overcorrection is evident in the first 7 to 10 days, local anesthetic is infiltrated as before, the wound is easily pulled apart, and often a single suture is identified as the cause of the overcorrection. The position of the eyelid is noted as the patient gazes at a cotton-tipped applicator. Then the suture is removed and the levator edge is separated from the tarsus, the tarsus is held with a forceps, and the patient is asked to look up, which recesses the levator slightly. The eyelid height is then observed as the patient gazes at a cotton-tipped applicator. The maneuver is repeated until the eyelid has been lowered the desired amount. The levator muscle may be resutured in the new recessed position, over the tarsus, or it may be left unsutured. The eyelid crease is re-formed.

If an undercorrection is identified in the first 7 to 10 days, again a Polaroid photograph is taken and an estimation of the undercorrection is made. The cause is insufficient advancement of the aponeurosis, and at the time of the revision all sutures are removed and the aponeurosis is separated from Müller's muscle by blunt dissection and readvanced and sutured. The height and contour is noted as the patient gazes at a cotton-tipped applicator. The lid crease is re-formed.

If significant swelling is present, this may be the cause of a slight undercorrection, and the eyelid level may be acceptable when the swelling resolves. If overcorrection or undercorrection is recognized after 7 to 10 days and significant swelling is present, it is best to reassure the patient and to plan for a revision in 4 to 6 weeks when all swelling is subsided. Swelling is rarely a factor in overcorrection, but revision can be delayed if the patient is not symptomatic from exposure symptoms. The disadvantage of a later revision is that tissue planes are not as easily identifiable and more dissection is required, more bleeding usually occurs, and the patient has to wait to obtain the desired result as well as undergo two episodes of swelling and healing. I prefer early revision when at all possible.

CONTOUR ABNORMALITY

The normal contour of the eyelid margin is one in which the lateral canthus is slightly higher than the medial canthus and the apex of the eyelid curve is between the light reflex and lateral limbus. Some alteration from this contour may be acceptable, but if the patient complains, it must be revised. A lateral "flaring," central peak, and flat central eyelid are common contour abnormalities. At the time of revision the offending suture is removed or replaced and special attention is given to restoring the normal contour. If a low contour is present, an alternative is either an anterior or posterior localized tarsectomy, in which tarsus is excised at its superior edge and resutured to the Müller muscle–conjunctiva–aponeurosis complex. Interrupted 7-0 Vicryl is used to approximate the edges of the excised tarsus to the levator complex. The skin is closed with absorbing gut suture. This technique is good for the central and lateral low eyelid, but a full-thickness excision may be required for the low medial eyelid. Skin, muscle, aponeurosis, and conjunctiva are excised in an ellipse medially, with a similar closure. In a very senile and lax eyelid, punctal ectropion can occur if conjunctiva is not excised. The punctal ectropion may not cause symptoms of epiphora, but it may be a cosmetic complaint. The cure would involve removing a "spindle" of conjunctiva just above the punctum, similar to what is done for punctal ectropion of the lower eyelid.

HIGH LID CREASE AND RESIDUAL PTOSIS

Once an eyelid crease is high, it is difficult to lower. An incision must be made in the desired crease location, fat must be either grafted over the exposed levator aponeurosis or teased down from the anterior orbit and placed over the levator aponeurosis. However, if residual ptosis and a high lid crease exist together, a full-thickness excision of the eyelid is performed. This "brings the eyelid" up to the lid crease. The superior edge of the resection is drawn at the present high lid crease, and the resection is marked essentially millimeter for millimeter of the amount of residual ptosis. Interrupted 7-0 Vicryl approximates the deep tissues, and the skin is closed with 6-0 fast-absorbing gut suture. No attempt is made to dissect tissue planes or re-form the lid crease.

SKIN EXCISION IN PTOSIS SURGERY

The most difficult revision in ptosis is correcting residual ptosis in the presence of lagophthalmos owing to shortening of the vertical skin dimension. This essentially becomes a two-stage reconstructive production in which first a skin graft is performed to allow the eyelid to close, then later a levator advancement is done. If the levator advancement is performed first, then the eyelid may look pretty but will not close and the patient's symptoms will be worsened. In ptosis surgery, conservative skin excision is the rule since revisions are so common. I quote a touch-up rate of 20% to my patients. A revision is much easier to perform if adequate or excess skin is left from the primary levator resection. Simple skin excision as a "touch-up" procedure is obviously more desirable than a skin graft.

REFERENCES

1. Beard C: Ptosis. St. Louis, CV Mosby, 1981.
2. Jones LT, Quickert MH, Wobig JL: The cure of ptosis by aponeurotic repair. Arch Ophthalmol 93:629–634, 1975.
3. Paris GL, Quickert MH: Disinsertion of the aponeurosis of the levator. Am J Ophthalmol 81:337–340, 1976.
4. Anderson RL: Aponeurotic ptosis surgery. Arch Ophthalmol 97:1123–1128, 1979.
5. Dortzbach RK, Sutula FC: Involutional blepharoptosis: A histopathological study. Arch Ophthalmol 98:2045–2049, 1980.
6. Schechter RJ: Ptosis with contralateral lid retraction due to excessive innervation of the levator palpebral superioris. Ann Ophthalmol 10:1324–1328, 1978.
7. Putterman AM, Urist MJ: Müller's muscle–conjunctival resection ptosis procedure. Ophthalmic Surg 9(3):27–32, 1978.
8. Fasanella RM, Servat J: Levator resection for minimal ptosis: Another simplified operation. Arch Ophthalmol 65:493–496, 1961.
9. Baylis HI, Shorr N: Anterior tarsectomy reoperation for upper eyelid blepharoptosis or contour abnormalities. Am J Ophthalmol 95:676, 1977.

C H A P T E R 4 2

Eyelid Trauma

Russell S. Gonnering

All ophthalmologists, regardless of the type of practice they have, will be called on to treat acute trauma to the eyelids. A systematic approach to the evaluation and management of eyelid trauma by the ophthalmologist will (1) maximize the results of primary treatment, (2) minimize the need for secondary reconstruction, and (3) lessen the exposure of the ophthalmologist to medicolegal risks.

Several factors make the management of trauma different from the medical or surgical treatment of disease or acquired or congenital abnormalities. No patient plans to be the victim of trauma. In most instances, the injury occurs suddenly and without warning. Eyelid trauma is highly visible, and in most cases, shocking in appearance to the patient (Figs. 42–1 and 42–2*A*). Anxiety about the possibility of loss of vision and disfigurement is high and must be dealt with skillfully. In most instances, the patient is grateful for expert care and attention and cooperates with the physician in the evaluation and treatment of the injury.

Some patients are an exception to this generalization, however. Patients who have been involved in an altercation that results in eyelid trauma are often belligerent and noncooperative because their primary aim is often to return to the altercation. Often, these patients are intoxicated, as are many victims of motor vehicular trauma. Both types of patients are most likely angry at whoever victimized them and may transfer this anger to the treating physician. In addition, legal actions often result from the injury, and possibly from the treatment, if the results are less than perfect.

EVALUATION

Most patients who suffer eyelid trauma significant enough to warrant the attention of an ophthalmologist go to an emergency facility. There, initial triage and stabilization begin. Although the diagnosis of associated injuries is usually made independent of the ophthalmologist's examination, a certain redundancy in evaluation is necessary for trauma to be treated appropriately and expeditiously (Fig. 42–3).

Mechanism of Injury

Even before seeing the patient, the ophthalmologist can anticipate the types of injuries that are likeliest to be encountered from a knowledge of the mechanism of injury. Traumatic injuries occur after contact with sharp or blunt objects, toxic substances, or sources of thermal or electromagnetic energy. Combination injuries may be present, such as those seen in motor vehicular trauma. This chapter considers injuries caused by mechanical energy.

Sharp Trauma

Eyelids can suffer lacerations either from contact of the moving patient with a sharp object, such as falling against a stick, or from contact of a moving sharp object with the stationary patient, such as receiving a knife wound. Sharp trauma tends to produce a clean wound of the eyelids without tissue loss, although amputation has been reported.[1] Sharp trauma can be associated with ocular injury, injury to extraocular muscles or other orbital structures, or, through penetration of the orbital walls, craniocerebral or upper respiratory tract injuries.[2] The ophthalmologist must evaluate for retained foreign bodies, especially in trauma caused by missiles.

Blunt Trauma

Blunt periorbital trauma, caused either by contact of a moving object, such as a fist, with the stationary patient or by contact of the moving patient with a stationary object, such as an automobile dashboard, can produce eyelid injuries.[3] Abrasions, irregular lacerations with tissue necrosis, and partial avulsions are commoner with blunt trauma than with sharp. Associated neurologic injury (intracranial or cervical), facial fractures, concussive ocular injury, or globe rupture must be ruled out (see Fig. 42–2).

Bites

Eyelid injuries caused by bites pose unique problems.[4–8] The injuries themselves can be a combination of

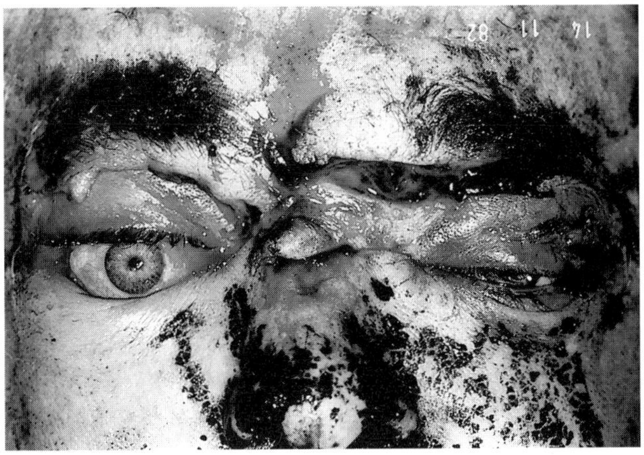

Figure 42–1. Bilateral eyelid lacerations with craniofacial fractures resulting from a motor vehicle accident.

sharp and blunt trauma, causing lacerations and tearing-type injuries and rarely, actual tissue loss (Figs. 42–4 and 42–5). In addition, all bite injuries are considered contaminated, and preventive measures against infection need to be employed.

Most periorbital bites are from the domestic dog.[9, 10] Facial and eyelid bites from other mammals, such as ferrets[11] and rats,[12] are extremely rare. Unfortunately, periorbital human bites, occurring as a result of passion or altercation, are not unheard of.[8, 13–15]

Patient Evaluation

Systemic Considerations

Evaluation of the patient with eyelid trauma is most expeditiously performed in an order slightly different from the normal history and physical examination.[16, 17] The potential injuries must be dealt with in their order of importance and severity. Resuscitation, if needed, and stabilization of vital signs are the initial goals for the treatment of any trauma patient. Although these responsibilities rarely fall on the shoulders of the ophthalmologist, any trauma patient has the potential of developing shock during the evaluation process as a result of occult serious or life-threatening injury.[18] Periodic monitoring of vital signs during the examination process is therefore prudent.

Once the patient is stabilized, the presence of life-threatening associated injury must be ruled out. Understanding the mechanism of injury is most helpful in this

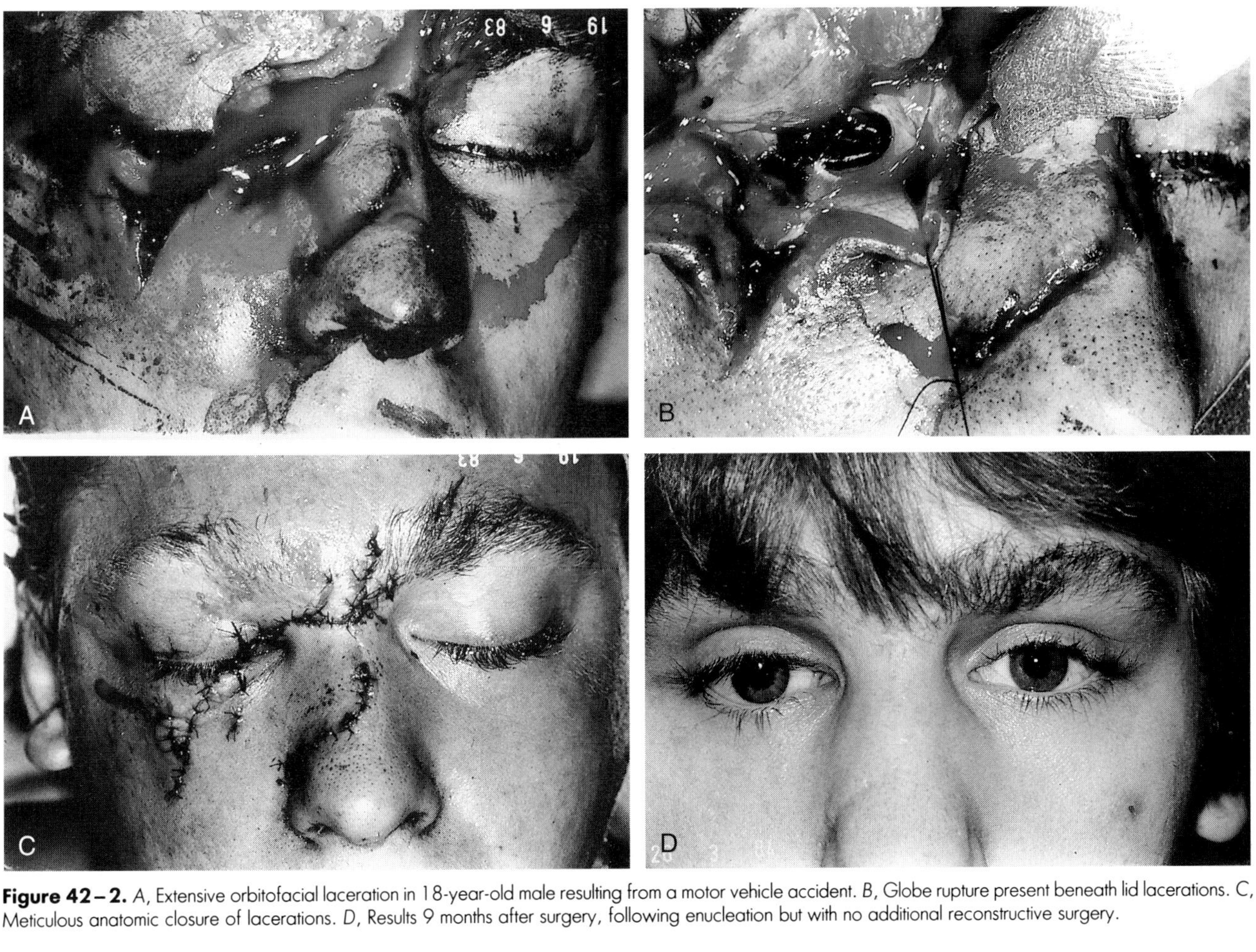

Figure 42–2. *A*, Extensive orbitofacial laceration in 18-year-old male resulting from a motor vehicle accident. *B*, Globe rupture present beneath lid lacerations. *C*, Meticulous anatomic closure of lacerations. *D*, Results 9 months after surgery, following enucleation but with no additional reconstructive surgery.

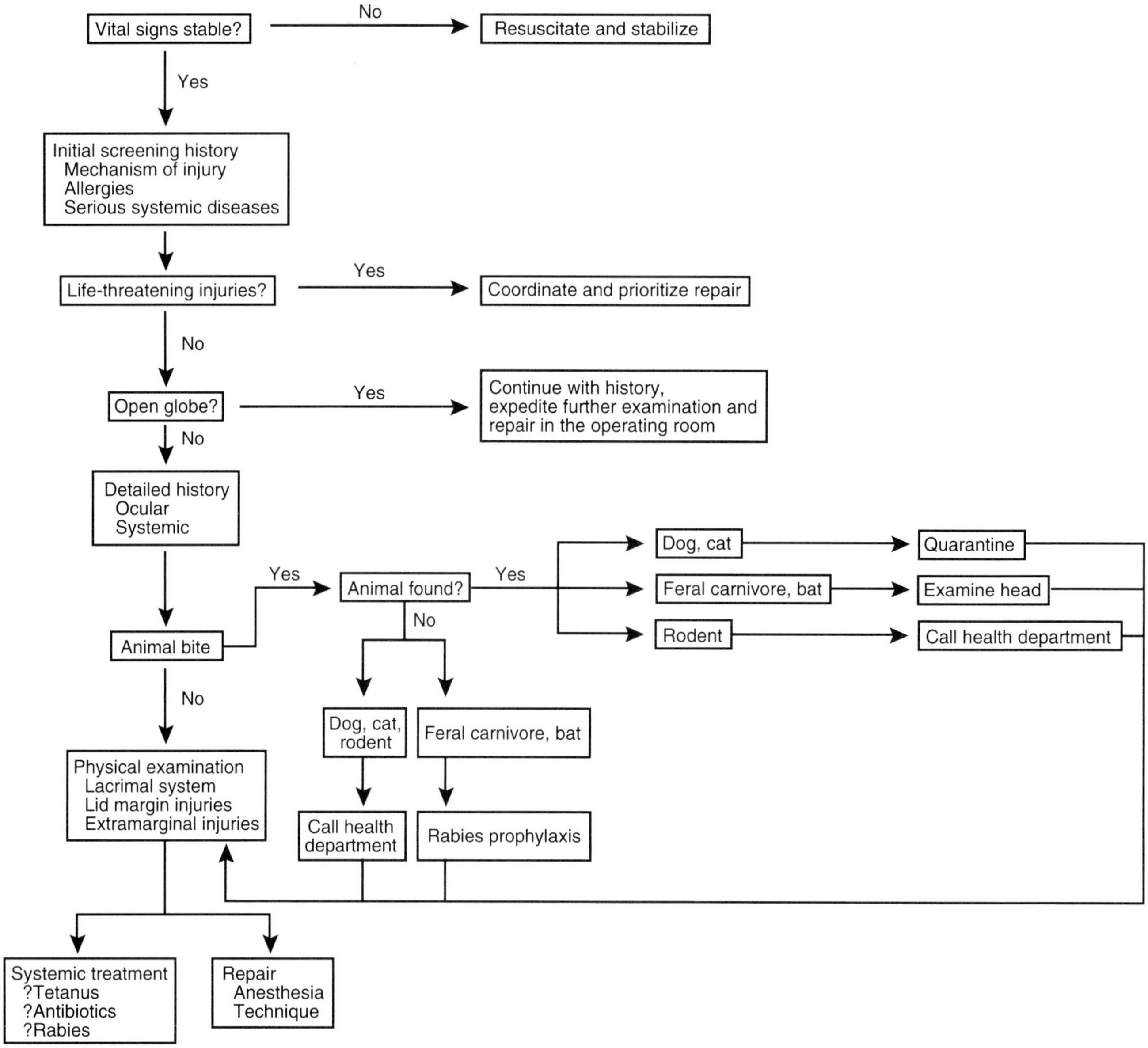

Figure 42–3. Evaluation of the patient with eyelid trauma.

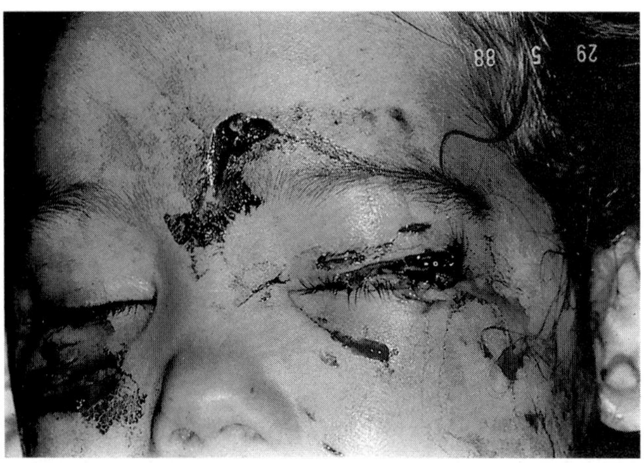

Figure 42–4. Dog bite injury with bilateral orbital involvement.

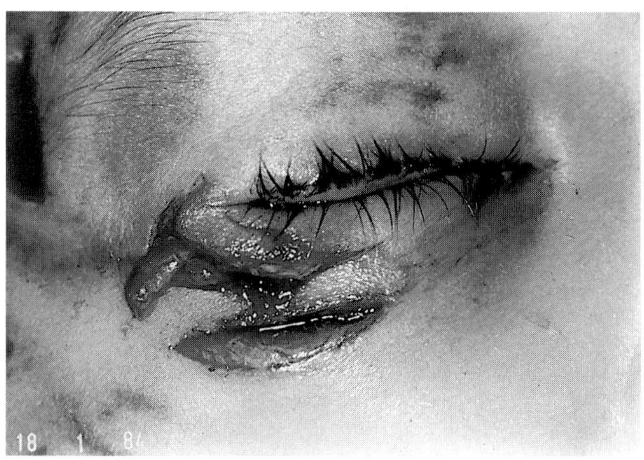

Figure 42–5. Dog (pit bull) bite injury with unilateral orbital involvement and extensive subsurface damage.

regard. An eyelid injury from a motor vehicle accident may be associated with central nervous system injury, either to the cranial or cervical spine; injury to the heart or aorta; abdominal injury; or pelvic fractures.

After life-threatening associated injuries have been ruled out, potential sight-threatening emergent conditions must be assessed. An open globe (see Fig. 42–2*B*) or massive orbital hemorrhage compressing the optic nerve requires emergency treatment, possibly at the expense of further evaluation of the trauma to the eyelids. Although normal visual acuity and absence of anterior segment injury on flashlight examination do not constitute a comprehensive evaluation, they allow the examination to proceed at a more methodical pace. All patients with significant eyelid trauma should receive a complete ophthalmic examination, but the order and venue for the examination (in the emergency department or the operating room) are dictated by the severity of associated ocular injury.

Concurrent with the screening examination for associated injury, an assessment of any complicating systemic factor can be performed. Potentially complicating systemic diseases, such as coronary artery disease or diabetes, should be identified. Medication use and allergies must be assessed, as should significant medical history, both ocular and systemic.

In patients with animal bites, the medical history must reveal whether or not immunocompromise, and particularly prior splenectomy, is present, so that increased risk of possible post-traumatic infection with unusual organisms can be assessed.[19–22] Of these fastidious, predominantly aerobic, gram-negative rods, *Capnocytophaga canimorsus* (formerly dysgonic fermenter-2), is the most well known and can cause life-threatening septicemia unless appropriate antibiotics are administered.[23–25] In addition, information regarding the biting animal must be collected at this time so that appropriate therapy may be instituted. In almost all instances of bites from the domestic dog, the animal is well known to the victim.[5] If the animal's rabies immunization status is not known, the animal should be quarantined with a veterinarian. If the dog cannot be found, advice on the institution of rabies prophylaxis should be sought from the local health department.

Bites from animals other than the domestic dog are more problematic. Rabies is becoming endemic in many species of feral carnivores. Bites from such animals as bats, skunks, raccoons, and foxes should be treated with rabies prophylaxis, unless the animal's head can be examined and found to be free of rabies by immunofluorescent testing.[26, 27] Bites from rodents, such as mice and chipmunks, carry a lower risk of rabies, but advice based on local risk factors for rabies prophylaxis should be sought from the local health department. After all potentially life- and sight-threatening associated injuries are anticipated and ruled out, evaluation of the eyelid injury can proceed.

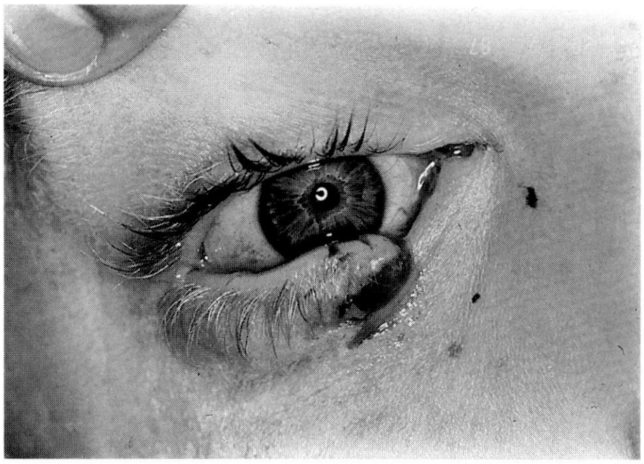

Figure 42–6. Full-thickness transmarginal eyelid laceration, with extension along the inferior edge of the tarsus.

Evaluation of Eyelid Injuries

Eyelid injuries can be conceptually divided into those involving the eyelid margin and those that do not, as well as those with tissue loss and those with none.

Marginal. Full-thickness transmarginal lid lacerations are in most cases easy to identify (Fig. 42–6). However, seemingly minor eyelid trauma, even to an area remote from the medial canthus, can result in rupture of the attachment of the medial canthal ligament to the tarsus, with resulting disruption of the canalicular system.[28] This is particularly true of animal bites, injuries from hook-like projections, and even finger pokes (Fig. 42–7).[29] All marginal trauma to the medial canthal region should be assumed to have damaged the canalicular system, unless proved otherwise. Assessing the lacrimal system may be difficult in a child with injury to the medial canthus, and in some situations, the patient must be sedated or anesthetized for the examination.

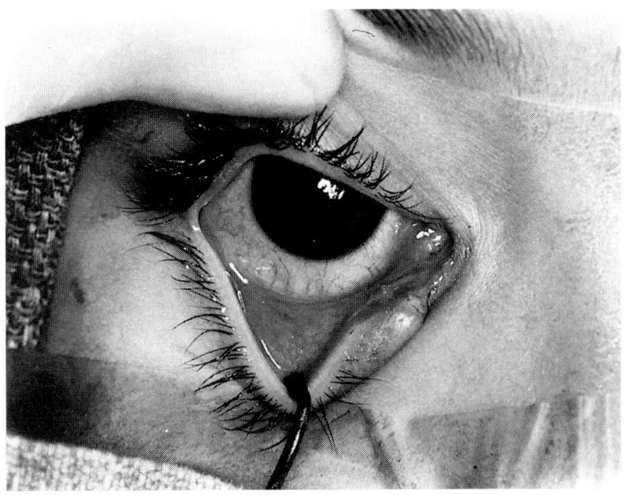

Figure 42–7. Minor finger poke to the eyelid with resulting disruption of medial canthal ligament and canalicular system.

Full-thickness transmarginal lid lacerations, particularly of the medial canthal region, can also be associated with tangential extensions at the level of the eyelid creases and distal borders of the tarsi (see Fig. 42–6). Disruption of the orbicularis muscle allows retraction of the cut edges, and gives the appearance of tissue loss; however, this is almost never the case, as is usually confirmed by measurement of the segments of the eyelid margin.

Extramarginal. In most instances, extramarginal lid lacerations tend to follow the relaxed skin-tension lines and are oriented parallel to the free margin of the eyelid. All such lacerations should be considered to be associated with possible underlying injury to the eye, the orbit, or contiguous structures, such as the cranial cavity or upper airway.[30] Depending on the mechanism of injury, appropriate clinical assessment, imaging studies, or both, should be undertaken to rule out the presence of retained foreign bodies. The wound should be gently explored to measure its depth. The presence of fat in the wound indicates that the wound has at least reached the level of the orbital septum. In the upper lid, the fat may represent an inferiorly displaced brow fat pad or orbital fat itself. In the lower lid, fat almost always indicates deeper orbital penetration. Likewise, significant orbital hemorrhage, as evidenced by proptosis, indicates damage to deeper structures.

Tissue loss is sometimes seen with extramarginal lacerations (Figs. 42–8), particularly in lacerations from a broken windshield, which produce a characteristic series of partial and sometimes full-thickness linear gouges together with irregular lacerations and abrasions, sometimes with loss of eyebrow cilia (Fig. 42–9).

In spite of the rich vascular supply to the periorbital area, most bleeding will have stopped by the time the patient is examined. Tissue manipulation may dislodge clots, and brisk bleeding may ensue. Care must be taken if thermal cauterization is needed in the emergency department so as not to damage the tear drainage system.

Formulation of Treatment Plans. After the nature of the injuries is assessed, treatment plans can be formulated. Although it has been stated that repair of eyelid injuries can be deferred for controlled repair in a nonemergency situation, repair is usually most easily performed as soon as possible after injury for the following reasons: (1) wound decontamination is more effective the earlier it is performed, (2) post-traumatic tissue edema increases during the first 24 hours after injury, and (3) repair becomes more technically difficult after the first 24 hours.

With a cooperative patient, many primary repairs can be undertaken in the emergency department with the patient under local anesthesia. This plan is predicated on the availability of proper lighting, magnification, instrumentation, suture material, and assistance. Repair of in-

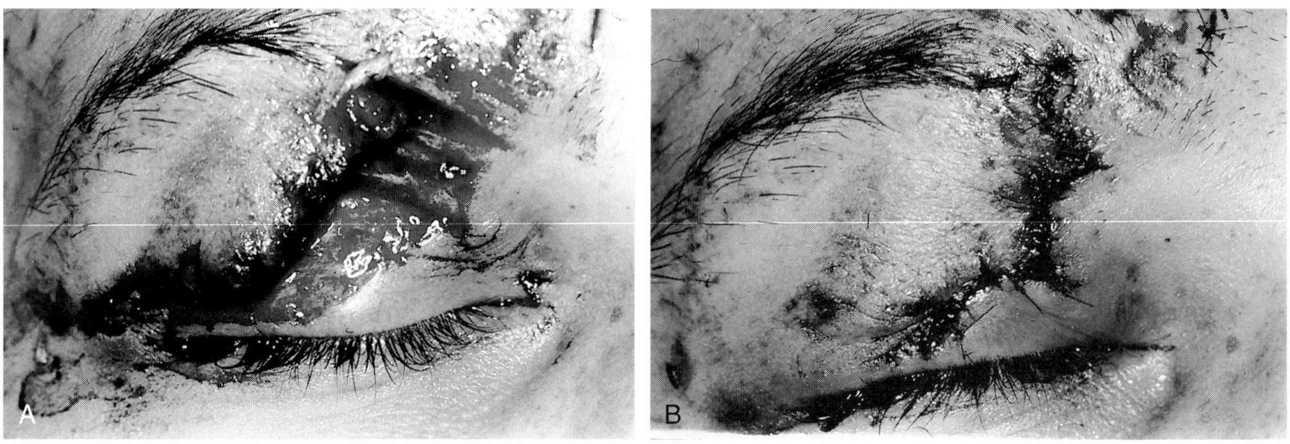

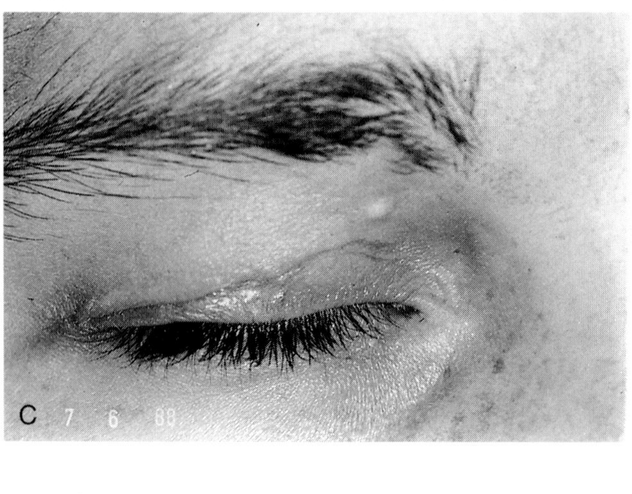

Figure 42–8. *A*, Extramarginal eyelid laceration from injury with broken bottle. Orbicular retraction suggests tissue loss. *B*, Unrolling of retracted flaps with anatomic repair. *C*, Results 2 months after repair. Note epidermal inclusion cyst.

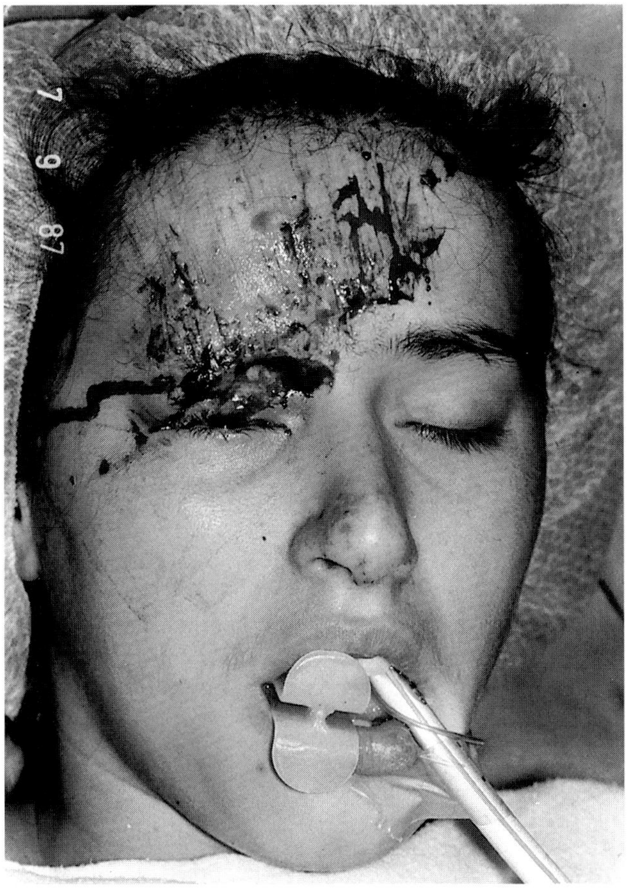

Figure 42–9. Characteristic injury from broken windshield with partial-thickness and full-thickness lacerations, scraping off eyebrow cilia and forehead gouges.

juries involving the eyelid margin in children are usually best performed with the patient under general anesthesia, even if the injuries do not involve the lacrimal system. If the ophthalmologist has doubt regarding the suitability of the facilities or the patient's cooperation, repair in the more controlled environment of the operating room, with the patient under general anesthesia or receiving intravenous relaxation, is the more prudent choice. If repair must be delayed because of anesthetic or logistical considerations, wound decontamination should be carried out, and a dressing should be applied until surgery can be performed.

Medicolegal Considerations

Documentation

Because many traumatic injuries will result in legal action being taken, either civil or criminal, accurate documentation of all information is essential.[31] Questions about the time and mechanism of injury are best answered as soon after the injury as possible, when events are fresh in the mind of the patient and accompanying individuals. In addition to written notes, a dictated summary of the history and physical examination, as well as the treatment, even if such documentation is not required by hospital policy, will serve the physician well should testimony concerning the injury be required in the distant future. In addition to covering the medical facts of the injury, this summary should record the time, place, and mechanism of injury; who was driving if the injury resulted from a motor vehicle accident; and any first aid or other care administered before the patient was evaluated by the treating physician. This summary must include a statement concerning the patient's vision, as well as a thorough description of the ocular examination and physical findings, even if they were unremarkable.

Photographs

Although not essential, photographic documentation of the nature and extent of the injuries is helpful to the physician in many ways: (1) objective documentation of how the patient appeared before the repair is useful in discussing postrepair appearance and possible need for further reconstructive measures; (2) objective documentation may be useful in supporting claims filed with the patient's health insurance; and (3) these same photographs can illustrate the physician's testimony should it be required in the future.

TREATMENT

Operative Repair

Wound Decontamination

The first element of a repair of a traumatic eyelid injury is adequate wound cleansing. The objective is to reduce bacterial contamination, as well as to remove foreign material from the wound. Particulate matter, particularly from contact with a pavement, otherwise becomes imbedded in the wound and produces a traumatic tattoo. Such a tattoo is extremely difficult to remove in a secondary procedure; thus, meticulous care should be given to its prevention.

Wound decontamination is best carried out with hydraulic pressure. Saline solution, irrigated by hand pressure on a 30-mL syringe with a 19-gauge needle (Fig. 42–10) produces up to 6 lb/in^2 of pressure and reduces bacterial counts by as much as 1.5 log units and experimental wound infection by 90%.[32] If irrigation is carried out over the globe, protection with a scleral contact lens prevents the production of a corneal abrasion.

The role of prophylactic antibiotic administration in the treatment of traumatic eyelid and facial wounds is controversial and by no means takes the place of wound decontamination.[33–35] Grossly contaminated wounds, wounds associated with significant tissue devitalization, wounds involving the orbit, and animal bites probably

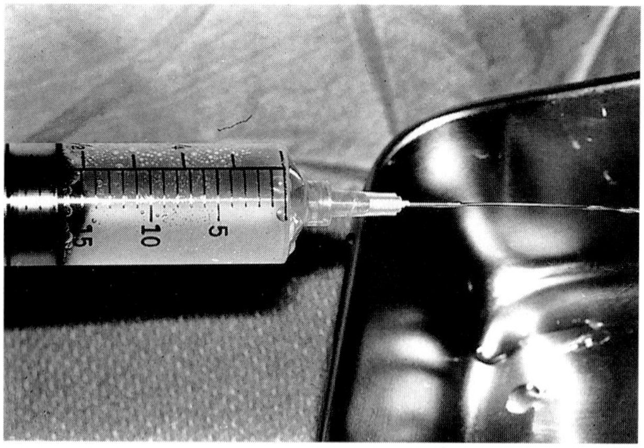

Figure 42–10. Thirty-five milliliter syringe and 19-gauge needle for hydraulic irrigation of traumatic wounds.

warrant antibiotic therapy, which should be started as early as possible.

In most instances, antibiotic therapy should begin against aerobic gram-positive organisms inhabiting the skin surface with first-generation cephalosporins, penicillinase-resistant penicillins, or amoxicillin-clavulanate. For a dog bite in an immunocompromised patient at risk for infection with *C. canimorsus*, or for a cat bite or scratch in a patient at risk for infection with *Pasteurella multocida*, penicillin should be used. Broad-spectrum prophylaxis should be instituted after human bites, or in wounds contaminated by vegetable matter.

Tetanus prophylaxis should be considered in all patients, according to the following guidelines[36]: in patients who have received prior complete immunization, clean wounds require no tetanus toxoid if fewer than 10 years have passed since the last injections. This criterion is reduced to 5 years for wounds with devitalized tissue or for contaminated wounds. Clean wounds in patients without prior immunization should be treated with tetanus toxoid. In patients with contaminated wounds or devitalized tissue, tetanus immune globulin should be given as well, using a separate syringe and injection site.

In the rare instance that rabies prophylaxis is indicated, it should be started at the time of repair, with a combination of active and passive immunization.[26, 37] On day 0 (the day of repair), 20 IU/kg of rabies immunoglobulin is administered, with half infiltrated at the site of injury and half given intramuscularly. In addition, 1 mL of human diploid cell rabies vaccine is given intramuscularly at days 0, 3, 7, 14, and 28. Immunocompromised patients should be tested to ensure adequate immune response.

Sequence of Repair (Figs. 42–11 and 42–12)

Canthal Injuries and Lacrimal System. After the wound has been decontaminated, it should be repaired in methodical fashion. First, if the lacrimal system is involved, it should be anatomically reconstructed.[29, 38] In the hands of a skilled surgeon, bicanalicular silicone intubation causes little if any iatrogenic trauma and offers numerous advantages over monocanalicular intubation: (1) when tightened, the silicone loop aids in anatomic repositioning of the medial canthal structures; (2) the loop of silicone at the medial canthus is more easily tolerated by the patient than currently available monocanalicular appliances; and (3) even for the occasional surgeon, the technique of passing bicanalicular silicone tubing, being akin to lacrimal probing, is easier than using the pigtail probe. Adequate nasal vasoconstriction will shrink the inferior turbinate and meatus and allow easy retrieval of the tubing from the nose.

With proper illumination and magnification, the cut proximal end of the lacrimal canaliculus can almost always be readily identified without the use of exotic maneuvers. It will be found very close to the conjunctival surface of the wound, and its lighter color makes it stand out against the surrounding orbicularis muscle. Gentle irrigation of the wound may help in its identification. No electrocautery or thermal cautery should be applied to the wound until it has been located and can be protected from damage.

After the silicone tubing has been passed, the medial canthal ligament should be reconstructed with a 5-0 or 6-0 permanent suture, with care being taken to avoid strangulation of the canaliculus. This suture should be drawn up to ensure its absolute anatomic placement, but then loosened so that microsurgical repair of the canaliculus itself can proceed. When possible, the canaliculus should be repaired with three equally spaced 10-0 nylon sutures placed through the substantia propria of the canaliculus. These sutures should be left untied until all three are placed. The silicone tubing can then be gently tightened and the suture reconstructing the canthal ligament tied. This action takes all tension off of the 10-0 sutures, which can then be tied blindly and cut. If the repair cannot be performed with 10-0 nylon because of the nature of the injury, repair of pericanalicular tissue with 7-0 synthetic absorbable suture can be performed as an alternative. Repair of the orbicularis muscle and lid margin completes the medial canthal repair.

Lateral canthal injuries are less common than medial and are approached in the same conceptual fashion, without the complicating factor of the lacrimal system. First, the lateral canthal ligament is reconstituted; then, the orbicularis muscle and lid margin are repaired.

Marginal Injuries. After the lacrimal system and associated eyelid injuries are repaired, the repair logically progresses to other marginal injuries. In most instances, no tissue loss has occurred, and primary repair is possible. If full-thickness tissue loss has occurred, primary reconstruction, using techniques outlined elsewhere in this book, can be performed.

Key elements to the primary repair of full-thickness

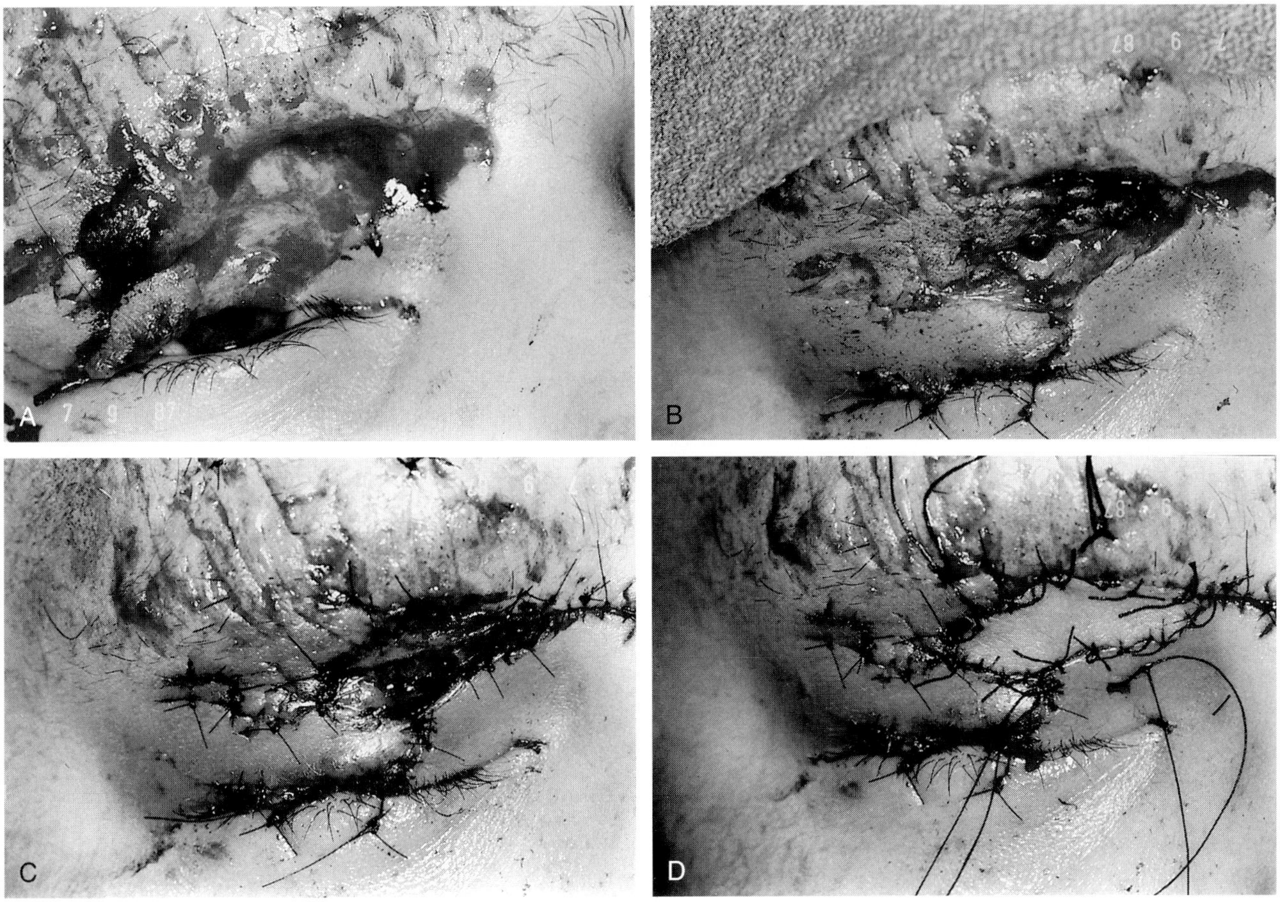

Figure 42–11. *A*, Extensive marginal and extramarginal lid lacerations, with tissue loss, following motor vehicle accident (same patient as in Fig. 42–8). *B*, Repair of marginal aspects of wound first. Temporary tarsorrhaphy sutures are in place. *C*, Extramarginal aspects of wound repaired. Tissue loss is apparent. *D*, Primary full-thickness skin graft placed.

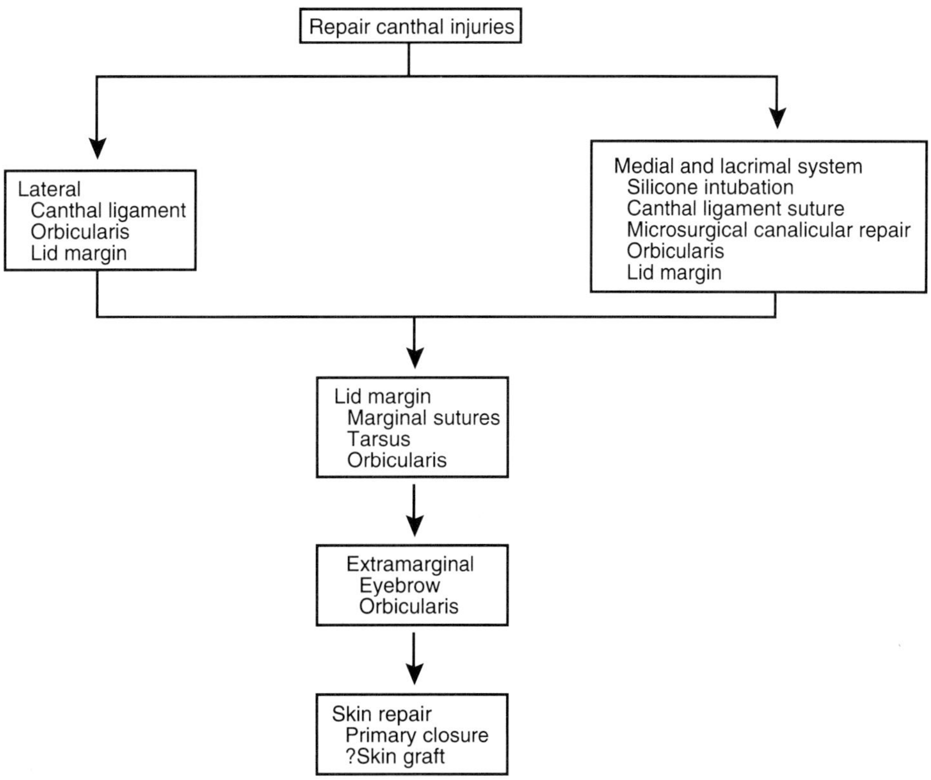

Figure 42–12. Sequence of operative repair.

transmarginal eyelid injuries are (1) absolute anatomic alignment of the lid margin and associated appendages, (2) restoration of structural integrity of the tarsus, (3) avoidance of vertical shortening of the eyelid and resulting postrepair lid malformation, and (4) limitation of cutaneous and deep scar formation. Specific technical maneuvers can be used to achieve these objectives.

Wound debridement should be kept to a minimum when primary repair of eyelid injuries is being performed (Fig. 42–13). Shredded tissue should be removed, but even dusky-appearing flaps in most cases survive because of the abundant vascular supply to that area. With magnification and appropriately sized sutures, anatomic alignment of tissue is possible, without the need for extensive debridement.

Three sutures can be used to anatomically align the eyelid margin. The first suture passes through the meibomian orifices, and additional sutures align the posterior and anterior lid margins. These sutures should be drawn up to check alignment, but they should not be tied at this point so as not to obstruct placement of the tarsal sutures. The marginal sutures should be left long so that they can be fixed to the drape with a hemostat to gently stretch the lid in the vertical dimension and to avoid foreshortening (Fig. 42–14).

In adults, 6-0 silk suture allows wound support with suppleness to avoid corneal abrasion. In children in whom general anesthesia may be needed for safe suture removal, 6-0 plain suture is adequate.

If a portion of the lid margin is missing, segmental excision of the involved area may be performed. If the extent of the missing lid margin is too great, and only a shallow loss is present, temporary tarsorrhaphy sutures may allow adequate reformation of the lid margin.

With the margin aligned and the lid gently stretched, the tarsus can be reconstructed with multiple sutures of 6-0 synthetic absorbable suture. The sutures should be passed partial thickness with the knots tied on the anterior surface to avoid corneal irritation. Beyond the peripheral border of the tarsus, the same suture can be used to repair vertical lacerations of the lower eyelid retractors or the levator muscle in the upper lid. The marginal sutures can then be tied but still left long and attached to the drape to aid in the rest of the repair.

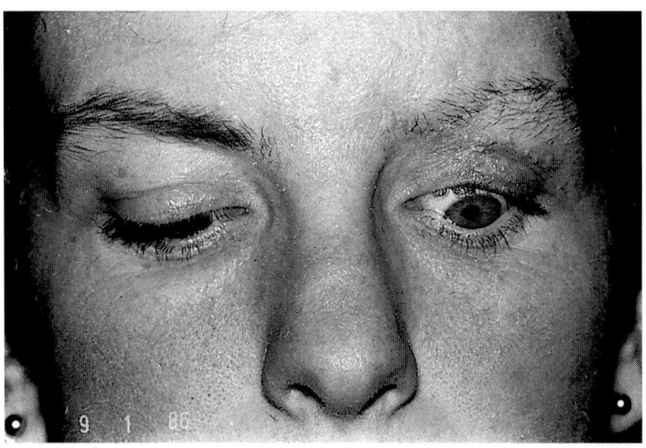

Figure 42–13. Lagophthalmos caused by overzealous débridement of an upper eyelid laceration.

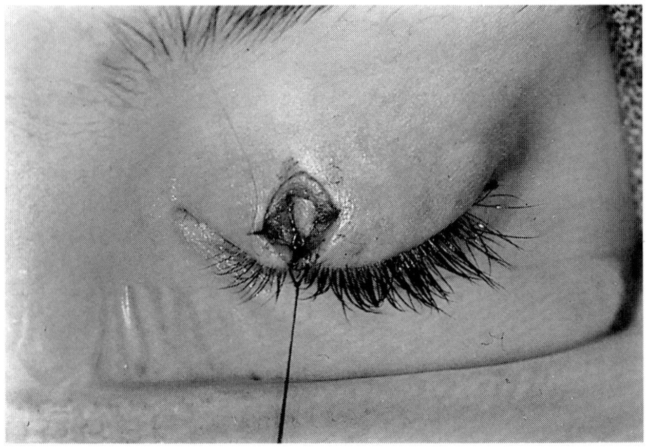

Figure 42–14. Traction on marginal sutures to prevent vertical shortening of lid during repair.

After the lid margin and tarsus are repaired, any horizontal disruptions of the lid retractors or levator muscle should be repaired. In the upper eyelid, lacerations of the orbital septum are best left unrepaired. In the lower lid, repair of septal injuries should be performed only in the region where the orbital septum is fused to the lower eyelid retractors and as part of a repair of those structures. Grossly contaminated orbital fat can be removed, but it should generally be left alone to prevent postoperative eyelid asymmetry.

Once the lid margin, tarsus, and deeper structures are repaired, the orbicularis and skin are dealt with. Although these can be closed in a single layer, a better aesthetic result can be achieved by closing them individually. In most instances, the surgeon is able to ascertain the proper place for the various elements of the cutaneous laceration. However, at times, this judgment may be difficult, akin to piecing together a jigsaw puzzle. Debridement of the numerous small flaps may at first glance appear to be a superior technique. However, loss of vertical lid height, particularly in a young patient, may induce significant lid malformation. If the marginal component of the laceration communicates with a significant extramarginal injury, cutaneous repair is best left until the end of the procedure.

Extramarginal Injuries. Key elements to the repair of extramarginal eyelid injuries are: (1) alignment of anatomic landmarks, particularly the eyebrow; (2) avoidance of vertical shortening and resulting eyelid malformation; and (3) optimization of cutaneous scar placement and formation.

In most instances, no actual tissue loss occurs in extramarginal injuries. However, long flaps both retract along their long axis and tend to roll along their short axis. The flaps must be carefully unrolled and tested as to their proper placement (see Figs. 42–8*A* and *B* and 42–11*A* through *C*). If the laceration extends to the eyebrow, repair should commence there, both to align the cilia and to properly place the thicker skin. Difficulty may arise if the cilia themselves have been sheared off, as in windshield injuries. In such cases, the thickness of the skin may be the best indicator of proper placement.

Tacking sutures of 6-0 plain suture in the orbicularis aids in alignment and takes tension off the cutaneous repair. Once the orbicularis has been positioned, skin repair is undertaken with 6-0 monofilament suture. From a practical standpoint, a blue suture is easier to remove from the eyebrow, particularly in a dark-haired individual. In linear wounds under no tension, a running suture can be used. However, with irregular or curvilinear wounds, interrupted sutures allow more exact wound approximation. As in all repairs, slight wound eversion minimizes scar formation. In young children in whom suture removal is likely to be traumatic, both psychologically and physically, repair with 6-0 fast-absorbing gut suture is acceptable.

If skin loss is present, primary skin grafting may be necessary (see Figs. 42–11*C* and *D*). This measure should be avoided if possible for many reasons. First, wound infection, although rare, would most likely cause loss of the graft and waste of limited donor material. Second, incomplete removal of epidermal elements from the wound results in implantation cysts (Fig. 42–15). Third, better aesthetic results may be attained by grafting the eyelid as an aesthetic unit, but the results can be judged only after primary healing has occurred.

After the cutaneous repair has been completed, the marginal sutures, if present, can be released from their attachment to the drape. In most instances, they can be tied into a suture on the skin surface that holds them away from the cornea. In instances in which vertical tension exists on the eyelid, or in which contraction of the eyelid retractors causes bunching of flaps with possible abnormal scar formation, these sutures can be taped to the cheek (upper eyelid) or forehead (lower eyelid) to provide vertical tension in the initial healing period.

Partial-Thickness Injuries. Perhaps the most difficult injuries to manage are extensive partial-thickness gouges of the type caused by contact with jagged windshield fragments. The resulting linear but irregular injuries may be extensive and very often run in a vertical fashion on the forehead, perpendicular to relaxed tension skin lines (see Fig. 42–8). If the injuries are few, the remaining dermis can be sharply excised with a razor blade fragment, and the wound closed primarily. However, when such injury is extensive, such an approach will likely produce more scarring, and the wounds are best allowed to heal by secondary intention, with reconstructive surgery performed after healing has been complete. At times, surprisingly good healing will result without the need for such reconstructive procedures (Fig. 42–16).

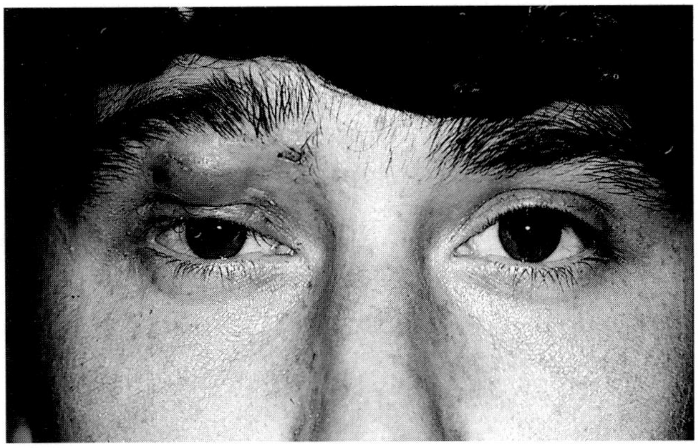

Figure 42–15. Large infected epidermal implantation cyst following primary skin grafting for traumatic eyelid injury.

Postoperative Care

Standard postoperative measures, such as elevation and the application of ice and topical antibiotic ointment, are used in the care of the patient after repair. In most instances, the eyepatch can be discontinued the first day after surgery, and the wound can be gently cleansed with warm water and cotton balls before daily reapplications of antibiotic ointment.

Prolonged patching should be avoided, especially in young children with eyelid injuries, to avoid the possibility of interference with fusion. The eyelid can be protected with a Fox shield, used without a patch. If the tape is placed along the edge of the shield, vision is still possible through the central holes.

Ideally, sutures should be removed in wounds not under tension on the fourth or fifth day after surgery, and adhesive strips should be used to support the wound for a few days more. In wounds under tension, such as marginal sutures in a full-thickness eyelid laceration, removal should be delayed until days 7 through 10.

Visual acuity should be checked on postoperative visits, to ensure that no delayed complications of the trauma are developing. Traumatic iritis may develop in the first week after injury and responds to appropriate treatment. Depending on the mechanism of injury, slit-lamp examination of the anterior segment, gonioscopy, and dilated fundus examination may need to be performed a few weeks after injury to document the presence or absence of associated ocular injuries.

Secondary Repair

The goal of primary repair is to avoid or minimize the need for secondary reconstructive procedures. In cases in

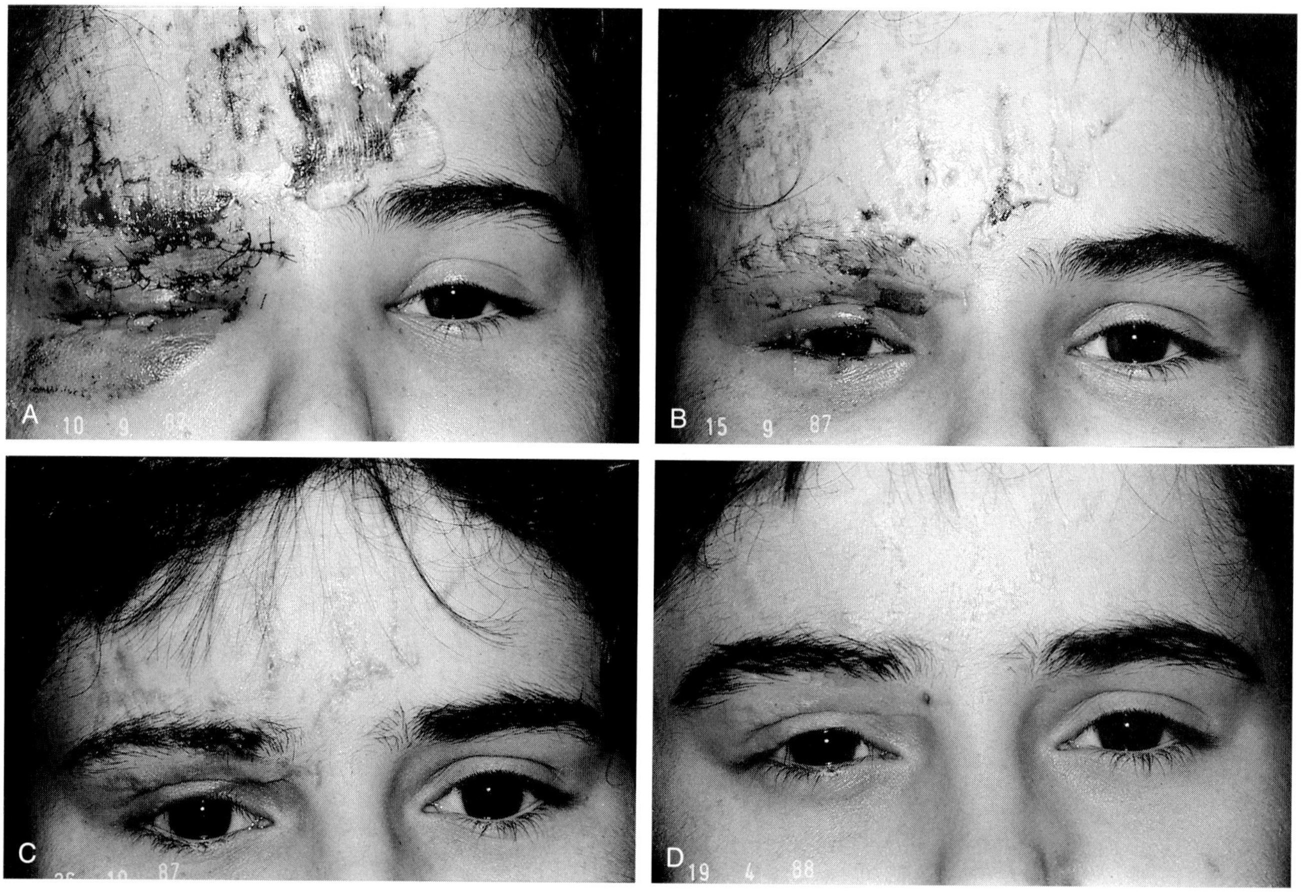

Figure 42–16. *A*, Patient in Figures 42–8 and 42–10, 3 days after injury at time of removal of tie-over dressing. *B*, Eight days after injury. *C*, Seven weeks after injury. *D*, Seven and one-half months following injury, with no further reconstructive surgery or scar revision.

which this is impossible, or when post-traumatic deformity is encountered, it is helpful to divide the reconstructive procedures into those that should be performed early, those that require some time after the injury for optimal evaluation or management, and those that are best deferred until late (3 to 6 months after injury).

Early

Secondary procedures that need to be performed early are primarily those dictated by instability of the cornea or reconstruction of severe anatomic deformities that if left untreated, would result in significant functional or aesthetic compromise (Figs. 42–17 and 42–18). Examples include exposure keratitis from lack of lid closure, mechanical keratitis from lid malposition, overlooking of injury to the canalicular system, lack of structural integrity to the medial or lateral canthal ligaments, or severe displacement of an anatomic landmark.

A general principle of secondary repair of post-traumatic deformities is to first recreate the injury by opening it along the lines of the original wound, and then anatomically repairing the underlying abnormality. An exception to this rule is the placement of a full-thickness skin graft into the anterior lamella of an eyelid that is shortened by loss of tissue or scar formation, in which case, a better result may follow the grafting of an esthetic unit.[39]

Intermediate

The eyelid reconstructive procedure that most often benefits from intermediate secondary repair is traumatic

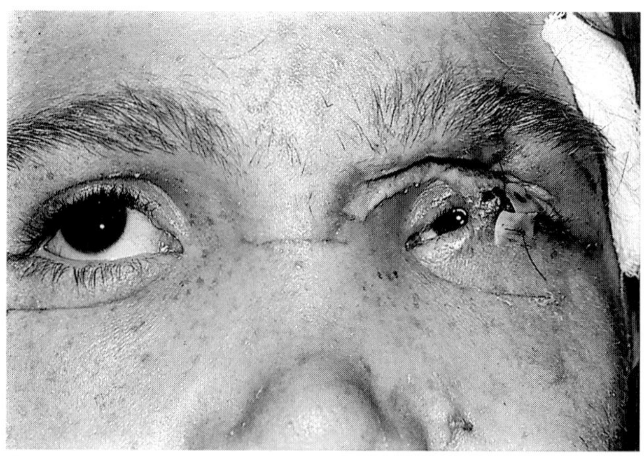

Figure 42–17. Severe post-traumatic deformity of upper lid requiring early reconstruction.

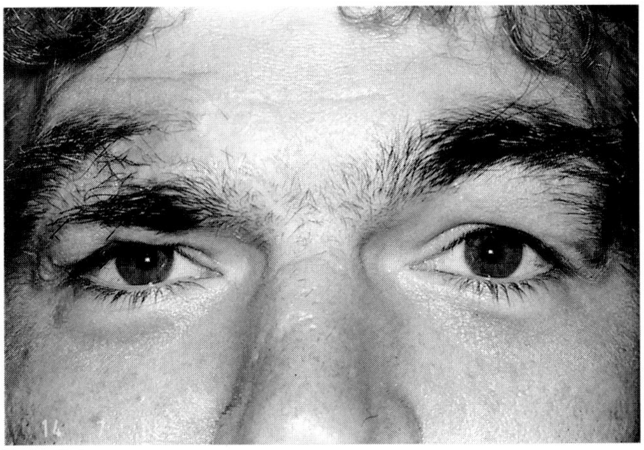

Figure 42–18. Result of inattention to eyebrow wound, with significant anatomic displacement.

ptosis. Injuries suspected of involving the levator should be explored at the time of the initial procedure, and any damage to the levator should be repaired at that time. However, patients are often seen with ptosis that follows blunt trauma to the eyelids. It is difficult to know if the ptosis has resulted from swelling and hematoma formation, from injury to the motor nerve supply of the levator, or from mechanical disruption of the levator aponeurosis.[40]

When intervention is delayed for 2 to 3 weeks after the injury, most swelling and hematoma will have subsided, and the differential cause of the ptosis narrows to mechanical versus neurologic damage. If the ptosis is significant but levator function poor, neurologic damage is probable, especially if an associated decrease in superior rectus function occurs. Definitive evaluation may need to be postponed for months to allow any levator function to return.

If levator function is good, lid crease is elevated, or significant scar tethering is present, mechanical ptosis, either from disruption of the levator or incorporation of the orbital septum in the scar, is likely and surgical intervention is indicated at that time.

Late

The timing of cutaneous scar revision is controversial. What appears as a significant cosmetic deformity 1 month after injury may fade to one that is inconspicuous 4 months later. Good results have been obtained with dermabrasion of post-traumatic facial scars 4 to 8 weeks after injury.[41] Borges also recommends surgical scar revision at 8 weeks after injury in adults and young children but postpones revision until 6 months after injury in patients under the age of 7.[42] He recommends (1) fusiform scar revision in unaesthetic scars running close to the relaxed skin tension lines; (2) W-plasty for long scars on the forehead temples, nose, cheeks, and chin when they run over 35 degrees from the relaxed skin tension line; (3) Z-plasty for antitension line scars on the eyelids, lips, and nasolabial folds as well as those on the forehead, temples, cheeks, nose, and chin that are at an angle of less than 35 degrees from the relaxed tension lines.

Local treatment with emollients and massage, especially in young patients, often results in improvement to the point that surgical intervention is not needed. If such intervention is needed, standard techniques of dermabrasion, dermal planing, and other techniques of scar revision can be employed.

REFERENCES

1. Aylward GW, Ohri R: Repair of an avulsed upper lid and partially severed lower lid. Br J Ophthalmol 73:39–41, 1989.
2. Brocheler J, Beer W: Head injuries: The treatment of combined injuries of the anterior cranial fossa, the nose and paranasal sinuses and the eyes. Neurosurg Rev 12(Suppl):81–87, 1989.
3. Joondeph BC: Blunt ocular trauma. Emerg Med Clinics North Am 6:147–167, 1988.
4. Herman DC, Bartley GB, Walker RC: The treatment of animal bite injuries of the eye and ocular adnexa. Ophthal Plast Reconstr Surg 3:237–241, 1987.
5. Gonnering RS: Ocular adnexal injury and complications in orbital dog bites. Ophthal Plast Reconstr Surg 3:231–235, 1987.
6. Gonnering RS: Periorbital animal bites. *In* Linberg JV (ed): Oculoplastic and Orbital Emergencies. Norwalk, CT, Appleton & Lange, 1990, pp 215–228.
7. Gonnering RS: Dog bite injuries. *In* Shingleton BJ, Hersh PS, Kenyon KR (eds): Eye Trauma. St. Louis, Mosby-Year Book, 1991, pp 347–353.
8. Avram DR, Hurwitz JJ, Kratky V: Dog and human bites of the eyelid repaired with retrieved autogenous tissue. Can J Ophthalmol 26:334–337, 1991.
9. Karlson TA: The incidence of facial injuries from dog bites. JAMA 251:3265–3267, 1984.
10. Palmer J, Rees M: Dog bites of the face: A 15-year review. Br J Plast Surg 36:315–318, 1983.
11. Paisley JW, Lauer BA: Severe facial injuries to infants due to unprovoked attacks by pet ferrets. JAMA 259:2005–2006, 1988.
12. Wykes WN: Rat bite injury to the eyelids in a 3-month-old child. Br J Ophthalmol 73:202–204, 1989.
13. Spinelli HM, Sherman JE, Lisman RD, Smith B: Human bites of the eyelid. Plast Reconstr Surg 78:610–614, 1986.
14. Aguirre Vila-Coro A, Bonafonte S, Fernandez del Cotero JN: Ocular human bite. Ann Ophthalmol 21:100–102, 1989.
15. Serrano F, Starck T, Esquenazi S: Surgical treatment of human bites of the upper eyelid. Ophthal Plast Reconstr Surg 5:127–130, 1989.
16. McNab AA, Collin JRO: Eyelid and canthal lacerations. *In* Linberg JV (ed): Oculoplastic and Orbital Emergencies. Norwalk, CT, Appleton & Lange, 1990, pp 1–13.
17. Hamill WB: Clinical evaluation. *In* Shingleton BJ, Hersh PS, Kenyon KR (eds): Eye Trauma. St. Louis, Mosby-Year Book, 1991, pp 3–24.
18. Morrissette MP: Rapid airway compromise following traumatic laceration of the facial artery. J Oral Maxillofac Surg 48:989–990, 1990.
19. Bailie WE, Stowe EC, Schmitt AM: Aerobic bacterial flora of oral and nasal fluids of canines with reference to bacteria associated with bites. J Clin Microbiol 7:223–231, 1978.
20. Saphir DA, Carter GR: Gingival flora of the dog with special reference to bacteria associated with bites. J Clin Microbiol 3:344–349, 1976.
21. Garre M, le Henaff C, Tande, et al: Fulminant *Eubacterium plautii* infection following dog bite in asplenic man. Lancet 338:384–385, 1991.
22. Homes B, Costas M, Wood AC: Numerical analysis of electrophoretic protein patterns of group EF-4 bacteria, predominantly from dog-bite wounds of humans. J Appl Bacteriol 68:81–91, 1990.

23. Findling JW, Pohlman GP, Rose HD: Fulminant gram-negative bacillemia (DF-2) following a dog bite in an asplenic woman. Am J Med 68:154–156, 1980.
24. Kalb R, Kaplan MH, Tenebaum MJ, et al: Cutaneous infection at dog bite wounds associated with fulminant DF-2 septicemia. Am J Med 78:687–690, 1985.
25. Hicklin H, Verghese A, Alvarez S: Dysgonic fermenter-2 septicemia. Rev Infect Dis 9:884–890, 1987.
26. Edlich RF, Spengler MD, Rodeheaver GT, et al: Emergency department management of mammalian bites. Emerg Med Clin North Am 4:595–604, 1986.
27. Jaffe AC: Animal bites. Pediatr Clin North Am 30:405–413, 1983.
28. Wulc AE, Arterberry JF: The pathogenesis of canalicular lacerations. Ophthalmology 98:1243–1249, 1991.
29. Hawes MJ, Segrest DR: Effectiveness of bicanalicular silicone intubation in the repair of canalicular lacerations. Ophthal Plast Reconstr Surg 1:185–190, 1985.
30. Mutlukan E, Fleck BW, Cullen JR, Whittle IR: Case of penetrating orbitocranial injury caused by wood. Br J Ophthalmol 75:374–376, 1991.
31. Shelton PA: Medicolegal considerations. *In* Shingleton BJ, Hersh PS, Kenyon KR (eds): Eye Trauma. St. Louis, Mosby-Year Book, 1991, pp 403–408.
32. Stevenson TR, Thacker JG, Rodeheaver GT, et al: Cleansing of the traumatic wound by high pressure syringe irrigation. J Am Coll Emerg Phys 5:17–21, 1976.
33. Zook EG, Miller M, Van Beek AL, Wavak P: Successful treatment protocol for canine fang injuries. J Trauma 20:243–247, 1980.
34. Guy RJ, Zook EG: Successful treatment of acute head and neck dog bite wounds without antibiotics. Ann Plast Surg 17:45–48, 1986.
35. Callaham M: Controversies in antibiotic choices for bite wounds. Ann Emerg Med 17:1321–1330, 1988.
36. Kunzwiler TP: Guidelines for tetanus prophylaxis. *In* Shingleton BJ, Hersh PS, Kenyon KR (eds): Eye Trauma. St. Louis, Mosby-Year Book, 1991, pp 409–410.
37. Flanigan TJ, Rippert ET, Nieusma GE: Rabies therapy for animal bites in the head and neck region. J Oral Maxillofac Surg 43:704–706, 1985.
38. Dortzbach RK, Angrist RA: Silicone intubation for lacerated lacrimal canaliculi. Ophthalmic Surg 16:639–642, 1985.
39. Maillard GF, Clavel PR: Aesthetic units in skin grafting of the face. Ann Plast Surg 26:347–352, 1991.
40. Arden RL, Moore GK: Complete post-traumatic ptosis: A mechanism for recovery? Laryngoscope 99:1175–1179, 1989.
41. Yarborough JM: Ablation of facial scars by programmed dermabrasion. J Dermatol Surg Oncol 14:292–294, 1988.
42. Borges AF: Timing of scar revision techniques. Clin Plast Surg 17:71–76, 1990.

CHAPTER 43

Facial Paralysis: Diagnosis and Management

Lawrence F. Handler, Steven L. Galetta, Allan E. Wulc, and Jeffrey C. Popp

Patients with acute facial paralysis may present to the ophthalmologist with irritative symptoms related to an inability to close the eye, often before the patients seek care from other physicians. Therefore, the ophthalmologist must be aware of the disorders that may cause facial paralysis, as well as the details of the evaluation of acute facial paralysis. In this section, the anatomy of the facial nerve is reviewed, and management related to the protection and reanimation of the eye is comprehensively discussed.

FACIAL NERVE ANATOMY

Supranuclear Pathways

Diagnosis of facial nerve disorders is greatly facilitated by a thorough understanding of facial nerve anatomy. The supranuclear neurons destined to innervate the facial nerve nucleus lie in the precentral gyrus of the frontal lobe.[1] Neural activity from this region initiates voluntary movements on command, such as smiling or puckering of the lips. Somatotopically, these supranuclear neurons are located most laterally in the frontal cortex just below the representation for the hand. On leaving the precentral gyrus, the axons of the facial motor area coalesce and become part of the corticobulbar tracts that descend through the middle of the internal capsule on their way to the medial part of the cerebral peduncle. Immediately below this midbrain level, most of the supranuclear fibers cross over to the opposite side of the pons to innervate the facial nerve nucleus. However, some fibers synapse in the ipsilateral facial nerve nucleus, providing the upper face with innervation from both cerebral hemispheres. This unusual anatomic feature explains why supranuclear lesions involving the descending motor pathways result in weakness of the contralateral lower face only (Fig. 43–1). Because lesions of the peripheral facial nerve may mimic those of the corticobulbar pathways, the supranuclear location of the facial weakness must be confirmed by documentation of the associated neurologic signs. Cortex and internal capsule lesions that produce lower facial weakness are usually associated with weakness of the ipsilateral arm. Because the facial nucleus also receives input from the basal ganglia region, a dissociation in voluntary facial movements compared with spontaneous ones may occur.

Pons

The motor nucleus of the facial nerve resides in the lateral midpons. This nucleus may be subdivided into four cell groups that innervate designated muscle groups. The dorsomedial cells supply the auricular and occipital muscles. Intermediate cells innervate the frontalis, orbicularis oculi, and corrugator muscles, whereas cells in the ventromedial location supply the platysma. Lateral cells innervate the buccinator and buccolabial muscles.[2]

Motor axons leaving the facial nucleus course dorsomedially toward the floor of the fourth ventricle to loop around the sixth nerve nucleus, thus forming the facial colliculus. After bending around the sixth nerve nucleus, the motor fibers extend laterally to exit the pons. The parasympathetic component of the facial nerve originates from the superior salivatory nucleus, which lies just superior to the facial motor nucleus. This nucleus supplies the sublingual, submandibular, and lacrimal glands and forms one part of the nervus intermedius (Fig. 43–2). The other component of the nervus intermedius is sensory and contains those fibers subserving taste to the anterior two thirds of the tongue, and somatic sensation to the external auditory meatus and postauricular region. Taste fibers synapse in the nucleus solitarius, whereas those of somatic sensation terminate in the spinal tract of the fifth nerve. Afferents to the facial nucleus are also derived from the trigeminal nucleus as part of the corneal reflex, and the acoustic pathways as part of the stapedius reflex. In the stapedius reflex, the eyes blink reflexively to a loud noise. Blinking also occurs in response to visual threat through ill-defined synapses from the visual pathways.

The separate locations of the parasympathetic, sensory, and motor fibers of the facial nerve help explain the sparing of taste and tearing in many congenital facial

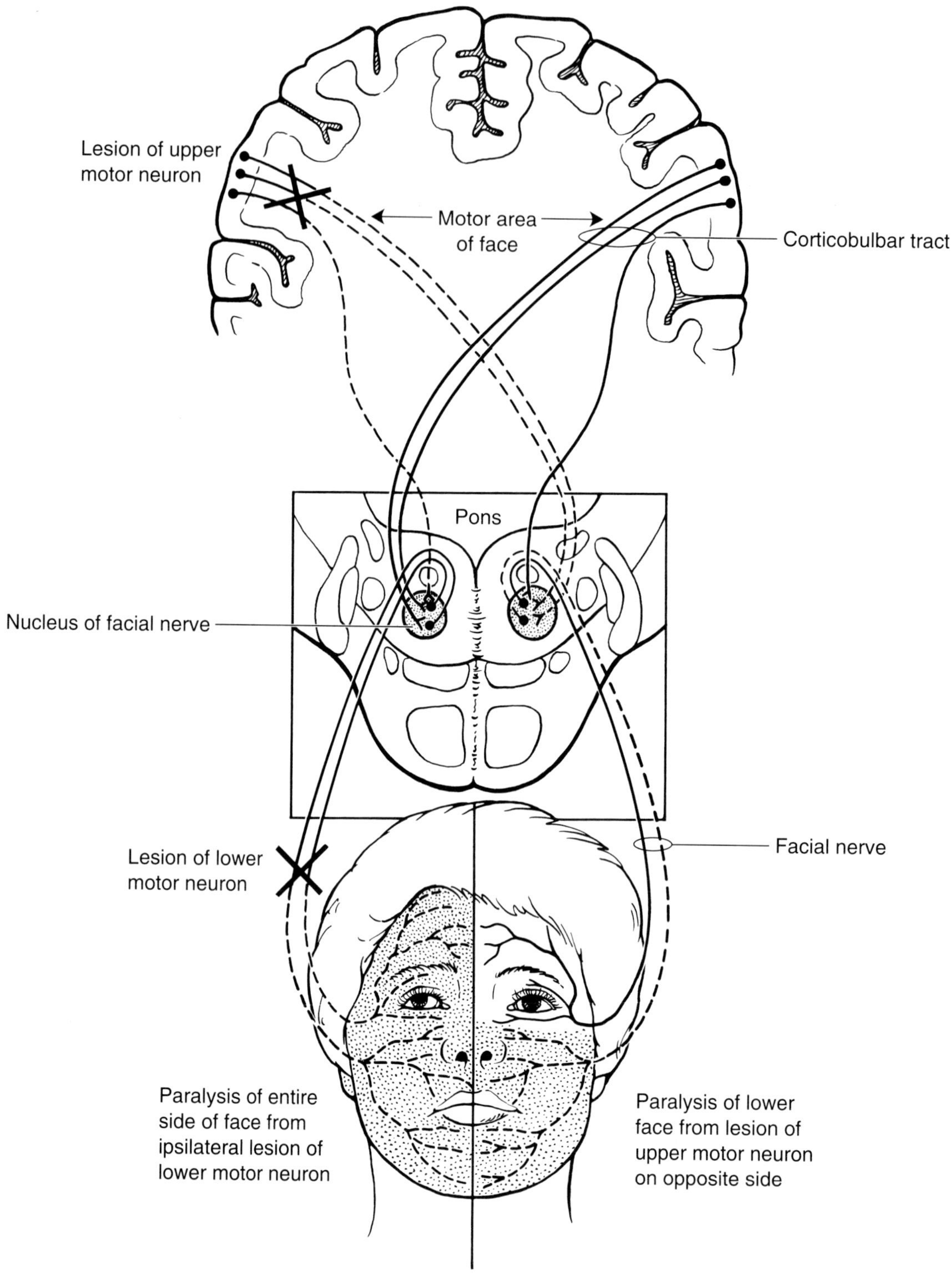

Figure 43–1. Facial motor axons descend from the precentral gyrus as part of corticobulbar tracts to the cerebral peduncle. Below midbrain level, most supranuclear fibers decussate to innervate the contralateral facial nerve nucleus. Some fibers destined to innervate the upper face synapse in the ipsilateral facial nucleus. Thus, the upper face is innervated by both hemispheres, which explains why supranuclear lesions result in weakness of the lower face only. (Modified from Gilman S, Newman SH: Manter and Gatz's Essentials of Clinical Neuroanatomy and Neurophysiology, 7th ed. Philadelphia, FA Davis, 1987, p 109.)

nerve palsies.[3] However, the proximity of the facial nerve to the abducens nucleus ties together the horizontal gaze palsy and facial weakness that characterize the Möbius syndrome. Diagnosis of pontine facial palsies is confirmed by detection of dysfunction of closely allied pontine structures. For example, the presence of facial weakness in combination with ipsilateral deafness, facial numbness, and Horner's syndrome signifies a lesion in the lateral pons. The presence of facial weakness and horizontal gaze palsy suggests injury to the facial colliculus region. More ventral pontine lesions may be associated with a contralateral hemiparesis (Fig. 43–3).

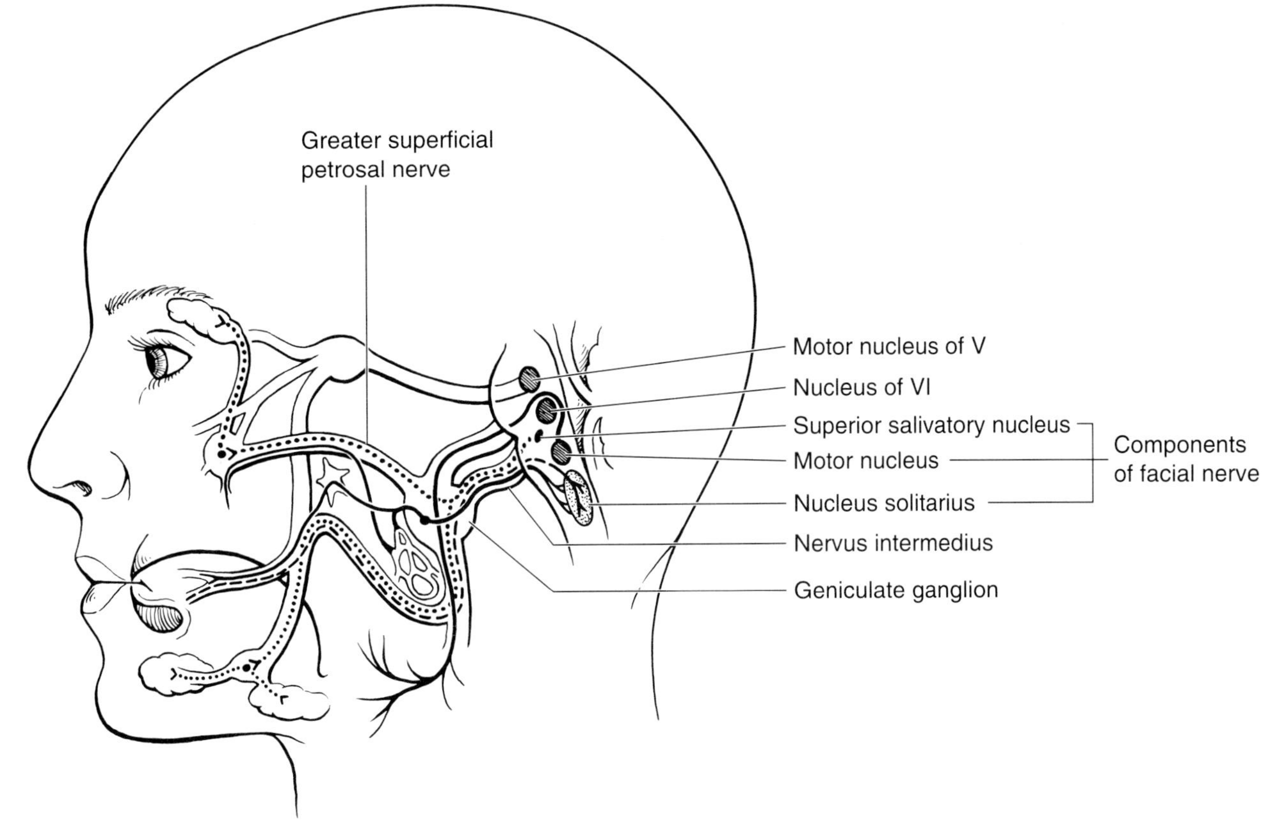

Figure 43 – 2. Facial nerve separated into motor fibers and nervus intermedius. The nervus intermedius contains both parasympathetic and sensory fibers. (Modified from Dejong RN: The Neurologic Examination, 4th ed. New York, Harper & Row, 1979, p 181.)

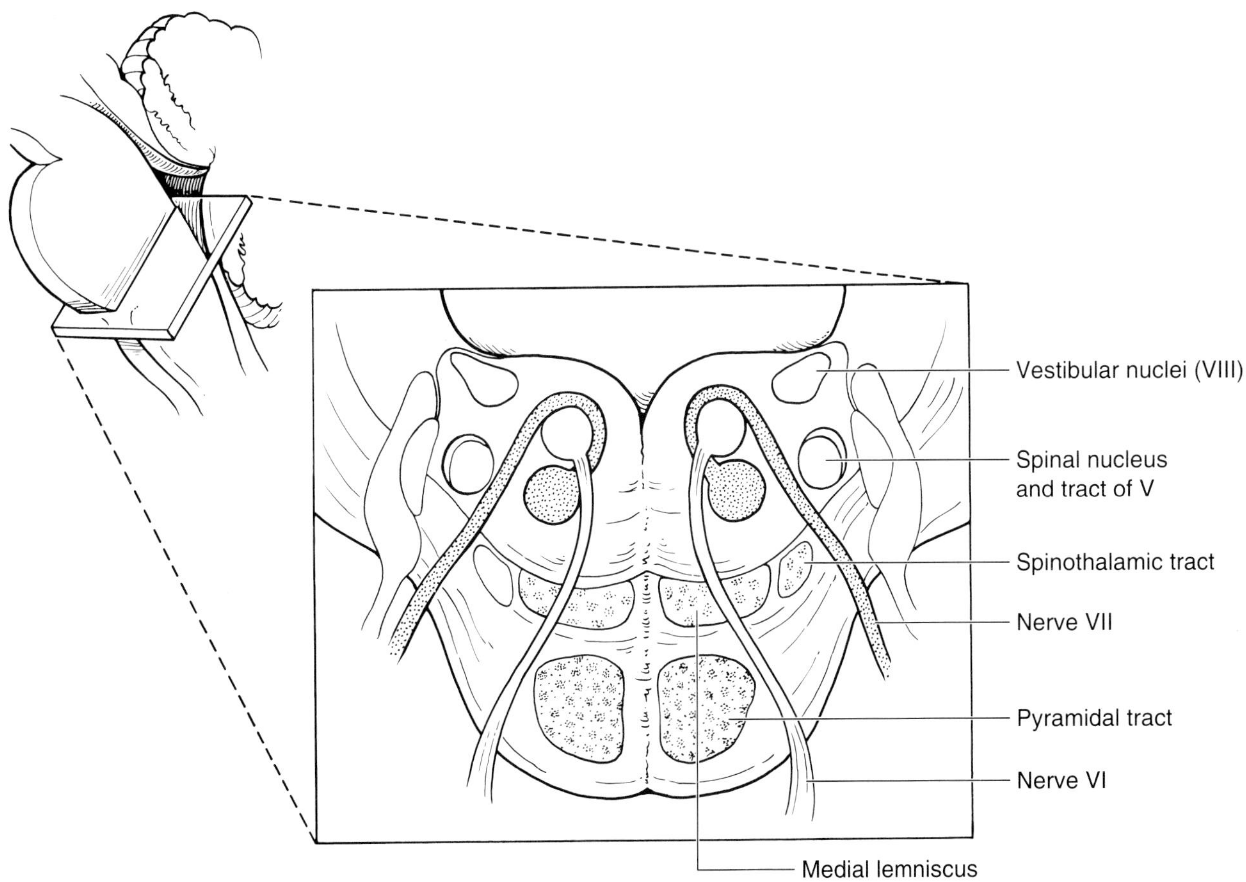

Figure 43 – 3. Cross section of the lower pons. There is close proximity of cranial nerve nuclei VI, VII, and VIII. Their location in relation to the pyramidal or corticospinal tracts should also be noted.

Cerebellopontine Angle

At the ventrolateral angle of the pons, the facial motor root and the vestibuloacoustic nerve exit the brain stem together. Between these two nerves lies the nervus intermedius, which carries facial nerve sensory and parasympathetic information. In the cerebellopontine angle, the anteroinferior cerebellar artery (AICA) courses between the seventh and eighth nerves to supply the lateral pons and anterior cerebellum.[4] A tortuous AICA is believed to be responsible for most cases of hemifacial spasm and provides the rationale for placement of a polytetrafluoroethylene (Teflon) sponge between the AICA and facial nerve in refractory cases of spasm. The proximity of the fifth, seventh, and eighth nerves in the cerebellopontine angle helps predict their involvement in tumors in this region, such as acoustic neuromas and tentorial meningiomas. As the facial nerve motor branch enters the internal auditory meatus, it is joined to the nervus intermedius and lies superior and anterior to the vestibuloacoustic nerve. After exiting the internal auditory meatus, the facial nerve separates from the acoustic nerve to enter its own canal, the fallopian, or facial, canal. The facial nerve runs a remarkable course in the fallopian canal, bending and changing directions to accommodate other structures in the temporal lobe. These changes in direction help subdivide the facial nerve into three parts, called the labyrinthine, tympanic, and mastoid segments (Fig. 43–4).[5] The facial nerve courses in the fallopian canal for approximately 30 mm. The labyrinthine segment is 3 to 5 mm long and incorporates the geniculate ganglion and the first branch of the facial nerve, also known as the greater superficial petrosal nerve.[3] This nerve travels forward along the floor of the middle cranial fossa to synapse in the sphenopalatine ganglion. Postganglionic parasympathetic fibers continue forward to innervate the lacrimal gland and nasopalatine glands.

At the geniculate ganglion, the facial nerve bends posteriorly to form the tympanic or horizontal segment. This portion is about 9 to 11 mm long and travels just above the oval window. The facial canal is very thin in this segment, and tiny dehiscences may appear over the oval window, an important anatomic feature for the middle ear surgeon to recognize and avoid.[6]

At the level of the lateral semicircular canal, the facial nerve takes a sharp downward course, marking the mastoid, or vertical, segment. The nerve to the stapedius originates at the proximal portion of this segment, and the chorda tympani nerve branches off more distally. The chorda tympani branch is approximately 5 mm above the stylomastoid foramen.[5] The chorda tympani nerve is a mixed nerve carrying taste fibers from the anterior two thirds of the tongue, parasympathetic fibers to the submaxillary and sublingual glands, and pain and temperature sensation from the external auditory meatus. The

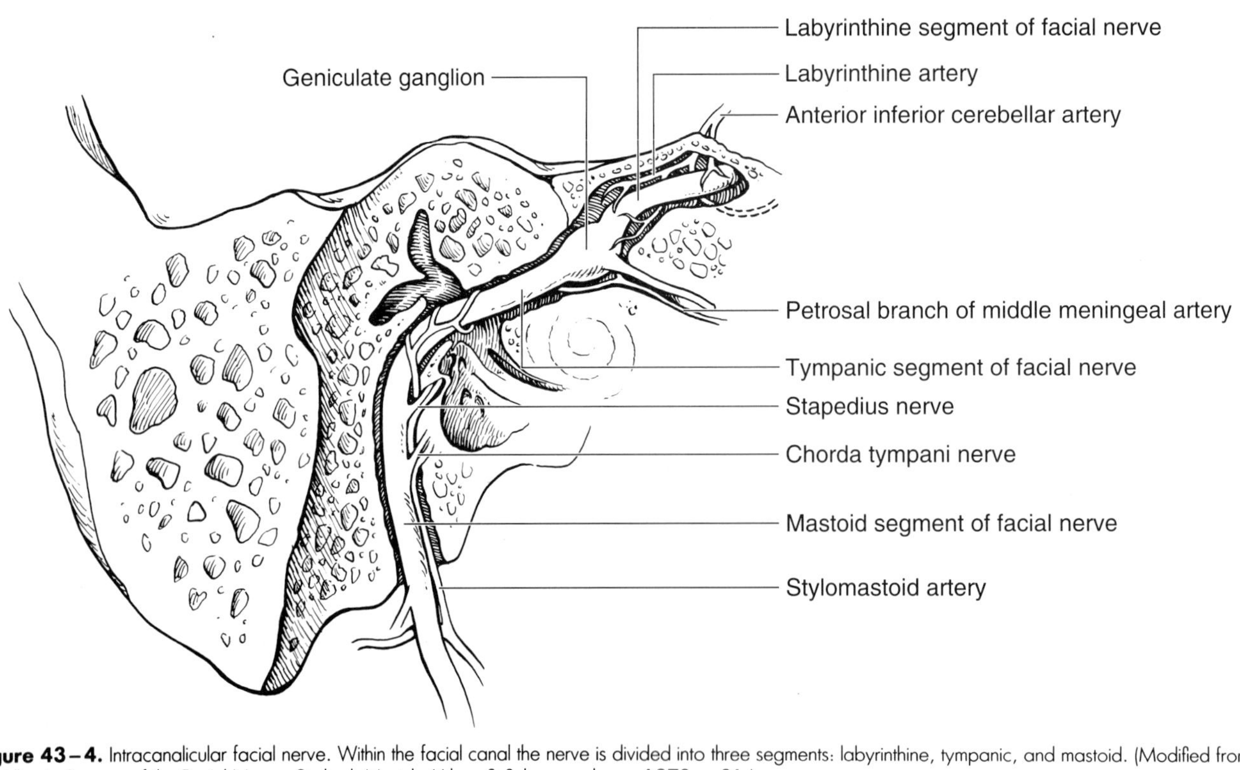

Figure 43–4. Intracanalicular facial nerve. Within the facial canal the nerve is divided into three segments: labyrinthine, tympanic, and mastoid. (Modified from Miehlke A: Surgery of the Facial Nerve, 2nd ed. Munich, Urban & Schwarzenberg, 1973, p 21.)

chorda tympani nerve may be seen coursing just underneath the tympanic membrane.[6]

Extracranial Course

The motor branches of the facial nerve exit the skull base via the stylomastoid foramen. Nerve twigs are immediately provided to the posterior auricular, the posterior belly of the digastric, and the stylohyoid muscles. The facial nerve then bends again to proceed forward to penetrate the posterior aspect of the parotid gland. Within the substance of the parotid gland, the facial nerve divides into upper and lower divisions, which may be further subdivided from top to bottom into the temporal, zygomatic, buccal, mandibular, and cervical branches (Fig. 43–5).[7] The vast interconnections among these branches provide the substrate for aberrant regeneration to ensue after facial palsy.[3] Common misdirection phenomena include eye closure on smiling or tearing in anticipation of eating food (crocodile tearing). In the latter case, nerve fibers destined to supply the salivary glands are misdirected to the lacrimal gland.

Blood Supply

From the brain stem to the internal auditory meatus, the facial nerve derives its blood supply from the AICA. The labyrinthine artery, a branch of the AICA, provides nourishment to the nerve in the internal auditory meatus. Moving distally, the petrosal branch of the middle meningeal artery enters the facial canal at the level of the geniculate ganglion and supplies blood to the tympanic portion of the nerve (see Fig. 43–4). Anastomotic connections are made to the tympanic region by the stylomastoid artery, which extends up the vertically oriented mastoid segment. The weakest link in the arterial supply to the facial nerve is just proximal to the geniculate ganglion, and this region is the likeliest site for ischemic injury to the nerve.[8]

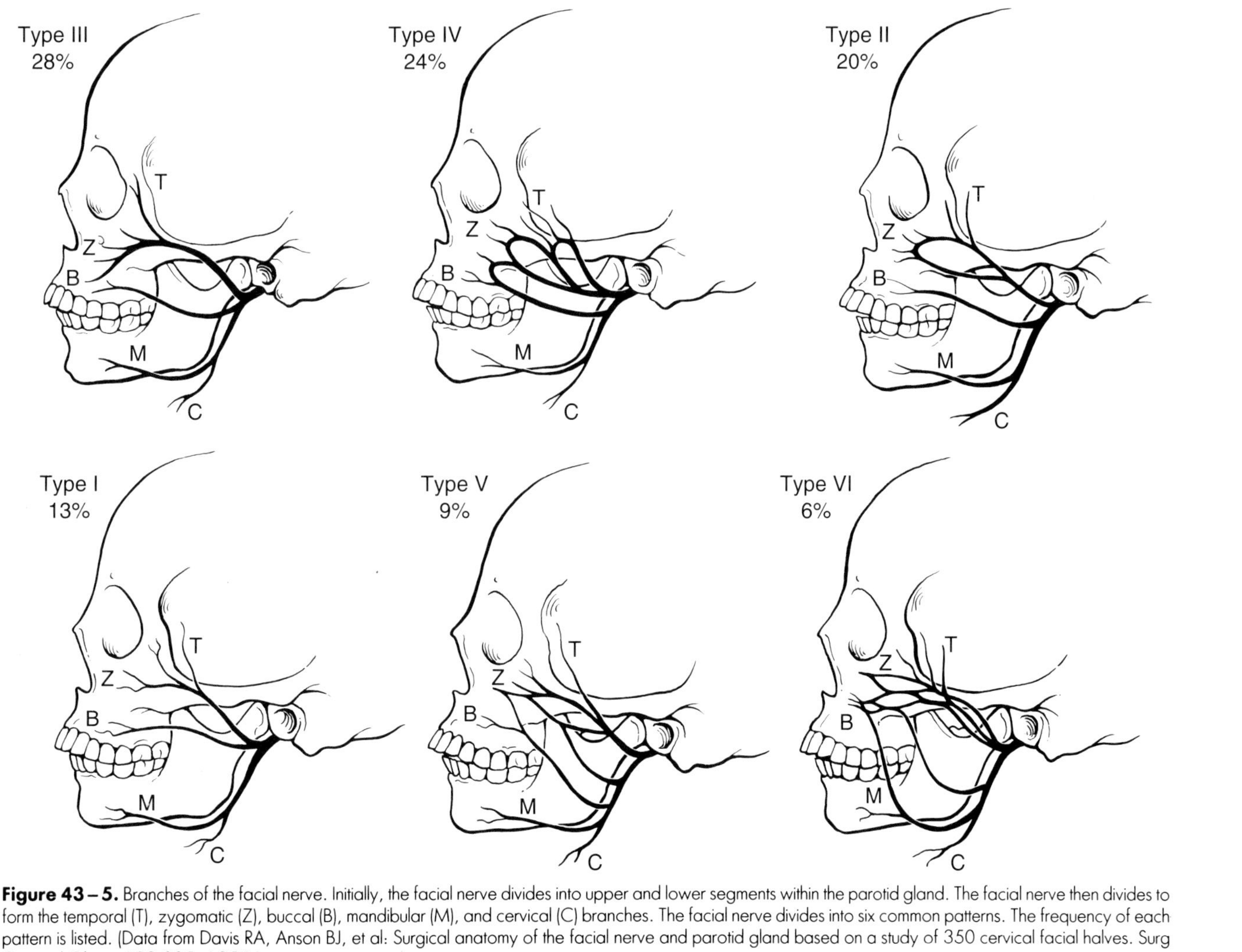

Figure 43–5. Branches of the facial nerve. Initially, the facial nerve divides into upper and lower segments within the parotid gland. The facial nerve then divides to form the temporal (T), zygomatic (Z), buccal (B), mandibular (M), and cervical (C) branches. The facial nerve divides into six common patterns. The frequency of each pattern is listed. (Data from Davis RA, Anson BJ, et al: Surgical anatomy of the facial nerve and parotid gland based on a study of 350 cervical facial halves. Surg Gynecol Obstet 102:385, 1956.)

HISTORY AND EXAMINATION

The ophthalmologist must take a full history and try to determine the cause and location of the palsy. The ophthalmologist should not presume that a patient with sudden facial weakness has Bell's palsy and will get better.

In the history, both the onset and the duration of facial palsy must be established. Facial weakness may be congenital or related to birth trauma from forceps delivery. A history of prior injury, either head trauma or regional trauma, should also be elicited, and information about facial or otologic surgery, which may have injured the seventh nerve, should also be obtained. Middle ear disease, such as otitis media, malignant external otitis, or cholesteatoma, may also cause seventh nerve palsy.

Pain obviously accompanies most ocular irritative symptoms, but occasionally pain precedes either Bell's palsy or herpes zoster. Symptoms of hyperacusis result from impairment of the stapedius muscle and are often seen in Bell's palsy. Decreased sense of taste may be involved in distal lesions. Symptoms of other cranial nerve dysfunction, such as numbness of the face, diplopia, anosmia, and difficulty swallowing, should also be sought. A thorough past medical history should exclude systemic illnesses, such as sarcoid, leprosy, and tuberculosis. It is equally important to ask about coexistent diseases, such as diabetes, an entity that is associated with an increased incidence of Bell's palsy. Recent immunizations for polio or influenza have been linked to facial palsy; thus, an immunization history should be obtained. Lyme disease is also an important consideration, especially in endemic areas for this tick-borne spirochetal disorder. Eliciting a history of the characteristic bull's-eye rash of erythema chronicum migrans may be helpful in confirming the diagnosis. Finally, a history of a periaural rash suggests the Ramsay Hunt syndrome (herpes zoster cephalicus).

The symptoms of facial palsy that bring the patient to the ophthalmologist relate to an inability to close the eye and include irritation, eye pain, and chronic red eye. Paralytic ectropion is seen in long-standing cases and may be a source of complaints. Paralytic drooping of the brow with obscuration of the visual field, drooling, and unilateral nasal airway obstruction may all be the result of chronic facial paralysis.

Facial palsy and facial paresis can often be diagnosed at a distance, but detection of subtle weakness, aberrant regeneration, and myokymia often requires careful observation. Analysis and examination of the face should begin with a determination of whether the palsy is central or peripheral. Asking the patient to look up allows the frontalis muscle to contract and, if unilaterally impaired, quickly reveals whether a palsy is central (intact frontalis function) or peripheral (impaired frontalis function) (see Fig. 43–1).

It is often helpful to observe the patient at rest. Facial palsy may affect either voluntary or involuntary movement, or both. At rest, all voluntary movement is eliminated. The position of the nasolabial fold and the nostrils should be noted because the nasolabial fold may disappear or be displaced in facial palsy, and the nostril may be ptotic or decreased circumferentially.

The ophthalmologist must determine whether the patient has a paralysis or a paresis. In Bell's palsy, for example, return of function may be likelier to occur if the facial weakness is incomplete.[9] The patient can be asked to smile, wrinkle the forehead, puff the cheeks, or wrinkle the nose. Aberrant regeneration as well as fasciculations of the involved muscles should be noted.

Examination of the skin should include the pinna and the auricle, in an attempt to detect the vesicular rash of herpes zoster oticus and cutaneous scars that might indicate an old facial nerve injury. The parotid gland should be palpated because infiltrative tumors often produce facial paralysis. Head and neck nodes are also readily accessible and may indicate an infectious or infiltrative cause of the facial paralysis. The lacrimal gland should be palpated because rarely, in sarcoid, lacrimal gland enlargement can occur in conjunction with facial diplegia.

With regard to the eye examination, assessment of visual acuity is routine. The degree of lid closure and the amount of lagophthalmos should be noted, as should orbicularis oculi strength, which is roughly assessed by measuring the force generated by the orbicularis with attempted eyelid closure. The two sides are compared as the examiner attempts to pry the patient's eyelids open. Ectropion, medial or lateral canthal laxity, and the degree of eyelid laxity should also be noted. The presence or absence of Bell's phenomenon should be observed because the cornea may be better protected during incomplete eyelid closure if the eyes roll upward.

Schirmer's test without anesthesia (Schirmer 1) can be performed. A normal Schirmer 1 test result (10 to 30 mm wetting of filter paper after 5 minutes) implies that the greater superficial petrosal nerve is intact and that the proximal facial nerve is spared.

The fifth cranial nerve function should be tested. Patients with seventh nerve palsy and exposure keratopathy may have chronic decreased corneal sensitivity. Consequently, a diminished corneal reflex is relatively nonspecific. However, when decreased corneal sensation exists in the presence of hypoesthesia of the adjacent skin of the eyelids and the nose, paresis of the fifth cranial nerve should be suspected.

Motility examination is critical in patients with seventh nerve palsy because the cranial nerves subserving eye movements lie in close anatomic proximity to the nucleus and fascicles of the seventh nerve. Sixth cranial nerve function may be impaired in infiltrative disorders, intracranial hemorrhage, stroke, or demyelinating syndromes. Central seventh nerve palsies are often accompanied by other neurologic sequelae, including eye movement impairment. In the Millard-Gubler syndrome, contralateral hemiparesis occurs along with a sixth and seventh nerve palsy. In Weber's syndrome, a lesion involves the ventral midbrain, resulting in an ipsilateral third nerve palsy and a contralateral central seventh nerve palsy and hemiparesis. Sixth nerve palsy can also occur in cryptogenic congenital syndromes affecting the facial nuclei, the fasciculi, or the facial nerve and muscles.

Eighth nerve testing can be performed at the patient's bedside by asking the patient to compare the examiner's whispering from one side to another. Sensorineural hearing loss in acoustic neuroma characteristically impairs speech discrimination before the pure tone range, and affected patients report an inability to distinguish speech before they complain of actual hearing loss. Testing of gait, coordination, and other cranial nerves may also be appropriate. Helpful clues in topographic diagnosis are listed in Table 43–1.

TABLE 43–1

Topical Diagnoses of Lesions of the Facial Nerve

Level	Signs	Probable Diagnosis
Supranuclear		
Cortex and internal Capsule	Tone and upper face intact, loss of volitional movement with intact spontaneous expression, slurred speech (tongue weakness), hemiparesis on side of facial involvement. Paresis of upper extremity begins with involvement of thumb, finger, and hand movement.	Lesion of motor cortex or internal capsule on side opposite facial involvement
Extrapyramidal	Increased salivary flow, impaired, spontaneous facial movement, intact volitional facial movement, masked face of parkinsonism or dystonia, progressive hemifacial spasm.	Tumor or vascular lesion of basal ganglia; parkinsonism, Meige's syndrome (cervical facial dystonia)
Midbrain	Involvement of face and oculomotor roots; loss of pupillary reflexes, external strabismus, and oculomotor paresis on side opposite facial paresis.	Weber's syndrome
	Bilateral facial paresis with other cranial nerve deficits, emotional lability, hyperactive gag reflex, marked hyperflexia associated with hypertension.	Pseudobulbar palsy associated with multiple infarcts
Pontine nucleus	Involvement of cranial nerves VII and VI on side of lesion with gaze palsy on side of facial paresis; associated ataxia, cerebellovestibular signs, and contralateral hemiparesis.	Involvement of pons at level of VII and VI nuclei by pontine glioma, multiple sclerosis, infection; infarction
	Cranial nerve VII and VI palsy noted from time of birth with or without other congenital anomalies. Facial motor involvement usually incomplete with sparing of corner of mouth or lower lip common. Involvement of the lower lip with complete or partial sparing of upper face. Anomalies of the pinna, canal, or mandible associated with facial palsy indicate developmental defect of facial nerve.	Developmental facial palsy (noted at birth); oculofacial syndrome, Möbius' syndrome; thalidomide toxicity; nondevelopmental facial or abducens nerve anomalies most often result from infranuclear lesions
Infranuclear		
Intracranial		
Cerebellopontine angle	Impairment of hearing, especially discrimination out of proportion to pure tone scores; possible ataxia, abnormalities of tearing or taste, stapes reflex decay, decreased corneal sensation; facial motor deficit (late sign).	Acoustic schwannoma
	Abnormalities in trigeminal, acoustic-vestibular, and facial nerve function, starting with facial pain or numbness. Lesion noted on CT (enhancement with contrast) may show evidence of calcification.	Meningioma
	Abnormalities of facial and acoustic-vestibular nerve function; may start with facial twitching; erosion or lytic area evident on plain radiographs of temporal bone	Cholesteatoma or facial schwannoma arising in temporal bone
	Abnormalities of cranial nerves VII, VIII, IX, X, XI, and XII; pulsatile tinnitus and purple-red pulsating mass bulging through the tympanic membrane.	Glomus jugulare tumor
	Abnormalities of abducens nerve in addition to above.	Glomus jugulare tumor extending to petrous apex to involve middle fossa
Skull base	Conductive or sensorineural hearing loss, acute or recurrent facial palsy; positive family history, abnormalities of bone density on skull radiograph.	Osteopetrosis
	Multiple cranial nerve involvement in rapid succession.	Carcinomatous meningitis, leukemia, Landry-Guillain-Barré, mononucleosis, diphtheria, tuberculosis, sarcoidosis, malignant external otitis

(Continued)

TABLE 43-1 *Continued*

Topical Diagnoses of Lesions of the Facial Nerve

Level	Signs	Probable Diagnosis
Transtemporal bone		
Internal auditory canal (IAC) and labyrinthine segment of facial nerve	Ecchymosis around pinna and mastoid prominence (Battle's sign); hematotympanum with sensorineural hearing loss (tuning fork lateralizes to normal side), vertigo, nystagmus (fast component away from involved side); sudden complete facial paralysis following head trauma; usually associated with basilar skull fracture, loss of consciousness, and CSF leak. Transection of facial nerve is likelier with this injury than with longitudinal fracture.	Temporal bone fracture (transverse, longitudinal, or combination)
Geniculate ganglion	Dry eye, decreased taste and salivation. Erosion of geniculate ganglion area or middle fossa is demonstrated by pluridirectional tomography and CT of temporal bone.	Schwannoma, meningioma, cholesteatoma, hemangioma, arteriovenous malformation
	Ear pain, vesicles on pinna, dry eye, decreased taste and salivary flow; sensorineural hearing loss, nystagmus, vertigo, red chorda tympani nerve. Facial palsy may be complete, incomplete, or progress to complete over 14 days.	Herpes zoster cephalicus (Ramsay Hunt syndrome)
	Same as above without vesicles, no other cause evident. Facial palsy may be complete, incomplete, or progress to complete over 10 days.	Idiopathic (Bell's) palsy (viral-inflammatory immune disorder)
	Same as above but no recovery in 6 months.	Tumor
	Ecchymosis around pinna and mastoid (Battle's sign), hematotympanum; conductive hearing loss (tuning fork lateralizes to involved ear); no vestibular involvement unless stapes subluxed into vestibule (causes fluctuating sensorineural hearing loss and vertigo with nystagmus).	Longitudinal fracture of temporal bone; may be proximal or at geniculate ganglion (dry eye), or distal to geniculate ganglion (tearing symmetric) (tear test valid only in acute injury)
Tympanomastoid	Decreased taste and salivation, loss of stapes reflex and symmetrical tearing; sudden-onset facial palsy, which may be complete or incomplete or may progress to complete.	
	Pain, vesicles, red chorda tympani.	Herpes zoster cephalicus
	Pain without vesicles, red chorda tympani.	Bell's palsy
	Red, bulging tympanic membrane, conductive hearing loss; usually history of URI. Lower face may be involved more than upper.	Acute suppurative otitis media
	Foul drainage through perforated tympanic membrane; history of recurrent ear infection, drainage, and hearing loss.	Chronic suppurative otitis media, most likely associated with cholesteatoma
	Pulsatile tinnitus, purple-red pulsatile mass noted through tympanic membrane.	Glomus tympanicum or jugulare
	Recurrent facial paralysis, positive family history, facial edema, fissured tongue; may present with simultaneous bilateral facial paralysis.	Melkersson-Rosenthal syndrome
Extracranial	Incomplete facial nerve paresis; hearing, balance, tearing, stapes reflex, taste, salivary flow spared.	Penetrating wound of face; sequelae of parotid surgery; malignancy of parotid, tonsil, or oronasopharynx; rarely, with benign lesion of parotid gland compressing facial nerve
	Uveitis, salivary gland enlargement, fever.	Sarcoidosis (Heerfordt's syndrome), Lyme disease, lymphoma
Various sites	Bilateral facial paralysis from birth.	Möbius' syndrome
	Bilateral facial paralysis, acquired.	Landry-Guillain-Barré syndrome, sarcoidosis, mononucleosis, leukemia, idiopathic (Bell's) palsy
	Facial paralysis, especially simultaneous bilateral facial paralysis with ascending areflexic quadriparesis; sensory changes usually mild with spinal fluid typically showing albuminocytologic dissociation (elevated protein without cells).	Landry-Guillain-Barré syndrome
	Deficits of cranial nerves VI and VII or VII, VI, and III, possibly in association with marked increase in jaw jerk or gag reflex.	Carcinoma of nasopharynx; metastatic carcinoma from breast, ovary, or prostate; meningitis; leukemia; diabetes mellitus
Pseudobulbar palsy	Inappropriate or exaggerated laughing or crying; may be associated with marked increase in jaw jerk or gag reflex.	Demyelinating, degenerative, or vascular lesion involving bilateral corticobulbar pathways

From May M, Galetta S: The facial nerve. *In* Tasman W, Jaeger EA (eds): Duane's Clinical Ophthalmology. Philadelphia, JB Lippincott, 1988, pp 5–7.
CSF, cerebrospinal fluid; CT, computed tomography; URI, upper respiratory infection.

DISORDERS

Bell's Palsy

All facial palsies are not Bell's palsy, as demonstrated in a study by May, in which only 53% of patients who were referred with the diagnosis of Bell's palsy had the disorder.[9] Approximately 10% had a treatable lesion. Bell's palsy is a diagnosis of exclusion. Table 43–2 lists the suggested evaluation for patients with facial palsies.

Bell's palsy is an idiopathic facial palsy that may have a viral cause. Presenting symptoms may include a combination of ipsilateral ear pain, numbness, or hyperacusis. Bell's palsy may recur in 10% to 20% of people. Diabetes may be a risk factor, as is pregnancy.[10] Fortunately, the prognosis is excellent in most cases of Bell's palsy, with full recovery of function occurring in approximately 84% of patients.[11] Most patients begin to recover within 3 weeks of onset. Prognostically, the sooner the palsy begins to recover, the better the outcome. As the palsy becomes more complete, the likelihood of aberrant regeneration increases.[9]

Regarding treatment options, it is a common misperception that the use of corticosteroids or facial nerve surgical decompression alters the natural course of idiopathic Bell's palsy. May and associates[12] have documented that no study to date can demonstrate an improvement in the natural course of idiopathic Bell's palsy with either surgical or corticosteroid intervention. Statistically significant patient numbers have yet to be recruited to accurately answer this treatment dilemma.

Ramsay Hunt Syndrome

Ramsay Hunt syndrome, or cephalic herpes zoster, is characteristically preceded by a prodrome of severe pain in the affected ear and is followed by a vesicular rash involving the pinna and external auditory canal.[13] The facial palsy may be accompanied by hearing loss, vestibular impairment, or encephalitis in severe cases. The prognosis for herpes zoster cephalicus is poorer than that for Bell's palsy in terms of complete recovery of facial function, with only 60% of patients having complete return of function.[14]

TABLE 43–2

Diagnostic Considerations in Facial Nerve Palsy

Clinical Problem	Test
Central facial palsy	Brain MRI
Peripheral facial palsy	
Bilateral palsy	Brain MRI, lumbar puncture, EMG (rule out Guillain-Barré syndrome, myotonia), Tensilon (rule out myasthenia)
Progressive palsy, dizziness, or associated hearing loss	MRI of cerebellopontine angle
Acute unilateral palsy	Blood glucose level, syphilis serology, and CBC; Lyme titer (endemic area or exposure history); angiotensin-converting enzyme (rule out sarcoid)
Chronic palsy	Chest radiograph (rule out sarcoid, tumor), brain MRI

CBC, complete blood count; EMG, electromyography; MRI, magnetic resonance imaging.

Acute Otitis Media

Acute otitis media with or without mastoiditis may occur and, when chronic, may affect the facial nerve as it courses through the temporal bone. In elderly diabetic patients, malignant external otitis is usually caused by a necrotizing *Pseudomonas* infection that progresses fulminantly. Both intravenous antibiotics and surgery, with wide debridement of necrotic bone and granulation tissue, are necessary. The facial nerve is vulnerable within the fallopian canal and can be affected by adjacent suppuration, abscess formation, or cholesteatoma. The association of a sixth cranial nerve palsy with facial palsy in petrous apex infection (Gradenigo's syndrome) is well described and usually responds to antibiotic treatment.[15]

Lyme Disease

Lyme disease, which is caused by the tick-borne spirochete *Borrelia burgdorferi,* may cause unilateral or bilateral facial palsy at some point in its course in approximately 10% of patients.[16] Approximately 60% of patients will recall the diagnostic skin lesion of erythema chronicum migrans lesion, an erythematous raised area that spreads centripetally, leaving a central clear zone and lasting several weeks if left untreated. Flu-like symptoms, including chills, fever, arthralgias, headaches, and myalgias, may occur concomitant with the lesion. The diagnosis may be made by finding a positive serum enzyme-linked immunosorbent assay titer and may be confirmed by the results of a Western blot. The facial palsy has an excellent prognosis regardless of the antibiotic regimen chosen.

Trauma

The facial nerve is vulnerable in its bony course within the temporal bone at its exit point from the stylomastoid foramen and along its course to innervate the muscles of facial expression. The nerve itself can be either lacerated or traumatized bluntly. Fractures parallel to the long aspect of the petrous portion of the temporal bone are often accompanied by fractures of the ossicles or the labyrinth.

The facial nerve may be injured by mandibular fractures or during surgery of the mandible. The facial nerve branches are particularly vulnerable to undermining in the vicinity of the zygoma and lateral orbit during a face lift.

Facial Nerve Tumors

Tumors of the facial nerve are rare. A facial neuroma often presents with hyperkinesis rather than palsy and can be diagnosed by magnetic resonance imaging. Surgery may consist of biopsy and resection with a cable graft.

Acoustic Neuroma

Acoustic neuromas usually present with a seventh cranial nerve palsy late in their course as the facial nerve is displaced and compressed by the expanding cerebellopontine tumor. Common symptoms of acoustic neuroma include tinnitus, hearing loss, and cerebellar and vestibular signs. Magnetic resonance imaging is essential for establishing the diagnosis and shows a cerebellopontine angle mass that is hypointense on T1-weighted imaging and hyperintense on T2-weighted sequences. When imaging is performed with gadolinium, this lesion is seen as a diffusely enhancing mass. Treatment consists of neurosurgical excision.

Metastatic Lesions

A history of cancer and the presence of a rapidly progressive facial palsy are highly suggestive of a metastatic lesion. The nerve or the meninges may be infiltrated. Magnetic resonance imaging with gadolinium may show enhancement of the dura, or disruption of the blood-brain barrier, or both. Serial lumbar punctures may be necessary for the cytologic diagnosis of meningeal carcinomatosis.

Related Disorders

Myotonic dystrophy is a hereditary bilateral distal myopathy that is associated with weakness of the muscles of the face and extremities. Other characteristic features include frontal baldness, testicular atrophy, and cataract. In addition to having ptosis, patients have bilateral weakness of the facial muscles.

Uncommon Disorders

Chickenpox, mumps, diphtheria, polio, Guillain-Barré syndrome, leprosy, and botulism are rare but may be infectious causes of facial weakness.

MEDICAL MANAGEMENT

The ophthalmologist's major concern in patients with facial paralysis is poor eyelid closure and resultant corneal exposure. Corneal problems range from mild punctate epithelial keratopathy to dellen to corneal ulceration and even perforation. It is not unusual for an ophthalmologist to see a young child with congenital facial nerve palsy or a young person with acquired palsy who completely adapts to the paralysis and requires no medical or surgical intervention. Conversely, an acute reduction of the quality and quantity of the tear film makes the older patient much more susceptible to exposure problems. Degrees of facial palsy range from partial to complete, and the severity of the palsy usually determines the severity of symptoms and signs.

The treatment of all patients with facial nerve palsy includes the application of topical lubricants. These drops should be a primary treatment. Some patients need topical lubrication throughout their course. Artificial tears administered four times a day and often more frequently are appropriate as an initial therapy. Patients should be urged to try several different tear preparations because their comfort level may vary widely between brands. Unpreserved lubricating drops can be used every half hour to hour. Initial therapy at night may also include a petrolatum-based ointment. Individuals with severe exposure keratitis may require the use of ointment during the day as well.

Additional factors that may further threaten visual integrity include ipsilateral corneal anesthesia, preexisting dry eye, or inflammatory lacrimal disease and sacrifice injury to the nervus intermedius, as occurs with acoustic neuroma surgery.

Additional protection of the eye at bedtime may be appropriate if drops and ointments are insufficient or if nocturnal lagophthalmos is present. A "moisture bubble" can be taped over the eye at night after ointment is applied. Figure 43–6 shows a commercially available protective ocular bubble obtained from Eagle Vision (no. 0088, Memphis, TN), and a similar device can be obtained from Concept Corporation (Largo, FL). Standard swimming goggles can also be used to create a moisture chamber while the patient is sleeping but are often bulky and impractical. A convenient alternative is the use of a small oval piece of plastic wrap measuring approximately 3 inches in diameter, placed from the brow to the cheek and encompassing the medial canthus and the lateral canthus; this often proves to be the most practical and efficacious means of shielding the cornea at night (Fig. 43–7). An additional technique involves closing the eyelid shut with adhesive tape. However, we have found that taping the eyelid closed also creates as many problems as therapeutic successes because the tape may come off or, if the patient is not skilled at taping the lid, the lids can be taped in an open position, thus abrading the cornea.

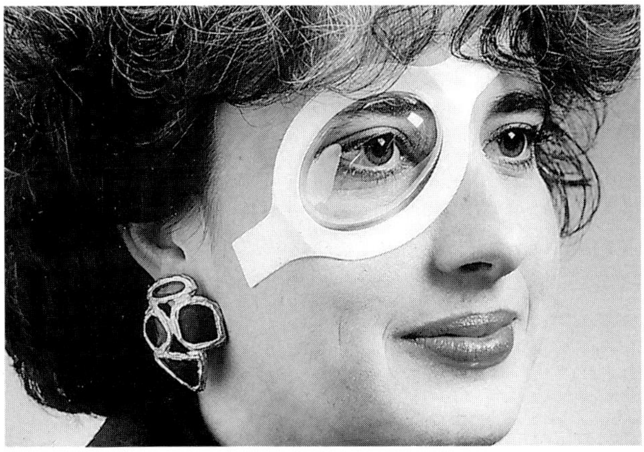

Figure 43–6. Protective ocular bubble (no. 0088). (Courtesy of Eagle Vision, Memphis, TN.)

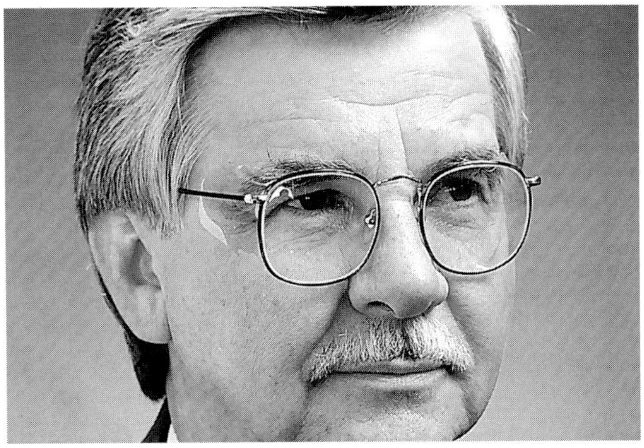

Figure 43–8. Moisture chamber glasses (no. 0070 or 0069). (Courtesy of Eagle Vision, Memphis, TN.)

A large percentage of patients with permanent facial nerve palsy require moisture chamber glasses. Moisture chambers (Fig. 43–8) (no. 0070 or 0069, Eagle Vision, Memphis, TN) are fitted to standard glass frames and molded to the face to create a tight seal. This method is equivalent to wearing swimming goggles but is much more aesthetically pleasing and allows the refraction to be placed in a normal spectacle frame. Moisture chamber glasses permit the patient to remain active in many activities that otherwise might be irritating. They also provide side protection from the elements. We encourage the early use of moisture chamber glasses because most palsy patients find them of great utility.

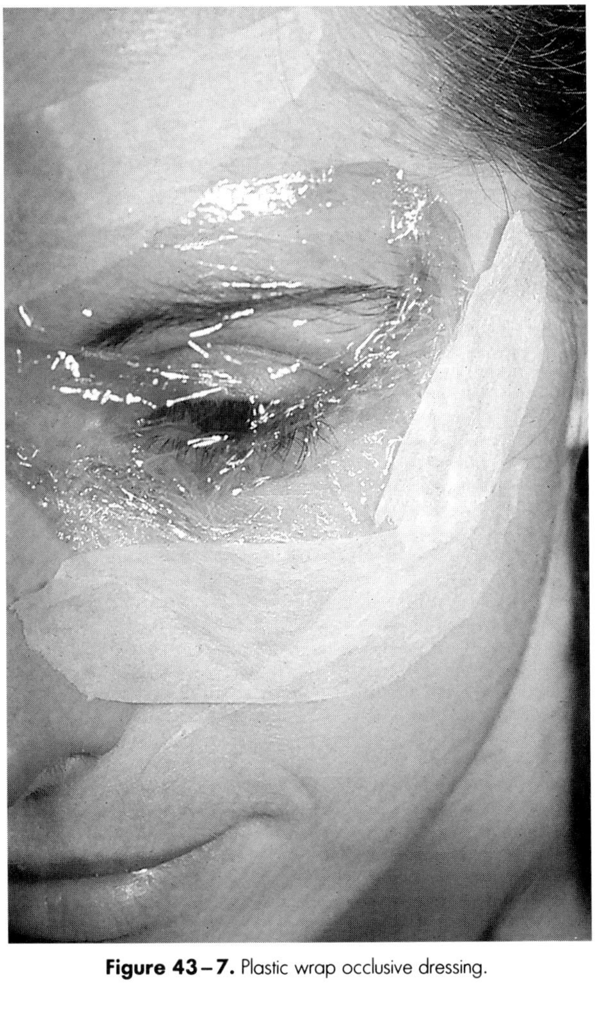

Figure 43–7. Plastic wrap occlusive dressing.

SURGICAL MANAGEMENT

Surgical intervention is primarily considered in cases in which medical management has failed and in the correction of malpositions and aesthetic deficiencies, such as ectropion, that occur in facial nerve palsy. Reanimation of the eyelid is a difficult problem, but it can be achieved in various ways.

Gold Weight

The surgical device most commonly used to protect the eye in instances of facial nerve palsy is the gold weight (Fig. 43–9). MedDev Corporation (Los Altos, CA) provides gold implants in various weights, and standard weights range from 0.6 to 1.6 g in increments of 0.2 g. These gold weights are intended for placement in the upper lid and easily work by a gravity effect during eyelid closure with levator relaxation (Fig. 43–10). The weight of the gold pulls the upper lid closed. The advantages of the gold weight are technical simplicity of surgery and low morbidity rate. The disadvantages are the unnatural slowed closure of the lid, lack of blink, and subtle thickening of the eyelid skin.

The size of the weight is determined preoperatively with the patient in the sitting position. One-eighth-inch Steri-Strips are used to tape gold weights on the lid; the ophthalmologist chooses the weight that provides the

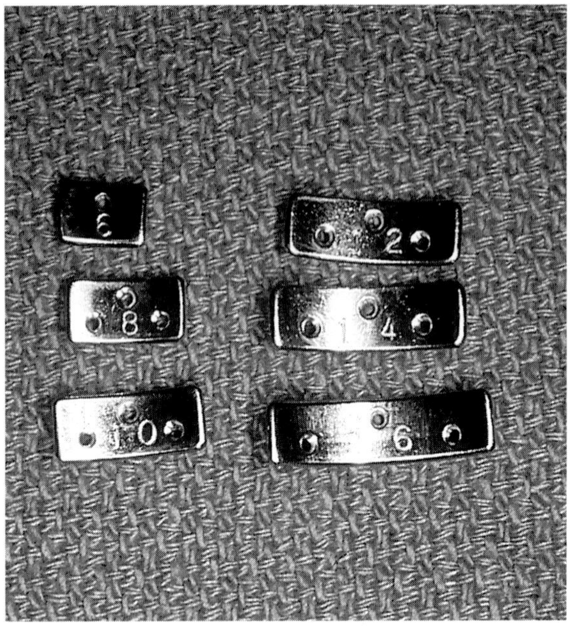

Figure 43–9. Series of gold weights. (Courtesy of MedDev, Los Altos, CA.)

greatest closure, but allows the eyelid to open as completely as possible, because the gold weight can cause mechanical ptosis. The same sized weight does not suffice in all individuals. In patients with a strong Bell's phenomenon, a small amount of lagophthalmos can be tolerated and at the same time allow the levator complex to lift the lid and the weight.

Surgical placement of the gold weight is usually performed on an outpatient basis with the patient under local anesthesia. An eyelid crease incision is made and carried through the orbicularis down to the tarsal plate (Fig. 43–11). Care is taken to avoid the upper border of the tarsus so that an artificial disinsertion of the aponeurosis and Müller's muscle is not created. A pocket is created within the orbicularis on the surface of the tarsus. All the gold weights have small holes in them for placement of sutures. A 6-0 polypropylene suture is passed through half-thickness tarsus and through the hole of the gold weight, securing it to the tarsal plate (Fig. 43–12). In

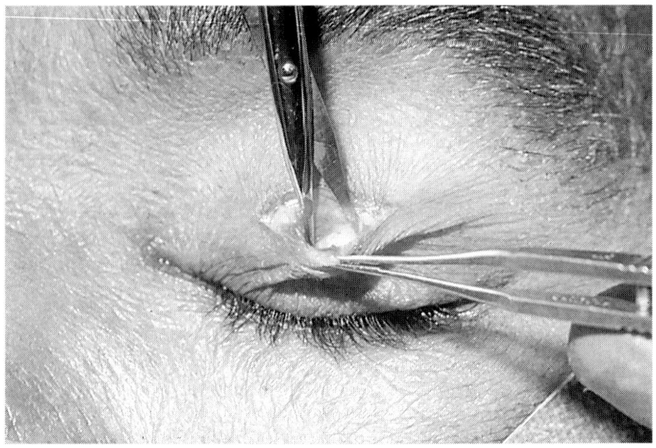

Figure 43–11. Eyelid crease incision, through the orbicularis down to the tarsal plate.

some instances, the gold weight is wrapped with a Dacron mesh to help secure it to the eyelid and prevent migration. The Dacron allows fibrovascular ingrowth around the weight to further stabilize its placement. Once the gold weight has been placed, the orbicularis is closed with interrupted 6-0 chromic sutures and the skin, with 6-0 polypropylene sutures (Fig. 43–13).

Palpebral Spring

Stainless steel springs can also be used to reanimate the upper eyelid. The advantages of the palpebral spring are as follows: retains a natural blink, allows for full eyelid closure, does not thicken the eyelid, and gives the most aesthetically pleasing result. Disadvantages, which are significant, include a more complicated process of placing the spring and the need for adjustments in the spring tension after surgery, as well as the potential for spring fatigue, fracture, and extrusion. As with the gold weight, the spring is formed before surgery.

A 0.1-mm-diameter stainless steel orthodontic dental wire is bent into a V shape with an approximately 3- to 5-mm diameter fulcrum (Fig. 43–14). Each limb of the spring can be curved to fit the natural curve of the eyelid

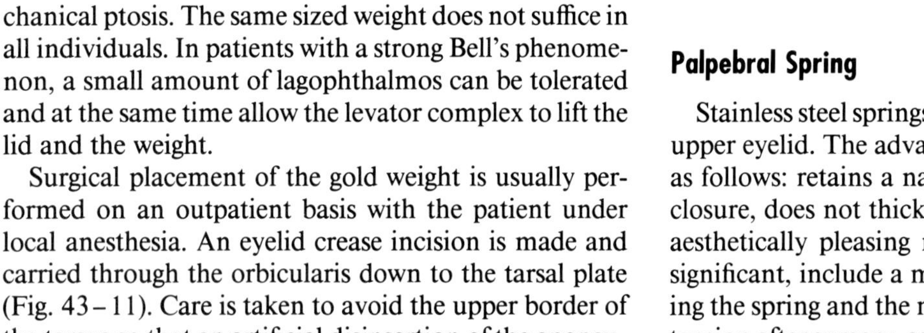

Figure 43–10. *A*, A trial gold weight is taped to the upper eyelid. The palpebral fissure opening is noted, both before and after placement of the gold weight. *B*, With the same trial gold weight as in *A*, the patient closes both eyes. An ideal weight will balance the amount of palpebral fissure opening and eliminate lagophthalmos. The severity of ocular symptoms, the presence of Bell's phenomenon, and the palpebral fissure opening on the contralateral side are additional considerations in selecting the appropriate weight.

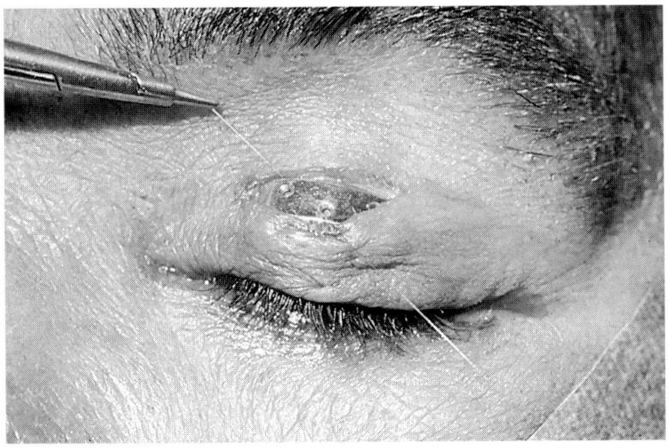

Figure 43–12. Gold weight sutured in place.

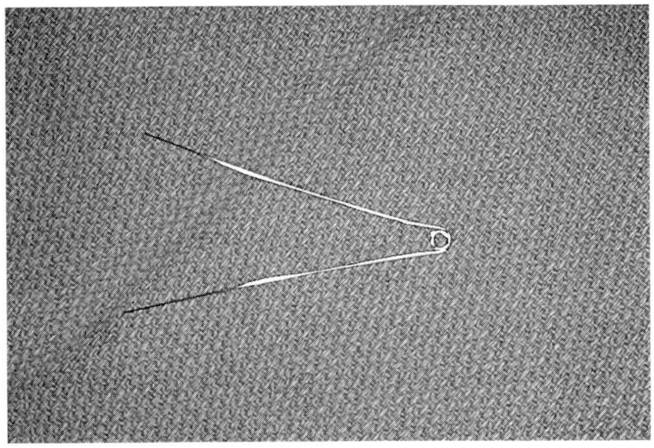

Figure 43–14. Orthodontic dental wire bent to the appropriate shape.

and orbital bony rim by use of the surgeon's fingernails stroked firmly over the limb to curve it around the eyelid. All these adjustments in size and shape are made most easily with orthodontic tools. Once adjusted, the spring is autoclaved. A local anesthetic is quite helpful in allowing the patient to aid the surgeon in establishing appropriate spring tension for maximum closure and eyelid opening.

An incision is made along the eyelid crease from the medial aspect of the lid extending out well into the lateral canthus. Through this incision, the tarsal plate is exposed, as is the periosteum at the lateral canthus and along the superior and lateral walls of the orbit (Fig. 43–15). Great care is taken not to interfere with the attachments of the aponeurosis. The tarsal limb of the spring should extend 2 mm past the midline medially. The sharp end is bent into a three-quarter curve so as to avoid end extrusion. A Dacron mesh measuring approximately 8 to 10 mm is folded in half to create an envelope that measures approximately 5 by 8 mm. The purpose of the Dacron mesh is to help secure the spring to the tarsal plate and to prevent extrusion. The Dacron is secured around the end of the tarsal limb and is sutured to the tarsal plate with multiple interrupted 6-0 polypropylene. Additional polypropylene can reinforce the Dacron if the Dacron is placed through the straight middle portion of the tarsal limb. The fulcrum of the spring is attached to the periosteum of the lateral orbit with 4-0 polypropylene (Fig. 43–16). Moving the fulcrum lateral or medial, up or down, alters the function of the spring. The fulcrum must be sutured into good position, and the patient must open and close the eyes so that this point can be adjusted appropriately.

Lid contour must also be taken into consideration in the bending of the spring because lateral eyelid ptosis can ensue if the tarsal limb is too straight rather than concave. Once the fulcrum has been fixated with adequate lid opening and maximum closure, the orbital limb is secured just inside the periosteum with multiple interrupted 4-0 polypropylene sutures along its entire length. The end of the limb can also be recurved into a three-quarter circle. The orbicularis is closed with interrupted 6-0 chromic sutures, and the skin, with 6-0 polypropylene sutures. Both topical and systemic antibiotics are instituted for 10 days. Some surgeons prefer to pass the eyelid portion of the spring by means of a trocar. However, exposure of the tarsal plate out to the lateral canthus allows the surgeon to titrate the curve and the tension of the spring, giving better functional and aesthetic results.

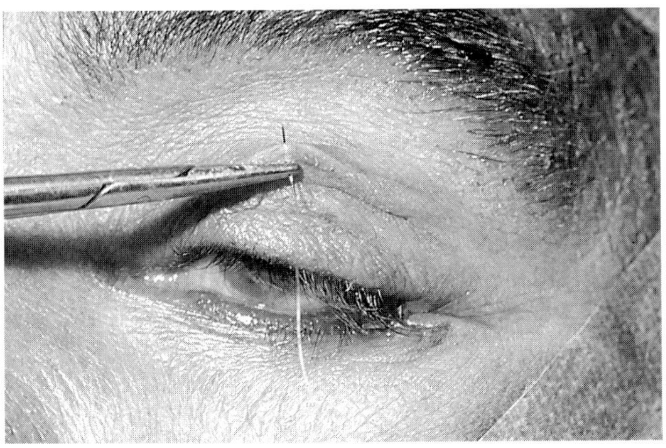

Figure 43–13. Both orbicularis and skin are sutured closed.

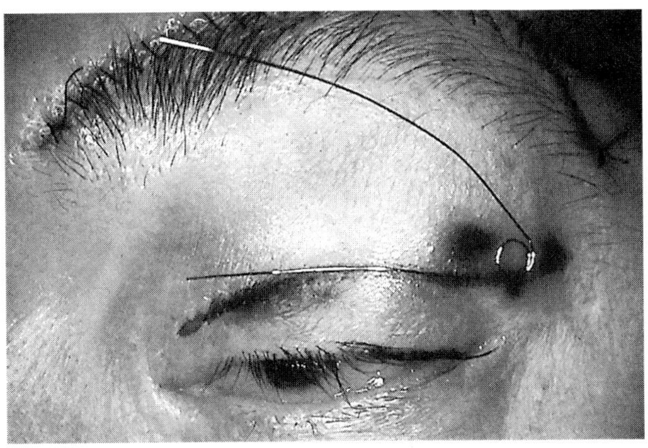

Figure 43–15. Incision for palpebral spring.

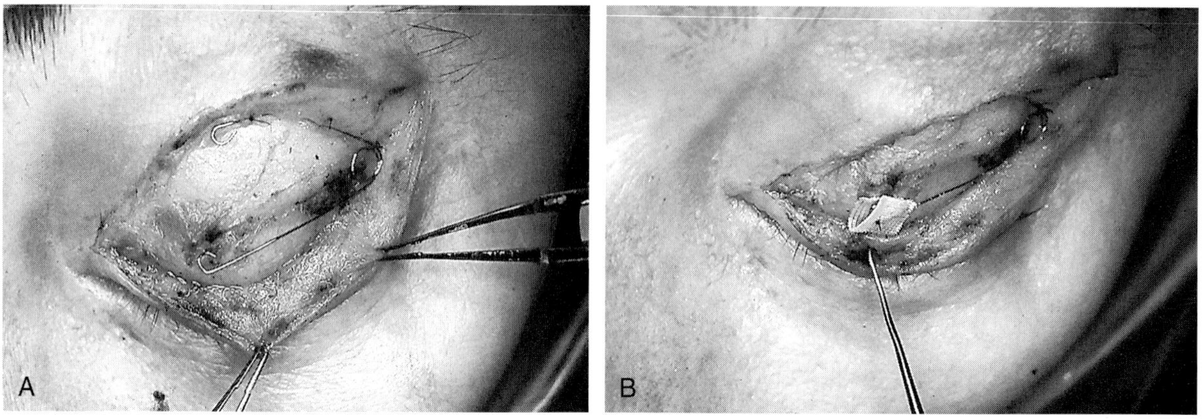

Figure 43–16. *A*, Palpebral spring positioned in the upper eyelid. *B*, Dacron mesh placed along the tarsal limb of spring.

Adjustments in spring tension in the postoperative period can be made by use of a 1 cm incision over the fulcrum of the spring in the physician's office with the patient under local anesthesia. The spring is then bent to either strengthen or weaken the closing effects of the device. The wound is then closed as in the primary procedure (Fig. 43–17).

Arion Silastic Sling

The Arion sling is used less frequently in Scheie Eye Institute but remains a third option for eyelid reanimation. Placement of a sling is technically more difficult than that of a gold weight, but it unquestionably provides a more natural movement to the lid. However, the overall functional and aesthetic results remain better with the palpebral spring than with the Arion sling.

The operation is performed with the patient under local anesthesia so that adjustments can be made in the tension of the Silastic. The Arion sling can be placed in the lower lid as well as the upper lid; however, many surgeons have abandoned the lower lid component because the sling may cause lower eyelid ectropion.

The technique described here characterizes our placement of the upper lid sling. A Dow Corning 1-mm diameter Silastic rod is used for this procedure. Older techniques provide for trocars or passers to thread the rod through the lid; direct suturing of the rod to the tarsus provides better aesthetic and functional results in our hands.

An upper eyelid crease incision is made for the length of the upper lid. A lateral and medial canthal incision is created to expose the lateral orbital rim and the medial canthal tendon (Fig. 43–18). Two holes are drilled at the level of the lateral orbital tubercle through the bone of the orbit (Fig. 43–19). A double strand of Silastic is placed in the upper lid. One end of the Silastic rod is passed around the anterior limb of the medial canthal tendon. The two ends are then passed over the tarsal plate to the drill holes in the orbital rim. The Silastic rods are passed from the inside of the rim to the outside. The rods are then sutured to the tarsal plate with 6-0 polypropylene close to the lower border of the tarsus in the upper lid to prevent ectropion. The tension on the knot can be manipulated to adjust the function of the spring so that maximal closure and maximal opening are achieved (Fig. 43–20). A small amount of lagophthalmos is acceptable and is desired in most cases because it will enhance the aesthetic result. Once satisfactory placement of the rods and tension have

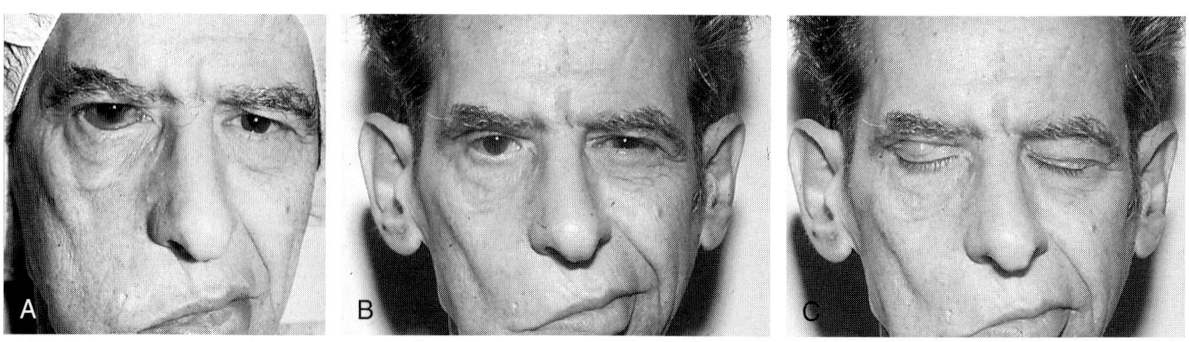

Figure 43–17. *A*, Patient with right-sided facial paralysis. Poor orbicularis muscle tone is causing significant ocular symptoms. *B*, Palpebral spring is placed into the right upper eyelid. Adjustments to the orthodontic wire are made, which result in good eyelid contour and proper palpebral fissure opening. A right lateral canthal tightening procedure has also been performed. *C*, The palpebral spring allows for full eyelid closure and aesthetically pleasing results.

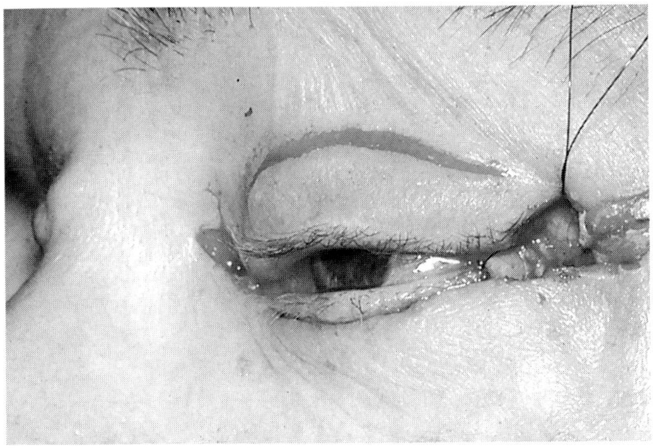

Figure 43–18. Incisions in preparation for placement of Arion sling. The current technique limits the placement of the Silastic to the upper eyelid.

been applied, multiple knots are tied on the ends of the Silastic thread outside the lateral orbital rim. The orbicularis is sutured with 6-0 chromic sutures, and the skin, with 6-0 polypropylene sutures. The patients then receive topical and systemic antibiotics.

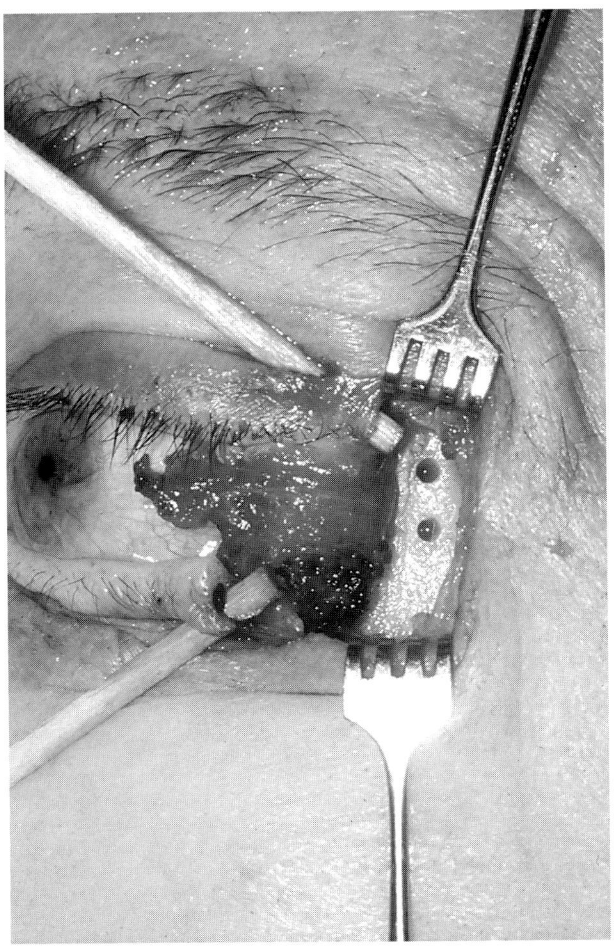

Figure 43–19. Holes drilled at lateral orbital rim to secure silicone.

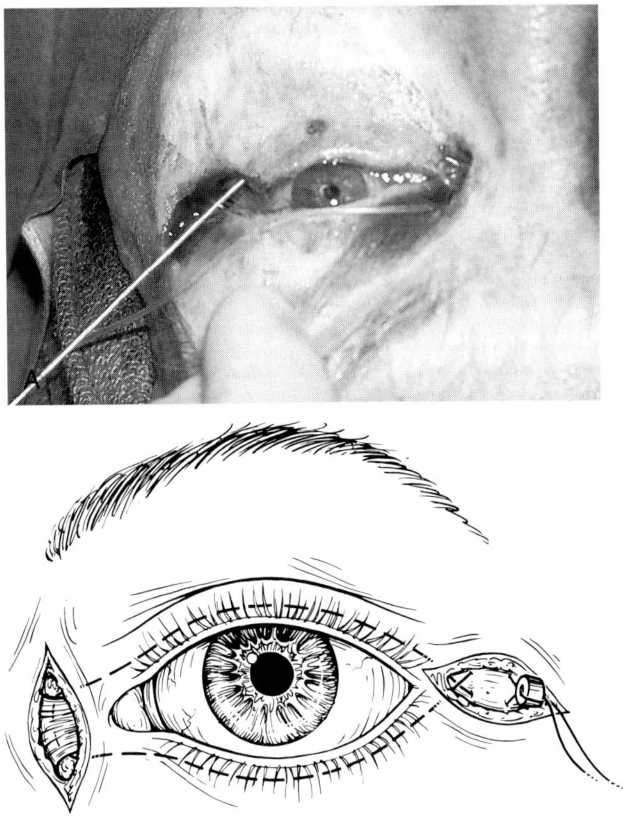

B

Figure 43–20. *A*, Silicone rod placed along the upper eyelid only. Both ends of the silicone are secured around the medial canthal tendon and drill holes through the lateral orbital rim. *B*, Silicone is placed in both upper and lower eyelids. Silicone rods are placed 2 to 3 mm from the upper and lower eyelid margins. A silicone sleeve can be used at the lateral orbital rim to ensure a secure knot. (Modified from McCord C, Tanenbaum M [eds]: Oculoplastic Surgery, 2nd ed. New York, Raven, 1987, p 320.)

Other Surgical Methods for the Upper Eyelid

Other surgical methods to reanimate the lids have selected applications. Transposition of temporalis muscle to the lids has been attempted to bring more resting tone to the eyelids as well as functional closure. The central third of the temporalis muscle is mobilized from the temporalis fossa and is brought over the lateral orbital rim. To achieve an optimal physiologic pull to the lids and to avoid external anatomic defects at the lateral orbital rim, a hole 1 to 2 cm in diameter is drilled in the orbital bone below the rim, at or about the area of the lateral orbital tubercle. The strip of temporalis muscle is passed through this hole and onto the lids. The strip of muscle is then split into two strands, one being passed along the anterior face of the upper tarsal border and the other along the anterior tarsal border of the lower lid. Extensions of the temporalis fascia are often needed to extend the muscle to the medial canthal tendon, to which the two strips are secured. Marked overcorrection is essential because the strips of muscle loosen with time. Despite the obvious

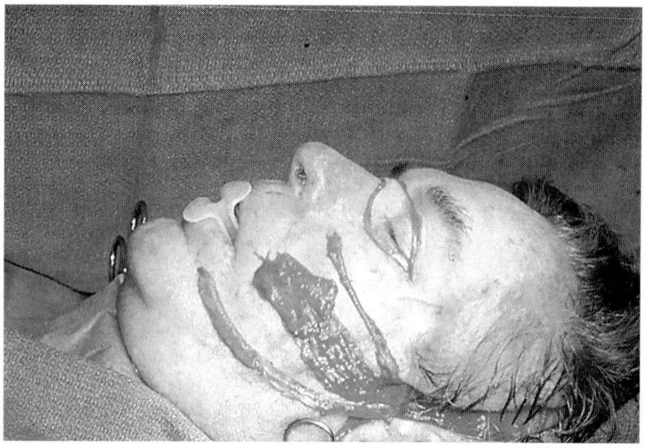

Figure 43–21. Preparation for transfer of temporal muscle, to reanimate the eyelids and face.

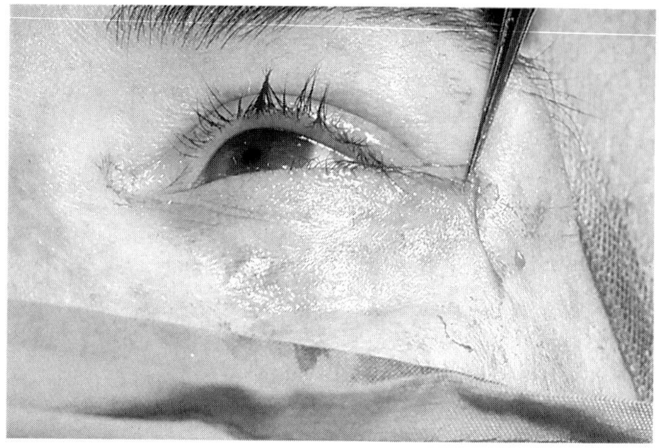

Figure 43–23. The amount of lower eyelid redundancy is determined by the degree of overlap at the lateral canthus.

appeal of using autogenous tissue and muscle transfer, results in our experience for reanimation of the eyelids with temporalis muscle are not as satisfactory as the results of the aforementioned techniques (Fig. 43–21). We reserve the use of temporalis muscle for reanimation of the lower face.

Lateral Canthal Tendon Reconstruction

In situations of true paralytic ectropion of mild-to-moderate degree in which the medial canthal tendon is intact, lateral canthal tendon tightening is employed. A lateral canthal incision is made along with lysis of the inferior crus of the lateral canthal tendon (Fig. 43–22). Once the entire lower lid has been freed from its attachments laterally, the lower lid is grasped with forceps, pulled laterally, and overlapped to appropriate tension (Fig. 43–23). The redundant full-thickness section of the eyelid is then cut. A 4-0 polypropylene suture is passed through the cut edge of the tarsus just inside the conjunctiva and parallel to it. The free ends are then passed inside the orbital rim into the periosteum near the level of the lateral orbital tubercle and is brought out externally. The lateral canthal angle is first re-formed by placement of 6-0 silk suture in the mucocutaneous junction and ciliary lines of the upper and lower lids. This action reforms the canthal angle. Next, the 4-0 polypropylene is tied securely, horizontally tightening the lower lid and reducing the ectropion (Fig. 43–24). The lateral canthal incision is closed with deep absorbable sutures of 5-0 or 6-0 chromic sutures, and the skin, with 6-0 fast chromic suture.

Fascial Strip

The lower-lid tightening procedure can be augmented by adding a strip of fascia across the entire lower lid from the medial canthal tendon to the lateral canthal incision if the original procedure fails or if medial canthal tendon laxity exists. Temporalis fascia can be easily harvested because it is close to the operative field.

A 1- to 2-inch incision is made just anterior to the hair line temporally. The dissection is carried down through

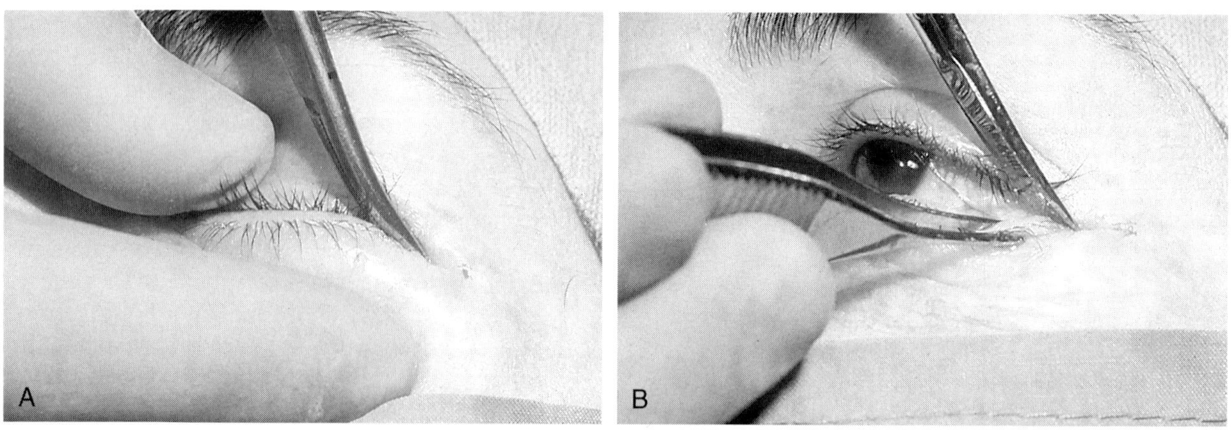

Figure 43–22. *A*, Lateral canthotomy. *B*, Lateral cantholysis.

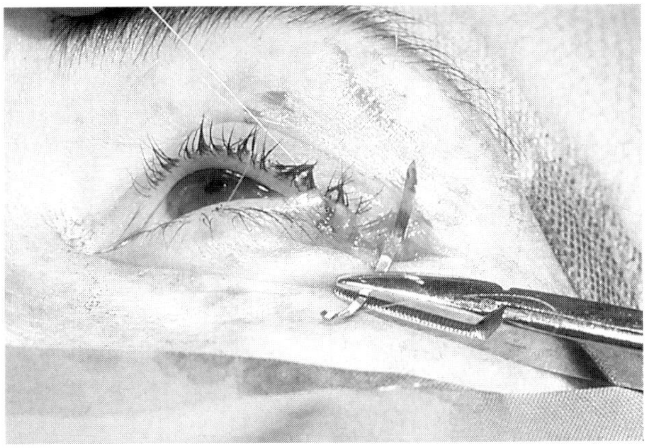

Figure 43–24. 4-0 polypropylene used to secure the tarsal strip to the lateral orbital rim.

skin and subcutaneous superficial fascia until the temporalis fascia is identified. A 40- × 10-mm strip of fascia is harvested. This donor site is closed with interrupted 6-0 subcutaneous polypropylene sutures, and the skin, with 6-0 nylon sutures.

After the lateral canthal reconstruction has been performed to the level of reattaching the lower lid to the lateral canthus, the fascia is placed. The entire lower lid tarsus must be exposed, as must the medial canthal tendon. The fascial strip must be placed high on the tarsus near the follicles of the cilia, to prevent ectropion. Tunneling can be used at the medial canthal incision with a large abdominal cutting needle or a Wright fascia needle. One end of the fascial strip is secured to the medial canthal tendon with multiple interrupted 5-0 polypropylene. Along the tarsus, the fascia is also reinforced with interrupted 5-0 polypropylene sutures. At the lateral canthal area, the lower lid is first tightened (as mentioned previously) before the fascial band is secured. The fascia can be attached to the superficial periosteum, or anterior drill holes can be made. Fascia is passed from the inner to the outer aspect of the rim, wrapped on itself, and secured with either absorbable or nonabsorbable sutures. The purpose of this step is to augment and further anchor the lower lid, in addition to securing it to the fixed points at the medial and lateral canthus.

Retractor Recession with Ear Cartilage Graft

In some patients, the lower lid will need not only tightening but also elevation, particularly in patients who continue to show signs of exposure despite maximal medical management and successful upper eyelid reanimation. In these instances, the inferior third of the cornea often continues to be exposed, especially in the presence of a weak Bell's phenomenon. Currently, our procedure of choice is supplementation of the posterior lamella with autogenous ear cartilage in combination with a lower lid retractor recession and lateral canthal tendon tightening.

The lateral canthal tightening procedure is completed to the point of suturing. Before suturing commences, an incision is made approximately 3 mm below the inferior tarsal border of the conjunctival surface. A conjunctival flap is created down to Tenon's fascia on the globe in a meticulous fashion to separate conjunctiva from the underlying lid retractors. Once this separation has been achieved along the entire aspect of the lower lid from an area below the inferior puncta to the lateral canthal incision, the lower lid retractors are dissected from the lower border of the tarsus. A surgical assistant places traction on the anterior skin surface to avoid button-holing through the skin. In long-standing facial nerve palsy, the orbicularis is atrophic and thin, and great attention must be paid to avoid cutting the skin; this care is facilitated by pulling of the skin away from the underlying muscle. The lower lid retractors, including some deep orbicularis fibers, are taken down to the level of the preaponeurotic fat pads posteriorly. The amount of lift given to the lid is measured in the preoperative examination. The surgeon determines the preoperative level of the lid and the postoperative level that he or she would like to achieve. A one-to-one or a one-to-two ratio is used to ensure proper postoperative lid height. Usually, in spite of the use of autogenous material, the authors use a one-to-two ratio of desired lid height to width of cartilage graft.

An anterior antihelix incision is made through the skin for approximately 2 inches (Fig. 43–25); a very thin layer of subcutaneous tissue exists between this and the perichondrium. Once skin rake retractors have been placed in the skin incision, the perichondrium can be removed from the cartilage with the blunt end of a Freer elevator. By using this method, the ophthalmologist does not cut into the cartilage graft. The grafts are usually approximately 30 mm long, and of course, the width varies according to the height of the lid desired. The graft usually has a concave and a convex surface. The concave surface is placed against the globe to contour to the natural convexity of the globe. The graft can be thinned and sculp-

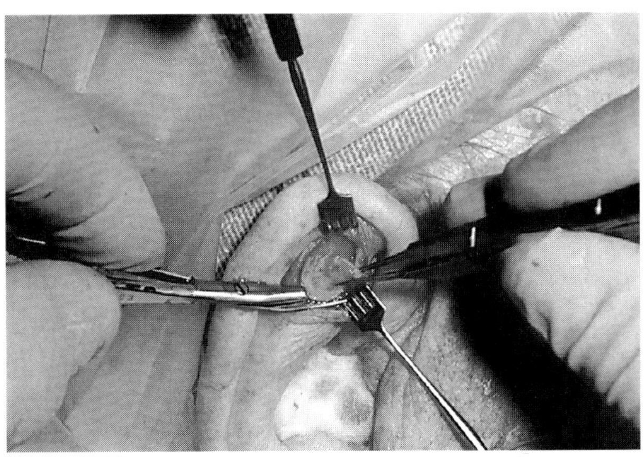

Figure 43–25. Cartilage graft obtained from the antihelix of the ear. (Courtesy of J. Foster, MD.)

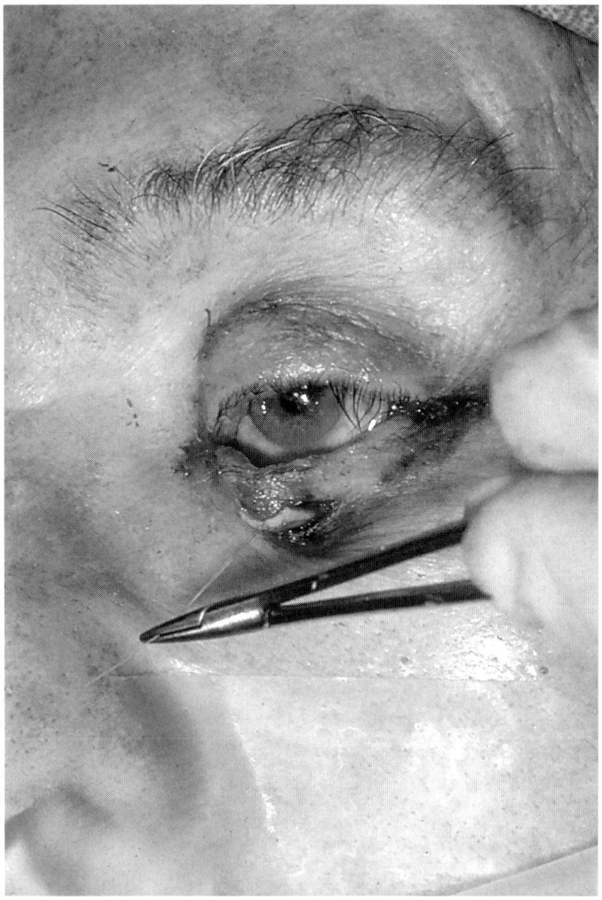

Figure 43–26. Cartilage graft sutured to host bed. (Courtesy of J. Foster, MD.)

tured by use of a point-tip monopolar cautery. The lower border of the cartilage graft is sutured to the upper border of the lower lid retractors, and the upper border of the cartilage graft is sutured to the lower border of the tarsus (Fig. 43–26). The graft is secured both superiorly and inferiorly with 6-0 absorbable sutures. The conjunctiva is then approximated over the graft by use of a running, 6-0 fast chromic suture. The completion of the procedure is the same as for a lateral canthal tendon reconstruction with horizontal tightening. At the completion of this procedure, however, a temporary tarsorrhaphy is usually placed anywhere for approximately 7 days to fix the graft in place. A mild pressure dressing is applied, and the patient is given systemic antibiotics.

Ancillary Surgical Techniques for the Eyelids

Other procedures can be useful in patients with facial nerve palsy who fail to respond to medical management or to other surgical intervention. The aforementioned procedures are geared toward functional rehabilitation first, with a strong emphasis on natural eyelid and facial aesthetics. Common ophthalmic approaches to exposure include a total or subtotal tarsorrhaphy to alleviate any exposure keratitis. However, the authors avoid this method because it is unaesthetic, disfiguring, and often further handicaps compromised eyelid closure. In addition, most patients, given the option, try to avoid undergoing this procedure.

If, however, all the above-mentioned surgical procedures do not alleviate the problem, then a 4- to 5-mm lateral and medial tarsorrhaphy could be performed. By "splitting" the tarsorrhaphy into medial and lateral procedures, the ophthalmologist still gets the desired lessening in exposed ocular surface without the gross physical deformity of a larger lateral tarsorrhaphy. The technique for the medial tarsorrhaphy involves denuding the lid margin with placement of buried interlid 5-0 polyglactin and horizontal mattress sutures of 6-0 or 5-0 polyglactin. No attempt is made to split the tarsus into a tongue-and-groove component because this measure is generally unnecessary.

Additional Operations for Facial Nerve Palsy

Unilateral brow ptosis is often significant in patients with facial nerve palsy, particularly in elderly patients. Unilateral problems are best corrected by direct brow lift or midforehead lift.

The amount of lift desired is measured with the patient sitting and staring in primary gaze; this amount of skin and subcutaneous tissue and fat is resected. Periosteal or subfrontalis fixation can be used, using nonabsorbable sutures, but this measure is often not necessary. Merely removing skin and superficial subcutaneous fat usually stabilizes the brow and achieves the desired results. A layered closure is required, using buried 5-0 polyglactin and polypropylene suture through the skin.

Problems of lower facial paralysis are sometimes as severe as eyelid problems. The details of reanimation of the lower face are not addressed in this section. The ophthalmic surgeon, however, must realize that several options are available to the patient with long-standing facial nerve paralysis involving the lower face. In particular, in patients in whom muscle and nerve function are attenuated to the point that nerve grafting is no longer practical, transposition of temporalis muscle, if the motor division of the fifth nerve is intact, allows the patient to avoid drooling during eating, to smile, and to balance the face through elevation of the lateral nares, the mouth, and the nasolabial fold.

REFERENCES

1. Crosby EC, DeJonge BR: Experimental and clinical studies of the central connections and the central relations of the facial nerve. Ann Otol 72:735–755, 1963.
2. Carpenter M: Core Text of Neuro-anatomy. Baltimore, Williams & Wilkins, 1985, p 151.

3. May M, Galetta SL: The facial nerve and related disorders of the face. *In* Glaser JS (ed): Neuro-ophthalmology. Philadelphia, JB Lippincott, 1990, pp 239–277.
4. Martin RG, Grant JL, Peace D, et al: Microsurgical relationship of the anterior inferior cerebellar artery and the facial vestibulocochlear nerve complex. Neurosurgery 6:483, 1980.
5. Malone B, Maisel RH: Anatomy of the facial nerve. Am J Otol 9:494–504, 1988.
6. Miehike A: Surgery of the Facial Nerve, 2nd ed. Philadelphia, WB Saunders, 1973, pp 7–21.
7. Davis RA, Anson BJ, Ruddinger JM, Kurth RE: Surgical anatomy of the facial nerve and parotid gland based upon a study of 350 cervical facial halves. Surg Gynecol Obstet 102:385–412, 1956.
8. Blunt MJ: The possible role of vascular changes in the etiology of Bell's palsy. J Laryngol 70:701–713, 1956.
9. May M: The Facial Nerve. New York, Thieme Stratton, 1986.
10. Paolino E, Granieri E, Tola MR, et al: Predisposing factor in Bell's palsy: A case control study. J Neurol 232:363–365, 1985.
11. Peitersen E: The natural history of Bell's palsy. Am J Otol 4:107–111, 1982.
12. May M, Klein SR, Taylor FH: Idiopathic (Bell's) facial palsy: Natural history defies steroid or surgical treatment. Laryngoscope 95:406–412, 1985.
13. Hunt JR: On herpetic inflammations of the geniculate ganglion. A new syndrome and its complications. J Nerv Ment Dis 34:73–96, 1907.
14. Portenoy RK, Duma C, Foley KM: Acute herpetic and postherpetic neuralgia. Clinical review and current management. Ann Neurol 20:651–664, 1986.
15. Gradenigo G: A special syndrome of endocranial otitic complications. Ann Otol Rhinol Laryngol 13:637, 1904.
16. Clark JR, Carlson RD, Sasak CT, et al: Facial paralysis in Lyme disease. Laryngoscope 95:1341–1345, 1985.

CHAPTER 44

Suborbital Augmentation

Kenneth D. Steinsapir and Norman Shorr

This chapter focuses on the functional and cosmetic aspects of augmentation of the suborbital region. Suborbital implants are distinct from cheek implants, which augment and enhance malar projection or fill in midcheek depressions. Suborbital implants offer the ability to alter the projection of the inferior and inferolateral orbital rim, thereby creating the potential for addressing lower eyelid problems that were uncorrectable with previous soft tissue techniques. The term *suborbital* is used to mean the region on the facial skeleton below the orbit, including all of the bony surfaces that underlie both the malar and the infraorbital regions together with the inferior orbital rim. This chapter focuses on two types of suborbital augmentation that are of interest to eyelid and orbit surgeons. One type of implant is for the correction of the pronounced nasojugal depression, also known as the tear trough deformity, caused by a flat or concave face of the maxillary bone. The second type of implant is the custom malar implant for correcting deficiencies in the inferior orbital rim projection. Correction of the tear trough deformity is a cosmetic concern. In contrast, custom rim and prefabricated implants for the correction of inadequate projection have significant functional importance.

The eyelid position, structure, function, and appearance depend on the relative globe prominence and relative rim projection. The eyelid and orbital surgeon has long been aware that greater globe prominence or lesser rim projection severely limits the results of eyelid surgery. Inferior and lateral orbital rim projection, contour, and topographic bony surface problems have been so difficult to correct that for practical purposes, the bony framework has been accepted as is. Surgical efforts have been limited to sometimes relatively futile attempts to make the eyelid function properly from an improper bony foundation. The recent development of alloplastic orbital rim and tear trough implants for the first time offers the eyelid and orbit surgeon a simple and reliable method of correcting or improving the bony structural foundation at the time of soft tissue reconstruction and esthetic eyelid surgery. Although obvious overlap exists, the two types of suborbital bony structural inadequacies are those relating to the anterior projection of the inferior orbital rim and those relating to the topography (convexity or concavity) of the face of the suborbital maxillary bone.

The inadequate rim projection deformity compromises the function of the eyelid. Augmentation of the anterior projection of the inferolateral orbital rim improves the relative globe and rim anterior projection disparity. These implants can be custom made or prefabricated and are used to correct injuries caused by trauma, to treat Graves' ophthalmopathy, and for normal variation reconstruction. Inadequate maxillary face deformity with associated soft tissue depression is also known as the tear trough deformity, which can be corrected in conjunction with, or independent of, orbital rim augmentation. The tear trough implant provides a beautiful esthetic correction to a cosmetic problem for which no reliable treatment was previously available.

ANATOMY

The lower eyelid cheek complex has many important landmarks that must be considered when the inferior orbital rim and subrim area are evaluated (Fig. 44–1). The orbitocheek fold is an important surface landmark that delineates the orbital rim; the fold is caused by a line of fusion between the deep and superficial planes of facial fascia, which in turn attach to the orbital rim. Laterally, this fold is also referred to as the *malar fold.* The medial aspect of the orbitocheek fold is referred to as the *nasojugal fold.* Below the nasojugal fold, a second fold may extend laterally as the midcheek fold. The nasojugal fold often lies in the center of a concavity referred to as the *tear trough* (Fig. 44–2). In part, the groove is created by the triangular gap between the orbicularis and the lateral border of the levator labii alaeque nasi muscle (Fig. 44–3). In youth, this gap is filled by fat. With the passage of time, atrophy of this fat occurs, and the groove can deepen to create the so-called tear trough deformity, which can impart a tired and haggard look to the face (Fig. 44–4). However, the medial suborbital bony contour may contribute significantly to the tear trough de-

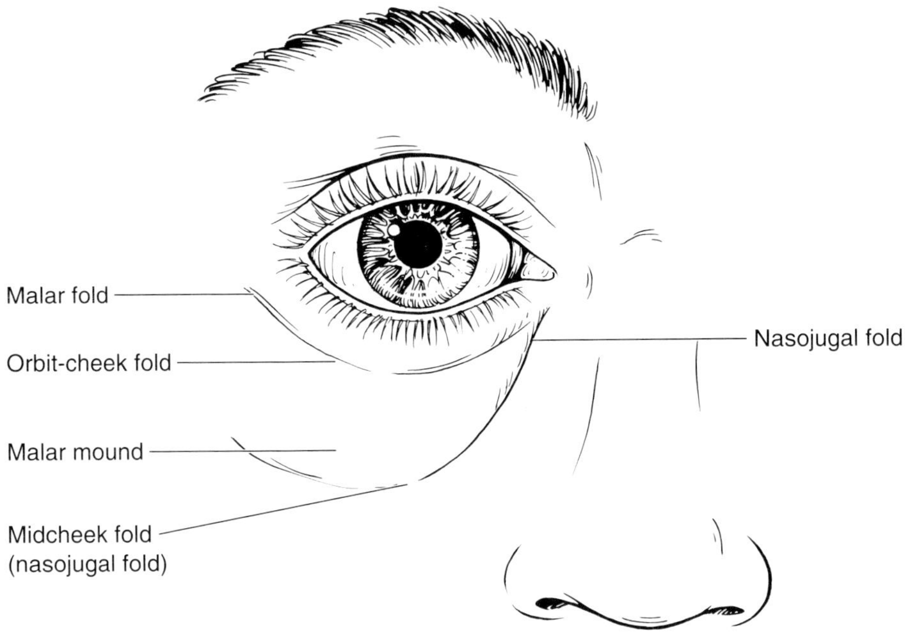

Figure 44 – 1. The orbitocheek fold is caused by a line of fusion between the deep and superficial planes of the facial fascia. The midcheek fold is seen below the orbitocheek fold.

formity, as is discussed later. The midcheek fold may extend laterally below the malar mound to the region of the zygomatic ligament. With sufficient gravitational changes, the midcheek fold may be the lower border of a malar festoon (Fig. 44–5).

Bony structure provides the support for the lower eyelid tissues. The bony contour creates the structural foundation over which the eyelid soft tissue drapes. Figure 44–6 illustrates the normal skeletal anatomy of the face. When the suborbital region is hypoplastic (Fig. 44–7), inadequate support for the lower eyelid often exists, leading to relative ocular prominence and inadequate support for the overlying soft tissues. As is discussed later, implants must be used to correct these deficits. Attempting to correct a problem by only addressing the soft tissues will never work. The effort expended by correcting the deficits themselves is more than rewarded by the results.

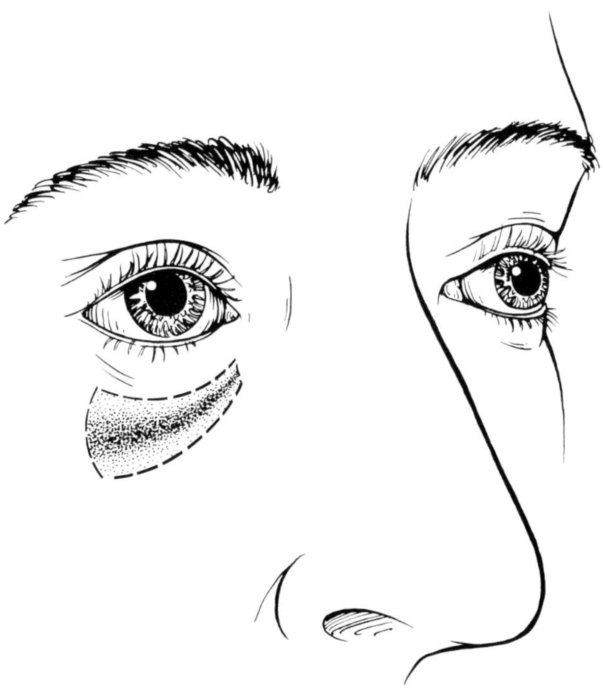

Figure 44 – 2. The geometric surface schematically represents the concavity known as the tear trough deformity.

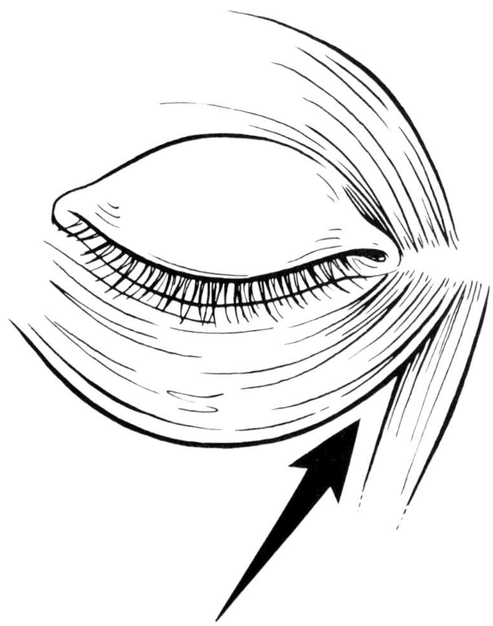

Figure 44 – 3. A depression can develop in the nasojugal region over the gap between the orbicularis and the levator labii alaeque nasi muscle and contributes to the tear trough deformity.

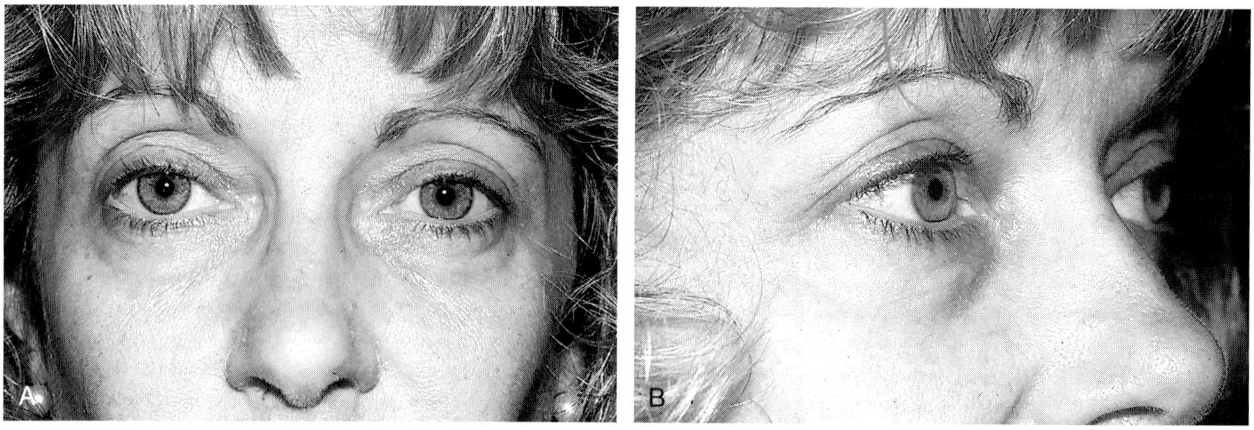

Figure 44–4. *A* and *B*, The tear trough deformity can create a tired appearance of the face.

ASPECTS OF SUBORBITAL DEFICIENCY

Prominent Globe

Support for the lower eyelid depends on the projection of the inferior orbital rim and the anterior projection of the maxillary face. Lack of suborbital bony projection can directly contribute to ocular prominence, and hollowness of the maxillary face contributes to the tear trough defect. Figure 44–8 illustrates the effect of orbital rim projection on ocular prominence. When the projection is limited, the globe effectively projects beyond the orbital rim, creating a prominent globe. The hypoplastic inferior orbital rim and suborbital region have a direct functional significance because limited support exists for the cheek and lower eyelid. Inferior scleral show is common in this setting. Lower eyelid surgery can be disappointing because any surgery performed on the lower eyelid often worsens lower eyelid retraction.

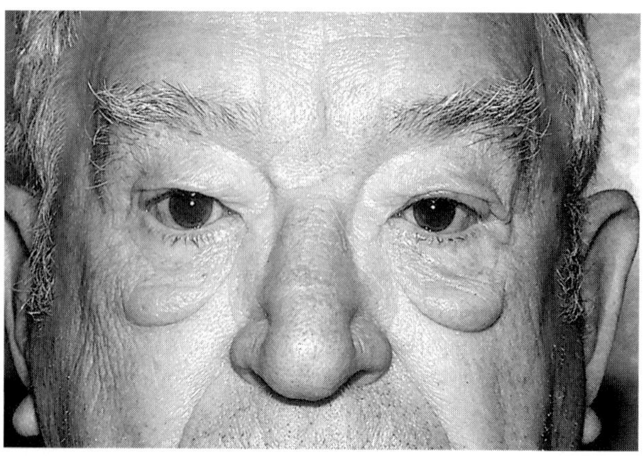

Figure 44–5. With sufficient gravitational changes, the midcheek fold can extend laterally as the inferior border of a malar festoon.

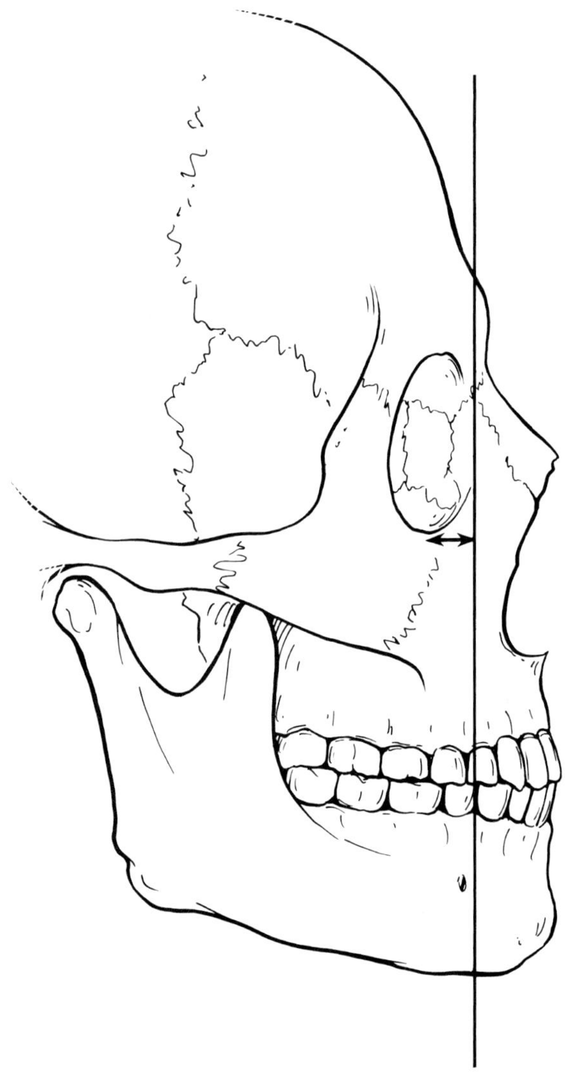

Figure 44–6. The normal skeletal anatomy of the face. Note the degree of suborbital projection (*double arrow*).

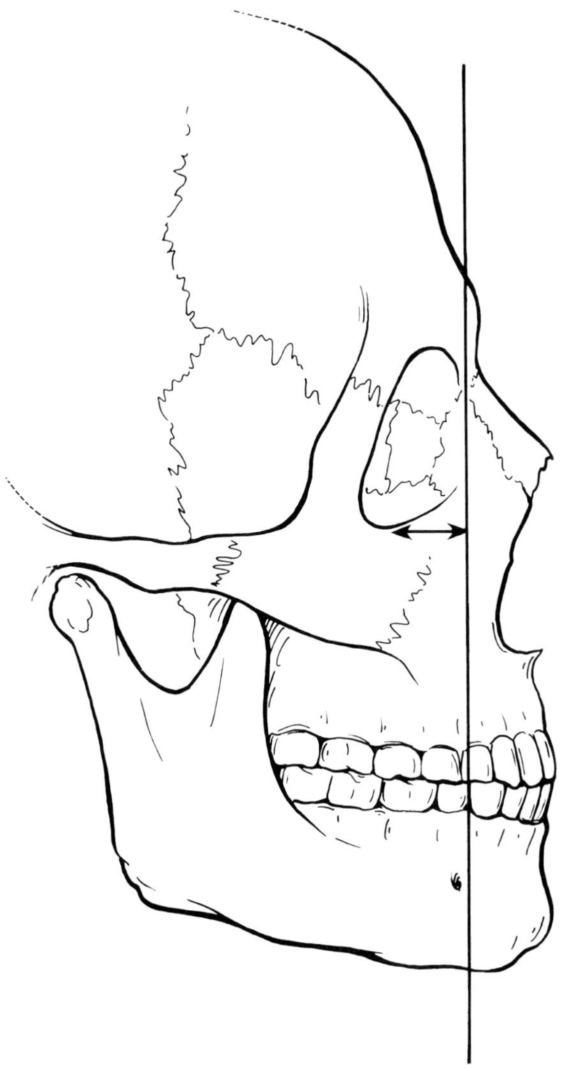

Figure 44–7. In contrast to the normal skeletal anatomy shown in Figure 44–6, note the relative lack of projection seen (*double arrow*) when the suborbital region is hypoplastic.

The two eyelid procedures that most commonly cause postsurgical lower eyelid retraction in patients with a prominent globe are transcutaneous lower eyelid blepharoplasty and lateral canthal resuspension surgery. Transcutaneous lower eyelid blepharoplasty creates a midlamellar eyelid scar that can tether the eye inferiorly. Lateral canthal resuspension of the lower eyelid with a tarsal strip procedure produces lower eyelid retraction by a different but important method. The tarsal strip procedure shortens the lower eyelid horizontally (Fig. 44–9). The situation is analogous to that of an obese man tightening his belt to support his pants. Tightening the belt on the rounded stomach forces the pants down under the curvature of the belly. Similarly, tightening the lower eyelid under the convex curvature of the prominent globe forces the eyelid inferiorly. Both of these circumstances are more profound when the lower eyelid has limited bony support.

In this instance, the globe is relatively prominent. The tarsoligamentous sling and the pretarsal orbicularis normally support the lower eyelid. However, when the globe is prominent, both the tarsoligamentous sling and the pretarsal orbicularis pull the eyelid under the curvature of the globe. When the rim hypoplasia is corrected, the forces of the tarsoligamentous sling are less likely to pull the eyelid below the globe curvature. Adequate correction of lower eyelid abnormalities in these situations can be optimally achieved only by first considering the underlying bony structure (see Fig. 44–8).

Tear Trough Deformity

When the medial suborbital region is flat or concave, the overlying soft tissues are not well supported, resulting in the tear trough depression. The tear trough deformity is a purely cosmetic problem. The tear trough deformity represents an exaggeration of the nasojugal fold or depression. It creates a haggard look in the face and can contribute to a lower eyelid dark circle. This is a very common cosmetic problem in patients desiring cosmetic blepharoplasty, yet it is seldom addressed. Until recently, no reliable method to address this problem existed. Surgeons used fat autografts or hand-carved subrim augmentation with unpredictable results. The Flowers tear trough implant (Implant Tech, Van Nuys, CA), which has been available for the past 2 years, provides a predictable method of correcting this cosmetic defect, often with dramatic results. It is particularly rewarding to correct a problem that has long been considered to be unfixable.

The implant is a prefabricated crescentic silicone implant with a premarked notch for the infraorbital nerve (Fig. 44–10). The implant sits just below the orbital rim (Fig. 44–11) and fills in the hypoplasia or concavity of the suborbital rim area. The implant can also be combined with functional lower eyelid reconstruction. For example, the placement of the Flowers tear trough implant could be combined with lower eyelid reconstruction using hard-palate graft material. This approach is effective in patients with postblepharoplasty lower eyelid retraction and tear trough depression or in patients with lower eyelid vertical inadequacy with mild suborbital hypoplasia. The topologic shape of the inferior orbital rim and the subrim region determines how the overlying tissue is draped. In contrast, orbital rim and subrim hypoplasia leading to globe prominence and inadequate lower eyelid support has important functional significance. There are variations on these structural abnormalities and they are often found in combination.

Inadequate Suborbital Projection

The prominent globe presents a difficult set of circumstances for the surgeon. Prominence may result from or-

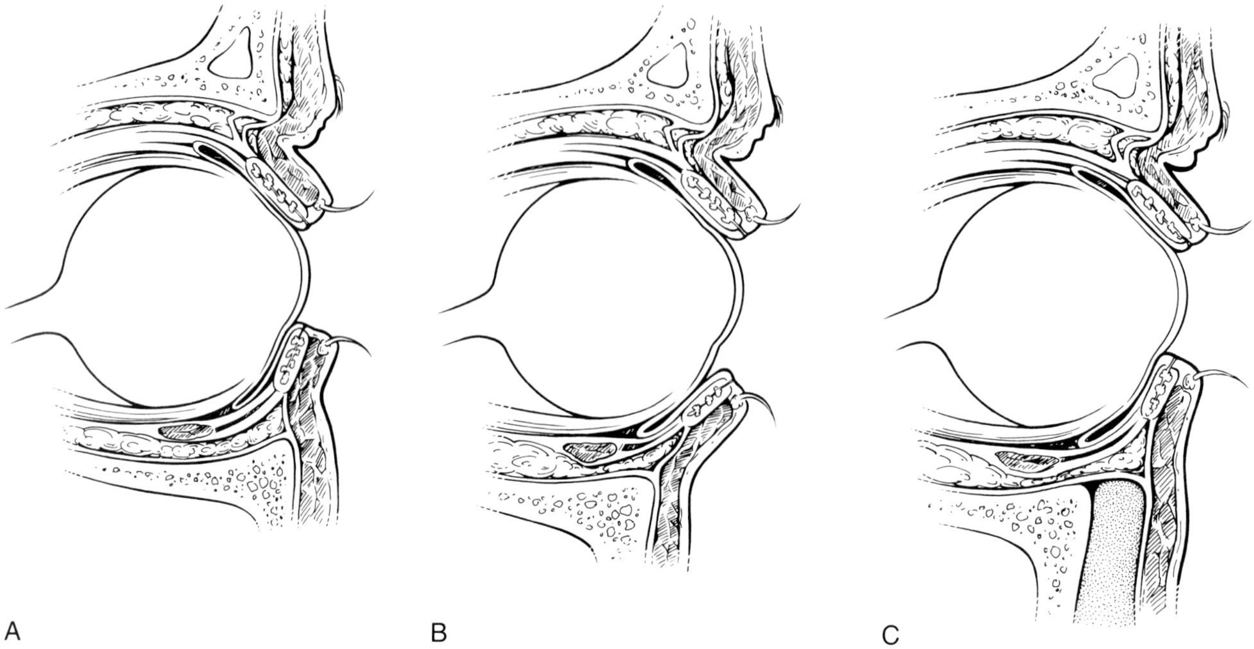

Figure 44–8. How the orbital rim supports the lower eyelid. *A*, Normal lower eyelid and inferior orbital rim relationship. Note the inferior orbital rim directly under the lower eyelid. There is no tendency for the tarsoligamentous sling and the pretarsal orbicularis to pull the eyelid below the curvature of the glove. *B*, Prominent globe with hypoplastic orbital rim. Note that because of the position to the orbital rim the tarsoligamentous sling and the pretarsal orbicularis tend to pull the lower eyelid under the curvature of the globe. C, With alloplastic augmentation of the orbital rim the lower eyelid can be supported, thereby counteracting the tendency of the lower eyelid to be pulled under the curvature of the globe.

bital contents that are large relative to their bony container, as is the case with thyroid-related orbitopathy or in craniofacial anomalies, such as Crouzon's syndrome. However, the commonest cause of ocular prominence is inadequate inferior orbital rim projection as a normal variation. A spectrum of normal inferior orbital rim projections exists that ranges from relatively more prominent to relatively less prominent. Beyond the relatively less prominent normal spectrum is the syndrome that has been referred to as *hemiexophthalmos*, or frank malar hypoplasia. In this disorder, lower eyelid support is often compromised in the absence of adequate orbital rim support, leading to disappointing blepharoplasty results. Blepharoplasty that is not tailored to the prominent eye may leave the patient with a "bug-eyed" appearance. Lower eyelid retraction with inferior scleral show is commonly associated with suborbital rim hypoplasia.

It is an axiom of facial surgery that success is possible only when tissue redraping is performed over a structurally correct foundation. The redraping of lower eyelid soft tissues alone never addresses bony deficiency. Consequently, these structural problems can be addressed only by augmentation of the underlying bony contour. The bone contour can be corrected with autografts, such as calvarial bone onlay grafts, or with allografts. The bone onlay is a natural material. However, harvesting bone for onlay grafts is time consuming and is associated with donor site morbidity. Controlling contour with onlay bone grafts is problematic. In contrast, controlling contour with prefabricated alloplastic materials is much easier. In the next section, two innovations in implant materials for the orbital rim and suborbital region are discussed.

SUBORBITAL RIM IMPLANTS

Prefabricated Implants

Prefabricated implants are available for numerous applications in the face. The number of suborbital implants is relatively limited. The most versatile of the prefabricated suborbital implants is the Flowers tear trough implant. The Goldberg Medpore lateral orbital rim implant (Porex Surgical, College Park, GA) is another example of a prefabricated suborbital implant. Figure 44–12 illustrates the Goldberg implant, which helps advance the soft tissue at the lateral orbital rim and addresses an excessively posterior lateral canthus when the globe is prominent. Figure 44–13 demonstrates the preoperative and postoperative appearance of a patient who received bilateral placement of this implant. Because of the versatility of the Flowers tear trough implant, discussion of prefabricated suborbital implants is primarily restricted to this particular device.

The Flowers tear trough implant is a solid silicone im-

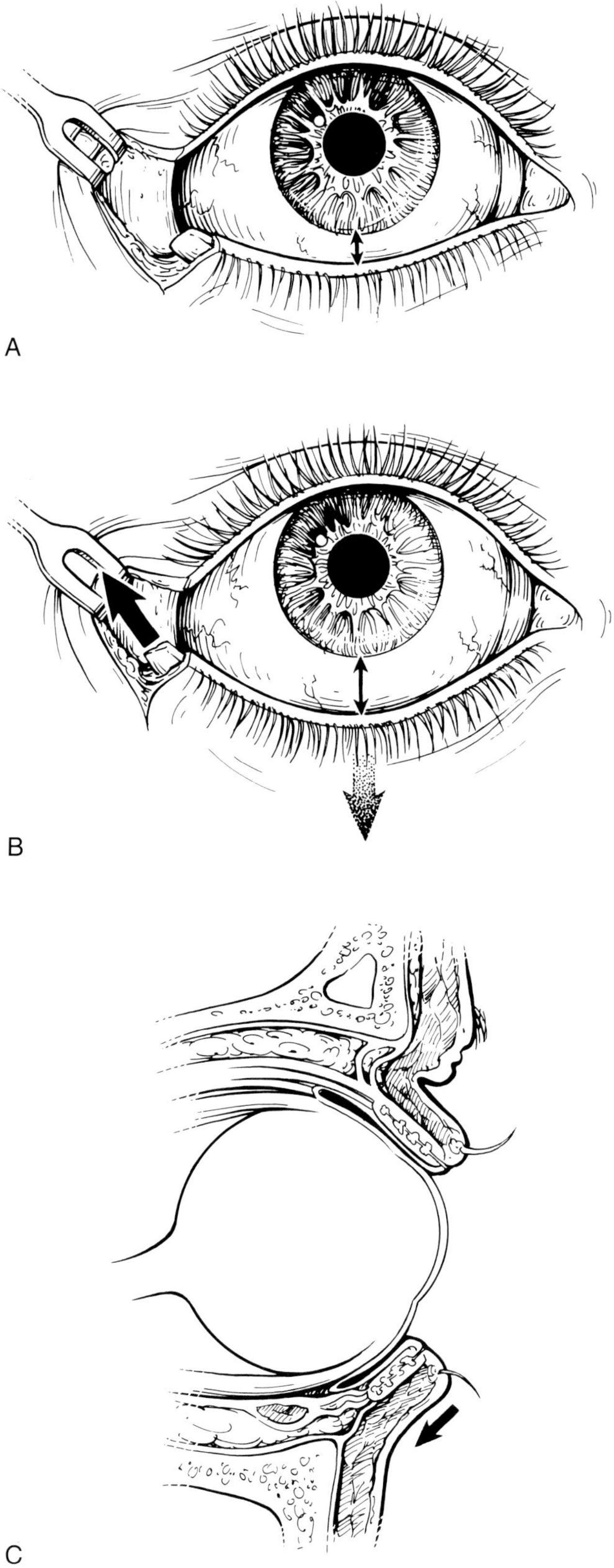

A

B

C

Figure 44–9. *A*, The effect of lateral canthal resuspension in the setting of the relatively prominent globe. *B*, When the lateral canthal tendon is tightened laterally, the lower eyelid tarsoligamentous sling is drawn below the curvature of the globe, worsening inferior scleral show. *C*, The same effect of lateral canthal tightening viewed sagittally.

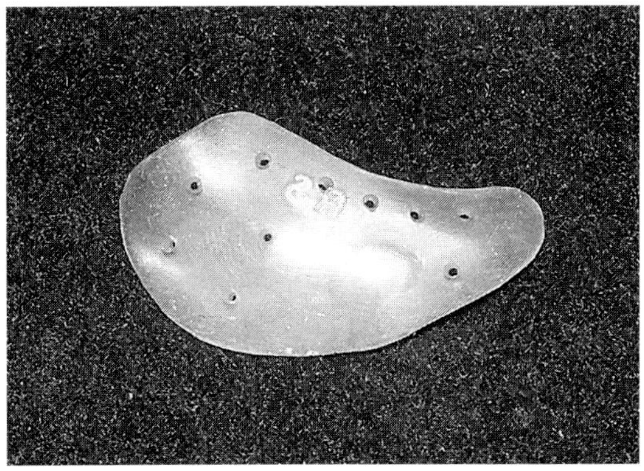

Figure 44–10. The Flowers tear trough implant. Note the outlined area on the implant for the creation of a notch for the infraorbital nerve.

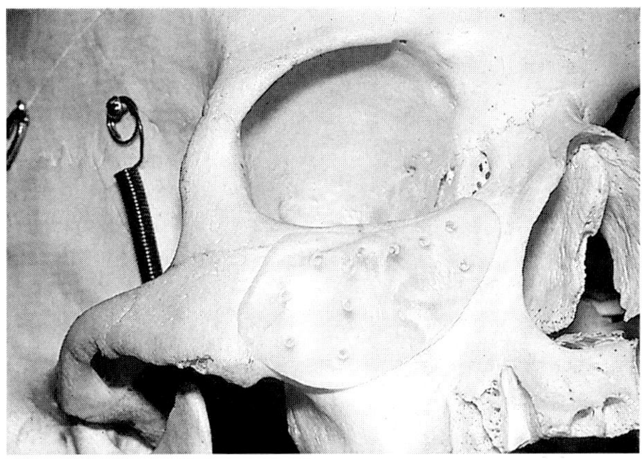

Figure 44–11. A Flowers tear trough implant in place on the orbital rim of a skull. Note that the tapered medial aspect of the implant extends to the base of the nose. Laterally, the implant extends to reach the zygoma.

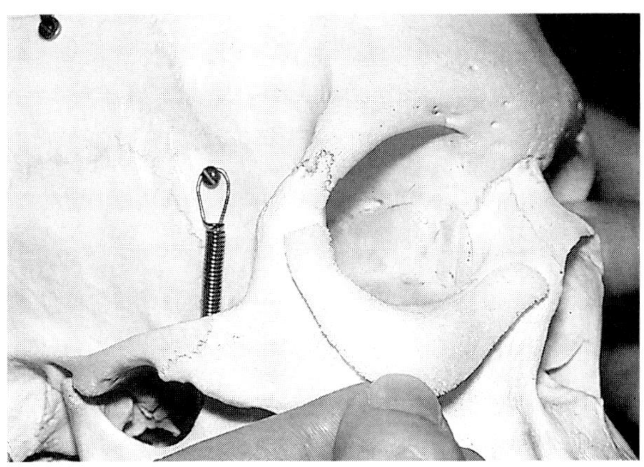

Figure 44–12. The Goldberg lateral orbital rim implant positioned on the orbital rim.

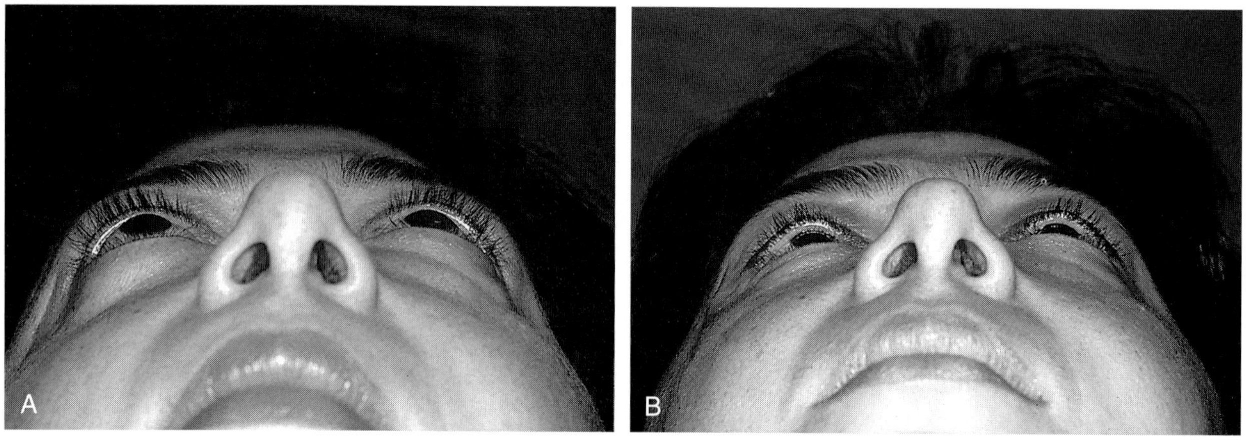

Figure 44–13. Placement of the Goldberg lateral orbital rim implant. *A*, Preoperative appearance. *B*, Postoperative appearance 2 months after surgery. Note the improved right orbital rim projection.

plant that is available in three sizes. The implant is designed as a subperiosteal implant. Its superior edge rests along the inferior orbital rim, its broad lateral end drapes the malar eminence, and its tapered medial end extends into the tear trough region between the medial orbital rim and the base of the nose. Inferiorly, a notch exists to accommodate the infraorbital neurovascular bundle (Fig. 44–14). Figure 44–15 demonstrates preoperative and postoperative appearance in a patient who underwent placement of a Flowers tear trough implant. As is described later, the implant is most advantageously placed transconjunctivally. The transcutaneous and intraoral approaches are also used for the placement of the Flowers tear trough implant.

Custom Suborbital Implants

Large degrees of suborbital hypoplasia are not adequately addressed by prefabricated implants; post-traumatic reconstruction, for example, often requires overcoming a significant volume deficit. Before the introduction of custom-made implants, volume deficiency of the suborbital region was addressed with onlay bone grafts, in situ fabricated implants using Cranioplast, or room temperature vulcanized (RTV) silicone. Each of these approaches has its limitations. Onlay bone grafting is time consuming and requires the morbidity of a donor site. Additionally, controlling the bony contour is difficult with in situ fabricated implants.

In situ fabricated implants are applied in a liquid state to fill a dissected soft tissue pocket. The materials then solidify. Once in solid form, the silicone or the methyl methacrylate may be removed for trimming if needed and then reinserted into the soft tissue pocket. Although these materials can address significant volume deficits,

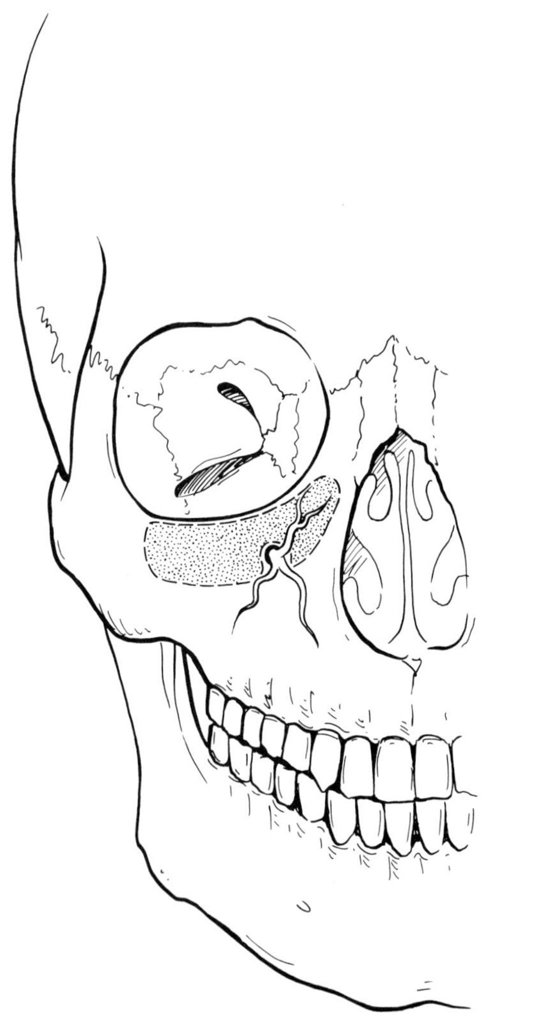

Figure 44–14. A Flowers tear trough implant in position on the skull. The superior edge is flush with the orbital rim. Medially, the implant extends to the base of the nose. Inferiorly, the notch in the implant places no pressure on the infraorbital neurovascular bundle.

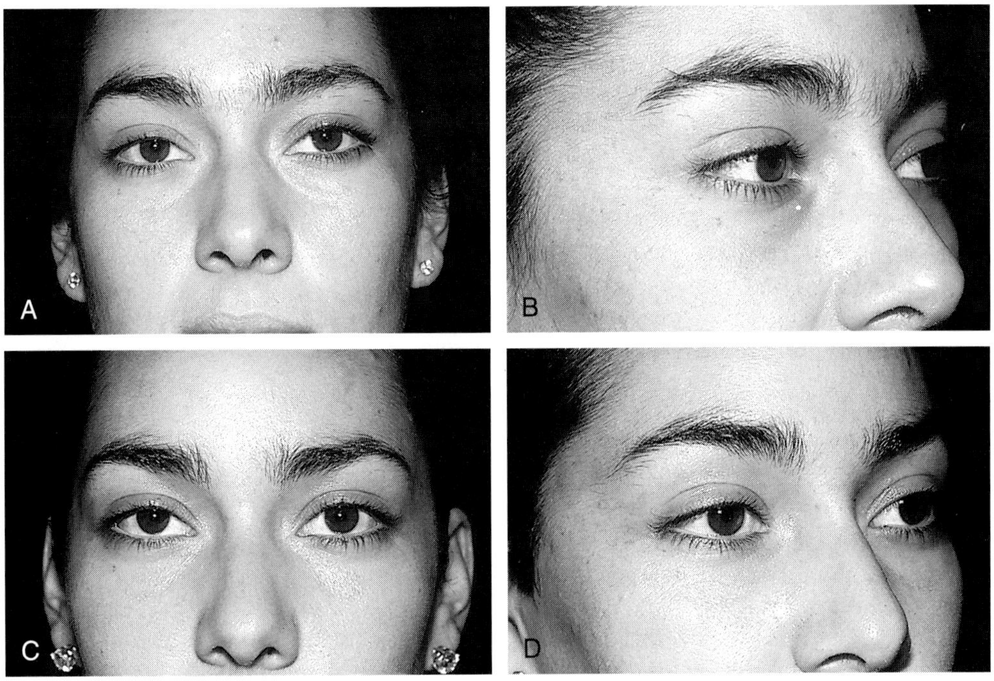

Figure 44 – 15. Preoperative and postoperative photographs of a patient with bilateral tear trough depression. *A* and *B*, Preoperative views. *C* and *D*, Three months postoperatively.

controlling the shape of the in situ fabricated implants is often difficult when larger suborbital bony defects and inadequacies are being treated. In these cases, custom-fabricated silicone implants have come to play an increasingly important role.

Suborbital hypoplasia often requires the use of customized orbital rim implants, which have the advantage of addressing significant volume deficits. These implants are created by use of computer-assisted design and computer-assisted manufacturing technology. High-resolution computed tomography of the patient is used to reconstruct the skull in three dimensions (Fig. 44 – 16). A computer-driven machining instrument then carves an anatomically correct life-sized model of the skull, which is used to sculpt a wax version of the desired implant (Fig. 44 – 17), which is then commercially fabricated in solid, medical-grade silicone for surgical implantation (Implant Tech, Van Nuys, CA). Obviously, this technique for the development of a customized subperiosteal implant can be used for many defects.

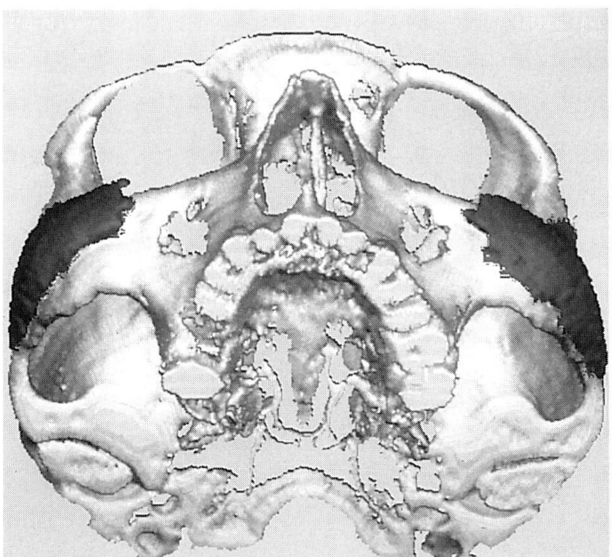

Figure 44 – 16. Three-dimensional computed tomographic reconstruction of a patient with cheek implants in place. This high-resolution image is the first step in the creation of custom suborbital implants.

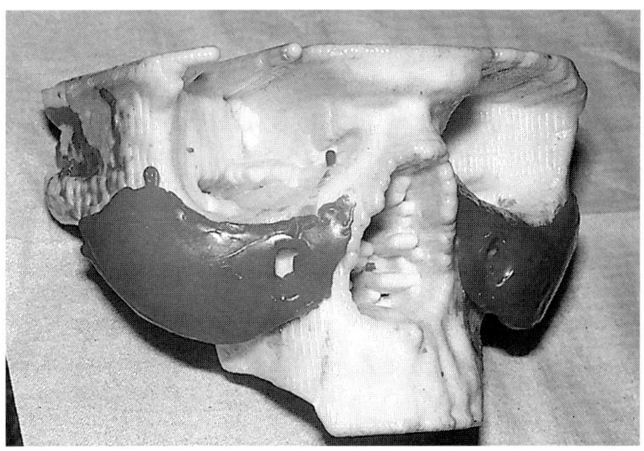

Figure 44 – 17. An anatomically correct model manufactured from a high-resolution computed tomographic scan serves as the basis for creating a wax model for a custom-made suborbital implant. The lost wax process is used to convert the wax model into a silicone implant that is ready for surgical use.

The Flowers Tear Trough Implant

The Flowers tear trough implant is designed to address the depression created by medial suborbital deficiency. Although this implant primarily addresses aesthetic concerns, it can correct mild-to-moderate degrees of suborbital hypoplasia because it lies on the maxillary face spanning the canine fossa between the alveolar process and the orbital rim and laterally on the zygoma. The concavity that creates the tear trough is filled in by the Flowers tear trough implant. The implant can be inserted by several routes. The method commonly used by the authors and described here is the transconjunctival approach. However, the implant may also be placed via an intraoral route or an infraciliary eyelid skin incision. Each of these incisions have advantages and disadvantages that must be weighed by the surgeon.

We prefer to use the transconjunctival approach combined with a canthotomy and inferior cantholysis for the placement of the tear trough implant. This approach does not violate the orbital septum and spares the orbicularis, thereby reducing the risk of iatrogenic lower eyelid retraction and lateral scleral show, which are all too frequent signs of lower eyelid surgery. The approach provides wide access to the orbital rim. The dissection creates the opportunity to expose the inferior orbital fat when removal of this tissue is part of the surgical plan.

In contrast to the transcutaneous approach, the transconjunctival approach is challenging because of the limited exposure of the suborbital region under the tunnel that is created when the subperiosteal pocket is dissected through the transconjunctival approach. This limited exposure makes lateral canthotomy and inferior cantholysis necessary. However, the disadvantage of limited exposure is outweighed by the benefit of avoiding the development of a tethering scar in the preseptal orbicularis and septum. Postoperatively, this type of cicatrix manifests as lower eyelid retraction, and it is responsible for the postsurgical pulled-down look often seen after transcutaneous blepharoplasty.

The principles of lateral canthal surgery must be adhered to as in any procedure involving the lateral canthus. Lateral canthal resuspension is an important aspect of this surgery, and it helps to support the eyelid after extensive lower eyelid dissection, counteracting any tendency for the eyelid to be pulled down postoperatively. Leaving the upper limb of the lateral canthal tendon intact when lateral canthotomy and inferior cantholysis are performed greatly facilitates lateral canthal resuspension. This method generally avoids the need to resuspend the superior limb of the lateral canthus when the lateral canthal angle is reconstructed. More importantly, it facilitates the reinsertion of the lower limb by helping locate the insertion of the inferolateral canthal limb.

Once cantholysis is performed, the conjunctiva and lower eyelid retractors are incised across the lower eyelid

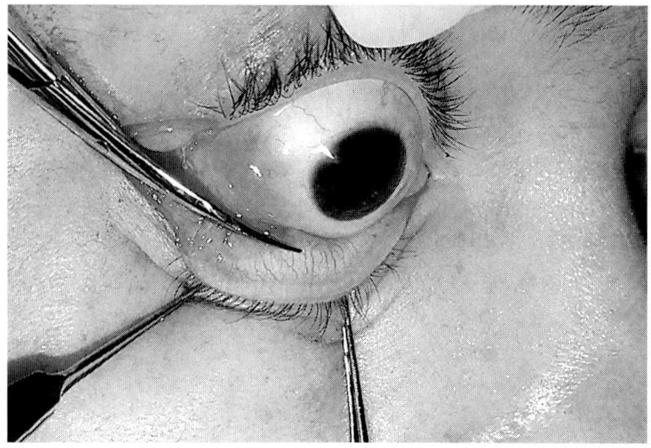

Figure 44–18. A step in the transconjunctival placement of a Flowers tear trough implant. After canthotomy and inferior cantholysis, a Stevens scissors is used to cut across the lower eyelid conjunctiva and lower eyelid retractor just inferior to the tarsus.

(Fig. 44–18). Dissection is carried down to the orbital rim, thereby developing a plane in the loose areolar tissue between the orbital fat and the orbital septum. At the inferior orbital rim, the septum inserts at the arcus marginalis. The septum is incised just above its insertion into the arcus marginalis. The subrim area is then widely exposed (Figs. 44–19 and 44–20). The periosteum is incised approximately 6 mm onto the suborbital face. This creates a cuff of periosteum at the orbital rim that is adherent to bone and provides a site for suturing of the Flowers tear trough implant. Below the periosteal incision, the periosteum is elevated with a periosteal elevator, and dissection is carried out onto the malar face to create a pocket large enough to accommodate the implant. The single critical structure in this area is the infraorbital neurovascular bundle, which must be carefully dissected out to avoid postoperative facial anesthesia or paresthesia (Figs. 44–21 and 44–22). The surgeon must carefully dissect the full extent of the neurovascular bundle and avoid damaging it.

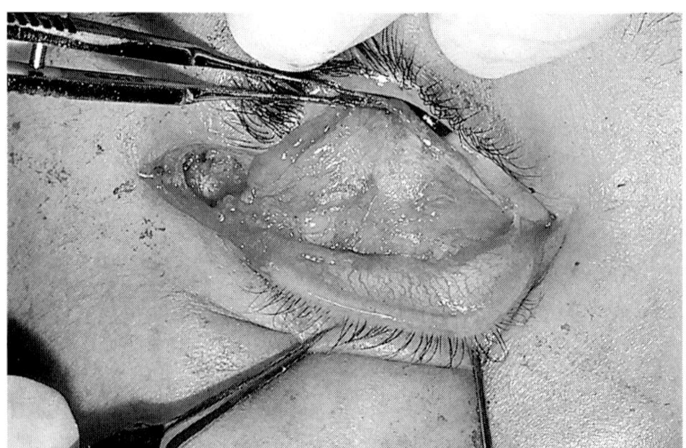

Figure 44–19. A step in the transconjunctival placement of a Flowers tear trough implant. A plane of dissection is followed anterior to the lower eyelid orbital fat and posterior to the orbital septum.

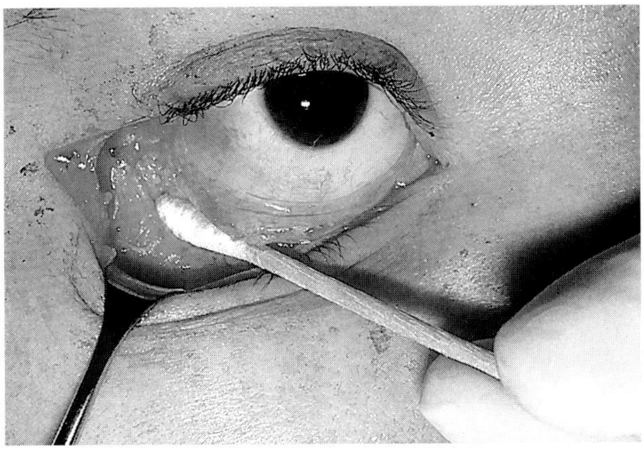

Figure 44–20. A step in the transconjunctival placement of a Flowers tear trough implant. The dissection plane is extended inferiorly to expose the inferior orbital rim.

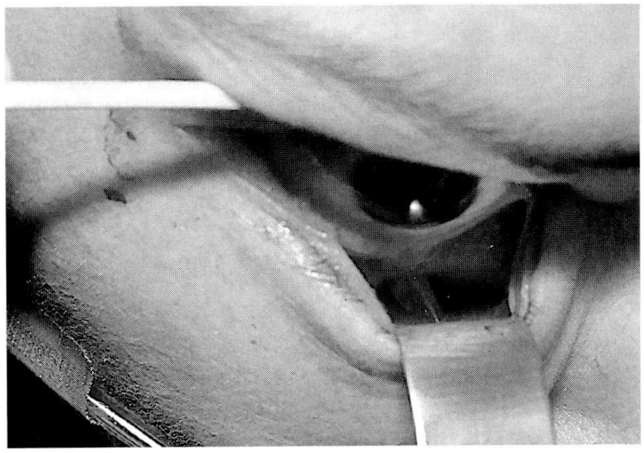

Figure 44–21. A step in the transconjunctival placement of a Flowers tear trough implant. The periosteum is opened just below the orbital rim, and a subperiosteal dissection is performed across the suborbital region with preservation of the infraorbital neurovascular bundle.

The Flowers implants are available in the right and left orientations. One end of the implant is tapered to fit along the orbital rim as it meets the base of the nose. On the implant is a premarked area for the infraorbital neurovascular bundle; this area must be cut out to accommodate the neurovascular bundle. A sterile wooden tongue blade makes a convenient cutting surface for this purpose (Fig. 44–23). The notch must be made large enough so that the implant does not impinge on the nerve. The implant is then ready for placement (Fig. 44–24). As is our routine when introducing an implant into the body, 1 g of cefazolin (Ancef) is administered 30 minutes before the implant is inserted, provided the patient has no history of cephalosporin allergy. Additionally, the implant is soaked in a gentamicin solution before it is implanted.

The implant is then inserted into the dissected subperiosteal pocket (Fig. 44–25), and the notch cut into the implant is seated around the neurovascular bundle (Fig. 44–26). Often, the implant does not lie flat when it is first inserted. In this case, the implant is removed and trimmed, or the subperiosteal pocket is enlarged as appropriate. When properly placed, the superior edge of the implant does not extend above the orbital rim, and the notch cut in the implant does not impinge on the neurovascular bundle. When the placement of the implant is satisfactory, the implant is sutured to the remaining cuff of periosteum along the orbital rim with 6-0 Dexon on a small half-circle needle. The conjunctiva is closed with interrupted 6-0 mild chromic sutures, the lateral canthus is resuspended (Fig. 44–27), and the lateral canthotomy incision is closed (Fig. 44–28). A lateral Frost suture is

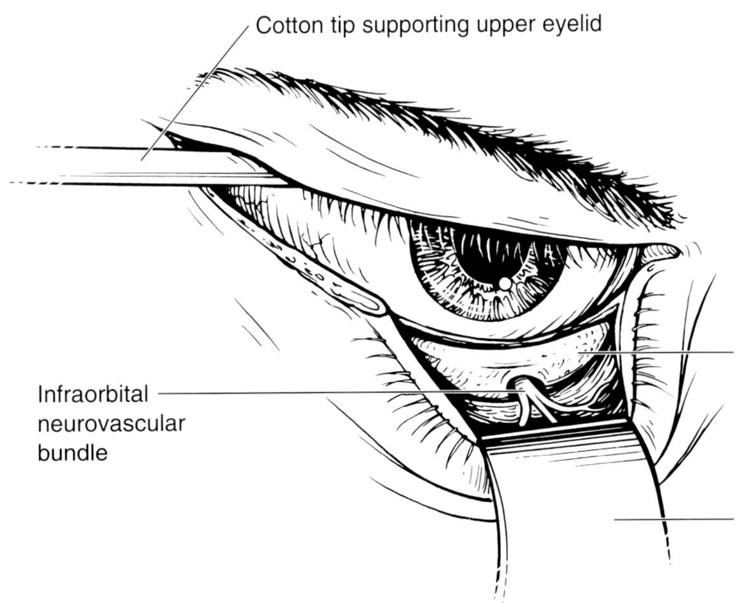

Figure 44–22. Schematic drawing of Figure 44–21. Note the exposure of the infraorbital neurovascular bundle.

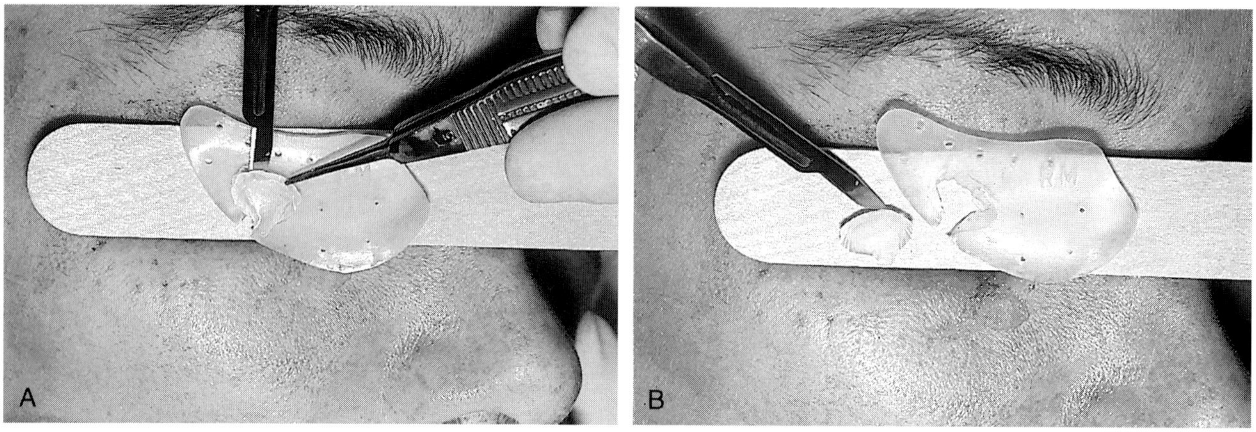

Figure 44–23. *A* and *B*, A step in the transconjunctival placement of a Flowers tear trough implant. Using a tongue blade for support, silicone is cut out of the implant to create a passageway for the infraorbital neurovascular bundle.

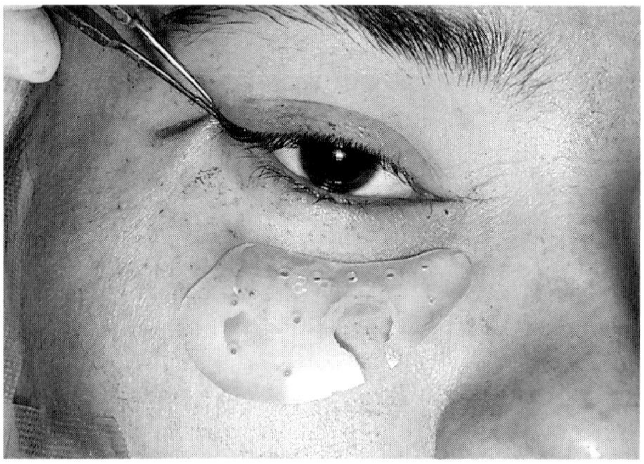

Figure 44–24. A step in the transconjunctival placement of a Flowers tear trough implant. A Flowers implant is ready for insertion.

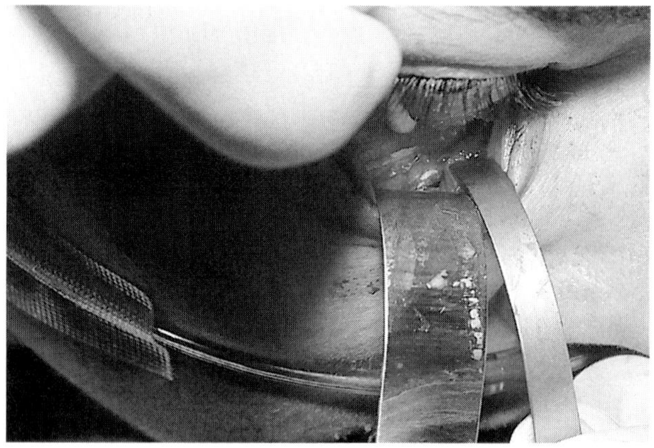

Figure 44–26. A step in the transconjunctival placement of a Flowers tear trough implant. The notch in the implant is carefully seated around the infraorbital neurovascular bundle.

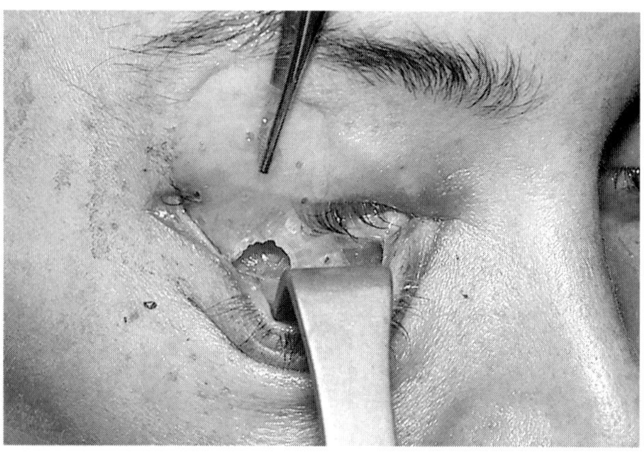

Figure 44–25. A step in the transconjunctival placement of a Flowers tear trough implant. The prepared implant is advanced into the dissected subperiosteal space.

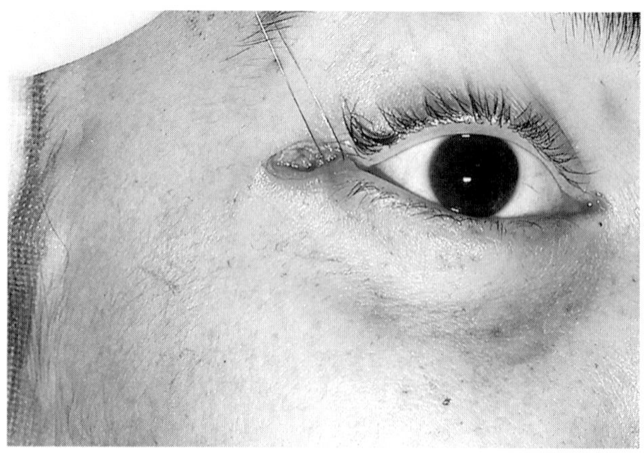

Figure 44–27. A step in the transconjunctival placement of a Flowers tear trough implant. The lateral canthus is resuspended.

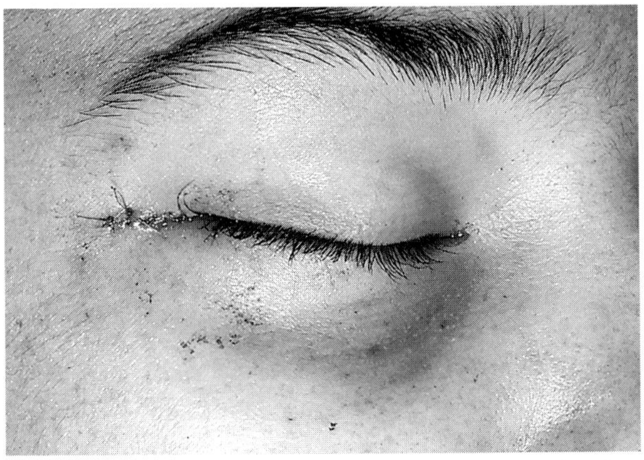

Figure 44–28. A step in the transconjunctival placement of a Flowers tear trough implant. Laterally, the orbicularis and skin are closed in separate layers.

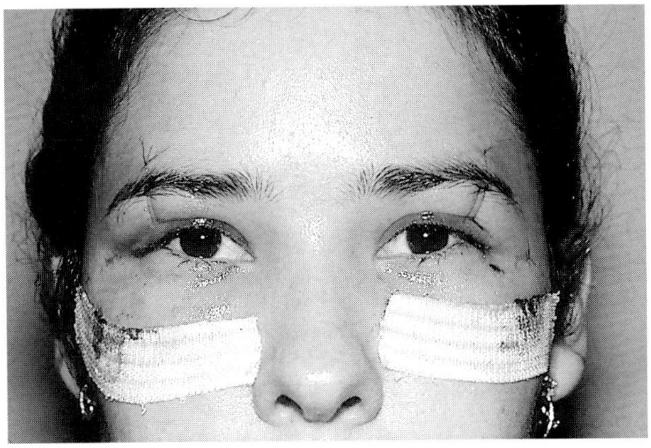

Figure 44–29. A step in the transconjunctival placement of a Flowers tear trough implant. The lower eyelid is supported with the placement of lateral Frost sutures and French elastic tape.

placed to help support the eyelid laterally, and elastic French tape is used to further support the lower eyelid (Fig. 44–29).

Patients are warned to expect postoperative swelling and bruising. Because a large flap is created by this surgery, healing can take much longer than it does in lower blepharoplasty. Additionally, some degree of postoperative anesthesia or paresthesia is common. Provided the neurovascular bundle was not frankly injured during surgery, recovery usually occurs quickly. Figure 44–30 demonstrates the preoperative and postoperative appearance of the patient illustrated in the operative series. Figure 44–15 shows the preoperative and postoperative photographs of this patient's sister, who also had bilateral Flowers tear trough implants. In both cases, the preoperative photographs document the presence of the tear trough deformity. Postoperatively, these deformities have been significantly addressed by the Flowers implant.

Custom Suborbital Implants

Prefabricated implants, such as the Flowers tear trough implant, the Binder submalar implant, or the Goldberg lateral orbital rim implant, are designed to address single problem areas. When significant rim or suborbital rim hypoplasia is present, the volume deficiency becomes too large to correct with the placement of a single standard implant. In this situation, a custom-made implant may be created to address the volume deficit. The decision to

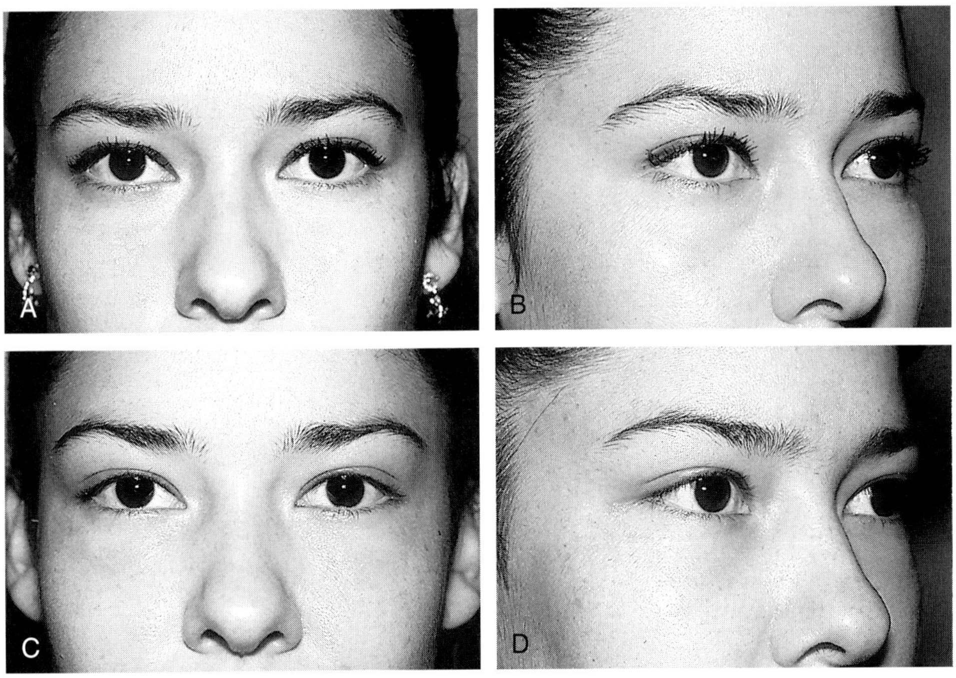

Figure 44–30. The effect of placing Flowers tear trough implants. *A* and *B*, Patient's preoperative appearance. *C* and *D*, Appearance 3 months after the placement of a Flowers tear trough implant.

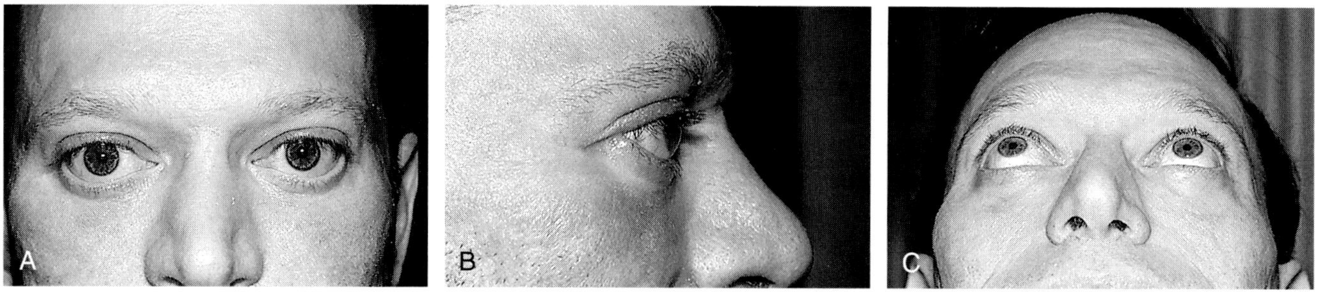

Figure 44–31. Preoperative series (*A* to *C*) of a patient with cheek implants. Note that the patient's cheek implants do not provide support for the suborbital region, which is flat. Additionally, ocular prominence and vertical inadequacy of the lower eyelids are present. Vertical inadequacy resulted from scarring in the lower eyelid and a lack of support for the lower eyelid tissues, a consequence of bony hypoplasia.

create a custom-made malar implant first begins with the definition of the problem, which is often obvious. The patient with late depression of the maxillary face resulting from trauma is a clear example. However, an equally important group of patients is that with globe prominence resulting from a hypoplastic infraorbital region with poor anterior projection. As was discussed earlier, inadequate lower eyelid support often has structural and functional consequences. Patients with this problem often present with dry eye and corneal exposure complaints. Careful evaluation can confirm superficial punctate keratopathy in the interpalpebral zone. Patients who fail to respond to maximal medical therapy with ocular lubrication often require eyelid reconstruction, particularly when the upper eyelids have been compromised by prior eyelid surgery. In these patients, structural support must be provided for the lower eyelids so that their function improves. Augmentation of the hypoplastic suborbital region is an essential component of this reconstruction.

The case of a patient with prior lower eyelid surgery and maxillary hypoplasia illustrates the creation of a custom-made malar implant and its placement. This patient had bilateral cheek implants placed through an infraciliary incision by a referring surgeon. The patient's baseline congenital facial morphology is an extreme in the normal spectrum because of prominent globes and hypoplastic development of the suborbital region and its anterior projection. Additionally, the patient had lower eyelid retraction resulting from significant lower eyelid scarring (Fig. 44–31). He had significant dry eye symptoms that failed to respond to medical management. Reconstruction of the lower eyelids was therefore felt to be necessary to address lower eyelid retraction that was contributing to corneal exposure. The patient had malar implants in place, which had been inserted by a well-meaning surgeon who addressed only the malar projection and not the functionally and aesthetically more important rim and suborbital projection. To provide adequate lower eyelid support, a customized malar implant was envisioned with the removal of the old cheek implants. Lower eyelid reconstruction with the placement of hard-palate graft material was also felt to be required for an optimal result.

The first step in the development of a customized malar implant is a high-resolution computed tomographic scan of the head. Three-dimensional reconstruction provides a representation of the patient's facial skeleton with his old cheek implants in place (Fig. 44–32). By use of digital subtraction methods, a three-dimensional

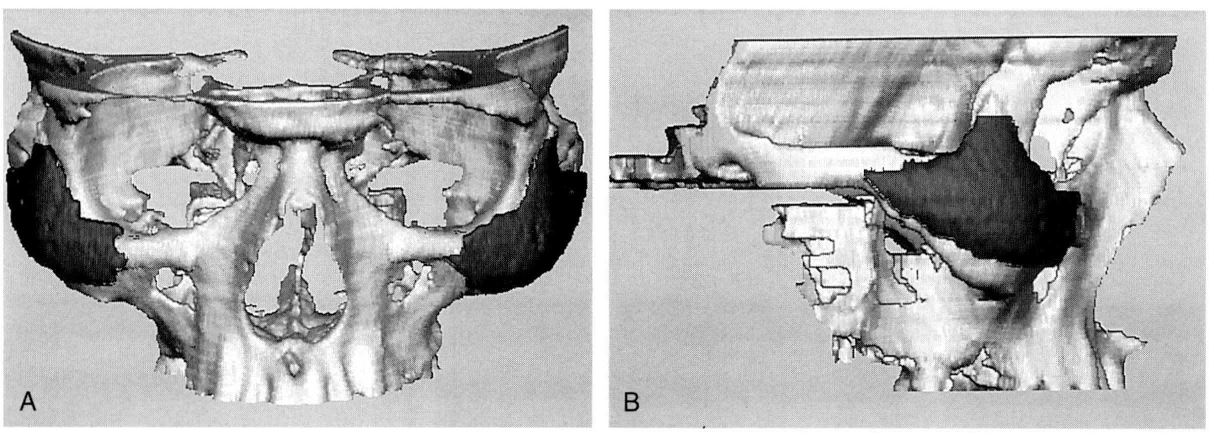

Figure 44–32. High-resolution three-dimensional computed tomographic reconstruction of the patient in Figure 44–31. Note the old cheek implants in place. *A*, Frontal view. *B*, Lateral view.

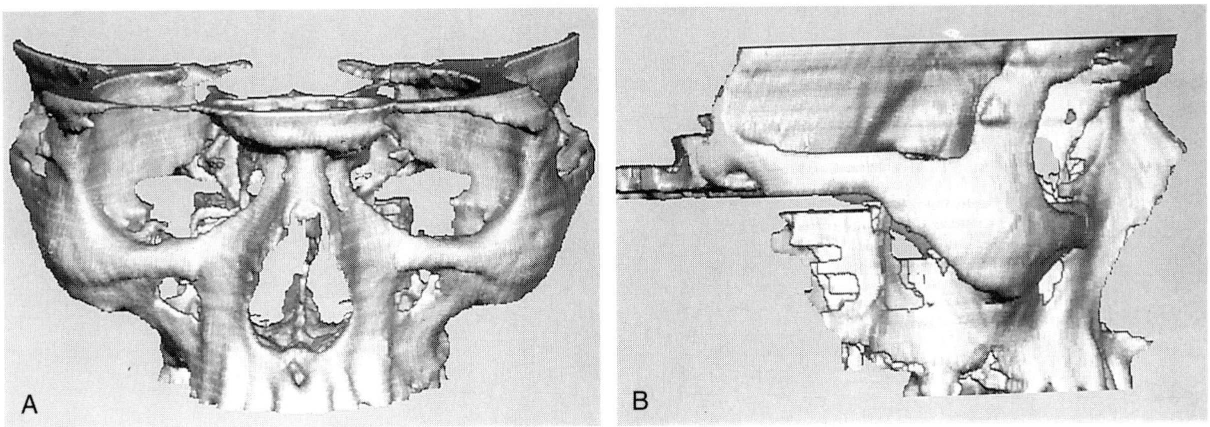

Figure 44–33. High-resolution three-dimensional computed tomographic reconstruction of the patient in Figure 44–31, with digital subtraction of the old cheek implants. Note the lace of projection in the suborbital bones. *A*, Frontal view. *B*, Lateral view.

representation of the facial skeleton without the old cheek implants can be generated (Fig. 44–33). Data from this study is used by computer-assisted machining tools to produce a life-sized plastic model of the patient's midfacial skeleton (Implant Tech, Van Nuys, CA).

In profile with a straight edge held sagittally to the skull, the lack of orbital rim projection and the inadequacy of the bony support for the malar and infraorbital regions are evident (Fig. 44–34). A skull with a normally positioned malar face is presented in Figure 44–35 for comparison.

The computer-generated model of the patient's facial skeleton is then used by the surgeon to create a version of the customized implant in dental wax (Fig. 44–36). On profile, the implant that will be created from the wax model will clearly provide the necessary bony contour (Fig. 44–37). When the desired shape is finalized on the skull model, the waxed implant models are removed from the skull model (Fig. 44–38) and cast in silicone by using a lost wax process. The lost wax process uses the volatility of the wax to create a mold for the final silicone implant.

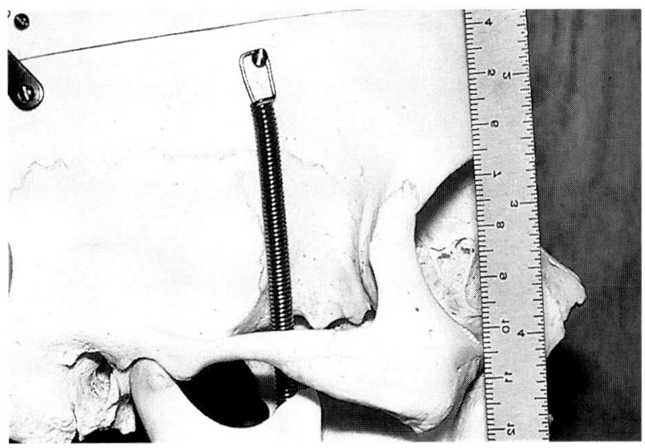

Figure 44–35. A straight edge held to a skull with normal suborbital projection.

To create a silicone implant with the lost wax process, the wax version of the implant is cast in plaster. Once the plaster is set, the plaster containing the wax model is brought to high temperature in a kiln. The wax vaporizes into the plaster, leaving a mold. Silicone is poured into

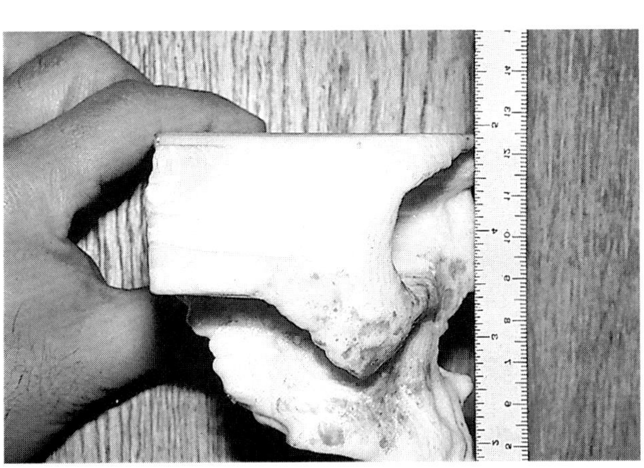

Figure 44–34. A straight edge held to the computer generated model created from the computed tomographic scans demonstrated the relatively poor projection of the suborbital region.

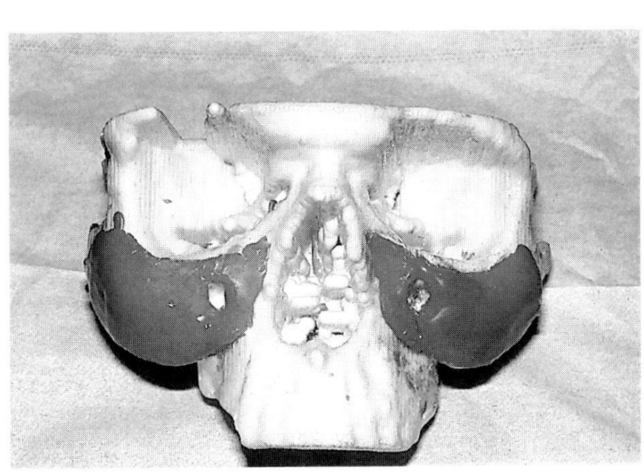

Figure 44–36. Wax models of the desired custom-made suborbital implants are made on the computer-generated model of the patient's skull.

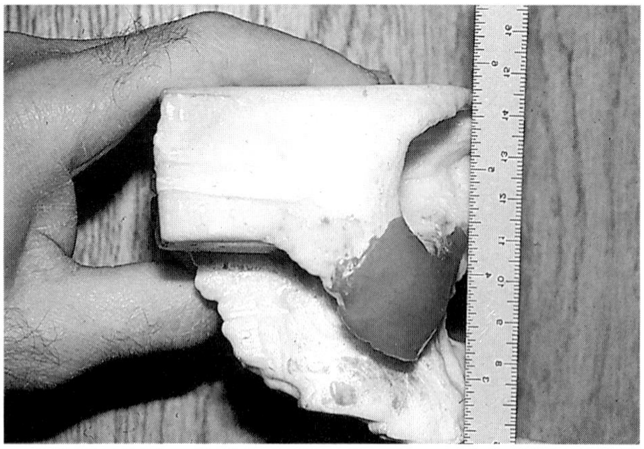

Figure 44–37. On profile the wax model provides the necessary anterior projection to create a normal bony profile. This projection will provide improved support for the lower eyelid.

the mold, and when this silicone polymerizes into a solid, it is in the exact shape of the desired implant. This customized implant is returned to the surgeon, and is then sterilized and is ready for surgical use. The final product is a customized implant made in medical-grade solid silicone.

In this patient, the resulting implant was placed via an intraoral route. The implant provides the necessary projection needed for the entire suborbital region (Fig. 44–39). Figure 44–40 shows the patient 3 months after the completion of all surgery, including bilateral lower eyelid reconstruction with hard-palate spacers, removal of the old cheek implants, and insertion of the customized cheek implants. The suborbital projection has significantly improved (Fig. 44–41). The difference could be achieved only by a comprehensive approach. This case demonstrates the powerful versatility of the custom-made malar implant in a clinical situation that was previously underrecognized or considered unsolvable.

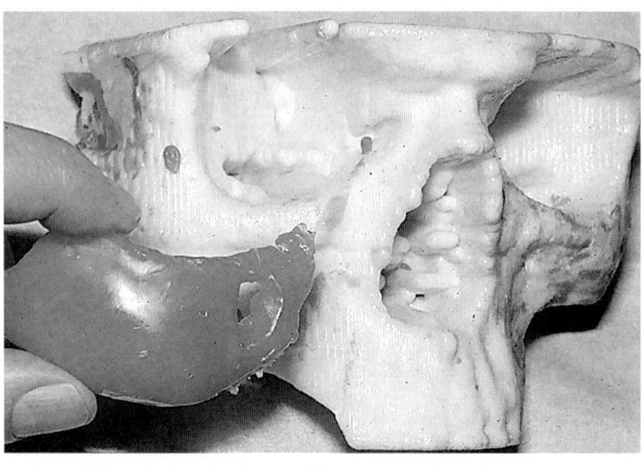

Figure 44–38. When the shapes of the wax models are finalized, the models are removed from the skull and sent for fabrication in silicone by a lost wax process.

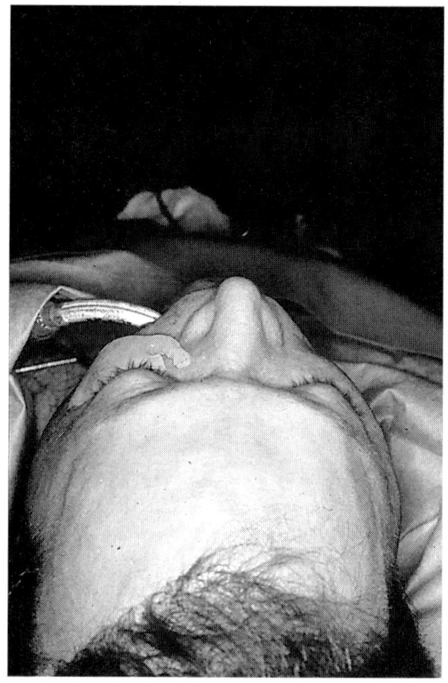

Figure 44–39. Intraoperative photograph with one of the custom-made cheek implants placed on the left cheek. Note the significant anterior projection of this implant.

VERTICAL EYELID AND SUBORBITAL AUGMENTATION

Suborbital hypoplasia is often associated with vertical inadequacy of the lower eyelid. Suborbital augmentation alone corrects vertical height inadequacy of the lower eyelid when it is the result of insufficient bony rim support. However, structural problems in the lower eyelid often contribute to the vertical inadequacy. When this is the case, suborbital augmentation alone does not solve the vertical inadequacy, and appropriate eyelid reconstruction and augmentation of the suborbit are required.

Patients with suborbital hypoplasia and a history of lower transcutaneous blepharoplasty commonly present with vertically inadequate lower eyelids resulting from cicatricial contracture of the middle lamella of the lower eyelid and inadequate bony support for the eyelid. Lysis of the middle lamellar scar in the lower eyelid and stenting of it with a spacer of hard-palate graft solves only part of the problem. Correction of the inadequate bony support must occur. We describe here a surgical approach for correcting both sets of problems by relying on the Flower tear trough implant for correcting the suborbital hypoplasia combined with reconstruction of the lower eyelid with hard-palate graft material. The method can be combined with either prefabricated or customized implants. In fact, the patient discussed in the section on customized implants also had lower eyelid reconstruction that incorporated hard-palate graft material (see Figs. 44–31, 44–40, and 44–41).

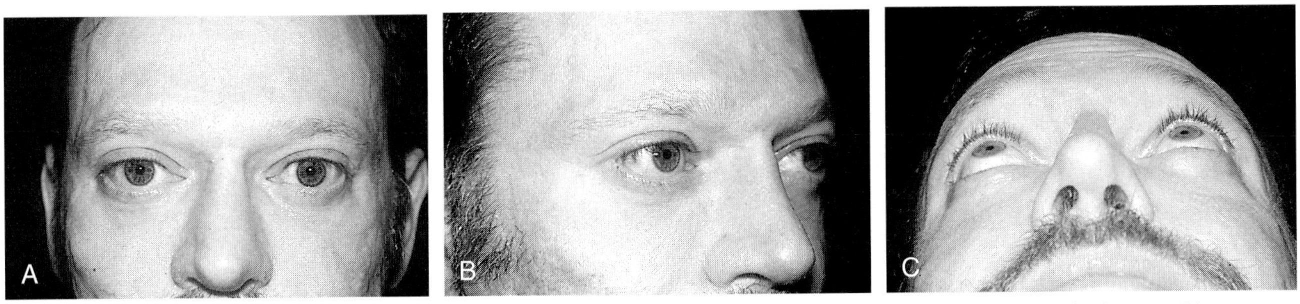

Figure 44–40. The patient 3 months after the placement of the custom-made suborbital rim implants (*A* to *C*). Note that the patient also has lower eyelid reconstruction with the placement of hard palate grafts as spacer to address the cicatricial lower eyelid retraction.

The surgical exposure required for placement of a Flowers tear trough implant via the transconjunctival approach permits the convenient placement of a tailored strip of hard palate mucoperiosteum in the lower eyelid as a spacer material. This procedure has been described in great detail. However, a description of the lower eyelid reconstruction facilitates an understanding of how these procedures are combined.

In brief, the height and length of vertical inadequacy in the lower eyelid are determined preoperatively. The mucoperiosteum of the hard palate has very little tendency to contract. Therefore, the desired strip of mucoperiosteum is harvested from the hard palate, with 1 mm added to the vertical height (Fig. 44–42). The mucoperiosteum is removed in a lamellar fashion (Fig. 44–43). Hemostasis is then obtained in the donor bed (Fig. 44–44), the hard-palate defect is filled with periodontal pack (Coe-Pak, Coe Laboratories, Chicago, IL) (Fig. 44–45), and surgical palatal stent prepared in advance by a dentist is placed in the mouth to protect the donor site after surgery (Fig. 44–46).

Next, a lateral canthotomy and inferior cantholysis are performed. The conjunctiva and lower eyelid retractors are severed with a Stevens scissors just below the inferior edge of the tarsus (Fig. 44–47). Dissection to the inferior orbital rim is performed as described earlier. However, many cases of lower eyelid vertical inadequacy are associated with significant lower eyelid midlamellar scarring. This cicatrix must be fully lysed to adequately free the lower eyelid (Fig. 44–48). Failure to completely lyse the scar prevents successful correction of lower eyelid retraction. After dissection of the midlamellar scars, dissection to expose the orbital rim is then performed.

With the inferior orbital rim exposed, the procedure for the placement of a Flowers tear trough implant proceeds as described earlier. Once the implant is in place, lateral canthal resuspension sutures are placed from the lateral edge of the lower eyelid tarsus to the point on the inside aspect of the lateral orbital rim that locates the lateral canthal angle in the optimal position. Typically, this point is 1 to 2 mm higher than the medial canthus (Fig. 44–49). In this situation, the surgeon must realize that a spacer of hard-palate mucoperiosteum will support the lower eyelid, not an overshortened lateral tarsal strip.

Before the lateral canthal resuspension suture is tied up, the lower eyelid is everted, and the hard palate graft is sutured across the lower eyelid between the cut edge of the conjunctiva and lower eyelid retractors on one side and the inferior edge of the tarsus on the other (Figs. 44–50 and 44–51). Great care must be taken in this suturing to avoid distorting the tissues or leaving exposed suture ends. Immobilizing the eyelid with Frost sutures is a critical step (Fig. 44–52), and the eyelids are typically left sutured and patched closed for a week. Often, a collagen-based dissolvable lens is placed to reduce the risk of suture-induced corneal abrasion. Given the necessity for patching the eye for 1 week, surgery on only one side at a time is performed.

Figure 44–53 schematically illustrates the relationship between the implant on the suborbital face and the hard palate graft in the eyelid. Figure 44–54 demonstrates the preoperative and postoperative appearance of a patient who underwent combined bilateral placement of a Flowers tear trough implant and lower eyelid reconstruction with a hard palate graft. Maximal rehabilitation of the lower eyelid vertical inadequacy has been achieved by

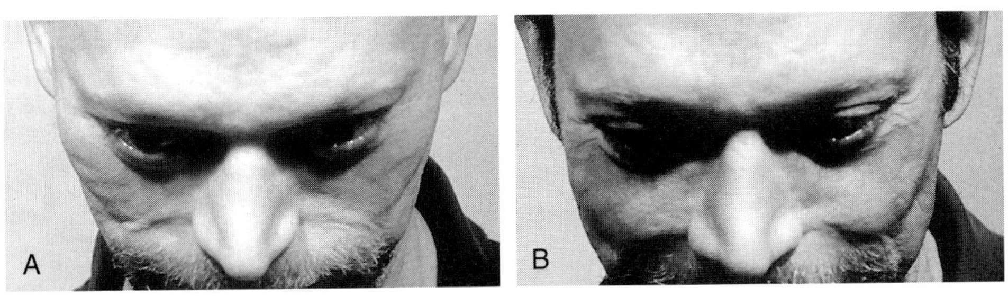

Figure 44–41. The effect of custom-made suborbital implants. *A*, Preoperative appearance. *B*, Postoperative appearance. Note the correction of the suborbital hypoplasia.

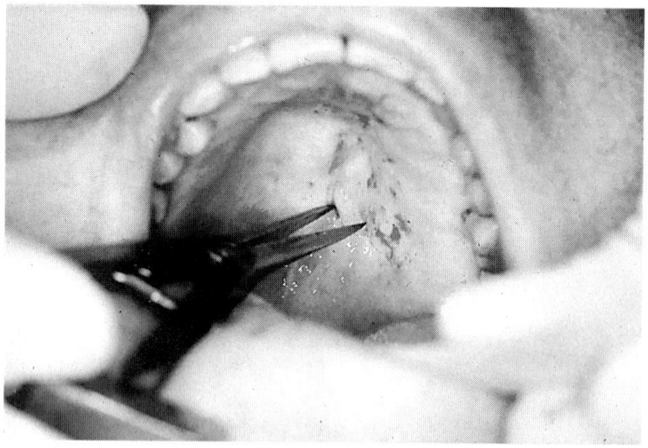

Figure 44–42. After infiltration with local anesthesia, the desired hard palate graft is marked out.

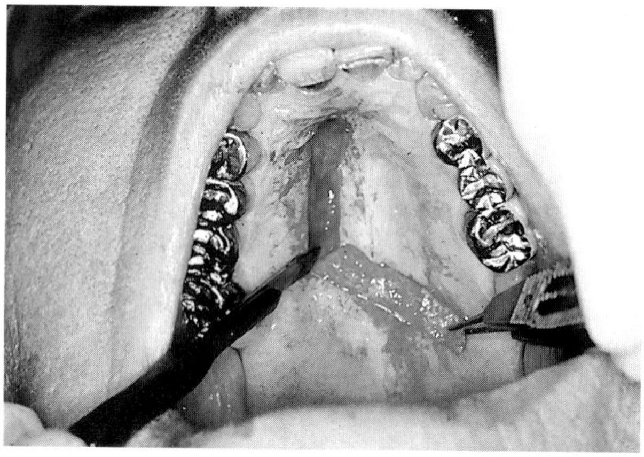

Figure 44–43. Using a no. 15 blade, the mucoperiosteum is excised in a lamellar fashion.

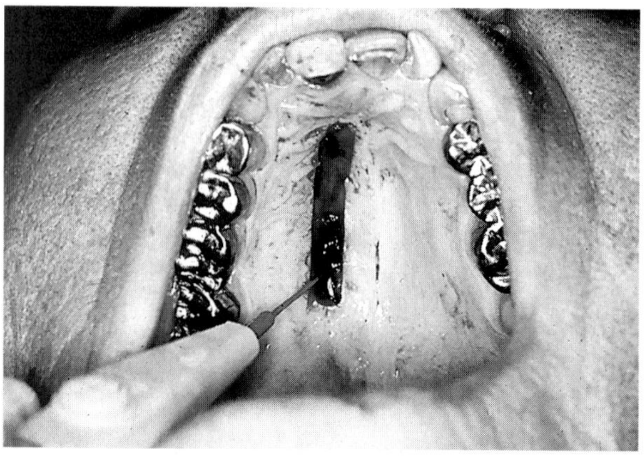

Figure 44–44. Meticulous hemostasis is obtained in the donor bed.

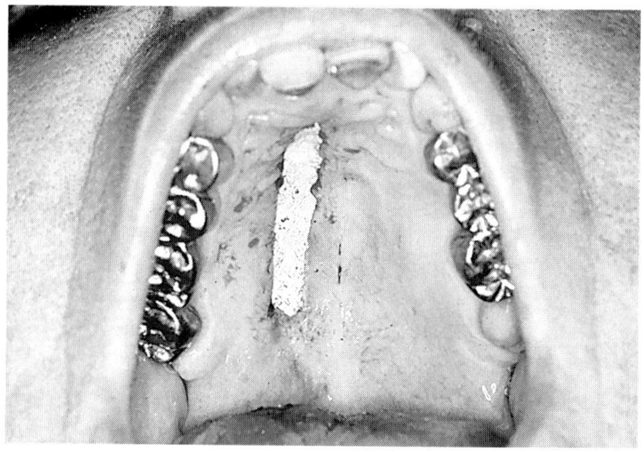

Figure 44–45. The donor bed is then covered with periodontal pack material.

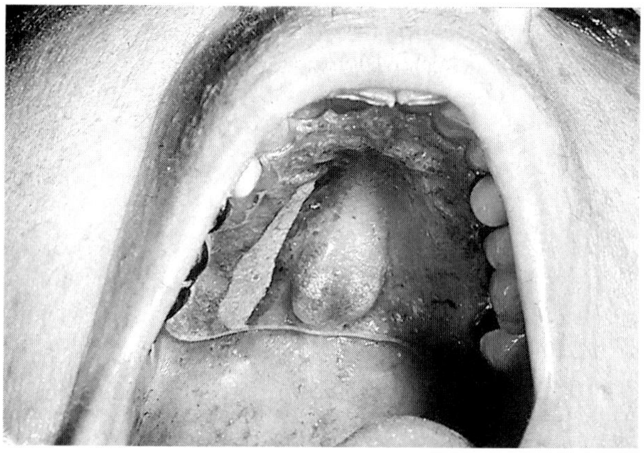

Figure 44–46. A surgical palatal stent prepared preoperatively by a dentist is placed in the mouth to further protect the donor site. The palatal stent is secured in the mouth with denture adhesive.

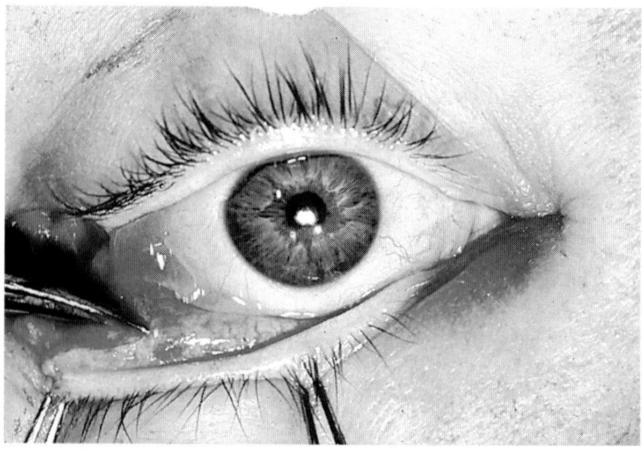

Figure 44–47. In preparation for the placement of the hard palate graft the conjunctiva and lower eyelid retractors are severed just inferior to the tarsus.

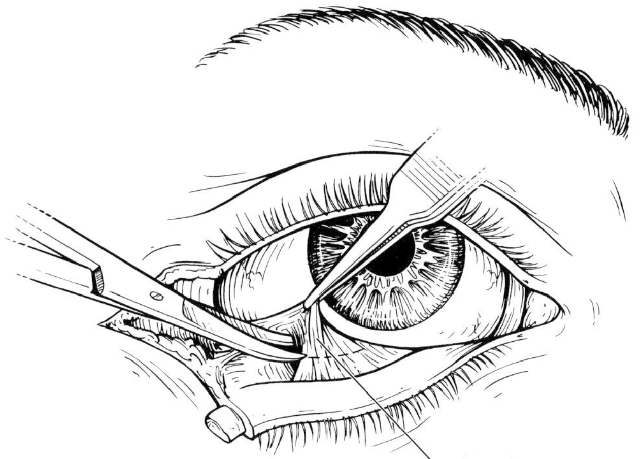

Figure 44–48. To permit elevation of the eyelid, all cicatrix present in the midlamella of the lower eyelid must be lysed. Once this is complete, dissection is performed to expose the orbital rim, and a Flowers tear trough implant is positioned as described earlier in the chapter.

providing improved lower eyelid support with a Flowers tear trough implant and reconstructing the lower eyelid by use of hard palate graft material. Full correction of this particular set of problems required addressing both the vertical inadequacy of the eyelids and the inadequate bony support. The choice of suborbital implant is determined by the nature of the suborbital hypoplasia. Therefore, this approach is flexible and makes it possible to correct a combination of problems that was previously impossible to satisfactorily address.

COMPLICATIONS

Both customized and prefabricated suborbital implants can be safely and reliably placed with minimal risk of complications, and both have an excellent safety

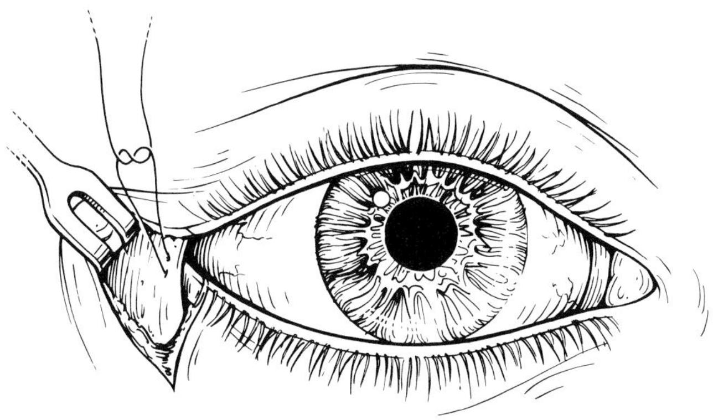

Figure 44–49. Just before the hard palate graft is sutured in place, the lateral canthus is resuspended. Typically, the lateral canthal angle is 1.5 mm superior to the medial canthal angle.

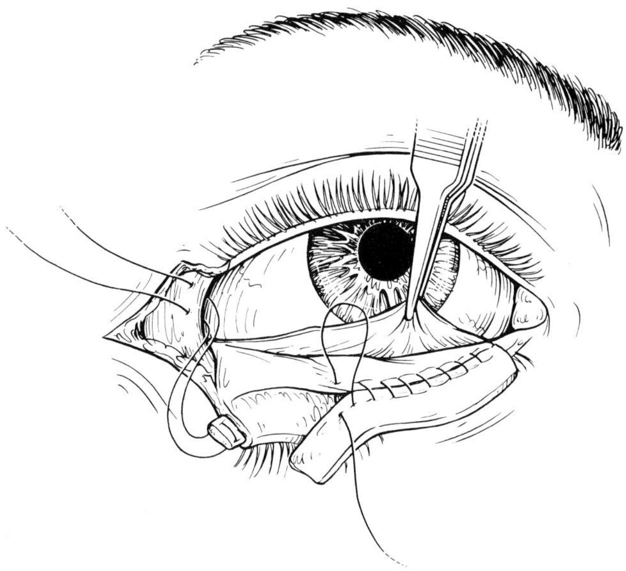

Figure 44–50. With the site of the lateral canthal angle fixed by sutures, the lower eyelid is pulled down to expose the recipient bed where the hard palate graft is to be sutured. The superior edge of the graft is first sutured to the inferior edge of the tarsus.

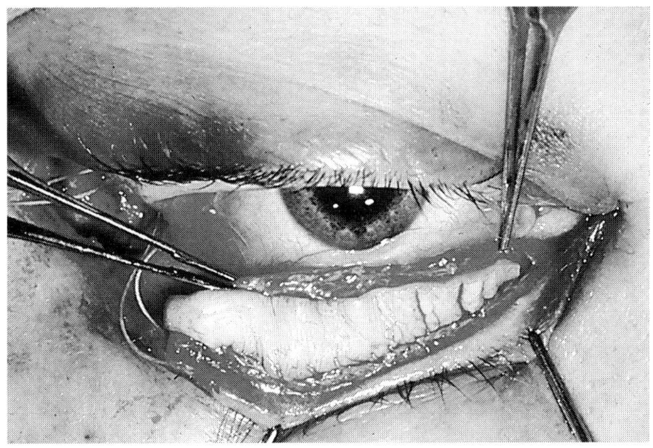

Figure 44–51. The hard palate graft in place in the recipient bed of the lower eyelid. Once suturing is complete, the lower eyelid resuspension suture will be tightened up and the orbicularis and skin closed in separate layers.

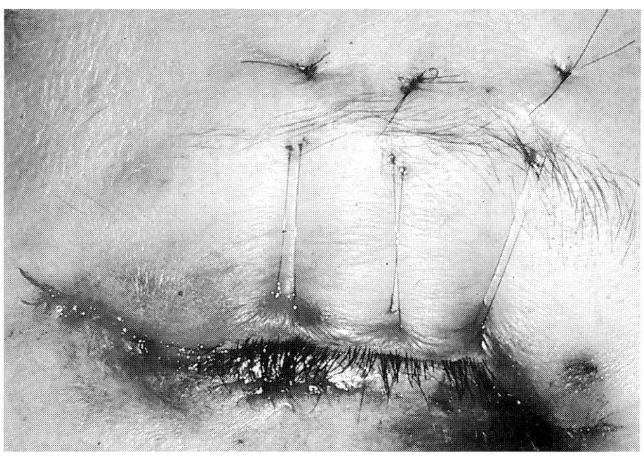

Figure 44–52. The eyelid is then supported with Frost sutures, and the eye is patched closed for a week.

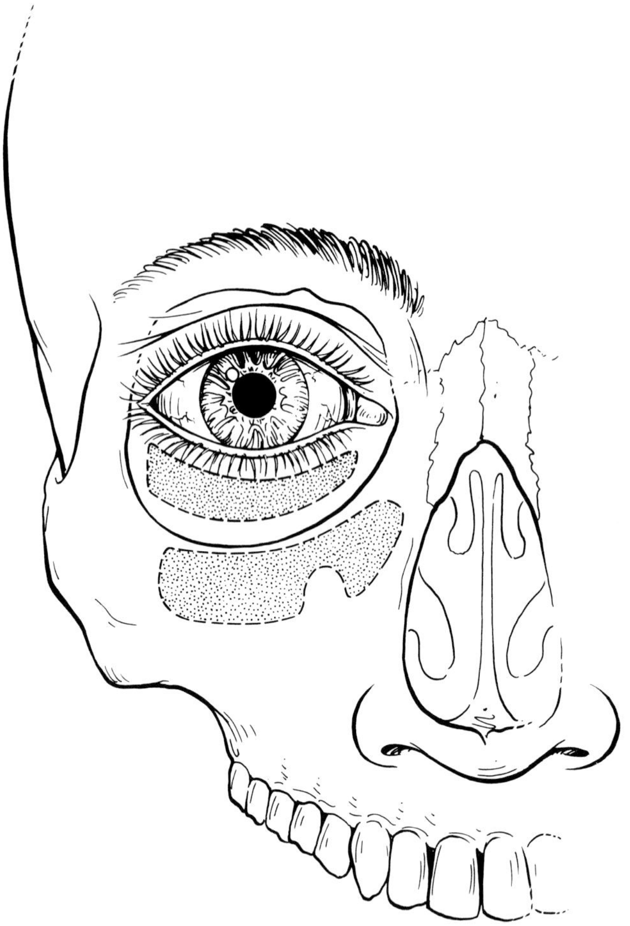

Figure 44–53. Schematic illustration of the relative positions of the hard palate graft and a Flowers tear trough implant.

record. However, many points are worth discussing regarding the eyelid and the orbit surgeon undertaking the placement of these implants. The complications of the procedure fall into two categories: (1) complications associated with lateral canthal surgery and (2) complications associated with suborbital dissection and implant placement. Because the potential complications of lateral canthal surgery are well known, this discussion focuses primarily on the complications associated with suborbital dissection and implant placement.

Another area of concern comes from the fact that many patients who need suborbital volume correction have had previous cosmetic eyelid surgery. Their expectations for postoperative healing are therefore conditioned by these previous experiences. They must be adequately prepared for postoperative swelling and bruising, which will typically last longer than that following simple cosmetic surgical procedures. Clear preoperative communication is essential so that patients have realistic expectations.

Meticulous avoidance of the use of anticoagulants reduces the risk of postoperative hematoma. The dissected pocket containing the implant is not closed until hemostasis is complete. Some surgeons advocate the routine placement of miniature drains at the end of the operation in the dissected subperiosteal pocket. The drain is evacuated by light suction that is typically applied by connecting the drain to a vacuum blood collection tube. We have not found the use of drains necessary and therefore do not routinely use them. If a hematoma does develop, it should be drained to reduce the risk of postoperative

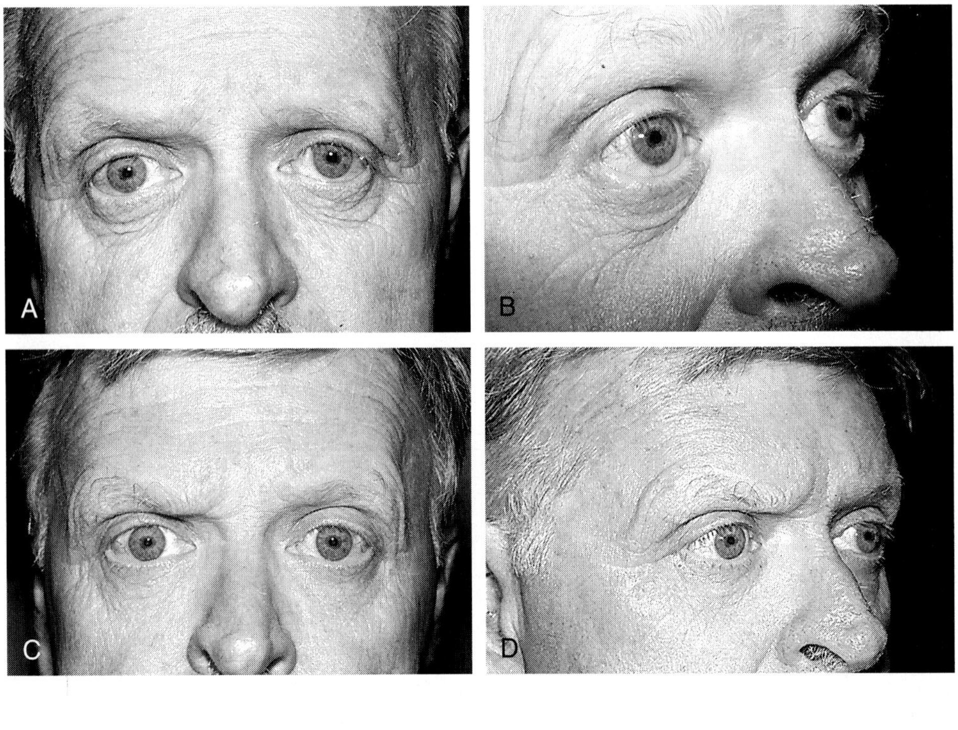

Figure 44–54. Preoperative and postoperative photographs of a patient who had the combination of a Flowers tear trough implant and lower eyelid reconstruction with hard palate grafts on each side. *A* and *B*, Preoperative appearance. *C* and *D*, Postoperative appearance.

contraction. Judicious use of triamcinolone (Kenalog) injections can be beneficial in these cases to minimize scar formation.

Postoperative malposition of the implant is perhaps the next most important concern. Fortunately, the risk of malposition can be minimized during surgery. An adequate dissection of the subperiosteal bed is essential. The implant should be carefully inspected once it has been seated in the subperiosteal pocket. If it does not seat well, the implant should be trimmed or the pocket enlarged. The implant must also be firmly secured. The Flowers implant is secured by suturing it to the cuff of periosteum preserved below the orbital rim; therefore, preserving a cuff of periosteum for this purpose is an important element of the procedure. Customized implants can also be secured in a similar fashion. Often, these implants are secured to bolsters brought out to the skin. When malposition does occur, triamcinolone injections can help minimize excess scarring. Eventually, the implant may need to be removed and a new implant inserted if the malposition creates an unsatisfactory result. It is helpful to warn patients of this unusual complication preoperatively.

The potential for nerve injury must be considered. During dissection of the cheek, a peripheral branch of the facial nerve may be injured. To minimize the risk of this injury, dissection should be kept to a minimum. Electrocautery may also damage the facial nerve. Bleeding in the depths of the dissection bed can usually be controlled by pressure or application of cotton pledgets soaked with 1:1000 epinephrine. A second potential site for nerve damage is at the infraorbital neurovascular bundle. Dissection of these structures should be carried out with care to avoid direct injury. An equally important potential cause of postoperative anesthesia is a poorly carved notch in the Flowers tear trough implant. If the implant rests on the nerve, postoperative anesthesia will occur. Transient anesthesia is common, and patients are counseled preoperatively about this possibility.

Perioperative antibiotics reduce the risk of postoperative infection and are routinely used in these cases. Lymphedema may occur in some patients for many weeks after surgery; this effect is often a function of the history of previous surgery in the lower eyelid. Steroids can be of benefit in this situation. However, the lymphedema, given sufficient time, will resolve on its own.

SUMMARY

1. The bony skeleton plays an important role in the structural support and the ultimate function of the lower eyelid.
2. Soft tissue abnormalities that result from hypoplasia of the underlying bone can be corrected only by treating the bony hypoplasia.
3. Mild and moderate suborbital volume deficiency can be managed with prefabricated implants.
4. The tear trough deformity, a particular type of suborbital volume deficiency, results from a flat or concave medial aspect of the infraorbital maxillary face.
5. The tear trough deformity can be satisfactorily treated with the Flowers tear trough implant.
6. More significant deficiencies in the suborbital region require a custom-made implant, but this approach can address problems that have previously been uncorrectable.
7. Combining the placement of a Flowers tear trough implant with reconstruction of the lower eyelid by use of a hard palate graft provides a method of solving significant lower eyelid problems in patients with bony hypoplasia without resorting to a custom implant.

REFERENCES

1. Flowers RS: Tear trough implants for correction of tear trough deformity. Clin Plast Surg 20:403–415, 1993.
2. Furnas DW: Festoons, mounds, and bags of the eyelid and cheek. Clin Plast Surg 20:367–385, 1993.
3. Shorr N: Madame butterfly procedure with hard palate graft: management of postblepharoplasty round eye and scleral show. Facial Plast Surg 10:90–118, 1994.

CHAPTER 45

Essential Blepharospasm and Hemifacial Spasm

John B. Holds

OVERVIEW OF FACIAL MOVEMENT DISORDERS

Abnormal eyelid and facial movements may cause great disability and distress to patients. Involuntary movements of the face, tongue and palate, pharynx, vocal cords, and neck are grouped into the broad classification of craniocervical dyskinesias.[1] A variety of lesions cause facial dyskinesias, and the pathogenesis of an anomalous facial movement may lie at any level of the motor pathway. Accurate diagnosis is vital to counsel and treat patients with these disorders.

The craniocervical dyskinesias of greatest interest to the ophthalmologist include essential blepharospasm, hemifacial spasm, and aberrant facial nerve regeneration following a Bell's or other facial palsy (Table 45–1). Essential blepharospasm, or benign essential blepharospasm, is a dystonic movement disorder characterized by involuntary spasm of the orbicularis oculi. The corrugator superciliaris and the procerus muscles, which are important protractor muscles of the medial eyebrow (Fig. 45–1), are also involved in this spasm. Dystonic movement disorders are characterized by slow, sustained twisting, pulling, or squeezing movements. *Meige's, Wood's,* and *Brueghel's syndromes* are eponyms used to refer to various degrees of dystonic oromandibular spasm. For purposes of this discussion, the term *Meige's syndrome* is used to describe dystonic facial or oromandibular spasm, with or without concomitant blepharospasm.

Dystonia, including essential blepharospasm, oromandibular dystonia, torticollis, and spastic dysphonia, is probably the most common form of spontaneous craniocervical dyskinesia. Involuntary contractions typically begin in one muscle group in craniocervical dystonia and spread over time to involve adjacent muscle groups. Areas of involvement in the head and neck region are frequently overlapping and appear to represent a similar disease process (idiopathic dystonia) with different levels and severity of involvement. It is common for patients who present with involvement in one area to progress and develop other manifestations of craniocervical dystonia.[2]

Hemifacial spasm is a unilateral facial spasm disorder that usually arises from extra-axial compression of the facial nerve in the cerebellopontine angle.[3] Hemifacial spasm is etiologically unrelated to the craniocervical dystonias, although it is reasonable to discuss it in the same section as essential blepharospasm and Meige's syndrome since similar treatments are employed.

ESSENTIAL BLEPHAROSPASM

Clinical Features

Essential blepharospasm is a progressively debilitating form of craniocervical dystonia characterized by chronic, forceful spasm of the orbicularis oculi (see Fig. 45–1). There is a 3:1 female-to-male predominance, with an average age at onset of 56 years and three fourths of cases beginning after age 50. The onset is heralded by an increased frequency of blinking that progresses to sustained, then forceful eyelid closure, culminating in uncontrollable eyelid spasm (see Table 45–1).[4] The course fluctuates, punctuated by spontaneous remissions and exacerbations. Symptoms generally progress for several years with a plateau reached 5 to 7 years after onset.

In essential blepharospasm the initial complaints may relate to photophobia, ocular pain, dry eyes, or other seemingly unrelated causes for uncontrollable eyelid closure.[5] Only after progression of the condition without other signs of pathology or after other facial dystonia is noted is the correct diagnosis made. Factors such as fatigue, bright lights, television watching, and interpersonal interactions may exacerbate the condition. Sensory and proprioceptive "tricks" such as whistling, humming, singing, or massaging a "pressure point" may temporarily relieve the spasm in some patients. Eyelid spasm typically remits during sleep. These factors, the fluctuating course, the lack of other organic signs, and the emotional

Supported in part by an unrestricted grant to the Department of Ophthalmology, St. Louis University Health Sciences Center, St. Louis, Missouri, from Research to Prevent Blindness, Inc.

TABLE 45–1

Diagnostic Features of Facial Spasm

Disorder	Female-to-Male Preponderance	Average Age at Onset (Years)	Laterality	Voluntary Control	Sleep Disturbance	Clinical Characteristics	Etiology	Diagnostic Studies*
Hemifacial spasm	3:2	45	Unilateral	No	May be present	Tonic-clonic movements in area of seventh cranial nerve innervation	Compression of seventh cranial nerve by dolichoectatic vessel, tumor, arteriovenous malformation	CT and/or MRI: dolichoectatic vessel, 80%; tumor, 2% EMG: arrhythmic discharge, 20–40/second
Essential blepharospasm	3:1	56	Bilateral	Minimal	Absent	Bilateral dystonic orbicularis oculi spasm	Usually idiopathic; lesion of basal ganglia or brain stem in secondary disease	CT and/or MRI: normal (in idiopathic form) EMG: normal
Meige's syndrome (idiopathic facial dystonia)	3:1	56	Bilateral	Minimal	Absent	As above, plus facial spasm	As above for essential blepharospasm	As above for essential blepharospasm
Facial synkinesis	Equally affected	Any	Unilateral	No	Present	Mass contraction with facial weakness	History of facial palsy, aberrant regeneration	CT and/or MRI: normal EMG: synkinesis, fibrillation potentials, reduced motor units
Facial myokymia	Equally affected	Any	Unilateral, segmental	No	Present	Rapid, undulating, flickering muscle	Transient: benign (caffeine, stress) Persistent: multiple sclerosis, intramedullary tumor	CT and/or MRI: perform only if persistent EMG: grouped fasciculations
Facial tic	Equally affected	Childhood	Unilateral or bilateral	Yes	Present	Brief, suppressible, stereotyped movements	Tourette's syndrome	CT and/or MRI: normal EMG: normal

CT, computed tomography; MRI, magnetic resonance imaging; EMG, electromyography.
*CT, MRI, and EMG are not indicated in the workup of every condition.
Adapted from Digre K, Corbett JJ: Hemifacial spasm: Differential diagnosis, mechanism, and treatment. Adv Neurol 49:151–176, 1988.

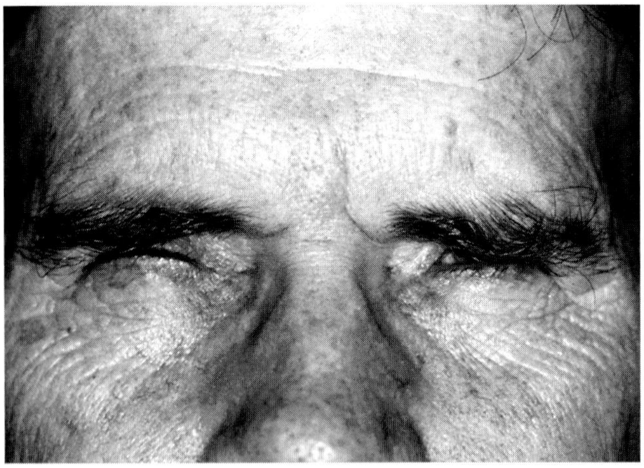

Figure 45–1. Patient with blepharospasm and Meige's syndrome showing marked degree of eyelid and brow spasm.

response to the disease often result in misinterpretation of the condition as psychogenic. In occasional patients, eyelid spasm is perceived as being unilateral. Most such patients have bilateral spasm and progress over time to display more symmetric eyelid spasm.

An ophthalmic examination is important in diagnosis to ensure that the eyelid closure is not secondary to a reflex blepharospasm from ocular disease such as uveitis, corneal disease, macular disease, and sometimes cataracts. Ocular disease, especially dry eyes, frequently exacerbates essential blepharospasm. Treatment of concurrent ocular conditions in essential blepharospasm may reduce the spasm to a level that the patient finds tolerable. Surveys and psychological profiles of patients with essential blepharospasm have pointed to the high incidence of depression in patients with this disorder[6] and a possible link to other personality traits, such as obsessive-compulsive behavior.[7] The depression and psychological distress associated with symptomatic essential blepharospasm validate the role of support groups (e.g., the Benign Essential Blepharospasm Research Foundation, Inc., P.O. Box 12468, Beaumont, TX 77726-2468) and psychological counseling for selected patients.

Pathogenesis

Areas of the basal ganglia involved in orofacial control may be particularly susceptible to aging and the effects of neuroleptic drugs, since the onset of many craniocervical dyskinesias seems to relate to advancing age or drug or other toxin exposure. Secondary dystonia may follow chronic neuroleptic administration (tardive dystonia) or may coexist with Parkinson's disease. Other secondary causes of blepharospasm or Meige's syndrome may include upper brain stem strokes or multiple sclerosis.[8] Gliosis and abnormal neurotransmitter levels have been demonstrated in midbrain and brain stem nuclei of patients with idiopathic facial dystonia.[4] Pontine level delays in the brain stem auditory-evoked potential in one third of patients with idiopathic Meige's syndrome or essential blepharospasm[9] provides noninvasive evidence of brain stem pathology in these disorders. The observation of prolonged saccadic latency[10] in patients with essential blepharospasm is additional evidence of the subcortical organic basis of essential blepharospasm, with the substantia nigra pars reticulata suggested as a common point of cranial motor control.[11] Other investigations of ocular movements in essential blepharospasm[12] showed no involvement of the oculomotor pathways, suggesting a selective involvement of motor pathways regulating the voluntary craniocervical musculature.

MEIGE'S SYNDROME

Dystonic oromandibular spasm with or without eyelid spasm was described as *spasme facial médian* by the French neurologist Henry Meige in 1910.[13] Despite recognition of this clinical syndrome by the American neurologist Horatio C. Wood in the 1870s, essential blepharospasm and Meige's syndrome were largely ignored in the English literature until the early 1970s. The lower facial spasm of Meige's syndrome can be disfiguring, although it is the frequently associated eyelid spasm that causes the greatest disability and distress in most patients. Approximately 75% of my patients presenting for the treatment of essential blepharospasm show evidence of dystonic spasm involving facial muscles other than the eyelid protractor muscles. Patients and even their families are often unaware of the oromandibular spasm, since the eyelid spasm is usually the focus of their complaints. All patients with dystonic spasm extending beyond the periocular region may be classified as having Meige's syndrome, although it is practical in terms of treatment and discussion to classify patients who are mainly bothered by their eyelid spasm as having essential blepharospasm and those patients with oromandibular dystonia alone, or in association with blepharospasm, as having Meige's syndrome.

Despite the evidence of brain abnormalities mentioned previously, the various forms of craniocervical dystonia remain clinical diagnoses. Imaging studies, such as computed tomography (CT) or magnetic resonance imaging (MRI), and other laboratory studies are generally unrevealing and are unnecessary for the workup of patients presenting with typical essential blepharospasm or Meige's syndrome. Atypical features, such as an acute onset, or the presence of other neurologic signs indicates a need for neurologic evaluation and imaging studies.[5]

MANAGEMENT OF ESSENTIAL BLEPHAROSPASM AND MEIGE'S SYNDROME

Unconventional Therapies

Poor understanding and inadequate therapy for facial spasm disorders have led to the use of a variety of unconventional therapies over the years. Patients with essential blepharospasm and Meige's syndrome uniformly report their disease to be extremely stressful. The tremendous amount of emotional overlay observed in these conditions led to a consensus for many years that these conditions were psychogenic and resulted in the referral of patients to psychiatrists. Discovery of an organic basis for these conditions over the past 2 decades has diminished the perception that dystonia is psychogenic. Nonetheless, unconventional therapies, including psychotherapy, biofeedback, acupuncture, and herbal and folk remedies, continue to be employed. These treatments may provide a brief period of perceived benefit but are generally of little objective value. Since essential blepharospasm and Meige's syndrome are aggravated by physical and psychological stress and are associated with a high incidence of depression, there is a role for psychological or psychiatric counseling in many patients. Patient support groups play an important role in counseling and informing affected patients and representing the interests of these patients.

General Eye Care

A variety of ocular and ocular adnexal conditions that cause reflex blepharospasm can contribute to the eyelid spasm in essential blepharospasm and Meige's syndrome. Conditions such as blepharitis and dry eye disorders should be aggressively managed, since control of these coexistent conditions often decreases the severity of the blepharospasm. Dry eye complaints are particularly common in the middle-aged and elderly female patient population prone to essential blepharospasm. The use of wraparound dark sunglasses or artificial tear drops may be mildly to moderately beneficial to many patients and are worthwhile nonspecific treatments to recommend. Occasional patients manage well with ptosis crutches on their eyeglasses.

Pharmacotherapy

Many drugs are reported to be effective in relieving essential blepharospasm and Meige's syndrome. Usually, relief is partial and short-lived, although occasional patients experience significant long-term relief with oral medications alone. The benzodiazepines, lorazepam (0.5 to 2 mg bid or tid), clonazepam (0.5 to 2 mg tid), or oxazepam (10 to 30 mg tid or qid), and the mild anticholinergics orphenadrine (1 tablet bid) and trihexyphenidyl (1 to 3 mg tid) are the medications that patients report to be the most effective.[6] Cyproheptadine, an antagonist of serotonin and histamine as well as an anticholinergic and sedative, has been recommended in doses of 4 mg orally two to four times daily for the treatment of essential blepharospasm.[14] Forty percent to 60% of patients obtain some relief of their facial spasm with one or more of these drugs. Oral medications are most useful in treating very mild essential blepharospasm or in suppressing the lower facial spasms in patients with Meige's syndrome after local treatment of the periorbital spasm. All medications should initially be used at low doses, increasing the dose as tolerated to obtain the desired effect. If objectionable side effects occur, the drug is ineffective after a trial of 2 to 6 weeks, or the effect is lost over weeks or months, the dosage should be tapered and the drug discontinued; then a different medication should be considered. I prefer to give motivated patients a trial of a benzodiazepine, an anticholinergic, and cyproheptadine before abandoning therapy with oral medications. Sometimes, low doses of drugs from two different pharmacologic groups provide added benefit.

Botulinum A Toxin (Botox) Injection

The A toxin serotype produced by *Clostridium botulinum* is a potent paralytic agent. Since the initial report by Frueh and associates,[15] botulinum toxin has been used extensively in the treatment of craniocervical dystonia, especially essential blepharospasm and the blepharospasm component of Meige's syndrome. Botulinum A toxin has been approved by the Food and Drug Administration and is commercially available (Botox, Allergan Pharmaceuticals, Irvine, CA). Subcutaneous injection of this toxin into the eyelids and brows provides relief from symptomatic blepharospasm for approximately 3 months in 85% to 90% of patients (Figs. 45–2 and 45–3).[6] The high efficacy of the injections and low risk of side effects have made this the preferred mode of therapy for disabling essential blepharospasm.

My preferred treatment pattern for patients with essential blepharospasm and eyelid spasm associated with Meige's syndrome is detailed in Figure 45–4 and Table 45–2. The injection over the glabellar crease denoted "a" is an important treatment point in patients with essential blepharospasm. It is vital, in patients with essential blepharospasm, to eliminate brow spasm, especially in the medial brow protractor muscles (corrugator and procerus). As much as one third of the total toxin dose may be needed at this site. The toxin administered over the pretarsal orbicularis at points "c," "d," "f," and "g" is given approximately 2 mm superior and inferior to the medial or lateral canthus. It is important to avoid injecting high

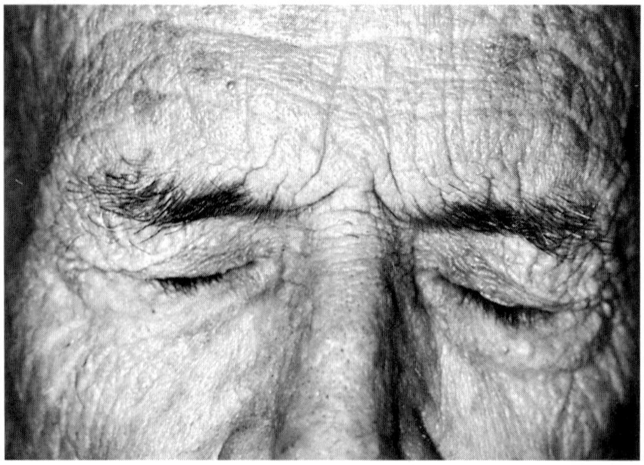

Figure 45–2. Patient with disabling essential blepharospasm before botulinum therapy.

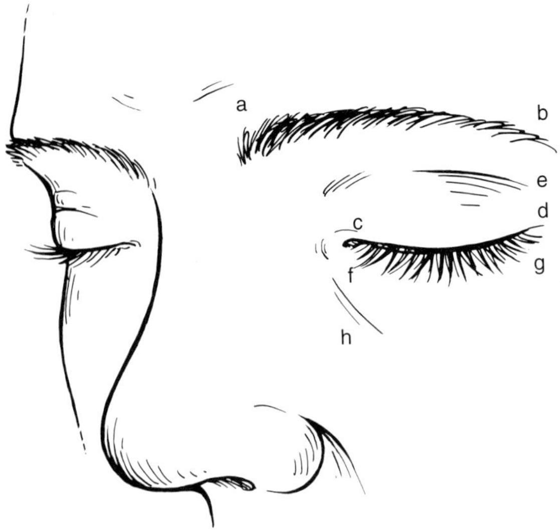

Figure 45–4. Typical injection points used in the treatment of essential blepharospasm and hemifacial spasm (see text for details).

doses of toxin at single points in the upper eyelid or over the central upper or lower eyelid to prevent ptosis or diplopia due to paralysis of the levator muscle or inferior oblique muscle. Spreading the toxin dose over multiple adjacent sites (as in "b," "d," and "e") appears to decrease the risk of ptosis. Toxin injections given over the pretarsal or preseptal orbicularis are given immediately subcutaneously to allow initial toxin diffusion in a subcutaneous plane and minimize the deeper diffusion of toxin.

Injections at points "h" and "i" are used to dampen upper facial spasm in patients with Meige's and hemifacial spasm. At point "h," one should avoid injecting inferior to a line halfway between the ala of the nose and the medial canthus. At point "i," toxin is not usually injected inferior to the midpoint of the malar prominence and is spread out over multiple sites if more than 2.5 units is given. Small doses of toxin given into the facial muscles dampen spasms in Meige's syndrome, although great caution is needed to avoid facial paralysis.

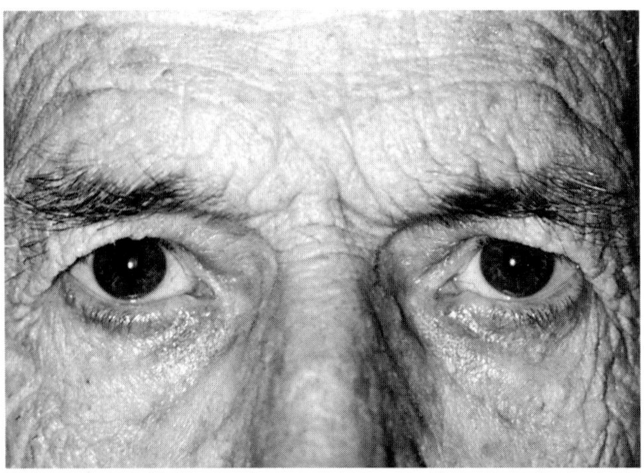

Figure 45–3. The same patient as in Figure 45–2, after botulinum injection, as detailed in Figure 45–4.

The side effects of botulinum A toxin are generally well tolerated. In a 4-year review of 1012 treatments, Dutton and Buckley[16] found a 7.5% incidence of symptomatic dry eye, a 7.3% incidence of ptosis, and less than a 1% incidence of diplopia due to inferior oblique or lateral rectus paresis. Mild exposure keratitis is frequent and can be prevented or controlled by providing patients prophylaxis with artificial tear drops four times daily and a nonmedicated ophthalmic ointment to the eyes at night for several weeks after the injections. The ptosis that may follow injection into the upper eyelids results from the diffusion of toxin into the levator palpebrae superioris. This ptosis is generally mild and improves markedly over the first month, with the toxin lasting an average of 3 months. Injections of the toxin into the lower face to control the oromandibular manifestations of Meige's syndrome must be done cautiously since facial drooping and drooling can result. A diagram is made after each treatment session to serve as a guide to future therapy.

In addition to its use in the treatment of essential blepharospasm, Meige's syndrome, and hemifacial spasm, botulinum A toxin has proved effective in the treatment of selected extraocular muscle disorders, spasmodic torticollis, and spastic dysphonia. Investigators are gaining experience in the treatment of other varied neuromuscular conditions including focal limb dystonias, vocal tremor, anismus, and urinary detrusor-sphincter dyssynergia.[17]

Surgical Therapy

The surgical treatment of blepharospasm has evolved from cutting a hole in the upper eyelid to variations of the current radical myectomy procedure originally described by Gillum and Anderson.[18] This procedure involves ex-

TABLE 45-2

Botulinum A (Botox) Toxin Injection Points

Injection Point*	Doses of Botulinum Typically Given		
	Essential Blepharospasm (Low Dose): 30 units total (15 U/side)	Essential Blepharospasm/ Meige's Syndrome (High Dose): 70 units total (35 U/side)	Hemifacial Spasm: 12.5 U total unilateral
a	5	7.5	0
b	0	2.5	0
c	2.5	5	2.5
d	2.5	5	2.5
e	0	2.5	0
f	2.5	2.5	2.5
g	2.5	5	2.5
h	0	2.5	0–2.5
i	0	2.5	0–2.5

*See Figure 45–4 for illustration of injection points.

tirpating the squeezing muscles around the eyelids (Fig. 45–5) and is the preferred treatment for functionally disabling essential blepharospasm resistant to other forms of therapy. It is possible at surgery to repair coexisting defects including brow ptosis, blepharoptosis, and lateral canthal laxity. It is vital in this surgery to perform a meticulous excision of the corrugator superciliaris, procerus, and orbicularis (Fig. 45–6). Good functional results can be obtained in approximately 80% of patients undergoing myectomy surgery.[19] The excellent results obtained with botulinum toxin injections have decreased the role of myectomy surgery in managing essential blepharospasm, although this treatment remains an option for selected patients.

Limited upper eyelid myectomy surgery has a role in the treatment of patients who respond well to botulinum toxin but have coexistent defects such as brow ptosis, blepharoptosis, or marked dermatochalasis with overhanging skin. Significant excision of orbicularis can be performed through an upper eyelid crease incision during upper blepharoplasty and ptosis repair with only a minimal increase in operative morbidity. This limited upper myectomy procedure is not recommended in patients in whom botulinum therapy may have failed, since these patients generally require a full radical myectomy procedure with aggressive extirpation of the orbicularis, corrugator superciliaris, and procerus muscles (see Figs. 45–5 and 45–6). Functional improvement is gained and the interval between botulinum injections extended in selected patients after limited upper myectomy surgery.

Future Directions

Wirtschafter,[20] in animal and human experiments, has demonstrated doxorubicin as a muscle-selective destructive agent in the eyelid. This approach cannot yet be considered clinically applicable, since Wirtschafter noted that the long-term safety and efficacy of the treatment are unproven. Complications of doxorubicin therapy have

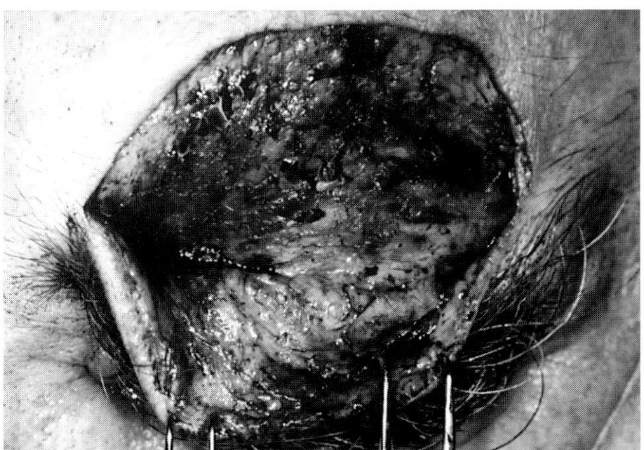

Figure 45–5. Surgical view through brow incisions at the time of surgical myectomy. The patient had disabling essential blepharospasm and had failed to respond adequately to botulinum injection. This patient had undergone three earlier surgical myectomy procedures.

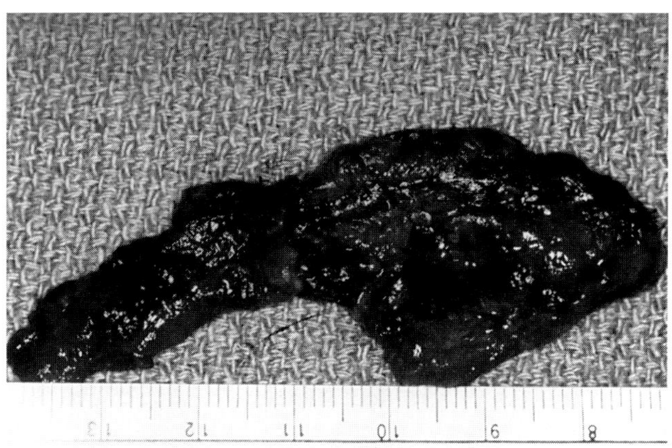

Figure 45–6. Orbicularis muscle specimen removed at the procedure shown in Figure 45–5, illustrating the inadequacy of earlier surgical myectomies.

included skin ulceration with scarring and ectropion, pain, and persistent edema. The degree of functional improvement in patients treated with experimental doxorubicin injection is debatable since these patients continued to require adjunctive botulinum therapy despite multiple doxorubicin treatment sessions.

The rate of sustained improvement in eyelid spasms after botulinum A toxin therapy has been reported as high as 97%.[16] Nonetheless, the "failure" rate following botulinum A toxin therapy and the potential for the development of "resistance" to further therapy has been debated in the literature.[21] Searches for functionally significant botulinum antibodies in patients receiving botulinum toxin have generally been unrevealing,[22] although more recent studies[22a] suggest that the frequent production of antibodies is of no clinical significance. Botulinum A toxin has been shown to cause long-term changes in the anatomy of terminal motor nerves and the motor end plates.[23,24] The functional significance of these changes remains unknown at this time. The toxin is distributed systemically,[25] causing jitter on single-fiber electromyographic recordings at sites distant to the point of injection. THe significance of this spread remains uncertain. The F serotype of botulinum toxin is being investigated as an alternative agent in patients who fail botulinum A therapy.

Patients with essential blepharospasm and Meige's syndrome frequently encounter misunderstanding of their condition. Inappropriate therapies are recommended despite recognition of focal dystonias as organic neurologic diseases and the availability of effective treatments. Continuing physician and public education is required to provide optimal treatment to people with these chronic, disabling conditions. Current approaches to therapy focus on treating the terminal manifestation of a dystonic spasm that appears to have a subcortical origin. It is hoped that continued research into the causative factors and organic basis of these conditions will yield treatments more specifically focused at the originating factors.

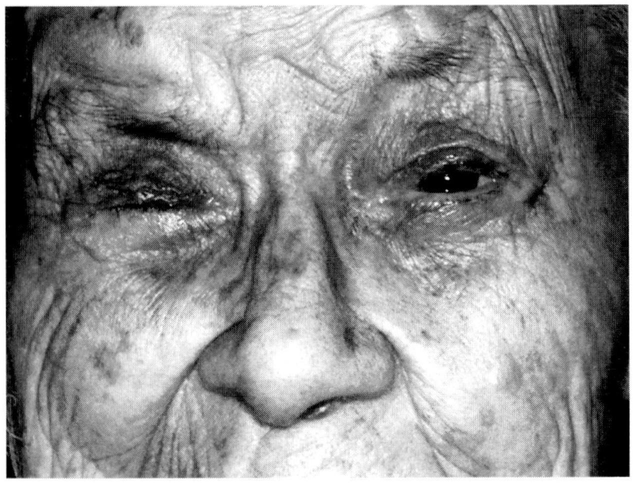

Figure 45–7. A patient with hemifacial spasm showing marked degree of contracture of her right hemiface. She had intermittent high-frequency twitches of her right face.

HEMIFACIAL SPASM

Clinical Features

Hemifacial spasm was described by Schultze in 1875 and elaborated on by Gowers.[26] This condition is characterized by involuntary paroxysmal bursts of tonic or clonic contraction of muscles innervated by the facial nerve. The average age at onset (45 years) and the female-to-male preponderance are less (3:2) than in the facial dystonias (see Table 45–1).[26] The condition typically begins with an intermittent twitching of one eyelid that progresses over months to years to involve other areas of ipsilateral facial nerve innervation (Fig. 45–7). Tension and fatigue are aggravating factors in many patients, although the spasm may occur during sleep. Associated findings include facial weakness, ipsilateral hearing loss, and, occasionally, vertigo.

The clinical examination alone usually separates hemifacial spasm from other unilateral squeezing disorders. Electromyography of the facial muscles and blink reflex testing distinguish hemifacial spasm from other conditions with a similar appearance (see Table 45–1), although a clinical diagnosis can generally be made. Conditions with an appearance similar to hemifacial spasm include facial synkinesis and hemifacial contracture in which a mass movement of the facial muscles results from aberrant nerve regeneration after a facial palsy (see Table 45–1). Transient myokymia is a frequent condition characterized by a rapid undulation or flickering contraction of individual fascicles of facial muscle. Myokymia usually follows stress or sleep deprivation, often in association with excessive alcohol or caffeine ingestion. Time and evolution of symptoms clearly distinguish the two conditions. A different and rare movement disorder termed *facial myokymia* is characterized by vermiform facial movements with progression and may be associated with multiple sclerosis or brain stem glioma. Hemifacial spasm may closely resemble benign transient eyelid myokymia very early in its course.

Etiology

Hemifacial spasm is thought to result from cross-compression of the facial nerve, generally by an anomalous vessel at the root entry zone of the nerve into the brain stem.[3] This pulsating compression damages the facial nerve, resulting in aberrant depolarization. A variety of theories have been proposed to explain the phenomenonology of hemifacial spasm and response to therapy.

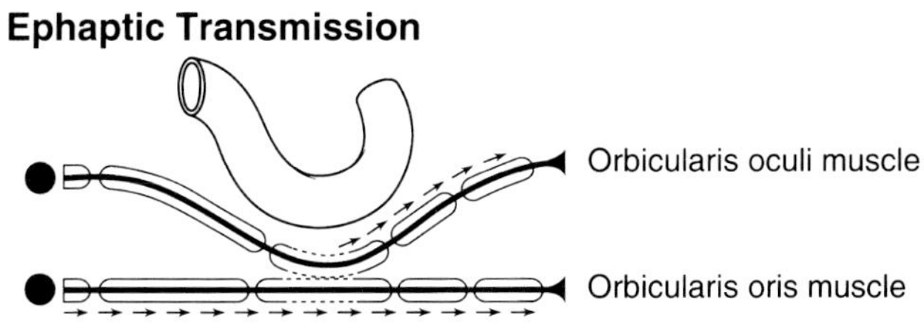

Figure 45-8. Ephaptic transmission, or "cross-talk," mechanism by which vascular compression damages axons that directly stimulate adjacent axons. The facial nucleus is to the left. (Adapted from the Archives of Neurology 1966, 14:149-156. Copyright 1966, American Medical Association.)

Ephaptic transmission or "cross-talk," popularized by Gardner,[27] postulates that damage to the axonal myelin sheath allows direct depolarization of adjacent axons (Fig. 45-8). Möller and Janetta have supported a "kindling" theory that proposes repeated antidromic (retrograde) stimulation of the motor neurons from the peripheral vascular cross-compression, resulting in altered excitability of motor neurons within the facial nucleus (Fig. 45-9).[28] Recent electrophysiologic observations suggest the interconnection of axons by unidirectional and bidirectional ephapses with self-sustained, repetitive axonal excitation occurring from both the site of cross-compression and within the motor nucleus.[29]

Surgeons report up to a 92% incidence of surgically demonstrable vascular cross-compression as the cause of hemifacial spasm,[3] with the anterior inferior cerebellar artery implicated in 34%, the posterior inferior cerebellar artery in 18%, and the acoustic or internal auditory artery in 7%. Arterial contact with the facial nerve in the root exit zone is found in 69% of autopsy brains in the absence of hemifacial spasm,[30] usually from the anterior inferior cerebellar artery or one of its branches. Many other lesions occasionally cause hemifacial spasm, including arteriovenous malformations, cholesteatoma, meningioma, and brain stem glioma. A compilation of several reports suggests that mass lesions that cause progressive systemic morbidity cause less than 1% of cases of hemifacial spasm.[26] A contrast CT scan or MRI scan has been recommended in the routine evaluation of patients with hemifacial spasm[26] because of the frequent radiologic finding of dolichoectasia of the vertebrobasilar system and this occasional association of hemifacial spasm with brain tumors. Sprik and Wirtschafter[30a] and others[5] noted the low incidence of unsuspected diagnostically significant intracranial mass lesions detected by routine neuroimaging and recommended neuroimaging only in patients with atypical clinical features.

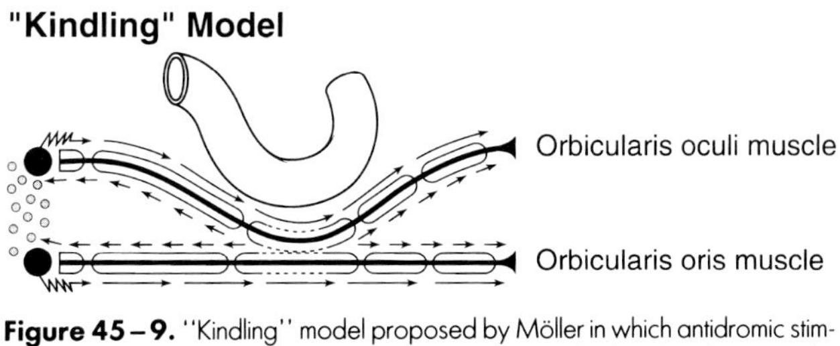

Figure 45-9. "Kindling" model proposed by Möller in which antidromic stimulation increases the excitability of the facial nucleus. The facial nucleus is to the left. (Adapted from Digre K, Corbett JJ: Hemifacial spasm: Differential diagnosis, mechanism, and treatment. *In* Jankovic J, Tolosa E [ed]: Advanced in Neurology, vol. 49: Facial Dyskinesias. New York, Raven Press, 1988, p 166.)

Pharmacotherapy

Anticonvulsants with membrane-stabilizing activities have been used in the treatment of hemifacial spasm by decreasing the excitability of the damaged facial nerve or hyperactive facial nucleus. Anticonvulsants such as phenytoin and carbamazepine[31] may occasionally control hemifacial spasm, although fewer than a fourth of patients benefit significantly from these therapies. The short-acting benzodiazepines and weak anticholinergics[32] recommended in the treatment of essential blepharospasm are sometimes effective in suppressing the facial spasm associated with mild hemifacial spasm not warranting more invasive therapy.

Botulinum A Toxin (Botox)

As in essential blepharospasm, the paralytic properties of botulinum A toxin have been exploited in treating the unilateral squeezing associated with hemifacial spasm. Excellent results have been noted in treating the periorbital manifestations of hemifacial spasm with botulinum A toxin, and few complications have been reported. Again, caution is urged in treating the lower facial involvement since a temporary lower facial palsy may be disconcerting to the patient. The response to botulinum A toxin injection is typically even better in hemifacial spasm than in essential blepharospasm, with a longer-lasting effect at lower doses. The typical doses of toxin used and injection pattern I use in the treatment of hemifacial spasm are detailed in Table 45-2 and Figure 45-4. Among the factors of importance in the treatment of hemifacial spasm is the intrinsic muscle weakness found in many patients.[33] Additional factors include the peripheral pathogenesis of hemifacial spasm and its unilaterality in contrast with essential blepharospasm. The high efficacy of botulinum A toxin in hemifacial spasm makes it nearly obligatory to try this mode of therapy before proceeding to surgery.

Surgical Treatments

Destructive procedures such as selective facial nerve avulsion have essentially been abandoned for the treatment of hemifacial spasm. The myectomy procedure, as described for essential blepharospasm, has been modified and successfully employed in the treatment of hemifacial spasm, with good functional results in 20 of 21 patients.[34] The scarring, postoperative edema, and numbness that occur after radical myectomy surgery must be considered before recommending such treatment to a patient with hemifacial spasm, given the generally excellent response to botulinum A toxin injection.

Microvascular decompression of the facial nerve by means of a submastoid craniectomy and microscopic manipulation of the vessels surrounding the facial nerve at its root entry zone in the cerebellopontine angle (Janetta procedure) is an effective treatment for hemifacial spasm. In a review of 433 patients,[3] 364 (84%) patients with hemifacial spasm were reported "cured" with one operation. Permanent complications, most often deafness or facial paralysis, were encountered in 70 (16%) patients. Early and late recurrences are possible, although intraoperative facial nerve monitoring may help ensure a successful decompression procedure.[35] Microvascular decompression provides a chance for permanent cure in patients with severe hemifacial spasm in whom other modes of therapy have failed and who are willing to risk neurosurgical complications.

SUMMARY

A number of facial movement disorders or dyskinesias may cause visual disability and are of interest to the ophthalmologist. Hemifacial spasm is a unilateral spasmodic contraction of muscles innervated by one facial nerve, usually beginning in the third and fourth decades. The craniocervical dystonias are a group of disorders, including essential blepharospasm, Meige's syndrome, and spasmodic torticollis, characterized by uncontrollable squeezing movements in the face and neck. Essential blepharospasm involves a waxing-and-waning progressive spasm of the orbicularis oculi. Patients typically present in their fifth or sixth decades with a variety of complaints and an otherwise unremarkable eye examination. In both essential blepharospasm and hemifacial spasm, symptoms are worse under stress, often leading to the misdiagnosis of a psychogenic disorder. Social embarrassment and functional deficits may lead to depression and reclusiveness. It is important to recognize, appropriately diagnose, and recommend appropriate therapy. Fortunately, most patients can be functionally and socially rehabilitated.

Botulinum A toxin injection is the primary mode of therapy for most patients with essential blepharospasm or hemifacial spasm. Three or more months of relief from eyelid spasm can be obtained by the direct injection of this neuromuscular toxin. Pharmacotherapy with benzodiazepines, anticholinergics, or other agents is a useful adjunctive treatment for many patients with essential blepharospasm, Meige's syndrome, and hemifacial spasm. Surgical therapy with radical myectomy for essential blepharospasm or microvascular decompression of the facial nerve (Janetta procedure) in hemifacial spasm is effective in treating patients whose eyelid or facial spasm cannot be adequately relieved with botulinum A toxin injection or pharmacotherapy. With a combination of these treatments, most patients with essential blepharospasm, Meige's syndrome, and hemifacial spasm can be functionally rehabilitated.

REFERENCES

1. Jankovic J: Cranial-cervical dyskinesias: An overview. *In* Jankovic J, Tolosa E (eds): Advances in Neurology, Vol 49, Facial Dyskinesias. New York, Raven Press, 1988, pp 2–13.
2. Patrinely JP, Anderson RL: Essential blepharospasm: A review. Geriatr Ophthalmol 2(4):27–33, 1986.
3. Loeser JD, Chen J: Hemifacial spasm: Treatment by microsurgical facial nerve decompression. Neurosurgery 13:141–146, 1983.
4. Jankovic J: Etiology and differential diagnosis of blepharospasm and oromandibular dystonia. *In* Jankovic J, Tolosa E (eds): Advances in Neurology, Vol 49, Facial Dyskinesias. New York, Raven Press, 1988, pp 103–116.
5. Holds JB, White GL, Thiese SM, Anderson RL: Facial dystonia, essential blepharospasm and hemifacial spasm. Am Fam Physician 43:2113–2120, 1991.
6. Holds JB, Anderson RL, Jordan DR: Essential blepharospasm: A patient survey. Presented before the 26th International Congress of Ophthalmology (abstracts, p 124). Singapore, March 17, 1990.
7. Bihari K, Pigott TA, Hill JL, Murphy DL: Blepharospasm and obsessive-compulsive disorder. J Nerv Ment Dis 180:130–132, 1992.
8. Jankovic J, Patel SC: Blepharospasm associated with brainstem lesions. Neurology 33:1237–1240, 1983.
9. Creel DJ, Holds JB, Anderson RL: Auditory brain-stem responses in blepharospasm. Electroencephalogr Clin Neurophysiol 86: 138–140, 1993.
10. Lueck CJ, Tanyeri S, Crawford TJ, et al: Saccadic eye movements in essential blepharospasm. J Neurol 237:226–229, 1990.
11. Hotson JR, Boman DR: Memory-contingent saccades and the substantia nigra postulate for essential blepharospasm. Brain 114:295–307, 1991.
12. Demer JL, Holds JB, Hovis LA: Ocular movements in essential blepharospasm. Am J Ophthalmol 110:674–682, 1990.
13. Meige H: Les convulsions de la face, une forme clinique de convulsion faciale, bilateral et mediane. Rev Neurol (Paris) 21:437–443, 1910.
14. Fasanella RM, Aghajanian GK: Treatment of benign essential blepharospasm with cyproheptadine. N Engl J Med 322:778, 1990.
15. Frueh BR, Felt DP, Wojno TH, Musch DC: Treatment of blepharospasm with botulinum toxin: A preliminary report. Arch Ophthalmol 102:1464–1468, 1984.
16. Dutton JJ, Buckley EG: Long-term results and complications of botulinum A toxin in the treatment of blepharospasm. Ophthalmology 95:1529–1534, 1988.
17. NIH Consensus Development Conference: Consensus Statement, vol 8, no. 8. U.S. Department of Health and Human Services, Public Health Service, National Institutes of Health, Bethesda, MD, 1990, pp 1–20.
18. Gillum WM, Anderson RL: Blepharospasm surgery: An anatomic approach. Arch Ophthalmol 99:1056–1062, 1981.
19. Anderson RL, Patrinely JR: Surgical management of blepharospasm. *In* Jankovic J, Tolosa E (eds): Advances in Neurology, Vol 49, Facial Dyskinesias. New York, Raven Press, 1988, pp 501–520.
20. Wirtschafter JD: Clinical doxorubicin chemomyectomy: An experimental treatment for benign essential blepharospasm and hemifacial spasm. Ophthalmology 98:357–366, 1991.
21. Holds JB, Fogg SG, Anderson RL: Botulinum A toxin injection: Failures in clinical practice and a biomechanical system for the study of toxin-induced paralysis. Ophthal Plast Reconstr Surg 6:252–259, 1990.

22. Biglan AW, Gonnering R, Lockhart LB, et al: Absence of antibody production in patients treated with botulinum A toxin. Am J Ophthalmol 101:232–235, 1986.
22a. Siatkowski RM, Tyntyunikov A, Biglan AW, et al: Serum antibody production to botulinum A toxin. Ophthalmology 100:1861–1866, 1993.
23. Holds, JB, Alderson K, Fogg SG, Anderson RL: Motor nerve sprouting in human orbicularis muscle following botulinum A injection. Invest Ophthalmol Vis Sci 31:964–967, 1990.
24. Alderson K, Holds JB, Anderson RL: Botulinum-induced alterations of nerve–muscle interactions in the human orbicularis oculi following treatment for blepharospasm. Neurology 41:1800–1805, 1991.
25. Sanders DB, Massey EW, Buckley EG: Botulinum toxin for blepharospasm: Single-fiber EMG studies. Neurology 36:545–547, 1986.
26. Digre K, Corbett JJ: Hemifacial spasm: Differential diagnosis, mechanism, and treatment. *In* Jankovic J, Tolosa E (eds): Advances in Neurology, Vol 49, Facial Dyskinesias. New York, Raven Press, 1988, pp 151–167.
27. Gardner WJ: Cross talk—the paradoxical transmission of a nerve impulse. Arch Neurol 14:149–156, 1966.
28. Möller AR, Janetta PJ: On the origin of synkinesis in hemifacial spasm: Results of intracranial recording. J Neurosurg 61:569–576, 1984.
29. Roth G, Magistris MR, Pinelli P, Rilliet B: Cryptogenic hemifacial spasm: A neurophysiological study. Electromyogr Clin Neurophysiol 30:361–370, 1990.
30. Matsushima T, Inoue T, Fukui M: Arteries in contact with the cisternal portion of the facial nerve in autopsy cases: Microsurgical anatomy for neurovascular decompression surgery of hemifacial spasm. Surg Neurol 34:87–93, 1990.
30a. Sprik C, Wirtschafter JD: Hemifacial spasm due to intracranial tumor: An international survey of botulinum toxin investigators. Ophthalmology 95:1042–1045, 1988.
31. Alexander GE, Moses H: Carbamazepine for hemifacial spasm. Neurology 32:286–287, 1982.
32. Hughes EC, Brackmann DE, Weinstein RC: Seventh nerve spasm: Effect of modification of cholinergic balance. Otolaryngol Head Neck Surg 88:491–499, 1980.
33. Frueh BR, Preston RA, Musch DC: Facial nerve injury and hemifacial spasm. Am J Ophthalmol 110:421–423, 1990.
34. Garland PE, Patrinely JR, Anderson RL: Hemifacial spasm: Results of unilateral myectomy. Ophthalmology 94:288–294, 1987.
35. Haines SJ, Torres FR: Intraoperative monitoring of the facial nerve during decompressive surgery for hemifacial spasm. J Neurosurg 74:254–257, 1991.

CHAPTER 46

The Eyelids in Graves' Ophthalmopathy

George B. Bartley

Eyelid malpositions, including retraction, ptosis, entropion, and lateral canthal obliquity, frequently cause functional impairment in patients with Graves' ophthalmopathy. Additionally, dermatochalasis, eyelid swelling, and lacrimal gland prolapse may be exacerbated by the orbital inflammation that accompanies the disorder and may result in cosmetic disfigurement. In this chapter I outline the clinical features of eyelid abnormalities associated with thyroid disease, review briefly the historical development of Graves' eyelid surgery, and describe the operative techniques I currently favor.

CLINICAL FEATURES

Eyelid retraction is the most common clinical sign of dysthyroid ophthalmopathy (Fig. 46–1*A*).[1, 2] Waller[3] proposed that upper lid retraction be graded as mild (1 to 2 mm), moderate (2 to 5 mm), or severe (more than 5 mm). Whereas mild and severe degrees of retraction tend to be relatively stable over time, moderate retraction tends to show much greater variability, often even from minute to minute.

If possible, it is preferable to determine the approximate eyelid level when the patient is not aware that a measurement is being made. Fairly accurate estimates of retraction may be made by carefully observing the patient's eyelid positions during casual conversation at the beginning of the examination. One should note the distance between the eyelid margin and the superior corneoscleral limbus and then add 1.5 mm to calculate the total amount of retraction, because most upper eyelids in adults rest 1 to 2 mm below the 12 o'clock limbus. Frequently, the lid fissures change (usually becoming more narrow) to some degree when a ruler is placed near the eyes or when photographs are taken; the patient may have become accustomed to "squinting" slightly to achieve a more normal appearance when he or she is aware that the eyes are being scrutinized.

Lower eyelid retraction may be categorized as mild (1 to 2 mm), moderate (3 mm), or severe (more than 3 mm). The lower lid normally rests approximately at the inferior corneoscleral limbus, and its position is less likely to vacillate than is the upper lid.

The pathophysiologic mechanisms that contribute to eyelid retraction may include adnexal fibrosis, contracture and scarring of the levator or lower eyelid retractors, abnormal sympathetic tone, proptosis, or overmedication with thyroid replacement hormone.[3] Additionally, contracture of the inferior rectus muscle may indirectly augment upper lid retraction as the ipsilateral superior rectus muscle "overcontracts" in an attempt to elevate the globe to the primary position; the levator is activated as well, and the eyelid elevates abnormally (Fig. 46–2). Likewise, the lower eyelid may retract in response to contracture of the ipsilateral superior rectus muscle. Lower eyelid retraction is a fairly frequent side effect of recession of the ipsilateral inferior rectus muscle, if the capsulopalpebral head of the lower eyelid retractors is simultaneously positioned posteriorly. Kushner[4] described a technique to reduce this complication of strabismus surgery.

Small[5, 6] postulated that enlargement of the levator muscle fibers contributes to upper eyelid retraction. Frueh,[7] however, found the evidence unconvincing, as did Feldon and Levin.[8] The latter authors believed that adherence of the levator to adjacent fixed orbital connective tissue and fat is the most plausible explanation for eyelid retraction and lid lag, as proposed by Grove.[9]

Lid lag and lagophthalmos are helpful diagnostic features of Graves' ophthalmopathy, but the terms are often used incorrectly. Harvey and Anderson[10] defined *lid lag* as a static sign in which an eyelid is higher or more retracted than normal when the globe is in downward gaze (see Fig. 46–1*B*). Von Graefe's sign, in contrast, describes the delayed descent of an eyelid as it follows the globe from primary gaze to downward gaze. *Lagophthalmos* refers to incomplete closure of the eyelids.

Although some patients are able functionally to tolerate lid retraction, lid lag, von Graefe's sign, and lagophthalmos, the eyelid malpositions frequently result in corneal exposure or alterations in the tear film, with the sequelae of ocular discomfort, photophobia, visual blur, superficial punctate keratopathy, or even corneal ulceration in severe cases. Globe subluxation is an uncommon

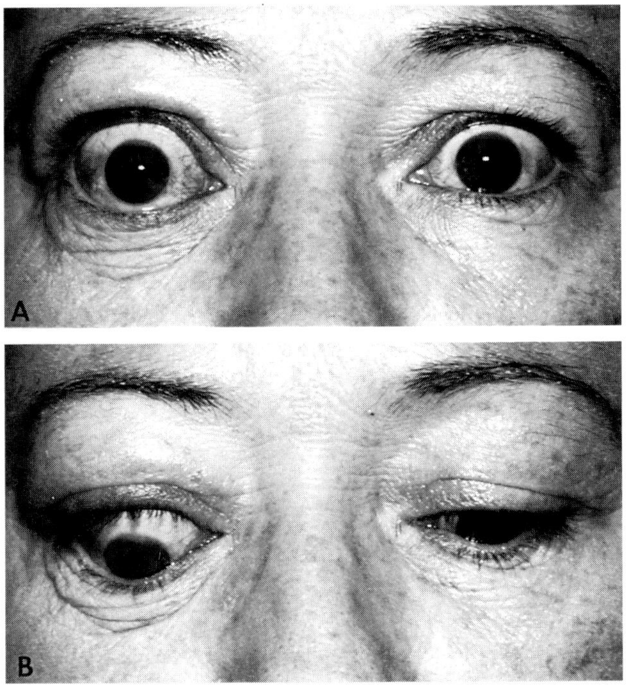

Figure 46–1. *A*, Severe retraction of the right upper eyelid, moderate retraction of the left upper eyelid, and mild retraction of the right lower eyelid. *B*, Lid lag of the right upper eyelid.

but dramatic complication of eyelid retraction, and it is most likely to occur when prominent exophthalmos is also present (Fig. 46–3). Prompt orbital decompression, with or without eyelid surgery, may be required if the lids cannot be repositioned manually.[11]

Other eyelid malpositions that may accompany Graves' ophthalmopathy include ptosis, entropion, and lateral canthal obliquity. Blepharoptosis in a patient with Graves' disease should lead the examiner to consider coexistent myasthenia gravis and to pursue the appropriate diagnostic evaluations (Fig. 46–4). In other patients, ptosis may result from weakness of the levator aponeurosis, either iatrogenically as a complication of eyelid retraction repair or secondary to lid swelling that may accompany the inflammatory phases of dysthyroid disease.[12] Waller[3] noted that blepharoptosis may be a temporary sequela of transantral orbital decompression or, rarely, may alternate rhythmically and idiopathically with eyelid retraction. Pseudoretraction of the eyelid of a nondominant eye may result from ptosis of the contralateral eyelid of the dominant eye because of Hering's law of equal innervation.[13–15]

Medial lower eyelid entropion (Fig. 46–5) and lateral canthal obliquity (Fig. 46–6) may result from decompression of the medial and inferior orbital walls, particularly when the operation is performed through the transantral route.[3, 16] Entropion presumably results from vertical traction between the medial lower lid retractors and the orbital tissues that prolapse inferomedially into the maxillary and ethmoidal sinuses. Lateral canthal obliquity, in which the lateral canthus appears to be abnormally high in relation to the medial canthus and globe, results from the posterior and inferomedial movement of the eye after orbital decompression into the maxillary and ethmoidal sinuses.[3] Goldberg and colleagues[17] advocated the retention of a bony strut at the maxillary-ethmoidal junction to prevent this complication.

Dermatochalasis, eyelid swelling, and lacrimal gland prolapse may result from or be worsened by orbital inflammation accompanying Graves' disease (Fig. 46–7). Although these clinical features usually cause more aesthetic concern than functional disease, they nevertheless

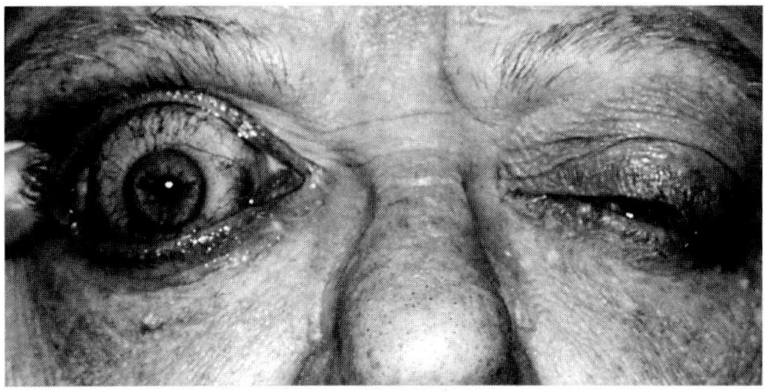

Figure 46–3. This patient with Graves' ophthalmopathy is demonstrating that her right eye subluxates anterior to the eyelids when mild pressure is applied to the right upper lid.

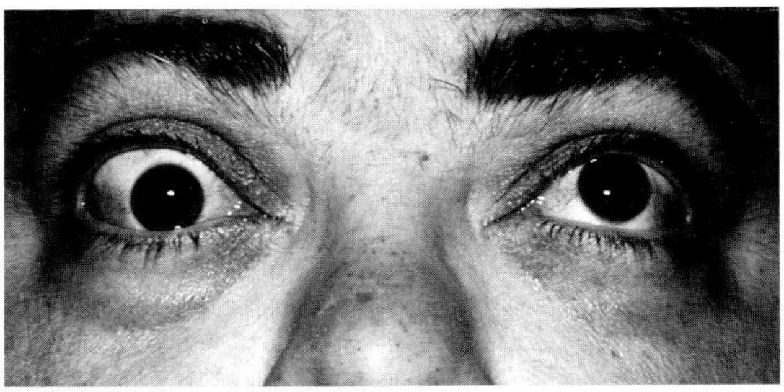

Figure 46–2. Because the right inferior rectus muscle is tight, right upper eyelid retraction is worsened when the patient attempts to look up.

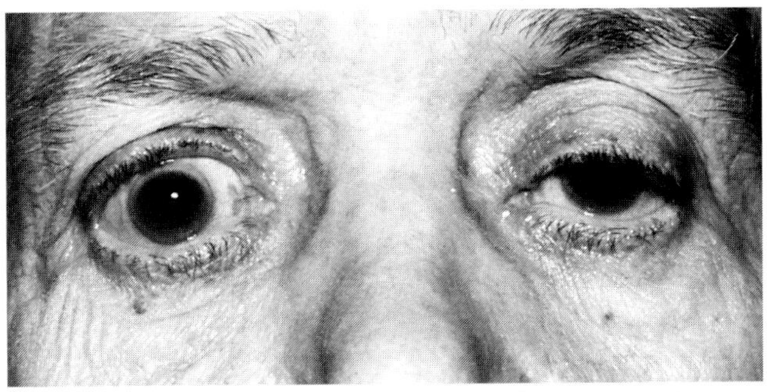

Figure 46–4. Concomitant eyelid retraction and blepharoptosis in a patient with Graves' disease; these findings should prompt the examiner to search for coexistent myasthenia gravis.

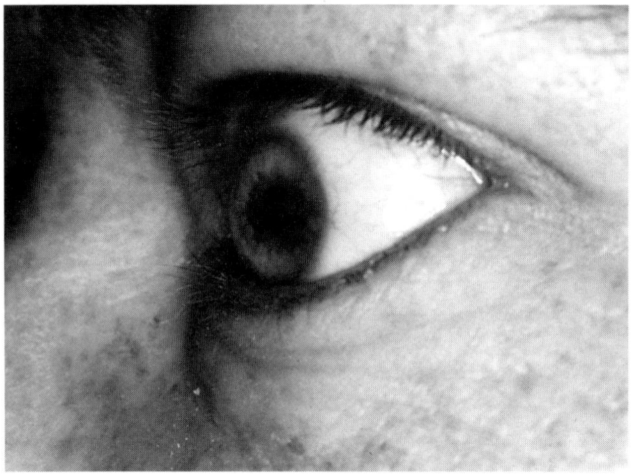

Figure 46–5. Entropion of the medial portion of the lower eyelid after transantral orbital decompression.

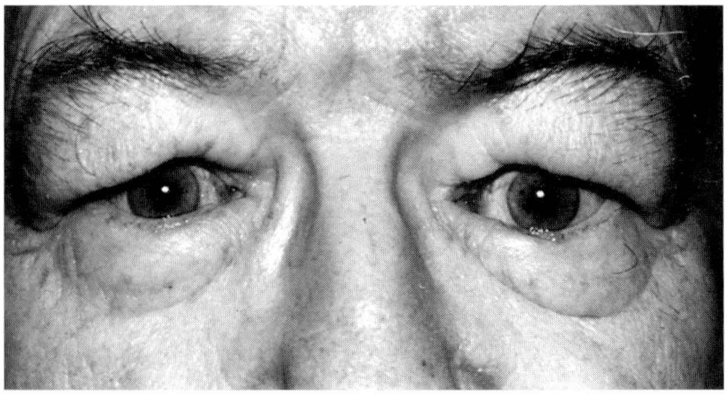

Figure 46–7. Bilateral upper eyelid dermatochalasis, edema, and lacrimal gland prolapse may mask underlying eyelid retraction.

contribute to the debilitation of patients afflicted with dysthyroid ophthalmopathy and warrant repair.

HISTORICAL BACKGROUND

Several topical sympatholytic drugs, including guanethidine, bethanidine, propranolol, and thymoxamine, diminish eyelid retraction, but long-term use has not been practical because of unacceptable side effects.[18–23] The mainstay of therapy for eyelid retraction, therefore, remains surgical. For many years the most common operation to reduce the eyelid fissure was to approximate portions of the lid margins with a blepharorrhaphy or tarsorrhaphy.[24] Although several procedures had been described that addressed the primary underlying problem, namely, functional overaction of the levator palpebrae superioris, Müller's muscle, or both, most ophthalmologists were unaware of these options until interest was revived by Henderson[25] in 1965. The operations outlined below do not represent an exhaustive survey of all reported approaches to Graves' eyelid surgery that preceded and followed Henderson's milestone, but rather they highlight some of the more notable advances and modifications in the evolution of the procedures.

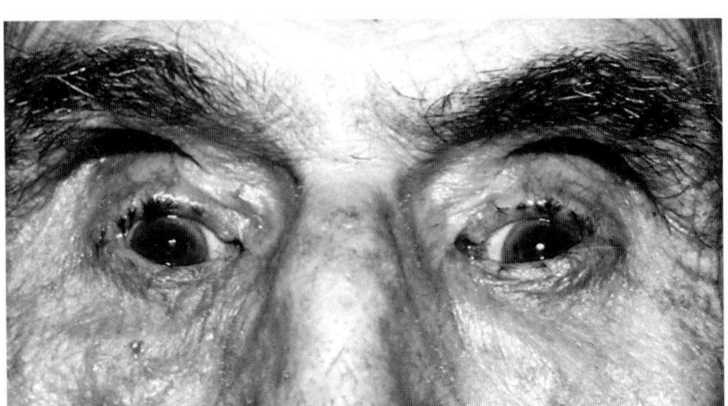

Figure 46–6. Lateral canthal obliquity secondary to hypoglobus and global recession after transantral orbital decompression.

Credit has been given to de Blaskovics for describing a relatively simple method of lowering a retracted eyelid by releasing the levator from its tarsal attachments through a conjunctival incision.[26] A review of the original cited report,[27] however, finds that de Blaskovics treated two patients with overcorrected ptosis operations by, in the author's words, "a more complicated procedure." First, a conjunctival incision was made. Next, through a skin incision, a 5-mm "bridgelike strip from the pretarsal fascia" was harvested and sewn with figure-eight sutures between the inferior edge of the eyelid retractors (distinction between the levator and Müller's muscle was not made) and the superior tarsal border. The sutures were tied on the skin surface and reportedly "the result was perfect."

Cusick and Sarrail[28] described an operation that also was used primarily to treat retraction resulting from an overcorrected ptosis procedure. The levator was approached through a conjunctival incision, and the muscle was isolated in a manner similar to an internal levator resection for blepharoptosis and was secured distally with three mattress sutures. After the levator was allowed to retract 1 mm for each desired millimeter of lid lowering, the sutures were passed through the tarsus and skin and tied anteriorly. The conjunctiva was then closed separately. Henderson[25] indicated that the "levator" described in these two early procedures described by de Blaskovics[27] and Cusick and Sarrail[28] actually may have been Müller's muscle.

Goldstein[29] treated eyelid retraction by a procedure performed with local anesthesia in which the conjunctiva was incised and recessed 10 mm, the superior 1 mm of "cartilage" (tarsus) was excised, and the levator was freed from "the underlying fascia" (by which presumably was meant Müller's muscle) and recessed 10 mm before being secured with mattress silk sutures to the skin surface. The conjunctiva was then closed. Goldstein noted that the operation also could be performed through a skin incision, apparently without excision of the superior tarsal edge.

Moran,[30] in 1956, described three variations that were used to treat 12 patients with upper lid retraction. The procedures were performed through a lid-crease incision with the use of local anesthesia in each instance. In the first four patients, the levator aponeurosis was divided 2 or 3 mm above the tarsal plate. Müller's muscle was incised but not divided, and the lateral horn of the levator was left intact. A pressure dressing was applied for 48 hours. Residual temporal flare was noted, so the operation was modified such that the lateral horn was released and a deliberate overcorrection was induced. The ptosis reportedly resolved in 4 to 6 weeks in every patient. A third variation was described in which the levator muscle (proximal to the aponeurosis) was incised to a depth of 80%, again with particular attention to weakening the temporal fibers.

Berke,[31] in a 1958 symposium on ptosis complications sponsored by the American Academy of Ophthalmology, described a method for lowering the upper eyelid that subsequently became known as a tarsotomy. A conjunctival incision was made through the tarsus approximately 1 mm from its superior border, and the incision was extended toward the skin until the wound gaped two or three times the amount one wanted to lower the eyelid. The conjunctiva was not closed. The lid then was placed on stretch with an intermarginal suture for 4 to 5 days. Although the procedure was presented as a method to treat overcorrected blepharoptosis, it later was adapted by others for the treatment of Graves' eyelid retraction.

Henderson[25] was the first surgeon to address Müller's muscle specifically in the repair of upper eyelid retraction. A conjunctival incision was made at the superior tarsal border, and Müller's muscle was released along the entire width of the tarsus. The procedure was helpful in treating 2 to 3 mm of retraction; if greater degrees of lid-lowering effect were desired, the dissection was carried inferiorly along the anterior face of the tarsus to release fibers of the levator aponeurosis. Tenzel[32] suggested that the levator aponeurosis could be weakened further by stretching the tissue vertically with forceps.

Schimek,[33] in 1972, found that the Berke tarsotomy method often produced undercorrections of upper eyelid retraction, leading him to advocate a block recession of levator, Müller's muscle, and conjunctiva. The tissues were approached posteriorly and were secured on a ptosis clamp before being recessed approximately 2 mm for each 1 mm of lid retraction. The exposed orbicularis posteriorly was left to be covered by conjunctival epithelialization. Immediate postoperative ptosis was expected from this procedure, but the final eyelid position in each of 12 described patients was reported to be either normal or residually retracted.

Putterman and Urist[34] described an operation for upper eyelid repair in which Müller's muscle was partially or completely excised through a conjunctival incision, coupled with partial tenotomy of the levator aponeurosis if needed. The conjunctiva was reapproximated at the conclusion of the procedure. The operation was performed with a sensory frontal nerve block to provide anesthesia without affecting eyelid motility. Postoperatively, the eyelid was stretched with a traction suture to minimize recurrent retraction. Putterman and coworkers[35-37] subsequently described modifications of the procedure: (1) using infiltrative anesthesia of 2% lidocaine with epinephrine rather than a frontal nerve block and (2) leaving Müller's muscle intact nasally, in some patients, to prevent segmental ptosis. Of 156 eyelids operated on, symmetry within 1.5 mm was achieved in 96% of cases.

Baylis and colleagues[38] advocated a recession of conjunctiva and Müller's muscle for mild (≤2 mm) amounts of eyelid retraction and an anterior recession of the levator for retraction that exceeded 2 mm. In each instance, the degree of recession was recommended to be twice the amount of lid-lowering effect desired. Additionally, placing the eyelid on stretch with a traction suture postoperatively was recommended.

Quickert and Dryden (at the 1971 meeting of the American Society of Ophthalmic Plastic and Reconstructive Surgery), Flanagan,[39] and Dryden and Soll[40] suggested that donor sclera be drafted as a spacer between the recessed eyelid retractors and the edge of the upper or lower eyelid tarsus to prevent readvancement of the levator and thus minimize the possible recurrence of retraction. A more comprehensive clinical and experimental work was subsequently presented by Flanagan.[41] In his experience, a scleral spacer measuring twice the amount of desired correction produced satisfactory results; the width of the graft should be greater temporally than nasally to counteract the greater degree of lateral eyelid retraction that is nearly always present in Graves' ophthalmopathy.

Harvey and Anderson,[42] in light of success in ptosis repair by aponeurotic adjustment, advocated an anterior approach to allow recession of the levator, division of the lateral horn of the aponeurosis, and extirpation of Müller's muscle. The advantages of the procedure included good visibility of important anatomic structures, less risk of damage to lacrimal gland ductules than with a posterior incision, and the avoidance of spacers. Results graded as good or satisfactory were achieved in 18 of 24 upper eyelid procedures. The authors recommended that operation for eyelid retraction be performed only after the patient's dysthyroid orbitopathy had been stable for 1 year.

The most common complication of the technique described by Harvey and Anderson was ptosis of the medial portion of the eyelid. Harvey and coworkers[43] subsequently described a modification of the procedure in which Müller's muscle, rather than being excised, was recessed in concert with the levator aponeurosis. Additionally, the eyelid retractors were not disinserted in the medial one fourth to one third of the eyelid. Good results were reported in 19 of 22 eyelids.

Levine and Chu[44] and Older[45] advocated maintaining the integrity of the orbital septum (unless removal of preaponeurotic fat is desired) during transcutaneous recession of the upper eyelid retractors. In an accompanying commentary of the latter article, Anderson noted that an intact orbital septum helps to prevent the eyelid crease from becoming elevated, which is particularly helpful in patients with unilateral retraction.

Waller[3] described a staged procedure comprising five options, any or all of which could be used to treat a retracted upper eyelid: (1) recession (without extirpation) of Müller's muscle and conjunctiva, (2) transection of the levator aponeurosis attachments to the anterior tarsus, (3) stretching of the aponeurosis, (4) release of the primary (subcutaneous) attachments of the levator aponeurosis, and (5) lateral tarsorrhaphy. The eyelid retractors were approached posteriorly, and the conjunctiva was not reapproximated at the conclusion of the procedure. In his extensive experience with more than 350 surgical repairs, the most effective combination of options included steps 1, 2, and 4, which resulted in an average reduction of eyelid retraction of 3.4 mm.

Bonavolontà[46] achieved an 80% success rate in treating upper eyelid retraction of 2 to 4 mm by incising the conjunctiva and Müller's muscle along the superior tarsal border, allowing the tissues to retract, teasing levator aponeurosis fibers apart if additional lid-lowering effect was needed, avoiding conjunctival closure, and applying a traction suture to the lid for 24 hours. It was his opinion that preserving Müller's muscle allows the surgeon to repair eyelid retraction "earlier without being obliged to wait for a stable hormonal condition."

A novel method of eyelid lowering, based on strabismus surgical principles, was presented by Grove[47, 48] in 1980. The levator and Müller's muscle were lengthened by myotomy incisions, coupled with dissection of the palpebral conjunctiva from the posterior surface of Müller's muscle for a distance of 15 to 20 mm from the superior tarsal border. A traction suture was applied to allow the levator to lengthen approximately one and one-half times the amount of upper lid retraction. The eyelid retractors were approached through a skin incision, which allowed adhesions between the levator and the overlying tissues to be released, if necessary.

Small[49] described a technique of upper eyelid retraction repair using adjustable 5-0 nylon "trombone sutures." The sutures were tied after the lid position was evaluated on the first postoperative day and were removed 2 weeks postoperatively. A subsequent modification of the operation involved dividing the levator proximal to Whitnall's ligament and securing the muscle with a 6-0 polypropylene suture that would allow postoperative adjustment of the eyelid level, if needed. The procedure was used in 25 eyelids of 14 patients, and it yielded postoperative eyelid symmetry within 1.5 mm in 13 patients.[5]

The surgical repair of lower eyelid retraction has not been associated with as many variations as have been described for the upper eyelid. Most surgeons have advocated a conjunctival approach to achieve maximal recession of the lower eyelid retractors. The correction of more than 2.5 mm of retraction usually requires the placement of a spacer of some sort between the edge of the recessed tissues and the inferior tarsal border.[42, 50] In addition to donor sclera, other materials that can be used as spacers include hard palate mucosa,[51, 52] polytetrafluoroethylene,[53] and cartilage. Traction sutures to stretch the lower lid superiorly for a few days nearly always are needed to counteract the effect of gravity.

SURGICAL TECHNIQUES AND COMPLICATIONS

This section describes the surgical techniques I currently favor to treat the eyelid malpositions and anatomic alterations that may result from dysthyroid disease. Additionally, complications that may be encountered are noted.

Patients who seek eyelid surgery to treat the sequelae of Graves' ophthalmopathy are often concerned about both eyelid retraction and the fullness of the eyelids that may result from dermatochalasis, orbital fat prolapse, lacrimal gland prolapse, or edema. Commonly, the patient brings photographs to the examination to demonstrate to the physician the appearance of his or her eyes before the onset of thyroid disease. The patient's request is usually straightforward and seemingly reasonable: "Can I be made to look as I did before all this started?" Unfortunately, even with excellent surgical technique and cooperative healing, an optimal surgical result in many, if not most, instances will be only an improvement of some of the eyelid abnormalities and not an absolute correction or reversal of the disease effects. Patient satisfaction with the ultimate outcome often relies considerably on realistic counseling and carefully cultivated rapport.

Upper Eyelid Retraction

In general, it is advisable to defer eyelid surgery until orbital decompression, radiation therapy, or strabismus procedures, if needed, have been completed.[12, 54, 55] Additionally, a stable endocrinologic status is preferable. When the timing for eyelid retraction repair is appropriate, the surgeon must decide whether to weaken the lid retractors through an anterior-external skin approach or through a posterior-internal conjunctival incision. Each route has advantages and disadvantages.

The external approach affords a more familiar display of anatomic structures, facilitates recession of the levator under direct visualization, and allows the surgeon concomitantly to suspend a prolapsed lacrimal gland or to excise preaponeurotic fat or prolapsed orbital fat, if desired. An anterior procedure usually requires more time than one performed transconjunctivally because of the more detailed dissection and the need to close the skin incision. The posterior or internal approach is generally a slightly quicker operation unless one elects to reapproximate the conjunctival incision after the eyelid retractors have been weakened. Disadvantages of the posterior route include a greater potential risk to the lacrimal gland ductules, the formation of pyogenic granulomas (to be discussed in greater detail later), more bleeding than the anterior approach, and the possibility of confusing tissue planes if the surgeon is inexperienced in approaching the dissection with the eyelid everted.[56]

The data reported by Waller[3] are important in helping to determine an appropriate surgical plan for treating upper eyelid retraction. Myotomy and recession of Müller's muscle (Fig. 46–8) usually lower an eyelid approximately 1.5 mm, which seems logical when one considers that Horner's syndrome, in which the effect of Müller's muscle is neutralized, commonly causes blepharoptosis of the same degree. Transection of the attachments of the levator aponeurosis to the anterior tarsal surface (Fig. 46–9) results in another 0.5 mm of lid lowering, on average. Therefore, mild upper eyelid retraction can usually be treated expeditiously with a posterior approach. In contrast to the technique described by Waller, I usually excise Müller's muscle (Fig. 46–10), rather than simply recess it, with hopes of reducing some of the minute-to-minute variability in eyelid position that perhaps is due to sympathetic innervation.

Waller showed that the greatest degrees of eyelid lowering are achieved by releasing the primary attachments of the levator to the subcutaneous tissues, and relief of eyelid retraction more than 2 mm usually requires this step in some form. The surgeon should release the primary attachments deliberately and incrementally, because considerable lid lowering may result from apparently minimal dissection. The levator slips may be divided equally well through either a posterior (Fig. 46–11) or an anterior (Fig. 46–12) approach, and the released tissue does not necessarily need to be sutured in its recessed position.

I prefer an external incision for severe retraction or in patients who have had previous operation. If lacrimal gland suspension or debulking of fat is desired, then an external route naturally is preferred. I agree, however, with Harvey and associates[43] that the excision of redundant skin at the same time as the correction of eyelid retraction probably should be avoided. The situation is similar to the myectomy procedure for essential blepharospasm: although preoperatively and intraoperatively it may seem that excess skin can be removed safely, the superficial tissues seem to contract postoperatively and

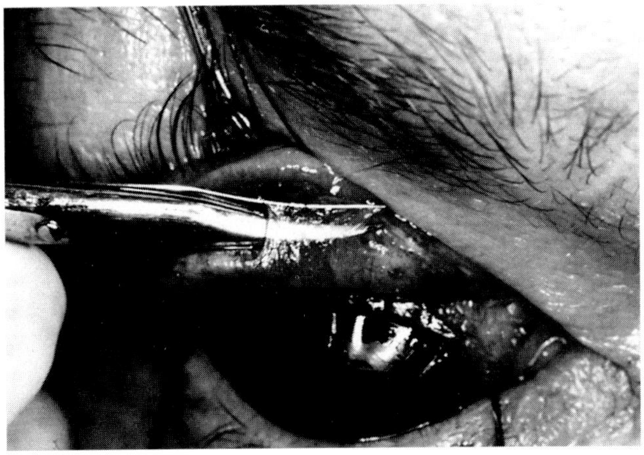

Figure 46–9. Releasing the attachments of the levator aponeurosis to the anterior surface of the tarsus lowers the eyelid approximately 0.5 mm.

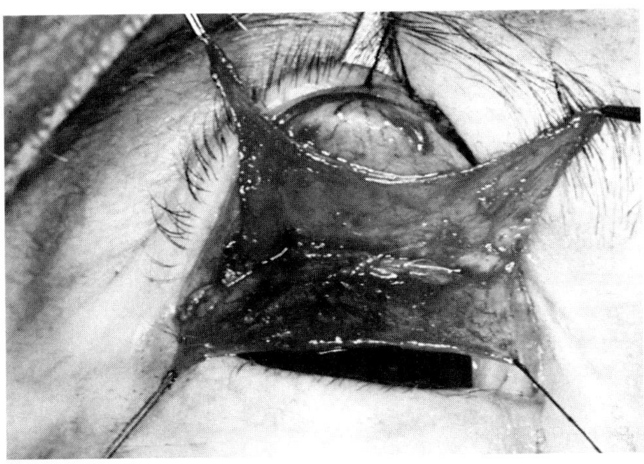

Figure 46–8. Through a conjunctival incision along the superior tarsal border, Müller's muscle has been dissected free from the underlying conjunctiva and the overlying levator aponeurosis. The sympathetic muscle may be either recessed or excised, depending on the preference of the surgeon.

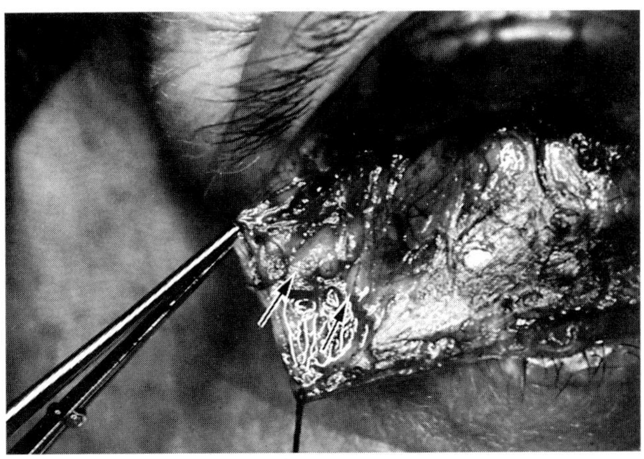

Figure 46–10. When Müller's muscle has been excised, as in this patient, care must be taken to avoid disturbing the lacrimal glands (arrows).

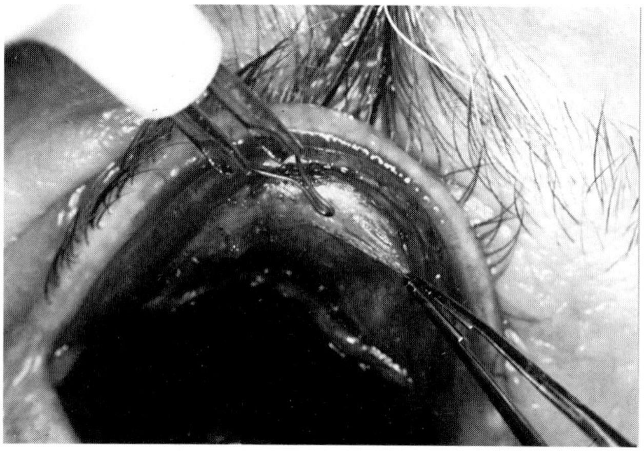

Figure 46–11. The primary attachments of the levator should be released slowly and incrementally, because large amounts of lid lowering may be achieved in some instances with minimal dissection. A thermal cautery is a useful dissection tool.

lagophthalmos may result. Additionally, patients with Graves' ophthalmopathy who initially request correction of both lid retraction and lid fullness are often sufficiently satisfied with the eyelid appearance after lid lowering alone that subsequent blepharoplasty is unnecessary. This result may be due to the increased postoperative visibility of the eyelid crease and the pretarsal portion of the eyelid, which are obscured when the lid is retracted but which "unfold" when the eyelid is restored to a more normal position (Fig. 46–13).

Lower Eyelid Retraction

Mild degrees of lower lid retraction may be corrected by making a conjunctival incision at the inferior tarsal border and maximally recessing the lower eyelid retractors into the inferior fornix (Fig. 46–14). If possible, the eyelid should be placed on stretch for at least 3 days. Although spacers are rarely needed in the repair of upper lid

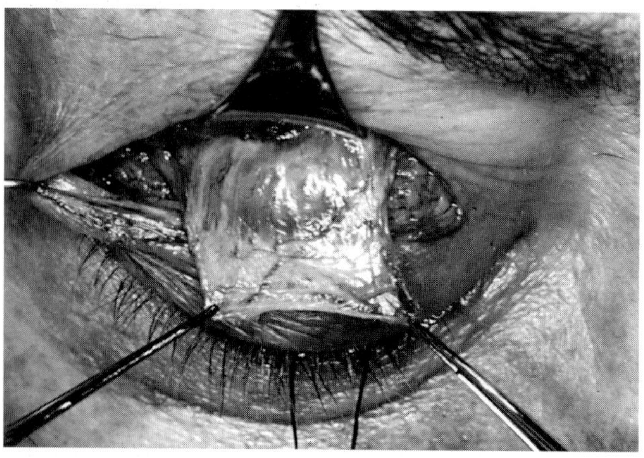

Figure 46–12. Complete disinsertion of the levator attachments and release of the lateral horn in a patient with severe retraction.

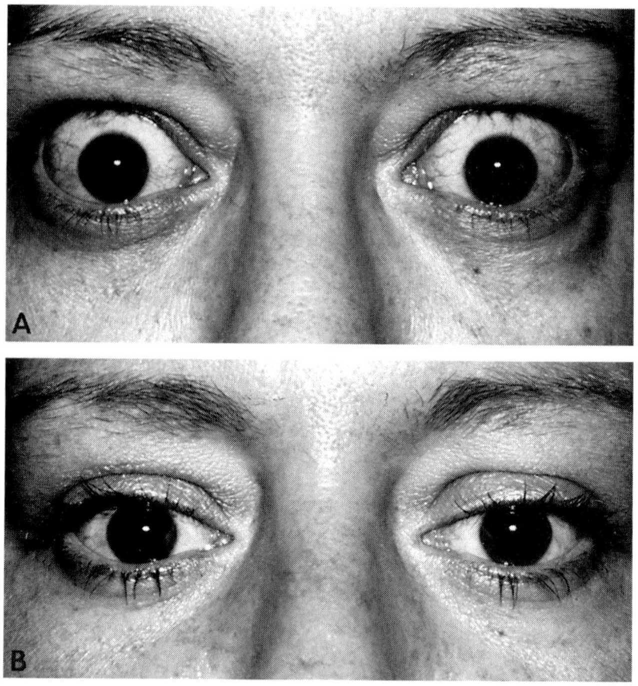

Figure 46–13. *A*, This patient wanted upper eyelid surgery to correct both retraction and eyelid fullness. *B*, The aesthetic result after eyelid retraction repair alone was satisfactory to the patient, precluding the need for blepharoplasty (see text for discussion).

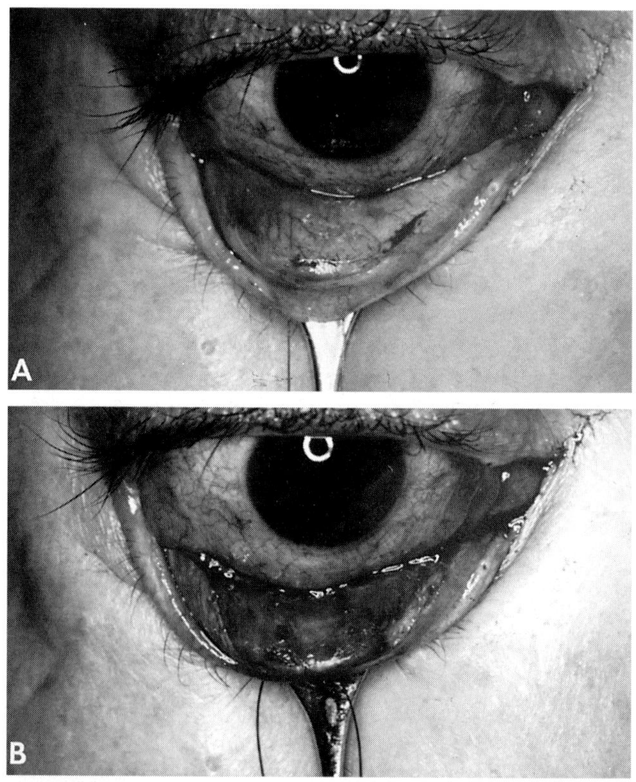

Figure 46–14. *A*, To treat mild lower eyelid retraction, a conjunctival incision is made along the inferior tarsal border. *B*, The lower eyelid retractors are then maximally recessed, and the eyelid is placed on stretch with a traction suture for several days postoperatively.

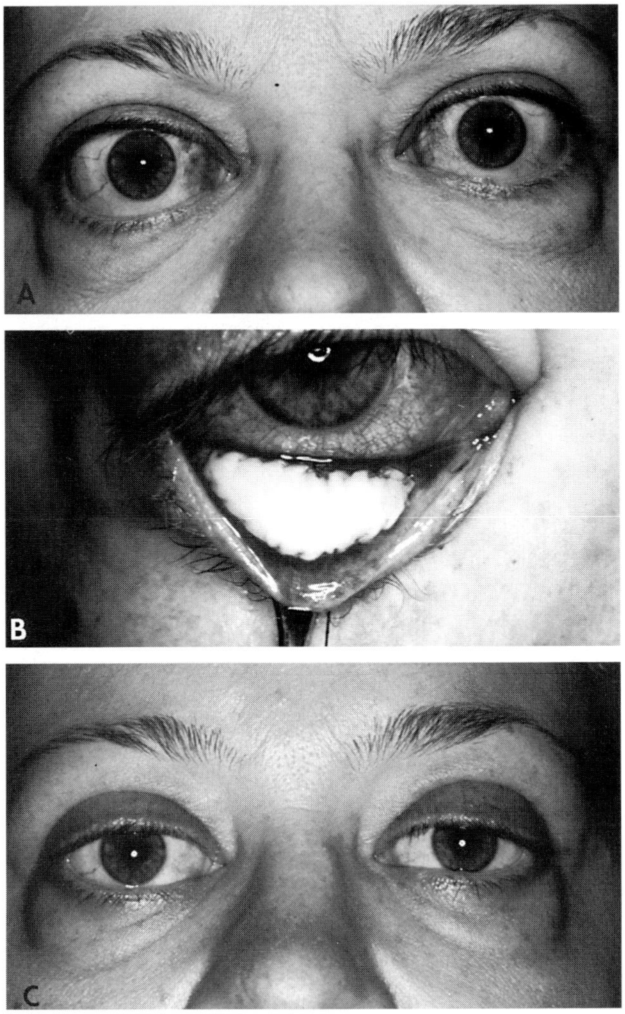

Figure 46–15. *A*, Bilateral upper and lower eyelid retraction. *B*, After the upper eyelid retraction had been corrected, the lower eyelid retractors were recessed and a spacer of hard palate mucosa was grafted between the inferior tarsal edge and the retractors. *C*, Postoperative appearance.

retraction, they are usually necessary to correct lower eyelid retraction of more than 2 mm. Hard palate mucosa (Fig. 46–15) has yielded satisfactory results in my practice; it is easily harvested, autologous, and epithelialized, and it does not result in a thickened lid (as may occur with implantation of cartilage or donor sclera).

A lateral tarsorrhaphy may be helpful in reducing both upper and lower eyelid retraction. Because a wide lid adhesion is usually cosmetically and optically objectionable, I prefer to use a tarsorrhaphy only as a minor supplement to recession of the eyelid retractors, rather than as a primary procedure. The technique described by Stamler and Tse[57] is simple and effective and has the advantage of being reversible even though it is designed to be permanent.

Medial Lower Eyelid Entropion

Entropion of the lower eyelid, as noted earlier, may result from medial decompression of the orbit. Correction may reliably be accomplished by recessing the nasal portion of the lower eyelid retractors; tarsal fracturing procedures should be avoided.[3]

Lateral Canthal Obliquity

The underlying mechanism for this abnormality is hypoglobus after decompression of the orbital floor. Treatment of the eyelid sequela is difficult and, fortunately, is not often required. In one patient, I disinserted the attachments of the lateral canthal tendons of both the upper and the lower eyelids to the lateral orbital rim and then secured the eyelids in a "tarsal strip"[58] manner to the rim at a lower position. The result was unsatisfactory, but perhaps it could have been better if the lids had been wired, rather than sutured, to the rim at the desired position. Subsequently, I have used a *Z*-plasty technique to reposition the lateral canthal angle; the postoperative results were improved but not optimal.

Complications

The most common and frustrating problem associated with the treatment of eyelid malpositions in Graves' ophthalmopathy is an imperfect postoperative eyelid level. To eliminate as many variables as possible and to gain experience in the lid-lowering effects of the various procedures, one should use consistent technique and the same anesthetic solution from case to case. My preference is 1 to 1.5 mL of lidocaine 2% with 1 : 100,000 epinephrine and hyaluronidase. When hyaluronidase is not used, it seems that Müller's muscle is stimulated for a longer period because the epinephrine does not diffuse as quickly.

Residual retraction is much more common than ptosis after operation for Graves' eyelids. The cause can be baffling (and maddening); identical procedures may be performed on the right and left upper eyelids in a patient with bilateral retraction and the intraoperative eyelid positions may be pleasing to both patient and surgeon, yet the postoperative results may be markedly asymmetric. In general, because patients are usually more forgiving of residual retraction than of postoperative ptosis and because it is probably easier and more predictable to recess the levator secondarily than it is to advance the levator if the eyelid retraction has been overcorrected, the intraoperative eyelid position should be at the desired final level or perhaps just slightly higher. If the eyelid is ptotic in the operating room, it almost always will remain so postoperatively. In this situation the levator aponeurosis should be advanced to elevate the eyelid to the proper position and then secured to the surrounding tissue (orbicularis in a posterior approach procedure; Müller's muscle or conjunctiva in a transcutaneous operation).

Abnormalities of the eyelid contour or crease may detract from an otherwise satisfactory result. Examples of

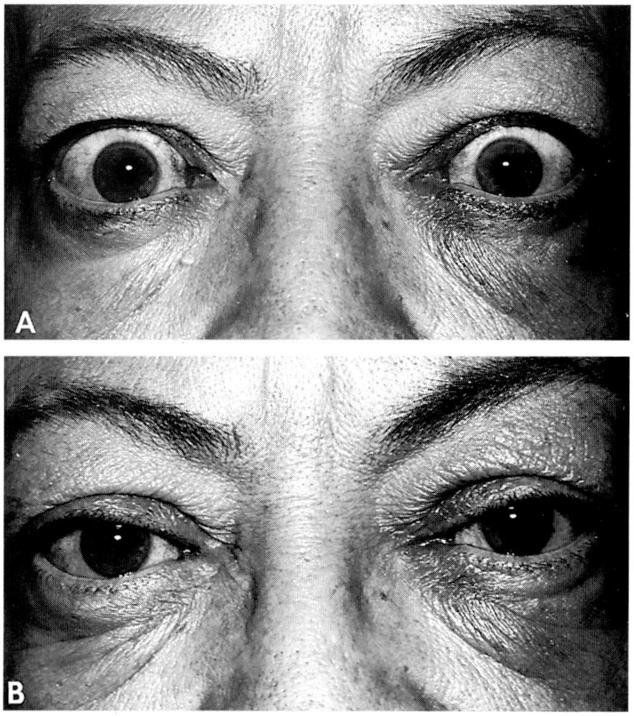

Figure 46–16. *A*, Preoperative appearance. *B*, Postoperative complication: mild bilateral nasal ptosis from excessive recession of the retractors nasally.

such problems include nasal ptosis, temporal flare, a flat lid contour, and asymmetric lid folds. Ptosis of the nasal portion of the eyelid (Fig. 46–16) occurs less frequently than might be expected from published reports, but the surgeon should err on the side of being too conservative rather than too aggressive when recessing the eyelid retractors in this portion of the lid. If a small nasal area of eyelid retraction persists postoperatively, it usually is a simple matter to perform a localized recession of Müller's muscle or the levator.

Residual temporal flare is a more common problem and can be treated by detaching the lateral horn of the levator aponeurosis (Fig. 46–17) or creating a small lateral tarsorrhaphy. Just as it is difficult to overcorrect blepharoptosis in a child with a congenitally droopy eyelid, it is unusual to overcorrect temporal flare in a patient with eyelid retraction from Graves' disease. A flat lid contour (Fig. 46–18) may result from excessive recession of the eyelid retractors in the central portion of the eyelid or from inadequate recession of the retractors nasally; this imperfection, unfortunately, rarely reveals itself intraoperatively but usually becomes apparent only after the postoperative inflammation has subsided.

Asymmetry of the eyelid creases may detract from an otherwise satisfactory result (Fig. 46–19). Waller[3] pointed out that greater degrees of retraction require greater degrees of levator recession; therefore, because

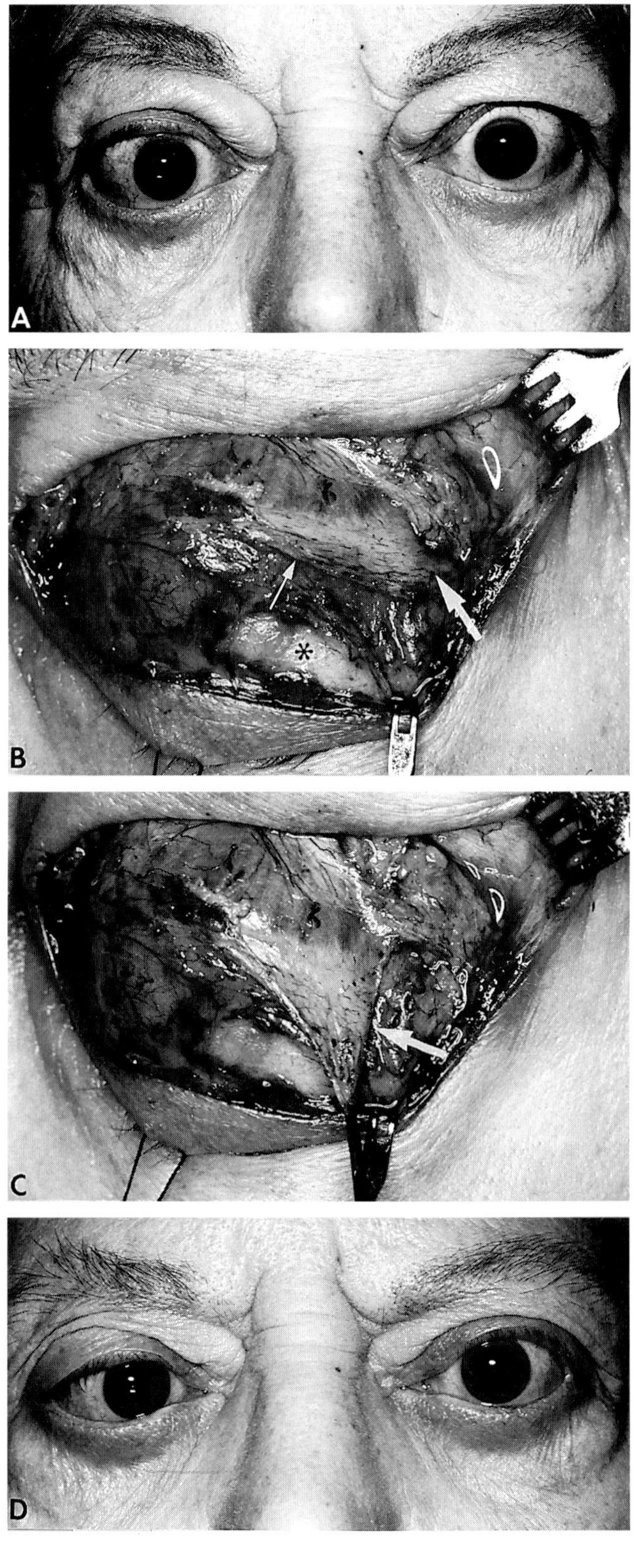

Figure 46–17. *A*, Preoperative appearance: bilateral upper eyelid retraction and marked temporal flare of the left upper lid. *B*, The left upper lid levator aponeurosis has been recessed *(small arrow)*, but the lateral horn remains intact *(large arrow)*. The tarsus is marked with an asterisk. *C*, The lateral horn of the levator has been partially released *(arrow)*. *D*, Postoperative complication: persistent temporal flare of the left upper lid; the lateral horn should have been weakened further, the lateral tarsorrhaphy should have been wider, or both.

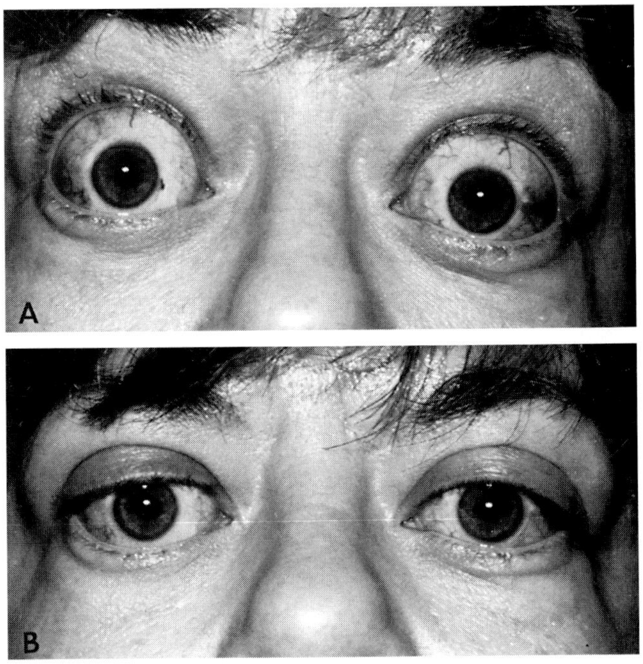

Figure 46–18. *A*, Preoperative appearance. *B*, Postoperative complication: the right upper eyelid margin contour is flat because of inadequate recession of the retractors nasally.

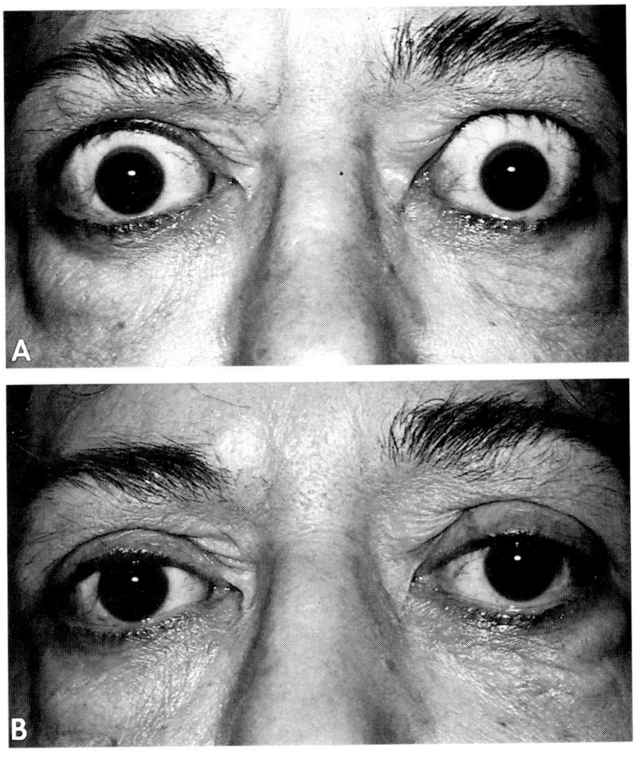

Figure 46–19. *A*, Preoperative appearance: asymmetric retraction. *B*, Postoperative complication: although the upper eyelid positions were symmetric after retraction repair by the posterior approach, the left upper eyelid appeared slightly ptotic to the patient because of its higher lid fold. Asymmetric preoperative retraction required greater recession of the left upper eyelid retractors. In circumstances such as this, it may be easier to equalize the eyelid creases by recessing the eyelid retractors through an anterior approach.

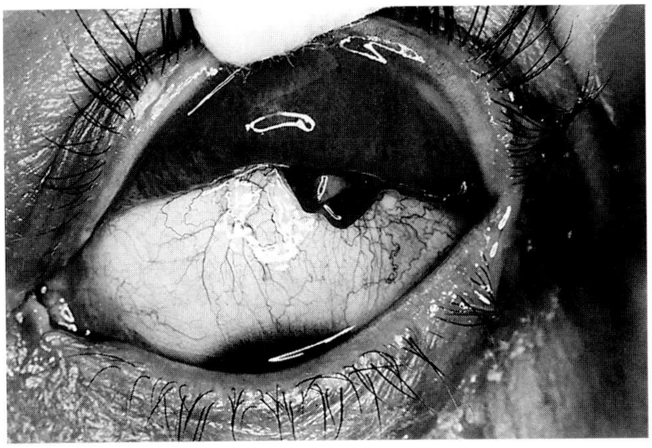

Figure 46–20. A "pyogenic granuloma" that formed along the conjunctival incision. This type of inflammatory mass causes persistent postoperative eyelid edema and mattering, but it responds to simple excision and the application of antibiotic-corticosteroid eyedrops.

the primary attachments of the levator determine the position of the lid crease, one may expect to alter the position of the fold if a large recession is performed. Weakening the retractors through a skin incision may allow for re-formation of the lid fold in a more predictable position.

A disadvantage of the conjunctival approach for repair of eyelid retraction is the occasional formation of a "pyogenic granuloma" along the incision (Fig. 46–20). Patients report persistent mild eyelid swelling and mattering and sometimes a subtle foreign body sensation when blinking. The inflammatory masses respond to simple excision and the application of antibiotic-corticosteroid eyedrops.

Hemorrhage and infection may complicate nearly any surgical procedure, but both are unusual in operations for Graves' eyelids. A small amount of blood-tinged oozing may occur during the first few hours after a posterior approach, however. Ice applied to the eyes postoperatively helps to reduce both bleeding and edema. The prescription of systemic antibiotics does not seem necessary unless a graft has been placed in an eyelid.

Acknowledgment

Supported in part by a grant from Research to Prevent Blindness, Inc., New York, NY.

REFERENCES

1. Day RM: Ocular manifestations of thyroid disease: Current concepts. Trans Am Ophthalmol Soc 57:572–601, 1959.
2. Bahn RS, Garrity JA, Bartley GB, Gorman CA: Diagnostic evaluation of Graves' ophthalmopathy. Endocrinol Metab Clin North Am 17:527–545, 1988.

3. Waller RR: Eyelid malpositions in Graves' ophthalmopathy. Trans Am Ophthalmol Soc 80:855–930, 1982.
4. Kushner BJ: A surgical procedure to minimize lower-eyelid retraction with inferior rectus recession. Arch Ophthalmol 110:1011–1014, 1992.
5. Small RG: Upper eyelid retraction in Graves' ophthalmopathy: A new surgical technique and a study of the abnormal levator muscle. Trans Am Ophthalmol Soc 86:725–793, 1988.
6. Small RG: Enlargement of levator palpebrae superioris muscle fibers in Graves' ophthalmopathy. Ophthalmology 96:424–430, 1989.
7. Frueh BR: Eyelid retraction in Graves' eye disease. Ophthalmology 96:1574–1575, 1989.
8. Feldon SE, Levin L: Graves' ophthalmopathy. Part V: Aetiology of upper eyelid retraction in Graves' ophthalmopathy. Br J Ophthalmol 74:484–485, 1990.
9. Grove AS Jr: Upper eyelid retraction and Graves' disease. Ophthalmology 88:499–506, 1981.
10. Harvey JT, Anderson RL: Lid lag and lagophthalmos: A clarification of terminology. Ophthalmic Surg 12:338–340, 1981.
11. Bahn RS, Bartley GB, Gorman CA: Emergency treatment of Graves' ophthalmopathy. Ballieres Clin Endocrinol Metab 6:95–105, 1992.
12. Frueh BR, Musch DC, Garber FW: Lid retraction and levator aponeurosis defects in Graves' eye disease. Ophthalmic Surg 17:216–220, 1986.
13. Lohman L, Burns JA, Penland WR, Cahill KV: Unilateral eyelid retraction secondary to contralateral ptosis in dysthyroid ophthalmopathy. J Clin Neurol Ophthalmol 4:163–166, 1984.
14. Gonnering RS: Pseudoretraction of the eyelid in thyroid-associated orbitopathy. Arch Ophthalmol 106:1078–1080, 1988.
15. Gay AJ, Salmon ML, Windsor CE: Hering's law, the levators, and their relationship in disease states. Arch Ophthalmol 77:157–160, 1967.
16. Goldberg RA, Christenbury JD, Shorr N: Medial entropion following orbital decompression for dysthyroid ophthalmopathy. Ophthal Plast Reconstr Surg 4:81–85, 1988.
17. Goldberg RA, Shorr N, Cohen MS: The medial orbital strut in the prevention of postdecompression dystopia in dysthyroid ophthalmopathy. Ophthal Plast Reconstr Surg 8:32–34, 1992.
18. Gay AJ, Wolkstein MA: Topical guanethidine therapy for endocrine lid retraction. Arch Ophthalmol 76:364–367, 1966.
19. Skinner SW, Miller JE: Permanent improvement of thyroid-related upper eyelid retraction from bethanidine. Am J Ophthalmol 67:764–766, 1969.
20. Cartlidge NEF, Crombie AL, Anderson J, Hall R: Critical study of 5% guanethidine in ocular manifestations of Graves' disease. Br Med J 4:645–647, 1969.
21. Dixon RS, Anderson RL, Hatt MU: The use of thymoxamine in eyelid retraction. Arch Ophthalmol 97:2147–2150, 1979.
22. Sneddon JM, Turner P: Adrenergic blockade and the eye signs of thyrotoxicosis. Lancet 2:525–527, 1966.
23. Gay AJ, Salmon ML, Wolkstein MA: Topical sympatholytic therapy for pathologic lid retraction. Arch Ophthalmol 77:341–344, 1967.
24. Mayo CH: The surgical treatment of exophthalmos. JAMA 63:1147–1149, 1914.
25. Henderson JW: Relief of eyelid retraction: A surgical procedure. Arch Ophthalmol 74:205–216, 1965.
26. King JH Jr, Wadsworth JAC: An Atlas of Ophthalmic Surgery, 3rd ed. Philadelphia, JB Lippincott, 1981.
27. de Blaskovics L: A new operation for ptosis with shortening of the levator and tarsus. Arch Ophthalmol 52:563–573, 1923.
28. Cusick P, Sarrail JA: Blepharoptosis modifications of Blaskovic's procedure, its indications, and management of its complications. *In* Smith JL (ed): Neuro-Ophthalmology Update. New York, Masson Publishing, 1977, pp 38–45.
29. Goldstein I: Recession of the levator muscle for lagophthalmos in exophthalmic goiter. Arch Ophthalmol 11:389–393, 1934.
30. Moran RE: The correction of exophthalmos and levator spasm. Plast Reconstr Surg 18:411–426, 1956.
31. Iliff CE, Berke RN, Crawford JS, Schimek RA: Ptosis complications: Discussion. Trans Am Acad Ophthalmol Otolaryngol 63:663–682, 1959.
32. Tenzel RR: Surgical treatment of upper lid. *In* Smith JL (ed): Neuro-Ophthalmology Update. New York, Masson Publishing, 1977, pp 17–18.
33. Schimek RA: Surgical management of ocular complications of Graves' disease. Arch Ophthalmol 87:655–664, 1972.
34. Putterman AM, Urist M: Surgical treatment of upper eyelid retraction. Arch Ophthalmol 87:401–405, 1972.
35. Putterman AM: Surgical treatment of thyroid-related upper eyelid retraction: Graded Müller's muscle excision and levator recession. Ophthalmology 88:507–512, 1981.
36. Chalfin J, Putterman AM: Müller's muscle excision and levator recession in retracted upper lid: Treatment of thyroid-related retraction. Arch Ophthalmol 97:1487–1491, 1979.
37. Putterman AM, Fett DR: Müller's muscle in the treatment of upper eyelid retraction: A 12-year study. Ophthalmic Surg 17:361–367, 1986.
38. Baylis HI, Cies WA, Kamin DF: Correction of upper eyelid retraction. Am J Ophthalmol 82:790–794, 1976.
39. Flanagan JC: Eye bank sclera in oculoplastic surgery. Ophthalmic Surg 5:45–53, 1974.
40. Dryden RM, Soll DB: The use of scleral transplantation in cicatricial entropion and eyelid retraction. Trans Am Acad Ophthalmol Otolaryngol 83:669–678, 1977.
41. Flanagan JC: Retraction of the eyelids secondary to thyroid ophthalmopathy—its surgical correction with sclera and the fate of the graft. Trans Am Ophthalmol Soc 78:657–685, 1980.
42. Harvey JT, Anderson RL: The aponeurotic approach to eyelid retraction. Ophthalmology 88:513–524, 1981.
43. Harvey JT, Corin S, Nixon D, Veloudios A: Modified levator aponeurosis recession for upper eyelid retraction in Graves' disease. Ophthalmic Surg 22:313–317, 1991.
44. Levine MR, Chu A: Surgical treatment of thyroid-related lid retraction: A new variation. Ophthalmic Surg 22:90–94, 1991.
45. Older JJ: Surgical treatment of eyelid retraction associated with thyroid eye disease. Ophthalmic Surg 22:318–323, 1991.
46. Bonavolontà G: A simplified technique for recession of the upper eyelid retractors. Ophthal Plast Reconstr Surg 2:113–115, 1986.
47. Grove AS Jr: Levator lengthening by marginal myotomy. Arch Ophthalmol 98:1433–1438, 1980.
48. Grove AS Jr: Eyelid retraction treated by levator marginal myotomy. Ophthalmology 87:1013–1018, 1980.
49. Small RG: Controlled recession of the upper eyelid. Adv Ophthalmic Plast Reconstr Surg 1:263–274, 1982.
50. Waller RR: Lower eyelid retraction: Management. Ophthalmic Surg 9:41–47, 1978.
51. Bartley GB, Kay PP: Posterior lamellar eyelid reconstruction with a hard palate mucosal graft. Am J Ophthalmol 107:609–612, 1989.
52. Kersten RC, Kulwin DR, Levartovsky S, et al: Management of lower-lid retraction with hard-palate mucosa grafting. Arch Ophthalmol 108:1339–1343, 1990.
53. Karesh JW, Fabrega MA, Rodrigues MM, Glaros DS: Polytetrafluoroethylene as an interpositional graft material for the correction of lower eyelid retraction. Ophthalmology 96:419–423, 1989.
54. Bartley GB, Waller RR: Graves' ophthalmopathy. *In* van Heerden JA (ed): Common Problems in Endocrine Surgery. Chicago, Year Book Medical Publishers, 1989, pp 25–29.
55. Simpson WAC, Downes RN, Collin JRO: Unusual complication of strabismus and lid surgery. Ophthal Plast Reconstr Surg 5:131–132, 1989.
56. Bartley GB, Waller RR: Retroaponeurotic fat. Am J Ophthalmol 107:301, 1989.
57. Stamler JF, Tse DT: A simple and reliable technique for permanent lateral tarsorrhaphy. Arch Ophthalmol 108:125–127, 1990.
58. Anderson RL, Gordy DD: The tarsal strip procedure. Arch Ophthalmol 97:2192–2196, 1979.

CHAPTER 47

Eyelid and Orbital Considerations in AIDS

Jan W. Kronish

Acquired immunodeficiency syndrome (AIDS) is a fatal disease of epidemic proportion caused by infection with human immunodeficiency virus (HIV). The syndrome is characterized by the presence of opportunistic infections and uncommon neoplasms in individuals with laboratory evidence of HIV infection who have no other known cause of immunodeficiency.[1, 2] Since the original reports of an acquired cellular immunodeficiency in homosexual men in 1981,[3, 4] more than 300,000 persons have developed this syndrome in the United States as of 1993, and an estimated 17 million persons worldwide have been infected with HIV.[2]

HIV is transmitted by intimate heterosexual or homosexual contact, by receipt of contaminated blood or blood products, and from mother to fetus or infant transplacentally or perinatally. An asymptomatic carrier state in HIV-infected individuals may last from 2 to 9 years, during which time transmission of the virus to others may occur. Groups at high risk for HIV infection include homosexual or bisexual men, heterosexual partners of HIV-infected persons, intravenous drug abusers, hemophiliacs and other recipients of blood product transfusions, and children with infected mothers. Recent epidemiologic studies have shown a decreasing proportion of homosexual men, an increasing frequency of heterosexual transmission, and a disproportionate number of minorities among those infected.[1]

HIV is a retrovirus that specifically attacks CD4-positive (CD4+) cells (mostly T helper cells) and copies its RNA-encoded genome into the host cell DNA with reverse transcriptase, a viral enzyme. Infection of these lymphocytes leads to either cell death, which lowers or reverses the CD4+/CD8+ (T helper/inducer cell to T suppressor/cytotoxic cell) ratio, or causes functional defects of the surviving cells. The progressive depletion of lymphocytes in the peripheral blood and impaired function of the surviving immune cells leads to profound immunosuppression.[5] Infection of other cells with CD4 receptors, such as macrophages, monocytes, endothelial cells of blood vessels, and glial cells, is thought to contribute to numerous clinical syndromes, such as neurologic illnesses, in AIDS.[5, 6] Antibodies to HIV may be detected 1 to 2 months after exposure by enzyme linked immunosorbent assay (ELISA) technique or the Western blot assay to confirm HIV infection.[1]

A wide spectrum of diseases may develop in HIV-infected persons, including an acute mononucleosis–like syndrome after initial infection, an asymptomatic carrier state, generalized lymphadenopathy and AIDS-related complex, and AIDS itself.[7] As a result of the derangement of the immune system, AIDS patients are susceptible to opportunistic infection and malignant tumor formation. The most common opportunistic pathogens include cytomegalovirus (CMV), *Candida* species, *Cryptococcus neoformans*, *Mycobacterium avium-intracellulare*, *Pneumocystis carinii*, herpes simplex virus, varicella-zoster virus, *Toxoplasma gondii*, and *Cryptosporidium* species. Non-Hodgkin's lymphoma (NHL) and Kaposi's sarcoma (KS) are the most frequently encountered neoplasms in AIDS patients.[8, 9] Ocular and adnexal manifestations are present in as many as 94% of patients and include opportunistic infections, such as CMV retinitis, a noninfectious microangiopathy, neoplasms of the conjunctiva, eyelids, and orbit, and neuro-ophthalmic disorders.[8, 10–19]

Management of HIV infection initially involves antiretroviral therapy and monitoring of patients' immune systems. Zidovudine halts the replication of HIV by inhibiting reverse transcriptase and has been effective in delaying progression to AIDS and partially restoring immune function with increased numbers of CD4+ (T helper) cells.[20] Other antiviral agents, such as didanosine and dideoxycytidine, are under study alone and in different combinations to establish a more effective treatment of HIV infection while minimizing side effects. A therapeutic regimen for prophylaxis of *P. carinii* pneumonia and certain viral infections may be initiated when CD4+ cell counts are rapidly falling or reach a critical level.[21] Treatment of complications of AIDS, such as infections and neoplasms, is improving and leading to prolonged survival. Psychosocial counseling regarding life-style changes and mental health issues should also be included in patient care.

EYELID MANIFESTATIONS

Infections

Infections in AIDS patients may be caused by opportunistic as well as nonopportunistic pathogens. An increased frequency or atypical manifestation of certain infections may develop in the HIV-seropositive patient as compared with an immunocompetent host. Impairment of the immune response may even be present in patients who are asymptomatic without a reduction in their cell counts.[1] Recognition of opportunistic infections or unusual characteristics of nonopportunistic infections involving the eyelids and orbit should alert the clinician to consider HIV infection and order appropriate serologic tests.

Molluscum Contagiosum

Molluscum contagiosum is a cutaneous infection caused by a DNA virus of the poxvirus group. The skin lesions are usually multiple, dome-shaped, umbilicated papules and are self-limited in immunocompetent hosts. A peak incidence is typically found in healthy children younger than 5 years old and young adults. In cases of eyelid involvement, an associated follicular conjunctivitis and keratitis may develop. Numerous effective treatments in immunocompetent hosts have been described, including incision and curettage, surgical excision, cryotherapy, electrodesiccation, and application of cantharidin.[22]

Disseminated molluscum contagiosum has been reported in patients with immune disorders.[11, 22–24] Severe and aggressive involvement of the eyelids and periocular region may occur in AIDS patients (Fig. 47–1).[11, 23, 24] Robinson and coworkers[24] reported recurrences in two patients with AIDS treated with surgical excision and cryotherapy of molluscum eyelid nodules within 6 to 7 weeks, the incubation period for this viral lesion. The atypical features of onset in adulthood, rapid proliferation, unusual distribution, large number and size, confluency, and resistance to therapy are indicators of an immunosuppressive state.[23, 24]

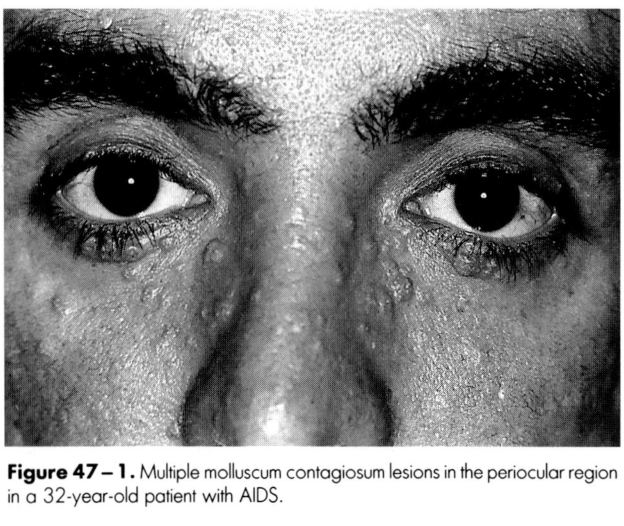

Figure 47–1. Multiple molluscum contagiosum lesions in the periocular region in a 32-year-old patient with AIDS.

Verruca Vulgaris

The lesions of verruca vulgaris are caused by a DNA-containing papillomavirus. These warts occur anywhere on the skin and occasionally develop on the eyelids. They appear as circumscribed, elevated growths with a hyperkeratotic, filiform surface. Treatment options include curettage, surgical excision, electrodesiccation, cryotherapy, and application of trichloroacetic acid.[25] The development of multiple warts in the periocular region have been described in patients with HIV infection.[11]

Herpes Zoster Ophthalmicus

The varicella-zoster virus is a herpesvirus that causes the ophthalmic sequelae of infection termed *herpes zoster ophthalmicus.* The disease most often affects immunocompetent patients in their fifth to seventh decade of life, and it is their advanced age that, perhaps, predisposes to latent virus reactivation. Patients typically develop a vesiculobullous rash in the distribution of the ophthalmic branch of the trigeminal nerve, including the upper eyelid, eyebrow, forehead, and, with involvement of the nasociliary branch, the side of the tip of the nose. Ocular diseases that may be associated with herpes zoster ophthalmicus include conjunctivitis, keratitis, scleritis, uveitis, retinitis, optic neuritis, and extraocular muscle palsies.[26]

A strong correlation exists between the development of herpes zoster ophthalmicus in young adults and HIV seropositivity. Herpes zoster may, in fact, represent the initial manifestation of HIV infection or AIDS, and this association should be suspected in individuals younger than 45 years of age. In addition, a more virulent course of disease ensues in this group of patients, including more severe skin lesions, keratitis, anterior uveitis, acute retinal necrosis, postherpetic neuralgia, and disseminated infection. These complications may be more refractory to standard therapy and lead to a prolonged course of disease.[12, 15, 27, 28] Treatment of immunocompromised patients should include parenteral or oral acyclovir in addition to appropriate topical agents to diminish the ocular sequelae of herpes zoster ophthalmicus.[11, 15]

Neoplasms

Kaposi's Sarcoma

Before the AIDS epidemic, KS was a disease that developed almost exclusively in older men of Mediterranean descent. This vascular, multicentric tumor most commonly involved the skin and soft tissues of the extremities and rarely progressed to an aggressive and disseminated life-threatening form. An "endemic" form of KS in equatorial Africa exists that manifests a more aggressive course with lymph node and visceral involvement.[13, 29]

KS was noted in the first reported cases of homosexual and bisexual men with opportunistic infections and immune system suppression in the early 1980s. It represents the most common malignancy associated with AIDS and occurs in approximately one third of these patients. The incidence of KS as the presenting manifestation of AIDS has been decreasing in recent years; however, its incidence as a later marker of HIV infection is increasing. The neoplasm is much more common in homosexual and bisexual men than in other AIDS risk groups.[13, 29, 30]

The course of disease varies from a limited form of cutaneous tumors with minimal or no progression to a very aggressive pattern of disseminated involvement of extracutaneous organs, such as liver, spleen, gastrointestinal tract, and pulmonary parenchyma. AIDS-related KS usually presents as plaque-like or nodular skin lesions that are single or multiple and range from pink to dark purple. Locally destructive fungating lesions and deep infiltrative tumors with bone invasion are encountered less frequently.[13, 29] KS may develop when immune competence is still relatively intact; however, rapid progression of disease and a poor prognosis is associated with low CD4+ cell counts, patients with systemic signs of symptoms, and the presence of concurrent opportunistic infection. The mortality rate is approximately 80% two years after the onset of KS in patients with opportunistic infections.[13, 31]

The pathogenesis of KS is controversial. An increased incidence of KS in renal transplant patients receiving immunosuppressive drugs in the 1970s established a direct link between KS and immune system function. The disproportionate number of homosexual and bisexual AIDS patients who develop KS raised speculation that another cofactor was involved. Evidence of viral DNA, RNA, and viral-encoded antigens in tumor specimens, as well as epidemiologic studies, suggest CMV may act as a promoter in the induction of KS.[13, 29, 30, 32] Finally, certain growth factors produced in AIDS patients may also play a role in tumorigenesis.[32]

The histogenesis of KS has been intensively studied to identify the cell of origin. The presence of factor VIII–related antigen on immunohistologic methods and Weibel-Palade bodies in the tumor cells on ultrastructural analysis supported an endothelial derivation.[33–35] More recent enzyme histochemical studies convincingly demonstrated that the tumor originates from lymphatic endothelium.[36]

Although extremely rare before the epidemic of HIV infection, ocular involvement of KS ranges from 5% to 24% of AIDS patients with systemic KS and may even represent the sole manifestation of this neoplasm.[12, 13, 37–39] The usual forms of ophthalmic KS include tumors of the eyelids and the palpebral and bulbar conjunctiva.[11, 13, 15, 28, 29, 33, 37, 39–43] Lesions of the caruncle, lacrimal sac,[13] and orbit[43] are less common. Eyelid cutaneous lesions are similar to skin tumors seen elsewhere in the body. They appear as single or multiple, nontender, dark red or purple nodules that, generally, progress slowly (Fig. 47–2). The upper or lower eyelids or both may be involved, and the condition is usually unilateral.[11, 13, 28, 29, 33, 40, 44] The tumors may result in visual compromise, owing to eyelid margin complications including trichiasis, entropion, ectropion, hemorrhage, and severe lid swelling.[13, 33, 38, 42] The mass effect of eyelid KS can also cause lagophthalmos and associated exposure keratopathy.[13, 38] Secondary infection of ulcerated lesions may lead to a severe blepharoconjunctivitis.[33, 42]

Histopathologically, nodular tumors consist of atypical, densely packed spindle-shaped cells with elongated oval hyperchromatic nuclei with abundant slit spaces often filled with erythrocytes (Fig. 47–3).[8, 13, 33, 37, 38]

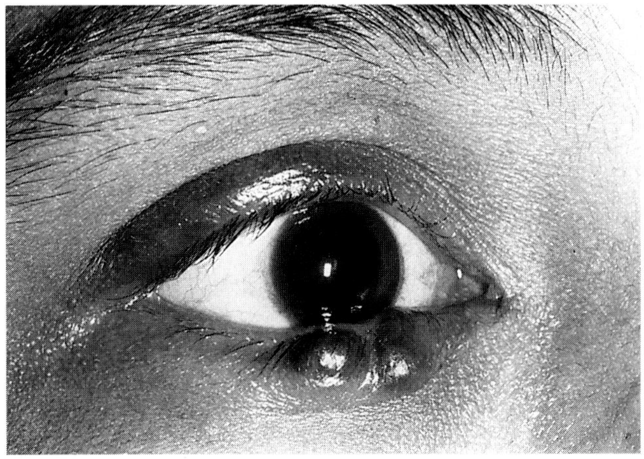

Figure 47–2. Kaposi's sarcoma of the right upper and lower eyelids. The upper eyelid lesion is relatively flat and diffuse in comparison to the nodular, elevated tumor in the lower eyelid. (Courtesy of Don S. Ellis, MD.)

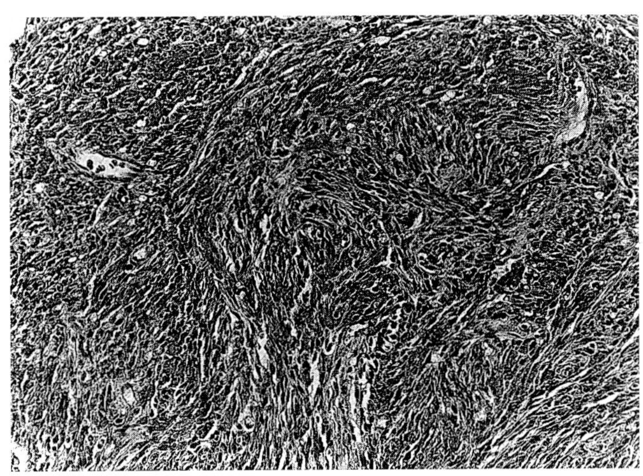

Figure 47–3. Kaposi's sarcoma is composed of spindle-shaped cells with nuclear atypia and slit-like spaces containing red blood cells and occasional inflammatory cells. (H & E, ×40.)

Patchy and flat tumors of the eyelids and conjunctiva are composed of flat endothelial cells lining dilated vascular channels or plump, fusiform endothelial cells with a few slit vessels.[38] A low-grade infiltrate of lymphocytes, macrophages, and plasma cells may also be present.[13, 38]

Therapeutic modalities available for treatment of patients with KS include surgery, cryotherapy, ionizing radiation, intralesional or systemic chemotherapy, and immunotherapy. The treatment regimen must be individualized according to the patient's stage of disease, with objectives established in the context of quality of life issues. AIDS-related KS is a multifocal neoplasm; therefore, local treatment of an ocular tumor will not affect the progression of involvement of the viscera and other mucocutaneous sites. For this reason, systemic therapy should be evaluated, particularly in cases of widespread disease. Before an aggressive treatment plan is instituted, a biopsy is mandatory to differentiate the tumor from other skin conditions. The goals of any form of therapy are palliation rather than cure.

Eyelid and conjunctival KS generally grow slowly and, when limited in size without visual compromise, may be best observed without therapeutic intervention. Specific treatment of ophthalmic tumors should be considered when they impair visual function or cause significant ocular surface or lid margin complications. Also, cosmetically objectionable lesions in exposed areas, such as the periocular region, should be addressed because of potential serious psychological and social effects.

Cryotherapy and local excision of small, well-circumscribed tumors of the eyelids and conjunctiva are effective methods of treatment of lesions that are limited in size. Lesions that are incompletely removed or treated typically recur[13]; therefore, complete excision with 1- to 2-mm margins free of tumor should be attempted when possible. Dugel and colleagues[45] recommended fluorescein angiography before the surgical excision of large bulbar conjunctival KS lesions to delineate blood vessels that emanate from or lead to the tumor. Alternative methods of treatment should be considered for more extensive lesions that would require complex or multiple-stage reconstructive techniques. Surgery on these immunocompromised patients must be approached cautiously because of the increased potential of secondary infection, poor wound healing, and scarring. It is also extremely important that appropriate methods during any interventional procedure be employed to protect the surgeon and health care professionals from exposure to infectious material.[46]

Radiation therapy is a relatively safe and effective treatment of AIDS-related KS. The tumor is highly radiosensitive to dosages in the range of 2000 to 3000 cGy.[8, 13, 39, 40] In one series by Shuler and associates,[40] 20 of 22 patients with conjunctival and eyelid KS treated with localized radiation with multiple-fraction regimens had total or near-total resolution of lesions with only three recurrences within 4 months. Ghabriel and coworkers[39] demonstrated similar response and recurrence rates in their comparison of single treatment of 800 cGy and multiple-fraction treatments with total doses between 1500 and 3600 cGy. An overall response rate of 98% was reported in their series, although only 30% of patients had a complete response and almost one third of the lesions recurred. Focal radiation may be used alone or in conjunction with systemic therapy for palliation of extensive lesions. Potential side effects include radiation dermatitis and conjunctivitis, hair loss, edema, hyperpigmentation, and optic neuropathy.[13, 39, 40]

A variety of systemic therapies are available for cutaneous and disseminated KS. Interferon alfa-2b has been found to limit the spread or result in regression of lesions in up to 40% of patients. The activity of alpha-interferons is attributed to direct antiproliferative effects and, perhaps, immunomodulating and antiviral properties.[13, 31] Side effects of interferon include a flu-like syndrome, transient neutropenia and thrombocytopenia, and neurologic disorders. Single-agent and combination chemotherapy protocols have also been studied; however, an already compromised immune system may limit their use. Doxorubicin, vinblastine, vincristine, and bleomycin are those agents that have been most commonly investigated.[13]

Non-Hodgkin's Lymphoma

NHL has been seen with increasing frequency in patients with HIV infection. Extranodal disease is relatively common, and most cases represent high-grade B cell proliferations with an associated poor prognosis. Goldberg and associates[47] reported a primary eyelid non-Hodgkin's lymphoma in an HIV-seropositive patient who presented with a rapidly enlarging, erythematous, tender, diffuse palpebral mass. In the absence of systemic lymphoma, the lesion was treated with local radiotherapy, resulting in remission throughout the 18-month follow-up interval. This case demonstrates the importance of obtaining a biopsy of all eyelid tumors in patients infected with HIV for proper identification and treatment planning.

Other Neoplasms

A variety of uncommon malignancies with atypical characteristics continue to be reported in association with HIV infection. A 36-year-old female HIV-infected patient was managed at the Bascom Palmer Eye Institute with a rapidly enlarging sebaceous cell carcinoma of the right lower eyelid (David T. Tse, MD, personal communication, June 10, 1991). This patient's presentation clearly differed from the common features of this eyelid tumor, which include onset in the fifth through ninth decade of life, involvement of the upper eyelid two to three times more frequently than the lower eyelid, and slow and insidious growth.[48] The development of tumors at an uncommonly young age that arise in atypical locations and progress rapidly with an aggressive growth pattern should alert physicians to suspect possible concurrent HIV infection.

ORBITAL MANIFESTATIONS

Infections

HIV produces a profound derangement of the host immune system. Immunologic abnormalities in AIDS patients include defective cell-mediated immunity with T cell lymphopenia, functional defects of CD4+ T cells, decreased cytotoxic responses, inadequate antigen-specific antibody response to new antigenic stimuli due to B cell dysfunction, and defective monocyte activity. These multiple alterations of the host defenses markedly enhance the susceptibility to opportunistic infections in HIV-infected patients.[5, 29] Bacterial, viral, fungal, and protozoan organisms have been associated with AIDS that may involve the orbit and contiguous structures.[49–52]

Bacterial Orbital Infections

The most common bacterial pathogens associated with AIDS include genera of the order Actinomycetales, *Salmonella typhimurium*, *Haemophilus influenzae*, *Campylobacter jejuni*, *Shigella* species, *Klebsiella pneumoniae*, *Legionella pneumophila*, *M. avium-intracellulare*, and *Mycobacterium tuberculosis*.[29] Orbital cellulitis and abscess due to paranasal sinusitis caused by unusual or opportunistic bacterial species have been reported in two patients with AIDS.[50, 51] One patient with AIDS-related complex presented with a rapidly progressive course of orbital inflammation leading to no light perception in the affected eye despite parenteral antibiotic therapy. *Propionibacterium acnes*, an opportunistic pathogen that is ubiquitous and may be found in the anaerobic flora of the nasal and sinus cavities,[53] was cultured from the orbital abscess. The second case occurred in a 47-year-old homosexual man with AIDS who developed a *Pseudomonas aeruginosa* ethmoidal sinusitis and contiguous subperiosteal orbital abscess that responded to surgical drainage and intravenous antibiotics. A third patient with AIDS was reported with an acute syphilitic orbital periostitis associated with a necrotizing vasculitis of the optic nerve.[51]

Orbital Pneumocystis carinii

Protozoan infections by such organisms as *P. carinii*, *T. gondii*, *Cryptosporidium* species, and *Entamoeba histolytica* are a hallmark of AIDS. *P. carinii* pneumonia is seen in more than half of AIDS patients[29] and, with the introduction of aerosolized pentamidine prophylaxis, extrapulmonary infection has become more prevalent. A 32-year-old man with AIDS who had a preceding episode of *P. carinii* pneumonia was reported by Friedberg and associates[49] to have developed orbital granulomatous inflammation attributed to *Pneumocystis* infection. The patient initially presented with blurred vision, pain on eye movement, and optic nerve swelling. Over a 7-month period, the visual acuity of the affected eye deteriorated to no light perception accompanied by progressive proptosis due to a diffuse orbital mass. *P. carinii* organisms were identified in a biopsy specimen, and the proptosis responded dramatically to treatment with trimethoprim-sulfamethoxazole.

Orbital Aspergillosis

Immunocompromised patients such as those with HIV infection are particularly susceptible to infection by fungi such as *Candida* species, *C. neoformans*, *Histoplasma capsulatum*, *Coccidioides immitis*, and *Aspergillus* species. Oropharyngeal and urinary candidiasis and cryptococcal meningitis are the most common fungal infections encountered in patients with AIDS.[8, 29] Five patients with AIDS have been reported with orbital aspergillosis and adjacent sinus infection.[50–52] One was a 29-year-old man with AIDS who had undergone numerous surgical procedures for bilateral pansinusitis over a 6-month period before presenting with diplopia and left periorbital pain worse with eye movement. Serial computed tomographic scans showed a progressively enlarging soft tissue mass in the inferomedial orbit and maxillary antrum associated with bony destruction of the orbital floor (Fig. 47–4). Necrotic bone, periorbita, and sinus mucosa were encountered and debrided during an anterior orbitotomy, and histopathologic examination revealed septate hyphae with acute angle branching. *Aspergillus fumigatus* was isolated with fungal cultures, and systemic amphotericin B therapy was initiated. Another patient had a more fulminant course with rapidly deteriorating vision to no light perception with an orbital mass and maxillary, ethmoidal, and sphenoidal sinus involvement. Two patients died with spread of the fungal infection to the central nervous system.[51] Invasive or fulminant aspergillosis of the orbit carries a poor prognosis, particularly when the immunosuppressed state cannot be reversed.

Inflammatory Diseases

Two patients have been reported with orbital inflammatory disorders as the initial manifestation of HIV infection. Fabricius and colleagues[54] managed a 30-year-old man with ocular myositis and episcleritis who presented with eyelid swelling, diplopia, and ocular pain. The presence of anti–smooth muscle antibodies and antinuclear antibodies suggested an autoimmune mecha-

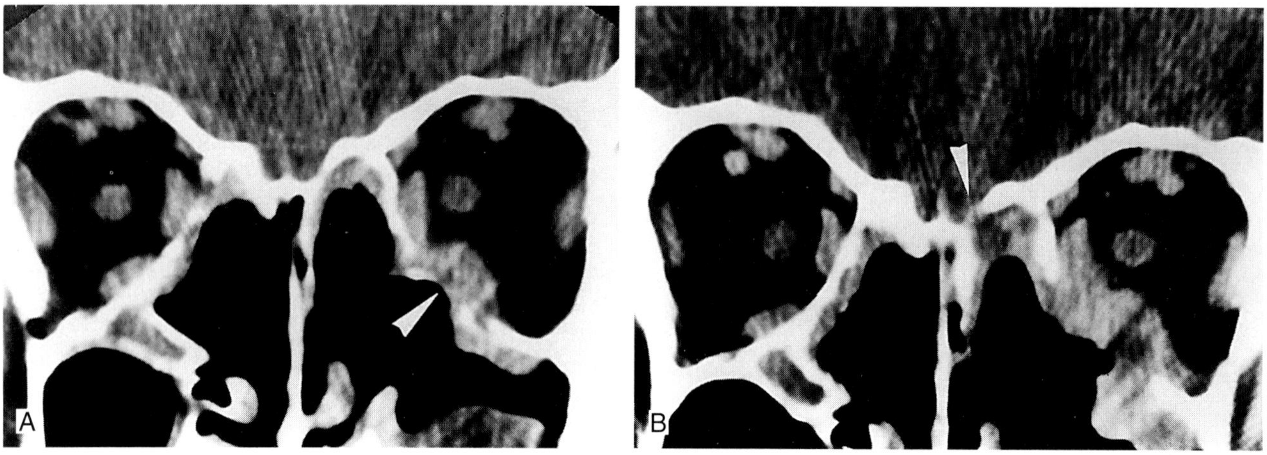

Figure 47–4. *A*, Coronal view of computed tomography of the orbits with soft tissue mass in the inferonasal orbit associated with bony erosion of the orbital floor (*arrowhead*). *B*, Computed tomography (coronal view) 4 months later demonstrates increased size of the soft tissue mass in orbit and maxillary antrum with more extensive bony destruction of the orbital floor. Progression of aspergillosis infection in ethmoidal sinus has led to a dehiscence in the cribriform plate (*arrowhead*).

nism. Interestingly, autoantibodies to lymphocytes, platelets, nerve tissue, and other cellular structures have been identified in patients infected with HIV. The second patient was a 22-year-old woman who was diagnosed with orbital pseudotumor based on a 2-day history of orbital pain, signs of acute orbital inflammation, and a mass in the lacrimal fossa.[9] Both patients had complete resolution of their inflammatory conditions in response to systemic corticosteroids.[9, 54] Steroids should be used cautiously to treat AIDS because of the patients' immunosuppressed state.

Lymphoproliferative Diseases

Non-Hodgkin's Lymphoma

NHL is the second most common neoplasm and a diagnostic feature of AIDS in patients who are seropositive for HIV. Three percent to 10% of AIDS patients develop lymphoma, and its rising incidence has been attributed to prolonged survival of patients with the introduction of antiretroviral therapy and prophylaxis of opportunistic infection.[55, 56] Unlike the NHLs that develop in immunocompetent individuals, AIDS-related lymphomas tend to occur at a younger age and are usually extranodal and widely disseminated. In addition, unusual sites of involvement are characteristic in AIDS patients, such as the kidneys, adrenal glands, and rectum, with an especially high incidence of primary central nervous system lymphomas.[55] A previous diagnosis of KS, herpes simplex virus or CMV infection, or oral hairy leukoplakia is associated with the development of NHL.[56]

The precise mechanisms of oncogenesis that lead to the development of NHL in AIDS patients remain speculative.The established association of Epstein-Barr virus (EBV) with African Burkitt's lymphoma and nasopharyngeal carcinoma, as well as the presence of EBV DNA in the AIDS-related lymphoma cell genomes, has provided evidence for an etiologic role of this herpesvirus. EBV has the ability to activate B lymphocytes in a polyclonal fashion, and in the setting of severe T cell immune deficiency, it may cause a cytogenetic change that results in a proliferating monoclonal cell line.[28, 55, 57–60] More recent studies, however, suggest that the c-*myc* oncogene plays a more frequent role in lymphomagenesis than EBV. Other potential causative factors that could induce AIDS-associated NHL include other viruses, not excluding HIV itself, other oncogenes, exposure to mutagenic drugs, and environmental agents.[55, 56, 58]

NHL is the most frequent orbital manifestation of AIDS,[50] yet it occurs relatively infrequently based on isolated case reports in the medical literature.[12, 43, 50, 57, 60–63] These tumors behave more aggressively with multiple atypical features in AIDS patients compared with immunocompetent persons. In the general population, orbital lymphoma classically presents as an insidious, painless, slowly progressive lesion in the superior orbit with mild axial or nonaxial displacement of the globe. Radiographic features typically include soft tissue density lesions with irregular margins that conform to the globe or encompass adjacent periocular structures without bony involvement.[61] In contrast, AIDS-related orbital lymphomas tend to develop more rapidly with painful eyelid swelling or mass, severe proptosis, diplopia, or visual compromise (Fig. 47–5*A*). Compression of the globe, destruction of the orbital bony walls, and involvement of the contiguous paranasal sinuses are not uncommon (see Fig. 47–5*B*).[43, 50, 59, 62, 63] Initial diagnostic evaluation should include neuroimaging studies, such as orbital computed tomography or magnetic resonance imaging, and needle aspiration or incisional biopsy.

NHLs associated with HIV infection are generally monoclonal B cell proliferations that exhibit an aggressive histologic pattern. More than 90% of AIDS-

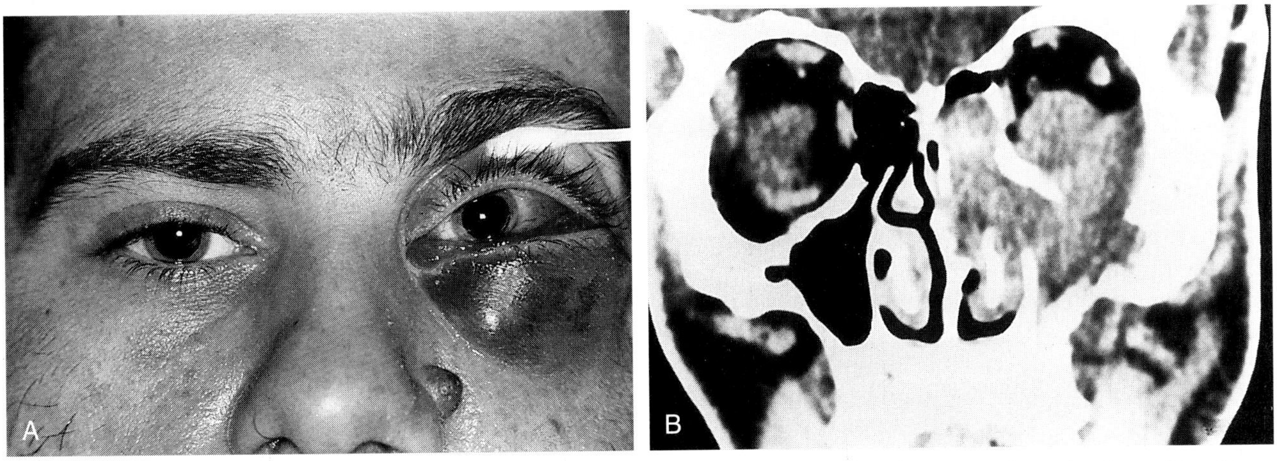

Figure 47 – 5. *A*, Clinical appearance of a 28-year-old patient with AIDS presenting with a visual acuity of hand motions, swelling and erythema of the left lower eyelid, proptosis, and superior displacement of the left eye. *B*, Computed tomography (coronal view) of the orbits and sinuses discloses a large mass involving the left maxillary sinus, nasal cavity, ethmoidal sinus, and inferior orbit and bony destruction of the orbital floor and maxilla.

related lymphomas are high- or intermediate-grade tumors.[55, 58, 61, 63] Six of the nine patients with orbital lymphoma in whom the pathologic features were described had immunoblastic, large cell high-grade lesions.[50, 57, 59–63] Histopathologically, monotonous infiltrates of large cells with abundant cytoplasm are seen with occasional mitotic figures and focal areas of necrosis (Fig. 47 – 6*A*). Two patients with orbital involvement had small, non – cleaved cell lymphomas, or "Burkitt's-like" tumors. These constitute the majority of high-grade lymphomas in AIDS patients[55, 58] and appear as undifferentiated, anaplastic lymphoid cells with numerous mitotic figures and scattered macrophages containing nuclear debris (see Fig. 47 – 6*B*).[64] Intermediate-grade tumors consist of large non – cleaved cell types, and this pattern was identified in one of the orbital lymphomas.[61]

Once a diagnosis of NHL is established, a prompt oncologic evaluation for staging of the disease should be obtained. This may include special studies such as gallium-67 scintigraphy, chest roentgenography, lumbar puncture with cerebrospinal fluid cytologic study, bone marrow aspiration and biopsy, and abdominal computed tomography.[59] Extranodal and widely disseminated disease is common and independent of CD4+ cell counts.[55]

Radiation therapy and chemotherapy are the two modalities of treatment available for NHL. Radiation therapy without systemic treatment is indicated for localized, low-grade lesions. High-grade tumors and disseminated disease are managed with chemotherapy and may be supplemented with local radiation for reduction of large tumors.[55, 59, 61] Bone marrow suppression and complicating opportunistic infections may limit the use of systemic therapy; however, the introduction of cytokines, such as colony-stimulating factors, may improve the success rate of chemotherapeutic regimens. In spite of these aggressive treatment protocols, however, the prognosis is generally dismal. Approximately half of the patients who

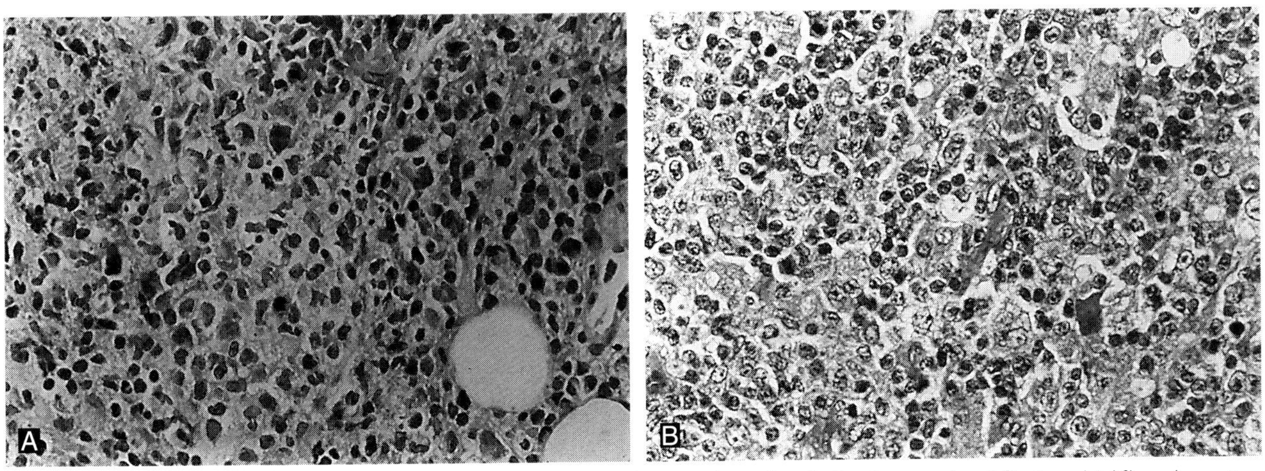

Figure 47 – 6. *A*, Large cell, diffuse pattern malignant lymphoma composed of mononuclear cells with abundant cytoplasm infiltrating orbital fibroadipose tissue. (H & E, ×40.) *B*, Burkitt's lymphoma is composed of undifferentiated lymphocytes with mitotic figures and scattered pale histiocytes containing phagocytic debris. (H & E, ×40.)

receive treatment achieve remission, but the majority develop a relapse after a short time interval[55] and have a 10% 2-year survival rate.[61]

Eosinophilic Granuloma

Eosinophilic granuloma represents the least aggressive form of the histiocytosis X syndromes that result from an abnormal proliferation of Langerhans' cells. Solitary infiltrates of eosinophilic granulocytes and mature histiocytes typically develop in bone and adjacent soft tissues and predominantly affect children. Gross and coworkers[65] reported a case of eosinophilic granuloma with an unusually aggressive behavior pattern causing a parasellar syndrome in an HIV-infected intravenous drug abuser. The patient was 35 years old and presented with painful ophthalmoplegia and compressive optic neuropathy. A mass lesion in the cavernous sinus with contiguous spread to the orbital apex was identified on computed tomography without bony destruction or erosion. Once the diagnosis was confirmed with tissue biopsy, radiation therapy was initiated, resulting in partial resolution of the extraocular motility defects. The authors suggest a possible association of the development of histiocytosis X in the setting of HIV infection based on increased numbers and activity of histiocytes and altered Langerhans' cell populations accompanying abnormal immune regulation.

Tumors

The most prevalent malignancy associated with HIV infection is KS. Two cases of orbital involvement of KS have been reported in the literature.[43, 66] Details are provided for only one of these cases in which bilateral periorbital lymphedema developed in conjunction with disseminated KS.[66] Since the orbit does not contain lymphatic channels and studies suggest that KS originates from lymphatic endothelium,[36] it would be unlikely to encounter primary KS in the orbit. On the other hand, anterior orbital involvement could potentially result from local invasion of tumor from the eyelid or conjunctiva.

Other malignancies have also been described in HIV-infected patients, such as cloagenic anorectal carcinoma[55, 60, 67]; squamous cell carcinoma of the head, neck, and oral cavity[55, 60, 67, 68]; Hodgkin's lymphoma; leukemia; and carcinoma of the testes, cervix, kidney, thyroid, bladder,[68] and lung.[29, 69] Gilberg and associates[50] managed a 56-year-old African American patient with AIDS who presented with a 6-month history of a progressively enlarging, painful, subcutaneous upper eyelid and anterior orbital mass (Fig. 47–7) that was found on biopsy to be squamous cell carcinoma. Human papillomavirus has been incriminated as the causative agent of squamous cell carcinoma in HIV-infected patients.[67] A

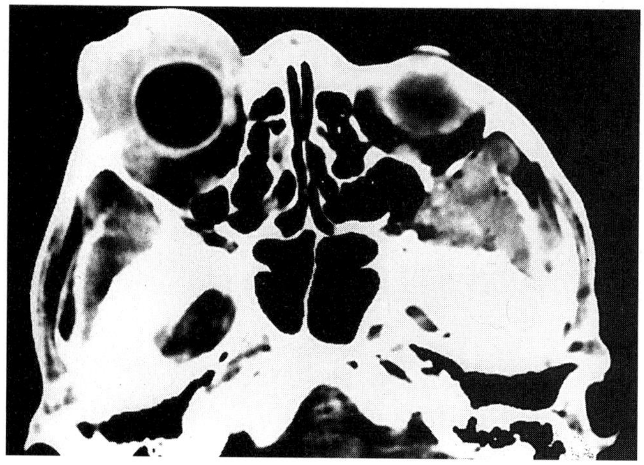

Figure 47–7. Computed tomography (axial view) of the orbits demonstrates a large eyelid and anterior orbital mass.

29-year-old patient with HIV infection has also been reported to have developed adenoid cystic carcinoma of the lacrimal gland.[50] Epidemiologic studies have not demonstrated an etiologic association between these tumors and AIDS; however, physicians should suspect HIV infection when neoplasms with atypical features are encountered.

OCULAR MANIFESTATIONS

Ocular disorders occur in as many as 94% of AIDS patients and include opportunistic infections, neoplasms, microvascular diseases, and neuro-ophthalmic signs of intracranial disease.[32] Some of these manifestations may be blinding and significantly contribute to the morbidity of this fatal syndrome. When managing eyelid and orbital diseases in patients with HIV infection, the clinician should be aware of the variety of ophthalmic disorders that are often present concurrently.

Approximately 18% of AIDS patients with KS have conjunctival involvement.[16] Conjunctival KS appears as a bright red, hemorrhagic, subconjunctival mass.[15, 32, 33] Tumors may originate on the bulbar or palpebral conjunctiva, but the majority develop in the inferior cul-de-sac.[15, 32, 40] The differential diagnosis of these lesions includes subconjunctival hemorrhage, pyogenic granuloma, hemangioma, and conjunctival inflammation.[40] Management of conjunctival KS, as discussed previously for KS of the eyelids, is based on accompanying ocular symptoms and systemic disease.

Other anterior segment disorders associated with AIDS include conjunctival microvasculopathy such as dilated capillaries, microaneurysms, and sludging of blood flow,[29, 32] nonspecific conjunctivitis,[14, 15] CMV conjunctivitis with keratitis sicca,[18] and squamous cell carcinoma of the conjunctiva.[70] Infectious keratitis due to herpes simplex and zoster viruses, microsporidia, and *Candida* species has also been reported.[11, 15, 32]

The most common opportunistic ocular infection is CMV retinitis, and it occurs in approximately one fourth of AIDS patients. Direct invasion of retinal cells by the virus leads to progressive, full-thickness retinal necrosis. Early retinal lesions usually affect the posterior pole and appear as irregular, granular white dots that eventually coalesce with associated hemorrhage. Without treatment, relentless progression of the retinitis, optic nerve involvement, and exudative retinal detachment usually lead to blindness.[29, 32, 42] Antiviral therapy with ganciclovir or forscarnet are effective in delaying the progression of CMV retinitis; however, their use is often limited by hematologic and renal toxicity, respectively.[32, 71]

Other intraocular infections include toxoplasmic retinochoroiditis,[29, 32] luetic retinitis[15, 28, 32] and uveitis,[11] *Candida* chorioretinitis,[12, 15, 28, 32] and atypical mycobacterial choroiditis.[12, 15] Noninfectious HIV-related retinopathy, which occurs in most patients with AIDS, is characterized by cotton wool spots, microaneurysms, telangiectasia, hemorrhages, perivasculitis, and ischemic maculopathy.[11, 12, 15–18, 19, 28, 29, 32] Finally, the posterior segment may be susceptible to the development of neoplasms such as intraocular malignant lymphoma.[57, 72]

Numerous neuro-ophthalmologic abnormalities, including optic nerve disease and cranial nerve palsies, may be a presenting manifestation of AIDS. Papilledema may occur due to intracranial disease, such as progressive multifocal leukoencephalopathy, cryptococcal meningitis, and other intracranial opportunistic infections.[12, 14, 15, 29, 33] CMV retinitis with optic nerve involvement and chronic papilledema may result in optic atrophy.[11, 14, 33] Luetic optic neuritis,[15, 32] anterior ischemic optic neuropathy,[28] visual field defects,[11, 15, 28] and cortical blindness[11] have also been described in HIV-infected patients. Extraocular motility disorders may also be an early sign of central nervous system disease in patients with AIDS. Cranial nerve palsies and gaze palsies have been associated with central nervous system lymphoma, toxoplasmosis, herpes zoster, HIV infection, CMV brain stem encephalitis, and cryptococcal meningitis.[17, 28]

REFERENCES

1. Schwartz LK: Epidemiology of AIDS and transmission of human immunodeficiency virus. Ophthalmol Clin North Am 1:1–13, 1988.
2. Centers for Disease Control and Prevention: Update: Trends in AIDS diagnosis and reporting under the expanded surveillance definition for adolescents and adults—United States, 1993. MMWR 43:826–831, 1994.
3. Gottlieb MS, Schroff R, Schander HM, et al: *Pneumocystis carinii* pneumonia and mucosal candidiasis in previously healthy homosexual men: Evidence of a new acquired cellular immunodeficiency. N Engl J Med 305:1425–1431, 1981.
4. Masur H, Michelis MA, Greene JB, et al: An outbreak of community-acquired *Pneumocystis carinii* pneumonia: Initial manifestation of cellular immune dysfunction. N Engl J Med 305:1431–1438, 1981.
5. Bloom JN, Nussenblatt RB: The immunology of AIDS and the pathogenesis of HIV infection. Ophthalmol Clin North Am 1:15–29, 1988.
6. Dalakas M, Wichman A, Sever J: AIDS and the nervous system. JAMA 261:2396–2399, 1989.
7. Centers for Disease Control: Human immunodeficiency virus infection in the United States. MMWR 366:801, 1987.
8. Freeman WR, Gross JG: Management of ocular disease in AIDS patients. Ophthalmol Clin North Am 1:91–100, 1988.
9. Benson WH, Linberg JV, Weinstein GW: Orbital pseudotumor in a patient with AIDS. Am J Ophthalmol 105:697–698, 1988.
10. Pepose JS, Holland GN, Nestor MS, et al: Acquired immunodeficiency syndrome: Pathogenic mechanisms of ocular disease. Ophthalmology 92:472, 1985.
11. Kestelyn P: Ocular problems in AIDS. Int Ophthalmol 14:165–172, 1990.
12. Jabs DA, Green WR, Fox R, et al: Ocular manifestations of acquired immune deficiency syndrome. Ophthalmology 96:1092–1099, 1989.
13. Herman DC, Palestine AG: Ocular manifestations of Kaposi's sarcoma. Ophthalmol Clin North Am 1:73–80, 1988.
14. Newsome DA: Noninfectious ocular complications of AIDS. Int Ophthalmol Clin 29:95–97, 1989.
15. Kreiger AE, Holland GN: Ocular involvement in AIDS. Eye 2:496–505, 1988.
16. Holland GN, Pepose JS, Pettit TH, et al: Acquired immune deficiency syndrome: Ocular manifestations. Ophthalmology 90:859–873, 1983.
17. Palestine AG, Rodrigues MM, Macher AM: Ophthalmic involvement in acquired immunodeficiency syndrome. Ophthalmology 91:1092–1099, 1984.
18. Khadem M, Kalish SB, Goldsmith J, et al: Ophthalmologic findings in acquired immune deficiency syndrome (AIDS). Arch Ophthalmol 102:201–206, 1984.
19. Rosenberg PR, Uliss AE, Friedland GH, et al: Acquired immunodeficiency syndrome: Ophthalmic manifestations in ambulatory patients. Ophthalmology 90:874–878, 1983.
20. Fujikawa LS: New therapies for HIV infection. Ophthalmol Clin North Am 1:111–121, 1988.
21. Masure H, Ognibene FP, Yarchoan R, et al: CD4 cell counts as predictors of opportunistic pneumonias in human immunodeficiency virus (HIV) infection. Ann Intern Med 11:223–231, 1989.
22. Gonnering RS, Kronish JW: Treatment of periorbital molluscum contagiosum by incision and curettage. Ophthalmic Surg 19:325–327, 1988.
23. Kohn SR: Molluscum contagiosum in patients with acquired immunodeficiency syndrome [letter]. Arch Ophthalmol 105:458, 1987.
24. Robinson MR, Udell IJ, Garber PF, et al: Molluscum contagiosum of the eyelids in patients with acquired immunodeficiency syndrome. Ophthalmology 99:1745–1747, 1992.
25. Font RL: Eyelids and lacrimal drainage system. *In* Spencer WH (ed): Ophthalmic Pathology: An Atlas and Textbook, 3rd ed, vol 3. Philadelphia, WB Saunders, 1986, pp 2260–2261.
26. De Luise VP, Wilson FM: Varicella and herpes zoster ophthalmicus. *In* Tasman W, Jaeger EA (eds): Duane's Clinical Ophthalmology, vol 4. Philadelphia, JB Lippincott, 1991, pp 1–21.
27. Cole EL, Meisler DM, Calabrese LH, et al: Herpes zoster ophthalmicus and acquired immune deficiency syndrome. Arch Ophthalmol 102:1027, 1984.
28. Ai E, Wong KL: Ophthalmic manifestations of AIDS. Ophthalmol Clin North Am 1:53–61, 1988.
29. Schuman JS, Orellana J, Friedman AH, Teich SA: Acquired immunodeficiency syndrome (AIDS). Surv Ophthalmol 31:384–410, 1987.
30. Drew WL, Mills J, Hauer LB, et al: Declining prevalence of Kaposi's sarcoma in homosexual AIDS patients paralleled by fall in cytomegalovirus transmission [letter]. Lancet 1:66, 1988.
31. Volberding PA, Mitsuyasu RT, Golando JP, Spiegel RJ: Treatment of Kaposi's sarcoma with interferon alfa-2b (Intron A). Cancer 59:620–625, 1987.

32. Holland GN, Pepose JS, Dinning WJ: Ophthalmic disorders associated with selected primary and acquired immunodeficiency disease. *In* Tasman W, Jaeger EA (eds): Duane's Clinical Ophthalmology, vol 5. Philadelphia, JB Lippincott, 1991, pp 1-20.
33. Rao NA, Biswas J: Ocular pathology in AIDS. Ophthalmol Clin North Am 1:63-72, 1988.
34. Macher AM, Palestine A, Masur H, et al: Multicentric Kaposi's sarcoma of the conjunctiva in a male homosexual with the acquired immunodeficiency syndrome. Ophthalmology 90:879-884, 1983.
35. Nadji M, Morales AR, Ziegles-Weissman J, Penneys NS: Kaposi's sarcoma: Immunohistologic evidence for an endothelial origin. Arch Pathol Lab Med 105:274-275, 1981.
36. Beckstead JH, Wood GS, Fletcher V: Evidence for the origin of Kaposi's sarcoma from lymphatic endothelium. Am J Pathol 119:294-300, 1985.
37. Soll DB, Redovan EG: Kaposi's sarcoma of the eyelid as the initial manifestation of AIDS. Ophthal Plast Reconstr Surg 5:49-51, 1989.
38. Dugel PU, Gill PS, Frangieh GT, Rao NA: Ocular adnexal Kaposi's sarcoma in acquired immunodeficiency syndrome. Am J Ophthalmol 110:500-503, 1990.
39. Ghabriel R, Quivey JM, Dunn JP Jr, Char DH: Radiation therapy of acquired immunodeficiency syndrome-related Kaposi's sarcoma of the eyelids and conjunctiva. Arch Ophthalmol 110:1423-1426, 1992.
40. Shuler JD, Holland GN, Miles SA, et al: Kaposi sarcoma of the conjunctiva and eyelids associated with the acquired immunodeficiency syndrome. Arch Ophthalmol 107:858-862, 1989.
41. Visser OHE, Bos PJM: Kaposi's sarcoma of the conjunctiva and CMV retinitis in AIDS. Doc Ophthalmol 64:77-85, 1986.
42. Holland GN: Acquired immunodeficiency syndrome. *In* Gold DH, Weingeist TA (eds): The Eye in Systemic Disease. Philadelphia, JB Lippincott, 1990, pp 240-243.
43. Mansour AM: Orbital findings in acquired immunodeficiency syndrome. Am J Ophthalmol 110:706-707, 1990.
44. McCluskey PJ, Wakefield D: Aust N Z J Ophthalmol 13:293-298, 1985.
45. Dugel PU, Gill PS, Frangieh GT, Rao NA: Treatment of ocular adnexal Kaposi's sarcoma in acquired immunodeficiency syndrome. Ophthalmology 99:1127-1132, 1992.
46. Centers for Disease Control: Guidelines for prevention of transmission of the human immunodeficiency virus and hepatitis B virus to healthcare and public safety workers. MMWR 38[Suppl 6]:1, 1989.
47. Goldberg SH, Fieo AG, Wolz DE: Primary eyelid non-Hodgkin's lymphoma in a patient with acquired immunodeficiency syndrome. Am J Ophthalmol 113:216-217, 1992.
48. Kass LG, Hornblass A: Sebaceous carcinoma of the ocular adnexa. Surv Ophthalmol 33:477-490, 1989.
49. Friedberg DN, Warren FA, Lee MH, et al: *Pneumocystis carinii* of the orbit. Am J Ophthalmol 113:595-596, 1992.
50. Gilberg SM, Kronish JW, Tse DT, Scott KR: Orbital manifestations of acquired immunodeficiency syndrome. Scientific poster, American Academy of Ophthalmology Annual Meeting, Dallas, October 1992.
51. Kronish JW, Johnson T, Gilberg SM, et al: Orbital infections in acquired immunodeficiency syndrome. Submitted for publication.
52. Vitale AT, Spaide RF, Warren FA, et al: Orbital aspergillosis in an immunocompromised host. Am J Ophthalmol 113:725-726, 1992.
53. Meisler DM, Mandelbaum S: *Propionibacterium*-associated endophthalmitis after extracapsular cataract extraction: Review of reported cases. Ophthalmology 96:54-61, 1989.
54. Fabricius EM, Hoegl I, Pfaeffl W: Ocular myositis as first presenting symptom of human immunodeficiency virus (HIV-1) infection and its response to high-dose cortisone treatment. Br J Ophthalmol 75:696-697, 1991.
55. Levine AM: Non-Hodgkin's lymphomas and other malignancies in the acquired immune deficiency syndrome. Semin Oncol 14:34-39, 1987.
56. Moore RD, Kessler H, Richman DD: Non-Hodgkin's lymphoma in patients with advanced HIV infection treated with zidovudine. JAMA 265:2208-2211, 1991.
57. Ziegler JL, Miner RC, Rosenbaum E, et al: Outbreak of Burkitt's-like lymphoma in homosexual men. Lancet 1:631-633, 1982.
58. Subar M, Neri A, Inghirami G, et al: Frequent c-*myc* oncogene activation and infrequent presence of Epstein-Barr virus genome in AIDS-associated lymphoma. Blood 72:667-671, 1988.
59. Brooks HL, Downing J, McClure JA, Engel HM: Orbital Burkitt's lymphoma in a homosexual man with acquired immune deficiency. Arch Ophthalmol 102:1533-1537, 1984.
60. Tien DR. Large cell lymphoma in AIDS [letter]. Ophthalmology 98:412, 1991.
61. Antle CM, White VA, Horsman DE, Rootman J: Large cell orbital lymphoma in a patient with acquired immune deficiency syndrome. Ophthalmology 97:1494-1498, 1990.
62. Turok DI, Meye DR: Orbital lymphoma associated with acquired immunodeficiency syndrome [letter]. Arch Ophthalmol 10:610-611, 1992.
63. Font RL, Laucirica R, Patrinely JR: Immunoblastic B-cell malignant lymphoma involving the orbit and maxillary sinus in a patient with acquired immunodeficiency syndrome. Ophthalmology 100:966-970, 1993.
64. Green WR: The uveal tract. *In* Spencer WH (ed): Ophthalmic Pathology: An Atlas and Textbook, 3rd ed, vol 3. Philadelphia, WB Saunders, 1986, pp 1671-1675.
65. Gross FJ, Waxman JS, Rosenblatt MA, et al: Eosinophilic granuloma of the cavernous sinus and orbital apex in an HIV-positive patient. Ophthalmology 96:462-467, 1989.
66. Freeman WR, Lerner CW, Mines JA, et al: A prospective study of the ophthalmologic findings in the acquired immune deficiency syndrome. Am J Ophthalmol 97:133-142, 1984.
67. Purtilo DT: Opportunistic cancers in patients with immunodeficiency syndromes. Arch Pathol Lab Med 111:1123-1129, 1987.
68. Farizo KM, Buehler JW, Chamberland ME, et al: Spectrum of disease in persons with human immunodeficiency virus infection in the United States. JAMA 267:1798-1805, 1992.
69. Irwin LE, Begandy MK, Moore TM: Adenosquamous carcinoma of the lung and the acquired immunodeficiency syndrome [letter]. Ann Intern Med 100:158, 1984.
70. Winward KE, Curtin VT: Conjunctival squamous cell carcinoma in a patient with human immunodeficiency virus infection. Am J Ophthalmol 107:554-555, 1989.
71. Studies of ocular complications of AIDS Research Group, in collaboration with the AIDS Clinical Trials Group. N Engl J Med 326:213, 1992.
72. Schanzer MC, Font RL, O'Malley RE: Primary ocular malignant lymphoma associated with the acquired immune deficiency syndrome. Ophthalmology 98:88-91, 1991.

CHAPTER 48

Micropigmentation and the Patient with Facial Burn and Facial Reconstruction

Richard W. Story and Darlene P. Story

> A postoperative hypopigmented area with or without a scar may negate any cosmetic improvement.[1]
>
> LARRY MILLIKAN

Reconstructive surgeons continue to research and advance the aesthetic treatment of burns and scars, with a particular emphasis on facial reconstruction. The use of new procedures has greatly enhanced the aesthetic look for patients with facial burns and scars.

Armed with scalpel and laser, the reconstructive surgeon can correct for texture, tension, and form but pigmentation remains a nemesis. Techniques such as skin grafts, melanocyte exchange grafts,[2] psoralens and ultraviolet A light (PUVA) therapy,[3] and laser surgery[4] have been employed to correct pigmentation problems inherent in burn and scar patients. These methods all have their limitations, and their success is unpredictable.

Micropigmentation, or medical tattooing, offers hope for the correction of pigmentation problems for the patient suffering facial burns and scars. This procedure offers the reconstructive surgeon total control and greater predictability of color correction and can be used to simulate the appearance of eyebrows, eyelashes, and lip borders.[5]

Tattooing conjures up the image of faddish body art performed in an unsterile back room and has met with disdain by the medical community.[6] Micropigmentation, or medical tattooing, is the surgical implantation of inert pigment granules in a clean surgical atmosphere by medically trained personnel for the purpose of cosmetic enhancement or medical pigment correction.[5] Although the purpose of a tattoo is to be seen, micropigmentation's purpose is one of concealment and camouflage.

HISTORY OF MICROPIGMENTATION

The first recorded use of micropigmentation was by Galen in the second century when he used copper sulfate to tattoo a cornea scar. Micropigmentation was used in the later part of the 1800s to treat congenital purple plaques and nevi and in the practice of cheiloplasty. It was also used for the cosmetic improvement of unsightly cornea scars from glaucoma.[7] In 1911, Kolle used micropigmentation to change the contour of scarred lips and to revise scars.[7] The landmark work of modern micropigmentation was performed by Conway, Hante Brown, Cannon, McDowell, and Robbins. Micropigmentation was performed on skin grafts and flaps as well as for the treatment of capillary hemangiomas. Beard, in 1960, described the use of micropigmentation to simulate eyelashes as an alternative to eyelash grafting.[7]

Micropigmentation experienced a leap in popularity with Angres' development of the blepharopigmentation procedure.[5] Blepharopigmentation is the cosmetic enhancement of the upper and lower eyelid by the implantation of pigment. Originally, this procedure was intended for women who had difficulty applying makeup (e.g., those with presbyopia, arthritis) or those who were allergic to cosmetic ingredients.

Micropigmentation has now found a place in the medical armamentarium. It is used to simulate brow hair for sparse brows; for alopecia and burn victims[8]; to camouflage scars after surgery, blend skin grafts, and mask skin defects (e.g., vitiligo)[3]; and for corneal tattooing.[9]

FACIAL MICROPIGMENTATION

Facial burns and scars pose a special challenge to reconstructive surgeons. Burns and scars are an impairment, but when they involve the face their visibility makes them a disfigurement. Facial reconstruction encompasses the objective of return of normal function, contour, and color.[10]

Pigmentary changes resulting from facial trauma most often occur in the form of keloids and hypertrophic, hyperpigmented, and hypopigmented scars.[4] The pigmentary management of keloids and hypertrophic and hyperpigmented scars can be obtained through various techniques with moderate success, such as surgery, pressure, irradiation, laser, dermabrasion, skin grafts, and pharmacologic treatment. Hypopigmented scars are characterized by a lightening of skin tone. Repigmenting techniques such as PUVA, melanocyte exchange, grafts, and cell growth have been employed with moderate success.[11] However, none of these techniques provides the surgeon with the predictability, flexibility, and control that micropigmentation offers.

The advantages of micropigmentation versus other repigmentation treatments can be characterized as its color simulation and ease of performance.

COLOR

Color Matching

In the past, the major obstacle to reconstructive micropigmentation was the need to get a proper color match. The difficulties of color matching were directly due to the limited number of available pigment colors. But in the past 5 years the number of pigment colors has tripled; 45 pigment shades are offered. It is now possible to obtain a near-perfect color match of any complexion or skin tone, and the color match obtained through micropigmentation is far superior than possible with any other method.

Color Adjusting

Scars are seldom one color; even hypopigmented scars reflect a variance of color.[12] The successful pigmentation of scars requires the ability to adjust for this variance. For example, hypopigmented scars may reflect pinkish undertones in certain areas and adjustments must be made to compensate for this pink hue, or else the undertone will show through. Micropigmentation offers the potential to make these adjustments and can be used to refine and maintain a near-perfect color match by performing periodic touch-ups.

Shading and Blending

The most dramatic aspect of a wide scar is the color of its outer edge, and the key aspect of thin scars is shape. The aesthetics of a scar are improved by lessening the color distortion between the outer edge of the scar and the surrounding tissue or the break-up of the shape of the scar.[13] The coloration of the scar's edges are shaded by a light brush stroke using a flat shading brush (several needles in a flat row). A scar's edge can be broken up using the same method, brushing across the entire width of the scar and in short intervals along the length of the scar (Figs. 48–1 and 48–2).

Blending is usually done on large grafted tissue to blur its distinctness. Blending merges the surrounding skin tone color to the graft with the depth of penetration, lessening as you move farther away from normal tissue. This is best done by implanting the pigment in a pointillistic fashion.

EYELINER RECONSTRUCTION

The eyelid, particularly the lid margin, is one of the most delicate and sensitive tissues on the face. Trauma to this area often results in partial or total loss of eyelashes. Lashes have a practical function, but their major value tends to be aesthetic. Without lashes, the eyes appear smaller and less defined. The best treatment for this disfigurement is blepharopigmentation, which is a micro-

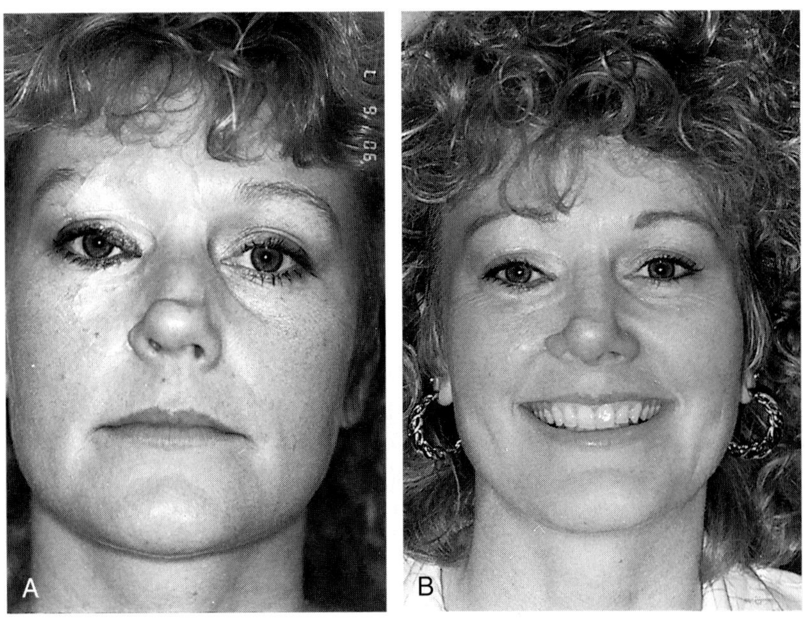

Figure 48–1. This patient was born with a hemangioma (port-wine stain). At age 2, the hemangioma was removed and replaced with a large graft. At age 32, the patient desired to improve the overall appearance of the graft, missing brow, and nose. *A*, Preoperative appearance. *B*, Postoperative appearance. (*A* and *B* courtesy of Joyce Miller, MPS.)

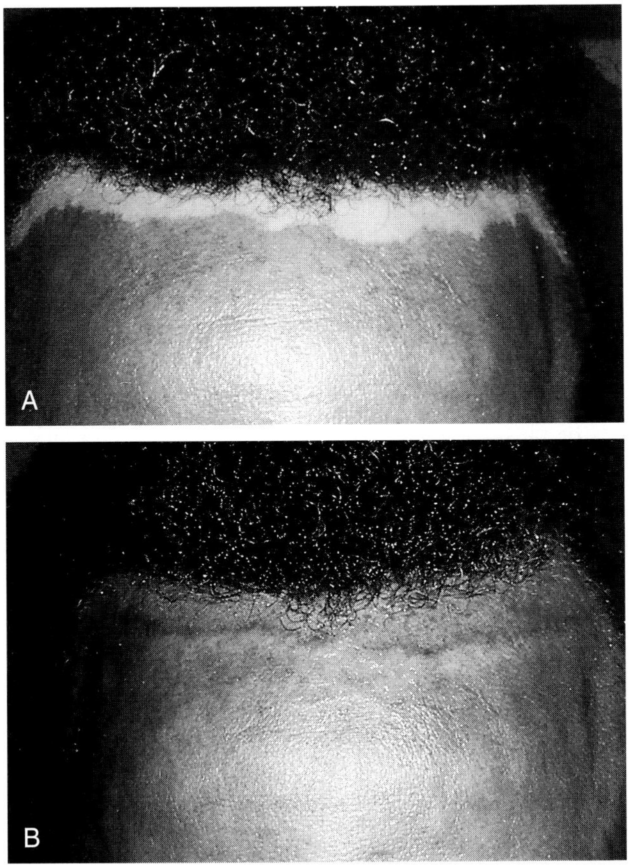

Figure 48 – 2. *A*, Patient with vitiligo. *B*, Same patient after treatment with forehead pigmentation. (*A* and *B* courtesy of Rebat Halder, MD.)

surgical procedure involving the implantation of pigment in a dot-like matrix into the base of the eyelashes. Because the pigment is placed in the dermis, the epidermis will cover it as the healing process takes place. This creates a translucent effect that looks very natural (Figs. 48 – 3 and 48 – 4).[5]

Suggestions to keep in mind for eyeliner reconstruction are presented here:

1. The medium brown pigments are suggested for a subtle appearance.
2. The dark brown pigments are suggested for a darker appearance.
3. The brown/black and gray pigments are suggested for a more dramatic appearance.
4. *Note*: Black pigment is not recommended for Caucasian patients.
5. *Note*: Organic pigments *must not* be used around the eyes.[14, 15]

EYEBROW RECONSTRUCTION

The partial or total loss of the eyebrows is a severe disfigurement and quite common for two reasons. First, due to their location at the ridge of the brow, they are particularly vulnerable to accidental abrasions and burns. Second, for cosmetic purposes, many women pluck their eyebrows. Over time, this can result in partial or full and permanent loss of brow hair (Figs. 48 – 5 and 48 – 6).[10]

Micropigmentation is increasingly being used as an alternative procedure to the traditional strip graft and hair punches for brow reconstruction. It eliminates the need for surgery, and the results are excellent, particularly in the case of partial brow loss. The micropigmentation procedure involves implantation of pigment in the brow line with a brush stroke technique that simulates strands of hair.

Suggestions for eyebrow reconstruction include the following:

1. Be conservative in the color choice; exact color match or 5% lighter shades are recommended.
2. The lighter shades of browns and taupe pigments are suggested for a more subtle and natural look.
3. On patients with fair skin, light hair, or light eyebrows, it is not recommended to use red tone pigments.

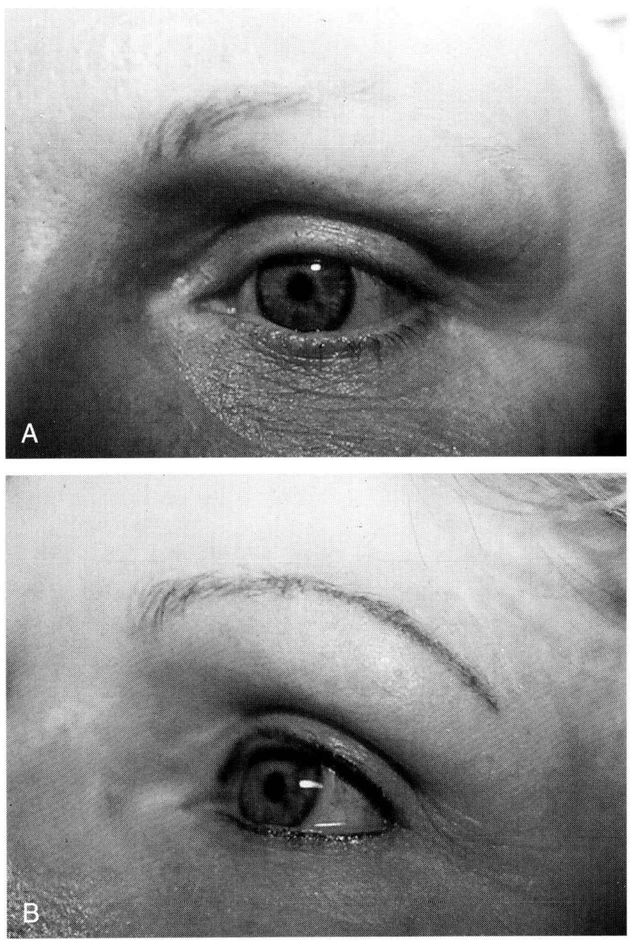

Figure 48 – 3. *A*, Patient with alopecia areata. *B*, Same patient after treatment with eyeliner and eyebrow pigmentation. (*A* and *B* courtesy of Harold Brody, MD.)

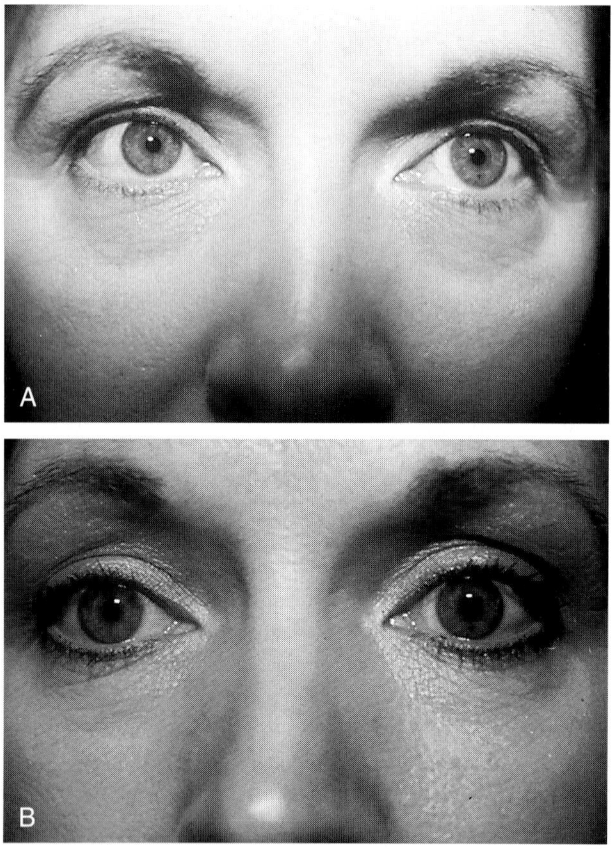

Figure 48–4. *A*, Preoperative appearance of patient. *B*, Patient after treatment with eyeliner pigmentation. (*A* and *B* courtesy of Harold Brody, MD.)

4. For highlighting and natural appearance, use of more than one color is recommended; for example, place a few strokes of a darker pigment among a predominantly lighter coloration within the brow area.[14, 16]

OTHER APPLICATIONS OF MICROPIGMENTATION

Although the usefulness of micropigmentation is obvious in facial plastic surgery, such as the simulation of eyebrows and eyelashes, its applications are much broader. It provides the surgeon with a color-correction system that eliminates the need to perform skin grafts and other surgery.[17] It also eliminates the need to select donor sites on the basis of the right skin tone. For example, the scalp is a popular location to harvest tissue for various facial reconstructions mainly because of its color. Micropigmentation permits the use of tissue obtained from more convenient and suitable sites of the patient's body. This is particularly important when large amounts of tissue are required.

Micropigmentation can also help to limit the extent of aesthetic reconstructive facial surgery. For example, without micropigmentation, the nose is typically resurfaced entirely because partial resurfacing results in a patched appearance as a result of the difficulty of matching skin colors.[10] Micropigmentation shading and blending can correct color differences, and this in turn permits the surgeon to simplify the surgical procedure.

Reconstructive surgery often necessitates the creation of a wound to correct another. The donor site for skin grafts is an example of this situation. Often this process results in scarring or hypopigmentation at the donor site.[12] Micropigmentation shading is ideal for correcting such defects. This corrective process is equally applicable in dermabrasion in which hypopigmentation is a common result.

In summary, pigmentary corrections of scars and burns (except for keloids and hypertrophic and hyperpigmented scars) by micropigmentation is only limited by the creativity and excellence of the person performing the procedure.

PIGMENT SELECTION

Various types of pigments are being used, from vegetable-based dyes and India ink to gold. Many of these pigments can cause an allergic reaction and result in pigment migration (pigment spreading) in the dermis or create more serious complications. Therefore, only high-quality, sterile, iron oxide pigments made from approved ingredients should be used.[18, 19]

The pigment molecule size should be 6 μm or more. Six micrometers is the ultimate particle size for pigment to be properly maintained in the dermis. If properly applied, there is less likelihood of rapid fading. If the pigment particle size is less than 6 μm, it can be readily enveloped by fixed tissue histiocytes or migrating macrophages and the pigment will be removed from the body through the process of phagocytolysis. However, if the pigment particle size is 6 μm or more, it is more difficult for the pigment to be engulfed, and migration and fading is therefore less likely.[7, 20–23]

PIGMENTATION COLOR MIXING PROCEDURE

It is best to perform the color mixing process during the patient consultation. This permits the patient to assist the physician with the color selection for optimal results.

1. Using a color chart, select two to three colors that match patient's skin and eyebrows.
2. Select and remove these same pigments from the mixer/tester kit (Fig. 48–7).
3. Remove one plastic slide and container with toothpicks.
4. Remove three toothpicks from toothpick container.
5. Open one of the pigment colors selected. Place a toothpick into the container and mix the pigment. (The pigment can also be mixed by shaking the container vigorously.)

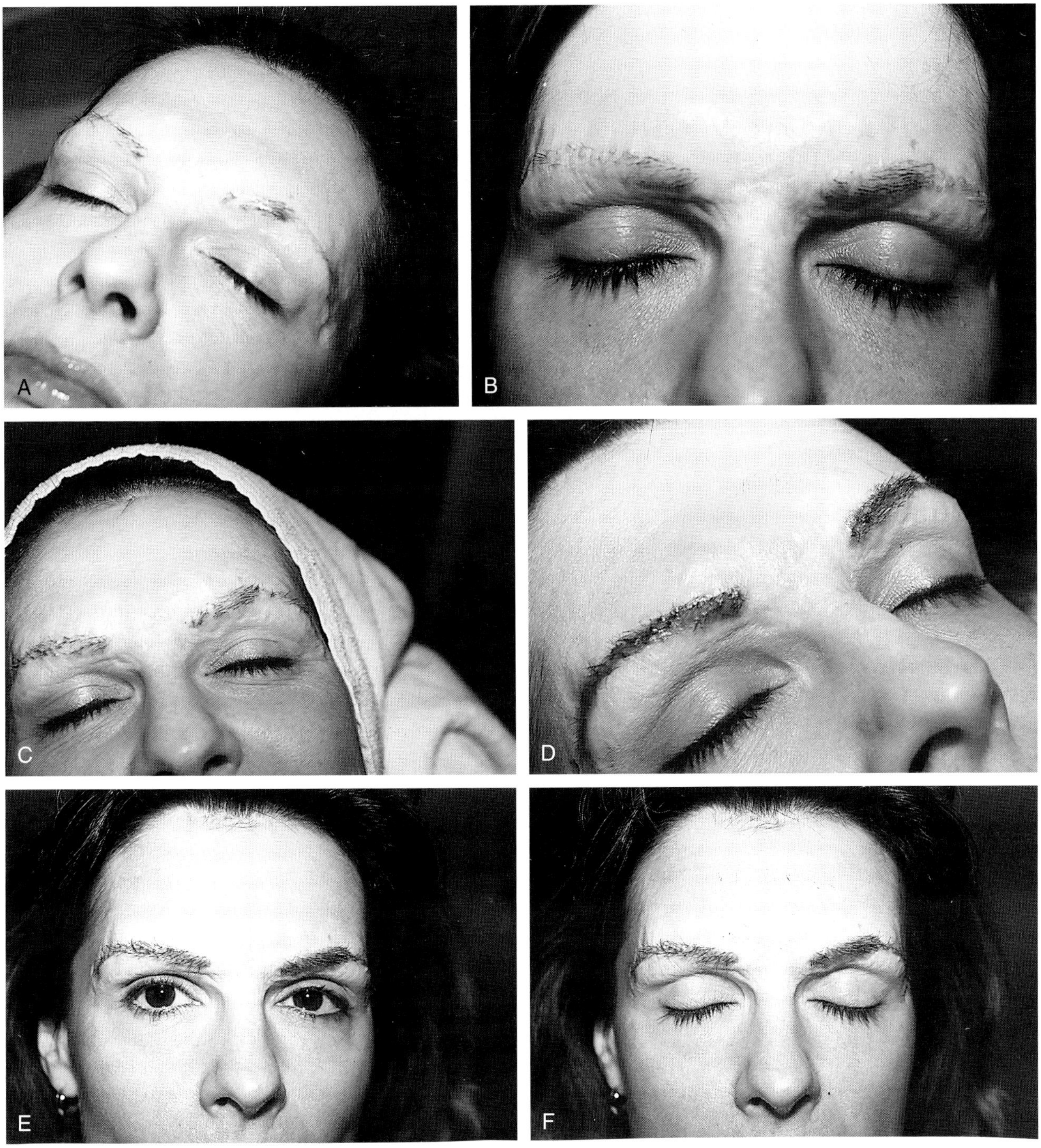

Figure 48–5. A 35-year-old Caucasian woman who sustained chemical burns to the supraorbital area bilaterally approximately 15 years earlier from using a cream depilatory agent on her eyebrows. The cream was left on overnight. *A*, Before treatment. *B*, After eyebrow transplant. C, Before pigmentation. *D*, After pigmentation. *E* and *F*, One month after pigmentation. (*A* to *F* courtesy of Theresa Wichtowski, CA, CPE.)

6. Place one small line of pigment on the plastic slide. Put the used toothpick aside.
7. Using a clean toothpick, open another of the selected pigment colors and repeat steps 5 and 6.
8. Take the slide with pigment and place it against the patient's skin. (*Note*: the slide is pliable plastic and can be contoured to any area of the patient's body.) If color selection is accurate, take a clean toothpick and place a dot of pigment from the slide directly on the patient's skin to see how well the color matches.
9. If color selection needs to be lightened, always start with the light color first and drop by drop add a darker color to properly achieve the results necessary. (To duplicate color with the larger pigment size, one drop of pigment on the toothpick is equivalent to one drop of pigment.)

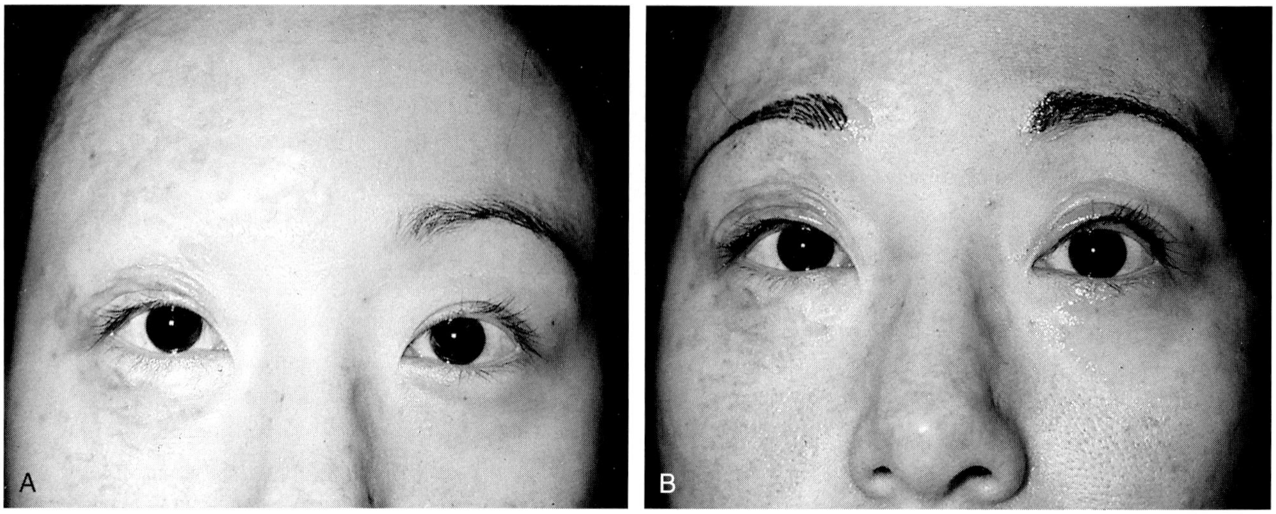

Figure 48–6. A 31-year-old burn survivor who permanently lost her right eyebrow and right upper and lower eyelashes as the result of a fire ignited upon impact during a car accident. She received second- and third-degree burns. *A*, Preoperative appearance. *B*, Postoperative appearance. (*A* and *B* courtesy of Yolanda Moore, MPS.)

10. Helpful hints:
    a. To "yellow up" color, use Yellow Modifier sparsely.
    b. To counteract red, use Green 2 sparsely.
    c. To counteract yellow, use Lavender Tint sparsely.
    d. To lighten gray pigment for eyebrows or eyeliner, try Brown 9, 10, or 11.
    e. To lighten dark pigment, try Beige 12 and add drop to a drop of a darker color.
    f. Caution is advised when mixing with white pigment—very little is required for mixing.
    g. Brown 8 is a truer brown and works well on eyebrows and patients with vitiligo.
11. If the area to be pigmented is large, use the oval/pointed applicator stick to spread the sample pig-

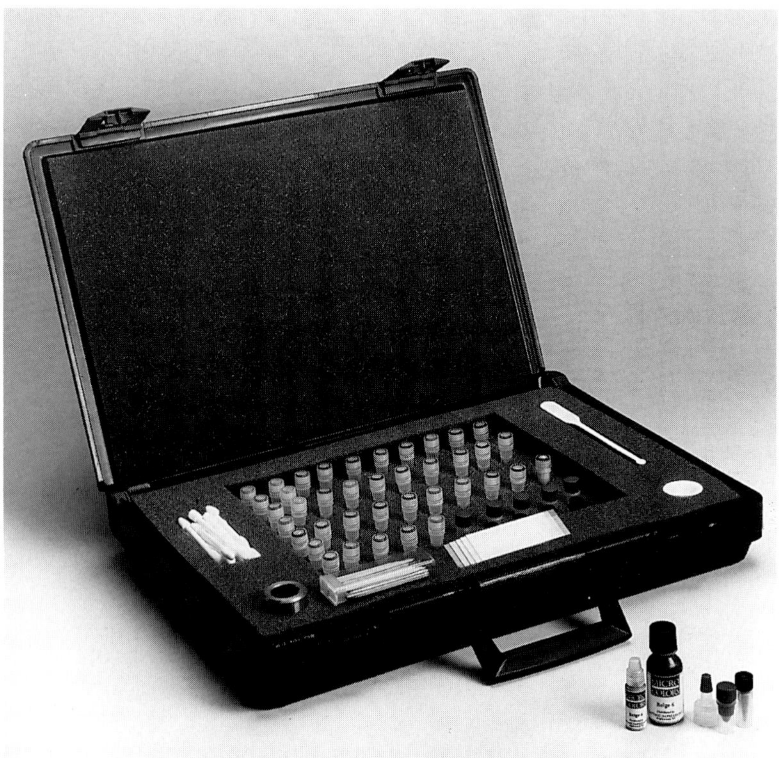

Figure 48–7. Mixer/tester kit for pigmentation color mixing.

ment on the patient to see how well the color matches.
12. To retrieve a larger amount of pigment from the vials, use a mix/dip spoon and place the desired amount onto a plastic slide or into a mixing pot. (Always first stir pigment well.)
13. A tester vial is used to perform a skin test. A 1-mL sterile syringe is used to draw a small amount of pigment. It is recommended that a patch test be performed directly on the pigmentation procedure site (e.g., eyebrows) and any reaction monitored.[14]

GUIDELINES FOR SKIN TESTING

Micropigmentation pigments can be subdivided into two categories: (1) inorganic and (2) organic pigments. Inorganic pigments consist of the relatively inert ingredients of iron oxide, glycerin, and alcohol. Organic pigments are commonly composed of red D&C dyes (drug and cosmetic dyes as listed in the FDA cosmetic additives) and coal tar derivatives.[24]

The iron oxide pigments are commonly used for eyeliner, eyebrow, and camouflaging procedures. The organic red dyes are commonly used for lip pigmentation.

In view of the invasive nature of micropigmentation and as a precaution against allergic reactions, it is recommended to conduct a thorough skin test before this procedure with any type of pigment to be used. The following skin test process is recommended for each patient.

1. Conduct a "scratch test" (depositing several dots of pigment on skin) on the back of the patient's ear. The back of the ear has sensitive tissue; therefore, any adverse reaction to the pigment to be used will more than likely appear here. Usually any adverse reaction is pruritic (intense itching of the skin without eruption) and is associated with erythema nodosum (abnormal redness of the skin with nodule-like characteristics).
2. Conduct an additional scratch test between the toes. Because this area is usually clothed, warm, and moist, its skin tissue is even more sensitive than the back of the ear. Therefore, any adverse reaction to the pigment to be used should more than likely appear here.
3. Conduct a "patch test" (depositing a series of dots of pigment on skin) in the area where the micropigmentation procedure will be performed. This will show if the specific site itself is susceptible to any adverse reaction.
4. *Note*: Each organic pigment has different ingredients; therefore, it is necessary to perform a separate patch test for each organic pigment. This is not necessary for different colors of inorganic pigment. The following test periods are recommended for skin patch tests[14]:
   a. Inorganic pigment: 5 to 7 days skin patch test.
   b. Organic pigment: 30 to 60 days skin patch test.

CONCLUSION

In terms of self-image, facial injuries are different from injuries elsewhere on the body. Whereas burns and scars on, for example, arms and legs are considered simply injuries, these same injuries on the face are viewed as disfigurements.

New techniques have evolved that are greatly improving the aesthetics of facial reconstruction. However, dyspigmentation and, particularly, hypopigmentation remain formidable obstacles.

With the micropigmentation procedure, these obstacles can be overcome completely. The introduction of new pigment skin colors makes it possible to match virtually every skin tone to correct dyspigmentation. In addition, micropigmentation is tremendously successful in simulating eyeliner and eyebrow.

Finally, micropigmentation used in combination with facial reconstructive surgery offers the unique advantage of allowing the surgeon to limit actual surgery and complement reconstruction with perfect coloration of critical facial features.

REFERENCES

1. Millikan LE: Surgical anatomy of the facial skin. *In* Thomas G, Holt J, Regan C (eds): Facial Scars: Incision, Revision & Camouflage. St. Louis, CV Mosby, 1989, p 4.
2. Robinson CM, Barnett AR, Leitch OWI: Prevention and treatment of post burn scars and contracture. World J Surg 16:87–96, 1992.
3. Halder RR, Pham HN, Breadon JY, Johnson BA: Micropigmentation for the treatment of vitiligo. J Dermatol Surg Oncol 15:1092–1098, 1989.
4. Henderson DL, Cromwell TA, Mes LG: Argon and carbon dioxide laser treatment of hypotrophic and keloid scars. Laser Surg Med 3:271–277, 1984.
5. Angres GG: Blepharo- and dermapigmentation techniques for facial cosmesis. Ear Nose Throat J 66:344–353, 1987.
6. Parry A: Tattoo, Secrets of Strange Art as Practiced among the Natives of the United States. New York, Simon & Schuster, 1933.
7. Zwerling CS, Christensen HF, Goldstein FN: Micropigmentation. State of the Art [Library of Congress No. 93-061357], 1993.
8. Patipa M: Eyelid tattooing. Adv Dermatol Surg 5:335–348, 1987.
9. Reed JW, Beran RF: Elimination of monocular diplopia by corneal tattooing. Ophthalmic Surg 19:437–439, 1988.
10. Young VL, Bartell HT: Burns of the face. *In* Thomas GR, Holt J, Regan C (eds): Facial scars: Incision, revision and camouflage. St. Louis, CV Mosby, 1989, pp 229–269.
11. Green H: Cultured cells for the treatment of disease. Sci Am 265:96, 1991.
12. Panke TW, McLeod CG Jr: Pathology of Thermal Injury: A Practical Approach. Orlando, FL, Grune & Stratton, 1985, p 111.
13. Thomas RJ, Bluestein JL: Cosmetics and hairstyling as adjuvants to scar camouflage. *In* Scar Revision. St. Louis, CV Mosby, 1989, pp 349–351.
14. Story DP, Story RW: Mixer/Tester Kit Booklet. Englewood, NJ, Lasting Impression I, 1992, pp 1–7.
15. Cristian S: Specific illustrations and guidelines for consulting on micropigmentation and eye cosmetics. *In* Understanding the Role of Eye Make Up in Today's Society. New York, The Facial Center, 1987.
16. Jackson C: Color Me Beautiful Make Up Book. New York, Ballantine Books, 1987.
17. Onur Erol O, Atabay K: The treatment of burn scar hypopigmen-

tation and surface irregularity by dermabrasion and thin skin grafting. Plast Reconstr Surg 85:754–758, 1990.
18. Story RW, Story DP: Focus spotlight. Skin January/February: 83, 1993.
19. Moore Y: Micropigmentation pigments. Adv Dermatol News 2(1):17, 1993.
20. Hurwitz JJ, Brownstein S, Mishkin SK: Histopathological findings in blepharopigmentation (eyelid tattoo). Can J Ophthalmol 23:267–269, 1988.
21. Tse DT, Folberg R, Moore K: Clinicopathologic correlate of a fresh eyelid pigment implantation. Arch Ophthalmol 103:1515–1517, 1985.
22. Patipa M, Jakobiec FA, Krebs W: Light and electron microscopic findings with permanent eyeliner. Ophthalmology 93:1361–1365, 1986.
23. Wolfley DE, Flynn KJ, Cartwright J, Tschen JA: Eyelid pigment implantation: Early and late histopathology. Plast Reconstr Surg 82:770–773, 1988.
24. Moore Y: Allergic reactions to organic cosmetic tattoo pigments. Adv Dermatol News 2(3), 1993.

SECTION

IV

Cosmetic Surgery

SECTION EDITORS

Ted. H. Wojno
Stephen L. Bosniak

Introduction

Stephen L. Bosniak

To perform cosmetic blepharoplasty in a satisfactory manner, the surgeon must be familiar with the normal eyelid and orbital anatomy and its variants as well as the technical options for their alteration. This type of surgery requires not only technical perfection but also the ability to perceive and understand the patients' desires. In addition, awareness of the comparative advantages of sophisticated surgical modalities, such as radio-frequency instrumentation (Fig. IV-1) and lasers (Fig. IV-2), is essential.

Blepharoplasty is not simply an operation for the removal of excess fat or hypertrophic muscle or redundant skin. When the cosmetic surgeon evaluates the patient, the diagnosis of any associated medical deformities must also be made.

When properly performed, cosmetic blepharoplasty can be the avenue for functional repair of congenital and involutional defects. Levator aponeurotic advancements, lateral canthal resuspensions, adjustments of lower lid margin malpositions, and laxity can all be conveniently incorporated into the blepharoplasty procedure. Adjacent facial tissue malformations, malpositions, and laxity must also be recognized and addressed either before or at the time of blepharoplasty. Browplasties and rhytidectomies are performed when necessary at the time of blepharoplasty.

Patient expectations are high. Patients may no longer be satisfied with mere structural correction of their eyelids; the surgeon must now address the need for resurfacing the eyelids with chemical peels or laser abrasions. In addition, because these patients demand accelerated results, the use of adjunctive techniques should be investigated. Currently, clinical studies are under way to examine the effectiveness of lymphatic drainage massage and a computerized cooling and healing mask that is capable of delivering iontophoresis and transcutaneous electrical nerve stimulation (Fig. IV-3). Continued technical developments will undoubtedly enhance the final result of cosmetic blepharoplasty in the future.

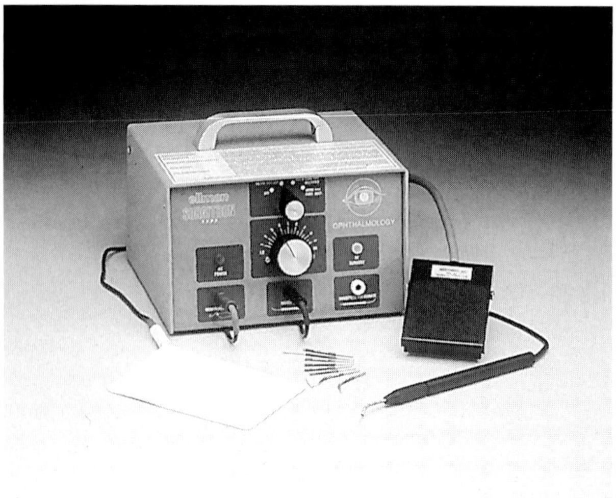

Figure IV – 1. A radio-frequency surgical unit that provides cutting, hemostatic, and blended cutting-hemostatic modes. (Courtesy of Ellman International, Hewlett, NY.)

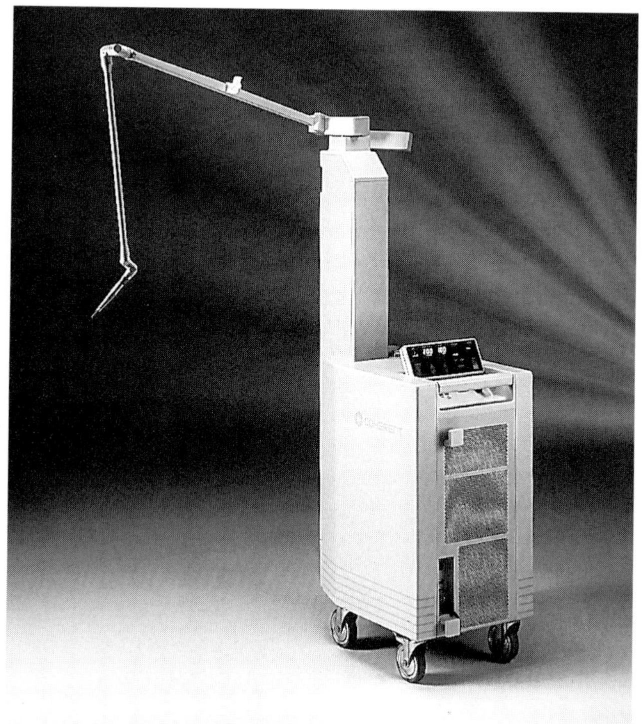

Figure IV – 2. An Ultrapulse carbon dioxide laser that may be used for blepharoplasty resections and laser abrasions. (Courtesy of Coherent, Inc., Palo Alto, CA.)

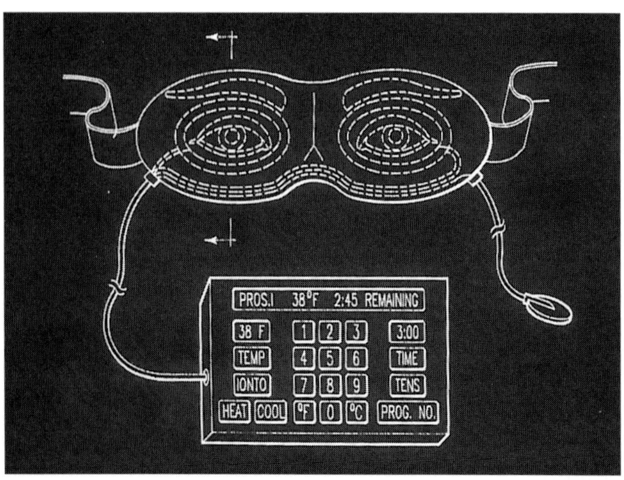

Figure IV – 3. The first proposal for the computer-controlled cooling-healing mask. (U.S. Patent Office, 1991; Bosniak, Kolen, U.S. patent no. 746, 658.)

CHAPTER 49

Preoperative Evaluation

Ted H. Wojno

Cosmetic blepharoplasty is, for many reasons, among the most challenging procedures performed by ophthalmologists. Truly outstanding results are difficult to obtain and are not always reproducible. Patient expectations are often very high or frankly unrealistic. Fortunately, most patients who seek blepharoplasty have reasonable requests for cosmetic improvement or may simply wish relief from visually disturbing hoods of upper lid skin. Such patients are grateful for properly performed surgery and become a source of future referrals.

Many patients seek cosmetic blepharoplasty without a clear idea of what they want corrected. They may simplistically request that the physician remove redundant skin when coexistent problems are present, such as brow or lid ptosis. Others instruct the physician to perform whatever surgery that he or she deems appropriate.

At the other end of the spectrum are patients who have agonized over the appearance of every wrinkle and can describe them with an almost microscopic attention to detail. Both types of patients may have unrealistic expectations for improvement and are bound to find fault with even the most expertly performed blepharoplasty.

An extensive discussion of blepharoplasty surgery and postoperative problems should therefore precede any surgical intervention. At this consultation, the physician should explore the patient's desires and set realistic goals for surgery. Preoperative counseling alleviates much anxiety and disappointment that could occur after completion of surgery.

A surgeon may be worried by a patient who has previously consulted other physicians. It is increasingly common for patients to obtain multiple opinions before having cosmetic surgery. It is hoped that such "comparison shopping" will lead to a better-educated patient. A physician who openly explains the surgery and potential complications before performing the surgery will project a favorable image to such an intelligent patient.

Cosmetic blepharoplasty is performed by physicians other than ophthalmologists, including plastic surgeons, otolaryngologists, oral surgeons, and dermatalogic surgeons. The ophthalmologist is obviously able to evaluate the visual system better than practitioners of the other specialties and should maintain a concern for visual function over cosmetic results. I stress this concept of "safe surgery" with every patient.

Virtually everyone, regardless of age, is a potential candidate for cosmetic surgery. I have operated on children in their early teens (usually "westernizing" procedures on adopted Asian children) and patients in their nineties (almost always functional blepharoplasty). The question arises, however, of whether one should perform blepharoplasty on a monocular patient. Despite the fact that the occurrence of blindness after blepharoplasty is exceptionally low,[1, 2] this risk must be carefully considered and the patient fully informed. Many monocular patients refuse surgery if informed of this rare complication.

The patient's overall health must be considered as it would be with any other surgery. Preoperative evaluation by an internist is appropriate if any doubt exists about the patient's health, especially when the surgery is performed in the physician's office.

EXAMINATION

A complete medical and ocular history should be obtained. The patient should be specifically questioned about all prescription and nonprescription medications that he or she is taking. The physician should also inquire about drug sensitivities and previous adverse reactions to surgery.

Thorough ophthalmic examination is necessary to rule out any unsuspected ocular pathology. It is critical to identify such problems because they may coincidentally manifest postoperatively and lead the patient to blame the surgical procedure for the problem.

Starting with the forehead, the physician should note the hairline. Patients with a high forehead or male pattern baldness may be poor candidates for a coronal lift, which would elevate the hairline even further or leave a visible scar. Prominent horizontal furrows on the midforehead can provide a suitable place to mask an incision line on such patients, although this approach is used infrequently.

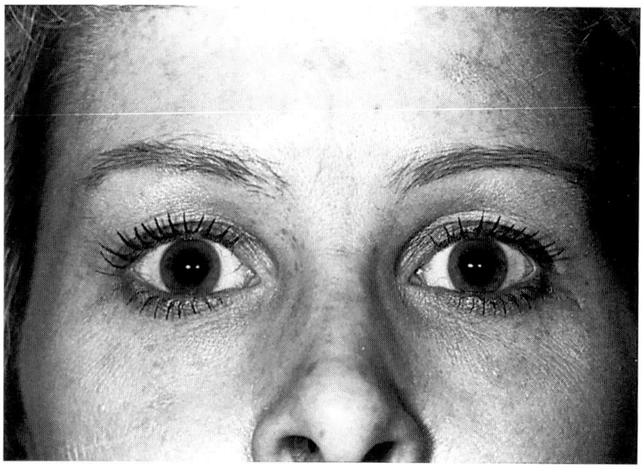

Figure 49–1. The normal female brow demonstrates a central arch that peaks between the lateral limbus and the lateral canthus.

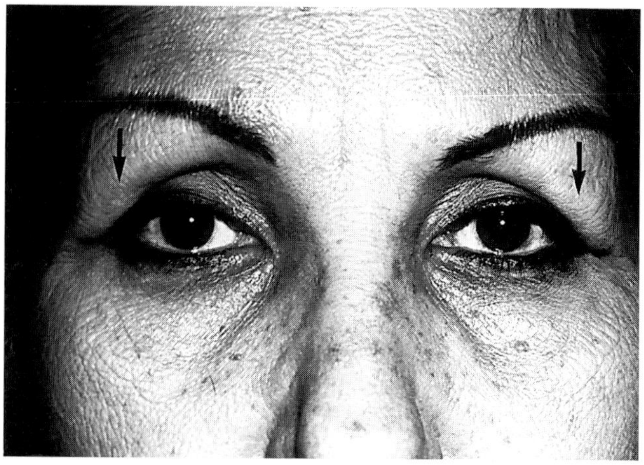

Figure 49–3. This patient has severe brow ptosis *(arrows)* but has plucked them and redrawn them at a higher level.

The physician should carefully evaluate the brow position. An aesthetically pleasing female brow sits above the supraorbital rim with a noticeable arch positioned between the lateral limbus and the lateral canthus (Fig. 49–1). The lateral half of the brow tapers downward only slightly. The male brow is somewhat flatter and positioned at the level of the supraorbital rim (Fig. 49–2). Brow ptosis should not be mistaken for upper lid dermatochalasis, because blepharoplasty only further lowers the brow position. In women, the physician should note if the lateral brow hairs have been plucked and redrawn at a higher level, camouflaging the true brow ptosis (Fig. 49–3).

The physician should note the contour of the brow. It may droop only segmentally in some patients. When marked, brow ptosis is usually much worse laterally, probably related to the lack of frontalis fibers on the lateral forehead (Fig. 49–4).[3] The physician should also look for asymmetry of brow position between the two sides; this feature may masquerade as excess skin on one upper lid as compared with the other (Fig. 49–5). Failure

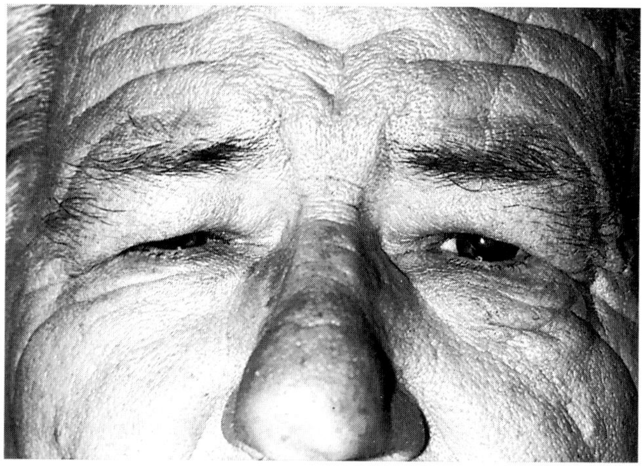

Figure 49–4. This patient demonstrates a severe brow ptosis that is much more marked laterally.

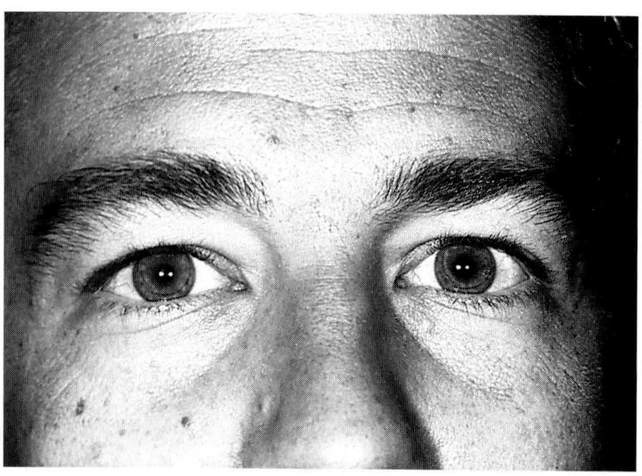

Figure 49–2. A typical male brow is flat and positioned at the level of the superior orbital rim.

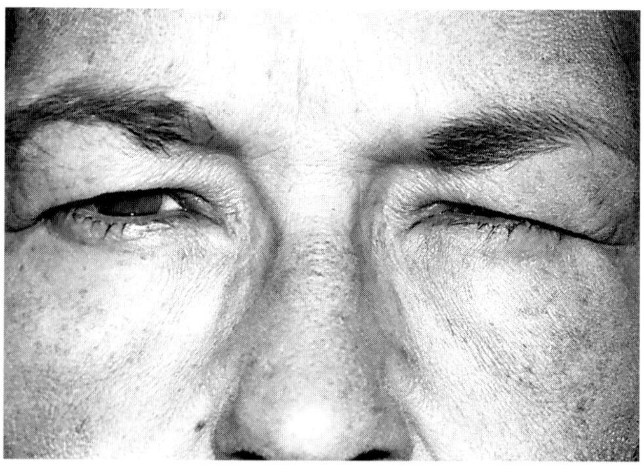

Figure 49–5. This patient demonstrates asymmetric brow ptosis that is worse on the left than on the right. This creates the impression of greater skin redundancy on the left eye.

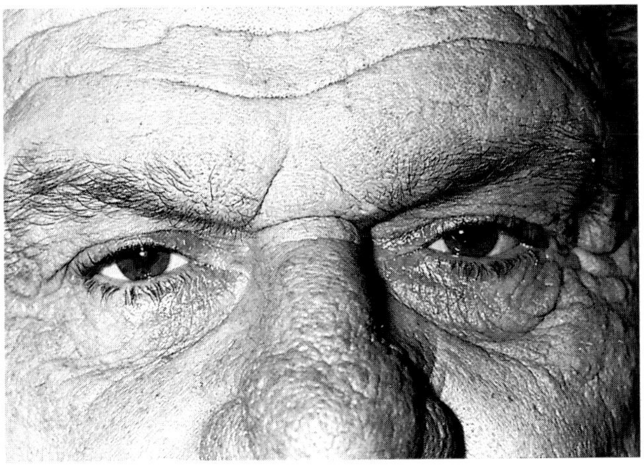

Figure 49–6. This patient demonstrates severe glabellar wrinkles between the eyebrows.

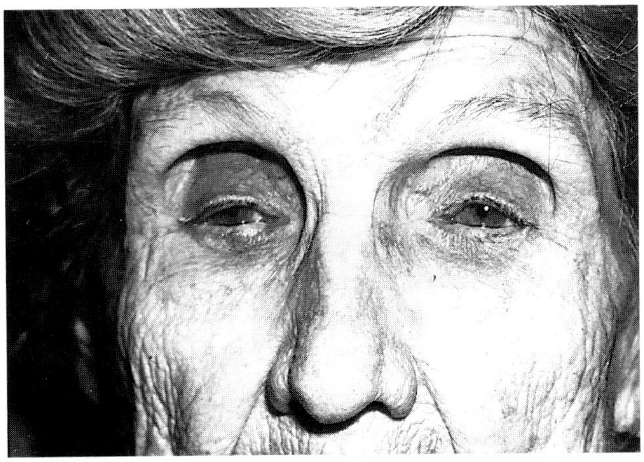

Figure 49–8. This patient demonstrates a severe atrophy of orbital fat as a consequence of aging.

to recognize this characteristic may lead to unequal supratarsal folds after surgery.

The physician should also look for glabellar wrinkles between the brows (Fig. 49–6). The vertical furrows result from the action of the corrugator muscles, and horizontal ones result from the action of the procerus muscle. Many patients mistakenly assume that these wrinkles can be corrected by blepharoplasty alone.

The brow may be excessively full because of the subbrow fat pocket, which lies behind the posterior frontal and orbicular muscle sheaths.[3] Alternatively, the bony supraorbital ridge may project excessively as a result of hyperpneumatization of the frontal sinus or cranial dysostosis.[4]

The physician should critically evaluate the amount of redundant upper lid skin and should note whether the upper lid crease is well formed and symmetrically placed in both upper lids. The physician should also determine the amount of redundant preaponeurotic fat in the medial and lateral compartments (Fig. 49–7). Light pressing against the closed upper lid will make the fat pockets clearly bulge. The physician should note any far lateral bulging, which is indicative of a prolapsed lacrimal gland that may require fixation to the orbital rim. Some patients may have very deep superior sulci owing to orbital fat atrophy; such individuals are obviously not candidates for blepharoplasty (Fig. 49–8).

The physician should check for true ptosis, which may be missed if dermatochalasis is marked. Uncorrected ptosis is more obvious after surgery, especially if the ptosis is unilateral. Lash ptosis, downward angulation of the lashes owing to relaxation of the anterior lamella of the eyelid, should also be noted and corrected during upper lid blepharoplasty.

In the lower lid, the physician should again note the amount of excess skin and fat. In this area, three fat pockets exist: medial, middle, and lateral (Fig. 49–7). Of these, the lateral is occasionally missed at surgery because of its more superior location. The physician should note the presence of any festoons, which are redundant skin folds along the inferior orbital rim that are sometimes filled with fluid (Fig. 49–9). These may have to be directly excised, sometimes as a separate procedure.

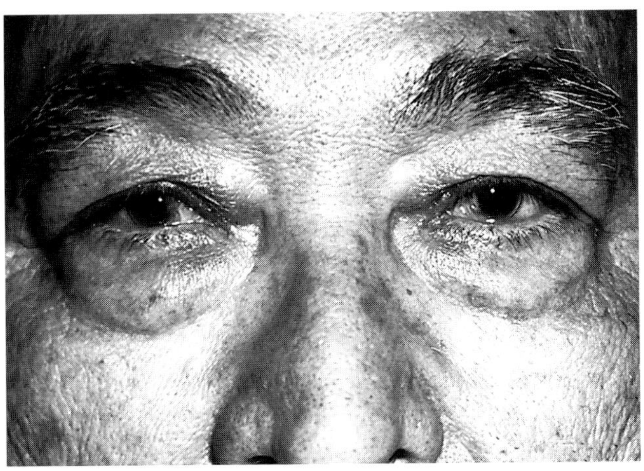

Figure 49–7. This patient demonstrates remarkable prolapse of the orbital fat in both the upper and lower eyelids.

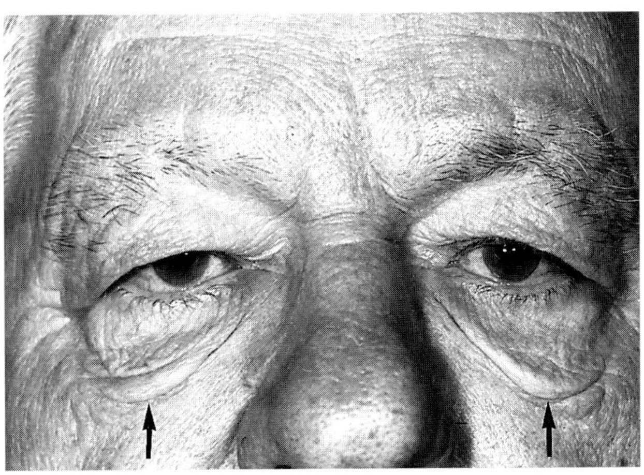

Figure 49–9. This patient has festoons in both lower eyelids *(arrows)*.

The physician should perform a lid distraction test to assess the degree of horizontal laxity and the strength of lateral canthal fixation to determine if the patient is likely to develop a postoperative ectropion or scleral show. In this procedure, the physician grasps the lid with the thumb and index finger and pulls it away from the globe. Lid distraction greater than 6 mm is at risk for postoperative ectropion or lagophthalmos if skin excision is aggressive. This complication is very likely to occur if lid distraction is greater than 10 mm. The physician performs the "snap back" test by pulling the lower lid inferiorly and then releasing it. A lid that fails to rapidly return to a snug position against the globe is also at risk for postoperative ectropion or lagophthalmos.

As much as 10% of the population may have naturally occurring scleral show unrelated to lower lid laxity.[5] This problem may result from slight hypoplasia of the maxilla and infraorbital rim, resulting in inadequate support of the lower lid. Alternatively, some patients have shallow sockets with relative physiologic exophthalmos. In young patients, slight inferior scleral show may actually be attractive, creating the appearance of large eyes (Fig. 49–10).[6] In older patients, these lids appear to have significant excess skin, but in reality the globe is pushing down on a poorly supported lid. It is a mistake to perform a horizontal shortening in these patients because the procedure will cause the lid to slip even further inferiorly and posteriorly under the globe, increasing scleral show. The importance of recognizing this entity preoperatively cannot be overemphasized.

The physician should look for subtle hints of Graves' ophthalmopathy. Mild cases often go unrecognized, and patients with such a condition may seek blepharoplasty for puffy eyelids (Fig. 49–11). In fact, the skin and subcutaneous tissues in these patients are thickened and infiltrated even after the disorder has resolved. The unsuspecting surgeon is surprised to find small fat pockets in patients with obviously puffy eyelids. It is best to operate

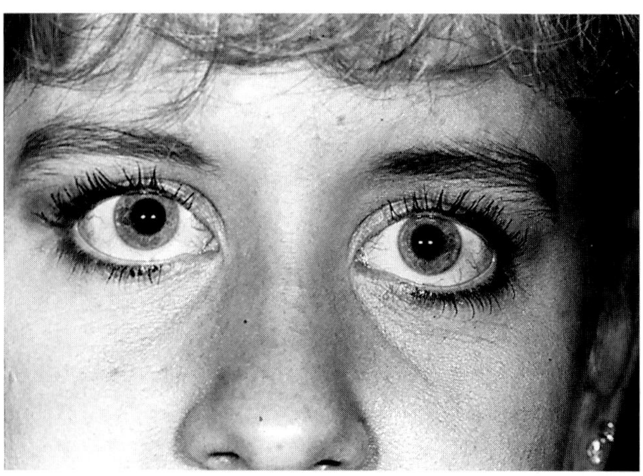

Figure 49–10. This patient has 2 mm of inferior scleral show as a normal anatomic variant. The effect, however, is pleasant and creates the appearance of large eyes.

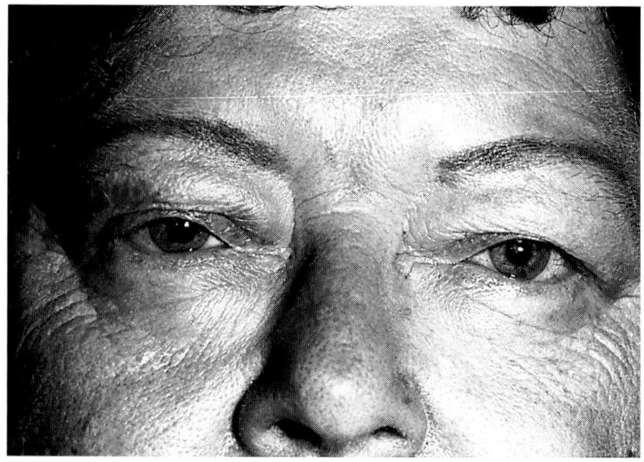

Figure 49–11. This patient presented for consideration of cosmetic blepharoplasty. A thorough ophthalmic and medical evaluation revealed Graves' eye disease.

on such patients only after they enter the inactive phase of the disease. Even so, these patients often have more bleeding and postoperative edema than would normally be expected.

The physician should suspect true blepharochalasis in patients with a history of episodic lid edema. Such patients have markedly thin, wrinkled skin that has been likened to cigarette paper. They have prominent telangiectatic vessels, severe fat atrophy, ptosis, and dehiscence of the lateral canthal tendon.[7] The lids of these patients may swell dramatically after blepharoplasty. For this reason, the surgeon may consider preoperative treatment with oral corticosteroids.

The physician should note the presence of lateral crow's-feet when the patient smiles. It is important to point out to the patient that crow's-feet are a natural part of facial expression and are not eliminated with blepharoplasty (Fig. 49–12). Even surgery aimed at direct excision of such lines is only minimally helpful. Collagen injection or chemical peel after surgery may decrease the prominence of these lines, and lateral brow lifting may also make them less noticeable.

Many patients complain of the presence of a thick roll of tissue below the lower lash line during smiling. Although sometimes thought to result from orbicular hypertrophy, this finding may also result from normal orbicular function in certain individuals (Fig. 49–12). With facial relaxation, this roll completely disappears.

Skin texture is an important consideration. Many older patients have very thin skin with little fixation to the underlying tissues. Overcorrection is easy in such patients because the skin can seemingly always be pulled tighter. The relatively thicker skin of younger patients is by contrast easier to contour, the lid creases easier to construct, and the fixation better maintained.

The physician should evaluate seventh nerve function. Occasionally, patients have mild weakness as a result of

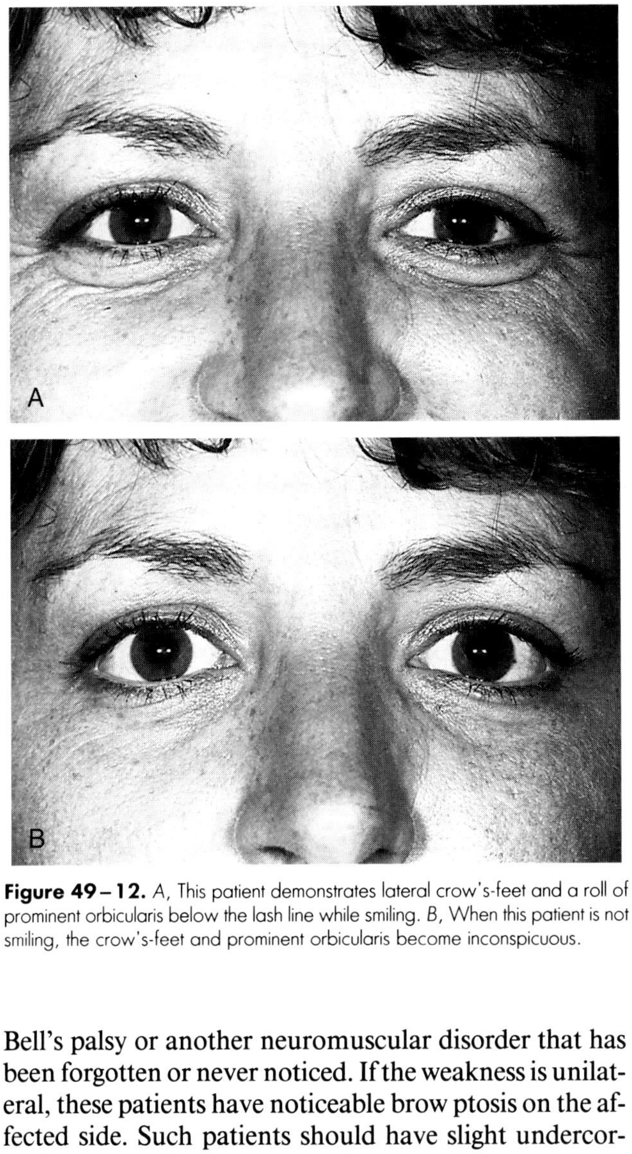

Figure 49 – 12. *A*, This patient demonstrates lateral crow's-feet and a roll of prominent orbicularis below the lash line while smiling. *B*, When this patient is not smiling, the crow's-feet and prominent orbicularis become inconspicuous.

Bell's palsy or another neuromuscular disorder that has been forgotten or never noticed. If the weakness is unilateral, these patients have noticeable brow ptosis on the affected side. Such patients should have slight undercorrection to avoid postoperative lagophthalmos.

The physician should determine the baseline tear function by performing a basic secretion tear test. Patients with severely dry eyes should have conservative skin excision to minimize the possibility of postoperative lagophthalmos. Even slight corneal exposure leads to severe symptoms in patients with true keratoconjunctivitis sicca.

DOCUMENTATION AND PATIENT INSTRUCTIONS

The physician should take preoperative photographs with the eyes in primary position to document the patient's appearance and any blockage of the pupillary axis.

The physician should perform a ptosis field to document any loss of the superior visual field resulting from the presence of redundant skin (Fig. 49 – 13). This test provides easily interpreted documentation of the degree of visual impairment to the insurance carrier. The test is best performed at a Goldmann-type perimeter using a large test object. Only the superior field need be tested.

It is often helpful to send a predetermination letter with photographs and visual fields to the patient's insurance carrier before surgery. No rigid or universally agreed on criteria exist by which the functional versus the cosmetic nature of blepharoplasty surgery can be determined. Predetermination, therefore, informs the patient in advance whether or not the claim will be covered and to what degree. This process usually takes 4 to 8 weeks.

I give all patients written instructions to refrain from taking any product containing aspirin or nonsteroidal anti-inflammatory drugs for 2 weeks before and 1 week after surgery. Both aspirin and nonsteroidal anti-inflammatory drugs have antiplatelet effects that increase bleeding and subsequent bruising. If the patient's general medical physician is unwilling to stop the administration of such drugs because the patient is at true cardiovascular risk, surgery can still be performed if the patient is aware of the increased risk of hemorrhage.

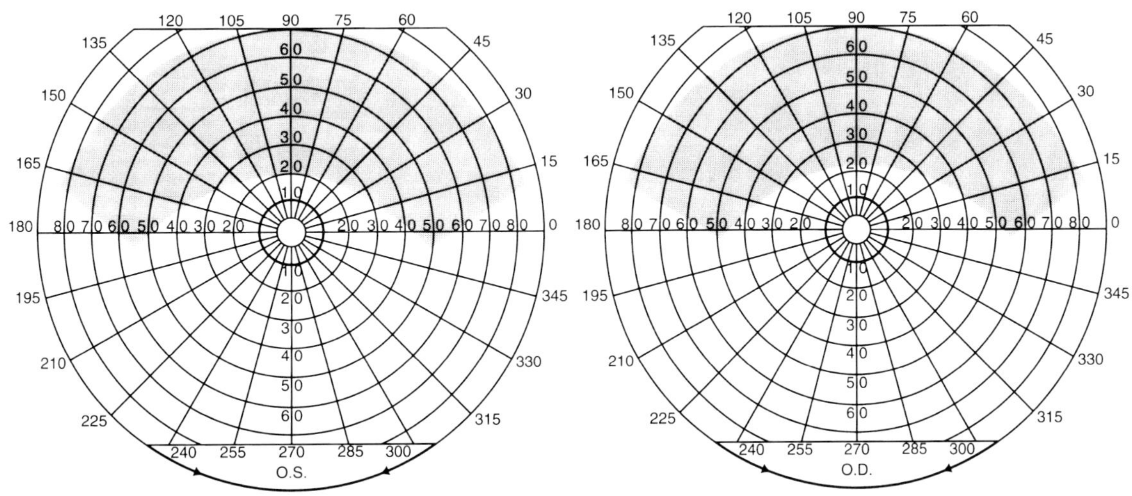

Figure 49 – 13. A typical ptosis field demonstrating the loss of visual field superiorly secondary to redundant skin.

Slight asymmetry of skin or fat removal is commonly found when the patient returns for suture removal. I counsel all patients, therefore, that a "touch up" may be necessary in the weeks following surgery. Patients who are forewarned of this possibility before surgery usually accept subsequent adjustments without any problem.

ANESTHESIA

I feel that local anesthesia, with or without sedation, is preferable to general anesthesia because local anesthesia allows for intraoperative adjustments of the surgery. In the upper lid, after skin and fat are removed and lid creases are formed, I place three to four temporary sutures across the incisions. The patient sits up on the operating table, allowing the surgeon to check for adequacy of skin and fat removal. The left and right sides are compared for symmetry, and if the sides are uneven, the sutures are removed, and modifications are made.

I prefer to use a one-to-one mixture of 2% lidocaine with epinephrine and 0.75% bupivacaine. I add 1 mL of hyaluronidase to 10 mL of this mixture. The hyaluronidase spreads the anesthetic through the tissues, decreasing the induced lid swelling. This measure increases the accuracy and precision of skin removal. The physician should use caution, however, when injecting beyond the lateral orbital rim. The hyaluronidase may actually spread the anesthetic to the superior branch of the facial nerve, resulting in temporary (up to 24 hours) paralysis of the ipsilateral frontal muscle.

UPDATE: ENDOSCOPIC BROW LIFT

At the time that this text was originally organized, the development of an endoscopic approach to brow and forehead lifts was unanticipated. For a detailed discussion of these techniques the reader is referred to an authoritative text.[8]

There are several advantages to the endoscopic brow lift. The entire surgery is performed through three small scalp incisions, thus minimizing scar formation, blood loss, and sensory loss normally associated with a coronal flap. The incisions are usually placed 1 to 2 cm posterior to the hairline to obviate the visible scar that results with a direct brow lift.

The corrugator and procerus muscles that are responsible for glabellar furrows can be directly excised under endoscopic visualization. Because these muscles are depressors of the brow, their resection results in relaxation of the opposing frontalis muscle, thereby reducing horizontal forehead wrinkles as well.

A single, midline, inverted T-shaped incision placed 1 to 2 cm behind the hairline is used to access the glabellar area. An elevator is used to develop an optical cavity beneath the periosteum inferiorly to the orbital rims and laterally to the anterior temporal crests. The lateral incisions are placed lateral to the temporal crests and go deep to both the temporoparietal fascia and the deep temporal fascia. An elevator is placed below the deep temporal fascia, thus freeing tissue down to the zygomatic arch and lateral orbital rim and then joining the dissection from the midline of the forehead.

The surgeon can incise the periosteum and expose the corrugator and procerus muscles, which are excised by using endoscopic visualization. The surgeon should use caution to avoid the supraorbital and supratrochlear vessels. A small amount of scalp is resected at each incision site, and these are closed to elevate the brows to the desired position and contour.

The obvious disadvantage to the technique is that it requires expensive endoscopic equipment, specialized instrumentation, and experience in a new surgical skill. The results, however, promise to be gratifying to both patient and surgeon.

REFERENCES

1. DeMere M, Wood T, Austin W: Eye complications with blepharoplasty or other eyelid surgery. Plast Reconstr Surg 53:634–637, 1974.
2. Wolfley DE: Blepharoplasty: The ophthalmologist's view. Otolaryngol Clin North Am 13:237–263, 1980.
3. Lemke BN, Stasior OG: The anatomy of eyebrow ptosis. Arch Ophthalmol 100:981–986, 1982.
4. Whitaker LA, Morales L, Farkas LG: Aesthetic surgery of the supraorbital ridge and forehead structures. Plast Reconstr Surg 78:23–32, 1986.
5. Mackinnon SE, Fielding JC, Dellon AL, Fisher DM: The incidence and degree of scleral show in the normal population. Plast Reconstr Surg 80:15–20, 1987.
6. Flowers RS: The art of eyelid and orbital aesthetics: Multiracial surgical considerations. Clin Plast Surg 14:703–721, 1987.
7. Custer P, Tenzel R, Kowalczyk A: Blepharochalasis syndrome. Am J Ophthalmol 99:424–428, 1985.
8. Bostwick J III, Eaves FF III, Nahai F: Endoscopic Plastic Surgery. St. Louis, Quality Medical Publishing, 1995.

CHAPTER 50

Photography of the Ophthalmic Plastic Surgery Patient

David A. B. Price

Photographing the external eye area can be a fairly simple matter if one has the correct equipment and some basic photographic knowledge. This chapter will take you beyond basic principles and, it is hoped, will help you to become a competent medical photographer.

The 35-mm single-lens reflex camera is probably the most practical camera for medical use because its viewfinder system is generally more than 95% accurate for making an image on film of exactly what is seen in the viewfinder. The single-lens reflex camera has the most accessories, such as lenses, viewfinders, and flashes, and perhaps the widest assortment of films to use.

I cannot recommend any of the medium-format cameras for medical work. These cameras provide film images of 2¼ × 2¼ inch or 2¼ × 2¾ inch. Medium-format cameras, such as the Hasselblad, can be clumsy and difficult to use. They are heavier than the 35-mm cameras and often have viewing systems through the top of the camera, which are very awkward to use when the camera is hand held or must be focused on a subject at head or shoulder height. These systems generally do not have the variety of lenses that are made for 35-mm cameras, and slide projectors for 2¼-inch square slides are not as readily available as 35-mm machines.

CAMERA FEATURES FOR MEDICAL PHOTOGRAPHY

The quality of a camera also must be considered carefully. The best professional 35-mm cameras are built to sustain a great deal of hard use. They are often designed for use in journalism and sports photography and are durably made. They often have high-strength alloy frames, titanium shutter systems, and strong gear components in the winding or film advance mechanisms. The shutters are often built to sustain at least 100,000 shots, whereas the less expensive cameras designed primarily for the amateur market sustain perhaps only one third of that number.

The Shutter and Shutter Speed

The camera's shutter is like a window shade that opens and closes quickly to let light in through the lens and onto the film plane. Shutter speeds are selected on the camera and can be made to open from several seconds to 1/4000 of a second on some cameras. All cameras have a certain shutter speed that is used to synchronize with the flash when it is used. This speed varies with the camera, but it is usually 1/60 to 1/250 of a second. For nonflash medical photography, one should not use a shutter speed below 1/125 of a second if one is holding the camera in one's hand because the slower speeds can result in blurring of the photograph and because it is very difficult to keep a camera steady at slow shutter speeds.

Automatic Film Advance

I believe that a camera with an automatic film advance sustains less abuse than a manually advanced camera because a mechanical advance executes a constant torque on the components, whereas a manual advance is often slammed by the user with considerable force, depending on how good—or how bad—a day the photographer is having.

I also prefer to use a film advance (called a motor drive or autowinder) that is detachable from the camera. In my experience, the motor drive mechanism absorbs considerable strain, and it is far likelier to malfunction than the camera itself. If the motor drive is detachable, then it alone goes into the shop, and one still has use of the camera; conversely, if the motor drive is integral to the camera, then one loses use of the camera entirely. I do not know of many amateur photographers—or surgeons—that have second cameras that are similar in quality and capability to their principal cameras. The motor drive is a luxury; the camera body itself is a necessity.

Flash-Cord Receptacle

It is also useful to have a flash-cord receptacle on the camera for use with an external or off-camera flash. Many of the new, completely automatic, flash-integral cameras do not have this feature, which is essential on a professional camera because it is used to trigger studio strobe lights.

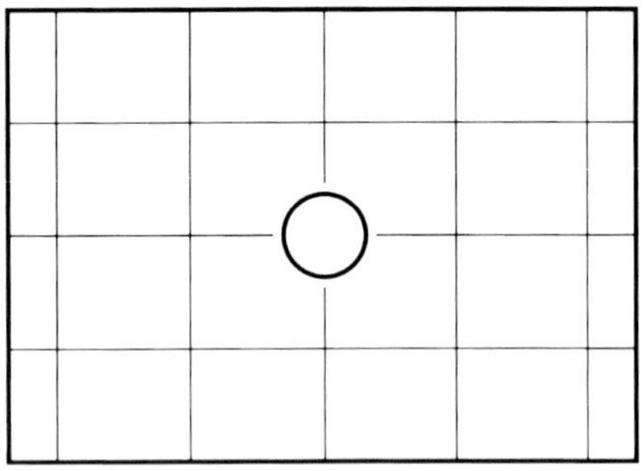

Figure 50–1. Diagram of a gridded split screen with focusing dot in the middle.

Focusing Screens

All professional cameras and most high-quality amateur cameras have interchangeable focusing screens—the ground glass fields on which the image that the film will record is seen by the viewer as he or she looks through the camera. I recommend changing the standard viewing (or focusing) screen for one that has a grid and a split-screen focusing dot in the middle (Fig. 50–1). All screens look sharp overall when an object is in focus, but when one is shooting at very close distances, focus is even more critical, and the split-screen dot in the middle is extremely accurate and may be used quickly.

A gridded screen enables the photographer to maintain a constant image size from patient to patient; for example, an image of an eye is the same size in every photo or slide. This feature greatly facilitates comparisons from patient to patient. If every eye photograph were of a slightly different size or were positioned differently in the picture, the visual effect would be distracting. Consistency in imaging is also most useful for before-and-after comparisons of surgical results.

Lens

The lens is the heart of the camera. Lenses for 35-mm cameras are vast in selection and type. These range from 6-mm, 220-degree, "fish-eye," wide-angle lenses to 2000-mm supertelephoto lenses. There are so-called zoom lenses with adjustable focal lengths (e.g., 43 mm to 86 mm, 80 mm to 200 mm), lenses that are very fast for low light conditions, lenses with circular (ring-light) flashes built into them, and lenses made especially for close-up photography.

Lens speed refers to how wide the aperture of a lens can be opened to allow in the most light. This aperture works similarly to the eye's iris: the lower the light level, the wider the iris opens to allow in light. The lower the aperture number, the faster the lens. Currently, the fastest lenses have apertures of about f/1.0 or 1.2. These apertures are adjustable via click stops down to f/32, which is the smallest opening for a 35-mm camera.

High-quality lenses should always be used, not just for the glass of the lens itself but for the tube that holds the lens elements and its aperture mechanism. The quality of the glass and the configuration of the elements that compose the camera lens are now uniformly excellent among all of the top camera manufacturers. The manufacturers even formulate their own glass compositions for nearly perfect clarity and color accuracy.

Our main concern is the quality of the aperture components because they take a lot of use. They are spring loaded to stay open at the largest aperture so that the image in the viewfinder is as bright as possible for the photographer. When the shutter release is pressed on the camera to take the picture, the aperture automatically "stops down" to the correct or selected aperture and then springs open again to the largest opening after the picture is made. This event happens in anywhere from a second or more (a time exposure) to 1/4000 of a second, so there is friction and strain on the aperture parts, in addition to the stress caused by the constant cranking in and out of the lens barrel while one is focusing. Higher-quality lenses are better able to withstand the wear caused by these activities.

The focal length of the lens is simply the distance in millimeters from the end of the lens to the plane of the film. Lenses with focal lengths of 6 to 35 mm are wide-angled lenses; lenses with lengths in the 50- to 75-mm range are the so-called normal lenses. These lenses are most similar in field of vision to the unaided human eye, although technically, the focal length of a normal lens is defined as the approximate length of the diagonal of the rectangular film area it is to cover. Lenses in the 80- to 135-mm range are medium telephoto lenses and are also known as "portrait" lenses because they give the most accurate, least distorted view of a person's head and shoulders. Long telephoto lenses can have focal lengths in excess of 2000 mm and can cause backgrounds to appear pulled up directly behind the subject and foreground elements to be similarly pushed back. With these lenses, the overall imaging can appear compressed.

Any wide-angle or normal lens is really unsatisfactory for full facial and close-up eye photographs. To fill the film frame with a picture of the face or eye area, the photographer must get close to the subject with the camera—50-mm lens will fill the film frame with a person's face with the camera held about 15 inches from the subject. The wide-angled and normal lenses used at distances as close as this will severely distort the photograph. The effect is as if the face "balloons" toward the camera: noses and lips seem to bulge out at the photographer. These images are not at all accurate and virtually all of the popularly available Polaroid cameras have fixed-medium wide-angled lenses. Many doctors use these types of cameras to document cases, and the results are usually unrealistic. One has to pull the camera back to include most of the head and torso before the distortion is diminished. The problem of close-up distortion persists until one uses lenses in excess of about 85 mm (Fig. 50–2).

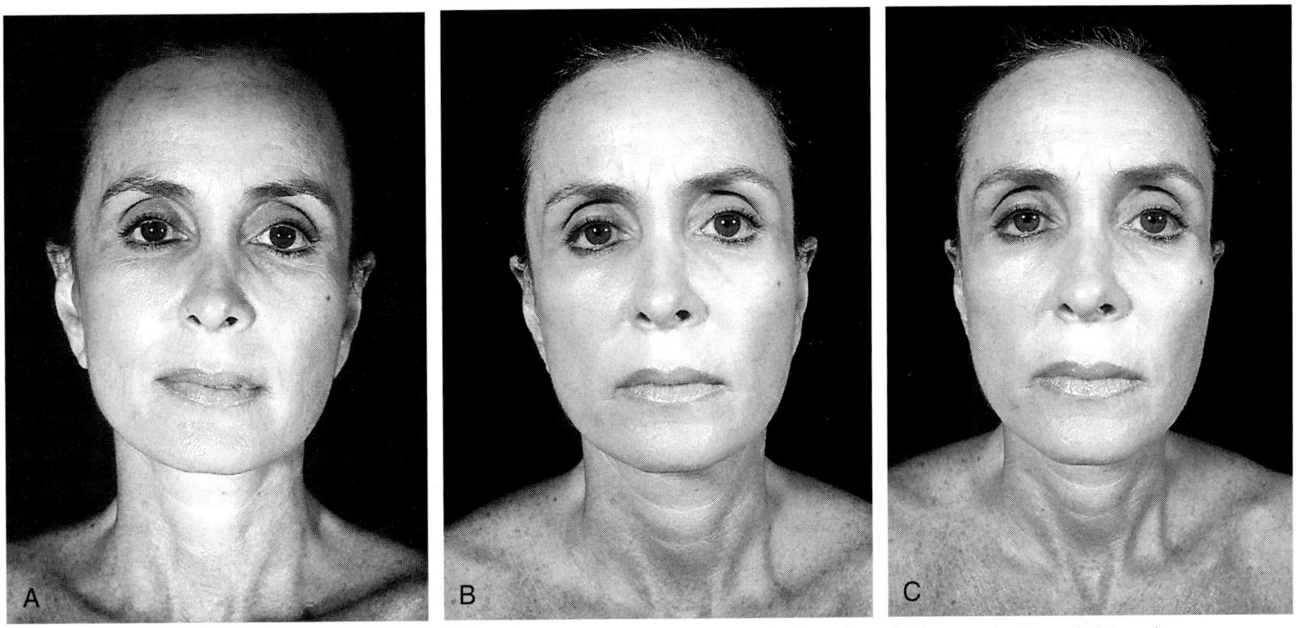

Figure 50–2. *A*, Photograph taken with 105-mm lens. *B*, Photograph taken with 55-mm lens. *C*, Photograph taken with 35-mm lens.

The best lenses for photographing the eyes are those in the 85- to 105-mm lengths. Actually, lenses longer than 105 mm are good, too, but they may be heavy and are hard to hand hold without shaking the camera. In fact, all lenses much longer than 105 mm should be firmly braced or used on a tripod. Long lenses are extremely sensitive to movement. A 200-mm lens that is hand held and used at a slow shutter speed, such as 1/60 of a second, almost certainly will move when the shutter is tripped; at slower shutter speeds, even heartbeat may cause the image to soften. Many amateur photographers buy 80- to 200-mm zoom lenses because the lenses are obviously versatile only to complain that the lens does not take photographs that are as sharp as the other, fixed focal length lenses they own. Frequently, the reason for this effect is that the photographer zooms to 150 or 200 mm while holding the camera in his or her hand, and the weight of the camera or a hard push on the shutter button causes a slight blur that is just enough to take the hard edge off the sharpness. Using a tripod almost always corrects this.

In addition to these limitations, not many lenses can focus closely enough to fit the image of just a single eye in the frame of the camera and also be able to pull back and focus to infinity, if need be. A special group of lenses is made to minimize distortion at close distances and is able to focus on objects from a few inches away to infinity. These macrofocusing lenses are lightweight and fairly compact. They are popularly available in 55-, 105-, and 200-mm focal lengths, and each length focuses closely enough to fill the film frame with a single human eye. I have always used the 105-mm length because at its closest focusing distance, it is about 10 inches from the subject, which is far enough back so I can put light from a non–camera-mounted flash or light source onto the subject without blocking the light. The 55-mm macrofocusing lens would be about 5 inches from the subject for the same shot, which is too close. The 200-mm macrofocusing lens should not be used, because it is too heavy to hold in the hand.

Macrofocusing lenses are not particularly fast, usually about f/2.8, but this characteristic is not really important to the medical photographer, who is in control of the light sources: the medical photographer can use a strong flash, artificial light, or even more sensitive film to compensate for low level of existing light.

Another reason why a fast lens is not especially important to the medical photographer is depth of field, which is the distance from the part of the subject closest to the camera to the part of the subject farthest from the camera that will be in sharp focus at a given lens aperture. A greater zone of sharp focus is achieved when the aperture is used at smaller apertures. At high reproduction ratios, that is, when one is holding the camera very close to the subject, the depth of field is rather shallow. Generally, for photographing the eye area an aperture of no larger than f/8 should be used. At the smaller apertures (f/8, 11, 16, 22, and 32), virtually everything important is in focus, even allowing for minor error in the perceived sharpness of the subject through the viewfinder.

Besides the aperture of the lens, the focal length of the lens also affects its depth of field. Shorter lenses, such as a 35-mm lens, set at a given aperture have much greater depth of field than would a longer lens, such as a 135 mm set at the same aperture.

For medical photography of the eye area, a 105-mm macrofocusing lens used at an aperture of f/8 or smaller gives excellent overall sharpness. The speed of the macrofocusing lens used in medical photography is consequently not very important, because medical photographers would never photograph with the lens at its widest (most open) aperture: depth of field at that point would be virtually nonexistent. Part of an eye would be in focus but another part, perhaps only 1/4 inch further in front or behind, would not be in focus, and it is extremely visually distracting when part of this sort of photograph is in focus and part is soft and fuzzy.

Film

Dozens of superb films are made for 35-mm cameras. Only color films for prints and slides are discussed here because the use of black and white prints for medical use is not a state-of-the-art choice. People are used to seeing the world in color, and for medical use, the nuance of color, the enhanced dimensional feeling, and the overall illusion of greater realism are invaluable. In addition, the cost of high-quality color prints is much less than the price of similarly sized black and white prints.

Color film comes in two varieties: one yields color prints and is called *negative* film, and the other produces color slides or transparencies and is sometimes called *reversal* film. Color transparency film is not flexible in terms of exposure error—virtually none exists—which is why professional photographers almost always "bracket" their exposures. In other words, they shoot several shots of the same subject but vary the exposure slightly, such as 1/3 of an f-stop, each time. A shot that is metered at f/11, for example, is shot at f/11, but also at f/8 1/3, f/8 2/3, f/11 1/3, and f/11 2/3. If the photographer is certain that the meter is perfectly accurate, that the lighting is totally consistent, and that all other variables are controlled, then he or she need not bracket. Film, however, is a cheap element in photography, and the subjects of medical photographs may not present themselves again. With a bracketed series of slides, some may be a bit light, some too dark, but one will be perfect.

Two types of color slide film exist. Some color slide film is for use only in outdoor lighting conditions and is referred to as *daylight* film. The other is called *tungsten-balanced* film and is for use indoors with tungsten lights. Tungsten light is derived from the filaments in lamps, has a different color temperature than daylight, and therefore requires a different film sensitivity.

Color temperature is based on the fact that a black element, heated until it glows, produces a color proportional to its temperature. This temperature, termed *color temperature*, is measured in degrees Kelvin (K). The highest color temperatures appear at the blue end of the spectrum and the lower temperatures, at the red. Daylight has a high color temperature (5500 to 6500 K) and artificial light (such as that emitted by tungsten bulbs and quartz iodine lamps), a lower color temperature (3200 to 3400 K). As a result, *daylight* reversal film and *tungsten* reversal film both exist. Flash units, attached to cameras or separate from them, all emit light balanced at daylight temperatures. Therefore, when flash is used, daylight balanced film is used.

Color negative film is also balanced for daylight and therefore works best with flash, but if a good color printer is used (some of the inexpensive 1-hour printers can produce high-quality prints), excellent prints can be made using illumination from a tungsten or quartz iodine light source. Negative film can also allow for a good deal of exposure error, plus or minus one to two f-stops, and still enable a competent printer to deliver good-quality photos. Black and white film, of course, can be used in any sort of light: indoors, outdoors, with or without flash, and even with fluorescent light. (Fluorescent light should be avoided with any color film.)

Film speed is a measure of the sensitivity of the film to light. The color films generally available have speeds from 25 ISO to 1600 ISO. The higher the ISO (an index of film speed), the faster the film; that is, the higher the ISO, the less light needed to shoot at our minimum of f/8 aperture. The speed of a film is also an indicator of the resolving power of the film, which is the capacity of a film to record fine detail. Slower films generally have higher resolving power. The resolving power and sharpness (also called *acutance*) of today's films is astonishing, and any softness or graininess is not apparent unless the images are enlarged in excess of 11 × 14 inches. We make 5 × 7-inch color prints for all of our client surgeons and use American-manufactured Kodacolor Gold Plus 100 ISO print film. The detail and color rendition of this film is superb. We have tested virtually every print film available and find that the 200 and 400 ISO films also work well. The films that are faster than 200 to 400 begin to compromise sharpness.

For color slides, I have long used Kodachrome 25, which is the best; it is virtually grainless (and therefore excellent for large-scale projection in lectures) and has fine color properties, especially in the skin tones. It is not a fast film, however, so if more speed is required, one can use Kodachrome 200, which is almost as grainless and will do the job if a tripod is not available, if the light is low, or if the photographer's hands shake.

LIGHTING

Lighting the subject is the most important and most difficult part of photography. For medical photography, a hard, evenly distributed light is required to show all of the lines, pores, indentations, scars, marks, and flaws that occur on and in the face and eyes.

Three light sources are available to the photographer. The first is daylight, or natural light; the second is tungsten or quartz iodine light; and the third is electronic flash or strobe light. Daylight or natural light is not an option for the medical photographer, who needs a controlled directional light source that is consistent from day to day.

Tungsten bulbs are inexpensive and have a consistent color temperature over their life span, which can be up to 60 hours. Quartz iodine lamps have even longer lives, up to 150 hours, and are small and powerful and emit the sort of hard, sharp light similar to the quality of light from an electronic flash that brings out all of the lines and pores in the skin. The problem with these light sources is that they are hot. A person sitting in front of a pair of these sort of lights is soon parboiled after only a couple of minutes, especially if the lights are usually fairly close to the subject. Another problem is that these lamps, particularly quartz lights, draw a lot of amperage. Because a pair of 250 to 500 watt lamps is required, fuses could be blown. However, this type of lamp can be arranged and adjusted for correct illumination of the subject very easily, and the effects of the lighting are readily visible to the photographer. This wide degree of control is a great advantage if one can stand the heat and the lights do not blow fuses. The printer can produce good-quality prints if color negative film is used.

With tungsten or quartz lights and an aperture of f/8 or smaller (on a 105-mm lens), shutter speeds of 1/125 or faster are recommended to avoid the effects of shaking or blurring caused by the subject's movement.

Electronic flash, or strobe, is the type of artificial light that most photographers use as a light source other than daylight. The flash tubes last for thousands of shots, they use batteries or very little amperage, and they stay cool even after extended use. When a flash is triggered, its duration is so short, 1/500 of a second or faster, that it freezes any movement from both the subject and the photographer. Therefore, as long as the camera shutter is set at the correct flash-synchronizing speed, small movement or shaking is no longer a problem.

The professional studio strobes even have small lamps, or modeling lights, in them that enable the photographer to observe the approximate effect of the lights when triggered. Studio strobes are expensive, however. A small generator (the electronic source for the flash heads or lights that are attached to it) and two flash heads can cost a couple of thousand dollars for a unit capable of emitting about 500 watt-seconds of power, which is about the amount needed to shoot at an aperture of f/8 or smaller. Some of the smaller amateur flash units that are meant to be attached to the camera, such as the Vivitar 283, can be mounted on light stands and used like studio strobes. They are inexpensive, dependable, and small. They do not have modeling lights, of course, but because a lighting set-up such as this would not generally be moved, this is not a problem.

A small office studio can be set up rather easily for ophthalmic plastic surgical preoperative and postoperative photographs. One needs a camera, a camera tripod, a pair of lights and stands, a revolving stool that is adjustable for height, and a piece of black material (felt is best) as a backdrop for the pictures. If black is used for the background, the subject can be seated immediately in front of the material, which saves space and eliminates shadows on the background. One can also have a window shade made of black material that can be mounted with brackets to the wall and rolled up or down as needed.

The camera should always be braced on a heavy tripod, like the Tiltall tripod. The tripod prevents camera movement and also allows the photographer to crop (compose) the photograph exactly. The view finders of high-quality 35-mm cameras are accurate, and the film used in these cameras records almost exactly what is seen.

The lights should be placed to the left and right of the camera, 2 to 3 feet to each side, and about 4 feet from the subject. The lights should be set at about the top of head height or a little higher and angled down to the eyes. If the lights are too close to the subject, 3 feet or less, then the lights' intensity illuminates the shadowing in the pores and creases of the skin that create the illusion of depth, creating a creamy, smooth-looking skin (this is an old trick of portrait and beauty photographers) (Fig. 50–3).

To determine the correct exposure, the photographer should use an exposure meter. In high-quality 35-mm cameras, built-in meters are accurate. If flash is used, then a separate flash meter must measure the light. A meter such as the Minolta Flashmeter IV can measure daylight, tungsten or quartz light, and flash, and it is accurate to 1/10 of an f-stop. I prefer to use separate meters rather than those in the camera. I prefer to measure the light that falls on the subject rather than the light that is reflected from the subject, as the in-camera meters do. This method is more accurate for our purposes.

The meter should be used to measure first one of the two lights, then the other to ensure that each is emitting the same amount of light on the subject. The photographer moves the lights forward or backward until they match the output on the subject. Then, the photographer turns both lights on, takes a reading, and uses the reading for the first exposure. The first shots are used to check whether the light balance and exposures are correct. If not, the lights are adjusted if one side is darker, or the aperture is adjusted if the image is too dark or too light overall. Once the lighting set-up is right, the light and subject positions do not move, so the photographs should be consistently correct. The distances from the lights to the subject should be marked in case the lights are moved inadvertently. The light output should also be checked occasionally with the meter. If these recommendations are followed, the photographer should have consistently good results (Fig. 50–4).

Preoperative and postoperative photographic comparisons should be essentially unchanged except for the surgical effects. A consistent set of lighting angles should be maintained preoperatively and postoperatively because otherwise the photographs can be misleading. Raising or lowering the lights or diffusing (softening) the light can alter the appearance of the subject: lower lid bags can be eliminated simply by lowering the lights a few inches. For example, if photographs are taken with the lights raised 8

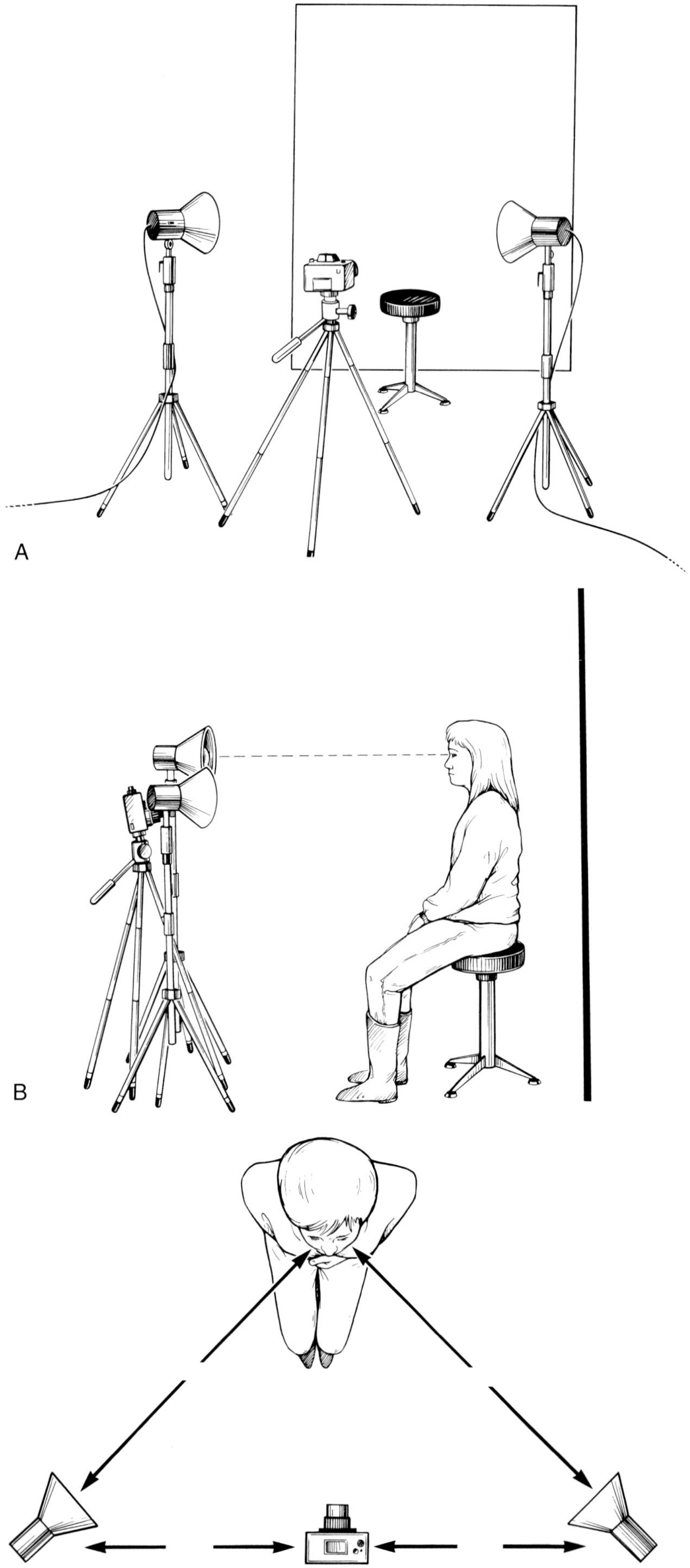

Figure 50 – 3. *A* to C, Proper lighting set up for photographing patients.

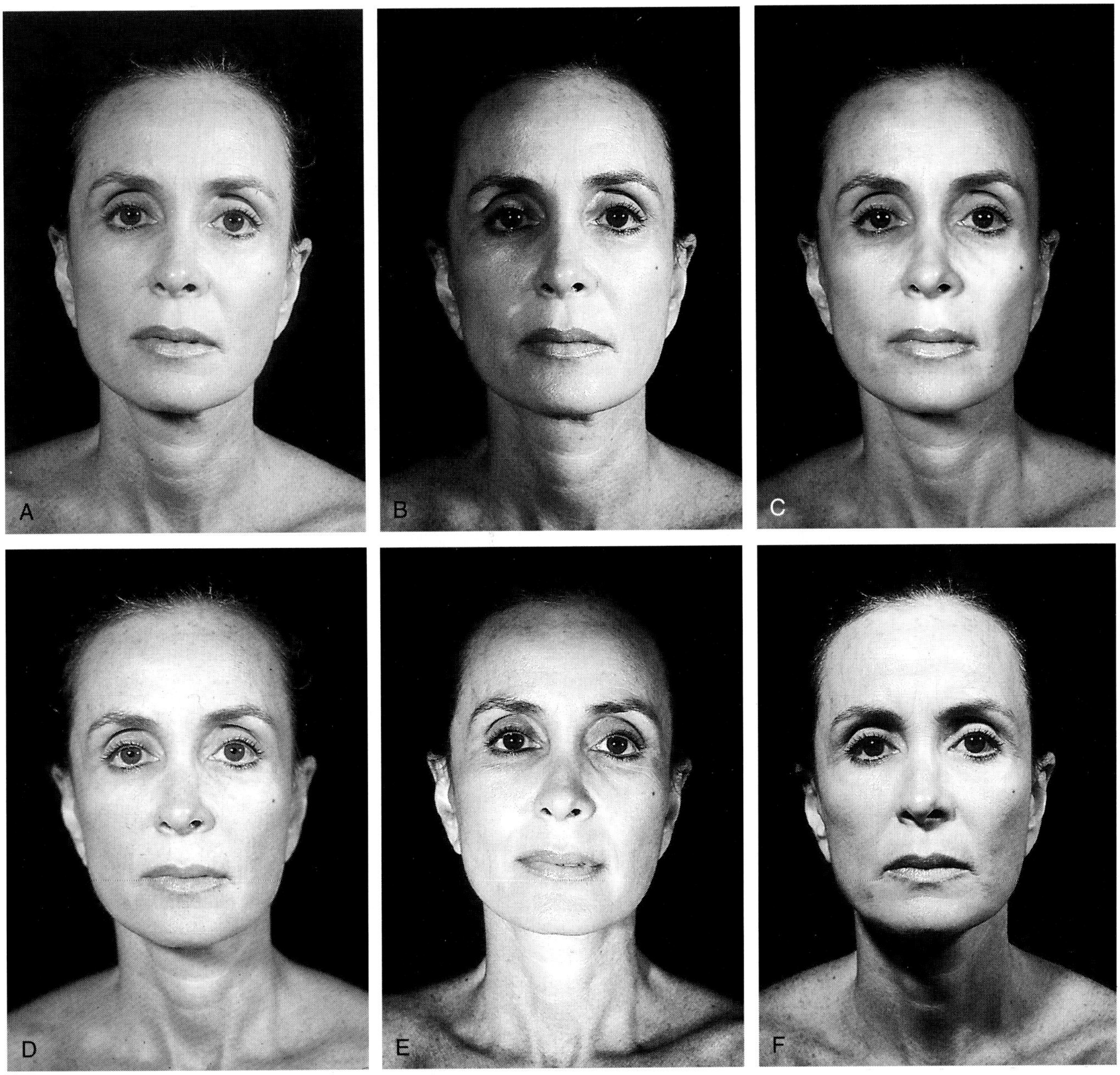

Figure 50–4. Photographs of patient with various light exposures. *A*, Correct light balance. *B*, Light too far away. *C*, Underexposure. *D*, Overexposure. *E*, Lights too low. *F*, Lights too high.

or 10 inches and again with the lights lowered to a straight-ahead position, the results would appear tangibly better even without surgical intervention.

Many on-camera flash accessories work well, and some even integrate electronically with the cameras to which they are dedicated. These accessories couple with virtually any lens in the system and operate automatically, regulating the amount of light needed as the flash senses the film speed, aperture, and distance from the camera to the subject. They are acceptable for medical use, but some limitations exist. Often, they cannot render correct readings at the close distances one needs for medical work. Each flash is different, but none seems to work well at distances closer than 2 to 3 feet. The exposure sensor gets confused and frequently underexposes or overexposes. This characteristic can be tested and the exact distances noted and the lens aperture adjusted to compensate. Of course, the close up distances must be same each time. If color print film is being used, enough exposure latitude exists so that some minor error will not ruin the shots. But this is not the case when slide film is used; in these situations, the photographer must bracket. Some on-camera flashes do give acceptable automatic exposures, even at distances as close as 6 or 7 inches, using a 105-mm macrofocusing lens. The problem I have found with these flashes is that they are usually mounted to one

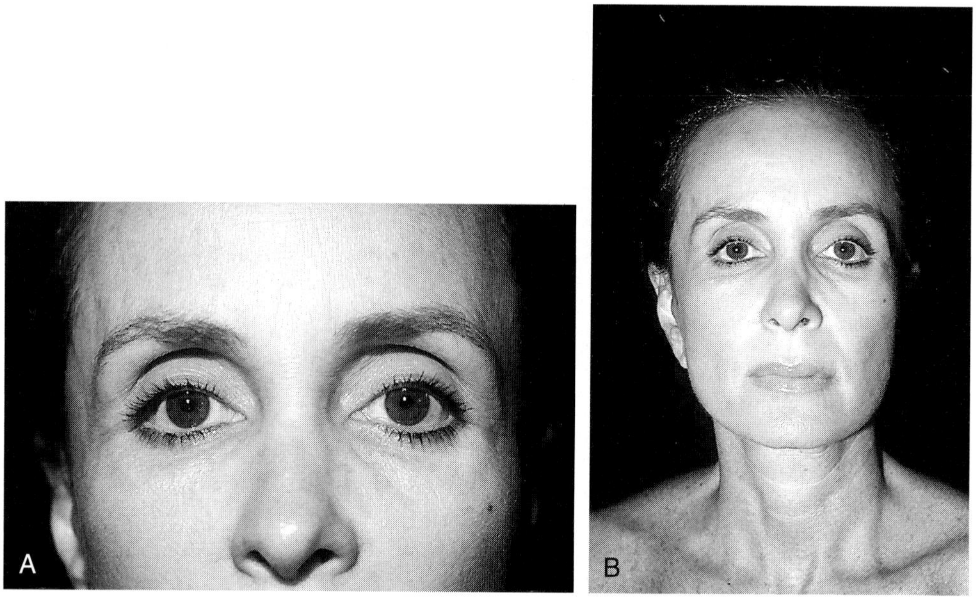

Figure 50–5. Shadowing of patient's face. *A*, On-camera strobe. Flash is mounted on the left side of the camera. *B*, On-camera strobe is mounted on the left side of the camera.

side of the camera and therefore tend to cause a bit of shadowing on the opposite side of the subject's face (Fig. 50–5).

Some flashes are made to work at very close distances and are called ring-light flashes. These are flashes that literally circle the end of the lens. They are designed for close work, such as that required for dental photography, and they are generally accurate. However, the light is rather "harsh" and often illuminates the shadows in the skin pores and lines. Some integrated camera/lens/ring light systems exist, such as the Yashica dental camera. However, with ring lights and dedicated dental cameras, the light source is fixed too straight onto the subject, and as a result, some angular definition that occurs with a light slightly above the subject is missing. Such photographs do not provide the surgeon with as much diagnostic input as would those obtained with other light sources.

To photograph procedures in the operating room itself, existing overhead lamps may be used for illumination. Usually, these lamps are high-quality quartz or halogen lights, and tungsten balanced film should be used if color slides are required. Tungsten films are available in ISO ratings from 64 to 320, so the photographer should not have a problem shooting at an f-stop–shutter speed combination that is satisfactory. Light may be measured with the camera's meter, but bracketing is necessary. Again, a hand-held meter is best because it can be used more easily to measure every quadrant of the area to be photographed. If any extreme variances exist in the light coverage—more than ¾ of an f-stop—then the lights can be repositioned. Ideally one would want light coverage of the overall area to be photographed to be consistent to half an f-stop. A motor drive enables shots to be taken very rapidly using the right hand to fire the shutter while the left hand moves the aperture ring for the bracketing. The photographer should bracket a lot for these shots. If a tripod cannot be used or the photographer is standing on a stool or chair for an overhead view, he or she should try to brace the camera by holding his or her elbows tightly against the rib cage. With an on-camera flash, the photographer does not have to worry as much about camera movement, but the use of the flash itself may be distracting to the rest of the surgical team. The use of color negative film would eliminate the need to bracket or even to be exact with the exposure, but an even distribution of the light over the subject area is still important.

Figure 50–6 shows the eight standard photographs provided to our client surgeons for eye surgery. At the surgeon's request, we furnish variations and additions to the basic series. We provide 5 × 7-inch borderless color prints and, when required, a set of 35-mm color transparencies. The grid on the focusing screen of the view finder allows every patient to be positioned similarly. If the photographer is exacting about this, then photographs taken

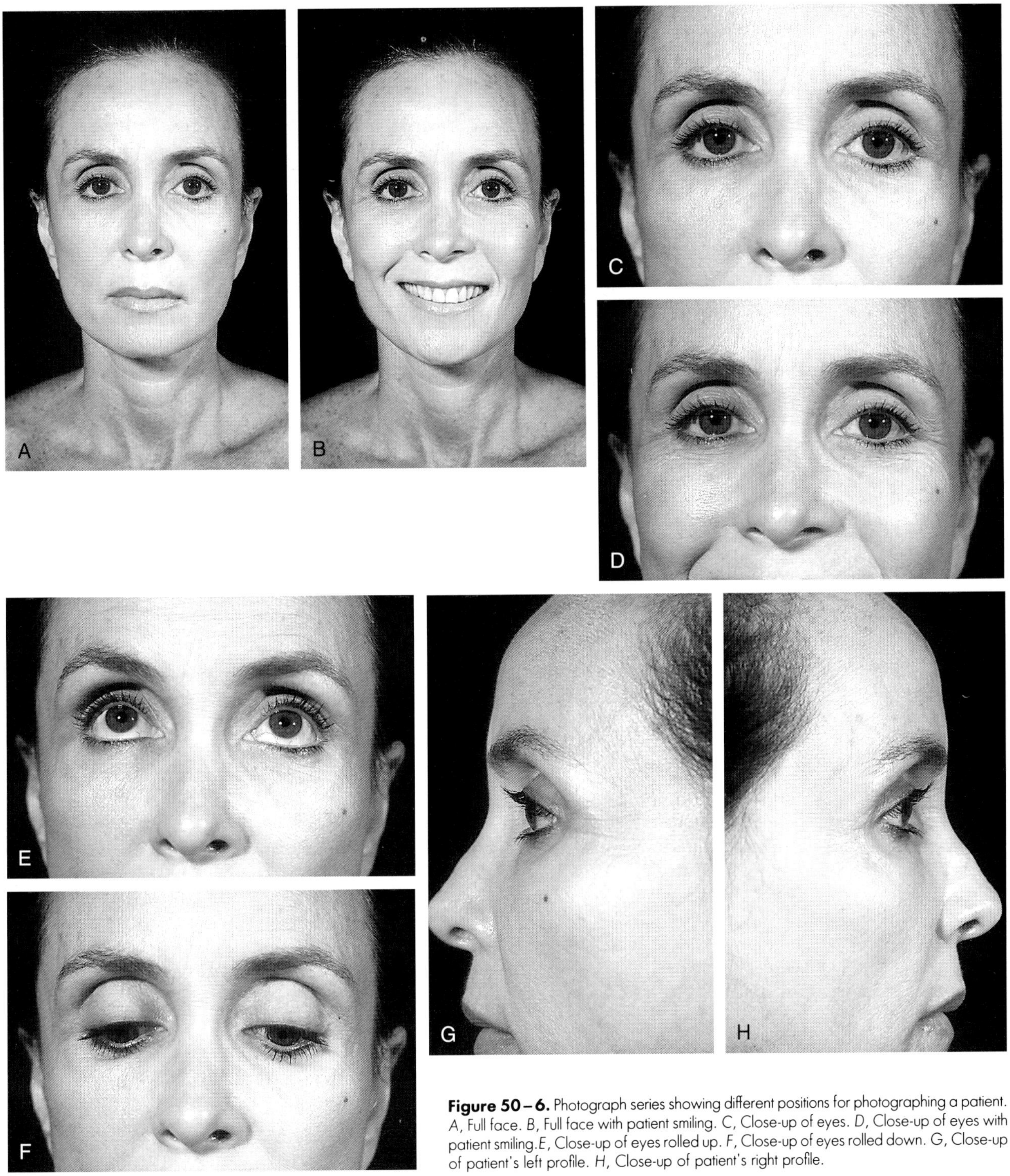

Figure 50–6. Photograph series showing different positions for photographing a patient. *A*, Full face. *B*, Full face with patient smiling. *C*, Close-up of eyes. *D*, Close-up of eyes with patient smiling. *E*, Close-up of eyes rolled up. *F*, Close-up of eyes rolled down. *G*, Close-up of patient's left profile. *H*, Close-up of patient's right profile.

months or even years later will match. The photographer can also take the preoperative photographs to the processor so that the postoperative or subsequent photograph series can be made to match the color tones and densities of the previous set of photographs.

Acknowledgment

I would like to express my gratitude to Julie Mardin, Elena Olivo, and J. Leslee Sosa-Basualdo for their help in preparing this chapter.

CHAPTER 51

Total Facial Rejuvenation

Nelson Lee Novick

Beauty, it is said, is in the eyes of the beholder. It is therefore a relative concept, representing the inherent quality of a person or object to be pleasing to the eye or mind. As such, the notion of what is beautiful often differs from one culture to another and even from one generation to the next. Although through the millenia, artists, philosophers, and scientists have attempted to define some of the elements contributing to physical beauty, it is perhaps only in our time, when so much can be done medically and surgically to enhance appearance, that this information has become critical. Whatever our sentiments about the issue, it is apparent that "in our culture the way one looks makes a difference in the response one gets," and, even more specifically, "it is the face that defines one's identity because it defines the reactions of others."[1]

The artist's rendering of the "ideal" face as seen in Figure 51–1 is based on what a sample of male American college students found most attractive in women when asked to judge a series of photographs.[2] The basic elements of this ideal include eyes high and wide, with a width of about one third of the face at eye level; high eyebrows and large pupils; a smile about half the width of the face at mouth level; and a small chin. Other aspects include wide cheekbones, their width about six tenths of the length of the face from the hairline to the chin, and a nose area smaller than 5% of the area of the entire face. The precise measurements aside, it is obvious that the two commanding aesthetic foci of the face are the eyes and the mouth. Clearly, then, anything that may be done to improve either or both of these aesthetic areas, as well as the regions surrounding them, can contribute significantly to rejuvenating the appearance of the face and achieving a more natural overall effect.

Experts agree that the many adverse effects that persons loosely call "aging" of the skin are really the sum of the interaction of five separate factors.[3] These are (1) intrinsic aging (i.e., each individual's genetic propensity to skin degeneration with the passage of time); (2) photoaging, primarily the accumulated effects through the years of damage from ultraviolet light on the collagen and elastin fibers and melanocytes; (3) gravity, which results in skin sagging; (4) muscle motion factors, such as squinting and smiling, that contribute to etched expression lines; and (5) mechanical factors, such as the way we position ourselves in sleep, leading to the development of "sleep lines." Of these, photoaging is by far the most significant factor, resulting in disfiguring precancers and skin cancers of all types; excessive dryness and coarseness; pigmentary changes (e.g., freckles, "liver spots," splotchy areas of irregular pigmentation, and melanoma); thinning of the skin; loss of elasticity; wrinkles; criss-cross, corrugated crepiness; and the development of telangiectases (what patients often call "broken blood vessels").[4, 5] These visible manifestations of photoaging correlate with the microscopic findings of a thickened horny layer, epidermal cellular atypia, melanocytic proliferation, and pronounced elastosis in the papillary and upper reticular dermis. Any attempt, therefore, to optimally improve appearance must be directed to ameliorating as many of these factors as possible.

Just as there is no debate that face-lift surgery is the best method for eliminating sagging and redundancy of the facial skin, there is little question that blepharoplasty and brow-lifts are the ideal procedures for dealing with the intrinsic and gravity-related problems of excessively lax and drooping skin and herniated fatty tissue in the upper and lower eyelids and brow. But surgically enhanced, more youthful lids and brows, for example, may look quite artificial against the backdrop of sallow, severely aged, weatherbeaten, and mottled skin on the forehead, cheeks, and temples. Fortunately, a variety of other simple topical measures and cosmetic procedures are available to improve overall facial appearance so that everything "fits."[6] When such a more global aesthetic approach is taken to complement face-lift or eyelid surgery, the entire process may be referred to quite appropriately as "total facial rejuvenation."

The following is an overview of some of the more frequent cosmetic problems of the aging face and their management. Although the removal of common premalignant conditions, such as atypical (dysplastic) moles or actinic keratoses, as well as true malignancies, such as basal and squamous cell skin cancer and malignant melanoma, may pose significant cosmetic problems, these are first and foremost medical conditions that require inter-

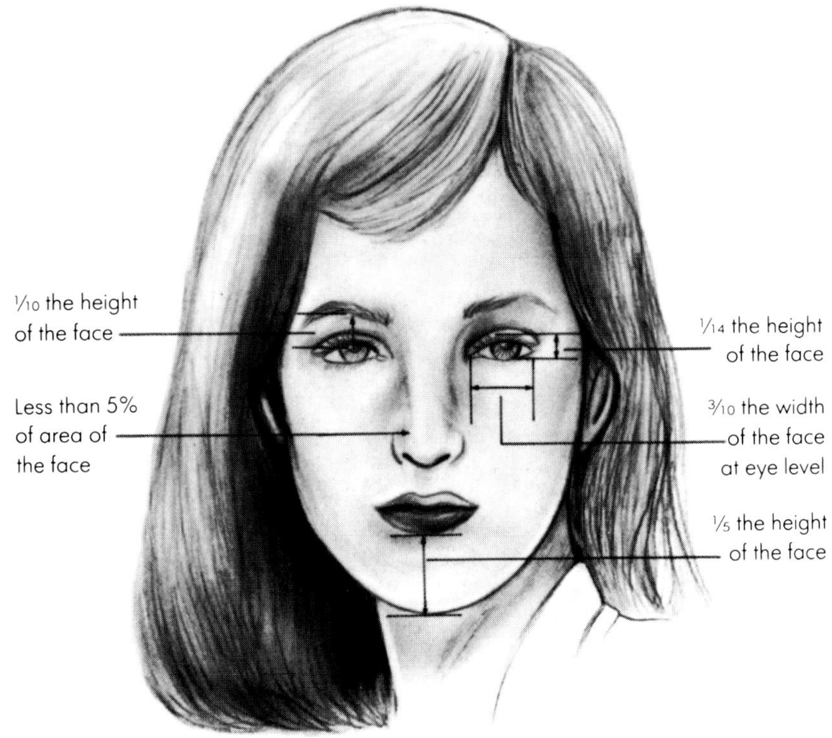

Figure 51 – 1. Aesthetic elements of the "ideal" face. (From Novick NL: Super Skin: A Leading Dermatologist's Guide to the Latest Breakthroughs in Skin Care. New York, Clarkson N. Potter, 1988, p 169.)

vention to preserve health; the cosmetic aspects are secondary, and, for that reason, the management of these problems has been excluded from this discussion of benign, exclusively cosmetic conditions.

PREVENTION

No discussion of total facial rejuvenation would be complete without at least a few words aimed at prevention. For some time now, we have known that despite its long-perceived beauty and health benefits and its implied link with "the good life" (popularized in the 1920s by Coco Chanel), the sun (and tanning parlors) is really a "wolf in sheep's clothing." The harmful effects of ultraviolet light exposure are insidious, however, often not being visible until somewhere between 5 and 20 years after damage has already taken place.[7] It has been estimated that protecting children from ultraviolet light exposure can reduce the lifetime risk of skin cancer by approximately 80%.[8] It would not be inconceivable that adequate sun protection during this same period could likewise reduce the ravages of photoaging by a similar percentage.

The best form of sun protection is obviously total avoidance. Nevertheless, for most active persons this advice would be impractical and would likely not be followed. However, educating patients, especially parents of young children and teenagers, to the long-term dangers of ultraviolet light exposure (both medical and cosmetic) and providing them with a few commonsense tips for reducing their exposure can potentially reap enormous future dividends.[9, 10] Suggestions include (1) rescheduling outdoor activities to before 10 A.M. or after 3 P.M., the periods of lower solar intensity; (2) using wide, ultraviolet light sunglasses; and (3) wearing broad-brimmed hats (preferably 4 inches in front and back), long-sleeved clothing, and long pants whenever possible.

Individuals should also be warned that nearly 70% of the sun's ultraviolet radiation may pierce the cloud layer on a cloudy day; that more than 70% of the rays may be reflected off sand, water, and concrete, mitigating much of the perceived benefit from sitting under beach umbrellas or the boardwalk; that ultraviolet light can penetrate up to 4 feet of water while swimming; and that increased heat and humidity can potentiate the harmful effects of ultraviolet light.[11]

Ordinary clothing, such as a T-shirt, provides about a sun protection factor (SPF) of 5 to 7, and even less when wet. Several manufacturers have introduced stylish, lightweight clothing lines made of specially woven nylon fabrics reportedly capable of providing protection in a range of at least SPF 30. They include Solar Protective Factor (800-786-2562), Frogwear (800-437-7055), and Sun Precautions (206-441-6688).

Sunscreens are another important means of protection.[12] They should be used routinely daily between mid-April and mid-October in northern latitudes and year-round in sunbelt regions. Fair-skinned persons should apply products providing at least an SPF 15 protection, and active individuals should look for waterproof products capable of withstanding heavy sweating or swimming for at least 1 or 2 hours. Consumers should also be reminded to apply the sunscreen to the nose, tops of the ears, and cheekbones, and with a cotton-tipped applicator even to the part line in the scalp. Persons with sensitive skin or allergies to *p*-aminobenzoic acid (PABA) should choose PABA-free sunscreens. Those who find difficulty with all chemical sunscreens may try a product containing micronized titanium dioxide, a physical blocking agent (e.g., Clinique Special Defense Sunblock [SPF 25]). Finally, the use of a wax stick sunscreen, such as Neutrogena Sunblock Stick (SPF 25) applied around the eyes eliminates the stinging and burning of the eyes that so commonly occurs when cream or lotion formulations are applied to that area.

WRINKLES

Wrinkles, or rhytides, and crepiness are probably the most disquieting hallmarks of the aging face. They are generally divided into three categories: fine, moderate, and coarse. Although coarse wrinkles are difficult to eliminate, more superficial wrinkles may be softened substantially or even improved dramatically by a variety of modalities, including the topical application of tretinoin and alpha-hydroxy acids, the use of chemical peeling agents, dermabrasion, and the injection of filler substances such as collagen or gelatin-matrix implants.

Tretinoin

Topical *trans*-retinoic acid, or tretinoin, a synthetic vitamin A derivative, commercially available by prescription as Retin-A, has been used successfully for the treatment of acne for more than 20 years. More recently, after several reports in clinical trials,[13-15] it has gained increasing popularity, even in the lay press, for its use in the long-term management of photoaging. It is one of a growing number of agents that have lately come to be known as "cosmeceuticals," topical preparations that straddle the line between a cosmetic, intended solely to beautify and enhance the skin, and a pharmacologic agent capable of affecting the structure and function of the skin.

Although the precise molecular and cellular mechanisms of action of tretinoin remain to be more fully understood, it has been observed to increase compaction of the stratum corneum and the rate of epidermal cellular turnover; reverse keratinocytic atypia (dysplasia); enhance new blood vessel formation in the dermis; disperse melanosomes; promote new collagen synthesis and deposition within the papillary dermis by its effects on dermal fibroblasts; and increase the amount of glycosaminoglycans within the dermis. Such changes would account for its apparent ability to smooth the texture of skin, restore a healthful pinkness, or "glow," diminish or eliminate so-called liver spots (solar lentigines), and lessen fine and moderate wrinkling. Coarse wrinkling tends to respond the least, although some decrease in wrinkling may be seen there, as well.

The optimum regimen for tretinoin use in photodamaged skin consists of nightly applications, usually 20 to 30 minutes after a gentle facewash, to minimize dryness.[16] The strongest concentration of the product is used (usually the 0.1% cream formulation) that does not result in undue irritation, although more than 90% of patients will experience early on some degree of redness and flaking, the so-called retinoid dermatitis. Fortunately, most persons will develop a tolerance to the irritation within a couple of weeks. When it is particularly severe, however, switching to the lower 0.025% concentration and adding a moisturizer to the regimen is usually sufficient to handle the problem. Occasionally, a mild topical corticosteroid, such as hydrocortisone 2.5%, may be needed temporarily to reduce irritation. Renova, a tretinoin product in an optimized moisturizing vehicle intended specifically for use in photoaged skin, awaits final approval by the Food and Drug Administration (FDA).

Although many patients report a more healthy, less sallow appearance after only 2 to 4 months of use, diminution of wrinkling is not usually observed for several months, and maximal effect is generally not seen until somewhere between 10 and 16 months of continuous nightly application of tretinoin 0.05% cream (Fig. 51–2). In most cases, visible improvement plateaus at 24 months.[14] In one study, digital image analysis of silicone rubber casts made from the crow's-feet region corroborated the clinical observation of diminished wrinkling.[15]

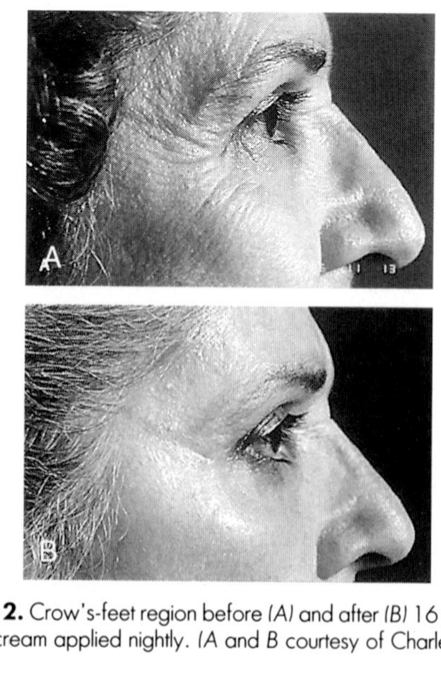

Figure 51–2. Crow's-feet region before *(A)* and after *(B)* 16 months of tretinoin 0.05% cream applied nightly. *(A and B courtesy of Charles Ellis, MD.)*

Once optimum improvement is achieved, a maintenance program of one to three times weekly applications may be initiated.[16]

Besides its potential for irritation, tretinoin slightly increases sensitivity to sun exposure and patients must be alerted to the possibility that they may sunburn more easily. Protective sunwear and the use of high SPF sunscreens should be advised. In general, contrary to a popular misconception, there is no need to discontinue tretinoin therapy during the sun season, as long as the proper precautions are taken. Tretinoin is best applied at night and with a sunscreen in the morning.

Interestingly, once-nightly application of tretinoin 0.1% cream initiated between 2 and 4 weeks before surgery has also been found to be useful for significantly speeding postoperative wound healing, particularly before chemical peeling and dermabrasion.[17, 18] Since there is some evidence suggesting that tretinoin may paradoxically slow wound healing when applied in the immediate postoperative period, it should be discontinued for 2 weeks *after* these procedures to allow for complete healing to take place.[19] After that, it may be restarted and continued as needed for photoaging.

Alpha-Hydroxy Acids

Alpha-hydroxy acids are another group of cosmeceuticals that have received considerable attention both in medical and lay circles. These chemicals, which include such naturally occurring acids as malic, citric, tartaric, lactic, and glycolic acids, among others, are nontoxic derivatives of many common products, including sour milk, sugar cane, and a variety of fruits.[20] For this reason, they are often referred to, particularly in the lay press, as "fruit acids," although these days, most alpha-hydroxy acids are actually synthesized in the laboratory. They are also byproducts of normal mammalian metabolism and as such are nontoxic. In concentrations generally ranging from 5% to 10%, alpha-hydroxy acids, particularly lactic acid preparations, have been used for many years to treat xerosis and icthyosis. In these concentrations they are generally available over the counter, with the exception of Lac-Hydrin lotion, a unique buffered form of ammonium lactate in a relatively high 12% concentration useful for treating especially resistant dry skin problems and the xerosis typically associated with eczema, psoriasis, and icthyosis.[21]

As in the case of tretinoin, the exact mechanism of action of these substances in photoaging is still not known. Some investigators contend that they function pharmacologically to enhance collagen, elastin, and ground substance synthesis.[22, 23] Others argue that the data suggest only that they function as chemical peeling agents, in low concentrations to effect decreased corneocyte cohesion and in much higher concentrations to promote true epidermolysis.[24] Whatever the case, patient satisfaction with these agents appears to run high and physicians typically observe smoother skin, diminution in fine and moderate wrinkling and crepiness, fading of brownish discolorations, and thinning or elimination of keratoses and other rough spots. Although, as in the case of tretinoin, glycolic acid creams are being used preoperatively to enhance postoperative wound healing, more research is needed to substantiate their benefits for this purpose.

Proprietary creams and lotions containing glycolic and lactic acids in concentrations ranging from 5% to 12% and applied once or twice daily at home have been the most frequently used alpha-hydroxy acids for photoaging.[25] In the main, these products are made available through smaller pharmaceutical firms to dermatology and plastic surgery practices. In my experience, however, the more potent preparations, such as ammonium lactate 12%, which have been shown to have pharmacologic effects on the skin,[26] offer the most consistent results. When needed, physicians may order from their pharmacists or chemical suppliers specially compounded formulations containing still higher percentages of alpha-hydroxy acids for home use than are otherwise available.

Although many cosmetic manufacturers have also gotten into the act by marketing glycolic acid in 1% to 4% creams through drug and department stores, there is no hard evidence that such low concentrations are effective. Moreover, sold as cosmetics, these items are exempted from the rigors of FDA scrutiny to which drugs must submit.

Benefits from home use of alpha-hydroxy acids for photoaging are reported after several weeks of use and consist of generally smoother, more lustrous, and less sallow skin. Although they may be used alone twice daily after a gentle washing, many dermatologists prefer to combine them with the use of tretinoin, usually prescribing alpha-hydroxy acids for morning application and tretinoin for bedtime use. Others prescribe both tretinoin and alpha-hydroxy acids twice daily. Whatever the regimen selected, the two agents, working by different mechanisms, are believed to act synergistically.[27]

The most significant side effects of alpha-hydroxy acid therapy are a transient stinging sensation that, in most cases, subsides in 15 to 30 seconds after application and, occasionally, persistent dryness and redness. If severe, the latter may be lessened by diluting the preparations with a little water or by the concurrent use of a hypoallergenic moisturizer, such as Moisturel cream or Vanicream. Alternate-day application of the alpha-hydroxy creams or lotions may also be tried to allow the skin to acclimatize to their use.

While the very low concentrations of alpha-hydroxy acids are of dubious value, very high concentrations may offer additional benefits in photoaging, as well as help for other problems. In concentrations of 40% to 50%, for example, glycolic acid has been useful in treating conventional acne and rosacea, and in 70% strength has been shown to be particularly beneficial in managing many of the manifestations of photoaging.

The procedure consists of degreasing the skin with alcohol and acetone, followed by the application of the acid with either a gauze pad or several cotton-tipped applicators. The solution is usually applied to the forehead first and then in a clockwise fashion worked downward to cover the entire face. The acid is generally left on for a period usually ranging from between 2 and 8 minutes, depending on the particular objective. It is then "neutralized" with plain water. In my experience, patients who complain of having "sensitive" skin tend to have a more intense reaction and require neutralization earlier. For optimal results, a series of between 6 and 12 treatments are ordinarily performed spaced at 2- to 4-week intervals (Fig. 51–3). Thereafter, maintenance treatments may be repeated every 3 to 4 months.

Patients typically complain of mild stinging or burning during application, but this quickly subsides and no prepeel sedation or anesthesia or postpeel analgesia is ordinarily necessary. They should be advised that the skin may be pink or red for 3 to 5 hours after treatment. Excessive irritation, scaling, and crusting, approaching that seen with a traditional chemical peel, is the main complication of the procedure but can usually be avoided by prompt neutralization. Minimal postpeel pigmentary side effects may also occur, but these usually resolve nicely even in individuals of black, Hispanic, or Asian backgrounds.[27]

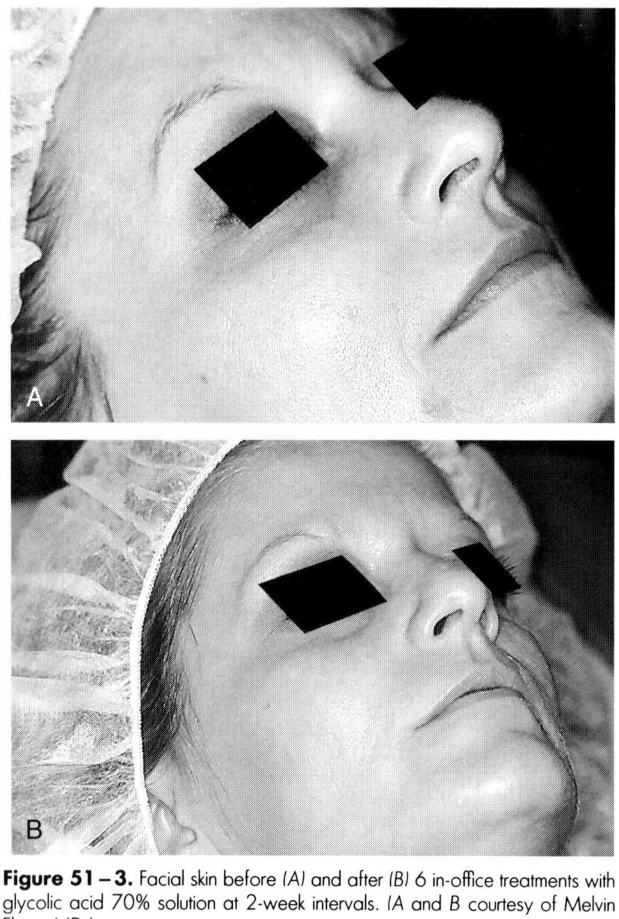

Figure 51–3. Facial skin before *(A)* and after *(B)* 6 in-office treatments with glycolic acid 70% solution at 2-week intervals. *(A and B courtesy of Melvin Elson, MD.)*

Individuals with photoaged skin may be treated with periodic high-concentration glycolic acid peels alone, but more commonly these treatments make up a part of an overall facial rejuvenation program. To maximize benefits, they are generally combined with the home application of tretinoin or alpha-hydroxy acid creams or lotions.[28] Fine wrinkling, thin keratotic lesions, and mottled discolorations of the skin respond especially well to this combination of therapies and the results, in my experience, have been quite gratifying.

Chemical Peels

Chemical peels, defined as the application of some form of exfoliating agent to the skin, have also been making a strong comeback in facial rejuvenation for the treatment of wrinkling, mottled discolorations, and acne scarring. New uses for old peeling agents, new combinations of agents, and refinements in techniques are contributing to the success of these procedures and the recent explosion of interest in them.

All chemical peels, regardless of the agents used or the manner of application, are methods of "wounding" the skin in a controlled manner so that after application the treatment areas may heal in a cosmetically more acceptable fashion. They may penetrate the epidermis or the dermis, and peels are generally classified as deep, medium, or superficial, according to the depth of wounding. The benefits of peels may last for several years. Phenol, as part of Baker's formula, a deep peeling agent, is less commonly used because of its risk of cardiac and systemic toxicity. Trichloroacetic acid in concentrations ranging from 20% to 50%, Jessner's solution, glycolic acid, and phenol remain the most widely used agents for the chemical peeling of wrinkling, as well as for other aspects of photoaged skin. Many excellent texts and reviews of chemical peeling have been published, and the reader is referred to these for details of patient selection, treatment, and postoperative care.[29, 30]

The current enthusiasm for combining peeling agents for medium-depth peels deserves special note, however. These two-stage peels combine the application of lower strengths of trichloroacetic acid, usually 35%, with the prior application of another agent, such as solid carbon dioxide, Jessner's solution, or glycolic acid 70% (kept on for no more than 2 minutes before neutralization).[31–33] Each approach has been reported to be as effective as straight 50% thrichloroacetic acid for superficial wrinkling and cross-hatching, depressed scars, blotchy pigmentation, and sun damage, but with less likelihood of scarring and generally fewer complications.

Dermabrasion

Dermabrasion (skin sanding or facial planing) using high-speed motor-driven wire brushes or diamond fraises is another modality for controlled wounding of the skin that is seeing a revival for the treatment of wrinkles, scars, and discolorations. Like chemical peels, with which it is often combined to improve the overall cosmetic result, dermabrasion is a subject that has been well reviewed, and the reader is invited to consult these references for the details of the technique and treatment.[34, 35]

A new technique, however, a modification of a procedure known as dermasanding, deserves special mention.[36, 37] Like traditional dermabrasion, this procedure has proven useful for dealing with fine and coarse wrinkling, as well as scarring. After standard premedication and the use of regional nerve blocks or topical anesthesia (e.g., EMLA), the skin is stretched and then sanded manually using small, 3 × 2-cm, sterilized, water-moistened (to enhance abrasiveness) squares of either commercial wallscreen or silicone-carbide sandpaper wrapped around two rolled 2 × 2-inch course-mesh gauze pads. The grade of sandpaper varies according to the problem being treated and the site. Medium and coarser grades are best reserved for deeper wrinkles and furrows, whereas the delicate areas around the eyes are best treated with fine grade no. 400. Once fine bleeding points are reached, the skin is next treated with trichloroacetic acid 25% to produce a light frost.

The entire technique, which has been colloquially called a "buff-peel," may be used for limited areas of scarring and wrinkling as well as for full-face treatment. Results in several hundred cases have proved comparable to those achieved with conventional dermabrasion (Fig. 51–4) but with several significant advantages[37]:

1. The technique allows for greater control in treating regions such as the upper lip or crow's-feet area where adequate control is often hard to achieve and more maneuverability restricted with conventional high-speed motor-driven dermabrading devices.
2. Because no skin refrigerants are needed, there is a substantially reduced risk of postinflammatory hypopigmentary changes.
3. Since no high-speed rotating device is required, there is essentially no risk of blood splattering—a distinct safety advantage in reducing risks to physician and staff from blood-borne pathogens.

Filler Substances

When wrinkles or scars are too deep to be adequately improved by the other measures already described, they may be significantly improved or softened by the use of injectable filler substances, a process known as soft tissue augmentation. Ice-pick acne scars (i.e., those that are deep and narrow), however, do not respond well to filler substances. Generally, any wrinkle (or scar) that improves significantly when the skin is stretched between the fingers can be reasonably expected to respond well to this method.

A common misconception by the lay public, in my experience, is that face-lifts and eyelid surgery are the ideal procedures for eliminating facial and crow's-feet wrinkling. Unfortunately, this notion is furthered by the fact that the medical term for a face-lift is a *rhytidectomy*, which literally means a wrinkle-removing procedure. Although it is true that some wrinkles, especially those located to the sides of the face, may be helped by the skin stretching involved in the procedure, a face-lift is far more effective for removing loose, hanging, and redundant skin. The public should be educated to this fact so that they do not plan to have extensive plastic surgical procedures unnecessarily when they could benefit significantly and less expensively from simple soft tissue augmentation. The only two approved filler substances are Zyderm and Fibrel.

Microlipoinjection or autologous fat transplantation, a procedure in which small amounts of the patient's own fat are harvested after surgery or drawn through a large-bore needle from the thigh or abdomen and reinjected into facial defects, is not indicated for intradermal filling. Filling a single wrinkle crease, even the deeper nasolabial folds, is rarely successful, and the procedure is generally reserved for filling and reshaping larger areas of loss.[38] Accordingly, it is not discussed in this section.

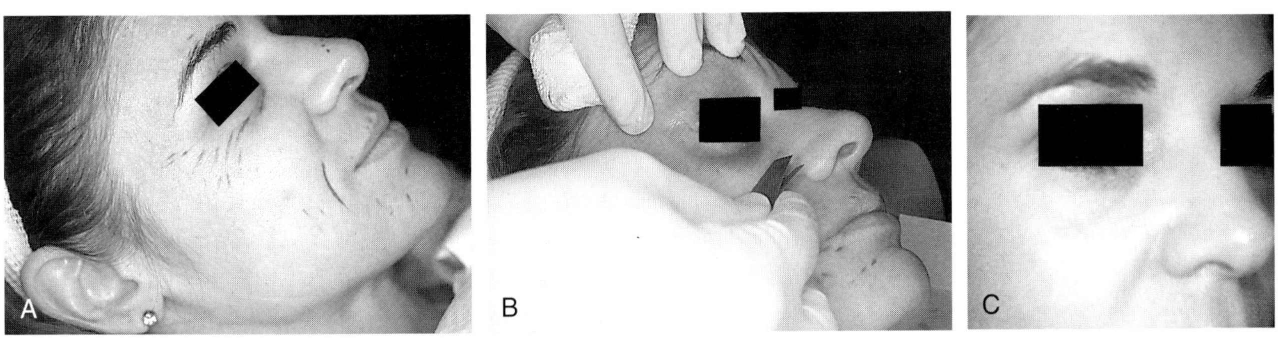

Figure 51–4. Before *(A)* intraoperatively *(B)*, and 24 months *(C)* after a "buff-peel." *(A to C courtesy of David Harris, MD.)*

Another common confusion is between silicon droplets and other filler substances. For nearly 3 decades silicone in microdroplet form was used by some practitioners without FDA approval for the treatment of wrinkles and scars. In fact, for many years before collagen was approved, silicone, an inorganic material, was the only substance available for these purposes. However, owing to growing numbers of reports of granuloma formation at the injection sites, migration, and other problems related in part to its lack of biodegradability, the FDA banned its use, and it is currently unavailable.[39] The confusion was compounded by the unrelated controversy over the dangers of silicone breast implants. Unfortunately, in the public's mind, these issues have left a lingering undercurrent of suspicion about all filler substances that must be addressed with each patient. It must be stressed that the currently available filler materials are in no way related to silicone microdroplets.

Zyderm Collagen

Approved by the FDA well over a decade ago, bovine collagen, by far, is the most frequently used substance for soft tissue augmentation. Although newer versions await approval, bovine collagen is available in three forms, each with its own specific recommended uses: Zyderm I, Zyderm II, and Zyplast. In generally, Zyderm I and Zyderm II, which differ only in that Zyderm II contains twice as much collagen material per unit as Zyderm I, are useful for more superficial wrinkles and scars. Zyplast, which is essentially a gluteraldehyde cross-linked Zyderm I, is more useful for elevating deeper wrinkles and furrows.

Approximately 3% of the general population is estimated to be allergic to collagen. Most often, this is manifested by persistent local redness, itching, and intermittent swelling at the injection sites. For this reason, two skin tests spaced at 2- to 4-week intervals, which will pick up approximately two thirds of all those who are potentially allergic, are now recommended before actual treatment is begun.[40]

The issue of the possible role of injectable collagen's role in promoting autoimmune diseases, such as polymyositis, has been raised on theoretical and legal grounds. Unfortunately, media hype about no more than a half-dozen cases allegedly connected to collagen augmentation (out of the more than 1 million persons who have been treated) contributed to some temporary public concern in this arena. However, reputable scientific inquiry into this question has shown no epidemiologic or scientific data to support the putative link between injectable collagen and autoimmune disease.[41]

The main drawback of any collagen filler procedure is the duration of correction. In general, the site loses approximately 30% in a matter of months, and corrections may last for somewhere between 6 months to a year, and occasionally as long as 2 years. On the other hand, the very biodegradability and lack of permanence of the filler is perhaps its greatest safety advantage. Anyone who experiences an allergic reaction can reasonably expect the allergic manifestations to entirely disappear in the same time frame as the correction. To prevent disappointment, patients should be advised of the periodic need for "touch-ups" before therapy is initiated.

The various techniques for injecting collagen have been well described elsewhere.[42] Two soft tissue augmentation techniques for treating the crow's-feet and the circles and bags under the eyes are particularly noteworthy. Changes in the manufacture of Zyderm I to ensure that all the collagen fibers are aligned have made the injection of material easier, smoother, and possible through a superfine 32-gauge needle. Although care must be taken not to overcorrect, the very fine lines of the crow's-feet area may now be treated with less chance for lumping or beading at the injection sites (Fig. 51 – 5).[43]

Zyderm I injected with a fine-gauge needle may be used for the dark circles and the bags under the eyes as well.[44] Placed in minute quantities under the bags (avoiding overcorrection), the filling material elevates the depression, thereby eliminating the infraorbital groove that accentuates the bag. In addition, collagen's

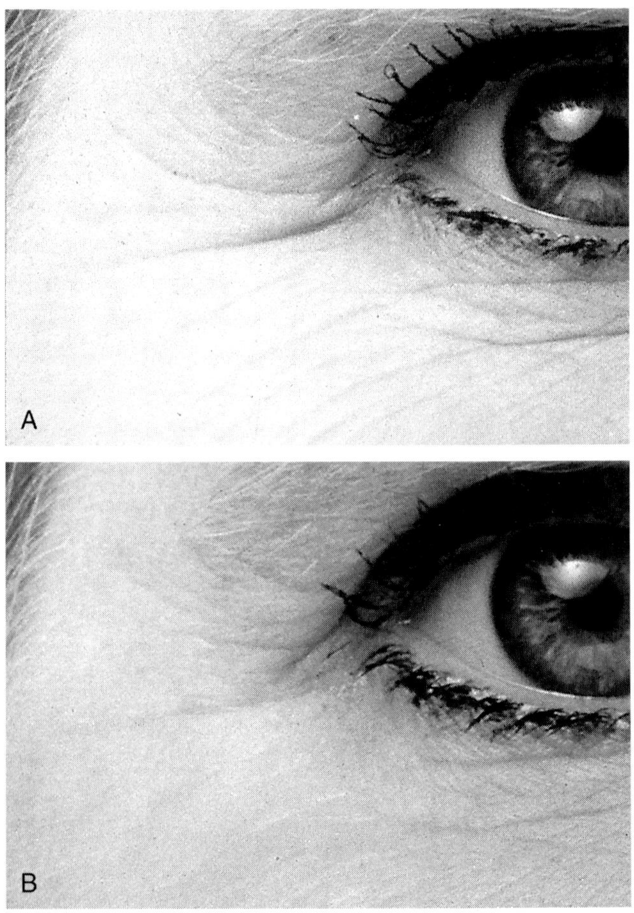

Figure 51 – 5. "Crow's-feet" region before *(A)* and after *(B)* treatment with Zyderm I collagen with a fine-gauge needle. *(A and B courtesy of Collagen Corporation, Palo Alto, CA.)*

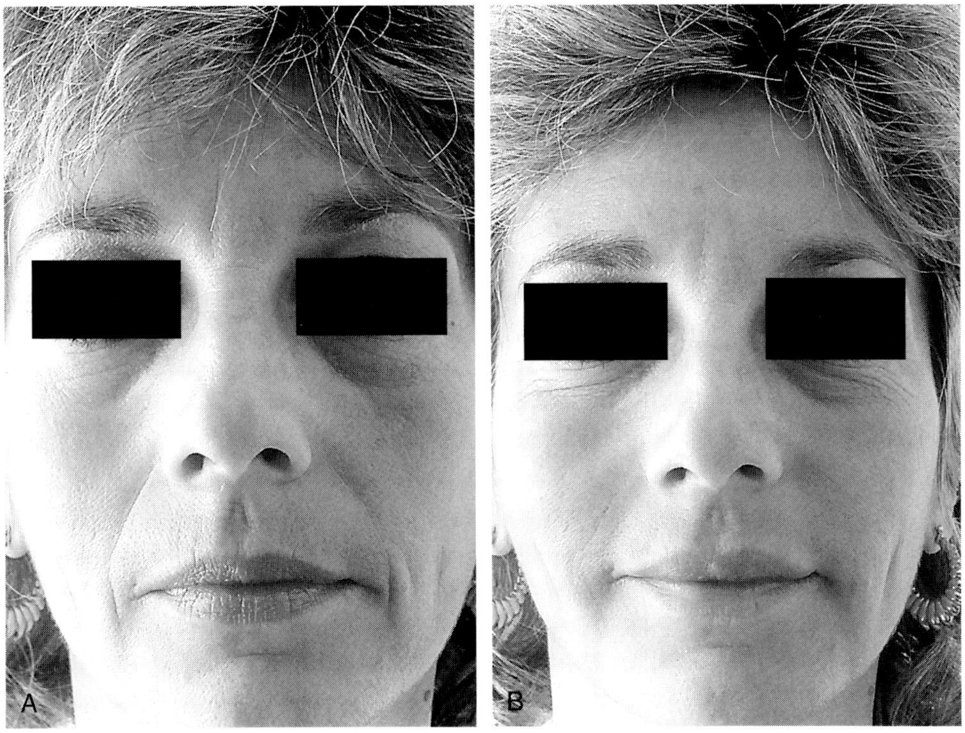

Figure 51 – 6. Nasolabial folds before *(A)* and after *(B)* treatment with Fibrel gelatin matrix implant. *(A* and *B* courtesy of Mentor Corporation, Santa Barbara, CA.)

whitish color when injected superficially into the skin acts very much like a cosmetic highlighter to lighten the color of the skin. Patients should be upright when treated, and the injection should begin at the midline with the needle directed toward the inner canthus. This should be followed by a gentle massage to mold and flatten the material.

Fibrel

Introduced in the mid 1980s, Fibrel gelatin matrix implant is the only other FDA-approved soft tissue filler substance for wrinkles and scars (Fig. 51 – 6). Fibrel contains a mixture of specially treated porcine collagen and epsilon-aminocaproic acid, and the evidence suggests that the implant combined with the patient's plasma and other tissue fluids reproduces the events that occur in normal wound repair to stimulate native collagen production. Although several other investigators and I have used Fibrel successfully without the addition of the patient's plasma, product recommendations call for mixing the material with a 0.5 mL of the patient's plasma, which must be drawn, centrifuged, and then mixed with the implant material before injection. For all intents and purposes, the uses of Fibrel roughly parallel those of Zyderm I. However, the techniques for delivery, which have been discussed thoroughly in the literature, differ somewhat from those suggested for collagen implants.[45]

Allergy to Fibrel has been noted in slightly less than 2% of the population. Nevertheless, double skin testing, although not formally recommended, is advisable. Allergy is indicated by persistent redness and swelling at the test sites longer than 24 to 48 hours. Interestingly, in one study, six patients with proven allergy to Zyderm collagen were treated with Fibrel without any evidence of cross allergenicity.[46] In addition, 10 patients in my own practice with documented collagen allergy have likewise been successfully treated with Fibrel without any evidence of allergy to the material. Although additional study is needed to determine the true extent of cross allergenicity between the two filler substances, the available evidence suggests that gelatin matrix implant may be a useful alternative in patients who have experienced allergy to collagen.

The duration of correction for wrinkles appears about the same as for collagen, although further studies are needed in this area. Accordingly, the necessity for periodic touch-ups must be explained to the patient before therapy is begun. However, a large study of Fibrel for scar treatment suggests that a significant degree of correction may be maintained for this condition for up to 5 years.[47]

PIGMENTARY PROBLEMS

Besides wrinkles, the aging face often possesses many types of benign blotchy discolorations of the skin, collectively known as dyschromia. These include freckles (ephelides), solar lentigines ("age or liver spots"), melasma ("mask of pregnancy"), and moles or even numerous tiny patches of pigment loss known as idiopathic guttate hypomelanosis.[48]

Topical therapy, while not always consistently effective, is by far the simplest means for dealing with a variety of blotchy discolorations. The several brands of hydroquinone 2% bleaching creams that are available over the counter usually do not prove particularly effective. However, prescription-strength bleaching agents containing hydroquinone in concentrations of 3% or 4% (e.g., Melanex, Solaquin Forte) applied twice daily may be effective in some cases after several months of continuous therapy coupled with diligent sun protection measures. In a double-blind study, single-agent therapy with tretinoin 0.1% cream applied once daily was found to promote a significant lightening of liver spots on the face and upper extremities.[49]

For more resistant cases, combination topical therapy may be tried. For example, the daily application of a mixture of hydroquinone 5%, tretinoin 0.1%, and dexamethasone 0.1% in hydrophilic ointment has been reported to be successful.[50] Others report satisfactory skin lightening using daily application of specially prepared combinations of hydroquinone in concentrations of up to 10% and glycolic acid in similar concentrations or with tretinoin combined with azelaic acid 20%, another well-known depigmenting agent.[51]

A number of minor surgical treatments may also be used to treat various pigmentary problems. Cryosurgery, especially the use of liquid nitrogen to destroy unwanted tissue, has been used for years to treat pigmented lesions, owing to the peculiar sensitivity of the skin's pigment cells to extreme cold.[52] The liquid nitrogen can be applied to the pigmented areas with either a cotton-tipped applicator or by spraying it on, without the need for fancy devices or thermocouples.[53] Owing to the numbing effect of the extreme cold, the procedure is only slightly uncomfortable and no local anesthesia is ordinarily required. The cosmetic results are generally good, but to prevent depigmentation of the surrounding normal skin, care must be taken to confine the freeze to the lesion. Curiously, scattered or isolated larger-sized spots appear to respond best to this form of therapy.

Chemical peeling agents and dermabrasion, as described earlier, whether for small or large problem areas, are also effective methods for dealing with unwanted pigmented lesions.[29-37]

Lasers likewise have been used successfully, particularly in the treatment of freckles and liver spots. Whereas not that long ago, the carbon dioxide and argon lasers were the workhorses of laser skin surgeons, the explosion in technology in this field has led to a whole new generation of lasers for specific uses.[54] Of those currently available, the Q-switched ruby laser, which emits a 69-nm wavelength visible red light; the Q-switched neodymium:yttrium-aluminum-garnet (Nd:YAG) laser, emitting a 1060-nm invisible near-infrared light; and the pulsed dye lasers, capable of outputs ranging in wavelengths from 400 to 1000 nm have proved best for treating hyperpigmented lesions. These lasers are capable of emitting energy in a range that is selectively absorbed by melanin, the skin's main pigment, leading to its destruction—a process known as selective photothermolysis. Damage to the pigment-laden melanosomes in this manner is responsible for the fading or disappearance of the unwanted discolorations.[55] The main drawbacks of laser therapy are the considerable expense of the treatments and the frequent necessity for multiple treatment sessions.

In my experience, comparable results for removing a variety of pigmentary abnormalities, including liver spots and keratoses, may be much more simply obtained with the use of a radiosurgical unit, the Ellman Surgitron (Fig. 51–7). Emitting at 3.8 MHz, the frequency of radiowaves, these units operate at a range of little tissue alteration. When used with local anesthesia and an extremely low, partially rectified cutting current, the outer rim of a sterilizable loop electrode or the broad base of a triangular one is drawn lightly across the unwanted tissue, literally melting it away. Wiping the treatment area gently with a moistened gauze pad will remove any residual material; wound care largely consists of repeated daily applications of silver sulfadiazine cream until complete healing occurs, usually in about 2 weeks.

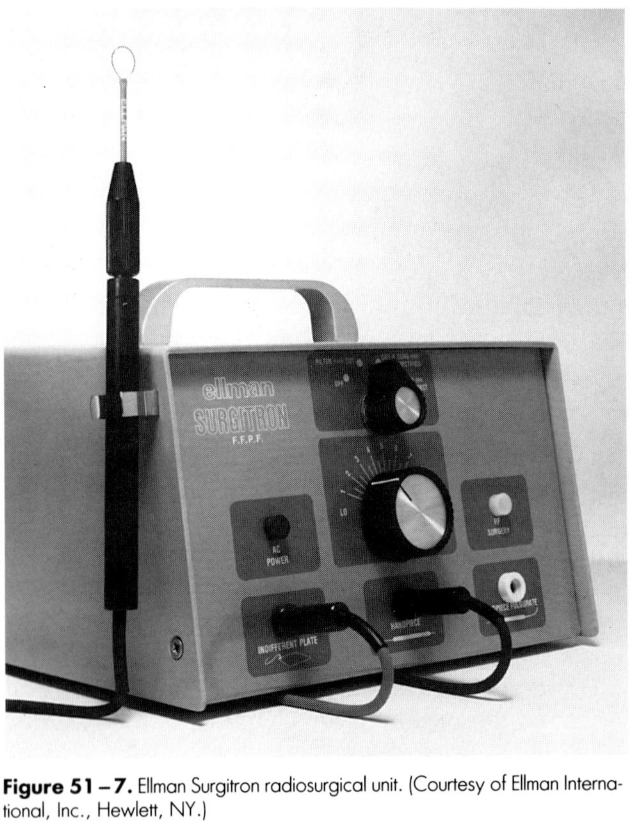

Figure 51–7. Ellman Surgitron radiosurgical unit. (Courtesy of Ellman International, Inc., Hewlett, NY.)

TELANGIECTASIA

Red linear telangiectasia of the face, which typically involves the nose and cheeks, is believed to be due to persistent arteriolar vasodilation. Often mistakenly referred to as "broken blood" vessels by most patients, unsightly, arborized networks of telangiectases may result from a variety of predisposing factors. They are commonly found in fair-complexioned persons who tend to be "flushers" (i.e., those who have a lifelong history of flushing easily when under emotional or physical stress or simply after eating hot or spicy foods or consuming alcohol). They also develop in sun-damaged skin and are quite commonly associated with rosacea.

Numerous methods of treatment have been tried through the years with varying success, including electrolysis and electrodesiccation. With either of these modalities some degree of superficial tissue damage invariably occurs, increasing the risk of developing multiple areas of white pinpoint scarring, especially in fair-skinned blonds and redheads.[56]

Laser therapy based on the selective photothermolysis of oxyhemoglobin, most recently with the tunable dye and copper vapor lasers, has also been used successfully to treat facial telangiectases.[57, 58] Although these lasers for treating telangiectases represent a significant advance over the nonselective carbon dioxide laser, or even the argon laser, such treatments are often expensive, and, overall, the typical postoperative complications of crusting and scabbing appear to be little different in most instances from those observed with the more conventional electrocautery and electrodesiccation devices.

A simple, but extremely effective radiosurgical method for obliterating facial and neck telangiectasia has been described, once again employing the Ellman Surgitron.[59] With the unit adjusted to a very low current setting, numerous telangiectases may literally be blanched in a matter of only a few minutes by lightly touching or "tapping" them in rapid succession while keeping the foot pedal continually depressed (Fig. 51–8). The low current and light touch required by this method is reported to significantly reduce the risk of post-treatment delling or depressions of the skin, which were common problems with the older electrosurgical units. Although a variety of needles are available for radiosurgical treatment of unwanted blood vessels, including insulated needles and 32- and 33-gauge needles with hub adaptors, I find the use of 32-gauge metal-hubbed needles bent at 30 degrees and fitted to the handpiece with a hub adaptor to be the most convenient method (Fig. 51–9).

In general, more than one treatment session is usually required for optimal results, especially if there is a good deal of arborization or networking of the blood vessels. Ordinarily, no prior topical or local anesthesia is required, and by using the partially rectified current setting on the device, patients generally experience at most a modestly annoying sensation on contact, another significant advantage over treatment with earlier electrosurgical devices. In my own experience treating thousands of telangiectases in this fashion, the results have been gratifying and overall patient satisfaction has been high.

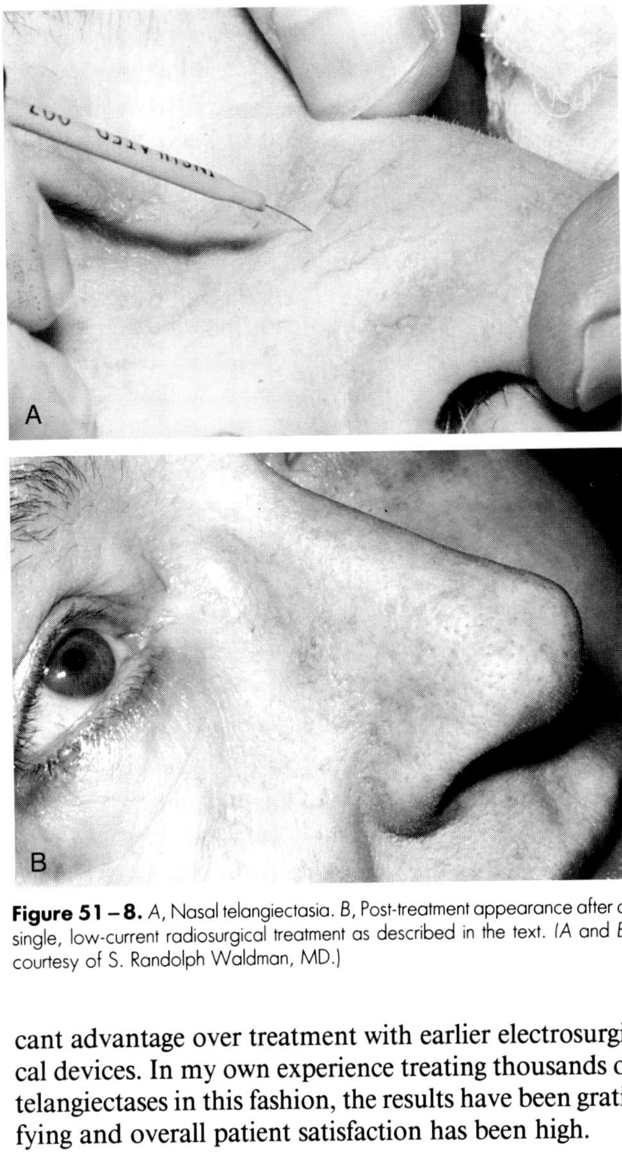

Figure 51–8. *A*, Nasal telangiectasia. *B*, Post-treatment appearance after a single, low-current radiosurgical treatment as described in the text. (*A* and *B* courtesy of S. Randolph Waldman, MD.)

COSMETIC TECHNIQUES

To exclude cosmetics from any discussion of total facial rejuvenation would be a significant omission. For

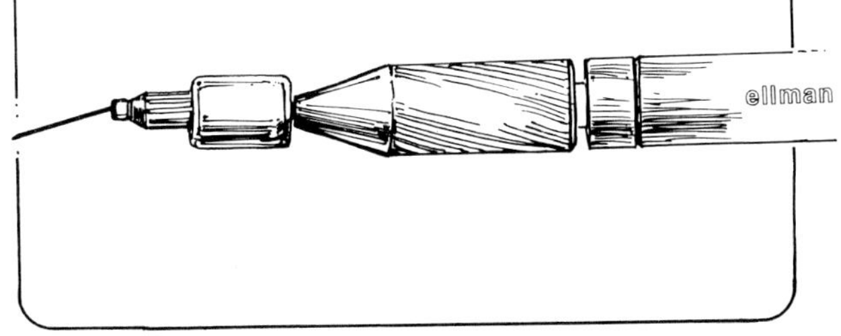

Figure 51–9. Disposable 30-gauge metal-hubbed needle bent at a 30-degree angle and attached by a special hub adapter. (Courtesy of Acuderm, Ft. Lauderdale, FL.)

most women, and many men these days, they represent the first line of "treatment" for a wide variety of skin deformities and irregularities, including wrinkling and discolorations of all sorts. Within the past decade, in fact, a whole new field, known as *paramedical cosmetic techniques*, has sprung up. This involves the use of make-ups for the appearance enhancement of persons with permanent disfigurement due to congenital defects, trauma, or disease, as well as cosmetic measures to more quickly normalize the appearance of persons with the temporary facial disfigurements that typically follow reconstructive or cosmetic surgery.[60]

A complete discussion of make-ups would take a book in itself. However, for the purposes of this chapter, it is important to at least have a working knowledge of two general categories of cosmetics that may complement any cosmetic medical or surgical work. These are camouflage make-ups and fashion make-ups.[61]

Camouflage Cosmetics

As the name implies, these make-ups are designed to mask, conceal, or disguise a wide variety of unsightly skin discolorations and scars, leaving the skin with a "normal" appearance. Companies specializing in camouflage make-ups include Covermark (800-524-1120), Dermablend (800-621-2158), and Coverderm (612-770-0611). Not sold as a rule in local drug stores or health aid stores, these products may be obtained at better salons or at the counters of some of the finer department stores.

To be effective, camouflage cosmetics are set apart from ordinary make-ups in a number of important ways. For one thing, they must be available in a broad range of colors and shades to cover ethnic variations and nuances in skin shading. Moreover, they must be opaque to conceal or mask even dark skin discolorations. They must also be water resistant, capable of withstanding not only rain, but also swimming and heavy perspiration. In addition, they must provide sufficient holding power to adhere to even nonporous surfaces, such as scar tissue, without sliding off. Finally, they must be long wearing, capable of providing full security throughout the entire day or night.

Because of their special nature, applications and removals of these products is a multistep process usually taking about 10 to 15 minutes each. I generally recommend that first-time users make an appointment with a cosmetologist or make-up specialist skilled in the selection and use of these items to ensure that the appropriate set of products are chosen and their use properly understood by the client. Because bumpy distortions of the skin are generally harder to conceal, masking make-ups are most useful for covering all kinds of flat discolorations and irregularities; and for some people with conditions such as port-wine stains or vitiligo of the face, they often make the difference between a devalued reclusive existence and a vibrant life in the productive mainstream.

Fashion Cosmetics

Make-ups for the mass market, otherwise known as consumer fashion cosmetics, comprise the largest category of cosmetics sold. Items in this array include among many others, toners, moisturizers, concealers, foundations, blushers, powders, lipsticks, make-up removers, eyeliners, eyebrow pencils, eye shadows, mascara, lash extenders, and false eyelashes.

In normal persons, each of these products is ordinarily used to produce a more "glamorous" look. However, in individuals with some form of facial disfigurement or those recently recovering from aesthetic surgery, they may be used to produce a more normal look. Selected properly, they may help in several ways. For example, they may be used for concealing dark discolorations (such as those around the eyes) or bruising by applying a slightly lighter-than-normal-toned concealer under the foundation. A greenish tinted underfoundation concealer may help disguise a ruddy complexion, telangiectases, or postoperative pinkness, and a purple-toned concealer is useful for decreasing sallowness.

By reflecting light, a process called *highlighting*, cosmetics may also be applied to certain facial planes, such as under the eyes, to reduce shadows. Conversely, light-absorbing darker shades may serve to diminish the appearance of a prominent surface irregularity or facial feature, a technique called *shadowing*. And finally, by *contouring*, which combines both shadowing and highlighting, cosmetics may be used, for example, to "narrow" a broad nose or "widen" narrowly spaced eyes.

Cosmetics experts agree that the general tendency on the part of the average consumer is to use too many products in an attempt to achieve a desired effect. Instead, they advise that the key to successful make-up is to limit the items to as few as absolutely necessary.[61] For this reason, it might be wise, even when it comes to selecting fashion cosmetics, to recommend at least one consultation with a reputable cosmetician to be certain that only the right kinds and the requisite minimum of cosmetics are purchased for the purpose.

One category of fashion cosmetic that has enjoyed a renaissance these past few years deserves special note: artificial tanning agents or sunless "tanning" products.[62] Containing the nontoxic, vital skin dye dihydroxyacetone (DHA), these agents rely on the harmless chemical reaction between the dye and skin surface proteins to impart a golden brown color to the skin. Today's lower concentrations of DHA and better vehicles have significantly improved the effect achieved by these products as compared with the artificial burnt orange color that characterized the first generation of sunless tanners more than 3 decades ago.

Available for light to dark skin tones in creams, lotions, and gels, sunless tanners usually require several successive applications to achieve the desired effect. Once this is achieved, these products usually need not be applied more than two to three times per week to maintain the effect, since the color is only gradually lost over several days as the skin's surface proteins are shed or washed away. Users must be warned, however, that no matter how deep the "tan" they get with these products, the color, unlike a real tan, offers no significant protection from the sun. To look their best and preserve their skin's health, they should be advised to apply sunless tanners to "tan" overnight and to use sunscreens every morning.

In summary, although it is certainly true that there is currently no substitute for procedures such as face-lifts and eyelid surgery to improve sagging and redundancy of skin, there are a wide array of relatively simple but extremely important preventive and treatment measures that may be used to complement these procedures. The routine use of sunscreens, the proper application of cosmetics and cosmeceuticals, and the adjunctive use of filler substances, chemical peels, and skin sanding, among other procedures that comprise total facial rejuvenation, can go a long way to enhancing and sustaining the effects of aesthetic surgery and ensuring maximal patient satisfaction.

REFERENCES

1. Macgregor FC: Insights and considerations. *In* After Plastic Surgery. New York, Praeger, 1979, p 115.
2. Novick NL: Super Skin: A Leading Dermatologist's Guide to the Latest Breakthroughs in Skin Care. New York, Clarkson N. Potter, 1988, pp 167–170.
3. Elson ML: Evaluation and treatment of the aging face. Cosmet Dermatol 3(6):11–14, 1990.
4. Finlay AY: Diagnosing Photoaged Skin. West Sussex, England, Cambridge Medical Publications, 1991, pp 1–14.
5. Lavker RM, Zeng P, Dong G: Morphology of aged skin. *In* Gilchrest BA (ed): Clinics in Geriatric Medicine, vol 5. Philadelphia, WB Saunders, 1989, pp 53–67.
6. Novick NL: Care of the aging face. *In* Bosniak SL (ed): Advances in Ophthalmic Plastic and Reconstructive Surgery, vol 2. New York, Pergamon Press, 1983, pp 209–215.
7. Kligman AM: Early destructive effect of sunlight on human skin. JAMA 210:2377–2380, 1969.
8. Taylor CR, Stern RS, Leyden JJ, et al: Photoaging photodamage and photoprotection. J Am Acad Dermatol 22:1–15, 1990.
9. Novick NL: Baby Skin: A Leading Dermatologist's Guide to Infant and Childhood Skin Care. New York, Clarkson N. Potter, 1991, pp 13–20.
10. Novick NL: Skin Care for Teens. New York, Franklin Watts, 1988, pp 16–20.
11. Owens DW, Knox JM: Influence of heat, wind, and humidity on ultraviolet radiation injury. NCI Monogr 50:161–167, 1978.
12. Sterling GB: Sunscreens: A review. Cutis 50:221–224, 1992.
13. Weinstein GD, Nigra TP, Pochi PE, et al: Topical tretinoin for treatment of photodamaged skin. Arch Dermatol 127:659–665, 1991.
14. Ellis CN, Weiss JS, Hamilton TA, et al: Sustained improvement with prolonged tretinoin (retinoic acid) for photoaged skin. J Am Acad Dermatol 23:629–637, 1990.
15. Leyden JJ, Grove GL, Grove MJ, et al: Treatment of photodamaged facial skin with topical tretinoin. J Am Acad Dermatol 21:638–644, 1989.
16. Kligman AM: Guidelines for the use topical tretinoin (Retin-A) for photoaged skin. J Am Acad Dermatol 21:650–654, 1989.
17. Hevia O, Nemeth AJ, Taylor JR: Tretinoin accelerates healing after trichloroacetic chemical peel. Arch Dermatol 127:678–682, 1991.
18. Mandy S: Tretinoin in the preoperative and postoperative management of dermabrasion. J Am Acad Dermatol 159[Suppl]:878–879, 1986.
19. Hung VC, Lee JY, Zitelli JA, et al: Topical tretinoin and epithelial wound healing. Arch Dermatol 125:65–69, 1989.
20. Van Scott EJ, Yu RJ: Alpha hydroxy acids: Therapeutic potentials. Can J Dermatol 1(5):108–112, 1989.
21. Rogers RS, Callen J, Wehr R, et al: Comparative efficacy of 12% ammonium lactate lotion and 5% lactic acid lotion in the treatment of moderate to severe xerosis. J Am Acad Dermatol 21:714–716, 1989.
22. Van Scott EJ, Yu RJ: Alpha hydroxy acids: Procedures for use in clinical practice. Cutis 43:222–228, 1989.
23. Moy LS: The use of glycolic acids in the treatment of various skin disorders. Communication at the 17th annual clinical and scientific meeting of the American Society for Dermatologic Surgery. Reported in the Canadian Medical News, July 27, 1990.
24. Van Scott EJ, Yu RJ: Hyperkeratinization, corneocyte cohesion and alpha-hydroxy acids. J Am Acad Dermatol 5:867–879, 1984.
25. Ridge JM, Siegle RJ, Zuckerman J: Use of alpha-hydroxy acids in the therapy of photoaged skin. J Am Acad Dermatol 23:932, 1990.
26. Lavker RM, Kaidbey K, Leyden JJ: Effects of topical ammonium lactate on cutaneous atrophy from a potent topical corticosteroid. J Am Acad Dermatol 26:535–544, 1992.
27. Moy LS, Murad H, Moy RL: Glycolic acid peels for the treatment of wrinkles and photoaging. J Dermatol Surg Oncol 19:243–246, 1993.
28. Elson ML: The utilization of glycolic acid in photoaging. Cosmet Dermatol 5(1):12–15, 1992.
29. Brody HJ: Chemical Peeling. St. Louis, Mosby–Year Book, 1992.
30. Matarasso SL, Glogau RG: Chemical face peels. Dermatol Clin 9:131–150, 1991.
31. Brody HJ, Hailey CW: Medium-depth chemical peeling of the skin: A variation of superficial surgery. J Dermatol Surg Oncol 12:1268–1273, 1986.
32. Monheit GD: The Jessner's and TCA peel: A medium-depth chemical peel. J Dermatol Surg Oncol 15:945–950, 1989.
33. Moy LS: Glycolic acid–TCA peel combination deemed consistent and predictable. Cosmet Dermatol 6(3):43–44, 1993.
34. Benedetto AV, Griffin TD, Benedetto EA, et al: Dermabrasion: Therapy and prophylaxis of the photoaged face. J Am Acad Dermatol 27:439–447, 1992.
35. Yarborough JM, Beeson WH: Dermabrasion. *In* Beeson WH, McCullough EG (eds): Aesthetic Surgery of the Aging Face. St. Louis, CV Mosby, 1986, pp 142–181.
36. Maliner JS: Regional hand dermabrasion. *In* Maliner JS (ed): Plastic and Reconstructive Surgery of the Head and Neck, the Third International Symposium, Vol 1, Aesthetic Surgery. New York, Grune & Stratton, 1981, pp 191–194.
37. Harris DR, Noodleman FR: Combining manual dermasanding with low-strength trichloroacetic acid to improve actinically injured skin. J Dermatol Surg Oncol 20:436–442, 1994.
38. Bircoll M: A nine-year experience with autologous fat transplantation. Am J Cosmet Surg 9(1):55–59, 1992.
39. Kessler D: Testimony of the FDA commissioner, before the House of Representatives Human Resources and Intergovernmental Relations Subcommittee, regarding "Promoting Drugs for Unapproved Uses," June 11, 1991.
40. Klein AW: In favor of double skin testing. J Dermatol Surg Oncol 15:263, 1989.
41. Elson ML: Injectable collagen and autoimmune disease. J Dermatol Surg Oncol 19:165–168, 1993.
42. Elson ML: Correction of dermal contour defects with injectable collagens: Choosing and using these materials. Semin Dermatol 6:77–82, 1987.
43. Elson ML: Soft tissue augmentation of periorbital fine lines and the orbital groove with Zyderm-I and fine-gauge needles. J Dermatol Surg Oncol 18:779–782, 1992.
44. Puissegur Lupo ML: A technique to correct undereye circles and bags. Cosmet Dermatol 6(3)14–16, 1993.
45. Monheit GD: Fibrel injection techniques in cutaneous scars for soft-tissue augmentation and wrinkles. Cosmet Dermatol 5(4):10–15, 1992.
46. Rosen T, Watkins HC: Use of gelatin matrix implant in patients hypersensitive to bovine collagen. J Am Acad Dermatol 22:848–849, 1990.
47. Millikan L, Banks K, Purkait B, et al: A 5-year safety and efficacy evaluation with Fibrel in the correction of cutaneous scars following one or two treatments. J Dermatol Surg Oncol 17:223–229, 1991.

48. Ortonne JP: Pigmentary changes of the aging skin. Br J Dermatol 122[Suppl 35]:21–28, 1990.
49. Rafal ES, Griffiths EM, Ditre CM, et al: Topical tretinoin (retinoic acid) treatment for liver spots associated with photodamage. N Engl J Med 326:368–374, 1992.
50. Kligman AM, Willis I: A new formula for depigmenting human skin. Arch Dermatol 111:40–48, 1975.
51. Harris DR: Several agents enhance effects of Retin-A, improve compliance. Communication at a Symposium on Problems of the Aging Skin, sponsored by Stanford University School of Medicine. Reported in Skin and Allergy News, June 1992, p 22.
52. Lubritz RR: Cryosurgery of benign lesions. Cutis 16:426–431, 1975.
53. Simon CA: A simple and accurate cryosurgical tool for the treatment of benign skin lesions: The "Hard Tail" dip-stick. J Dermatol Surg Oncol 12:680–682, 1986.
54. Alster TS, Kohn SR: Dermatologic lasers: Three decades of progress. Int J Dermatol 3:601–610, 1992.
55. Margolis RJ, Dover JS, Polla LL, et al: Visible action spectrum for melanin-specific selective photothermolysis. Lasers Surg Med 9:389–397, 1989.
56. Goldman MP, Bennett RG: Treatment of telangiectasia: A review. J Am Acad Dermatol 17:167–182, 1987.
57. Polla LL, Tan OT, Garden JM, et al: Tunable pulsed dye laser for the treatment of benign cutaneous vascular ectasia. Dermatologica 174:11–17, 1987.
58. Key JM, Waner M: Selective destruction of facial telangiectasia using a copper vapor laser. Arch Otolaryngol Head Neck Surg 118:509–513, 1992.
59. Harris DR, Noodleman R: Using a low current radiosurgical unit to obliterate facial telangiectasias. J Dermatol Surg Oncol 17:382–384, 1991.
60. Westmore MG: The use of cosmetics in facial rehabilitation, post surgery. Presented before the Annual Meeting of the American Society of Plastic and Reconstructive Surgeons, San Francisco, CA, 1974.
61. Westmore MG: Make-up as an adjunct and aid to the practice of dermatology. Dermatol Clin 9:81–88, 1991.
62. Novick NL: Saving Face: A Dermatologist's Guide to Maintaining a Healthier and Younger-Looking Face. Los Angeles, The Body Press, 1986, pp 33–465.

CHAPTER 52

The Practical Application of Aestheticians in the Plastic and Reconstructive Surgeon's Office

Susanne S. Warfield

For an accurate description of an aesthetician, the definition of aesthetics should be examined: "pertaining to beauty, or the improvement of appearance." Across the United States, the use of the word aesthetician is synonymous for the person who performs beautifying services. However, this description may be outdated because the field of aesthetics has now moved into the medical arena not just to beautify patients but to deal with many other physical and psychological aspects as well. In some states, the name for this new branch of medicine or aesthetic therapy may be called by different names, such as paramedical aesthetician, medical aesthetician, beauty therapist, facial technologist, and clinical aesthetician. The focus of this chapter is to give an overview of what an aesthetician can do in a medical office and how this new field of skin care will enhance the surgical and reconstructive patient's care.

The types of treatments offered by these specialists are varied, and some aestheticians have chosen to practice in a medical setting.

Treatments offered by skin care specialists are

- Preoperative and postoperative skin care
- Exfoliation treatments, which may include superficial chemical exfoliation
- Lymphatic drainage massage to assist the postoperative patient with edema
- Cosmetic camouflage therapy
- Dermal micropigmentation
- Preoperative removal of comedone impactions to facilitate wound healing
- Electrolysis and unwanted hair removal

These treatments are not limited to the facial area and may include other body areas, such as in the surgical reconstruction of the breast after a mastectomy or in burn disfigurement therapy.

Integration of skin care services into an established surgical practice requires time and energy. The most difficult task in starting a skin care practice is finding a skin care specialist whose methods and philosophies are compatible with those of the physician and also who has, or is willing to learn, the necessary medical knowledge. The alliance of physicians and skin care practitioners is so new that few postgraduate training classes or facilities are available. At time of publication, no state-accredited institution or recognized license existed for a clinical or medical aesthetic course. However, private schools, skin care companies, and associations offer certification courses in medical aesthetics, cosmetic camouflage therapy, and dermal micropigmentation. Table 52–1 lists the various associations and postgraduate training facilities available.

BENEFITS FOR THE PHYSICIAN

Several benefits exist for the physician incorporating skin care services into an existing medical practice.

Generation of New Patient Base

The addition of ancillary services offers patients a wider variety of treatments ranging from conservative therapy to surgery. The ability of the physician's office to cater to all patients' needs and desires for self-improvement can increase the physician's patient base. The reconstructive surgery patient who has undergone psychological trauma may feel more comfortable receiving cosmetic or skin care therapy in medical surroundings.

Development of Patient Loyalty Through Extended Visits

Once patients have undergone a surgical procedure that was accompanied by skin care treatments, their need for continued advice and guidance does not stop. The patient's results speak to the fact that the adjuncts of skin care and cosmetic therapy provided much-needed and effective treatment.

Increase in Patient's Confidence in Care

Patients who are concerned about their appearance or who have undergone a traumatic event, such as an acci-

TABLE 52-1

Skin Care Associations and Postgraduate Training Facilities

Aesthetics International Association
4447 McKinney Avenue
Dallas, TX 75205
(214) 526-0752
Fax (214) 526-2925

Alliance of Medical Estheticians
Attention: Lori Bridgeford
105 North Eastwood
Suite 5
Inglewood, CA 90301
(310) 540-3636
Fax (310) 540-9787

American Aestheticians Education Association, Inc.
Contact Bonnie Day
AAEA Headquarters
P.O. Box 117896
Carrollton, TX 75011-7896
(214) 394-1740
Fax (214) 492-9630

American Electrology Association
106 Oak Ridge Road
Trumbull, CT 06611
(203) 374-6667

American Society of Esthetic Medicine
Michelle Palmer, Chairperson
734 N. LaSalle
Suite 1109
Chicago, IL 60610-3539
(312) 789-0003
(312) 751-2031
(312) 248-6530

International Guild of Professional Electrologists, Inc.
202 Boulevard Street
Suite B
High Point, NC 27262
(910) 841-6631
(910) 841-5187

Medical Aesthetic Foundation
Dennis M. Everton, M.D.
Facial Surgery Institute
1215 E. Brown Road
Mesa, AZ 85203
(602) 844-8544

National Cosmetic Tattooing Association
P.O. Box 453
Tehacahpi, CA 93581
(805) 822-1508

Scott & White Hospital
2401 South 31st Street
Temple, TX 76508
(817) 774-0255

Society of Clinical and Medical Electrologists Inc.
132 Great Road
Suite 200
Stow, MA 01775
(508) 461-0313
Fax (508) 897-5442

Society of Cosmetic Professionals
P.O. Box 446
Vallejo, CA 94590
(707) 557-1012

Society of Plastic Surgical Skin Care Specialists
C/O The Aesthetic Society
3922 Atlantic Avenue
Long Beach, CA 90807
(310) 595-4275
Fax (310) 427-2234

Advanced Skin Care and Training Center
450 Sutter Street
Suite 1723
San Francisco, CA 94108
(415) 398-6013

dent, need to believe that they are receiving the best treatment available. Through the possibly long recuperation period, patients need additional advice on how to care for their skin and how to cover bruising and healing. They also seek the psychological support that can be provided by a skin care specialist who listens to a patient's concerns.

Integration of Office Space and Use in Off-Peak Hours

From a profitability standpoint, the addition of an aesthetician to a plastic and reconstructive surgery practice need not add substantially to the surgeon's overhead. The aesthetician can see patients in the office during offpeak office hours. During peak office hours, the skin care specialist can be available for consultation and advice for patients who need aesthetic services.

BENEFITS FOR THE PATIENT

Education of Patient on Skin Physiology

Education is key to patient compliance, and preoperative and postoperative instructions and understanding of the procedure are vital for optimal results. During this education process, the aesthetician can also find out if patients have a realistic understanding of the aesthetic results of the surgical procedure.

Increases Time Spent with Patient

Most of the additional services offered by a skin care or dermal micropigmentation specialist take a minimum of 1 hour. During this time, much education on home care can be covered with the patient. The patient then feels that he or she is receiving comprehensive and personalized care.

Reinforces Home Care Instructions on Treatment

The postoperative healing phase can be a very frightening time for many patients. During this time, compliance with home care instructions is vital for the best surgical outcome. The skin care specialist can also keep a watchful eye on wound healing.

Addresses Psychological Concerns that the Patient Might Not Have Brought to the Physician's Attention

The longer the time spent with a patient, the likelier it is that concerns will surface that might not have been brought to the physician's attention. Communication between the patient and skin care specialist can often lead to revealing information that would be useful to the physician. Under no circumstances should the skin care specialist be giving psychological counseling to the patient, but often an empathetic ear can help alleviate anxieties associated with reconstructive surgeries.

CONCLUSION

Physicians who incorporate a skin care specialist into their practice are able to offer a new dimension in the care of the surgical patient. Many plastic and reconstructive surgery practices will benefit from the presence of an aesthetician on their staff; this burgeoning field can improve patients' perception of their care as well as the aesthetics of their surgical results.

REFERENCE

1. Dorland's Illustrated Medical Dictionary. Philadelphia, WB Saunders, 1988, p 583.

CHAPTER 53

The Role of the Aesthetician Before and After Surgery

Catherine Atzen

As a higher and more scientific level of education becomes available to the aesthetic professional, the aesthetician's role in treating the surgical patient is becoming more prominent. The aesthetician is actively involved in improving the skin's appearance and can prepare the patient psychologically for the surgery and provide comfort and reassurance. The aesthetician can

Advise the patient on how to properly remove eye makeup, correctly shape the eyebrows, and use skin care products at home.
Listen to the patient's concerns and needs.
Select safe and efficient skin care products.
Communicate and discuss critical topics with the surgeon.
Select and perform skin care procedures before and after surgery to prepare the skin and improve its condition. These procedures may activate the healing process and may reduce postoperative swelling and bruising.
Explain the benefits of regular skin care procedures that may maximize the results of surgery.

As more and more women and men seek out professional aestheticians for facials, body treatments, and advice on proper home skin care, the demand for skin care services by licensed aestheticians has increased at a rate of 14% to 15% per year, one of the highest increases of any consumer industry. Informed and educated consumers are drifting away from department store and drugstore sales counters because they want professional advice from someone who understands the specific needs of their skin. These are the same individuals who seek cosmetic surgery.

When surgery is planned, it is the perfect time to consider a fresh approach to the patient's skin care program. Skin care treatments may improve the final appearance of surgery by reducing postoperative bruising and swelling, improving skin tone, reducing fine wrinkling, and rehydrating the skin.

The most important role of the aesthetician is to advise clients on the best skin care regimen that will maintain their skin in excellent condition. Aestheticians cleanse their client's skin, extract comedones, and exfoliate dead skin cells to prevent a thick, leathery, and uneven skin texture. Aestheticians warn their clients about the risk of sun exposure and recommend sun block creams not only for summer but also for daily use.

A skin care regimen is a complex and personalized program that is constantly evolving according to season, climate, age, stress level, and environmental and pollution factors, as well as the general health of the client. The client's commitment to the prescribed skin care regimen is essential for optimal results. Skin care regimens usually include regular treatments performed at the skin care salon and use of skin care products for maintenance at home between treatments. In addition to cleansing facials, electrotherapy, electrocosmetology, lymphatic drainage, and mild peeling methods may be offered.

The aesthetician should establish contact with the patient before surgery to explain the treatment and to schedule appointments at the patient's convenience. These consultations allow the aesthetician to ask questions about the patient's skin condition and sensitivities (allergies to, or irritations from, some products), the products the patient is currently using to cleanse and protect the skin, sun protection, and other lifestyle habits. The aesthetician then informs the patient about product ingredients and recommends products for home use.

The aesthetician reassures the patient and reinforces the surgeon's recommendations. Whether working in an independent skin care practice or within the surgeon's facility, the aesthetician is an "outsider," to whom the patient may be more open in discussing expectations and fears. The aesthetician provides emotional and physical support to the patient and shares the patient's concerns with the surgeon or surgeon's assistant.

Ideally, the aesthetician gives a consultation 2 or more weeks before the surgery is planned and schedules the skin care program according to the needs of the patient. During the first consultation, the aesthetician evaluates the condition of the patient's skin, particularly around the eyes to determine if the skin is dehydrated, irritated or sensitive, sun damaged, or has lost elasticity, or if dark circles or swelling appears. In addition, to best prepare

the patient's skin for surgery, the aesthetician gives lymphatic drainage treatments (manual or mechanical) to the patient on each of the 3 days before the operation.

The aesthetician discusses the patient's lifestyle, being especially concerned with lack of sleep, consumption of alcohol, nutrition, use of fragrance and oil-based (e.g., baby oil) or alcohol-based eye make-up remover, which could cause irritation or swelling. The patient is warned against using products that could cause sensitivity or inflammation, and the aesthetician demonstrates gentle and efficient skin cleansing methods that rely on a water-soluble cleanser or water-based tonic lotion. The aesthetician explains that soap may cause irritation and dryness, and how some heavy creams and oils can clog pores and make the eyes puffy. Strong eye make-up removers, such as those used for waterproof mascara, can cause the eyes to water and make the eyelids red and irritated. Sun exposure before surgery may cause dehydration and retard healing. Sleeping while wearing eye make-up is drying and irritating to the eyes as well as to the eyelids. The aesthetician can recommend a light, water-based eye gel that keeps make-up from running into the eyes, as well as a water-based sun block gel containing titanium dioxide for ultraviolet protection and as a base for make-up.

The aesthetician reviews the make-up and skin care products the patient is using and makes recommendations as necessary. One concern is the fact that many patients use bacteria-filled mascara and other make-up items. The aesthetician advises the patient on the hygienic use of make-up and advises against putting fingers into jars and experimenting with make-up at department store counters. Obviously, the last thing the patient desires is an eye infection just before surgery. Replacing make-up on a regular basis and disinfecting make-up brushes are explained. The aesthetician can supply disposable make-up brushes, sponges, and mascara applicators for the patient's use. These steps can help prevent allergic reactions, infections, and irritations.

Depending on the needs of the patient, other services are recommended, such as eyebrow shaping. The eyebrow shape that is appropriate for the proportions of the face is helpful to the surgeon. Aestheticians often see too much hair removed at the wrong places. With the eyebrow properly shaped, a person with a sad, angry, or tired appearance can look rested and happy. Aestheticians can teach proper eyebrow shaping to the patient, or patients can visit the aesthetician monthly for professional care. Men may see an aesthetician to improve the appearance of bushy brows. Aestheticians often wax the hair line as well, which brightens the face when the forehead is small and the hairline uneven.

During the early postoperative period, skin treatments are very relaxing and promote a feeling of well being in the patient. This effect is especially helpful for patients who have difficulty sleeping. Lymphatic drainage may help reduce edema more rapidly when the regimen is offered daily for a few days starting the day after surgery. The aesthetician offers camouflage make-up, if needed. Aestheticians who have extensive training in color can also advise the patient on what colors are appropriate for make-up and clothing and refer the patient to a hair colorist or stylist if needed.

In addition, aestheticians retain thousands of files on potential patients for cosmetic surgery. The surgeon can benefit from referrals from these clients, and the aesthetician benefits from surgeon referrals.

SUMMARY

A good skin care program is a lifetime commitment. Skin care is not yet well understood in the United States, just as nutrition, exercise, and preventive dentistry were virtually ignored only a few years ago. Skin care clinics are part of the hospital settings in many European countries, where aestheticians are recognized as health practitioners. By working together, surgeons and aestheticians can create an environment that increases patients' feelings of confidence and well being, help them overcome their fears, and ensure optimal results.

CHAPTER 54

Brow Ptosis

Robert A. Weiss

Early signs of the aging face are often manifest by forehead soft tissue wrinkles, brow ptosis, and mechanical or true myogenic involutional blepharoptosis. These changes result from age-related loss of the skin's normal elasticity and from lifelong effects resulting from the forces of gravity on the facial soft tissues. In addition, "fibrosclerosis" of the muscles of facial expression may contribute to these apparent aging changes.[1, 2]

An understanding of the anatomy and appreciation of the pathophysiology of eyebrow position is integral to cosmetic and functional upper eyelid blepharoplasty and ptosis surgery.[3] Eyebrow laxity or brow ptosis often contributes to the development of mechanical ptosis in the patient with cosmetic and functional dermatochalasis. Brow ptosis may develop from normal aging changes, after trauma, or iatrogenically as the result of blepharoplasty. Although eyebrows may be in good anatomic position before upper eyelid surgery, especially blepharoplasty, frequently a lax eyebrow tends to assume a more ptotic position after this surgery. Postoperative brow ptosis often results in the recurrence of dermatochalasis with a suboptimal cosmetic result manifest as a full-appearing upper eyelid or recurrent mechanical ptosis.

The importance and necessity of surgically addressing the forehead soft tissues in aesthetic and functional surgery is certainly not a new concept, as is validated by medical literature reports dating to 1919.[4] For example, when glabellar folds develop above the nasal bridge from depression of the medial aspect of the eyebrows resulting, in turn, from the action of the corrugator supercilii muscles, the facial expression of "pain and suffering" typically results. Similarly, when the frontalis muscle contracts, the eyebrows elevate and the anterior scalp depresses, resulting in the facial appearance that communicates "attention or surprise."[5] In addition to contributing to facial expression and facial aesthetics, the eyebrow and its adjacent soft tissues may be directly responsible for functional ptosis by mechanically obstructing the superior visual field.

Patients with eyebrow ptosis frequently present with complaints of ocular fatigue and frontal region headaches. In addition, cosmetic patients frequently present with a complaint of large transverse furrows in the prefrontal region. These furrows develop from the continuous action of the frontalis muscle to elevate the ptotic brow. During clinical examination, the patient is asked to relax the frontalis muscle. At this time, it usually becomes apparent to both the patient and examiner that the action of the frontalis muscle was unconscious and compensatory to elevate the lax brow that may be weighing the lid down.

Anthropologically, individual variations in the frontal and brow regions have been noted for their usefulness in differentiation of the sexes.[6–11] Frontal bossing or prominence of the frontal bone[12] or subcutaneous tissues[13] over the bone, a typically male characteristic, may be particularly bothersome to the female patient. Women tend to have a soft curve extending from the superior orbital rim to the upper forehead. In some women, the soft contour may be absent because of a prominent sub-brow fat pad.

Surgical correction of a ptotic brow or a prominent sub-brow fat pad may be undertaken by several different approaches. As always, each has specific advantages and disadvantages and each must be individualized for the particular case. Brow ptosis may be corrected by use of a standard suprabrowpexy. Alternatively, midforehead and coronal brow lifts may be employed. A prominent sub-brow fat pad may be contoured and softened surgically by either a trans-lid browplasty or a coronal forehead approach, or the bony structures may be sculpted and adjusted by a superolateral orbital rim ostectomy. Of note, the sub-brow fat pad may be directly responsible for persistent post upper eyelid blepharoplasty fullness in appearance, as well as for the development of brow ptosis.

Since brow ptosis can be asymmetric, the brows may be uneven. In addition to asymmetry between the brows, areas of uneven or irregular ptosis may exist within each brow. To determine the vertical extent of planned excision for suprabrowplasty or suprabrowpexy, the brow is elevated to the desired position with the patient sitting upright and the amount of necessary elevation is measured and documented. These measurements are made along the entire width of the brow to ensure even elevation of the brow ptosis. In many cases, the brow ptosis is limited to the lateral third of the brow. As such, the area of necessary elevation should correspond to the specific area of ptosis present. Measurements must be made preoperatively, since the brow position changes once the patient is placed into a supine position.

With the patient lying in a flat supine position on the operating room table, an incision line is delineated across the edge of the uppermost row of brow cilia, parallel to their direction of growth. For brow ptosis limited to the lateral aspect of the brow, a simple ellipse centered appropriately may suffice (Fig. 54–1). When most or all of the brow is ptotic, a soft S-shaped incision should be demarcated, with the lateral aspect of the incision line curving upward away from the brow (Fig. 54–2). This is necessary to camouflage the postoperative scar since an incision line that directly corresponds to the curvature of the brow, especially laterally, looks very surgical and does not blend into the transverse furrows that may be present across the remainder of the prefrontal region. Once the inferior limb of the incision line is delineated, a parallel vertical line is delineated several millimeters superiorly, based on preoperative measurements. To the preoperative measurements, I typically add a correction factor of 2 mm to compensate for the effect of contraction during wound healing and from the effects of gravity when the patient is sitting erect. The superior and inferior incision lines are joined medially by downward sloping of the superior line to meet the brow. The lateral aspect of the incision is joined by a 30-degree gentle upward sloping of the suprabrow line over a 3- to 4-mm course. As mentioned previously, this upper angulation of the line in a soft S fashion will optimize postoperative cosmesis.

With the incision lines appropriately demarcated, 1% lidocaine (Xylocaine) with epinephrine and hyaluronidase (Wydase) is infiltrated as a frontal block. This is followed by local infiltration of the soft tissues to be excised.

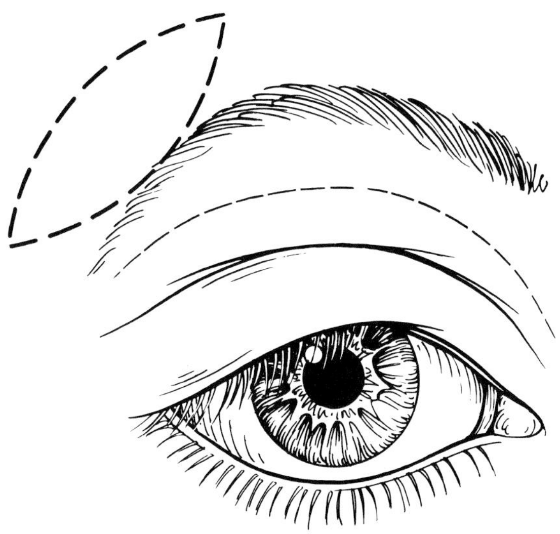

Figure 54–1. A simple elliptical incision may be delineated over the area of focal brow ptosis.

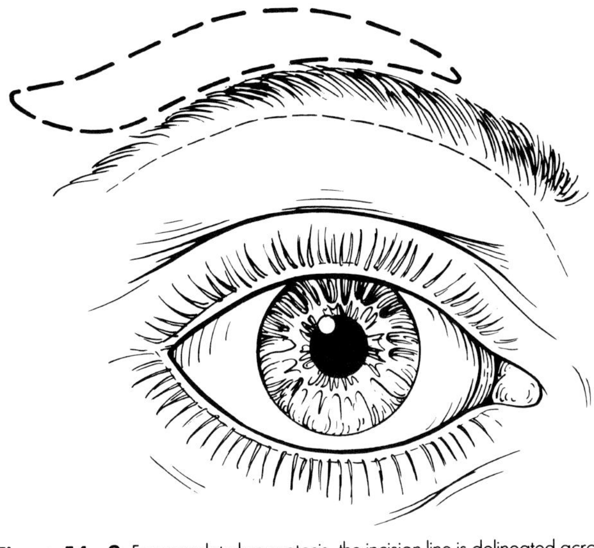

Figure 54–2. For complete brow ptosis, the incision line is delineated across the edge of the uppermost row of brow cilia, parallel to the direction of growth. A soft S-shaped incision should be demarcated with the lateral aspect of the incision line curving upward away from the brow to camouflage the postoperative scar.

Excessive amounts of local anesthesia are to be avoided since they distort the tissues and are unnecessary. Adequate time should be allowed to elapse for the optimal hemostatic effect of the injected epinephrine to occur. Once appropriate vasoconstriction of the highly vascular brow soft tissues has occurred, significantly less capillary oozing will develop.

The surgical incision is created with a no. 15 blade. The dissection is carried down through deep subcutaneous tissue with a needlepoint foot-controlled bovie until the fibers of the frontalis muscle are encountered. Although sharp surgical instruments can be used to incise these tissues, hemostasis is superior and surgical excision is greatly facilitated by the use of either an electrocautery or radiofrequency cutting device. Surgical laser cutting instruments also work well; however, I do not believe their high cost justifies their use in this type of surgery. The entire demarcated area is dissected free from underlying frontalis muscle and excised en bloc. Significant oozing may develop from the prominent vasculature in this area as well as from potential disruption of the frontalis muscle fibers. Hemostasis is best obtained with bipolar cautery forceps or an appropriate electrocautery device. Bipolar cauterization of the underlying frontalis muscle may be performed.

Careful layered closure of the wound defect is necessary to prevent the excessive scarring that frequently develops in this area. If the patient has a facial paresis with paralytic brow ptosis, the lower aspect of the brow must be elevated to join the superior aspect of the wound defect with deep permanent sutures that anchor the brow to underlying periosteum. Use of a permanent, relatively inert suture such as 4-0 polypropylene (Prolene) is pre-

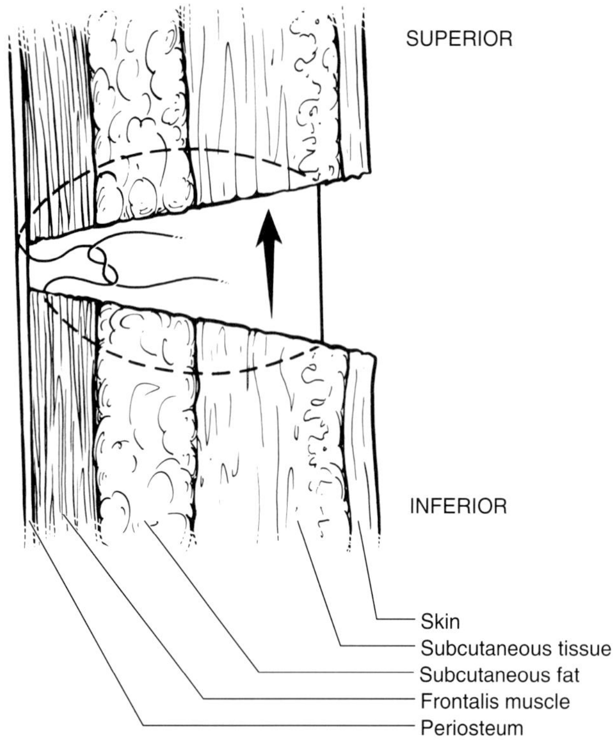

Figure 54–3. Permanent 4.0 polypropylene sutures may be used to perform a browpexy suspension. The suture must pass through cutaneous and subcutaneous tissue as well as the anterior edge of frontalis muscle along the inferior aspect of the incision site and then to deep periosteum at the superior margin of the incision site before coursing through overlying frontalis muscle and subcutaneous tissue. The suture should be placed such that the knot is deeply buried.

fewer layers and greater ease by use of a running vertical mattress suture using 5-0 or 6-0 silk sutures. Interrupted 6-0 silk sutures may be used to close any small wound gaps in the skin edges. In general, a cosmetically superior surgical scar results from use of a vertical mattress closure. Sutures should be removed in 5 to 7 days. The wound may be reinforced with Steri-Strips, if necessary, once the sutures are removed. A topical antibiotic ointment should be applied across the surgical site once or twice daily while the sutures are in place.

Although the suprabrowplasty/suprabrowpexy approach to eyebrow ptosis is technically easy, the postoperative scarring is frequently disturbing to the patient and surgeon. To avoid this scarring, a midforehead or coronal lift may be superior. In addition to leaving a prominent scar by a direct brow surgical approach, suprabrowplasty/suprabrowpexy does not allow appropriate correction of glabellar folds, which may be quite prominent and cosmetically significant. A coronal forehead lift is particularly useful to elevate ptotic brows; however, patients with male-pattern baldness, thinning hair, or a high hairline are not appropriate candidates for the coronal approach because of the resultant cosmetically unacceptable scarring. In these patients, a midforehead approach is ideal.[14] The scarring is significantly less apparent as compared with scars from a standard suprabrowpexy, and the incision line may be fairly cleanly hidden in a

ferred. Several brow suspension sutures must be placed to ensure that the brow is appropriately and evenly elevated. The anchor sutures must go through subcutaneous tissues along the inferior aspect of the wound and periosteum with overlying subcutaneous tissues at the superior aspect of the wound to allow appropriate elevation and not cause significant contraction and scar prominence along the incision line (Fig. 54–3). In my experience, browpexy periosteum suspension sutures may be used in patients with nonparalytic brow ptosis with excellent functional results. In fact, browpexy suspension sutures that involve periosteal fixation ensure an excellent postoperative result without rapid recurrence of brow ptosis. It has been reported that browpexy anchor sutures may prevent normal excursion of the brow in a nonparalytic patient. I have not found that problem to be the case.

The deep layers of brow region soft tissues may be closed with interrupted permanent sutures such as 4-0 nylon or polypropylene or with dissolving sutures such as 4-0 polyglactin (Vicryl). The more superficial subcutaneous tissues may be closed with interrupted 5-0 polyglactin or 5-0 chromic sutures. These sutures are tied such that their knots are buried to prevent suture reaction below the skin line. The overlying soft tissues may be closed with interrupted 5-0 or 6-0 nylon or polypropylene sutures (Fig. 54–4). The wound may be closed with

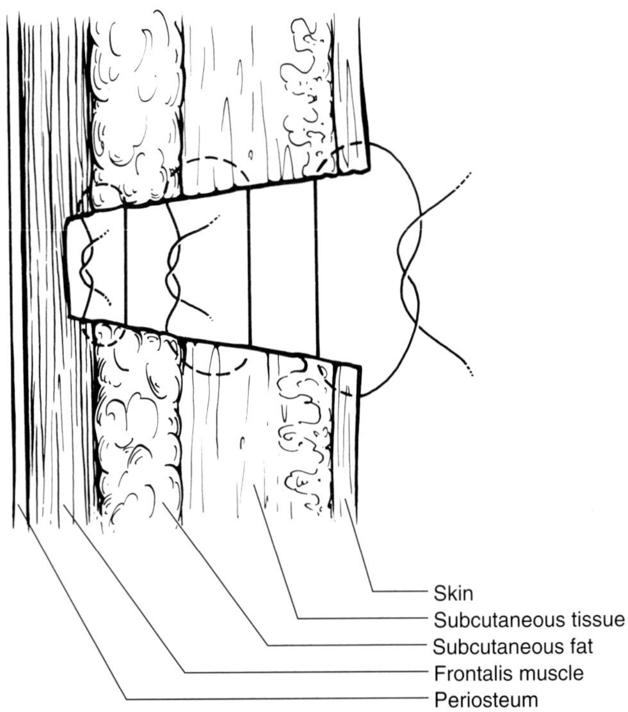

Figure 54–4. Careful layered closure of the wound defect is necessary to prevent excessive scarring. Layered closure should include use of a buried knot 4-0 nylon or polypropylene suture to repair and fix the brow to deep frontalis muscle. The subcutaneous tissue can be closed with a 5-0 polyglactin or 5-0 chromic suture with the knot buried. The skin and superficial subcutaneous tissue is closed with interrupted 5-0 nylon sutures.

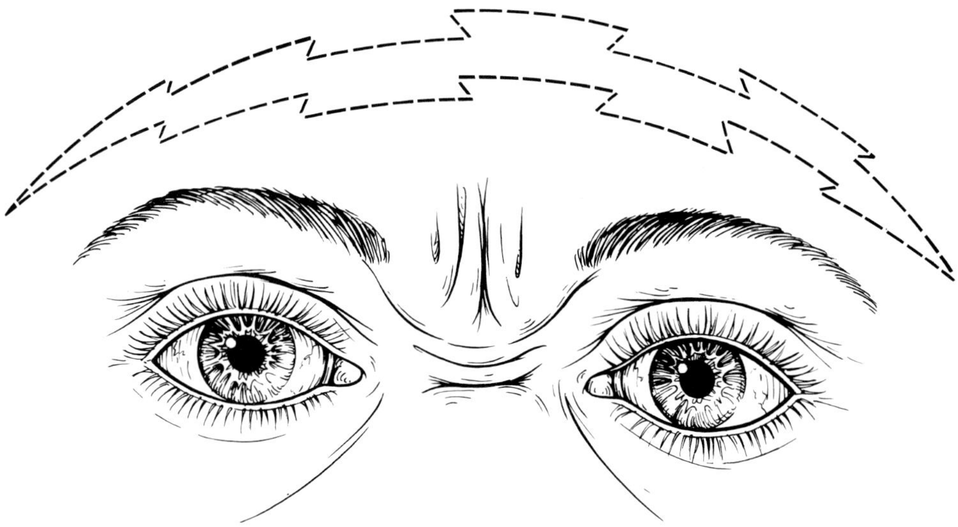

Figure 54–5. A broken geometric incision line or soft W-plasty incision may significantly help hide a midforehead incision scar.

normal skinfold or transverse furrow. In addition, prominent glabellar furrows may be corrected easily through this approach. The incision line delineated should follow a forehead crease line, even if the line appears asymmetric and irregular. This tends to help mask the surgical scar. In select patients, an interrupted incision at two different crease or furrow levels on the corresponding right and left side may even further hide the surgical incision scar. A broken geometric incision line or soft W-plasty incision may also help hide a midforehead incision scar (Fig. 54–5).

As previously described, the vertical dimension of the incision should reflect the desired amount of elevation of the brown and glabellar region tissues. However, a greater degree of overcorrection is required in this area as compared with direct brow elevation to compensate for changes in the tissues once the patient is in an erect position. For the midforehead region, 5 to 10 mm of overcorrection is appropriate. As with a direct brow lift procedure, the area of elevation should correspond to the area of brow ptosis (Figs. 54–6 and 54–7). The skin and subcutaneous tissues should be incised and removed in a manner similar to that already described for the direct brow lift approach (Fig. 54–8). Again, the underlying frontalis muscle is left intact. Skin flaps are then elevated inferiorly to the edge of the supraorbital rim and superiorly for 0.5 cm, staying just above the underlying musculature. If the corrugator muscles are to be disinserted to address prominent glabellar fold lines, a transverse incision is created in the frontalis muscle and its fascia approximately 4 cm above the nasal root and the medial aspects of the superior orbital rims (Fig. 54–9). This incision should not extend as far lateral as the meridian of the supraorbital notches. Care must be exercised to avoid disruption of the underlying neurovascular structures, including the supratrochlear vessels and nerves. The flap is dissected inferiorly along the galea plane, just above the periosteum. The medial ends of the corrugator muscle are identified and isolated to avoid disruption of the adjacent neurovascular structures. The procerus and corrugator muscles may then be disinserted with use of an electrocautery or radiofrequency cutting unit. Superiorly, dissection can be carried out in the subgaleal plane to the level of the hairline. Once this dissection is complete, a portion of frontalis muscle and fascia may be excised to elevate the glabellar and medial brow tissues if

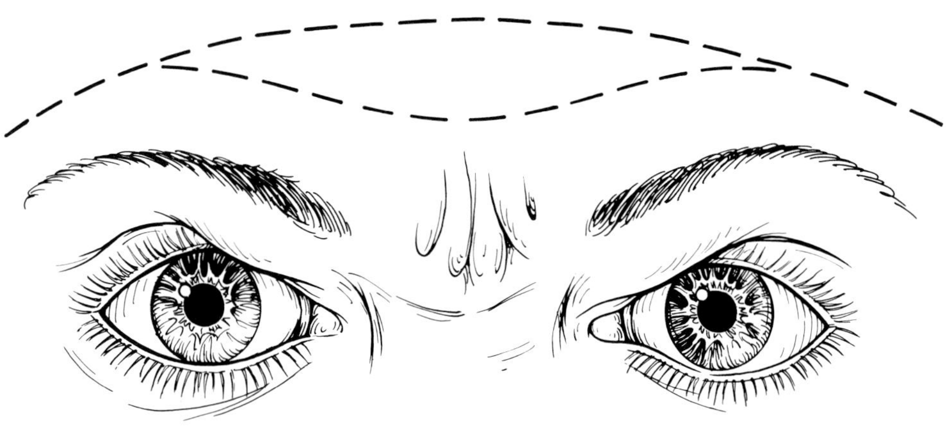

Figure 54–6. The midforehead incision line delineated is designed to elevate ptotic medial brow and glabellar regions.

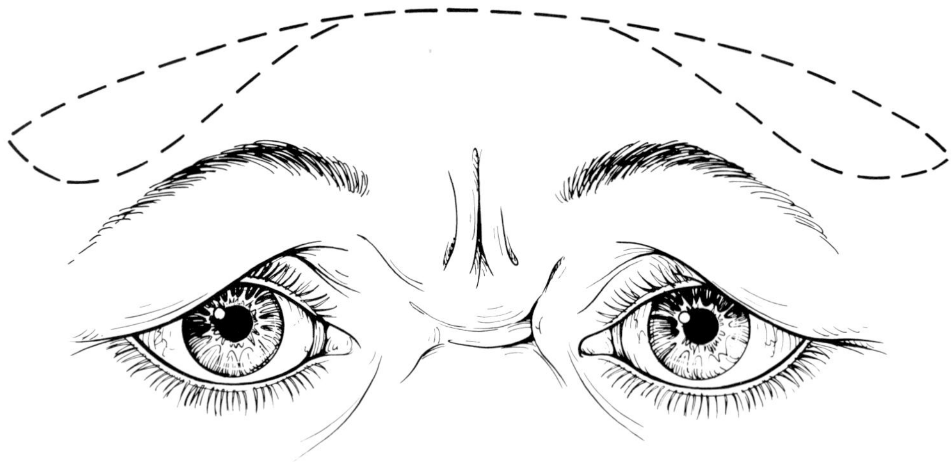

Figure 54–7. The midforehead incision line delineated is designed to elevate ptotic lateral brow regions.

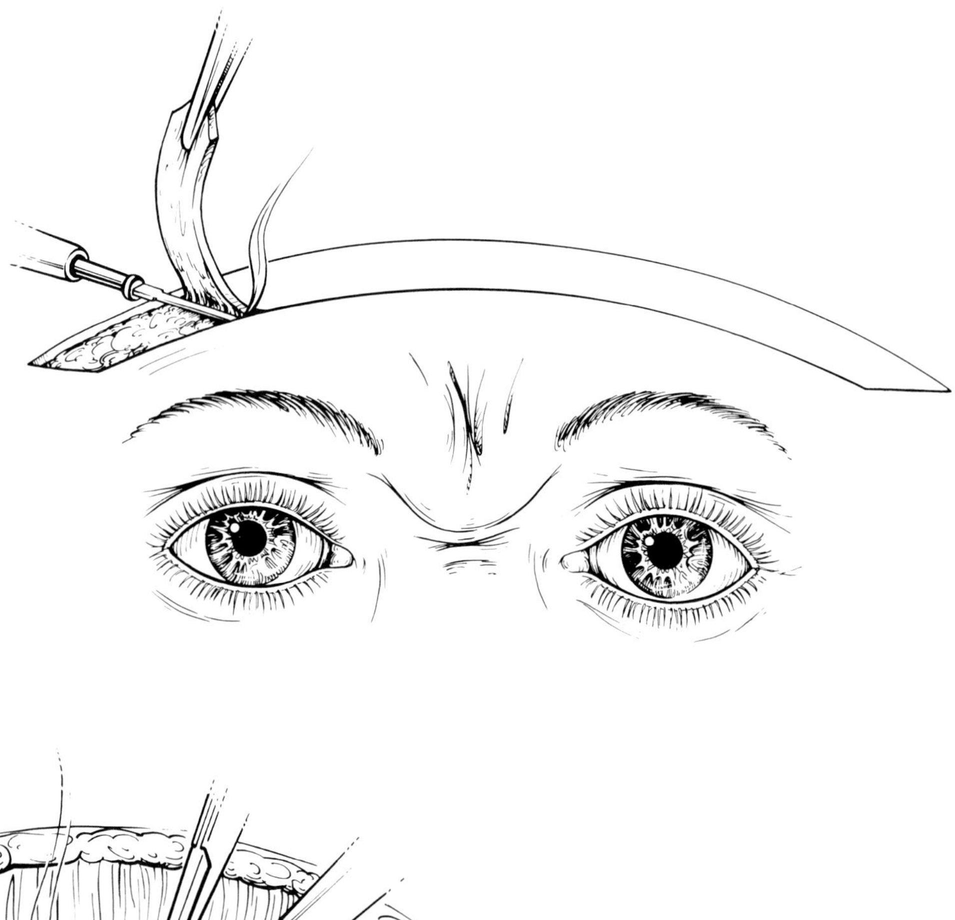

Figure 54–8. After the skin is incised with a surgical scalpel, the deep subcutaneous tissue and fat is incised and separated from underlying frontalis muscle with an electrocautery or radiofrequency cutting device.

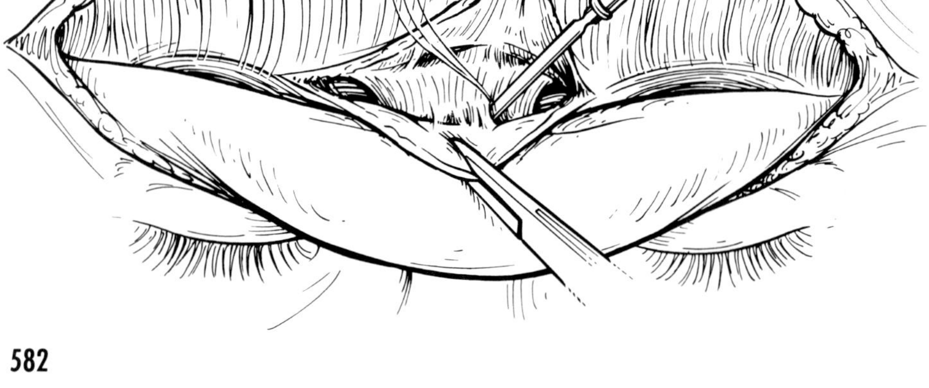

Figure 54–9. A transverse incision line is created in the frontalis muscle and its fascia approximately 4 cm above the nasal root to provide exposure of the corrugator supercilii and procerus muscles.

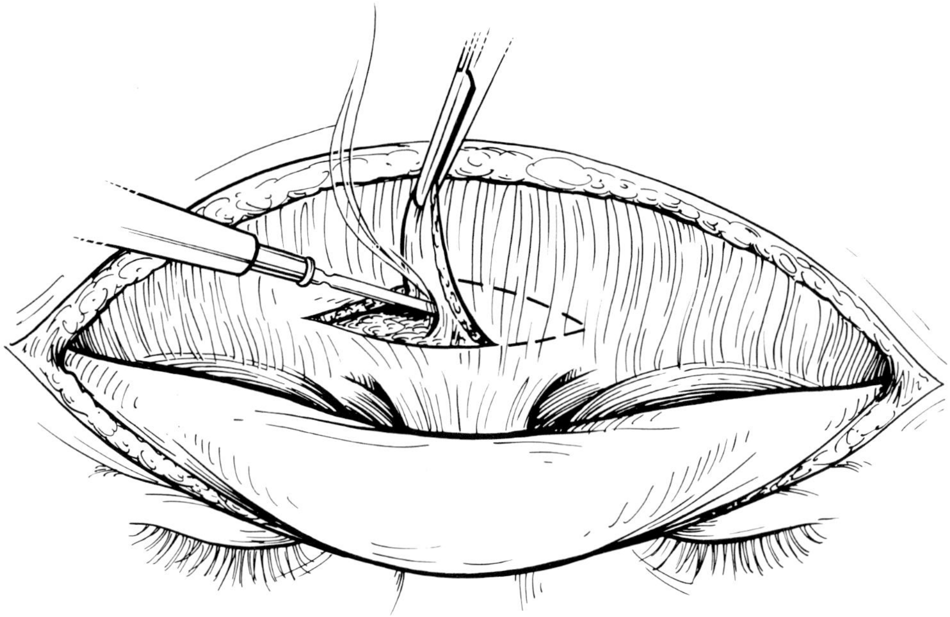

Figure 54 – 10. A portion of the frontalis muscle and its fascia may be excised to elevate the glabellar and medial brow tissues.

necessary (Fig. 54 – 10). Some authors believe this minimal disruption of the frontalis muscle is the optimal approach to this surgery since significant frontalis muscle scarring may cause a localized flattened or shiny appearance to the overlying forehead soft tissues. This incision site should be closed with interrupted, nonabsorbable, inert sutures such as 4-0 nylon or polypropylene. The upper margin of orbicularis oculi may be anchored to periosteum, as described in the direct brow elevation procedure, to stabilize the tissues and prevent recurrent brow ptosis. Closure of the deep and overlying soft tissues can be accomplished in a manner identical to that described for the direct brow lift approach.

The coronal incision forehead lift approach, including brow fixation, is an excellent surgical approach to correct brow ptosis. In general, this technically superior approach to correction of brow and forehead laxity achieves the best possible cosmetic and functional results, except in those cases in which the surgical scar is contraindicated as previously described.[15, 16]

Preoperative preparation for coronal approach surgery is particularly important. The patient is instructed to shampoo his or her hair with an iodine-based surgical scrub the evening before surgery. This surgery if often best performed with the use of general anesthesia, although it can easily be performed with local anesthesia as well by using both local and regional blocks. The patient is placed in a supine position on the operating room table in a flat or 10 to 15-degree reverse Trendelenburg (head-up) position. A neurosurgical headrest (e.g., Mayfield headrest) is useful to optimize surgical exposure to the head.

The hair is parted along the planned incision line with a surgical scrub brush (Fig. 54 – 11). A small portion of the hair in the planned incision site may be shaved at this point. Although shaving the hair makes the scalp flap somewhat easier to manage surgically, it is not necessary for cosmetic cases, since the risk of infection is extremely low. The face and scalp are prepped with an iodine-based surgical scrub solution. With the hair appropriately parted along the planned scalp incision line, the hair is

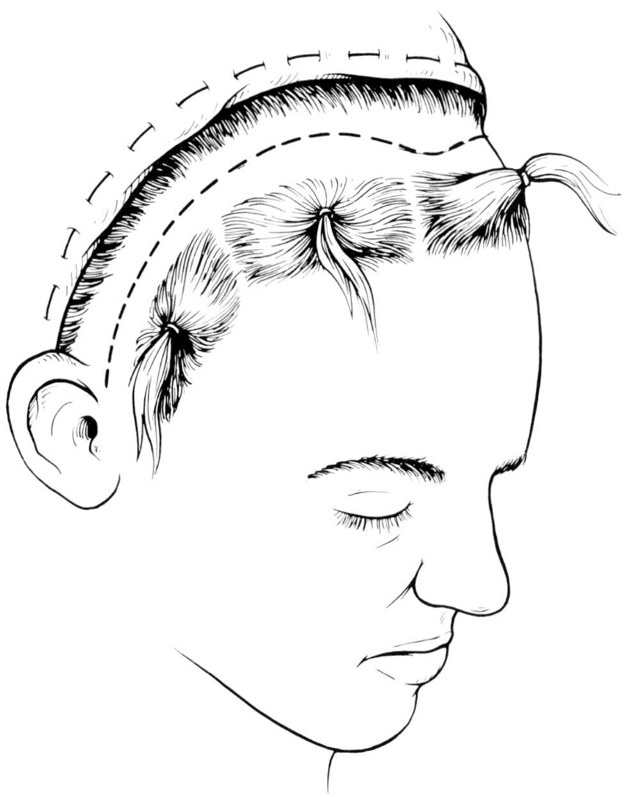

Figure 54 – 11. The coronal incision line is delineated extending from the ear root to the anterior midline of the scalp.

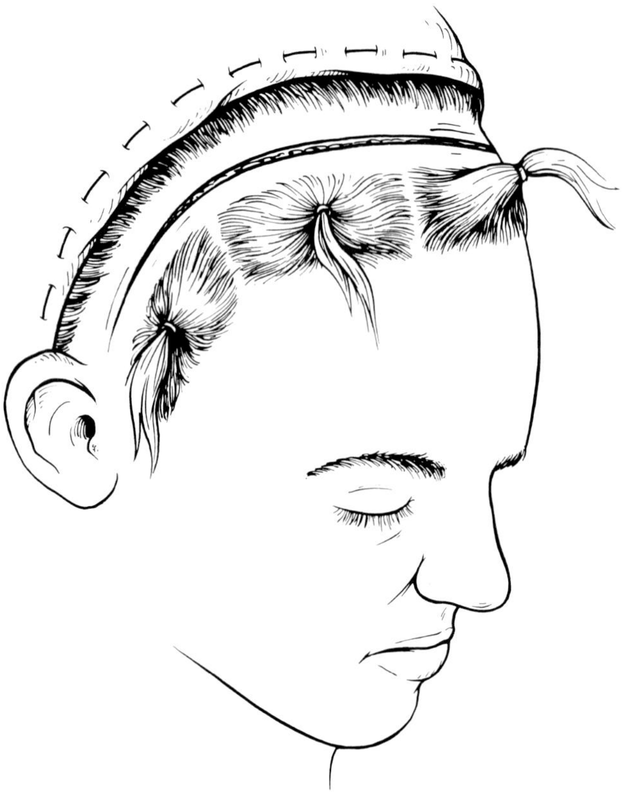

Figure 54–12. The hair is tied in multiple corn rows with sterile rubber bands. A surgical scrub towel is sutured to the scalp several centimeters posterior to the proposed incision line. With the hair appropriately parted (and shaved if desired), excellent, clean exposure of the planned incision site is afforded.

tied in multiple corn rows with sterile rubber bands. Surgical scrub towels are sutured or stapled to the scalp several centimeters posterior to the proposed incision line (Fig. 54–12). Sterile cotton balls or surgical sponges are placed in the external auditory canal meatus to prevent blood from pooling in the ear. The planned incision site, along with the scalp, forehead, and glabellar regions, is infiltrated with local anesthetic. I prefer the use of 2% lidocaine with epinephrine at a concentration of 1 : 100,000 and 150 units of hyaluronidase. The same anesthetic mixture may be used with general anesthesia, except 1% lidocaine in place of 2% is used. Adequate time should be allowed to elapse for the optimal hemostatic effect of the injected epinephrine to occur. An incision line is delineated extending from the anterior superior edge of the helix of one ear to the same position on the other ear. Incision lines that are placed more posterior to this area increase the technical difficulty of mobilizing and elevating the scalp tissues. Incision lines that are delineated more anterior to this position tend to approach the anterior edge of the hairline and may result in a cosmetically apparent scar. To avoid this potential complication, the surgical incision line should always be placed at least 5 cm posterior to the midfrontal hairline. A curvilinear or W-plasty cutaneous incision line may be created to further hide the scar, although this incision is probably unnecessary except in individuals with very fine, thin hair. The W-plasty tips should be at 90-degree angles with 1-cm legs (Fig. 54–13).[17] After the cutaneous tissues are incised, the underlying galea aponeurotica should be incised separately. If a W-plasty skin incision is created, the underlying galea should not be incised in a similar manner; rather, a clean curvilinear incision should be created through the galea. Of note, the surgeon should be prepared to extend the incision inferiorly along the ear root if difficulty is encountered when trying to mobilize the coronal forehead flap. The lateral aspect of the incision is best created with sharp scissors rather than a scalpel blade to avoid accidental incision of the temporalis fascia since significant secondary bleeding may result from the underlying temporalis muscle. This oozing may be surprisingly difficult to control. Care should be exercised to avoid disruption of the superficial temporal vessels, since these vessels contribute to the blood supply of the forehead, scalp, and frontalis muscles.

Once the galea is appropriately incised and retracted to expose the underlying pericranium, hemostasis may be obtained with use of a bipolar cautery forceps, direct pressure, indirect pressure from injection of additional anesthetic, and use of neurosurgical hemostatic clamps (e.g., Rainey clips). If hemostatic pressure clips are used, they should incorporate the galea since the blood supply to the scalp is carried in the galea itself. Frequently, the clips are not necessary for cosmetic procedures since the procedures are relatively short with minimal blood loss.

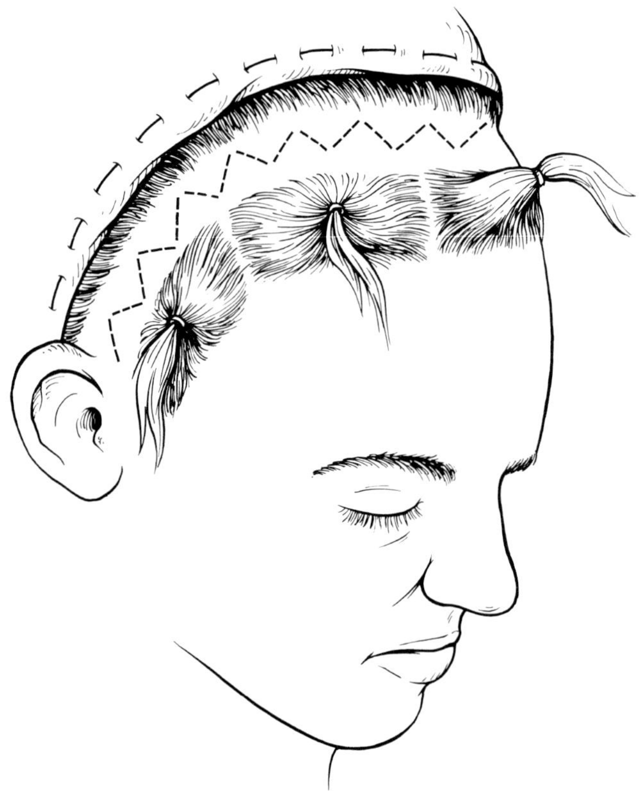

Figure 54–13. The planned coronal incision line can be delineated in a W-plasty manner to further camouflage the postoperative scar. This incision approach should be considered only in patients with very fine or thin hair.

Once hemostasis is achieved, sharp and blunt techniques are used to elevate the coronal flap to the supraorbital ridges. The orbital cavities should not be violated. To elevate the flap, blunt dissection with the use of a peanut dissector or the surgeon's finger is particularly effective. Passive retraction of the flap by the surgeon's assistant facilitates its elevation. Care should be exercised to avoid accidental trauma to the terminal branches of the facial nerve from retractors placed in the region of the superior and lateral orbital rims.[18] Since these facial nerve branches innervate the frontalis muscle, surgical trauma may result in a transient and, in some cases, permanent brow ptosis. This is a disastrous complication in a cosmetic surgical case. As previously mentioned, when developing the flap in the avascular subgaleal plane, care must be exercised laterally in the region of the temporalis fascia to avoid disruption of the frontal branch of the facial nerve since this nerve runs just superficial to the fascia and just deep to the superficial musculoaponeurotic system. Again, damage in this area may result in postoperative brow paresis or paralysis.

To allow clean elevation of the brows, the corrugator supercilii and procerus muscles should be disinserted even if prominent glabellar folds are not present preoperatively. The fibers of these muscles are readily identified as they blend with the vertically oriented fibers of the frontalis muscle. A portion of these muscles should be excised. Some authors recommend complete excision of these muscles, although this may result in a focal depression in the glabellar region. It is especially important to meticulously dissect these muscles from the dermis to avoid direct injury to the dermis itself. To assist in hemostasis, an electrocautery or radiofrequency cutting device may be employed (Fig. 54–14). It is impossible to completely dissect the supraorbital and supratrochlear neurovascular bundles from the surrounding orbicularis oculi, corrugator supercilii, and procerus muscle fibers; therefore, these structures are invariably damaged. Nevertheless, care should be exercised to try to dissect a portion of the structures from the muscles, if possible, to minimize postoperative anesthesia. Since postoperative cutaneous anesthesia always develops after this surgery, it is important to warn the patient of this expected result preoperatively. Although the forehead and prefrontal region anesthesia improves over time, it may not fully recover. During the recovery period, patients usually develop pruritus and related discomfort along the pathway of the regenerating nerves.

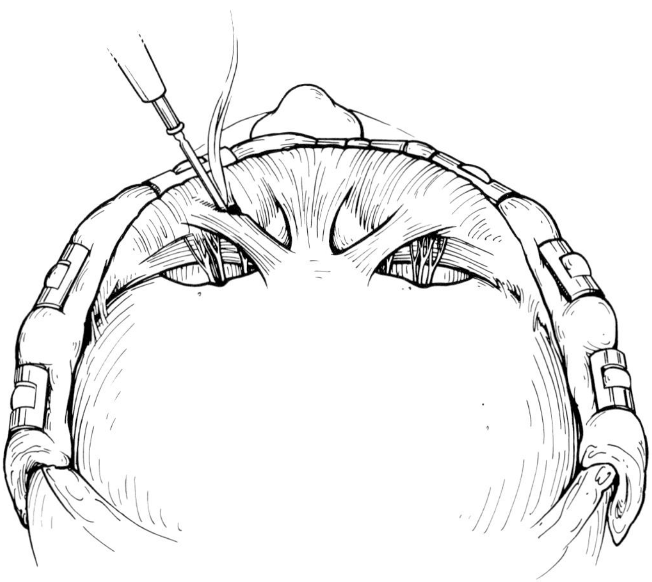

Figure 54–14. The eyebrow protractors including the corrugator supercilii, the procerus, and a portion of the orbicularis oculi are disinserted with a cutting electrocautery or radiofrequency device. The associated frontalis muscle fibers should be left undisturbed.

The flap should be bluntly dissected from the orbital rims to allow for appropriate brow and forehead elevation. However, the superior orbital septum along the superior arcus marginalis should not be surgically violated at this time. With hemostasis achieved and the flap fully mobile, the flap should be reflected to its normal anatomic position. If hemostatic clamps were applied, they should be removed, and a conservative elevation of the forehead soft tissues should be completed. To determine the amount of cutaneous tissue for removal, the flap is pulled superiorly, such that it overlaps the posterior aspect of the original incision line. The amount of tissue to be resected is typically in the range of 2 to 2.5 cm. When the amount of tissue to be resected is determined, multiple vertical incisions are created anteriorly in the coronal flap, corresponding to the amount of skin to be excised. This causes the hairline to be moved posteriorly. Patients should be informed preoperatively of this expected change in their hairline. The apex of each vertical incision line is then sutured to the posterior skin, subcutaneous tissue, and galea with interrupted 3-0 or 4-0 polypropylene sutures (Fig. 54–15). To achieve the optimal cosmetic results, the deep galea and overlying cutaneous tissues should be closed separately. Although some surgeons believe it is not necessary to close the galea itself, significant tension is placed across the cutaneous closure site if the galea is not closed directly. Deep galeal closure may be accomplished with 3-0 polypropylene or nylon on a taper needle. It is best not to use a slow dissolving suture, such as 3-0 polyglactin, since unwanted, avoidable postoperative inflammation develops in the surgical site as the suture dissolves. The overlying cutaneous tissue is best closed with a surgical stapler. Staples tend to do less damage to the hair follicles than sutures, thereby minimizing potential postoperative alopecia along the incision line. The skin staples are left in place for approximately 2 weeks. Before the final staples are placed, a flat Jackson-Pratt section drain can be positioned to actively remove accumulated serous fluid and blood. This drain needs to be left in place for only 24 hours. The patient should be informed preoperatively of the plan to place this drain during surgery. During the healing period, a standard cutaneous antibiotic ointment is placed along

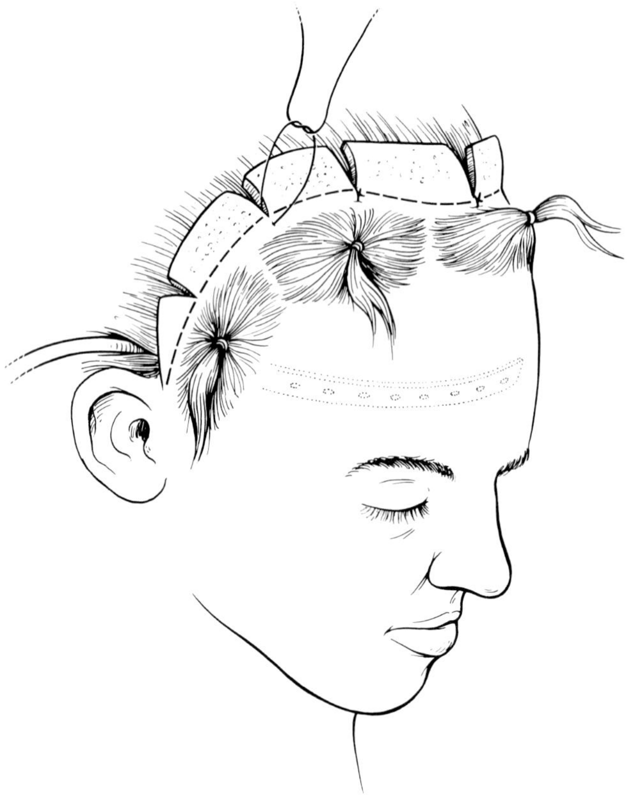

Figure 54–15. The coronal flap is returned to its normal anatomic position. Vertical relaxing incisions are created to assist in determining the degree of cutaneous tissue to be excised. Typically, 2.0 to 2.5 cm of tissue is excised. The apex of each vertical incision line is sutured to the posterior skin, subcutaneous tissue, and galea with interrupted 3-0 or 4-0 polypropylene sutures. The adjacent deep galea and overlying subcutaneous tissues should be closed in separate layers. Skin staples are the best way to close the superficial tissues since they cause less damage to the hair follicles, thereby minimizing posteroperative alopecia.

the staple line once or twice daily to keep the wound clean and to minimize the risk of local cutaneous infection.

For patients who do not wish posterior displacement of their hairline, the coronal flap incision line may be created at the anterior hairline; however, a fine scar does develop in this area even with meticulous, tedious cosmetic closure of the skin. As such, this approach should be considered only for patients who wear their hair in a forward manner, such as with bangs. Once the coronal portion of the surgery is complete, upper lid blepharoplasty may be performed. It is essential to perform all forehead and brow work before the blepharoplasty, since the amount of hooding dermatochalasis and redundant myocutaneous upper lid tissue will be significantly affected by surgical elevation of the brow and prefrontal soft tissues.

To address a prominent sub-brow fat pad, especially in cases of the marked frontal bossing, the standard surgical technique employed to address this problem involves superolateral orbital rim ostectomy.[19, 20] Although this technique is very effective, it does not address what is frequently the true anatomic cause, the sub-brow fat pad. A trans-lid approach to superolateral orbital rim ostectomy can be performed in select cases, but the optimal approach for the surgery necessitates the use of relatively involved surgical procedures such as midforehead or coronal flaps. These approaches are often more than what the cosmetic patient has in mind. In addition, a patient who is undergoing a blepharoplasty for cosmetic or functional reasons can have his or her prominent brow corrected by the relatively simple translid approach to browplasty surgery. In some cases, this procedure can result in significant softening of forehead wrinkles with results similar to those obtained with a standard coronal brow lift (Fig. 54–16). However, this procedure requires only minimally more involved surgical dissection than the standard upper eyelid blepharoplasty itself.

The trans-lid operative technique to surgically address a prominent sub-brow fat pad is relatively simple.[12, 21, 22] After standard upper eyelid blepharoplasty, the upper edge of the incised tissues is mechanically elevated to expose the sub-brow fat pad after appropriate dissection in the submuscular postorbicular fascial plane.[3] This anatomic plane of dissection is readily identified between the muscular and brow fat pad soft tissues. The appropriate lateral region of the sub-brow fat to be delineated for excision is identified by marking the corresponding overlying skin with methylene blue or a surgical marking pen. The overlying brow soft tissues are further elevated with

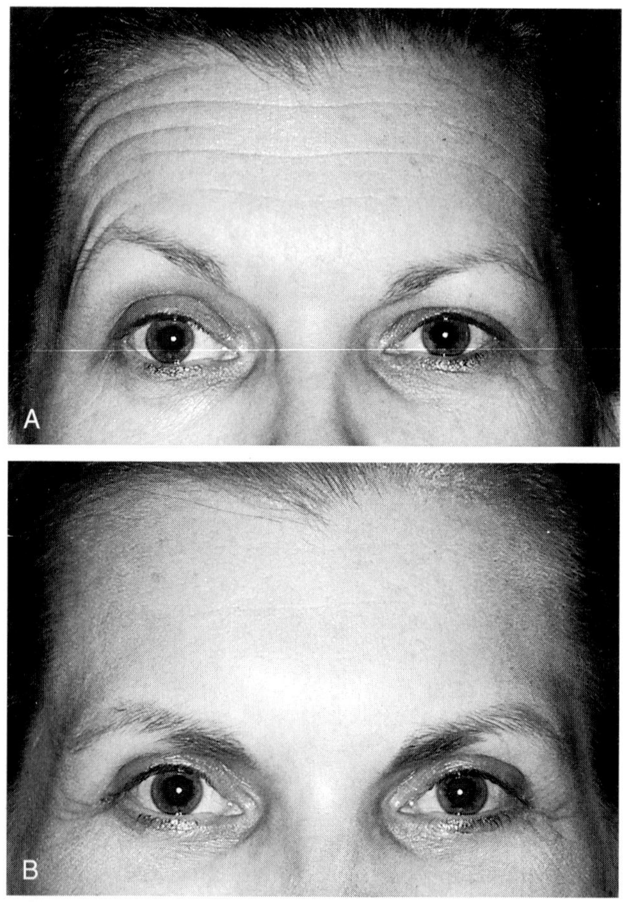

Figure 54–16. *A*, Clinical photograph of a patient with prominent transverse forehead furrows. *B*, Dramatic improvement after translid browplasty and blepharoplasty.

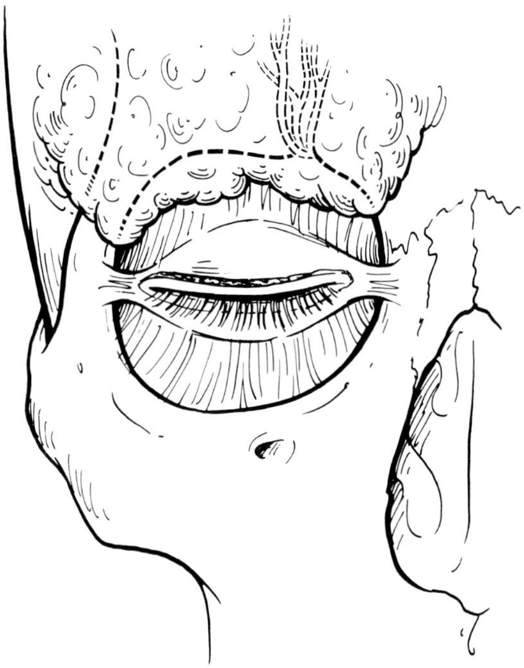

Figure 54–17. Artist's illustration of the prominent deep neurovascular structures evident deep to the cutaway portion of sub-brow fat. Care must be exercised to avoid disruption of the structures during the browplasty procedures.

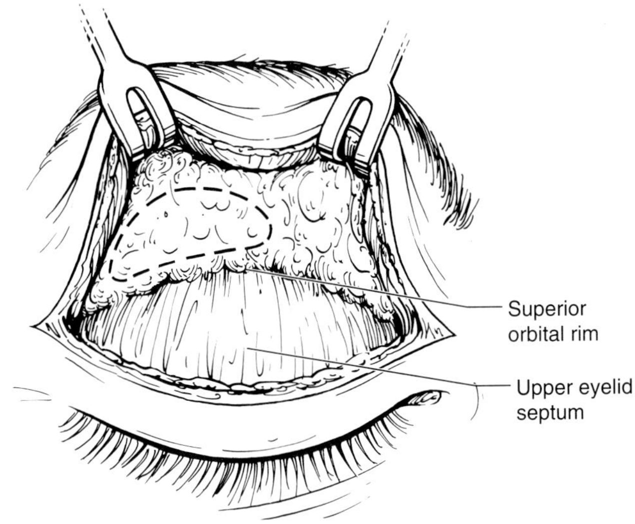

Figure 54–18. The sub-brow fat is exposed by retracting the myocutaneous tissues above the brow after a standard blepharoplasty. The area of sub-brow fat to be excised is demarcated and then gingerly excised in a downward beveled fashion with an electrocautery or radiofrequency device. Again, care is exercised to avoid disruption of the deep underlying neurovascular structures.

retractors to fully expose the appropriate area to be delineated for excision. Care should be exercised to avoid delineation of sub-brow fat overlying the supraorbital neurovascular structures (Fig. 54–17). As such, this area of excision should be limited to the lateral portion of the sub-brow region. An electrocautery or radiofrequency cutting device is used to cleanly elevate and excise the demarcated portion of the sub-brow fat pad (Fig. 54–18). The ellipse of the fat should be excised in a manner such that there is appropriate medial and lateral taper to ensure a soft postoperative contour. Again, care must be exercised. Deep excision will damage the underlying neurovascular structures. The overlying muscular tissues should be avoided to prevent unnecessary bleeding, irregular scarring, or contracture and potential loss of overlying brow cilia. Similarly, the underlying periosteum should be avoided to prevent irregular and unpredictable scarring and unnecessary postoperative discomfort. Once the sub-brow fat pad is appropriately removed, the overlying myocutaneous tissues are reapproximated in a standard blepharoplasty closure. If the brow is lax, deep anchor sutures may be placed medially, centrally, and laterally, or in those points clinically indicated, to stabilize the brow. I prefer the use of a 4-0 polypropylene suture. The sutures should be passed through the subcutaneous tissues immediately below the superior aspect of the brow cilia. The suture is then passed through underlying frontalis muscle and deep periosteum to anchor the brow in a mattress fashion (Figs. 54–19 and 54–20). To determine the position of periosteal fixation, a caliper is used to measure the appropriate height desired from the superior orbital rim. Attempts to physically elevate a ptotic brow by supraplacement of the fixation suture are generally met with poor results since the elevated brow tissue causes buckling and folding of the overlying more superior cutaneous tissues.

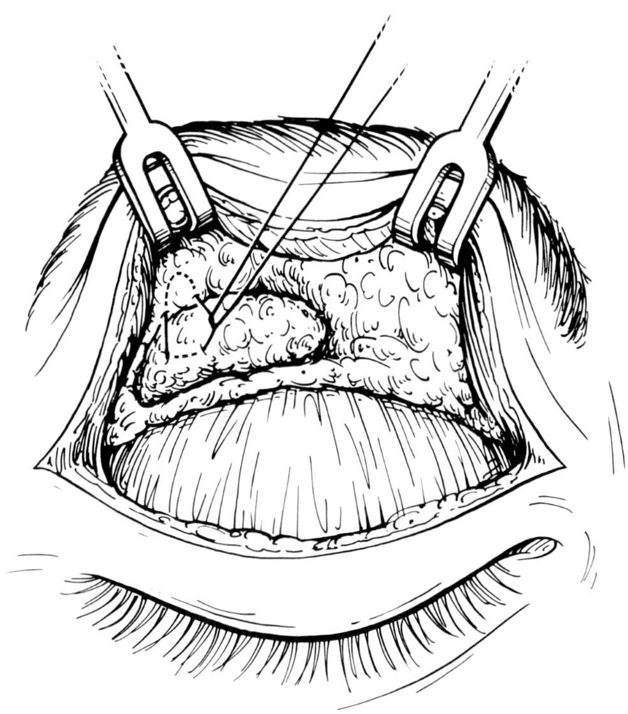

Figure 54–19. A translid browpexy procedure may be performed to stabilize the brow in its current position in an attempt to prevent secondary brow ptosis after blepharoplasty or translid browplasty. The brow should be anchored in its current position with the patient in a supine position by using a permanent 4-0 polypropylene suture that is passed in a mattress fashion through the subcutaneous tissues deep to the superior aspect of the brow cilia and into the underlying frontalis and deep periosteum.

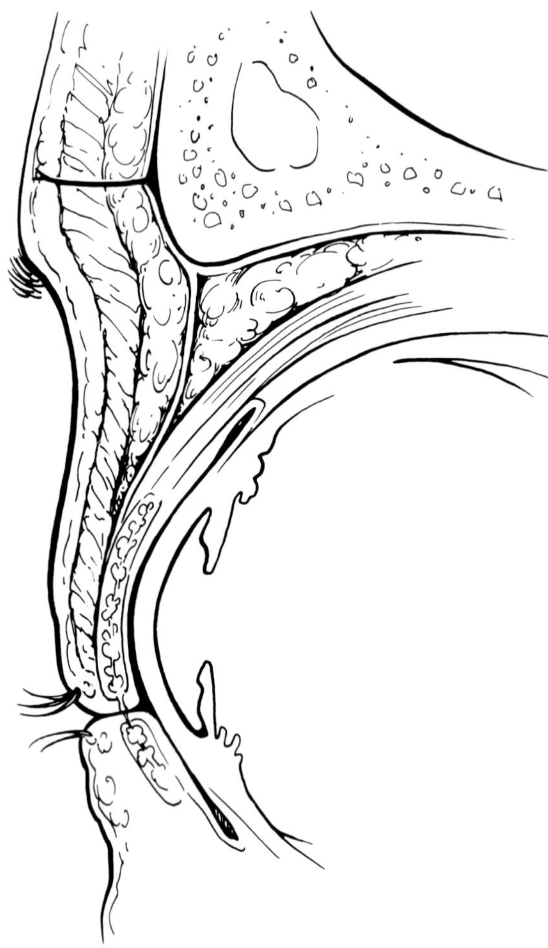

Figure 54–20. Sagittal view demonstrating proper placement of the browpexy periosteal anchor suture. These sutures should be placed in a manner that ensures that the knot is buried.

REFERENCES

1. Dingman RO, Peled I, Izenberg P: Forehead and brow lifts and their relationship to blepharoplasty. Ann Plast Surg 2:32, 1979.
2. Hinderer UT: Blepharocanthoplasty with eyebrow lift. Plast Reconstr Surg 56:402, 1975.
3. Lemke BN, Stasior OG: The anatomy of eyebrow ptosis. Arth Ophthalmol 100:981, 1982.
4. Passot R: La chirurgie esthetique des rides du visage. Presse Med 27:258, 1919.
5. Castanares S: Forehead wrinkles, glabellar frown and ptosis of the eyebrows. Plast Reconstr Surg 344:406, 1964.
6. Edgerton MT: Feminization of forehead: Contour changing to improve facial aesthetics (discussion). Plast Reconstr Surg 79:712, 1987.
7. Giles E, Elliot O: Sex determination by discriminant function analysis of crania. Am J Phys Anthropol 21:53, 1963.
8. Ousterhout DK: Contour changing to improve facial aesthetics. Plast Reconstr Surg 79:701, 1987.
9. Snow CC, Gatliff BP, McWilliams KR: Reconstruction of facial features from the skull: An evaluation of its usefulness in forensic anthropology. Am J Phys Anthropol 33:221, 1970.
10. Steward TD: Sex determination of the skeleton by guess and by measurement. Am J Phys Anthropol 12:385, 1954.
11. Whitaker LA, Pertschuk M: Facial skeletal contouring for aesthetic purposes. Plast Reconstr Surg 69:245, 1982.
12. McCord CD, Doxanas MT: Browplasty and browpexy: An adjunct to blepharoplasty. Plast Reconstr Surg 86:248, 1990.
13. Guyuron B: Soft-tissue frontal bossing. Plast Reconstr Surg 80,2:296, 1987.
14. Johnson C: The brow lift 1978. Arch Otolaryngol 105:124, 1979.
15. Brennan HG: The frontal lift. Arch Otolaryngol 104:26, 1978.
16. Kaye BL: The forehead lift. Plast Reconstr Surg 60:161, 1978.
17. Newman J, Dolsky RL, Imber P: Thin haired coronal lift W-plasty incision. Laryngoscope 94:407, 1984.
18. Liebman EP, Webster RC, Berger AS, et al: The frontal nerve in the temporal brow lift. Arch Otolaryngol 108:232, 1982.
19. Lassus C: Ostectomy of superior orbital rim in cosmetic blepharoplasty. Plast Reconstr Surg 63:481, 1979.
20. Whitaker LA, Morales L Jr, Farkas LG: Aesthetic surgery of the supraorbital ridge and forehead structures. Plast Reconstr Surg 78:23, 1986.
21. Castanares S: Forehead wrinkles, glabellar frown, and ptosis of the eyebrows. Plast Reconstruct Surg 31:106, 1964.
22. Weiss RA, McCord CD, Tanenbaum M: Translid browplasty: Anatomy and surgical techniques. Presented at the American Society of Oculoplastic and Reconstructive Surgery XVIII Clinical Conference, Dallas, Texas, November 7, 1987.

CHAPTER 55

Electrology and Eyebrow Contouring

Wallace A. Roberts and Cora Buggea

The three modalities that are accepted by the medical profession as being valid and effective means of removing hair safely and permanently are electrolysis; short wave, or thermolysis; and the blend.

A practical understanding of these modalities is needed to safely and effectively operate any brand of epilator while simultaneously achieving maximal patient comfort. The first use of an electrical means of permanent epilation was accomplished in 1875 by Charles E. Michel, a Saint Louis ophthalmologist.[1] The first modality used to permanently epilate hair was single-needle galvanic electrolysis. Michel successfully used the process of electrolysis to remove an ingrown eyelash. Gradually, the practitioners of permanent removal of superfluous hair came to be called electrologists, and the process of permanent hair removal came to be known as electrolysis. Today, with the use of nonelectrolytic methods, such as short wave or thermolysis, the more contemporary term for the practice of permanent hair removal is electrology. The word electrologist, however, generically refers to the practitioner who performs permanent hair removal and will likely never change, regardless of the modality used.

ELECTROLYSIS (GALVANIC) SINGLE-NEEDLE METHOD

Electrolysis is a chemical process that can be used for permanent hair removal. The classic definition of electrolysis is "the chemical decomposition of a substance by passing through that substance a unidirectional current of electricity."[2]

Permanent hair removal by electrolysis is the chemical decomposition, caused by sodium hydroxide (lye), of the matrix area of the hair follicle by passing a galvanic current of electricity through the follicle and its surrounding tissue. The substance in the classic definition of electrolysis is the body tissue, comprising the hair follicle and its surrounding tissue, and the unidirectional (one way) current of electricity is direct current. Because the amount of direct current used is small, it is called galvanic current.

Polar Effects of Current

The chemical effects of galvanic current are polar.[3] When we connect a patient to a galvanic epilator, two connections must be made to form a complete circuit. These electrodes, or poles, are called the active electrode and the indifferent electrode. The needle is the active electrode because it is at the needle that the desired activity is achieved, namely the production of sodium hydroxide. The indifferent electrode is needed in galvanic electrolysis because the current used is direct current, and direct current can travel only on a wire or a conductor. The indifferent electrode can take several forms; it may be a sponge moistened with tap water (distilled water is not a good conductor of electricity), a metal rod, or a cylinder, covered with a sponge moistened with tap water.

Whatever form the indifferent electrode takes, its physical surface area is much greater than that of the needle. Because the effect of the current is polar, chemicals are created at both electrodes, and the effects of the current must be diluted, or lessened, at the indifferent electrode. This effect is achieved by making the physical size of the indifferent electrode much larger than that of the needle. This is the principle of current density, which is discussed later.

Removal of Metal Jewelry

Because the effect of the current is polar, the chemicals created are in a high concentration only in proximity to each pole or electrode. The effect of the current (production of chemicals) varies inversely with the square of the distance from the electrode.[4] This means that the chemicals produced will drop off precipitously as the distance from the electrode increases, which is a benefit of the use of this modality for epilation around the eye.

The practitioner must have the patient remove jewelry from the area being treated and from the area where the indifferent electrode will be attached or held, which is generally the hand or wrist. This is done to avoid interaction of the chemicals produced with the metal of the jewelry, causing an irritation to the skin.

When using galvanic current, one must determine during the taking of the patient case history if the patient has any metal in his or her mouth in the form of fillings, bridge work, or braces. Naturally, these items cannot be removed, and no danger exists in the treatment of such patients. Chemicals are created in small quantities in the mouth during work on the face, and the patient gets a metallic taste. The quantity of chemicals created is small because of the polar effect of the current, and the chemicals created are diluted by the saliva in the mouth. The practitioner should tell such patients being treated for the first time to expect a metallic taste in their mouth soon after the treatment begins. Psychologically, preparing patients in advance is much better than telling them nothing and having them ask what is happening when they begin to get the metallic taste. One disadvantage of galvanic current is that the patient can interfere with the treatment, if he or she chooses, by merely letting go of the indifferent electrode.

Current Density

The current density, or concentration, of the current as well as its concomitant chemical effects is determined by the surface area of each electrode. As previously stated, this is the reason for making the indifferent electrode very much larger than the active needle electrode.

Chemical and Physiologic Effects

Opposite chemical and physiologic effects occur at the electrodes, which is an important feature of galvanic electrolysis. When the polarity of the needle electrode is negative, sodium hydroxide, which is alkaline, is formed in the follicle from the chemical breakdown of the body tissue by electrolysis. When the polarity of the needle is negative, the indifferent electrode is positive, and hydrochloric acid is formed at this electrode. The effect of this acid in the area of the indifferent electrode is minimized by the low current density (due to the large surface area of the electrode). Similarly, hydrogen gas is created and released in the area of the negative electrode, whereas oxygen gas is created and released in the area of the positive electrode.

Without fail, the needle electrode must always be the negative electrode when any form of galvanic current is used for epilation. The reason for this rule is that hydrochloric acid will be created in the follicle close to the needle should the operator inadvertently connect the needle to the positive pole of the epilator. The acid will attack the metal needle, creating metal oxides that will in turn permanently and visibly tattoo the patient. The sodium hydroxide created when the needle has a negative polarity will not attack the metal needle, and therefore no tattoo will be formed. Either sodium hydroxide or hydrochloric acid will effectively destroy the matrix area of the follicle, but only sodium hydroxide will accomplish the task without the side effect of a tattoo.

Principle of Time and Intensity

The practical range of current used to epilate hair using galvanic current is generally accepted to be between 0.3 and 1.0 mA.[2] There is no such thing as an average hair; however, if one assumes that a given coarse-textured hair will be satisfactorily epilated after 1 mA of galvanic current flows in the follicle for 1 minute, a sufficient amount of sodium hydroxide (lye) was created in the follicle. The production of lye is a function of the product of the amount of current flowing multiplied by the time that the current flows.[1] In other words, the quantity of lye equals the milliamperes multiplied by the time. We can epilate the same theoretical hair from the previous example using 0.5 mA of current and 2 minutes of time. Most electrologists would agree that patients would prefer the latter rather than the former because 1 mA of current is at the higher end of the generally acceptable range for galvanic epilation. The patient must decide whether he or she prefers a shorter, more intense sensation or a longer, less intense sensation. The hair is just as well epilated either way.

Multiple-Needle Galvanic Electrolysis

Most electrologists would agree that galvanic electrolysis is the most efficient modality for permanent hair removal. This modality is also the slowest.

The use of multiple needles speeds up the process. Multiple-needle galvanic epilators with anywhere from 6 to 24 needles have been produced. Modern multiple-needle galvanic epilators even have computer-controlled circuits to keep track of how many needles are inserted at any given time and to automatically adjust the current to keep the level constant in each follicle as needles are inserted and removed. Although this process somewhat solves the slowness problem, it creates new problems because some patients fear needles, and because of concerns about infectious diseases and acquired immunodeficiency syndrome.

Advantages and Disadvantages of Galvanic Electrolysis

Advantages

One advantage of galvanic electrolytes is that the accuracy of insertion of the electrode is not as critical as with the short-wave modality, because with galvanic electrolysis, chemicals are created from the body tissue wherever the current flows in the follicle. Even with a relatively shallow insertion, sodium hydroxide will flow to the base of the follicle.

Another advantage is that distorted hair follicles are easier to treat than with the short-wave modality because the chemicals created by electrolysis will find their way to the matrix area of the follicle, regardless of the position of the needle.

In addition, galvanic electrolysis offers the highest percentage of permanent epilation. The reasons for this success are related to the fact that the chemicals created during the treatment go home with the patient and continue to do their destructive work in the follicle.

Disadvantages

The first disadvantage is that galvanic current produces caustic chemicals in the follicle. If the current is excessively strong or if it is left on for too long, the caustic chemicals can spill over from the orifice of the follicle and could damage the eye.

The second disadvantage is that galvanic electrolysis is a slow process because it takes time for the process of electrolysis to break down the body tissue and to create the chemicals.

In addition, the sensation of the current is more lingering than sensations produced by other methods. The reason for this effect is that the current is flowing for a longer time, and with multiple-needle galvanic electrolysis, the patient receives multiple sensations of the current.

Another disadvantage is that the after effects of the treatment are more lingering because the body systems must absorb the chemicals created by the galvanic process and must excrete them as foreign substances in the body. With the short-wave modality, the heat created is more readily absorbed by the body.

The last disadvantage is that, as previously stated, the patient has control over the process by being able to release the indifferent electrode.

SHORT-WAVE OR THERMOLYSIS METHOD

In 1923, Bordier, from Paris, France, was credited with being the first to use high-frequency current to permanently epilate hair.[1] At that time, the technology of electronics was very crude by today's standards, and the short-wave modality did not gain wide acceptance, in spite of its dramatic improvement in speed over the galvanic method. A hair could now be epilated in a fraction of a second.

Not until after World War II, when better vacuum tubes and the transistor were developed, did practitioners begin to embrace this modality. Although the obvious benefit of short-wave epilation was its speed, its disadvantage was the fact that short-wave energy by its very nature did not need a wire to travel from point A to point B. Short-wave energy, unlike galvanic current, can travel through the air just like radio and television signals. In the early days of the use of short-wave energy to epilate hair, it would escape from the needle cord on its way to the needle and caused wild fluctuations and unpredictable results for the practitioners attempting to master this new technology. Patient movement or the position of the needle cord with respect to the patient or the practitioner caused the current at the needle to either increase or decrease as radio-frequency energy was being absorbed and was escaping from the wire.

In the early 1960s, epilator manufacturers realized this problem and provided what was undoubtedly the biggest advance to the taming of the short-wave modality—the shielded needle cord.[2] With this development, all of the energy programmed by the setting of the controls of the epilator was kept on the needle cord wire and was delivered without fluctuation to the hair follicle.

REGULATORY AGENCIES

Because radio-frequency short-wave energy can escape into the atmosphere and can travel without benefit of wires, it became necessary for the government to regulate the use of this type of electrical energy to protect the safety of the public and to minimize interference between users of this type of energy. In the United States, this regulatory body is called the Federal Communications Commission (FCC). In Canada, it is the Department of Transport, which looks after the regulation of radio waves. By international treaties, most countries agree to the use of specific frequencies for specific purposes because radio waves know no international borders. Specific frequencies are assigned for such uses as AM radio, FM radio, television stations, radar, fire, and police. Radio-frequency epilators fall into a medical band of frequencies reserved for the heating of body tissue, called the medical diathermy band. In North America, the lowest frequency available in this band is 13.56 MHz, and most epilators manufactured in the United States and Canada operate on this frequency.

Short-wave epilators used in the United States must have FCC-type approval indicating that they operate on a medical diathermy approved frequency. Similar approval is needed in Canada from the Department of Transport. FCC-type approval has nothing to do with safety or effectiveness as to epilators; the government agency concerned with safety and effectiveness is the Food and Drug Administration.

The primary and most significant difference between the galvanic and short-wave modalities is that short-wave epilation is a heat process, whereas galvanic epilation is a chemical process.

Another important difference is that short-wave energy is a form of alternating current, as opposed to galvanic current, which is a form of direct current. As has already been discussed, galvanic current creates chemical effects when it is applied to the body. Alternating current in any of its forms does not. The reason is that whatever chemical effects would be created when the electrons go in one direction would be canceled out when the electrons go in the opposite direction.

Heating Effects of Radio-Frequency Current

There is nothing magical about the frequency of 13.56 MHz that most radio-frequency epilators use to create a heating effect in body tissue. When the reversals of the alternating current energy reach approximately 1 million cycles/sec, or hertz, the heating effect begins to take place.[4] What this means is that if we could disregard the FCC, we could use epilators that operated at any frequency above 1 million cycles/sec and expect to achieve similar results in the hair follicle.

The radio-frequency epilator works on the same basic principle as the microwave oven. The rapid fluctuations or reversals of the electrical energy emanating from the needle in the follicle cause the molecules of body tissue surrounding the needle (especially the tip) to rapidly vibrate. Because of the molecular attraction (friction), heat is created in the tissue. This heat causes the area of the follicle in proximity to the needle to electrocoagulate; in other words, the tissue cooks itself with electricity.

Bundle of Energy Theory[2]

When the foot switch used in short-wave epilation is depressed, a bundle of short-wave energy is delivered into the follicle by way of the needle. With radio-frequency epilation, the needle is actually an antenna, and the radio-frequency energy actually emanates from the tip of the needle in much the same way that concentric circles form on a still pond of water when a rock is thrown in. The tissue in the area of the needle is heated by the needle. The needle itself does not get hot other than by the heat that is conducted back to it from the heated tissue.

The bundle of energy that is released when the foot switch is depressed has dimensions. Its length, or duration, is determined either by the length of time that the foot switch is held depressed in manual mode or by the setting of the automatic timing control on the epilator. Its height, or magnitude, is determined by the setting of the intensity control on the epilator. Therefore, the bundle of energy will have dimensions that will vary as determined by the settings on the epilator. Embodied within the dimensions of the bundle of energy is the radio-frequency current that provides the heating effect for electrocoagulation.

The amount of heating effect in the follicle is determined by the product of the length (timing) and height (intensity) of the bundle of energy (Fig. 55–1). This principle is very similar to the principle that the amount of lye created in the follicle using galvanic current is determined by the product of the magnitude of the current in milliamperes and the time that the current is applied. In

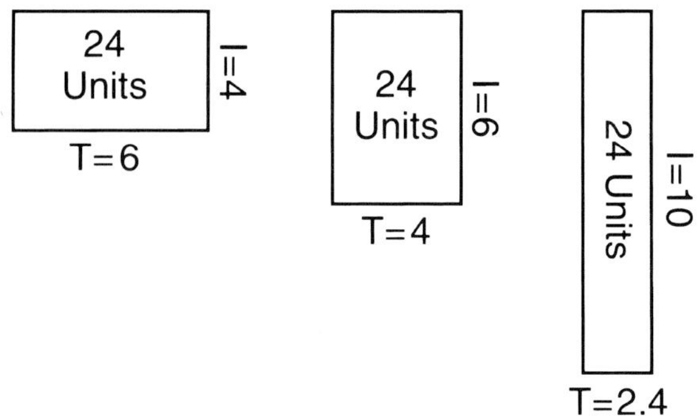

Figure 55–1. Bundle of energy. I, intensity setting. T, timing setting. Units, qualitative radio-frequency sources.

short-wave epilation, especially that using automatic timing, the amount of energy released in the follicle is best expressed in joules or watt-seconds, the joule being the smaller equivalent of the kilowatt hour.

What this means is that on a given epilator, a timing setting of 6 and an intensity setting of 4 will produce a product of 24. Any combination of settings producing the same product will provide the same heating effect in the follicle. In other words, a timing setting of 4 and an intensity setting of 6 will also produce a product of 24. Most practitioners would agree that the latter setting is more comfortable to the patient than the former. This does not mean that the practitioner has to sit beside the epilator with a calculator; rather, it is a way to understand that the timing control has just as much to do with the amount of heat energy released into the follicle as does the intensity control (see Fig. 55–1).

Various Configurations for the Bundle of Energy

The practitioner can usually optimize the patient's comfort level by first using the necessary amount of intensity, and then introducing more timing, as needed. This is commonly called the flash technique.[1] Carrying the previous example to its ultimate, we could then assume that if a given hair needs a product of 24 for proper epilation, and if our epilator has a maximum intensity setting of 10, then we could set the intensity to 10, and increase the timing setting to 2.4 to achieve the desired product of 24 units of heat in the follicle.

Cautions for Short-Wave Energy Use

The previous examples are idealized and are presented to achieve an understanding of the principles of timing and intensity and their interrelationship. One might wonder, if practitioners generally agree that a shorter burst of higher intensity provides less sensation than longer timing and lower intensity, why manufacturers do not use higher and higher intensities to create the theoretical painless epilator. The answer is that intensity, or magnitude, of the radio-frequency energy has a practical limit beyond which it is unsafe to use. As the intensity increases, we reach a point at which the radio-frequency energy will cause the sebum and moisture on the surface of the skin and within the follicle to vaporize with a puff of smoke that smells like burning tissue. Although tissue is not burning, the smell is the same because when tissue does burn, part of the resultant smell is the oil, or sebum. Timing, no matter how long, does not cause this phenomenon because the duration of the current has nothing to do with the flash point of the sebum. Therefore, on some patients with fine hair, and oily, moist skin, a point can be reached, if the insertion is relatively shallow, at which this flash point phenomenon will occur. In this case, the practitioner must reduce the intensity to a level beneath this flash point and must compensate by adding sufficient timing to achieve the desired result.

Point Effect

When students are just beginning to learn to epilate hair using the short-wave modality, they will have more success if they use settings with higher timing and commensurately lower intensity. The reason for this is a phenomenon of short-wave transmission called the point effect. When radio-frequency energy leaves a wire, it radiates outwardly from the point. That is why radio and television antennas are tall, straight structures either placed on the ground or on the tops of tall buildings. With a short-wave epilator, the needle is the antenna, and the energy builds from the tip back toward the surface of the skin, conforming to the shape of the needle. In addition, when the timing is longer with respect to the intensity, the heating pattern at the tip of the needle is broader.[1] For these reasons, a student who at the beginning of training cannot make a very accurate insertion will have better success using more timing and less intensity.

When distorted follicles are treated using the short-wave modality, we can compensate for not being able to get the needle point exactly at the matrix of the follicle by broadening the heating pattern by using more timing and less intensity. It should always be the goal of the practitioner wishing to achieve maximum efficiency and patient comfort to use less timing and more intensity as he or she becomes more proficient at making an accurate insertion. The short-wave modality delivers the fastest results, depending on the ability of the practitioner to make an accurate insertion.

BLEND MODALITY

The blend is not a modality itself, but rather a combination of the galvanic and short-wave modalities. In 1948, a patent was granted to Henri E. St. Pierre from San Francisco for the blend epilator.[1] He worked in close collaboration with Arthur Hinkel. St. Pierre was the practitioner; Hinkel, who later became an electrologist, was the engineer. St. Pierre correctly concluded that a type of epilator could be built that would embrace the benefits of both the galvanic and short-wave currents. The basic concept was that the heat of the short-wave current could be used to heat up the chemicals produced by the galvanic method and consequently speed up the whole process. St. Pierre and Hinkel were able to combine both currents and the technique known as the blend method was born.

Many theories of how to use blend epilation exist, and today, automatic, computer-controlled blend epilators are on the market that sense the insertion of the needle and even help the practitioner with the settings of the two currents and how they are sequenced. This discussion is confined to the basic blend epilator using two foot switches, one for the galvanic current and the other for the short-wave current.

A basic blend epilator is a single-needle galvanic epilator whose current flow is started and stopped by means of a foot switch. This mechanism is combined with a manual short-wave epilator whose short-wave energy is started and stopped by means of a second foot switch. All of this equipment is contained in a single cabinet. With the blend epilator, the practitioner has the option and the flexibility to use each type of modality in various sequences, such as

Galvanic, short wave, galvanic
Short wave, galvanic, short wave
Galvanic, short wave and galvanic, short wave

Of course, several other possible combinations exist, and each has its proponents.

COMPARISONS OF GALVANIC, SHORT-WAVE, AND BLEND TECHNIQUES

For the purposes of understanding the relative speed and the efficiency of each modality, some generalizations and assumptions must be made. Let us first assume that a given type of hair can be effectively epilated using a single-needle galvanic current of 1 mA over a period of 1 minute. Let us also assume that every hair that we epilate is permanently epilated (100% efficiency). Most experts would agree the same hair would be epilated using the blend modality in about 20 seconds. Let us assume the same 100% efficiency for the blend modality. If we now treat the same type hair using the short-wave modality exclusively, we would treat each hair for only a fraction of a second. If we assume that the short-wave modality has only a 50% efficiency, eventually every other hair will grow back.

The question then becomes how many hairs can be treated with the short-wave modality in the same 1 minute that the galvanic modality needs, and how many hairs can be treated during the 20 seconds that the blend method needs. If the practitioner using short-wave epilation can treat only one hair in each 5-second period and can permanently epilate only 50% of the hairs, then one can assume that the practitioner using only short-wave epilation has successfully treated twice as many hairs in the 20 seconds that the blend modality took, and six times as many hairs as the single-needle galvanic method.

Although this discussion seems to strongly favor the short-wave modality, in the final analysis, the modality to use depends on the preference of the practitioner. Generally, practitioners who are capable and willing to achieve the skill and technique to make an accurate insertion of the needle will fare best with the short-wave modality. Clearly, the galvanic and blend modalities are the most forgiving regarding the accuracy of the insertion.

EYEBROW CONTOURING

The eyebrows consist of hairs, called the supercilia, growing on the transverse elevation at the junction of the forehead and the upper eyelid.

The supercilia are classified as asexual hair, whose type is secondary. Secondary hair is considered to be that of the eyebrows, eyelashes, nose, and ears. The function of the supercilia is to protect the eye area by preventing liquids from entering the eye. In addition to protection, the eyebrow offers the eye more definition.

Eyebrows differ from person to person; their pattern may be to grow together in the middle of the face, creating what appears to be one long eyebrow. The shaping of eyebrows is an interesting subject. Teenagers begin to shape their eyebrows by removing unwanted hairs according to fashion and likes and dislikes.

Adults continue to shape their eyebrows to enhance the expression of their eyes. Persons who have undergone eyelid surgery realize the importance of eyebrow shaping. Unfortunately, not everyone can define their eyebrows properly or permanently. For this reason, electrology should be considered. A well-trained electrologist shapes the eyebrow hair appropriately and permanently. A carefully trained electrologist uses a special technique to determine a shapely and balanced eyebrow.

First, the excess hair on the bridge of the nose is removed. It is important not to overtreat the skin. Once this hair has been removed, the electrologist proceeds with the shaping of the eyebrow (Fig. 55–2). To establish the beginning of the eyebrow, the electrologist draws an imaginary straight line connecting the beginning of the eyebrow to the inner corner of the eye. The line then connects to the outer edge of the nostril (see Fig. 55–2, *line A*).

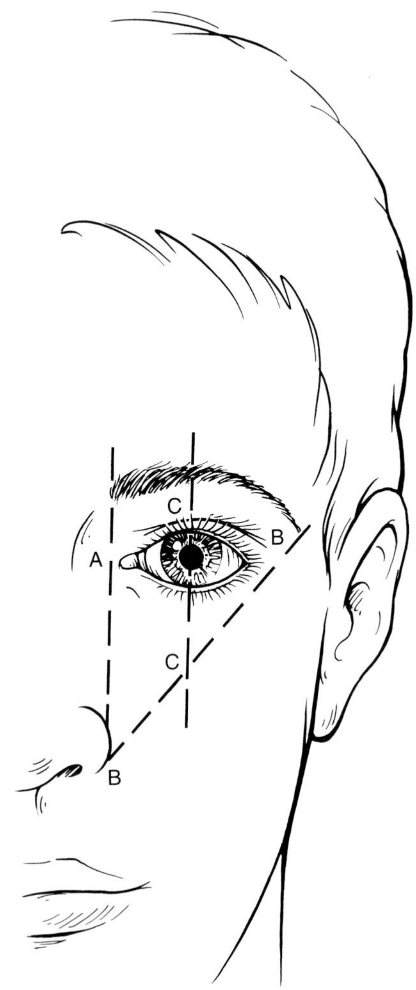

Figure 55–2. By using the eyebrow, eye, and corner of the nose, the electrologist determines the new shape of the eyebrow.

To determine where the arch of the eyebrow should begin, the electrologist draws an imaginary straight line from the center of the pupil, moving up into the eyebrow, and then down into the cheek (see Fig. 55–2, *line C*).

The length of the eyebrow is found by drawing an imaginary straight line from the outer edge of the nostril to connect with the outer corner of the eye and then to connect with the length of the eyebrow (see Fig. 55–2, *line B*).

The excess hair is then removed. By using an eyebrow comb to comb the eyebrow hair, the electrologist combs the hair in an upward motion, and any excess hairs that do not follow the natural line of the eyebrows are then removed. The combing procedure is repeated in a downward motion, and any excess hairs that do not follow the natural line of the eyebrow are removed. Naturally, the patient must be apprised of the process and consent to the entire procedure.

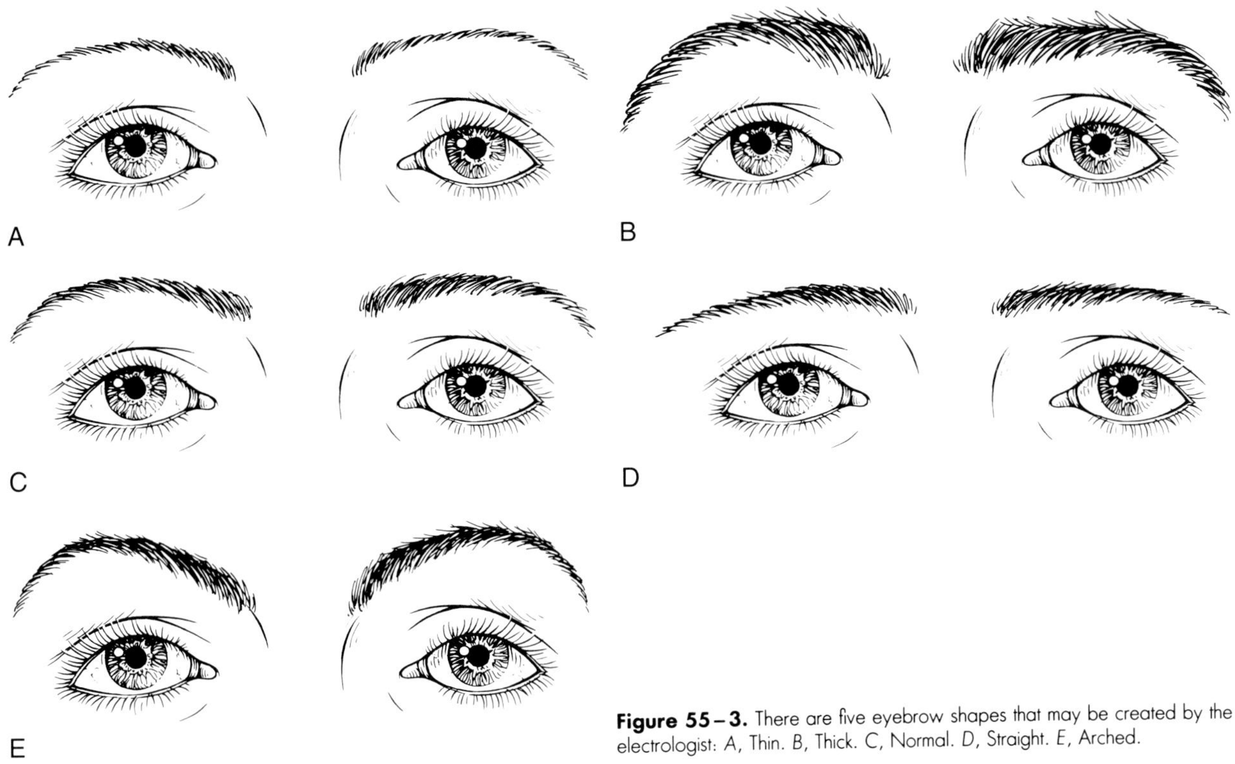

Figure 55–3. There are five eyebrow shapes that may be created by the electrologist: *A*, Thin. *B*, Thick. *C*, Normal. *D*, Straight. *E*, Arched.

As a result of aging, the eyebrow hair growth cycle changes. As we age, our hair becomes thicker and longer. The electrologist should remove only the hair that is necessary to achieve the desired result. The rest should be trimmed to avoid having the eyebrow appear too sparse.

There are five eyebrow shapes that may be created, depending on the wishes of the patient. These shapes—thin, thick, normal, straight, and arched—are indicated in Figure 55–3. Patients may consider undergoing permanent eyebrow contouring after undergoing eyelid surgery because once electrology removes hair permanently and successfully, the patient is relieved from using temporary methods of hair removal.

REFERENCES

1. Hinkel AB, Lind RW: Electrolysis Thermolysis and the Blend, 5th ed. Los Angeles, Arroway, 1983.
2. Roberts WA: Electricity and Modalities for Electrologists. Bellingham, MA, WA Roberts, 1989.
3. Kovacs R: Electrotherapy and Light Therapy, 5th ed. Philadelphia, Lea & Febiger, 1946.
4. Watkins AL: A Manual of Electrotherapy. Philadelphia, Lea & Febiger, 1958.

CHAPTER 56

Upper Eyelid Blepharoplasty

David M. Reifler

The evaluation of the patient undergoing blepharoplasty is summarized in Chapter 49. Ocular, general medical, and psychological considerations and their extreme practical importance have been described in detail. In this chapter, further attention is given to the clinical evaluation of patients being considered for upper eyelid blepharoplasty, with an emphasis on functional versus cosmetic considerations. This is followed by a discussion of surgical techniques. Complications of upper eyelid blepharoplasty are described in Chapter 61.

Upper eyelid blepharoplasty is a surgical procedure with many technical nuances and either pleasing or untoward consequences arising from every surgical step. This chapter therefore attempts to outline the author's personal philosophies and preferred techniques, followed by commentary on the blepharoplasty literature. Thus, in addition to a description of surgical technique, a literature review is provided that catalogues modern trends in the approach to upper eyelid blepharoplasty for each surgical step. One must recognize that the modern approaches to blepharoplasty rest on foundations laid down by great observers and innovators of the past. Katzen[1] historically reviewed the literature concerning blepharoplasty from the first century writings of Cornelius Celsus to the twentieth century (Table 56–1). As Katzen noted, Castanares' contributions to the classification of the "baggy eyelid deformity"[2, 3] should be acknowledged and studied (Table 56–2). Attention to this history will provide the blepharoplasty surgeon with a greater appreciation of his or her art.

FUNCTIONAL INDICATIONS FOR BLEPHAROPLASTY

Patients who present with a need or desire for upper eyelid blepharoplasty often have questions regarding functional versus cosmetic indications for surgery. This issue often determines whether or not the patient is eligible for third-party reimbursement.

A widely accepted criterion for functionally necessary upper eyelid blepharoplasty is a roll of skin lying on the eyelashes. A more detailed statement on the functional indications for blepharoplasty has been provided by the Ophthalmic Procedures Assessment Committee of the American Academy of Ophthalmology, which was adopted June 24, 1990.[4] The review and formal action by the Academy was prompted by several inquiries from insurance companies. The author served as one of the consultants in the preparation of this statement, excerpts of which follow:

> The most common functional indication for blepharoplasty is a superior visual field defect secondary to redundant upper eyelid tissue (dermatochalasis) that overhangs the eyelid margin. This condition is one cause of 'pseudoptosis' as described by Beard:[5] The upper eyelids may be abnormally low because of the mechanical weight of the excess upper eyelid tissues, but there may also be concomitant levator aponeurosis dehiscence or disinsertion.[6] 'Myogenic' (including aponeurotic) or neurologic factors are usually found in true blepharoptosis.[5] Since dermatochalasis and true ptosis often coexist, blepharoplasty at the time of ptosis repair is often indicated.[5, 7–10] Failure to excise redundant tissues at the time of ptosis repair may result in accentuating the overhanging of skin and muscle at the eyelid margin.[7–9] Excision of redundant skin and muscle is often performed concurrently with ptosis repair utilizing a frontalis sling technique,[8] internal approach for tarsectomy or Muellerectomy,[9] external tarsectomy[10] or levator aponeurosis advancement.[11, 12] In the latter instances where the coexisting problems of dermatochalasis and ptosis are corrected using an aponeurotic approach, the surgeon may excise redundant skin and/or orbicularis muscle at the time of initial skin incision[11] or toward the end of the operation.[12]
>
> Visual field loss from malpositioned upper eyelids has been confirmed by Cahill and associates[13] and quantified by Linberg and co-workers.[14] Impairment of the superior visual field ranged from 20% for mild ptosis to 64% in advanced cases where the eyelid crosses the middle of the pupil. Excessive upper eyelid skin also may produce asthenopic symptoms and persistent blepharoconjunctivitis ('functional dermatochalasia').[15]
>
> In addition, blepharoplasty may be indicated to treat the sequelae of several inflammatory disorders of the orbit or eyelids. For example, a common feature of Graves' ophthalmopathy is edema and fullness of the eyelids with anterior prolapse of orbital fat and lacrimal gland tissue. Blepharoplasty may be included in the surgical rehabilitation of these patients, and can often be performed concomitantly with repair of eyelid retraction.[16] Blepharochalasis (not to be confused with dermatochalasis) is an unusual disease affecting primarily young persons in which recurrent episodes of idiopathic eyelid edema result in stretching and redundancy of the eyelid tissues; blepharoplasty, usually in combination with advancement of the levator aponeurosis, is frequently indicated.[17, 18] Floppy eyelid syndrome, another

TABLE 56-1

Historic Landmarks in Upper Eyelid Blepharoplasty

Year	Investigator	Contribution
1817	Beer	First illustration of dermatochalasis
1818	von Graefe	Introduction of the term *blepharoplasty*
1896	Fuchs	Introduction of the term *blepharochalasis*
1907	Miller	First textbook of cosmetic surgery
1911	Kolle	Preoperative marking of the skin
1926	Noel	Emphasis of clinical photography
1929	Brouguet	Upper eyelid fat excision
1952	Fox	Introduction of the term *dermachalasis*
1954	Sayoc	Cosmetic alteration of Asian eyelid crease
1974	Sheen	Introduction of the term *supratarsal fixation*
1978	Dryden	Combined blepharoplasty and aponeurosis advancement

Data from Katzen LB: The history of cosmetic blepharoplasty. *In* Putterman A (ed): Cosmetic Oculoplastic Surgery. New York, Grune & Stratton, 1982, p 2.

unusual disorder that may be related to blepharochalasis[19] and which causes a chronic papillary conjunctivitis[20, 21] is effectively treated with surgery that may include blepharoplasty.[22, 23]

Trauma to the eyelids and orbit may result in the need for a functional blepharoplasty. Blowout fractures of the orbit commonly lead to loss or atrophy of orbital fat, resulting in enophthalmos and a deep superior palpebral sulcus. Putterman[24] has emphasized that it is possible to camouflage the orbital asymmetry by performing an upper eyelid blepharoplasty on the contralateral side in lieu of more extensive surgery on the traumatized orbit. An additional traumatic setting in which blepharoplasty may be useful is when skin grafts are required to replace or cover avulsed or burned eyelid tissue; subsequent trimming of the healed grafts (in effect a blepharoplasty) may be required.

PREOPERATIVE CONSIDERATIONS IN COSMETIC BLEPHAROPLASTY

The preoperative evaluation of the blepharoplasty patient has been extensively covered in Chapter 49. The importance of having and communicating objective criteria that clearly define cosmetic versus functional surgery should be further emphasized.[25, 26] In any oculoplastic procedure, the surgeon strives for a pleasing cosmetic result, yet in functionally indicated surgery, the cosmetic result is not the primary goal. Conversely, the absence of functional indications for upper eyelid blepharoplasty defines what is generally accepted as cosmetic (or aesthetic[27]) upper eyelid blepharoplasty. Baker[28] stated that most upper eyelid blepharoplasties in the United States are performed for cosmetic reasons. However, functional blepharoplasties may actually predominate in a practice confined to ophthalmic plastic and reconstructive surgery.

The various components of eyelid deformity as well as individual anatomic variations must be appreciated by the blepharoplasty surgeon. Castanares[2, 3] was among the first to attempt to provide a classification of the baggy eyelids deformity (see Table 56-2). Individualized plans for surgery should be based on the types and extent of the existing deformities. Preoperatively, the goals of cosmetic blepharoplasty must be mutually agreed on between the patient and the surgeon. After cosmetic blepharoplasty alone, patients may not necessarily look younger, but they are apt to appear more rested, alert, and healthy. For many other patients, upper eyelid blepharoplasty is only one component of cosmetic facial plastic surgery that may include lower eyelid blepharoplasty, browplasty, or face lift.

TABLE 56-2

Castanares' Classification of Baggy Eyelids Deformity

1. Blepharochalasis
2. Dermachalasis* (or ptosis adiposa of Sichel, or pseudoptosis)
3. Hypertrophy of the orbicularis
4. Protrusion of intraorbital fat
5. Combination of any of the above conditions
6. Hooding of upper lids due to ptosis of the brows

*The term *dermatochalasis* is more commonly used.

Data from Castanares S: Classification of baggy eyelids deformity. Plast Reconstr Surg 59:629-633, 1977.

SURGICAL TECHNIQUES

Many differences exist in the general approach to upper eyelid blepharoplasty, and the technical variations that have been adopted in its performance are categorized here. We begin with the author's favored surgical techniques (Table 56-3), followed by a discussion of technical variations. Although the author's techniques are described in an instructive cookbook style, the intent was not to establish a standard of care for upper eyelid blepharoplasty. In fact, variations in general approach and in specific techniques are also presented. Although the author performs upper eyelid blepharoplasty in an operating room, many surgeons perform this procedure in an office without extensive monitoring or patient preparation. However, the administration of supplemental oxygen and the use of a pulse oximeter, blood pressure cuff, and electrocardiogram are consistent with a strategy that includes giving profound intravenous sedation to the patient.

TABLE 56-3

Surgical Steps in Upper Eyelid Blepharoplasty

1. Preparation and draping of the patient
2. Skin marking
3. Local anesthetic infiltration
4. Excision of skin and muscle
5. Excision and incision of orbital septum
6. Excision of fat
7. Repair of prolapsed lacrimal gland
8. Concurrent ptosis repair
9. Eyelid crease formation and skin closure
10. Postoperative care

Preparation and Draping of the Patient

The physician instills tetracaine (Pontocaine) 0.5% solution in both eyes. This agent reduces ocular discomfort and the resulting eyelid spasm from antiseptics. The physician cleans away any residual make-up and prepares the face and eyelids with povidone solution. Next, the physician applies drapes with self-contained adhesive strips, exposing the entire face without producing tension on the eyelids or brows.

Skin Marking

The physician identifies and marks the upper eyelid crease with a fine-tipped gentian violet marking pen after retracting the eyelid fold with a finger. The patient is instructed to look superiorly and inferiorly to assist in confirming the location of the eyelid crease or the "dominant crease" when multiple creases are present. Extra care should be taken when the normal eyelid crease is obliterated by levator aponeurosis disinsertion, or fat herniation, or both. The physician draws the eyelid crease 10 mm superior to the central eyelid marking in women and 7 to 8 mm in men. The physician draws the medial extent of the incision about 5 mm superior to the superior punctum, and the lateral extent of the incision, at least 5 mm superior to the lateral canthus. In cases of lateral hooding, the eyelid crease marking is carried up to 1.5 cm lateral to the lateral canthus. This lateral portion is angled slightly superiorly, to produce a "happy" rather than a "sad" postoperative appearance (Fig. 56–1). Contrary to older textbook descriptions, the physician should not hesitate to extend the incision beyond the lateral orbital rim if required.

The patient is instructed to close the eyes. The central upper eyelid crease and redundant fold superior to it are gently grasped with a smooth or 0.5-mm toothed Castroviejo forceps. The amount of tissue grasped is increased or decreased until excessive skin is eliminated, while no more than 0.5 mm of separation is produced between the upper and lower eyelids. A mark is made at the site of the superior forceps blade (Fig. 56–2). This procedure is repeated medially and laterally, and the medial and lateral markings are connected to each other and to the ends of the eyelid crease marking (Fig. 56–3). If the amount of redundant skin is unequal between the two sides, the skin markings will necessarily be asymmetric. However, careful measurements of the distance from the eyebrow to the superior skin marking must be made to assess resulting symmetry after tissue resection. If marked redundancy of skin medially exists, a W-plasty design is marked, as is discussed later. The physician should consult preoperative clinical photographs while in the operating room to assess subtle nuances, such as eyelid symmetry and localized redundancy of skin.

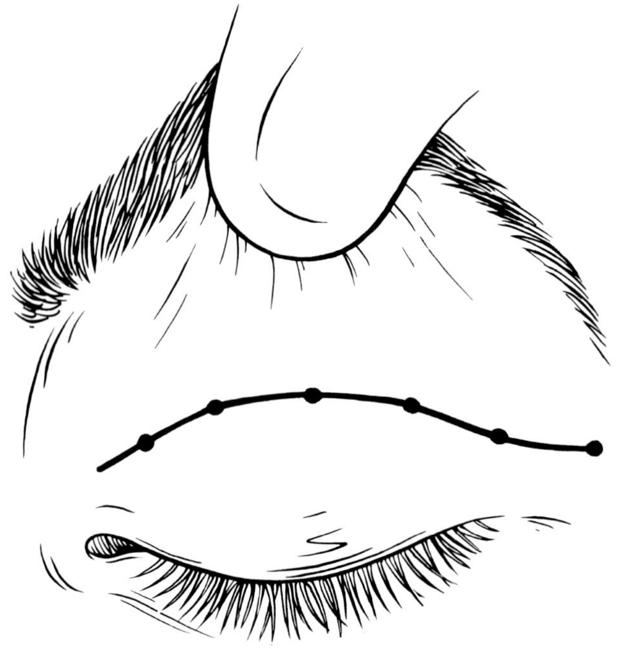

Figure 56–1. Marking of the inferior incision. Preliminary dot markings are connected into a continuous line. The marking begins superior to the punctum; it extends laterally as far as 1.5 cm beyond the lateral canthal angle, staying at least 0.5 cm superior to the lateral extension of superior lower eyelid laugh line to avoid connection with any subsequent lower eyelid blepharoplasty incision. With the eye open and in supraduction, the eyelid marking usually falls within the eyelid crease.

Local Anesthetic Infiltration

When the skin marking process is nearing completion, the anesthetist is notified to induce a brief, profound sedation for local anesthetic infiltration. When the desired

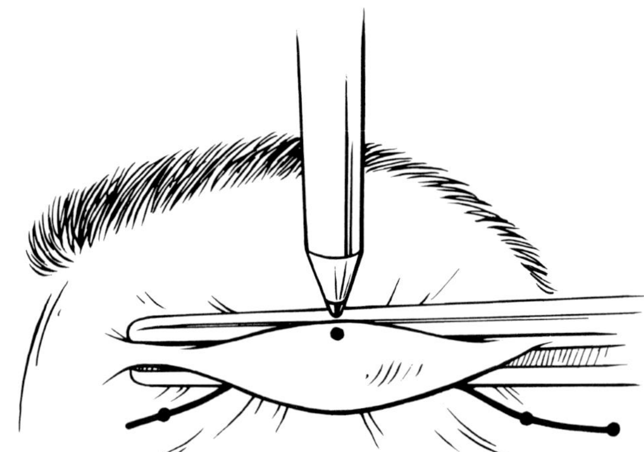

Figure 56–2. Grasping technique to assist in marking the superior incision. The position of the forceps is adjusted to produce only slight separation of the eyelids and slight eversion of the eyelashes. A small mark is made centrally at the edge of the superior forceps blade.

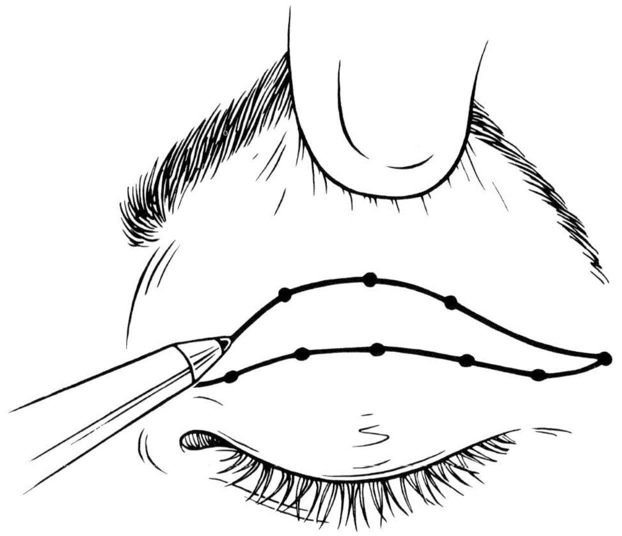

Figure 56–3. Marking of the superior incision is completed. Continuous marking line is completed between the medial and lateral markings determined by the grasping technique; they are connected with the medial and lateral extent of the lower incision markings at fairly acute angles.

level of sedation is achieved, 2 to 3 mL of local anesthetic is infiltrated subcutaneously in several locations in each upper lid using a 27- or 30-gauge disposable needle (Fig. 56–4). I prefer to use lidocaine (Xylocaine) 2% with 1 : 100,000 epinephrine. Because the skin is marked before the injections are made, the addition of hyaluronidase (Wydase) is unnecessary and serves only as a potential source of medication or dilution error. To derive some hemostatic benefit from the epinephrine, the physician should allow 10 minutes to elapse before proceeding with the skin excision. For this reason, the skin should be marked before the surgeon scrubs and the patient's face is prepared and draped.

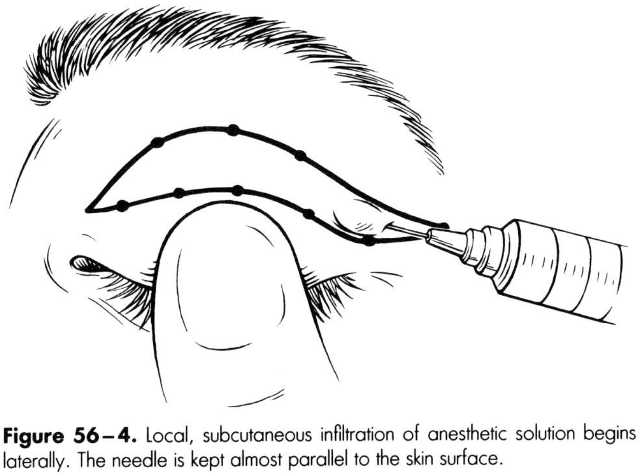

Figure 56–4. Local, subcutaneous infiltration of anesthetic solution begins laterally. The needle is kept almost parallel to the skin surface.

Excision of Skin and Muscle

The eyelid can be stabilized by finger-tip countertraction in most routine blepharoplasties. In cases of extreme dermatochalasis, eyelid laxity, or blepharoptosis, a 4-0 black silk traction suture is placed in the upper eyelid margin, parallel and deep to the gray line. With the eyelid stabilized, the skin is incised in a nasal-to-temporal direction along the premarked lines with a no. 15 scalpel blade. Each of the inferior and superior lines is incised with one smooth stroke to avoid irregularities. The incisions follow the skin markings as closely as possible, including the crisp, acute angles medially and laterally.

Skin excision alone suffices in thin eyelids without orbicularis hypertrophy or herniated orbital fat. In this case, demarcated skin is excised with Westcott scissors, and the blades are kept between the skin and the orbicularis (Fig. 56–5). When eyelid heaviness and fat are slightly more prominent, a thin strip of preseptal orbicularis is removed separately after the skin has been excised (Fig. 56–6). The skin and orbicularis are excised simultaneously in cases of heavy eyelids characterized by subcutaneous fat, hypertrophied orbicularis, and herniated orbital fat. In this case, the dissection is kept superficial, with minimal disruption of the orbital septum; this method avoids blind cutting into retroseptal fat or the levator aponeurosis. In each of the types of excision techniques described (skin only, separate muscle strip, skin–muscle), the assistant stretches the wound apart as tissue is resected with Westcott scissors. The lateral edge of the tissue being resected is lifted with a toothed Adson or 0.5-mm Castroviejo forceps to provide a third point of countertraction. The blade of a monopolar Bovie hand piece is applied to a 0.5-mm toothed Castroviejo (or fine Bonac-

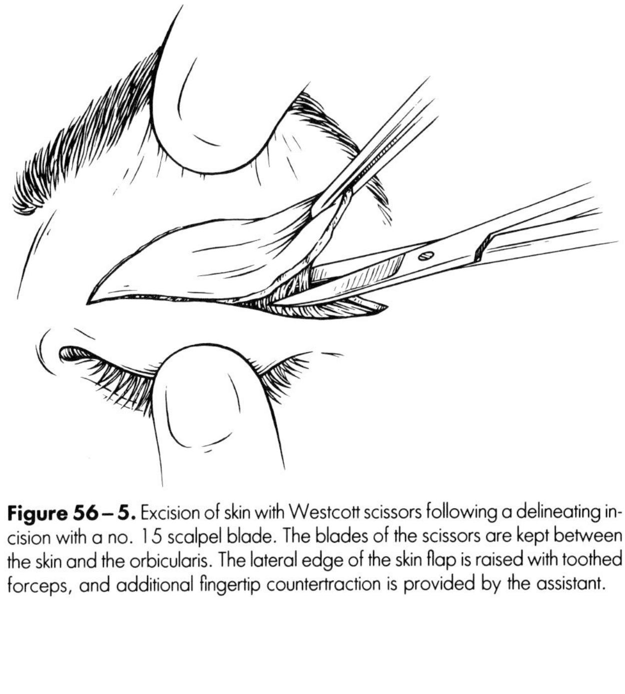

Figure 56–5. Excision of skin with Westcott scissors following a delineating incision with a no. 15 scalpel blade. The blades of the scissors are kept between the skin and the orbicularis. The lateral edge of the skin flap is raised with toothed forceps, and additional fingertip countertraction is provided by the assistant.

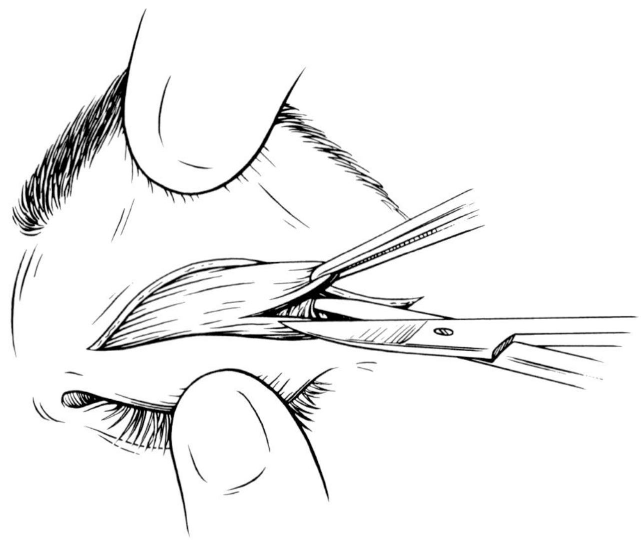

Figure 56–6. Removal of preseptal orbicularis with Westcott scissors as the lateral edge of the tissue resected is raised with a toothed forceps. The assistant provides fingertip countertraction.

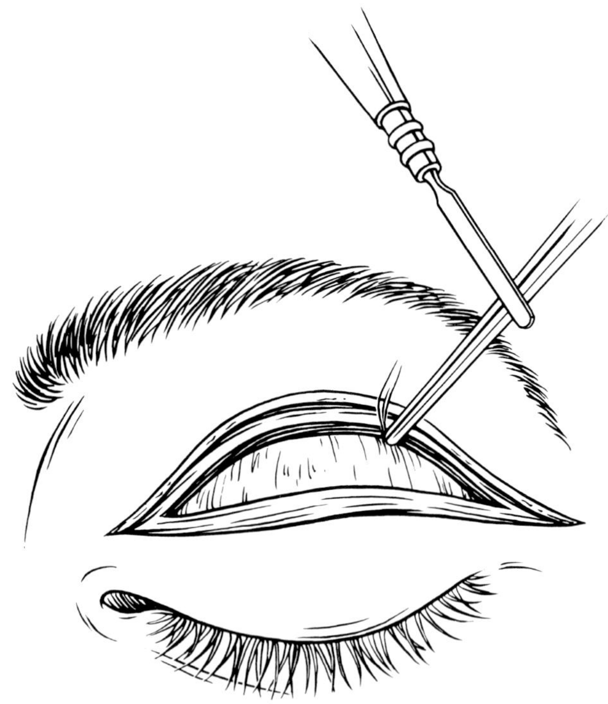

Figure 56–7. Pinpoint cauterization of fine bleeding vessels on the orbicularis using a monopolar Bovie hand piece applied to a fine forceps.

colto) forceps while individual points of bleeding on the orbicularis are grasped until hemostasis is achieved (Fig. 56–7).

Excision and Incision of Orbital Septum

In cases with significant obribularis excision, the well-exposed orbital septum is excised across the horizontal length of the wound in an "open-sky" fashion that fully exposes orbital fat in the medial and central compartments, and the lacrimal gland in the lateral compartment if this too has prolapsed anteriorly (Fig. 56–8). If fat herniation is minimal and mostly medial, the alternative method of a smaller button-hole through the septum (and orbicularis if not resected) is used to prolapse retroseptal fat into the wound for excision.

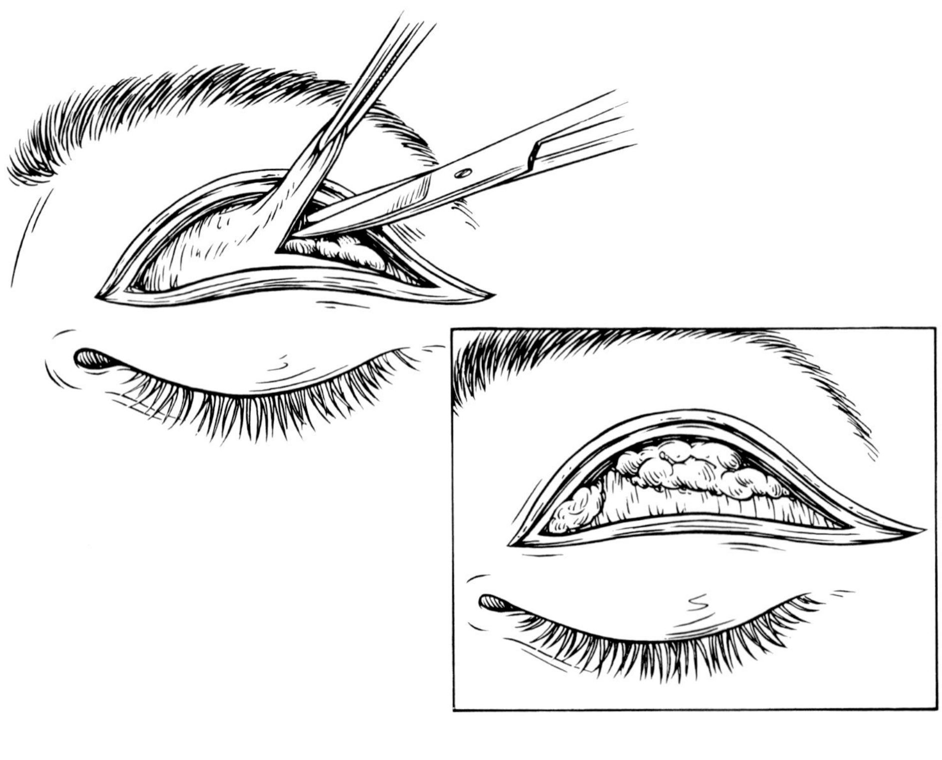

Figure 56–8. Excision of the orbital septum across the entire upper eyelid. *Inset,* Open-sky exposure of the orbital fat pockets.

Excision of Fat

Central fat exposed in the open skin technique is carefully mobilized away from the levator aponeurosis by gentle wiping with a cotton-tipped applicator and cutting of filamentary attachments with a Westcott scissors as necessary. After preaponeurotic fat is fully visualized and distinguished from lacrimal gland, the relatively avascular central fat is excised without first clamping it with a hemostat. The excision is carried up to the superior orbital rim (Fig. 56–9).

Excision of medial fat is omitted if there was very little medial bulging preoperatively. When medial fat is excised, care is taken to avoid cutting of the upper medial palpebral vessels, which course over the medial fat. When prominent vessels are present in the orbital fat or surrounding connective tissue cannot be avoided, the tissue is first clamped with a curved hemostat before it is excised (Fig. 56–10). To first produce anterior prolapse of the fat, the physician should have the assistant apply gentle digital pressure to the globe through the upper eyelid. Anterior traction should not be applied on the orbital fat when the hemostat is placed so as to avoid injury to deeper vasculature. The fat is excised almost flush with the anterior concave surface of the hemostat jaws, which are cauterized with the blade of a monopolar Bovie. Strategic placement of cotton-tipped applicators can insulate the skin from the hemostat or Bovie blade tip (Fig. 56–11).

The orbital septum is not closed, because doing so offers no functional or cosmetic advantage and only predisposes to lagophthalmos and upper eyelid lag in down gaze. Also, in the rare event of a postoperative orbital hemorrhage, retroseptal sequestration of hemorrhage would pose a threat to visual function.

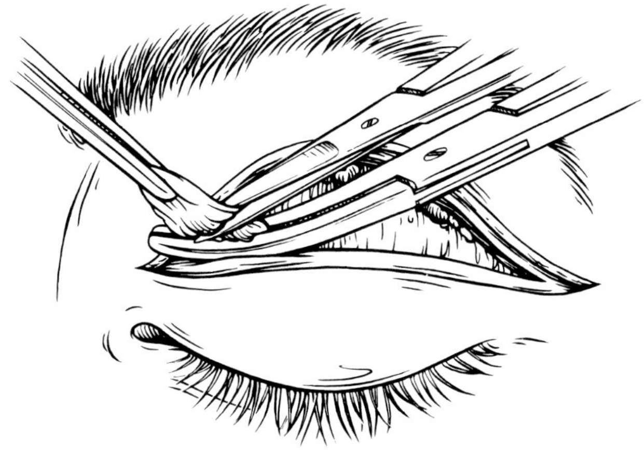

Figure 56–10. Excision of medial orbital fat clamped within the jaws of a curved hemostat.

Any brow fat that presents as a discrete structure in the lateral upper eyelid is excised, but such excision is limited to the retro-orbicularis-preseptal plane and the border of the wound. In routine cases, subcutaneous fat should not be further thinned or debulked in the eyelid fold, because this practice carries a risk of localized depressions of surface contour. However, if this aesthetic feature is of significant importance to the patient, more aggressive fat excision can be considered at this point.

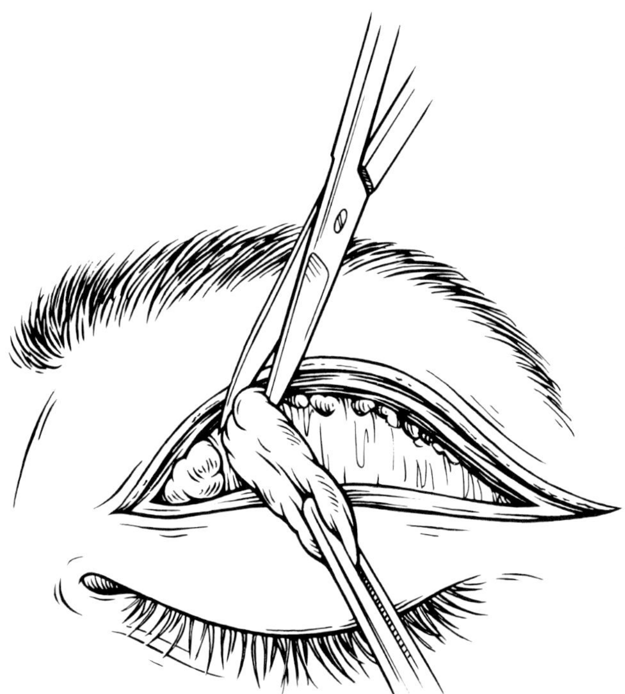

Figure 56–9. Excision of preaponeurotic fat without clamping.

Repair of Prolapsed Lacrimal Gland

Before surgery, a prolapsed orbital lobe of the lacrimal gland presents as a moderately firm bulge in the lateral

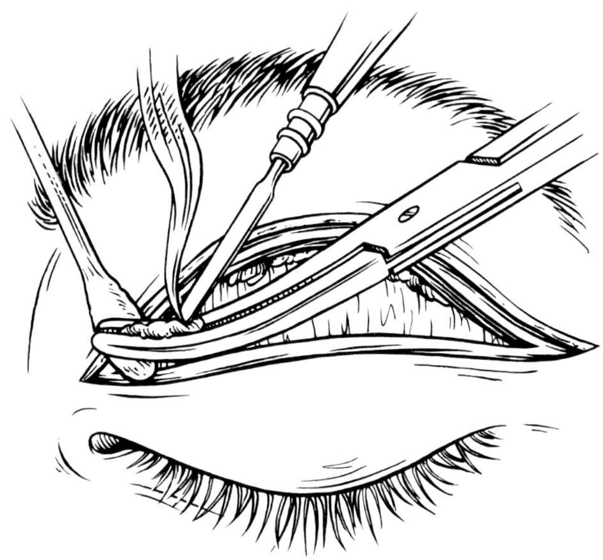

Figure 56–11. Insulation of the hemostat from skin with a cotton-tipped applicator. Monopolar Bovie cautery is applied to the hemostat and the stump of medial orbital fat.

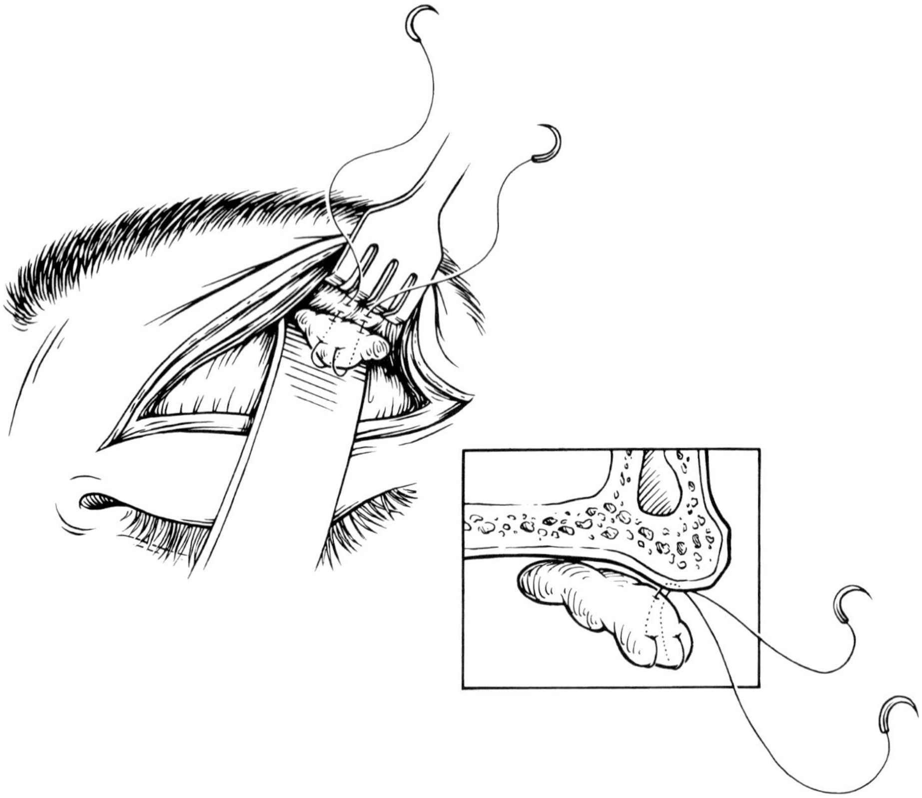

Figure 56–12. Repositioning of a prolapsed lacrimal gland. A double-armed 4-0 chromic suture is passed in a whipstitch fashion at the central inferior pole of the gland. Each arm of the suture is then brought through to the superior surface of the gland and then passed through the periosteum posterior to the orbital rim. Exposure of the lacrimal fossa is achieved with a lacrimal rake at the superior edge of the blepharoplasty wound as a malleable retractor gently displaces the anterior orbital structures inferior to the lacrimal gland. *Inset*, Side view showing position of periosteal attachment in the lacrimal fossa.

upper lid that can be moved back into the lacrimal gland fossa. If no enlargement or other suspected pathology exists, repair is indicated without the need for biopsy. At the time of blepharoplasty, a prolapsed lacrimal gland presents in the superolateral upper eyelid as a firm, pink-gray, and glandular structure that is easily distinguished from the adjacent soft, yellow orbital fat.

After excess fat is excised, both arms of a double-armed 4-0 chromic gut suture are passed through the gland from the inferior to superior surface and then through the periosteum of the lacrimal gland fossa posterior to the orbital rim (Fig. 56–12). A second suture can be added to reinforce the suspension.

Concurrent Ptosis Repair

After the aforementioned steps are completed, cosmetically or functionally significant ptosis is repaired. The amount of ptosis serves as a general guide for the types of surgical repair that are outlined below.

Mild Ptosis

A concurrent Fasanella-Servat procedure is used for cases of mild ptosis without much orbicularis hypertrophy or fat prolapse. The upper eyelid is everted and two hemostats applied across the upper tarsal border, incorporating 2 to 3 mm of tissue. A 5-0 black monofilament nylon suture is passed from the medial superior edge of the skin wound to the medial palpebral conjunctiva. Then, a serpentine whip stitch is passed along the superior border of the hemostats to the lateral palpebral conjunctiva, and the suture is externalized to the lateral superior edge of the skin wound. The hemostats are removed, and the tarsus and conjunctiva are excised with Westcott scissors, with the blades being kept within the crush marks. The eyelid is returned to its natural position, and the suture is gently drawn back and forth as the undersurface is smoothed. The 5-0 nylon suture is tied to itself with a surgeon's knot only after the skin wound is closed.

As an alternative to the Fasanella-Servat technique, an observable aponeurosis dehiscence that exposes Müller's muscle is repaired by including the superior edge of the dehiscence in a supratarsal fixation suture. A more extensive disinsertion discovered at surgery is advanced cautiously to fascia or the posterior edge of the orbicularis muscle near the upper tarsal border with 6-0 Vicryl suture. The sutures are tied temporarily with slip knots. Eyelid height and contour are assessed with the patient in both the supine and the sitting positions. The suture placement is adjusted accordingly and the sutures tied with square surgeon's knots.

Moderate Ptosis

For moderate ptosis noted preoperatively, the levator aponeurosis is advanced onto the tarsal plate. The ante-

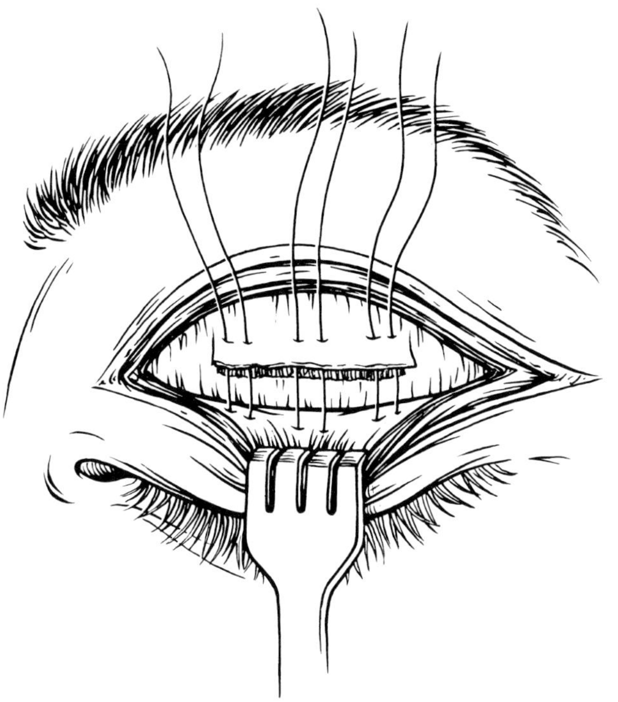

Figure 56–13. Correction of aponeurotic ptosis during blepharoplasty. Preplaced double-armed 6-0 polyglactin 910 sutures are brought up through the levator aponeurosis, which is then advanced onto the tarsus. The sutures are (1) tied with a slip knot to asses the eyelid height and contour, (2) tied permanently with square surgeon's knots, and (3) secured to the orbicularis by passing only one arm of the suture through the cut inferior edge of the orbicularis before tying a second surgeon's knot.

rior tarsal surface is exposed with Westcott scissors. Three double-armed 6-0 polyglactin 910 (Vicryl) sutures on spatula needles are passed partial thickness through the anterior surface of the tarsus 1 to 2 mm below its superior border. The sutures are brought up through the levator aponeurosis, and each is tied with a slip knot. Again, the eyelid height and contour are assessed in both the supine and the sitting positions and are adjusted accordingly before the slip knots are converted to square surgeon's knots (Fig. 56–13). One arm of the suture is passed through the inferior edge of the orbicularis wound and tied with a second knot to help form the eyelid crease. Alternatively, each arm of the suture is brought through both the superior and inferior skin wound edges, and they are tied permanently to produce an even more pronounced crease.

Severe Ptosis

Preoperatively, when the ptosis overshadows the dermatochalasis (e.g., severe ptosis, poor levator function, associated ophthalmoplegia), the ptosis correction is performed first by the appropriate technique. The redundant skin is treated after a satisfactory eyelid height and contour has been achieved.

Eyelid Crease Formation and Skin Closure

If the levator aponeurosis has been advanced onto or near the tarsus with 6-0 polyglactin 910 sutures and secured to the orbicularis as described earlier, further reconstruction or supraplacement of the eyelid crease is not attempted. When supratarsal fixation is appropriate, a closely spaced, running 6-0 black silk suture is used, and small bites of the aponeurosis are taken 1 mm superior to the tarsus as part of the skin wound closure (Fig. 56–14). Only a few aponeurosis bites may be required, each separated by several millimeters, but each is checked for depth and vertical placement to avoid blepharoptosis or a lid crease that is higher than desired.

If a W-plasty was part of the original preincision design, the apex is advanced 5 to 6 mm laterally with an interrupted 6-0 black silk suture, and interrupted sutures are added medially (Fig. 56–15). If a W-plasty was not part of the original preincision design and an excess amount of medial canthal skin is still present, a base-down Burrow triangle is excised from the superior edge of the wound 5 mm from its medialmost extent (Fig. 56–16).

Postoperative Care

At the conclusion of the procedure, ophthalmic antibiotic ointment is applied to the wounds and to the eyes. Ice-cold compresses are applied to the closed eyelids (e.g., an Invotec Swiss Therapy eye mask or iced, wet, gauze compresses). These therapies are continued postoperatively in a recovery area for 1 hour or longer. The compresses are soaked in ice water at the bedside. Alternatively, if a 4×4 gauze sponge is used, the nurse or attendant places ice chips between layers of the folded

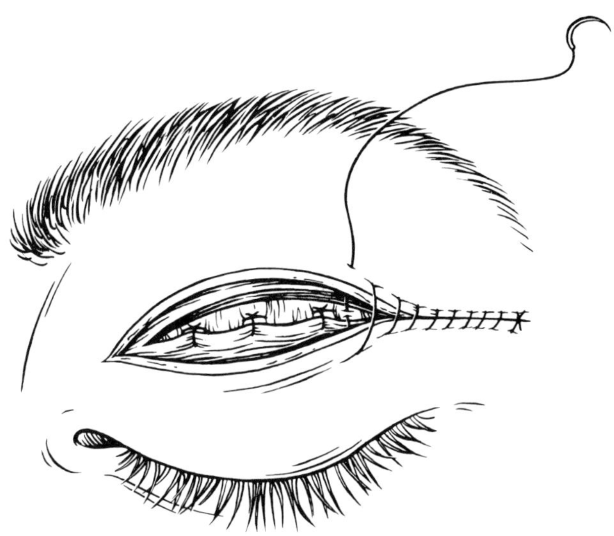

Figure 56–14. The skin wound is closed with a running 6-0 black silk suture. Small bites of the aponeurosis, each 1 mm superior to the tarsus, are taken at 5- to 6-mm intervals.

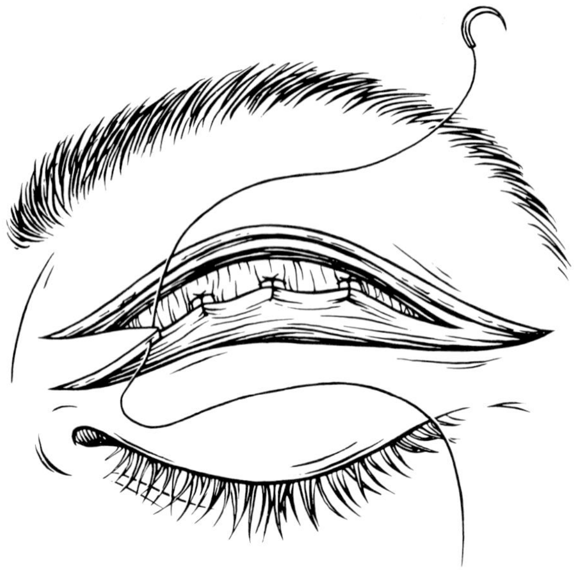

A

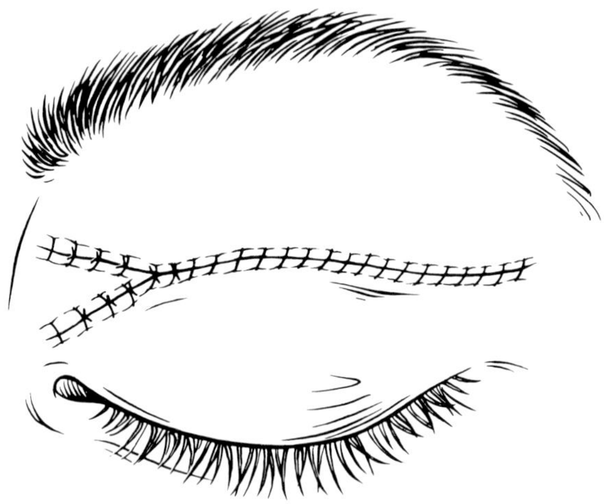

B

Figure 56–15. Closure of the medial portion of the wound when a W-plasty has been delineated. *A*, The W-plasty is advanced 5 to 6 mm laterally with a 6-0 black silk interrupted suture that passes subcutaneously beneath the apex of the small flap. *B*, Interrupted 6-0 black silk sutures are added medially as needed, whereas the lateral portion of the wound is closed with running 6-0 black silk.

sponge. A terrycloth towel placed behind the patient's head and neck helps keep the pillow dry.

The patient is discharged with detailed written instructions. Ice-cold compresses are resumed at home during waking hours for the remainder of the day and the following morning. The patient is instructed to immediately contact the physician if the eyelid swells shut or if bleeding occurs. The patient is called later that day to ensure that he or she clearly understands all instructions and is experiencing no difficulties.

At home, the patient cleans the wounds twice daily and as needed with a clean washcloth or cotton balls wet with warm tap water. Also, the patient applies antibiotic ointment onto the wounds twice daily and instills artificial tears in the eyes four times daily or more frequently if indicated. The sutures are removed in the physician's office four days after the surgery. Sutures may be left in place for 8 to 9 days, but the wounds must be kept clean and moist with ointment to reduce the probability of suture tracts.

TECHNICAL VARIATIONS

Most authorities agree that the upper eyelids should be repaired before the lower eyelids are repaired.[29, 30] Gradinger[31] pointed out that a planned forehead lift need not be performed before upper eyelid blepharoplasty to

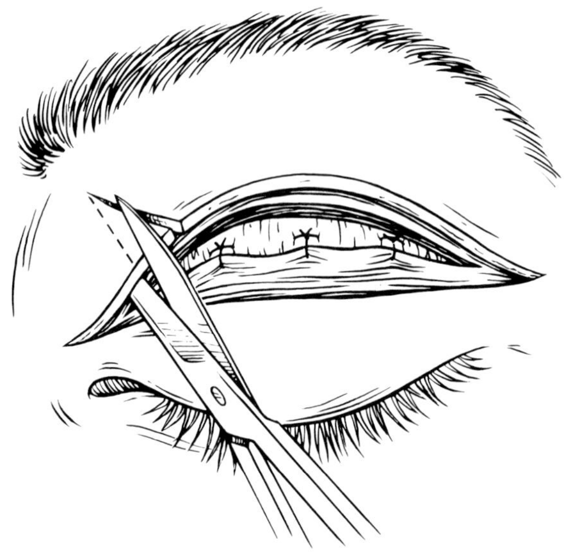

A

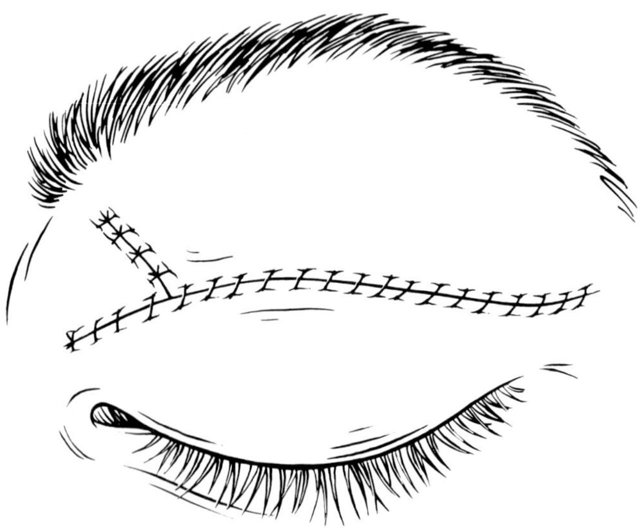

B

Figure 56–16. Treatment of redundant medial eyelid skin with a base-down Burrow triangular excision. *A*, After an initial vertically oblique incision, tangenital to the medial superior edge of the wound, the redundant skin is drawn laterally and excised about 5 mm lateral to the medial-most extent of the blepharoplasty wound. *B*, Interrupted 6-0 black silk sutures are placed as needed to close the medial portion of the wound. A running 6-0 black silk suture is used to close laterally.

avoid removing too much eyelid skin. If the blepharoplasty is to be performed first, Gradinger recommends stabilizing the eyebrow in the anticipated elevated position and marking the upper lid excess skin in the usual fashion.

The following review is confined to basic and adjunctive techniques in upper eyelid blepharoplasty, again following the sequence of surgical steps that have been outlined. A further discussion of standard brow lift techniques can be found in Chapter 54.

Preparation and Draping of the Patient

Antiseptic preparation of the skin in upper eyelid blepharoplasty is most commonly performed with povidone. Courtiss[27] believes that infection is rare in blepharoplasty; therefore, a mild colorless antiseptic, such as benzalkonium chloride (Zephiran), is sufficient.

It is very important to converse with the patient while preparations for surgery are taking place in the operating room. The patient is informed of each preparatory step while pleasant conversation is interspersed. Lynch[32] points out that gentleness is an art when inducing and sustaining a pain-free unconscious state. He emphasizes that the surgeon can attend entirely to the surgical endeavor by sharing responsibility for a semiconscious or unconscious patient with the anesthesiologist. As Katzen and Karvelis[33] noted, the anesthesiologist is in a position to provide calming human contact (e.g., holding the patient's hand) while carefully monitoring the patient during surgery.

Leaving the entire face exposed also reduces any feelings of isolation or claustrophobia the patient may have. Bosniak[30] mentions the possible distortion of the brow or lid crease by surgical drapes and his avoidance of plastic Steri-Drapes. Commercially available eyes, ears, nose, and throat paper drapes with self-contained adhesive can almost always be applied without distorting the patient's anatomy. The head drape can be wrapped around the patient's head or simply applied high over the forehead. In either case, the drapes should be secure enough to remain in place if the patient is brought temporarily to a sitting position.[12]

The most likely potential systemic complication of upper eyelid blepharoplasty is respiratory depression produced by preoperative medications or intravenous narcotics (e.g., fentanyl) and sedatives (e.g., midazolam [Versed] or thiamylal [Surital]). A pulse oximeter enables the surgeon and anesthesiologist to anticipate problems before they occur.[31]

The patient's clinical photographs taken in the office[34] are commonly in clear view of the surgeon. They may be referred to when incisions are planned and skin, muscle, and fat are removed.[31] Review of office notes and photographs should only reinforce the planning that has already taken place preoperatively. As Courtiss[27] notes, "Determining for the first time in the operating room what and how much to do is a gamble."

Skin Marking

Dyes may be used in marking the skin. Brilliant green mixed in an acetone base[28] or methylene blue applied with tooth picks will resist removal when applied before the skin is prepared.[30] A wide selection of sterile gentian violet marking pens are commercially available. Because accurate skin marking is crucial, a fine tip must be used to draw any line on the skin. A scalpel blade may be used to sharpen the blunt tip of a prepackaged marking pen.[30]

The design of the skin markings in upper eyelid blepharoplasty varies depending on the morphology of the patient. The final scar should fall naturally into the supratarsal crease.[30] At the lateral canthus, the incision should angle upward and outward, parallel to, or in, a normal skin crease.[31] Rees[35, 36] did much to popularize wide lateral extensions of the blepharoplasty incisions to correct lateral skin folds and wrinkles. Within reason, the lateral incision should indeed be carried as far as necessary to remove the excess skin.[31] Shorr and Seiff[37] stated that placement of the surgical scar in a superior "laugh line," provides a "happy" rather than "sad" appearance. However, many authors[30, 36] point out that carrying the surgery beyond the lateral orbital rim in patients with no lateral hood of skin may be unnecessary. The use of a double W-plasty, as described by Courtiss and colleagues,[38] is a variation that is apparently not routinely practiced by its originator.[27] The W-plasty configuration has only limited applications laterally, although medially it may be helpful.

Other techniques go well beyond the standard upper eyelid blepharoplasty in dealing with lateral rhytids. A Z-plasty technique, transposing a triangular flap from the upper to the lower lateral canthus, has been proposed by Lewis.[39] Rees[29] pointed out that the additional resulting scars may be relatively inconspicuous but may interfere with future secondary operations. Another, more involved, method aimed at the lateral crow's-feet involves division of the lateral ring of the orbicularis oculi and transposition of the muscle flaps superiorly and inferiorly away from the horizontal raphe.[40, 41] This latter approach is more an extension of face-lift surgery than simply a blepharoplasty technique.

Based on the surgeon's preferences and variations in patient morphology, marking of the medial portion of the upper eyelid blepharoplasty incision may also be variable. A conservative approach is to not carry the incision more medial than a point superior to the superior punctum.[37, 42] Baylis[43] routinely carries the skin marking about 5 mm medial to the punctum (halfway between the medial canthus and the punctum). Gradinger[31] also uses a rather medial incision, which also angles superiorly. He states that this method helps to avoid a skin contractures, which can look like an epicanthal fold. Other techniques that have been devised for skin resections medial to the superior punctum include a medial W-plasty[38, 42] or Burrow triangle.[30, 42]

The actual measured distances between the crease (or lower incision) and margin of the eyelid vary, depending on the amount of manual eyelid fold and eyebrow retraction performed by the surgeon. Most descriptions of upper eyelid blepharoplasty include this step of digital retraction to mark the lower incision. Surgeons who do not stretch the eyelid measure a shorter crease-margin distance,[43] usually only 7 to 8 mm in the vertical midpupillary axis. In any case, the surgeon performing blepharoplasty must have an accurate technique of skin marking that is reproducible.[31]

Grasping of excess skin, such that the eyelid margin elevates slightly, is widely practiced in upper eyelid blepharoplasty. This technique should be distinguished from the pinch technique described later. Rees and colleagues[29, 44] and Tenzel[45] have illustrated a grasping technique with a Green forceps that has wide opposing jaws. Others prefer a smaller smooth forceps that is horizontally placed and allows the surgeon to more easily regrasp and mark at different locations across the upper lid.[42] Baylis[43] "mildly" objected to the grasping technique because it implies that a correct amount of skin exists to excise and it under emphasizes the importance of orbicular muscle and fat excision. However, the value of this technique in avoiding excessive resection of skin should be appreciated.

Another method of determining how much skin to remove in upper eyelid blepharoplasty is the so-called pinch technique of Parkes and associates.[46] A key part of this technique is the injection of hyaluronidase mixed with the local anesthetic at least 30 minutes before surgery. No more than 1 to 2 mL of the anesthetic mixture should be injected.[47] The small volume combined with the hyaluronidase virtually ensures that the edema from the injection will almost completely resolve, enabling the surgeon to accurately determine the amount of excess skin to be removed. About 30 minutes after the injection, the excess skin is pinched with the hope that the subcutaneous layers in the base will adhere into a ridge. The amount of skin that is pinched is increased until an eversion of the lid is about to be produced. The ridge that remains standing is then excised with a scissors. Where suitable, the authors also advocated proceeding with an orbicularis-septal button-hole followed by orbital fat removal.

Beard[48] stated that the pinch technique "cannot be used on every eyelid, but it can be useful on many." He advocated its use in patients with thin, parchment-like skin of old age. He also stated that if the pinching does not readily work, the surgeon can then convert to the routine method of skin excision.

Instead of premarking tissue for upper eyelid tissue excision, Silver[49] chose to prepare a superiorly based skin flap and excision of the apron of skin that drapes over the supratarsal wound and eyelid margin. A similar approach is often adopted in ptosis surgery in which levator aponeurosis is first repaired or advanced and redundant skin and orbicular muscle are resected subsequently.[12]

Local Anesthetic Infiltration

Topical instillation of tetracaine 0.5% onto both corneas eliminates discomfort from antiseptic scrub solutions and allows the patient to tolerate corneoscleral protective shields if these are used by the surgeon. The disadvantage of tetracaine use is that the medication itself may produce transient discomfort, and the patient should be warned of this effect in advance. The advantage of tetracaine over proparacaine (Ophthaine, AK-Taine, Alcaine) is that the former is available in sterile vials for intraoperative use. Tetracaine has a rapid onset (under 30 seconds) and a duration of action of 15 to 20 minutes.[50]

Various types, concentrations, and combinations of anesthetic solutions have been advocated for use in upper eyelid blepharoplasty. Currently, the most commonly employed agents probably are lidocaine with epinephrine (1%/1 : 200,000 or 2%/1 : 100,000). The onset of anesthesia occurs within minutes and lasts approximately 90 minutes. Mixing bupivacaine (Marcaine) 0.5% to 0.75% with lidocaine will prolong the duration of anesthesia for 4 to 12 hours while maintaining a rapid onset. However, prolonged postoperative orbicular weakness and lagophthalmos may also result. If upper eyelid blepharoplasty alone is being performed, the addition of bupivacaine is probably not necessary. If a brow lift or lower eyelid blepharoplasty is being performed concurrently with upper eyelid blepharoplasty, the prolonged anesthesia from bupivacaine is helpful. Etidocaine (Duranest) is gaining popularity because of its short onset of action and its prolonged anesthetic effect.[50] It is available in 0.5% to 2% solutions.

The vasconstrictive effects of epinephrine are also invaluable and may prolong anesthesia. Because the hemostatic vasoconstriction of epinephrine begins in about 10 minutes, many surgeons routinely mark and inject the eyelids before proceeding with their scrub.[27, 30, 37, 43] Still, I sometimes prefer to scrub and have the patient prepared and draped before local anesthetic is injected. This method ensures that the patient will be settled comfortably and that the anesthetist will have finished attaching monitoring devices and is fully prepared to administer sedatives or analgesics.

Solutions of epinephrine that are more dilute than 1 : 100,000 or 1 : 200,000 can give equally good vasoconstriction as more concentrated ones.[51] I usually prefer to avoid any possibility for dilutional errors by using pre-mixed solutions. In patients with controlled hypertension, Courtiss[27] recommended using 1:400,000 epinephrine; those with uncontrolled hypertension are not offered surgery. Many surgeons have offered various recipes for anesthetic solutions used in blepharoplasty. In addition to possible errors in dilution, large volumes of anesthetic are wasted when only a few milliliters are actually injected. Gradinger[31] follows a standard recipe for dilution of epinephrine to 1:500,000, made by mixing 50 mL of 0.5% lidocaine with 0.1 mL of 1:100,000 epinephrine; he uses only 2 to 3 mL of this solution.

During surgery, epinephrine-soaked pledgets may also be placed on an open wound while excision is performed on the opposite side.[45] When the ophthalmologist comes back to the side of the first skin excision, less bleeding is present.

In addition to hastening the resolution of distortion from anesthetic solution, the addition of hyaluronidase in the injected mixture may also speed and enhance the effect of anesthesia and the vasoconstrictive effect of epinephrine.[27] It may also lessen edema occurring after surgery. The use of hyaluronidase is almost indispensable for determining the amount of tissue to be resected if the injection precedes the skin marking or if the pinch technique is used. Various recommendations have appeared regarding the appropriate amount of time to wait after injection before a quantified diagnosis of redundant skin can be made: Wilkins and coworkers[52] recommend a 10-minute wait; Shorr and Seiff,[37] 15 minutes; and Baylis,[43] 20 minutes. Devotees of the pinch technique advocate waiting 30 minutes.[47, 48]

Various recipes have been mentioned for the addition of hyaluronidase to the anesthetic solution. Beard[48] adds 150 U of hyaluronidase to every 30 mL of anesthetic, whereas Courtiss[27] adds 300 U of hyaluronidase to every 30 to 50 mL of anesthetic.

Bosniak[30] listed various techniques that may be used to reduce patient discomfort during injection of local anesthetic. A 30-gauge needle penetrates the skin almost imperceptibly and decreases the rate of volume distortion, thereby reducing discomfort. Buffering the solution with sodium bicarbonate solution and warming the solution to room temperature also may reduce patient discomfort.

For injection of the eyelids, it is convenient to start laterally,[27, 30, 31] keeping the needle parallel to the skin surface. I find that superficial subcutaneous injection[30] is sufficient to achieve excellent anesthesia; augmentation of the anesthesia into the medial orbital fat may subsequently be given, if necessary, under direct visualization when the ophthalmologist is preparing to excise herniated orbital fat in that region. Other surgeons initially inject deep to the preseptal portion of the orbicular muscle, hoping to better anesthetize sensory nerves that lie deep to the muscle.[31] Initial deep injection into the fat compartments[27] seems to pose a greater risk of ocular penetration.

Excision of Skin and Muscle

An accurate skin incision must be made on a completely stable eyelid. During the smooth pass of the incision, the assistant must understand not to reposition fingers that are placing traction on the skin.[31] A clean, full-thickness incision through the skin brings the fibers of the orbicularis into view. Various instruments, such as a razor blade fragment[27, 45] or permanent diamond knife[44] may be used for the skin incision but offer little or no advantage over a no. 15 Bard-Parker scalpel blade. Scissors are commonly used instead when the blepharoplasty is performed with the pinch technique or when a skin muscle flap is draped over the wound.

As mentioned earlier in the presentation of the author's standard techniques, excision of redundant anterior eyelid tissue may be characterized as skin only,[42] skin-muscle,[27, 31, 37] or skin excision with a separate muscle strip.[28, 53] Especially when skin is excised together with orbicularis, it is easiest to excise tissue in a lateral-to-medial direction using scissors of the surgeon's preference (e.g., a Westcott, Kaye, or Stevens scissors).

Tenzel[45] described grasping the corner of the flap of skin along with an open gauze sponge and applying traction on the skin by pulling it over his index finger. The surgeon begins with the medial edge of the skin excision, and the underlying attachments to the orbicularis are cut by just placing a no. 15 Bard-Parker blade perpendicular to the bands and pressing on them. This technique excises the skin but very little subcutaneous tissue.

Excision of muscle with the skin or in a separate strip exposes the orbital septum and allows the surgeon to proceed with an open-sky excision of that structure and the underlying orbital fat. It also allows the option of placing deeper fixation sutures to prevent late loss of the eyelid crease, as is discussed later. Many surgeons believe that excision of a horizontal strip of orbicularis alone produces an upper eyelid crease just as well as more complex levator fixation techniques.[28, 53] Zide[54] stated that the strip of orbicularis should be at least 3 to 5 mm wide because removal of a thinner strip would diminish the probability of crease formation.

Baker and colleagues,[55] David and Sanders,[56, 57] Mittelman and Apfelberg,[58] and others have used a carbon dioxide laser to make incisions in skin and deeper tissues in blepharoplasty. Putterman[59] and others have also used the scalpel neodymium:yttrium-aluminum-garnet laser in blepharoplasty. However, the application of lasers in routine blepharoplasty is not currently in widespread use.

Excision and Incision of Orbital Septum

The orbital septum is a critical landmark in blepharoplasty because through it, the surgeon gains access to the bulging orbital fat that has been targeted for excision.[54]

However, the pathologic changes in the orbital septum that cause anterior bulging of fat have been a matter of controversy. Through surgical dissections, Putterman and Urist[60] viewed the orbital septum as a firm, strong, inelastic fibrous sheet of connective tissue that, in some cases, was found to be detached from the levator aponeurosis with encapsulated fat protruding forward. They maintained that baggy eyelids occur as a true hernia resulting from the separation of the orbital septum from the levator aponeurosis in the upper lid.[61] They believed that thin suborbicularis fascia may be mistaken for orbital septum. Castanares[2] also referred to the protrusion of orbital fat as a "herniation." However, he later emphasized, "It is not a hernia in the true sense of the word—not comparable, for example, to an inguinal hernia where there is a definite break or rent of the fascia and musculature."[3]

A technique of reducing fat herniation by tightening the orbital septum through the application of cautery has been described,[30] but it is apparently not commonly practiced.

To gain access to protruding orbital fat, the ophthalmologist can make a buttonhole with scissors in the overlying orbicular muscle and orbital septum. Alternatively, the septum may be excised across the horizontal length of the wound (open-sky approach). This approach not only allows superior visibility of the medial blood vessels but also allows careful dissection of fascial connections between the central fat and the levator. Excision of fat by these two methods is further discussed in the next section.

Broad resection of the orbital septum may be considered one component of achieving a concave, high supratarsal (orbitopalpebral) sulcus.[62] The ophthalmologist should be mindful of the variations in patient morphology and the goals of blepharoplasty for the individual patient. In some cases, less debulking of the eyelid is indicated, and the orbital fat and the septum need not be excised.

Excision of Fat

The classic descriptions of medial and lateral fat compartmentalization in the upper eyelid have already been mentioned.[2, 3] Although this concept has been challenged,[63, 64] it remains clinically useful.[54, 65] Surgically, one may appreciate the central, preaponeurotic fat pad that is horizontally elongated and butter-yellow in color. The central fat may extend laterally and may surround a prolapsed lacrimal gland, and it may also extend medially. In many patients, this medial extension is responsible for an observable medial bulge.[66] However, a truly distinct medial fat pocket also exists; in contrast, it is white and may be more multilobulated. This "true" medial fat pad has been described as arising from a portion of muscle cone fat that prolapses around the medial edge of the levator aponeurosis[66] and extending superiorly to engulf the superior oblique tendon-trochlea complex.[67] The varying descriptions of the fat compartments should not obscure the importance of these fat pads in upper eyelid blepharoplasty. From a practical standpoint, localized or generalized bulging of fat must be adequately recognized and treated as part of the blepharoplasty procedure to achieve a satisfactory result.

When the septal buttonhole technique is used, Tenzel[45] cautioned that the fat pocket should be opened superficially because thrusting instruments into the orbit may cause hemorrhage or other intraorbital injury. Because of the possibility of insufficient cauterization of vessels within the clamp, fixation forceps are used to keep the residual stump presenting through the buttonhole, allowing further inspection and cautery before its release.[42, 45, 66, 69]

With an open-sky approach, the relatively avascular central fat permits simple scissors excision without clamping. Gaining sufficient access to the medial fat may require incision of multiple septa. A Desmarres retractor gives adequate exposure in the central eyelid, but hooks or a lacrimal rake may be required medially to properly expose the fat in this area. Courtiss[27] stated that traction is required to deliver the medial fat, which is then excised (without clamping) with a monopolar cutting electric current. Many authors have cautioned against placing anterior traction on fat excised during blepharoplasty to avoid tearing deeper orbital vessels and causing serious orbital hemorrhage.[37, 45] Whether a septal buttonhole[2, 34, 40, 43, 62] or an open-sky technique[37, 62] is used, gentle pressure on the globe by an assistant facilitates the protrusion of both the central and the medial fat pads, greatly minimizing the need for traction on the fat.

In addition to simple excision of fat, electrosurgical methods may also be used to reduce fat volume. Methods used to reduce orbital fat include additional cauterization after initial fat excision with scissors.[70] In addition, lipolytic diathermy alone has been used through an intact septum to shrink orbital fat.[30, 71]

Owsley[72] described a lateral fat pad deep to the orbicular muscle, but superficial to the orbital septum, in patients who had marked bagginess of the upper lid and a bulky hood of tissue extending beyond the lateral canthal region. Although he noted that this fat is separate from the fusiform central fat pad, he advocated its resection to completely correct the lateral hood in such individuals. May and associates[73] termed this fibrofatty soft tissue *retro-orbicularis oculus fat* and confirmed the ability to soften and flatten a bulky lateral upper orbital region with resection of this fatty tissue in conjunction with blepharoplasty. Of course, lateral preseptal fat excision is mainly limited to patients undergoing blepharoplasty for cosmetic reasons alone. However, other techniques, such as brow lift or repair of a prolapsed lacrimal gland, should also be assessed as possible alternatives or adjunctive approaches in these patients. Interestingly, Lassus[74] advocated the use of partial ostectomy of the superolateral orbital rim to reduce lateral fullness in exceptional cases of a prominent bony brow.

Repair of Prolapsed Lacrimal Gland

Relaxation of the suspensory ligaments of the orbital septum may result in prolapse of the lacrimal gland.[75, 76] Subtle subconjunctival prolapse of the palpebral lobe is common, whereas a herniated orbital lobe presenting as a bulge beneath the skin is unusual. Orbital lobe herniation may be seen in the elderly and in younger patients who have undergone trauma or who develop blepharochalasis.[77]

Although this point is not emphasized in the literature, patients with shallow orbits may be predisposed to lacrimal gland prolapse. In acquired orbital diseases, orbital contents that are displaced anteriorly may include not only the globe and orbital fat but also the lacrimal gland. In addition to weakening of ligaments and the septal barrier, a shallow orbital configuration also predisposes to lacrimal gland prolapse. The exaggerated condition of lacrimal gland prolapse may occur as a congenital defect in craniosynostosis syndromes.[78]

On examination, lacrimal gland prolapse presents as a well-defined mass that can be easily palpated and reduced into the lacrimal fossa. Leone[79] noted that a tumor or inflammatory pseudotumor is not as easily reducible as lacrimal gland prolapse and is usually larger in bulk; if it is an inflammatory process, the gland may be tender. Petrelli[80] summarized other benign and malignant conditions that must be differentiated from lacrimal gland herniation and reviewed indications for biopsy.

Gradinger[31] and others have noted that lacrimal gland prolapse may also be encountered during surgery after the orbital septum has been incised. In blepharoplasty, differentiation of herniated lacrimal gland from orbital fat is especially important to avoid the serious complication of lacrimal gland excision.

The surgical repair of prolapsed lacrimal glands generally follows techniques devised in the late 1970s. Through a high lateral incision in the orbital septum, Smith and Petrelli[75] passed a double-armed 4-0 chromic catgut suture through the anterior margin of the gland and tied this securely before suspending the gland to the periosteum. Meticulous hemostasis and closure of the orbital septum were emphasized. Horton and coworkers,[76] described using a similar approach but did not detail their suturing technique. Courtiss[27] advocated the use of 4-0 Vicryl to reposition the lacrimal gland. Bosniak[30] recommended double-armed, nonabsorbable 4-0 suture (Polydek, Prolene, or Mersilene). Leone[79] has used double-armed sutures of 5-0 polypropylene (Prolene), approaching the gland through a standard blepharoplasty incision and leaving the orbital septum unsutured. Bosniak[30] also mentioned the possibility of pulling sutures through holes drilled posterior to the orbital rim if periosteal fixation does not seem adequate.

Scherz and Dohlman[81] condemned any surgical procedure that totally eliminates the main lacrimal gland for cosmetic reasons. They reviewed several cases of keratoconjunctivitis sicca that occurred after lacrimal gland excision. Such problems have not been reported after simple repositioning of the lacrimal gland without excision.

Concurrent Ptosis Repair

Hornblass[9] reviewed several operations for mild ptosis that may be used in conjunction with blepharoplasty, including the Fasanella-Servat procedure[82] and the Müller muscle-conjunctiva resection.[83]

In reviewing the history of cosmetic oculoplastic surgery, Katzen[1] noted that significant recent contributions have centered on the levator aponeurosis and crease-fold complex (see Table 56–1).

Aponeurotic defects, such as dehiscence near the upper tarsal border, are common in elderly patients undergoing blepharoplasty. Sheen[84] noted that an inadvertent tuck of the levator aponeurosis could produce an unexpected postoperative lid retraction. Kahn[85] recommended levator plication to correct senile ptosis during cosmetic blepharoplasty. Dryden and Liebsohn[86] emphasized that the exposure of the levator aponeurosis during blepharoplasty affords an opportunity for repair of any defect in the aponeurosis; it may prophylactically defer the development of acquired ptosis or reverse an early unrecognized ptosis. They emphasized reattachment of the inferior edge of the aponeurosis to the upper edge of the tarsus rather than to relatively weak, adjacent connective tissue only. Wilkins and Patipa,[87, 88] Leone,[89] and Millay and Larrabee[90] have also emphasized the recognition and management of ptosis in the blepharoplasty patient.

Eyelid Crease Formation and Skin Closure

The initial steps of skin markings ensure proper positioning of the eyelid crease. Additional steps for attempting to enhance the eyelid crease include excision of a strip of orbicular muscle and various suture fixation techniques.

Supratarsal Fixation

The term *supratarsal fixation* was introduced by Sheen,[91] who sutured the levator aponeurosis to the tarsus and the overlying cut edge of the orbicular muscle. The technique was a modification of Asian eyelid operations[92–96] used to create a permanent supratarsal fold. Sheen[84] later recommended a change in his technique, fixing levator only to the lower cut edge of the orbicular muscle in patients whose skin fold is lower than

10 mm from the lid margin. Flowers[97] also adapted the Asian eyelid procedure to Caucasians, fixing the levator and tarsus to the skin.

Both Sheen[91] and Flowers[97] excised a strip of orbicular muscle as part of their technique. Baker and colleagues,[53] Gradinger,[31] and others have maintained that orbicular muscle excision alone is responsible for improved results in creating the upper eyelid crease; interestingly, this step was included in many of the original Asian eyelid operations.[93, 95] Still, with some dissenting opinions, the usefulness of supratarsal fixation in selected patients has been widely accepted.

Beyond the original techniques described by Sheen,[84, 91] the term supratarsal fixation has been commonly used in generic sense, with descriptions of many technical variations.[98] In 1977, Small[99] pointed out that various forms of supratarsal fixation have been used by ophthalmic plastic surgeons for many years, not only in standard blepharoplasty but also in more complex eyelid reconstruction.[100] Tenzel[101] distinguished the basic techniques as follows: "In the supratarsal fixation technique, the lower skin (orbicularis) edge is fixed to the levator aponeurosis, whereas in the anchor blepharoplasty, the aponeurosis is incised and the lower skin (orbicularis) edge is attached to the tarsus and usually to the superior incised edge of the aponeurosis."

Various suture materials and techniques have been recommended in supratarsal fixation. Sheen[91] originally used several interrupted 7-0 silk sutures spaced about 5 to 6 mm apart. Other buried sutures that have been recommended include interrupted 6-0 polyglactin 910[62]; horizontal mattress 6-0 polypropylene[45] or braided polyester (Mersilene)[101, 102]; and running, locked 7-0 polypropylene or 8-0 virgin silk.[103] Alternatively, the levator aponeurosis may be incorporated into a final skin closure with interrupted or running sutures.[30, 37, 66, 104] Here, only a small bite of the levator aponeurosis should be taken in three or more locations, but no higher than 1 mm superior to the tarsus.[37, 104] Preferences for suture materials reported for this technique have included 5-0 or 6-0 silk or gut,[104] 6-0 silk or nylon,[30] 6-0 nylon or mild chromic gut,[37] and 7-0 polypropylene.[66]

Many ophthalmic plastic surgeons, including McCord,[62] Small,[99] and Tenzel,[101] have noted that supratarsal fixation can minimize the amount of skin that is required to be excised, introducing a safety factor in the prevention of postoperative lagophthalmos. This is especially true for patients with a low or asymmetric lid crease, but less for patients with preoperatively normal lid creases. Therefore, McCord,[62] Rees,[29] and others have considered supratarsal fixation to be an advanced technique and have cautioned the surgeon who performs blepharoplasty only occasionally to proceed cautiously with appropriate patient selection. The pleasing results from simple orbicular strip excision[28–31] and the potential complications of eyelid malposition and lagophthalmos from supratarsal fixation[84] should certainly guide the novice blepharoplasty surgeon to the simpler approach.

As an alternative to suture fixation, several authors[30, 105, 106] have described thermal cauterization to induce fixation of the eyelid crease. Cautery may be applied to reappose the inferior and superior edges of resected orbicularis[30] or to fuse the inferior skin edge of the orbicularis to epitarsal tissue.[106] These techniques are not recommended in cases in which an eyelid crease must be reconstructed de novo.

Skin Closure

Techniques and material for eyelid skin closure are almost as numerous as the number of surgeons performing blepharoplasty. Interrupted sutures allow the greatest precision and security of wound closure, whereas running sutures may be placed and subsequently removed more quickly. Wilkins and coworkers[52] recommended the use of interrupted 6-0 nylon sutures; Iliff[68] recommended the use of interrupted 8-0 black silk sutures. Both of these publications mentioned starting the wound closure centrally to ensure symmetry and to avoid puckers. Even advocates of subcuticular running suture generally have recommended reinforcing interrupted sutures centrally and especially in the lateral portion of the wound, as is discussed later.

Examples of simple running sutures in upper blepharoplasty wound closure include 6-0 nylon,[62] 6-0 silk, polyglactin 910, or polyglycolic (Dexon).[102] Running sutures may also be placed in a locked fashion, as illustrated by Bosniak[30] and Gavaris.[103] Putterman[102] stated a preference for running 6-0 black silk, finding certain characteristics of other sutures less desirable: greater difficulty in handling stiffer nylon and polypropylene, rapid dissolution of catgut, and slow absorption of polyglactin 910 or polyglycolic sutures. The main drawback of silk is an increased incidence of suture cysts or tracts, which is managed by early removal of sutures.[29, 62, 102]

For an interrupted or simple running closure technique, McCord[62] recommended using several subcuticular sutures of 6-0 polyglactin 910 to align the skin edges. Callahan and Callahan[104] objected to the use of subcutaneous sutures, citing an absence of wound tension and the probability of extrusion through the thin upper eyelid skin.

The use of subcuticular running suture is a popular method of closing the upper blepharoplasty wound.[29, 38, 107] It has mainly been recommended to avoid epithelial cysts and tracts. Rees[29] and Hornblass[9] favored closure with a running, subcuticular 6-0 nylon medially and centrally, with interrupted sutures laterally and elsewhere for reinforcement as needed. Guy and Liverett[107] advocated the use of subcuticular 5-0 nylon but also used 6-0 nylon interrupted sutures laterally as well as centrally for reinforcement. Courtiss[27] recommended using running subcuticular 5-0 polypropylene, which he considered easier to remove than nylon. In 6-0 nylon subcuticular closures, Bosniak[30] recommended that a suture stent be placed under a suture loop in the midline of the wound. If the surgeon has any difficulty removing the subcuticular suture postoperatively, the stent and suture can be elevated and the suture cut in the midline to facilitate its removal.

Methods of nonsuture skin closure have also been applied to upper eyelid blepharoplasty. Kosko[108] used butyl-2-cyanoacrylate (Histaacryl glue) after using a modified pinch technique. Although this material has been variously used in ophthalmic and aesthetic facial plastic surgery,[109] the cyanoacrylates have not been approved by the Food and Drug Administration for wound closure.[110] Mandel[110] used autologous fibrin glue (and a few sutures only). In the fibrin glue technique, fibrinogen was prepared from autologous blood by a cryoprecipitate technique. The simultaneous application of fibrinogen and thrombin to the wounds produced a thin layer of instant clot with sufficient strength to close the wound. One notes with great relief that staples have not been reported in the closure of blepharoplasty wounds.

Postoperative Care

The postoperative period is the final test of the patient-physician relationship. Because the patient is ambulatory, most of his or her time is spent away from medical supervision. The immediate postoperative period of observation usually lasts no longer than 1 to 3 hours.[31, 42] Detailed written instructions and follow-up telephone conversations reinforce the specific details of the postoperative regimen while conveying a sense of genuine concern and empathy.

Gradinger[31] stated, "Everything we do for the patients and ask them to do for themselves is designed to minimize swelling and bruising and decrease the risk of bleeding and corneal or ocular complications." Because the orbicularis has been weakened by excision and residual anesthesia, the application of ophthalmic ointment to the eye is immediately started to protect the cornea from dessication. Subsequently, lubricating eyedrops and ointment at nighttime are usually recommended. Iliff[68] noted that the application of bland ophthalmic ointment to the wound can prevent drying and crusting. I usually give the patient the tube of ophthalmic antibiotic ointment for use on both the eyelid and the eye. The use of commonly sensitizing antibiotics, such as neomycin, should be avoided, and topical steroids also have a theoretic risk in the patient with corneal exposure. Tenzel,[45] however, recommended the use of topical steroid-antibiotic ointment after blepharoplasty.

Elevating the head of the bed in the immediate postoperative period has been mentioned by several authors.[27, 31, 42] Iced compresses area also begun immediately, although the methods have varied between authors. Putterman[42] recommended resoaking 4 × 4 gauze pads in a bucket of iced saline as needed to keep the compresses cold. McCord[62] recommended placing crushed ice in 4 × 4 gauze pads to form an "ice sandwich," which is held in position with a wrap-around head towel. Courtiss[27] recommended the use of iced witch hazel compresses. The duration of treatment with cold compresses has also varied between authors from 24 hours[42] or 48 hours[27, 45] to as long as 72 hours.[37] Switching to a regimen of hot compresses on the fourth postoperative day has also been recommended.[37]

Because of the risk of retrobulbar hemorrhage and blindness, numerous authors have stressed the avoidance of pressure dressings at the completion of blepharoplasty.[62] Conversely, Rees[27] has vacillated about bandaging the eyes because, theoretically, a moderate pressure dressing for the first few hours after surgery would be beneficial in helping to control oozing, edema, and hematoma. However, these problems are less of a concern in the patient receiving local anesthesia. Iliff[68] used a mild pressure dressing of a dry nonadherent type (Telfa) for 24 hours. Only a mild amount of pressure is applied by a wrap around towel that McCord[62] has recommended to keep iced gauze compresses in place. Any complaint of severe pain warrants an immediate check for light perception and removal of any dressing.[45]

Variations in the timing of suture removal depend mainly on the types of suture materials used. Absorbable sutures dissolve, and residual material is simply cleaned away. Nonabsorbable sutures are removed relatively early to prevent suture cysts and tracts. Very early removal of some sutures has been advocated at 1 to 2 days after surgery by Rees[29] and at 2 to 3 days by Guy and Liverett[107] when the subcuticular nylon closure technique is used. Also the medial end of subcuticular nylon is cut and partially retracted to prevent pustule formation; the subcuticular and lateral sutures are removed at 4 to 7 days after surgery.[29, 107] Putterman[42] recommended removing running 6-0 silk sutures 4 days after surgery but would apply Steri-Strips to the wound for an additional 3 days.

At the time of suture removal, the patient should be questioned regarding any symptoms of ocular discomfort. An ocular slit-lamp examination after instillation of fluorescein dye can reveal the extent of any microscopic corneal erosions (superficial punctate keratopathy). The regimen of lubricating eyedrops and ointment can be adjusted accordingly.

RESULTS

Usually, the cosmetic or functional improvement from upper eyelid blepharoplasty may be appreciated almost immediately. Edema and ecchymosis is most noticeable on the first and second postoperative days, this effect subsides remarkably quickly. Persistent edema can

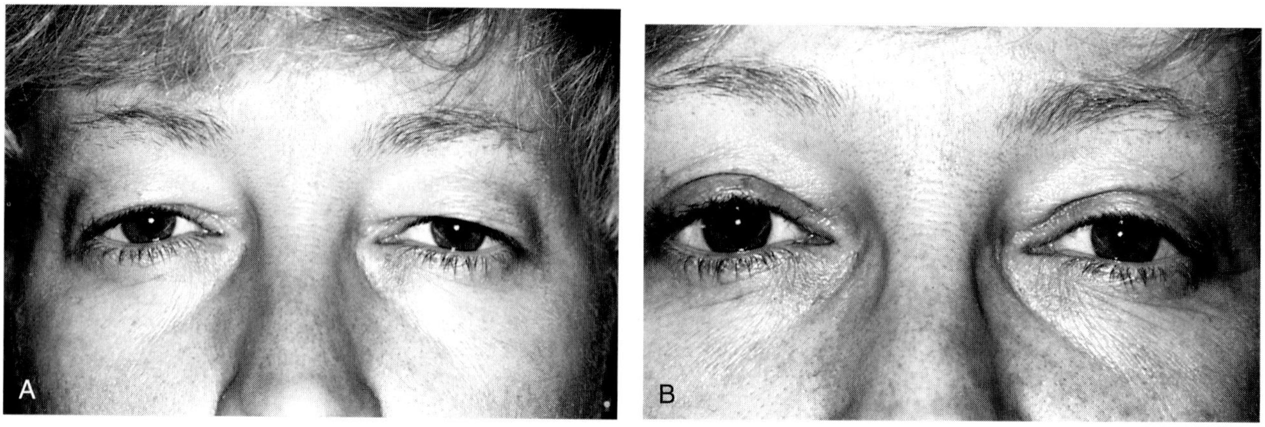

Figure 56–17. *A*, Preoperative photograph of a 41-year-old woman with hereditary hooded dermatochalasis. Even when wide awake, her friends would ask her if she were falling asleep. An open-sky bilateral upper eyelid blepharoplasty was performed. To achieve symmetry, a greater amount of skin was resected from the left upper lid, but an equal amount of preaponeurotic and medial orbital fat excision was done on each side. *B*, Postoperative photograph 7 weeks after surgery. Note the symmetry of the eyelid folds.

be expected to occur in cases of true blepharochalasis or posttraumatic deformities. Blepharoptosis often persists for a few weeks after supratarsal fixation, and the patient may require reassurance during this time.

Blepharoplasty does not always give a stereotypic result. The eyelids may be surgically modified, but the process relies on individual anatomy and tissue characteristics. Distinctive individual features, such as the skeletal framework, the overall appearance of the face, and the texture and color of the skin, remain the same, yet a relative improvement is the key to a satisfactory result. Clinical examples of this truism are well illustrated by comparative preoperative and postoperative photographs (Figs. 56–17 through 56–22).

Although patients should be warned preoperatively of a possible need for revision, such revision surgery is only occasionally necessary. With such early and lasting improvement, patient satisfaction is high.

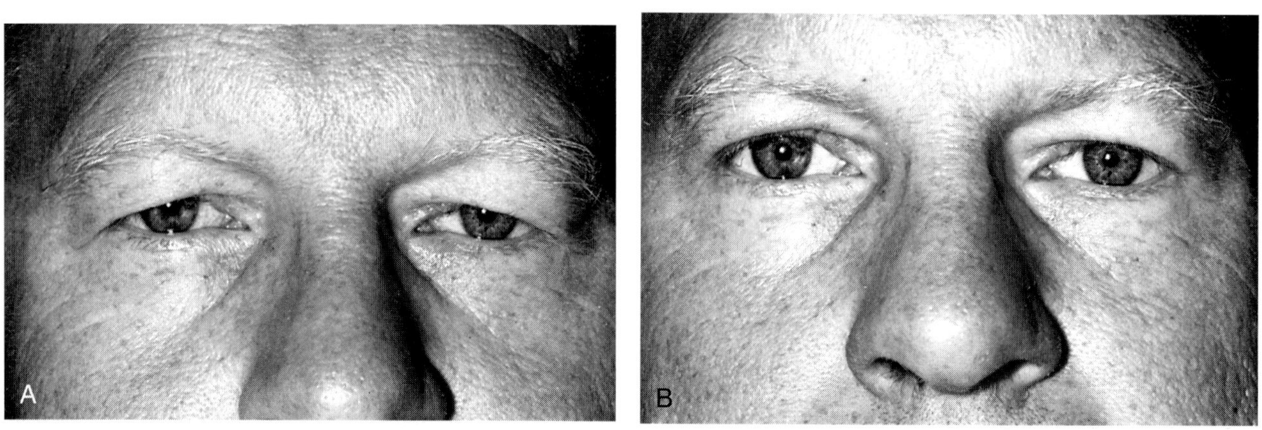

Figure 56–18. *A*, Preoperative appearance of a 51-year-old man with a low, prominent brow and heavy upper eyelid folds that were obstructing vision. The patient wished to avoid "feminizing" browplasty or debulking of fat. Bilateral upper eyelid blepharoplasty consisted of the excision only of skin. *B*, Postoperative appearance 8 months after surgery. Visual function was restored, and a good cosmetic result was achieved.

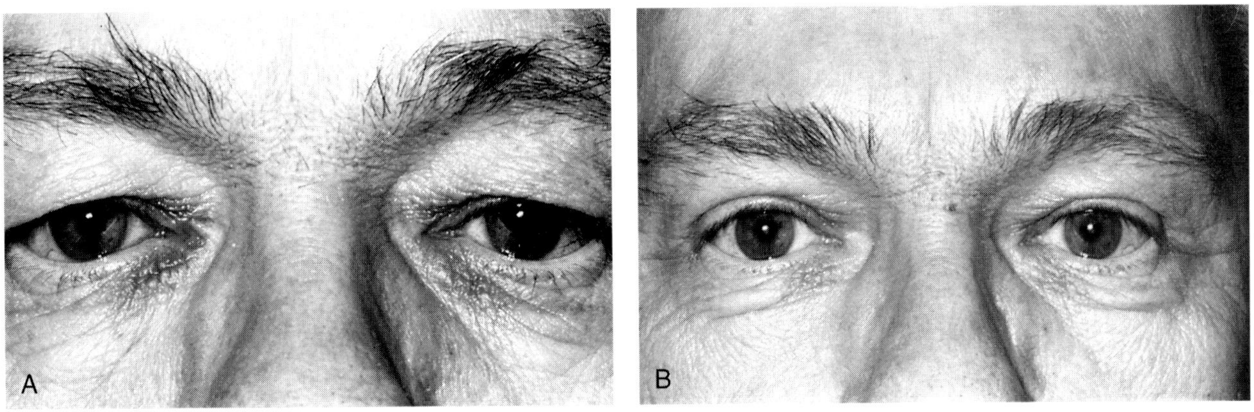

Figure 56–19. *A*, Preoperative appearance of a 64-year-old man with moderately heavy upper eyelid folds that draped over the eyelid margins. The patient wished to have significant debulking of the eyelids. A bilateral open-sky upper eyelid blepharoplasty included excision of preaponeurotic fat, a small amount of levator aponeurosis advancement, and supratarsal fixation. *B*, Postoperative appearance 2 months after surgery. The patient was pleased with the cosmetic and functional result.

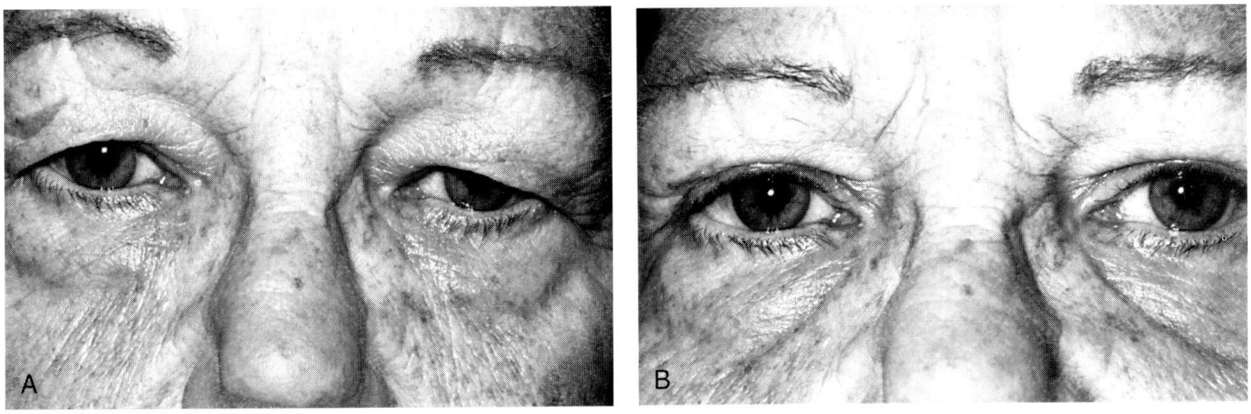

Figure 56–20. *A*, Preoperative appearance of a 68-year-old woman with asymmetric bilateral upper eyelid dermatochalasis. There was an old post-traumatic scar in the lateral right upper lid that probably reduced the upper eyelid fold. A prolapsed lacrimal gland was present in the lateral left upper lid. Bilateral upper eyelid blepharoplasty included suspension of the prolapsed lacrimal gland to the superior orbital rim periosteum. *B*, Postoperative appearance 8 weeks after surgery. Bilateral symmetry is restored, and visual fields are improved.

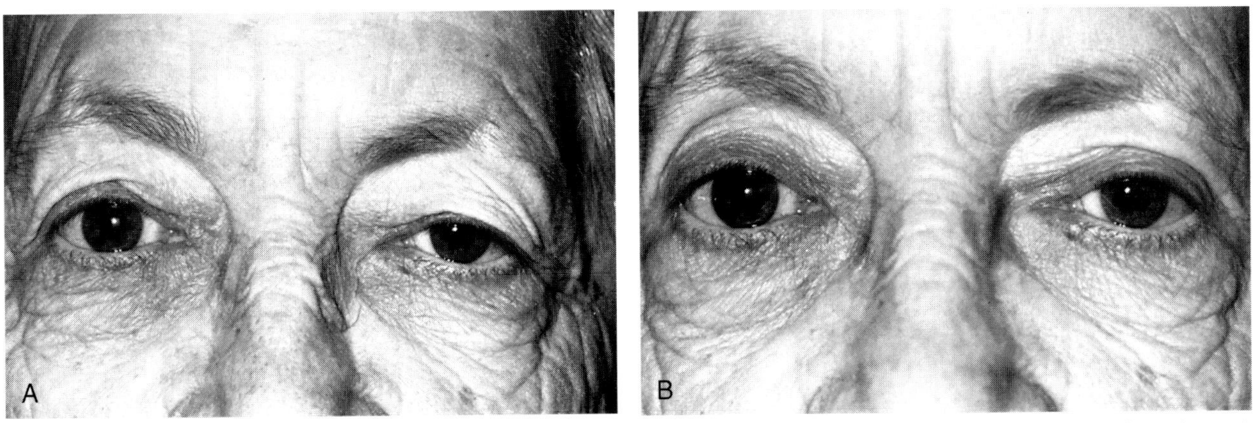

Figure 56–21. *A*, Preoperative appearance of a 76-year-old woman with bilateral upper eyelid dermatochalasis and a mild acquired ptosis of the left upper lid. There was also a loose, redundant fold of skin on the left side of the nasal bridge. A posterior tarsectomy-Müllerectomy (modified Fasanella-Servat procedure) of the left upper lid was combined with a bilateral upper eyelid blepharoplasty. The redundant nasal skin was also simply excised and the wound closed primarily. *B*, Postoperative appearance 10 weeks after surgery. Symmetry is much improved.

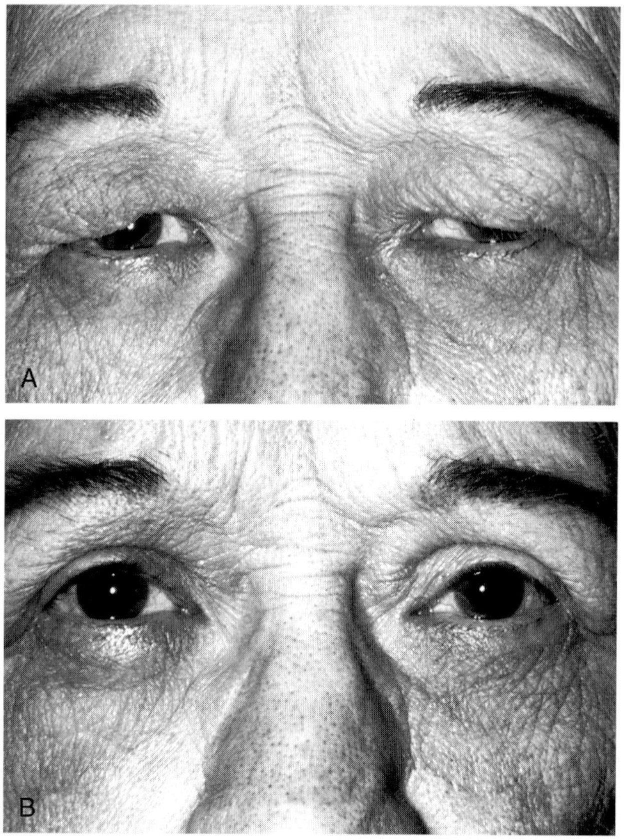

Figure 56–22. *A*, Preoperative appearance of a 73-year-old woman with severe, bilateral dermatochalasis and mild to moderate blepharoptosis that interfered with vision. A bilateral "open-sky" upper eyelid blepharoplasty was combined with levator aponeurosis advancement and supratarsal fixation. *B*, Postoperative appearance 8 months after surgery. Visual function was restored and a good cosmetic result was achieved.

REFERENCES

1. Katzen LB: The history of cosmetic oculoplastic surgery. *In* Putterman A (ed): Cosmetic Oculoplastic Surgery. New York, Grune & Stratton, 1982, p 2.
2. Castanares S: Blepharoplasty for herniated intraorbital fat: Anatomical basis for a new approach. Plast Reconstr Surg 8:46–58, 1951.
3. Castanares S: Classification of baggy eyelids deformity. Plast Reconstr Surg 59:629–633, 1977.
4. American Academy of Ophthalmology: Ophthalmic procedures assessment: Functional indications for upper and lower blepharoplasty. Ophthalmology 98:1461–1463, 1991.
5. Beard C: Ptosis, 3rd ed. St Louis, CV Mosby, 1981, p 74.
6. Callahan MA: Pseudoptosis. *In* Bosniak SL (ed): Advances in Ophthalmic Plastic and Reconstructive Surgery, vol 1. New York, Pergamon Press, 1982, p 32.
7. Beard C: Blepharoptosis. *In* Soll DB (ed): Management of Complications in Ophthalmic Plastic Surgery. Birmingham, AL, Aesculapius, 1976, p 218.
8. Crawford JS: Congenital blepharoptosis. *In* Smith BC, Della Rocca RC, Nesi FA, Lisman RD (eds): Ophthalmic Plastic and Reconstructive Surgery, vol 1. St. Louis, CV Mosby, 1987, p 631.
9. Hornblass A: Ptosis and pseudoptosis and blepharoplasty. Clin Plast Surg 8:811–830, 1981.
10. McCord CD: An external minimal ptosis procedure: External tarsoaponeurectomy. Trans Am Acad Ophthalmol Otolaryngol 79:683–686, 1975.
11. Older JJ: Acquired ptosis. *In* Hornblass A (ed): Oculoplastic, Orbital and Reconstructive Surgery. Baltimore, Williams & Wilkins, 1988, p 341.
12. Anderson RL, Dixon RS: Aponeurotic ptosis surgery. Arch Ophthalmol 97:1123–1128, 1979.
13. Cahill KV, Burns JA, Weber PA: The effect of blepharoptosis on the field of vision. Ophthal Plast Reconstr Surg 3:121–125, 1987.
14. Meyer DR, Linberg JV, Powell SR, et al: Quantitating the superior visual field loss associated with ptosis. Arch Ophthalmol 107:840–843, 1989.
15. Carroll RP: Functional dermatochalasia. Minn Med 59:15–17, 1976.
16. Waller RR: Eyelid malpositions in Graves' ophthalmopathy. Trans Am Ophthalmol Soc 80:855–930, 1982.
17. Custer PL, Tenzel RR, Kowalcyzk AP: Blepharochalasis syndrome. Am J Ophthalmol 99:424–428, 1985.
18. Bergin DJ, McCord CD, Berger T, et al: Blepharochalasis. Br J Ophthalmol 72:863–867, 1988.
19. Goldberg R, Seiff S, McFarland J, et al: Floppy eyelid syndrome and blepharochalasis. Am J Ophthalmol 102:376–381, 1986.
20. Culbertson WW, Ostler HB: The floppy eyelid syndrome. Am J Ophthalmol 92:568–575, 1981.
21. Schwartz LK, Gelender H, Forster RK: Chronic conjunctivitis associated with "floppy eyelids." Arch Ophthalmol 101:1884–1888, 1983.
22. Dutton JJ: Surgical management of floppy eyelid syndrome. Am J Ophthalmol 99:557–560, 1985.
23. Moore MB, Harrington J, McCulley JP: Floppy eyelid syndrome: Management, including surgery. Ophthalmology 93:184–188, 1986.
24. Putterman AM: Late management of blow-out fractures of the orbital floor. Trans Am Acad Ophthalmol Otolaryngol 83:650–659, 1977.
25. Anderson RL, Holds JB: Does anyone know how to differentiate a "functional" defect from a cosmetic one? Arch Ophthalmol 108:1685–1686, 1990.
26. Small RG: Functional vs cosmetic ophthalmologic defects [letter]. Arch Ophthalmol 109:1194, 1991.
27. Courtiss EH: Selection of alternatives in esthetic blepharoplasty. Clin Plast Surg 8:739–755, 1981.
28. Baker TJ: Upper blepharoplasty. Clin Plast Surg 8:635–641, 1981.
29. Rees TD: Blepharoplasty. *In* Rees TD (ed): Aesthetic Plastic Surgery, vol 2. Philadelphia, WB Saunders, 1980, pp 459–580.
30. Bosniak SL: Cosmetic Blepharoplasty. New York, Raven Press, 1990.
31. Gradinger GP: Cosmetic upper blepharoplasty. Clin Plast Surg 15:289–297, 1988.
32. Lynch S: Anesthesia. *In* Rees TD (ed): Aesthetic Plastic Surgery. Philadelphia, WB Saunders, 1989, p 40.
33. Katzen LB, Karvelis JJ: Anesthesia, analgesia, and amnesia. *In* Putterman A (ed): Cosmetic Oculoplastic Surgery. New York, Grune & Stratton, 1982, p 89.
34. Silver B: Photographing the blepharoplasty patient. *In* Putterman A (ed): Cosmetic Oculoplastic Surgery. New York, Grune & Stratton, 1982, p 53.
35. Rees TD: Blepharoplasty. *In* Rees TD, Wood-Smith D (eds): Cosmetic Facial Surgery. Philadelphia, WB Saunders, 1973.
36. Rees TD, Guy CL: Patient selection and techniques in blepharoplasty and rhytidoplasty. Surg Clin North Am 51:353–370, 1971.
37. Shorr N, Seiff SR: Cosmetic Blepharoplasty: An Illustrated Surgical Guide. Thorofare, NJ, Slack, 1986.
38. Courtiss EH, Webster RC, White MF: Use of double W-plasty in upper blepharoplasty. Plast Reconstr Surg 53:25–28, 1974.
39. Lewis JR: The Z-blepharoplasty. Plast Reconstr Surg 44:331–335, 1969.
40. Aston SJ: Orbicularis oculi muscle flaps: A technique to reduce crow's feet and lateral canthal skin folds. Plast Reconstr Surg 65:206–216, 1980.
41. Chi-Tsung S, Morgan RF, Manson PN, Hoopes JE; Technique for division and suspension of the orbicularis oculi muscle. Clin Plast Surg 8:673–678, 1981.
42. Putterman A: Surgical treatment of upper eyelid dermatochalasis and orbital fat. *In* Putterman A (ed): Cosmetic Oculoplastic Surgery. New York, Grune & Stratton, 1982, p 99.
43. Baylis HI: Upper Blepharoplasty. Oculoplastic Newsletter. Los Angeles, No. 3, 1989.
44. Rees TD, Aston SJ, Thorne CHM: Blepharoplasty and facialplasty including forehead-brow lift. *In* McCarthy JG (ed): Plastic

Surgery: The Face, vol 3. Philadelphia, WB Saunders, 1990, p 2320.
45. Tenzel RR: Cosmetic blepharoplasty. Int Ophthalmol Clin 18:87-99, 1978.
46. Parkes M, Fein W, Brennan HG: Pinch technique for repair of cosmetic eyelid deformities. Arch Ophthalmol 89:324-328, 1973.
47. Parkes M, Fein W: Further experience with the pinch technique for repair of eyelid deformities. Arch Ophthalmol 94:1534-1536, 1976.
48. Beard C: The pinch technique for skin removal in blepharoplasty. *In* Putterman A (ed): Cosmetic Oculoplastic Surgery. New York, Grune & Stratton, 1982, p 233.
49. Silver HL: A new approach to the operation of blepharoplasty. Br J Plast Surg 22:253-256, 1969.
50. Epstein GA: Anesthesia in ophthalmic plastic surgery. *In* Hornblass A (ed): Oculoplastic, Orbital, and Reconstructive Surgery. Baltimore, Williams & Wilkins, 1988, p 42.
51. Siegel RJ, Vistnes LM, Iverson RE: Effective hemostasis with less epinephrine. Plast Reconstr Surg 51:129-133, 1973.
52. Wilkins RB, Hunter GJ, McCord CD, Tanenbaum M: Blepharoplasty: Cosmetic and functional. *In* McCord CD, Tanenbaum M (eds): Oculoplastic Surgery, 2nd ed. New York, Raven Press, 1987, p 451.
53. Baker TJ, Gordon HI, Mosienko P: Upper lid blepharoplasty. Plast Reconstr Surg 60:692-698, 1977.
54. Zide BM: Anatomy of the eyelids. Clin Plast Surg 8:623-634, 1981.
55. Baker SS, Muenzler WS, Small RG, Leonard JE: Carbon dioxide laser blepharoplasty. Ophthalmology 91:238-244, 1984.
56. David LM, Sanders G: CO_2 laser blepharoplasty: A comparison to cold steel and electrocautery. J Dermatol Surg Oncol 13:110-114, 1987.
57. David LM: The laser approach to blepharoplasty. J Dermatol Surg Oncol 14:741-746, 1988.
58. Mittelman H, Apfelberg DB: Carbon dioxide laser blepharoplasty—Advantages and disadvantages. Ann Plast Surg 24:1-6, 1990.
59. Putterman AM: Scalpel neodymium : YAG laser in oculoplastic surgery. Am J Ophthalmol 581-584, 1990.
60. Putterman AM, Urist MJ: Surgical anatomy of the orbital septum. Ann Ophthalmol 6:290-294, 1974.
61. Putterman AM, Urist MJ: Baggy eyelids—A true hernia. Ann Ophthalmol 5:1029-1032, 1973.
62. McCord CD: Techniques in blepharoplasty. Ophthalmic Surg 10:40-55, 1979.
63. Tobin HA: Electrosurgical blepharoplasty: A technique that questions conventional concepts of fat compartmentalization. Ann Plast Surg 14:59-63, 1985.
64. Hugo NE, Stone E: Anatomy of a blepharoplasty. Plast Reconstr Surg 53:381-385, 1978.
65. Barker DE: Dye injection studies of intraorbital fat compartments. Plast Reconstr Surg 59:82-85, 1977.
66. Baylis HI: Upper Blepharoplasty II—Oculoplastic Newsletter. Los Angeles, No. 4, 1989.
67. Beard C: Blepharoplasty. *In* Symposium on Surgery of the Orbit and Adnexa. Transactions of the New Orleans Academy of Ophthalmology. St. Louis, CV Mosby, 1974.
68. Iliff CE: Dermatochalasis and blepharochalasis of the upper lids. Trans Am Acad Ophthalmol Otolaryngol 85:709-711, 1978.
69. Beyer CK, McCarthy RW, Webster RC: Baggy lids: A classification and newer aspects of treatment to avoid complications. Ophthalmic Surg 11:169-174, 1980.
70. Leone CR, Glover AT: Lipocauterization and thermal fixation in blepharoplasty. Am J Ophthalmol 106:635-637, 1988.
71. Sachs ME, Bosniak SL: Nonsurgical fat removal in cosmetic blepharoplasty: A new technique. Ann Plast Surg 16:516-520, 1986.
72. Owsley JQ: Resection of the prominent lateral fat pad during upper lid blepharoplasty. Plast Reconstr Surg 65:4-9, 1980.
73. May JW, Fearon J, Zignarelli P: Retro-orbicularis oculus fat (ROOF) resection in aesthetic blepharoplasty: A 6-year study in 63 patients. Plast Reconstr Surg 86:682-689, 1990.
74. Lassus C: Ostectomy of superior orbital rim in cosmetic blepharoplasty. Plast Reconstr Surg 63:481-484, 1979.
75. Smith B, Petrelli R: Surgical repair of prolapsed lacrimal glands. Arch Ophthalmol 96:113-114, 1978.
76. Horton CE, Carraway JH, Potenza AD: Treatment of a lacrimal bulge in blepharoplasty by repositioning the gland. Plast Reconstr Surg 61:701-702, 1978.
77. Duke-Elder S: The ocular adnexa: Diseases of the eyelids. *In* Duke-Elder S (ed): System of Ophthalmology, vol 13, part 1. St. Louis, CV Mosby, 1975, p 350.
78. Jordan DR, Germer BA, Anderson RL, Morales L: Lacrimal gland prolapse in craniosynostosis syndromes and poor function congenital ptosis. Ophthalmic Surg 21:97-101, 1990.
79. Leone CR Jr: Treatment of a prolapsed lacrimal gland. *In* Putterman A (ed): Cosmetic Oculoplastic Surgery. New York, Grune & Stratton, 1982, p 210.
80. Petrelli RL: Management of prolapsed lacrimal glands. *In* Hornblass A (ed): Oculoplastic, Orbital, and Reconstructive Surgery. Baltimore, Williams & Wilkins, 1988, p 532.
81. Scherz W, Dohlman C: Is the lacrimal gland dispensable? Arch Ophthalmol 93:281-283, 1975.
82. Fasanella RM, Servat J: Levator resection for minimal ptosis: Another simplified operation. Arch Ophthalmol 65:493-496, 1961.
83. Putterman AM, Urist MJ: Müller muscle-conjunctiva resection: Technique for treatment of blepharoptosis. Arch Ophthalmol 93:619-623, 1975.
84. Sheen JH: A change in the technique of supratarsal fixation in blepharoplasty. Plast Reconstr Surg 59:831-834, 1977.
85. Kahn S: Correction of senile blepharoptosis during cosmetic blepharoplasty. Plast Reconstr Surg 60:725-729, 1977.
86. Dryden R, Leibsohn J: The levator aponeurosis in blepharoplasty. Ophthalmology 85:718-725, 1978.
87. Wilkins RB, Patipa M: The recognition of acquired ptosis in patients considered for upper eyelid blepharoplasty. Plast Reconstr Surg 70:431-432, 1982.
88. Patipa M, Wilkins RB: Acquired ptosis in patients undergoing upper eyelid blepharoplasty. Ann Ophthalmol 16:266-270, 1984.
89. Leone CR: Management of the blepharoplasty patient with ptosis. Ophthalmic Surg 19:515-522, 1988.
90. Millay DJ, Larrabee WF: Ptosis and blepharoplasty. Arch Otolaryngol Head Neck Surg 115:198-201, 1989.
91. Sheen JH: Supratarsal fixation in upper blepharoplasty. Plast Reconstr Surg 54:424-431, 1974.
92. Sayoc BT: Plastic construction of the superior palpebral fold. Am J Ophthalmol 38:556-559, 1954.
93. Millard DR: Oriental peregrinations. Plast Reconstr Surg 16:319, 1955.
94. Pang RP: Surgical formation of upper lid fold. Arch Ophthalmol 65:783-784, 1961.
95. Boo-Chai K: Plastic construction of the superior palpebral fold. Plast Reconstr Surg 31:74-78, 1963.
96. Fernandez LR: Double eyelid operation in the Oriental in Hawaii. Plast Reconstr Surg 25:257-264, 1960.
97. Flowers RS: Anchor blepharoplasty. *In* Transactions of the Sixth International Congress of Plastic Surgeons. Paris, Masson et Cie, 1976.
98. Hinderer UT: Aesthetic surgery of the eyelids and periocular region. *In* Smith JW, Aston SJ (eds): Grabb and Smith's Plastic Surgery, 4th ed. Boston, Little, Brown & Company, 1991, p 565.
99. Small RG: Supratarsal fixation in ophthalmic plastic surgery. Ophthalmic Surg 9:73-84, 1978.
100. Putterman AM, Urist MJ: Reconstruction of the upper eyelid crease and fold. Arch Ophthalmol 94:1941-1954, 1976.
101. Tenzel RR: Upper eyelid crease formation. *In* Putterman A (ed): Cosmetic Oculoplastic Surgery. New York, Grune & Stratton, 1982, p 179.
102. Putterman AM: Upper eyelid blepharoplasty. *In* Hornblass A (ed): Oculoplastic, Orbital, and Reconstructive Surgery. Baltimore, Williams & Wilkins, 1988, p 474.
103. Gavaris PT: The eyelid crease. *In* Hornblass A (ed): Oculoplastic, Orbital, and Reconstructive Surgery. Baltimore, Williams & Wilkins, 1988, p 505.
104. Callahan MA, Callahan A: Ophthalmic Plastic and Orbital Surgery. Birmingham, AL, Aesculapius, 1979, pp 124-133.
105. Rogers BO: Cosmetic blepharoplasty using an electrocauterization technique. Aesthetic Plast Surg 1:263, 1977.

106. Leone CR, Glover AT: Lipocauterization and thermal fixation in blepharoplasty. Am J Ophthalmol 106:635–637, 1988.
107. Guy CL, Liverett DM: Upper and lower blepharoplasty. Clin Plast Surg 8:663–671, 1981.
108. Kosko PI: Upper lid blepharoplasty: Skin closure achieved with butyl-2-cyanocrylate. Ophthalmic Surg 12:424–425, 1981.
109. Kamer FM, Joseph JH: Histoacryl: Its use in aesthetic facial plastic surgery. Arch Otolaryngol Head Neck Surg 115:193–197, 1989.
110. Mandel MA: Closure of blepharoplasty incisions with autologous fibrin glue. Arch Ophthalmol 108:842–844, 1990.

CHAPTER 57

Lower Eyelid Blepharoplasty

Philip L. Custer

The indications for lower eyelid blepharoplasty are generally cosmetic and not functional. The desire for an improved appearance motivates patients to pursue surgery that may not necessarily be in their best medical interest. It is thus the physician's responsibility to determine which patients are reasonable surgical candidates and to select the appropriate operative technique to achieve each patient's goals.

Lower eyelid blepharoplasty is performed to remove redundant skin and orbital fat. The procedure may be indicated solely for cosmetic reasons, or it may be combined with the repair of various functional eyelid abnormalities, such as entropion, ectropion, or eyelid retraction. The blepharoplasty incision and surgical dissection may also be used to facilitate the exposure of the inferior orbit for such procedures as blow-out fracture repair.

EVALUATION

The initial evaluation of the cosmetic blepharoplasty patient is intended to clarify patients problems, identify patients who are at an increased risk of developing postoperative complications, and educate patients about the nature of blepharoplasty surgery. The ophthalmologist initiates the evaluation by eliciting the individual's complaints. The ideal patient presents with a clear understanding of his or her cosmetic deformity or simply reports he or she wants a more youthful or rested appearance. Further questioning by the physician often prompts a more detailed description of the patient's problem. The patient should be encouraged to be specific about the features that he or she does not like. Patients who are excessively vague or simply prefer the physician to determine what is wrong may also have ill-defined expectations and thus be poor surgical candidates. Some may have a history of multiple prior cosmetic procedures, an indication that they may be striving for an unattainably perfect body image and appearance. Others seek cosmetic procedures to improve interpersonal relationships or job performance. Assisting patients in the recognition of the specific features of their aesthetic eyelid deformity serves to focus the ensuing evaluation and initiates the patients' understanding of realistic surgical results. They will begin to recognize that the blepharoplasty procedure is intended to address specific anatomic abnormalities.

The ophthalmologist ascertains the duration of the eyelid deformity, which can be documented by examination of old photographs. Changes of recent onset may be related to associated problems, such as allergies, endocrine disorders, and orbital masses. Orbital imaging may be necessary to ensure that the patient has normal orbital anatomy.

The ophthalmologist obtains a detailed medical history. Anticoagulant use or bleeding diathesis are relative contraindications to cosmetic eyelid surgery, and a history of chronic dermatologic conditions or multiple skin malignancies is a concern in patients desiring eyelid skin resection. Redundant cutaneous tissue may prove to be functionally necessary, should future dermatologic disease develop. Patients with a history of thyroid abnormalities have a limited risk of developing future dysthyroid ophthalmopathy. Excessive skin resection in such individuals contributes to the development of corneal exposure.

The ophthalmologist reviews the patient's ocular history and documents symptoms of dry eyes, ocular irritation, or tearing, which may indicate either a pre-existing corneal disorder or a predisposition to the development of such a condition after surgery. Prior blepharoplasty or eyelid procedures may also increase the risk of postoperative complications.

The ophthalmologist performs a complete ophthalmic examination with detailed attention to the position and function of the eyelids and eyebrow. The lower eyelid margin is normally positioned near the inferior corneal limbus with the eye in primary gaze. A significantly lower position of the lid margin results in visualization of the inferior sclera, so-called scleral show. Although some degree of scleral show may be physiologic, this finding raises the suspicion of pathologic lower eyelid retraction secondary to previous surgery, trauma, or Graves' disease. High myopia, prominent globes secondary to shallow orbits or flat malar eminences, and true proptosis may also result in scleral show. Standard blepharoplasty with skin resection may be hazardous in such patients unless the procedures are combined with eyelid retraction repair or horizontal eyelid suspension.

Varying degrees of redundant eyelid skin develop as part of the normal aging process. Although a certain amount of eyelid skin is needed to allow full eyelid excursion, any excess over this amount can theoretically be excised without adversely affecting eyelid function. The ophthalmologist estimates the redundant lower eyelid skin by directing the patient to look in far up-gaze and noting the remaining loose tissue. Alternatively, the ophthalmologist inferiorly stretches the excess skin at the base of the lower eyelid. Initial inferior displacement of the eyelid margin indicates the end point of possible skin resection. Redundant skin ("festoons") may also be present below the orbital rim, requiring special surgical techniques for improvement.[1] The ophthalmologist notes the character of the lower eyelid skin. Unusually thick skin may lead to prominent incisional scars. Deeply pigmented skin is often present in the medial aspect of the lids. Standard methods of lower eyelid blepharoplasty fail to correct this finding, although resection of large medial fat pockets may offer some improvement by diminishing the shadowing of this area. Fine wrinkles often remain after surgery, whereas deeper creases are usually softened with eyelid skin resection. Wrinkles that significantly deepen during smiling or other facial expressions are often related to the action of the underlying orbicular muscle and may persist after blepharoplasty. Occasionally, patients have a roll of skin in the pretarsal region that results from a redundant or overactive orbicular muscle. The offending muscle can be thinned during surgery, if the patient considers this objectionable. Thickened, edematous eyelids are often associated with underlying thyroid abnormalities or allergic conditions. The cosmetic appearance often improves when the systemic condition is treated.

Anterior prolapse of the orbital fat often occurs with age, as progressive laxity of the orbital septum and anterior eyelid tissue develops. Occasionally, patients note the prominence of the normal orbital fat pockets presumably resulting from hereditary factors, at a much younger age. The ophthalmologist notes the degree of orbital fat prolapse and grades each fat pocket on a scale from 0 to 4+. The patient is directed to look in up-gaze to facilitate the visualization of the inferior fat pockets (Fig. 57–1). Any or all of the three fat pockets in each lower eyelid may be affected, and the findings are remarkably symmetric. Significant asymmetry in the amount of prolapsed orbital fat should raise the suspicion of an occult orbital process causing anterior displacement of the adipose tissue. An abnormally hollow lower eyelid may be present in conditions that result in bony orbital expansion, such as unrepaired orbital wall fractures. Fullness below the inferior orbital rim usually results from a prominent cheek fat pad and is not corrected with typical blepharoplasty surgery.

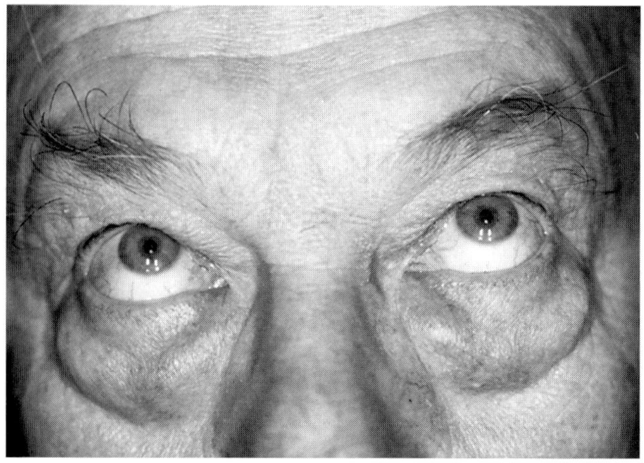

Figure 57–1. Directing the patient to look in far up-gaze facilitates the visualization of the lower eyelid fat pockets and the amount of redundant skin.

The ophthalmologist critically evaluates the horizontal tension of the lower eyelid margin before performing the blepharoplasty. Uncorrected, preexisting eyelid laxity creates a significant risk of postoperative ectropion in patients undergoing skin resection. Eyelid margin laxity is detected with the manual distraction test.[2] The surgeon grasps the central portion of the eyelid and pulls it away from the globe (Fig. 57–2*A*), thus determining the ability

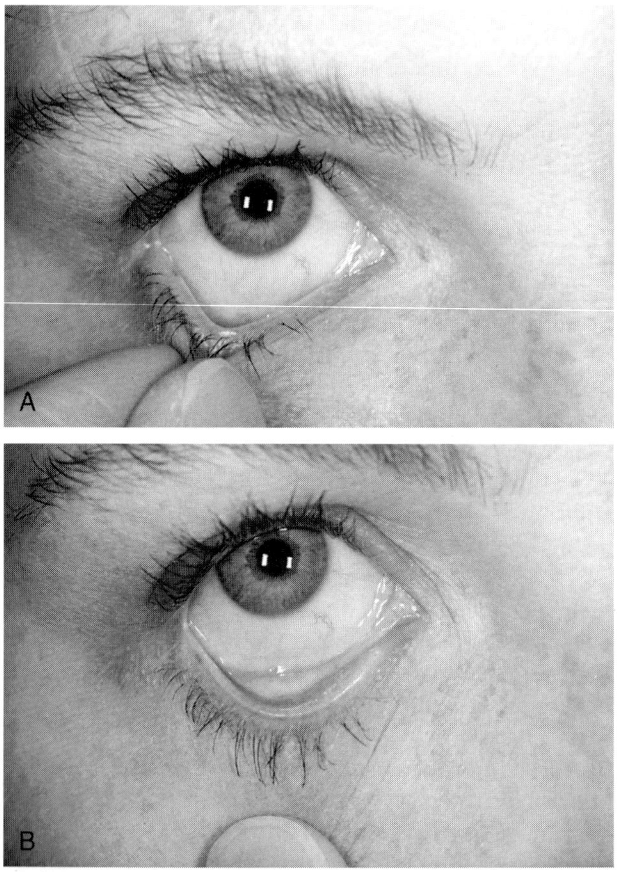

Figure 57–2. Estimate the tension of the lower eyelid margin with either the manual distraction test (*A*) or the inferior traction test (*B*).

to anteriorly displace the lid. The inferior traction test is a second method used to detect lower eyelid laxity. The lower lid margin is pulled inferiorly and released (see Fig. 57–2*B*). An eyelid with adequate lid margin tension immediately snaps back to its normal anatomic position, re-establishing close contact with the globe. Eyelids with significant laxity tend to sag away from the cornea, returning to their original position slowly or only after the patient blinks. Patients with very flat malar eminences and eyelid laxity are at particular risk of postoperative ectropion or eyelid retraction secondary to poor bony support of the eyelid and orbital tissue.

The ophthalmologist assesses ocular motility with attention to the presence or absence of Bell's phenomenon. An absent Bell's phenomenon predisposes the patient to exposure keratitis, should any lagophthalmos develop after surgery. The ophthalmologist examines the anterior segment of the eye with the binocular microscope to determine the adequacy of the tear film or the presence of pre-existing keratitis, or ocular inflammation. Any abnormality requires evaluation before surgery is performed.

Abnormally low tear production is another risk factor for the development of exposure keratitis in patients with postoperative lagophthalmos or eyelid retraction. The ophthalmologist obtains a quantitative measurement of tear production by using the basic secretory test. The ophthalmologist administers topical anesthesia, gently blots the eyes dry, and places Schirmer's test strips in each lower eyelid cul-de-sac for 5 minutes. Although fewer than 10 mm of wetting may be considered abnormal, the basic secretory rate is often an inaccurate predictor of clinically significant dry eye states. The results of this test are most useful when they are considered in conjunction with the patient's symptoms and tear film evaluation.

At the completion of the examination, the physician will have clarified the patient's particular eyelid abnormality, which generally consists of isolated redundant skin, orbital fat, or combined skin and fat excess. Some patients have associated findings that require special consideration during the planning of the blepharoplasty procedure. Significant lower eyelid laxity may necessitate repair to minimize the risk of postoperative ectropion. A limited basic secretory rate, a history of thyroid abnormality or skin malignancy, and an absent Bell's phenomenon may indicate the need to minimize skin resection or may render some patients poor candidates for blepharoplasty. A frank explanation of this recommendation is generally accepted because most individuals appreciate hearing the physician's honest opinion.

The ophthalmologist should thoroughly discuss the proposed surgical technique with the patient. A hand mirror facilitates the demonstration of both the incision site and the eyelid abnormalities to be addressed at surgery. Patients requiring only fat excision may be approached via a conjunctival (fornix, posterior) incision, but combined skin and fat removal requires a cutaneous (anterior) approach. The ophthalmologist notes findings that will not be improved by standard blepharoplasty, such as fine wrinkles, hyperpigmentation, or prominent cheek fat pad. The postoperative treatment regimen is outlined, including timing of office visits and suture removal. Patients are instructed to avoid using facial cosmetic products on the day of their procedure.

Fully informed consent requires a complete discussion of the operative risks. Objectionable cutaneous scarring is a concern with any facial surgery and significant hemorrhage or postoperative infection are also possible, although they are uncommon in eyelid procedures. Loss of vision remains a devastating, although rare, complication of blepharoplasty. Postoperative ectropion, eyelid retraction, and lagophthalmos are among the most frequent operative complications. Patients should be informed that an asymmetric eyelid appearance may occur after surgery, and additional "touch-up" procedures may be necessary to obtain the most ideal surgical results in such cases.

DRAPING AND ANESTHETIC INJECTION

A standard full-face preparation and drape are performed, and care is taken to ensure that no traction exists on the periocular tissue from the drape. Supplemental oxygen is used only when necessary and with great caution to minimize the risk of drape fires during thermal cauterization. The upper eyelid portion of the procedure is generally performed first in patients undergoing combined upper and lower eyelid blepharoplasty. Blepharoplasty surgery is generally best performed with local infiltrative anesthesia, although sedation may be necessary in certain cases. General anesthesia is only rarely indicated in simple cosmetic eyelid surgery, because it adds to the potential operative risks and prevents active patient involvement during the procedure. An equal mixture of 2% lidocaine (Xylocaine) and 0.75% bupivacaine provides early onset and prolonged duration of anesthesia. Using epinephrine in the local anesthesia further prolongs the anesthetic action and facilitates hemostasis. Warming the anesthetic mixture, adding buffering solutions, and employing a 30-gauge needle improve patient comfort. The anesthetic may be effectively administered by injection through the conjunctival surface after a 45-degree bend is placed in the needle to aid in passing the needle over the globe. The conjunctiva is entered midway between the lower edge of the tarsus and the inferior fornix, and the needle tip is directed anterior to the inferior orbital rim. A preoperative topical conjunctival anesthetic eliminates the discomfort of initial needle entry. Effective anesthesia is generally obtained with 1 to 3 mL of anesthetic in each lower eyelid. This method of lower eyelid anesthesia minimizes ecchymosis because the needle does not pass through the vascular skin and orbicular muscle. Excellent anesthesia is usually obtained with this method because it combines local infiltration with a partial regional block of the infraorbital nerve. Many patients move or develop voluntary blepharospasm during local anesthetic administration. The risk of globe penetration is minimized with this technique because the needle is always directed away from the eye.

SKIN FLAP APPROACH

The physician may use either a skin or combined skin-muscle flap in the lower eyelid blepharoplasty procedure. The simple skin flap may be useful in cases requiring minimal skin resection or segmental thinning of the orbicular muscle. However, this approach can be time consuming and often results in extensive bruising. Hyperpigmentation and subcutaneous irregularity may be noted in the early postoperative period.[3] The lower eyelid incision is placed in an infraciliary location, at least 2 mm below the lashes (Fig. 57–3). This spacing is important because unusually close approximation of the resultant scar to the lash line results in an unnaturally appearing crease in selected patients. A Superblade or razor knife is used to begin the infraciliary incision several millimeters temporal to the punctum, following the lid margin to the lateral canthus (see Fig. 57–3), then orienting the incision in a more horizontal direction. This lateral extension ideally falls in a pre-existing wrinkle (crows-feet line) and should not extend in a superior direction so that damage to the periocular lymphatic system is avoided. At least 5 to 10 mm of intact skin is left between the lateral aspects of the upper and lower lid incisions because closer approximation may result in cicatrization and lymphedema. The horizontal extent of the lower eyelid incision depends on the amount of skin resection necessary but usually ends near the lateral orbital rim.

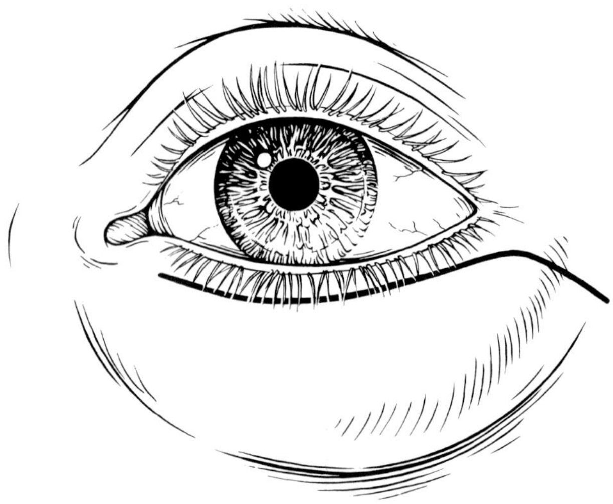

Figure 57–3. The infraciliary incision is marked several millimeters below the lashes, starting just temporal to the punctum. The lateral extension of the incision falls in a natural skin crease.

An alternative incision uses the position of the normal lower eyelid crease. This location should be avoided in cases requiring horizontal eyelid tightening. The eyelid crease incision may be problematic in patients with marked redundancy of skin because significant skin resection may lower the postoperative position of the crease. The local anesthetic injection may create difficulty visualizing the crease; therefore, marking this incision before anesthetic is administered is justified.

The flap to the inferior orbital rim is raised with sharp Wescott's microscissors. Blunt dissection is minimized because the thin eyelid skin is easily traumatized. The skin flap is retracted with a blunt-tipped rake because sharp skin hooks may perforate and lacerate the tissue. Areas of orbicular muscle hypertrophy are thinned. The orbicularis fibers over the orbital fat pockets requiring resection are separated, the septum is divided, and the orbital fat is removed.

The goal of the careful blepharoplasty surgeon is to avoid alteration of normal eyelid function. Before skin removal, the patient is directed to look in up-gaze. The skin flap is draped in a superolateral direction over the dissection bed, and the skin is allowed to follow the eyelid contour without inferior traction. Asking the patient to widely open their mouth during skin excision provides additional insurance against excessive skin removal. Redundant skin extending above the infraciliary incision is removed. Additional skin resection places the patient at an increased risk for postoperative ectropion, lid retraction, or lagophthalmos. First, the wedge of redundant skin is removed above the infraciliary portion of the incision, and then a second triangle of excess skin is removed above the lateral extension of the incision. The excised tissue should be kept moist on the operative field until the procedure is completed because a portion could be replaced as a full-thickness graft should it later be determined that too much skin had been resected.

Redundant skin in the malar region (festoons) may be reduced during lower eyelid blepharoplasty by extending the skin flap below the inferior orbital rim. Alternatively, these festoons may be directly resected in an elliptical fashion. The skin flap technique may also be used to partially resect hyperpigmented skin in the medial aspect of the lower eyelids. The surgeon elevates a flap by extending a second incision inferiorly, near the nasojugal fold. The surgeon advances the skin flap in a superomedial direction, allowing partial resection of the unsightly medial eyelid tissue. Care is taken to avoid excessive skin resection and postoperative ectropion.[4]

SKIN–MUSCLE FLAP APPROACH

The combined skin–muscle flap provides the advantages of rapid dissection, optimal exposure of the orbital fat, and ability to shorten the entire anterior eyelid lamella. The dissection is performed in a natural plane,

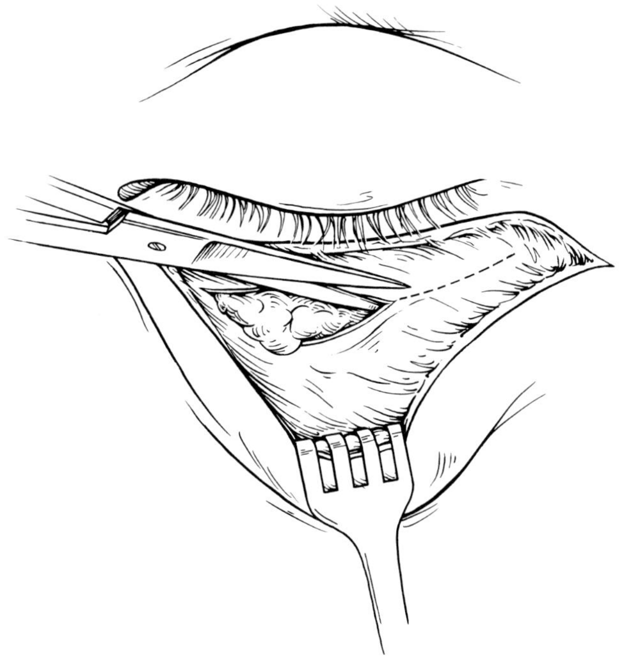

Figure 57–4. The skin–muscle flap is retracted, exposing the orbital septum.

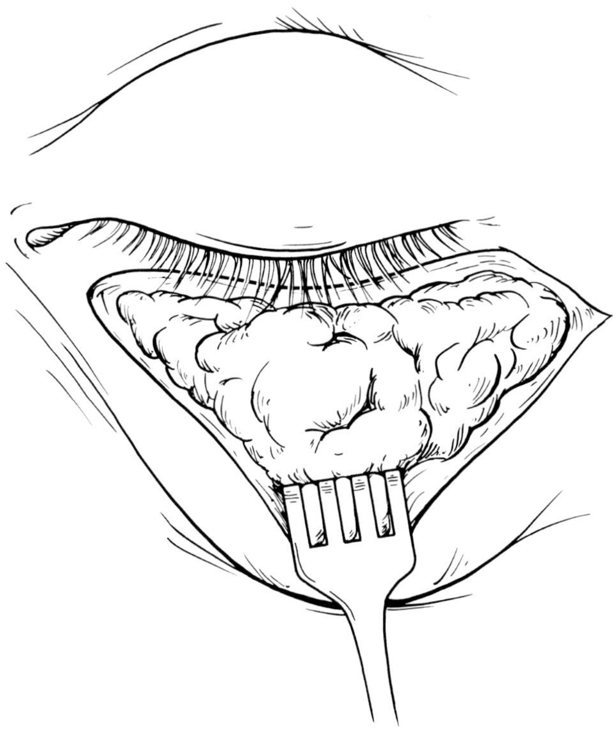

Figure 57–5. The three fat pockets are visualized after the septum is divided.

minimizing intraoperative bleeding and postoperative ecchymosis. The skin–muscle flap may be raised with a beveled dissection, starting at the infraciliary incision (see Fig. 57–3). An alternative method involves beginning the procedure in the lateral portion of the eyelid, where the incision extends in a crow's-feet line (see Fig. 57–3). The orbicularis is divided, thereby exposing the lateral portion of the orbital septum. The orbicularis is bluntly dissected from the underlying septum and the incision is extended medially in the infraciliary line, completing the development of the anterior lamellar (skin–muscle) flap (Fig. 57–4). Areas of orbicularis hypertrophy on the undersurface of the flap are thinned.

Prolapsed orbital fat may be managed by various techniques. Some surgeons advocate tightening the orbital septum with sutures or thermal cautery in an effort to reposition the displaced fat.[5–7] This technique may lead to lid retraction from excessive scar formation or a return of fat prolapse should septal laxity recur.

Most surgeons prefer to excise the prolapsed tissue. The orbital septum is divided with sharp scissors, and the thin capsule surrounding the orbital fat is opened. This fat is usually compartmentalized into three spaces, although the division between the central and lateral pockets may be indistinct (Fig. 57–5). Gentle pressure on the globe aids in exposing the redundant fat. The surgeon should avoid forceful grasping and traction so that the risk of damage to vessels and nerves within the orbital fat is minimized. The fat is clamped with a hemostat and is divided with scissors (Fig. 57–6). The remaining stump of fat is cauterized. A battery-powered, high-temperature cautery is effective for this purpose. A monopolar cautery may also be used, but this device may increase tissue necrosis. Bipolar cautery may not provide adequate hemostasis in adipose tissue. Supplemental oxygen should be discontinued during fat cauterization because flaming can occur because of the risk of drape ignition. The fat pedicle is grasped before the clamp is released, and the tissue is inspected for complete hemostasis (Fig. 57–7). Patients may occasionally experience pain or retro-ocular aching during fat excision, a manifestation

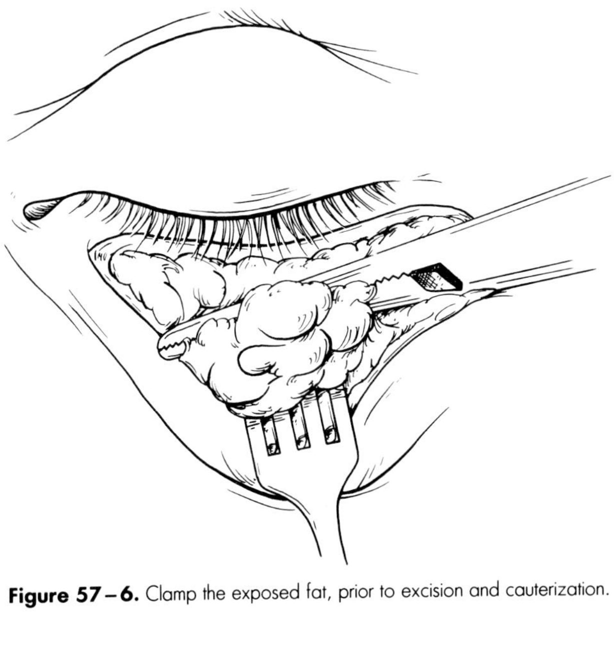

Figure 57–6. Clamp the exposed fat, prior to excision and cauterization.

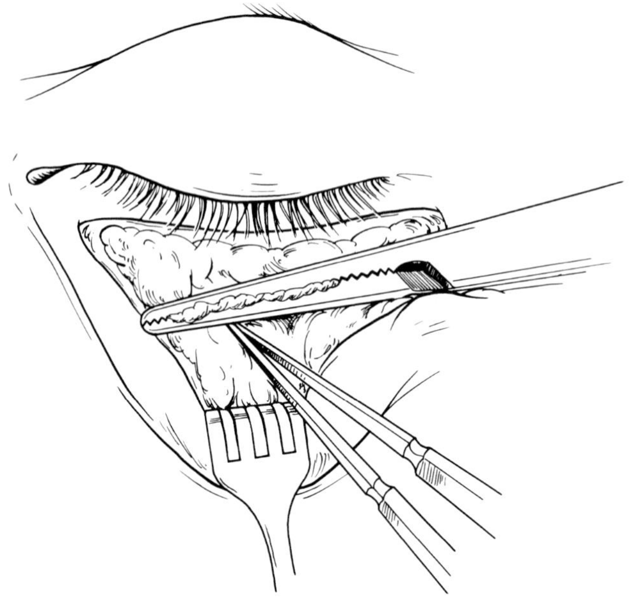

Figure 57–7. Grasp the fat pedicle to prevent posterior retraction of the tissue when the hemostat is released, allowing adequate observation to ensure that complete hemostasis has been achieved.

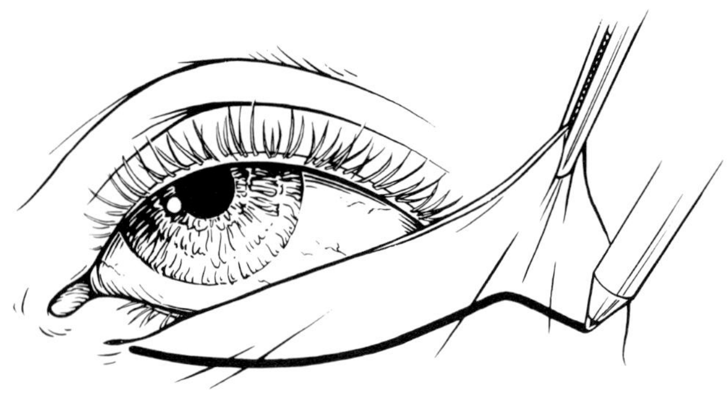

Figure 57–8. Drape the excess skin–muscle flap superiorly and laterally and resect the redundant tissue above the infraciliary portion of the incision. Then remove the triangle of skin above the lateral portion of the incision.

of referred pain. The fat pockets may be individually injected with local anesthetic to relieve this discomfort. Fat resection should continue until an ideal eyelid contour is achieved. The patient is placed in a sitting position to confirm that sufficient tissue has been removed. Special attention should be paid to the lateral compartment because the amount of fat is commonly underestimated in this location. Care is taken to avoid the inferior oblique muscle as it passes deeply between the medial and central fat pockets. Direct visualization of this muscle may be wise in cases requiring significant fat resection.

Skin resection is performed in a method identical to that used in the skin flap technique. The skin-muscle flap is draped over the eyelid, while the patient looks in upgaze (Fig. 57–8). Excess tissue is removed by resection of the full-thickness flap. A small (2- to 4-mm) strip of orbicular muscle is excised from the edge of the flap, preventing postoperative fullness of the pretarsal region. Both eyelids are checked for symmetry of skin, orbital fat, and lid margin position. The patient is placed in a sitting position to facilitate this determination. The wound is examined for complete hemostasis. The orbital septum should not be sutured so that postoperative contracture and resultant lid retraction are minimized. The skin is closed with a running 6-0 or 7-0 monofilament suture (Fig. 57–9). The pretarsal orbicularis should not be closed. If any tension exists at the lateral aspect of the incision, the orbicularis should be closed with 6-0 polyglycolic sutures or with mattress skin sutures. The function and position of the eyelid should be checked; eyelid retraction or ectropion indicates either excessive skin resection or uncorrected eyelid laxity.

REPAIR OF EYELID LAXITY

Patients with preoperative eyelid laxity require concomitant horizontal lid shortening after fat removal and before skin excision. The lid may be shortened in an intramarginal location or at the lateral canthus. A block resection of the central lid margin necessitates complex closure and retention of the marginal eyelid sutures for 10 to 14 days, possibly resulting in a lid notch or trichiasis. Central eyelid resection fails to correct lateral canthal tendon laxity and may draw the dehisced canthal angle medially, resulting in horizontal shortening of the palpebral fissure.

By contrast, a block resection of the lateral eyelid removes the dehisced tendon, preserving the tarsal support of the central lid margin. Any resulting notch or trichiasis is isolated to the inconspicuous lateral canthus. After the fat is removed, a short (2- to 4-mm) lateral canthotomy is performed to expose the intact portion of the canthal tendon. A vertical cantholysis is performed that divides the lid margin from the canthal angle (Fig. 57–10). The patient is asked to gaze upward and draw the lid margin laterally to determine the amount of tissue resection necessary (Fig. 57–11). Caution should be exercised in pa-

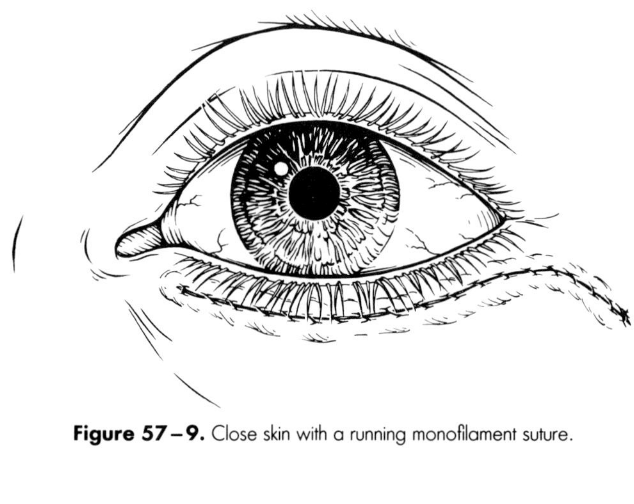

Figure 57–9. Close skin with a running monofilament suture.

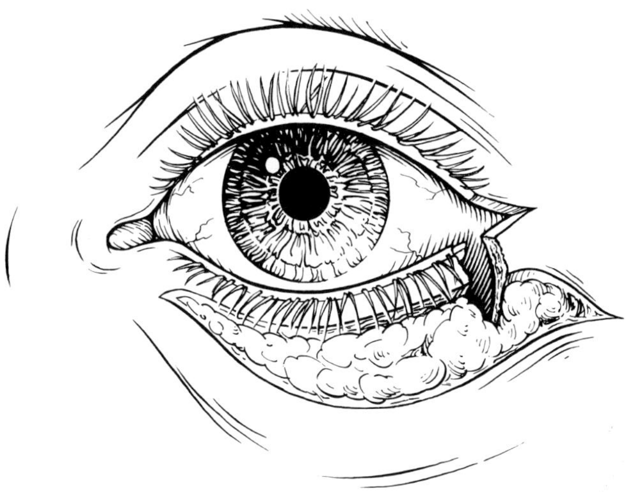

Figure 57–10. Block resection of the lateral eyelid margin begins with a short lateral canthotomy. A vertical cantholysis divides the inferior arm of the tendon.

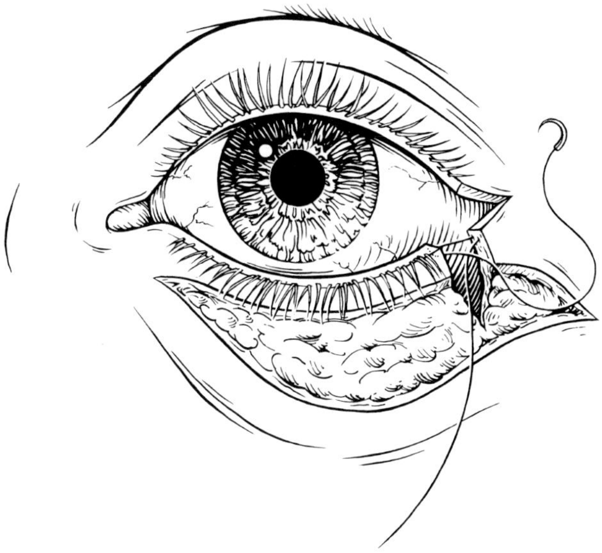

Figure 57–12. Reattach the tarsus to the canthal tendon with buried sutures.

tients with poor malar support or proptotic eyes because excessive shortening may result in lid retraction. The redundant lid margin is resected, and the cut edge of the tarsus is sutured to the intact remnants of the lateral canthal tendon with buried interrupted 6-0 or 7-0 polyglycolate (Fig. 57–12). The orbicularis is closed in a similar fashion. An acute, well-aligned canthal angle is reestablished by placing a buried 6-0 polyglycolate suture between the lateral upper and lower eyelid margins (Fig. 57–13). The skin is resected and closed as in simple lower eyelid blepharoplasty.

An alternative method of lateral lid tightening is the tarsal strip procedure which is useful in eyelids with marked laxity or ectropion.[8-10] A lateral canthotomy is performed after orbital fat is removed (see Fig. 57–5). The inferior arm of the lateral canthal tendon is disinserted from the lateral orbital wall with sharp-tipped scissors. With the eyes open, the eyelid is drawn laterally to determine the amount of redundant lid margin by placing varying degrees of tension on it. Excessive horizontal traction may draw the eyelid below the globe or force the eye posteriorly. When the correct amount of horizontal tension has been achieved, the point at which the lower lid crosses the canthal angle is marked. A tendon-tarsal strip is fashioned from the excess eyelid by excising the lid margin and lash follicles, and the strip is sutured to the inner surface of the lateral periorbita with a mattress, 5-0 nylon suture (Fig. 57–14). The correct point of attachment depends on the amount of lateral suspension needed and the patient's anatomy. The lateral canthal angle is reformed by joining of the tarsal strip to the superior crus of the canthal tendon with a buried 6-0 polyglycolic suture. The orbicularis is closed and the skin excised as previously discussed.

Entropion repair may also be performed during blepharoplasty. In addition to lateral eyelid shortening by one of the aforementioned techniques, the dehisced lower

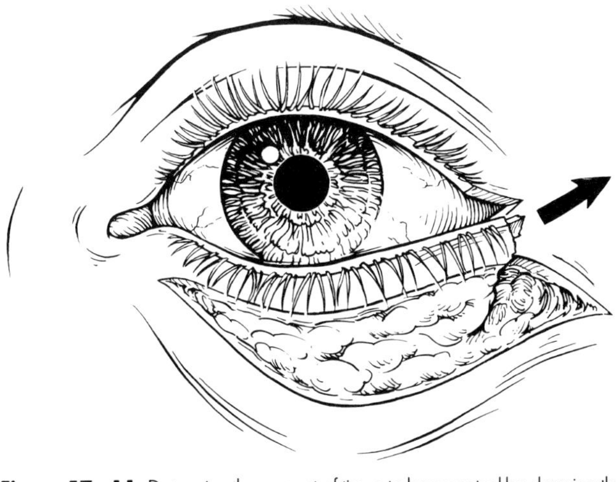

Figure 57–11. Determine the amount of tissue to be resected by drawing the lid margin laterally until the desired tension and position of the lower lid are achieved.

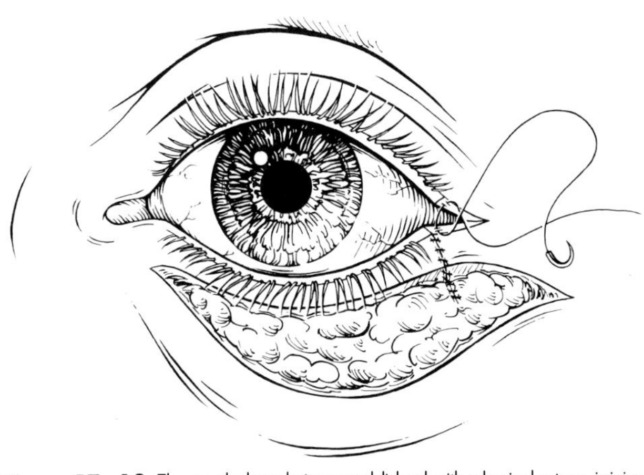

Figure 57–13. The canthal angle is reestablished with a buried suture, joining the lateral aspects of the upper and lower eyelid margins.

eyelid retractors can be isolated and reattached to the inferior edge of the tarsus.

POSTOPERATIVE CARE

Patients are observed after surgery, with the goal of confirming that complete hemostasis has been achieved. Pressure patches are avoided to facilitate the early detection of bleeding or other complications. Postoperative instructions direct the patient to inform the surgeon of significant discomfort, bleeding, or visual disturbance. Ice packs or cold compresses are initiated during waking hours for the first 36 hours, and a head-elevated position is maintained to help minimize postoperative edema. An ophthalmic antibiotic ointment is placed on the incision three to four times daily until the sutures have been removed. This medication reduces the incidence of suture infection and aids in cleansing the wound. This same ointment is applied to the eye to relieve the minor ocular surface irritation that often follows surgery. Wet and warm compresses are applied several days after surgery, and the patient is encouraged to shower daily to assist in cleansing the incision. Occasionally, patients develop significant conjunctival chemosis after eyelid surgery. An antibiotic-steroid ointment is often beneficial in these cases, although subsequent examinations are needed to detect any ocular side effects caused by the medication. Blepharoplasty patients may resume nonexertional activities immediately after surgery. Athletics, swimming, ocular cosmetics, and contact lenses are generally avoided for 2 weeks. The patient is examined on the day after surgery to confirm that no postoperative problems are developing. Sutures are removed on the fourth to seventh postoperative day. Eyelid edema and bruising generally resolve within 2 to 3 weeks after surgery. The patient is examined at that time to detect the development of any unusual eyelid healing or scar formation. The patient is examined several months after blepharoplasty to confirm patient satisfaction and to obtain postoperative photographs (Fig. 57–15).

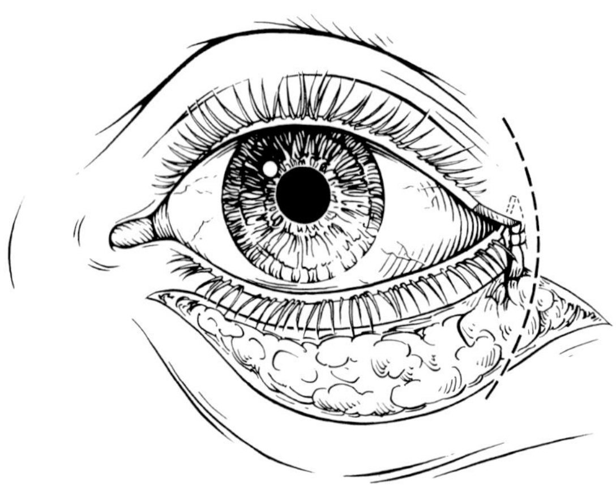

Figure 57–14. Create a tendon-tarsal strip by excising the epithelial surfaces and lash follicles of the excess eyelid margin. The tendon-tarsal strip is attached to the inner surface of the periorbita with a permanent suture.

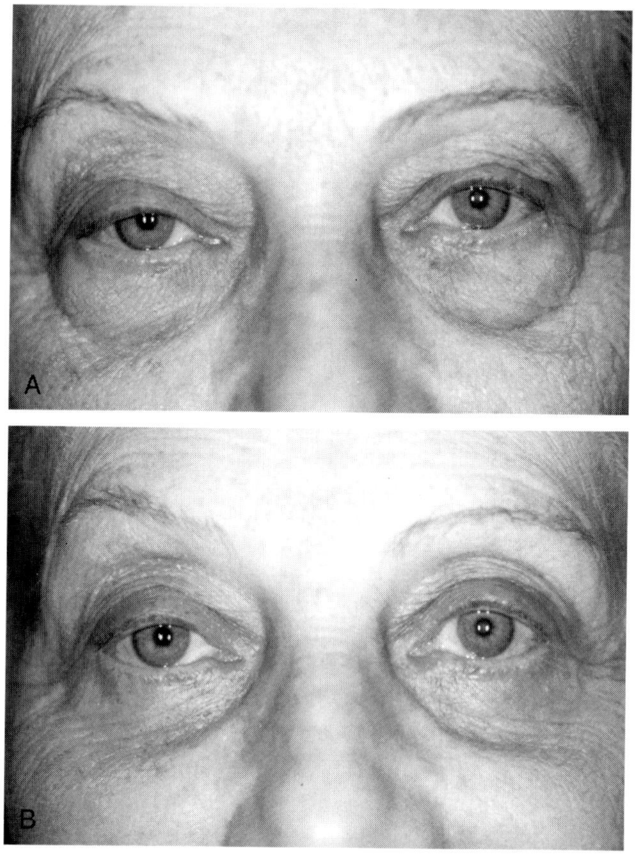

Figure 57–15. Preoperative (A) and postoperative (B) appearance of a patient with a typical lower eyelid blepharoplasty.

SUMMARY

Successful lower eyelid blepharoplasty often results in dramatically improved cosmesis, but inappropriate or poorly performed surgery may result in an adverse cosmetic result or may place the patient at risk for developing vision-threatening complications. The physician is responsible for effectively screening potential surgical candidates, and patients must be educated regarding the nature and potential risks of blepharoplasty surgery.

REFERENCES

1. Avelar JM: Reverse lower blepharoplasty: A new approach. Aesthetic Plast Surg 12:45–50, 1988.
2. Hill JC: Treatment of epiphora owing to flaccid eyelids. Arch Ophthalmol 97:323, 1979.
3. Massiha H: Combined skin and skin–muscle flap technique in lower blepharoplasty: A 10-year experience. Ann Plast Surg 25:467–476, 1990.
4. Putterman AM: Simultaneous treatment of lower eyelid dermatochalasis and abnormal-appearing skin. Am J Ophthalmol 96:69, 1983.
5. Cook TA, Derebery J, Harrah ER: Reconsideration of fat pad man-

agement in lower lid blepharoplasty surgery. Arch Otolaryngol Head Neck Surg 110:521–524, 1984.
6. de la Plata R, Arroyo JM: A new technique for the treatment of palpebral bags. Plast Reconstr Surg 81:677–685, 1988.
7. Sachs ME, Bosniak SL: Correction of true periorbital fat herniation in cosmetic lower lid blepharoplasty. Aesthetic Plast Surg 10:111–144, 1986.
8. Tenzel RR: Treatment of lagophthalmos of the lower eyelid. Arch Ophthalmol 81:366–368, 1969.
9. Anderson RL, Gordy DD: The tarsal strip procedure. Arch Ophthalmol 97:2192, 1979.
10. Lisman RD, Rees T, Baker D, et al: Experience with tarsal suspension as a factor in lower lid blepharoplasty. Plast Reconstr Surg 79:897–905, 1987.

CHAPTER 58

Transconjunctival Lower Blepharoplasty

Robert Alan Goldberg, Henry I. Baylis, and Stacia H. Goldey

The transconjunctival approach to lower blepharoplasty is an excellent operation for diminishing fullness of the lower eyelids while maintaining lower eyelid position and contour. Additional advantages of transconjunctival blepharoplasty over the traditional transcutaneous approach are the low incidence of overcorrection and the lack of an external scar postoperatively. Transcutaneous blepharoplasty is frequently complicated by an alteration of lower eyelid margin contour and even frank lower eyelid retraction with only a modest chance of reducing lower skin wrinkles or folds.[1-5] Therefore, the transconjunctival approach is our procedure of choice for all patients desiring lower blepharoplasty, perhaps combined with a "skin pinch" direct excision of skin folds or chemical peel to soften wrinkles. In this chapter, we describe our current surgical technique and discuss complications of transconjunctival lower blepharoplasty.

LOWER EYELID SURGICAL ANATOMY

Inspection of the anatomy of the lower eyelid reveals that removal of orbital fat through a transconjunctival approach avoids an incision through the orbital septum, thereby reducing the possibility of middle lamellar cicatricial lid retraction.[5] The lower eyelid is composed of skin and underlying orbicularis that continues past the lower orbital rim onto the face. Behind the orbicularis near the lid margin is the tarsal plate. The orbital septum fuses to the inferior border of the tarsus and continues caudally to attach to the crest of the inferior orbital rim at the arcus marginalis. Just behind this orbital septum are the lower eyelid orbital fat compartments. The orbital fat is bordered posteriorly and superiorly by the lower eyelid retractors, which arise from the terminal muscle fibers and tendon of the inferior rectus muscle. The lower lid retractors fuse with the orbital septum approximately 5 mm inferior to the inferior tarsal border before inserting on the tarsal plate. Posteriorly, the lower eyelid retractors are closely adherent to the palpebral conjunctiva of the lower lid (Fig. 58-1).

The orbital fat is surrounded by many fine connective tissue septa (septa of Koorneef).[6] A fascial extension of the sheath of the inferior oblique muscle and Lockwood's ligament called the arcuate expansion inserts on the anterolateral orbital rim and separates the central from the lateral fat compartments.[7] The inferior oblique muscle originates from the anteromedial orbital floor and separates the medial fat compartment from the central fat compartment as it passes posteriorly and laterally beneath the equator of the globe. As shown in Figure 58-2, the orbital fat is easily reached by incising the conjunctiva and lower lid retractors in the fornix; the orbital septum remains well anterior to these structures, captured beneath the eyelid retractor, and is not violated (and, in fact, typically not even visualized) in transconjunctival blepharoplasty.

PREOPERATIVE EVALUATION AND CONSIDERATIONS

The preoperative evaluation of each patient begins with the identification and localization of prominent lower lid fat. The most common deformity is prominent fat in the medial two thirds of the lid, but there is wide variation and frequent asymmetry. The extent and the amount of fat to be removed is estimated at this time, and photographs are taken. Before surgery, the surgeon should plan how much fat to take out of each compartment. Achieving symmetry is more important than absolute amounts of fat to be removed, so an attempt is made to excise the same amount of fat from each compartment except in cases of obvious preoperative asymmetry. The position of the planned incision can be demonstrated to patients by pulling down their eyelid to expose the conjunctival surface. Our philosophy is for conservative fat removal with the patient understanding that if he or she is dissatisfied with the results, more fat can be removed at a second operation several months later in which the physician's fee is waived. The concept of such an "enhancement" surgery is now commonplace in association with radial keratotomy and is well accepted by patients. We would rather anticipate possible

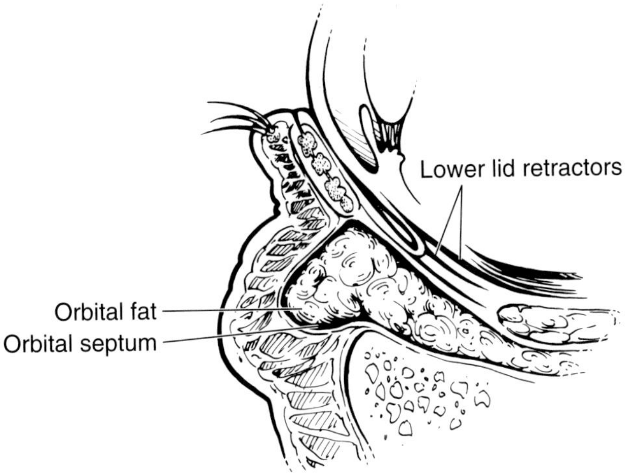

Figure 58–1. Sagittal section of the lower eyelid depicting the relationship of the conjunctiva, lower lid retractors, and orbital septum to the orbital fat. (Adapted from Baylis HI, Long JA, Groth MJ: Transconjunctival lower eyelid blepharoplasty: Techniques and complications. Published courtesy of Ophthalmology [1989; 96:1027–1032].)

additional surgery for undercorrections than to overcorrect the problem in one procedure.

The lower eyelid skin should be evaluated for wrinkles and folds of skin and orbicularis. Discrete folds of skin and orbicularis can be removed by a skin pinch technique; fine wrinkles are best removed with a chemical peel that can be performed at the time of blepharoplasty. In general, we advise patients the lower lid wrinkles cannot be improved with surgery. The position and tension of the lower eyelid lid is also evaluated preoperatively. In patients with extreme lower lid laxity, retraction, ectropion, or entropion, consideration may be given to performing a lateral canthal tightening procedure or transconjunctival entropion surgery at the time of transconjunctival fat excision.

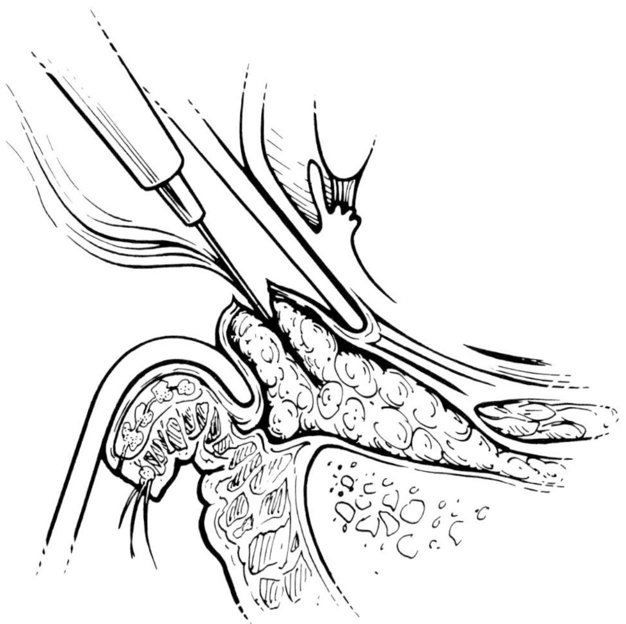

Figure 58–2. Sagittal section of the lower eyelid showing eversion of the lid with Desmarres retractor, ballottement of the globe with a lid plate, and placement of conjunctival incision 1 to 2 mm posterior to the orbital rim. (Adapted from Baylis HI, Long JA, Groth MJ: Transconjunctival lower eyelid blepharoplasty: Techniques and complications. Published courtesy of Ophthalmology [1989; 96:1027–1032].)

LOCAL ANESTHESIA

Local anesthesia for transconjunctival blepharoplasty is somewhat different from that for other lower lid procedures. The injection must be made through the conjunctiva since the sensory nerves of the conjunctiva and orbital fat originate in the orbit. First, a drop of proparacaine 0.5% is placed on the conjunctiva. Then, a cotton-tipped applicator soaked in 10% cocaine is held on the conjunctival surface for 1 to 2 minutes without touching the cornea. This step may be omitted if the patient has deep intravenous sedation. Two percent lidocaine with 1:100,000 epinephrine and hyaluronidase (one vial of hyaluronidase per 50 mL bottle of lidocaine) is then injected with a 27- or 30-gauge needle. The surgeon sits at the head of the table and tents up the eyelid so that the injection can be delivered through the conjunctival fornix under direct visualization. The needle is directed slightly posterior to the inferior orbital rim behind the orbital septum and then walked posteriorly until the needle literally touches the floor of the orbit. One milliliter of anesthetic is injected in this fashion medially, centrally, and laterally to anesthetize each individual fat pocket. The hyaluronidase in the injection allows for posterior spread, and it is not uncommon to see pupillary dilation and weakness of the extraocular muscles, causing temporary diplopia after the injection. Gentle intermittent pressure is applied to the lids, and 15 minutes is allowed for the hemostatic properties of epinephrine to become effective.

SURGICAL TECHNIQUE

After sterile preparation with povidone-iodine solution and open-face draping of awake patients, the surgery begins with the transconjunctival incision. An assistant retracts the medial third of the lower lid downward with a medium or small Desmarres retractor to expose the cul-de-sac. A nonconductive eyelid plate (a Pyrex plate is available from Weiss Glass Blowing Company in Portland, Oregon, which also makes Jones tubes) is placed over the globe into the inferior fornix and is used to ballotte the globe posteriorly (Fig. 58–3). This action with the lid plate prolapses the orbital fat over the orbital rim. If the lower eyelid is too tight to allow adequate exposure, a lateral canthotomy and inferior cantholysis can be performed. This is rarely necessary, however. A needle-tip monopolar cutting cautery unit on a low setting is then

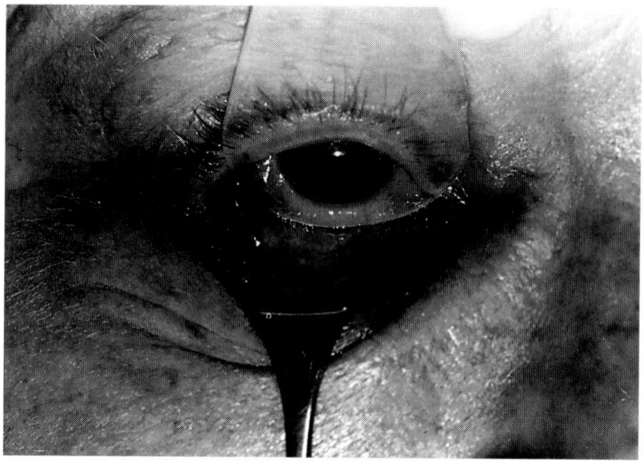

Figure 58–3. A Desmarres retractor is used to retract the lower eyelid and septum, while a glass eyelid plate protects the cornea and ballottes the globe.

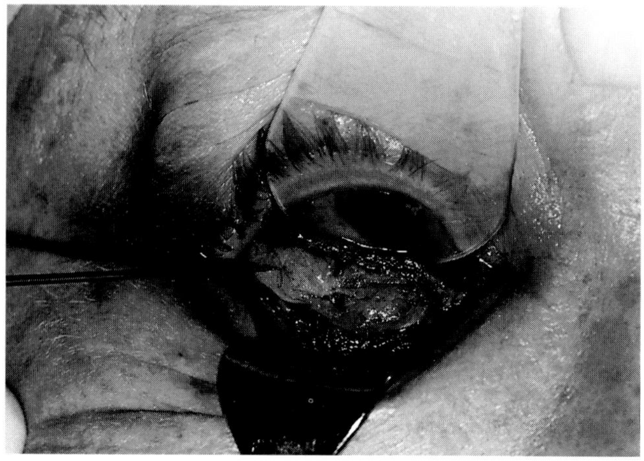

Figure 58–5. As the conjunctival incision is elongated, encapsulated pockets of orbital fat prolapse into the surgical field. The fine capsule surrounding the fat is teased open using the needle tip, resulting in a billowing of yellow orbital fat.

used to palpate the medial, inferior orbital rim (see Fig. 58–2). We prefer a monopolar electrocautery unit set on 1.5 to 2.0 W and an insulated Colorado MicroDissection needle tip (available from Colorado Biomedical, Evergreen, CO). If the insulated cutting cautery needle tip is not available, a 19-gauge Intracath catheter can be placed over any cautery needle tip to avoid inadvertently cauterizing adjacent structures.

The conjunctiva and lower lid retractors are incised directly over the fat with the needle tip directed 1 to 2 mm posterior to the inferior orbital rim (Fig. 58–4). The incision may be made from medial to lateral beginning at the apex of the caruncle and extending to the lateral canthus if necessary to expose the lateral fat. The incision should be made at least 4 mm inferior to the inferior punctum to avoid damage to the canaliculus. An alternative technique is to make several small (5–7 mm) incisions over the individual fat pockets and connect them as necessary for full exposure. After excising the conjunctiva and lower lid retractors, yellow orbital fat can be seen bulging into the field. Once the fat is noted, the connective tissue septa can be dissected away with the needle tip or toothed forceps until a tuft of fluffy yellow fat is exposed (Fig. 58–5). At this point, the glass lid plate is removed and the assistant grasps the posterior edge of the wound (lower lid retractors) with a 0.5 mm Castroviejo forceps and lifts it up and over the globe (Fig. 58–6). This maneuver protects the globe and further prolapses the fat into the surgical field. The Desmarres retractor can now be repositioned so that the blade is in the wound itself, providing wider exposure. With the connective tissue septa on stretch, the cutting cautery can then be used to open the fat compartments widely. The closer the fat compartment is opened to the orbital rim, the easier the exposure and the less chance of encountering bleeding or damage to the inferior oblique.

Laterally, the arcuate expansion of the inferior oblique separates the central from the lateral fat pockets. Incision

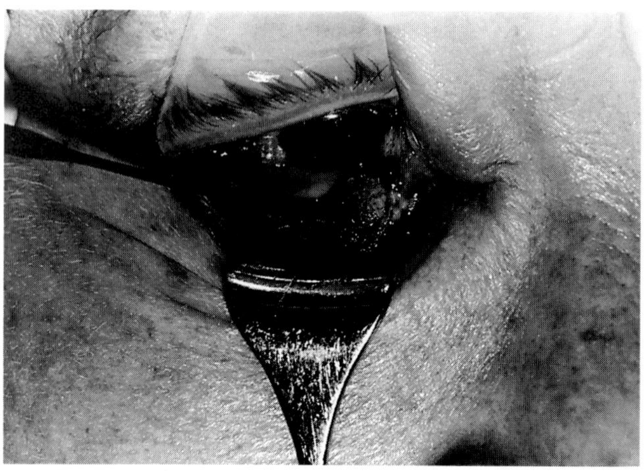

Figure 58–4. Needle-tip cautery incision is made through conjunctiva and lower eyelid retractors, exposing orbital fat.

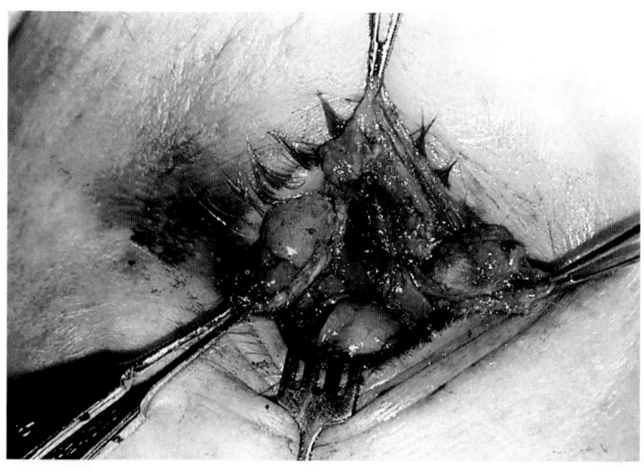

Figure 58–6. The lower eyelid retractors are grasped and lifted with a toothed forceps. Identification of the arcuate expansion of the inferior oblique separating central from lateral fat pads (left band) and inferior oblique muscle separating the central from medial fat pads (right band).

of this fascial band at its attachment to the orbital rim with scissors or cutting cautery makes the central fat pad continuous with the lateral fat pad. This permits identification and exposure of the lateral fat pocket. The lateral fat pad is covered with more septa than the central fat pad and may not spring forward as easily. With excision of the superficial portion of the lateral pad, the fat posterior to this comes forward more freely. Medially, the valley of the inferior oblique separates the central and medial fat compartments. It is important to identify this valley, especially when learning this technique, to ensure that both medial and central fat compartments are excised and to avoid injury to the inferior oblique muscle.

The medial fat compartment is the most difficult to locate, and partial resection of the central fat may be necessary to identify the medial fat. After exposure of the central fat, the medial fat may be totally obscured or may present as a slight bulge in the superomedial aspect of the wound. The glass lid plate can be replaced at this point and pressure placed on the globe to ballotte the fat forward. The needle tip can be used to sharply dissect the overlying septa. The medial fat is different from the central and lateral fat in that it appears white and membranous, may not be postseptal at all, but may come around the edge of the retractor of the lower lid from the muscle cone. Just as in the upper eyelid, the medial prominence of the lower lid probably represents primarily the medial aspect of the central fat pad rather than a prominent medial fat pad. The only difference between this fat pad and the medial fat pad in the upper lid is that the palpebral vessels go directly through this fat pad as opposed to the upper eyelid where the medial vessels lie on the surface of the fat pad. Once the central and medial fat pads are excised, the inferior oblique muscle can be seen.

Once all of the fat is exposed as described previously, the fat is excised in a careful graded fashion with cutting monopolar cautery or scissors. A small hemostat or clamp can be used to help define the line of excision when the exposure is tight. Before any excision of fat, it is useful to expose the fat of both lower eyelids, especially when beginning to use this technique, to allow for more symmetric fat excision. The end point of fat excision is reached when the anterior border of the fat is flush with the orbital rim while applying light pressure on the globe simulating upright posture. This results in a slight concavity of the lower lid in the supine position. Meticulous hemostasis is necessary during the procedure. The blood vessels associated with each fat compartment should be directly visualized by means of blunt dissection with applicator tips and cauterized with the monopolar cautery unit (Valley Labs cautery unit on coagulation mode set at 2.0 to 2.5 W).

After excising the fat (Fig. 58–7), the lower lid margin is pulled superiorly to release any adhesions that might result in lid retraction and to realign the tissue planes. With the lid on stretch, gentle pressure on the globe reveals any residual fat bulges. If necessary, further fat can be excised at this point. In our experience, it is not necessary to close the conjunctival and lower lid retractors at all, however, a single interrupted 6-0 absorbable suture is used to close the conjunctiva centrally if the tissues do not appear well opposed (Fig. 58–8).

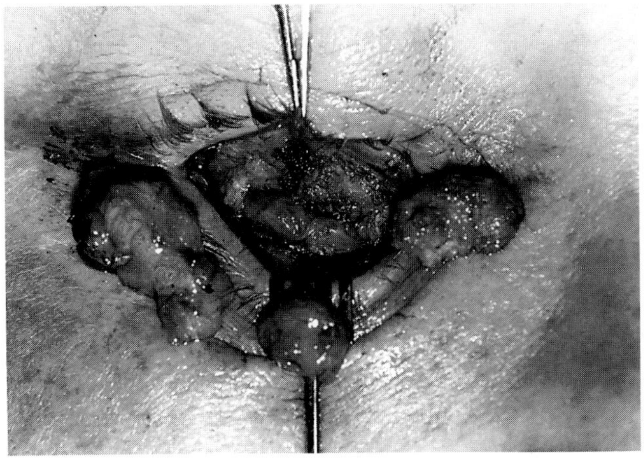

Figure 58–7. Fat that has been removed in graded fashion from the medial, central, and lateral fat pockets is laid out on the eyelid skin. The volume of removed fat is compared with the volume of fat removed from the opposite side: symmetric amounts of fat should be excised from each pocket.

POSTOPERATIVE CARE AND COMPLICATIONS

Antibiotic ophthalmic ointment is applied to the conjunctiva, and ice compresses are immediately applied to the lower lids and used as much as tolerated for the first 48 hours postoperatively. After the first 48 hours, warm compresses are used four times per day for another 7 to 10 days. Antibiotic drops or ointments may be used for patient comfort postoperatively but we have found them unnecessary and use only artificial tears as needed in the postoperative period. The conjunctival incision makes

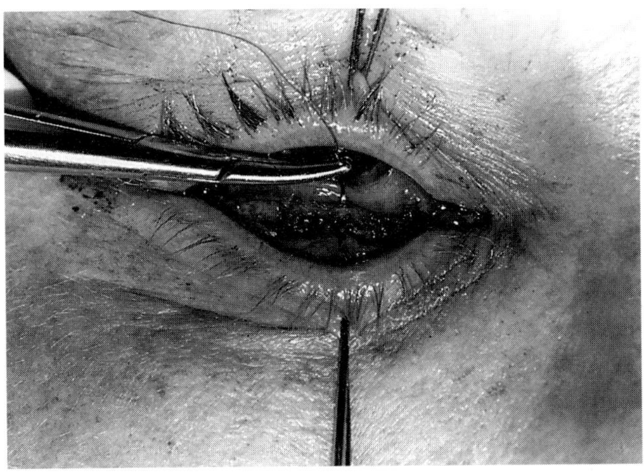

Figure 58–8. After fat removal, the conjunctiva is closed with a single 6-0 mild chromic suture if desired.

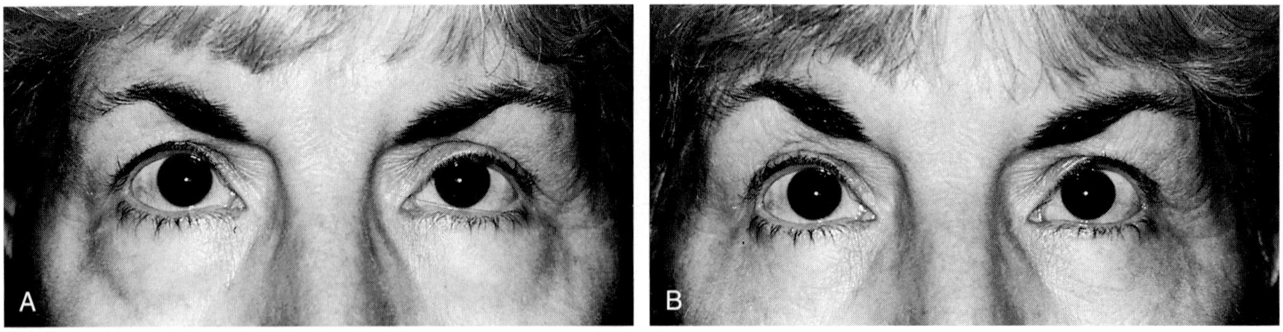

Figure 58 – 9. *A*, Preoperative photograph of a 45-year-old female patient with prominent lower eyelid fat. *B*, After transconjunctival blepharoplasty there is marked reduction in lower eyelid fullness with no alteration of lower eyelid contour or position.

soft contact lens wear difficult for the first 1 or 2 weeks, but generally, wearing soft contact lenses can be successfully resumed within 10 days. Wearing hard contact lenses can be resumed after 3 to 4 days. Postoperative bruising lasts 10 to 14 days in general, and patients should be warned that postoperative ecchymosis may increase or appear first on the third postoperative day with the switch to warm compresses.

The most common complication of transconjunctival blepharoplasty reported in the five series in the literature is inadequate fat excision ranging from 0% to 20% of cases.[8] As previously stated, we do not consider this a complication at all, rather an expected sequela given our conservative philosophy of graded fat excision. No cases of overexcision of fat have been reported, but we have had one case of an overcorrection severe enough to warrant a postoperative dermis fat graft. Lower eyelid malpositions have not previously been reported; however, we have seen several cases of lower eyelid retraction and malposition. Increased skin wrinkling and redundant lower eyelid skin were reported as complications in 1.6% to 3.3% of patients in the literature, although one small series of seven patients reported redundant skin in two of seven (28.6%) of cases.[9] Again, this is easily remedied with careful patient preoperative evaluation and counseling along with a skin pinch excision[10] or chemical peel at the time of transconjunctival fat excision.

No cases of permanent inferior oblique palsy have been reported after this procedure, but transient inferior oblique weakness has been noted. We have seen two cases of restrictive strabismus with diplopia in extremes of gazes due to conjunctival symblepharon that did not completely resolve with surgery to release the symblepharon. Additionally, we had seen one bizarre case of inadvertent disinsertion of the inferior rectus muscle from the globe during transconjunctival blepharoplasty. Fortunately the muscle was retrieved in the anterior orbit 3 months later and reattached with resolution of diplopia. We have reported one postoperative wound hemorrhage that resolved spontaneously without permanent ocular sequelae.[5] Additionally, we have seen several cases of persistent conjunctival chemosis after transconjunctival blepharoplasty that resolved over several months. Persistent chemosis was thought to be a direct result of incision placement too close to the globe.

SUMMARY

Transconjunctival lower blepharoplasty is extremely effective at reducing lower lid "bags" due to prominent orbital fat (Figs. 58–9 through 58–11). Tranconjunctival and transcutaneous approaches are similarly effective in achieving this goal. However, the transconjunctival

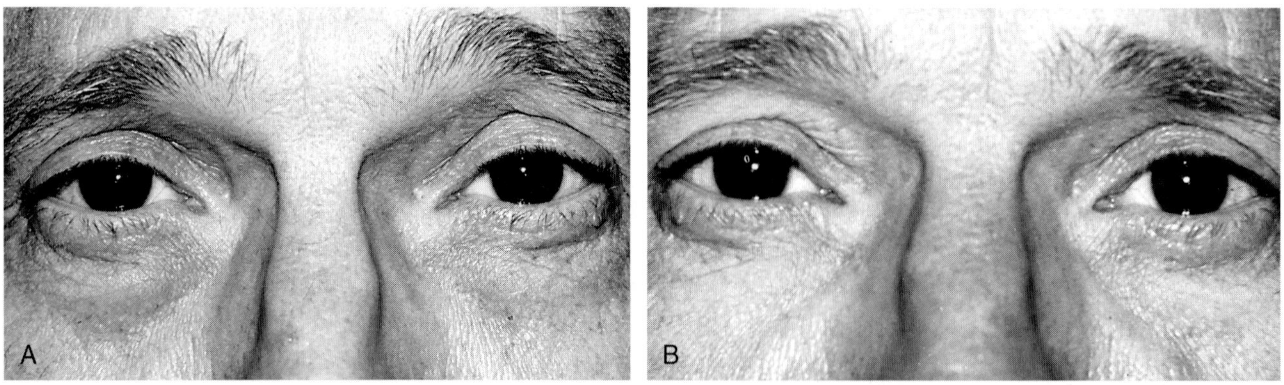

Figure 58 – 10. *A*, Preoperative photograph of a 50-year-old male patient with prominent lower eyelid fat. *B*, After transconjunctival blepharoplasty there is marked reduction in lower eyelid fullness with no alteration of lower eyelid contour or position.

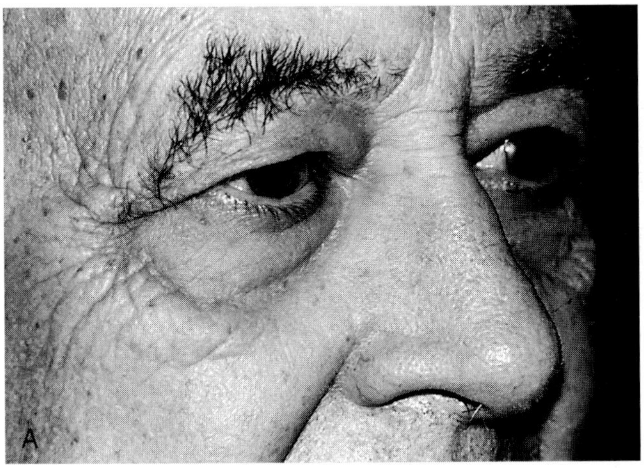

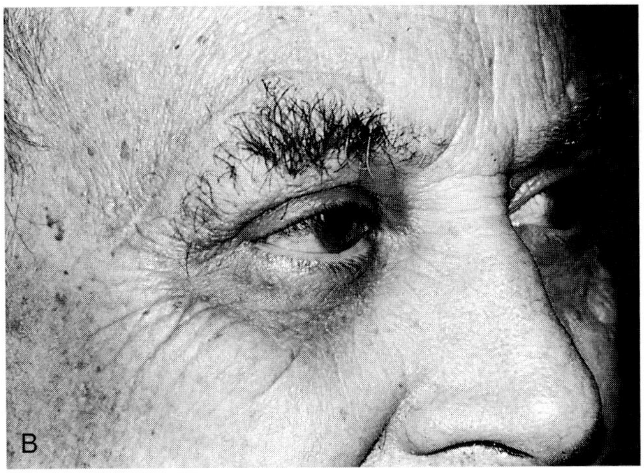

Figure 58 – 11. *A*, Preoperative photograph of a 75-year-old male patient with prominent lower eyelid fat. *B*, After transconjunctival blepharoplasty there is marked reduction in lower eyelid fullness with no alteration of lower eyelid contour or position.

approach offers several advantages over the transcutaneous approach. These include a reduced incidence of lower eyelid malposition or contour alteration and the lack of a cutaneous scar. The main disadvantage of the transconjunctival approach is that it is more foreign to most surgeons and takes longer to learn. However, with knowledge of the anatomy and the technique described, exposure of orbital fat is superb through the transconjunctival approach. It provides an elegant access to lower blepharoplasty that reduces complications compared with cutaneous approaches. The fact that skin is not removed is generally an advantage; misguided attempts to remove lower eyelid wrinkles by excising skin rarely achieve significant cosmetic improvement in our experience and are fraught with risk of subtle or overt lower eyelid retraction or rounding of the lateral canthal angle. Skin wrinkles in the lower eyelid are better addressed in our hands with chemical peel. Very few patients actually have excess lower eyelid skin; when it is present, skin pinch techniques can be combined with transconjunctival blepharoplasty, avoiding violation of the orbital septum. In all age groups and both men and women, the transconjunctival approach is overwhelmingly our most commonly used surgery for lower blepharoplasty.

REFERENCES

1. Baylis HI, Wilson MC, Groth MJ: Complications of lower blepharoplasty. *In* Putterman AM (ed): Cosmetic Oculoplastic Surgery, 2nd ed. Philadelphia, WB Saunders, 1993, pp 356–388.
2. Levine MR, Boyton J, Tenzell RR, Miller GR: Complications of blepharoplasty. Ophthalmic Surg 6:53–57, 1975.
3. Edgerton MT Jr: Causes and prevention of lower eyelid ectropion following blepharoplasty. Plast Reconstr Surg 49:367–373, 1972.
4. Hamako C, Baylis HI: Lower eyelid retraction after blepharoplasty. Am J Ophthalmol 9:517–521, 1980.
5. Baylis HI, Long JA, Groth MJ: Transconjunctival lower eyelid blepharoplasty: Technique and complications. Ophthalmology 96:1027–1032, 1989.
6. Koorneef L: Orbital septa: Anatomy and function. Ophthalmology 86:876–880, 1979.
7. Warwick R: Eugene Wolff's Anatomy of the Eye and Orbit: Including the Central Connections, Development and Comparative Anatomy of the Visual Apparatus, 7th ed. Philadelphia, WB Saunders, 1976, p 273.
8. Palmer FR, Rice DH, Churukian MM: Transconjunctival blepharoplasty complications and their avoidance: A retrospective analysis and review of the literature. Arch Head Neck Surg 119:993–999, 1993.
9. Tomlinson FB, Hovey LM: Transconjunctival lower blepharoplasty for removal of fat. Plast Reconstr Surg 56:314–318, 1975.
10. Parkes M, Fein W, Brennan HG: Pinch technique for repair of cosmetic eyelid deformities. Arch Ophthalmol 89:324–328, 1973.
11. Shorr N, Morrow D: Complications of lower blepharoplasty. *In* Putterman AM (ed): Cosmetic Oculoplastic Surgery, 2nd ed. Philadelphia, WB Saunders, 1993, pp 300–315.

CHAPTER 59

Male Blepharoplasty

Hector M. Marines and James R. Patrinely

The appearance of the eyes and eyelids reflects the well-being, character, and youthfulness of a person. Social interaction begins with the eyes. When natural eyelid shapes are impaired, a coexistent impairment of function and alteration of facial appearance usually exist that may affect the quality of the person's social relations and self-esteem. This is particularly important to individuals who have a great deal of social interaction and authority.

Excess eyelid skin (dermatochalasis) or pseudoherniation of orbital fat (bags) may occur at any age and may result from many predisposing conditions; among the most common are recurrent eyelid edema (e.g., resulting from allergy or thyroid disease), heredity, and aging.

People undergo elective surgery to rejuvenate and restore their eyelids and facial appearance for many different reasons. Performing blepharoplasty and eyebrow surgery in males is a decidedly different surgical quest than in females. Anatomic differences as well as subtle social and cultural factors must be considered for optimal results to be achieved.

PSYCHOSOCIAL ISSUES

Social, ethnic, and cultural factors are important considerations for the surgeon performing blepharoplasty in men. Some surgeons have proclaimed that blepharoplasty is not a procedure for men. This, however, is an oversimplified statement when one considers the number of male patients with upper eyelid problems causing functional or appearance changes that significantly benefit from surgical correction.

Men and women handle the stress of changes in appearance differently. Women are accustomed to radical changes in appearance that occur via drastic hairstyle, make-up, and clothing alterations, whereas men are far more rigid in maintaining a constant appearance. This has been culturally reinforced because changes in appearance (such as hairstyle, make-up, and clothing) are accepted throughout a woman's life. In the past, men have had no psychosocial support for accepting alterations in appearance. Typically, the more professional stature and responsibility a man acquires in his career, the more rigid he is about making any significant appearance changes. Also, in some societies, cosmetic surgery in males is in conflict with masculinity standards.

Regardless of societal standards, improvement in an individual's appearance after surgery often results in a sense of well-being and optimal physical appearance, which usually translate positively in his relations with others. A newfound self-esteem from the improved appearance may also promote professional advancement and employability and therefore be sufficient justification for some men to undergo aesthetic surgery.

Expectations from cosmetic eyelid surgery must be completely understood and discussed with patients. Most men seek eyelid surgery more for functional than for cosmetic reasons, although an increasing number of men over the past 10 years have sought purely cosmetic procedures. However, many men are unable to accept the concept of undergoing surgery for purely aesthetic reasons. Thus, dramatic changes in appearance may not be well accepted. A more natural (non-surgically appearing) outcome therefore is more desirable and more easily accepted by males. The "postblepharoplasty look" (round eye with scleral show, lateral brow ptosis, deep sulcus, high eyelid crease), which may be acceptable to some women, should be avoided in men. Also, men rarely elect to have chemical peels to remove fine rhytids (wrinkles) or surface blemishes.

Because men are not prepared to camouflage the ecchymosis and scars postoperatively, they should be counseled differently so that immediate postoperative expectations and stress are minimized. Those who must return to "normal" appearance as soon as possible because of professional responsibilities may benefit from instructions from a professional cosmetologist to achieve optimal results with postoperative make-up. Others simply wear darker glasses or work from home in the early postoperative period.

For all of these reasons, the surgeon should take care to select the right patient for blepharoplasty, which at times may be more difficult than selecting the right procedure. Realistic expectations of the patient and the surgeon are the key for a good relationship and for surgical success.[1, 2]

ANATOMIC DIFFERENCES

Some anatomic differences between men and women should be considered when aesthetic eyelid surgery is performed in males. These differences may be very subtle but must always be considered for optimal aesthetic and physiologic results.

The first major difference is the prominence of the supraorbital rim and the glabella. This is more pronounced in the male skull, thus creating a brow ridge and apparent depression, which has continuity with the frontal bone superiorly. The female skull usually displays a much softer and less prominent or even indistinct orbital rim and glabella, creating a smoother profile (Fig. 59–1). Also, the lateral orbital rim is characteristically stronger and more prominent in the male and is less conspicuous in the female.[3]

Another important difference is that male eyebrows are placed in a lower position and have a straighter configuration (brow pseudoptosis) than do female eyebrows. Women tend to have thin, arching brows that peak at the lateral canthal area (Fig. 59–2). The eyebrow shape and position are important masculine features that must be preserved when upper eyelid and eyebrow surgery is performed in men. In men, the eyebrow is acceptable in a lower position, just at the level of the superior orbital rim, preferably without causing undue crowding of the eyelids. Male eyebrow hairs are also more numerous and more irregularly arranged.[1–4]

In the upper eyelids, the location of the crease is closer to the eyelid margin in males than in females. This characteristic together with the lower position of the eyebrows are the main anatomic features that are culturally accepted as standards of masculinity. In women, the higher location of the eyebrows and eyelid crease is considered to be an attractive feminine feature. Together, these features highlight the contour of the eyelids and are enhanced by the eyelashes. The more exposed pretarsal skin in women provides a larger skin surface for make-up use. In men, the supratarsal fold should be visible in primary gaze and partly covering the pretarsal eyelid skin.[1–4]

The thickness of the epidermis and dermis is greater in men than in women. Furthermore, male skin is richer in capillaries and has more hair follicles than female skin. In addition, smoking, which is still commoner in men than in women, tends to toughen the skin and damage the microcirculation, which may cause suboptimal scarring. Also, males are more prone to have acne rosacea, which can cause more intraoperative cutaneous bleeding, postoperative swelling, and hypertrophic scar formation resulting from the increased vascularity and sebaceous gland hyperplasia.[5, 6]

Aging changes common to men and women are the decrease in the synthesis of collagen and elastic fibers, causing wrinkling and loss of elasticity, and a relative dehydration and thinning of the epidermis.[6]

Women have learned that sun exposure increases aging and wrinkling, and they usually take appropriate measures for protection. However, men are more cavalier about sun protection and generally have more advanced actinic skin damage. Factors that may alter these findings and gender differences are industrial exposures, eye rubbing, genetics, and overall health of the person.

PREOPERATIVE EVALUATION OF THE PATIENT

Three types of patient evaluation must be performed: first, an evaluation of the patient's morphologic alter-

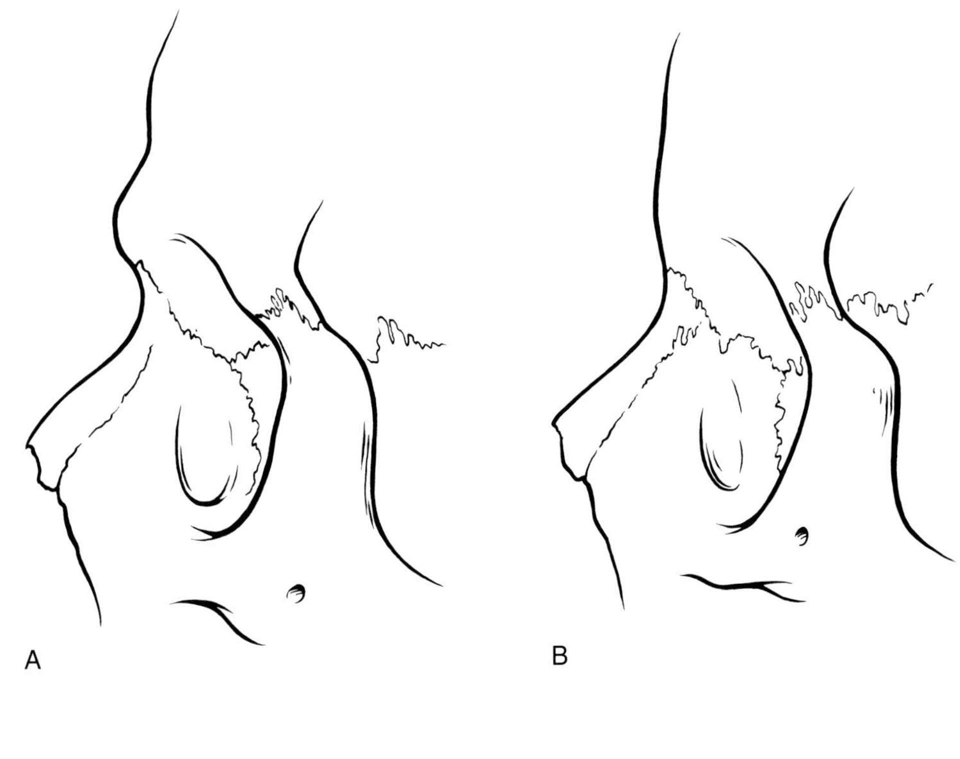

Figure 59–1. *A*, Lateral view of the male orbital bones, demonstrating a prominent and thickened supraorbital rim and glabella. *B*, Profile of the female orbital bones, demonstrating a smoother, rounded supraorbital ridge; a flatter glabella region; and a less defined lateral orbital rim.

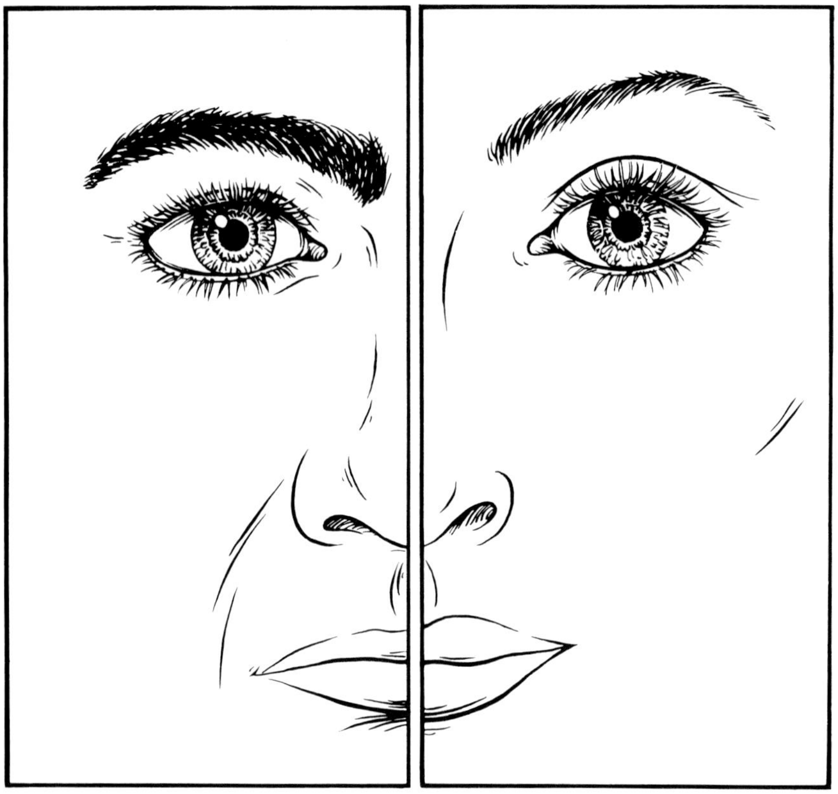

Figure 59–2. Contrasting view of the periorbital soft tissue features of men *(left)* and women *(right)*. The male brow is lower, straighter, and heavier than the female brow, which arches to peak between the lateral limbus and the lateral canthus. The male supratarsal fold is fuller and covers more of the pretarsal skin creating a lower apparent eyelid crease. Also, the female eyelid skin is thinner and contains fewer sebaceous glands and eyelid cilia.

ations; second, an evaluation of the patient's general health; and third, a complete ophthalmologic examination.

A thorough preoperative evaluation of morphologic changes is essential in the male blepharoplasty candidate. Every patient must be individually evaluated to allow for variations and changes in the surgical technique.

The surgeon should consider the differences between the younger patient with familial eyelid deformities (minimal skin excess but predominant fat herniation) and the older patient with involutional changes. In younger men, a low-positioned eyebrow can be considered very handsome but may be more problematic with aging. With aging, the eyebrows tend to slide inferiorly, and the supporting collagenous network relaxes. The inferiorly displaced eyebrows can result in mechanical blepharoptosis via accentuated dermatochalasis in the upper eyelids. The secondary visual obstruction requires constant contraction of the frontal muscle so that the patient can see. This action provides a forehead with deeply etched transverse furrows. Also, the corrugator muscles are usually hyperactive, resulting in marked glabellar furrowing. Attenuation of the orbital septum and adjacent subcutaneous periorbital tissue with age allows the orbital fat to bulge forward and create "bags." Lower eyelid atonicity with manifest or impending ectropion or scleral show also increases with age. Senile blepharophimosis caused by attenuation of the canthal tendons leads to the diminution of the horizontal eyelid aperture.[1, 2]

For some older men, the rugged, sunburned, "outdoorsy" look with low masculine brows (as seen in the "Marlboro man") is attractive. This rugged appearance, however, can also project images of fatigue and weariness. Also, male pattern baldness increases with age and may influence the choice of forehead lifting procedure, if indicated.[1, 2]

In younger men, hereditary factors are important in the development of morphologic eyelid alterations. Recurrent periorbital edema is another common condition that may exacerbate morphologic eyelid changes in younger patients. This edema may occur in blepharochalasis, which is idiopathic but commoner in women. In men, recurrent eyelid edema may result from allergies, thyroid imbalance, alcoholism, cardiovascular disease, and renal dysfunction.

A distinction must be made between patients who mainly seek cosmetic improvement and those who require functional correction because of conditions like blepharoptosis that cause visual field impairment or contact lens intolerance. This distinction is particularly important for insurance carriers, who have for too long minimized the functional importance of periorbital restorative surgery.

The patient seeking aesthetic surgery may present more of a challenge than the patient seeking functional correction because the former's expectations may not be realistic. Also, because no pre-existing disease is present in aesthetic surgery patients, they may minimize the possibility of complications. Because cosmetic surgery in men is usually performed more conservatively than in women, the patient should be informed that radical changes are not planned so that a natural, nonfeminized look will be maintained. Fortunately, most men seeking cosmetic eyelid surgery today prefer a discreet change.[7]

The man with a functional disturbance, such as reduction of superior visual fields caused by dermatochalasis and secondary blepharoptosis, is the type most frequently seen by the ophthalmic plastic surgeon. These patients commonly present with eyebrow ptosis as an aggravating factor; however, they rarely complain about this being a cosmetic problem. Actually, the low-set eyebrows, as previously noted, are very well accepted as masculine features. Sometimes, however, correction of the eyebrow ptosis must be simultaneously performed to achieve a more satisfying functional result.

A quantitative evaluation of the orbital fat bulging in the upper and lower eyelids is important. A careful assessment of the amount of skin excess and horizontal eyelid laxity is mandatory to determine the appropriate surgical techniques. Other features that should be checked during the surgical planning of lower eyelid blepharoplasty are as follows:

1. Malar hypoplasia that may allow postoperative downward displacement of the face and lower eyelid, resulting in scleral show with the classic postoperative round eye. This complication is unacceptable in men.
2. Lower eyelid hypotonia, which is a predisposing factor for postoperative ectropion or retraction.
3. Pseudoherniation of orbital fat, which should be checked with the patient in sitting and supine positions. Malar adiposity and edema can also be confused with orbital fat. The lower eyelid bulges resulting from orbital fat pseudoherniation usually improve in recumbency, whereas eyelid edema and malar subcutaneous adiposity do not change with position. Distinction between these features is important because the latter two are not correctable with a routine blepharoplasty and may actually get worse postoperatively. Different surgical procedures are usually necessary for correction of these problems.[1, 2, 8, 9]

The characteristics of the skin should also be taken into consideration when evaluating the male candidate for blepharoplasty. As already noted, male skin is typically thicker and more vascular than female skin, particularly in areas where hair follicles are more numerous. These features are more pronounced in patients with actinic skin damage and in heavy smokers.

The preoperative evaluation is not complete without a detailed ophthalmologic examination. Blepharoplasty has a denervating effect on eyelid blinking that may take several months to resolve and may cause an exacerbation in the dry eye patient. Of particular interest is the tear production test (Schirmer's test) for detection of patients who are at risk for dry eye syndrome postoperatively. This test cannot diagnose dry eye syndrome but can have significant medicolegal significance. Most of the patients who are prone to develop this condition, however, typically have a history of dry eye complaints or related symptoms. Other pertinent information sought is the presence of Bell's phenomenon, blink rate or completeness, subtle corneal changes (epitheliopathy, mucous microfilaments), and punctal position and patency.

A general health evaluation with a complete workup is advisable because certain systemic conditions, like hypertension and cardiovascular disease, are commoner in males. Blepharoplasty should not be considered simple skin surgery that does not require the same approach and care as other "major" surgeries.[2]

SURGICAL TECHNIQUE

In the authors' experience, men generally tend to be more difficult patients than women during surgery because of lower pain thresholds and intolerance to physical stress. They may require more weight-adjusted anesthesia for sedation and may become more restless and intolerant of laying still for long periods.

The key to postoperative success of upper eyelid blepharoplasty is accurate skin marking. The selection of the upper eyelid crease and the design of the incisions must be very carefully planned. Most men do not use cosmetics postoperatively; therefore, occlusive make-up concealment of scars may not be an option. Thus, placement of incisions for maximum invisibility is essential for men. The lower line of the ellipse of skin to be excised is placed along the natural eyelid crease. In men, this crease is usually located 7 to 8 mm from the ciliary border. The surgeon should expect about a 1- to 2-mm upward displacement of the crease postoperatively, particularly in older patients with loose pretarsal skin. When the creases are not symmetric, it is sometimes helpful to ask the patient which of the two heights is more desirable by using a hand-held mirror. Women used to prefer a high eyelid crease and a sunken superior sulcus, but now a lower crease with a more natural look is more desirable. In men, it is crucial to preserve a supratarsal fold that gives the appearance of a lower apparent crease so that the standards of masculinity are maintained.

With the patient in the sitting position, the amount of excess skin to be excised is determined by placing the lower arm of a toothless forceps at the crease line and gently pinching the excess skin enough to cause discrete eversion of the eyelashes. Forces that act on the face and eyelids change dramatically when the patient is supine. The lower eyelid position and tone, brow position, secondary eyelid skin excess, and orbital fat prominence are all underestimated when vertical gravitational forces are removed. The lateral extent of the incision should stay within the thin eyelid skin, which usually ends about 1 to 1.5 cm inferior to the eyebrow. The maneuver is repeated in different points across the eyelid to design the ellipse of skin and orbicular muscle to be excised. The lateral extension of the ellipse is often gull winged to correct the common lateral hooding present. Generally, men require less of a skin operation and more of a deeper tissue (muscle, septum, aponeurosis) resection and plication than women.

The skin is cleaned with an alcohol wipe, and a fine-tipped gentian violet skin marking pen is used to draw the incision lines. Gentian violet is the preferred dye because it is water and blood resistant, but alcohol or lidocaine erases it when necessary.

If orbital fat excision is in the surgical plan, it is convenient to localize and mark the fat pads to be excised by encircling and shadowing the selected areas, with the patient sitting up. This measure is particularly helpful in lower eyelid blepharoplasty.

Blepharoplasty of the upper and lower eyelids is performed by most surgeons on an outpatient basis with the patient under local anesthesia with intravenous sedation. This method avoids the potentially disastrous nausea and vomiting (which may cause an intraorbital hemorrhage) that can occur after general anesthesia. However, for difficult patients, general anesthesia can be used, although it is not advisable if blepharoptosis or eyelid retraction correction is in the surgical plan, because intraoperative adjustments cannot be made. A common cause of nausea is hypoxia, which can be minimized by preparing and draping the whole face or using an oxygen cannula. Numerous techniques for local anesthesia exist, and every surgeon has preferences.

We routinely use 1% lidocaine (Xylocaine) with 1 : 100,000 epinephrine, mixed in equal amounts with 0.75% bupivacaine, and 1 mL of hyaluronidase to enhance the diffusion in the tissues with minimal secondary tissue distortion. This regimen allows the surgeon to better estimate the final result and make subtle intraoperative adjustments. A preblock with saline-diluted (1 : 10) local anesthetic or bicarbonate-buffered anesthetic is advisable for a relatively painless injection. This method normalizes the acidic pH of the anesthetic, which lessens the painful burning sensation it causes and provides adequate anesthesia for the full-strength injection. A small-caliber needle (30 gauge) and a slow injection minimize discomfort. The needle can be slightly bent at the hub to avoid its direct pointing toward the eye should an inadvertent release of the needle from the syringe occur.

If a lower eyelid transconjunctival blepharoplasty is planned, a cotton pledget soaked in topical tetracaine and 4% lidocaine is packed in the inferior conjunctival fornix before the subconjunctival and subcutaneous injections are performed.

For male upper eyelid blepharoplasty, skin and muscle are simultaneously excised. Because the muscle is usually redundant and hypotonic, most surgeons recommend excision of skin and muscle as a unit to obtain a more natural look by facilitating the skin closure. Also, this technique allows wide exposure of the septum, which makes removal of orbital fat easier. Fullness of the lateral portion of the eyelid is usually not related to orbital fat but to suborbicularis adipose tissue. This fat pad is located toward the tail of the eyebrow. Another cause of fullness in the lateral third of the eyelid is ptosis of the lacrimal gland, which can be resuspended to the lacrimal fossa with double-armed, 6-0 nonabsorbable horizontal mattress sutures.

After the fat has been excised and meticulous hemostasis achieved, the skin is closed with a 7-0 nylon or 6-0 rapidly absorbing plain gut suture. The excision of orbicular muscle will contribute to the formation of a natural crease. Crease fixation is avoided if possible in men because this may result in a deep, feminized crease (Fig. 59-3). Sometimes, however, fixation of crease is desirable. When this is necessary, the orbicular muscle edges are anchored to the levator aponeurosis with a plain gut suture. Because the skin edge is not incorporated in the crease fixation, the crease will appear more natural and disappears in down-gaze, which is a more natural appearance for men.

Correction of the lower eyelid is the most challenging part of male blepharoplasty, and it provides the fewest postoperative effects but the highest rate of complications. The commonest complication is lower eyelid re-

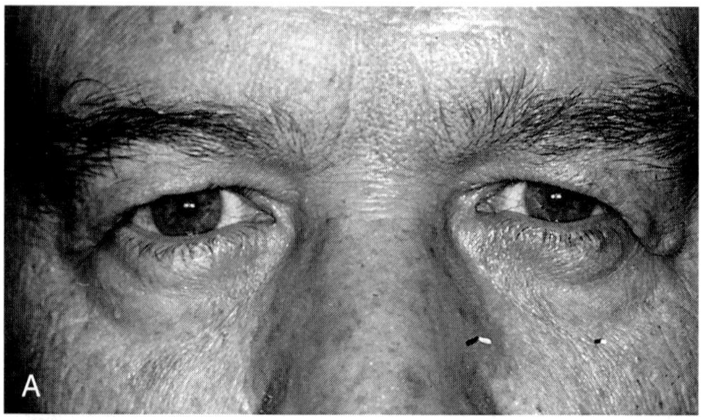

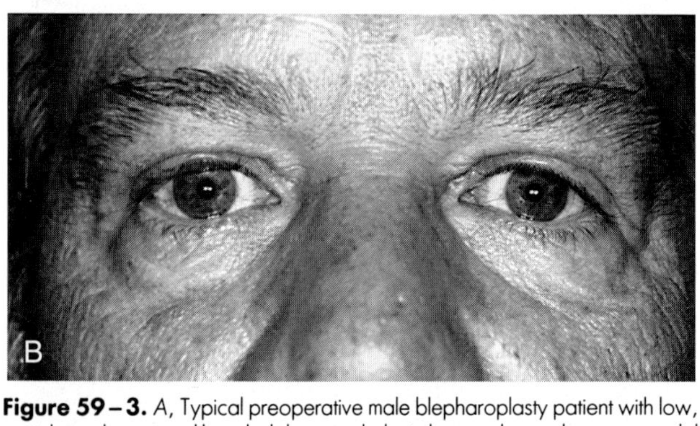

Figure 59-3. *A*, Typical preoperative male blepharoplasty patient with low, straight eyebrows and hooded dermatochalasis that overhangs the upper eyelid margin. The skin is thickened by sun exposure and tobacco use and demonstrates early acne rosacea with sebaceous gland hyperplasia. *B*, Six months after conservative upper eyelid blepharoplasty performed with skin–muscle resection and minimal fat resection. The low-positioned masculine upper eyelid creases and heavy, straight brows are maintained.

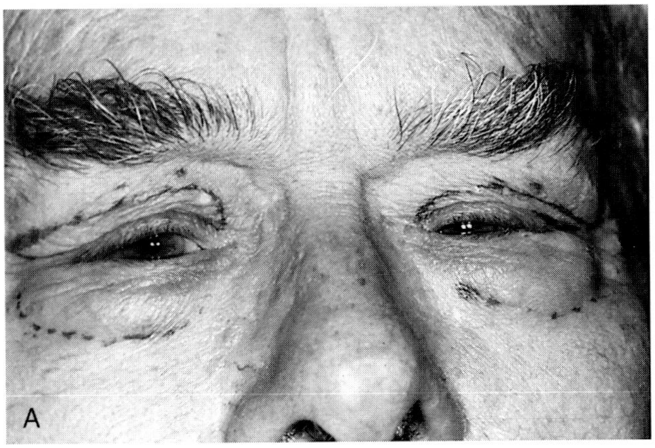

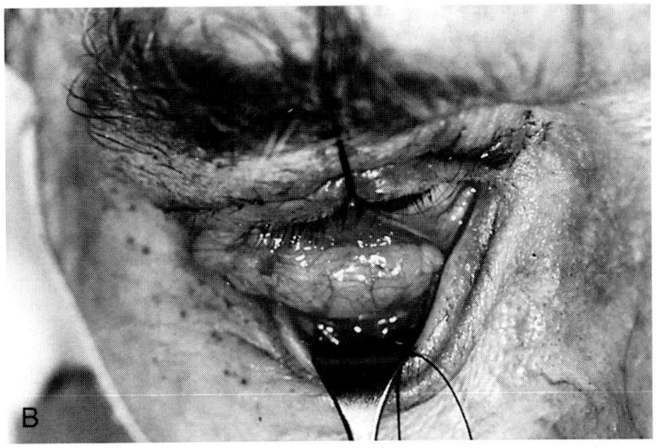

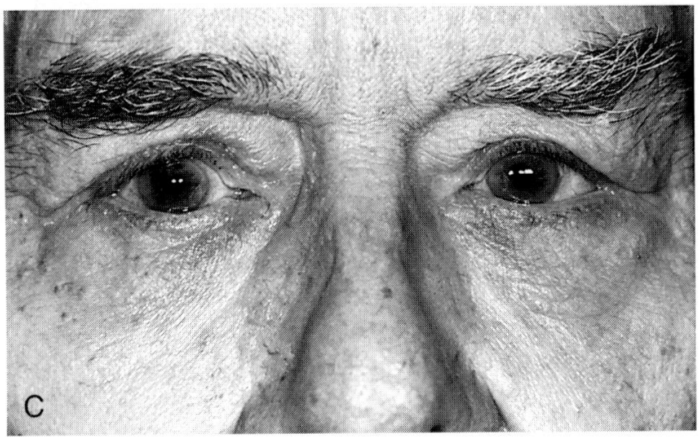

Figure 59–4. *A*, Preoperative markings *(dotted lines)* outlining pseudoherniation of lower orbital fat ("bags") in an 80-year-old cosmetic surgery patient. The upper eyelid skin redundancy is conservatively marked to minimize postoperative dry eye complaints. *B*, Transconjunctival delivery and resection of lower eyelid orbital fat. C, Six months after conservative upper eyelid blepharoplasty and lower eyelid fat resection. No lower eyelid skin has been resected. The apparent skin "excess" noted in *A* is distributed evenly by the decrease in preseptal convexity after the fat resection.

traction or ectropion. In addition, lower eyelid blepharoplasty is usually performed for purely cosmetic reasons.

Different techniques have been described for lower eyelid blepharoplasty. The commonest technique is the anterior transcutaneous approach, with a subciliary incision and development of a skin muscle flap. This is the technique of choice for simultaneous correction of truly redundant lower eyelid skin. However, most patients have a predominant pseudoherniation of orbital fat without a true excess of skin. For this reason, we frequently use a posterior transconjunctival approach, which avoids cutaneous scars and eyelid malposition complications (Fig. 59–4). We prefer to use the transconjunctival route in most patients.[8, 9] When moderate skin excess is also present, the procedure can be combined with a limited external skin excision (pinch technique) without violating the orbicularis. A form of lateral canthoplasty or tarsal strip procedure can be performed simultaneously to restore eyelid tone and position and to prevent postoperative retraction and scleral show. Malar bags or festoons are best managed by plication of an extended orbicular muscle flap to the lateral orbital rim in addition to the aforementioned procedures.

REFERENCES

1. Courtiss EH: Objectives of aesthetic surgery. *In* Courtiss EH (ed): Male Aesthetic Surgery. St. Louis, CV Mosby, 1991, pp 3–5.
2. Flowers RS: Periorbital aesthetic surgery for men. Eyelids and related structures. Clin Plast Surg 18:689–729, 1991.
3. Doxanas MT, Anderson RL: Clinical Orbital Anatomy. Baltimore, Williams & Wilkins, 1984, pp 19–88.
4. Graham WP, Davis TS, Miller SH: Physiology of maleness. *In* Courtiss EH (ed): Male Aesthetic Surgery. St. Louis, CV Mosby, 1991, pp 36–40.
5. Moretti G, Ellis RA, Mescon H: Vascular patterns in the skin of the face. J Invest Dermatol 33:103, 1959.
6. Bentley JP: Aging of collagen. J Invest Dermatol 73:80, 1979.
7. Jacobson WE, Meyer E, Edgerton MT: Psychiatric evaluation of male patients seeking cosmetic surgery. Plast Reconstr Surg 26:356, 1960.
8. Dortzbach R: Lower eyelid blepharoplasty by the anterior approach: Prevention of complications. Ophthalmology 90:223, 1983.
9. Baylis HI, Long JA, Groth MJ: Transconjunctival lower eyelid blepharoplasty. Techniques and complications. Ophthalmology 96:1027, 1989.

CHAPTER 60

Alternative Techniques of Fat Removal

Stephen L. Bosniak, Timothy F. McDevitt, and Ted H. Wojno

To attain the goal of cosmetic blepharoplasty—smooth eyelid contours, appropriate lid levels, and undisturbed or improved physiologic eyelid function—various surgical techniques must be used. A thorough preoperative evaluation determines the location and quantity of the tissues to be resected.

A significant concern, however, is the possibility of a postoperative eyelid contour that does not fulfill preoperative expectations. The patient will most certainly object to residual eyelid contour irregularities caused by inadequate or excessive fat resection. Any technique that enhances the accuracy of fat resection is of obvious benefit.

Resecting the fat pockets is also often uncomfortable for the patient because of traction applied to the deep orbital tissues. Here again, any technique that more gently manipulates the fat and minimizes deep orbital traction has a clear advantage. This chapter discusses alternative techniques that can effectively and safely remove fat during cosmetic blepharoplasty.

CLAMP—CUT—CAUTERIZE

Before removing fat, the ophthalmologist should be certain that the pocket is properly anesthetized. Subcutaneous infiltration of local anesthesia is frequently inadequate for pain control during fat resection, causing the patient to complain of discomfort referred to the retrobulbar area. In such cases, the fat pockets must be injected under direct visualization with 0.5 to 1.0 mL of anesthetic to obtain adequate analgesia. Occasionally, patients develop temporary extraocular muscle palsy owing to spread of the anesthetic to the rectus or oblique muscles, but this problem resolves a few hours after surgery. During resection, traction on the orbital fat is kept to a minimum; excessive traction anteriorly can lead to hemorrhage deep within the orbit. Many surgeons have been taught the dictum of "clamp-cut-cauterize" for the resection of orbital fat. The wisdom of this basic technique cannot be overemphasized (Fig. 60–1). After the remaining stump is cauterized thoroughly, the clamp is released slowly while the surgeon inspects for bleeders before the fat retracts into the orbit. With this technique, the fat may be cauterized with a bipolar forceps, unipolar Bovie electrocautery, disposable high-temperature cautery, contact neodymium:yttrium-aluminum-garnet (Nd:YAG) laser, or radio-frequency instrumentation. Lateral spread of electrical current is lowest with the bipolar cautery, but coagulation of fat is most rapid and complete with a high-temperature disposable cautery. The surgeon should be mindful, however, that excessive electrical cauterization can lead to postoperative lid retraction or "malignant cicatrization."[1]

MONOPOLAR MICRODISSECTION

Monopolar electromicrodissection (Colorado needle; Colorado Biomedical, Evergreen, CO) with a very sharp tip can also be used for orbital fat resection. Cutting can begin with an initial power setting of 5 W. If tissue drag occurs, the power can be increased slowly. When pure coagulation is needed, the power setting should begin at 11 W and be increased slowly.

LIPOCAUTERIZATION

Direct lipocauterization of fat pockets with bipolar cautery can be performed without any fat excision.[2] The orbital septum is opened, the preaponeurotic fat is prolapsed, and cautery is applied directly to the fat (Fig. 60–2).

The fat pockets liquify and contract. This technique is most useful for small amounts of fat, such as that in the medial pocket of the upper eyelid. A high-temperature disposable cautery or monopolar electrical cautery also works well when used in this manner.

CARBON DIOXIDE LASER

Fat can also be vaporized with the carbon dioxide laser (wave length 1056 nm). Baker and coworkers[3] described using this technique as part of a carbon dioxide laser blepharoplasty. The technique has the advantage of cau-

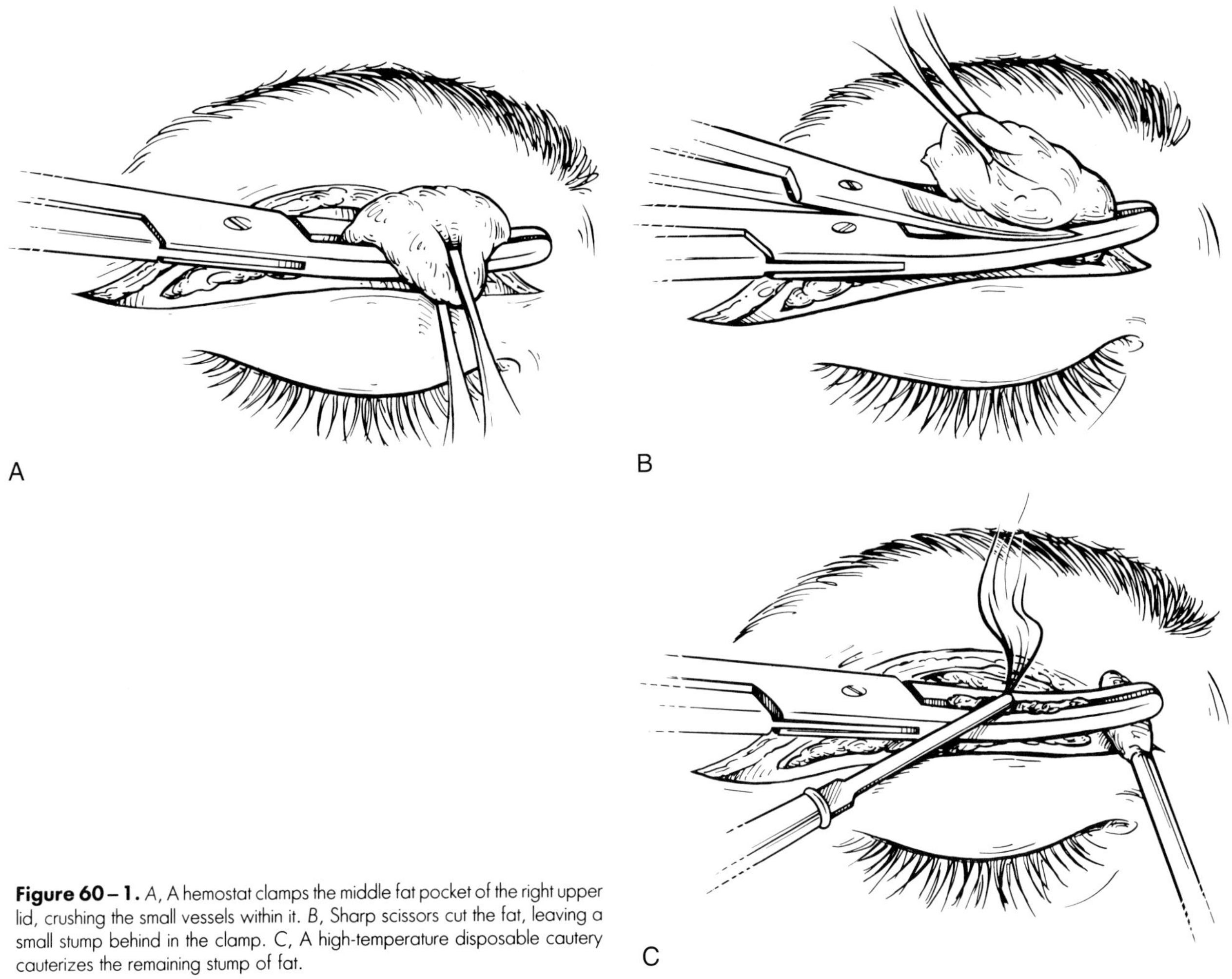

Figure 60 – 1. *A*, A hemostat clamps the middle fat pocket of the right upper lid, crushing the small vessels within it. *B*, Sharp scissors cut the fat, leaving a small stump behind in the clamp. C, A high-temperature disposable cautery cauterizes the remaining stump of fat.

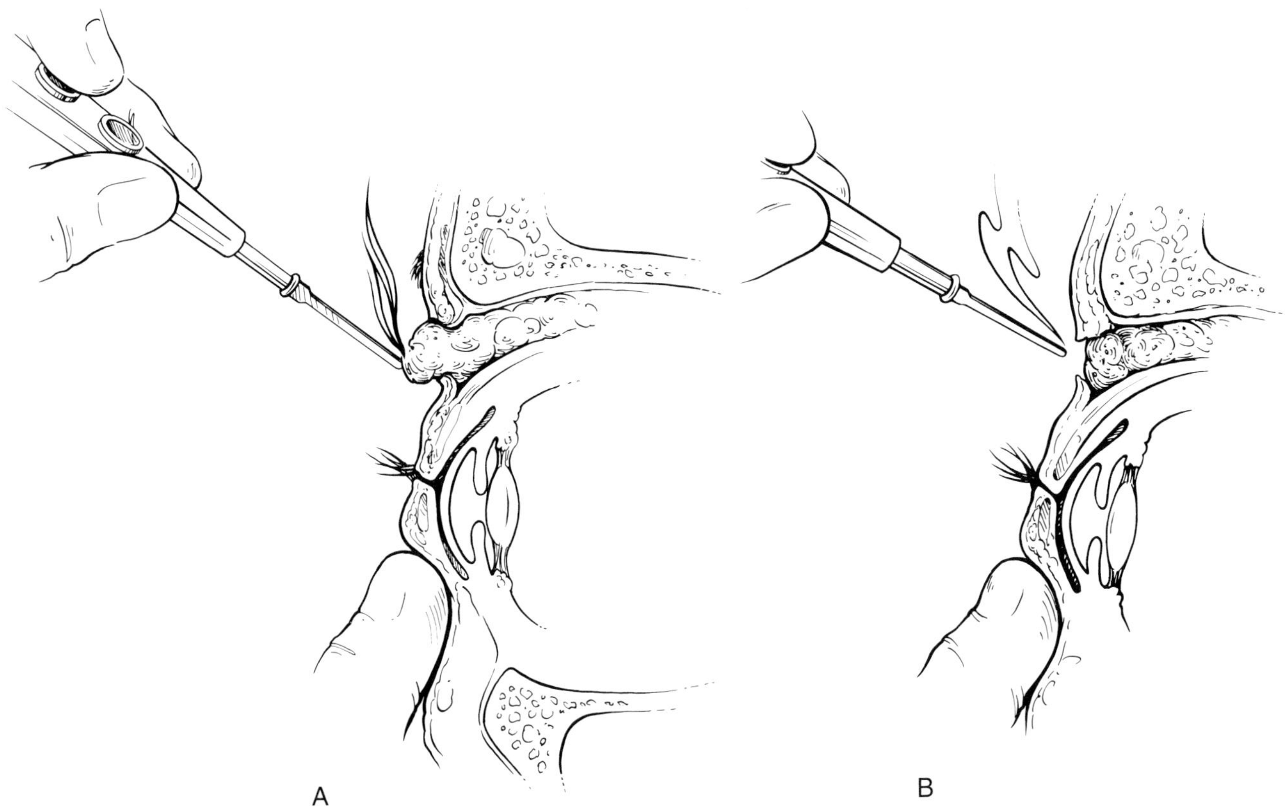

Figure 60 – 2. *A* and *B*, Direct lipocauterization of the medial fat pocket of the upper lid with the bipolar cautery, causing liquefaction and shrinkage of this pocket.

terizing vessels up to 0.5 mm in diameter during cutting. The authors felt that this procedure resulted in decreased postoperative ecchymosis, edema, and discomfort.

Although potential apparently exists for decreasing the operative time needed to perform cosmetic blepharoplasty and increasing the safety with which it can be performed, several obvious disadvantages of this technique remain. The instrumentation is expensive. Routine operating room procedures must be altered when the carbon dioxide laser is in use: all operating room personnel must wear protective goggles, and all sterile drapes must be moistened to avoid inadvertent ignition. The articulated area of the hand piece is cumbersome to use. The surgeon must learn to hold instruments away from the tissue being vaporized and to avoid inadvertent reflection of the beam with resultant reflected burn of nonoperative sites or the surgical assistant. Because treated tissue yields DNA-containing vapors, powerful vapor evacuation systems are necessary. But the most significant disadvantage is that for all the effort, the hemostatic effect is not complete. Large vessels are not sealed with the carbon dioxide laser; rather, their walls are punctured, and they bleed. Skin incised with the carbon dioxide laser does not heal well — wound strength may be decreased and wound erythema prolonged. Baker and coworkers[3] also felt that cutaneous scar formation was greater in patients who underwent carbon dioxide laser blepharoplasty for skin resection than in those who had conventional cold knife surgery.

The new Ultra-Pulse laser (Coherent, Palo Alto, CA) provides an improved hemostatic effect and, when combined with the transconjunctival approach, obviates the need for a lower lid subciliary incision.

LIPOLYTIC DIATHERMY

Lipolytic diathermy was originally described by Bosniak and Sachs as a technique that used monopolar electrical cautery.[4] Although the technique was effective in cases of mild fatty prolapse with mild lid contour irregularities, the theoretic potential existed for electrical conduction of monopolar cautery through the optic nerve. This technique was replaced with bipolar lipolytic diathermy technique using a customized bipolar forceps (Mentor, Norwall, MA). The sharp tips of the forceps can be used to pierce the orbital septum and the prolapsed fat pockets (Fig. 60 – 3). The bipolar forceps are applied just as the conductive 30-gauge needle was applied, and the same precautions are followed. However, the area cauterized is more controlled, and no potential exists for optic nerve conduction. These forceps can also be used

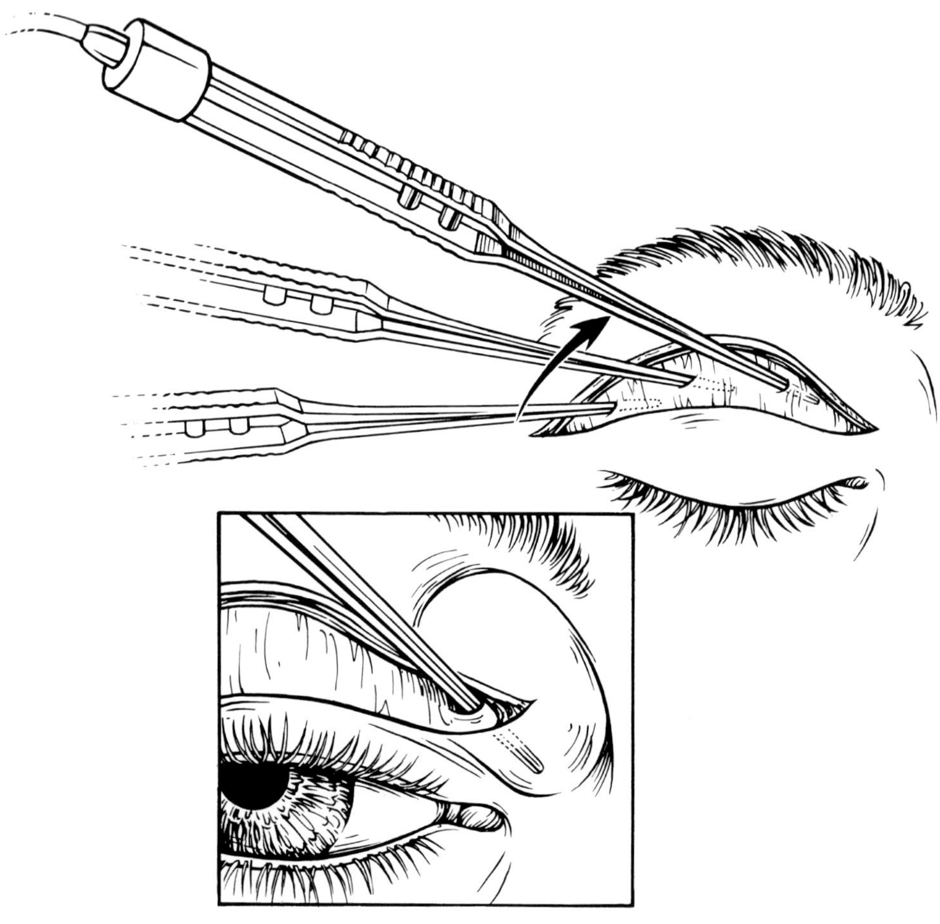

Figure 60 – 3. Sharp-pointed bipolar lipolytic diathermy forceps pierce the orbital septum and reduce the volume of orbital fat. In the upper lid this action may facilitate contouring of the nasal fat pocket medial to the skin incision *(inset)*. (From Bosniak SL (ed): Cosmetic Blepharoplasty. New York, Raven Press, 1990.)

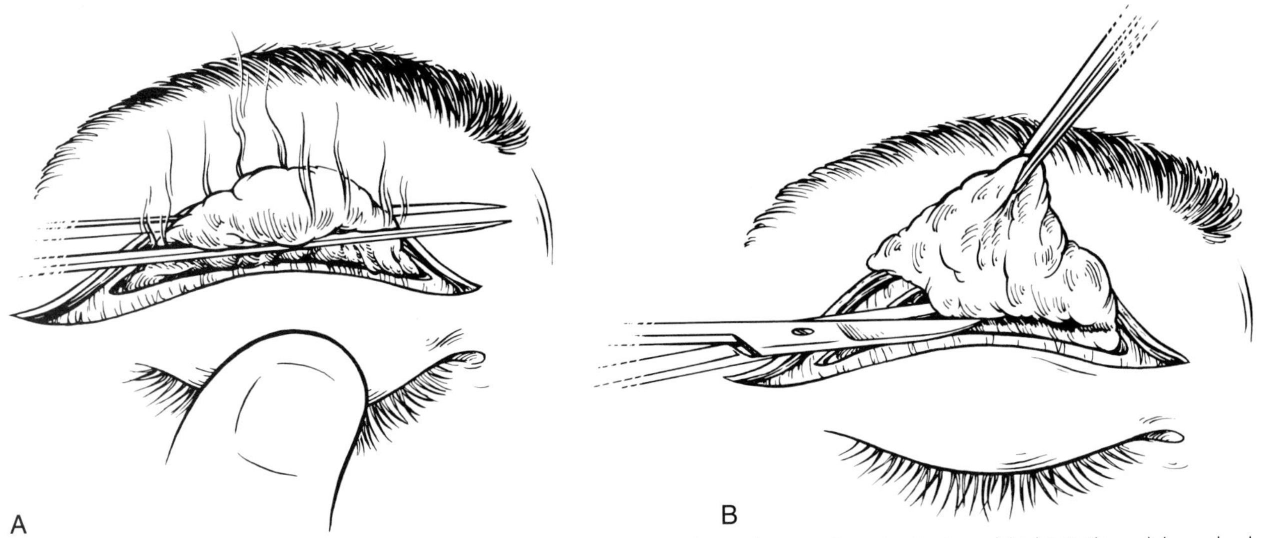

Figure 60 – 4. *A*, Once the septum is opened, the bipolar lipolytic diathermy forceps can be used to grasp the prolapsing fat and shrink it. *B*, This pedicle can then be resected without bleeding. (From Bosniak SL (ed): Cosmetic Blepharoplasty. New York, Raven Press, 1990.)

for direct lipocauterization (Fig. 60 – 4*A*) or as a cauterizing clamp. In cases of more generously prolapsing orbital fat when trans-septal techniques do not completely recontour the eyelids and sulci, the septum is opened, the residual fat is grasped with the forceps, cautery is applied, and the fat is resected in the line of cautery (see Fig. 60 – 4*B*).

FAT REPOSITIONING

Fat excision increases the risk of intraoperative or postoperative hemorrhage, as well as the risk of inadvertent damage to the levator and oblique muscles. Obviously, therefore, any technique that eliminates fat excision has multiple theoretic advantages. Such a technique was described by de la Plaza and Arroyo.[5] Instead of resecting, they reposited fat deeper within the orbit. They secured it by suturing the capsulopalpebral fascia to the periosteum at the inferior orbital rim with a running, nonabsorbable suture. This method was later described by Sachs and Bosniak but was discarded because of its potential for tethering the lower lid to the orbital rim, resulting in lagophthalmos and scleral show.[6]

CONTACT YTTRIUM-ALUMINUM-GARNET LASER

The contact Nd:YAG laser (Surgical Laser Technologies, Oaks, PA) is a 1060-nm, continuous-wave focused laser that uses a sapphire scalpel tip. The size of this tip is changeable; the GRP 2 tip has a diameter of 200 μm and is the smallest tip that offers the finest focus. Power density is defined as power per unit tip area; it is also the property that vaporizes tissue. The advantage of a small tip diameter is increased power density.

In the free-beam mode, the YAG laser light is absorbed by hemoglobin. In contrast, the carbon dioxide laser light is absorbed by water, instantly vaporizing the cell. The YAG laser's reacting with hemoglobin allows for deeper penetration through tissue and creates a thermal effect as well. The heating of this probe provides excellent hemostasis as well as the ability to resect fat. A noncontact YAG laser is a poor instrument to resect fat because this mode essentially "boils" the fat. As fat boils, it becomes very reflective, and much thermal energy scatter is evident. The frosted side of the sapphire-tip contact YAG laser is used to resect fat because this area provides thermal energy from conduction combined with radiant energy from scattered YAG light (Fig. 60 – 5). Blood vessels

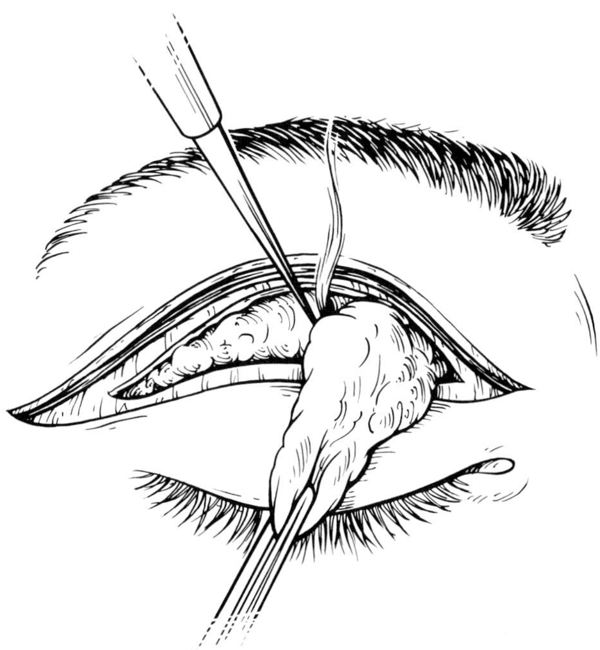

Figure 60 – 5. The contact Nd:YAG laser being used to excise orbital fat.

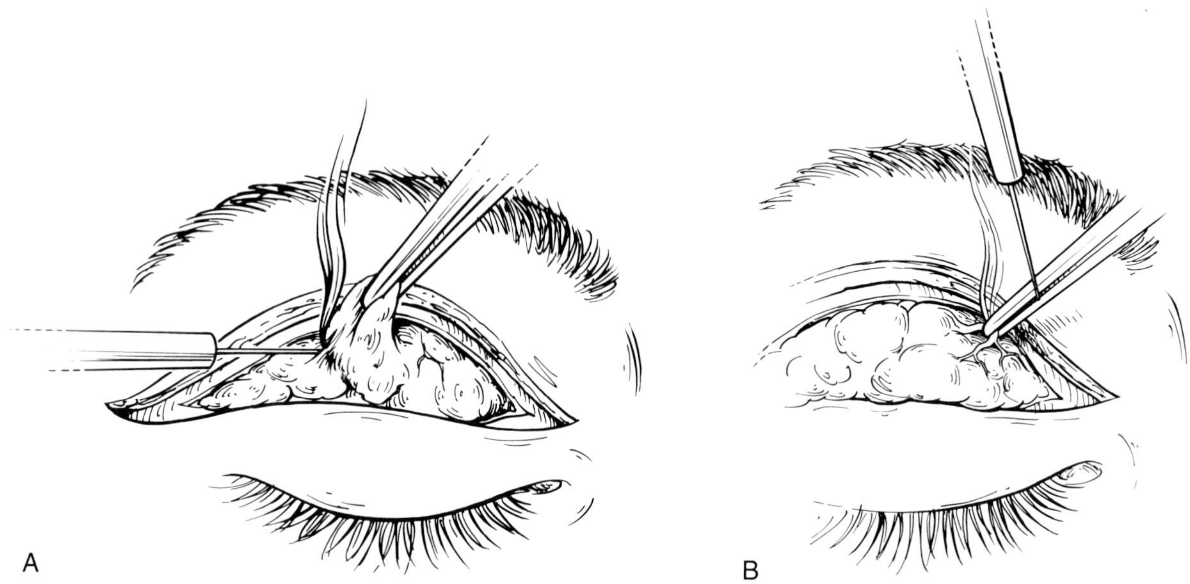

Figure 60–6. *A*, Radiosurgery lipocontouring. *B*, Large blood vessels within the fat and coagulating by grasping them with forceps and touching the electrode to the forceps.

are sealed with a combination of these two efforts, unlike the carbon dioxide laser, which simply provides immediate vaporization and may perforate, not seal, larger-diameter vessels. The YAG laser may not be useful in making a skin incision because of its tendency to char tissue while making this incision. The manufacturer reports that multiple rapid light strokes with the instrument may provide a burn-free skin incision, but this has not been our experience. For fat resection and lipocontouring, settings starting at approximately 15 W are effective.

RADIO-FREQUENCY INSTRUMENTATION

Radio-frequency units, such as the Ellman Unit (Ellman Company, New York, NY) use high-frequency radio waves to volatilize (boil) water in each cell. The Ellman unit uses a 4.8 MHz radio wave; the wave form changes depending on which setting is used. The first setting is a continuous, filtered wave form that results in a cutting current. The second setting is a fully rectified wave form. It has an evenly dispersed interruption in wave form to give a 50% coagulation. This setting would be most useful for fat resection, using a power setting of 1.5 to 2. On the cutting mode, the radio-frequency unit does not provide complete hemostasis. Large-caliber vessels must be grasped with forceps; the radio-frequency probe can then be placed in contact with the forceps to cauterize the vessel (Fig. 60–6). This instrument is comparable to the carbon dioxide laser in its hemostatic effectiveness when cutting the orbital fat. By using a fine wire electrode, with a quick, smooth stroke, little lateral spread of thermal energy occurs,[7] making this instrument ideal for skin incisions as well.

REFERENCES

1. Bosniak SL: Cosmetic Blepharoplasty. New York, Raven Press, 1990, p 107.
2. Leone CR, Glover AT: Lipocauterization and thermal fixation in blepharoplasty. Am J Ophthalmol 106:635–637, 1988.
3. Baker SS, Muenzler WS, Small RG, Leonard JE: Carbon dioxide laser blepharoplasty. Ophthalmology 91:238–244, 1984.
4. Bosniak SL, Sachs ME: Lipolytic diathermy. Orbit 4:157–165, 1985.
5. de la Plaza R, Arroyo JM: A new technique for the treatment of palpebral bags. Plast Reconstr Surg 81:677–685, 1988.
6. Sachs ME, Bosniak SL: Correction of true periorbital fat herniation in cosmetic lower lid blepharoplasty. Aesthetic Plast Surg 10:111–114, 1986.
7. Hurwitz JJ, Johnson D, Howarth D, Molgat Y: High-frequency radio wave electrosection of full-thickness eyelid tissues. Can J Ophthalmol 28(1):28–31, 1993.

CHAPTER 61

Management of Blepharoplasty Complications

Ted H. Wojno

Chapter 60 outlined precautions and surgical techniques aimed at prevention of complications after blepharoplasty. Problems are inevitable, however, even in the hands of the most careful surgeon. This chapter discusses the complications of blepharoplasty surgery and their management.

VISUAL LOSS

Blindness is undoubtedly the most serious complication of blepharoplasty surgery. Although exceedingly rare, it can have a devastating effect in the context of cosmetic surgery.

The incidence of blindness after blepharoplasty is difficult to determine accurately because of its relative rarity and the natural reluctance of surgeons to discuss its occurrence. Attesting to the infrequency of the event is the fact that most reports in the literature are of isolated events or small series.[1-15] The most comprehensive report is that of DeMere and coworkers,[16] who polled 16,000 ophthalmologists and plastic surgeons in 1973, inquiring as to the frequency of this event. From the 3000 who responded, the investigators found 40 cases of blindness in 98,514 surgeries over a 1-year period, which was an incidence of 0.04%. Although the statistical significance of this study is questionable, it points out that a small but finite risk of blindness exists after cosmetic blepharoplasty, something that every prospective patient should be told. In three cases,[12,13,15] transient bilateral visual loss occurred.

The usual cause of blindness after blepharoplasty is thought to be retrobulbar hemorrhage. In support of this theory is the fact that blindness has never been reported in a "skin-only" blepharoplasty. Retrobulbar hemorrhage may arise from inadequately cauterized orbital fat pockets or from rebound vasodilation from uncauterized vessels after the vasoconstrictive effect of epinephrine wears off. Of particular concern are the medial pockets of the upper and lower lids, which often contain the large medial palpebral arteries. Orbital hemorrhage may also result from vigorous traction on orbital fat that tears deeper orbital vessels or from orbicularis bleeding that finds its way posteriorly through an open septum. With loculated hemorrhage, orbital pressure rises and is perhaps compounded by edema from surgical manipulation or from pressure patches. Increased intraorbital pressure may cause a central retinal artery occlusion or ischemia of the microcirculation of the optic nerve.[5,7] Increased intraorbital pressure may also raise intraocular pressure, which, in patients with preexisting vascular disease or glaucoma, could damage an already compromised ocular circulation or optic nerve head.[2]

Other, less frequent, causes of visual loss include precipitation of narrow-angle glaucoma,[2] organic coagulopathy, remote effects of cautery on the optic nerve,[17-19] globe perforation with the anesthetic needle,[17] coincidental occurrence of an unrelated blinding ocular disease,[5] or preoperative blindness that was unknown to the patient.[20]

Because orbital hemorrhage is the likely cause of most cases of blindness after blepharoplasty, measures should be taken to reduce the probability of orbital bleeding. As stated in the introductory chapter of this section, administration of all medication with anticoagulant properties should be discontinued 2 weeks before surgery, if pos sible. The physician should keep in mind that patients with preexisting retinal vascular disease, glaucoma, or optic nerve disorders are already compromised and are therefore more susceptible to increased intraorbital pressure from any cause. The surgeon should not put undue pressure on the globe when attempting to prolapse orbital fat into the field and should take care not to put excessive traction on the orbital fat to avoid inadvertent damage to vessels deep within the orbit. Many surgeons feel that it is wise to cauterize the stump of fat that remains after resection or at least inspect it for bleeding before allowing it to retract back into the orbit. Before final closure, the surgeon checks for bleeding vessels that may have opened after the effect of epinephrine has worn off. The surgeon avoids pressure patches because they can raise intraorbital and intraocular pressure and can prevent the early diagnosis of visual loss.[7] Iced compresses and head elevation for the first 2 days help to reduce edema.[15] Patients are instructed to avoid strenuous physical activity after surgery that might increase venous pressure, which could lead to hemorrhage from the orbital vessels. Avoidance of coughing or Valsalva maneuvers may also be helpful.[17] Patients are instructed to call immediately if they note visual loss, obvious hemorrhage, or severe pain.

If visual loss occurs as a result of retrobulbar hemorrhage, the wound edges are opened to release increased intraorbital pressure, and any blood that may have accumulated is evacuated. Lateral canthotomy with superior and inferior crus cantholysis may also be helpful. If possible, the wound is explored thoroughly to locate and cauterize any bleeding vessels. The surgeon may also choose to start intravenous mannitol and acetazolamide and instill a topical beta-blocker to lower intraocular pressure. If a central retinal artery occlusion occurs, paracentesis or breathing of a mixture of 5% carbon dioxide and 95% oxygen may be helpful.[2] The surgeon may choose to leave a drain in place for 24 to 48 hours to ensure that any bleeding has access to the surface.

DIPLOPIA

Patients commonly experience transient diplopia immediately after blepharoplasty, especially if the fat pockets were directly injected with anesthetic and if hyaluronidase was used in the anesthetic mixture. Such diplopia, which is caused by diffusion of the anesthetic to the extraocular muscles, usually resolves within several hours of the surgery. Likewise, diplopia resulting from minor orbital hemorrhage and edema resolves within a few days of surgery.

Persistent diplopia after blepharoplasty is distinctly unusual. This condition may be secondary to direct trauma to the inferior oblique, inferior rectus, or superior oblique muscle during fat resection,[21–25] or it may result from a Volkmann-type contracture from edema and hemorrhage into the muscle sheath.[26] Rarely, persistent diplopia may represent decompensation of a phoria, especially if patches were used.[27] Patients who undergo a repeat blepharoplasty are at an especially increased risk of this complication because scar tissue from the original surgery makes the dissection more difficult and trauma to the muscles more likely.[24]

Diplopia may be prevented by minimizing traction on the orbital fat, avoiding orbital hemorrhage, and taking care to avoid direct damage to the muscles. Fortunately, most cases of diplopia eventually resolve spontaneously.[28] If, however, a muscle is known to have been transected or forced ductions remain positive, early treatment is appropriate. Therapy depends on the type of problem (restrictive versus paralytic) and the muscle involved.

PTOSIS

Mild ptosis immediately after blepharoplasty is relatively common and results from lid edema. This mechanical ptosis is short lived and resolves in a few days. Edema and hematoma can result in persistent ptosis by stretching or dehiscence of the levator aponeurosis (Fig. 61–1). Alternatively, the levator may be directly damaged during fat excision, or it may be transected at the lower border of the skin muscle excision where the levator fibers merge with the tarsal plate, septum, and orbicular muscle.[29]

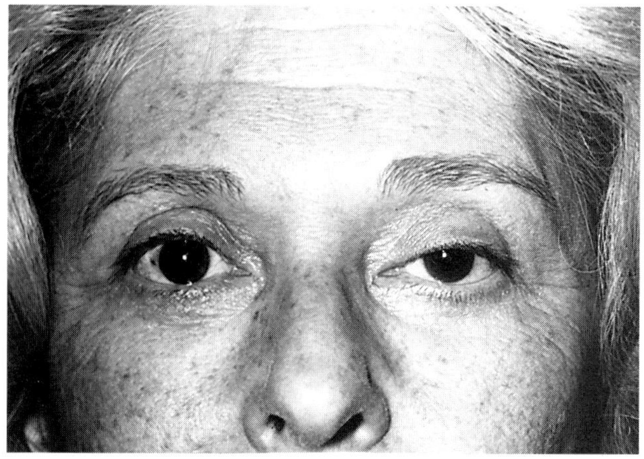

Figure 61–1. This patient developed ptosis of the left upper eyelid immediately after blepharoplasty. At surgery, a thinned levator aponeurosis was found.

Excessively high supratarsal fixation can also result in ptosis by mechanical limitation of the upward movement of the eyelid via its attachments to the medial and lateral canthal tendons.[29] Incorporation of the orbital septum into the closure can likewise cause a mechanical ptosis and can limit the upward movement of the eyelid.

The surgeon should take care to note any ptosis preoperatively that may be unmasked by removal of the redundant skin. This point deserves special emphasis because surprisingly large degrees of ptosis can be hidden by overhanging upper eyelid skin. Cautious dissection prevents direct levator damage. If the orbital septum is incarcerated or the crease stitches are placed excessively high, the wound should be reopened and the traction released. Persistent ptosis with good levator function and no obvious cause should be followed up for at least 3 to 4 months because many of these cases spontaneously improve.[30] For the cases that do not improve, levator aponeurosis surgery is usually curative.

LOWER LID MALPOSITION

Lower lid malposition (lid retraction or ectropion) (Fig. 61–2) most commonly results from excessive skin excision or failure to recognize horizontal laxity.[17,20] Other possible causes include inadvertent incorporation of the orbital septum into the skin sutures, scarring of the lid to the orbital floor,[31] orbicularis paresis, gravitational drag by the cheeks,[32] and inflammation in the fat pockets.[33] Some eyes are anatomically predisposed, such as those with exophthalmos (caused by Graves' disease,

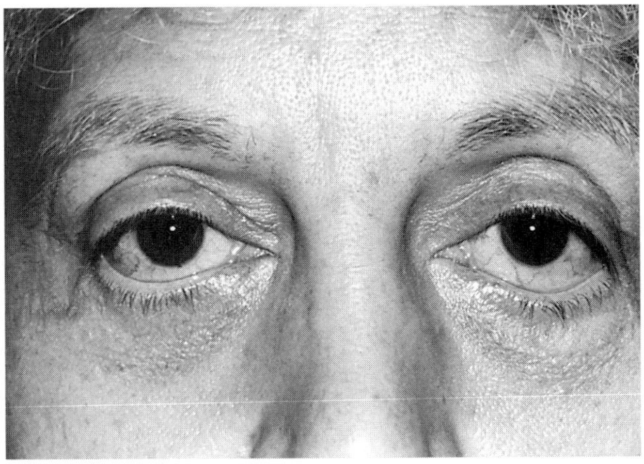

Figure 61 – 2. This patient was referred because of severe lower eyelid retraction after lower blepharoplasty. Skin excision was excessive, and excess horizontal laxity was present.

high myopia, shallow orbits) or flat malar eminences that render inadequate support to the lower lid.

As was discussed in Chapter 49, excessive horizontal laxity should be noted preoperatively and corrected at the time of blepharoplasty with a lid shortening procedure. When skin is excised, the excess is draped superolaterally and not just superiorly so that tension is placed not only on the lid margin but also on the more stable lateral canthus. Although generalizing is difficult, no more than 6 mm of skin usually needs to be resected in a vertical direction in most cases.[20]

Mild ectropion noted within the first week after surgery may be treated by removing the sutures and teasing the wound edges apart. This action releases the traction on the lid margin, allowing it to return to a normal position. The wound epithelizes spontaneously a few weeks later, yielding surprisingly good functional and cosmetic results (Fig. 61 – 3). Although originally described for the lower lid[31] I have used this procedure in the upper eyelid on one occasion with good results, as has Lisman.[17]

For more severe ectropion resulting from unrecognized horizontal laxity, reoperation is necessary, consisting of a horizontal eyelid shortening procedure, as described previously. If the problem results from excess skin excision, the surgeon may reoperate and perform the "Madame Butterfly" procedure, as described by Shorr and Fallor.[34] This procedure consists of extensive undermining of the cheek at the level of periosteum, lysis of any adhesions in the septum, horizontal lid shortening, and suspension of the cheek to the periosteum lateral to the lateral canthal angle. The procedure gives the eyes a mongoloid slant, which resolves over several months.

If the skin shortage is severe, a skin graft is necessary. Generally, no skin is available from the upper eyelids because this was also removed at the time of blepharoplasty. The next best choice is a retroauricular skin graft, which can be used with satisfactory results in the lower eyelid if it is appropriately thinned.[33]

Inflammation in the fact pockets causes a severe ectropion that begins 2 to 3 days after surgery that is associated with a remarkable degree of lid inflammation.[28] Palpation of the fat pockets reveals a firm mass. Treatment consists of injection of 1 mL of triamcinolone into the fat pockets and support of the lid with tape or with a suture to the brow (Fig. 61 – 4).

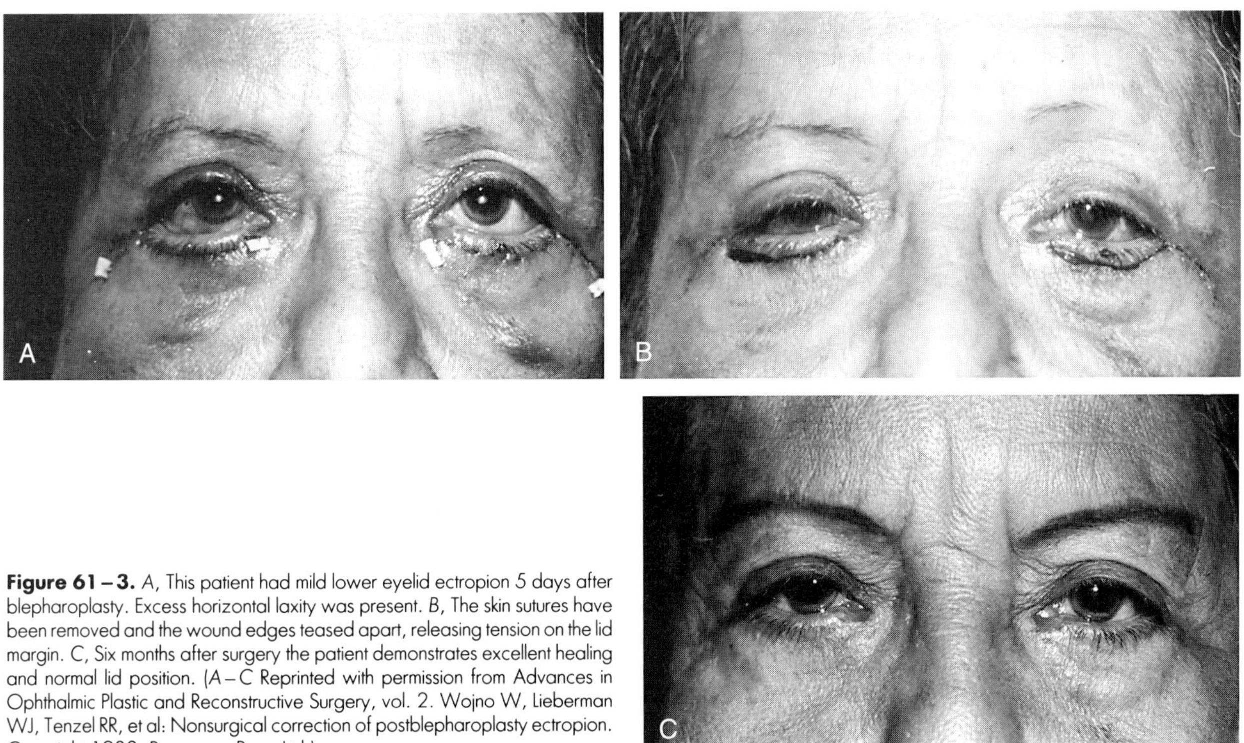

Figure 61 – 3. *A*, This patient had mild lower eyelid ectropion 5 days after blepharoplasty. Excess horizontal laxity was present. *B*, The skin sutures have been removed and the wound edges teased apart, releasing tension on the lid margin. C, Six months after surgery the patient demonstrates excellent healing and normal lid position. (*A – C* Reprinted with permission from Advances in Ophthalmic Plastic and Reconstructive Surgery, vol. 2. Wojno W, Lieberman WJ, Tenzel RR, et al: Nonsurgical correction of postblepharoplasty ectropion. Copyright 1983, Pergamon Press Ltd.)

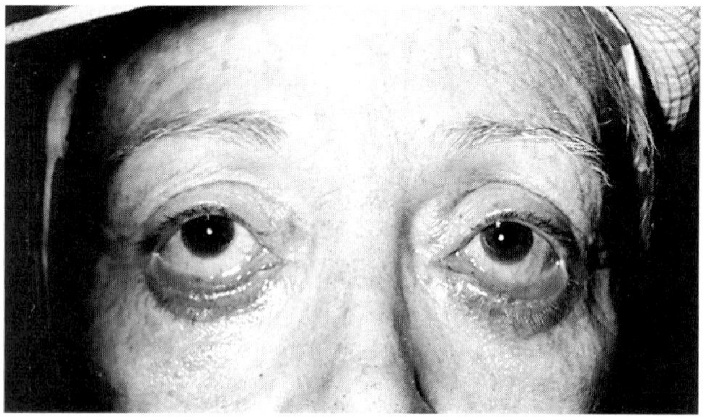

Figure 61–4. This patient developed severe ectropion due to inflammation within the orbital fat pockets. This problem resolved rapidly after injection of triamcinolone into each lid and taping of the lids back into position. (Courtesy of Dr. Richard R. Tenzel.)

ROUND EYE DEFORMITY

Rounding of the lateral canthus is essentially a variation of ectropion (Fig. 61–5) and results from unrecognized lateral canthal tendon laxity, excessive skin excision laterally, or a combination of the two. The vertical tension placed on the lateral canthus is too great for the thinned tendon and results in a conversion of the acute lateral canthal angle to a rounded shape. The lateral canthus is slightly medially and inferiorly displaced. Most cases respond well to fixation of the lateral canthal tendon or tarsal plate to the periosteum at the lateral orbital rim.

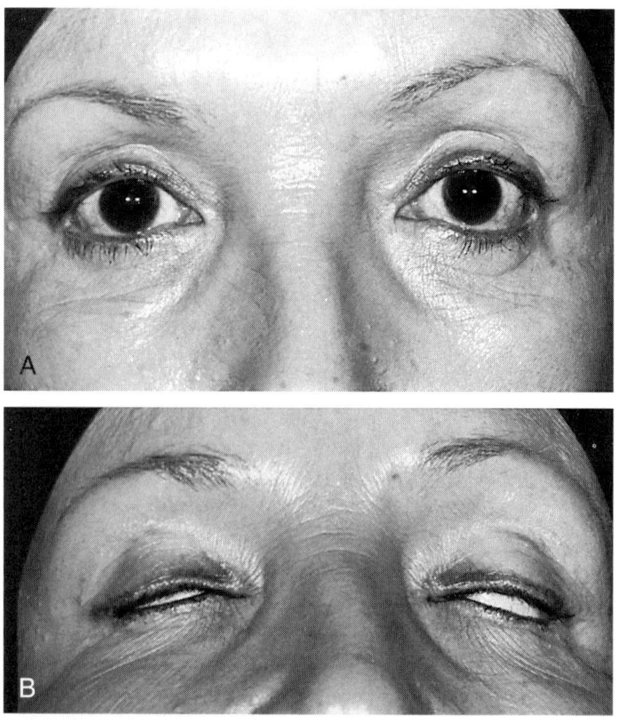

Figure 61–5. *A*, This patient was referred after a four-lid blepharoplasty. She has a round eye deformity that is slightly worse on the left. *B*, With passive closure there is noticeable lagophthalmos due to excess excision from upper and lower lids.

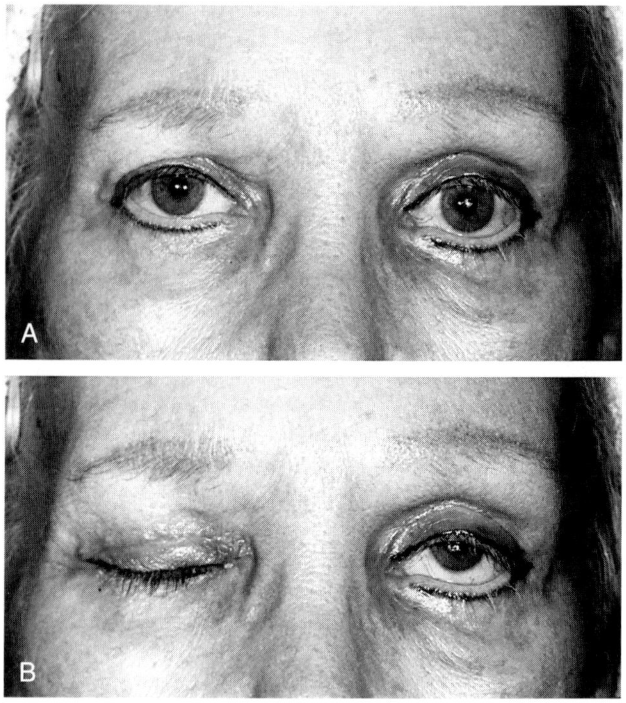

Figure 61–6. *A*, This patient was referred after a four-lid blepharoplasty, face lift, and forehead lift. *B*, Passive closure shows a complete lagophthalmos due to palsy of the superior division of the seventh nerve.

LAGOPHTHALMOS

Transient mild lagophthalmos is common immediately after surgery and results from edema and orbicularis anesthesia. Persistent lagophthalmos usually results from excess skin excision in the upper eyelid, lower eyelid, or both. It may also result from incorporation of the orbital septum in the closure of either lid. Partial damage to the peripheral branches of the seventh nerve occurs occasionally, especially if a forehead lift was also performed (Fig. 61–6).

If lagophthalmos is mild and the symptoms are not severe, the patient can be treated with lubrication. More severe cases may require skin grafts to the responsible eyelid.[28] If the orbital septum was incarcerated in the closure, it should be released. Orbicularis paresis is treated symptomatically if transient and surgically as appropriate and discussed elsewhere in this text.

INCOMPLETE OR EXCESSIVE ORBITAL FAT REMOVAL

In the lower eyelid, the lateral fat pocket is occasionally missed because of its more superior location (Fig. 61–7). The medial fat pocket of the upper and lower lids may also be missed if the incision is not carried far enough to expose these pockets. The relatively smaller medial fat pockets have a tendency to drop posteriorly into the orbit

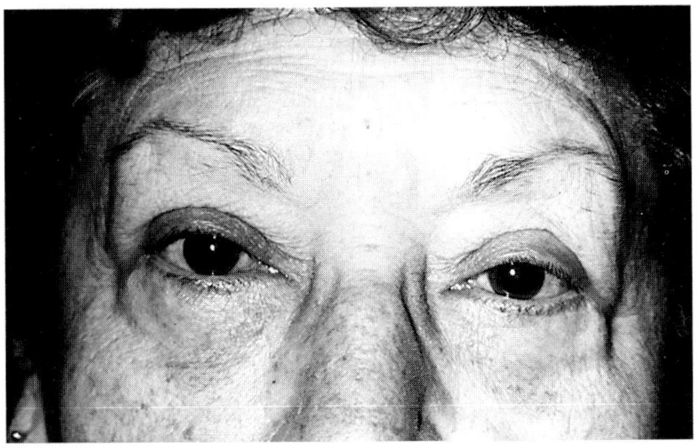

Figure 61 – 7. This patient was referred after a four-lid blepharoplasty because of "lumps" in the lower lids, which are the lateral fat pockets.

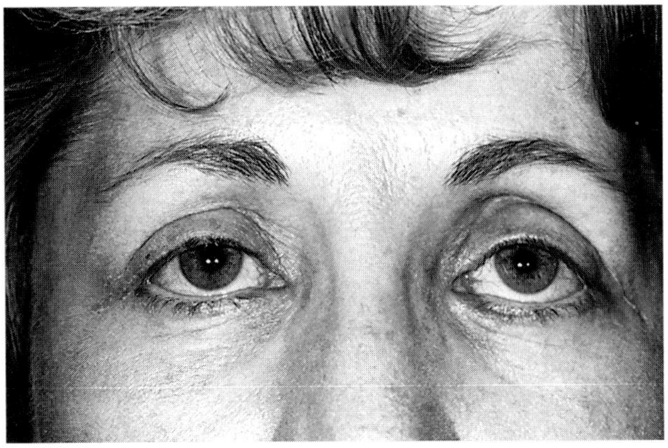

Figure 61 – 8. This patient was referred after a four-lid blepharoplasty. The left superior sulcus is unpleasantly deep due to excessive fat resection.

when the patient is supine, contributing to the difficulty in finding them. If discovered postoperatively, this situation is easily remedied by reopening the incision line directly over the remaining fat pocket and excising it.

Excessive fat resection in the upper eyelid results in a displeasingly shallow superior sulcus (Fig. 61 – 8). If excessive fat is resected from the lower eyelid, the inferior orbital rim may appear unusually prominent. Treatment of this deformity is most difficult. Tenzel described a technique of overlapping small flaps of orbicular muscle from medial and lateral to the defect in an attempt to fill it (Fig. 61 – 9). This technique is useful for relatively mild cases of overcorrection. Larger defects can be filled with a buried dermis graft placed at the level of the orbital septum.[35] Such grafts shrink approximately 25% and thus should be slightly oversized.

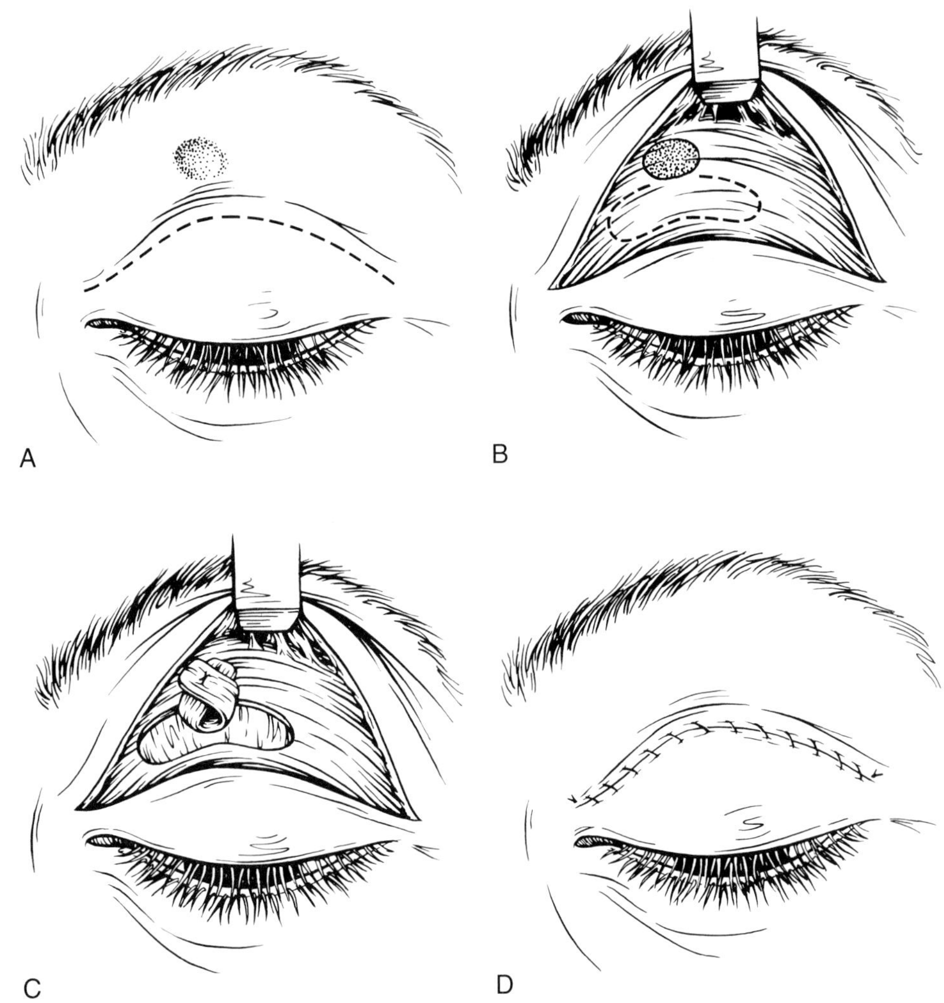

Figure 61 – 9. The technique of Dr. Richard R. Tenzel for the correction of mild fat overexcision. *A* and *B*, After opening the skin in the old incision line free up flaps of orbicularis on each side of the depression in the superior sulcus. *C* and *D*, Overlap and suture the flaps together over the defect. Close the skin. (*A – D* from Tenzel RR: Cosmetic blepharoplasty. *In* Soll DB (ed): Management of Complications in Ophthalmic Plastic Surgery. Birmingham, AL, Aesculapius, 1976, p 128.)

SKIN ASYMMETRY

Asymmetric appearance of the upper eyelid skin is caused by unequal removal of skin, failure to note unilateral brow ptosis, or failure to form symmetric lid creases.[36] In the case of unequal skin removal, the surgeon can simply excise more skin from the side with some remaining redundancy if this process does not result in lagophthalmos. Most patients accept this "touch-up" of their original surgery very well.

Unilateral brow ptosis is easy to miss during surgery with the patient supine because both brows rest at the same level in this position. If equal amounts of skin were excised from both the left and the right upper eyelids, the side with brow ptosis appears to have more skin after surgery. The surgeon can elevate the ptotic brow or excise more skin from the lid on this side, on the condition that neither procedure will cause lagophthalmos.

If the lid creases are formed at different levels, the side of the lower crease appears to have more skin. The lower crease should be elevated to match the other side, as long as this action does not place the new crease higher than 10 mm. Trying to elevate a low crease is easier than trying to lower a high one.

DOUBLE CREASE

Very rarely, a second crease may form just superior to the surgically created eyelid crease (Fig. 61–10). Although double or even triple creases occur naturally, one that forms after upper lid blepharoplasty is a source of patient dissatisfaction. I have seen this situation on only two occasions, once in a referred patient and once in my own patient. In the first patient, the referring doctor unsuccessfully tried three times to undermine the abnormal superior crease to break any adhesions to the deeper tissue that may have caused the crease. In my own patient, I excised the redundant fold of skin that resulted from the second crease with good results. I took a small amount of skin from the opposite upper eyelid for symmetry.

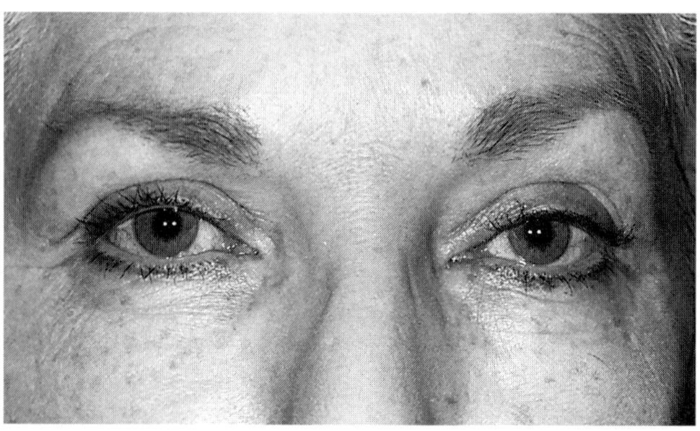

Figure 61–10. This patient returned 2 months after an upper lid blepharoplasty and left ptosis repair. The patient reported a second crease that developed laterally on the left upper lid.

INFECTION

Because of the good vascular supply to the eyelids, wound infections are fortunately very rare.[37,38] Any cellulitis that develops after blepharoplasty should be cultured and treated appropriately.

WOUND DEHISCENCE

Patients may inadvertently rub the operated eyelids, especially on awakening in the morning.[20] They should be cautioned to treat the incision lines carefully because a traumatically dehiscenced wound may scar excessively or become infected. If mild, the wound edges may be left to heal spontaneously. If severe, the edges should be resutured.

PROMINENT SCARS

Cosmetically objectionable scar formation is uncommon after blepharoplasty, although the incision line may remain detectable, especially in the upper lid. The incision usually falls into a natural skin crease and therefore blends well. If an incision line remains prominent, injection of triamcinolone is appropriate.[27]

PIGMENTATION

The naturally occurring pigmentation of the lower eyelids sometimes seems more prominent after blepharoplasty. Removal of bulging orbital fat pockets and tightening of the redundant, wrinkled skin now focuses the patient's attention on the pigmentation. The surgeon should remind the patient preoperatively that such pigmentation will not be removed with blepharoplasty. Ecchymosis of the eyelid may result in hemosiderin deposition in the skin, but this condition usually resolves gradually over several months. Rare cases may persist up to 1 year.

LACRIMAL DISORDERS

Many patients complain of transient symptoms of ocular dryness immediately after blepharoplasty performed to treat lagophthalmos. Slit lamp examination often discloses an inferior punctate epithelial keratopathy. Symptoms may be marked if the basic secretion test is low ($<$10 mm) in patients with only 1 to 2 mm of lagophthalmos. Such patients may have been asymptomatic before blepharoplasty surgery but suddenly become symptomatic with slight corneal exposure. Even without lagophthalmos, blepharoplasty may increase the vertical width of the palpebral fissure and may increase corneal drying, causing more subtle dry eye symptoms. Despite opinions to the contrary, patients with a low basic secretion of tears are at increased risk of developing dry eye symptoms if they are left with lagophthalmos and corneal exposure. Every effort should be made, therefore, to avoid exposure in such patients. If corneal exposure occurs immediately after blepharoplasty, the patient can be treated symptomatically with artificial tears or ophthalmic ointment. If the basic secretion test result is low, a trial of temporary punctal occlusion may suggest that permanent occlusion or silicone plug occlusion may be helpful. If symptomatic lagophthalmos persists or the cornea begins to decompensate, the surgeon should take the necessary steps for correction of this problem as outlined in Chapters 56 and 57.

Some patients may report having epiphora in the immediate postoperative period as a result of loss of pump function from orbicularis resection and lid swelling. Edema may temporarily occlude the canaliculi,[27] but this problem resolves rapidly in the first few days to weeks after surgery. If the medial skin excision was excessive, punctal ectropion may be the cause of the epiphora. This problem may require skin grafting for correction.

I have seen one patient in whom the main lobe of the lacrimal gland was excised when it was mistaken for a fat pocket. The main lobe of the lacrimal gland is pink, as opposed to the yellow color of the orbital fat pockets. If it prolapses into the field, it should be sutured inside the superior orbital rim, as described in Chapter 56.

MEDIAL CANTHAL FOLDS

A pseudoepicanthal fold may result from excessive skin excision in the medial upper eyelid or from an incision that extends too close to the lid margin. A V-Y plasty usually corrects the problem.[28]

BROW DISPLACEMENT

Many older patients have poor fixation of the eyelid and brow skin to the subcutaneous tissues. When skin is pinched together for upper lid blepharoplasty measurements, it is seemingly very easy to take more and more skin. In fact, this effect results from inferior displacement of the brow and forehead tissues from traction by the surgeon's forceps. This inferior displacement of the brow is often difficult to appreciate in the supine patient but is obvious after surgery (Fig. 61–11). To avoid this complication, the surgeon should fix the brow in position with a finger when determining the amount of upper lid skin to be excised.

SUTURE TRACTS

Suture tracts may form in the incision line as a result of epithelialization of the suture tunnels. Tracts occur more frequently with silk than with monofilament sutures. A fine-pointed scissors is inserted through the tract, the tract is cut through, the two small remaining tags of the skin are excised down to the level of the skin surface.[39]

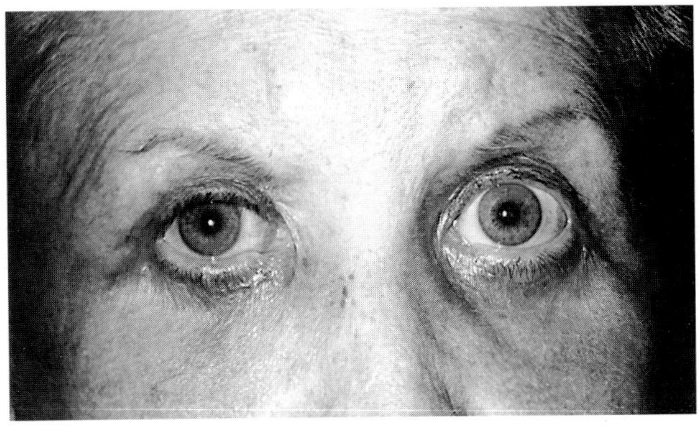

Figure 61–11. This patient presented with multiple complaints after a four-lid blepharoplasty performed by another surgeon. Note the medial canthal fold on the right, the left upper lid retraction, and the inferior displacement of the medial brows. All of these complications result from excess skin excision from the upper lids.

LASH LOSS OR MISDIRECTION

Dissection down to the base of the lash can injure the buds, resulting in lash loss or misdirection. Lost lashes usually regrow in several months. Misdirected lashes are treated as discussed in Chapter 15 on trichiasis.

POSTERIOR LID MARGIN DISEASE (MEIBOMIANITIS)

My impression is that any lid surgery, including blepharoplasty, can increase the symptoms of posterior lid margin disease. This effect may result from some mechanical factor induced by manipulation of the tissues around the tarsal plate; it should be treated with lid scrubs, topical medications, or oral tetracycline, as appropriate.

REFRACTIVE CHANGES

Lid tightening, edema, and changes in the position of the lid margin may induce a temporary refractive change that resolves within the first few weeks after surgery. Rarely, surgery induces a permanent refractive change, usually a plus cylinder at 90 degrees, requiring a change in the patient's eyeglass prescription.

SENSORY NERVE DAMAGE

Patients may report having small areas of anesthesia of the eyelids that results from cutting of the sensory nerves during orbicularis excision. This effect is relatively common in the upper eyelid in the area just inferior to the incision line. The nerves quickly regrow, or the patient learns to ignore the area of numbness. I have seen one case of unilateral supraorbital nerve anesthesia that probably resulted from damage during dissecting of the medial fat pocket of the upper lid.

LID NECROSIS

One case of inadvertent formalin injection into an upper eyelid has resulted in complete necrosis of that eyelid.[40]

OCULOCARDIAC REFLEX

Traction on the orbital fat pockets can produce the oculocardiac reflex with resultant profound bradycardia.[41] If noted, the traction on the orbital fat pocket should be released.

REFERENCES

1. Heinze JB: Blindness after blepharoplasty. Mechanism and early reversal. Plast Reconstr Surg 51:364–370, 1973.
2. Hartley JH, Lester JS, Schatten W: Acute retrobulbar hemorrhage during elective blepharoplasty. Pathophysiology and management. Plast Reconstr Surg 52:8–11, 1973.
3. Jafek BW, Kreiger AE, Morledge D: Blindness following blepharoplasty. Arch Otolaryngol Head Neck Surg 98:366–369, 1973.
4. Lemoine AN, Rees TO, Newell FW: Commentary on retrobulbar hemorrhage following cosmetic blepharoplasty. Plast Reconstr Surg 52:12–15, 1973.
5. Moser MH, DiPirro E, McCoy FJ: Sudden blindness following blepharoplasty. Report of seven cases. Plast Reconstr Surg 51:364–370, 1973.
6. Hueston JT, Heinze JB: Successful early relief of blindness occurring after blepharoplasty. Plast Reconstr Surg 53:588–592, 1974.
7. Putterman AM: Temporary blindness after cosmetic blepharoplasty. Am J Ophthalmol 80:1081–1083, 1975.
8. Helper RS, Sugimura GI, Straatsma BR: On the occurrence of blindness in association with blepharoplasty. Plast Reconstr Surg 57:233–235, 1976.
9. Hueston JT, Heinze JB: A second case of relief of blindness following blepharoplasty. Plast Reconstr Surg 59:430–431, 1977.
10. Heinze JB, Hueston JT: Blindness after blepharoplasty. Mechanism and early reversal. Plast Reconstr Surg 61:347–354, 1978.
11. Waller RR: Is blindness a realistic complication in blepharoplasty procedures? Trans Am Acad Ophthalmol Otolaryngol 85:730–735, 1978.
12. Rafaty FM: Transient total blindness during cosmetic blepharoplasty. Ann Plast Surg 3:373–375, 1979.
13. Anderson RL, Edwards JJ: Bilateral visual loss after blepharoplasty. Ann Plast Surg 5:288–292, 1980.
14. Stasior OG: Blindness associated with cosmetic blepharoplasty. Clin Plast Surg 8:793–795, 1981.
15. Lloyd WC, Leone CR: Transient bilateral blindness following blepharoplasty. Ophthal Plast Reconstr Surg 1:29–34, 1985.
16. DeMere M, Wood T, Austin W: Eye Complications with blepharoplasty or other eyelid surgery. Plast Reconstr Surg 53:634–637, 1974.
17. Lisman RD, Hyde K, Smith B: Complications of blepharoplasty. Clin Plast Surg 15:309–335, 1988.
18. Feldstein M: Discussion of Jafek BW, Kriegar AE, Morledge D: Blindness following blepharoplasty. Arch Otolaryngol 98:369, 1973.
19. Liu O, Stasior OG: Thermal orbital injuries from disposable cauteries. Plast Reconstr Surg 74:1–9, 1984.
20. Castanares S: Complications in blepharoplasty. Clin Plast Surg 5:139–165, 1978.
21. Levine MR, Boynton J, Tenzel RR, et al: Complications of blepharoplasty. Ophthalmic Surg 6:53–57, 1975.
22. Wesley RE, Pollard ZF, McCord CD: Superior oblique paresis after blepharoplasty. Plast Reconstr Surg 66:283–287, 1980.
23. Alfonso E, Levada AJ, Flynn JT: Inferior rectus paresis after secondary blepharoplasty. Br J Ophthalmol 68:535–537, 1984.
24. Harley RD, Nelson LB, Flanagan JC, et al: Ocular motility disturbances following cosmetic blepharoplasty. Arch Ophthalmol 104:542–544, 1986.
25. Neely KA, Ernest JT, Mottier M: Combined superior oblique paresis and Brown's syndrome after blepharoplasty. Am J Ophthalmol 109:347–348, 1990.
26. Hayworth RS, Lisman RD, Muchnick RS, Smith B: Diplopia following blepharoplasty. Ann Ophthalmol 16:448–451, 1984.
27. Smith B, Nesi FA: The complications of cosmetic blepharoplasty. Trans Am Acad Ophthalmol Otolaryngol 85:726–729, 1978.
28. Tenzel RR: Surgical treatment of complications of cosmetic blepharoplasty. Clin Plast Surg 5:517–523, 1978.
29. Baylis HI, Sutcliffe T, Fett DR: Levator injury during blepharoplasty. Arch Ophthalmol 102:570–571, 1984.
30. Tenzel RR: Cosmetic blepharoplasty. *In* Soll DB (ed): Management of Complications in Ophthalmic Plastic Surgery. Birmingham, AL, Aesculapius, 1976, pp 119–131.
31. Wojno T, Lieberman WJ, Tenzel RR, et al: Non-surgical correction of post-blepharoplasty ectropion. Adv Ophthal Plast Reconstr Surg 2:113–118, 1983.
32. Edgerton MT: Causes and prevention of lower lid ectropion following blepharoplasty. Plast Reconstr Surg 49:367–373, 1972.
33. Tenzel RR; Complications of blepharoplasty. Orbital hematoma, ectropion, and scleral show. Clin Plast Surg 8:797–802, 1981.
34. Shorr N, Fallor MK: "Madame Butterfly" procedure: Combined cheek and lateral canthal suspension procedure for post-blepharoplasty, "round eye" and lower eyelid retraction. Ophthal Plast Reconstr Surg 1:229–234, 1985.
35. Wojno T, Tenzel RR: Dermis grafts in socket reconstruction. Ophthal Plast Reconstr Surg 2:7–14, 1986.
36. Tenzel RR: Upper eyelid crease formation. *In* Putterman AM, (ed): Cosmetic Oculoplastic Surgery. New York, Grune & Stratton, 1982, pp 179–186.
37. Morgan SC: Orbital cellulitis and blindness following a blepharoplasty. Plast Reconstr Surg 64:823–826, 1979.
38. Rees TD, Craig SM, Fisher Y: Orbital abscess following blepharoplasty. Plast Reconstr Surg 73:126, 1984.
39. Converse JM: Clinical note: Treatment of epithelialized suture tracts of the eyelid by marsupialization. Plast Reconstr Surg 38:576, 1966.
40. Smith B, Nesi FA: Upper lid loss due to formalin injection: Surgical reconstruction. Trans Am Acad Ophthalmol Otolaryngol 86: 1951–1955, 1979.
41. Matarasso A: The oculocardiac reflex in blepharoplasty surgery. Plast Reconstr Surg 83:243–248, 1989.

CHAPTER 62

Lymphatic Drainage Massage

Peter T. Pugliese and Linda Garofallou

Lymphatic drainage massage is a physical technique that assists the movement of lymphatic fluid in the body tissues. The earliest use of gravity to assist lymphatic drainage by elevation of the extremities is lost in antiquity, but it continues to be a simple and very effective method to move lymphatic fluid. A system of massage techniques has been developed over the past 60 years that incorporates both art and science into an effective treatment modality little known to most physicians. This system is called manual lymphatic drainage (MLD), commonly know as the Vodder method.

Emil Vodder and his wife Estrid observed during the early 1930s that individuals with lymphadenopathy secondary to upper respiratory infections could benefit by gentle massage of these swollen lymph nodes. Experimenting with various techniques involving combinations of pressure and motions, the Vodders found that not only did the swelling of the lymph nodes decrease but also the upper respiratory infection symptoms disappeared. After many years of trials and observations, the Vodders established a training school for their system, where many technicians have been trained in MLD.

ANATOMY AND PHYSIOLOGY OF THE LYMPHATIC SYSTEM

A thorough knowledge of the anatomy and physiology of the lymphatic system is crucial to understanding and appreciating the benefits derived from MLD. The lymphatic system is a primitive method of moving fluid through the body of animals. It is however, an evolutionary marvel when the details of the structure are closely examined. Every cell in the body must be supplied with nutrition, oxygen, hormones, water, essential ions, and other material. The metabolic process requires not only the delivery of these essentials but also the removal of their byproducts, as waste. Each cell is not contiguous with its neighbor but is surrounded by a thin fluid layer that provides the contact with the fluid stream that is essential to the metabolic process. The task of the lymphatic system is to remove these waste products and return them to the blood stream, where they may be recycled or destroyed. We assume that the reader is generally familiar with the gross anatomy of the lymphatic system, so a general description is not included here.

The system starts with the tiny subcutaneous lymph vessels (Fig. 62–1). The lymphatic system can be viewed as drains that remove metabolic debris. The best description of the function of the lymphatic system has been provided by Ryan:

> The lymphatics are the drains that take away the debris and excesses of daily wear and tear in the tissues. While there are incinerators everywhere in the form of macrophages, even these need a disposal system for their ashes. The lymphatics, by draining into lymph nodes, ensure that any kind of peripheral pollution is monitored and adequately dealt with by the mobile team of specifically programmed cells. The lymphatics are essential channels for the return of protein and cells from the tissues into the blood stream.[1]

LYMPHATIC FLUID

The lymphatic fluid contains most of the constituents of the blood plasma. The protein content of lymphatic fluid averages 4.9 g/dL, but the glucose level may be 20% to 25% higher than the blood plasma glucose level, which is 130 to 140 mg/dL.[2] Cholesterol, uric acid, and nonprotein nitrogen content are present in about the same concentration in lymphatic fluid as in the blood plasma. The amount of lymph drained each day as measured in the thoracic duct ranges from 2 to 4 L/day, or 2 to 3 mL/minute.[3] Lymphatic fluid is usually colorless, except when it flows from the intestinal region after a meal.

LYMPHATIC VESSELS

The smallest lymphatic vessels are actually cavities, or pools of fluid, lined with endothelial cells that become interconnected channels. A unidirectional flow, toward the heart, is maintained by valves and smooth muscle walls. Interestingly, these fluid-filled tissue spaces are early nutritional supply systems that continue as cerebral

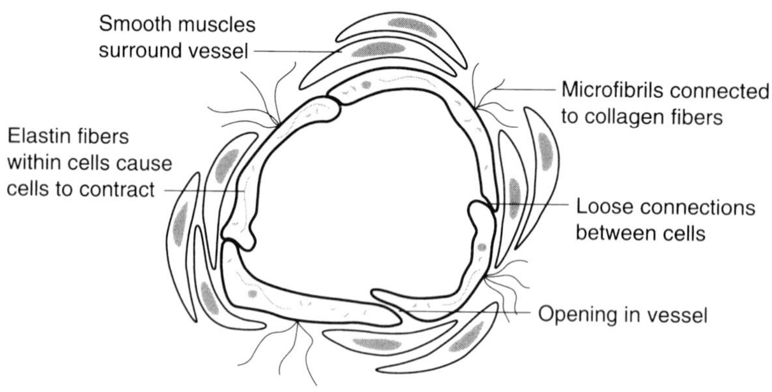

Figure 62–1. Diagram of a cross-section (end view) of a small lymphatic vessel. Note the loose approximation of the cells and the microfibrils attached to the cells. These microfibers attach to collagen fibers in the interstitium.

fluid. The endothelial cell of the lymphatic vessel is flatter and almost featureless.[4, 5] The mitochondria and endoplasmic reticula are fewer in number, although the Golgi apparatus is of normal size. Elastic fibers are located just under the endothelial cells. Numerous gaps are present in the vessel because cell-to-cell contact occurs only at isolated points at the periphery of the cell. When the vessels are stretched, these openings become even wider because of the collagen fibers that are attached to these endothelial cells; moving the tissue moves the attached vessel (see Fig. 62–1).

In the skin, the lymphatic vessels are located in the papillary dermis. They are not visible under light microscopy. Figure 62–2 is a diagram of the lymphatic vessels that shows the endothelial cells and the valves. The segment between valves is called a lymphangion, the size of which may vary from 1 to 15 mm, the latter being in the thoracic duct. These vessels are composed of loosely joined cells with the remarkable ability of containing fluid while at the same time being able to admit fluid and propel it in a directional manner (Fig. 62–3).

PUMPING ACTION OF THE LYMPHATIC VESSELS

Blood capillaries pass nutrient fluids into the interstitial spaces, which are at very low pressure, around −6 mm Hg. The increase in fluid in the interstitial space raises the interstitial pressure, forcing the collagen and elastin fibers to move apart. Because the endothelial cells of the lymphatic vessels are anchored to the interstitium by the connecting microfilaments, these cells move outward, widening the lumen of the lymphatic vessel. As the lumen widens, the endothelial cells separate, allowing interstitial fluid to pass into the lumen. Increased hydrostatic pressure in the lumen of the vessel causes the endothelial cells to tighten by contraction of the cytoplasmic actin–like filaments, and as a result, the lymphatic valves close. This process sets the stage for the next step, which is the propulsion of the fluid toward the heart.

FORWARD PROPULSION OF LYMPHATIC FLUID

This seemingly simple filling process provides the mechanism for the movement of fluid into the lymphatics and triggers the forward propulsion of the fluid. Although a great deal of attention has been paid to external auxilliary forces as the major contributors to the forward movement of lymphatic fluid, we now know that the real propulsive force is provided by elastic and smooth muscle fibers. These fibers surround the lymphatic vessels between the lymphangions, and they contract in a rhythmic pattern. Although each lymphangion appears to be independent, the contraction rhythm allows the forward lymphangion to relax while the distal

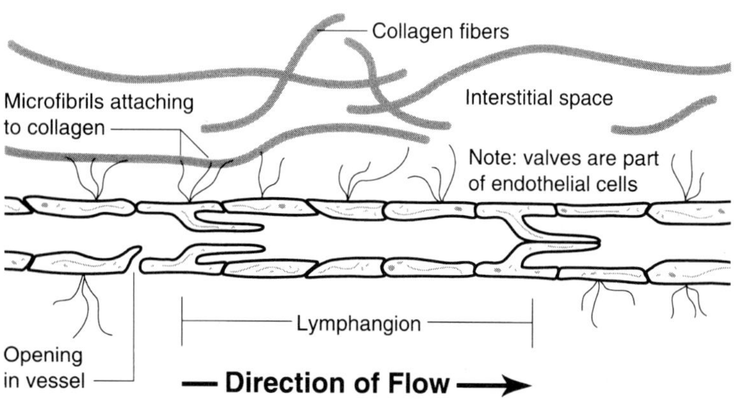

Figure 62–2. Diagram of a lymphatic vessel and lymphangion. Note the valves at both ends of the lymphangion: one is open and the other is closed. The openings in the vessel close when the lymphangion is filled with fluid and a high tension is placed on the vessel walls. The contracting smooth muscles are not shown in this diagram.

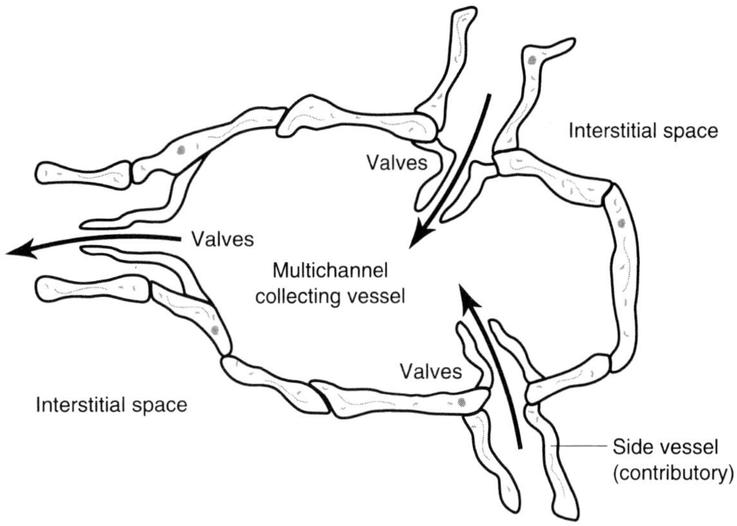

Figure 62–3. Diagram of a multichannel collecting vessel. Multiple vessels empty into one larger collecting chamber. When the chamber is filled and tension is at the right level, the two posterior, or contributing, vessels will be shut off by their valves and the fluid will be propelled forward.

one is contracting.[6] During this period, the valves of the forward lymphangion are open while the distal lymphangion valves are closed (see Fig. 62–2).

The concept of tissue compliance is at the heart of MLD, and an understanding of this concept assists in the appreciation of the applications of MLD. Compliance is a term used in physics to describe the strain, or movement, of an elastic material that is subjected to a given force. In the case of tissue, which has viscoelastic properties, a force transmitted by a pulsation of a blood vessel through that tissue is greater if the compliance is less. In other words, as compliance increases, elasticity decreases and vice versa. In the case of lymphedema, the compliance is greatly increased so that the effective pumping action of the vessels is decreased. In tissues with elastosis, abnormally dilated vessels have been observed that suggest widened lymphatic vessels. For example, in acne rosacea, which is characterized by elastosis, marked lymphedema is present.[7]

PULSE-WAVE NATURE OF LYMPHATIC FLOW

Numerous studies have shown that the flow of lymphatic fluid is rhythmic, with pulsations occurring at various intervals. The pulse rate varies from 1 to 30 pulses per minute. The pressure produced by these pulses ranges from 1 to 25 mm Hg.[4] Interestingly, as the pressure rises in the lymphatic vessels, the number of contractions increases so that the volume of fluid moved is related to both the pressure and the number of contractions. Even more interesting is that these same investigators found that the rate of formation of lymphatic fluid is the controlling factor in both the frequency and the force of the pulse and pressure in the vessels.[4] The contraction of associated muscles and the transmitted impulses from contracting arteries have very little influence on the movement of the lymphatic fluid. Only in the thoracic duct did any association exist between volume of fluid moved and respiratory effort; a direct correlation was noted. These studies indicate that the major forces moving the lymphatic fluid are (1) the formation of the fluid in the interstitial spaces, (2) the intrinsic pressure within the lymphatic vessels, and (3) the force and number of contractions produced by the vessel.

In summary, the flow of lymph proceeds stepwise as follows. Increased formation of lymph in the tissue increases interstitial pressure, which causes the endothelial cells of the lymphatic vessels to open and receive the new fluid. As the fluid enters the vessels, the vessels fill, stretching the endothelial cells and causing the actin-like cytoplasmic fibers to contract and close the inlet valves between the cells. The proximal valves then open, and the distal valves close as the expanded lymphangion contracts and the lymph is moved forward (see Fig. 62–3).[8]

PERIOCULAR SOFT TISSUE AND POSTOPERATIVE EDEMA

Because the globe rests in a compartment of fat within the bony socket of the skull, it is well equipped to handle most mild traumatic insults, including the trauma of eyelid surgery. The eyelids, however, are not so well equipped. Considering the histologic structure of the eyelid, a great deal of soft tissue space waits to be filled with interstitial fluid. The orbicularis oculi muscle is sandwiched in the center of the eyelid, with soft connective tissue present both anteriorly and posteriorly. The amount of collagen and elastic is quite small; therefore, any increase in interstitial fluid results in a marked swelling of the eyelids. The lymphatic vessels are not overly abundant in the eyelids; most of the vessels are in the posterior portion. Generally, the distribution of lymphatic vessels about the lids parallels the course of the facial vein and its tributaries.

After surgery, the inflammatory process is typical of most post-traumatic inflammatory states. Vasodilation occurs, plasma seeps from the capillaries, and interstitial fluid increases within the interstitial spaces. The soft, thin eyelids are easily swollen to a considerable size, frequently obscuring vision. Fortunately, the thinness of the eyelids allows the interstitial fluid to be moved into the lymphatic system with gentle lymphatic drainage.

PROTEIN AND OSMOTIC PRESSURE

The protein concentration of the lymphatic fluid is higher than that of the tissue fluid, as noted earlier. The large protein molecules enter the lymphatic vessels along with lymphatic cellular elements, such as lymphocytes and macrophages. A colloidal osmotic pressure difference is built up along the length of the lymphatic vessels; this concentration difference increases as the vessels move proximally. This increased osmotic pressure at the larger end of the vessels is unlikely to play a great role in the movement of lymphatic fluid. A combination of hydrostatic pressure and osmotic pressure controls the flow of lymph from the tissue spaces, but these forces appear to be more important at the capillary end.

LYMPHATIC DRAINAGE MASSAGE

The anatomy and physiology of the lymphatic system provide the foundation for the methods used in MLD. Lymphatic massage has a scientific basis, as indicated by the many articles related to this system in the scientific literature.[9-14] MLD is usually presented by a practitioner skilled in this area or through a training course.

The amount of pressure used in MLD is very important. Vodder recommends using 30 to 40 mm Hg, or 8 to 12 ounces per square inch, but even lighter pressure, as low as 1 ounce per square inch, may be used. The direction of the massage is consistent with the direction of the lymphatic flow. For superficial edema of the skin, a series of six to seven strokes per minute over a 1-square-inch area is repeated until the tissue is perceptibly different. The degree of edema determines the amount of pressure to be applied. Tissue that is distended from edema requires lighter pressure; excess pressure causes the lymphatic flow to stop flowing. Lymphatic vessels can dilate 10 to 15 times their normal size when the interstitial fluid increases, and not very much additional external pressure is required to collapse these dilated vessels. Light pressure applied externally to the tissues is sufficient to induce contraction of the vessels via the intrinsic elastic fiber network within the lymphatic vessels. The intermittent application and removal of pressure produces the pumping action of MLD, duplicating the body's own lymphatic pumping mechanism.

The application of pressure in the Vodder technique[15] requires four hand movements: stationary circles, pump techniques, scoop technique, and rotary technique. All of these movements apply light pressure and stretching action to the tissue surrounding the lymphatic vessels. The treatment durations are usually 30 to 45 minutes, but sessions as long as 1.5 hours may be needed. The description of the movements follows.

Stationary Circles. Using the palms of the hands or the pads of the fingertips, the practitioner makes a circular motion that is sufficient to move the skin. This motion is used mainly for the head and neck.

Pumping. The cupped wrist is flexed and extended with the palmar surface on the skin to contact and stretch the skin. This motion is used mainly on the arms and legs.

Scooping. The wrist is flexed and extended, using the thumb as a pivot, while the forearm is supinated. In this motion again, the palmar surface contacts the skin and stretches it. This motion is used on the arms and legs.

Rotary. Flexion and extension of the wrist is applied in a rotary motion with the palmar surface contacting and stretching the skin. This motion is used on large surface areas, such as the buttocks, back, and abdomen.

HAUSCHKA LYMPHATIC STIMULATION

The Hauschka modification of the Vodder technique was developed for the treatment of the head and neck. It was developed to encourage the spontaneous activation of the lymph system. This goal is achieved through a series of rhythmic hand and brush movements that stimulate the lymph nodes and lymphatic fluid to initiate the inherent and spontaneous activity of the lymph. The gentle and rhythmic movements stimulate the lymph flow, not directly by conducting manual manipulation, but by setting up the conditions to initiate the spontaneous contractility of the lymphangions, thereby activating the flow of the lymphatic fluid. In this way, the lymphatic stimulation method helps the lymphatic system to help itself.

The rhythmic hand and brush movements used in Hauschka lymphatic stimulation are performed in a series of rhythmic repetitions. They begin by opening the nodes in the neck and then follow the natural flow lines, leading the lymph downward from the forehead to the chest area, where the lymph returns to the venous system. The effectiveness of the stimulation is achieved through the gentle but precise pressure of the fingers, hands, and brushes and the rhythmic quality of the movements. The rhythm inherent in these movements stimulates a parallel rhythmic activity in the lymphangion that results in the lymph flow. Interestingly, the term *rhythm* comes from the Greek word "rhythmos," which means "to flow."

Treatments using lymphatic stimulation are recommended preoperatively to help clear the lymph nodes and to prepare the skin and lymphatic system for the surgical procedure. Because of the subtle and gentle nature of the hand and brush movements, treatments postoperatively can begin the day after surgery and should be performed two times per week for the first 2 weeks and thereafter on an individual basis, depending on the speed of wound healing. Direct contact over the surgical site is avoided until the sutures have been removed.

Other Features of Lymphatic Drainage Massage. Pressure bandages are recommended as additional therapy when MLD is used on the extremities.[16] This added measure increases the duration of the benefit desired from MLD. Pressure must be maximal at the distal end of the extremities and less at the proximal end of the extremities. Special types of sleeve garments with correct pressures are available for this therapy in Europe.[16] The article by Harris is an excellent introduction to MLD and some of its applications.[17]

MECHANICAL METHODS OF LYMPHATIC DRAINAGE

Some mechanical devices have been reported to be beneficial in assisting the flow of lymph fluid. Evidence suggests that mechanical devices may be of benefit in lymphatic drainage. Only three physical modalities provide movement of the tissues that aid in lymph flow. The first of these is direct external pressure, which occurs with MLD. A device that is capable of delivering a well-controlled pressure in a repetitive manner could be helpful, if it were versatile enough to mimic the action of the fingertips. The second means is an intermittent suction device that could lift the skin and produce movement in the interstitial tissue indirectly. This type of device may have a serious drawback in areas where the tissue is less resilient. The third method is a vibration device that delivers a series of intermittent pulses to the skin's surface. The method has been tested by Ryan and Salter and, to our knowledge, is the only method that is supported by a clinical trial proving both the efficacy and safety of this technique.[18]

All mechanically assisted devices are designed to make the application of lymphatic drainage easier to perform by providing a standardized force to the skin along with a highly regulated rhythm. Such devices may be of benefit in extending the use of lymphatic drainage, but at present more clinical trials are needed to provide supportive data for the use of these devices.

INDICATIONS FOR MANUAL LYMPHATIC DRAINAGE

Just as in any art or science, the more one is familiar with a method, the more applications one can see. The dangers in MLD arise from (1) use by inexperienced, although well-meaning, practitioners, (2) failure to understand the scientific basis of the method, and (3) assumptions that the method is a panacea for all the human ills. Some of the indications and contraindications for MLD are listed in Tables 62–1 and 62–2, respectively.

TABLE 62–1

Indications for Manual Lymphatic Drainage
Trauma-induced swelling
Injuries such as sprains, strains, hematomas, and bruises
Postsurgical edema, particularly postmastectomy lymphedema
Edema of the extremities, radiation edema
Chronic inflammatory disorders
Arthritic swellings, bursitis, tendinitis
Cellulitis
Scar tissue
Dermatologic conditions
Acne
Noninflammatory, atopic dermatitis
Rosacea

PHARMACOLOGY OF LYMPHATIC VESSELS

In the excellent report by Wang and Zhong,[9] an extensive study on the lymphatic system of the rat provided corroboration with studies on the lymphatic system from other species, including humans. These investigators feel that the main propulsive force of lymphatic flow is the smooth muscles in the vessels. By using various pharmacologic agents, they studied the effects of stimulation of both alpha- and beta-receptors on the smooth muscles. When applied to smooth muscle, epinephrine caused a spasmodic contraction of the lymphatic vessel immediately after application. This action was blocked by phentolamine, an α-adrenergic blocking agent that is also a vasodilator. The effect of isoproterenol, a beta-receptor stimulator, is blocked effectively by the beta-blocker propranolol. This result indicates that as are blood vessels, the lymphatic vessels are also subject to neurohumoral factors.[9] While pharmacologic effects are present, the underlying tension in the tissues as new lymphatic fluid is formed dilates the vessels and triggers the contraction of the smooth muscles via the reflex arc. Wang and Zhong also observed that above a certain tension, the lymphatic vessel failed to contract.[9] This effect is observed in lymphedema, in which tissue pressure may be high.

TABLE 62–2

Contraindications for Manual Lymphatic Drainage
Any acute inflammatory condition
Metastatic carcinoma
Cardiac edema
Thrombosis
Certain metabolic disorders, such as thyroid disease
Hypotension

SUMMARY

MLD has long been used in Europe, but only recently has the technique been used in the United States. As with any new drug or technique in medicine, it will take time to learn the applications and use of MLD. We are at the early stages of our understanding of the lymphatic system, even though great advances have been made in the past 20 years. In spite of the vast complexity of the immune aspects of the lymphatic system, we now have a physical modality that promises relief in conditions that do not respond to conventional treatments. Although not a panacea, MLD is a useful treatment modality that deserves serious attention.

REFERENCES

1. Ryan TJ: Lymphatics of the skin. *In* Jarrett A (ed): The Physiology and Pathophysiology of the Skin, vol 5. London, Academic Press, 1978, p 1756.
2. Altman PL: Lymph. *In* Dittmer DS (ed): Handbook of Blood and Other Body Fluids. Washington, DC, Federation of American Societies for Experimental Biology, 1961.
3. Hall JG, Morris B, Woolley G: Intrinsic rhythmic propulsion of lymph in the sheep. J Physiol 180:336–349, 1965.
4. Casely-Smith JR: Lymph and lymphatics. *In* Kaley G, Altura BM (eds): Microcirculation. Baltimore University Park Press, 1977, pp 423–502.
5. Wilson-Jones E: Malignant vascular tumors. J Clin Exp Dermatol 1:297–312, 1976.
6. Mislin H: Active contractility of the lymphangion and coordination of lymphangion chains. Experientia 37:820, 1976.
7. Marks R, Harcourt-Webster JN: Histopathology of rosacea. Arch Dermatol 100:683–691, 1969.
8. Smith RO: Lymphatic contractility, a possible intrinsic mechanism of lymphatic vessels for transport of lymph. J Exp Med 90:497, 1949.
9. Wang G, Zhong S: Experimental study of lymphatic contractility and its clinical importance. Ann Plast Surg 15:278, 1985.
10. MacMaster PD: Conditions in the skin influencing interstitial fluid movement, lymph formation and lymph flow. Ann NY Acad Sci 46:743, 1976.
11. Caener JS, Pflug JJ, Reig NO, et al: Lymphatic pressures and the flow of lymph. Br J Plast Surg 232:305, 1970.
12. Olszewski WL, Engeset A: Intrinsic contractility of prenodal lymph vessels and lymph flow in the human leg. J Physiol 239:H775, 1980.
13. Emmett AJJ, Barron NJ, Veal N: Clinical assessment of patients with lymphedema. J Plast Reconstr Surg 20:1–15, 1967.
14. Godat S, Leduc A, Delacave G: De L'influence du massage lymphatique sur la progression de la lymphe. Angeiolorie 23:214–218, 1973.
15. Wittinger H, Wittinger G: Textbook of Dr Vodder's Manual Lymph Drainage, vol 1, Basic Course. 3rd ed revised. Translated by Harris RH. UK, Haug, Heidelberg, Appl Bio, 1990.
16. Hutzschenreuter PO, Wittlinger H, Wittlinger G, et al: Post-mastectomy arm lymphaedema: Treated by manual lymph drainage and compression bandage therapy. Eur J Phys Med Rehabil 1:166–170, 1991.
17. Harris R: An introduction to manual lymph drainage. Massage Ther J 31:55–66, 1992.
18. Ryan TJ, Salter DC: The effect of vibration on the skin blood flow. Bibl Anat 16:180–184, 1977.

CHAPTER 63

Principles of Camouflage Make-up and the Postoperative Patient

Annette Hanson and Nancy Dugan

Camouflage make-up therapy is increasingly gaining recognition as an adjunctive service recommended by dermatologists and cosmetic surgeons after elective surgery. There are many facilities offering training in camouflage therapy; and, as a result, there are qualified camouflage therapists working in clinics who are available to assist physicians. The aim of camouflage make-up is to conceal the incisions, ecchymosis, and edema during the early postsurgical period (Figs. 63–1 through 63–3). This helps to normalize the patient's appearance as quickly as possible, as well as to minimize the postsurgical anxiety that frequently results; it also allows the patient to return to work and social activities as soon as possible.

PATIENT MANAGEMENT

If referral of a patient to a camouflage therapist is considered by a surgeon, the patient should consult with the therapist before surgery so that he or she will realistically understand what can be achieved. Not all ecchymoses and edema can be disguised perfectly, and it is important that the patient know in advance what to expect. The patient's anxiety can be minimized with the use of a series of preoperative and postoperative photographs of other patients demonstrating the healing and camouflaging processes.

WHEN TO USE CAMOUFLAGE MAKE-UP

The surgeon must determine the best time to camouflage each patient on a case-by-case basis. Usually, however, one can apply camouflage cosmetics to cover discoloration or to disguise swelling 1 to 2 days after surgery. If the surgical procedure required a skin incision, once the incision is completely closed and the sutures have been removed, make-up can be applied 24 hours later.

CHOOSING A CAMOUFLAGE MAKE-UP

The camouflage product itself should be waterproof, should be long lasting, and should contain a total sun block to protect damaged or sensitive areas (Table 63–1). It should be opaque to provide complete coverage, yet remain lightweight to ensure a natural look. The cream should not be chalky or waxy and should spread easily so it does not drag on the skin. The product should be nonirritating, be fragrance free, and feature a number of colors available to easily match a wide variety of skin tones.

Camouflage make-up is more occlusive than regular make-up and therefore requires special products to accompany its usage: a cleanser that will thoroughly remove camouflage make-up and prevent product buildup on the skin; a toning lotion to ensure that no oil is left on the skin before application; and a translucent, hypoallergenic finishing powder to ensure that the make-up sets properly.

CHOOSING THE CORRECT COLORS FOR CAMOUFLAGE

The best camouflage is achieved by choosing the proper colors to offset the skin's discoloration. With ecchymosis the bruise is initially a dark purple in the center, surrounded by a yellow area. As the bruise heals, the yellow area increases while the purple area fades. Occasionally, erythema will surround the bruise. To camouflage, one must consider color theory to be able to successfully offset discoloration.

All colors are based on the three primary colors: red, blue, and yellow (Fig. 63–4*A*). By mixing together two adjoining primary colors in equal proportions, we arrive at the secondary colors: orange, green, and violet (see Fig. 63–4*B*). By using a color wheel, we can see the opposite of each color, better known as its complementary color.

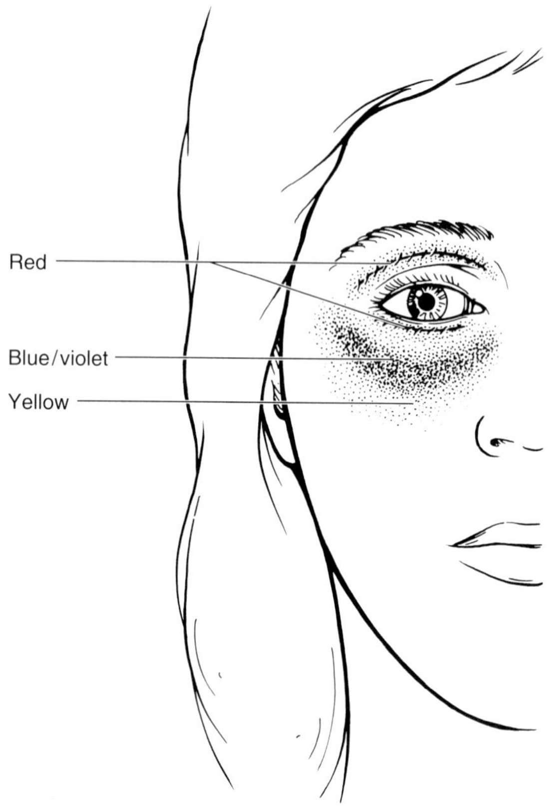

Figure 63–1. Illustration of the postoperative patient with erythema and the various colors of ecchymosis indicated. The aim of camouflage make-up is to effectively reduce postoperative anxiety and minimize the disruption of the patient's work and social schedules.

In the diagram, green is the complement of red, orange the complement of blue, and violet the complement of yellow. The understanding of complements is essential to be able to neutralize the skin's discoloration effectively (Fig. 63–5).

NEUTRALIZING SKIN DISCOLORATIONS

Selecting or blending the base coat to match the patient's skin is extremely important. The base color is the preoperative color of the skin (the patient's natural skin tone). Skin contains elements of all the primary colors. The addition of black or white may be necessary to help match the skin tone. A good camouflage line will frequently contain skin tone colors crossing the spectrum from light, medium, to dark skin tones and will include warm and cool colors (warm colors are those with a yellow, rose, or orange cast; cool are those with a bluish, green, or violet cast). Most of the time achieving a good match with the skin tone is simply a matter of blending two skin tone colors together. The goal is to make the procedure as easy as possible so the patient can get the same results at home.

APPLYING COLOR PRINCIPLES

To neutralize the purple in a bruise, use yellow pigment; for a yellowish area, violet; for a reddened area, green. One method of coverage is to add small amounts of these offsetting pigments to the base color. Another method is to first apply a thin layer of the pigment required to neutralize the bruise, followed by the base color to cover. When layering, each layer must be powdered separately before proceeding to the next layer. There are no absolute rules for coverage; each case must be judged separately depending on the color of the patient's natural skin tone as well as on the depth of discoloration (Fig. 63–6).

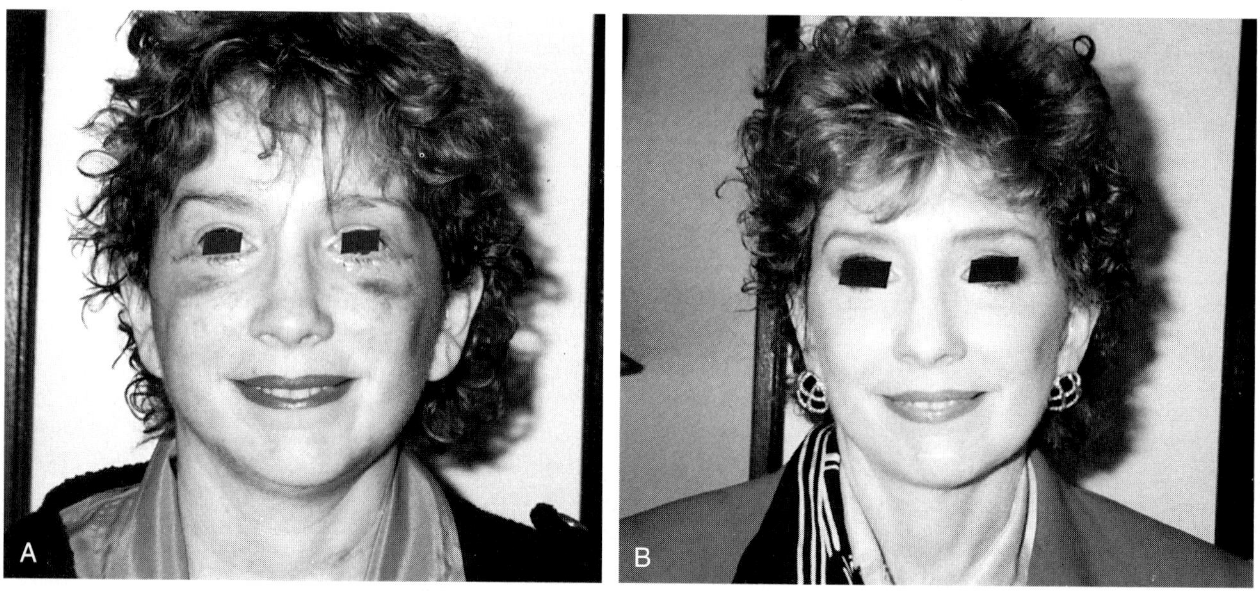

Figure 63–2. *A*, A 50-year-old woman 1 week after transcutaneous lower lid blepharoplasty. *B*, The same patient after camouflage make-up. (*A* and *B* courtesy of Lillian Lang, Lang Institute of Philadelphia; make-up by Jacqueline Leftwich of Xanadoo, Philadelphia, PA.)

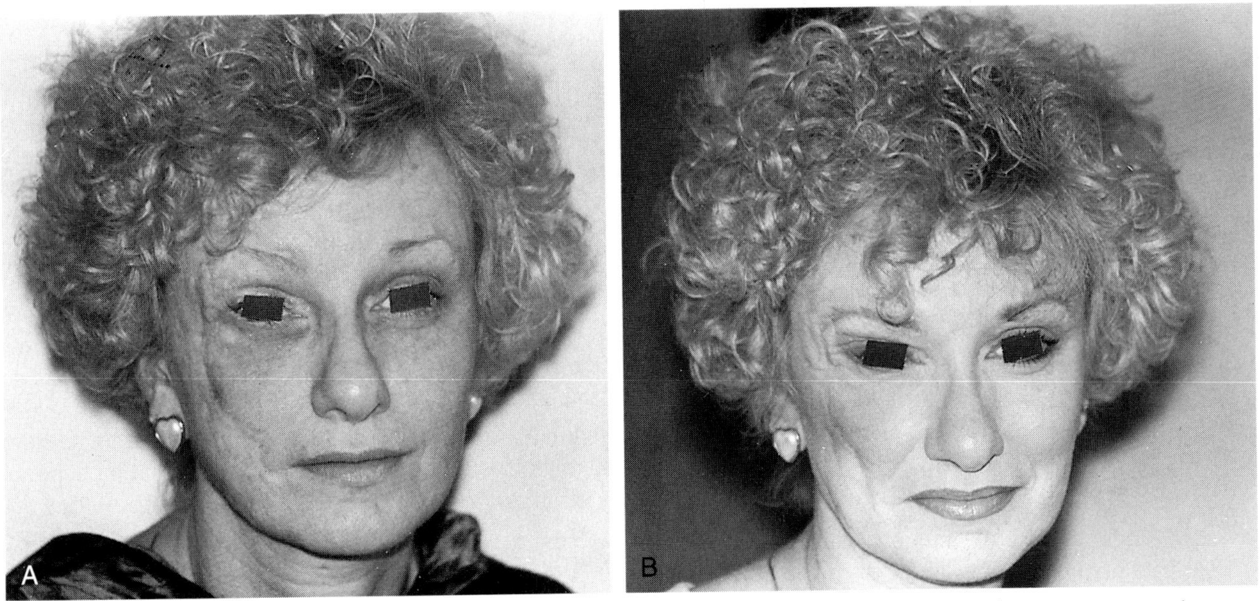

Figure 63–3. *A*, A 49-year-old woman 15 years after multiple traumatic facial injuries and multiple facial reconstructive procedures. *B*, Improvement after camouflage make-up. (*A* and *B* courtesy of Lillian Lang, Lang Institute of Philadelphia; make-up by Jacqueline Leftwich of Xanadoo, Philadelphia, PA.)

LIGHTING

Another consideration to ensure undetectable coverage is lighting. The best results will come from working under natural sunlight. Because this is not always possible, be aware that the worst light to work under is incandescent light (standard light bulb), which adds too much yellow; fluorescent light is too blue/green to allow an accurate match. However, some full-spectrum light bulbs are available, as well as full-spectrum tubes that are second to sunlight in their accuracy. A brief discussion of color principles should help patients to understand how to alter their own color results in the light that they will be working under at home.

APPLICATION PRINCIPLES

To apply camouflage make-up, use a small brush (e.g., lip brush) for the smaller areas and a finger or latex wedge for the larger ones. It is essential to start with clean, oil-free skin, because any moisturizers, oils, or make-up will negatively affect the occlusive ability of the camouflage products.

Proper aim is of paramount importance when camouflaging an area with a hard edge. The make-up must be applied accurately, within the boundaries of the discol-

TABLE 63–1
Selected List of Camouflage Make-up Lines

DERMACOLOR 32 Ninth Street c/o Kryolan Corporation San Francisco, CA 94103-2603 (415) 863-9684
VEIL c/o ATELIER ESTHETIQUE 386 Park Avenue South—Suite 1409 New York, NY 10016 (800) 626-1242

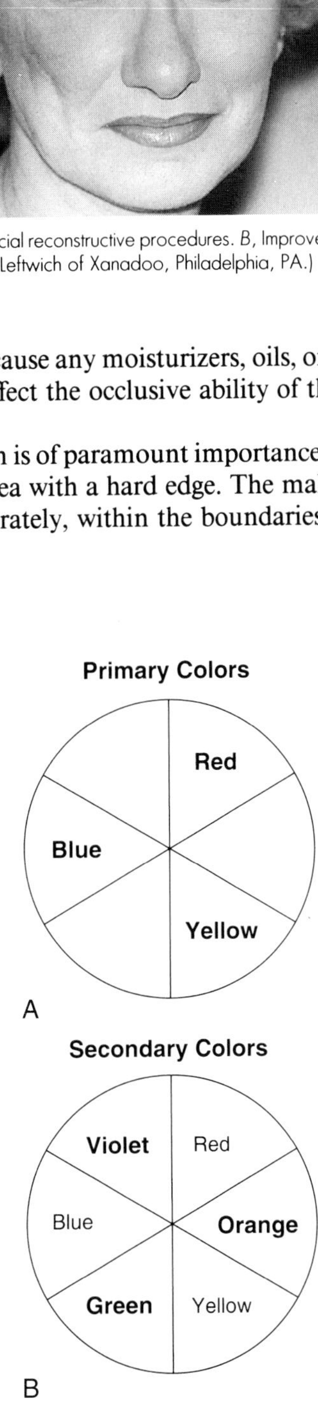

Figure 63–4. *A*, Primary colors. *B*, Secondary colors.

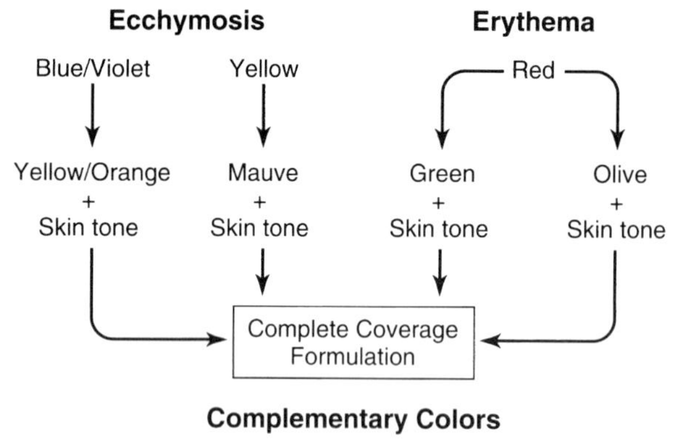

Figure 63–5. Complementary color scheme. This is essential in neutralizing skin discoloration effectively.

ored area, or the camouflaged area may be left surrounded by a light or odd-colored ring. The camouflage therapist may need to "fan out" the base color to gradually blend the camouflaged area with the unaffected surrounding skin. The make-up coverage should be thin and even; two thin layers are better than one thick one. If the colors have been selected properly, there is no need to apply a thick unnatural-looking layer of make-up to the skin; an even texture should be maintained wherever possible.

After the camouflage cream product is applied, it must be set immediately with a camouflage finishing powder. The use of powder is imperative to give the camouflaged area a matte (nonoily) appearance, to prevent the camouflage make-up from "slipping," and to ensure long-lasting, waterproof coverage. If multiple layers of camouflage cream are being used, the powder must go between each layer so as not to dislodge the previously applied layer. The final layer must also be set with powder.

Enhancement make-up (regular fashion make-up) can follow the camouflage, but it is highly recommended, especially after eyelid surgery, that the patient purchase new make-up products to ensure that they are free of bacteria. Using powdered blushes and eyeshadows is recommended since cream products could disturb the camouflage products. If an eyeliner pencil is used, it must be soft enough not to drag on the skin. Mascara should be water soluble and fiber free. Foundations should be water based.

LIGHT AND DARK: HIGHLIGHTING AND CONTOURING

Camouflaging hypertrophic and hypotrophic areas is considerably more difficult than camouflaging discolorations. Although the discoloration in these areas can be effectively camouflaged, there are certain limitations.

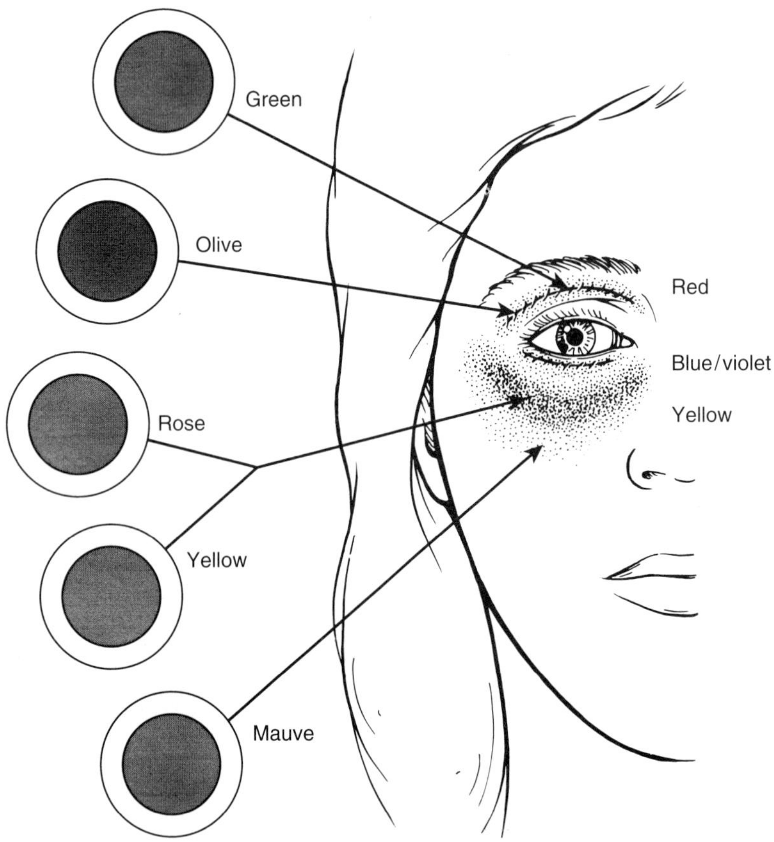

Figure 63–6. Illustration indicating the neutralization of skin discoloration using pigments.

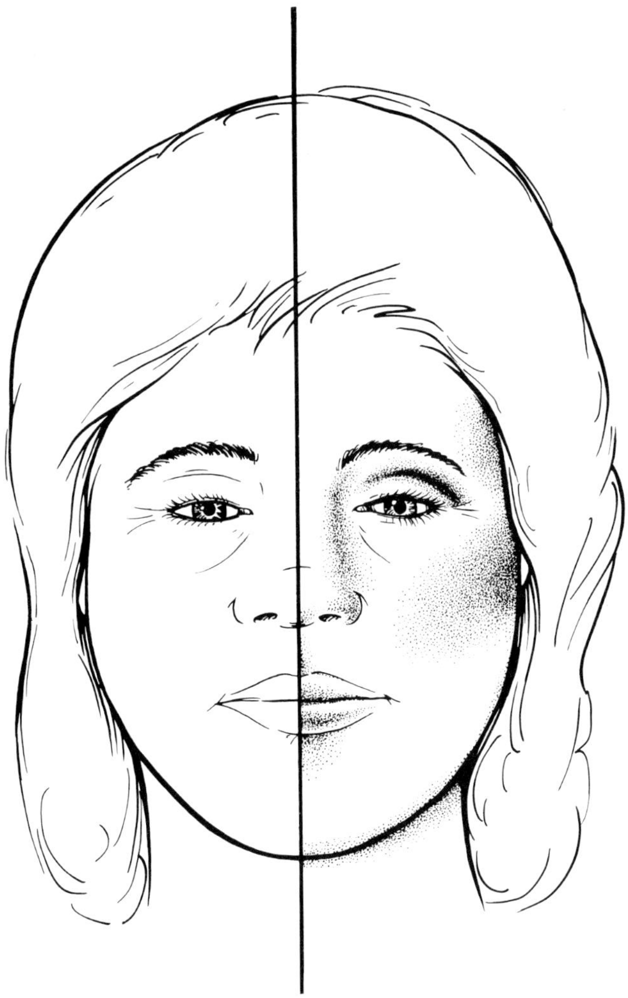

Figure 63–7. This diagram illustrates both a swollen face *(left)* and a contoured face *(right)* created by camouflage make-up.

For instance, shape is dramatically affected by the light to which it is subjected. Humans are constantly moving in and out of doors; and, as a result, camouflaged areas appear differently in the varying lighting. The rule to keep in mind when attempting to alter the perceived shape of an area is that light "brings out" or "highlights" and dark "recedes" or "contours." For example, when camouflaging edema or swelling, a slightly darker base than usual is used in the areas where bone structure would normally allow the skin to sink in (i.e., underneath the cheekbone, at the temples, at the superior sulcus, under the lower lip, at the sides of the nose, under the jawbone). By doing this, a shadow is created and the appearance of swelling is reduced (Fig. 63–7).

REALISM: FAKING FAULTS

Since camouflage make-up has a tendency to obliterate all "faults" in the skin as it covers, it may be necessary to employ the technique known as "faking faults," in which the natural look of freckles, moles, undereye circles, visible capillaries, and beard hair is replaced with make-up. Faking faults is done over an already powdered area and is then followed by a final powdering. The process is easy: simply re-create with camouflage make-up colors or an eyebrow pencil the natural pattern of any freckles, moles, capillaries, beard hair, and so on.

BIBLIOGRAPHY

Allsworth J: Skin Camouflage: A Guide to Remedial Techniques. London, Stanley Thornes, 1985.

Rayner V: Clinical Cosmetology: A Medical Approach to Esthetic Procedures. New York, Milady Publishing, 1993.

CHAPTER 64

Chemical Peels

Howard Murad and Nita Patel

Chemical peeling of the eyelid area employs many of the same principles as chemical peeling in other locations, but there are some significant differences as well. We must first begin by understanding the specific anatomy of the area being peeled. Eyelid skin has a relatively flat dermoepidermal junction with a thinner but denser dermis. There is a great reduction of pilosebaceous units, and the dermis is composed of a spongy fibrous connective tissue.[1] Only a small amount of fat is present, which is closer to the surface along with muscle. Thus, eyelid skin is very thin and delicate. Any chemical peel plan must therefore take this into consideration.

DEPTHS OF CHEMICAL PEELS

There are three depths of chemical peels (Table 64–1). Deep peels are performed using Baker's phenol. They can penetrate to the midreticular dermis.[2] Twenty percent to 50% trichloroacetic acid, pyruvic acid, 88% phenol, and 70% unbuffered glycolic acid are most commonly used to obtain medium-depth peels. They can modify the papillary and upper reticular dermis.[2] The superficial peels include the trichloroacetic acids (10% to 20%) and the alpha-hydroxy acids (most commonly the glycolic acids). They affect the epidermis and the upper regions of the papillary dermis.[2]

INDICATIONS FOR CHEMICAL PEELS

Photodamage

Chemical peels have been used for the entire photodamage spectrum; this includes solar elastosis, actinic keratoses, fine wrinkles, and irregular pigmentation in the periorbital area. The extent of photodamage is influenced by the skin type, which is characterized according to the Fitzpatrick classification (Table 64–2).

Fitzpatrick types I to III are ideal for chemical peeling, whereas persons with types IV or VI can develop problems with postinflammatory hyperpigmentation. Photoaging can also be evaluated according to Glogau's classification (Table 64–3).

The extent of photoaging will also determine the depth of chemical peel required. Histologically, sun-exposed skin shows accumulation of an elastotic substance. Fibroblasts damaged by ultraviolet radiation are thought to be responsible for the abnormal deposition of collagen and elastin.[4] This elastotic material lacks structural integrity, which leads to sagging and wrinkling. Chemical peels can improve photodamaged skin by stimulating deposition of new collagen on top of or in place of the elastotic deposits in the upper papillary dermis.[5] This can be performed using superficial and medium-depth chemical peels. More severe photodamage requires deeper chemical peels.

Crow's-Feet

Photodamage includes crow's-feet, which are the fine and deep wrinkles seen at the lateral aspect of the orbit. These can result from long-term sun exposure, aging, expression lines, and genetic predisposition. The dynamic action of puffing and squinting of smokers also contributes to wrinkles in the perioral and periorbital area. Smoking can contribute to the wrinkling caused by photodamage since compounds in smoke may activate enzymes that damage elastin and collagen.[6] Persons with Fitzpatrick skin types I and II can also have an increased predisposition for the development of wrinkles. Medium-depth chemical peels can be used to stimulate new collagen deposition within the wrinkle lines.

Melasma

Hyperpigmentation around the periorbital area is seen commonly in melasma after an inflammatory process or genetic predisposition. This pigmentation can respond to chemical peels provided that the melanocytic pigment is within the depth of the chemical peel. Melasma is the blotchy, irregularly bordered hyperpigmentation seen in

TABLE 64-1

Depths of Chemical Peels

Superficial (stratum granulosum–papillary dermis)
Buffered glycolic acid 70%
Unbuffered glycolic acid 50%
Trichloroacetic acid 10%–20%
Jessner's solution
Solid CO_2
Tretinoin
Medium depth (upper reticular dermis)
Unbuffered glycolic acid 70%
Pyruvic acid 50%–70%
Trichloroacetic acid 20%–50%
Combination solid CO_2 and trichloroacetic acid 15%–25%
Combination Jessner's and trichloroacetic acid 20%–35%
Full-strength phenol 88%
Deep depth (midreticular dermis)
Baker's phenol, unoccluded
Baker's phenol, occluded

young to middle-aged women that can clinically appear on the upper cheeks, forehead, and upper lip areas. The deposition of melanin pigment can be in the epidermis, primarily in the basal and superbasal layers, and can be in the dermis, where melanin-engulfed macrophages are found perivascularly in the superficial and mid-dermis.[7] The pathogenesis of melasma is unknown, but estrogen and progesterone are thought to be principally responsible, especially during pregnancy and with the use of oral contraceptives.

The standard treatment of melasma involves using hydroquinone in concentrations of 1% to 4%. Hydroquinone acts as a bleaching agent by interfering in the tyrosinase pathway of melanin synthesis.[8] However, the dermal component of melasma can be resistant to topical therapy. Dermabrasion has been used in the past, but the risks for scarring are high. Chemical peels using glycolic acid in 50% to 70% concentrations have been shown to be effective in patients with more resistant melasma.

Periorbital Hyperpigmentation

Periorbital hyperpigmentation is seen commonly in Fitzpatrick skin types III and IV. This includes those with a Middle Eastern, Indian, or Mediterranean background.

TABLE 64-2

Fitzpatrick Skin Types

Skin Type	Color	Reaction to First Summer Exposure
I	White	Always burn, never tan
II	White	Usually burn, tan with difficulty
III	White	Sometimes mild burn, tan average
IV	Moderate brown	Rarely burn, tan with ease
V	Dark brown*	Very rarely burn, tan easily
VI	Black	No burn, tan very easily

*Asian, Indian, Hispanic, or light-skinned African descent, for example.

TABLE 64-3

Evaluation of Photoaging According to Glogau's Classification

Group I—Mild (usually age 28–35)
No keratoses
Little wrinkling
No scarring
Little or no make-up
Group II—Moderate (usually age 35–50)
Early actinic keratoses—slight yellow skin discoloration
Early wrinkling—parallel smile lines
Mild scarring
Little make-up
Group III—Advanced (usually age 50–65)
Actinic keratoses—obvious yellow skin discoloration with telangiectasia
Wrinkling—present at rest
Moderate acne scarring
Wears make-up always
Group IV—Severe (usually age 65–70)
Actinic keratoses and skin cancers
Wrinkling—much cutis laxa of actinic, gravitational, and dynamic origin
Severe acne scarring
Wears make-up that does not cover but cakes on

The hyperpigmentation is within a 2-cm circumferential area around the palpebral fissure. The cause of this discoloration is thought to be melanin deposition. Thus, periorbital hyperpigmentation can be treated very similarly to melasma. Denny's lines, or infraorbital hyperpigmentation, are seen commonly in children and adults with atopic diatheses. They result from chronic rubbing and irritation. Chemical peels may also improve their clinical appearance.

Actinic Keratoses

Superficial chemical peels can be used to treat mildly hypertrophic actinic keratoses. This treatment modality is an alternative to liquid nitrogen, which can cause hypopigmented scars. 5-Fluorouracil is used to treat diffuse actinic damage, but it can produce an intense inflammatory reaction. Seventy percent glycolic acid can be used to cause epidermolysis and discohesiveness of cells, eventually thinning actinic keratoses.[9] Trichloroacetic acid at 30% to 35% can also be used to effectively treat actinic keratoses when it is applied locally to specific lesions.

Lentigines

Chemical peels can also be used to treat lentigines. Lentigines are brown macules on sun-exposed areas, such as the upper cheeks and temples. They are due to an increase of melanocytes and melanocytic activity at the epidermal basal layer.[9] Fifty percent to 70% glycolic acid can be used to perform a superficial peel. Multiple peels can be performed to gradually fade the lentigines. Fifteen percent to 20% trichloroacetic acid can also be used to increase the depth of penetration, which can be effective on the hands, chest, and back.[6]

EVALUATION OF PATIENT FOR CHEMICAL PEEL

The patient must first be evaluated to determine the desired objective of the chemical peel and to select the most appropriate agent and concentration. For example, pigmentation is generally superficial and epidermal, therefore requiring a superficial peel for removal; deep wrinkles are more dermal and require a deeper peeling agent. During an evaluation of a patient for a chemical peel, a complete history is necessary to prevent certain complications after the peel. If the patient has a history of recurrent herpes simplex, a prophylactic course of acyclovir should be given before a medium-depth or deep peel. A dose of 400 mg three times daily is usually adequate for 2 days before the peel, as well as 3 days after. Patients with a tendency to form a hypertrophic scar or keloids are also at risk to form scars with deep peels compared with medium-depth peels.

Mapping and detailing defects before the peel can further provide insight into potential treatment areas for future peels.[10] Photographs before and after peeling indicate treatment areas and can document improvement after treatment. Complete assessment of the patient ensures a good relationship between patient and physician. This is important to prevent unrealistic expectations in the post-healing period. A consent form should be signed listing the expectations of the peel (Table 64–4).

Multiple factors determine the depth of a chemical peel (Table 64–5). This includes the preoperative care weeks before the peel, the skin preparation immediately before the peel, the concentration and peel agent, the length of time the agent is in contact with the skin, and the method of removal of the agent and postoperative care.[11]

SKIN PREPARATION OF CHEMICAL PEEL

At least two weeks before the actual chemical peel, the patient is prepared with topical therapy with retinoids (Retin-A 0.025% cream at bedtime) and/or glycolic acid 8% to 10% every morning or glycolic acid twice daily. This is to promote fast post–chemical peel healing. The patient is also instructed to use sunscreens on a daily basis. A sunscreen with a sun protection factor of at least 15 and containing protection against ultraviolet light A and B blocking agents should be used.

Skin preparation immediately before the peel is important in obtaining a uniform result. The patient is first instructed to remove any make-up or sunscreen.[3] Various agents are used to remove any additional debris on the skin. These include chlorhexidine, acetone, alcohol, prepping solution, and Jessner's solution. A variable amount of stratum corneum is also removed, depending on the prep material and the extent of scrubbing or pres-

TABLE 64–4

Chemical Peel Consent

Patient Expectations
1. A stinging sensation of the area that lasts 30 to 60 minutes occurs. Regular Tylenol, or medication prescribed by the doctor if needed, should control any more persistent pain. Swelling and erythema also occur. Initially, freckles and pigmentation will seem more noticeable.
2. For the first few days, use a mild nondrying cleanser. Do not peel any of the superficial dead skin. Apply mild moisturizers and sunscreens.
3. Often bleeding points occur in areas. These bleeding points are a normal response and usually heal in 4 to 7 days. Persistent redness may last for up to 3 months.
4. Chemical peels gradually improve your skin. As with many cosmetic procedures, the "quick fix" dramatic effects do not occur. However, safely and effectively, the skin improves.
5. Avoid sun exposure for at least 6 weeks after the facial peeling. Sun exposure incurs the risk of pigmentation of the face.
6. There are no dietary restrictions with this treatment; however, occasionally the swelling may make it difficult to open the mouth. The first 1 or 2 days, the initial diet may consist of liquids only. Talking and mouth movements should be restricted so as not to disrupt the crust. During the entire time of the process (5–10 days), physical activity should also be restricted.
7. Occasionally the face will have a blotchy appearance after the peel. This generally fades with time. A prescribed ointment is beneficial.
8. Because of the swelling that occurs, residual wrinkles are hidden and the face may present a smoother appearance initially then subsequently. The face overall, however, will be smoother and more youthful looking.
9. After the healing phase, the peeled area may be lighter in color than the unpeeled region because some skin pigment that lies in the epidermal layers has been removed.
10. Infrequently, a person with a history of cold sores (herpes simplex) will have an outbreak after a peel. Notify the doctor if you have a history of such infections.

I understand that patient responsibility and proper performance of the postoperative care and regular office visits are critical to the success of the chemical peel. I have read and understand the postoperative instructions.

I also understand that rare complications of color changes, infection, and scarring can occur. It is possible that this procedure will not help you. Further, even if your procedure is successful initially, the results may not be permanent.

I CERTIFY: I have read or had read to me the content of this form; I understand the risks and alternatives involved in this procedure; I have had the opportunity to ask any questions that I had and all of my questions have been answered.

Date: ____________ Signature: ______________________________

(patient)

TABLE 64-5

Factors That Determine Depth of Chemical Peel

Preoperative care weeks before peel
Tretinoin
Alpha-hydroxy acids
Sunscreen
Facials
Skin preparation immediately before chemical peel
Chlorhexidine
Alcohol
Acetone
Jessner's solution used as a superficial peel
Prepping agents such as salicyclic acid
Agent and concentration used
Length of time in contact with skin
Method of application
Cotton-tipped applicators
Gauze pads
Cotton balls
Pressure applied by the surgeon
Method of removal
Cleanse with water
Scrubbed off
Postoperative care
Occlusion
Lubricants
Topical corticosteroids
Systemic corticosteroids
Long-term postoperative care
Glycolic acid
Tretinoin
Sunscreens
Facials

sure used to apply the agent. Jessner's solution removes most of the stratum corneum, whereas acetone only partially removes the stratum corneum.[12] Chlorhexidine probably only removes surface debris and oils. It should also not be used in the periorbital area because it has been reported to cause corneal scarring. Degreasing with acetone or Jessner's solution is very important since even a small amount of oil can prevent penetration of the chemical peel.[6]

APPLICATION TECHNIQUE

The periorbital area is prepared as described with alcohol and acetone. Care should be used to avoid any contact with the eye. Saline syringes should be prepared for flushing in case of accidental introduction into the eyes. The head should be kept in an upright position since wrinkles are accentuated with gravity. Tears should be wiped away during peeling with a cotton-tipped applicator to avoid pulling the agent into the eye by capillary action.[6]

A cotton-tipped applicator is used to apply the Jessner's solution or prepping agent. The skin is gently stretched between two fingers to ensure an even application. Throughout the area the agent is applied within 1 mm of the lower lid margin and it is feathered into the surrounding hairline at the periphery.[6] The peel of the upper lid can be performed with the patient's eyes closed and in the direction of the lateral canthus below the eyebrow to the inner canthal area. Upper eyelid skin should be peeled only to the superior border of the tarsal plate to minimize edema.[6]

When trichloroacetic acid is used as the chemical peel agent, a 5% higher concentration is placed within the furrows of crow's-feet with a broken sharp end of a cotton-tipped applicator. The trichloroacetic acid solution is applied so that a frosted appearance is present after application (Fig. 64-1). The patient is asked to smile during application to accentuate the wrinkles. This technique can be used in any defects on the face, including acne scars, perioral wrinkles, or depressed scars.

Postoperatively, the patient is instructed to use only a gentle cleanser and to avoid scrubbing the peeled area. Moisturizers should be applied twice a day to protect the skin barrier. Sunscreens should be continued on a daily basis to prevent postinflammatory hyperpigmentation. Tretinoin and glycolic acid can be continued 1 week after the chemical peel or when the erythema from the peel subsides.

CHEMICAL PEEL AGENTS

Tretinoin

Tretinoin used consistently in a concentration of 0.1% for more than 4 months produces a compaction of actinically damaged stratum corneum.[13] Electron microscopy

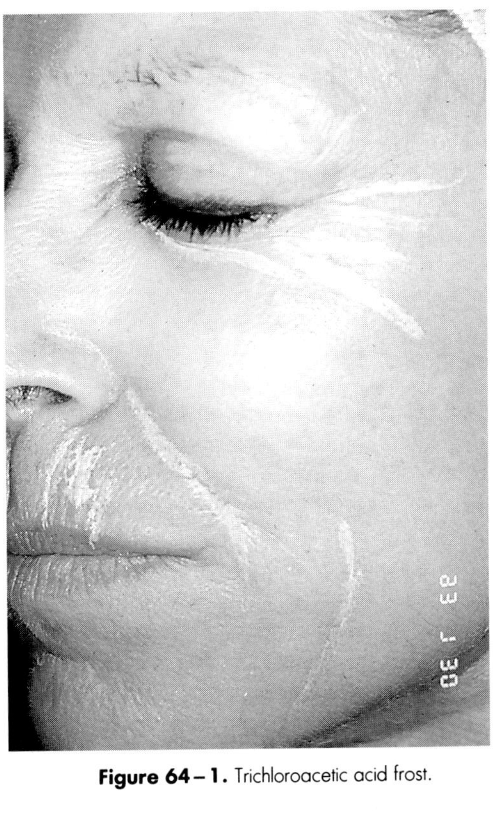

Figure 64-1. Trichloroacetic acid frost.

TABLE 64-6

Jessner's Solution or Combes' Formula

Resorcinol, 14 g
Salicylic acid, 14 g
Lactic acid (85%), 14 g
Ethanol (95%) qs* 100 mL

*qs = quantity sufficient to add up to.

reveals increased collagen formation with increased fibroblasts.[1] Continued treatment beyond 1 year widens the papillary dermal grenz zone and pushes down the old elastotic tissue.[1]

Jessner's Solution

Jessner's solution, also called a Combes' peel, consists of a combination of resorcinol, salicylic acid, and lactic acid in an alcohol solution (Table 64-6).[12] It is used in preparation of another chemical peel by acting as a debriding agent. Jessner's solution can also be used as a superficial peeling agent. It shows only stratum corneum separation with upper epidermal intraepithelial and intercellular edema.[12] No dermal changes are apparent. A light coat of the solution can be applied using a small cotton-tipped applicator. The depth of the peel is determined by the number of coats applied. A slightly frosted appearance is apparent after deeper penetration is obtained. Application of Jessner's solution is limited to the face to avoid potential toxicity from resorcinol.[14]

Azelaic Acid

Other peel agents include azelaic acid, which is a naturally occurring, straight-chained, saturated dicarboxylic acid.[11] Azelaic acid inhibits tyrosinase and may have a cytotoxic effect on hyperactive melanocytes.[11] Fifteen to 20% azelaic acid is applied twice a day to treat acne and pigmentary changes.[15] It produces a mild inflammatory response with minimum scaling and slow improvement in 6 months.

Solid Carbon Dioxide

Solid carbon dioxide (dry ice) has been used for treatment of acne for more than 50 years. Carbon dioxide slush is prepared by releasing the gas from a cylinder through a chamois leather bag.[16] This is then compacted into a ball and is placed in the center of a 4 × 4-inch gauze pad. The carbon dioxide slush is then dipped into acetone, which serves to dissolve sebum and lower the temperature of the carbon dioxide by accelerating the change of carbon dioxide from solid to gas.[17]

This carbon dioxide slush is then applied with even pressure so that a trail of light frost is seen immediately and then disappears. This treatment can be repeated on a weekly basis. Carbon dioxide applied to the skin for 15 seconds produces complete epidermal necrosis with pronounced dermal edema.[1] A mixed inflammatory infiltrate is seen, but there is no collagen destruction.[18] This is a more superficially aggressive modality than Jessner's solution.

Alpha-Hydroxy Acids

Alpha-hydroxy acids are used predominantly as a superficial peeling agent. These acids are derived from food sources, for example, glycolic acid (sugar cane), lactic acid (sour milk), malic acid (apples), citric acid (citrus fruits), and tartaric acid (grapes) (Table 64-7).[19] In low concentrations up to 20%, alpha-hydroxy acids can disrupt corneocyte cohesion just above the stratum granulosum, whereas epidermolysis below the level of the stratum corneum is caused by concentrations of 70% or higher.[9]

Lactic acid is slower to cause epidermolysis.[11] It is physiologically converted to pyruvic acid, an alpha-ketoacid. A 5% to 20% concentration of lactic acid causes corneocyte detachment, resulting in desquamation.[11] Fifty to 70% alpha-hydroxy acid, most commonly glycolic acid, is applied with a small or soaked cotton-tipped applicator. The peel agent is left on for 1 to 5 minutes or until erythema accompanied by a burning sensation develops, and then it is neutralized by using water-soaked gauze pads or by having the patient splash water on the face.

Factors that determine whether an alpha-hydroxy acid peel will result in desquamation depend on the concentration of the acid, the type of formulation, the frequency of application, and the duration that the acid remains on the skin.[11] The mechanism of alpha-hydroxy acids in improving wrinkles is believed to be enhancement of the synthesis of intercellular ground substances, glycosaminoglycans, or collagen.[15]

Seventy percent glycolic acid can be applied to acne lesions with a cotton ball by using a gloved hand. After 3 to 5 minutes acne papules will blanch and acne pustules and comedones become unroofed.[11] Rinsing with water then

TABLE 64-7

Sources of Alpha-Hydroxy Acids

Type of Acid	Source
Glycolic acid	Sugar cane
Malic acid	Apples
Tartaric acid	Grapes
Citric acid	Citrus fruits
Lactic acid	Sour milk
Pyruvic acid	Citrus fruits

prevents further penetration. The same concentration of glycolic acid is used to treat wrinkles. After the skin is prepped to remove cutaneous oils, the glycolic acid is applied to the skin with cotton-tipped applicators or slightly damp cotton balls. The acid is kept on for 1 to 3 minutes or until slight erythema or a burning sensation develops. Then the area is rinsed with water. This procedure can be repeated on a weekly basis. Patients can use 5% to 15% glycolic acid–based products twice daily between treatments.

Trichloroacetic Acid (Figs. 64–2 to 64–4)

Trichloroacetic acid is a versatile peeling agent that can be used as a superficial peel in strengths ranging from 15% to 20% or as a medium-strength peel (25%–35%) or a deep peel (40%–70%). It is thought that there are differences in skin metabolism in various regions of body skin that account for variability in reaction. The reaction is slower on extensor surfaces compared with flexor surfaces.[11] Stimulation of new collagen formation within furrows and fine wrinkles occurs at deeper strengths between 40% and 50%. Seventy percent trichloroacetic acid can also be used for very thick hyperkeratotic lesions. Higher concentrations are also required on the lower extremities.

Trichloroacetic acid acts to precipitate epidermal proteins and causes necrosis and sloughing of both normal and actinically damaged skin. The acidity of the agent is neutralized by serum in the superficial dermal vessels after application and is nontoxic to internal organs.[11] An aqueous solution must be prepared by mixing the desired concentration in grams of trichloroacetic acid crystals with up to 100 mL of distilled water so that adequate penetration of the skin occurs.[20] Stock solutions of trichloroacetic acid are stable for at least 6 months.[21] They should be kept in dark glass bottles to prevent degradation.[22] Refrigeration of samples also maintains stability of the concentration of the solution.[22] The solution should be poured from the stock bottle into a small medication cup for use.

Once the trichloroacetic acid solution has been applied, a whitish film or frost appears within minutes. This indicates that the effect of the agent has taken place. Trichloroacetic acid does not require inactivation with water, but water can be splashed on for comfort. A slightly higher strength concentration of trichloroacetic acid can be used within furrow lines, acne scars, and depressed areas to stimulate additional collagen production. The frosted appearance will then evolve into an erythema after an hour of application. Light exfoliation equivalent to a mild sunburn begins the second day and lasts 3 to 6 days with superficial peels.[11] Patients with medium- to deep-strength peels may develop intense erythema, swelling, and crusting, which can last up to 2 weeks. Most superficial peels can be repeated every 2 to 3 weeks until the desired result is achieved. Medium- to deep-strength peels are usually repeated every 6 months.

Pyruvic Acid

Preliminary findings show pyruvic acid, an alpha-ketoacid, as a peeling agent.[23] Epidermolysis occurs in 30 to 60 seconds with dermal penetration occurring rapidly within 1 to 2 minutes with 100% pyruvic acid.[24] Although pyruvic acid and lactic acid convert physiologically to each other, it is a very potent chemical peel agent.[24] Further research is necessary to understand the penetration of this agent and its scar capability. This agent should not be used in the periorbital area.

Baker's Phenol Peel

Deeper chemical peels include the Baker's phenol solution. These peels are usually not recommended for olive- or dark-skinned patients. The periorbital area should be avoided since, histologically, the dermis is

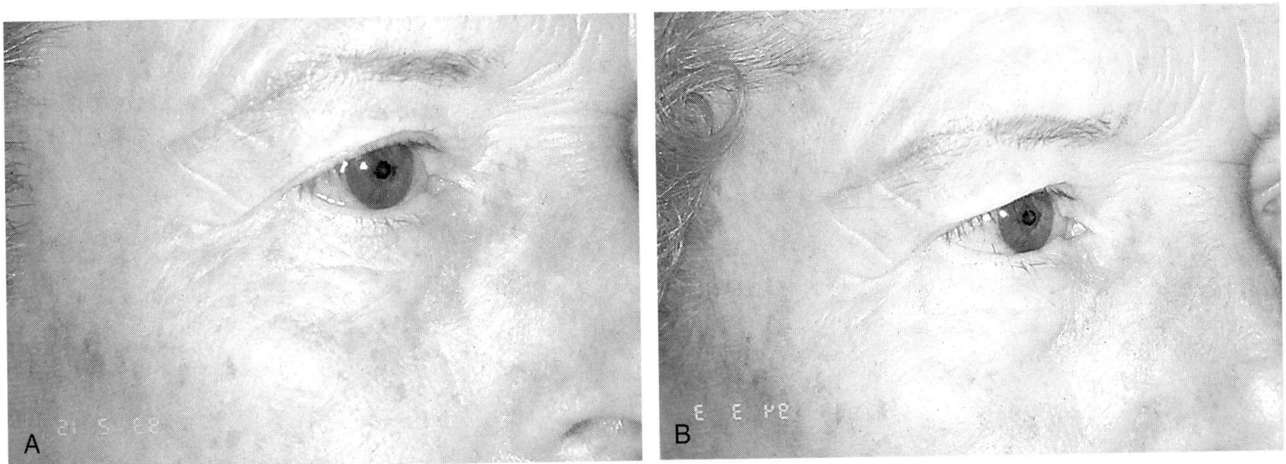

Figure 64–2. *A*, Eye area before chemical peel with trichloroacetic acid. *B*, Eye area after peel.

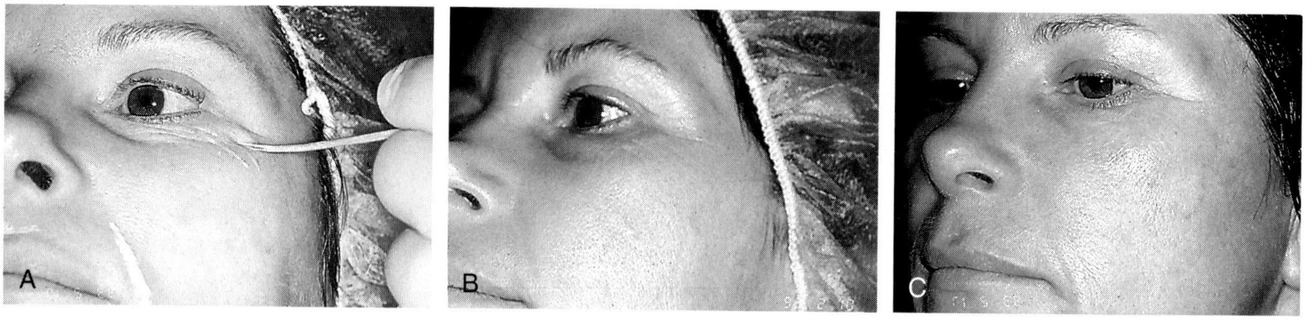

Figure 64–3. *A*, Tricholoroacetic acid chemical peel procedure. *B*, Eye area before peel. *C*, Eye area after peel.

thinner. Using a phenol peel in this area could result in atrophy. The full-strength, unoccluded 88% phenol peel is comparable to a medium-depth chemical peel. It causes immediate coagulation of epidermal keratin proteins, preventing further penetration of phenol.[25] This concentration can give a uniform appearance with barely noticeable hypopigmentation. The Baker's phenol peel consists of phenol, distilled water, septisol liquid soap, and croton oil.[25] It usually produces a white complexion and hypopigmentation but can achieve deeper penetration and more effectively treat wrinkles and furrows. Phenol can also be absorbed percutaneously.[25] The application of waterproof tape after the peel increases penetration of the agent due to maceration.[25] This process increases the wound depth of the phenol. Patients under consideration for a phenol peel must have an adequate hepatorenal status since phenol is detoxified in the liver and renally cleared.[25] A recent electrocardiogram and blood studies are also needed as well as cardiac monitoring during the chemical peel since cardiotoxicity in the form of arrhythmias is a possibility.[25]

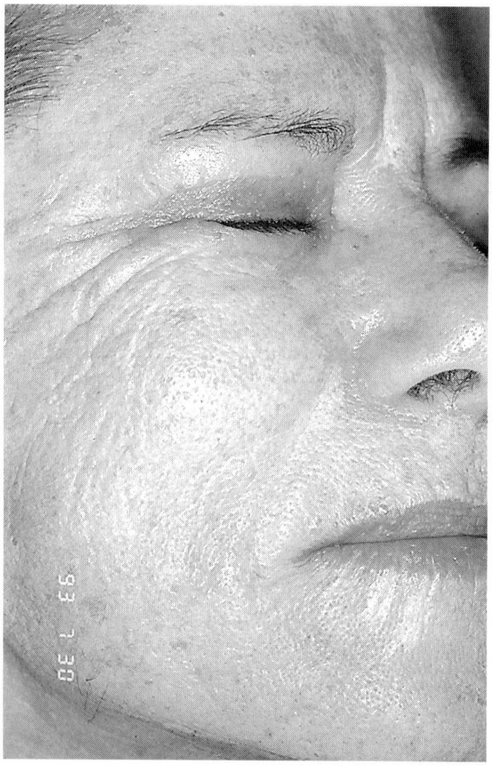

Figure 64–4. Tricholoroacetic acid frost eye area.

COMPLICATIONS

Chemical peels can be used to produce a controlled defect to promote elimination of pigmentary changes, hyperkeratotic lesions, and scars. However, different types of complications can occur with chemical peels (Table 64–8).

When a single cosmetic unit is peeled, the solution should be feathered beyond the natural boundaries to prevent demarcation lines. A superficial peel can also be used in surrounding areas so that the peeled area is less noticeable.

Although hyperpigmentation can occur with any depth peel, it is most likely to occur with Fitzpatrick types IV through VI. Other complications include scarring especially with medium-depth peels and with greater than 50% trichloroacetic acid peels.[7] Lower lid ectropion after chemical peel and in conjunction with a blepharoplasty may resolve spontaneously in 3 to 4 months.[26] Infections can also develop after chemical peels and can include *Pseudomonas* infection,[27] toxic shock syndrome,[28] herpes simplex infections,[29] and Epstein-Barr keratitis.[30]

TABLE 64–8

Complications from Chemical Peels
Hypopigmentation
Hyperpigmentation
Ectropion
Hypertrophic scarring
Demarcation of treatment areas
Persistent erythema
Infection—bacterial and viral
Prurigo
Milia
Atrophy
Textural changes
Peau d'orange with enlarged pores
Systemic toxicities with phenol

Patients can also develop prolonged erythema, pruritus, textural changes, atrophy, or milia.[31] Although many potential complications exist, they are minimal when patients are evaluated and instructed on proper postoperative care.

Chemical peels can thus be used as an alternative for treatment of lesions in the periorbital area. This includes photodamage, crow's-feet, hyperpigmentation, melasma, lentigines, and hyperkeratotic actinic keratoses. Chemical peels can thus produce a controlled effect that can stimulate new collagen production, eliminating unwanted surface and pigment changes with minimal potential complications.

REFERENCES

1. Brody HJ: Histology and classification. *In* Brody HJ: Chemical Peeling. St. Louis, Mosby-Year Book, 1992, pp 7–31.
2. Brody HJ: Update on chemical peels. *In* Advances in Dermatology. St. Louis, Mosby-Year Book, 1992, p 276.
3. Murad H, Moy LS: Use of AHA's add new dimensions to chemical peeling. Cosmet Dermatol 3:32–34, 1990.
4. Uitto J, Fazio MJ, Olsen DR: Cutaneous aging: Molecular alterations in elastic fibers. J Cutan Aging Cosmet Dermatol 1:13–26, 1988.
5. Ayers S: Dermal changes following application of chemical cauterants to aging skin. Arch Dermatol 82:578, 1960.
6. Brody HJ: General peeling concepts. *In* Brody HJ: Chemical Peeling. St. Louis, Mosby–Year Book, 1992, pp 33–52.
7. Sanchez NP, Pathak MA, Sato S, et al: Melasma: A clinical, light microscopic, ultrastructural, and immunofluorescence study. J Am Acad Dermatol 4:698–710, 1981.
8. Pathak MA, Fitzpatrick TB, Parish JA: Treatment of melasma with hydroquinone. J Invest Dermatol 76:324, 1981.
9. Van Scott EJ, Yu RJ: Alpha-hydroxy acids: Procedures for use in clinical practice. Cutis 43:222–229, 1989.
10. Brody HJ: The art of chemical peeling. J Dermatol Surg Oncol 15:918–921, 1989.
11. Brody HJ: Superficial peeling. *In* Brody HJ: Chemical Peeling. St. Louis, Mosby–Year Book, 1992, pp 53–73.
12. Brody HJ: Variations and comparisons in medium-depth chemical peeling. J Dermatol Surg Oncol 15:953–963, 1989.
13. Weiss JS, Ellis CN, Headington JT, et al: Tropical tretinoin improves photoaged skin: A double-blind, vehicle-controlled study. JAMA 259:527–532, 1989.
14. Pascher F: Systemic reactions to topically applied drugs. Bull NY Acad Med 49:613–627, 1973.
15. Murad H, Moy LS: Use of AHA's add new dimensions to chemical peeling. Cosmet Dermatol 3:32–34, 1990.
16. Rook A, Wilkinson DS, Ebling FJG: Textbook of Dermatology. Oxford, England, Blackwell Scientific Publications, 1972, p 2099.
17. Moseley JC, Katz SI: Acne vulgaris: Treatment with carbon dioxide slush. Cutis 10:429–431, 1972.
18. Montagna W, Kirchner S, Carlisle K: Histology of sun-damaged human skin. J Am Acad Dermatol 21:907–918, 1989.
19. Van Scott EJ, Yu RJ: Hyperkeratinization, corneocyte cohesion and alpha-hydroxy acids. J Am Acad Dermatol 11:867, 1984.
20. Resnick SS: Chemical peeling with trichloroacetic acid. J Dermatol Surg Oncol 10:549, 1984.
21. Spinowitz AL, Dumsfield J: Stability-time profile of trichloroacetic acid at various concentrations and storage conditions. J Dermatol Surg Oncol 15:974–975, 1989.
22. Doelzal JF: Stability study of trichloroacetic acid [letter]. J Dermatol Surg Oncol 16:489–490, 1990.
23. Griffin TD, Van Scott EJ, Maddin S: The use of pyruvic acid as a chemical peeling agent [abstract]. J Dermatol Surg Oncol 15:1316, 1989.
24. Brody HJ: General peeling concepts. *In* Brody HJ: Medium-Depth Peeling. St. Louis, Mosby–Year Book, 1992, pp 75–97.
25. Brody HJ: General peeling concepts. *In* Brody HJ: Deep Peeling. St. Louis, Mosby–Year Book, 1992, pp 99–120.
26. Wojno T, Tenzel R: Lower eyelid ectropion following chemical face peeling. Ophthalmic Surg 15:596–597, 1984.
27. Stegman SJ, Tromvitch TA, Glogau RG: Chemical Peeling. *In* Cosmetic Dermatology Surgery. St. Louis, Mosby–Year Book, 1990, pp 35–58.
28. Dytryshyn JR: Chemical face peel complicated by toxic shock syndrome. Arch Otolaryngol 109:170, 1983.
29. Rapaport MJ, Kamer F: Exacerbation of facial herpes simplex after phenolic face peels. J Dermatol Surg Oncol 10:57–58, 1984.
30. Pflugfelder SC, Huang A, Crouse C: Epstein-Barr virus keratitis after a chemical face peel. Am J Ophthalmol 110:571–573, 1990.
31. Brody HJ: Complications of chemical peels. *In* Brody HJ: Chemical Peeling. St. Louis, Mosby–Year Book, 1992, pp 121–145.

CHAPTER 65

Autologen: Autologous, Injectable Dermal Collagen

Dale P. DeVore, Charles D. Kelman, Steven Fagien, and Phillip Casson

There has yet to be a perfect material for replacing or repairing damaged or defective tissue. However, it is generally accepted that an autologous material would be best for such purposes.[1,2] Autologous tissue preparations theoretically should be devoid of allergic reaction and tissue rejection. In fact, such complications have not been observed after autotransplantation of human tissues.[3] Homologous or allograft tissue would be less desirable due to concerns of viral transmission and potential immunologic reactions. Heterologous material carries an even greater risk of immunogenic and associated tissue reactions. Inflammation accompanying tissue reactions would result in elevated levels of active proteases, which could accelerate the degradation of biologic replacement materials.

Autologous materials are commonly, and successfully, used to replace or augment body tissues. For example, autologous conjunctival tissue has been used as an autotransplant to restore the ocular surface,[4] particularly for reconstruction after pterygium or tumor removal. Autologous pericardium has been used to repair or patch damaged mitral valve tissue,[5] and autologous veins are used for infrainguinal reconstruction.[6] Autologous bone replacement is used to treat bone defects (i.e., after trauma or for orbital and maxillofacial reconstruction),[7,8] and autologous skin, if available, is still preferred for grafting to full-thickness burn sites[9] and is the treatment of choice in ophthalmic plastic and facial surgery. The list of autograft materials also includes fascia grafts for orbital, eyelid, and facial reconstruction[10] and autologous muscle transplants.[11] Autologous material is preferred and used if available in facial reconstruction: autologous septal cartilage for augmenting the nasal dorsum,[12,13] temporoparietal fascia for nasal and facial augmentation,[14] and hard palate grafting or ear cartilage for eyelid reconstruction.

The availability and use of autologous dermal fillers to smooth wrinkle lines and scars has been limited to intact dermal grafts and injectable fat. The former requires surgical implantation of a harvested dermal strip into the skin. The latter requires harvesting and processing of fat. Both procedures require extraction and processing of tissues in a clinical setting. Sterility testing of the implant may not be performed before implantation. Resorption rates up to 20% have been reported for autologous dermal grafts[15] and up to approximately 60% with autologous dermis fat grafts.[16] Fat grafts and injectable processed fat have provided disappointing long-term correction.[17,18] In addition, injectable fat is predominantly a subcutaneous filler and may not be appropriate for fine lines and wrinkles.[19]

A commercial process for preparing intact collagen fibers from dermal tissue has been made available. This process is being used to prepare a sterile, injectable dispersion of autologous collagen fibers (Autologen) for smoothing dermal defects. Autologen appears to fulfill the criteria for the next generation of injectable filler materials. That is, it is a preparation that is safe and longer lasting than current injectable materials.

INJECTABLE FILLER MATERIALS

Several injectable materials have been available as fillers to smooth facial wrinkles and depressed scars. These include (1) silicone oils; (2) reconstituted bovine collagen (Zyderm I, Zyderm II, and Zyplast, which is glutaraldehyde cross-linked Zyderm I); (3) porcine gelatine enhanced with autologous plasma and epsilon-aminocaproic acid (Fibrel); and (4) autologous fat preparations. Each material has certain deficiencies, making it less than ideal for tissue augmentation. Silicone is not approved by the Food and Drug Administration (FDA), and use of silicone injections is prohibited.[20] Reconstituted bovine collagen has been used in more than 500,000 individuals. Adverse reactions and complications resulting from reconstituted collagen, although infrequent,[3,21] have somewhat quelled the enthusiasm initially generated for this filler material. Probably of more importance is the apparent rapid resorption of these collagen preparations and the disappointing long-term correction requiring multiple reinjections to maintain correction.[8] The porcine gelatin product Fibrel generally suffers the same deficiencies as reconstituted bovine collagen suspensions.[3,8] In addition, preparation of Fibrel requires an aliquot of the patient's plasma and the addition of epsilon-aminocaproic acid that must be mixed with the porcine gelatin powder. This must be performed in the physician's office using aseptic techniques and requires more time than using prepackaged injectable filler products. Both reconstituted bovine products and the porcine gelatin product contain a heterologous biologic material and are subject to potential tissue and immunologic reactions as discussed earlier.

Autologous fat transplantation is not a new concept, being performed in the late nineteenth century and the early twentieth century.[22] However, this method of correcting soft tissue deformities received limited use. Surgical excisions were required to harvest donor fat, and the longevity of correction was limited because of rapid resorption of the transplant. The use of autologous fat preparations to correct dermal defects appeared to be revived with the advent of suction lipectomy. A number of procedures have been developed for preparing autologous fat for injection. In most procedures, fat is aspirated from the abdominal subcutaneous space and washed with saline or lactated Ringer's solution. In some cases, the fat extract is frozen and then thawed and placed plunger-up in a sterile syringe to allow the oily fraction to separate from the "fibrous collagen" fraction.[3] Other procedures wash the extracted fat with lactated Ringer's solution and then filter through a fine mesh stainless steel strainer before being placed in the syringe[19] or simply reinject aspirated fat without washing or addition of other components, such as insulin.[22] In still other cases, the fat globules are ruptured by passing through an orifice with decreasing diameter (i.e., a series of syringe needles starting with an 18-gauge needle and continuing through a 27-gauge needle). The emulsion is then centrifuged to recover the "fibrous debris" fraction, which is used as the injectable filler. The pellet is then injected mid-dermally to correct dermal defects. Fat extraction and processing is conducted in the office by the clinician, and sterility testing of injectable material is not conducted before injection. Autologous fat injections appear, in general, to be resorbed and provide only short-term correction.[23]

AUTOLOGEN: AUTOLOGOUS COLLAGEN DISPERSION

A new, autologous collagen material, Autologen, has become available for use in filling dermal imperfections. This material is composed of intact collagen fibers dispersed from the dermal layer of skin specimens obtained from the donor-recipient. The collagen fibers are suspended in a neutral pH phosphate buffer. Autologen can be prepared to contain a range of collagen concentrations generally from 25 mg/mL (2.5%) to as high as 100 mg/mL (10%), in some cases. Autologen provides two significant advantages: (1) it is an autologous preparation and therefore allergic and tissue reactions should not occur and (2) it contains intact dermal collagen fibers with natural cross-links inherently formed during collagen fibril formation in the body. These characteristics should contribute to the durability of Autologen as an injectable filler to smooth wrinkle lines and depressed scars. The main disadvantage of Autologen is that tissue specimens, primarily skin, must be obtained from the donor-recipient. However, access to tissue does not appear to be a significant drawback to most plastic and reconstructive surgeons. For example, in 1990 more than 300,000 surgical procedures were performed in which tissue was removed and generally discarded. Interestingly enough, the majority of the procedures were eyelid surgery. The American Society of Plastic and Reconstructive Surgery reported nearly 80,000 blepharoplasties performed by society members in 1990. For patients not undergoing aesthetic plastic surgery but who want Autologen, skin can easily be removed from an inconspicuous area such as the suprapubic region or the inner gluteal fold.

Autologen Preparation

Autologen is prepared from intact dermal tissue. Skin specimens are dissected to remove epidermis and subcutaneous tissues, leaving only the dermal layer of skin. The dermis is minced and then mechanically pulverized in sterile buffer into a dispersion of intact collagen fibers. The dispersed collagen fibers are extensively washed in sterile phosphate buffer and concentrated by centrifugation. A range of collagen concentrations can be prepared by controlling centrifugation speed. The final concentrate is then placed into sterile, 1-mL Luer-Lok syringes and hand labeled with the donor-recipient's identification codes. All procedures are aseptically performed, and each processed tissue lot is tested for sterility. Processing and analysis generally require 3 to 4 weeks, including testing for sterility and receipt of a certificate of sterility.

Tissue Source for Autologen Preparation

Several sources of dermal tissue have been used to prepare Autologen. In most cases, tissue removed during routine cosmetic surgical procedures is provided for processing into Autologen. This tissue would otherwise be discarded. Sources include abdominal skin from abdominoplasty surgery, suprapubic excisions, and abdominal excisions during other routine surgery; gluteal region skin excisions or punch biopsies; scalp and brow skin removed during hair transplants and brow-lifts; facial skin removed during face-lift surgery; eyelid tissue removed during blepharoplasty; breast tissue from breast reduction procedures; and skin removed from the upper arm during surgical procedures (brachioplasty or arm-lift). Autologen can be prepared from virtually any dermal tissue removed from the body. The yield of Autologen having an average solids content of 50 mg/mL (5%) is

TABLE 65-1

Average Yield of Autologen (n = 25)

Skin Weight (g)	Dermis weight (g)	Yield (mL)
5.76 ± 2.41	5.10 ± 1.26	3.4 ± 1.3

Note: Average yield = 0.6 mL/g of skin.

TABLE 65-3

Autologen From Blepharoplasty Specimens (Averages from 18 Specimens)

	Skin Weight (g)	Hydrated Dermis Weight (g)	Autologen Yield (mL)
	1.49 ± 0.94	1.31 ± 1.00	0.65 ± 0.48
Range	0.31-3.60	0.2-2.10	0.1-1.90

shown in Table 65-1: 5.76 g of full-thickness skin yields about 3.4 mL of Autologen. The area of skin needed to prepare 1 mL of Autologen has been calculated from numerous skin excisions taken specifically for Autologen preparation. As shown in Table 65-2, 1.28 square inches of abdominal skin yields 1 mL of Autologen at about 50 mg/mL solids. The yield of Autologen varies depending on the source of tissue. Eyelid skin is thinner than abdominal skin. The average yield of Autologen from eyelid skin taken during routine blepharoplasty procedure is shown in Table 65-3. An average of 1.49 g of skin has been provided from upper eyelid tissue. This has provided 1.31 g of dermis, which has yielded an average of 0.65 g of Autologen.

Collagen Fibers in Autologen

Collagen fibers in Autologen exhibit normal banding and banding periodicity, as shown in Figure 65-1. Banding patterns are absent or only partially observed in reconstituted, bovine collagen preparations (Figs. 65-2 and 65-3). Reconstituted collagen fibers are formed from solubilized, atelopeptide collagen molecules. Telopeptide fragments are nonhelical, terminal peptides of collagen molecules that exhibit the most prominent antigenic determinants.[24-26] These peptides are routinely removed when using heterologous collagen as a human implant material, since their presence could increase the risk of allergic or tissue reaction. However, they are also essential to the quarter stagger formation of collagen fibers and to formation of intermolecular cross-links between adjacent collagen molecules.[27,28] In Autologen, the in vivo architecture of collagen fibers is maintained, including the presence of intermolecular, enzymically catalyzed cross-links. It is anticipated that these natural collagen fibers will exhibit greater resistance to protease degradation than will reconstituted collagen fiber units, especially when telopeptides have been removed.

Clinical Use of Autologen

Autologen has been used by more than 30 plastic surgeons and dermatologists to treat wrinkle lines and depressed, distensible scars. More than 300 units of Autologen have been injected into 200 individuals. Since the preparation is strictly autologous, skin testing for hypersensitivity reactions has not been necessary. Injection is typically through a 30-gauge needle into the mid-dermis, generally with minimal or no overcorrection. Autologen contains less collagen than dermal tissue (about 30%), and several injections are likely to be required to attain full correction. Clinicians using a "layering" technique appear to obtain long-term correction after three to four injections. Postinjection sequelae are negligible and primarily include transient redness at the injection site. Blanching is not observed. Autologen does not contain an anesthetic agent, and some physicians have pretreated the injection area with a local anesthetic 10 to 15 minutes before Autologen injection, particularly when multiple units or a high concentration requiring the use of a

TABLE 65-2

Excised Skin Specimens (Abdominal): Correlation of Autologen Yield to Skin Size (sq in) (n = 10)

Skin Size (sq in)	Skin Weight (g)	Dermis Weight (g)	Autologen Yield (mL)
1.0	3.34	2.20	1.0
1.4	2.74	1.65	1.2
0.6	0.99	0.60	0.5
0.5	0.64	0.42	0.7
4.0	4.08	2.91	3.0
5.0	5.05	3.53	3.5
0.9	3.65	1.06	1.5
2.5	5.20	3.37	2.5
5.0	8.13	3.24	3.0
6.0	6.75	3.77	4.1
x = 2.69± SD = 2.11	4.05± 2.35	2.28± 1.27	2.10± 1.28

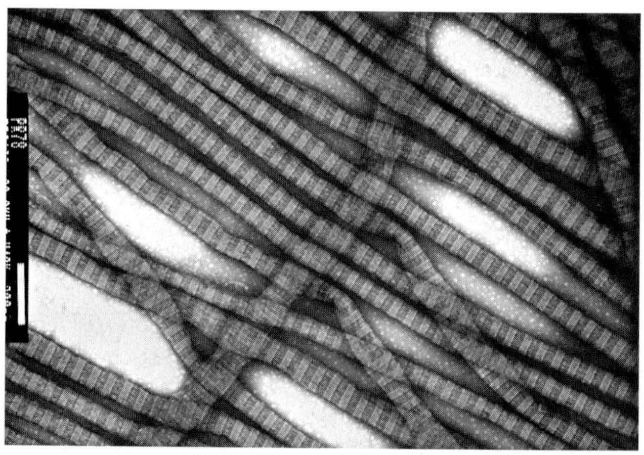

Figure 65-1. Transmission electron microscopy of Autologen collagen fibers stained with phosphotungstic acid. Note the uniform fiber diameter and the consistent banding pattern.

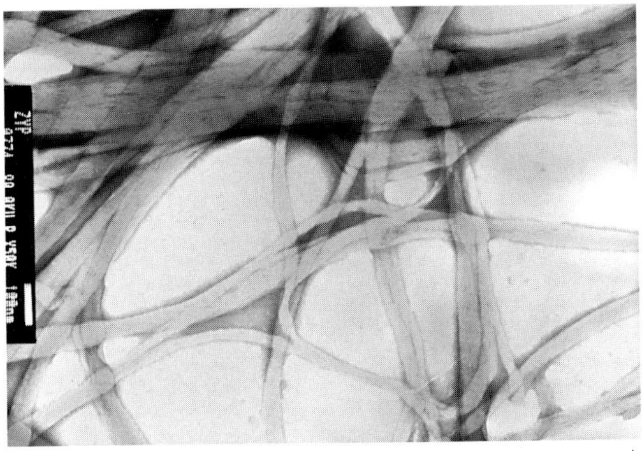

Figure 65–2. Transmission electron micrograph of cross-linked, reconstituted collagen fibers (Zyplast) stained with phosphotungstic acid. Note the absence of typical collagen banding.

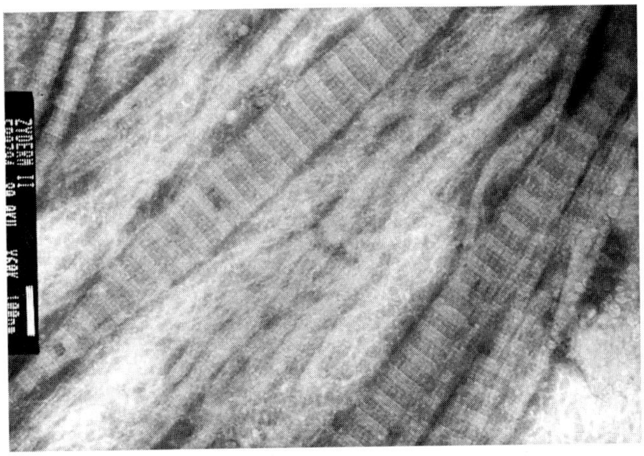

Figure 65–3. Transmission electron micrograph of reconstituted collagen fibers (Zyderm II) stained with phosphotungstic acid. Note the background of poorly organized collagen units and the variable diameter of the few fibers observed in this field.

larger-gauge needle is being administered. Regional nerve blocks such as the supraorbital for glabellar frown lines and the infraorbital, or "dental," block for the nasolabial area or upper lip are also useful and would not distort tissue planes.[29] Higher-concentration Autologen (e.g., greater than 70 mg/mL) may not flow through a 30-gauge or even a 27-gauge needle. Since Autologen is custom prepared, the consistency can be adjusted, within limits, to meet specific needs.

Clinical Results

There is little question among the physicians using Autologen that it lasts longer than reconstituted bovine collagen (Zyderm I and Zyderm II) and degraded porcine collagen (Fibrel). In addition, only one minor incident of tissue reaction has been reported, this being transient erythema along the injection track for several days after injection. It is suspected that this redness may have resulted from bleeding during the injection. Most clinical results have been subjective in which the physician rates the degree of correction from 0 to 4, where 0 is no correction, 1 is 25% correction, 2 is 50% correction, 3 is 75% correction, and 4 is 100% correction. One of us (Dr. Casson) has conducted followup evaluations of the safety and efficacy of Autologen in more than 25 patients receiving multiple treatments. Results from this study are presented in Figure 65–4. The patients were given from one to three injections of Autologen to treat wrinkle lines in various locations. Followup evaluations ranged from 1 month to more than 1 year. Volumes from 0.5 to 1.0 mL were injected, per session, into the mid-dermis with slight overcorrection. As shown in Figure 65–4, a single injection provided 50% to 75% correction up to 3 months and 50% correction up to 6 months. Two injections provided 75% correction up to 6 months. Three or more injections in this series provided greater than 75% correction beyond 12 months. There were no reports of adverse reactions in any of the patients in this study.

Excellent correction after multiple Autologen injections has been supported by another of us (Dr. Fagien). Figures 65–5 and 65–6 show a deep glabellar furrow before treatment and 3 months after the two injections to-

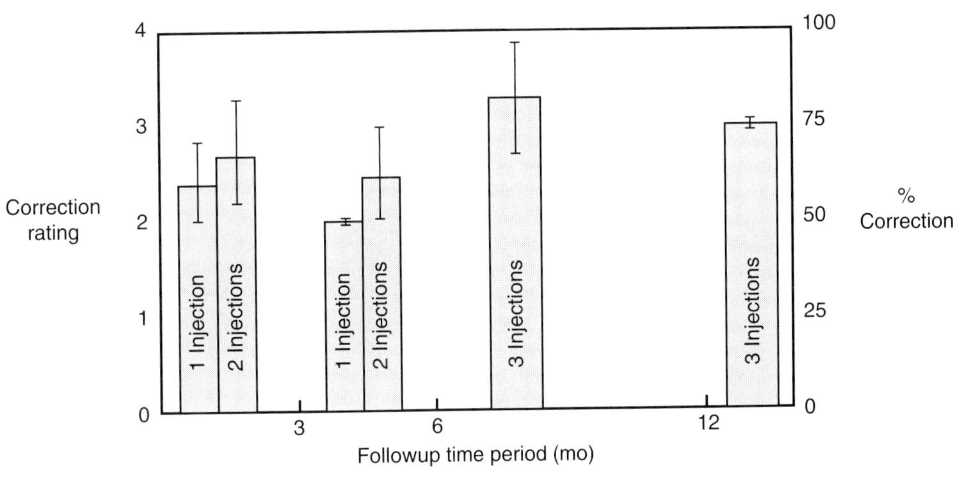

Figure 65–4. Autologen followup scores in clinical evaluations (see text for details).

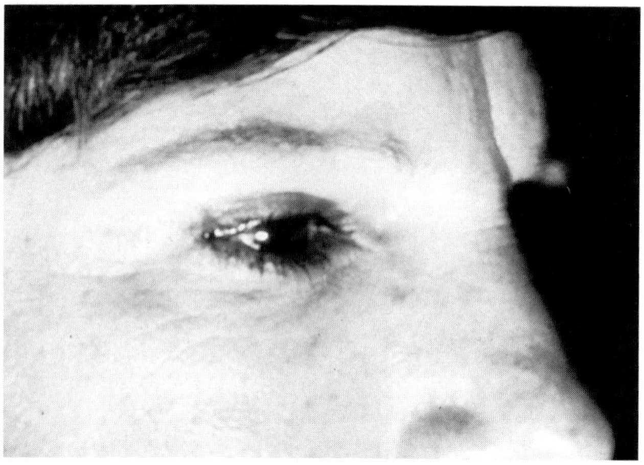

Figure 65–5. Deep glabellar furrow: pretreatment.

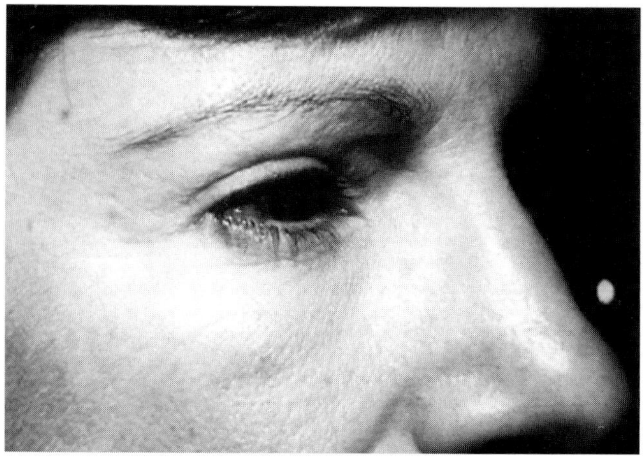

Figure 65–7. Glabellar correction 8 months after the fourth Autologen injection. Total volume is 1.5 mL.

taling 0.8 mL of Autologen. Figure 65–7 shows the same patient 8 months after two additional injections totaling 0.7 mL of Autologen. Correction of the glabellar furrow has now been maintained 12 months after the final treatment with Autologen. In total, four small injections totaling 1.5 mL were administered over a period of 6 months. Most of the Autologen injected into this patient was processed from eyelid tissue removed during a routine blepharoplsty.

Other clinical reports, primarily based on subjective observations, clearly indicate that Autologen is long lasting (beyond 12 months in the patients followed for this time period).

Histopathology of Implant Sites

Small aliquots (0.1 mL) of Autologen and Zyderm II were injected into the mid-dermis of the forearm of a volunteer. The injection site was photographed and the location carefully recorded using visible dermal markers. At 1 month, the injection sites were visibly examined and palpated to determine the presence of the implant. Biopsy specimens of about 2 mm were removed, fixed in formalin, sectioned, and subjected to hematoxylin and eosin and to trichrome staining.

Clinically, both injection sites were unremarkable with no evidence of inflammation or irritation. The presence of Autologen was detected by palpation. Zyderm II could not be detected by palpation. Histopathologic examination of stained specimens revealed normal orthokeratosis, although the Zyderm II specimen shown in Figure 65–8 contains a thin layer of compact keratin at the deepest level of the corium. This specimen also shows evidence of epidermal thickening and disorganization with epithelial cell regeneration, indicative of a mild inflammatory reaction. The Autologen specimen (Fig. 65–9) shows no indication of epidermal disorganization, and the epidermis is of normal thickness with clear cells.

In general, the 1-month biopsy specimens show histopathologic changes in the epithelium of the Zyderm II injection site indicative of a mild response to injury. Al-

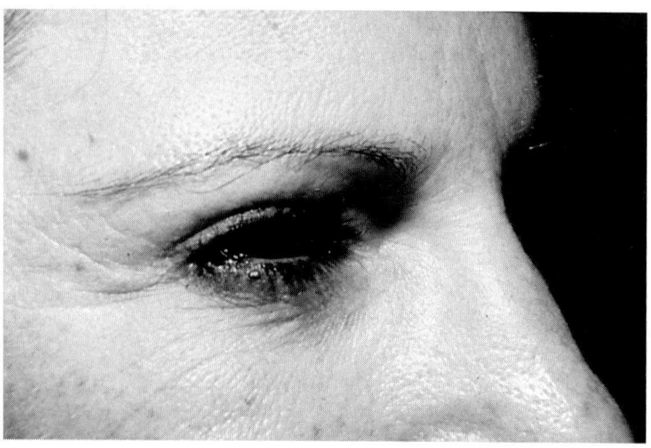

Figure 65–6. Glabellar correction 3 months after the second Autologen injection. Total volume is 0.8 mL.

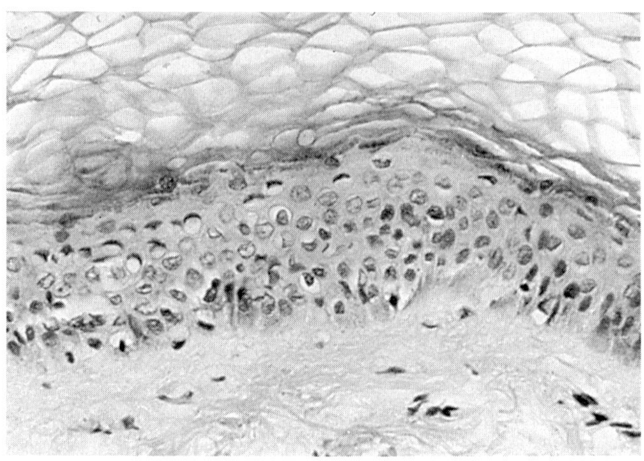

Figure 65–8. Zyderm II biopsy site: epidermal layer.

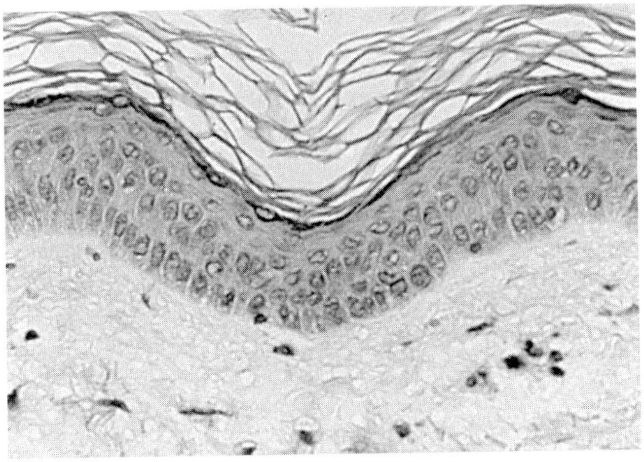

Figure 65–9. Autologen biopsy site: epidermal layer.

though both materials seem to be well tolerated, Autologen appears to be devoid of any tissue reaction.

REFERENCES

1. Leaf N, Zarem HA: Correction of contour defects of the face with dermal and dermal-fat grafts. Arch Surg 105:715, 1972.
2. Spira M, Rosen T: Injectable soft tissue substitutes. Clin Plast Surg 20:181, 1993.
3. Hanke CW, Coleman WP III: Collagen filler substances. *In* Coleman WC III, Hanke CW, Alt TH, Asken BC (eds): Cosmetic Surgery of the Skin—Principles and Techniques. Philadelphia, BC Decker, 1991, p 89.
4. Clinch TE, Goins KM, Cobo LM: Treatment of contact lens-related ocular surface disorders with autologous conjunctival transplantation. Ophthalmology 99:634, 1992.
5. Chauvard S, Jebara V, Chachaques JC, et al: Valve extension with glutaraldehyde-preserved autologous pericardium: Results in mitral valve repair. J Thorac Cardiovasc Surg 102:171, 1991.
6. Schulman ML, Schulman LG, Lledoperez AM: Unusual autogenous vein grafts. Vasc Surg 26:257, 1992.
7. Tenbruggenkate CM, Kraaijenhagen HA, Vanderkwast WAM, et al: Autogenous maxillary bone grafts in conjunction with placement of ITI endosseous implants: A preliminary report. Int J Oral Maxillofac Surg 21:81, 1992.
8. Boyce RG, Toriumi DM: Considerations in the use of biological grafts and alloplastic implants in facial plastic and reconstructive surgery. J Long-term Effects Med Implants 2(4):199, 1992.
9. Nanchahal J, Ward CM: New grafts for old? A review of alternatives to autologous skin. Br J Plast Surg 45:354, 1992.
10. Wiggs EO: Extrusion of enucleated implants: Treatment with secondary implants and autogenous temporalis fascia or fascia lata patch grafts. Ophthalmic Surg 23:472, 1992.
11. Hakelius L, Olsen L: Free autogenous muscle transplantation in children: Long-term results. Eur J Pediatr Surg 1:353, 1991.
12. Gunter JP, Rohrich RJ: Augmentation rhinoplasty: Dorsal onlay grafting using shaped autogenous septal cartilage. Plast Reconstr Surg 86:39, 1990.
13. Endo T, Nakayama Y, Ito Y: Augmentation rhinoplasty: Observations on 1200 cases. Plast Reconstr Surg 87:54, 1991.
14. Miller TA: Temporalis fascial grafts. Plast Reconstr Surg 65:236, 1980.
15. Beekhius GJ: Saddle nose deformity: Etiology, prevention, and treatment: Augmentation rhinoplasty with polyacrylamide. Laryngoscope 83:368, 1989.
16. Nunnery WR, Hetzler KJ: Dermal fat graft as a primary enucleation. Ophthalmology 92:1256, 1985.
17. Illouz YG: Present results of fat injection. Aesthet Plast Surg 12:175, 1988.
18. Fredericks S: Fat-grafting injection for soft-tissue augmentation. Plast Reconstr Surg 84:935, 1989.
19. Churukian M: Autologous fat transplantation. *In* Glasgold AI, Silver FH (eds): Applications of Biomaterials in Facial Plastic Surgery. Boca Raton, FL, CRC Press, 1991, p 257.
20. Dow Corning Silicone Injection Study Questioned by Rep. Weiss. MDDI Rep June 17, 1991, p 5.
21. Clark DP, Hanke CW, Swanson NA: Dermal implants: Safety of products injected for soft tissue augmentation. J Am Acad Dermatol 21:992, 1989.
22. Teimorourian B, Chajchir A, Gotkin R, et al: Semiliquid autologous fat transplantation. Adv Plast Reconstr Surg 5:57, 1989.
23. Parsons RW: Editor's comment. Adv Plast Reconstr Surg 5:83, 1989.
24. Timpl R: Immunological studies on collagen. *In* Ramachandran GN, Reddi AH (eds): Biochemistry of Collagen. New York, Plenum Press, 1976, p 319.
25. Furthmayr H, Timpl R: Immunochemistry of collagens and procollagens. Int Rev Connect Tissue Res 7:61, 1976.
26. Linsenmayer TE: Immunology of purified collagens and their use in localization of collagen types in tissues. *In* Weiss JB, Jayson MIV (eds): Collagen in Health and Disease. Edinburgh, Churchill Livingstone, 1982, p 244.
27. Capaldi MJ, Chapman JA: The C-terminal extrahelical peptide of type I collagen and its role in fibrillogenesis in vivo. Biopolymers 21:2291, 1982.
28. Brennan M, Davison PF: Influence of the telopeptides on type I collagen fibrillogenesis. Biopolymers 20:2195, 1981.
29. Fagien S, Kelman CD, DeVore DP, et al: Soft tissue augmentation with autologous injectable dermis. Presented at the Annual Meeting of the American Society of Ophthalmic Plastic and Reconstructive Surgery, Dallas, TX, November 1992.

CHAPTER 66

Electropigmentation and the Cosmetic Surgery Patient

Holla'e Ploof

Blepharopigmentation is an ancient art. Cleopatra's attendants implanted cobalt blue dye into her eyelid margins utilizing gold needles. Later, in the Orient, bamboo sticks forced permanent dyes and inks into the eyelids of geishas. This technique was crude, leaving ink mixed with congealed blood and often placed at variable depths. It eventually became known as sailors' art or tattooing. In the 1980s, surgically applied microimplantation known as permanent eyeliner was introduced. For this technique, local infiltration of anesthetic and a blepharostat, to stabilize the lid margin and protect the globe, are used.

INDICATIONS (Table 66–1)

Lash Enhancement. Electropigmentation *does not replace conventional cosmetics.* It should be implanted so as to appear natural and not overdone. Traditional make-up can then be applied to allow for changes of moods, hair styles, weight changes, and changes in skin coloration.

Scar Camouflage. Electropigmentation can be used to cover conspicuous hyperpigmented or hypopigmented scars.

Lash Regrowth. Cases of lash alopecia have been observed in which significant regrowth occurred after electropigmentation; stimulation of the hair matrix with papillary regeneration has been postulated.

Brow Alopecia. Thin, absent, or malpositioned brows can be augmented or recontoured (Fig. 66–1).

PATIENT EVALUATION

Before a patient undergoes electropigmentation the general condition of the skin must be evaluated. Any congenital, localized, or systemic conditions must be identified. All medications that the patient may be taking must also be considered. Any anticoagulants or vasodilators may adversely affect the final result. The patient's desired outcome and realistic expectations must be discussed; I call this subjective complaint analysis. The oculoskeletal facial planes (Fig. 66–2) are identified and evaluated. The electropigmentologist must remember that the procedure does not take the place of surgical intervention. The past and future surgical options must be considered. Rapport with your plastic surgical colleagues is essential. For example, a patient with brow ptosis, upper lid redundancy, and a marked deficiency in hair density index may be well served with a combination of surgical correction and electropigmentation. A patient with brow ptosis who undergoes electropigmentation of the ptotic brow without surgical correction may find that the newly pigmented brows appear inappropriately elevated after corrective brow surgery performed at a later date.

TECHNIQUE

Tattoo machines traditionally utilize a mini jack hammer technique as the tattooist uses a writing movement against the skin. Multiple needles are often used simultaneously—frequently 3 to 14 (Fig. 66–3). Slight bleeding and excoriation are not uncommon while this procedure is performed. The result may be a smudged look caused by fanning of the pigment.

Electropigmentation is a procedural concept based on electrolysis. Small amounts of pigment are deposited into the very shallow reticular dermis using a single-needle technique (Fig. 66–4). There is a disposable needle chamber; the needle, pigment cone, and the chamber are disposed of after each treatment. The stainless steel shaft is autoclaved. Although specialized single needles are designed expressly for camouflage procedures, the best needle for lid and eyebrow procedure is 80 gauge of medium length without any irregular surfaces to excoriate the tissue. Insertion skill is a prerequisite. The epidermal thickness is a factor that will determine pigment resolution and retention. Average epidermal layer thickness is between 0.07 and 0.12 mm. It is crucial that pigment is deposited into the upper level of the reticular layer to both promote retention and ensure against migration (Fig. 66–5). This is particularly true in the upper lid where

TABLE 66-1

Indications and Contraindications of Electropigmentation

Indications
- Lash enhancement
- Scar camouflage
- Lash regrowth
- Brow alopecia

Contraindications
- Any active lid pathologic process
  - Blepharitis
  - Chalazia
  - Benign or malignant lesions in the area to be treated
- Positive skin test to the pigment demonstrating allergy to pigment
- Recent eye or lid surgery
- Unrealistic expectations
- Psychological disorders
- Bleeding tendencies or medications that promote bleeding (aspirin, warfarin, heparin)
- Excessive sun exposure

fanning or spreading of the pigment line has been described. A fairly simple way to determine tissue depth is to grip a terminal hair shaft with forceps at the skin surface and lift upward. The distance between the forcep and the beginning of the hair bulb sheath is a good indication of the epidermal thickness (usually about 1 mm). Since the eyelashes on each individual patient will differ in density, the number of lashes per centimeter should be counted (hair density index). In the average patient there are three rows of lashes on the upper lid and one or two rows on the lower lid.

On the morning of the procedure and again just before the procedure is performed the patient is instructed to cleanse the eye area with pHisoDerm or a cleansing solution that does not leave residue. A topical anesthetic (benzocaine) is applied to the eyelid skin. The lid margin is held away from the globe for 6 to 8 seconds until the anesthetic dries. Electropigmentation begins from the lateral canthus (Fig. 66-6).

An easy gliding motion affords gentle entry into the skin to a depth of 1 to 2 mm, depositing pigment at the lash line without tissue maceration (Fig. 66-7). There should be no bleeding and little discomfort. Edema and inflammation should be minimal. Overpenetration is avoided since it will cause discomfort and bleeding.

Pooling pigment is wiped away with a surgical sponge. Generally, the pigment should be thicker laterally and thinner medially (Fig. 66-8). Pigment insertion should end 1 to 2 mm temporal to the punctum. The patient and electropigmentologist should be aware that the final result will not be as dark as it appears immediately after the procedure. The pigment will lighten 15% to 20% during 7 to 12 days after implantation.

Undercorrection is useful in that a preliminary line is created and the patient and electropigmentologist can assess its position. Additional pigment is easily applied. The highest percentage of patients will make the decision to "go darker and more dramatic."

The application of pigment may be modified if a change in the shape or size of the eyes is desired. In patients with close-set eyes the insertion of pigment is most intense at the lateral canthi and will give the appearance of more widely spaced eyes. In patients with deep-set eyes pigment is applied most heavily from the midportion of the lid to the lateral canthus. To bring wide-set eyes closer together the pigment is implanted evenly from the medial canthus and ends nasal to the lateral canthus. To make the eyes appear larger, pigment is inserted below the lower lid lash line and a heavier application is applied to the midportion of the upper lid lash line. In patients with prominent eyes, if there is a desire to minimize the size of the eyes in relation to the rest of the face and provide a balance and softening to the face, a softer more lateral application of pigment is required. In Asian patients desiring more oval-shaped eyes, the pigment is applied above the top row of lashes in the upper lid and below the bottom row of lashes in the lower lid (Fig. 66-9).

TATTOO PIGMENTS

Unsuccessful pigment coloration has been a problem historically. Often reds and rose colors turned blue-black or brownish and blacks often appear faded blue-gray. Tattoo pigments have primarily an India ink base. A thinner ink is used for detailed line and a heavier one for shading. Permanent cosmetic pigments are usually concentrated iron oxide. However, because of possible inter-

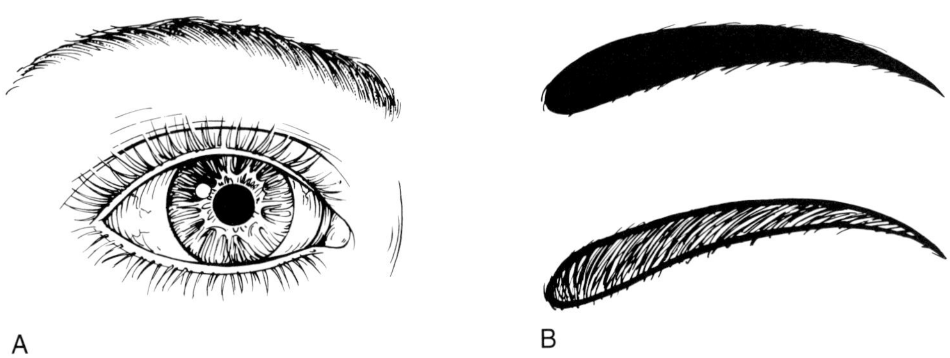

Figure 66-1. *A*, Simulation of natural brow hairs. *B*, Eyebrows with permanent make-up, including solid-filled brow shape and solid outline of brow shape.

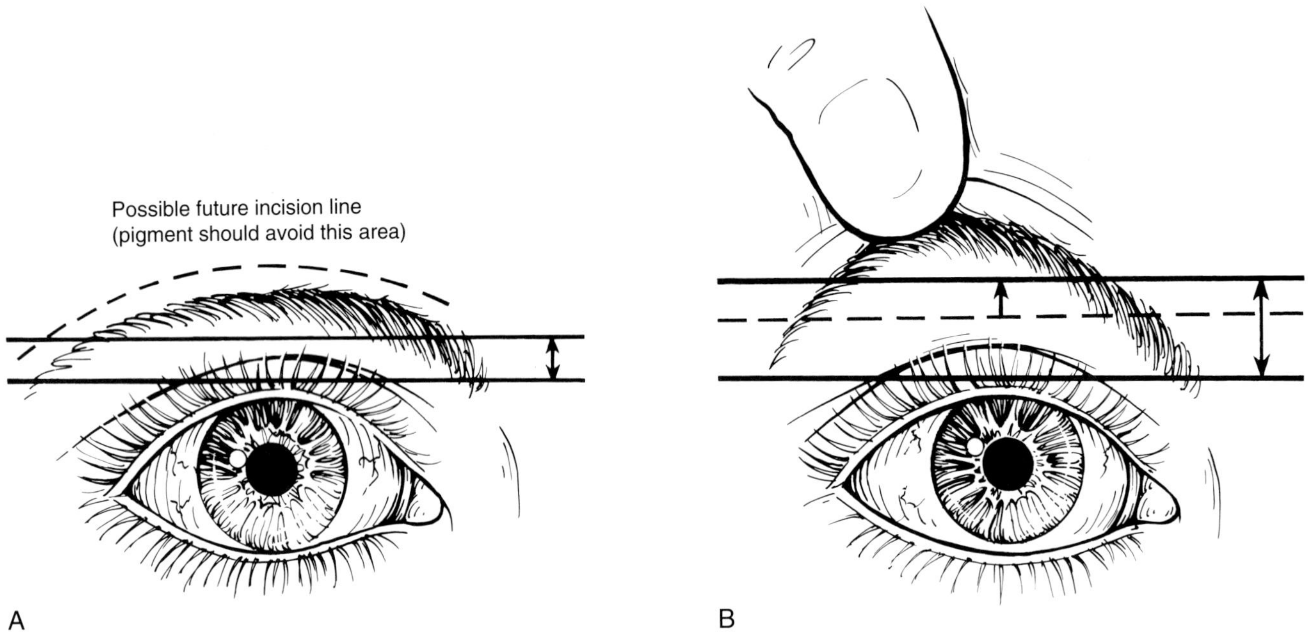

Figure 66–2. *A*, Ptotic brow position. *B*, Manual elevation of eyebrow demonstrates brow ptosis.

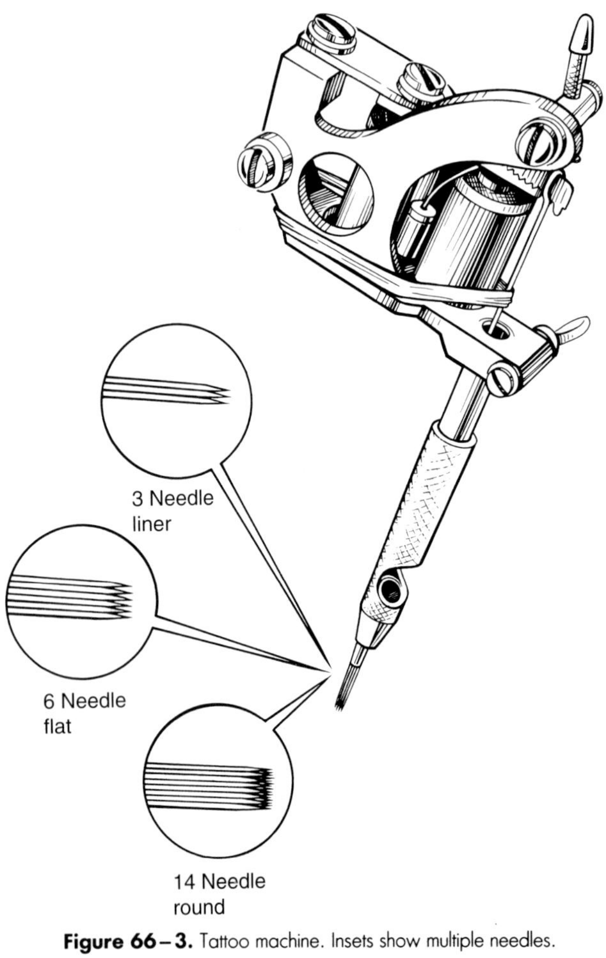

Figure 66–3. Tattoo machine. Insets show multiple needles.

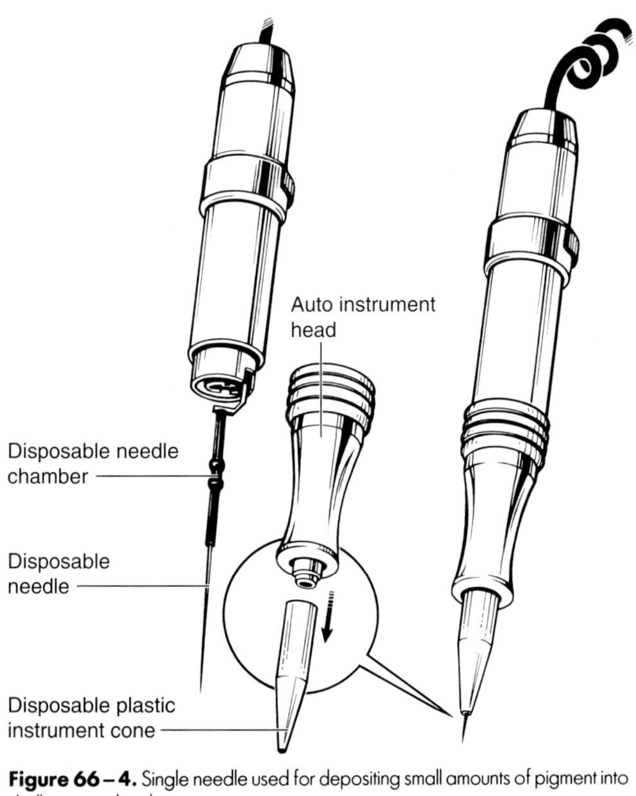

Figure 66–4. Single needle used for depositing small amounts of pigment into shallow reticular dermis.

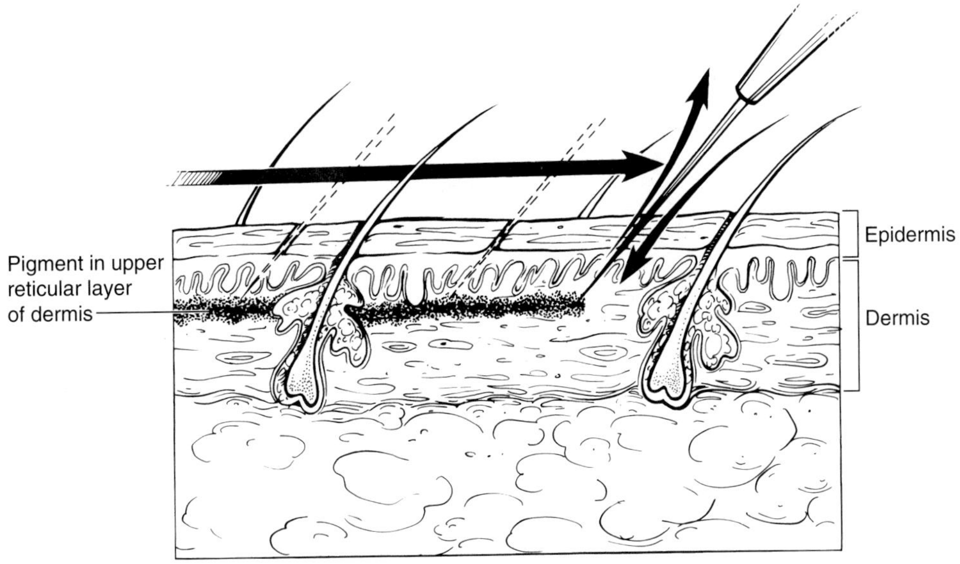

Figure 66–5. Rolling insertion technique for depositing pigment into the upper level of the reticular layer of the skin.

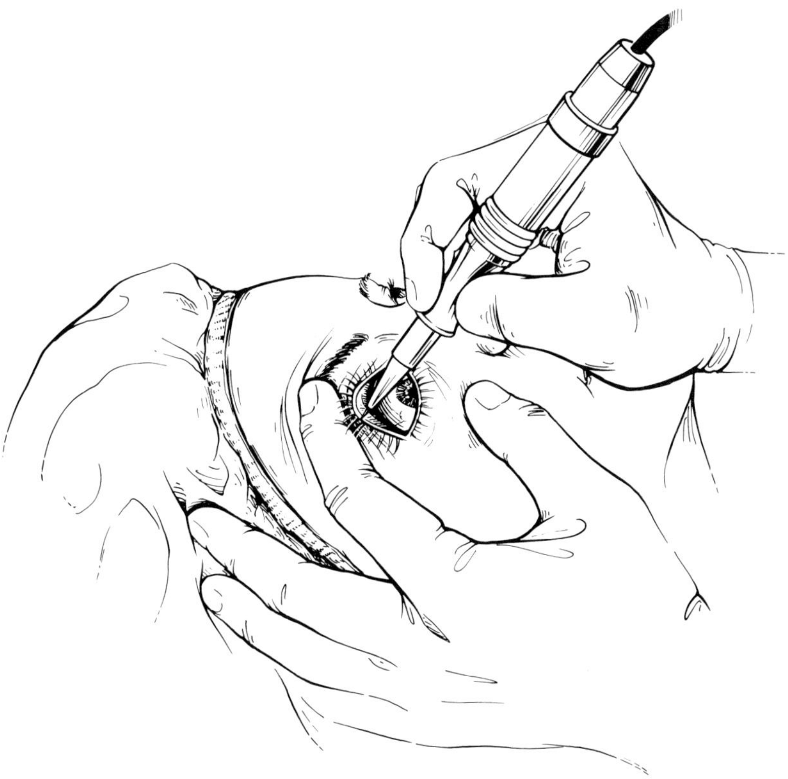

Figure 66–6. Electropigmentation around the eye begins from the lateral canthus.

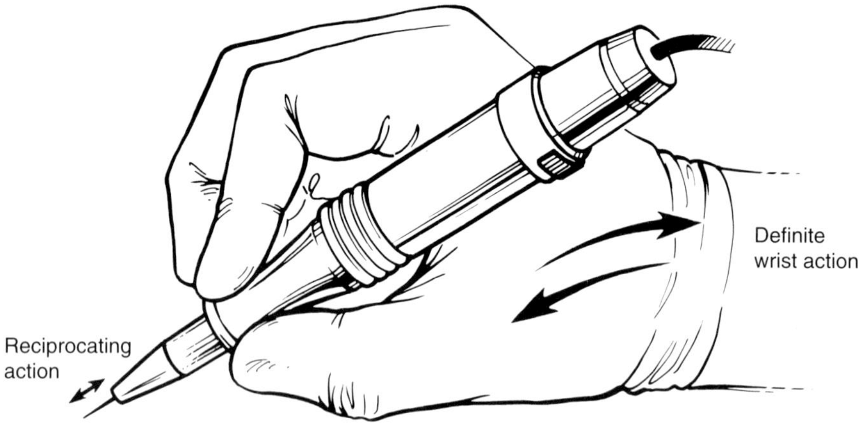

Figure 66–7. An easy gliding motion allows gentle entry into the skin to deposit pigment at the lash line without tissue maceration.

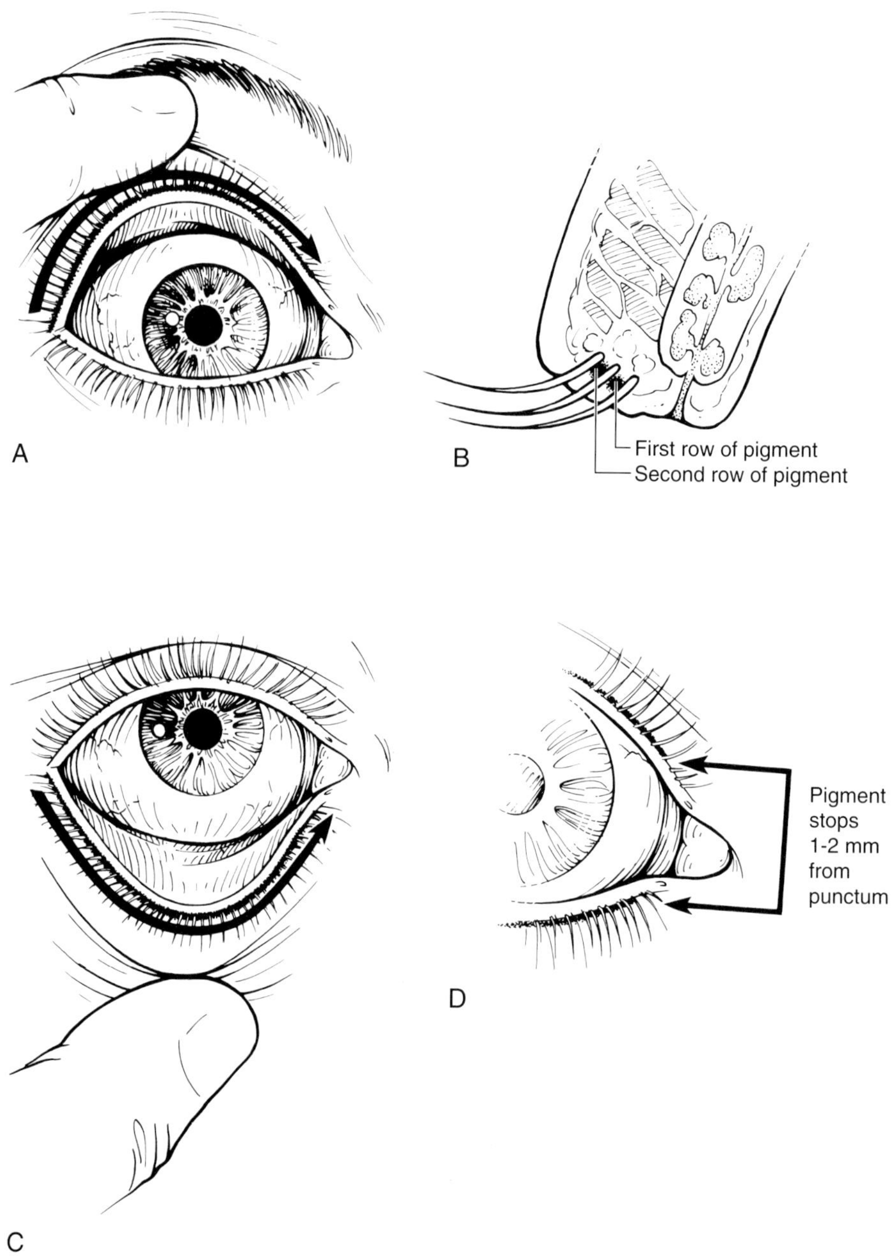

Figure 66–8. *A* to *D*, Generally, the pigment should be thicker laterally and thinner medially.

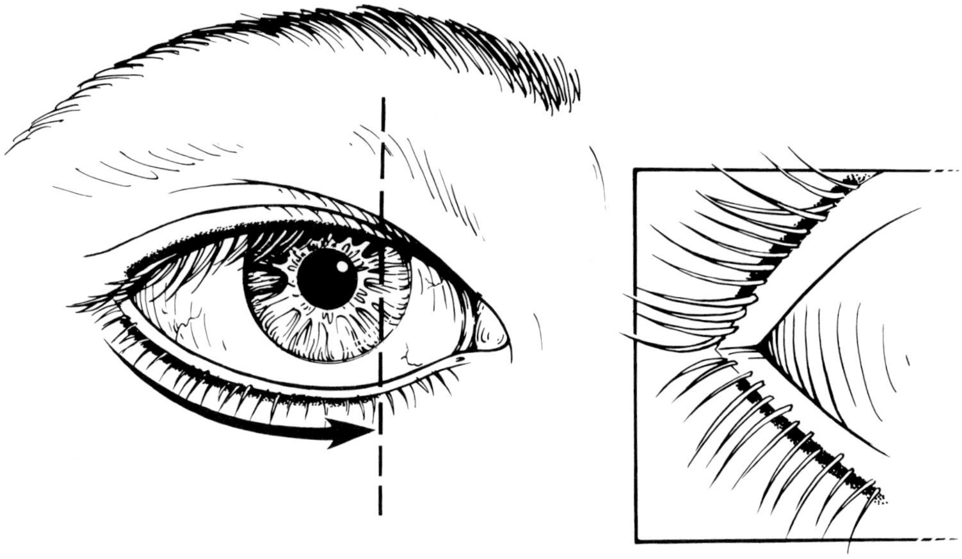

Figure 66–9. In Asian patients who desire more oval-shaped eyes, the pigment is applied slightly above the top lashes and slightly below the lower lashes *(inset)*.

ference with magnetic resonance imaging a plant extract pigment may be substituted. The basic available colors are black, blue, yellow, beige, white, red, light brown, dark brown, and gray. Custom formulated colors can be mixed for individual patients. Although allergy to the pigments is exceptionally rare (red pigment being the most sensitizing), strict mandates for pigment testing are followed. Each patient is given a subcutaneous test dose of pigment behind the ear or between the toes and observed for 72 hours. A second test of base pigment may be implanted in the eyelid. Erythema and induration at the test site indicate sensitivity.

Before selection of the pigment, the patient's natural melanin base must be evaluated. For instance, patients of Mediterranean descent may make implanted brown and black pigments appear purple if their natural base pigment is not blocked or neutralized.

PIGMENT REMOVAL

If the pigment is implanted inappropriately or too densely, it can be removed if the correction is undertaken *immediately* after implantation. Late removal of eyelid pigment is difficult, requiring direct resection or tunable dye laser ablation; neither of these techniques is a guarantee of complete removal. The best treatment is to avoid the complication by conservatively implanting the pigment, saturating cautiously, and constantly reassessing the pigmentation, thus avoiding the creation of large areas that need to be corrected. This will allow for a darker enhancement to be achieved during recoloration after the initial procedure.

If correction is necessary, the area is topically anesthetized. A sterile needle is used to remove the pigment from the dermis. If the area is oversaturated, a lighter shade can be inserted over the implanted area.

COMPLICATIONS

Inexact pigment depth penetration may contribute to pigment migration and a smudged look. Pigment color selection may be inappropriate and there may be failure to block underlying pigment. Inappropriate brow and eyelid pigment placement occurs without regard for preexisting brow ptosis or lidfold redundancy. Overapplication of pigment may be too dark (oversaturated) or implanted in a line that is too thick and unnatural.

CONCLUSION

An open dialogue and communication between the cosmetic surgeon, aesthetician and electropigmentologist can enhance the final result of cosmetic eyelid patients.

CHAPTER 67

Blepharopigmentation: Techniques, Indications, and Comparison of Modalities

Joseph F. Mazza, Jr., and Cynthia Rager

The use of micropigmentation for cosmetic and reconstructive procedures is well established. Medical use of tattooing began in the 1940s primarily to camouflage skin grafts and port-wine stains. Current use has been expanded to include cosmetic micropigmentation for the eyelids, eyebrows, and lips.

Reconstructive micropigmentation includes traumatic and surgical scars, alopecia, vitiligo, and nipple areolar reconstruction. The focus in this chapter includes micropigmentation of the eyelids and eyebrows.

PATHOPHYSIOLOGY

Properly placed pigment should be within the dermis, most of which gets incorporated by macrophages with minimal inflammatory reactions. Fading of pigment over the long term may occur by migration within macrophages to the lymphatics.

PIGMENTS

Most medical-grade pigments are sterilized iron oxide and titanium dioxide in a glycerol and alcohol base. These inorganic pigments tend toward neutral colors such as grays, browns and blacks, rust reds, and skin tone pinks and beiges. In addition, organic pigment or dye is available as tattoo ink. Ingredients are usually red dyes, barium sulfate in suspension, vegetable dyes, and India ink. These colors tend to retain their brightness. Care must be taken when using these dyes since they tend to be more reactive and have a higher rate of allergic reactions. Allergies to paints, crayons, and certain cosmetics would indicate relative contraindications to the use of these pigments. Regardless of the choice of pigment, a patch test is injected behind the ear in the hairline before the procedure. A test of 7 days is used for inorganic pigments, and a test of 30 days is used for the organic pigments or dyes. Each pigment manufacturer will make recommendations for patch testing their pigments.

If you chose to create new colors by blending pigments, care must be taken. Product liability provided by the manufacturer may be forfeited when mixing pigments. Some general rules toward blending pigments exist. If pigment is too dilute because of the proportion of alcohol and glycerin to iron oxides, heavy fading may occur. Pigments of various particle sizes must be constantly remixed to keep particles from settling out. Some manufacturers suggest blending only the same particle size. For this reason, it is important to be knowledgeable about pigments. Gray and black organics exhibit a bluish hue in Caucasian skins after initial fading. Many ash tone beiges for brow color will fade to a pinkish hue. The half-tone of the pigment may be important to note, since pigments sometime fade to the strongest component of their base color, which shows up with half dilution to white. Theoretically, this problem should not occur if a suspension of pigment blended from the same particle size is used.

Pigment choice may define this procedure as a permanent or "extended wear" procedure. An inorganic pigment is not permanent as dyes or India inks. Remember also that India ink can lead to permanent migration. Fading of pigment and individual color acceptance varies from patient to patient after it has been introduced intradermally. Some anatomic areas tend toward more fading than others. In our experience, eyebrows will fade more readily than lash liner. The thickness or transparency of the skin may alter the appearance of the color as well. Primarily, proper technique affects the longevity of the procedure. Many factors affect pigment retention and stability of color when introduced into the skin. Because of the unpredictability of the pigment, patch testing for color is a necessity. We recommend using sterilized pigments in all situations. This may be done by gamma-radiation or autoclaving. Sterile pots of pigments are available to use for blending. Once open, pigment may be sterilized.

Particles must be implanted within the dermis for optimal ingestion by macrophages. It is suggested by most pigment manufacturers that particle size is important and should be no greater than 6 μm. There is some indication that particles of less than 6 μm may be reabsorbed. The suspension of pigment particles must be concentrated enough to leave sufficient particles within the dermis to produce the desired intensity of color.

Allow for a 15% to 20% fading over the first 4 weeks after the procedure and a gradual overall fading of up to 50% over the next several years.

EQUIPMENT

There are a number of available equipment choices. They range from tiny handheld motor-in-pen units to heavier, more elaborate handpieces with separate power units. Several considerations to keep in mind when choosing equipment include variable-depth penetration and speed, visibility of the needle for accuracy, and a unit relatively free of noise and vibration. It is very important to know if the handpiece can be completely sterilized. Some units have an inherent design flaw that allows pigment and fluids to enter the motor housing through the pigment well when the pen is held at an angle greater than 45 degrees. This may freeze the bearings and allow for potential cross contamination. We prefer a power unit that allows for high revolutions of the needle for less drag on the skin. Needle changing should be easy. There are several methods of implantation of pigment. In this chapter we refer to equipment that is used with the "pointilist" method, or the placing of pigment dots very close together.

Needles are available in cluster combination as well as combs and single needles. Usually, they are 26 to 28 gauge. Some manufacturers suggest that the needles are reusable through sterilization, but cluster and comb units have the potential to retain tissue within their prolonged arrangement and may not be totally sterilizable. We recommend using needles only once since they tend to dull with use.

AESTHETIC GOALS

An individual's natural coloring plays an important part in choosing the correct colors for pigmenting. Several considerations are level of values, contrast and undertone of a patient's body, and harmony colors found in hair and skin tones. The color choice should enhance appearance rather than be too obvious and distracting. As a general rule, lighter values of skin tones and eye color (i.e., blond hair, blue eyes) require softer pigment colors. Deeper levels of skin tone, hair, and eye color can carry darker, more vibrant colors (Table 67–1). We recommend a color analysis by a well-trained aesthetician to help in determining suitable undertones. This is especially important if customizing a pigment color by blending is attempted.

Morphology of facial features helps decide placement and width of the pigment. Rounded or angular facial features can help determine the style of the eyebrows. One should look at the contour, width, and depth of the orbit, along with bony prominences and overall facial projection. The arch of the eyebrow is created in accordance with the angularness of the features for balance. Placement of the pigment must be accurately measured from established landmarks to provide for good symmetry.

Eye contour is important in determining pigment placement for the lateral one third of the eyelid. Eyes that have an upward curvature toward the lateral canthus should have pigment thickened and slightly extended into this area. This achieves the illusion of a more almond-shaped eye, which is considered aesthetically pleasing. Pigment dots that are placed beyond the eyelashes in the medial aspect will be highly visible and should be done with extreme care. Pigment in this area should not end abruptly. If the intercanthal distance appears to be decreased, pigment may start several millimeters in the lateral direction from the first lash. Placing pigment in the lateral canthus and connecting the upper and lower lid lines in a V shape may be aesthetically pleasing if the patient wants the pigment to look like a cosmetic line. Take care not to retract the skin too tightly, or the extended line may have a downward droop when released.

CONSULTATION AND PREOPERATIVE TEACHING

A patient's first visit to the office for a consultation regarding micropigmentation can be used to achieve the following:

1. Establish the patient's aesthetic goals
2. Establish a good patient relationship
3. Evaluate the patient's medical history
4. Discuss pretreatment medication and teaching
5. Explain the procedure and the risks
6. Explain general postoperative instructions

A new patient fills out the usual medical history with close attention to any allergies to paints, crayons, or dyes, since this would be a relative contraindication and to a history of any previous eye surgery (especially any recent implantation) or of blepharitis. A documentation of visual acuity is highly recommended. We usually discontinue any therapy with anticoagulants or blood thinning products 1 week before the procedure. This includes warfarin, aspirin, ibuprofen, vitamin E, and alcohol. We also explore any history of iron-deficient anemia, since these patients will tend to reabsorb the iron portions of their pigments.

TABLE 67 – 1

Color Chart for Eyelining Pigment*

Skin Tones	Hair Color: / Eye Colors:	Blonde: Blue	Blonde: Green	Blonde: Brown	Medium Brown: Blue	Medium Brown: Green	Medium Brown: Brown	Dark Brown/Black: Blue	Dark Brown/Black: Green	Dark Brown/Black: Brown	Red: Blue	Red: Green	Red: Brown
Light Values													
Pale beige		Gray	Charcoal	—	Gray/ash brown	Charcoal	Brown/ brown/ black	Charcoal	Charcoal	Brown/ black	—	—	—
Ivory		Light/ medium browns	Light/ medium browns	Medium red	—	—	—	Dark brown	Dark brown	—	Light/ medium brown	Medium gold brown	Medium gold/ dark brown
Medium Values													
Rose beige		Gray/ charcoal	Gray/ charcoal	Medium brown/ charcoal	Gray	Charcoal	Dark brown/ charcoal	Charcoal	Charcoal	Brown/ black	—	—	—
Medium beige		Gray/ charcoal	Gray/ charcoal	Medium brown/ charcoal	Gray	Charcoal	Dark brown/ charcoal	Charcoal	Charcoal	Charcoal	Dark brown	Dark red/ brown	Dark red gold/ brown/ black
Pale olive		Gray/ charcoal	Gray/ charcoal	Medium brown/ charcoal	Gray	Charcoal	Dark brown/ charcoal	Charcoal	Charcoal	Charcoal	—	—	—
Deep Values													
Deep gold beige		Gray w/color	Gray w/color	Dark red/gold brown	Dark brown	Dark brown	Brown/ black	Brown/ black	Brown/ black	Brown/ black	Dark brown	Dark red/ gold brown	Dark gold/ brown black
				Dark brown	Brown/ black charcoal	Brown/ black charcoal	Charcoal	Brown/ black	Brown/ black	Brown/ black	Brown/ black	—	—
Dark Skin Tones Indian, Hispanic, Mediterranean, Asian, African	—	—	—	—	—	—	Brown/ black	Brown/ black	Black	—	—	—	

*Eyebrow colors should be two shades darker than hair color.

Aesthetic considerations are discussed based partly on life-style and age. Diagrams and pictures are helpful, and color match is agreed on.

The procedure is discussed in depth at this time and the risks of the procedure including color fading, nonspecific color guarantee, possibility for alopecia, infection, pigment migration, interference with magnetic resonance imaging, and allergies are discussed. It is stressed that this procedure is not a permanent procedure and touch-ups will be necessary at some later time.

General postoperative care is reviewed with the patient, including the length of recovery time (2 to 3 days) for reduction of edema and resolution of the ecchymosis so that the patient can plan the postoperative period. Swimming and sunbathing are avoided for 1 week, and make-up should not be worn for at least 3 days postoperatively.

At this point a good patient relationship and sense of trust should be established. The patient is encouraged to ask questions and is also referred to patients who have had the procedure.

A patch test is usually performed during the first encounter. This is usually done in the hairline behind the ear but can also be done between the toes.

Managing patient expectations is critical. An exact color or shade is never promised because of the variability of the pigments. Before the procedure the patient will sign his or her operative consent and photographs are always taken. A view of the full face and a close-up of both eyes and each individual eye are obtained.

Postoperatively, the patient is instructed not to rub or vigorously wash the pigmented area. It is important to stress the importance of not picking any scabs or crusts. The patient may gently wipe the area with a cotton swab for the first 48 hours. Some blood-tinged tears are normal for the first day after eye-lining procedures.

Once the procedure is completed, application of ice and head elevation are required for the next 24 hours. The patient returns to the office approximately 1 month after the procedure for a postoperative check. Occasionally, a touch-up is required because of insufficient retention or loss of pigment when healing. We offer touch-ups at no charge for the first 3 months, at which time additional work becomes a new procedure.

TECHNIQUES

Eyelid Blepharopigmentation

Once the color and shape have been agreed on, the eyelids are prepped by removing all make-up. Most patients are premedicated with an oral dose of diazepam approximately 45 minutes before the injection of anesthesia. Two to three drops of proparacaine (Alcaine) 0.5% are placed in the lower lid cul-de-sac. A cotton swab moistened with 4% lidocaine (Xylocaine) is placed over the proposed injection site. We prefer using 0.5% bupivacaine (Marcaine) with epinephrine 1 : 200,000 since there is no delay of onset in this setting. Approximately 6 mL of local anesthetic is required to anesthetize all four lids. The lower eyelid is distracted from the globe and a 27- or 30-gauge needle is placed through the conjunctiva just below the tarsus. The first injection is directed medially, to be followed with a lateral injection of 1 to 1.5 mL per eyelid.

Next the upper eyelid is inverted using a Desmarres eyelid retractor. The first injection is subconjunctival just above the tarsus and placed centrally. One to 1.5 mL is infiltrated, and then a second injection is used laterally to anesthetize the lateral canthal region.

Loupe magnification is highly recommended during placement of the pigment. Tension and protection of the globe is provided by employing a Jaegar lid plate. An alternate method is to use a corneal protector. A three-cluster needle is most commonly employed since this will provide a very distinct dot. A single needle can be used for thinner lines or to taper the medial aspect of the eyelid. Needle power and penetration will vary according to the manufacturer's recommendation. The needles enter the skin at a 90-degree angle to achieve best penetration of the dermis and to avoid any tearing or masceration of the skin. Actual application may follow a template that is created with the first dots and then filled in. The area is wiped frequently with a cotton-tipped applicator and antibiotic ointment to achieve a clean field. A small amount of blood encountered during the procedure ensures proper placement within the dermis. Epidermal placement will desquamate in approximately 5 days. Pigment placed too deep will spread within the tarsus.

Pigment is often extended into the lateral canthus to create a flattering sweep (Fig. 67 – 1). Some patients will prefer complete separation of the lines or only one lid done per side. The procedure is often done simultaneously with an upper and lower blepharoplasty. Pigmentation is placed first to avoid unsightly pigmented blepharoplasty scars. Procedure time is approximately 45 minutes for a lid blepharopigmentation. Local ecchymosis and edema lasting 2 to 3 days are almost universal. Iced compresses are used during the first 24 to 36 hours. Ointment is reapplied as needed.

EYEBROW PIGMENTATION

Anesthesia to the eyebrow may be provided by one of two methods. The first is direct subcutaneous infiltration with 1% lidocaine with epinephrine 1 : 200,000. The second is application of EMLA cream 2 hours before the procedure with an occlusive dressing. We have found the latter technique to be highly effective.

Eyebrow pigmentation is done carefully using reference points at the intercanthus as well as a line drawn from the nasal ala through the lateral canthus to give lat-

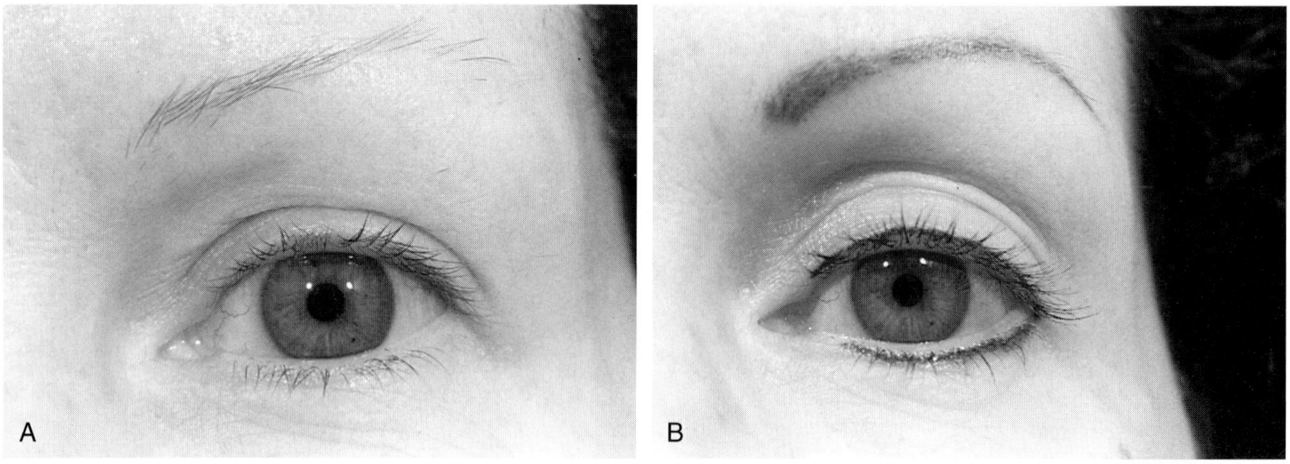

Figure 67–1. Cosmetic application of eyeliner and eyebrow. *A*, Preoperative photograph. *B*, Postoperative photograph.

eral margins. Predesigned templates may be useful to help the patient visualize the desired effect. A template is created by dotting or scraping with a needle until the entire shape has been lightly outlined. Next, using a stroking technique, a single needle is used to mimic each individual cilium. Depending on your equipment and the available needle clusters, a two-needle comb or a three-needle cluster may also be used to simulate hair strokes. We recommend setting the rpms on high when using a stroking technique to avoid tearing of the tissue. Care must be taken over the lateral eyebrow since tearing is common over this bony prominence. Tension of the skin during the micropigmentation procedure is provided by the nondominant hand. Some skin tones should be visible through the strokes to create a dimensional effect. Dark blond, beige, taupe, light brown, and gray are preferable colors used for the eyebrows. In general, eyebrows should be approximately two shades darker than natural hair tones.

Procedure time is 30 to 45 minutes for both eyebrows (Figs. 67–2 and 67–3). Once complete, the area is cleaned and the eyebrows are painted with pigment using a Copland applicator for further absorption. Ice and antibiotic ointment are applied after 2 to 3 hours. Patients are instructed not to pick or remove scabs since this may also remove pigment. The patient's pigment is labeled with a date and refrigerated for any possible future touch-ups. This pigment may be sterilized before its use.

Most complications for this procedure will pertain to the pigmentation itself. Postoperative alopecia (Fig. 67–4) has been encountered in one case when the procedure was performed in conjunction with a blepharoplasty. Approximately 4 mm of lashes from the medial aspect were lost. Some subsequent lash growth spontaneously recurred. The area was repigmented. There have been no encounters with actual allergies to the inorganic pigments, but we have seen loss of pigmentation secondary to anemia in these patients. Allergies to the organic dyes

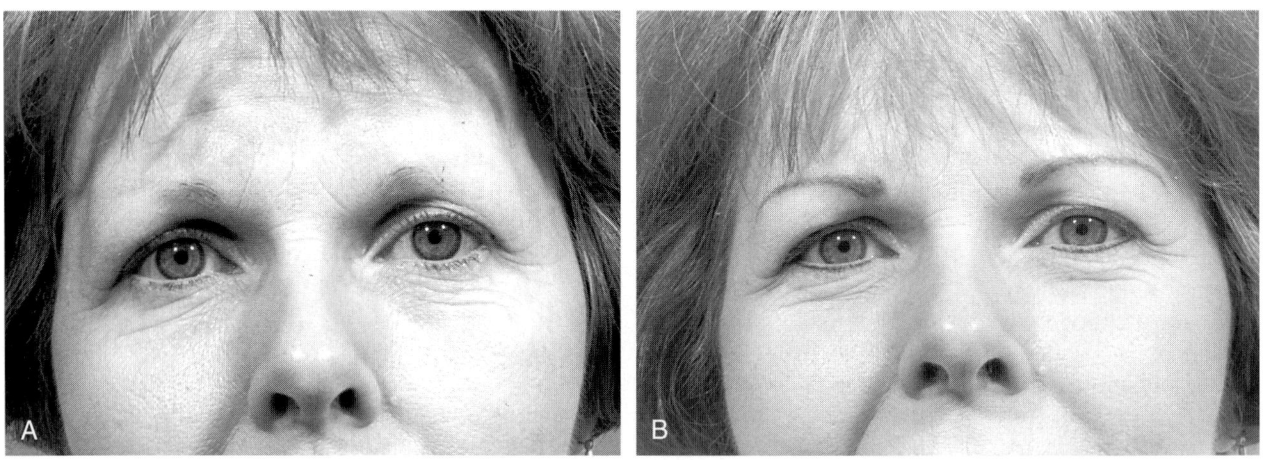

Figure 67–2. Brow pigment and eyelash pigmentation. *A*, Preoperative photograph. *B*, Postoperative photograph.

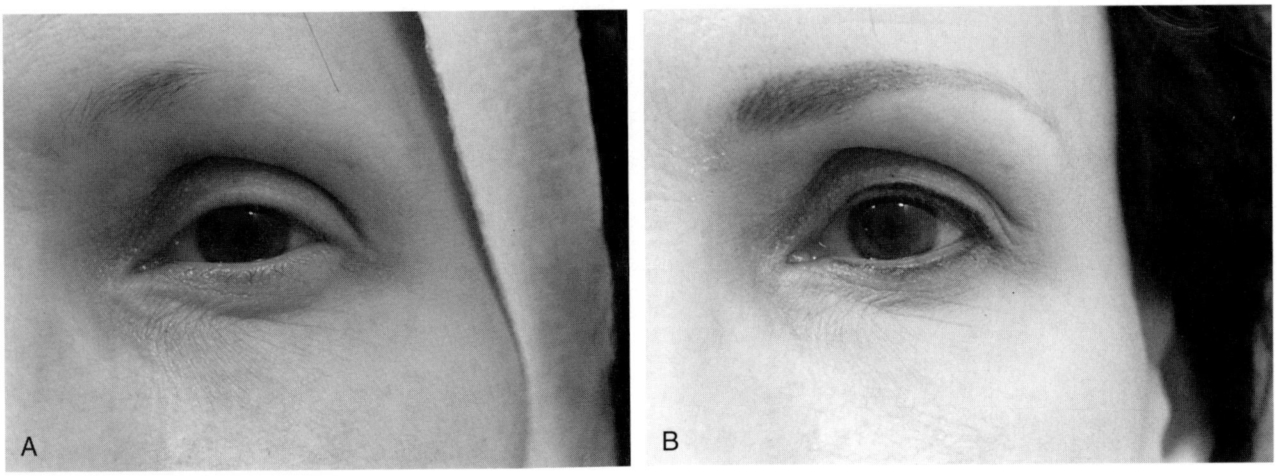

Figure 67 – 3. Alopecia areata is one indicator for microdermal pigmentation for eyeliner and brows. *A*, Preoperative photograph. *B*, Postoperative photograph.

or inks have been encountered in the patch test, and these patients were not candidates for the procedure. Careful placement of the pigment is imperative to avoid asymmetries and the need for removal of any pigment, since this procedure is difficult and painstaking. In the event that pigment is misplaced, multiple modalities can be helpful in correction. Some success has been found by abrading the area with a clean needle and then applying alcohol for dilution. Another technique that may be successful immediately after pigment placement is hydrogen peroxide applied to the area after abrasion. A mixture of glycerol and tannic acid has been applied to abraded areas by tattoo artists for removal of their organic dyes. This forms a scab, and the scab is removed early and at multiple times, taking away most of the pigment. An obvious complication of this method is scarring. Phenol along with trichloroacetic acid have also been used for this purpose. Laser therapy has been shown to be effective in removing pigment, along with direct surgical excision.

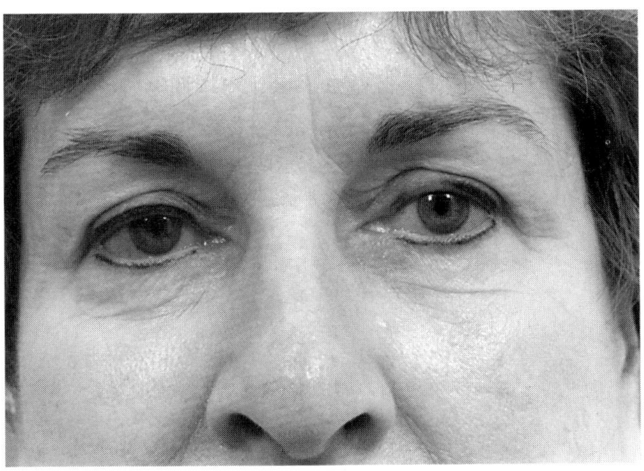

Figure 67 – 4. Postoperative alopecia has been encountered. The area has been repigmented.

New pigment may be placed over a previously implanted area to correct color. Gray-based pigment tends to leave a blue or violet shade when faded. This can be corrected with an organ-based pigment. Many brown pigments will fade to a pinkish hue, which can be corrected with an olive-based green pigment applied directly to the faded area. Several patients have presented themselves to us for correction after having the procedure improperly placed or colored. We have had some success in blending flesh tones to match the patient's natural coloring and stroking this pigment through the old pigment that was darkly applied (Fig. 67 – 5).

Orange tone pigment will help neutralize unwanted bluish casts, and green pigment will do the same for tones that are too pink.

Excess exfoliation may occur as a result of pigment that is placed in the epidermis. Check gauge settings on the handpiece for proper depth of the reciprocating needle, which should be implanted 1.6 to 1.8 mm in the eyelid area. We find that some skin is extremely thin and that pigment is rapidly accepted into the dermis, while other surfaces are tougher to penetrate. Holding the implanting device at 90 degrees to the skin or not less than at a 45-degree angle will help find the proper depth penetration. The longer the needle is actually allowed to stay under the epidermal barrier, the more pigment will be retained. However, care must be taken not to allow the needle to stay too long on the dermis or streaking of the pigment may occur underneath the skin.

Pigment will only be accepted in the areas where other pigment does not reside. Therefore, total masking of unwanted pigment is not possible with this method. However, an acceptable blending effect is achieved in the observer's eye somewhat like a Seurat painting.

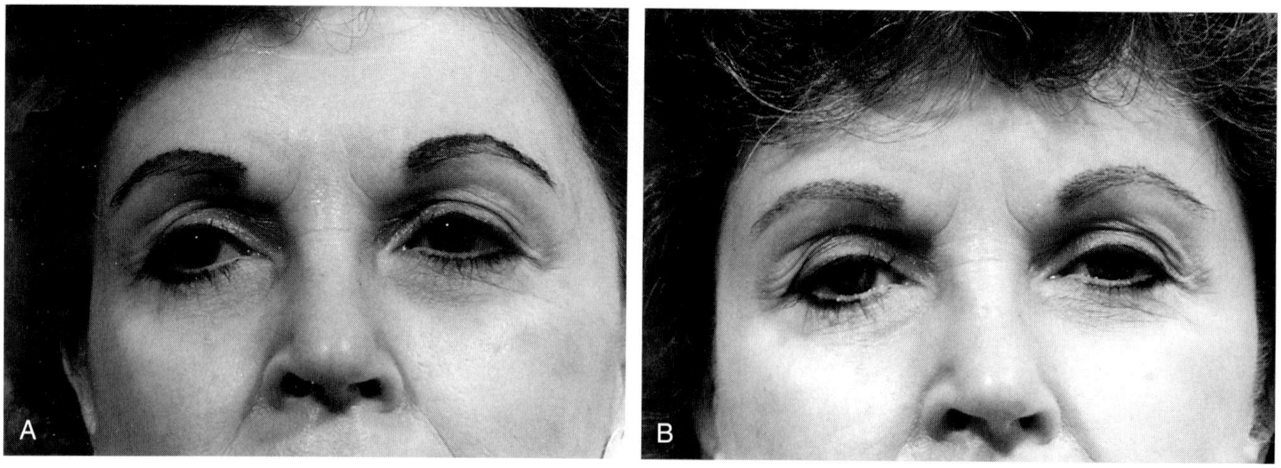

Figure 67 – 5. Eyebrow pigmentation correction. *A*, This pigment was improperly placed and too dark. *B*, Correction was achieved by adding skin-toned pigment.

Because of the method of application (dots versus stroking), eyeliner pigment is usually retained more strongly than brow pigment. Using more than one method of placement may help pigment retention. Using a single color as a base, then stroking a second similar but darker color may achieve a more dimensional looking brow. On placing pigment for corrective purposes or to touch up an existing line, the color should always be applied to the entire area to ensure an even nonsegmented color application.

Index

Note: Page numbers in *italics* refer to illustrations; page numbers followed by t refer to tables.

Abducens nerve, anatomy of, 845
Abducens nerve palsy, eyelid retraction associated with, 74, *75*
  in diabetic patient, 139
Abscess, subperiosteal, diagnostic and therapeutic features of, 941t–942t
    MRI scan of, 889–890, *890*
  with preseptal cellulitis, 310, *310*
Absorbable suture(s), 284, 284t
Acantholysis, in pemphigus, 103
Acanthosis nigricans, *23,* 23–24
  differential diagnosis of, 24
  disorders associated with, 23t
  drug-induced, 23
  in diabetic patient, 140
  malignant, 23–24
ACE (angiotensin-converting enzyme), in sarcoidosis, 108
Acetylcysteine, to reduce ulceration, after chemical injury, 225
ACLE (acute cutaneous lupus erythematosus), 4. See also *Lupus erythematosus (LE).*
  diagnosis of, 6
  ocular complications of, 4–5, 5t
  revised criteria for, 4t
  treatment of, 6–7
Acne rosacea, 38, *38*
Acoustic neuroma, 474
Acquired immunodeficiency syndrome (AIDS), 525–533
  conjunctival Kaposi's sarcoma in, 236, 242, *243*
  eyelid manifestation(s) of, 526–529
    herpes zoster ophthalmicus in, 526
    infection as, 526
    Kaposi's sarcoma as, 526–528, *527*
    molluscum contagiosum in, 526, *526*
    non-Hodgkin's lymphoma as, 528
    sebaceous cell carcinoma as, 528–529
    verruca vulgaris in, 526
  management of, 525
  ocular manifestation(s) of, 532–533
    cytomegalovirus retinitis as, 533
    Kaposi's sarcoma as, 532
  orbital manifestation(s) of, 529–532
    aspergillosis as, 529, *530*
    eosinophilic granuloma as, 532
    infection as, 529
    inflammatory diseases as, 529–530
    non-Hodgkin's lymphoma as, 530–532, *531*
    Pneumocystis carinii infection and, 529
    tumors as, 532, *532*
Acquired immunodeficiency syndrome (AIDS) *(Continued)*
  seborrheic dermatitis in, *37,* 38
  transmission of, 525
  virus causing, 525
Acrochordon (skin tag), of eyelid, 324, *324*
Acromegaly, 142–143
Acrospiroma, eccrine, of eyelid, 334
Actinic keratoses, chemical peels for, 663
Actinomycosis, involving eyelids, 314
Acuity, visual. See *Visual acuity.*
Acupuncture, 695
  auricular, equipment for, 719
    for blepharospasm, 718–720, 719t
    mapping studies in, 718
    point localization in, 718–719, *719*
    preparation for, 718
    technique of, 719, *720*
Acute cutaneous lupus erythematosus (ACLE), 4. See also *Lupus erythematosus (LE).*
  diagnosis of, 6
  ocular complications of, 4–5, 5t
  revised criteria for, 4t
  treatment of, 6–7
Acute disseminated epidermal necrosis (ADEN), 35, 106
Addison's disease, 141
ADEN (acute disseminated epidermal necrosis), 35, 106
Adenoacanthoma (adenoid squamous carcinoma), of eyelid, 350
Adenocarcinoma, metastatic, to eyelid, *54*
  of lacrimal glands, 999, *1000*
    treatment of, 1004
Adenoid cystic carcinoma, of lacrimal glands, 68–69, *69,* 303, *304*
    metastasis from, 1004, *1006*
    prognosis for, 1004–1005, *1005*
    radiologic features of, 1001, *1001–1002*
    treatment of, 1005
  of orbit, 68–69, *69*
Adenoid squamous carcinoma (adenoacanthoma), of eyelid, 350
Adenoma, pleomorphic, of eyelid, 334, *334*
    of lacrimal glands, epidemiology of, 999, 1001
      malignant transformation of, 1002, 1003
      natural history of, 1002
      presentation of, *1000,* 1001
      radiologic features of, 1001, *1001–1002*
      treatment of, 1004
Adenoma *(Continued)*
  sebaceous, in tuberous sclerosis, 27
    of eyelid, 337, *337*
Adie's pupil, 877
Adipose tumor(s), of orbit, 996–997
Adult pleomorphic rhabdomyosarcoma, 995
Aesthetician, role of, before and after surgery, 576–577
Aesthetics, definition of, 573
  in plastic and reconstructive surgery, 573–575
    patient benefits of, 574–575
    physician benefits of, 573–574
  medical, certification courses in, 574t
African American(s), exophthalmometry in, 699t
  oculoplastic surgery in, considerations for, 715–717, *716–717,* 717t
Age, osteotomy and, 1053
Age distribution, of orbital lesions, 854t–856t, *857–858,* 858t
AIDS. See *Acquired immunodeficiency syndrome (AIDS).*
Alfentanil, as anesthetic agent, 296
Alginate impression, used in design and making of prosthesis, 1138, *1138*
Alkali burns, 222–230. See also *Chemical injury(ies).*
Alkylating agents, pharmacology of, 97
Allergic granulomatous angiitis, 113
Allergic reaction(s), to anesthesia, 297
Allergy, causing tearing, 751
  pseudonasolacrimal duct obstruction secondary to, 751–752
"Alligator" tears, 735
Alloplasty, and spontaneous epithelialization, in conjunctival mucous membrane replacement, 171–172, *171–172*
Alopecia, brow, electropigmentation for, 676
Alopecia areata, *44,* 44–45
Alopecia mucinosa, 44, *44*
Alopecia totalis, 44
Alopecia universalis, 44, *44*
Alpha-hydroxy acids, for wrinkles, 563–564, *564*
  used in chemical peels, 666t, 666–667
Alveolar rhabdomyosarcoma, 995
Amebiasis, involving eyelids, 317
Amphotericin B, for phycomycosis, 138
Ampicillin, for sinus infections, 939
Amyloid A, 18, 238
Amyloid AA, 944

Amyloid fibrils, cause and structure of, 944–945
Amyloid L, 18, 238
Amyloidosis, *17,* 17–19, 944–947
classification of, 18t, 945
conjunctival, *65,* 65–66, 238–240
classification of, 238, 239t
primary localized, 238–239, 239t
amyloid in, 239, *239–240*
management of, 239–240
ptosis due to, 240
secondary localized, 239t, 240
differential diagnosis of, 19
eyelid as site of, *65,* 65–66
localized forms of, 238, 239t
myeloma-associated, 18
ocular presentation of, 945–946, *945–946*
pathology of, 946–947, *947*
secondary systemic form of, 238, 239t
systemic manifestations of, 945
Anaphylactic response (hypersensitivity type I), 96
Anesthesia, "balanced," 297
for blepharoplasty, 706
for enucleation, 1038
for harvesting of tissue grafts, 1080, 1083
for oculoplastic surgery, 294–299
commonly used agents in, 296–297
in pediatric patients, 298–299
intraoperative problems in, 298
local or monitored approach to, advantages and disadvantages of, 297–298
management of concurrent medications with, 295–296
monitoring during, 298
preoperative evaluations and screening tests in, 294–295
for tarsal polishing with mucous membrane grafting, 203
for transantral approach to orbital decompression, 974
for transorbital antroethmoidal orbital decompression, 969
general, agents for, 297
monitored care during, 296–297
regional, advantages of, 297
for eyelid surgery, 278–279, 442, 550
for lower eyelid blepharoplasty, 619–620, 627
for male blepharoplasty, 636
for pterygia removal, 212
for upper eyelid blepharoplasty, 589–599, *599*
variations in, 606–607
Anesthetic agents, allergy to, 297
anxiolytics as, 296
barbiturates as, 297
for general anesthesia, 297
narcotics as, 296–297
use of, monitored care during, 296–297
Angiitis, allergic granulomatous, 113
orbital, 966
Angioedema, 40, *40*
Angiolymphoid hyperplasia, with eosinophilia, 949–950, *949–950*
of eyelid, 332
Angiotensin-converting enzyme (ACE), in sarcoidosis, 108
Angular vein, anatomy of, 275, *276*
Animal bite(s), eyelid injury caused by, 453, 455
Anisocoria, in Horner's syndrome, 78
Ankyloblepharon, congenital, 409
Annulus of Zinn, anatomy of, 847, *847,* 848
Anophthalmic orbit syndrome, 1105. See also *Anophthalmos, acquired.*
Anophthalmic socket, 1127–1133
complications associated with, evaluation and management of, 1105–1125
enucleation vs. evisceration procedures and, 1129–1130
ideal, condition of socket in, 1131, *1131*
evaluation of, 1130–1131
eye symmetry in, 1131, *1131*
head structure in, 1130, *1130*
implant location in, 1131, *1131*
implant mobility in, 1131, *1132*
surgical conditions leading to, 1128–1129, *1128–1130*
volume loss in, 1131, *1131*
lax, 1106–1108
new mobility implants for, 1132, *1133*
nonsurgical monocular conditions of, 1127–1128, *1128*
postsurgical considerations for, 1131–1132
severe contracture in, repair of, 1121, *1122–1125*
split-thickness skin grafts for, 167–168
surgical approach to, 1053–1054
Anophthalmos, 905
acquired, 1105–1125, *1106–1108.* See also *Enucleation.*
enophthalmos in, 1108–1111, *1108–1112*
implant complication(s) following, 1119–1121
exposure or extrusion as, 1119–1121, *1120*
migration as, 1119, *1119*
lax socket in, 1106–1108
lower lid malposition in, 1113–1114, *1115–1118,* 1116–1118
orbital deformity after, 1121
ptosis in, *1118,* 1118–1119
socket contraction after, 1121, *1122–1125*
sulcus deformity in, 1111–1113, *1112–115*
congenital, 1105, *1106*
volume replacement in, 1043
Anterior chamber, paracentesis of, following chemical injury, 223–224
Anthrax, causing necrotic eschars of eyelid, 313
Antibiotics, for orbital cellulitis, 148
for preseptal cellulitis, in children, 310
for sinus infections, 939
Antibody(ies), 95
monoclonal, 96
Antibody-dependent cell-mediated cytotoxicity, 95
Anticholinergics, for essential blepharospasm and Meige's syndrome, 507
Anticonvulsants, chronic patient use of, anesthetic considerations with, 295
for hemifacial spasm, 511
Antigen(s), epidermolysis bullosa acquisita, 105
factor VIII–related, in Kaposi's sarcoma, 242
histocompatibility, 96
Antihypertensives, chronic patient use of, anesthetic considerations with, 295
Antimetabolites, pharmacology of, 97
Anti-Ro/SSA, in subacute cutaneous lupus erythematosus, 5–6
Antrostomy, Caldwell-Luc, 974
Anxiolytics, as anesthetic agents, 296
Aorta, irradiated, used in upper eyelid reconstruction, 365
Apert's syndrome, brachycephaly associated with, 1181, *1183*
subcranial approach to, 1170, *1172–1173*
results of, 1176t
with cranial vault and midface dysplasia, anterior cranial base approach to, 1193, *1196–1197*
Apocrine sweat gland(s), 273, *273,* 324
benign adnexal lesions originating in, 334–335, *334–335*
Aqueous humor, accumulation of inflammatory products in, glaucoma resulting from, 222–223
Aqueous layer, and precorneal tear film, 736
Argon laser, postoperative use of, for pterygia, 219
Arion sling, in surgical management of facial paralysis, 478–479, *479*
Arlt's line, 203
Arterial arcades, tarsal, *275*
Arteriovenous malformation(s), of eyelid, 331
Arteritis, temporal, 112
Artery(ies). See also specific artery, e.g., *Ophthalmic artery.*
of ocular region, 273–274, *274–275*
Arthropod venom, disruption of neuromuscular transmission by, 83
Ascorbate, to reduce corneal ulceration, after chemical injury, 229
Asian patient(s), anatomic differences among, 696t, 696–700, 697t, 698t, 699t, 700t
blepharoplasty in, 702–713. See also *Blepharoplasty, in Asian patients.*
Chinese view of medicine and, *692–694,* 692–695, 693t
cultural background of, 691–692
eyelid tumor(s) in, 721–727
basal cell carcinoma as, 723, *723*
lid reconstruction with donor sclera for, 724–727, *725–727*
sebaceous gland carcinoma as, 721–722, *727*
squamous cell carcinoma as, 721, *727*
statistics on, 723–724
Aspergillosis, orbital, diagnostic and therapeutic features of, 941t–942t
in AIDS patients, 529, *530*
Aspirin, chronic patient use of, anesthetic considerations with, 296
Asteroid bodies, 65
Astrocytoma, juvenile pilocytic, imaging of, 899–900, *899–900*
Atenolol, for thyrotoxicosis, 125, 128
Atopic dermatitis, 41–42, *42*
treatment of, 42
Atrial fibrillation, evaluation of, prior to oculoplastic surgery, 294–295
Atypia, definition of, 179
Auricular cartilage, used in upper eyelid reconstruction, 364, *364*
Auricular prosthesis, osseointegrated, 1159
Auspitz's sign, in psoriasis vulgaris, 39
Autograft(s). See also *Graft(s).*
bone, harvesting of, 1077–1080, *1078–1082*
conjunctival, for management of pterygia, 214–215, *216–217,* 217
complications of, 217
graft harvesting in, 215, *216*
for repopulation of corneal epithelium,

Autograft(s) *(Continued)*
indications for, 249–250
surgical technique of, 250, *250*
Autoimmune syndrome(s), cicatricial pemphigoid associated with, 199
polyglandular, 141
Autologen, 670–675
clinical results with, 673–674, *673–674*
clinical use of, 672–673
collagen dispersion in, 671
collagen fibers in, 672, *672–673*
injection implant site and, histopathologic changes at, 674–675, *674–675*
preparation of, 671
tissue source for, 671–672, 672t
Avitene, for hemostasis in wound repair, 283
Avulsion, in pterygia removal, 211
Azathioprine, for cicatricial pemphigoid, 199
pharmacology of, 97
Azelaic acid, used in chemical peels, 666

B cell(s), 94–95
Bacillus anthracis infection, 313
Bacterial infection(s), causing nasolacrimal duct obstruction, 797–799, 798t, *799*
of eyelid, 313–315
of orbit, in AIDS patients, 529
Baker's phenol solution, used in chemical peels, 667–668
Balloon cell nevus, of eyelid, 338
Barbiturates, as anesthetic agents, 297
Bare-sclera technique (BST), concept of, 212
of pterygia removal, 212–214, *213*
administration of beta radiation after, 217–218
Bartonellosis, of eyelid, 314
Basal cell carcinoma, of eyelid, 300
clinical presentation of, 342–343
histologic features of, 343, *344*
in African American patients, 716, *717*
in Asian patients, 723, *723*
morphea pattern of, 344, *345*
nodular pattern of, 343, *344*
orbital invasion of, 300, *301*
superficial spreading (multicentric) pattern of, 344–345, *345*
ulcerative pattern of, 344, *344*
Basal cell nevus syndrome, of eyelid, 67, *68*
Basilar hyperplasia, definition of, 179
Basophil(s), 95
Bell's palsy, 470, 473
in diabetic patient, 139
ptosis following, 91, *91*
Benign reactive lymphoid hyperplasia, involving orbit, 61–62
Benzodiazepines, for essential blepharospasm and Meige's syndrome, 507
for hemifacial spasm, 511
Béraud valve, 742, *743*
Beta radiation, as adjunct to surgery for pterygia, 217–218
Beta-adrenergic antagonists, for thyroid storm, 130
for thyrotoxicosis, 125, 128
Bianchi valve, 742, *743*
Biologic agents, for metastatic renal cell carcinoma, 1012
Biopsy, diagnostic, of neurogenic tumors of orbit, 984
excisional, for conjunctival lymphoid tumors, 236, *236*
for idiopathic orbital inflammation, 955
Biopsy *(Continued)*
indications for, 1046
of eyelid, for suspected sebaceous gland carcinoma, 193
Birbeck granules, 64
Bite(s), eyelid injury caused by, 452–453, *454,* 455
spider, eyelid necrosis due to, 313
Blastomycosis, of eyelid, 318
Blend modality, used in eyebrow contouring, 593
vs. other techniques, 593–594
Blending, of skin color tone, in micropigmentation, 536
Blepharoconjunctivitis, chronic, sebaceous gland carcinoma masquerading as, 346
sebaceous carcinoma presenting as, 301, *303*
Blepharophimosis syndrome, 411, *411*
Blepharopigmentation, 535, 536–537, *537–538.* See also *Electropigmentation; Micropigmentation.*
Blepharoplasty, complication(s) of, 643–650
brow displacement as, 649, *649*
diplopia as, 644
double crease as, 648, *648*
eyelash loss or misdirection as, 649
incomplete or excessive fat removal as, 646–647, *647*
infection as, 648
lacrimal disorders as, 648–649
lagophthalmos as, 646, *646*
lid necrosis as, 650
lower lid malposition as, 644–645, *645–646*
medial canthal folds as, 649
meibomianitis as, 649
oculocardiac reflex as, 650
prominent pigmentation as, 648
ptosis as, 644, *644*
refractive changes as, 649
round eye deformity as, 646, *646*
scarring as, 648
sensory nerve damage as, 649–650
skin asymmetry as, 648
suture tracts as, 649
visual loss as, 643–644
wound dehiscence as, 648
cosmetic, 543–550
anesthesia for, 550
documentation and patient instructions for, *549,* 549–550
fat excision in, 638, *639–642,* 640–642. See also *Fat excision.*
patient examination prior to, 545–549
baseline tear function in, 549
blepharochalasis in, 548
brow contour in, *546,* 546–547
brow position in, 546, *546*
crow's feet in, 548, *549*
glabellar wrinkles in, 547, *547*
Graves' disease in, 548, *548*
ptosis in, 547
redundant upper and lower lid skin in, 547, *547*
scleral in, 548, *548*
seventh nerve function in, 548–549
surgical modalities used in, *544*
in African American patients, 715–716, *716*
in Asian patients, 702–713
anesthesia for, 706
determination and marking of lid crease in, 706, *706*
Blepharoplasty *(Continued)*
incision techniques in, 706–708, *707–708*
complications of, 709
postoperative care following, 708–709
preoperative evaluation in, 705–706
procedures in, 706–713
suture technique(s) in, 709–713
buried mattress, 710–711, *710–711*
combined buried sutures and small incisions as, 712, *713*
complications of, 712–713
continuous suturing as, 711–712, *712*
postoperative care following, 712
lower eyelid, 617–624
anesthetic injection for, 619–620
draping of patient for, 619
evaluation for, 617–619, *618*
postoperative care in, 624, *624*
repair of lid laxity in, 622–624, *623–624*
skin flap approach to, 620, *620*
skin-muscle flap approach to, 620–622, *621–622*
transconjunctival approach to, 626–631
complications of, 630
inspection of anatomy in, 626, *627*
local anesthesia for, 627
postoperative care in, 629–630
preoperative evaluation and considerations in, 626–627
surgical technique of, 627–629, *628–629*
male, 632–637
anatomic differences in, 633, *633–634*
anesthesia for, 636
lower eyelid correction in, 636–637, *637*
preoperative evaluation in, 633–635
psychosocial issues in, 632
surgical technique in, 635–637, *636*
variations in, 637, *637*
upper eyelid, 596–614
concurrent ptosis repair with, 602–603, *603*
variations of, 609
crease formation and skin closure in, 603, *603–604*
variations of, 609–610
excision and incision of orbital septum in, 600, *600*
variations of, 607–608
excision of fat in, 601, *601*
variations of, 608–609
excision of skin and muscle in, 599–600, *599–600*
variations of, 607
functional indications for, 596–597
historical landmarks in, 597t
local anesthetic infiltration for, 598–599, *599*
variations in, 606–607
postoperative care in, 603–604
variations of, 611
preoperative considerations in, 597, 597t
preparation and draping of patient for, 598
variations in, 605
repair of prolapsed lacrimal gland in, 601–602, *602*
variations of, 609
results of, 611–612, *612–614*
skin closure in, variations of, 610–611
skin marking for, 598, *598–599*
variations in, 605–606
surgical steps in, 597t

Blepharoplasty *(Continued)*
surgical techniques in, 597t, 597–604
variations of, 604–611
Blepharoptosis, in Graves' ophthalmopathy, 515, *515*
Blepharosis, moniliform, 20
Blepharospasm, 89
atypical, 90
auricular acupuncture for, 718–720, 719t, *719–720*
essential, 89, *89*
clinical features of, 504, 506, *506*
diagnostic features of, 505t
management of, 507–510
botulinum A toxin injection in, 507–508, *508*, 509t
future directions in, 509–510
general eye care in, 507
pharmacotherapy in, 507
surgery in, 508–509, *509*
pathogenesis of, 506
management of, 90
Blindness, after blepharoplasty, 643–644
Blood cyst(s), drainage of, 925
Blood supply, to conjunctiva, 161
to facial nerve, *468*, 469
to lacrimal gland, 734, 849
to orbit, 843–844, *843–844*
Blue nevus, of eyelid, 338–339
Bochdalek valve, 742, *743*
Bone(s), craniofacial, abnormality of, 1178–1182, *1179–1185*. See also specific anomaly, e.g., *Brachycephaly.*
male vs. female, 633, *633*
Paget's disease of, causing nasolacrimal duct obstruction, 813
Bone graft(s), autogenous, harvesting of, 1077–1080, *1078–1082*
Bone removal, in orbital surgery, 1048
in transorbital antroethmoidal decompression, *971*, 971–972
Bone wax, for hemostasis in wound repair, 283–284
Bone-anchored hearing aids, 1159
Borrelia burgdorferi, 473
Botryoid rhabdomyosarcoma, 995
Botulinum A toxin, injection of, for essential blepharospasm and Meige's syndrome, 507–508, *508*, 509t
for hemifacial spasm, *508*, 509t, 511
Botulism, cranial nerve paresis in, 152
ptosis from, 83, *84*
Bournville's disease, 26–27, 27t
Brachycephaly, 1180–1181, *1182*
associated with Apert's and Crouzon's syndromes, 1181, *1183–1184*
Bradycardia, during oculoplastic surgery, 298
Breast carcinoma, metastatic orbital disease from, *1009*, 1009–1010
Brightness desaturation, in optic nerve dysfunction, 874–875
Brittle hair (trichothiodystrophy), in ichthyosis, 46
Brow ptosis. See *Ptosis, brow.*
Brown tumor (osteoclastoma), in hyperparathyroidism, 133–134, *134–135*
Browpexy procedure, translid, 587, *587–588*
Brueghel's syndrome, 504
BST (bare-sclera technique), concept of, 212
of pterygia removal, 212–214, *213*
administration of beta radiation after, 217–218
Buccal mucous membrane graft(s), for cicatricial entropion and trichiasis, 203–206
anesthesia and, 203
complications of, 205
harvesting of lower lip membrane in, 204–205, *205*
results of, 205, *206*
surgical methods of, 203–205, *204–206*
for pterygia, 217
"Buff-peel," for wrinkled skin, 565, *565*
Bulbar conjunctiva, 159. See also *Conjunctiva.*
Bulla(e), 29
Bullous disease(s), 98–106. See also specific disease for details.
cicatricial pemphigoid as, 98–100
epidermolysis bullosa as, 103–105
erythema multiforme as, 100–102
pemphigus as, 102–103
toxic epidermal necrolysis as, 105–106
Bullous pemphigoid, vs. cicatricial pemphigoid, 198–199
Bundle of energy theory, *582*, 592
Burkitt's lymphoma, Epstein-Barr virus associated with, 530, 959
Burn(s), alkali, 222–230. See also *Chemical injury(ies).*
facial, micropigmentation for, 535. See also *Micropigmentation.*
thermal, 222

Café-au-lait spots, in neurofibromatosis, 25
Calcification, orbital, dystrophic, differential diagnosis of, 887t
metastatic, differential diagnosis of, 887t
Calcifying epithelioma, Malherbe's, of eyelid, 336, *336*
Calcinosis cutis, in childhood dermatomyositis, 7
Calcium metabolism, regulation of, 132
Caldwell-Luc antrostomy, 974
Caliper(s), used in ophthalmic plastic surgery, *290*
Calymmatobacterium granulomatis infection, 314
Camera, for medical photography, 551–554
automatic film advance in, 551
film in, 554
flash-cord receptacle on, 551
focusing screens of, 552, *552*
lens of, 552–554, *553*
shutter and shutter speed of, 551
Camouflage make-up, 657–661, *658–659*
application principles in, 659–660
choice of, 657, 659t
color principles in, application of, 658, *660*
colors in, choice of, 657–658, *659*
cosmetics used in, 569–571
"faking faults" in, 661
good lighting for, 659
highlighting and contouring in, 660–661
in neutralization of skin discoloration, 658
referral of patient for, 657
use of, 657
in facial rejuvenation, 570–571
Canaliculitis, 153
diagnosis of, 826, *828*
treatment of, 827–829
Canaliculodacryocystorhinostomy, for canalicular stenosis, 830–831
Canaliculus(i), 739–740, *739–741*
agenesis of, 782
Canaliculus(i) *(Continued)*
anatomy of, 821
congenital malformations of, 740, *740*, 821–822, *822*
treatment of, *822*, 822–823
elastic properties of, 745
lower eyelid defects involving, 406
physiology of, 821
stenosis of, 829–831
epiphora due to, 751, *752*
trauma to, 824–825
repair of, 825–826, *826–828*
tumors of, 823–824, *824*
upper eyelid lacerations of, repair of, 359–361, *362*
Candidal infection(s), of eyelid, 318
Cantalano stents, for nasolacrimal duct obstruction, 780
Canthal folds, medial, after blepharoplasty, 649
Canthal ligament(s), medial, 265, *267*
Canthal obliquity, in Graves' ophthalmopathy, surgical techniques for, 521
Canthal tendon, injuries to, repair of, 361–363, *363*
medial, anatomy of, 744
fixation/reconstruction of, 388–390
cantilevered miniplates in, 389–390, *390*
creation of new tendon in, 388, *389*
Nelson screw in, 389, *390*
suturing in, 388–389, *390*
transnasal wiring with dacryocystorhinostomy in, 388, *389*
reconstruction of, in surgical management of facial paralysis, 480, *480–481*
Cantholysis, inferior, in transorbital antroethmoidal orbital decompression, 970, *970*
lateral, in lower eyelid reconstruction, 400, *401*
Canthoplasty, lateral, for paralytic ectropion, 432, *433–435*
Canthotomy, lateral, in transorbital antroethmoidal orbital decompression, 970, *970*
Canthus, injury to, sequence of repair following, 458, *459*
lateral, migration of, as complication of medial reconstruction, 398
rounding of, after blepharoplasty, 646, *646*
medial, laxity of, plication for, 426–427, *426–427*
reconstruction of, 387–398
complications of, 398
composite graft in, 391
direct closure in, 388
glabellar flap in, 391, 393, *395*
goals in, 387
insertion of pretarsal muscles in, 387, *388*
island forehead flap in, 393, *396*
lacrimal involvement in, 396, 398
midline forehead flap in, 393, *396*
Mustardé flap in, 390–391, *392*
myocutaneous flap in, 390, *391*
pedicle flap in, 391, *395*
skin grafts in, 393, 396, *397*
sliding tarsoconjunctival flap in, 391, *394*
spontaneous granulation in, 387
tendon fixation in, 388–390, *388–390*
Tenzel flap in, 391, *393*

Cantilevered miniplates, in fixation/reconstruction of canthal tendon, 389–390, *390*
Capillary hemangioma. See *Hemangioma, capillary.*
Capnography, monitoring of, during anesthesia, 298
Carbon dioxide, solid, used in chemical peels, 666
Carbon dioxide laser, fat removal by, 638, 640
  treatment of lymphangioma with, 926
  ultrapulse, used in blepharoplasty, *544*
Carcinoembryonic antigen (CEA), in diagnosis of metastatic disease, 1008
Carcinoid tumor(s), metastatic, to orbit, 57, *58*
Carcinoma, adenoid cystic, of lacrimal glands. See *Adenoid cystic carcinoma, of lacrimal glands.*
    of orbit, 68–69, *69*
  adenoid squamous, of eyelid, 350
  basal cell. See *Basal cell carcinoma.*
  breast, metastatic orbital disease from, *1009,* 1009–1010
  gastrointestinal, metastatic orbital disease from, 1012
  lung, metastatic orbital disease from, 1010
  mucoepidermoid, of lacrimal glands, 68, *69,* 999
    of orbit, 68, *69*
  of sebaceous glands. See *Sebaceous gland carcinoma.*
  prostate, metastatic orbital disease from, 1010–1011, *1011*
  renal cell, metastatic orbital disease from, 1012
  squamous cell. See *Squamous cell carcinoma.*
  thyroid, metastatic, to rectus muscle, *55*
Carotenemia, in diabetic patient, 141
Carotid artery, to eyelids, 273–274, *274–275*
Carotid cavernous fistula, CT scan of, 897, *898*
Cartilage, auricular, used in upper eyelid reconstruction, 364, *364*
Cartilage graft(s), harvesting of, 1080, 1082
  in surgical management of facial paralysis, 481–482, *481–482*
Cartilage-mucosal compound graft(s), 176
Caruncle, of conjunctiva, 159
Castanares' classification, of baggy eyelid deformity, 597, 597t
Cataract surgery, for cicatricial pemphigoid, 201
Cat-scratch disease, 149
Caucasian(s), exophthalmometry in, 699t
  orbits in, 696, 696t
Cautery, thermal, for hemostasis in wound repair, 282–283
Cavernous hemangioma. See *Hemangioma, cavernous.*
Cavernous lymphangioma (cystic hygroma), of eyelid, 331
Cavernous sinus thrombosis, diagnostic and therapeutic features of, 941t–942t
CCLE (chronic cutaneous lupus erythematosus), 4. See also *Lupus erythematosus (LE).*
  common form of, 6
CEA (carcinoembryonic antigen), in diagnosis of metastatic disease, 1008
Ceftriaxone, for sinus infections, 939
Cell(s). See also named cell.
  of immune system, 94–95
Cellulitis, eyelid, 313
  orbital, 146–148, *147,* 889
    bacteriology of, 146–147
    complications of, 148
    diagnostic and therapeutic features of, 941t–942t
    medical management of, 148
    radiographic diagnosis of, 147–148, *148*
    role of paranasal sinus disease in, 935–940, 941t–942t
    signs and symptoms of, 147t
  postseptal, 146, *147*
  preseptal, 144, *147,* 310–312, 889
    CT scan of, *148*
    diagnostic and therapeutic features of, 941t–942t
    in children and neonates, 310
    post-traumatic, 311
    treatment of, 311–312
    with abscess formation, 310, *310*
Centigray (cGy), 1023
Central core myopathy, ptosis in, 84, *85*
Centronuclear (myotubular) myopathy, ptosis in, 84
Cerebellar artery, anteroinferior, 468, *468*
Cerebellopontine angle, *468,* 468–469
Cervicofacial nerve, anatomy of, 277, *277*
Cestode infection(s), of eyelid, 317–318
cGy (centigray), 1023
Chagas' disease, of eyelid, 316–317
  periorbital edema in, 152
Chalazion, development of, 308
  marginal, 308
  recurrent, sebaceous gland carcinoma masquerading as, 346
  sebaceous carcinoma presenting as, 190, 301, *303*
  surgical removal of, 168, 309
  treatment of, 308–309
Chancroid, of eyelid, 314
Chemical agents, topically applied, for hemostasis in wound repair, 283–284
Chemical injury(ies), 222–230
  aqueous component of tear film after, reduced, 226
  classification of, 223, *224*
  emergency care for, 223–225
  epidemiology of, 222–223
    clinical history in, 222–223
    natural repair in, 223
  intermediate care for, 225
  nature of, 222
  perilimbal epithelial loss after, influence of, 226–227, *227*
  prognosis of, 223
  reevaluation of conjunctiva and tear frame after, 226
  treatment of, epidermal growth factor in, 229–230
    fibronectin in, 229
    orthomolecular approaches to, 229
  visual rehabilitation after, 227–228, *228*
Chemical peel(s), 662–669
  agents used in, 665–668, 666t, *667–668*
  application technique for, 665, *665*
  complications of, 668t, 668–669
  consent for, 664t
  depths of, 662, 663t
  evaluation of patient for, 664, 664t, 665t
  for wrinkles, 564
  indications for, 662–664, 663t
  skin preparation for, 664–665
Chemosis, 160
Chemotherapy, causing secondary acquired nasolacrimal duct obstruction, 804
  for lymphoid tumors, 961–962
  for metastatic breast carcinoma, 1010
  for metastatic gastrointestinal carcinoma, 1012
  for metastatic lung carcinoma, 1010
  for metastatic melanoma, 1012
  for non-Hodgkin's lymphoma, 531
  for orbital metastatic disease, 1008
  for orbital metastatic tumors, 57
  for rhabdomyosarcoma, 995–996
Chest radiography, for sarcoidosis, 108
  prior to oculoplastic surgery, 294
Chiasmal syndrome, anterior, 883, *884*
Chickenpox, 152
Child(ren), myasthenia gravis in, acquired, 80–81
    Prostigmin test for, 82, *82*
  oculoplastic surgery in, anesthesia for, 298–299
  orbital deformities in, anterior cranial base approach to, access to tumors in, 1188
      indications for, 1188–1207
      surgical refinement for, 1187–1188. See also *Craniofacial surgery, pediatric.*
  orbital rhabdomyosarcoma in. See *Rhabdomyosarcoma, orbital.*
  preseptal cellulitis in, 310
Chinese, epicanthal folds in, prevalence of, 699, 700t, 705t
  exophthalmometry measurements in, 698, 698t
  eyelid dimensions of, 698–700, 699t, 700t
  lacrimal fossa in, 696–698, 697t, 698t
  optic nerve foramen in, 696–697
  orbits in, 696, 696t, 697t, 698t
    male vs. female, 696, 696t
  tarsus and fat pad in, 699, 700t
Chinese culture, and medicine, *692–694,* 692–695, 693t
Chinese diet, in balance of yin and yang, 695
Chlamydia trachomatis, 154
  lymphogranuloma venereum caused by, 315
  trachoma caused by, 314
Chloroma (granulocytic sarcoma), orbital, 61, *61*
Chocolate cyst, 926, *926*
Chondrodysplasia punctata syndrome(s), 46
Chondroid syringoma, of eyelid, 334, *334*
Choristoma, of eyelid, *327,* 327–328
  phakomatous, 328, *328*
Choroidal detachment, imaging of, 906–907, *906–907*
Choroidal folds, presence of, in orbital disease, 881, *881*
Choroidal hemangioma, imaging of, 910–911, *910–911*
Chromic gut suture, 284, 284t
Chronic cutaneous lupus erythematosus (CCLE), 4. See also *Lupus erythematosus (LE).*
  common form of, 6
Chronic progressive external ophthalmoplegia (CPEO), 86–88
  neurologic deficits associated with, 88
  pigmentary retinopathy in, 87–88, *88*
  ptosis in, 87, *87*
  ragged-red fibers in, 86
Churg-Strauss syndrome, 11
  criteria for classification of, 11t
  ocular abnormalities of, 10t

Cicatricial ectropion, as cause of tearing, 765, 767–768, *767–769*
Cicatricial entropion. See *Entropion, cicatricial.*
Cicatricial pemphigoid, *31,* 31–32
associated with secondary acquired nasolacrimal duct obstruction, 801, 802, *803*
clinical stages of, 99
cutaneous manifestations of, 196
differential diagnosis of, 100, 198t, 198–199
disorders associated with, 199
drug-induced, *197,* 197t, 197–197
epidemiology of, 98
general aspects of, 196–199
histopathology of, 99, 198
immunopathology of, 198
nonocular mucous membrane manifestations of, 196
ocular manifestations of, 98, 196–197
staging of, 196–197, *197,* 197t
pathogenesis of, 99–100
systemic manifestations of, 98–99
treatment of, 32, 100, 199–201
medical, 199–200
surgical, *200,* 200–201
Ciliary ganglion, 846, *847*
CIN (conjunctival intraepithelial neoplasia), 231–232
recurrence rates for, 232
Cirrhosis, hepatic, eyelid retraction associated with, 75, *76*
Citrate, to reduce corneal ulceration, after chemical injury, 229
Clamp(s), used in ophthalmic plastic surgery, *290*
Clamp-cut-cauterize technique, of fat removal, 638, *639*
Clavulanate, for sinus infections, 939
Clear cell hidradenoma, of eyelid, 334
Cleft, craniofacial, with orbital and facial hypertelorism, anterior cranial base approach to, 1193, *1198,* 1199
Clindamycin, for sinus infections, 939
Clonazepam, for essential blepharospasm and Meige's syndrome, 507
Clostridial myonecrosis (gas gangrene), of eyelid, 312
Clostridium botulinum, 83, 152
Clostridium tetani, 83, 152
Closure, direct, of eyelid defect, 366
Coats' disease, CT scan of, 908, *910*
Cocaine test, for Horner's syndrome, 79, *79*
Coccidioidomycosis, of eyelid, 318–319
Collagen, autologous dermal, for wrinkles, 670–675. See also *Autologen.*
Zyderm, for wrinkles, *566,* 566–567, 670
Collagen fibers, in Autologen, 672, *672–673*
Collagen vascular disease(s), 3–12. See also specific disease for detail.
Churg-Strauss syndrome as, 10t, 11, 11t
dermatomyositis as, 7, 7t
lupus erythematosus as, 3–7, *4,* 4t, 5t
lymphomatoid granulomatosis as, 10t, 11–12
scleroderma as, 7–9, *8,* 8t
Wegener's granulomatosis as, 9–11, 10t
Collier's sign, in dorsal mesencephalic syndrome, 72, *73*
Coloboma, congenital, 407–409, *408*
creation of, 408–409
definition of, 407
in Goldenhar's syndrome, 407–408
management of, 409
imaging of, 905
Color(s), correct, for camouflage, 657–658, *659*
Color adjustment, in micropigmentation, 536
Color desaturation, in optic nerve dysfunction, 874
Color film, photographic, 554
Color matching, in micropigmentation, 536
of prosthesis, 1138, 1139, *1140*
Color mixing procedure, in micropigmentation, 538–541, *540*
Color perception, altered (dyschromatopsia), 860
Combined nevus, of eyelid, 339
Comedones, nodular elastosis with, of eyelid, 327, *327*
Complement system, 95–96
Complexion-associated melanosis, clinical features of, 180–181, *180–181*
Composite graft(s), used in medial canthal reconstruction, 391
used in upper eyelid reconstruction, 382, *383*
Compound nevus, of eyelid, 337, *337*
Compton effect, 1023, *1025*
Computed tomography (CT), diagnostic, for tearing, 760
of capillary hemangioma, 893, *893*
of carotid cavernous fistula, 897, *898*
of cavernous hemangioma, 894, *894*
of cellulitis, 147–148, *148*
of choroidal detachment, 906–907, *906–907*
of Coats' disease, 908, *910*
of dermoid cyst, 886–888, *888*
of hemangiopericytoma, 895–896, *896*
of idiopathic orbital inflammation, 954, *954*
of lacrimal gland lesions, 903, *904*
of lacrimal gland tumors, 1001, *1001–1002*
of lymphoid tumor, 957, *957*
of lymphoma, *892,* 892–983
of mucoceles, in paranasal sinuses, 1016
of neurofibroma, *990*
of neurogenic tumors, 984
of optic nerve glioma, *899,* 899–900
of optic nerve meningioma, *987,* 987–988
of optic nerve sheath meningioma, 897, *898*
of orbit, 885–886
of pseudotumor, *890,* 890–891
of retinoblastoma, *907,* 907–908
of rhabdomyosarcoma, 902, *903*
of schwannoma, *991,* 992
of subperiosteal phlegmon, *889,* 889–890
of thyroid orbitopathy, 891, *892*
of uveal malignant melanoma, 909, *910*
of varices, 896, *897*
Computer-controlled cooling-heating mask, used in blepharoplasty, *544*
Congenital anomaly(ies), craniofacial. See *Craniofacial congenital anomaly(ies).*
of eyelids, 407–411. See also specific anomaly, e.g., *Coloboma, congenital.*
Congenital dacryocystocele, *781,* 781–782
Congenital erythropoietic porphyria, 29
Congenital ichthyosiform erythroderma, 45, *45*
Congenital nevus, of eyelid, 338, *339*
Conjunctiva, 159–161
alkali burns to, 222–230. See also *Chemical injury(ies).*
amyloidosis of, 65–66, 238–240. See also *Amyloidosis, conjunctival.*
anatomy of, 178, *179*
macroscopic, 159–160
Conjunctiva *(Continued)*
microscopic, *160,* 160–161
blood supply to, 161
bulbar, triangular tumor of. See *Pterygium(ia).*
embryology of, 159
epithelium of, 160, *160*
loss of, 170, *171.* See also *Conjunctival mucous membrane(s), replacement of.*
glandular structure of, 160–161
lacerations of, 168–169
lymphatic supply to, 161
neoplasms of. See *Conjunctival neoplasm(s).*
nerve supply to, 161
physiology of, 161
prolapse of, management of, 253–254
reevaluation of, after chemical injury, 226
sarcoidosis of, 65, *65*
scarring of, in cicatricial pemphigoid, 98
stroma of, 160
thermal burns to, 222
tissue of, handling of, 161
xeroderma pigmentosum of, 66–67, *67*
Conjunctival autograft(s), for management of pterygia, 5, *214–215,* 216–217
complications of, 217
graft harvesting in, 215, *216*
for repopulation of corneal epithelium, indications for, 249–250
surgical technique of, 250, *250*
Conjunctival flap(s), 163–165
complete, 164–165, *166*
disadvantages of, 165
for management of pterygia, 214, *215*
Gundersen-type, 248, *249*
partial, 163–164, *164–165*
transpositional, 163, *164*
types of, 163
Conjunctival graft(s), 165–168
free, 165–167
mucous membrane, full-thickness, 167
split-thickness, 167
skin, split-thickness, 167–168
Conjunctival intraepithelial neoplasia (CIN), 231–232
recurrence rates for, 232
Conjunctival mucous membrane(s), replacement of, 170–176
alloplastic grafting and spontaneous epithelization in, 171–172, *171–172*
cartilage-mucosal compound grafts in, 176
free tarsoconjunctival grafts in, 175, *175–176*
oral mucous membrane grafts in, 172–175, *173–174*
spontaneous granulation in, 170–171
transplantation in, 172
Conjunctival neoplasm(s), 231–237
complexion-associated melanosis as, clinical features of, 180–181, *180–181*
intraepithelial, 231–232
recurrence rates for, 232
Kaposi's sarcoma as, 236–237, 242, *243,* 532
lymphoid tumors as. See *Lymphoid tumor(s), of conjunctiva.*
malignant melanoma as, 233–235, *234*
clinical features of, 183, *183*
treatment of, 187t, 187–188, *188,* 188t
nevi as, clinical features of, 181–182, *181–182*

Conjunctional neoplasm(s) *(Continued)*
differential diagnosis of, 181, *182*
histopathological classification of, 181
treatment of, 185
pigmented, 178–189
classification of, 179–180, 180t
clinical evaluation of, 183t, 183–185
examination in, *184,* 184–185
history in, 183–184, *184*
clinical features of, 180–183
management of, *185–186,* 185–188
terminology used for, 178–179
primary acquired melanosis as, clinical features of, 182, *182–183*
treatment of, 185–187, *186*
squamous cell carcinoma as, 231–232, *232–233*
squamous papilloma as, 68, *69,* 251, *252*
treatment of, 251–252
Conjunctival surgery, 163–169
flaps in, 163–165, *164–166*
for superior limbic keratoconjunctivitis, indications for, 248–249
technique in, 249
grafts in, 165–168
miscellaneous techniques in, 168–169
Conjunctival-retractor excision, for involutional ectropion, 425, *425*
Conjunctivitis, ligneous, 20
Connective tissue, orbital, 840–842, *842*
Connective tissue disease(s). See *Collagen vascular disease(s);* specific disease.
Contact dermatitis, *42,* 42–43
treatment of, 43
Contact yttrium-aluminum-garnet (YAG) laser, fat removal by, *641,* 641–642
Contouring, as cosmetic technique, used in facial rejuvenation, 570
Contrast sensitivity testing, for optic nerve dysfunction, 874, *875*
Cooling-heating mask, computer-controlled, used in blepharoplasty, *544*
Cornea, alkali burns to, 222–230. See also *Chemical injury(ies).*
thermal burns to, 222
Corneal disease, conjunctival procedure(s) for, 248–250
autografting as, 249–250
Gundersen flap as, 248, *249*
resection as, 248–249
Corneal epithelium, repopulation of, conjunctival autograft for, indication for, 249–250
surgical technique of, 250, *250*
Corneal transplantation, after chemical injury, 228, *228*
Corneal ulcer(s), prevention of, after chemical injury, 225, 229
Corneoscleral graft(s), lamellar, in management of pterygia, 214, *214*
Coronal flap, for brow ptosis, 585–586, *586*
Coronal synostosis, unilateral, 1179–1180, *1181*
Corrugator supraciliaris muscle, 262, *263,* 264
contraction of, 262
Cortical tubers, in tuberous sclerosis, 27
Corticosteroids, chronic patient use of, anesthetic considerations with, 295
for capillary hemangioma, 919–920
for lymphoid tumors, 961
for orbital floor fractures, 1088
pharmacology of, 97
topical, for pterygia, 211, 219
Corynebacterium diphtheriae infection, 313
Cosmeceutical(s), alpha-hydroxy acids as, 563–564
tretinoin as, 562–563
Cosmetic(s), camouflage. See *Camouflage make-up.*
Cosmetic blepharoplasty. See *Blepharoplasty, cosmetic.*
Costal rib graft(s), harvesting of, 1077–1078, *1079*
Cowpox, involving eyelids, 316
CPEO. See *Chronic progressive external ophthalmoplegia (CPEO).*
Cranial arteritis, 112
Cranial base–orbital tumor(s), pediatric, anterior cranial base approach to, 1199, 1202–1204, *1203–1206*
Cranial bone graft(s), harvesting of, 1079–1080, *1080–1082*
Cranial nerve(s). See also specific nerve, e.g., *Facial nerve.*
assessment of, in orbital disease, 877–878, *878–879*
function of, testing, 470–471
Cranial nerve palsy(ies), in diabetic patient, 138t, 138–139
infectious diseases causing, 152
Cranial suture(s), premature closure of, 1178–1182, *1179–1185*
Craniocervical dyskinesia(s), 504. See also specific disorder, e.g., *Blepharospasm, essential.*
Craniofacial cleft, with orbital and facial hypertelorism, anterior cranial base approach to, 1193, *1198,* 1199
Craniofacial congenital anomaly(ies), 1163–1207
anterior cranial base approach to, 1187–1207. See also *Craniofacial surgery, pediatric.*
historical perspective on, 1187
indications for, 1189–1207
refinements in, 1187–1188
brachycephaly as, 1180–1181, *1182–1184*
diagnosis of, 1178
evaluation of, 1178–1185
lambdoidal synostosis as, 1182
multiple suture synostosis as, 1182, *1185*
preoperative evaluation of, 1182, 1184
sagittal synostosis as, 1178–1179, *1179–1180*
subcranial approach to, 1163–1177
advantages of, 1163
results of, 1170, 1176t
surgical procedures in, 1163–1164, *1164–1169,* 1170, *1171–1176*
trigonocephaly as, 1181–1182, *1184*
unilateral coronal synostosis as, 1179–1180, *1181*
Craniofacial surgery, pediatric, anterior cranial base approach to, access to tumors in, 1188
for congenital orbital anomalies, 1189, 1193, *1194–1198,* 1199, *1200–1202*
for traumatic upper orbital deformities, 1188–1189, *1190–1192*
for tumors and neoplasms, 1199, 1202–1204, *1203–1206,* 1207
indications for, 1188–1207
refinements in, 1187–1188
Cranio-orbital neurofibromatosis, anterior cranial base approach to, 1204, *1206,* 1207
Cranio-orbital trauma, pediatric, anterior cranial base approach to, 1188–1189, *1190–1192*
Craniotomy, modified, for transcranial approach to tumors, 985
CREST syndrome, 9
Cretinism, 14
"Crocodile" tears, 735
Crouzon's syndrome, brachycephaly associated with, 1181, *1184*
subcranial approach to, results of, 1176t
Crow's feet, chemical peels for, 662
Cruveilhier valve, 742, *743*
Cryoablation, for districhiasis and trichiasis, 201
Cryotherapy, care following, 188t
complications of, 187t
excision with, for conjunctival malignant melanoma, 235
for conjunctival squamous cell carcinoma, 232
for hyperpigmented facial lesions, 568
for Kaposi's sarcoma, 528
for pagetoid spread of sebaceous gland carcinoma, 348
for pigmented conjunctival neoplasms, *185–186,* 185–188
for sebaceous gland carcinoma, 193–194, *194*
Cryptophthalmos, 407, *408*
Crypts of Henle, 160, *273*
CT. See *Computed tomography (CT).*
Curette(s), used in ophthalmic plastic surgery, *290*
Current, in electrolysis, density of, 590
polar effects of, 589
radio-frequency, heating effects of, 592
Customized suborbital implant, 490–491, *491,* 495–498, *496–499*
Cutaneous. See also *Skin* entries.
Cutaneous horn, of eyelid, 326, *326*
Cutler-Beard flap, used in upper eyelid reconstruction, technique of, 374–375, *375–378*
Cyclophosphamide, for cicatricial pemphigoid, 199
pharmacology of, 97
Cyclosporine, pharmacology of, 97–98
Cylindroma (turban tumor), of eyelid, 334–335, *335*
Cyproheptadine, for essential blepharospasm and Meige's syndrome, 507
Cyst(s), blood, drainage of, 925
chocolate, 926, *926*
dermoid, nasal, with intracranial extension, anterior cranial base approach to, 1199, *1200*
of eyelid, *327,* 327–328
of orbit, 886–888, *888–889*
epidermal inclusion, of eyelid, 326–327, *327*
epidermoid, of orbit, 886–888, *888*
horn, 325
hydatid, 151
Moll's, 334, *334*
nodular elastosis with, of eyelid, 327, *327*
pseudohorn, 325
L-Cysteine, to reduce ulceration, after chemical injury, 225
Cystic hygroma (cavernous lymphangioma), of eyelid, 331
Cysticercosis, 151
Cytomegalovirus retinitis, in AIDS patients, 533

Cytotoxic response (hypersensitivity type II), 96
Cytotoxicity, antibody-dependent cell-mediated, 95

Dacron suture, 284
Dacryoadenitis, 965
associated with infection, 153, *153*
clinical manifestations of, 964–966
diagnostic evaluation of, 954
Dacryocystitis, chronic, in primary acquired nasolacrimal duct obstruction, 785, *785*
Dacryocystocele, congenital, *781,* 781–782
Dacryocystography, in evaluation of tearing, 759, *759–760*
Dacryocystorhinostomy, for canalicular stenosis, 830–831
for nasolacrimal duct obstruction, 781
for primary acquired nasolacrimal duct obstruction, *786–792,* 786–794
endonasal, 792–794, *793–795*
history in, 786–787
incisions in, 788, *789*
Kerrison rongeur for bone removal in, 789–790, *790*
lacrimal sac flaps in, 790–792, *791–792*
nasal packing for, 787, *788*
sedation for, 787
transnasal wiring with, in fixation/reconstruction of canthal tendon, 388, *389*
Dacryolith(s), causing nasolacrimal duct obstruction, 812
Dapsone, for cicatricial pemphigoid, 199
Darier's disease (keratosis follicularis), 21
Darier's sign, in mastocytoma, 43
Daylight, for photography, 554
Daylight film, photographic, 554
DDAVP (desmopressin), for hemostasis in wound repair, 283
de Hertoghe's sign, in atopic dermatitis, 42
Decompression, optic nerve sheath, 1056–1059
complications of, 1059
indications for, 1047
mechanism of action of, 1056
postoperative care following, 1059
technique of, 1056–1059, *1057–1059*
orbital, for Graves' disease, 967–982. See also *Graves' disease, orbital decompression for.*
indications for, 1047
Dehiscence(s), wound, after blepharoplasty, 648
Zuckerkandl's, 935
Delayed reaction (hypersensitivity type IV), 96
Dendritic cell(s), of eyelid, 323
Dengue fever, involving eyelids, 316
Dennie-Morgan fold, in atopic dermatitis, 42
Dermabrasion, for wrinkles, 565, *565*
Dermal fillers, autologous, for wrinkles, 670. See also *Autologen.*
Dermatitis, atopic, 41–42, *42*
treatment of, 42
contact, *42,* 42–43
treatment of, 43
seborrheic, *37,* 37–38
Dermatochalasis, in Graves' ophthalmopathy, 515–516, *516*
Dermatofibroma, of eyelid, 333
Dermatomyositis, 7
diagnostic criteria for, 7t
Dermatoses, 37–46. See also specific type.
Dermis. See also *Skin.*
of eyelid, 324
benign lesions of, 328–333. See also under *Eyelid tumor(s).*
Dermoid cyst, nasal, with intracranial extension, anterior cranial base approach to, 1199, *1200*
of eyelid, *327,* 327–328
of orbit, 886–888, *888–889*
Dermolipoma(s), 255–257, *256*
complications of, 255–256
treatment of, 256–257
excision of, 256
Desmopressin (DDAVP), for hemostasis in wound repair, 283
"Devil's eye," 1179
Dexamethasone, for thyroid storm, 130
Diabetes mellitus, complication(s) of, 137–141, 138t
acanthosis nigricans as, 140
carotenemia as, 141
eruptive xanthomas as, 140–141
granuloma annulare as, 140
hemochromatosis as, 141
idiopathic optic disc edema as, 138–139
malignant external otitis as, 138
necrobiosis lipoidica diabeticorum as, 139–140
phycomycosis as, 137–138
rhinoscleroma as, 138
vitiligo as, 140
Diathermy, lipolytic, fat removal by, 640–641, *640–641*
Diazepam, as anesthetic agent, 296
DIDMOAD (Wolfram) syndrome, in diabetic patient, 138t, 139
Diet, Chinese, in balance of yin and yang, 695
Diffuse cutaneous leishmaniasis, of eyelid, 150, *150*
Digoxin, chronic patient use of, anesthetic considerations with, 295
Diphtheria, involving eyelids, 313
Diplopia, after blepharoplasty, 644
persistent, as complication of orbital floor fractures, 1091, *1092*
Discoid lupus erythematosus (DLE), 3. See also *Lupus erythematosus (LE).*
characteristic features of, 6
Dissection, in orbital surgery, 1049
Disseminated neonatal hemangioma, 920t, 920–921, *920–921*
Distichiasis, congenital, 409, *409*
in cicatricial pemphigoid, correction of, 201
Diuretics, chronic patient use of, anesthetic considerations with, 295–296
DLE (discoid lupus erythematosus), 3. See also *Lupus erythematosus (LE).*
characteristic features of, 6
Documentation, for medicolegal considerations with eyelid trauma, 457
Dog bite(s), eyelid injury caused by, 453, *454*
Dolichocephaly, 1178
Doll's eye maneuver, 72
Donor sclera, for eyelid reconstruction, 364
in Asian patients, 724–727
histology of homograft and, 726, *726–727*
immunopathology of homograft and, 726–727
results with, 727, *727*
surgical technique and, 725, *725*
Dorsal mesencephalic syndrome, eyelid retraction in, 72–73, *73*
Dorsonasal artery, anatomy of, 274, *275*
Down syndrome, epicanthal folds associated with, 411
Doxycycline, for trachoma, 155
Drainage, indications for, 1046
of blood cysts, 925
of orbital abscess, 939–940
Dressing(s), eyelid, 384
Drug(s). See also specific drug or drug group.
associated with cicatricial pemphigoid, *197,* 197–198
chronic patient use of, anesthetic considerations with, 295
disruption of neuromuscular transmission by, 83–84
for hemostasis in wound repair, 283
Dry eye, treatment of, after chemical injury, 226
Dye disappearance test, in tearing, 753–754, *754*
Dyschromatopsia, 860
Dysplastic nevus syndrome, 67–68, *68*

Ear cartilage, used in upper eyelid reconstruction, 364, *364*
Eaton-Lambert syndrome, 83
EBV (Epstein-Barr virus), associated with Burkitt's lymphoma, 530
Ecchymosis, due to blepharoplasty, 709
Eccrine sweat gland(s), *273,* 323–324
benign adnexal lesions originating in, 333–334, *333–334*
Ecthyma gangrenosum, of eyelid, 312–313
Ectropion, 422–437
after blepharoplasty, 644–645, *645–646*
as complication of medial canthal reconstruction, 398
cicatricial, as cause of tearing, 765, 767–768, *767–769*
congenital, 410, *410*
infection causing, 308t
involutional, 422–429
as cause of tearing, 762–765, *763–764, 766–767*
etiology of, 422, *423–424*
medical treatment of, 424
preoperative evaluation of, 422–424, *424*
surgical treatment of, 424–429, 763–765
conjunctival-retractor excision in, 425, *425*
horizontal full-thickness eyelid shortening in, 427, *428,* 764–765
inferior punctoplasty in, 424–425, *425*
lateral tarsal strip procedure in, 427, 429, *429–430,* 765, *766–767*
medial plication for canthal laxity in, 425–427, *426–427*
posterior lamellar shortening procedure in, 763–764, *764*
Smith lazy-T procedure in, 425, *426*
paralytic, 429–437
as cause of tearing, 768–770, *769*
etiology of, 429
medical management of, 430
pathology of, 429, *430*
preoperative evaluation of, 429–430
surgical management of, 430–437
eyelid sling procedure in, 432, 434, *435*
indications for, 430
lateral canthoplasty in, 432, *433–435*
tarsorrhaphy in, 430–432, *431–432*
temporalis transfer in, 434, 436–437, *436–437*

Edema, due to blepharoplasty, 709
eyelid, in Graves' ophthalmopathy, 515–516, *516*
optic disc, in diabetic patient, 138t, 138–139
periorbital, diseases and organisms associated with, 308t
infectious causes of, 151–152
postoperative, manual lymphatic drainage for, 653–654
preseptal, in sinus disease, 938–939
Edinger-Westphal nucleus, preganglionic fibers from, 846
EDTA (ethylenediaminetetra-acetic acid), to reduce ulceration, after chemical injury, 225
Electrocardiography, prior to oculoplastic surgery, 294, 295
Electrocautery, for hemostasis in wound repair, 283
Electrology, and eyebrow contouring, 589–595
Electrolysis, 589–591
and current density, 590
and polar effects of current, 589
chemical and physiologic effects of, 590
galvanic, advantages of, 590–591
disadvantages of, 591
multiple-needle, 590
single-needle, 589
principle of time and intensity in, 590
removal of metal jewelry before, 589–590
vs. other epilating techniques, 593–594
Electronic flash, for photography, 555
Electropigmentation, 676–681. See also *Micropigmentation.*
and pigment removal, 681
complications of, 681
contraindications to, 677t
indications for, 676, 677t
patient evaluation for, 676, *677*
tattoo pigments used in, 677, 681
technique of, 676–677, *678–681*
Elephantiasis neuromatosa, 25
ELISA (enzyme-linked immunosorbent assay), 97
Ellman Surgitron radiosurgical unit, used in removal of hyperpigmented facial lesions, 568, *568*
used in treatment of telangiectasia, 569
Embolus, cerebral, ptosis caused by, 75–76, *77*
Embryonal rhabdomyosarcoma, 995
Encephalocele, frontonasalethmoidal, anterior cranial base approach to, 1199, *1201–1202*
Endocrine disease. See also specific disease.
non–thyroid-related, ocular manifestations of, tarsal polishing with, 137–143
Endophthalmitis, sclerosing, imaging of, 908–909
Endoscope(s), used for endonasal dacryocystorhinostomy, 793, *793*
Endoscopic sinus surgery kit, *292*
Endoscopy, in evaluation of tearing, 760
Endothelial hyperplasia, intravascular papillary, of eyelid, 332
Enophthalmos, 1108–1111, *1108–1112*
as complication of orbital floor fracture, 1091, *1092–1093*
associated with orbital disease, 881
Entamoeba histolytica infection, 317
Entropion, 413–421
cicatricial, 414, *415*
as cause of tearing, 771
Entropion *(Continued)*
buccal mucous membrane grafting for, 203–206
anesthesia in, 203
complications of, 205
results of, 205, *206*
surgical methods of, 203–205, *204–206*
correction of, *200,* 200–201
surgical approach to, 417–421, *418*
technique in, 418–419, *419–420,* 421
congenital, 409, *410,* 413
in Graves' ophthalmopathy, 515, *516*
surgical techniques for, 521
involutional, 414–415
as cause of tearing, 770–771, *772–773*
surgical approach to, 415–416, *416–417*
spastic, 414
as cause of tearing, 771, *773*
Enucleation, 1035–1043. See also *Anophthalmos, acquired.*
care following, 1041
eye protection following, 1037–1038
hydroxyapatite implant and, 1041–1042. See also *Prosthesis.*
contraindications to, 1042
indications for, 1035–1037
lax socket following, 1106–1108
preoperative counseling for, 1037
presurgical set-up for, 1038
psychological impact of, 1037
surgical anatomy for, 1038
surgical steps in, 1038
vs. evisceration, 1129–1130
with myoconjunctival attachments, 1039, *1040–1042,* 1041
Enucleation and evisceration kit, *290*
Enzyme-linked immunosorbent assay (ELISA), 97
Eosinophil(s), 95
Eosinophilia, angiolymphoid hyperplasia with, 949–950, *949–950*
of eyelid, 332
Eosinophilic granuloma, of orbit, 62, *63*
in AIDS patients, 532
Ephelides (freckles), in neurofibromatosis, 25
of eyelid, 339, *339*
Epiblepharon, as cause of tearing, 775, *775*
congenital, 409–140
Epiblepharon fold(s), 261
Epicanthal fold(s), 261, 704–705
congenital, 410–411
prevalence of, 699, 700t, 705t
Epidermal growth factor (EGF), wound healing with, after chemical injury, 229–230
Epidermal inclusion cyst, of eyelid, 326–327, *327*
Epidermal necrolysis, toxic. See *Toxic epidermal necrolysis (Lyell's syndrome).*
Epidermal nevus, linear, of eyelid, 327
Epidermis. See also *Skin.*
of eyelid, 323
benign lesions of, 324–328. See also under *Eyelid tumor(s).*
Epidermoid cyst, of orbit, 886–888, *888*
Epidermolysis bullosa, 29–31, 103–105
classification of, 103
epidemiology of, 104
immunohistopathology of, 104–105
ocular manifestations of, 30t, 104
subgroups and types of, 30–31
systemic manifestations of, 104
treatment of, 31, 105
types of, 30
Epidermolysis bullosa acquisita antigen, 105
Epilation, permanent, of eyelashes, radiation therapy and, 1031
Epinephrine, for hemostasis in wound repair, 283
Epiphora, 729–730, 749, 751, *752.* See also *Tearing.*
age of onset of, 730
causes of, 751–752
definition of, 729
Episcleritis, in AIDS patients, 529
Epithelial eyelid tumor(s), malignant, 342–350. See also *Eyelid tumor(s), malignant.*
Epithelialization, in wound repair, 281, 282t
spontaneous, alloplastic grafting and, in conjunctival mucous membrane replacement, 171–172, *171–172*
Epithelioid (spindle) nevus, of eyelid, 338
Epithelioma, Malherbe's calcifying, of eyelid, 336, *336*
Epithelium, conjunctival, 160, *160*
loss of, 170, *171*
corneal, repopulation of, conjunctival autograft for, 249–250, *250*
perilimbal, loss of, after chemical injury, 226–227, *227*
Epstein-Barr virus (EBV), associated with Burkitt's lymphoma, 530
Erdheim-Chester disease, of orbit, 64, *64*
xanthogranulomas of, 948
Eruptive xanthoma, in diabetic patient, 140–141
Erythema multiforme, *34–35,* 34–37
causes of, 36t
differential diagnosis of, 36–37
epidemiology of, 100
immunohistopathology of, 101
major (Stevens-Johnson syndrome), *34,* 34–35, 100
minor, 34, 100
ocular manifestations of, 100–101
pathogenesis of, 101–102
systemic manifestations of, 101
toxic epidermal necrolysis form of, 34, 35, *35*
drugs causing, 35, 36t
treatment of, 37, 102
Erythema nodosum, in sarcoidosis, 16
Erythroderma, congenital ichthyosiform, 45, *45*
exfoliative, 41
Erythromycin, for trachoma, 155
Erythropoietic porphyria, congenital, 29
Erythropoietic protoporphyria, 29
Ethmoidal sinus(es), anatomy of, 1014–1015
mucoceles in, *1018,* 1018–1019
radiographic findings in, 1018, *1019*
treatment of, 1018–1019
Ethylenediaminetetra-acetic acid (EDTA), to reduce ulceration, after chemical injury, 225
Euthyroid Graves' disease, 121
Euthyroid hyperthyroxinemia, 129
causes of, 129t
Evisceration, enucleation and, kit for, *290*
presurgical set-up for, 1043
surgical steps in, 1043–1044, *1044*
vs. enucleation, 1129–1130
Excimer laser, postoperative use of, for pterygia, 219
Excision, conjunctival-retractor, for involutional ectropion, 425, *425*
for rhabdomyosarcoma, 995
indications for, 1046
of capillary hemangioma, 918–919
of cavernous hemangioma, 928–929

Excision *(Continued)*
of conjunctival lymphoid tumors, 236, *236*
of hemangiopericytoma, 931–932, *932*
of lymphangioma, 925
of sebaceous gland carcinoma, 348
of skin, in ptosis surgery, 450–451
with cryotherapy, for conjunctival malignant melanoma, 235
for conjunctival squamous cell carcinoma, 232
Exenteration, for conjunctival malignant melanoma, 235
indications for, 1047
orbital, indications for, 1070, 1071t
reconstructive and prosthetic options in, 1073–1075, *1074*
technique of, 1071–1073, *1071–1073*
osseointegration following, 1150–1159. See also *Osseointegration, for exenterated orbit.*
Exfoliative erythroderma, 41
Exophthalmometry, in Caucasian and African American adults, 699t
in Chinese and Taiwanese adults, 698, 698t
Exophthalmos, systemic diseases associated with, 13t
Exposure, adequate, in orbital surgery, 1048
Extraocular muscles, anatomy of, 841
enlarged, causes of, 886t
Extremity(ies), manual lymphatic drainage of, pressure bandages with, 655
Eye(s), "devil's," 1179
dry, treatment of, after chemical injury, 226
enucleation of, 1035–1043. See also *Enucleation.*
ocular protection following, 1037–1938
evisceration of. See *Evisceration.*
wet, 726–730. See also *Epiphora.*
Eyebrow(s), 262, *263–265,* 264. See also *Hair; Hair follicles.*
contouring of, 594–595, *594–595*
technique(s) used in, 589–595
blend modality as, 593
comparison of, 593–594
electrolysis as, 589–591
regulatory agencies and, 591–593
short-wave or thermolysis method as, 591
displacement of, after blepharoplasty, 649, *649*
elevation of, endoscopic approach to, 550
for ptosis, 585, *585.* See also *Ptosis, brow.*
male vs. female, 633, *634*
reconstruction of, electropigmentation in, 676
micropigmentation in, 537–538, *539–540,* 685–688, *686–688*
Eyelash(es), 273. See also *Hair; Hair follicles.*
epilation of, permanent, radiation therapy and, 1031
loss or misdirection of, after blepharoplasty, 649
misdirected. See *Trichiasis.*
pigmentary treatment of, 536–537, *537–538,* 676
sebaceous glands of, 323. See also *Sebaceous gland(s).*
Eyelid(s), 261–279
acquired immunodeficiency syndrome affecting, 526–529. See also *Acquired immunodeficiency syndrome (AIDS), eyelid manifestation(s) of.*
amyloidosis of, 65–66
anatomy of, 261, *262,* 413, *414*

Eyelid(s) *(Continued)*
ancillary techniques involving, in management of facial paralysis, 482
and precorneal tear film, 738
apraxia of, *89,* 90
arterial supply to, 273–274, *274–275*
basal cell carcinoma of. See *Basal cell carcinoma, of eyelid.*
basal cell nevus syndrome of, 67, *68*
chalazion of. See *Chalazion.*
chancroid of, 314
changes of, in orbital disease, 865–868, *867–868*
congenital anomaly(ies) of, 407–411. See also specific anomaly, e.g., *Ectropion.*
ankyloblepharon as, 409
blepharophimosis syndrome as, 411, *411*
coloboma as, 407–409, *408*
cryptophthalmos as, 407, *408*
distichiasis, 409, *409*
ectropion as, 410, *410*
entropion as, 409, *410*
epiblepharon as, 409–410
epicanthal folds as, 410–411
lid retraction as, 411, *411*
crease in. See *Eyelid crease(s).*
dimensions of, in Chinese adults, 698–700, 699t, 700t
disorders of, 72–91. See also specific disorder, e.g., *Ptosis.*
injury to. See *Eyelid trauma.*
innervation of, 275, 277–278, *277–278*
lower, blepharoplasty for, 617–624. See also *Blepharoplasty, lower eyelid.*
bony support of, 485, *486–487*
defects in, closure of, 400, *401*
involving canaliculus, 406
lacerations of, 455–456, *455–457*
malposition of, after blepharoplasty, 644–645, *645–646*
correction of, 1113–1114, *1115–1118,* 1116–1118
muscles retracting, anatomy of, 269–272, *270–272*
reconstruction of, 400–406. See also *Eyelid reconstruction, lower.*
retraction of, 438–446. See also *Eyelid retraction, lower.*
transconjunctival approach to, complications of, 630
lymphatic drainage of, 275, *276*
margins of. See *Eyelid margin.*
mycosis fungoides of, 62
necrosis of, after blepharoplasty, 650
nodular eruptions of, infectious causes of, 149–150, *150*
pseudoptosis of, *88–91,* 89–91
retraction of, 72–75. See also *Eyelid retraction.*
sebaceous glands of, benign lesions originating in, 336–337, *337*
carcinoma of, 190–194, 301–303. See also *Sebaceous gland carcinoma.*
inflammation of, 307–310, *309*
causes of, 308t
shortening of, after chemical injury, 226
horizontal full-thickness, for involutional ectropion, 427, *428*
skin folds (laugh lines) around, 261–262, *263*
skin of, 262
histology of, 323–324
symmetry of, anophthalmic socket and, 1131, *1131*
tumors of. See *Eyelid tumor(s).*

Eyelid(s) *(Continued)*
ulcerative lesion of, causes of, 308t
upper, blepharoplasty for, 596–614. See also *Blepharoplasty, upper eyelid.*
components of, 356
double, 703–704, *704,* 705t
prevalence of, 705t
horizontal section through, *266*
lacerations of, repair of, 359–361, *362*
protractors of, anatomy of, 264–265, 267–269, *267–269*
reconstruction of, 356–384. See also *Eyelid reconstruction, upper.*
single, 703, *704*
venous supply to, 274–275, *276*
vertical, and suborbital augmentation, 498–499, *499–502,* 501
xeroderma pigmentosum of, 66–67
Eyelid crease(s), 261, *262–263*
double, after blepharoplasty, 648, *648*
formation of, in upper eyelid blepharoplasty, 603, *603–604*
variations of, 609–610
high, surgery for, 450
male vs. female, 633
upper, determination and marking of, 706, *706*
Eyelid deformity, baggy, Castanares' classification of, 597, 597t
Eyelid dressings, 384
Eyelid edema, in Graves' ophthalmopathy, 515–516, *516*
Eyelid lag, definition of, 514
in Graves' ophthalmopathy, 514
in orbital disease, 866–867
Eyelid laxity, as complication of medial canthal reconstruction, 398
in involutional ectropion, 762–763, *763,* 764
pinch test for, 762, *763*
repair of, 622–624, *623–624*
Eyelid margin, 272–273, *273*
contour of, abnormal, 450
injury to, evaluation of, *455,* 455–456
sequence of repair following, 458, 460, *460*
inward rotation of. See *Entropion.*
outward rotation of. See *Ectropion.*
pigmentary treatment of, 536–537, *537–538*
reapproximation of, following injury, 357–358, *359–360*
Eyelid necrosis, *312,* 312–313
causes of, 308t, 312
Eyelid reconstruction, donor sclera for, in Asian patients, 724–727, *725–727*
results with, 727, *727*
lower, 400–406
closure of defects in, 400, *401*
Hughes flap for, 402–404, *403–404*
severing of, 404, *405*
lateral cantholysis in, 400, *401*
Mustardé flap for, 404–405, *405*
Tenzel rotation flap for, 400–402, *401–402*
Trepier flap (rotated myocutaneous) for, 403, *403–404*
upper, 356–384
dressings used in, 384
objectives of, 356
technique(s) used in, 363–384
auricular cartilage for, 364, *364*
autogenous tarsus for, 363–364
composite grafting as, 382, *383*

Eyelid reconstruction *(Continued)*
Cutler-Beard flap as, 374–375, *375–378*
direct closure as, 366
donor sclera for, 364
hard palate mucosa for, 364–365
irradiated tarsal plates and aorta for, 365
lateral transpositional skin flap as, 371, *372*
median forehead flap as, 371, *373*
myocutaneous flap as, 369, *369–370*
nasochondral tissue for, *356,* 365
nasojugal myocutaneous flap as, 373–374, *374*
oral mucosa for, 365
pedicle flap from lower lid to upper lid as, 382–383, *383*
semicircular flap as, 366, *367*
skin grafting as, 366–367, *368,* 369
sliding tarsal flap as, 380, 382, *382*
split-level full-thickness grafts as, 384, *384*
tarsal rotational flap as, 375–378, *379–380*
tarsal substitutes for, 363
tarsoconjunctival flap as, 378–380, *381*
traumatic injury requiring, 356–363, *357*
canalicular lacerations as, 359–361, *362*
canthal tendon injury as, 361–363, *363*
extensive, 358–359, *360–361*
lid margin reapproximation and, 357–358, *359–360*
with no tissue loss, 357, *358*
with tissue loss, 357
Eyelid retraction, 72–75
as complication of orbital floor fractures, 1091, *1091*
congenital, 411, *411*
in Graves' disease, 514–523. See also *Graves' disease, eyelid retraction in.*
lower, 438–446
anterior lamellar defects in, 438
surgical repair of, 439–440, *440*
causes of, 438
functional and cosmetic complaints associated with, 438–439
middle and posterior lamellar defects in, 438
surgical repair of, 440–446
greater palatine nerve block in, 442
hard palate graft in, 441–442, *442*
harvesting of, 442–444, *443–444*
nasopalatine nerve block in, 442
technique of, 444–446, *444–446*
myopathic, 74–75, *76*
neuromuscular, 74, *76*
neuropathic, nuclear and infranuclear lesions causing, 73–74, *74–76*
supranuclear lesions causing, 72–73, *73*
pseudoptosis and, 89–91
upper, in orbital disease, 867, *867*
Eyelid retractor(s), lower, with spacers, 440
used in ophthalmic plastic surgery, *290*
Eyelid sling procedures, for paralytic ectropion, 432, 434, *435*
Eyelid sulcus, *262*
Eyelid surgery, anesthesia for, 278–279
cosmetic. See *Blepharoplasty.*
hemostasis in, 282–284
pharmacologic agents for, 283
Eyelid surgery *(Continued)*
pressure tamponade for, 282
thermal cautery and electrocautery for, 282–283
topically applied chemical agents for, 283–284
lower, greater palatine nerve block for, 442
hard palate graft for, 441–442, *442*
harvesting of, 442–444, *443–444*
nasopalatine nerve block for, 442
technique of, 439–440, 444–446, *444–446*
ophthalmic plastic instruments used in, 289, *290–292*
suture material used in, 284, 284t
suture needles used in, 284–285, *285*
suturing techniques used in, 285–286, *285–289,* 288
wound healing following, primary, 281, 282t
secondary, 281–282
Eyelid trauma, 452–463
bites causing, 452–453, *454,* 455
blunt, 452
evaluation of, 452–457, *454*
mechanism of injury in, 452
patient evaluation in, 453, 455–457
extramarginal injuries and, 456, *456–457*
formulation of treatment plans and, 456–457
marginal injuries and, *455,* 455–456
medicolegal considerations and, 457
systemic considerations and, 453, 455
sharp, 452
treatment of, 457–463
surgical, 457–461
care following, 461
secondary procedures in, 461–463
sequence of repair in, 458, *459–462,* 460–461
wound decontamination in, 457–458, *458*
upper, canalicular lacerations in, 359–361, *362*
canthal tendon injuries in, 361–363, *363*
penetrating injuries in, 357–359
lid margin reapproximation and, 357–358, *359–360*
with no tissue loss, 357, *358*
with tissue loss, 357
reconstruction for, 356–363
techniques used in, 363–384. See also *Eyelid reconstruction, upper, technique(s) used in.*
Eyelid tumor(s), benign, 323–340
classification of, 342, 343t
diagnosis and management of, 324
of dermis, 328–333
angiolymphoid hyperplasia with eosinophilia as, 332
arteriovenous malformation as, 331
capillary hemangioma (strawberry nevus) as, 330, *330*
cavernous hemangioma as, 330
dermatofibroma as, 333
glomus tumor as, 332
granular cell tumor as, 329
intravascular papillary endothelial hyperplasia as, 332
juvenile xanthogranuloma as, 64, 333
leiomyoma as, 329
lymphangioma as, 331, *331*
neurilemoma (schwannoma) as, 328–329
Eyelid tumor(s) *(Continued)*
neurofibroma as, 328, *329*
neuroma as, 329
nevus flammeus (port wine stain) as, *329,* 329–330
pyogenic granuloma as, 331, *331*
varix as, 330–331
xanthelasma as, 332, *332*
xanthoma as, 332
of epidermis, 324–328
acrochordon (skin tag) as, 324, *324*
cutaneous horn lesion as, 326, *326*
dermoid cyst as, *327,* 327–328
inclusion cyst as, 326–327, *327*
inverted follicular keratosis as, 326, *326*
keratoacanthoma as, 325–326, *326*
linear nevus as, 327
milia as, *324,* 324–325
nodular elastosis with cysts and comedones as, 327, *327*
oncocytoma as, 328
phakomatous choristoma as, 328, *328*
seborrheic keratosis as, 325, *325*
pigmented, 337–339
blue nevus as, 338–339
congenital nevus as, 338, *339*
freckles as, 339, *339*
lentigo simplex as, 339
nevocellular nevi as, 337–338, *337–338*
Ota's nevus as, 339
solar lentigo as, 339, *340*
in Asian patients, 721–727
basal cell carcinoma as, 723, *723*
lid reconstruction with donor sclera for, 724–727, *725–727*
sebaceous gland carcinoma as, 721–722, *722*
squamous cell carcinoma as, 721, *722*
statistics on, 723–724
malignant, 300–306, 342–350
basal cell carcinoma as, 300, 342–345, *343–345*
in African American patients, 716, *717*
in Asian patients, 723, *723*
classification of, 342, 343t
metastatic, *54,* 56
sebaceous gland carcinoma as. See *Sebaceous gland carcinoma.*
squamous cell carcinoma as, 300–301, *302,* 349–350, *349–350*
in Asian patients, 721, *722*
low-grade, 325
types of, 343t
painless, diseases and organisms associated with, 308t
Eyelid twitch response, in myasthenic patients, 80
Eyeliner reconstruction, with micropigmentation, 536–537, *536–537*

Face, "ideal," artist's rendition of, 560, *561*
skin tension lines in, 285, *285*
Face-lift (rhytidectomy), 565
Facial anomaly(ies), anomalies of nasolacrimal drainage system with, 783
Facial expression, muscles of, 262, *263,* 264
Facial movement, disorders of. See also specific disorder, e.g., *Hemifacial spasm.*
overview of, 504
Facial myokymia, 510
diagnostic features of, 505t

Facial nerve, aberrant regeneration of, 91, *91*
anatomy of, 275, 277, *277*
blood supply to, *468*, 469
disorders of, 473–474
injury to, 473–474
lesions of, 474
diagnosis of, 471t–472t
motor branches of, 469, *469*
motor nucleus of, 465–466, *467*
supranuclear pathways of, 465, *466*
Facial paralysis, 465–482
diagnostic considerations in, 473t
examination of, 470–471, 471t–472t
history of, 470
medical management of, 474–475, *475*
pontine, diagnosis of, 465–466, *467*
surgical management of, 475–482
ancillary eyelid techniques in, 482
Arion sling in, 478–479, *479*
fascial strip in, 480–481
gold weight in, 475–476, *476–477*
lateral canthal tendon reconstruction in, 480, *480–481*
palpebral spring in, 476–478, *477–478*
retractor recession with ear cartilage graft in, 481–482, *481–482*
transposition of temporalis muscle to lids in, 479–480, *480*
unilateral brow ptosis and, 482
symptoms of, 470
Facial rejuvenation, 560–571
cosmetic technique(s) used in, 569–571
camouflage, 570
fashion, 570–571
for pigmentary problems, 567–568, *568*
for telangiectasia, 569, *569*
for wrinkled skin, 562–567
alpha-hydroxy acids used in, 563–564, *564*
chemical peels used in, 564
dermabrasion used in, 565, *565*
Fibrel used in, 567, *567*
filler substances used in, 565–567
tretinoin used in, *562*, 562–563
Zyderm collagen used in, *566*, 566–567
harmful effects of ultraviolet light and, prevention of, 561–562
Facial spasm(s), diagnostic features of, 505t
Facial synkinesis, diagnostic features of, 505t
Facial tic, diagnostic features of, 505t
Facial vein, anatomy of, 275, *276*
Factor VIII–related antigen, in Kaposi's sarcoma, 242
Familial periodic paralysis, ptosis in, 85–86, *86*
Fasanella-Servat procedure, 448
Fascia, orbital, anatomy of, 841–842, *842*
Fascial strip, in surgical management of facial paralysis, 480–481
Fasciitis, necrotizing, of eyelid, 312
nodular, of orbit, 997
Fashion cosmetics, used in facial rejuvenation, 570–571
Fat excision, in cosmetic blepharoplasty, technique(s) of, 638–642
carbon dioxide laser as, 638, 640
clamp, cut, and cauterize as, 638, *639*
contact yttrium-aluminum-garnet laser as, *641*, 641–642
fat repositioning as, 641
lipocauterization as, 638, *639*
lipolytic diathermy as, 640–641, *640–641*
monopolar dissection as, 638
radio-frequency lipocontouring as, 642, *642*
Fat excision *(Continued)*
in transconjunctival lower blepharoplasty, inadequate, 630
in upper eyelid blepharoplasty, 601, *601*
variations of, 608–609
incomplete or excessive, 646–647, *647*
Fat pad, orbital, 269, *269*
anatomy of, 842, *842*
pseudoherniation of, evaluation of, 635
removal of. See *Fat excision.*
repositioning of, 640–641, *640–641*
sub-brow, surgical management of, 586–587, *586–588*
tarsus and, in Chinese adults, 699, 700t
Fat transplantation, autologous, for wrinkles, 565
Favre-Racouchot syndrome, 327, *327*
Fc receptors, 95
Fenestration, indications for, 1047
Fentanyl, as anesthetic agent, 296
Fibrel, for wrinkles, 567, *567*, 670
Fibroblastic phase, of wound repair, 281, 282t
Fibroma, orbital, 997
Fibromatosis, orbital, 997
Fibronectin, wound healing with, after chemical injury, 229
Fibrosarcoma, orbital, 997
Fibrous tissue, benign eyelid tumors derived from, 333
Fibrous tissue tumor(s), of orbit, 997
Filamentary keratitis, associated with dry eye, 226
Filler substance(s), for wrinkles, 565–567
Fibrel as, 567, *567*
Zyderm as, *566*, 566–567
Film, photographic, automatic advance of, 551
color, 554
speed of, 554
radiographic, 1023, *1024*
Fissure, orbital. See *Orbital fissure.*
Fistula, carotid cavernous, CT scan of, 897, *898*
lacrimal sac, 782–783, *783*
naso-orbital, as complication of medial canthal reconstruction, 398
Fitzpatrick classification, of photodamage, 662, 663t
Flap(s), conjunctival. See *Conjunctival flap(s).*
coronal, for brow ptosis, 585–586, *586*
skin, used in lower eyelid blepharoplasty, 620, *620*
skin-muscle, used in lower eyelid blepharoplasty, 620–622, *621–622*
used in lower eyelid reconstruction, Hughes, 402–404, *403–404*
severing of, 404, *405*
Mustardé, 404–405, *405*
Tenzel rotation, 400–402, *401–402*
Trepier (rotated myocutaneous), 403, *403–404*
used in medial canthal reconstruction, 390–391, 393
composite, 391
glabellar, 391, 393, *395*
island forehead, 393, *396*
midline forehead, 393, *396*
Mustardé, 390–392, *392*
myocutaneous, 390, *391*
pedicle, 391, *395*
tarsoconjunctival, 391, *394*
Tenzel, 391, *393*
used in upper eyelid reconstruction, Cutler-Beard, 374–375, *375–378*
forehead, 371, *373*
Flap(s) *(Continued)*
lateral transpositional, 371, *372*
myocutaneous, 369, *369–370*
nasojugal, 373–374, *374*
pedicle, from lower lid to upper lid, 382–383, *383*
semicircular, 366, *367*
sliding tarsal, 380, 382, *382*
tarsal rotational, 375–378, *379–380*
tarsoconjunctival, 378–380, *381*
sliding, 380, 382, *382*
Flash-cord receptacle, of camera, 551
Flower tear trough implant, 488, *489*, 492–493, *492–495*, 495
Focusing screen, of camera, 552, *552*
Fogo selvagem, 33
Follicles, hair. See *Hair follicles.*
Follicular keratosis, inverted, of eyelid, 326, *326*
Foltz valve, 742, *743*
Forceps, used in ophthalmic plastic surgery, *290*
Forehead flap, used in medial canthal reconstruction, island, 393, *396*
midline, 393, *396*
used in upper eyelid reconstruction, technique of, 371, *373*
Forehead fracture, unilateral, orbital fracture and, anterior cranial base approach to, 1188–1189, *1190*
Foreign body(ies), causing secondary acquired nasolacrimal duct obstruction, 812
removal of, 1047
surgical approach in, 1054
Fornical conjunctiva, 159. See also *Conjunctiva.*
Foster's classification, of cicatricial pemphigoid, 197, 197t
Four-wall orbital decompression, for Graves' disease, combined transorbital-neurosurgical, 980. See also *Graves' disease, orbital decompression for.*
Fracture(s), orbital. See *Orbital fracture(s).*
Francisella tularensis, 149
tularemia caused by, 313
Freckles (ephelides), in neurofibromatosis, 25
of eyelid, 339, *339*
Free thyroxine index (FTI), in thyrotoxicosis, 124
Fresh tissue technique, for removal of skin cancer, 352
advantages of, 354–355
steps in, 352–354, *353–355*
Frontal nerve, anatomy of, 277, *278*
Frontal sinus(es), anatomy of, 1015
mucoceles in, *1017*, 1017–1018
radiographic findings in, 1017, *1017–1018*
treatment of, 1018
Frontalis muscle, *263*, 264, *266*
contraction of, 262
Frontobasal fracture(s), 1096–1098
complications of, 1097–1098
treatment of, 1097, *1097*
Frontonasalethmoidal encephalocele, anterior cranial base approach to, 1199, *1201–1202*
Fronto-orbital asymmetry, subcranial approach to, results of, 1176t
Fronto-orbital fracture, cerebrospinal fluid leak with, anterior cranial base approach to, 1189, *1192*
Fronto-orbital osteotomy, subcranial approach to, 1163–1164, *1165–1167*
Frost-type sutures, in eyelid surgery, 439, *440*

FTI (free thyroxine index), in thyrotoxicosis, 124
Fuchs, islets of, 208
Fungal infection(s), of eyelid, 318–319

Gangrene, gas, of eyelid, 312
progressive synergistic, of eyelid, 312
Gas gangrene (clostridial myonecrosis), of eyelid, 312
Gastrointestinal carcinoma, metastatic orbital disease from, 1012
Gelfoam, for hemostasis in wound repair, 283
Giant cell arteritis, 112
Glabellar flap, used in medial canthal reconstruction, 391, 393, *395*
Glanders, involving eyelids, 313
Glaucoma, development of, following alkali burn, 222–223
in cicatricial pemphigoid, 98
Glioma, midbrain, ptosis caused by, 76
optic canal, 881–882, *882*
optic nerve, 985–987, *986*
clinical presentation of, 986–987
imaging of, 899–900, *899–900*
radiographic findings in, 987
treatment of, 987
Globe, anatomy of, 846–847, *847*, 904
examination of, evidence of orbital disease in, 868–870, *869–870*
malignant melanoma of, 909, *910–911*
metastasis of, *911*, 911–912
neuroradiologic imaging of, 904–912
techniques in, 904–905
ocular pathology of, 905–909
position and movement of, in orbital disease, 861–862, *863–865*
prominent, 486–487, *488–489*
cause of, 487–488
Glogau's classification, of photodamage, 662, 663t
Glomus tumor, of eyelid, 332
Glucocorticoids, for thyroid storm, 130
for thyrotoxicosis, 128
Gold weight, in surgical management of facial paralysis, 475–476, *476–477*
Goldberg lateral orbital rim implant, 488, *489*
Goldenhar's syndrome, 255
congenital colobomas in, 407–408
Goldmann perimetry, kinetic, 860
Gottron's papules, in dermatomyositis, 7
Gradenigo's syndrome, 473
Graft(s). See also *Autograft(s); Homograft(s).*
alloplastic, and spontaneous epithelialization, in conjunctival mucous membrane replacement, 171–172, *171–172*
bone, harvesting of, 1077–1080, *1078–1082*
buccal mucous membrane. See *Buccal mucous membrane graft(s).*
cartilage, harvesting of, 1080, 1082
in surgical management of facial paralysis, 481–482, *481–482*
cartilage-mucosal compound, 176
composite, used in medial canthal reconstruction, 391
used in upper eyelid reconstruction, 382, *383*
conjunctival. See *Conjunctival graft(s).*
hard palate, harvesting of, 442–444, *443–444*, 1082–1083
harvesting of, 1077–1083
for eyelid surgery, 440
lamellar corneoscleral, in management of pterygia, 214, *214*
Graft(s) *(Continued)*
nasal septal mucosa, harvesting of, 1080, 1082
oral mucosal. See *Oral mucosal graft(s).*
skin, used in medial canthal reconstruction, 393, 396, *397*
used in upper eyelid reconstruction, 366–367, *368*, 369
split-level full-thickness, used in upper eyelid reconstruction, 384, *384*
tarsoconjunctival, free, 175, *175–176*
Granular cell tumor, of eyelid, 329
Granulation, spontaneous, in conjunctival mucous membrane replacement, 170–171
of medial canthal area, 387
Granulocyte(s), 95
Granulocytic sarcoma, involving orbit, 61, *61*
Granuloma, eosinophilic, of orbit, 62, *63*
in AIDS patients, 532
in sarcoidosis, 107
lethal midline, 114
midline idiopathic, of orbit, 66, *66*
pyogenic, of eyelid, 331, *331*
Granuloma annulare, 43, *43*
in diabetic patient, 140
Granuloma faciale, 43
Granuloma inguinale, involving eyelids, 314
Granulomatosis, lymphomatoid, 10t, 11–12, 113–114
Wegener's. See *Wegener's granulomatosis.*
Granulomatous angiitis, allergic, 113
Graves' disease, *12*, 12–14
canthal obliquity in, surgical techniques for, 521
euthyroid, 121
eyelid retraction in, clinical features of, 514–516, *515–516*
historical background to, 516–518
lower, surgical techniques for, 520–521, *520–521*
surgical techniques for, 518–521
complications of, 521–523, *522–523*
upper, surgical techniques for, 518–520, *519–520*
lower eyelid entropion in, surgical techniques for, 521
orbital decompression for, 967–982
four-wall, combined transorbital-neurosurgical, 980
in patients with compressive optic neuropathy, *973*, 973–974
indications for, 968
overview to surgery in, *968*, 968–969
preoperative evaluation in, 967–968
three-wall, transorbital approach to, 976–980, *976–980*
tissue compliance impacting on, 969
transantral approach to, 974–976, *974–976*
transorbital antroethmoidal, 969–973, *970–973*
orbital expansion for, complications of, 981–982
craniofacial approach to, 980–981
postoperative management in, 981
Graves' ophthalmopathy, 13–14
Gray (Gy), defined, 1023
Ground substance, of wound repair, 281
Gundersen conjunctival flap(s), contraindications to, 248
indications for, 248
postoperative management of, 248, *249*
surgical technique of, 248, *249*
Gundersen flap, 164–165
Günther's disease, 29
Guttate, in scleroderma, 8
Gy (gray), defined, 1023

Haemophilus ducreyi, chancroid caused by, 314
Hair. See also *Eyebrow(s); Eyelash(es).*
direction of, in adult, 264, *265*
in infant, 264, *264*
permanent removal of, 589–594
blend modality in, 593
comparison of techniques in, 593–594
electrolysis in, 589–591
regulatory agencies and, 591–593
short-wave or thermolysis method in, 591
Hair follicles, 268, 324
benign adnexal lesions originating in, 335–336, *335–336*
Hand-Schüller-Christian disease, 62
Hansen's disease (leprosy), 153–154
involving eyelids, 313
Hard palate, anatomy of, 441, *442*
mucosa of, used in upper eyelid reconstruction, 364–365
Hard palate graft(s), harvesting of, 442–444, *443–444*, 1082–1083
Hard palate surgery, 441–442
Harlequin fetus, 45, *45*
Harvesting, of auricular cartilage, technique in, 364, *364*
of autogenous bone grafts, 1077–1080, *1078–1082*
of hard palate graft(s), 442–444, *443–444*, 1082–1083
of mucous membrane grafts, 173, *173*, 1080, 1082–1083
of nasochondral tissue, technique in, 365, *365*
Hasner valve, 742, *743*
Hasner's membrane, 777
rupture of, 778, 780
Hasner's valve, 777
Hauschka technique, of lymphatic drainage, 654–655
Head structure, anophthalmic socket and, 1130, *1130*
Hearing aids, bone-anchored, 1159
Heerford's syndrome, 16, 901
Heliotrope, 7
Helminthic infection(s), of eyelid, 317–318
Hemangioendothelioma, benign, imaging of, 893, *893–894*
malignant, 929
Hemangioma, capillary, of eyelid, 330, *330*
of orbit, 913–920
clinical course of, 913–916, *915–916*
complications of, 917, *918*
corticosteroids for, 919–920
diagnostic testing for, 916–917, *916–917*
histopathology of, 913, *914–915*
imaging of, 893, *893–894*
radiation therapy for, 919
surgical excision of, 918–919
treatment of, 917–920
indications for, 917–918
cavernous, of eyelid, 330
of orbit, 926–929
clinical course of, 927–928
diagnostic testing for, 928, *928–929*
histopathology of, 926–927, *927*
imaging of, 894, *894–895*
treatment of, 928–929
choroidal, imaging of, 910–911, *910–911*
disseminated neonatal, 920–921

Hemangioma *(Continued)*
clinical course of, 921, *921*
histopathology of, 920, *920*
ocular and ophthalmic manifestations of, 920t
treatment of, 921
eruptive (pyogenic granuloma), of eyelid, 331, *331*
retinal, 910–911
Hemangiopericytoma, 929–932
clinical course of, 930, *931*
diagnostic testing for, 930–931, *931*
histopathology of, 930, *930–931*
orbital, imaging of, 895–896, *896*
treatment of, 931–932, *932*
Hematoma, as complication of medial canthal reconstruction, 398
Hemiexophthalmos, 488
Hemifacial spasm, 90, *90*, 510–512
botulinum A toxin injection for, *508*, 509t, 511
clinical features of, 510, *510*
diagnostic features of, 505t
drug therapy for, 511
etiology of, 510–511, *511*
management of, 90
surgical therapy for, 511–512
Hemochromatosis, in diabetic patient, 141
Hemorrhage, as complication of orbital decompression surgery, 981–982
retrobulbar, causing blindness, 643
surgical approach to, 1054
Hemostasis, in orbital surgery, 1049
in wound repair, 282–284
pharmacologic agents for, 283
pressure tamponade for, 282
thermal cautery and electrocautery for, 282–283
topically applied chemical agents for, 283–284
Hemostats, used in ophthalmic plastic surgery, *290*
Hepatic cirrhosis, eyelid retraction associated with, 75, *76*
Hepatoblastoma, metastatic, to orbit, *56*
Hereditary hemorrhagic telangiectasia (Osler-Weber-Rendu disease), 9
Hering's law of equal innervation, 878
eyelid retraction secondary to, 74, *76*
Herpes simplex infection, of eyelid, 315, *315*
treatment of, 315
Herpes zoster infection, 152
of eyelid, 315
treatment of, 315–316
Herpes zoster ophthalmicus, of eyelid, in AIDS patients, 526
Hidradenoma, clear cell, of eyelid, 334
Hidrocystoma, apocrine (Moll's cyst), of eyelid, 334, *334*
Highlighting, as cosmetic technique, used in facial rejuvenation, 570
Highlighting and contouring, with camouflage make-up, 660–661
Histiocytes, benign eyelid tumors derived from, *332*, 332–333
Histiocytic disorder(s), involving orbit, 62, *63*, 64
Histiocytosis, Langerhans' cell, 62
sinus, associated with secondary acquired nasolacrimal duct obstruction, 801
Histiocytosis X. See *Eosinophilic granuloma.*
Histocompatibility leukocyte antigen (HLA), 96
HIV (human immunodeficiency virus), 525
infection by. See *Acquired immuno-deficiency syndrome (AIDS).*
HLA (histocompatibility leukocyte antigen), 96
HMB-45 marker, for malignant melanoma, 57
Hollow bulb prosthesis, 1143–1144, *1143–1145*. See also *Prosthesis.*
Homograft(s). See also *Graft(s).*
scleral, for eyelid reconstruction, 724–727
results with, 727, *727*
histology of, 726, *726–727*
immunopathology of, 726–727
Hordeolum (stye), 307, *309*
treatment of, 307–308
Hormonal therapy, for orbital metastatic disease, 57, 1008
Horn cyst, 325
Horner's muscle, *850*, 744850
Horner's syndrome, 77–79
anisocoria in, 78
cocaine test for, 79, *79*
evaluation of, 78–79
Paredrine test for, 79
postganglionic, orbital disease causing, 877
ptosis in, 77–78, *78*
Hrytl valve, 742, *743*
Hudson-Stähli line, 208
Hughes flap, in lower eyelid reconstruction, 402–404, *403–404*
severing of, 404, *405*
Human immunodeficiency virus (HIV), 525
infection by. See *Acquired immuno-deficiency syndrome (AIDS).*
Huschke valve, 742, *743*
Hutchinson's freckle (lentigo maligna), definition of, 179
of eyelid, 339
Hyalinosis cutis et mucosae, 20–21
Hyaloid detachment, posterior, MRI of, 905, *905*
Hydatid cyst, 151
Hydralazine lupus, 5, 5t. See also *Lupus erythematosus (LE).*
Hydrocystoma, eccrine, of eyelid, 334
Hydroxyapatite implant. See also *Prosthesis.*
enucleation with, 1036, 1041–1042
complications of, 1042
contraindications to, 1042
Hygroma, cystic (cavernous lymphangioma), of eyelid, 331
Hypercalcemia, causes of, 133t
evaluation of, parathyroid hormone in, 132–133
hyperparathyroidism causing, 132
severe, definition of, 135
treatment of, 135–136
Hyperparathyroidism, 132–136
clinical manifestations of, 133–135, *134–135*
diagnostic considerations in, 132–133, 133t
management of, 135–136, 136t
Hyperpigmentation, periorbital, chemical peels for, 663
Hyperplasia, angiolymphoid, with eosinophilia, of eyelid, 332
intravascular papillary endothelial, of eyelid, 332
sebaceous gland, of eyelid, 336–337
Hypersensitivity reaction(s), types of, 96
Hypertelorism, subcranial approach to, results of, 1176t
Hyperthyroidism, 12–14
in pregnancy, 129–130
thyrotoxicosis vs., 123
Hyperthyroxinemia, euthyroid, 129
causes of, 129t
Hypertropia, as complication of orbital floor fractures, 1091, *1092*
Hypothalamic-pituitary-thyroid axis, physiologic regulation of, 122–123, *123*
Hypothyroidism, associated with myxedema, 14, *14*
due to ^{131}iodine therapy, 128
Hypotonia, lower lid, evaluation of, prior to male blepharoplasty, 635

"Ice pack" test, for myasthenia gravis, 82
Ichthyosis, *45*, 45–46
treatment of, 46
Ichthyosis vulgaris, 45
Idiopathic midline destructive disease, of orbit, 66, *66*
Idiopathic optic disc edema, in diabetic patient, 138t, 138–139
Idiopathic orbital inflammation, 952–956
acute form of, 952–953, *953*
biopsy of, 955
CT scans of, 954, *954*
diagnosis of, 953–954
histopathology of, 954–955, *955*
historical perspective on, 952
imaging of, 890–891, *890–891*
immunopathogenesis of, 955
subacute, 953
treatment of, 955–956
Idiopathic orbital pseudotumor, 965
IgA (immunoglobulin A), 95
IgD (immunoglobulin D), 95
IgE (immunoglobulin E), 95
IgG (immunoglobulin G), 95
IgM (immunoglobulin M), 95
Iliac bone graft(s), harvesting of, 1077, *1078–1079*
Immune complex reaction (hypersensitivity type III), 96
Immune disease, ocular manifestation(s) of, 94–114
allergic granulomatous angiitis and, 113
cicatricial pemphigoid and, 98–100
epidermolysis bullosa and, 103–105
erythema multiforme and, 100–102
lethal midline granuloma and, 114
lymphomatoid granulomatosis and, 113–114
pemphigus and, 102–103
polyarteritis nodosa and, 111–112
polymorphic reticulosis and, 113–114
sarcoidosis and, 106–108
temporal arteritis and, 112
toxic epidermal necrolysis and, 105–106
Wegener's granulomatosis and, 109–111
Immune reaction(s), classic, 96
Immune system, 94–98
cells of, 94–95
histocompatibility antigens of, 95
hypersensitivity reactions of, 95
monoclonal antibodies of, 95
Immunity, cell-mediated, 94, 96
Immunoglobulin(s), classes of, 95
Immunosuppressive therapy, for cicatricial pemphigoid, 199
complications of, 199–200
goal of, 200
Imperforate punctal membrane, 782, *782*
Implant(s). See *Prosthesis.*

Impression(s), alginate, used in design and making of prosthesis, 1138, *1138*
Incision(s), for blepharoplasty, 707–708, *707–708*
  for brow ptosis, 579, *579*, 581, *581–583*, 583
  for orbital surgery, 1060, *1061*
Infection(s). See also specific infection.
  after blepharoplasty, 648
  causing nasolacrimal duct obstruction, 797–799, 798t, *798–800*
  of eyelid, 313–319
    bacterial, 313–315
    fungal, 318–319
    in AIDS patients, 526
    parasitic, 317–318
    viral, 315–316, *315–316*
  of orbit, 146–155, 888–891
    causing edema, 151–152
    causing nodular eruptions, *140*, 149–150
    cellulitis due to, 146–148, 147t, *147–148*
    Chlamydia trachomatis causing, 154t, 154–155, *155*
    dacryoadenitis associated with, 153, *153*
    herpes zoster virus causing, 152
    in AIDS patient(s), 529
    in diabetic patient, 137–138, 138t
    miscellaneous, 150–151, *151*
    Mycobacterium leprae causing, 153–154
    Mycobacterium tuberculosis causing, 152–153
    syphilis and, 153
Infiltrative myopathy, 88
Inflammation, of eyelid, 307–310, *309*
  causes of, 308t
  of orbit, idiopathic. See *Idiopathic orbital inflammation.*
    in AIDS patients, 529–530
Inflammatory cause(s), of secondary acquired nasolacrimal duct obstruction, 799, 801t, 801–804, *802–804*
Inflammatory myopathy, 88
Inflammatory phase, of wound repair, 281, 282t
Infranuclear factor(s), tearing due to, 750
Infranuclear lesion(s), eyelid retraction caused by, 73–74, *74–76*
  ptosis caused by, 77, *78*
Injury. See *Trauma.*
Inorganic pigment, 541. See also *Pigment(s).*
Insulin, chronic patient use of, anesthetic considerations with, 295
Intensity, principle of, in electrolysis, 590
Interferon(s), for Kaposi's sarcoma, 528
Interrupted suture(s), deep, 286, *287*
  simple, 286, *286*
Intracranial hypertension, benign, optic nerve decompression for, 1056–1059, *1057–1059*
Intradermal nevus, of eyelid, 337–338, *338*
Intravascular papillary endothelial hyperplasia, of eyelid, 332
Iodide, oral (Lugol's solution), for thyroid storm, 130
  for thyrotoxicosis, 128
^{131}Iodine therapy, for thyrotoxicosis, 128
  side effects of, 128
Irrigation, immediate, following chemical injury, 223
Islets of Fuchs, 208

Jaw winking phenomenon, Marcus Gunn, 73, *74*
Jessner's solution, used in chemical peels, 666, 666t
Jewelry, metal, removal of, before electrolysis, 589–590
Jones I test, in tearing, 754–755
Jones II test, in tearing, 755
Jones' muscle, 744
Junctional nevus, of eyelid, 337
Juvenile melanoma, of eyelid, 338
Juvenile pilocytic astrocytoma, imaging of, 899–900, *899–900*
Juvenile xanthogranuloma, of eyelid, 64, 333
  of orbit, 64

K (killer) cell(s), 95
Kaposi's sarcoma, of conjunctiva, in AIDS patients, 236–237, 242, *243*, 532
  of eyelid, in AIDS patients, 526–528, *527*
Kearns-Sayre syndrome, 87
  in diabetic patient, 138t, 139
  pigmentary retinopathy in, 87–88, *88*
Keloid(s), in African American patient, 715–716, *716*
  pigmentary management of, 535–536
  vs. hypertrophic scarring, 717t
Keratinocyte(s), of eyelid, 323
Keratoacanthoma, of eyelid, 325–326, *326*
Keratoconjunctivitis, superior limbic, conjunctival resection for, indications for, 248–249
    surgical technique of, 249
Keratosis, actinic, chemical peels for, 663
  of eyelid, inverted follicular, 326, *326*
    seborrheic, 325, *325*
Keratosis follicularis (Darier's disease), 21
KID syndrome, 46
Kiem test, for sarcoidosis, 108
Killer (K) cell(s), 95
Kimura's disease (angiolymphoid hyperplasia with eosinophilia), 949–950, *949–950*
  of eyelid, 332
Kissing nevus, of eyelid, 337, *337*
Klebsiella rhinoscleromatis, 138
  rhinoscleroma caused by, 314
Kleeblatt-Schaedel's anomaly, 1182
Koenen's tumors, in tuberous sclerosis, 27
Krause gland(s), 161, *273*, 732, *732*, *737*
Krause (Béraud) valve, 742, *743*
Krönlein-Berke orbitotomy, technique of, 1056–1059, *1057–1059*
Kuhnt-Szymanowski procedure, Smith modification of, for involutional ectropion, 427, *428*
Kveim test, for sarcoidosis, 65

Laceration(s), conjunctival, 168–169
  lower eyelid, evaluation of, 455–456, *455–457*
  upper eyelid, repair of, 359–361, *362*
Lacrimal artery, anatomy of, 274, *274–275*
Lacrimal diaphragm, 744
Lacrimal ductule(s), destruction of, treatment for, 255
Lacrimal fossa, 731
  in Chinese skulls, 696–698, 697t, 698t
Lacrimal gland(s), 273, *273*, 731–736
  adenoid cystic carcinoma of, 68–69, *69*, 303, *304*
Lacrimal gland(s) *(Continued)*
  anatomy of, 731–732, *732–733*
  blood supply to, 849
  direct stimulation of, tearing and, 750–751
  disorders of, after blepharoplasty, 648–649
  embryology of, 731
  histology of, 732–734, *734*
  innervation of, 734–736, *735*
  lesions of, imaging of, 902–904, *904*
  mucoepidermoid carcinoma of, 68, *69*
  prolapse of, in Graves' ophthalmopathy, 515–516, *516*
    repair of, in upper eyelid blepharoplasty, 601–602, *602*
      variations of, 609
  pseudocapsule of, 732
  secretion of, 735–736
  tumor(s) of, 999–1006
    benign, 999
    differential diagnosis of, 1003t, 1003–1004
    epidemiology of, 999, 1001
    malignant, 999
    natural history of, 1002
    presentation of, 1001
    prognosis for, 1006
    radiologic features of, *1000–1002*, 1001
    secondary, 999
    treatment of, 1004–1006, *1005–1006*
      principles and problems in, 1002–1003
  vascular supply to, 734
Lacrimal nerve, 849
  anatomy of, 277, *278*
Lacrimal nucleus, stimulation of, tearing due to, 750
Lacrimal probes, for nasolacrimal duct obstruction, 778, *779*
  for ophthalmic plastic surgery, *290*
Lacrimal pump, disorders of, epiphora due to, 751
  integrity of, affecting tearing, 762
Lacrimal pump mechanism, composition of, 267
Lacrimal sac, 740–741, *742*
  anatomy of, 268, *268*, 850
  fistula of, 782–783, *783*
  tumors of, 304–305, *305*
Lacrimal surgery, for altered tear production, 201
Lacrimal system, 731–746
  anatomy of, 784, *785*
  congenital abnormalities of, 777–783. See also specific anomaly, e.g., *Nasolacrimal duct obstruction, congenital.*
  excretory, 738–746, *739*
    anatomy of, 849–850, *850*
    canaliculi of, 739–740, *739–741*
    embryology of, *738*, 738–739
    lacrimal sac in, 740–741, *742*
    nasolacrimal duct in, 741–745, *743–746*
    pump system in, 744–745, *746*
    puncta of, 739
  glands in, 731–738
    anatomy of, 731–72, *732–733*
    embryology of, 731
    histology of, 732–734, *734*
    innervation of, 734–736, *735*
    vascular supply to, 734
  injury to, sequence of repair following, 458
  involvement of, in medial canthal reconstruction, 396, 398
  secretory, anatomy of, 849

Lacrimation. See also *Tearing.*
afferent and efferent pathways of, 734, *735*
causes of, 750–751
Lagophthalmos, after blepharoplasty, 646, *646*
in Graves' ophthalmopathy, 514
Lambdoidal synostosis, 1182
Lamellar corneoscleral graft(s), in management of pterygia, 214, *214*
Langerhans' cell histiocytosis, 62
Large cell lymphoma, 959
Laser(s), carbon dioxide, fat removal by, 638, 640
treatment of lymphangioma with, 926
ultrapulse, used in blepharoplasty, *544*
in treatment of endonasal dacryocystorhinostomy, 794
in treatment of hyperpigmented facial lesions, 568
in treatment of telangiectasia, 569
postoperative use of, for pterygia, 219
YAG, fat removal by, *641,* 641–642
treatment of lymphangiomas with, 926
Laugh line (skin folds), around eyelids, 261–262, *263*
LE. See *Lupus erythematosus (LE).*
LeFort fracture(s), 1095, *1095*
Leiomyoma, of eyelid, 329
of orbit, 996
Leiomyosarcoma, metastatic, to orbit, *58*
of orbit, 996
Leishmaniasis, diffuse cutaneous, of eyelid, 150, *150*
involving eyelids, 316
Lens, of camera, 552–554, *553*
Lentigines, chemical peels for, 663–664
Lentigo maligna (Hutchinson's freckle), definition of, 179
of eyelid, 339
Lentigo maligna melanoma, 179
of eyelid, 339
Lentigo senilis, of eyelid, 339, *340*
Lentigo simplex, of eyelid, 339
Leprosy (Hansen's disease), 153–154
involving eyelids, 313
Lethal midline granuloma, 114
Leukemia, involving orbit, 60
Leukocoria, 907
Levator aponeurosis, applied anatomy of, 448
Levator palpebrae superioris muscle, anatomy of, 270–271, 849
superior view of, *272*
Lichen planus, 40–41
treatment of, 41
Lichen simplex chronicus, 41
Lid(s). See *Eyelid(s).*
Lidocaine (Xylocaine), for aponeurotic surgery, 448
for lower eyelid blepharoplasty, 619, 627
for male blepharoplasty, 636
for transantral approach to orbital decompression, 974
for transorbital antroethmoidal orbital decompression, 969
for upper eyelid blepharoplasty, 599
recommended maximal dosage of, 298
Lighting, for orbital surgery, 1048
for photography, 554–555, *556–559,* *557–559*
proper set-up of, *556*
sources of, 554–555
Ligneous conjunctivitis, 20
Limbal tumor(s), 69–70
Lipocauterization, in fat removal, 638, *639*
Lipocontouring, radio-frequency, in fat removal, 642, *642*
Lipodermoid(s). See *Dermolipoma(s).*
Lipoid proteinosis, 20–21
differential diagnosis of, 21
Lipolytic diathermy, fat removal by, 640–641, *640–641*
Lipoma, orbital, 996
Liposarcoma, orbital, 996–997
Lisch nodules, in neurofibromatosis, 25
Lithium, for thyroid storm, 130
for thyrotoxicosis, 128
Loa loa infection, of eyelid, 317
Local anesthesia. See *Anesthesia, regional.*
Lockwood's ligament, anatomy of, 841–842, *842*
Löfgren's syndrome, 16
Lorazepam, for essential blepharospasm and Meige's syndrome, 507
Lubricants, topical, for facial paralysis, 474
Lugol's solution, for thyroid storm, 130
for thyrotoxicosis, 128
Lung carcinoma, metastatic orbital disease from, 1010
Lupus erythematosus (LE), 3–7, *4*
acute cutaneous, 4
chronic cutaneous, 4
common form of, 6
clinical manifestations of, 3–4
discoid, 3
characteristic features of, 6
drug-related, 5, 5t
mucocutaneous lesions of, classification of, 4t
subacute cutaneous, 3
serologic marker for, 5–6
systemic manifestations of, 5
systemic, 3
diagnosis of, 6
ocular complications of, 4–5, 5t
revised criteria for, 4t
treatment of, 6–7
Lupus miliaris disseminatus faciei, 38, *38*
treatment of, 39
Lupus panniculitis, 6
Lupus profundus, 6
Lutzner's cells, 62
Lyell's syndrome. See *Toxic epidermal necrolysis (Lyell's syndrome).*
Lyme disease, 473
Lymphadenopathy, sinus histiocytosis with, of orbit, 62, *62*
Lymphangioma, 921–926
clinical course of, 923–924, *923–924*
diagnostic testing for, 924–925, *924–926*
histopathology of, *922,* 922–923
of eyelid, 331, *331*
orbital, imaging of, 894–895, *895*
treatment of, 925–926, *926*
Lymphangion, 652, *652*
Lymphatic drainage, manual, 651–656
contraindications to, 655t
features of, 655
Hauschka technique of, 654–655
indications for, 655, 655t
mechanical methods of, 655
of extremities, pressure bandages with, 655
Vodder technique of, 654
of conjunctiva, 161
of eyelid, 275, *276*
Lymphatic flow, pulse-wave nature of, 653, *653*
Lymphatic fluid, 651
forward propulsion of, *652,* 652–653
osmotic pressure of, 654
protein concentration of, 654
Lymphatic system, anatomy and physiology of, 651, *652*
Lymphatic vessels, 651–652, *652–653*
pharmacology of, 655
pumping action of, 652
Lymphoblastic lymphoma, 959
Lymphocyte(s), subpopulations of, 94–95
Lymphocytic lymphoma, small cell, 959
Lymphogranuloma venereum, involving eyelids, 315
Lymphoid cells, gene rearrangement unique to, 960
Lymphoid granulomatosis, ocular abnormalities of, 10t
Lymphoid hyperplasia, benign reactive, involving orbit, 61–62
Lymphoid tumor(s), of conjunctiva, 58–59, 235–236, *235–236,* 244–246, 956–957
classification of, 244
clinical features of, 244, *245*
demographics and, 245
histology of, 244
histopathologic analysis of, 244
immunophenotypic analysis of, 244–245
molecular genetic analysis of, 245
patient evaluation for, 245–246
prognosis for, 245
treatment of, 246
of orbit, 58–60, *59,* 303–304, 956–962
benign, 958
classification of, 956
clinical course of, 960
clinical presentation of, 956–957, *956–957*
differential diagnosis of, 960–961
historical perspective on, 952
laboratory evaluation of, 957–960, *958*
malignant, 958–959
treatment of, 961–962
Lymphoma, 58–60, *59,* 303–304
Burkitt's, Epstein-Barr virus associated with, 530, 959
imaging of, 892–983, *893*
large cell, 959
lymphoblastic, 959
mantle cell, 959
non-Hodgkin's. See *Non-Hodgkin's lymphoma.*
of lacrimal glands, natural history of, 1002
radiologic features of, 1001, *1001*
treatment of, 1004
small cell lymphocytic, 959
Lymphomatoid granulomatosis, 11–12, 113–114
Lymphoproliferative disease(s), of orbit, in AIDS patients, 530–532, *531*

MacCallan classification, of trachoma, 314–315
Macrophage(s), 94
Macrophthalmia, 905
"Madame Butterfly" procedure, for ectropion, 645
Magnetic resonance imaging (MRI), of capillary hemangioma, 893, *894*
of cavernous hemangioma, 894, *895*
of choroidal hemangioma, 910, *911*
of dermoid cyst, 886–888, *889*
of epidermoid cyst, 886–888, *888*
of hemangiopericytoma, 895–896, *896*
of lacrimal gland lesions, 904, *904*
of lymphangioma, 894–895, *895*
of lymphoid tumor, 957

Magnetic resonance imaging (MRI) *(Continued)*
of lymphoma, 892–983, *893*
of mucoceles, in paranasal sinuses, *1016,* 1016–1017
of neurofibroma, *991*
of neurogenic tumors, 984
of optic nerve glioma, 900, *900, 986,* 987
of optic nerve meningioma, 988, *988*
of optic nerve sarcoidosis, 900–901, *902*
of optic nerve sheath meningioma, 899, *899*
of optic neuritis, 900, *900*
of orbit, 885–886
of persistent hyperplastic primary vitreous, 908, *909*
of posterior hyaloid detachment, 905, *905*
of pseudotumor, 890–891, *891*
of retinal detachment, 905–906, *906*
of retinoblastoma, 907–908, *908*
of rhabdomyosarcoma, 902, *903*
of schwannoma, 992, *992*
of sphenoid wing meningioma, *989,* 990
of subperiosteal abscess, 889–890, *890*
of uveal malignant melanoma, 909, *910–911*
of uveal metastatic disease, *911,* 911–912
Magnification, in orbital surgery, 1048
Maier's sinus, 740, *742,* 850
Make-up, camouflage. See *Camouflage make-up.*
Malar fold, *262–263,* 484
Malar hypoplasia, evaluation of, prior to male blepharoplasty, 635
Malherbe's calcifying epithelioma (pilomatricoma), of eyelid, 336, *336*
Malignancy. See also specific neoplasm.
acanthosis nigricans associated with, 23–24
dermatomyositis associated with, 7
life-threatening, orbital exenteration for, 1070, 1071t
Malignant external otitis, in diabetic patient, 138
Malignant hemangioendothelioma, 929
Malignant melanoma, metastatic orbital disease from, 1012
of conjunctiva, 233–235, *234*
clinical features of, 183, *183*
primary acquired melanosis associated with, 233, 234
treatment of, 187–188, *188*
care following, 188t
complications of, 187t
of lacrimal sac, 305
of orbit, 57–58, *58,* 992
imaging of, 909, *910–911*
of uvea, anterior cranial base approach to, 1202–1204, *1204–1205*
Mantle cell lymphoma, 959
Manual lymphatic drainage, 651–656
contraindications to, 655t
features of, 655
Hauschka technique of, 654–655
indications for, 655, 655t
mechanical methods of, 655
of extremities, pressure bandages with, 655
Vodder technique of, 654
Manz gland(s), 160, *273,* 736, 737, *737*
Marcus Gunn jaw winking phenomenon, 73, *74*
Marcus Gunn pupil, 876
reverse, 876, *877*
Marcus Gunn swinging light test, 860–861
Mask, computer-controlled cooling-heating, used in blepharoplasty, *544*
Masquerade syndrome, in sebaceous gland carcinoma, 190
Massage techniques, of lymphatic drainage, 651–656. See also *Manual lymphatic drainage.*
Mast cell(s), 95
Mastocytoma, 43
Mastocytosis, 43
Mattress suture(s), buried, 710–711, *710–711*
combined with small incisions, 712, *713*
horizontal, 288, *288*
half-buried, 288, *289*
vertical, 288, *289*
Maturation phase, of wound repair, 281, 282t
Maxillary nerve, anatomy of, 278
Maxillary sinus(es), anatomy of, 1015
mucoceles in, 1021, *1021*
as complication of orbital floor fracture, 1091, *1093*
Maxillary vein, anatomy of, 275
McReynolds operation, for pterygia removal, 211
Mechanical cause(s), of nasolacrimal duct obstruction, 812t, 812–813, *812–813*
Mechanobullous disease(s), 29–31, 30t
Medical device, migrated or retained, causing nasolacrimal duct obstruction, 812, *812*
Medical photography, 551–559
camera feature(s) for, 551–554
automatic film advance as, 551
film as, 554
flash-cord receptacle as, 551
focusing screens as, 552, *552*
lens as, 552–554, *553*
shutter and shutter speed as, 551
lighting for, 554–555, *556–559,* 557–559
daylight as, 554
electronic flash or strobe as, 555
proper set-up and, *556*
tungsten bulbs as, 555
Medical tattooing. See *Micropigmentation.*
Medicine, Chinese view of, *692–694,* 692–695, 693t
Meibomian gland(s), 273, *273,* 736, *737*
carcinoma arising in, 190. See also *Sebaceous gland carcinoma.*
hyperplasia of, 336–337
inflammation of, 307, *309*
Meibomitis, acute, 307
after blepharoplasty, 649
chronic, 307, *309*
Meige's syndrome, 89–90, 504, 506
diagnostic features of, 505t
management of, 90, 507–510
botulinum A toxin injection in, 507–508, *508,* 509t
future directions in, 509–510
general eye care in, 507
pharmacotherapy in, 507
surgery in, 508–509, *509*
unconventional therapies in, 507
Melanocytosis, oculodermal, of eyelid, 339
Melanoma, choroidal, 182, *182*
juvenile, of eyelid, 338
malignant. See *Malignant melanoma.*
nodular, 179
superficial spreading, 179
Melanosis, complexion-associated, clinical features of, 180–181, *180–181*
definition of, 178–179
primary acquired. See *Primary acquired melanosis (PAM).*
Melasma, chemical peels for, 662–663
Melkersson-Rosenthal syndrome, 15–16
differential diagnosis of, 16
MEN I (Wermer's syndrome), 22, 142
MEN II (Sipple's syndrome), 22, 142
MEN III (multiple endocrine neoplasia III), 21–23, 22t, 142
Meningioma, optic nerve, 882, *883,* 987–989
management of, 988–989
radiographic findings in, 987–988, *987–988*
optic nerve sheath, imaging of, 897, *898–899,* 899
sphenoid wing, 989–990
radiographic findings in, *989,* 990
treatment of, 990
Metabolic disease(s). See *Systemic and metabolic disease(s).*
Metabolism, calcium, regulation of, 132
Metal jewelry, removal of, before electrolysis, 589–590
Metastatic disease, causing nasolacrimal duct obstruction, 804, *805–810,* 806–807
from adenoid cystic carcinoma, of lacrimal glands, 1004, *1006*
of eyelid, *54,* 56
of orbit, 53–56, *54–57,* 1007–1013. See also *Orbital tumor(s), metastatic.*
prevalence of, 53
of uvea, *911,* 911–912
progressive palsy and, 474
Methimazole, for thyroid storm, 130
for thyrotoxicosis, 125
Methohexital, as anesthetic agent, 297
for aponeurotic surgery, 448
Methotrexate, pharmacology of, 97
Methyl methacrylate rings, insertion of, following chemical injury, 225
Metoprolol, for thyrotoxicosis, 125, 128
Microabscess, Pautrier's, 62
Microdissection, monopolar, fat removal by, 638
Microphthalmia, 905
severe, volume replacement in, 1043
Micropigmentation, 535–541. See also *Electropigmentation.*
aesthetic goals of, 683, 684t
consultation and preoperative teaching concerning, 683, 685
equipment for, 683
eyebrow reconstruction with, 537–538, *539–540*
technique of, 685–688, *686–688*
eyeliner reconstruction with, 536–537, *537–538*
technique of, 685, *686*
facial, 535–538
color adjusting in, 536
color matching in, 536
shading and blending in, 536, *536–537*
history of, 535
pigment color matching procedure in, 538–541, *540*
pigments for, 682–683
inorganic and organic, 541
selection of, 538
skin testing prior to, guidelines for, 541
techniques of, 685
Midazolam, as anesthetic agent, 296
Midbrain, glioma of, ptosis caused by, 76
Midbrain ptosis, *77*
Mikulicz's cells, in rhinoscleroma, 138
Mikulicz's syndrome, 107
Milia, of eyelid, *324,* 324–325
Miliary sarcoid, 16
Millard-Gubler syndrome, 470

Mini-driver, used in ophthalmic plastic surgery, *291*
Miniplates, cantilevered, in fixation/reconstruction of canthal tendon, 389–390, *390*
Miosis, ipsilateral, and unilateral ptosis. See *Horner's syndrome.*
Mitomycin C, as adjunct to surgery for pterygia, 218–219
Mixed eccrine tumor, of eyelid, 334, *334*
Mobility prosthesis, new, 1132, *1133*
Mohs' surgery, for periorbital malignancy, 352–355
  advantages of, 354–355
  drawbacks to, 352
  fresh tissue technique in, 352–354, *353–355*
Moisture bubble, for facial nerve palsy, 474, *475*
Moisture chamber glasses, for facial nerve palsy, 475, *475*
Moll's cyst (apocrine hidrocystoma), of eyelid, 334, *334*
Moll's gland(s), 273, *273,* 324, 737, *737*
Molluscum contagiosum, involving eyelids, 316, *316*
  in AIDS patients, 526, *526*
Mondino and Brown classification, of cicatricial pemphigoid, 196–197, 197t
Monoamine oxidase inhibitors, chronic patient use of, anesthetic considerations with, 296
Monoclonal antibody(ies), 96
Monocular condition(s), nonsurgical, for anophthalmic socket, 1127–1128, *1128*
Mononucleosis, periorbital edema in, 151
Monopolar microdissection, fat removal by, 638
Morning glory anomaly, 905
Moxibustion, 695
MRI. See *Magnetic resonance imaging (MRI).*
Mucin, 160
  reduced production of, after chemical injury, 226
Mucin layer, and precorneal tear film, 737
Mucocele(s), causing secondary acquired nasolacrimal duct obstruction, 813, *813*
  in paranasal sinuses, 1014–1021, *1015*
    as complication of orbital floor fracture, 1091, *1093*
    diagnostic imaging of, 1014–1017, *1016,* 1017–1018, *1017–1021,* 1020–1021
    histopathology of, 1014
    pathophysiology of, 1014
    treatment of, 1018–1019, 1021
Mucoepidermoid carcinoma, of lacrimal glands, 68, *69,* 999
Mucopyocele, 1014
Mucormycosis (phycomycosis), diagnostic and therapeutic features of, 941t–942t
  in diabetic patient, 137–138, 138t
    treatment of, 138
  rhinocerebral, 150–151, *151*
Mucosa, used in upper eyelid reconstruction, hard palate, 364–365
  oral, 365
Mucosal graft(s), oral. See *Oral mucosal graft(s).*
Mucous glands, conjunctival, 160–161
Mucous membrane(s), conjunctival, replacement of. See *Conjunctival mucous membrane(s), replacement of.*
  nonocular, involvement of, in cicatricial pemphigoid, 196
Mucous membrane graft(s), harvesting of, 1080, 1082–1083
Mular lesions, of eyelid, 314
Mulberry lesion, in squamous cell carcinoma of conjunctiva, *232*
Müller's muscle, anatomy of, 272, *273*
  in aponeurotic surgery, 448
Multicore disease, ptosis in, 84
Multiple endocrine neoplasia I (Wermer's syndrome), 22, 142
Multiple endocrine neoplasia II (Sipple's syndrome), 22, 142
Multiple endocrine neoplasia III (MEN III), 21–23, 22t, 142
Multiple mucosal neuroma syndrome, 21–23
  differential diagnosis of, 22–23
  ocular manifestations of, 22, 22t
  treatment of, 23
Multiple myeloma, of orbit, 62, *63*
Multiple suture synostosis, 1182, *1185*
Multiple-needle galvanic electrolysis, 590. See also *Electrolysis.*
Muscle(s). See also specific muscle, e.g., *Orbicularis oculi muscle.*
  excision of, in upper eyelid blepharoplasty, 599–600, *599–600*
    variations in, 607
  extraocular, enlarged, causes of, 886t
  of facial expression, 262, *263,* 264
Muscle of Riolan, 268
Muscle retraction, in orbital surgery, 1048
Muscular dystrophy, 84
Mustardé flap, in lower eyelid reconstruction, 404–405, *405*
  in medial canthal reconstruction, 390–391, *392*
Myasthenia gravis, 79–83
  acquired, in children, 80–81
  autoimmune disorders associated with, 83
  clinical findings in, 79–80
  eyelid retraction in, 74, *76*
  "ice pack" test for, 82
  ophthalmoparesis of, 80
  Prostigmin test for, in children, 82, *82*
  ptosis in, 80, *80–81*
  sleep test for, 82, *82*
  Tensilon test for, *80,* 81
    advantages and disadvantages of, 81–82
Myasthenic syndrome(s), 83
Mycobacterial infection(s), of eyelid, 313–314
Mycobacterium leprae, 153
  Hansen's disease caused by, 313
Mycosis cells, 62
Mycosis fungoides, of eyelid, 62
Myeloma, multiple, of orbit, 62, *63*
Myocutaneous flap, nasojugal, used in upper eyelid reconstruction, technique of, 373–374, *374*
  rotated, used in lower eyelid reconstruction, 403, *403–404*
  used in medial canthal reconstruction, 390, *391*
  used in upper eyelid reconstruction, 369, *369–370*
Myokymia, facial, 510
  diagnostic features of, 505t
Myonecrosis, of eyelid, clostridial, 312
  streptococcal, 312
Myopathy(ies), structural, ptosis caused by, 84, *85*
Myositis, ocular, in AIDS patients, 529
  orbital, 965–966
Myotonia, ptosis in, 85–86, *85–86*
Myotonic dystrophy, facial nerve disorders and, 474
  ptosis in, 85, *85–86*
Myxedema, 14, *14*

Narcotics, as anesthetic agents, 296
  reversal of, 296–297
Nasal dermoid, with intracranial extension, anterior cranial base approach to, 1199, *1200*
Nasal septal mucosa graft(s), harvesting of, 1080, 1082
Nasal telangiectasia, treatment of, 569, *569*
Nasochondral tissue, used in upper eyelid reconstruction, 365, *365*
Nasociliary nerve, anatomy of, 277, *278*
Nasoethmoidal fracture(s), 1095–1096
  treatment of, 1096
Nasojugal fold, *262–263,* 484
Nasojugal myocutaneous flap, used in upper eyelid reconstruction, technique of, 373–374, *374*
Nasolabial fold, *263*
Nasolacrimal duct, 741–745, *743–746,* 850
  congenital malformations of, 742–743, *743*
  stenosis of, epiphora due to, 751
  valves of, 742, *743*
Nasolacrimal duct obstruction, congenital, 777–778, *779,* 780
    probing of, 778, *779*
      failed, 780–781
    variant of, 780–781, *782*
  primary acquired, 784–796
    cause of, 784–785
    clinical presentation of, *785,* 785–786
    dacryocystorhinostomy for, *786–792,* 786–794
      endonasal, 792–794, *793–795*
      history in, 786–787
      incisions in, 788, *789*
      nasal packing for, 787, *788*
      procedure in, 787–792, *788–792*
      sedation for, 787
  secondary acquired, 797–813
    infectious causes of, 797–799, 798t, *798–800*
    inflammatory causes of, 799, 801t, 801–804, *802–804*
    mechanical causes of, 812t, 812–813, *812–813*
    neoplastic causes of, 804, 805t, *805–810,* 806–807
    traumatic causes of, 809–811, 810t, *810–812*
Nasolacrimal excretory system, dimensions of, 268, *268*
Nasolacrimal sac, narrowing of, epiphora due to, 751
Naso-orbital fistula, as complication of medial canthal reconstruction, 398
Naso-orbital fracture(s), 1095–1096
  treatment of, 1096
Naso-orbitoethmoid fracture, with associated brain and dural injury, anterior cranial base approach to, 1189, *1191*
Nasopalatine nerve block, 442
Natural killer (NK) cell(s), 95
Necrobiosis lipoidica diabeticorum, in diabetic patient, 139–140
Necrobiotic xanthogranuloma, 19–20
Necrosis, eyelid, *312,* 312–313
  causes of, 308t, 312

Necrotizing fasciitis, of eyelid, 312
Needle(s), suture, 284–285, *285*
Needle holder(s), used in ophthalmic plastic surgery, *290*
Nelson stainless steel screw, in fixation/reconstruction of canthal tendon, 389, *390*
Nemaline myopathy, ptosis in, 84
Nematode infection(s), of eyelid, 317
Neodymium:yttrium-aluminum-garnet (Nd:YAG) laser(s), used in removal of hyperpigmented facial lesions, 568
Neonate(s), disseminated hemangioma in, 920t, 920–921, *920–921*
  preseptal cellulitis in, 310
Neoplasm(s). See *Tumor(s);* specific neoplasm.
Nerve(s). See also specific nerve, e.g., *Facial nerve.*
  conjunctival, 161
  lacrimal, 734
  of ocular region, 275, 277–278, *277–278*
Nerve block(s), for eyelid surgery, 442
Nerve tissue, benign eyelid tumors derived from, 328–329, *329*
Neurilemoma (schwannoma), of eyelid, 328–329
  of orbit, 991–992, *991–992*
Neuritis, optic, MRI scan in, 900, *900*
Neuroblastoma, metastatic orbital disease from, 1011–1012
Neurodermatitis circumscripta (lichen simplex chronicus), 41
Neurofibroma, of eyelid, 328, *329*
  of orbit, 990, *990–991*
    diffuse, 991
    isolated, 991
    plexiform, 991
Neurofibromatosis, *24,* 24–26, 990–991
  cranio-orbital, anterior cranial base approach to, 1204, *1206,* 1207
  diagnostic criteria for, 24t
  ocular features of, 25–26, 26t
  types of, 25
Neurogenic tumor(s), of orbit, 983–992. See also *Orbital tumor(s), neurogenic.*
Neuroma, acoustic, 474
  of eyelid, 329
Neuromuscular toxin(s), ptosis caused by, 83–84, *84*
Neuropathy, optic, transorbital decompression for, *973,* 973–974
Neuroradiologic imaging. See also specific imaging technique, e.g., *Computed tomography (CT).*
  of globe, 904–912
  of orbit, 885–904
Neutrophil(s), 95
Nevocellular nevus, of eyelid, 337–338, *337–338*
    variants of, 338
Nevoxanthoendothelioma (juvenile xanthogranuloma), of eyelid, 64, 333
Nevus(i), definition of, 179
  of conjunctiva, clinical features of, *181,* 181–182
    differential diagnosis of, 181, *182*
    histopathological classification of, 181
    treatment of, 185
  of eyelid, blue, 338–339
    combined, 339
    compound, 337
    congenital, 338, *339*
    intradermal, 337–338, *338*
    junctional, 337
    kissing, 337, *337*
Nevus(i) *(Continued)*
    linear epidermal, 327
    nevocellular, 337–338, *337–338*
      variants of, 338
    Ota's, *181,* 339
    strawberry, 330, *330.* See also *Hemangioma, capillary.*
Nevus flammeus (port wine stain), of eyelid, *329,* 329–330
Nevus ichthyosiformis, 20–21
Newton's groove, in surgical management of pterygia, 214
Nicotinic acid, chronic patient use of, anesthetic considerations with, 296
Nikolsky's sign, 29
  in pemphigus, 34, 102
  in toxic epidermal necrolysis, 35, 105
Nodular elastosis, with cysts and comedones, of eyelid, 327, *327*
Nodular fasciitis, of orbit, 997
Nodular melanoma, 179
Nonabsorbable suture(s), 284
Non-Hodgkin's lymphoma, of eyelid, in AIDS patients, 528
  of orbit, 60
    in AIDS patients, 530–532, *531*
Nonsteroidal anti-inflammatory drugs (NSAIDs), chronic patient use of, anesthetic considerations with, 296
Nose, evaluation of, tearing and, 755, 757–758, *758*
NSAIDs (nonsteroidal anti-inflammatory drugs), chronic patient use of, anesthetic considerations with, 296
Nuclear lesion(s), eyelid retraction caused by, 73–74, *74–76*
  ptosis caused by, 77, *77*
Null cell(s), 95
Nylon suture, 284

Oblique muscle(s), inferior, 849
  superior, 848
Ocular adnexa. See also specific part, e.g., *Eyelid(s).*
  benign lesion(s) of, apocrine sweat gland origin of, 334–335, *334–335*
    eccrine sweat gland origin of, 333–334, *333–334*
    hair follicle origin of, 335–336, *335–336*
    sebaceous gland origin of, 336–337, *337*
  collagen vascular disease(s) affecting, 3–12
    Churg-Strauss syndrome as, 10t, 11, 11t
    dermatomyositis as, 7, 7t
    lupus erythematosus as, 3–7, *4,* 4t, 5t
    lymphomatoid granulomatosis as, 10t, 11–12
    scleroderma as, 7–9, *8,* 8t
    Wegener's granulomatosis as, 9–11, 10t
  dermatosis(es)/hypersensitivity disorder(s) affecting, 37–46
    alopecia areata as, 44–45
    alopecia mucinosa as, 44, *44*
    angioedema as, 40, *40*
    atopic dermatitis as, 41–42, *42*
    contact dermatitis as, *42,* 42–43
    exfoliative erythroderma as, 41
    granuloma annulare as, 43, *43*
    granuloma faciale as, 43
    ichthyosis as, *45,* 45–46
    lichen planus as, 40–41
    lichen simplex chronicus as, 41
    mastocytoma and mastocytosis as, 43
    pityriasis rubra pilaris as, 39
Ocular adnexa *(Continued)*
    psoriasis as, 39–40, *39–40*
    rosacea as, *38,* 38–39
    seborrheic dermatitis as, *37,* 37–38
    ulerythema ophryogenes as, 43–44
    urticaria as, 40
  systemic and metabolic disease(s) affecting, 12–29
    acanthosis nigricans as, *23,* 23t, 23–24
    amyloidosis as, *17,* 17–19, 18t
    congenital erythropoietic porphyria as, 29
    Darier's disease as, 21
    erythropoietic protoporphyria as, 29
    hyperthyroidism as, *12,* 12–14, 13t
    ligneous conjunctivitis as, 20
    lipoid proteinosis as, 20–21
    Melkersson-Rosenthal syndrome as, 15–16
    multiple mucosal neuroma syndrome as, 21–23, 22t
    myxedema as, 14, *14*
    necrobiotic xanthogranuloma as, 19–20
    neurofibromatosis as, *24,* 24t, 24–26, 26t
    sarcoidosis as, *16,* 16–17, 17t
    scleredema as, 15
    scleromyxedema as, *14,* 14–15
    tuberous sclerosis as, 26–28, 27t
    variegate porphyria as, 28
  vesicobullous disease(s) affecting, 29–37
    cicatricial pemphigoid as, *31,* 31–32
    epidermolysis bullosa as, 29–31, 30t
    erythema multiforme as, *34–35,* 34–37, 36t
    pemphigus as, 33–34
Oculocardiac reflex, after blepharoplasty, 650
Oculodermal melanocytosis (Ota's nevus), of eyelid, 339
Oculofacial prosthesis, following orbital exenteration, *1074,* 1075
Oculoglandular syndrome of Parinaud, 149
Oculomotility disorder(s), in orbital disease, 877–878, *878–879,* 880
Oculomotor nerve, anatomy of, 277, 844–845
Oculomotor nerve palsy, in diabetic patient, 139
  ptosis caused by, 77, *78*
Oculopharyngeal dystrophy, 86
Oculoplastic surgery. See also specific procedure, e.g., *Blepharoplasty.*
  aesthetician in, patient benefits of, 574–575
    physician benefits of, 573–574
  anesthesia for, 294–299
    commonly used agents in, 296–297
    in pediatric patients, 298–299
    intraoperative problems in, 298
    local or monitored care approach to, 297–298
    management of concurrent medications with, 295–296
    monitoring during, 298
    preoperative evaluation and screening tests in, 294–295
  in African American patient, considerations for, 715–717, *716–717,* 717t
  in Asian patient, cultural background and anatomic considerations for, 691–700
  medical photography for, 551–559. See also *Medical photography.*
  role of aesthetician in, before and after surgery, 576–577

Oil layer, and precorneal tear film, 737–738
Onchocerca volvulus infection, of eyelid, 317
Onchocercomata, of eyelid, 317
Oncocytoma, of eyelid, 328
Ophthalmia, sympathetic, enucleation for, 1035
Ophthalmic artery, anatomy of, 274, *275,* 843, *843*
Ophthalmic nerve, anatomy of, 277, *278*
Ophthalmic plastic instrument(s), 288, *290–292*
Ophthalmic vein(s), anatomy of, 275, *276,* 844, *844*
Ophthalmoparesis, of myasthenia gravis, 80
Ophthalmopathy, Graves,' 13–14
  thyroid-associated, 121–122
    clinical features of, 122
    management of, 122
Ophthalmoplegia, painful, 892
Ophthalmoscopy, in orbital disease, 875, *875*
Optic canal, decompression of, indications for, 1047
  glioma of, 881–882, *882*
  orbital disease invasion via, 881–882, *882–883*
Optic disc(s), edema of, in diabetic patient, 138t, 138–139
Optic nerve, anatomy of, 844
  function of, index of, 860
    status of, orbital disease and, 874–876, *875–876*
  glioma of. See *Optic nerve glioma.*
  meningioma of. See *Optic nerve meningioma.*
  nontumoral enlargement of, 900
  sarcoidosis of, MRI scan of, 900–901, *902*
Optic nerve decompression, subcranial approach to, 1164, *1166*
Optic nerve foramen, in Chinese skulls, 696–697
    measurement of, 697t
Optic nerve glioma, 985–987, *986*
  clinical presentation of, 986–987
  imaging of, 899–900, *899–900*
  radiographic findings in, 987
  treatment of, 987
Optic nerve meningioma, 882, *883,* 987–989
  management of, 988–989
  radiographic findings in, 987–988, *987–988*
Optic nerve sheath, meningioma of, imaging of, 897, *898–899,* 899
Optic nerve sheath decompression, 1056–1059
  care following, 1059
  complications of, 1059
  indications for, 1047
  mechanism of action of, 1056
  technique of, 1056–1059, *1057–1059*
Optic neuritis, MRI scan in, 900, *900*
Optic neuropathy, compressive, transorbital decompression for, *973,* 973–974
Oral mucosa, used in upper eyelid reconstruction, 365
Oral mucosal graft(s), in conjunctival mucous membrane replacement, 172–175, *173–174*
    complications of, 174–175
    harvesting and storage of, 173, *173*
  technique of, 173–174, *174*
Orbicularis oculi muscle, 261, *263*
  contraction of, 262
  shortening of, laugh lines caused by, 261, *263*
  superficial relations of, 264–265, *266*
Orbit. See also *Orbital* entries.
  acquired immunodeficiency syndrome affecting, 529–532. See also *Acquired immunodeficiency syndrome (AIDS), orbital manifestation(s) of.*
  adenoid cystic carcinoma of, 68–69, *69*
  amyloidosis affecting, *65,* 65–66
  anatomy of, 146, *147,* 837–849
  anterior structures of, parasagittal section of, 270, *271*
  basal cell carcinoma of, 300, *301*
  basal cell nevus syndrome affecting, 67, *68*
  benign reactive lymphoid hyperplasia of, 61–62
  blood supply to, 843–844, *843–844*
  cellulitis of. See *Cellulitis, orbital.*
  compartments of, 885, 886t, 887t
  connective tissues of, 840–842, *842*
  deformity(ies) of, after acquired anophthalmos, management of, 1121
    anterior cranial base approach to, 1187–1207
      historical perspective on, 1187
      in children, surgical refinement for, 1187–1188. See also *Craniofacial surgery, pediatric.*
        access to tumors in, 1188
        indications for, 1188–1207
  dysplastic nevus syndrome affecting, 67–68, *68*
  embryology of, 850–851, *851*
  exenteration of, 1070–1077. See also *Exenteration, orbital.*
  fibrous dysplasia of, presenting as blindness, anterior cranial base approach to, 1202, *1203*
  idiopathic inflammation of. See *Idiopathic orbital inflammation.*
  infections of, 146–155, 888–891. See also *Infection(s), of orbit.*
  leukemia involving, 60
  mucoepidermoid carcinoma of, 68, *69*
  mycosis fungoides of, 62
  neoplastic and related condition(s) affecting, 53–70
    diagnosis of, 53–57, *54–57*
    Erdheim-Chester disease as, 64, *64*
    histiocytic disorders as, 62, *63,* 64
    idiopathic midline destructive disease as, 66, *66*
    laboratory tests for, 57
    treatment of, 57
  neuroradiologic imaging of, 885–904
    anatomic and developmental considerations on, 885, *886*
  of Caucasian adult, 696, 696t
  of Chinese adult, male vs. female, 696, 696t
    relationship between lacrimal fossa and ethmoidal cells in, 697t
    relationship between lacrimal fossa and middle turbinate in, 698t
  osteology of, 837–840, *838–840*
    shape and dimensions in, 837, *838*
  paraneoplastic syndromes affecting, 58
  pathology of, epidemiology of, 853, 854t–856t, 856, *857–858,* 858t, 859
  prosthesis for. See *Prosthesis.*
  pseudorheumatoid nodules of, 67
  pseudotumor of. See *Pseudotumor(s), orbital.*
  sarcoidosis of, 64–65, *64–65*
  sinus histiocytosis with lymphadenopathy affecting, 62, *62*
  soft tissue of, *842–845,* 842–849, *847–848*
  squamous cell carcinoma of, 300–301, *302*
Orbit *(Continued)*
  vascular conditions of, imaging of, 893–897, *893–898*
  xeroderma pigmentosum affecting, 66–67, *67*
Orbital and lacrimal kit, *291*
Orbital apex, anatomy of, 839–840, *840*
  fractures of, 1099–1100, *1100*
    treatment of, 1100
Orbital apex inflammatory syndrome, 965
Orbital apex syndrome, 148
Orbital calcification, dystrophic, differential diagnosis of, 887t
  metastatic, differential diagnosis of, 887t
Orbital cyst, 886–888. See also *Dermoid cyst; Epidermoid cyst.*
Orbital decompression, for Graves' disease, 967–982. See also *Graves' disease, orbital decompression for.*
Orbital disease, 860–873
  clinical signs of, 860
  evidence of, within globe, 868–870, *869–870*
  extent of, 862–863, 865, *866*
  eyelid changes in, 865–868, *867–868*
  globe position and movement in, 861–862, *863–865*
  neuro-ophthalmic conditions in, 874–884
    clinical method(s) of assessment of, 874–880
      motility disorders as, 877–878, *878–879*
      pupillary function as, 876–877, *877*
      status of optic nerve function as, 874–876, *875–876*
      trigeminal function as, *879,* 879–880
    localization of disease process(es) in, 880–883
      choroidal folds and, 881, *881*
      enophthalmos and, 881
      oculomotility disturbances and, 880
      perturbation of acuity and visual field and, 880
      proptosis and, 880–881
      pupillary disturbances and, 880
  periorbital function changes in, 868
  periorbital injury and, 871, *873*
  pupillary reflex changes in, 868
  radiation therapy in, 1023–1032
  systemic signs of, 870–871, *871–872*
Orbital expansion, craniofacial approach to, 980–981
Orbital fascia, anatomy of, 841–842, *842*
Orbital fat pad, 269, *269*
  anatomy of, 842, *842*
  pseudoherniation of, evaluation of, 635
  removal of. See *Fat excision.*
Orbital fissure, inferior, neuroradiologic imaging of, 885
  superior, neuroradiologic imaging of, 885
    orbital disease invasion via, 882–883, *884*
Orbital floor, fractures of, 1087–1091
    blow-out, 1087
    complications of, 1090–1091, *1090–1093*
    management of, *1088–1089,* 1088–1090
Orbital fracture(s), 1085–1100
  evaluation of, 1085–1086, *1086*
  fixation of, principles in, 1086–1087
  incidence of, 1085
  management of, 1047
  site of, 1087–1100. See also specific site, e.g., *Orbital floor, fractures of.*

Orbital fracture(s) *(Continued)*
surgical approach to, 1054
unilateral forehead fracture and, anterior cranial base approach to, 1188–1189, *1190*
Orbital lesion(s), age distribution of, *857–858,* 858t
clinicopathologic classification of, 854t–856t
extraconal, 887t
intraconal, 886t
pathology of, epidemiology of, 853, 856, 859
subperiosteal, 887t
Orbital margins, anatomy of, 837, *838*
Orbital nerve(s), anatomy of, 844–846, *845*
paresis involving, 152
Orbital rim, sulcus of, sculpturing and recontouring of, 707, *707*
Orbital roof, fractures of, *1098,* 1098–1099
treatment of, 1099
Orbital septum, anatomy of, 268–269, *269*
excision and incision of, in upper eyelid blepharoplasty, 600, *600*
variations of, 607–608
Orbital surgery. See also specific procedure, e.g., *Orbitotomy.*
anatomic planes and exposure of different routes during, 1051, 1051t, *1052*
approach(es) to, 1050–1051
anophthalmic socket and, 1053–1054
associated with paranasal sinus disease, 1055, *1055*
based on pathologic process, 1051–1055
neoplasms and, 1051–1053, *1052–1053*
trauma and, 1054
dissection in, 1049
exposure in, 1048
general principles in, 1050
hemostasis in, 1049
incisions utilized in, 1060, *1061*
indications for, 1046–1047
instrumentation for, 1050, *1051*
operative principles in, 1048–1049
Orbital tumor(s). See also specific tumor.
adipose, 996–997
carcinoid, 57, *58*
fibrous, 997
in AIDS patients, 532, *532*
lymphoid, 58–60, 303–304, 956–962
malignant, 300–306
surgical approach to, 1053
metastatic, 1007–1013
clinical features of, 1007–1008, 1008t
from breast carcinoma, *1009,* 1009–1010
from gastrointestinal carcinoma, 1012
from lung carcinoma, 1010
from melanoma, 1012
from neuroblastoma, 1011–1012
from prostate carcinoma, 1010–1011, *1011*
from renal cell carcinoma, 1012
pathologic features of, 1008
primary sites of, 1008t
tests for, 1008
treatment of, 1008
myogenic, 994–996
neurogenic, 983–992
biopsy of, 984
clinical examination of, 983–984
general approach to, 983–984
noninvasive imaging of, 984
transcranial approach to, 984–985
preparation for, 984
Orbital tumor(s) *(Continued)*
technique of, 984–985
treatment of, 984
pediatric, anterior cranial base approach to, 1199, 1202–1204, *1203–1206*
resection of, 1060–1068
anterior approach to, 1060–1061, *1061–1062*
combined procedures in, 1065, *1067–1068,* 1068
lateral approach to, 1063, *1064*
medial approach to, 1063, 1065, *1065–1067*
secondary, 68
surgical approach to, 1051–1053, *1052–1053*
vascular, 913–932
Orbital varices, CT scan of, 896, *897*
Orbital wall(s), anatomy of, 837–839, *838–839*
medial, fractures of, 1092
Orbitocheek fold, *485*
Orbitoethmoidal osteotomy, transcranial approach to tumors via, 985
Orbitopathy, thyroid, CT scan of, 891, *892*
Orbitotomy, 1051
anterior extraperiosteal approach to, 1060–1061, *1062*
anterior transseptal approach to, 1060, *1062*
combined lateral and inferior, 1065, *1067–1068*
combined superior and lateral, 1068, *1068*
Krönlein-Berke, technique of, 1056–1059, *1057–1059*
lateral approach to, 1063, *1064*
medial approach to, 1063, *1065–1067*
transconjunctival approach to, 1060, *1061*
Orchiectomy, for metastatic prostate carcinoma, 1011
Orf, involving eyelids, 316
Organic pigment, 541. See also *Pigment(s).*
Oriental sore, 150
Orphenadrine, for essential blepharospasm and Meige's syndrome, 507
Osler-Weber-Rendu disease (hereditary hemorrhagic telangiectasia), 9
Osmotic pressure, of lymphatic fluid, 654
Osseointegration, biology of, 1155–1156, 1158–1159
effects of irradiation on, 1158–1159
for exenterated orbit, 1150–1159
abutment installation in, 1151, *1156–1157*
implant installation in, 1150–1151, *1152–1155*
technique of, 1150–1151, *1151*
placement of bone-anchored implants by, 1159
Osteoclastoma (brown tumor), in hyperparathyroidism, 133–134, *134–135*
Osteotomy, age and, 1053
fronto-orbital, subcranial approach to, 1163–1164, *1165–1167*
orbitoethmoidal, transcranial approach to tumors via, 985
Ota's nevus, of eyelid, 339
Otitis, malignant external, 138
Otitis media, acute, 473
Oxycel, for hemostasis in wound repair, 283
Oxymetazoline, for hemostasis in wound repair, 283
P component, of amyloid fibrils, 944
Pagetoid spread, definition of, 179
of sebaceous gland carcinoma, 190, *191,* 347, *347*
management of, 348
Paget's disease of bone, causing nasolacrimal duct obstruction, 813
Palate, hard. See *Hard palate* entries.
Palatine nerve block, 442
Palpebral conjunctiva, 159. See also *Conjunctiva.*
Palpebral spring, in surgical management of facial paralysis, 476–478, *477–478*
Palsy(ies). See also *Paralysis.*
abducens nerve, eyelid retraction associated with, 74, *75*
in diabetic patient, 139
Bell's, 470, 473
in diabetic patient, 139
ptosis following, 91, *91*
cranial nerve, in diabetic patient, 138t, 138–139
oculomotor nerve, in diabetic patient, 139
ptosis caused by, 77, *78*
progressive, metastatic lesions in, 474
PAM. See *Primary acquired melanosis (PAM).*
PANDO. See *Nasolacrimal duct obstruction, primary acquired.*
Panfacial fracture(s), 1100
Papillary endothelial hyperplasia, intravascular, of eyelid, 332
Papilloma, of eyelid, 324, *324*
squamous, of conjunctiva, 68, *69,* 251, *252*
treatment of, 251–252
of orbit, 68, *69*
Papillomavirus, warts caused by, eyelid presentation of, 316
Papular sarcoid, 16
Paracentesis, of anterior chamber, following chemical injury, 223–224
Paracoccidioidomycosis, of eyelid, 318
Paralysis, 469, *469.* See also *Palsy(ies).*
facial, 465–482. See also *Facial paralysis.*
familial periodic, ptosis in, 85–86, *86*
partial, involving orbital nerves, 152
Paranasal sinus(es). See also *Sinus* entries.
anatomy of, 935, *936–938,* 937, 1014–1015
disease of, approach to orbital surgery associated with, 1055, *1055*
role of, in orbital cellulitis, 935–943
mucoceles in, 1014–1021, *1015*
diagnostic imaging of, 1014–1017, *1016*
histopathology of, 1014
pathophysiology of, 1014
Parasitic infection(s), of eyelid, 317–318
Parathyroid hormone (PTH), calcium regulation by, 132
Paredrine test, for Horner's syndrome, 79
Parinaud's syndrome, 149
Patch test, for micropigmentation, 541
Patient, evaluation of, for chemical peels, 664, 664t, 665t
for electropigmentation, 676, *678*
pediatric. See *Child(ren).*
preparation and draping of, for lower eyelid blepharoplasty, 619
for upper eyelid blepharoplasty, 598
variations in, 605
Pautrier's microabscess, 62
Pediatric patient. See *Child(ren).*
Pedicle flap, upper eyelid, used in medial canthal reconstruction, 391, *395*
used in upper eyelid reconstruction, from lower lid to upper lid, 382–383, *383*

Pemphigoid, cicatricial. See *Cicatricial pemphigoid.*
Pemphigus, 33–34
differential diagnosis of, 103
epidemiology of, 102
immunohistopathology of, 103
ocular manifestations of, 102
pathogenesis of, 103
systemic manifestations of, 102–103
treatment of, 34, 103
variants of, 33
Pemphigus vulgaris, vs. cicatricial pemphigoid, 198
Penetrating trauma. See also *Trauma.*
to upper eyelid, 357–358
extensive, 358–359, *360–361*
lid margin reapproximation following, 357–358, *359–360*
with no tissue loss, 357, *358*
with tissue loss, 357
Perilimbal epithelial loss, after chemical injury, 226–227, *227*
Periorbita, anatomy of, 840–841
changes in function of, in orbital disease, 868
vascularization of, 841
anatomy of, 841
Periorbital edema, diseases and organisms associated with, 308t
infectious causes of, 151–152
Periorbital hyperpigmentation, chemical peels for, 663
Periorbital malignancy, Mohs' surgery for, 352–355
advantages of, 354–355
drawbacks to, 352
fresh tissue technique in, 352–354, *353–355*
Persistent hyperplastic primary vitreous, imaging of, 908, *909*
Phakoma, in tuberous sclerosis, 27
Pharmacologic testing, for myasthenia gravis, *80,* 81–82, *82*
Pharmacology, of therapeutic agents, 97–98
Phenol solution, Baker's, used in chemical peels, 667–668
Phenylephrine, for hemostasis in wound repair, 283
Pheochromocytoma(s), 141–142
Phlegmon, subperiosteal, CT scan of, *889,* 889–890
Photodamage, chemical peels for, 662, 663t
Photoelectric effect, 1023, *1025*
Photographs, for medicolegal considerations with eyelid trauma, 457
Photography. See *Medical photography.*
Phycomycosis. See *Mucormycosis (phycomycosis).*
Pigment(s), changes in, management of, 535–541. See also *Micropigmentation.*
resulting from facial trauma, 535–536
for micropigmentation, 682–683
inorganic, 541
organic, 541
removal of, 681
selection of, for micropigmentation, 538
tattoo, used in electropigmentation, 677, 681
Pigmentary retinopathy, in Kearns-Sayre syndrome, 87–88, *88*
Pigmentation, prominent, after blepharoplasty, 648
Pigmented lesion(s). See also specific lesion, e.g., *Nevus(i).*
of aging skin, treatment for, 567–568, *568*
Pigmented lesion(s) *(Continued)*
of conjunctiva, 179–189, 183t, *184–186*
of eyelid, benign, 337–339, *337–340*
Pilocytic astrocytoma, juvenile, imaging of, 899–900, *899–900*
Pilomatricoma (Malherbe's calcifying epithelioma), of eyelid, 336, *336*
Pinch test, for lid laxity, 762, *763*
Pinta, involving eyelids, 314
Pityriasis rubra pilaris, 39
Plagiocephaly, 1179
subcranial approach to, results with, 1176t
Plague, involving eyelids, 314
Plain gut suture, 284, 284t
Plasma cell tumor(s), of orbit, 62, *63*
Plastic instrument(s), ophthalmic, 288, *290–292*
Plastic wrap, creation of moist chamber with, following chemical injury, 225
Plastic wrap occlusive dressing, for facial nerve palsy, 474, *475*
Pleomorphic adenoma, of eyelid, 334, *334*
of lacrimal glands, 999–1004
Pleomorphic rhabdomyosarcoma, in adults, 995
Plica semilunaris, of conjunctiva, 159. See also *Conjunctiva.*
Plication, medial, for canthal laxity, in involutional ectropion, 426–427, *426–427*
PMNs (polymorphonuclear neutrophil leukocytes), role of, in injured eye repair, 223
Pneumatic drill, used in ophthalmic plastic surgery, *291*
Pneumocystis carinii infection, of orbit, in AIDS patients, 529
Poliomyelitis, cranial nerve paresis in, 152
Polyarteritis nodosa, differential diagnosis of, 112
epidemiology of, 111
laboratory findings in, 111–112
ocular manifestations of, 111
pathogenesis of, 112
systemic manifestations of, 111
treatment of, 112
Polyclonal antibody(ies), 96
Polydioxanone suture, 284, 284t
Polyendocrine disease, acromegaly as, 142–143
Addison's disease as, 141
MEN syndromes as, 142
pheochromocytoma as, 141–142
polyglandular autoimmune syndromes as, 141
polyostotic fibrous dysplasia as, 143
Polyglactin suture, 284, 284t
Polyglandular autoimmune syndrome(s), 141
Polymethyl methacrylate acrylic, for prosthesis, 1135–1136
Polymorphic reticulosis, 114
Polymorphonuclear neutrophil leukocytes (PMNs), role of, in injured eye repair, 223
Polyostotic fibrous dysplasia, 143
Polypropylene suture, 284
Polytetrafluoroethylene (polytef) graft, and spontaneous epithelialization, in conjunctival mucous membrane replacement, 171–172, *171–172*
Polyurethane sheet, for prosthesis, 1136–1137
Pons, cross section of, *467*
Porphyria, 28–29
congenital erythropoietic, 29
variegate, 28–29
Porphyria cutanea tarda, 27–28
Port wine stain (nevus flammeus), of eyelid, *329,* 329–330
Potassium abnormality(ies), evaluation of, prior to oculoplastic surgery, 294
Pott's puffy tumor, 1017, *1017*
Prednisone, for capillary hemangioma, 919
for idiopathic orbital inflammation, 955–956
for orbital floor fractures, 1088
in preoperative treatment of malignant melanoma, 187
with dapsone, for cicatricial pemphigoid, 199
Pregnancy, hyperthyroidism in, 129–130
Premature ventricular contraction, evaluation of, prior to oculoplastic surgery, 295
Preseptal cellulitis, 310–312
CT scan of, *148*
in children and neonates, 310
post-traumatic, 311
treatment of, 311–312
with abscess formation, 310, *310*
Preseptal muscles, anatomy of, 744
Pressure bandages, with manual lymphatic drainage of extremities, 655
Pressure tamponade, for hemostasis in wound repair, 282
Pretarsal muscles, anatomy of, 744
insertion of, in medial canthal area, 387, *388*
Primary acquired melanosis (PAM), of conjunctiva, classification of, 79–180, 180t
clinical features of, 182, *182–183*
malignant melanoma arising from, 233
treatment of, 185–187, *186*
types of, 234
Probing, in evaluation of tearing, 755, *756–757*
Procerus muscle, 262, *263,* 264
Progressive synergistic gangrene, of eyelid, 312
Prolapse, conjunctival, management of, 253–254
lacrimal gland, repair of, in upper eyelid blepharoplasty, 601–602, *602*
variations of, 609
Propofol, as anesthetic agent, 297
Propranolol, for thyroid storm, 130
for thyrotoxicosis, 125, 128
Proptosis, in orbital disease, 880–881
Propulsion, forward, of lymphatic fluid, *652,* 652–653
Propylthiouracil (PTU), for hyperthyroidism, 129–130
for thyrotoxicosis, 125
Prostate carcinoma, metastatic orbital disease from, 1010–1011, *1011*
Prosthesis, 1134–1149
after enucleation, 1036–1037
hydroxyapatite, 1036, 1041–1042
complications of, 1042
contraindications to, 1042
anatomically retained, design of, 1143–1144, *1143–1145*
auricular, osseointegrated, 1159
bulb-style, 1143–1144, *1143–1145*
challenges regarding, 1144–1146, *1146–1148*
design, making, and fitting of, treatment plan in, 1137–1139, *1138–1141,* 1141
for acquired anophthalmos, complications of, *1119–1120,* 1119–1121
functions of, 1134–1135, *1135–1136*

Prosthesis *(Continued)*
installation of, for exenterated orbit, 1150–1151, *1152–1155*
location of, in anophthalmic socket, 1131, *1131*
magnet attachments to, 1155, *1158*
material(s) for, 1135–1137
polymethyl methacrylate acrylic as, 1135–1136
polyurethane sheet as, 1136–1137
silicone elastomer as, 1135
silicone foam as, 1137
silicone gels as, 1137
mobility, new, 1132, *1133*
mobility of, in anophthalmic socket, 1131, *1131*
ocular component of, 1138, *1139*
oculofacial, following orbital exenteration, *1074,* 1075
optimal results with, surgical nuances for, 1141–1143, *1142–1143*
suborbital rim, 488, 490–498
complications associated with, 501–503
customized, 490–491, *491,* 495–498, *496–499*
Flower tear trough, 488, *489,* 492–493, *492–495,* 495
Goldberg lateral, 488, *489*
malposition of, 503
prefabricated, 488, *489–491,* 490
surgical considerations for, 1135
Prosthetist, challenges for, 1144–1146, *1146–1148*
Prostigmin test, for myasthenia gravis, in children, 82, *82*
Protein, concentration of, in lymphatic fluid, 654
Proteinosis, lipoid, 20–21
Protoporphyria, erythropoietic, 29
Pseudocapsule, of lacrimal gland, 732
Pseudo-Graefe's sign, 74, *75*
Pseudoherniation, of orbital fat pad, evaluation of, 635
Pseudohorn cyst, 325
Pseudomelanocytic lesion, *184*
Pseudomonas aeruginosa, 138
Pseudomonas mallei, glanders caused by, 313
Pseudo-ocular pemphigoid syndrome, 203
Pseudoporphyria, 28
Pseudopterygium, vs. true pterygium, 209
Pseudoptosis, and eyelid retraction, 89–91
associated with vertical strabismus, *88,* 89
Pseudorheumatoid nodule(s), of orbit, 67
Pseudotumor(s), idiopathic inflammatory, associated with nasolacrimal duct obstruction, 801–802
orbital, classification of, 890
imaging of, 890–891, *890–891*
in AIDS patients, 530
Pseudotumor cerebri, optic nerve decompression for, 1056–1059, *1057–1059*
Psoriasis vulgaris, 39–40, *39–40*
treatment of, 40
Psychosocial issues, in male blepharoplasty, 632
Pterygium(ia), 208–220
adjunctive therapy for, 217–219
argon laser in, 219
beta radiation in, 217–218
corticosteroids in, 219
excimer laser in, 219
mitomycin C in, 218–219
thiotepa in, 218
aggressive, 210
anatomy of, 208
differential diagnosis of, 209–210
Pterygium(ia) *(Continued)*
general considerations concerning, 219–220
histopathology of, 208–209
inactive, 210
nonsurgical management of, 210–211
pathogenesis of, 209
prognosis for, 210
recurrent, 209, 210
surgical management of, anesthesia in, 212
bare-sclera technique in, 212–214, *213*
buccal mucous membrane graft in, 217
conjunctival autograft in, 214–215, *216–217,* 217
conjunctival flaps in, 214, *215*
current, 211–217
historical, 211
indications for, 210
lamellar grafts in, 214, *214*
preoperative evaluation in, 211
treatment alternatives in, 211
vs. pseudopterygium, 209
Pterygoid plexus, venous drainage into, 275, *276*
PTH (parathyroid hormone), calcium regulation by, 132
Ptosis, 75–88
after blepharoplasty, 644, *644*
after dermolipoma excision, treatment of, 256
aponeurotic, 447–451
evaluation of, 447
residual, 450
correction of, 450–451
surgery for, applied anatomy used in, 448
choice of, 448
complications of, 449
contour abnormality in, 450
overcorrection in, 449–450
skin excision in, 450–451
undercorrection in, 450
as complication of conjunctival amyloidosis, 240
brow, 578–588
asymmetric, 578–579
in facial paralysis, surgical management of, 482
presenting complaints in, 578
surgical management of, 579–581, *579–588,* 583–587
coronal flaps in, 585–586, *586*
incisions in, 579, *579,* 581, *581–583,* 583
prominent sub-brow fat pad and, 586–587, *586–588*
correction of, *1118,* 1118–1119
following Bell's palsy, 91, *91*
myopathic, 84–88
in chronic progressive external ophthalmoplegia, 86–88, *87–88*
in inflammatory and infiltrative myopathies, 88
in muscular dystrophy, 84
in myotonia and myotonic disorders, 85–86, *85–86*
in structural myopathies, 84, *85*
neuromuscular, 79–84
in myasthenia gravis, 79–83, *80–82*
in myasthenic syndromes, 83
toxins causing, 83–84, *84*
neuropathic, 75–77
infranuclear lesions causing, 77, *78*
nuclear lesions causing, 77, *77*
supranuclear lesions causing, 75–77, *76–77*
sympathetic lesions causing, 77–79, *78–79*
Ptosis *(Continued)*
repair of, concurrent with upper eyelid blepharoplasty, 602–603, *603*
variations of, 609
PTU (propylthiouracil), for hyperthyroidism, 129–130
for thyrotoxicosis, 125
Pulmonary function test(s), for sarcoidosis, 108
Pulse oximetry, monitoring of, during anesthesia, 298
Pulse-wave flow, of lymph, 653, *653*
Pumping action, of lymphatic vessels, 652
Punctoplasty, inferior, for involutional ectropion, 424–425, *425*
Punctum(a), 739
anatomy of, 268, *268,* 821
atresia of, 782, *782*
congenital abnormalities of, 740, *740,* 821–822, *822*
treatment of, 822–823
imperforate membrane of, 782, *782*
physiology of, 821
stenosis of, 829, *829*
supernumerary, *741*
trauma to, 824–825
tumors of, 823–824, *824*
Pupil(s), Adie's, 877
Marcus Gunn, 876
reverse, 876, *877*
Pupillary function, in orbital disease, assessment of, 876–877, *877*
disturbances of, 880
Pupillary reflex, changes in, with orbital disease, 868
Pyogenic granuloma, of eyelid, 331, *331*
Pyruvic acid, used in chemical peels, 667

Quartz iodine lamp, for photography, 555

R (roentgen), defined, 1023
Rabies, cranial nerve paresis in, 152
prophylaxis for, 458
Rad (radiation absorbed dose), 1026, *1027–1029,* 1030
Radiation, beta, as adjunct to surgery for pterygia, 217–218
ultraviolet, exposure to, pterygia due to, 209
Radiation absorbed dose (rad), 1026, *1027–1029,* 1030
Radiation therapy, 1023–1032
causing nasolacrimal duct obstruction, 803–804
clinical applications of, *1030,* 1030t, 1030–1031
complications of, 1031, *1032*
diagnostic energies in, 1023, 1024t
film in, 1023, *1024*
for capillary hemangioma, 919
for conjunctival lymphoid tumors, 246
for idiopathic orbital inflammation, 956
for Kaposi's sarcoma, 242, 528
for lacrimal gland tumors, 1005–1006
for lymphangioma, 925
for lymphoid tumors, 961
for metastatic breast carcinoma, 1009–1010
for metastatic gastrointestinal carcinoma, 1012
for metastatic lung carcinoma, 1010
for metastatic melanoma, 1012

Radiation therapy *(Continued)*
for metastatic prostate carcinoma, 1011
for non-Hodgkin's lymphoma, 531
for orbital metastatic disease, 57, 1008–1012
for rhabdomyosarcoma, 303, 996
for sebaceous gland carcinoma, 302–303, 348
measurement of dose in, 1023
photoelectric or Compton effect in, 1023, *1025*
practical applications of, 1026
prior to osseointegration, effects of, 1158–1159
rad in, 1026, *1027–1029,* 1030
side effects of, incidence of, 1030t
Radioactive iodine therapy, for thyrotoxicosis, 128
Radiobiology, 1023–1026. See also *Radiation therapy.*
long-term complication rates in, 1024–1025
radiosensitivity in, 1025, *1025*
redistribution in, 1026
reoxygenation in, 1025, *1026*
repopulation in, 1025–1026
Radio-frequency current, heating effects of, 592
Radio-frequency lipocontouring, in fat removal, 642, *642*
Radio-frequency surgical unit, used in blepharoplasty, *544*
Radiography, chest, for sarcoidosis, 108
prior to oculoplastic surgery, 294
of mucoceles, in paranasal sinuses, 1016
Radiosensitivity, in radiobiology, 1025, *1025*
Radiosurgical unit, Ellman Surgitron, used in removal of hyperpigmented facial lesions, 568, *568*
used in treatment of telangiectasia, 569
Ramsay Hunt syndrome, 470, 473
RAPD (relative afferent pupillary defect), 860–861
Rappaport classification, of non-Hodgkin's lymphoma, 60
Reconstructive plan, in orbital exenteration, 1073–1075, *1974*
goals of, 1073
Rectus muscle(s), horizontal, 847
inferior, 848
capsulopalpebral head of, 269–270, *270*
medial, 848
metastasis of thyroid carcinoma to, *55*
superior, 841, 848
Redistribution, in radiobiology, 1026
Reflex, oculocardiac, after blepharoplasty, 650
pupillary, changes in, with orbital disease, 868
Reflex tearing, 750
Refraction, changes in, after blepharoplasty, 649
Refsum's disease, 46
Regional anesthesia. See *Anesthesia, regional.*
Regulatory agency(ies), 591–593
Rehabilitation, visual, after chemical injury, 227–228, *228*
Rejuvenation, facial, 560–571. See also *Facial rejuvenation.*
Relative afferent pupillary defect (RAPD), 860–861
Renal cell carcinoma, metastatic orbital disease from, 1012
Reoxygenation, in radiobiology, 1025, *1026*
Repopulation, in radiobiology, 1025–1026
Reptile venom, disruption of neuromuscular transmission by, 83
Reticulosis, polymorphic, 114
Retinal detachment, MRI of, 905–906, *906*
Retinal hemangioma, 910–911
Retinitis, cytomegalovirus, in AIDS patients, 533
Retinoblastoma, enucleation for, 1035–1036
imaging of, 907–908, *907–908*
Retinopathy, pigmentary, in Kearns-Sayre syndrome, 87–88, *88*
Retraction, skin and muscle, in orbital surgery, 1048
Retrobulbar hemorrhage, causing blindness, 643
Rhabdomyoma, orbital, 996
Rhabdomyosarcoma, alveolar, 995
botryoid, 995
embryonal, 995
orbital, 303, *303,* 994–996
differential diagnosis of, 994, 995
epidemiology of, 994
histopathology of, 994–995
imaging of, 901–902, *903*
presentation of, 994
prognosis of, 996
treatment of, 995–996
pleomorphic, in adults, 995
Rhinocerebral mucormycosis, 150–151, *151*
Rhinoscleroma, in diabetic patient, 138
of eyelid, 314
Rhinosporidiosis, of eyelid, 319
Rhinosporidium seeberi, rhinosporidiosis caused by, 319
Rhytidectomy (face-lift), 565
Rhytides. See *Wrinkles (rhytides).*
Rib graft(s), costal, harvesting of, 1077–1078, *1079*
Rickettsial disease, involving eyelids, 313
Riley-Day syndrome, 736
"River blindness," caused by *Onchocerca volvulus,* 317
Rod myopathy, ptosis in, 84
Roentgen (R), defined, 1023
Romaña's sign, 152
in Chagas' disease, 316
Rosacea, *38,* 38–39
treatment of, 39
Rose bengal testing, of tearing, 759
Rosenmüller valve, 744
Round eye deformity, after blepharoplasty, 646, *646*
Ruby laser(s), used in removal of hyperpigmented facial lesions, 568
Running suture(s), percutaneous, 286, *286*
subcuticular, 288, *288*
Russell body(ies), in rhinoscleroma, 138

Sagittal synostosis, 1178–1179, *1179–1180*
SALDO. See *Nasolacrimal duct obstruction, secondary acquired.*
"Salmon patches," in conjunctival lymphoid tumors, 235, *235*
Sarcoid, 106
miliary (papular), 16
Sarcoidosis, 106–108
associated with secondary acquired nasolacrimal duct obstruction, 801, *803*
diagnosis of, 108
differential diagnosis of, 108
epidemiology of, 106–107
Sarcoidosis *(Continued)*
erythema nodosum in, 16
immunohistopathology of, 107–108
ocular manifestations of, 16–17, 17t, 107
of conjunctiva, 65, *65*
of optic nerve, MRI scan of, 900–901, *902*
of orbit, *64,* 64–65
systemic manifestations of, 107
treatment of, 17, 108
Sarcoma, granulocytic, involving orbit, 61, *61*
Kaposi's, of conjunctiva, in AIDS patients, 236–237, 242, *243,* 532
of eyelid, in AIDS patients, 526–528, *527*
Sawdust, exposure to, pterygia due to, 209
Scaphocephaly, 1178
Scar(s), facial, electropigmentation for, 676. See also *Electropigmentation.*
micropigmentation for, 535. See also *Micropigmentation.*
hypertrophic, vs. keloids, 717t
prominent, after blepharoplasty, 648
Schaumann's bodies, 65
Schirmer's test, of tearing, 758–759
without anesthesia, 470
Schistosomiasis, of eyelid, 318
Schwannoma (neurilemoma), of eyelid, 328–329
of orbit, 991–992
radiographic findings in, *991–992,* 992
treatment of, 992
Scintillography, lacrimal, in evaluation of tearing, 759–760
Scissors, used in ophthalmic plastic surgery, *290*
SCLE (subacute cutaneous lupus erythematosus), 3. See also *Lupus erythematosus (LE).*
serologic marker for, 5–6
systemic manifestations of, 5
Sclera, donor. See *Donor sclera.*
Scleredema, 15
Scleroderma, 7–9
facial linear, *8,* 8–9
ocular manifestations of, 8t
localized, 8
systemic, 9
treatment of, 9
Scleromyxedema, *14,* 14–15
differential diagnosis of, 15
treatment of, 15
Sclerosis, systemic, 9
tuberous, 26–27
diagnostic criteria for, 27t
ocular manifestations of, 27t
Scratch test, for micropigmentation, 541
Sebaceous gland(s), of eyelid. See also specific gland, e.g., *Zeis gland(s).*
benign lesions originating in, 336–337, *337*
carcinoma of. See *Sebaceous gland carcinoma.*
inflammation of, 307–310, *309*
Sebaceous gland carcinoma, 190–194, 345–348
clinical features of, 190–192, *191–192*
clinicopathologic features of, 346, *346*
diagnosis of, 347–348
excision with cryotherapy for, 302, 348
histopathologic features of, 346–347, *347*
in AIDS patients, 528–529
in Asian patients, 721–722, *722*
management of, 193–194, *194,* 348
metastasis of, 194
mortality rates in, 301

Sebaceous gland carcinoma *(Continued)*
  multicentric, 347
  pagetoid involvement of epithelium in, 190, *191,* 347, *347*
    management of, 348
  pathology of, 192-193, *192-193*
  prognosis of, 193, 348
  radiation therapy for, 302-303, 348
Sebaceous gland hyperplasia, of eyelid, 336-337
Seborrheic dermatitis, *37,* 37-38
Seborrheic keratosis, of eyelid, 325, *325*
Secondary tumor(s), from ocular lesions, 68
Sedation, "startle reaction" following, 298
Seizure(s), ptosis caused by, 75, *76*
Semicircular flap, used in upper eyelid reconstruction, 366, *367*
Senear-Usher syndrome, 33
Sensory nerve, damage to, after blepharoplasty, 649-650
Septum, orbital. See *Orbital septum.*
Shading, of color distortion, in micropigmentation, 536, *536-537*
Shadowing, as cosmetic technique, used in facial rejuvenation, 570
Shagreen patches, in tuberous sclerosis, 27
Short-wave modality, for epilation, 591
  cautions associated with, 592-593
  point effect in, 593
  vs. other techniques, 593-594
Shutter, of camera, 551
Silicone droplets, for wrinkles, 566
Silicone elastomer, for prosthesis, 1135
Silicone foam, for prosthesis, 1137
Silicone gels, for prosthesis, 1137
Silicone intubation, for canalicular stenosis, 830
  for nasolacrimal duct obstruction, 780-781
Silk suture, 284
Single-needle galvanic electrolysis, 589. See also *Electrolysis.*
Sinus(es), Maier, 740, *742,* 750
  maxillary. See *Maxillary sinus(es).*
  paranasal. See *Paranasal sinus(es).*
  sphenoidal. See *Sphenoidal sinus(es).*
Sinus histiocytosis, with lymphadenopathy, of orbit, 62, *62*
Sinus infection(s), bacterial, 937-940, *938*
  fungal, complications of, 940
  orbital extension of, 937-943
  preseptal edema associated with, 938-939
  surgical exploration and drainage for, 939-940
Sinus surgery kit, endoscopic, *292*
Sinus thrombosis, cavernous, diagnostic and therapeutic features of, 941t-942t
Sinusitis, causing orbital cellulitis, 889
Sipple's syndrome (multiple endocrine neoplasia II), 22, 142
Sjögren-Larsson syndrome, 46
Sjögren's syndrome, 736
Skeletal muscle tumor(s), of orbit, 994-996
Skin, aging of, factors contributing to, 560
    pigmentary problems in, treatment of, 567-568, *568*
  asymmetry of, after blepharoplasty, 648
  disorders of, in diabetic patient, 138t, 139-141
  excision of, in ptosis surgery, 450-451
    in upper eyelid blepharoplasty, 589-599, 599-600, *599-600*
      variations in, 607
  facial, rejuvenation of, 560-571. See also *Facial rejuvenation.*
Skin *(Continued)*
  inflammation of. See *Dermatitis.*
  involvement of, in cicatricial pemphigoid, 196
  of eyelid, 262
    histology of, 323-324
  wrinkled. See *Wrinkles (rhytides).*
Skin cancer, removal of, Mohs' fresh tissue technique in, 352
    advantages of, 354-355
    steps in, 352-354, *353-355*
Skin closure, in upper eyelid blepharoplasty, 603, *603-604*
  variations of, 609-610, 610-611
Skin discoloration, neutralization of, application of color principles in, 658, *660*
Skin flap(s), used in lower eyelid blepharoplasty, 620, *620*
Skin folds (laugh lines), around eyelids, 261-262, *263*
Skin graft(s), for eyelid surgery, harvesting of, 439
  for medial canthal reconstruction, 393, 396, *397*
  for upper eyelid reconstruction, 366-367, *368,* 369
Skin marking, for upper eyelid blepharoplasty, 598, *598-599*
  variations in, 605-606
Skin retraction, in orbital surgery, 1048
Skin staples, 284
Skin tag (acrochordon), of eyelid, 324, *324*
Skin tension lines, in face, 285, *285*
Skin testing, for anesthetic allergies, 297
  for micropigmentation, guidelines in, 541
Skin wrinkling, in transconjunctival lower blepharoplasty, 630
Skin-muscle flap(s), used in lower eyelid blepharoplasty, 620-622, *621-622*
Skull base, fibrous dysplasia of, presenting as blindness, anterior cranial base approach to, 1202, *1203*
SLE. See *Systemic lupus erythematosus (SLE).*
Sleep test, for myasthenia gravis, 82, *82*
Sliding tarsal flap, used in upper eyelid reconstruction, technique of, 380, 382, *382*
Small cell lymphocytic lymphoma, 959
Smallpox, involving eyelids, 316
Smith lazy-T procedure, for involutional ectropion, 426, *426*
Smooth muscle, benign eyelid tumors derived from, 329
Smooth muscle tumor(s), of orbit, 996
Soemmering's ligament, 732
Soft contact lens, corneal reepithelialization with, following chemical injury, 225
Soft tissue, orbital, *842-845,* 842-849, *847-848*
Solar lentigo, of eyelid, 339, *340*
Sore, oriental, 150
Spasm(s), eyelid. See *Blepharospasm.*
  facial, diagnostic features of, 505t
  hemifacial. See *Hemifacial spasm.*
Sphenoid wing meningioma, 989-990
  radiographic findings in, *989,* 990
  treatment of, 990
Sphenoidal sinus(es), anatomy of, 1015
  mucoceles in, 1019-1021
    radiographic findings in, *1020,* 1020-1021
    treatment of, 1021
Spider bite(s), eyelid necrosis due to, 313
Spindle (epithelioid) nevus, of eyelid, 338
Spiradenoma, eccrine, of eyelid, 333-334
Spiral of Tillaux, *847,* 847-848
Spirochetal infection(s), of eyelid, 314
Split-level full-thickness graft, used in upper eyelid reconstruction, technique of, 384, *384*
Sporotrichosis, of eyelid, 150, *150,* 319
Squamous cell carcinoma, of conjunctiva, 231-232, *232-233*
    recurrence rates for, 232
    treatment of, 232, *233*
  of eyelid, 300, 349-350
    clinical presentation of, 349, *349*
    histologic features of, 349-350, *350*
    in Asian patients, 721, *722*
    low-grade, 325
    management of, 350
    metastatic potential of, 350
    orbital invasion by, 300-301, *302*
    radiotherapy as etiologic factor in, 349
    variation of, 350
  of lacrimal sac, 305, *305*
Squamous papilloma, of conjunctiva, 68, *69,* 251, *252*
    treatment of, 251-252
  of orbit, 68
Stainless steel screw, Nelson's, in fixation/reconstruction of canthal tendon, 389, *390*
Stainless steel wire suture, 284
"Startle reaction," following sedation, 298
Stenosis. See under anatomy, e.g., *Canaliculus(i), stenosis of.*
Steroids, topical, after chemical injury, 225
Stevens-Johnson syndrome, *34,* 34-35, 100
  and ocular pemphigoid, 203
  definition of, 35
  differential diagnosis of, 36
  treatment of, 37
  vs. cicatricial pemphigoid, 198
  vs. toxic epidermal necrolysis, 35
Stocker's line, in corneal epithelium, 208
Strabismus, after dermolipoma excision, treatment of, 256
  vertical, pseudoptosis associated with, *88,* 89
Strawberry nevus. See also *Hemangioma, capillary.*
  of eyelid, 330, *330*
Streptococcal myonecrosis, of eyelid, 312
Strobe lighting, for photography, 555
Stroma, conjunctival, 160
Strontium 90, as source of beta radiation, 217
ST-T segment, changes in, evaluation of, prior to oculoplastic surgery, 295
Stye (hordeolum), 307, *309*
Subacute cutaneous lupus erythematosus (SCLE), 3. See also *Lupus erythematosus (LE).*
  serologic marker for, 5-6
  systemic manifestations of, 5
Subcutaneous suture(s), buried, 286, *287*
Suborbital region, anatomy of, 484-485, *485-487*
  augmentation of, 484-503
    implants in, 484, 488, 490-498
      complications associated with, 501-503
      custom, 490-491, *491,* 495-498, *496-499*
      Flower tear trough, 488, *489,* 492-493, *492-495,* 495
      Goldberg lateral, 488, *489*
      malposition of, 503

Suborbital region *(Continued)*
prefabricated, 488, *489–491,* 490
vertical eyelid and, 498–499, *499–502,* 501
deficiency of, inadequate projection in, 487–488
prominent globe in, 486–487, *488–489*
tear trough deformity in, *486,* 487, *489*
Substantia propria, of conjunctiva, 160, *160,* 178
Sulbactam, for sinus infections, 939
Sulcus, deformity of, 1111–1113, *1112–1115*
Summerskill's sign, *76*
Sunscreen(s), use of, 561–562
Supranuclear lesion(s), eyelid retraction caused by, 72–73, *73*
ptosis caused by, 75–77, *76–77*
Supraorbital artery, anatomy of, 843
Supratarsal fixation technique, of eyelid crease creation, 708, *708*
Surgery, role of aesthetician before and after, 576–577
Surgicel, for hemostasis in wound repair, 283
Suture(s), buried mattress, 710–711, *710–711*
combined with small incisions, 712, *713*
continuous, 711–712, *712*
cranial, premature closure of, 1178–1182, *1179–1185*
Frost-type, in eyelid surgery, 439, *440*
horizontal mattress, 288, *288*
half-buried, 288, *289*
in fixation/reconstruction of canthal tendon, 388–389, *390*
interrupted, deep, 286, *287*
simple, 286, *286*
running percutaneous, 286, *286*
running subcuticular, 288, *288*
subcutaneous, buried, 286, *287*
used in blepharoplasty, 709–713, *710–713*
used in brow ptosis, 580, *580*
vertical mattress, 288, *289*
Suture material, absorbable, 284, 284t
nonabsorbable, 284
Suture needle(s), 284–285, *285*
Suture tracts, after blepharoplasty, 649
Sweat gland(s), apocrine, 273, *273,* 324
benign adnexal lesions originating in, 334–335, *334–335*
eccrine, *273,* 323–324
benign adnexal lesions originating in, 333–334, *333–334*
Symblepharon, conjunctival, treatment of, 226
Sympathetic innervation, to orbit, 846
Sympathetic lesion(s), ptosis caused by, 77–79, *78–79*
Synkinesis, facial, diagnostic features of, 505t
physiologic, 74, *74*
Synostosis(es), lambdoidal, 1182
multiple suture, 1182, *1185*
sagittal, 1178–1179, *1179–1180*
unilateral coronal, 1179–1180, *1181*
anterior cranial base approach to, 1193, *1194–1195*
Synthes mini- and microplating kit, *292*
Syphilis, 153
involving eyelids, 314
Syringocystadenoma papilliferum, of eyelid, 335
Syringoma, of eyelid, 333, *333*
chondroid, 334, *334*
Systemic and metabolic disease(s), 12–29. See also specific disease for detail.
Systemic and metabolic disease(s) *(Continued)*
acanthosis nigricans as, *23,* 23t, 23–24
amyloidosis as, *17,* 17–19, 18t
congenital erythropoietic porphyria as, 29
Darier's disease as, 21
erythropoietic protoporphyria as, 29
hyperthyroidism as, *12,* 12–14, 13t
ligneous conjunctivitis as, 20
lipoid proteinosis as, 20–21
Melkersson-Rosenthal syndrome as, 15–16
multiple mucosal neuroma syndrome as, 21–23, 22t
myxedema as, 14, *14*
necrobiotic xanthogranuloma as, 19–20
neurofibromatosis as, *24,* 24t, 24–26, 26t
porphyria cutanea tarda as, 27–28
sarcoidosis as, *16,* 16–17, 17t
scleredema as, 15
scleromyxedema as, *14,* 14–15
tuberous sclerosis as, 26–27, 27t
variegate porphyria as, 28
Systemic lupus erythematosus (SLE), 3. See also *Lupus erythematosus (LE).*
diagnosis of, 6
ocular complications of, 4–5, 5t
revised criteria for, 4t
treatment of, 6–7

T cell(s), 94–95
T_3 (triiodothyronine), in thyrotoxicosis, 124
T_4 (thyroxine), in thyrotoxicosis, 124
Taenia solium, 151
Taillefer valve, 742, *743*
Taiwanese, epicanthal folds in, prevalence of, 705t
exophthalmometry in, 698, 698t
Takayasu's arteritis, 112
Tamoxifen, for metastatic breast carcinoma, *1009,* 1009–1010
Tamponade, pressure, for hemostasis in wound repair, 282
Taoist view, of medicine, 692–693, *692–693*
Tarsal arterial arcades, *275*
Tarsal flap, rotational, in upper eyelid reconstruction, 375–378, *379–380*
sliding, in upper eyelid reconstruction, 381–382, *382*
Tarsal strip procedure, lateral, for involutional ectropion, 427, 429, *429–430*
Tarsal substitutes, used in upper eyelid reconstruction, 363
Tarsoconjunctival flap, in upper eyelid reconstruction, 378–380, *381*
sliding, in medial canthal reconstruction, 391, *394*
in upper eyelid reconstruction, 380, 382, *382*
Tarsoconjunctival graft(s), free, 175, *175–176*
Tarsoconjunctival polishing, with mucous membrane grafting, for cicatricial entropion and trichiasis, 203–205, *204–206*
Tarsorrhaphy, for paralytic ectropion, 430–432, *431–432*
Tarsus, and submuscular fat pad, in Chinese adults, 699, 700t
used in upper eyelid reconstruction, autogenous, 363–364
irradiated, 365
Tattoo machine, 676, *678*
Tattoo pigments, used in electropigmentation, 677, 681
Tattooing, medical. See *Micropigmentation.*
Tear(s), "alligator" or "crocodile," 735
artificial, in management of pterygia, 211
drainage of, 762
Tear break-up time, 759
Tear film, abnormalities in, pterygia due to, 209
precorneal, *736–737,* 736–738
aqueous layer of, 736
eyelids and, 738
mucin layer of, 737
oil layer of, 737–738
quantity and quality of, after chemical injury, 226
Tear frame, reevaluation of, after chemical injury, 226
Tear production, altered, lacrimal surgery for, 201
Tear trough, 484, *485*
deformity of, *486,* 487, *489*
Tear trough implant, Flower, 488, *489,* 492–493, *492–495,* 495
Tearing, anatomic location responsible for, 749–750
cause(s) of, 750–751
eyelid, cicatricial ectropion as, 765, 767–768, *767–769*
cicatricial entropion as, 771
epiblepharon as, 775, *775*
involutional ectropion as, 762–765, *763–764, 766–767*
involutional entropion as, 770–771, *772–773*
paralytic ectropion as, 768–770, *769*
spastic entropion as, 771, *773*
trichiasis as, 771, *774,* 774–775
evaluation of, 748–760
from blocked outflow. See *Epiphora.*
history of, 748–752, *749*
physical examination of patient with, 752–760, *753*
computed tomography in, 760
dacryocystography in, 759, *759–760*
dye disappearance test in, 753–754, *754*
endoscopy in, 760
Jones I test in, 754–755
Jones II test in, 755
lacrimal scintillography in, 759–760
nasal evaluation in, 755, 757–758, *758*
probing in, 755, *756–757*
rose bengal testing in, 759
Schirmer testing in, 758–759
tear break-up time in, 759
ultrasonography in, 760
reflex, 750
Teflon-coated Dacron suture, 284
Telangiectasia, treatment of, 569, *569*
Temporal arteritis, 112
Temporal nerve, anatomy of, 277, *277*
Temporalis muscle transfer, for paralytic ectropion, 434, 436–437, *436–437*
in surgical management of facial paralysis, 479–480, *480*
TEN. See *Toxic epidermal necrolysis (Lyell's syndrome).*
Tendon(s). See also named tendon, e.g., *Canthal tendon.*
creation of, in fixation/reconstruction of canthal tendon, 388, *389*
Tensilon test, for myasthenia gravis, *80,* 81–82

Tenzel flap, in lower eyelid reconstruction, 400–402, *401–402*
  in medial canthal reconstruction, 391, *393*
Tetanus, 83
  cranial nerve paresis in, 152
Tetracycline, for hordeolum, 308
  for rosacea, 39
  for trachoma, 155
Therapeutic agent(s), pharmacology of, 97–98
Thermal cautery, for hemostasis in wound repair, 282–283
Thermal injury, 222. See also *Chemical injury(ies).*
Thermolysis method, of epilation, 591
Thiopental, as anesthetic agent, 297
Thiotepa, as adjunct to surgery for pterygia, 218
Thiourea drug(s), for thyroid storm, 130
  for thyrotoxicosis, 125
Three-wall orbital decompression, for Graves' disease. See also *Graves' disease, orbital decompression for.*
    transorbital approach to, 976–980, *976–980*
Thrombin, for hemostasis in wound repair, 283
Thrombophlebitis, orbital, 966
Thrombosis, cavernous sinus, diagnostic and therapeutic features of, 941t–942t
Thyroid carcinoma, metastatic, to rectus muscle, *55*
Thyroid drugs, chronic patient use of, anesthetic considerations with, 296
Thyroid dysfunction, ocular manifestations of, 13
Thyroid orbitopathy, CT scan of, 891, *892*
Thyroid storm, management of, 129–130
Thyroid-associated ophthalmopathy, 121–122
  clinical features of, 122
  management of, 122
Thyroidectomy, subtotal, for thyrotoxicosis, 128–129
Thyroid-stimulating hormone (TSH), in thyrotoxicosis, 124
Thyrotoxicosis, 121–130
  "apathetic," 124
  biochemical diagnosis of, 124–125
  causes of, 125t
  clinical manifestations of, 123–124
  during pregnancy, management of, 129–130
  etiology of, characteristic test results in, 126t–127t
    determination of, 125
  management of, 125, 128–129
    drug therapy in, 125, 128
    radioactive iodine therapy in, 128
    subtotal thyroidectomy in, 128–129
  signs and symptoms associated with, 123t
  thyroid storm and, management of, 129–130
  vs. hyperthyroidism, 123
Thyroxine (T_4), in thyrotoxicosis, 124
Tic, facial, diagnostic features of, 505t
Ticarcillin, for sinus infections, 939
Tillaux, spiral of, *847*, 847–848
Time, principle of, in electrolysis, 590
Tissue, conjunctival, handling of, 161
Tissue flap(s). See *Flap(s).*
Tissue graft(s). See also *Graft(s).*
  harvesting of, 1077–1083
Tolosa-Hunt syndrome, 882, 892, 965
Torre's syndrome, 337, *337*
Touton giant cell, 64
Toxic epidermal necrolysis (Lyell's syndrome), 34, 35, *35*
  differential diagnosis of, 36–37, 106
  drug-induced, 35, 36t
  epidemiology of, 105
  immunohistopathology of, 105–106
  ocular manifestations of, 105
  pathogenesis of, 106
  systemic manifestations of, 105
  treatment of, 37, 106
  vs. Stevens-Johnson syndrome, 35
Toxin(s), neuromuscular, ptosis caused by, 83–84, *84*
Toxocariasis, ocular, imaging of, 908–909
Trachoma, bacteriology of, 154
  clinical presentation of, 155, *155*
  diagnosis of, 155
  epidemiology of, 154
  eyelid retraction caused by, 315
  MacCallan classification of, 314–315
  pathogenesis of, 154–155
  staging system for, 154t
  treatment of, 155
Transnasal wiring, with dacryocystorhinostomy, in fixation/reconstruction of canthal tendon, 388, *389*
Transplantation, corneal, after chemical injury, 228, *228*
  fat, autologous, for wrinkles, 565
  in conjunctival mucous membrane replacement, 172
Transpositional skin flap, in upper eyelid reconstruction, 371, *372*
Trauma. See also specific anatomic site, e.g., *Eyelid trauma.*
  causing nasolacrimal duct obstruction, 809–811, 810t, *810–812*
  chemical, 222–230. See also *Chemical injury(ies).*
  facial nerve, 473–474
  orbital, surgical approach to, 1054
Trepier flap, in lower eyelid reconstruction, 403, *403–404*
Treponema carateum, pinta caused by, 314
Treponema pallidum, syphilis caused by, 314
Treponema pertenue, yaws caused by, 314
Tretinoin, for wrinkles, *562*, 562–563
  used in chemical peels, 665–666
Triamcinolone, for capillary hemangioma, 919
Trichiasis, as cause of tearing, 771, *774*, 774–775
  cicatricial, buccal mucous membrane grafting for, 203–206
    anesthesia in, 203
    complications of, 205
    results of, 205, *206*
    surgical methods of, 203–205, *204–206*
  correction of, 201
  infection causing, 308t
Trichilemmoma, of eyelid, 336
Trichinella spiralis, causing periorbital edema, 151
Trichloroacetic acid, used in chemical peels, 667, *667–668*
Trichoepithelioma, of eyelid, *335*, 335–336
Trichofolliculoma, of eyelid, 336
Trichothiodystrophy (brittle hair), in ichthyosis, 46
Trigeminal nerve, anatomy of, 277–278, *278, 845*, 845–846
  function of, assessment of, in orbital disease, *879*, 879–880
Trigonocephaly, 1181–1182, *1184*
Trihexyphenidyl, for essential blepharospasm and Meige's syndrome, 507
Triiodothyronine (T_3), in thyrotoxicosis, 124
Trochlea, *848*, 848–849
Trochlear nerve, anatomy of, 845
Trypanosoma cruzi, 152
  Chagas' disease caused by, 316
TSH (thyroid-stimulating hormone), in thyrotoxicosis, 124
Tuberculosis, 152–153
  eyelid involvement due to, 313
Tuberous sclerosis, 26–27
  diagnostic criteria for, 27t
  ocular manifestations of, 27t
Tularemia, 149
  involving eyelids, 313–314
Tumor(s). See also specific tumor.
  causing nasolacrimal duct obstruction, 804, 805t, *805–810*, 806–807
  conjunctival. See *Conjunctival neoplasm(s).*
  eyelid, benign, 323–340
    malignant, 300–306, 342–350
  facial nerve, 474
  lacrimal gland, 999–1006
  orbital. See *Orbital tumor(s).*
  pediatric, anterior cranial base approach to, 1199, 1202–1204, *1203–1206*
  prognosis of, markers in, 53
Tungsten light, for photography, 555
Tungsten-balanced film, photographic, 554
Turban tumor (cylindroma), of eyelid, 334–335, *335*

Ulcer(s), corneal, prevention of, after chemical injury, 225, 229
  eyelid, causes of, 308t
Ulerythema ophryogenes, 43–44
Ultrapulse carbon dioxide laser, used in blepharoplasty, *544*
Ultrasonography, diagnostic, for tearing, 760
  of mucoceles, in paranasal sinuses, 1015–1016, *1016*
  of neurogenic tumors of orbit, 984
Ultraviolet light, harmful effects of, prevention of, 561–562
Ultraviolet radiation, exposure to, pterygia due to, 209
Unilateral coronal synostosis, 1179–1180, *1181*
  anterior cranial base approach to, 1193, *1194–1195*
Urbach-Wiethe disease, 20–21
  differential diagnosis of, 21
Urticaria, 40
Urticaria pigmentosa, 43
Uvea, malignant melanoma of, anterior cranial base approach to, 1202–1204, *1204–1205*
  metastatic disease of, *911*, 911–912
Uveoparotid fever (Heerfordt's syndrome), 16, 901

Varicella zoster. See *Herpes zoster infection.*
Variegate porphyria, 28–29
Varix (varices), of eyelid, 330–331
  of orbit, CT scan of, 896, *897*
Vascular tissue, benign eyelid tumors derived from, *329–331*, 329–332
Vascular tumors, of orbit, 913–932. See also specific tumor, e.g., *Hemangioma.*

Vasculitic disease(s). See also specific disease for detail.
  allergic granulomatous angiitis as, 113
  lethal midline granuloma as, 114
  lymphoid granulomatosis as, 113–114
  polyarteritis nodosa as, 111–112
  polymorphic reticulosis as, 113–114
  temporal arteritis as, 112
  Wegener's granulomatosis as, 109–111
Vein(s). See also specific vein, e.g., *Facial vein.*
  of ocular region, 274–275, *276*
Venom, arthropod and reptile, disruption of neuromuscular transmission by, 83
Ventricular contraction(s), premature, evaluation of, prior to oculoplastic surgery, 295
Verruca vulgaris lesions, of eyelid, in AIDS patients, 526
  papillomavirus-induced, 316
Vesicle(s), 29
Vesicobullous disease(s). See also specific disease for detail.
  affecting ocular adnexa, 29–37
    cicatricial pemphigoid as, *31,* 31–32
    epidermolysis bullosa as, 29–31, 30t
    erythema multiforme as, *34–35,* 34–37, 36t
    pemphigus as, 33–34
Viral infection(s), causing nasolacrimal duct obstruction, 798t, 799, *799–800*
  of eyelid, 315–316, *315–316*
Visual acuity, and orbital disease, 860–861, *861,* 880
  in optic nerve dysfunction, 874, *875*
Visual field, in orbital disease, 875–876, *876,* 880
Visual field defect(s), screening for, 860–861, *861*
Visual loss, after blepharoplasty, 643–644
  after surgery for orbital floor fractures, 1090–1091
Visual rehabilitation, after chemical injury, 227–228, *228*
Vitiligo, in diabetic patient, 140
Vitreous, persistent hyperplastic primary, imaging of, 908, *909*
Vodder technique, of lymphatic drainage, 654
Von Graefe's sign, in Graves' ophthalmopathy, 514
Von Recklinghausen's disease. See *Neurofibromatosis.*

Warburg disease, imaging of, 908, *909*
Warfarin, chronic patient use of, anesthetic considerations with, 296
Wart(s), eyelid, in AIDS patients, 526
  papillomavirus-induced, 316
Wax model, of prosthesis, 1138–1139, *1139*
Weber's syndrome, 470–471
Wegener's granulomatosis, 9–11
  associated with secondary acquired nasolacrimal duct obstruction, 799, 801, *802*
  criteria for classification of, 10t
  differential diagnosis of, 11, 110–111
  epidemiology of, 109
  laboratory findings in, 110
  ocular abnormalities of, 10t
  ocular manifestations of, 109–110
  of orbit, 66, *66*
  systemic manifestations of, 109
  treatment of, 11, 110
Weibel-Palade body(ies), in Kaposi's sarcoma, 242
Wermer's syndrome (multiple endocrine neoplasia I), 22, 142
Whitnall's ligament, 270–271, *272,* 732
Wickham's striae, in lichen planus, 40
Wiring, transnasal, with dacryocystorhinostomy, in fixation/reconstruction of canthal tendon, 388, *389*
Wolfram (DIDMOAD) syndrome, in diabetic patient, 138t, 139
Wolfring gland(s), 161, *273,* 732, *732, 737*
Wood's syndrome, 504
Wound decontamination, after eyelid trauma, 457–458, *458*
Wound dehiscence, after blepharoplasty, 648
Wound repair, 281–282
  after chemical injury, epidermal growth factor for, 229–230
    fibronectin for, 229
  phases of, approximate times for, 282t
  primary, 281, 282t
  secondary, 281–282
Wrinkles (rhytides), alpha-hydroxy acids for, 563–564, *564*
  chemical peels for, 564
  dermabrasion for, 565, *565*
  filler substance(s) for, 565–567
    autologous, 670. See also *Autologen.*
    Fibrel as, 567, *567,* 670
    injectable, 670–671
Wrinkles (rhytides) *(Continued)*
    Zyderm collagen as, *566,* 566–567, 670
  tretinoin for, *562,* 562–563

Xanthelasma, of eyelid, 332, *332*
Xanthogranuloma, juvenile, of eyelid, 64, 333
    of orbit, 64
  necrobiotic, 19–20, *947,* 947–948
  orbital, 948, *948–949*
Xanthoma, eruptive, in diabetic patient, 140–141
  of eyelid, 332
Xeroderma pigmentosum, of conjunctiva and eyelid, 66–67, *67*
Xylocaine. See *Lidocaine (Xylocaine).*

Yaws, involving eyelids, 314
Yersinia pestis, plague caused by, 314
Yin and yang, 692, 693
  balance of, Chinese diet in, 695
  symbol of, *692*
Yttrium-aluminum-garnet (YAG) laser, fat removal by, *641,* 641–642
  treatment of lymphangiomas with, 926

Zeis gland(s), 273, *273,* 736, *737*
  carcinoma arising in, 190. See also *Sebaceous gland carcinoma.*
  infection of, 307, *309*
Zinn, annulus of, anatomy of, 847, *847,* 848
Zosteriform herpes, 315
Z-plasty conjunctival flap, 163, *164*
Zuckerkandl's dehiscences, 935
Zyderm collagen, for wrinkles, *566,* 566–567, 670
Zygomatic fracture(s), 1093
  complications of, 1094, *1094*
  treatment of, 1093–1094
Zygomatic nerve, anatomy of, 277, *277*
Zygomaticofacial nerve, anatomy of, 846
Zygomaticotemporal nerve, anatomy of, 846
Zygomycosis. See *Mucormycosis (phycomycosis).*

PRINCIPLES AND PRACTICE OF

Ophthalmic Plastic and Reconstructive Surgery

VOLUME II

PRINCIPLES AND PRACTICE OF

Ophthalmic Plastic and Reconstructive Surgery

Stephen Bosniak, M.D.
Associate Clinical Professor, State University of New York at Stony Brook;
Director, Ophthalmic Plastic and Reconstructive Surgery, Nassau County Hospital and Kings County Hospital;
and Associate Attending Surgeon, Manhattan Eye, Ear, and Throat Hospital and
New York Eye and Ear Infirmary, New York, New York

Section Editors

Giulio Bonavolontà, M.D.
Professor and Chairman of Ophthalmology (Eye Institute),
University of "Federica II" School of Medicine,
University of Naples,
Naples, Italy

Stephen Bosniak, M.D.
Associate Clinical Professor,
State University of New York at Stony Brook;
Director, Ophthalmic Plastic and Reconstructive Surgery,
Nassau County Hospital and Kings County Hospital;
and Associate Attending Surgeon, Manhattan Eye, Ear, and
Throat Hospital
and New York Eye and Ear Infirmary,
New York, New York

Robert Alan Goldberg, M.D.
Associate Professor of Ophthalmology,
University of California, Los Angeles, School of Medicine;
and Chief, Orbital and Ophthalmic Plastic Surgery,
Jules Stein Eye Institute,
Los Angeles, California

Russell S. Gonnering, M.D.
Associate Professor of Ophthalmology,
University of Wisconsin School of Medicine;
and Active Staff, St. Luke's Medical Center,
Milwaukee, Wisconsin

James W. Karesh, M.D.
Assistant Professor, Johns Hopkins University School of
Medicine, Wilmer Ophthalmologic Institute
and the University of Maryland School of Medicine;
Director, Ophthalmic Plastic and Reconstructive Surgery,
Krieger Eye Institute, Sinai Hospital of Baltimore,
Baltimore, Maryland

Don Liu, M.D.
Associate Professor, Department of Ophthalmology,
University of Southern California School of Medicine,
Los Angeles, California

Jeffrey A. Nerad, M.D.
Professor of Ophthalmology,
University of Iowa College of Medicine;
and Director, Oculoplastic, Orbital, and Oncology Service,
University of Iowa Hospitals and Clinics,
Iowa City, Iowa

Robert A. Weiss, M.D.
Clinical Associate Professor of Ophthalmology,
Oculoplastic and Reconstructive Surgery
and Ophthalmic Oncology, University of Illinois at Chicago,
and the Chicago Eye Institute, Chicago, Illinois

Ralph E. Wesley, M.D.
Director, Ophthalmic Plastic and Orbital Surgery, and
Clinical Professor of Ophthalmology,
Vanderbilt University Medical Center;
Chief of Ophthalmology, Baptist Medical Center,
Nashville, Tennessee

Ted H. Wojno, M.D.
Associate Professor of Ophthalmology,
Emory University School of Medicine;
and Director, Oculoplastic and Orbital Surgery,
Emory Clinic, Atlanta, Georgia

W.B. SAUNDERS COMPANY
A Division of Harcourt Brace & Company
Philadelphia London Toronto Montreal Sydney Tokyo

W.B. SAUNDERS COMPANY
A Division of Harcourt Brace & Company

The Curtis Center
Independence Square West
Philadelphia, Pennsylvania 19106

Library of Congress Cataloging-in-Publication Data

Principles and practice of ophthalmic plastic and reconstructive surgery / [edited by] Stephen Bosniak. — 1st ed.

p. cm.

ISBN 0-7216-3559-8

1. Ophthalmic plastic surgery. I. Bosniak, Stephen
[DNLM: 1. Eye—surgery. 2. Surgery, Plastic. WW 168 P957 1996]
RE87.P75 1996 617.7′1—dc20
DNLM/DLC 95-12616

Principles and Practice of Ophthalmic Plastic and Reconstructive Surgery
Volume 1 ISBN 0-7216-6033-9
Volume 2 ISBN 0-7216-6034-7
Two-Volume Set ISBN 0-7216-3559-8

Printed in the United States of America

Last digit is the print number: 9 8 7 6 5 4 3 2 1

Dedication

For **Marian,** *who changed my life.*

S.B.

Contributors

Ronald G. Amedee, M.D.
Associate Professor of Otolaryngology, Department of Otolaryngology, Tulane University Medical School; Chief of Surgical Services, Eye, Ear, Nose, and Throat Hospital, New Orleans, Louisiana.
Ophthalmic Manifestations of Mucoceles

Catherine Atzen, P.M.A., CIDESCO Diplomat
Catherine Atzen Laboratories; Vice-President, Aesthetics International Association, Campbell, California.
The Role of the Aesthetician Before and After Surgery

John C. Baer, M.D.
Assistant Professor, Department of Ophthalmology, University of Maryland School of Medicine; Staff, Veterans Affairs Medical Center, Baltimore, Maryland.
Ocular Manifestations of Systemic Immune Disease

George B. Bartley, M.D.
Chair, Department of Ophthalmology, Mayo Clinic and Mayo Foundation; Associate Professor of Ophthalmology, Mayo Medical School, Rochester, Minnesota.
The Eyelids in Graves' Ophthalmopathy; Secondary Acquired Lacrimal Drainage Obstruction

Henry I. Baylis, M.D.
Clinical Professor of Ophthalmology, University of California, Los Angeles, School of Medicine; Founding Chief, Orbital and Ophthalmic Plastic Surgery, Jules Stein Eye Institute, University of California, Los Angeles, Los Angeles, California.
Transconjunctival Lower Blepharoplasty

Fred S. Bodker, M.D.
Private Practice, Kansas City Eye Clinic, Overland Park, Kansas.
Harvesting and Use of Biological Tissue Grafts

Giulio Bonavolontà, M.D.
Professor and Chairman of Ophthalmology (Eye Institute), University "Federico II" School of Medicine, University of Naples, Naples, Italy.
Surgical Approaches to the Orbit; Anterior, Medial, Lateral, and Combined Surgical Approaches for Orbital Tumor Resection

Stephen Bosniak, M.D.
Associate Clinical Professor, State University of New York at Stony Brook; Director, Ophthalmic Plastic and Reconstructive Surgery, Nassau County Hospital and Kings County Hospital; and Associate Attending Surgeon, Manhattan Eye, Ear, and Throat Hospital and New York Eye and Ear Infirmary, New York, New York.
Alternative Techniques of Fat Removal

Jeffrey Bruce, M.D.
Assistant Professor of Clinical Neurosurgery (in Pathology), Columbia University; Assistant Attending Physician in Neurological Surgery, Columbia Presbyterian Medical Center, New York, New York.
Neurogenic Tumors

Cora Buggea
Electrolysis Instructor, Gina's School of Aesthetics and Electrology, Toronto, Ontario, Canada.
Electrology and Eyebrow Contouring

Richard C. Cape, M.D.
Private Practice; Staff, Methodist Hospital, Dyersburg, Tennessee.
Surgical Intervention in Conjunction with Medical Treatment of Cicatricial Pemphigoid

Keith D. Carter, M.D.
Associate Professor of Ophthalmology, Oculoplastics, Orbital and Oncology Services, Associate Professor, University of Iowa Hospitals and Clinics, Iowa City, Iowa.
Primary Acquired Nasolacrimal Duct Obstruction

Phillip Casson, M.D.
Associate Professor of Surgery (Plastic), New York University School of Medicine; Assistant Attending Surgeon, Tisch Hospital, Bellevue Hospital, New York Eye and Ear Infirmary, and Veterans Affairs Medical Center, New York, New York.
Autologen: Autologous, Injectable Dermal Collagen

William P. Chen, M.D.
Assistant Clinical Professor of Ophthalmology, Jules Stein Eye Institute, University of California, Los Angeles, School of Medicine; Associate Clinical Professor of Ophthalmology, University of California, Irvine, College of Medicine; Senior Attending Surgeon, Ophthalmic Plastic Surgery Service, Harbor-UCLA Medical Center, Torrance, California.
Tarsoconjunctival Polishing with Mucous Membrane Grafting for Cicatricial Entropion and Trichiasis; Enucleation and Evisceration

David B. Christie, M.D.
Instructor in Ophthalmology, Tufts University School of Medicine, Boston, Massachusetts.
Basic Surgical Techniques, Technology, and Wound Repair

Jonathan Christenbury, M.D.
Attending Physician, Presbyterian Hospital, Carolinas Medical Center, Charlotte, North Carolina.
Aponeurotic Ptosis

Chieh Chung, M.D.
Assistant Professor of Ear, Nose, and Throat Medicine, Yang Ming Medical School, Taipei, Taiwan.
Auricular Acupuncture in the Treatment of Blepharospasm

Michael Clarke, M.A., M.B., B.Chir., D.O., F.R.C.S., F.R.C.Ophth.
Acting Head, Department of Ophthalmology, Medical School, University of Newcastle; Consultant Paediatric Ophthalmologist, Royal Victoria Infirmary, Newcastle Upon Tyne, England.
Mesenchymal and Fibro-osseous Tumors

Marc S. Cohen, M.D.
Assistant Professor, Thomas Jefferson University School of Medicine; Assistant Surgeon, Wills Eye Hospital, Philadelphia, Pennsylvania.
Lower Eyelid Retraction and Cicatricial Ectropion; Optic Nerve Sheath Decompression

Harvey P. Cole III, M.D.
Clinical Instructor of Ophthalmology, Emory University School of Medicine; Staff, Southeastern Oculoplastic Center, Piedmont Hospital, Atlanta, Georgia.
Conjunctiva: Structure and Function; Basic Techniques of Conjunctival Surgery; Treatment of Squamous Papillomas of the Conjunctiva

M. Ronan Conlon, M.D., F.R.C.S.C.
Assistant Clinical Professor of Ophthalmology, University of Saskatchewan; Staff, Saskatoon City Hospital, Saskatoon, Saskatchewan, Canada.
Pigmented Conjunctival Neoplasms; Benign Eyelid Tumors

Philip L. Custer, M.D.
Associate Professor of Ophthalmology, Washington University School of Medicine; Director, Orbital Center, Barnes Hospital, St. Louis, Missouri.
Lower Eyelid Blepharoplasty

Roger A. Dailey, M.D.
Assistant Professor of Ophthalmology, Casey Eye Institute, Oregon Health Sciences University; Active Staff, Oregon Health Sciences University, Veterans Affairs Medical Center, Good Samaritan Hospital, St. Vincent Hospital, and Emanuel Hospital, Portland, Oregon.
Medial Canthal Reconstruction

Carlo de Conciliis, M.D.
Staff, Ophthalmic Plastic Reconstructive and Orbital Surgery, Department of Ophthalmology and Visual Science, Scientific Institute H. S. Raffaele, Milan, Italy.
Epidemiology of Orbital Pathology

Robert D. Deitch Jr., M.D.
Assistant Clinical Professor, Department of Ophthalmology, Indiana University School of Medicine, Indianapolis, Indiana.
Management of Pterygia

Dale P. DeVore, Ph.D.
Chief Scientific Officer, Autogenesis Tech, Inc., Acton; Managing Director, Organogenesis, Inc., Canton, Massachusetts.
Autologen: Autologous, Injectable Dermal Collagen

Marcos T. Doxanas, M.D.
Staff, Department of Ophthalmology, Greater Baltimore Medical Center, Baltimore, Maryland.
Malignant Epithelial Eyelid Tumors

Steven C. Dresner, M.D.
Associate Clinical Professor of Ophthalmology, Jules Stein Eye Institute, University of California, Los Angeles, Los Angeles, California.
Reconstruction of the Lower Eyelid and Lateral Canthus

Nancy Dugan, B.A.
Paramedical Camouflage Consultant
Principles of Camouflage Make-up and the Postoperative Patient

Jonathan J. Dutton, M.D., Ph.D.
Professor, Duke University Eye Center, Durham, North Carolina.
Replacement of Conjunctival Mucous Membrane

Steven Fagien, M.D., F.A.C.S.
Boca Raton Center for Ophthalmic Plastic and Reconstructive Surgery; Director, Boca Raton Center for Ophthalmic Plastic and Reconstructive Surgery, Boca Raton, Florida.
Autologen: Autologous, Injectable Dermal Collagen

James C. Fleming, M.D.
Assistant Professor, Department of Ophthalmology, University of Tennessee Center for the Health Sciences, University of Tennessee, Memphis, Tennessee.
Surgical Intervention in Conjunction with Medical Treatment of Cicatricial Pemphigoid

Jill A. Foster, M.D.
Director of Oculoplastic and Orbital Surgery Service, Division of Ophthalmology, Cleveland Clinic Foundation, Cleveland, Ohio.
Congenital Eyelid Anomalies

Tamara R. Fountain, M.D.
Clinical Instructor and Clinical Fellow, Department of Ophthalmic Plastic and Reconstructive Surgery, Doheny Eye Institute, University of Southern California, Los Angeles, California.
Considerations for Oculoplastic Surgery in the African American Patient

Craig D. Friedman, M.D.
Staff, Department of Otolaryngology, Yale University Medical Center, New Haven, Connecticut.
Harvesting and Use of Biological Tissue Grafts

Constance L. Fry, M.D.
Clinical Professor of Oculoplastics and Orbital Disease, Tulane University; Staff, Oculoplastics and Orbital Surgery Service, Ochsner Clinic, and Eye, Ear, Nose, and Throat Hospital, New Orleans, Louisiana.
Eyelid Infections and Inflammations

Steven L. Galetta, M.D.
Associate Professor and Director, Neuro-ophthalmology Service, Department of Neurology and Ophthalmology, University of Pennsylvania School of Medicine, Philadelphia, Pennsylvania.
Facial Paralysis: Diagnosis and Management

Linda Garofallou, B.S.
Director of Training, Dr. Hauschka Skin Care, USA; Authorized International Trainer, WALA Heilmittel, GmbH, Germany.
Lymphatic Drainage Massage

Steven M. Gilbard, M.D.
Consultant, Ophthalmic Plastic Surgery, St. Joseph's Hospital and Medical Center and Barrow Neurological Institute, Phoenix, Arizona.
Involutional and Paralytic Ectropion

Gregory G. Gion, B.A., B.S., C.M.I.
Adjunct Faculty, Department of Biomedical Communications, Graduate School of Biomedical Sciences, University of Texas Southwestern Medical Center, Dallas, Texas.
Orbital Prostheses

Robert Alan Goldberg, M.D.
Associate Professor of Ophthalmology, University of California, Los Angeles, School of Medicine; Chief, Orbital and Ophthalmic Plastic Surgery, Jules Stein Eye Institute, University of California, Los Angeles, Los Angeles, California.
Entropion; Transconjunctival Lower Blepharoplasty

Stacia H. Goldey, M.D.
Attending Surgeon, Florida Hospital, Eustis; and Leesburg Regional Medical Center, Leesburg, Florida.
Transconjunctival Lower Blepharoplasty

Russell S. Gonnering, M.D.
Associate Clinical Professor, University of Wisconsin School of Medicine; Active Staff, St. Luke's Medical Center, Milwaukee, Wisconsin.
Eyelid Trauma

Holly Gore, M.D.
Clinical Instructor, Department of Ophthalmology, Tulane University School of Medicine, New Orleans; Corneal Specialist, North Lake Eye Center, Slidell, Louisiana.
Vascular Tumors of the Orbit

Diana Habrich
Staff, Sunnyside Medical Office, Kaiser Permanente, Clackamas, Oregon.
Medical Canthal Reconstruction

Barrett G. Haik, M.D.
Professor and Chairman, Department of Ophthalmology, University of Tennessee School of Medicine, Memphis, Tennessee.
Vascular Tumors of the Orbit; Ophthalmic Manifestations of Mucoceles

Lawrence F. Handler, M.D.
Clinical Instructor, Scheie Eye Institute, University of Pennsylvania School of Medicine, Philadelphia, Pennsylvania.
Facial Paralysis: Diagnosis and Management

Annette Hanson, B.A.
President, Atelier Esthétique, Inc., New York, New York.
Principles of Camouflage Make-up and the Postoperative Patient

Will Harms, M.D.
Former Office Medical Director, Anchor Norridge Medical Office, Norridge, Illinois.
Pseudotumors

Ramzi K. Hemady, M.D.
Assistant Professor, Department of Ophthalmology, University of Maryland School of Medicine; Chief, Ophthalmology Section, Baltimore Veterans Affairs Medical Center, Baltimore, Maryland.
Ocular Manifestations of Systemic Immune Disease

John B. Holds, M.D., F.A.C.S.
Associate Professor of Ophthalmology and Otolaryngology, St. Louis University Health Sciences Center, Anheuser-Busch Eye Institute, St. Louis, Missouri.
Essential Blepharospasm and Hemifacial Spasm; The Role of Paranasal Sinus Disease in Orbital Cellulitis

Anne R. Horan, M.D.
Instructor in Ophthalmology, Vanderbilt University Department of Ophthalmology and Visual Sciences, Vanderbilt University Medical Center, and Nashville Veterans Affairs Medical Center, Nashville, Tennessee.
Conjunctival and Limbal Neoplasia: Diagnosis and Management

Wen Ming Hsu, M.D.
Associate Professor, Department of Ophthalmology, Yang Ming-University School of Medicine; Director, Oculoplastic Section, Department of Ophthalmology, Veterans General Hospital–Taipei, Taipei, Taiwan.
Auricular Acupuncture in the Treatment of Blepharospasm

William D. James, M.D.
Chief, Dermatology Service, Walter Reed Army Medical Center, Washington, D.C.
Cutaneous and Multisystemic Processes Affecting the Ocular Adnexa

Walter J. Johnson
Board-Certified Ocularist, Fellow, American Society of Ocularists, Denver Optic Company, Englewood, Colorado.
The Perfect Socket: The Ocularist's View

Kelly Jones, M.D.
Staff, Department of Ophthalmology, University of Maryland School of Medicine, Baltimore, Maryland.
Neoplastic and Related Conditions of the Orbital and Adnexal Structures

David R. Jordan, M.D., F.A.C.S., F.R.C.S.(C)
Associate Professor, University of Ottawa Eye Institute, Ottawa, Ontario, Canada.
Reconstruction of the Upper Eyelid; Evaluation of the Tearing Patient

Sara A. Kaltreider, M.D.
Associate Professor of Ophthalmology, University of Virginia School of Medicine, Charlottesville, Virginia.
Orbital Fractures

Leonard P. Kapcala, M.D., F.A.C.P.
Associate Professor of Medicine and Physiology, University of Maryland School of Medicine; Attending Physician, Endocrinology Division, University of Maryland Hospital, Baltimore, Maryland.
Diagnosis and Management of Thyrotoxicosis; Diagnosis and Management of Hyperparathyroidism

James W. Karesh, M.D.
Assistant Professor, Johns Hopkins University School of Medicine, Wilmer Ophthalmologic Institute and the University of Maryland School of Medicine; Director, Ophthalmic Plastic and Reconstructive Surgery, Krieger Eye Institute, Sinai Hospital of Baltimore, Baltimore, Maryland.
Neoplastic and Related Conditions of the Orbital and Adnexal Structures; The Ocular Manifestations of Non–Thyroid-Related Endocrine Disease

James A. Katowitz, M.D.
Associate Professor of Ophthalmology (Children's Hospital), University of Pennsylvania School of Medicine; Attending Physician, Hospital of the University of Pennsylvania, Philadelphia, Pennsylvania.
Congenital Eyelid Anomalies

Jonathan Kay, M.D.
Staff, Department of Anesthesiology, St. Luke's Medical Center, Milwaukee, Wisconsin.
Anesthetic Considerations for Oculoplastic Surgery: An Update for the 1990s

Michael Kazim, M.D.
Assistant Professor of Clinical Ophthalmology and Clinical Surgery, Columbia University College of Physicians and Surgeons and Columbia-Presbyterian Medical Center, New York, New York.
Neurogenic Tumors

Charles D. Kelman, M.D.
Clinical Professor, New York Medical College, Valhalla; Attending Surgeon, New York Eye and Ear Infirmary, New York, New York.
Autologen: Autologous, Injectable Dermal Collagen

Robert C. Kersten, M.D.
Assistant Professor of Ophthalmology, Department of Ophthalmology, University of Cincinnati College of Medicine, Cincinnati, Ohio.
Congenital Lacrimal Abnormalities

Don O. Kikkawa, M.D.
Assistant Professor and Director of Orbital and Oculoplastics Service, Department of Ophthalmology, University of California, San Diego, LaJolla; Attending Staff, Surgical Service, Veterans Affairs Medical Center, San Diego, California.
Orbital Anatomy and Embryology

Jan W. Kronish, M.D.
Clinical Assistant Professor, Department of Ophthalmology, Bascom Palmer Eye Institute, University of Miami School of Medicine, Miami; Delray Eye Associates, Delray Beach, Florida.
Eyelid and Orbital Considerations in AIDS; Metastatic Tumors

Kurt Laedrach, M.D., D.M.D.
Assistant Professor, University Hospital of Bern, Bern, Switzerland.
Craniofacial Congenital Anomalies: The Subcranial Approach

Brian Leatherbarrow, B.Sc., M.B.Ch.B., F.R.C.S., F.R.C.Ophth.
Honorary Lecturer, University of Manchester; Consultant Ophthalmic, Oculoplastic, and Orbital Surgeon, Manchester Royal Eye Hospital, Manchester, United Kingdom.
Benign Eyelid Tumors

Bradley N. Lemke, M.D.
Clinical Professor, Department of Ophthalmology and Visual Sciences, University of Wisconsin, Madison; Staff, Davis Duehr Dean Clinic, Madison, Wisconsin.
Clinical Eyelid Anatomy; Orbital Anatomy and Embryology

Peter S. Levin, M.D.
Director, Ophthalmic Plastic and Orbital Surgery, Stanford University School of Medicine, Stanford, California.
Orbital Exenteration

Richard D. Lisman, M.D., F.A.C.S.
Clinical Associate Professor of Ophthalmology, New York University School of Medicine; Clinic Chief, Division of Ophthalmic Plastic Surgery, Manhattan Eye and Ear Hospital, New York, New York.
Diagnosis and Management of Sebaceous Gland Carcinoma

Don Liu, M.D.
Associate Professor, Department of Ophthalmology, University of Southern California School of Medicine; Head of Oculoplastics, Doheny Eye Institute, Los Angeles, California.
An Overview: Cultural Background and Anatomic Considerations in the Asian Patient; Asian Blepharoplasty; Eyelid Tumors in Chinese

John A. Long, M.D.
Clinical Assistant Professor, University of Alabama, Birmingham, Alabama.
Entropion

Mahmood F. Mafee, M.D.
Professor of Radiology, University of Illinois at Chicago Medical Center; Director, MRI Center, and Director, Radiology Section, Eye and Ear Infirmary, University of Illinois at Chicago, Chicago, Illinois.
Neuroradiologic Imaging of the Orbit and Globe

Hector M. Marines, M.D.
Assistant Professor of Ophthalmic Plastic and Orbital Surgery, and Ocular Pathology, Department of Ophthalmology, Hospital San Jose, Instituto Tecnologico y de Estudios Superiores de Monterrey; Associate Member, Instituto de Oftalmologia, S.C., Monterrey, N.L. Mexico.
Male Blepharoplasty

Alice Y. Matoba, M.D.
Associate Professor, Baylor College of Medicine; Chief, Ophthalmology Service, Houston Veterans Affairs Medical Center, Houston, Texas.
Conjunctival Procedures for Corneal Disease

Joseph F. Mazza, Jr., M.D.
Private Practice, Ft. Myers, Florida.
Blepharopigmentation: Techniques, Indications, and Comparison of Modalities

Steven A. McCormick, M.D., F.C.A.P.
Associate Professor of Pathology, Ophthalmology and Otolaryngology/Head and Neck Surgery, New York Medical College, Valhalla; Director of Pathology and Laboratory Medicine, New York Eye and Ear Infirmary, New York, New York.
Idiopathic Orbital Inflammation and Lymphoid Tumors of the Orbit

Timothy F. McDevitt, M.D.
Staff Ophthalmologist, Faulkner Institute, Honolulu, Hawaii.
Alternative Techniques of Fat Removal

Michael E. Migliori, M.D., F.A.C.S.
Clinical Assistant Professor of Ophthalmology, Brown University; Director of Ophthalmic Plastic and Reconstructive Surgery, Rhode Island Hospital, Providence, Rhode Island.
Evaluation and Management of the Anophthalmic Socket

James P. Milite, M.D.
Associate Adjunct Attending Ophthalmologist and Fellow in Ophthalmic Pathology, New York Eye and Ear Infirmary, New York, New York.
Idiopathic Orbital Inflammation and Lymphoid Tumors of the Orbit

Neil R. Miller, M.D.
Professor of Neuro-ophthalmology, Johns Hopkins Medical Institutions, Baltimore, Maryland.
Disorders of Eyelid Function Caused by Systemic Disease

Ronald L. Moy, M.D.
Assistant Professer, University of California, Los Angeles, School of Medicine; Director of Dermatologic Surgery, Veterans Affairs Medical Center—West Los Angeles, Los Angeles, California.
Mohs' Surgery for Periorbital Malignancies

Howard Murad, M.D.
Assistant Clinical Professor of Dermatology, University of California, Los Angeles, California.
Chemical Peels

Brent A. Murphy, M.D.
Assistant Professor of Ophthalmology and Director of Ophthalmic Plastic and Orbital Surgery, University of South Alabama College of Medicine, Mobile, Alabama.
Management of Conjunctival Amyloidosis; Kaposi's Sarcoma of the Conjunctiva; Lymphoid Tumors of the Conjunctiva

Marjorie Murphy, M.D.
Former Resident, Wills Eye Hospital, Philadelphia, Pennsylvania.
Lower Eyelid Retraction and Cicatricial Ectropion

Jeffrey A. Nerad, M.D.
Professor of Ophthalmology, University of Iowa College of Medicine; Director, Oculoplastic, Orbital, and Oncology Service, University of Iowa Hospitals and Clinics, Iowa City, Iowa.
Benign Eyelid Tumors; Eyelid Causes of Tearing; Primary Acquired Nasolacrimal Duct Obstruction; Osseointegration for the Exenterated Orbit

Russell W. Neuhaus, M.D.
Clinical Professor of Ophthalmology, University of Texas Health Science Center at San Antonio, San Antonio, Texas.
Eyelid Infections and Inflammations

Nelson Lee Novick, M.D., F.A.C.P., F.A.A.D.
Associate Clinical Professor of Dermatology, Mount Sinai School of Medicine; Associate Attending Physician, Mount Sinai Medical Center, New York, New York.
Total Facial Rejuvenation

Thaddeus S. Nowinski, M.D.
Clinical Associate Professor, Jefferson Medical College; Associate Surgeon, Oculoplastics Service, Wills Eye Hospital, Philadelphia, Pennsylvania.
Anatomy and Physiology of the Lacrimal System

William R. Nunery, M.D., F.A.C.S.
Clinical Associate Professor of Ophthalmology, Indiana University School of Medicine; Staff, Methodist Hospital, Indiana University Hospital, Wishard Hospital, and Meridian Plastic Surgery Center, Indianapolis, Indiana.
Enucleation and Evisceration

Denis M. O'Day, M.D.
Chairman and George Weeks Hale Professor, Vanderbilt University Department of Ophthalmology and Visual Sciences; Professor of Ophthalmology, Vanderbilt University Medical Center, Nashville Veterans Affairs Medical Center, Nashville, Tennessee.
Conjunctival and Limbal Neoplasia: Diagnosis and Management

Brian Patrick O'Donnel, M.D.
Private Practice, Portland, Maine.
Cutaneous and Multisystemic Processes Affecting the Ocular Adnexa

Nita Patel, M.D.
Affiliated Dermatology, Inc., Los Angeles, California.
Chemical Peels

James R. Patrinely, M.D.
Associate Professor of Ophthalmology and Plastic Surgery, Baylor College of Medicine; Clinical Assistant Surgeon of Ophthalmology and Clinical Assistant Professor in the Division of Surgery, Department of Head and Neck Surgery, University of Texas, M.D. Anderson Cancer Center, Houston, Texas.
Male Blepharoplasty

Jay M. Pensler, M.D.
Associate Professor, Northwestern University Medical School; Attending Plastic Surgeon, Children's Memorial Hospital, Evanston Hospital, and Northwestern Memorial Hospital, Chicago, Illinois.
Diagnostic and Presurgical Evaluation of Congenital Craniofacial Anomalies

Roswell R. Pfister, M.D.
Clinical Professor, University of Alabama School of Medicine; Director of Eye Research, Brookwood Medical Center, Birmingham, Alabama.
Chemical and Thermal Injuries of the Cornea and Conjunctiva

Phillip F. Pierce, M.D.
Associate Professor of Medicine and Microbiology, Georgetown University School of Medicine, Washington, D.C.
Infections of the Orbit and Orbital Structures

Holla'e Ploof, B.A.
Director, Training Clinical Electropigmentation, The Holla'e Methode Inc., Tucson, Arizona.
Electropigmentation and the Cosmetic Surgery Patient

Jeffrey C. Popp, M.D., F.A.C.S.
Assistant Clinical Professor and Director, Oculoplastic Orbital Oncology Service, University of Nebraska School of Medicine, Omaha, Nebraska.
Facial Paralysis: Diagnosis and Management

Jeffrey C. Posnick, D.M.D., M.D.
Associate Professor, Division of Plastic Surgery; Department of Periodontics; and Department of Ear, Nose, and Throat, Georgetown University Medical Center, Washington, D.C.
Orbital Deformities: Anterior Cranial Base Approach

David A. B. Price, B.A.
Medical Photographer, David Price Photography, New York, New York.
Photography of the Ophthalmic Plastic Surgery Patient

Peter T. Pugliese, M.D.
Chairman and Chief Scientific Officer, Milmar Research, Inc., Bernville, Pennsylvania.
Lymphatic Drainage Massage

Cynthia Rager, C.P.M.E.
Adjunct Staff, Edison Community College, Ft. Myers, Florida.
Blepharopigmentation: Techniques, Indications, and Comparison of Modalities

Sankaran Rajagopalan, M.D.
Staff, Department of Ophthalmology, University of Maryland School of Medicine, Baltimore, Maryland.
Neoplastic and Related Conditions of the Orbital and Adnexal Structures

Joram Raveh, M.D., D.M.D.
Head and Professor, University Hospital of Bern, Bern, Switzerland.
Craniofacial Congenital Anomalies: The Subcranial Approach

David M. Reifler, M.D., F.A.C.S.
Clinical Associate Professor of Surgery/Ophthalmology, Michigan State University College of Human Medicine (GRAMEC); Attending Physician, Butterworth Hospital and Blodgett Memorial Medical Center, Grand Rapids, Michigan.
Upper Eyelid Blepharoplasty

Daniel Rivlin, M.D.
Chief, Mohs' Surgery Unit, Mt. Sinai Medical Center, Miami Beach, Florida.
Mohs' Surgery for Periorbital Malignancies

Wallace A. Roberts, A.S.E.E.
Electrology Instructor, Newbury College, Brookline, Aquinas College, Milton, and Roberts Institute, Brookline, Massachusetts.
Electrology and Eyebrow Contouring

Merlyn M. Rodrigues, M.D., Ph.D.
Professor, University of Maryland Medical School, Baltimore, Maryland.
Neoplastic and Related Conditions of the Orbital and Adnexal Structures

Geoffrey E. Rose, B.S., M.B.B.S., M.S., M.R.C.P., F.R.C.S., F.R.C.Ophth.
Honorary Lecturer in Ophthalmology, Institute of Ophthalmology, University of London; Consultant Ophthalmic Surgeon, Moorfields Eye Hospital, London; Honorary Consultant Ophthalmic Surgeon, Hospital for Sick Children, London, United Kingdom, and Royal Victoria Hospital, Belfast, Northern Ireland.
Clinical Examination in Orbital Disease; Lacrimal Gland Neoplasia

Marian Rubenfeld, M.D.,Ph.D.
Clinical Associate Professor, Department of Ophthalmology, University of Minnesota School of Medicine; Subsection Chief, Minneapolis Veterans Affairs Medical Center, Minneapolis, Minnesota.
Neuro-ophthalmic Considerations in Orbital Disease

Peter A.D. Rubin, M.D.
Assistant Professor, Department of Ophthalmology, Harvard Medical School; Director, Eye Plastics and Orbital Surgery, Massachusetts Eye and Ear Infirmary, Boston, Massachusetts.
Pigmented Conjunctival Neoplasms

Steven J. Rubin, M.D.
Assistant Professor, Department of Radiation and Cellular Oncology, University of Chicago School of Medicine; Instructor, University of Illinois at Chicago, Chicago, Illinois.
Radiation Therapy in Orbital Disease

Evan H. Sacks, M.D.
Assistant Attending Physician, Manhattan Eye, Ear and Throat Hospital and Beth Israel Medical Center, New York, New York.
Diagnosis and Management of Sebaceous Gland Carcinoma

Curt P. Samlaska, M.D.
Assistant Professor of Medicine, University of Hawaii; Chief, Dermatology Service, Tripler Army Medical Center, Honolulu, Hawaii.
Cutaneous and Multisystemic Processes Affecting the Ocular Adnexa

Jeffrey Schiller, M.D.
Professor of Ophthalmology, Chairman of Ophthalmology University "Federico II" of Naples School of Medicine, Institute of Ophthalmology, Naples, Italy.
Translator for *Surgical Approaches to the Orbit; Anterior, Medial, Lateral, and Combined Surgical Approaches for Orbital Tumor Resection*

Norman Shorr, M.D., F.A.C.S.
Clinical Professor of Ophthalmology and Director, Fellowship in Orbital and Ophthalmic Plastic and Reconstructive Surgery, Jules Stein Eye Institute, University of California, Los Angeles, Los Angeles, California.
Suborbital Augmentation

Joseph P. Shovlin, M.D.
Associate in Ophthalmology; Director, Division of Ophthalmic Plastic and Reconstructive Surgery, Geisinger Medical Center, Danville, Pennsylvania.
Clinical Eyelid Anatomy; Amyloidosis and Idiopathic Orbital Conditions

David I. Silbert, M.D.
Active Staff, Lancaster General Hospital, Lancaster; and Courtesy Staff, Wills Eye Hospital, Philadelphia; Lancaster General Hospital, Lancaster; and Wills Eye Hospital, Philadelphia, Pennsylvania.
Malignant Eyelid and Orbital Tumors

Mary A. Stefanyszyn, M.D.
Assistant Professor, University of Pennsylvania Hospital; Clinical Instructor, Thomas Jefferson University; Associate Surgeon, Wills Eye Hospital, Lankenau Hospital, and Thomas Jefferson University Hospital, Philadelphia; Associate Surgeon, Lankenau Hospital, Wynnewood, Pennsylvania.
Malignant Eyelid and Orbital Tumors

Kenneth D. Steinsapir, M.D.
Visiting Assistant Professor of Ophthalmology, Jules Stein Eye Institute, University of California, Los Angeles, School of Medicine, Los Angeles, California.
Suborbital Augmentation

Darlene P. Story, B.A.
President, Lasting Impression I, Inc., Englewood, New Jersey.
Micropigmentation and the Patient with Facial Burn and Facial Reconstruction

Richard W. Story, B.A.
Lasting Impression I, Inc., Englewood, New Jersey.
Micropigmentation and the Patient with Facial Burn and Facial Reconstruction

Gerald G. Striph, M.D.
Clinical Assistant Professor, Medical College of Ohio, Toledo, Ohio.
Disorders of Eyelid Function Caused by Systemic Disease

Nancy C. Swartz, M.D.
Instructor, Wills Eye Hospital, Philadelphia, Pennsylvania.
Lower Eyelid Retraction and Cicatricial Ectropion

Myron Tanenbaum, M.D., F.A.C.S.
Assistant Clinical Professor, Department of Ophthalmology, Bascom Palmer Eye Institute, University of Miami School of Medicine, Miami, Florida.
Orbital Decompression for Graves' Orbitopathy

Thierry Vuillemin, M.D., D.M.D.
Assistant Professor, University Hospital of Bern, Bern, Switzerland.
Craniofacial Congenital Anomalies: The Subcranial Approach

Susanne S. Warfield, B.S.
President, Paramedical Consultants, Inc., Ridgewood, New Jersey.
The Practical Application of Aestheticians in the Plastic and Reconstructive Surgeon's Office

Robert A. Weiss, M.D.
Clinical Associate Professor of Ophthalmology, Oculoplastic and Reconstructive Surgery and Ophthalmic Oncology, University of Illinois at Chicago and the Chicago Eye Institute, Chicago, Illinois.
Brow Ptosis; Harvesting and Use of Biological Tissue Grafts

Ralph E. Wesley, M.D.
Director, Ophthalmic Plastic and Orbital Surgery and Clinical Professor of Ophthalmology, Vanderbilt University Medical Center; Chief of Ophthalmology, Baptist Medical Center, Nashville, Tennessee.
Conjunctiva: Structure and Function; Basic Techniques of Conjunctival Surgery; Management of Conjunctival Amyloidosis; Kaposi's Sarcoma of the Conjunctiva; Lymphoid Tumors of the Conjunctiva; Treatment of Squamous Papillomas of the Conjunctiva; Management of Conjunctival Prolapse; Conjunctival Dermolipoma Surgery

William White, M.D.
Clinical Instructor of Ophthalmology, Children's Mercy Hospital, University of Missouri; Staff, Baptist Medical Center, Kansas City, Missouri.
Disorders of the Canaliculus and Punctum

Fred M. Wilson II, M.D.
Professor of Ophthalmology, Department of Ophthalmology, Indiana University School of Medicine, Indianapolis, Indiana.
Management of Pterygia

Jonathan D. Wirtschafter, M.D.
Professor, Departments of Ophthalmology, Neurology, and Neurosurgery; Director, Neuro-ophthalmology, Orbit, and Oculoplastics Service, University of Minnesota, Minneapolis, Minnesota.
Neuro-ophthalmic Considerations in Orbital Disease

Ted H. Wojno, M.D.
Associate Professor of Ophthalmology, Emory University School of Medicine; Director of Oculoplastic and Orbital Surgery, Emory Clinic, Atlanta, Georgia.
Preoperative Evaluation; Alternative Techniques of Fat Removal; Management of Blepharoplasty Complications; Indications for Orbital Surgery; Operative Principles and Instrumentation

John J. Woog, M.D.
Clinical Associate Professor, Tufts University School of Medicine; Clinical Instructor, Harvard Medical School; Co-Director, Eye Plastics and Orbit Service, New England Eye Center; Staff, Ophthalmic Consultants of Boston, Boston, Massachusetts.
Basic Surgical Techniques, Technology, and Wound Repair; Disorders of the Canaliculus and Punctum

Allan E. Wulc, M.D., F.A.C.S.
Assistant Professor and Director, Oculoplastic Orbital Service, Scheie Eye Institute, University of Pennsylvania School of Medicine, Philadelphia, Pennsylvania.
Facial Paralysis: Diagnosis and Management

Nai Jiang Xu, M.D.
Professor, Division of Ophthalmic Plastic and Reconstructive Surgery, Ninth People's Hospital, Shanghai, China.
Eyelid Tumors in Chinese

Guang-Xi Zhao, M.D.
Professor of Ophthalmology, Beijing Medical University; Vice Chief Editor, Chinese Language Edition of *Archives of Ophthalmology*; Editor, *Chinese Journal of Ophthalmology*, Beijing, China.
Eyelid Tumors in Chinese

Foreword

It has become obvious that the borders of our oculoplastic surgery discipline have now been expanded further with this magnum opus by Stephen Bosniak. Not too long ago an authoritative text on ophthalmic plastic surgery would be considered complete if it contained the requisite number of chapters dealing with the standard periorbital problems of ectropion, entropion, ptosis, and lid reconstruction. *Principles and Practice of Ophthalmic Plastic and Reconstructive Surgery*'s 112 chapters force us to realize that from now on much more will be expected of an oculoplastic textbook and an oculoplastic surgeon than previously.

The first section teaches us that, above all, we oculoplastic surgeons are physicians and thus must be diagnostically alert to the periorbital manifestations of systemic disease. Conjunctiva, the "Rodney Dangerfield" of the orbit because it "gets no respect," is handsomely treated in the second section with 100 pages of text, starting with an elegantly written chapter on anatomy. The third and fourth sections, which discuss the eyelids, are textbooks within themselves, especially the relevant sections on cosmetic procedures. In this decade of declining remuneration by third party insurers, cosmetic oculoplastic surgery, a "fee-for-service business," is becoming more a part of everyone's practice—patients also desire this kind of surgery more now then ever before. As such, the chapters on preoperative and postoperative aesthetics will be somewhat of a surprise to most ophthalmologists, but they should be read. Section 5 is a well-written, fascinating glimpse into the Eastern mind and culture with respect to eyelid surgery and, together with other chapters in this section, makes us realize that our practice will be more internationally based in future years.

The closing sections on lacrimal surgery, orbital disease and fractures, and the ophthalmic socket are updated and germane to modern oculoplastic surgery. The final small section of craniofacial disorders is excellent, but proportional in length to its relevance in our specialty.

It is often said that a multidiscipline-author book suffers from uneven writing, inconsistent illustration material, and the inability to mesh different styles of writing, not to mention the archenemy of all textbooks—repetition. Dr. Bosniak's book has none of this. On the other hand, obvious advantages of a multiauthor text show in that different cross sections of oculoplastic surgery practice are presented in one source—how else can you find a chapter written by authors in private practice who see the "regular" patients of an unskewed population and thus provide insight to those who work "in the trenches?" At the same time, institutional studies have great merit in that by analyzing referred series of patients they bring together the experience of professors combined.

To become an oculoplastic surgeon of the 1990s, we can no longer be content that we know several versions of operations for entropion or a handful of classic techniques for ptosis correction. We must have more than a passing knowledge of the use of endoscopic surgery, and we certainly must know of the indications for

diagnostic procedures like flow cytometry in tumor analysis. With the influx of immigrants we must be aware of the social and cultural differences of our patients, and we must be ready to diagnose the systemic diseases that many of the immigrants bring with them. It also can be said that if we wish to survive in the era of managed care, we all must become more familiar with cosmetic eyelid surgery, which does not just mean "how to do a blepharoplasty," but the indications for brow lifting and the different ways to do it, cosmetology consultation, and even the method for performing a skin peel.

Principles and Practice of Ophthalmic Plastic and Reconstructive Surgery will never be an obsolete book. The wealth of information contained herein is encyclopedic and well referenced. With its multitude of illustrations it presents a systematized approach to oculoplastic surgery, and many of us will spend the better part of our remaining careers attempting to read and retain all the facts contained herein.

Dr. Bosniak and all the section editors have truly left what Longfellow penned as "footprints in the sands of time."

MICHAEL A. CALLAHAN, M.D.

Preface

Writing books and sharing information with physicians and surgeons who have interests in common with me have been driving forces in my life. W.B. Saunders Company has provided me with the opportunity to present a magnum opus. With this book, I have had the luxury and pleasure of working with Giulio Bonavolontà, Robert Goldberg, Russell Gonnering, James Karesh, Don Liu, Jeffrey Nerad, Robert Weiss, Ralph Wesley, and Ted Wojno— a new generation of creative minds.

During the years spent organizing and compiling this project, dramatic advances in technology have become available to the ophthalmologist. Ophthalmic plastic and reconstructive surgeons have sought the most effective and appropriate applications of this technology. In this book we have strived to incorporate these latest advances and to describe the indications for their use.

In *Principles and Practice of Ophthalmic Plastic and Reconstructive Surgery,* we have emphasized an approach to the patient as a whole. We have allotted a complete section to systemic diseases and a discussion of systemic perioperative preparation of the surgical patient, including postoperative treatment to enhance and accelerate wound healing. Current and historical surgical advances in eyelid reconstruction, ptosis correction, and entropion and ectropion repair are thoroughly presented and documented. A separate section on conjunctival diseases and surgery has been included to highlight their importance and the necessity for alternative techniques in handling conjunctival tissue. The orbital section is voluminous to accommodate the current advanced status of diagnosing and documenting orbital pathology. The anatomic and physiologic distinctions of ethnic ophthalmic patients are also represented in a separate section. In addition, the significance of a multidisciplinary approach to the orbit in selected cases is clearly established. The state-of-the-art techniques of socket reconstruction are also presented in a separate section.

Ophthalmic plastic surgeons are endeavoring to competitively enter into the arena of aesthetic surgery. The section on cosmetic surgery not only provides the surgical principles but also introduces adjunctive techniques essential to a cosmetic surgical practice: topical home care products, in-office peeling agents, camouflage make-up, and lymphatic drainage massage. New surgical modalities have been introduced: radiosurgery and ultra-pulse laser surgery.

I am joined with the section editors in the commitment to a totally new presentation of the state-of-the-art ophthalmic plastic surgery. Not only is the content updated but the presentation is revitalized. The two-volume presentation of the text lends itself to easy accessibility and logical organization of material.

STEPHEN BOSNIAK

Acknowledgments

This book would not have been possible without the diligence of the section editors and authors. Our editors at W.B. Saunders, Nellie McGrew and Kim Kist, have facilitated and coordinated this complex project. Drs. Marian Cantisano Zilkha, Charles Crane, and Ferdinand Tan have been of invaluable assistance in the preparation, editing, and proofreading of the manuscripts. I also would like to thank my office staff, Barbara Bozzone, Sharon Murphy, June Hummel, and Rene Harris, for their secretarial support.

S.B.

Contents

VOLUME 1

SECTION I

Orbital and Periorbital Manifestations of Systemic Diseases 1

James W. Karesh

Introduction 1

James W. Karesh

CHAPTER 1

Cutaneous and Multisystemic Processes Affecting the Ocular Adnexa 3

Curt P. Samlaska, Brian Patrick O'Donnel, and William D. James

CHAPTER 2

Neoplastic and Related Conditions of the Orbital and Adnexal Structures 53

Merlyn M. Rodrigues, Sankaran Rajagopalan, Kelly Jones, and James W. Karesh

CHAPTER 3

Disorders of Eyelid Function Caused by Systemic Disease 72

Gerald G. Striph and Neil R. Miller

CHAPTER 4

Ocular Manifestations of Systemic Immune Disease 94

John C. Baer and Ramzi K. Hemady

Ocular Manifestations of Systemic Endocrine Diseases 121

CHAPTER 5

Diagnosis and Management of Thyrotoxicosis 121

Leonard P. Kapcala

CHAPTER 6

Diagnosis and Management of Hyperparathyroidism 132

Leonard P. Kapcala

CHAPTER 7

The Ocular Manifestations of Non–Thyroid-Related Endocrine Disease 137

James W. Karesh

CHAPTER 8

Infections of the Orbit and Orbital Structures 146

Phillip F. Pierce

SECTION II

Conjunctiva 157

Ralph E. Wesley

Introduction 157

Ralph E. Wesley

CHAPTER 9

Conjunctiva: Structure and Function 159

Harvey P. Cole III and Ralph E. Wesley

CHAPTER 10

Basic Techniques of Conjunctival Surgery 163

Harvey P. Cole III and Ralph E. Wesley

CHAPTER 11

Replacement of Conjunctival Mucous Membrane 170

Jonathan J. Dutton

CHAPTER 12

Pigmented Conjunctival Neoplasms 178

M. Ronan Conlon and Peter A. D. Rubin

CHAPTER 13

Diagnosis and Management of Sebaceous Gland Carcinoma 190

Evan H. Sacks and Richard D. Lisman

CHAPTER 14

Surgical Intervention in Conjunction with Medical Treatment of Cicatricial Pemphigoid 196

James C. Fleming and Richard C. Cape

CHAPTER 15

Tarsoconjunctival Polishing with Mucous Membrane Grafting for Cicatricial Entropion and Trichiasis 203

William P. Chen

CHAPTER 16
Management of Pterygia 208
Robert D. Deitch, Jr., and Fred M. Wilson II

CHAPTER 17
Chemical and Thermal Injuries of the Cornea and Conjunctiva 222
Roswell R. Pfister

CHAPTER 18
Conjunctival and Limbal Neoplasia: Diagnosis and Management . . . 231
Anne R. Horan and Denis M. O'Day

CHAPTER 19
Management of Conjunctival Amyloidosis 238
Brent A. Murphy and Ralph E. Wesley

CHAPTER 20
Kaposi's Sarcoma of the Conjunctiva 242
Brent A. Murphy and Ralph E. Wesley

CHAPTER 21
Lymphoid Tumors of the Conjunctiva 244
Brent A. Murphy and Ralph E. Wesley

CHAPTER 22
Conjunctival Procedures for Corneal Disease 248
Alice Y. Matoba

CHAPTER 23
Treatment of Squamous Papillomas of the Conjunctiva 251
Ralph E. Wesley and Harvey P. Cole III

CHAPTER 24
Management of Conjunctival Prolapse 253
Ralph E. Wesley

CHAPTER 25
Conjunctival Dermolipoma Surgery 255
Ralph E. Wesley

SECTION III
Eyelids 259
Robert Alan Goldberg and Russell S. Gonnering
Introduction 259
Robert Alan Goldberg and Russell S. Gonnering
Basic Sciences 261

CHAPTER 26
Clinical Eyelid Anatomy 261
Joseph P. Shovlin and Bradley N. Lemke

CHAPTER 27
Basic Surgical Techniques, Technology, and Wound Repair 281
David B. Christie and John J. Woog

CHAPTER 28
Anesthetic Considerations for Oculoplastic Surgery: An Update for the 1990s 294
Jonathan Kay

CHAPTER 29
Malignant Eyelid and Orbital Tumors 300
Mary A. Stefanyszyn and David I. Silbert

Clinical Sciences 307

CHAPTER 30
Eyelid Infections and Inflammations 307
Constance L. Fry and Russell W. Neuhaus

CHAPTER 31
Benign Eyelid Tumors 323
M. Ronan Conlon, Brian Leatherbarrow, and Jeffrey A. Nerad

CHAPTER 32
Malignant Epithelial Eyelid Tumors 342
Marcos T. Doxanas

CHAPTER 33
Mohs' Surgery for Periorbital Malignancies 352
Daniel Rivlin and Ronald L. Moy

CHAPTER 34
Reconstruction of the Upper Eyelid 356
David R. Jordan

CHAPTER 35
Medial Canthal Reconstruction 387
Roger A. Dailey and Diana Habrich

CHAPTER 36
Reconstruction of the Lower Eyelid and Lateral Canthus 400
Steven C. Dresner

CHAPTER 37
Congenital Eyelid Anomalies 407
Jill A. Foster and James A. Katowitz

CHAPTER 38
Entropion 413
John A. Long and Robert Alan Goldberg

CHAPTER 39
Involutional and Paralytic Ectropion 422
Steven M. Gilbard

CHAPTER 40
Lower Eyelid Retraction and Cicatricial Ectropion 438
Nancy C. Swartz, Marjorie Murphy, and Marc S. Cohen

Foreword

It has become obvious that the borders of our oculoplastic surgery discipline have now been expanded further with this magnum opus by Stephen Bosniak. Not too long ago an authoritative text on ophthalmic plastic surgery would be considered complete if it contained the requisite number of chapters dealing with the standard periorbital problems of ectropion, entropion, ptosis, and lid reconstruction. *Principles and Practice of Ophthalmic Plastic and Reconstructive Surgery*'s 112 chapters force us to realize that from now on much more will be expected of an oculoplastic textbook and an oculoplastic surgeon than previously.

The first section teaches us that, above all, we oculoplastic surgeons are physicians and thus must be diagnostically alert to the periorbital manifestations of systemic disease. Conjunctiva, the "Rodney Dangerfield" of the orbit because it "gets no respect," is handsomely treated in the second section with 100 pages of text, starting with an elegantly written chapter on anatomy. The third and fourth sections, which discuss the eyelids, are textbooks within themselves, especially the relevant sections on cosmetic procedures. In this decade of declining remuneration by third party insurers, cosmetic oculoplastic surgery, a "fee-for-service business," is becoming more a part of everyone's practice—patients also desire this kind of surgery more now then ever before. As such, the chapters on preoperative and postoperative aesthetics will be somewhat of a surprise to most ophthalmologists, but they should be read. Section 5 is a well-written, fascinating glimpse into the Eastern mind and culture with respect to eyelid surgery and, together with other chapters in this section, makes us realize that our practice will be more internationally based in future years.

The closing sections on lacrimal surgery, orbital disease and fractures, and the ophthalmic socket are updated and germane to modern oculoplastic surgery. The final small section of craniofacial disorders is excellent, but proportional in length to its relevance in our specialty.

It is often said that a multidiscipline-author book suffers from uneven writing, inconsistent illustration material, and the inability to mesh different styles of writing, not to mention the archenemy of all textbooks—repetition. Dr. Bosniak's book has none of this. On the other hand, obvious advantages of a multiauthor text show in that different cross sections of oculoplastic surgery practice are presented in one source—how else can you find a chapter written by authors in private practice who see the "regular" patients of an unskewed population and thus provide insight to those who work "in the trenches?" At the same time, institutional studies have great merit in that by analyzing referred series of patients they bring together the experience of professors combined.

To become an oculoplastic surgeon of the 1990s, we can no longer be content that we know several versions of operations for entropion or a handful of classic techniques for ptosis correction. We must have more than a passing knowledge of the use of endoscopic surgery, and we certainly must know of the indications for

diagnostic procedures like flow cytometry in tumor analysis. With the influx of immigrants we must be aware of the social and cultural differences of our patients, and we must be ready to diagnose the systemic diseases that many of the immigrants bring with them. It also can be said that if we wish to survive in the era of managed care, we all must become more familiar with cosmetic eyelid surgery, which does not just mean "how to do a blepharoplasty," but the indications for brow lifting and the different ways to do it, cosmetology consultation, and even the method for performing a skin peel.

Principles and Practice of Ophthalmic Plastic and Reconstructive Surgery will never be an obsolete book. The wealth of information contained herein is encyclopedic and well referenced. With its multitude of illustrations it presents a systematized approach to oculoplastic surgery, and many of us will spend the better part of our remaining careers attempting to read and retain all the facts contained herein.

Dr. Bosniak and all the section editors have truly left what Longfellow penned as "footprints in the sands of time."

MICHAEL A. CALLAHAN, M.D.

CHAPTER 41
Aponeurotic Ptosis 447
Jonathan Christenbury

CHAPTER 42
Eyelid Trauma 452
Russell S. Gonnering

CHAPTER 43
Facial Paralysis: Diagnosis and Management 465
Lawrence F. Handler, Steven L. Galetta, Allan E. Wulc, and Jeffrey C. Popp

CHAPTER 44
Suborbital Augmentation 484
Kenneth D. Steinsapir and Norman Shorr

CHAPTER 45
Essential Blepharospasm and Hemifacial Spasm 504
John B. Holds

CHAPTER 46
The Eyelids in Graves' Ophthalmopathy 514
George B. Bartley

CHAPTER 47
Eyelid and Orbital Considerations in AIDS 525
Jan W. Kronish

CHAPTER 48
Micropigmentation and the Patient with Facial Burn and Facial Reconstruction 535
Richard W. Story and Darlene P. Story

SECTION IV
Cosmetic Surgery 543
Ted H. Wojno and Stephen Bosniak
Introduction 543
Stephen Bosniak

CHAPTER 49
Preoperative Evaluation 545
Ted H. Wojno

CHAPTER 50
Photography of the Ophthalmic Plastic Surgery Patient 551
David A. B. Price

CHAPTER 51
Total Facial Rejuvenation 560
Nelson Lee Novick

CHAPTER 52
The Practical Application of Aestheticians in the Plastic and Reconstructive Surgeon's Office 573
Susanne S. Warfield

CHAPTER 53
The Role of the Aesthetician Before and After Surgery 576
Catherine Atzen

CHAPTER 54
Brow Ptosis 578
Robert A. Weiss

CHAPTER 55
Electrology and Eyebrow Contouring 589
Wallace A. Roberts and Cora Buggea

CHAPTER 56
Upper Eyelid Blepharoplasty 596
David M. Reifler

CHAPTER 57
Lower Eyelid Blepharoplasty 617
Philip L. Custer

CHAPTER 58
Transconjunctival Lower Blepharoplasty 626
Robert Alan Goldberg, Henry I. Baylis, and Stacia H. Goldey

CHAPTER 59
Male Blepharoplasty 632
Hector M. Marines and James R. Patrinely

CHAPTER 60
Alternative Techniques of Fat Removal 638
Stephen Bosniak, Timothy F. McDevitt, and Ted H. Wojno

CHAPTER 61
Management of Blepharoplasty Complications 643
Ted H. Wojno

CHAPTER 62
Lymphatic Drainage Massage 651
Peter T. Pugliese and Linda Garofallou

CHAPTER 63
Principles of Camouflage Make-up and the Postoperative Patient . . 657
Annette Hanson and Nancy Dugan

CHAPTER 64
Chemical Peels 662
Howard Murad and Nita Patel

CHAPTER 65
Autologen: Autologous, Injectable Dermal Collagen 670
Dale P. DeVore, Charles D. Kelman, Steven Fagien, and Phillip Casson

CHAPTER 66
Electropigmentation and the Cosmetic Surgery Patient 676
Holla'e Ploof

CHAPTER 67
Blepharopigmentation: Techniques, Indications, and Comparison of Modalities . . . 682
Joseph F. Mazza, Jr., and Cynthia Rager

VOLUME 2

SECTION V
Ethnic Ophthalmic Plastic Surgery . . . 689
Don Liu
Introduction . . . 689
Don Liu

CHAPTER 68
An Overview: Cultural Background and Anatomic Considerations in the Asian Patient . . . 691
Don Liu

CHAPTER 69
Asian Blepharoplasty . . . 702
Don Liu

CHAPTER 70
Considerations for Oculoplastic Surgery in the African American Patient . . . 715
Tamara R. Fountain

CHAPTER 71
Auricular Acupuncture in the Treatment of Blepharospasm . . . 718
Chieh Chung and Wen Ming Hsu

CHAPTER 72
Eyelid Tumors . . . 721
Don Liu, Guang-Xi Zhao, and Nai Jiang Xu

SECTION VI
Lacrimal Surgery . . . 729
Jeffrey A. Nerad
Introduction . . . 729
Jeffrey A. Nerad

CHAPTER 73
Anatomy and Physiology of the Lacrimal System . . . 731
Thaddeus S. Nowinski

CHAPTER 74
Evaluation of the Tearing Patient . . . 748
David R. Jordan

CHAPTER 75
Eyelid Causes of Tearing . . . 762
Jeffrey A. Nerad

CHAPTER 76
Congenital Lacrimal Abnormalities . . . 777
Robert C. Kersten

CHAPTER 77
Primary Acquired Nasolacrimal Duct Obstruction . . . 784
Keith D. Carter and Jeffrey A. Nerad

CHAPTER 78
Secondary Acquired Lacrimal Drainage Obstruction . . . 797
George B. Bartley

CHAPTER 79
Disorders of the Canaliculus and Punctum . . . 821
William White and John J. Woog

SECTION VII
The Orbit . . . 835
Robert A. Weiss and Giulio Bonavolontà
Introduction . . . 835
Robert A. Weiss and Giulio Bonavolontà

CHAPTER 80
Orbital Anatomy and Embryology . . . 837
Don O. Kikkawa and Bradley N. Lemke

CHAPTER 81
Epidemiology of Orbital Pathology . . . 853
Carlo de Conciliis

CHAPTER 82
Clinical Examination in Orbital Disease . . . 860
Geoffrey E. Rose

CHAPTER 83
Neuro-ophthalmic Considerations in Orbital Disease . . . 874
Marian Rubenfeld and Jonathan D. Wirtschafter

CHAPTER 84
Neuroradiologic Imaging of the Orbit and Globe . . . 885
Mahmood F. Mafee

CHAPTER 85
Vascular Tumors of the Orbit . . . 913
Barrett G. Haik and Holly Gore

Orbital Inflammatory Disorders . . . 935

CHAPTER 86
The Role of Paranasal Sinus Disease in Orbital Cellulitis . . . 935
John B. Holds

CHAPTER 87
Amyloidosis and Idiopathic Orbital Conditions . . . 944
Joseph P. Shovlin

CHAPTER 88
Idiopathic Orbital Inflammation and Lymphoid Tumors of the Orbit . . . 952
James P. Milite and Steven A. McCormick

CHAPTER 89
Pseudotumors 964
Will Harms

CHAPTER 90
Orbital Decompression for Graves' Orbitopathy 967
Myron Tanenbaum

Orbital and Periorbital Neoplasia 983

CHAPTER 91
Neurogenic Tumors 983
Michael Kazim and Jeffrey Bruce

CHAPTER 92
Mesenchymal and Fibro-osseous Tumors 994
Michael Clarke

CHAPTER 93
Lacrimal Gland Neoplasia 999
Geoffrey E. Rose

CHAPTER 94
Metastatic Tumors 1007
Jan W. Kronish

CHAPTER 95
Ophthalmic Manifestations of Mucoceles 1015
Barrett G. Haik and Ronald G. Amedee

CHAPTER 96
Radiation Therapy in Orbital Disease 1023
Steven J. Rubin

Orbital Surgery 1035

CHAPTER 97
Enucleation and Evisceration 1035
William R. Nunery and William P. Chen

CHAPTER 98
Indications for Orbital Surgery 1046
Ted H. Wojno

CHAPTER 99
Operative Principles and Instrumentation 1048
Ted H. Wojno

CHAPTER 100
Surgical Approaches to the Orbit 1050
Giulio Bonavolontà

CHAPTER 101
Optic Nerve Sheath Decompression 1056
Marc S. Cohen

CHAPTER 102
Anterior, Medial, Lateral, and Combined Surgical Approaches for Orbital Tumor Resection 1060
Giulio Bonavolontà

CHAPTER 103
Orbital Exenteration 1070
Peter S. Levin

CHAPTER 104
Harvesting and Use of Biological Tissue Grafts 1077
Craig D. Friedman, Fred S. Bodker, and Robert A. Weiss

Orbital Trauma 1085

CHAPTER 105
Orbital Fractures 1085
Sara A. Kaltreider

SECTION VIII
Anophthalmic Socket 1103
Robert A. Weiss and Stephen Bosniak

CHAPTER 106
Evaluation and Management of the Anophthalmic Socket 1105
Michael E. Migliori

CHAPTER 107
The Perfect Socket: The Ocularist's View 1127
Walter J. Johnson

CHAPTER 108
Orbital Prostheses 1134
Gregory G. Gion

CHAPTER 109
Osseointegration for the Exenterated Orbit 1150
Jeffrey A. Nerad

SECTION IX
Craniofacial Deformities 1161
Robert A. Weiss

CHAPTER 110
Craniofacial Congenital Anomalies: The Subcranial Approach 1163
Joram Raveh, Kurt Laedrach, and Thierry Vuillemin

CHAPTER 111
Diagnostic and Presurgical Evaluation of Congenital Craniofacial Anomalies 1178
Jay M. Pensler

CHAPTER 112
Orbital Deformities: Anterior Cranial Base Approach 1187
Jeffrey C. Posnick

Index i

SECTION V

Ethnic Ophthalmic Plastic Surgery

SECTION EDITOR

Don Liu

Introduction

Don Liu

As we approach the twenty-first century, the buzz word is "global," whether dealing with geopolitical issues, economic competition, or scientific cooperation. It is no different for medicine. To practice good medicine, which is an art as a science, the physician's understanding of the patient's particular cultural background greatly facilitates communication, and knowledge of diseases unique to a region and of conditions especially prevalent in a group of people definitely aids in establishing a diagnosis and in making therapeutic decisions.

Demographically, the population of the United States is changing dramatically, with immigrants from the Asian-Pacific region leading the influx. Economically, also, the Pacific Rim has been the most vibrant and energetic region. In other words, the world is getting smaller and our contact with people from other parts of the world and of different cultural backgrounds is increasing. American ophthalmologists routinely care for patients of diverse backgrounds, but with the current immigration trend and the geopolitical and economic development of many Asian countries, it is especially important that practicing ophthalmologists understand the anatomic differences and appreciate the cultural background and unique needs of these people.

This section is included to meet these needs. Chapter 68, "An Overview: Cultural Background and Anatomic Differences in the Asian Patient," introduces the reader to the centuries-old practice of traditional Chinese medicine. Fact is separated from myth, and the readers are encouraged to examine these concepts with an open mind. Valuable information on Asian anatomy is presented that is rarely known outside Chinese literature. Some very helpful and practical tips for treating and simply communicating with Asian patients are also offered. Similarly, Chapter 72 on eyelid tumors gives the reader a new perspective and emphasizes the very different incidence rates of various tumors in the Chinese population. Some surgical techniques that have been found to be particularly useful and effective when dealing with the unique anatomy of Chinese patients are also discussed.

Chapter 69 on Asian blepharoplasty is most authoritative, coauthored by some of the most respected and experienced surgeons in that part of the world. The sociopsychological aspects and the nuances of the surgical techniques are masterfully presented. To illustrate the point that global thinking requires bridging cultural gaps, in both space and time, Chapter 71 on the treatment of blepharospasm by means of acupuncture is most appropriate. This procedure, which is time honored in the Orient but often looked on askance in the West, provides ophthalmologists and their patients an alternative treatment and suggests a challenging research project for academicians.

I am sure that discriminating readers will find these chapters fascinating to read and most helpful in their clinical practice of ophthalmic plastic and reconstructive surgery.

CHAPTER 68

An Overview: Cultural Background and Anatomic Considerations in the Asian Patient

Don Liu

With the lowering of political barriers and changes toward more worldwide economic parity, the demographics of the United States are undergoing profound changes. Asian-Americans, for over 100 years a large ethnic minority in certain areas of the United States, are now among the fastest growing ethnic minority in this country. Furthermore, newly arrived immigrants from the Pacific Rim countries account for the recent large increase, in contrast to the higher birth rates that account for increases in some other ethnic groups. These newcomers have brought to this country their values, customs, and philosophies. In addition to their obviously different physical appearance and subtle anatomic variations, there are also differences in their views of and approaches to health care, which present new challenges to clinicians born and trained in the United States. An understanding of the patient's needs, perspective, and expectations is of great help to any physician attending the patient, and an understanding of the patient's cultural background allows for more empathy and better communication. In this chapter an overview is provided of the Asian culture and philosophy as it affects the approach to health care of these patients and some of the subtle anatomic differences that the physician may encounter are discussed.

Asian patients are no different from any others when it comes to their human nature and basic needs. Most of them are loyal and cooperative patients, follow their physician's directions faithfully, and show great appreciation. On the other hand, a few can be very difficult to deal with; they may be noncompliant or demanding and may go from office to office doctor shopping. These differences, to a large extent, depend on the individual's personality, educational level, and socioeconomic background. Regardless of ethnicity, when the patient is told that the diagnosis is life threatening or will result in blindness, there are four stages of psychiatric adjustment: shock, denial, anger, and acceptance. Despite these similarities, however, there are indeed some obvious and some subtle behavioral differences between Asian patients and American patients. These differences are especially apparent when it becomes awkward, uncomfortable, or even stressful—for patient and surgeon. If the physician is offended, or even worse, displays a loss of temper, the patient's confidence may be lost. To better understand these differences, and to avoid the pitfalls that can result, the patient's cultural background must be taken into consideration. As a general rule, a patient who is a newly arrived immigrant can be expected to be deeply rooted in the traditions and beliefs of his or her country of birth. On the other hand, when the patient has been in this country (or some other Western country) for a long time or is "second generation" and has become Americanized, many of these traditions and beliefs may be just as foreign to the patient as they are to the physician.

Almost all Asian countries have been influenced, to one degree or another, by China and its culture. Taoism, Confucianism, and Buddhism, the guiding forces of the Chinese way of life, have greatly influenced the lives of all Asians; although regional variations and interpretations are evident, the general principles apply. In other words, regardless of national origin, ethnicity, and religious preference, much of the way of thinking, customs, traditions, behaviors, and values is essentially the same. For example, both Taoist and Confucian scholars emphasize reverence for ancestors and the aged; according to traditional teachings, ancestors are the origin of our being and age implies experience and wisdom. Thus age, per se, is a status symbol. Understandably, Asian patients prefer older physicians; to them, the older the physician, the more experienced. Furthermore, coming from a traditionally patriarchal society, Asians tend to prefer male physicians. When a patient of Asian origin is referred to a physician, they each may experience any of various scenarios. In the "worst case" scenario, a 71-year-old Chinese man is referred for surgery to a 32-year-old female urologist. But in the majority of cases, one of the following two scenarios will take place. In the first, the patient is afraid of surgery and is not willing to accept such a suggestion. The patient may not flatly refuse surgery but will certainly show signs of hesitation, perhaps politely inquiring about alternative treatment plans (e.g., is there a medicine or a shot that can be taken, a dietary regimen, an exercise scheme, an acupuncture treatment, or even radiation therapy that can yield the same result as surgery). In short, the patient does not want to have surgery and is suggesting everything possible to avoid it. This should not be taken personally by the physician; such behavior can be explained easily by the patient's belief in Confucian values, which hold that one of the highest virtues is reverence for one's ancestors and that one can best practice this by protecting and preserving the physical body that has been received from them. Surgery, especially elective surgery, which "cuts up" the body and sometimes even removes a part of the body, is therefore to be avoided at all costs. This same belief also accounts for the severe shortage of cadavers for teaching or for research purposes and for the scarcity of donor organs in most Asian countries. These same people are otherwise very agreeable, open to suggestion, and generous; in fact, they are often the most grateful patients and almost never litigious. In many cases these patients will eventually return to their physician after trying out various other "traditional" remedies or "unorthodox" methods. I would like to suggest that the physician remain firm in the conviction that surgery is needed but also maintain an open mind to alternative treatment plans.

In the second scenario, the patient is quite receptive to surgery. This notwithstanding, the physician soon realizes a subtle but very important point: the patient expects a 100% success and does everything possible to avoid a discussion of any possible complications! Interestingly, this also has its roots in Confucianism and Taoism. In that framework, the physician who attends the patient is the "authority" in charge, who is bound by duty to do the very best possible job and who is not to betray the trust bestowed by others. The patient is saying in effect, if this physician cannot do it right, no one else can; the patient is giving the highest respect and total trust to the physician. At the same time, the patient does not want to bring bad luck by talking about potential complications; spoken words can influence the outcome. I would recommend, however, that the physician discuss the benefits and risks realistically but not elaborate on all of the possible complications. More importantly, the physician should suggest having these discussions with the family members as well and, as always, to document these meetings on the patient's chart. Such a suggestion may be unacceptable to westerners and imply a breach of confidentiality, but in Confucianism there is no "private" matter within a family. A major decision, such as one regarding surgery, is a family matter, and such a family discussion with the physician is not only expected but most welcome. In all likelihood the proposed surgery will be successful and the patient and the entire extended family will be most grateful.

For most elective surgical procedures it is possible to plan a date ahead of time. Often, an Asian patient may insist on a particular date or time that has to do with his or her religious belief and the Chinese calendar. The belief is rooted in Taoism, and the goal is to achieve harmony in all endeavors and undertakings by properly choosing the time, place, and persons who are involved. In addition, diet, attire, spoken words, and even numbers all play a part. The physician is expected to be open to such discussions and to answer many questions, especially in regard to postoperative medications and physical and dietary restrictions.

The previous discussion is pertinent to elective surgery. These same patients and their families would voice no objection to surgery in an emergency situation. A more detailed discussion of how the Asian patient approaches cosmetic surgery is presented in Chapter 69.

THE CHINESE VIEW OF MEDICINE

Yin and yang, a concept of Taoist origin, permeates the Chinese life. It is an idea that is to surpass all ideas and a phenomenon that explains all phenomena. Yin and yang are opposing life forces of nature; they are dynamic, constantly interacting and ever changing. Yin represents inertia, passivity, and negativity, while yang symbolizes dynamism, action, and positivity. From the constant interaction between these two opposing forces, all known phenomena are produced: chaos and order, good and bad, male and female, health and sickness, and so on. Tao means, among other things, to flow with nature and to keep yin and yang in balance. A healthy life is a life in harmony with nature, and good health is to have yin and yang in balance with one's body. Illness is an imbalance in the dynamic exchange of yin and yang in the total picture: it is the result of improper interaction of the body with weather, diet, environment, and emotions (Fig. 68–1).

In the Taoist view of cosmology and medicine, there are five elements (wood, fire, earth, metal, and water) and eight trigrams (in addition to yin and yang) that help to describe or explain all of the phenomena in the universe, both physically and metaphysically. These five elements are arranged in a cyclic fashion, so that in one direction one element "creates" the next; when arranged in a different way, one element "destroys" the next. This may be looked upon as five stages of constant change or transfor-

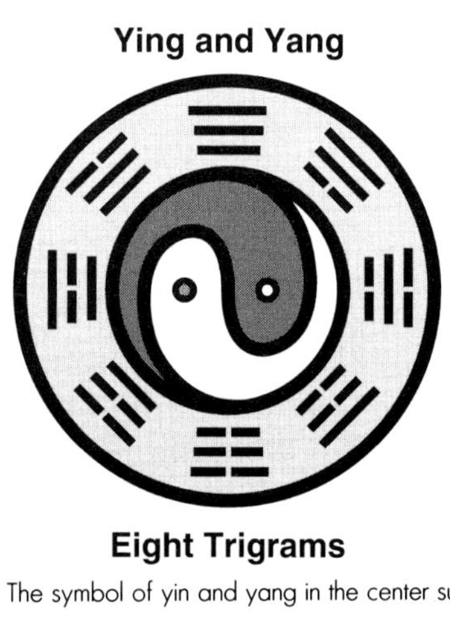

Figure 68–1. The symbol of yin and yang in the center surrounded by the eight trigrams.

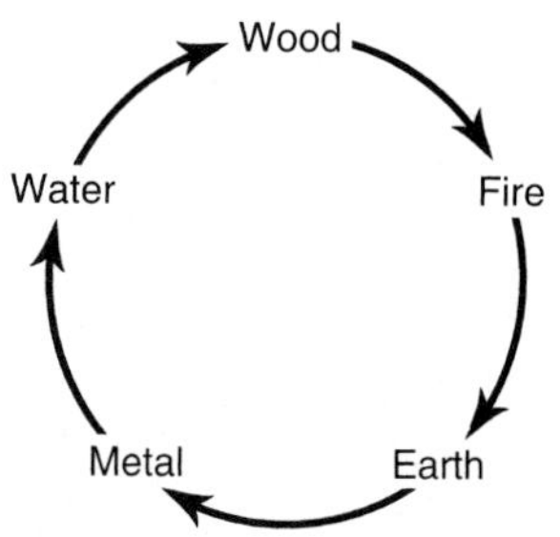

The Five Elements and the Cycle of Creation

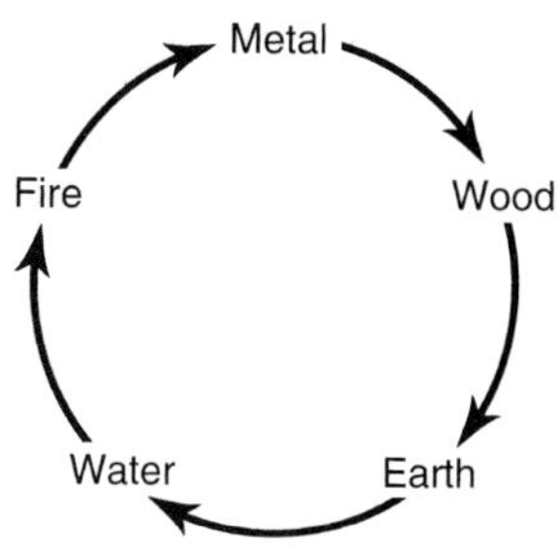

The Five Elements and the Cycle of Destruction

Figure 68 – 2. *Upper,* The five elements and the cyclic relationship of creation. *Lower,* The five elements and the cyclic relationship of destruction.

mation in the continuing cosmic cycle. Specifically, wood creates fire, which creates earth, which creates metal, which creates water, which creates wood. In a simplistic manner, this can be depicted in the following natural phenomena. Fire is created from rubbing two pieces of wood together; from the burning fire, ashes or earth is created. Metal, of course, comes out of the earth, and on the surface of cold metal water droplets are produced, and water gives life to wood. A different arrangement gives the relationship of destruction. A metal axe destroys wood; wood and plants subdue earth. Earth contains water, water extinguishes fire, and fire melts metal (Fig. 68 – 2). Although these relationships may appear to be arbitrary and artificial, they make perfect sense within the Taoist framework of the universe.

The familiar design of yin and yang, as well as the eight trigrams (see Fig. 68 – 1), is attributed to Fushi, a legendary figure from 300 B.C. The eight trigrams are the earliest binary codes, and perhaps the earliest computer. Starting with an intact and a broken line arranged in combinations of 3s, eight possible arrangements can be arrived at (2^3). Further combinations and permutations of these basic elements yield thousands and millions of possibilities. Each trigram is an ideogram, and as such has intrinsic meaning, both explicit and implicit. When two, three, or more trigrams are combined as a unit, a new meaning or phenomenon is produced. From yin to yang, there is a constant but smooth, sometimes almost imperceptible, subtle change. Within yin, there is the seed of yang, and within yang there is harbored the nucleus of yin. Using the concepts and complex relationships of yin and yang, the five elements, and the eight trigrams, practically all phenomena in the universe can be categorized, classified, explained, or even predicted.[1, 2]

The Chinese culture views the human body as a small and insignificant, albeit integral, part of nature. It is constantly interacting with and is influenced by other forces in nature. Similarly, an organ such as an eye, being only a small part of the body, is expected to constantly interact with other parts of the body, and a dynamic exchange of influence continuously takes place both internally (within the body with the other organs) and externally (other exogenous factors without). In other words, the body is a microcosmos: for whatever goes on within the body, a corresponding phenomena can be found in the macrocosmos. Conversely, some natural phenomena in the macrocosmos can be used as examples or as a reflection of what goes on inside the body. Just as humans are able to harvest energy from nature or manipulate some of nature's forces, within the human body one can adjust or manipulate these forces or elements to produce the desired result, thereby promoting continued good health or curing a disease. Indeed, it was because of this philosophy that the Chinese were the first to recognize and to emphasize the effects that emotion, diet, weather, and exercise have on one's health and their importance in the prevention of disease.

As an example, the five senses of the human body have their corresponding elements; the internal organs, bones, muscles, and skin all have their corresponding elements modified by yin and yang. The acupuncture meridians and points similarly have their corresponding five elements, modified or complemented by yin and yang; emotions, feelings, activities, foods, and time (the year, month, day, and hour) also have corresponding elements that are modified by yin and yang (Table 68 – 1).

TABLE 68 – 1
Corresponding Elements

Elements	Seasons	Directions	Organs	Ocular Anatomy	Parts or Tissues
Wood	Spring	East	Liver	Cornea	Extremities
Fire	Summer	South	Heart	Canthus	Blood
Earth		Center	Spleen	Lids	Muscles
Metal	Autumn	West	Lung	Sclera	"Chi" or breath*
Water	Winter	North	Kidney	Pupil	Large bones

*Not the usual breath but an intangible energy that flows along the acupuncture meridians.

In the Chinese view, Western medicine, although technologically "advanced," is too compartmentalized, often overlooks the obvious, and neglects the human factor. An unavoidable tendency is seeing the tree but missing the forest, or improving the part while letting the whole deteriorate. On the other hand, despite an enormous body of clinical information and sometimes impressive results, Westerners view Chinese medicine as unscientific, outdated, illogical, and irrational. Much of what Chinese medicine has to provide has, at least to the Western mind, no rhyme or reason and cannot be explained by rigorously controlled scientific studies.

Fanciful, mysterious, or arbitrary as all this may seem, Chinese medicine has worked for more than 5000 years. In fact, it is within this framework that the Chinese made many important observations and contributions to medicine centuries ahead of the West. For example, the circulation of blood had become an accepted fact and was well described by Chinese physicians by the second century B.C., long before William Harvey's work in 1628. In the *Yellow Emperor's Canon of Medicine* (Huang Dee Nay Jing), written by an unknown author or authors in 2697 B.C., the heart was recognized as a pump and a distinction was made between arterial and venous blood flow (Fig. 68–3). A "closed circuit" circulation, the distance that blood has to travel to complete this circuit, and the flow rates were also calculated. Sphygmology was highly developed, and hundreds of diagnostic pulse rates were described. In the same classic manual also appeared passages that clearly described the circadian rhythm, although the existence of such a biologic clock had long been accepted by the Chinese as a matter of fact. As a result, timing of the treatment, whether medicine, acupuncture, or surgery, was most important. The acupuncture meridians and techniques and the importance of exercise and of emotion (psychosomatic) were discussed in detail.

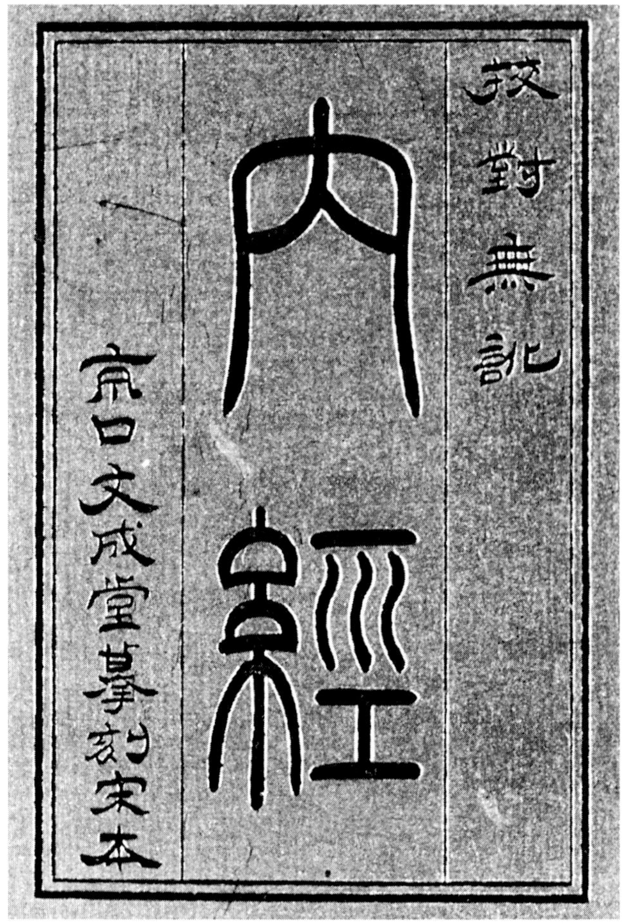

Figure 68–3. Yellow Emperor's Canon of Medicine by an unknown author or authors, circa 2697 B.C. This is a copy printed in the tenth century A.D.

In addition to describing hundreds of recipes for herbal medicines, Shen Nong, by 2737 B.C., stressed the importance of diet, both as a means of preventing disease and as a means of preserving, promoting, and restoring good health. By 3000 B.C., Bien Chiao described plastic surgery for what appears to be a harelip and the use of general anesthesia. Definitely by A.D. 115, general anesthesia induction by *Cannabis indica* was available and was used by Whua Tuo, a surgeon who performed a laparotomy and splenectomy, among other operations.[3]

It is perhaps most remarkable that the Chinese anticipated modern biochemistry to such an extent that, by the second century B.C., they had isolated sex and pituitary hormones from human urine and, indeed, had used these for medicinal purposes. A distinction between male and female urine was emphasized, and several methods to extract hormones from the urine were meticulously described. The first was sublimation, a method in which the Chinese alchemists and physicians were well versed. A second technique was the use of the beans of *Gleditschia sinensis* to precipitate the hormones out of urine, and a third method was natural evaporation.[1, 3, 4]

In the seventh century, Chinese physicians described techniques for treating goiters. Thyroid glands of gelded rams were defatted, soaked in warm water, dried, and chopped up to be taken with jujube dates. In addition, seaweed, now known to be rich in iodine, was prescribed for the patient as a necessary part of the diet. In the tenth century, the Taoist alchemists, who had guarded the secret of smallpox vaccination, perhaps for many centuries, began to make it public knowledge. It is truly amazing that they already appreciated a distinction between variola major and variola minor. Without any modern laboratory equipment, they attenuated this deadly virus before inoculation. Two such methods were carefully described so that the chances of getting the disease were minimized and the desired effect of immunization was maximized.[1, 4]

In the West, it was not until the nineteenth century that the medical world recognized that many diseases, such as beriberi, scurvy, and rickets, were deficiency diseases; that is, they were caused by the lack of certain crucial elements. The Chinese awareness of deficiency diseases dates back to antiquity, which is not surprising given their views of the importance of the balance of nature and, consequently, balance in diet. Written evidence of this knowledge of dietary deficiency diseases dates to A.D. 200. Although Chinese physicians did not yet have a knowledge of vitamins, the foods and the diet that they recommended would have been rich in the vitamins necessary to cure these deficiency-related conditions. One of the most prominent authors on the subject of diet was Hu, an imperial dietitian in the Yuan Court between 1314 and 1330. He wrote a book entitled *The Principles of Healthy Diet*, which was subtitled *Many Diseases Can Be Cured by Diet Alone.* In this volume he not only collected many widely known and time-tested recipes but also added new ones, analyzing and explaining their effectiveness according to the principles of yin and yang. He emphasized the role of the diet and of the dietitian in the management of all patients.[4]

Diabetes was described at length in the *Yellow Emperor's Canon of Medicine*, and three distinct forms were recognized. In modern terminology, the first type is the common diabetes mellitus, and the second type is secondary to consumption of large quantities of sweets and fatty foods; the third type may be referred to simply as diabetes in obese patients. In 655, Sun wrote that, among other things, salt, wine, and starch cereal products should be avoided and suggested that diabetes might even be cured by avoiding these things and following a well-balanced diet. The "sweetness" of the patient's urine was well described in a text by Chen in the early seventh century.[1, 3, 4]

In some classic Chinese medical writings, the clinical findings in the eyes are correlated with systemic diseases. For example, yellowish discoloration of the sclera was recognized as being the result of an imbalance of the yin and yang in the liver and gallbladder. Many remedies and acupuncture points have been described to treat various eye conditions. These remedies consist mainly of herbs, animal parts and derivatives, and minerals and are aimed primarily at the associated or related organs, depending on the diagnosis. In other words, they are aimed at "strengthening the liver," "enhancing the function of the spleen," or "clearing the lungs." Conditions that reportedly responded very well to these remedies include blepharitis, styes, and pterygia.[5]

The Chinese diet, considered by many to be one of the best balanced and most healthy, is prepared using ingredients and in a manner that will best ensure the balance of yin and yang and that will best suit the individual's needs. For example, when a person has too much "fire" combined with yang, the recommended diet would likely include cucumbers, bamboo shoots, mushrooms, and seafood—foods of the "water" category; whether conceptually or from real experience, foods from this water category would "destroy" the "fire" and restore the balance of yin and yang. Garlic, a constant condiment in Chinese cuisine, was thought to have many important medicinal properties. These properties, which in modern terminology would include antimicrobial and antioncogenic activities, were well described and well accepted in China but only recently have been verified in the laboratory to be present.[6–12] One of the most common diet ingredients, mushrooms, comes in many varieties and, together with other favorites such as asparagus, chives, and celery, is supposed to "improve circulation." Indeed, some of these effects have been verified and the active pharmacologic ingredients identified. Schiller and coworkers[13] performed a study on a group of Chinese patients who had been observed to bleed more during surgery than anticipated, despite normal preoperative laboratory results. They found that these patients had all had mo-er in their diets preoperatively. Mo-er, a form of fungus or mushroom, indeed "improves circulation" by inhibiting the aggregation of platelets.

Acupuncture and moxibustion have been used as adjunct therapy for many centuries. The exact mechanism by which these treatments work still defies explanation by modern technology, but clinical effectiveness in treating certain diseases is evident. In addition to diet, acupuncture and moxibustion, exercise, physical therapy, and psychological counseling all have been used by the Chinese with the emphasis on prevention of disease and the promotion of good health.

It is extremely difficult to evaluate individually the therapeutic effects of the various aspects of the Chinese medical regimen. This regimen not only consists of pharmaceutical agents, dietary control, exercise, and acupuncture, but also involves emotions and beliefs; in the Chinese framework, no one part can be analyzed in isolation from the whole. Thus, to design a scientific study to simultaneously evaluate these many variables would be almost impossible. Nonetheless, the Chinese experience is the largest body of clinical information available, involving millions of patients over the centuries, and some conclusions can be drawn: what continues to be used must work or it would not survive, even though we do not quite understand why and how it works.

Acupuncture is being investigated in the treatment of blepharospasm and dry eyes. Chung and Hsu have studied many patients with essential blepharospasm; two different acupuncture treatment plans were tested, and each yielded satisfactory results (see Chapter 71). At the Doheny Eye Institute, I am conducting a study on the effectiveness of acupuncture in the treatment of dry eyes. This study grew out of the observation that some dry eye conditions, while recalcitrant to known modern treatment modalities, respond very well to acupuncture. This intriguing observation raised many questions. Does acupuncture alleviate the condition by neurally stimulating increased tear production or by dilating lacrimal gland ductules? Does it restore yin and yang of the lacrimal system or of another part of the body? Is this a placebo effect?

TABLE 68-2

Comparison of Male and Female Orbits

	Width (mm)		Height (mm)		Depth (mm)		Volume (mL)		Orbital Index*	
	M	F	M	F	M	F	M	F	M	F
No. of orbits	669	346	669	346	663	345	320	200	669	346
Average value	39.1	38.5	35.4	34.8	48.3	47.0	28.0	25.1	88.3	90.4
Range	35.0–47.0	34.2–43.7	29.8–40.5	29.3–40.5	41.0–55.5	40.0–52.5	21.0–34.0	19.0–32.0	71.3–109.0	71.5–102.0

*Orbital Index by Broca = $\frac{\text{Orbital height}}{\text{Orbital width}} \times 100$.

Data from Cui M, Zhang CY, Liang SJ: Measurements and observations of Chinese orbits. Chin J Ophthalmol 4:208–211, 1959.

ANATOMIC DIFFERENCES

In a study published in 1959, Cui and colleagues[14] analyzed the dimensions of the orbits in Chinese males and females. Their study consisted of 482 skulls (315 males and 167 females) and 51 half skulls (39 males and 12 female), for a total of 1015 orbits. Some of the important conclusions reached were (1) there is very little difference (less than 0.2 mm) between the right and left orbits in both males and females in all of the orbital measurements and in average values; (2) all measurements obtained for males are greater than are those for the females, the only exception being the orbital index; (3) the measurements for these Chinese skulls are different from those reported for Caucasians by Whitnall[15] and Wolff (revised by Warwick)[16] (Tables 68–2 and 68–3). Clinically, the most important difference is in the orbital volume. The average is 26.9 mL (range, 19.0 to 34.0 mL) in Chinese and 30 mL in Caucasians. Another important difference is in the depth of the orbit. These authors found an average depth of 47.8 mm in the Chinese skulls, while the accepted average value in Caucasians is 40 mm, according to Whitnall[15] and Warwick.[16]

At first glance it appears that, on the average, the Chinese has a deeper orbit. On closer examination, however, we find that the Chinese authors measured the depth of the orbit from the inferior orbital rim all the way to the orbital apex, while the average value for the Caucasian orbits represents only the posterior extent of the floor of the orbit. Many authors believe that the depth of the orbit in Caucasians, if measured to the apex, would be at least 50 mm.[17, 18] This study thus provides anatomic information regarding Chinese patients that can have important clinical bearing, especially when giving retrobulbar injections, in planning orbitotomies, and in reconstructing the orbit or socket. As a general rule, the dimensions of the orbit are smaller in Chinese. Therefore, when giving a retrobulbar injection in a Chinese patient, the physician should consider inserting the needle less far into the orbit than might be done in Caucasian patients and consider also not giving as much local anesthetic. Similarly, when the surgeon is planning an orbitotomy for removal of a lesion, for drainage of an abscess, or for insertion of a subperiostal implant, awareness of these smaller dimensions will facilitate dissection and possibly help to avoid complications. After enucleation, fracture of the orbital wall, or other major orbital reconstruction, the physician with this knowledge could obtain the appropriate size bone graft or carve out the appropriate size alloplastic material, and would be more likely to select the appropriate size of implant or dermis-fat graft to reconstruct the socket.

In a 1984 study, Cui and Li[19] studied 194 orbits of 97 male Chinese skulls. Using plaster of Paris casts, calipers, and statistical analyses, they measured the following: (1) the dimensions of the optic foramen, both vertically and horizontally; (2) the distance between the medial walls of the optic canal, both within the orbit and within the skull; and (3) the dimensions of the superior and inferior orbital fissures and their distance to the orbital rim. The average distance between the inner walls of the optic foramen within the orbit is 27.9 mm, whereas the average distance within the skull is 13.5 mm. In their study, a superior orbital notch was noted in 51 right orbits and 46 left orbits; a foramen was observed in 46 of the right orbits and 51 left orbits. A bilateral foramen was noted in 37 skulls, and a bilateral superior orbital notch was seen in 47 skulls. Twenty-seven skulls had a foramen on one side and a notch on the other (Table 68–4). The "normal" findings and the variations that they reported are extremely helpful in the clinical situation when a coronal flap is planned, an anterior orbitotomy is contemplated, or a brow incision is used. With this knowledge, the surgeon can best avoid cutting or avulsing the supraorbital nerves

TABLE 68-3

Average Values of the Orbit in Caucasians

Width (mm)	Height (mm)	Depth (mm)	Volume (mL)	Interorbital Distance (mm)
40	35	40	30	25

From Warwick R: Eugene Wolff's Anatomy of the Eye and Orbit, 7th ed. Philadelphia, WB Saunders, 1976.

TABLE 68-4

Measurements of Optic Nerve Foramen in Chinese Males

	No. of Orbits	Average Vertical Dimension (mm)	Average Horizontal Dimension (mm)	Average Superior Wall Length (mm)	Average Inferior Wall Length
Right	97	5.98	5.20	7.48	5.10
Left	97	5.96	4.93	7.45	5.01

$P > .05$.
Data from Cui M, Li FC: Measurements and observation of Chinese orbits. Chin J Ophthalmol 20:304–306, 1984.

and vessels. When the surgeon is planning an optic canal decompression via the ethmoidal sinus, being aware of the average dimensions described in this study will also be of great help.

Clinicians are often frustrated when performing nasal lacrimal reconstructive surgery on an Asian patient: either the procedure appears to be especially difficult or the results are not as good as expected. In such instances, variation in the nasal structures and sinus cavities can be a contributing factor. A 1964 study by Zhang and Luo[20] may be helpful in avoiding these difficulties because these researchers discuss the anatomic variations that may be encountered. Their study involved 50 skulls (100 orbits and lacrimal fossa); they used adult skulls only and made no distinction between the sexes. Using calipers, they measured the vertical and horizontal dimensions of the lacrimal fossa, the depth of the lacrimal fossa, and the thickness of the anterior lacrimal crest. More importantly, they further defined the relationship between the lacrimal fossa and the ethmoidal sinus and the relationship between the lacrimal fossa and the middle turbinate. In 56 of the orbits they noted that ethmoidal cells extended to the lacrimal fossa; in 7 orbits these reached the upper third of the lacrimal fossa, in 40 orbits the ethmoidal cells reached the middle third of the fossa, and in 9 orbits they reached the level of the lower third. Ethmoidal cells also reached the posterior lacrimal crest in 44 orbits: in 6 orbits they reached the upper third of the lacrimal fossa, in 36 orbits the middle third, and in 2 orbits the level of the lower third. In 21 orbits, the middle turbinate reached the frontal process of the lacrimal fossa: in 15 orbits it reached the level of the upper third of the fossa, while in 6 orbits it reached the middle third. In 76 orbits of the specimens studied, the middle turbinate extended to the lacrimal fossa itself. Of these, in 21 orbits it was at the level of the upper third and in 55 orbits at the level of the middle third. In only 3 orbits was the middle turbinate observed to have reached the posterior lacrimal crest, and in each of these orbits it was at the level of the upper third (Tables 68–5 through 68–7). Hsu of Taiwan measured the thickness of the lacrimal bone during dacryocystorhinoplasty in 386 patients and found the average thickness in males to be 5.8 ± 0.9 mm, and the average thickness in females to be 4.2 ± 0.8 mm. He noticed also that in 8% of the study population the ethmoidal cells reached the middle turbinate.

Zhang and Luo emphasized that in 56% of the specimens the lacrimal fossa was occupied by ethmoidal cells, and in 76% of the specimens studied this area was occupied also by the anterior portion of the middle turbinate. Therefore, in procedures that involve the paranasal sinuses or nasal cavities, such as dacryocystorhinostomy or a medial approach to the orbit, the surgeon must be aware of these anatomic variations. For example, in performing dacryocystorhinostomy it is likely that the surgeon will enter the ethmoidal cells rather than the nasal cavity in the majority of cases. In addition, when anastomosing the nasal mucosa with the lacrimal sac, or when inserting a Pyrex tube, chances are that the anterior portion of the middle turbinate will be in the way. Similarly, when draining paranasal sinuses the surgeon has to be aware of the anterior extension of these ethomoidal cells. When planning endoscopic nasal surgery, or when planning to enter the orbit through the ethmoidal sinuses or to decompress the ethmoidal sinuses, these variations should be kept in mind.

Blaylock and associates,[21] in 1990, published their study of the relationship between ethmoidal cells and the lacrimal sac fossa. This study presumably involved both Caucasians and African Americans and was based on analysis of computed tomographic scans of 190 orbits. In 93% of the orbits, they found that the anterior ethmoidal air cells lay adjacent to the lacrimal sac fossa and that the

TABLE 68-5

Average Dimensions of the Lacrimal Fossa in 50 Adult Chinese Skulls (100 orbits)

Long Axis (Vertical) (mm)	Short Axis (Horizontal) (mm)	Thickness (mm)
17.88	3.40	4.65

Data from Zhang GH, Luo WB: The lacrimal fossa: Measurements of 100 Chinese orbits. Chin J Ophthalmol 11:253–257, 1964.

TABLE 68-6

Relationship Between the Lacrimal Fossa and the Ethmoidal Cells in 100 Adult Chinese Orbits*

Lacrimal Fossa	Lacrimal Bone	Posterior Lacrimal Crest
Upper third	7	6
Middle third	40	36
Lower third	9	2

*Number of specimens with ethmoidal cells reaching various anatomic landmarks.
Data from Zhang GH, Luo WB: The lacrimal fossa: Measurements of 100 Chinese orbits. Chin J Ophthalmol 11:253–257, 1964.

TABLE 68-7

Relationship Between Lacrimal Fossa and the Middle Turbinate in 100 Chinese Adult Orbits*

Lacrimal Fossa	Frontal Process	Lacrimal Bone	Posterior Lacrimal Crest
Upper third	15	21	3
Middle third	6	55	0

*Number of specimens with middle turbinate reaching various anatomic landmarks.
Data from Zhang GH, Luo WB: The lacrimal fossa: Measurements of 100 Chinese orbits. Chin J Ophthalmol 11:253–257, 1964.

anterior to exterior extension of the air cells was most pronounced under the superior half of the lacrimal sac fossa. They emphasized the clinical importance of these findings, although they did not comment on the relationship between the middle turbinate and the lacrimal fossa or the anterior ethmoidal cells. Nevertheless, the contrasting statistics are of great value to clinicians.

In 1959, Luo and Deng[22] determined the "normal" position of the globe by measuring 3102 normal subjects with the aid of a Hertel exophthalmometer. The study population included 2811 males and 291 females of Han ethnicity, with ages ranging from 15 to 23 years. These authors found that, in the males, the average proptosis was 13.19 ± 0.03 mm (range, 9 to 18 mm), with an average base of 98.59 ± 0.10 mm. Eighty-one percent of the male population had a reading of between 12 and 15 mm. In the females, proptosis had an average value of 13.94 ± 0.07 mm, with an average base of 97.33 ± 0.08 mm. Eighty-seven percent of the female population had a reading of between 12 and 15 mm. Hsu, in 1990, studied 860 Taiwanese, and reported similar findings. By comparison, Caucasians have an average value of 16 mm of proptosis, with a range from 10 to 20 mm, according to Duke-Elder and MacFaul.[23] A slightly higher reading in males (17 mm in males, compared with 16 mm in females) has also been observed and confirmed by several authors.[23] Migliori and Gladstone,[24] in 1984, also determined the normal range of exophthalmometric values for black adults and for Caucasian adults. They found the mean normal value of proptosis to be 16.5 mm in Caucasian males, 18.5 mm in African American males, 15.4 mm in Caucasian females, and 17.8 mm in African American females. In addition, they found that the upper limits of normal were 21.7 mm for Caucasian males, 24.7 mm for African American males, 20.1 mm for Caucasian females, and 23.0 mm for African American females. They also stressed that no individual had more than 2 mm of asymmetry between eyes, and the differences between African Americans and Caucasians, both males and females, are statistically significant. These racial differences should be kept in mind when evaluating patients for proptosis (Tables 68-8 and 68-9).

A large study that examined the external eyelid dimensions of Chinese people was conducted by Feng and colleagues in 1964.[25] A total of 1677 normal individuals, 636 males and 1041 females, was included; ages ranged from 1 to 78 years. These investigators used specially fabricated transparent rulers. They found no statistical difference between the left eye and the right eye. Their measurements of the Chinese people are similar to those obtained for Japanese and Koreans but are smaller than the known values for Caucasians. They also found that the peak values of all of these measurements tend to occur between the ages of 11 and 25. The differences between the male patients and female patients are not statistically significant. The palpebral fissure dimensions in males are 27.78 × 8.98 mm and in females are 27.66 × 8.92 mm. The inner intercanthal distance is 33.09 mm for males and 32.87 mm for females; the outer intercanthal distance is 88.61 mm in males and 87.97 mm in females. The interpupillary distance in males is 60.90 mm and is 58.30 mm in females.

A similar study in 1987 by Xu and colleagues[26] comprised 300 normal males and 300 normal females from Southern China, with ages ranging from 11 to 50 years. The techniques they used to obtain the measurements were similar to those used by Feng and coworkers. The palpebral fissure measurements in the males were

TABLE 68-8

Exophthalmometry Measurements in Chinese and Taiwanese

	Chinese*		Taiwanese†	
	Males	Females	Males	Females
Number of patients	2811	291	380	340
Hertel base average	98.59 ± 0.10	97.3 ± 0.08	104.3 ± 4.6	100.7 ± 4.7
Range	87–119	87–107		
Exophthalmometry measurements average	13.19 ± 0.03	13.94 ± 0.07	14.1 ± 1.4	13.2 ± 1.3
Range	9–18	1–17	10.5–17.0	9.5–16.5

*N = 3102.
†N = 720.
Data from Luo WB, Deng YP: Measurements and statistics of exophthalmometry in Chinese. Chin J Ophthalmol 4:200–202, 1959; and Hsu WM, personal communication.

TABLE 68-9

Exophthalmometry in Caucasians and African Americans

	Caucasian Males	African American Males	Caucasian Females	African American Females
Number of patients	127	113	200	241
Base	98.39 ± 3.86	101.42 ± 3.70	95.41 ± 3.83	98.49 ± 3.57
Right eye	16.55 ± 2.57	18.56 ± 3.08	15.46 ± 2.34	17.90 ± 2.61
Left eye	16.47 ± 2.60	18.41 ± 3.08	15.36 ± 2.33	17.73 ± 2.53
Range	11.31–21.71	12.30–24.65	10.74–20.8	12.60–23.04

Values given in millimeters; mean ± 1 SD for base and right and left eyes; mean ± 2 SD for range.
Adapted from Migliori ME, Gladstone GJ: Determination of the normal range of exophthalmometric values for black and white adults. Am J Ophthalmol 98:438–442, 1984. Published with permission from The American Journal of Ophthalmology. Copyright by The Ophthalmic Publishing Company.

28.96 × 8.51 mm and were 28.42 × 8.62 mm in the females. In their study, they found 40% of the population to have a single eyelid and 60% to have a double eyelid. The measurement of the double lid crease was 2 to 3 mm at the inner canthus and 2.5 to 3.5 mm at the outer canthus; it was highest centrally, where it usually measured between 4.5 and 6 mm. Statistically, Xu and colleagues reached the same conclusions, as did other authors, that there was no significant difference between the left and the right eyes or between males and females and that some of the values tend to peak at adolescence and in the mid 20s. Xu and colleagues believe that the differences between their findings and those previously reported represent regional variations only, since they studied only southern Chinese; furthermore, the differences were not statistically significant. They also reported the measurement of skin thickness in these patients; skin was pinched with a caliper and the value divided by two. The average thickness in males was 0.64 mm, whereas in females it was 0.63 mm. Another interesting measurement that they obtained was the distance between the inferior border of the brow and the upper eyelid crease at the midpupillary point. This distance in the male, on the average, is 17.88 mm, and it is 18.32 mm in the female. Liang and Zhang,[27] in 1981, studied a total of 888 northern Chinese; there were 512 males and 376 females, and ages ranged from 18 to 26. Their palpebral measurements were 27.23 × 8.53 mm in males and 26.10 × 8.73 mm in females (Table 68-10).

To determine the thickness of the eyelid in normal Chinese, He,[28] in 1982, studied 555 males and 445 females from all over China. The thickness of the upper eyelid ranged from 1.5 to 3.0 mm with an average of 2.0 mm; the lower eyelids ranged from 1.0 to 2.0 mm in thickness, with an average of 1.0 mm. Liu and Hsu,[29] in 1986, reported the upper eyelid skin thickness as determined both clinically and histologically. They found that in the Chinese population the upper eyelid skin thickness ranged from 0.30 to 0.80 mm, depending on the age of the patient, with an average of 0.65 mm. In addition, they found that, in nearly 85% of the population studied, a submuscular fat pad was present. In addition, they reported the incidence of various types of double eyelids, single eyelids, and the epicanthal fold. Some of their interesting findings of clinical relevance are summarized in Tables 68-11 through 68-13.

TABLE 68-10

Eyelid Dimensions in Chinese

Factor	Feng et al (1964)	Xu et al (1987)	Liang and Zhang (1981)	Liu and Hsu (1986)	Hsu (1991)
Number of patients	636 males 1041 females	300 males 300 females	512 males 376 females	1792 males 1848 females	1380 males 1220 females
Palpebral length × height in males	27.78 × 8.92	28.96 × 8.51	27.23 × 8.53	}27.2 × 8.5	27.6 × 8.7
Palpebral length × height in females	27.78 × 8.92	28.42 × 8.62	26.10 × 8.73		26.3 × 8.3
Inner intercanthal distance	33.09 males 32.87 females	34.47			35.8 males 35.1 females
Outer intercanthal distance	88.61 males 87.97 females	34.03			
Upper lid crease height		5.09*		6.50	6.5 males 6.6 females
Skin thickness		0.64 males 0.63 females		0.65	
Other comments		Southern Chinese†	Northern Chinese	Submuscular fat pad 84.5%	Submuscular fat pad 76.5%

*Crease height at inner canthus 2.43 mm, outer canthus 2.80 mm, and centrally 5.09.
†Brow and crease distance of 17.88 mm in males and 18.22 mm in females.

TABLE 68-11

External Eye Findings in Chinese

Upper tarsal plate height	7–10 mm males 6–8 mm females
Lower tarsal plate height	5 mm males and females
Double eyelid	70%–80% Northern China
Central crease height	3–5 mm
Lash angle eyes open	110°–130° males 140°–160° females
Lash angle eyes closed	110°–120° males 100°–110° females

Data from Wei ZX: Oculoplastic Surgery. Helungjiang, China, Helungjiang Publishing Co, 1981, pp 1–20.

The incidence of the epicanthal fold (i.e., the presence of an upper eyelid fold; double eyelid vs. single eyelid) in Asians varies in the literature. Understandably, a number of these discrepancies are due to differences in ethnic background of the study group and regional variations. The incidence of double eyelid ranges from 40% to 90%, and the incidence of epicanthal fold ranges from 30% to 90%.[28, 30] The presence and absence of an eyelid crease is related to fusion of the levator aponeurosis and orbital septum. This is discussed in more detail in Chapter 69.

Wang and Bian[31] dissected 40 eyelids of 20 Chinese cadavers in 1986. They found that the level of the fusion of the orbital septum with the levator aponeurosis was below the superior margin of the tarsus in 90% of the specimens. This fusion level in single eyelids was lower than in the double eyelids. Double eyelids were present in 18 (45%) of the upper eyelids in this study, and height of the crease ranged from 3.0 to 6.5 mm above the lid margin, with an average of 4.6 ± 1.0 mm above the lid margin. Among these 18 double eyelids, fusion of the orbital septum with the aponeurosis was 1.8 to 3.3 mm above the superior margin of the tarsal plate in 4 and was 1.6 to 4.8 mm below the margin in 14. The average was 2.4 ± 1.9 mm below the margin for all of these double eyelids. In 22 single eyelids, fusion of the orbital septum with the aponeurosis was 2.1 to 5.9 mm below the margin of the superior tarsus, with an average of 3.9 ± 1.0 mm. The difference in fusion level between single and double eyelids was statistically significant ($t = 6.12$, $P < .01$). This study by Wang and Bian, together with those of Hisatomi and Fujino[32] and Doxanas and Anderson,[33] have provided an anatomic basis for the differences in the appearances of Asians and Caucasians.

TABLE 68-12

Prevalence of Epicanthal Fold and Eyelid Crease in 2800 Taiwanese

Epicanthal Fold	Single Eyelid (No Lid Crease)	Double Eyelid Outer	Double Eyelid Inner	Double Eyelid Partial
48.8%	26.8%	78.2%	17.2%	7.8%

From Hsu WM, personal communication, 1991.

TABLE 68-13

Measurements of Tarsus and Incidence of Submuscular Fat Pad During Primary Lid Procedures

	Upper Lid	Lower Lid
Number of patients	268	184
Tarsus height (mm)	8.2	3.6
Submuscular fat	76.5%	0%

From Hsu WM, personal communication, 1991.

Acknowledgments

Many of the original Chinese references of anatomy were furnished by Dr. Nai Jiang Xu of Shanghai. Dr. Guang Xi Zhao of Beijing and Dr. Wen Ming Hsu of Taipei also provided some valuable data of their own.

REFERENCES

1. Needham J: The Grand Titration: Science and Society in East and West. London, George Allen and Unwin, 1969, pp 15, 142, 229.
2. Chan WT: A Source Book in Chinese Philosophy. Princeton, NJ, Princeton University Press, 1963, pp 244–250.
3. Ancient China's Technology and Science, an Anthology. Beijing, Foreign Language Press, 1983.
4. Temple RKG: The Genius of China: 3,000 Years of Science, Discovery, and Invention. New York, Simon & Schuster, 1986.
5. Liu JC (ed): The Practice of Ophthalmology, Traditional Chinese Medicine. Beijing, People's Health Publishing Co, 1982, pp 782–807.
6. Belman S: Onion and garlic oils inhibit tumor promotion. Carcinogenesis 4:1063–1065, 1983.
7. Block E, Ahmad S, Jain MK, et al: (E,Z)-Ajoene: A potent antithrombotic agent from garlic. J Am Chem Soc 106:8295–8296, 1984.
8. Feldberg RS, Chang SC, Kotik AN, et al: In vitro mechanism of inhibition of bacterial cell growth by allicin. Antimicrob Agents Chemother 32:1763–1768, 1988.
9. Mayeux PR, Agrawal KC, Tou JS, et al: The pharmacological effects of allicin, a constituent of garlic oil. Agents Actions 25:182–190, 1988.
10. Makheja AN, Bailey JM: Identification of the antiplatelet substance in Chinese black tree fungus. N Engl J Med 304:175, 1981.
11. Makheja AN, Bailey JM: Antiplatelet constituents of garlic and onion. Agents Actions 29:360–363, 1990.
12. Scharfenbert K, Wagner R, Wagner KG: The cytotoxic effect of ajoene, a natural product from garlic, investigated with different cell lines. New York, Elsevier, 1990, pp 103–108.
13. Schiller J, Bosniak S, Ko W: Why do Chinese patients bleed more during ophthalmic plastic surgery: Presented at the 22nd annual symposium of the American Society of Ophthalmic Plastic and Reconstructive Surgery, Anaheim, California, October 12, 1991.
14. Cui M, Zhang CY, Liang SJ: Measurements and observations of Chinese orbits. Chin J Ophthalmol 4:208–211, 1959.
15. Whitnall SE: Anatomy of the Human Orbit and the Accessory Organs of Vision, 2nd ed. London, Oxford University Press, 1932, p 95.
16. Warwick R: Eugene Wolff's Anatomy of the Eye and Orbit, 7th ed. Philadelphia, WB Saunders, 1976.
17. Rootman J: Disease of the Orbit: A Multidisciplinary Approach. Philadelphia, JB Lippincott, 1988, pp 3–18.
18. Doxanas MT, Anderson RL: Clinical Orbital Anatomy. Baltimore, Williams & Wilkins, 1984.
19. Cui M, Li FC: Measurements and observation of Chinese orbits. Chin J Ophthalmol 20:304–306, 1984.
20. Zhang GH, Luo WB: The lacrimal fossa: Measurements of 100 Chinese orbits. Chin J Ophthalmol 11:253–257, 1964.

21. Blaylock WK, Moore CA, Linberg JV: Anterior ethmoid anatomy facilitates dacryocystorhinostomy. Arch Ophthalmol 108:1774–1777, 1990.
22. Luo WB, Deng YP: Measurements and statistics of exophthalmetry in Chinese. Chin J Ophthalmol 4:200–202, 1959.
23. Duke-Elder S, MacFaul PA: The ocular adnexa: Lacrimal, orbital and para-orbital diseases. *In* Duke-Elder S (ed): System of Ophthalmology, vol 13, pt 2. St. Louis, CV Mosby, 1973, pp 780–782 and 785.
24. Migliori ME, Gladstone GJ: Determination of the normal range of exophthalmometric values for black and white adults. Am J Ophthalmol 98:438–442, 1984.
25. Feng BH, Zhu DQ, Chang JK, Kang XH: Measurements and observations of the external eye lids. Chin J Ophthalmol 11:101–104, 1964.
26. Xu JD, Tang FS, Huang FM: Normal values of the eyelids: Observations and clinical significance. Chin J Ophthalmol 23:253–255, 1987.
27. Liang ZY, Zhang YT: Measurements and statistics of the eyelids. Chin J Ophthalmol 18:282–285, 1981.
28. He L: Measurements of eyelid thickness. Chin J Ophthalmol 18:178, 1982.
29. Liu D, Hsu WM: Oriental eyelids: Anatomic difference and surgical consideration. Ophthalmic Plast Reconstr Surg 2:59–64, 1986.
30. Duke-Elder S: System of Ophthalmology, vol 3. St. Louis, CV Mosby, 1963, p 849.
31. Wang HM, Bian CJ: The anatomy of the upper eyelid and its clinical significance. Chin J Plast Surg Burns 2:273–275, 1986.
32. Hisatomi C, Fujino T: Anatomical considerations concerning blepharoplasty in the Oriental patient. Adv Ophthalmic Plast Reconstr Surg 2:151–165, 1983.
33. Doxanas MT, Anderson RL: Oriental eyelids: An anatomic study. Arch Ophthalmol 102:1232–1235, 1984.

CHAPTER 69

Asian Blepharoplasty

Don Liu

The appreciation, glorification, and pursuit of beauty is basic to human nature. In one way or another, and to varying degrees, everyone attempts to enhance his or her appearance. When it comes to appreciation or beautification of human facial features, the eyes are almost invariably the focus of attention. Since antiquity, men and women of all cultures and societies have tried everything possible, from cosmetics to surgical procedures, to enhance the beauty of their eyes. From Egypt to China, from Greece to India, despite differences in the cultural standards and values, this same desire has always been, and continues to be, shared by all. Over the past several decades there has been a notably increased interest in the construction of an upper eyelid crease in Asians. To understand why this is so, it is necessary to begin with an examination of the Asian cultural background in a historic context. Certainly, standards of beauty are greatly influenced by traditions and customs and thus vary greatly from culture to culture; furthermore, these standards are subject to change as times change.

To begin with, it should be kept in mind that the Mongolian race is the largest family of the human race and is distributed widely over several continents; over time, there have developed numerous divisions and subgroups of ethnicity, and, consequently, large regional variations are apparent. This discussion is limited to the Chinese, although the principles of the procedures discussed herein are applicable to other Asian populations, such as the Japanese and Korean peoples.

The Chinese people, with a glorious history and a highly refined culture, have one of the oldest continuous civilizations and have made remarkable contributions to world civilization. As the Middle Kingdom, China's culture and influence spread to the neighboring countries, and for centuries it was held that the more these neighbors became Chinese-like, the more civilized they became. These neighbors adopted, to various degrees, Confucianism, Taoism, and Buddhism; they use the Chinese lunar calendar, follow Chinese customs, and practice medicine within the Chinese framework. As a consequence, Chinese standards of beauty easily became their standards of beauty. Traditionally, one of the most prominent features of a classic beauty is the "almond" eye (Fig. 69-1). From literary descriptions, paintings, and sculptures, these eyes are like a pair of almonds set slightly obliquely, with the larger end toward the nose and the pointed end laterally. This means the presence of an epicanthal fold that gives the rounded off appearance medially and a typical Mongolian slant. Only very rarely is an eyelid crease noted; and, if present, this crease is generally an extension of the epicanthal fold. In today's nomenclature, this is either a single eyelid or an inner double eyelid. Such eyes supposedly convey an impression of kindness and wisdom and an aura of mysteriousness. A benevolent emperor has these eyes, as does a brilliant scholar and a wealthy merchant. In contrast, a barbarian or a nomad from the central Asian steppe would usually be depicted with large eyes with creases around them. These eyes convey (to the Chinese and other Asians) the impression that the possessor is energetic, untamed, and fearsome (Fig. 69-2). Such notions were widely held until the nineteenth century when the western powers came to Asia.

Over the past 200 years, the military might and the economic influence of the West have changed the world. Since World War II there has been an especially accelerated global spread of Western influence, with the Western way of living, values, and standards being further disseminated through motion pictures and television. As a consequence, some of the Western standards of beauty have become accepted as standards in the East. In many Asian cities, hair styles and fashions keep pace with those in New York, Paris, and London; and, in fact, cities such as Tokyo, Taipei, and Singapore are beginning to set the pace. As the standard of living continues to rise, and the tireless pursuit of beauty goes on, a most notable change in the East is the acceptance and appreciation of the typical Western type of upper eyelid. To a lesser degree, other facial features characteristic of Caucasians, such as a narrow and long nose, are now considered desirable by many Asians.

To be sure, there are many differences in the facial features of an Asian of the Mongolian race and of a Caucasian. In general, the Asian has a rounder face; the frontal bone tends to be wider and the supraorbital ridge less

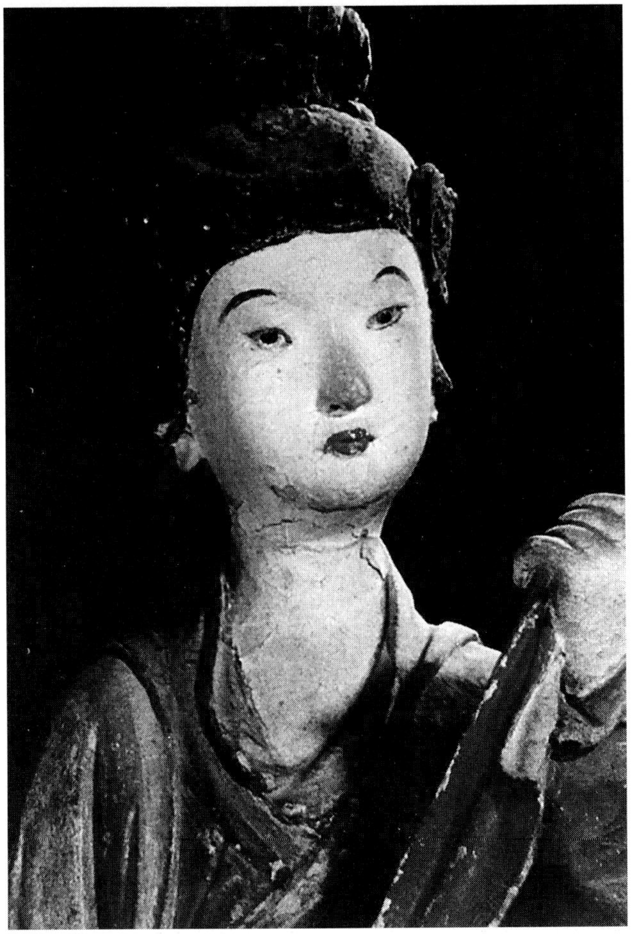

Figure 69–1. A Chinese ceramic figurine of the seventh century A.D. depicting a typical much-admired almond-shaped eye. It has a typical exaggerated Mongolian slant, an epicanthal fold, and no eyelid crease.

prominent; the bridge of the nose tends to be wider and flatter and the tip of the nose and the nostrils more rounded; and the lips tend to be thicker and less pointed at the mucocutaneous junction. In the periorbital region, there is fullness in the area of the superior sulcus. Frequently, an eyelid crease is absent and an epicanthal fold is apparent. When compared with those of a Caucasian, the palpebral fissure is narrower and the eyelashes are shorter and straighter. On the other hand, the face of a Caucasian will typically have a relatively narrow frontal bone with a more prominent supraorbital ridge, a long and narrow nose with a pointed tip, narrow alae, and small nostrils. The cheek bones are high, and the periorbital area, by contrast, is sunken. There is a deep superior sulcus with a distinct upper eyelid crease. There is no epicanthal fold, the lashes are long and curved, and the palpebral fissures are wide.

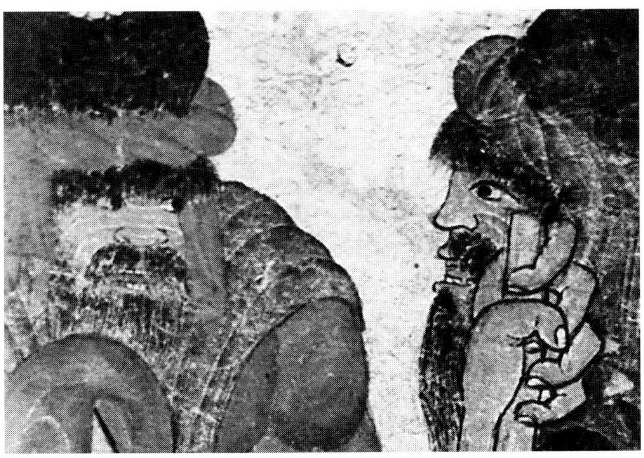

Figure 69–2. A small portion of a Chinese painting from the eleventh century A.D. depicting the northern barbarians. Note the large round eyes with a crease, the large nose, and the bushy mustache and beard.

For the past several decades the double eyelid operation has been the single most popular cosmetic procedure in many Asian countries; it is requested by both men and women and by persons of all walks of life, not so much to westernize their eyelids but rather to enhance the "natural" beauty of the Asian face; furthermore, many of these individuals will also inquire about a simultaneous rhinoplasty. A very interesting phenomenon has been observed. On the one hand, this procedure is looked on by many as a simple, routine procedure that can be performed by even nonmedical personnel. Many techniques, including the use of tapes, glue, and buried sutures, are performed by beauticians and paramedical personnel in many Asian cities. Consequently, the procedure is perceived as a "quick fix" in which pain, scarring, infection, and temporary results are often expected. These patients tend to be bargain hunters, who go from one practitioner to the next looking for the best price. Long-term follow-up of these patients is next to impossible; once the surgery is performed, these patients tend to disappear, regardless of the outcome. On the other hand, it is considered by others to be a most serious and challenging surgical procedure that only the most accomplished surgeon can perform. Members of the latter group tend to be of the upper socioeconomic echelon who believe in the concept of "you get what you pay for." Money is of no object to them, and they want the perfect result. Unlike other situations, where the patient disappears when the word "surgery" is brought up, these patients tend to be very sophisticated, well educated, and demanding. In the United States, Asian patients seeking cosmetic surgery are usually newly arrived, wealthy immigrants; only rarely are they second-generation American citizens. It is advisable that surgeons avoid terms such as "westernization of the Oriental eyelid," or "correction or revision of the Oriental eyelid." In fact, a good way to win the heart of these patients is for the surgeon to use terms that are familiar to them. *Double eyelid* is a term used by all Asians to describe an upper eyelid with a crease, and *single eyelid* is a term to describe an eyelid without a crease (Fig. 69–3). Written in Chinese idiogram these terms make perfect sense but defy good translation. Many terms have been used in the English literature to describe various types of upper eyelid creases in Asians, but I believe that these terms and classifications

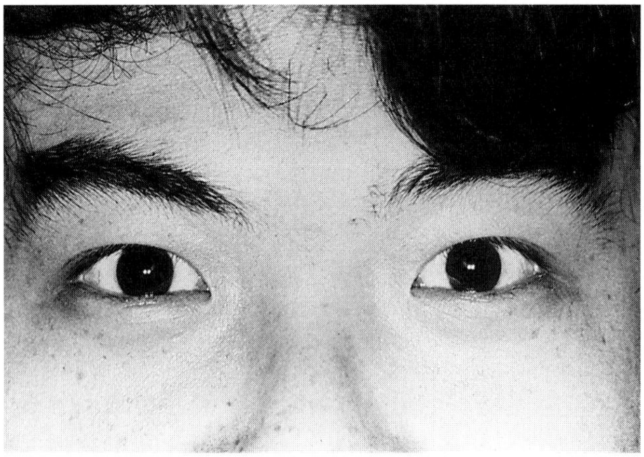

Figure 69–3. A single eyelid with a noticeable epicanthal fold.

only add to the confusion. The fact is, only two types of double eyelids are of clinical significance: the outer and inner double eyelids. The others are essentially variations of these two basic types, and the goal of surgery is to create one or the other of these.

Hsu and Liu studied the lid crease in more than 3600 Chinese patients and classified the double eyelids into these two clinically significant groups.[1] The first, the outer (outside or external) double eyelid, is a distinct upper eyelid crease located 7 to 10 mm above the lash margin. Many authors use the term *parallel type* to describe it because, in general, the crease parallels the lid margin. Associated with this type of double eyelid is a minimal or absent epicanthal fold. This lid crease very much resembles that of the Caucasian lid. The second type of double eyelid, the "inner" (inside or internal) double eyelid, has a crease located from 3 to 5 mm above the lash margin centrally. This type of double eyelid is usually associated with a minimal or moderately prominent epicanthal fold. The lid crease is obscured when the patient looks up, as the overlying skin fold touches the eyelashes. Some authors use the term *unfolded fan* to describe this type of eyelid crease because it follows the curvature of the epicanthal fold and is a natural extension of the epicanthus tarsalis (Fig. 69–4). Variations of these two types of lid creases include a lateral flare, a medial dip, and multiple or secondary creases. Hsu and Liu also find that the majority of our patients prefer the inner double eyelid because of its "natural" look.

Hu[2] studied 2320 normal eyelids of healthy Chinese in Shanghai and found that the incidence of a single eyelid was 44.5%. He also found that 70% of those with single eyelids are children younger than 10 years of age, and only 28.2% are adults older than 20 years of age. In his study, the single eyelid was bilateral in most cases and was unilateral in only 3.9% of the children and 1.7% of the adults. Other investigators have shown that the mode of heredity of the single eyelid is autosomal dominant.[3]

Wang and Bian,[4] in 1986, dissected 40 eyelids in 20 cadavers of Chinese origin and very nicely correlated the anatomic studies with clinical findings. First, in contrast to the Caucasian anatomy, the fusion level of the orbital septum and the levator aponeurosis was below the superior margin of the tarsal plate in 90% of the specimens. This fusion level in single eyelids was much lower than that found in double eyelids. Double eyelids were present in 18 of the upper lids (40%), and the fusion level in 4 eyelids was above the superior margin of the tarsus and in 14 eyelids it was below the margin. A statistically significant difference was found also between the fusion level in the single eyelids and in the double eyelids, the former being much lower. Wang and Bian also made the very interesting and important observation that the average upper eyelid crease in live patients is at least 2 mm higher than that found in the cadavers. Tables 69–1 through 69–3 summarize many of these eyelid findings.

EPICANTHAL FOLD

This anatomic entity was first described by Schon in 1828,[5] and the term *epicanthal fold* was coined by Van Ammon in 1860.[6] The epicanthal fold consists of a semilunar fold of skin extending from the upper eyelid across the medial canthal area to the margin of the lower eyelid. It is apparent beginning between the third and sixth

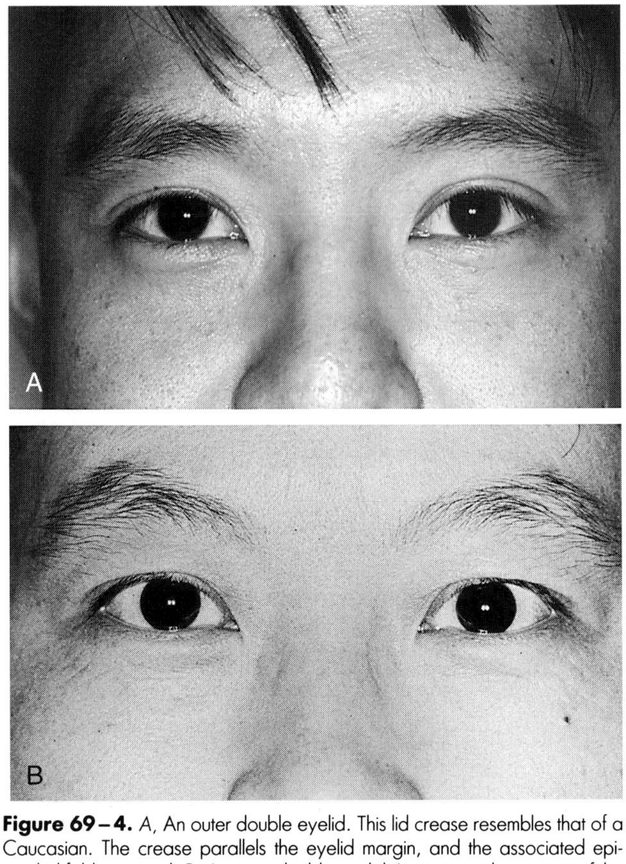

Figure 69–4. *A*, An outer double eyelid. This lid crease resembles that of a Caucasian. The crease parallels the eyelid margin, and the associated epicanthal fold is minimal. *B*, An inner double eyelid. It is a natural extension of the epicanthus tarsalis. The crease is at a lower level compared with the outer type.

TABLE 69-1

Level of Fusion of Orbital Septum and the Levator Aponeurosis and the Measurements of Lid Crease Height in 40 Chinese Cadavers

	Fusion Level (Below Superior Tarsal Margin)	Range of Crease Height	Average Crease Height
Double eyelid (18)	2.4 ± 1.9 mm	3.0 ± 6.5 mm	4.6 ± 1.0 mm
Single eyelid (22)	3.9 ± 1.0 mm	0	0

$P < .01$; $t = 6.12$.
Data from Wang HM, Bian CJ: The anatomy of upper eyelid and its clinical significance. Chin J Plast Surg Burns 2:273–275, 1986.

months of gestation in all races. In Caucasians, African Americans, and some Inuits, it usually disappears before birth. In the Mongolian race, however, it remains as a characteristic feature and is present in an estimated 40% to 90% of that race, but in only 2% to 5% of Caucasians.[7] These variations depend, to a great extent, on geographic location and the ethnic background of the population studied.

The epicanthal fold is almost invariably bilateral, but it may be asymmetric; only rarely is it unilateral. In the Mongolian race, the combination of an epicanthal fold and a relatively flat nose results quite often in an esotropic appearance. In Caucasians, the epicanthus may be an isolated anomaly or may be associated with ptosis or blepharophimosis.

PREOPERATIVE EVALUATION

As is true for all cosmetic surgery, careful patient selection is the first step toward successful surgery. The surgeon should ascertain the patient's expectations of and motivations for the surgery. Although these cosmetic procedures can most certainly improve the appearance of these patients, they will not help them find an ideal companion, restore a failing marriage, land a new job, or get a promotion. These underlying psychosocial factors must be carefully scrutinized, and a candid discussion between the physician and the patient should define what can be realistically expected. In short, the surgeon should make sure that there is no psychiatric contraindication to surgery.

Cosmetic eyelid surgery should be considered only after thyroid, cardiac, and renal disorders have been ruled out and only if the patient is not known to form keloids. In addition to a pertinent medical history, the eye evaluation should include visual acuity, funduscopic examination, slit lamp examination, and a lacrimal function evaluation. Photographic documentation and sketches are a necessary part of the record. The upper eyelid height and contour and the direction of the lashes should be noted. If brow ptosis, eyelid ptosis, or an epicanthal fold is present, this should be taken into consideration in planning the surgery. If the patient desires a deeper superior sulcus, or removal of orbital fat and subcutaneous tissues, this aspect of the procedure should be considered during the planning stages.

It is advisable to avoid surgery in the medial canthal area whenever possible because this region exhibits a biologic predisposition to hypertrophic scar formation, and even the most meticulously performed procedure in this area may be complicated by an aesthetically unpleasing scar. If the patient does not specifically request removal of the epicanthal fold, such surgery should be avoided. If the patient does bring up the subject, the effect of removal of these folds can be demonstrated by pulling the nasal skin medially, providing the patient with a realistic approximation of what to expect. Occasionally, young

TABLE 69-2

Prevalence of Double Eyelid, Mongolian Slant, and Epicanthal Fold

Total no. of patients: 2248
Males: 1432
Females: 816
- Double eyelids
  - Males, 75.41%
  - Females, 81.98%
  - Overall average, 77.80%
- Single eyelids
  - Males, 24.59%
  - Females, 18.02%
  - Overall average, 22.20%

Total no. of patients: 1020
- Mongolian slant, 13.23%
- Anti-Mongolian slant, 4.71%
- Leveled, 82.06%
- Epicanthal fold, 53.50%

Data from Jee MD: Chin Ophthalmol J 5:285, 1958.

TABLE 69-3

Prevalence of Epicanthal Fold and Double Eyelids of Chinese and Taiwanese

	Liu and Hsu (1986)	Hsu (1992)
Total no. of patients	3640	2800
Epicanthal fold	40.7%	48.8%
Single eyelid*	23.2%	26.8%
Double eyelid	76.8%	73.21%

*Sixty percent of these patients prefer the inner double eyelid.
Adapted from Liu D, Hsu WM: Oriental eyelids: Anatomic difference and surgical consideration. Ophthalmic Plast Reconstr Surg 2:59–64, 1986, and from Hsu WM, personal communication, 1992.

children are brought in by parents who believe them to have esotropia. Similar digital manipulation of the nasal skin will eliminate the child's esotropic appearance, which will demonstrate to the parents that removal of the epicanthal fold is the appropriate surgery. The parents should be advised, however, that a temporary, hypertrophic scar may result.

It is not uncommon for an Asian patient undergoing blepharoplasty to request a simultaneous rhinoplasty. Only rarely does an Asian exhibit a large nose with a dorsal hump formation that requires reduction rhinoplasty. A high, narrow nasal bridge is an aesthetically desirable feature in most Asian cultures, apart from a desire for "westernization." Details of the anatomic differences, surgical indications and techniques, and potential complications are beyond the scope of this chapter. The ophthalmologist should consult with an otolaryngologist or with a plastic surgeon if a patient desires rhinoplasty. Candidates for any surgical procedure who are taking aspirin or warfarin are instructed to discontinue taking these drugs for at least 2 weeks before the scheduled surgery. In addition, these patients should refrain from mo-er, Chinese chives, and other Chinese herbs that they may be using to "improve circulation." As described in Chapter 68, it is generally appreciated by the patient and by the patient's family when the physician includes family members in these discussions. The doctor–patient relationship will be off to a much better start if the physician has at least some understanding of the cultural background and religious teachings of the patient.

DETERMINATION AND MARKING OF THE LID CREASE

It is most helpful to demonstrate to the patient what can be achieved, which is easily done with the aid of some simple, readily available devices. For example, the patient looks in a mirror while the surgeon uses a small paper clip to gently press on the medial aspect of the upper eyelid (Fig. 69–5); this usually results in a natural eyelid crease that extends from the epicanthal fold. A more elaborate means of demonstrating the expected result is the use of a sterile strip or glues; photographs and sketches may also be helpful.

As stated before, a preference for the location of the new upper eyelid crease may vary from patient to patient. If an inner double eyelid is preferred, the curvature and the location of such a crease are determined by gently depressing the upper lid skin nasally (such as with a small paper clip) to accentuate the epicanthal fold. The surgeon can follow the epicanthal fold superiorly and laterally, and thereby determine the location of the new crease. Occasionally, this can be achieved also by direct and arbitrary measurement.

If the patient desires an outer double eyelid, the position and the curvature of the crease should be agreed on

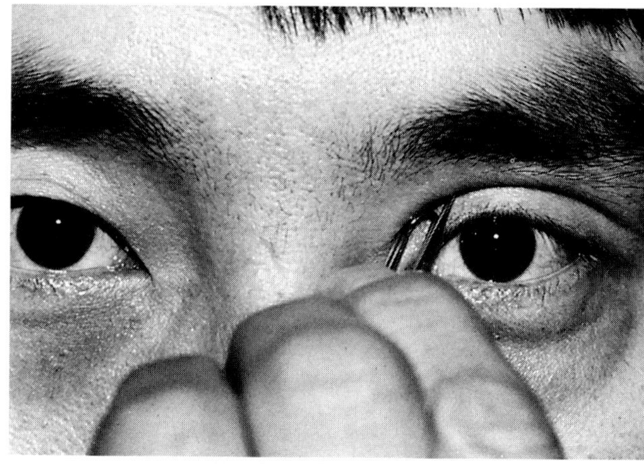

Figure 69–5. When a small paper clip is used to gently press on the upper eyelid skin medially, an upper eyelid crease is created.

preoperatively and the markings made accordingly. For most Asians, the crease will be situated 5 to 8 mm above the lash margin. In general, a lid crease placed higher in an Asian does not look natural and is not. Finally, if the patient has an existing unilateral double eyelid, the proposed crease in the fellow eye should match the existing crease, for symmetry.

ANESTHESIA

Local anesthesia supplemented by intravenous sedation is preferred. Usually, an intravenously administered bullous dosage of propofol (30 to 40 mg) is given just before the local injection. After the measurements and the necessary markings have been made, and the patient is sufficiently sedated, local anesthesia is achieved by means of 2% lidocaine with epinephrine 1:100,000 which is injected with a 25-gauge needle inserted immediately beneath the skin. This facilitates dissection of the tissue planes and improves hemostasis.

SURGICAL PROCEDURES*

Incision Techniques

An incisional technique is used when an extensive change in the overall appearance of the periorbital region is desired. This procedure is necessary when the patient has much redundant skin and an abundant amount of subcutaneous and orbital fat. The superior sulcus can be deepened, the periorbital region recontoured, and the brow lifted. Depending on the final objectives and the contour desired, various amounts of skin, muscle, subcutaneous tissue, and orbital fat can be removed. Further-

*Drs. Wen Ming Hsu, Nai Jiang Xu, and Guang Xi Zhao have contributed to this section.

more, this technique yields a more permanent result even if the only goal is to create a new eyelid crease.

Technique

The location of the proposed eyelid crease is first marked. Repeated measurements are made to ensure symmetry of the two eyelids. The marked lid crease is used as the inferior border of the area to be excised. The superior border is determined by the pinch technique: with one blade at the eyelid crease, the skin is grasped with a smooth forceps; the amount of skin that can be grasped when the lashes first evert is the amount that can be safely excised (Fig. 69–6). To avoid damage to the punctum and to preclude webbing, the medial markings should be at least 3 mm from the lid margin. The angle at the junction of the inferior and superior incisions is 30 degrees or less, to avoid a dog-ear and extension of the incision. At the lateral canthus, the lower incision should be at least 5 mm above the horizontal midline and should form an angle of 30 degrees or less when it joins with the superior incision. This precludes damage to the lymphatics and unsightly scarring. Both upper eyelids should be marked at the same time to ensure symmetry. After the induction of local anesthesia, the patient's face is gently prepared and draped. Using a no. 15 blade, the surgeon makes an incision first along the lid crease, leaving the superior marking intact. The skin is undermined superiorly for a few millimeters beyond the marking, and with this skin reflected, a small strip underlying orbicularis is removed. If a submuscular fat pad is present, it is also removed to ensure formation of a deep, permanent, and distinct eyelid crease. Unless brow fixation is intended, no extensive dissection superiorly should be performed.

The extent of sculpturing or recontouring of the superior sulcus of the orbital rim that is required must be determined preoperatively. If minor recontouring is planned, removal of skin, orbicularis, and submuscular fat will usually suffice. If still deeper contour is desired, more submuscular fat pad and orbital fat pad need to be removed. A brow fixation can be accomplished by using a 4-0 Mersilene suture to anchor the subcutaneous tissue of the eyebrow to the periosteum at the desired level. Generally, either a posterior eyebrow fixation technique or a coronal approach is used. The curvature of the eyebrow is controlled by the placement of these sutures at different positions or by the amount of coronal lift.

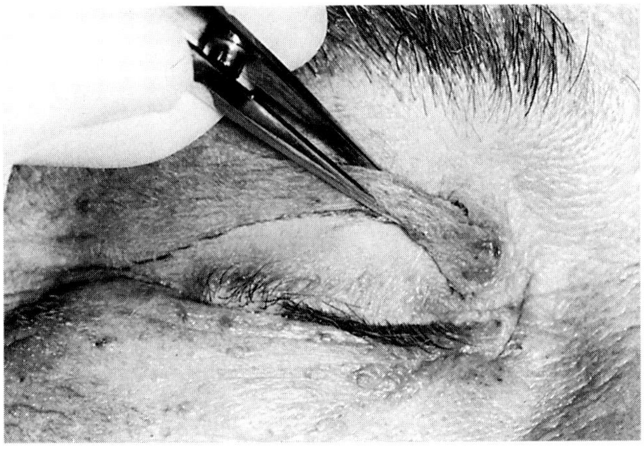

Figure 69–6. The desired upper eyelid crease is marked, and the skin is grasped with a smooth forceps until the lashes begin to evert.

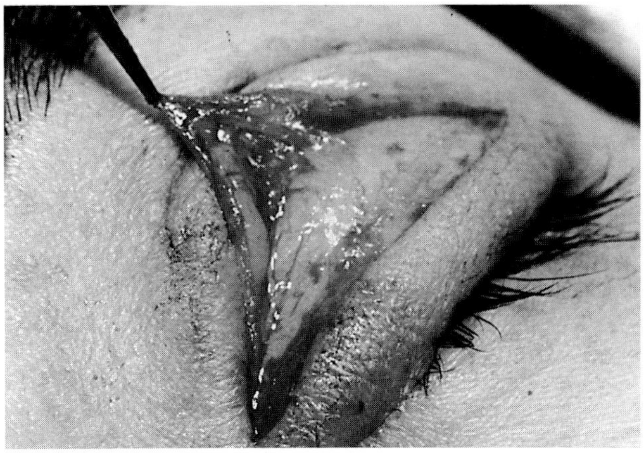

Figure 69–7. Note the small submuscular fat pad attached to the underside of the muscle. Its color and consistency are different from those of the large lobule of the orbital fat pad anterior to the tarsus seen in the wound.

In the majority (76% to 85%) of Asian patients, a submuscular fat pad is present.[1, 8] This is easily identified by its anatomic location because it lies immediately beneath the orbicularis layer anterior to the orbital septum. In addition, the consistency, color, and size of the fat globules are somewhat different from those of the orbital fat pad; the submuscular fat pad is more like a subcutaneous fat pad, with harder consistency, smaller globules, and a more yellowish color (Fig. 69–7).

To remove orbital fat, an incision is made into the orbital septum and the fat pad is gently prolapsed and grasped with a small mosquito clamp; it is then excised and the pedicle cauterized lightly. The fat pad is allowed to retract into the orbit and then the area is inspected to be certain that there is no further bleeding. If there is no medical contraindication, the operated area is irrigated with a few drops of Neosporin solution and triamcinolone suspension. Superiorly, the central fat pad is found along with a smaller medial fat pad; the lateral pad is the smallest of all and sometimes cannot be found in an Asian patient.[9] When excising tissue laterally, the surgeon should take care to avoid damage to the lacrimal gland. Gentle pressure on the globe will usually tease out more fat medially. These fat pads tend to bleed more and should be carefully ligated or cauterized before allowing them to retract into the orbit.

Putting aside and comparing the excised fat and subcutaneous tissue from both sides helps to ensure symmetry. When the desired result is achieved, the superior skin flap is gently draped over the lower skin edge. The previous

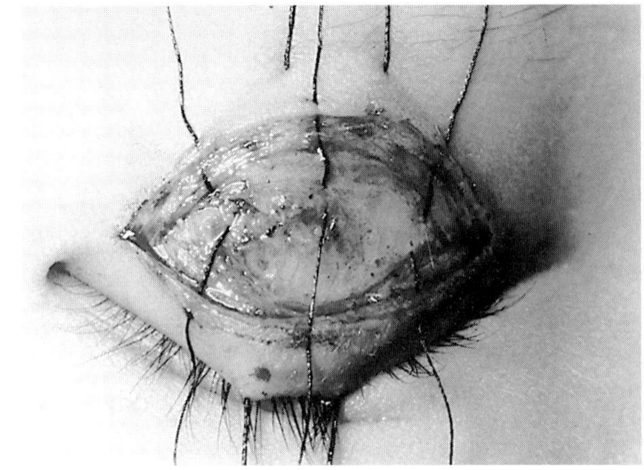

Figure 69–8. Supratarsal fixation technique; 6-0 silk suture is used. In addition to approximating the wound edges, the suture is anchored in the levator aponeurosis above the tarsal plate.

marking is used as a guide, and the redundant skin is excised. As a result of the removal of large amounts of subcutaneous tissue from the eyelid and orbit, a new contour is carved out. Since there is very little skin redundancy, to cover this new contour without exerting tension on the skin the surgeon should perform skin resection very conservatively. The orbital septum and orbicularis layer are not closed with sutures.

One way to create the eyelid crease is use of the supratarsal fixation technique.[10] The levator aponeurosis is first identified, and a 6-0 silk suture is placed along the midpupillary line through the lower skin edge, taking a bite through the muscular layer. Next, a small horizontal bite is taken into the aponeurosis at the superior border of the tarsal plate; the same needle is then brought out through the muscle and then the upper skin edge. Two additional sutures are placed in a similar manner on either side of the first one about 5 mm away. These sutures, which are tied tight and cut long, are the crease sutures and will be left in place for 10 to 14 days. The remaining skin wound can be approximated with 6-0 nylon in an interrupted fashion. Using sutures of a different material or color makes identification of the crease sutures easier (Fig. 69–8).

At the conclusion of the procedure, the surgeon should once again inspect the lid crease for its curvature and height and assess symmetry and closure of the lids (Fig. 69–9). Maxitrol ointment (a combination product of dexamethasone and neomycin) is placed over the incision and in the eye. The eyes are left unpatched, but cold compresses are applied immediately in the recovery room.

POSTOPERATIVE CARE

All of our cosmetic blepharoplasty procedures are done on an outpatient basis. The patient's vision is

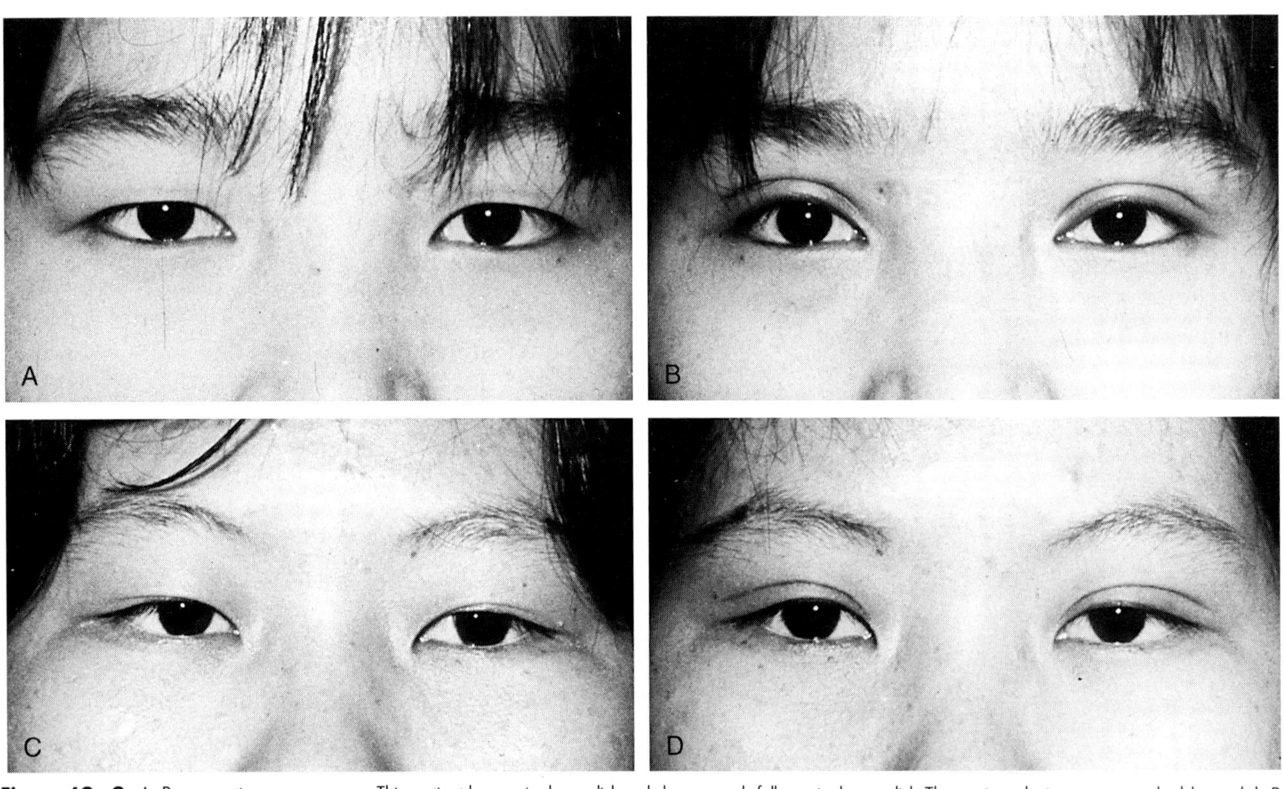

Figure 69–9. *A*, Preoperative appearance. This patient has a single eyelid and shows much fullness in the eyelid. The patient desires an outer double eyelid. *B*, Postoperative appearance of the same patient. An outer double eyelid is created by using the incisional technique. Note the change in the contour and the distinct lid crease. *C*, Preoperative appearance of a patient who desires a higher and more distinct inner double eyelid. Some fullness in the upper eyelids is noted. The patient also has a noticeable epicanthal fold. *D*, Postoperative appearance of the same patient. Note the higher and more distinct inner double eyelid with a lateral flare.

checked and the wound is inspected in the recovery room. Before discharge the patient is instructed to apply cold compresses over the wound for the next 48 hours, and the patient and relatives are instructed to be alert for possible signs of an orbital hemorrhage; if such signs or symptoms develop, they are to alert the physician immediately. The first postoperative visit is scheduled usually on the fifth day, at which time visual acuity is recorded, the cornea examined with the slit lamp, and the wound inspected. Symmetry of eyelid contour and closure and the directions of the lashes are assessed. The nonabsorbable skin sutures are removed at this time, but the eyelid crease sutures are left in place for an additional 7 to 10 days. The wound may be dressed with a sterile strip.

COMPLICATIONS

The best management of complications is their prevention, which is best achieved by careful planning, atraumatic surgical techniques, and meticulous closure. Complications of blepharoplasty that have been reported include blindness, ectropion, entropion, ptosis, extraocular muscle palsy, ocular muscle palsy, epiphora, unacceptable scarring, asymmetry, overcorrection, undercorrection, dry eyes, and loss of lashes, although the very serious complications are quite rare.[9, 11]

Edema or ecchymosis is a commonly seen postoperative sequela, especially when a large amount of tissue has been resected. This complication can be minimized, however, by making certain that the patient is not taking aspirin, warfarin, mo-er, or other anticoagulants (see Chapter 68) and by atraumatic surgical technique, good hemostasis throughout the procedure, meticulous wound closure, and immediate postoperative application of cold compresses to the eyelids. Subconjunctival hemorrhage is seen occasionally when there has been extensive removal of orbital fat. Wound gaping may result from excessive swelling, undue tension on the wound, or faulty closure techniques; this can usually be amended by approximating the wound and applying a sterile strip.

Asymmetry can be prevented by careful planning, precision in measuring, and surgical techniques. Exposure keratitis or ectropion can be prevented by conservative resection of skin and soft tissue. In addition, the muscle layer and orbital septum should not be closed with sutures. Abnormal folds can result from overaggressive undermining of the skin, removal of the subcutaneous tissues, or both and from overzealous application of cautery and faulty suture techniques.

Formation of a shallow eyelid crease or a temporary crease has been reported. Understandably, a hematoma or edema immediately after surgery may disrupt some or all of the sutures that are used to create the adhesion between the skin and the deeper sutures. Additionally, the sutures may not be tied tightly enough or be left in long enough to form a good adhesion. It has been suggested that, at least in some cases, the lower skin flap may be anchored to the orbital septum; with the passage of time, the supraorbital fat pushes the septum forward and downward and eventually removes all of the adhesions that were formed between the skin and the deeper tissues.

SUTURE TECHNIQUES

The principles of the suture techniques are based on the development of adhesions of cicatricial changes between the skin and deeper tissue that are induced by the suture material. These techniques do not involve any incising of the skin. They are simple to perform and can be repeated when necessary. For those patients who do not want extensive surgery, or in whom radical surgery is not indicated, the suture techniques are very effective in creating an upper eyelid crease. The ideal candidates for these procedures are young persons who have taut skin and relatively little or no orbital and submuscular fat.

As mentioned earlier, suture techniques are frequently used by even nonmedical personnel. The earliest description of a suture technique to create a double eyelid is by Mikamo in 1896, according to Shirakabe and colleagues.[12] Other Japanese and Chinese authors also described their suture techniques in their own native language. Perhaps the first suture technique described in English was by Koo in 1964.[13] Koo used only three nylon sutures extending from the conjunctival surface toward the skin surface to create an eyelid crease. Mutou and Mutou,[14] in 1972, used two silk or catgut sutures, placing them horizontally from the conjunctival surface and parallel to the superior tarsal border and burying the ligatures on the conjunctival side; they claim a 99.9% success rate.

Pang's[15] technique uses three double-armed silk sutures that are placed in a mattress fashion through the full thickness of the eyelid tissue. The lid crease thus created tends to be somewhat temporary, and the exposed sutures on the conjunctival side can cause corneal irritation. Mutou, on the other hand, uses double-armed 6-0 buried silk sutures, but again some small skin incisions are necessary. In 1988, I described a suture technique using a 5-0 chromic suture.[16] This suture is placed in the lid substance in a continuous fashion from one end of the proposed lid crease to the other. The suture is entirely buried within the eyelid substance, thereby causing no irritation to the cornea. Back and colleagues,[17] in 1989, described a one-stitch suture technique using 6-0 Prolene. In this large combined series of 762 patients, and with followup ranging from 2 months to 5 years, these authors reported a success rate of 95.8%. Only 32 of the 762 patients needed a reoperation, and of these 32 there were 22 who had disappearance of the newly created lid crease.

All of the various suture techniques are performed with the use of local anesthesia on an outpatient basis. Some patients may benefit from the use of a mild sedative, which may be given orally, intravenously, or intramuscularly. Once the proposed eyelid crease is determined and marked, a small amount of 2% lidocaine with epinephrine is used; this is injected along these markings both on the skin and on the conjunctival sides just above the superior border of the tarsal plate. Some surgeons advocate the use of a bone plate to protect the globe or traction sutures along the lid margin to facilitate exposure or dissection.

Technique 1: Buried Mattress Suture Technique

The upper eyelid is everted after being marked and injected. A double-armed 6-0 nylon suture is inserted on the conjunctival side 2 mm above the superior tarsal border. Aiming at the skin marking, this needle is pushed through the substance of the eyelid to emerge on the skin side. The second arm of the suture is inserted through the same needle hole but traverses horizontally for 2 mm, very close to the conjunctival surface, before exiting on the skin side 2 mm away from the first. The second suture arm now reenters the skin through its own exit hole on the skin; it takes a 2-mm subcutaneous bite before exiting from the same hole from which the first arm exits. The two arms are then tied tight and cut short; the knot is buried beneath the skin. Before tying the suture, this exit hole is enlarged slightly with the needle. Three or four such mattress sutures are placed along the skin marking (Fig. 69–10).

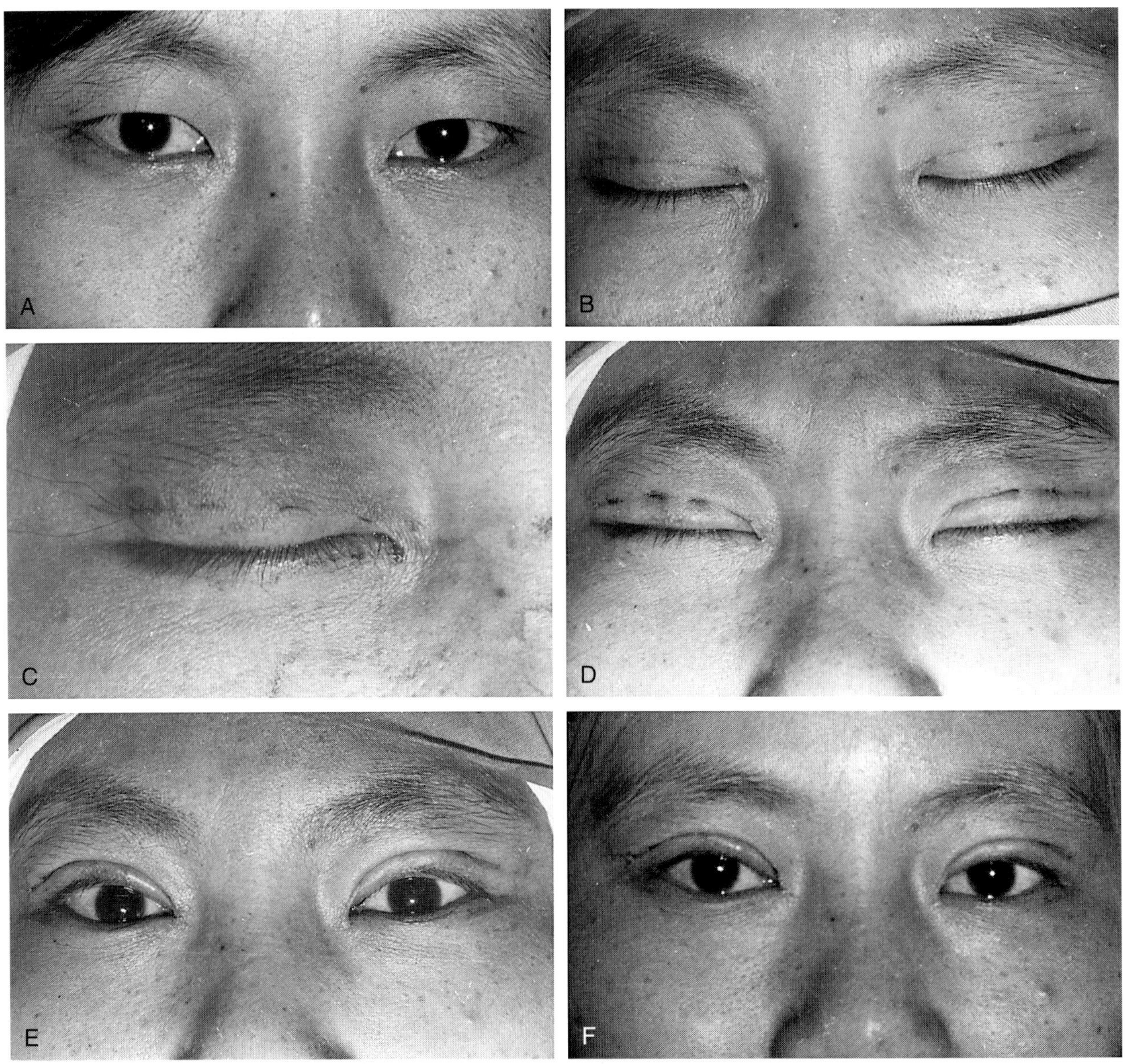

Figure 69–10. *A*, The patient has a single eyelid and desires an inner double eyelid. She does not have much orbital or submuscular fat and also has tight skin. A suture technique is ideal. *B*, The desired eyelid crease is marked, and four points are selected along this proposed crease where the sutures will be buried. *C*, This demonstrates the placement of a buried suture laterally. *D*, At the conclusion of the procedure, only minimal swelling is noted. No suture is exposed. *E*, The appearance at the end of the procedure. *F*, Postoperative appearance 2 months later.

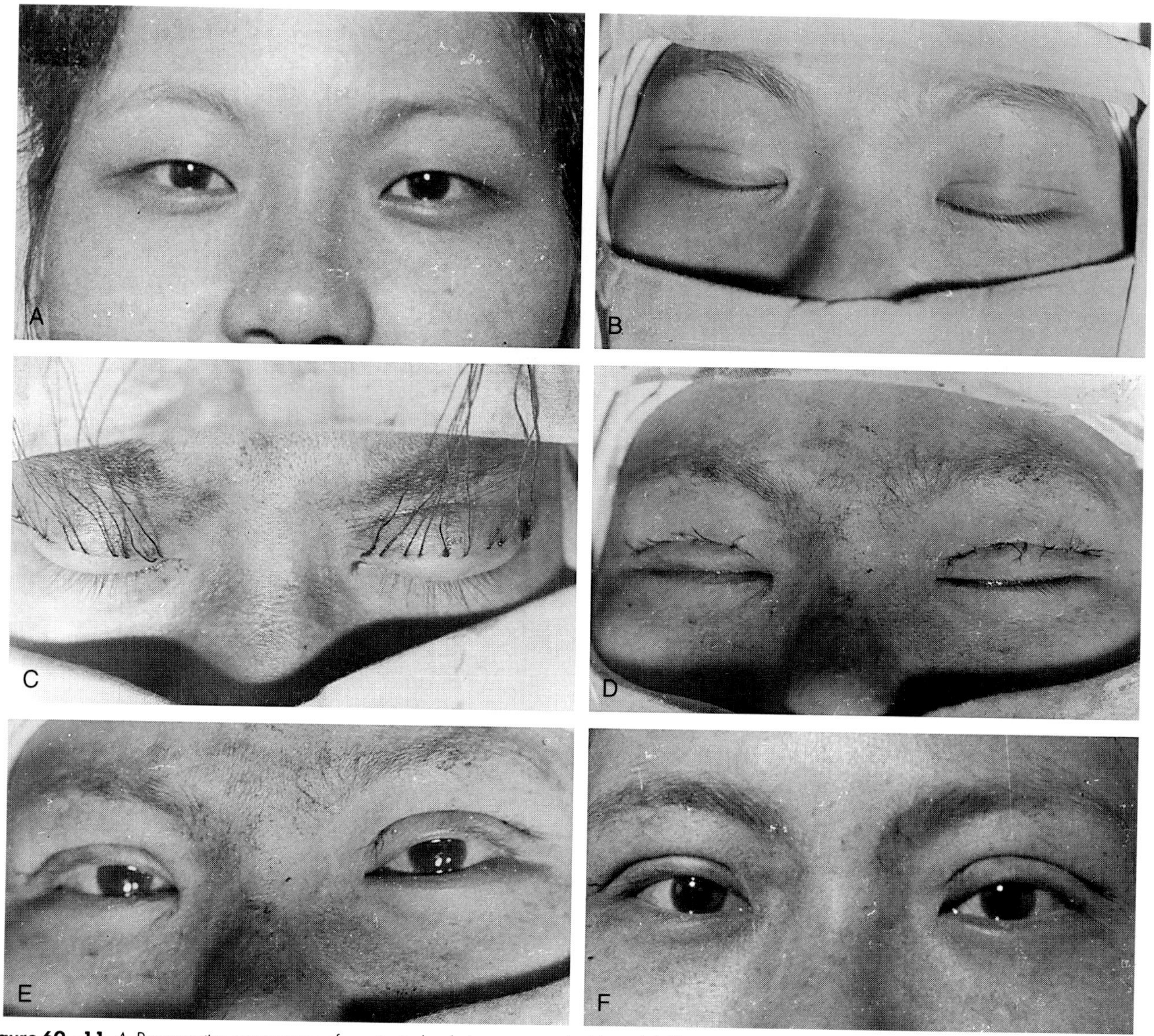

Figure 69–11. *A,* Preoperative appearance of a patient who desires an outer double eyelid. She does not have much fullness in the upper eyelid, and she has tight skin. A suture technique is good for this patient. *B,* The desired lid crease is marked and injected. *C,* Five mattress sutures are placed along the desired lid crease, evenly spaced and exteriorized. *D,* These sutures are tied tight and cut short. *E,* Appearance when the patient is still on the operating table at the conclusion of the procedure. *F,* Postoperative appearance of the patient 7 days later, at the time of suture removal.

If the surgeon finds these maneuvers to bury the sutures difficult, he or she can exteriorize the sutures and achieve almost the same results. These sutures need to be removed 10 to 12 days postoperatively (Fig. 69–11).

Technique 2: Continuous Suture Technique

The proposed lid crease is marked and a local anesthetic is administered along this marking on the skin side and on the conjunctival side. A bone plate is used to protect the globe. Beginning laterally, a single-armed 6-0 nylon suture of ⅜ circle is inserted from the skin side, taking a large bite of all of the tissues except the conjunctiva itself before it exits on the skin side some 5 mm more medially. The needle is then reentered into the skin through the previous exit wound, in a medial direction, taking a 5-mm shallow subcutaneous bite and exiting 5 mm away. The same needle again reenters the substance of the eyelid to include all tissues except the conjunctiva and exits 5 mm away. The next step is a shallow subcutaneous bite. This alternating process is repeated several times until the needle exits on the skin side at the medial end of the marking after a deep bite. Then, beginning at the medial end of the crease, the process is reversed. The same needle is reentered through the previous exit wound on the skin, going in the lateral direction to take a shallow bite of the subcutaneous tissue. It exits 5 mm laterally, through the previous puncture wound. Reentering this puncture wound, the needle takes a deep bite of lid tissues. This process is repeated until the needle fi-

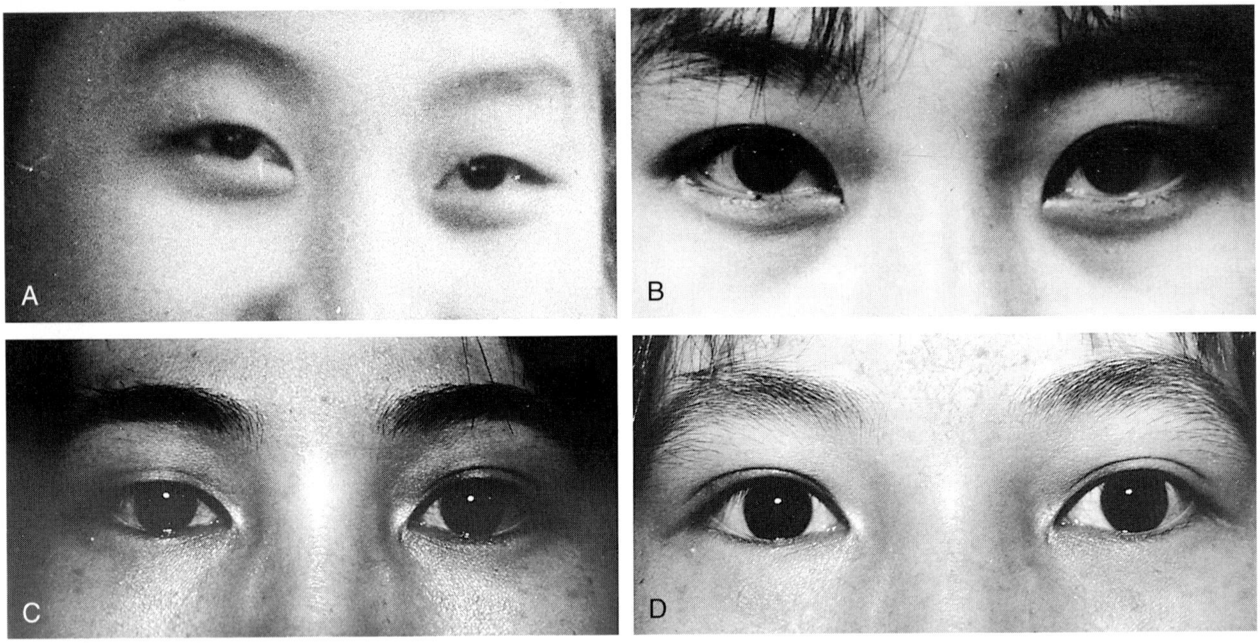

Figure 69–12. *A*, Preoperative appearance of a patient with a single eyelid who desires an inner double eyelid. She does not have much fullness or skin redundancy in the upper eyelids. *B*, Postoperative appearance of the same patient. A continuous buried suture technique was used. *C*, Preoperative appearance of a patient with an indistinct right upper eyelid crease. This patient desires an accentuation of this crease. *D*, Postoperative appearance of the same patient. A continuous buried suture technique was used.

nally reaches the lateral end of the lid crease, where the process was first begun. Where the needle has previously taken a large bite of all lid tissues, it is now taking a very shallow, subcutaneous bite. Now, over the first puncture wound, the suture is tied tight and cut short; the knot is then tucked in subcutaneously with a forceps. At the conclusion of the procedure, only a few needle puncture wounds are seen, in addition to the newly formed eyelid crease (Fig. 69–12).

This technique is a very useful intermediate procedure between the full incisional technique and the suture techniques. It is applicable when a small degree of recontouring of the eyelid is necessary but a full eyelid crease incision and deep tissue dissections are to be avoided. Such a situation can be seen in a relatively young patient with very little orbital fat and requires a short recovery course. When using this technique, it should be kept in mind that only a small amount of orbital fat may be removed through these stab incisions.

Technique 3: Combined Buried Sutures and Small Incisions

The crease is marked, injected, and everted. Three 3-mm-long incisions are made on the crease marking, at the center and at the lateral and medial ends of the crease. A stab incision is made through the orbicularis and the orbital septum. A small amount of orbital fat may be prolapsed through these incisions with gentle pressure applied to the globe; these are clamped, cut, and cauterized. A small amount of orbicularis can also be grasped, pulled out through these small incisions, and excised. Buried mattress sutures, using 6-0 nylon to include all of the deep substance of the eyelid, except the skin and the conjunctiva, are placed through these small incisions. The skin incisions may be closed with a single suture or left unsutured (Fig. 69–13).

Postoperative Care

Careful examination should be made of both the skin side and the conjunctival side to make sure that the sutures are buried entirely. Antibiotic ointment is placed in the eye and over the skin, and a cold compress is immediately placed over the eyelids. In most instances these patients are able to return to their usual work the next day. The first postoperative visit is usually 7 days later, at which time visual acuity is recorded and the status of the cornea is carefully assessed.

Long-term followup of these patients is relatively poor except at major medical centers, where patients with surgical complications after surgery performed elsewhere are often seen.

Complications

Disappearance of the lid crease is the most common complication seen with the suture technique.[1, 15, 18] Although the exact incidence is difficult to estimate, it is relatively high, especially when absorbable sutures are used. As these techniques have been refined, and the use of per-

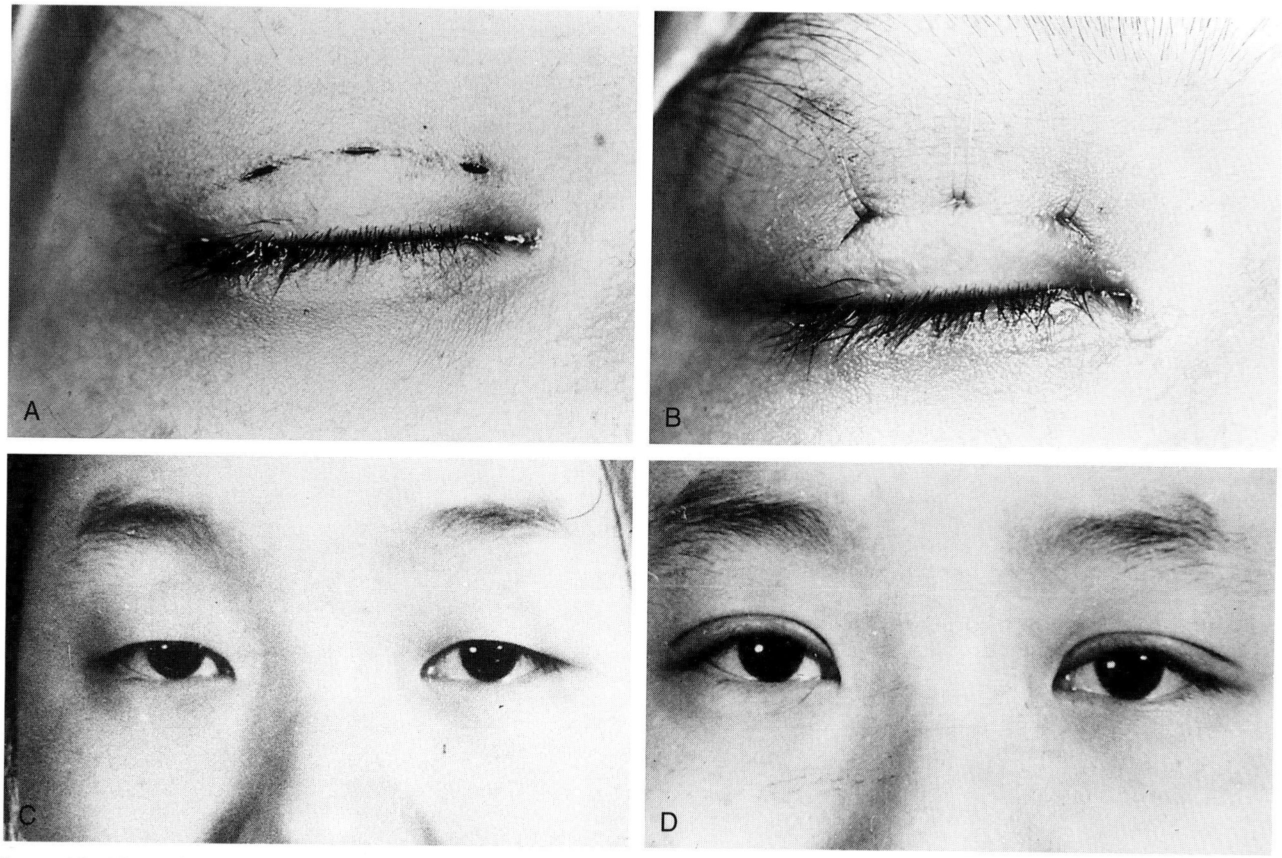

Figure 69–13. *A*, Three small stabbing incisions are made along the proposed crease. *B*, After the removal of a small amount of orbital fat by means of these incisions, three mattress sutures were used to create the eyelid crease. *C*, Preoperative appearance of a patient with a single eyelid. *D*, Postoperative appearance of the same patient as in C. A combined buried suture with a small incision technique was used.

manent sutures introduced, this rate is apparently on the decline. Similarly, other complications, such as corneal abrasion, which was a fairly common complication when these procedures were first described, is rarely seen now. Pang,[15] Koo,[13] and others have used either nylon or chromic sutures placed through the conjunctival fornix and have tied off the skin in a mattress fashion. Understandably, when these sutures are placed relatively low on the conjunctival side or are left fairly long, corneal abrasion can occur. These techniques have been modified so that the placement of the suture is relatively higher on the conjunctival side and the surgeon makes sure that the suture is tied tight; in addition, an antibiotic ointment instilled in the eye decreases such incidents. Granuloma formation has been seen with the buried suture technique, although the exact incidence of this complication is unknown. Asymmetry of the lid crease can occur also with the suture techniques but is due mainly to faulty surgical techniques. Other complications include hematoma and persistent edema. Complications in patients whose surgery was performed by nonmedical personnel include unsightly scarring, infection, hypertrophic scarring, ptosis, and preseptal cellulitis. Mutou and Mutou[14] reported that cyst formation is the most common complication, but loss of the eyelid crease, asymmetry, neurosis syndrome, and eyelid infections have also been reported by these authors.

REFERENCES

1. Liu D, Hsu WM: Oriental eyelids: Anatomic differences and surgical consideration. Ophthal Plast Reconstr Surg 2:59–64, 1986.
2. Hu DL: Heredity in Ophthalmology. Shanghai, Shanghai Scientific and Technical Publishing House, 1988, pp 105–109.
3. Xu ZS: Preliminary report on distribution and mode of inheritance of single and double eyelid in Han people. Transactions of the Second Conference of Chinese Genetic Ophthalmology, p 174.
4. Wang HM, Bian CJ: The anatomy of upper eyelid and its clinical significance. Chin J Plast Surg Burns 2:273–275, 1986.
5. Schon HB: Hb path anat d Auges. Hamburg 60:1882.
6. von Ammon FA: Epicanthus und das Epiblepharon. Behr Hildebr J Kinder 34:313–393, 1860.
7. Duke-Elder S: System of Ophthalmology, vol 3. St. Louis, CV Mosby, 1963, p 849.
8. Hsu WM: Personal communication, 1990.
9. Liu D, Stasior OG: Cosmetic blepharoplasty. Prospect Ophthalmol 5:203–209, 1981.
10. Sheen JH: Supratarsal fixation in upper blepharoplasty. Plast Reconstr Surg 54:424–431, 1974.
11. Smith B, Nesi FA: The complications of cosmetic blepharoplasty. *In* Symposium: Blepharoplasty Procedures. Ophthalmology 85:726–729, 1979.

12. Shirakabe Y, Dinugasa T, Kawata M, et al: The double-eyelid operation in Japan: Its evolution as related to cultural changes. Ann Plast Surg 15:224–241, 1985.
13. Koo BC: Plastic construction of the superior palpebral fold. Plast Reconstr Surg 111:149–153, 1985.
14. Mutou Y, Mutou H: Intradermal double eyelid operation and its follow-up results. Br J Plast Surg 25:285, 1972.
15. Pang HG: Surgical formation of upper lid fold. Arch Ophthalmol 63:783–784, 1961.
16. Liu D: Oriental eyelids: Anatomic difference and surgical consideration. *In* Hornblass A (ed): Oculoplastic, Orbital and Reconstructive Surgery, Volume 1, Eyelids. Baltimore, Williams & Wilkins, 1988, pp 513–524.
17. Baek SM, Kim SS, Tokunaga S, Bindinger A: Oriental blepharoplasty: Single-stitch, non-incision technique. Plast Reconstr Surg 83:236–242, 1989.
18. Hin LC: Oriental blepharoplasty—a critical review of technique and potential hazards. Ann Plast Surg 7:362–372, 1981.

CHAPTER 70

Considerations for Oculoplastic Surgery in the African American Patient

Tamara R. Fountain

The literature of ophthalmic reconstructive surgery is based overwhelmingly on procedures performed in patients who are Caucasian. Considerable attention has been devoted to surgery of the Asian lid owing to its unique anatomic features. However, there has been much less reported on cosmetic and reconstructive surgery in the African American. Structural or biochemical distinctions between African Americans and Caucasians are few, but these differences can have profound implications on clinical management. The most important feature for the surgeon to consider in African American patients is the potential for dyspigmentation and keloid formation in the postoperative period.

The density of cutaneous melanocytes is the same in African Americans and Caucasians. The greater pigmentation in African Americans is due to a greater production of melanin, which in turn is degraded more slowly. Melanocytes of African American patients may respond unpredictably to a variety of insults, including trauma, infection, and inflammation. Melanin production may shut down in some settings, causing hypopigmentation; increase in others, leading to hyperpigmentation; or undergo both processes, thus producing irregular mottling. The ophthalmic surgeon is more likely to encounter dyschromic changes after subcutaneous corticosteroid injections, cryotherapy, dermabrasion, and chemical peels or along postoperative wound closure lines. Modifications of some of these procedures to minimize pigmentary disturbances have been described. One author performs cryotherapy for trichiasis by approaching the hair follicle from the palpebral conjunctiva, thus avoiding application of the cryoprobe to the pigmented cutaneous surface.[1] Others have continued to perform dermabrasion but take care to limit its application to the most superficial skin layers.[2] Although these procedures may not be absolutely contraindicated in most African Americans, a thorough and detailed explanation of the potential for dyspigmentation must be provided in the course of preoperative evaluation and documented with informed consent.

Perhaps the most significant feature to consider when surgically manipulating black skin is the possibility of inciting keloid formation. Although this is a widely recognized complication of wound healing in African Americans, the actual risk is surprisingly low. The incidence of keloid formation in the general population ranges from 0.09% in England to 16% in Zaire.[3] A survey of 464 African Americans revealed a history of keloid formation in only 5.4%.[4] Although keloids pose a frustrating and chronic challenge to both patient and surgeon alike, the overwhelming majority of African American patients are not keloid formers.

Descriptions of keloids date back over 1000 years,[3] yet much about their etiology and pathogenesis remains uncertain. They are benign proliferative tumors that form in response to cutaneous insults such as infection, inflammation, burns, and penetrating trauma. They affect predominantly nonwhite races and are most prevalent in African Americans. The degree of pigmentation within a race does not correlate with keloid formation since light-skinned blacks are just as susceptible as those with dark complexions. Keloid formation has been shown to run in families, and both autosomal recessive and autosomal dominant patterns have been reported.[3] No consistent mode has been documented, however, and keloid risk is probably inherited in a multifactorial fashion.

Very rarely a keloid may arise in the absence of antecedent injury. These spontaneous lesions are typically confined to the presternal chest area. Secondary keloids form on many parts of the body, particularly the chest, back, and shoulders, but are rarely found on the palms or soles. Some authors have noted a female predilection, but this more likely represents a greater number of earlobe keloids in response to ear piercing than a true sexual predisposition. Fortunately for the oculoplastic surgeon, keloids are exceedingly rare on the eyelids, and one author has reported uneventful blepharoplasty in a known keloid former.[5]

As a rule, if blepharoplasty incisions are kept within the confines of the orbit, hypertrophic scarring and keloid formation will be avoided (Fig. 70–1). Although direct brow resections and incisions extending beyond the lateral orbital rims should be avoided in known keloid formers, they can be performed without consequence in other African American patients (Fig. 70–2).

Pathologically, keloids demonstrate exuberant dermal

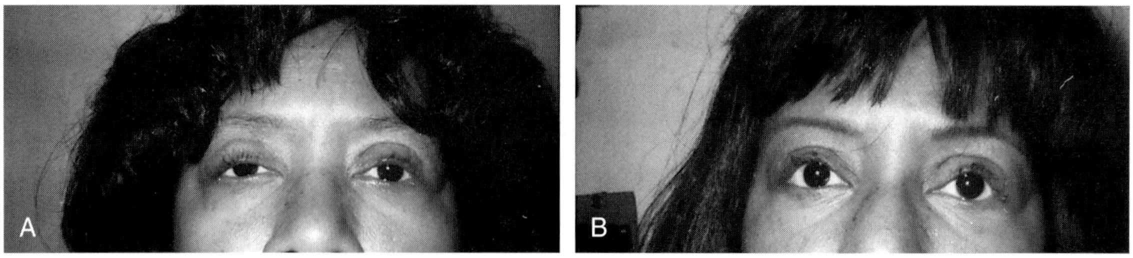

Figure 70–1. *A,* This 42-year-old African American woman has asymmetries of palpebral apertures and upper lid crease-fold complexes after numerous operations performed by several surgeons. *B,* Following levator aponeurotic advancements, her palpebral apertures are symmetric. There was no keloid formation or hypertrophic scarring. (*A* and *B* courtesy of Stephen Bosniak.)

proliferation of thick, randomly oriented collagen bundles. Fibroblasts are few, and there are increased amounts of hyaluronic acid and sulfated glycosaminoglycans. Keloids should be distinguished from hypertrophic scars, which unlike keloids, have no racial predilection, remain confined to the original area of trauma, and tend to regress over 12 to 18 months (Table 70–1). Histologically, numerous fibroblasts are present, and the collagen in hypertrophic scars is aligned parallel to the long axis of the scar.[6] Like keloids, hypertrophic scars very rarely occur on the eyelids.

Treatment of keloids is primarily surgical. Intralesional triamcinolone acetate may promote partial regression but rarely effects a complete cure. In this manner, corticosteroid injections are useful in debulking large tumors before surgical excision. Patients should be informed of possible depigmentation before initiating treatment.

As in the management of any cutaneous tumor, the surgical approach must take into account the keloid's shape, size, and location. Small tumors may be removed with a shave incision and the skin edges closed primarily. If the defect is too large to be closed without excessive tension, rotational flaps may be necessary or, alternatively, a tissue expander can be inserted several weeks preoperatively. Distal earlobe lesions can be excised through a wedge resection, followed by reapproximation of the wound edges.

To prevent or delay keloid recurrence, intraoperative and postoperative triamcinolone injections may be used. In addition, pressure devices applied over the wound several hours a day for the first 3 to 4 months will help inhibit new keloid formation. Most cases of recurrent keloids present within a year of removal.

Another oculoplastic consideration in evaluating the African American patient is bilateral herniation of the lacrimal glands, which occurs more commonly in African Americans and is often associated with blepharochalasis.[6] Additionally, when an African American patient presents with a skin tumor, one must still consider basal cell and squamous cell carcinoma in the differential diagnosis. These tumors tend to be pigmented in African American patients,[7] and it is this pigmentation along with the deeply ingrained misconception that African Americans are protected from ultraviolet light–associated skin tumors that can contribute to unfortunate and unnecessary delays in diagnosis.

Cosmetic surgery continues to appeal to a growing and more diverse population. As more African American patients seek the services of the oculoplastic surgeon, the following unique features must be considered:

1. The patient must be made aware of the potential for postoperative hyperpigmentation, hypopigmentation, or mottling. This is particularly important when dermabrasion, chemical peels, corticosteroid injec-

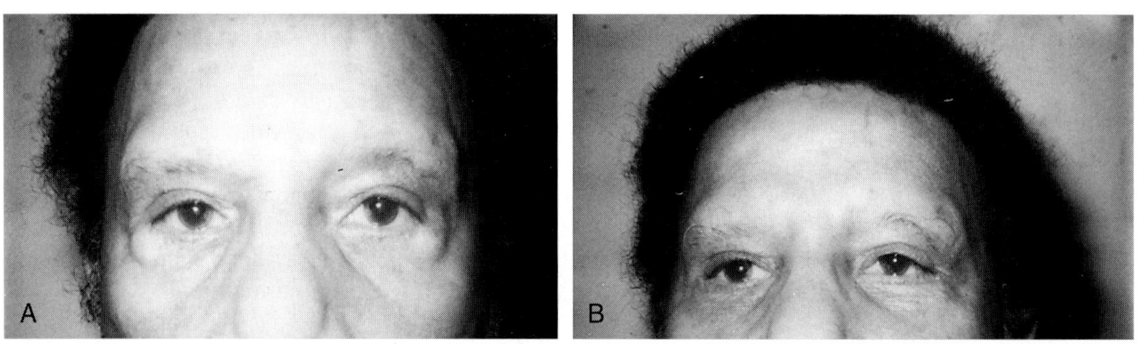

Figure 70–2. *A,* After previous blepharoplasties, this 70-year-old African American man had residual prolapse of his lateral lower lid, fat pockets, and mild right upper lid temporal hooding secondary to a mild right brow ptosis. *B,* This patient healed with hypertrophic scarring or keloid formation after direct blow resection and transconjunctival lipocontouring of the lower lids. (*A* and *B* courtesy of Stephen Bosniak.)

tions, or cryosurgery is contemplated. Some physicians advise against the elective use of these procedures in African Americans or reserve them for severe cases of disfigurement.

2. The minority of African American patients who are keloid formers must be identified by questioning each patient about previous wound healing responses and by examining all scars. Some keloid experts do not consider an isolated earlobe lesion as a predictor of future keloid risk. Patients who have developed keloids in the past should be advised of the likelihood of recurrence. However, given the very rare incidence of keloid formation on the eyelid, most oculoplastic procedures can be performed safely.
3. Ultraviolet light–associated tumors should not be excluded from the differential diagnosis of cutaneous lesions in African Americans. Although rare, basal cell and squamous cell carcinomas do occur and often present as atypically pigmented tumors (Fig. 70–3).

It is a misconception that all, or even most, African Americans will respond to surgical procedures with dyspigmentation, keloid formation, or both. In reality, the overwhelming majority of patients will not suffer either of these consequences. African Americans can therefore continue to enjoy all the physical, emotional, and social benefits that the oculoplastic surgeon has to offer.

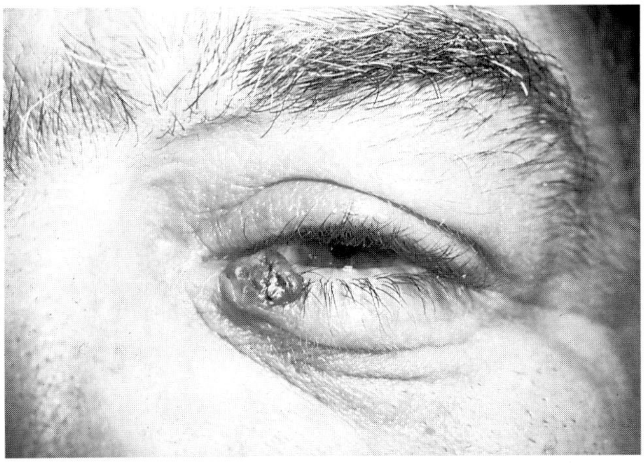

Figure 70–3. This 68-year-old light complexioned African American woman has a pigmented basal cell carcinoma of the left lower lid. (Courtesy of Stephen Bosniak.)

TABLE 70–1

Comparison of Hypertrophic Scars and Keloids

Hypertrophic Scar	Keloid
No racial predilection	Nonwhites
Confined to borders of original	Extends beyond borders of original trauma
Trauma tends to regress	Grows slowly, thens stabilizes
Collagen aligned parallel to original scar	Collagen randomly oriented
Many fibroblasts	Few fibroblasts

REFERENCES

1. Peart D, Hill J: Cryosurgery for trichiasis in black patients. Br J Ophthalmol 70:712–714, 1986.
2. Grimes PE, Hunt SG: Considerations for cosmetic surgery in the black population. Clin Plast Surg 20:27–34, 1993.
3. Kelly AP: Keloids. Dermatol Clin 6:413–424, 1988.
4. Moreno FG, Pennington FR, Bond WR Jr, Morrison WV: Facial keloids and their management. Ear Nose Throat J 60:43–49, 1981.
5. Chrisman BB: Blepharoplasty and browlift with surgical variations in non-white patients. J Dermatol Surg Oncol 12:58–66, 1986.
6. Smith B, Petrelli R: Herniation of the lacrimal glands. Trans Am Acad Ophthalmol Otolaryngol 84:988–990, 1977.
7. Mora RG: Surgical and aesthetic considerations of cancer of the skin in the black American. J Dermatol Surg Oncol 12:24–31, 1986.

CHAPTER 71

Auricular Acupuncture in the Treatment of Blepharospasm

Chieh Chung and Wen Ming Hsu

Blepharospasm is an intermittent or persistent involuntary bilateral eye closure due to spasmodic contraction of the entire length of each orbicularis oculi. This may or may not be accompanied by deep pain or by retro-orbital discomfort or may be associated with dystonic movement of other muscles of the neck and head.

The etiology and the neuroanatomic localization of blepharospasm are still unknown. However, because of the abnormal blinking rates and various associated extrapyramidal disorders, it has been suggested that (1) the basal ganglia are primarily involved or that (2) a mesencephalic-diencephalic dysfunction or a combined cerebellar and brain stem dysfunction is involved. The relationship between blepharospasm and the central nervous system and the endocrine system has been considered.[1] The mechanism of acupuncture is based on a neurohumoral response through mechanical stimulation of some special triggering sites of the human body. Although the cause of blepharospasm is unknown, we are able to use acupuncture on an empiric basis.

A preliminary report of 19 cases of blepharospasm treated with acupuncture was published in 1985[2]; subsequently, studies using other acupuncture techniques, such as auricular acupuncture, laser acupuncture, and electric acupuncture, have been performed.

In 1988, a heretofore unknown relationship between the external ear and the cranial nerves was discovered in the acupuncture clinic of Veterans General Hospital—Taipei.[3] This newly discovered relationship was satisfactorily used for the treatment of facial palsy, trigeminal neuralgia, and facial neuralgia. In 1989, we applied this new technique to the treatment of blepharospasm. Seven patients, ranging in age from 40 to 62 years, were treated. All required multiple treatments at various intervals of from 1 to 10 days. Only two of these patients exhibited a satisfactory response, two others showed some improvement, and three had no response (Tables 71–1 and 71–2) in spite of the addition of the regular acupuncture method that we used from 1980 to 1984.

MAPPING

Based on the initial observation of a relationship between the external ear and cranial nerves, we performed mapping studies and found that there was a band area around the middle of the tragus from the edge of the crus of the helix to the incisure of the incisura tragica superioris that was related to the 12 pairs of cranial nerves; another area in the region of the antitragus was related to the forehead and cheek. Stimulation of the appropriate points might thus result in immediate arrest or remarkable decrease of severe blepharospasm.

PREPARATION

The ear is cleansed about 30 minutes before beginning the auricular therapy for blepharospasm. The patient should be kept calm and cautioned against rubbing or irritating the ear for at least 20 minutes so as to maintain the natural electric resistance of the ear skin and to minimize the influence of electric conductivity to identify the sites related to the blepharospasm. The room temperature should be about 20°C. If the room temperature is much higher, the auricle will perspire; if it is much lower, the blood vessels of the auricle will contract. Either condition can affect conductivity and can lead to incorrect identification of relevant points.

LOCALIZATION

We use an auriculoelectric resistance detector called Ear Master (Fig. 71–1) to search for the related point. The detecting pressure should be light and even, and the probe tip should be needle sharp; the diameter of the tip should be no more than 1 mm. However, the contacting time can be doubled when a reacting point is located. Meanwhile, close attention should be paid to the flashing frequency of the indicator light on the Ear Master, which

TABLE 71-1

Spasm Intensity Scale

Scale	Spasm Intensity
0	None
1	Increased blinking caused by external disease
2	Mild, noticeable fluttering (without actual spasm); not incapacitating
3	Moderate, very noticeable spasm; mildly incapacitating
4	Severely incapacitating (e.g., unable to drive, read)

acts as a guide for finding the related points; the locations for subsequent treatment are then marked (Fig. 71-2).

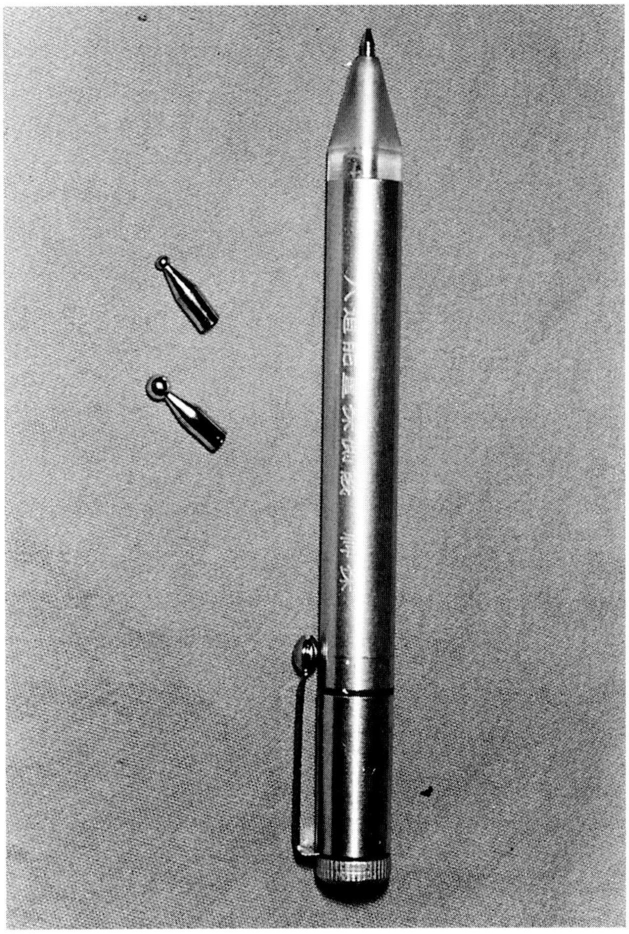

Figure 71-1. Ear Master.

EQUIPMENT

The equipment required for auricular therapy is very simple:

1. An ear point detector, which is an electric device used to differentiate the skin resistance in the range of 20 to 500 K Ohm.
2. Cosmetic acupuncture needles (i.e., 1-cm-long 32-gauge needles).

TECHNIQUE

The needle is inserted into the related point identified by the detector deep to the cartilage. It is turned clockwise 15 degrees using the thumb and index finger and then left in place (Fig. 71-3) for 30 minutes; electric stimulation is not necessary. Any bleeding that may occur after needle removal is controlled by compression.

CONCLUSION

Despite the many advances in ophthalmology in recent years, there is still no satisfactory method for the

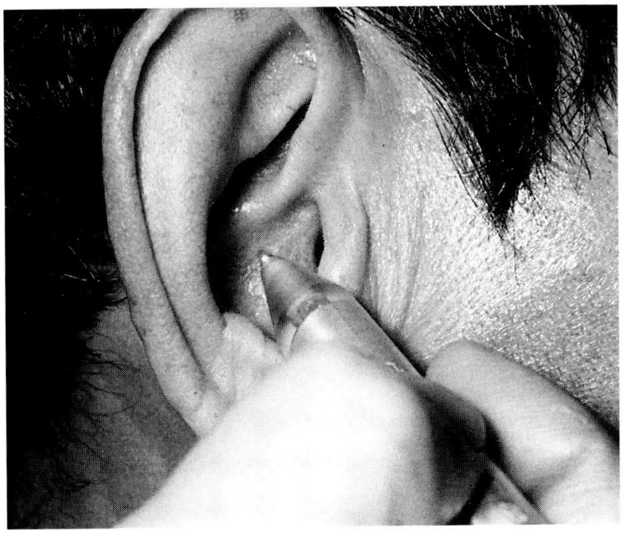

Figure 71-2. Detecting the related point with an Ear Master.

TABLE 71-2

Effect of Auricular Acupuncture on Blepharospasm

Case	Preacupuncture SIS	Postacupuncture SIS	Response
1	3	1	Improvement
2	2	2	None
3	3	0	Satisfactory
4	4	1	Satisfactory
5	3	3	None
6	4	2	Improvement
7	2	2	None

SIS, Spasm Intensity Scale.

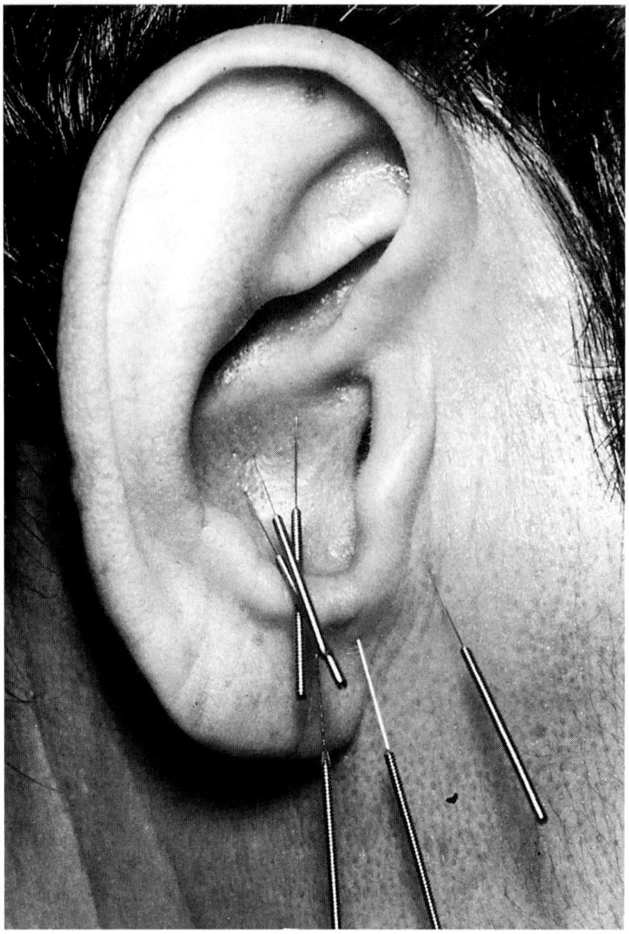

Figure 71 – 3. Needles stay on the auricle during treatment.

treatment of blepharospasm. Acupuncture therapy, however, has been shown to be beneficial to some patients. Furthermore, it is simple, convenient, cost effective, and free from side effects. Accordingly, pending discovery of the definitive effective treatment of this condition, we suggest that acupuncture be considered as an alternative treatment modality.

REFERENCES

1. Henderson JW: Essential blepharospasm. Adv Ophthalmic Plast Reconstr Surg 4:13–66, 1985.
2. Chung C, Hsu WM: Acupuncture in the treatment of blepharospasm: A preliminary report. Adv Ophthalmic Plast Reconstr Surg 4:241–242, 1985.
3. Chung C, Chung FWT: The golden law of auricular therapy. Natl Med 1990.

CHAPTER 72

Eyelid Tumors

Don Liu, Guang-Xi Zhao, and Nai Jiang Xu

The diagnostic workup and the subsequent management of eyelid tumors are discussed in detail elsewhere in the book. In this chapter we highlight the differences in the rates of occurrence of various eyelid tumors in Chinese as compared with those of Caucasians. A technique using donor sclera in eyelid reconstruction is also presented.

SQUAMOUS CELL CARCINOMA

Squamous cell carcinoma, capable of metastasizing to regional lymph nodes, is a potentially lethal neoplasm. Sun exposure, chronic skin injury, and genetics are important factors in the development of this tumor, which occurs most commonly in parts of the world where fair-skinned persons are exposed to large amounts of ultraviolet light from the sun.[1, 2] Other conditions that may predispose to the development of squamous cell carcinoma of the eyelid include Bowen's dermatosis and keratosis resulting from arsenic tar or irradiation.[1–4] Patients with xeroderma pigmentosa, which is a rare premalignant dermatosis inherited in an autosomal recessive manner,[3, 4] have a genetic predisposition to squamous cell carcinoma. There is certainly a racial predisposition, since the incidence of eyelid tumors in Asians is much higher than in Caucasians.

In general, it appears that tumors develop in the lower eyelid slightly more often than is the upper eyelid, with most studies reporting a ratio of about 1.1 : 1.[2, 7] These tumors arise de novo or from a precancerous dermatosis. They begin as a rough, scaly patch that slowly but eventually forms crusts and fissures; this patch usually has an erythematous base and is well defined, with indurated, elevated borders (Fig. 72–1). The erosion or the ulceration is typically very shallow. Orbital involvement by the tumor results from local extension into the dermis, muscle, or connective tissue, and eventually the periosteum. When the orbit is invaded by tumor, the orbital nerves are usually involved early and severely and ptosis and ophthalmoplegia may precede the development of proptosis. Involvement of the orbital nerves also provides a route for intracranial extension of the tumor. These tumors are further disseminated through the lymphatic drainage system; the parotid nodes are involved when the tumor is in the upper eyelid or the lateral canthus, and the submaxillary nodes are involved when the tumor is in the lower eyelid or in the medial canthus.[1, 2, 8]

The clinical diagnosis of squamous cell carcinoma of the eyelid is not always easy since other benign and malignant tumors can mimic it. These lesions include actinic keratosis, inverted follicular keratosis, keratoacanthoma, pseudoepitheliomatous hyperplasia, Bowen's disease, and basal cell carcinoma. Although squamous cell carcinoma of the eyelid presents most commonly as an ulcerative lesion, it can also present as a papillomatous growth or as a nodular or cyst-like lesion. To further complicate the matter, patients with squamous cell carcinoma tend also to have other tumors of the skin, including Bowen's disease, senile keratosis, and basal cell carcinoma.[1, 9, 10] These conditions, and keratoacanthoma, can be mistaken histologically for squamous cell carcinoma. Therefore, to make the correct diagnosis, an adequate biopsy specimen showing the characteristic cytologic features and evidence of dermis invasion should be obtained.

Pathologists generally grade the degree of malignancy of squamous cell carcinoma in a semiquantitive manner by describing each tumor as well differentiated, moderately differentiated, or poorly differentiated. In contrast to tumors of the nasopharynx or sinuses, most squamous cell carcinomas of the eyelids are well differentiated.[11] In tumors of low-grade malignancy, keratin formation is retained by the malignant epidermal cells; in tumors of higher-grade malignancy, keratin pearls are less frequent and evidence of increasing cellular anaplasia is found. Squamous cells may invade the dermis at various levels; and because the dermis of the eyelids is very thin, deep penetration of these tumors is possible and the potential for local extension and for regional metastases is great.[1, 11–13]

SEBACEOUS GLAND CARCINOMA

The cause of sebaceous gland carcinoma is unknown, but predisposing factors may include age, a prior history

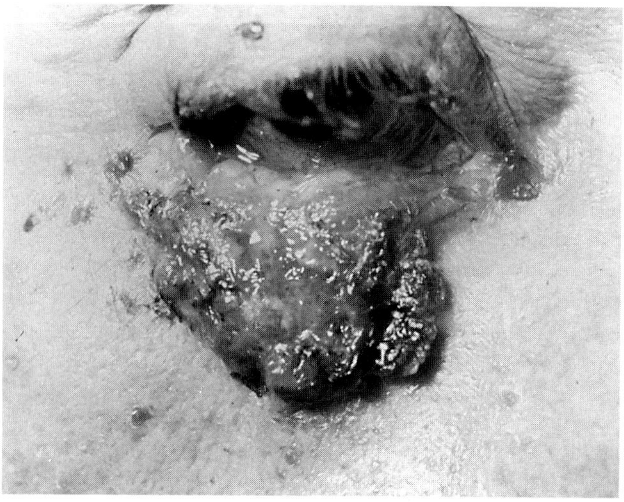

Figure 72–1. Squamous cell carcinoma of the eyelid. This lesion had been present in the eyelid for 3 years and at this point is fairly well defined and indurated and has elevated borders. Some crust and fissures are seen.

of radiation therapy, and race. There is a relatively increased incidence in the elderly,[14] although those patients who develop eyelid sebaceous gland carcinoma after irradiation for a benign condition or for treatment of retinoblastoma tend to be much younger.[15, 17–20] Although sebaceous gland carcinoma of the eyelid is worldwide in distribution, there appears to be a significant difference in the reported incidence between the eastern and western hemispheres: Asians have a much higher incidence of sebaceous gland carcinoma than do Caucasians.[16, 21]

All sebaceous glands of the ocular adnexa, including the meibomian glands and the glands of Zeis and Moll, can give rise to neoplasms, but the meibomian glands are the most common site for sebaceous carcinoma in the eyelids. This tumor, which can be multicentric, is an aggressive malignant neoplasm with metastatic and lethal potential.

Since the tarsal plate of the upper lid is larger and has more meibomian glands, it is more likely for sebaceous gland carcinoma to occur in the upper than in the lower eyelid (Fig. 72–2). These tumors usually begin insidiously, as a nontender lump. The lesion gradually enlarges and eventually produces thickening and distortion of the eyelid. Because the tarsus and deeper structures of the eyelid are involved, there is very little evidence of erosion or ulceration of the skin. In fact, all too commonly these tumors are misdiagnosed and treated as a chalazion.[15, 16, 20, 22] Loss of eyelashes invariably occurs, and sometimes an ulceration of the eyelid margin is noted; a papillomatous growth or, more rarely, a cutaneous horn may be observed.[15, 16, 20, 23] On the conjunctival side, the tumor presents a characteristic yellowish white appearance and lobular architecture. Follicular changes are seen frequently adjacent to the mass.[24] Evidence of metastases is most frequently heralded by the enlargement of preauricular or cervical lymph nodes or of the parotid gland.[14, 21, 25] Other sites of distant metastases include lung, liver, brain, pleura, pericardium, lip, ethmoidal sinus, and skull.[14, 26, 27] Orbital extension occurs in 6% to 16% of cases and is associated with a mortality rate that has been reported to be as high as 76%.[14, 21]

Sebaceous gland carcinoma is perhaps the most lethal of all eyelid tumors because of its ability to metastasize and because it is so often misdiagnosed. Clinically, it is often misdiagnosed as a recurrent chalazion, blepharoconjunctivitis, granuloma, papilloma, or a cutaneous horn, and in rare cases as a pigmented lesion.[15, 16, 23] Recurrent or persistent unilateral blepharoconjunctivitis or chalazion should raise suspicion. Material removed from such a recurrent lesion, especially in an elderly patient, should always be examined histopathologically. Full-thickness eyelid biopsy should be considered in atypical cases since superficial skin or conjunctival biopsy specimens may be misleading. Sebaceous gland carcinoma can present, albeit rarely, as a primary orbital process with proptosis, and it can arise from ectopic sebaceous glands or from a lacrimal gland.

Histologically, sebaceous gland carcinoma may be confused with basal or squamous cell carcinoma or, more rarely, malignant melanoma. Rao and associates identified various clinical and pathologic features of sebaceous gland carcinoma that are associated with a poor prognosis. These include vascular, lymphatic, and orbital invasion; involvement of both the upper and lower eyelids; poor differentiation; mulitcentric origin; duration of symptoms greater than 6 months; tumor diameter exceeding 10 mm; a highly infiltrative pattern; and pagetoid invasion of the overlying epithelia of the eyelid. They also found that sebaceous gland carcinoma of the upper eyelid has a 28% mortality, but none of the patients with lower eyelid tumor died as a result of the tumor during the same period of time. In cases in which both upper and lower eyelids were involved, the mortality rate rose to 83%.[14, 16, 28, 29]

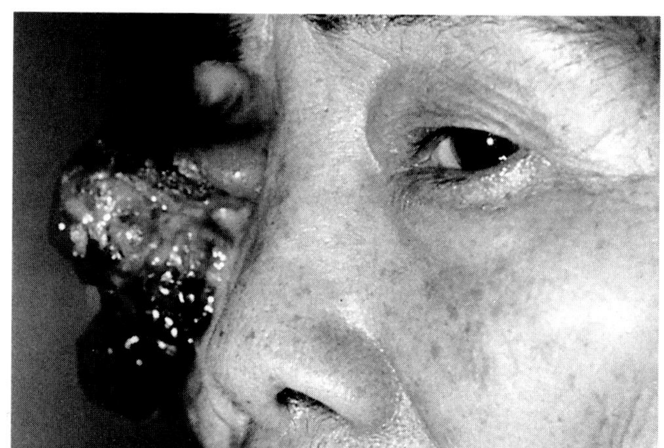

Figure 72–2. Sebaceous gland carcinoma of the right lower eyelid. This patient neglected this eyelid lesion for 2 years.

BASAL CELL CARCINOMA

Basal cell carcinoma is the most common malignant tumor of the eyelids in the United States, where it accounts for over 90% of all epitheliomas of the lids. The sites at which this most commonly occurs are the lower eyelid, followed by the medial canthus and then the lateral canthus; the tumors occur commonly in the upper eyelid.[30, 31] Basal cell carcinomas can present as nodular, diffuse, ulcerative, or multicentric lesions. Most commonly seen is the nodular type, which accounts for approximately 60% of all basal cell carcinomas of the eyelid. These usually present as a chronic, indurated, nontender raised lesion with an erythematous base and a crater-like center. Telangiectatic vessels are generally present, and, if the lesion occurs at the eyelid margin, lashes are invariably missing (Fig. 72–3). The diffuse type or amorphous form of basal cell carcinoma is most difficult to treat because it does not have clinically distinct margins. These tumors are likely to have deeply invasive or clinically distinct margins. Very rarely, basal cell carcinoma can be heavily pigmented, leading to a mistaken impression of a nevus or melanoma.[30, 32]

Basal cell carcinomas spread by local extension and rarely metastasize. Orbital involvement is secondary to local extension and is generally manifest as an orbital mass fixed to the bone, as a frozen globe, or both. It has been estimated that up to 4% of basal cell carcinomas of the lids have orbital extension that necessitates an orbital exenteration.[33] Distant metastases from basal cell carcinoma are exceedingly rare, but these tumors have been seen to spread to lymph nodes, lungs, and bones. Basal cell carcinomas occur worldwide and have no predilection for any race or sex; sun exposure, however, is definitely a predisposing factor.

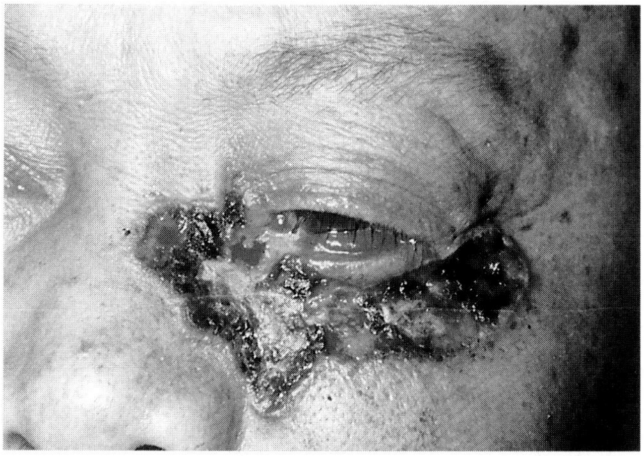

Figure 72–3. Basal cell carcinoma of the lower eyelid. The medial canthus and deep orbital tissues are involved by local extension. Clinically, this lesion may be difficult to differentiate from squamous cell carcinoma.

CONTRASTING STATISTICS

In the western hemisphere, basal cell carcinoma is the most common cutaneous malignancy and accounts for 85% to 95% of all eyelid malignancies.[22, 34, 35] Squamous cell carcinoma is relatively rare and accounts for 2.4% to 7.2% of all eyelid malignancies,[16, 22, 32, 36] while sebaceous gland carcinoma is still rarer, accounting for 0.5% to 5.5% of all eyelid malignancies.[16, 21, 22] In the older literature, the ratio of basal cell carcinoma to squamous cell carcinoma was roughly 40 : 1. However, many authors believe that this may be an underestimation of squamous cell carcinoma. More recent studies have shown that the ratio may be 11.4 to 12.7 : 1. The ratio of basal cell carcinoma to sebaceous gland carcinoma is roughly 15 to 20 : 1.

Ni of Shanghai (in eastern China) reviewed a series of 2590 eyelid tumors and found the ratio between benign and malignant lesions to be about 2 : 1.[37] In his large series there were 360 basal cell carcinomas (36.99% of the malignant tumors), 308 meibomian gland carcinomas, (31.65%), 194 squamous cell carcinomas (19.98%), 52 melanomas (5.43%), and 59 other malignant lesions (6.05%). The ratio of basal cell carcinoma to squamous cell carcinoma was about 1.86 : 1, and the ratio of basal cell carcinoma to meibomian gland carcinoma was 1.17 : 1.

Hu, of central China, reported a series of 110 eyelid tumors, of which 77 were malignant.[38] These included 25 (32.5%) basal cell carcinomas, 24 (31.2%) squamous cell carcinomas, 15 (19.3%) meibomian gland carcinomas, and 4 melanomas (5.2%). The remaining lesions consisted of other rare malignancies, such as lymphosarcoma, vascular endothelioma, papillary carcinoma, reticulum cell carcinoma, fibrocarcinoma, and basal-squamous cell carcinoma. The ratio of malignant to benign tumors was 3 : 7 or 2.3 : 1. The ratio of basal cell carcinoma to squamous cell carcinoma is almost 1 : 1, while the ratio of basal cell carcinoma to meibomian gland carcinoma is 1.67 : 1. Liao[39] reported a consecutive series from northern China of 373 cases of eyelid tumors. In his series, the ratio between the benign and malignant tumors was 4 : 1, and the ratios of basal cell to squamous cell or sebaceous gland carcinomas were similar to those reported by Ni. Zhang and Du[40] analyzed 130 malignant tumors of the eyelid in central China. They found 60 cases of basal cell carcinoma (46.2%), 29 meibomian carcinomas (22.3%), 28 squamous cell carcinomas (21.5%), and 13 melanomas (10%). The ratio of basal cell carcinoma to squamous cell carcinoma in their series was 2.14 : 1, and the ratio of basal cell carcinoma to meibomian gland carcinoma was 2.07 : 1.

Authors from other regions of China have reported slightly different incidences or ratios of these tumors. Qian and Liang[41] reported the ratio of basal cell carcinoma to squamous cell carcinoma to be about 1 : 1. Fu[42] analyzed 35 malignant tumors of the eyelid seen in the

Uygur ethnic group in China; he found the ratio of basal cell to squamous cell carcinoma to be 5.75 : 1 in this particular minority group, which has its origin in central Asia. Hsu, of Taiwan, reporting a series of 78 cases of eyelid malignancy, found that basal cell carcinoma accounted for 48.7% of the total tumors, meibomian gland carcinoma for 29.5%, and squamous cell carcinoma for 10.3%. The ratio of basal cell to squamous cell carcinomas in Hsu's series was 4.73 : 1, while the ratio of basal cell carcinoma to meibomian gland carcinoma was 1.65 : 1.

Despite the regional, ethnic, and practice pattern variations, it is clear that the incidences of these various eyelid tumors in China are quite different from those in the United States. In China, basal cell carcinoma accounts for 50% to 80% of all eyelid malignancies, followed by meibomian gland carcinoma at 17.5% to 33.3%; squamous cell carcinoma accounts for 8% to 10% of the total.

The ratio of lower to upper eyelid involvement is 1 : 1 for basal cell carcinoma, whereas the ratio is 3 to 5 : 1 for squamous cell carcinoma. Both of these tumors have a propensity for the medial canthal area. From the various series reported in China, sebaceous gland carcinoma involves the upper lid in 65% to 69% of the cases, while the lower eyelid is involved in only 24% to 30% of the cases. The ratio of the upper to lower eyelid involvement is 2 to 3 : 1.[16, 37]

In a collaborative study of eyelid malignancies seen in Boston and in Shanghai,[16] the relatively increased incidence of sebaceous carcinoma in Asians was emphasized. In the Boston population, this accounts for only 1.5% of all lid malignancies, while in the Shanghai population it accounts for 32.7%. The relative incidence of basal cell carcinoma in the Boston group was 92.5%, but in Shanghai it was 42%. Sebaceous gland carcinoma is perhaps the most lethal of all eyelid tumors, with an overall mortality rate of between 23% and 41%. The highest rate of mortality, 41%, was reported by Ni and Kuo[43] and probably reflects a higher incidence of advanced cases, a referral pattern, or perhaps a more aggressive course in Asians. In this collaborative study, the average age at the time of diagnosis was 57 in Shanghai and 67 in Boston, and in both groups women were predominantly affected. The propensity of upper eyelid involvement is in agreement with previous reports. The authors of this collaborative study thought that race and environmental factors are important. However, the reasons for such a striking difference in frequency remain unknown. At the present time there is no information available for comparing tumor incidences in first-, second-, and third-generation Chinese Americans. Similarly, the role of chalazion in the causation of this tumor has been questioned.

Wang and Lei[44] treated 52 patients with various eyelid tumors with radiation. More specifically, all 19 patients (100%) with basal cell carcinoma had a 3-year survival rate, 17 (89.5%) had a 5-year survival rate, and 10 (52.6%) had a 10-year survival rate. In their series, 24 patients with squamous cell carcinoma were treated with radiation therapy; all 24 were alive after 3 years, 21 (87.5%) were alive at 5 years, and 7 (29.2%) were alive at 10 years. There were only two patients with meibomian gland carcinoma in this study, and only one of these received radiation therapy. This patient had radiation therapy first to shrink the tumor to half of its original size, then underwent complete surgical excision under frozen section control; no recurrence was found 11 years after exenteration.

Wang and associates[45] reported the longest followup of patients with sebaceous carcinoma. They had 24 patients who were treated and followed during the period of 1960 to 1990; 11 were male and 13 were female. Ages ranged from 25 to 72 years, with an average age of 50. Fifteen lesions (62.5%) were in an upper lid, and nine (37.5%) were in a lower eyelid; Wang and associates found no difference between the right eye and the left eye. Duration of the disease ranged from 4 months to 15 years before the patient sought care. Twelve cases were misdiagnosed as chalazion. Recurrences were noted in 26.3% of the cases. The 3-year survival rate was 92.8%, the 5-year survival rate was 90.9%, and the 10-year survival rate was 71.4%.

EYELID RECONSTRUCTION WITH DONOR SCLERA

Full-thickness eyelid defect involving less than a fourth to a third of the eyelid can usually be closed primarily. When necessary, a lateral canthalysis or canthotomy may be performed to mobilize the eyelid and to facilitate the closure. When the full-thickness eyelid defect is greater than one third of the length of the lid, various methods of reconstruction are available: sliding flaps, rotation flaps, and grafts using auricular cartilage, nasal septum cartilage, tarsal plate from the contralateral eye, periosteum, or hard palate. Hugh's method, the Cutler-Beard technique, Tenzel's semicircular flap, or a Mustardé flap can be used.[46–49] Donor sclera has also been used in reconstruction of the eyelid.[50–55] Over the past 10 years, one of us (Zhao, of Beijing) has successfully used donor sclera in repairing 50 cases of extensive full-thickness eyelid defect. The causes for the defect included trauma in 21 patients, 22 cases of neoplasm, congenital deformities in 6 patients, and a purulent eyelid infection in 1 patient. There was involvement of the upper eyelid in 28 patients, the lower eyelid in 16 patients, unilateral upper and lower eyelids in 5 patients, and bilateral upper eyelids in 1 patient. The extent of the defect was one third of the dimension of the lids in 10 patients, one half in 12 patients, three fourths in 8 patients, and a total loss in 26 patients. The age of the patients ranged from 4 to 71 years, with an average age of 37.5 years. The scleral homografts were obtained from enucleated eyes of unrelated patients with absolute glaucoma or who had sustained trauma. All donors were free of infectious disease and malignancy and had negative hepatitis B surface antigen tests. The donor tissue was prepared by removing the cornea, optic nerve, and ocular contents from the eye. The sclera was soaked in 95% alcohol for 3 days, with daily changes of the alcohol, and then immersed in 75% alcohol and stored in a refrigerator. The material was reconstituted in normal saline for 15 minutes before use.

Surgical Technique

A full-thickness upper eyelid defect involving the entire dimension of the tarsal plate will serve as an example. With the use of local anesthesia, the edges of the upper eyelid defect are freshened, the skin undermined, and the remaining orbicularis mobilized. The lower eyelid margin is incised (1 – 2 mm deep) along the gray line for a distance equal to the upper eyelid defect, and the epithelial layer of the posterior lip is removed. Both the medial and lateral canthal tendons are dissected and identified from the eyelid defect at these respective locations. A piece of the preserved sclera of the appropriate size and shape is anchored to the canthal tendon at both ends, with appropriate permanent sutures. Superiorly, through the eyelid defect, the levator complex is dissected and identified. The superior margin of the sclera graft is then sutured to the remnants of the levator complex, and the lower margin is sutured to the lower eyelid within the groove. The anterior surface of the sclera graft is covered with the remaining orbital portion of the orbicularis. A free skin graft or a local flap is advanced to cover the muscle. The reconstructed eyelid is dressed for 10 days before removal of the sutures. The upper eyelid is separated from the lower lid after 3 to 6 months.

Zhao has used the following grading system to assess the clinical results. "Excellent" implies that both functional and cosmetic results are optimal; "good" is used when the functional result is excellent but a cosmetic defect, such as minimal exposure or ptosis, is present; "fair" is used when a lagophthalmos of 3 mm or greater or a ptosis of 3 mm or greater is present; "failure" means sloughing of the graft or that a severe eyelid deformity is present (Fig. 72–4).

In 30 patients (60%) Zhao's results were excellent, in 15 (30%) the results were good, and 5 (10%) had fair results; none of the cases were considered failures. Postoperative complications included partial dehiscence of the surgical wound in four cases; this was associated with early removal of the sutures or poor blood circulation. There was mild ectropion of the lower eyelid in two cases, which was associated with inadequate fixation of the canthal tendon attachment. In this particular study, no attempt was made to correlate the results of surgery with the primary cause of the defect, sex of the patient, or location of the defect. Followup ranged from 1 to 5 years, with an average followup of more than 3 years.

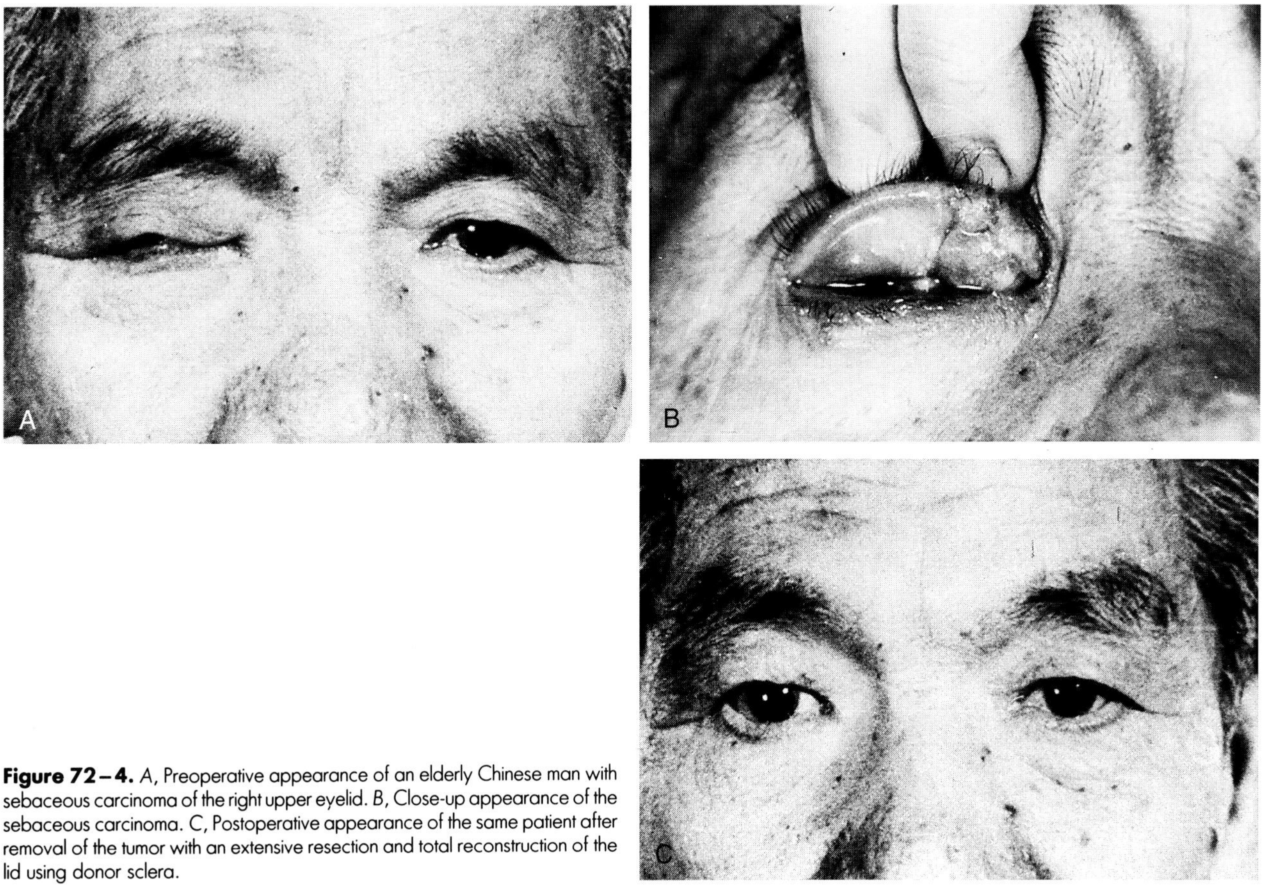

Figure 72–4. *A*, Preoperative appearance of an elderly Chinese man with sebaceous carcinoma of the right upper eyelid. *B*, Close-up appearance of the sebaceous carcinoma. *C*, Postoperative appearance of the same patient after removal of the tumor with an extensive resection and total reconstruction of the lid using donor sclera.

Histology of Scleral Homograft

One of us (Zhao) has investigated the fate of scleral homografts by implanting them into the eyelids of 30 rabbits and into the backs of 8 rabbits. The specimens were removed for microscopic examinations at 1 week, 2 weeks, 1 month, 2 months, 3 months, and 4 months after the implantation. By the end of the first week, a thin layer of connective tissue began to form around the implant, with slight infiltration of monocytes, plasma cells, eosinophilic leukocytes, foreign body megalocytes, and fibroblasts. By the end of the third week, the fibroblasts increased remarkably in number with ingrowth of small blood vessels and a decrease in numbers of other cells. Two to 4 months after implantation, the new connective tissue began to mature and replace the scleral fibers. These changes were observed to take place much faster in the eyelids than in the back. Under transmission electron microscopy, the marginal collagen fibers of the implant began to show lysis by the end of the second week and the invading fibroblasts manifested signs of enhanced functional activity. The rich rough endoplasmic reticulum expanded into pools, and mitochondria were enlarged and oval with a dense stroma. The collagenolytic process was still in evidence 4 months after implantation, with most fibroblasts by now transformed into fibrocytes, and the implant became a dense, clear structure of collagen fibers that varied greatly in diameter. On vertical sectioning, the periodic striations showed no alterations, indicating that the implanted sclera was replaced by fibrous connective tissue rather than being absorbed or remaining as a long-term foreign body (Figs. 72–5 through 72–9).

Immunopathology of Homograft

Further investigation (by Zhao) of the immunopathology of scleral homografts was done using 15 adult albino rabbits that were divided equally into three groups. Rabbits in group 1 had scleral grafts implanted into both the

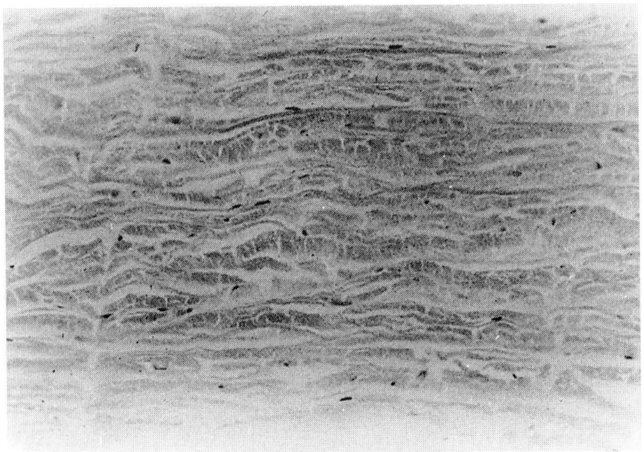

Figure 72–5. Normal rabbit sclera. H & E, ×40.

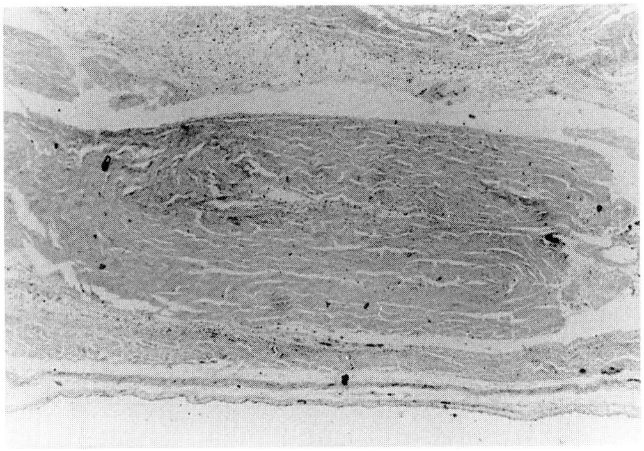

Figure 72–6. Appearance of a scleral homograft in a rabbit eyelid 1 week after surgery. Infiltration of monocytes, plasma cells, occasional foreign body megalocyte fibroblasts, and eosinophilic leukocytes is seen. H&E, ×40.

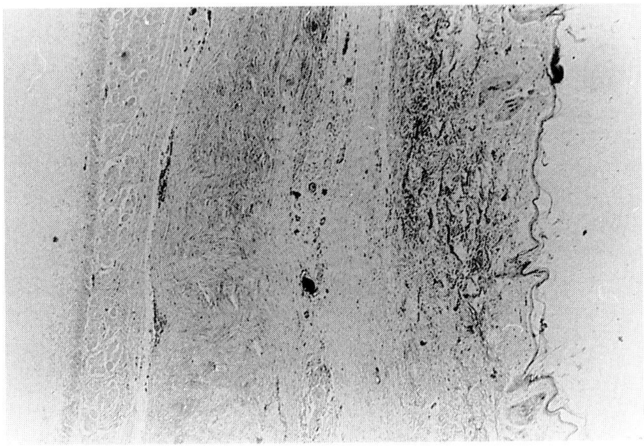

Figure 72–7. Rabbit scleral homograft at the end of the third week. The inflammatory response has subsided, and there is an increase in the number of fibroblasts and ingrowth of small blood vessels. H&E, ×100.

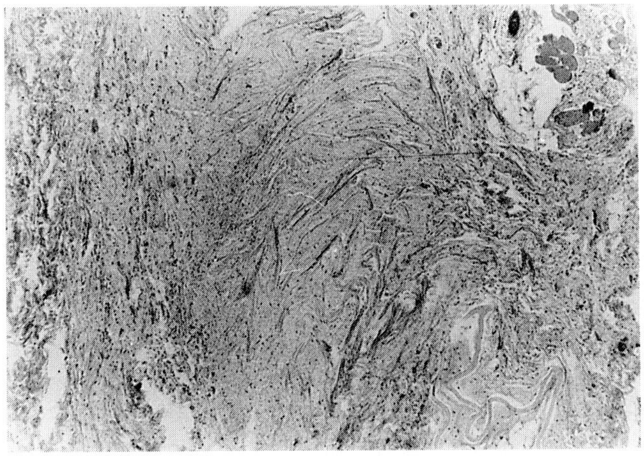

Figure 72–8. Scleral homograft in a rabbit eyelid at 4 months. Replacement of the sclera fibers by the growth of new connective tissue is evident. H&E, ×100.

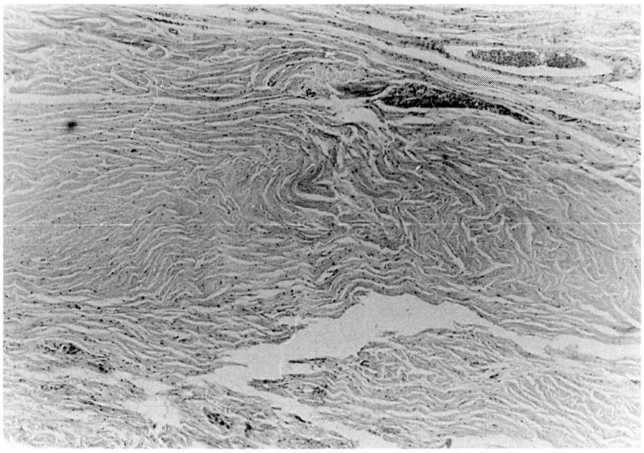

Figure 72–9. Scleral homograft in a rabbit eyelid at 9 months. The homograft appears to be almost completely replaced by fibrous connective tissue. No foreign body reaction is seen.

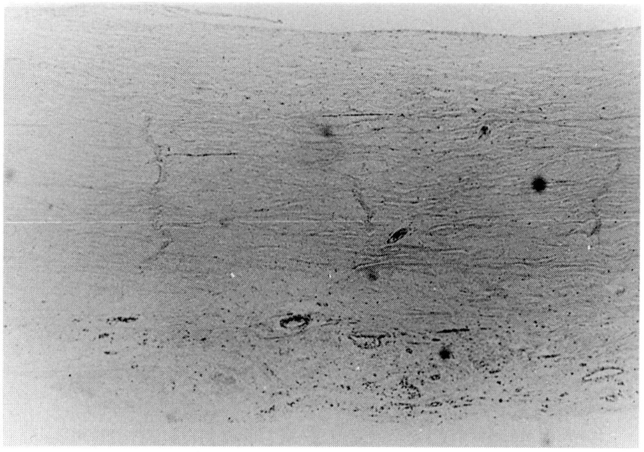

Figure 72–10. Scleral homograft in a human eyelid at 2 years. The donor graft has been entirely replaced by new connective tissue. No inflammatory response or foreign body reaction is seen.

eyelid and the back; rabbits in group 2 had absorbable sutures placed in the eyelid and in the back; group 3 underwent no surgical procedure whatsoever and served as controls. Five days after the procedure, 1% trypan blue was injected in an ear vein of each rabbit and the animals were sacrificed 2 hours later by air bubble emboli. The periauricular lymph nodes were removed immediately and fixed in 4% methyl alcohol for 24 hours, dehydrated with ethyl alcohol, and stained by methyl green–pyronine. The number of lymphoblasts per millimeter at 10 randomly selected sites from the pericortical area of the lymph node was determined for comparison among the three groups, and the differences between group 1 and the other two groups were very significant ($P < .05$). In light of the microscopic observations and the immunopathologic findings, cellular immune reactions after implantation of the scleral grafts were evident but were of short duration and did not lead to tissue rejection, as was demonstrated clinically as well.

Donor Sclera

Donor sclera has been used in eyelid reconstruction, in the repair of eyelid retraction secondary to dysthyroid ophthalmopathy, in reconstruction of the socket, and for wrapping other ocular implants. Experimental and clinical results reported so far have been satisfactory. The experiments with rabbits and the clinical results have further confirmed this. It was concluded that sclera is indeed a satisfactory substitute for the missing tarsal plate and can be used with gratifying results in reconstruction of eyelids. The sclera is a tough material with pliable tenacity. It is easily acquired, stored, and used. The animal experiments showed that the evolution of grafted sclera is faster in the eyelid, which has a rich supply of blood, than in the back, where fewer blood vessels exist. The ingrowth of new blood vessels is also faster in the eyelid than in the back. Apparently good circulation during the surgery was conducive to improved wound healing. It was also found that grafted sclera does not appear to contract very much shortly after transplantation because of the scarcity of elastic fibers. However, after replacement by connective tissue, the potential for contraction is increased, and one is cautioned against undercorrection (Fig. 72–10).

REFERENCES

1. Stoll HL Jr: Squamous cell carcinoma. *In* Fitzpatrick TB, Eisen AZ, Wolff K, et al (eds): Dermatology in General Medicine: Textbook and Atlas, 2nd ed. New York, McGraw-Hill, 1979, pp 362–377.
2. Yanoff M, Fine BS: Ocular Pathology: A Text and Atlas, 2nd ed. Hagerstown, MD, Harper & Row, 1982.
3. Stout AP: Malignant manifestations of Bowen's disease. NY J Med 39:801–809, 1939.
4. Montgomery H: Precancerous dermatosis and epithelioma in situ. Arch Dermatol Syph 39:387–408, 1939.
5. Mortada A: Incidence of lid, conjunctival and orbital malignant tumors in xeroderma pigmentosa in Egypt. Bull Ophthalmol Soc Egypt 61:231–236, 1968.
6. Whitmore PV: Skin and mucous membrane disorders. *In* Tasman W, Jaeger EA (eds): Duane's Clinical Ophthalmology, vol 5, chap 27. Philadelphia, JB Lippincott, 1991, pp 1–27.
7. Jakobiec FA: Tumors of the lids. *In* Symposium on Diseases and Surgery of the Lids, Lacrimal Apparatus and Orbit: Transactions of the New Orleans Academy of Ophthalmology. St. Louis, CV Mosby, 1982, pp 264–307.
8. Hogan MJ, Zimmerman LE (eds): Ophthalmic Pathology: An Atlas and Textbook, 2nd ed. Philadelphia, WB Saunders, 1962, p 214.
9. Caya JG, Hidayat AA, Weiner JM: A clinicopathologic study of 21 cases of adenoid squamous cell carcinoma of the eyelid and periorbital region. Am J Ophthalmol 99:291–297, 1985.
10. Boniuk M: Differentiation of squamous cell carcinoma from other epithelial tumors of the eyelid. *In* Boniuk M (ed): Ocular and Adnexal Tumors: New and Controversial Aspects. St. Louis, CV Mosby, 1964, p 75.
11. Jakobiec FA, Rootman J, Jones IS: Secondary and metastatic tumors of the orbit. *In* Tasman W, Jaeger EA (eds): Duane's Clinical Ophthalmology, vol 2, chap 46. Philadelphia, JB Lippincott, 1991, pp 1–67.

12. Broders AC: Practical points on the microscopic grading of carcinoma. NY J Med 32:667–671, 1932.
13. Lever WF, Schaumburg-Lever G: Histopathology of the Skin, 5th ed. Philadelphia, JB Lippincott, 1975, p 537.
14. Rao NA, Hidayat M, McLean IW, Zimmerman LE: Sebaceous carcinoma of the ocular adnexa: A clinicopathologic study of 104 cases, with five-year follow-up data. Hum Pathol 13:113–122, 1982.
15. Boniuk M, Zimmerman LE: Sebaceous carcinoma of the eyelid, eyebrow, caruncle, and orbit. Trans Am Acad Ophthalmol Otolaryngol 72:619–642, 1968.
16. Ni C, Searl SS, Kuo PK, et al: Sebaceous cell carcinomas of the ocular adnexa. Int Ophthalmol Clin 22:23–61, 1982.
17. Khalil MK, Dario WC, Lorenzetti, MD: Sebaceous gland carcinoma of the lid. Can J Ophthalmol 15:117–121, 1980.
18. Forrest AW: Tumors following radiation about the eye. Trans Am Acad Ophthalmol Otolaryngol 65:694–717, 1961.
19. Lemos LB, Santa Cruz DJ, Baba N: Sebaceous carcinoma of the eyelid following radiation therapy. Am J Surg Pathol 2:305–311, 1978.
20. Straatsma BR: Meibomian gland tumors. Arch Ophthalmol 56:71–93, 1956.
21. Ginsberg J: Present status of meibomian gland carcinoma. Arch Ophthalmol 73:271–277, 1965.
22. Kwitko ML, Boniuk M, Zimmerman LE: Eyelid tumors with reference to lesions confused with squamous cell carcinoma: I. Incidence and errors in diagnosis. Arch Ophthalmol 69:693–697, 1963.
23. Brauninger GE, Hood CI, Worthen DM: Sebaceous carcinoma of the lid margin masquerading as cutaneous horn. Arch Ophthalmol 90:380–381, 1973.
24. Tenzel RR, Stewart WB, Boynton JR, Zbar M: Sebaceous carcinoma of the eyelid: Definition of surgical margins. Arch Ophthalmol 95:2203–2204, 1977.
25. Maniglia AJ: Meibomian gland adenocarcinoma of the eyelid with neck metastasis. Laryngoscope 88:1421–1426, 1978.
26. Magnus JA: Adenocarcinoma of meibomian gland with secondaries in the liver. Trans Ophthalmol Soc UK 67:432–435, 1947.
27. Gowey RJ, Kern WH: Metastasizing adenocarcinomas of the tarsal glands. Calif Med 103:126–130, 1965.
28. Cavanagh HD, Green WR, Goldberg HK: Multicentric sebaceous adenocarcinoma of the meibomian gland. Am J Ophthalmol 77:326–332, 1974.
29. Doxanas MT, Green WR: Sebaceous gland carcinoma: Review of 40 cases. Arch Ophthalmol 102:245–249, 1984.
30. Milverton EJ: A survey of basal cell carcinoma of the eyelid. Aust J Ophthalmol 5:106–108, 1977.
31. Lund HZ: Tumors of the skin, section 1, fascicle 2. Washington, DC, Armed Forces Institute of Pathology, 1957, pp 205–234.
32. Aurora AL, Blodi FC: Lesions of the eyelids: A clinicopathological study. Surv Ophthalmol 15:94–104, 1970.
33. Payne JW, Duke JR, Butner R, Eifrig DE: Basal cell carcinoma of the eyelids: A long-term follow-up study. Arch Ophthalmol 81:553–558, 1969.
34. Martin HE: Cancer of the eyelids. Arch Ophthalmol 22:1–20, 1939.
35. Henkind P, Friedman A: Cancer of the lids and ocular adnexa. *In* Andrade R, Gumport SL, Popkin GL, Rees TD (eds): Cancer of the Skin: Biology—Diagnosis—Management. Philadelphia, WB Saunders, 1976.
36. Doxanas MT, Iliff WJ, Iliff NT, Green WR: Squamous cell carcinoma of the eyelids. Ophthalmology 94:538–541, 1987.
37. Ni C: Pathologic classification and erroneous diagnosis in 2590 cases of eyelid tumors. Pract J Tumor 3:207–210, 1988.
38. Hu DL: Heredity in Ophthalmology. Shanghai, Shanghai Scientific and Technical Publishing House, 1988, pp 105–109.
39. Liao SL: Clinicopathological analysis of 465 biopsy specimens of the eyelid lesion. Chin J Ophthalmol 18:156, 1982.
40. Zhang SX, Du VZ: Clinical analysis of 130 cases of malignant tumors of eyelids. Pract J Ophthalmol 7:91–93, 1989.
41. Qian YZ, Liang DY: Extension and metastasis of squamous cell carcinoma and basal cell carcinoma of eyelid. Chin J Ophthalmol 16:232, 1980.
42. Fu L: Analysis on 308 cases of malignant tumors of eyelids. Pract J Ophthalmol 8:591–592, 1990.
43. Ni C, Kuo P: Meibomian gland carcinoma: A clinical pathological study of 156 cases with long-term follow-up of 100 cases. Jpn J Ophthalmol 23:388–401, 1979.
44. Wang CY, Lei YF: Long-term follow-up of carcinoma of eyelids after radiotherapy (in press).
45. Wang CY, Xu XL, Liu SZ: Surgical treatment of meibomian gland carcinoma: A long-term follow-up study (24 case reports) (in press).
46. Callahan A: Reconstructive Surgery of the Eyelids and Ocular Adnexa. Birmingham, AL, Aesculapius, 1977.
47. Mustardé JC: Repair and Reconstruction in the Orbital Region. Edinburgh, Churchill Livingstone, 1971.
48. Tenzel RR: Reconstruction of the central one-half of an eyelid. Arch Ophthalmol 93:215, 1975.
49. Jelks GW, Smith BC: Reconstruction of the eyelids and associated structures. *In* McCarthy JG (ed): Plastic Surgery. Philadelphia, WB Saunders, 1990, pp 1671–1784.
50. Doxanas MT, Dryden RM: The use of sclera in the treatment of dysthyroid eyelid retraction. Ophthalmology 88:887–894, 1981.
51. Beyer CK, Albert DM: The use and fate of fascia lata and sclera in ophthalmic plastic and reconstructive surgery. Ophthalmology 88:869–886, 1981.
52. Flanagen JC: Eye bank sclera in oculoplastic surgery. Ophthalmic Surg 53:45–53, 1974.
53. Dryden RM, Soll DB: The use of scleral transplantation in cicatricial entropion and eyelid retraction. Trans Am Acad Ophthalmol Otolaryngol 83:669–678, 1977.
54. Frueh BR, Felker GV: Baseball implant: A method of secondary insertion of an intraorbital implant. Arch Ophthalmol 94:429–430, 1976.
55. Soll DB: The anophthalmic socket. *In* Soll DB (ed): Management of Complications in Ophthalmic Plastic Surgery. Birmingham, AL, Aesculapius, 1976.

SECTION VI

Lacrimal Surgery

SECTION EDITOR

Jeffrey A. Nerad

Introduction

Jeffrey A. Nerad

Epiphora is a common complaint among ophthalmic patients. In its simplest form, tears overflowing the eyelids may interfere with the patient's quality of life. The vision may be blurred because of a large tear lake or tears drying on the inside of the glasses. Mucopurulent discharge resulting from infection secondary to stasis of tears may develop, causing crusting of the eyelashes. An associated irritation of the eyelid skin may occur. This irritation is worsened by constant wiping of the eyelids, an action that may, in turn, contribute to stretching of the lower eyelid and eventual ectropion. In some cases, infection progresses in the lacrimal sac, causing an acute dacryocystitis that requires urgent drainage and antibiotic therapy.

Causes of epiphora include ocular and eyelid problems, congenital nasolacrimal duct obstruction, canalicular disease resulting from infection or trauma, and several types of acquired nasolacrimal duct obstruction. In rare cases, epiphora may be associated with a life-threatening tumor of the lacrimal sac, nasal cavity, or orbit. An appropriate understanding of the anatomy and physiology of the lacrimal system is essential for a full evaluation of the patient with epiphora. An accurate history and physical examination will lead to the correct cause and treatment.

Tears are produced in the lacrimal gland and provide a protective coating of the ocular surface. The distribution and drainage of the tears depend on normal eyelid anatomy and function. Tears enter the puncta and travel to the lacrimal sac in the canaliculi. The tears drain into the nasal cavity through the nasolacrimal duct. Any mechanical or functional abnormality in the production, distribution, and drainage of tears disrupts this process.

The exact abnormality can usually be determined through a detailed history and physical examination. Several points of the patient's history should be stressed. Epiphora is defined as tears overflowing the eyelids onto the cheek. Most patients complaining of epiphora have an identifiable cause, and appropriate treatment is available. In contrast, patients who report having a "wet eye" frequently have a tear film abnormality as opposed to a true disorder of lacrimal drainage. Unilaterality frequently suggests nasolacrimal duct obstruction. A history of periocular facial trauma, dacryocystitis, or conjunctivitis also suggests nasolacrimal system obstruction.

Age of onset is an important clue in the identification of the cause of nasolacrimal duct obstruction. Congenital nasolacrimal duct obstruction usually presents in the first few weeks of life as a large tear lake. In unusual cases, obstruction of the lacrimal sac may present as a medial canthal mass at birth or within the first few days of life. More commonly, epiphora develops in the first few weeks of life. Both of these presentations are caused by a membrane that blocks the entrance of the nasolacrimal duct into the nose, at Hasner's valve. A young adult who reports having frequent tearing has suffered trauma to the canaliculus or facial bones. In other cases, a preceding viral conjunctivitis is identified that has led to obstruction of the canaliculus. Middle-aged adults may complain of intermittent epiphora, suggesting nasolacrimal duct obstruction due to the presence of stones in the lacrimal sac or nasolacrimal duct. Most frequently, older adults complain of tearing or mucopurulent discharge resulting from idiopathic obstruction of the nasolacrimal duct.

The physical examination is aimed at identifying the presence and location of any obstruction in the lacrimal drainage system. The examination begins with a complete ophthalmic examination to rule out ocular or eyelid problems that may contribute to epiphora. The most useful test in the evaluation of the tearing patient is the dye disappearance test. This simple test quickly confirms or denies presence of the tearing. The dye disappearance test may be the only test that can be used in a small child. In adults, irrigation of the lacrimal system and palpation of the canaliculus identify any possible obstruction.

The cause of the epiphora is usually related to an anatomic abnormality that is identified during the physical examination. Abnormalities in the tear film or eyelid problems, such as entropion or trichiasis, may cause reflex tearing. Punctal ectropion or ectropion of the entire eyelid may prevent tears from entering the lacrimal drainage apparatus. A canalicular obstruction may be present as a result of viral infection or trauma. A more indolent cause of epiphora and mucopurulent discharge is canaliculitis. Obstruction of the common canaliculus may be present as an isolated finding or in association with nasolacrimal duct obstruction. Nasolacrimal sac and duct obstruction may be caused by stones or scar tissue. In congenital cases, the only obstruction may be an imperforate membrane at Hasner's valve.

For every cause of nasolacrimal duct obstruction, an appropriate treatment exists. Fortunately, the results of treatment are usually successful and gratifying for both the patient and the surgeon. In some cases, treatment may be as simple as observation in cases of congenital nasolacrimal duct obstruction because the natural history is one of resolution as the child grows. In cases in which spontaneous resolution does not occur, nasolacrimal duct probing or intubation is usually curative. In adults with acquired nasolacrimal duct obstruction, a dacryocystorhinostomy is required. Nearly 100 years of refinement have made dacryocystorhinostomy one of the most predictable and successful procedures in ophthalmic surgery. Refinements in technique and newer technologies, including nasal endoscopy and laser surgery, may speed patient recovery and maintain the same high degree of success as that achieved with traditional external dacryocystorhinostomy. Canalicular laceration may occur as a single laceration or in the setting of multiple facial injuries. Repair involves the use of sophisticated microsurgical techniques and silicone tube intubation. These reconstructions yield a high success rate. In cases in which the canaliculus cannot be anatomically reconstructed, a Jones tube may be required. In cases in which the trauma is extensive, surgical correction may require significant soft tissue or bony reconstruction. In cases of tumor involving the lacrimal sac, maxillectomy and radiation therapy may be necessary.

Most patients who report having epiphora can look forward to an accurate diagnosis and successful treatment of their tearing. An understanding of the anatomy and physiology of the lacrimal system is required to appreciate all the possible causes of epiphora. In most cases, an accurate history and physical examination identify a precise cause of tearing. A successful treatment plan is available for all causes of tearing. Once the principles outlined in this section are absorbed, the ophthalmologist will see many successes in the management of epiphora.

CHAPTER 73

Anatomy and Physiology of the Lacrimal System

Thaddeus S. Nowinski

The lacrimal system comprises two components: the main and accessory lacrimal glands and their secretions and the lacrimal excretory system. An understanding of applied clinical anatomy and pathophysiology is essential for the evaluation of a tearing or tear film abnormality and for the development of predictable and functional medical and surgical treatments.

MAIN AND ACCESSORY LACRIMAL GLANDS

Embryology

The main lacrimal gland develops from a series of buds of ectodermal origin from the superior fornix of the conjunctiva.[1, 2] These epithelial buds, usually eight in number, grow into the underlying mesenchyma of the superotemporal orbit and migrate to the area of the eventual lacrimal gland fossa. The path is evident by the excretory ducts, which later canalize to form secretory units and multiple ducts. However, recent evidence proposes a possible neural crest origin of the lacrimal acini.[3] Development of the levator palpebrae superioris divides the gland into orbital and palpebral portions. The levator muscle and aponeurosis may develop abnormally, resulting in congenital blepharoptosis. Many cases of congenital ptosis demonstrate an obvious abnormality in the temporal portion of the eyelid that is secondary to a lack of support, or even prolapse, of the palpebral lobe.[4] The accessory lacrimal glands (Krause, Wolfring) probably develop from an epithelial invagination from the tarsal conjunctiva. Tears are usually not produced until the second or third month after birth.

Anatomy

The serous exocrine lacrimal gland is composed of a larger almond-shaped orbital lobe and a smaller palpebral lobe that are continuous posteriorly around the lateral edge of the levator aponeurosis (Fig. 73–1). The orbital portion lies anterolateral to the globe in the superolateral orbit, pressing against the frontal bone and producing a slight shallowing in the anterior and lateral roof of the orbit just inside the rim of the orbit, known as the *lacrimal gland fossa* (fossa glandulae lacrimalis). The orbital portion of the gland measures approximately $20 \times 12 \times 5$ mm in the adult and weighs 0.78 g, two to three times the size of the palpebral portion.[5, 6] The superior surface is convex and somewhat flattened against the lacrimal fossa. The most anterior border lies behind the orbital septum, and the anterior medial edge abuts the preaponeurotic (central) fat pad. The grayish-pink color of the lacrimal gland can usually be easily clinically distinguished from the yellow orbital fat. The mildly concave inferior surface lies above the levator aponeurosis, is molded by the globe, and extends laterally over the lateral rectus muscle to the level of the zygomaticofrontal suture. The posterior medial edge rests over a portion of the superior rectus muscle. The posterior portion of the orbital lobe presses into the orbital fat and lies in approximately the same coronal plane as the posterior pole of the globe.

The palpebral lobe rests below the levator aponeurosis, which provides its superior border (Fig. 73–2). The palpebral lobe extends into the posterior upper eyelid and can be seen on eyelid eversion near the lateral part of the superior fornix of the conjunctiva. The orbital and palpebral lobes are continuous around the lateral edge of the levator aponeurosis. This continuous portion of the gland between the lobes, along with the ductules, occupies an oval opening in the fascial support that is known as the lacrimal foramen.[7] The palpebral lobe is firmly attached to the conjunctiva. Prolapse of the palpebral portion of the lacrimal gland may occur with age or as the result of trauma.[8]

Two to six ducts from the orbital lobe pass through the palpebral lobe, where they are joined by ducts of the palpebral lobe to form eight to twelve ducts. The ducts then enter the postaponeurotic space, pass through Müller's muscle and conjunctiva, and enter the superolateral conjunctival fornix approximately 4 to 5 mm above the convex lateral margin of the upper eyelid tarsus. The palpebral lobe also sends additional independent ducts into the

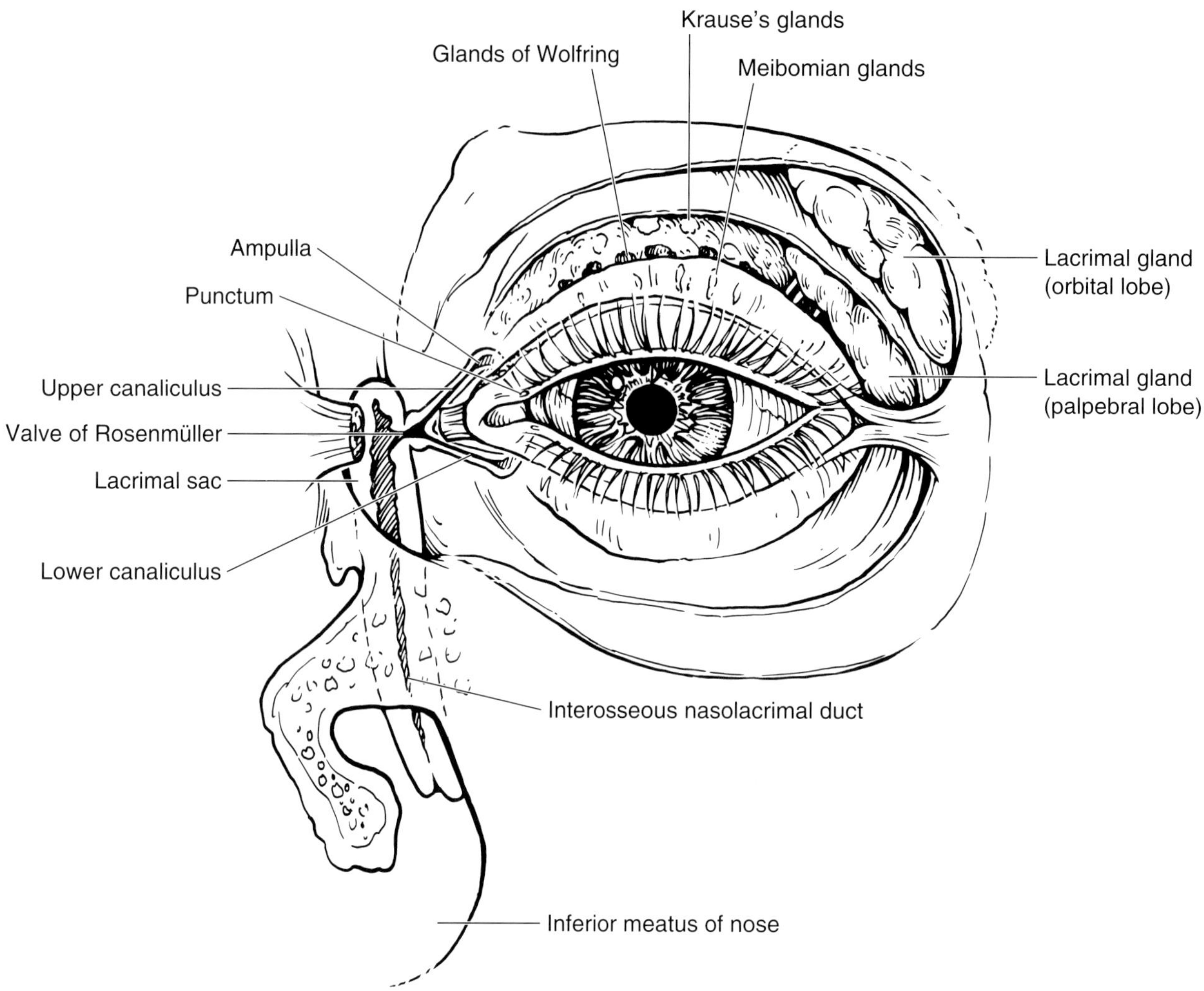

Figure 73–1. Lacrimal secretory and excretory systems.

superior fornix, and some may extend to the lateral canthus. Removal or damage of the palpebral lobe practically eliminates secretion of the main lacrimal gland.

The lacrimal gland has no definite capsule but possesses a thin, connective tissue pseudocapsule that is continuous with the tissue between the glandular lobules. This thin pseudocapsule is clinically distinct and provides an important anatomic landmark in the management of lacrimal tumors.[9] Many fascial strands (improperly called ligaments) attach to the lacrimal gland to provide support.[7] The superior transverse ligament of the orbit (Whitnall's ligament) probably provides the most support to the orbital lobe, along with help of the lateral edge and the horn of the levator aponeurosis. Whitnall's ligament inserts on the superlateral orbital wall, intermingles with the connective tissue of the gland, and connects via a small attachment to the lateral orbital tubercle.[10] Loose connective tissue strands also pass superiorly and laterally from the stroma of the gland to the periorbita (Soemmering's ligament). The inferior ligament of Schwalbe surrounds the hilus of the gland and inserts above the lateral orbital tubercle, helping to form the fascial lacrimal foramen, also providing some posterior support.

The accessory lacrimal glands are scattered around the conjunctival sac in the connective tissue of the conjunctiva, their ducts opening directly to the free surface of the conjunctiva. The 20 to 40 Krause's glands of the upper eyelid are situated in the superior fornix, mostly at the apex. Krause's glands were likened in structure to a continuation of the palpebral lobe by some earlier anatomists. A much smaller number are present in the fornix of the lower eyelid and are concentrated laterally.[11] A few glands of Wolfring are located just above and adjacent to the superior edge of the upper eyelid tarsus, and occasionally just below the lower eyelid tarsus.[12] An occasional accessory lacrimal gland may also be found in the plica or caruncle.

Histology

The lacrimal gland is a lobulated tubuloacinar structure on gross evaluation that is similar in appearance to

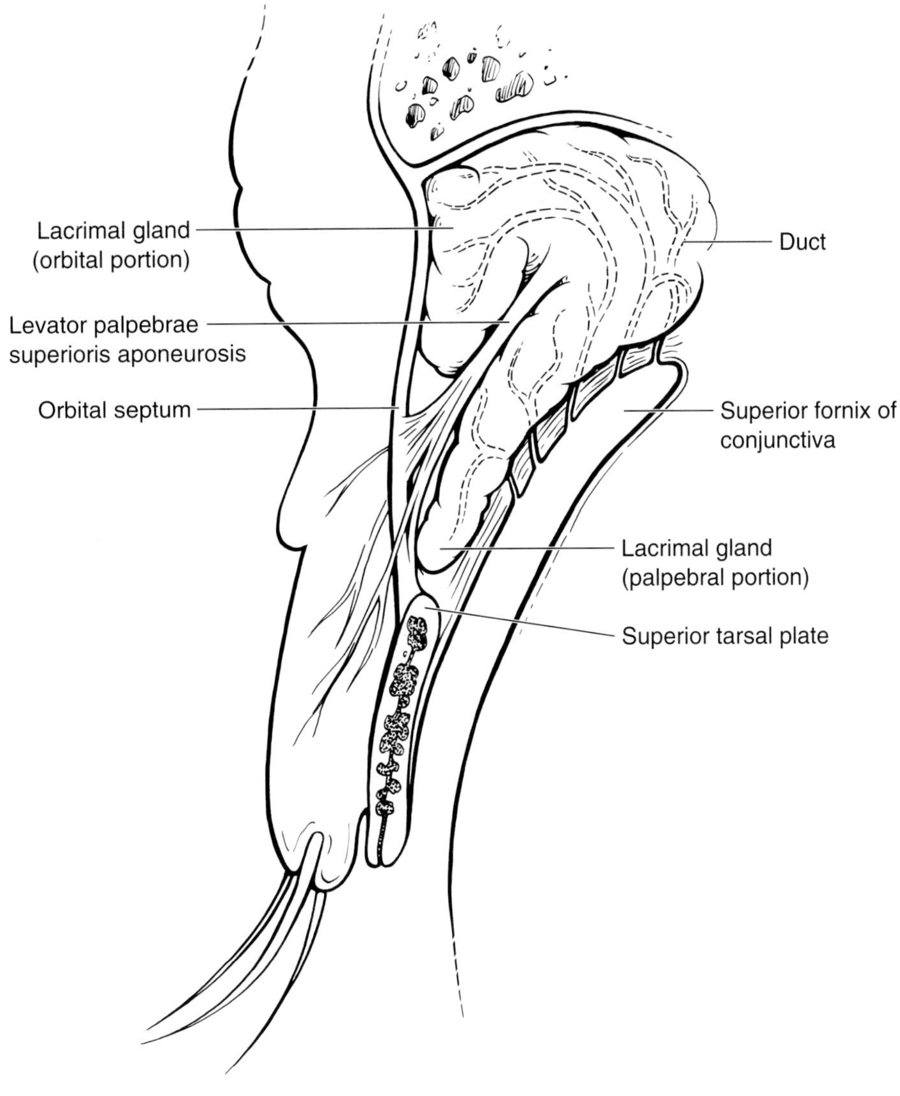

Figure 73–2. Relationship of the levator aponeurosis to the lacrimal gland.

the parotid gland. Each lobule is the size of a pinhead, and the lobules are separated by loose connective tissue. The palpebral lobe is 15 to 40 loosely knit lobules, and the orbital lobe contains two to three times as many. The acinus is the basic secretory unit of the lacrimal gland (Fig. 73–3). Microscopically, the acini are round or tube-shaped masses of columnar cells in an irregular circular arrangement with central lumens. The acini are composed of two layers of cells on a thin basement membrane: the inner cylindrical secretory cells with their retained granules and the incomplete outer flat and contractile basal myoepithelial layer. Contraction of the myoepithelial cells lining the acini forces secretions into the central canal. Acini join to form intralobular, then interlobular, ducts, which progressively join to form the definitive excretory ducts. The smallest intralobular ducts are lined with a single layer of low columnar or cuboidal cells with peripheral myoepithelial cells, whereas larger ducts have a two- to four-layer epithelial lining.

Electron microscopy characterizes the truncated-conical shape of the epithelial secretory cells of the acini surrounded by a discontinuous layer of myoepithelial cells. Microvilli are present on the luminar apical surface. The nucleus is located at the base, and scattered junction complexes and scattered desmosomes are present laterally. Narrow extensions known as canaliculi are found between adjacent cells. The apical cytoplasm contains a well-developed, rough endoplasmic reticulum and Golgi apparatus, as well as a moderate number of mitochondria, free ribosomes, and lipid droplets and vacuoles. A large number of secretory granules dominate the apical and middle regions. These round-to-ovoid, membrane-bound granules may be homogeneous or finely granular and may represent different stages in one or two distinct cell types. The dense granules are mainly serous, but staining for acid mucopolysaccharides shows that mucus is also produced.[11–13] A small amount of the mucoid layer of the precorneal tear film is of lacrimal gland origin.

Plasma cells represent the predominant mononuclear

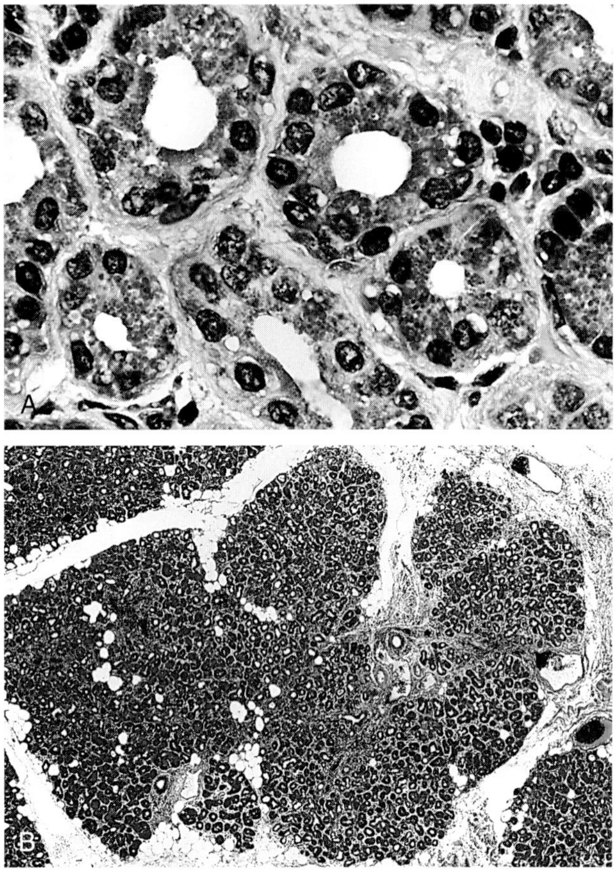

Figure 73–3. Lacrimal gland histology. *A*, The acinus, the basic secretory unit of the lacrimal gland. Acini are composed of inner, cylindrical cells and outer, flatter myoepithelial cells that form numerous excretory ducts. *B*, Low-power view showing multiple acini in a chronically inflamed gland. (*A* and *B* courtesy of Dr. Ralph Eagle.)

cell population of the normal lacrimal gland.[14] Most of these plasma cells contain gamma A immunoglobulin. Suppressor-cytotoxic T cells, followed by helper T cells, represent the next common cell types found. These findings help support a concept that the lacrimal gland belongs to the mucosa-associated lymphoid system.

Vascular Supply

The main blood supply to the gland is through the "lacrimal artery," a branch of the ophthalmic artery and therefore a branch of the internal carotid artery. The lacrimal artery penetrates the gland posteriorly. Branches of the transverse facial or infraorbital arteries may supply the gland in some patients, thus connecting the external and internal carotid branches. The lacrimal artery often anastomoses with the anterior division of the middle meningeal artery (external carotid) through the distal tip of the superior orbital fissure. Terminal branches of the lacrimal artery also anastomose in the eyelid with the anterior deep temporal artery (external carotid). The venous drainage of the gland is usually into the superior ophthalmic vein. The lymphatic drainage of the gland passes to the preauricular (superficial parotid) lymph nodes.

Nerve Supply

The lacrimal nerve, part of the ophthalmic branch of the trigeminal (fifth cranial) nerve, is the afferent reflex pathway for the main and palpebral lobes of the lacrimal gland, and the facial (seventh cranial) is the efferent pathway.[15] Sometimes, branches of the zygomatic nerve also carry sensory afferents. The ophthalmic division of the fifth nerve supplies sensation to the eye. This reflex arc may be stimulated by disorders of the cornea and conjunctiva, as well as by pain or irritation from iritis, glaucoma, or other causes. Stimulation of the retina with bright lights or some other stimuli to the posterior globe may also produce lacrimation, possibly from the same pathway. Direct inflammation or tumor of the lacrimal gland may cause hypersecretion or hyposecretion by different mechanisms on the afferent pathway.

The lacrimal nucleus of the seventh nerve lies in the pons, close to the salivatory nucleus (Fig. 73–4).[16] This nucleus is distinct from that of the main facial nerve, and some feel that this nerve should be considered a separate cranial nerve. Parasympathetic preganglionic fibers run through the pons as the nervus intermedius to the ventrolateral cerebellopontine angle, between the motor root of the seventh and eighth nerves. These nerves enter the internal auditory meatus to the geniculate ganglion. Here the greater superficial petrosal nerve is formed, which runs along the petrous bone. This is joined by the deep petrosal nerve from the carotid artery to form the nerve of the pterygoid canal (vidian nerve) to synapse in the sphenopalatine ganglion.[17] Postganglionic parasympathetic fibers travel through the foramen lacerum to join the maxillary nerve. These fibers then pass via the short pterygopalatine nerves into the maxillary nerve's zygomatic branch and the zygomaticotemporal nerve, which reach the lacrimal gland through the infraorbital groove to send a branch to join the lacrimal nerve. The zygomatic nerve bifurcates, with the sensory branch ending in the upper eyelid and superior conjunctival fornix. The efferent branch lies firmly attached to the inferior surface and then enters the orbital lobe of the lacrimal gland midway on its superolateral surface and penetrates to the hilus. It then follows each excretory duct backward in the orbital lobe and downward into the palpebral gland. Some terminal branches become cutaneous in the lateral canthal and supraorbital regions. Removal or damage of the orbital lobe of the lacrimal gland may eliminate the efferent supply and activation of the palpebral lobe.

Sympathetic innervation to the gland may arise from several routes. The superior cervical ganglion provides postganglionic fibers that travel in the plexus around the internal carotid artery. They join the deep petrosal nerve,

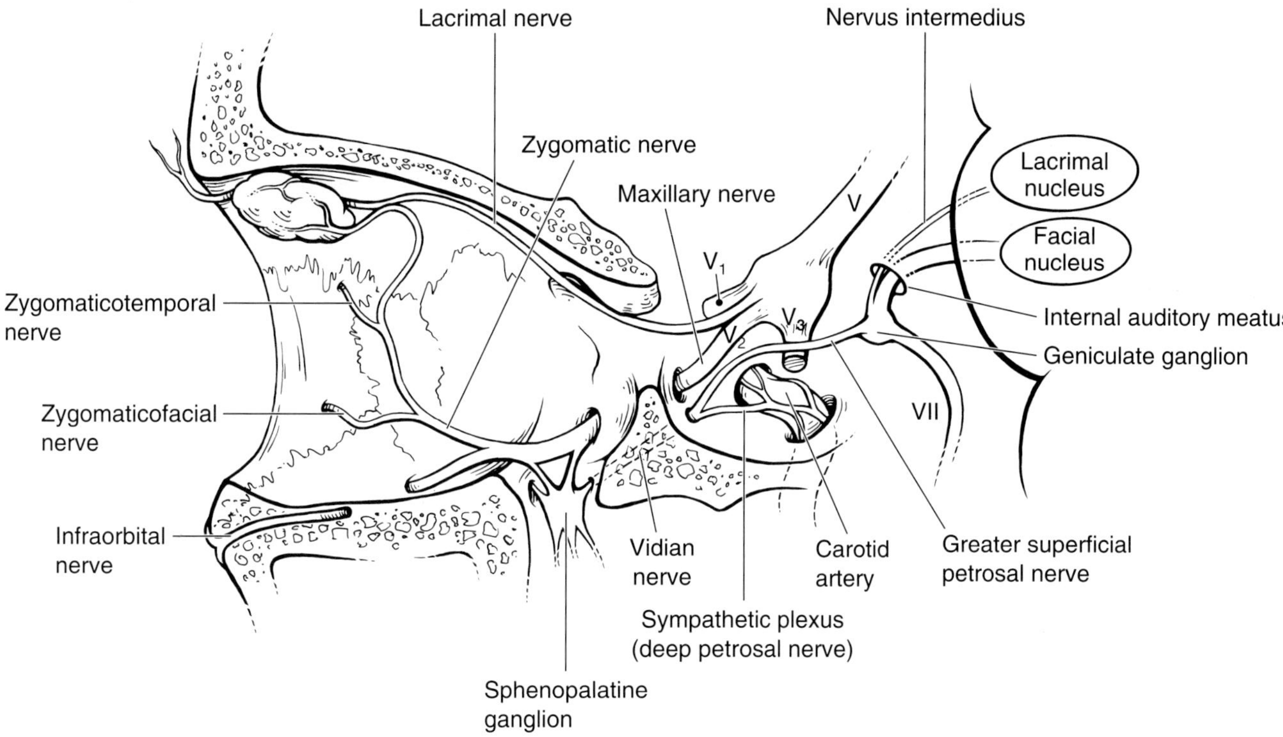

Figure 73–4. Afferent and efferent pathways of lacrimation.

the nerve of the pterygoid canal, synapse in the sphenopalatine ganglion, and travel along the maxillary nerve, the zygomatic nerve, the zygomaticotemporal nerve, and finally the lacrimal nerve. Additional sympathetic fibers may follow a path from the internal carotid artery along the ophthalmic artery and enter via the lacrimal artery. The role of the sympathetic fibers in tear production is unknown.

Higher (supranuclear) centers influence the aforementioned pathways. The seventh nerve lacrimal nucleus receives afferent fibers from the hypothalmus from the reticular formation, which may explain tearing from an emotional or psychological response. Also, a similar pathway may connect the olfactory system with the lacrimal nucleus. Stimuli that initiate tearing may come from such varied sources as the frontal cerebral cortex, the basal ganglia, the thalamus, the hypothalmus, and the cervical sympathetic ganglia.[18] Humans alone appear to possess the psychogenic type of reflex secretion. Graves' disease, as well as some other endocrine abnormalities, appears to affect lacrimal secretion, but the mechanism of this effect remains vague.

Reflex secretion appears to have only one afferent nerve supply, often incompletely established at birth. Sensory fibers are carried by the lacrimal nerve to the trigeminal ganglion (fifth cranial nerve) cell bodies. The superior division of the lacrimal nerve provides most of the input from the gland and pierces the orbital septum to supply the afferent innervation to the lateral conjunctiva and skin. The inferior division of the lacrimal nerve joins the zygomaticotemporal branch of the zygomatic nerve, providing sensation to the temple. Tearing occurs after stimulation of the zygomaticotemporal trunk or any of its branches. The sensory nuclei of the trigeminal nerve are connected to the lacrimal nucleus by internuncial neurons. Blocking the sphenopalatine ganglion stops the flow of reflex tears.

Excessive lacrimation may also occur with Bell's palsy, tumors, or other disorders of the cerebellopontine angle that stimulate the nervus intermedius. Misdirected regenerating salivatory axons to the otic ganglion may grow back into the greater superficial petrosal portion of the seventh nerve, which innervates the lacrimal gland, producing "crocodile or alligator tears,"[19, 20] a gustatory-lacrimal reflux stimulated by eating or even thinking of food.

The secretion of the lacrimal gland includes the watery tears, an antibacterial enzyme (lysozyme), gamma A immunoglobulin, a bactericidal protein (B-lysin), and a small amount of mucin.[20, 21] Fifty times more acini are present in the main lacrimal gland than in all of the accessory lacrimal glands combined. The main function of the lacrimal glands is to keep the corneal epithelium moist to preserve refraction; secondarily, the glands lubricate the eyeball so that it moves freely beneath the eyelids. Controversy exists as to whether the orbital and palpebral lobes are important in the maintenance of baseline tear production. Some feel that the main lacrimal gland is an integral component of baseline production, whereas others cite the accessory glands as the main or only source of aqueous tear production.[7, 22–24] Variations of both theories probably exist in certain patients. Dacryoadenectomy of the main or palpebral gland may produce severe keratoconjunctivitis sicca in some patients, whereas in many others, no alteration of baseline tear production occurs.[24]

PRECORNEAL TEAR FILM

The precorneal tear film is composed of aqueous, mucinous, and oily components and is necessary for the maintenance of the refractive power of the cornea as well as the maintenance of the functional integrity of the corneal and conjunctival epithelium (Fig. 73–5).[17, 25] The accessory exocrine lacrimal glands of Krause and Wolfring provide aqueous production. The glands of Zeis and the meibomian glands provide the oil layer. Moll's glands, Manz's glands and Henle's crypts provide the mucin layer (Fig. 73–6).

Aqueous Layer

In most people, the aqueous layer is the thickest part of the tear film, measuring 6.5 to 7.5 μm. This watery layer contains inorganic salts, bicarbonate ions, glucose, urea, enzymes, proteins, and glycoproteins.[26, 27] There appears to be no demonstrable efferent nerve supply to the basic secretors; however, some recent evidence implies that all tear secretion may be reflex. Baseline tear production seems to diminish with age. Aqueous tear deficiency (keratoconjunctivitis sicca) is the commonest abnormality of the tear film. It is most often idiopathic and usually involves all of the basic secretors. Fibrocystic changes may occur in the glands, most frequently in women in the fifth or sixth decade of life. Systemic medical diseases, especially collagen vascular disorders such as rheumatoid arthritis, may cause an aqueous deficiency problem. When this problem occurs as part of a general systemic involvement, it is usually called Sjögren's syndrome and consists of the triad of dry eyes, dry mouth, and arthritis, although multiple-system involvement may also be present. Lupus erythematosus, scleroderma, sarcoidosis, lymphoproliferative disorders, and other systemic medical disorders may be associated with aqueous deficiency.[25] Congenital alacrima, paralytic hyposecretion, and Riley-Day syndrome are less common causes of aqueous deficiency.

Hypersecretion is almost always the result of reflex tearing. Reflex secretion owing to keratoconjunctivitis sicca is a common cause of symptoms of excess tearing, as are inflammation, allergies, or infections of the eye, orbit, or adnexae. External pollutants, noxious chemicals or gases, or ocular medications may also be responsible for reflex tearing.

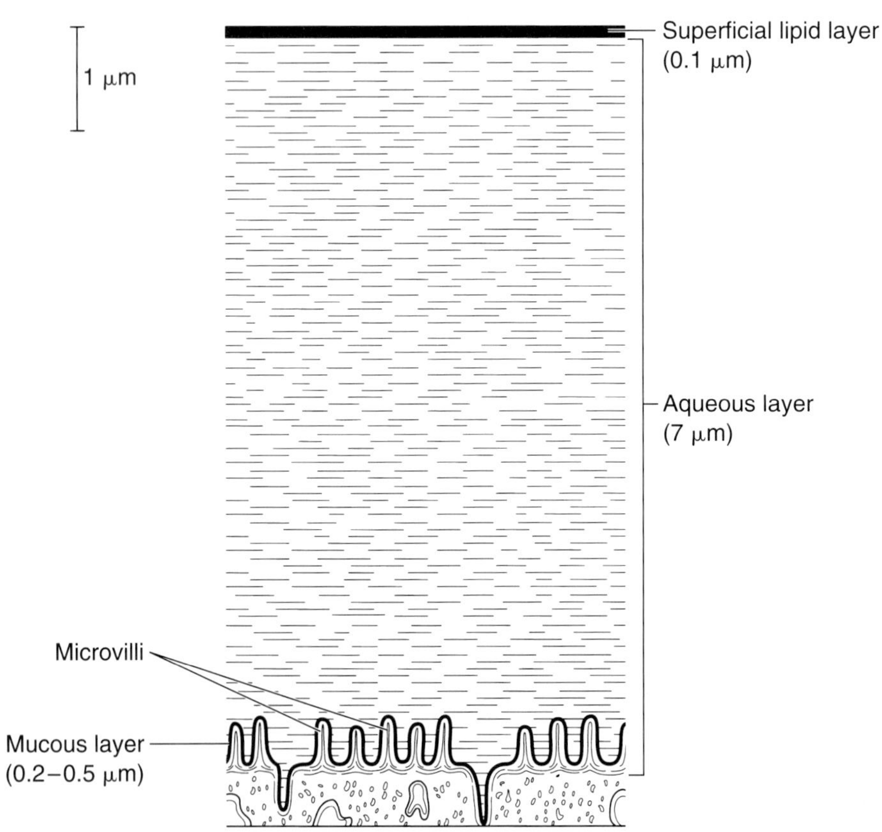

Figure 73–5. Precorneal tear film.

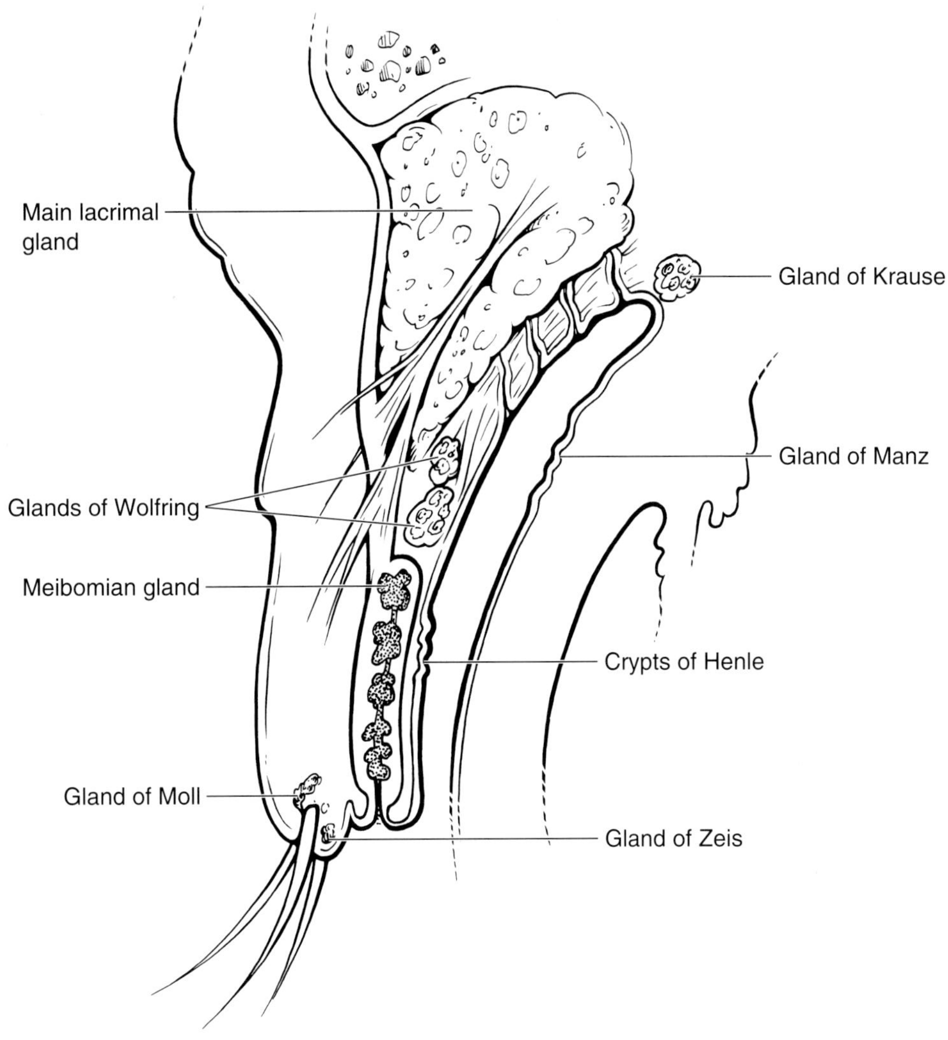

Figure 73–6. Accessory lacrimal glands of basic secretion.

Mucin Layer

The very thin mucinous component of the tear film is the innermost layer. It measures 0.2 to 0.5 μm and is probably provided mainly by the unicellular goblet cells of the conjunctiva, which are most abundant in the fornices. The complex Henle's crypts are located in the palpebral conjunctiva near the peripheral third of the tarsal margin of the upper and lower eyelids. These provide some mucinous secretion, as does the circumcorneal ring of Manz's glands, which are located in the limbal conjunctiva. A small amount of mucin originates from main lacrimal gland.

Mucin secretion increases in response to inflammation. Mucin production appears to be relatively increased in aqueous deficiency problems, even though recent evidence shows that the actual total mucin production may decrease.[28] The mucinous component of the precorneal tear film is in a highly hydrated, semisolid state and wets the microvilli of the corneal epithelium to convert the hydrophobic corneal epithelium to a wettable surface. Abnormal break-up time of the tear film is a direct measure of the functioning ability of the mucous layer of the tear film but is not necessarily related to a quantitative volume deficiency.[29] Ocular pemphigoid, Stevens-Johnson syndrome, trachoma, hypovitaminosis A, and chemical burns may interfere with mucin production by goblet cells.

Oil Layer

The specialized (holocrine) sebaceous meibomian glands of the tarsus produce the superficial, oily lipid layer of the tears, which measures only 0.1 μm. This layer is mainly composed of low-polarity lipids, including waxy and cholesterol esters.[30] High-polarity triglycerides, free fatty acids, and phospolipids are present in negligible amounts.[31] The meibomian glands open perpendicular to the lid margin just behind the mucocutaneous junction and number 25 to 30 in the upper and 15 to 20 in the lower eyelids. The less common sebaceous glands of Zeis are present in the palpebral margin, whereas the sweat (apocrine) glands of Moll are associated with the roots of the eyelashes. No known deficiency of tear film lipid exists, but alterations in lipid composition may occur as a result of certain microbes in such conditions as chronic blepharitis.

The lipid layer helps maintain tear film stability and prevent its evaporation by preserving the surface tension balance. The surface tension of the tear film also relies on the width of the horizontal palpebral fissure and is responsible for the 1-mm inferior marginal tear strips' position over the inferior cornea.[32]

Less specialized sebaceous glands of the skin elsewhere are usually associated with a hair shaft. Lack of sebaceous gland specialization in the eyelid may result in a congenital extra row of lashes from the meibomian gland orifices, known as distichiasis. Acquired distichiasis may occur from metaplasia of normal glands secondary to trauma or inflammations, such as that from Stevens-Johnson syndrome, ocular pemphigoid, or chemical burns. In this condition, lashes grow from the meibomian gland orifices that were previously normal. Blockage of the meibomian or Zeis gland orifices results in a back-up of fatty material, which may elicit a lipogranulomatous inflammation, resulting in a chalazion. Acute staphylococcal infection or inflammation of Moll's or Zeis's glands or lash follicles may form external hordeola (styes). When they occur in meibomian glands, they are known as internal hordeola.

Eyelids

The eyelids are essential for the proper wetting action of the cornea during blinking. After each blink, the first monolayer of lipids spreads quickly, limited by the speed of the eyelid (approximately 8 cm/second).[19] This action is followed by spreading of excess lipid, and eventually by areas of local thinning (break-up). Reflex aqueous tear production causes tears to flow across the cornea, diminishing its refractive efficiency.[33] Seventh nerve palsy, with resultant weakening of the orbicularis oculi muscles, or any disorder that results in a decreased blink may greatly interfere with the normal tear-spreading apparatus. Proper position and function of the eyelids are essential for the normal tear lake. Many eyelid malpositions may disturb the delicate balance and result in excess tearing. Scarring of the eyelids or conjunctiva or formation of symblepharon may limit eyelid movement and interfere with tear film dynamics. A decreased blink interval or infrequent blinking may result in inadequate inferior corneal wetting.[34, 35] Nocturnal lagophthalmos may result in morning irritation or tearing.[36, 37]

LACRIMAL EXCRETORY SYSTEM

Embryology

The nasolacrimal drainage system begins as an invagination of ectodermal cells along the cleft between the lateral nasal process and the maxillary process of the face (Fig. 73–7).[1] This fold extends into the mesenchyma, forming the naso-optic fissure, and detaches from the surface to form a solid cord of cells between the medial canthus and the nasal cavity. This ectodermal bud elon-

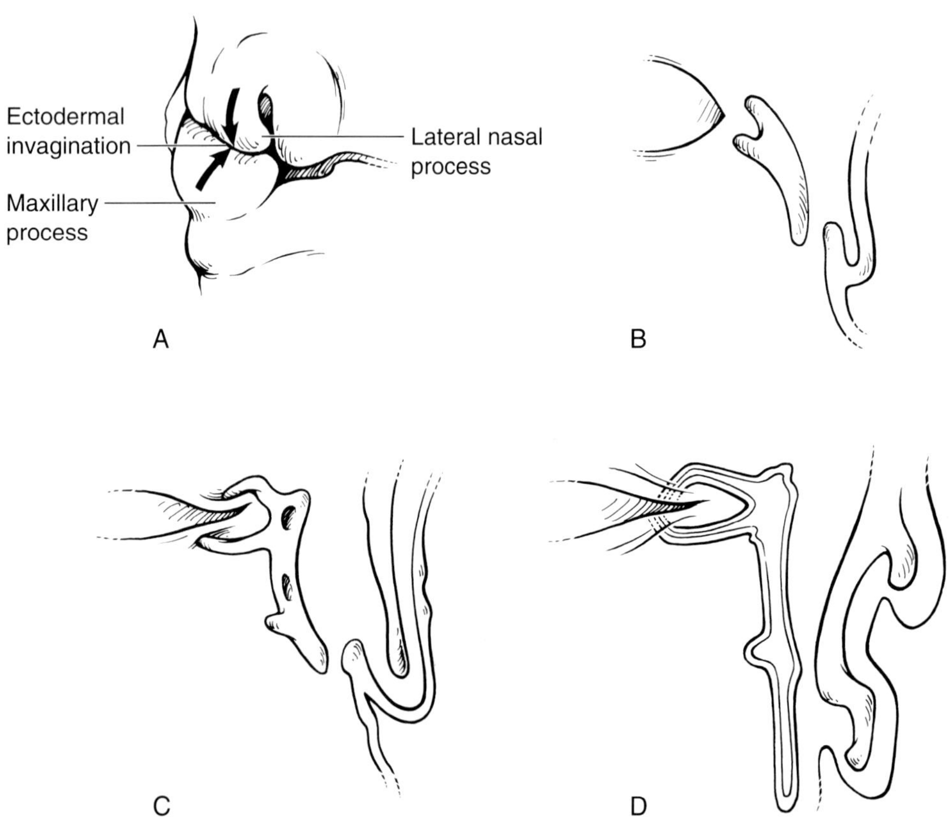

Figure 73–7. Embryology of the lacrimal excretory system. *A*, Invagination between the lateral nasal process and the maxillary process. *B*, Solid ectodermal cord. *C*, Canalization of solid bud. *D*, Canalized system prior to final patency into the nasal meatus.

gates and extends both toward the medial canthus and the nasal cavity during the 6th and 12th week of gestation. Laterally, the cord splits to conform to the medial canthal angle and later extends to the eyelid margin. Another cord of epithelial cells emerges from the primitive nasal cavities and remains separate from the other cord for some time. A proliferation of cells also begins to form a lacrimal sac rudiment.

Central necrosis occurs in this solid epithelial cord during the third month, forming isolated cavities that later coalesce. The upper cord begins canalization at the lateral end and progresses nasally. The lower cord begins to form a canal that opens into the inferior meatus. A dilation of this cord of tissues at its superior end becomes the lacrimal sac. The puncta later become patent onto the eyelid margins just before the eyelids separate at the 7th month of gestation. The two epithelial rods coalesce, and cell necrosis establishes a continuation between the lacrimal duct and the nose, usually between the 6th month and birth, or later.

Puncta

The lacrimal punctum sits on the summit of the lacrimal papilla, a small projection that is in line with the mucocutaneous junction, which separates the ciliated and nonciliated portions of the eyelid margin. The tone of the orbicularis helps push the punctum inward, thus maintaining its position against the lacus lacrimalis. The punctum of the upper eyelid lies slightly more medial than the lower, approximately 6.0 mm versus 6.5 mm from the medial canthus in the lower eyelid.[17] The round-to-oval orifices measure 0.2 to 0.3 mm in diameter. The size of the puncta may vary considerably from person to person, but the lower punctum is consistently larger than the upper.[38] The normal puncta are tilted posteriorly toward the globe and are visible only if the eyelid margin is everted during examination. Malpositions of eyelids may cause misdirection by turning the eyelid outward (ectropion) or inward (entropion). Normal drainage from the tear lake is then impossible and usually results in overflow tearing. The puncta glide in a groove between the plica semilunaris and the globe at the medial end of the marginal tear strip. The punctal openings are surrounded by a ring of elastoid dense connective tissue and appear to be the only portion of the lacrimal passages that is rigid enough to produce capillary attraction. The tissue surrounding the punctum is relatively avascular, giving a paler appearance than that of the surrounding tissue. This variation in color is valuable for the search for a clinically stenosed punctum, or when a congenital punctal membrane exists. The tarsal meibomian glands end 0.5 to 1.0 mm lateral to the punctum.

Canaliculi

The canaliculi, which average 0.5 to 2.0 mm in diameter and 10 to 12 mm in length, join the puncta with the lacrimal sac (Fig. 73–8). The initial 2-mm portion of the

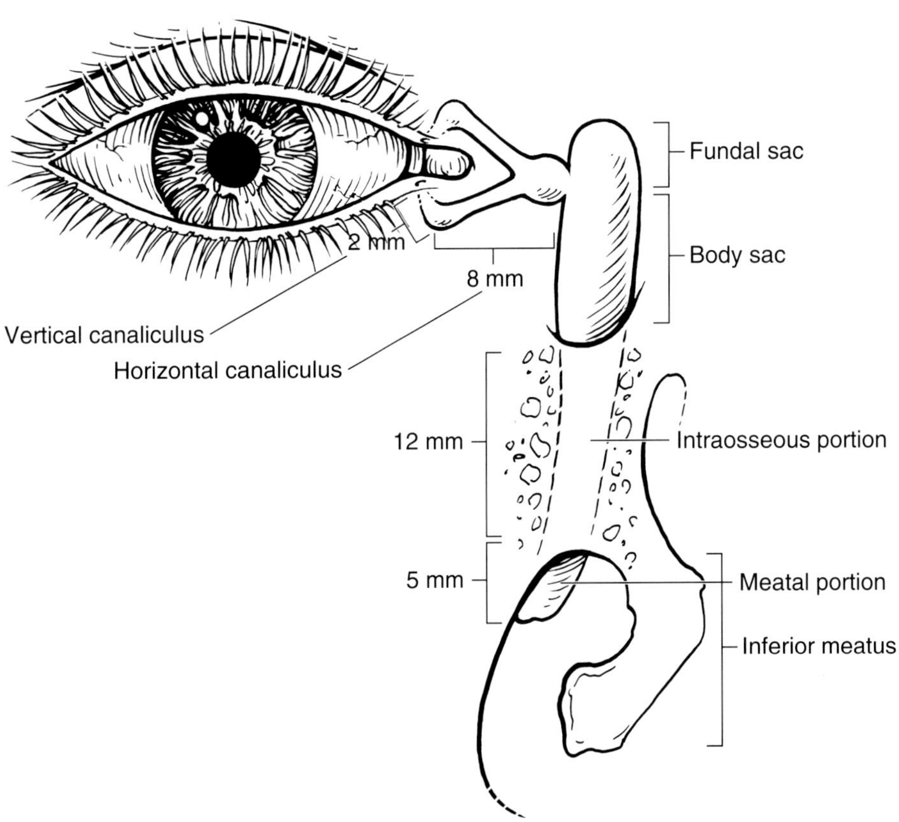

Figure 73–8. Lacrimal excretory system.

canaliculus begins at the lacrimal punctum and travels vertically, perpendicular to the eyelid margin. The canaliculus dilates 2 to 3 mm horizontally at this point, turning sharply medially, almost at a right angle, to travel 8 mm horizontally to the lacrimal sac. The two canaliculi pierce the periorbita (lacrimal fascia) and, in 90% of patients, unite to form the common canaliculus (internal common punctum) 2 to 5 mm before entering the lacrimal sac through the common punctum (internal common punctum). The canaliculi enter separately in the remaining 10% of cases.[39] The angle between the upper and lower canaliculi has been recently meticulously calculated down to 0.5-mm distances.[40] A small diverticulum of the lacrimal sac (Maier's sinus) is situated at the site of entry and precedes or replaces the common punctum. This canalicular opening is guarded by a fold of mucosa known as Rosenmüller's valve, which prevents reflux from the sac into the canaliculus. This one-way valve may cause the distention and subsequent pain seen in acute dacryocystitis. Massage of the sac may be unsuccessful in allowing expression of the tight sac contents. Decompression of the sac may be possible by probing to force the valve to open, thus relieving the increased pressure inside the sac. The canaliculi enter the lacrimal sac on the posterosuperior portion of its lateral wall 2 to 3 mm below its apex. At the medial canthus, the medial third of each canaliculus passes behind the medial canthal tendon and is surrounded by fibers of the pretarsal orbicular muscle. The common canaliculus lies directly beneath the central portion of the medial canthal tendon.

Congenital malformations may occur in the puncta and the canaliculi and may range from a small membrane of the punctum with a normal underlying system, to stenosis, duplication, fistulas, or complete abscence (Fig. 73–9). Atresia of the puncta may be produced by a failure in the opening of the conjunctival epithelium. Agenesis or atresia of the canalicular system may be caused by the failure of the anlage in the lacrimal passages to proliferate in the sixth to twelfth week of gestation, or by failure of canalization of the solid epithelial cords. Additional openings to the eyelid may occasionally exist along the canaliculi. True supernumerary canaliculi and puncta, also called lacrimal anlage ducts, may exist. These structures result from abnormal budding or proliferation of the superior portion of the epithelial cord of the lacrimal system, either as isolated abnormalities or associated with facial abnormalities.[41] This anomaly may also represent canalization of a rod of epithelial cells extending from the lacrimal sac. These anlage ducts usually form below the inferior canaliculus and may open onto the skin several millimeters below the caruncle (Figs. 73–10 and 73–11). Anlage ducts may drain to the skin as a congenital malformation, or a fistula may be acquired from chronic dacryocystitis.[42]

Histologically, a gradual transition occurs at the punctum from conjunctival epithelium to the nonkeratinizing stratified squamous epithelium of the canaliculi. The canalicular epithelium is 3 to 8 cells thick on a delicate basement membrane and is surrounded by dense, collagenized connective tissue that helps maintain resiliency of the apparatus. An abrupt transition to stratified columnar epithelium of the lacrimal sac and nasolacrimal duct occurs at the junction of the common canaliculus and the lacrimal sac. Many goblet cells are present in this modified nonciliated respiratory epithelium. The most distal portions of the duct closely resemble typical nasal mucosal epithelium.

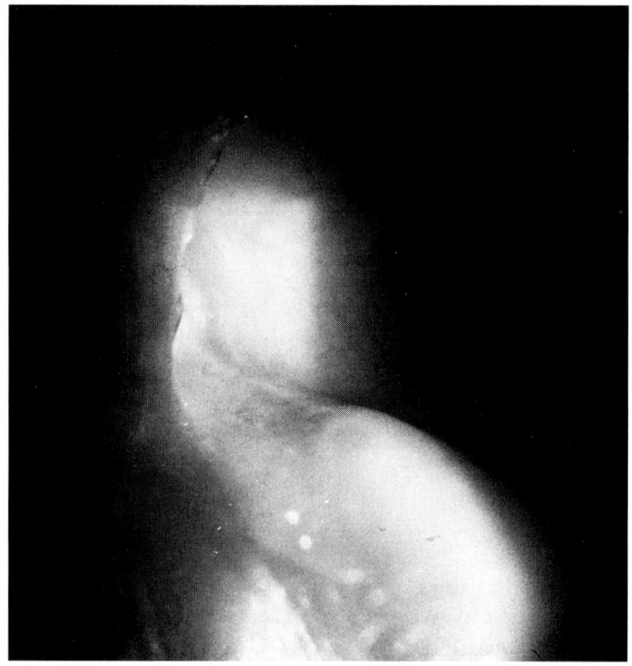

Figure 73–9. Membrane covering the lacrimal punctum (imperforate punctum).

Lacrimal Sac

The lacrimal sac is the widest portion of the drainage system. The lacrimal sac is situated in the lacrimal fossa in the anterior portion of the medial orbital wall. The sac is approximately 12 to 15 mm long vertically, with 3 to 5 mm of the sac situated above the medial canthal tendon (fundus). The lumen is 4 to 8 mm in anteroposterior diameter and 1 to 2 mm in lateral diameter. The main portion, or body (10 mm), of the lacrimal sac is located from the medial canthal tendon to the beginning of the bony nasolacrimal canal below. At this portion, the sac narrows, forming an isthmus. The sac is usually flattened and irregular in contour, with a normally collapsed lumen. The sac usually receives the canaliculus just behind the middle of the lateral surface of the sac approximately 2.5 mm from the apex. The anlage of the lacrimal duct normally involutes after the formation of ectoder-

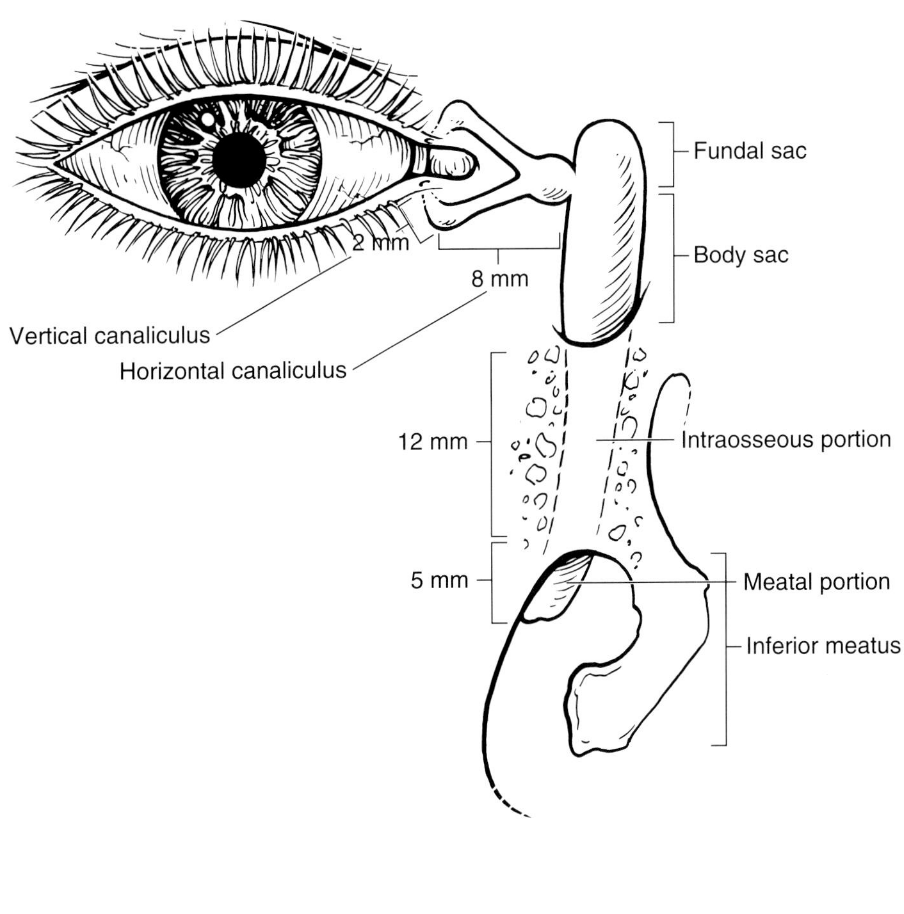

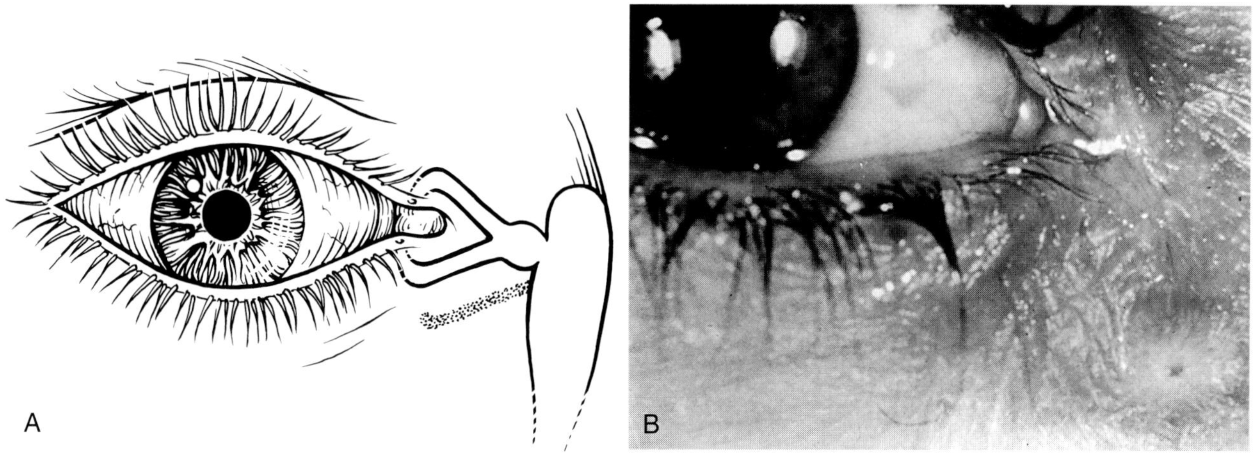

Figure 73–10. *A*, Normal involution of the lacrimal anlage duct. *B*, Persistence of the lacrimal anlage duct. (*B* courtesy of Dr. Robert Penne.)

mal cords after its invagination along the cleft between the lateral nasal process and the maxillary process.

The lacrimal sac is loosely surrounded by a fascial sheath (diaphragm) derived from the periorbita, which is attached to the posterior lacrimal crest of the lacrimal bone and to the anterior lacrimal crest of the maxilla. Between the lacrimal fascia and the mucosa there exists a potential plane, which must be recognized during lacrimal surgery. The lateral wall of the sac attaches firmly to the periorbita. This lacrimal fascia is related to the medial palpebral ligament (medial canthal tendon) anteriorly and to the deep heads of the preseptal and pretarsal orbicular muscle posteriorly, thus forming a potential space to create the pressures necessary for the lacrimal pump.

The lacrimal fossa is formed at the point of fusion between embryonic maxillary and nasal processes and is marked by a small sulcus or a lacrimal tubercle in many patients. This vertically placed landmark may run midway between the anterior and posterior crests or is often more posterior, with predominance of the maxillary bone. Located in the anterior portion of the medial orbital wall, the fossa measures approximately 15 mm high, 4 to 8 mm wide, and 2 mm deep (Fig. 73–12). Superiorly, the fossa is shallow and blends into the frontal bone's angular process. Inferiorly, the fossa deepens and takes a more oval shape. The front edge of the fossa, the thick anterior lacrimal crest, is continuous with the inferior orbital rim. A narrow sulcus, the so-called sutura notha, is 2 to 3 mm anterior to the anterior lacrimal crest. A small nutrient artery in this groove may cause bleeding during lacrimal surgery. The sutura notha is a good landmark for identifying the anterior lacrimal crest.[20] The floor of the lacrimal fossa becomes very thin in the area of the lacrimal bone before it thickens at the more prominent posterior lacrimal crest. This crest terminates inferiorly at the nasolacrimal duct, where the hamular process of the lacrimal bone articulates in the lacrimal notch of the orbital surface of the maxillary bone. The superior portion of the fossa is related medially to the anterior ethmoidal air cells, and the larger inferior portion abuts the anterior portion of the middle meatus of the nose. In some patients, large ethmoid air cells (agger nasi) may extend under the entire lacrimal fossa. In this anatomic situation, the lacrimal surgeon may fail to distinguish thin, friable, gray ethmoid air cell mucosa from the thicker, pink nasal mucosa.

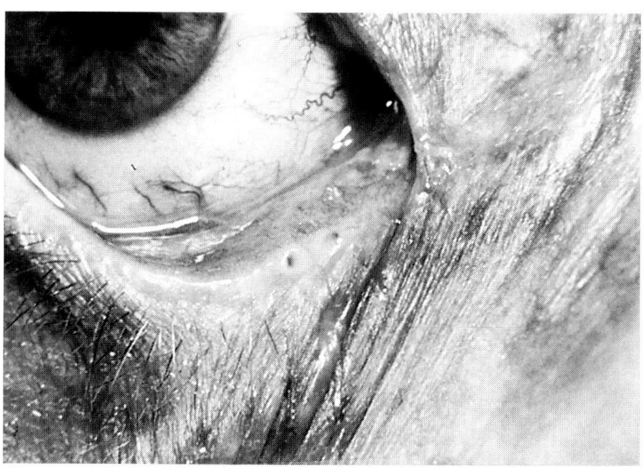

Figure 73–11. Supernumerary punctum.

The angular vessels, from the supratrochlear and supraorbital systems, cross the anterior surface of the medial canthal tendon approximately 8 mm nasal to the medial canthus. After crossing the medial canthal tendon, this vein continues inferiorly as the facial vein. Tributaries may also cross the tendon between the medial canthus and the main vein. A venous plexus exists between the lacrimal sac and the lacrimal fascia in the fibroelastic tissue of the wall of the sac.

Nasolacrimal Duct

The nasolacrimal duct is 12 to 18 mm long and connects the lower portion of the sac with the inferior nasal

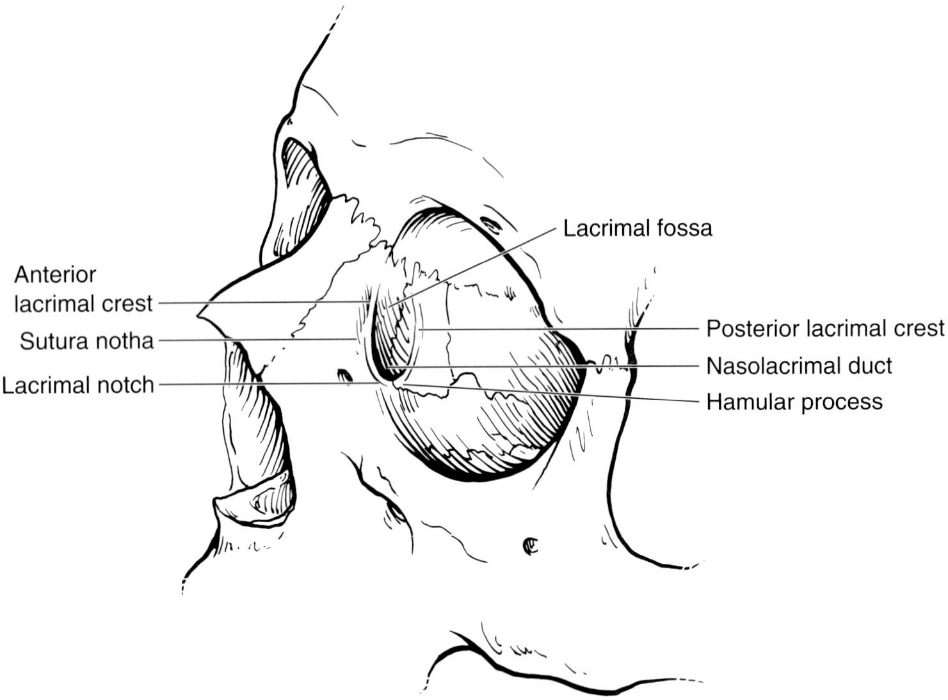

Figure 73–12. Medial bony orbit and lacrimal fossa.

meatus. It is composed of a longer intraosseous component (10 to 12 mm) and a shorter, membranous meatal duct (3 to 5 mm). The bony nasolacrimal canal is formed by a groove in the maxilla, the lacrimal bone, and the lacrimal process of the inferior nasal concha between the maxillary sinus and the middle meatus.[43-46] An angular bend may exist between the duct and the lacrimal sac. The nasolacrimal canal curves dorsomedially in most cases, bending an average of 15 to 20 degrees, but sometimes as much as 37.5 degrees.[47] The duct then generally continues downward, posteriorly, and laterally and is narrower in the middle than at either end. The distal portion of the duct bends medially in an irregular J shape in many neonates. The infantile pattern tends to straighten with normal growth.[48] The duct extends into the inferior meatus before penetrating the nasal mucosa, producing the meatal portion of the duct. The duct ends under the inferior turbinate (ostium lacrimale) and empties into the inferior meatus 5 mm below the vault of the anterior end of the inferior nasal meatus approximately 3 cm from the external nares in the adult. Many anatomic variations may exist in this opening and its location.[49] Diseases, fractures, or surgery of the sinuses or nose may involve and obstruct the lacrimal sac or nasolacrimal canal.

The membranous duct may have many folds, incorrectly called valves (Fig. 73–13). Krause's (Béraud's) valve may be present at the upper end of the nasolacrimal duct, whereas other narrowing mucosal folds, Hrytl's and Taillefer's valves, are located near the middle of the interosseous part of the duct, usually the narrowest portion of the duct. The best-developed fold (plica lacrimalis) guards the inferior end and represents the remains of the fetal septum, Hasner's (Cruveilhier's, Bianchi's) valve. The mucosa is closely adherent to the mucoperiosteum in the inferior portion of the nasolacrimal canal, but it is easily separated from the bone superiorly. A strong familial correlation may exist for the incidence of Hasner's membrane.[50] Less-developed valves of Bochdalek, Foltz, Huschke, and others have been described, and their functional significance is unclear.[17] The valves of the entire drainage system help present the retrograde passage of air through the puncta during nose blowing or sneezing.

Failure of complete canalization of the duct into the nasal meatus is common at birth, most commonly as a result of persistence of Hasner's membrane at the duct's outlet. Most ducts become patent within the first few months of life. Some cases may have a deep bend in the nasolacrimal duct just before entering the nasal cavity, making routine probing procedures inadequate. An angular bend at the sac-duct junction may also be difficult to adequately probe, leading to false passage. Hasner's membrane is especially soft, and high-pressure irrigation after infraction of the inferior turbinate may be successful in cases in which routine probing fails.

Multiple congenital malformations may occur in the nasolacrimal duct. In addition to an imperforate Hasner's membrane, many anatomic variations have been identified (Fig. 73–14). The severest defects may result from failure of fusion between the lateral nasal and maxillary processes and result in absence of the lacrimal excretory system. The duct may extend to the floor of the nose lateral to the nasal mucosa, or somewhere in between, without an opening.[7] The duct may end blindly in

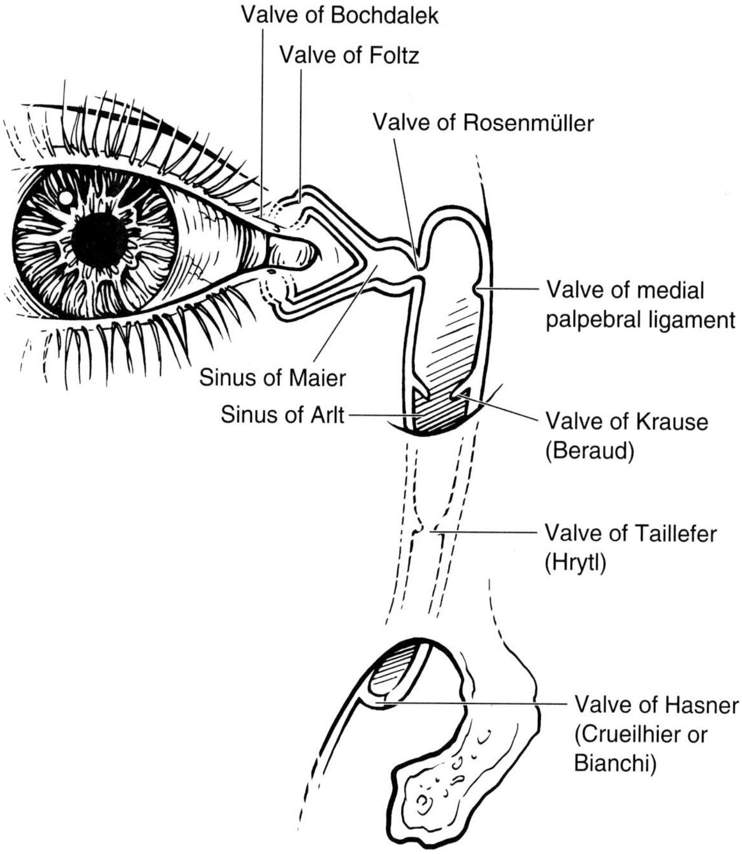

Figure 73–13. Valves of the lacrimal excretory system.

the medial wall of the maxillary sinus, in the anterior end of the inferior turbinate, or it may be blocked by an impacted anterior end of the inferior turbinate. The bony nasolacrimal canal may extend to the floor of the nose without an opening. In rare cases, the duct may be almost completely absent. A combination of a nasolacrimal obstruction below the sac and at the common canaliculus can be associated with the trapping of amniotic fluid and mucus and can result in a dilated lacrimal sac at birth without infection (amniotocele, or mucocele of sac).[51] Intranasal extension beneath the inferior turbinate (Fig. 73–15) may require nasal endoscopy for definitive diagnosis and treatment.

The medial canthal area contains numerous anasto-

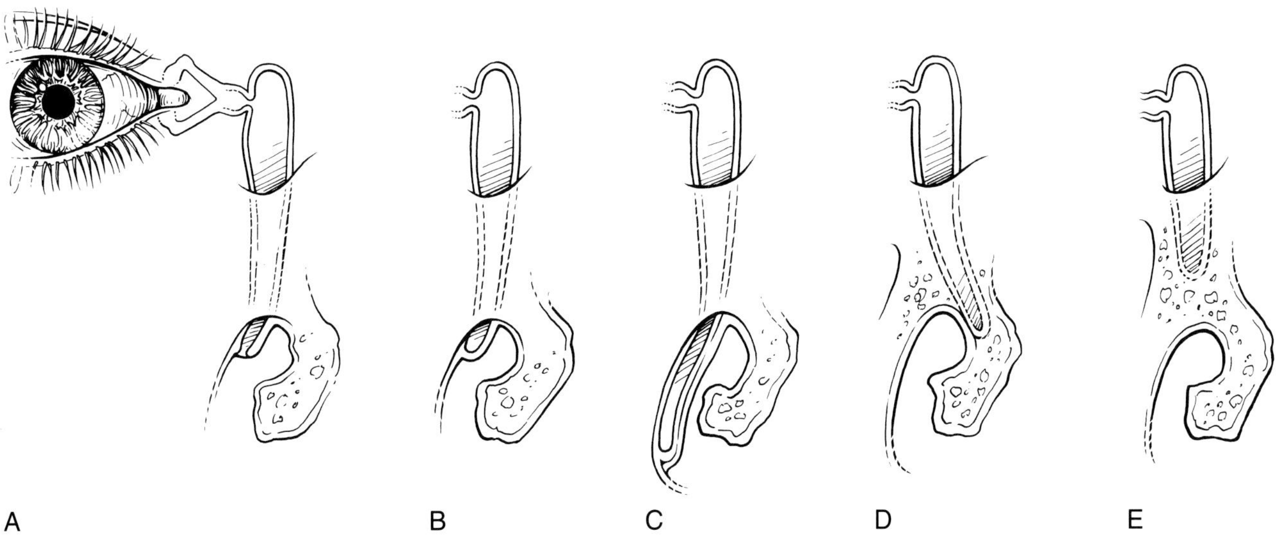

Figure 73–14. *A*, Patent nasolacrimal canal. *B–E*, Congenital obstruction of the nasolacrimal canal.

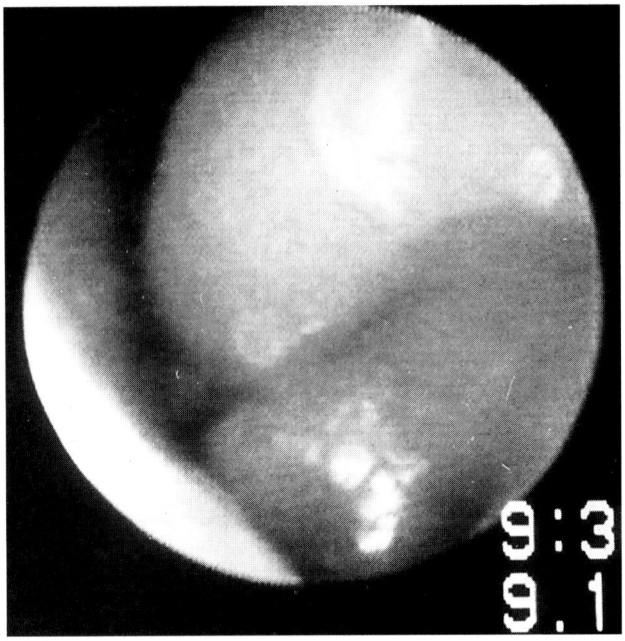

Figure 73 – 15. Intranasal extension of amniotocele into the nose as seen during intranasal endoscopy.

moses of the internal and external carotid circulations. The ophthalmic artery supplies the superior and inferior medial palpebral branches, the facial artery supplies the angular branch, and the infraorbital and sphenopalatine branches supply the richly vascular area. The venous drainage is similarly complex, with the angular and infraorbital branches providing the main branches. The infratrochlear branch of the first division of the trigeminal nerve and the anterior superior alveolar branch of the second division of the trigeminal nerve provide the nerve supply to the lacrimal sac. A rich plexus of veins (erectile tissue) is present around the nasolacrimal duct. Within the walls is a venous plexus continuous with the lacrimal sac plexus above and the veins of the nasal mucosa below. Engorgement of this erectile tissue may result in temporary obstruction of the nasolacrimal excretory system.

The medial canthal tendon (palpebral ligament) is a complex structure in its components and insertions and plays a major role in tear outflow dynamics. All components of the orbicularis oculi contribute to the strong superficial (anterior limb) head of the medial canthal tendon. The pretarsal and preseptal orbicularis oculi insert medial to the anterior lacrimal crest (anterior to the lacrimal fossa) near the nasomaxillary suture on the frontal process of the maxillary bone. Superiorly, these fibers fan out to cover the fundus of the lacrimal sac.[52] Inferiorly, below the ligament, only a few strands of the orbicularis insert. This structure offers very little resistance to distensions or swellings of the sac. Clinically, the sac distends below the medial canthal tendon with dacryocystitis, and this site is also a common site for the development of a fistula from the sac to the skin in chronic or neglected cases. In fact, swelling above the medial canthal tendon suggests a neoplastic rather than an infectious process. The pretarsal portion of the orbicularis oculi is firmly attached to the entire length of the tarsus. The preseptal portion is adherent to the orbital septum and laterally forms a continuous layer with the pretarsal and orbital portions.[53] The anterior limb lies anterior to the canaliculus.

The pretarsal and preseptal muscles also have thinner deep extensions (posterior limb) that insert on the posterior lacrimal crest (Fig. 73 – 16). Extensions from the pretarsal (tensor tarsi or Horner's muscle) and preseptal (Jones' muscle) blend with portions of the orbital periosteum, the posterior lacrimal crest, and other components of the lacrimal diaphragm. The deep head of the lower eyelid preseptal muscle may insert on the anterior wall of the sac, whereas the deep head of the pretarsal muscle appears to insert posterolateral to the sac.[53] The deep insertions pass posterior to the canaliculus. The lacrimal sac is thus uniquely separate from the orbit and the adnexa. The multiple fascial attachments isolate the sac, and any distention of the sac may cause severe pain and pressure owing to lack of planes to accommodate expansion.

Jones, based on in vitro anatomic observations, postulated a dynamic pump system that integrated three components of interaction (Fig. 73 – 17).[19, 39, 55] First, contracture of the superficial and deep heads of the pretarsal muscle closes the ampulla and compresses and shortens the canaliculi to pump tears toward the lacrimal sac. This important function has been confirmed by intubation and manometric studies that have documented a positive pressure peak in the canaliculus with each blink.[56–58] Second, contracture of the deep heads of the pretarsal muscle (Horner's muscle) and the preseptal muscle (Jones' muscle) causes a negative pressure in the lacrimal sac and expands it during lid closure. This effect has not been confirmed by the methods mentioned earlier, and positive peaks were documented. In fact, Doane[59] postulated that the lacrimal sac and canaliculi all are compressed and collapse at time of maximum eyelid closure. High-speed cinematic studies have given evidence that a negative-pressure phase may exist at the end of the blink. Tears were observed to rush into the canalicular system just after eyelid opening.[57] Third, the multiple fascial attachments around the lacrimal sac, especially those covering the lateral wall of the sac, and their relationship to the deep heads of the orbicularis were called the *lacrimal diaphragm*. Pulling the lacrimal diaphragm laterally creates negative pressure within the sac. Reflux is prevented by Rosenmüller's valve.

More than 90% of the lacrimal fluid is removed by the

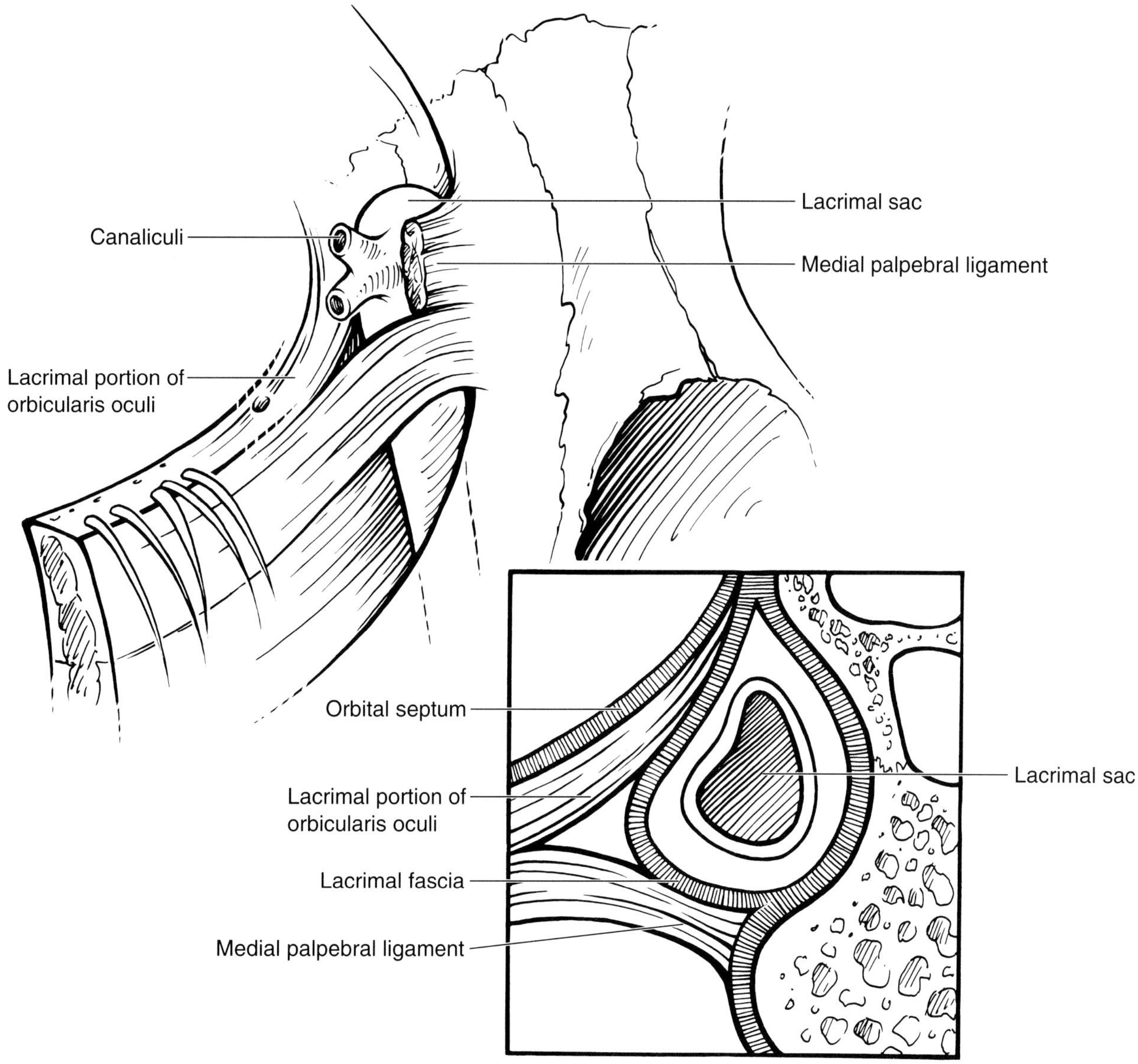

Figure 73–16. Deep and superficial insertions of the orbicularis oculi.

excretory system, whereas less than 10% evaporates between blinks.[19] The orbicularis oculi pumping action may be disturbed by facial paralysis from Bell's palsy, surgery (e.g., for acoustic neuroma), or other interferences with the cerbellopontine angle. Elimination of the lacrimal pump causes overflow tearing if tear production remains normal. Overstimulation of the orbicularis oculi as is seen in blepharospasm or hemifacial spasm, may also disrupt the normal lacrimal pump mechanism. Any eyelid malposition may also disrupt this pump, resulting in tearing.

The elastic properties of the canaliculi and the surrounding tissues expand after compression, creating a partial vacuum. Tears are thus drawn into the lacrimal excretory system after each blink. This canalicular pump and drainage by capillary action appears to be clinically significant because lacrimal drainage remains functionally intact even after the lacrimal sac is surgically removed as well as during sleep. Loss of canalicular resiliency, known as flaccid or floppy canalicular syndrome, may occur in the elderly and may prevent normal tear flow in a patent system.[60] The passage of tears down the nasolacrimal duct is influenced by gravity, evaporation in the nose, and inspiration and expiration.

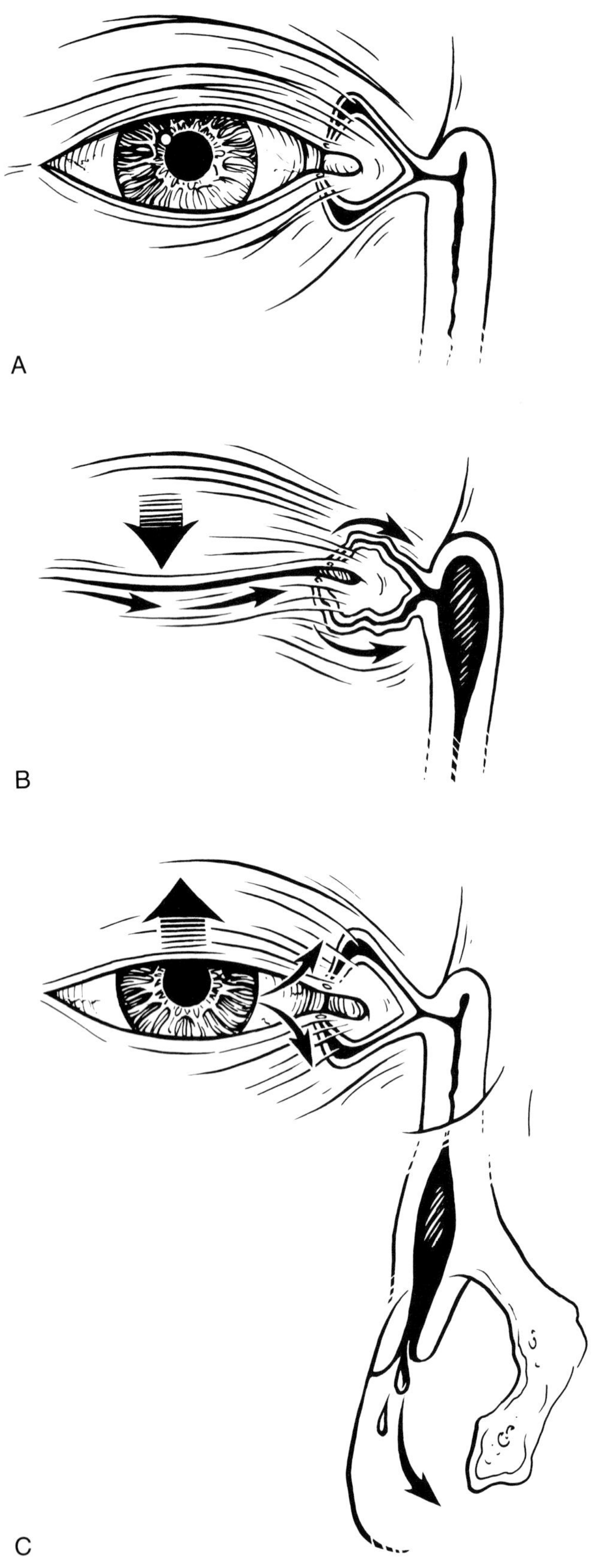

Figure 73–17. Lacrimal pump. *A*, Eyelids open. Tears enter the canaliculi by capillary attraction and gravity into the expanded ampulla and canaliculi. The lacrimal sac is collapsed. Tears flow through the duct into the nose. *B*, Eyelids close. Compression of ampulla and canaliculi, along with expansion of the lacrimal sac, pulls tears into the sac by negative pressure. *C*, Eyelids open. Lacrimal sac is collapsed; tears flow from the sac down the nasolacrimal canal.

REFERENCES

1. Duke-Elder S, Cook C: Normal and abnormal development: Part 1. Embryology. *In* Duke-Elder S (ed): System of Ophthalmology, vol 3, St. Louis, CV Mosby, 1963.
2. Patten BM: Human Embryology, 3rd ed. New York, McGraw Hill, 1968.
3. Tripathi BJ, Tripathi RC: Evidence for the neuroectodermal origin of the human lacrimal gland. Invest Ophthalmol Vis Sci 31:393, 1990.
4. Anderson RL, Dixon RS: Role of Whitnall's ligament in ptosis surgery. Arch Ophthalmol 97:705, 1979.
5. Whitnall SE: The Anatomy of the Human Orbit and Accessory Organs of Vision, 2nd ed. London, Oxford University Press, 1932.
6. Snell RS, Lemp MA: Clinical Anatomy of the Eye. Boston, Blackwell, 1989.
7. Jones LT, Wobig JL: Surgery of the Eyelids and Lacrimal System. Birmingham, AL, Aesculapius, 1976.
8. Smith B, Petrelli R: Surgical repair of the prolapsed lacrimal gland. Arch Ophthalmol 96:113, 1978.
9. Stewart WB, Krohel GB, Wright J: Lacrimal gland and fossa lesions. Ophthalmology 86:886, 1979.
10. Doxanas M, Anderson RL: Clinical Orbital Anatomy. Baltimore, Williams & Wilkins, 1984.
11. Egeberg J, Jensen OA: The ultrastructure of the acini of the human lacrimal gland. Acta Ophthalmol (Copenh) 47:400, 1969.
12. Orzales N, Riva A, Testa F: Fine structure of the human lacrimal gland. Part I: The normal gland. J Submicrosc Cytol Pathol 3:283, 1971.
13. Iwamoto T, Jackobiec FA: Lacrimal glands. *In* Duane TD, Jaeger EA (eds): Biomedical Foundations of Ophthalmology, vol 1. Philadelphia, Harper & Row, 1982, p 20.
14. Wieczorek R, Jakobiec FA, Sacks EH, Knowles DM: The immunoarchitecture of the normal human lacrimal gland. Ophthalmology 95:100, 1988.
15. Ruskin SL: Control of tearing by blocking the nasal ganglion. Arch Ophthalmol 4:208, 1930.
16. Crosby DG, Humphrey T, Lauer EW: Correlative Anatomy of the Nervous System. New York, Macmillan, 1962.
17. Wolff E: The Anatomy of the Eye and Orbit, 4th ed. New York, Blakiston, 1954.
18. Czermak W: Die topographischen Beziehumgem der Augenelohle, Augn. Anzliche Unterrichtstafeln (Magnus). Breslau, 1895, IX.
19. Jones LT: The lacrimal secretory system and its treatment. Am J Ophthalmol 62:47, 1966.
20. Linberg JV: Lacrimal Surgery. New York, Churchill Livingstone, 1988.
21. Ford LC, DeLange RJ, Petty RW: Identification of a non-lysozymal bactericidal factor (beta lysin) in human tears and aqueous humor. Ophthalmology 81:30, 1976.
22. Jordan A, Baum J: Basic tear flow: Does it exist? Ophthalmology 87:920, 1980.
23. Linberg JV, Slade S: Lacrimal secretion after sphenopalatine ganglion block. Ophthalmic Plast Reconstr Surg 2:97, 1986.
24. Scherz W, Dohlman CH: Is the lacrimal gland dispensable? Arch Ophthalmol 93:281, 1975.
25. Holly FJ, Lemp MA: Tear physiology and dry eyes. Surv Ophthalmol 22:69, 1977.
26. Mishima S: Some physiological aspects of the precorneal tear film. Arch Ophthalmol 73:233, 1965.
27. van Haeringern NJ: Clinical biochemistry of tears. Surv Ophthalmol 26:84–96, 1981.
28. Ralph RA: Conjunctival goblet cell density in normal subjects and in dry eye syndromes. Invest Ophthalmol 14:299, 1975.
29. Lemp MA, Dohlman CH, Kuwabara T, et al: Dry eye secondary to mucin deficiency. Trans Am Acad Ophthalmol Otolaryngol 75:1223, 1971.
30. Andrew JS: Human tear film lipids: Part I: Composition of the principal nonpolar component. Exp Eye Res 10:223, 1970.
31. Holly FJ, Lemp MA (eds): The preocular tear film and dry eye syndromes. Int Ophthalmol Clin 13:1, 1973.
32. Holly FJ: Formation and rupture of the tear film. Exp Eye Res 15:515, 1973.
33. Berger RE, Corrsin S: A surface tension gradient mechanism for driving the precorneal tear film after blinking. J Biomech 7:227, 1974.

34. Doane MG: Blinking and the mechanics of the lacrimal drainage system. Ophthalmology 88:844, 1981.
35. Doane MG: Interactions of eyelids and tears in corneal wetting and the dynamics of the normal human eyeblink. Am J Ophthalmol 89:507, 1980.
36. Katz J, Kaufman HE: Corneal exposure during sleep (nocturnal lagophthalmos). Arch Ophthalmol 95:449, 1977.
37. Sturrock GD: Nocturnal lagophthalmos and recurrent erosion. Br J Ophthalmol 60:97, 1976.
38. Carter KD, Nelson CC, Martony CL: Size variation of the lacrimal punctum in adults. Ophthalmic Plast Reconstr Surg 4:231, 1988.
39. Jones LT: An anatomical approach to problems of the eyelids and lacrimal apparatus. Arch Ophthalmol 66:111, 1961.
40. Corin SM, Hurwitz JJ, Jaffer N, Botta EP: The true canalicular angle: A mathematical model. Ophthalmic Plast Reconstr Surg 6:42, 1990.
41. Whitaker LA, Katowitz JA, Randall P: The nasolacrimal apparatus in congenital facial abnormalities. J Craniomaxillofac Surg 2:59, 1974.
42. Masi AV: Congenital fistula of the lacrimal sac. Arch Ophthalmol 81:701, 1969.
43. Whitnall SE: The nasolacrimal canal: The extent to which it is influenced by the maxilla and the influence on its caliber. Ophthalmoscope 10:557, 1912.
44. Duke-Elder S, Wybar KC: The anatomy of the visual system. *In* Duke-Elder S (ed): System of Ophthalmology, vol 2. St. Louis, CV Mosby, 1961, p 562.
45. Kuribayshi Y: Observations of the opening of nasolacrimal duct. Report 2. Jpn J Ophthalmol 1:96, 1957.
46. Calhoun KH, Rotzler WH, Stiernberg CM: Surgical anatomy of the lateral nasal wall. Otolaryngol Head Neck Surg 102:156, 1990.
47. Peters A: Zur Behandlung der Tranenschlauchatresie der Neugeborenen. Klin Monatsbl Augenheilkd 30:363, 1892.
48. Busse H, Muller KM, Kroll P: Radiologic and histologic findings of the lacrimal passages of newborns. Arch Ophthalmol 43:203, 1957.
49. Schaeffer JP: Types of ostia nasolacrimalis in man and their genetic significance. Am J Anat 13:183, 1913.
50. Fernández-Valencia R, Gómez Pellico L: Functional anatomy of the human saccus lacrimalis. Acta Anat (Basel) 139:54, 1990.
51. Weinstein GS, Biglan AW, Patterson JH: Congenital lacrimal sac mucoceles. Am J Ophthalmol 94:106, 1982.
52. Anderson RL: Medial canthal tendon branches out. Arch Ophthalmol 95:2051, 1977.
53. Howes MJ, Dortzbach RK: The microscopic anatomy of the lower eyelid retractors. Arch Ophthalmol 100:1313, 1982.
54. Rosengren B: On lacrimal drainage. Ophthalmologica 164:409, 1972.
55. Jones LT: Epiphora II. Its relationship to the anatomic structures and surgery of the medial canthal region. Am J Ophthalmol 43:203, 1957.
56. Hill JC, Bethell W, Smirmaul HJ: Lacrimal drainage—A dynamic evaluation. Can J Ophthalmol 9:411, 1974.
57. Maurice DM: The dynamics and drainage of tears. Int Ophthalmol Clin 13:103, 1973.
58. Steinkogler FJ, Burian M, Mayr R, Lischka M: Morphological observations of the nasolacrimal canal. Orbit 5:239, 1986.
59. Doane MG: Blinking and the mechanics of the lacrimal drainage system. Ophthalmology 88:844, 1981.
60. Hill JC: Treatment of epiphora owing to flaccid eyelids. Arch Ophthalmol 97:323, 1979.

CHAPTER 74

Evaluation of the Tearing Patient

David R. Jordan

A thorough history and a physical examination are essential for patients with tearing. A patient may be producing too many tears, as in those patients with dry eyes and reflex secretions of tears, or not adequately draining the normal amount of tears produced because of a problem in the outflow pathway, which is by far the more common situation.

The focus in this chapter is on the evaluation of the tearing patient by initially discussing important points to consider during history taking. The physical examination, including office testing, is discussed and examples of tearing problems are illustrated. It is important to appreciate that appropriate drainage of tears depends on a complex interplay of anatomy and physiology. A variety of features have to be considered, including volume of tear production, eyelid position, anatomic status of the nasolacrimal system, as well as the patency of the nasal passageway. There is no single test that will pinpoint the anatomic site or physiologic basis for a tearing problem. After listening to the history, examining the patient, and carrying out some simple office tests, the physician can usually arrive at a diagnosis. Sophisticated nasolacrimal testing may be required at times and is also discussed.

HISTORY

The evaluation of a tearing patient begins as the patient walks into the office. The patient holding a facial tissue in his or her hand presents with a tell-tale sign of significant tearing that can be seen almost immediately when the patient enters the examining room. As the patient sits down and begins to talk about the tearing problem, the physician should watch the patient while he or she is describing the symptoms. Facial nerve paralysis, congenital developmental anomalies, traumatic scars, ectropion and entropion, signs of aging skin (indicative of a possible poor tear pump mechanism), excoriation of lid skin (dermatitis), lacrimal sac swelling or fistula, and even an increased tear lake may be noticed within 30 seconds of the onset of the interview and may help diagnose the problem quickly (Figs. 74–1 through 74–4).

Without any of these tell-tale clues one needs to pursue the patient's tearing history and get a feel for how symptomatic the patient is. At times, the patient may not actually complain of tearing but may relate trouble with reading vision (looking through a pool of water), blurring of vision or mattering due to a build-up of mucopurulent discharge. On most occasions, the patient with a nasolacrimal blockage of some degree will have tears that run down onto the cheek either medially or laterally. The time of onset, duration, and frequency (steady versus intermittent) and whether the tears are clear or contain a discharge are good initial features to inquire about. Some persons will experience tearing all day; in others tearing is intermittent. Some tear only in the presence of an aggravating factor (e.g., wind, cold, weather, sunlight), while others will tear only very episodically (e.g., weekly or monthly), such as in those individuals with a dacryolith. The patient with a dacryolith is commonly between the ages of 20 and 40 and presents with very intermittent symptoms of tearing (i.e., lasting 1 to 2 weeks and then gone for 6 to 12 months only to return in a similar fashion). There may be associated pain from dacryocystic retention. Diagnostic testing may show normal dye passage, a functional type block, or complete obstruction, depending on how the dacryolith is blocking the passage.

If the nasolacrimal sac is filling up and becoming distended with the discharge, the patient may learn to push on the area of the sac to express the contents. The patient may describe associated symptoms such as itching and burning, as with allergies (see Fig. 74–4) and blepharitis, or pain and photophobia, as with iritis. The patient with lacrimal drainage insufficiency may give a past history of recurrent dacryocystitis or may relate having sustained an injury or had surgery to the eyes or nose in past years. Past and present ocular history is important to ask about since both the eye disease and drops being used to treat the eye disease may be responsible for tearing. Previous midfacial fractures and nasal surgery (polyp removal, turbinate reduction, Caldwell-Luc procedures) may damage the nasolacrimal outflow system. A general review of systems should be carried out to determine if other medical conditions exist that may contribute to the patient's tearing (e.g., past history of Bell's palsy, stroke history, or Wegener's granulomatosis).

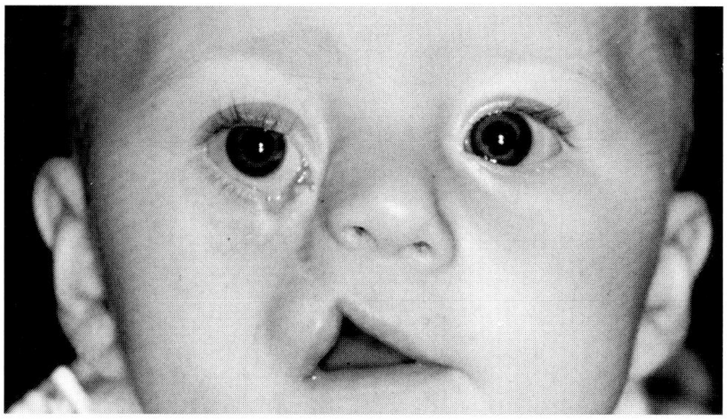

Figure 74–1. Young infant with cleft lip and palate as well as a medial eyelid coloboma presents with tearing. The tearing may be secondary to the lid defect or a nasolacrimal outflow obstruction as a result of an incomplete embryologic development in the area.

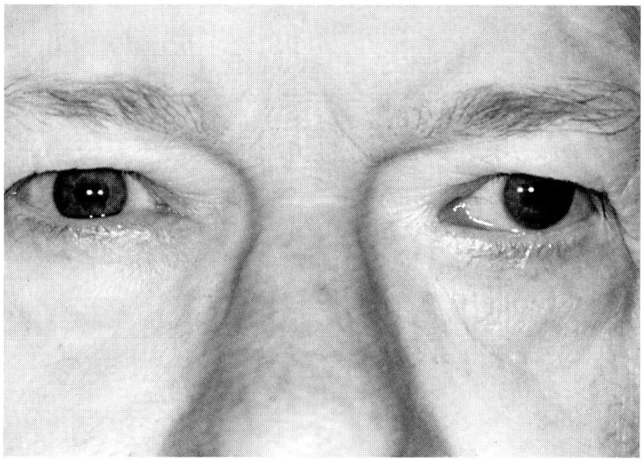

Figure 74–2. Middle-aged man, with previous trauma to left medial canthus, has rounding at left medial canthal angle. The left lower lid is pulled away from globe, exposing the conjunctiva medially.

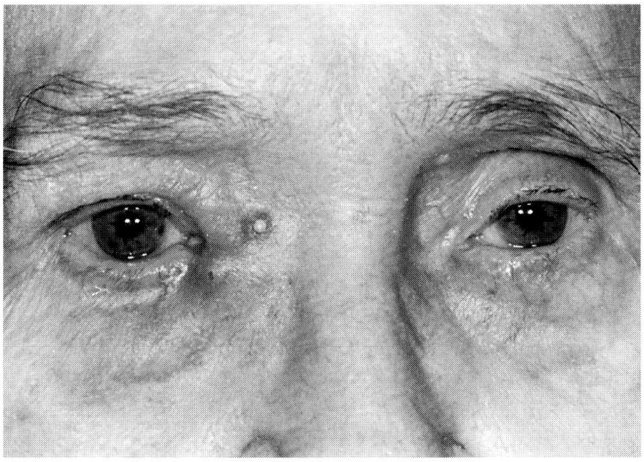

Figure 74–3. Elderly woman with swelling over right nasolacrimal sac and fistula tracking onto skin.

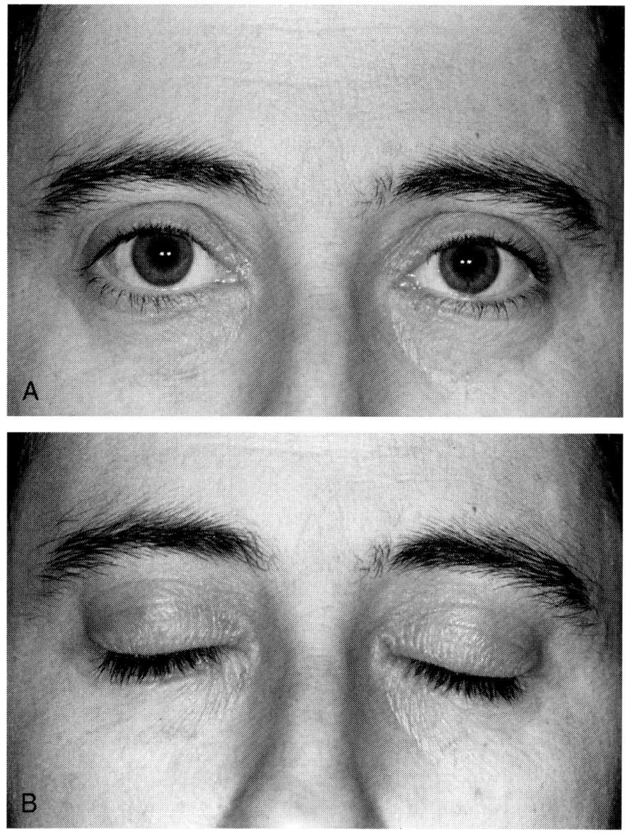

Figure 74–4. *A* and *B*, A 20-year-old person presents with red itchy eyelid and tearing secondary to allergy. Eyelid skin is red and thickened from rubbing.

It is helpful during the history-taking to try to determine if the patient's complaints are from excessive lacrimation (increased production of tears) or from blocked outflow (epiphora). Patients with lacrimal drainage insufficiency (complete or incomplete block) may have unilateral or bilateral complaints. Unilateral epiphora is more often associated with an outflow obstruction than bilateral complaints. The patient with bilateral complaints may have outflow obstruction as well, but other causes such as reflex tearing due to a dry eye, an inadequate tear pump, blepharitis, or excessive production of tears (in some stroke patients), which are usually bilateral diseases, need to be considered. Overall, when looking at the etiology of tearing, outflow obstruction is far more common than increased production of tears.

Anatomy

An appreciation of the neurologic pathways responsible for tear production is important to help one decide the anatomic location responsible for causing tearing in each patient. The lacrimal nerve (a division of the ophthalmic division of the trigeminal nerve) provides sensory innervation to the lacrimal gland. The lacrimal gland secretion is produced by stimulation of a reflex arc as well as central stimulation. The afferent limb of the reflex pathway is supplied by the trigeminal nerve. The efferent limb runs a complicated course via the facial nerve. Stimulation of any branches of the trigeminal nerve results in activation of the reflex arc, and tearing is the result. For example, defects of the corneal epithelium or spasms of the ciliary body (iritis) stimulate the ophthalmic division of the trigeminal nerve and trigger the reflex arc, and the lacrimal gland produces tears. The pathways responsible for central stimulation (emotional, psychogenic) are poorly understood, but stimuli directed toward parts of the frontal cortex, basal ganglia, and hypothalamus are thought to cause tearing.[1]

The efferent pathway to the lacrimal gland follows a complicated course.[1, 2] The efferent pathway of this reflex arc is made up of parasympathetic fibers that originate in the pons (the so-called lacrimal nucleus area)[1] adjacent to the superior salivatory nucleus (in the region of the facial nerve nucleus). These fibers arise outside the facial nucleus and then travel through the facial nucleus where facial nerve sensory and motor fibers originate. This portion of the nerve has been referred to as the nervous intermedius and believed by some to be a separate cranial nerve.[1] Thus, as the facial nerve exits the brain stem, it is composed of motor fibers, sensory fibers, and parasympathetic fibers destined for the lacrimal gland. At the geniculate ganglion, these parasympathetic fibers, without synapsing, exit from the rest of the facial nerve and travel through a small passageway in the petrous temporal bone, entering onto the anterior aspect of the temporal ridge. The nerve is referred to as the greater superficial petrosal nerve at this point. This nerve then travels along the petrous temporal ridge toward the carotid artery. In the area of the carotid artery, these parasympathetic fibers (greater superficial petrosal nerve) join with sympathetic fibers that are traveling alongside of the carotid artery. These sympathetic fibers are referred to as the deep petrosal nerve. Therefore, we have the joining of the greater superficial petrosal nerve with the deep petrosal nerve in the area of the carotid artery as it comes intracranially. This new nerve is known as the vidian nerve and passes through the pterygoid canal in the sphenoid bone. Some persons refer to this nerve as the nerve of the pterygoid canal. This nerve, after passing through the pterygoid canal, joins the sphenopalatine ganglion. At this point, the parasympathetic nerve fibers synapse. The sympathetic fibers have previously synapsed in the superior cervical ganglion of the sympathetic chain. From the sphenopalatine ganglion the parasympathetic postganglionic fibers and sympathetic fibers join the maxillary nerve and travel by means of the zygomatic nerve toward their destination of the lacrimal gland. As this zygomatic nerve travels along the lateral wall, it splits into zygomaticofacial and zygomaticotemporal branches. The fibers we are interested in continue up the lateral wall to anastomose with the lacrimal nerve just posterior to the lacrimal gland and then enter the gland along with the lacrimal nerve. The lacrimal nerve therefore carries sensory, sympathetic, and parasympathetic fibers.

Causes of Lacrimation

Lacrimation (increased production of tears) may result from stimulation of the lacrimal gland by a number of possible routes.

Supranuclear (Central Mechanisms). Stimulation of the so-called lacrimal nucleus (that area of the brain stem where the parasympathetic fibers originate that will eventually stimulate the lacrimal gland) may occur with emotions or after insults to the central nervous system, such as an ischemic episode (stroke). The pathways for psychogenic or emotional tearing are not entirely known, although the frontal lobes, basal ganglia, and hypothalamus play a role.[3, 4]

Reflex Tearing. Stimulation to the ophthalmic division of the trigeminal nerve, which supplies sensation to the eye, in turn stimulates the lacrimal nucleus to increase nerve impulses through the parasympathetic fibers running with the facial nerve to the main lacrimal gland. The result is increased tear production. This reflex may be stimulated by pain after a corneal abrasion or by irritation from iritis, glaucoma, contact lenses, dry eye, or other diseases of the cornea or conjunctiva. For example, in the dry eye patient with decrease in tear production, the cornea becomes dry and irritated, stimulating the trigeminal nerve and triggering this reflex. These patients may be recognized by inquiring about burning or a dry, gravel feeling in the eye as well as a history of arthritis or autoimmune disorder, which may suggest Sjögren's syndrome. If the cornea is kept moist with artificial tears, this reflex arc is not stimulated and the patient will be relieved of the epiphora. Other reflex arcs for lacrimation that are not as well understood include retinal stimulation from bright lights, yawning, or laughing. Whatever the stimulant to lacrimation, the efferent pathway appears to be parasympathetic via the facial nerve fibers and the sphenopalatine ganglion.[3, 4]

Infranuclear Factors. Tumors of the cerebellopontine angle can cause irritation of the nervous intermedius and result in excess lacrimation. After Bell's palsy, a patient may have misdirection of regenerating salivary nerve axons in the peripheral portion of the seventh nerve. These fibers grow along the nerve, innervating the lacrimal gland and producing a gustatory lacrimal reflex or "crocodile tears" when the patient eats or thinks of food.[2, 5]

Direct Stimulation of the Lacrimal Gland. An inflammatory process or tumors of the lacrimal gland may cause either an increase or a decrease in tear production. Parasympathetic drugs such as methacholine, which mimics the neurotransmitter of the facial nerve, or cholinesterase inhibitors such as physostigmine may cause increased lacrimation.

Allergy. The possibility that tearing is primarily from the direct reaction of allergens at the conjunctival level must be considered.[4, 6, 7] In sensitized individuals, allergies bind with IgE antibody attached to mast cells in the surrounding tissue. The activated mast cell then releases histamine and other mediators of inflammation into the surrounding tissue, leading to itching, vasodilation, edema of tissue, and subsequent tearing. The tearing is presumably secondary to lacrimal hypersecretion. These patients may have a history of atopy and have other allergy-associated diseases such as asthma. Allergens may be seasonal, as in the case of pollen, or perennial, as seen with dust, animal danders, and mold spores. Seasonal allergies often slowly evolve into perennial or year-round presence of allergy symptoms, which then may wax and wane but never fully resolve.[7]

Causes of Epiphora (Blockage of Tear Outflow)

Abnormalities may be detected in the lacrimal pump mechanism or anywhere from the punctal opening to the nasolacrimal duct and nasal passage. Outflow obstruction is by far the most common cause of tearing in the pediatric and adult age group. Many causes are seen.

Lacrimal Pump. The orbicularis is intimately related to the canalicular system and nasolacrimal sac. Contraction of the pretarsal and preseptal orbicularis components on these structures are believed to serve a "lacrimal pump" that opens and closes the canaliculi and nasolacrimal sac.[7–12] In the aging eyelid with laxity of the skin, the orbicularis, and the eyelid support structures (medial and lateral canthal tendon, capsulopalpebral fascia), the lid loses some of its tone and thus pumping action. With facial nerve weakness or paralysis, the tear pumping will also be reduced. This most commonly occurs with Bell's palsy or after neurosurgery in the area of the cerebellopontine angle. Although there is much debate over the details of the lacrimal pump theory, it is clear that normal eyelid function is essential for tear drainage.

Punctal. There may be a congenital absence of the puncta, keeping the tears from entering the nasolacrimal system. This may consist of a fine membrane occluding the opening or total absence of the punctum and canaliculus (punctal and canalicular atresia) (Fig. 74–5*A* and *B*). A double punctum may be seen, indicative of an embryologic maldevelopment in the system (see Fig. 74–5*C*). One or both of these puncta may be functional. The punctum may be everted (ectropic) and sitting away from the tear lake. Conjunctiva may be overriding the lid and preventing normal tear flow or may be blocking the punctal opening. This is referred to as conjunctivochalasis (see Fig. 74–5*D*).

Canalicular. There may be stenosis of the punctum or canaliculus from viral infections or drugs such as idoxuridine and phospholine iodide. The canaliculus may be occluded from canaliculitis secondary to *Actinomyces* or mycotic infections (Fig. 74–6). There may be scarring in the canaliculus from previous injuries or lacerations. Wojno[6] has also described allergy, with intense itching in the medial canthal area, as a temporary cause of tearing secondary to canalicular narrowing. He postulates that sensitized individuals come in contact with allergens, have pruritic medial canthal areas, and rub the area intensely, setting up edema in the surrounding tissues. Mucosal edema narrows and occludes the canaliculus and perhaps part of the nasolacrimal sac.[6]

Nasolacrimal Sac. The sac may be narrowed or obstructed from traumatic insults to the nasolacrimal region (Le Fort II, midfacial smash injuries) and also by the surgery to correct these various fractures. For example, a mini plate with screw fixation over the frontal process of maxilla may injure the sac. Supramid or Teflon plates used during orbital floor and medial wall fractures may impinge on the nasolacrimal sac and compress it. Transnasal wiring may compress the nasolacrimal sac. Other abnormalities that may lead to narrowing or obstruction of the sac include nasolacrimal stones (dacryoliths), inflammation, or sludge (e.g., hair, mucus), and rarely tumors.

Nasolacrimal Duct. The duct may be stenosed from idiopathic inflammation (primary acquired nasolacrimal duct obstruction[13]), scarring following injuries, previous probings or surgery in the nose, as well as tumors.

Valve of Hasner. The distal opening of the nasolacrimal duct may be congenitally imperforate or obstructed by the inferior turbinate impinging on it. This is the main cause of tearing in children. Previous nasal surgery may also be responsible for narrowing or obstruction at this level.

Pseudolacrimal Duct Obstruction Secondary to Nasal Allergy. Primary changes in the nasal cavity can cause symptoms that may mimic mechanical obstruction. Although in its most common form allergic rhinitis causes bilateral rather than unilateral epiphora, it nonetheless may produce changes that resemble mechanical obstruction.[14, 15] The basic pathophysiology of nasal allergy is the antibody–antigen reaction and the subsequent tissue change that results from this reaction.[16] These allergenic substances are usually airborne. The release of histamine and other vasoactive substances causes vasodilation with edema and tissue swelling.[14] The swelling of the nasal mucosa can block the valve of Hasner at the opening of the nasolacrimal duct in the nose, unilaterally or bilaterally depending on the individual's nasal anatomy, and prevent the drainage of tears away from the eye. Mucosal swelling can also occur around the ostomy site from pre-

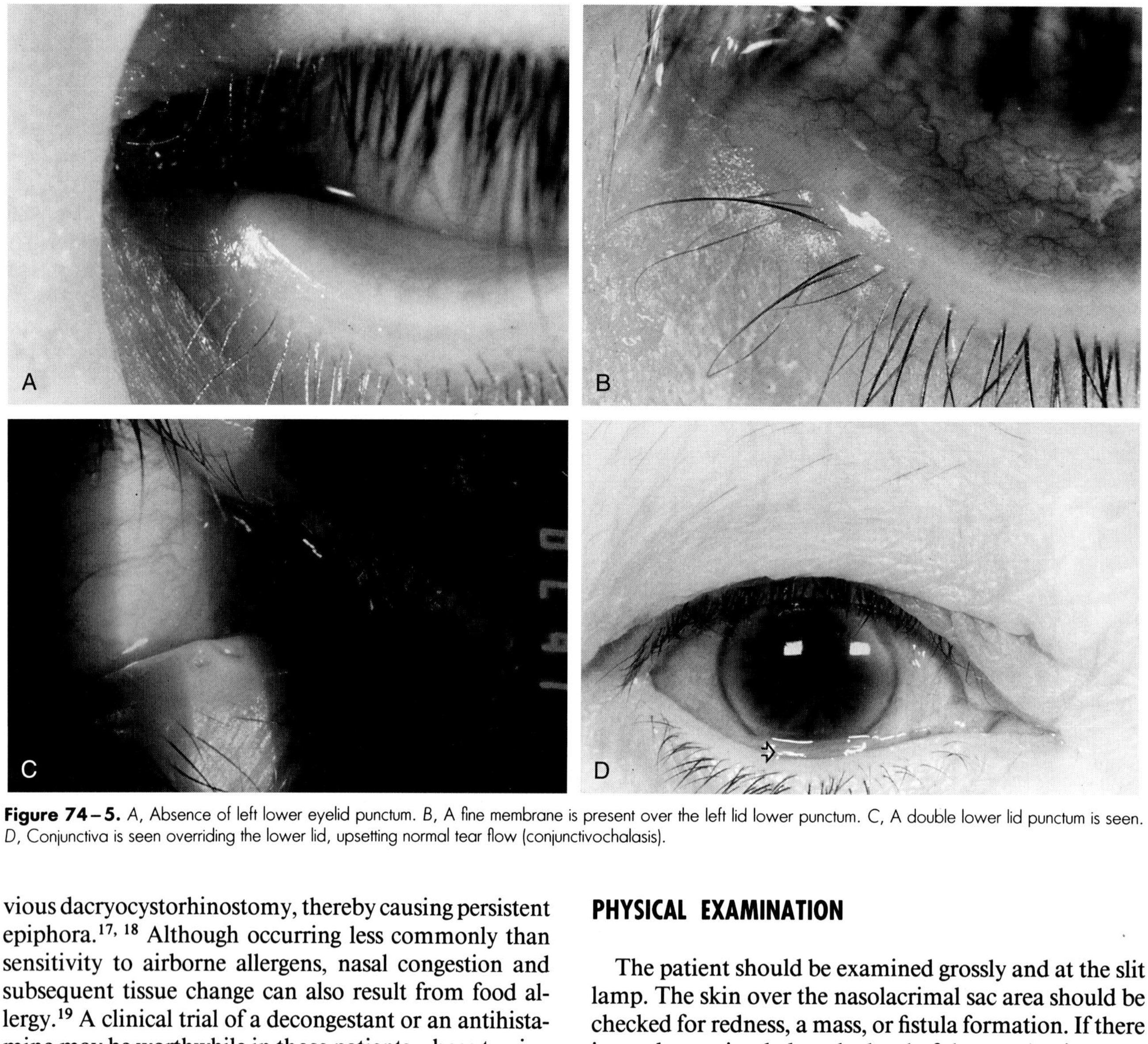

Figure 74–5. *A*, Absence of left lower eyelid punctum. *B*, A fine membrane is present over the left lid lower punctum. *C*, A double lower lid punctum is seen. *D*, Conjunctiva is seen overriding the lower lid, upsetting normal tear flow (conjunctivochalasis).

vious dacryocystorhinostomy, thereby causing persistent epiphora.[17, 18] Although occurring less commonly than sensitivity to airborne allergens, nasal congestion and subsequent tissue change can also result from food allergy.[19] A clinical trial of a decongestant or an antihistamine may be worthwhile in those patients whose tearing may have an allergic component.

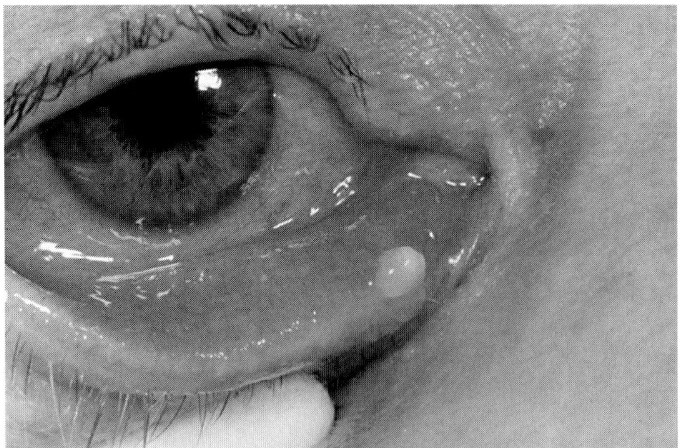

Figure 74–6. With pressure over the prominent lower punctum (pouting punctum), concretions are extruded, indicating that a canaliculitis is present.

PHYSICAL EXAMINATION

The patient should be examined grossly and at the slit lamp. The skin over the nasolacrimal sac area should be checked for redness, a mass, or fistula formation. If there is an obstruction below the level of the nasolacrimal sac and the sac is distended, one frequently can express mucopurulent material out of one of the puncta with gentle pressure. If this occurs, further diagnostic tests are rarely needed since the diagnosis of nasolacrimal duct obstruction has been documented by clinical examination. The patient may demonstrate weakness of the orbicularis by decreased muscle strength on forced lid closure or by lagophthalmos. An assessment of eyelid laxity may be obtained by gently pulling the lower eyelid away from the globe. If the lid can be retracted more than 6 mm from the globe, it is lax. If the lid does not immediately snap back to its position but tends to hang downward until a blink, it is also lax (snap back test). In addition, if lateral traction on the lid displaces the punctum temporally to the pupil edge, the medial canthal tendon is lax. Conjunctivochalasis (conjunctiva overriding lid margin and blocking the punctal opening), vertical punctum, punctal stenosis, and ectropion with punctal eversion should be noted. Entropion, trichiasis, or distichiasis may cause irritation

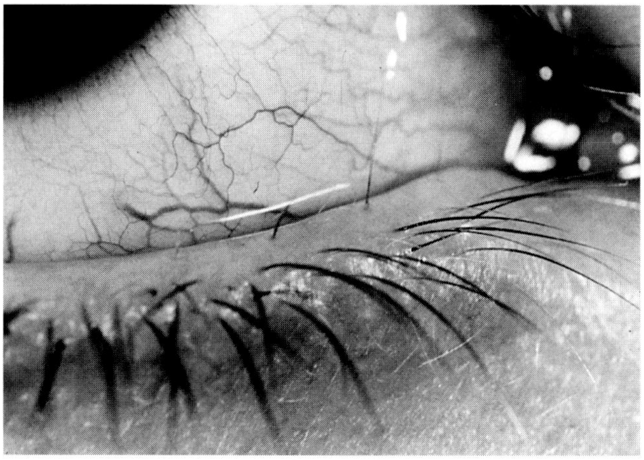

Figure 74–7. Congenital distichiasis. A find second row of lashes located posterior to the normal lashes is seen coming out of the meibomian gland orifices.

and reflex lacrimation (Fig. 74–7). Aberrant lacrimal gland ductules, which usually open near the lateral canthus (Fig. 74–8*A*) or a persistent nasolacrimal duct anlage (see Fig. 74–8*B*), may be indicative of faulty embryologic development and should be searched for. Careful slit lamp examination may uncover disease of the lid margin, conjunctiva, cornea, or anterior chamber that may cause reflex lacrimation.

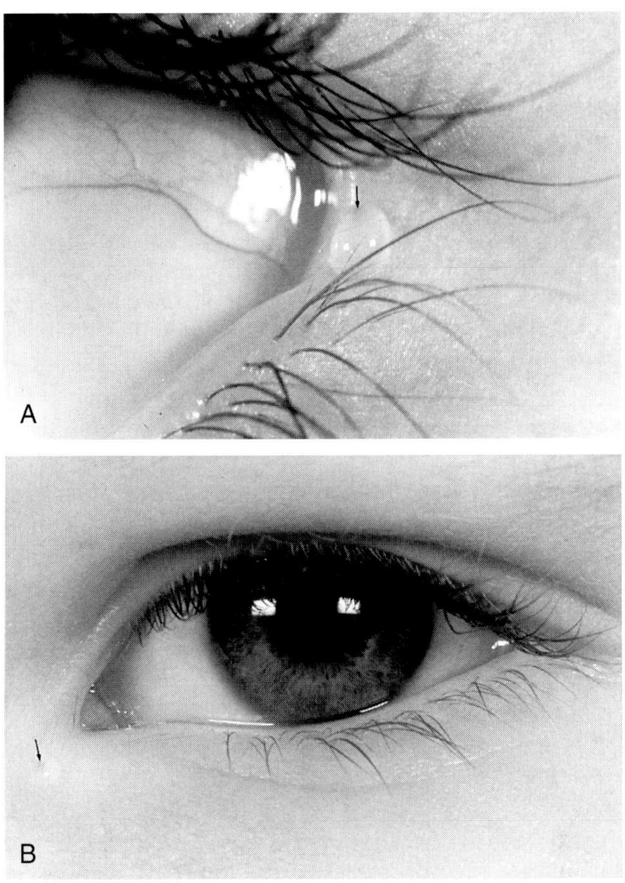

Figure 74–8. *A*, Aberrant lacrimal gland ductule with a tear exiting from it (arrow). *B*, Persistent nasolacrimal anlage (arrow) with intermittent tears coming from the opening.

A nasal examination is very important during the assessment of a tearing patient and is best performed during the diagnostic testing part of the examination. It is discussed later in this chapter.

Diagnostic Testing

Appropriate drainage of tears depends on a large variety of factors, including the volume of tear production, eyelid position, normal pump mechanisms, anatomic status of the drainage passages, gravity, and nasal air convection currents. There is no single test that will pinpoint the anatomic site or physiologic basis for tear production and drainage imbalances. A number of tests have been described over the years. In this section, we describe those tests we find most practical in assessing the tearing patient. Like many diagnostic tests in medicine, most of those to be described will require some subjective interpretation to determine the probable cause of the tearing. The mere demonstration of lacrimal system pathology, either anatomic or physiologic, does not indicate lacrimal dysfunction. Patients with significant degrees of partial or even complete outflow obstruction may be asymptomatic as long as the tear production and drainage balance are maintained.

The simplest, most widely used testing that will lead to an accurate diagnosis in over 95% of the tearing patients involves a series of three tests done sequentially. These tests can be completed within 5 to 10 minutes and include the dye disappearance test and Jones I and Jones II tests.[4, 19–24] These tests should be run sequentially.

The equipment required to perform this part of the examination includes topical anesthesia, 2% fluorescein dye, calcium alginate swabs, nasal speculum, head light or indirect ophthalmoscope, lacrimal irrigating syringe, punctal dilator, and lacrimal probe.

Dye Disappearance Test

The patient is asked to sit quietly, with the head in the normal upright position, looking straight ahead. A drop of topical anesthetic is placed in the patient's fornix and then the eyes are dabbed with a tissue. This is done to decrease any irritating effect from 2% fluorescein dye, which will be used subsequently. One drop of 2% fluorescein dye is placed into the inferior fornix bilaterally, and as this is done a timer is turned on. A second drop may be put in at 30 seconds. This test should always be done as a bilateral test. In those with only unilateral symptoms, the normal asymptomatic eye serves as a control (i.e., what happens on the uninvolved side is normal for that patient). The dye is observed for 5 minutes, and the examiner should notice how it disappears and whether it overflows. The rate of disappearance of the dye from the conjunctival sac is used as an indirect estimate of the patency of the drainage system. The patient is not to touch the eyelids during the examination. At the end of the 5 minutes in a normal patient, the dye should be almost completely gone. At this point, the examiner makes a subjective assessment of how much is remaining and writes it down (+1 to +4). If there was no decrease in color intensity, the residual dye is designated as +4 (Fig. 74–9), while +1 or 0 represents minimal or no residual dye. Residuals of +2 or +3 are determined by repeated experience and clinical observation of numerous tests.[23] With +4, there is often overflow onto the cheek, and this can be written in beside the +4 (i.e., +4 with overflow) to indicate what is happening (Fig. 74–10). A residual dye designation of 0 or +1 at 5 minutes indicates normal disappearance, whereas one of +2 to +4 indicates inadequate lacrimal excretion. This is subjective, but the value of this test lies in looking for asymmetry with the opposite side. For example, one may find that the dye disappeared equally well from each eye or that one side is obviously retaining more dye than the other.

The dye disappearance test part of the examination should run for 5 minutes, followed by the second portion, referred to as the Jones I Test.[20, 22]

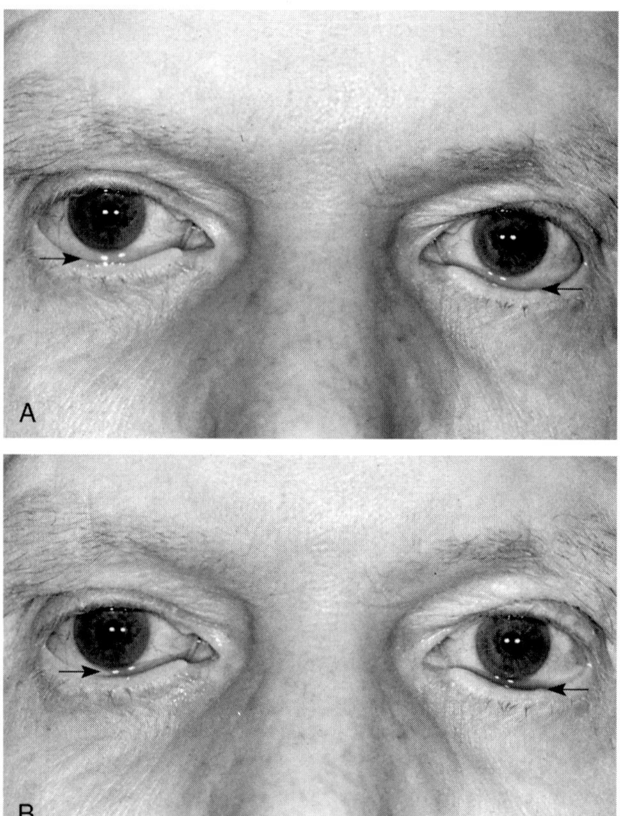

Figure 74–9. *A*, Time 0: one drop of 2% fluorescein dye has been placed into each conjunctival fornix. Arrows point to increased tear lake. *B*, Time 5 minutes: the same amount of dye remains, indicating a lack of passage of dye into the nasolacrimal system. Arrows point to increased tear lake.

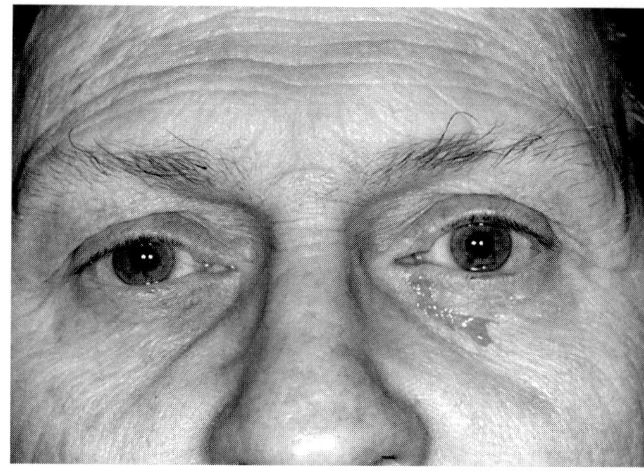

Figure 74–10. During a dye disappearance test, a drop of dye runs onto the eyelid skin, indicating significant overflow of tears on this side while the dye on the opposite side is disappearing normally.

Jones I Test

The Jones I test is a physiologic evaluation of the nasolacrimal system (i.e., can the dye travel on its own from the conjunctival fornix into the nose). During this portion of the examination, the patient is asked to blow each side of the nose separately. In the normal population, dye should have reached the nasal passageway and be seen on the tissue, confirming patency. If no dye is visualized on the tissue, a nasal speculum is placed into the nasal vestibule and one examines the inferior meatus for the presence of dye. If none is seen, a calcium alginate swab is placed into the inferior meatus to see if dye is present. This part of the testing must be done very slowly and carefully since the inside of one's nose is very sensitive to any external stimulation. A 5% cocaine spray can be used to help anesthetize the mucosa, but we have found this not to be necessary if one talks to the patient as the nose is being examined and if the calcium alginate swab is moved slowly. This concludes this portion of the test. It is important to realize that 22% of the normal adult population will not have any dye present in the inferior meatus at this stage despite having a patent system and lack of tearing.[22] Thus, if dye is recovered, the system is patent, whereas if dye is not recovered, the system may still be patent but not allowing passage of fluid at the time of the examination. If dye is recovered, one does not have to go onto Jones II testing since it is known that the system is passing tears. If no dye is recovered, the Jones II test is essential.

It is important, at this point, to comment on "positive tests" and "negative tests." A "positive Jones I" test could be positive because dye was found in the nose or could be positive because no dye was recovered, indicating that a nasolacrimal sac obstruction may be present (i.e., what is interpreted as positive for one investigator may not refer to what is positive for another investigator). It is therefore much more helpful to record the result of a Jones I test as "dye recovered" or "no dye recovered."

Jones II Test

The Jones II test uses irrigation through the canaliculus to evaluate the anatomic patency of the lacrimal system.[23] This test involves rinsing out any residual dye in the conjunctiva with balanced salt. The lower puncta are dilated. With the patient sitting forward and holding either a tissue or a small catch basin under the nose, the nasolacrimal system is irrigated and the examiner first looks to see if any fluid drips from the nose and then assesses its color (clear or dye stained). While the irrigating cannula is in the canaliculus, the fluid may be immediately regurgitated, indicating canalicular obstruction. Fluid irrigation into the lower canaliculus and regurgitated through the upper canaliculus, without mucous debris, suggests obstruction at the level of the common canaliculus or internal common punctum. If fluid is irrigated through the lower canaliculus and the lacrimal sac distends, either visibly or palpably, and mucous debris is present in the fluid regurgitated through the upper canaliculus, the nasal lacrimal duct is likely obstructed. A patient with acute dacryocystitis should not be irrigated since the obstruction must be present at the nasolacrimal duct. Irrigation provides no additional information and may spread the infection.

If fluid can be irrigated into the nose, a complete blockage of the lacrimal excretory system cannot be present. The fluid irrigated to the nose should always be examined to see if it is clear or stained with dye. Dye-stained fluid is important since it indicates that fluorescein used for the Jones I test got into the nasolacrimal sac. The puncta, canaliculus, common canaliculus, and internal common puncta are patent in this circumstance. A relative obstruction, partial obstruction, or physiologic or "functional" block is said to be present at the nasolacrimal duct when dye has disappeared well on the dye disappearance test (N→ +2), no dye is recovered on the Jones I test, but dye is recovered on the Jones II test (i.e., dye has gotten into the system but not out unless it is irrigated out). This may be due to inflammation at the nasolacrimal duct level, causing a stenosis, a narrow bony canal, internal mucosal strictures, or flaps blocking tear flow.[13] Whether this will require surgical intervention will depend on how symptomatic the patient is.

Clear fluid irrigated into the nose indicates a failure of the fluorescein dye to have reached the lacrimal sac. This may be due to eyelid, punctal, or canalicular problems or to a failure of the lacrimal pump to function, as in a facial nerve palsy.

Probing

When the previous testing indicates a canalicular block may be present, the canaliculi can be probed gently (to the level of the lacrimal sac) to appreciate where the block is and whether it is complete or is a stenotic passageway. This should be done after punctal dilation and slowly because it can be uncomfortable when done briskly.

The results of the dye disappearance, Jones I, Jones II, and probing tests are recorded in a chart format, and an assessment of why the patient is tearing can be arrived at in the vast majority of patients at this stage. By knowing the various patterns of test results, the examiner can get a mental image of where the block is likely to be (Fig. 74–11).

Nasal Examination

The nasal passageway should always be examined in the tearing patient. This may be done during the Jones I testing. It is important to assess the mucosal health and the presence of a pathologic process that may be responsible for intranasal obstruction of the nasolacrimal duct. One also wants to be sure there is enough space available in the nasal passageway for any possible nasolacrimal procedure (Fig. 74–12).

The lateral wall of the nose has three turbinates or conchae. The turbinates have a thin, bony framework and are covered with highly vascular mucosal tissue that is composed of a dense arterial network and venus plexuses (lakes) similar to erectile tissue. This covering is particularly evident on the inferior turbinate. The turbinates (particularly the inferior) periodically swell by means of vascular engorgement and can lead to variation in size of the nasal airway.

Beneath each turbinate lies a meatus. The inferior meatus receives drainage from the nasolacrimal duct only, at a point about one third of the way back from its anterior margin. The middle meatus receives drainage from the nasofrontal duct and anterior ethmoidal cells anteriorly, from the middle ethmoidal cells and maxillary sinus ostium medially and from the posterior ethmoidal cells posteriorly. Mucopurpulent material may be seen draining from these regions during acute sinus infections. The superior turbinate is very small, is located high and posterior, and cannot ordinarily be seen on clinical examination.

The nasal septum is formed by cartilage anteriorly and by bone posteriorly. The septum may grow irregularly or may be traumatized so that it obstructs breathing on one or both sides of the nose. If the deviation is severe enough, it will inhibit proper drainage or will obstruct sinus ostia by putting pressure on the turbinate. The deviated sep-

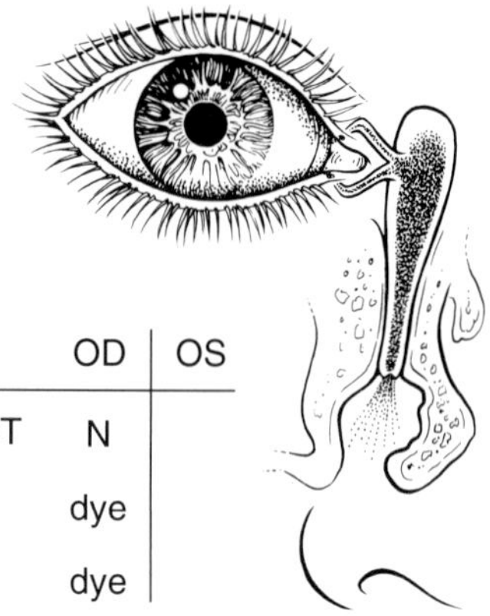

	OD	OS
DDT	N	
J1	dye	
J2	dye	

A

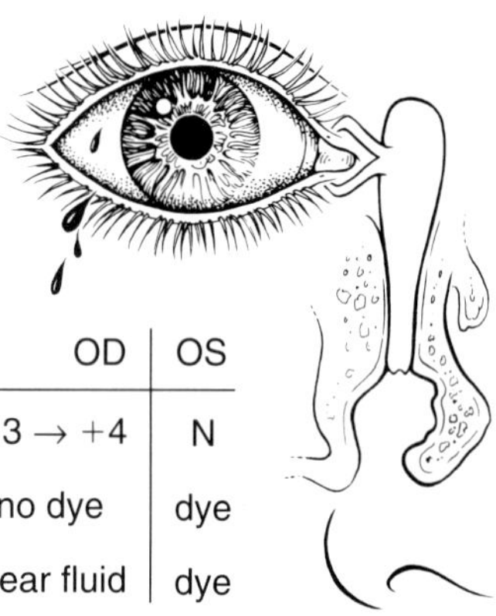

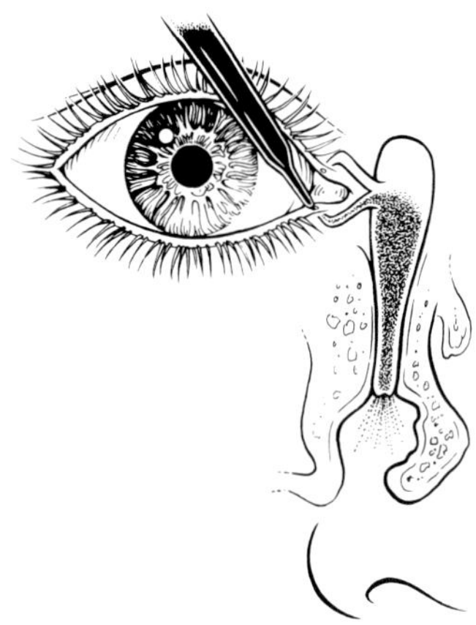

	OD	OS
DDT	+3 → +4	N
J1	no dye	dye
J2	clear fluid	dye

B

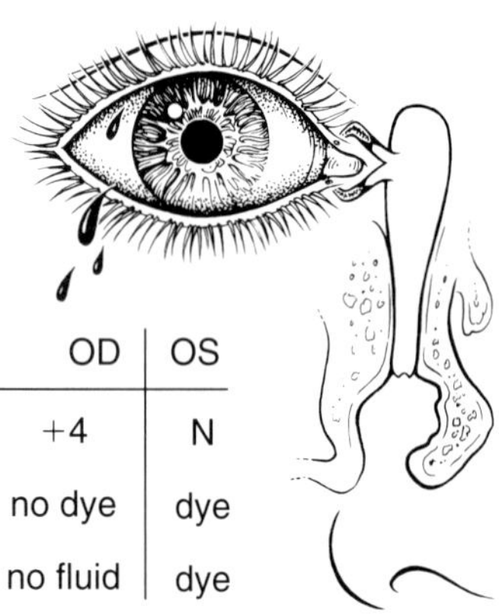

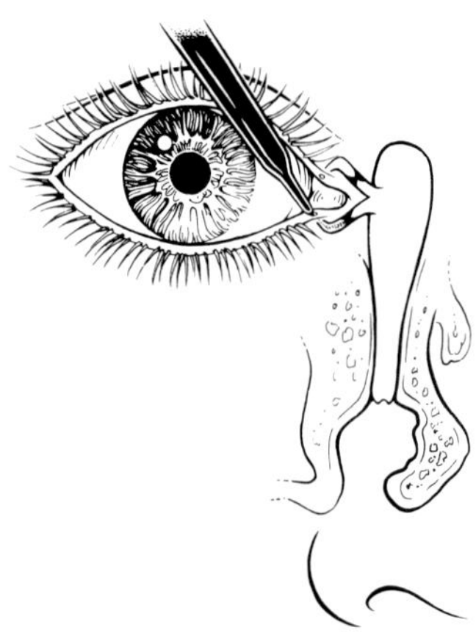

	OD	OS
DDT	+4	N
J1	no dye	dye
J2	no fluid	dye

C

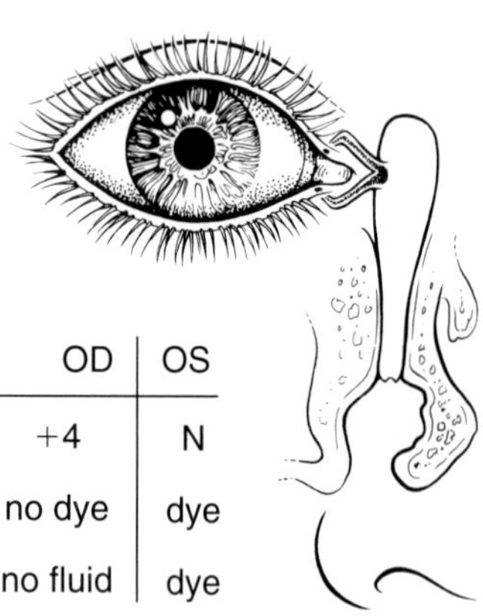

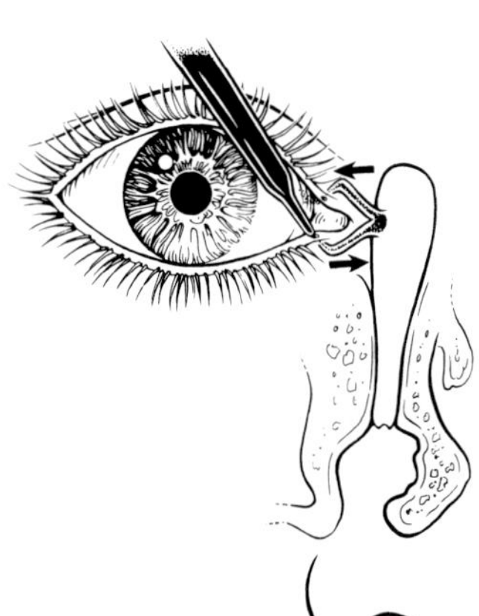

	OD	OS
DDT	+4	N
J1	no dye	dye
J2	no fluid	dye

D

Figure 74–11. *A*, Normal dye studies on the right nasolacrimal system. N = normal result, that is, most of the dye has disappeared into the sac with only a small trace sitting along the lid margin. *B*, Punctal stenosis of right eye. Patient's tearing is intermittent, aggravated by wind and cold. There is dye retention with no dye seen on the Jones I test. Once puncta dilated on Jones II test, clear fluid will pass into system. If stenosis is less severe, some dye may be seen on Jones I. *C*, Canalicular stenosis or occlusion of right eye. Patient has tearing constantly or intermittently depending on the degree of block. With complete occlusion, no dye or fluid will get through. If canaliculi stenosed, some clear fluid may be seen on Jones II test if syringe overcomes stenosis. *D*, Common canalicular stenosis or occlusion. Patient has tearing constantly or intermittently depending on degree of block. With complete occlusion, no dye or fluid will get through and fluid will irrigate with reflux out opposite canaliculus. If common canaliculus is stenosed, some clear fluid may be seen on Jones II test if syringe overcomes stenosis.

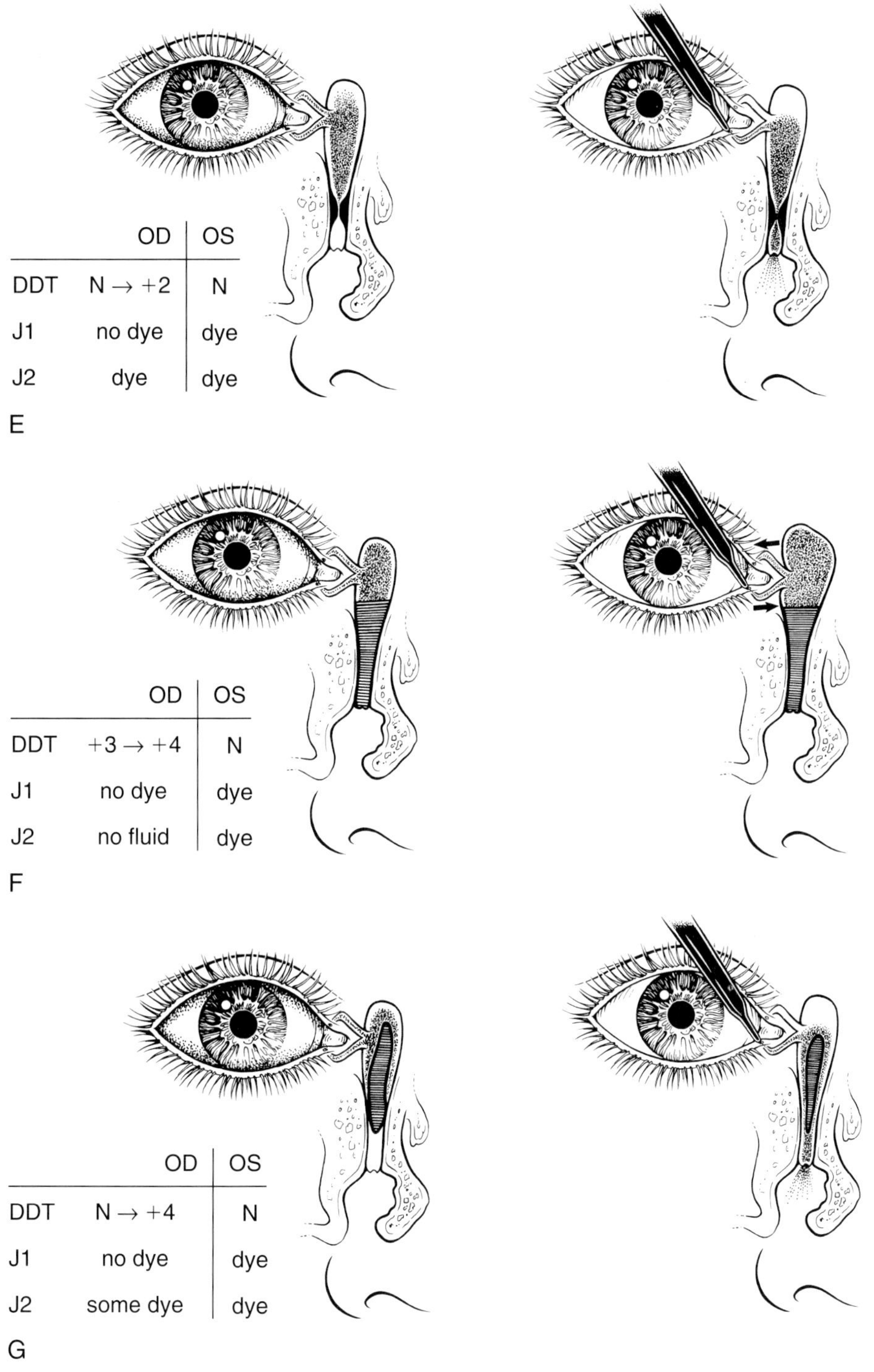

	OD	OS
DDT	N → +2	N
J1	no dye	dye
J2	dye	dye

E

	OD	OS
DDT	+3 → +4	N
J1	no dye	dye
J2	no fluid	dye

F

	OD	OS
DDT	N → +4	N
J1	no dye	dye
J2	some dye	dye

G

Figure 74–11 *Continued. E*, Dacryostenosis or nasolacrimal duct stenosis. Patient has intermittent tearing. Dye disappearance testing may be normal or show some retention (+2). No dye is seen on the Jones I test, yet on the Jones II test dye comes out. The studies show that dye gets into system but not out unless irrigated. This is referred to as a "functional block." N = normal. *F*, Complete or anatomic nasolacrimal block. Patient tears regularly and may have recurrent infection or distention of nasolacrimal sac. Dye studies confirm complete block with no dye into nose either passively (Jones I) or with irrigation (Jones II). *G*, Dacryolith in system. Patient has episodic tearing and may have intermittent painful distention of sac. Dye disappearance is variable and may be anywhere from normal (N) to lots of dye retained (+4). Tear studies show a functional block but may show normal patency or a complete obstruction depending on whether the stone has caused complete or partial block.

tum, if severe, needs to be identified and corrected before contemplating dacryocystorhinostomy.

The nasal and sinus mucosa is pseudostratified columnar epithelium. Like the skin, the mucosa has free nerve endings that respond to chemicals and to changes in temperature, humidity, and pressure. These receptors serve to alert and protect the lower airway after exposure to extremes of temperature or to pollutants. They stimulate vasodilation, mucus production, and bronchial constriction.

Explanation and proper patient positioning are the keys to successful examination of nasal passage. The patient should be sitting erect and slightly forward with the back away from the chair. The examiner sits close to one side of the patient with the patient's nose at eye level. Basic equipment for intranasal examination consists of a strong focused light source (an indirect ophthalmoscope or a fiberoptic headlight generally works fine) and a nasal speculum. The speculum is gently inserted into the nasal vestibule and opened without exerting pressure on the

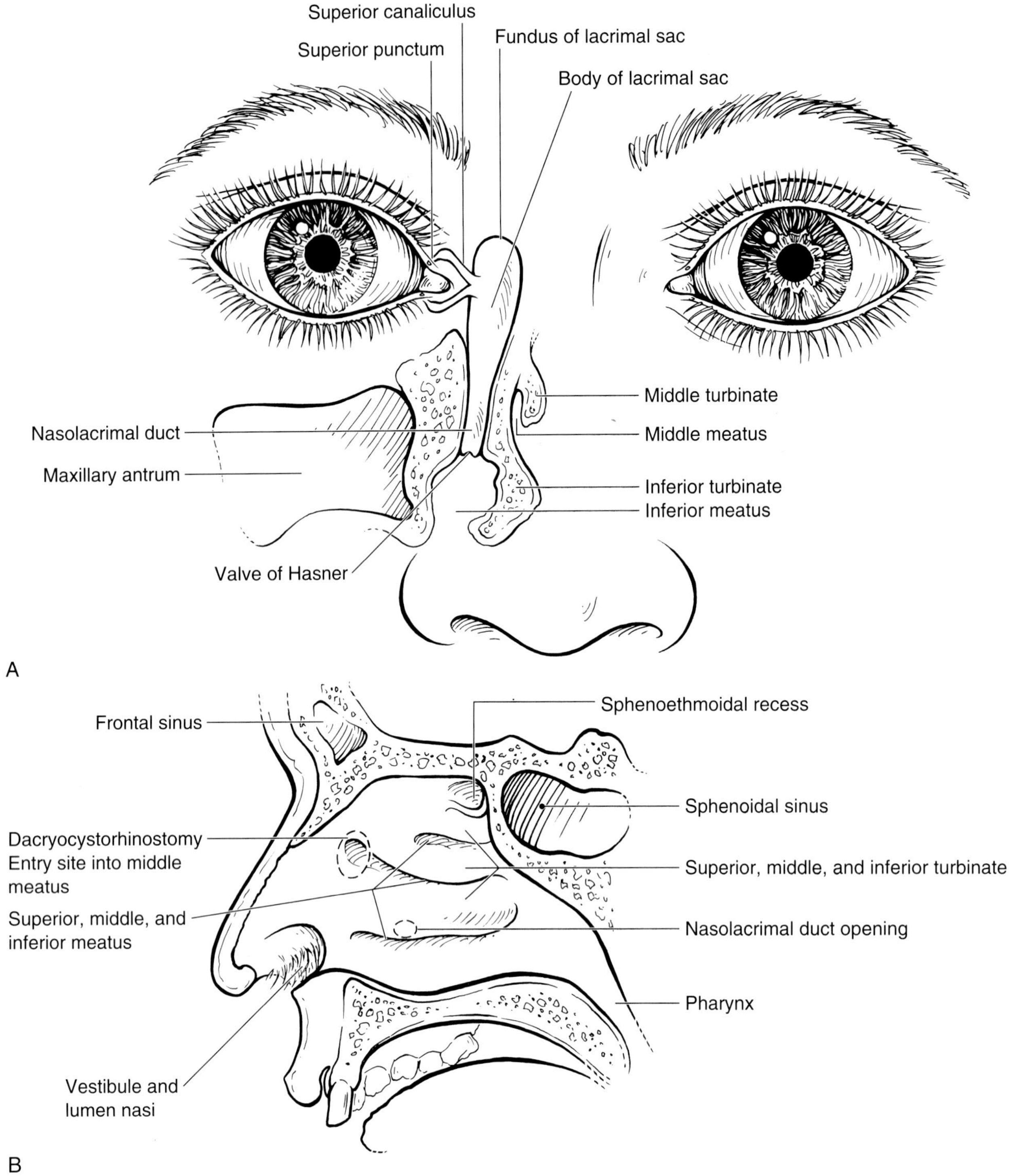

Figure 74–12. *A*, Coronal drawing illustrating the nasal anatomy as it relates to the nasolacrimal system. *B*, Sagittal drawing illustrating the lateral wall of the nose.

highly sensitive nasal septum. Examination proceeds by looking at the nasal floor, inferior turbinate and lower septum, and upward at the middle meatus, middle turbinate, and superior septum.

The mucosa is generally moist and deep pink. Inflammation results in erythema, edema, and ulceration if severe. Areas of crusting may also be noted. The nasal septum is rarely perfectly straight and may be so deviated as to block the proposed area of a dacryocystorhinostomy. One may note adhesions between the septum and turbinate, indicating previous trauma.

Other Tests

Schirmer Testing. If the examiner is suspicious that a patient may have a dry eye with reflex tearing, a Schirmer test is very valuable. This test (devised by Schirmer in 1903[3]) uses a 5 × 30-mm strip of no. 41 Whatman filter paper. If the strip is simply put into the conjunctival fornix, because of a possible irritant effect an outpouring of reflex tears will occur. This will be eliminated or minimized by instilling topical anesthetic (e.g., proparacaine or tetracaine anesthetic eye drops) before placing the strip into position. The strip is put in place, and a 5-minute time period is given to see how much of the strip is filled. The moistening of the exposed portion of the paper strip over a 5-minute period is believed to be a measure of the basic secretion mechanism. The normal range of Schirmer finding is from 10 to 25 mm at 5 minutes. Although the Schirmer test leaves much to be desired as a quantitative test, it is rapid, simple, and generally repeatable in a given subject. The results must be interpreted in terms of the patient's symptoms and objective findings. Results of less than 5 mm are generally associated with symptoms such as burning, scratchiness, and a dry feeling, indicative of a reflex cause for the patient's tearing. Although the Schirmer test is a useful device for evaluating tear flow, it actually measures the aqueous component of the tear film.

Tear Break-up Time. Deficiencies of the mucus layer can be detected by another test, referred to as the tear film "break-up time" test. The uniform normal wetting of the corneal surface depends on even spreading of the absorbed mucin layer. The rapidity of appearance of dry spots on the cornea between blinks becomes an index of the adequacy of the mucin layer.[3, 25, 26] Break-up time can be defined as the interval between a complete blink and the appearance of the first randomly distributed dry spot.[26] The break-up time is measured by instilling fluorescein solution into the conjunctival sac and scanning the cornea with cobalt blue illumination at the slit lamp microscope for the first sign of dry areas (fluorescein free). The normal tear film break-up time is 15 to 35 seconds. A break-up time of less than 10 seconds suggests mucin deficiency. The test is reproducible for a given eye.

Rose Bengal Testing. Rose bengal stains devitalized epithelial cells. If tear secretion is deficient, the application of a 1% solution of rose bengal to the eye will result in staining of the abnormal epithelium of the conjunctiva, particularly in the interpalpebral space. Thus, the rose bengal test is indirectly a measure of tear secretion.

Dacryocystography and Modified Dacryocystography. Sophisticated nasolacrimal tests are available to help determine the cause of an individual's tearing but in my experience these are only occasionally required since a diagnosis and treatment plan can be arrived at with the previously mentioned tests in approximately 95% of patients.

Dacryocystography involves injecting a radiopaque dye into the lacrimal sac (through a cannula) and simultaneously taking radiographs to demonstrate the lacrimal sac cavity. Modified dacryocystography includes radiologic subtraction techniques and macrography.[27-30]

For these tests, the patient is lying down in front of an x-ray machine with one or both of the canalicular systems intubated with tubing. A control film is taken before injection and then the radiopaque dye is injected. Serial radiographs are taken during injection. The technique of macrography is used to increase the image size. Subtraction eliminates background detail and allows better visualization of structures. Modified dacryocystography is very accurate in localizing areas of obstruction within the nasolacrimal outflow pathway. It is useful in showing the size of the sac and its displacement, which one may see in trauma, stones (dacryoliths), and tumors of the lacrimal sac or the nearby ethmoidal sinus. Modified dacryocystography may help to determine strictures of the common canaliculis and whether a common canalicular obstruction is located at the medial or the lateral end of the common canaliculus.[27] After dacryocystorhinostomy, modified dacryocystography is useful in showing the size of the remaining sac after an unsuccessful dacryocystorhinostomy (Figs. 74–13 and 74–14).

The modified dacryocystography defines the lacrimal anatomy but cannot reproduce true lacrimal physiology. Because of instrumentation in the system, it is not a reflection of the true nasolacrimal physiology. It is useful in certain situations when clinical examination cannot find an anatomic cause for obstruction, after dacryocystorhinostomy in the patient with tearing who may have a residual sac pooling tears (sump syndrome), or when a dacryolith or tumor is suspected.

Lacrimal Scintillography (Technetium Scan). The lacrimal technetium scan is a physiologic test that images the passage of the tears through the lacrimal excretory passages without instrumenting the system.[27] Technetium scanning does not provide the detailed anatomic visualization available with dacryocystography. In standard nuclear studies, the palpebral aperture is well seen and the proximal canalicular system is usually poorly

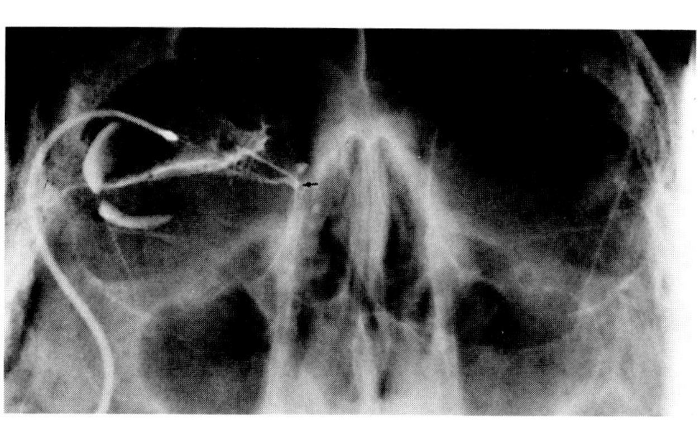

Figure 74–13. After dacryocystorhinostomy, the patient returned with tearing. Clinical testing suggested blockage at common duct. Standard dacryocystogram confirmed dye was being held up at common duct level (*arrow*) with little dye entering the nose.

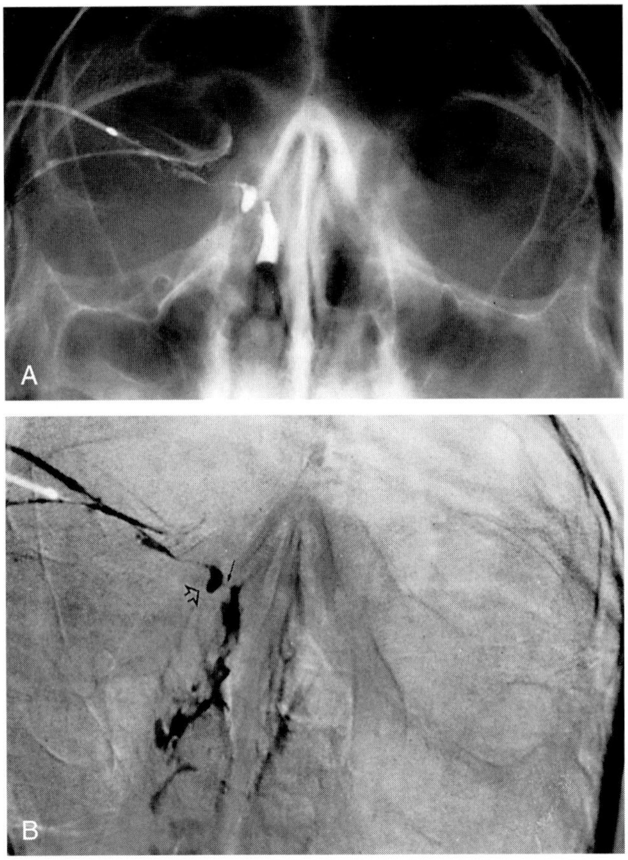

Figure 74–14. *A*, After dacryocystorhinostomy patient had persistent tearing. Clinical tests suggested patency. Standard dacryocystogram revealed a residual tear sac "sump syndrome." *B*, A subtraction dacryocystogram of the same patient allows excellent visualization of the residual sac (*open arrow*) and tract into the nose (*small arrow*) by eliminating the bone in the background of the radiograph.

imaged unless dilated. The sac and duct are generally well outlined. Complete blocks in the sac or duct can be detected, although precise localization of the obstruction may be difficult. The technetium scan can yield considerable information concerning physiologic function, and this is the real value of this test. Generation of dynamic activity curves for specific regions (conjunctival sac, lacrimal sac, lacrimal duct, and nose) will demonstrate incomplete anatomic obstructions as well as subtle degrees of functional impairment.[30–35] This information may then be useful in deciding whether the patient has a lacrimal pump dysfunction or a delay in tear flow elsewhere in the system. Technetium scanning has also been quite helpful in quantitatively studying the lacrimal drainage in the superior and inferior canaliculi, for example, a difference in tear flow rate between the normal (both canaliculi patent) and obstructed (one canaliculus patent) states.[32–35]

The patent is required to be sitting upright in front of a pinhole collimeter of a gamma camera.[30] Technetium sulfur colloid is placed on the marginal tear strip on each lower lid. Pictures are then taken every 10 seconds for the first minute and then every 1 minute for 20 minutes. The information is kept on computer so that it may be used later. Rapid-sequence display is possible so that the sequence may be shown as a moving picture.[33]

Computed Tomography. Computed tomography, with and without the use of radiopaque contrast dye, is occasionally useful when investigating the tearing patient.[38–40] This is particularly so when a mass is palpable in the area of the sac, when the patient has had midfacial trauma and nasolacrimal involvement, or when dacryocystorhinostomy fails.

Diagnostic Ultrasonography. The techniques of A- and B-mode ultrasonography are noninvasive methods to evaluate gross anatomic abnormalities of the lacrimal drainage system. Physiologic dysfunction or the precise site of anatomic obstruction cannot be evaluated. However, a dilated lacrimal sac can easily be distinguished from one of normal dimensions, and mucus within the sac can be differentiated from air or concretions. Lacrimal sac neoplasms can also be detected.[40]

Endoscopy. Nasal endoscopy may be useful when investigating a patient after dacryocystorhinostomy who still has tearing.[38, 39] The nasal ostium and surrounding tissue may be viewed readily with this instrument, and one can then get an idea if there is common canalicular scarring, adhesions, blocking due to one of the turbinates, and so on.

CONCLUSIONS

For most tearing patients, a diagnosis can be arrived at after a thorough history and a few relatively simple office procedures. A small number of cases will require more sophisticated studies to confirm the site of anatomic block or region of physiologic dysfunction. With the various tests available, appropriate medical or surgical management can be determined in the vast majority of patients with tear production and drainage imbalance. There are occasional patients with tearing who seem to have normal tear production and a patent system on standard clinic examination as well as sophisticated testing. These are puzzling findings and when faced with this situation a second opinion may be worthwhile to gain another individual's assessment of the problem.

REFERENCES

1. Doxanas MT, Anderson RL: The lacrimal system. *In* Clinical Orbital Anatomy. Baltimore, Williams & Wilkins, 1984, pp 89–107.
2. Jacklin HN: The gusto-lacrimal reflex (syndrome of crocodile tears): Report of case with tear analysis. Am J Ophthalmol 61:1521–1526, 1966.
3. Milder B: The lacrimal apparatus. *In* Moses RA (ed): Adler's Physiology of the Eye, 8th ed. St. Louis, CV Mosby, 1987, pp 15–35.
4. Jones LT: The lacrimal secretory system and its treatment. Am J Ophthalmol 62:47–60, 1966.
5. Golding-Wood PH: Crocodile tears. Br Med J 1:1518–1521, 1963.

6. Wojno TH: Allergic lacrimal obstruction. Am J Ophthalmol 106:48-52, 1988.
7. Jones LT: An anatomical approach to problems of the eyelids and lacrimal apparatus. Arch Ophthalmol 66:111-124, 1961.
8. Jones LT: Epiphora: II. Its relationship to the anatomic structures and surgery of the medial canthal region. Am J Ophthalmol 43:203-212, 1957.
9. Doane MG: Blinking and the mechanics of the lacrimal drainage system. Ophthalmology 88:844-851, 1981.
10. Hill JC, Bethell W, Smirmaul HJ: Lacrimal drainage: A dynamic evaluation: I. Mechanics of tear transport. Can J Ophthalmol 9:411-416, 1974.
11. Maurice DM: The dynamics and drainage of tears. Int Ophthalmol Clin 13:103-116, 1973.
12. Rosengren D: On lacrimal drainage. Ophthalmologica 164:409-421, 1972.
13. Linberg JV, McCormick SA: Primary acquired nasolacrimal duct obstruction: A clinicopathologic report and biopsy technique. Ophthalmology 93:1055-1063, 1986.
14. Tennenbaum JI: Allergic rhinitis. *In* Patterson R (ed): Allergic Diseases: Diagnosis and Management. Philadelphia, JB Lippincott, 1980, pp 179-203.
15. Sanke RF: Pseudonasolacrimal duct obstruction caused by nasal allergy. Ophthalmic Surg 20:63-67, 1989.
16. Altman LC: Basic immune mechanisms in immediate hypersensitivity. Med Clin North Am 65:941-957, 1981.
17. Osguthorpe JD, Calcaterra TC: Nasolacrimal obstruction after maxillary sinus and rhinoplastic surgery. Arch Otolaryngol 105:264-266, 1979.
18. Welham RAN, Henderson PH: Results of dacryocystorhinostomy analysis of causes for failure. Trans Ophthalmol Soc UK 93:601-609, 1973.
19. Nagy SM: Evaluation and management of chronic nasal symptoms. *In* Gershwin ME, Nagy SM (eds): Evaluation and Management of Allergic and Asthmatic Disease. New York, Grune & Stratton, 1979, pp 33-48.
20. Jones LT: The cure of epiphora due to canalicular disorders, trauma and surgical failure on the lacrimal passages. Trans Am Acad Ophthalmol Otolaryngol 66:506-524, 1962.
21. Jones LT, Marquis MD: Lacrimal function. Am J Ophthalmol 73:658-659, 1972.
22. Zappia RJ, Milder B: Lacrimal drainage function: I. The Jones fluorescein test. Am J Ophthalmol 74:154-159, 1972.
23. Zappia RJ, Milder B: Lacrimal drainage function: II. The fluorescein dye disappearance test. Am J Ophthalmol 74:160-162, 1972.
24. Wright MM, Bersani TA, Frueh BR, Musch DC: Efficacy of the primary dye test. Ophthalmology 94:481-483, 1989.
25. Lemp MA, Hamill JR: Factors affecting the tear film breakup in normal eyes. Arch Ophthalmol 89:103-105, 1973.
26. Vanley GT, Leopold IH, Gregg TH: Interpretation of the tear film breakup. Arch Ophthalmol 95:445-448, 1977.
27. Hurwitz JJ, Victor WH: The role of sophisticated radiological testing in the assessment and management of epiphora. Ophthalmology 92:407-413, 1985.
28. Montanara A, Mannino G, Contestabile MT: Macrodacryocystography and echography in diagnosis of disorders of the lacrimal pathways. Surv Ophthalmol 28:33-41, 1983.
29. Lloyd GAS, Welham RAN: Subtraction macrodacryocystography. Br J Radiol 47:379-382, 1974.
30. Amanat LA, Hilditch TE, Kwok CS: Lacrimal scintigraphy: II. Its role in the diagnosis of epiphora. Br J Ophthalmol 67:720-728, 1983.
31. Hilditch TE, Kwok CS, Amanat LA: Lacrimal scintigraphy: I. Compartmental analysis of data. Br J Ophthalmol 67:713-719, 1983.
32. Hurwitz JJ: Investigation and treatment of epiphora due to lid laxity. Trans Ophthalmol Soc UK 98:67-70, 1978.
33. Doucet TW, Hurwitz JJ, Chin-Sang H: Lacrimal scintillography: Advances and functional applications. Surv Ophthalmol 27:105-113, 1982.
34. Daubert J, Nik N, Chandeyssoun PA, el-Choufi L: Tear flow analysis through the upper and lower systems. Ophthalmic Plast Reconstr Surg 6:193-196, 1990.
35. Chavis RM, Welham RAN, Maisey MN: Quantitative lacrimal scintillography. Arch Ophthalmol 96:2066-2068, 1978.
36. Glatt HJ, Cahn AC: Lacrimal obstruction after medial maxillectomy. Ophthalmic Surg 22:757-758, 1991.
37. Zinreich SJ, Miller NR, Freeman LN, et al: Computed tomographic dacryocystography using topical contract media for lacrimal system visualization: Preliminary investigations. Orbit 9:79-87, 1990.
38. Orcutt JC, Hillel A, Weymueller EA: Endoscopic repair of failed dacryocystorhinostomy. Ophthalmic Plast Reconstr Surg 6:197-202, 1990.
39. Allen KM, Berlin AJ, Levine HL: Intranasal endoscopic analysis of dacryocystorhinostomy failure. Ophthalmic Reconstr Surg 4:143-145, 1988.
40. Dutton JJ: Diagnostic tests and imaging techniques. *In* Lindberg JV (ed): Lacrimal Surgery. New York, Churchill Livingstone, 1988, pp 19-48.

CHAPTER 75

Eyelid Causes of Tearing

Jeffrey A. Nerad

When evaluating the patient with tearing, the surgeon must recognize and treat any eyelid abnormalities before recommending surgery on the lacrimal sac or the nasolacrimal duct. Changes in the eyelid anatomy and function as result of aging, trauma, or disease may affect the normal drainage of tears. Subtle scarring, loss of tone, or paralysis of the eyelid may alter the function of the lacrimal pump. Eversion of the punctum or ectropion of the eyelid may prevent tears from reaching the canaliculi. Entropion and trichiasis can cause corneal exposure, resulting in reflex tearing that surpasses the capacity for normal tear drainage.

LACRIMAL PUMP

Tear drainage depends on normal eyelid anatomy and function as well as on an intact nasolacrimal sac and duct. The eyelid skin is the thinnest skin of the body. The redundancy of the skin fold and the delicate nature of the skin allow movement of the underlying muscle with little resistance. The orbicularis is intimately related to the lacrimal sac via fascial and tendinous connections around the sac, known as the lacrimal diaphragm. Movements of the eyelids caused by orbicularis contraction have been suggested to serve as a lacrimal pump that opens and closes the sac, contributing to the drainage of tears. Eyelid malpositions, deformities, paralysis, abnormal stiffness, or contracture of the eyelids affect the integrity of the lacrimal pump and may prevent normal drainage of tears.

ECTROPION

Ectropion of the eyelid is characterized by a turning of the eyelid margin away from the eyeball, a condition that is usually associated with a separation of the eyelid from the globe. As the eyelid turns outward, conjunctival exposure occurs, and the patient reports a red eyelid margin that is often accompanied by symptoms of tearing. Chronic exposure causes metaplastic changes in the palpebral conjunctiva, which lead to keratinization (Fig. 75–1). Corneal irritation results in inferior punctate keratopathy and, in rare cases, corneal ulceration. Epiphora increases as exposure worsens as a result of increased reflex tearing. Rubbing the eyes and wiping away the tears pull the lid away from the eye and exacerbate the ectropion. The tear meniscus enlarges and flows over the margin onto the cheek. Often, patients report that their vision, particularly their reading vision, is disturbed as though they are looking through water. Mucus and debris in the tear lake may cause intermittent blurring of vision.

Involutional

By far, the commonest form of lower lid ectropion is the involutional form. The primary mechanism is laxity of the eyelid associated with stretching of the canthal tendons. The tarsal plate is thought to remain unchanged in length.

The onset of involutional ectropion is gradual. The first sign of lid laxity may present medially as punctal eversion. At the slit lamp, the punctum should appose the globe and should not be easily seen without slight manual eversion of the lid. If the punctum is pointing straight up or outward, punctal ectropion is present. As the lid laxity increases, the medial portion of the lid sags and turns outward. Medial ectropion (Fig. 75–2) is commoner than localized lateral ectropion; however, ectropion may occur anywhere on the lid. Gradual worsening of the condition leads to ectropion of the entire lid.

Lid laxity may be demonstrated by the pinch test (Fig. 75–3).[1] If the lower lid can be distracted more than 6 mm from the globe, the lid is lax. An approximation of eyelid elasticity can be made by pulling the lid down from the globe and allowing it to snap back into place.[2] If the lid returns to normal position without blinking, lid laxity is not present. If one or more blinks are required to place the lid into normal position, laxity is present. With these tests, a qualitative estimation of the eyelid laxity can be made. In some instances, eyelid laxity, without any overt ectropion, may be a cause of epiphora. If lacrimal examination results are normal and persistent tearing occurs, repair of lid laxity alone may improve symptoms.

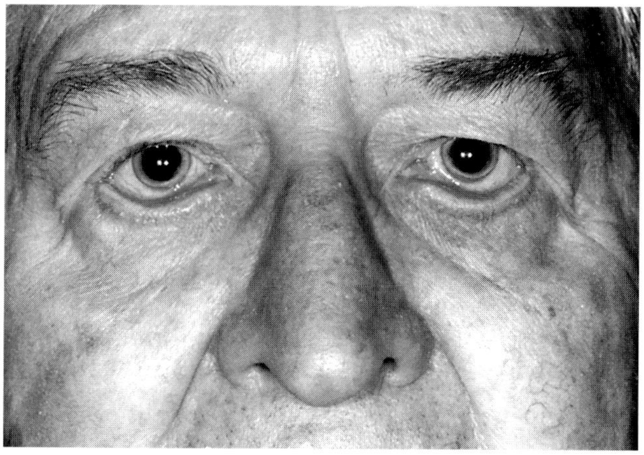

Figure 75–1. Bilateral lower lid involutional entropion with chronic conjunctival changes.

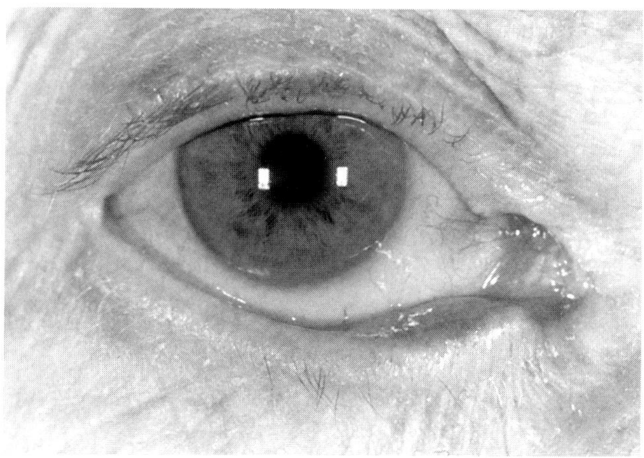

Figure 75–2. Medial ectropion. Note that the punctum and the medial half of the eyelid are everted.

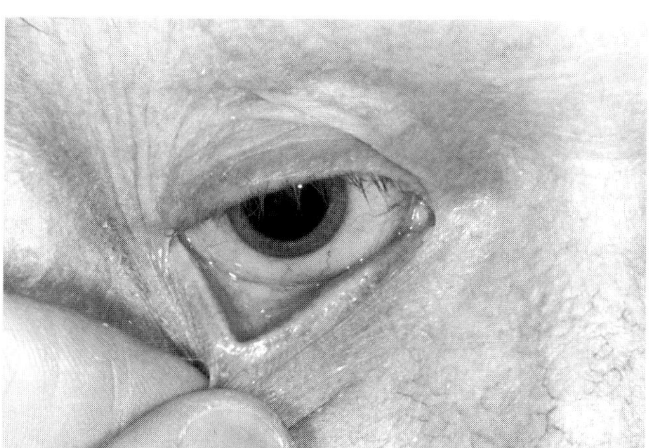

Figure 75–3. Pinch test demonstrating lower lid laxity.

Lid laxity associated with involutional ectropion is thought to result from stretching of the canthal tendons rather than from elongation of the tarsal plate. Older patients may complain that their eyes appear smaller (phimosis of the eyelids) than when they were young. Narrowing of the vertical measurements of the palpebral fissures results from stretching or dehiscence of the levator aponeurosis and lower lid retractors. Similarly, the horizontal dimensions of the palpebral fissures narrow as a result of canthal tendon lengthening. Lateral tendon laxity is evidenced by rounding or blunting of the lateral canthus as well (Fig. 75–4). Medial canthal tendon laxity is demonstrated when pulling the lid laterally causes the punctum to be displaced at, or lateral to, the nasal limbus (Fig. 75–5).

The choice of treatment of ectropion is based on the location of the ectropion and the degree of laxity. In cases of only punctal eversion or minimal medial ectropion, little lid laxity may be present. In these cases, a posterior lamellar shortening procedure with inverting sutures, the medial spindle operation (Fig. 75–6), reapposes the punctum,[3, 4] to the globe without need for horizontal lid shortening. The procedure is as follows. A diamond of conjunctiva below the punctum is excised (see Fig. 75–6*A*). The lower lid retractors (which are often difficult or impossible to identify) are grasped deep within the dia-

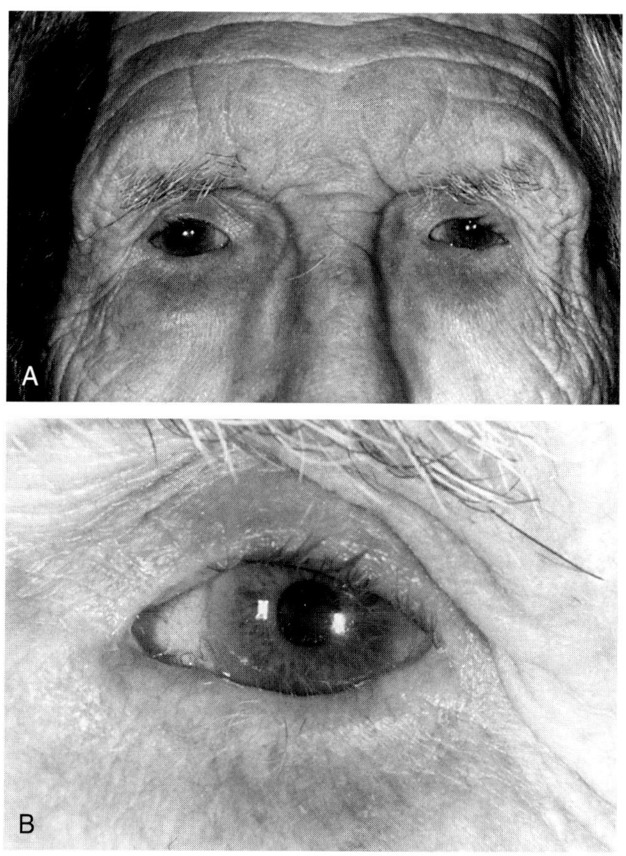

Figure 75–4. *A*, Phimosis of the eyelids due to stretching of the medial and lateral canthal tendons. *B*, Note associated ptosis of lower and upper lids.

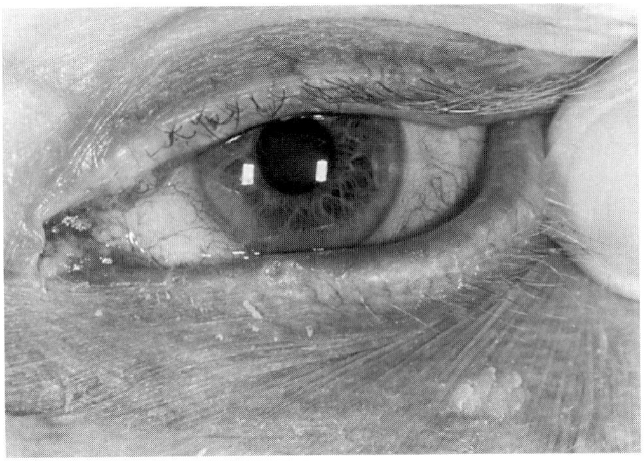

Figure 75–5. Medial canthal tendon laxity demonstrated by pulling the punctum lateral to the limbus.

mond-shaped wound. A horizontal mattress suture is placed backhanded through the retractors using a double-armed 4-0 chromic suture. The needles are then passed through the upper apex of the diamond (adjacent to the punctum) from the anterior aspect of the wound through to the conjunctiva. The last pass of the sutures is made through the conjunctiva of the lower apex of the diamond and continues through the eyelid to emerge from the skin 10 to 15 mm below the punctum. The arms of the suture are tied on themselves, adjusting the degree of inward turning of the punctum (see Fig. 75–6*B*). A small overcorrection or punctal inversion is desirable at the end of the operation. If the punctum is stenosed, dilation may be performed. When the lid is apposed to the globe, the punctum generally remains open. A punctoplasty is usually not necessary. When the diamond of conjunctiva is excised, care must be taken not to cut the vertical portion of the canaliculus, which extends 1 to 2 mm inferior to the lid margin. If anterior lamellar cicatricial changes are causing the punctal eversion, the medial spindle operation may be ineffective, and a small full-thickness skin graft is required.

If lid laxity is present with medial ectropion, as is usually the case, a horizontal lid shortening operation is performed. The degree of success in reapposing the punctum can be anticipated at the slit lamp. As the lid is pulled temporally, the punctum should revert to its normal position. If complete apposition is not accomplished with this maneuver, a medial spindle operation is combined with a horizontal lid-shortening procedure. When combined, the medial spindle operation must be performed before the lid shortening. If the horizontal shortening is performed first, access to the posterior lamella is limited. For horizontal lid shortening, a lateral tarsal strip procedure is preferred, as is discussed later.

For generalized lower lid involutional ectropion, horizontal lid shortening at the lateral canthus is performed. Although pentagonal resections of the lid, as in the Bick procedure and the Kuhnt-Szymanowski operation, tighten the lid, they unnecessarily shorten the tarsus and do not correct the lateral canthal blunting associated with elongation of the lateral canthal tendon. Similarly, the "lazy-T"[5] operation for medial ectropion, which combines a diamond resection of posterior lamella with a

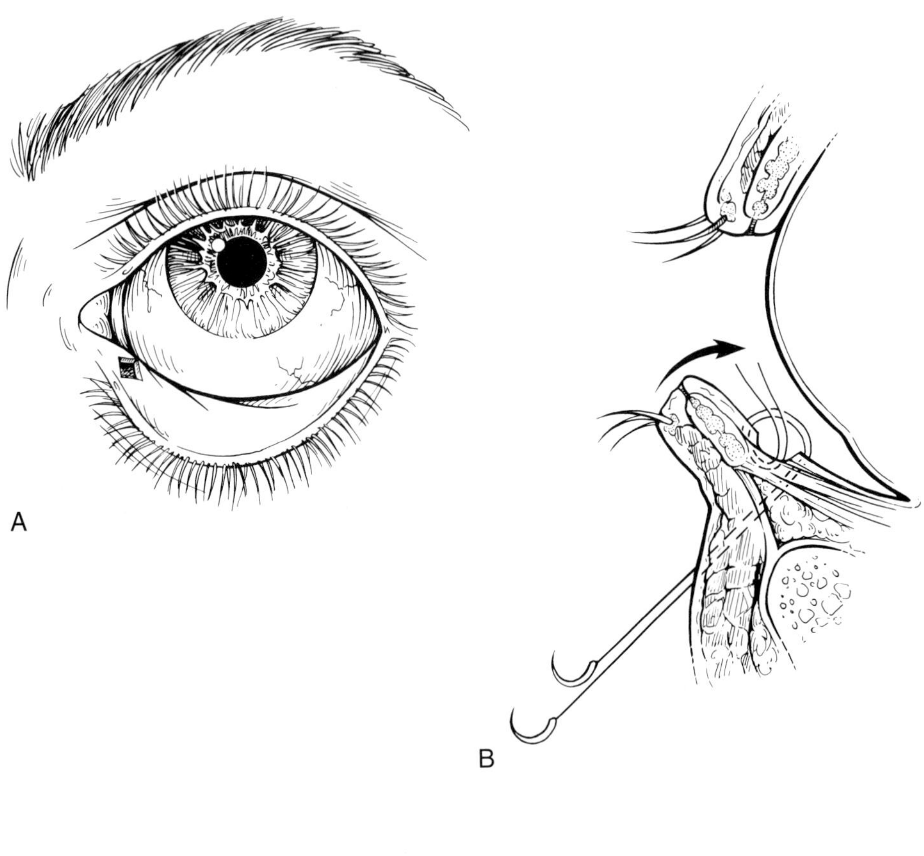

Figure 75–6. Medial spindle operation. *A*, A diamond of conjunctiva is excised. *B*, Double-armed suture attaches the lower lid retractors, shortens the diamond vertically, and mechanically inverts the lid.

pentagonal wedge resection of tarsus, does not attack the problem of lid laxity at its origin, the canthal tendons.

In 1979, Tenzel and colleagues[6, 7] described the lateral canthal tendon sling for repair of ectropion. Anderson and Gordy modified this procedure and termed it the *tarsal strip procedure*.[8] This operation is very effective in correcting ectropion and is the author's choice for horizontal lid shortening because it does not shorten a normal tarsus; rather, it shortens the lateral canthal tendon and corrects any rounding of the lateral canthus. The tarsal strip operation is recommended for the correction of ectropion caused by lid laxity.

The lateral tarsal strip operation is performed as an outpatient procedure using 2% lidocaine (Xylocaine) with 1 : 100,000 epinephrine mixed with an equal part of 0.75% bupivacaine (Marcaine). The local anesthetic solution is injected into the lateral canthus and then into the periosteum near the attachment of the lateral canthal tendon at Whitnall's tubercle. Additional local anesthetic is injected subconjunctivally in the lateral lower conjunctival cul-de-sac. The local anesthetic should be injected at least 10 minutes before the operation begins, to allow the vasoconstriction from the epinephrine to take effect. A small canthotomy is performed with straight iris scissors. The deep tissues are dissected with Westcott's scissors to clearly expose the lateral orbital rim. The white periosteum should be visible. The periosteum must not be violated because this is where the sutures will be passed to reattach the lid. Small, double-pronged skin hooks or a Freer periosteal elevator may assist with exposure, if necessary. The temporal portion of the eyelid is grasped, and lateral and upward traction is applied. A cantholysis is performed using curved iris scissors. Strumming the inferior limb of the canthal tendon and the septum with scissors identifies the tissues that must be cut to allow the entire lid to be pulled temporally. The cantholysis should be adequate to allow the lid to move temporally, but not so large to allow fat prolapse through the cut septum. Bipolar cautery should be applied at this point to stop any bleeding.

A strip of tarsus devoid of skin and conjunctiva is then prepared. The skin and muscle are separated from the anterior surface of the tarsal plate using sharp, curved iris scissors (Storz no. 3347). A cut just below and parallel to the inferior border of tarsus is made through the conjunctiva and lower lid retractors; the length of this cut should be the same as the estimated amount of shortening needed. The mucocutaneous lid margin is trimmed off using Westcott's scissors. The conjunctiva is scraped off the back of tarsus using a scalpel blade. An appropriate length of tarsus and lateral canthal tendon then is trimmed off. Conservative resection of tarsus is recommended if necessary.

A small half-circle needle (P-2 Ethicon) is used to sew the tarsal strip to the inner (medial) aspect of the lateral rim at or slightly above midpupil height with a 4-0 Vicryl or polydioxanone suture. A slightly high overcorrection is desired. If the eyelid is not tight against the eyeball, the sutures are removed and slightly more tarsus is resected. Excess anterior lamella including lashes is trimmed off, and a minimal number of canthal sutures, using 7-0 Vicryl or fast-absorbing 6-0 gut, are placed to close the canthotomy (Fig. 75–7). Care should be taken to not overtighten lower lids in eyes with scleral show, maxillary hypoplasia, or proptosis because tightening may cause the lid to slide inferiorly on the globe. As mentioned earlier, a medial spindle may be combined with the tarsal strip operation if horizontal shortening does not place the punctum against the globe.

A severe form of ectropion (which Fox termed *tarsal ectropion*) occurs where the entire lid is everted and the tarsus is essentially turned upside down (Fig. 75–8).[9] This problem may sometimes be seen in the absence of horizontal lid laxity, perhaps associated with a retractor disinsertion. Wesley[10] described conjunctival excision beneath the tarsal border with closure including the retractors. We have successfully used similar resections with inverting sutures, as described in the medial spindle procedure, in combination with horizontal lid shortening to correct tarsal ectropion. A similar procedure was described by Tse and coworkers[11] and is useful in correcting tarsal ectropion.

The correction of horizontal lid laxity that results from medial canthal tendon laxity is difficult. A medial canthal tendon plication operation can be performed; however, the results are often unsatisfactory—bunching of the canaliculus and distraction of lid off the globe occur because all the shortening is of the anterior limb of the medial canthal tendon. Many surgeons prefer not to perform the medial canthal tendon plication operation. In patients with mild-to-moderate medial canthal tendon laxity, a lateral tarsal strip is performed alone. A wedge resection medial to the punctum and canalicular reanastomosis over silicone stents, as suggested by McCord and colleagues,[12] can be performed if severe medial canthal tendon laxity is present, but this procedure is rarely necessary.

Cicatricial

Shortening of the anterior lamella of the eyelid may cause a cicatricial ectropion. The onset of the symptoms and signs may be gradual in disease conditions affecting the skin or may be sudden after surgery or accidental trauma. Shortening of the skin and muscle may result from irradiation, burns, tumors, chemical injury, or cicatricial skin diseases. Iatrogenic causes include skin removal for skin cancer excision, xanthelasma removal, or blepharoplasty.

The cause of the cicatricial changes should be treated, if possible. In cicatrizing skin disease, topical steroid lotion may be helpful; however, if scarring is permanent, as is often the case, replacement of the shortened skin must

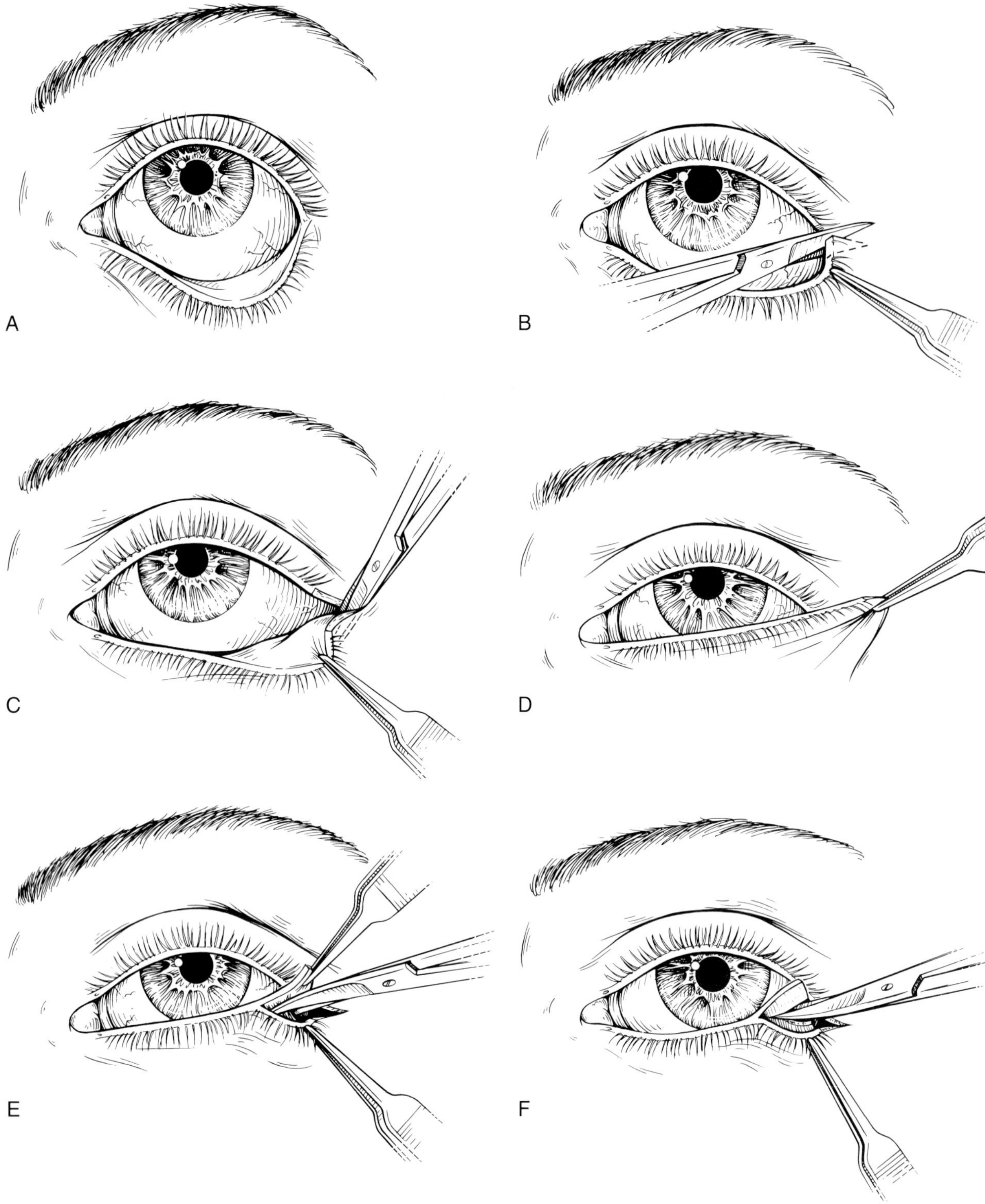

Figure 75–7. The lateral tarsal strip operation. *A*, Lower lid ectropion. *B*, A small lateral cathotomy is performed exposing the periosteum of the lateral orbital wall. *C*, A cantholysis is performed, severing the inferior crus of the lateral canthal tendon, the lower lid retractors, and the orbital septum. *D*, The lid is pulled laterally to estimate the amount of shortening. *E*, The anterior and posterior lamellae are split along the gray line. *F*, The conjunctiva and lower lid retractors are cut from the bottom edge of tarsus, forming a tarsal strip.

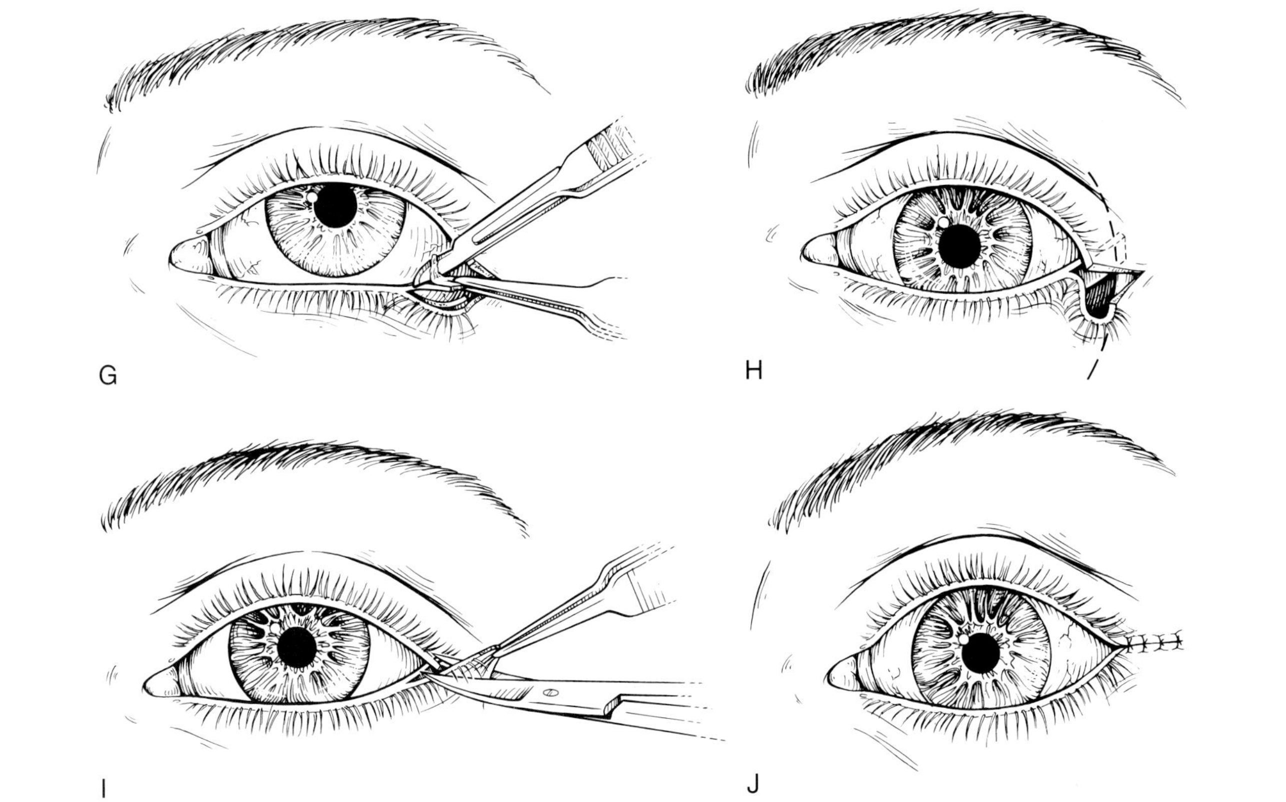

Figure 75–7 *Continued. G*, The mucosa is cut off the lid margin with scissors and is scraped off the back of the tarsus with a blade. *H*, The tarsal strip is shortened a conservative amount and suture on the inner aspect of lateral orbital rim. A small half-circle needle such as a P-2 needle with 4-0 Vicryl suture is essential for this step. *I*, Redundant anterior lamella including lashes is removed. *J*, The canthotomy is closed with 7-0 Vicryl or gut sutures.

be performed. Often, no local tissue is available for flap formation, and full-thickness skin grafting is necessary.

The best source for eyelid skin grafts is the upper lid skin fold. Eyelid skin is the thinnest and most flexible skin on the body, and only skin from another lid matches in texture and mobility. When redundant upper lid skin exists, one or both upper lid folds may be used as donor sites. Bilateral harvesting generally offers the best symmetry. Practical considerations often prevent bilateral upper lid fold harvesting. Alternative choices for full-thickness graft donor sites are the retroauricular or the preauricular skin.[13] Preauricular skin is useful (Fig. 75–9) because of its convenient location for harvesting. A piece as large as 15 × 40 mm can be obtained and is generally the correct size and shape for correcting cicatricial changes in the lower lid. A skin–muscle flap for correction of cicatricial medial ectropion of the lower lid can be made by mobilizing skin and muscle just above the upper lid skin crease and hinging it at the medial canthus.[14] This method works well if redundant upper lid skin exists and the cicatricial forces in the lower lid are medial. Other alternative donor sites include the supraclavicular area and the inner aspect of the arm. Split-thickness skin grafts should be avoided because significant contracture usually occurs, often leaving more cicatricial problems to deal with.

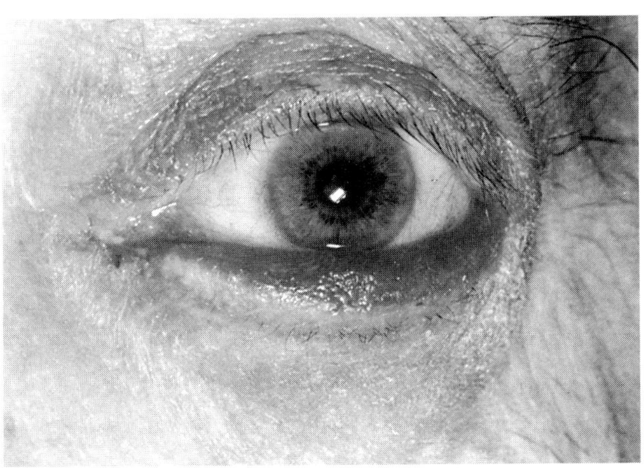

Figure 75–8. Tarsal ectropion.

A full-thickness skin grafting operation of the lower lid starts with two transmarginal lid traction sutures placed temporally and medially to the limbus. The scar bands are cut, or tight skin is released. The lid is allowed to fall back into normal position against the globe. In most cases, a lateral tarsal strip is performed to prevent possible ectropion. All bleeding sites are cauterized. A template of the defect is made and transferred to the graft donor site. The size of the graft is outlined with a surgical marking pen or with gentian violet applied with a sharpened broken cotton swab. The graft is slightly oversized

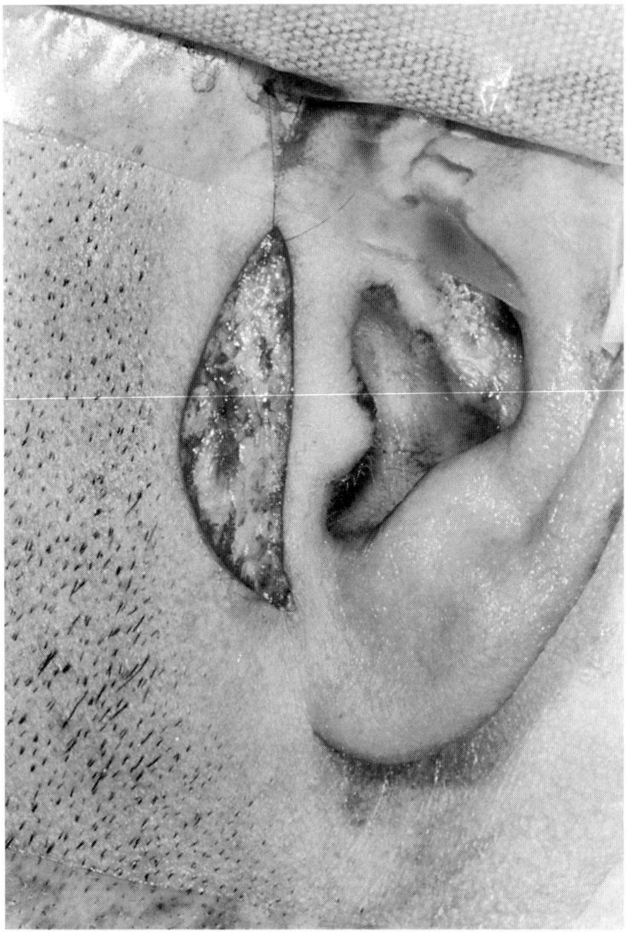

Figure 75–9. Harvest site for preauricular skin. Note area of non–hair-bearing skin.

to compensate for contracture. The graft is harvested using sharp dissection with scissors or a scalpel placed directly beneath the skin. During harvesting of preauricular skin, the facial nerve is easy to avoid because it is deep to the parotid fascia. Any remaining subcutaneous fat is removed from the graft before it is sutured into position. Cardinal sutures tack the graft in place, and then the wound is closed with a running absorbable suture. No pie crusts are made. A bolster of surgical sponge is tied into position with the long ends of the cardinal sutures. The traction sutures are taped to the brow. A firm eye patch is then placed for 1 week. Postoperatively, a moderate overcorrection usually occurs that reduces spontaneously (Fig. 75–10).

Paralytic

Facial nerve palsy causes a weakening or paralysis of the orbicularis oculi and other muscles of facial expression. The decreased tone of the orbicularis oculi muscle causes loss of support of tarsoligamentous sling of the lower lid. In elderly individuals in whom lid laxity preexists, a paralytic ectropion will develop. In younger individuals with tight lids, ectropion is often not a consequence of the paralysis. Lagophthalmos or abnormalities in the lacrimal pump, such as an incomplete blink, often cause exposure and tearing.

Facial nerve paralysis may occur as a result of trauma, tumor growth, tumor resection, or inflammatory conditions. Paralysis secondary to tumor growth, resection of tumor, or trauma is often permanent and severe. Removal of cerebellopontine angle tumors, such as acoustic neuromas, may cause trigeminal nerve damage as well as facial nerve paralysis because of the proximity of these nerves to the eighth nerve. Ectropion secondary to facial nerve paralysis in association with an anesthetic cornea is a dangerous situation because a neurotrophic keratitis may coexist. Exposure may progress to ulceration without the symptoms of pain or irritation. Bell's palsy or idiopathic facial palsy is the commonest inflammatory condition affecting the facial nerve. Viral, inflammatory, and immune factors have been implicated. Seventy to 80% of patients with Bell's palsy have a complete or satisfactory return of function.[12]

Signs and symptoms of facial nerve paralysis differ widely in degree. A subtle brow ptosis, an incomplete blink, and a shallowing of the nasolabial fold may be the only sign of a mild or nearly resolved facial nerve paralysis. Other patients may develop a complete facial paralysis with severe ectropion, brow ptosis obscuring the vision, and difficulty speaking owing to orbicularis oris involvement (Fig. 75–11). Severe aberrant regeneration may follow, with resultant cocontraction of the facial muscle. Eye findings vary from minimal inferior epithelial keratopathy to frank corneal ulceration. Tearing may result from inadequate lacrimal pump function, punctal eversion, or ectropion.

Mild cases often resolve and can be managed conservatively with lubricants. Nonincisional tarsorrhaphy with temporary 5-0 prolene sutures may be helpful.[14] A temporary tarsorrhaphy may be performed by simply denuding of the eyelid margins and simple suturing.[12] A more permanent technique involves splitting the anterior and posterior lamella and suturing denuded tarsal edges together with mattress sutures of 5-0 Vicryl. This procedure serves as either a temporary or permanent tarsorrhaphy. Many other permanent tarsorrhaphies have been described.[12] Medial and lateral tarsorrhaphies are useful in combination in cases in which a lateral tarsorrhaphy alone does not prevent exposure. Combined small medial and lateral tarsorrhaphies correct exposure better and yield more attractive results than does a larger lateral tarsorrhaphy. Ectropion can be corrected using the tarsal strip operation sometimes in association with a medial spindle procedure.

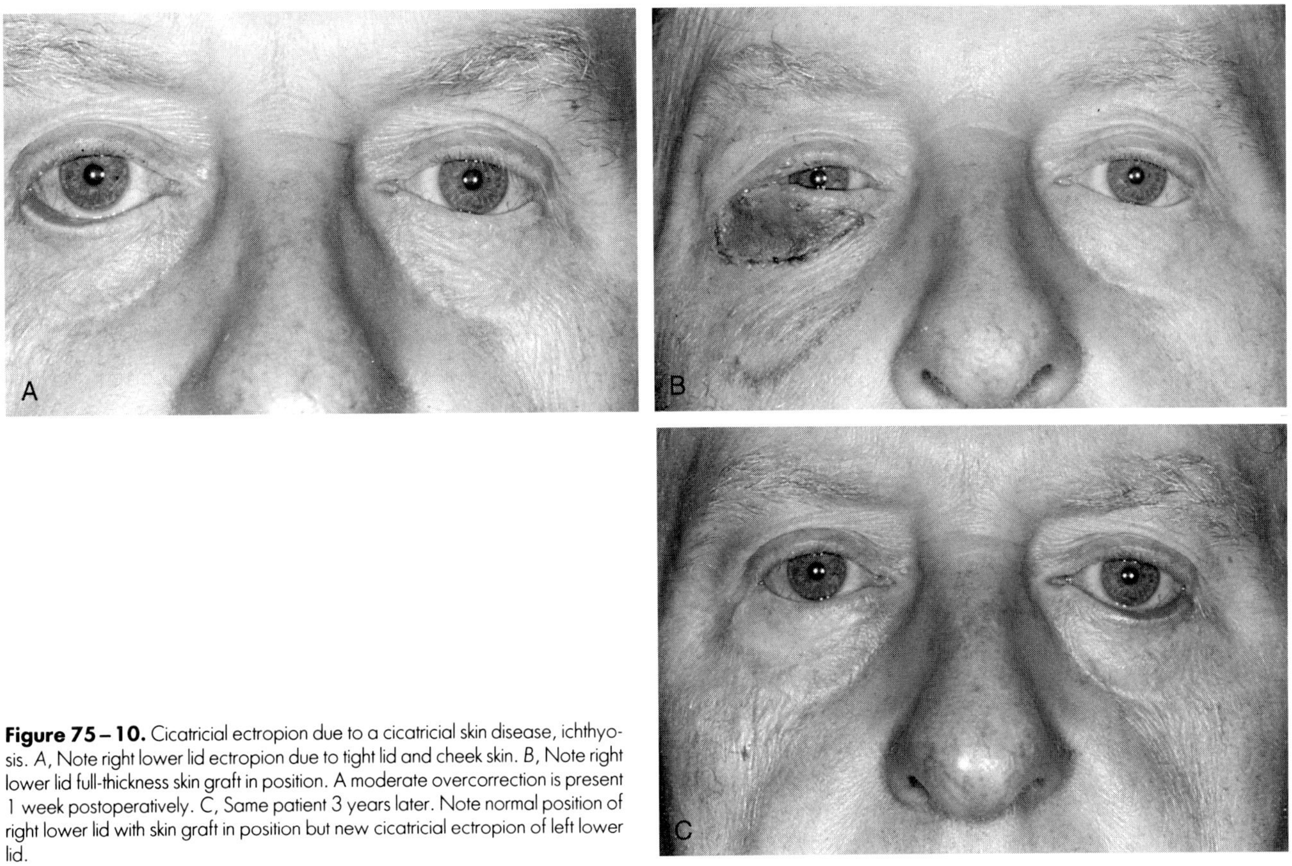

Figure 75–10. Cicatricial ectropion due to a cicatricial skin disease, ichthyosis. *A*, Note right lower lid ectropion due to tight lid and cheek skin. *B*, Note right lower lid full-thickness skin graft in position. A moderate overcorrection is present 1 week postoperatively. *C*, Same patient 3 years later. Note normal position of right lower lid with skin graft in position but new cicatricial ectropion of left lower lid.

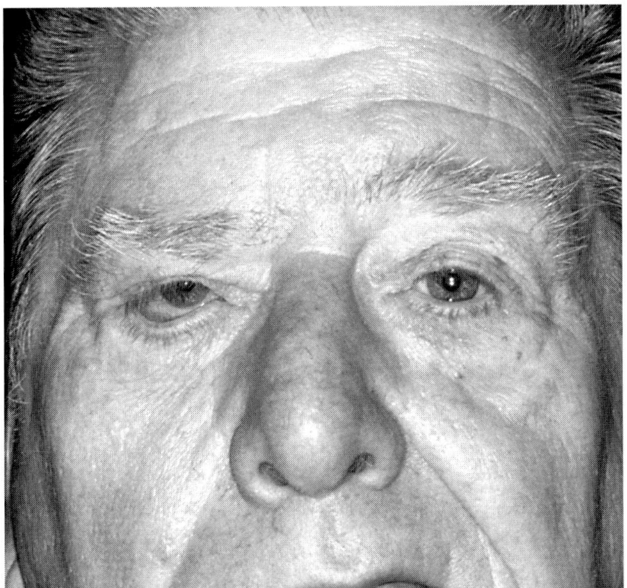

Figure 75–11. Paralytic ectropion due to facial nerve paralysis. Note right brow ptosis, loss of forehead wrinkles, ectropion, and shallowing of nasolabial fold.

Various mechanical devices have been suggested to augment orbicularis function. Upper lid gold weights are frequently successful.[15, 16] Muhlbauer described the use of palpebral magnets, which aid in eyelid closure.[17] Arion[18] suggested the use of a silicone band encircling the lids in the pretarsal space as an aid to lid closure (Arion sling). Morel and colleagues[19] devised a palpebral spring that would push the upper eyelid closed as the levator muscle relaxed. The Arion sling and the palpebral spring are useful techniques; however, over a period of time, they may extrude. The placement of upper lid gold weights, sometimes combined with elevation of the lower lid using hard-palate mucosa or ear cartilage, are the current procedures of choice.[20]

Reinnervation and reanimation procedures have been described.[21] Direct nerve suturing or facial nerve grafting is useful in cases of laceration or iatrogenic injury to peripheral facial nerve. In cases in which facial paralysis results from intracranial lesions or disorders of the temporal bone and no spontaneous recovery is observed, nerve crossovers employing the glossopharyngeal, accessory, phrenic, or hypoglossal nerves or the contralateral

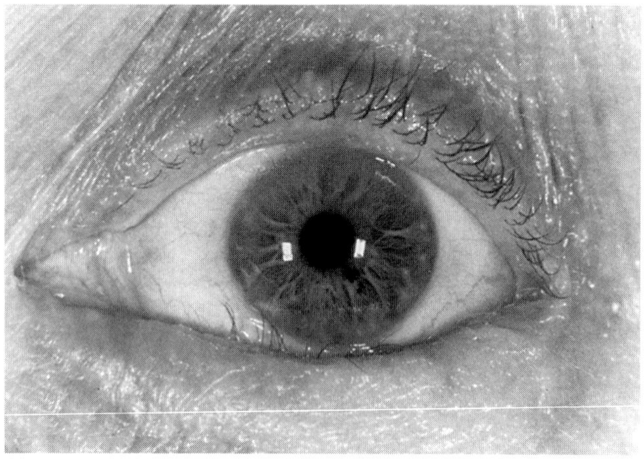

Figure 75–12. Involutional entropion of lower lid. Note that the lid margin is rotated inward.

facial nerve may be useful. Muscle transpositions with intact nerve supply have been performed with the temporalis and masseter muscles. Good results have been obtained in a high percentage of cases in which patients were carefully selected.

ENTROPION

Entropion of the eyelid is characterized by turning of the eyelid margin toward the eyeball (Fig. 75–12). Lashes and lid skin turn against the eye, causing a foreign body sensation and corneal exposure problems. Once irritation begins, lid spasm follows, and a vicious cycle of increasing entropion may follow. Because of pain and irritation, patients with entropion tend to seek medical attention sooner than do these with ectropion. Epiphora is often a symptom of entropion. The entropion may be intermittent and therefore a cause of intermittent epiphora.

Epiblepharon and forms of trichiasis, including distichiasis and misdirected lashes, are often confused with entropion. Similarities exist in that lashes abrade the cornea in all of these conditions and may be the source of irritation and tearing. However, the eyelid margin remains in anatomic position in epiblepharon and trichiasis, as is discussed later. In entropion, the eyelid margin is always rotated toward the globe.

Three forms of entropion are seen: the involutional form is the commonest in the United States, an intermittent spastic form may also occur, and a cicatricial form results from scarring of the conjunctiva and tarsus.

Involutional

The causes of involutional entropion include lid laxity; disinsertion or stretching of the lower lid retractors; spasm of the preseptal orbicularis, causing overriding onto the pretarsal orbicularis; age-related enophthalmos.

Involutional changes leading to horizontal lid laxity allow the eyelid to become unstable. This instability may be exacerbated by age-related enophthalmos such that the eye can no longer offer support for the lid in the normal position. The accompanying laxity of the lower lid retractors allows the eyelid margin to rotate inward (Fig. 75–13).

More than 100 procedures and modifications have been devised to correct involutional entropion and to prevent its recurrence, but most of these procedures address only one or two causal factors associated with entropion. Vertical anterior lamellar shortening was at-

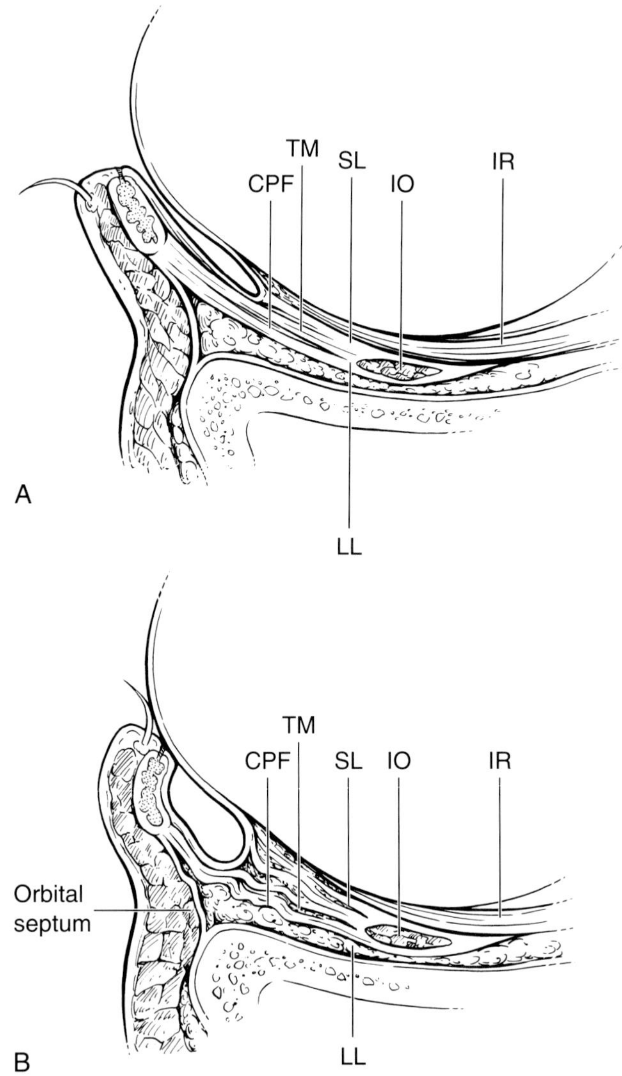

Figure 75–13. Involutional entropion. *A*, Normal lower lid anatomy. IR, inferior rectus muscle; IO, inferior oblique muscle; LL, Lockwood's ligament; TM, inferior tarsal muscle; SL, suspensory ligament of the fornix; CPF, capsulopalpebral fascia. The lower lid retractors consisting of Lockwood's ligament and the inferior tarsal muscle hold the lower eyelid in normal position. *B*, Involutional entropion exists as a result of lax lower lid retractors, overriding preseptal orbicularis (*PO*), horizontal lid laxity, and age-related enophthalmos.

tempted by use of Ziegler cautery,[22] and by excision of a horizontal ellipse of skin by Hotz.[23] Horizontal lid tightening was suggested by Butler,[24] Fox,[25] and Bick.[26] Fibrosis or tightening of the orbicularis was described by Wies[27] and Wheeler.[28] Jones was the first to suggest tightening of the inferior lid retractors.[28] All of these procedures work for some time, but they often lead to recurrence when used alone. Collin and Rathbun reported a combination of horizontal lid shortening, orbicularis fibrosis, and retractor reattachment using the "four-snip procedure,"[29] which was originally devised by Quickert. The concept of combining a horizontal lid shortening operation with a retractor reinsertion operation, as conceived by Jones, is used by many surgeons today.

An effective repair for involutional entropion is a combination of a reinsertion of the lower lid retractors and a lateral tarsal strip operation. The reinsertion is performed as follows. A subciliary skin incision is marked, and the lid is infiltrated with local anesthesia that contains epinephrine. A 4-0 silk traction suture is placed through the lid margin. A scalpel is used to incise the skin, and the muscle layer is opened with Westcott's scissors. Dissection of a myocutaneous flap is carried out inferiorly until the preaponeurotic fat is seen. The septum is opened, and the fat is retracted to expose the lower lid retractors, which are identified as a white, fibrous sheet. A strip of orbicularis is cleared from the lower margin of tarsus, and the retractors are separated free from the underlying conjunctiva (Fig. 75-14). The free edge of the retractors is sutured to the inferior edge of the tarsus with four 5-0 Vicryl sutures spaced across the tarsus. Generally, the lid is mildly ectropic at this point. If gross ectropion is seen, the sutures are removed, and the retractors are allowed to recess some. A tarsal strip operation is performed to further stabilize the lid. Very little or no ectropion should exist at this point. The skin is closed with a running suture of 7-0 Vicryl or 6-0 fast-absorbing gut. Three of the four causes of entropion are corrected with this procedure. Theoretically, the subciliary incision causes a blockade of preseptal fibers onto the pretarsal muscle. The retractors are tightened, thereby rotating the lid margin outward. The horizontal laxity is corrected, providing a stable lid. Any age-related enophthalmos is not addressed.

Spastic

Acute ocular inflammation or lid swelling accompanied by lid spasm may cause entropion, as is often seen after retinal or anterior segment surgery. Lid and retractor laxity probably predispose patients to this condition, although spastic entropion may occur in young adults. It is not uncommon for a surgeon to operate on a patient for unilateral entropion only to find while the patient is being prepared that the sting of topical anesthetic in the "normal" eye will cause a spastic entropion.

In cases in which a reversible cause of the spasm is recognized, Quickert sutures are a good temporizing measure to eliminate the entropion.[30] Double-armed 4-0 chromic sutures (medial, central, and lateral) are passed from deep in the inferior conjunctival fornix anteriorly through the lid to exit 2 mm below the eyelashes (Fig. 75-15). Sutures are tied tightly enough to produce a mild overcorrection of the entropion. The technique is simple and works well temporarily as the ocular irritation resolves. Although the technique is generally reserved for spastic entropion, it may be useful in bedridden or ill patients with involutional entropion who are unable to withstand a more involved entropion repair. In cases of spastic entropion in which no reversible cause can be identified, the patient is assumed to have intermittent involutional entropion, and a retractor reinsertion and lateral tarsal strip operation is performed.

Cicatricial

Shortening of the posterior lamella may cause cicatricial entropion, which pulls the lashes against the eyeball. Inflammatory processes, including chronic blepharitis, acne rosacea, chronic allergy, ocular pemphigoid and Stevens-Johnson syndrome, are common causes. Trauma or chemical injuries may be causes of posterior lamellar shortening or cicatricial entropion. Trachoma is the leading cause of entropion outside the Western world.

Antimetabolites or steroids may be useful in Stevens-Johnson disease and ocular pemphigoid. In most cases, surgical redirection or replacement of damaged tissue is necessary. Procedures that redirect the lower eyelid margin and lashes are the Wies procedure, or transverse tarsotomy,[27] and the tarsal fracture operation, or tarsotomy[31] (discussed further in the trichiasis section). Upper lid entropion may be repaired by anterior tarsal wedge resection or anterior lamellar advancement. Severe posterior lamellar scarring may be released surgically, and the length of the posterior lamella may not be restored using buccal mucosa, hard-palate mucosa,[20] or nasochondral mucosa. Hard-palate mucosa should not be used in the upper lid. Autogenous ear cartilage or sclera can be used; however, these materials cause ocular irritation while epithelialization occurs. Sclera exhibits variable degrees of resorption.[12]

Sporadic cases of true congenital entropion and ectropion are seen rarely and therefore are not described in this chapter.

TRICHIASIS

Trichiasis is a condition in which misdirected lashes arise from a normally positioned lid and rub against the

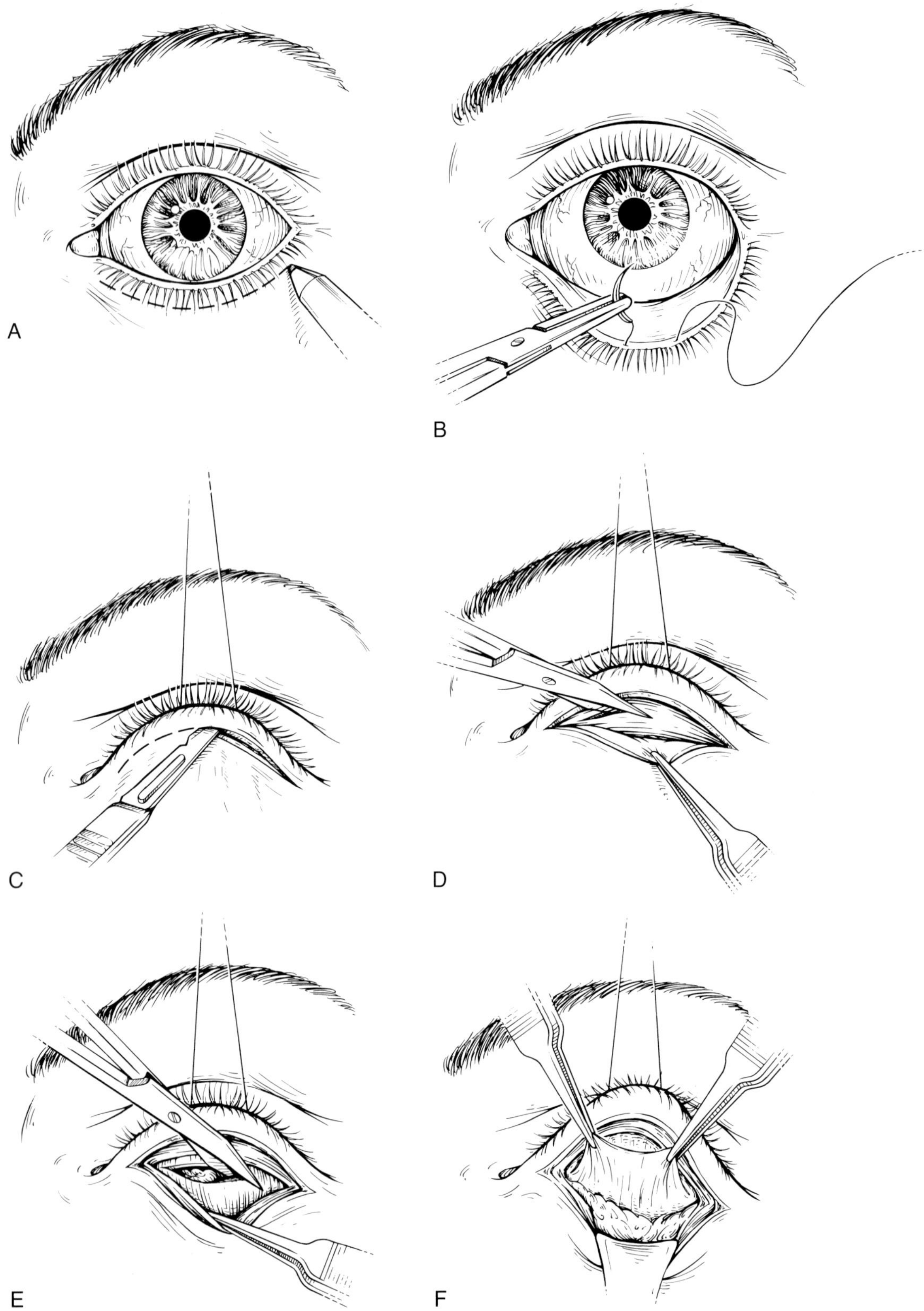

Figure 75–14. The retractor reattachment operation. *A*, A subciliary incision is marked 2 mm below the lashes. *B*, After injection of local anesthetic, a 4-0 black silk suture is passed through the lid margin for retraction. C, A skin incision is made using a no. 15 blade. *D*, The orbicularis is incised and opened medially and laterally. *E*, The preaponeurotic fat is identified. The lower lid retractors are seen posterior to the fat. *F*, The retractors are dissected free from the underlying conjunctiva and the preaponeurotic fat.

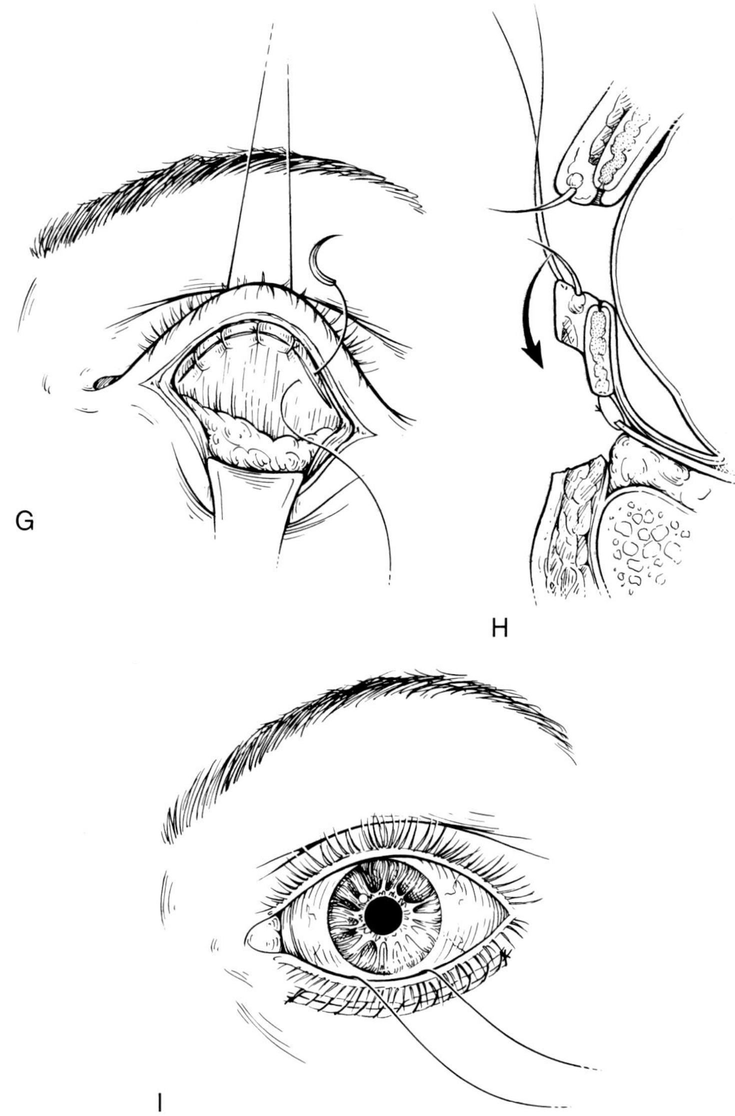

Figure 75–14 *Continued.* *G*, The retractors are advanced and sutured to the inferior tarsal margin using 5-0 Vicryl sutures. *H*, Cross section of lower lid showing reattachment of retractors and resultant outward rotation of lid margin. *I*, The skin is closed with a running suture of 7-0 Vicryl or 6-0 gut.

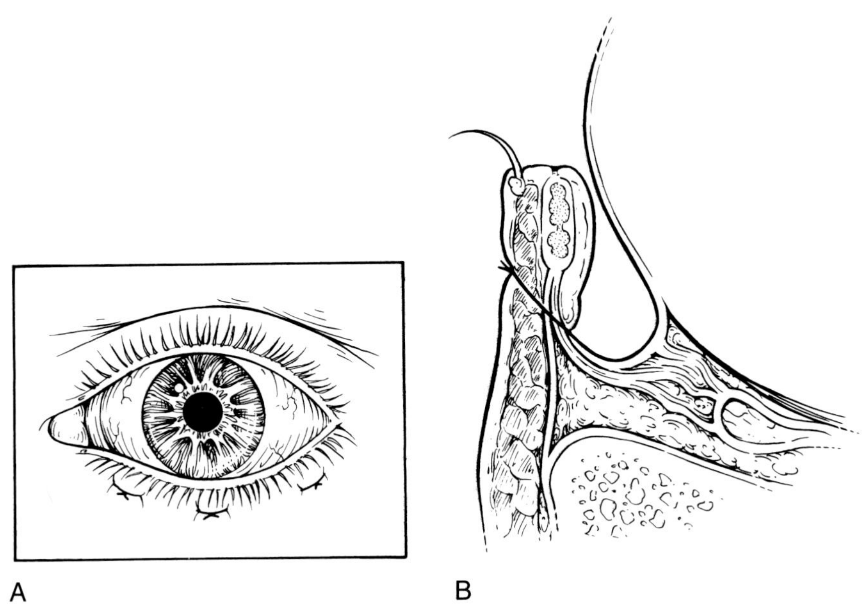

Figure 75–15. Quickert sutures. *A*, Double-armed 4-0 chromic sutures are passed from deep in the fornix out through the lid, emerging just below the lashes. *B*, Medial, central, and lateral sutures are placed, leaving the lid in a slightly overcorrected position.

cornea and conjunctiva. Reflex tearing occurs along with conjunctival and corneal irritation. Four processes can be categorized under trichiasis: distichiasis, aberrant lashes, marginal entropion, and metaplastic lashes. Each category may have a distinct cause and treatment. Often, overlap between the latter three types occurs.

Distichiasis is an uncommon congenital abnormality in which the multipotential meibomian gland cells of the tarsus develop into hair follicles and form a second row of eyelashes along the posterior margin of the eyelid. The extra row may be complete or incomplete. Often, the lashes grow upward and cause exposure keratitis. Anderson and Harvey[32] described performing lid splitting and posterior lamellar cryotherapy; the procedure was successful in destroying the abnormal lashes and preserving the normal lashes.

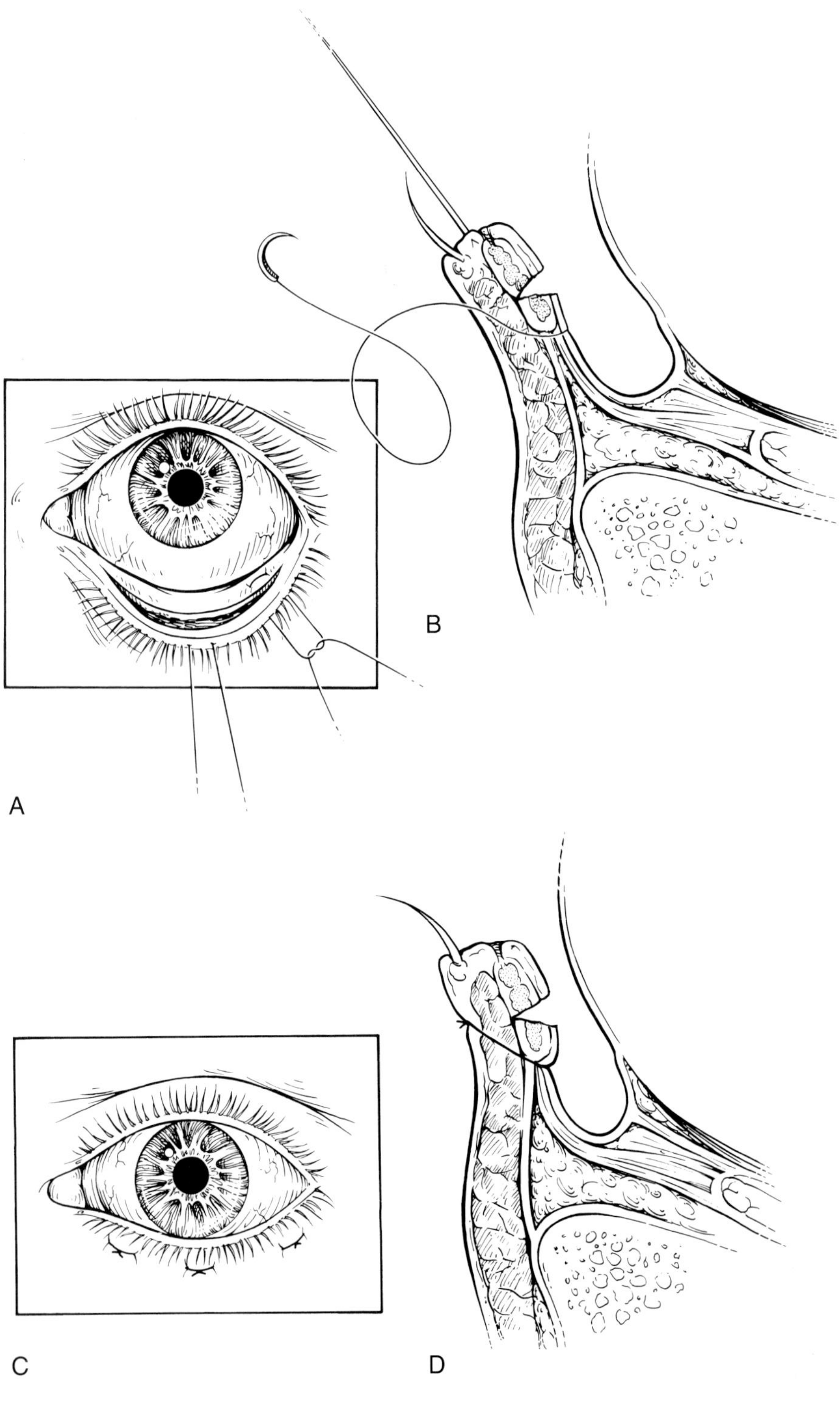

Figure 75–16. Inferior tarsotomy, or the tarsal fracture operation. *A*, A 4-0 black silk suture is passed through the lid margin and the lid is everted. A no. 15 blade is used to incise the tarsus horizontally along its entire length. *B*, Double-armed 4-0 chromic sutures are passed from just beneath the tarsal plate to emerge just beneath the lashes. *C*, Medial, central, and lateral sutures are passed. *D*, The sutures are tied, leaving the lid in a slightly overcorrected position. The tarsotomy is allowed to granulate closed.

Aberrant lashes may arise after trauma or after eyelid reconstruction following tumor excision. However, in many cases, no cause can be identified. Often, the aberrant lashes may be localized and cured by a wedge resection with primary closure of the involved eyelid. More diffuse areas of aberrant lashes should be treated with cryotherapy. For diffuse areas of trichiasis in the lower lid, the tarsal fracture operation, or tarsotomy, is useful to reposition the lashes without destroying large areas of follicles. In this operation, a horizontal incision is made half-way down on the tarsal plate and extending to the orbicularis. The "fractured" tarsal margin is everted and held in eversion using double-armed sutures (Fig. 75-16).[31]

Marginal entropion[33] is a subtle in-turning of the lid margin resulting from mild scarring of the posterior lamella. In these cases, lashes against the cornea are recognized more readily than the cicatricial entropion. The condition is evidenced by a posterior migration or conjunctivalization of the meibomian glands and a rounding of the lid margin. Cryotherapy, or preferably, lid margin rotations, such as the tarsal fracture procedure, are recommended.

Metaplastic lashes are a rare form of trichiasis that follows chronic eyelid inflammation. Metaplasia of the meibomian glands causes hair follicles to be produced. In most cases, eyelid margin irregularities resulting from scarring are present. This scarring may misdirect normal lashes, and a cycle of increasing irritation and metaplastic lash production may ensue. Lid hygiene and topical antibiotics with or without mild steroids should be tried to stop the cycle. Misdirected lashes causing corneal or conjunctival changes should be treated; cryotherapy or other lid procedures used for aberrant lashes may be required to correct the problem.

Epiblepharon may be confused with trichiasis. Epiblepharon (Fig. 75-17) is a condition in children (usually Asian) in which an extra roll of lower lid skin pushes the lashes against the cornea. The eyelid margin is in normal position. Surprisingly, minimal symptoms and signs of corneal exposure, such as photophobia, tearing, or epitheliopathy, are often seen despite significant numbers of lashes against the cornea. Generally children outgrow the disease by age 10 as the face assumes more adult features. If symptomatic, the condition can be cured by a horizontal excision of the extra roll of skin and muscle.[23]

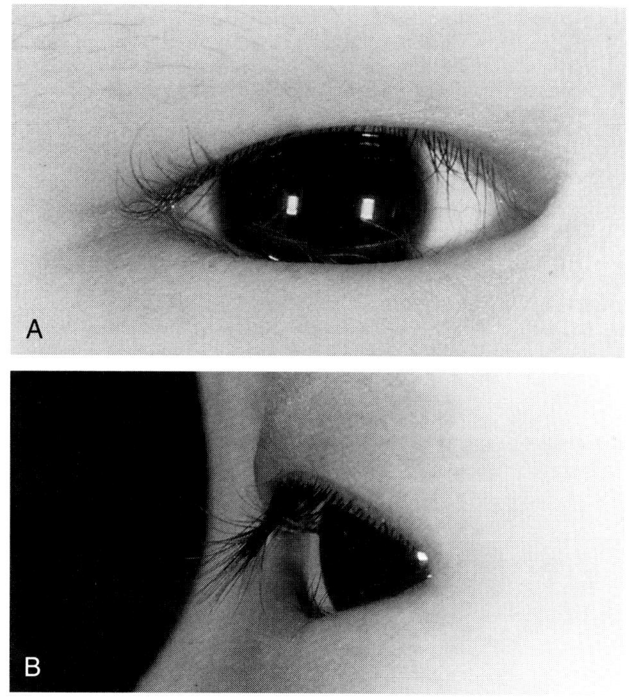

Figure 75-17. *A*, Epiblepharon. *B*, Note the extra roll of skin that is pushing the lashes against the cornea.

CONCLUSION

Eyelid malpositions and related conditions are common causes of epiphora. Lacrimal pump failure resulting from lid laxity or orbicularis paresis may be helped by horizontal lid shortening. Involutional punctal eversion, medial ectropion, or more advanced cases of ectropion may be relieved by lid shortening, often performed in combination with the medial spindle operation. Involutional entropion can be treated with anatomic reinsertion of the lower lid retractors and the tarsal strip operation. Cicatricial causes of ectropion and entropion are repaired by restoring normal length to the shortened lamella using appropriate grafts. Reflex tearing resulting from trichiasis is managed by excision or cryodestruction of the lash follicles or by repositioning of the lashes using the tarsal fracture operation or a similar operation. Recognition and appropriate treatment of these conditions relieves the patient's symptoms of epiphora.

REFERENCES

1. Hill JC: Analysis of senile changes in the palpebral fissure. Trans Ophthalmol Soc UK 95:49-53, 1975.
2. Schaefer AJ: Lateral canthal tendon tuck. Ophthalmology 86:1879-1882, 1979.
3. Tse DT: Surgical correction of punctal malposition. Am J Ophthalmol 100:339-341, 1985.
4. Nowinski TS, Anderson RL: The medial spindle procedure for involutional medial ectropion. Arch Ophthalmol 103:1750-1753, 1985.
5. Smith B: The "lazy-T" correction of ectropion of the lower punctum. Arch Ophthalmol 94:1149-1150, 1976.
6. Tenzel RR: Treatment of lagophthalmos of the lower lid. Arch Ophthalmol 81:366-368, 1969.
7. Tenzel RR, Buffam FV, Miller GR: The use of the "lateral canthal sling" in ectropion repair. Can J Ophthalmol 12:199-202, 1977.
8. Anderson RL, Gordy DD: The tarsal strip procedure. Arch Ophthalmol 97:2192-2916, 1979.
9. Fox SA: Marginal (tarsal) ectropion. Arch Ophthalmol 63:660, 1960.
10. Wesley RE: Tarsal ectropion from detachment of the lower eyelid retractors. Am J Ophthalmol 93:491-495, 1982.
11. Tse DT, Kronish JW, Buus D: Surgical correction of lower-eyelid tarsal ectropion by reinsertion of the retractors. Arch Ophthalmol 109:427-431, 1991.

12. McCord CD, Tanenbaum M, Dryden RM, Doxanas MT: Eyelid malpositions: Entropion, eyelid margin deformity and trichiasis, ectropion, and facial nerve palsy. *In* McCord CD, Tanenbaum M (eds): Oculoplastic Surgery, 2nd ed. New York, Raven Press, 1987.
13. Anderson RL, Hatt MU, Dixon R: Medial ectropion: A new technique. Arch Ophthalmol 97:521–524, 1979.
14. Dryden RM, Adams JL: Temporary nonincisional tarsorrhaphy. Ophthal Plast Reconstr Surg 1:119–120, 1985.
15. Smellie GD: Restoration of the blinking reflex in facial palsy by a simple lid-load operation. Br J Plast Surg 19:279–283, 1966.
16. Barclay TL, Roberts AC: Restoration of movement to the upper eyelid in facial palsy. Br J Ophthalmol 22:257, 1969.
17. Muhlbauer WD: Palpebral magnets for paretic lagophthalmos. *In* Fredericks S, Brady GS (eds): Symposium on the Neurologic Aspects of Plastic Surgery. St. Louis, CV Mosby, 1978.
18. Arion HG: Dynamic closure of the lids in paralysis of the orbicularis muscle. Surg 57:48–50, 1972.
19. Morel J, Fatio D, LeLardie JP: Palliative surgical treatment of facial paralysis. The palpebral spring. Plast Reconstr Surg 33:446–456, 1964.
20. Kersten RC, Kulwin DR, Levartovsky S, et al: Management of lower-lid retraction with hard-palate mucosa grafting. Arch Ophthalmol 108:1339–1343, 1990.
21. Baker DC: Facial paralysis. Ophthalmic Plast Reconstr Surg 1:580, 1987.
22. Ziegler SL: Galvanocautery puncture in ectropion and entropion. JAMA 53:183–186, 1909.
23. Hotz FC: Eine neue operation fur entropium and trichiasis. Arch fur Aufenhix 68–80, 1879–1880.
24. Butler JBV: A simple operation for entropion. Arch Ophthalmol 40:665–667, 1948.
25. Fox SA: Correction of senile entropion: Modification of technique. Arch Ophthalmol 48:624–626, 1952.
26. Bick MW: Surgical management of orbital tarsal disparity. Arch Ophthalmol 75:386–389, 1966.
27. Wies FA: Surgical treatment of entropion. J Int Coll Surg 21:758–760, 1954.
28. Wheeler JM: Spastic-entropion correction by orbicularis transplantation. Am J Ophthalmol 22:477–483, 1939.
29. Collin JRO, Rathbun JE: Involutional entropion: A review with evaluation of a procedure. Arch Ophthalmol 96:1058–1064, 1978.
30. Quickert MH, Rathburn E: Suture repair of entropion. Arch Ophthalmol 85:304–305, 1971.
31. Kersten RC, Kleiner FP, Kulwin DR: Tarsotomy for the treatment of cicatricial entropion with trichiasis. Arch Ophthalmol 110:714, 1992.
32. Anderson RL, Harvey JT: Lid splitting and posterior lamella cryosurgery for congenital and acquired distichiasis. Arch Ophthalmol 99:631–634, 1981.
33. Barber K, Dabbs T: Morphological observations on patients with presumed trichiasis. Br J Ophthalmol 72:17–22, 1989.

CHAPTER 76

Congenital Lacrimal Abnormalities

Robert C. Kersten

Congenital lacrimal system abnormalities are related to defects in embryogenesis. The embryology of the lacrimal system has been covered in previous chapters. In brief, the lacrimal excretory system is formed as an ectodermal invagination from the conjunctiva when a solid epithelial cord is buried beneath the mesoderm. This cord then thickens and extends proximally to form the canaliculi and inferiorly to form the nasolacrimal duct. This solid cord then undergoes canalization, which begins from the canaliculi proximally toward the sac and then down through the duct to the inferior meatus. Failure in normal development or complete canalization of the epithelial cord will result in obstruction to the normal flow of tears from the lacrimal lake into the nose.

CONGENITAL NASOLACRIMAL DUCT OBSTRUCTION

The most common congenital lacrimal system dysfunction is caused by failure of the nasolacrimal duct cord to completely canalize. This is noted to be symptomatic in 5% to 6% of infants.[1] However, postmortem examination of term and premature infants suggests that the incidence at the time of birth is much higher. Busse and associates[2] found that only 37% of term infants had patent nasolacrimal ducts, with 20% exhibiting bilateral nasolacrimal duct obstruction and 44% having unilateral nasolacrimal duct obstruction. Their postmortem examination of mature infants dying within the first month of birth revealed a slightly lower incidence of obstruction, but still 52% had either unilateral or bilateral obstruction. They attributed obstruction to persistence of a fine membrane at the distal nasolacrimal duct, which they referred to as Hasner's membrane in analogy to Hasner's valve, which is normally present at that location. The obstructing membrane consists of opposing fused layers of lacrimal duct epithelium and overlying nasal mucosa. When still present at birth, the membrane will usually spontaneously canalize within the first 2 months of life. By this time it will persist in only about 5% of infants.

Symptoms of congenital nasolacrimal duct obstruction consist of epiphora and dacryocystitis. Symptomatic occlusion occurs unilaterally 75% of the time and bilaterally 25% of the time.[3] The diagnosis is easily made in the office by observing epiphora and mattering of the eyelashes. It can be confirmed by compression over the nasolacrimal sac, which results in regurgitation of mucopurulent material in those patients who have developed chronic dacryocystitis. Instillation of 2% fluorescein dye and observation of abnormally delayed passage from the cul-de-sac is helpful in confirming the diagnosis in cases in which dacryocystitis is not present.[4] It is important to visualize the puncta in both lids for patency and to look for other lacrimal system abnormalities such as a lacrimal fistula before concluding that the tearing and dye delay are due to obstruction at the distal nasolacrimal duct.

The timing of treatment of congenital lacrimal duct obstruction has been somewhat controversial.[3, 4] However, it has not been well established by a number of large surveys that in the large majority of patients the symptomatic nasolacrimal duct obstruction will spontaneously resolve as spontaneous canalization of the distal nasolacrimal duct becomes complete. In 90% of obstructed infants this process will be completed by 13 months of age.[3, 5, 6] Beyond this age the duct may still continue to spontaneously canalize, but the rate of improvement tends to plateau. I have observed one patient with congenital nasolacrimal duct obstruction that spontaneously resolved at the age of 4 years. Nonetheless, it is generally thought that if obstruction has failed to resolve by 13 months of age that the likelihood of spontaneous remission is quite low.

Because the large majority of symptomatic obstructions will canalize and resolve by 13 months of age the current standard of care is to treat patients symptomatically before this age. Surgical intervention is not recommended unless acute dacryocystitis intervenes or a chronic dacryocystitis is so problematic that the parents are insistent.[6] Paul[7] studied a population of 62 eyes of 55 infants in an attempt to calculate the "odds of a cure" by 12 months of age by medical management alone. He found that patients presenting at age 3 months had an 80% chance of spontaneous resolution by 12 months.

Those presenting at 6 months had a 70% chance of resolution by 12 months, and even those patients presenting at 9 months of age had a 52% chance of spontaneous canalization if observed over the ensuing 3 months. Although some surgeons have proposed 9 months of age as a cutoff for the likelihood of spontaneous resolution, it is clear that over 50% of these patients will still be cured if managed expectantly.

During the first 12 to 13 months of expectant observation, "massage" of the affected nasolacrimal system has been recommended.[3] In this maneuver compression with one index finger is used to occlude the superior and inferior canaliculus while the thumb is used to forcefully press downward from the fundus of the lacrimal sac attempting to expel the sac contents down through the nasolacrimal duct to hydraulically burst the imperforate Hasner membrane. It is unclear whether this maneuver materially speeds the canalization of the imperforate membrane, but it does allow the anxious parent to participate in "treatment." Topical antibiotic drops or ointment is usually utilized for symptomatic dacryocystitis. Rarely a congenital lacrimal duct obstruction may lead to development of acute dacryocystitis and lacrimal sac abscess formation. In these circumstances appropriate treatment with systemic antibiotics and surgical incision and drainage may be needed. When this does occur it is advisable to proceed with probing of the nasolacrimal system either concurrently if general anesthesia is required for drainage of an abscess or shortly after resolution of the acute dacryocystitis.

If a patient reaches 13 months of age and continues to have some symptomatic nasolacrimal duct obstruction, most surgeons would recommend that surgical opening of the persistent membrane be undertaken. Rupture of the imperforate membrane with a probe passed down the nasolacrimal duct is a highly effective means of relieving congenital nasolacrimal duct obstruction. It has been the procedure of choice for many decades. Probing is usually carried out under insufflation general anesthesia. A nasal packing of well-wrung out 0.5% Neo-Synephrine-soaked gauze or cotton packing is placed beneath the middle turbinate. A no. 1-0 Bowman probe is most desirable since smaller probes increase the likelihood of false passage and have been reported to break off within the nasolacrimal duct leaving a residual foreign-body obstruction.[8] The probe is bent to a slight curve and the tip coated with ointment to lubricate its passage. Surgeons vary as to whether they recommend probing through the inferior or superior canaliculus.[9–11] I think it makes very little difference but have found it slightly easier to probe through the superior system when directing the probe inferiorly through the duct. Therefore, I introduce the probe through the vertical and horizontal limbs of the superior canaliculus and through the internal common punctum (Fig. 76–1). Continuous lateral traction is applied to the lid to keep the canaliculus on stretch and prevent its bunching up in front of the probe tip. In this fashion the probe is directed against the medial wall of the lacrimal sac and a "hard stop" is encountered as the probe abuts the underlying lacrimal bone. The probe is then rotated superiorly until it lies over the supraorbital notch at the superior orbital rim. The curve of the probe is directed posteriorly and is gently directed inferiorly. As it passes down the duct the probe tip must travel slightly posteriorly and laterally, following the direction of the nasolacrimal duct. It is important to perform this maneuver very gently, and if significant resistance is encountered the probe should be withdrawn and the procedure restarted. The approximate distance from the punctum to the level of the inferior meatus in the infant is 10 to 15 mm. Although occasionally one may feel resistance as the probe passes through the imperforate membrane, often the membrane is so thin that no significant resistance is felt as the probe passes through it. At this point the packing is removed from beneath the inferior turbinate. I prefer to directly observe the probe within the nose and to see that it is, in fact, exiting from the inferior meatus. This can be done with a nasal speculum and fiberoptic headlight. Other surgeons recommend passing a larger Bowman probe beneath the inferior meatus and relying on a feel of "metal on metal" to ensure that the probe has passed down through the duct. Unfortunately this will fail to detect false passages where the probe has lacerated through mucosa in a spot other than the inferior meatus. Once the probe is withdrawn, patency of the duct can be confirmed by irrigation with saline mixed with fluorescein. A Frazier-tipped suction catheter placed beneath the inferior meatus should retrieve the dye-tinged saline. Failure to readily irrigate through the system after probing usually requires a careful repeat of the steps of the probing and reexamination beneath the inferior turbinate to ensure that the probe has properly passed through the inferior meatus. Postoperatively, it is common to prescribe a topical corticosteroid antibiotic combination for 1 to 2 weeks, although there is no vigorous rationale for this step.

Probing in this fashion will cure better than 90% of those congenital nasolacrimal duct obstructions that are persisting at 13 months of age. Some authors have suggested that if the initial probing has delayed beyond 13 months it will have a lower success rate.[4] This is attributed to fibrosis of the nasolacrimal system caused by recurring infections. Others, however, have suggested that delayed probing beyond 13 months continues to enjoy a very high rate of success,[12] and I have personally seen success with initial probing as late as 6 years of age.

Because the "Hasner membrane" responsible for the vast majority of congenital nasolacrimal duct obstructions is very thin and tenuous, some investigators have argued that it can be readily ruptured by insufflating a bolus of air through the system.[13] In this procedure an air-filled syringe attached to a lacrimal irrigating cannula is used to force 1.5 to 2 mL of air into the lacrimal sac while occluding the opposing punctum. The increased

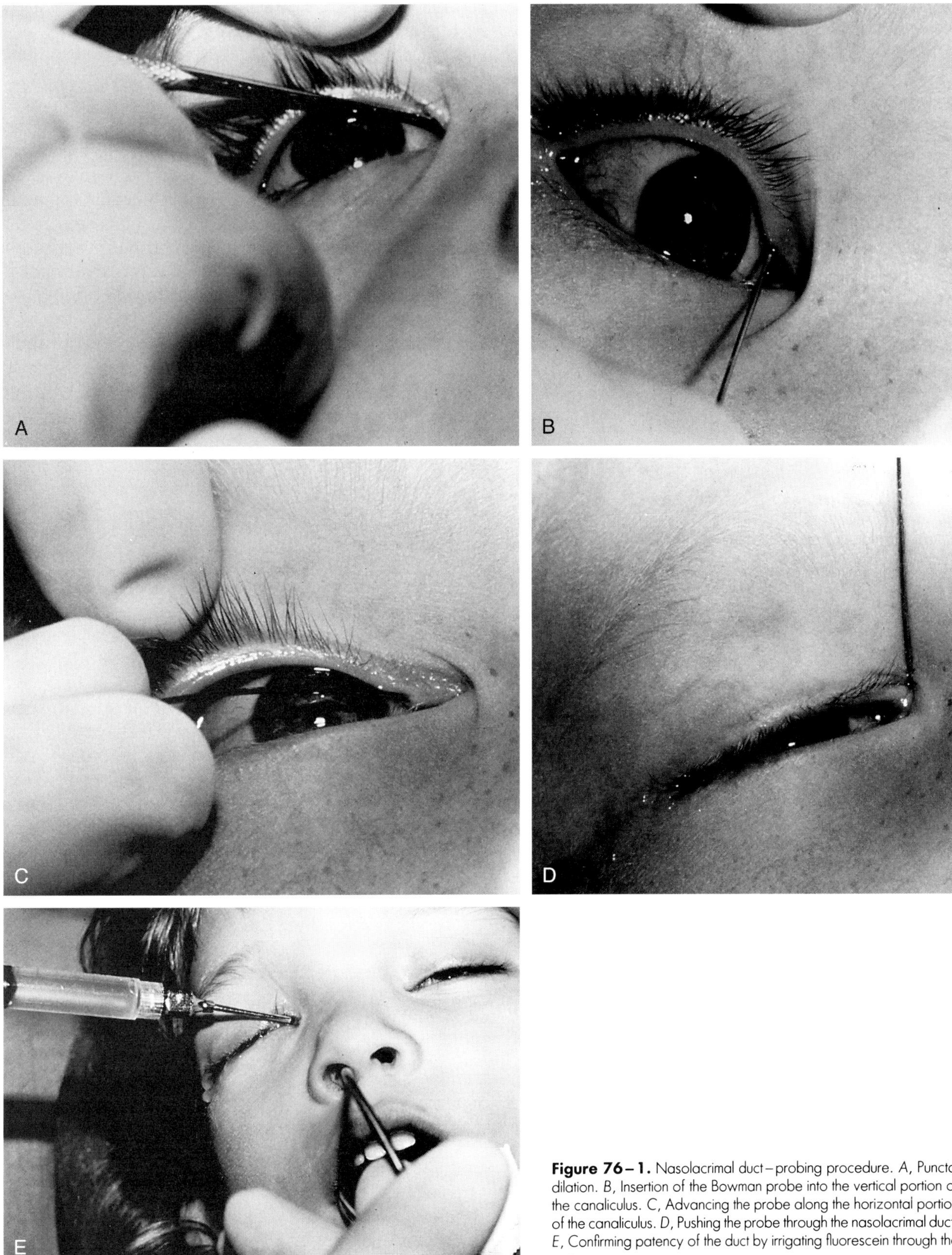

Figure 76–1. Nasolacrimal duct–probing procedure. *A*, Punctal dilation. *B*, Insertion of the Bowman probe into the vertical portion of the canaliculus. *C*, Advancing the probe along the horizontal portion of the canaliculus. *D*, Pushing the probe through the nasolacrimal duct. *E*, Confirming patency of the duct by irrigating fluorescein through the system.

hydrostatic pressure within the lacrimal system then causes rupture of the membrane into the nose. The purported advantage of this procedure is that it should avoid damage to the mucosa of the nasolacrimal duct and subsequent scarring. Most surgeons believe this problem is insignificant and that manipulation of the air syringe while occluding the opposing canaliculus may be somewhat difficult. For this reason the technique has not received widespread acceptance.

FAILED NASOLACRIMAL DUCT PROBING

Virtually all authors have reported a better than 90% success rate with probing for congenital nasolacrimal duct obstruction. In a small percentage of patients, however, the initial probing will fail to provide symptomatic relief. These patients can be divided into roughly three groups. In the first group there is a more extensive underlying anatomic abnormality that prevents initial passage of the probe through Hasner's membrane and into the nose. In addition to the common nasolacrimal duct obstruction where the duct extends to the nose but fails to perforate the nasal mucosa leaving an intact imperforate membrane, Jones and Wobig[14] described seven other types of lower nasolacrimal duct obstruction. These include a nasolacrimal duct that remains buried beneath the lateral nasal mucosa extending to the floor of the nose, an absent duct because of failure of the osseous canal to form, or a duct that ends blindly in the medial wall of the maxillary sinus or anterior end of the inferior turbinate. These situations should all be discovered at the time of initial probing because the probe will not be visualized exiting the inferior meatus beneath the inferior turbinate. In those cases in which the nasolacrimal duct remains buried beneath the lateral nasal mucosa, the probe can often be seen beneath the mucosa and a cutdown can be performed to expose it. In this situation, placement of indwelling silicone stents is usually advised to maintain patency of the duct. In cases in which there is lack of development of the bony canal or misdirection into the maxilla or turbinate it is usually necessary to perform a dacryocystorhinostomy. This will be discussed further later.

The second and most common group of patients are those in whom the probe is passed through the duct and into the inferior meatus with ready irrigation of fluid but which in the postoperative period again scars closed. This is often associated with a laterally displaced inferior turbinate bone compromising the opening of the inferior meatus. In those patients in whom an initial probing appeared to reveal an anatomically normal nasolacrimal duct but whose symptoms persist, a repeat probing is combined with therapeutic infracture of the inferior turbinate.[15, 16] In this procedure the inferior turbinate bone is rotated medially and superiorly, causing an increase in the space in the inferior meatus. Although some surgeons have recommended using a hemostat to grasp and infracture the turbinate, this may traumatize the mucosa along the medial wall of the turbinate and may cause septal adhesions. A preferable method is to place a Freer elevator beneath the lateral wall of the middle turbinate and to use this to lever the turbinate medially and superiorly. This avoids trauma to the mucosa along its medial wall. Turbinate infracture has been reported to markedly increase the success rate of repeat probings, and some surgeons[16] have suggested that it should obviate the need for silicone stent intubation in failed probings. Because infracture is simple, is quick, and has very low morbidity, it is now included as part of the initial lacrimal probing and irrigation by many surgeons.

Repeat probing in combination with therapeutic infracture of the turbinate will cure 90% of those patients with normal anatomic nasolacrimal ducts who have failed initial probing. In 10% of patients, however, repeat probing and infracture is still unsuccessful in providing relief. It is presumed that fibrosis at the inferior meatus has resulted in reocclusion of the nasolacrimal duct. In these patients placement of indwelling silicone stents through the superior and inferior canaliculus and down to the nasolacrimal duct is recommended.[17–19] This dilates the inferior meatus and stents it open during the postoperative period. This procedure is carried out under general anesthesia and requires endotracheal intubation. Packing beneath the inferior turbinate with 0.5% Neo-Synephrine will shrink the inferior turbinate and allow visualization of the stents as they exit the inferior meatus. Many different lacrimal stents are available, and all consist of silicone tubing wedged to a metal probe. I prefer Catalano stents, which have a very flexible silver amalgam tip. This allows for atraumatic passage through the canaliculus and duct and ready retrieval beneath the inferior turbinate. One limb of the stent is introduced through the superior canalicular system and down to the nose in a fashion identical to that previously described for probing. The packing is then removed from beneath the inferior meatus, and the tip of the probe is visualized beneath the inferior meatus. If visualization is obscured, then the inferior turbinate should be infractured as previously described. A long, straight hemostat is then used to grasp the tip under direct observation and withdraw it. It is helpful once the probe tip has been observed to withdraw the metal probe partially back through the nasolacrimal duct so that the tip is no longer in contact with the mucosa of the nasal floor. This allows for more atraumatic removal. Once one limb of the stent has been passed in this fashion the opposing limb is then passed through the opposing canaliculus and again visualized beneath the inferior turbinate, grasped, and withdrawn. Some surgeons recommend that the stent be tied with a square knot so that when it is removed it can be withdrawn back up through the nasolacrimal duct and sac and through the canaliculus. Alternately, others recommend suturing of the stent to the lateral wall of the nose so that it can be easily identified and removed.[18] I prefer to pass both limbs of the silicone stent through a silicone encircling element (no. 42 band) and to then tie the stent. This silicone band serves as a stop to prevent inadvertent traction on the silicone tube from displacing the stent up into the duct. Although this prevents inadvertent prolapse of the stent, the disadvantage of this approach is that the stents then have to be removed from within the nose and in young children this requires repeat mask ventilation.

The success rate of silicone intubation for refractory congenital nasolacrimal duct obstruction is reported to be between 83% and 100%.[17-19] The duration of stent employment ranges from 6 weeks[18] to 6 months.[17] Silicone stents are usually very well tolerated but rarely may cause irritation, chronic conjunctivitis, or pyogenic granuloma formation. In addition, if the stents are tied too tightly beneath the inferior meatus they can erode or "cheesewire" through the punctum and cause slit elongation of the canaliculus.

Dacryocystorhinostomy is usually reserved for patients who have failed silicone intubation or those patients with anatomic abnormalities that prevent probing or silicone intubation because of inadequate development of the nasolacrimal duct. The advent of endoscopic assisted transnasal laser dacryocystorhinostomy has proved particularly helpful in the pediatric age group in whom the external scar associated with a standard dacryocystorhinostomy and the possibility of blood loss may be problematic. (This topic is covered elsewhere.) I have found this procedure particularly helpful in dealing with pediatric patients.

CONGENITAL DACRYOCYSTOCELE

Congenital dacryocystocele is a rare variant of nasolacrimal duct obstruction in which there is a coexistent functional block at the valve of Rosenmüller and the valve of Hasner so that fluid within the sac cannot egress back through the internal common punctum or down the duct. When blocked both proximally and distally, fluid accumulates within the sac, causing distention. This condition is also referred to as a dacryocele, mucocele, lacrimal sac cyst, or amniotocele.[20-23] The last term incorrectly suggests that the fluid within the sac is amniotic fluid. In fact, the fluid is respiratory epithelial secretions and the lesion is therefore more like a mucocele. These congenital dacryocystoceles present as a distended lacrimal sac within the first 2 weeks of life. The dacrocystocele manifests itself as a bluish swelling below the medial canthal area (Fig. 76–2). The sac is filled with mucoid material and may become secondarily infected.

Controversy exists whether conservative management or early probing for decompression are preferable. Often the distended dacryocystocele is associated with a "dumbbell" dilation of the distal end of the nasolacrimal duct into the nose presenting as a nasal cyst (Fig. 76–3). This has been reported to occur in between 12% and 87% of patients with congenital dacryocystocele.[22, 23] These nasal extensions of the dacryocystocele may reach sufficient size that they cause respiratory obstruction.[22]

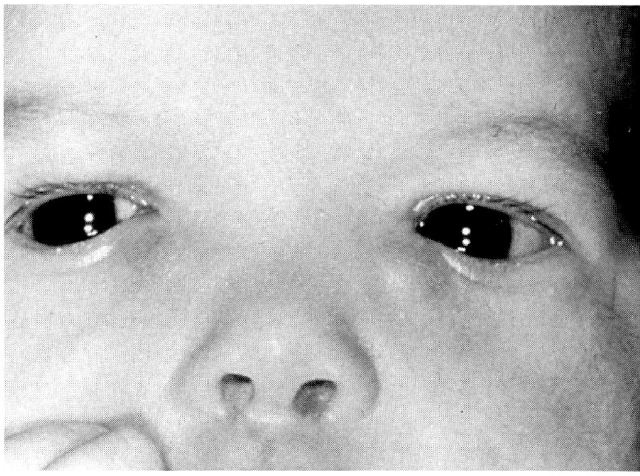

Figure 76–2. Congenital dacryocystocele.

Although the dacryocystocele may spontaneously resolve with canalization of the nasolacrimal duct, secondary infection may develop in up to 75% of cases.[22] Manual compression over the medial canthal distention may allow hydraulic pressure to rupture through into the nose or may allow decompression of the cyst contents back through the canaliculi.

Surgical intervention in the form of probing with or without marsupialization of the intranasal component of the cyst is recommended in cases with dacryocystitis; cellulitis; large dacryocele, which may cause astigmatism and narrowing of the palpebral fissure; recurrent dacryoceles; respiratory difficulty from nasal cysts; or nonreso-

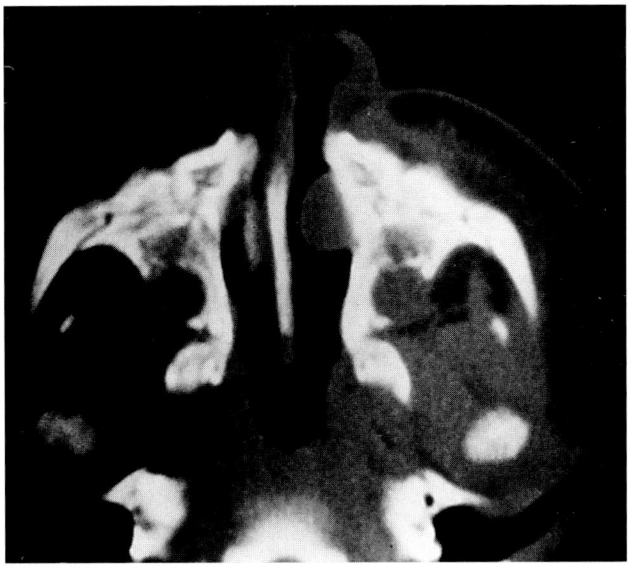

Figure 76–3. Computed tomographic scan of congenital dacryocystocele demonstrating cystic structure in the inferior meatus.

lution of the cyst after initial trial of local massage.[23] Recurrence of the dacryocele has been recorded to occur in 22% of a large series of patients after initial probing. In these cases a second probing was curative.

PROXIMAL NASOLACRIMAL SYSTEM ABNORMALITIES

Although the large majority of congenital lacrimal problems consist of disorders of the distal nasolacrimal duct, embryologic abnormalities during formation of the proximal canaliculi and puncta may also rarely occur. These are usually due to failure of migration of the epithelial cord from the lacrimal sac out to the eyelids or failure of this cord to canalize.

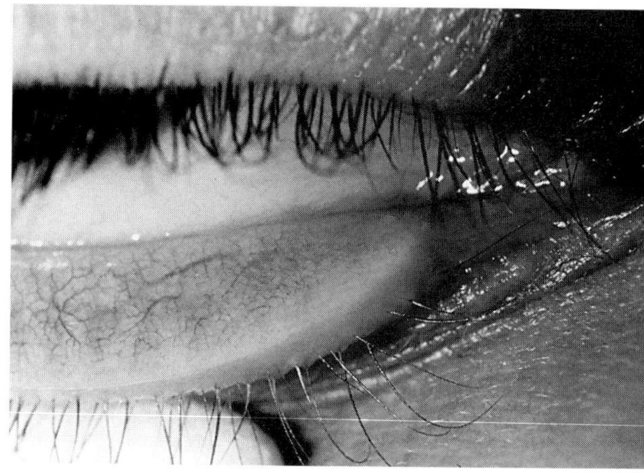

Figure 76–5. Punctal atresia. (Courtesy of Dr. Jeff Nerad.)

PUNCTAL MEMBRANE

An imperforate punctal membrane is a not uncommon cause of epiphora. This occurs when the canalicular epithelium develops and canalizes, but a thin membrane of conjunctiva persists over the punctum (Fig. 76–4). With the aid of the slit lamp it is usually possible to see the patent canaliculus beneath the membrane. Treatment consists of rupture of the membrane with a punctal dilator. Irrigation can then usually be readily accomplished through the remainder of the system.[24]

PUNCTAL AND CANALICULAR AGENESIS

A much more troublesome problem occurs when the canaliculus and punctum fail to develop or canalize. In this circumstance a punctal papillae may or may not be present but no punctal opening can be discerned (Fig. 76–5). When there is agenesis of the punctum, it is not possible to know whether the underlying canaliculus has also failed to develop. Although some surgeons have reported success with microscopic cutdown overlying the anticipated course of the canaliculus in the proximal eyelid, Welham and Hughes[24] reported that 17 of 19 patients with punctal agenesis also had canalicular agenesis. Because patients with punctal or canalicular agenesis are not at risk for dacryocystitis (since their obstruction is above the level of the sac) it may be preferable to delay any surgery until the patient is approximately 10 years of age. If microscopic cutdown and exploration for a proximal canalicular remnant is unsuccessful (as it will be in 90% of cases), then a conjunctival dacryocystorhinostomy with a Pyrex glass tube can be performed under the same anesthesia. Alternately, one may attempt to outline a residual canaliculus by injecting methylene blue dye into the sac and looking for retrograde flow of the dye into the canalicular remnant. In those patients in whom one punctum is present and the opposing punctum is absent, Cahill and Burns[25] have suggested various methods for attempted recanalization and intubation. As a general rule, however, as long as one punctum in the canalicular system is patent, 90% of patients will be asymptomatic and not require treatment.

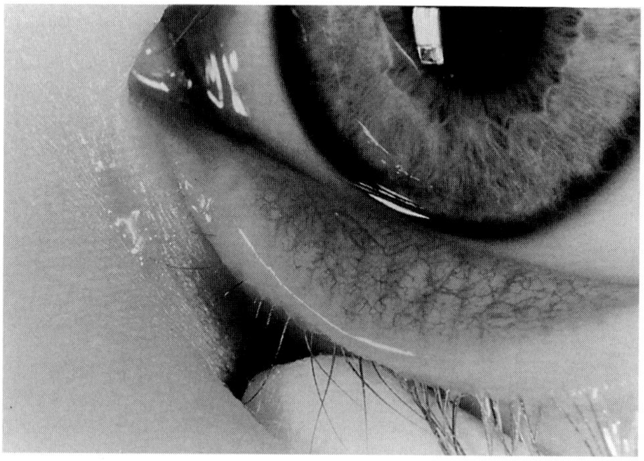

Figure 76–4. Congenital imperforate punctum. (Courtesy of Dr. Jeff Nerad.)

LACRIMAL SAC FISTULA

Congenital lacrimal sac fistulas occur in approximately 1 in 2000 births. They consist of an epithelial-lined fistula track that connects the skin to the common canaliculus or to the lacrimal sac (Fig. 76–6). The fistula is usually asymptomatic and nonprogressive and may be easily overlooked. It occurs just inferonasal to the medial canthal angle and is usually noted only when increased lacrimation may cause tears to exit the fistula and run down the cheek. The pathogenesis is uncertain and is believed to represent either an overdevelopment or outbudding of the lacrimal duct or incomplete closure of the embryonic facial fissure. It is also referred to as an anlage

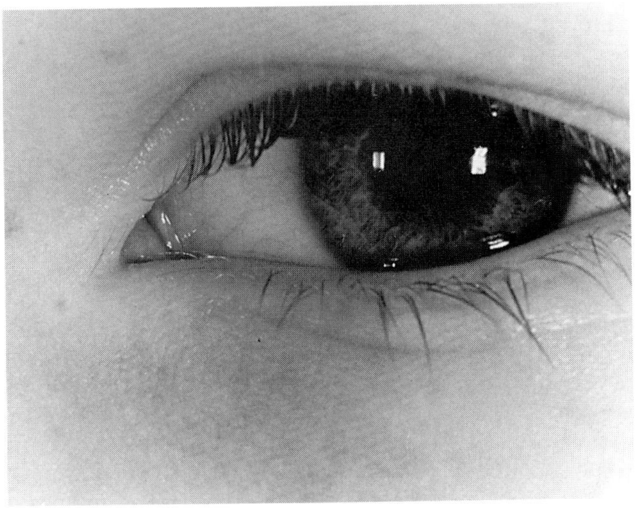

Figure 76–6. Congenital lacrimal fistula. (Courtesy of Dr. Jeff Nerad.)

duct fistula. Approximately one third of patients will have an underlying nasolacrimal duct obstruction.[26] In this case, chronic mucoid discharge may be noted to exit from the fistula, draining the underlying chronic dacryocystitis.

Treatment consists of excision of the epithelial-lined track and closure.[26] This is aided by placement of a Bowman probe into the fistula so that dissection can be carried out proximally toward the lacrimal sac. The excisional site is then sutured closed. In those cases with underlying lacrimal duct obstruction, fistula excision is combined with intubation with indwelling silicone stents. Although other surgeons have advocated this procedure be performed in conjunction with dacryocystorhinostomy,[27] I have not found this necessary.[26]

FACIAL ANOMALIES

Patients with congenital facial anomalies also have an increased incidence of anomalies of the nasolacrimal drainage system. In one large series of patients with facial clefts, 12% were found to have absent puncta, canalicular problems, or nasolacrimal duct obstructions.[28] These various problems usually fall into those categories already described and are handled appropriately on a case-by-case basis. Very severe facial clefting or deformities caused by amniotic band syndrome may be more difficult to treat and may require Jones' tube bypass surgery.

REFERENCES

1. Guerry DP III, Kendig EL Jr: Congenital impatency of the nasal lacrimal duct. Arch Ophthalmol 39:193–204, 1948.
2. Busse H, Muller K, Kroll P: Radiological and histological findings of the lacrimal passages of newborns. Arch Ophthalmol 98:528–532, 1980.
3. Nelson LB, Calhoun JH, Menduke H: Medical management of congenital nasal lacrimal duct obstruction. Ophthalmology 92:1187–1190, 1985.
4. Katowitz JA, Welsh MG: Timing of initial probing and irrigation in congenital nasal lacrimal duct obstruction. Ophthalmology 94:698–705, 1987.
5. Petersen RA, Robb RM: The natural course of congenital obstruction of the nasal lacrimal duct. J Pediatr Ophthalmol Strabismus 15:246–250, 1978.
6. Robb RM: Probing and irrigation for congenital nasal lacrimal duct obstruction. Arch Ophthalmol 104:378–379, 1986.
7. Paul TO: Medical management of congenital nasal lacrimal duct obstruction. J Pediatr Ophthalmol Strabismus 22:68–70, 1985.
8. Yeatts DL, Crum SO: Nasal lacrimal duct probing. Ophthalmic Surg 20:490–493, 1989.
9. Flanagan J: Diseases of the lacrimal apparatus. *In* Harley RD (ed): Pediatric Ophthalmology. Philadelphia, WB Saunders, 1975, pp 224–237.
10. Helveston EM, Ellis FD: The nasolacrimal system. *In* Pediatric Ophthalmology Practice. St. Louis, CV Mosby, 1980, pp 104–107.
11. Putterman AM: Basic oculoplastic surgery. *In* Peyman GA, Sanders DR, Goldberg MF (eds): Principles and Practice of Ophthalmology, 3rd ed. Philadelphia, WB Saunders, 1980, pp 2277–2279.
12. El-Mansoury J, Calhoun JH, Nelson LB, Harley RD: Results of late probing for congenital nasal lacrimal duct obstruction. Ophthalmology 93:1052–1054, 1986.
13. Sevel D: Insufflation treatment of occluded nasal lacrimal apparatus in the child. Ophthalmology 89:329–334, 1982.
14. Jones LT, Wobig JL: Surgery of the Eyelids in Lacrimal System. Birmingham, AL, Aesculapius, 1976, p 160.
15. Havins WE, Wilkins RB: A usual alternative to silicone intubation in congenital nasal lacrimal duct obstructions. Ophthalmic Surg 14:666–670, 1983.
16. Wesley RE: Inferior turbinate fracture in the treatment of congenital nasolacrimal duct obstruction and congenital nasolacrimal duct anomaly. Ophthalmic Surg 16:368–371, 1985.
17. Welsh MG, Katowitz JA: Timing of Silastic tubing removal after intubation for congenital nasal lacrimal duct obstruction. Ophthalmic Plast Reconstr Surg 5:43–48, 1985.
18. Migliori ME, Putterman AM: Silicone intubation for the treatment of congenital lacrimal duct obstruction: Successful results removing the tubes after six weeks. Ophthalmology 95:792–795, 1988.
19. Kraft ST, Crawford JS: Silicone tube intubation in disorders of the lacrimal system in children. Am J Ophthalmol 94:298–299, 1982.
20. Harris GJ, Diclementi D: Congenital dacryocystocele. Arch Ophthalmol 100:1763–1765, 1982.
21. Weinstein GS, Biglan AW, Patterson JH: Congenital lacrimal sac mucoceles. Am J Ophthalmol 94:106–110, 1982.
22. Grin TR, Mertz JS, Stass-Isern M: Congenital nasal lacrimal duct cysts in dacryocystocele. Ophthalmology 98:1238–1242, 1991.
23. Mansour AM, Cheng KP, Mumma JV, et al: Congenital dacryocele: A collaborative review. Ophthalmology 98:1744–1751, 1991.
24. Welham RA, Hughes SM: Lacrimal surgery in children. Am J Ophthalmol 99:27–34, 1985.
25. Cahill KV, Burns JA: Management of epiphora in the presence of congenital punctal and canalicular atresia. Ophthalmic Plast Reconstr Surg 7:167–172, 1991.
26. Birchansky LD, Nerad JA, Kersten RC, Kulwin DR: Management of congenital lacrimal sac fistula. Arch Ophthalmol 108:388–390, 1990.
27. Welham RA, Bergin DJ: Congenital lacrimal fistulas. Arch Ophthalmol 103:545–548, 1985.
28. Whitaker LA, Katowitz JA, Randall P: The nasal lacrimal apparatus in congenital patient anomalies. J Maxillofac Surg 2:59–61, 1974.

CHAPTER 77

Primary Acquired Nasolacrimal Duct Obstruction

Keith D. Carter and Jeffrey A. Nerad

Primary acquired nasolacrimal duct obstruction is a common challenge for ophthalmologists. Patients with this problem frequently present with only epiphora but can have clinical evidence of a chronic, or more severe, acute dacryocystitis. Irrespective of the clinical presentation, most patients do not have an obvious cause for their nasolacrimal duct obstruction. They commonly have no history of facial trauma, sinus disease, and nasal or sinus surgery. Contrary to congenital nasolacrimal duct obstruction, this type of lacrimal obstruction typically presents in the fifth to seventh decade of life, affecting women approximately three times more frequently than men.[1-5] Proper evaluation of these patients requires a careful attention to clinical history, a comprehensive clinical examination, and occasionally further ancillary tests to determine the anatomic site of the tear drainage obstruction. Only after the anatomic site of lacrimal obstruction is identified can the appropriate treatment modality be determined.

LACRIMAL ANATOMY

The excretory portion of the lacrimal system is divided into an upper and lower system. The upper system begins at the punctum and ends at the lacrimal sac. The drainage of tears begins at the punctum, located at the medial portion of both the upper and lower eyelids. The punctal opening is approximately 0.3 mm^2,[6] lies in the plica semilunaris of the conjunctiva, and is inverted against the globe. The normally positioned punctum should not be visible without slight eversion of the eyelid. The upper eyelid punctum rests slightly medial to the lower eyelid punctum. The canaliculus begins with a vertical 2 mm section, which then turns horizontally across the eyelid for 8 to 12 mm. Each canaliculus terminates at the lacrimal sac, forming a common canaliculus in most patients before it enters the lateral wall of the lacrimal sac.

The lower system begins at the lacrimal sac and ends at the opening of the nasolacrimal duct beneath the inferior turbinate. The lacrimal sac rests in a fossa composed of the lacrimal bone and the frontal process of the maxilla. The sac extends 3 to 5 mm above the level of entry of the canaliculi. The body of the sac is 10 mm long and drains into the nasolacrimal duct. The nasolacrimal duct carries tears 12 mm through the intraosseous portion of the maxilla and empties into the superior aspect of the inferior meatus (Fig. 77–1).

The anterior ethmoid air cells represent another important anatomic area in lacrimal surgery. These cells are commonly encountered during dacryocystorhinostomy surgery, and their proper identification is required to avoid draining the lacrimal sac into the ethmoid sinuses. These air cells have been shown to extend anteriorly to lie adjacent to the lacrimal sac fossa in 93% of orbits, with 40% of the cells extending into the frontal process of the maxilla (Fig. 77–2).[7] These air cells are usually encountered during the phase of the operation that involves the superior portion of the lacrimal sac fossa.

CAUSE

The cause of primary acquired nasolacrimal duct obstruction remains unknown. Past work focused on the osseous canal and attempted to explain its possible contribution to the nasolacrimal duct narrowing. Autopsy series have demonstrated that the nasolacrimal duct is longer and narrower in women and Caucasians[8, 9]; however, other work has demonstrated interpersonal variation in the size of the canal.[10] In addition, radiographic evidence indicates that the size of the inlet of the duct is comparable between normal patients and patients with nasolacrimal duct obstruction.[11] These studies show that osseous changes alone are not the principal cause for duct narrowing.

The pathogenesis of primary acquired nasolacrimal duct obstruction is currently thought to be secondary to involutional narrowing of the membranous nasolacrimal duct. Linberg and McCormick[12] coined the term PANDO for primary acquired nasolacrimal duct obstruction. They showed that the narrowing is attributable to a chronic inflammatory process within the nasolacrimal duct. This process causes compression of the duct by

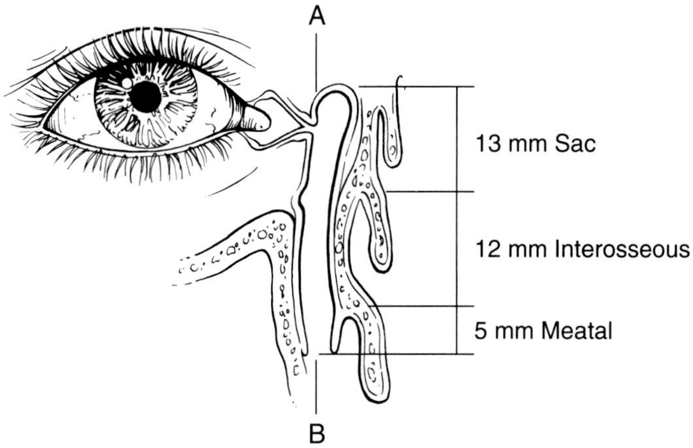

Figure 77 – 1. The anatomy and dimensions of the upper and lower lacrimal system. *A*, Valve of Rosenmüller; *B*, valve of Hanser.

inflammatory infiltrates and edema, but the duct remains partially patent. The lacrimal system of patients with obstruction at this stage can be irrigated and a functional block can be demonstrated. As this inflammatory process continues, the duct is obliterated by a fibrotic reaction (anatomic block), and the patient displays symptoms of epiphora or chronic dacryocystitis. This inflammatory process and resultant fibrosis appear to involve the entire course of the duct.

CLINICAL PRESENTATION

Patients with primary acquired nasolacrimal duct obstruction most commonly present with a history of epiphora. This tearing is often variable but may be bothersome daily. A chronic dacryocystitis owing to tear stasis can show a mucopurulent discharge at the punctum, or pus can be expressed from the punctum by massage of the lacrimal sac (Fig. 77 – 3*A*). Signs of acute dacryocystitis with an enlarged lacrimal sac and erythema of the skin overlying the lacrimal sac may also appear (see Fig. 77 – 3*B*).

The presence of epiphora alone requires a complete ocular and lacrimal examination because other ocular pathology, such as ocular surface problems, eyelid malpositions, facial palsy, or canalicular stenosis, may be the cause. Signs and symptoms of chronic or acute dacryocystitis indicate a nasolacrimal duct obstruction. When

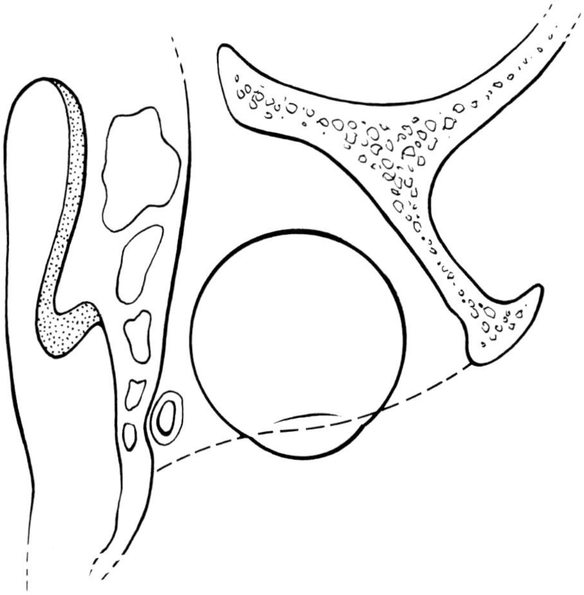

Figure 77 – 2. Schematic diagram showing the relationship of the lacrimal sac, middle turbinate, and anterior extension of ethmoidal air cells.

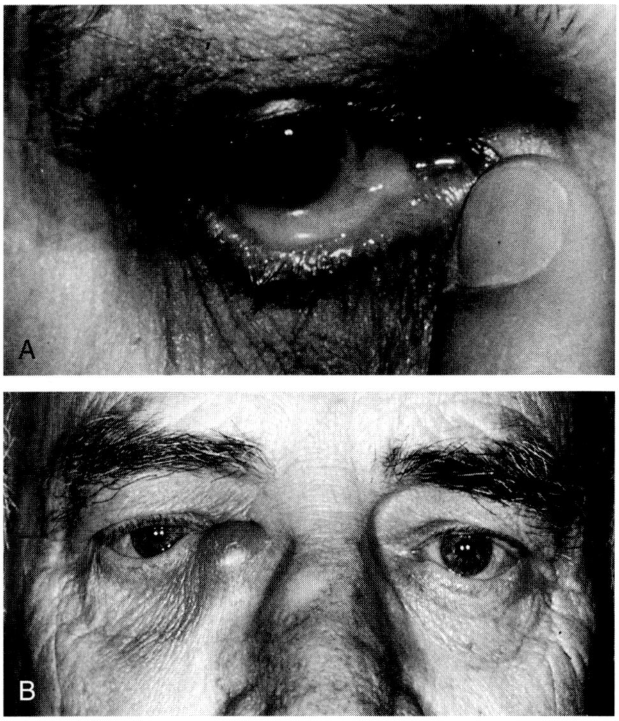

Figure 77 – 3. *A*, Chronic dacryocystitis. Note mucopurulent discharge, but no surrounding cellulitis. *B*, Acute dacryocystitis in a 47-year-old man. Note the enlarged lacrimal sac with associated erythema.

acute or chronic dacryocystitis is present, lacrimal irrigation should not be performed.

In the tearing patient with a functional block, irrigation of the lacrimal system is possible because the irrigating syringe can generate a pressure that is high enough to force water beyond a partial obstruction. The physiologic pressure generated by the lacrimal pump, however, is inadequate, leading to epiphora. More commonly, clinical testing shows delayed dye disappearance, negative Jones primary and secondary dye tests (no dye recovered), and reflux of fluid from the canaliculus when the lacrimal system is irrigated. These findings are all compatible with a complete, or anatomic, lacrimal duct obstruction.

Evaluation of the nose is imperative to ensure that nasal pathology is not the cause of the lacrimal drainage problem. Any pathologic condition, such as a deviated septum, nasal polyps, or a mucosal mass or erosion, should be treated before definitive lacrimal surgery is attempted. Checking for adequate space between the lateral wall of the nose, the middle turbinate, and the septum is important if surgical treatment is to be successful. Adhesions between the created ostium and the middle turbinate or nasal septum are a common cause of dacryocystorhinostomy failure.

Signs of acute dacryocystitis (see Fig. 77–3*B*) represent an inflammatory response in the lacrimal sac that results from tear stasis and bacterial overgrowth. The commonest cause in adults is primary acquired nasolacrimal duct obstruction. Externally, swelling in the medial canthal area occurs below the medial canthal tendon overlying the lacrimal sac, with associated erythema. Frequently, the mass may be fluctuant and may represent an abscess. Severe pain is common. Initial treatment is directed toward resolution of the infection. Warm compresses should be applied to the affected area as often as the patient can tolerate. If the abscess is localized and fluctuant, it should be incised and drained. We attempt to place the drainage site in the location of the future dacryocystorhinostomy incision to decrease the likelihood of development of a draining skin fistula, a complication that is associated with lacrimal sac abscesses. Cultures are taken for a causative organism and antibiotic sensitivity. Common causative organisms include *Staphylococcus*, *β*-hemolytic *Streptococcus*, and *Streptococcus pneumoniae*. The abscess cavity is then packed with one half-inch iodoform gauze. Antibiotic coverage should include penicillinase-producing organisms. If the infection is considered mild, oral antibiotics may be used, but most patients require parenteral antibiotics to control the infection. Once the acute event is resolved, these patients require a dacryocystorhinostomy.

Patients with chronic dacryocystitis report having epiphora, recurring conjunctivitis, and reflux of a mucopurulent discharge on palpation of the lacrimal sac on the side of the obstruction (see Fig. 77–3*A*). These patients do not have pain, and many say that they have learned to decompress their lacrimal sac daily to decrease the amount of discharge. Medical treatment consists of topical antibiotic administration and massage to decrease the bacterial flora, but this is only a temporizing measure. Definitive treatment of chronic dacryocystitis is dacryocystorhinostomy.

DACRYOCYSTORHINOSTOMY

History

Correcting blockage of tear flow and subsequent infections dates back to Celsus (25 B.C.), who excised the involved tissue down to bone and burned it with a hot iron.[13] Archigenes (second century A.D.) destroyed the lacrimal sac with caustics and bored several holes into the nose.[13] The original external dacryocystorhinostomy was described by Toti in 1904. This procedure involved the placement of an external skin incision that exposed the lacrimal sac. The sac was then opened with its medial wall excised, the nasal bone was removed with a hammer and chisel, and the adjacent nasal mucosa was excised. The skin incision was then closed. Toti's success was approximately 50%.[14] The creation of anterior and posterior flaps was introduced by Ohm[15] and Dupuy-Dutemps and Bourguet.[16] Their addition to Toti's work was to create anterior and posterior flaps of the lacrimal sac and nasal mucosa and to suture these flaps together. This modification improved the procedure's success rate to 94%.[16] This method is basically the procedure that is employed today. Mosher also modified Toti's procedure by enlarging the lacrimal sac opening, excising the nasal mucosa to the edge of the ostium, and intranasally removing the anterior portion of the middle turbinate. This modification did not use flaps, but the anterior margin of the lacrimal sac was sutured to tissue above the bony ostium. The success rate was 90%.[17] The debate about the use of flaps continues today, with successful results of better than 90% with or without their use.[1, 18–20]

Lacrimal sac transplantation, in which the sac is excised from the nasolacrimal duct, rotated into a bony ostium, and secured with nasal sutures, has also been successfully performed[21, 22] but is not a common practice.

The bony ostium has been created in many ways, using instruments such as dental burrs, bone chisels, rongeurs, oscillating saws, and trephines (Iliff trephine).[23] The size of the ostium created was once thought to relate to the success of the procedure. The size of the healed ostium can be approximately 2% of that of the original surgical ostium without affecting the success of the procedure.[24, 25] Apparently, the ostium need be only large enough to allow the anastomosis of the lacrimal sac with the nasal passage. Failures in dacryocystorhinostomy surgery are primarily the result of ostium occlusion from membranous closure or synechiae formation between the ostium and the middle turbinate or a deviated nasal septum. Other causes are malpositioned bony ostia and canalicular obstructions.[26–28]

Attempts to improve on this successful surgical procedure have centered on placement of stenting material, such as gauze, suture, rubber catheter,[23] nasal catheter,[29] silicone tubes,[30] and inflatable catheters,[31] across the lacrimal sac–nasal mucosal anastomosis to prevent recurrent obstruction. It is apparent that the basic technique of the dacryocystorhinostomy surgery is good and has provided excellent results. Improving on this success by using flaps of lacrimal sac and nasal mucosa, or by stenting this anastomosis, has failed to provide an absolute method of cure. The procedure of choice continues to evolve.

Procedure

Proper preoperative evaluation of patients undergoing a dacryocystorhinostomy is important. The commonest problem with this procedure is bleeding. Talking with the patient about his or her medical history allows detection of preventable causes of bleeding. Any past history of excessive bleeding during surgery is important. A history of cardiac problems, such as a previous myocardial infarction, cardiac valve dysfunction, or cerebral vascular insufficiencies, might indicate the possible need for anticoagulants. Administration of drugs such as warfarin sodium (Coumadin), aspirin or aspirin-containing products, and nonsteroidal anti-inflammatory agents decreases the patient's coagulation status. Consultation with the patient's prescribing physician assists in the determination of how to properly handle these medications.

Generally, a patient taking warfarin sodium should discontinue taking it for 3 to 4 days before surgery, and a prothrombin time should be obtained. The prothrombin time should have decreased to a normal range before the procedure is performed. If the patient's medical condition precludes discontinuation of anticoagulation therapy, then heparin should be substituted for warfarin sodium. The heparin should be stopped approximately 6 hours before the surgery. A partial thromboplastin time should be checked to monitor the effects of the heparin on coagulation. The heparin and the warfarin sodium therapy should be resumed postoperatively until the prothrombin time is adequate for the heparin to be discontinued.

Aspirin and aspirin-containing products (e.g., Anacin, Ecotrin, Bufferin, Alka-Seltzer) inhibit platelet function and should not be taken 2 to 3 weeks before surgery. If concern exists about the coagulation state preoperatively, a bleeding time should be obtained. Nonsteroidal anti-inflammatory agents (e.g., Feldene, Motrin, Indocin) have a shorter duration of action on platelet function, but they should not be taken 3 days before surgery. Often, patients taking these medications do not consider them to be as important as other prescription medicines and do not include them in the medical history. For this reason, specific inquiries should be made with regard to these medications.

The patient can elect to be under either general or local anesthesia during the dacryocystorhinostomy. We perform most of our procedures with the patient under local anesthesia unless he or she desires general anesthesia. Our local anesthetic consists of a mixture of 2% lidocaine (Xylocaine) with 1 : 100,000 epinephrine and 0.75% bupivacaine (Sensorcaine-MPF). If general anesthesia is used, we use only 1% lidocaine with 1 : 100,000 epinephrine for the hemostatic effect of the epinephrine. The surgeon should use a fiberoptic headlight source and surgical loupes to facilitate visualization of the surgical field.

Three important steps exist in the dacryocystorhinostomy procedure: (1) the skin incision and identification of the lacrimal sac, (2) the formation of the ostium and flaps, and (3) the proper closure of the wound. The surgical approach, cutting instruments, flap formation, and use of stents is based on the preference of the surgeon. Our approach follows.

The patient is placed in the supine position with the operating table at 10 to 15 degrees in reverse Trendelenburg's position. This position decreases venous bleeding. Intravenous sedation of midazolam hydrochloride (Versed) or another sedative of choice is given. The nasal mucosa is decongested through spraying with 5% cocaine solution or oxymetazoline hydrochloride 0.05% (Afrin) if cocaine administration is contraindicated. Because oxymetazoline is an effective vasoconstrictor, but unlike cocaine, it lacks local anesthetic properties; therefore, its use is limited to general anesthesia cases. The use of the general anesthesia halothane is relatively contraindicated with cocaine because both agents sensitize the myocardium. The nose is packed with neurosurgical cottonoids (0.5 × 3 inch) that have been soaked in the same vasoconstricting solution and then wrung dry. Packing the nose properly is very important in controlling bleeding during the procedure. The physician will see the inferior turbinate by looking straight into the nose, parallel to the plane of the hard palate. The physician must look above this landmark to find the middle turbinate. The cottonoid is placed anterior and lateral to the tip of the middle turbinate (Fig. 77–4).

The skin is marked with gentian violet after being defatted using isopropyl alcohol. The incision line is located midway between the bridge of the nose and the medial canthus (Fig. 77–5). We place this incision closer to the medial canthus if the patient has a high nasal bridge. This incision should be close to the anterior lacrimal crest, but not on eyelid skin or crossing a concavity so to avoid excessive scarring or webbing. The subcutaneous tissue is infiltrated with local anesthetic (Fig. 77–6). The injection is extended down to the level of the periosteum under the skin incision. Next, the local anesthetic is injected into the lacrimal sac, and care is taken not to push the needle into the nose (see Fig. 77–6). The injection should be performed at least 10 minutes before the start

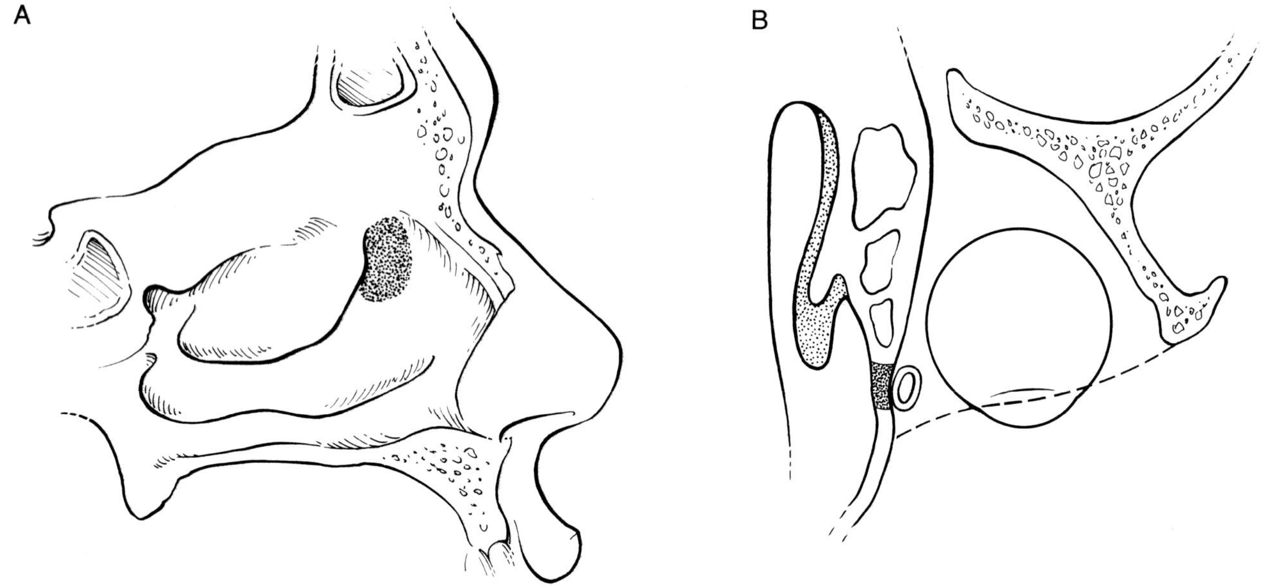

Figure 77–4. Sagittal (A) and axial (B) view of the nasal cavity showing the relationship of the ostium formed during the dacryocystorhinostomy and the middle turbinate. Anterior to the middle turbinate is the proper site for the nasal packing.

of the procedure to allow for the hemostatic action of epinephrine to take effect. The patient's surgical preparation and draping are then performed.

The procedure begins with a full-thickness skin incision using a no. 15 Bard-Parker blade. We do not make this initial incision down to periosteum but use Stevens scissors to bluntly dissect through the orbicularis to the level of the periosteum. The scissors tips are placed on the periosteum, and the blades are spread open, parallel to the orbicularis fibers (Fig. 77–7). This maneuver does not damage the angular vessels. If bleeding is encountered, a bipolar cautery is used to coagulate these vessels. We maintain retraction by placing four 4-0 black silk sutures through skin and muscle on the edges of the wound and securing the suture to the surgical drape. Once the periosteum is in view, it is incised using the sharp end of a Freer periosteal elevator in the surgeon's dominant hand. A suction tip in the nondominant hand is used to keep the surgical field bloodless. The periosteum is reflected off the frontal process of the maxilla to identify the anterior lacrimal crest. The innominate suture (sutura notha)

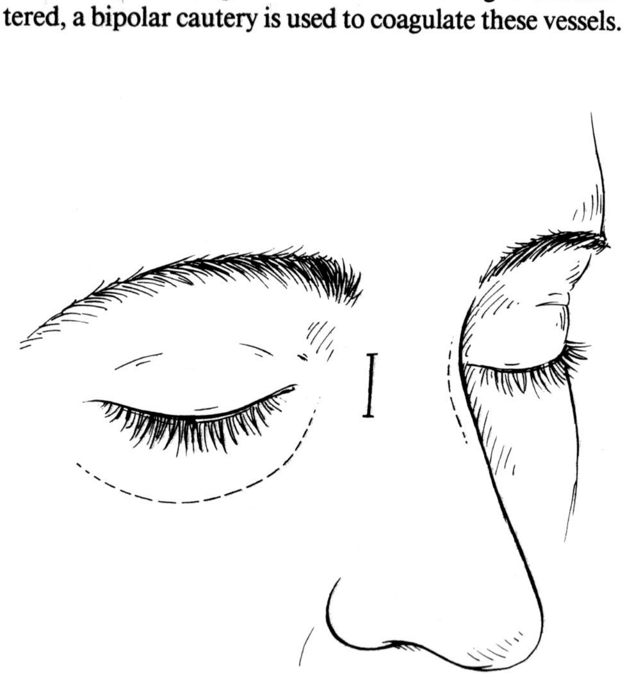

Figure 77–5. The incision is drawn midway between the bridge of the nose and the medial canthus. The direction is toward the lateral cartilage of the nose and is 1 to 1.5 cm.

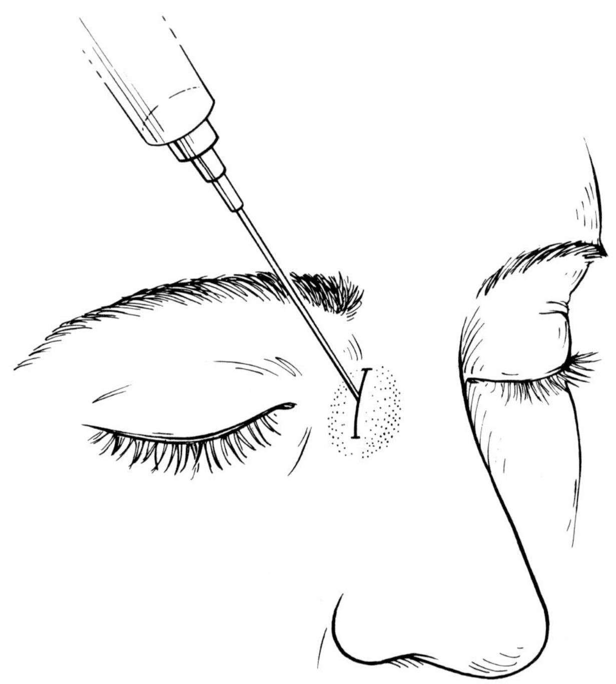

Figure 77–6. The local anesthetic is initially injected throughout the incision site, followed by injection of the lacrimal sac.

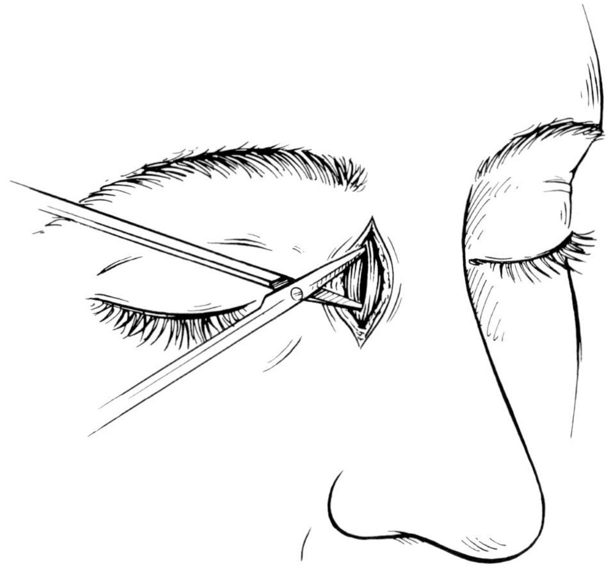

Figure 77–7. Stevens scissors are used to bluntly dissect the orbicularis to expose the periosteum.

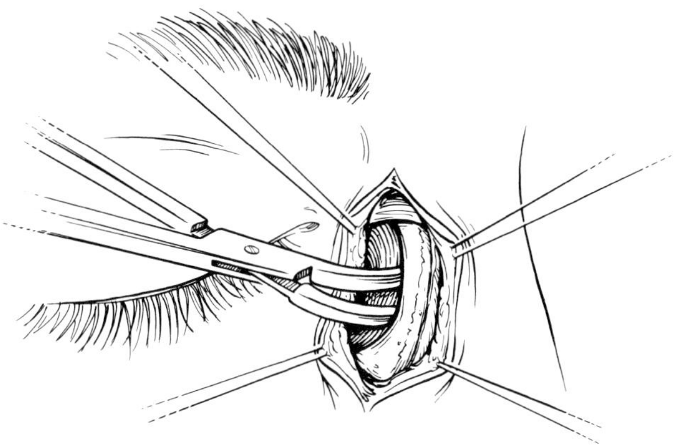

Figure 77–9. The curved hemostat is used to break the thin bone of the lacrimal sac fossa. The hemostat is opened to enlarge this break to enable entry of a Hardy sella punch.

is found 1 to 2 mm anterior to the anterior lacrimal crest. A branch of the infraorbital artery runs in this groove and can lead to bleeding that requires unipolar cautery or bone wax for control. Once the anterior lacrimal crest is located, the periorbita of the lacrimal sac is elevated from the floor of the lacrimal sac fossa, with care being taken not to damage the lacrimal sac (Fig. 77–8).

Once the lacrimal sac fossa is visualized, the thin area in the floor of the lacrimal fossa is punctured with a curved hemostat or Freer elevator. Care is taken to avoid damaging the underlying nasal mucosa (Fig. 77–9). The hole in the bone is carefully enlarged. The lacrimomaxillary suture is located at the posterior two thirds of the fossa floor. Generally, this area is the thinnest in the fossa and the easiest area to enter. Penetrating the fossa inferiorly makes it less likely that the hemostat or Freer elevator will enter ethmoidal air cells if present.

Occasionally, a drill with a small burr may be used to fashion the ostium if the bone is thick (Fig. 77–10). This measure is more frequently necessary when the patient has a history of trauma with thickened or loose pieces of bone. In most cases, the ostium formation is begun using an up-biting Hardy sella punch until the osteotomy is large enough to introduce an up-biting Kerrison rongeur. These rongeurs come in various sizes and are used to enlarge the osteotomy to approximately 15 × 15 mm. The blunt tip of the rongeur is placed against the nasal mucosa and then rotated, dissecting the nasal mucosa from the underlying bone. This process allows the cutting edge to slip behind the bone without damaging the nasal mucosa (Fig. 77–11). Damage to the mucosa will lead to persistent bleeding and, interfere with surgical exposure and flap formation.

The anterior border of the ostium is made 3 to 4 mm anterior to the anterior lacrimal crest. The superior border is at the medial canthal tendon, which we do not remove. The superior bone is carefully cut, not cracked, thereby avoiding fractures of the cribriform plate and a

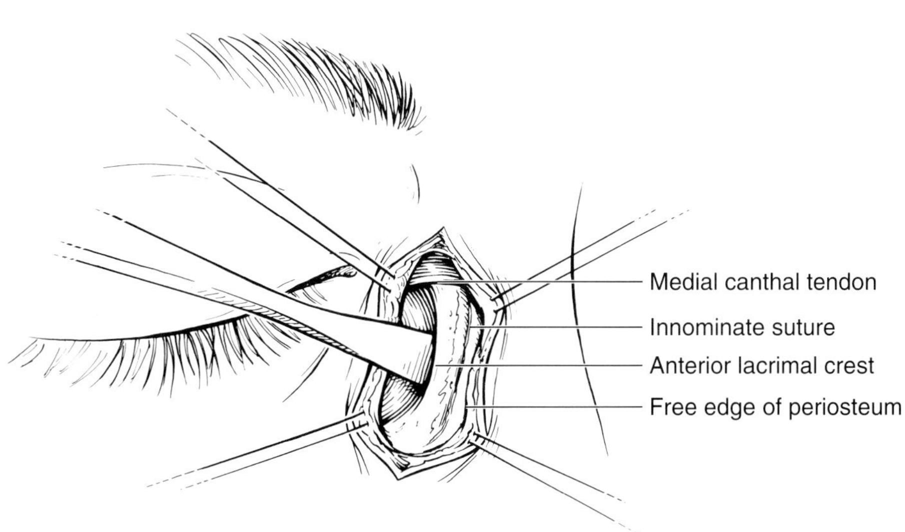

Figure 77–8. The skin edges are retracted using 4-0 silk sutures for exposure and hemostasis. The Freer elevator separates the lacrimal sac from the fossa.

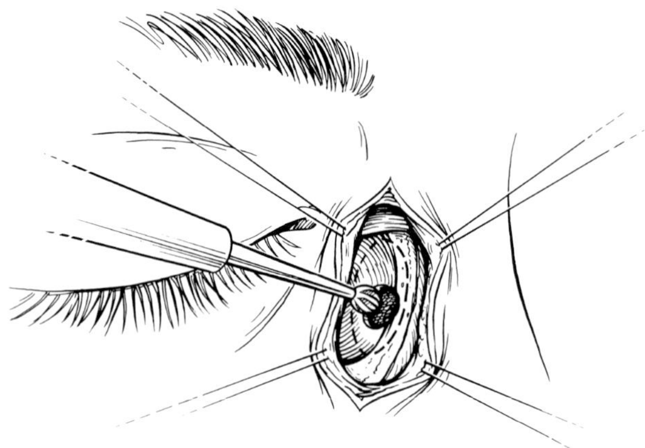

Figure 77–10. A bone bur may be used for thinning thick bone before forming the ostium. Care is taken to avoid cutting the underlying nasal mucosa.

cerebrospinal fluid leak.[32] Some surgeons disinsert the medial canthal tendon to provide better access to the superior portion of the sac. This measure is generally unnecessary; however, any bone adjacent to or near the common internal punctum should be removed. The inferior border of the ostium is formed using a curved Belz lacrimal rongeur to allow removal of approximately 3 mm of the spine of bone between the nasal mucosa and the nasolacrimal duct. Occasionally, removal of anterior ethmoidal air cells between the sac and nasal mucosa is necessary. The ethmoid mucosa is very thin, in contrast to the thicker nasal mucosa. The exact size of the ostium varies from patient to patient but should be sufficient for adequate flap formation. An average dimension is 12 to 15 mm on each side.

After the ostium is complete, the anterior and posterior flaps of the lacrimal sac and the nasal mucosa are formed. Before the nasal flap is formed, the nasal mucosa is injected with local anesthetic that contains epinephrine. This action promotes hemostasis initially by swelling the nasal mucosa and later by imparting the effects of the epinephrine. If bleeding becomes a problem, the source of the bleeding determines the best method of control. Light bleeding from the mucosa stops with bipolar cautery or injection of the mucosa with local anesthetic and epinephrine. Diffuse vigorous bleeding may indicate that the original nasal packing was improperly placed. We occasionally repack the nose or pack the surgical site with cocaine-soaked neurosurgical cottonoids. Other options include temporarily packing the surgical site with absorbable gelatin sponge (Gelfoam or Surgicel) soaked in a thrombin solution.

The lacrimal sac flaps are formed by first placing a no. 0 or no. 1 Bowman nasolacrimal probe through the canalicular system until the tip of this probe tents the sac toward the nasal mucosa (Fig. 77–12). The incision in the lacrimal sac is made using a no. 66 Beaver blade. This incision is positioned over the previously placed probe. The incision extends from the superior border of the sac vertically to the neck of the sac into the nasolacrimal duct. Once this vertical incision is made, the probe is exposed. The blade is turned to form a perpendicular incision at the superior and inferior extent of the sac, allowing the mucosa to open anteriorly and form the anterior lacrimal sac flap. The posterior lacrimal sac flap is made using Westcott scissors. The nasolacrimal probe should be visible in the open sac.

The probe should be advanced until it apposes the nasal mucosa. This point marks the location for the vertical nasal mucosal incision with the no. 66 Beaver blade. The nasal packing is removed. This incision is a repeat of the one in the lacrimal sac. It extends from the superior margin of the ostium to the inferior margin. Perpendicular incisions are made at the margins to form the anterior nasal flap. A small skin hook can be used to elevate the anterior nasal flap and to allow visualization before the posterior nasal flap is cut. Occasionally, additional bone

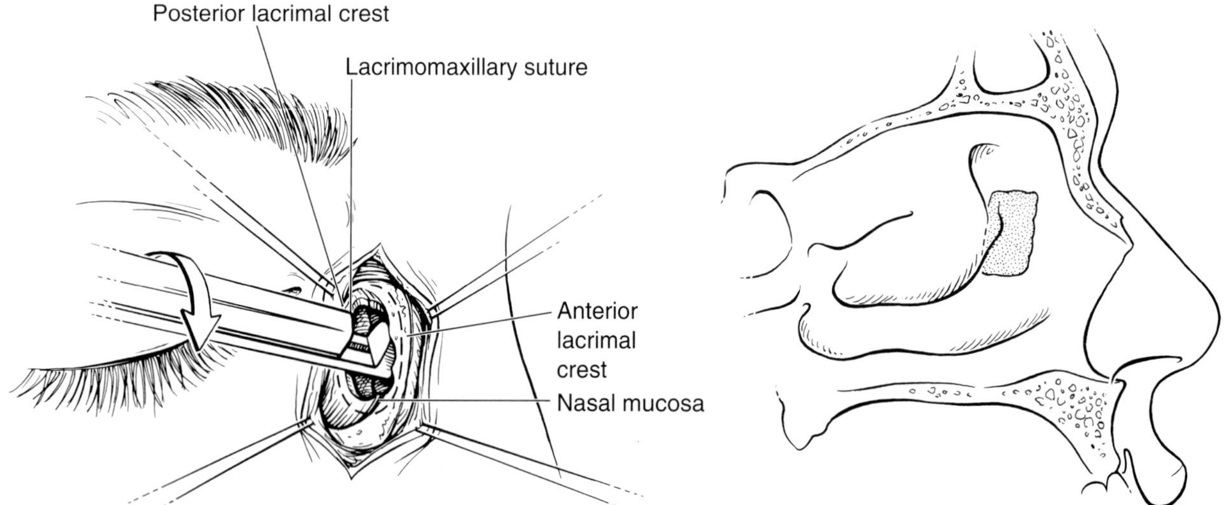

Figure 77–11. *A*, Kerrison rongeurs are used for bone removal. The blunt end of the instrument is placed against the nasal mucosa, and then the cutting edge is rotated behind the bone. This process provides protection for the nasal mucosa. *B*, Sagittal view of the middle turbinate and the ostium.

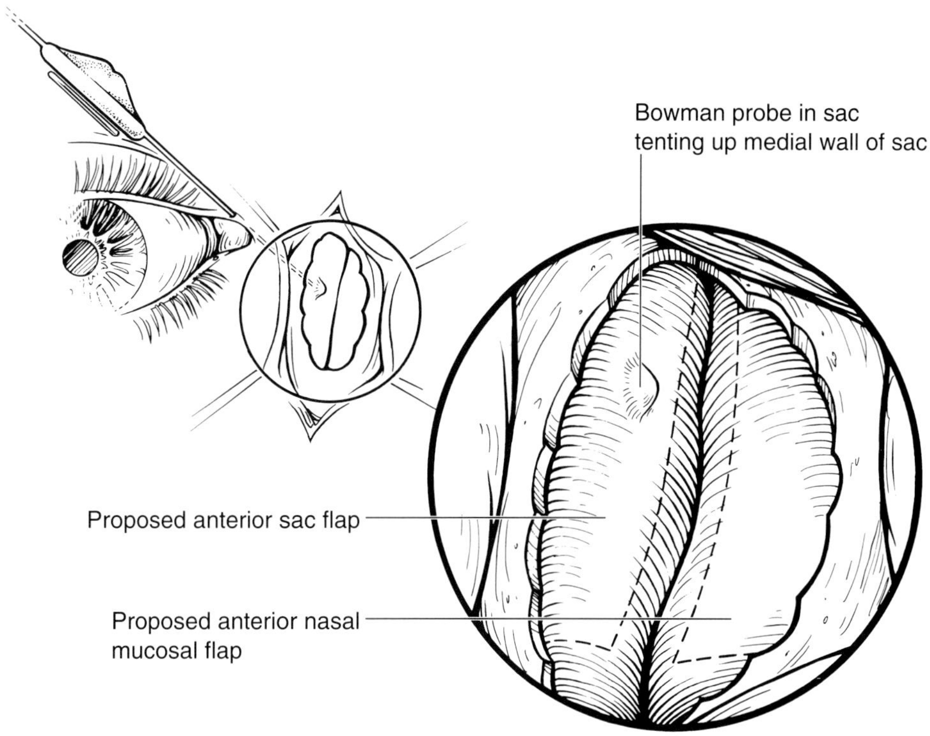

Figure 77–12. Intact lacrimal sac lying next to the nasal mucosa. The lacrimal probe tents the medial wall of the lacrimal sac, indicating the level to incise the sac for flap formation. The intact lacrimal sac is lying next to the nasal mucosa. The nasal flap is positioned at the same level.

removal is necessary to allow mobilization of the anterior nasal flap. These suggestions for flap formation generally work well. In some cases, especially if any of the flaps have been damaged, adjustments must be made when the flaps are cut to ensure that the flaps will easily touch each other to allow suturing of the flaps.

Once the nasal passage is visualized, the position of the middle turbinate should be evaluated. Occasionally, this turbinate may be positioned anteriorly such that it can obstruct the inferior margin of the ostium and lead to postoperative adhesion and subsequent failure (Fig. 77–13). The anterior portion of the turbinate should be injected with the local mixture for hemostasis. By use of rongeurs, the anterior portion of the turbinate is resected until the ostium is cleared. Bleeding is usually minimal.

The posterior flaps are sutured together first. By use of a small-toothed forceps, the posterior flap of nasal mucosa is grasped. A 4-0 polyglactin suture on a P-2 needle is passed from the posterior nasal mucosa flap through the posterior lacrimal sac flap (Fig. 77–14). The small half-circled needle is essential for this step. To decrease friction on these mucosal surfaces, this suture is coated with bone wax before it is passed. The silicone stents are passed through the upper and lower canaliculi into the lacrimal sac, through the bony ostium (Fig. 77–15*A*) and out of the nose, guided with a grooved director that is

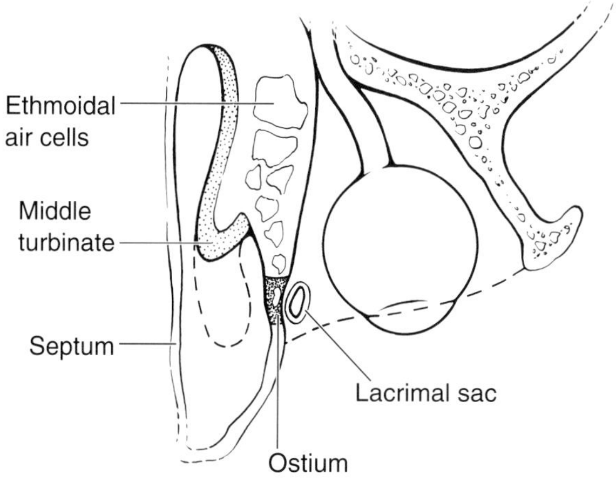

Figure 77–13. Axial view showing relationship of the nasal passage, lacrimal sac, and globe. An enlarged middle tubinate may obstruct the ostium (*dashed line*).

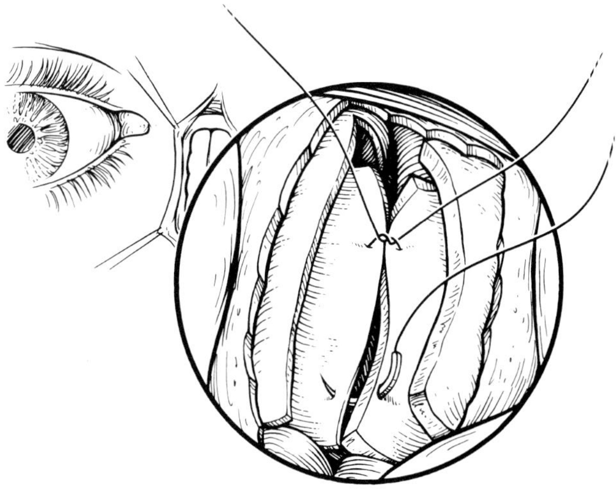

Figure 77–14. The posterior flaps are sutured using a half-circled needle.

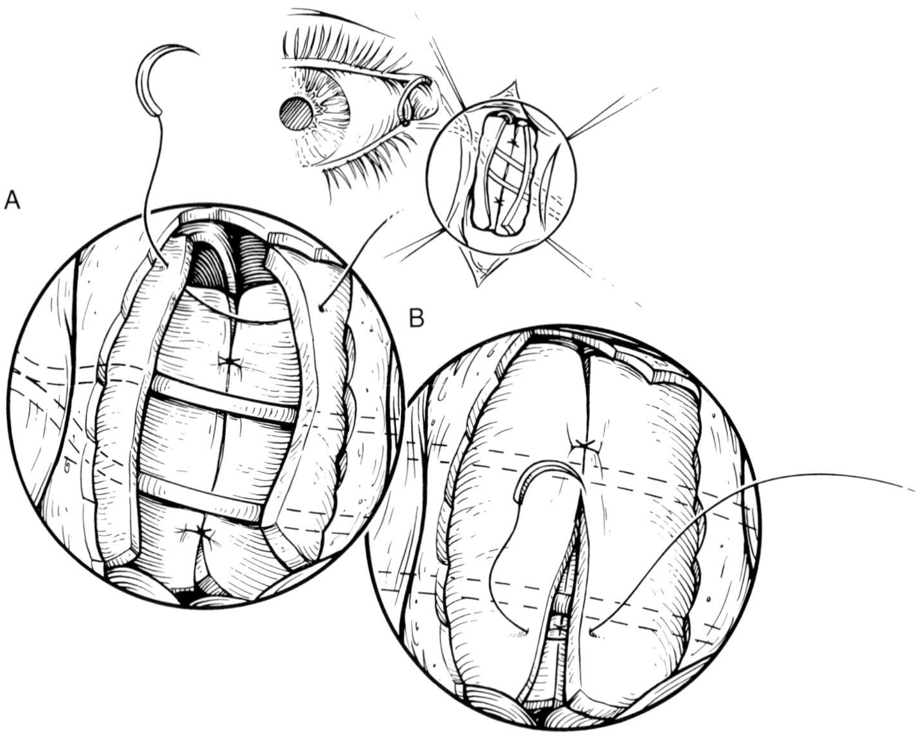

Figure 77 – 15. *A*, Silicone stents are passed through the canaliculi and ostium above the posterior flaps into the nose. *B*, The anterior flaps are closed covering the silicone stents. The stents are positioned between these flaps.

placed up through the nostril. The stents are pulled out of the nose for tying. Some surgeons tie a suture around the stents near the ostium to prevent prolapse of the stent.[33] Once the stent is passed the anterior flaps are sutured together in a similar manner (see Fig. 77 – 15*B*). Because the nasal mucosa flap lacks support, passage of the suture from the anterior lacrimal flap to the nasal mucosal flap allows support of the nasal flap with the needle.

The silicone stent should now be positioned in the space created between the closed posterior and anterior flaps. By use of a Castroviejo needle holder, the silicone stent is grasped within the nasal vestibule at the level where the knot is to remain. The stent is tied using three to four single throws. The silicone knot is allowed to retract within the nose, and the ends are trimmed. Care is taken to check the amount of tension that the stent places on the puncta, so as to prevent punctal stretching or slitting of the canaliculus, which occurs in up to 11% of cases.[3, 4]

The 4-0 silk traction sutures are removed. The subcutaneous tissue is closed with interrupted 5-0 polyglactin sutures. The skin margin is closed with a 7-0 polyglactin suture in a running fashion or using interrupted vertical mattress sutures (Fig. 77 – 16). An antibiotic ointment should be used three times daily for 1 week after surgery. Oral antibiotics are not used unless a resolving acute dacryocystitis is present. Patients should be warned against blowing their nose or sneezing the first few weeks postoperatively. We recommend that patients sneeze with their mouth open to decrease the intranasal pressure. This action prevents tearing of the mucosal flaps and possible orbitopalpebral emphysema. The stents are left in place for up to 1 year and are removed by cutting the stent in the medial canthus and pulling it out of the nose.

Endonasal Dacryocystorhinostomy

Recently, interest has focused on the intranasal approach to dacryocystorhinostomy surgery. The performance of a dacryocystorhinostomy by an endonasal ap-

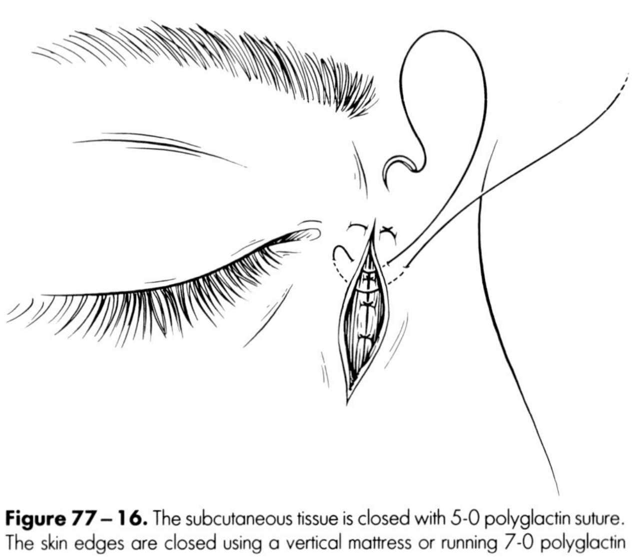

Figure 77 – 16. The subcutaneous tissue is closed with 5-0 polyglactin suture. The skin edges are closed using a vertical mattress or running 7-0 polyglactin suture.

proach provides a direct internal route to the lacrimal sac, thereby eliminating the need for a skin incision and decreasing periorbital ecchymosis and recovery time.

Nasal approaches for dacryocystorhinostomy were described long ago, but direct visualization was limited because of the anterior location of the lacrimal sac and a limited area of the nasal cavity.[35, 36] To improve visualization of the lacrimal sac, an intranasal trans-septal technique was developed that allowed the surgeon to view the involved lacrimal sac from the uninvolved side through a large opening in the nasal septum. These techniques were described by otolaryngologists and have had reported success. Endonasal dacryocystorhinostomy using a microscope for improved visualization has also been described.[37]

The introduction of rigid nasal endoscopes for sinus surgery has allowed visualization of the entire intranasal anatomy. The availability of these endoscopes is excellent because of the interest otolaryngologists have for these instruments in the treatment of sinus disease. These small-diameter endoscopes, which have angled fields of view, are suitable for ophthalmologists to perform endonasal dacryocystorhinostomy surgery under excellent visualization (Fig. 77–17*A* and *B*).

The performance of endonasal dacryocystorhinostomy begins in the same manner as the standard external approach. The patient can elect to have general or local anesthesia. Meticulous hemostasis is important; bleeding interferes with the view through the endoscope and increases the difficulty of this procedure. A nasal packing, consisting of cottonoids soaked in 5% cocaine or 0.05% oxymetazoline hydrochloride and then wrung dry, is placed anterior to the middle turbinate. Later, under endoscopic visualization, the nasal mucosa is infiltrated with 1% lidocaine with epinephrine 1 : 100,000 along the lateral nasal wall, anterosuperior to the middle turbinate. The patient is prepared and draped.

A zero- or 30-degree Hopkins rigid endoscope attached to a video camera is used to provide both the surgeon and the assistant with a view of the operative site. A vertical incision is made that extends from the mucosa over the agger nasi inferiorly for approximately 1 cm using the cutting blade of choice (see Fig. 77–17*C*). The agger nasi is the bony protrusion lying in front of the anterior insertion of the middle turbinate. The mucosa is dissected posteriorly to form a flap and is then excised. The underlying bone is removed with a forceps, curette, or small drill bit until an adequate bony ostium is present. A Bowman lacrimal probe is placed through the canaliculus into the lacrimal sac; this measure will cause the sac to bulge through the bony defect and serve as a guide for the location of the ostium. The size and position of the ostium can be modified after the lacrimal sac is clearly identified. The lacrimal sac is opened with an incision in the center of the exposed sac. The sac flaps are removed with Takahashi forceps. The interior lacrimal sac, with the lacrimal probe extending into the nose through the bony ostium, should be visible. Silicone intubation of the lacrimal system is used to improve patency.[38–40]

Revisions of failed external dacryocystorhinostomies

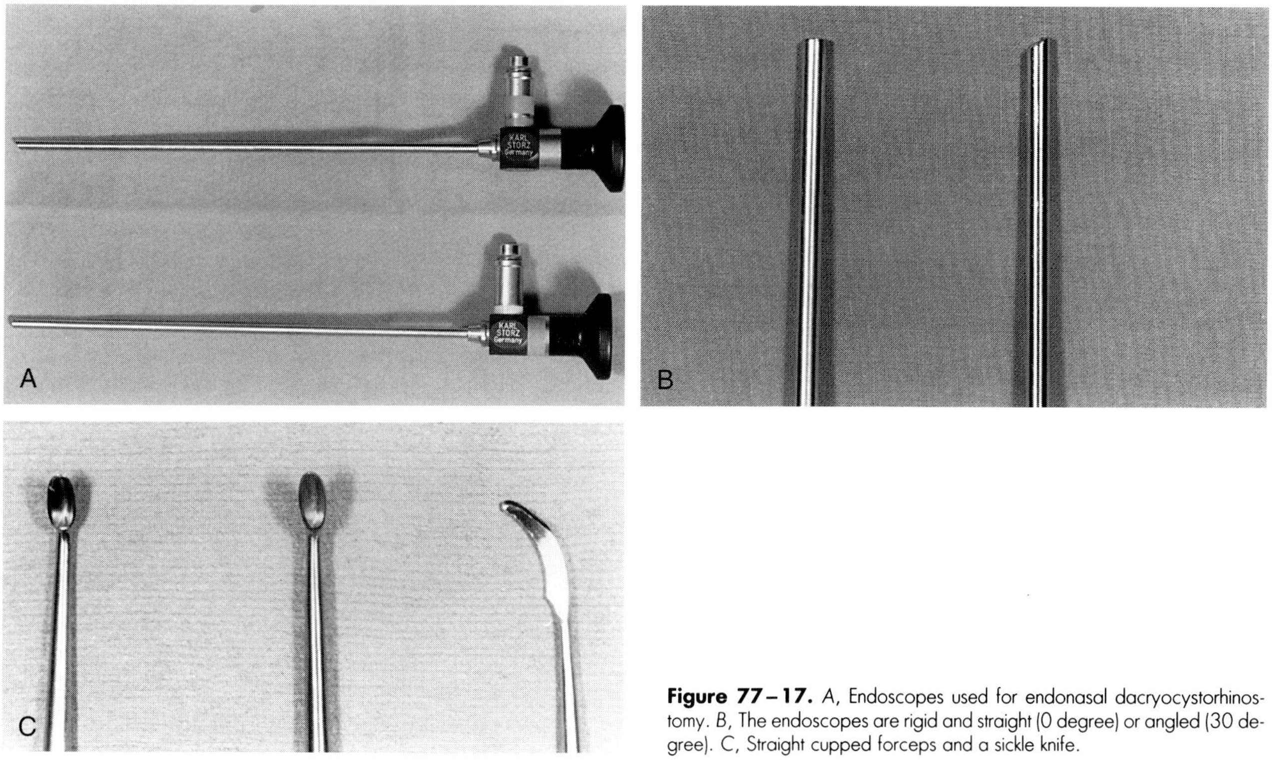

Figure 77–17. *A*, Endoscopes used for endonasal dacryocystorhinostomy. *B*, The endoscopes are rigid and straight (0 degree) or angled (30 degree). *C*, Straight cupped forceps and a sickle knife.

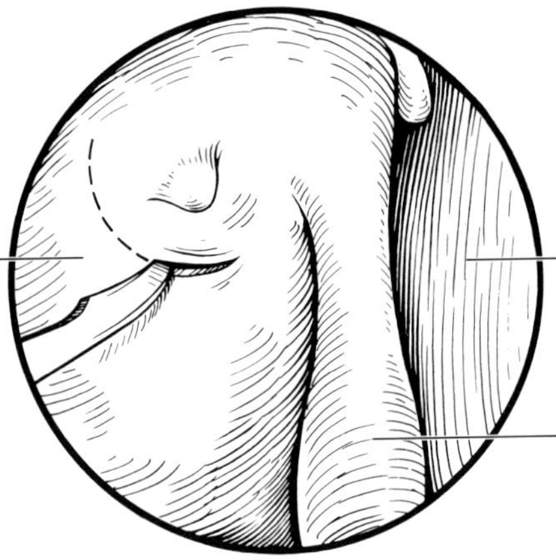

Figure 77–18. Endoscopic view showing the lacrimal probe tenting the occlusive membrane of the lateral nasal wall. A sickle knife is used to open the tissue anterior to the probe.

have been performed endoscopically.[41, 42] Because most failed dacryocystorhinostomies result from membranous occlusion of the ostium or synechiae of the rhinostomy to the middle turbinate or nasal septum, the endoscope can be used to visualize these obstructed areas. The bony ostium is identified by placement of a lacrimal probe through the canaliculus into the lacrimal sac, which pushes the mucosa of the lateral nasal wall into the nasal cavity. An incision is made anterior to the probe, sufficient to open the previously formed ostium (Fig. 77–18). The mucosa or occluding tissue is reflected posteriorly. This dissection is continued until the lacrimal probe is exposed. The scar tissue is removed to provide a final opening of 8 to 10 mm. Care should be taken not to damage the common canaliculus while opening the occluded ostium. The probe should be in full view with adequate space surrounding it when completed. Again, to ensure prolonged patency, silicone intubation is performed. Endoscopically, the mucosa appears to heal within 8 weeks.[41] In two small series for revision of failed external dacyrocystorhinostomies, the success rate was 75% to 87%.[41, 42] When failure of dacryocystorhinostomy results from an inappropriately sized or positioned ostium, a more extensive revision is required.

Recently, lasers were introduced for the creation of endonasal dacryocystorhinostomy. The effect of lasers on tissue depends on the laser's wavelength and power, the beam diameter, and the exposure time. Currently, four lasers are used for endonasal dacryocystorhinostomy: the argon blue-green (488 and 514 nm), potassium titanyl phosphate:yttrium-aluminum-garnet (KTP:YAG [532 nm]), carbon dioxide (10,600 nm), and the holmium:YAG laser (2140 nm). Each of these lasers has unique properties that provide distinct benefits in endonasal surgery. These lasers are capable of tissue coagulation, cutting, and vaporization. Modifications of the spot size and power influence the physical effect that these lasers have on tissue. The carbon dioxide laser has primarily cutting and vaporizing capabilities. When this laser is used, a dry operative field is required because a portion of the laser's energy is absorbed by fluid. The KTP:YAG laser has all three capabilities but has a greater ability to coagulate blood vessels. The holmium:YAG also has the good soft tissue properties mentioned earlier, along with the added feature of bone ablation. All of these except the carbon dioxide laser can be delivered by a flexible fiberoptic system that facilitates endonasal surgery. The carbon dioxide laser has a cumbersome delivery system, which makes its use less desirable in the operating room.

Patient preparation is the same as for a standard dacryocystorhinostomy. Laser precautions are important. Assistants should wear protective eye wear. The endotracheal tube and the patient's eyes should be covered. To avoid flash fires, oxygen should not be given to the patient under local anesthesia during laser use.[43, 44]

The involved side of the nose is entered with the Hopkins rigid endoscope attached to a video camera. The location of the lacrimal sac in the posteroinferior portion of the lacrimal sac fossa is determined by placing a 20-gauge fiberoptic light source through the canaliculus to illuminate the sac. A laser attached to suction catheter is introduced into the nose. These lasers are primarily used in a noncontact or near-contact mode. With the selected laser, the nasal mucosa surrounding the point of illumination is ablated. This tissue ablation is accomplished by the heating of tissue, leading to vaporization of its water content. Care is taken to heat only the involved area and not to produce laser damage to adjacent surfaces. A suction device is required to remove the resulting plume of vapor that is created. Caution must be taken to properly dispose of these vapors because of their potential biologic hazard.[45]

Any char that is created is removed with curettes. Charring is the carbonization of tissue from overheating. Excess charring is avoided by use of appropriate energy levels at the site of action for ablation while avoiding the accumulation of energy that produces charring at the tissue periphery. Once the bone is exposed, the ostium can be formed with the laser or with rongeurs. After a rhinostomy of approximately 5 mm is produced, silicone stents are placed to maintain the patency of the ostium (Fig. 77–19).[43, 46]

Laser technology in lacrimal surgery continues to evolve, and its role in lacrimal surgery will be better defined when increased use allows long-term evaluation of its effectiveness.

SUMMARY

The anatomy and physiology of the lacrimal drainage system are well understood. The cause of primary acquired nasolacrimal duct obstruction appears to be related to a process of acute and chronic inflammation that

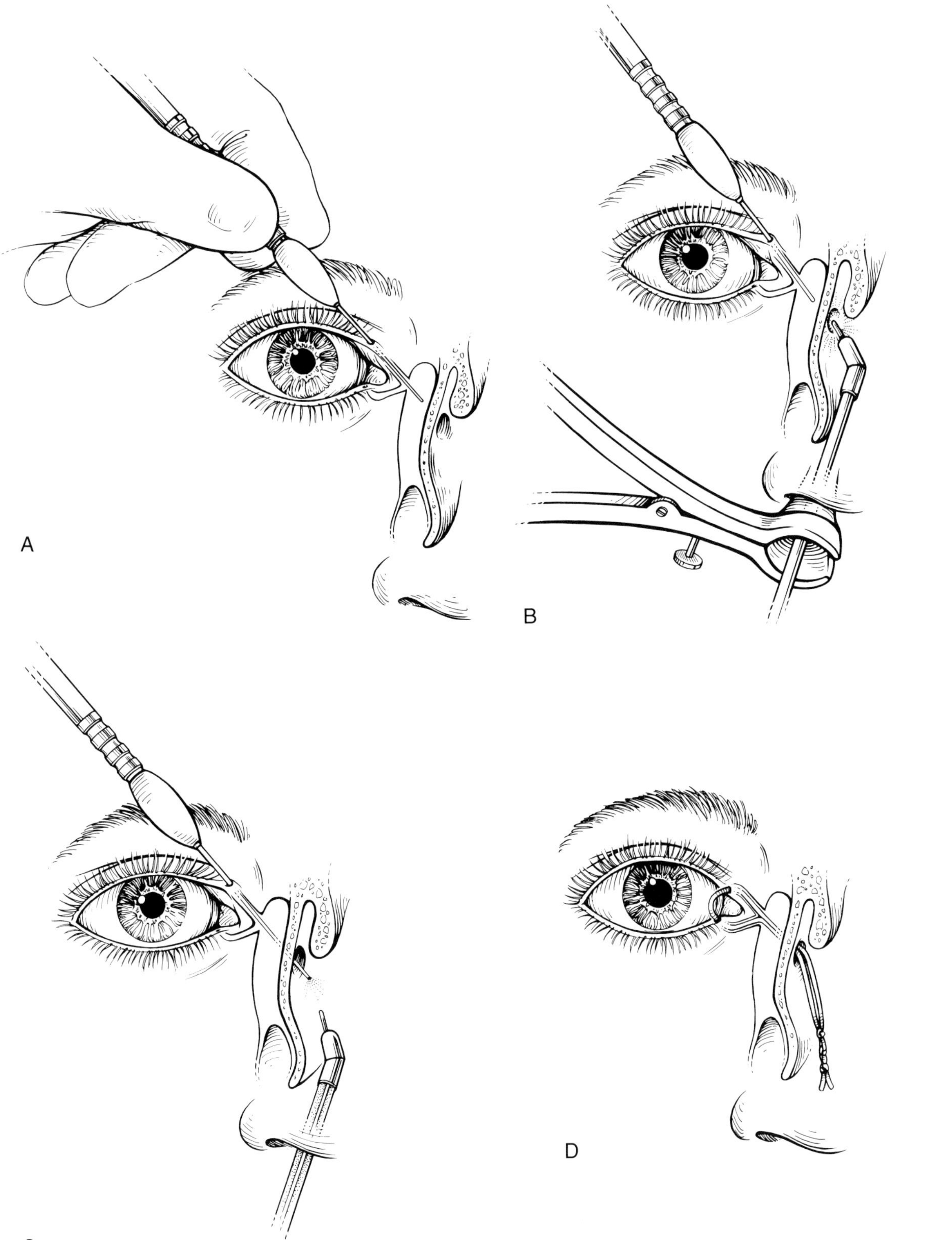

Figure 77 – 19. Performing endonasal laser dacryocystorhinostomy. *A*, Fiberoptic light source identifies the lacrimal sac. *B*, Under endoscopic view the laser with suction catheter is used to ablate tissue. C, The ostium is formed. *D*, Ostium completed with silicone stents in place. (*A* through *D* adapted from Massaro BM, Gonnering RS, Harris GJ: Endonasal laser dacryocystorhinostomy: A new approach to nasolacrimal duct obstruction. Arch Ophthalmol 108(8):1172 – 1176, 1990; Copyright 1990, American Medical Association.)

leads to fibrous occlusion of the duct. Patients with nasolacrimal duct obstruction may present with tearing alone, mucopurulent discharge associated with chronic dacryocystitis, or signs and symptoms of acute dacryocystitis. Although medical treatment controls the infection, surgical treatment is required to provide a long-term cure. Refinements in traditional external dacryocystorhinostomy, use of silicone stents, and use of local anesthesia have provided a high success rate with low morbidity. Innovative new intranasal procedures that use laser technology may prove successful with the promise of a quicker recovery and no requirement for a skin incision.

REFERENCES

1. Burns JA, Cahill KV: Modified kinosian dacryocystorhinostomy: A review of 122 cases. Ophthalmic Surg 16:710–716, 1985.
2. Berryhill BH, Dorenbusch AA: Twenty years experience with intranasal transseptal dacryocystorhinostomy. Laryngoscope 92: 379–381, 1982.
3. McPherson SD, Egleston D: Dacryocystorhinostomy: A review of 106 cases. Am J Ophthalmol 47:328–331, 1959.
4. Iliff CD: A simplified dacryocystorhinostomy: 1954 to 1970. Arch Ophthalmol 85:586–591, 1971.
5. Zolli CL, Shannon GM: Dacryocystorhinostomy: A review of 119 cases. Ophthalmic Surg 13:905–910, 1982.
6. Carter KD, Nelson CC, Martonyi CL: Size variation of the lacrimal punctum in adults. Ophthal Plast Reconst Surg 4:231–233, 1988.
7. Blaylock WK, Moore CA, Linberg JV: Anterior ethmoid anatomy facilitates dacryocystorhinostomy. Arch Ophthalmol 108:1774–1777, 1990.
8. Santos-Fernandez J: The measurements of the nasal canal according to the race. Am J Ophthalmol 4:32–37, 1921.
9. Meller J: Diseases of the lacrymal apparatus. Trans Ophthalmol Soc UK 49:233–311, 1929.
10. Whitnall SE: The naso-lacrimal canal: The extent to which it is formed by the maxilla, and the influence of this upon its calibre. Ophthalmoscope 10:557–558, 1912.
11. Phillips CI, George M. Epiphora and the bony nasolacrimal canal. Br J Ophthalmol 40:673–680, 1956.
12. Linberg JV, McCormick SA: Primary acquired nasolacrimal duct obstruction: A clinicopathologic report and biopsy technique. Ophthalmology 93:1055–1063, 1986.
13. Duke-Elder S, MacFaul PA: Diseases of the lacrimal passages. *In* Duke-Elder S (ed): System of Ophthalmology. The Ocular Adnexa. St. Louis, CV Mosby, 1974, pp 714.
14. Toti A: Nuovo motodo conservatore di cura radicale delle suppurazioni chroniche del sacco lacrimale (dacriocistorinostomia). Clin Mod (Fireze) 10:385–387, 1904.
15. Ohm J: Bericht uber 70 Totische operationen. Zeitschrift fur Auganheilkande 46:37–49, 1921.
16. Dupuy-Dutemps L, Bourguet J: Procede plastique de dacryocystorhinostomy et ses resultats. Ann Oculist 158:241–261, 1921.
17. Mosher HP: The combined intranasal and external operation on the lacrimal sac (Mosher-Toti). Ann Otol Rhinol Laryngol 32:1–14, 1923.
18. Kinosian HJ: A new technique for dacryocystorhinostomy. Arch Ophthalmol 70:33–37, 1963.
19. Romanes GJ: Dacryocystorhinostomy: Clinical report of fifty cases. Br J Ophthalmol 39:237–240, 1955.
20. Becker BB: Dacryocystorhinostomy without flaps. Ophthalmic Surg 19:419–427, 1988.
21. Forsmark E: On dacryocystorhinostomien. Hygiea 73.2:1432–1435, 1911.
22. Gifford HJ: Dacryocystitis, the transplantation operation. Arch Ophthalmol 32:485–487, 1944.
23. Iliff CE: A simplified dacryocystorhinostomy. Trans Am Acad Ophthalmol Otolaryngol 58:590–592, 1954.
24. Bumsted RM, Linberg JV, Anderson RL, et al: External dacryocystorhinostomy: A prospective study comparing the size of the operative and healed ostium. Arch Otolaryngol 108:407–410, 1982.
25. Linberg JV, Anderson RL, Bumsted RM, Barreras R: Study of intranasal ostium external dacryocystorhinostomy. Arch Ophthalmol 100:1758–1762, 1982.
26. Welham RAN, Wulc AE: Management of unsuccessful lacrimal surgery. Br J Ophthalmol 71:152–157, 1987.
27. McLachlan DL, Shannon GM, Flanagan JC: Results of dacryocystorhinostomy: Analysis of the reoperations. Ophthalmic Surg 11:427–430, 1980.
28. Allen KM, Berlin AJ, Levine HL: Intranasal endoscopic analysis of dacryocystorhinostomy failure. Ophthal Plast Reconstr Surg 4:143–145, 1988.
29. Griffiths JD: Nasal catheter use in dacryocystorhinostomy. Ophthal Plast Reconstr Surg 7:177–186, 1991.
30. Quickert MH, Dryden RM: Probes for intubation in lacrimal drainage. Ophthal Plast Reconstr Surg 74:431–433, 1970.
31. Vila-Coro AA, Sevilla MAG, Guijo MdCR-B, et al: Inflatable catheter for dacryocystorhinostomy. Arch Ophthalmol 106:692–694, 1988.
32. Neuhaus R, Baylis H: Cerebrospinal fluid leakage after dacryocystorhinostomy. Ophthalmology 90:1091–1095, 1983.
33. Jordan DR, Anderson RL: Prevention of prolapsed silicone stents in dacryocystorhinostomy surgery. Arch Ophthalmol 105:455, 1987.
34. Anderson RL, Edwards JJ: Indications, complications, and results with silicone stents. Ophthalmology 86:1474–1487, 1979.
35. West J: Eine Fensterresektion des Ductus naso-lacrimalis in Fällen von stenose. Arch Laryngol Rhinol 24-25:62–64, 1911.
36. Halle M: Zur intranasalen operation am Tranensack. Arch Laryngol Rhinol 28:256–266, 1914.
37. Jokinen K, Kärjä J: Endonasal dacryocystorhinostomy. Arch Otolaryngol Head Neck Surg 100:41–44, 1974.
38. Rice DH: Endoscopic intranasal dacryocystorhinostomy: Results in four patients. Arch Otolaryngol Head Neck Surg 116:1061, 1990.
39. Rice DH: Endoscopic intranasal dacryocystorhinostomy: A cadaver study. Am J Rhinol 2:127–128, 1988.
40. McDonogh M, Meiring JH: Endoscopic transnasal dacryocystorhinostomy. J Laryngol Otol 103:585–587, 1989.
41. Metson R: The endoscopic approach for revision dacryocystorhinostomy. Laryngoscope 100:1344–1347, 1990.
42. Orcutt JC, Hillel A, Ernest A, Weymuller J: Endoscopic repair of failed dacryocystorhinostomy. Ophthal Plast Reconstr Surg 6:197–202, 1990.
43. Gonnering RS, Lyon DB, Fisher JC: Endoscopic laser-assisted lacrimal surgery. Am J Ophthalmol 111:152–157, 1991.
44. Selkin SG: Pitfalls in intranasal laser surgery and how to avoid them. Arch Otolaryngol Head Neck Surg 112:285–289, 1986.
45. Kokosa JM, Eugene J: Chemical composition of laser-tissue interaction smoke plume. J Laser Applications 1(3):59–63, 1989.
46. Massaro BM, Gonnering RS, Harris GJ: Endonasal laser dacryocystorhinostomy: A new approach to nasolacrimal duct obstruction. Arch Ophthalmol 108:1172–1176, 1990.

CHAPTER 78

Secondary Acquired Lacrimal Drainage Obstruction*

George B. Bartley

Secondary acquired lacrimal drainage obstruction (SALDO) may be categorized into five groups: infectious, inflammatory, neoplastic, traumatic, and mechanical (Table 78–1). Infections leading to lacrimal drainage obstruction may be of bacterial, viral, fungal, or parasitic origin. Inflammatory disorders associated with blockage of the tear outflow channel may be divided into those that arise endogenously, such as sarcoidosis or Wegener's granulomatosis, and inflammation that results from exogenous stimuli, such as eyedrops, radiation, and allergens. Various neoplasms can occlude the nasolacrimal drainage system and may be classified by site of origin: primary tumors, secondary invaders, or cancers that have metastasized to the lacrimal drainage region. Traumatic causes of lacrimal drainage obstruction include both iatrogenic and noniatrogenic events. Finally, mechanical obstruction of the outflow system may result from objects within the lumen of the tract or from external blockage or compression.

INFECTIOUS CAUSES OF SECONDARY ACQUIRED LACRIMAL DRAINAGE OBSTRUCTION

Bacteria, viruses, fungi, and parasites have been implicated as underlying causes of lacrimal drainage obstruction (see Tables 78–1 and 78–2).

Most cases of dacryocystitis probably are associated with primary acquired nasolacrimal duct obstruction (PANDO, a term coined by Linberg and McCormick[1] in their landmark report). Because the theme of this chapter is the causes rather than the consequences of lacrimal drainage obstruction, the discussion is focused more on the organisms that have been implicated in the development of blockage than on the myriad varieties of bacteria that have been cultured once a lacrimal sac abscess forms.[2–6]

Actinomyces typically causes canalicular obstruction and inflammation rather than blockage of the nasolacrimal duct. Canaliculitis is classically associated with *Actinomyces israelii*, a gram-positive aerotolerant rod that demonstrates true branching.[7–19] Although *Actinomyces* organisms are sensitive to penicillin, topical antibiotic therapy is usually ineffective and surgical removal of the canalicular dacryoliths is required. The stones, which typically are yellow or white and have been described as "sulfur granules" (Fig. 78–1), are not unique to canaliculitis and may be found within actinomycotic purulent loculations elsewhere in the body. In addition, they occasionally may be seen in infections from *Nocardia*, *Streptomyces*, and *Staphylococcus*.[20] Previously named *Streptothrix israelii*, *Actinomyces* is an obligate parasite whose only host is humans.[7]

I have treated one patient with canaliculitis secondary to *Actinomyces meyeri*, an uncommon pathogen that resides principally in the periodontal sulcus.[7] When an infection occurs, it usually is localized to the lung, skeleton, neck, brain, dentoalveolar region, or breast; disseminated disease is rare.[21–23] In addition to differing from *A. israelii* in a few of its fermentation characteristics, *A. meyeri* microcolonies are nonfilamentous, and branching may be difficult to demonstrate.[7] A review[24] of ocular actinomycosis had no examples associated with *A. meyeri*.

Propionibacterium propionicus (formerly, *Arachnia propionica*) also may be associated with canaliculitis. *Propionibacterium* shares many similarities with *Actinomyces*—both are gram positive and have a branching, rod-shaped morphology. Although facultatively anaerobic, carbon dioxide is not necessary for growth, unlike *Actinomyces*.[25] Berlin and coworkers[15] identified *Arachnia* in dacryoliths from five patients with canaliculitis; *Fusobacterium*, *A. israelii*, and *Bacteroides* were isolated from other stones. Weinberg and associates[26] emphasized that some cases of presumed (from results of Gram stain) actinomycotic canaliculitis are probably infections by *Fusobacterium*. Canaliculitis usually responds to simple, thorough curettage.[27]

Several species of mycobacteria have been implicated as causative agents of dacryocystitis: *Mycobacterium for-*

*Portions of this chapter are from Bartley GB: Acquired lacrimal drainage obstruction: An etiologic classification system, case reports, and a review of the literature. Parts I, II, and III. Ophthal Plast Reconstr Surg 8:237–249, 1992; 9:11–26, 1993.

TABLE 78-1

Causes of Acquired Lacrimal Drainage Obstruction

Primary acquired nasolacrimal drainage obstruction (PANDO)
Secondary acquired lacrimal drainage obstruction (SALDO)
- Infectious
  - Bacterial
  - Viral
  - Fungal
  - Parasitic
- Inflammatory
  - Endogenous
  - Exogenous
- Neoplastic
  - Primary
  - Secondary
  - Metastatic
- Traumatic
  - Iatrogenic
  - Noniatrogenic
- Mechanial
  - Internal
  - External

From Bartley GB: Acquired lacrimal drainage obstruction: An etiologic classification system, case reports, and a review of the literature. Parts I, II, and III. Ophthal Plast Reconstr Surg 8:237–249, 1992; 9:11–26, 1993.

tuitum,[28] *Mycobacterium leprae* (Fig. 78-2),[29, 30] and *Mycobacterium tuberculosis*.[31-33] In a report by Rootman and colleagues,[34] canaliculitis was caused by *Mycobacterium chelonei*; this bacterium is not included in the outline of SALDO, however, because the infection appeared to be a response to nasolacrimal intubation rather than the underlying cause of obstruction.

Punctal occlusion, canalicular scarring, and nasolacrimal duct obstruction may result from infection by *Chlamydia trachomatis*.[35-38] To determine whether antitrachomatous antibiotics should be used after dacryocystorhinostomy in a susceptible population, Rice and Kersten[39] examined biopsy specimens of the lacrimal sac

TABLE 78-2

Infectious Causes of Secondary Acquired Lacrimal Drainage Obstruction

Bacterial
- *Actinomyces* sp.
  - *A. israelii*
  - *A. meyeri*
- *Propionibacterium propionicus* (formerly, *Arachnia propionica*)
- *Fusobacterium* sp.
- *Bacteroides* sp.
- *Mycobacterium* sp.
  - *M. fortuitum*
  - *M. leprae*
  - *M. tuberculosis*
- *Chlamydia trachomatis*
- *Nocardia asteroides*
- *Enterobacter cloacae*
- *Aeromonas hydrophilia*
- *Treponema pallidum*
- *Staphylococcus aureus*

Viral
- Herpes simplex virus
- Herpes zoster virus
  - Varicella
- Adenovirus
- Vaccinia virus
- Epstein-Barr virus
- Variola virus (smallpox)

Fungal
- *Aspergillus* sp.
  - *A. fumigatus*
  - *A. niger*
- *Candida* sp.
  - *C. albicans*
  - *C. parapsilosis*
- *Pityrosporum* sp.
  - *P. orbiculare*
  - *P. pachydermatis*
- *Rhinosporidium seeberi*
- *Sporothrix schenckii*
- *Streptomyces somaliensis*
- *Trichophyton rubrum*

Parasitic
- *Ascaris lumbricoides*

From Bartley GB: Acquired lacrimal drainage obstruction: An etiologic classification system, case reports, and a review of the literature. Parts I, II, and III. Ophthal Plast Reconstr Surg 8:237–249, 1992; 9:11–26, 1993.

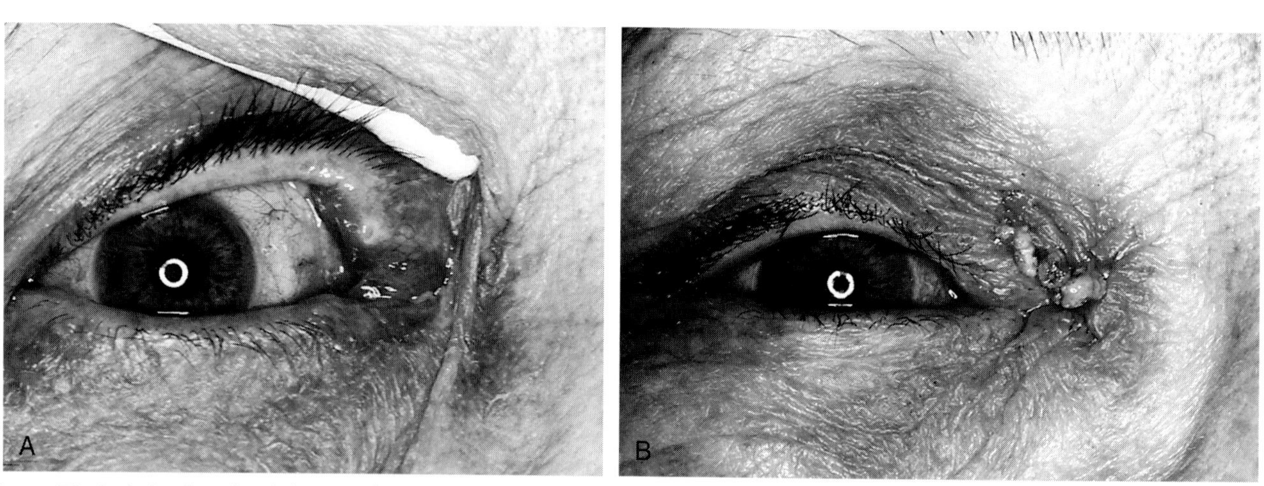

Figure 78-1. *A*, Swelling of medial portion of the right upper eyelid and a "pouting" punctum due to canaliculitis. *B*, The stones that were removed from the canaliculus.

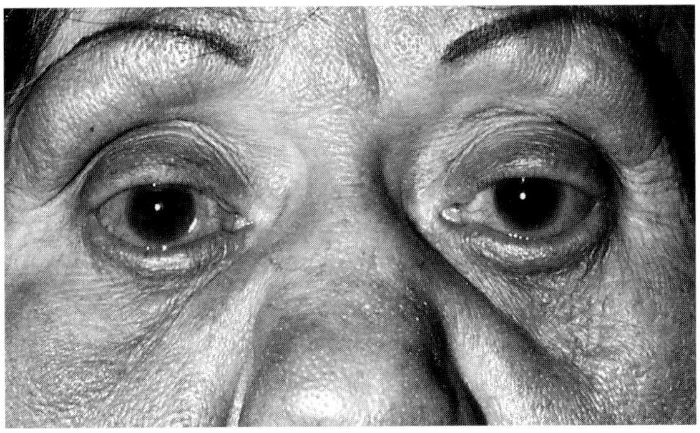

Figure 78–2. A 48-year-old woman with unusually thick and immobile skin from lepromatous leprosy. She had bilateral lacrimal obstruction, possibly related to her systemic disease.

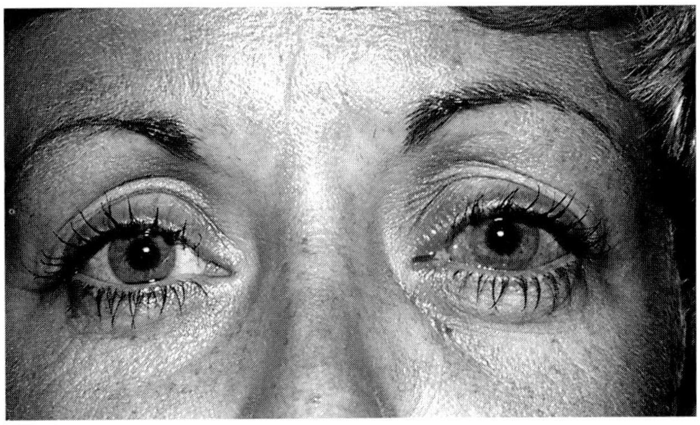

Figure 78–4. A woman with lacrimal obstruction secondary to epidemic keratoconjunctivitis; this photograph was taken during a recurrence of the viral infection.

with the direct-smear fluorescent antibody test. All specimens were negative in patients with presumed trachoma; the authors therefore concluded that postoperative adjunctive therapy was not necessary.

Other bacteria that have been associated with lacrimal drainage obstruction include *Nocardia asteroides*,[40] *Enterobacter cloacae*,[41] *Aeromonas hydrophila*,[42] *Treponema pallidum*,[31, 43] and *Staphylococcus aureus*.[18] Dacryocystitis usually requires dacryocystorhinostomy.

A viral causation of lacrimal drainage obstruction, especially canalicular stenosis, is most common with herpetic infections (including herpes simplex [Fig. 78–3], herpes zoster, and chickenpox) and epidemic keratoconjunctivitis (Fig. 78–4).[18, 36, 44–54] Obstruction appears to result from damage to the elastic tissue of the substantia propria rather than to the canalicular epithelium alone.[49, 54] Another contributory mechanism may be the adherence of raw epithelial surfaces due to overlying inflammatory membranes.[54] Lacrimal obstruction has also been associated with vaccinia virus,[46] the Epstein-Barr

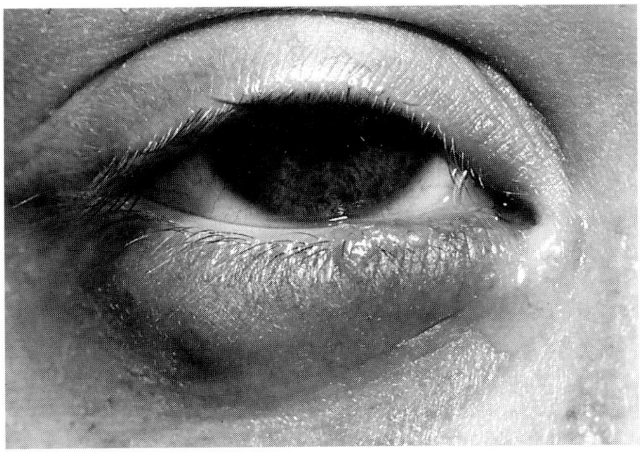

Figure 78–3. A young girl with a history of recurrent herpes simplex blepharoconjunctivitis who eventually required dacryocystorhinostomy. The silicone tubing is left in place indefinitely to prevent lacrimal stenosis from subsequent episodes of viral reactivation, as occurred in this case.

virus,[55] and smallpox.[56] Intubation of the lacrimal drainage system with silicone tubing may be attempted in patients with mild stenosis of the canaliculi. Severe or diffuse canalicular obstruction, however, usually necessitates placement of a Jones tube.

When fungi occlude the lacrimal drainage system, it is usually by formation of a stone or cast. The fungal concretions in some instances pass through the system spontaneously, in others they are expelled through irrigation, and in some patients they are discovered during dacryocystorhinostomy. Recurrences are unusual. Obstruction has been associated with *Aspergillus fumigatus* (Fig. 78–5),[57] *Aspergillus niger*,[58] *Candida albicans*,[59–62] *Candida parapsilosis*,[63] *Pityrosporum orbiculare*,[64] *Pityrosporum pachydermatis*,[65] *Streptomyces somaliensis*,[66] and *Trichophyton rubrum*.[67] Two cases of lacrimal sac involvement with *Rhinosporidium seeberi* were included in a series of 15 patients from India, but details were sketchy.[68] Similarly, the case described by Gifford[69] in 1922 of dacryocystitis associated with *Sporothrix schenckii* lacks specific information about the lacrimal examination.

Parasitic obstruction of the lacrimal outflow tract is unusual; when reported, it is usually associated with the nematode *Ascaris lumbricoides*.[70–72] The worm gains entrance to the nasolacrimal system through the valve of Hasner, ascends through the duct and sac, and then emerges from the punctum, prompting immediate medical evaluation. Simple extraction has proved successful.

INFLAMMATORY CAUSES OF SECONDARY ACQUIRED LACRIMAL DRAINAGE OBSTRUCTION

The nasolacrimal passages may become occluded secondary to inflammation resulting from numerous disorders (Table 78–3; see Table 78–1). Diseases of endogenous origin will be considered first.

Wegener's granulomatosis is a systemic vasculitis with

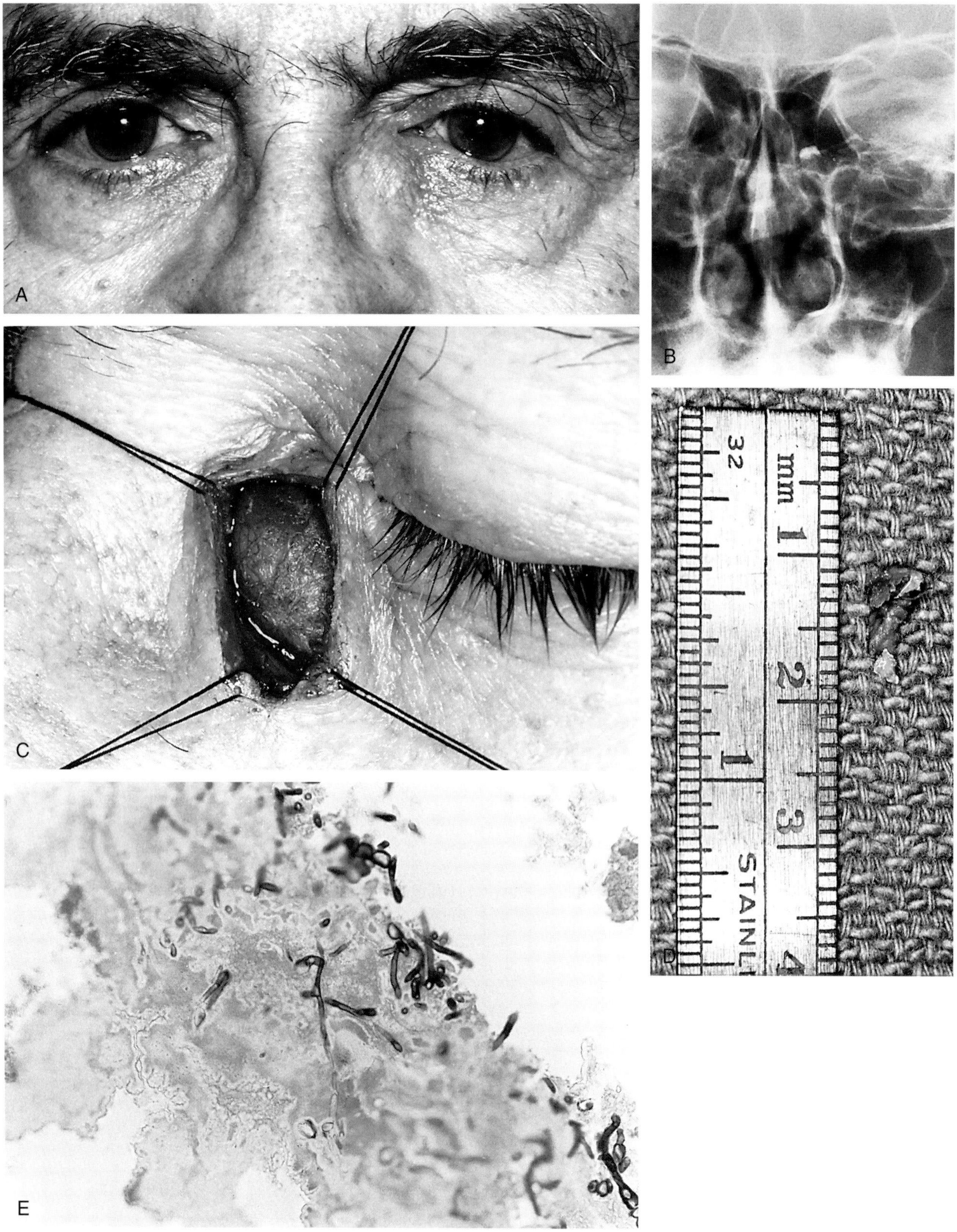

Figure 78 – 5. *A*, Left dacryocystitis with an enlarged lacrimal sac. *B*, Dacryocystogram was suggestive of a dacryolith. *C*, Intraoperative appearance of the swollen sac. *D*, The obstructing dacryolith. *E*, Silver chromate stain of the dacryolith demonstrated *Aspergillus*. Original magnification, ×100.

TABLE 78-3

Inflammatory Causes of Secondary Acquired Lacrimal Drainage Obstruction

Endogenous
- Wegener's granulomatosis
- Sarcoidosis
- Cicatricial pemphigoid
- Stevens-Johnson syndrome (erythema multiforme)
- Toxic epidermal necrolysis
- Sinus histiocytosis
- "Pseudotumor"
- Kawasaki's disease (mucocutaneous lymph node syndrome)
- Porphyria cutanea tarda
- Epidermodysplasia verruciformis, ichthyosis, scleroderma
- Idiopathic punctal stenosis

Exogenous
- Eyedrops
  - Antiviral agents
    - Idoxuridine
    - Vidarabine
    - Trifluridine
    - Acyclovir
  - Antiglaucoma medications
    - Demecarium
    - Echothiophate
    - Isoflurophate
    - Furmethide
    - Neostigmine
    - Physostigmine
    - Epinephrine
  - Silver nitrate, silver protein, colloidal silver
  - Thiotepa
- Radiation therapy
- Fluorouracil (systemic)
- Graft-versus-host disease
- "Pyogenic granuloma"
- Foreign body granuloma
- Allergy
  - Ocular
  - Nasal
- Burns
  - Thermal
  - Chemical

From Bartley GB: Acquired lacrimal drainage obstruction: An etiologic classification system, case reports, and a review of the literature. Parts I, II, and III. Ophthal Plast Reconstr Surg 8:237–249, 1992; 9:11–26, 1993.

diverse clinical manifestations. Classically, the disease involves the triad of the upper respiratory tract, the lung, and the kidneys, although limited forms of the disorder may occur.[73-75] The disease was uniformly fatal before effective immunosuppressive therapy became available.[76]

In a comprehensive review of the ophthalmic manifestations of Wegener's granulomatosis in 140 patients,[77] nasolacrimal obstruction was present in 10 patients. Nasolacrimal obstruction is typically associated with advanced nasal disease and is a late manifestation of Wegener's granulomatosis in most instances. Treatment of nasolacrimal obstruction by dacryocystorhinostomy was complicated by wound necrosis and a nasal-cutaneous fistula in two patients described by Jordan and coworkers.[78] The authors recommended a conservative approach and suggested the use of systemic corticosteroids if operation is required when inflammation is active. In a subsequent report, Holds and associates[79] proposed dacryocystectomy as an alternative to dacryocystorhinostomy to treat dacryocystitis in patients with Wegener's granulomatosis in whom tearing is not problematic. Glatt and Putterman[80] subsequently described two patients with inactive disease who had excellent results from dacryocystorhinostomy. Success with a conjunctivodacryocystostomy has been reported in one patient.[81]

My colleagues and I reviewed our experience with 13 lacrimal bypass operations in 9 patients with Wegener's granulomatosis.[82] Adequate follow-up data were available for 10 patients, of whom 6 had a satisfactory surgical outcome. Operative failure was related to the presence of a dacryopyocele or active nasal, upper airway, or sinus disease, concurrent use of nonmaintenance immunosuppressive therapy, or a history of prior operation. No patient developed a nasal-cutaneous fistula postoperatively. We recommend that operation be deferred if possible until the inflammation is quiescent, that trimethoprim-sulfamethoxazole be included in the medical therapy,[83] and that testing for anticytoplasmic autoantibodies be done to help monitor disease activity.[84-86] Figure 78-6 illustrates a patient in whom the surgical outcome was satisfactory despite concurrent active inflammation.

Obstruction of the nasolacrimal sac and duct by sarcoidosis (Fig. 78-7) is probably more common than has been reported.[87-96] Karma[91] noted that 5 of 281 patients with sarcoidosis had lacrimal drainage obstruction. In a subsequent review of these five cases, he emphasized that an initially successful dacryocystorhinostomy is at risk for late failure because of progression of the inflammatory process within the nasal and lacrimal sac mucosa.[93] Because tear production is often reduced in sarcoidosis as a result of lacrimal gland infiltration, Karma treated two of his patients with dacryocystectomy rather than with lacrimal bypass surgery.

Cicatricial pemphigoid (Fig. 78-8), Stevens-Johnson syndrome, and toxic epidermal necrolysis[98] are uncommon disorders that may cause lacrimal drainage obstruction with advanced disease.[18, 36, 81, 99-105]

Lacrimal drainage obstruction has been reported in association with sinus histiocytosis with massive lymphadenopathy.[106, 107] The disorder is considered to be benign even though many of the clinical features of the disease suggest neoplasia. The underlying cause is unknown but may be related to an allergy or an immunologic abnormality of histocytes. A comprehensive review of the ophthalmic manifestations of the disorder included "increased lacrimation" as a symptom, but further specifics were not provided.[108]

Idiopathic inflammatory pseudotumor has been reported to cause lacrimal obstruction,[97, 109, 110] as has Kawasaki's disease (mucocutaneous lymph node syndrome).[111] Obstruction of the distal nasolacrimal system is known to coexist with lower eyelid ectropion,[112] which often has an inflammatory or cicatricial component and may be associated with systemic diseases.[113] Sober and

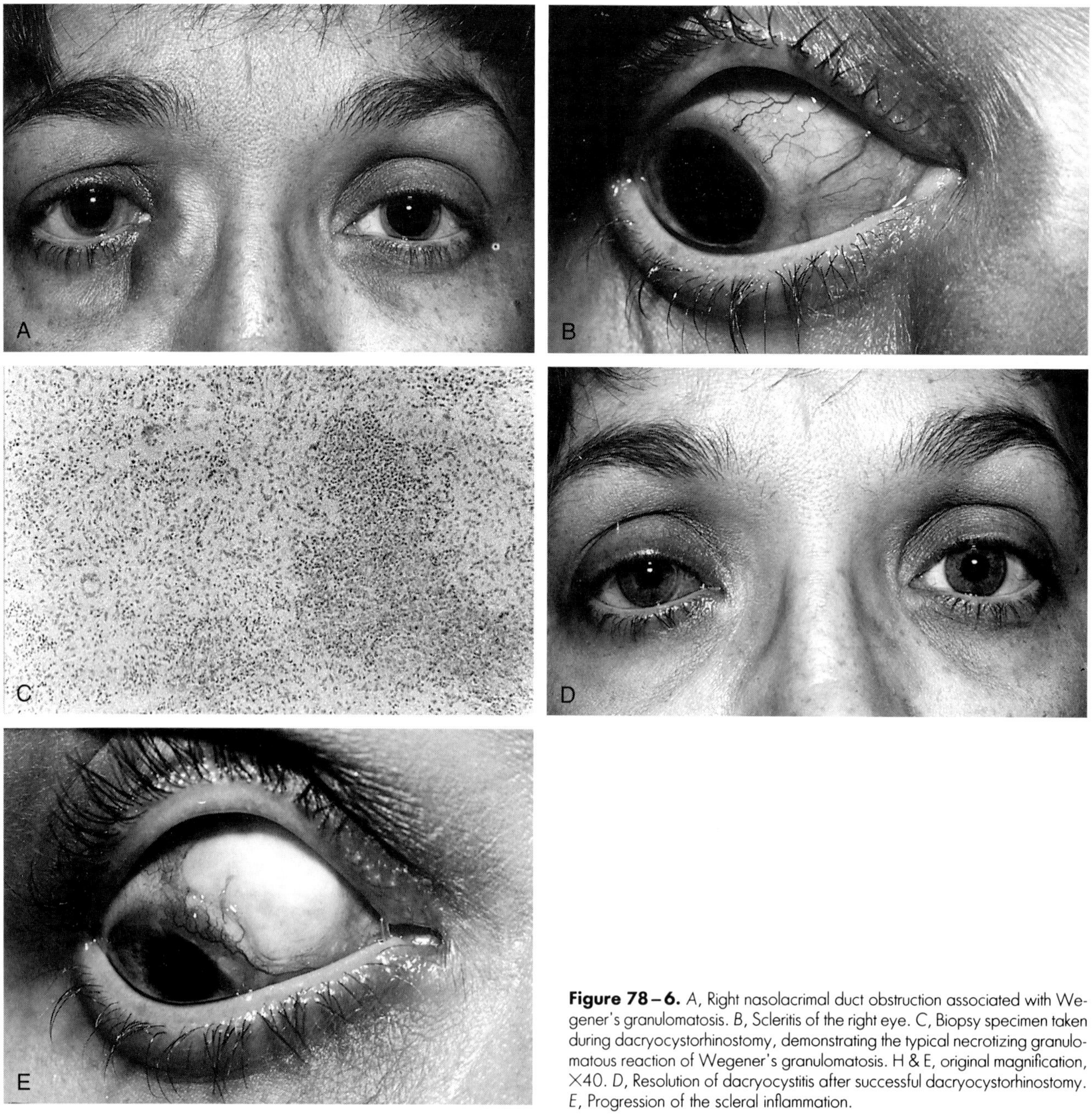

Figure 78–6. *A*, Right nasolacrimal duct obstruction associated with Wegener's granulomatosis. *B*, Scleritis of the right eye. *C*, Biopsy specimen taken during dacryocystorhinostomy, demonstrating the typical necrotizing granulomatous reaction of Wegener's granulomatosis. H & E, original magnification, ×40. *D*, Resolution of dacryocystitis after successful dacryocystorhinostomy. *E*, Progression of the scleral inflammation.

associates[114] described a patient with punctal and canalicular stenosis and cicatricial ectropion that was associated with the sclerodermoid variant of porphyria cutanea tarda. I have evaluated a similar patient who had ectropion and left lacrimal obstruction at the level of the proximal lacrimal sac or common canaliculus in the setting of epidermodysplasia verruciformis, ichthyosis, and scleroderma. Finally, punctal stenosis occasionally may occur spontaneously.[115–117]

All of the disorders described previously may be classified as inflammations that arise endogenously, although external stimuli that are as yet unidentified may be responsible for initiating the body's response. Lacrimal obstruction that is related to known exogenous factors is considered next.

Cicatricial lacrimal drainage obstruction has been reported to result from various modalities, including eyedrops, radiation therapy, systemic chemotherapy, and bone marrow transplantation.

Iatrogenic punctal or canalicular scarring has been associated with idoxuridine, vidarabine, trifluridine, acyclovir, demecarium, echothiophate, isoflurophate, furmethide, neostigmine, physostigmine, epinephrine, silver preparations, and thiotepa.[36, 81, 102, 118–129] Drops

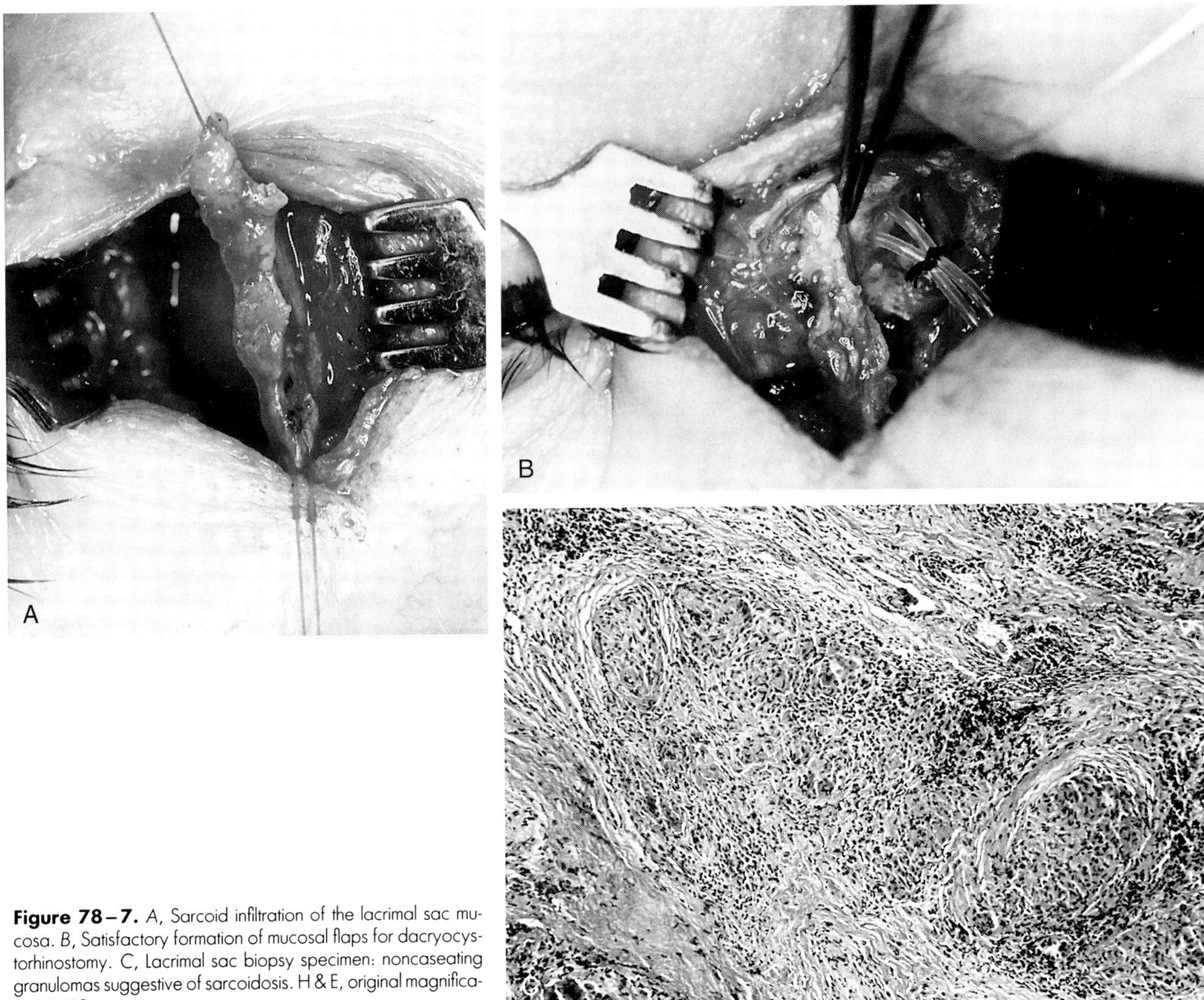

Figure 78–7. *A*, Sarcoid infiltration of the lacrimal sac mucosa. *B*, Satisfactory formation of mucosal flaps for dacryocystorhinostomy. *C*, Lacrimal sac biopsy specimen: noncaseating granulomas suggestive of sarcoidosis. H & E, original magnification, ×63.

used to treat glaucoma, in particular, may induce conjunctival cicatrization that may be clinically indistinguishable from cicatricial pemphigoid.[130]

External radiation for the treatment of neoplasia can incite sufficient inflammation to occlude the lacrimal drainage passages (Fig. 78–9).[36, 104, 131–135] Call and Welham[133] stated that canalicular stenosis may result from as little as 1800 rad (cGy); a report in the radiology literature, in contrast, indicated that "the membranous lacrimal passages are relatively immune to radiation therapy" at significantly higher doses.[136] Lovato and colleagues,[137] in a prospective study of the effect of prophylactic nasolacrimal intubation with silicone tubing on epiphora in patients undergoing helium ion therapy for uveal melanoma, found that 11 of 12 patients in the intubation group maintained lacrimal drainage patency, whereas 10 of 12 patients in the control group (no silicone intubation) had punctal closure. Epiphora appears to result from a combination of anatomic lacrimal obstruction, conjunctival epithelial alterations, and damage to conjunctival goblet cells and glands; the authors recommended that "intubation should be considered in any patient with a medial canthal tumor that requires irradiation." Topical corticosteroid therapy also may be helpful in preventing punctal occlusion.[138]

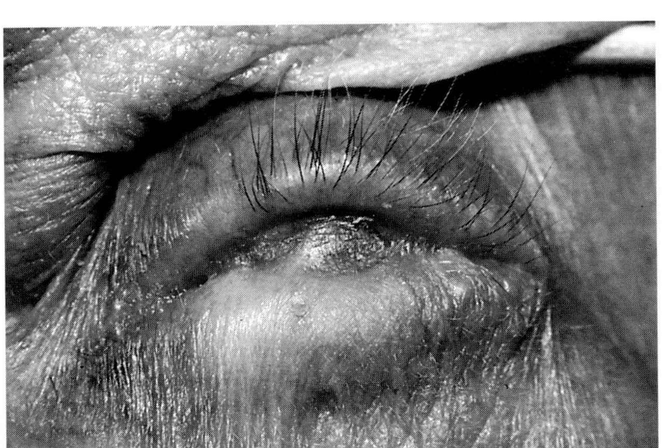

Figure 78–8. Stage IV cicatricial pemphigoid.

In addition to external beam radiation, severe derma-

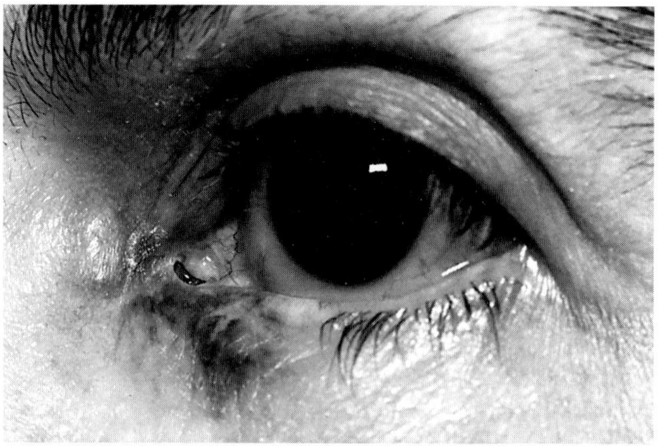

Figure 78–9. Pigmentary skin changes and obstruction of the puncta and canaliculi after external beam radiation; a Jones tube is in place.

titis and lacrimal drainage stenosis may result from cobalt[139] or iridium[140] brachytherapy. Punctal and canalicular occlusion has not been observed at the Mayo Clinic as a complication of radioactive iodine plaque therapy (Robertson DM, personal communication, February 19, 1991), probably because of the desirable rapid spatial radiation decay characteristics of the isotope.[141, 142]

Systemic chemotherapy with 5-fluorouracil is well known to be associated with occlusion of the puncta or canaliculi[143–147]; in severe cases, ankyloblepharon may occur.[148] Contemporary oncologic regimens use lower doses of the drug for shorter periods than in past years; therefore, one would expect that lacrimal drainage problems related to fluorouracil should become less frequent. Indeed, a review from the Mayo Clinic of 210 patients found no examples of lacrimal stenosis.[149]

An intriguing case of bilateral nasolacrimal duct obstruction with dacryocystitis was reported in a 3½-year-old boy who 18 months previously had undergone bone marrow transplantation.[150] Because the child had not had tearing before transplantation, the authors concluded that the nasolacrimal ducts were a target "organ" for graft-versus-host disease.

Two final causes of treatment-related inflammatory lacrimal drainage obstruction relate to silicone intubation of the nasolacrimal system. I have operated on several patients in whom either "pyogenic granulomas" (granulation tissue)[151] or foreign body granulomas formed in response to silicone tubes, resulting in SALDO. Although medical-grade silicone rubber is generally considered to be biologically and immunologically inert, physically stable, and well tolerated by host tissues,[152–154] inflammatory responses, both granulomatous and nongranulomatous, to the material occasionally occur.[155–158] Secondary inflammatory lacrimal obstruction is not unique to silicone; Stallard[159] described a case more than 50 years ago in which a granulation tissue mass formed around a silver style that had been placed to stent the nasolacrimal duct.

Allergens may contribute to lacrimal drainage obstruction in patients with atopic disease,[160] nasal inflammation,[161, 162] or both a local and a systemic allergic response.[163] Oral antihistamines were effective in improving the symptoms of nasolacrimal duct obstruction in approximately 50% of patients in one study,[164] and a comparable success rate was reported by Italian investigators who injected corticosteroid-antibiotic ointment intracanalicularly on alternate days for 2 to 3 months for nasolacrimal obstruction from various causes.[165] Although such a labor-intensive approach is probably impractical in contemporary American medical practice, it is prudent to avoid surgical intervention in patients with allergic lacrimal obstruction unless medical therapy has proved to be ineffective.[161]

Finally, inflammatory lacrimal obstruction may occur in association with either thermal or chemical burns.[102, 166, 167]

NEOPLASTIC CAUSES OF SECONDARY ACQUIRED LACRIMAL DRAINAGE OBSTRUCTION

Tumors involving the lacrimal drainage system may be classified into lesions that arise primarily within the puncta, canaliculi, lacrimal sac, or nasolacrimal duct; neoplasms that secondarily infiltrate or compromise the drainage passages; and malignancies that metastasize to the nasolacrimal region and obstruct tear flow (Table 78–4; see Table 78–1).

Primary tumors of the lacrimal drainage anatomy are relatively uncommon.[4, 168, 169] Neoplasms of epithelial origin, in particular papillomas and squamous cell carcinomas (Fig. 78–10), are the most frequent in published reports.[109, 170–196] Tumors arising from other tissue types have been described, usually as single cases: adenoid cystic carcinoma,[197] angiofibroma,[198] angiosarcoma,[176, 179] cavernous hemangioma,[199] lacrimal sac cyst,[200] dermoid cyst,[201] fibroma,[202] fibrous histiocytoma,[203, 204] hemangioendothelioma,[6] hemangiopericytoma,[191, 205–208] lymphoma (Fig. 78–11),[97, 175, 186, 209–211] melanoma,[179, 212–218] mucoepidermoid carcinoma,[219–221] neurofibroma,[222] neurilemmoma,[223] oncocytic adenoma,[187, 224–226] oncocytic adenocarcinoma,[182, 225, 227] and pleomorphic adenoma.[228, 229] A glomus tumor of the lacrimal sac has been reported.[230] The lesion apparently arose within the fascial covering of the sac, so it has been included in the outline as a primary tumor.

Obstruction of the lacrimal drainage passages by tumors that arise in nearby tissues and secondarily invade or compromise the system is much more common than blockage by primary lesions. Secondary lesions that have been reported in the literature include adenoid cystic carcinoma (Fig. 78–12),[231] basal cell carcinoma, capillary hemangioma,[232] esthesioneuroblastoma (Fig. 78–13),[233] fibrous dysplasia,[234] fibrosarcoma,[235] intraos-

TABLE 78-4

Neoplastic Causes of Secondary Acquired Lacrimal Drainage Obstruction

Primary	Secondary
Adenoid cystic carcinoma	Adenoid cystic carcinoma
Angiofibroma	Basal cell carcinoma
Angiosarcoma	Capillary hemangioma
Cavernous hemangioma	Esthesioneuroblastoma
Cyst	Fibrous dysplasia
Dermoid cyst	Fibrosarcoma
Fibroma	Intraosseous cavernous hemangioma
Fibrous histiocytoma	Leukemia
Glomus tumor	Lymphoma
Hemangioendothelioma	Mucoepidermoid carcinoma
Hemangiopericytoma	Osteoma
Lymphoma	Papilloma
Melanoma	Conjunctival
Mucoepidermoid carcinoma	Inverted ("schneiderian")
Neurofibroma	Rhabdomyosarcoma
Neurilemmoma	Sebaceous gland carcinoma
Oncocytic adenoma	Squamous cell carcinoma
Oncocytic adenocarcinoma	**Metastatic**
Papilloma	Breast carcinoma
Pleomorphic adenoma	Melanoma
Squamous cell carcinoma	Prostate carcinoma

From Bartley GB: Acquired lacrimal drainage obstruction: An etiologic classification system, case reports, and a review of the literature. Parts I, II, and III. Ophthal Plast Reconstr Surg 8:237–249, 1992; 9:11–26, 1993.

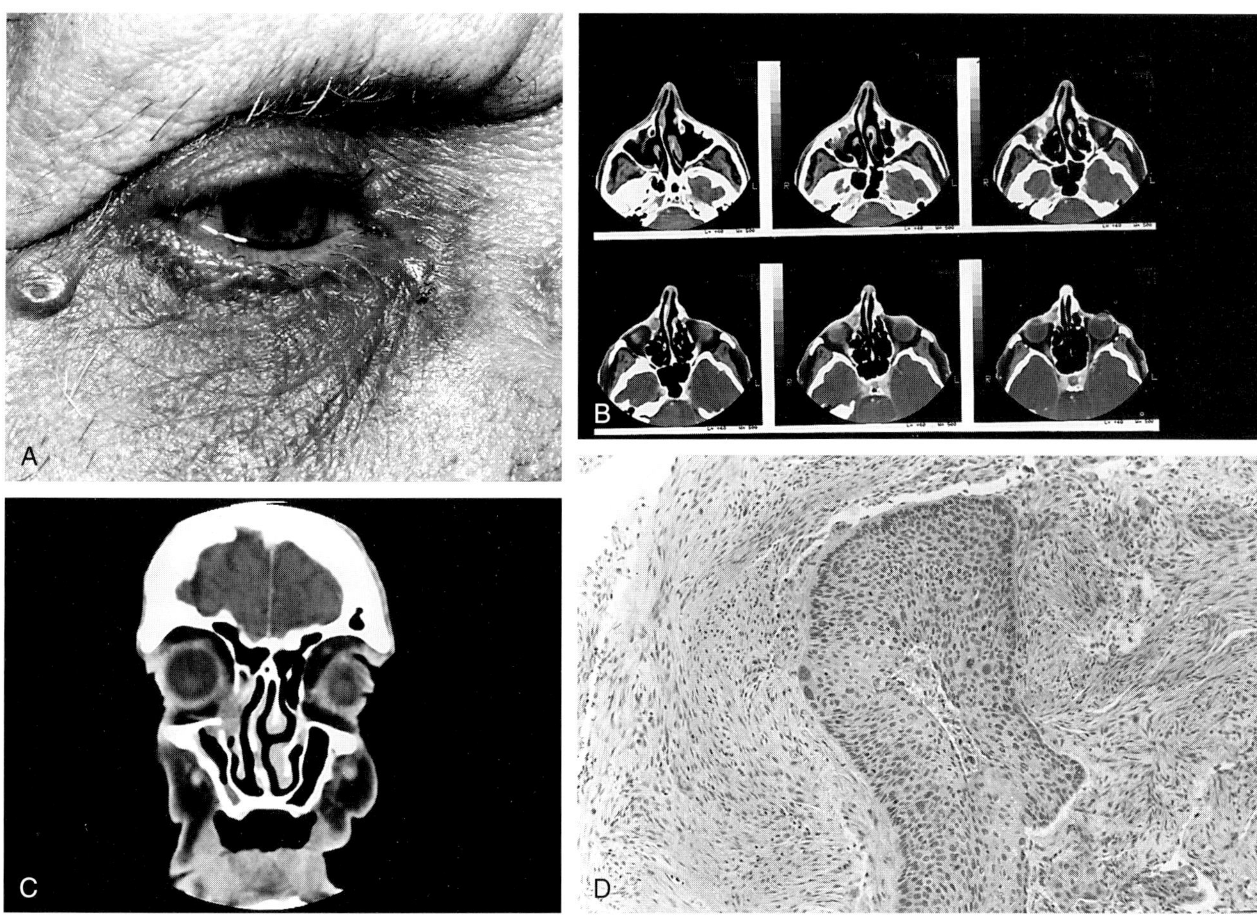

Figure 78–10. *A*, Primary squamous cell carcinoma of the lacrimal sac with extension through the skin. *B* and *C*, Computed tomograms, axial (*B*) and coronal (*C*) planes, demonstrating a soft tissue mass that originates in the lacrimal sac and extends into the anterior orbit. *D*, Grade 3 invasive squamous cell carcinoma of the lacrimal sac. H & E, original magnification, ×40.

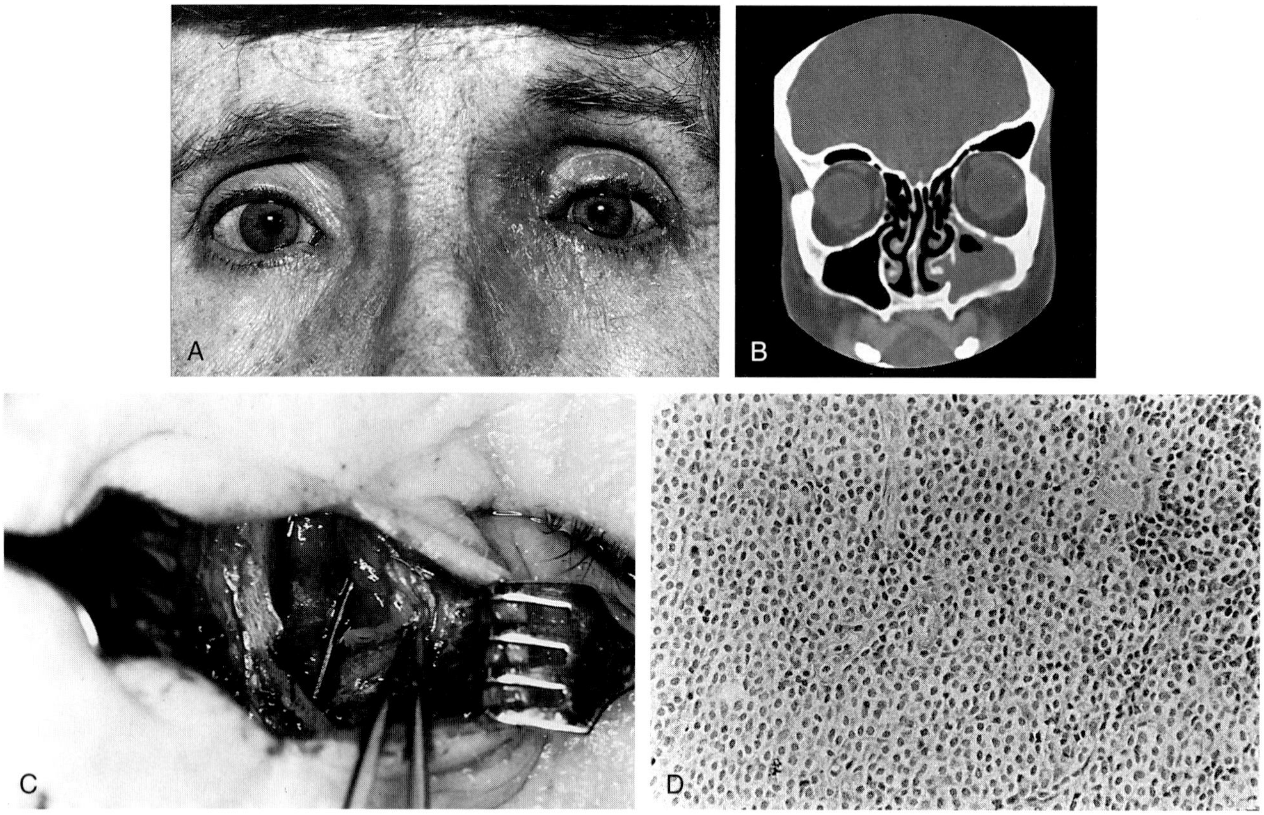

Figure 78–11. *A*, Lymphoma of the left lacrimal sac; the lacrimal system had been intubated with silicone tubing 2 years previously to treat epiphora. *B*, Computed tomogram, coronal plane, demonstrating opacification of the left maxillary sinus and a bony defect at the inferior meatus; biopsy specimens from this area demonstrated only inflammation. *C*, The lacrimal sac and nasolacrimal duct were infiltrated with lymphoma. The previously placed silicone tubing is visible. *D*, Diffuse small B-cell lymphoma with plasmacytic differentiation. H & E, original magnification, ×100.

seous cavernous hemangioma (Fig. 78–14),[236] leukemia,[237–240] lymphoma (Fig. 78–15),[210, 241] mucoepidermoid carcinoma, osteoma,[31, 242] conjunctival papilloma,[243] inverted papilloma (Fig. 78–16),[244] sebaceous gland carcinoma,[245] and squamous cell carcinoma. Kersten has examined an infant with lacrimal drainage obstruction secondary to external compression by rhabdomyosarcoma (Kersten RC, personal communication, February 19, 1991).

The most frequent secondary invaders are probably eyelid cancers, particularly basal cell carcinoma. A case of dacryocystitis caused by a basal cell carcinoma that allegedly arose within the lacrimal sac has been described; the evidence, however, is tenuous and it is probable that

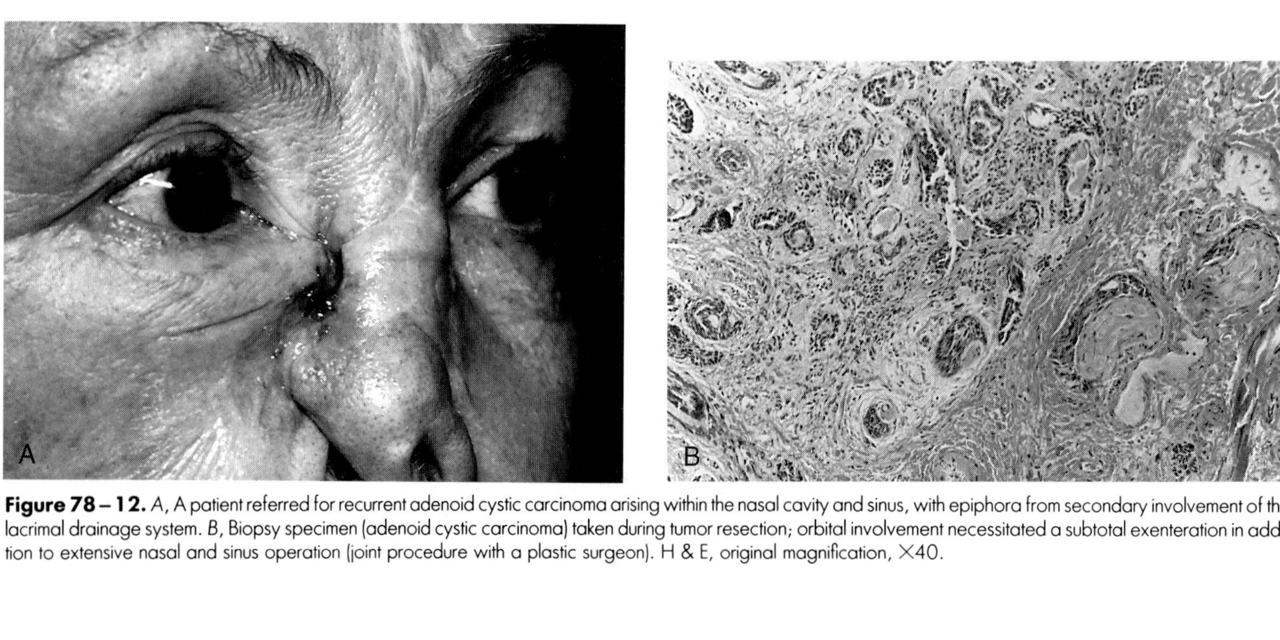

Figure 78–12. *A*, A patient referred for recurrent adenoid cystic carcinoma arising within the nasal cavity and sinus, with epiphora from secondary involvement of the lacrimal drainage system. *B*, Biopsy specimen (adenoid cystic carcinoma) taken during tumor resection; orbital involvement necessitated a subtotal exenteration in addition to extensive nasal and sinus operation (joint procedure with a plastic surgeon). H & E, original magnification, ×40.

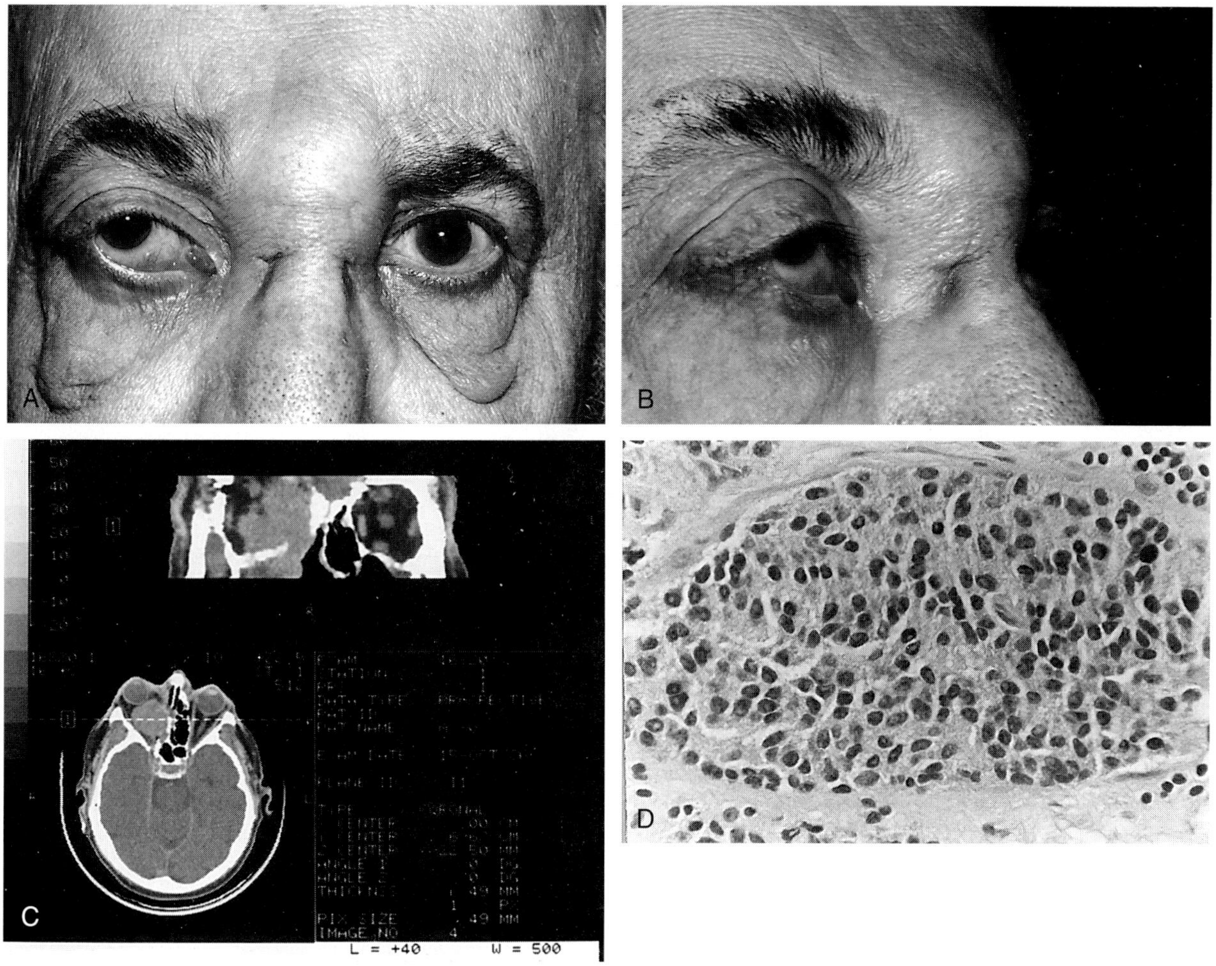

Figure 78 – 13. *A* and *B*, A patient with a massive but slowly progressive esthesioneuroblastoma. Proptosis, the right lower eyelid malposition, and tumor extension to the lacrimal drainage system all contributed to tearing. *C*, Computed tomograms, axial and coronal sections, demonstrated a large orbital component to the tumor. Other sections showed invasion of the lacrimal drainage system. *D*, Biopsy specimen (esthesioneuroblastoma) obtained during a debulking procedure. H & E, original magnification, ×160.

the tumor arose from the skin and invaded the lacrimal sac secondarily.[246] Squamous cell carcinoma and, less frequently, sebaceous carcinoma may also arise within proximity to the puncta and canaliculi. Of the pigmented eyelid tumors, either benign or malignant, that I have treated, none have invaded the lacrimal drainage system. Scott and coworkers[247] emphasized that peripunctal melanocytic nevi do not cause epiphora.

Tumors that arise within the maxillary antrum may compromise the nasolacrimal duct, and of these lesions squamous cell carcinoma is the most common.[173, 235, 248–251] Smith and Wheliss[252] showed that lesions arising from the nasopharynx, in contrast, are more likely to be lymphomatous; one patient in their series had dacryocystitis, but the tissue type of the invading tumor was not specified. A case of nasopharyngeal squamous cell carcinoma has been reported in which the initial symptom was tearing.[253]

Metastatic disease is an extraordinarily rare cause of acquired lacrimal drainage obstruction. A choroidal melanoma with metastasis to the lacrimal sac has been reported,[186] but the reference is a brief summary of a patient with an epibulbar lymphoma and bilateral lymphoma of the lacrimal glands.[254] In 1987, a patient with prostate carcinoma that metastasized to the region of the lacrimal sac was reported.[255] A subsequent report by the same authors[256] indicated that 2 of 35 patients with metastatic tumors to the orbit had as the initial symptom unilateral epiphora from external tumor compression of the lacrimal drainage system; both patients had metastatic prostate carcinoma (Shields CL, personal communication, March 11, 1991). Additional examples are conspicuously absent from recent reviews of metastatic orbital disease.[257–259]

I have treated two patients who had acquired lacrimal drainage obstruction from metastatic tumors. The neoplasms involved were breast carcinoma (Fig. 78 – 17) and malignant melanoma (Fig. 78 – 18).

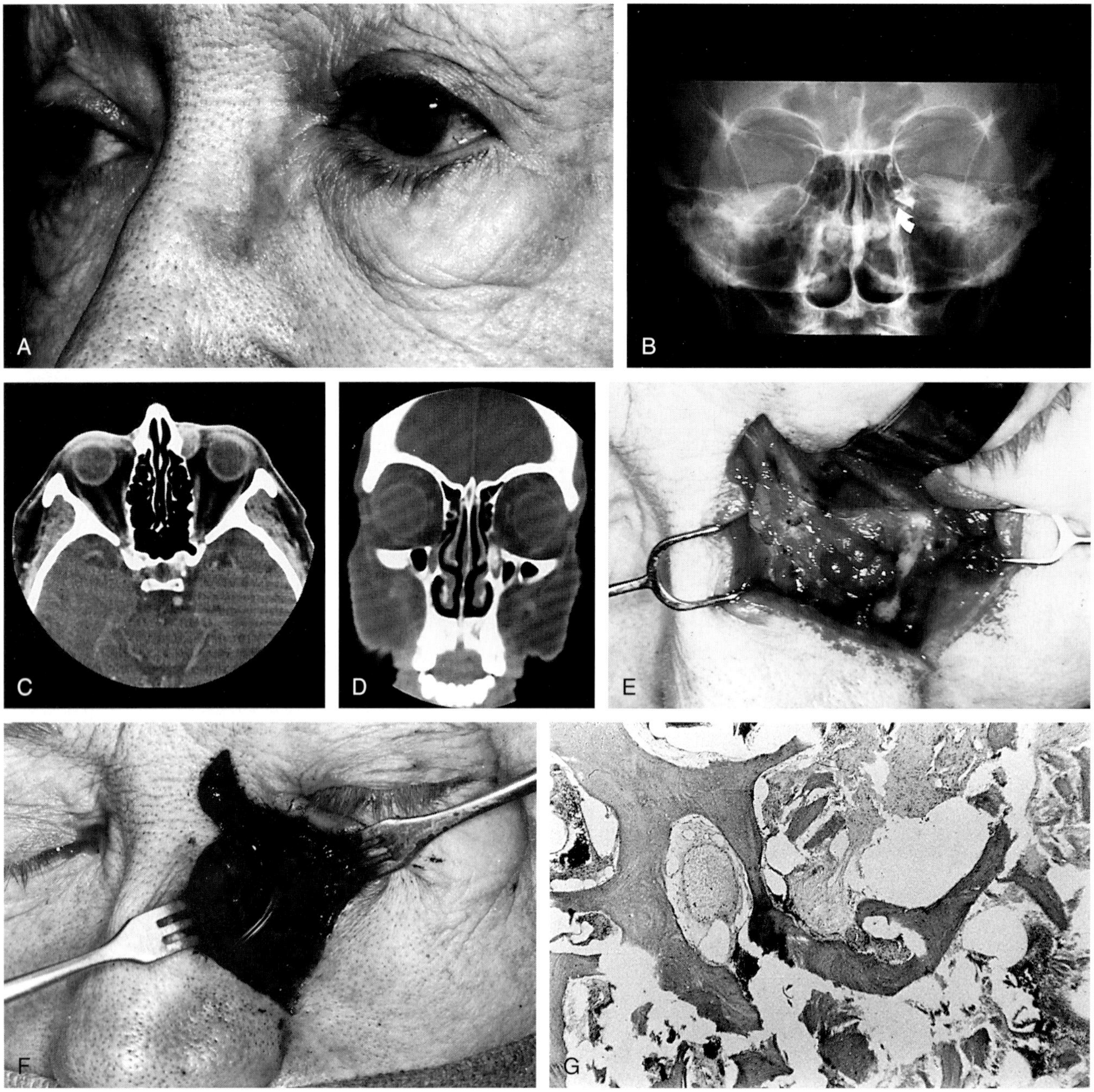

Figure 78–14. *A*, A firm, slowly enlarging mass was palpable along the left inferior medial orbital rim. *B*, Dacryocystogram, demonstrating obstruction of the left lacrimal drainage system (*arrow*). *C* and *D*, Computed tomograms, axial (*C*) and coronal (*D*) planes, identifying a bony lesion in the region of the frontal process of the maxilla and the nasolacrimal canal. *E*, The tumor was exposed by means of a lateral rhinotomy. *F*, After en bloc excision, the lacrimal drainage system was stented with silicone tubing. *G*, Histopathologic analysis showed a hemangioma of bone. H & E, original magnification, ×160. (*A*, *B*, *D*, and *E* published courtesy of *Ophthalmology* [1991;98:541–7].)

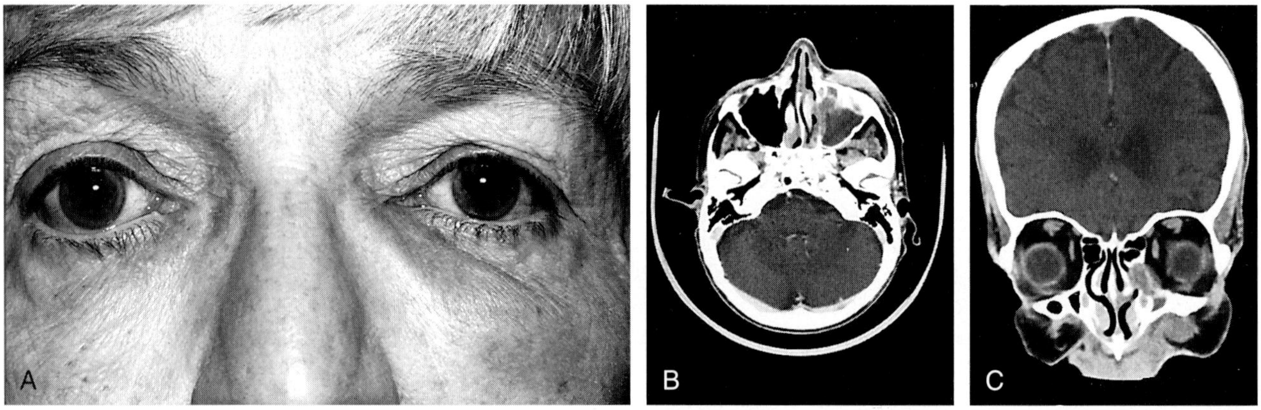

Figure 78–15. *A*, Secondary involvement of the left lacrimal drainage system by lymphoma arising within the left maxillary sinus. *B* and *C*, Computed tomograms, axial (*B*) and coronal (*C*) planes, demonstrating complete opacification of the antrum with lymphoma and secondary nasolacrimal duct encroachment.

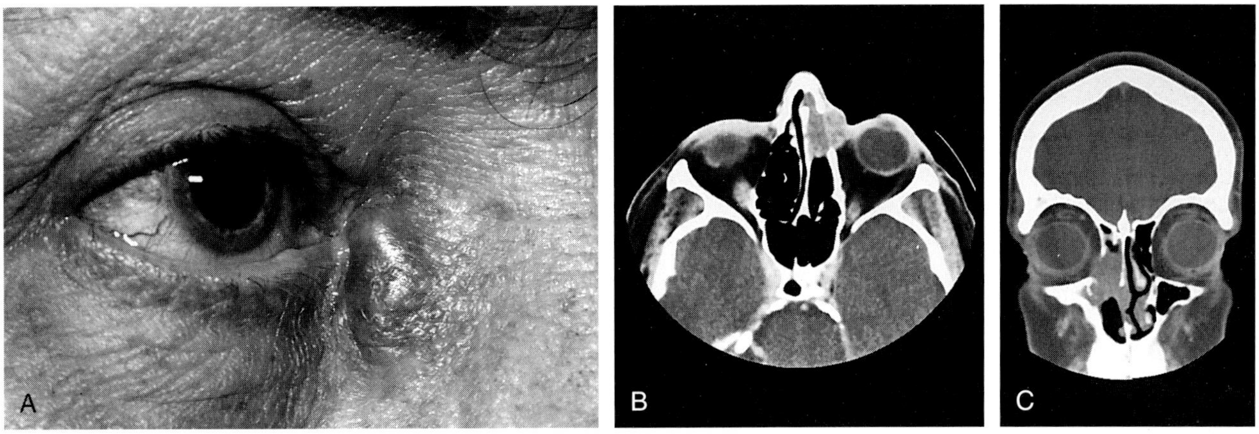

Figure 78–16. *A*, Inverted papilloma with secondary invasion of the lacrimal drainage system and extension through the skin. *B* and C, Computed tomograms, axial (*B*) and coronal (C) planes, demonstrating nasal, sinus, and orbital extension of the inverted papilloma. (From Bartley GB: Acquired lacrimal drainage obstruction: An etiologic classification system, case reports, and a review of the literature. Parts I, II, and III. Ophthal Plast Reconstr Surg 8:237–249, 1992; 9:11–26, 1993.)

TRAUMATIC CAUSES OF SECONDARY ACQUIRED LACRIMAL DRAINAGE OBSTRUCTION

Lacrimal drainage obstruction is a frequent sequela of trauma. Such causes may be classified into those related to medical therapy and those that result from accidental trauma (Table 78–5; see Table 78–1).

Iatrogenic obstruction of the lacrimal drainage system with symptomatic tearing may result from many procedures. The first cause to be considered is punctal occlusion, which is commonly used to treat severe keratoconjunctivitis sicca. The lacrimal openings may be closed intentionally in various manners,[260–264] and it is significant that few patients subsequently have epiphora.[265]

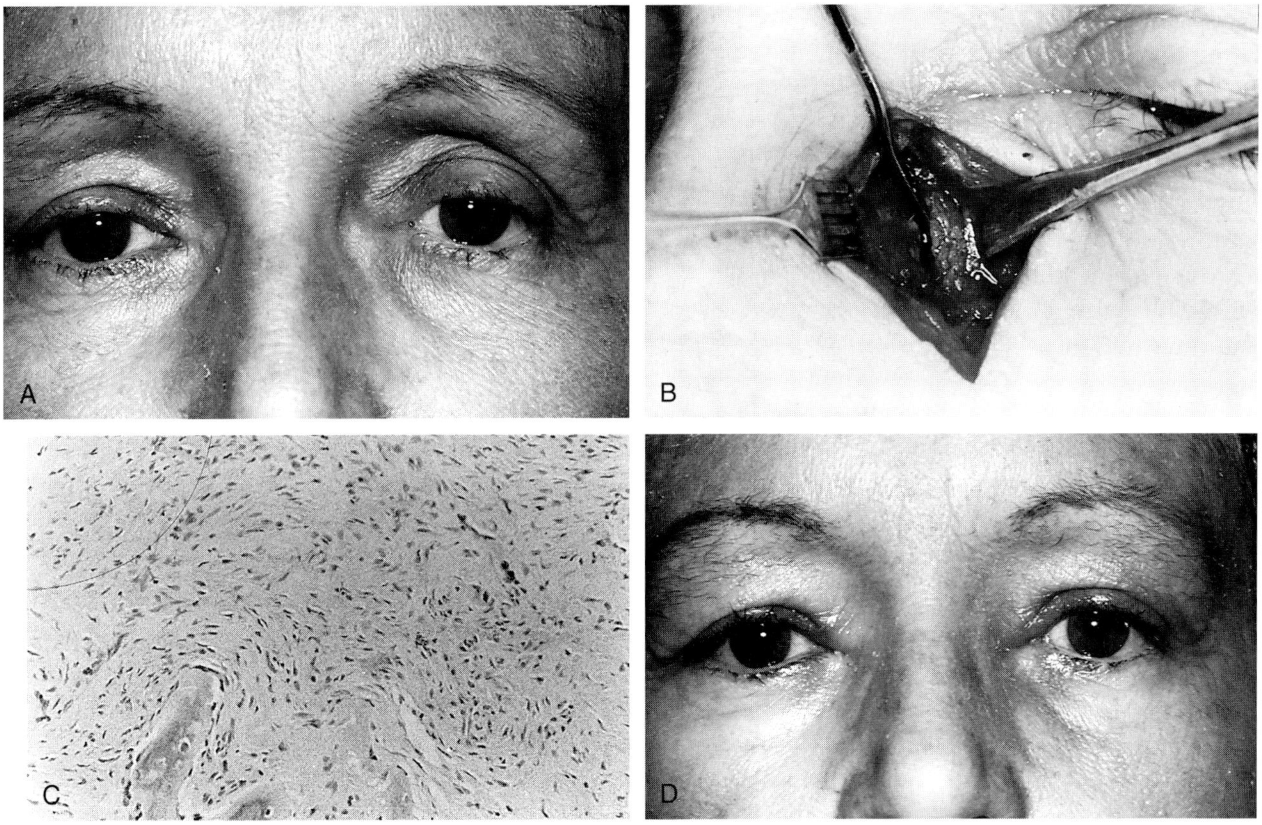

Figure 78–17. *A*, Left dacryocystitis secondary to metastatic breast carcinoma. *B*, At dacryocystorhinostomy, the lacrimal crest (identified between the periosteal elevators) was found to be putty-like from metastatic tumor. C, Biopsy specimen of the lacrimal crest showed infiltration with metastatic breast carcinoma. H & E, original magnification, ×63. *D*, Appearance of the patient 4 months after dacryocystorhinostomy and radiation therapy to the left lacrimal drainage region. (*A*, *B*, and *D*, from Bartley GB: Acquired lacrimal drainage obstruction: An etiologic classification system, case reports, and a review of the literature. Parts I, II, and III. Ophthal Plast Reconstr Surg 8:237–249, 1992; 9:11–26, 1993.)

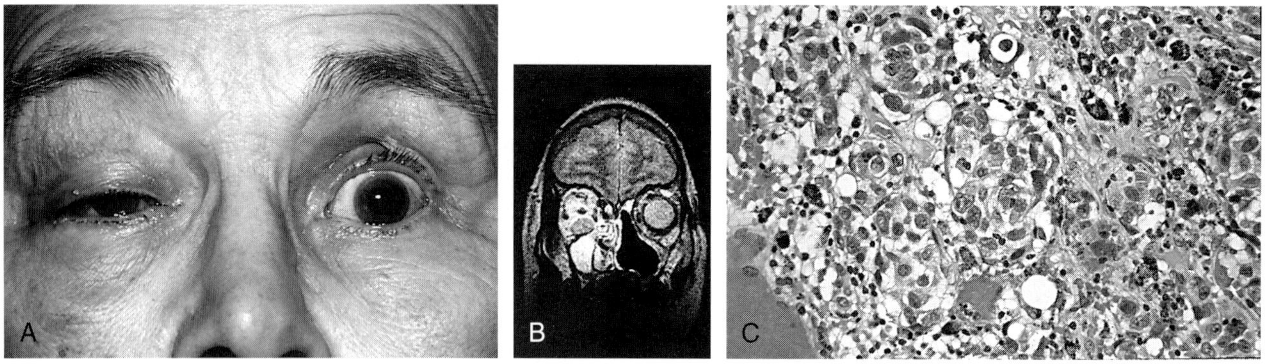

Figure 78 – 18. *A*, A patient with metastatic malignant melanoma from the left nasal cavity to the right orbit, medial canthal region, and maxillary sinus. *B*, Magnetic resonance imaging demonstrated the metastatic tumor. *C*, Highly anaplastic malignant melanoma; biopsy specimen taken during palliative orbital exenteration. H & E, original magnification, ×400. (*A* and *B* from Bartley GB: Acquired lacrimal drainage obstruction: An etiologic classification system, case reports, and a review of the literature. Parts I, II, and III. Ophthal Plast Reconstr Surg 8:237–249, 1992; 9:11–26, 1993.)

Glatt,[266] however, described a patient in whom acute dacryocystitis developed 11 weeks after occlusion of all four puncta for dry eyes, and he emphasized the need for a lacrimal examination to exclude nasolacrimal duct obstruction before obliteration of the puncta. The use of punctal plugs may be complicated by scarring of the punctal openings (Fig. 78 – 19).[267, 268]

Probing of the nasolacrimal duct is highly successful in the treatment of congenital dacryostenosis, but it occasionally is complicated by the formation of a false passage with subsequent scarring of the lacrimal drainage passages.[18, 52, 166]

Because the pigtail probe[269–272] has been associated with frequent secondary damage to the lacrimal drainage anatomy, some authorities advise against its use.[273] Jordan and associates,[274] however, have argued cogently that with improved instrumentation and refined techniques the tool can be useful in canalicular reconstruction. In inexperienced hands, nevertheless, the pigtail probe is a potentially harmful device, as illustrated in Figure 78 – 20, which shows a child in whose care I consulted. A single canalicular laceration had been stented with silicone tubing that had been placed with a pigtail probe. Obstruction of both the superior and the inferior canaliculi subsequently developed, complicated by the formation of several "pyogenic granulomas."

Despite the favorable success rate for dacryocystorhinostomy, secondary lacrimal obstruction may occur.[102, 104, 128, 134, 275–281] In most cases, failure is due to persistent stenosis at the common internal punctum or to an improperly fashioned osteotomy (Fig. 78 – 21). Conjunctivodacryocystorhinostomy with placement of a Jones tube is the definitive lacrimal bypass procedure,[36, 81, 102, 104, 128, 134, 282–286] yet secondary obstruction of the lacrimal drainage system may occur.[287]

Nasolacrimal duct obstruction complicated transantral orbital decompression for Graves' ophthalmopathy in 9 of the first 200 patients who underwent this procedure at the Mayo Clinic.[288, 289] Seiff and Shorr,[290] in a review of 123 decompressions in 63 patients, found that 14 of 90 cases (16%) had epiphora postoperatively, presum-

TABLE 78 – 5

Traumatic Causes of Secondary Acquired Lacrimal Drainage Obstruction

Iatrogenic
Punctal occlusion for dry eyes
After nasolacrimal duct probing with or without silicone intubation
After canalicular repair with pigtail probe
After dacryocystorhinostomy
After conjunctivodacryocystorhinostomy
After transantral orbital decompression
After sinus surgery (conventional or endoscopic)
After rhinoplasty, rhinotomy, or other nasal surgery
After craniofacial surgery
Noniatrogenic
Laceration of canaliculus
Laceration of lacrimal sac
Fractures involving nasolacrimal duct

From Bartley GB: Acquired lacrimal drainage obstruction: An etiologic classification system, case reports, and a review of the literature. Parts I, II, and III. Ophthal Plast Reconstr Surg 8:237–249, 1992; 9:11–26, 1993.

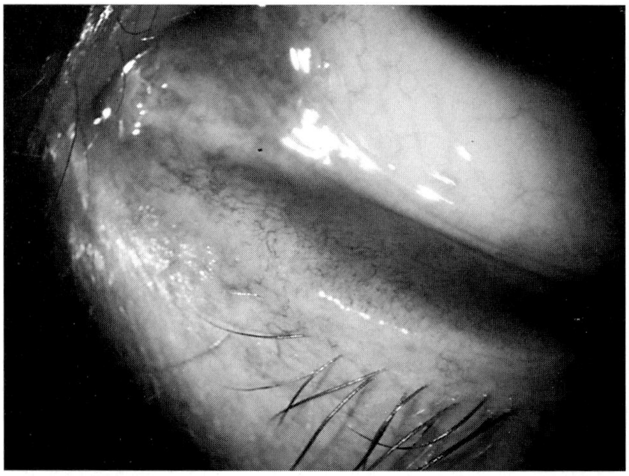

Figure 78 – 19. Stenosed left inferior punctum 1 week after removal of a Freeman punctal plug. (From Maguire LJ, Bartley GB: Complications associated with the new smaller size Freeman punctal plug [letter to the editor]. Arch Ophthalmol 107:961 – 962, 1989. Copyright 1989, Mayo Foundation.)

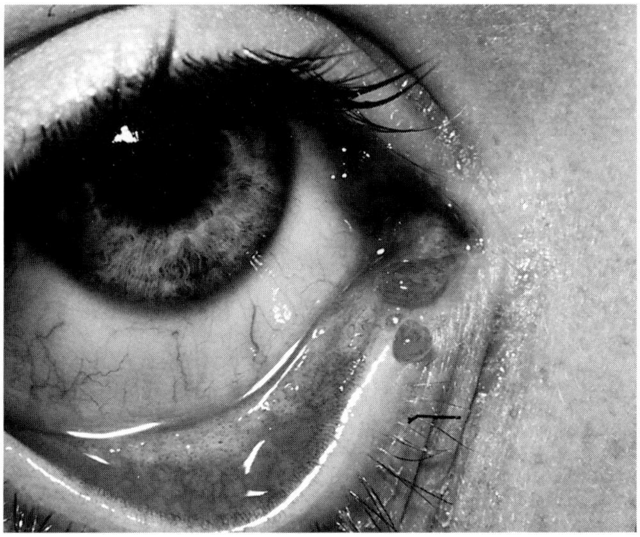

Figure 78–20. Bicanalicular obstruction and granulation tissue after a single canalicular repair with a pigtail probe.

ably from delayed scarring around the nasoantral window. My colleagues and I reviewed our group's experience with nearly 500 patients who have undergone orbital decompression; 2.5% had persistent nasolacrimal obstruction. Preliminary results from this study have been reported.[291] Damage to the nasolacrimal duct may be reduced by careful placement of the nasoantral window,[290] performing the procedure without an opening between the nose and the sinus (Seiff SR, personal communication, September 13, 1988), placement of a Bowman probe within the nasolacrimal duct to identify its position during the operation,[292] or approaching the orbital floor through an eyelid or conjunctival fornix incision.[293]

In addition to the ophthalmic procedures described previously, nasolacrimal obstruction may occur as a complication of paranasal sinus surgery (either conventional or endoscopic), nasal procedures, or craniofacial operations.[128, 166, 294–302]

Accidental, noniatrogenic trauma is a frequent cause of lacrimal drainage obstruction.* The nasolacrimal drainage system is usually violated at one of three sites: the canaliculus, the lacrimal sac, or the nasolacrimal duct.

Because studies have shown that both the superior and the inferior canaliculi are important for tear drainage, surgical repair of an isolated canalicular laceration is indicated.[309–311] The anastomosed canaliculus should be stented to prevent obstructive scarring, and various devices have been fashioned for this purpose. The Veirs rod[312, 313] and the Johnson wire[314, 315] were popular previously, but they have been largely supplanted in contemporary practice by silicone lacrimal intubation.[155, 316–323] Although bicanalicular stenting is preferred, in some instances it is not possible technically or anatomically. In such cases, monocanalicular intubation can be accomplished by various techniques.[324–332] In unusually difficult cases, a dacryocystotomy may be performed to allow retrograde canalicular intubation.[333] Another variation on the theme of canalicular repair was described by Hawes and Shawbitz,[334] who used a segment of angular vein to repair an avulsed common canaliculus.

Midfacial fractures frequently involve the nasolacrimal canals, and lacrimal drainage obstruction may ensue (Fig. 78–22).[335–339] If the nasolacrimal system clearly is violated, prophylactic intubation of the system with silicone tubing should be considered to prevent subsequent occlusion.

*References 18, 36, 81, 95, 102, 128, 166, 284, 285, 303–308.

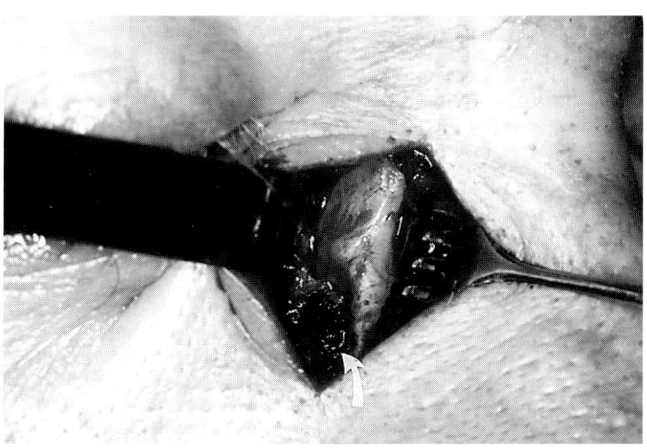

Figure 78–21. Failure of a previous dacryocystorhinostomy due to an inadequate and improperly placed osteotomy (*arrow*). The bony opening should have been made more posteriorly and superiorly.

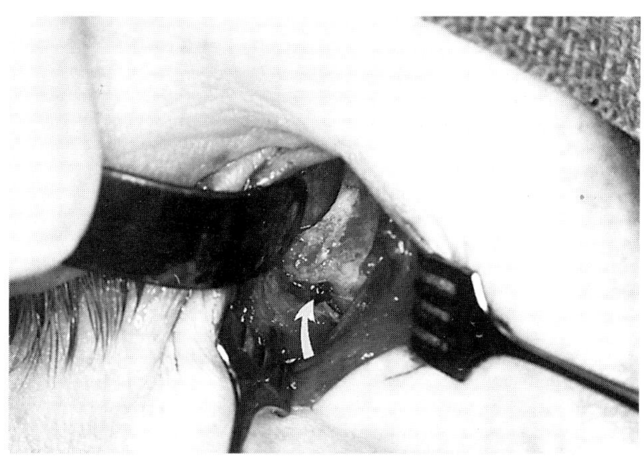

Figure 78–22. Nasolacrimal duct obstruction and dacryocystitis after a midfacial fracture (*arrow*) that violated the duct's bony canal.

MECHANICAL CAUSES OF SECONDARY ACQUIRED LACRIMAL DRAINAGE OBSTRUCTION

SALDO may result from mechanical blockage of the drainage passages, either from an intraluminal foreign body or from external compression or occlusion of the system (Table 78–6; see Table 78–1).

Dacryoliths are by far the most common cause of internal mechanical lacrimal drainage obstruction.[30, 95, 340–349] In my colleagues' and my review of 200 consecutive dacryocystorhinostomies, a dacryolith was found to be the underlying cause for nasolacrimal drainage in approximately 10% of patients[350]; this prevalence is comparable with that in other published reports. Although some dacryoliths are associated with fungal infections, as described previously in the section on infectious causes of SALDO, the underlying reason for most stones is indeterminate. In 1976, Jay and Lee[342] described a patient in whom an eyelash was found in the center of the dacryolith, presumably serving as a nidus. My colleagues and I have treated two similar patients and have speculated that migrated cilia may contribute to stone formation in a higher percentage of cases than has been reported.[350]

Medications, in particular epinephrine[351–353] and quinacrine,[118] may contribute to the formation of lacrimal drainage system casts.

Migrated or retained medical devices may cause lacrimal drainage obstruction. Freeman punctal plugs, particularly the newer, small size (model 003), have been reported to migrate or become displaced into the canaliculus.[267, 268, 354]

Two reports have described the retention of a Veirs rod[355] and a fragment of a Bowman probe.[356] I treated a patient with SALDO secondary to a modified myringotomy tube that had been placed by an otorhinolaryngologist in the right superior canaliculus to assist tear drainage from the lacrimal lake to the lacrimal sac. Apparently the device had migrated through the canaliculus to the lacrimal sac, causing obstruction (Fig. 78–23).

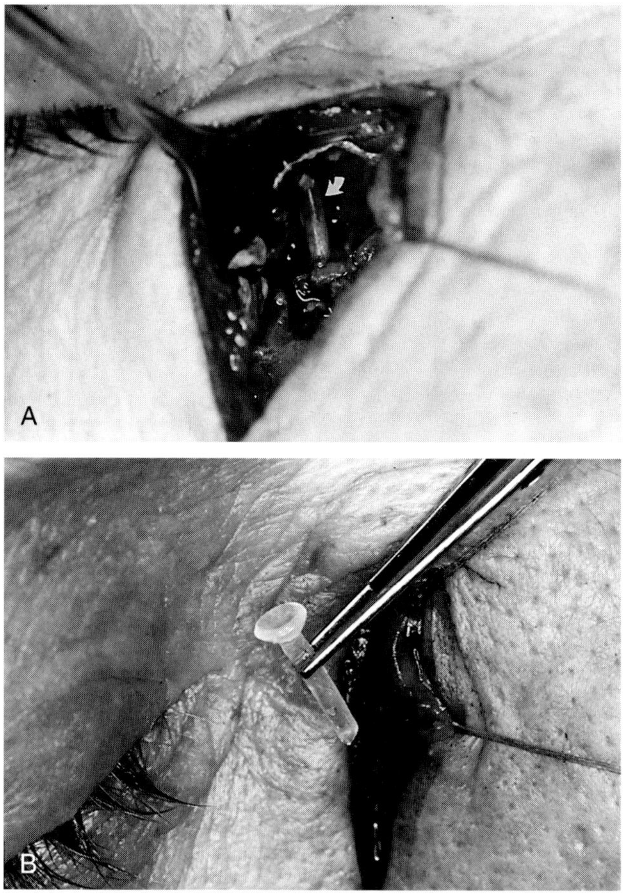

Figure 78–23. *A*, Obstruction of the lacrimal drainage system by a modified myringotomy tube (arrow) that had been placed within the right superior canaliculus 17 years previously. *B*, The device was removed, and a dacryocystorhinostomy was fashioned to reestablish lacrimal drainage. (*A* and *B* from Bartley GB: Acquired lacrimal drainage obstruction: An etiologic classification system, case reports, and a review of the literature. Parts I, II, and III. Ophthal Plast Reconstr Surg 8:237–249, 1992; 9:11–26, 1993.)

TABLE 78–6

Mechanical Causes of Secondary Acquired Lacrimal Drainage Obstruction

Internal
Dacryolith
Idiopathic
Eyelash nidus
Epinephrine cast
Quinacrine deposits
Migrated or retained medical device
Punctal plug
Veirs rod
Fragment of nasolacrimal probe
Modified myringotomy tube
Bullet (BB)
External
"Kissing puncta"
"Conjunctivochalasis"
Mucocele
Migrated silicone implant after repair of orbital floor fracture
Paget's disease
Osteopetrosis
Rhinolith or other nasal foreign bodies
Suture stent after esophagocolostomy

From Bartley GB: Acquired lacrimal drainage obstruction: An etiologic classification system, case reports, and a review of the literature. Parts I, II, and III. Ophthal Plast Reconstr Surg 8:237–249, 1992; 9:11–26, 1993.

Rarely, internal mechanical lacrimal drainage obstruction may be caused by foreign bodies that do not arise within the sac or that are not intentionally placed within the lacrimal drainage system. Such a case was reported by Felt and Frueh,[357] who described a patient who had a BB within the lacrimal sac.

Mechanical lacrimal obstruction with resultant epiphora may be associated with several external forces, from the level of the puncta to the valve of Hasner. Proximal obstruction is common with "kissing puncta," which customarily can be treated satisfactorily with appropriate eyelid procedures.[358] In "conjunctivochalasis,"[359] redundant bulbar conjunctiva rests on the lower eyelid margin and may cover the inferior punctum.

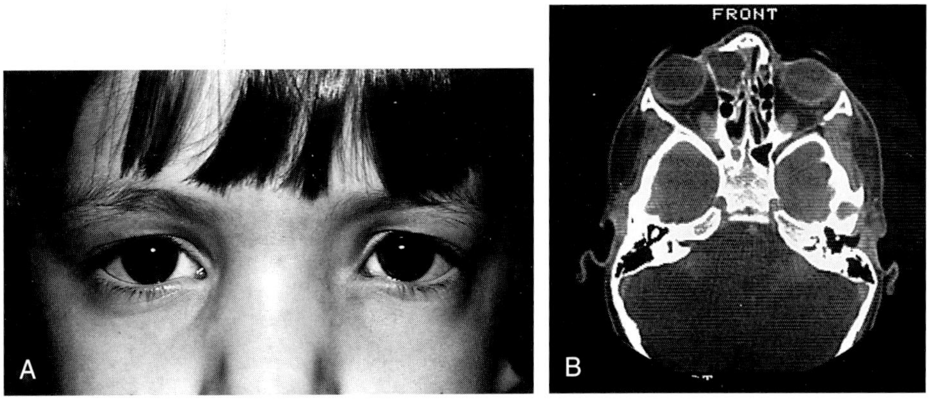

Figure 78-24. *A*, A 3-year-old girl with recent signs and symptoms of right lacrimal obstruction. (*A*, Courtesy of James A. Garrity, MD) *B*, An ethmoidal mucocele, demonstrated by computed tomography, was compressing the nasolacrimal drainage system. The lacrimal obstruction was relieved by drainage of the mucocele.

Some patients experience a foreign body sensation from the excess tissue, and rose bengal staining of the eyelid margin may be seen. Simple excision of an ellipse of the redundant conjunctiva is usually helpful in eliminating both epiphora and ocular discomfort.

Mucoceles arising from the paranasal sinuses may compress the lacrimal sac or compromise the nasolacrimal duct (Fig. 78-24).[360-362] External compression of the lacrimal sac or nasolacrimal duct by a migrated orbital floor implant has been reported.[363, 364]

Paget's disease of bone has been cited as a cause of dacryocystorhinostomy failure by Hurwitz,[365] who advised placement of a Jones tube after creation of an adequate bony window. I have treated a similar patient with Paget's disease by dacryocystorhinostomy alone. Although the operation has been successful during a followup period of 2½ years, future disease-related bone changes may compromise the osteotomy. Osteopetrosis has been reported as a cause of acquired lacrimal drainage obstruction.[366] Finally, mechanical external lacrimal drainage obstruction can occur distally, at the valve of Hasner. Although uncommon, rhinoliths or other nasal foreign bodies may occlude the inferior meatus.[367, 368] I have described an unusual case in which a silk suture that had been placed beneath the inferior turbinate after esophagocolostomy caused partial, reversible, mechanical nasolacrimal obstruction (Fig. 78-25).[369]

CONCLUSION

Secondary acquired lacrimal drainage obstruction may result from many causes, both common and obscure. In some instances, information gained from lacrimal evaluations and procedures was important in the overall care of the patient. Biopsy of the lacrimal sac or nasolacrimal duct, as described by Linberg and McCormick,[1] seems prudent when operation is required.

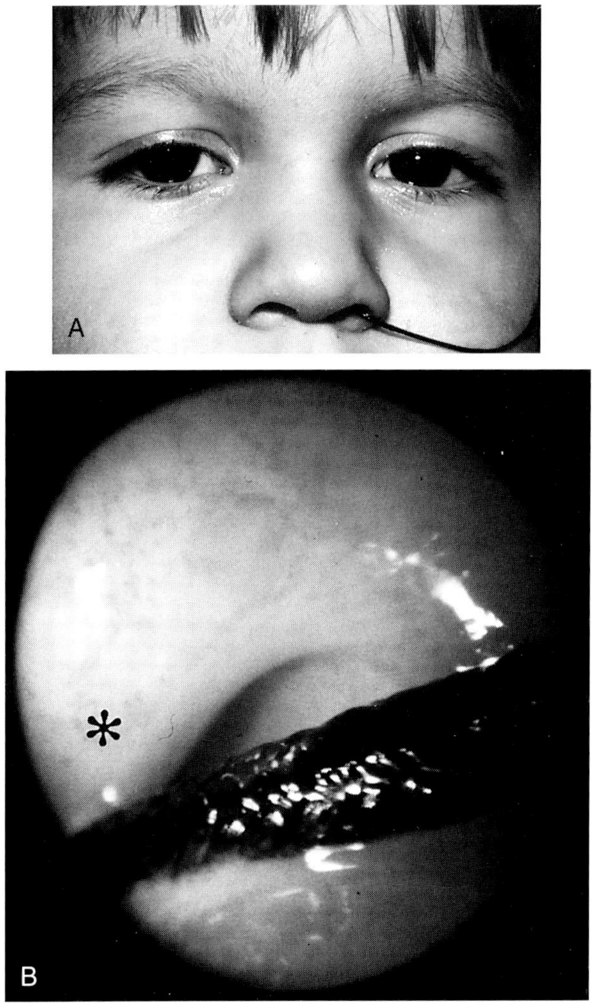

Figure 78-25. *A*, A no. 2 silk suture placed as a "guidewire" stent to facilitate dilation of the esophagocolostomy. *B*, The suture caused mechanical partial obstruction at the valve of Hasner; the inferior turbinate is indicated by the asterisk. Epiphora was relieved by removal of the suture. (*A* and *B* from Bartley GB, Moir CR, McCaffrey TV: Acquired partial nasolacrimal obstruction due to a suture stent following esophagocolostomy. Arch Ophthalmol 108:1074, 1990. Copyright 1990, American Medical Association.)

Acknowledgment

The work for this chapter was supported in part by an unrestricted grant from Research to Prevent Blindness, Inc., New York, New York.

REFERENCES

1. Linberg JV, McCormick SA: Primary acquired nasolacrimal duct obstruction: A clinicopathologic report and biopsy technique. Ophthalmology 93:1055-1062, 1986.
2. Traquair HM: Chronic dacryocystitis: Its causation and treatment. Arch Ophthalmol 26:165-180, 1941.
3. Scott GI, Summerskill WH: Discussion on treatment of chronic dacryocystitis. Trans Ophthalmol Soc UK 69:477-505, 1949.
4. Dalgleish R: Idiopathic acquired canaliculus obstruction. Trans Ophthalmol Soc UK 85:191-195, 1965.
5. Dalgleish R: Idiopathic acquired lacrimal drainage obstruction. Br J Ophthalmol 51:463-468, 1967.
6. Duke-Elder S, MacFaul PA: The Ocular Adnexa, vol 13, part 2. St. Louis, CV Mosby, 1974, pp 675-770.
7. Schaal KP: Genus *Actinomyces* harz 1877, 133[AL]. *In* Sneath PHA, Mair NS, Sharpe ME, Holt JG (eds): Bergey's Manual of Systemic Bacteriology, vol 2. Baltimore, Williams & Wilkins, 1986, pp 1383-1418.
8. von Graefe A: Konkretionen im unteren Thränenröhrchen durch Pilzbildung. Arch Ophthalmol 1:284-288, 1854.
9. McClanahan R: Fungus infection of the lacrimal canaliculi. Am J Ophthalmol 19:418-419, 1936.
10. Smith CH: Ocular actinomycosis. Proc R Soc Med 46:209-212, 1952.
11. Pine L, Hardin H: *Actinomyces israelii*, a cause of lacrimal canaliculitis in man. J Bacteriol 78:164-170, 1959.
12. Pine L, Hardin H, Turner L, Roberts SS: Actinomycotic lacrimal canaliculitis: A report of two cases with a review of the characteristics that identify the causal organism, *Actinomyces israelii*. Am J Ophthalmol 49:1278-1288, 1960.
13. Richards WW: Actinomycotic lacrimal canaliculitis. Am J Ophthalmol 75:155-157, 1973.
14. Demant E, Hurwitz JJ: Canaliculitis: Review of 12 cases. Can J Ophthalmol 15:73-75, 1980.
15. Berlin AJ, Rath R, Rich L: Lacrimal system dacryoliths. Ophthalmic Surg 11:435-436, 1980.
16. Smith RL, Henderson PN: Actinomycotic canaliculitis. Aust J Ophthalmol 8:75-79, 1980.
17. Joseph TA, Paniker CKJ, Kumari S, et al: Actinomycotic lacrimal canaliculitis. Indian J Ophthalmol 28:157-159, 1980.
18. Welham RAN, Hughes SM: Lacrimal surgery in children. Am J Ophthalmol 99:27-34, 1985.
19. Ritleng P, Loubiere R, Marcelet B: Suppurative pseudolithiasic canaliculitis. Ophtalmologie 3:1-3, 1989.
20. George WL: Actinomycosis. *In* Finegold SM, George WL (eds): Anaerobic Infections in Humans. San Diego, Academic Press, 1989, pp 535-536.
21. Rose HD, Varkey B, Kutty CPK: Thoracic actinomycosis caused by *Actinomyces meyeri*. Am Rev Respir Dis 125:251-254, 1982.
22. Lentino JR, Allen JE, Stachowski M: Hematogenous dissemination of thoracic actinomycosis due to *Actinomyces meyeri*. Pediatr Infect Dis 4:698-699, 1985.
23. Marty HU, Wüst J: Disseminated actinomycosis caused by *Actinomyces meyeri*. Infection 17:154-155, 1989.
24. Roussel TJ, Olson ER, Rice T, et al: Chronic postoperative endophthalmitis associated with *Actinomyces* species. Arch Ophthalmol 109:60-62, 1991.
25. Schaal KP: Genus *Arachnia* pine and george. *In* Sneath PHA, Mair NS, Sharpe ME, Holt JG (eds): Bergey's Manual of Systemic Bacteriology, vol 2. Baltimore, Williams & Wilkins, 1986, pp 1332-1342.
26. Weinberg RJ, Sartoris MJ, Buerger GF Jr, Novak JF: *Fusobacterium* in presumed *Actinomyces* canaliculitis. Am J Ophthalmol 84:371-374, 1977.
27. Pavilack MA, Frueh BR: Thorough curettage in the treatment of chronic canaliculitis. Arch Ophthalmol 110:200-202, 1992.
28. Katowitz JA, Kropp TM: *Mycobacterium fortuitum* as a cause for nasolacrimal obstruction and granulomatous eyelid disease. Ophthalmic Surg 18:97-99, 1987.
29. Weerekoon L: Ocular leprosy in Ceylon. Br J Ophthalmol 53: 457-465, 1969.
30. Werb A: Unusual causes of epiphora. Br J Ophthalmol 55:559-564, 1971.
31. Garfin SW: Etiology of dacryocystitis and epiphora. Arch Ophthalmol 27:167-188, 1942.
32. Andersen SR: Tuberculous dacryocystitis and lupus of the nose diagnosed as Boeck's disease. Acta Ophthalmol 25:455-459, 1947.
33. Csüllög F, Gát G, Gát L, Kelemen JT: Über die Tuberkulose der Bindehaut und des Tränensackes. Klin Monatsbl Augenheilkd 148:79-86, 1966.
34. Rootman DS, Insler MS, Wolfley DE: Canaliculitis caused by *Mycobacterium chelonae* after lacrimal intubation with silicone tubes. Can J Ophthalmol 24:221-222, 1989.
35. Postic S: Remarques sur le trachome lacrymal: Étude comparative. Arch Ophtal (Paris) 17:749-768, 1957.
36. Welham RAN: Canalicular obstructions and the Lester Jones tube: What to do when all else fails. Trans Ophthalmol Soc UK 93:623-632, 1973.
37. Dawson CR: Lids, conjunctiva, and lacrimal apparatus: Eye infections with *Chlamydia*. Arch Ophthalmol 93:854-862, 1975.
38. Tabbara KF, Bobb AA: Lacrimal system complications in trachoma. Ophthalmology 87:298-301, 1980.
39. Rice CD, Kersten RC: Absence of *Chlamydia* in trachomatous lacrimal sacs. Am J Ophthalmol 105:203-206, 1988.
40. Penikett EJK, Rees DL: *Nocardia asteroides* infection of the nasal lacrimal system. Am J Ophthalmol 53:1006-1008, 1962.
41. Chumbley LC: Canaliculitis caused by *Enterobacter cloacae*: Report of a case. Br J Ophthalmol 68:364-366, 1984.
42. Garweg J, Bialek R, Guthoff R: *Aeromonas hydrophila*-Dakryozystitis. Klin Monatsbl Augenheilkd 193:189-191, 1988.
43. McPherson SD Jr, Egleston D: Dacryocystorhinostomy: A review of 106 operations. Am J Ophthalmol 47:328-331, 1959.
44. Bouzas A: Canalicular inflammation: In ophthalmic cases of herpes zoster and herpes simplex. Am J Ophthalmol 60:713-716, 1965.
45. Sanford-Smith JH: Herpes simplex canalicular obstruction. Br J Ophthalmol 54:456-460, 1970.
46. Bouzas AG: Virus aetiology of certain cases of lacrimal obstruction. Br J Ophthalmol 57:849-851, 1973.
47. Coster DJ, Welham RAN: Herpetic canalicular obstruction. Br J Ophthalmol 63:259-262, 1979.
48. Harris GJ, Hyndiuk RA, Fox MJ, Taugher PJ: Herpetic canalicular obstruction. Arch Ophthalmol 99:282-283, 1981.
49. Harley RD, Stefanyszyn MA, Apt L, Nelson LB: Herpetic canalicular obstruction. Ophthalmic Surg 18:367-370, 1987.
50. Nasr AM, Beyer-Machule CK, Yeatts RP: Cicatricial ectropion secondary to herpes zoster. Ophthalmic Surg 14:763-765, 1983.
51. Sanke RF, Welham RAN: Lacrimal canalicular obstruction following chickenpox. Br J Ophthalmol 66:71-74, 1982.
52. Nagashima K: "Silicone-octopus repair" of lacrimal obstructions in children. Ophthalmic Surg 14:766-769, 1983.
53. Panda A, Vasisht S, Patnaik NK: Lacrimal canalicular obstruction following herpes zoster ophthalmicus. Indian J Pediatr 53:817-819, 1986.
54. Hyde KJ, Berger ST: Epidemic keratoconjunctivitis and lacrimal excretory system obstruction. Ophthalmology 95:1447-1449, 1988.
55. Atkinson PL, Ansons AM, Patterson A: Infectious mononucleosis presenting as bilateral acute dacryocystitis. Br J Ophthalmol 74:750, 1990.
56. Saxena RC, Garg KC, Ramchand S: Ankyloblepharon following smallpox. Am J Ophthalmol 61:169-171, 1966.
57. Brightbill FS, Fraser LK: Unilateral keratoconjunctivitis: With canalicular obstruction by *Aspergillus fumigatus*. Arch Ophthalmol 91:421-422, 1974.
58. Donahue HC: Unusual mycotic infection of the lacrimal canaliculi and conjunctiva. Am J Ophthalmol 32:207-210, 1949.
59. Fine M, Waring WS: Mycotic obstruction of the nasolacrimal duct (*Candida albicans*). Arch Ophthalmol 38:39-42, 1947.
60. Wolter JR, Stratford T, Harrell ER: Cast-like fungus obstruction

of the nasolacrimal duct: Report of a case. Arch Ophthalmol 55:320–322, 1956.
61. Newton JC, Tulevech CB: Lacrimal canaliculitis due to *Candida albicans*: Report of a case and a discussion of its significance. Am J Ophthalmol 53:933–936, 1962.
62. Wolter JR, Deitz MR: Candidiasis of the lacrimal sac. Am J Ophthalmol 55:153–155, 1963.
63. Hanssens M, Rysselaere M, Domen F: *Candida parapsilosis* associated with dacryoliths in obstructive dacryocystitis. Bull Soc Belge Ophtalmol 201:71–81, 1982.
64. Wolter JR. *Pityrosporum* species associated with dacryoliths in obstructive dacryocystitis. Am J Ophthalmol 84:806–809, 1977.
65. Romano A, Segal E, Blumenthal M: Canaliculitis with isolation of *Pityrosporum pachydermatis*. Br J Ophthalmol 62:732–734, 1978.
66. Savir H, Henig E, Lehrer N: Exogenous mycotic infections of the eye and adnexa. Ann Ophthalmol 10:1013–1018, 1978.
67. Bergaust B, Eng J: Obstruction of the lacrimal passage due to *Trichophyton rubrum* infection: Report of a case. Acta Ophthalmol (Copenh) 43:708–713, 1965.
68. Jain SC, Darbari BS, Bhatnagar BS: Ocular rhinosporidiosis. Eye Ear Nose Throat Mon 47:380–382, 1968.
69. Gifford SR: Ocular sporotrichosis. Arch Ophthalmol 51:540–547, 1922.
70. Kaplan CS, Freedman L, Elsdon-Dew R: A worm in the eye: A familiar parasite in an unusual situation. South Afr Med J 30:791–792, 1956.
71. Roche PJL. *Ascaris* in the lacrimal duct [letter to the editor]. Trans R Soc Trop Med Hyg 65:540, 1971.
72. Cunha MC, Veloudios A, Dantas PEC, Eagle RC Jr: Obstruction of the nasolacrimal duct by *Ascaris lumbricoides*. Ophthalmic Plast Reconstr Surg 5:141–143, 1989.
73. Carrington CB, Liebow AA: Limited forms of angiitis and granulomatosis of Wegener's type. Am J Med 41:497–527, 1966.
74. Cassan SM, Coles DT, Harrison EG Jr: The concept of limited forms of Wegener's granulomatosis. Am J Med 49:366–379, 1970.
75. DeRemee RA: Extrapulmonary manifestations of Wegener's granulomatosis and other respiratory vasculitides. Semin Respir Med 9:403–408, 1988.
76. Fauci AS, Wolff SM: Wegener's granulomatosis: Studies in eighteen patients and a review of the literature. Medicine (Baltimore) 52:535–561, 1973.
77. Bullen CL, Liesegang TJ, McDonald TJ, DeRemee RA: Ocular complications of Wegener's granulomatosis. Ophthalmology 90:279–290, 1983.
78. Jordan DR, Miller D, Anderson RL: Wound necrosis following dacryocystorhinostomy in patients with Wegener's granulomatosis. Ophthalmic Surg 18:800–803, 1987.
79. Holds JB, Anderson RL, Wolin MJ: Dacryocystectomy for the treatment of dacryocystitis patients with Wegener's granulomatosis. Ophthalmic Surg 20:443–444, 1989.
80. Glatt HJ, Putterman AM: Dacryocystorhinostomy in Wegener's granulomatosis. Ophthalmic Plast Reconstr Surg 6:207–210, 1990.
81. Chandler AC Jr, Wadsworth JAC: Conjunctivodacryocystostomy. Am J Ophthalmol 77:830–836, 1974.
82. Hardwig PW, Bartley GB, Garrity JA: The surgical management of nasolacrimal duct obstruction in patients with Wegener's granulomatosis. Ophthalmology 99:133–139, 1992.
83. DeRemee RA, McDonald TJ, Weiland LH: Wegener's granulomatosis: Observations on treatment with antimicrobial agents. Mayo Clin Proc 60:27–32, 1985.
84. Specks U, Wheatley CL, McDonald TJ, et al: Anticytoplasmic autoantibodies in the diagnosis and follow-up of Wegener's granulomatosis. Mayo Clin Proc 64:28–36, 1989.
85. Kalina PH, Garrity JA, Herman DC, et al: Role of testing for anticytoplasmic autoantibodies in the differential diagnosis of scleritis and orbital pseudotumor. Mayo Clin Proc 65:1110–1117, 1990.
86. Pulido JS, Goeken JA, Nerad JA, et al: Ocular manifestations of patients with circulating antineutrophil cytoplasmic antibodies. Arch Ophthalmol 108:845–850, 1990.
87. Lund S: Boecks Sarcoid i Taaresaekken. Hospitalstid 81 (Suppl):46–51, 1938.
88. Neault RW, Riley FC: Report of a case of dacryocystitis secondary to Boeck's sarcoid. Am J Ophthalmol 70:1011–1013, 1970.
89. Fisher OE, Burton GG, Bryan WF: Sarcoidosis involving the lacrimal sac. Am Rev Respir Dis 103:708–710, 1971.
90. Coleman SL, Brull S, Green WR: Sarcoid of the lacrimal sac and surrounding area. Arch Ophthalmol 88:645–646, 1972.
91. Karma A: Ophthalmic changes in sarcoidosis. Acta Ophthalmol Suppl (Copenh) 141:1–94, 1979.
92. Harris GJ, Williams GA, Clarke GP: Sarcoidosis of the lacrimal sac. Arch Ophthalmol 99:1198–1201, 1981.
93. Karma A: Sarcoidosis of the lacrimal sac [letter to the editor]. Arch Ophthalmol 100:664, 1982.
94. Weingarten R, Goodman EF: Late failure of a dacryocystorhinostomy from sarcoidosis. Ophthalmic Surg 12:343–346, 1981.
95. Nik NA, Hurwitz JJ, Sang HC: Mechanism of tear flow after dacryocystorhinostomy and Jones' tube surgery. Arch Ophthalmol 102:1643–1646, 1984.
96. Lauer M, Reim H, Reim M: Vielfältige okuäre Manifestationen bei Morbus Boeck. Klin Monatsbl Augenheilkd 195:183–186, 1989.
97. Radńot M, Gáll J: Tumoren des Tränensackes. Ophthalmologica 151:1–22, 1966.
98. Leahey AB, Wulc AE, Day D, et al: Canalicular obliteration from toxic epidermal necrolysis. Am J Ophthalmol 112:469–470, 1991.
99. Mamelok AE, Laval J: Stenosis of the lacrimal canals and puncta: Caused by the Stevens-Johnson syndrome. Am J Ophthalmol 40:83–86, 1955.
100. Hardy KM, Perry HO, Pingree GC, Kirby TJ Jr: Benign mucous membrane pemphigoid. Arch Dermatol 104:467–475, 1971.
101. Arstikaitis MJ: Ocular aftermath of Stevens-Johnson syndrome: Review of 33 cases. Arch Ophthalmol 90:376–379, 1973.
102. Callahan A, Callahan MA: Conjunctivodacryocystorhinostomy: Emplacement of the Jones Pyrex glass tube. *In* Anderson RL, Blodi FC, Boniuk M, et al (eds): Symposium on Diseases and Surgery of the Lids, Lacrimal Apparatus, and Orbit. St. Louis, CV Mosby, 1982, pp 123–128.
103. Wright P, Collin JRO: The ocular complications of erythema multiforme (Stevens-Johnson syndrome) and their management. Trans Ophthalmol Soc UK 103:338–341, 1983.
104. Welham RA, Guthoff R: The Lester-Jones tube: A 15-year follow-up. Graefes Arch Clin Exp Ophthalmol 223:106–108, 1985.
105. Auran JD, Hornblass A, Gross ND: Stevens-Johnson syndrome with associated nasolacrimal duct obstruction treated with dacryocystorhinostomy and Crawford silicone tube insertion. Ophthalmic Plast Reconstr Surg 6:60–63, 1990.
106. Karcioglu ZA, Allam B, Insler MS: Ocular involvement in sinus histiocytosis with massive lymphadenopathy. Br J Ophthalmol 72:793–795, 1988.
107. Dolman PJ, Harris GJ, Weiland LH: Sinus histiocytosis involving the lacrimal sac and duct: A clinicopathologic case report. Arch Ophthalmol 109:1582–1584, 1991.
108. Foucar E, Rosai J, Dorfman RF: The ophthalmologic manifestations of sinus histiocytosis with massive lymphadenopathy. Am J Ophthalmol 87:354–367, 1979.
109. Cole JG, Brackup A, Hanley JS, Higgins GK: Pseudotumor of lacrimal sac. Am J Ophthalmol 55:136–138, 1963.
110. Heathcote JG, Allen LH, Willis NR: Plasma cell granuloma of the lacrimal sac. Can J Ophthalmol 22:387–390, 1987.
111. Mauriello JA Jr, Stabile C, Wagner RS: Dacryocystitis following Kawasaki's disease. Ophthalmic Plast Reconstr Surg 2:209–211, 1986.
112. O'Donnell FE Jr: Medial ectropion: Association with lower lacrimal obstruction and combined management. Ophthalmic Surg 17:573–576, 1986.
113. Bartley GB, Bullock JD, Waller RR: Eyelid manifestations of connective tissue disorders. *In* Hornblass A, Hanig CJ (eds): Oculoplastic, Orbital, and Reconstructive Surgery, vol 1, Eyelids. Baltimore, Williams & Wilkins, 1988, pp 181–189.
114. Sober AJ, Grove AS Jr, Muhlbauer JE: Cicatricial ectropion and lacrimal obstruction associated with the sclerodermoid variant of porphyria cutanea tarda. Am J Ophthalmol 91:396–400, 1981.
115. Hughes WL, Maris CSG: A clip procedure for stenosis and eversion of the lacrimal punctum. Trans Am Acad Ophthalmol Otolaryngol 71:653–654, 1967.

116. Fein W: Cautery applications to relieve punctal stenosis. Arch Ophthalmol 95:145-146, 1977.
117. Kristan RW: Treatment of lacrimal punctal stenosis with a one-snip canaliculotomy and temporary punctal plugs [letter to the editor]. Arch Ophthalmol 106:878-879, 1988.
118. Fraunfelder FT: Drug-Induced Ocular Side Effects and Drug Interactions, 3rd ed. Philadelphia, Lea & Febiger, 1989, pp 580-581.
119. Shaffer RN, Ridgway WL: Furmethide iodide in the production of dacryostenosis. Am J Ophthalmol 34:718-720, 1951.
120. Jones BR: Prospects in treating viral disease of the eye. Trans Ophthalmol Soc UK 87:537-579, 1967.
121. Patterson A, Jones BR: The management of ocular herpes. Trans Ophthalmol Soc UK 87:59-83, 1967.
122. Romano A, Barishak R, Stein R: Obstruction of lacrimal puncta caused by topical epinephrine. Ophthalmologica 166:301-305, 1973.
123. Laibson PR: Current therapy of herpes simplex virus infection of the cornea. Int Ophthalmol Clin 13(Winter):39-52, 1973.
124. McGill J, Williams H, McKinnon J, et al: Reassessment of idoxuridine therapy of herpetic keratitis. Trans Ophthalmol Soc UK 94:542-551, 1974.
125. Binder PS: Herpes simplex keratitis. Surv Ophthalmol 21:313-330, 1977.
126. Wilson F II: Adverse external ocular effects of topical ophthalmic medications. Surv Ophthalmol 24:57-88, 1979.
127. Wood JR, Anderson RL, Edwards JJ: Phospholine iodide toxicity and Jones' tubes. Ophthalmology 87:346-349, 1980.
128. Lamping K, Levine MR: Jones' tubes: How good are they? Arch Ophthalmol 101:260-261, 1983.
129. Lass JH, Thoft RA, Dohlman CH: Idoxuridine-induced conjunctival cicatrization. Arch Ophthalmol 101:747-750, 1983.
130. Fiore PM, Jacobs IH, Goldberg DB: Drug-induced pemphigoid: A spectrum of diseases. Arch Ophthalmol 105:1660-1663, 1987.
131. Levitt SH, Bogardus CR Jr, Brandt EN Jr: Complications and late changes following radiation therapy for carcinoma of the eyelid and canthi. Radiology 87:340-347, 1966.
132. MacFaul PA, Bedford MA: Ocular complications after therapeutic irradiation. Br J Ophthalmol 54:237-247, 1970.
133. Call NB, Welham RAN: Epiphora after irradiation of medial eyelid tumors. Am J Ophthalmol 92:842-845, 1981
134. Hurwitz JJ, Howcroft MJ: Use of Lester Jones tubes: A review of 40 cases. Can J Ophthalmol 16:176-177, 1981.
135. Wilder RB, Kittelson JM, Shimm DS: Basal cell carcinoma treated with radiation therapy. Cancer 68:2134-2137, 1991.
136. Brizel HE, Sheils WC, Brown M: The effects of radiotherapy on the nasolacrimal system as evaluated by dacryoscintigraphy. Radiology 116:373-381, 1975.
137. Lovato AA, Char DH, Castro JR, Kroll SM: The effect of silicone nasolacrimal intubation on epiphora after helium ion irradiation of uveal melanomas. Am J Ophthalmol 108:431-434, 1989.
138. English FP: Epiphora after irradiation of medial eyelid tumors [letter to the editor]. Am J Ophthalmol 93:804, 1982.
139. Shields JA, Augsburger JJ, Brady LW, Day JL: Cobalt plaque therapy of posterior uveal melanomas. Ophthalmology 89:1201-1207, 1982.
140. Kronish JW, Mieler WF, Dortzbach RK: Eyelid phimosis and chronic radiation dermatitis associated with iridium brachytherapy [letter to the editor]. Am J Ophthalmol 105:431-432, 1988.
141. Packer S, Rotman M, Fairchild RG, et al: Irradiation of choroidal melanoma with iodine 125 ophthalmic plaque. Arch Ophthalmol 98:1453-1457, 1980.
142. Robertson DM, Fountain KS, Anderson JA, Posthumus GW: Radioactive iodine-125 as a therapeutic radiation source for management of intraocular tumors. Trans Am Ophthalmol Soc 79:294-303, 1981.
143. Hamersley J, Luce JK, Florentz TR, et al: Excessive lacrimation from fluorouracil treatment [letter to the editor]. JAMA 225:747-748, 1973.
144. Haidak DJ, Hurwitz BS, Yeung KY: Tear-duct fibrosis (dacryostenosis) due to 5-fluorouracil. Ann Intern Med 88:657, 1978.
145. Caravella LP Jr, Burns JA, Zangmeister M: Punctal-canalicular stenosis related to systemic fluorouracil therapy. Arch Ophthalmol 99:284-286, 1981.
146. Seiff SR, Shorr N, Adams T: Surgical treatment of punctal-canalicular fibrosis from 5-fluorouracil therapy. Cancer 56:2148-2149, 1985.
147. Imperia PS, Lazarus HM, Lass JH: Ocular complications of systemic cancer chemotherapy. Surv Ophthalmol 34:209-230, 1989.
148. Insler MS, Helm CJ: Ankyloblepharon associated with systemic 5-fluorouracil treatment. Ann Ophthalmol 19:374-375, 1987.
149. Loprinzi CL, Love RR, Garrity JA, Ames MM: Cyclophosphamide, methotrexate, and 5-fluorouracil (CMF)-induced ocular toxicity. Cancer Invest 8:459-465, 1990.
150. Hanada R, Ueoka Y: Obstruction of nasolacrimal ducts closely related to graft-versus-host disease after bone marrow transplantation. Bone Marrow Transplant 4:125-126, 1989.
151. Margo CE, Grossniklaus HE: Ocular Histopathology: A Guide to Differential Diagnosis. Philadelphia, WB Saunders, 1991, pp 3-7.
152. Stewart WB, Gelender H, Miller GR, Tenzel RR: Silicone in ophthalmic plastic and reconstructive surgery: A review and laboratory trial. Ophthalmic Surg 9:92-101, 1978.
153. Snead JW, Rathbun JE, Crawford JB: Effects of the silicone tube on the canaliculus: An animal experiment. Ophthalmology 87:1031-1036, 1980.
154. Bartley GB, Buettner H, Campbell RJ: Scanning electron-microscopic study of Silastic scleral sponges. Retina 5:42-46, 1985.
155. Anderson RL, Edwards JJ: Indications, complications and results with silicone stents. Ophthalmology 86:1474-1487, 1979.
156. Dresner SC, Codère F, Brownstein S, Jouve P: Lacrimal drainage system inflammatory masses from retained silicone tubing. Am J Ophthalmol 98:609-613, 1984.
157. Travis WD, Balogh K, Abraham JL: Silicone granulomas: Report of three cases and review of the literature. Hum Pathol 16:19-27, 1985.
158. Jordan DR, Nerad JA: An acute inflammatory reaction to silicone stents. Ophthalmic Plast Reconstr Surg 3:147-150, 1987.
159. Stallard HB: A case of chronic granuloma of the lacrymal sac. Br J Ophthalmol 24:457-459, 1940.
160. Wojno TH: Allergic lacrimal obstruction. Am J Ophthalmol 106:48-52, 1988.
161. Sanke RF: Pseudonasolacrimal duct obstruction caused by nasal allergy. Ophthalmic Surg 20:63-67, 1989.
162. Reifler DM: Allergic nasolacrimal obstruction [letter to the editor]. Arch Ophthalmol 106:172-173, 1988.
163. Nolan J: Granuloma of lacrimal sac: Simulating a neoplasm. Am J Ophthalmol 62:756-757, 1966.
164. Cinotti AA, Siliquini JJ: Antihistaminic therapy of chronic dacryocystitis. Am J Ophthalmol 62:1116-1118, 1966.
165. Missiroli A, Novacco V, Polli NSA: Treatment of obstructive epiphora with intralacrimal ointment: Clinical pattern. Orbit 5:217-218, 1986.
166. Katowitz JA: Silicone tubing in canalicular obstructions: A preliminary report. Arch Ophthalmol 91:459-462, 1974.
167. Huang TT, Blackwell SJ, Lewis SR: Burn injuries of the eyelids. Clin Plast Surg 5:571-581, 1978.
168. Font RL: Eyelids and lacrimal drainage system. *In* Spencer WH (ed): Ophthalmic Pathology, 3rd ed, vol 3. Philadelphia, WB Saunders, 1986, pp 2141-2336.
169. Flanagan JC, Zolli CL: Lacrimal sac tumors: Surgical management. *In* Linberg JV (ed): Lacrimal Surgery. New York, Churchill Livingstone, 1988, pp 203-226.
170. Ayres SC: Polyps of the lower canaliculus. Arch Ophthalmol 32:369-371, 1903.
171. Libby GF: Polyps in the lower canaliculus. Ophthalmic Rec 13:368-370, 1904.
172. Hird RB: Papilloma of the lacrymal sac. Br J Ophthalmol 16:416-417, 1932.
173. Tennent JN III: Diseases of lids and lacrymal apparatus: I. Carcinoma of the lacrymal sac: Report of two cases. Trans Ophthalmol Soc UK 53:93-101, 1933.
174. Burke JW: Papilloma lying within lower canaliculus. Am J Ophthalmol 21:189, 1938.
175. Ashton N, Choyce DP, Fison LG: Carcinoma of the lacrimal sac. Br J Ophthalmol 35:366-376, 1951.
176. Jones IS: Tumors of the lacrimal sac. Am J Ophthalmol 42:561-566, 1956.
177. Spaeth EB: Carcinomas in the region of the lacrimal sac. Arch Ophthalmol 57:689-693, 1957.

178. Anderson DR: Unilateral epiphora caused by a papilloma of the lower canaliculus. Arch Ophthalmol 78:618-620, 1967.
179. Harry J, Ashton N: The pathology of tumours of the lacrimal sac. Trans Ophthalmol Soc UK 88:19-34, 1968.
180. Milder B, Smith ME: Carcinoma of lacrimal sac. Am J Ophthalmol 65:782-784, 1968.
181. Paxton BR, Davidorf FH, Makley TA Jr: Carcinoma of lacrimal canaliculi and lacrimal sac. Arch Ophthalmol 84:749-753, 1970.
182. Ryan SJ, Font RL: Primary epithelial neoplasms of the lacrimal sac. Am J Ophthalmol 76:73-88, 1973.
183. Schenck NL, Ogura JH, Pratt LL: Cancer of the lacrimal sac: Presentation of five cases and review of the literature. Ann Otol Rhinol Laryngol 82:153-161, 1973.
184. Schindler R, Watson TA, Oliver G: Carcinoma of the lacrimal sac. Can J Ophthalmol 8:161-163, 1973.
185. Juler FA: A papilloma in the upper canaliculus. Trans Ophthalmol Soc UK 35:243-244, 1915.
186. Flanagan JC, Stokes DP: Lacrimal sac tumors. Ophthalmology 85:1282-1287, 1978.
187. Hornblass A, Jackobiec FA, Bosniak S, Flanagan J: The diagnosis and management of epithelial tumors of the lacrimal sac. Ophthalmology 87:476-489, 1980.
188. Khalil MK, Lorenzetti DWC: Epidermoid carcinoma of the lacrimal sac: A clinicopathological case report. Can J Ophthalmol 15:40-43, 1980.
189. Kohn R, Nofsinger K, Freedman SI: Rapid recurrence of papillary squamous cell carcinoma of the canaliculus. Am J Ophthalmol 92:363-367, 1981.
190. Nunziata BR, Horbeek JH, Gombos GM: Lacrimal sac papilloma: Presentation of an unusual case. Ophthalmic Surg 13:920, 1982.
191. Ni C, D'Amico DJ, Fan CQ, Kuo PK: Tumors of the lacrimal sac: A clinicopathological analysis of 82 cases. Int Ophthalmol Clin 22(Spring):121-140, 1982.
192. Bonder D, Fischer MJ, Levine MR: Squamous cell carcinoma of the lacrimal sac. Ophthalmology 90:1133-1135, 1983.
193. Karcioglu ZA, Caldwell DR, Reed HT: Papillomas of lacrimal drainage system: A clinicopathologic study. Ophthalmic Surg 15:670-676, 1984.
194. Williams R, Ilsar M, Welham RAN: Lacrimal canalicular papillomatosis. Br J Ophthalmol 69:464-467, 1985.
195. Spira R, Mondshine R: Demonstration of nasolacrimal duct carcinoma by computed tomography. Ophthalmic Plast Reconstr Surg 2:159-161, 1986.
196. George JL, Heymann V, Vignaud JM, Barthelme A: Carcinome épidermoïde du sac lacrymal après dacryocystite aiguë post-traumatique. J Fr Ophthalmol 10:515-517, 1987.
197. Kincaid MC, Meis JM, Lee MW: Adenoid cystic carcinoma of the lacrimal sac. Ophthalmology 96:1655-1658, 1989.
198. Hanselmayer H, Becker H: Tränensackfibrom: Klinik und Pathologie. Klin Monatsbl Augenheilkd 157:676-682, 1970.
199. Ferry AP, Kaltreider SA: Cavernous hemangioma of the lacrimal sac [letter to the editor]. Am J Ophthalmol 110:316-318, 1990.
200. Hornblass A, Gross ND: Lacrimal sac cyst. Ophthalmology 94:706-708, 1987.
201. Hurwitz JJ, Rodgers J, Doucet TW: Dermoid tumor involving the lacrimal drainage pathway: A case report. Ophthalmic Surg 13:377-379, 1982.
202. Howcroft MJ, Hurwitz JJ: Lacrimal sac fibroma. Can J Ophthalmol 15:196-197, 1980.
203. Cole SH, Ferry AP: Fibrous histiocytoma (fibrous xanthoma) of the lacrimal sac. Arch Ophthalmol 96:1647-1649, 1978.
204. Marback RL, Kincaid MC, Green WR, Iliff WJ: Fibrous histiocytoma of the lacrimal sac. Am J Ophthalmol 93:511-517, 1982.
205. Gurney N, Chalkley T, O'Grady R: Lacrimal sac hemangiopericytoma. Am J Ophthalmol 71:757-759, 1971.
206. Carnevali L, Trimarchi F, Rosso R, Stringa M: Haemangiopericytoma of the lacrimal sac: A case report. Br J Ophthalmol 72:782-785, 1988.
207. Roth SI, August CZ, Lissner GS, O'Grady RB: Hemangiopericytoma of the lacrimal sac. Ophthalmology 98:925-927, 1991.
208. Rubin PA, Shore JW, Jakobiec FA, To K: Hemangiopericytoma of the lacrimal sac. Ophthalmic Surg 23:562-563, 1992.
209. Carlin R, Henderson JW: Malignant lymphoma of the nasolacrimal sac. Am J Ophthalmol 78:511-513, 1974.
210. Benger RS, Frueh BR: Lacrimal drainage obstruction from lacrimal sac infiltration by lymphocytic neoplasia. Am J Ophthalmol 101:242-245, 1986.
211. Jordan DR, Nerad JA: Diffuse large-cell lymphoma of the nasolacrimal sac. Can J Ophthalmol 23:34-37, 1988.
212. Eitrem E: Innocent, pigmented naevus-cell tumor (melanoma) of the lacrimal sac. Acta Ophthalmol (Copenh) 31:283-285, 1953.
213. Duguid IM: Malignant melanoma of the lacrimal sac. Br J Ophthalmol 48:394-398, 1964.
214. Farkas TG, Lamberson RE: Malignant melanoma of the lacrimal sac. Am J Ophthalmol 66:45-48, 1968.
215. Yamade S, Kitagawa A: Malignant melanoma of the lacrimal sac. Ophthalmologica 177:30-33, 1978.
216. Schreinzer W, Breitfellner G: Primäres malignes Melanom des Tränensackes. Klin Monatsbl Augenheilkd 176:262-265, 1980.
217. Lloyd WC III, Leone CR Jr: Malignant melanoma of the lacrimal sac. Arch Ophthalmol 102:104-107, 1984.
218. Glaros D, Karesh JW, Rodrigues MM, Hirsch DR, Zimmerman LE: Primary malignant melanoma of the lacrimal sac. Arch Ophthalmol 107:1244-1245, 1989.
219. Bambirra EA, Miranda D, Rayes A: Mucoepidermoid tumor of the lacrimal sac. Arch Ophthalmol 99:2149-2150, 1981.
220. Ni C, Wagoner MD, Wang W-J, et al: Mucoepidermoid carcinomas of the lacrimal sac. Arch Ophthalmol 101:1572-1574, 1983.
221. Blake J, Mullaney J, Gillan J: Lacrimal sac mucoepidermoid carcinoma. Br J Ophthalmol 70:681-685, 1986.
222. Milder B: Neurofibroma of the lacrimal sac. Am J Ophthalmol 53:1016-1018, 1962.
223. Sen DK, Mohan H, Chatterjee PK: Neurilemmoma of the lacrimal sac. Eye Ear Nose Throat Mon 50:179-180, 1971.
224. Radnót M: Aus Onkocyten bestehende adenomartige Hyperplasie in der Tränensackwand. Ophthalmologica 101:95-100, 1941.
225. Biggs SL, Font RL: Oncocytic lesions of the caruncle and other ocular adnexa. Arch Ophthalmol 95:474-478, 1977.
226. Aurora AL: Oncocytic metaplasia in a lacrimal sac papilloma. Am J Ophthalmol 75:466-468, 1973.
227. Peretz WL, Ettinghausen SE, Gray GF: Oncocytic adenocarcinoma of the lacrimal sac. Arch Ophthalmol 96:303-304, 1978.
228. White JP, Michaelson IC, Heggie JF: VI. Diseases of the lacrymal sac apparatus: I. Tumour of lacrymal sac of cellular mixed parotid type associated later with tumour of parotid region of same histological character. Trans Ophthalmol Soc UK 58:159-163, 1938.
229. McCool JL: Mixed-cell tumor of the lacrimal sac. Am J Ophthalmol 22:734-743, 1939.
230. Zolog N: Glomustumor der Pralakrimalgegend. Klin Monatsbl Augenheilkd 149:347-352, 1966.
231. Miller CL, Offutt WN, Kielar RA: Adenoid cystic carcinoma of the antrum and epiphora. Am J Ophthalmol 83:582-586, 1977.
232. Jamieson IW: Haemangioma in lacrimal sac region, a case report. Trans Ophthalmol Soc NZ 27:71, 1975.
233. Rakes SM, Yeatts RP, Campbell RJ: Ophthalmic manifestations of esthesioneuroblastoma. Ophthalmology 92:1749-1753, 1985.
234. Calhoun KH, Stiernberg CM, Clark WD, Bailey BJ: Unusual presentation of fibrous dysplasia. Tex Med 83:47-48, 1987.
235. Johnson LN, Krohel GB, Yeon EB, Parnes SM: Sinus tumors invading the orbit. Ophthalmology 91:209-217, 1984.
236. Relf SJ, Bartley GB, Unni KK: Primary orbital intraosseous hemangioma. Ophthalmology 98:541-546, 1991.
237. Stokes WH: Dacryocystitis in lymphatic leukemia. Arch Ophthalmol 20:85-87, 1938.
238. Cant JS: Dacryocystitis in acute leukaemia. Br J Ophthalmol 47:57-59, 1963.
239. Kincaid MC, Green WR: Ocular and orbital involvement in leukemia. Surv Ophthalmol 27:211-232, 1983.
240. Slonim CB, Older JJ: Bilateral lymphocytic infiltrates causing dacryostenosis after bilateral successful dacryocystorhinostomies. Ophthalmic Plast Reconstr Surg 4:105-108, 1988.
241. Spalton DJ, O'Donnell PJ, Graham EM: Lethal midline lymphoma causing acute dacryocystitis. Br J Ophthalmol 65:503-506, 1981.
242. Sternberg I, Levine MR: Ethmoidal sinus osteoma: A primary cause of nasolacrimal obstruction and dacryocystorhinostomy failure. Ophthalmic Surg 15:295-297, 1984.
243. Migliori ME, Putterman AM: Recurrent conjunctival papilloma causing nasolacrimal duct obstruction. Am J Ophthalmol 110: 17-22, 1990.

244. Campbell CH, Apt RK, Schimek RA: Compression of lacrimal sac by inverted papilloma arising in the maxillary sinus. South Med J 67:773–775, 1974.
245. Khan JA, Grove AS Jr, Joseph MP, Goodman M: Sebaceous carcinoma: Diuretic use, lacrimal system spread, and surgical margins. Ophthalmic Plast Reconstr Surg 5:227–234, 1989.
246. Barton D: A case of basal-cell carcinoma of the lacrimal sac presenting as chronic dacryocystitis. Trans Ophthalmol Soc UK 69:523–527, 1949.
247. Scott KR, Jakobiec FA, Font RL: Peripunctal melanocytic nevi: Distinctive clinical findings and differential diagnosis. Ophthalmology 96:994–998, 1989.
248. Conley JJ: Sinus tumors invading the orbit. Trans Am Acad Ophthalmol Otolaryngol 70:615–619, 1966.
249. Mohan H, Sen DK, Gupta DK: Orbital affection in nasal and paranasal neoplasms. Acta Ophthalmol (Copenh) 47:289–294, 1969.
250. Henderson JW, Farrow GM: Orbital Tumors, 2nd ed. New York, BC Decker, 1980, pp 67–74 and 425–450.
251. Bartley GB, Bullock JD, Waller RR: Secondary neoplasms of the orbit. *In* Hornblass A, Hanig CJ (eds): Oculoplastic, Orbital, and Reconstructive Surgery, vol 2, Orbit and Lacrimal System. Baltimore, Williams & Wilkins, 1990, pp 1053–1067.
252. Smith JL, Wheliss JA: Ocular manifestations of nasopharyngeal tumors. Trans Am Acad Ophthalmol Otolaryngol 66:659–664, 1962.
253. Cohan BE: Epiphora: As the initial manifestation of a malignant nasopharyngeal tumor. Am J Ophthalmol 50:644–649, 1960.
254. Rollet E: Episcleral lymphoma and double-sided lymphoma of the lacrymal gland. Arch Ophthalmol 34:194, 1905.
255. Kaden IH, Shields JA, Shields CL, Rose LJ: Occult prostatic carcinoma metastatic to the medial canthal area: Diagnosis by immunohistochemistry. Ophthalmic Plast Reconstr Surg 3:21–24, 1987.
256. Shields CL, Shields JA, Peggs M: Tumors metastatic to the orbit. Ophthalmic Plast Reconstr Surg 4:73–80, 1988.
257. Bartley GB, Bullock JD, Waller RR: Metastatic tumors of the orbit. *In* Hornblass A, Hanig CJ (eds): Oculoplastic, Orbital, and Reconstructive Surgery, vol 2, Orbit and Lacrimal System. Baltimore, Williams & Wilkins, 1990, pp 1068–1078.
258. Goldberg RA, Rootman J, Cline RA: Tumors metastatic to the orbit: A changing picture. Surv Ophthalmol 35:1–24, 1990.
259. Goldberg RA, Rootman J: Clinical characteristics of metastatic orbital tumors. Ophthalmology 97:620–624, 1990.
260. Freeman JM: The punctum plug: Evaluation of a new treatment for the dry eye. Trans Am Acad Ophthalmol Otolaryngol 79:OP874–OP879, 1975.
261. Dohlman CH: Punctal occlusion in keratoconjunctivitis sicca. Ophthalmology 85:1277–1281, 1978.
262. Lamberts D: Punctal occlusion. Int Ophthalmol Clin 27:44–46, 1987.
263. American Academy of Ophthalmology: Punctal occlusion for the dry eye. Ophthalmology 95(Suppl):71–73, 1988.
264. Knapp ME, Frueh BR, Nelson CC, Musch DC: A comparison of two methods of punctal occlusion. Am J Ophthalmol 108:315–318, 1989.
265. Tuberville AW, Frederick WR, Wood TO: Punctal occlusion in tear deficiency syndromes. Ophthalmology 89:1170–1172, 1982.
266. Glatt HJ: Acute dacryocystitis after punctal occlusion for keratoconjunctivitis sicca [letter to the editor]. Am J Ophthalmol 111:769–770, 1991.
267. Maguire LJ, Bartley GB: Complications associated with the new smaller size Freeman punctal plug [letter to the editor]. Arch Ophthalmol 107:961–962, 1989.
268. Nelson CC: Complications of Freeman plugs. Arch Ophthalmol 109:923–924, 1991.
269. Worst JGF: Method for reconstructing torn lacrimal canaliculus. Am J Ophthalmol 53:520–522, 1962.
270. Simons JN: Useful instrument for repair of lacerated lacrimal canaliculus. Plast Reconstr Surg 43:78–80, 1969.
271. Adams AD: Silicone-loop repair of the torn canaliculus. Arch Ophthalmol 94:1958–1960, 1976.
272. Walter WL: The use of the pigtail probe for silicone intubation of the injured canaliculus. Ophthalmic Surg 13:488–492, 1982.
273. Saunders DH, Shannon GM, Flanagan JC: The effectiveness of the pigtail probe method of repairing canalicular lacerations. Ophthalmic Surg 9:33–40, 1978.
274. Jordan DR, Nerad JA, Tse DT: The pigtail probe, revisited. Ophthalmology 97:512–519, 1990.
275. Welham RAN, Henderson P: Failed dacryocystorhinostomy. Trans Am Acad Ophthalmol Otolaryngol 78:OP824–OP828, 1974.
276. Older JJ: Routine use of a silicone stent in a dacryocystorhinostomy. Ophthalmic Surg 13:911–915, 1982.
277. Burns JA, Cahill KV: Modified Kinosian dacryocystorhinostomy: A review of 122 cases. Ophthalmic Surg 16:710–716, 1985.
278. Hurwitz JJ, Rutherford S: Computerized survey of lacrimal surgery patients. Ophthalmology 93:14–19, 1986.
279. Welham RAN, Wulc AE: Management of unsuccessful lacrimal surgery. Br J Ophthalmol 71:152–157, 1987.
280. Rosen N, Sharir M, Moverman DC, Rosner M: Dacryocystorhinostomy with silicone tubes: Evaluation of 253 cases. Ophthalmic Surg 20:115–119, 1989.
281. Allen K, Berlin AJ: Dacryocystorhinostomy failure: Association with nasolacrimal silicone intubation. Ophthalmic Surg 20:486–489, 1989.
282. Jones LT: The cure of epiphora due to canalicular disorders, trauma and surgical failures on the lacrimal passages. Trans Am Acad Ophthalmol Otolaryngol 66:506–524, 1962.
283. Jones LT: Conjunctivodacryocystorhinostomy. Am J Ophthalmol 59:773–783, 1965.
284. Medgyesi S: Tear drainage: Reconstruction by implantation of a glass tube prosthesis a.m. Lester T. Jones: Case report. Scand J Plast Reconstr Surg 11:83–85, 1977.
285. Steinsapir KD, Glatt HJ, Putterman AM: A 16-year study of conjunctival dacryocystorhinostomy. Am J Ophthalmol 109:387–393, 1990.
286. Sekhar GC, Dortzbach RK, Gonnering RS, Lemke BN: Problems associated with conjunctivodacryocystorhinostomy. Am J Ophthalmol 112:502–506, 1991.
287. Bartley GB, Gustafson RO: Complications of malpositioned Jones tubes. Am J Ophthalmol 109:66–69, 1990.
288. Colvard DM, Waller RR, Neault RW, DeSanto LW: Nasolacrimal duct obstruction following transantral-ethmoidal orbital decompression. Ophthalmic Surg 10:25–28, 1979.
289. DeSanto LW: The total rehabilitation of Graves' ophthalmopathy. Laryngoscope 40:1652–1678, 1980.
290. Seiff SR, Shorr N: Nasolacrimal drainage system obstruction after orbital decompression. Am J Ophthalmol 106:204–209, 1988.
291. Garrity JA, Bartley GB, DeSanto LW, et al: Orbital decompression: Long-term results. *In* Wall JR, How J (eds): Graves' Ophthalmopathy. Cambridge, MA, Blackwell Scientific Publications, 1990, pp 171–182.
292. Migliori ME: Nasolacrimal drainage system obstruction after orbital decompression [letter to the editor]. Am J Ophthalmol 107:91, 1989.
293. Hornblass A: Nasolacrimal drainage system obstruction after orbital decompression [letter to the editor]. Am J Ophthalmol 107:92, 1989.
294. Flowers RS, Anderson R: Injury to the lacrimal apparatus during rhinoplasty. Plast Reconstr Surg 42:577–581, 1968.
295. Cies WA, Baylis HI: Epiphora following rhinoplasty and Caldwell-Luc procedures. Ophthalmic Surg 7:77–81, 1976.
296. Freedman HM, Kern EB: Complications of intranasal ethmoidectomy: A review of 1,000 consecutive operations. Laryngoscope 89:421–432, 1979.
297. Osguthorpe JD, Calcaterra TC: Nasolacrimal obstruction after maxillary sinus and rhinoplastic surgery. Arch Otolaryngol 105:264–266, 1979.
298. Maniglia AJ, Chandler JR, Goodwin WJ Jr, Flynn J: Rare complications following ethmoidectomies: A report of eleven cases. Laryngoscope 91:1234–1242, 1981.
299. Dutton JJ: Orbital complications of paranasal sinus surgery. Ophthalmic Plast Reconstr Surg 2:119–127, 1986.
300. Kennedy DW, Zinreich SJ, Shaalan H, et al: Endoscopic middle meatal antrostomy: Theory, technique, and patency. Laryngoscope 97(Suppl 43):1–9, 1987.
301. Neuhaus RW: Orbital complications secondary to endoscopic sinus surgery. Ophthalmology 97:1512–1518, 1990.

302. Serdahl CL, Berris CE, Chole RA: Nasolacrimal duct obstruction after endoscopic sinus surgery. Arch Ophthalmol 108:391-392, 1990.
303. Jones BR: The surgical cure of obstruction in the common lacrimal canaliculus. Trans Ophthalmol Soc UK 80:343-353, 1960.
304. Billson FA, Taylor HR, Hoyt CS: Trauma to the lacrimal system in children. Am J Ophthalmol 86:828-833, 1978.
305. Zolli CL, Shannon GM: Dacryocystorhinostomy: A review of 119 cases. Ophthalmic Surg 13:905-910, 1982.
306. Nowinski TS, Flanagan JC, Mauriello J: Pediatric dacryocystorhinostomy. Arch Ophthalmol 103:1226-1228, 1985.
307. Dryden RM, Wulc AE: Pseudoepiphora from cerebrospinal fluid leak: Case report. Br J Ophthalmol 70:570-574, 1986.
308. Harris GJ: Canalicular laceration at birth [letter to the editor]. Am J Ophthalmol 105:322-323, 1988.
309. Linberg JV, Moore CA: Symptoms of canalicular obstruction. Ophthalmology 95:1077-1079, 1988.
310. White WL, Glover AT, Buckner AB, Hartshorne MF: Relative canalicular tear flow as assessed by dacryoscintigraphy. Ophthalmology 96:167-169, 1989.
311. Daubert J, Nik N, Chandeyssoun PA, El-Choufi L: Tear flow analysis through the upper and lower systems. Ophthalmic Plast Reconstr Surg 6:193-196, 1990.
312. Veirs ER: Malleable rods for immediate repair of the traumatically severed lacrimal canaliculus. Trans Am Acad Ophthalmol Otolaryngol 66:263-264, 1962.
313. Veirs ER: Aids in restoring patency in obstructions of the lacrimal drainage system. Am J Ophthalmol 56:977-982, 1963.
314. Johnson CC: A canaliculus wire. Am J Ophthalmol 78:854-855, 1974.
315. Nasr A, Johnson CC, Beyer-Machule CK: Repair of the lacerated canaliculus using a modified silver wire lacrimal rod. Ophthalmic Surg 14:601-603, 1983.
316. Quickert MH, Dryden RM: Probes for intubation in lacrimal drainage. Trans Am Acad Ophthalmol Otolaryngol 74:431-433, 1970.
317. Guibor P: Canaliculus intubation set. Trans Am Acad Ophthalmol Otolaryngol 79:OP419-OP420, 1975.
318. Crawford JS: Intubation of obstructions in the lacrimal system. Can J Ophthalmol 12:289-292, 1977.
319. Baylis HI, Axelrod R: Repair of the lacerated canaliculus. Ophthalmology 85:1271-1276, 1978.
320. Pashby RC, Rathbun JE: Silicone tube intubation of the lacrimal drainage system. Arch Ophthalmol 97:1318-1322, 1979.
321. Hawes MJ, Segrest DR: Effectiveness of bicanalicular silicone intubation in the repair of canalicular lacerations. Ophthalmic Plast Reconstr Surg 1:185-190, 1985.
322. Dortzbach RK, Angrist RA: Silicone intubation for lacerated lacrimal canaliculi. Ophthalmic Surg 16:639-642, 1985.
323. Kennedy RH, May J, Dailey J, Flanagan JC: Canalicular laceration: An 11-year epidemiologic and clinical study. Ophthalmic Plast Reconstr Surg 6:46-53, 1990.
324. Lauring L: Silicone intubation of the lacrimal system: Pitfalls, problems and complications. Ann Ophthalmol 8:489-498, 1976.
325. Older JJ: Treatment of the lacrimal excretory system after resection of medial canthal and eyelid tumors. Ophthalmic Surg 10:29-34, 1979.
326. Romano PE: Single silicone intubation for repair of single canaliculus laceration. Ann Ophthalmol 18:112-113, 1986.
327. Braverman DE, Brown RE Jr: Externalized silicone tube in single canalicular intubation [letter to the editor]. Am J Ophthalmol 103:335-336, 1987.
328. Gonnering RS: Simplified monocanalicular silicone intubation [letter to the editor]. Arch Ophthalmol 105:1024, 1987.
329. Patrinely JR, Anderson RL: Monocanalicular silicone intubation [letter to the editor]. Arch Ophthalmol 106:579-580, 1988.
330. Long JA: A method of monocanalicular silicone intubation. Ophthalmic Surg 19:204-205, 1988.
331. Haik BG: Teflon sleeve canalicular splints [letter to the editor]. Am J Ophthalmol 106:367, 1988.
332. Jordan DR, Anderson RL, Patrinely JR: Unicanalicular stent for nasolacrimal duct obstruction. Can J Ophthalmol 24:251-253, 1989.
333. Neuhaus RW: Silicone intubation of traumatic canalicular lacerations. Ophthalmic Plast Reconstr Surg 5:256-260, 1989.
334. Hawes MJ, Shawbitz SD: Repair of acute common canalicular avulsion by angular vein grafting. Ophthalmic Plast Reconstr Surg 2:197-200, 1986.
335. Smith B: Late bilateral naso-orbital fracture and dacryostenosis. Trans Am Acad Ophthalmol Otolaryngol 76:1378-1379, 1972.
336. Gruss JS, Hurwitz JJ, Nik NA, Kassel EE: The pattern and incidence of nasolacrimal injury in naso-orbital-ethmoid fractures: The role of delayed assessment and dacryocystorhinostomy. Br J Plast Surg 38:116-121, 1985.
337. Harris GJ, Fuerste FH: Lacrimal intubation in the primary repair of midfacial fractures. Ophthalmology 94:242-247, 1987.
338. Balle VH, Andersen R, Siim C: Incidence of lacrimal obstruction following trauma to the facial skeleton. Ear Nose Throat J 67:66-70, 1988.
339. Dufresne CR, Manson PN, Iliff NT: Early and late complications of orbital fractures. Clin Plast Surg 15:239-253, 1988.
340. Jones LT: Tear-sac foreign bodies. Am J Ophthalmol 60:111-113, 1965.
341. Smith B, Tenzel RR, Buffam FV, Boynton JR: Acute dacryocystic retention. Arch Ophthalmol 94:1903-1904, 1976.
342. Jay JL, Lee WR: Dacryolith formation around an eyelash retained in the lacrimal sac. Br J Ophthalmol 60:722-725, 1976.
343. Herzig S, Hurwitz JJ: Lacrimal sac calculi. Can J Ophthalmol 14:17-20, 1979.
344. Maltzman BA, Favetta JR: Dacryolithiasis. Ann Ophthalmol 11:473-475, 1979.
345. Wilkins RB, Pressly JP: Diagnosis and incidence of lacrimal calculi. Ophthalmic Surg 11:787-789, 1980.
346. Hawes MJ: The dacryolithiasis syndrome. Ophthalmic Plast Reconstr Surg 4:87-90, 1988.
347. Gonnering RS, Bosniak SL: Recognition and management of acute noninfectious dacryocystic retention. Ophthalmic Plast Reconstr Surg 5:27-33, 1989.
348. Daxecker F, Philipp W, Müller-Holzner E, Tessadri R: Analyse eines Dakryolithen. Ophthalmologica 195:125-127, 1987.
349. Kaye-Wilson LG: Spontaneous passage of dacryolith. Br J Ophthalmol 75:564, 1991.
350. Baratz KH, Bartley GB, Campbell RJ, Garrity JA: An eyelash nidus for dacryoliths of the lacrimal excretory and secretory systems. Am J Ophthalmol 111:624-627, 1991.
351. Spaeth GL: Nasolacrimal duct obstruction caused by topical epinephrine. Arch Ophthalmol 77:355-357, 1967.
352. Barishak R, Romano A, Stein R: Obstruction of lacrimal sac caused by topical epinephrine. Ophthalmologica 159:373-379, 1969.
353. Bradbury JA, Rennie IG, Parsons MA: Adrenaline dacryolith: Detection by ultrasound examination of the nasolacrimal duct. Br J Ophthalmol 72:935-937, 1988.
354. Levenson JE, Hofbaver J: Problems with punctal plugs [letter to the editor]. Arch Ophthalmol 107:493-494, 1989.
355. Becker BB: Retained Veirs rod and canaliculitis [letter to the editor]. Am J Ophthalmol 111:251-252, 1991.
356. Yeatts RP, Crum B: An unusual complication of nasolacrimal duct probing. Ophthalmic Surg 20:490-493, 1989.
357. Felt DP, Frueh BR: Exogenous ball valve in the lacrimal sac. Ophthalmic Plast Reconstr Surg 1:115-117, 1985.
358. Glatt HJ: Epiphora caused by blepharoptosis [letter to the editor]. Am J Ophthalmol 111:649-650, 1991.
359. Liu D: Conjunctivochalasis: A cause of tearing and its management. Ophthalmic Plast Reconstr Surg 2:25-28, 1986.
360. Perrin C, Friot J-M, Bacri D: Mucocèle du sinus maxillaire de forme pseudo-néoplastique avec blocage palpébral supérieur. Rev Otoneuroophtalmol 46:23-27, 1974.
361. Ormerod LD, Weber AL, Rauch SD, Feldon SE: Ophthalmic manifestations of maxillary sinus mucoceles. Ophthalmology 94:1013-1019, 1987.
362. Kaltreider Sa, Dortzbach RK: Destructive cysts of the maxillary sinus affecting the orbit. Arch Ophthalmol 106:1398-1402, 1988.
363. Kohn R, Romano PE, Puklin JE: Lacrimal obstruction after migration of orbital floor implant. Am J Ophthalmol 82:934-936, 1976.

364. Mauriello JA Jr, Fiore PM, Kotch M: Dacryocystitis: Late complication of orbital floor fracture repair with implant. Ophthalmology 94:248–250, 1987.
365. Hurwitz JJ: Failed dacryocystorhinostomy in Paget's disease. Can J Ophthalmol 14:291–293, 1979.
366. Orengo SD, Patrinely JR: Dacryocystorhinostomy in osteopetrosis. Ophthalmic Surg 22:396–398, 1991.
367. Gillissen JPA: The lacrimal system and the ENT surgeon. Orbit 5:169–174, 1986.
368. Udovicki J: Rhinolithiasis complicated by purulent dacryocystitis. Med Pregl 42:329–331, 1989.
369. Bartley GB, Moir CR, McCaffrey TV: Acquired partial nasolacrimal obstruction due to a suture stent following esophagocolostomy. Arch Ophthalmol 108:1074, 1990.

CHAPTER 79

Disorders of the Canaliculus and Punctum

William White and John J. Woog

A pathologic process originating from the canaliculus and punctum is seldom sight or life threatening, but it can be extremely annoying for the affected person. Two of the more common presenting symptoms seen in patients with problems in this area are epiphora and ocular discharge. Such complaints should initiate a systematic evaluation of the lacrimal system, including inspection of the tear film (e.g., evaluating the tear lake height and observing for signs of corneal irritation), inspecting the eyelids (taking special care to note the lid position in relationship to the globe), observing the punctum (noting its diameter and relationship to the tear lake), and evaluating the patency of the lacrimal system. The following discussion pertains only to disorders affecting the upper portion of the lacrimal system, that is, the punctum and canaliculus. A variety of disorders may affect this area, including congenital lesions, benign and malignant neoplasms, involutional changes, iatrogenic problems (both medical and surgical), trauma, and infections. A thorough knowledge of the anatomy and physiology of the lacrimal system is necessary to diagnose and treat these problems effectively.

ANATOMY

The puncta and canaliculi constitute the first anatomic sections of the lacrimal drainage system. The punctal orifice averages 0.3 mm^2, with the lower punctum being slightly larger than the upper.[1] The puncta are surrounded by a dense ring of connective tissue.[2] The puncta and canaliculi are lined internally by stratified squamous epithelium. The canaliculi extend vertically from the punctum to the ampulla, which is approximately 2 mm in length. They then turn horizontally and extend for about 8 mm before entering the lacrimal sac. In most cases there is a common canaliculus and a single internal punctum entering the lacrimal sac, although in some individuals the canaliculi enter the sac independently. The relaxed intraluminal diameter of the canaliculi is 0.5 to 1 mm.[3] There have been numerous valves described throughout the lacrimal drainage system, although they are not a constant finding.[4] The canaliculi are covered posteriorly by the deep heads of the pretarsal orbicularis oculi and anteriorly by the superficial heads of the pretarsal orbicularis oculi. In their most medial extent the canaliculi are covered by the medial canthal tendon.[5, 6]

PHYSIOLOGY

Until this century tears were thought to drain primarily by gravitational forces.[5] Numerous investigators have more recently observed that tear drainage is a dynamic process, although the exact mechanism is still speculative.[5-9] The relative importance of the canaliculi in tear drainage has also been a topic of recent research. The practical significance of this matter is primarily in regard to the need or lack thereof for surgical repair of an isolated superior canalicular injury. The inferior canaliculus was previously thought to transport the majority of tears while the superior canaliculus was only of secondary importance. Based on recent studies, however, the roles of the two canaliculi appear to be of approximately equal importance.[10-12] It can be anticipated that about half of all patients with a single functioning canaliculus will experience epiphora under conditions of increased tear secretion (such as reflex or stress epiphora), while few will have epiphora under baseline conditions.[13]

CONGENITAL ABNORMALITIES

Congenital absence of the lacrimal puncta and canaliculi can be unilateral or bilateral and likely represents a failure of the system to canalize during embryogenesis (Fig. 79-1). The "absence" can be partial or total and involve the upper, lower, or both canalicular systems.[14] In some cases only the puncta are absent and canaliculi are present in their normal location.[15] This may occur because embryologically the puncta are formed after the canaliculi.[16] Congenital absence of the lacrimal puncta and canaliculi is usually a sporadic finding, although autosomal dominant inheritance has also been reported.[14, 17] It may be seen as an isolated condition, but it

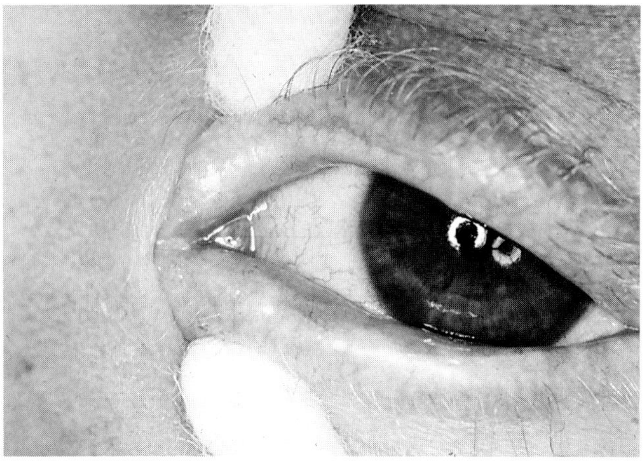

Figure 79–1. Punctal agenesis.

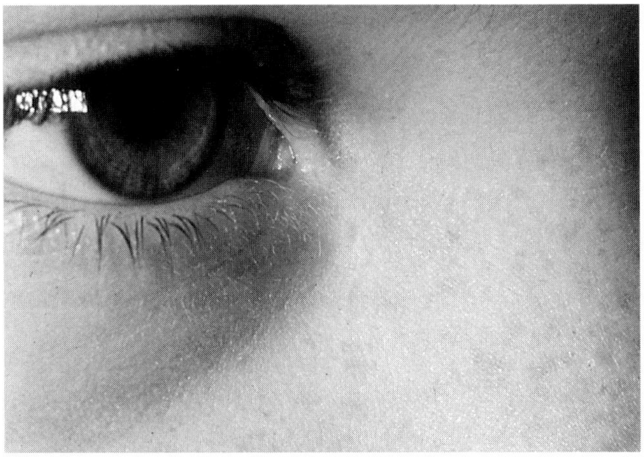

Figure 79–3. Lacrimocutaneous fistula inferior to the medial commissure.

has also been reported with concomitant alacrima and aptyalism (lack of salivation).[17, 18] In addition, it has been observed as a part of several other syndromes, including mandibulofacial dysostosis (Treacher Collins syndrome), dyskeratosis congenita, ectrodactyly–ectodermal dysplasia–clefting syndrome, and the blepharophimosis syndrome.[19–23]

Reduplication of the lacrimal punctum and canaliculus is an unusual finding and may be entirely asymptomatic. The duplicated system is usually located in the lower eyelid medial to the normally situated lacrimal punctum.[24, 25]

Congenital lacrimal fistulas may be unilateral or bilateral, and there may be more than one fistulous tract per side.[26] The patency of each system may sometimes be assessed by observation of reflux from each orifice while pressing on the lacrimal sac after the instillation of fluorescein. Congenital lacrimal fistulas may arise off of the lacrimal sac, but more often they originate from the common canaliculus (Figs. 79–2 and 79–3).[26, 27] Congenital lacrimal fistulas appear not to have a familial tendency.[27]

Treatment

The mere finding of an anatomic abnormality in the lacrimal drainage system does not mean surgical intervention is necessary, since some patients will be entirely asymptomatic.[24, 25] Specific indications for surgery in patients with congenital lacrimal fistulas include infection or mass in the fistula and lacrimal outflow obstruction.

If the lacrimal system is functioning, the fistulous tract may be excised. This can be done under local or general

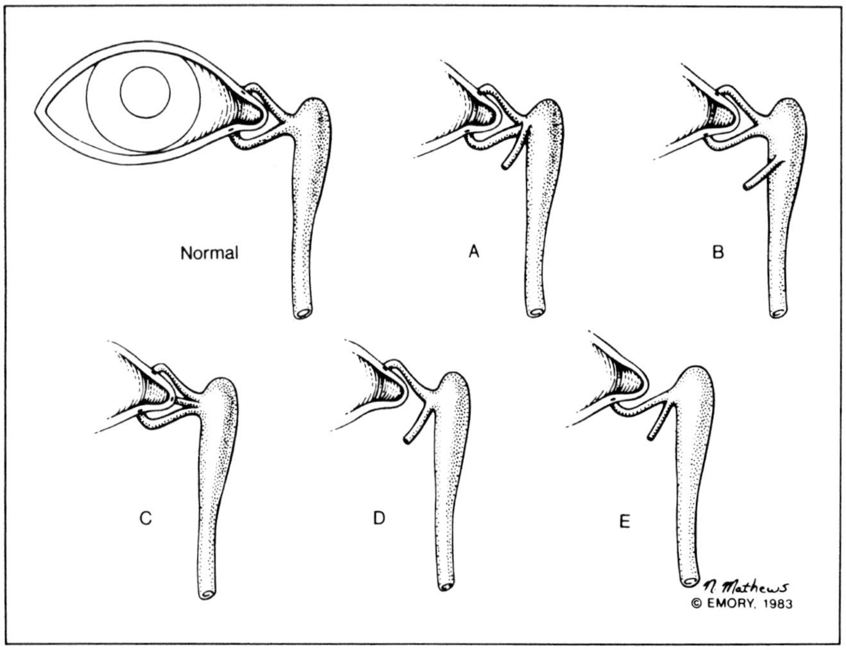

Figure 79–2. Congenital lacrimocutaneous fistulas. *A*, Originates at the common canaliculus. *B*, Originates in the lacrimal tear sac. *C*, Canaliculi have separate openings into the lacrimal sac. *D*, Absent inferior canaliculus. *E*, Absent superior canaliculus. (Modified from Welham R, Bergin D: Congenital lacrimal fistulas. Arch Ophthalmol Apr 103[4]:545–548, 1985. Copyright 1985, American Medical Association.)

anesthesia, primarily depending on the age of the patient. The surgery may be done either under the operating microscope or with the aid of loupe magnification. The fistulous tract along with the normally located system are each intubated with lacrimal probes that are left in place throughout the surgery that follows. Sharp dissection of the fistulous tract is then accomplished, removing it en bloc after placement of a purse-string suture across its medial end. The normally functioning system should be left intact. If there is concern regarding canalicular patency at the end of the case, silicone intubation of the canaliculi may be performed.[28]

It may sometimes be necessary in patients with congenital lacrimal fistula and lacrimal obstruction to perform a dacryocystorhinostomy (DCR) with silicone intubation,[27] although usually simple fistula excision with selective silicone stenting is sufficient.[28] If DCR is required, surgery may be done under either local or general anesthesia and typically with loupe magnification. A standard DCR incision is placed 8 mm medial to the medial canthus and carried down to the anterior lacrimal crest. The lacrimal sac is reflected laterally, and a generous osteotomy is performed. The lacrimal sac is then opened vertically, and the canaliculi are intubated with silicone tubing, which is passed through the nasolacrimal duct and into the nose. Anterior and posterior mucosal flaps are then constructed and closed with a 4-0 absorbable suture. The fistulous tract is then intubated with a lacrimal probe, and the skin is incised around the fistula perpendicularly to the DCR incision so that the skin may be closed later in a T. The fistulous tract is then gently dissected out and a 6-0 absorbable purse-string suture is placed across its base before its removal en bloc. The skin is then closed with fine sutures, and the silicone tubing is secured in the nose. The silicone tubing should be left in place for 3 to 6 months.

Due to the spectrum of clinical findings seen in atresia of the lacrimal puncta and canaliculus, a single surgical approach cannot be recommended. In pediatric patients, best results are probably achieved by delaying surgery until at least 18 months of age to allow for growth of lacrimal and nasal structures.[15] The procedure may be done under loupe magnification or the operating microscope, using either general or local anesthesia, and must be tailored to the individual findings for a given case. The surgery begins with a diligent search for the lacrimal punctum in its usual anatomic location at the medial aspect of the ciliated eyelid margin. Rotating the eyelid externally can sometimes make this task easier.[29, 30] If the punctum is located, it should be entered with either a 20-gauge needle or a sharp punctum dilator. If the remaining system is patent to probing, the punctal ostium is enlarged by dilation or by making a 2-mm vertical incision on its conjunctival surface and intubation with silicone tubing is done.[31] A punctal incision is usually unnecessary if a canalicular stent is placed.

When the punctum cannot be found, other options may be pursued. If one punctum and canaliculus is patent, a round-tipped pigtail probe may be gently passed in an attempt to locate the other canaliculus. If the cannulation is successful and the canaliculus is present, a wedge of tissue can be removed from the margin of the eyelid and the system subsequently intubated with silicone tubes. The punctal ostia may also be made with a Holth sclerectomy punch, which creates a uniform opening in the eyelid margin.[30] Alternatively, the patent canaliculus may be used to irrigate methylene blue into the lacrimal sac. The material will sometimes enter the blind canaliculus, and an appropriate location can be identified to cut down on the eyelid and create a lacrimal punctum. When neither punctum nor canaliculus can be located, methylene blue may be percutaneously injected into the lacrimal sac to identify the canalicular system.[15] Although these maneuvers are theoretically helpful, frequently no canaliculus is found.

If the previous steps do not lead to the localization or establishment of the canalicular system, a standard DCR incision is performed and the lacrimal sac retracted laterally. The bony ostia and nasal mucosal flaps are constructed in a standard fashion. The sac is then incised vertically, and the lateral portion of the sac is inspected for any evidence of a canalicular opening. A no. 0 lacrimal probe is frequently helpful in identifying canalicular openings into the sac when they are present without creating false openings in the sac. If a canaliculus is identified, it is intubated and a punctum is created by cutting down on the eyelid.

Finally, if all of the previously mentioned maneuvers are unsuccessful, an 18-gauge intravenous catheter may be passed from the eyelid margin vertically 4 mm and then horizontally to the lacrimal sac. The sac is entered at least 2 mm away from any functioning canalicular opening into the sac to minimize the chance of iatrogenic canalicular injury. After silicone intubation the mucosal flaps and superficial closure are accomplished in the standard fashion. The silicone tubes should be left in place for approximately 6 months.[15]

NEOPLASMS

Tumors affecting the lacrimal puncta and canaliculi may be divided into two general categories. The first type are those tumors that arise from within the tissues of the puncta and canaliculi themselves. The second and more common variety are those that arise from outside the puncta and canaliculi and only secondarily involve the lacrimal drainage system.

Primary Tumors

Tumors of the lacrimal canaliculi and puncta are exceedingly rare. The epithelial lining in these structures may produce squamous cell or transitional cell papillomas that are capable of transforming into carcinomas. Papillomas of the canalicular system in general may be of either neoplastic or viral origin, similar to conjunctival papillomas.[32] A dacryocystogram may be helpful in evaluating the extent of these lesions. By such testing it can be determined whether the visible lesion represents a continuation of a mass in the lacrimal sac or one limited to the canaliculus. Suspicious lesions are best treated initially with a biopsy for precise histologic diagnosis. For malignant lesions, wide local excision with microscopic confirmation of clear surgical margins is the procedure of choice. Similar lesions in the past have been treated by incomplete excision with postoperative irradiation, but rapid regrowth of a histologically more malignant tumor has been reported in this scenario.[33] Pyogenic granuloma formation may be noted in the punctum, canaliculus, or both (Fig. 79–4).

The punctum may also be affected by pigmented lesions. Melanomas are more common than nevi and usually obliterate the punctal lumen. They should be treated surgically with wide local excision. Peripunctal nevi are rarer and may cause the punctum to gape or pout rather than causing punctal obstruction. Histologic confirmation of nevi can usually be accomplished by performing a shave excision, possibly with temporary placement of a silicone punctum plug[34] or stent to maintain punctal and proximal canalicular patency.

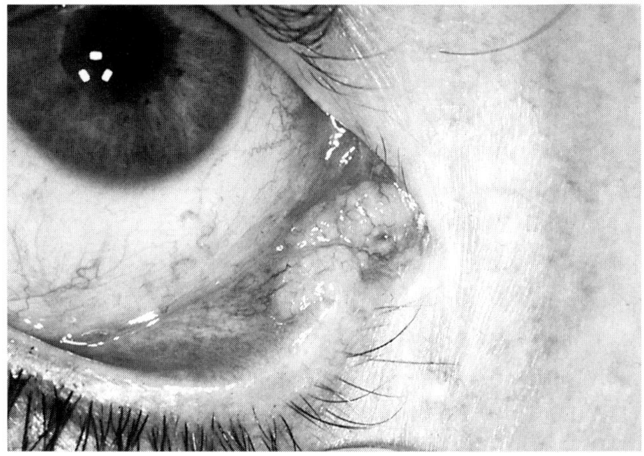

Figure 79–5. Basal cell carcinoma surrounding the punctum.

Secondary Tumors

The lacrimal punctum and canaliculus are frequently affected by tumors of the medial eyelid skin and conjunctiva, such as basal cell carcinoma, squamous cell carcinoma, and sebaceous cell carcinoma (Fig. 79–5).[35] The appearance of such tumors in the canaliculus or punctum should in no way limit the resection of these malignant tumors. By submitting mapped frozen section margins of the tumor bed, the extent of lacrimal system loss may be limited. A new canalicular drainage system may be constructed if at least one fourth of the resected canaliculus remains after tumor removal. This is accomplished by first creating vertical margins for routine eyelid closure. Both canaliculi are intubated with silicone tubing, but not secured in the nose until the end of the case. The annular margins of the resected canaliculus are marsupialized and secured to the eyelid margin with 7-0 or 8-0 absorbable suture as the eyelid is repaired in a standard fashion.[36] The silicone tubing is then secured and should be left in place for 3 to 6 months.

One of the possible complications of surgery on or around the punctum is punctal occlusion. Silicone intubation or, for smaller lesions, silicone punctum plug placement may decrease the incidence of postoperative lacrimal occlusion. It has also been observed that silicone intubation of the lacrimal system before irradiation of uveal tumors decreases the incidence of lacrimal obstruction.[37] Excellent results have also been achieved using the carbon dioxide laser for surgery on peripunctal lesions without lacrimal intubation, but this therapeutic modality may not be readily available.[38]

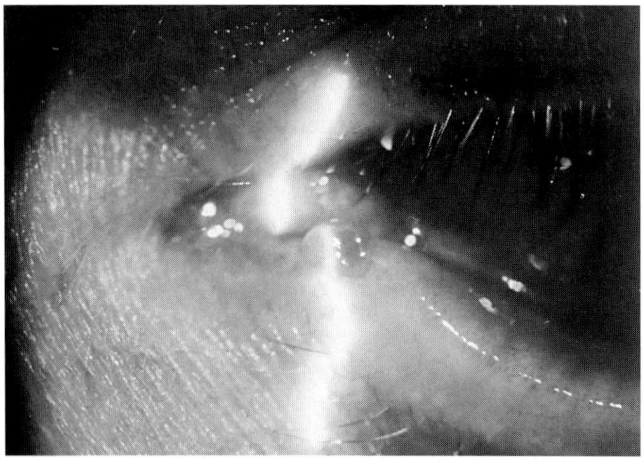

Figure 79–4. Pyogenic granuloma emanating from the punctum.

TRAUMA

Injuries to the lacrimal canaliculus, usually in the form of a canalicular laceration, are relatively common in facial trauma. While some canalicular lacerations are caused by a sharp object and are true lacerations, most of these injuries are better referred to as avulsions and occur secondary to indirect or diffuse trauma rather than a laceration per se. Canalicular avulsions probably occur because the eyelid ruptures at its weakest point (the canaliculus) when it is stretched past its internal elastic limit against the fixed tendinous attachments.[39] The punctum is only rarely involved.[40] Epidemiologically, the highest frequency of these injuries occurs in young adults and the majority are males. There have been cases reported in preschool-aged children (in which dog bites are a frequent mechanism) and even at birth.[41,42]

Although no one would propose that an eyelid avulsion in general should not be repaired, there are some who have argued that an isolated, especially superior, canalicular laceration is best not repaired. This is because of the risk of jeopardizing the patency of the intact canalicular system with operative instrumentation and because some patients will not experience epiphora with a single functioning canaliculus.[43,44] It has been observed, though, that some patients will experience epiphora if they have only a single functioning canaliculus. Since we cannot predict which patients will experience epiphora, we prefer to attempt repair of all canalicular lacerations.[13]

One way to avoid manipulation of the uninjured canaliculus is through the use of a monocanalicular stent, although these may be cumbersome in the postoperative period and are less familiar to many surgeons.[45–47] Given the instrumentation available, adequate magnification, fine suture material, and an adequate knowledge of lacrimal and eyelid anatomy, however, iatrogenic injury to the intact canaliculus should be rare.[44]

Repair of Canalicular Lacerations

Before initiation of repair of the injured eyelid, the patient must be examined for associated nonocular injuries and for ocular injuries such as penetration of the globe. These injuries take priority in the planning of surgical repair. We prefer to repair all canalicular lacerations within 24 to 36 hours of injury, when possible, although good results have been achieved when circumstances have necessitated the delay of surgical repair for up to 5 days. Iced saline compresses applied over the affected area until surgery assists in limiting edema of eyelid tissues, which theoretically should make isolation of the medial end of the lacerated canaliculus easier. The repair can be done under loupe or operating microscope control; magnification is particularly useful during the identification, cannulation, and reapproximation of the lacerated canalicular tissues. Since the repair of canalicular lacerations can be lengthy and tedious, it is often preferable to perform the surgery the morning after the injury under optimal conditions rather than during the night of the trauma. Surgery may be done with the use of local anesthesia, although general anesthesia is preferred because it eliminates the soft tissue distortion that follows local anesthetic injection and ensures patient comfort during silicone intubation of the nasolacrimal system.

The punctum of the injured system is dilated with a punctum dilator, and a silicone intubation set is used (such as Crawford, Quickert-Dryden, Jackson, or Guibor) to pass the metal probe of the set to the site of the canalicular disruption. There are many methods that may provide assistance in locating the injured medial segment of the canaliculus. The canaliculus is usually pink or gray when compared with the surrounding orbicularis oculi and the pericanalicular soft tissues. Frequently the probe from the cannulated lateral system will point directly to the medial segment. Passing a lacrimal probe through the uninjured canaliculus can also give the surgeon a better idea of where to look for the injured medial segment. Various substances have been used to irrigate through the canalicular system in an attempt to identify the medial segment. Recently used agents include viscoelastic materials usually used during intraocular surgery.[48,49] The viscous nature of these substances ensures slow movement of the fluid from the end of the injured segment once passed. Although any of these techniques may be of great assistance in an individual case, meticulous examination using the operating microscope is usually sufficient to locate the medial segment.

After the medial segment of the canaliculus is localized, the metal probe from the intubation set is passed gently through it into the nose and retrieved. The silicone tube is then passed through the uninjured canalicular system and retrieved from the nasal cavity (Fig. 79–6*A*). The posterior limb of the medial canthal tendon is then reconstructed, if necessary, with placement of a nonabsorbable suture such as 4-0 Polydek between the medial border of the tarsal plate and the periosteum overlying the posterior lacrimal crest (see Fig. 79–6*B*). The orbicularis surrounding the canaliculus is subsequently approximated using 5-0 or 6-0 Vicryl sutures in the pericanalicular tissues to transfer the force of lid closure from the compromised canaliculus. The canalicular mucosa itself is reapproximated with two or three interrupted 8-0 Vicryl sutures (Fig. 79–7). The eyelid is repaired as appropriate with attention directed at creating an everted lid margin using vertical mattress sutures (Fig. 79–8). The silicone tubing is then secured in the nose and left in place for 6 months.

The pigtail probe is an instrument that has stirred considerable controversy in the repair of canalicular lacerations. In its earlier form, the Worst pigtail probe had a barb on its distal end, similar to the end of a crochet hook, and was capable of causing considerable damage to the entire canalicular system during its outward rotation. The currently used probes have rounded, eyed, blunt tips rather than the distal hook of the Worst probe. Some authors have reported considerable success with the instrument,[50] while others recommend not using it.[51–53] The pigtail probe can be especially useful in identifying the cut medial end of the canaliculus as it is passes from the intact to the cut canaliculus. This technique has at least theoretical merit because nasolacrimal duct intubation is not necessary in cases of localized disruption of the canaliculus. The use of the pigtail probe is demonstrated in Figures 79–9 through 79–14. If the pigtail probe is to be used, it is passed slowly through the dilated punctum of the uninjured canaliculus. Slight resistance is sometimes felt at the level of the common canaliculus. If it does not pass smoothly, however, an alternative method

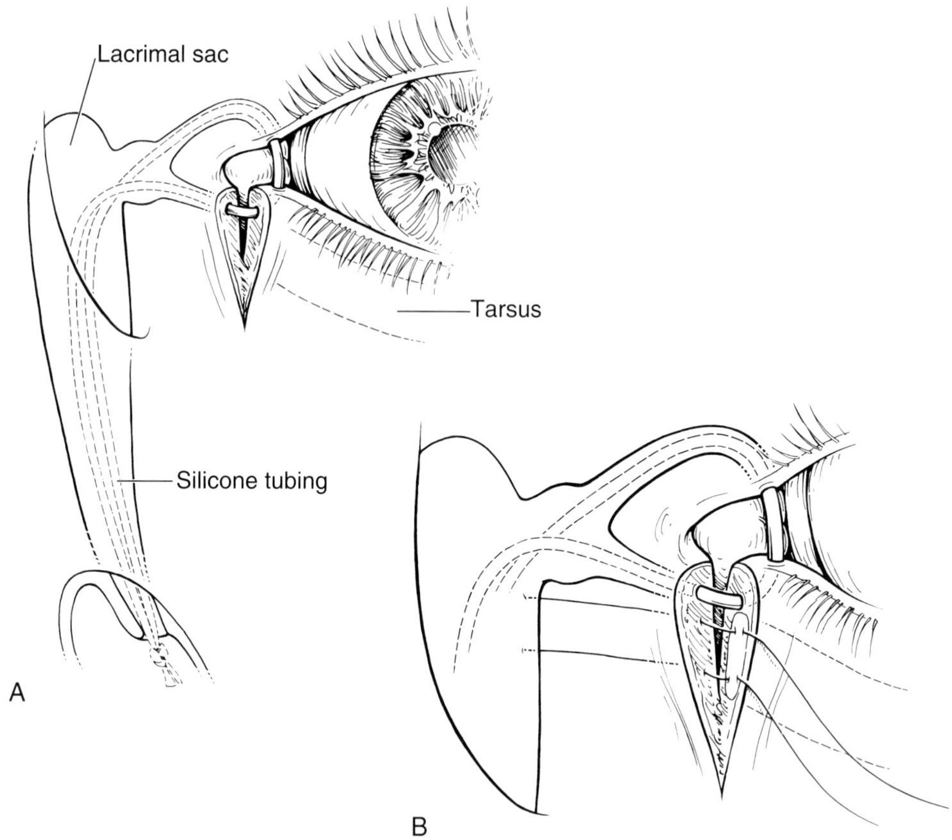

Figure 79–6. *A*, Placement of a silicone tubing stent across the site of canalicular laceration with passage of tubing down the nasolacrimal duct. *B*, Reconstruction of the medial canthal tendon.

of canalicular isolation should be pursued. After intubation, a single 6-0 nylon suture can be threaded through the canalicular system, and a 20- to 25-mm segment of silicone tubing is passed over the nylon suture. The lacerated segment of the canaliculus is then reapproximated as described earlier. The 6-0 nylon suture in the silicone tube is then secured with three single throws, making a continuous ring of silicone tubing in the canalicular system. The nylon knots will then retract into the lumen of the silicone tubing.[50] The system is once again left intubated for 6 months.

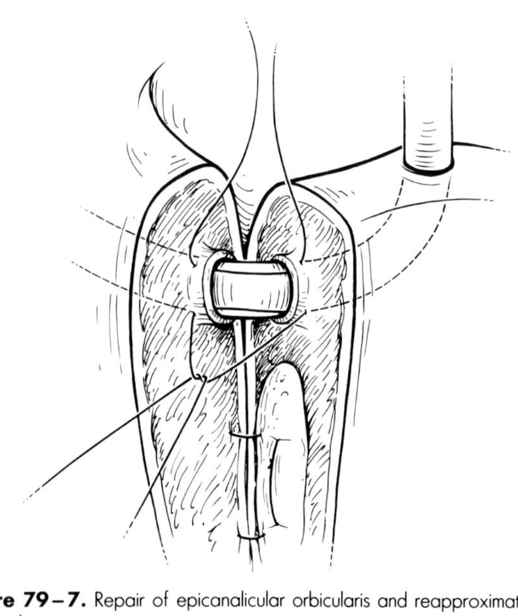

Figure 79–7. Repair of epicanalicular orbicularis and reapproximation of canalicular mucosa.

CANALICULITIS

Diagnosis

Canaliculitis is a well-known clinical entity despite its relative rarity in ophthalmic practice.[54] Symptoms of canaliculitis include purulent discharge, epiphora, tenderness and edema over the canaliculus, and punctal pouting (Fig. 79–15). It most commonly occurs in the lower canaliculus, although it may occur in the upper canaliculus or both canaliculi simultaneously.[55, 56] Canaliculitis may be caused by a variety of organisms, including bacteria such as *Actinomyces israelii*,[55, 57] *Enterobacter cloacae*,[58] *Fusobacterium*,[59] *Arachnia propionica*,[60] and *Mycobacterium*[61, 62]; spirochetes such as syphilis[61]; and fungi such as *Aspergillus*, *Candida*, *Trichosporon*, *Scopulariopsis*, *Cephalosporium*, *Pityrosporum pachydermatis*,[54] and *Eikenella corrodens*. Other causes include herpes simplex and herpes zoster viruses,[63, 64] Stevens-Johnson syndrome,[63] silicone intubation,[62] and retained Veirs rods.[65]

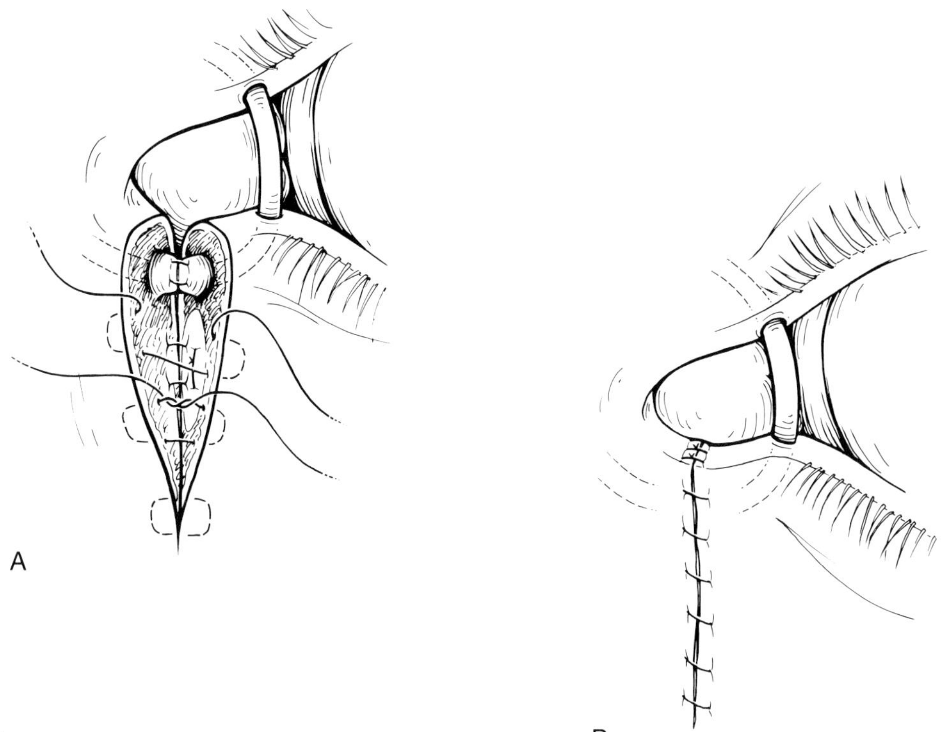

Figure 79–8. *A* and *B*, Closure of eyelid margin.

Treatment

There are several options available to the ophthalmologist in the treatment of canaliculitis. We prefer to utilize expression and curettage of concretions in conjunction with appropriate antimicrobial therapy for initial treatment, with reservation of canaliculotomy for cases that fail curettage.

Canalicular curettage begins with the infiltration of the soft tissues adjacent to the offending canaliculi with a local anesthetic mixture containing epinephrine. A punctum dilator is then used to maximally dilate the puncta so that a 1 to 2-mm chalazion curette can comfortably be passed. The curette is then used to remove all

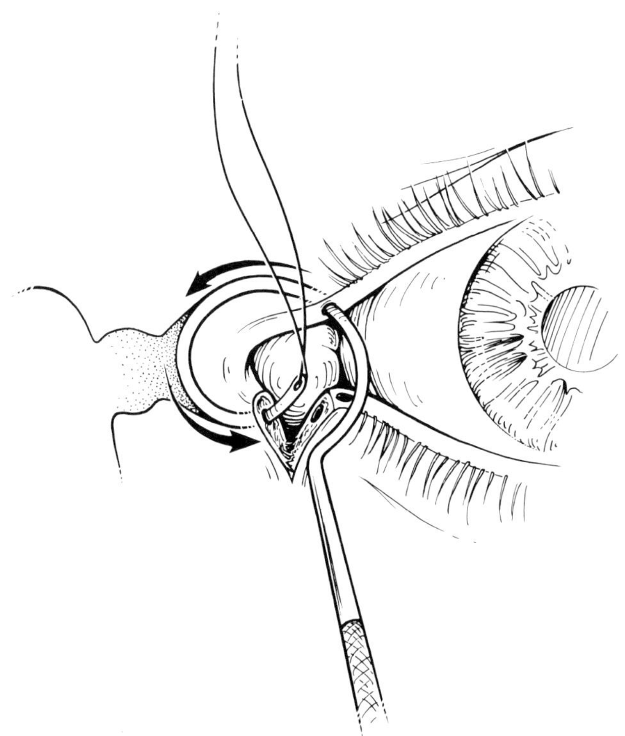

Figure 79–9. The blunt-tipped pigtail probe is introduced through the proximal cut end of the canaliculus.

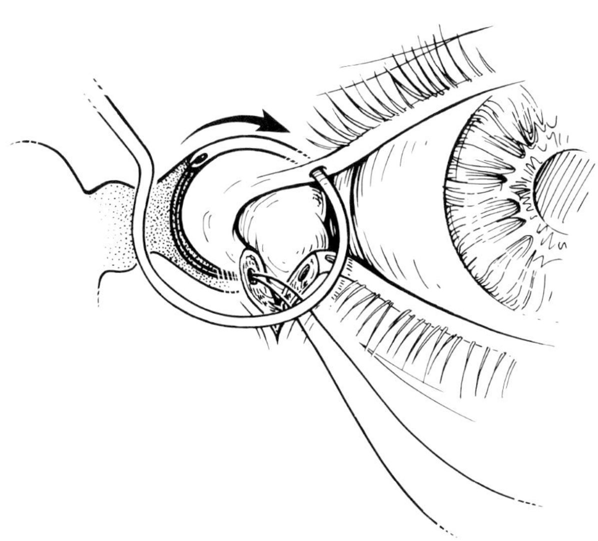

Figure 79–10. A 20- to 25-mm length of silicone tubing containing a 6-0 nylon suture is withdrawn through the intact canaliculus, the common canaliculus, and the proximal end of the lacerated canaliculus.

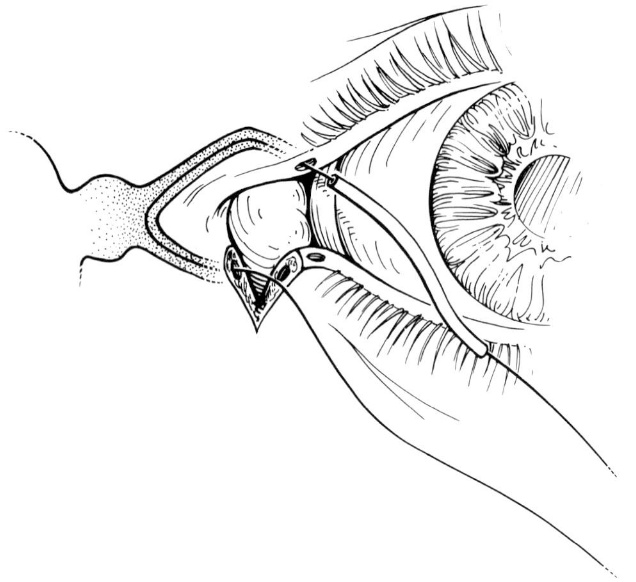

Figure 79–11. The pigtail probe is introduced through the punctum and brought out the distal cut end of the canaliculus.

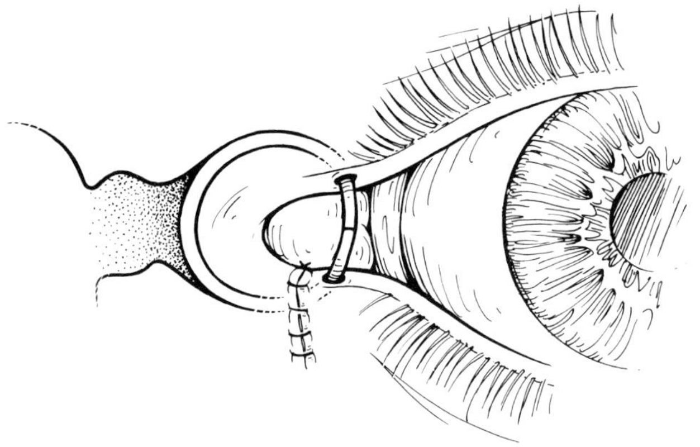

Figure 79–14. The nylon suture is tied, completing ring intubation of the canalicular system. Closure of the eyelid margin is completed.

of the debris from the canaliculus. To assure that all of the debris possible is removed from the canaliculi, approximately six nonproductive passes should be made before declaring the procedure complete.[56] Aerobic and anaerobic culture and sensitivity analysis along with histologic review of the debris should be performed. After curettage, either an antibiotic solution or saline should be irrigated through the canaliculus to prove lacrimal system patency. A topical antibiotic solution may be used for 7 to 10 days after curettage and should be altered if necessary based on culture and sensitivity reports, but surgical débridement appears to be primarily responsible in achieving cure.

If simple curettage and topical antibiotic administration fails to improve the patient's symptoms, then the procedure should be repeated and the canaliculus surgically opened. A Vannas scissors may be used to make a vertical cut through the ampulla of the canaliculus on the conjunctival surface, followed by a 1 to 2-mm horizontal cut. A chalazion curette or a small (5 F) suction tip is used to remove all of the debris possible before irrigation of saline or antibiotic solution through the canaliculus.[55]

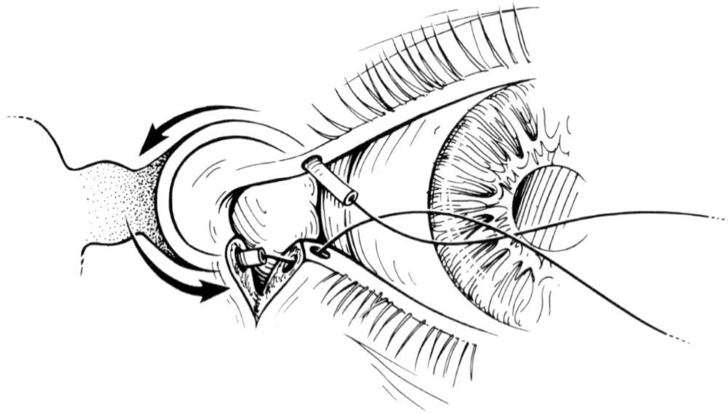

Figure 79–12. The silicone tubing is withdrawn through the distal cut end of the canaliculus.

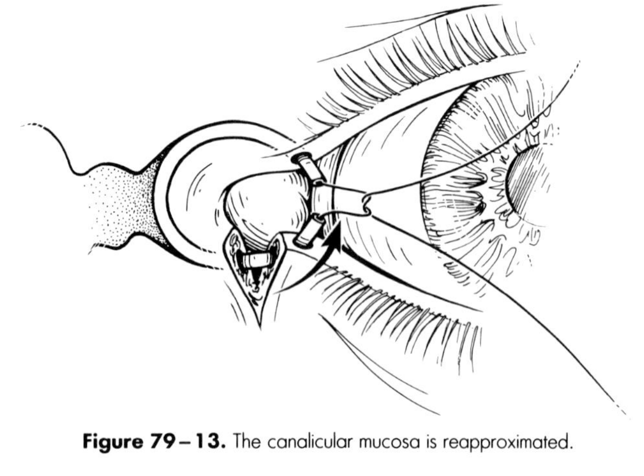

Figure 79–13. The canalicular mucosa is reapproximated.

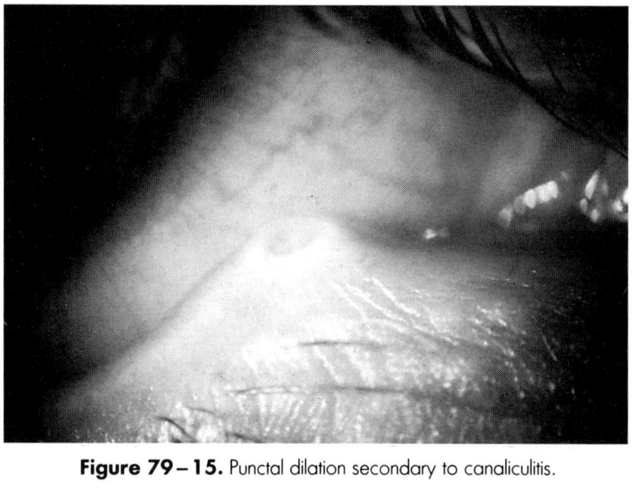

Figure 79–15. Punctal dilation secondary to canaliculitis.

Once again, the material obtained is sent for culture and sensitivity testing and histologic analysis. Topical antibiotic solution is prescribed for 10 to 14 days. Refractory cases may respond to canaliculotomy followed by canalicular marsupialization. Regardless of therapy, recurrence of symptoms is common, and treatment may need to be repeated periodically.

PUNCTAL STENOSIS

Diagnosis

The diagnosis of punctal stenosis is a visual one usually made at the slit lamp. During the routine evaluation of the tearing patient, after the resting position of the eyelids is noted, the medial upper and lower eyelids are everted to inspect the lacrimal papillae. The patient with punctal stenosis may have a pinpoint opening at the apex of the puncta or no visible opening at all (Fig. 79–16).

There are a number of causes of acquired punctal stenosis. The dense fibrous ring around the punctum and the surrounding orbicularis fibers can change with aging and result in senescent punctal stenosis.[66] It can also be caused by infections such as *Chlamydia trachomatis* and herpes simplex.[67–70] Punctal stenosis may be induced by topical ocular medications such as epinephrine, idoxuridine, vidarabine, trifluridine, thiotepa, furmethide, or echothiophate iodide and also by systemic medications such as 5-fluorouracil.[22, 71–73] Systemic conditions such as acrodermatitis enteropathica and Stevens-Johnson syndrome have also been reported to cause punctal stenosis.[74–76]

Treatment

Although there are many different causes of punctal stenosis, the treatment is generally the same. After local infiltration anesthesia has been achieved, the punctum is dilated with a punctal dilator. One blade of a Vannas scissors is introduced into the punctum vertically for approximately 2 mm, and a vertical cut is made on the conjunctival surface of the punctum and canaliculus. In some patients a single incision in each punctum is sufficient to allow normal tear flow. In others, a second short (1–2 mm) cut may be made from the base of the first incision horizontally through the canaliculus.[31] A third cut may be made to excise a triangle of tissue between the two previous cuts. Maneuvers to aid in punctal patency include the placement of a temporary silicone punctum plug, a cutaneous traction suture to draw the medial aspect of the lid more medially, cautery around the peripunctal tissues, or silicone intubation.[66, 77, 78] Postoperative medications generally include an antibiotic corticosteroid eyedrop for 7 to 10 days.

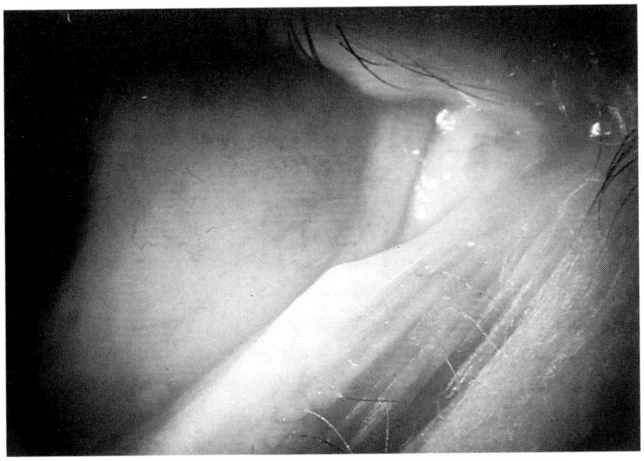

Figure 79–16. Punctal stenosis.

CANALICULAR STENOSIS

Diagnosis

Canalicular stenosis or obstruction is suspected during the evaluation of the patient with epiphora when it is not possible to irrigate through a canaliculus with a normal amount of pressure. In some cases, a reduced lumen may be relatively overcome by high hydrostatic pressure exerted through the irrigation syringe, but frequently such pressure will merely push the eyelid more medially and cause the irrigation canula to be forced from the punctum. A canalicular obstruction can also be suspected during routine probing. The probe can catch on the narrowed or occluded segment and cause a "soft stop" as the probed canaliculus gathers the soft tissue between the occluded segment and the normal bony "hard stop." The phenomenon can also be appreciated externally where a wrinkle is seen in the skin of the eyelid medial to the canalicular obstruction.[79]

Canalicular stenosis, similar to punctal stenosis, has many potential causes. Canalicular scarring following canaliculitis has been reported from viral infections such as epidemic keratoconjunctivitis, herpes simplex, herpes zoster, varicella, vaccinia, and infectious mononucleosis.[68, 80, 81] Previously there was some concern that medical treatment of viral infections was the cause of the obstructions in the lacrimal system rather than the infection itself, but there have been cases reported in which no antiviral medications were administered before the onset of canalicular stenosis.[68] It has been observed that the site of canalicular obstruction after viral canaliculitis is typically in the mid or distal portion of the canaliculus, and less frequently at more proximal locations.[68, 81]

Other infectious causes of canalicular obstruction include *Chlamydia trachomatis*, *Aspergillus*, *Streptococcus*, *Corynebacterium diphtheriae*, and *Actinomyces*.[67] Bacterial infections do not seem to be associated as frequently with canalicular obstruction as viral infections. One proposed hypothesis for this observation is that viral infections extend deeper in the canaliculus to the elastic layer while bacterial infections remain more localized to the epithelium. The resultant cicatrization in the elastic layer could lead to a greater rate of obstruction than simple epithelial involvement.[81]

Medications capable of inducing canalicular stenosis include idoxuridine, trifluridine, vidarabine, phospholine iodide, epinephrine, pilocarpine, and fluorouracil.[72, 81, 82] Iatrogenic canalicular obstruction has occurred secondary to a retained Veirs rod[65] and following unsuccessful probing of the lacrimal system for congenital nasolacrimal duct obstruction.[83] Trauma is likewise a common cause of canalicular stenosis.[84] Systemic conditions such as Stevens-Johnsons syndrome, porphyria cutanea tarda, graft-versus-host disease following bone marrow transplantation, and ocular cicatricial pemphigoid all have been associated with canalicular obstruction.[74, 85, 86] Idiopathic canalicular stenosis can also occur as a consequence of aging.[87] Infrequently the involutional changes in the canaliculi lead to canalicular cystocele formation (canaliculops), which can be associated with canalicular obstruction.[88, 89]

Overall, the most common causes of canalicular obstruction appear to be trauma and idiopathic, followed by congenital abnormalities, tumors, medications, and viral infections.[84]

Treatment

The treatment of symptomatic canalicular obstruction generally entails one of three categories: silicone intubation, canaliculodacryocystorhinostomy (CLDCR), and conjunctival dacryocystorhinostomy (CJDCR). The choice of procedure depends to some degree on the nature and cause of the canalicular compromise. If the obstruction is incomplete or associated with a temporary condition (such as a viral infection or treatment with a drug that can be discontinued), silicone intubation may be performed to maintain patency of the system.[72] Unless a contraindication to topical corticosteroid therapy exists, an antibiotic-corticosteroid combination is generally administered for 7 to 10 days after tube placement. The tube should be left in place for 3 to 6 months after the offending agent has been removed or the infection subsided.

If the obstruction is located at the level of the common canaliculus, then a DCR with silicone intubation of the canaliculi may be considered. During the procedure, the area of the common canaliculus may be inspected directly after the lacrimal sac is opened and adhesions involving the common canaliculus may be sharply divided.

If the obstruction is located within 2 mm of the lacrimal sac, lacrimal reconstruction by means of a CLDCR may be performed. A standard DCR incision is made and the orbicularis oculi and subcutaneous tissues are retracted. The medial canthal tendon is identified incised at its periosteal attachment and retracted laterally. Lacrimal probes are then passed that will identify the common canaliculus posterior to the medial canthal tendon. The scarred canaliculi are then microscopically separated from the posterior limb of the medial canthal tendon with a periosteal elevator. The canaliculi are then opened over the medial end of lacrimal probes, and the scar tissue between this area and the lacrimal sac is excised. Silicone tubes are then passed through the shortened canaliculi. A generous rhinostomy is then performed, and standard mucosal flaps are fashioned. The posterior mucosal flaps are secured, following which a 2- to 3-mm vertical incision is made in the lateral nasolacrimal sac in the area of the common canaliculus. The silicone tubes are passed through the lateral wall of the sac into the nose. The new medial canaliculi are then secured in the lateral wall of the nasolacrimal sac with 5-0 chromic sutures, and the anterior mucosal flap is subsequently approximated. The incision is then closed in a standard fashion, and the silicone tubes are secured. The lacrimal system should remain intubated for approximately 6 months. This procedure has also been used for relief of common canalicular obstruction.[90, 91]

In the case of a complete canalicular obstruction, an obstruction involving the lateral 6 mm of the canaliculi, or an obstruction that has recurred following silicone tube placement, we prefer to perform a CJDCR.[92] This procedure was originally described by Jones and referred to as a conjunctivorhinostomy.[93] It involves the placement of a hollow Pyrex glass tube (Jones tube) from the medial inferior tear lake into the nasal cavity. The procedure can be done with a silicone tube, but the canaliculi do not drain well partly because of the poor capillary attraction of the silicone.[84]

A CJDCR begins with the same steps as a standard DCR, including the skin incision, bony opening, and nasal mucosal window. Following this, attention is turned to the caruncle, which is excised. A standard 18-gauge intravenous catheter with a metal introducer is used to create a tract from the site of the caruncle directed medially, posteriorly, and inferior through the ostia created in the nasal mucosa. The catheter should be placed at a 45-degree angle from vertical to maximize the tear drainage through the tube. The metal trochar is removed from the intravenous catheter leaving the outer flexible sleeve in place. A lacrimal probe is placed through the intravenous catheter, and then the catheter is removed, leaving the lacrimal probe in place.

The length from the conjunctival surface to the nasal cavity is estimated, and a glass Jones tube is directed over the lacrimal probe into the previously made tract. Tubes used typically have flanges that are 3.5 to 4.0 mm in diameter and 15 to 25 mm in length. The surgeon should have a wide assortment of tubes available. Attention is given to ensure that undue pressure is not placed on the glass tube since fracture of the glass is possible. If the tube will not pass, the tract may be gently enlarged with blunt scissors dissection. The passageway should not be too large, however, since this may allow the glass tube to become buried postoperatively in the soft tissue rather than staying in the tear lake. Nasal mucosa is excised as necessary to ensure that the nasal opening of the tube will not be occluded. A properly selected tube will pass from the inferior medial fornix to the middle meatus with a clearance of at least 2 mm from the nasal septum and lateral nasal wall.

If irrigation solution is dripped onto the eye when the glass tube is properly placed, fluid will flow freely into the nose. Direct inspection of the tube using a headlight should be performed to ascertain the exact location of the tube in its resting state. Nasal endoscopy is useful for this task, especially when direct visualization is difficult. After the surgeon is satisfied with the length and angle of the tube, it is secured in place with a 6-0 nylon suture, which can be removed 10 to 14 days postoperatively. This ensures that the tube protrudes into the nasal cavity but does not migrate against the nasal septum. As in a standard DCR, the patient should be instructed not to blow his or her nose for 2 weeks postoperatively. An antibiotic-corticosteroid solution is administered for 7 to 10 days after CJDCR. Function of the tube postoperatively may be assessed by fluorescein dye disappearance testing, free irrigation into the nose, or a positive sniff test (air flowing through the tube when the patient gently sniffs with the nostrils occluded).[84]

Numerous postoperative problems may be encountered after otherwise successful CJDCR surgery. The tubes may be displaced medially or laterally and even completely extruded. The length of time from surgery to tube displacement is also quite variable and can occur any time from immediately postoperatively to years after the procedure. Tubes that become dislodged laterally are typically too long and should be replaced by shorter tubes. It may be difficult to distinguish between medial (intranasal) tube migration from tube extrusion. If the patient presents with an unclear history, and did not actually see the tube extrude, a diligent search should be made to ensure that it is not just medially displaced. Sometimes even if the tube is extruded, the patient will not have epiphora. Despite the frequent occurrence of postoperative problems, most CJDCRs can be made to function adequately.[84]

CONCLUSION

Pathology involving the canaliculus and punctum is commonly encountered in clinical practice. Most problems in this area can be easily addressed after a systematic evaluation of the lacrimal system has been conducted. By utilizing a flexible approach to the repair of these disorders, functional results should generally be obtained.

REFERENCES

1. Carter KD, Nelson CC, Martonyi CL: Size variation of the lacrimal punctum in adults. Ophthalmic Plast Reconstr Surg 4:231–233, 1988.
2. Sevel D: Developmental and congenital abnormalities of the nasolacrimal apparatus. J Pediatr Ophthalmol Strabismus 18:13–29, 1981.
3. Busse H, Kuchle HJ, Greul G: Microsurgical reconstruction of the destroyed canaliculus. Aust NZ J Surg 50:343–346, 1980.
4. Kurihashi KK, Imada M, Yamashita A: Anatomical analysis of the human lacrimal drainage pathway under an operating microscope. Int Ophthalmol 15:411–416, 1991.
5. Zide BM, Jelks GW: Surgical Anatomy of the Orbit. New York, Raven Press, 1985.
6. Norman CA, Hill JC: Horner's muscle and the lacrimal system. Arch Ophthalmol 100:488–493, 1982.
7. White WL, Glover AT, Buckner AB: Effect of blinking on tear elimination as evaluated by dacryoscintigraphy. Ophthalmology 98:367–369, 1991.
8. Hill JC, Apt R, Smirmaul HJ: Lacrimal pump pressure patterns. Can J Ophthalmol 10:25–31, 1975.
9. Lemp MA, Weiler HW: How do tears exit? Invest Ophthalmol Vis Sci 24:619–622, 1983.
10. White WL, Glover AT, Buckner AB, Hartshorne MF: Relative canalicular tear flow as assessed by dacryoscintigraphy. Ophthalmology 96:167–169, 1988.
11. Daubert J, Nik N, Chandeyssoun PA, El-Choufi L: Tear flow analysis through the upper and lower systems. Ophthalmic Plast Reconstr Surg 6:193–196, 1990.
12. Meyer DR, Antonello A, Linberg JV: Assessment of tear drainage after canalicular obstruction using fluorescein dye disappearance. Ophthalmology 97:1370–1374, 1990.
13. Linberg JV, Moore CA: Symptoms of canalicular obstruction. Ophthalmology 95:1077–1079, 1988.
14. Town AE: Congenital absence of lacrimal puncta in three members of a family. Arch Ophthalmol 29:767–771, 1943.
15. Cahill KV, Burns JA: Management of epiphora in the presence of congenital punctal and canalicular atresia. Ophthalmic Plast Reconstr Surg 7:167–172, 1991.
16. Leone CR: The management of pediatric lacrimal problems. Ophthalmic Plast Reconstr Surg 5:34–39, 1989.
17. Caccamise WC, Townes PL: Congenital absence of the lacrimal puncta associated with alacrima and aptyalism. Am J Ophthalmol 89:62–65, 1980.
18. Blackman FB: Congenital atresia of all lacrimal puncta with absence of salivary glands. Am J Ophthalmol 8:139–140, 1925.
19. Kohn R: Additional lacrimal findings in the syndrome of blepharoptosis, blepharophimosis, epicanthus inversus and telecanthus. J Pediatr Ophthalmol Strabismus 20:98–100, 1983.
20. Wang FM, Millman AL, Sidoti PA, Goldberg RB: Ocular findings in Treacher Collins syndrome. Am J Ophthalmol 110:280–286, 1990.
21. Bartley GB: Lacrimal drainage anomalies in mandibulofacial dysostosis. Am J Ophthalmol 109:571–574, 1990.
22. Woog JJ, Dortzbach RK, Wexler SA, Shahidi NT: The role of aminocaproic acid in lacrimal surgery in dyskeratosis congenita. Am J Ophthalmol 100:728–732, 1985.
23. Mawhorter LG, Ruttum MS, Koenig SB: Keratopathy in a family with the ectrodactyly-ectodermal dysplasia-clefting syndrome. Ophthalmology 92:1427–1431, 1985.
24. Solomon A, Feiler-Ofry V, Lazar M: Congenital reduplication of the lacrimal punctum and canaliculus. Ann Ophthalmol 13:727, 1981.
25. Chignell AH: Double punctum and canaliculus. Am J Ophthalmol 65:736–739, 1968.
26. Wormald RP, Wulc AE, Welham AN: Congenital double lacrimal fistula. Ophthalmic Plast Reconstr Surg 4:109–110, 1988.
27. Welham RAN, Bergin DJ: Congenital lacrimal fistulas. Arch Ophthalmol 103:545–548, 1985.
28. Birchansky LD, Nerad JA, Kersten RC, Kulwin DR: Management of congenital lacrimal sac fistula. Arch Ophthalmol 108:388–390, 1990.
29. Putterman AM: Treatment of epiphora with absent lacrimal puncta. Arch Ophthalmol 89:125–127, 1973.

30. Putterman AM: Reconstruction of the absent lacrimal puncta. Ophthalmic Surg 10:20–24, 1979.
31. Jones LT, Wobig JL: Surgery of the Eyelids. Birmingham, AL, Aesculapius, 1976, p 176.
32. Slade CS, Katz NNK, Whitmore PV, Bardenstein DS: Conjunctival and canalicular papillomas and ichthyosis vulgaris. Ann Ophthalmol 20:251–255, 1988.
33. Kohn R, Nofsinger K, Freedman SL: Rapid recurrence of papillary squamous cell carcinoma of the canaliculus. Am J Ophthalmol 92:363–367, 1981.
34. Scott KR, Jakobiec FA, Font RL: Peripunctal melanocytic nevi. Ophthalmology 96:994–998, 1989.
35. Khan JA, Grove AS, Joseph MP, Goodman M: Sebaceous carcinoma: Diuretic vs. lacrimal system spread and surgical margins. Ophthalmic Plast Reconstr Surg 5:227–237, 1989.
36. McCord CA: Canalicular resection and reconstruction by canaliculostomy. Ophthalmic Surg 11:440–444, 1980.
37. Lovato AA, Char DH, Castro JR, Kroll SM: The effect of silicone nasolacrimal intubation on epiphora after helium ion irradiation of uveal melanoma. Am J Ophthalmol 108:461–464, 1989.
38. Korn EL: Use of the carbon dioxide laser for removal of lesions adjacent to the punctum. Ann Ophthalmol 22:230–234, 1990.
39. Wulc AE, Arterberry JF: The pathogenesis of canalicular laceration. Ophthalmology 98:1243–1249, 1991.
40. Hurwitz JJ, Corin SM, Tucker SM: Punctal and vertical canaliculus lacerations. Ophthalmic Surg 20:514–515, 1989.
41. Hawes MJ, Segrest DR: Effectiveness of bicanalicular silicone intubation in the repair of canalicular lacerations. Ophthalmic Plast Reconstr Surg 1:185–190, 1985.
42. Harris GJ: Canalicular laceration at birth. Am J Ophthalmol 105:322–323, 1988.
43. Reifler DM: Management of canalicular laceration. Surv Ophthalmol 36:113–132, 1991.
44. Patrinely JR, Anderson RL: A review of lacrimal drainage surgery. Ophthalmic Plast Reconstr Surg 2:97–102, 1986.
45. Long JA: A method of monocanalicular silicone intubation. Ophthalmic Surg 19:204–205, 1988.
46. Dibble RF, Friedel SD: A simplified method of monocanalicular silicone intubation. Ophthalmic Surg 21:134–135, 1990.
47. Romano PE: Single silicone intubation for repair of single canaliculus laceration. Ann Ophthalmol 18:112–113, 1986.
48. Seiff SR, Ahn JC: Locating cut medial canaliculi by direct injection of sodium hyaluronidase into the lacrimal sac. Ophthalmic Surg 20:176–178, 1989.
49. Vila-Coro AA, Vila-Coro AA, Garcia PZ: Hyaluronate in the identification of the cut end in lacerations of the lacrimal canaliculi. Am J Ophthalmol 105:214–215, 1988.
50. Jordan DR, Nerad JA, Tse DT: The pigtail probe, revisited. Ophthalmology 97:512–519, 1990.
51. Dortzbach RK, Angrist RA: Silicone intubation for lacerated lacrimal canaliculi. Ophthalmic Surg 16:639–642, 1985.
52. Kennedy RH, May J, Dailey J, Flanagan JC: Canalicular lacerations, an 11-year epidemiologic and clinical study. Ophthalmic Plast Reconstr Surg 6:46–53, 1990.
53. Saunders DH, Shannon GM, Flanagan JC: The effectiveness of the pigtail probe method of repairing canalicular lacerations. Ophthalmic Surg 9:33–40, 1978.
54. Romano A, Segal E, Blumenthal M: Canaliculitis with isolation of *Pityrosporum pachydermatis*. Br J Ophthalmol 62:732–734, 1978.
55. Demant E, Hurwitz JJ: Canaliculitis: Review of 12 cases. Can J Ophthalmol 15:73–75, 1980.
56. Pavilack MA, Frueh BR: Thorough curettage in the treatment of chronic canaliculitis. Arch Ophthalmol 110:200–202, 1992.
57. Richards WW: Actinomycotic lacrimal canaliculitis. Am J Ophthalmol 75:155–157, 1973.
58. Chumbley LC: Canaliculitis caused by *Enterobacter cloacae*: Report of a case. Br J Ophthalmol 68:364–366, 1984.
59. Weinberg FJ, Sartoris MJ, Buerger GF, Novak JF: *Fusobacterium* in presumed *Actinomyces* canaliculitis. Am J Ophthalmol 84:371–374, 1977.
60. Seal DV, McGill J, Flanagan D, Purrier B: Lacrimal canaliculitis due to *Arachnia (Actinomyces) propionica*. Br J Ophthalmol 65:10–13, 1981.
61. Specific inflammatory diseases of the lacrimal system. *In* Wilson FM II (chairperson): Basic and Clinical Science Course, External Disease and Cornea, Book 7A. San Francisco, American Academy of Ophthalmology, 1987, pp 136–137.
62. Rootman DS, Insler MS, Wolfley DE: Canaliculitis caused by *Mycobacterium chelonei* after lacrimal intubation with silicone tubes. Can J Ophthalmol 24:221–222, 1989.
63. Welham RAN, Hughes SM: Lacrimal surgery in children. Am J Ophthalmol 99:27–34, 1985.
64. de Koning EWJ, van Bijsterveld OP: Herpes simplex virus canaliculitis. Ophthalmologica 186:173–176, 1983.
65. Becker BB: Retained Veirs rod and canaliculitis. Am J Ophthalmol 111:251–252, 1991.
66. Kristan RW: Treatment of lacrimal punctal stenosis with a one-snip canaliculotomy and temporary punctal plugs. Arch Ophthalmol 106:878–879, 1988.
67. Tabbara KF, Bobb AA: Lacrimal system complications in trachoma. Ophthalmology 87:298–301, 1980.
68. Harris GJ, Hyndiuk RA, Fox MJ, Taugher PJ: Herpetic canalicular obstruction. Arch Ophthalmol 99:282–283, 1981.
69. Patterson A, Jones BR: The management of ocular herpes. Trans Ophthalmol Soc UK 87:59–84, 1967.
70. Laibson PR, Hyndiuk R, Krachmer JH, Schutz RO: Ara-A and IDU therapy of human superficial herpetic keratitis. Invest Ophthalmol 14:762–763, 1975.
71. Romano A, Stein R: Obstruction of lacrimal puncta caused by topical epinephrine. Ophthalmologica 166:301–305, 1973.
72. Caravella LP Jr, Burns JA, Zangmeister M: Punctal-canalicular stenosis related to systemic fluorouracil therapy. Arch Ophthalmol 99:284–286, 1981.
73. Shaffer RN, Ridgway WL: Furmethide iodide in the production of dacryostenosis. Am J Ophthalmol 34:718–720, 1951.
74. Auran JD, Hornblass A, Gross ND: Stevens-Johnson syndrome with associated nasolacrimal duct obstruction treated with dacryocystorhinostomy and Crawford silicone tube insertion. Ophthalmic Plast Reconstr Surg 6:60–63, 1990.
75. Arstikaitis M: Ocular aftermath of Stevens-Johnson syndrome: Review of 33 cases. Arch Ophthalmol 90:376–379, 1973.
76. Matta CS, Felker GV, Ide CH: Eye manifestations in acrodermatitis enteropathica. Arch Ophthalmol 93:140–142, 1975.
77. Dolin SL, Hecht SD: The punctum pucker procedure for stenosis of the lacrimal punctum. Arch Ophthalmol 104:1086–1087, 1986.
78. Fein W: Cautery applications to relieve punctal stenosis. Arch Ophthalmol 95:145–146, 1977.
79. Burns JA, Penland WR, Cahill KV: The wrinkle sign in tear duct obstruction. Ophthalmic Surg 15:930–931, 1984.
80. Hyde KJ, Berger ST: Epidemic keratoconjunctivitis and lacrimal excretory system obstruction. Ophthalmology 95:1447–1449, 1988.
81. Harley RD, Stefanyszyn MA, Apt L, Nelson LB: Herpetic canalicular obstruction. Ophthalmic Surg 18:367–370, 1987.
82. Zimmerman TJ: Pilocarpine. Ophthalmology 88:85–88, 1981.
83. Lyon DB, Dortzbach RK, Lemke BN, Gonnering RS: Canalicular stenosis following probing for congenital nasolacrimal duct probing. Ophthalmic Surg 22:228–232, 1991.
84. Sekhar GC, Dortzbach RK, Gonnering RS, Lemke BN: Problems associated with conjunctivodacryocystorhinostomy. Am J Ophthalmol 112:502–506, 1991.
85. Sober AJ, Grove AS Jr, Muhlbauer JE: Cicatricial ectropion and lacrimal obstruction associated with the sclerodermoid variant of porphyria cutanea tarda. Am J Ophthalmol 91:396–400, 1981.
86. West RH, Szer J, Pedersen JS: Ocular surface and lacrimal disturbances in chronic graft-versus-host disease: The role of conjunctival biopsy. Aust NZ J Ophthalmol 19:187–191, 1991.
87. Steinsapir KD, Glatt HJ, Putterman AM: A 16-year study of conjunctival dacryocystorhinostomy. Am J Ophthalmol 109:387–393, 1990.
88. Weinstein GS, Tse DT, Anderson RL: Canalicular cystocele. Ophthalmologica (Basel) 189:64–68, 1984.
89. Sacks E, Jakobiec FA, Dodick J: Canaliculops. Ophthalmology 94:78–81, 1987.

90. Doucet TW, Hurwitz JJ: Canaliculodacryocystorhinostomy in the treatment of canalicular obstruction. Arch Ophthalmol 100:306–309, 1982.
91. Doucet TW, Hurwitz JJ: Canaliculodacryocystorhinostomy in the management of unsuccessful lacrimal surgery. Arch Ophthalmol 100:619–621, 1982.
92. Seiff SR, Shorr N, Adams T: Surgical treatment of punctal-canalicular fibrosis from 5-fluorouracil therapy. Cancer 56:2148–2149, 1985.
93. Jones LT: The cure of epiphora due to canalicular disorders, trauma, and surgical failures of the lacrimal passages. Trans Am Acad Ophthalmol Otolaryngol 66:506–524, 1962.

SECTION VII

The Orbit

SECTION EDITORS

Robert A. Weiss
Giulio Bonavolontà

Introduction

Robert A. Weiss and Giulio Bonavolontà

The diagnosis and management of orbital pathologic conditions continue to move toward the state of the art as refinements are made in neuroradiologic imaging, surgical techniques, and instrumentation, and as an understanding of the underlying pathophysiologic mechanisms of orbital disorders progresses. A small group of pioneers in orbital disease and surgery began to accumulate knowledge and understanding of these diseases years in the past. Their knowledge and experience was passed on to their students in an apprenticeship approach to medicine. This approach was particularly important to gain the requisite knowledge as well as to develop an understanding of the nuances necessary for the appropriate diagnosis and management of orbital disorders. The orbital specialist's clinical skills were profoundly advanced in the 1970s with the development of computed tomographic scanning and, more recently, with the advent of magnetic resonance imaging. As the result of these technologic advances, the need for diagnostic exploratory surgery of the orbit has essentially vanished. In the vast majority of cases, the exact location of the lesion, the specific tissues involved, and, many times, the underlying histologic nature of an orbital disorder can be diagnosed preoperatively. This knowledge combined with knowledge derived from the experiences of neurosurgery, craniofacial surgery, and head and neck/maxillofacial surgery allows the orbital surgeon to approach surgery in a manner that optimizes the anatomic exposure and avoids unnecessary morbidity as a result of surgery.

As orbital surgery has ultimately developed into a complete subspecialty, national and international societies on orbital disorders have come into being, and scientific journals now exist specifically on this subject. The following chapters on the orbit have been written by recognized experts and their "apprentices" from around the globe. These chapters reflect how close we have actually come toward achieving state of the art in the diagnosis and management of orbital disorders. The chapters in this text have been written with emphasis on surgical approaches to management of orbital disorders.

CHAPTER 80

Orbital Anatomy and Embryology

Don O. Kikkawa and Bradley N. Lemke

Comprehension of orbital anatomy is crucial in the study of disease processes affecting the orbit and provides a primary base of information to the operating surgeon. Surgical approaches, avoidance of complications, and successful orbital surgery are all founded in a firm knowledge of anatomy in this complex region.

ORBITAL ANATOMY

Osteology

Orbital Shape and Dimensions

The bony orbit most closely resembles a four-sided pyramid that becomes three-sided approaching the orbital apex. The absence of the orbital floor posteriorly causes this change in geometry, and this is accounted for by the upward slope of the lateral wall toward the medial wall.[1] The medial orbital walls are separated in the adult by 25 mm and are essentially parallel, converging as they near the orbital apex. The lateral orbital walls in the adult each diverge 45 degrees from the sagittal midline, together forming a 90-degree angle. The visual axis of the orbit is thus 22.5 degrees (Fig. 80–1). The divergence of the visual axes necessitates constant tone in the medial rectus muscles to maintain globe alignment.

The orbital entrance is rectangular, measuring horizontally 40 mm and vertically 32 mm, and its maximal width occurs 1 cm behind the anterior orbital rim. Although the depth from orbital rim to apex in adults varies from 40 to 45 mm, safe subperiosteal dissection may be accomplished along the lateral wall and the orbital floor for 25 mm and along the medial wall and orbital roof for 30 mm before vital neurovascular structures are encountered.[2] The orbital volume varies with race and sex but is approximately 30 mL.

Orbital Margins

The orbital margin is a discontinuous ring due to the lacrimal sac fossa medially and therefore forms a quadrilateral spiral (Fig. 80–2). The frontal bone alone gives rise to the superior orbital rim. The supraorbital notch or foramen is located at the junction of the medial one third with the lateral two thirds of the superior rim and transmits the supraorbital nerve and vessels. The superior orbital rim becomes rounded medially and is continuous with the posterior aspect of the medial rim. Three bones, the frontal bone, the posterior lacrimal crest of the lacrimal bone, and the anterior lacrimal crest of the frontal process of the maxillary bone, form the medial orbital rim. The lacrimal sac fossa is an indentation between the anterior lacrimal crest, which is continuous with the inferior orbital rim, and the posterior lacrimal crest, which is continuous with the superior orbital rim.

The maxillary bone and zygomatic bone form the inferior orbital rim. At the joining of the medial one third and lateral two thirds of the inferior orbital rim lies the zygomaticomaxillary suture. The infraorbital foramen is approximately 1 cm from the orbital margin in the adult, but at birth it is much closer to the orbital rim. When dissecting along the inferior orbital rim in children, this relationship should be noted and avoided. The lateral orbital rim is formed by the zygomatic process of the frontal bone superiorly and by the frontal process of the zygomatic bone inferiorly. Articulation of these two bones occurs at the frontozygomatic suture, where a stepoff can be palpated in fractures. The zygoma is often referred to as the "facial buttress," owing to its strong resistance to fracture.

Orbital Walls

The orbital plate of the frontal bone forms the orbital roof primarily with a small contribution posteriorly from the lesser wing of the sphenoid bone (Fig. 80–3). During growth, the orbital roof convexly molds around the globe. Significant frontal trauma to the superior rim is usually required to fracture the orbital roof, which is comparatively stronger compared with the medial wall and orbital floor. The fossae for the lacrimal gland and trochlea are found anterolaterally and anteromedially. The recurrent meningeal artery traverses the meningeal foramen, which can be found near the frontosphenoidal suture. Communicating with the lacrimal artery, these

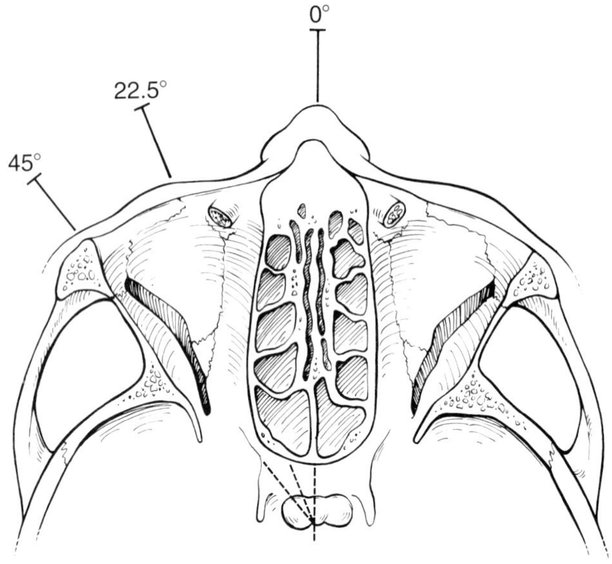

Figure 80–1. Horizontal section through orbits. Lateral orbital walls diverge 45 degrees from midline, while visual axes diverge 22.5 degrees.

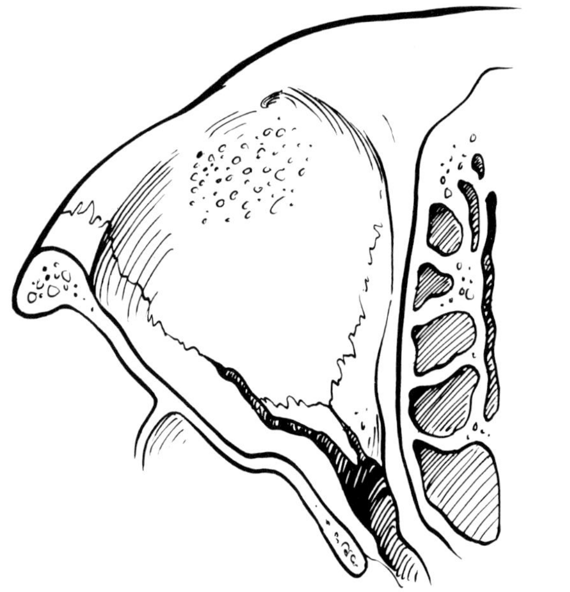

Figure 80–3. Orbital roof showing frontal bone and small contribution from sphenoid bone.

vessels provide for reversal of blood flow during the internal carotid artery stenosis.

The medial orbital wall comprises four bones: the maxillary, lacrimal, ethmoid, and sphenoid (Fig. 80–4). The anterior medial wall is relatively thick anteriorly owing to the frontal process of the maxilla. Posteriorly, the lacrimal fossa and posterior lacrimal crest of the lacrimal bone are encountered. Becoming progressively thinner nearing the ethmoid bone, pneumatized ethmoidal air cells may be visible beneath the lamina papyracea. Medial wall blow-out fractures frequently occur in this region. Nearing the body of the sphenoid bone, the wall thickens posteriorly. The anterior and posterior ethmoidal foramina, which transmit branches of the ophthalmic artery and nasociliary nerve, are located 20 mm and 35 mm posterior to the anterior lacrimal crest at a level just superior to the medial canthal ligament.[3] Posteriorly, the

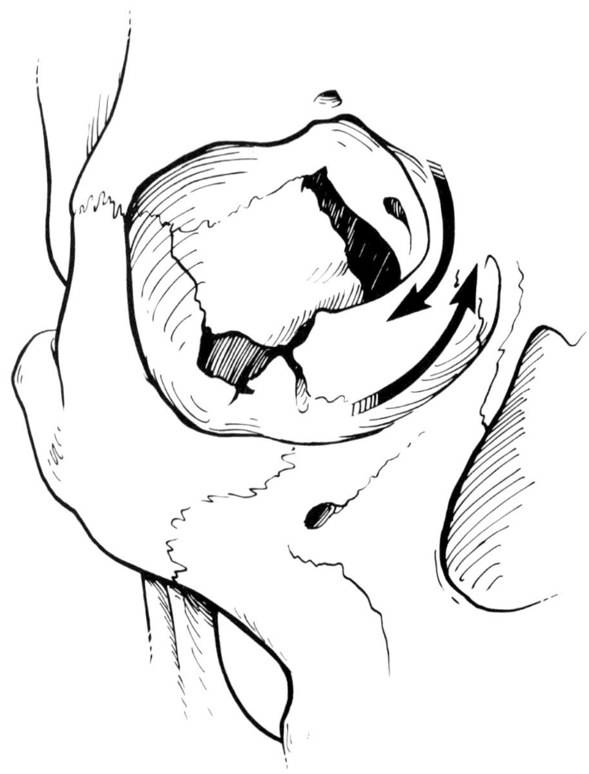

Figure 80–2. Orbital margin showing spiral and discontinuity from lacrimal sac fossa.

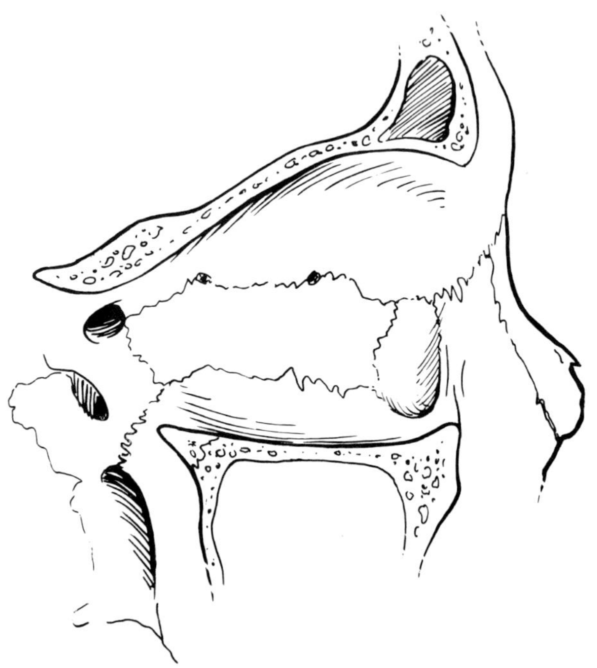

Figure 80–4. Anterolateral view of medial orbital wall. The anterior and posterior ethmoidal foramina and optic foramen are located 20 mm, 35 mm, and 50 mm posterior to the anterior lacrimal crest.

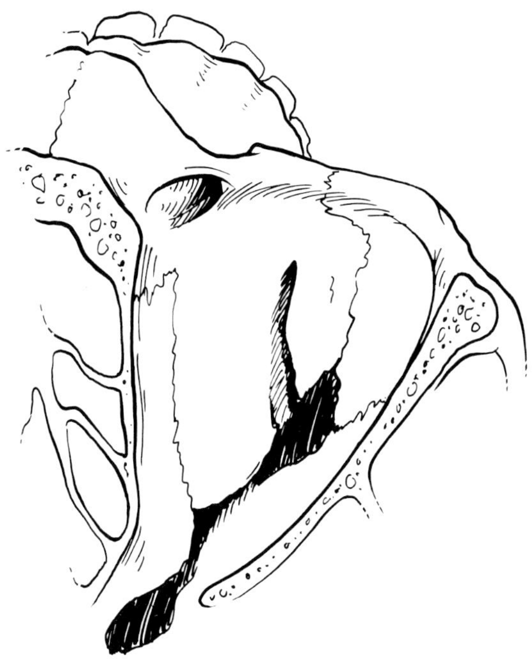

Figure 80–5. Anterior view of the orbital floor. It is formed primarily by the orbital plate of the maxillary bone with small contributions from the palatine and zygomatic bones.

optic foramen is located approximately 50 mm from the anterior lacrimal crest.

The orbital floor is formed from three bones—the orbital plate of the maxillary bone, which forms the majority of the floor, along with the palatine bone posteriorly and the zygoma anterolaterally (Fig. 80–5). The infraorbital groove houses the infraorbital nerve and artery and becomes the infraorbital canal anteriorly. The infraorbital nerve, as it courses from posterior to anterior, is not housed within the bone of the orbital floor until it enters the infraorbital canal and is susceptible to injury in a subperiosteal dissection plane. Medially and posteriorly to the infraorbital nerve is the thinnest area of the orbital floor, where blow-out fractures most frequently occur. Being the only extraocular muscle not to originate from the orbital apex, the inferior oblique muscle arises from a shallow fossa lateral to the opening of the nasolacrimal canal.

The thickest of the orbital walls is the lateral wall. It is formed anteriorly by the zygoma and posteriorly by the greater wing of the sphenoid (Fig. 80–6). Posteriorly, the superior orbital fissure and inferior orbital fissure form the boundaries of the lateral wall. Located anteriorly along the lateral wall are the zygomaticotemporal and zygomaticofacial canals, which transmit arterial and nerve branches of the lacrimal artery and lacrimal and zygomatic nerves, respectively. Three to four mm behind the orbital rim and 11 mm inferior to the frontozygomatic suture lies the lateral orbital tubercle of Whitnall.[4] The lateral canthal ligament, the deep pretarsal orbicularis insertion, the lateral horn of the levator aponeurosis, the check ligament of the lateral rectus muscle, the superior (Whitnall's) and inferior (Lockwood's) transverse ligaments, and an expansion of the superior rectus muscle sheath all attach to the lateral orbital tubercle of Whitnall.[5]

The lateral orbital rim and wall are removed during lateral orbitotomy. During the dissection the zygomaticofacial and zygomaticotemporal nerves and vessels should be identified. The zygomaticosphenoid suture provides a vertical breaking point for bone removal during osteotomy. The middle cranial fossa is in close proximity to the superior osteotomy made in lateral orbitotomy. This distance has been studied in cadavers and is only 12 to 13 mm in males and the distance may be 5 to 6 mm shorter in females.[6]

Orbital Apex

The optic foramen, the superior orbital fissure, and inferior orbital fissure (Fig. 80–7) provide passages to and from the orbit with the intracranial cavity, pterygopalatine fossa, and paranasal sinuses. Multiple functional deficits may be seen with pathologic processes affecting this region because of the high concentration of blood vessels and nerves in this confined area. An orbital apex syndrome consists of multiple cranial nerve palsies with diminished vision and an afferent pupillary defect and localizes the disease process to the posterior orbit.

The superior orbital fissure averages 22 mm in length and is located between the greater and lesser wings of the sphenoid bone. The fissure width is variable, but it is usually largest medially beneath the optic foramen and narrowed supratemporally where the lacrimal, frontal, and

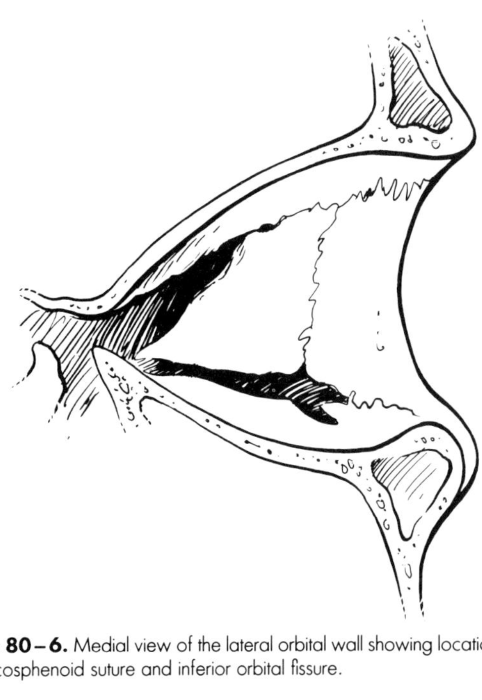

Figure 80–6. Medial view of the lateral orbital wall showing location of zygomaticosphenoid suture and inferior orbital fissure.

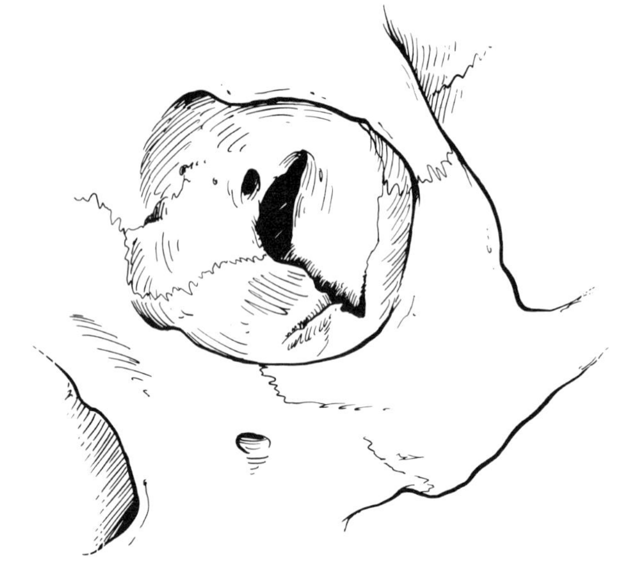

Figure 80–7. Anterolateral view of the orbital apex, showing optic foramen and superior and inferior orbital fissures.

trochlear nerves enter it. Passing through the fissure in addition are the superior and inferior divisions of the oculomotor nerve, the abducens nerve, the nasociliary branch of the ophthalmic division of the trigeminal nerve, sympathetic nerve fibers, and the superior orbital veins. With the use of immunoperoxidase techniques, sympathetic nerve anatomy has been studied in the cynomolgus monkey, and it was found that sympathetic nerves enter the orbit exclusively through the superior orbital fissure and none entered through the optic canal.[7]

Aneurysm, meningioma, chordoma, pituitary adenoma, and tumors may cause enlargement of the superior orbital fissure that may be seen radiologically.[8] Blunt trauma may cause a superior orbital fissure syndrome in which contusion occurs to the structures within the fissure with resultant partial or total ophthalmoplegia with eyelid and forehead anesthesia. In rare cases of fracture, medial displacement of the greater wing of the sphenoid may mask involvement of the optic nerve.[9] The superior orbital fissure may also be affected by granulomatous inflammation causing painful ophthalmoplegia (Tolosa-Hunt syndrome).

The inferior orbital fissure is bounded by the greater wing of the sphenoid laterally and by the palatine and maxillary bones medially. The fissure averages 20 mm in length, and its axis parallels that of the optic canal. Dissection in a subperiosteal plane along the orbital floor is limited posteriorly by the inferior orbital fissure. The inferior orbital fissure communicates with both the pterygopalatine and infratemporal fossae posteriorly, and trauma to the temporalis muscle can result in orbital hemorrhage through this communication.

The maxillary division of the trigeminal nerve, the infraorbital artery, the inferior orbital vein, and autonomic branches from the pterygopalatine ganglion traverse the inferior orbital fissure. The infraorbital nerve, a branch of the maxillary division of the trigeminal nerve, travels with the infraorbital artery, a terminal branch of the maxillary artery, into the infraorbital groove and canal, supplying innervation to the lower eyelid, cheek, lateral nose, upper lip, and upper anterior gingiva. Orbital branches arising from the infraorbital artery, which supply the inferior rectus and inferior oblique, should be avoided or cauterized and divided during inferior orbitotomy.[10]

The optic foramen is housed in the lesser wing of the sphenoid and is the opening of the optic canal into the orbit. The axis of the optic canal is lateral and downward 38 degrees from the sagittal and horizontal planes. The optic canal transmits the optic nerve and ophthalmic artery; and as they traverse the canal, they shift positions. This causes a change in canal width, posteriorly being more horizontally oval and anteriorly more vertically oval. The canal exhibits symmetry between the two sides and reaches adult size by the age of 3. The optic canal diameter is 6.5 mm, and it is 8 to 10 mm long in the adult. Optic nerve gliomas can cause enlargement of the optic canal, and the foramina should be examined bilaterally when considering this diagnosis. Sarcoidosis, neurofibromas, chronic hydrocephalus, adhesive arachnoiditis, and arachnoidal cysts can also affect and enlarge the optic canal, while fibrous dysplasia and ossifying fibroma can narrow and compress its width, causing impingement on the intracanalicular optic nerve.

The optic foramen is separated from the superior orbital fissure by the bony optic strut, and it is susceptible to distortion by optic nerve gliomas, infraclinoid aneurysms, and intracranial chiasmal tumors that spread anteriorly.[11] The portion of the optic nerve that resides within the optic canal is particularly susceptible to injury. Blunt forehead pressure may cause injury indirectly,[12] or injury may occur directly from impingement of bony spicules on the nerve from adjacent fractures.[13] While the medial aspect of the optic canal is formed by the body of the sphenoid bone, in approximately 50% of cases, posterior ethmoidal air cells are in contact with the ipsilateral optic canal.[1, 14] The relationship must be considered when performing extracranial optic canal decompression.

Orbital Connective Tissues

Periorbita

The periorbita lines the bony orbit and is a continuous fibrous membrane. Firm attachments are found to the bone at the orbital margins, the trochlear fossa, suture lines, fissures, the arcus marginalis, and the lacrimal crest. It can be easily lifted from the underlying bone other than these places in which it is firmly attached, creating a potential subperiosteal space. Blood or inflammatory exudates may accumulate within this potential space.

The periorbita is directly continuous with the periosteum of the frontal, zygoma, and maxillary bones. This area of continuity forms a ridge, the arcus marginalis, which is the origin of the orbital septum. The periorbita lines the lacrimal sac fossa medially; and the lacrimal fascia, which is an extension of the periorbita, covers the lacrimal sac between the anterior and posterior lacrimal crests. Thickened periorbita lines the superior orbital fissure and optic canal, and posteriorly it is continuous with the intracranial periosteal dura mater. Inferiorly, through the inferior orbital fissure, the periorbita is continuous with the sphenopalatine and temporal fossae; however, the smooth orbital muscle of Müller covers the inferior orbital fissure itself.

Vascularization of the periorbita is derived from orbital soft tissue internally and orbital bones externally. The interconnection of these blood supplies is linked such that the periorbita itself does not serve as a vascular border.[15] The regional branches of the intraorbital trigeminal nerve provide sensory innervation to the periorbita. The periorbita limits the spread of infections and tumors by providing a boundary that protects intraorbital contents from external disease processes involving the adjacent bone and sinuses. As a surgical plane, the subperiorbital space is an attractive surgical plane because of the ease with which the periorbita can be dissected from the bone and its little resultant bleeding. When dissecting around certain orbital tumors, such as benign mixed tumor of the lacrimal gland, this plane should not be violated for fear of surgical dissemination of the tumor. The periorbita, however, may be opened in certain instances, for example, during orbital decompression for thyroid-related orbitopathy, in which prolapse of orbital fat into sinus cavities is desired.

Orbital Fascia

A highly complex and organized connective tissue skeleton supports and suspends the intraorbital contents. Koorneef's studies of thick orbital serial sections[16, 17] and gross anatomic descriptions have contributed immensely to understanding these intricate interconnections. This intraorbital network is divided for practical purposes into three parts: (1) Tenon's capsule (fascia bulbi), (2) the extraocular muscle fascial sheaths, and (3) the extensions and check ligaments that connect the muscle sheaths to the periorbita and eyelids.

Tenon's capsule is a fibroelastic layer that extends posteriorly from the optic nerve and anteriorly to join the bulbar conjunctiva approximately 2 mm behind the corneoscleral limbus. It is attached to the globe loosely and is attached to fibrous septa externally, which divide and partition the orbital fat. Tenon's capsule is penetrated by nerves, blood vessels, and extraocular muscles to reach the globe. Elastic fibers within the fascial planes and orbital fat septa allow distensibility and mobility of the globe. Tenon's capsule provides the strongest barrier to extrusion of an orbital implant placed after enucleation and evisceration and should be carefully closed surgically to prevent extrusion.

Each extraocular muscle is encompassed within a fascial sheath for its entire length. They are denser anteriorly and thinner posteriorly.[18] The muscle sheaths are attached externally to the orbital walls and internally to the intraconal fat septa.[19] The extraocular muscles are connected to the surrounding fascia along the anterior one third of their length and especially at their globe insertions. These attachments, if not severed, limit retraction of the extraocular muscles far posteriorly in the orbit if lost during strabismus surgery. The medial rectus muscle is the most frequently lost muscle,[20] and it has been speculated that the medial rectus muscle sheath may be less well fixated in the orbit owing to lack of juxtaposition to an oblique muscle sheath.

The intermuscular septum is formed by fusion of the rectus muscle sheath extensions before their insertion on the globe. A common muscle sheath separating the intraconal from extraconal space cannot be identified posterior to this septum, and thus there is no anatomic boundary creating a true muscle cone.[16]

Each muscle is connected through an extension to its adjacent orbital wall. They become prominent anteriorly and are known as check ligaments. The most developed check ligaments are those of the lateral and medial rectus muscles. The lateral rectus check ligament inserts on Whitnall's tubercle and also to the conjunctival fornix laterally and the orbital septum. The medial rectus check ligament inserts behind the posterior lacrimal crest and also to the orbital septum, to the caruncle, and to the plica semilunaris.

The superior rectus muscle sheath is connected with that of the levator palpebrae superioris by an intermuscular fascia.[21] The superior transverse ligament of Whitnall[22] originates from the levator palpebrae fascial sheath and is located just posterior to the area of transition from aponeurotic to muscular portions of the muscle. Medially it attaches to the periorbita in the trochlear region, and laterally it travels between the lobes of the lacrimal gland to reach the lateral orbital wall. It appears to limit the posterior longitudinal movement of the muscle, acting as a check ligament.[23] Also located in muscular septa of the levator–superior rectus muscle complex is the superior ophthalmic vein.

Lockwood's ligament, a hammock-like suspensory ligament, is formed from the fused fascia of the inferior rectus and inferior oblique muscles.[24] This ligament is strongest anterior to the inferior oblique muscle,[25] and it will support the globe after floor removal and maxillectomy, as long as its medial and lateral attachments are intact. After decompression and removal of the orbital floor, however, globe ptosis can occur. Studies suggest

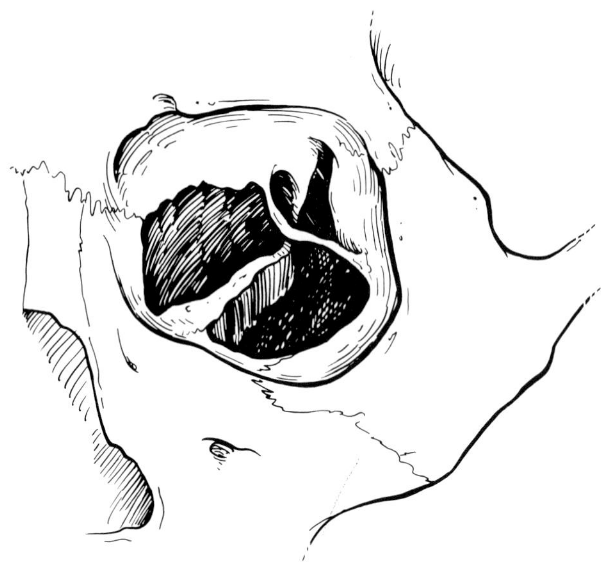

Figure 80–8. Anterolateral view of left orbit showing inferomedial orbital strut remaining after bony removal. The strut is located at the junction of the maxillary and ethmoidal sinuses.

that a ledge of bone between the maxillary and ethmoidal sinuses, the medial orbital strut (Fig. 80–8),[26] and the periorbita,[27] together play a role in sustaining the globe, preventing post-decompression dystopia.

Knowledge of the intricate fascial framework of the orbit was largely advanced by Koorneef's studies. His studies of orbital thick serial sectioning showed that the interrelation of all fibrous structures within the orbit is variable between individuals but fairly constant between orbits of the same individual. Venous channels appear to be supported within the fibrous framework, but the arterial system travels independently.

Orbital Soft Tissues

Orbital Fat

The remainder of the space in the orbit that is not filled with fascia, globe, muscles, nerves, vessels, and glandular structures is occupied by orbital fat. The character of the fat anteriorly is fibrous and posteriorly is more lobular owing to the decrease in the fibrous framework in that region. The orbital fat provides the globe with the medium for a wide range of movement and also cushions, stabilizes, and supports it. Surgically, the orbital fat is a valuable landmark; however, it can be a hindrance, causing obstruction of the operative view when dissecting posteriorly in the orbit.

Distinct fat compartments can be identified anteriorly in the orbit (Fig. 80–9). The preaponeurotic fat pad, an important surgical landmark, lies just posterior to the orbital septum in the upper eyelid. The medial fat pad is located medial to the preaponeurotic fat pad and inferior to the trochlea and is firmer and whiter compared with the preaponeurotic fat pad. It is associated with the medial palpebral artery and the infratrochlear nerve. Removal of this fat pad during blepharoplasty usually requires anesthetic placement deeper in the medial orbit. Careful attention when dissecting surgically in this region is necessary because of the close relationship of the medial fat pad to the trochlea and the medial palpebral artery. Superior oblique palsy and Brown's syndrome have been reported after upper eyelid blepharoplasty.[28]

Clinically, the inferior orbital fat may be divided into three compartments (see Fig. 80–9).[29] The inferior oblique muscle divides the medial third of the fat from the central third. In the cadaver the medial and central fat pads are found to be continuous, but clinically a valley can be seen dividing the two fat pads and in its depths lies the inferior oblique muscle. The central fat is divided from the lateral fat by an arcuate expansion of the inferior oblique muscle sheath that courses inferotemporally toward the orbital floor. The inferior orbital fat provides an excellent surgical landmark for the transconjunctival approach in inferior orbitotomy. The dissection plane should proceed through the conjunctiva and lower eyelid retractors and remain anterior to the orbital fat to identify the orbital rim and floor.

The orbital fat is relatively resistant to loss in dietary deficiency syndromes. It does, however, become attenuated in senescence, resulting in enophthalmos and superior sulcus deepening. Studies in anophthalmic primate sockets have shown that orbital fat, however, does not atrophy when compared with nonenucleated normal controls.[30]

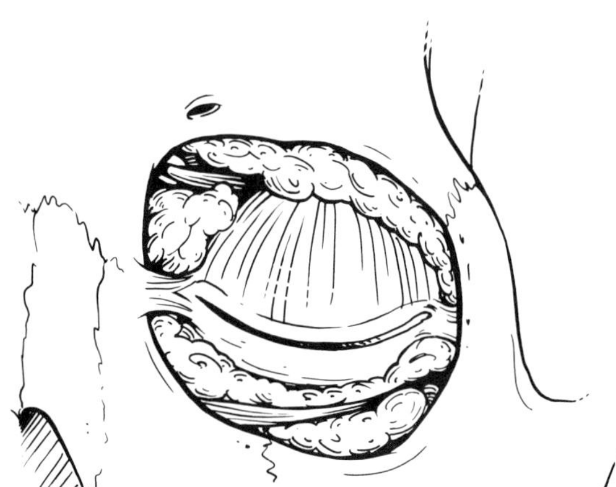

Figure 80–9. Anterior view showing dissection of orbital fat. The trochlea divides the fat pads in the superior orbit, while the inferior oblique muscle and its fascial attachments divide the inferior orbital fat.

Vasculature

The major orbital blood supply is derived from the ophthalmic artery, the first branch of the internal carotid artery, with contributions from the middle meningeal and maxillary branches of the external carotid artery. Bergen's studies of Koorneef's serial sections noted that orbital arteries traveled within the fat compartments and remained independent of the fibrous septa, only crossing them to enter another fat pad.[31-35] Three radially arranged conical planes that are coaxial with the orbital axis may be used to categorize the orbital arteries (Fig. 80-10). The inner cone represents the posterior ciliary arteries, the middle cone represents the muscular arteries, and the outer cone represents the lacrimal, supraorbital, and ophthalmic arteries.

The ophthalmic artery enters the orbit from the intracranial cavity through the optic canal and lies inferior and lateral to the optic nerve.[36] The ophthalmic artery crosses superior to the optic nerve and is attached to the optic nerve sheath in approximately 80% of orbits. In the remaining 20%, the artery crosses inferiorly to the nerve and affects its branching pattern.[37] The central retinal artery is the first branch of the ophthalmic artery and travels beneath the optic nerve to enter its dural sheath approximately 10 mm posterior to the globe. It penetrates the nerve substance to lie centrally. The posterior ciliary arteries typically arise as two trunks from the ophthalmic artery but may consist of a group of 6 to 8 vessels. These vessels then subdivide into 15 to 20 smaller branches, which surround the optic nerve and enter the sclera posteriorly as the short posterior ciliary arteries. Two branches, the medial and lateral long posterior ciliary arteries, enter the globe axially and supply the ciliary body and iris. These vessels are often encountered when performing optic nerve sheath fenestration and should be avoided.

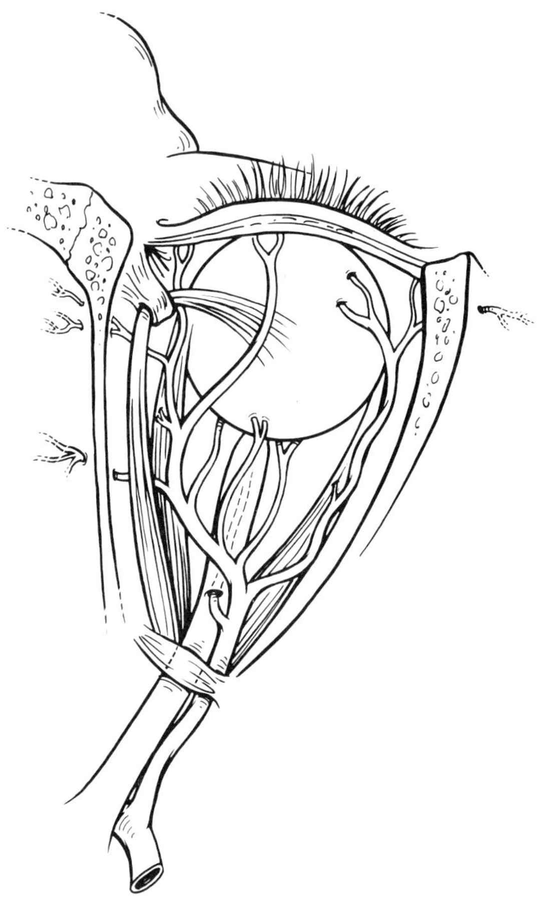

Figure 80-10. Most common branching pattern of ophthalmic artery. Of these three radially arranged conical planes as described by Bergen, the innermost cone represents the posterior ciliary vessels, the middle cone represents the muscular arteries, and the outermost cone represents the lacrimal, supraorbital, and ophthalmic arteries.

The muscular branches usually arise from two trunks of the ophthalmic artery and supply the extraocular muscles. Each muscular artery divides anteriorly into two anterior ciliary arteries, except the lateral rectus, in which there is only one. These vessels enter the sclera anterior to the rectus muscle insertions and anastomose with the long posterior ciliary arteries. The lacrimal artery arises from the ophthalmic artery lateral to the optic nerve and travels with the lacrimal nerve along the upper aspect of the lateral rectus anteriorly to reach the lacrimal gland. It communicates with the middle meningeal branch of the external carotid artery by means of the recurrent meningeal artery, which usually passes through the superior orbital fissure. The lacrimal artery also gives off zygomatic branches, which enter the zygomaticofacial and zygomaticotemporal foramina, and the lateral palpebral branch, which supplies the lateral aspect of the eyelids.

The supraorbital artery arises from the ophthalmic artery superior to the optic nerve and travels medially then superiorly between the levator muscle and the orbital roof. It then exits the orbit through the supraorbital notch with the supraorbital nerve to supply the eyebrow and forehead. The anterior and posterior ethmoidal arteries branch from the ophthalmic artery as it courses along the medial wall between the superior oblique and medial rectus muscles. The larger anterior ethmoidal artery supplies the middle and anterior air cells, frontal sinus, and lateral wall of the nose and nasal septum while the posterior ethmoidal artery supplies only the posterior ethmoidal air cells. The ophthalmic artery gives off the medial palpebral branch, which contributes to the marginal arcade of the eyelid before dividing into its terminal branches, the dorsal nasal and supratrochlear arteries.

The external carotid contributes to orbital blood supply through the maxillary artery and the middle meningeal artery, which communicates with the lacrimal artery through the recurrent meningeal artery as previously mentioned. The maxillary artery passes deep to the mandible and enters the pterygopalatine fossa through the infratemporal fossa.[38] The infraorbital artery, a terminal branch of the maxillary artery, enters the orbit through the inferior orbital fissure. It continues into the infraorbi-

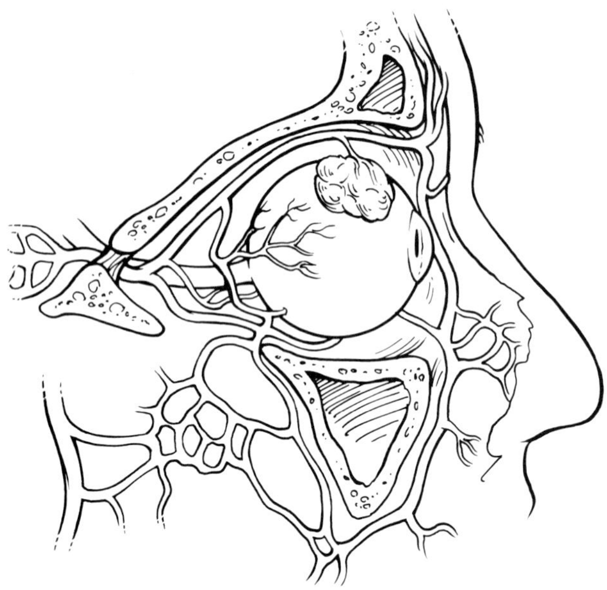

Figure 80–11. Parasagittal view of orbit showing superior and inferior ophthalmic veins and their relation to the cavernous sinus, pterygoid plexus, and facial vein.

tal sulcus and supplies the inferior rectus and inferior oblique muscles, the lacrimal gland, and orbital fat and then emerges from the infraorbital foramen. The facial artery also provides some collateral blood flow to the eyelids and anterior orbit with its anastomoses to the dorsal nasal artery and the infraorbital artery after it exits the infraorbital foramen.

The venous drainage system of the orbit is largely through the superior and inferior ophthalmic veins (Fig. 80–11). The superior ophthalmic vein is the larger of the two and is formed anteromedially near the superior oblique tendon by the confluence of the angular, supraorbital, and supratrochlear veins. It courses along the medial border of the superior rectus muscle and then enters the muscle cone and receives branches from the ciliary veins and the superior vortex veins. The vein continues beneath the superior rectus muscle laterally to lie along the lateral border of the muscle, where it then enters the superior orbital fissure to drain into the cavernous sinus. The more variable inferior ophthalmic vein is derived anteriorly from a plexus along the orbital floor and receives contributions from the inferior rectus and inferior oblique muscles and vortex veins. The vein then travels posteriorly along the inferior rectus muscle and either empties into the superior ophthalmic vein or drains independently into the cavernous sinus. It may also communicate with the pterygoid plexus through the inferior orbital fissure.

Endothelial cell–lined true lymphatic vessels have not yet been identified in the orbit. The presence of lymphoid aggregates and lymph nodes is considered pathologic. In spite of this, lymphatic drainage is thought to slowly occur in the orbit. Although lymphatic drainage of the eyelids and conjunctiva is documented draining into the preauricular and submaxillary lymph nodes, there is only one case report of an ectopic orbital lymph node.[39] Primate studies using India ink and radioactive colloid injections have shown that injections of these tracers spread along the orbital fibrous septa.[40] Injections that were outside the muscle cone traveled anteriorly and were removed by conjunctival and eyelid lymphatics, while those injected in the retrobulbar space did not reach lymph nodes over a 24-hour period. Some tracer did leave the orbit posteriorly through the optic canal and was detected in the contralateral orbit.

Orbital Nerves

Five cranial nerves supply the orbit with innervation. Along with the sympathetic and parasympathetic contributions, these nerves converge and enter the orbit through the orbital apex. Structural lesions in this region will most likely affect a multitude of neurovascular structures, causing a variety of functional deficits.

The optic nerve (cranial nerve II) is essentially an extending neural tract from the brain into the orbit. Unlike other orbital nerves, it is unique in that it is covered by meninges, is surrounded by circulating cerebrospinal fluid, and contains neuroglial cells. It is divided into intraocular, intraorbital, intracanalicular, and intracranial segments.

Axons of retinal ganglion cells give rise to the optic nerve, which exits the globe at the lamina cribrosa. This intraocular segment within the lamina cribrosa is 1 mm in length, and its diameter is 3 mm as it exits from the globe, where myelination begins.[41] The intraorbital portion of the optic nerve is surrounded by intraconal orbital fat, which allows for its freedom of movement. The length of the intraorbital segment is 24 mm, which is 6 mm longer than the direct length between the posterior sclera and the optic foramen. This excess length allows some margin of safety if proptosis occurs and also permits unrestricted globe movement within the orbit. With severe proptosis, the nerve is tethered from the globe, creating a radiologic sign referred to as globe tenting.[42] Cerebrospinal fluid freely bathes the nerve and communicates with the fluid surrounding the midbrain and explains the sudden respiratory collapse, which can be seen with inadvertent nerve sheath penetration in retrobulbar injections.[43] Clinically, during optic nerve sheath fenestration, this fluid can be seen to flow through incisions made in the perioptic meninges.

The oculomotor nerve (cranial nerve III) divides into superior and inferior divisions within the cavernous sinus, just behind the annulus of Zinn. The two divisions enter the orbit, separated by the nasociliary nerve, through the superior orbital fissure within the annulus of Zinn. The superior division travels within the muscle cone and supplies the superior rectus on its internal side, 15 mm from the orbital apex. The levator palpebrae superioris is then innervated by terminal branches of the superior division that have passed around the medial border of the superior rectus muscle or through it. The inferior division gives rise to three branches as it traverses the intraconal space under the optic nerve. One branch enters the medial rectus on its inner surface one third of its length posteriorly, while another branch innervates the inferior rectus in a similar fashion. The third branch travels along the lateral border of the inferior rectus and innervates the inferior oblique near its crossing of the inferior rectus. This branch carries parasympathetic fibers, including pupillomotor fibers, to the ciliary ganglion. Postoperative pupillary dilation has been described in patients with normal pupils undergoing repair of orbital floor fractures from injury to these fibers.[44]

The trochlear nerve (cranial nerve IV) enters the orbit supratemporal to the annulus of Zinn through the superior orbital fissure. It is the only motor nerve of the extraocular muscles that does not enter the muscle cone. Clinically, this relationship is seen by the continued action of the superior oblique muscle after retrobulbar anesthesia. The trochlear nerve courses anteriorly and medially a short distance to innervate the superior oblique muscle superiorly in the orbit. The trochlear nerve is also unique in that it is the longest intracranial nerve, the only cranial nerve that is completely decussated, and the only motor nerve to exit dorsally from the brain stem. Resulting from its long intracranial course, it is the nerve most susceptible to injury in closed-head trauma.

The abducens nerve (cranial nerve VI) enters the orbit through the superior orbital fissure within Zinn's annulus. It travels between the optic nerve and the lateral rectus muscle and innervates the muscle along its inner surface near the junction of the posterior one third and anterior two thirds. The abducens nerve is susceptible to compression with increased intracranial pressure due to the sharp angle with which it crosses the taut petrosphenoidal ligament intracranially.

The ophthalmic and maxillary divisions of the trigeminal nerve (cranial nerve V) supply cutaneous and deep sensory innervation to the upper two thirds of the face, including the orbit (Fig. 80–12). The ophthalmic division has three branches (lacrimal, frontal, and nasociliary), and all enter the orbit through the superior orbital fissure. The lacrimal nerve is the smallest branch and passes along the superior border of the lateral rectus muscle supratemporally, with the lacrimal artery, to supply the lacrimal gland. On reaching the lacrimal gland, it sends a branch to anastomose with the zygomaticotemporal nerve. The lacrimal nerve supplies the lacrimal gland, conjunctiva, and lateral upper eyelid. The frontal nerve, the largest branch, travels anteriorly between the

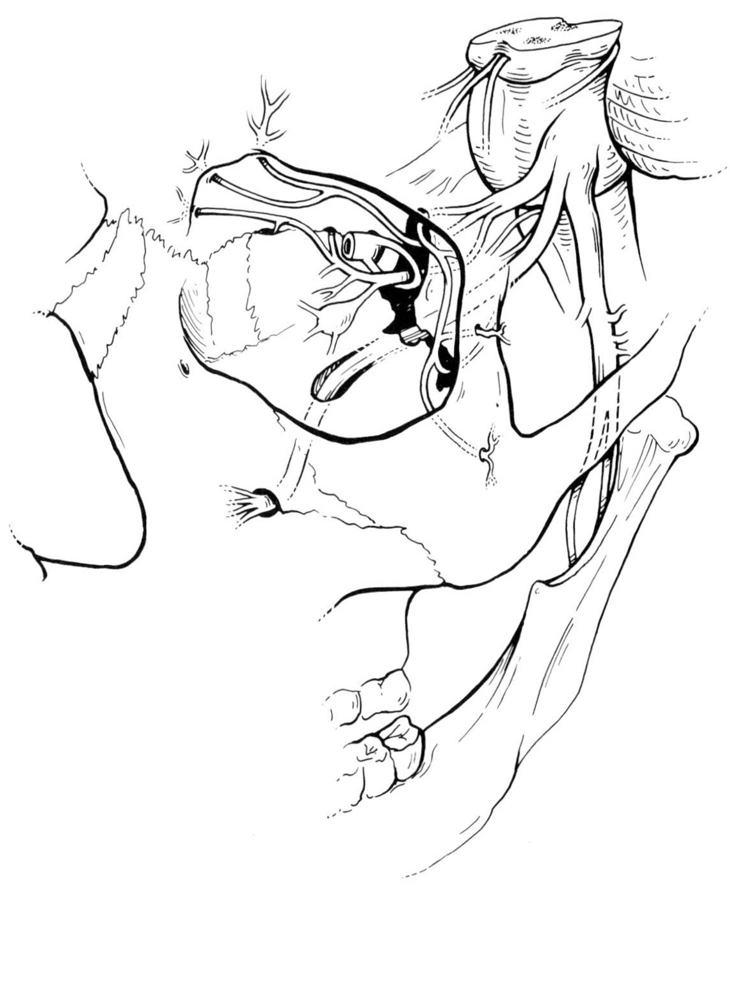

Figure 80–12. Orbital branches of the trigeminal nerve.

periorbita and the levator and divides into the supraorbital and supratrochlear nerves. The supratrochlear nerve courses medially toward the trochlear region and innervates the medial upper eyelid and forehead regions. The supraorbital nerve exits the orbit through the supraorbital notch and supplies the majority of the forehead. The nasociliary nerve, the only branch to pass through the annulus of Zinn, passes over the optic nerve to travel between the superior oblique and medial rectus muscles. The nasociliary nerve terminates as the infratrochlear nerve, after giving rise to the posterior and anterior ethmoidal nerves, two or three long ciliary nerves to the globe, and a sensory root to the ciliary ganglion. Most regional nerve blocks in the orbital region target these ophthalmic division branches.

The maxillary division exits the intracranial cavity through the foramen rotundum and enters the pterygopalatine fossa. Within the pterygopalatine fossa, it gives rise to the zygomatic, sphenopalatine, and posterosuperior alveolar nerves, but most of the nerve continues into the inferior orbital fissure and enters the infraorbital sulcus as the infraorbital nerve. An anterior superior alveolar branch is given off within the infraorbital canal. The zygomatic nerve divides into zygomaticofacial and zygomaticotemporal nerves. The former travels along the inferolateral orbit and passes through the zygomaticofacial foramen to supply the skin of the cheek, while the latter exits the orbit through a small fissure into the temporal fossa to innervate the lateral forehead. The infraorbital nerve emerges through the infraorbital foramen and its terminal branches are the inferior palpebral, the lateral nasal, and the superior labial. These innervate the skin and conjunctiva of the lower eyelid, the skin and septum of the nose, and the skin and mucosa of the upper lip.

Sympathetic innervation to the orbit results in pupillary dilation, constriction of eyelid smooth muscle, vasoconstriction, and hidrosis. Sympathetic nerve fibers originate in the superior cervical ganglion and enter the cavernous sinus surrounding the internal carotid artery. These sympathetic fibers join nerve branches within the cavernous sinus that will ultimately enter the orbit. The sympathetic fibers may travel with some or all of the cranial nerves. Wolff states that the pupillomotor fibers are carried within the nasociliary nerve[41]; however, the exact pathway to end organs in the orbit is not well known. Although pathways for sympathetic nerve entry into the orbit have been described through the optic canal, superior orbital fissure, and inferior orbital fissure,[1] studies in primates have shown that they may enter exclusively through the superior orbital fissure.[7] Pathways for sympathetic innervation to the superior and inferior tarsal muscles are also unknown, but some evidence has shown that sympathetic nerves may travel along with the motor nerves that supply the extraocular muscles within the perimysium of the extraocular muscles.[45]

The ciliary muscle, pupillomotor fibers, lacrimal gland innervation, and vasodilatory fibers are supplied by parasympathetic nerves to the orbit. These fibers originate from the Edinger-Westphal nucleus, the facial nerve nucleus, and the parasympathetic ganglia serving the orbital region. Preganglionic fibers from the Edinger-Westphal nucleus destined for the orbit travel with the inferior division of the oculomotor nerve. The fibers then synapse in the ciliary ganglion, and postganglionic fibers then enter the globe as short posterior ciliary nerves. The majority of these fibers (90%) supply the ciliary body, and the remainder innervate the iris sphincter. Traditionally, the lacrimal gland is thought to be innervated by the nervus intermedius portion of the facial nerve. After exiting the internal acoustic meatus and passing through the geniculate ganglion, these preganglionic parasympathetic nerve fibers arrive in the pterygopalatine ganglion as the vidian nerve, joining sympathetic fibers from the carotid plexus. The supply to the lacrimal gland from this point occurs as postganglionic parasympathetic nerve fibers travel from the pterygopalatine ganglion to the maxillary nerve through sphenopalatine nerves, then leave the maxillary nerve with the zygomatic branch. The zygomatic nerve then anastomoses with the lacrimal nerve to supply the lacrimal gland or travels independently along the periorbita to innervate the gland directly. Some evidence in primates has shown that branches directly from the pterygopalatine ganglion, rami orbitales, enter the orbit directly through the inferior orbital fissure and directly enter the lacrimal gland as rami lacrimales.[46]

The ciliary ganglion is located between the lateral rectus and the optic nerve approximately 10 mm from the orbital apex and varies in its size and shape (Fig. 80–13). Three roots typically enter the ciliary ganglion: a sensory root from the nasociliary nerve, a parasympathetic root from the nerve to the inferior oblique, and a sympathetic root that is less predictable in presence and origin.[47] Parasympathetic fibers synapse in the ganglion, while sympathetic and sensory axons do not. Five to six short ciliary nerves enter the globe from the ciliary ganglion, most of which enter lateral to the optic nerve.

Globe and Extraocular Muscles

The eye is located in the anterior orbit, slightly superior and lateral to the center of the orbit. The front surface of the eye lies in the same plane formed by the superior, medial, and inferior orbital rims. It is anterior to the lateral rim by 12 to 18 mm if measured by exophthalmometry. The volume of the eye is 6.5 mL in the adult, and it measures 24 mm anteroposteriorly, 23 mm vertically, and 23.5 mm horizontally. The anteroposterior diameter of the eye at birth is approximately 16 mm and by 20 months of age reaches 90% of its adult size.

Changes in eye position in children and adults have been studied with respect to Hertel exophthalmometry, orbital width, and interpupillary distance.[48] Hertel read-

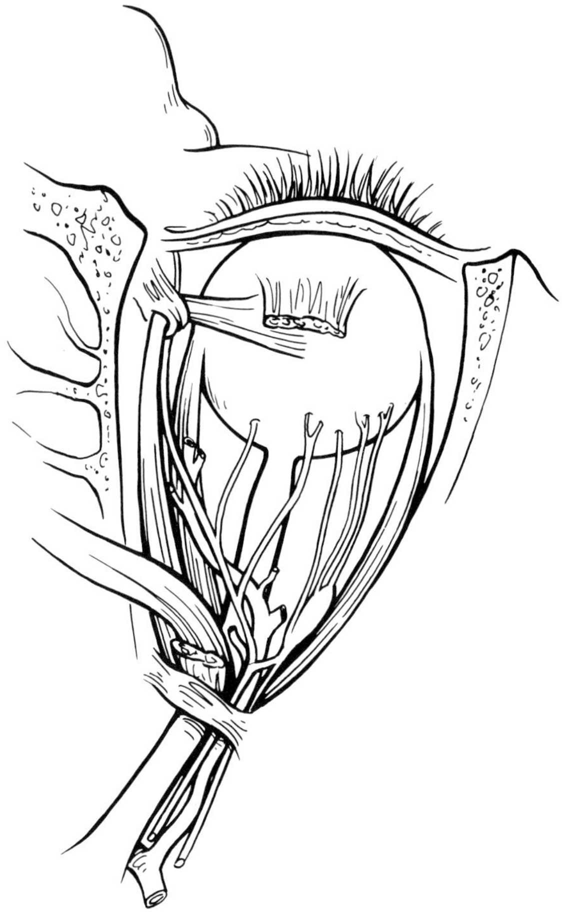

Figure 80–13. Superior view of orbit to show location of ciliary ganglion. (Superior rectus muscle has been removed.)

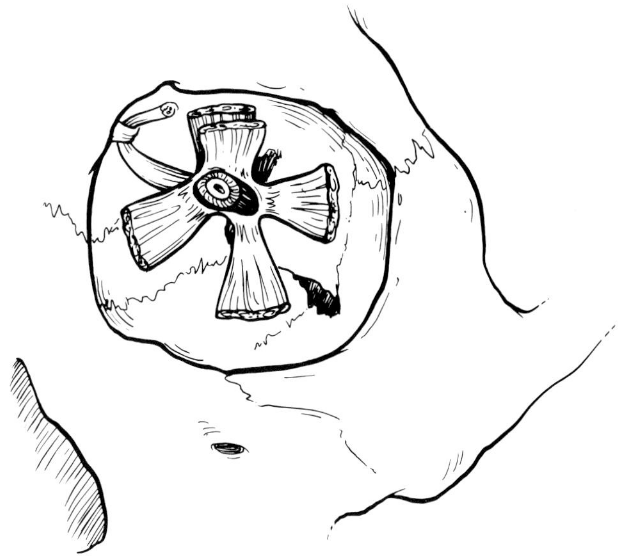

Figure 80–14. Schematic drawing of annulus of Zinn and extraocular muscle insertions.

ings have been shown to increase until age 20 and then stabilize, and interpupillary distance increases in the elderly. A relatively divergent eye position was seen with senescence, primarily from the increased interpupillary distance and increase in orbital width. This was thought to reflect age-related laxity and atrophy of orbital tissues.

Lockwood's ligament supports the eye inferiorly and Tenon's fascia covers the eye from posteriorly to the corneoscleral limbus. Tenon's fascia is penetrated by the six extraocular muscles, the optic nerve, the ciliary nerves and vessels, and the four to seven vortex veins as they enter or exit the globe.

All of the extraocular muscles originate from the orbital apex except the inferior oblique (Fig. 80–14). The four rectus muscles arise from a tendinous ring, the annulus of Zinn. The annulus of Zinn is posteriorly connected to the dura and spans the optic foramen and central superior orbital fissure. The levator and superior oblique originate from the lesser wing of the sphenoid superomedially, while the inferior oblique arises from the orbital floor anteriorly, just lateral to the nasolacrimal sac.

The horizontal rectus muscles average 40.5 mm in length, with the superior rectus being slightly longer and the inferior rectus being slightly shorter. The medial rectus has the greatest mass of the four recti muscles and the superior rectus the least. The muscles insert onto the globe with progressively increasing distance posterior to the limbus, starting with the medial rectus in the spiral of Tillaux (Fig. 80–15). This spiral is in a clockwise fashion in the right eye and a counterclockwise fashion in the left

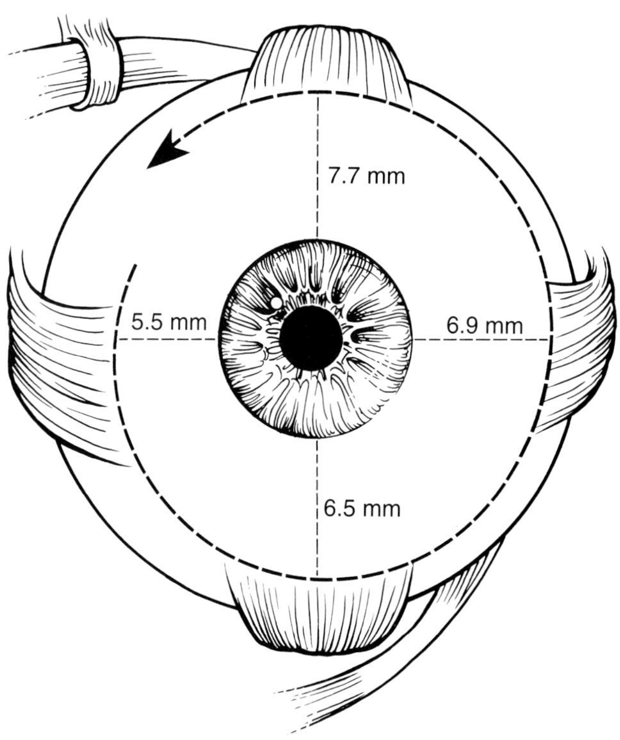

Figure 80–15. Anterior view of right globe depicting spiral of Tillaux and superimposed ora serrata.

eye. The distances for each rectus muscle insertion may vary by as much as 3 mm.[49]

The medial rectus travels closely to the lamina papyracea of the medial wall until the anterior third of its length, where it angles to insert on the globe. Adduction is the sole action of the medial rectus. Terminal branches of the nasociliary and ophthalmic artery lie along the superior border of the medial rectus muscle. The medial rectus is prone to entrapment in medial orbital wall fractures within the thin lamina papyracea.

The inferior rectus lies close to the orbital floor posteriorly and is separated anteriorly from it by the orbital fat. Orbital floor fractures may entrap the inferior rectus muscle sheath and the series of fibrous septa that radiate from it toward the orbital floor. This may restrict infraduction or supraduction of the globe. The nerve bound for the inferior oblique muscle travels closely along the lateral border of the inferior rectus. Infraduction is the primary action of the inferior rectus. Its secondary actions are excyclotorsion and adduction due to the axis, with which it angles to reach the globe from the orbital apex.

Posteriorly, within the annulus of Zinn, the lateral rectus is separated from the optic nerve by the nerves traveling within the annulus. Anteriorly, the ciliary ganglion separates it from the optic nerve. The lacrimal gland, as well as the lacrimal artery and nerve, lie superior to the muscle. The lateral rectus is separated from the lateral orbital wall by orbital fat. The sole action of the lateral rectus is abduction.

The superior rectus and levator palpebrae superioris originate from the same embryonic mesenchyme and have a fused fascial sheath medially. Hence, the primary superior relationship of the superior rectus is its intimate contact with the levator palpebrae. The nasociliary nerve and ophthalmic artery are also related to the superior rectus and cross beneath it from lateral to medial as they course anteriorly in the orbit. The primary action of the superior rectus is supraduction, and its secondary actions are intorsion and adduction.

The superior oblique muscle travels anteriorly and superiorly, closely applied to the superomedial orbital wall. This round muscle narrows to 1 to 2 mm in diameter, passing through the trochlea and then making a 54-degree angle to continue posteriorly, laterally, and inferiorly toward the globe. The reflected superior oblique tendon is 2.8 cm long and begins 10 mm behind the globe. The tendon then fans out beneath the superior rectus to insert on the posterolateral aspect of the globe. This insertion is variable and can be 10 mm in width. The average distance between temporal insertions of the superior rectus and superior oblique muscles is 4.7 mm.[50] The superior oblique depresses, intorts, and abducts the globe.

The trochlea is located on the anteromedial orbital roof in a shallow fossa. It is composed of a crescent-shaped cartilage connected to the periorbita by fibrous pillars laterally (Fig. 80–16). The superior oblique tendon within the trochlea is separated from the surrounding cartilage by a bursa-like structure. Its purpose is to reduce friction and allow maximal sliding action of the tendon.[51] Centrally, the thicker tendinous fibers display few attachments to surrounding fibers. Peripherally, however, the thinner fibers appear related to each other. The attachment of the trochlea to the periorbita provides

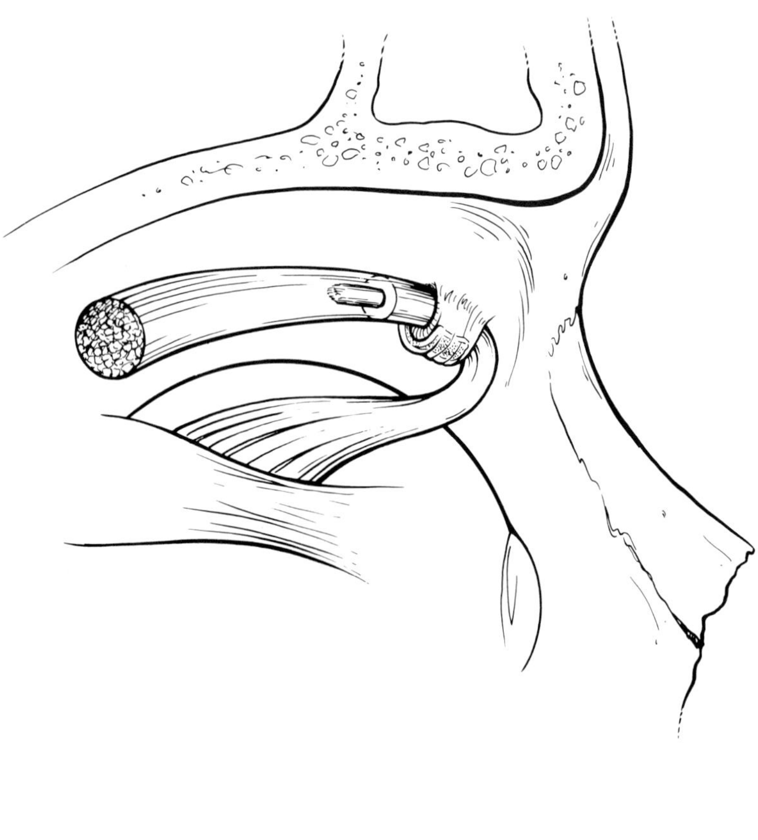

Figure 80–16. Schematic drawing of right trochlea. Tendon is supported by cartilage, which is attached to the periorbita by a fibrous hammock. (Modified from Helveston EM, Merriam WW, Ellis FD, et al: The trochlea: A study of the anatomy and physiology. Published courtesy of *Ophthalmology* [89:124–133, 1982].)

some margin of safety when elevating this complex during subperiosteal surgical dissection.

The inferior oblique arises posteriorly from its insertion on the orbital floor and courses toward the globe in a similar fashion to the reflected superior oblique. The inferior oblique passes inferior to the inferior rectus, and together their fascial sheaths give rise to the suspensory ligament of Lockwood. The inferior oblique remains muscular until it inserts on the globe, 2.2 mm inferior and lateral to the macula and 9.5 mm posterior to the lateral rectus insertion. The nerve to the inferior oblique enters the muscle along the lateral border of the inferior rectus muscle. Elevation, excyclotorsion, and abduction are the actions of the inferior oblique.

The levator palpebrae superioris arises from the lesser wing of the sphenoid, above the annulus of Zinn and medial to the superior oblique. It courses anteriorly, separated from the orbital roof by a thin layer of orbital fat, the supraorbital artery, the frontal nerve, and the trochlear nerve. It lies directly above the superior rectus and can be easily separated from it except medially, where they share a common fascial sheath. The superior division of the ophthalmic nerve innervates both muscles and enters them approximately 12 mm from the orbital apex. Ptosis and superior rectus underaction are frequently associated due to their shared embryonic mesenchymal origin.[52]

The muscular levator continues anteriorly until it attaches to the superior transverse ligament of Whitnall, 36 mm from its origin from the orbital apex. Its attachments to the transverse ligament are strongest medially and laterally, but centrally it can be separated from the muscle. The muscle thins, fans out, and becomes more fibrous as the aponeurosis is formed at the level of the superior transverse ligament of Whitnall. Its width at this point measures 18 mm, and it continues to widen horizontally as the medial and lateral horns insert into the medial and lateral retinacula. The distance from Whitnall's ligament to the tarsal border is 14 to 20 mm.[53]

LACRIMAL SYSTEM ANATOMY

Lacrimal Secretory System

The main lacrimal gland and the accessory lacrimal glands of Krause and Wolfring compose the lacrimal secretory system. They produce the aqueous component of the tear film. The main lacrimal gland is located in the superotemporal orbit in the shallow lacrimal fossa. The lateral horn of the levator aponeurosis divides the gland into a larger orbital lobe and a smaller palpebral lobe; however, because of shared parenchyma posteriorly, the division is not complete. The lacrimal gland measures 20 × 12 × 5 mm and weighs approximately 80 g.[9]

The orbital lobe conforms to the space between the globe and the lateral orbital wall. It extends from the lateral border of the levator aponeurosis to the frontozygomatic suture, and medially it is bound by the intermuscular membrane between the superior and lateral rectus muscles. Anteriorly its boundaries are the orbital septum and the preaponeurotic fat pad. The palpebral lobe lies beneath the levator aponeurosis in the subaponeurotic space, and it is separated from the conjunctiva by Müller's muscle. Attachments to the periorbita, the lateral horn of the levator aponeurosis, the orbital septum, the conjunctiva, and the lacrimal fascial attachments to Whitnall's ligament support the lacrimal gland in its fossa. Lacrimal gland prolapse inferiorly may be present as a bulge in the lateral upper eyelid due to laxity of the attachments.

Secretory ducts (10 to 12) from the main lobe pass through the palpebral lobe or remain tightly bound to its capsule. From the palpebral lobe they open into the superotemporal conjunctival fornix, 4 to 5 mm from the superior tarsal border. Palpebral dacryoadenectomy will therefore interrupt tear secretion from the larger orbital lobe. Scarring in the fornix superotemporally from surgery may also affect gland secretion.

Blood supply to the lacrimal gland is from the lacrimal artery, from a branch of the ophthalmic artery, and also from a branch of the infraorbital artery. The lacrimal vein arises from the gland and travels with the artery to drain into the superior ophthalmic vein. The artery and vein are located posteriorly within the lacrimal gland. The lacrimal nerve supplies the gland with sensory innervation, and parasympathetic secretomotor fibers innervate the gland from the facial nerve complex. Sympathetic innervation provides vasomotor innervation, but the exact pathway to the gland is uncertain.

The accessory lacrimal glands of Krause and Wolfring lack parasympathetic innervation, differing from the lacrimal gland. Approximately 20 accessory lacrimal glands are present in the superior conjunctival fornix, and about half that number are present in the lower eyelid. Due to their lack of parasympathetic innervation, the accessory glands are thought to be basic secretors, with the main gland being responsible for reflex tearing.[54] Surgical removal or injury to these glands may affect basal tear secretion.

Lacrimal Excretory System

Tears flow medially across the eye and enter the lacrimal excretory system through the upper and lower eyelid puncta. The dynamic action of blinking eyelids creates the positive and negative pressure within the lacrimal excretory system necessary for efficient tear drainage.

The upper and lower puncta are located 5 to 7 mm laterally from the medial canthal angle in each eyelid. The lower punctum is usually located 1 to 2 mm lateral to the upper punctum. The punctal opening measures 0.3 mm in diameter. The lacrimal papilla surrounds the punctal

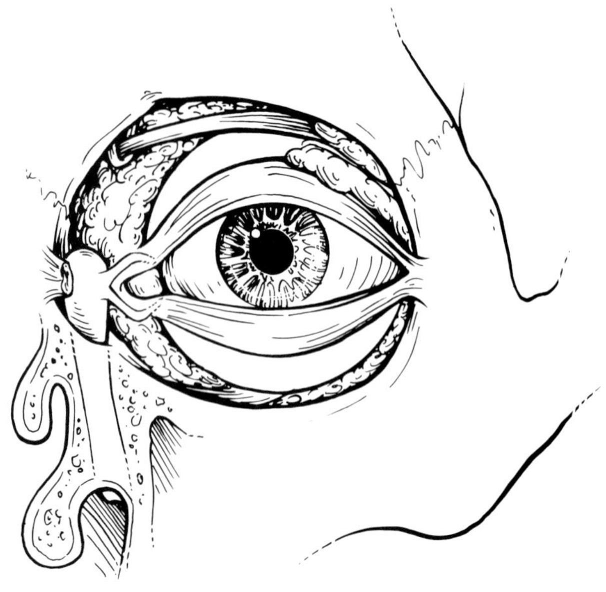

Figure 80–17. Lacrimal excretory system.

os and is an elevated mound of fibrous tissue. The puncta are normally well opposed to the globe and, if visible on external examination, represent punctal ectropion by definition.

The canaliculi represent the palpebral portion of the excretory system (Fig. 80–17). Each canaliculus is 2 mm long vertically and ends at a right angle in the ampulla. The canaliculi continue medially buried within the orbicularis muscle, just beneath the eyelid margin. The horizontal canalicular length is 8 mm, and each canaliculus angles before entering the lacrimal sac. The superior canaliculus angles inferiorly and the inferior canaliculus angles superiorly to reach the lacrimal sac. Ninety percent of the time the canaliculi join to form a common canaliculus. The common canaliculus is located within the central portion of the medial canthal tendon and is a diverticulum of the lacrimal sac. If the common canaliculus is dilated, it is termed the *sinus of Maier.* The valve of Rosenmüller is located where the distal end of the common canaliculus joins the lacrimal sac and prevents reflux. If the valve becomes incompetent, it will allow air to escape from the nose through the puncta with increased pressure during nose blowing.

The lacrimal sac fills the bony lacrimal fossa and is sheathed in thick periorbita and the surrounding fascia. The sac measures 12 mm vertically and 4 to 8 mm in width. A 4-mm segment vertically is superior to the medial canthal ligament. The walls of the sac are usually apposed unless filled with fluid or air. In females, the lacrimal fossa is narrower and this may explain the increased percentage of females who undergo dacryocystorhinostomy. The nasolacrimal duct measures 12.5 mm vertically within the nasolacrimal canal and extends an additional 2 to 5 mm into the inferior meatus.

Anteriorly, the lacrimal sac is bound by the anterior limb of the medial canthal ligament, which inserts on the anterior lacrimal crest. Posteriorly, the smaller posterior limb of the medial canthal ligament inserts on the posterior lacrimal crest. Horner's lacrimal muscle, the deep head of the pretarsal and preseptal orbicularis oculi, and the orbital septum insert posterior, superior, and inferior to insertion of the posterior limb of the medial canthal ligament (Fig. 80–18). The lacrimal sac is thus, technically, external to the orbit. Swelling of the lacrimal sac, which is seen in dacryocystitis, occurs inferiorly, in the area of the sac not bound by the medial canthal ligament.

The nasolacrimal duct conforms to the bony nasolacrimal canal and can be easily separated from the canal superiorly. Inferiorly within the bony canal, the duct acquires characteristics of nasal mucosa and becomes more adherent. During nasolacrimal duct probing, a greater resistance is usually felt inferiorly if false passages are created. Biopsy of the nasolacrimal duct in this region also requires sharp dissection to separate the duct from the surrounding canal.

The nasolacrimal duct typically opens beneath the inferior turbinate but may extend to the nasal floor or remain imperforate.[55] Its opening into the nose may consist of a slit or a mucosal valve (valve of Hasner). At birth, membranous obstructions at the inferior aspect of the duct have been reported to persist from 35% to 73% of the time.[56]

EMBRYOLOGY

The human orbit and face start developing in the third gestational week. Growth of the optic pits begins at 24 days, with their axes separated 180 degrees. The optic pits are derived from neural ectoderm, surface ectoderm, and cells of neural crest origin and develop lateral to the forebrain. The optic pits become pouch-shaped vesicles at 25 days and then invaginate to form optic cups. Mesoderm migrates to and enters the optic cup fissure shortly thereafter, from which the extraocular muscles and vascular endothelium arise.[57]

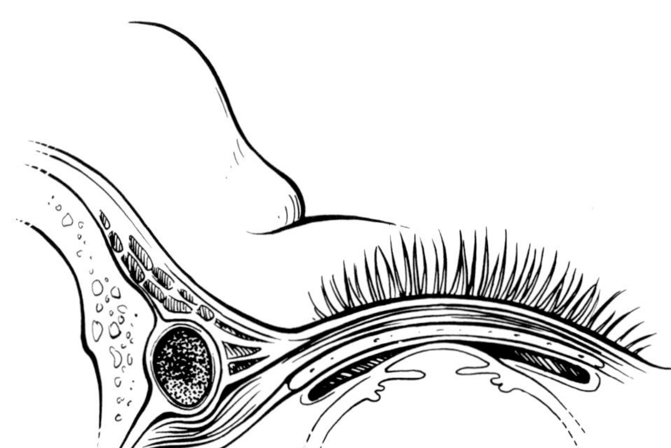

Figure 80–18. Horizontal section through right upper eyelid near palpebral margin to show relations of lacrimal sac and insertion of Horner's muscle.

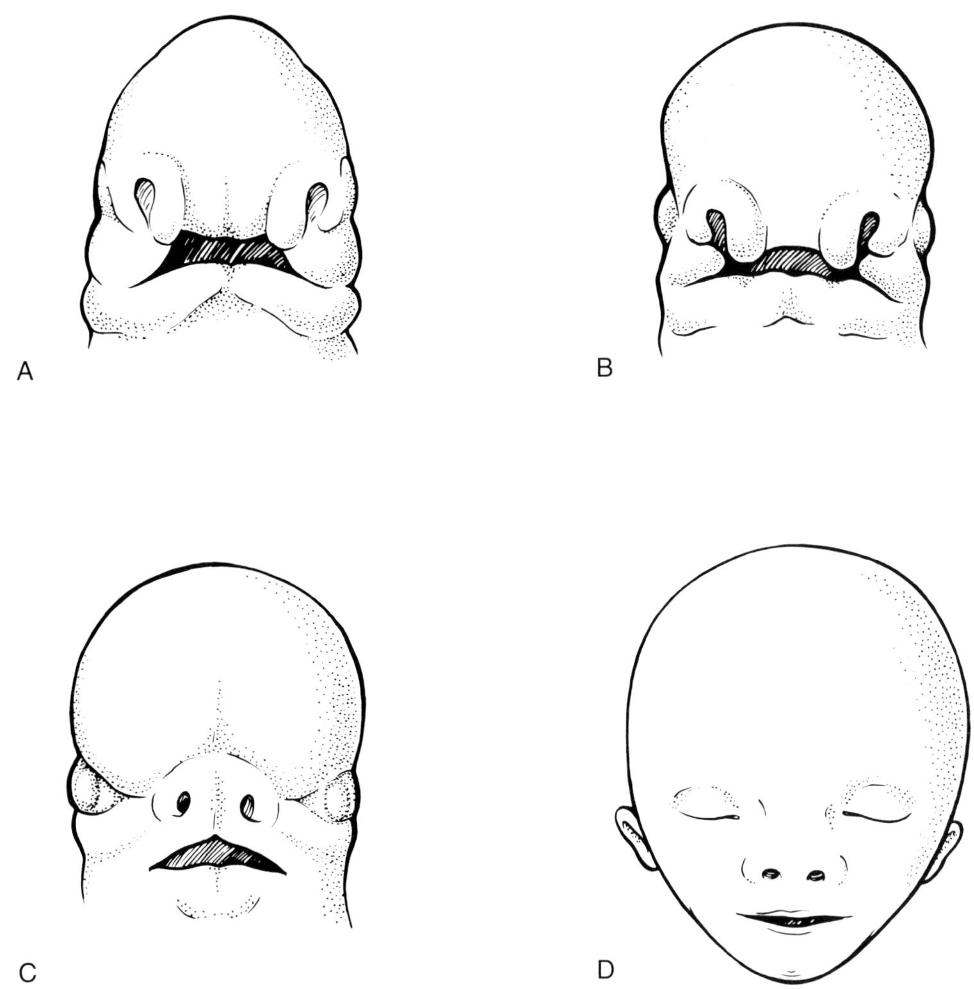

Figure 80–19. Sequential facial development. *A*, Frontonasal and mandibular processes separated by maxillary processes and mouth. *B*, Lacrimal groove develops between lateral nasal and maxillary processes. C, Lateral wall and floor of orbit formed by medial expansion of maxillary processes. Lateral nasal process and frontal process give rise to medial wall and roof, respectively. *D*, Upper lip and hard palate are formed from fusion of medial nasal processes.

The osseous structures of the orbit, which are derived from neural crest cells, migrate and surround the developing optic cups. Ossification centers are formed that give rise to the orbital walls, while orbital and facial soft tissues develop from the frontonasal, maxillary, and mandibular processes (Fig. 80–19). The orbit is completely ossified at birth, with the exception of the orbital apex (lesser wing of the sphenoid).[58] Neural crest cells give rise to all connective tissue in the orbit, which includes the connective tissue septa, the periorbita, and orbital fibroadipose tissue.

In the sixth week, mesenchymal condensations in the frontonasal and maxillary processes give rise to the upper and lower eyelid folds, which grow toward each other. The eyelids begin to fuse at 8 weeks, while the specialized structures of the eyelids, including the orbicularis oculi, tarsal plates, and lacrimal excretory structures continue to develop. At 5 months, separation of the eyelids takes place and innervation of the eyelid muscles continues until birth.[59]

REFERENCES

1. Whitnall SE: Anatomy of the Human Orbit and Accessory Organs of Vision. London, Oxford University Press, 1932.
2. Zide BM, Jelks GW: Surgical Anatomy of the Orbit. New York, Raven Press, 1985.
3. Lemke BN, Della Rocca RC: Surgery of the Eyelids and Orbit, an Anatomical Approach. Norwalk, CT, Appleton & Lange, 1990.
4. Whitnall SE: On a tubercle on the malar bone, and on the lateral attachments of the tarsal plates. J Anat Physiol 45:426, 1911.
5. Jones LT: A new concept of the orbital fascia and rectus muscle sheaths and its surgical implications. Trans Am Acad Ophthalmol Otolaryngol 72:755, 1968.
6. Simonton JT, Garber PF, Ahl N: Margins of safety in lateral orbitotomy. Arch Ophthalmol 95:1229–1231, 1977.
7. Lyon DB, Lemke BN, Wallow IH, Dortzbach RK: Sympathetic nerve anatomy in the cavernous sinus and retrobulbar orbit of the cynomologus monkey. Ophthalmic Plast Reconstr Surg 8:1, 1992.
8. Rischbieth RHC, Bull JWD: The significance of enlargement of the superior orbital fissure. Br J Radiol 31:125, 1958.
9. Rootman J: Diseases of the Orbit. Philadelphia, JB Lippincott, 1988.
10. Coulter VL, Holds JB, Anderson RL: Avoiding complications of orbital surgery: The orbital branches of the infraorbital artery. Ophthalmic Surg 21:141, 1990.
11. Cares HL, Bakay L: The clinical significance of the optic strut. J Neurosurg 34:355, 1971.
12. Anderson RL, Panje WR, Gross CE: Optic nerve blindness following blunt forehead trauma. Ophthalmology 89:445, 1982.
13. Seiff SR, Berger MS, Guyon J, Pitts LH: Computed tomographic evaluation of the optic canal in sudden traumatic blindness. Am J Ophthalmol 98:751, 1984.
14. Bansberg SF, Harner SG, Forbes G: Relationship of the optic nerve to the paranasal sinuses as shown by computed tomography. Otolaryngol Head Neck Surg 96:331, 1987.
15. Lang J: The vascularization of the periorbita, Medline (abstract). Gegenbaurs Morphol Jahrb 121(2):174, 1975.

16. Koorneef L: New insights in the human orbital connective tissue: Results of a new anatomic approach. Arch Ophthalmol 95:1269, 1977.
17. Koorneef L: Orbital septa: Anatomy and function. Ophthalmology 86:876, 1979.
18. Hargiss JL: Surgical anatomy of the eyelids. Trans Pacif Coast Otolaryngol Soc 44:193, 1963.
19. Sutton JE: The fascia of the human orbit. Anat Reconstr 18:141, 1920.
20. Plager DA, Parks MM: Recognition and repair of the "lost" rectus muscle. Ophthalmology 97:131, 1990.
21. Fink WH: An anatomical study of the check mechanism of the vertical muscles of the eyes. Am J Ophthalmol 44:800, 1957.
22. Whitnall SE: On a ligament acting as a check to the action of the levator palpebrae superioris muscle. J Anat Physiol 14:131, 1910.
23. Lemke BN, Stasior OG, Rosenberg PN: Surgical relations of the levator palpebrae superioris muscle. Ophthalmic Plast Reconstr Surg 4:24, 1988.
24. Lockwood CB: The anatomy of the muscles, ligaments, and fascia of the orbit, including an account of the capsule of Tenon, the check ligaments of recti, and of the suspensory ligament of the eye. J Anat Physiol 20:1, 1886.
25. Hawes MJ, Dortzbach RK: The microscopic anatomy of the lower eyelid retractors. Arch Ophthalmol 100:1313, 1982.
26. Goldberg RA, Shorr N, Cohen MS: The medial orbital strut in the prevention of postdecompression dystopia in dysthyroid ophthalmopathy. Ophthalmic Plast Reconstr Surg 8:32, 1992.
27. Long JA, Baylis HI: Hypoglobus following orbital decompression for dysthyroid ophthalmopathy. Ophthalmic Plast Reconstr Surg 6:185, 1990.
28. Neely KA, Ernest JT, Mottier M: Combined superior oblique palsy and Brown's syndrome after blepharoplasty. Am J Ophthalmol 109:347, 1990.
29. Castanares S: Blepharoplasty for herniated intraorbital fat: Anatomical basis for a new approach. Plast Reconstr Surg 8:46, 1951.
30. Kronish JW, Gonnering RS, Dortzbach RK, et al: The pathophysiology of the anophthalmic socket: II. Analysis of orbita fat. Ophthalmic Plast Reconstr Surg 2:88, 1990.
31. Bergen MP: Microvessels in the human orbit in relation to the connective tissue system. Acta Morphol Neerl Scand 20:139, 1982.
32. Bergen MP: Relationship between the arteries and veins and the connective tissue system in the human orbit: I, II, and III. Acta Morphol Neerl Scand 28:1, 1982.
33. Bergen MP: A spatial reconstruction of the orbital vascular pattern in relation with the connective tissue system. Acta Morphol Neerl Scand 20:117, 1982.
34. Bergen MP, Los JA: Vascular patterns in the human orbit in relation to the connective tissue septa. *In* Proceedings of the Third International Symposium on Orbital Disorders, Amsterdam, 1977. The Hague, Dr. W Junk Publishers, 1978, pp 197–201.
35. Bergen MP: A literature review of the vascular system in the human orbit. Acta Morphol Neerl Scand 19:273, 1981.
36. Hayreh SS: The ophthalmic artery: II. Origin and intracranial and intracanalicular course. Br J Ophthalmol 46:65, 1962.
37. Hayreh SS: The ophthalmic artery: III. Branches. Br J Ophthalmol 46:212, 1962.
38. Pearson BW, Mackenzie RG, Goodman WS: The anatomical basis of transantral ligation of the maxillary artery in severe epistaxis. Laryngoscope 79:969, 1969.
39. Wolter JR, Rosenberg RJ: Ectopic lymph node of the orbit simulating a lacrimal gland tumor. Am J Ophthalmol 83:908–914, 1977.
40. McGetrick JJ, Wilson DG, Dortzbach RK, et al: A search for lymphatic drainage of the monkey orbit. Arch Ophthalmol 107:255–260, 1989.
41. Warwick R: Eugene Wolff's Anatomy of the Eye and Orbit, 7th ed. Philadelphia, WB Saunders, 1976.
42. Dalley RW, Robertson WD, Rootman J: Globe tenting: A sign of increased orbital tension. Am J Neuroradiol 10:181, 1989.
43. Drysdale DB: Experimental subdural retrobulbar injection of anesthetic. Ann Ophthalmol 16:716, 1984.
44. Hornblass A: Pupillary dilatation in fractures of the floor of the orbit. Ophthalmic Surg 10:44, 1979.
45. Manson PN, Lazarus RB, Morgan R, Iliff N: Pathways of sympathetic innervation to the superior and inferior (Müller's) muscles. Plast Reconstr Surg 78:33, 1986.
46. Ruskell GL: The distribution of autonomic postganglionic nerve fibers to the lacrimal gland in monkeys. J Anat 109:229, 1971.
47. Simreich Z, Nathan H: The ciliary ganglion in man (anatomical observations). Anat Anz 150:287, 1981.
48. Fledlius HC, Stubgaard M: Changes in eye position during growth and adult life based on exophthalmometry, interpupillary distance, and orbital distance measurements. Acta Ophthalmol 64:481, 1986.
49. Apt L: An anatomic reevaluation of rectus muscle insertions. Trans Am Ophthalmol Soc 78:365, 1980.
50. Fink WH: The surgical anatomy of the superior oblique muscle. Trans Am Ophthalmol Soc 46:154, 1948.
51. Helveston EM, Merriam WW, Ellis FD, et al: The trochlea: A study of the anatomy and physiology. Ophthalmology 89:124, 1982.
52. Sevel D: Ptosis and underaction of the superior rectus muscle. Ophthalmology 91:1080, 1984.
53. Anderson RL, Dixon RS: The role of Whitnall's ligament in ptosis surgery. Arch Ophthalmol 97:705, 1979.
54. Jones LT: The lacrimal secretory system and its treatment. Am J Ophthalmol 62:47, 1966.
55. Jones LT, Wobig JL: Surgery of the Eyelids and Lacrimal System. New York, Aesculapius, 1976.
56. Ffooks OO: Dacryocystitis in infancy. Br J Ophthalmol 46:422, 1962.
57. Jakobiec FA, Ozanics V: Prenatal development of the eye and its adnexa. *In* Jakobiec FA (ed): Ocular Anatomy, Embryology, and Teratology. New York, Harper & Row, 1982, pp 11–96.
58. Lemke BN: Anatomy of ocular adnexa and orbit. *In* Smith BC (ed): Ophthalmic Plastic Reconstructive Surgery, vol 1. St. Louis. CV Mosby, 1987, pp 3–74.
59. Sevel D: A reappraisal of the development of the eyelids. Eye 2:123, 1988.

CHAPTER 81

Epidemiology of Orbital Pathology*

Carlo de Conciliis

Although the incidence of orbital pathology in general ophthalmic practice is low, the gravity of these potentially life-threatening diseases has justified the creation of a subspecialty of its own.

By studying the relative frequencies of diseases of the orbit and their incidence in various age groups, we can extrapolate data that are useful to nonspecialists. Although the study of these parameters may seem to be of marginal importance, in reality this effort constitutes the first and easiest step in the differential diagnosis of these rare diseases.

The diagnostic dilemma presented by orbital diseases is complicated by the great number of pathologic entities involving the orbit. This extreme richness in such a localized anatomic site can be readily understood, considering that all three embryologic layers are well represented in the formation of the eye and the ocular adnexa. Developmental anomalies, neoplastic processes, and inflammatory pathology can result in clinical and pathologic pictures that differ, depending on the type of structures affected. Moreover, the continuity of the orbit with the surrounding cranial cavities and facial regions via the various fissures, foramina, and canals explains the frequency with which the orbit becomes involved in pathology originating in these neighboring regions. The thin osseous walls that delimit the orbit are frequently insufficient to block the extension of infectious, inflammatory, or neoplastic processes to the soft tissue of the orbit. Finally, tumors from distant organs that metastasize to the orbit are common, probably because of the rich vascularization of the cervicofacial region.

The histogenic classification of orbital tumors is used most commonly. This classification is based on the histopathologic examination of the cellular type. This lends itself particularly well to neoplastic lesions, in which the pathologic process is based on a single cellular component. However, it is not altogether useful when used for non-neoplastic lesions and can be confusing when the progenitor cell is in dispute or when the lesion is composed of many cell populations. In clinical practice, a mixed clinicopathologic classification is used, which provides a clear organization for non-neoplastic pathology.

In reading the numerous and broad series of cases reported in the literature,[1-11] one must always take into account the specialty of the authors (e.g., ophthalmology, neurosurgery, otolaryngology, or pathology), the material from which the study was derived (e.g., series of clinic charts, surgical series, or pathology series), the type of institution that generated the data (e.g., university, private practice, large city, or small center), and the population that makes up the sample, including race and age.

We wish to report the accrued experience of 15 consecutive years (1976 to 1991) of the Orbital Unit of the IInd Medical School, University of Naples, Italy.

Ours is a large university center that receives patients from the entire Italian peninsula. For this reason, the data presented can be considered a valid sample of a homogeneous Mediterranean caucasian ethnic group. However, because of the size and reputation acquired by our group over the years, our data reflect a relatively greater frequency of cases that call for complex surgical approaches and a greater frequency of rare diseases, compared with series from a standard ophthalmologic practice.

From more than 2000 clinical records, 1703 cases were selected, excluding those lost to follow-up or those with insufficient histopathologic information. Most of the patients underwent surgery, except for a few with benign tumors or some who underwent medical treatment without biopsy. The list of all cases and their diagnoses is reported in Table 81 – 1. The clinicopathologic type of classification has been adopted, except for pseudotumors, for which a slightly different classification has been used.

Orbital pathologies have been divided into six principal groups: thyroid orbitopathy (16%), neoplasia (34.6%), structural (31.8%), inflammatory (12.7%), vascular (3.8%), and degenerative (1.1%). The neoplasia group includes benign and malignant lesions divided by histogenesis into neurogenic, lymphoproliferative, vascular, lacrimal gland, mesenchymal, secondary and metastatic categories. Included in the structural group are cystic, congenital and acquired, and traumatic le-

*Original manuscript translated by Jeffrey Schiller, M.D.

TABLE 81-1

Age Distribution of Orbital Lesions Seen at the Orbital Unit, University of Naples, Italy (1976–1991)

	Incidence by Decade of Life									
Type of Lesion	**1**	**2**	**3**	**4**	**5**	**6**	**7**	**8**	**9**	**Total**
Thyroid Orbitopathy	3	11	41	62	66	55	23	11	1	273 (16.0%)
Neoplasia										
Neurogenic										
Optic nerve glioma	8	4	—	—	1	—	—	—	—	13
Meningioma										
Optic nerve	1	3	2	7	5	10	2	2	—	32
Other	—	—	1	3	14	7	5	—	1	31
Other optic nerve tumors										
Optic nerve cyst	1	—	—	—	—	—	—	—	—	1
Peripheral nerve sheath										
Neurofibroma										
Plexiform	6	—	1	—	—	—	2	—	—	9
Solitary	—	—	—	2	1	—	3	—	—	6
Schwannoma	1	1	1	5	1	—	—	—	—	9
Total neurogenic	17	8	5	17	22	17	12	2	1	101
Lymphoproliferative										
Lymphocytic										
Lymphomas	2	2	1	3	9	17	21	13	5	73
Plasma cell tumors										
Myeloma	—	—	—	—	4	2	—	1	1	8
Other										
Leukemias	1	1	—	—	2	—	1	—	—	5
Histiocytoses										
Histiocytosis X	6	2	—	1	1	1	—	—	—	11
Malignant histiocytosis	1	—	—	—	—	—	—	—	—	1
Total lymphoproliferative	10	5	1	4	16	20	22	14	6	98
Vascular neoplasias										
Capillary hemangioma	46	5	1	1	1	—	—	—	—	54
Cavernous hemangioma	—	1	2	15	13	7	6	—	—	44
Lymphangioma	9	7	4	—	1	—	—	2	—	23
Hemangiopericytoma	—	2	—	—	—	—	—	—	—	2
Hemangioendothelioma	—	—	1	—	—	—	—	—	—	1
Total vascular neoplasias	55	15	8	16	15	7	6	2	0	124
Secondary tumors										
Ethmoid	—	—	1	1	1	2	1	—	1	7
Maxilla	—	—	—	2	2	5	3	4	—	16
Nasopharynx										
Carcinoma	—	—	—	1	—	—	3	1	—	5
Angiomyofibroma	—	3	—	—	—	—	—	—	—	3
Esthesioneuroblastoma	—	—	—	—	2	—	—	—	—	2
Eyelids										
Basal cell	1	—	1	—	1	5	23	11	5	47
Squamous	—	—	—	—	—	1	2	5	1	9
Melanoma	—	—	—	—	—	—	1	1	—	2
Adenocarcinoma	—	—	—	—	—	—	1	—	—	1
Lacrimal sac										
Squamous	—	—	—	—	1	—	—	—	—	1
Conjunctiva										
Melanoma	—	—	—	—	—	—	2	—	—	2
Ocular										
Melanoma	—	—	—	—	1	3	1	2	3	10
Total secondary tumors	1	3	2	4	8	16	37	24	10	105
Mesenchymal										
Striated muscle										
Rhabdomyosarcoma	15	7	2	—	—	—	—	—	—	24
Histiocytic										
Fibrous histiocytoma	—	1	1	—	—	1	2	1	—	6
Bone tumors										
Fibrous dysplasia	5	5	2	2	—	—	—	2	—	16
Ossifying fibroma	1	1	—	—	—	—	—	—	—	2
Cholesterol granuloma	—	—	—	—	1	—	1	—	—	2
Aneurysmal bone cyst	—	—	—	1	—	1	—	—	—	2

TABLE 81-1

Age Distribution of Orbital Lesions Seen at the Orbital Unit, University of Naples, Italy (1976–1991) *Continued*

	Incidence by Decade of Life										
Type of Lesion	**1**	**2**	**3**	**4**	**5**	**6**	**7**	**8**	**9**	**Total**	
Neoplasia											
Ewing's sarcoma	1	—	1	—	—	—	—	—	—	2	
Osteoma	2	9	1	4	2	3	1	—	1	23	
Osteogenic sarcoma	—	—	—	1	—	—	—	—	—	1	
Chondromyxoma	—	—	—	—	—	1	—	—	—	1	
Total mesenchymal	24	23	7	8	3	6	4	3	1	79	
Metastastic											
Breast	—	—	—	2	1	5	4	2	—	14	
Lung	—	—	—	—	1	2	2	—	1	6	
Prostate	—	—	—	—	—	—	1	1	—	2	
Skin melanoma	—	—	—	1	2	2	3	1	—	9	
Ewing's sarcoma	2	—	—	—	—	—	—	—	—	2	
Kidney	—	—	—	—	1	1	—	—	—	2	
Parotid gland	—	—	—	1	—	—	—	—	—	1	
Liver	—	—	—	—	—	—	1	—	—	1	
Uterus	—	—	—	—	—	—	—	1	—	1	
Skin squamous cell carcinoma	—	—	—	—	—	—	—	—	1	1	
Neuroblastoma	1	1	—	—	—	—	—	—	—	2	
Unknown	—	—	—	—	—	1	1	1	—	3	
Total metastatic	3	1	0	4	5	11	12	6	2	44	
Lacrimal											
Benign mixed tumor	—	1	7	2	1	1	5	—	—	17	
Malignant mixed tumor	—	—	—	—	1	1	—	—	—	2	
Adenoid cystic	—	2	2	—	3	3	—	1	—	11	
Adenocarcinoma	—	—	—	—	—	—	1	—	—	1	
Mucoepidermoid	—	—	—	—	—	1	—	—	—	1	
Squamous cell	—	—	—	—	—	2	1	2	—	5	
Acinic cell	—	—	—	—	—	1	—	—	—	1	
Total lacrimal	0	3	9	2	5	9	7	3	0	38	
Total neoplasias	110	58	32	55	74	86	100	54	20	589	(34.6%)
Structural Lesions											
Congenital											
Cystic											
Dermoids and epidermoids	61	36	21	12	1	1	2	2	—	136	
Serous	1	2	1	2	1	—	—	—	1	8	
Hematic	—	1	—	—	—	—	1	—	—	2	
Maxillary	1	3	—	—	2	1	—	—	—	7	
Meningocele	—	1	1	—	—	—	—	—	—	2	
Bony anomalies											
Asymmetry and micro-orbitism	9	9	6	4	6	5	1	—	—	40	
von Recklinghausen	3	5	3	1	1	1	2	—	—	16	
Crouzon	1	2	—	1	—	—	—	—	—	4	
Craniostenosis	1	1	—	—	—	—	—	—	—	2	
Ectopia											
Dermolipoma	5	6	—	1	—	—	—	—	—	12	
Acquired											
Cystic											
Mucocele	3	5	4	4	9	11	20	13	2	71	
Lacrimal	—	—	—	—	1	—	2	—	—	3	
Polyposis	—	—	—	—	2	—	—	—	—	2	
Pneumatocele	—	—	1	—	—	—	—	—	—	1	
Echinococcus cyst	—	—	—	1	—	—	—	—	—	1	
Trauma											
Fractures	17	47	47	34	33	21	5	—	—	204	
Soft tissues	3	7	3	1	1	1	2	1	—	19	
Foreign bodies	4	1	2	1	1	2	—	—	—	11	
Total structural lesions	109	126	89	62	58	43	35	16	3	541	(31.8%)
Inflammatory Lesions											
Infectious lesions											
Microbial											
Cellulitis	3	3	5	3	1	1	1	—	—	17	
Sinusitis	—	—	—	—	1	—	1	—	—	2	

(Continued)

TABLE 81-1

Age Distribution of Orbital Lesions Seen at the Orbital Unit, University of Naples, Italy (1976–1991) *Continued*

Type of Lesion	Incidence by Decade of Life									
	1	2	3	4	5	6	7	8	9	Total
Nonspecific inflammation										
Inflammatory pseudotumors										
Fasciitis	4	5	5	6	4	2	7	2	—	35
Fibrous	—	—	1	2	3	3	3	1	—	13
Tenonitis	5	3	5	3	7	7	9	4	—	43
Myositis	—	1	2	6	11	2	4	3	1	30
Dacryoadenitis	3	8	8	8	8	9	11	2	1	58
Pseudolymphoma	—	1	—	—	3	8	1	—	—	13
Other inflammations										
Sarcoidosis	—	—	—	—	—	1	2	—	—	3
Wegener's granulomatosis	—	1	—	—	—	—	—	—	—	1
Tolosa-Hunt syndrome	—	—	—	—	—	1	—	—	—	1
Total inflammatory lesions	15	22	26	28	38	34	39	12	2	216 (12.7%)
Vascular lesions										
Arteriovenus shunts										
Malformations	1	2	3	—	—	7	—	3	—	16
Carotid-cavernous fistula	1	3	—	1	4	5	7	1	—	22
Venous										
Varix	1	5	6	5	3	—	—	2	—	22
Cavernous sinus thrombosis	—	—	—	—	—	—	1	2	2	5
Total vascular lesions	3	10	9	6	7	12	8	8	2	65 (3.8%)
Degenerative lesions										
Myopia	—	3	3	2	5	—	2	1	—	16
Fat prolapse	—	1	1	—	—	—	—	—	—	2
Progressive external ophthalmoplegia	—	—	—	—	—	—	1	—	—	1
Total degenerative lesions	0	4	4	2	5	0	3	1	0	19 (1.1%)
Overall Total	240	231	201	215	248	230	208	102	28	1703 (100%)
	471		894				338			

sions. The inflammatory group includes infective and noninfective and specific and aspecific lesions. The vascular group includes nonneoplastic vascular lesions of arterious, venous, or mixed origin. Finally, the degenerative lesions include those secondary to degenerative pathologies and those not included elsewhere.

The graph of the incidence of orbital diseases (Fig. 81–1) in relation to age of presentation shows that all ages are affected, with a greater incidence in the first and fifth decades of life and progressive diminution in the seventh and eighth decades.

Graphing each group separately (Figs. 81–2 and 81–3) shows that each age group has its own incidence of disease. Structural lesions are more often seen in children and peak in the second decade, an effect that is related to the prevalence of congenital cystic lesions and to orbital trauma among the young. Neoplastic lesions have two peaks, in the first and seventh decades, which correspond to the presence of primary tumors of infancy and the prevalence of secondary tumors in older patients. Thyroid orbitopathy has a bell-shaped curve, with the maximum incidence in the fourth and fifth decades. Inflammatory lesions have an almost constant incidence throughout life, with a slight increase in the fifth, sixth, and seventh decades. Vascular and degenerative lesions show no particular age preference, although their low numbers prevent strong conclusions from being drawn.

Examination of the incidence of single subgroups within the neoplastic lesions reveals that a peak incidence of vascular tumors, consisting of congenital hemangiomas and lymphangiomas, occurs in the first decade, followed by a stable low incidence at other ages. Similarly, mesenchymal tumors have a more modest peak in the first and second decades, corresponding to the incidence of rhabdomyosarcoma. Neurogenic and lymphoproliferative tumors have similar incidences, presenting a peak in the first decade and another area of greater incidence in older age, respectively, centered in the fifth as well as the seventh decades. Secondary (and to a lesser extent metastatic) tumors have a maximum incidence in

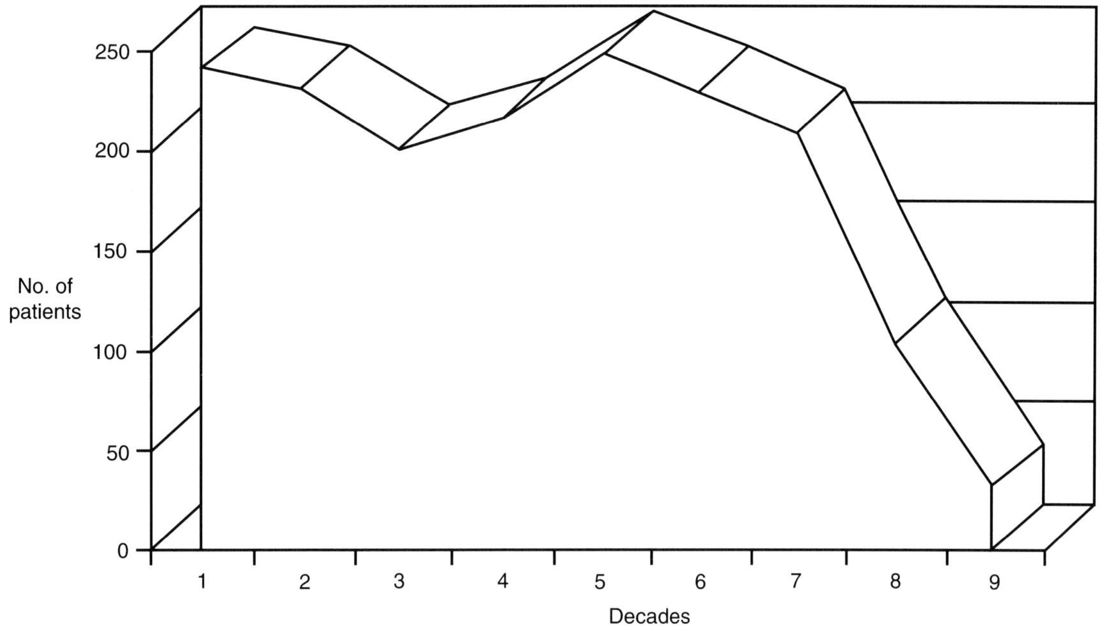

Figure 81–1. Age distribution of 1703 cases of orbital lesion seen from 1976 through 1991 at the Orbital Unit, University of Naples, Italy.

the seventh decade. Tumors of the lacrimal gland have a bimodal curve of incidence, with a peak in the third decade and another broader peak in the sixth.

The commonest pathologic entities in our survey are listed in Table 81–2. Tables 81–3 through 81–5 describe the most common pathology by patient age.

In the pediatric age group, from birth to age 20, in a total of 471 cases (28% of the total cases), the commonest lesions are dermoid cysts, trauma with or without fracture, and infantile hemangiomas. Among the tumors, hemangiomas are followed by rhabdomyosarcomas, lymphangiomas, lymphoproliferative lesions (lym-

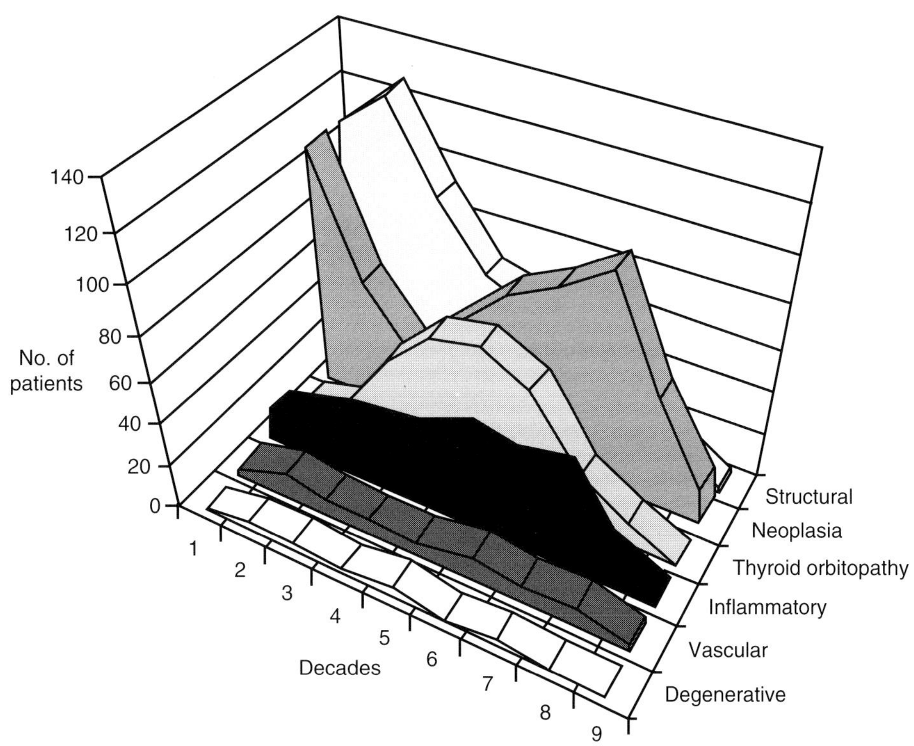

Figure 81–2. Age distribution by groups of orbital lesion seen from 1976 through 1991 at the Orbital Unit, University of Naples, Italy.

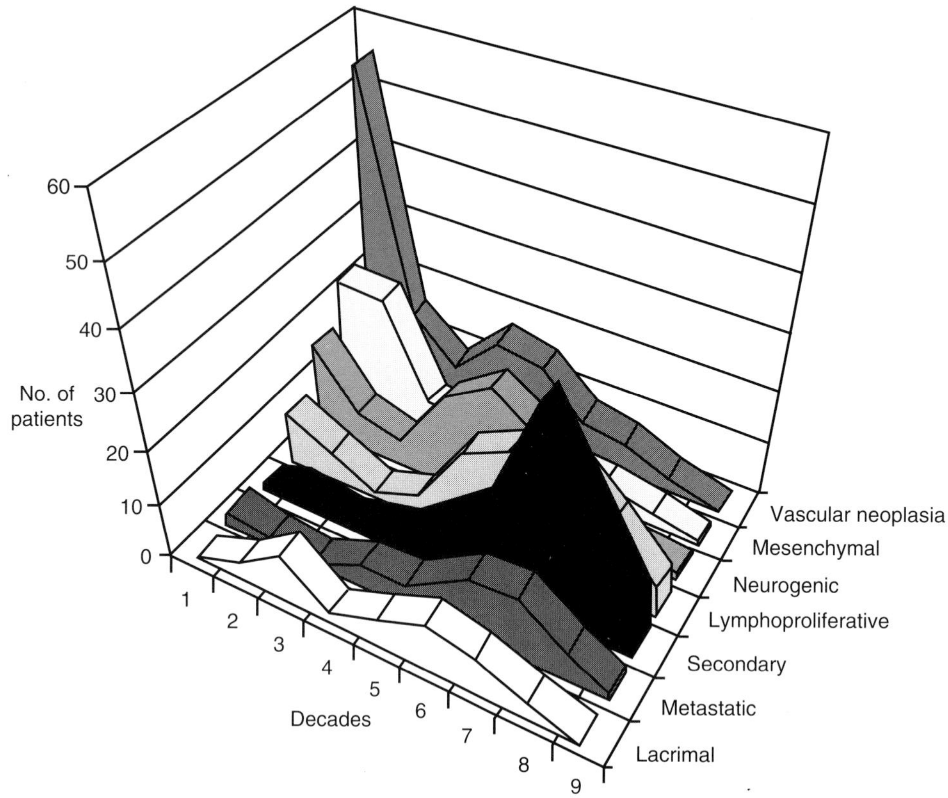

Figure 81 – 3. Age distribution in the neoplasia group (total neoplasia, 589 cases).

TABLE 81 – 2

Commonest Orbital Lesions in Patients of All Ages

Lesion	n(%)
Thyroid orbitopathy	273(16.03)
Trauma	234(13.74)
Pseudotumor	192(11.27)
Dermoids	136(7.99)
Secondary neoplasia	105(6.17)
Lymphoma	73(4.29)
Mucocele	71(4.17)
Vascular lesion	65(3.82)
Capillary hemangioma	54(3.17)
Metastatic neoplasia	44(2.58)
Cavernous hemangioma	44(2.58)

TABLE 81 – 3

Commonest Orbital Lesions in Patients Aged 0 to 20 Years

Lesion	n(%)
Dermoid	97(20.59)
Trauma	79(16.77)
Capillary hemangioma	51(10.83)
Pseudotumor	30(6.37)
Rhabdomyosarcoma	22(4.67)
Micro-orbitism	18(3.82)
Lymphangioma	16(3.40)
Lymphoproliferative neoplasia	15(3.18)
Thyroid orbitopathy	14(2.97)
Vascular lesion	13(2.76)
Optic nerve glioma	12(2.55)
Osteoma	11(2.34)
Dermolipoma	11(2.34)

TABLE 81 – 4

Commonest Orbital Lesions in Patients Aged 21 to 60 Years

Lesion	n(%)
Thyroid orbitopathy	224(25.06)
Trauma	147(16.44)
Pseudotumor	113(12.64)
Cavernous hemangioma	37(4.14)
Dermoid	35(3.91)
Vascular lesion	34(3.80)
Lymphoma	30(3.36)
Secondary neoplasia	30(3.36)
Mucocele	28(3.13)
Other meningiomas	25(2.80)
Lacrimal neoplasia	25(2.80)
Optic nerve meningioma	24(2.68)
Metastatic neoplasia	20(2.24)

TABLE 81 – 5

Commonest Orbital Lesions in Patients Aged over 60 Years

Lesion	n(%)
Secondary neoplasia	71(21.01)
Pseudotumor	49(14.50)
Lymphoma	39(11.54)
Mucocele	35(10.36)
Thyroid orbitopathy	35(10.36)
Metastatic neoplasia	20(5.92)
Vascular lesion	18(5.33)

phoma, leukemia, histiocytosis), and gliomas of the optic nerve.

In the adult age group, from 21 to age 60, in a total of 894 cases (52% of the total cases), the commonest lesions are dysthyroid orbitopathy, trauma, and pseudotumor. Among the neoplastic lesions, cavernous hemangiomas, lymphomas, secondary neoplasias, meningiomas of the optic nerve and of other sites, epithelial tumors of the lacrimal gland, and metastic tumors are the commonest.

In the group over the age of 60, who represent the remaining 338 cases (20% of the total), secondary tumors, followed by pseudotumor, lymphoma, mucocele of the paranasal sinuses, thyroid orbitopathy, and metastatic tumors, constitute the commonest lesions.

From these data, we can see that at different ages, different groups of lesions predominate, starting with congenital malformations and trauma in the young, and progressing to neoplastic and malignant lesions in the elderly.

REFERENCES

1. Duke-Elder S: System of Ophthalmology. Volume 13: The Ocular Adnexa. London, Henry Kimpton, 1976.
2. Henderson JW, Farrow GM: Orbital Tumors, 2nd ed. New York, Brian C Decker, 1980.
3. Iliff WD, Green WR: Orbital tumors in children. *In* Jakobiec FA (ed): Ocular and Adnexal Tumors. Birmingham, Aesculapius, 1978, p 669.
4. Jones IS, Jakobiec FA: Diseases of the Orbit. Philadelphia, Harper & Row, 1979.
5. Kennedy RE: An evaluation of 820 orbital cases. Trans Am Ophthalmol Soc 82:134, 1984.
6. Krohel GB, Stewart WB, Chavis RM: Orbital Disease: A Practical Approach. New York, Grune & Stratton, 1981.
7. Moss HM: Expanding lesions of the orbit: A clinical study of 230 consecutive cases. Am J Ophthalmol 54:761, 1962.
8. Reese AB: Expanding lesions of the orbit: Bowman Lecture. Trans Ophthalmol Soc UK 91:85, 1971.
9. Rootman J: Diseases of the Orbit. Philadelphia, JB Lippincott, 1988.
10. Shields JA, Bakewell B, Augsburger JJ, et al. Classification and incidence of space-occupying lesions of the orbit. Arch Ophthalmol 102:1606, 1984.
11. Silva D: Orbital tumors. Am J Ophthalmol 65:318, 1968.

CHAPTER 82

Clinical Examination in Orbital Disease

Geoffrey E. Rose

Together with an accurate history, the clinical examination of the patient with orbital disease can provide a strong indication of the likely cause and extent of the illness. Clinical evidence of the extent of disease is valuable in directing the course of further investigation and treatment.

Clinical signs of orbital disease are caused by changes in the normal position and function of orbital structures. Because the orbit is largely bounded by bone, normal orbital structures are generally displaced away from tumor masses; where an orbital mass lies alongside compressible, air-filled paranasal sinuses, however, the thin bone separating the orbit and sinus may slowly yield to an expansile mass. Changes of function, such as visual loss or reduced ocular motility, result from either direct injury by the disease or indirect injury with impairment of the vascular or more rarely, the nervous, supply to the orbital tissues.

The clinical examination of patients with orbital disease should gather an accurate but practical record of changes in the function and position of orbital structures and should elicit any relevant systemic signs related to the orbital disease.

VISUAL FUNCTIONS

A measure of corrected visual acuity, such as a Snellen test or an equivalent, should be readily available and may be supplemented with the assessment of acuity for near vision. Axial compression of the globe by an orbital mass, with induced axial hypermetropia or presbyopia, can cause symptoms early in orbital disease.

Color discrimination is a sensitive index of optic nerve function, and the examiner should seek a history of altered color perception (dyschromatopsia); this problem is generally appreciated by the patient as a difference in color saturation between the two eyes or as a drabness of color hues in the affected eye. With appropriate reading correction and good lighting, Ishihara (or similar) test plates provide the most practical assessment of color discrimination; the results should be recorded in terms of accuracy and speed of testing. After an adequate and simple explanation, most patients are able to subjectively assess the desaturation of color hues in the affected eye as compared with those in the unaffected eye; a neurologic test pin with a bright red head is useful for this examination, and it should be stressed that the *redness,* not brightness, is being tested.

It is convenient to screen for visual field defects once the patient has gained experience in judging the saturation and hue of a test target. Through accepted methods of confrontational testing, clinical screening for field defects should be directed toward certain common deficits in orbital disease. On the affected side, the examiner should look particularly for the presence of an enlarged blind spot, a central or centrocecal scotoma, or a peripheral constriction of the field (Fig. 82–1). A junctional scotoma within the visual field for the contralateral eye (Fig. 82–2) suggests extension of the optic nerve or orbital disease to the optic chiasm on the affected (ipsilateral) side. In cases in which postchiasmal disease is suspected, the presence of quadrantic or hemianopic field defects, either bitemporal or homonymous, should be sought, and tests of cortical visual function, such as visual sensory inattention, should also be performed.

Mechanically assisted visual field testing, such as kinetic Goldmann perimetry, should be used to record field loss shown by clinical screening or to determine where mild defects might be expected on the basis of clinical history or other signs. Such formal visual field testing provides an objective and more accurate assessment of the status or progression of orbital or intracranial disease and is imperative in the monitoring of patients with primary optic nerve tumors, such as gliomas or meningiomas.

The relative afferent pupillary defect (RAPD), or Marcus Gunn swinging light test, is an essential clinical test; if it cannot be accurately performed, this fact should be recorded in the patient's clinical case notes. Because of the bright light used for testing the RAPD, the test is best performed after other tests of visual function—particularly tests of acuity and color discrimination—have been performed. The patient should have undisturbed fixation of a nonaccommodative distant target. A bright light is directed alternately into the right and left

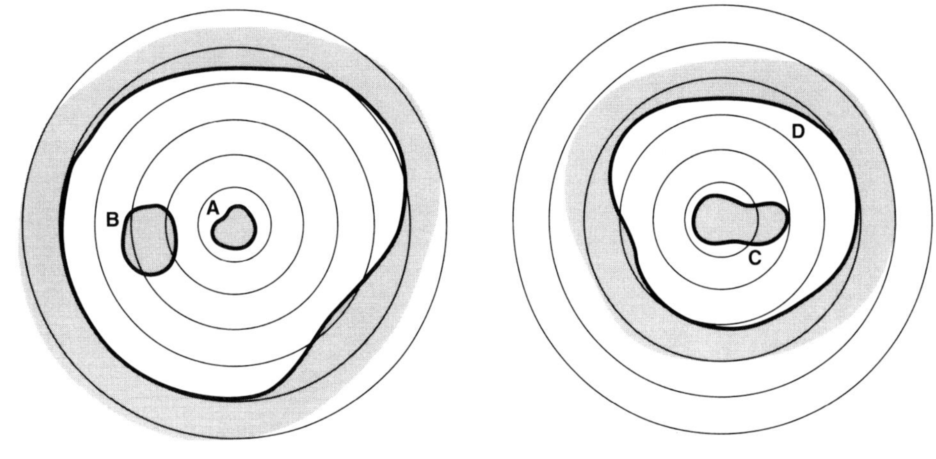

Figure 82–1. Composite illustration showing some defects of visual field that may occur with orbital disease: optic nerve disease may lead to a central scotoma (A), enlarged blind spot (B), centrocecal scotoma (C), or generalized constriction of peripheral visual field (D).

pupils, for about 1 second at each eye, and the pupillary reaction is assessed; the degree of spontaneous pupillary oscillation (hippus) should also be noted.

In cases in which both pupils are reactive to light, either may be used to monitor the clinical test, and a positive response is represented by anomalous pupillary dilation occurring when light is shone into the affected eye. The extent of the anomalous dilation can be approximately graded as "mild," "moderate," or "dense." The test is hardly affected by opacities in the ocular media, but retinal detachments or extensive macular disease produce a positive RAPD. Impairment of optic nerve function generally produces a positive RAPD, which implies reduced transmission of the visual stimulus along the affected afferent pathway, relative to the contralateral afferent pathway. This valuable sign can also be assessed from a single reactive pupil (a "consensual" RAPD). In cases in which both pupils are nonreactive, the patient's subjective appreciation of the brightness of the light in the affected eye relative to the other eye can provide a subjective assessment of the RAPD.

The loss of a relative afferent pupillary defect, if it had been present at a previous examination, has two distinct interpretations: either the disease causing the original ipsilateral neuropathy has resolved or a newly acquired impairment of conduction by the contralateral afferent pathway has occurred, such contralateral impairment being of a degree similar to that seen on the ipsilateral side.

POSITION AND MOVEMENT OF THE GLOBE

Abnormalities in the position or movement of the globe may present symptomatically; intermittant diplopia is often one of the first symptoms of orbital disease and may indicate a recent onset. In some patients, diplopia disappears if, for example, optic nerve function is damaged by progression of orbital disease or if the visual axis is obstructed by the onset of ptosis.

The globe, being very mobile within the orbit, tends to be displaced by an orbital mass, and the pattern of such displacement can suggest the location of the disease. However, abnormalities of the osseous orbit should also be considered when the position of the globe is assessed (Fig. 82–3).

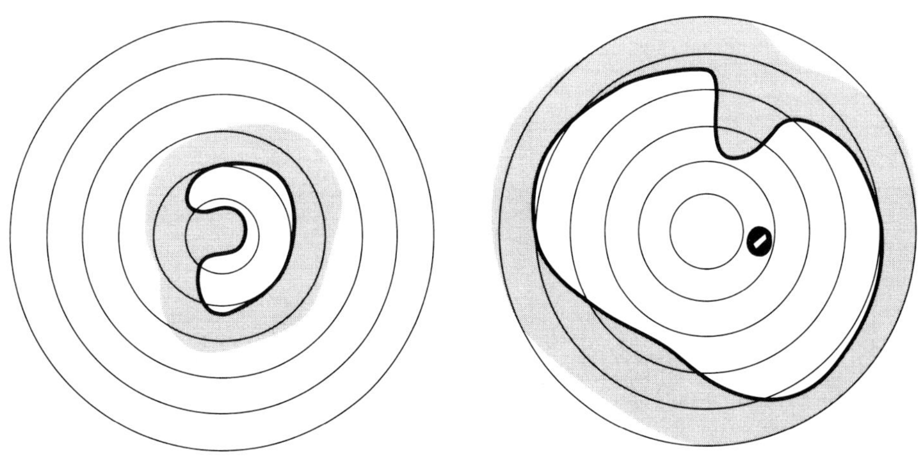

Figure 82–2. Diagrammatic representation of a junctional scotoma of Traquair, with a left optic nerve lesion (causing grossly reduced peripheral visual field) and an early superotemporal field loss in the opposite (right) eye.

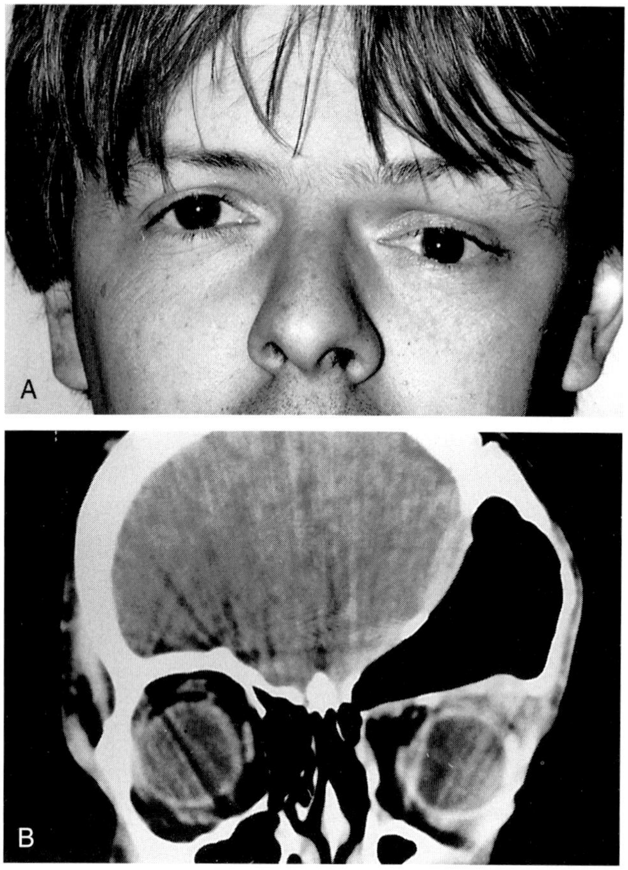

Figure 82–3. Clinical examination suggested downward displacement of the left globe (*A*), possible due to a mass on the roof of the orbit. Radiologic investigation (*B*) showed the whole of the left osseous orbit to be displaced downward by massive enlargement of the frontal sinus.

The position of the globe in the coronal plane may be readily estimated by placing a ruler horizontally across the nasal bridge of the patient, parallel to the normal lateral canthi. While the patient fixates the examiner's nasal bridge, the horizontal distance from the facial midline to the center of the pupil is assessed; this assessment is simplified if a convenient ruling, such as the 150-mm mark, is placed at the midpoint of the patient's nose (Fig. 82–4*A*). The vertical position of each globe can be estimated at the same time, and the magnitude and direction of the difference between the two sides can be recorded (Fig. 82–4*B*).

Proptosis, or displacement of the globe along the anteroposterior axis of the orbit, may be estimated clinically (Fig. 82–5), or it can be assessed more accurately by use of one of the several designs of exophthalmometer; Hertel's exophthalmometer is simple to use and has good reproducibility of measurement. During exophthalmometry, the patient should fixate either the examiner's nasal bridge or to the corresponding (nearest) eye, and the instrument must rest accurately and firmly on the patient's lateral orbital rim.

Errors of measurement, resulting from parallax, may arise during the assessment of ocular position; such errors can be minimized by the examiner's using the right eye while assessing the patient's left eye and vice versa. Likewise, manifest ocular deviations (tropias) can cause apparent displacement of the globe (Fig. 82–6*A*), and the true ocular displacement must be estimated during occlusion of the dominant eye (see Fig. 82–6). A diagnosis of pseudoproptosis resulting from unilateral axial myopia should be considered in cases in which the apparent axial proptosis is mild (≤ 4 mm); A-mode ultrasound estimates of axial length for both eyes can resolve this issue.

Variability in the ocular position occurs with some orbital diseases and should be specifically sought during examination. Variation in synchrony with the peripheral pulse implies either an orbital vascular malformation with a major arterial supply or a breach of bone between the orbit and the dura mater, with transmitted intracranial pulsation; such absence of bone may be congenital (as with sphenoid dysplasia of neurofibromatosis) or acquired (as with damage to the orbital roof caused by trauma or by malignant tumors). Ocular displacement resulting from low-pressure vascular malformations of the orbit, such as primary varices, tends to increase with the passive venous engorgement that occurs during prolonged bending or the Valsalva maneuver (Fig. 82–7). Retraction of the globe (enophthalmos) during an attempted duction implies a restrictive fibrosis or entrapment of the ipsilateral antagonist muscle (Fig. 82–8); exceptions to this principle are the retraction that occurs with co-contraction syndromes, such as Duane's syndromes, or with aberrent reinnervation. Muscular restriction may be differentiated from a neurogenic cause by a positive result (resistance to passive global movement) during forced duction testing.

Assessment of eye movement in patients with orbital disease should follow accepted practice—the clinical estimation of the range of ductions in each eye and, if binocular, an examination for the presence of manifest or latent ocular deviations. The location of orbital disease may be indicated by specific patterns of ocular deviation (Fig. 82–9) or movement (Fig. 82–10).

EXTENT OF ORBITAL DISEASE

The position, extent, surface characteristics, and hardness of an intraorbital mass should be assessed by palpation, and the opposite orbit should be used for comparison when possible. Displacement of the globe may suggest the site of an orbital mass and direct palpation. Fixation to the deep orbital structures can indicate the origin of the mass, as with orbital extension of intraocular melanoma (attached to the globe), or it may indicate a mass involving the orbital bones, as with malignant

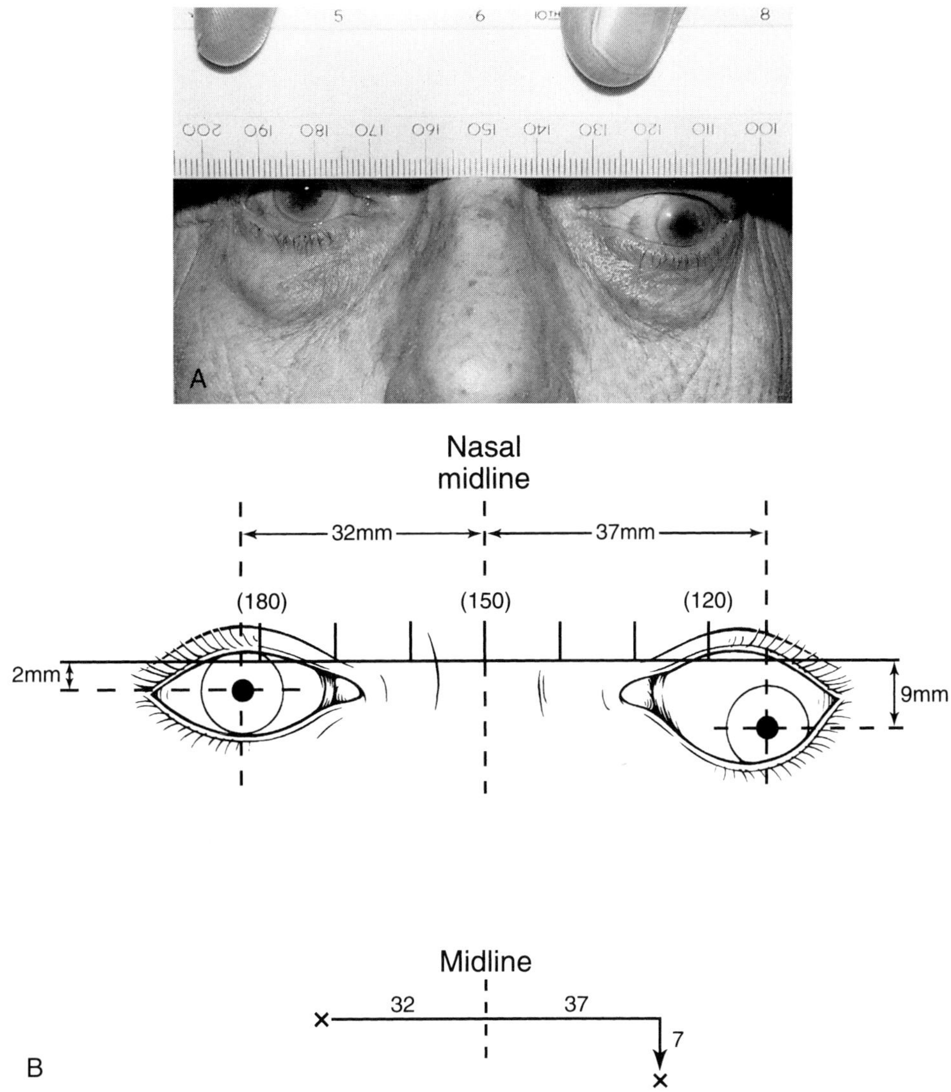

Figure 82–4. Clinical estimation of the displacement of the globe in a patient with left orbital mass. A ruler is placed horizontally with a convenient mark at the midpoint of the nose (*A*) and the position of the pupillary axis estimated for each eye (*B, top*). The measurements can be recorded in the notes using simple notation (*B, bottom*).

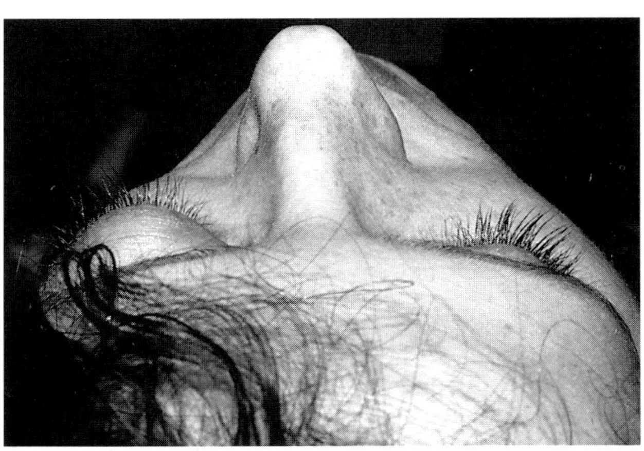

Figure 82–5. A simple clinical assessment of proptosis in a patient with left proptosis due to an orbital tumor.

tumors invading the orbit. Similarly, fixation of a mass to the eyelids influences the diagnosis and affects the clinical management.

If a mass is not evident on palpation, then the procedure should be repeated with the patient looking away from the area of palpation; masses attached to the extraocular muscles or levator muscle occasionally are demonstrated with this technique. Some masses can be palpated only when the globe is firmly ballotted backward in the orbit; this action displaces forward other orbital tissues and is particularly useful with small or mobile masses in the anterior part of the orbit. Orbital varices may be impalpable unless the patient performs a Valsalva maneuver.

Displacement of normal orbital structures must be

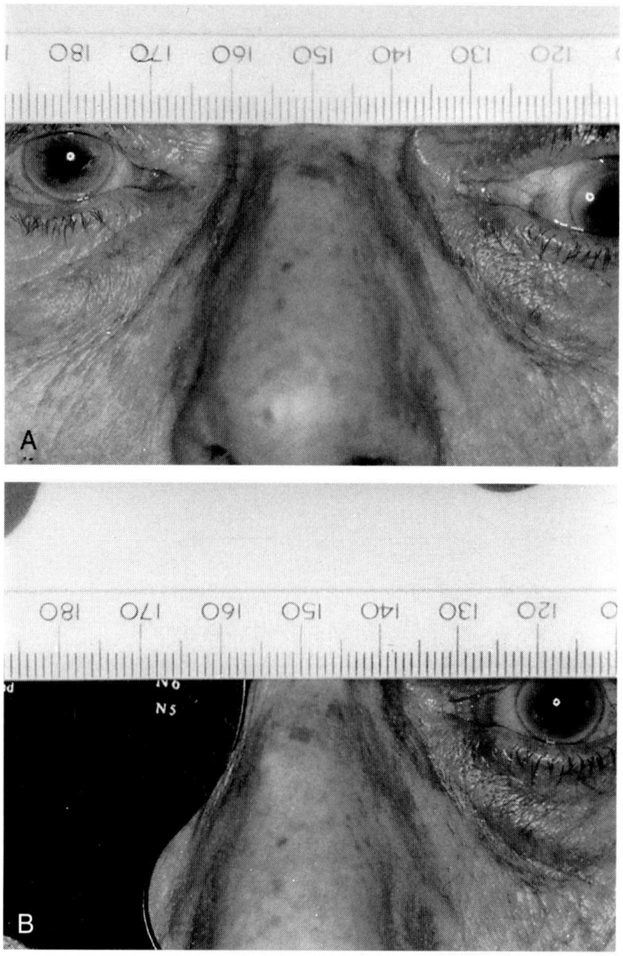

Figure 82–6. Errors in the estimation of globe position, due to the presence of a left hypoexotropia: in the absence of a cover test (*A*), the left eye appears to be displaced by about 7 mm laterally and 6 mm inferiorly, relative to the right eye. However, cover-testing (*B*) shows the true displacement of the left globe to be only 2 mm laterally.

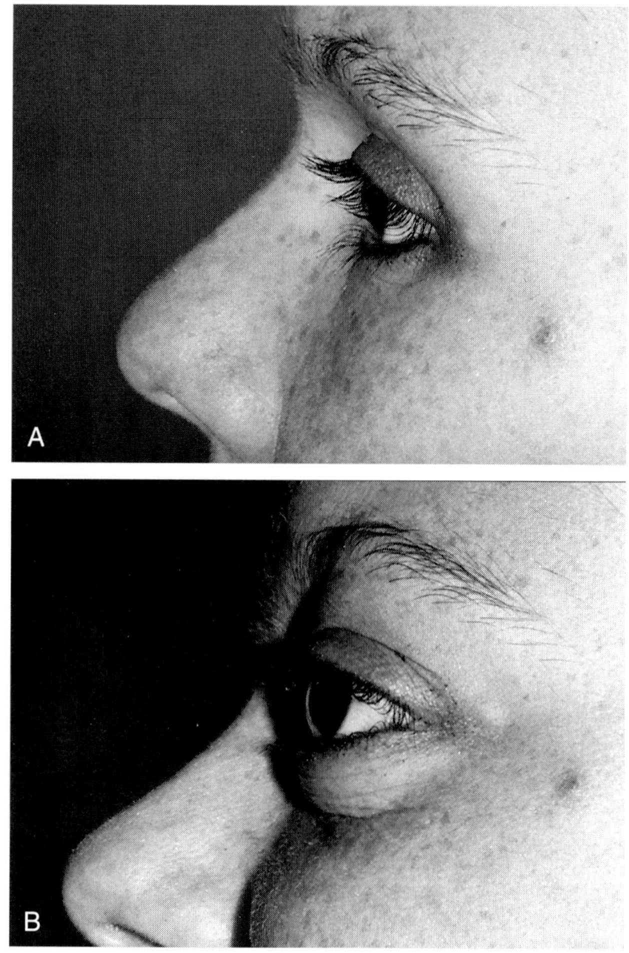

Figure 82–7. Variation of proptosis in a patient with primary varices situated posteriorly in the left orbit: lateral view before (*A*) and after (*B*) a Valsalva maneuver.

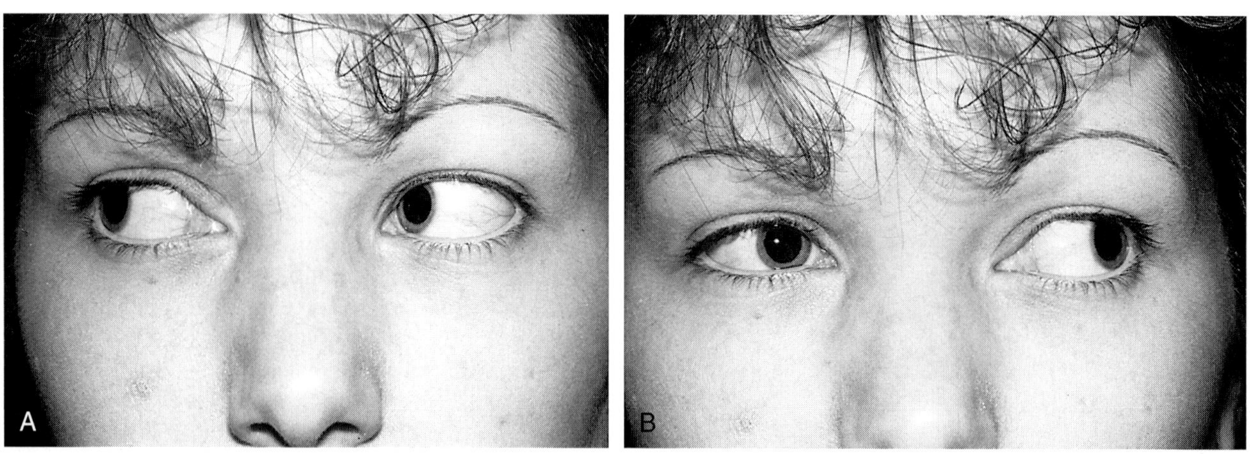

Figure 82–8. Patient after a severe episode of myositis affecting predominantly the right lateral rectus. Postinflammatory fibrosis restricts relaxation of this muscle and shift of the gaze from right (*A*) to left (*B*) causes globe retraction and narrowing of the palpebral fissure on the right.

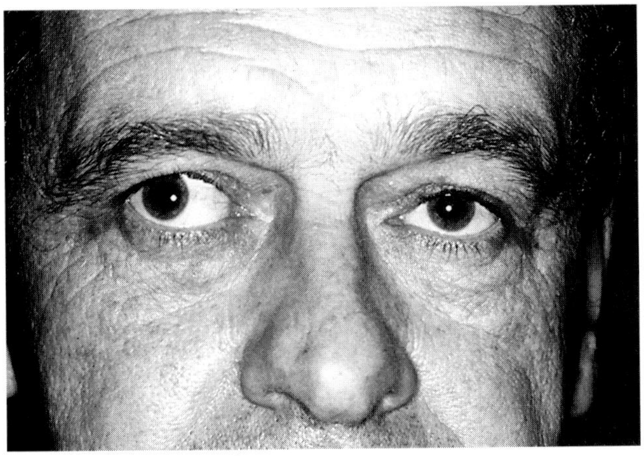

Figure 82–9. Orbital disease affecting the inferior branch of the right third cranial nerve, with a right hyperexotropia and an internal ophthalmoplegia.

noted and may be indicative of a posteriorly located orbital mass. Apart from the globe, the most frequently affected structures are the lacrimal gland and the orbital fat; displacement of fat manifests as changes in the profile of the eyelids.

Extraorbital extension of orbital disease may appear as an alteration in the contour of the temporalis fossa (Fig. 82–11), as an enlargement of the regional lymph nodes (Fig. 82–12), or as metastatic (or multifocal) masses; these metastases can be clinically evident or occult (Fig. 82–13*A*). Intracranial extension of orbital disease (see Fig. 82–13*B*) may cause symptoms and signs appropriate to lesions in the anterior or middle cranial fossa.

CHANGES WITHIN THE EYELIDS

The profile of the eyelids, particularly that of the upper eyelid, is frequently affected by orbital disease. Characteristics that should be assessed include contour, position and movement of the eyelid margins; profile and color of the eyelid sulci; and the form of the upper eyelid skin crease.

Loss of the normal smooth contour of the eyelid margin may indicate a tarsal mass with orbital extension (Fig. 82–14). The position of the lid margins in relation to the corneal limbus and the central corneal light reflex should be recorded and compared with the contralateral eyelids.

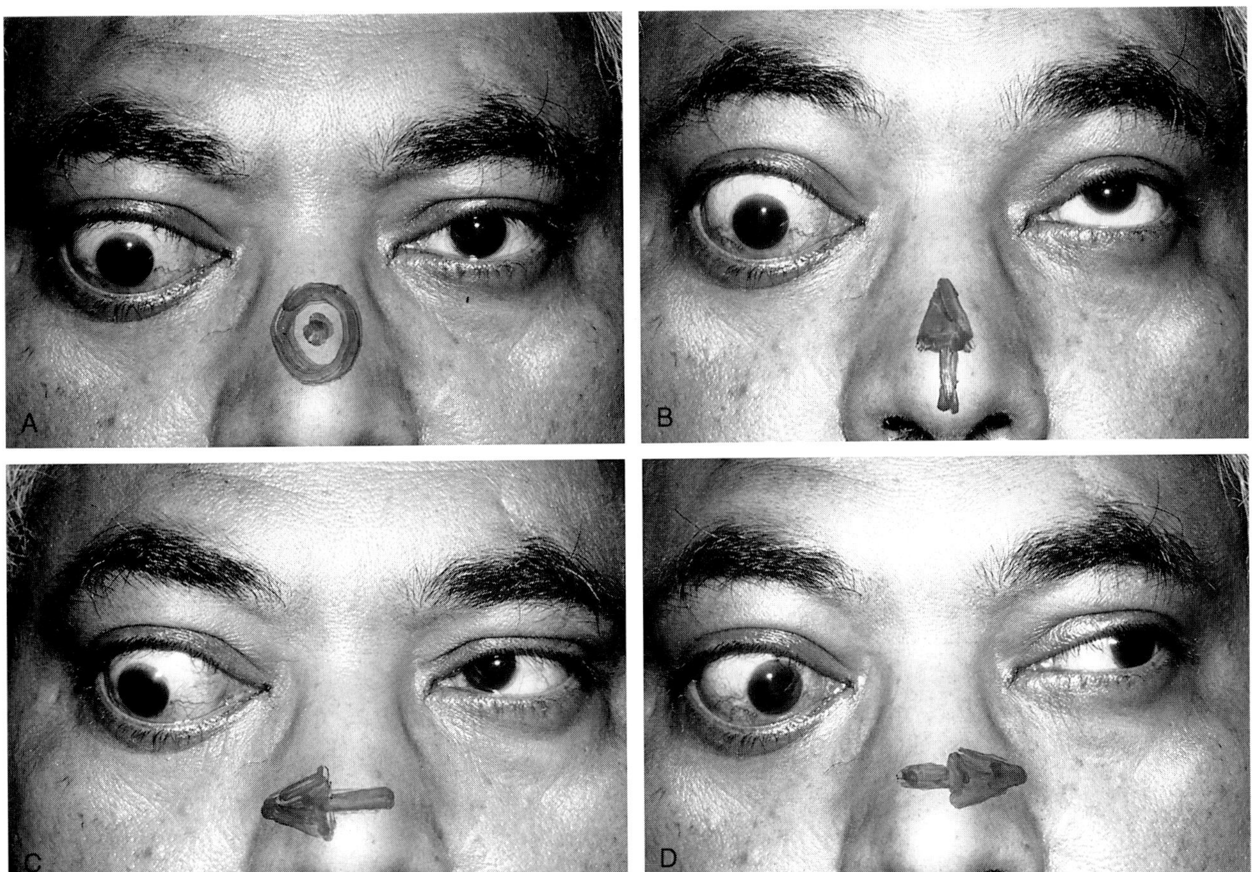

Figure 82–10. Severe right unilateral dysthyroid orbitopathy. Fibrosis of the inferior rectus causes right hypotropia in all positions of gaze (*A* through *D*), but relatively greater in abduction (*C*)—the field of maximum inferior rectus action. Upward gaze is restricted (*B*), with increased retraction of the upper eyelid as compared with the primary position (*A*). Horizontal movements of the right eye are also limited due to medial rectus disease (*C, D*).

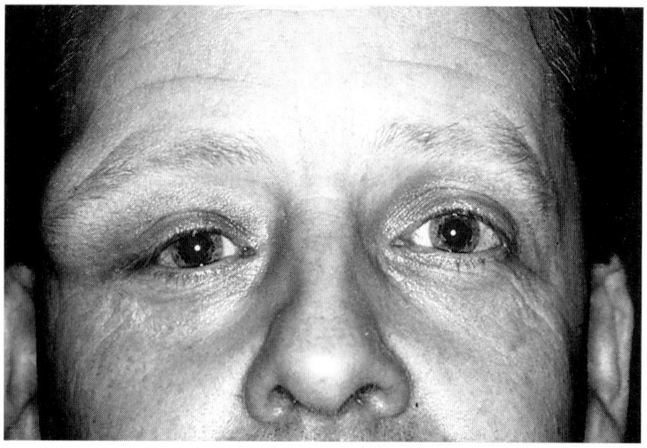

Figure 82–11. Alteration of the contour of the right temporalis fossa due to a large orbital dermoid extending through the lateral orbital wall and into the temporalis muscle.

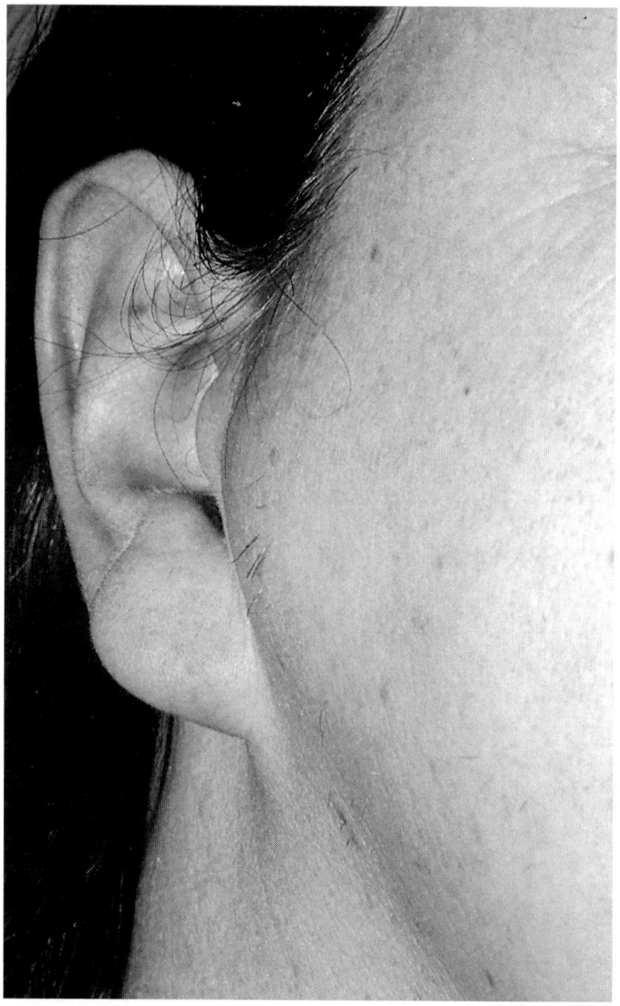

Figure 82–12. Clinically visible enlargement of the preauricular lymph nodes in a patient with metastatic orbital melanoma.

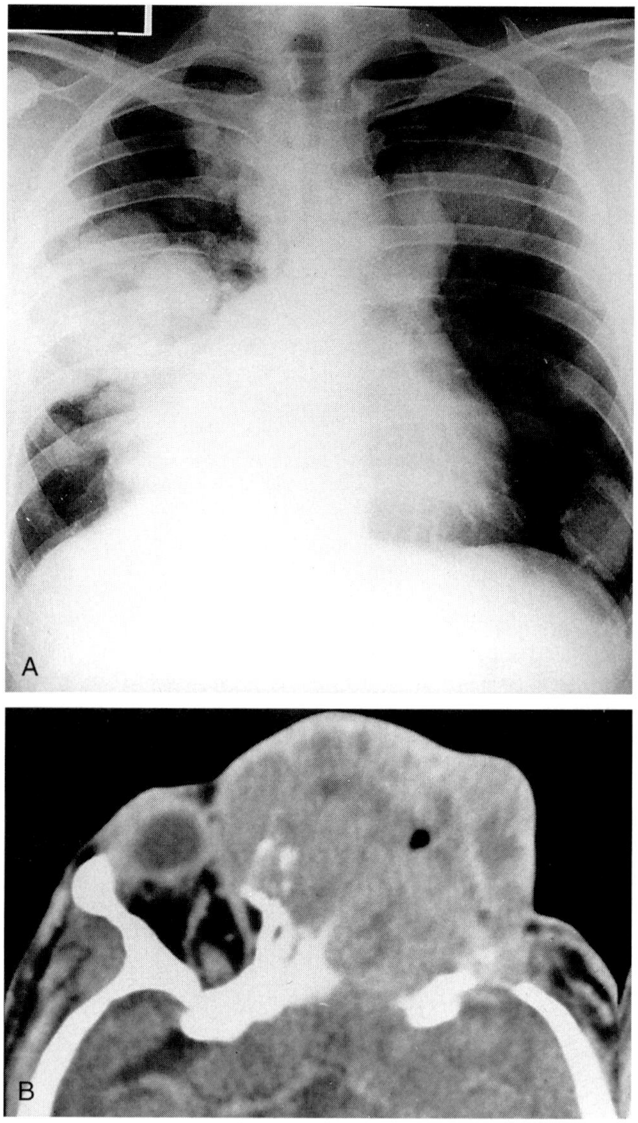

Figure 82–13. Multiple pulmonary metastases (*A*) and local tumor recurrence involving the face and the middle and anterior cranial fossae (*B*) in a patient with lacrimal gland carcinoma.

Upper lid retraction may occur with levator muscle overaction or fibrosis, as in dysthyroid eye disease (Fig. 82–15), or with tumors infiltrating the levator muscle. In these cases, upper lid retraction tends to be greater on downward gaze, and in cases in which fibrosis is marked, the eyelid shows marked resistance to downward traction. Retraction of the lower eyelid, particularly when it is associated with restricted upgaze, implies fibrosis, tethering, or infiltration of the inferior rectus muscle and the lower lid retractors (see Fig. 82–10); in such cases, any retraction of the upper eyelid tends to be greater in upward gaze.

Eyelid lag is a clinical sign that is evident only during ocular movement, in contrast to lid retraction, which is

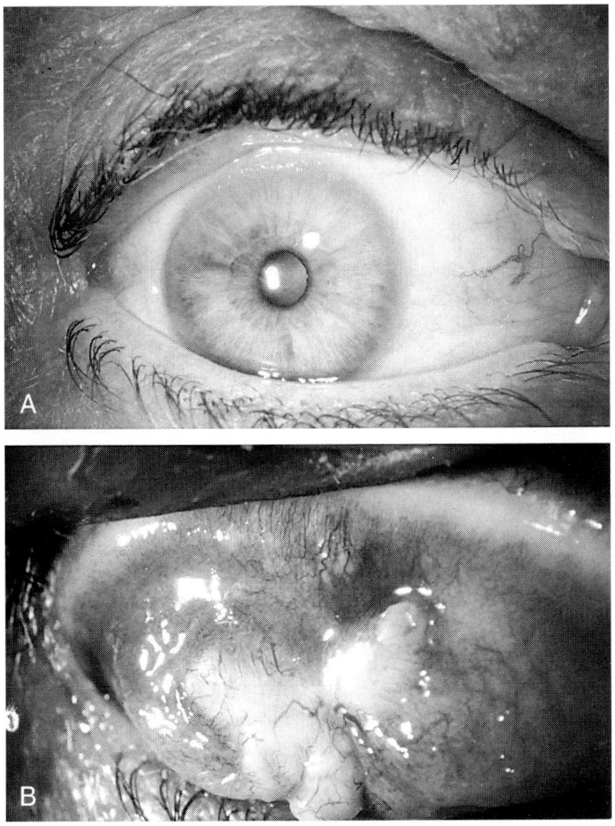

Figure 82–14. Notching of the upper eyelid (*A*) was the major outward manifestation of a large meibomian cell carcinoma (*B*).

assessed during ocular fixation. To examine for the presence of eyelid lag, the examiner should instruct the patient to follow a target moving from upward to downward gaze over about 3 to 4 seconds; lag is present when the upper eyelid margin falls behind (i.e., "lags") its normal position relative to the cornea. Eyelid lag is demonstrable in almost all patients with dysthyroid orbitopathy.

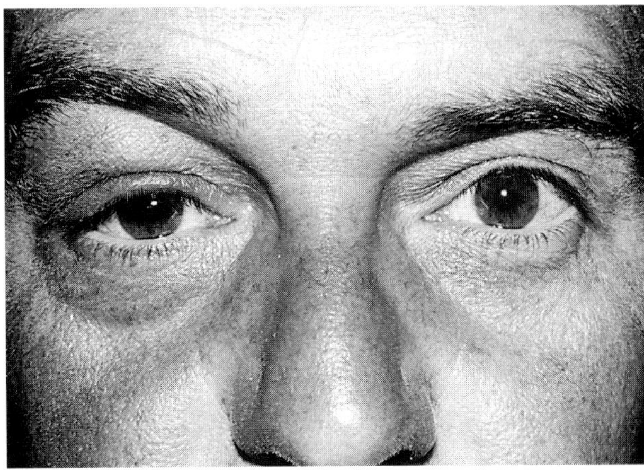

Figure 82–16. A mass in the superior part of the right orbit is causing "fullness" of the upper eyelid sulcus and asymmetry of the upper eyelid skin crease.

The profile of the upper eyelid depends on the position of the tarsal plate relative to the globe, the bulk of extraconal tissues in the upper part of the orbit, the integrity of the orbital septum, and the position of the upper eyelid skin crease. Retraction of the upper eyelid causes a greater degree of overhanging of the upper lid skin crease, with apparent asymmetry of the skin fold (see Fig. 82–15); this overhang is reduced somewhat by the coexistence of proptosis. Increased tissues in the superior part of the orbit result in a fullness of the upper eyelid sulcus and skin fold (Fig. 82–16), in prolapse of orbital fat through defects in the orbital septum (Fig. 82–17), or in loss of the skin crease. Changes in position or definition of the upper eyelid skin crease often provide the earliest sign of orbital disease and may be recorded clinically and photographically (Fig. 82–18). The coloration and texture of the eyelid skin can be strongly suggestive of the diagnosis (Fig. 82–19) or can indicate a vascular origin for an orbital mass (Fig. 82–20).

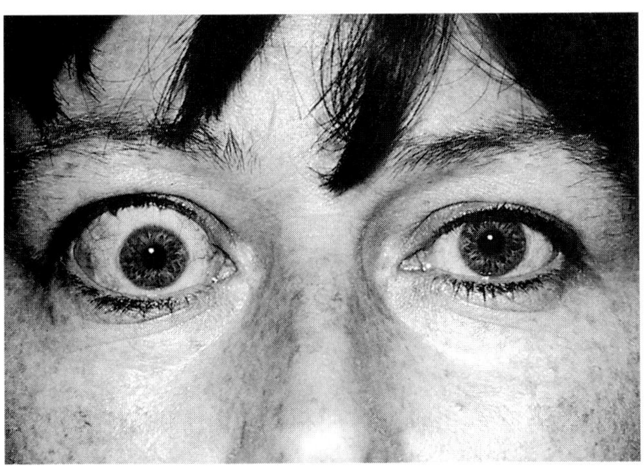

Figure 82–15. Marked retraction of the upper eyelid and mild lower lid retraction with right dysthyroid orbitopathy.

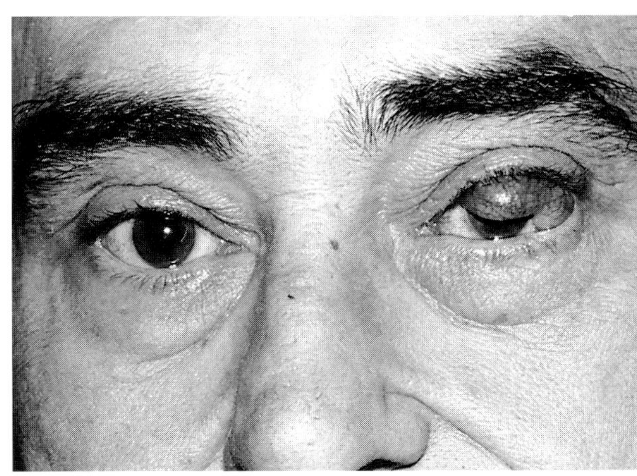

Figure 82–17. Displacement of orbital fat through the septum or at the palpebral aperture (as shown) may rarely be caused by an orbital mass.

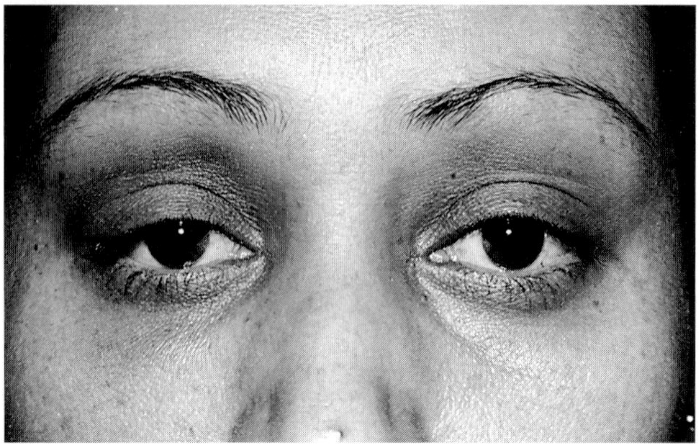

Figure 82–18. Changes in the upper eyelid skin crease may provide the earliest sign of orbital disease: here the lateral end of the right crease is effaced owing to lacrimal gland disease.

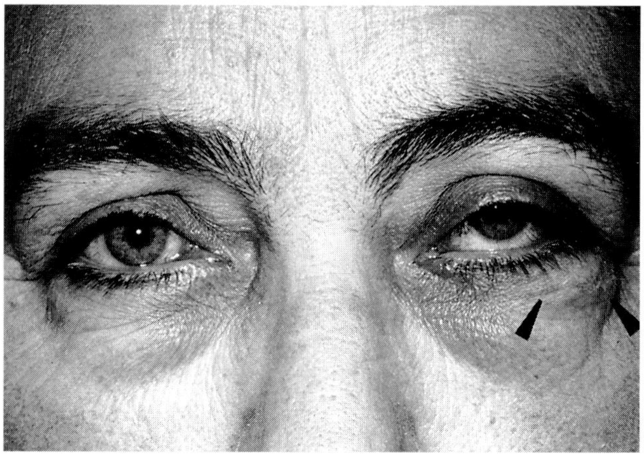

Figure 82–21. An orbital floor lymphoma is displacing the left globe upward, with "scleral show" below the inferior limbus and a minor alteration in the contour of the left lower eyelid sulcus (*arrowheads*).

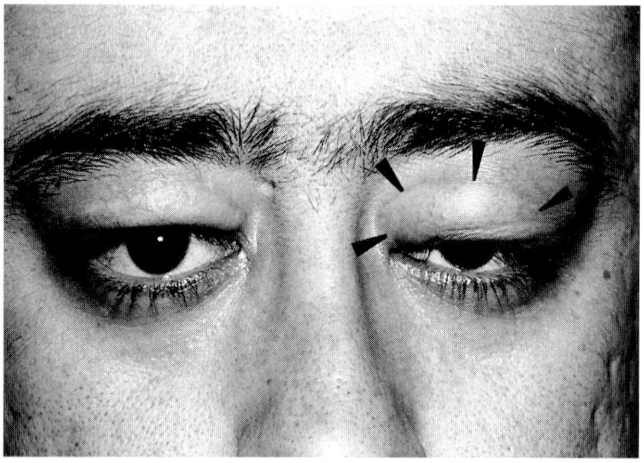

Figure 82–19. A typical large, smooth, shiny yellow plaque (*arrowheads*) in the upper eyelids of a patient with orbital xanthogranuloma.

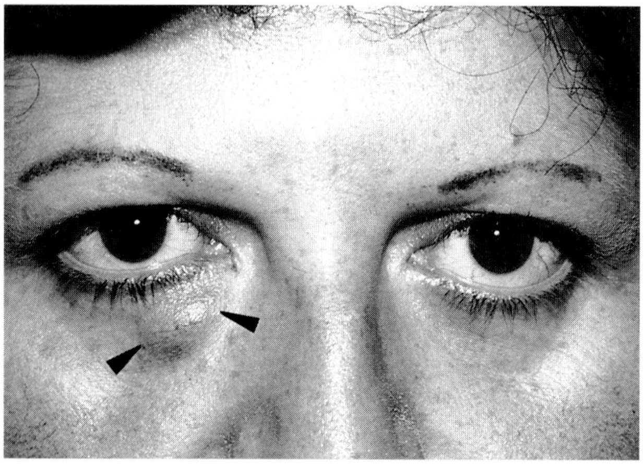

Figure 82–20. The purple coloration and soft texture of the lower eyelid mass (*arrowheads*) were typical of the anterior extension of primary orbital varices.

Tumors on the orbital floor often cause inferior scleral show, resulting from upward displacement of the globe or lower lid retraction, and a fullness of the lower eyelid sulcus (Fig. 82–21).

CHANGES IN PERIORBITAL FUNCTIONS AND PUPILLARY REFLEXES

Sensory nerves to the periorbital and eyelid skin pass through the extraconal orbital space or along the orbital floor, and orbital disease can impair sensory function by compression or infiltration of the nerves. Such impairment is, however, relatively rare. The function of these nerves should be tested, by use of standard clinical neurologic methods, and any asymmetry of the corneal sensory reflexes should be sought.

Examination of the lacrimal drainage system is imperative when disease effects the medial part of the orbit, and appropriate symptoms should be ascertained by direct questioning. Objective evidence is gained by the use of dye tests, diagnostic syringing, and dacryocystography.

Pupillomotor nerves pass through the ciliary ganglion and along the inferior division of the third cranial nerve. Damage to the orbital portion of the third cranial nerve may result in a pupillary dilation or a sectoral (vermiform) contraction of the pupil; the latter sign is best assessed with the aid of a slit-lamp biomicroscope.

EVIDENCE OF DISEASE WITHIN THE GLOBE

Examination of the globe can provide valuable evidence for the nature and extent of orbital disease, or it can prove intraocular disease to be the origin for orbital symptoms.

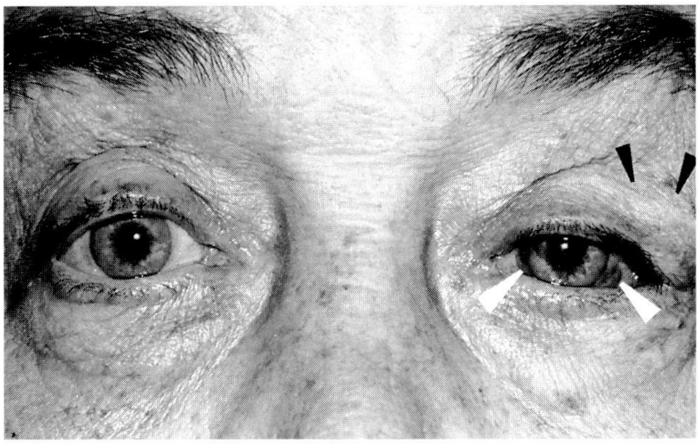

Figure 82–22. Orbital malignant melanoma (*black arrowheads*) in a patient with acquired conjunctival malanosis (*white arrowheads*).

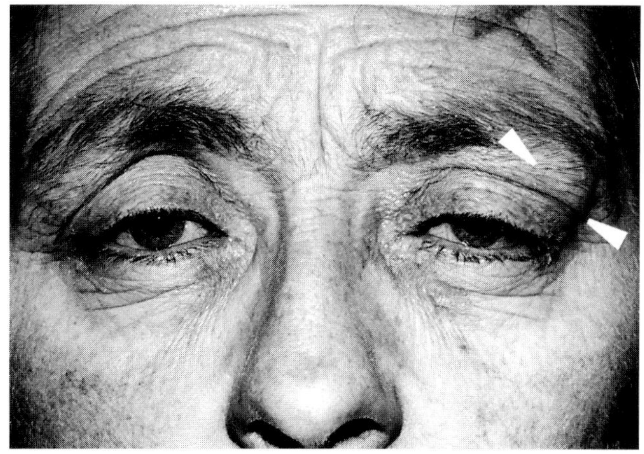

Figure 82–24. Left lacrimal gland lymphoma (*arrowheads*) in a patient with chronic Sjögren's syndrome.

The origin of orbital tumors should be sought specifically within the eyelids and within the structures of the globe. The conjunctiva and episclera may display melanosis (Fig. 82–22), invasive melanoma (Fig. 82–23), or other epithelial malignancies. Keratoconjunctivitis sicca may be the result of chronic dacryoadenitis, and lacrimal gland lymphoma is a known risk for patients with Sjögren's syndome (Fig. 82–24). Similarly, small primary uveal melanomas may present with orbital invasion; therefore, thorough examination of the fundus through a dilated pupil is mandatory. A diagnosis of neurofibromatosis is suggested by the presence of Lisch nodules of the iris.

Choroidal striae or visible indentation of the posterior segment may indicate compression of the globe by an orbital mass, either discrete or diffuse (Fig. 82–25); choroidal striae can, however, occur with small meningiomas of the optic nerve or in the absence of orbital disease. Dilation of episcleral veins, which indicates raised pressure in the orbital venous system, may have an acute presentation (Fig. 82–26) or may follow a more indolent course (Fig. 82–27); raised orbital venous pressure results from compression of posterior orbital veins (by an orbital mass) or from an arteriovenous communication, either intraorbital or intracranial. Secondary venous dilation should be readily distinguished from primary orbital varices, which often cause symptoms by subconjunctival

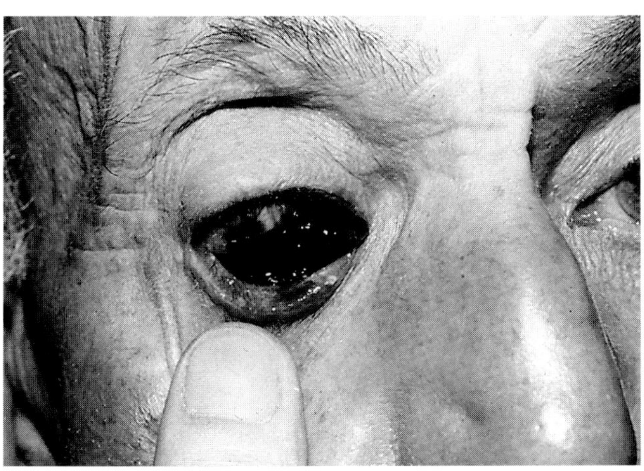

Figure 82–23. Conjunctival melanoma invading the orbit and eyelid.

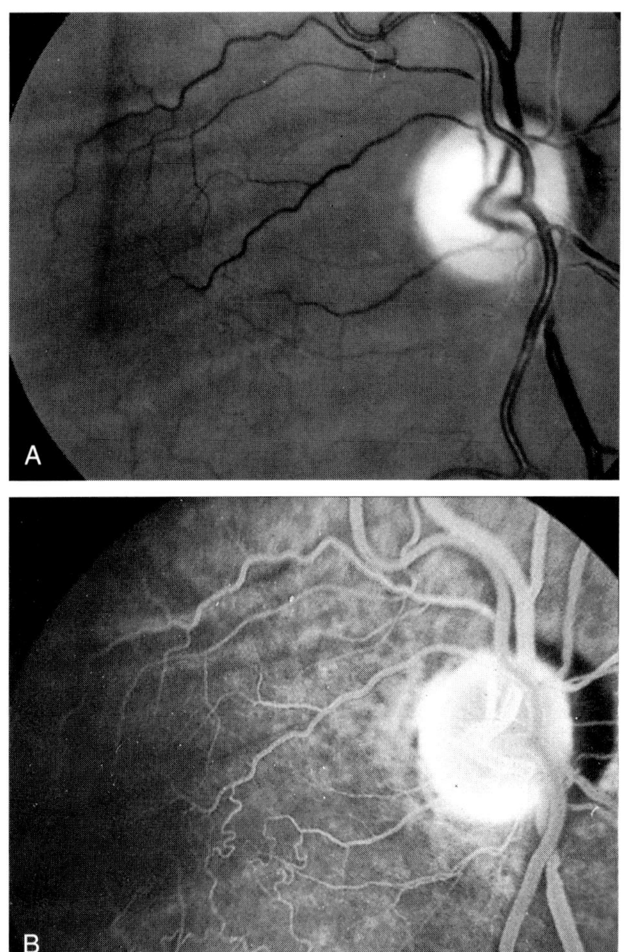

Figure 82–25. Red-free fundus photograph (*A*) and fluorescein angiogram (*B*) showing macular choroidal striae secondary to an orbital mass.

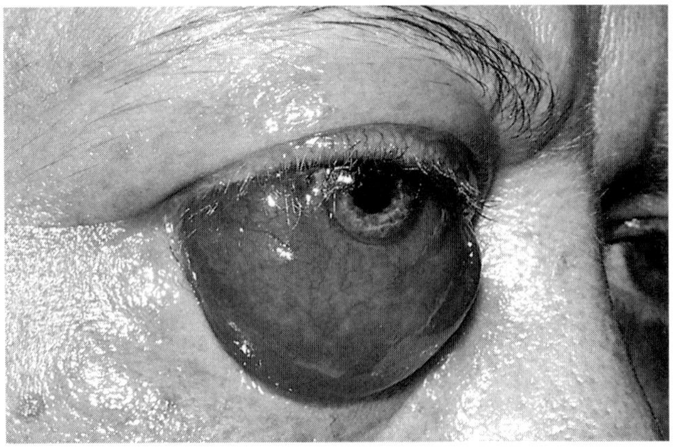

Figure 82–26. Gross chemosis with prolapse of the lower fornix, caused by the acute onset of a carotid cavernous fistula.

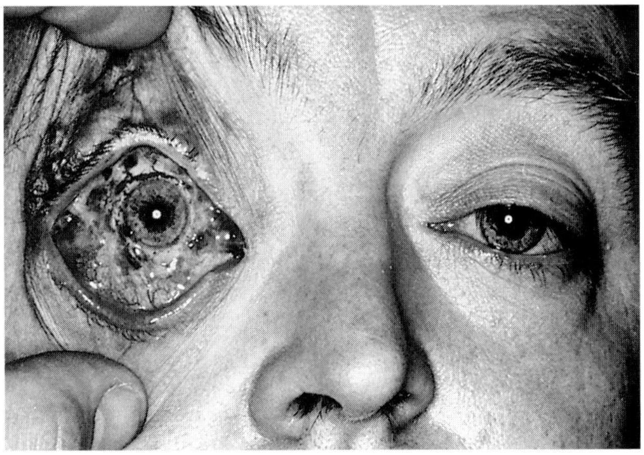

Figure 82–28. Widespread primary orbital varices affecting the eyelids, conjunctiva, episclera, and deep orbital tissues.

extension (Fig. 82–28) and can rarely involve the intraocular vasculature (Fig. 82–29).

Compression of posterior orbital tissues is associated with engorgement of retinal venules, loss of the spontaneous pulsation of the central retinal vein, partial blurring of the optic disc margins, or even frank papilledema; all of these signs should be accurately assessed, particularly the degree of asymmetry between the two sides. With longstanding optic nerve compression, papilledema may progress to optic atrophy and the development of optociliary shunt vessels (Fig. 82–30).

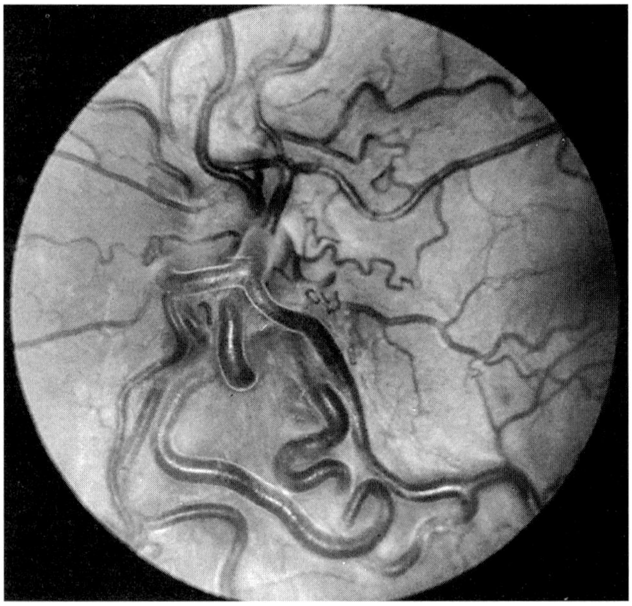

Figure 82–29. Congenitally abnormal fundal vessels may rarely be associated with orbital vascular anomalies.

EVIDENCE OF SYSTEMIC DISEASE AND PERIORBITAL INJURY

Systemic signs can support or refute a provisional diagnosis based on orbital and ocular examination and should form part of the routine clinical investigation of patients with orbital disease.

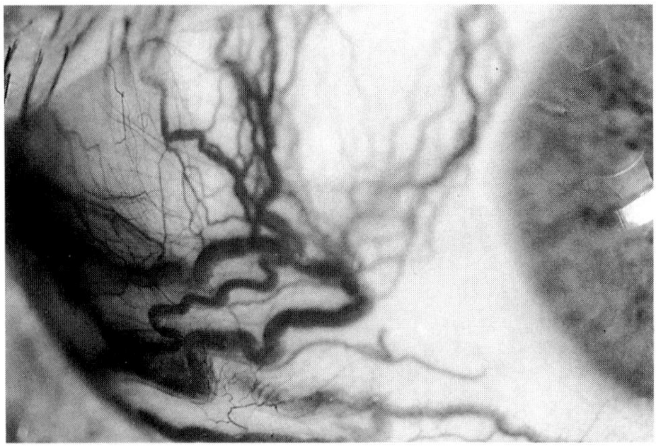

Figure 82–27. Low-flow dural arteriovenous shunt causing dilated and tortuous episcleral veins in the absence of chemosis.

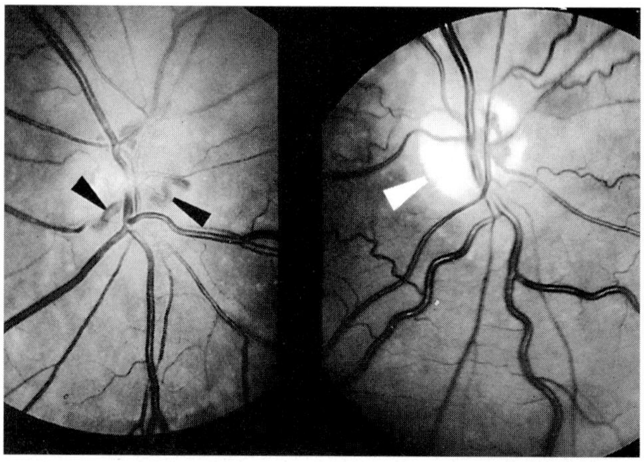

Figure 82–30. Optociliary shunt vessels (*black arrowheads*) and marked optic atrophy (*white arrowhead*) in a patient with bilateral optic nerve meningioma.

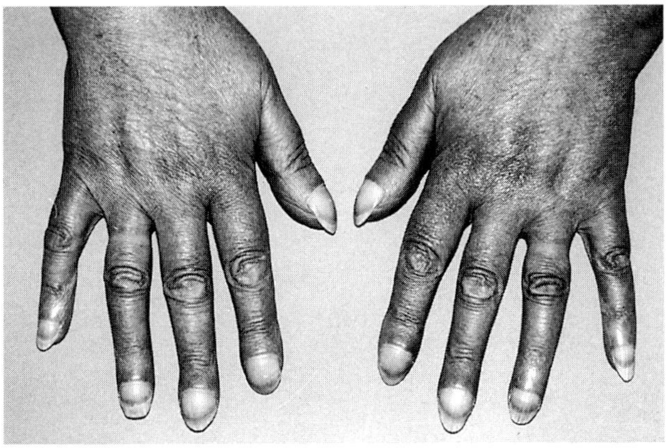

Figure 82–31. Thyroid acropachy in a thyrotoxic patient; acropachy is characterized by clubbing and the development of tight and shiny skin on the dorsum of the fingers.

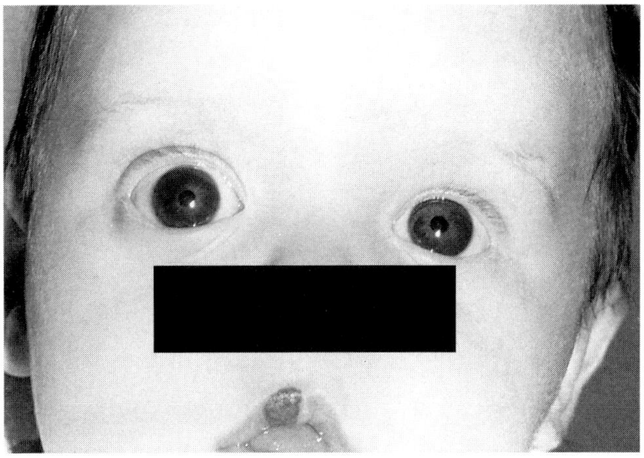

Figure 82–33. The "strawberry nevus" on the right half of the upper lip strongly suggests a diagnosis of orbital capillary hemangioma causing the right proptosis.

The neurologic and cardiologic signs of the hyperthyroid or hypothyroid state should be sought in patients with signs of dysthyroid orbitopathy; evidence of a goiter, thyroid acropachy (Fig. 82–31), or pretibial myxedema may also be present.

In patients with an orbital mass, clinical assessment should particularly include examination of the nasopharynx, paranasal sinuses, mouth (Fig. 82–32), skin (Fig. 82–33), major lymph nodes, abdomen (Fig. 82–34), neck, and breasts. Examination may indicate an underlying cause, such as neurofibromatosis (Fig. 82–35) or sarcoidosis (Fig. 82–36), or may reveal a primary or multifocal malignancy, such as lymphoma. Other systemic signs of malignancy, such as neurologic degenerations or clubbing (Fig. 82–37), should be noted.

After trauma, systemic injury should be ruled out. The clinical examination may then be directed toward the assessment of visual function, especially acuity and the presence of an RAPD, and the ocular movements; restriction of ductions may conform to a mechanical or a neurologic pattern. Displaced fractures of the orbital margin or zygoma are generally visible, and palpable discontinuities may be present in the bones. Blow-out fractures of the orbital floor frequently cause infraorbital neuropraxia, manifested as reduced ipsilateral cutaneous sensation in the upper lip and cheek. After trauma, visible subconjunctival emphysema (Fig. 82–38) suggests fracture of the orbital walls involving, most commonly, the maxillary or ethmoid sinuses.

In patients with signs of orbital inflammation or abscess, a particular search should be made for a previous breach of periorbital skin. At the time of injury, the unrecognized entrance of a foreign body may have occurred, and some patients dismiss or forget a previous injury that may have occurred months before (Fig. 82–39).

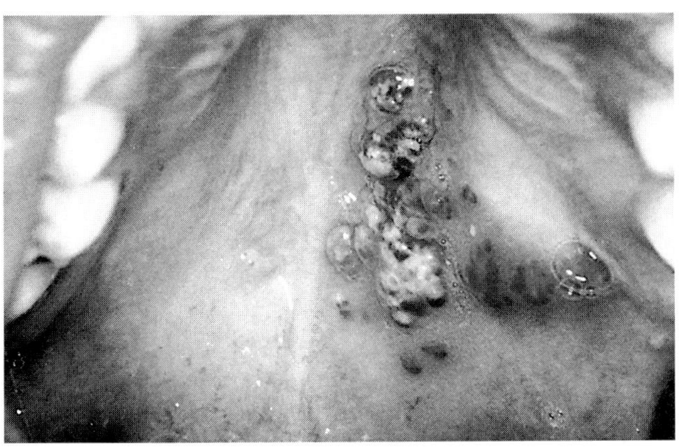

Figure 82–32. Varices on the left half of the hard palate in a patient with primary varices in the left orbit and maxilla.

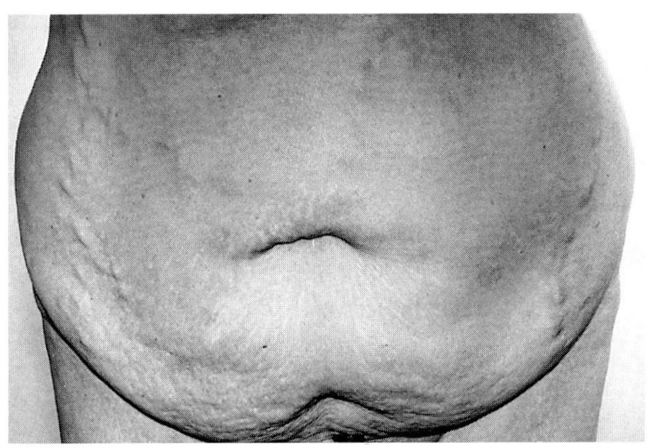

Figure 82–34. Hepatomegaly and markedly dilated abdominal veins (due to inferior vena caval thrombosis) provide evidence of disseminated malignancy in a patient with an orbital tumor.

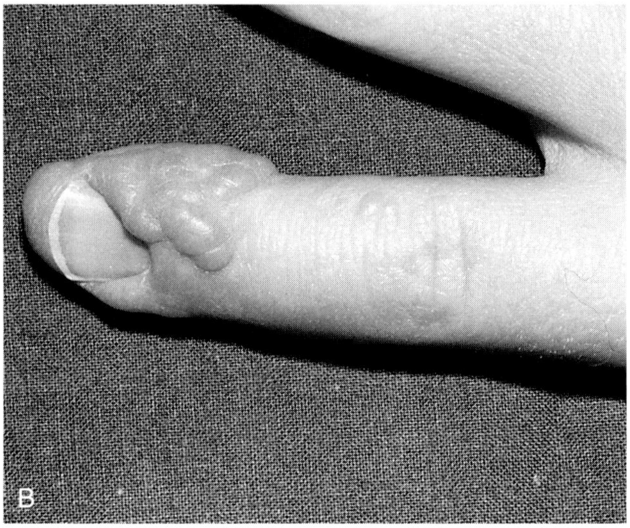

Figure 82–35. Systemic signs of neurofibromatosis may include café-au-lait spots or widespread cutaneous freckles (*A*) and periungual, or other, neurofibromas (*B*).

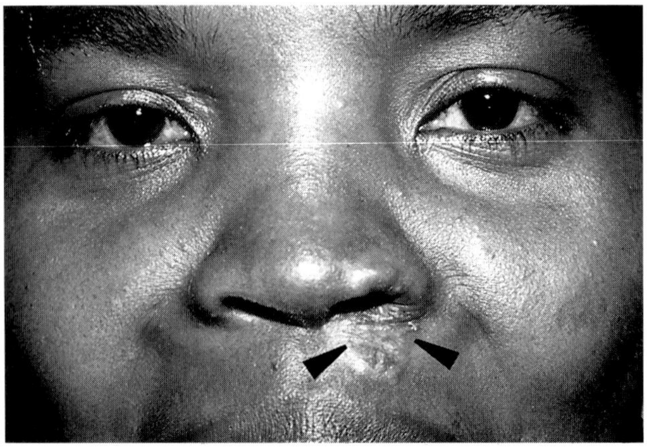

Figure 82–36. Bilateral lacrimal gland enlargement due to sarcoid may be associated with cutaneous sarcoid infiltration (*arrows*).

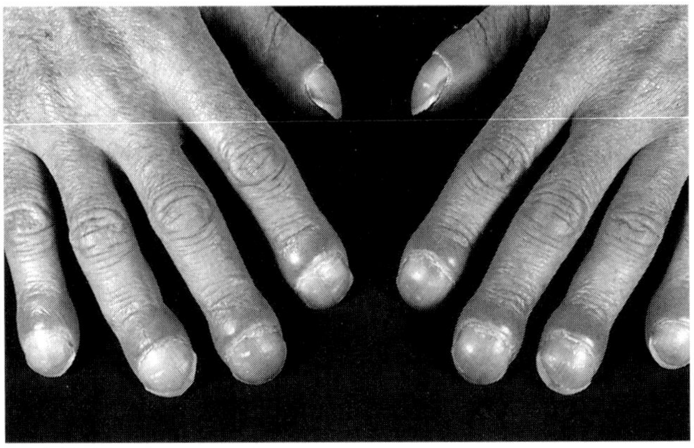

Figure 82–37. Gross clubbing in a patient with orbital metastases from a bronchogenic carcinoma.

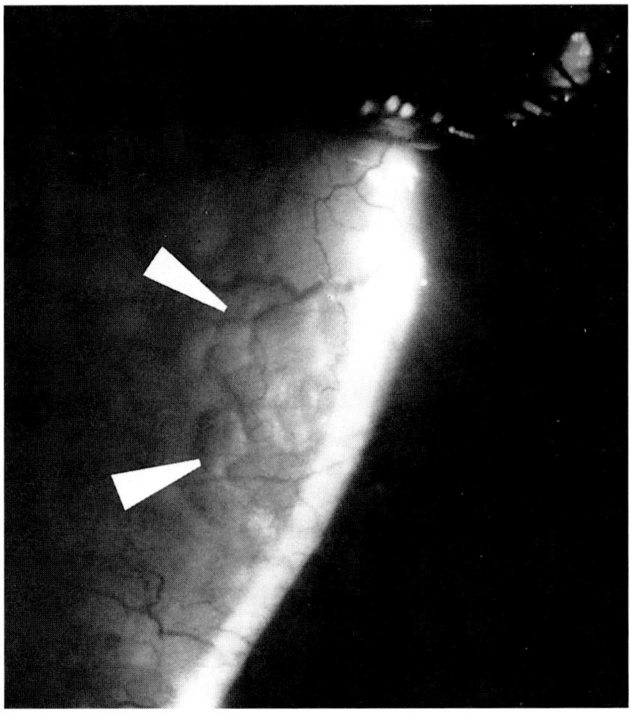

Figure 82–38. Subconjunctival emphysema (*arrows*) due to a blowout fracture of the ethmoidal sinuses.

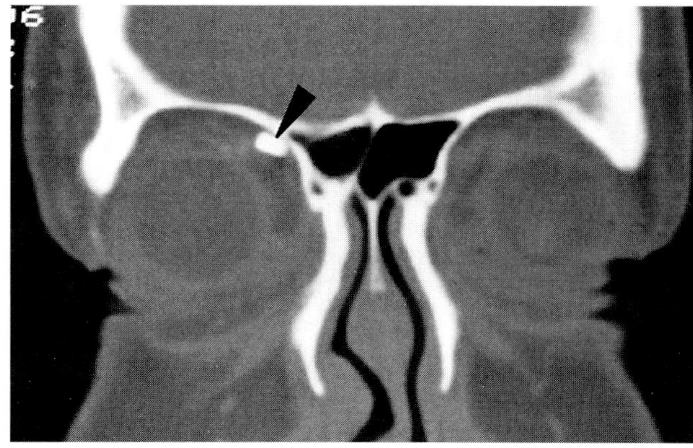

Figure 82–39. Unrecognized epitrochlear foreign body (glass) in a patient presenting late after a vehicular accident.

CHAPTER 83

Neuro-ophthalmic Considerations in Orbital Disease

Marian Rubenfeld and Jonathan D. Wirtschafter

The anatomic contiguity and functional integration of orbital structures with the nervous system requires that the adept clinician master concepts of neuro-ophthalmic diagnosis and localization. The current expansion and refinement of optic nerve sheath fenestration techniques to treat pseudotumor cerebri most dramatically underscores this point. Endoscopic decompression of the optic canal for traumatic optic neuropathy is also an emerging technique, and extended orbital decompression requires similar knowledge.

The purpose of this chapter is to reacquaint the clinician with techniques of neuro-ophthalmic assessment that are particularly useful for interpreting the signs and symptoms of orbital disease. It also discusses these signs and symptoms, localization of lesions, and particular clinical entities that encompass the realms of both orbit and neuro-ophthalmology. These latter topics are those that have received emphasis in the recent ophthalmic and neurologic literature and should be helpful to the clinician. For practical purposes, given the nature of this volume, the chapter covers disease to the level of the optic chiasm.

CLINICAL METHODS OF ASSESSMENT

Status of Optic Nerve Function

Visual Acuity

The commonest first approach for discerning the level of optic nerve function is the Snellen visual acuity chart. However, other techniques are available that can provide more information.

Contrast sensitivity testing is a much more sensitive and quantitative mode for appreciating optic nerve dysfunction than the Snellen chart. The test may reveal that the functional channels carrying specific ranges of spatial frequencies are faulty. The test can be performed with charts either at distance from or near the patient (Fig. 83–1). The patient's best refraction is required to optimize results, so that refractive blur is not confused with optic nerve disease. The test is simple to administer and requires only about 5 minutes to complete. Several systems are currently available; they require uniformity of testing conditions (e.g., lighting levels) during sequential tests for the results to be meaningful. This method is so sensitive that we have even been able to detect defects so subtle that threshold perimetry was unable to detect them. One caveat is that contrast sensitivity testing is necessarily subjective; results of testing in those in whom hysteria or malingering is suspected must be viewed with due caution.

Finally, the visually evoked potential test is available, both in flash and checkerboard pattern form. The former does not require assiduous cooperation on the part of the patient, whereas the latter does. Thus, the pattern visually evoked potential test may not be the wisest choice if one is testing a patient in whom malingering or hysteria is suspected, despite its potential for visual acuity determination. In most patients with orbital disease, resorting to these techniques is rarely necessary; contrast sensitivity is usually adequate.

Color and Brightness Saturation

Appreciation of color desaturation in the absence of fundal lesions is often an early and prominent sign of optic nerve dysfunction. This problem is particularly marked in detection of the color red, which is often more profoundly depressed than the Snellen acuity would have predicted. In other words, although the patient may have a Snellen acuity of 20/25 or even 20/20, he or she may have pronounced red desaturation. This effect is a hallmark of optic nerve dysfunction. Assessment of this problem is most frequently performed by presenting a red bottle cap to the eyes in succession and asking if significant wash-out is notable. It is often useful to attempt to quantitate degree of wash-out; we suggest percentages to the patient, calling the red perceived by the unaffected eye "100% red." During the course of recovery, the clinician may follow the improvement of red desaturation along with other parameters. This desaturation is relative; damage to both optic nerves may cause the patient to deny having desaturation.

A similar technique would be the brightness desaturation assessment, in which the patient compares the in-

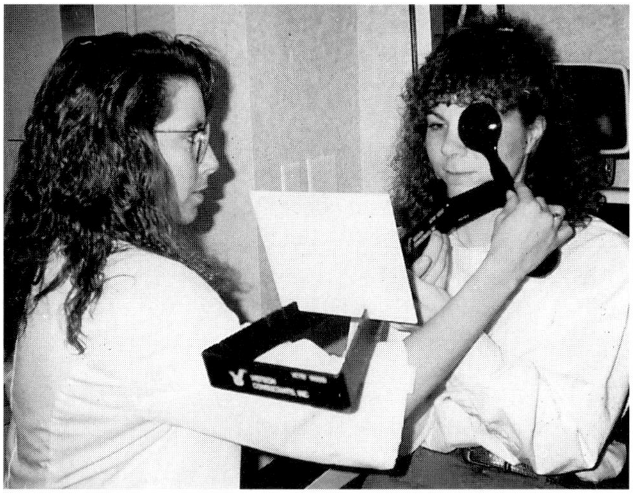

Figure 83–1. Technique for determining contrast sensitivity near the patient. The patient should be wearing the appropriate near-vision correction, and lighting should be standardized, for maximal reproducibility.

tensity of light perceived in the two eyes. This test could be combined with the macular light stress test, to help differentiate optic nerve disease from subtle retinal dysfunction. Here, the clinician records the best corrected visual acuity for each eye, shines a bright light (e.g., a direct ophthalmoscope or a muscle light) in each eye for 30 seconds, and notes the time in seconds required by each eye to recover to one line less than the previously recorded acuities. Prolongation of recovery time beyond the normal 45 to 50 seconds, especially if recovery is asymmetric, suggests retinal disease. Retinal disease is also suggested if the patient has a lengthy delay between reading of successive lines of the acuity chart.

An important caveat should be noted here. In the aforementioned assessments, the clinician should be aware of the issue of ocular dominance. Many people have a markedly dominant eye, usually the same side as their handedness. The dominant eye sometimes perceives colors and brightness more intensely than does the other eye. For this reason, we require patients to tell us if a significant difference exists between the two eyes. If only a small difference exists, we check for ocular dominance as the reason. The easiest way to perform this check is to ask the patient to point with one finger at a small, distant object. Without moving the patient's hand, we cover the suspected dominant eye. The patient then reports that he or she is no longer pointing directly at the target; had the other eye been covered, the pointing finger would still seem to be directly on the target.

Ophthalmoscopy

It is always essential to examine the appearance of the optic nerve head when its competence is in question. Some processes do not produce a notable change in the nerve head, such as retrobulbar optic neuritis, posterior ischemic optic neuropathy, or even early compression. However, many others deface the nerve head.

We consider evaluation of the nerve by indirect ophthalmoscopy to be inadequate. The direct ophthalmoscope provides a highly magnified view but cannot add accurate stereopsis to the view. We currently prefer to use either a 78- or 90-diopter hand-held lens at the slit lamp to examine the nerve head (Fig. 83–2). The 78-diopter lens provides more magnification than does the 90 diopter, albeit with less surrounding field. It is also easier to handle than the smaller, 90-diopter lens. Both of these lenses afford an easy evaluation of such attributes as cupping, slope, color of the neuroretinal rim, nerve fiber layer edema, hemorrhage depth, and choroidal folds.

Visual Fields

The art and science of topographic identification of lesions in the visual pathway are extensive subjects that are encyclopedically treated elsewhere.[1] For our purposes, we briefly describe helpful techniques and later describe the nature of defects that are able to be localized to the region from the optic disc to the chiasm.

Confrontation visual fields are crude but often helpful, especially at the patient's bedside. They are most accurately performed by moving the fingers or hands because kinetic targets are more readily seen than static ones. This technique can be enhanced by the addition of the red bottle cap; this combination can be particularly useful when hemianopic or quadrantic defects are being sought. The clinician applies the concept of red desaturation to the various portions of the visual field and ascertains whether a marked difference in the perception of red exists, for example, on either side of the vertical meridian.

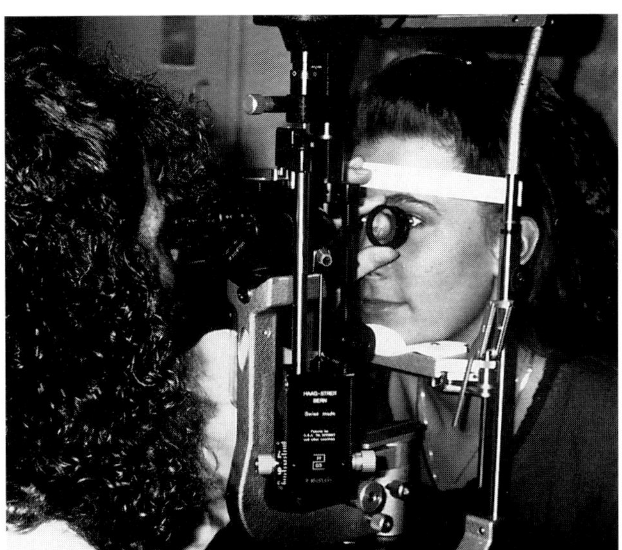

Figure 83–2. Use of the 78-diopter lens at the slit lamp.

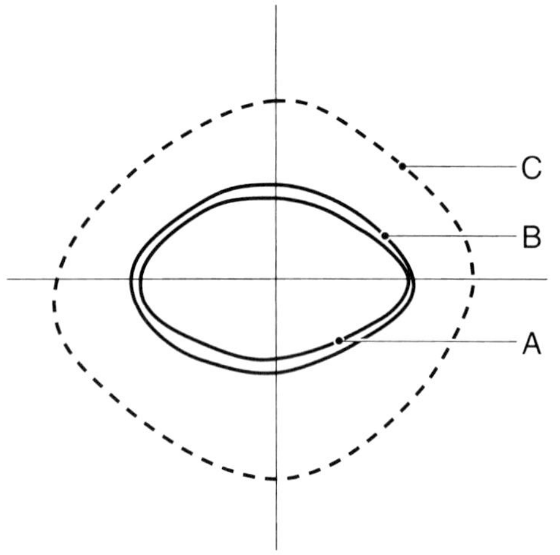

Figure 83–3. Nonphysiologic, hysterical visual fields. The isopter marked A was determined at the tangent screen with a 2-mm white target at a 1-meter testing distance. Isopter B was obtained with a 4-mm white target at 2 meters. The two isopters are collapsed down on one another, the so-called tubular visual field. A normal response to the 4-mm target is shown by dashed isopter C, which should almost double in size the area demarcated by isopter A.

The tangent screen visual field is useful for the detection of defects within 30 degrees of fixation and is invaluable in the detection of malingering or hysteria. The visual field is assessed with a 2-mm white target with the patient 1 meter away from the screen, and then with a 4-mm white target with the patient 2 meters away. If the resultant fields are tubular and superimposable, the diagnosis is a truly nonphysiologic field (Fig. 83–3). The normal result is a not-quite doubling of the 2-mm field with the 4-mm/2-m set-up. We find it helpful, if we suspect either hysteria or malingering, to point out to the patient the circles of eccentricity sewn into the standard tangent field that we use as an aid to our plotting the field. The patient may then use these landmarks too, making the task simple.

Automated perimetry is now the predominant technique for examining the visual field. It relies on the principle of static-kinetic dissociation to identify focal depressions in afferent visual function. However, the Goldmann perimeter still has many uses, even in the age of the automated perimeter. Many patients demonstrate a so-called rim effect with the automated perimeters that can easily be confused with arcuate defects. The Goldmann perimeter can more accurately determine if these are truly arcuate effects. Additionally, the Goldmann perimeter can rapidly screen for the inferonasal isopter constriction, which is characteristic of the visual loss of papilledema. Examining this region selectively is not convenient with automated perimetry, and a 30- to 60-degree program adds substantially to test time, subject fatigue, and, hence, the clinician's insecurity about data so collected.

Because automated perimeters are vastly preferred today, not only because of their excellent sensitivity but also because of the incontrovertible fact that less skill is necessary to operate them than the Goldmann, the user must recall the rim effect and attempt to overcome it. The effect may be overcome in many ways: use a set of trial lenses that have little or no metal rims around the lenses; make sure that the trial lens holder is as close to the patient's eye as possible during the test; chart the 30- to 60-degree field if a rim effect may be occurring; and finally, be aware that the tubular hysterical or malingering field can be mistaken for a double arcuate—correlate your clinical impressions with the print-out of the automated perimeter.

Assessment of Pupillary Function

Because the components of the automatic nervous system controlling pupillary size traverse the orbital cavity, orbital disease frequently results in abnormalities of pupillary function. Many techniques are helpful in ascertaining such problems.

Pupils are best tested in the semidilated state; hence, dim room lighting is best. The examiner should have some method of ensuring that the same degree of illumination is used for prepharmacologic and postpharmacologic testing. The most important pupillary test for the assessment of orbital disorders is that for the afferent pupillary defect, or the Marcus Gunn pupil. The clinician should use a bright flashlight to perform the swinging flashlight test; many clinicians have missed subtle afferent pupillary defects by testing with a direct ophthalmoscope emitting a dim, yellowed light. The patient should be directed to gaze at a distant target to control for accommodation. The light is held in front of and slightly below the pupillary axis of one eye for 2 to 3 seconds, and then quickly transferred to a similar position in front of the contralateral eyes. No relative change should occur in overall pupillary size. Younger subjects may demonstrate hippus, or oscillatory pupillary unrest, that should not be confused with an afferent pupillary defect. The development of an afferent pupillary defect where heretofore none existed in an orbital condition reflects an increase in pressure on the optic nerve and may be an indication for surgery.

In our society, many of the elderly have had cataract surgery performed, or some trauma or intraocular disease may have contributed to an irregular or immobile pupil. In this case, the reverse Marcus Gunn effect can be elicited: a beam of light is shone into the reactive eye first, and then into the other eye. The first eye is observed: if the contralateral eye is normal, not much change will occur, but if it is damaged, the first pupil will dilate (Fig. 83–4). The presence of an afferent pupillary defect does not explain an anisocoria; generally, anisocoria of greater than 1.5 mm is suggestive of pathologic (versus physiologic) anisocoria.

If pupils do not seem very reactive to the light, light-near dissociation should be evaluated. In this assessment,

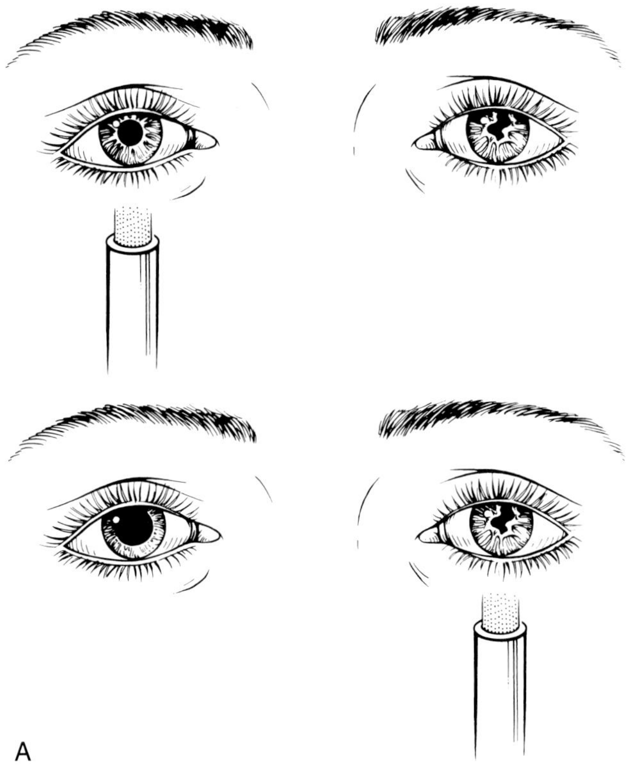

A

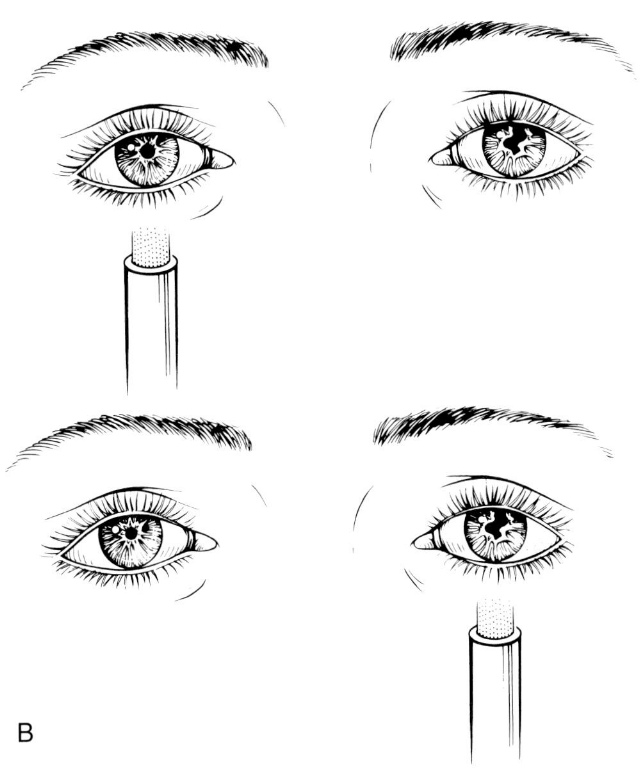

B

Figure 83–4. The reverse Marcus Gunn pupil. This test is crucial for detecting an afferent pupillary defect when the patient has one pupil that does not respond normally (e.g., from trauma, cataract surgery). After shining the light stimulus into the eye with the normal pupil, quickly shine it into the other eye. If the second eye, with the defective iris, has an afferent defect, the pupil of the first eye will *dilate* (*A*). If the first eye had an afferent defect, the first eye's pupil will not *constrict* as the second eye is illuminated (*B*).

the patient focuses on an accommodative target nearby. This test determines whether the near reflex is intact.

Orbital damage may cause a tonic, or Adie's pupil. This effect is more frequently noted in young women and is thought to be of viral origin. However, if orbital disease damages the ciliary body, Adie's pupil may result. This pupil is more dilated than the other, reacts tonically, and the iris may demonstrate vermiform movements when it is examined with a narrow beam at the slit lamp. The pharmacologic test can be performed by diluting 1% pilocarpine to ⅛% with sterile saline or artificial tear solution, and checking for denervation hypersensitivity in the affected eye. A normal eye does not constrict when exposed to ⅛% pilocarpine, whereas one with an Adie's pupil does.

Orbital disease may also cause an acquired postganglionic Horner's syndrome. The clinical presentation of miosis and ptosis may suggest such a diagnosis; anhydrosis is not found in orbital Horner's syndrome. Sympathetic anisocoria is accentuated and is thus best observed in a dark or dimly lit room. If Horner's syndrome is suspected, it should first be confirmed by the use of 4% to 10% cocaine drops; the clinician should wait 60 minutes after the drops are administered before gauging the full effect. A positive test result consists of the suspected pupil failing to dilate. The next test, the hydroxyamphetamine test, must be performed on a different day. If Horner's syndrome is known to be present, the cocaine test can be deleted altogether, and the hydroxyamphetamine test can be performed on the first examination. In the case of postganglionic Horner's syndrome, the suspected pupil does not dilate. Although hydroxyamphetamine was not available in the United States for a time recently, it is now being produced again, owing to its status as an orphan drug.

The combined presence of postganglionic sympathetic paresis and oculomotor nerve palsy causes a fixed, mid-position pupil that neither dilates to dark nor constricts to light. Such cases are almost always the result of disease at the orbital apex or within the cavernous sinus, as is discussed later.

Assessment of Cranial Nerves III, IV, and VI: Motility Disorders

The control of the extraocular muscles is through cranial nerves III, IV, and VI. Orbital disease frequently causes derangement of oculomotility, through interference either with the cranial nerves or with the muscles themselves. Hence, the clinician must become proficient in tests of oculomotility.

First, the clinician examines ductions, movements of one eye, then versions, with both eyes attempting a conjugate gaze. The eyes are examined in all six cardinal positions of gaze. In each of these positions, one extraocular muscle is predominantly responsible for the position of the eye. Hering's law of motor correspondance states that yoke muscles receive equal and simultaneous innervation. This effect is the basis of observing for secondary deviation while having the paretic eye fixate. In that case, the nonparetic eye will overact, which may be more readily visible than the underaction of the paretic muscle otherwise.

In recent years, ophthalmic plastic surgeons have stressed the importance of Hering's law in the evaluation of eyelid position ("pseudoretraction" of the normal upper eyelid when ptosis of the contralateral lid is present). For example, excessive elevation of the left upper eyelid may result from (1) restrictive myopathy of the right inferior rectus muscle, (2) paresis of the right superior rectus muscle, and (3) paresis of the right levator palpebrae superioris muscle. Recognition of these conditions can contribute to a more successful surgical result in conditions such as Graves' ophthalmopathy.

The examiner should make use of the cover-uncover test to distinguish between tropias and phorias, and the alternate cover test to quantitate the deviations horizontally. Similarly assessing for a vertical malalignment is difficult unless the malalignment is a large one; the Maddox rod is much more useful in these cases. The Maddox rod is a red glass with high-power parallel cylinders placed adjacent to each other (Fig. 83–5). It generates an image of a red line that is oriented perpendicularly to the direction of the cylinder axis. Although it does not distinguish between phorias and tropias, it is invaluable for detecting and quantifying the vertical deviation with

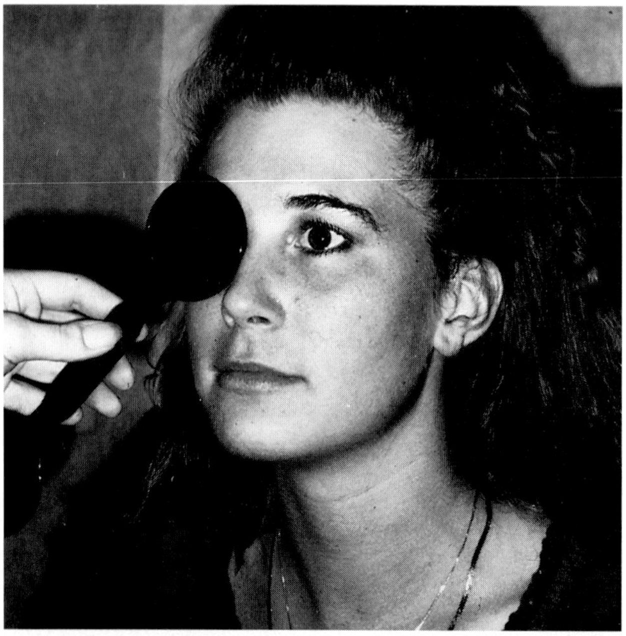

Figure 83–5. Use of the Maddox rod. In this situation, the rod is positioned to seek a vertical malalignment, with its parallel cylinders oriented vertically. Horizontal malalignment can be determined with the cylinders placed horizontally, although other techniques are superior for assessing horizontal malalignment (see text).

prisms. The double Maddox rod test is used to quantitate torsional deviations that accompany vertical strabismus. Most present-day phoropters contain both a white and red Maddox rod. The line images they create can be separated by inducing a few diopters of vertical prism, and the patient then aligns the two lines so that they are parallel. One may then read off the dial to determine the direction and degrees of torsional malalignment.

The doll's head reflex, or oculocephalic maneuver, is helpful in adults as well as infants. With the patient fixating on a target, the head is moved horizontally and vertically. The eyes should move in a direction opposite to that in which the head is turning. With infants, the examiner should hold the baby and spin appropriately. Caloric tests are not normally applied in patients with orbital disease. Furthermore, the head movements employed in oculocephalics are contraindicated in cases of trauma, in which they may actually be dangerous. These movements are reserved for assessment of paresis in nontraumatic instances.

If a paretic muscle is identified, forced ductions and force generations should be performed in the physician's office. Application of a cocaine-soaked pledget over the affected muscle for 5 minutes allows even the squeamish patient to be examined. For forced ductions, the patient should direct his or her gaze toward the field of action of the paretic muscle. The clinician uses toothed forceps to grasp not only the conjunctiva but also the underlying episcleral tissue; the clinician then tugs in the same direction. Grasping in this fashion reduces the risk of conjunctival laceration and bleeding, but the patient should be forewarned that some degree of bruising may be unavoidable. Restriction is easily appreciated, as in the case of dysthyroid ophthalmopathy or orbital fractures.

For force-generation testing, the patient gazes away from the presumed paretic field, and the clinician grasps the tissue overlying the muscle insertion and then asks the patient to look in the paretic direction. The clinician should appreciate a tug denoting the muscle activity, unless it is totally paralyzed. This tug can then be compared with that produced by the same muscle in the contralateral eye. It is important to distinguish the paretic muscle from the restricted muscle; the same condition may produce both problems, as in an orbital fracture. Entrapment of an extraocular muscle is necessarily treated differently than a paretic extraocular muscle. Entrapment and paresis may coexist after an orbital floor fracture. Late changes after surgical intervention to release tissues are most likely paretic.

The examiner should check saccadic and pursuit movements, especially in patients with such disorders as ocular myasthenia. Good use is made here of an opticokinetic nystagmus tape or drum (Fig. 83–6). Associated lid status, pain, and head turns and tilts all are important. Combining all the aforementioned techniques should allow a clear delineation of the nature and extent of the cranial nerve or oculomotility problem.

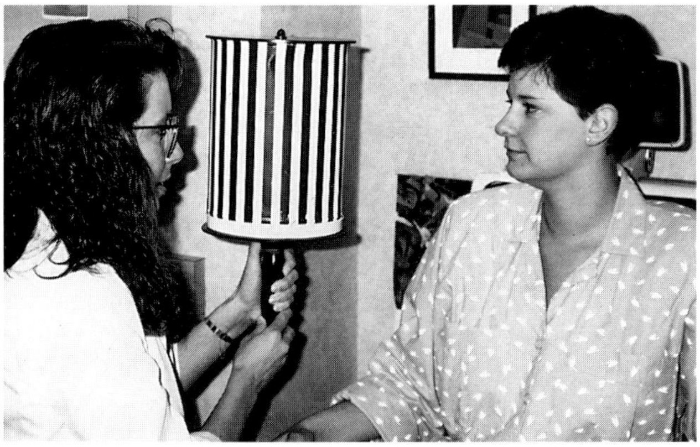

Figure 83–6. Use of the opticokinetic drum, testing horizontal saccadic and pursuit movement. Changing the orientation of the drum 90 degrees allows testing of vertical saccades and pursuit.

Assessment of Trigeminal Function

All branches of the trigeminal nerve pass through the cavernous sinus, and the first division branch enters the orbit through the superior orbital fissure. Thus, orbital and periorbital disease may produce derangement of the function of this cranial nerve as well.

Pain is a common symptom in orbital disorders and can also appear as a result of processes located in areas as diffuse as the cranial cavity, the cervical spine, and the occipital nerves. Pain (especially pain on movement of the globe) is a presenting symptom in almost all cases of optic neuritis, so this symptom does not serve to differentiate demyelinating from other inflammatory disorders. The absence of pain when it might be expected is usually a sign of carcinomatous infiltration of the sensory nerves. Involvement of the lacrimal nerve by adenocystic carcinoma of the lacrimal gland can cause acceleration of symptoms. Finally, when an abducens palsy is complicated by pain or anesthesia of the maxillary nerve, one should be suspicious of tumor infiltration from the posterior nasopharynx into the inferior portion of the cavernous sinus.

The three divisions of the trigeminal nerve should thus be tested for integrity of cutaneous sensation. Although one can assess also for temperature, clinical testing for touch and pain usually suffices and is more expeditious. A cotton-tipped applicator is used to gently stroke the face on either side of the midline in the distributions of V, branches 1 to 3. The patient is asked to report any substantial difference in sensation. Then, the applicator stick is broken in two, and a sharply pointed edge is used to test for pain in a similar manner.

Finally, corneal sensation to touch is assessed. Many clinicians have invented esoteric gadgets, such as the aesthesiometer, to quantitate this sensation. Especially in these days of human immunodeficiency virus infection, we prefer to use an easily disposable system that does not require laborious sterilization procedures (Fig. 83–7). The terminal cotton from a cotton-tipped applicator is twisted into a short but sturdy wick. The clinician prepares the patient by explaining that he or she will not be hurt; the patient is then instructed to look away from the initial test site. The testing is begun in the temporal bulbar conjunctiva, and the wick is slowly dragged toward and then onto the cornea. The patient is asked to indicate when he or she feels the wick touch the eye. Frequently, the clinician must rely on nonverbal signs of perception, such as blinking of the eyelids or aversive movements of the head. The clinician can get an estimate of sensitivity by noting the millimeters of excursion onto the cornea necessary to evoke a response. The same quadrants should be tested in each eye because sensitivity varies

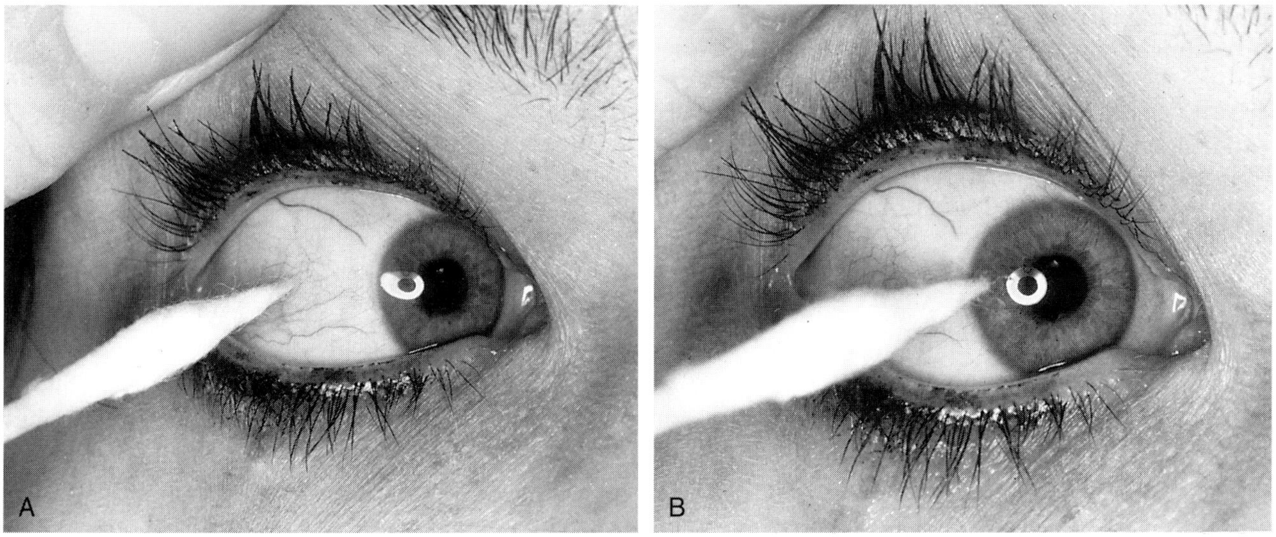

Figure 83–7. Testing of corneal sensation. The patient gazes away from the stimulus to avoid withdrawal reflex. Begin as in A, a few millimeters away from the corneoscleral limbus, and slowly and gently drag the stimulus toward the limbus. A blink is normally elicited at or near the limbus, or the patient can note the onset of sensation verbally. Multiple corneal axes can thus be quickly assessed for trigeminal nerve function.

geographically. The central cornea is more sensitive than the peripheral cornea, and the area around the horizontal meridian is more sensitive than that around the vertical meridian. The clinician should also be alert to reasons for focal areas of decreased sensation, such as herpes zoster infection, past or present. Short-latency somatosensory evoked potentials can now be assessed,[2] but such physiologic esoterica is seldom necessary for the screening of orbital disease.

Because posterior orbital disease frequently may extend to the cavernous sinus, motor function as well as sensory function should be assessed. Having the patient exert forceful jaw closure tests the integrity of the masseter and temporal muscles; asking the patient to alternately deviate the jaw sideways tests the internal and external pterygoid muscles. Weakness of pterygoids causes weakness of deviation to the contralateral side.

LOCALIZATION OF DISEASE PROCESSES

Perturbation of Acuity or Visual Field

A loss in visual acuity limits the pathologic process to a prechiasmal position, except when both occipital lobes are damaged. If loss of acuity exists, one should ascertain whether an afferent pupillary defect, color or brightness desaturation, and contrast sensitivity loss are also present. Ophthalmoscopy should be performed to look for signs of optic nerve swelling or atrophy. The presence of a unilateral swollen optic nerve head is a harbinger of orbital or unilateral optic nerve disease. Intracranial processes that ultimately produce raised intracranial pressure usually produce bilaterally swollen papillae. A famous exception to this is the Foster-Kennedy syndrome, wherein unilateral papilledema and contralateral optic atrophy exist. Today, most such presentations actually represent acute anterior ischemic optic neuropathy occurring in the second eye.

The presence of optociliary shunt vessels should also be sought ophthalmoscopically. These shunts from the retinal to the choroidal circulation are usually found after long-term compression of the optic nerve and central retinal vein (e.g., after central retinal vein occlusion). Shunts from the choroidal circulation to the retinal vessels are congenital variants and may be differentiated by fluorescein angiography.

Unilateral optic nerve head disc swelling may be seen in the absence of a decrease in vision, afferent pupillary defect, or color desaturation.[3] The presence of this condition would still indicate interference with the axoplasmic flow anterior to the lateral geniculate body.

The presence of intermittent visual loss localizes to the orbit if it is truly gaze evoked. In this case, blood flow obstruction is caused by the combination of a mass lesion and its compression of the optic nerve only when a particular gaze direction is employed. The commonest causes of such gaze-evoked amauroses are cavernous hemangiomas and optic nerve sheath meningiomas.[4] It is of course imperative to differentiate this condition from amaurosis fugax, which is not gaze or position dependent.

A comprehensive course on the topographic localization of visual field defects is beyond the scope of this chapter. However, several pertinent points should be made. First, attention should be directed to whether the field defects respect the vertical meridian. If so, a lesion at or posterior to the optic chiasm may be present. Orbital diseases produce defects including central, paracentral, arcuate, and altitudinal scotomas as well as enlargement of the blind spot. One must consider such entities as glaucoma, demyelinating disease, or vasculopathic causes before one concludes that the cause is an orbital process.

Pupillary Disturbances

The diagnoses of orbitally induced Adie's and Horner's pupils have already been discussed. A special note should be made of the case of the isolated sixth nerve palsy with ipsilateral Horner's syndrome. This condition usually indicates the presence of a lesion impinging on the sympathetic neurons as they leave the cavernous portion of the internal carotid artery to run briefly with the abducens nerve. If, however, a mass lesion increases in size, it eventually impinges on other constitutents of the cavernous sinus as well.

Disturbances of Oculomotility

Diplopia may be caused by interference with the innervation of the extraocular muscles or by physical impairment of the muscles themselves. Use of the techniques elaborated earlier will reveal whether one muscle or more are disabled. The use of forced ductions and force generations is then essential to seek signs of orbital pathology. Other clinical signs should also be sought, such as proptosis, orbital congestion, and pupillary abnormalities to aid localization. An increase in intraocular pressure on sustained upward gaze is valuable for detecting an increase in orbital restrictive disease; it is no longer considered pathognomonic of Graves' ophthalmopathy. Suspicion of orbital disease then warrants an imaging study to seek confirmation of the condition.

Proptosis, Enophthalmos, and Choroidal Folds

The development of absolute indices for the criteria for proptosis is difficult because the degree of protrusion of the globe in the orbit varies by gender as well as by race.[5] Although excursion of the eye more than 21 mm beyond the lateral orbital rims may be considered to denote proptosis, it is more helpful from the standpoint of orbital disease to seek signs of differential excursions of an individual's two eyes. Various forms of exophthalmometers exist to measure this effect; a rapid and surprisingly sensitive assessment can be performed by looking downward at the eyes from above the patient's head. A difference of excursion of more than 2 mm between the eyes is considered pathologic.

If a mass exists within the extraocular muscle cone, it usually produces an axial proptosis. Here, the globe is displaced straight ahead. Extraconal masses displace the globe in a direction opposite to the position they occupy.

Proptosis may be either constant or intermittent. The latter translates to a vascular or skeletal cause. For example, patients with neurofibrosis type I often display pulsatile proptosis owing to the agenesis of a portion of the sphenoid wing and contiguous bone. Finally, the clinician must be careful not to mistake eyelid retraction for true proptosis.

Enophthalmos is most associated with orbital fractures, especially with induced defects in the orbital floor. Acutely, the cause is herniation or entrapment of orbital contents into the defect. Whether, with time, atrophy of fat contributes to this effect is controversial. Insidious progressive enophthalmos in the absence of trauma should alert the clinician to the possibility of scirrhous carcinoma of the breast, both in females and in males.

The presence of choroidal folds may indicate pressure on the posterior portion of the globe by a mass lesion (Fig. 83–8). However, one must be aware that these lesions have been seen in diverse conditions, such as hypotony, epiretinal membranes, or intraocular inflammation, or after intraocular surgery. The combination of proptosis with choroidal folds is a hallmark of true orbital disease.

Localizing Neuro-ophthalmic Syndromes

This section is concerned mainly with conditions that invade or extend from the orbit via the optic canal or superior orbital fissure. We briefly discuss disorders that cause cranial contents to enter the orbits via other routes.

Optic Canal

Osteopetrosis can effect the optic canal's becoming inhospitable to the optic nerve because of progressive narrowing. Although the disorder has a wide spectrum of presentation,[6] the infantile form can cause blindness, deafness, even death. The optic canal can also become narrowed in the syndrome of fibrous dysplasia of bone. Thus, early surgical decompression may be essential to preserve structure and function.

Anterior visual pathway gliomas may subtly change the configuration of the optic canal. Thin-section axial computed tomographic scanning with bone windows are thus the optimal screen should this condition be suspected. Standard head scan angles are inadequate for diagnosis and may even miss large (1-cm) tumors. An anterior visual pathway glioma that begins in the chiasmal region may extend anteriorly to create a bullet-headed enlargement of the posterior aspect of one or both optic canals (Fig. 83–9). Soft tissue aspects of optic nerve tumors are best seen with contrast-enhanced magnetic resonance imaging obtained with fat-suppression techniques. Such tumors can involve both orbits, even leading to mechanical restriction of ocular movement and proptosis. In children, these tumors are usually slow growing, and thus rarely benefit from surgical intervention other than biopsy. If treatment is required, they are usually treated by radiation or chemotherapy. Occasionally, an optic nerve glioma may extend outside the con-

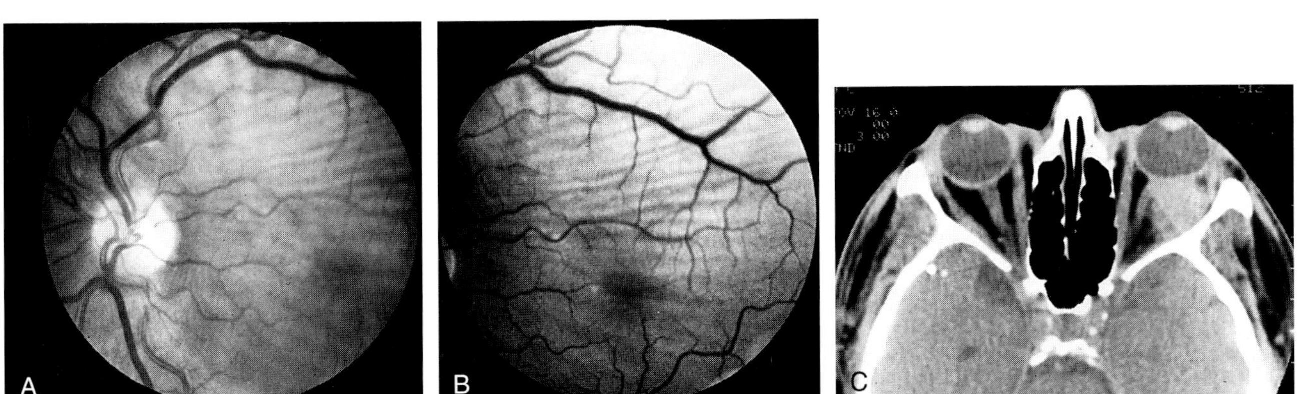

Figure 83–8. Choroidal folds. Ophthalmoscopic changes seen with a retrobulbar tumor, metastatic renal adenocarcinoma in a 50-year-old man. *A*, Ophthalmoscopic findings as seen with white light; choroidal folds extend in the horizontal plane temporal to a normal-appearing optic nerve head. *B*, Choroidal folds in the horizontal plane extending through the macular region as seen with red-free light. The border of the optic nerve head is at the left margin of the photograph. Choroidal folds are sometimes better appreciated with red-free ophthalmoscopic illumination. *C*, Axial CT scan showing metastases in orbit between the left lateral rectus muscle and the optic nerve. (Courtesy of Mark W. Balles, MD.)

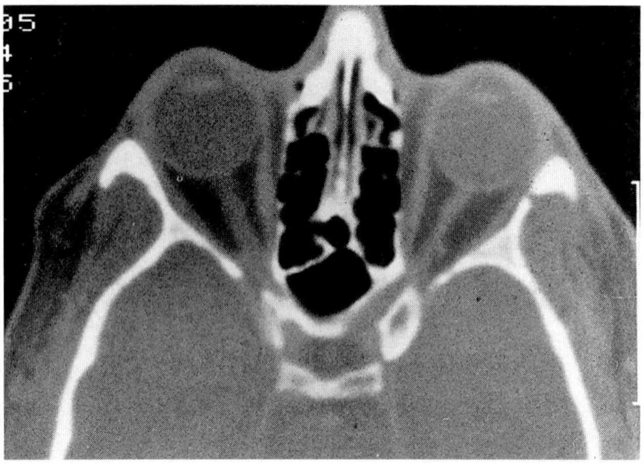

Figure 83–9. Bullet-head enlargement of posterior left optic canal due to anterior visual pathway glioma enlarging posterior portion of left optic nerve. Although the plane of the unenhanced axial computed tomographic scan is slightly tilted (as is usually the case with 5-year-old children), the asymmetric and bullet-head enlargement can be easily defined on this bone window scan. The intracranial optic chiasm is not well appreciated because of lack of inherent contrast. The orbital optic nerves are seen to be normal in size and are naturally contrasted with regard to the adjacent orbital fat.

fines of the nerve (exophytic growth pattern) sufficiently that decompression is required to relieve proptosis or to debulk tumor mass before other treatment commences. Should a glioma arise posterior to the globe, it is usually observed until it causes blindness or unacceptable proptosis or threatens the optic chiasm. Unilateral optic nerve gliomas that do not extend posteriorly through the optic canal at the time of presentation may never do so. In contrast, optic nerve gliomas in adults are rapidly progressive and malignant tumors. Orbital biopsy is usually performed for identification, but these tumors are usually too far advanced for complete excision.

Meningiomas may directly extend into the orbit from the intracranial cavity by way of the optic canal. Intracranial meningiomas may also seed the intraorbital optic nerve meninges via the cerebrospinal fluid, thus producing one or more masses that are discontinuous from the primary tumor. An intracranial meningioma can invade the sphenoid bone and thus compress the optic canal. Such tumors show bone thickening and may require both contrast-enhanced computed tomography and magnetic resonance imaging for accurate diagnosis.

Meningiomas may also originate within the intraorbital optic nerve. Such meningiomas are fortunately rare in childhood; but if they do occur, they may show rapid progression. Primary optic nerve meningiomas in adults progress slowly. The classical computed tomographic hallmark of these lesions is the "railroad track" sign, which results from calcification patterns. Intracranial extension via the optic canal can lead to a dumbbell-shaped tumor, the thin portion occupying the canal itself (Fig. 83–10). These tumors cannot be removed without serious risk of visual compromise. Thus, the usual management is to perform a biopsy of the tumor and treat it with radiation. Occasionally, debulking or removal after the eye becomes blind may be required.

Finally, the optic canal can be destroyed by tumor involving the adjacent paranasal sinuses or by enlargement of an intracavernous carotid aneurysm.

Superior Orbital Fissure

The superior orbital fissure is bounded medially and laterally by the lesser and greater wings of the sphenoid bone, and it is continuous inferiorly with the inferior orbital fissure. As such, it and the adjacent bone can become distorted by such disorders as fibrous dysplasia, meningioma, and metastatic tumors (e.g., prostate and breast). Pathologic processes can move either way through the fissure, but the preponderant direction is posteroanterior. Rarely will orbital pseudotumors, tumors, or granulomatous disease enter the cavernous sinus.

The nerves passing through the fissure can harbor primary tumors of their myelin sheaths, or schwannomas. These usually involve the trigeminal nerve and are usually anesthetic. Conversely, meningiomas of the cavernous sinus are likelier to compress the trigeminal nerve and produce pain.

The didactic separation of cavernous sinus, superior orbital fissure, and orbital apex syndromes is somewhat artificial but may be useful for an understanding of where to focus diagnostic studies. Tumors, inflammations, and vascular lesions may cause symptomatology that suggests that the anatomic problem is more or less widespread than it is. Tumors may be large and may displace nerves without interfering with their function, or a small lesion can invade a nerve or compromise its blood supply, yielding major clinical findings. The most reliable indicator of cavernous sinus involvement is dysfunction of the mandibular or maxillary divisions of the trigeminal nerve. Sympathetic involvement is also suggestive of this involvement. Common pathologic conditions of the cavernous sinus include carotid-cavernous fistulas, intracavernous carotid aneurysms, cavernous sinus thrombosis, meningiomas, extension of adjacent adenomas, metastatic tumors, and inflammatory conditions, such as Tolosa-Hunt syndrome.

Arterial communication with the cavernous sinus raises the venous pressure in the orbit and sometimes in the eye. Carotid-cavernous fistulas, whether traumatic or spontaneous, tend to be relatively high-flow systems and usually can be diagnosed on the basis of a bruit combined with positive findings on magnetic resonance imaging or angiography. Conversely, dural arteriovenous fistulas are often occult, low-flow systems that may give suggestive symptoms but defy diagnostic efforts.

The nerves and vessels of the cavernous sinus are separated by fibrous and somewhat fatty connective tissue,

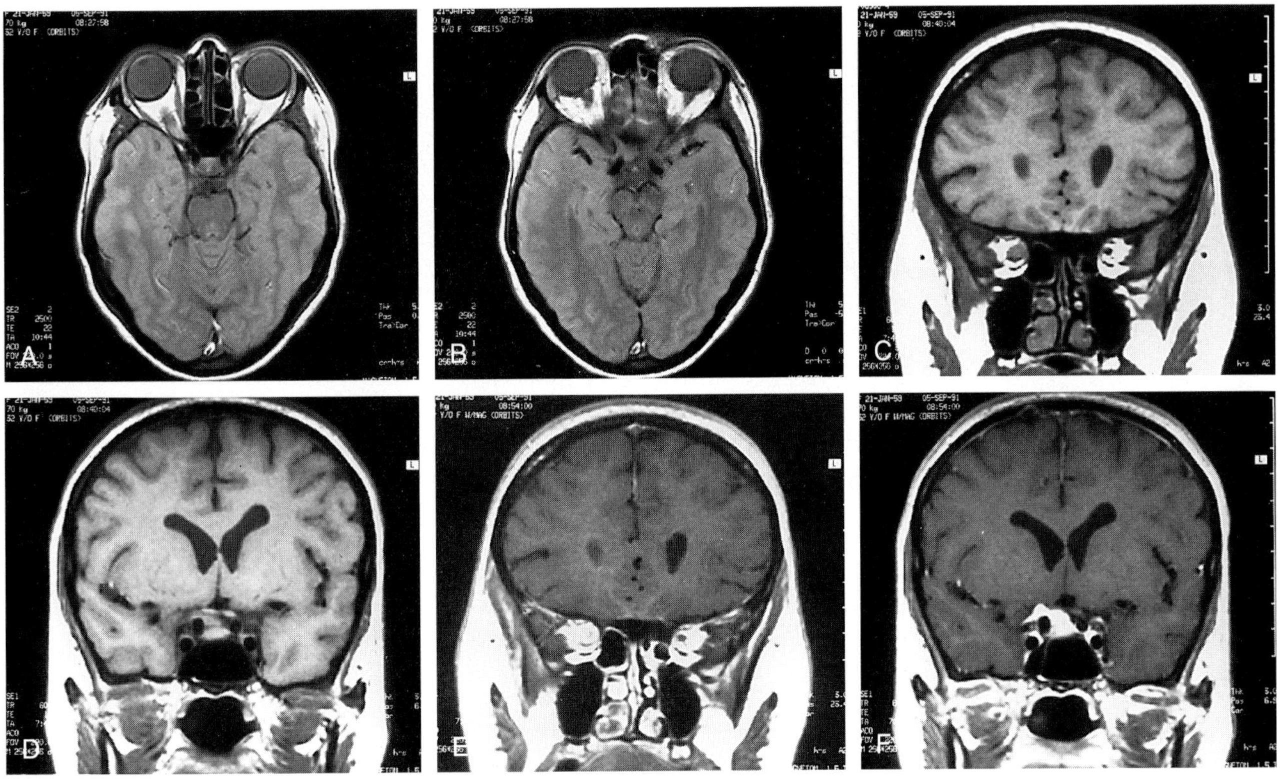

Figure 83–10. Right optic nerve meningioma extending with dumbbell-shaped intracranial extension through optic canal in a 52-year-old woman. *A*, Axial MRI scan with normal head angulation showing a thickened optic nerve extending from the upper plane of the lens to the anterior optic canal. The left optic nerve (as seen to the viewer's right) is normal width. *B*, Section 4.5 mm higher showing thickened optic nerve extending through posterior portion of optic canal and asymmetry of the tuberculum sellae region just anterior and medially to the internal carotid artery. *A* and *B* are second echo scans with TR = 2500, TE = 22. *C*, Coronal scan of posterior orbit showing the right optic nerve as about five times thicker than the left optic nerve (TR = 600, TE = 15, this scan would be described as T1-weighted without contrast medium enhancement). *D*, Coronal MRI 14.5 mm posterior to C showing upward displacement of the optic chiasm by the tumor of the nerve and tuberculum sellae. *E*, Gadolinium-enhanced coronal scan of the orbit with ring-like enhancement of the optic nerve due to the tumor. *F*, Coronal scan at same plane as *D* but with enhancement easily showing the intracranial dumbbell extension of the tumor. As shown, unenhanced T1-weighted coronal images are more useful for identifying the orbital portion of the tumor, whereas the enhanced T1-weighted images are more useful for identifying the intracranial portion of the tumor.

and these structures extend through the superior orbital fissure. The superior ophthalmic vein may be compressed by tumors at this location, although considerable developmental variation exists in the venous drainage of the orbital compartments. Moreover, the slow development of impaired flow in the superior ophthalmic vein allows for the rerouting of venous drainage to such vessels as the inferior ophthalmic vein and the tributaries of the facial veins. Thus, both developmental and acquired differences in venous flow may explain the relative lack of symptoms in some cases of cavernous sinus thrombosis or orbital apex syndrome.

Cranial nerves III, IV, V1 and VI all enter the orbit through the superior orbital fissure, with the oculomotor nerve usually dividing just within the orbit into its superior and inferior branches. In the past few years, magnetic resonance imaging of the brain has indicated that some cases of divisional paralysis of the oculomotor nerve may arise from small strokes or other lesions within the midbrain. For example, an acquired paralysis of the superior division of the third cranial nerve would usually be considered to arise within the orbit or in the rootlets or fascicles of the nerve as it exits from the midbrain. Recently, it has been demonstrated that the fibers of the levator and superior rectus muscles traverse the midbrain lateral to the red nucleus, and thus a lesion at this location can create dysfunction that might otherwise be interpreted as pathology at the superior orbital fissure.[7–9]

Finally, the orbital specialist must recognize the localizing signs of the anterior chiasmal syndrome (Fig. 83–11). Tumors are the commonest cause of the syndrome, especially meningiomas, gliomas, and metastatic disease. It can also occur in cases of retrodisplaced chiasm with a pituitary adenoma or craniopharyngioma. This syndrome combines signs of an optic neuropathy (e.g., decreased visual acuity, afferent pupillary defect, color desaturation, and central or paracentral scotoma) on the affected side with a depression of the superotemporal visual field of the contralateral side. This effect results from compression not only of the most distal optic nerve on the affected side, but also of the crossing inferonasal fibers located in von Willebrandt's knee.

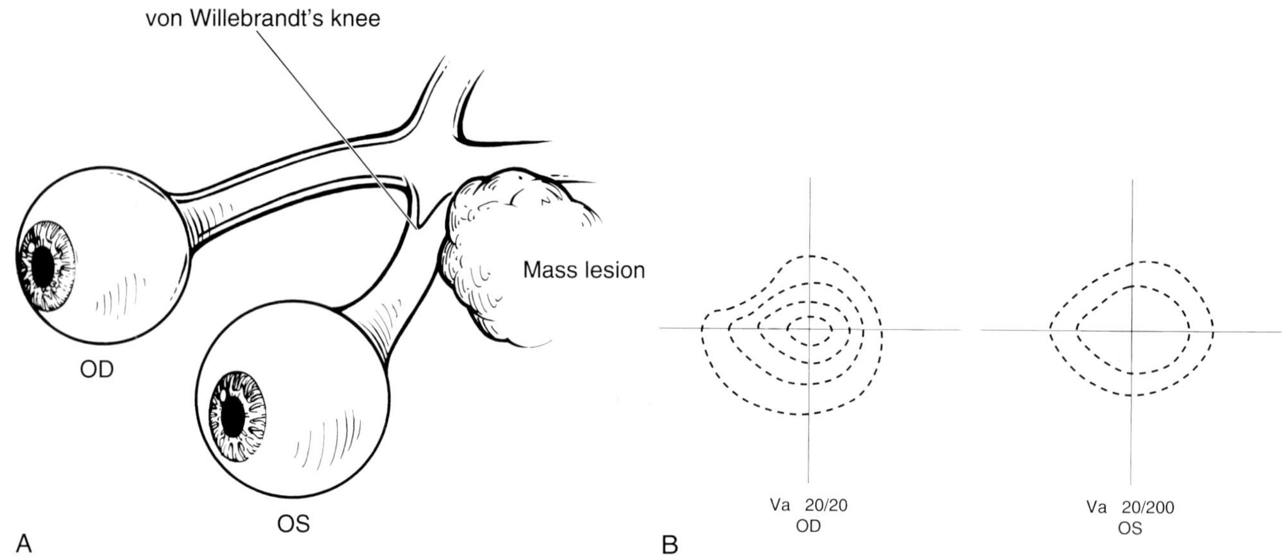

Figure 83–11. The anterior chiasmal syndrome. A mass lesion encroaching on this region that injures von Willebrandt's knee as well as the ipsilateral optic nerve (*A*) will cause a marked decrease in Snellen acuity and a variation on the theme of central scotoma on the side of the lesion and a superotemporal depression in the contralateral field (*B*).

CONCLUSION

It is our hope that the preceding chapter will serve the orbital specialist in his or her evaluation of clinical signs and symptoms in this complicated region. We hope that we have added to and underscored the clinical tools available for study and assessment herein.

REFERENCES

1. Miller N: Topical diagnosis of lesions in the visual sensory pathway. *In* Walsh and Hoyt's Clinical Neuro-ophthalmology, 4th ed. Baltimore, Williams & Wilkins, 1982, pp 108–152.
2. Singh N, Sachdev K, Brisman R: Trigeminal nerve stimulation: Short latency somatosensory evoked potentials. Neurology 32:97–101, 1982.
3. Sibony P, Krauss H, Kennerdell JS, et al: Optic nerve sheath meningiomas: Clinical manifestations. Ophthalmology 91:1313–1326,1984.
4. Orcutt J, Tucker W, Mills R, et al: Gaze-evoked amaurosis. Ophthalmology 94:213–218, 1987.
5. Bogren H, Franti C, Wilmarth S: Normal variations of the position of the eye in the orbit. Ophthalmology 93:1072–1077, 1986.
6. Wirtschafter J: Osteopetrosis. *In* Fraunfelder F, Roy F (eds): Current Ocular Therapy, 3rd ed. Philadelphia, WB Saunders, 1990, pp 220–221.
7. Hopf H, Gutmann L: Diabetic third nerve palsy: Evidence for a mesencephalic lesion. Neurology 40:1041–1045, 1990.
8. Ksiazek S, Repka M, Maguire A, et al: Divisional oculomotor paresis caused by intrinsic brainstem disease. Ann Neurol 26:714–718, 1989.
9. Castro O, Johnson L, Mamourian A: Isolated inferior oblique paresis from brain-stem infarction: Perspective on oculomotor fascicular organization in the ventral midbrain tegmentum. Arch Neurol 47:235–237, 1990.

CHAPTER 84

Neuroradiologic Imaging of the Orbit and Globe

Mahmood F. Mafee

ORBIT

Anatomic and Developmental Considerations

The orbits are two recesses that contain the globes, muscles, blood vessels, lymphatics, cranial nerves (II, III, IV, V, and VI), adipose and connective tissues, and most of the lacrimal apparatus. Each orbit is bordered by the periosteum and separated from the globe by Tenon's capsule. Anteriorly are the orbital septum and the lids. The orbital cavity is pyramidal; its apex is directed posteriorly and medially and its base anteriorly and laterally as the orbital opening. Its bony walls separate it from the anterior cranial fossa superiorly, the ethmoidal air cells and nasal cavity medially, the maxillary sinus inferiorly, and the lateral surface of the face and temporal fossa laterally and posteriorly (Fig. 84–1).[1, 2]

Bony Orbit

Each orbit presents a roof, floor, medial and lateral walls, a base or orbital opening, and an apex. At the posterior end of the junction of the roof with the medial wall, the optic canal and optic foramen establishes communication between the orbit and the middle cranial fossa. The optic canal contains the optic nerve, ophthalmic artery, and sympathetic fibers (see Fig. 84–1).

Superior Orbital Fissure

Just lateral and inferolateral to the optic canal, and separated from it by the optic strut, is the superior orbital fissure. It communicates with the middle cranial fossa and transmits the oculomotor, trochlear, and abducens nerves and the terminal branches of the ophthalmic nerve and the superior ophthalmic vein.[2]

Inferior Orbital Fissure

At the posterior aspect of the orbit the inferior and lateral walls of the orbit are separated by the inferior orbital fissure. The fissure is bounded above by the greater wing of the sphenoid, below by the maxilla and the orbital process of palatine bone, and laterally by the zygomatic bone or the zygomaticomaxillary suture. In fact, the inferior orbital fissure extends obliquely as a gently curving continuation of the more medial pterygopalatine fossa. The maxillary nerve is the most important structure traversing the inferior orbital fissure. In addition to the maxillary nerve, the inferior orbital fissure transmits the infraorbital vessels, the zygomatic nerve, and a few minute twigs from the pterygopalatine ganglion. Through the anterior part of the inferior orbital fissure, a vein passes to communicate the inferior ophthalmic vein with the pterygoid venous plexus.[2]

Orbital Compartments

In descriptive terms, the orbit has been divided into the extraperiosteal, subperiosteal, extraconal, conal, and intraconal spaces. The intraconal space is separated from the other spaces by the rectus muscles and their intermuscular septae, which are denser in the anterior orbit and best seen on coronal scans. Certain lesions have a predilection to present in specific or various orbital spaces (Tables 84–1 through 84–4). Some orbital and ocular pathology may show dystrophic calcifications (Tables 84–5 and 84–6). The concept of various orbital spaces serves some practical value that will be very useful for surgical planning for surgeons and differential diagnosis for radiologists.[1]

Computed Tomography and Magnetic Resonance Imaging

Because of its high-contrast resolution and ability to define hard and soft tissues, computed tomography (CT) had become the imaging method of choice for many orbital disorders. Magnetic resonance imaging (MRI), on the other hand, is a noninvasive technique that has remarkable sensitivity in differentiating various normal and abnormal soft tissues. MRI is the imaging modality of choice for many intracranial pathologic entities. Except for foreign bodies, retinoblastomas (calcification),

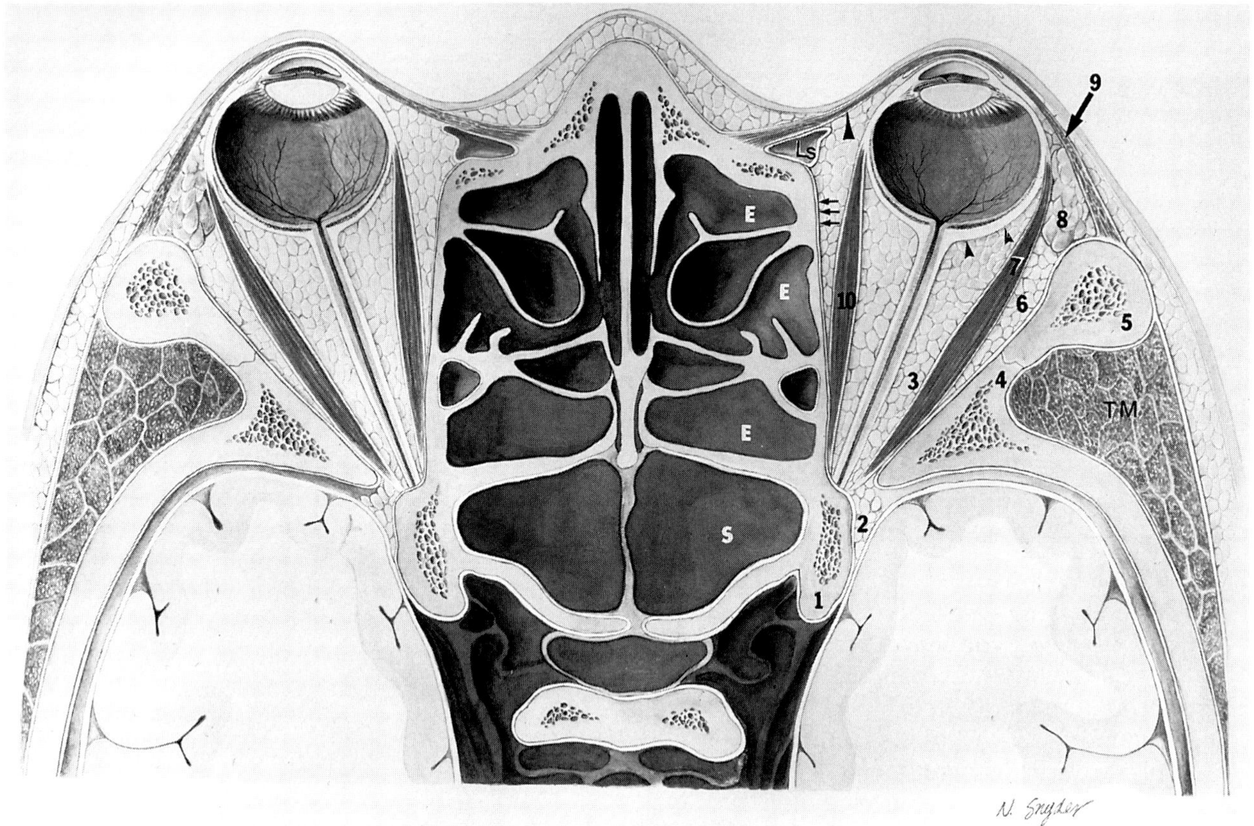

Figure 84 – 1. Diagram of an axial section of the orbits at the level of optic nerves. Note periorbital periosteum (*three black arrows*). The periorbita splits at the level of the lacrimal sac and then forms the orbital septum (*arrowhead*). Note Tenon capsule (*arrowheads*). 1, anterior clinoid; 2, superior orbital fissure; 3, central orbital fat; 4, greater wing of sphenoid; 5, zygomatic bone; 6, peripheral orbital fat; 7, lateral rectus muscle; 8, lacrimal gland; 9, fibers of orbicularis oculi; 10, medial rectus muscle; E, ethmoidal air cells; Ls, lacrimal sac; s, sphenoidal sinus; TM, temporalis muscle. (Reprinted with permission from Valvassori G [ed]: Imaging of the Head and Neck. Thieme Medical Publishers, 1995. Copyright Thieme Medical Publishers, Inc.)

and osseous lesions, MRI has proved superior to CT for many orbital and intraocular applications.

In keeping with the purpose of this chapter, selective common intraconal, conal, extraconal, subperiosteal, and intraocular lesions are presented and their imaging findings emphasized.

TABLE 84 - 1

Intraconal (Central) Orbital Lesions

More Common	Less Common
Cavernous hemangioma	Capillary hemangioma
Optic nerve meningioma	Peripheral nerve tumors
Optic nerve glioma	Neurofibroma
Optic nerve granulomatous disease (sarcoid)	Schwannoma
Optic neuritis (multiple sclerosis)	Fibrous histiocytoma
Lymphoma	Leukemia
Pseudotumor	Hematocele
Lymphangioma	Optic nerve sheath cyst
Venous angioma	Colobomatous cyst
Varix	Hemangioblastoma (optic nerve)
Arteriovenous malformation	Chemodectoma (ciliary ganglion)
Carotid cavernous fistula	Necrobiotic xanthogranuloma
Hemangiopericytoma	Lipoma
Rhabdomyosarcoma	Amyloidosis
Metastasis (breast, lung, carcinoid tumors)	
Orbital cellulitis and abscess	

Developmental Orbital Cysts

The most frequent developmental cysts involving the orbit and periorbital structures are the dermoid and epidermoid cysts. Both result from the inclusion of ectodermal elements during closure of the neural tube. The dermal elements that are pinched off along the cranio-orbitofacial suture lines, diploë, or within the meninges or scalp in the course of embryonic development give rise to these cysts. Both have a fibrous capsule of varying degrees of thickness. The epidermoid has a lining of keratinizing, stratified epithelium. The dermoid contains one or more dermal adnexal structures, such as sebaceous glands and hair follicles. Teratomas are choristomatous

TABLE 84 - 2

Common Causes of Enlarged Extraocular Muscle
Graves' myositis
Inflammatory myositis, including cysticercosis
Granulomatous myositis (less common)—sarcoidosis
Pseudotumor (myositic type)
Lymphoma
Vascular lesions (hemangioma, arteriovenous malformation)
Acromegaly
Pseudorheumatoid nodule
Metastasis (breast, lung)

TABLE 84-3

Extraconal (Peripheral) Orbital Lesions

More Common	Less Common
Capillary hemangioma	Amyloidosis
Cholesterol granuloma	Hemangiosarcoma
Dermoid and epidermoid	Hemangiopericytoma
Fibrous histiocytoma	Hematic cyst
Lacrimal gland lesions	Lipoma
Inflammation	Orbital encephalocele
Lymphoma	Wegener's granulomatosis
Pseudotumor	
Sarcoidosis	
Epithelial tumors	
Lymphangioma	
Peripheral nerve tumors	
Plasmacytoma	
Rhabdomyosarcoma	
Sarcoidosis	

TABLE 84-4

Common Orbital Subperiosteal Lesions

Subperiosteal cellulitis	Extension of:
Subperiosteal abscess	Lacrimal gland tumors
Infiltration of neoplastic lesions of paranasal sinuses	Dermoid and epidermoid
	Hematoma and hematic cyst
Infiltration of meningiomas (en plaque meningiomas)	Cholesterol granuloma
	Fibrous histiocytoma
Lymphomas	Primary osseous or cartilaginous tumors
Leukemia	
Plasmacytomas	Metastasis (neuroblastoma)

TABLE 84-5

Differential Diagnosis of Metastatic Orbital Calcification

- Congenital
  - Fanconi's syndrome (proximal renal tubular dysfunction)
  - Milk-alkali syndrome
  - Renal tubular acidosis
- Endocrine
  - Hyperparathyroidism, primary or secondary
  - Hypoparathyroidism
  - Pseudohypoparathyroidism
- Idiopathic—sarcoidosis
- Infectious
  - Cytomegalovirus
  - Leprosy
  - Osteomyelitis
  - Syphilis
  - Toxoplasmosis
  - Tuberculosis
- Toxic
  - Excessive ingestion of calcium phosphate or alkali
  - Vitamin D intoxication
- Traumatic—immobilization
- Neoplastic
  - Bronchogenic carcinoma
  - Metastatic involvement of bone
  - Multiple myeloma
  - Parathyroid adenoma
  - Parathyroid carcinoma

Adapted from Ragozzino MW, DeLuca SA: Orbital calcifications. Am Fam Physician 34:121-125, 1986.

TABLE 84-6

Differential Diagnosis of Dystrophic Orbital Calcification

Intraocular

- Cataract
- Endophthalmitis
- Granulomas (sarcoid, *Toxocara* infection)
- Hyaline plaques
- Idiopathic sclerochoroidal calcification
- Optic nerve drusen
- Phthisis bulbi
- Retinal detachment
- Retinal dysplasia
- Retinoblastoma
- Retinopathy of prematurity
- Tuberous sclerosis
- von Hippel-Lindau disease

Extraocular

Within the lacrimal gland fossa:
- Amyloid
- Choristoma
- Dermolipoma
- Malignant and benign tumors of the lacrimal gland (more common in malignant tumor)
- Plasmacytoma
- Pleomorphic adenoma
- Varix

Extrinsic to the lacrimal gland fossa:
- Amyloid
- Arteriovenous shunt or malformation
- Calcified trochlea
- Cartilaginous tumors
- Cysticercosis (cestode or tapeworm: *Taenia solium*)
- Glioma
- Hemangioma
- Hemangiopericytoma
- Hemorrhage
- Idiopathic inflammatory "pseudotumor"
- Lymphangioma
- Lymphoma
- Melanoma
- Meningioma
- Metastatic colonic carcinoma
- Mucocele
- Neuroblastoma
- Neurofibroma
- Orbital bone fragment after trauma
- Teratoma
- Trichinosis (nematode: *Trichinella spiralis*)
- Varix

From Froula PD, Bartley GB, Garrity JA, et al: The differential diagnosis of orbital calcifications, as detected on computed tomographic scans. Mayo Clinic Proc 68:256-257, 1993.

tumors that contain tissue representing two or more germ layers. Endodermal derivatives such as gut or respiratory epithelium, ectodermal tissues such as skin and its appendages, and neural and mesodermal tissues such as connective tissues, smooth muscles, cartilage and bone, and vessels may be present. Teratomas are evident at birth as grossly visible cystic orbital masses. The dermoid and epidermoid cysts favor the upper portion rather than the lower quadrants of the orbit for their growth. They grow slowly, but at times these cysts can grow significantly, particularly in adults.[3] Epidermoids are seen on CT scans as nonenhancing masses (hypodense or isodense to adjacent soft tissues). There may be compres-

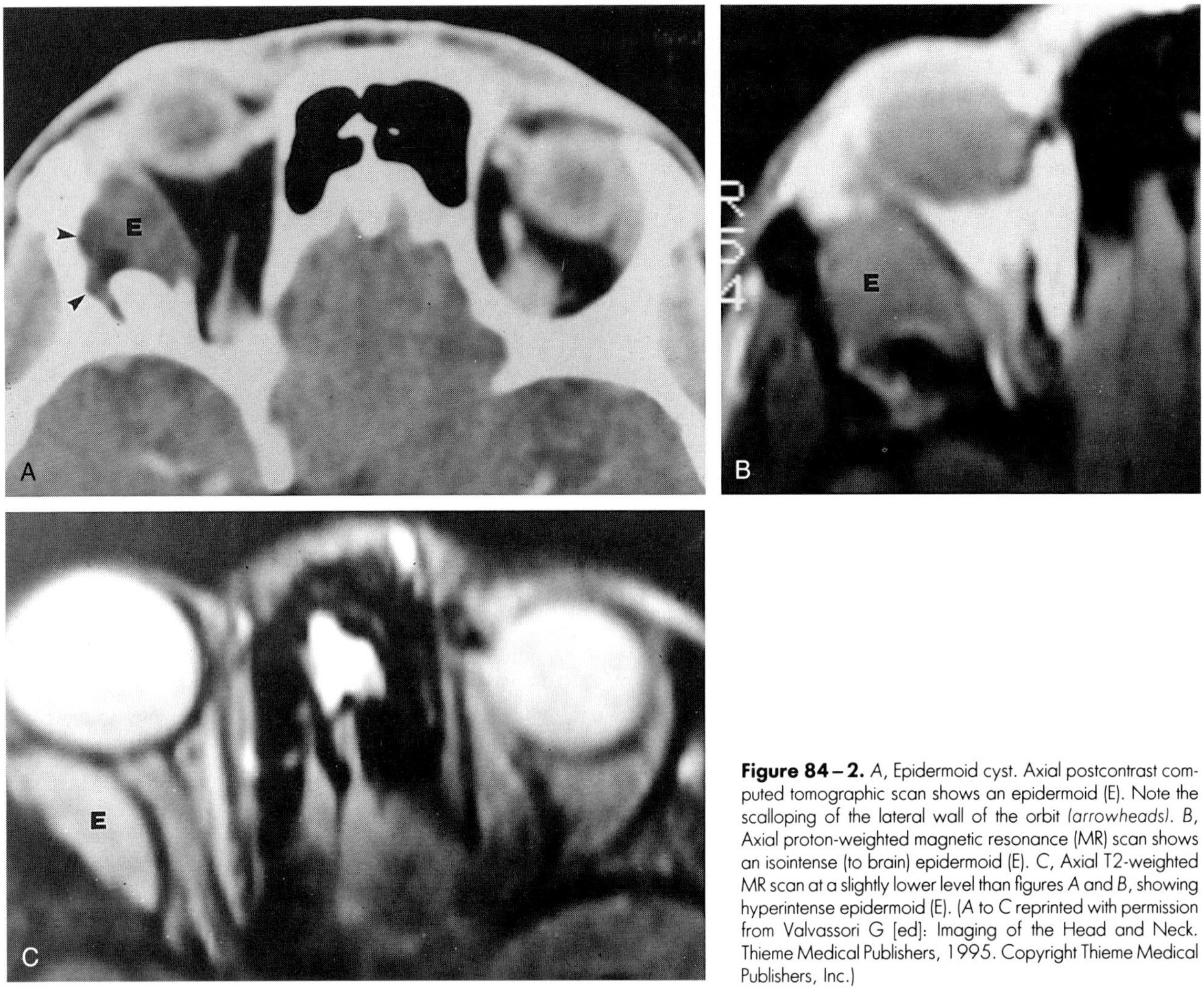

Figure 84–2. *A*, Epidermoid cyst. Axial postcontrast computed tomographic scan shows an epidermoid (E). Note the scalloping of the lateral wall of the orbit *(arrowheads)*. *B*, Axial proton-weighted magnetic resonance (MR) scan shows an isointense (to brain) epidermoid (E). *C*, Axial T2-weighted MR scan at a slightly lower level than figures *A* and *B*, showing hyperintense epidermoid (E). (*A* to *C* reprinted with permission from Valvassori G [ed]: Imaging of the Head and Neck. Thieme Medical Publishers, 1995. Copyright Thieme Medical Publishers, Inc.)

sion atrophy or significant scalloping of the adjacent bony orbital wall (Fig. 84–2). Dermoids have similar CT findings. At times, fat density, fluid–fluid level, and calcification may be present in dermoids (Fig. 84–3). The MRI characteristics of epidermoids include hypointensity in regard to brain in T1-weighted and hyperintensity in T2-weighted images (see Fig. 84–2*A* and *B*). The fat component of dermoids shows short T1-weighted and short T2-weighted characteristics (Fig. 84–4). These characteristics include brightness on T1-weighted images and darkness on T2-weighted images.

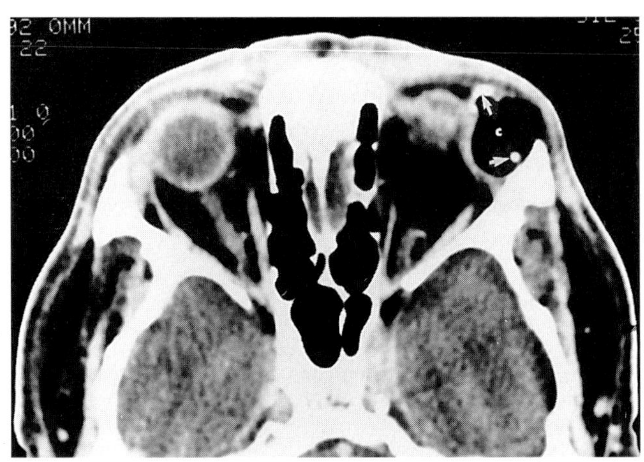

Figure 84–3. Dermoid cyst. Axial postcontrast computed tomographic scan shows a fat-containing cyst compatible with dermoid cyst (c). Note calcifications *(arrow)*. (Reprinted with permission from Valvassori G [ed]: Imaging of the Head and Neck. Thieme Medical Publishers, 1995. Copyright Thieme Medical Publishers, Inc.)

Inflammatory Diseases of the Orbit

Orbital infections account for about 60% of primary orbital disease processes. The process may be acute, subacute, or chronic. The majority of acute inflammatory

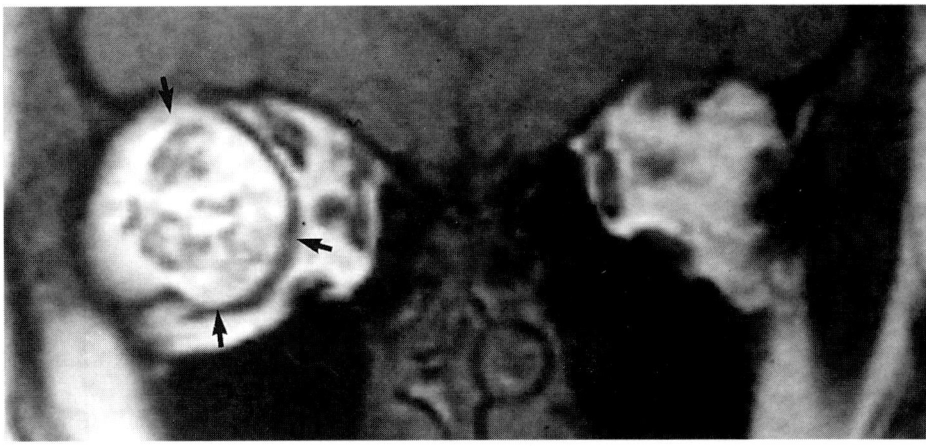

Figure 84–4. Dermoid cyst. Coronal T1-weighted magnetic resonance scan shows a large dermoid cyst *(arrows)*. (Reprinted with permission from Valvassori G [ed]: Imaging of the Head and Neck. Thieme Medical Publishers, 1995. Copyright Thieme Medical Publishers, Inc.)

disorders are of sinus origin. However, inflammation may develop from an infectious process of the face or pharynx, from trauma, or from foreign bodies or it may be secondary to septicemia. The bacteria most commonly involved are *Staphylococcus*, *Streptococcus* (including *S. pneumoniae*), *Pseudomonas*, *Neisseria*, *Haemophilus*, and *Mycobacterium*. Herpes simplex and herpes zoster are the major viral infections of the orbit. In immune-suppressed patients and poorly controlled diabetic patients, opportunistic infections such as fungal and parasitic pathogens may be responsible for severe sinonaso-orbital infections.[4, 6]

Orbital Cellulitis and Sinusitis

Sinusitis is the most common frequent cause of orbital cellulitis. Pathophysiologically, infection originating within the sinuses can spread readily to the orbit through the thin and often dehiscent bony walls and its many foramina or by means of the interconnecting valveless venous system of the face, sinus, and orbit. The classification of orbital cellulitis includes five categories or stages of orbital involvement from sinusitis. These are (1) inflammatory edema, (2) subperiosteal phlegmon and abscess, (3) orbital cellulitis, (4) orbital abscess, and (5) ophthalmic vein and cavernous sinus thrombosis. Limiting a particular inflammatory lesion to one of these categories is difficult, because they tend to overlap.[5]

Inflammatory Edema or Preseptal Cellulitis

Preseptal cellulitis is the first stage; it is often misdiagnosed as orbital or periorbital cellulitis. The infection in this early stage actually is still confined to the sinus. This is characterized by swelling of the eyelids. A slightly more advanced stage includes chemosis. CT or MRI at this stage will demonstrate the edema of the eyelids and inflammatory changes of the infected sinus or sinuses.

Subperiosteal Phlegmon and Abscess

As the reaction of the orbital periosteum begins and gradually advances, the edema of the eyelids and conjunctivae becomes more generalized and the eye begins to protrude. Inflammatory tissue and edema collects beneath the periosteum to form a subperiosteal phlegmon (Fig. 84–5). Subsequently, pus may form to represent a subperiosteal abscess (Fig. 84–6). As the disease progresses, the inflammatory process may infiltrate the periorbital and retro-orbital fat to give rise to a true orbital cellulitis.[4]

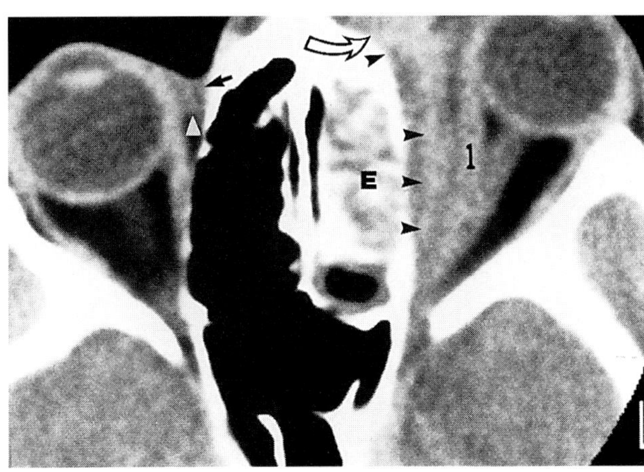

Figure 84–5. Subperiosteal phlegmon. Axial postcontrast computed tomographic scan shows opacification of ethmoidal air cells (E) and subperiosteal infiltration (granulation tissue) *(arrowheads)*, resulting in lateral displacement of the medial rectus muscle (1). Note the right medial check ligament *(white arrowhead)* and medial palpebral ligament *(arrow)*. The orbital septum at this level may not be seen as a discrete image, owing to partial volume averaging of the lacrimal sac. The orbital septum is anterior to the medial check ligament and posterior to the medial palpebral ligament. Note the thickened left orbtial septum *(curved arrow)*. (Reprinted with permission from Valvassori G [ed]: Imaging of the Head and Neck. Thieme Medical Publishers, 1995. Copyright Thieme Medical Publishers, Inc.)

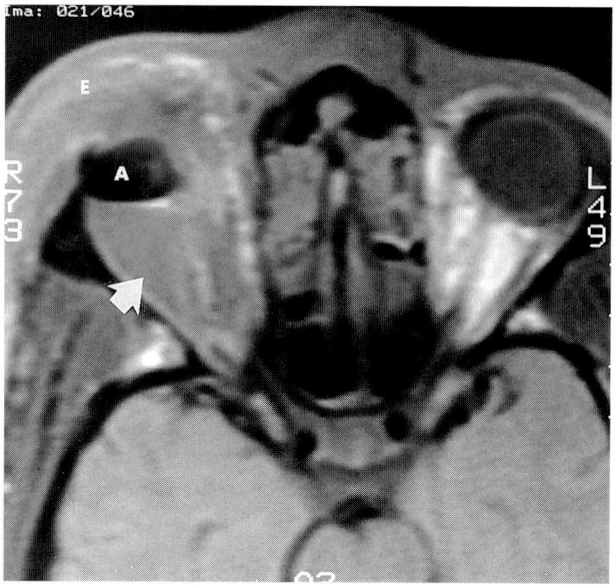

Figure 84–6. Subperiosteal abscess. Axial proton-weighted magnetic resonance scan shows opacification of bilateral ethmoidal air cells, edema of right eyelid, and a large subperiosteal abscess *(arrow)* with air (A) and fluid collection within the abscess cavity. (Reprinted with permission from Valvassori G [ed]: Imaging of the Head and Neck. Thieme Medical Publishers, 1995. Copyright Thieme Medical Publishers, Inc.)

Ophthalmic vein thrombosis and cavernous sinus thrombosis are very serious complications of the orbital and sinonasal infections.[6] Cavernous sinus thrombosis is heralded by profound central nervous system (CNS) deficit and orbital functional impairment.

Acute and Subacute and Chronic Idiopathic Orbital Inflammatory Disorders (Pseudotumors)

Idiopathic inflammatory syndromes are usually referred to as orbital "pseudotumors," a clinically and histologically confusing category of lesions. In general, orbital pseudotumor comprises a broad category of orbital inflammatory diseases. It is defined as a nonspecific, idiopathic inflammatory condition for which no local identifiable cause or systemic disease can be found.[7]

Pseudotumors may be classified as (1) acute and subacute idiopathic anterior orbital inflammation, (2) acute and subacute idiopathic diffuse orbital inflammation, (3) acute and subacute idiopathic myositic orbital inflammation, (4) acute and subacute idiopathic apical orbital inflammation, (5) idiopathic dacryoadenitis, and (6) perineuritis (optic nerve).[7]

Of the various CT and MRI characteristics associated with different features of pseudotumors, the most common CT and MRI findings include enhancement with intravenous contrast medium (95%) (Fig. 84–7), infiltration of the retrobulbar fat (76%) (Fig. 84–8), proptosis (71%), extraocular muscle enlargement (57%) (Fig. 84–9), apical fat infiltration and edema (48%), muscle tendon and sheath enlargement (43%), and optic nerve thickening (38%).

We have found no specific imaging findings nor are there any specific clinical signs to establish the diagnosis of pseudotumors with absolute certainty. Classically, the rapid development of unilateral, painful ophthalmoplegia, proptosis, and chemosis, and a rapid and lasting response to corticosteroid therapy in an otherwise

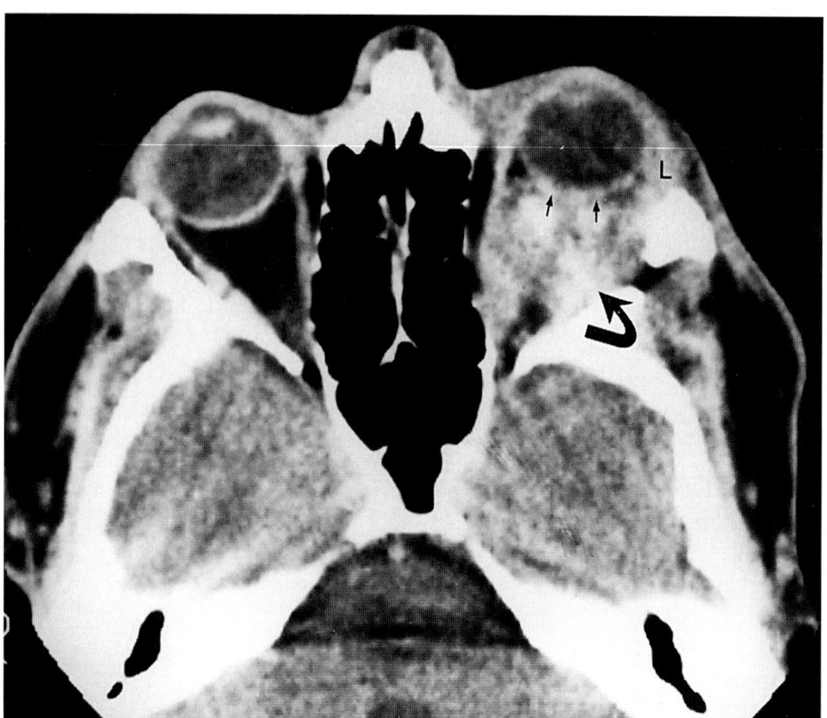

Figure 84–7. Pseudotumor. Axial postcontrast computed tomographic scan shows an infiltrative process involving the lacrimal gland (L), Tenon space *(arrows)*, and retrobulbar space *(curved arrow)*. Note the osteotomy defect, the site for biopsy. (Reprinted with permission from Valvassori G [ed]: Imaging of the Head and Neck. Thieme Medical Publishers, 1995. Copyright Thieme Medical Publishers, Inc.)

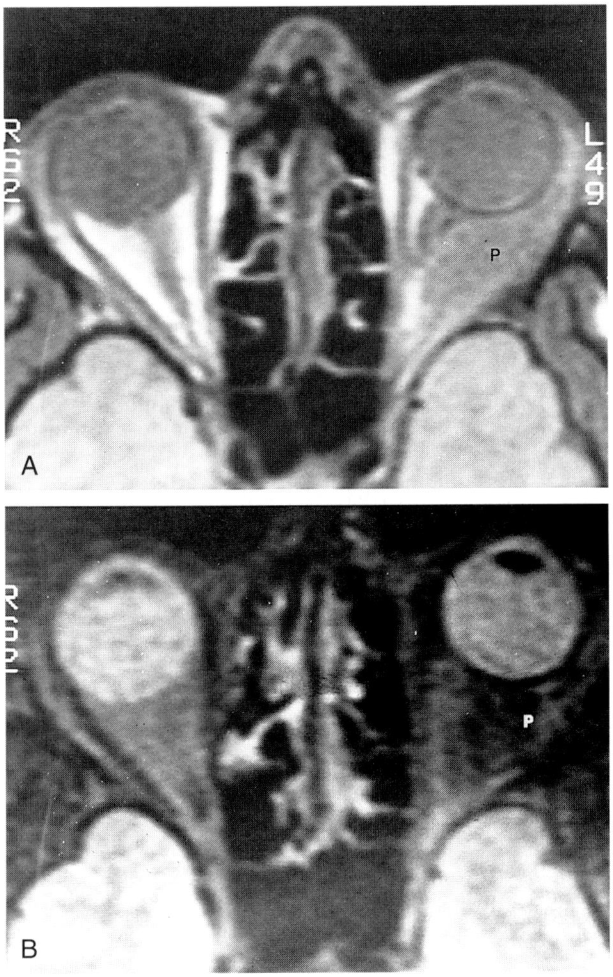

Figure 84–8. *A*, Pseudotumor. Axial proton-weighted magnetic resonance (MR) scan shows an infiltrative process due to pseudotumor (P). *B*, Axial T2-weighted MR scan shows orbital pseudotumor (P). The process appears hypointense as compared with normal retrobulbar tissue on the right side. (Reprinted with permission from Valvassori G [ed]: Imaging of the Head and Neck. Thieme Medical Publishers, 1995. Copyright Thieme Medical Publishers, Inc.)

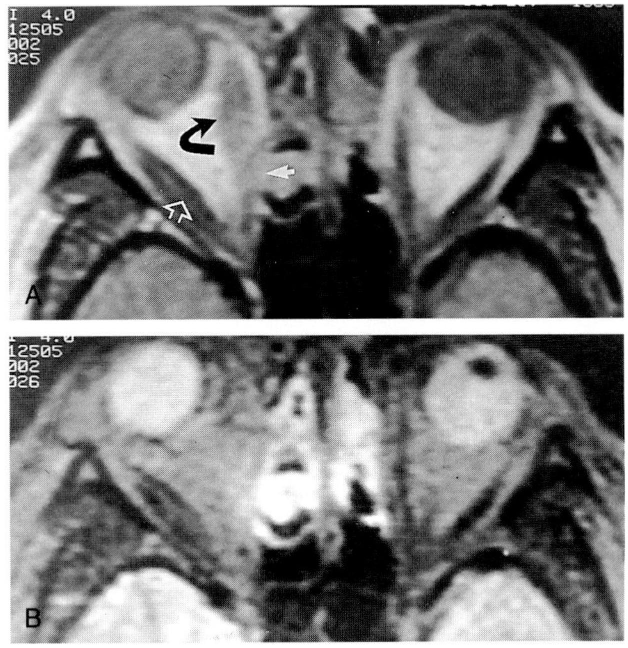

Figure 84–9. Myositic orbital pseudotumor. Axial proton-weighted *(A)* and T2-weighted *(B)* magnetic resonance scans show enlargement of the right medial *(curved arrow)* and lateral *(open arrow)* rectus muscles. The medial rectus shows markedly increased signal intensity on the T2-weighted image. Note inflammatory changes in the ethmoidal sinuses. This myositic pseudotumor is most likely a reaction to sinus infection. The edema of the right medial rectus is more at the site where the medial wall of the orbit is poorly defined *(white solid arrow)*. (*A* and *B* reprinted with permission from Valvassori G [ed]: Imaging of the Head and Neck. Thieme Medical Publishers, 1995. Copyright Thieme Medical Publishers, Inc.)

healthy patient, is highly suggestive of pseudotumor. In the absence of a characteristic clinical presentation of pseudotumor or poor responsiveness to corticosteroids, biopsy is necessary.

Thyroid Orbitopathy

Thyroid orbitopathy occurs most commonly in middle-aged women. It is ophthalmologically characterized by exophthalmos and in some patients by the gradual onset of diplopia, usually the vertical type. Initially, in the acute congestive phase, the retrobulbar orbital contents are markedly swollen and congested. Later, a more chronic, noncongestive phase follows, in which a restrictive type of limited eye movement often develops, secondary to infiltration of the extraocular muscles and to subsequent loss of elasticity. The involvement can be unilateral or bilateral; when it is bilateral it is often fairly symmetric. The inferior rectus muscle is most commonly involved, leading to a limitation of elevation of the involved eye. The medial and superior rectus muscles are also frequently involved, and the lateral rectus and superior oblique muscles are less commonly affected. The forced duction test result is almost always abnormal. The myopathy may occur at any time in the course of Graves' disease; laboratory evaluation may reveal hyperthyroidism, hypothyroidism, or euthyroidism. Extraocular muscle enlargement in Graves' disease and associated compressive neuropathy, if any, can be visualized by CT and MRI (Fig. 84–10). Typically, enlargement involves the muscle belly, sparing its tendinous portion. However, there are rare patients who show thickening of the tendinous portion.[8] Another helpful finding in thyroid myopathy is the presence of low density areas within the muscle bellies. These are probably the result of focal accumulation of lymphocytes and mucopolysaccharide deposition and fatty degeneration. Other CT and MRI findings in thyroid orbitopathy are increased orbital fat, enlargement (engorgement) of the lacrimal glands, edema (fullness) of the eyelids, proptosis, and stretching of the optic nerve with or without associated "tenting" of the posterior globe.

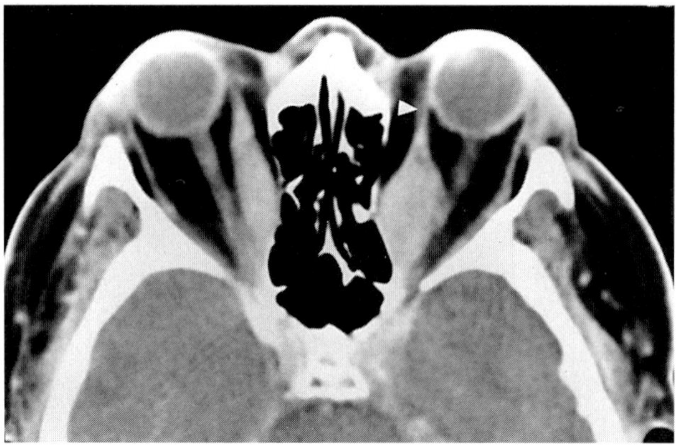

Figure 84–10. Thyroid ophthalmopathy. Axial computed tomographic scan shows enlargement of both medial rectus muscles. Note that the tendinous portion *(arrowhead)* is not involved. (Reprinted with permission from Valvassori G [ed]: Imaging of the Head and Neck. Thieme Medical Publishers, 1995. Copyright Thieme Medical Publishers, Inc.)

Painful External Ophthalmoplegia (Tolosa-Hunt Syndrome)

Painful external ophthalmoplegia, or Tolosa-Hunt syndrome, is considered an idiopathic inflammatory process and a regional variant of idiopathic orbital pseudotumors that, because of its anatomic location, produces typical clinical manifestations. Pathologically, there is an infiltration of lymphocytes and plasma cells along with thickening of the dura mater. The condition generally responds to systemic corticosteroid therapy. It is important to exclude the possibility of a neoplastic, inflammatory (particularly mycotic), and vasculogenic lesion. Carotid angiography and MRI are most useful in excluding aneurysm as a cause of the clinical signs and symptoms. Certain parasellar lesions such as pituitary adenomas, meningiomas, craniopharyngiomas, neurogenic tumors, dermoid cysts, lymphoma, leukemic infiltration, sinonasal and nasopharyngeal carcinomas, and metastatic lesions (e.g., melanoma, lung, breast, kidney, thyroid, prostate) may produce similar symptoms.

Orbital Lymphomas

Lymphomas are solid tumors of the immune system. The extranodal presentation of non-Hodgkin's lymphoma is common, with an incidence ranging from 21% to 64%. Roughly 10% of non-Hodgkin's lymphomas present in the head and neck region. Lymphoid tumors account for 10% to 15% of orbital masses.[9]

Lymphoid neoplasms of the orbit span a large continuum of various classifications from the malignant lymphomas to the benign pseudolymphomas or pseudotumors to the reactive and atypical lymphoid hyperplasias. There are no absolute imaging, clinical, or even laboratory tests that delineate all types of benign orbital lymphoid lesions from orbital lymphomas or lesions, which can simulate them. A pleomorphic cellular infiltrate is correlated with the more benign biologic activity. The more uniform the cellular appearance, the greater the likelihood that malignancy is present. Of all patients with orbital lymphoma, 75% have or will have systemic lymphoma. There is extensive overlap histologically from one type to another, and some forms of the benign process can transform over time into a more aggressive variety of lymphoma. True lymphoid tissue in the eye is found in the subconjunctiva and lacrimal gland. These two areas account for most orbital lymphoreticuloses.[9]

Ultrasonography, CT, and MRI can be used to evaluate orbital lymphomas. CT and MRI have made it possible to make a strong presumptive diagnosis of orbital lymphoma, especially when CT and MRI features are examined in conjunction with the clinical characteristics. The CT and MRI are usually nonspecific and at times it can be impossible to differentiate orbital lymphoma from orbital pseudotumors, lacrimal gland tumors, optic nerve tumors, Graves' orbitopathy, primary orbital tumors, and orbital cellulitis. Orbital lymphomas are homogeneous masses of relatively high density and sharp margins, which are more often seen in the anterior portion of the orbit (Fig. 84–11), retrobulbar areas, or the superior orbital compartment. Generally, the lesions mold themselves to pre-existing structures without eroding the bone or enlarging the orbit.[10] Mild to moderate enhancement is present.[9]

A bulky lesion in the region of the lacrimal fossa that does not produce any bony erosion is most likely to be inflammatory or lymphoid. However, the aggressive malignant lymphomas can produce frank destruction of bone.

MRI has proved to be as sensitive as CT for the diagnosis of orbital lymphoma and pseudotumors. Both pseudotumor and lymphoma may have an intermediate or hypointense signal in T1- and proton-weighted MR images and appear isointense to fat in T2-weighted MR images (Fig. 84–12). Lymphomas may be more hypointense in T1-weighted images than pseudotumors. Lym-

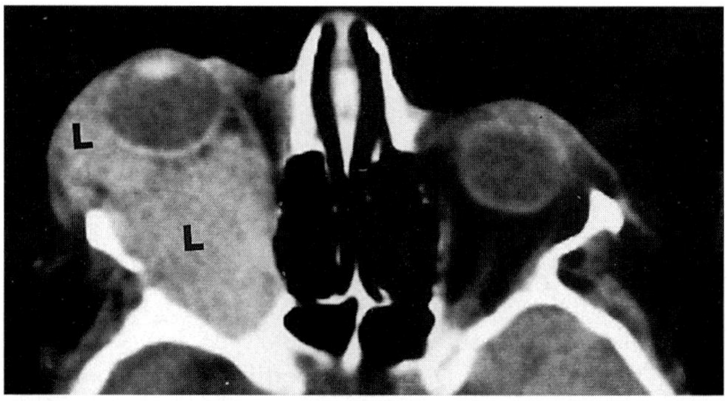

Figure 84–11. Orbital lymphoma. Axial computed tomographic scan shows a large orbital mass, which proved to be lymphoma (L) involving the lacrimal gland and entire retrobulbar space. Note that the mass molds itself with the globe rather than invading it. (Reprinted with permission from Valvassori G [ed]: Imaging of the Head and Neck. Thieme Medical Publishers, 1995. Copyright Thieme Medical Publishers, Inc.)

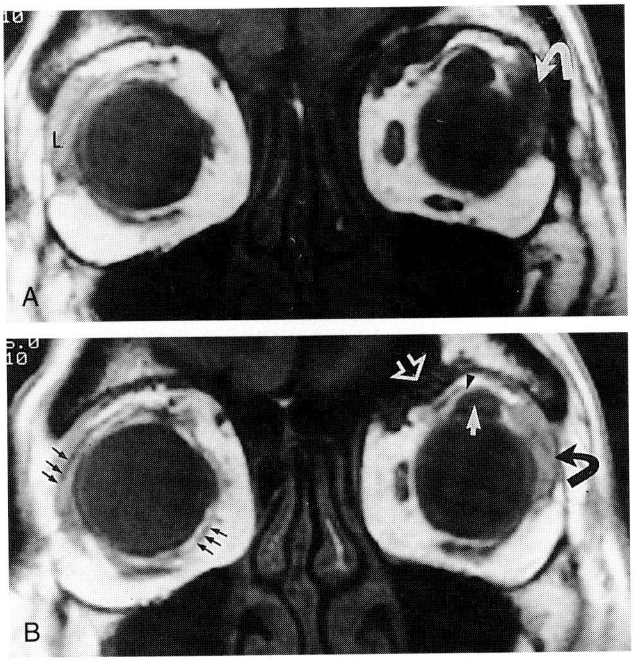

Figure 84–12. *A* and *B*, Applied anatomy of the orbital compartments. Coronal T1-weighted magnetic resonance scan shows the tendinous insertions of the rectus muscles and their intermuscular septae (*small black arrows*), outlining the space. Note the normal lacrimal gland (L). There is enlargement of the left superior rectus muscle (*white solid arrow*), extraconal infiltration (subperiosteal) adjacent to the roof of the orbit (*hollow arrow*), and enlargement as well as abnormal signal of the left lacrimal gland (*curved arrows*). The levator palpebrae superioris is displaced upward (*arrowhead*). (*A* and *B* reprinted with permission from Valvassori G [ed]: Imaging of the Head and Neck. Thieme Medical Publishers, 1995. Copyright Thieme Medical Publishers, Inc.)

phomatous lesions may be hyperintense in T2-weighted images. Leukemic infiltration has similar MR appearances to those of lymphomatous lesions. All criteria used for CT in the diagnosis of orbital pseudotumors and lymphoma in terms of morphology, location, homogeneity, contouring, and contrast enhancement with gadolinium (Gd-DTPA) are to be used for MRI in the diagnosis of these conditions.

Vascular Conditions of the Orbit

Capillary Hemangiomas

Capillary hemangiomas (benign hemangioendotheliomas) are tumors that occur primarily in infants during the first year of life. The tumors often increase in size for 6 to 10 months and then gradually involute. They most commonly occur in the superior nasal quadrant. Involution generally commences by the 10th month of life. Microscopically, each tumor is composed of endothelial and capillary vessel proliferation with benign endothelial cells surrounding small, capillary-sized vascular spaces. Capillary hemangiomas in and around the orbit usually have an arterial supply from the external and/or internal carotid arteries, and are capable of bleeding profusely. These angiomas may extend intracranially through the superior orbital fissure, optical canal, and orbital roof. On CT scans, these lesions are seen as fairly well-marginated to poorly marginated, irregular, enhancing lesions (Fig. 84–13). Most of those seen by my colleagues and I were extraconal, although some of these lesions may be seen in the intraconal space (Fig. 84–14). On dynamic CT study, these capillary hemangiomas characteristically show an intense, homogeneous enhancement (see Fig. 84–13*B*).[11] MRI features of capillary hemangiomas are characteristic of long T1 (hypointense in T1-weighted) and long T2 (hyperintense in T2-weighted) lesions. There will be marked contrast enhancement after intravenous administration of Gd-DTPA contrast material.

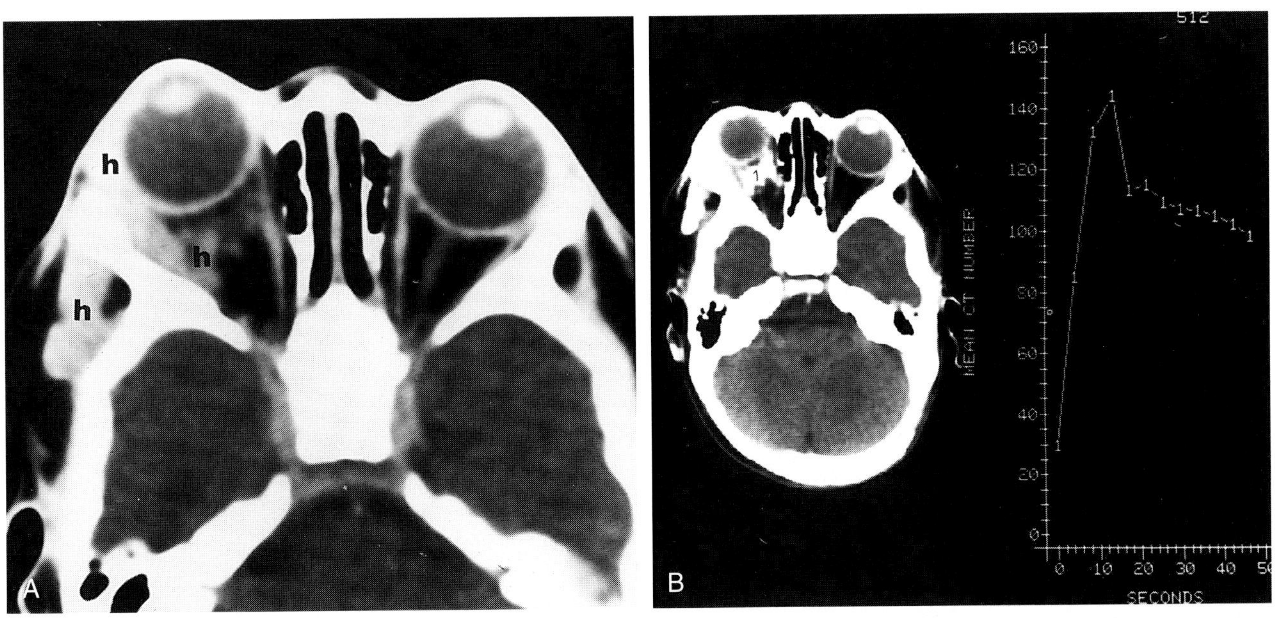

Figure 84–13. Capillary hemangioma. *A*, Axial postcontrast computed tomographic (CT) scan shows a diffuse intraorbital and extraorbital hemangioma (h). *B*, Dynamic CT study shows the rapid wash-in, high peak, and rapid wash-out phase characteristic of highly vascular lesions. (*A* and *B* reprinted with permission from Valvassori G [ed]: Imaging of the Head and Neck. Thieme Medical Publishers, 1995. Copyright Thieme Medical Publishers, Inc.)

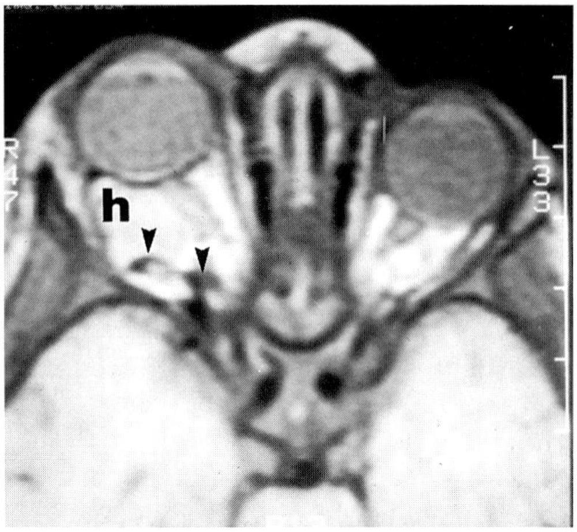

Figure 84–14. Intraconal capillary hemangioma. Axial proton-weighted magnetic resonance scan in a 5-month-old girl shows a large retrobulbar mass compatible with a capillary hemangioma (h). Note signal voids due to prominent vessels *(arrowheads)*. (Reprinted with permission from Valvassori G [ed]: Imaging of the Head and Neck. Thieme Medical Publishers, 1995. Copyright Thieme Medical Publishers, Inc.)

Cavernous Hemangiomas

Cavernous hemangiomas of the orbit, the most common orbital vascular tumors in adults, have distinctive clinical and histopathologic features.[12] They tend to occur in the second to fourth decades of life. These tumors show a slowly progressive enlargement distinct from capillary hemangiomas, which gradually diminish in size. A prominent arterial supply is usually absent, in contrast to capillary hemangiomas. Cavernous hemangiomas possess a distinct fibrous pseudocapsule and therefore appear as well-defined masses. Histologically, cavernous hemangiomas are composed of large dilated vascular channels (sinusoid-like spaces) lined by thin, attenuated endothelial cells.[12, 13] These hemangiomas may be located anywhere in the orbit but frequently (83%) occur within the retrobulbar muscle cone. On the CT scans, cavernous hemangiomas appear as well-defined, smoothly marginated, homogeneous, rounded, ovoid, or lobulated soft tissue of increased density with variable degrees of contrast enhancement (Fig. 84–15*A*). The MRI features of these cavernous hemangiomas are indicative of a lesion with long T1 and T2 relaxation time characteristics (Fig. 84–15*B* and *C*). There will be moderate to marked enhancement after intravenous administration of Gd-DTPA contrast material (Fig. 84–16).

Lymphangiomas

Orbital lymphangiomas occur in children and young adults. In contrast to rapid, self-limited growth of infan-

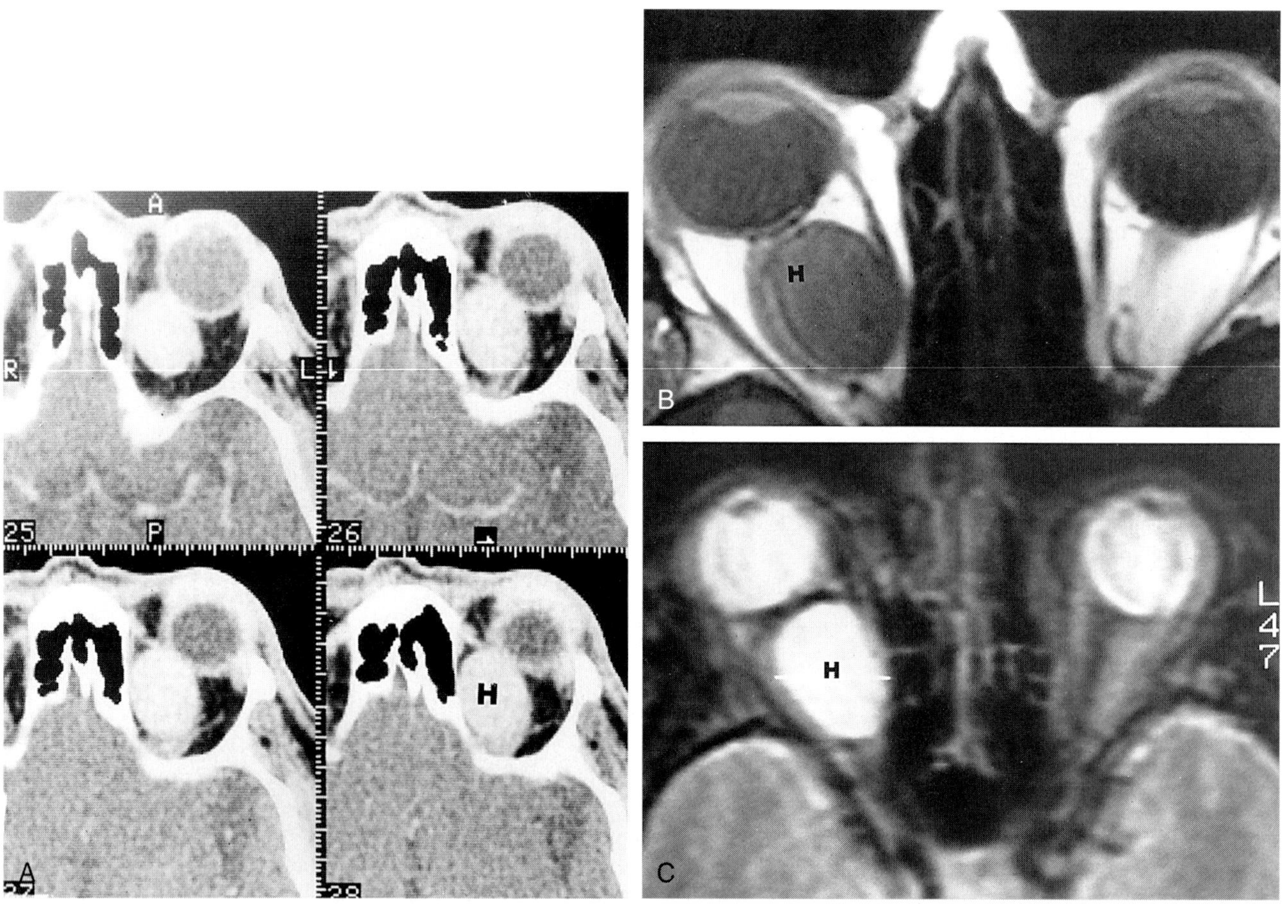

Figure 84–15. Cavernous hemangioma. *A*, Serial axial postcontrast computed tomographic scans show a well-defined intraconal enhancing mass compatible with a hemangioma (H). *B* and C, Axial T1-weighted *(B)* and T2-weighted *(C)* magnetic resonance scans show a well-defined intraconal mass compatible with cavernous hemangioma (H). (*A* to C reprinted with permission from Valvassori G [ed]: Imaging of the Head and Neck. Thieme Medical Publishers, 1995. Copyright Thieme Medical Publishers, Inc.)

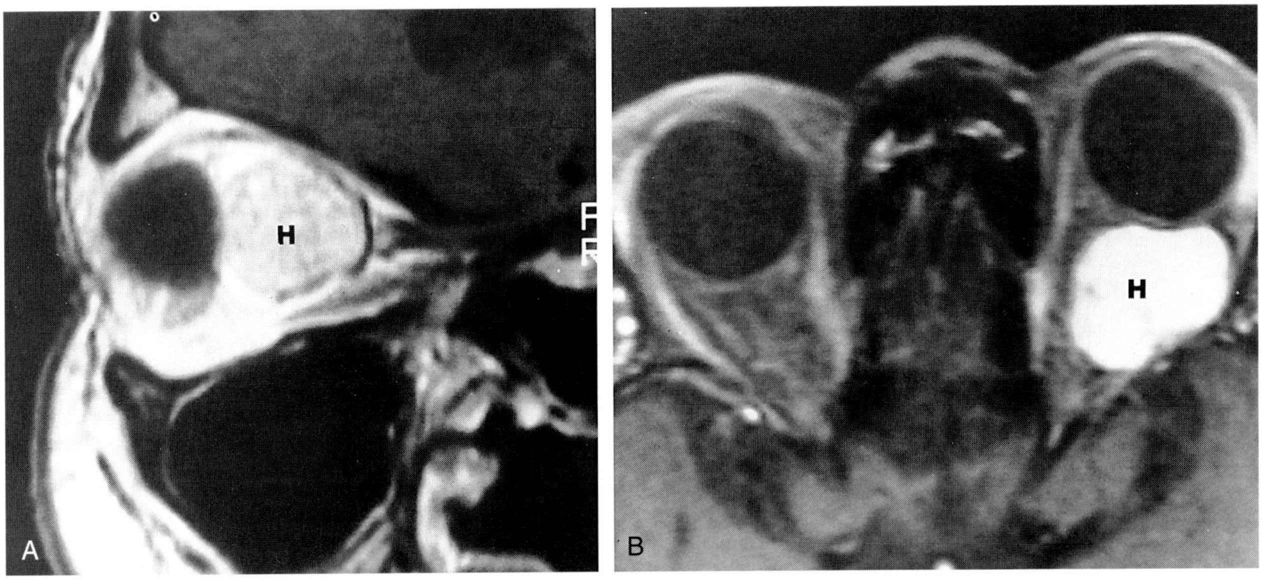

Figure 84–16. Cavernous hemangioma. Sagittal postcontrast *(A)* and axial postcontrast fat-suppressed *(B)* magnetic resonance scans show a well-defined intraconal mass compatible with cavernous hemangioma (H). The lesion is better outlined with the fat-suppression technique. (*A* and *B* reprinted with permission from Valvassori G [ed]: Imaging of the Head and Neck. Thieme Medical Publishers, 1995. Copyright Thieme Medical Publishers, Inc.)

tile capillary hemangiomas, lymphangiomas gradually and progressively enlarge during the growing years. Cavernous lymphangiomas are composed of delicate, endothelium-lined, lymph-filled sinuses (filled with clear fluid or chocolate-colored unclotted fluid) that invade the surrounding connective tissue stroma. The interstitial tissue often shows lymphoid follicles and lymphocytic infiltration. Spontaneous hemorrhage within the lesion is common. Lymphangiomas may have distinct borders but are typically diffuse and not well capsulated, with portions of the lesion infiltrated within normal tissues of the lid and orbit.[12, 13] They are usually multilobular, complete surgical excision is seldom accomplished, and recurrence is common. These tumors are more common in the extraconal space. On CT scans, these lymphangiomas appear as poorly circumscribed, often heterogeneous masses of increased density in the extraconal or intraconal space. Bony expansion may be present, calcification is rare, and minimal to marked contrast enhancement may be present. On MR scans, lymphangiomas are seen as relatively hyperintense images on T1-weighted scans and usually very hyperintense on T2-weighted MR scans. Some lymphangiomas may be hypointense on T1-weighted MR scans. Their MRI characteristics should help to differentiate them from pseudotumors, hemangiomas, and many other lesions (Fig. 84–17). Fluid–fluid level and areas of hemorrhage may be present in lymphangiomas.

Hemangiopericytomas

Hemangiopericytomas are rare, slow-growing vascular neoplasms that arise from the pericytes of Zimmermann that normally envelop capillaries and postcapillary venules of practically all types of tissues. Histologically, these tumors are composed of scattered, capillary-like spaces surrounded by proliferating pericytes.[14] Hemangiopericytomas may be divided into lobules by fibrovascular

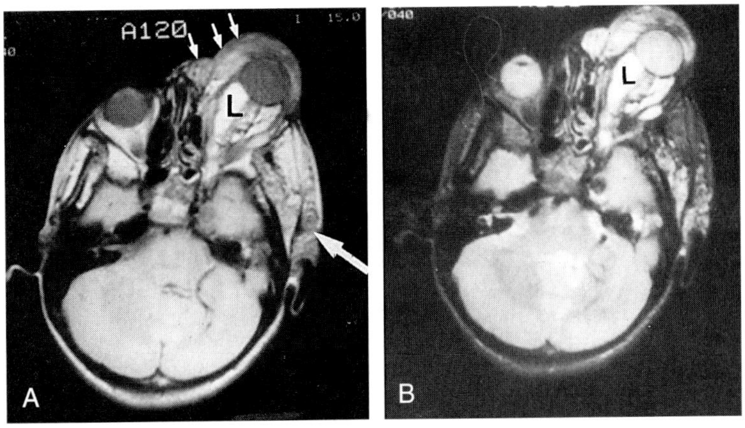

Figure 84–17. Lymphangioma in a 10-year-old girl. *A*, Axial proton-weighted magnetic resonance (MR) scan shows a large lymphangioma involving the eyelid *(short arrows)*, intraconal space (L), and temporal fossa *(arrow)*. *B*, In axial T2-weighted MR scan lymphangioma (L) appears hyperintense. (*A* and *B* reprinted with permission from Valvassori G [ed]: Imaging of the Head and Neck. Thieme Medical Publishers, 1995. Copyright Thieme Medical Publishers, Inc.)

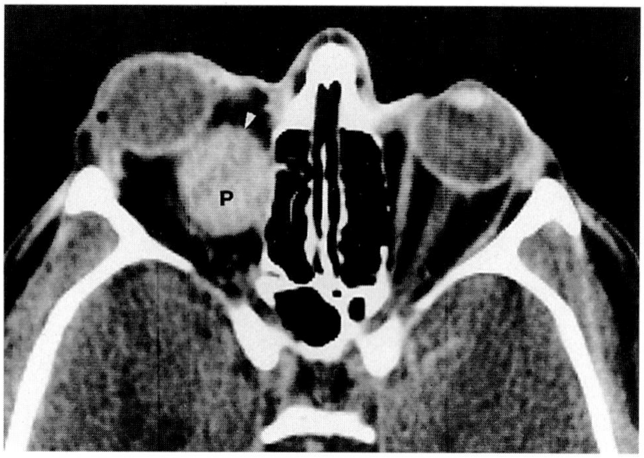

Figure 84–18. Hemangiopericytoma. Axial postcontrast computed tomographic scan shows an intraconal mass compatible with hemangiopericytoma (P). Note the irregularity of the medial portion *(arrowhead)* of the lesions. Cavernous hemangiomas have a very smooth border. (Reprinted with permission from Valvassori G [ed]: Imaging of the Head and Neck. Thieme Medical Publishers, 1995. Copyright Thieme Medical Publishers, Inc.)

septa. About 50% of the cases are malignant, and distant metastases, although uncommon, occur by means of the vascular and lymphatic routes; the lungs are the most common sites for them.[1, 14] These lesions tend to recur if not excised completely. Wide surgical excision is the treatment of choice.

On CT, the margins of orbital hemangiopericytomas (particularly when the tumor is large) in contrast to cavernous hemangiomas may be slightly less distinct owing to their tendency to invade the adjacent tissues (Fig. 84–18). Erosion of the underlying bone may be present. Marked contrast enhancement is often present. Calcifications, if present, favor hemangiopericytomas rather than cavernous hemangiomas. The MR features are indicative of lesions with long T1 and T2 relaxation times (Fig. 84–19). MR scans may not differentiate them from cavernous hemangiomas, neurogenic tumors, meningiomas, and other lesions. Angiography may be very helpful to differentiate the tumors from cavernous hemangiomas, meningiomas, and schwannomas. Hemangiopericytomas usually have an early florid blush, and cavernous hemangiomas show late minor pooling of the contrast medium or often behave as avascular masses. Meningiomas may show multiple tumor vessels and a late blush, and schwannomas may show no tumor blush. Hemangiopericytomas may be difficult to differentiate from other vasculogenic tumors such as angioleiomyomas, from malignant hemangioendotheliomas (angiosarcomas), and from fibrous histiocytomas.

Orbital Varices

Primary orbital varices are congenital venous malformations characterized by proliferations of venous elements and massive dilation of one or more orbital veins presumably associated with congenital weakness in the venous wall. Orbital varices are the most common cause of spontaneous orbital hemorrhage. The CT appearance of orbital varices may be normal in axial sections but quite abnormal in coronal sections, particularly those obtained in a prone position because of increased venous pressure. Any time an orbital varix is suspected, additional CT sections during Valsalva maneuver are recommended.[1] In suspected patients, MRI should also be performed with the patient in a prone position. MRI of orbital varices in one of our patients with bilateral varices showed hyperintense lesions in T1-weighted, proton-weighted, and T2-weighted images. Orbital varices may be seen as several round or tubular images with associated calcifications (Fig. 84–20).

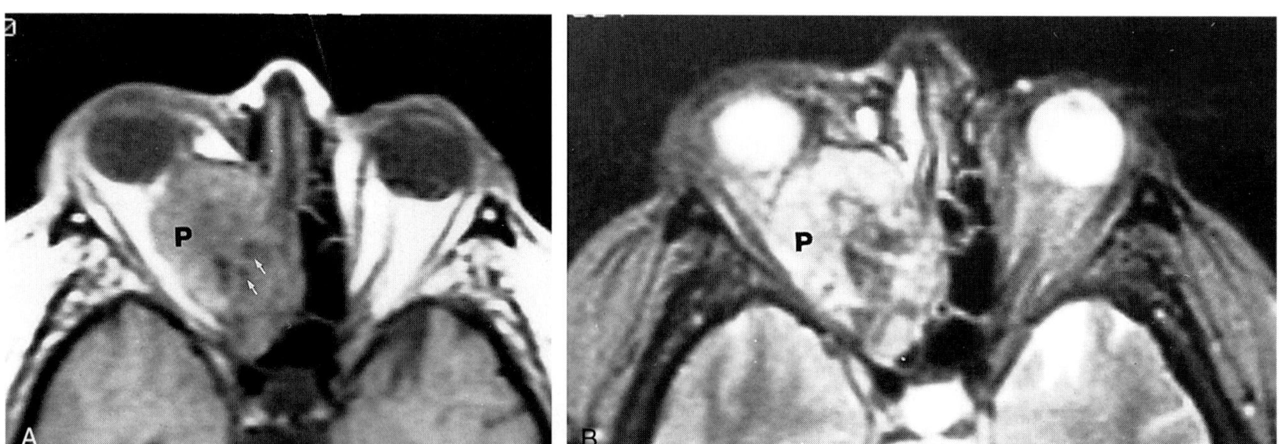

Figure 84–19. Hemangiopericytoma. *A*, Axial T1-weighted magnetic resonance (MR) scan shows a large hemangiopericytoma (P) invading the adjacent ethmoid sinus. The hypointense areas *(arrows)* were due to calcifications seen on computed tomography, not shown here. *B*, Axial T2-weighted MR scan shows the hemangiopericytoma (P). (*A* and *B* reprinted with permission from Valvassori G [ed]: Imaging of the Head and Neck. Thieme Medical Publishers, 1995. Copyright Thieme Medical Publishers, Inc.)

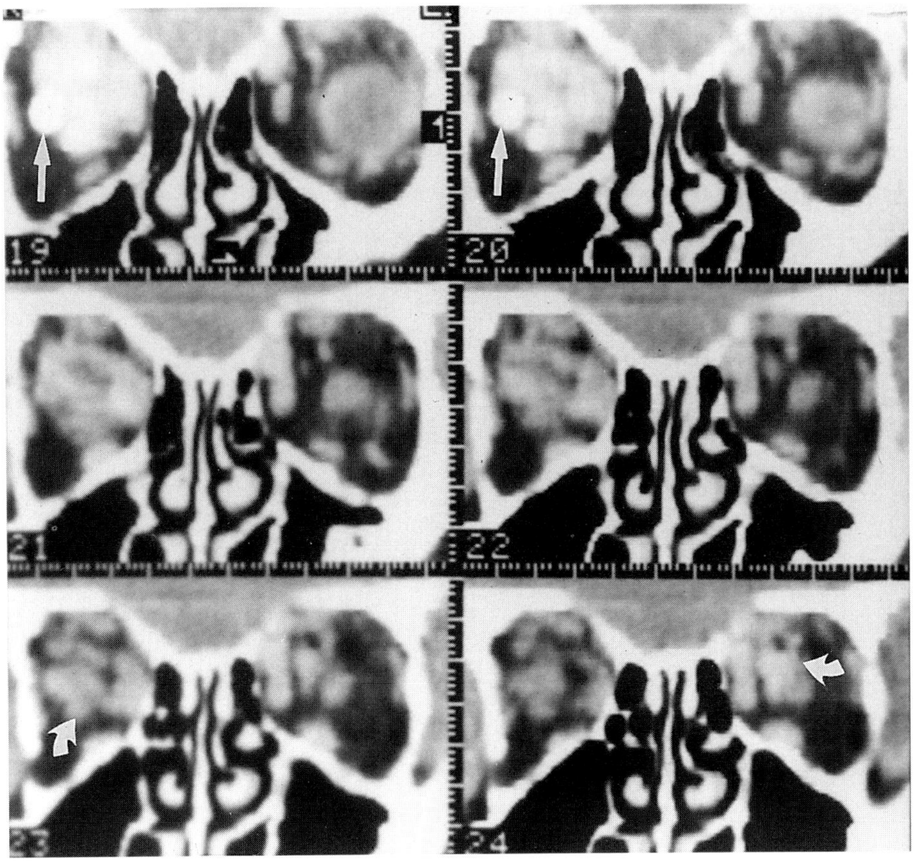

Figure 84–20. Orbital varix. Serial reformatted postcontrast computed tomographic scan shows multiple bilateral enhancing masses *(curved arrows)*. Note the round calcifications *(straight arrows)*. (Reprinted with permission from Valvassori G [ed]: Imaging of the Head and Neck. Thieme Medical Publishers, 1995. Copyright Thieme Medical Publishers, Inc.)

Carotid-Cavernous Fistulas

Carotid-cavernous fistulas produce proptosis, chemosis, venous engorgement, pulsating exophthalmos, and an auscultatable bruit. Ischemic ocular necrosis resulting from carotid-cavernous fistula has been reported. A carotid-cavernous fistula may result from trauma or surgery or may occur spontaneously. Spontaneous carotid-cavernous fistulas have been reported in patients with osteogenesis imperfecta, Ehlers-Danlos syndrome, and pseudoxanthoma elasticum, probably caused by weakness of the vessel walls related to connective tissue disease. CT and MRI will demonstrate proptosis with engorgement of the superior ophthalmic vein and frequent enlargement of the ipsilateral extraocular muscles (Fig. 84–21). There may be CT or MRI evidence of venous thrombosis in the lumen of the superior ophthalmic vein or cavernous sinus. Angiographic demonstration of the exact location of the carotid-cavernous fistula is essential and aids in planning definitive therapy.

Optic Nerve Sheath Meningiomas

Optic nerve meningiomas arise from either the arachnoid cells covering the optic nerve or extension into the orbit from an intracranial meningioma.[15] Meningiomas are usually seen in middle-aged women. Childhood optic nerve meningiomas are much more aggressive than the adult form. Bilateral optic nerve meningiomas may occur in patients with or without neurofibromatosis. Bilateral optic nerve gliomas, however, always occur in patients with neurofibromatosis type 1.

CT is presently the most informative radiologic study used to evaluate optic nerve meningiomas. CT is best obtained with and without infusion of iodinated contrast media. Thin sections (1.5 to 3 mm) are essential to visualize the actual extent of the tumor. Since optic nerve meningiomas are confined to the dura mater, they appear as well-defined tubular thickenings in 64% of the cases. Optic nerve sheath meningiomas are commonly seen as localized eccentric expansion, often at the orbital apex (Fig. 84–22). After injection of contrast media, meningiomas often show homogeneous and well-defined enhancement. The "tram-track" sign originally described with optic nerve meningioma, where enhanced CT shows lucency in the center of an enlarged optic nerve–sheath complex with peripheral enhancement, is not a specific finding. This pattern of enhancement may be seen in pseudotumors, lymphoma, leukemia, and optic neuritis. On CT images, linear or granular calcifications within an optic nerve mass are almost always an indication of optic nerve meningioma. Large optic glioma,

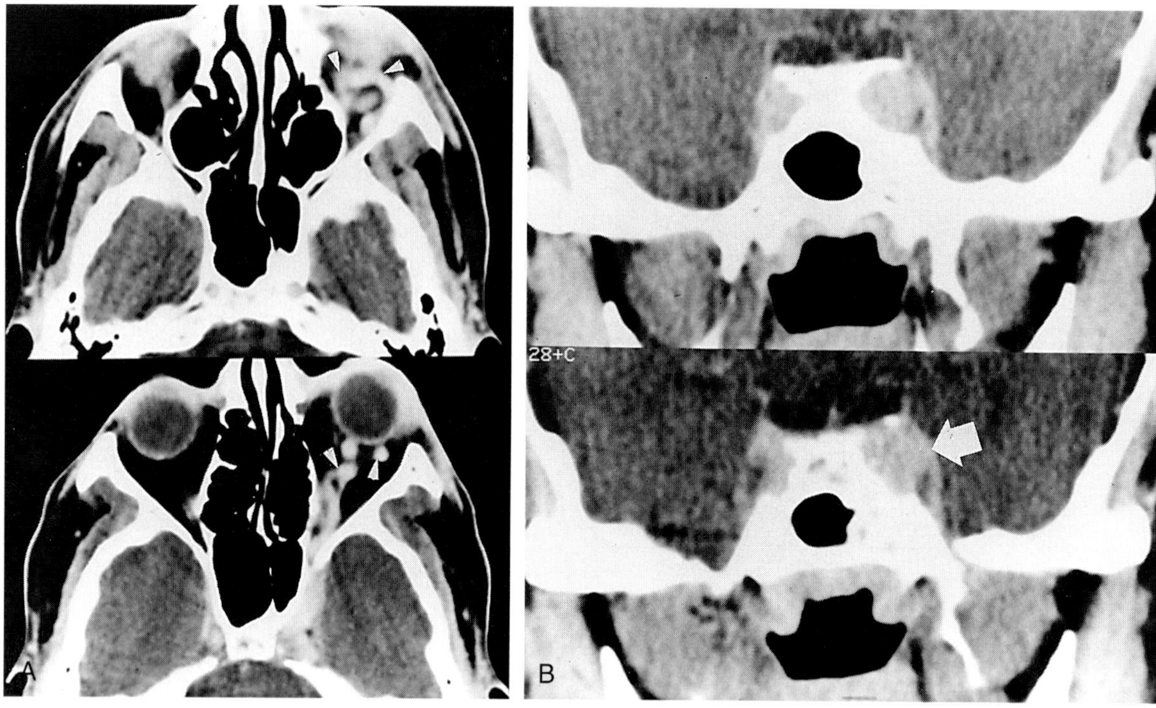

Figure 84–21. *A*, Carotid-cavernous fistula. Axial postcontrast computed tomographic (CT) scans show marked engorgement of orbital veins *(arrowheads)*. *B*, Coronal postcontrast CT scans show marked engorgement of the left cavernous sinus *(arrow)*. (*A* and *B* reprinted with permission from Valvassori G [ed]: Imaging of the Head and Neck. Thieme Medical Publishers, 1995. Copyright Thieme Medical Publishers, Inc.)

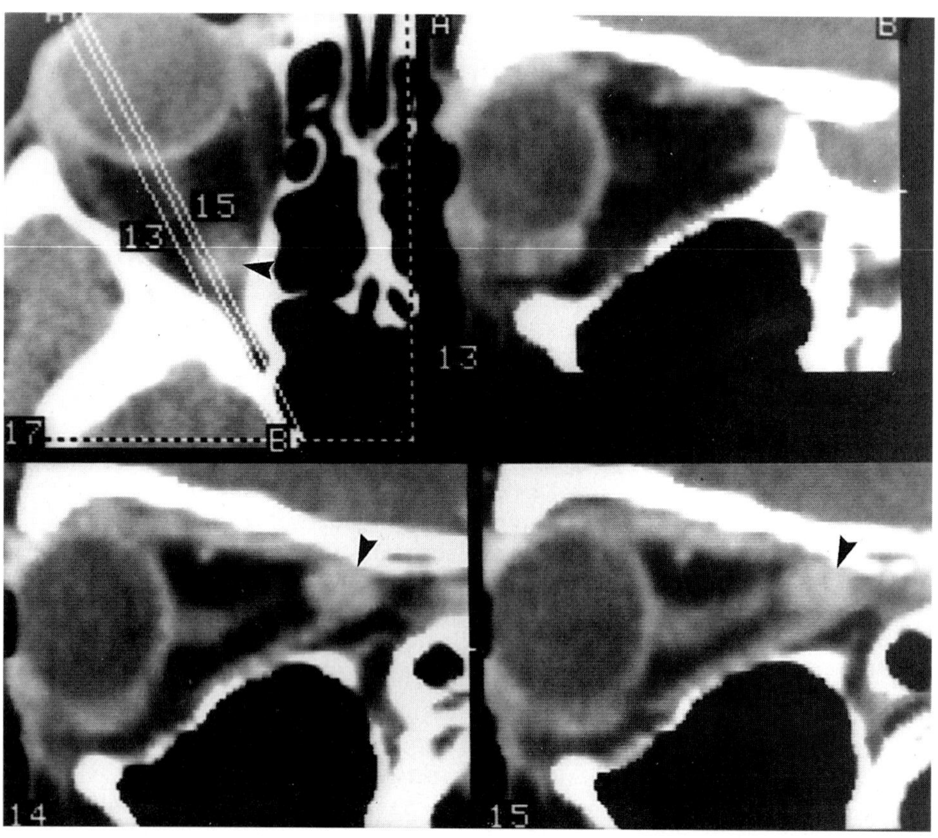

Figure 84–22. Optic sheath meningioma. Serial reformatted sagittal computed tomographic scan shows a meningioma involving the apical segment of the optic nerve *(arrowheads)*. (Reprinted with permission from Valvassori G [ed]: Imaging of the Head and Neck. Thieme Medical Publishers, 1995. Copyright Thieme Medical Publishers, Inc.)

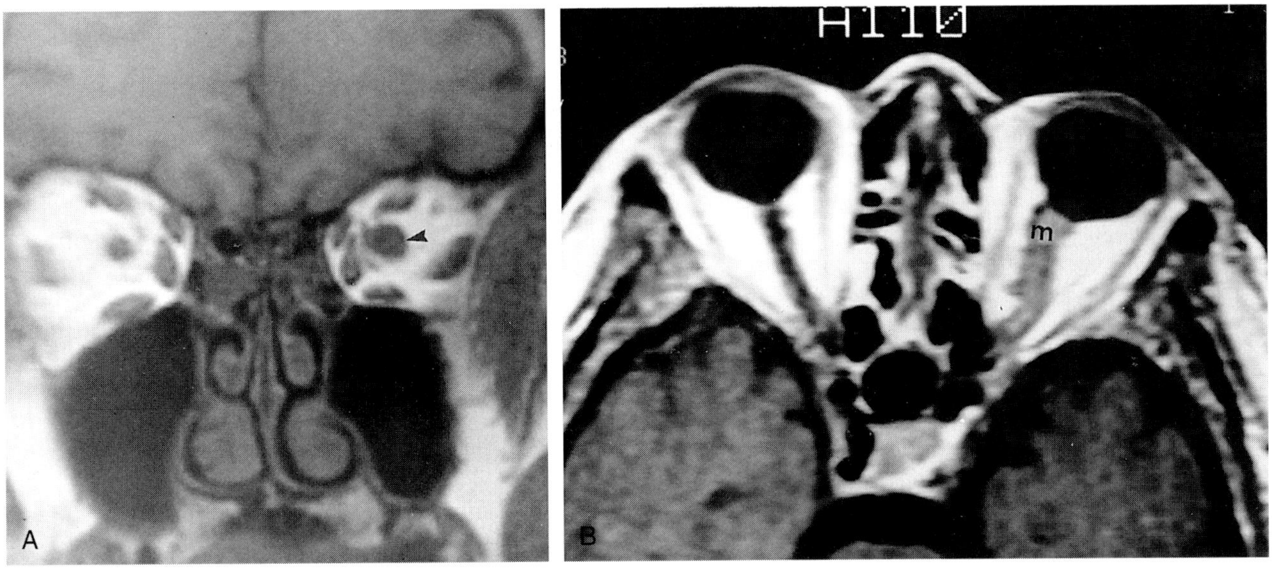

Figure 84–23. *A*, Coronal T1-weighted magnetic resonance (MR) scan. The meningioma (*arrowhead*) is isointense to the normal left optic nerve and brain. *B*, Axial postcontrast T1-weighted MR scan shows moderate enhancement of the meningioma (m). (*A* and *B* reprinted with permission from Valvassori G [ed]: Imaging of the Head and Neck. Thieme Medical Publishers, 1995. Copyright Thieme Medical Publishers, Inc.)

however, may rarely show focal calcification. MRI can make multiple contributions to the imaging evaluation of optic nerve meningiomas. On MR scans, meningioma can be seen as a uniform or round enlargement of the optic nerve (Fig. 84–23). Meningiomas may be hypointense to brain in T1-weighted and proton-weighted scans and hyperintense in T2-weighted scans. Intravenous injection of paramagnetic gadolinium contrast usually results in marked enhancement of meningiomas. When intravenous gadolinium is used, additional T1-weighted fat suppression pulse sequence may prove very valuable for enhancing meningiomas.

Optic Nerve Gliomas (Juvenile Pilocytic Astrocytomas)

Optic nerve gliomas are tumors arising from the neuroglia.[2, 13, 16] Although they are usually tumors of childhood (2–6 years), they can be seen at birth and rarely in the adult years. Nine of 10 cases are symptomatic in the first 2 decades. Optic nerve gliomas in children are benign, well-differentiated, and slow-growing tumors. Bilateral optic nerve gliomas are characteristic of type I neurofibromatosis. The natural history of childhood optic glioma does not involve malignant transformation or systemic metastasis. Local invasion into the extraocular muscles rarely occurs. Thickening of perineural tissue seems to be responsible for the fusiform shape of optic nerve glioma. The primary sequela of this tumor is atrophy that results from damage to the optic nerve fibers and the optic nerve nutrient arteries. Malignant optic gliomas are primarily seen in adults. They are rare and fatal and usually extend from an intracranial glioma (glioblastoma multiforme).

Unenhanced axial CT shows well-defined fusiform enlargement of the optic nerve. Diffuse, tortuous enlargement of the optic nerve with characteristic kinking and buckling (sinusoid) appearance is a characteristic feature of the childhood form of optic glioma. Calcification is rare in optic nerve gliomas. After intravenous contrast medium administration these tumors may show homogeneous or nonhomogeneous enhancement (Fig. 84–24). The inhomogeneity is probably the result of tumor

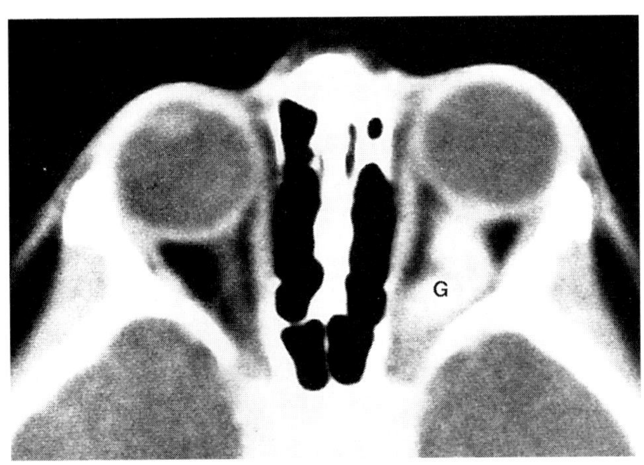

Figure 84–24. Optic nerve glioma. Axial postcontrast computed tomographic scan shows marked enhancement of an optic nerve glioma (G) in this 5-year-old boy with no history of neurofibromatosis. Note the characteristic kinking and tortuosity of the tumor. (Reprinted with permission from Valvassori G [ed]: Imaging of the Head and Neck. Thieme Medical Publishers, 1995. Copyright Thieme Medical Publishers, Inc.)

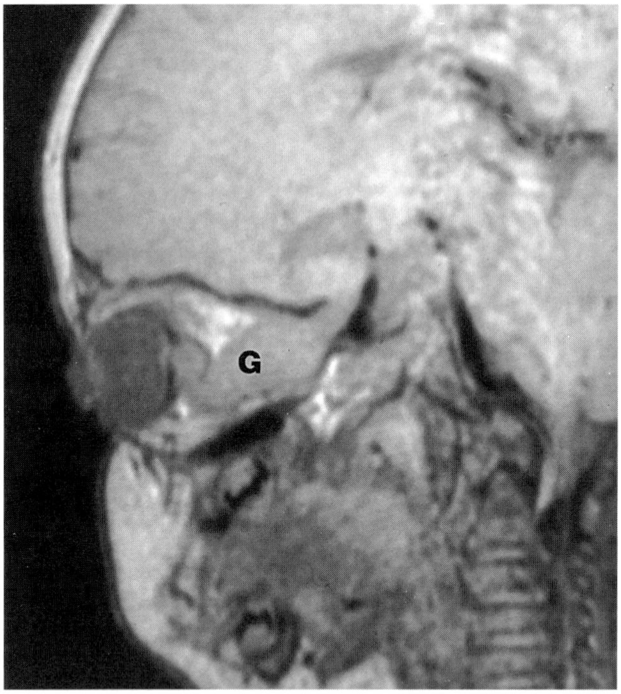

Figure 84–25. Optic nerve glioma. Sagittal proton-weighted magnetic resonance scan shows a large optic nerve glioma (G). (Reprinted with permission from Valvassori G [ed]: Imaging of the Head and Neck. Thieme Medical Publishers, 1995. Copyright Thieme Medical Publishers, Inc.)

infarction secondary to obliteration of the small nutrient arteries of the optic nerve.[15]

MRI also readily demonstrates an enlarged fusiform and kinked optic nerve. On T1-weighted images, the optic glioma will appear isointense or slightly hyperintense compared with the white matter (Fig. 84–25). On T2-weighted images, the lesion may show greater variability in intensity, but it may appear hyperintense compared with the white matter. Intracranial extension of optic nerve gliomas can be better appreciated on MRI.[15] The use of paramagnetic contrast media results in enhancement of gliomas, although less than meningiomas.

Nontumoral Enlargement of the Optic Nerve and Sheath

Primary or secondary involvement of the optic nerve in cases of lymphoma, sarcoid, leukemia, tuberculosis, toxoplasmosis, and syphilis has been reported.

Optic Neuritis

Optic neuritis is an acute inflammatory process involving the optic nerve and may present as optic nerve enlargement. It is sometimes an early manifestation of multiple sclerosis. In optic neuritis, CT may show an enlarged optic nerve with some degree of contrast medium enhancement. On MRI, the optic neuritis may appear as hyperintense image on T2-weighted MR scans. MR visualization of optic neuritis may be accentuated by post–Gd-DTPA, T1-weighted with or without fat suppression technique (Fig. 84–26).

Optic Nerve Sarcoidosis

Certain inflammatory conditions, such as syphilis, tuberculosis, or sarcoidosis, may be responsible for a chronic and progressive loss of vision. Chronic optic neuropathy, however, is more frequently due to a compressive lesion such as meningioma (intracanalicular or tuberculum sellae), pituitary tumor, or paraclinoid aneurysm.

Sarcoidosis frequently involves the nervous system and can present as abrupt or very chronic visual loss, with or without disc changes. In one series of 11 patients with sarcoidosis of the optic nerve ranging in age from 16 to 48 years, only 2 patients were previously known to have the disorder. Four patients showed disc granulomas, 4 had optic nerve granulomas, and 5 had posterior uveitis and retinitis. In this series, chest radiographs were characteristically abnormal in 8 of the 11 patients. Only one third had elevated serum levels of angiotensin converting enzyme. CT scans in these 11 patients infrequently showed enlarged nerves or other findings. Although sarcoidosis is

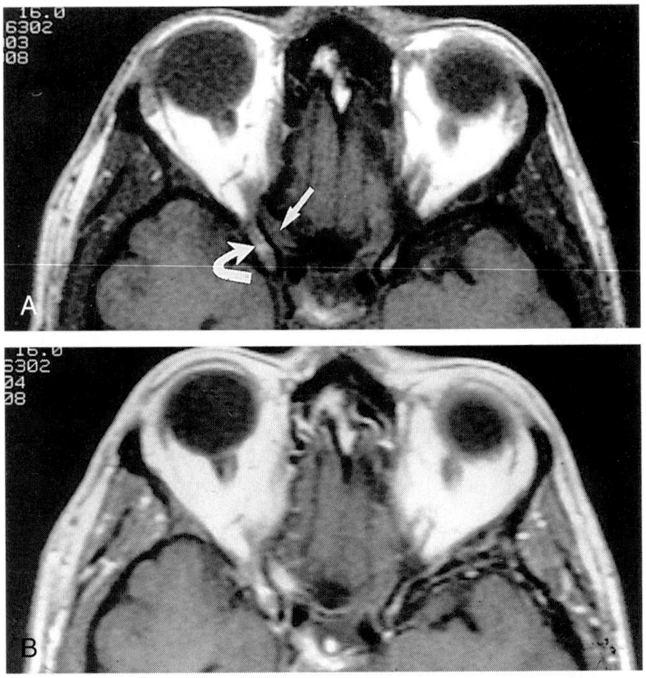

Figure 84–26. Optic neuritis. Axial T1-weighted magnetic resonance scans before *(A)* and after *(B)* administration of Gd-DTPA show enhancement of only the intracanalicular segment of the right optic nerve *(straight arrow)*. The left optic nerve shows no enhancement. The curved arrow points to the marrow portion of the anterior clinoid process. (From Mafee MF: Case 35: Optic nerve sheath meningioma. Head and Neck Disorders [Fourth Series] Test and Syllabus. American College of Radiology, 1992.)

classically believed not to involve the optic nerves commonly, we have seen increasing numbers of cases of presumed optic nerve sarcoidosis on MR and CT scans, some of them with histologic confirmation.

Sarcoidosis is an idiopathic, multisystemic, granulomatous inflammation, often involving the mediastinal and peripheral lymph nodes, the lungs, liver, spleen, bone marrow, parotid glands, eyes, lacrimal glands, and many other organs. In the United States, the disease is more prevalent in young adult African Americans and more common in women than men. In ophthalmologic series, up to 50% of patients with sarcoidosis have ocular involvement. Thirty percent of cases of posterior uveitis are associated with sarcoidosis. Neurologic involvement with sarcoidosis takes two forms. In acute sarcoidosis, there tends to be involvement of a peripheral nerve, especially a cranial nerve and in particular the facial nerve. The optic nerve (which is not a peripheral nerve) is involved next most frequently. Sarcoid uveitis, in combination with a facial nerve palsy and fever, is known as Heerfordt's syndrome or uveoparotid fever. The second form of nervous system sarcoid occurs in the chronic form of the disease, with CNS involvement. Involvement of the optic nerve is more common in this form. The involvement may be at the chiasm or in the intracanalicular or intraorbital segments of the nerve head. Orbital pseudotumor could easily be mistaken for sarcoidosis. Sarcoidosis-like lesions can be found in patients with syphilis, lymphogranuloma venereum, leprosy, tularemia, torulosis, histoplasmosis, blastomycosis, and coccidioidomycosis.

The early lesions of sarcoidosis are much more likely to respond to corticosteroid therapy than are the late, fibrotic hyalinized lesions. Lesions that demand systemic corticosteroid therapy are uveitis, optic neuritis, pulmonary and CNS lesions, facial palsy, persistent hypercalcemia, and cutaneous lesions.

When an ophthalmologist or neurologist suspects that an optic nerve is involved by sarcoidosis or that there is sarcoid of the CNS, a chest radiograph can be very useful. Active pulmonary sarcoidosis shows bilateral hilar adenopathy, with or without parenchymal disease. The nodes characteristically stand out from the right-sided heart border, and there is associated right paratracheal nodal involvement. Chest abnormalities are found in about 80% of patients with ocular sarcoidosis (uveitis). Gallium scintigraphy is more sensitive than chest radiography for showing pulmonary involvement in patients with sarcoidosis. It lacks specificity, however, because other pulmonary diseases also show similar uptake. Lacrimal gland uptake of gallium-67 also occurs in more than 80% of patients with active sarcoidosis. This uptake is also nonspecific.

CT and MR scans in patients with optic nerve sarcoidosis may show no significant findings; however, not infrequently, they may show enlargement of the optic nerve, as well as expansion of the optic canal, mimicking an optic nerve sheath meningioma or glioma on orbital imaging (Fig. 84–27).

The optic nerve may be secondarily involved by various inflammatory lesions of surrounding tissues, including the orbit, paranasal sinuses, base of the skull, and meninges. Idiopathic inflammatory cuffing of the orbital and intracranial optic nerve may present as progressive visual deterioration and thus mimic an optic nerve sheath meningioma clinically. In general, acute and subacute idiopathic inflammatory orbital syndromes have been designated as pseudotumors, a clinically and histologically ill-defined category of lesions that were discussed before in detail. In patients with orbital pseudotumor, the main focus of inflammation may involve the anterior orbit and adjacent globe with and without perineural infiltration (cuffing). The major features on presentation are pain, proptosis, lid swelling, injection, and decreased vision. Other findings may include uveitis, sclerotenonitis, papillitis, and exudative retinal detachment. The characteristic CT and MR findings are of a diffuse anterior orbital infiltration intimately related to the globe, producing thickening of the choroid, sclera, and Tenon's capsule. There may be fluid (exudate) in Tenon's space, producing a characteristic semilunar configuration around the posterior globe with obscuration of the junction of the globe and the optic nerve, and there may be variable extension along the optic nerve sheath. The optic nerve involvement may be seen in patients with other types of orbital pseudotumors, including diffuse, myositic, and apical types of pseudotumors, as well as in those in orbital lymphoma and orbital leukemic infiltration. In patients with optic nerve pseudotumor (perineuritis), optic nerve involvement is rarely an isolated finding. There are other CT and MR findings in the retrobulbar and extraconal spaces characteristic of pseudotumor. CT shows variable enhancement. MRI shows a ragged, edematous enlargement of the optic nerve sheath complex, as well as enhancement.Rapid corticosteroid responsiveness is almost pathognomonic for pseudotumors. CT and MR scanning are useful, particularly for assessing resolution after therapy. Failure of resolution should suggest alternative diagnoses, and a biopsy may be necessary.

Rhabdomyosarcomas

Rhabdomyosarcomas are the most common primary orbital malignancy in children. Clinically, their occurrence involves the differential diagnosis of acute and subacute proptosis of childhood. Changes in chemotherapy over the past decade have markedly improved the prognosis, particularly in orbital cases. Rhabdomyosarcomas arise in the orbit from extraocular muscles or from pluripotential mesenchymal elements. On the basis of their histopathologic features, most can be classified into one of the three histologic types: embryonal, differentiated,

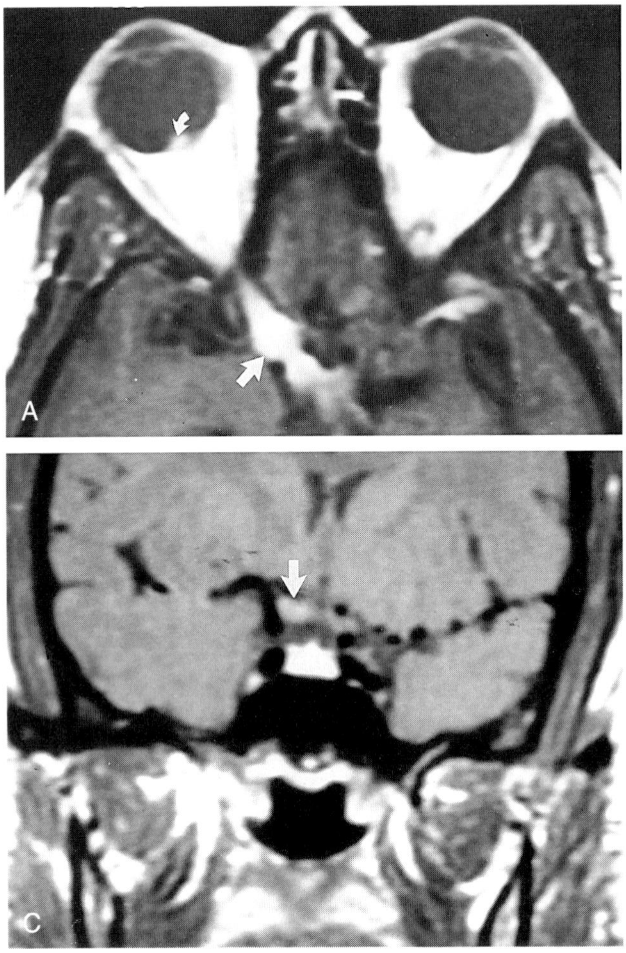

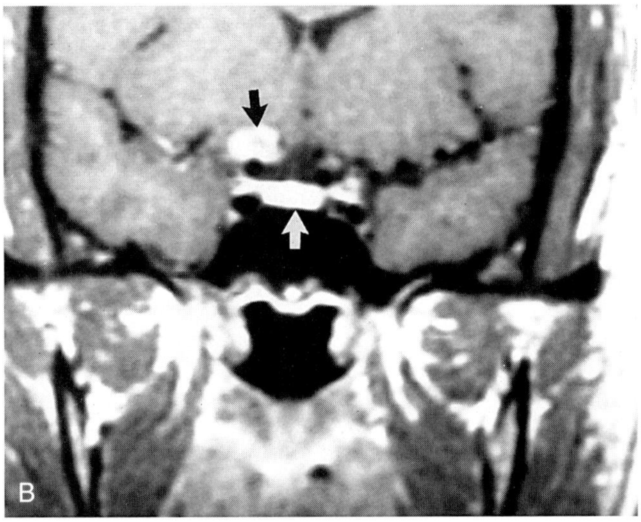

Figure 84–27. Sarcoidosis of optic nerve. *A*, Axial postcontrast T1-weighted magnetic resonance (MR) scan shows marked enhancement of the intracanalicular and intracranial segments of the right optic nerve (*straight arrow*). There is also an enhancing intraocular mass (*curved arrow*), indicative of intraocular granuloma. These MR findings were initially believed to be compatible with either optic nerve glioma or meningioma in this 28-year-old African American woman. However, because of the enhancing lesion in the globe and the clinical setting, sarcoidosis was suggested as the primary consideration, and the patient was placed on corticosteroid therapy. Followup MR findings are shown in *B*. *B*, Coronal postcontrast T1-weighted MR scan shows marked enhancement of the intracranial portion of the right optic nerve (*black arrow*). Enhancement of the pituitary gland (*white arrow*) is normal. *C*, Coronal postcontrast T1-weighted MR scan after steroid therapy showing marked improvement. There is asymmetry and slight thickening and enhancement of the right side of the chiasm (*arrow*). (From Mafee MF: Case 35: Optic nerve sheath meningioma. Head and Neck Disorders [Fourth Series] Test and Syllabus. American College of Radiology, 1992.)

or alveolar rhabdomyosarcoma. The embryonal type is the most common, and the differentiated is the least frequent type.

Rapidly progressing unilateral proptosis is the hallmark of orbital rhabdomyosarcomas. Congenital proptosis in infants is most likely to be caused by a rhabdomyosarcoma, hemangioma, or optic glioma if primary or by a neuroblastoma or leukemic deposit if secondary.

Clinically the differential diagnosis of orbital rhabdomyosarcoma includes progressive, rapidly developing tumors and inflammatory conditions of childhood. These include neuroblastoma, chloroma, lymphangioma, infantile hemangioma, teratoma, dermoid cysts, Langerhans' histiocytosis, and orbital cellulitis.

CT and MRI provide information about the orbital soft tissue structures and the relationship among them and adjacent bone, cranial fossae, and paranasal sinuses. Rhabdomyosarcomas are aggressive malignant tumors capable of bone destruction. On CT scans, these tumors are seen as enhancing masses within the orbit. There may be associated bone destruction (Fig. 84–28). The MRI features of orbital rhabdomyosarcoma are characteristic of lesions with long T1 and T2 relaxation times (Fig. 84–29). There will be moderate to marked enhancement after intravenous injection of Gd-DTPA contrast material. CT and MRI can accurately define the anatomic location of the orbital mass, the involvement of various intraorbital structures, and the extension of tumor into the surrounding structures. Biopsy should be performed to establish the diagnosis. Rhabdomyosarcomas are sensitive to radiation therapy and chemotherapy.

Lacrimal Gland and Fossa Lesions

Lesions of the lacrimal gland and fossa present special problems in diagnosis and management. The excellent prognosis for benign mixed tumors, provided they are completely excised at first surgery, necessitates that these lesions should not undergo incisional biopsy but require en bloc excision along with adjacent tissues. Because of the importance of preoperative diagnosis, all clinical ancillary findings should be integrated in the assessment of individual cases. In general, epithelial tumors represent

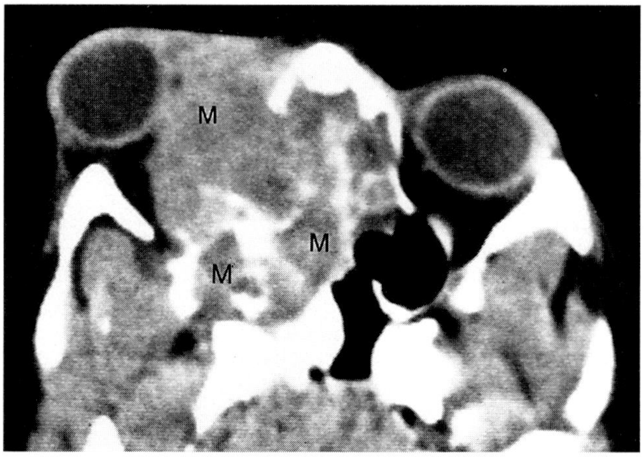

Figure 84–28. Rhabdomyosarcoma in a 17-year-old patient. Axial post-contrast computed tomographic scan shows a large destructive mass (M) involving the right orbit and extending into the ethmoid sinuses. (Reprinted with permission from Valvassori G [ed]: Imaging of the Head and Neck. Thieme Medical Publishers, 1995. Copyright Thieme Medical Publishers, Inc.)

50% of masses involving the lacrimal gland. The remaining 50% of lacrimal gland masses are the lymphoid-inflammatory type. Metastases to the parenchyma of the lacrimal gland are rare. Dermoid cysts are not true lacrimal gland tumors, but rather arise from epithelial rests located in the orbit, particularly in the superolateral quadrant. Epithelial cysts, on the other hand, are intrinsic lesions that result from dilation of the lacrimal ducts.

Lymphomatous lesions of the lacrimal gland include a broad spectrum from reactive lymphoid hyerplasia to malignant lymphomas of various types. Inflammatory or lymphoid lesions of the lacrimal gland show diffuse enlargement of the gland. Contrast enhancement on CT or

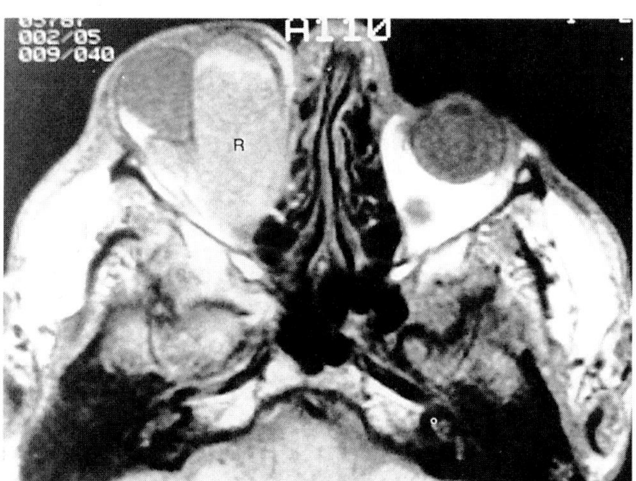

Figure 84–29. Rhabdomyosarcoma in a 60-year-old patient. Axial proton-weighted magnetic resonance scan shows a large orbital mass compatible with rhabdomyosarcoma (R). The "senile" rhabdomyosarcoma is very rare. The differential diagnosis should include lymphoma, metastasis, primary orbital melanoma, malignant histiocytoma, and hemangiopericytoma. (Reprinted with permission from Valvassori G [ed]: Imaging of the Head and Neck. Thieme Medical Publishers, 1995. Copyright Thieme Medical Publishers, Inc.)

MRI may be marked, and there may be associated acute lateral rectus muscle myositis. In chronic dacryoadenitis, the gland also shows diffuse oblong enlargement. The glands may be massively enlarged in case of sarcoidosis or other conditions such as Mikulicz' syndrome, pseudotumors, and Wegener's granulomatosis.

Benign and malignant lymphoid tumors situated in the lacrimal gland also display diffuse enlargement with oblong contouring of the gland; however, these lesions are bulkier and have more frequent evidence of anterior and posterior extension and molding and draping on the globe. In general, inflammatory processes and lymphomas tend to involve all aspects of the lacrimal gland, often including its palpebral lobe. However, neoplastic lesions of the gland rarely originate in the palpebral lobe of the gland, and therefore there is often a tendency for posterior extension rather than for extension anteriorly beyond the orbital rim.

Since the lacrimal gland is histologically similar to the salivary gland, it is involved by similar disease processes. Epithelial tumors represent 50% of masses involving the lacrimal gland. Half of these are pleomorphic (benign mixed) adenomas; the other half are malignant. Of the malignant tumors, the adenoid cystic (adenocystic) type is the most common, followed by pleomorphic (malignant mixed), mucoepidermoid, adenocarcinoma, squamous cell carcinoma, and undifferentiated (anaplastic) carcinoma. A significant number of these tumors arise within pleomorphic adenomas.

Jakobiec and associates[17] reviewed by CT 39 patients with solid masses in the lacrimal gland: 16 had parenchymal benign and malignant tumors, 6 had benign mixed, 1 had a schwannoma, and 9 had malignant epithelial tumors. Tumors exhibited rounded or globular soft tissue outlines and were frequently associated with continuous bone changes. Benign tumors had smooth encapsulated outlines, whereas the malignant tumors displayed microserrations indicative of infiltration. Calcifications are more common in malignant tumors of lacrimal gland. Inflammatory conditions in this series demonstrated diffuse, compressed, and molded enlargement of the lacrimal gland in an oblong fashion, and there were no associated bone defects. They concluded that well-capsulated, rounded masses of long duration are likely to be benign mixed tumors (Fig. 84–30). In contrast, inflammatory and lymphoid lesions of lacrimal gland were seen as diffuse expansion of the lacrimal gland and the lesions molded themselves to preexisting orbital structures without eroding bone or enlarging the orbit.

Bone changes in the lacrimal gland fossa may be produced by benign or malignant epithelial tumors, other parenchymal lacrimal gland tumors, such as schwannomas, and lesions originating within the subperiosteal space or bone, including benign orbital cyst, cholesterol granuloma, hematic cyst, eosinophilic granuloma, dermoid cyst, and metastatic carcinoma. Lymphoid and inflammatory processes may rarely produce bone change.

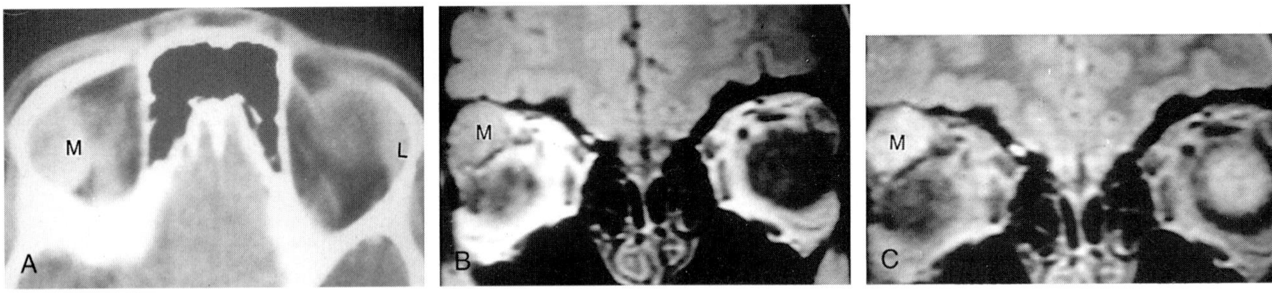

Figure 84–30. Benign lacrimal gland tumor. *A*, Axial postcontrast computed tomographic scan shows a well-defined right lacrimal gland mass (M), compatible with a benign mixed tumor. Note the normal left lacrimal gland (L). Coronal proton-weighted (*B*) and T2-weighted (*C*) magnetic resonance scans show the lacrimal mass (M) compatible with a benign mixed tumor. (*A* to *C* reprinted with permission from Valvassori G [ed]: Imaging of the Head and Neck. Thieme Medical Publishers, 1995. Copyright Thieme Medical Publishers, Inc.)

The MRI features of benign and malignant epithelial tumors of the lacrimal gland are characteristic of lesions with long T1 and long T2 relaxation times (Figs. 84–31 and 84–32). These tumors demonstrate moderate to marked enhancement following intravenous injection of Gd-DTPA contrast material.[18]

GLOBE

Normal Anatomy of Globe

The eye consists of three primary layers: (1) the sclera, or outer layer, is composed primarily of collagen-elastic tissue; (2) the uvea, or middle layer of the eye, is richly vascular and contains pigmented tissue consisting of three components—the iris, ciliary body, and choroid; and (3) the retina, or inner layer, which is the neural, sensory stratum of the eye. The sclera is covered by the Tenon capsule. The Tenon capsule (bulbar fascia) is a fibroelastic membrane that envelops the eyeball from the optic nerve to the level of ciliary muscle.

Imaging Techniques

CT of the globe should be performed using 1.5-mm collimation. Contiguous slices should be obtained. The major application of CT for lesions of the globe include detecting foreign bodies and intraocular calcification. For intraocular tumors and other intraocular pathology, we prefer MRI as the initial study of choice.

MRI of the globe requires focused imaging techniques. Three-millimeter thick sections with 0 to 0.6-mm interslice gap is recommended. Single-echo spin-echo (SE) pulse sequences, using a surface or head coil as the receiving coil, are needed with a repetition time (TR) of 400 to 800 ms and an echo time (TE) of 20 to 25 ms (TR/TE = 400–800/20–25 ms). Multiple echoes SE pulse sequences are recommended with a TR of 1500 to

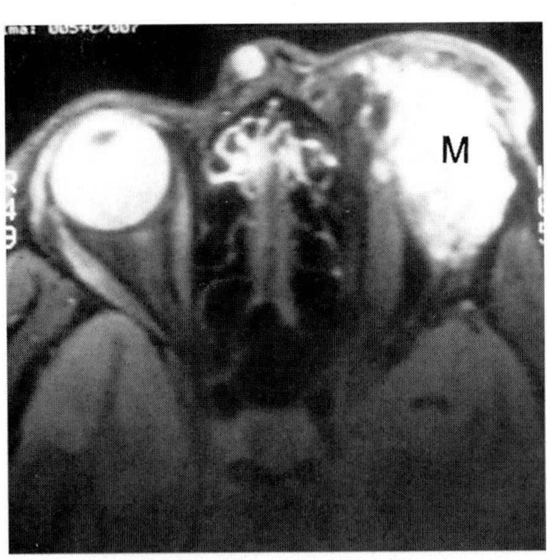

Figure 84–31. Axial short inversion time inversion recovery (1700/25/160, TR/TE/TI) shows a large hyperintense mass (M) compatible with a mixed tumor. (Reprinted with permission from Valvassori G [ed]: Imaging of the Head and Neck. Thieme Medical Publishers, 1995. Copyright Thieme Medical Publishers, Inc.)

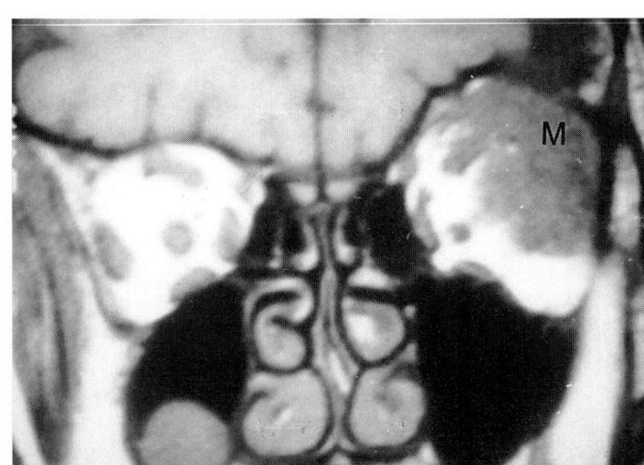

Figure 84–32. Adenoid cystic carcinoma of the lacrimal gland. Coronal magnetic resonance scan shows an irregular infiltrative mass (M) invading the adjacent superior and lateral rectus muscles as well as the extraconal and intraconal fatty reticulum. (Reprinted with permission from Valvassori G [ed]: Imaging of the Head and Neck. Thieme Medical Publishers, 1995. Copyright Thieme Medical Publishers, Inc.)

2500 ms and a TE of 20 to 100 ms. In our institution, the studies are most often performed with one number of excitation (NEX), a 256 × 256 matrix, and a 12- to 16-cm field of view. For shorter TR (400–800 ms), the studies are often performed with two excitations. We use Gd-DTPA (0.1 mmol/kg) for all suspected intraocular masses and infectious and infiltrative processes. Post Gd-DTPA T1-weighted fat suppression pulse sequences are recommended for intraocular tumors and inflammatory processes.

Ocular Pathology

Congenital Lesions

Anophthalmia. Bilateral anophthalmia is a rare condition. There may be rudimentary tissue or no globe present on CT or MRI. The extraocular muscles, lacrimal glands, and eyelids are present.

Microphthalmia. Microphthalmia may occur as an isolated disorder or may be associated with other craniofacial anomalies. Congenital rubella syndrome, persistent hyperplastic primary vitreous, and retinopathy of prematurity are other causes of microphthalmia.

Macrophthalmia. Macrophthalmia is seen in patients with axial myopia, in patients with Sturge-Weber syndrome with juvenile glaucoma, and at times in patients with neurofibromatosis.

Coloboma and Morning Glory Anomaly. A coloboma is a notch, gap, hole, or fissure that is congenital or acquired and in which a tissue or portion of a tissue is lacking. A variety of ocular and systemic abnormalities may be seen with an optic nerve coloboma. Microphthalmia with cyst is an anomaly in which an eye with a retinochoroidal coloboma also has a cyst, which is usually attached to the inferior aspect of the globe.

Morning glory disc anomaly was first characterized by Kindler in 1970. He described a unilateral congenital anomaly of the optic nerve head in 10 patients. Because of the similarity in appearance between the nerve head and a morning glory flower, he referred to the anomaly as the morning glory syndrome. Ophthalmoscopically, the abnormal nerve head has several characteristic findings. The disc is enlarged and excavated and has a central core of white tissue.

The CT and MR appearance of optic nerve head coloboma and the morning glory anomaly is quite characteristic, corresponding to its clinical appearance as a large funnel-shaped disc. The colobomatous cyst associated with coloboma of the optic nerve can be easily identified on CT and MR scans. Any retroglobal cyst associated with a microphthalmic eye should be suspected for a colobomatous cyst.

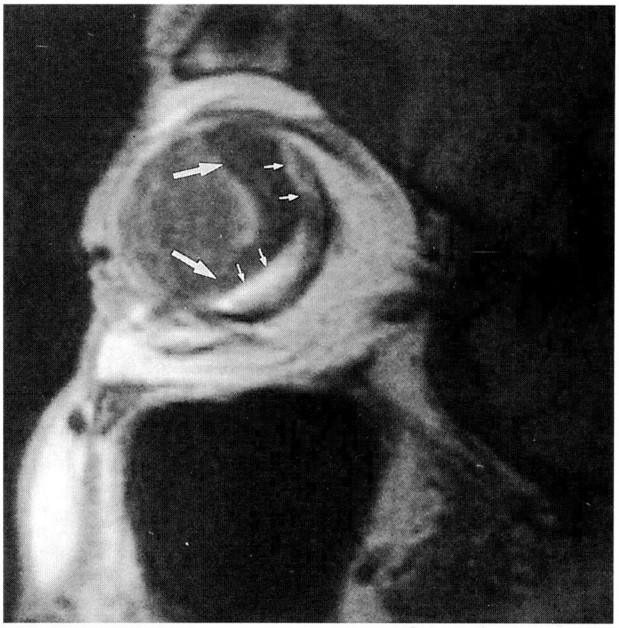

Figure 84–33. Posterior hyaloid and retinal detachments. T1-weighted sagittal magnetic resonance scan. The detached posterior hyaloid membrane (*large arrows*) is seen anterior to the detached retina (*short arrows*). The hypointensity in the subhyaloid space is due to acute hemorrhage; the hyperintensity in the subretinal space is due to chronic hemorrhage. (Reprinted with permission from Valvassori G [ed]: Imaging of the Head and Neck. Thieme Medical Publishers, 1995. Copyright Thieme Medical Publishers, Inc.)

Ocular Detachments

Posterior Hyaloid Detachment. Posterior hyaloid detachment usually occurs in adults older than the age of 50 years, but it may occur in children with persistent hyperplastic primary vitreous. Posterior hyaloid detachment in adults is usually caused by liquefaction of the vitreous and may be associated with macular degeneration (Fig. 84–33).[19]

Retinal Detachment. Retinal detachment occurs when the sensory retina is separated from the retinal pigment epithelium. Fluid in the subretinal space can be detected by both CT and MR scans. Retinal detachment is usually the result of retraction caused by a mass or a fibroproliferative disease in the vitreous such as vitreoretinopathy of prematurity or vitreoretinopathy of diabetes. Retinal detachment may be due to a choroidal mass or to acute (viral) or chronic inflammatory process such as larval granuloma of *Toxocara* endophthalmitis. Retinal detachment may also occur because of retinal vascular leakage, which is seen in patients with Coats' disease, a primary vascular anomaly of the retina characterized by telangiectasia.

When a retinal detachment is identified, the principal question that must be answered is what is the cause of it. Retinal detachment and primary underlying disease can often be differentiated from each other by CT, and in particular by MRI.[19] In an axial CT or MRI scan taken below or above the optic disc, the retinal detachment will appear as homogeneous increased density or increased intensity of the globe. The retina is very thin and therefore is beyond the limits of resolution of CT and MRI scanners. However, it may be shown when it is outlined by significant contrast differences between subretinal effusion and the vitreous cavity. The imaging appearance of retinal detachment varies with the amount of exudation and organization of subretinal materials. In a section taken at the level of the optic disc, retinal detachment is seen with a characteristic indentation at the optic disc. When total retinal detachment is present and the entire vitreous cavity ablated, the leaves of the detached retina may not be detected clearly. Retinal detachment is seen on coronal MR scans as a characteristic folding membrane. The subretinal fluid in the exudative retinal detachment is rich in protein, giving higher CT numbers and stronger MR signals than subretinal fluid (transudate) seen in rhegmatogenous detachment. Retinal detachment is characteristically seen on CT or MRI as a V-shaped image, with its apex at the optic disc and its extremities toward the ciliary body (Fig. 84–34).[19] This appearance of retinal detachment may be confused with the appearance of posterior choroidal detachment; however, posterior choroidal detachment, in the region of the optic disc and macula involves detachment of the choroid that is restricted by the anchoring effect of the short posterior ciliary arteries and nerves as well as the vortex veins. This restriction usually results in a characteristic appearance that the leaves of the detached choroid, unlike the detached retina, do not extend to the region of the optic disc.

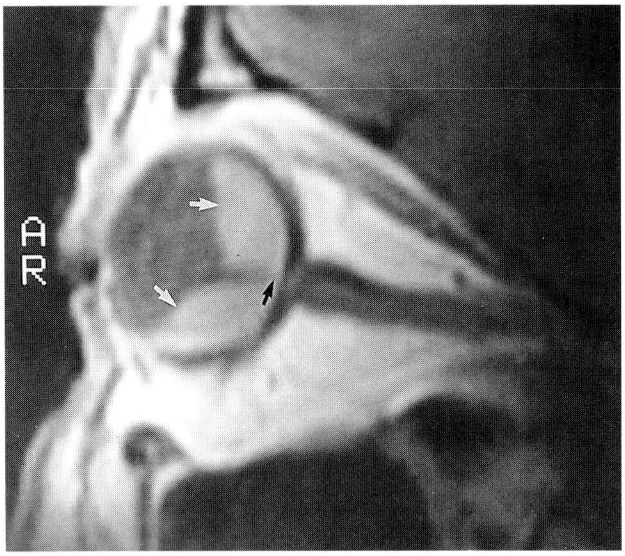

Figure 84–34. Exudative retinal detachment. Proton-weighted axial magnetic resonance (MR) scan shows the leaves of the detached retina (*white arrows*). The retina cannot be detached from the optic disc (*black arrow*). (Reprinted with permission from Valvassori G [ed]: Imaging of the Head and Neck. Thieme Medical Publishers, 1995. Copyright Thieme Medical Publishers, Inc.)

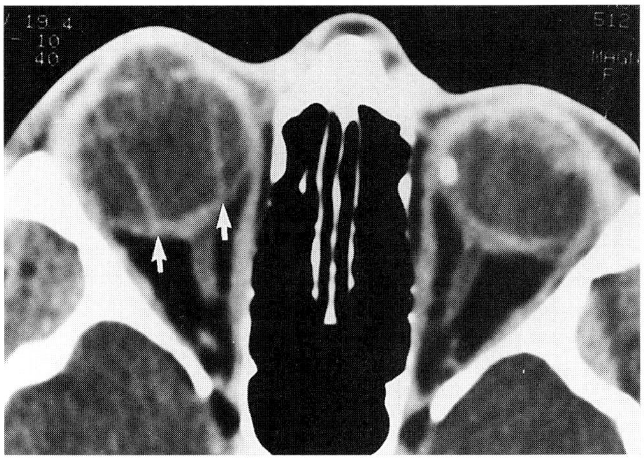

Figure 84–35. Serous choroidal detachment. Axial computed tomographic scan shows the detached choroid (*arrows*). Because of the anchoring effect of the short posterior ciliary arteries and nerves, the detached leaves do not extend toward the optic disc. The hypodensity in the suprachoroidal space indicates serous rather than acute hemorrhage. (Reprinted with permission from Valvassori G [ed]: Imaging of the Head and Neck. Thieme Medical Publishers, 1995. Copyright Thieme Medical Publishers, Inc.)

Choroidal Detachment, Choroidal Effusion, and Ocular Hypotony. Choroidal detachment is caused by the accumulation of fluid (serous choroidal detachment) or blood (hemorrhagic choroidal detachment) in the potential suprachoroidal space.[20] Serous choroidal detachment frequently occurs after intraocular surgery, penetrating ocular trauma, or inflammatory choroidal disorders. Hemorrhagic choroidal detachment often occurs after a contusion, after a penetrating injury, or as a complication of intraocular surgery (ocular hypotony). Such detachment significantly influences the prognosis of the involved eye. Serous choroidal detachment appears on CT scans as a semilunar or ring-shaped area of variable attenuation (Fig. 84–35). The degree of attenuation depends on the cause but is generally greater with inflammatory disorders of the eyeball. Hemorrhagic choroidal detachments appear as a high or low mound-like image of high intensity on CT, which can be quite large and irregular (Fig. 84–36).[20] MRI shows choroidal hematoma as a focal, well-damarcated, lenticular mass in the wall of the eyeball. The signal intensity of the choroidal hematoma depends on its age. Within the first 48 hours, the hematoma is isointense to slightly hypointense relative to the normal vitreous body on T1-weighted and proton-weighted MR images but is markedly hypointense on T2-weighted images. After about 5 days, its signal intensity characteristics are different, being relatively confused with choroidal melanoma. The hematoma usually continues to increase in signal intensity on T1-weighted, proton-weighted, and T2-weighted images and usually becomes markedly hyperintense by 2 to 3 weeks on all MR pulse sequences. Serous choroidal detachment and choroidal effusion has a different appearance on CT and MRI from that of choroidal hematoma. A choroidal

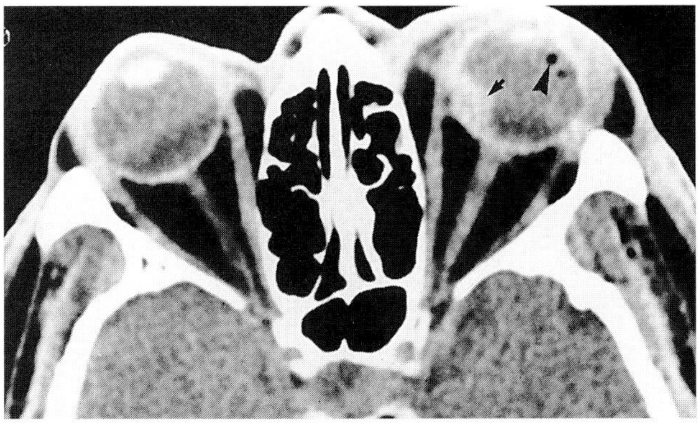

Figure 84–36. Hemorrhagic choroidal detachment. Axial computed tomographic scan shows post-traumatic choroidal hematoma (*arrow*). Note the intraocular air (*arrowhead*) due to ocular laceration. (Reprinted with permission from Valvassori G [ed]: Imaging of the Head and Neck. Thieme Medical Publishers, 1995. Copyright Thieme Medical Publishers, Inc.)

effusion is usually seen as a crescentic or ring-shaped lesion on both CT and MR scans. It does not resemble the lenticular appearance of a hematoma. Finally, it is not always possible to differentiate retinal detachment and choroidal detachment.

Leukocoria. Leukocoria is a white, pink-white or yellow-white pupillary reflex (cat's eye). It is a sign that results from any intraocular abnormality that reflects the incident light back through the pupil toward the observer. This reflection of light is the result of a white or light-colored intraocular mass, membrane, or retinal detachment or from retinal storage disease.

When examining a child with leukocoria, the major diagnostic considerations are retinoblastoma, persistent hyperplastic primary vitreous, retinopathy of prematurity, congenital cataract, Coats' disease, toxocariasis, total retinal detachment, and a variety of other nonspecific causes of leukocoria.

Retinoblastoma. Retinoblastoma, the most common intraocular tumor of childhood, is a highly malignant, primary retinal tumor that arises from neuroectodermal cells (nuclear layer of the retina) that are destined to become retinal photoreceptors. The manner of intraocular and extraocular extension, patterns of metastasis and recurrence, ocular complications, and associated malignancies make the diagnosis of retinoblastoma one of the most challenging problems of pediatric ophthalmology and radiology.

Retinoblastoma accounts for about 1% of all deaths from childhood cancer in the United States. It must be differentiated from a host of benign lesions that simulate retinoblastoma to ensure appropriate therapy.

The diagnosis of retinoblastoma can usually be made by an ophthalmoscopic examination; however, the detection and clinical differentiation of retinoblastoma from a host of benign simulating lesions may be difficult. Imaging modalities should be used on all patients suspected of harboring a retinoblastoma to determine the presence of gross retrobulbar spread, intracranial metastasis, and secondary tumor.

Imaging techniques may allow differentiation of retinoblastoma from lesions such as persistent hyperplastic primary vitreous, Coats' disease, retinopathy of prematurity, toxocariasis, retinal detachment, organized subretinal hemorrhage, organized vitreous, endophthalmitis, retinal dysplasia, retinal astrocytoma (hamartoma), retinal gliosis, myelinated nerve fibers, choroidal hemangioma, coloboma, morning glory anomaly, congenital cataract, choroidal osteoma, drusen of optic nerve head, and other so-called pseudogliomas and leukocorias. These lesions may have a clinical appearance similar to that of retinoblastoma.

Ultrasonography, CT, and MRI are the most useful imaging techniques in the evaluation of these lesions. The tumor and calcification can be diagnosed by ultrasonography. However, the accuracy of ultrasonography for this condition is only 80%.

Over 90% of retinoblastomas show evidence of calcification on CT scan (Fig. 84–37). The DNA released from necrotic cells in retinoblastomas has a propensity to form a DNA-calcium complex.[21]

The presence of intraocular calcification in children younger than 3 years of age is highly suggestive of retinoblastoma. In children older than 3 years of age, some of the simulating lesions, including retinal astrocytoma, retinopathy of prematurity, toxocariasis, and optic nerve head drusen can produce calcification.

In the diagnosis of retinoblastoma, MRI is not as specific as CT scanning, owing to its lack of sensitivity in de-

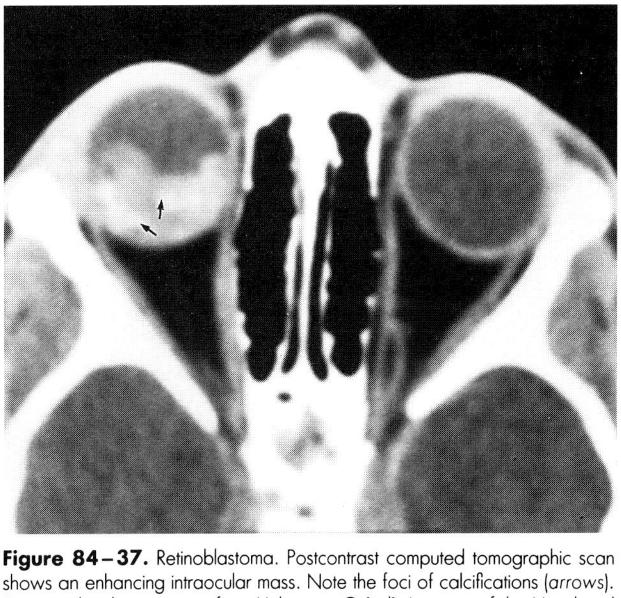

Figure 84–37. Retinoblastoma. Postcontrast computed tomographic scan shows an enhancing intraocular mass. Note the foci of calcifications (*arrows*). (Reprinted with permission from Valvassori G [ed]: Imaging of the Head and Neck. Thieme Medical Publishers, 1995. Copyright Thieme Medical Publishers, Inc.)

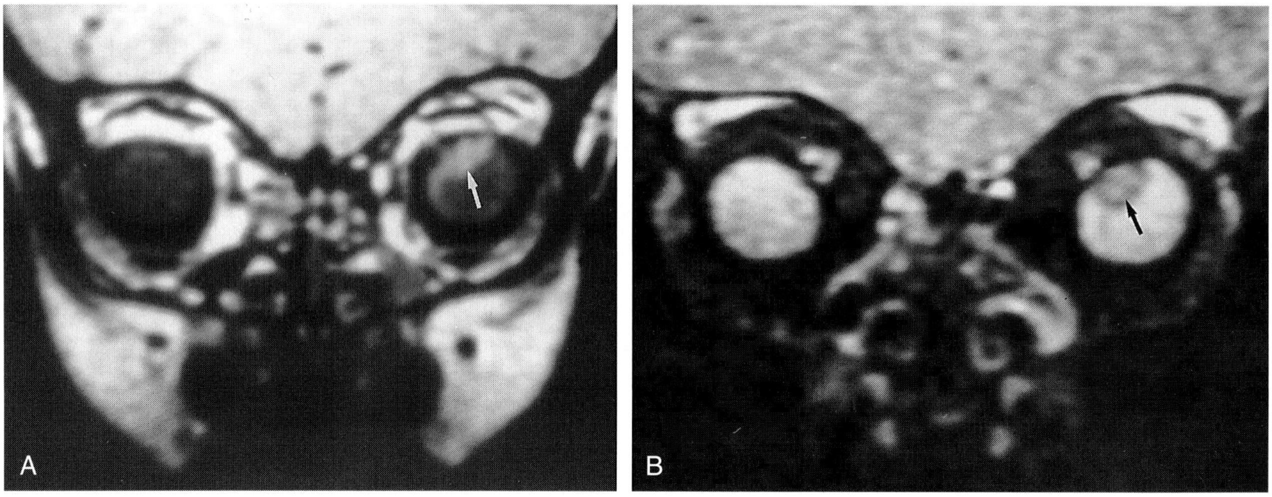

Figure 84 – 38. Retinoblastoma. Proton-weighted (*A*) and T2-weighted (*B*) magnetic resonance (MR) scan show a retinoblastoma (*arrows*). The tumor appears moderately hypointense on T2-weighted MR images. (*A* and *B* reprinted with permission from Valvassori G [ed]: Imaging of the Head and Neck. Thieme Medical Publishers, 1995. Copyright Thieme Medical Publishers, Inc.)

tecting calcification. However, the MR appearance of retinoblastoma may be specific enough to differentiate retinoblastoma from simulating lesions.

Retinoblatomas appear slightly or moderately hyperintense in relation to normal vitreous on T1-weighted and proton-weighted MR images. On T2-weighted MR images, they appear as areas of markedly to moderately low signal intensity (Fig. 84–38). Tumors elevated 3 to 4 mm in height may not be definitely identified on MR scans. Lesions less then 3 mm in height are not recognized by present MRI technology.

In the diagnosis of retinoblastoma, CT is the study of choice because of its superior sensitivity for detecting calcification. Calcification as small as 2 mm can be reliably detected by CT scan. MRI, however, has superior contrast resolution and provides more information for differentiation of leukocoric eyes.

Persistent Hyperplastic Primary Vitreous. Persistent hyperplastic primary vitreous is caused by the failure of the embryonic hyaloid vascular system to regress normally. The basic lesion is caused by a persistence of various portions of the primary vitreous and tunica vasculosa lentis with hyperplasia and extensive proliferation of the associated embryonic connective tissue. The diagnosis is often made difficult by its extremely broad array of clinical manifestations, etiologic heterogeneity, and frequently opaque ocular media. The CT findings include the following:

1. Microphthalmos is usually detectable.
2. Calcification is absent within or around the globe.
3. Generalized increased density of the entire vitreous chamber may be visible, although minimally affected cases may show normal attention values in the vitreous chambers.
4. Enhancement on the CT image of abnormal intravitreal tissue may be seen after intravenous administration of a contrast media.
5. Tubular, cylindrical, triangular, or other discrete intravitreal densities suggest the persistence of fetal tissue in Cloquet's canal or congenital nonattachment of the retina.

The MR appearance of different types of causes of persistent hyperplastic primary vitreous may be different. Early experience with MRI in patients with persistent hyperplastic primary vitreous has revealed marked hyperintensity of the vitreous chamber on T1-weighted, proton-weighted, and T2-weighted MR scans (Fig. 84–39).

Coats' Disease. Coats' disease is a primary vascular anomaly of the retina characterized by idiopathic retinal telangiectasia and exudative retinal detachment (exudative retinopathy). The condition occurs more frequently in boys than in girls. The condition is also seen in adults, and it is almost always unilateral.

The CT and MRI findings in Coats' disease vary with the stages of progression of the disease. At early stages, both techniques may yield little information. In the later stages of the disease, retinal detachment accounts for all the pathologic findings in CT and MRI (Fig. 84–40). Enhancement of the detached leaves of the retina along with enhancement of the peripheral retina may be shown on post Gd-DTPA contrast-enhanced MR scans.

Ocular Toxocariasis (Sclerosing Endophthalmitis). The granuloma of *Toxocara canis* is actually an eosinophilic abscess with the second-stage larva of *Toxocara* within the abscess. The infection results from ingestion of eggs of the nematode *Toxocara canis*. In these patients,

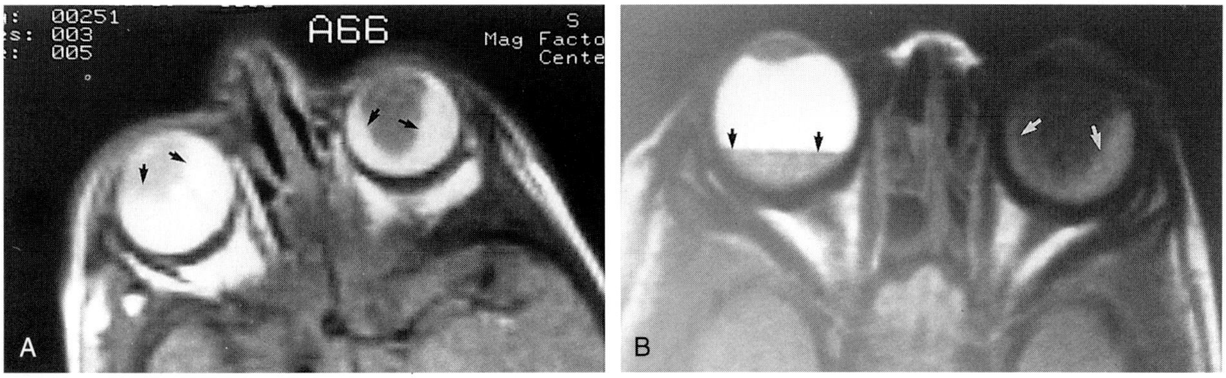

Figure 84–39. Warbung disease. *A*, T1-weighted axial magnetic resonance (MR) scan showing bilateral chronic hemorrhagic retinal detachments (*arrows*). *B*, Followup proton-weighted axial MR scan shows the unchanged appearance of left retinal detachment (*white arrows*). Note the fluid–fluid level on the right side (*black arrows*) related to recent hemorrhage in the right eye. (*A* and *B* reprinted with permission from Valvassori G [ed]: Imaging of the Head and Neck. Thieme Medical Publishers, 1995. Copyright Thieme Medical Publishers, Inc.)

the death of the larva results in a wide spectrum of intraocular inflammatory reactions.

CT findings consist of a nonhomogeneous intravitreal density that corresponded to detached retina, organized vitreous, and inflammatory subretinal exudate.

In general, the proteinaceous subretinal exudate produced by inflammatory response to larval infiltration is seen as variable hyperintense image on T1-, proton-, and T2-weighted MR scans. Gd-DTPA MRI study may delineate one or more foci (abscesses) of enhancement.

Malignant Uveal Melanoma

The uvea (iris, ciliary body, and choroid) is derived from the mesoderm and neuroectoderm and may harbor tumors of both origins. Since it is the most highly vascular portion of the eyeball, it provides a suitable substrate for tumor cells. Most primary and metastatic ocular neoplasms involve the choroid, with the most common being malignant melanoma. Malignant melanomas of the uvea are unusual in African Americans; the ratio of Caucasian to African American patients is about 15:1. Those involving the ciliary body and choroid are thought to originate from preexisting nevi.

Although uveal melanomas can be accurately diagnosed by ophthalmoscopy, fluorescein angiography, or ultrasonography, misdiagnosis continues to occur, particularly when opaque media preclude direct visualization. CT scanning has proved to be useful for demonstrating uveal melanoma and a wide variety of pathologic conditions. Most uveal melanomas are seen on CT scans as elevated, hyperdense, sharply marginated lesions (Fig. 84–41).

MRI has been used to diagnose various intraocular lesions. On T1- and proton-weighted MR scans, uveal melanomas are seen as areas of moderately high signal (greater signal intensity than vitreous). On T2-weighted images, melanomas are seen as areas of moderate to marked low signal intensity (lesser intensity than vitreous) (Fig. 84–42). These MR characteristics of uveal melanomas are very similar to retinoblastomas.[22, 23]

Associated retinal detachment is better visualized by MRI than CT scanning, particularly after intravenous administration of Gd-DPTA contrast medium. Exudative retinal detachment is usually depicted on MR scans as a dependent area of moderate to very high signal intensity in T1-, proton-, and T2-weighted images. Total retinal detachment may be present. Chronic retinal detachment and hemorrhagic subretinal fluid have varied MR appearances. Most uveal melanomas appear as well-defined solid masses. At times, atypical features of ocular melanoma may be present. When necrotic or hemorrhagic foci are present within the uveal melanoma, the inhomogeneity present within the tumor can be problematic. Some melanomas may be seen better in T2-weighted MR images. Other uveal melanomas may show no significant hypointensity on T2-weighted MR images.

Discoid melanomas or ring melanomas may not be detected if they are flat. Invasion of the sclera, extension of tumor into the optic disc and Tenon capsule, and extraocular invasion can be easily detected by MR scan.

The MRI diagnosis of uveal melanomas is greatly enhanced by the use of gadolinium contrast material. Uveal melanomas will show moderate enhancement (Fig. 84–43).

A number of benign and malignant lesions of the eye may be confused with malignant uveal melanomas. The main ocular conditions that may be mistaken for a malignant uveal melanoma include metastatic tumors, choroidal detachment, choroidal nevi, choroidal hemangioma, choroidal cyst, neurofibroma, schwannoma of the uvea, leiomyoma, adenoma, medulloepithelioma, retinal detachment, and disciform degeneration of the macula.

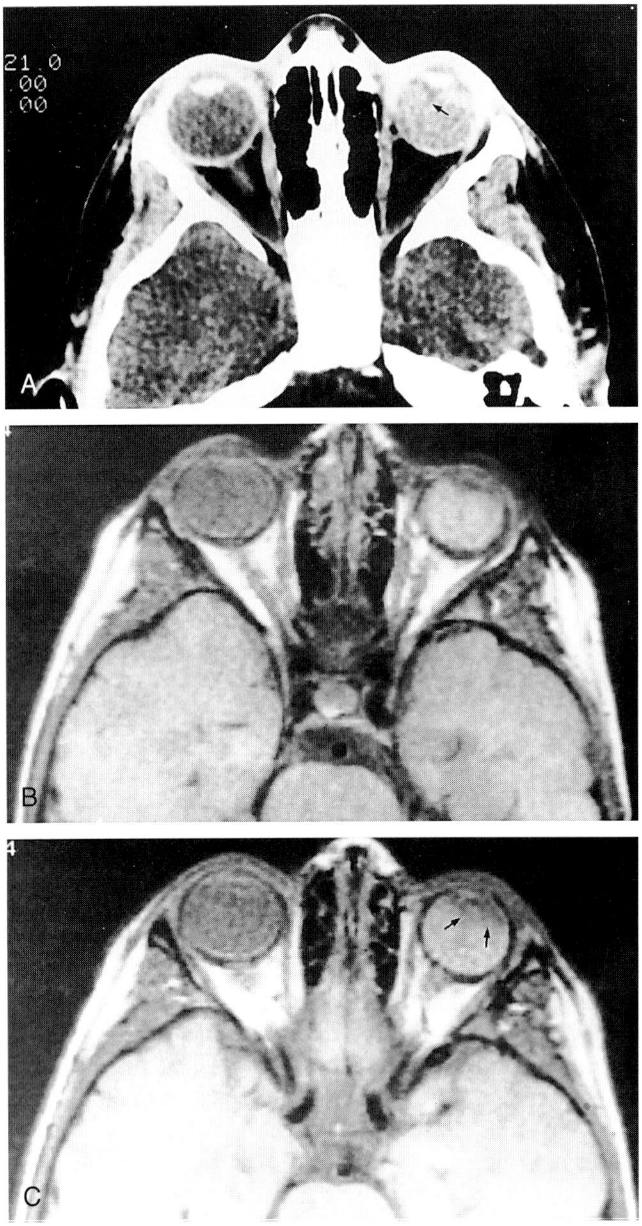

Figure 84–40. Coats' disease. *A*, Computed tomographic scan shows changes compatible with retinal detachment. Note the folded retina (*arrow*). *B* and *C*, Proton-weighted magnetic resonance scans show increased intensity of the left globe. Note the detached retina. Increased intensity is due to subretinal exudate. (*A* and *B* reprinted with permission from Valvassori G [ed]: Imaging of the Head and Neck. Thieme Medical Publishers, 1995. Copyright Thieme Medical Publishers, Inc.)

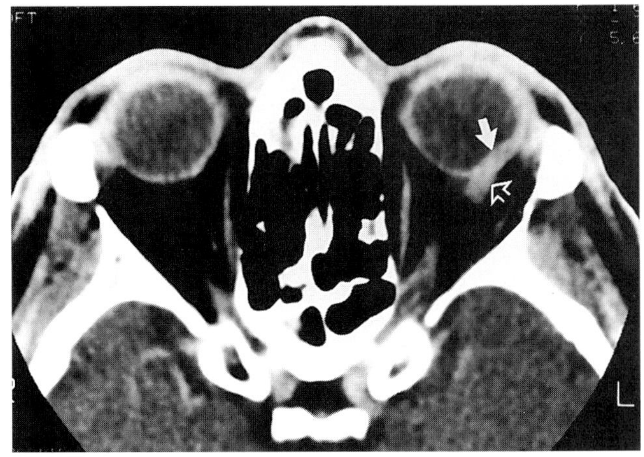

Figure 84–41. Choroidal melanoma. Computed tomographic scan shows a melanoma (*solid arrow*) and its extraocular extension (*open arrow*). (Reprinted with permission from Valvassori G [ed]: Imaging of the Head and Neck. Thieme Medical Publishers, 1995. Copyright Thieme Medical Publishers, Inc.)

Although choroidal hemangiomas can be diagnosed by ophthalmoscopy, fluorescein angiography, or ultrasonography, this is a lesion in which at times diagnosis on clinical grounds presents some difficulty.

Choroidal hemangiomas are seen on plain CT scans as ill-defined images. They demonstrate intense enhancement on contrast infusion and dynamic CT scans.[22]

On MRI, choroidal hemangiomas may be seen as hypointense areas on T1-weighted images and as hyperin-

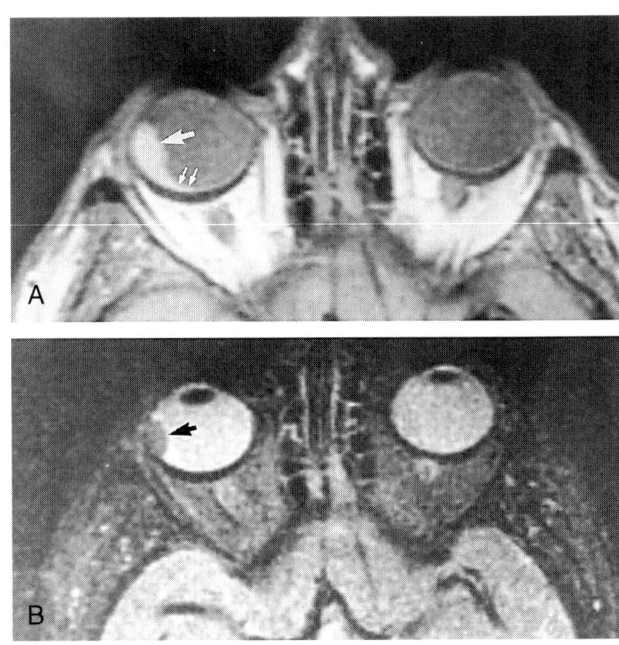

Figure 84–42. Choroidal melanoma. Proton-weighted (*A*) and T2-weighted (*B*) magnetic resonance scans show a melanoma (*large arrows*). The detached retina over the slope of the tumor with minimal subretinal exudate is seen on the proton-weighted image (*short arrows*) and can be differentiated from the tumor on the T2-weighted image. (*A* and *B* reprinted with permission from Valvassori G [ed]: Imaging of the Head and Neck. Thieme Medical Publishers, 1995. Copyright Thieme Medical Publishers, Inc.)

Choroidal and Retinal Hemangiomas

Choroidal hemangiomas are usually seen in association with Sturge-Weber disease, which consists of capillary or cavernous hemangiomas with the cutaneous distribution of the trigeminal nerve and of a predominantly venous hemangioma of the leptomeninges. Retinal angiomas, on the other hand, occur in patients with von Hippel-Lindau disease.

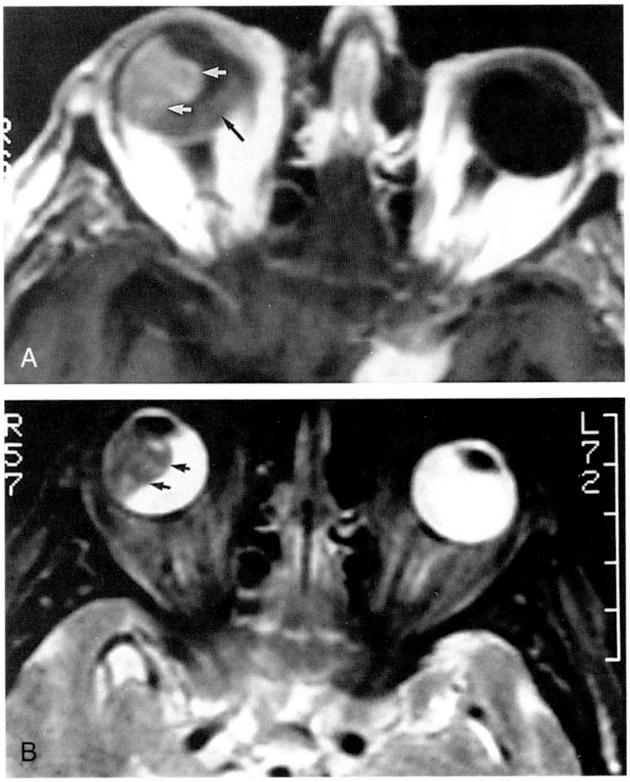

Figure 84–43. Choroidal melanoma. *A*, Post–Gd-DTPA contrast T1-weighted axial magnetic resonance (MR) scan shows a large melanoma (*white arrows*). Because of the enhancement, the tumor can be differentiated from the subretinal exudate (*black arrow*). *B*, T2-weighted axial MR scan shows a large hypointense mass (*arrows*) compatible with melanoma. (*A* and *B* reprinted with permission from Valvassori G [ed]: Imaging of the Head and Neck. Thieme Medical Publishers, 1995. Copyright Thieme Medical Publishers, Inc.)

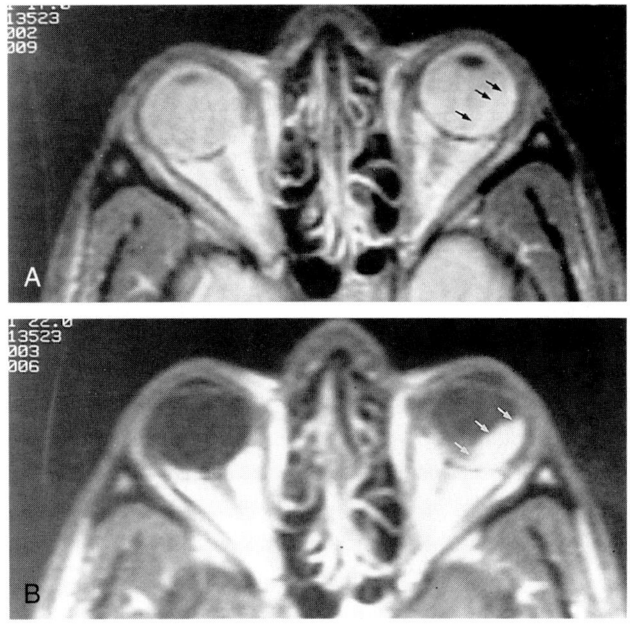

Figure 84–44. Presumed choroidal hemangioma. Axial proton-weighted (*A*) and post–Gd-DTPA contrast T1-weighted (*B*) magnetic resonance scans show a slightly hyperintense mass (*black arrows*). Note the intense enhancement (*white arrows*). (*A* and *B* reprinted with permission from Valvassori G [ed]: Imaging of the Head and Neck. Thieme Medical Publishers, 1995. Copyright Thieme Medical Publishers, Inc.)

tense areas on T2-weighted images. Some choroidal hemangiomas are seen as moderately intense areas in T1-, proton-, and T2-weighted images. Choroidal hemangiomas show intense enhancement after intravenous administration of Gd-DTPA contrast medium (Fig. 84–44).

Uveal Metastasis

Uveal metastasis can be clinically and from an imaging point of view confused with uveal melanoma. Metastatic lesions of the uvea extend chiefly in the plane of the choroid and with relatively little increase in thickness. Unlike uveal melanomas that tend to form a protuberant mass, the metastatic lesions often have a mottled appearance and a diffuse outline. The malignant cells (emboli) get access to the eye by the blood stream by means of the short posterior ciliary arteries, and this may be the reason why the site of the majority of the metastases is in the posterior half of the eye. The most common source of secondary carcinoma within the eye is from breast or lung. Tumor metastasis may occur in both retina and choroid, with both eyes being affected in about one third of the cases. Uveal metastasis and lymphoreticular involvement of the choroid may have similar MRI characteristics as uveal melanomas. A mucin-producing metastatic lesion (adenocarcinoma) may simulate uveal melanoma as well because the proteinaceous fluid tends to decrease

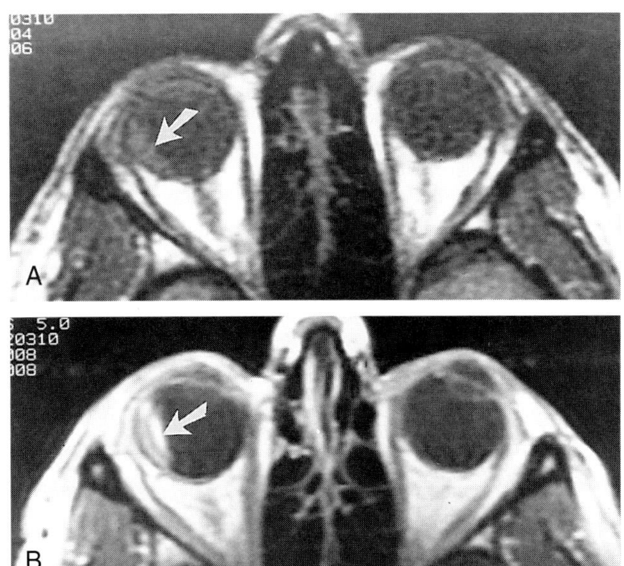

Figure 84–45. Choroidal metastasis. Axial precontrast T1-weighted (*A*) and postcontrast (Gd-DTPA) T1-weighted (*B*) magnetic resonance scans show an ill-defined mass (*A*, *arrow*) with marked enhancement (*B*, *arrow*) in this patient with a primary breast lesion. There was a small enhancing nodule in the left eye as well as in other sections not shown. (*A* and *B* reprinted with permission from Valvassori G [ed]: Imaging of the Head and Neck. Thieme Medical Publishers, 1995. Copyright Thieme Medical Publishers, Inc.)

T1 and T2 relaxation times of the lesion. Metastatic lesions demonstrate moderate to marked enhancement after intravenous injection of Gd-DTPA. The MRI contrast study increases the detection of metastatic foci (Fig. 84–45).

REFERENCES

1. Mafee MF, Putterman A, Valvassori GE, et al: Orbital space-occupying lesions: Role of CT and MRI: An analysis of 145 cases. Radiol Clin North Am 25:529–559, 1987.
2. Rootman J (ed): Diseases of the Orbit. Philadelphia, JB Lippincott, 1988.
3. Grove AS: Giant dermoid cysts of the orbit. Ophthalmology 86:1513–1520, 1979.
4. Mafee MF, Dobben GD, Valvassori GE: Computed tomography assessment of paraorbital pathology. *In* Gonzalez CA, Becker MH, Flanagan JC (eds): Diagnostic Imaging in Ophthalmology. New York, Springer-Verlag, 1985, pp 281–302.
5. Hawkins DD, Clark RW: Orbital involvement in acute sinusitis. Clin Pediatr 16:464–471, 1977.
6. Weber AL, Mikulis DK: Inflammatory disorders of the paraorbital sinuses and their complications. Radiol Clin North Am 25:615–630, 1987.
7. Flanders AE, Mafee MF, Rao VM, et al: CT characteristics of orbital pseudotumors and other orbital inflammatory processes. J Comput Assist Tomog 13 (1):40–47, 1989.
8. Trokel SL, Hilal SK: Recognition and differential diagnosis of enlarged extraocular muscles in computed tomography. Am J Ophthalmol 87:503–512, 1979.
9. Flanders AE, Espinosa GA, Markiewicz DA, et al: Orbital lymphoma. Radiol Clin North Am 25:601–612, 1987.
10. Yeo JH, Jakobiec FA, Abbott GF, et al: Combined clinical and computed tomographic diagnosis of orbital lymphoid tumors. Am J Ophthalmol 94:235–245, 1982.
11. Mafee MF, Miller MT, Tan WS, et al: Dynamic computed tomography and its application to ophthalmology. Radiol Clin North Am 25:715–731, 1987.
12. Henderson JW: Orbital Tumors. Philadelphia, WB Saunders, 1973, pp 116–123.
13. Shields JA (ed): Diagnosis and Management of Orbital Tumors. Philadelphia, WB Saunders, 1989.
14. Bockwinkel KD, Diddams JA: Haemangiopericytoma: Report of case and comprehensive review of literature. Cancer 25:896–901, 1970.
15. Azar-Kia B, Naheedy MF, Elias DA, et al: Optic nerve tumors: Role of MRI and CT. Radiol Clin North Am 25:561–581, 1987.
16. Hoyt WF, Baghdassarian SA: Optic glioma of childhood: Natural history and rationale for conservative management. Br J Ophthalmol 53:793–798, 1969.
17. Jakobiec FA, Yeo JH, Trokel SL, et al: Combined clinical and computed tomographic diagnosis of primary lacrimal fossa lesions. Am J Ophthalmol 94:785–807, 1982.
18. Mafee MF, Haik BG. Lacrimal gland and fossa lesions: Role of computed tomography. Radiol Clin North Am 25:767–779, 1987.
19. Mafee MF, Peyman GA: Retinal and choroidal detachments: Role of MRI and CT. Radiol Clin North Am 25:487–507, 1987.
20. Mafee MF, Peyman GA: Choroidal detachment and ocular hypotony: CT evaluation. Radiology 153:697–703, 1984.
21. Mafee MF, Goldberg MF, Cohen SB, et al: Magnetic resonance imaging versus computed tomography of leukocoric eyes and use of in vitro proton magnetic resonance spectroscopy of retinoblastoma. Ophthalmology 96:965–976, 1989.
22. Mafee MF, Peyman GA, Grisolano JE, et al: Malignant uveal melanoma and simulating lesions: MR imaging evaluation. Radiology 160:773–780, 1986.
23. Mafee MF, Peyman GA, Peace JH, et al: Magnetic resonance imaging in the evaluation and differentiation of uveal melanoma. Ophthalmology 94:341–348, 1987.

CHAPTER 85

Vascular Tumors of the Orbit

Barrett G. Haik and Holly Gore

Vascular tumors constitute one of the largest, most frequently encountered groups of orbital lesions in both the pediatric and adult populations. Although the majority of these tumors are benign, the mere physical presence of the tumor may significantly affect vision, motility, and cosmesis. Because treatment of vascular tumors varies, an accurate diagnosis is essential; neuroradiologic, clinical, and sometimes surgical studies are needed. Depending on the histologic character of the tumor, its size and growth patterns, and associated ocular complications, treatment may vary from observation to exenteration with postoperative radiation therapy and chemotherapy. Understanding the natural history of the lesion, as well as its response to various therapeutic modalities, is the basis for instituting appropriate management.[1]

CAPILLARY HEMANGIOMA

Capillary hemangioma is the most common adnexal and orbital vascular lesion of childhood[2] and is among the most common pediatric orbital tumors.[3, 4] This analogue of primitive vasoproliferative tissue is a hamartoma rather than a true neoplasm. The tumor has been amply described by several names, including infantile hemangioma, juvenile hemangioma, hemangioblastoma, benign hemangioendothelioma, and hypertrophic hemangioma; yet the term *capillary hemangioma* remains the most accurate, since the lesion consists of true capillaries with endothelial cells surrounded by pericytes.[5]

Histopathology

Anastomosing, blood-filled, endothelial-lined channels compose the tumor mass. In some cases, the capillary lumina are ectatic; in others, plump endothelial cells occlude the vascular lumina. Lobular proliferations of solid nests of endothelial cells with a variable miotic index may be seen separated by fibrous septa (Fig. 85–1). Large feeding and draining vessels are interspersed throughout these fibrous septa, and an infiltrative growth pattern with no encapsulation is evident.[1]

The true nature of a capillary hemangioma may be seen more clearly when a reticulum stain is used to outline the basement membranes surrounding the vascular channels (Fig. 85–2) or when ultrastructural studies define the pericytes (Fig. 85–3) enveloping the endothelial cells (see Fig. 85–3).[5] The histology differs from the ultrastructural characteristics of cavernous hemangiomas of adults, in which multilaminar smooth muscle cells surround the ectatic endothelial cells.[1]

Capillary hemangioma can occasionally be confused with a malignant process, especially on frozen section. Vascular channels may not be apparent. The cells at the tumor perimeter may be compressed into a spindle morphology, and a high number of mitotic cells may be seen. It is important, therefore, to have an adequate tissue sample for histologic study; an experienced pathologist, with the capability of performing reticulum stains and electron microscopy, should review the specimen.[1]

Clinical Course

With rare exceptions, capillary hemangiomas present in the first 6 months of life, and one third are clinically obvious at birth. Pregnancy and birth history are typically normal. Although capillary hemangiomas of the skin are thought by many to be more common in low-birth-weight infants, we have not found evidence in periocular capillary hemangiomas to support this finding.[6] We also have found no strong statistical evidence to support the early speculations that capillary hemangiomas and retrolental fibroplasia are related in more than a coincidental manner.[6, 7] Typically, there is no clear hereditary pattern to this tumor, and while we occasionally have noted a history of nonfacial capillary hemangiomas in siblings, these have not been more com-

This study was supported by the St. Giles Foundation, New York, New York.

Portions of this text and photographs are reprinted with permission from Haik BG, Jones IS, Ellsworth RM: Vascular tumors of the orbit. *In* Hornblass A (ed): Oculoplastic, Orbital, and Reconstructive Surgery, © 1988, the Williams & Wilkins Company, Baltimore.

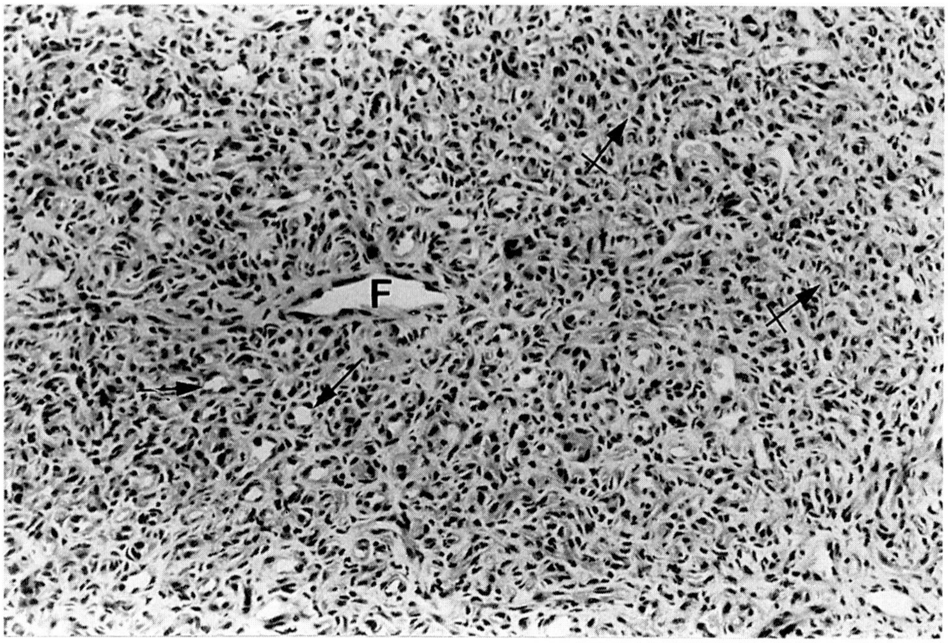

Figure 85–1. Photomicrograph of a capillary hemangioma consisting of closely packed units of capillary-type vessels. Some lumina are open (*arrow*), while others are closed (*crossed arrow*). F, feeder vessel. H & E, ×200.

mon than the incidence in the general population. None of the siblings of the twins or triplets we have evaluated had lesions similar to those seen in other patients. There is a female-to-male ratio of 3:2 in the occurrence of periocular capillary hemangiomas. No racial, ethnic, or national patterns have been found.[1]

Although the superior orbit and lids are most commonly involved clinically,[6] periocular capillary hemangiomas may manifest in one of three ways. Most frequently a bluish purple, subcutaneous mass is noticed with relatively normal overlying skin in the anterior orbit (Fig. 85–4). Approximately one third of patients will have an obvious superficial component consisting initially of "herald spots," which are small, red, macular lesions that later develop into an overlying strawberry hemangioma (Fig. 85–5).[8] Five percent of patients will present with a deep orbital mass and no signs suggesting the diagnosis (Fig. 85–6). The latter group of patients is by far the most clinically perplexing and diagnostically important since the differential diagnosis of deep orbital tumors in an infant includes such malignancies as rhabdomyosarcoma and metastatic neuroblastoma. Fortunately, this situation is rare, and the diagnosis of capillary hemangioma can usually be made on clinical grounds alone without the necessity of biopsy.[1]

There are several valuable clinical signs that assist in

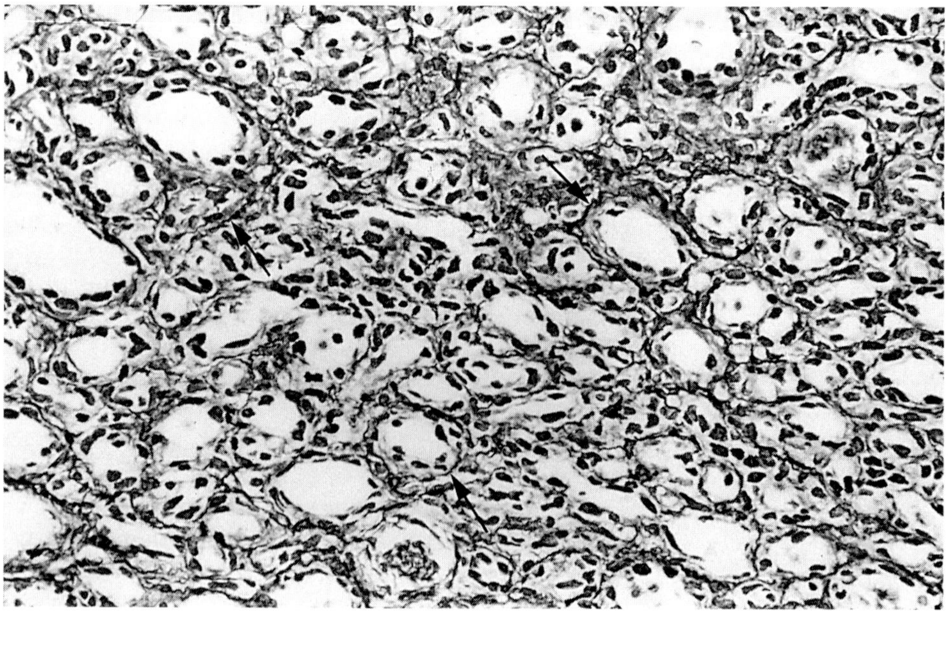

Figure 85–2. Photomicrograph of a capillary hemangioma. Reticulum stain (*arrow*) outlines the outer surface of capillary-type units. Lumina, whether closed or opened, are always within the reticulum-positive circles. Reticulum stain, ×400.

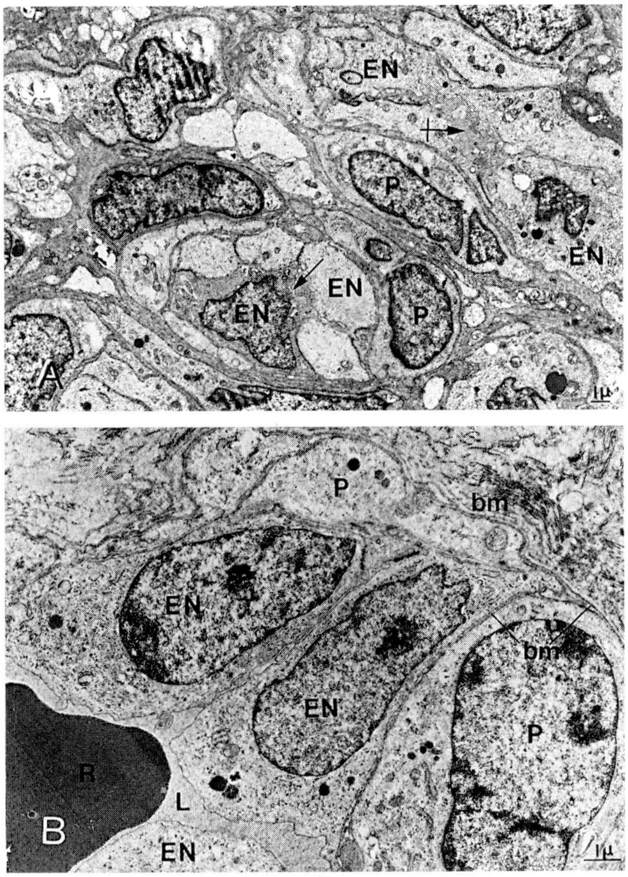

Figure 85–3. Electron micrographs of capillary hemangioma. *A,* Low magnification showing two capillary-type units, each consisting of endothelial cells (EN) and pericytes (P). One unit has an entirely closed lumen (*arrow*), while the other has a slightly opened lumen (*crossed arrow*). ×4600. *B,* Higher magnification of another capillary unit with widely opened lumen (L). EN, endothelial cell; P, pericytes; R, red blood cell; arrow indicates basement membrane. ×8500. (Courtesy of Dr. Takeo Iwamoto.)

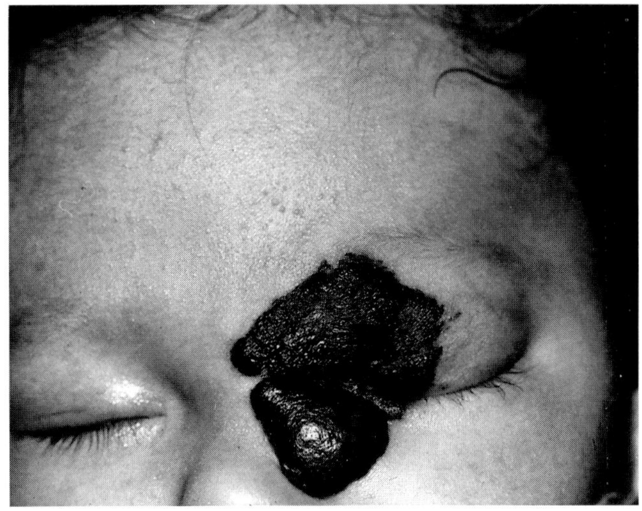

Figure 85–5. A 2-month-old infant with orbital hemangioma and an obvious superficial strawberry mark.

differentiating capillary hemangiomas. The superficial component will lighten upon digital pressure, unlike the port-wine stain,[9] and a Valsalva maneuver will easily demonstrate the highly expansive nature of this vascular tumor.[1]

Evidence of superficial hemangiomatosis involving the conjunctiva (Fig. 85–7) or palpebral lobe of the lacrimal gland itself is noted in 40% of patients. Approximately 25% of all patients with periocular capillary hemangiomas have multiple superficial hemangiomas on other parts of the body (Fig. 85–8). This is not a pathognomonic sign, however, since 1% of all normal children will have a strawberry mark somewhere on their skin.[1]

Capillary hemangiomas follow a characteristic clinical course, with a period of rapid hypertrophy for 3 to 12 months, followed by a period of stabilization and eventual involution[10, 11]; 50% will involute by 5 years of age

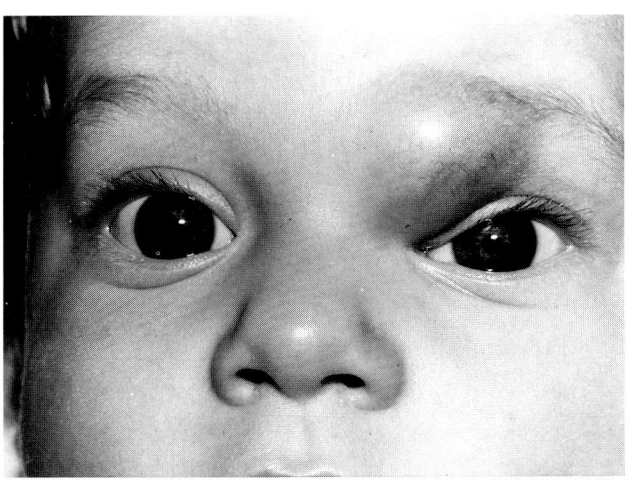

Figure 85–4. A 4-month-old child presenting with a large superior nasal orbital mass and globe displacement. A bluish purple subcutaneous mass was seen through the upper lid skin. Several small telangiectatic vessels are present in the epidermis.

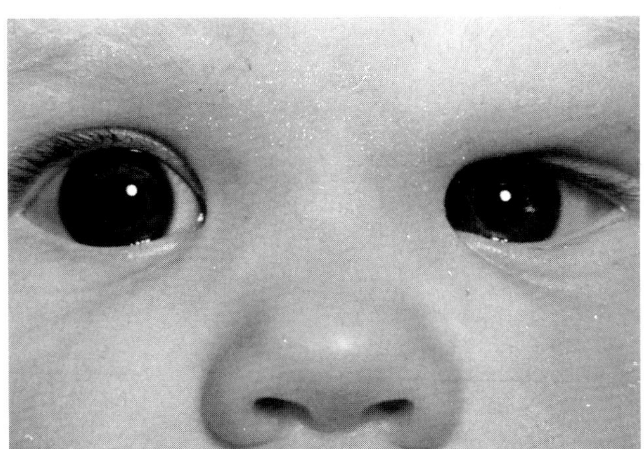

Figure 85–6. Infant presenting with unilateral proptosis and no anterior orbital, cutaneous, or conjunctival signs of hemangioma.

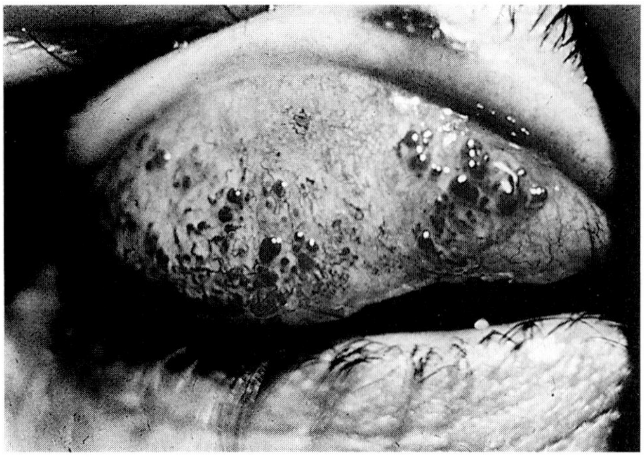

Figure 85–7. Diffuse hemangiomatosis of the tarsal conjunctiva.

and 75% to 90% by 7 years of age.[12] In the majority of cases, tumor regression will be complete, with no significant cosmetic sequelae. However, in some large lesions, especially those with a combined superficial subcutaneous component, it is not uncommon to observe cosmetically disturbing defects. Although large capillary hemangiomas are benign in that they do not metastasize and only extremely rarely have they been reported to undergo malignant degeneration, they are by nature quite disruptive to normal ocular development.[1]

When these tumors occur in the orbit, they tend to be more aggressive and disruptive to the tissues than similar strawberry hemangiomas occurring elsewhere in the body. They are associated with a high degree of complications, such as cosmetic deformities and amblyopia, which occur in both treated and untreated cases. Proptosis occurs in 30% to 40% of patients, with the possible development of corneal exposure.[16] Several series have shown amblyopia occurring secondary to papillary occlusion, anisometropia, or strabismus in 50% to 75% of patients with orbital and adnexal capillary hemangioma.[6, 13–15] Other ocular complications include optic atrophy, occlusion of the nasolacrimal system, diplopia, and ptosis.[16]

Systemic complications may also occur. In large lesions, the tumor may ulcerate and cause secondary infections.[16] Airway obstruction due to a hemorrhagic supraglottic hemangioma during intubation has been reported.[17] Large hemangiomas may shunt a significant volume of blood causing congestive heart failure.[9] The rare Kasabach-Merritt syndrome of hemangioma with thrombocytopenia may be life threatening.[16]

Diagnostic Testing

There are many available ancillary tests to aid in diagnosis, treatment planning, and subsequent management of capillary hemangiomas. Plain radiography and computed tomography reveal diffuse enlargement of the orbit without evidence of bony erosion (Fig. 85–9). Computed tomography with contrast enhancement (Fig. 85–10), angiography, digital intravenous subtraction angiography, and magnetic resonance angiography reveal the existence and extent of the diffusely infiltrating vascular tumor, as well as outline the major feeding vessels supplying this tumor. Ultrasonographic studies are valuable in determining the presence and extent of orbital involvement and provide a safe, noninvasive method of monitoring tumor growth and regression.[18] On T1-weighted magnetic resonance images the tumor is isointense to brain and muscle (Fig. 85–11). On T2-weighted studies

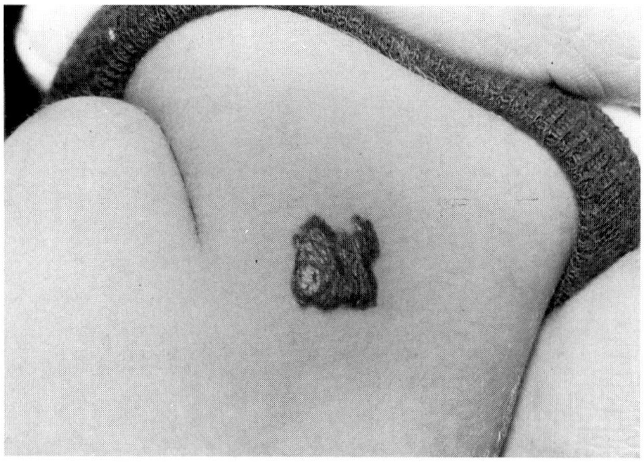

Figure 85–8. Hemangioma on limb of patient with periocular hemangioma and other superficial hemangiomas on the limbs and trunk.

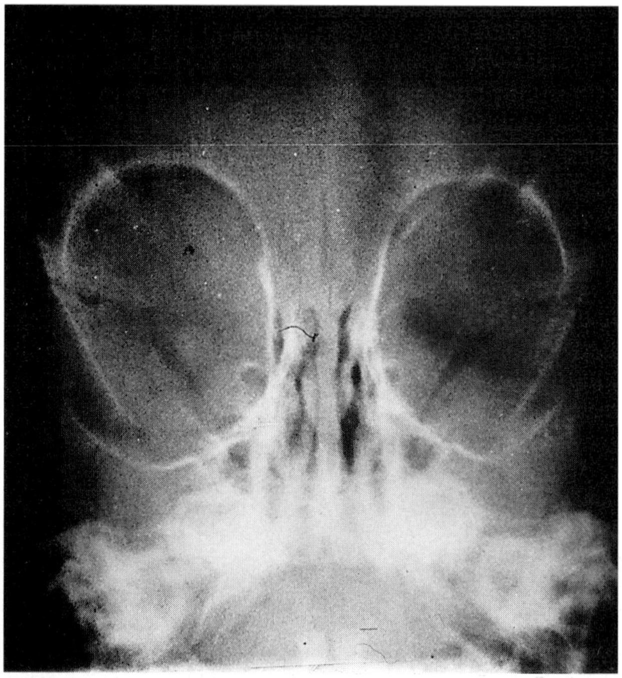

Figure 85–9. Plain radiograph demonstrates enlargement of the orbit without evidence of bony erosion.

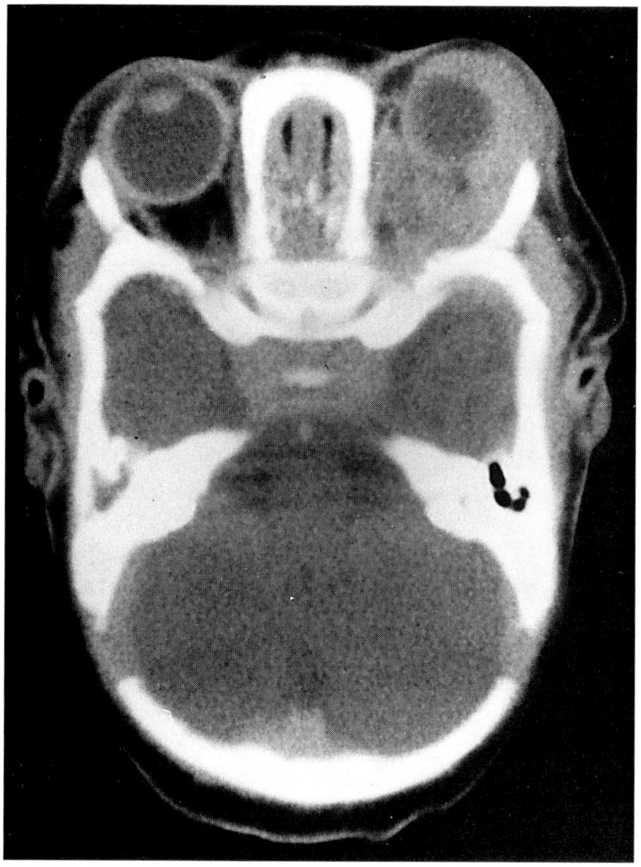

Figure 85–10. Contrast-enhanced axial computed tomographic scan of the orbit demonstrates right orbital enlargement and a diffusely infiltrating, enhancing mass.

the mass becomes hyperintense. The tumor mass enhances following gadolinium-DTPA administration (Fig. 85–12); therefore, fat suppression is advantageous in differentiating the tumor from orbital fat on T1-weighted enhanced images.

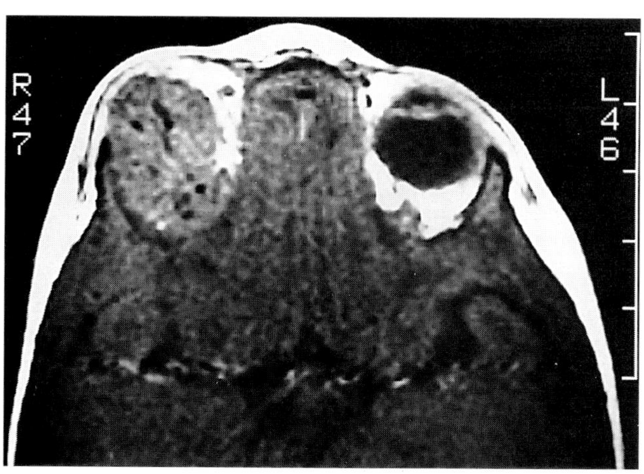

Figure 85–11. T1-weighted axial magnetic resonance scan demonstrates right superior orbital mass isointense to brain. Feeding vessels are seen as dark serpiginous or circular structures depending on the angle of transection.

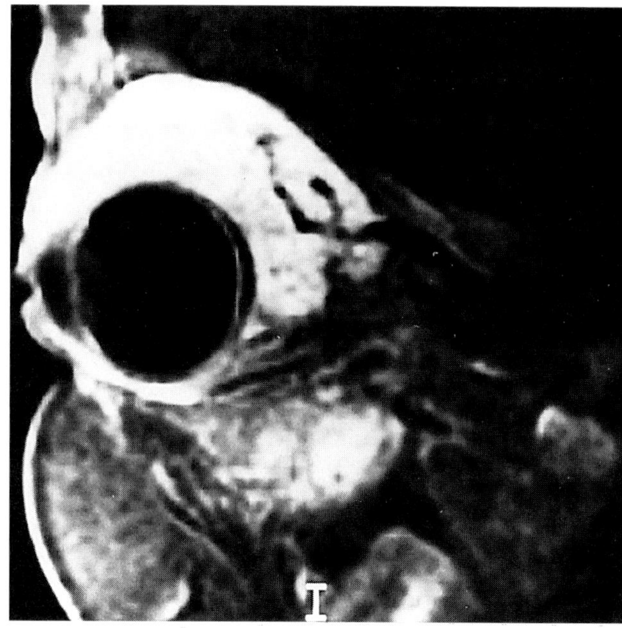

Figure 85–12. T1-weighted gadolinium-DTPA enhanced sagittal magnetic resonance scan depicts the caliber and location of the major feeding blood vessels.

Treatment Alternatives

The great majority of capillary hemangiomas undergo significant spontaneous regression. Although it is well established that therapy can speed regression of these tumors, it will not significantly affect the final amount of tumor involution nor the cosmetic result. Therefore, unless there are specific ocular, dermatologic, or systemic indications for rapid resolution, treatment should be withheld; all of the available therapeutic modalities have significant real or theoretical risks.[19] It is generally of great value to discuss the natural history of the tumor with the family and to explain the advantages and disadvantages of administering or withholding therapy in any particular case. It is also often advantageous to allow parents to study photographs of children who have undergone spontaneous regression and to speak to parents of children who have reached the stage of maximal tumor regression.[1]

The rate of complications in adnexal and orbital capillary hemangioma is very high. Therapy may be instituted for ocular, dermatologic, or systemic problems.[1]

Ocular indications for treatment include occlusion of the visual axis by tumor infiltrating the lid and periorbita (Fig. 85–13), compression of the optic nerve by rapidly growing tumor, or corneal exposure secondary to severe proptosis. Although there is no evidence that tumor-induced anisometropia disappears with treatment, it seems logical that treatment that minimizes ocular distortion will minimize the resultant amount of anisometropia[1] with patching and optical correction in the meantime.[8]

Dermatologic indications for therapy are severe hypertrophy of the epidermal and subcutaneous tissues

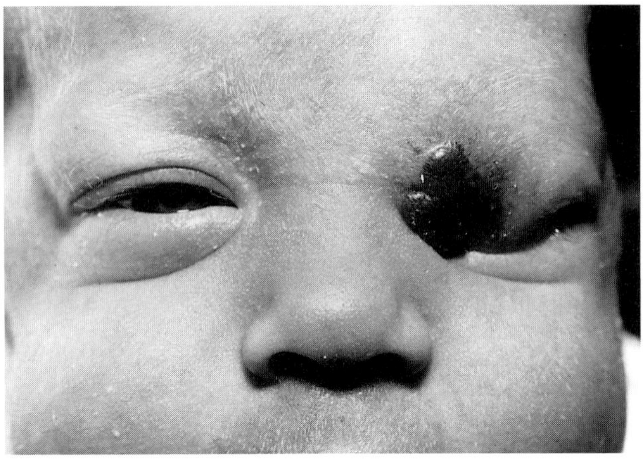

Figure 85–13. Occlusion of the visual axis had occurred in this infant secondary to a large upper lid and orbital hemangioma.

leading to maceration and erosion of the epidermis (Fig. 85–14). The skin is thereby predisposed to secondary infections and potential disfigurement.[1]

The systemic indications for treatment include the following complications: cardiovascular (high-output congestive heart failure); hematologic (thrombocytopenia and hemolytic anemia); and obstructive (nasopharyngeal, oral, or subglottic extensions of the hemangioma).[1]

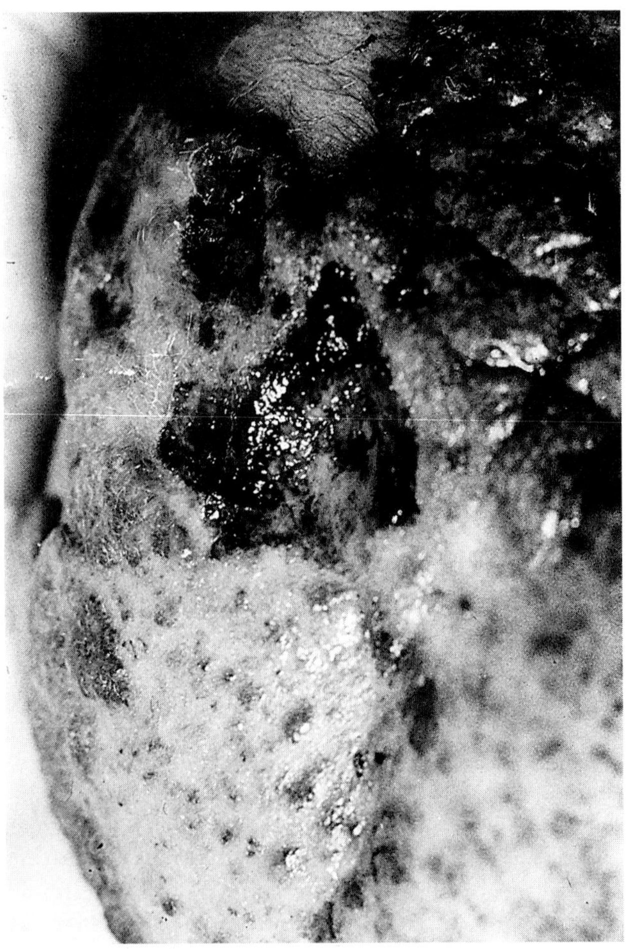

Figure 85–14. Extensive superficial facial hemangioma demonstrating macerated tissue and superficial erosion of the epidermis.

Many effective techniques may be employed in the treatment of capillary hemangiomas, such as vascular occlusive modalities, surgical excision, irradiation, and corticosteroid therapy. Each has its share of complications.[2]

Before any major surgery, children and infants should be thoroughly evaluated to avoid any systemic abnormalities that may complicate therapy. A pediatrician should examine the patient for any signs of heart anomalies, anemias, or potential airway obstruction. A presurgical plan should be made by the surgeon based on the preoperative evaluation and all radiographic data to decrease blood loss and obtain the desired goal with the least intervention. Typed and cross-matched blood must be readily accessible. Hypotensive anesthesia may be used to minimize blood loss and permit more accurate visualization of orbital structures during surgery.[1]

Various surgical procedures exist that attempt to reduce tumor size through either compromise of the major arterial feeding vessels, constriction and sclerosing of the smaller vascular channels, or primary surgical excision of the mass.[20] Occlusion of afferent vessels either surgically or through intra-arterial embolization can be an effective means of decreasing blood flow to the tumor mass. Involution is stimulated with decreased vascularity before excisional surgery. Accurate radiographic visualization of the major vascular channels supplying the tumor is required. This is often difficult because of the complex configurations and anastomosis assumed by major feeding vessels to such tumors. Cryotherapy, diathermy, and injections of both sclerosing solutions and boiling water may destroy the smaller vascular channels stimulating the natural regression. Tumor involution is rapid, but often more significant cosmetic and functional deformities occur than would have with less destructive forms of therapy or natural involution.[1]

Surgical excision is occasionally effective in small, relatively localized adnexal hemangiomas and for the excision of fibrovascular remnants after regression. Primary surgical excision of large actively growing tumors has limited value; these lesions are diffusely infiltrative, lack encapsulation, and are difficult to differentiate from critical orbital structures. A preoperative arteriogram or magnetic resonance angiography to delineate the major vascular channels of the tumor is often recommended when surgery is necessary. Complications of surgery include inevitable scar formation and excision of critical vascular, muscular, and neurogenic components of the orbit.[1]

The approach to the orbit can be made in any of the standard manners, including the conjunctival, anterior, or lateral orbital approaches. When the incision is through the skin, care should be taken to place the incision in a natural lid or skin crease and to minimize excision of skin. One should carefully identify all critical ocular structures visible in the field, such as the lacrimal gland, lacrimal drainage apparatus, and extraocular muscles, so that they can be avoided during dissection. A canalicular stent is often helpful when dissecting or suturing in the area of the canaliculus, and a black silk traction suture is routinely passed under the insertions of the rectus muscles so that they can be localized during the procedure. When the conjunctiva is involved, great care should be taken to spare all uninvolved tissue for later closure and reconstruction of the fornices. Careful sharp and blunt dissection under coaxial illumination and magnification is carried out in a meticulous manner to dissect free the tumorous tissue while also avoiding the sacrifice of adjacent critical orbital structures. When surgery is being performed for diagnostic reasons, a frozen section can be obtained to establish the diagnosis, thus allowing confirmation of the macroscopic diagnosis. Intralesional injection of corticosteroids, when indicated, may then be used under direct visualization during the same surgical procedure. When a mass of highly vascular tumor is isolated for excision, a curved hemostat is used to crush the base of the tumor and a razor or scissors is used to cut free the distal segment. Diathermy is then applied to the tumor pedicle before the clamp is removed, and the tumor retracts posteriorly. This simple maneuver aids in reducing the possibility of immediate blood loss and decreases the possibility of postoperative orbital hemorrhage. After the surgical objectives are achieved, the orbital incision is closed in any standard manner the surgeon prefers. When the surgery is performed with the use of hypotensive anesthesia, it is advisable to raise the blood pressure levels to normal before complete closure of the wound. This normotensive procedure reduces the possibility of postoperative orbital hemorrhage.[1]

Because of the risk and complications inherent in surgical therapy, we prefer nonsurgical means of patient management, such as radiation therapy or corticosteroid therapy.[1]

Radiation therapy can be highly effective in the management of capillary hemangioma. Low-level radiation can help to create microembolic episodes in these vascular tumors and speed regression of the mass.[21, 22] Either supervoltage or orthovoltage radiation therapy in the 150- to 250-cGy range is administered in a single treatment, with appropriate shielding of the globe and adjacent uninvolved tissues. An involution response is usually noted with 1 to 2 weeks in the majority of patients. These treatments may be repeated to achieve additional resolution. Only rarely should doses over 1000 cGy be employed. Both radioactive needles and seeds have been effectively used in the treatment of deep-seated hemangiomas. This requires more complex planning since shielding of uninvolved structures is impossible. In the past, when large doses of radiation were administered and methods of delivery and shielding were less exact, radiation-induced complications of the skin, orbit, and eye were commonplace.[23] At present, with appropriate radiation precautions and shielding, direct damage from radiation should not occur. It is, however, possible to induce a radiation cataract with 200 to 600 cGy when the anterior segment has not been adequately shielded.[1]

Our primary concern in the radiation treatment of these benign tumors in the pediatric population is the potential susceptibility to late radiation oncogenesis. Although we are unaware of patients in our treatment group developing secondary cancers in the field of therapeutic irradiation, the possibility of radiation oncogenesis must nevertheless be considered.[1]

Systemic corticosteroids have been shown to be effective in significantly speeding natural tumor involution.[13, 14, 24] In 1963, a child with Kasabach-Merritt syndrome was treated with corticosteroids with resultant regression of the tumor at Johns Hopkins Hospital. In 1967, Zarem and Edgerton reported successful responsiveness of seven infants with large capillary hemangiomas.[24] The exact mechanism of their inhibitory effect is now known but appears to be related to vasoconstrictor effect. Sasaki and colleagues found there to be elevated levels of estradiol-17β binding capacity in pathologic specimens. Corticosteroids may inhibit estradiol-17β binding capacity with resultant tumor involution.[25] Others have noted an increase in antihemophilic globulin that may cause tumor regression by clot formation.[26]

The typical oral dosage of corticosteroids is either 2 mg/kg of prednisone daily or 4 mg/kg on an alternate-day basis. A significant reduction in size is usually noted within 1 week after administration. Unfortunately, after the corticosteroids are discontinued or reduced, rebound growth often occurs. It can be quite difficult to taper the dose of corticosteroids, and prolonged administration may induce complications.[1]

The undesired effects of sustained administration of systemic corticosteroids include delayed growth, iatrogenic Cushing's syndrome, and adrenal suppression. These systemic complications from corticosteroid usage generally follow relatively high-dose, long-term use but should not result from "pulsed" treatment of several weeks' duration. All children receiving systemic or intralesional corticosteroids should be exempted from routine pediatric immunizations with live attenuated viruses during and for 2 weeks before and after administration of corticosteroids.[1]

The use of intralesional corticosteroids has been the recent treatment of choice.[9, 27] It is suggested that a combination of the rapid-acting betamethasone sodium phosphate and the long-acting triamcinolone be injected into the tumor mass with a 27- to 30-gauge needle of 1.5 inches in a deep and radial manner.[1, 28, 29] The tumor may enlarge for the 24 hours after injection, followed by a significant reduction in size over the subsequent week.[9] This injection may be performed as a primary form of treatment or after biopsy or partial excision in deeper orbital areas when direct visualization of the mass is obtained.[1]

Intralesional corticosteroids are not without complications. Eyelid depigmentation may occur,[1, 30] or solid corticosteroid in carrier complexes beneath the skin may persist for several months after injection.[1] Adrenal suppression has occurred[1, 2] with resultant decrease in growth and weight in an infant.[2] Full-thickness eyelid necrosis has resulted from injection.[31] Fat atrophy in a linear formation following the lymphatic vessels has been noted distal to the infection site.[32] The most dreaded complication of central retinal artery occlusion has been reported[28]; the depo-steroid carrier complexes are of sufficient size to occlude vascular channels after introduction into the arterial system. It is recommended, therefore, to use a small-gauge needle with low pressure injections while slowly withdrawing the needle.[1, 28] Firm digital pressure after injection should be avoided.[1]

Multiple other modalities have been utilized in the treatment of capillary hemangioma, including interferon and laser therapy. Each therapy must be evaluated as to the risk–benefit ratio to the child, in the context of the clinical course of this tumor. At times, modalities may be combined in a synergistic fashion during the treatment of complex tumors that are not responsive to conventional therapy. Rarely, a tumor will be extremely resistant to all therapeutic modalities, resulting in an extremely difficult situation for the patient's family and the treating physician.[1]

All forms of treatment should include periodic evaluation of refractive errors and the institution of amblyopia therapy when indicated. Amblyopia therapy is difficult in these patients because anisometropia, obstruction of the visual axis, and mechanical restriction of motility may exist individually or in combination. Patient compliance with patching regimens is often poor, since this technique occludes the normal side of the patient's face and serves to accentuate the cosmetic defects associated with the hemangioma.[1]

DISSEMINATED NEONATAL HEMANGIOMATOSIS

Disseminated neonatal hemangiomatosis is a rare, nonhereditary disorder first described by Ramdohr in 1878.[33] Holden and Alexander[34] titled the condition disseminated neonatal hemangiomatosis (DNH) with three criteria: (1) neonatal onset of visceral hemangiomas involving (2) three or more viscera with (3) no malignancy of the hemangiomas. DNH should be differentiated from benign neonatal hemangiomatosis, which has only skin involvement and no related mortality. There have been 33 cases of DNH in the literature (Table 85–1).[35–46]

TABLE 85-1

Summary of Ocular and Neuro-ophthalmic Manifestations in Disseminated Hemangiomas (N = 33)

Finding	No. Patients	%
Ocular involvement	11/33	33
Iris hemangioma	6/11	55
Conjunctival hemangioma	3/11	27
Abnormal chorioretinal vasculature	4/11	36
Lid hemangioma	3/11	27
Microphthalmia	3/11	27
Glaucoma	1/11	9
Ocular/neuro-ophthalmic involvement	3/11	27
Sixth nerve palsy secondary to central nervous system hemangioma	2/11	18
Third nerve palsy secondary to central nervous system hemangioma	1/11	9
Cortical blindness	1/11	9

Histopathology

The hamartomatous nodules consist of multiple blood-filled vascular channels.[34] The vessels of the tumors are endothelial lined and supported by a fibrous stroma (Fig. 85–15).[1]

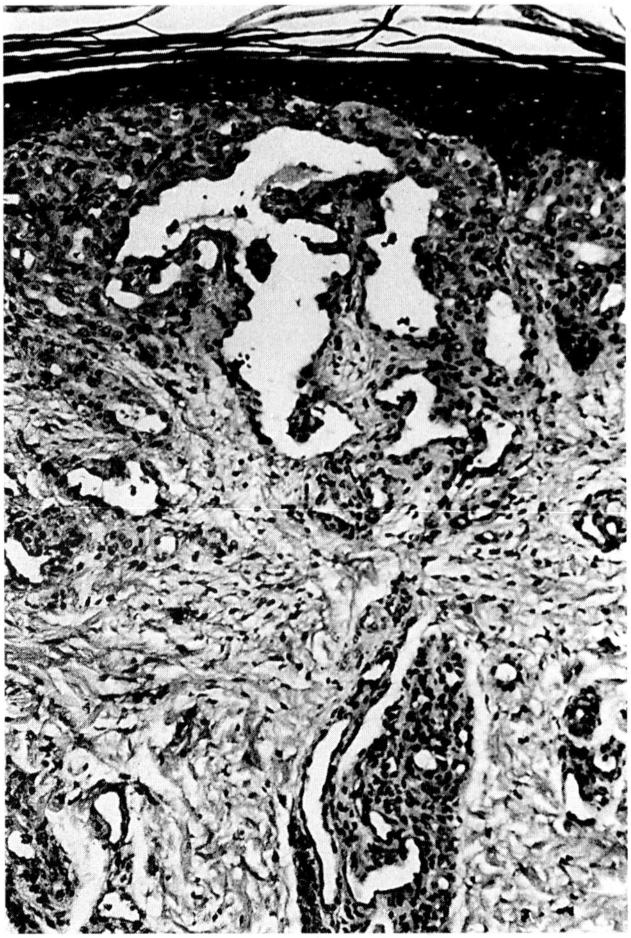

Figure 85–15. Nodule from the trunk of a patient with disseminated neonatal hemangiomatosis, demonstrating blood-filled, endothelial-lined vascular channels.

Clinical Course

The onset at birth or in infancy, tendency to spontaneously grow, and eventual involution of the hemangiomas in DNH seem to be similar to that of other benign hemangiomas. Unfortunately, survival past the first few months of life is rare, owing to the complications of the multiple organ systems involved. Congestive heart failure is the most common cause of mortality secondary to massive arteriovenous shunting in extensive liver hemangiomas.[1] The patient may also experience seizures, hydrocephalus, gastrointestinal hemorrhaging, dyspnea,[35] thrombocytopenia, and anemia.[34] DNH has also been reported to be associated with the cluster of findings of tricuspid atresia, absent corpus callosum, and ectopia cordis (sternal agenesis).[36]

Since the hemangiomas involve most major organ systems (Fig. 85–16), the eye and orbit have been no exception. In reviewing the literature, the incidence of ocular involvement in reported cases is 33% and is summarized in Table 85–1. (The actual incidence may be higher, since an ocular examination is frequently not mentioned).

A significant number of patients with ocular involvement have anterior segment abnormalities characterized primarily by iris hemangiomatosis (Fig. 85–17). Unfortunately, the natural history of these ocular lesions is not well understood, owing to the poor survival rate of these infants. The hemangiomas characteristically occur after birth and undergo a period of hypertrophy, followed by spontaneous regression. Therefore, the goal of therapy is to minimize secondary complications from the abnormal iris vessels before involution. In three patients surviving with DNH and iris involvement, only one developed secondary glaucoma.[1] The predisposition to glaucoma exists and is supported by autopsy findings in one patient in whom significant vascular and anatomic defects in the iris and angle were noted, apparently causing eventual intraocular pressure elevation.[47] Although the exact mechanism of the glaucoma is unclear, it appears that the vascular abnormality is a significant component in its etiology.[1]

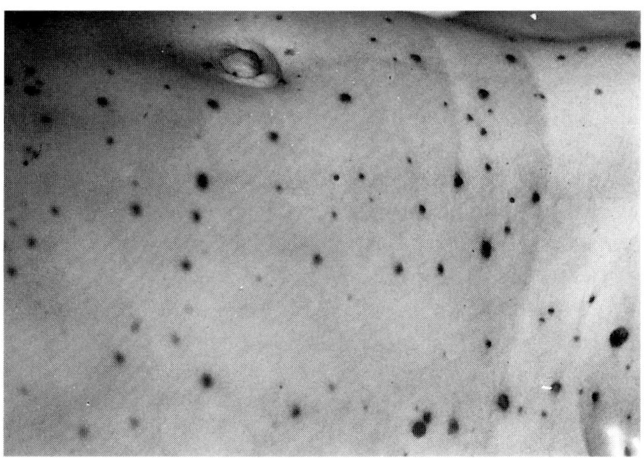

Figure 85–16. Abdomen of patient revealing multiple miliary hemangiomas ranging from 1 to 5 mm in diameter.

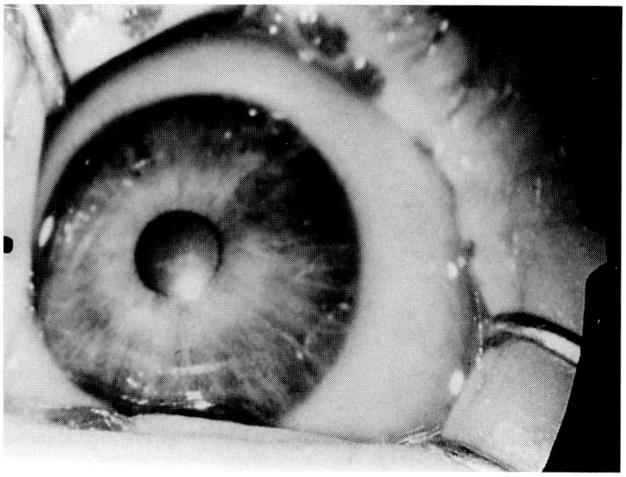

Figure 85–17. Segmental areas of iris hemangiomatosis and multiple miliary hemangiomas of the eyelids.

Neurologic complications involving the eye may also exist, and a thorough examination should be performed. In newborns, papilledema will not manifest, since increased intracranial pressure will be displaced through the fontanelles.[35] It is, therefore, advised that patients with DNH be observed closely not only for systemic but also for ocular and neurologic complications.

Treatment Alternatives

Reports[46, 47] suggest that early initiation of corticosteroid therapy is conducive to speeding regression and may avert serious system compromise in infants. Systemic corticosteroid therapy is a reasonable form of treatment for both systemic and ocular complications of the hemangiomas. The effectiveness of corticosteroids in stimulating involution elsewhere in the body is well documented,[21–23] and indeed their use appears justified for purely ocular anomalies when a functional threat exists.[1]

LYMPHANGIOMA

Lymphangioma is a controversial and sometimes confusing tumor in its etiology, terminology, histopathology, and treatment. The lesion presents commonly in the head and neck regions but is a rare tumor of the orbit.[48] It occurs in 3% of all[49] and 8% of expanding orbital tumors,[50] and Jones estimates the occurrence to be 3.4 patients of 100,000 in the general population.[51]

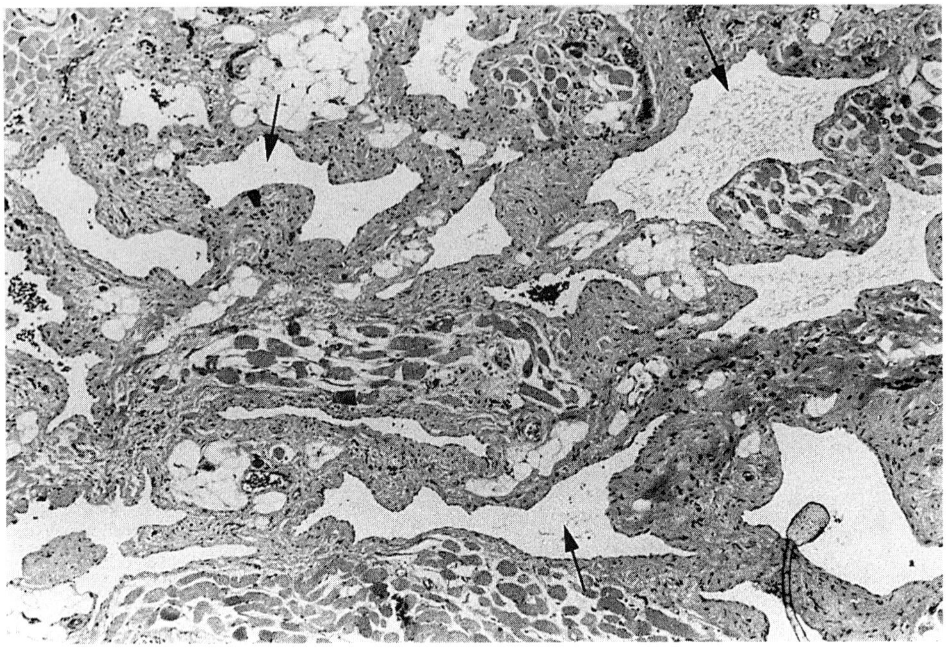

Figure 85–18. Lymphangioma demonstrating multiple thin-walled vessels of varying sizes *(arrows)*. Typically, the lumina contain no red blood cells. H & E, ×80. (Courtesy of Takeo Iwamoto, MD.)

Lymphangioma is not a true neoplasm but rather a hamartomatous proliferation. This mesodermal tissue appears to be pleuripotent, possessing the ability to differentiate into either lymphatic or vascular tissue.[52, 53] Lymphatic tissue is not known to be present in the orbit except in small aggregates of lymph tissue in the conjunctival fornices, lacrimal gland,[52] and possibly the perineural or perivascular sheaths. If indeed there are no lymphatic channels in the orbit, this tumor should be classified as a choristoma.[1] Jones,[51] however, has suggested that embryonic nests of lymphatics do exist and give rise to these abnormalities. He has also demonstrated that particulate matter injected into the extravascular spaces of cat orbits eventually will appear in the cervical lymph nodes, thus suggesting some form of lymphatic drainage.

It is the ambiguous nature of this tumor with its vascular and lymphatic characteristics over which many have debated. Histopathology, clinical examination, and diagnostic testing demonstrate its dual nature.

Histopathology

The term *lymphangioma* may be considered by some to be a misnomer, since the histology is variable, containing both lymphatic and vascular components.

Several histologic characteristics favor a lymphatic classification. The channels of the tumor are often lined by a single layer of flattened endothelial cells (Fig. 85–18) surrounded by an interrupted basal lamina (Fig. 85–19). An eosinophilic proteinaceous fluid, usually free of erythrocytes, fills the vessels. The supporting stroma may be infiltrated with variable amounts of lymphocytes and occasionally well-formed germinal lymphoid follicles.[1]

Conversely, the tumor also has evidence of vascular influences. The lining often has areas of overlapping endothelial cells with tight junctions. The basement membrane in these regions is continuous, and pericytes are present. Smooth muscle fibers are located in the walls.[54] In Harris and coworkers' study of 30 cases of orbital lymphangioma with microscopic correlation, the lymphocytes were not indigenous but rather had migrated in response to hemorrhage. The lymphoid pattern was more typically perivascular than follicular.[55]

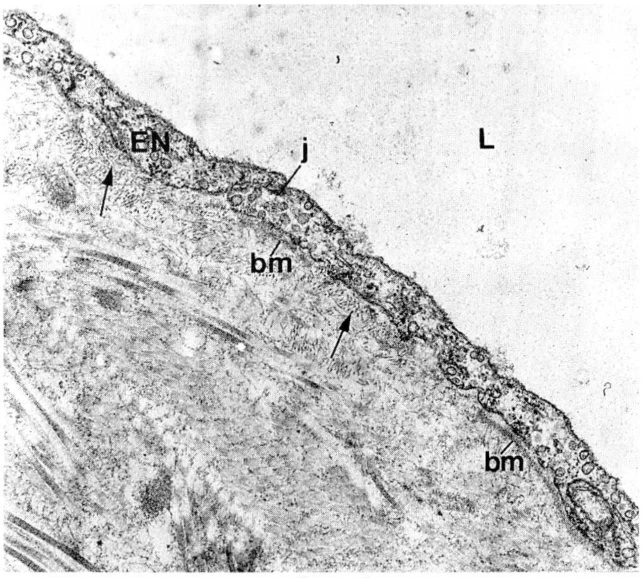

Figure 85–19. Electron micrograph of a portion of the wall of a vascular lumen (L) of a lymphangioma. Attenuated endothelial cells (EN) are joined by a poorly developed junctional complex (j) and are surrounded by an interrupted basement membrane (bm) and anchoring thin filaments *(arrows)*. ×23,800. (Courtesy of Takeo Iwamoto, MD.)

Lymphangioma has been classified according to the size of the channels into three groups: (1) capillary or simple lymphangiomas have lumina the dimensions of a capillary; (2) cavernous lymphangiomas have larger channels; and (3) cystic lymphangiomas have large multicystic areas of variable sizes.[56] In Graeb and coworkers' correlation of histopathology with 11 orbital lymphangioma patients, the majority of the tumors were found to be of the cavernous type.[54]

With time, scar tissue, hemosiderin-laden macrophages, and free hemosiderin, as well as occasional thrombi, calcifications, and deposits of cholesterol may be seen. After treatment or trauma, spontaneous fibrovascular growth and progressive vascularization may be noted. When small blood vessels rupture, blood is spilled into the endothelial-lined channels. Since the tumor is unencapsulated, large blood-filled "chocolate" cysts may readily expand, compromising a large amount of the tumor volume.[1]

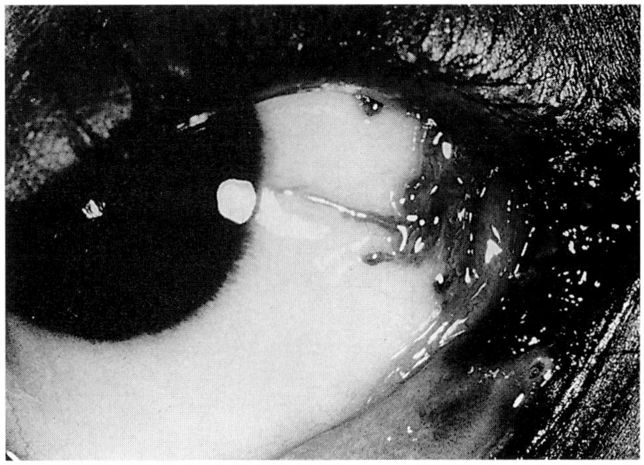

Figure 85–21. Conjunctival lymphangioma outlined by spontaneous hemorrhage into the vascular spaces.

Clinical Course

Orbital lymphangiomas most commonly appear in the first decade of life. They typically grow at the same rate as the child's body (Fig. 85–20). Mulliken and Glowacki[57] were able to demonstrate this by using [^{3}H]-thymidine to measure the turnover rate of the endothelial cells of the lymphangioma. The turnover rate was found to be normal as opposed to the increased rate in a proliferating capillary hemangioma. The tumor occasionally can have exuberant growth. Often, by the third decade, the orbital lymphangioma will stabilize in size.[1]

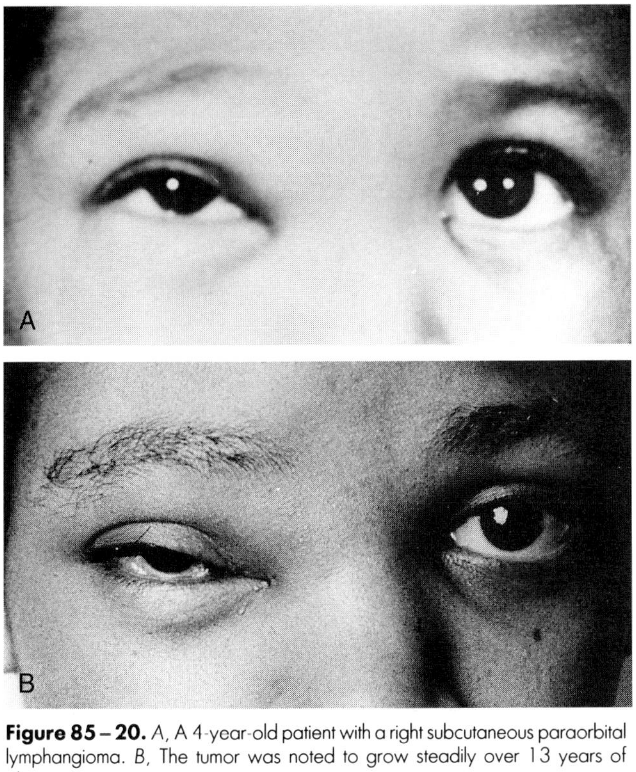

Figure 85–20. *A*, A 4-year-old patient with a right subcutaneous paraorbital lymphangioma. *B*, The tumor was noted to grow steadily over 13 years of observation.

Orbital lymphangiomas usually show no tendency for spontaneous regression and are frequently associated with severe cosmetic and functional abnormalities.[58] The mass is most often conjunctival (Fig. 85–21)[51] but may also be subcutaneous or deep orbital (Fig. 85–22). It typically infiltrates diffusely throughout multiple tissue planes in the orbit. At times, the tumor is found to be also present in other facial compartments, such as the maxillary or mandibular areas, or even intraorally (Fig. 85–23).[1]

Orbital lymphangioma patients most frequently present as proptosis. The proptosis does not increase with the Valsalva maneuver or head position. No bruits are present.[54] In two situations, a dramatic increase in tumor volume can occur. The first is a reactive hyperplasia of the lymphoid tissue within the tumor in response to an upper respiratory tract infection. This immunologic re-

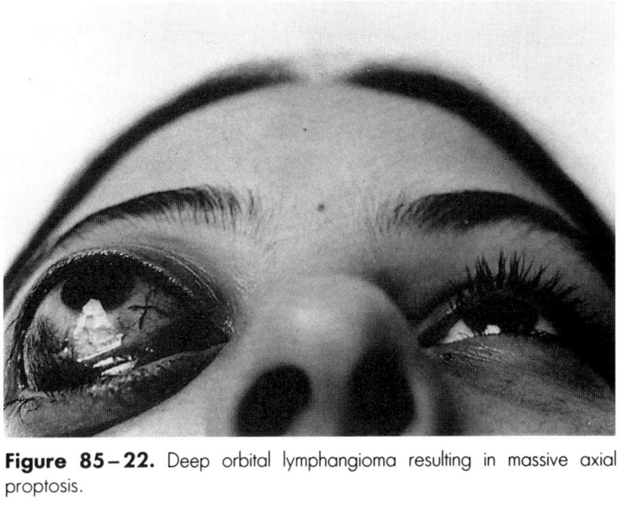

Figure 85–22. Deep orbital lymphangioma resulting in massive axial proptosis.

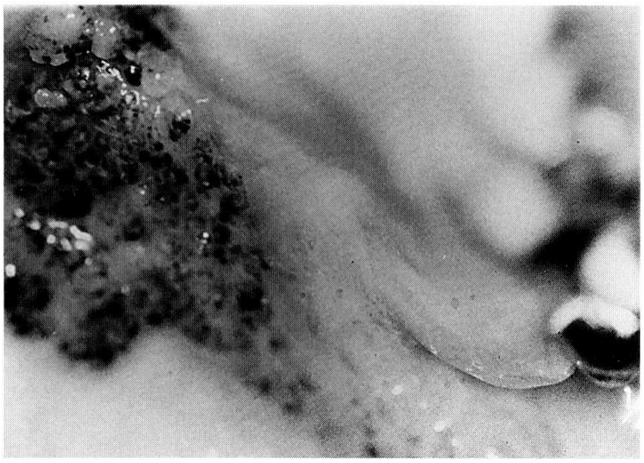

Figure 85–23. Intraoral involvement with lymphangiomatous tissue.

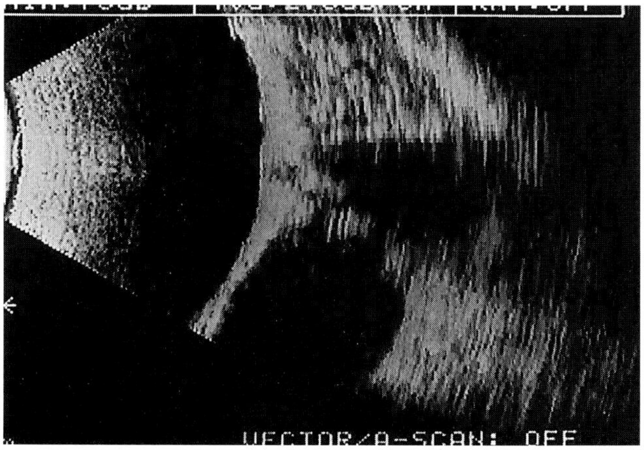

Figure 85–24. Contact B-scan ultrasonogram revealing a large blood cyst in the temporal orbit.

sponse usually subsides with a subsequent decrease in tumor volume. The second cause of rapid tumor growth, which must be differentiated from rhabdomyosarcoma, is blood cyst formation. In this more dramatic situation, massive tumor growth can occur within hours. Blood cyst formation is often heralded by massive proptosis, subconjunctival hemorrhage, or ecchymosis. These conditions result from hemorrhage of one of the poorly supported blood vessels projecting into a lymph channel. Blood cysts may occur spontaneously after accidental trauma or may be secondary to scarring after surgery on the tumor mass. In patients who have had repeated anatomic disruptions from surgery, trauma, or blood cyst formation, extensive fibrovascular proliferation may occur, as well as secondary arterialization of the tumor mass.[1]

Diagnostic Testing

The diagnosis is made primarily on clinical inspection; however, ancillary imaging techniques produce various characteristic findings. Plain radiographic analysis often reveals diffuse orbital enlargement typical of any benign, expanding tumor of the orbit that is present in infancy. The unencapsulated nature of the tumor and its ability to cross tissue planes is evident. Lymphatic and blood cysts scattered throughout the orbital cavity display a characteristic appearance on both ultrasonography and computed tomography. Diffuse infiltration of orbital fat with tumor results in a coarser-than-normal appearance of the tissue. Cyst formation produces discrete round or oval foci interrupting the heterogeneous fat pattern; these are seen clearly on A- and B-scan ultrasonography (Fig. 85–24).[1] On computed tomography in the past, cysts were typically nonenhancing (Fig. 85–25). In Graeb's series of 10 using second- and third-generation scanners with contrast material, all lesions showed rim enhancement.[54]

The imaging modality of choice for this lesion is magnetic resonance imaging. Magnetic resonance imaging can precisely delineate the extent and character of the mass, identify specific tissue planes, and determine the duration of the hemorrhage.[59] The superior contrast resolution of magnetic resonance imaging allows facilitation in separating normal and abnormal tissue planes and choosing the surgical approach. Since hemoglobin is paramagnetic, areas of old intraorbital hemorrhage or stagnated blood seen in lymphangiomas are depicted and outlined with great sensitivity using magnetic resonance imaging (Fig. 85–26).[1] As the blood breaks down from deoxyhemoglobin and oxyhemoglobin to methemoglobin and eventually to hemosiderin and ferritin, the paramagnetic qualities change. One can, therefore, not only more easily differentiate these lesions from other orbital

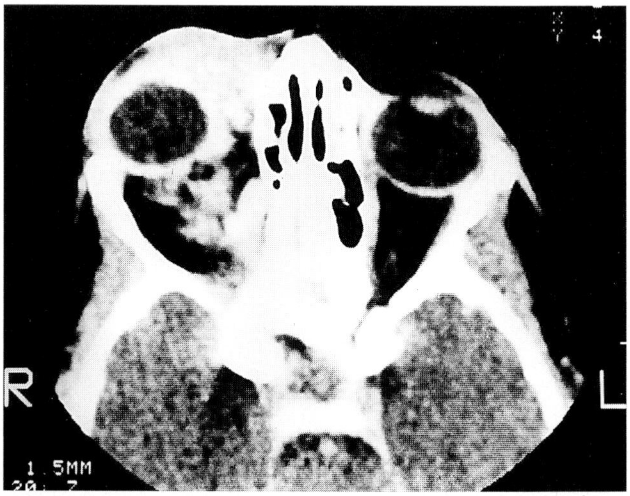

Figure 85–25. Contrast-enhanced axial computed tomographic scan demonstrates a diffusely enlarged right orbit and ocular proptosis and displacement in a patient with diffusely infiltrating orbital lymphangioma. The enhancing mass involves both the preseptal and postseptal regions of the orbit. Multiple, discrete, nonenhancing cysts are seen outlined by the fibrovascular tissues.

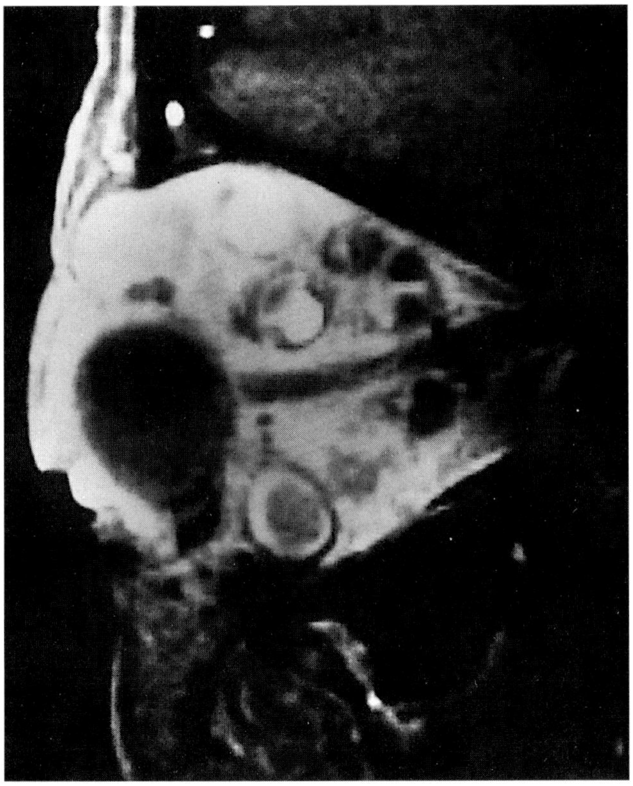

Figure 85–26. T1-weighted sagittal magnetic resonance scan reveals multiple blood cysts with variable stages of organization.

masses but also define the chronicity of the hemorrhage.[59] Magnetic resonance imaging also has the advantage over arteriography and contrast-enhanced computed tomography of detecting any major feeder vessels in a noninvasive manner with no exposure to ionizing radiation.[60]

Although Wright[61] has argued convincingly that these abnormalities are congenital varices based on venographic studies, Iliff and Green[49] and Jakobiec and Jones[62] report patients with the clinical diagnosis of lymphangioma who do not show similar venous anomalies. Many of our patients have undergone detailed vascular studies before treatment. Most of the studies revealed no associated abnormality. However, in several notable exceptions, major venous abnormalities were noted intraorbitally and intracranially.[1]

Therapeutic Alternatives

In contrast to capillary hemangiomas, the primary form of therapy in the management of lymphangiomas is often surgical. It should be noted, however, that medical, including conservative, management with observation[63] and minor surgical therapy can be effective in the management of specific complications. These means may achieve the desired therapeutic goal without major surgical intervention or revision.

Medical therapy is limited to shrinking the lymphoid portion of the tumor. The lymphoid tissue and follicles characteristic of the tumor hypertrophy after an antigenic stimulus such as an upper respiratory tract infection. This acute inflammatory component of the tumor is usually quite responsive to systemic corticosteroid therapy. Moderate doses for several days are usually adequate to carry the patient through this period. Unfortunately, the lymphoid portion is usually a relatively small percentage of the tumor volume and corticosteroid therapy has no significant effect on the remaining fibrovascular portion of the tissue.[1]

Radiation therapy is also effective in minimizing the lymphoid component of the lymphangioma; at safe therapeutic levels, however, it has little effect on the size or growth of its fibrovascular component. It is thus rarely indicated in the treatment of lymphangiomas.[1]

Conservative management has also been used successfully in acute proptosis. Wilson and coworkers[63] report on a series of six pediatric orbital lymphangiomas (biopsy proven in five). All six patients presented with acute proptosis and decreased visual acuity but none had an afferent pupillary defect. The patients were monitored for changes in vision and pupillary response. The proptosis resolved uneventfully in all with a return to 20/20 vision.

Surgical excision is a difficult and often frustrating task. Because of the diffusely infiltrative nature of the tumor with no encapsulation and its bountiful blood supply, extraction is extremely challenging.[1] In fact, the first reported surgical case[64] resulted in enucleation to allow for removal of the lesion.

Blood cysts may be drained effectively. If a large blood cyst is detected on ultrasonography and computed tomography, a large-bore needle can be passed into the hemorrhagic cavity and blood can be aspirated to reduce the tumor. Surgical drainage is less effective when blood has clotted or is secondarily organized, but it may achieve sufficient orbital decompression to obviate further immediate treatment. One must be aware, however, of a possible consequence of this procedure. While attempting to drain a "chocolate" cyst with a large-bore needle, the surgeon may traumatize other vascular channels within the tumor and cause an iatrogenic hemorrhage.[1]

When surgery is anticipated, careful preoperative evaluation of the eyelids, conjunctiva, and orbital adnexa must be performed, as well as a careful evaluation of present ocular function. It is unrealistic to anticipate total removal of the tumor mass and, in most cases, the goal is reduction of the most disfiguring or functionally disruptive portion. Since the tumor characteristically infiltrates many planes of the orbit and recurs, surgery is typically staged so that the results of each procedure can be assessed before additional excision is contemplated. In a significant percentage of patients, staging permits more appropriate management of both residual and new tumor components.[1]

The tumor often becomes significantly arterialized

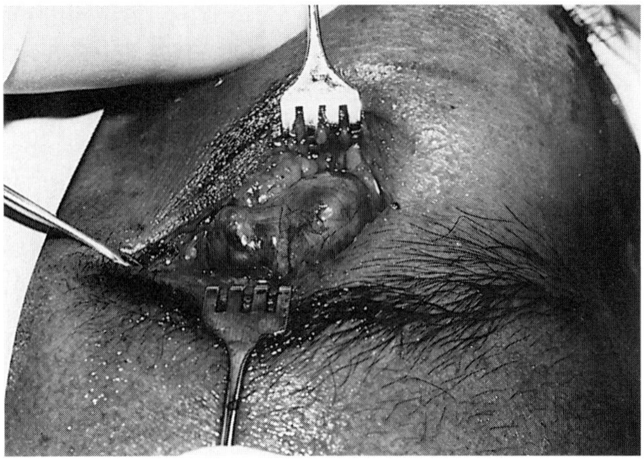

Figure 85–27. Surgical photograph demonstrating several large "chocolate cysts" resulting from previous hemorrhage.

spontaneously or after trauma. It is therefore advantageous to obtain preoperative radiographic studies of the vascular supply. If preoperative studies show no significant arterial feeders, surgery carries less risk and is hence more justifiable. If the tumor has significantly arterialized spontaneously, or after trauma or surgery, it may be advantageous to embolize or ligate major feeding vessels before excision. Hypotensive, hypothermic anesthesia serves to minimize bleeding during surgery, thereby reducing risk to the patient and improving the surgeons' visualization. Additionally, it is advisable (especially in young children or infants) to have cross-matched and typed blood available for use during the procedure.[1]

Sharp and blunt dissection is carried out to isolate and excise large masses of fibrovascular tissue after the excision and decompression of blood cysts (Fig. 85–27). Henderson[4] suggests that cryotherapy may be valuable in destroying the vascular channels in the tumor, minimizing the need for extensive primary excision. We have little experience with this concept but do occasionally apply cryotherapy to disrupted cysts that are not easily excisable in an attempt to stimulate fibrosis of the cyst cavity.[1]

We presently employ a Bovie electrocautery needle or carbon dioxide laser in the management of lymphangiomas. Others have used the yttrium-aluminum-garnet (YAG)–tipped laser successfully.[65] These techniques permit meticulous dissection while maximizing hemostasis. An additional, recent advance in the management of these tumors is the injection of soluble and insoluble corticosteroids into the residual tumor mass at the termination of surgery. This usually will increase postoperative comfort and decrease the postoperative inflammation.

When adequate cosmetic and functional results cannot be obtained by tumor excision alone, a decompression of the bony orbit should be considered. Decompression is similar to the procedure used for thyroid ophthalmopathy. A lateral and/or inferomedial orbital decompression, combined with controlled excision of the tumor mass, permits significant retroplacement of the globe in all but the most extreme cases.[1]

Unfortunately, there are usually residual cosmetic abnormalities in these patients, even after repeated operations. In large tumors, this may be quite disfiguring and create a complex management problem. Many of the patients are also amblyopic secondary to mechanical obstruction at the visual axis, anisometropia, and/or strabismus. Supportive measures, such as refractive correction and occlusion therapy, should be instituted. These are often disappointing in this patient group because of the complex regimens required and poor patient compliance.[1]

CAVERNOUS HEMANGIOMA

Cavernous hemangioma is among the most common primary orbital tumor of adults.[1] It is a benign vascular hamartoma that occurs more commonly in women and usually presents in the third to fifth decade of life.[66] It can occur in any portion of the orbit but usually develops in the muscle cone[1] on the temporal side.[67] The majority of cavernous hemangiomas are isolated lesions, although multiple tumors have been reported simultaneously or sequentially, separated by long time intervals. Cavernous hemangioma may occur bilaterally,[68] and the orbital tumor may be associated with lesions elsewhere in the body.[69, 70] Mafucci's syndrome (multiple soft tissue hemangiomas and enchondromas) should be considered in the patient with simultaneous, bilateral orbital cavernous hemangiomas.[70]

Histopathology

The tumor is round or oval with a slightly nodular (Fig. 85–28) or "mulberry"[71] surface and a purplish red color. It is typically well circumscribed and contained within a firm fibrous capsule, with only small vessels penetrating the tumor surface.[1] These small vessels have been noted to be incorporated into the mass as enlargement occurs.[72] Microscopically, a cavernous hemangioma is composed of large blood-filled vascular channels that are lined by flattened endothelial cells and are often separated by multiple fibrous septa (Figs. 85–29 and 85–30). Multilayered smooth muscle cells surround these endothelial cells, as seen with the electron microscope (Fig. 85–31).[1]

The pathogenesis of cavernous hemangioma is unknown.[73] The tumor is not believed to develop from a capillary hemangioma. The capillary lesions are distinct with no encapsulation, a more superficial location in the dermis, and a tendency to involute. Cavernous hemangiomas that occur in the pediatric age show no signs of involution. Others believe that with frequent enlargement of the orbital cavity, and the slowly progressive na-

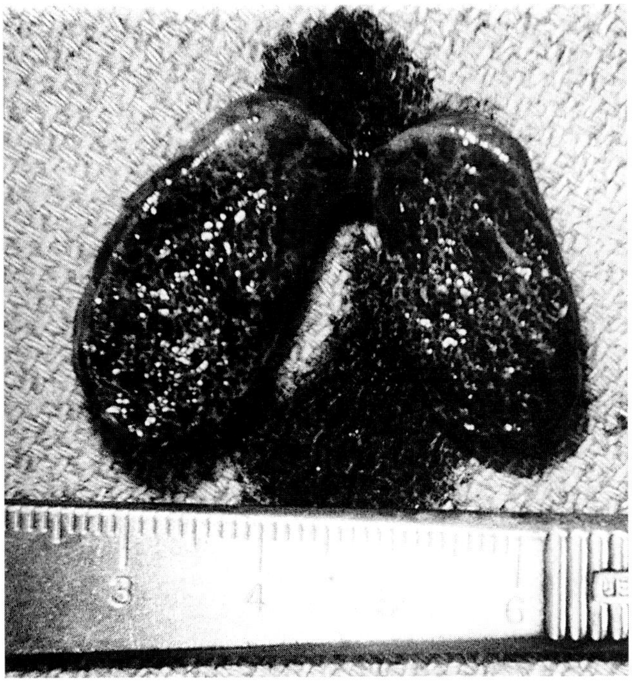

Figure 85–28. Macroscopic photograph of a transected, oval cavernous hemangioma demonstrating the well-circumscribed nature of this tumor.

ture of the tumor, which may span a decade, the tumor is most likely congenital or long standing.[74] There is, however, one reported case of a cavernous hemangioma occurring de novo 4 years after an enucleation for a melanoma.[73]

Clinical Course

The clinical course is characteristic: slow progressive enlargement, possibly associated with ophthalmologic findings related to compression or displacement of ocular or orbital structures.[66] The tumor may, however, have

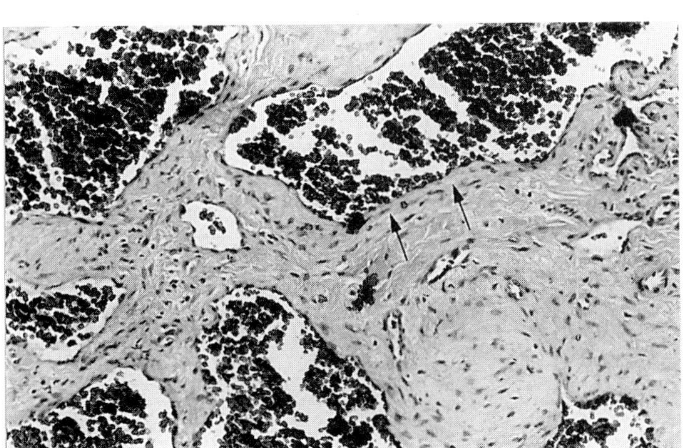

Figure 85–29. Cavernous hemangioma. Large vascular lumina filled with red blood cells are lined by a single layer of endothelial cells, which is further surrounded by mural smooth muscle cells *(arrows)*. H & E, ×200. (Courtesy of Takeo Iwamoto, MD.)

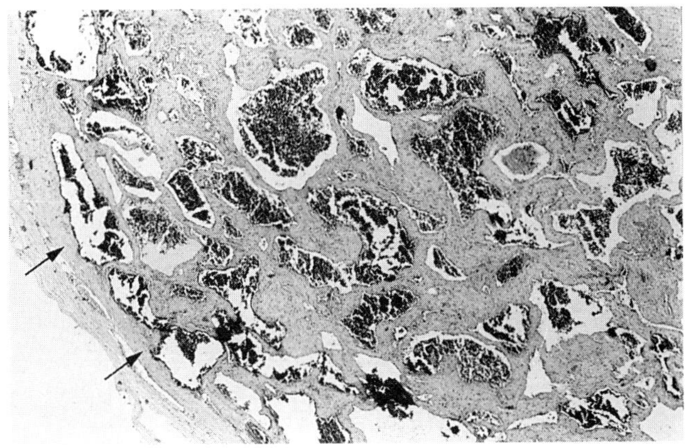

Figure 85–30. Photomicrograph of a cavernous hemangioma, which consists of large vascular spaces lined by flattened endothelial cells and separated by fibrous septa and surrounded by a fibrous capsule *(arrows)*. H & E, ×40. (Courtesy of Takeo Iwamoto, MD.)

a variable growth pattern. In a case of an incompletely removed cavernous hemangioma that was followed over an 18-year period, the tumor progressively enlarged over 11 years, stabilized over 2, and eventually involuted.[67] Many asymptomatic lesions have been found incidentally on computed tomography and were found to remain stable.[75] Growth of the tumor has also reportedly accelerated with the beginning of menses and during pregnancy, thus implicating hormonal influences.[76, 77]

The clinical sign at the time of diagnosis is generally proptosis of the affected eye. Commonly, the proptosis is not severe, being 5 mm or less[74]; it is usually axial, but occasionally the condition can present with associated horizontal or vertical displacement. Additionally, the tumor can exert sufficient pressure on the posterior sclera to cause hyperopia and choroidal folds. Restrictions of extraocular motility may be present, as well as diplopia in extreme positions of gaze. There are reports of headaches

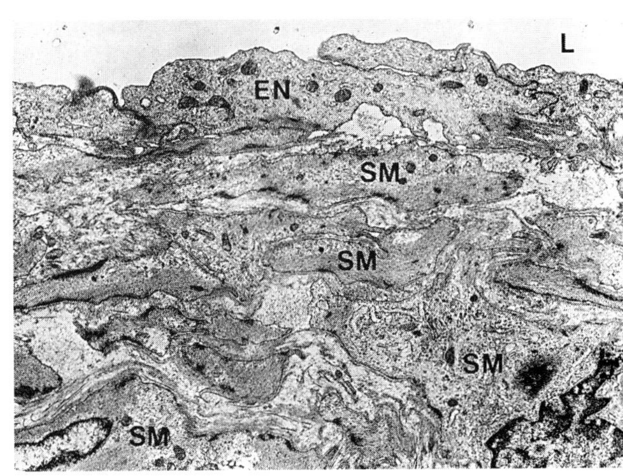

Figure 85–31. Electron micrograph of a wall of a vascular lumen of cavernous hemangioma showing a single layer of endothelium (EN) lining the lumen (L) and multilayered mural smooth muscle cells (SM). ×8500. (Courtesy of Takeo Iwamoto, MD.)

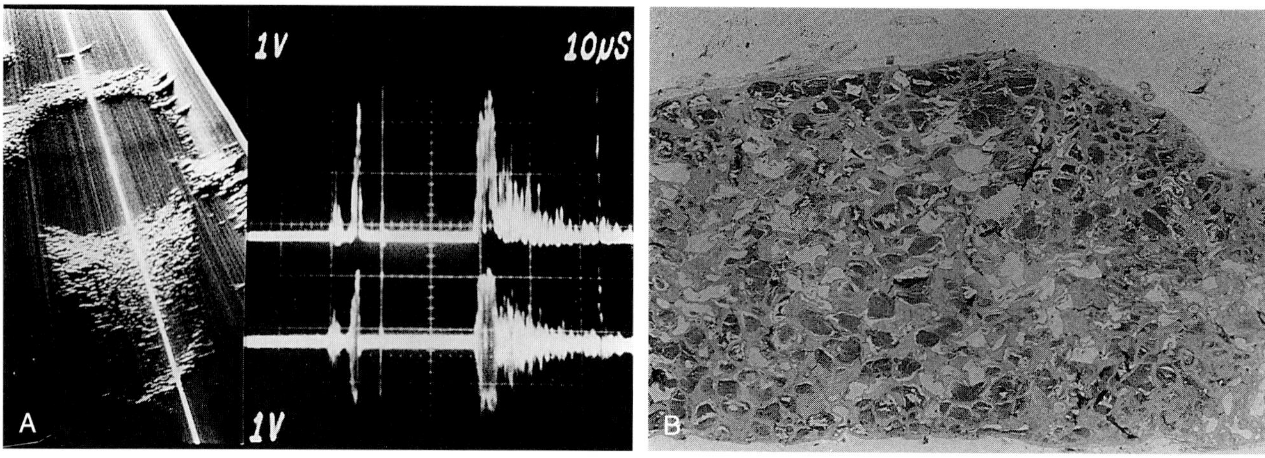

Figure 85–32. *A*, B- and A-scan ultrasonogram demonstrating a well-circumscribed intraconal mass. A-scan ultrasonogram demonstrates good sound transmission with multiple internal echoes produced by blood–septa interfaces. *B*, Microscopic section of the tumor demonstrates the origin of the internal echoes, demonstrated on both B- and A-scan ultrasonograms.

on the side of the orbital tumor, as well as recurrent subconjunctival hemorrhages in the affected eye.[1]

Diagnostic Testing

Ancillary diagnostic tests often aid in differentiating cavernous hemangiomas from other benign and malignant orbital conditions. Plain orbital radiographs may show an increase in soft tissue density and, more rarely, phlebolith formation. Additionally, orbital asymmetry secondary to diffuse orbital enlargement, local fossa formation, or hyperostosis may be detected after chronic pressure on the orbital bone. B- and A-scan ultrasonography can reveal the presence and location of a circumscribed mass in the orbit.[18] Sound transmission through the tumor is usually good, with a high degree of internal reflectivity produced by the blood–septa interfaces of these vascularized lesions (Fig. 85–32).

On computed tomography, a discrete circumscribed orbital mass may be detected and localized. The rounded or oval contour of the mass is well portrayed (Fig. 85–33). When the mass is adjacent to the optic nerve, a distinct separation may not be possible. Internal heterogeneity and location of the mass are often noted. Enhancement of the tumor mass after intravenous contrast injection is usually present but can be totally absent in some cases.[1]

Magnetic resonance imaging[78] easily outlines the typical isolated, discrete intraconal cavernous hemangioma and its relationship to the surrounding orbital structures (Fig. 85–34). The lesions are encapsulated, and while the capsule itself is beyond the limits of resolution, it provides a clear-cut boundary in imaging these lesions. The internal vascular components provide the basis of the different signal intensities. The longitudinal relaxation time of cavernous hemangiomas is greater than fat and less than the longitudinal relaxation time of brain.[1]

Treatment Alternatives

The primary treatment modality is surgical excision.[66, 79] Nonsurgical means of treatment, such as irradiation or pharmacologic therapy, have been ineffective. Surgical therapy optimally consists of total excision of the tumor mass using whichever standard orbital approach is dictated by the tumor location. In selected cases, the use of single or dual cryoprobes will secure the tumor during removal.[80] In certain cases when the tumor abuts the optic nerve or other neurovascular structures in the orbital apex, incomplete excision may be acceptable. Cavernous hemangiomas seldomly recur even after incomplete excision[1, 67]; it is assumed that the residual

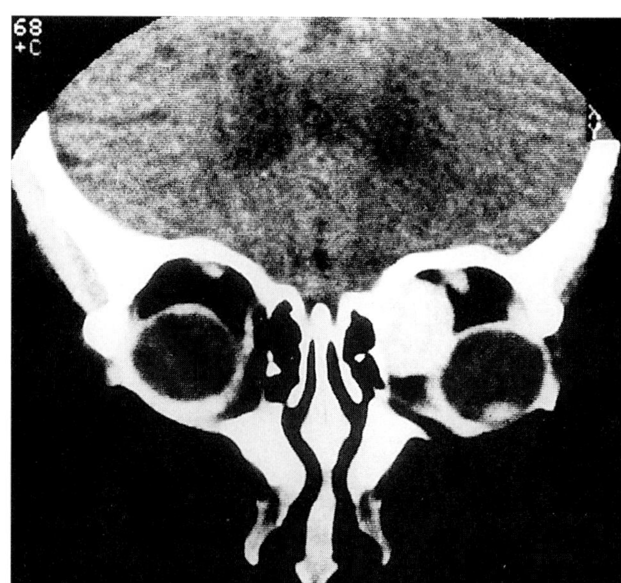

Figure 85–33. Contrast-enhanced direct coronal computed tomographic study reveals a discrete, oval mass in the superior nasal orbit causing proptosis and displacing the globe laterally.

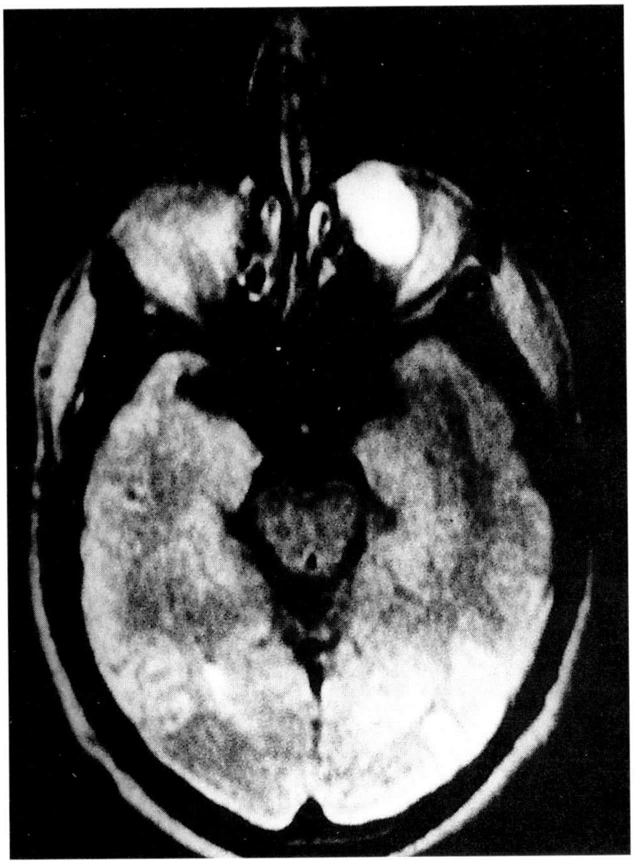

Figure 85–34. T2-weighted magnetic resonance scan of a patient with a discrete, isolated, oval cavernous hemangioma, well separated from the surrounding orbital structures.

mass of incompletely excised tumor is obliterated by postsurgical fibrosis. Some advocate observation in asymptomatic lesions as an alternative to surgery.[75] We believe that in the rare cases where a secure clinical diagnosis can be established without surgery and the tumor is adjacent to the critical orbital structures, observation alone may be indicated. In such cases, even subtotal excision may present a significant risk of visual complications, which outweighs the benefit of surgery. The period of observation should include not only clinical examination but also serial computed tomograms, ultrasonograms, and visual fields to dictate if and when surgical intervention should take place.

MALIGNANT HEMANGIOENDOTHELIOMA

Malignant hemangioendothelioma of the endothelial cell is an extremely rare tumor in the orbit; therefore, only limited information is available on its natural history and response to treatment. In 1942 and 1943, Stout and Murray[81, 82] revised the histopathologic classification of vascular tumors and documented a detailed report of a patient with this condition. A 40-year-old woman presented with a mass in the upper nasal quadrant of the orbit, which had caused unilateral proptosis and diplopia of several months' duration. At surgery, the tumor was found to be 2 cm long and to extend beneath the roof of the orbit posteriorly. The mass was partially resected during the original surgical procedure and recurred within 3 years, with such extensive growth that additional surgery was required. The patient was followed for 3 additional years without significant recurrence; however, no detailed long-term follow-up is available.[1]

Histopathology

These vascular tumors are characterized histopathologically by clusters of proliferating endothelial cells displaying cellular atypia and anaplasia.[62] Individual endothelial cells are found to proliferate within the lumina of the capillary and can totally obliterate the lumina, in some cases even extending outside the vascular tube. The use of reticulum staining will demonstrate the limiting membrane of reticulum outlining the lumina. This stain demonstrates the endothelial cells proliferating in a lumen-forming fashion (pseudoglandular). Because the malignant hemangioendothelioma is so rare, we have been unable to evaluate its appearance using computed tomography[1]; however, earlier reports describe successful imaging of the tumor using ultrasonography.[83]

Clinical Course

In two large ophthalmic centers (Mayo Clinic, Columbia-Presbyterian Medical Center)[4, 62] where several thousand patients with orbital disease have been evaluated, there is not a single case on file that corresponds to the description of orbital hemangioendothelioma as defined by Stout. Jakobiec and Jones[62] report that six cases exist in the Armed Forces Institute of Pathology, but scant detail is provided. Isolated reports[84, 85] exist in the Japanese literature: one of a child and one of an adult. In other parts of the body, these tumors have been found to be locally aggressive and to have a high metastatic potential.[82]

Treatment Alternatives

Owing to scant information on the malignant hemangioendothelioma and its response to treatment in the orbit, it is difficult to make appropriate therapeutic recommendations. It appears that total surgical excision is the treatment of choice.[1]

HEMANGIOPERICYTOMA

Hemangiopericytoma is a rare tumor of the pericyte. This contractile cell closely envelops the endothelial cells of capillaries and postvenous channels. Stout and Murray originally described the neoplasm in 1942.[81] The lesion usually occurs in the soft tissues surrounding the musculoskeleton and was not described as a primary orbital tumor until 1955 by Fox[86] and Goodman[87] independently. Hemangiopericytoma has an incidence of 3.14% of all primary orbital neoplasms.[88] Aside from primary involvement, the orbit may be affected from extension through an adjacent sinus or metastasis. Three major clinicopathologic reports provide our understanding of the behavior of hemangiopericytoma in the orbit.[88-90]

Histopathology

Macroscopically, hemangiopericytoma is purplish red and typically is encapsulated and oval. It may have a nodular surface and occasionally may be locally infiltrative without a well-defined capsule. This vascular tumor originates from pericytes and typically has a varying number of capillary-like spaces scattered throughout it. Surrounding these spaces outside its reticulum sheath are closely packed, crowded aggregates of pericytes (Fig. 85–35). When silver impregnations are performed, the presence of heavy deposits of reticular fibers confirms that the cells are primarily outside the basement membrane of the capillaries and are, therefore, of pericyte origin (see Fig. 85–35). The cells do not form lumina, as typically occurs in the hemangioendothelioma (see Fig. 85–2). Electron microscopy has shown that the tumor consists of cells with features ranging from pericytes to smooth muscle cells (Fig. 85–36).[91]

On the basis of Henderson's findings,[4, 88] some histologically benign-appearing tumors metastasize while patients with other, more malignant-appearing tumors survive for many years after diagnosis. In the small series by Geisinger and coworkers,[92] it has been suggested that DNA aneuploidy may be a prognostic indicator for a more malignant course. A definite relationship between the clinical course and histopathologic classification cannot be made in these limited series.[1]

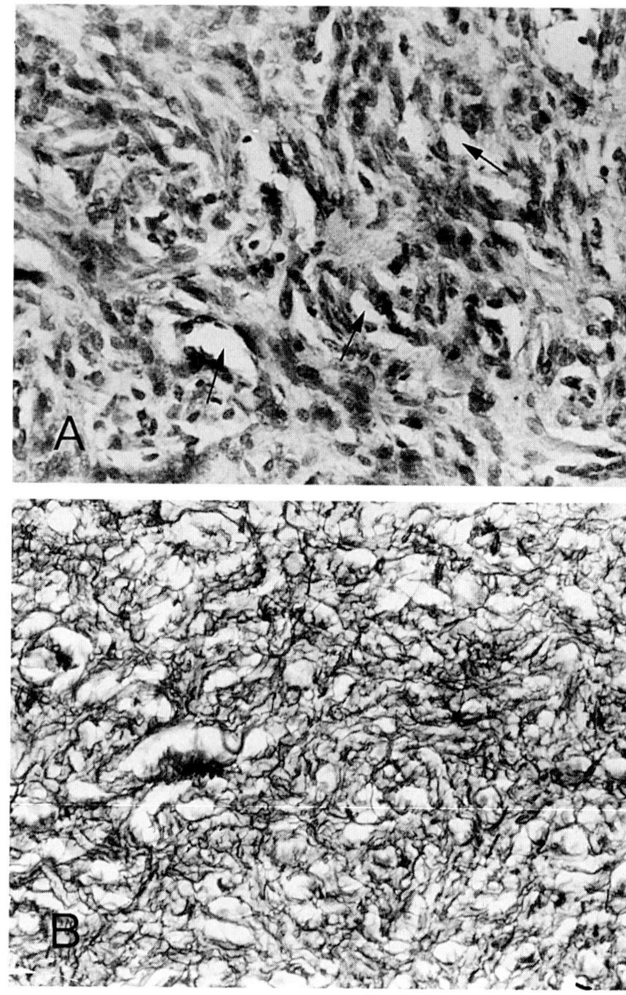

Figure 85–35. Hemangiopericytoma. *A*, Oval to spindle-shaped tumor cells occupy the spaces between scattered capillary-type blood vessels *(arrows)*. H & E, ×400. *B*, Reticulum stain delineates individual or small groups of tumor cells that do not themselves contain lumina. Reticulum stain, ×400. (Courtesy of Takeo Iwamoto, MD.)

Clinical Course

Hemangiopericytoma usually occurs in adults and presents as a slow-growing, circumscribed, painless orbital mass (Fig. 85–37). The tumor may occur in infancy with a more benign course.[93] It can occur in any part of the orbit but is usually located in the superior quadrants[88, 90]; other sites, including the muscle cone and lacrimal sac,[94] have been reported. The common presenting features of diplopia and proptosis are both secondary to the mass effect of the tumor.[1]

Hemangiopericytoma recurs in approximately 30% of orbital cases[90] and may metastasize.[88] Close follow-up is necessary, since the neoplasm has been noted to recur up to 33 years after excision.[95] Incomplete removal and duration of the tumor before excision have been correlated with recurrence.[88] Metastasis is often preceded by a recurrence and is most often to the lung and bone regardless of the primary location.[96]

Diagnostic Testing

Plain radiographs of the orbit may be normal or may demonstrate diffuse orbital enlargement without bony destruction. This is typical of any slow-growing tumor and is not a specific sign. On ultrasonography and computed tomography (Fig. 85–38), the circumscribed spherical or oval mass can be detected, in addition to any associated orbital enlargement. Unfortunately, there are no pathognomonic characteristics of hemangiopericytoma on either of the tests that permit differentiation of this mass from other well-encapsulated orbital tumors

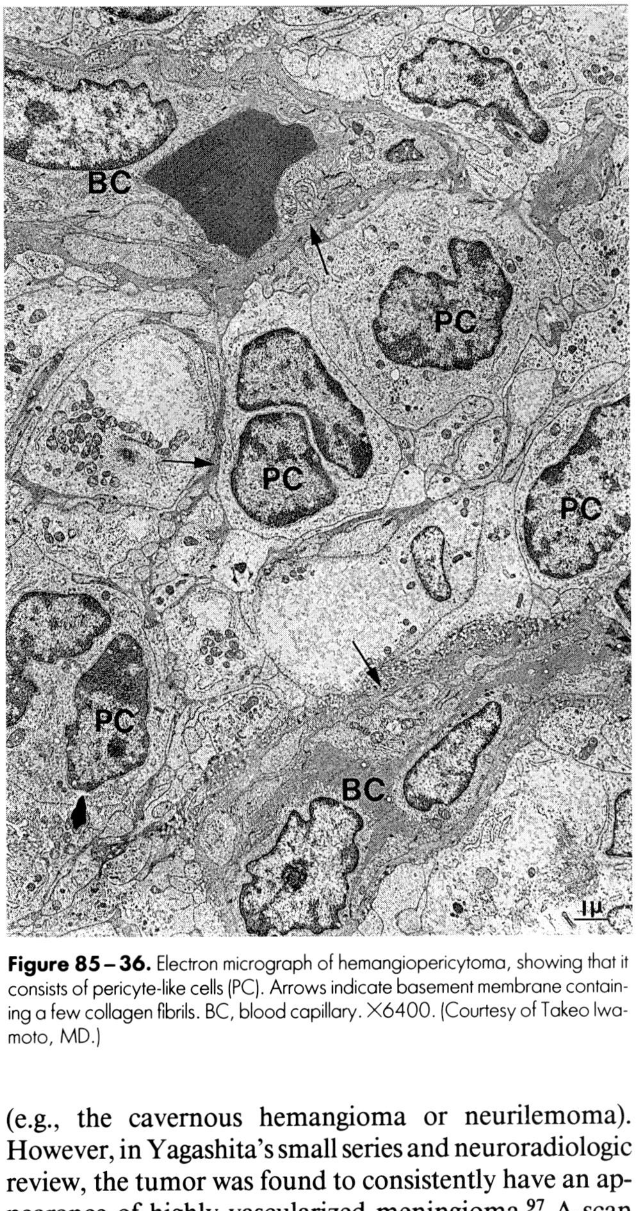

Figure 85–36. Electron micrograph of hemangiopericytoma, showing that it consists of pericyte-like cells (PC). Arrows indicate basement membrane containing a few collagen fibrils. BC, blood capillary. ×6400. (Courtesy of Takeo Iwamoto, MD.)

(e.g., the cavernous hemangioma or neurilemoma). However, in Yagashita's small series and neuroradiologic review, the tumor was found to consistently have an appearance of highly vascularized meningioma.[97] A-scan ultrasonography reveals the internal homogeneity of the

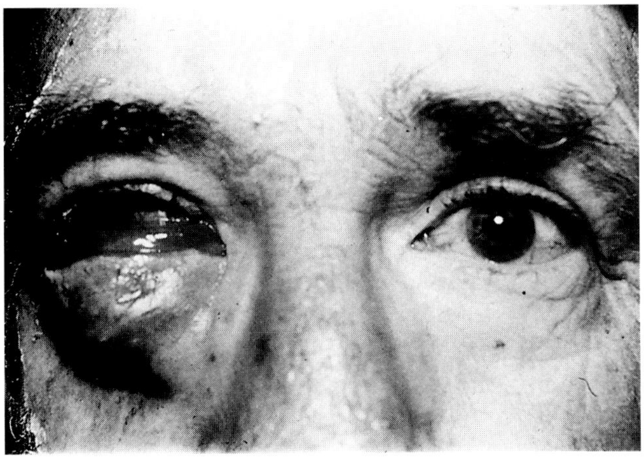

Figure 85–37. A 60-year-old patient presented with painless, enlarging, right inferior orbital hemangiopericytoma.

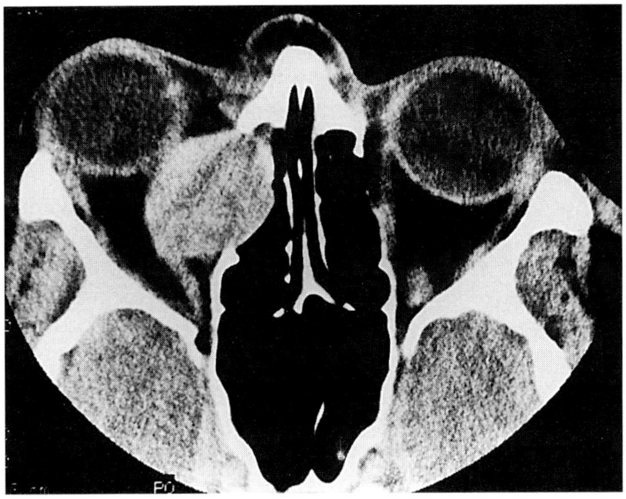

Figure 85–38. Contrast-enhanced computed tomographic scan demonstrates a well-circumscribed, enhancing orbital hemangiopericytoma in the medial orbit displacing the globe laterally.

tumor with minimal internal reflectivity. These findings can be expected to vary slightly, depending on the internal architecture of the tumor and on the size and distribution of the internal vascular channels. The tumor has also been noted to have areas of calcification.[98] Magnetic resonance imaging experience in orbital hemangiopericytoma is extremely limited. In our initial impression, the tumor behaves in a fashion similar to the cavernous hemangioma (Fig. 85–39).

Treatment Alternatives

Radiation therapy and chemotherapy have not been well established as primary treatment options for these tumors[88, 99]; the treatment of choice is total surgical excision.[4, 89] Extreme care should be taken to excise the

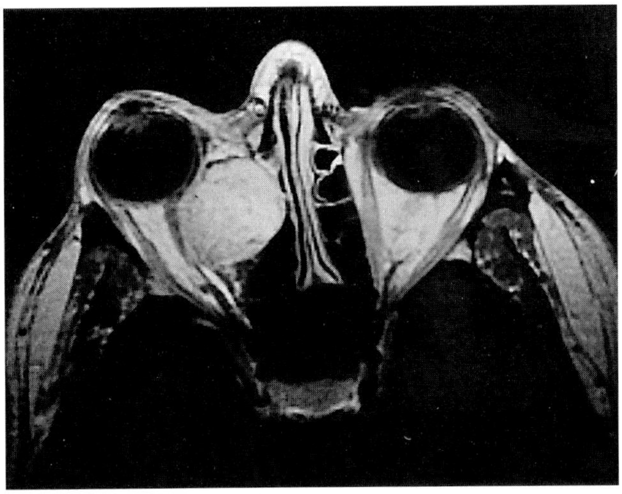

Figure 85–39. T1-weighted gadolinium-DTPA contrast-enhanced magnetic resonance scan demonstrates a well-circumscribed enhancing mass.

tumor completely within its pseudocapsule. The pseudocapsule is fragile and at times adherent to surrounding tissues, making complete removal impossible. In general, wedge biopsies are not recommended, since any transection of the tumor or interruption of the delicate pseudocapsule may permit tumor recurrence. The recurrent tumor can be locally infiltrative, can metastasize to distant sites, or both (Fig. 85–40). Since death may result from intracranial spread due to direct extension or metastases, one should consider extensive surgery (including exenteration) or radiation therapy when recurrent hemangiopericytomas are detected. Henderson,[4, 88] however, has shown that thorough piecemeal excision of the tumor mass occasionally results in an apparent recurrence-free period, similar to that of patients with total excision of the tumor. The unusual ability of the neoplasm to recur as long as 33 years after initial excision (Fig. 85–41)[95] or metastasize more than 30 years after the onset[88] should emphasize the need for careful postoperative monitoring. Doxorubicin (Adriamycin) used alone or in combination is the drug of choice in the treatment of metastatic disease.[100]

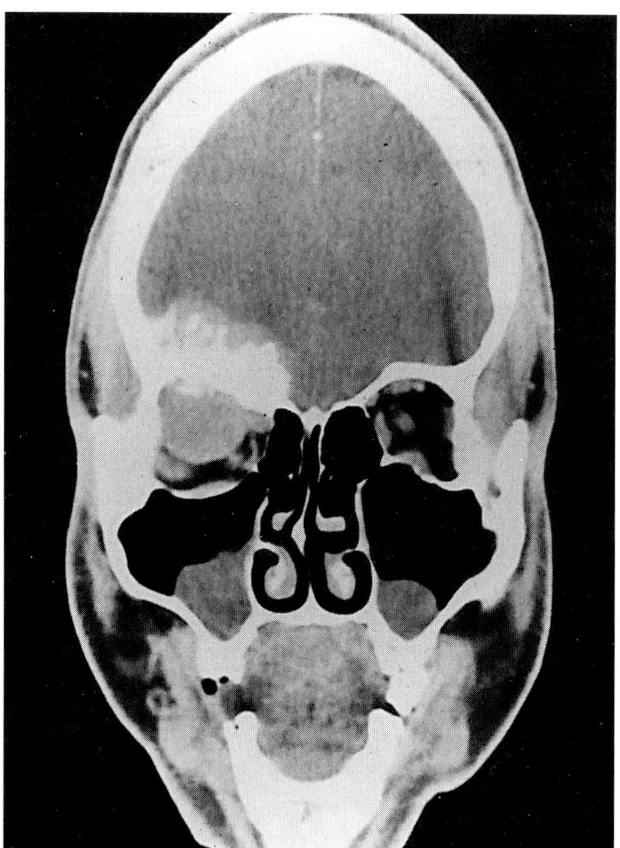

Figure 85–40. Coronal computed tomographic scan of a patient with recurrent hemangiopericytoma after incomplete excision.

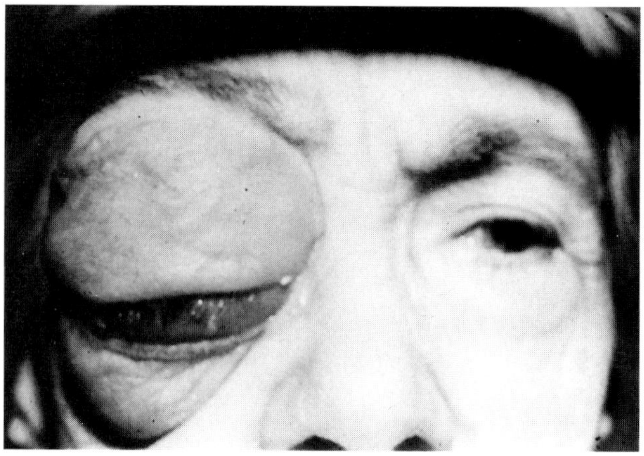

Figure 85–41. A 65-year-old patient who had undergone partial excision of hemangiopericytoma 7 years previously. There was massive recurrence of the tumor, with malignant degeneration.

REFERENCES

1. Haik BG, Jones IS, Ellsworth RM: Vascular tumors of the orbit. *In* Hornblass A (ed): Oculoplastic, Orbital, and Reconstructive Surgery. Baltimore, Williams & Wilkins, 1988.
2. Weiss AH: Adrenal suppression after corticosteroid injection of periocular hemangiomas. Am J Ophthalmol 107:518–522, 1989.
3. Reese AB: Tumors of the Eye, 3rd ed. Hagerstown, MD, Harper & Row, 1976.
4. Henderson JW: Orbital Tumors, 2nd ed. New York, Thieme-Stratton, 1980.
5. Iwamoto T, Jakobiec FA: Ultrastructural comparison of capillary and cavernous hemangiomas of the lids and orbit: An analysis of the clinical features and therapeutic results in 101 cases. Ophthalmology 86:760–788, 1979.
6. Haik BG, Jakobiec FA, Ellsworth RM, Jones IS: Capillary hemangioma of the lids and orbit: An analysis of the clinical features and therapeutic results in 101 cases. Presented before the American Academy of Ophthalmology, May 1979.
7. Andrews GC, Domankos AW: Skin hemangioma and retrolental fibroplasia. Arch Dermatol 68:320–323, 1953.
8. Haik BG, Karcioglu ZA, Gordon RA, Pechous B: Capillary hemangioma. Surv Ophthalmol 38:399–426, 1994.
9. Haik BG, Weiss R, Ellsworth RM: Capillary hemangioma of the orbit. Ophthalmic Pract 5:2, 1987.
10. Margileth AM, Museles M: Cutaneous hemangiomas in children. JAMA 194:523–526, 1965.
11. Bowers RE, Graham EA, Tomlinson KM: The natural history of strawberry nevus. Arch Dermatol 82:667–680, 1960.
12. Cohen BA: Hemangiomas in infancy and childhood. Pediatr Annu 16:17, 1987.
13. Holland VG: Hemangioma der Lider. Klin Monatsbl Augenheilkd 152:365–372, 1968.
14. Robb RM: Refractive errors associated with hemangiomas of the eyelids and orbit in infancy. Am J Ophthalmol 83:52–58, 1977.
15. Stigmar G, Crawford JS, Ward CM, et al: Ophthalmic sequelae of infantile hemangiomas of the eyelids and orbit. Am J Ophthalmol 85:806–813, 1978.
16. Haik BG, Lum B: Capillary hemangiomas. *In* Gold DH, Weingeist TA (eds): The Eye in Systemic Disease. Philadelphia, JB Lippincott, 1989.
17. Yee RD, Hepler RS: Congenital hemangiomas of the skin with orbital and subglottic hemangiomas. Am J Ophthalmol 75:876–879, 1973.
18. Coleman DJ, Jack RL, Frazen LA: Ultrasonography: II. Hemangiomas of the orbit. Arch Ophthalmol 80:368–374, 1972.
19. Haik BG: Capillary hemangioma. *In* Fraunfelder FT, Roy FH (eds): Current Ocular Therapy, 2nd ed. Philadelphia, WB Saunders, 1985, pp 189–190.

20. Haik BG: Advances in the surgical managements of capillary hemangiomas. *In* Jakobiec FA, Sigelman J (eds): Advanced Techniques in Ocular Surgery. Philadelphia, WB Saunders, 1984, pp 659–666.
21. Nordberg UB, Sundberg J: Indications and methods for radiotherapy of cavernous hemangiomas. Acta Radiol 1:257–274, 1962.
22. McEldresh AE, Robbins R: Radiation therapy of hemangiomas. J Pediatr 59:311–312, 1961.
23. Haik BG, Jereb B, Abramson DH, Ellsworth RM: Ophthalmic radiotherapy. *In* Iliff NT (ed): Complications in Ophthalmic Surgery. New York, Churchill Livingstone, 1983, pp 449–485.
24. Zarem HA, Edgerton MT: Induced resolution of cavernous hemangioma following prednisolone therapy. Plast Reconstr Surg 39:76–83, 1967.
25. Sasaki GH, Pang CY, Wittliff JL: Pathogenesis and treatment of infant skin strawberry hemangiomas: Clinical and in vitro studies of hormonal effects. Plast Reconstr Surg 73:359–370, 1984.
26. Ozsoylus S, Strauss HS, Diamond LK: Effects of corticosteroids on coagulation of the blood. Nature 195:1214–1215, 1962.
27. Kushner BJ: Intralesional corticosteroid injection for infantile adnexal hemangioma. Am J Ophthalmol 93:496–506, 1982.
28. Shorr N, Seiff SR: Central retinal artery occlusion associated with periocular corticosteroid injection for juvenile hemangioma. Ophthalmic Surg 17:229–231, 1986.
29. Haik BG, Ellsworth RM: Pediatric orbital tumors. *In* Pediatric Ophthalmology and Strabismus. Transactions of the New Orleans Academy of Ophthalmology. New York, Raven Press, 1986.
30. Cogen MS, Elsas FJ: Eyelid depigmentation following corticosteroid injection for infantile ocular adnexal hemangioma. J Pediatr Ophthalmol Strabismus 26:35–38, 1989.
31. Satula FC, Glover AT: Eyelid necrosis following intralesional corticosteroid injection for capillary hemangioma. Ophthalmic Surg 18:103–105, 1987.
32. Droste PJ, Ellis FD, Sondhi N, Helveston EM: Linear subcutaneous fat atrophy after corticosteroid injection of periocular hemangiomas. Am J Ophthalmol 105:65–69, 1988.
33. Ramdohr M: Ein Fall von angeborenem multiple Angiosarcoma. Virchows Arch [Pathol Anat] 73:459, 1878.
34. Holden KR, Alexander F: Diffuse neonatal hemangiomatosis. Pediatrics 46:411–421, 1970.
35. Golitz LE, Rudikoff J, O'Meara OP: Diffuse neonatal hemangiomatosis. Pediatr Dermatol 3:145–152, 1986.
36. Geller JD, Topper SF, Hashimoto K: Diffuse neonatal hemangiomatosis: A new constellation of findings. J Am Acad Dermatol 24:816–818, 1991.
37. Haik BG, Clancy P, Ellsworth RM, et al: Ocular manifestations in diffuse neonatal hemangiomatosis. J Pediatr Ophthalmol Strabismus 20:101–105, 1983.
38. Stillman AE, Hansen RC, Hallinan V, Strobel C: Diffuse neonatal hemangiomatosis with severe gastrointestinal involvement. Clin Pediatr 22:589–591, 1983.
39. Teillac D, Pariente D, Latouche X, et al: Hemangiomatose neonate diffuse. Ann Dermatol Venereol 112:765–766, 1985.
40. Colin A, Castel Y, LeFoll J, Toudic L: Diffuse neonatal hemangiomatosis: Clinical and therapeutic aspects. Ann Pediatr (Paris) 31:401–402, 405–406, 1984.
41. Davanzo R, Riosa R, Longo F: Emangiomatosi neonatale diffusa: Rapida risposta clinica al trattamento steroideo. Pediatr Med Chir 9:483–486, 1987.
42. Hendriks JJ, van de Staak FH, Vio PM, Tolboom JJ: Neonatal hemangiomatosis with prolonged icterus. Tijdschr Kindergeneeskd 57:29–31, 1989.
43. Montgomery SP, Guillot AP, Barth RA: MRI of disseminated neonatal hemangiomatosis: Case report. Pediatr Radiol 20:204–205, 1990.
44. Poirier VC, Ablin DS, Frank EH: Diffuse neonatal hemangiomatosis: A case report. Am J Neuroradiol 11:1097–1099, 1990.
45. Sayama K, Higaki T, Ohtsuka H, et al: Diffuse neonatal hemangiomatosis with a giant cutaneous hemangioma of the axilla. J Dermatol 18:286–290, 1991.
46. Haik BG, Clancy P, Ellsworth RM, et al: Ocular manifestations in diffuse neonatal hemangiomatosis. J Pediatr Ophthalmol 20: 101–105, 1983.
47. Schiliro G, Guarneri B, Russo A: A case of multiple neonatal hemangiomatosis with favorable outcome following steroid therapy. Acta Pediatr Scand 65:257–270, 1976.
48. Hemmer KM, Marsh JL, Milder B: Orbital lymphangioma. Ophthalmic Plast Reconstr Surg 82:340–343, 1986.
49. Iliff WJ, Green WR: Orbital lymphangiomas. Ophthalmology 86:914–929, 1979.
50. Reese AB: Expanding lesions of the orbit. Trans Ophthalmol Soc UK 91:85–104, 1971.
51. Jones IS: Lymphangiomas of the ocular adnexa: An analysis of 62 cases. Trans Am Ophthalmol Soc 57:603–662, 1959.
52. Jones IS, Jakobiec FA: Diseases of the Orbit. New York: Harper & Row, 1979.
53. Enzinger FM, Weiss SW: Soft Tissue Tumors. St. Louis, CV Mosby, 1983.
54. Graeb DA, Rootman J, Robertson WD, et al: Orbital lymphangiomas: Clinical, radiologic, and pathologic characteristics. Radiology 175:417–421, 1990.
55. Harris GJ, Sakol PJ, Bonavonta G, DeConcilis C: An analysis of thirty cases of orbital lymphangioma: Pathophysiologic considerations and management recommendations. Ophthalmology 97:1583–1592, 1990.
56. Landing BH, Faber S: Tumors of the Cardiovascular System. *In* Atlas of Tumor Pathology. Washington, DC, Armed Forces Institute of Pathology, 1956.
57. Mulliken JB, Glowacki J: Hemangiomas and vascular malformations in infants and children: A classification based on endothelial characteristics. Plast Reconstr Surg 69:412–420, 1982.
58. Rootman J, Hay E, Graeb D: Orbital-adnexal lymphangiomas. Ophthalmology 93:1558, 1986.
59. Bond JB, Haik BG, Francis BA, et al: Magnetic resonance imaging of orbital lymphangioma with and without gadolinium contrast enhancement. Presented at the annual meeting of the American Academy of Ophthalmology, Anaheim 1991.
60. Haik BG, Saint Louis L, Smith ME, et al: Magnetic resonance imaging of orbital lymphangiomas. Am J Ophthalmol 103:724–725, 1987.
61. Wright JE: Orbital vascular anomalies. Trans Am Acad Ophthalmol Otolaryngol 78:606, 1974.
62. Jakobiec FA, Jones IS: Vascular tumors, malformations, and degenerations. *In* Duane TD (ed): Clinical Ophthalmology. Philadelphia, Harper & Row, 1981.
63. Wilson ME, Parker PL, Chavis RM: Conservative management of childhood orbital lymphangioma. Ophthalmology 96:484–489, 1989.
64. Ayres SC: Lymphangioma cavernosum of the orbit, with an original case. Am J Ophthalmol 12:321–331, 1895.
65. Hornblass A: The use of YAG-tipped contact laser in removing orbital lymphangiomas [letter]. Plast Reconstr Surg 83:397, 1989.
66. Harris GJ, Jakobiec FA: Cavernous hemangioma of the orbit: A clinicopathologic analysis of sixty-three cases. *In* Jakobiec FA (ed): Ocular and Adnexal Tumors. Birmingham, AL, Aesculapius, 1980.
67. Henderson JW, Farrow GM, Garrity JA: Clinical course of an imcompletely removed cavernous hemangioma of the orbit. Ophthalmology 97:625–628, 1990.
68. Fries PD, Char DH: Bilateral orbital cavernous hemangioma. Br J Ophthalmol 72:871–873, 1988.
69. Bisaria KK, Misra UC: Haemangioma of the orbit and cheek. Br J Ophthalmol 52:628–630, 1968.
70. Johnson TE, Nasr AM, Nalbandian RM, Cappelen Smith J: Enchondramatosis and hemangioma (Mafucci's syndrome) with orbital involvement. Am J Ophthalmol 110:153–159, 1990.
71. Wolin MJ, Holds JB, Anderson RL, Mamalis N: Multiple orbital tumors were cavernous hemangioma. Ann Ophthalmol 22:426–428, 1990.
72. Hood CI: Cavernous hemangioma of the orbit: A consideration of pathogenesis with illustrative case. Arch Ophthalmol 83:49–53, 1970.
73. Harnett AN, Thorpe P, Hungerford J: Cavernous hemangioma presenting as an orbital mass after enucleation for a choroidal melanoma: Case report. Br J Ophthalmol 72:618–620, 1988.
74. Jakobiec FA, Jones IS: Vascular tumors, malformations, and degenerations. *In* Duane TD, Jaeger EA (eds): Clinical Ophthalmology, vol 2. Philadelphia, JB Lippincott, 1991.

75. Orcutt JC, Wulc AE, Mills RP, Smith CH: Asymptomatic orbital cavernous hemangiomas. Ophthalmology 98:1257–1260, 1991.
76. Watson WL, McCarthy WD: Blood and lymph vessel tumors. Am J Ophthalmol 24:386–394, 1941.
77. Zauberman H, Feinsow M: Orbital hemangioma with growth during pregnancy. Acta Ophthalmol 48:929–933, 1970.
78. Haik BG, Saint Louis L, Smith ME: Nuclear magnetic resonance imaging in orbital disease. Ophthalmol Forum 3:31–34, 1985.
79. Haik BG: Cavernous hemangioma. *In* Fraunfelder R: Current Ocular Therapy, 2nd ed. Philadelphia, WB Saunders, 1985, pp 190–191.
80. Henderson JW, Neault RW: The use of the cryoprobe in removal of the tumor of the orbit and ocular adnexa. Am J Ophthalmol Surg 7:45–47, 1976.
81. Stout AP, Murray MR: Hemangiopericytoma: A vascular tumor featuring Zimmermann's pericytes. Ann Surg 116:26–33, 1942.
82. Stout AP, Murray MR: Hemangio-endothelioma: A tumor of blood vessels featuring vascular endothelial cells. Ann Surg 118:445–464, 1943.
83. Coleman DJ, Lizzi FL, Jack RL: Ultrasonography of the Eye and Orbit. Philadelphia, Lea & Febiger, 1977
84. Tsuda N, Tukaku I: A case report of malignant vascular tumor of the orbit in the newborn. Folia Ophthalmol Jpn 22:728, 1970.
85. Sekimoto T, Nakaseko H, Kondo K, et al: A case of malignant hemangioendothelioma in the orbit. Folia Ophthalmol Jpn 22:535, 1971.
86. Fox SA: Hemangiopericytoma of the orbit. Am J Ophthalmol 40:786–789, 1955.
87. Goodman SA: Hemangiopericytoma of the orbit. Am J Ophthalmol 40:237–243, 1955.
88. Henderson JW, Farrow GM: Primary orbital hemangiopericytoma: An aggressive and potentially malignant neoplasm. Arch Ophthalmol 96:666–673, 1978.
89. Jakobiec FA, Howard GM, Jones IS, Wolff M: Hemangiopericytoma of the orbit. Am J Ophthalmol 78:816–834, 1974.
90. Croxatto JO, Font RL: Hemangiopericytoma of the orbit: A clinicopathologic study of 30 cases. Hum Pathol 13:210–218, 1982.
91. Hahn MJ, Dawson R, Esterly JA, Joseph DJ: Hemangiopericytoma and ultrastructural study. Cancer 31:255–261, 1973.
92. Geisinger KR, Silverman JF, Cappellari JO, Dabbs DJ: Fine-needle aspiration cytology of malignant hemangiopericytomas with ultrastructural and flow cytometric analysis. Arch Pathol Lab Med 114:705–710, 1990.
93. Boyle J, Kennedy C, Berry J, Mott MG: Congenital hemangiopericytoma. J R Soc Med 78(suppl 11):10–12, 1985.
94. Roth SI, August CZ, Lissner GS, O'Grady RB: Hemangiopericytoma of the lacrimal sac. Ophthalmology 98:925–927, 1991.
95. Rice CD, Kersten RC, Mark RE: An orbital hemangiopericytoma recurrent after 33 years. Arch Ophthalmol 107:552–556, 1989.
96. Enzinger FM, Smith BH: Hemangiopericytoma: An analysis of 106 cases. Hum Pathol 7:61–82, 1976.
97. Yagishita A, Hussoun D, Vincentelli F, et al: Neuroradiologic study of hemangiopericytomas. Neuroradiology 27:420–425, 1985.
98. Garrity JA, Kennerdell JS: Orbital calcification associated with hemangiopericytoma. Am J Ophthalmol 102:126, 1986.
99. Setzkorn RK, Lee D, Iliff NT, Green R: Hemangiopericytoma of the orbit treated with conservative surgery and radiotherapy. Arch Ophthalmol 105:1103–1105, 1987.
100. Wong PP, Yogada A: Chemotherapy of malignant hemangiopericytoma. Cancer 41:1256–1260, 1978.

Orbital Inflammatory Disorders

CHAPTER 86

The Role of Paranasal Sinus Disease in Orbital Cellulitis

John B. Holds

A variety of bacterial, fungal, parasitic, and other infectious processes may invade the eyelids and orbit with devastating consequences. Invasive eyelid and orbital infections are a common group of disorders and are of importance when the potential for morbidity is considered. This chapter examines infectious orbital processes, with attention given to orbital infection secondary to sinus infection. The differential diagnosis, evaluation, and treatment of these clinical syndromes are presented in detail. A thorough knowledge of the signs and symptoms of eyelid and orbital infectious processes allows appropriate decisions to be made regarding radiologic and laboratory workup, subspecialty consultation, antimicrobial therapy, and surgical intevention.

RELEVANT ANATOMY

The varied structural elements and anatomic relationships of the orbit cause a wealth of distinctive pathology with unique clinical syndromes. Knowledge of regional anatomy is vital in understanding and treating infectious orbital processes. The orbit is bounded anteriorly by the eyelids, superiorly and posteriorly by the intracranial space, and medially and inferiorly by the paranasal sinuses (Fig. 86 – 1). For purposes of discussion, it is useful to divide the orbit into extraperiosteal, extraconal, and intraconal spaces because disease processes may arise within or be confined to one of these spaces. The latter two spaces are separated by the rectus muscles and intermuscular septae. The periosteum of the orbit, or periorbita, is loosely adherent to bone except at the anterior orbital margin and margins of the fissures. The orbital septum arises from the arcus marginalis of the anterior orbital rim and fuses with the aponeurotic structures of the upper and lower eyelids near the lid margins, delimiting the orbit anteriorly.[1]

The paranasal sinuses are the most important sources of pyogenic orbital infections, and a knowledge of their anatomy is of utmost importance in the recognition and treatment of infectious orbital processes. The ethmoidal and maxillary sinuses are present at birth and undergo initial rapid enlargement, reaching adult size in the late teenage years. The ethmoidal sinus is most frequently involved in the extension of sinus infection into the orbit. The thin lamina papyracea that separates the ethmoidal sinuses from the medial orbit has several neurovascular canals and random bone defects (Zuckerkandl's dehiscences) (Fig. 86 – 2) that provide a ready route for pyogenic processes into the medial orbit and subperiosteal space.[2] Intracranial communication through neurovascular canals traversing the orbit may allow extension of infectious processes intracranially. The maxillary sinus has somewhat less potential for orbital extension of sinusitis. Nonetheless, the maxillary sinus is a common initial site of infection in fungal sinusitis or for orbital extension of bacterial sinusitis, when associated with traumatic or surgical injury. Bacterial and fungal infections of the sphenoidal sinuses may invade the posterior orbit with no clinical involvement in the more anterior and accessible ethmoidal and maxillary sinuses. The indentation of

This chapter was supported in part by an unrestricted grant to the Anheuser-Busch Eye Institute of St. Louis University, St. Louis, Missouri, from Research to Prevent Blindness, Inc.

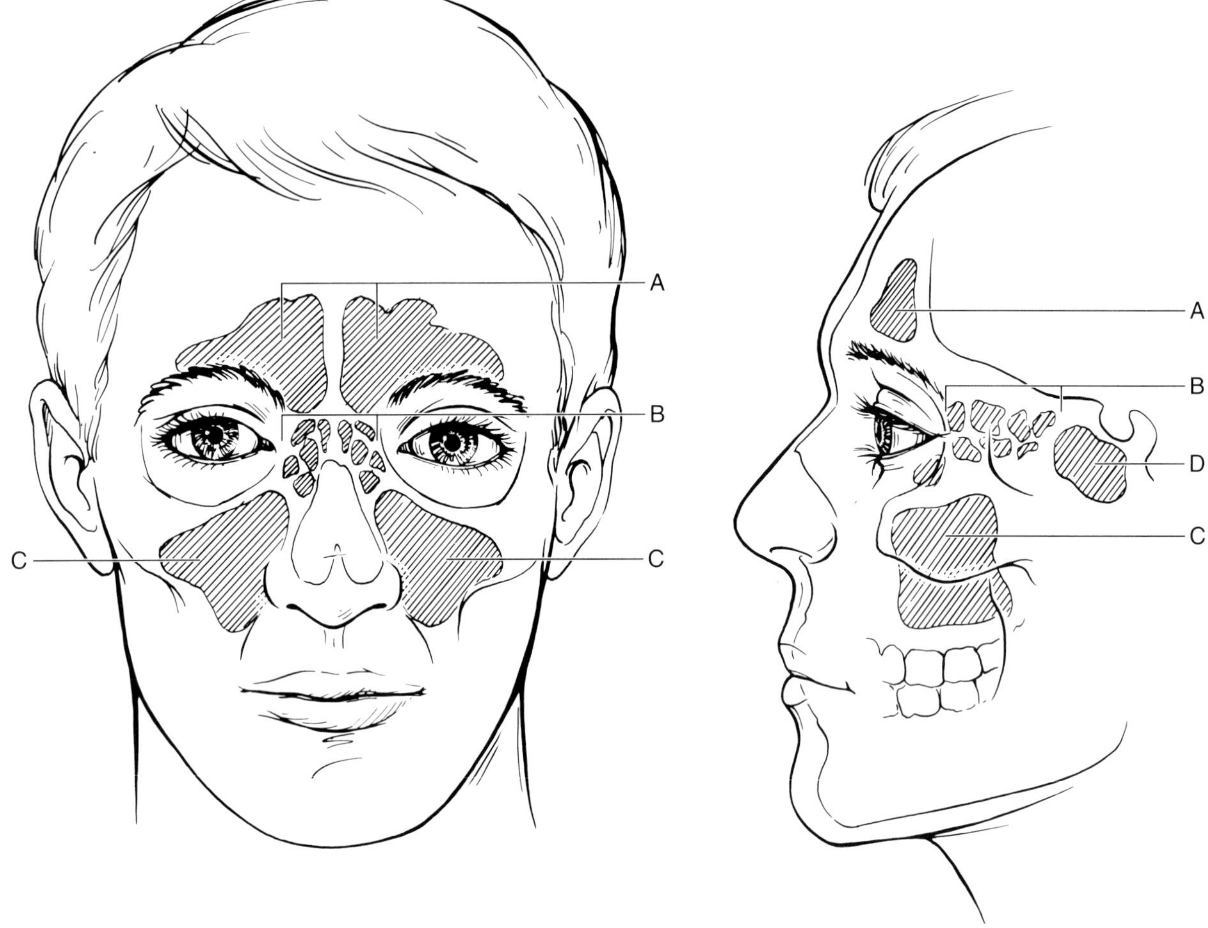

Figure 86–1. Relationships of the orbits to the paranasal sinuses. *A*, frontal; *B*, ethmoidal; *C*, maxillary; *D*, sphenoidal. (From Doxanas MT, Anderson RL: Clinical Orbital Anatomy. © 1984, the Williams & Wilkins Co., Baltimore.)

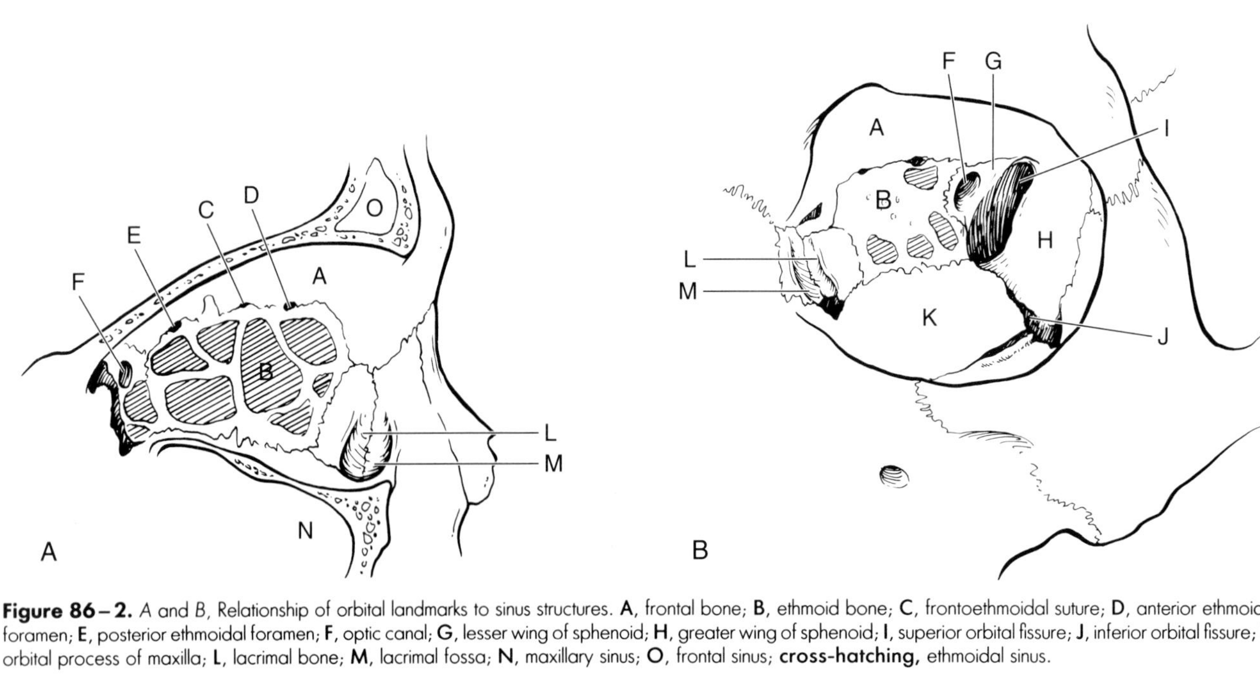

Figure 86–2. *A* and *B*, Relationship of orbital landmarks to sinus structures. **A**, frontal bone; **B**, ethmoid bone; **C**, frontoethmoidal suture; **D**, anterior ethmoidal foramen; **E**, posterior ethmoidal foramen; **F**, optic canal; **G**, lesser wing of sphenoid; **H**, greater wing of sphenoid; **I**, superior orbital fissure; **J**, inferior orbital fissure; **K**, orbital process of maxilla; **L**, lacrimal bone; **M**, lacrimal fossa; **N**, maxillary sinus; **O**, frontal sinus; **cross-hatching**, ethmoidal sinus.

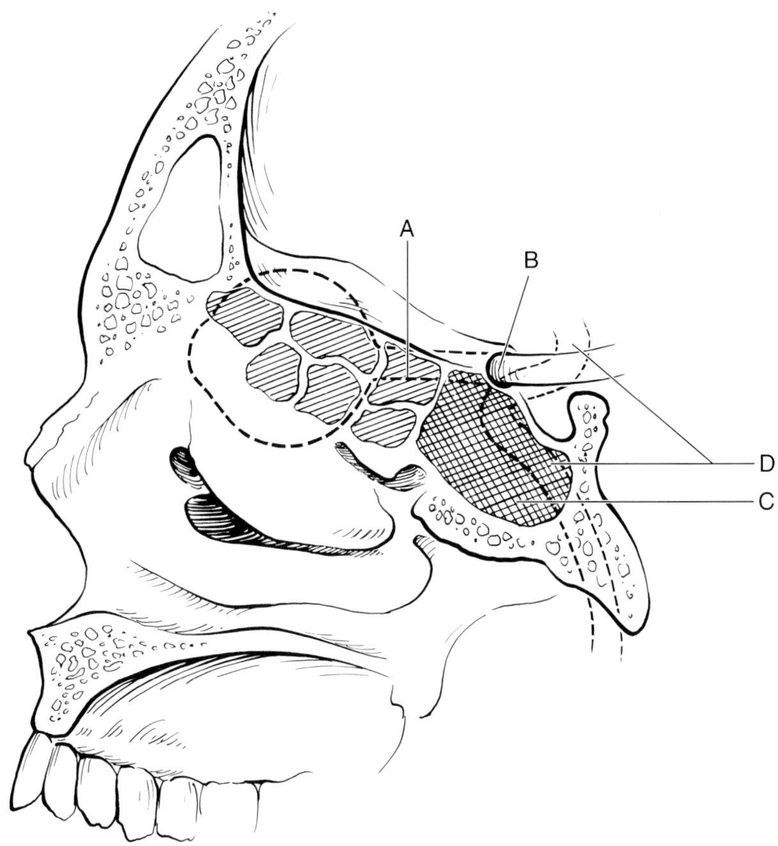

Figure 86–3. Relationship of the posterior ethmoidal air cells and sphenoidal sinus to the optic canal. **A**, posterior ethmoidal air cells; **B**, optic nerve; **C**, sphenoidal sinus; **D**, internal carotid artery.

the lateral sphenoidal sinus by the optic nerve and frequent bony dehiscences overlying this nerve (Fig. 86–3) explain the rapid, irreversible visual loss that may occur following orbital extension of sphenoidal sinusitis.[3] The frontal sinuses appear as extensions of the ethmoidal air cells, usually passing above the orbital roof between 4 and 10 years of age (average of 8 years).[4] The frontal sinuses generally overlie the anterior part of the orbital roofs and superior orbital rim. Orbital extension of frontal sinus mucopyocele is not uncommon.

The valveless veins of the middle third of the face, paranasal sinuses, orbit, and brain allow free venous communication.[5] Facial and orbital structures drain into the pterygoid plexus and cavernous sinus (Fig. 86–4). Intracranially, communicating veins may allow extension to the contralateral venous system or surrounding meninges. This communication is important to remember because infectious processes can readily access any one of these anatomic spaces from the others. Not only can direct extension occur but infections may leapfrog through venous channels from the face or sinuses to the brain or orbit (Figs. 86–5 and 86–6).

ORBITAL EXTENSION OF SINUS INFECTIONS

Bacterial Sinus Infections

Most cases of orbital cellulitis result from the extension of bacterial ethmoidal sinusitis into the orbit (Fig. 86–7). Usually, this presents with acute proptosis due to a subperiosteal abscess (Fig. 86–8). A classification of orbital complications of acute sinusitis was proposed by Hubert in 1937, and updates and modifications of this scheme were undertaken by Smith and Spencer in 1948 and by

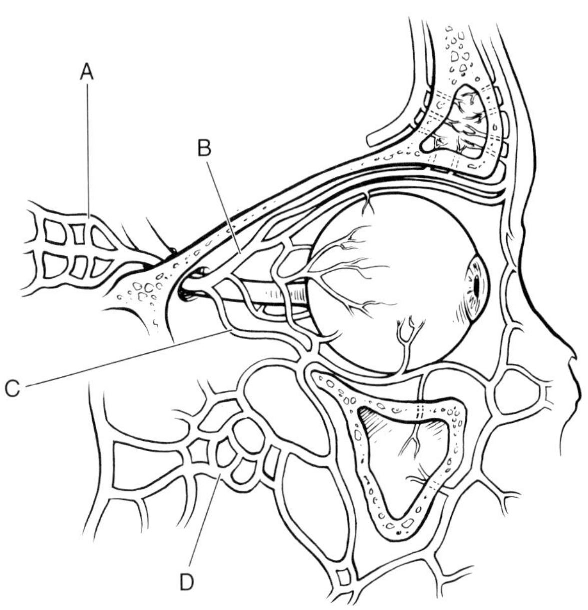

Figure 86–4. Facial and intracranial connections of the orbital venous system. **A**, cavernous sinus; **B**, superior ophthalmic vein; **C**, inferior ophthalmic vein; **D**, pterygoid venous plexus.

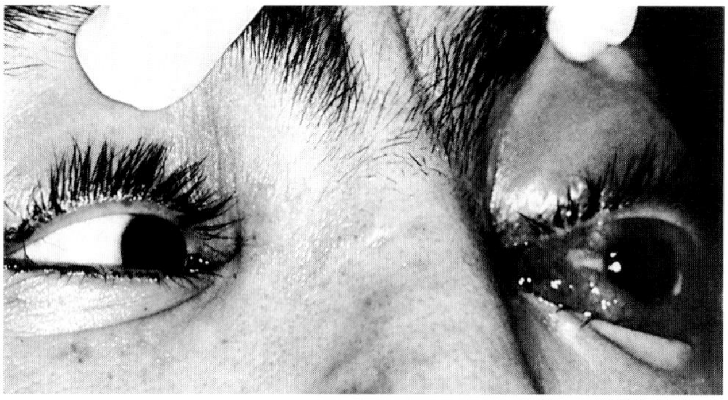

Figure 86–5. A 34-year-old male suddenly developed left proptosis while on antibiotic therapy for a premaxillary abscess occurring after dental extraction. Patient is seen in left gaze showing left sixth cranial nerve palsy. Partial deficits were also seen in third, fourth, and fifth cranial nerve function.

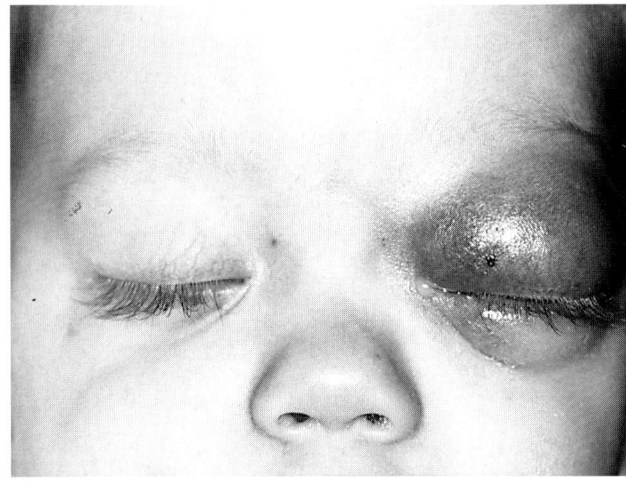

Figure 86–7. A 2-year-old boy presented with subperiosteal orbital abscess secondary to ethmoidal sinus disease. Complete recovery followed surgical drainage and antibiotic therapy.

Chandler[6] in 1970. The classification groups are presumably arranged in increasing order of severity, with group 1 comprising inflammatory preseptal edema and cellulitis, group 2 orbital cellulitis without abscess, group 3 subperiosteal abscess, group 4 orbital abscess, and group 5 cavernous sinus thrombosis.[6] The suggestion of clinical severity or orderly progression that one might gain from such a stepped classification is false, because a group 2 orbital cellulitis may entail much greater morbidity than a group 3 or 4 subperiosteal and orbital abscess, for example. Also, because of the anatomic factors discussed previously, any stage of infection may evolve into any other stage. Other than serving as a list of potential complications of acute sinus disease, I have not found this classification scheme to be clinically useful.

Preseptal edema may occur in sinus disease with swollen eyelids but a nondisplaced eye with normal motility. Conjunctival chemosis may occur even in the absence of orbital or preseptal extension of infection, although other orbital signs should not be present. The initial location of this preseptal erythema and edema may help localize the acutely infected sinus, with swelling above the medial canthal tendon in the upper eyelid pointing to the ethmoidal sinus, the upper eyelid the frontal sinus, and the lower eyelid the maxillary sinus. Preseptal cellulitis may

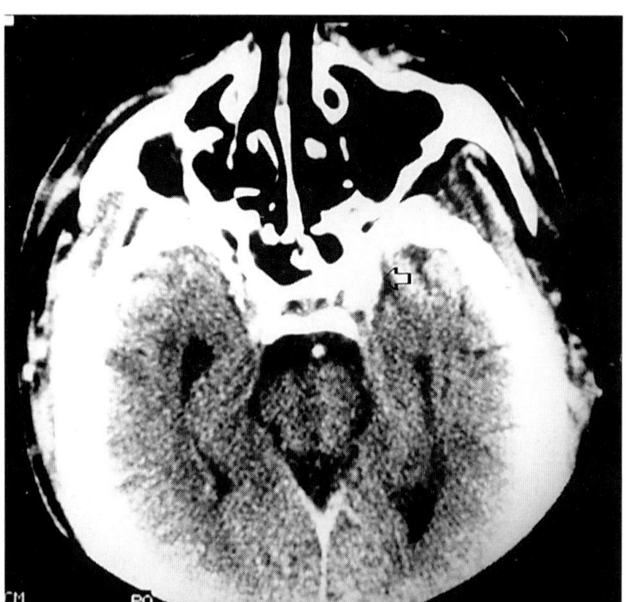

Figure 86–6. Computed tomographic scan of the same patient as in Figure 86–5 showing lateral bulging of the left cavernous sinus (*arrow*). Septic cavernous sinus thrombosis was diagnosed. Proptosis and deficits resolved after broad-spectrum antibiotic and intravenous heparin therapy. Infection occurred by the hematogenous extension of bacteria from the maxilla into the cavernous sinus.

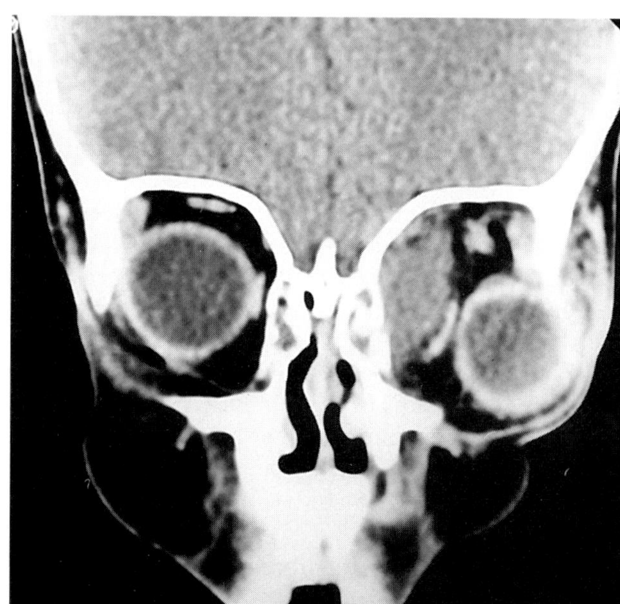

Figure 86–8. Computed tomographic scan of the patient shown in Figure 86–7. Note the large subperiosteal mass displacing the left globe and opacification of the adjacent ethmoidal sinus. Maxillary sinus opacification was also present.

evolve by either direct extension of infection or inoculation of the preseptal space through the valveless veins. Preseptal abscess may occur by the acute exacerbation of chronic sinus disease with mucopyocele formation. In these syndromes, appropriate evaluation and treatment of the underlying sinus pathology resolve the preseptal inflammation.

Schramm and coworkers[7] reported acute sinusitis as the cause of 84% of cases of acute orbital or periorbital cellulitis requiring hospitalization. They also reported an incidence of abscess formation of 21%, with all such patients requiring incision and drainage. Their study reviewed routine sinus roentgenograms and hospital records made in the pre–computed tomography (CT) era. Subsequent series have reported an incidence of orbital abscess formation as high as 79%.[8] Accurately distinguishing between subperiosteal abscess and intraorbital abscess in reviewing published series and case reports is difficult because the authors' reporting criteria, preoperative imaging, and surgical approach are often unclear.[9] True intraorbital abscess is uncommon in my experience; I have treated more than 20 patients with subperiosteal abscess or inflammation related to sinus disease, confirmed by CT scan and echography, but none with intraorbital abscess. Gold and colleagues[10] commented on the occasional unreliability of CT scanning in diagnosing subperiosteal abscess formation in acute orbital cellulitis, with periosteal edema and subperiosteal hematoma being found at surgery. Harris,[11] noting the discrepancy between imaging studies suggesting subperiosteal abscess and surgical findings, has proposed the term *subperiosteal inflammation* to describe orbital periosteal elevation in association with infection. The use of this term to describe patients who do not have operative proof of abscess formation may help diffuse the implications of the term *abscess.*

Most patients presenting with an acute orbit in association with sinus disease have had an upper respiratory infection in the preceding 2 weeks.[7] Three fourths of these patients are younger than 16 years of age, with about one third being younger than 4 years of age.[7] Antibiotic therapy prior to hospitalization is frequent. Typical signs and symptoms of orbital cellulitis include a 1- to 4-day history of symptoms with fever, lid swelling and chemosis, proptosis or globe displacement, and possibly diplopia or decreased vision. Patients with subperiosteal abscess often develop orbital signs very rapidly, possibly from drainage of the ethmoidal or other involved sinus into the subperiosteal space. Harris[12] has suggested that increased intraorbital pressure is the primary and reversible mechanism of visual loss in subperiosteal abscess. Patients with abscesses that resolve with medical therapy alone may acutely drain their abscess, demonstrating that spontaneous or surgical drainage of the involved sinus may resolve the orbital abscess without direct orbital intervention.

The literature is confusing regarding recommendations for surgical drainage of the orbit and involved sinuses. Rubin and colleagues[13] have reported on the successful nonsurgical treatment of nine patients with subperiosteal abscess diagnosed by CT criteria. The composition of this patient group is interesting, because the authors noted an additional three patients who required surgical drainage, and three of their patients who resolved on medical therapy had neither proptosis nor limitation of ocular motility but were thought to have subperiosteal abscess based only on CT findings from scans obtained for other reasons.

Blood cultures are positive in 30% of children but are seldom positive in adults.[7] Bacteriology of orbital cellulitis and abscesses is determined by the source of the infection. This is generally the bacteriology of acute sinusitis: *Haemophilus influenzae* is the most frequently identified pathogen in children younger than 5 years of age. Above age 5, *Streptococcus pneumoniae*, *Staphylococcus aureus*, beta-hemolytic or microaerophilic streptococci, and a variety of non–spore-forming anaerobes predominate. Mixed infections are frequent, especially in adult patients with chronic sinusitis.[11] Aerobic and anaerobic blood, nasal, sinus, and orbital cultures are indicated, as obtainable. Gram's stains also should be performed on any abscess or other purulent material obtained. Broad-spectrum antibiotic therapy should be initiated following blood and nasal cultures. Harris[14a] recommends ceftriaxone sodium (50 mg/kg intravenously [IV] daily) in children younger than age 9, with the addition of clindamycin sodium 20 mg/kg IV divided every 6 hours in children older than age 9. Alternate drug regimens include ampicillin sodium/sulbactam sodium (Unasyn) 75 mg/kg IV divided every 8 hours or ticarcillin/clavulanate potassium 250 mg/kg IV divided every 4 to 6 hours. Therapy may be modified pending results of culture and sensitivity. When orbital cellulitis occurs in patients older than 5 years of age, *H. influenzae* is a decreasing concern, and therapy with cefuroxime (750 mg IV every 8 hours) alone is usually adequate. Therapy with a penicillinase-resistant semisynthetic penicillin or vancomycin can be added in appropriate cases. Harris[11] has pointed out that the presence of anaerobes should be presumed in patients 10 years of age and older and that mixed aerobic-anaerobic infections and beta-lactamase–producing organisms frequently occur with a more prolonged and potentially complicated course. In odontogenic infections, therapy with clindamycin or metronidazole is an excellent addition. Given the frequent changes and advances in infectious disease with shifting patterns of drug resistance, consultation with an infectious disease specialist is often appropriate.

Various criteria have been used in deciding to perform surgical exploration and drainage in a patient with subperiosteal inflammation of the orbit. Many authors such as Schramm and associates[7] surgically drained all demonstrable orbital abscesses. It is clear that some patients with subperiosteal abscess improve with medical therapy alone.[13] In my experience, these patients may improve in a stepwise fashion as the ethmoidal sinus re-establishes normal drainage. Harris[14a] has suggested the criteria of no visual compromise, medial location, no intracranial or frontal sinus involvement, and children younger than age 9 for medical treatment alone for subperiosteal abscess. It may sometimes be possible to adequately drain the orbital abscess by intranasal drainage of the affected sinus alone. Because the orbit should not be entered in this situation transnasally, I have generally decided to use an external approach to the orbital abscess and ethmoidal sinus in these cases, with temporary placement of an external drain.

The proximity of the posterior ethmoidal and sphenoidal sinuses to the orbital apex (see Fig. 86–3) allows early invasion of the optic nerve with acute, irreversible visual loss. Slavin and Glaser[3] termed this syndrome *"posterior" orbital cellulitis.* It is possible in this syndrome for visual loss to overshadow or precede any other signs, such as proptosis, restricted ocular motility, and chemosis. Slavin and Glaser[3] proposed a combination of intracanalicular optic nerve edema and vasculitis as the cause of visual loss in this syndrome. This "posterior" orbital cellulitis also may occur with mycotic infections,[15, 16] sinus obstructive disease,[17] or inflammatory[18] diseases of the orbital apex. These syndromes share common anatomic predisposing factors and an acute and usually irreversible course of visual loss. Common treatment approaches in these syndromes include prompt neuroimaging and surgical sinus ventilation, débridement, and biopsy, with aggressive control of infection or inflammation.

Orbital Complications of Fungal Sinusitis

Several clinical syndromes may result from fungal sinus infections caused by *Aspergillus* genera or by several species from the genera *Absidia, Mucor,* and *Rhizopus* of the family Mucoraceae. The inhalation of fungal spores into the nasopharynx and paranasal sinuses and an altered host environment and response to the fungus are common factors in these infections. Sinus aspergillosis is especially common in hot, humid climates. *Aspergillus fumigatus* and *Aspergillus flavus* are the most frequent species in both immunocompetent and immunoincompetent patients. A variety of other saprophytic fungi including *Sporothrix schenckii, Pseudallescheria boydii, Alternaria, Candida*, and *Paecilomyces* species, among others, may cause similar clinical syndromes.[19] Patients with invasive aspergillosis may have an obscure presentation, delaying diagnosis and contributing to the eventual high morbidity rates.[20] In immunocompetent patients, sinus ventilation alone with excision of the fungal mass and treatment of any concurrent bacterial sinusitis is generally adequate therapy. In patients who are immunoincompetent or if soft tissue invasion of the *Aspergillus* organisms has occurred, sinus ventilation and débridement of involved soft tissue should be performed in conjunction with administration of systemic amphotericin B and possibly hyperbaric oxygen.[21] Appropriate identification of the involved fungus with tissue histology and cultures is important in invasive cases, because *P. boydii* exhibits in vitro resistance to amphotericin B.[19]

The pathogenic fungi of the genera *Absidia, Mucor,* and *Rhizopus* are ubiquitous organisms that cause a devastating rhino-orbitocerebral infection in immunocompromised hosts. As most such infections result from *Rhizopus* species, the term *phycomycosis* has been suggested as a more accurate and less confusing term.[22] Nonetheless, the term *mucormycosis* has remained in common usage. Infections rarely occur in otherwise healthy people. Inoculation occurs through the inhalation of airborne fungal spores. A failure of the local cellular immune response allows the infection to establish itself. Orbital signs develop through the direct invasion of orbital tissues and by perivascular extension with ischemic tissue necrosis. Patients with diabetes who are in ketoacidosis are the most commonly affected group, probably due to changes in pH, glucose concentration, and oxygen tension that favor fungal growth and invasion. The increase in numbers of immunosuppressed patients (because of disease or treatment) during the past decade has led increasingly to the appearance of this infection in new groups.

Facial pain and rhinorrhea are the initial symptoms. These are followed by orbital pain and edema and then progressive orbital neurologic deficits. These findings in an appropriate immunocompromised host should alert the clinician to the possibility of rhino-orbital mucormycosis and prompt CT scans of the orbit, sinuses, and anterior skull base and brain. A fever or black eschar in the nose or palate should be looked for but may be a late sign.[22] Aggressive surgical débridement of involved tissues has been standard in the management of these patients for some years.[21] This recommendation has often equated to radical sinusectomy with orbital exenteration, because the orbit is usually involved at the time of diagnosis. Early recognition followed by prompt local débridement of necrotic tissue and histologic verification of the infection may allow better tissue preservation and function. With early recognition and treatment with local débridement, sinus ventilation and daily orbit and sinus packing with amphotericin B, and systemic amphotericin B, Kohn and Hepler[23] have reported successful management of rhino-orbital mucormycosis without exenteration. Hyperbaric oxygen therapy can reduce the tissue acidosis and hypoxia associated with the ischemic necrosis in rhino-orbital mucormycosis and may have an adjunct role in the treatment of this condition.[24]

TABLE 86–1

Diagnostic and Therapeutic Features of Orbital Infectious Processes Originating in Sinuses

	Condition						
	Preseptal Cellulitis	Orbital Cellulitis Without Abscess	Subperiosteal Abscess	Cavernous Sinus Thrombosis	"Posterior" Orbital Cellulitis	Orbital Aspergillosis	Mucormycosis (Phycomycosis)
Typical Patient	Spontaneous: children <6 yr. Trauma: any age. Patients have direct or transvenous extension of infection from adjacent area	Any age, most common in adolescents and children. Less common than subperiosteal abscess	Most common in children. Adults have mixed infections associated with chronic sinus disease	Adult with focal infection of face (especially furuncles near the nose), paranasal sinuses, orbit, ear, or mastoid region	Usually adult with chronic sinus disease. Chronic sinus pathogens or pathogenic fungi usual cause	Adult with chronic sinus disease. More aggressive in immunocompromised patients	Diabetic or immunocompromised adult. Metabolic alteration common (diabetic ketoacidosis)
Initial Presentation	Unilateral eyelid edema and hyperemia; normal vision with absence of orbital signs. Fever and leukocytosis in children	Usually rapidly progressive with pain, fever, proptosis and eyelid edema, painful limitation of motion, and conjunctival chemosis	Rapid or stepwise progression with pain, fever, proptosis, painful limitation of motion, and conjunctival chemosis	Eyelid edema and chemosis with rapidly progressive proptosis, ophthalmoplegia, visual loss, high fever, meningeal signs, and confusion	Sudden or subacute visual loss with pain and variable orbital signs (proptosis, chemosis, limitation of ocular motility)	Usually patients from hot, humid climates. Chronic or subacute onset of pain, proptosis, limitation of ocular motility, and visual loss	Sinusitis, pharyngitis, nasal discharge, and periorbital pain followed by proptosis, visual loss, and black eschar in nose
Evaluation	Blood and conjunctival cultures. Wound cultures and lumbar puncture if indicated	Blood and nasal cultures followed immediately by IV antibiotic therapy. Neuroimaging of orbit and adjacent sinuses	Blood and nasal cultures followed immediately by IV antibiotic therapy. Neuroimaging of orbit and adjacent sinuses	Prompt neuroimaging, lumbar puncture, blood and cerebrospinal fluid cultures, and antibiotic therapy	Immediate neuroimaging, cultures and histology of adjacent sinus tissues	Neuroimaging followed by cultures and biopsy of involved adjacent sinus and sinus ventilation	Neuroimaging of orbit and sinuses. Diagnostic biopsy and débridement of involved sinus and orbital tissues
Microbiology	*Haemophilus influenzae* predominates <5 yr. *Streptococcus pneumoniae*, *Staphylococcus aureus*, others >5 yr	*S. pneumoniae*, other streptococci, *S. aureus*, non–spore-forming anaerobes, and *H. influenzae* in children	Sinus pathogens for age group: *S. pneumoniae*, *H. influenzae*, *Moraxella catarrhalis*, less frequent than would be expected compared with sinusitis	Most frequently *S. aureus*, but *Streptococcus* species, gram-negative, fungi, and other sinus pathogens occasional causes	Fungi such as *Aspergillus* species and Mucoraceae, other indolent sinus pathogens	Usually *Aspergillus fumigatus* or *Aspergillus flavus*. Rarely *Sporothrix schenckii*, *Pseudallescheria boydii*, *Alternaria*, *Paecilomyces*, other *Aspergillus* or *Candida* species	*Rhizopus* species most frequent. Occasionally *Mucor* or *Absidia* species

(continued)

TABLE 86 – 1

Diagnostic and Therapeutic Features of Orbital Infectious Processes Originating in Sinuses (*Continued*)

	Condition						
	Preseptal Cellulitis	Orbital Cellulitis Without Abscess	Subperiosteal Abscess	Cavernous Sinus Thrombosis	"Posterior" Orbital Cellulitis	Orbital Aspergillosis	Mucormycosis (Phycomycosis)
Pathophysiology	Direct inoculation with trauma or spread from adjacent upper airway or sinus infection. Preseptal edema and inflammation with normal eye	Usually extension of acute infection from ethmoidal or maxillary sinuses. Neurovascular canals and bony dehiscences allow orbital spread	Usually extension of acute infection of ethmoidal or maxillary sinuses. Neurovascular canals and bony dehiscences allow orbital spread	Venous extension of regional infection causes local thrombophlebitis within the cavernous sinus	Direct extension of infection or inflammation from sphenoid or posterior ethmoidal sinus into orbital apex	Poorly aerated sinus aids fungal growth. Much more aggressive in immuno-incompetent patients	Airborne spores grow in nasal airway or sinus. High blood glucose levels and acidosis speed growth. Thrombosing vasculitis and tissue necrosis result
Complications	Abscess formation, eyelid necrosis, progression to orbital cellulitis	Blindness, corneal exposure, intraorbital abscess, cavernous sinus thrombosis, meningitis, brain abscess, death	Blindness, corneal exposure, cavernous sinus thrombosis, brain abscess, meningitis, death	Cranial neuropathy (50%) and visual loss (15%), stroke, pituitary necrosis, meningitis, brain abscess, and death	Acute or subacute visual loss, intracranial invasion, and death	Orbital progression with visual loss, intracranial extension and death	Visual loss and orbital necrosis. Intracranial extension and death are frequent
Treatment	Ceftriaxone 50 mg/kg/day IV (children), cefuroxime 750 mg every 8 hours IV (adult); oral medications in mild cases; other regimens as indicated	Ceftriaxone 50 mg/kg/day IV (children), cefuroxime 750 mg every 8 hours IV (adult); other regimens as indicated. Surgical exploration to rule out abscess if uncertain	Ceftriaxone 50 mg/kg/day IV (children <9 yr); clindamycin for anaerobes (children >9 yr). Alternative regimens: ampicillin sodium/sulbactam sodium (Unasyn) or ticarcillin/clavulanate potassium (Timentin); other regimens as indicated. Surgically drain sinus and abscess for visual loss	Penicillinase-resistant semisynthetic penicillin + third-generation cephalosporin or chloramphenicol. Modify regimen by culture results or clinical situation. Heparin or corticosteroid therapy controversial	Diagnostic sinusotomy and sinus biopsy. Appropriate antimicrobial regimen and tissue débridement as indicated	Sinus ventilation adequate in healthy patient without orbital tissue invasion. Systemic amphotericin B and aggressive débridement needed in immunocompromised patient with invasive disease	Débridement of affected tissues with systemic amphotericin B. Local irrigation with amphotericin B and hyperbaric oxygen may be helpful

SUMMARY

A number of other infectious processes may affect the orbit (Table 86-1). Bacterial infectious processes may extend from the preseptal space into the orbit. Traumatic injuries or infections of ocular adnexal structures also may result in orbital extension of infection, with different characteristic features for each infection. This chapter has presented orbital infections resulting from the most frequent source, the extension of sinusitis. Characteristic clinical syndromes result depending on the bacteriology, host age and physical condition, and location of the sinus infection. Prompt recognition of these characteristic clinical syndromes with aggressive early therapy limits morbidity in these life-threatening infections.

REFERENCES

1. Doxanas MT, Anderson RL: Clinical Orbital Anatomy. Baltimore, Williams & Wilkins, 1984.
2. Jones DB, Steinkuller PG: Microbial preseptal and orbital cellulitis. *In* Tasman W, Jaeger EA (eds): Duane's Clinical Ophthalmology, vol. 4. Philadelphia, JB Lippincott, 1989.
3. Slavin ML, Glaser JS: Acute severe irreversible visual loss with sphenoethmoiditis: "Posterior" orbital cellulitis. Arch Ophthalmol 105:345-348, 1987.
4. Maresh MM: Paranasal sinuses from birth to late adolescence. Am J Dis Child 60:55, 1940.
5. Batson OV: Relationship of the eye to the paranasal sinuses. Arch Ophthalmol 16:322-323, 1936.
6. Chandler JR, Langenbrunner DJ, Stevens ER: The pathogenesis of orbital complications of acute sinusitis. Laryngoscope 80:1414, 1970.
7. Schramm VL, Myers EN, Kennerdell JS: Orbital complications of acute sinusitis: Evaluation, management, and outcome. Trans Am Acad Ophthalmol Otolaryngol 86:221, 1978.
8. Morgan PR, Morrison WV: Complications of frontal and ethmoid sinusitis. Laryngoscope 90:661, 1980.
9. Hornblass A, Herschorn BJ, Ster K, Grimes C: Orbital abscess. Surv Ophthalmol 29:169-178, 1984.
10. Gold SC, Arrigg PG, Hedges TR: Computerized tomography in the management of acute orbital cellulitis. Ophthalmic Surg 18:753-756, 1987.
11. Harris GJ: Subperiosteal inflammation of the orbit: A bacteriological analysis of 17 cases. Arch Ophthalmol 106:947-952, 1988.
12. Harris GJ: Subperiosteal abscess of the orbit. Arch Ophthalmol 101:751-757, 1983.
13. Rubin SE, Rubin LG, Zito J, et al: Medical management of orbital subperiosteal abscess in children. J Pediatr Ophthalmol Strab 26:21-26, 1989.
14. Sanford JP: Guide to Antimicrobial Therapy 1994. Dallas, Antimicrobial Therapy, Inc., 1994, p 7.

14a. Harris GJ: Age as a factor in the bacteriology and response to treatment of subperiosteal abscess of the orbit. Trans Am Ophthalmol Soc 91:441-516, 1993.

15. Slavin ML: Primary aspergillosis of the orbital apex. Arch Ophthalmol 109:1502, 1991.
16. Miyazaki S, Izaki A, Shimo-Oku, Harui M: Optic neuritis due to *Aspergillus* infection. Neuro-ophthalmology 11:183-187, 1991.
17. Johnson LN, Hepler RS, Yee RD, Batzdorf U: Sphenoid sinus mucocele (anterior clinoid variant) mimicking diabetic ophthalmoplegia and retrobulbar neuritis. Am J Ophthalmol 102:111-115, 1986.
18. Newman NM, KiLoreto DA, Ho JT, et al: Bilateral optic neuropathy and osteolytic sinusitis: Complications of cocaine abuse. JAMA 259:72-74, 1988.
19. Morgan MA, Wilson WR, Neel HB, Roberts GD: Fungal sinusitis in healthy and immunocompromised individuals. Am J Clin Pathol 82:597-601, 1984.
20. Green WR, Font RL, Zimmerman LE. Aspergillosis of the orbit: Report of ten cases and review of the literature. Arch Ophthalmol 82:302-313, 1969.
21. Stevens MH: Primary fungal infections of the paranasal sinuses. Am J Otolaryngol 2:348, 1981.
22. Ferry AP, Abedi S: Diagnosis and management of rhino-orbitocerebral mucormycosis (phycomycosis): A report of 16 personally observed cases. Ophthalmology 90:1096, 1983.
23. Kohn R, Hepler R: Management of limited rhino-orbital mucormycosis without exenteration. Ophthalmology 92:1440-1444, 1985.
24. Ferguson BJ, Mitchell TG, Moon R, et al: Adjunctive hyperbaric oxygen for treatment of rhinocerebral mucormycosis. Rev Infect Dis 10:551, 1988.

CHAPTER 87

Amyloidosis and Idiopathic Orbital Conditions

Joseph P. Shovlin

AMYLOIDOSIS

Amyloidosis is a condition characterized by deposition of amorphous proteinaceous material with a beta pleated sheet secondary structure. This secondary structure not normally found in vertebrates is common in invertebrates. This unique structure provides amyloid with its staining characteristics and resistance to enzymatic degradation. The inability of enzymes to metabolize amyloid proteins allows for their accumulation in tissues.

Amyloid may deposit in any organ of the body. Systemic manifestations of amyloidosis include hepatomegaly, splenomegaly, nephropathy, neuropathy, and pulmonary deposition. Amyloid may deposit in any portion of the orbit, globe, or ocular adnexa. Rather than a single clinical entity, amyloidosis represents a spectrum of disease characterized by abnormal protein deposition. The processes that result in amyloid deposition may have little in common. In this chapter, we attempt to unify the approaches to the ocular conditions involved with amyloid.

Cause and Structure of Amyloid Fibrils

The tinctorial properties and clinical syndromes associated with amyloid result from its protein structure, the beta pleated sheet. This structure resists digestion by mammalian enzyme systems. When disease processes lead to the production of amyloid proteins, accumulation in tissues results.

Our understanding of the production of amyloid protein is still in its infancy.[1] Most studies on the ultrastructure of amyloid have been performed on cases of primary systemic amyloidosis, and the findings have been generalized to other forms of amyloidosis. Routine hematoxylin and eosin preparations demonstrate amyloid as an eosinophilic amorphous hyaline material located extracellularly. Amyloid deposits tend to be perivascular in distribution and may give an onion skin appearance to small arteries and arterioles. These deposits are often associated with a variable inflammatory infiltrate. Human amyloid consists of nonbranching fibrils that measure 10 nm in diameter by electron microscopy. Distinct staining characteristics identify amorphous material as amyloid. The unique staining characteristics have become pathognomonic of amyloid and result from the beta pleated sheet structure of the fibrillar protein component. The fibrillar component binds to planar Congo red molecules along the long axis of the fiber, resulting in blue-green birefringence with polarizing microscopy. These deposits may also be defined histochemically by metachromasia with crystal violet or fluorescence in ultraviolet light after staining with thioflavin T.

A pentagonal unit known as the P component comprises approximately 10% of the amyloid deposit. The P component is a plasma glycoprotein related to C-reactive protein but does not behave as an acute-phase reactant. Radioimmunoassay shows the P component to be a normally occurring plasma protein not directly related to the deposition of amyloid. The P component does not contribute to the staining characteristics of amyloid with Congo red or thioflavin T but does render the deposits positive on periodic acid–Schiff staining.

Biochemical studies of amyloid deposits in primary systemic amyloidosis have demonstrated the fibrillar component to be a homogeneous intact immunoglobulin light polypeptide chain.[2] Amino acid sequences identical to that of the variable region of the immunoglobulin light chain polymerize to form the amyloid fibrils. Even though the fibrillar portion of the amyloid deposit has been shown to be composed of immunoglobulin light chains, no peculiarity could identify which light chains were likely to produce amyloid. Antibody studies have demonstrated immunologically identical amyloid deposits from different locations in the same patient with no cross-reactivity with amyloid from other patients.[1] A second form of amyloid protein has been described in patients with secondary forms of systemic amyloidosis. This protein, designated AA, may also be related to immunoglobulin. An acute-phase serum component antigenically related to AA has been found in human serum (SAA). SAA behaves as an acute-phase reactant and is elevated in aging, infection, and inflammation. SAA appears to suppress antibody response and function as an immunoregulator. Which SAA proteins are amyloidogenic has not been determined.

Classification and Systemic Manifestations

Attempts have been made to classify amyloid proteins based on their immunochemical composition. The most clinically useful classification based on the pattern of the disease was established by Reimann and coworkers[3] in 1935. The classification divides amyloidosis into four categories, based on the distribution of deposits and the presence of underlying disease:

1. Primary systemic amyloidosis
2. Amyloidosis associated with myeloma
3. Secondary amyloidosis
4. Tumor-forming amyloid

Primary systemic amyloidosis demonstrates nodular deposition in mesenchymal organs, such as the myocardium, blood vessels, and skeletal muscle, with inconsistent involvement of the gastrointestinal tract. By definition, there is no underlying predisposing factor to amyloid deposition, such as preceding or concurrent disease. Primary systemic amyloidosis includes familial forms, with their tendency toward peripheral neuropathy. Amyloidosis associated with multiple myeloma resembles primary systemic amyloidosis in composition and distribution of amyloid fibrils; however, the osteolytic lesions and hypergammaglobulinemia of a plasma cell dyscrasia are present. Immunoglobulin light chains compose the deposits in these conditions and are termed *AL amyloid.*

A concurrent disease process that is usually inflammatory may result in secondary acquired systemic amyloidosis. Rheumatoid arthritis is the commonest cause, with amyloid deposits present in approximately 10% of patients with this condition.[4] Other conditions linked to the deposition of amyloid include leprosy, osteomyelitis, dermatomyositis, scleroderma, and lung abscess. SAA, a serum protein that functions as an acute-phase reactant, contributes to the formation of the amyloid protein in secondary amyloidosis. The precursor SAA behaves as an acute-phase reactant, and concentrations of this protein increase in infection, inflammation, and aging.[5] Chronic hyperstimulation of the immune system underlies the pathophysiologic process in secondary amyloidosis, leading to amyloid deposition in parenchymal organs, such as the liver, spleen, and kidneys. The fourth type of amyloidosis, designated as tumor-forming amyloid, deposits locally without systemic involvement. The cause and chemical composition of the tumor-forming amyloid remain enigmas. Amyloid deposits of the eye, orbit, and ocular adnexa most commonly fall into this category. Other organ-limited depositions, such as neuritic plaques in the central nervous system and senile cardiomyopathy, are considered to be tumor-forming amyloid.

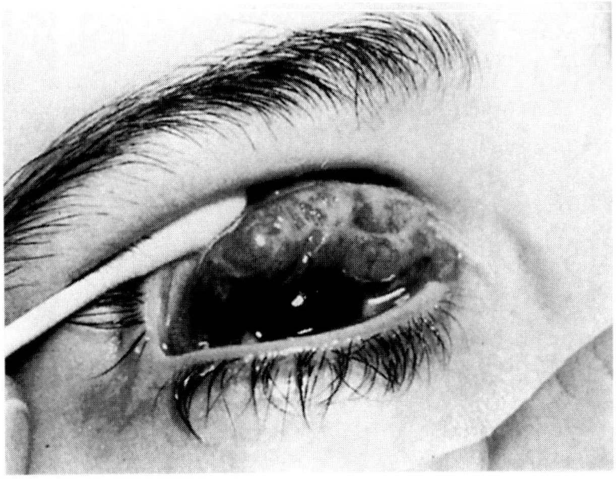

Figure 87–1. Amyloid deposit of the tarsal and supratarsal regions. (From Jakobiec FA, Font RL: Orbit. *In* Spencer WH, Font RL, Green WR [eds]: Ophthalmic Pathology: An Atlas and Textbook, 3rd ed, vol 3. Philadelphia, WB Saunders, 1986, pp 2459–2860.)

Ocular Presentations

Amyloid deposits may involve any portion of the eye or ocular adnexa. The propensity for perivascular deposition imparts a fragility to blood vessels. Amyloid deposits of the eyelid skin appear as slightly raised, waxy papules that are similar to xanthelasma and may become ecchymotic with minor trauma. Involvement of eyelid skin indicates systemic disease.[6] Amyloid deposits in the conjunctiva as nodules that show variable degrees of injection (Fig. 87–1). Episcleral injection or enlargement of the deposits that results in mechanical ptosis may cause patients thus affected to visit the ophthalmologist. Corneal amyloidosis has been reported in eyes with phlyctenular keratoconjunctivitis, uveitis, and lipoid dystrophy.[7] This pattern of corneal amyloidosis is a localized secondary form of amyloidosis that is associated with a chronic inflammatory state. Lattice dystrophy is an autosomal dominant form of localized corneal amyloidosis whose underlying biochemical abnormality remains unknown.

Deposition of amyloid within the confines of the orbit can occur in the lacrimal gland,[8, 9] the extraocular muscles,[10–13] the orbital fat,[14–16] and the optic nerve sheath.[17] Orbital involvement seldom suggests systemic disease; however, cases associated with multiple myeloma, lymphosarcoma, and Bence Jones proteinuria have been reported.[6, 12, 14] Amyloid deposits within the lacrimal gland present similarly to other lacrimal gland masses with proptosis and inferomedial displacement of the globe. The proptosis may be slowly progressive over years without acute inflammatory signs. In a description

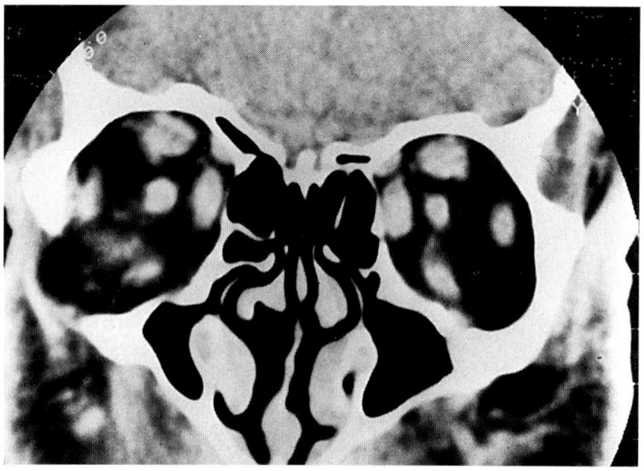

Figure 87 – 2. Coronal computed tomographic scan demonstrating enlarged extraocular muscles. (Courtesy of Dr. Russell S. Gonnering.)

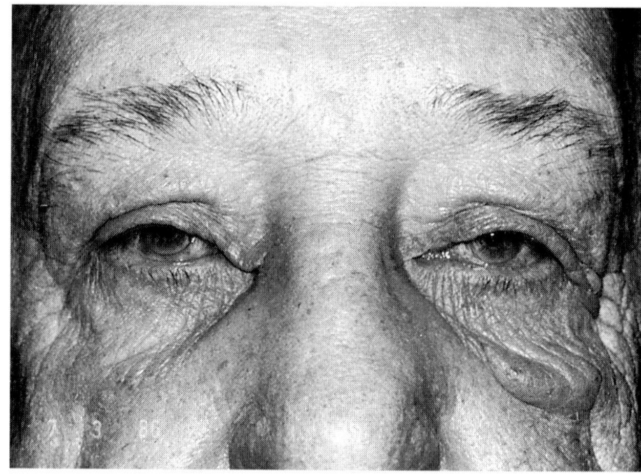

Figure 87 – 4. Dermatochalasis and ptosis in a patient with a plasma cell dyscrasia and periocular amyloidosis. (Courtesy of Dr. Russell S. Gonnering.)

of the computed tomographic findings in localized amyloidosis of the lacrimal gland, Levine and Buckman[8] reported bony changes in the lacrimal fossa similar to those seen in benign mixed tumors. These authors also noted multiple calcifications initially believed to be phleboliths.

Several cases of extraocular muscle involvement have been reported.[10–13] Presentations varied from complete ophthalmoplegia to proptosis with restrictive ocular motility akin to patterns seen in Graves' orbitopathy. Computed tomography demonstrated fusiform enlargement of the recti muscles with involvement of the tendinous insertions (Figs. 87 – 2 and 87 – 3). At surgery, the muscles were enlarged and infiltrated by a waxy yellow material. Histopathology revealed amyloid deposits within the connective tissue and the blood vessel walls. Restrictive motility patterns resulting from muscle involvement respond favorably to strabismus surgery.

Diffuse infiltration of the orbital tissues with amyloid presents with blepharoptosis and an anteriorly located firm mass (Fig. 87 – 4). The yellowish deposits may be visualized beneath the conjunctiva in the fornices. The amyloid deposits have a predilection for the anterior portion of the orbit, where they are amenable to biopsy. Involvement of the optic nerve sheath has been reported.[17] Enlargement of the mass produced compressive optic neuropathy that did not respond to surgical intervention. Involvement of the pial vessels supplying the nerve may compromise the vascular supply and render the nerve more susceptible to damage by compression.

Pathology of Orbital Cases

Orbital cases of amyloidosis present as localized orbital masses without acute inflammatory changes. When mass effect becomes problematic, these deposits may be removed by excisional biopsy. Amyloid deposits involving the lacrimal gland must be removed to rule out an epithelial tumor of the lacrimal gland because clinical and radiographic studies cannot distinguish these with any degree of certainty.

At surgery, the deposits appear a waxy yellow with a consistency of firm rubber. Excessive hemorrhage similar to that seen during debulking of neurofibromas may indicate amyloid. The pathologist should perform special stains to detect amyloid. Histopathologically, amyloid replaces the normal surrounding tissues with an affinity for involvement of the blood vessel wall (Fig. 87 – 5). In the advanced stages of the process, large masses of amyloid entrap, and in time destroy, the cellular constituents of the involved organ. On light microscopy, plasma cells are uniformly present in a mixed inflammatory cell infiltrate, and occasionally foreign body giant cells may be seen. Russell bodies, which represent plasma cells overloaded with immunoglobulin, may also be present.

Amyloid exerts its deleterious effects through mass effect, pressure necrosis, and replacement of functioning tissues. Because host protein comprises amyloid deposits

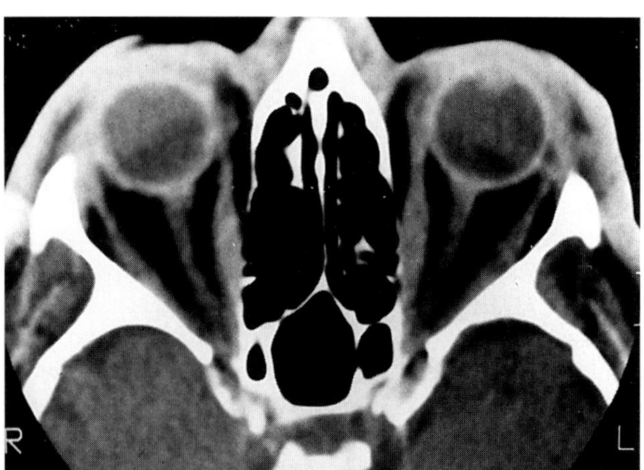

Figure 87 – 3. Axial computed tomographic scan showing enlarged extraocular muscles and periorbital infiltration of amyloid. (Courtesy of Dr. Russell S. Gonnering.)

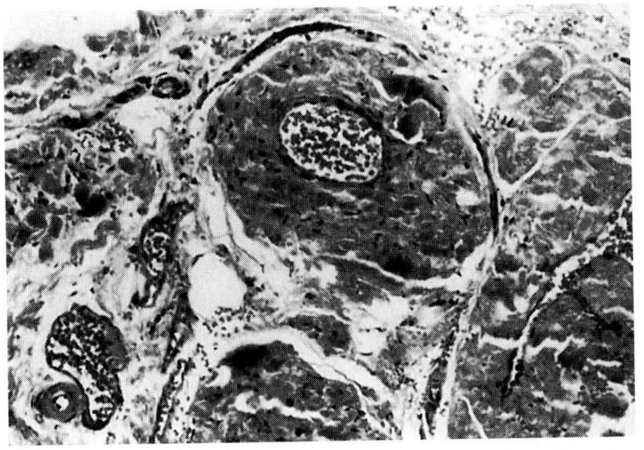

Figure 87 – 5. Orbital amyloidosis with typical perivascular deposition. H & E, ×160. (From Jakobiec FA, Font RL: Orbit. *In* Spencer WH, Font RL, Green WR [eds]: Ophthalmic Pathology: An Atlas and Textbook, 3rd ed, vol 3. Philadelphia, WB Saunders, 1986, pp 2459–2860.)

an acute inflammatory response does not occur. Treatment consists of excisional biopsy of orbital masses and strabismus surgery for motility disorders. The tumor may recur if it is incompletely excised. Systemic steroid therapy has not been effective. Orbital involvement seldom indicates systemic disease. Evaluation should include a physical examination to detect skin involvement or lymphadenopathy. Laboratory studies including erythrocyte sedimentation rate, serum protein electrophoresis, serum immunoprotein electrophoresis, and urinalysis for Bence Jones protein. A bone marrow aspirate and biopsy may be indicated in patients suspected of having plasma cell dyscrasia. If an underlying condition is detected, treatment may reduce the amyloid deposits; however, the prognosis is poor in patients with systemic disease, regardless of the therapy used.

NECROBIOTIC XANTHOGRANULOMA

Necrobiotic xanthogranuloma is a granulomatous inflammatory condition that involves the eyelid skin and may affect the extraocular muscles and orbit. The presence of eyelid plaques has been reported in all cases. These plaques resemble xanthelasma but tend to be firmer and involve the deeper dermis. The lesions appear either as firm, superficial, waxy yellow plaques with prominent telangiectases, as deeper violaceous plaques, or as flesh-colored nodules (Fig. 87–6).[18] A peripheral inflammatory margin may be present. Skin lesions located in the periorbital region, trunk, and proximal limbs produce disfigurement and may become chronic ulcerations. Lesions begin small and tend to progress with time. They may multiply, expand, and ulcerate after biopsy. Ocular abnormalities include scleritis, episcleritis, uveitis, orbital infiltration, and exposure keratitis from cicatricial changes of the eyelid skin.[19] Ulcerative keratitis may lead to ocular perforation.[20] The clinical and histopathologic differential diagnosis includes sarcoidosis, chalazion, xanthalasma, xanthoma tuberosum, necrobiosis lipoidica, granuloma annulare, rheumatoid nodules, juvenile xanthogranuloma, systemic amyloidosis, and Erdheim-Chester disease. Discussion of these conditions is beyond the scope of this chapter; however, necrobiotic xanthogranuloma can be identified by the combination of clinical and histopathologic findings.

Myeloma, lymphoma, and chronic lymphocytic leukemia are systemic abnormalities that are associated with necrobiotic xanthogranuloma. Monoclonal gammopathy detected by serum immunoprotein electrophoresis constituted a universal finding in reported cases of necrobiotic xanthogranuloma. The paraprotein detected consists of either kappa or gamma light chains.[21] Other

Figure 87 – 6. Periorbital and supraclavicular plaques (*A* and *B*) in an elderly patient with necrobiotic xanthogranuloma and plasma cell dyscrasia. The plaques resolved following treatment with chlorambucil. (Courtesy of Dr. Bradley N. Lemke.)

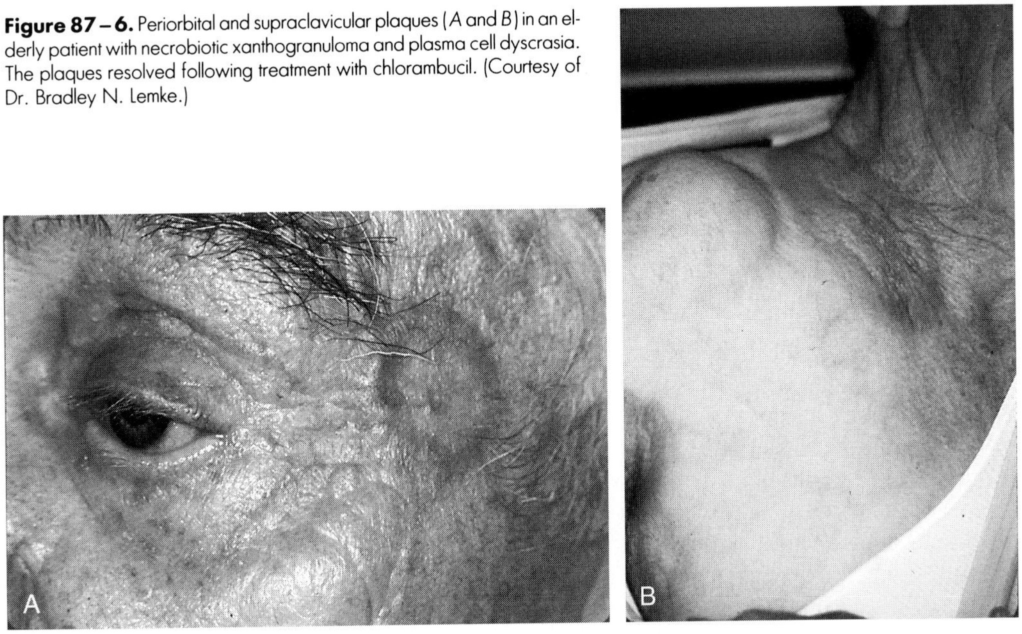

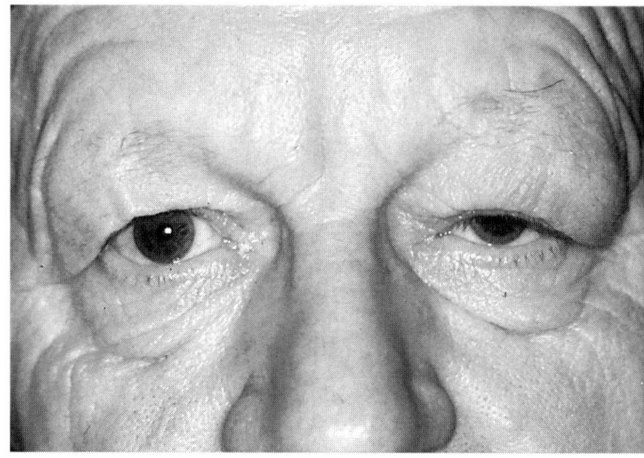

Figure 87–7. Patient with orbital xanthogranuloma presenting with a left ptosis and palpable mass in the left upper eyelid.

laboratory abnormalities include elevated erythrocyte sedimentation rate, cryoglobulinemia, leukopenia, elevated serum viscosity, and low hemolytic complement levels. Bone marrow biopsies may reveal frank multiple myeloma, abnormal plasma cell hyperplasia, or a lymphoproliferative process.

Lesions tend to recur and may become more aggressive after excision or biopsy. Histopathologically, lesions show diffuse inflammation with lymphocytes, histiocytes, foreign body giant cells, Touton's giant cells, and prominent eosinophilic collagen degeneration, known as necrobiosis. Cholesterol clefts may also be present. Skin lesions exhibit prominent involvement of the reticular dermis and subcutis. Immunoperoxidase stain of an orbital specimen demonstrated extracellular deposition of kappa light chains.[22] Transmission electron microscopy shows lipid-laden multinucleated histiocytes within a dense collagenous matrix.

The cause of the lesions in necrobiotic xanthogranuloma remains unknown. Proposed causes include an autoimmune reaction with secondary histiocytic response,[23] small-vessel damage from sludging of red cells that allows deposition of immune complexes,[19] and serum immunoglobulins complexing with lipids depositing within the skin with subsequent foreign body reaction.[22] The association remains between necrobiotic xanthogranuloma, gammaglobulinemia, and histiocytic inflammation; however, the inter-relationship requires further definition.

The results of treatment of patients with necrobiotic xanthogranuloma remain disappointing. A thorough evaluation must be performed to rule out active hematologic proliferation. Patients require continued evaluation to ensure early detection in case malignancy later develops. Patients with benign monoclonal gammopathy have approximately a 10% risk of developing myeloma, amyloidosis, or macroglobulinemia.[24] Treatments show a variable response and include excision of lesions, local injections of triamcinolone, administration of systemic corticosteroids, and cytotoxic chemotherapy. Patients require prolonged follow-up by hematologists, dermatologists, and ophthalmologists.

ADULT ORBITAL XANTHOGRANULOMA

Isolated xanthogranulomas may involve the anterior orbit of patients without an underlying systemic disease (Figs. 87–7 and 87–8). Histopathologically, the xanthogranulomas contain lipid-laden histiocytes and Touton giant cells (Fig. 87–9). They do not possess the eosinophilic collagen degeneration demonstrated by necrobiotic xanthogranulomas. Patients with orbital xanthogranulomas may present with yellowish periorbital plaques and an orbital mass located in the anterior, usually superior, orbit. The clinical and radiographic presentations may mimic an orbital lymphoma. At biopsy the waxy yellowish appearance of the xanthogranuloma readily distinguishes it from a lymphoid lesion.

Following histologic confirmation of an orbital xanthogranuloma, a workup for systemic involvement is required. Erdheim-Chester disease is an idiopathic condition characterized by infiltration of the heart, lungs, retroperitoneum, bones, and other soft tissues by a fibrosing xanthogranulomatous process.[25] Although the xanthogranulomas of Erdheim-Chester disease rarely affect the orbit, the condition is often fatal owing to cardiomyopathy, lung disease, and renal failure. Patients with isolated orbital xanthogranulomas and no evidence of systemic involvement have been treated with corticosteroids, radiation therapy, and chemotherapy with various degrees of success.[26] Although eradication of the xanthogranuloma may be difficult, the prognosis for long-term survival in patients with isolated xanthogranulomas of the orbit appears to be excellent. Continued surveillance for development of a hematologic malignancy is mandatory.

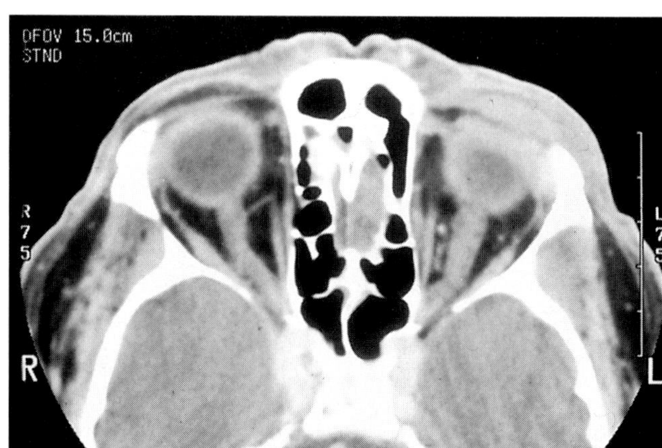

Figure 87–8. Computed tomographic scan of the orbits showing diffuse infiltration of the tissue of the left upper eyelid with xanthogranuloma.

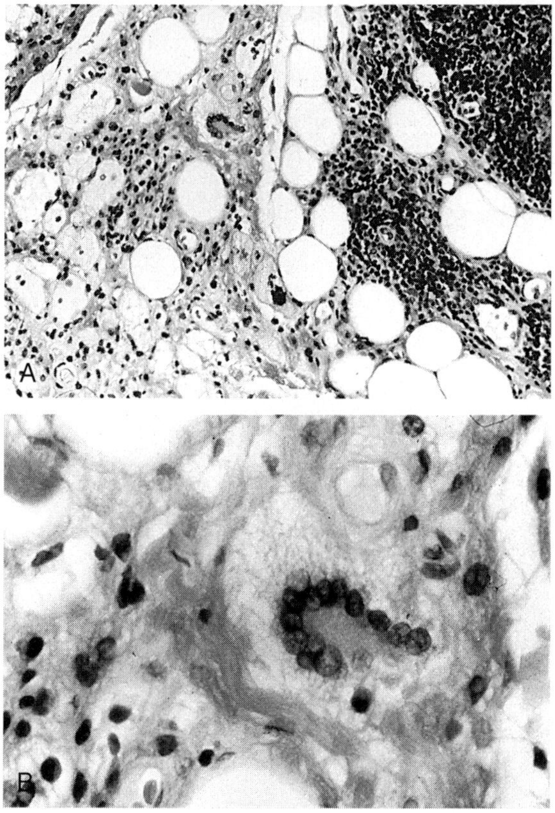

Figure 87–9. *A*, Histopathology of xanthogranuloma demonstrating intense inflammatory infiltrate arranged in a follicular pattern surrounded by fat lobules. H & E, ×4. *B*, Foamy macrophages surrounding a Touton giant cell. H & E, ×40.

KIMURA'S DISEASE AND ANGIOLYMPHOID HYPERPLASIA WITH EOSINOPHILIA

The terms *Kimura's disease* and *angiolymphoid hyperplasia with eosinophilia* have been used interchangeably in the ophthalmic literature. The pathology literature attempts to differentiate these conditions based on clinical and histologic characteristics. Cases reported involving the orbit and ocular adnexa appear similar and may be considered as one clinical entity.

In 1948, Kimura and colleagues described a syndrome characterized by granulation tissue associated with hyperplastic changes in lymphatic tissue.[27] Clinically, lesions appear as single or multiple angiomatous papules or nodules involving the head and neck. The preauricular and submandibular regions are the commonest locations, but lesions have been reported on the radial artery,[28] buttock,[29] popliteal fossa,[30] and penis.[31] The precise cause of the lesions remains unknown, but an association of the lesions with peripheral blood eosinophilia, elevated immunoglobulin E, and lesions developing at the site of intramuscular injections[32] point to the immunologic nature of the disease.

Clinicians seldom diagnose Kimura's disease preoperatively, and the histopathology has been mistaken for angiosarcoma[33] and recurrent malignant melanoma,[34] leading to radical surgery. Kimura's disease is a benign condition that responds well to local excision. The clinical and histopathologic differential diagnosis includes foreign body granuloma, sarcoid, orbital pseudotumor, lymphoma, Wegener's granulomatosis, and primary angiosarcoma.

Patients with adnexal or orbital involvement with Kimura's disease present with localized masses without inflammatory signs (Fig. 87–10). Tumors involving the orbit are usually situated in the anterosuperior aspect and are asymptomatic apart from the mass effect. Neuroimaging studies demonstrate lesions with indistinct borders molding to the contour of the globe and bony orbital walls. All reported cases have been extraconal except a case associated with an Iowa implant after enucleation for ocular melanoma.[34] Two cases have involved the lacrimal gland,[35, 36] and these cases showed prior parotid gland involvement. Regional lymphadenopathy has not been reported in Kimura's disease involving the orbit.

Proliferation of plump, vesicular endothelial cells, tissue eosinophilia, and lymphoid aggregates characterizes

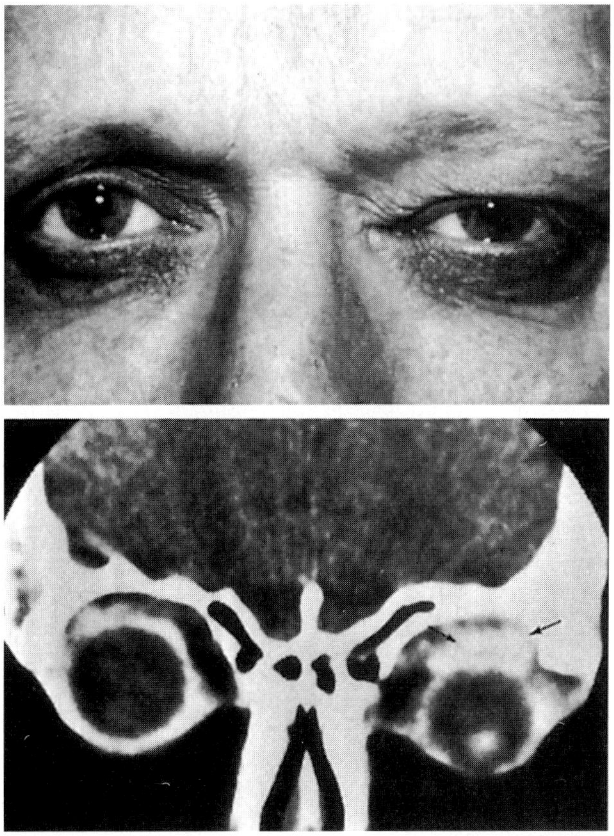

Figure 87–10. Orbital angiolymphoid hyperplasia with eosinophilia. The patient presented with left-sided proptosis and a palpable mass above the globe. Coronal computed tomographic scan shows a well-circumscribed lesion above the globe. (From Hidayat A, Cameron J, Font RL, Zimmerman LE: Angiolymphoid hyperplasia with eosinophilia [Kimura's disease] of the orbit and ocular adnexa. Am J Ophthalmol 96:176–189, 1983. Published with permission from *The American Journal of Ophthalmology*. Copyright by the Ophthalmic Publishing Company.)

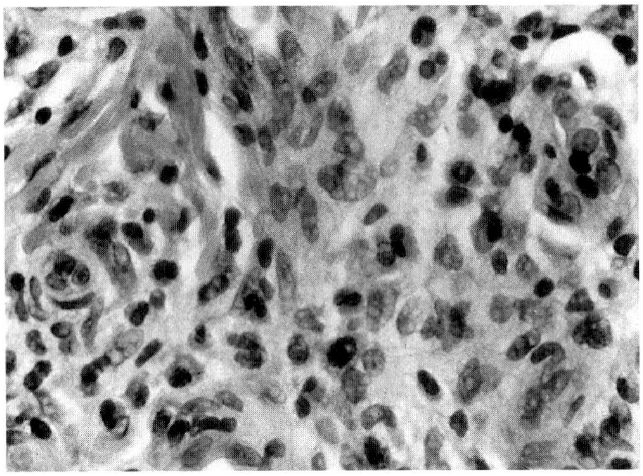

Figure 87–11. Histopathology of angiolymphoid hyperplasia with eosinophilia showing proliferation of histiocytoid endothelial cells with mixed inflammatory infiltrate.

the histopathology of Kimura's disease (Fig. 87–11). Blood vessels with histiocytoid or epithelioid endothelial cells may be present along with lymphoid follicles containing active germinal centers (Fig. 87–12). Eosinophilic deposits with infiltration of the germinal centers by eosinophils causing folliculolysis is also observed.[37] Adjacent lymph nodes may also be involved in the process and demonstrate similar histologic changes.

Medical conditions that may coexist with Kimura's disease include obstructive airway disease,[38] nephrotic syndrome,[39–41] and hypertension secondary to renin production by the tumor.[42] Systemic abnormalities reported include lymphadenopathy, peripheral eosinophilia, and elevated serum immunoglobin E levels.

Various modalities, including radiotherapy, laser photocoagulation, and surgical excision, have been used in the treatment of Kimura's disease with variable degrees of success. Corticosteroids and cytotoxic chemotherapy have been ineffective in most cases.[43] Tumors may recur after incomplete excision, but malignant degeneration has not been reported. Surgery alone is the most effective treatment, provided the excision is complete.

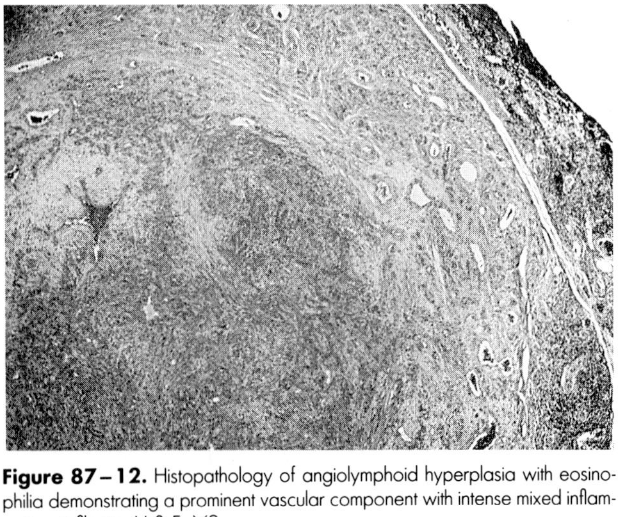

Figure 87–12. Histopathology of angiolymphoid hyperplasia with eosinophilia demonstrating a prominent vascular component with intense mixed inflammatory infiltrate. H & E, ×2.

REFERENCES

1. Glenner GG: Amyloid deposits and amyloidosis: The beta fibriloses. N Engl J Med 302:1283, 1333, 1980.
2. Glenner GG, Terry W, Harada M, et al: Amyloid fibril proteins: Proof of homology with immunoglobulin light chains by sequence analysis. Science 172:1150–1151, 1971.
3. Reimann HA, Koucky RF, Eklund CM: Primary amyloidosis limited to tissue of mesodermal origin. Am J Pathol 11:977–988, 1935.
4. Arapakis G, Tribe CR: Amyloidosis in rheumatoid arthritis investigated by means of rectal biopsy. Ann Rheum Dis 56:256–262, 1963.
5. Cohen AS: Amyloidosis. *In* Harrison's Principles of Internal Medicine, 10th ed. 1983, p 368.
6. Knowles DM, Jakobeic FA, Rosen M, Howard G: Amyloidosis of the orbit and adnexa. Surv Ophthalmol 19:367–384, 1975.
7. Garner A: Amyloidosis of the cornea. Br J Ophthalmol 53:73–81, 1969.
8. Levine MR, Buckman G: Primary localized orbital amyloidosis. Ann Ophthalmol 18:165–167, 1986.
9. Radnot M, Lapis K, Feher J: Amyloid tumor in the lacrimal gland. Ann Ophthalmol 3:727–742, 1971.
10. Holmstrom GE, Nyman KG: Primary orbital amyloidosis localized to an extraocular muscle. Br J Ophthalmol 71:32–33, 1987.
11. Erie JC, Garrity JA, Norman ME: Orbital amyloidosis involving the extraocular muscles. Arch Ophthalmol 107:1429, 1989.
12. Raflo GT, Farrell TA, Sioussat RS: Complete ophthalmoplegia secondary to amyloidosis associated with multiple myeloma. Am J Ophthalmol 92:221–224, 1981.
13. Gonnering RS, Sonneland PR: Ptosis and dermatochalasis as presenting signs in a case of occult primary systemic amyloidosis. Ophthalmic Surg 18:495–497, 1987.
14. Raab EL: Intraorbital amyloid. Br J Ophthalmol 54:445–449, 1970.
15. Jensen OA: Bilateral amyloidosis of the orbit. Ophthalmologica 173:70–78, 1976.
16. Patrinely JR, Koch DD: Surgical management of advanced ocular adnexal amyloidosis. Arch Ophthalmol 110:882–885, 1992.
17. Leone CR, Wissenger JP: Surgical approaches to diseases of the orbital apex. Ophthalmology 95(3):391–397, 1988.
18. Codere F, Lee RD, Anderson RL: Necrobiotic xanthogranuloma of the eyelid. Arch Ophthalmol 101:60–63, 1983.
19. Robertson DM, Winkelman RK: Ophthalmic features of necrobiotic xanthogranuloma with paraproteinemia. Am J Ophthalmol 97:173–183, 1984.
20. Cornblath WT, Dotan SA, Trobe JD, Headington JT: Varied clinical spectrum of necrobiotic xanthogranuloma. Ophthalmology 99(1):103–107, 1992.
21. Kossard S, Winkelman RK: Necrobiotic xanthogranuloma with paraproteinemia. Am Acad Dermatol 3(3):257–269, 1980.
22. Bullock JD, Bartley GB, Campbell RJ, et al: Necrobiotic xanthogranuloma with paraproteinemia: Case report and a pathogenic theory. Ophthalmology 93(9):1233–1236, 1986.
23. Rendall JRS, Vanhegan RI, Robb-Smith AHT: Atypical multicentric reticulohistiocytosis with paraproteinemia. Arch Dermatol 113:1576–1582, 1977.
24. Kyle RA: Monoclonal gammopathy of undetermined significance: Natural history in 241 cases. Am J Med 64:814–826, 1978.
25. Shields JA, Karcioglu ZA, Shields CL, et al: Orbital and eyelid involvement with Erdheim-Chester disease. Arch Ophthalmol 109:850–854, 1991.
26. Rose GE, Patel BC, Garner A, et al: Orbital xanthogranulomas in adults. Br J Ophthalmol 75:680–684, 1991.
27. Reed RJ, Terayakis N: Subcutaneous angioblastic lymphoid hyperplasia with eosinophilia (Kimura's disease). Cancer 29(2):489–497, 1972.

28. Morton K, Robertson AJ, Hadden W: Angiolymphoid hyperplasia with eosinophilia: Report of a case arising from the radial artery. Histopathology 11(9):963–969, 1987.
29. BeHinato G, Insabato L, DeChiara A, et al: Fine needle aspiration cytology of angiolymphoid hyperplasia with eosinophilia: A case report with electron microscopy and immunohistochemistry. Diagn Cytopathol 5(1):88–94, 1989.
30. Moeshu J, Pallesen R, Rensen B: Angiolymphoid hyperplasia with eosinophilia (Kimura's disease): A case with dermal lesions in the knee region and a popliteal arteriovenous fistula. Arch Dermatol 117(10):650–653, 1981.
31. Rao RN, Spurlock BO, Witherington R: Angiolymphoid hyperplasia with eosinophilia: Report of a case with penile lesions. Cancer 47(5):944–949, 1981.
32. Hallam LA, MacKinlay GA, Wright AM: Angiolymphoid hyperplasia with eosinophilia: Possible etiologic role for immunization. J Clin Pathol 42(9):944–949, 1989.
33. Calhoun KH, Newton RC, Sanchey RL: Angiolymphoid hyperplasia with eosinophilia: A case report and review of the literature. Arch Otolaryngol Head Neck Surg 114(12):1474–1476, 1988.
34. Smith DL, Kincaid MC, Nicolitz E: Angiolymphoid hyperplasia with eosinophilia (Kimura's disease) of the orbit. Arch Ophthalmol 106(6):793–795, 1988.
35. Cook HT, Stafford ND: Angiolymphoid hyperplasia with eosinophilia involving the lacrimal gland: Case report. Br J Ophthalmol 72:710–712, 1988.
36. Eisenberg E, Lowlicht R: Angiolymphoid hyperplasia with eosinophils: A clinicopathologic conference. J Oral Pathol 14:216–223, 1985.
37. Ku TT, Shih LY, Chan HL: Kimura's disease: Involvement of regional lymph nodes and distinction from angiolymphoid hyperplasia with eosinophilia. Am J Surg Pathol 12(11):843–854, 1988.
38. Sheren SB, Custer PL, Smith ME: Angiolymphoid hyperplasia of the orbit associated with obstructive airway disease. Am J Ophthalmol 108(2):353–356, 1989.
39. Whelan TV, Maher JF, Krogel P, et al: Nephrotic syndrome associated with Kimura's disease. Am J Kidney Dis 11(4):353–356, 1988.
40. Quinibi WY, Al-Sibai MB, Akhtar M: Mesangioproliferative glomerulonephritis associated with Kimura's disease. Clin Nephrol 30(2):111–114, 1988.
41. Sonkodi S, Jarmay K, Korcron I, et al: Membranous nephropathy accompanied by angiolymphoid hyperplasia of the skin. Nephron 47(1):320, 1987.
42. Fernandez LA, Olsen TG, Barurick KW, et al: Renin in angiolymphoid hyperplasia with eosinophilia: Its possible effect on vascular proliferation. Arch Pathol Lab Med 110(12):1131–1135, 1986.
43. Hidayat AA, Cameron JP, Font RL, Zimmerman LE: Angiolymphoid hyperplasia with eosinophilia (Kimura's disease) of the orbit and ocular adnexa. Am J Ophthalmol 96:176–189, 1983.
44. Ramsey MS, Fine BS, Cohen SW: Localized corneal amyloidosis. Case report with electron microscopic observations. Am J Ophthalmol 73:560–565, 1972.

BIBLIOGRAPHY

Howard GM: Amyloid tumors of the orbit. Br J Ophthalmol 50:421–425, 1966.

Kaiser-Kupfer MI, McAdam KPWJ, Kuwabara T: Localized amyloidosis of the orbit and upper respiratory tract. Am J Ophthalmol 84(5):721–728, 1977.

Kossard S, Goellner JR, Daniel Su WP: Subcutaneous necrobiotic granulomas of the scalp. J Am Acad Dermatol 3(2):180–185, 1980.

Ratnakar KS, Mohan M: Amyloidosis of the iris. Can J Ophthalmol 11:256–257, 1976.

Rootman J: Disease of the Orbit. Philadelphia, JB Lippincott, 1988, p 569.

Savino P, Schatz N, Rodrigues M: Orbital amyloidosis. Can J Ophthalmol 11:252–255, 1976.

CHAPTER 88

Idiopathic Orbital Inflammation and Lymphoid Tumors of the Orbit

James P. Milite and Steven A. McCormick

HISTORICAL PERSPECTIVE

Historically, idiopathic orbital inflammation and lymphoid tumors of the orbit were often grouped together under the nonspecific term *pseudotumor*.[1] Coined by Birch-Hirschfeld in 1930, this term was employed to describe a wide range of pathologic processes due to lack of understanding of their underlying pathogenesis. His definition encompassed any swelling of the orbital contents or mass lesion that caused proptosis and simulated a neoplasm. With the development of more sophisticated laboratory and clinical techniques, precise diagnosis of specific local and systemic pathologic processes previously referred to as pseudotumor has been facilitated. Consequently, today this imprecise term has little usefulness and should be avoided in clinical usage.[2, 3]

For example, as microbiologic techniques developed, isolation of *Mycobacterium tuberculosis* from certain granulomatous inflammatory processes allowed specific diagnosis of tuberculosis involving the orbit in some patients. Similarly, with establishment of sarcoidosis as a definable clinical entity in the 1930s, orbital involvement was realized to be a prominent feature of this disease, particularly within the lacrimal gland.[4–6] Each of these diseases had previously been considered examples of orbital "pseudotumor." Even as recently as 25 years ago, Graves' disease, or thyroid-related orbitopathy, was not well characterized clinically. As imaging and laboratory techniques developed, however, the characterization of Graves' disease as a specific disease entity was clarified and this condition was carved out of the "pseudotumor" category.

By the mid 1960s, *pseudotumor* had become a general term to describe any idiopathic inflammatory condition or lymphoid proliferation and even included frank malignant lymphoma of the orbit. Even as recently as the 1970s, the various lymphoid tumors, both benign and malignant, had been classified as lymphoid pseudotumors.[7] By using current exhaustive clinical, radiographic, and pathologic modalities of these various processes, more precise classification of these disease entities previously considered as orbital lymphoid pseudotumors has become possible.[8]

IDIOPATHIC ORBITAL INFLAMMATION

In large series of orbital inflammatory processes, many cases can be attributed to a specific pathologic diagnosis such as sarcoidosis, tuberculosis, thyroid-related orbitopathy, and other infectious processes. In addition, retained foreign bodies, ruptured dermoid cysts, hemorrhagic lymphangiomas, and other specific disease processes may lead to an inflammatory presentation.[9] However, a large group of patients remains in which no underlying cause of the inflammatory process is elucidated, leading to a diagnosis of orbital "inflammatory pseudotumor" or, more correctly, idiopathic orbital inflammation. In fact, this category of patients often presents with clinical and histopathologic findings that, to the experienced clinician, suggest this diagnosis a priori.

Idiopathic orbital inflammation may present acutely, subacutely, or chronically in adults and, less commonly, in children.[10, 11] The disease may present as unilateral or bilateral involvement or may even alternate between the two orbits. Bilateral involvement is more common in children. In addition, this entity can be further characterized radiographically and histologically by which orbital structure is predominantly involved, such as the extraocular muscles (idiopathic myositis), the lacrimal gland (idiopathic dacryoadenitis), the periscleral or epibulbar tissues, or perineural tissues. More commonly, these lesions are diffuse, involving more than one structure, including the orbital adipose tissue. Frequently, the site of orbital involvement is largely either anterior or posterior, with anterior involvement being more common in our experience. In one clinical series, idiopathic orbital inflammation was the second most frequent cause of orbital disease after thyroid-related orbitopathy (Graves' disease).[12]

The acute form of idiopathic orbital inflammation (Fig. 88 – 1) has a dramatic clinical presentation, allowing it to be readily distinguished from less strikingly symptomatic orbital conditions such as thyroid-related orbitopathy and lymphoid tumors. The typical clinical features of acute idiopathic orbital inflammation include acute, and sometimes severe, proptosis, pain, injection, che-

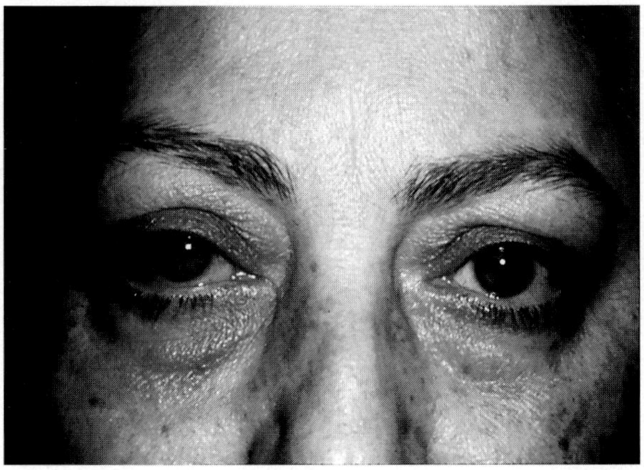

Figure 88–1. Clinical presentation of acute anterior idiopathic orbital inflammation, right eye. Conjunctival injection, mild chemosis, erythema, and edema are present.

mosis, and lid swelling. The significant pain and prominent inflammatory signs associated with this disease may mimic infectious orbital cellulitis, from which it must be differentiated.

A less fulminant onset characterizes subacute idiopathic orbital inflammation, in which symptoms and signs develop more slowly over a period of several weeks to a few months. The inflammatory signs are much less impressive than those seen in the acute form, and the patients describe symptoms of orbital discomfort that are slowly progressive. In the chronic variety of idiopathic orbital inflammation, patients complain of gradually increasing proptosis, diplopia, and decreased vision, usually in the absence of significant pain or inflammatory signs.

In addition to classification of idiopathic orbital inflammation based on disease duration, identification of the main anatomic site of involvement provides a complementary system of organization of these lesions. Although anatomic classification of idiopathic orbital inflammation does not address the underlying pathogenic mechanisms of these conditions, it has utility in formulating an approach to the diagnosis and management of these lesions.

Anterior idiopathic orbital inflammation primarily involves Tenon's fascia and the periscleral tissues, with occasional secondary involvement of the sclera. Other terms used to describe this entity include sclerotenonitis, periscleritis, and anterior idiopathic pseudotumor.[13] Symptoms of anterior idiopathic orbital inflammation typically include pain and tenderness of the eyelids and ocular adnexa, with local edema and erythema. Examination of these patients may reveal proptosis, ptosis, and abnormally increased resistance to retrograde displacement of the globe. Signs of ocular involvement include conjunctival injection and anterior chamber cell and flare in the anterior segment, as well as choroidal effusions, chorioretinal striae, exudative retinal detachment, and cystoid macular edema in the posterior segment.[14, 15] Glaucoma is possible secondary to either uveitis or reactive choroidal effusions. Intraocular findings are more common when inflammation of the posterior sclera is a feature of the disease.

In addition to the globe, the inflammatory response typical of anterior idiopathic orbital inflammation may involve other tissues contiguous with Tenon's fascia. Inflammation of the extraocular muscle insertions may be a feature of anterior idiopathic orbital inflammation, often causing a painful restrictive strabismus. Similarly, the sheath of the optic nerve may be infiltrated with inflammatory cells, giving rise to a perineuritis or even papillitis.

Diagnosis of anterior idiopathic orbital inflammation relies on clinical presentation and ophthalmic examination, with other important information provided by adjunctive imaging procedures. Computed tomography often reveals an infiltrative process with poorly defined borders partially surrounding the globe and involving the tissues of the anterior orbit. B-scan ultrasonography typically shows thickening of the uvea and sclera in cases in which posterior scleral inflammation accompanies the anterior orbital inflammatory response.[16] Another ultrasonographic feature of these lesions is the detection of fluid in sub-Tenon's space posteriorly, represented on B-scan ultrasonography as an echolucent zone between the sclera and the orbital fat (the so-called T-sign).[17]

Due to the marked inflammatory presentation of patients with acute anterior orbital inflammation, the differential diagnosis must include infectious orbital cellulitis, especially in cases with exuberant chemosis, erythema, and lid edema. Absence of sinus disease on computed tomography usually excludes an infectious cause from the differential diagnosis. Cases with a prominent uveitic component may be initially mistaken as a purely intraocular inflammatory process, with failure to recognize the accompanying orbital inflammation. Systemic inflammatory diseases, such as Wegener's granulomatosis and Erdheim-Chester disease, must also be considered when evaluating these patients. Additionally, sudden structural changes in noninflammatory lesions, such as hemorrhage into a preexisting orbital lymphangioma or rupture of a dermoid cyst, may cause acute proptosis with pain and ocular motility abnormalities.

Idiopathic orbital inflammation that is largely confined to the lacrimal gland may be referred to as noninfectious dacryoadenitis. Typically, these patients present with pain, swelling, and erythema without induration localized to the superotemporal orbit. Examination may reveal a secondary ptosis, and often an S-shaped deformity is imparted to the upper eyelid. Proptosis is unusual, but inferonasal displacement of the globe is possible in cases with exuberant inflammation involving the lacrimal gland. The palpebral lobe of the gland is frequently enlarged and is easily visible in the superotemporal conjunctival fornix on lid eversion and may display adjacent chemosis and conjunctival hyperemia. Contiguous involvement of the lateral rectus muscle is possible, causing a painful, restrictive strabismus. In addition to this acute form, subacute and chronic varieties of dacryoadenitis are recognized.

Diagnostic evaluation of dacryoadenitis includes computed tomography, which typically reveals lacrimal gland enlargement and elongation with conformation to the borders of adjacent orbital structures. Infiltration of the lateral rectus or Tenon's fascia in the vicinity of the lacrimal gland may be identified. Erosion or remodeling of bone is not typically encountered. B-scan ultrasonography reveals enlargement of the gland with a homogeneous internal acoustic structure.[13] In many cases of dacryoadenitis, biopsy may be required to differentiate idiopathic orbital inflammation from a primary epithelial or lymphoid neoplasm within the gland.

Idiopathic inflammation primarily involving the extraocular muscles is called orbital myositis. Symptoms heralding the acute form of this disease are diplopia and painful ophthalmoplegia. Examination is remarkable for restrictive strabismus in the field of action of the affected extraocular muscles, with positive forced duction testing. Localized injection of the insertions of the involved extraocular muscles is often discernible on slit lamp examination. Proptosis may be a feature, with pain and increased resistance on retrograde displacement of the globe. Tenderness in the vicinity of the trochlea may be noted in cases involving the superior oblique muscle (peritrochleitis).[18] Numerous systemic associations with orbital myositis have been recognized, including viral upper respiratory tract infection, allergic rhinitis, sinusitis, asthma, inflammatory bowel disease (particularly Crohn's disease), trauma, and serum sickness.[19, 20]

Computed tomographic images can be critical in differentiating idiopathic orbital myositis from thyroid-related orbitopathy, which can be identical in clinical presentation. Orbital myositis (Fig. 88–2) is characterized by diffuse enlargement of the extraocular muscles inclusive of their tendons, in contradistinction to the tendon-sparing, fusiform muscle enlargement of thyroid-related orbitopathy.[21] A predilection for involvement of the superior and medial rectus muscles has been noted in idiopathic myositis, in contrast to thyroid-related orbitopathy's predilection for inferior rectus involvement.[6] Spillover of the inflammatory infiltrate into the adjacent orbital tissues is often noted on computed tomography.

Another localized form of idiopathic orbital inflammation involves the posterior orbit. Cases of posterior idiopathic orbital inflammation usually present with ophthalmoplegia and optic neuropathy (orbital apex syndrome). These patients complain of pain, proptosis, diplopia, and symptoms of optic nerve dysfunction, including dyschromatopsia, reduced visual acuity, and visual field defects. Examination reveals an afferent pupillary defect, papillitis, and restrictive strabismus, owing to inflammation of the extraocular muscle origins in the orbital apex. The optic neuropathy results from either direct inflammation of the optic nerve sheath or compression of the nerve by an adjacent inflammatory mass in the orbital apex. The computed tomographic images obtained in these cases directly reflect the clinical picture, with an infiltrate found in the orbital apex involving the extraocular muscle origins and enlargement of the optic nerve sheath.[22, 23]

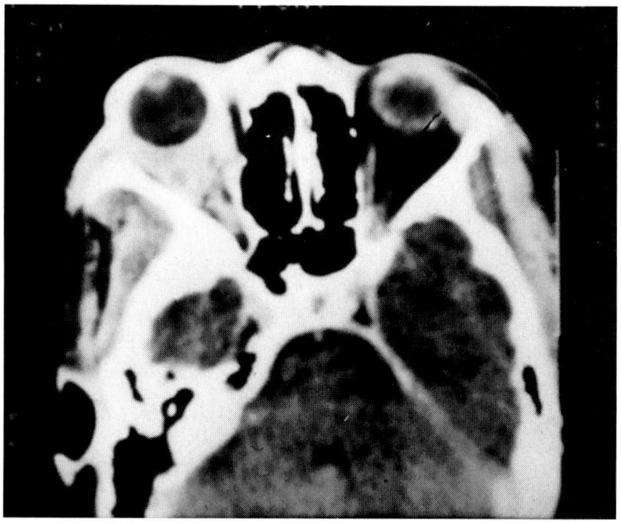

Figure 88–2. Axial computed tomographic scan of patient with idiopathic orbital inflammation with a myositic component affecting the right orbit. A diffuse infiltrate is seen in the right orbit with enlargement of the bodies of the extraocular muscles.

The histopathologic picture in most cases of idiopathic orbital inflammation is not only dependent on the location of the inflammation but is also largely determined by the stage of the disease process at the time of biopsy (Fig. 88–3). Early in the disease, a polymorphous inflammatory infiltrate is present, composed of a mixture of lymphocytes, plasma cells, neutrophils, and eosinophils. The eosinophilia may be especially striking in children.[24] As the process progresses there is increasing fibrosis, with the inflammatory cells separated into islands by bundles of nascent collagen. This generalized desmoplastic response is paralleled by alterations in the connective tissue arrangement of the orbital structures specifically involved. For example, the connective tissue of the extraocular muscles thickens and the fibrous septa of the lacrimal gland become hyperplastic as the glandular architecture atrophies. In some cases, lymphoid follicles with germinal centers may be found scattered throughout these lesions. Vessels involved in these lesions may have a perivascular lymphocytic cuffing, rather than a true vasculitis. Inflammation may lead to necrosis of orbital fat with a secondary lipogranulomatous reaction.

Two less common histologic forms of idiopathic orbital inflammation exist: granulomatous and chronic sclerosing. As its name indicates, granulomatous idiopathic orbital inflammation features a granulomatous

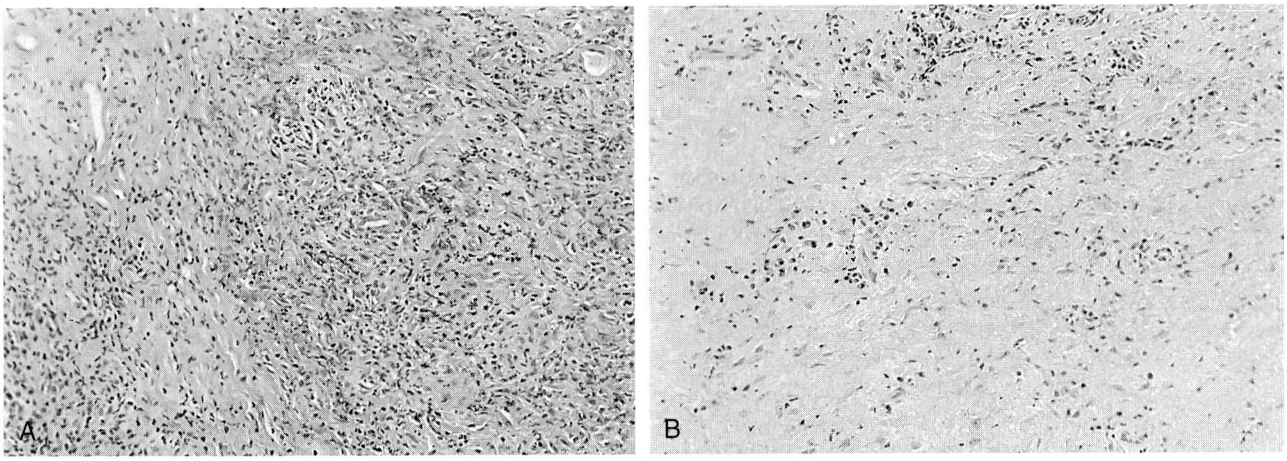

Figure 88–3. Histopathology of idiopathic orbital inflammation. *A*, Acute idiopathic orbital inflammation. A heterogeneous, hypocellular inflammatory infiltrate is present, including neutrophils, lymphocytes, plasma cells, and macrophages superimposed on a background of vascular proliferation and early fibrosis. H & E, ×20. *B*, Chronic idiopathic inflammation. Replacement of normal orbital soft tissues by dense fibrosis is seen. Note the minimal, scattered polymorphous inflammatory infiltrates. H & E, ×10.

inflammatory infiltrate. This diagnosis can only be made after systemic workup has ruled out the presence of infectious or systemic granulomatous disease (e.g., sarcoidosis, tuberculosis, fungal infection). Chronic sclerosing idiopathic orbital inflammation is characterized histologically by a polymorphous inflammatory infiltrate with an exuberant desmoplastic response. Not only does this form of idiopathic orbital inflammation differ from other types histologically, but the clinical presentation is also unusual. Consistent with other forms of idiopathic orbital inflammation, clinical signs of the chronic sclerosing type include proptosis, restrictive strabismus (usually severe), and decreased vision if the orbital apex is involved. However, unlike typical idiopathic orbital inflammation, erosion of the orbital bones with intracranial extension of the mass lesion has been reported.[25, 26] Chronic sclerosing idiopathic orbital inflammation may rarely be associated with other systemic sclerosing disorders involving the thyroid gland, mediastinum, retroperitoneum, and meninges.[27–29]

The immunopathogenesis of idiopathic orbital inflammation is enigmatic, but the presence of some form of autoimmunity or immune complex deposition has been suggested by numerous authors. Based on several series, it has been estimated that the incidence of underlying systemic disease in idiopathic orbital inflammation is less than 10%, with a slightly higher incidence in cases of bilateral idiopathic orbital inflammation. Due to the possible complications of an undetected underlying systemic condition, medical workup by the internist or rheumatologist is indicated in most cases of idiopathic orbital inflammation to rule out sarcoidosis, periarteritis nodosa, Wegener's granulomatosis, multifocal fibrosclerosis, Erdheim-Chester disease, or other systemic inflammatory diseases.

When a patient with suspected idiopathic orbital inflammation is encountered, diagnostic evaluation can be initiated to a great extent by the ophthalmologist. Laboratory evaluation includes complete blood cell count with differential, erythrocyte sedimentation rate, thyroid function tests, antinuclear antibodies, serum protein electrophoresis, and VDRL and fluorescent treponemal antibody absorption testing. Imaging of the orbital soft tissues in this condition by either computed tomography or magnetic resonance imaging provides useful diagnostic information. Although magnetic resonance images may provide better soft tissue definition and visualization of the orbital apex, computed tomography is superior for evaluation of the bones of the orbit. Thus, the choice of imaging modality is determined largely by the patient's clinical presentation in view of the previously described considerations.

Biopsy of idiopathic orbital inflammation is generally not necessary in typical acute and subacute cases.[8, 29] Indications for biopsy include chronicity, failure to respond to treatment, involvement of bone, and extraorbital extension. When a tissue diagnosis is required, incisional biopsy is performed. Excision of idiopathic orbital inflammation is not routine and is usually only performed in an effort to debulk large lesions causing compression of the optic nerve. Fine needle aspiration biopsy of accessible lesions may provide adequate tissue for diagnosis, but experience with this technique is limited.[30, 31]

The primary goal of treatment in idiopathic orbital inflammation is suppression of the orbital inflammation. Systemic corticosteroids are the first line of therapy after infectious causes have been ruled out. As stated earlier, empiric treatment without biopsy is acceptable in cases in which the diagnosis is straightforward based on clinical and radiographic presentation. Prednisone in oral doses of 60 to 100 mg daily often leads to marked improvement in 48 to 72 hours.[30, 32] Depending on the degree of inflammation, this dosage may be continued for 2 to 3 weeks, followed by a slow taper in 10-mg increments on a weekly basis.

Lack of response of the inflammation to oral corticosteroid therapy is an indication for incisional biopsy of the lesion. If the biopsy result remains consistent with idiopathic orbital inflammation, then other therapeutic modalities must be considered. Low-dose external beam radiation therapy with shielding of the globe in doses of 1000 to 3000 cGy is often helpful in treating these corticosteroid-refractory cases. In selected cases, cytotoxic agents may also be used. When the diagnosis is sclerosing idiopathic orbital inflammation, treatment is frequently more difficult and may require a combination of the above therapies with functional surgical excision of the mass to achieve a satisfactory result.[30]

ORBITAL LYMPHOID TUMORS

Clinical Presentation

The other broad category of orbital lesions formerly referred to as pseudotumors are the orbital lymphoproliferative tumors. These are reactive or neoplastic lymphoid proliferations and are not related to idiopathic orbital inflammation. Because the normal human orbit has no native lymphatic system or lymph nodes, any lymphoid process of the orbit is by definition extranodal and pathologic. In classification schemes, extranodal lymphoid proliferations are often problematic to both the pathologist and the clinician in arriving at a diagnosis and in determining prognosis and appropriate therapy. Advances in immune system physiology and development of modern immunologic diagnostic techniques have allowed better understanding of this group of lymphoid lesions.

The current preferred classification for orbital and ocular adnexal lymphoid tumors divides them into three principal categories: (1) reactive lymphoid hyperplasia, (2) atypical lymphoid hyperplasia, and (3) malignant lymphoma. Distinction between benign and malignant lymphoproliferative lesions of the orbit and ocular adnexa cannot be made solely on clinical or radiologic criteria. Diagnosis, and therefore prognosis, is dependent on histopathologic features, coupled with immunophenotypic and molecular genetic data when indicated. Therefore, when clinically suspicious, the lesions must be biopsied. Fine needle aspiration is of limited usefulness because the tissue architecture is the single most important parameter needed to classify these lesions.

Lymphoid tumors are typically insidious in onset and lack inflammatory signs and symptoms. Most patients are in their sixth to seventh decade, especially those with malignant lymphoma, and there is a slight female predominance.[33, 34] Lymphoproliferative lesions of the orbit are extremely rare in children, and any lymphoid infiltrate in this age group should be considered a tissue manifestation of leukemia until proved otherwise. These lesions may be either unilateral or bilateral, but bilateral involvement does not necessarily increase the likelihood of the development of systemic lymphoproliferative disease.[35]

Patients typically complain of slowly developing, mild proptosis with little or no disturbance in visual function. Diplopia may result from mass effect of the tumor with secondary alteration of ocular motility or from direct infiltration of the extraocular muscles.[36] Involvement of the levator complex may also cause ptosis. The lack of pain and of severe symptoms often causes a significant delay in prompting patients to seek treatment, with many patients presenting 6 months or more after the onset of proptosis.

The most common site of involvement of lymphoid tumors is the superior orbit, with greater than 30% occurring in the lacrimal gland. Lesions in this location result in proptosis with downward displacement of the globe. When palpable, these tumors are rubbery, firm, and conform to the orbital septum. Lymphoid tumors occurring in the superior orbit may also interfere with the function of the superior rectus–levator complex (Fig. 88–4). Involvement of the retrobulbar soft tissues causes axial displacement of the globe. The high incidence of primary lymphoid tumors in the lacrimal gland may be related to its normal standing population of lymphocytes. These lesions may be difficult to differentiate clinically from epithelial tumors of the lacrimal gland, which is a vital distinction given the marked difference in treatment of these two groups of tumors.

Lymphoproliferative lesions involving the conjunctiva usually have the classic "salmon patch" appearance but may also appear pink or flesh colored. This appearance is due to their dense cellularity, fine microvasculature, and scant interstitium. Conjunctival lymphoid

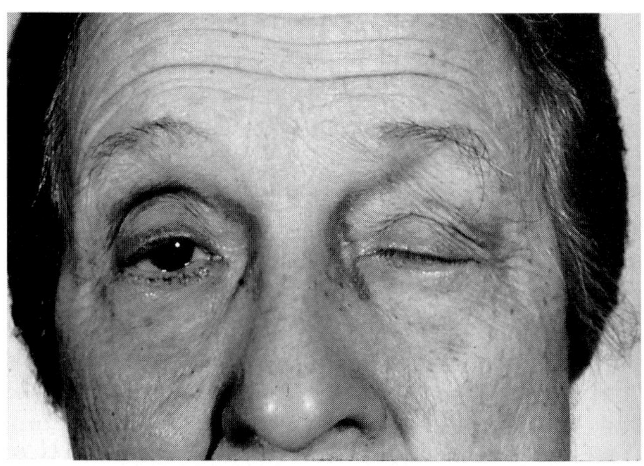

Figure 88–4. Malignant lymphoma of the left orbit involving the superior rectus–levator palpebrae superioris complex, causing a secondary ptosis.

tumors are usually moderately dense, nontender masses that are mobile over the bulbar surface, in contrast to tumors that are fixed to the sclera, which probably represent extraocular extension of uveal lymphoproliferative processes.[37] Occasionally, conjunctival salmon patches may be the initial manifestation of an orbital lymphoid tumor that has spread into the subconjunctival space, rather than a primary conjunctival tumor.[38] Similarly, salmon patches may present as lesions distinct from an occult orbital process. In this situation, the histologies may differ; therefore, biopsy of the orbital lesion is indicated despite the fact that the conjunctival process is more accessible.

Lymphoid tumors in the preseptal eyelid are rare in comparison to other sites of presentation but cause readily palpable masses. Lesions in this location may cause ptosis and mild ocular irritation. Affected eyelids have a mildly edematous appearance and a doughy consistency.

Radiologic evaluation of orbital lymphoproliferative disease is well served by both magnetic resonance imaging and computed tomography. Although both of these imaging modalities reveal features suggestive of their histopathology, there are no reliable radiographic signs that allow differentiation among benign lymphoid hyperplasia, atypical lymphoid hyperplasia, and malignant lymphoma.[39–41]

The radiologic hallmark of orbital lymphoid disease is a soft tissue mass of homogeneous density that molds or conforms to adjacent orbital structures (Fig. 88–5). This behavior reflects the underlying histology of these lesions, which are composed of a relatively monomorphic cell population with a paucity of stroma. These tumors are not invasive, resulting in the visualization of sharply

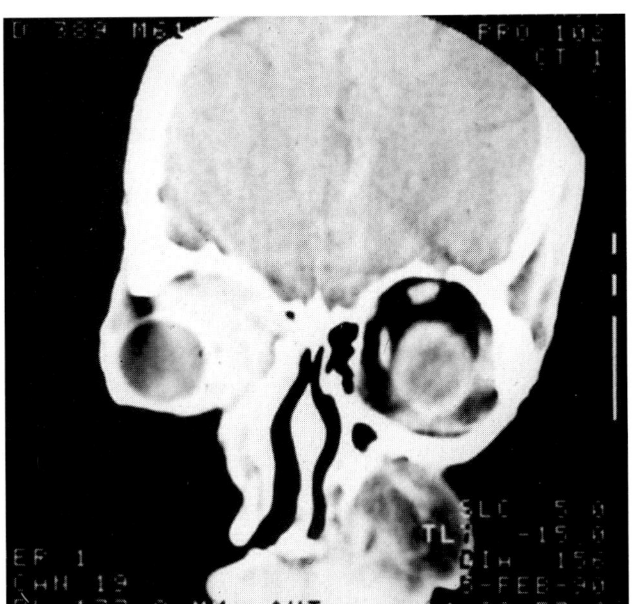

Figure 88–5. Coronal computed tomographic scan of malignant lymphoma involving the right orbit. A soft tissue infiltrate is present in the medial aspect of the right orbit, conforming to the globe.

demarcated borders where they contact normal orbital structures. Bone destruction and orbital enlargement are rare. When located in the intraconal space, or elsewhere within the orbital fat, the edge of the tumor typically has finely irregular borders, corresponding to the fascial septations of the orbital fat.[42]

Although the previous features are certainly highly suggestive of lymphoid tumors, differentiation from other orbital pathologic processes can be difficult based on radiologic features alone. Mild enhancement with injection of contrast dye is exhibited by orbital lymphoproliferative lesions, and based on computed tomography alone it may be difficult to distinguish them from idiopathic orbital inflammation. Helpful findings that are indicative of idiopathic orbital inflammation include multifocality and the presence of more diffuse, "fuzzy" borders than those seen in lymphoid tumors. Although extraocular muscle infiltration is a characteristic of several orbital processes, muscle enlargement in lymphoproliferative disease is usually greater than that seen in orbital myositis or thyroid-related orbitopathy.[36]

Certain radiologic features of lymphoid tumors of the lacrimal gland help distinguish them from epithelial neoplasms. Lymphoid lacrimal gland tumors usually appear as an elongation and thickening of the gland, which makes acute angles with the orbital walls. In contrast, epithelial tumors are usually more globular and form obtuse angles with adjacent bone. Additionally, changes in bone structure are more commonly a feature of epithelial neoplastic disease.

Magnetic resonance imaging is comparable to computed tomography in identification of orbital lymphoid tumors, but it offers no improvement in determination of the malignant potential of a given lesion. T2-weighted images are often most helpful since lymphoid lesions yield a high relative signal intensity and have improved contrast with surrounding orbital fat in these images. Definition of orbital bone anatomy with magnetic resonance imaging is inferior to that with computed tomography, and, overall, magnetic resonance imaging offers no clear advantages in the imaging of lymphoproliferative lesions.

When clinical and radiographic data point to the presence of an orbital lymphoid tumor, biopsy is indicated. Although there are no clinical or radiographic features that are indicative of a benign or malignant diagnosis, recurrent lesions and lesions with bilateral presentation may be suggestive of malignancy. However, histopathologic evaluation is required to determine the exact tissue diagnosis in a case of suspected orbital lymphoproliferative disease and to predict patient prognosis.

Laboratory Evaluation and Classification

Essential to correctly diagnosing an orbital lymphoid tumor is evaluation of the cell population comprising a

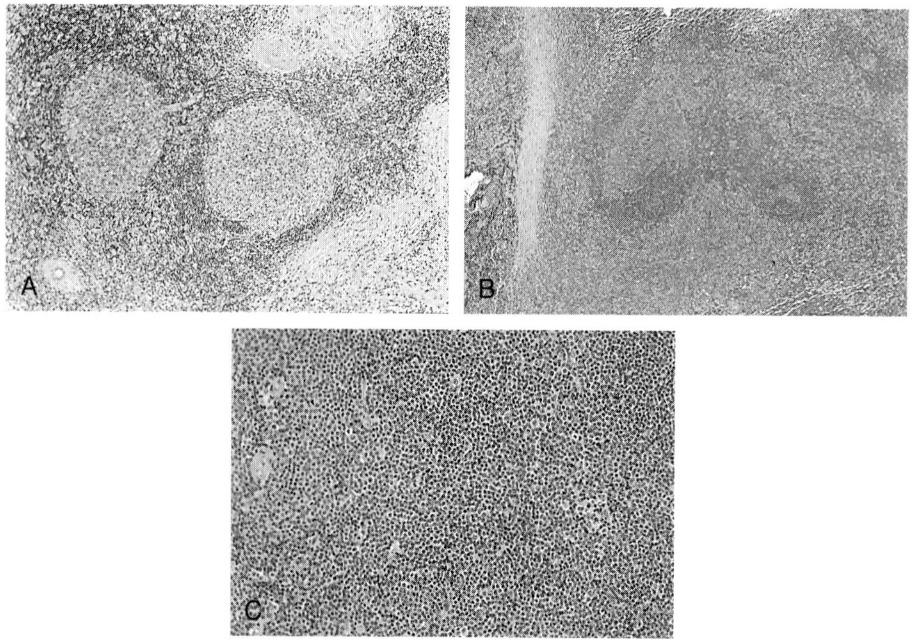

Figure 88–6. Histopathologic features of orbital lymphoproliferative disease. *A*, Benign lymphoid hyperplasia. Discrete, well-formed lymphoid follicles are present. Germinal centers are well developed and discrete, displaying a mixture of small and large lymphocytes in varying stages of maturity. H & E, ×20. *B*, Atypical lymphoid hyperplasia. Large and more irregular, focally coalescent follicles are present. These also display less sharp borders. H & E, ×10. *C*, Malignant lymphoma. A diffuse infiltrate of monomorphous, atypical lymphocytes is present with no follicular architecture. H & E, ×20.

given lesion (Fig. 88–6). The presence of lymphoid follicles indicates a mixed B- and T-cell population and is a feature of the architecture of both benign and atypical lymphoid hyperplasia. In comparison, malignant lymphomas are composed of a predominantly uniform cell population, usually B cells in the case of orbital lymphomas.[33, 34] Primary T-cell lymphomas and Hodgkin's lymphomas are exceedingly rare in the orbit.[43–45] Thus, when a lesion lacks a follicular arrangement and contains a diffuse infiltrate of atypical lymphocytes, the diagnosis of malignant lymphoma is relatively straightforward.

However, many lesions are more difficult to interpret histologically, possessing features of both benign and malignant lymphoid proliferations. These "borderline" lesions, the atypical lymphoid hyperplasias, may contain vague follicular arrangements or regions consistent with benign lymphoid hyperplasia and malignant lymphoma admixed within the same lesion. The difficulty in diagnosing such tumors is compounded by small biopsy specimens, crush artifact, and specimen sampling errors. Thus, immunophenotypic and genetic analyses of these tumors have improved diagnostic accuracy in cases in which the histology of a tumor is borderline.

Benign lymphoid hyperplasia is typified by discrete, well-formed lymphoid follicles resembling a reactive lymph node. The follicles may vary considerably in size and may occasionally be coalescent. The follicles house germinal centers composed of a mixture of small and large lymphocytes, with the normal range of lymphocyte maturity from immunoblast to mature differentiated lymphocyte represented. The germinal centers are surrounded by a zone of small lymphocytes, the mantle zone, which clearly demarcates the germinal center from the intervening tissue. Mitotic activity is frequently observed within the germinal centers but is rarely seen in the surrounding tissue. Other inflammatory cells, including macrophages containing debris (tingible bodies) scattered within the germinal centers, complete the histologic picture of these lesions.

The histologic architecture of atypical lymphoid hyperplasia mimics that of benign lymphoid hyperplasia, but the follicles are less distinctly formed and more irregularly shaped.[46] The follicles in these lesions are also more likely to be coalescent and larger than in benign lymphoid hyperplasia. Mitoses may be seen outside the follicles as well as in the germinal centers. Diffuse areas of lymphocytic infiltration without follicle formation may compose large portions of these tumors. Although many of the cells in these tumors may appear mature, a subpopulation of lymphocytes displaying cytologically atypical features, such as irregular nuclear contours, prominent nuclear membranes, and a more monomorphic appearance, is present.

Although its general architecture reflects that of benign lymphoid hyperplasia, atypical lymphoid hyperplasia and malignant lymphoma of the orbit also share common features. Hemosiderin deposition, a curious feature of orbital lymphomas, is often present within these tumors. Also, collections of multiple nuclei with ill-defined cell borders, known as polykaryocytes, are frequently noted. These are unique characteristics that are not seen in benign lymphoid hyperplasia of the orbit nor usually in systemic lymphoid infiltrates.

Orbital malignant lymphomas typically present as diffuse atypical lymphocytic infiltrates. These cells are usually monomorphous, although mixed cell lymphomas, composed of small and large cells, are recognized. In the orbit, lymphomas of B-cell origin overwhelmingly predominate, though a reactive benign T-cell population may be present, comprising up to 15% of the total component lymphocytes in many cases. Although the presence of follicles usually indicates a mixed B- and T-cell population and, therefore, the diagnosis of benign or atypical lymphoid hyperplasia, follicular lymphomas may exist.[47] We believe that many examples previously classified as follicular lymphoma were, in fact, atypical lymphoid hyperplasia. In our experience, true follicular lymphoma in the orbit is very rare.

Classification of malignant lymphoma has been subject to repeated modification over the past few decades. Improved understanding of lymphocyte morphology and maturation has allowed improved identification of subtypes of non-Hodgkin's lymphoma. Malignant lymphomas of the orbit are clinically classified as low, intermediate, or high grade according to the scheme proposed by the National Cancer Institute for non-Hodgkin's lymphoma (the "Working Formulation").[48] Given the rarity of Hodgkin's lymphoma and, in our experience, follicular and mixed cell lymphoma of the orbit, the majority of orbital lymphomas can usually be organized into a few distinct subtypes.

Small cell lymphocytic lymphoma, including the lymphoplasmacytic variant, is a low-grade tumor displaying sheets of monotonous small lymphocytes in a diffuse infiltrating pattern. Tumors in this subgroup with plasmacytoid differentiation feature cells with nuclear characteristics similar to small lymphocytes but containing moderate amounts of amphophilic cytoplasm as well as cells with the appearance of mature plasma cells. In less mature small cell lymphocytic lesions, foci of larger, immunoblast-like cells (known as prolymphocytes) may be clustered throughout the lesion.[49] Collections of these cells are termed *proliferation centers*, and they may impart a pseudofollicular pattern to the tumor when studied at low-power light.[50] The presence of periodic acid–Schiff-positive inclusions within the cytoplasm (Russell's bodies) or of pseudonuclear inclusions in the lymphocytes of these lesions is frequently noted and represents intracellular retention of immunoglobulin.[51]

A subtype of lymphoma that has been recognized with increasing frequency in the orbit is mantle cell lymphoma (lymphocytic lymphoma of intermediate differentiation). Although this tumor has been well characterized only recently in the medical literature, it comprises nearly 40% of our overall series of conjunctival and orbital lymphomas. Histologically, these tumors are composed of monotonous intermediate-sized lymphoid cells with irregular nuclear contours, nuclei with condensed chromatin, and scant cytoplasm.[52] No prolymphocytes, proliferation centers, or large lymphoid cells are present in these lesions. Macrophages with granular and eosinophilic cytoplasm may be scattered throughout these tumors, imparting a "starry sky" pattern at low power.[53]

Large cell lymphomas and immunoblastic lymphomas are high-grade tumors that also occur in the orbit. In immunosuppressed patients, particularly those with the acquired immunodeficiency syndrome, immunoblastic lymphoma and Burkitt's lymphoma are becoming increasingly common. Although orbital lymphoma of childhood is rare, orbital Burkitt's lymphoma may occur in young children in endemic areas in association with Epstein-Barr virus infection.[54, 55] Large cell and immunoblastic lymphomas contain cells with nuclei larger than those of benign histiocytes. These cells resemble the large cells that are normally present in the germinal centers of a reactive lymphoid follicle. The mitotic rate of these tumors tends to be higher than lower-grade lymphomas, and a "starry sky" pattern may also occasionally be noted.

Burkitt's lymphomas often differ from other lymphomas in their growth patterns, displaying expansile growth with compression of adjacent tissues, rather than by diffuse infiltration. The starry sky pattern is a classic and prominent feature with numerous faintly staining macrophages scattered against a background of dark staining malignant lymphoid cells.[56] These macrophages contain abundant cytoplasmic cellular debris, reflective of the high rate of cell turnover within these tumors.[57]

Although the above classification has some clinical value, the inability of histopathologic evaluation to predict the ultimate clinical course of lymphoid tumors of the ocular adnexa, particularly in cases of atypical lymphoid hyperplasia, has placed greater importance on the development of other tests to determine clonality.[58] Immunophenotypic analysis allows characterization of a lymphoid infiltrate based on expansion of cell surface antigens. More recently, genotypic analysis employing Southern blot techniques allows detection of monoclonal cell populations by detecting gene rearrangements that direct immunoglobulin and T-cell receptor production in lymphocytes.

Numerous lymphocyte cell surface antigens have been identified, some of which allow distinction between T cells and B cells, while others provide a means of identifying subpopulations of B cells and T cells.[59] For instance, among the surface markers housed on B-cell membranes are endogenous immunoglobulins (composed of heavy and light chains), with each different clone of B cells expressing a unique immunoglobulin. Utilization of immunohistochemical stains, typically using enzyme-based reagents, allows identification of the constituent cells in a lymphoid lesion as T cells or B cells. In addition, expression of the same surface marker by a majority of cells in a lesion, for example, immunoglobulin kappa light chain, can provide evidence of monoclonality and therefore support a diagnosis of malignancy. Marker studies have shown that reactive lymphoid hyperplasia of the ocular adnexa are T-cell–rich lesions (comprising up to 60% of a given lesion), with an associated polyclonal B-cell proliferation.[60–62] Orbital lesions that have a histopathologic appearance consistent with malignant lymphoma are almost always monoclonal B-cell tumors. It is important that the surgeon submit tissue obtained at biopsy to the pathology laboratory in unfixed, fresh state if lymphoma is suspected, because formalin fixation destroys many of the antigenic markers detected by immunohistochemical techniques.

The presence of monoclonal cell populations in orbital lymphoproliferative lesions can also be detected using genotypic analyses. These techniques employ DNA hybridization, restriction endonucleases, and Southern blot techniques[63] in an effort to identify clonal gene rearrangements manifested by monoclonal expansions of lymphocytes within these tumors. To understand these methods, one must realize that gene rearrangement is the physiologic mechanism by which lymphocytes are enabled to produce T-cell receptors and immunoglobulins of unique antigenic specificity.[64, 65]

The process of gene rearrangement unique to lymphoid cells involves splicing and reassembling a group of noncontinuous gene segments. Both the T-cell receptor and the immunoglobulin germline genes contain variable (V), diversity (D), joining (J), and constant (C) segments that can be combined to generate sequence diversity in the variable regions of the polypeptides they encode. Because the DNA rearrangement present within each T cell or B cell is unique, serving as a virtual fingerprint of the lymphocyte, very specific characterization of the cells in a lymphoid lesion is possible.[65–67] In a benign lymphoid tumor, containing a polyclonal cell population by definition, myriad gene rearrangements would be present, with no single clone predominating. However, in malignant lymphoma, an identically rearranged gene will be present in all constituent cells, allowing identification of the tumor as a monoclonal neoplasm of genotypically identical lymphocytes.

In addition to identification of malignant lymphoma of the orbit, detection of monoclonal gene rearrangements may allow isolation of "premalignant" lymphocytic lesions that appear histologically benign but may harbor unsuspected monoclonal subpopulations of cells.[68, 69] In a series of 14 orbital lymphoid tumors compiled over the past 2 years, we identified two cases of histologically defined atypical lymphoid hyperplasia that harbored a monoclonal cell population detected by gene rearrangement studies. These findings corroborate the work of other investigators[68, 69] that suggests that polyclonal lymphoproliferative lesions may be precursors to orbital lymphoma. If this concept is correct, identification of DNA rearrangements in otherwise histologically benign tumors may identify those patients who may benefit from more aggressive treatment in an effort to prevent potential evolution to frank malignant behavior.

Clinical Course and Management

The core clinical issue in caring for patients with orbital lymphoproliferative disease is determining the concomitant presence or predicting future development of systemic lymphoma. The diagnosis of frank malignant lymphoma of the orbit portends a significant risk for development of systemic lymphoma; some sources cite up to a 60% risk within 5 years of initial diagnosis.[70] Knowles and associates have also noted the predictive value of cell type. High-grade lymphomas were associated with the highest rate of systemic disease in their series of 108 patients.[34] However, even benign lymphoid hyperplasia has a 20% to 25% risk of developing systemic lymphoma after 5 years.[47] The accurate prediction of which seemingly benign lymphocytic infiltrates are harbingers of malignancy may be aided by the use of immunohistochemistry and DNA rearrangement studies, but this scenario is not yet completely resolved.[71] Because of the potential risk of malignant lymphoma elsewhere, systemic evaluation is advised for each patient with the diagnosis of any orbital or adnexal lymphoproliferative lesion, regardless of the histologic type.

The anatomic location of a lymphoid infiltrate is an important factor in determining risk for developing systemic disease. The overall rate of systemic disease in all lymphoid proliferations of the orbit, including the lacrimal gland, is 30% to 35%.[72] Surprisingly, this figure holds true for bilateral as well as unilateral lesions. Lymphoid tumors of the conjunctiva, however, are associated with an excellent prognosis. The great majority of these conjunctival lesions are histologically diagnosed as benign lymphoid hyperplasia, and well over 90% of patients show no evidence of systemic disease. This improved prognosis may be related to earlier diagnosis of these lesions due to their immediate visibility. Another consideration is that the conjunctiva, unlike the orbit, contains a native population of lymphocytes that may be more likely to undergo reactive hyperplasia.

Lymphoproliferative disease originating in the preseptal eyelid is associated with the poorest prognosis; systemic lymphoma occurs in approximately 67% of cases.[72] This finding correlates with the histology of these lesions, which display the highest rate of malignancy among the adnexal lymphoid tumors. Fortunately, the eyelid is also the rarest site of presentation, with only 5% to 10% of ocular adnexal lymphoproliferative disease presenting there.

Clinically, the differential diagnosis of lymphoid tumors of the orbit and ocular adnexa is broad. As previously stated, true lymphoid tumors must be distinguished from idiopathic orbital inflammation. Most cases are readily diagnosed based on the clinical presentation and, when sampled, on the histopathology. Accurate differentiation becomes increasingly difficult in subacute cases of idiopathic orbital inflammation with a less typical clinical course or when biopsy samples reveal secondary fibrosis or increased numbers of lymphocytes.

Another orbital pathologic process that may mimic orbital lymphoma is acute leukemic infiltration of the orbit. Orbital "lymphoma" in a child should be considered a leukemic infiltrate until proved otherwise, and soft tissue involvement with acute leukemia should be suspected in any child whose orbital biopsy is interpreted as an "undifferentiated round cell" tumor. Leukemic infiltrates, whether lymphoid or myeloid, can be best detected with monoclonal antibodies against lineage and differentiation-associated antigens. It must be again stressed that detection of these antigens by either immunohistochemistry or flow cytometry requires submission of fresh, unfixed biopsy tissue. A bone marrow aspirate and biopsy should be performed in any suspected case, even if the white blood cell count is normal. Some patients do not show bone marrow involvement for up to a year after presentation with leukemic involvement of the orbit.[73]

Plasma cell tumors, such as multiple myeloma and plasmacytoma, while related to lymphoma, behave in clinically distinct fashions. Orbital involvement in multiple myeloma is rare,[74] and plasmacytoma, when it occurs in the orbit, tends to produce lytic lesions of the orbital bones with spillover of the tumor into the adjacent soft tissues. Patients with these tumors require thorough systemic evaluation, including bone survey, serum and urine electrophoresis, and quantitative measurement of serum immunoglobulins.

Two additional entities that may occasionally mimic orbital lymphoma are the Langerhans' granulomatoses (comprising eosinophilic granuloma, Hand-Schüller-Christian disease, and Letterer-Siwe disease) and sinus histiocytosis with massive lymphadenopathy. The Langerhans' granulomatoses consist of proliferations of benign histiocytes affecting any organ system. On clinical grounds, these lesions are usually easily differentiated from orbital lymphoma because they typically affect children and often cause lytic bone lesions, uncommon in orbital lymphoid tumors. Sinus histiocytosis is distinguishable from lymphoma only on histopathologic examination, which reveals a proliferation of large histiocytes in a background of lymphocytes and plasma cells. The cytoplasm of the histiocytes often contains lymphocytes or hematopoietic cells, a phenomenon called emperipolesis.

Early systemic evaluation and clinical staging is most predictive of development of later systemic lymphoma and overall survival in patients with orbital and adnexal lymphoma. The large series of Knowles and coworkers and Mederios and associates both indicate that a relatively small percentage of patients (13% to 19%)[33, 34] have a known past history of systemic lymphoma on presentation with ocular adnexal or orbital disease. Patients with a negative workup for systemic lymphoma on presentation and who remained disease free at 1 year followup have an 87% chance of remaining disease free.[34] Thus, prompt systemic workup allows accurate staging that is predictive of disease survival.

Management of any case of suspected lymphoproliferative disease of the orbit or ocular adnexa begins with obtaining tissue for histopathologic diagnosis. Complete excision of these tumors is generally not necessary, but adequate tissue should be taken to ensure that all diagnostic modalities can be employed. When localized to the orbit, these tumors typically respond well to low-dose irradiation and their infiltrative growth pattern makes complete extirpation difficult if not impossible. Therefore, incisional biopsy is indicated in most cases and is facilitated by the predilection of these tumors to occur in the more accessible superior and anterior aspects of the orbit. The surgical approach to suspected lymphoid lesions elsewhere in the orbit is dictated by the site of presentation. Fine-needle aspiration biopsy has been used with some success and may be attempted for tumors that are less easily accessible. The only cases in which suspected lymphoid tumors of the orbit should be completely excised are those involving only the lacrimal gland. Occasionally these tumors may be epithelial neoplasms, rather than lymphoproliferative lesions, for which incisional biopsy is contraindicated.

At our institution, all patients with biopsy-proven orbital or ocular adnexal lymphoproliferative disease undergo systemic oncologic workup. This includes complete blood cell count, serum chemistry panel, computed tomography of the chest and abdomen, and bone marrow biopsy.[74] Other imaging modalities, such as liver-spleen and bone scanning may occasionally be indicated. Serum protein electrophoresis may be helpful, particularly in low-grade lymphoplasmacytic lymphomas.

The treatment of orbital and ocular adnexal lymphoproliferative disease is dictated both by the histologic diagnosis and the results of systemic evaluation. Local irradiation with shielding of the globe is indicated for tumors confined to the orbit or ocular adnexa. One thousand to 2000 cGy in divided doses is given for histologically benign tumors, while 2000 to 4000 cGy is suggested for lesions with phenotypic or genotypic evidence of malignancy.[75, 76] Corticosteroids should not be used as primary treatment of suspected lymphoproliferative tumors because, although transient reduction in the size of the lesions will be seen, rebound occurs on cessation of the corticosteroids. Continued ophthalmologic and oncologic followup examinations should be scheduled at least every 6 months for 2 years after primary treatment to rule out development of systemic disease.

Chemotherapy is reserved for patients with evidence of systemic disease on the initial workup and is not indicated for tumors that lack a defined systemic component. Local side effects of radiation on the eye and ocular adnexa are potentiated by systemic chemotherapy. Concomitant local irradiation and systemic chemotherapy are typically reserved for those cases in which the mass effect of the orbital lesion must be immediately alleviated to avoid loss of vision or other secondary effects.

REFERENCES

1. Birch-Hirschfeld A: Zur Diagnostic and Pathologic der orbital Tumoren. Ber Dtsch Ophthalmol Ges 32:127–135, 1905.
2. Blodi FC, Gass JD: Inflammatory pseudotumor of the orbit. Trans Am Acad Ophthalmol Otolaryngol 71:303–322, 1967.
3. Chavis RM, Garner A, Wright JE: Inflammatory orbital pseudotumor: A clinicopathological study. Arch Ophthalmol 96:1817–1822, 1978.
4. Crick RP, Hoyle C, Smellie H: The eyes in sarcoidosis. Br J Ophthalmol 45:461–481, 1961.
5. Melmon K, Goldberg J: Sarcoidosis with bilateral exophthalmos as the presenting symptom. Am J Med 33:158, 1962.
6. Snebold NG: Noninfectious orbital inflammations and vasculitis. *In* Albert DM, Jakobiec FA (eds): Principles and Practice of Ophthalmology. Philadelphia, WB Saunders, 1994, pp 1933–1942.
7. Henderson JW, Farrow GM: Orbital Tumors. New York, Thieme-Stratton, 1980.
8. Mauriello JA, Flanagan JC: Pseudotumor and lymphoid tumor: Distinct clinicopathologic entities. Surv Ophthalmol 34:142–148, 1989.
9. Mauriello JA, Flanagan JC: Management of Orbital and Ocular Adnexal Tumors and Inflammations. New York: Field & Wood, 1990, p 20.
10. Mottow LS, Jakobiec FA: Idiopathic inflammatory orbital pseudotumor in childhood. Arch Ophthalmol 96:1410–1417, 1978.
11. Levine MR: Pseudotumor in a three month old child. Paper presented at the spring meeting of the American Society of Ophthalmic Plastic and Reconstructive Surgery, 1984.
12. Dallow RL, Pratt SG: Approach to orbital disorders and frequency of disease occurrence. *In* Albert DM, Jakobiec FA: Principles and Practice of Ophthalmology. Philadelphia, WB Saunders, 1994, pp 1881–1889.
13. Rootman J, Nugent R: The classification and management of acute orbital pseudotumors. Ophthalmology 89:1040–1048, 1982.
14. Bertelsen TI: Acute sclerotenonitis and ocular myositis complicated by papillitis, retinal detachment, and glaucoma. Acta Ophthalmol 38:136–152, 1960.
15. Allen JC, France TD: Pseudotumor of the orbit and peripheral uveitis. J Pediatr Ophthalmol 14:33–34, 1977.
16. Benson WE: Posterior scleritis. Surv Ophthalmol 32:297–316, 1988.
17. Kenny AH, Hafner JN: Ultrasonic evidence of inflammatory thickening and fluid collection within the retrobulbar fascia: The T sign. Ann Ophthalmol 91:1557–1563, 1977.
18. Tychsen L, Tse D, Ossoinig K, et al: Trochleitis with superior oblique myositis. Ophthalmology 91:1075–1079, 1984.
19. Purcel JJ, Taulbee WA: Orbital myositis after upper respiratory tract infection. Arch Ophthalmol 99:437–438, 1981.
20. Slavin ML, Glaser JS: Idiopathic orbital myositis: Report of six cases. Arch Ophthalmol 100:1261–1265, 1982.
21. Trokel SL, Jakobiec FA: Correlation of CT scanning and pathologic features of ophthalmic Graves' disease. Ophthalmology 88:553–564, 1981.
22. Trokel SL, Hilal SK: Submillimeter resolution CT scanning of orbital diseases. Ophthalmology 87:412–417, 1980.
23. Nugent RA, Rootman J, Robertson WD, et al: Acute orbital pseudotumors: Classification and CT features. Am J Radiol 137:957–962, 1981.
24. Mottow-Lippa L, Jakobiec FA, Smith M: Idiopathic pseudotumor in childhood. Ophthalmology 88:565–574, 1981.
25. Edwards MK, Zauel DW, Gilmore RL, et al: Invasive orbital pseudotumor—CT demonstration of extension beyond the orbit. Neuroradiology 23:215–217, 1982.
26. Frohman LP, Kupersmith MJ, Lang J, et al: Intracranial extension and bone destruction in orbital pseudotumor. Arch Ophthalmol 104:380–384, 1986.
27. Berger JR, Snodgrass S, Glaser J, et al: Multifocal fibrosclerosis with hypertrophic intracranial pachymeningitis. Neurology 39: 1345–1349, 1989.
28. Coming DE, Shubi KB, van Eyes J, et al: Familial multifocal fibrosclerosis: Findings suggesting that retroperitoneal fibrosis, mediastinal fibrosis, sclerosing cholangitis, Riedel's thyroiditis, and pseudotumor of the orbit may be different manifestations of a single disease. Arch Ophthalmol 98:1617–1620, 1980.
29. Rootman J: Disease of the Orbit. Philadelphia, JB Lippincott, 1988, pp 143–204.
30. Kennerdell JS: Management of nonspecific inflammatory and lymphoid orbital lesions. Int Ophthalmol Clin 31:7–15, 1991.
31. Warren FA, Kennerdell JS: Orbital fine needle aspiration biopsy. *In* Hornblass A (ed): Oculoplastic, Orbital, and Reconstructive Surgery. Baltimore, Williams & Wilkins, 1990, p 803.
32. Leone CR, Lloyd WC: Treatment protocol for orbital inflammatory disease. Ophthalmology 92:1325–1331, 1985.
33. Mederios LJ, Harris NL: Lymphoid infiltrates of the orbit and conjunctiva: A morphologic and immunophenotypic study of 99 cases. Am J Surg Pathol 13:459–471, 1989.
34. Knowles DM, Jakobiec FA, McNally L, Burke JS: Lymphoid hyperplasia and malignant lymphoma occurring in the ocular adnexa (orbit, conjunctiva, and eyelids): A prospective multiparametric analysis of 108 cases during 1977–1987. Hum Pathol 21:959–973, 1990.
35. McNally L, Jakobiec FA, Knowles DM: Clinical, morphologic, immunophenotypic, and molecular genetic analysis of bilateral ocular adnexal lymphoid neoplasms in 17 patients. Am J Ophthalmol 103:555–568, 1987.
36. Hornblass A, Jakobiec FA, Riefler DM, et al: Orbital lymphoid tumors located predominantly within extraocular muscles. Ophthalmology 94:688–697, 1987.
37. Jakobiec FA, Sacks E, Kronish JW, et al: Multifocal static creamy choroidal infiltrates: An early sign of lymphoid neoplasia. Ophthalmology 94:397–406, 1987.
38. Malis N, Mackman G, Holds J, et al: Simultaneous and bilateral conjunctival and orbital lymphoma presenting as a conjunctival lesion. Ophthalmol Surg 19:662–663, 1988.
39. Jakobiec FA, Yeo JH, Trokel SL, Abbott GF: Combined clinical and computed tomographic diagnosis of primary lacrimal fossa lesions. Am J Ophthalmol 94:785–807, 1982.
40. Yeo JH, Jakobiec FA, Abbott GF, Trokel SL: Combined clinical and computed tomographic diagnosis of orbital lymphoid tumors. Am J Ophthalmol 94:235–245, 1982.
41. Flander AE, Espinosa GA, Marciewicz DA, Howell DD: Orbital lymphoma: Role of CT and MRI. Radiol Clin North Am 25:601–614, 1987.
42. Korneef L: New insights into human orbital connective tissue. Arch Ophthalmol 95:1269–1273, 1977.
43. Patel S, Rootman J: Nodular sclerosing Hodgkin's disease of the orbit. Ophthalmology 90:1433, 1983.
44. Fratkin JD, Shammas HF, Miller SD: Disseminated Hodgkin's disease with bilateral orbital involvement. Arch Ophthalmol 96:102–104, 1978.
45. Stenson S, Ramsay DL: Ocular findings in mycosis fungoides. Arch Ophthalmol 99:272–277, 1981.
46. Jakobiec FA, Iwamoto T, Knowles DM: Ocular adnexal lymphoid tumors: Correlative ultrastructural and immunologic marker studies. Arch Ophthalmol 100:84–98, 1982.
47. Knowles DM, Jakobiec FA: Orbital lymphoid neoplasms: A clinicopathologic study of 60 cases. Cancer 46:576–589, 1980.
48. Rosenberg SA: National Cancer Institute–sponsored study of classification of non-Hodgkin's lymphomas: Summary and description of a working formulation for clinical usage. Cancer 49:2112–2135, 1982.
49. Dick FR: Chronic lymphocytic leukemia and related small lymphocytic malignancies. *In* Jaffe ES (ed): Surgical Pathology of the Lymph Nodes and Related Organs. Philadelphia, WB Saunders, 1994, pp 205–220.
50. Lennert K, Mohri N, Stein H, Kaiserling E: The histopathology of malignant lymphoma. Br J Hematol 31[Suppl]:193–205, 1975.

51. Dutcher T, Fahey J: Immunohistochemical demonstration of intranuclear localization of 18S gamma macroglobulin in macroglobulinemia of Waldenström. Proc Soc Exp Biol Med 193:452–455, 1960.
52. Weisenburger DD, Kim H, Rappaport H: Mantle zone lymphoma: A follicular variant of intermediate lymphocytic lymphoma. Cancer 49:1429–1438, 1982.
53. Bookman MA, Lardelli P, Jaffe ES, et al: Lymphocytic lymphoma of intermediate differentiation: Morphologic, immunophenotypic, and prognostic factors. J NCI 83:742–748, 1990.
54. Burkitt D: A sarcoma involving the jaws in African children. Br J Surg 46:218–223, 1958.
55. Epstein MA, Achong BG, Barr YM: Virus particles in cultured lymphoblasts from Burkitt's lymphoma. Lancet 1:252–253, 1964.
56. Berard C, O'Conor GT, Thomas LB, Torloni H: Histopathological definition of Burkitt's tumor. Bull WHO 40:601–607, 1969.
57. Burkitt D, O'Conor GT: Malignant lymphoma in African children: I. A clinical syndrome. Cancer 14:258–269, 1961.
58. Jakobiec FA, Antonino N, Knowles DM: Genotypic monoclonality in immunophenotypically polyclonal orbital lymphoid tumors: A model of tumor progression in the lymphoid system. Ophthalmology 94:980–994, 1987.
59. Roitt I, Brostoff J, Male D: Immunology, 2nd ed. London, Gower Publishing, 1989.
60. Knowles DM, Jakobiec FA, Halper JP: Immunologic characteristics of ocular adnexal lymphoid neoplasms. Am J Ophthalmol 87:603–619, 1979.
61. McNally L, Jakobiec FA, Burke JS, Knowles DM: A prospective, correlative clinical, morphologic, and immunophenotypic investigation of 100 ocular adnexal lymphoid neoplasms. Lab Invest 56:49A, 1987.
62. Jakobiec FA, Font RL: Orbital lymphoid tumors. *In* Spencer WH (ed): Ophthalmic Pathology: An Atlas and Textbook. Philadelphia, WB Saunders, 1986, p 2663.
63. Southern EM: Detection of specific sequences among DNA fragments separated by gel electrophoresis. J Mol Biol 98:503–517, 1975.
64. Tonegawa S: Somatic generation of antibody diversity. Nature 302:575–581, 1983.
65. Hoo L, Kronenburg M, Hunkapiller T: T cell antigen receptors and the immunoglobulin supergene family. Cell 40:225–229, 1985.
66. Cossman J, Uppenkamp M, Sundeen J, et al: Molecular genetics and the diagnosis of lymphoma. Arch Pathol Lab Med 112:112–127, 1988.
67. Waldmann TW, Davis MM, Bongiovanni KF, Forsmeyer SJ: Rearrangements of genes for the antigen receptor on T cells as markers of lineage and clonality in human lymphoid neoplasms. N Engl J Med 313:776–783, 1985.
68. Jakobiec FA, Neri A, Knowles DM: Genotypic monoclonality in immunophenotypically polyclonal orbital lymphoid tumors: A model of tumor progression in the lymphoid system. Ophthalmology 94:980–994, 1987.
69. Mederios LJ, Andrade RE, Harris NL, Cossman J: Lymphoid infiltrates of the orbit and conjunctiva: Comparison of immunologic and gene rearrangement data. Lab Invest 660:614, 1989.
70. Jakobiec FA, McLean I, Font RL: Clinicopathologic characteristics of orbital lymphoid hyperplasia. Ophthalmology 86:948–960, 1979.
71. Mederios LJ, Harris NL: Immunohistologic analysis of small lymphocytic infiltrates of the orbit and conjunctiva. Hum Pathol 21:1126–1131, 1990.
72. Jakobiec FA, Knowles DM: An overview of ocular adnexal lymphoid tumors. Trans Am Ophthalmol Soc 87:420–444, 1989.
73. Rodman RM, Font RL: Orbital involvement in multiple myeloma. Review of the literature and report of three cases. Arch Ophthalmol 87:30–35, 1972.
74. Rubin PAD, Jakobiec FA: Orbital and ocular lymphoid neoplasms. *In* Albert DM, Jakobiec FA (eds): Principles and Practice of Ophthalmology. Philadelphia, WB Saunders, 1994, p 2015.
75. Bessell EM, Henk JM, Wright JE, et al: Orbital and conjunctival lymphoma treatment and prognosis. Radiother Oncol 13:2237–2244, 1988.
76. Reddy EK, Bhata P, Evans RG: Primary orbital lymphomas. Int J Radiat Oncol Biol Phys 15:1239–1241, 1988.

CHAPTER 89

Pseudotumors

Will Harms

Pseudotumors of the orbit comprise a variable and indistinct group of diseases. Birch-Hirschfeld[1] is credited with being the first to use the term *pseudotumor* to describe the occurrence of this group of orbital entities. He defined it as proptosis that appeared to be caused by a neoplasm but resulted instead from orbital inflammation. He included three types of "pseudotumor" in his classification: (1) proptosis that resolves spontaneously without surgery, (2) proptosis that at operation demonstrates an orbital mass that when sampled shows nonspecific chronic inflammation, and (3) exophthalmos that at the time of surgery demonstrated no causative orbital mass but a sample of orbital tissue that shows nonspecific chronic inflammation.

The term *pseudotumor* has been broadly applied and generally lacks precision beyond that of *pseudoneoplasm*—the determination that proptosis, thought to be caused by a neoplastic orbital mass, is due to a nonspecific orbital inflammatory process rather than a true neoplasm. As such it is essentially a diagnosis made by exclusion of more well-defined orbital phenomena.

It may be most appropriate to restrict the usage of the term pseudotumor to describe idiopathic, nonspecific, chronic, polymorphous, orbital inflammatory processes that may be localized as a distinguishable mass or may be diffuse, and for which no local or systemic cause can be identified.[2, 3] This would exclude orbit inflammation due to thyroid-related orbitopathy; neoplastic processes; unsuspected infections from bacteria, fungi, or parasites; nonresorbing blood products; ruptured dermoid cysts; retained orbital foreign bodies; amyloidosis; sinusitis; sarcoidosis, tuberculosis; syphilis; and well-defined vasculitides (such as Wegener's granulomatosis and polyarteritis nodosa).[4]

The symptomatology of orbital inflammation in general depends on the acuteness of the disease process. In an acute process such as idiopathic inflammatory orbitopathy, the prominent presenting symptoms are usually pain and proptosis developing over several hours to days. Periorbital edema and erythema, conjunctival injection and chemosis, eyelid ptosis, extraocular motility disturbances, reduced visual acuity, and intraocular inflammation may also be present.

The presentation of a subacute inflammatory process generally occurs over weeks or months. The same collection of symptoms may occur, but their quality, quantity, and sequence of progression is more moderate. Chronic inflammatory ocular disease may not be associated with significant symptomatology early in its presentation, though, over time, proptosis, motility disturbances, and eyelid and conjunctival edema will likely occur. Pain is not commonly a symptom of chronic orbital phenomena.[5–8]

The spectrum of presentations of idiopathic orbital inflammatory pseudotumor is broad. Any site or tissue or group of tissues within the orbit can be involved in the inflammatory process. Myositis, trochleitis, scleritis, tenonitis, dacryoadenitis, or perioptic neuritis describe inflammation of specific tissues and structures.[6] If the inflammatory process is localized to the superior orbital fissure or cavernous sinus, the Tolosa-Hunt syndrome may be described.[9] In addition to localized or diffuse involvement of the orbit, the inflammatory process may cause bony destruction and extend intracranially or to adjacent sinuses.[7, 10, 11]

CLINICAL MANIFESTATIONS

The most common presenting features of idiopathic orbital inflammatory pseudotumor are pain and proptosis. These symptoms usually present and progress over a few hours to days. Additionally, conjunctival chemosis and injection (particularly over the extraocular muscle insertions), periorbital edema, and ptosis may be present. Occasionally, the symptoms evolve over a longer period of time or painless, quiet proptosis may occur. Depending on the specific orbital tissues involved, the prominence of the presenting signs may vary. If the lacrimal gland is the site of inflammation, proptosis may well be lacking and a painful mass may be palpable in the lateral eyelid. Disturbances of ocular motility are common when inflammation occurs diffusely in the orbit and involves the superior orbital fissure, or the muscle or muscles directly but are uncommon when the inflammatory process is more localized.[2, 7, 12, 13] Visual loss, although unusual, may occur secondary to intraocular inflammation or to perineuritis of the ocular nerve.[2] Patients with pseudotumor may also complain of generalized feelings of malaise and distress.[14]

The occurrence of pseudotumor is most common in the third through fifth decades but can affect children as well as those in their 70s.[15] Males and females are equally affected, and there is no racial preference. Bilateral disease has been reported but is rare. Infrequently, the inflammation may even alternate between one orbit and the other.[16] There may also be occasional presentations of multiple recurrences or of resistant disease despite appropriate therapy.

Given that the diagnosis of idiopathic inflammatory orbital pseudotumor is one of exclusion, several distinctive clinical presentations have been described. *Dacryoadenitis* is an inflammatory enlargement of the lacrimal gland in the superior lateral aspect of the orbit.[6, 13] The mass is usually palpable and tender and results in an S-shaped curve of the upper eyelid on the affected side. If the mass effect is great enough, inferonasal proptosis may result. A similar presentation may be manifest in infections of the lacrimal gland, sarcoidosis, Sjögren's syndrome, lymphoma, and neoplasm. It is particularly important to differentiate a neoplastic process, involving the lacrimal gland, from inflammation, on computed tomography. Dacryoadenitis usually shows somewhat indistinct enlargement of the lacrimal gland in all dimensions with extension of the inflammatory process into proximate orbital soft tissue. The adjacent bony structures are usually uninvolved.[5, 13] A neoplastic process involving the lacrimal gland is frequently nodular and more distinct, and erosion of bone is common.

A localized inflammatory process may occur more deeply in the orbit as a solitary "neoplastic" phenomena and is termed *focal idiopathic orbital pseudotumor*. The characteristic presenting sign is proptosis.[6, 7] Depending on the acuteness of the process, periorbital edema and conjunctival injection and chemosis may or may not be present. Extraocular muscle involvement from inflammation or secondary edema may cause diplopia. Again, neoplastic orbital processes must be excluded when considering this clinical picture.

Superior orbital fissure and orbital apex inflammatory syndrome results from idiopathic inflammation of the orbital apex. The distinctive presenting signs are a boring, persistent retrobulbar pain and pronounced restriction of ocular motility.[17, 18] An afferent pupillary defect and decreased vision frequently are present and secondary to perineural inflammation or edema. There are usually few other signs of inflammation. Periorbital edema, chemosis, and proptosis are usually minimally present. Evaluation of the orbit by computed tomography usually reveals a diffuse inflammatory process in the posterior orbit with variable anterior extension.[5, 10]

The Tolosa-Hunt syndrome is a specific entity involving idiopathic inflammation of the superior orbital fissure and the cavernous sinus.[9, 17–20] The presentation is acute and generally unilateral. All structures passing through the superior orbital fissure are involved, including the third, fourth, and sixth cranial nerves and the first division of the fifth as well as the superior orbital vein. The patient with this syndrome presents complaining of headache and a deep, unrelenting pain.[18] Chemosis and periorbital edema result from venous compromise.[20] Involvement of the sympathetic innervation to the pupil may result in mydriasis and decreased pupillary motility. It is thought that the inflammatory process begins in the cavernous sinus and progresses anteriorly to the superior orbital fissure. Because of the cavernous sinus involvement, structures passing through the inferior orbital fissure and the optic nerve may also be affected.

When the inflammatory process affects primarily the anterior globe, especially the sclera, Tenon's capsule, and the surrounding orbital tissues, the entity may be described as *acute anterior orbital inflammation*. The patient typically presents with pain that may radiate to the temple, eyelid edema, conjunctival and episcleral injection, chemosis, and decreased vision. The reduced vision may either be due to uveitis, possibly associated with an exudative retinal detachment, or to optic nerve inflammation.[5, 7, 21, 22] To be considered in the differential diagnosis of anterior orbital inflammation are rupture of a dermoid cyst, hemorrhage from lymphangioma, scleritis, rhabdomyosarcoma, leukemic infiltration, orbital cellulitis, and collagen vascular disease.[5] If uveal effusion and associated exudative retinal detachment are prominent findings, Wegener's granulomatosis, uveal effusion syndrome, choroidal melanoma, metastatic disease, or lymphoma should be considered in the differential diagnosis.[23]

Diffuse idiopathic orbital inflammation presents with similar but generally more severe symptoms as compared with anterior orbital inflammation. In addition to significant visual loss secondary to optic nerve involvement and exudative retinal detachment, limitation of extraocular motility and possibly diplopia are prominent symptoms. Erosion of bone and extension into adjacent sinus cavities can also rarely occur.[5, 10, 11] The differential diagnosis includes the consideration of orbital cellulitis, sarcoidosis, and orbital neoplastic processes.

Another idiopathic orbital inflammatory phenomena, *orbital myositis*, presents as diplopia, painful ocular motility, and focal conjunctival injection overlying the involved extraocular muscle.[7, 16, 24] Eyelid edema, ptosis, proptosis, and multiple extraocular muscle involvement are present much less commonly. The superior and medial rectus muscles are the most common to be involved, and forced duction testing is usually positive. The differential diagnoses include particularly thyroid orbitopathy and metastatic infiltration of an extraocular muscle and also infectious infiltration, myasthenia gravis, and arteriovenous malformations. Thyroid and metastatic involvement are usually confined exclusively to the muscle belly while idiopathic orbital inflammation involves the entire muscle, tendon, and adjacent fat.[25, 26] Additionally, thyroid-related orbitopathy and metastatic infiltration are rarely associated with pain. Thyroid function testing, computed tomography, clinical evaluation, and pharmaceutical testing are all helpful in making the diagnosis. Although most commonly idiopathic, orbital myositis has also been reported to occur following upper respiratory tract infections and in association with collagen vascular diseases, periarteritis nodosa, and myocarditis.

Idiopathic inflammation affecting primarily orbital arteries and arterioles has been termed *orbital angiitis*.[6, 8] The acute inflammation involving the small vessels of the orbit and adjacent connective tissue is similar to that seen in connective tissue disease but without systemic involvement. Patients present with nonspecific signs and symptoms typical of acute inflammation, including pain, eyelid edema and ptosis, proptosis, chemosis, and conjunctival injection. Histopathologically, the inflammatory infiltrate consists of neutrophils, lymphocytes, monocytes, and plasma cells. Destruction and necrosis of vessel walls leads to perivascular hemorrhage.

Nonspecific inflammation of the orbital veins and venules has been termed *orbital thrombophlebitis*. Presenting signs include acute pain, ocular motility disturbances, chemosis, and decreased vision.[5] Additionally, spontaneous orbital hemorrhage is common and thrombosis of the central retinal artery has also been reported.[27] The orbital pain is somewhat characteristic of this condition. It is unilateral and boring in nature and is more intense on eye movements and exposure to cold temperatures. Orbital thrombophlebitis, although localize to the orbit, may be associated with systemic diseases, including connective tissue diseases, polyarteritis nodosa, mucormycosis, and various parasitic infestations.

Histopathologic evaluation of tissue from orbital thrombophlebitis demonstrates a predominance of neutrophils and lymphocytes but without any significant granulomatous component. The inflammation is centered around veins, is usually segmental, and may be associated with thrombosis. As the inflammation resolves, fibrous tissue replaces smooth muscle in the wall of affected veins.[5]

REFERENCES

1. Birch-Hirschfeld A: Die Krankheiten der Orbita. *In* Graefe A, Saemisch T (eds): Handbuch der Gesamten Augenheilkunden. Berlin, Springer, 1930.
2. Blodi F, Gass JD: Inflammatory pseudotumour of the orbit. Br J Ophthalmol 52:79, 1968.
3. Coop M: Pseudotumour of the orbit. Br J Ophthalmol 45:513, 1961.
4. Jakobiec R, Jones I: Orbital inflammations. *In* Duane's Clinical Ophthalmology, vol 2, chap 35. Philadelphia, JB Lippincott, 1994.
5. Jakobiec FA, Font RL: Orbit. *In* Spencer WH (ed): Ophthalmic Pathology, 3rd ed, vol 3. Philadelphia, WB Saunders, 1986.
6. Kennerdell JS, Dresner SC: The nonspecific orbital inflammatory syndromes. Surv Ophthalmol 29:93, 1984.
7. Nugent RA, Rootman J, Robertson WD, et al: Acute orbital pseudotumors: Classification and CT features. AJR 137:957, 1981.
8. Jakobiec F: Orbital inflammations and lymphoid tumors. Proc New Orleans Acad Med 52, 1982.
9. Aron-Rosa D, Doyon D, Salamon G, Michotey P: Tolosa-Hunt syndrome. Ann Ophthalmol 10:1161, 1978.
10. Edwards M, Zanel D, Gilkor R, Muller J: Invasive orbital pseudotumor: CT demonstration of extension beyond orbit. Neuroradiology 23:215, 1982.
11. Eshagian J, Anderson R. Sinus involvement in inflammatory orbital pseudotumor. Arch Ophthalmol 99:627–630, 1981.
12. Frohman LP, Kupersmith MJ, Lang J, et al: Intracranial extension and bone destruction in orbital pseudotumor. Arch Ophthalmol 104:380, 1986.
13. Jakobiec FA, Yeo JH, Trokel SL, et al: Combined clinical and computed tomographic diagnosis of lacrimal fossa lesions. Am J Ophthalmol 94:785, 1982.
14. Jellinek EH: The orbital pseudotumor syndrome and its differentiation from endocrine exophthalmos. Brain 92:35, 1969.
15. Jakobiec F, Mottow L: Pediatric orbital pseudotumor. *In* Jakobiec F (ed): Ocular and Adnexal Tumors. Birmingham, AL, Aesculapius, 1978.
16. Keane JR: Alternating proptosis. A case report of acute orbital myositis defined by the computerized tomographic scan. Arch Neurol 34:642, 1977.
17. Fowler T, Earl C, McAllister V, McDonald W: Tolosa-Hunt syndrome. Br J Ophthalmol 59:149, 1975.
18. Kline L: Tolosa-Hunt syndrome. Surv Ophthalmol 27:79, 1982.
19. Andersson BI: Unusual course of painful ophthalmoplegia. Report of a case. Acta Ophthalmol 58:841, 1980.
20. Spirn FH, Wolintz AH, Tenner MS, Gombos GM: Tolosa-Hunt syndrome. Ann Ophthalmol 7:1087, 1975.
21. Hatsuda TA, Tanaka J: Bilateral necrotizing scleritis. Am J Ophthalmol 86:710, 1978.
22. Spoor TC, Hartel WC: Orbital myositis. J Clin Neuro Ophthalmol 3:67, 1983.
23. Bullen CL, Liesegang TJ, McDonald TJ, DeRemee RS: Ocular complications of Wegener's granulomatosis. Ophthalmology 90:279, 1983.
24. Ross WH: Myositic pseudotumor of the orbit. Can J Ophthalmol 18:199, 1983.
25. Trokel S, Jilal S: Recognition and differential diagnosis of enlarged extraocular muscles in computed tomography. Am J Ophthalmol 87:503, 1979.
26. Trokel S, Jakobiec R: Correlation of CT scanning and pathologic features of ophthalmic Graves' disease. Ophthalmology 88:553, 1981.
27. Zimmerman L, Rodgers J: Idiopathic thrombophlebitis of orbital veins simulating primary tumor of orbit. Trans Am Acad Ophthalmol Otolaryngol 6:609, 1957.

CHAPTER 90

Orbital Decompression for Graves' Orbitopathy

Myron Tanenbaum

Graves' orbitopathy is an inflammatory disorder affecting the orbital and periocular tissues. Hallmark features of this condition include exophthalmos, lid retraction, and enlarged extraocular muscles. More severe forms can involve visual loss due to compressive optic neuropathy. Patients with Graves' orbitopathy can be hyperthyroid, hypothyroid, or euthyroid based on appropriate thyroid laboratory study.

The material in this chapter includes indications and goals for surgery, orbital decompression techniques, postoperative management, and complications of surgery. The main emphasis is on surgical recommendations for orbital decompression. The topic of orbital decompression for Graves' orbitopathy is an evolving one. Decompression techniques will no doubt continue to evolve in the future.

PREOPERATIVE EVALUATION

A thorough discussion of the signs and symptoms of Graves' orbitopathy, as well as the laboratory evaluation of thyroid abnormalities, is presented in Chapter 46.

The first part of the evaluation of the patient for orbital decompression pertains to history. The surgeon must be sure that the signs and symptoms of the patient's Graves' orbitopathy are remaining stable over at least a 6-month period. The patient should be questioned regarding the prominence of the eyes, the degree of eyelid retraction, and any new or changing symptoms of double vision. The patient should be asked to bring in old photographs when necessary. Other members of the family or close friends can be contacted for further impressions. In the absence of compressive neuropathy, visual loss, or severe exposure keratopathy, all other patients being considered for decompression can be approached on a relatively elective basis. If necessary, the surgeon should follow this patient for 6 to 12 months to verify that the ophthalmic findings of Graves' orbitopathy are remaining stable.

Visual function must, of course, be thoroughly assessed. This includes visual acuity, color vision testing, and formal visual field testing in both eyes. Patients with significant ocular irritation, excess tearing, and exposure keratopathy may have diminished visual acuity. The examiner must separate these etiologies of decreased visual acuity from compressive optic neuropathy. It is here that color vision testing and formal visual field perimetry can detect abnormal optic nerve function. The complete examination should, of course, include pupillary testing to detect a possible afferent pupillary defect and, after dilation, examination of the fundus with specific attention to the optic nerve and posterior pole of the fundus. The demonstration of delayed or decreased visual evoked response may be very useful in select patients in confirming a diagnosis of optic neuropathy.

Careful measurement of the amount of exophthalmos is very important. The standard for this is through use of an exophthalmometer. The examiner must be cautious to always examine the patient using the same base measurement for that particular patient, that is, the distance from outer canthus to outer canthus.

Careful documentation and examination should be made of the eyelid position, amount of lid lag, and lagophthalmos on each side. The motility examination should thoroughly document the degree, if any, of restrictive strabismus, symptomatic diplopia, or both. Photographs are helpful in documenting the amount of exophthalmos, the amount of eyelid retraction, and any motility abnormalities. Photographs can be taken from a frontal view, a side view, as well as a coronal view with the photographer standing over the patient. Photographs can be used to demonstrate the patient's motility pattern in various fields of gaze.

Computed tomographic scans of the orbits in the axial and coronal views remain an important part of the preoperative workup in candidates for orbital decompression. They anatomically demonstrate the posterior muscle belly enlargement and the actual degree of crowding and compression of the optic nerve at the orbital apex. Computed tomographic scans are invaluable for imaging the periorbital sinuses, especially the anatomy of the ethmoidal air cells and their relation to the orbit and orbital apex. The view of the sinuses, of course, rule out any acute or chronic sinus disease—maxillary sinusitis would typically require treatment before embarking on antroethmoidal decompression surgery. Overall, these scans remain a much more useful preoperative test than magnetic resonance imaging. Orbital echography is of great value in evaluating extraocular muscle size and in diagnosing subtle cases of Graves' orbitopathy. Although diagnostically of great use, its role in assessing candidates for orbital decompression is less important.

INDICATIONS FOR SURGERY

The indications for orbital decompressive surgery include decreased vision associated with compressive optic neuropathy, severe exophthalmos, corneal exposure, and significant unilateral asymmetry. Compressive optic neuropathy has been a well-established indication for surgical decompression of the orbit. I would emphasize for the reader that the "other" indications for orbital decompression that do not involve compressive neuropathy are nonetheless quite legitimate. Many patients with severe lid retraction and exophthalmos will ultimately do better, from the standpoint of eyelid repair, if surgical decompression is first performed. Severe disfiguring unilateral exophthalmos, significant bilateral exophthalmos with exposure, irritation, tearing, and entrapment of the eyelids behind the globe are all significant functional problems for the patient. With an operation of this magnitude, however, the goals and indications for surgery, as well as the potential risks and benefits of surgery, must be carefully evaluated in the context of each individual patient.

For patients with compressive optic neuropathy, the foremost goal of surgery is posterior apical orbital decompression to relieve pressure and restore vision. The potential untoward side effects of a worsened postoperative motility imbalance must remain a secondary consideration. In the patient with significant exophthalmos with good visual function and good motility, the goals of decompression are to achieve appropriate retrodisplacement of the globe with all possible efforts made to avoid inducing a postoperative motility imbalance. The surgical techniques presented in this chapter cover pertinent details related to these specific surgical goals.

OVERVIEW TO SURGERY

In its simplest terms, the orbital tissues are encompassed by four walls: the orbital roof, the lateral orbital wall, the medial orbital wall, and the orbital floor. Orbital decompressive surgery has been attempted by means of removal of each of the individual orbital walls or by various combinations of these walls (Fig. 90–1).[1–4] Additional surgical decompressive efforts have involved removal of the intraorbital fat, either through both extraperiosteal posterior orbitotomies as well as trans-lid anterior orbitotomies.[5,6] The surgeon must try to clearly

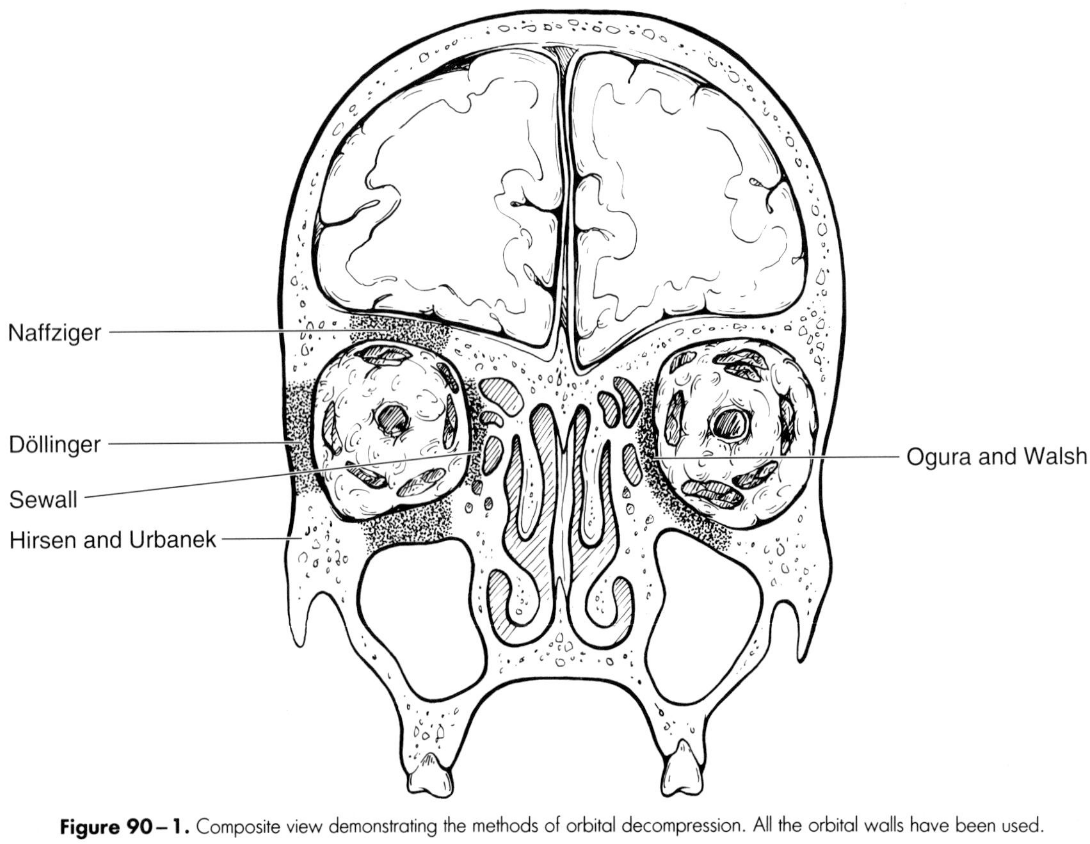

Figure 90–1. Composite view demonstrating the methods of orbital decompression. All the orbital walls have been used.

analyze the anatomic and pathophysiologic problem of each patient and make a logical treatment decision based on this assessment. For compressive optic neuropathy, the single important goal of the surgery is to achieve posterior decompression of the orbital apex. From the list of basic decompression choices just presented, the clear and logical choice is to achieve apical decompression by removal of the medial ethmoidal structures and medial orbital wall. No other side of the orbit offers such ready access as the medial wall (transconjunctival,[7] transorbital,[8] transantral,[9] Lynch incision,[10] coronal flap,[11] and transnasal endoscopic[12]).

For significant symptomatic exophthalmos with compliant orbital tissues, the two-wall antroethmoidal decompression remains my procedure of choice. In patients with significant bilateral exophthalmos, the orbital decompression surgery is typically performed on both sides at the same time.

Conventional antroethmoidal decompression in patients with severe restrictive motility problems and noncompliant orbital tissues can yield highly disappointing results. The surgery may not achieve the desired retrodisplacement effect or the postoperative hypoglobus, and severe motility problems may be quite undesirable.[13,14] In these patients, orbital expansion techniques may be the best choice.

ORBITAL COMPLIANCE

The compliance of the orbital tissues in any given patient with Graves' orbitopathy will have a significant impact on the results of surgical decompression. Preoperatively, these patients tend to have prominent exophthalmos, good ocular motility with little or no diplopia symptoms, and a full range of extraocular motion or perhaps mild limitation in upward gaze and abduction only. Digital pressure on the globes results in a ready amount of retrodisplacement, and the globes can be seen to spontaneously retrodisplace when these patients are changed from an upright to a supine position. These patients typically have prominent fatty tissue prolapse into the upper and lower eyelids. Patients with good compliance of the orbital tissues will tend to show the best postoperative globe retrodisplacement after surgical decompression.

The patient with good compliance of the orbital tissues is in marked contradistinction to the patient in whom the orbital tissues have extensive fibrosis and thus poor compliance. The extraocular motility shows a severe restrictive pattern in all fields of gaze, and these patients often have severe symptomatic diplopia. Intraocular pressures typically show a significant increase when measured in upward gaze versus intraocular pressure in primary gaze. Palpation of the orbital reveals indurated noncompliant tissues, and ballottement of the globes shows minimal ability to retrodisplace them. Surgical decompression in these patients would likely have much less retrodisplacement effect yet carries a significant risk of worsening the motility imbalance (i.e., the globes sink down and in after antroethmoidal decompression).

The previous examples illustrate the obvious extremes of "good compliance" and "poor compliance." In reality, many patients fall between these two extremes. Clinical estimation or resistance to retropulsion is notoriously unreliable,[15] and more accurate means of reassuring these forces are not yet widely available.[16] Orbital compliance influences the management decisions in Graves' orbitopathy patients, and for now, the assessment of orbital compliance remains relatively crude.

TRANSORBITAL ANTROETHMOIDAL ORBITAL DECOMPRESSION

The transorbital approach provides excellent surgical exposure for the two-wall or antroethmoidal orbital decompression. I generally prefer an inferior fornix transconjunctival incision combined with a lower eyelid lateral canthotomy and cantholysis. Very similar excellent transorbital exposure can be achieved through a subciliary transcutaneous incision as well. The transorbital antroethmoidal decompression is best suited for exophthalmic patients with good motility and compliant orbital tissues. This technique can usually achieve 4 to 6 mm of retrodisplacement of the globe postoperatively. This transorbital approach to decompression has a much less adverse effect on ocular motility than surgical decompression procedures of the posterior orbit.

Preoperatively, orbital CT scans are obtained to evaluate the patient for possible sinus disease or variations in the normal anatomy (Fig. 90–2). Significant blood loss is a potential risk of this surgery, and attention must be paid to any blood clotting abnormalities, including medicines that affect clotting. Aspirin is typically discontinued 10 to 14 days before orbital decompression. The night before surgery, the patient is given oral corticosteroids and decongestants to help reduce mucosal inflammation and edema.

The surgery is performed under general anesthesia with endotracheal intubation. The patient should be positioned in a reverse Trendelenburg position with the head elevated. All arm boards are omitted from the operating room table to allow the surgeon better positioning and mobility. Lidocaine 2% with 1 : 100,000 epinephrine and hyaluronidase is infiltrated transconjunctivally along the floor of the orbit, over the lateral canthal region, and transconjunctivally into the ethmoidal sinus. An adequate amount of time is allowed to elapse for the vasoconstrictive effect of the epinephrine. It is mandatory that the surgeon wear a fiberoptic headlight during this procedure. A nasal speculum and bayonet forceps are used to pack the nasal cavity on the operative side, or on both sides if the surgery is bilateral. Nasal packing is placed up into the superior nasal cavity and the packing

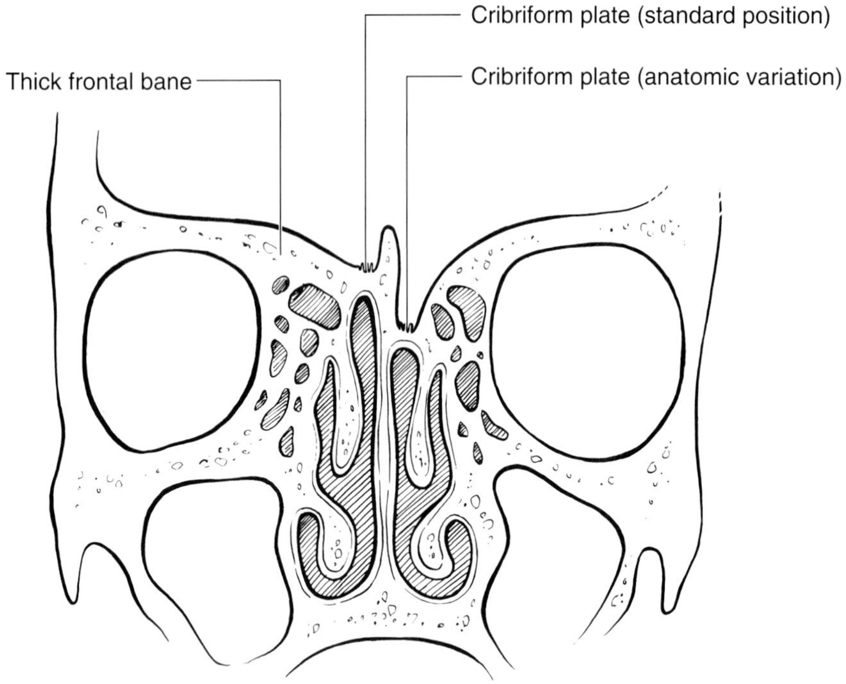

Figure 90 – 2. Coronal view of the anatomic variations or the cribriform plate in relation to the orbits and ethmoidal air cells.

continued all the way to the tip of the inferior turbinate. I prefer plain gauze packing soaked in a mixture of 0.25% phenylephrine (Neo-Synephrine) and oxymetazoline (Afrin). Nasal packing gauze soaked in 4% cocaine solution is also suitable. Moistened gelatin sponge (Gelfoam) pads are helpful for protecting the cornea during surgery because protective scleral shells often do not remain in place in these patients with severe exophthalmos.

To begin the inferior fornix approach, a lateral canthal incision line is made with a marking pen and a no. 15 blade is used to perform the superficial lateral canthotomy. The needle-tip unipolar electrosurgical unit (e.g., Bovie) is used to complete the lateral canthotomy and inferior cantholysis of the inferior crus of the lateral canthal tendon (Fig. 90 – 3). Small rake retractors are used to evert the lower eyelid and hold it down under tension (Fig. 90 – 4). The needle-tip unit is used to incise the inferior fornix conjunctiva and lower eyelid retractors (Fig. 90 – 5). At this point, somewhat larger rake retractors can typically be used to evert the lower eyelid downward. An exuberant amount of prolapsing inferior orbital fatty tissue may be encountered at this point. If excessive fatty tissue obscures the surgical field, it may be clamped, excised, and carefully cauterized. This partial debulking of fatty tissue will allow the surgeon to proceed with less interference. Blunt dissection with malleable ribbon retractors is performed down to the level of the inferior orbital rim. The needle-tip electrosurgical unit is used to

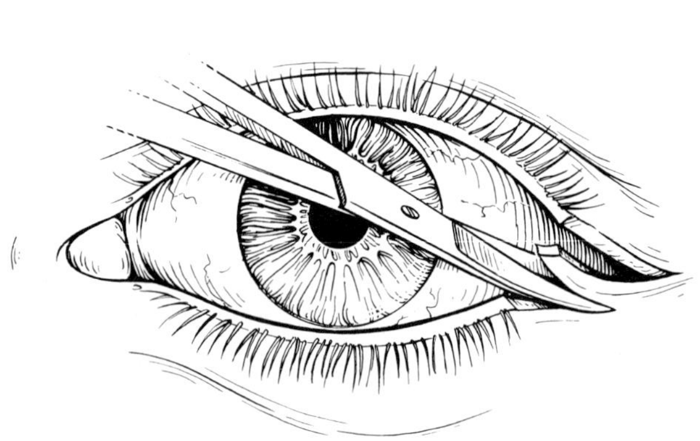

Figure 90 – 3. A lateral canthotomy and inferior cantholysis is performed.

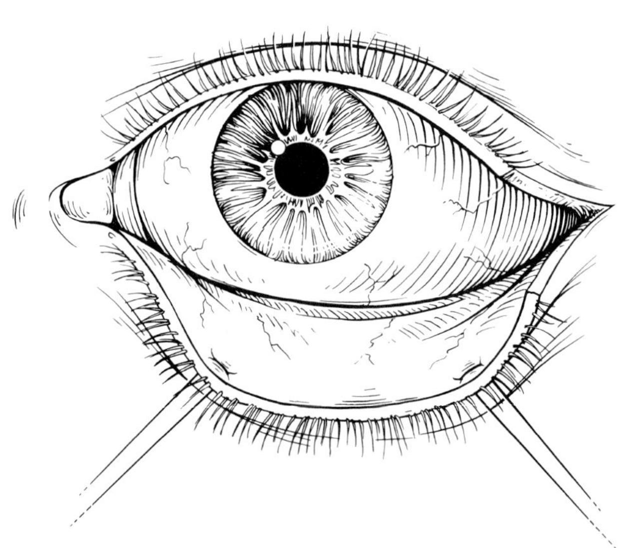

Figure 90 – 4. The lower lid is reflected downward to expose the inferior fornix conjunctiva.

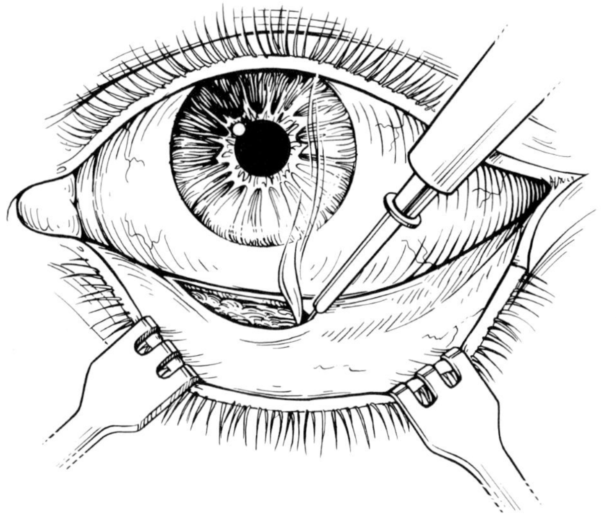

Figure 90–5. The needle-tip unipolar cutting-cautery unit is used to incise the inferior fornix conjunctiva and lower lid retractors.

incise the periosteum across the entire width of the inferior orbital rim. A sharp periosteal elevator is used to reflect the periosteum and periorbita off of the entire floor of the orbit as well as off the inferior ethmoidal area medially (Fig. 90–6). Great care must be taken anteromedially to avoid injuring the lacrimal sac or nasolacrimal duct. The inferior oblique muscle originates at a posterolateral point adjacent to the nasolacrimal canal. This muscle insertion may be disinserted carefully to enhance exposure. Along the medial orbital wall, the periosteal and periorbital reflection should extend to but not beyond the frontoethmoidal bony suture line. This represents the superior boundary beyond which medial orbital wall and ethmoidal sinus tissue should not be resected. Dissection above this level could injure the cribriform plate region and risk cerebrospinal fluid leakage.

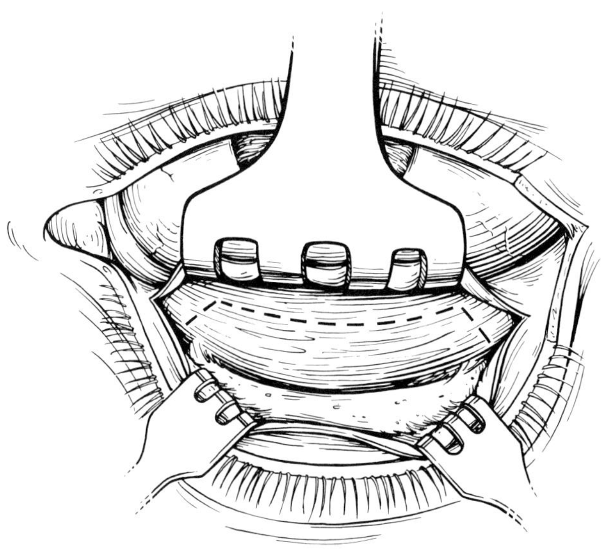

Figure 90–6. Retractors are used to maintain good exposure of the orbit after elevation of periosteum from the orbital floor and medial wall.

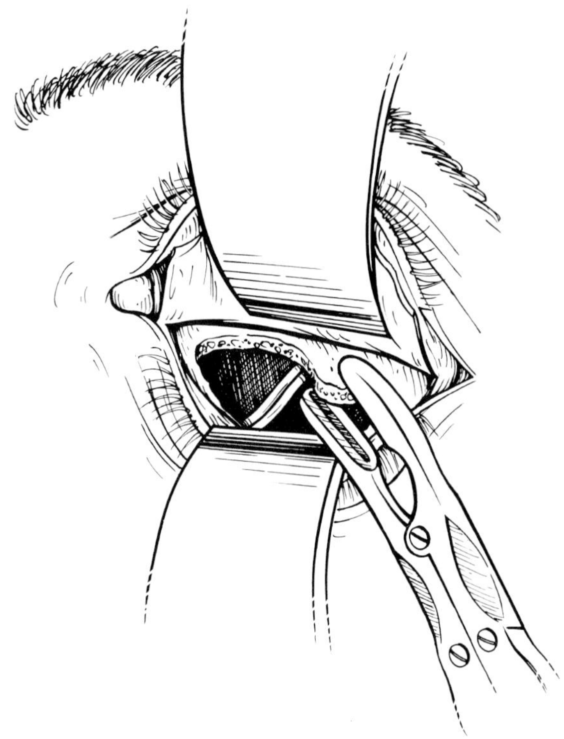

Figure 90–7. Rongeurs are used to remove bone from the orbital floor. Care is taken to avoid trauma to the infraorbital neurovascular bundle. The orbital floor is removed before performing medial orbital wall and ethmoidal sinus resection.

The bone removal most easily begins in the thin medial portion of the floor of the orbit. A thin osteotome and mallet is used to puncture through this very thin portion of the orbital floor. Pituitary forceps and Kerrison rongeurs are used to remove the floor of the orbit in piecemeal fashion (Fig. 90–7). The infraorbital neurovascular complex appears as a dark line coursing through the floor of the orbit in a posterolateral-to-anteromedial direction. For decompression of exophthalmos in the patient with good motility, the surgeon should remove bone up to and overlying the infero-orbital neurovascular complex, but the remainder of the lateral portion of the floor of the orbit should remain intact. An aggressive resection of the entire orbital floor would greatly increase the chances of developing an unwanted hypoglobus postoperatively. There is a moderately thick junction of bone between the orbital floor and the medial orbital wall. A portion of this junctional bone must be resected to achieve adequate exposure of the remainder of the medial orbital wall and ethmoidal sinus air cells. I have typically left the anterior portion of this bony strut in place for theoretical support considerations for the orbital tissues and the globe. The pituitary forceps is used to proceed with the ethmoidectomy. A suction-cautery instrument is helpful for controlling some of the oozing of blood from the ethmoidal air cell mucosa. The ethmoidal sinus mucosa itself should be resected along with bony ethmoidal air cells. From this anterior transorbital approach, it is difficult to complete a full ethmoidal air cell resection back to the actual orbital apex. In the exophthalmic patient without compressive neuropathy, resecting the majority of the medial ethmoidal sinus is adequate. The following sections in this chapter describe additional specific techniques for decompression of the posterior portions of the orbit. With the orbital floor, medial orbital wall, and ethmoidal sinus spaces resected, a few minutes is spent obtaining hemostasis. It is helpful to simply pack the single unified ethmoidal sinus space with a hemostatic substance. Commonly used materials include oxidized cellulose (Surgicel) packing or 1/2-inch plain gauze soaked in thrombin or soaked in 1:100,000 epinephrine solution. Several minutes waiting time is typically adequate to significantly help with hemostasis of this region. If the orbital decompression is bilateral, this ethmoidal packing is left in place while the surgeon proceeds with decompression on the opposite orbit. After removal of hemostatic packing, attention is turned to opening the periorbita. For bilateral cases, it is preferable that bone removal has been performed on both sides so that "simultaneous" openings can then be made in the periorbita of each orbit.

A fine-toothed forceps is used to tent the periorbita, and a sharp Westcott scissors is used to make an incision. Periorbital fat will typically prolapse through this small incision. A thin malleable retractor or thin periosteal elevator can be inserted into this hole and help further elevate the more posterior portions of periorbita. A no. 15 blade can be used to cut down directly onto the malleable ribbon, or a Westcott scissors sharp blade can be inserted between the malleable ribbon and the periorbita. Relaxing incisions are made in the periorbita. A hemostat is then used to grasp and tear the periorbital opening (Fig. 90–8). I have not found that making multiple slits in the periorbita is any more accurate in quantitating or titrating the decompression effect. With the periorbita opened, gentle pressure is placed directly on the globe to

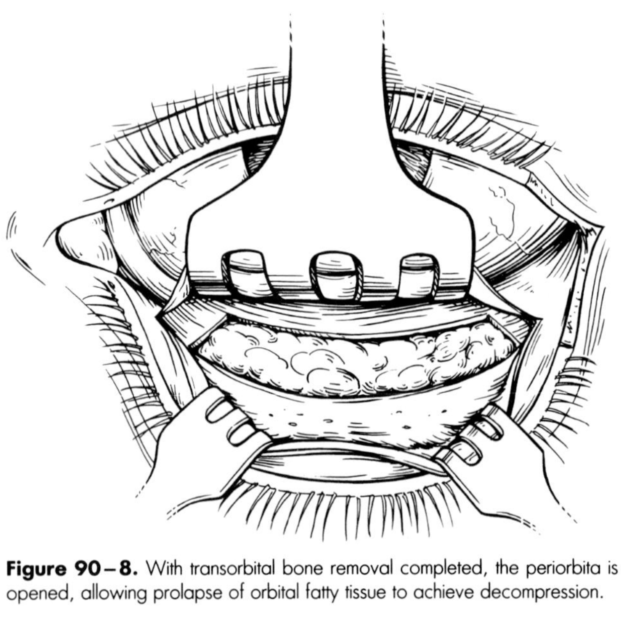

Figure 90–8. With transorbital bone removal completed, the periorbita is opened, allowing prolapse of orbital fatty tissue to achieve decompression.

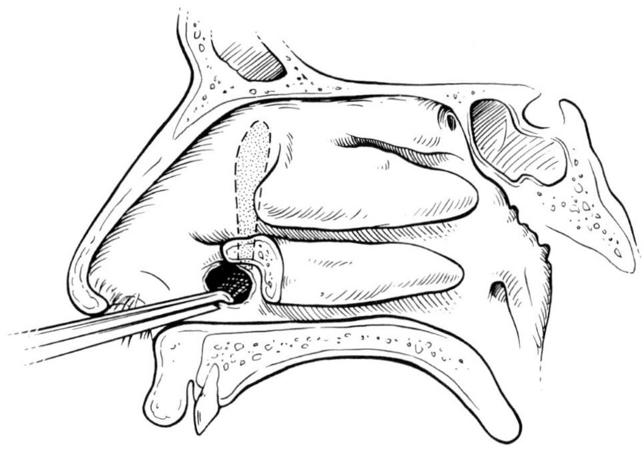

Figure 90–9. Sagittal view of the intranasal space. The tip of the inferior turbinate can be resected to facilitate the fashioning of a nasoantral window for drainage after Caldwell-Luc surgery. Note the close proximity of the nasolacrimal duct.

help retrodisplace the globe and force the orbital fat into the enlarged opening or openings. Overcorrections (i.e., enophthalmos) are uncommon, although possible. Thus, the surgeon should avoid overvigorous pressure and retrodisplacement of the globe. In general, it is not necessary to resect the readily available anterior portions of prolapsed orbital fatty tissue to achieve the desired orbital decompression effect. Several authors have recommended removal of orbital fatty tissue as a means of retrodisplacing the globe.[5,6] This orbital fatty tissue resection has been performed either as an adjunct procedure to bony decompression or as the principal surgical procedure that has been designed.

In unilateral, or bilateral, cases the surgeon should observe the immediate decompressive effect observable on the operating room table. The periosteal opening or openings can be enlarged and further retrodisplacement pressure placed on the globe if necessary. Again, the surgeon should be aware of the potential for overcorrection.

If there is still a moderate amount of oozing of blood from the sinus mucosa, the surgeon should create a nasoantral window to ensure adequate postoperative drainage. This is an elective maneuver on the transorbital decompression and is only performed if deemed necessary. The nasal packing is removed, and a small portion of the tip of the inferior turbinate is excised. The nasolacrimal duct can be probed if there is any question as to the location of the distal nasolacrimal duct. With the use of a nasal speculum for direct visualization, a sharp pointed rasp is punctured through the nasal mucosa and bone into the maxillary sinus. Gentle enlargement of the opening is performed. A drainage catheter is inserted through the nose into the maxillary sinus (Fig. 90–9). It is typically secured to the lateral wall of the nose with a single 6-0 nylon suture. The catheter is cut flush with the external nare and remains in place for the first postoperative week or as long as drainage through the nasoantral window is required.

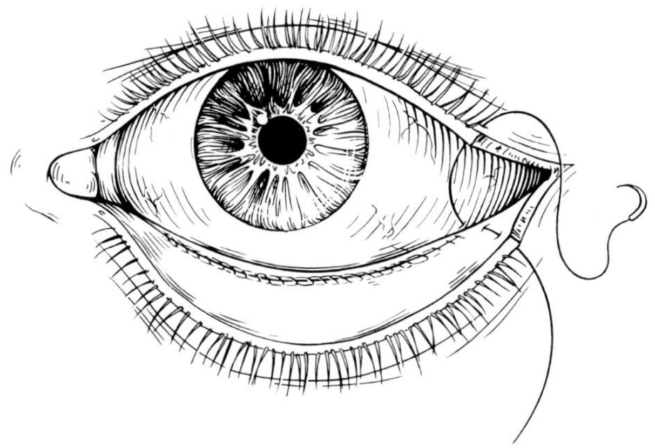

Figure 90–10. A running fast absorbable suture is used to close the inferior fornix conjunctiva. A permanent suture is used to refixate the lateral edge of the lower lid to periosteum at the lateral orbital tubercle.

The inferior fornix conjunctival incision is closed with a running 6-0 plain gut suture (Fig. 90–10). It is not necessary to reattach or suture the lower lid retractors. Lateral canthal fixation is performed attaching the lower eyelid lateral edge of the tarsus to periosteum inside the lateral orbital rim. The surgeon should match the opposing side in unilateral decompression and strive for good symmetry of the two sides in bilateral cases. The tendency to overly tighten the lower lid during refixation should be avoided. It is not uncommon to actually "sling" the eyelid slightly using a 4-0 Prolene suture with buried knot. The upper and lower lid lateral margin is secured with 6-0 nylon suture, and the remainder of the lateral canthal incision is closed with interrupted sutures.

The anesthesiologist should make every effort to extubate the patient atraumatically and avoid heavy episodes of coughing or Valsalva maneuvers. Cool compresses with crushed ice are lightly applied to the periorbital region after the decompression.

TRANSORBITAL DECOMPRESSION IN PATIENTS WITH COMPRESSIVE OPTIC NEUROPATHY

As emphasized earlier, orbital decompression for the purposes of relieving compressive neuropathy must include a decompression of the most posterior aspects of the orbital apex. The most suitable of the four orbital walls to achieve this decompression is through complete resection of the posterior aspect of the medial orbital wall and ethmoidal sinus. The majority of the orbital decompression can be accomplished with the transconjunctival inferior fornix approach as detailed earlier. To complete the ethmoidectomy and medial orbital wall resection, a second surgical incision may be used to enhance exposure and ensure the completeness of the superior and posterior ethmoidectomy. For this purpose, a modified Lynch incision[10] is used.

A curvilinear incision is marked in methylene blue in the superonasal orbit (Fig. 90–11). The modification of the standard Lynch incision is to make sure that the incision extends far enough inferiorly between the inner canthus and paranasal region. As with all orbital approaches, the skin and subcutaneous tissues are previously infiltrated with local anesthetic with epinephrine and hyaluronidase. A skin incision is made with a no. 15 blade and sharp dissection is carried down to the level of periosteum where a periosteal incision is made. In the area of the superior oblique tendon, the trochlea and periorbita should be reflected carefully as an intact unit. As the dissection proceeds posteriorly, the periorbita is reflected laterally away from the medial orbital wall (Fig. 90–12). This extraperiosteal orbitotomy approach

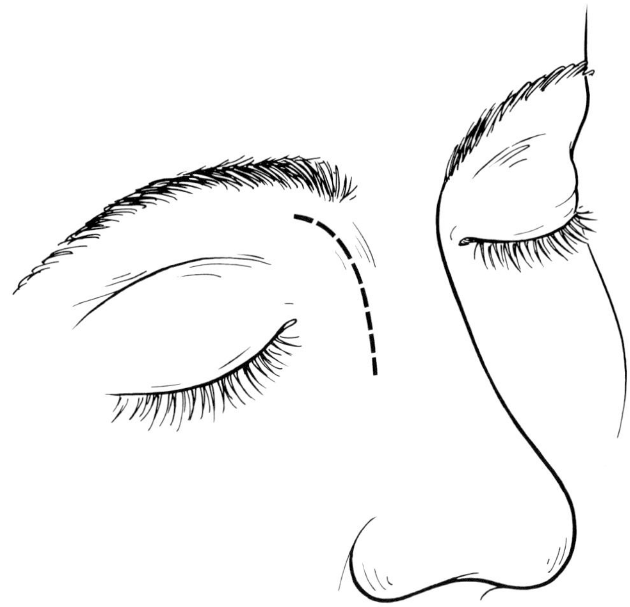

Figure 90–11. Modified Lynch incision for extranasal ethmoidectomy and medial orbital wall decompression.

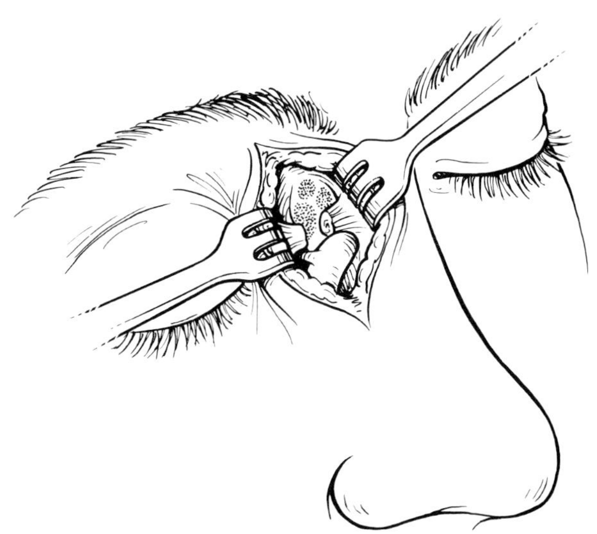

Figure 90–12. The medial periorbita is reflected laterally away from the medial orbital wall and ethmoidal sinus air cells. The anterior and posterior ethmoidal arteries should be cauterized when encountered during the dissection.

should quickly become continuous with the transorbital extraperiosteal approach, which has been made by means of the transconjunctival inferior fornix approach. By using this combined approach, the frontoethmoidal suture line as well as the anterior and posterior ethmoidal arteries are quite apparent. The anterior and posterior ethmoidal arteries may be cauterized meticulously with bipolar cautery and then severed to maximize exposure. This second separate surgical incision from above will supplement the orbital decompression of the orbital floor and inferior portions of the medal orbital wall and ethmoidal sinus air cells. The pituitary forceps is used to resect ethmoidal sinus bony septa and mucosa back to the level of the thicker sphenoid bone surrounding the optic foramen. As stated previously, the frontoethmoidal bony suture line is the superior limit of the orbital decompression bone resection.

The anatomy of the midfacial region and sinus passages is different in each patient. This secondary adjunct surgical incision is to be used in patients in whom a posterior orbital decompression cannot be adequately achieved by either the transconjunctival inferior fornix approach or the transcutaneous subciliary lower eyelid incision.

For posterior decompression, the periorbita should be opened as has been previously described. A small opening is made in the anterior portion of the periorbita. This opening is extended posteriorly using a malleable retractor or periosteal elevator to protect the interorbital contents. Once the slit opening has been extended to the posterior aspects of the orbit, the periorbita, which is typically thin and attenuated, can be grasped with a hemostat and gently torn to release the posterior orbital tissues from the confines of the periorbita.

For closure, if the trochlea has been disinserted, this portion of the periorbita should be reattached to periosteum. A 4-0 or 5-0 Vicryl suture is suitable. The remainder of the superonasal orbitotomy incision is closed in layered fashion with deep 6-0 Vicryl sutures and multiple interrupted 6-0 nylon cutaneous everting sutures for final closure.

ANTROETHMOIDAL DECOMPRESSION BY TRANSANTRAL APPROACH

The transantral approach for orbital decompression offers excellent exposure of the orbital apex and posterior extent of the ethmoidal sinus. This posteriormost orbital decompression has a significant risk of patients developing new diplopia after surgery. Those patients with preoperative restrictive strabismus have a significant chance of developing a worsened motility pattern after decompression.[1,14] The transantral decompression technique is recommended for patients with compressive optic neuropathy only. All other patients, and some patients with compressive neuropathy, can be treated successfully with the transorbital approach to antroethmoidal decompression.

The patient is positioned in a semirecumbent position for surgery. The operating room table should not have any armboards, which could restrict the movement or vantage point of the surgeon, and the endotracheal tube should be positioned midline or toward the opposing orbit. Orbital decompression for compressive optic neuropathy is typically performed as a unilateral operation. In patients with bilateral compressive optic neuropathy, surgery for the second orbit may be safely performed a few days after the first orbit has undergone surgery.

Lidocaine 2% with 1:100,000 epinephrine and hyaluronidase is infiltrated into the ethmoidal air cells, the floor of the orbit, and the buccogingival mucosa. The surgeon must wear a headlight during this procedure (an operating microscope with a 300-mm lens and coaxial illumination may also be used). It is extremely helpful to have a surgical assistant for this procedure, beyond the presence of the scrub nurse. Large blunt retractors are used to elevate the upper lip on the involved side. A buccogingival sulcus incision is made with a no. 15 blade and the dissection carried down to the level of periosteum (Fig. 90–13). An adequate cuff of gingiva should be left above the tooth line. The periosteum is incised and reflected to expose the anterior wall of the maxillary antrum. The infraorbital nerve should be identified and preserved. An osteotome and mallet is used to make a standard Caldwell-Luc antrostomy through the canine fossa and anterior maxillary wall. Rongeurs are used to widely enlarge the antrostomy as much as possible medially and laterally. Laterally, care must be taken to avoid injury to Stenson's duct. Superiorly, the surgeon must

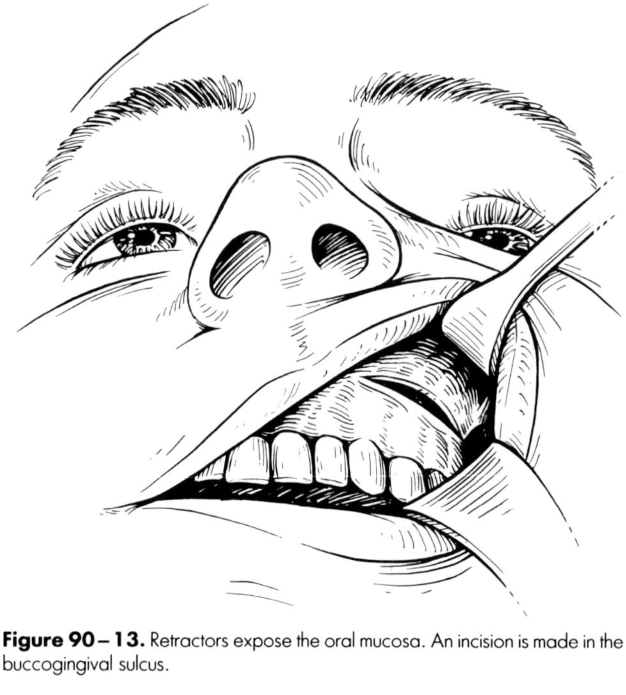

Figure 90–13. Retractors expose the oral mucosa. An incision is made in the buccogingival sulcus.

avoid injury to the infraorbital nerve. The mucosal lining of the superior and nasal aspects of the maxillary sinus is removed with a curette. A suction cautery instrument using unipolar cautery is helpful in maintaining good hemostasis.

The initial part of the orbital decompression is to perform the ethmoidectomy. The inferior portion of the ethmoidal sinus can typically be entered with the scratching motion of a Frazier suction tip or curette. A good point of entry is midway between the inferior orbital rim and posterior wall of the maxillary sinus. In some patients, the nasolacrimal canal may be quite prominent and obstruct the surgeon's view of the ethmoidal air cells. In these patients, the nasolacrimal canal can be compressed with the surgeon's finger to enhance exposure. This inward fracturing of the nasolacrimal canal does not cause nasolacrimal duct obstruction. The ethmoidectomy is performed with patient suctioning and curetting of the ethmoidal air cells (Fig. 90 – 14). The pituitary forceps is helpful in removing larger pieces of the bony septa. When ethmoidal air cell removal is complete, the thicker white frontal bone is seen at the superior aspect of the ethmoidal sinus space. The surgeon must remain aware of the anatomy at all times (see Fig. 90 – 2). Injury to the cribriform plate can occur if the curetting and bone removal veers nasally; premature penetration of the medial orbital wall and periorbita can occur if the surgical dissection veers laterally. If the suction cautery instrument is inadequate to obtain the desired degree of hemostasis, 1/2-inch plain gauze or cottonoid sponges can be soaked in 1:100,000 epinephrine solution and packed

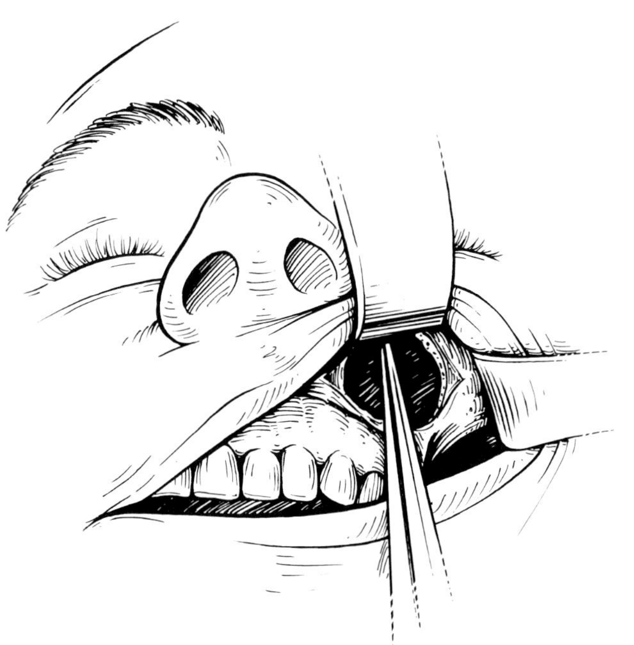

Figure 90 – 14. Pituitary forceps is introduced through a large maxillary sinus antrostomy. The transantral ethmoidectomy is completed *before* removal of the medial orbital wall and orbital floor (roof of the maxillary sinus).

into the ethmoidectomy space. With the ethmoidectomy completed, the bone of the medial orbital wall is removed.

Attention is now turned to the floor of the orbit. The first step is to identify the infraorbital groove, which contains the infraorbital neurovascular complex. The surgeon should aim the fiberoptic headlight at the roof of the maxillary antrum (i.e., the floor of the orbit) and identify a dark line coursing through the orbital floor in a posterolateral to anteromedial direction. The thinner medial bone of the orbital floor is removed initially (Fig. 90 – 15). The bone resection continues laterally to the approximate level of the infraorbital neurovascular complex. As much bone as possible from the orbital floor should be removed from the inferior orbital rim to the posterior apex of the maxillary sinus. From a transantral approach it is very difficult to visualize the anterior portion of the orbital floor: this bone must be removed slowly and cautiously. For purposes of orbital decompression to relieve compressive neuropathy, it is not necessary to remove bone lateral to the infraorbital neurovascular complex. Removal of this latter portion of the orbital floor would do little to enhance the decompressive effect of the surgery and would significantly increase the risk of postoperative hypoglobus.

Periorbita is opened along the anteroposterior length of the orbit. If possible, hinged incisions are made on each end. Care must be taken whenever slitting open the periorbita to avoid inadvertent injury to the intraorbital soft tissues. A hemostat is then used to grasp and tear the periorbita. The surgeon should generally widely open this hinged flap of periorbita medially and inferomedially. Gentle pressure and retrodisplacement of the globe will help tense and identify any remaining strands of periorbita. These are all carefully cut so that no further restricting bands contain the orbital fat and extraocular muscles. With gentle pressure applied to the globe, a blunt instrument can be used to gently tease the orbital fat into the enlarged sinus openings. In some patients with compressive optic neuropathy, the chronically enlarged extraocular muscles and orbital fat contain indurated fibrotic changes that prevent ready prolapse of the orbital soft tissues through the periorbital openings. The surgeon must recognize the inherent limitations and inelasticity of the orbital tissues in these patients and avoid the temptation to aggressively dissect these fibrotic tissues. Such attempts could carry significant risk of hemorrhage or damage to one of the extraocular muscles or optic nerve.

A nasoantral window should be fashioned in virtually all cases of orbital decompression through the transantral approach. The nasoantral window technique is described in the transorbital approach section. It is helpful to fashion this nasoantral drainage window before closure so that direct transantral visualization can be made of any drainage catheters or packing that is placed. With the nasoantral window formed, and good hemostasis obtained,

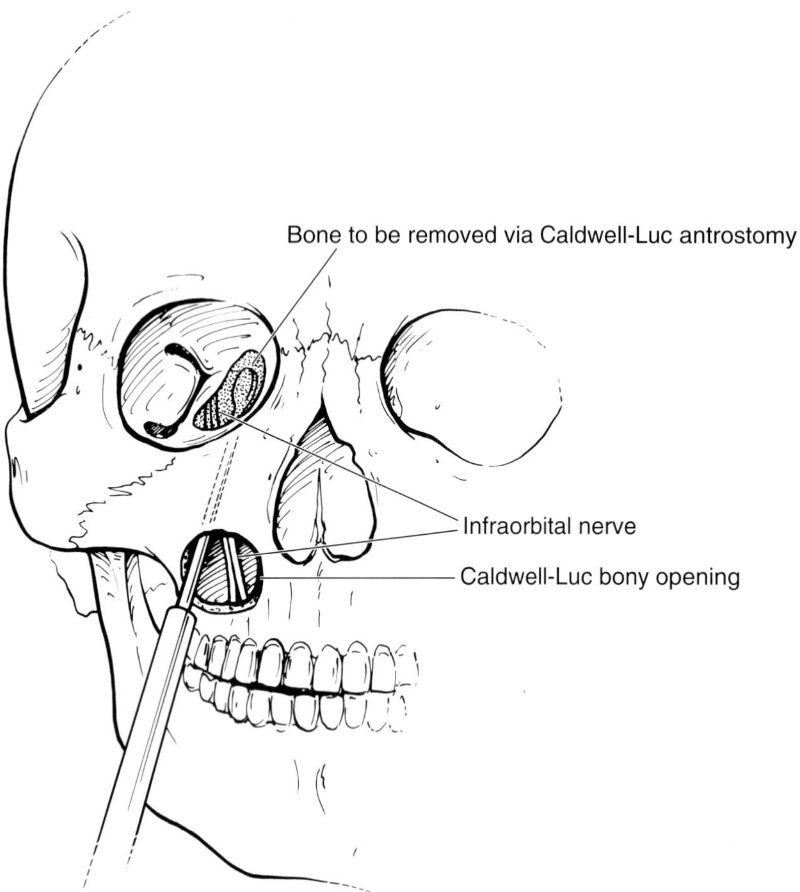

Figure 90–15. Composite illustration of bony skull demonstrating Caldwell-Luc antrostomy for antroethmoidal orbital decompression.

the buccal gingival mucosal incision is closed with interrupted absorbable sutures.

TRANSORBITAL APPROACH TO THREE-WALL DECOMPRESSION

The so-called three-wall orbital decompression, which offers the most advantages at present, is the standard antroethmoidal two-wall decompression combined with a lateral orbital wall valgus osteotomy, which achieves both orbital expansion as well as orbital decompression laterally.[17] This technique offers distinct advantages over simple removal of the lateral orbital bone. Unlike extensive craniofacial procedures or combined orbital-neurosurgical procedures,[3, 18, 19] this modified valgus osteotomy of the lateral orbital wall can readily be performed by the knowledgeable orbital surgeon.

In this three-wall decompressive procedure, the antroethmoidal two-wall decompression is performed as outlined previously. In patients with compressive optic neuropathy, a posterior medial orbital wall removal and ethmoidectomy has already been emphasized as an important part of the surgery. In these patients, performing the lateral orbitotomy and lateral orbital wall removal first can greatly enhance exposure of the posterior medial orbit since the globe and orbital contents can be retracted laterally to a greater degree. This combined orbitotomy method of enhancing orbital surgical exposure has been well described in the literature.[20, 21]

The lateral canthal and temporalis region should be infiltrated with local anesthetic with epinephrine and hyaluronidase. A 2.5 to 3-cm incision line is marked from the lateral canthal angle toward the ear (Fig. 90–16). A superficial skin incision is followed by subcutaneous tis-

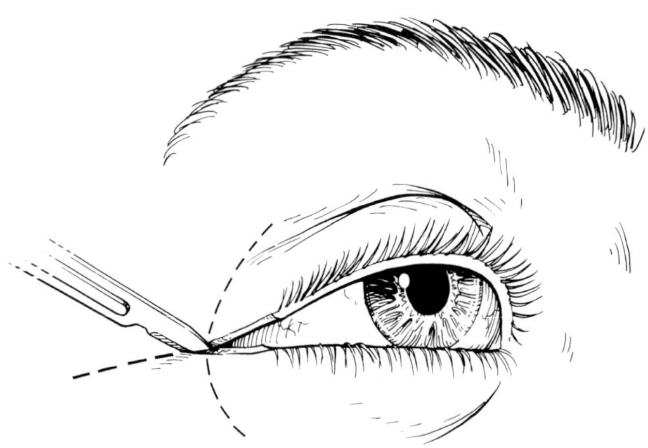

Figure 90–16. A no. 15 blade is used to make the lateral orbitotomy skin incision.

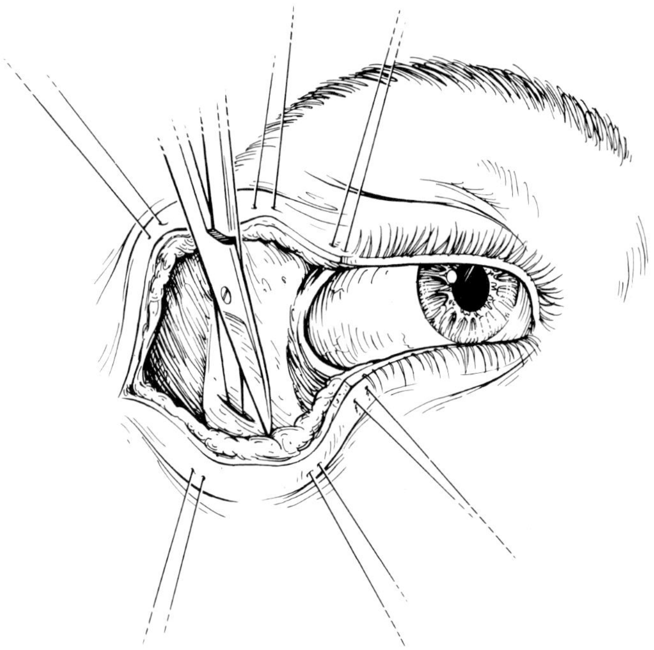

Figure 90–17. After the superior and inferior cantholysis of the lateral canthal tendon, the pretemporalis fascia plane is broadly undermined.

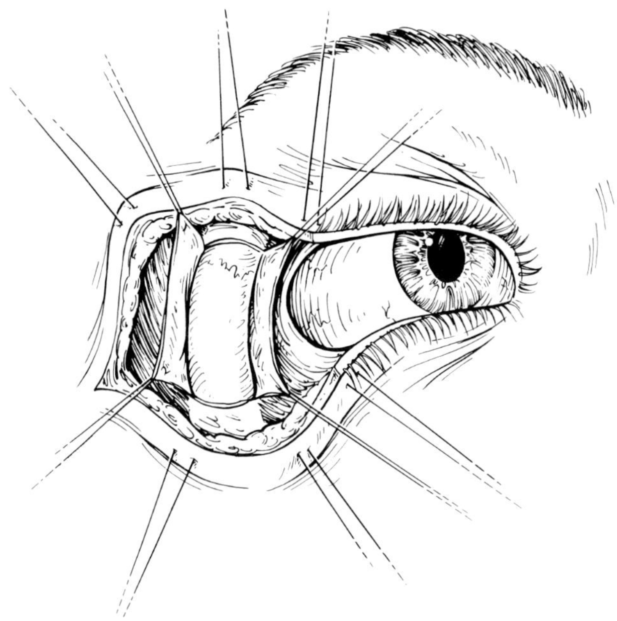

Figure 90–18. The outer layer of periosteum and temporalis muscle is carefully reflected laterally away from the lateral orbital bony rim. The inner layer of periorbita is reflected medially.

sue dissection down to the level of the superficial temporalis fascia. The needle-tip monopolar cutting-cautery unit is helpful for this dissection. A superior and inferior lateral cantholysis is performed and the subcutaneous tissues broadly undermined to expose the lateral orbital wall (Fig. 90–17). The periosteum of the lateral orbital wall is incised 2 to 3 mm outside the orbital rim. Relaxing incisions are made superiorly and inferiorly. The temporalis muscle can be reinfiltrated with local anesthetic, and some blunt dissection is performed with a heavy periosteal elevator to separate portions of the temporalis muscle from the lateral orbital bone. A fine orbital periosteal elevator is then used to elevate periorbita from the lateral orbital wall and superolateral orbit (Fig. 90–18). An oscillating saw is used to make two osteotomies in the lateral orbital wall. A broad malleable retractor should be held at all times between the lateral orbital bone and the periorbita, such that the orbital soft tissues are protected. The superior horizontal osteotomy can be made a few millimeters above the frontozygomatic suture line (Figs. 90–19 and 90–20). The inferior osteotomy is made at the superior portion of the zygomatic arch. The oscillating saw should be used to cut through the thicker portion of the lateral orbital wall until the thinner posterior portions are reached. Slow, steady saline drip irrigation is used throughout the sawing of the bone to reduce buildup of heat and prevent unnecessary bone necrosis. A large bone rongeur is then used to grasp, fracture, and remove this segment of lateral orbital bone. This bony specimen, which should measure 3 to 3.5 cm in length, is kept in a saline-soaked gauze pad on the sterile operative field.

A rongeur is used to remove all of the thin sphenoid bone along the lateral orbit (Fig. 90–21). Posteriorly, as the thicker aspects of the greater wing of the sphenoid are encountered, bone wax can be used to control oozing of blood. Resection of lateral orbital bone is complete at this time.

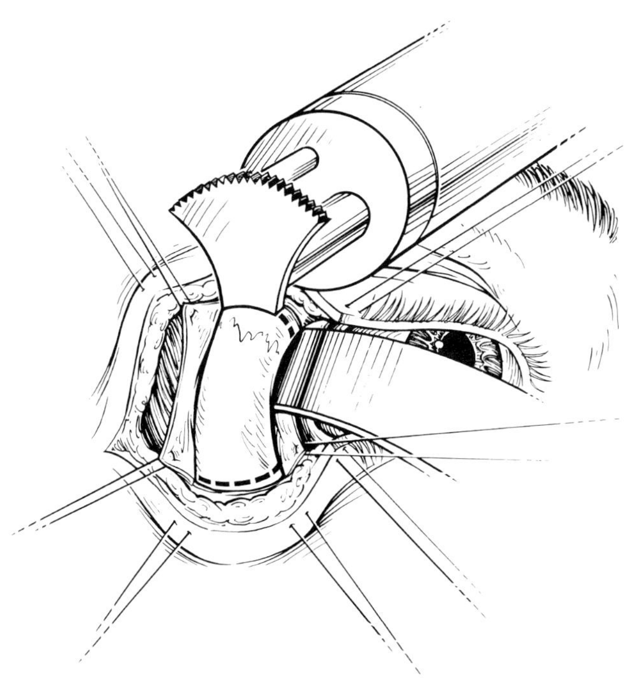

Figure 90–19. An oscillating Stryker saw is used to cut the lateral orbital rim. A broad malleable retractor remains between the lateral orbital bone and the reflected periorbita at all times.

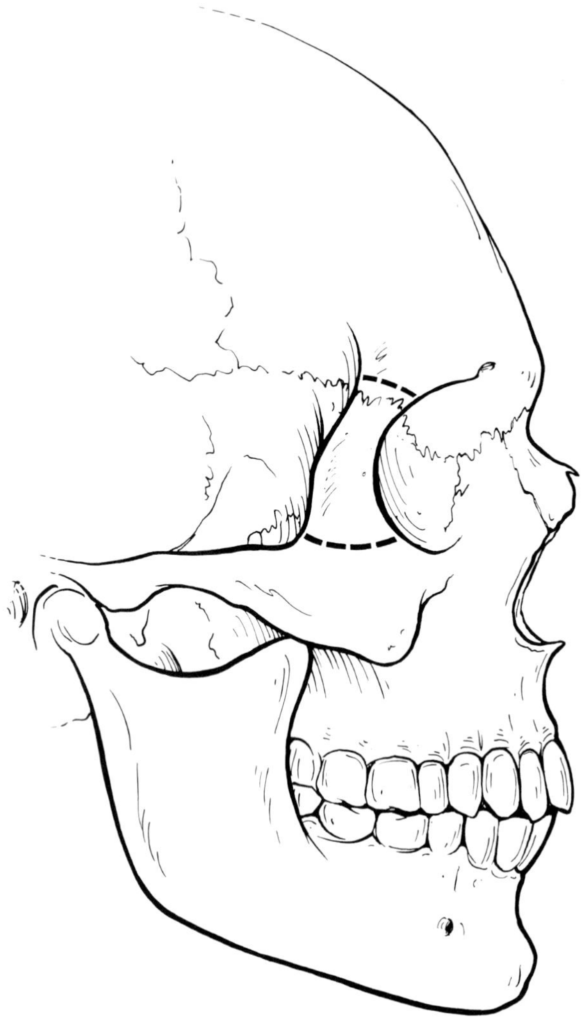

Figure 90–20. Bony skull view demonstrating incision sites through lateral orbital bony rim.

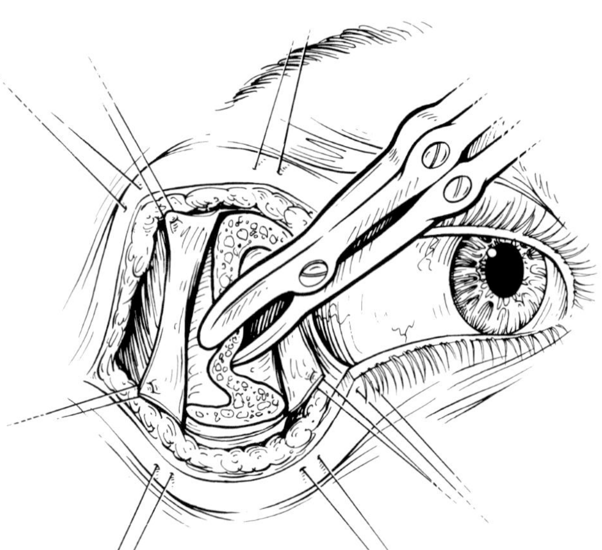

Figure 90–21. A rongeur is used to remove the thin portions of sphenoid bone and enlarge the lateral orbitotomy opening.

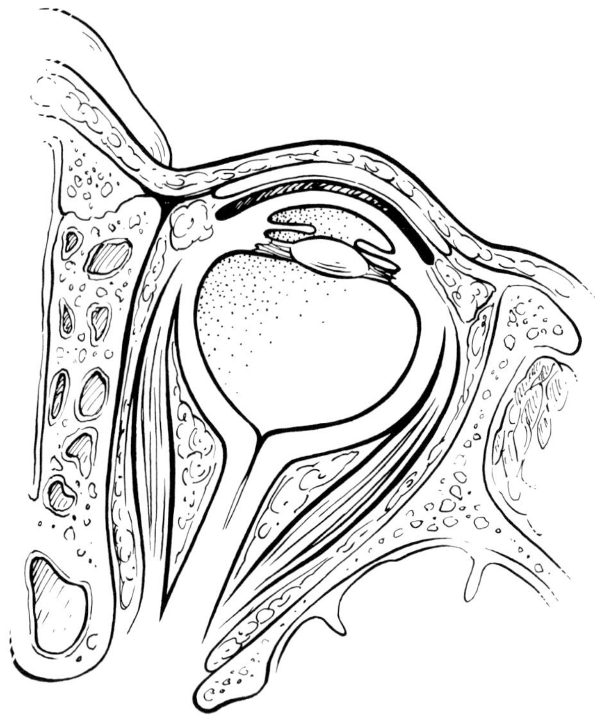

Figure 90–22. Axial view illustration of the globe, lateral wall, and medial wall–ethmoidal sinus air cells.

As stated earlier, the lateral orbitotomy combined with the lateral cantholysis and some release of periorbita will greatly enhance outward rotation of the globe and orbital tissues (Fig. 90–22). This can certainly aid the ease with which the ensuing antroethmoidal decompression can be performed, especially with regard to the posterior aspects of the orbital decompression, which are performed as needed for the patients with compressive neuropathy (Figs. 90–23 and 90–24).

Attention can now be turned to restoration of the lateral orbital wall. The previously resected piece of bone can be thinned along its posterior surface. This still allows a very adequate piece that can be advanced anteriorly and outwardly rotated to achieve an orbital expansion while still allowing lateral orbital decompression (Fig. 90–25). The key to this part of this procedure is to achieve accurate, rigid fixation of the advanced rotated piece of bone using titanium miniplates.[22–24] These miniplates allow for very secure and accurate fixation of the bone, though this requires meticulous technique on the part of the orbital surgeon. The lateral orbital bone specimen should be advanced anteriorly 3 to 4 mm and rotated laterally approximately 2 mm (Fig. 90–26). The miniplate system templates are used to accurately bend the actual titanium miniplates. Micro drill holes are made, followed by 1.5-mm self-tapping titanium screws. This will rigidly fixate the lateral orbital bone fragment to the superior orbital rim and zygomatic arch inferiorly. This repositioning of the lateral orbital bone increases the entrance width to the bony orbit as well as expanding the

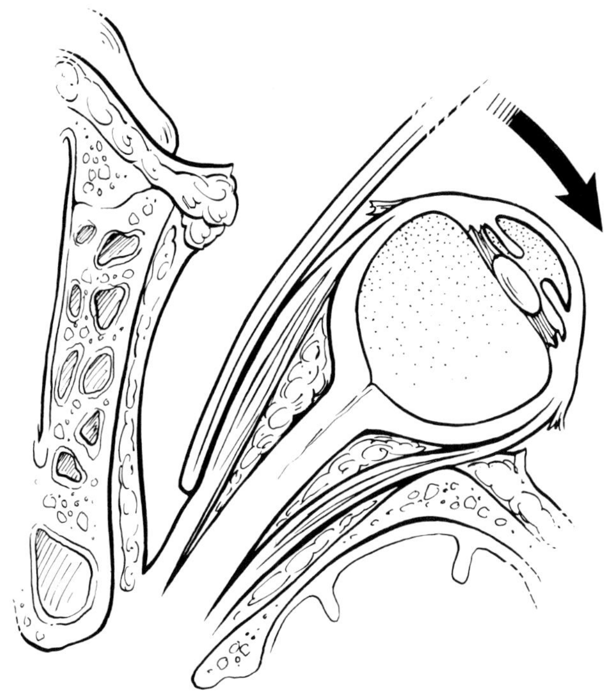

Figure 90–23. Combined orbitotomy. Removal of the lateral orbital wall allows for lateral rotation of the globe with enhanced exposure of the medial orbit.

sagittal length. A stepoff deformity is created at the superior lateral orbit. A power-driven drill with a 5.0- to 6.0-mm bone cutting bur can be used to polish down this stepoff deformity superiorly. The space created behind the refixated lateral orbital bone, due to the outwardly rotated position of the bone, allows for some decompressive effect of the lateral orbital tissues (through periorbital openings) to supplement the decompressive effect gained through the medial and inferior wall decompressions. If other significant contour gaps are present after the lateral orbital bone refixation, the surgeon may consider the use of autogenous bone grafts (e.g., iliac crest bone) or alloplastic materials (e.g., bone cement).

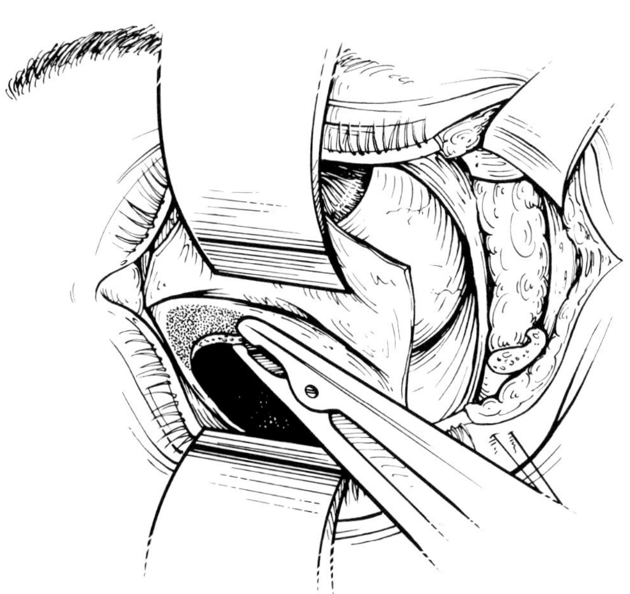

Figure 90–24. With the combined orbitotomy approach, the lateral orbital rim is removed first. Enhanced exposure can then be achieved of the medial orbit, including the medial apex for removal of posterior bone and ethmoidal air cells.

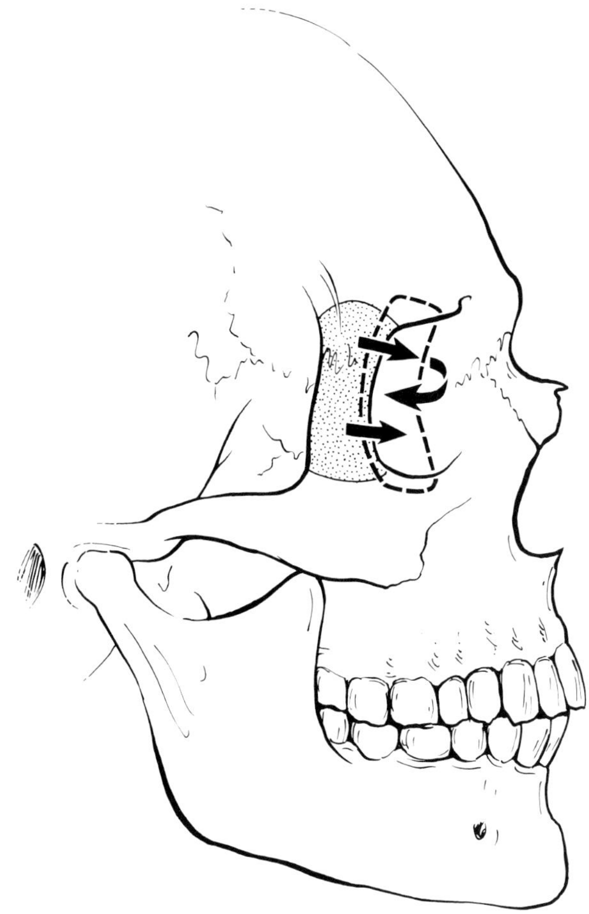

Figure 90–25. Proposed advancement and outward rotation of lateral orbital wall segment.

The most important aspect of closure is refixation of the upper lid and lower lid lateral canthal angle. The chosen fixation point must be appropriate in terms of superoinferior placement as well as anteroposterior placement. The outer canthus may be located at the level of, or slightly superior to, the level of the medial canthal angle. The anteroposterior placement should be appropriate so that the eyelids follow the curvature of the globe. If adequate periorbita has been preserved laterally, a permanent suture (e.g., 4-0 Prolene suture) can be used to fixate both the upper and lower eyelid lateral canthal tendons and lateral edge of tarsus. Care should be taken to avoid overtightening of the eyelids. In some cases, the nonabsorbable suture can be used to "sling" the eyelids from a periorbital fixation point. If adequate periorbita is not present, a small drill hole can be made through an appro-

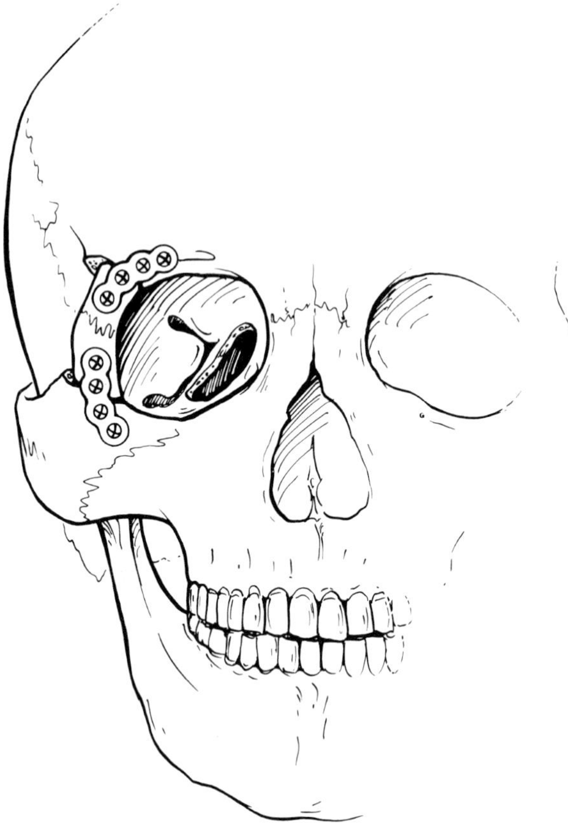

Figure 90–26. Titanium miniplates are used to rigidly fixate the advanced, outwardly rotated lateral orbital bone segment.

priate point in the refixated lateral orbital bone piece. A suture can be used to secure the lateral edges of the upper and lower eyelid and is then brought through the bony drill hole for external fixation to the soft tissues. Again, the surgeon must take care to observe that the eyelids have proper position and contour, as well as correct horizontal tension.

Smaller 6-0 nylon sutures are then used to pinch the upper and lower lid margin together laterally. The remainder of the lateral closure is performed in layered fashion with 6-0 Vicryl sutures in the subcutaneous layers and 6-0 nylon sutures superficially.

COMBINED TRANSORBITAL-NEUROSURGICAL FOUR-WALL ORBITAL DECOMPRESSION

So-called four-wall orbital decompression is generally reserved for the most severe cases of Graves' orbitopathy with severe exophthalmos. This procedure is performed by an experienced orbital and neurosurgical team. The results reported in the literature generally show a more significant reduction in exophthalmos than has been achieved by more conservative orbital decompressive procedures.[3]

After the standard lateral orbitotomy incision is made the elevation of lateral periorbita is extended into the superior orbit. A 3 to 3.5-cm piece of lateral orbital bone is removed in standard fashion. Rongeurs, combined with the power-driven drill, are used to remove the posterior portions of the lateral orbital wall. The bone-cutting drill is used to remove superolateral portions of the sphenoid wing down to the level of the dura overlying the temporal lobe of the brain. This is a most delicate portion of the procedure, and cerebrospinal fluid leakage can occur as a complication. Kennerdell and Maroon[3] have found cerebrospinal fluid leakage to be especially common in older patients, in whom the dura tends to be quite attenuated. They generally recommend that this procedure of decompression of the superolateral portion of the orbit not be performed in patients older than 65 years old.

As bone is removed from the superolateral orbit and orbital roof, computed tomographic scans should be available for review in the operating room. The surgeons must be aware of the size and position of the frontal sinuses so as to avoid entering the lateral portion of the frontal sinus space with the Kennerdell-Maroon decompression. Other descriptions of four-wall decompression techniques emphasize the transcranial removal of the floor of the frontal sinus to specifically create an extra empty space in addition to the temporal, inferior, and medial decompression spaces.[4]

After removal of the lateral orbital wall and portions of the orbital roof and sphenoid wing, the anterior piece of lateral orbital bone can be thinned and refixated. The miniplate system of rigid fixation of the lateral orbital bone in an anteriorly advanced and outwardly rotated position is suitable as part of the four-wall decompression.

The antroethmoidal portions of this decompression are performed as have been previously described. In these severe cases of exophthalmos, a larger portion of the orbital floor can be removed lateral to the infraorbital neurovascular bundle.

CRANIOFACIAL APPROACH TO ORBITAL EXPANSION

As described in this chapter, standard transorbital decompressive techniques attempt to enlarge the area of the bony orbit posterior to the orbital rim and allow for expansion and decompression of the retrobulbar orbital fat into the contiguous sinus spaces. Orbital expansion is a surgical technique that moves the position of the orbital rim anteriorly in an attempt to compensate for abnormal exophthalmos seen in Graves' orbitopathy.[18, 19] There are two basic settings in which I generally refer Graves' orbitopathy patients for cranofacial consultation:

1. Patients with extremely severe exophthalmos. Ophthalmic surgeons should carefully assess their decompressive goals. I believe that there is such a thing as at-

tempting to "push too far" the effects of standard transorbital decompression. Patients who would otherwise require extreme amounts of antroethmoidal, as well as lateral, bone removal to adequately retrodisplace the globe, would likely be better served by orbital expansion. Expansion of the bony orbit would likely be able to better address the problem of exophthalmos with lesser risks of postoperative globe malpositions or motility problems. This recommendation does not apply to patients with compressive optic neuropathy and visual loss—these patients still require surgical decompression of the orbital apex to alleviate pressure on the apical portions of the optic nerve.

2. Patients with severely noncompliant orbits and indurated periorbital tissues and fat. These patients will generally not respond well to standard transorbital decompression. The basic problem is that despite decompression of the orbital walls and opening of the periorbita, the orbital soft tissues retain their shape and position. This subset of patients will generally do better with bony orbital expansion. In the future, there may be better means of more accurately identifying this group of patients. For now, some of these patients will invariably be identified after unsuccessful transorbital antroethmoidal decompression.

Much has been written in the ophthalmic and nonophthalmic literature regarding orbital expansion. I would refer the interested reader to these references for more thorough details of these craniofacial techniques.[18, 19, 25–27]

In its most aggressive form, orbital and midfacial expansion can be performed by Le Fort III osteotomies with anterior expansion of the entire orbital rim, with removal of the medial orbital wall, and lowering of the orbital floor. This technique is typically performed by a craniofacial surgeon working with a neurosurgeon. The use of autogenous bone grafts to fill in the expanded space is an important part of this technique.

Modifications of the Le Fort III osteotomy technique confine themselves to significant expansion of the lateral orbit, including the superolateral and inferolateral orbital space. These techniques also combine the skills of a craniofacial surgeon and neurosurgeon. They offer greater potential for orbital expansion than could be achieved with the more simple three-wall transorbital decompression with simple lateral wall advancement as described earlier in this chapter.

POSTOPERATIVE MANAGEMENT

Cool compresses with crushed ice should be lightly applied to the involved orbit after surgery. The crushed-ice compresses should be used as much as possible during the first 48 postoperative hours. Beyond that, cool compresses are used approximately four times per day for 1 hour each time for the first week after surgery. The patient is instructed to remain indoors and avoid overexertion and vigorous straining. The patients should not be outside in the sun or in other warm areas that could promote swelling.

The patient will typically have received intravenous cephalosporin antibiotics (e.g., cefazolin [Ancef] 1 g) as well as intravenous corticosteroids. Postoperatively, the patient is continued on a tapering dosage of corticosteroids for 5 to 7 days. While the patient is in the hospital for 1 to 3 days after surgery, intravenous corticosteroids may be used at an intermediate dosage (e.g., dexamethasone [Decadron] 20–40 mg in divided daily doses or methylprednisolone [Solu-Medrol] 250–500 mg in divided daily doses). On an outpatient basis, oral prednisone in a range of 40 to 80 mg may be used in a tapering dosage. Oral decongestants (e.g., pseudoephedrine) taken twice daily are used for 1 month after surgery.

The nasoantral window drain is typically removed 1 week after surgery if the patient is doing well.

Ophthalmic antibiotic ointments are applied inside the eyelids at bedtime, and antibiotic-corticosteroid eye drops are used during the day.

COMPLICATIONS OF SURGERY

Orbital decompression is a surgery of considerable magnitude, and all candidates for this procedure should have potential risks, complications, and side effects of the procedure carefully explained to them.

Common associated features or side effects of the surgery can include a downward settling of the globes or, in some cases, severe hypoglobus. The patient should be told that the upper eyelid retraction may appear to worsen after decompressive surgery due to this settling effect of the globes. Some patients may experience a change or a worsening of their diplopia. Patients' gaze restriction in upward gaze may worsen. Other side effects of the surgery can include infraorbital nerve numbness, periorbital and lid edema, and ipsilateral facial edema and discomfort after Caldwell-Luc surgery.

Beyond the above potential side effects of surgery, a number of very serious complications are possible. Cerebrospinal fluid leakage could occur from injury to the area of the cribriform plate during ethmoidectomy and medial wall decompression. The patient would be at risk for meningitis, and neurosurgical consultation is usually obtained. Management of these patients must be individualized and done on a case-by-case basis.

Severe hemorrhage and blood loss can occur with this surgery. It would be unusual to require blood transfusion, though the surgeon should be aware of this possibility. Considerable bleeding can occur from the anterior or posterior ethmoidal arteries or from the infraorbital artery should inadvertent injury to this structure occur.

The ethmoidal sinus air cells and mucosa will ooze quite a bit of blood, though not nearly the amount of rapid bleeding that can occur with arterial injury.

The posterior decompression of the orbital apex poses the greatest potential risk of direct injury to either the medial rectus muscle or the optic nerve. The orbital structures are all crowded together in the orbital apex. It is typical for the periorbita to be quite thin and attenuated, and the surgeon must avoid "incising into" a bulging medial rectus muscle when opening the periorbita. Direct visualization of structures will minimize the potential for direct optic nerve injury.

In the anteromedial orbit, the surgeon should be aware of the location of the lacrimal sac and nasolacrimal duct. These structures, as well as the origin of the inferior oblique, should be avoided during bone removal. If inadvertently incised or transsected, the lacrimal sac and nasolacrimal duct tissues should be reopposed and sutured in one or two places, as well as internally stented with silicone lacrimal tubing.

Inadequate sinus drainage or frank sinusitis can develop immediately after orbital decompression. The surgeon should generally have a low threshold for performing nasoantral drainage windows as part of the decompression procedure. If this has not been performed during the primary surgery, it can certainly be performed secondarily if significant fluid buildup proves to be a problem in the maxillary sinus.

REFERENCES

1. McCord CD Jr: Current trends in orbital decompression. Ophthalmology 92:21–33, 1985.
2. Ogura JH, Lucente FE: Surgical results of orbital decompression for malignant exophthalmos. Laryngoscope 84:637–644, 1974.
3. Kennerdell JS, Maroon JC: An orbital decompression for severe dysthyroid exophthalmos. Ophthalmology 89:467–472, 1982.
4. Stranc M, West M: A four-wall orbital decompression for dysthyroid orbitopathy. J Neurosurg 68:671–677, 1988.
5. Olivari N: Transpalpebral decompression of endocrine ophthalmopathy (Graves' disease) by removal of intraorbital fat: Experience with 147 operations over 5 years. Plast Reconstr Surg 87:627–641, 1991.
6. Hecht SD, Guibor P, Wolfley D, Wiggs EO: Orbital dissection defatting technique for Graves' disease. Ann Ophthalmol 16:314–315, 1984.
7. McCord CD Jr: Orbital decompression for Graves' disease: Exposure through lateral canthal and inferior fornix incision. Ophthalmology, 88:533–541, 1981.
8. Anderson RL, Linberg JV: Transorbital approach to decompression in Graves' disease. Arch Ophthalmol 99:120–124, 1981.
9. Walsh TE, Ogura JH: Transantral decompression for malignant exophthalmos. Laryngoscope 67:544–568, 1957.
10. Lynch RC: The technique of a radical frontal sinus operation which has given me the best results. Laryngoscope 31:1–5, 1921.
11. Maarten M, Koornneef L, Wiersinga WM, et al: Orbital decompression for Graves' ophthalmopathy by inferomedial, by inferomedial plus lateral, and by coronal approach. Ophthalmology 97:636–641, 1990.
12. Kennedy DW, Goodstein ML, Miller NR, Zinnreich SJ: Endoscopic transnasal orbital decompression. Arch Otolaryngol Head Neck Surg 116:275–282, 1990.
13. Long JA, Baylis HI: Hypoglobus following orbital decompression for dysthyroid ophthalmopathy. Ophthalmic Plast Reconstr Surg 6:185–189, 1990.
14. Shorr N, Neuhaus RW, Baylis HI: Ocular motility problems after orbital decompression for dysthyroid ophthalmopathy. Ophthalmology 89:323–328, 1982.
15. Kearns TP, Henderson TW, Haines SF: Clinical orbitometry in Graves' disease. Am J Ophthalmol 36:45–55, 1953.
16. Frueh BR, Musch DC, Grill R, et al: Orbital compliance in Graves' eye disease. Ophthalmology 92:657–665, 1985.
17. Wulc AE, Popp JC, Bartlett SP: Lateral wall advancement in orbital decompression. Ophthalmology 97:1358–1369, 1990.
18. Tessier P: Expansion of the orbital cavity. *In* Tessier P (ed): Plastic Surgery of the Orbit and Eyelids. New York, Masson, 1981, pp 107–112.
19. Wolfe SA: Surgical treatment of exophthalmos and enophthalmos. Ann Ophthalmol 13:995–1002, 1981.
20. Smith JL: Anterolateral approach to the orbit. Trans Am Acad Ophthalmol Otolaryngol 75:1059–1064, 1961.
21. McCord CD: A combined lateral and medial orbitotomy for exposure of the optic nerve and orbital apex. Ophthalmic Surg 9:58–66, 1978.
22. Glassman RD, Manson PN, Vandercock CA, et al: Rigid fixation of external orbital fractures. Plast Reconstr Surg 86:1103–1109, 1990.
23. Luhr HG: Indications for use of a microsystem for internal fixation in craniofacial surgery. J Craniofac Surg 1:35–52, 1990.
24. Rubin PAD, Shore JW, Yaremchuk MJ: Complex orbital fracture repair using rigid fixation of the internal orbital skeleton. Ophthalmology 99:553–559, 1992.
25. Tessier P: Expansion chirurgicale de l'orbite. Ann Chir Plast 14:207–214, 1969.
26. Wolfe SA: Modified three-wall orbital expansion to correct persistent exophthalmos or exorbitism. Plast Reconstr Surg 64:448–455, 1979.
27. Whitaker LA, Bartlett SP: The craniofacial dysostoses: Guidelines for management of symmetric and asymmetric disease. Clin Plast Surg 14:73–81, 1987.

Orbital and Periorbital Neoplasia

CHAPTER 91

Neurogenic Tumors

Michael Kazim and Jeffrey Bruce

Developments in noninvasive imaging and surgical instrumentation have permitted more accurate diagnosis and effective treatment of neurogenic tumors. Noninvasive images refine otherwise nonspecific constellations of clinical signs. Computed tomography (CT) and ultrasonography were the first modalities to be used to image lesions previously viewed only by "diagnostic orbitotomy." Newer CT technology provides three-dimensional reconstructions that may assist in surgical planning. More recent application of magnetic resonance imaging (MRI) to orbital diseases renders unparalleled soft tissue detail.

Surgical technologic advances include use of the operating microscope, which provides superior intraoperative visualization. Mounted on a free-floating frame, the neurosurgical microscope permits identification of critical structures that might otherwise be sacrificed during tumor resection. Surgical lasers, in particular the carbon dioxide (CO_2) and neodymium:yttrium-aluminum-garnet (Nd:YAG), are valuable tools for tumor excision. The CO_2 laser can be targeted through the operating microscope with a micromanipulator. Shallow energy penetration spares underlying normal tissue from damage while meticulously vaporizing the tumor.

The most important benefit has come from a multidisciplinary team approach to these lesions, which increases the opportunity for successful tumor excision while limiting surgical morbidity.

GENERAL APPROACH TO NEUROGENIC TUMORS

The approach to this group of tumors combines a detailed clinical neuro-ophthalmic and systemic evaluation, radiologic examination guided by clinical findings, and surgical intervention for diagnosis or treatment when indicated.

Clinical Examination

Neurogenic tumors may exist in both the intracranial and intraorbital compartments. Measures of optic nerve function, including visual acuity, color vision, pupil reactivity, and visual fields, should be recorded. A refraction (cycloplegic if appropriate) may be critical to the assessment of visual function or proptosis. Ocular motility to assess the function of the oculomotor (III), trochlear (IV), and abducens (VI) nerves should be tested, along with evaluation of the trigeminal (V_1, V_2, V_3), facial (VII), auditory (VIII), and olfactory (I) nerves. External examination should identify thickening of the eyelids, ptosis (with or without impairment of levator function), engorgement of the episcleral blood vessels, and proptosis. Particular attention should be paid to the direction in which the globe is displaced. Axial proptosis suggests an intraconal mass, whereas displacement of the globe off-axis suggests a lesion in one of the orbital quadrants. Intraocular pressure measurements should be recorded. Asymmetry may herald orbital venous outflow obstruction. Slit lamp examination should note the presence of iritis, iris nodules, or cataract formation. A dilated fundoscopic examination should reveal retinal or choroidal lesions, choroidal folds as well as papilledema, optic atrophy, or optociliary shunt vessels.

If a systemic process is suspected (e.g., neurofibromatosis or malignancy), evaluation by an internist or pediatrician is indicated.

Noninvasive Imaging

It is not uncommon for lesions to bridge the orbital, sinus, and intracranial compartments. Noninvasive imaging is required in all cases. The clinical picture guides the selection of the imaging modality.

Ultrasonography provides a simple, safe, and readily available method to evaluate the orbit. It can detail the location of a lesion and its solid or cystic characteristics, and in skilled hands it can provide a high level of diagnostic information. A standard 10-mHz probe is limited by the lack of penetration beyond approximately 20 mm into the orbit. Lower-frequency probes have greater depth of penetration but sacrifice resolving power. We generally employ ultrasonography as the initial imaging tool for anterior orbital lesions.

The CT scan, rendered in the axial and coronal projections with and without contrast medium enhancement, remains the best single imaging choice for orbital pathology. It remains unparalleled in providing bony detail and has excellent soft tissue resolution. All cases that require a neurosurgical approach are imaged with CT. The sole disadvantage is the associated ionizing radiation.

MRI produces the highest resolution of soft tissue detail without ionizing radiation. It provides superior detail in the region of the optic canal, superior ophthalmic fissure, and intracranial space. The paramagnetic contrast material gadolinum (Gd-DTPA) is particularly helpful in selected cases. Fat suppression techniques and surface coils have been used to enhance orbital details. Fat suppression eliminates the bright signal produced by orbital fat on T1-weighted sequences that may obscure intraorbital lesions. Surface coils may provide greater detail in the anterior orbit but have limited resolution at the orbital apex and intracranial space where the field effect falls off. The development of new paramagnetic contrast dyes and higher-tesla magnets may produce still greater resolution.

Highly vascular tumors are imaged angiographically to detail blood flow and to identify those lesions that may be embolized either in lieu of surgery or as a preoperative adjunct.

Diagnostic Biopsy

Tumor biopsy is required when the clinical and radiologic information are inadequate to construct a treatment plan. Fine-needle aspiration biopsy has been a valuable technique in our experience. It is best suited to the diagnosis of lymphoid lesions, and it has limited value in cases of neurogenic tumors and should be used only in those cases in which surgery must be avoided because of patient wishes or medical necessity. The shortcomings of fine-needle aspiration biopsy include sampling error, cytologic misinterpretation, orbital hemorrhage, and globe perforation.

Several technical details should be emphasized. The biopsy needle (22-gauge, 1.55-inch) is introduced through one of the four orbital quadrants chosen based on tumor location. When possible, the superotemporal quadrant is avoided, since passing the needle through the lacrimal gland can confound cytologic interpretation by introducing normal glandular tissue in the specimen. If an orbital hemorrhage is produced, pressure on the globe is generally adequate to control the bleeding. However, the surgeon should be prepared to proceed with decompressive techniques if indicated.

Treatment

Treatment is individualized to the tumor type and clinical picture. The approach to each tumor is discussed below. Surgical details are discussed elsewhere in this text. Here we limit ourselves to the technique we apply to the transcranial approach to the orbit.

TRANSCRANIAL APPROACHES TO THE ORBIT

For tumors located in the superior quadrant of the orbital apex or extending intracranially, the transcranial fronto-orbitotomy provides maximal exposure for the intraorbital, intracanalicular, and intracranial segments of the optic nerve.

Preparation

Intravenous antibiotics are given preoperatively and continued for 48 hours after surgery. If retraction of the frontal lobe is anticipated, a spinal drain is placed intrathecally at the L3–L4 interspace and cerebrospinal fluid is removed to facilitate brain relaxation. Mannitol may be used as an adjunct to provide further brain relaxation. High-dose corticosteroids are used to reduce cerebral and orbital edema. Prophylactic anticonvulsants are necessary only if the mass extends intradurally and direct manipulation of the cerebral cortex is anticipated.

Opening

The patient is placed supine on the operating table and a Mayfield three-point head holder, or similar device, is used to secure the head. The head is extended to allow the frontal lobe to fall away from the orbital roof. A bicoronal incision is made 1 to 2 cm behind the hairline extending from the tragus on the ipsilateral side to the superior temporal line on the contralateral side. A similar incision extending only to the midline can be used if the orbital rim is not removed and medial exposure is not required. The incision is made through the pericranium, leaving the temporalis muscle and fascia undisturbed. The pericranium remains attached to the scalp to preserve its blood supply since it may be required for reconstruction at the end of the operation. If the lateral orbital rim and zygoma are to be removed or exposed, the temporalis fascia should be brought forward with the scalp flap to ensure that the frontal branches of the facial nerve are preserved. The scalp flap is advanced to expose sufficient frontal bone to allow the inferior portion of the craniotomy to be flush with the floor of the anterior cranial fossa. If the supraorbital rim is to be removed, the scalp flap should be advanced farther to expose the supraorbital rim and periorbita, which is continuous with the pericranium and can be dissected from the orbital roof. The dissection must avoid damage to the supraorbital nerve as it exits the supraorbital foramen. A fine osteotome or rongeur may be required to unroof the foramen if the nerve is completely enclosed by bone.

A small bur hole is placed in the posterolateral portion of the frontal bone, and a craniotome is used to create a bone flap extending to the floor of the anterior fossa lateral to the sagittal sinus. A median frontal craniotomy provides sufficient exposure for the majority of orbital cases. Modifications of the craniotomy are made to alter the degree of exposure. If the orbital lesion is anterior, the supraorbital rim is removed. In such cases the orbital rim should be removed in continuity with the orbital roof to minimize the bony defect that must be repaired at the conclusion of the surgery. The orbital roof is opened with a drill, and an oscillating or Gigli saw is threaded through the opening to make a medial and lateral cut through the orbital rim. The cut should be narrow to minimize the gap in the rim after it is replaced.

If the lesion extends laterally in the orbit, or into the cavernous sinus, or parasellar region through the optic foramen or superior orbital fissure, a frontotemporal exposure is required. The temporalis muscle is incised and advanced with the scalp to expose the inferotemporal area. The craniotomy should include the temporal bone and pterion. To expose the cavernous sinus, the lateral wing of the sphenoid bone is removed with a drill, unroofing the optic foramen and superior orbital fissure. The anterior clinoid is also generally removed.

If the lesion extends medially into the ethmoidal sinus and wide exposure is required, an orbitoethmoidal osteotomy can be utilized by making cuts through the supraorbital rim, frontonasal suture, and the contralateral, medial orbital rim. The frontal craniotomy in this situation must extend across the midline, exposing the sagittal sinus. Although this opening invariably sacrifices the ipsilateral olfactory nerve, the contralateral olfactory nerve should be preserved if possible. When the olfactory nerve is cut at its sheath, the ensuing dural opening must be repaired primarily. To complete the orbitoethmoidal osteotomy, additional cuts are made through the cribriform plate and orbital roof. An osteotome is used to release the final attachment through the ethmoid bone.

If the frontal sinus is opened with the craniotomy, the mucosa is exenterated and the sinus obliterated with a fat graft, pericranium, temporalis muscle, or temporalis fascia. At the end of the procedure, a flap of vascularized pericranium is brought over the frontal sinus defect and sutured to the dura, cordoning off the sinus.

After the craniotomy, the orbital roof is carefully exposed extradurally and the orbit is unroofed with a high-speed cutting drill. Depending on the location of the lesion, it may be necessary to open the optic foramen. In this situation a diamond drill bit is used with copious irrigation to avoid thermal injury to the nerve. Once the orbit is exposed, the lesion may be removed using the techniques previously described.

If the ethmoidal sinus is entered, it must be covered with vascularized tissue. A pericranial flap is most convenient and should be developed and separated from the scalp, while preserving its blood supply anteriorly. If the olfactory nerve has been sacrificed, the pericranium should be sutured behind the area of the closure of dural sleeve, completely covering it. If the dura has been torn or intentionally opened to remove an intradural lesion, a watertight dural repair is required to prevent cerebrospinal fluid leakage. If the dural opening is small, this can be accomplished primarily, but a larger opening must be covered with a graft taken from either the pericranium or the temporalis fascia.

In the case of small orbital roof defects, the vascularized pericranium flap is usually sufficient to provide support and no further reconstruction is needed. If the orbital defect is large, reconstruction to avoid enophthalmos or pulsatile proptosis is desirable. We generally prefer to reconstruct the orbital defect with bone from the inner table of the craniotomy flap plated to the orbital rim. If the defect is large, a cancellous bone graft may be taken from the iliac crest. Although defects may be repaired with titanium mesh, autologous bone is generally preferred to reduce the risk of infection and degradation of postoperative radiographic imaging quality.

The craniotomy flap is replaced with wires or titanium plates. The orbital rim is replaced first and secured with plates or wire. The galea and skin are closed in separate layers. A subgaleal Hemovac is placed for 24 hours. A tight head wrap will discourage the accumulation of subcutaneous or subgaleal fluid. If a spinal drain has been used, it is removed immediately unless there has been a significant dural repair with potential for cerebrospinal fluid leakage postoperatively. Under these conditions the spinal drain may be left on continuous drainage (5–10 mL/h) for up to 5 days to allow the leaks to seal.

TUMORS

Optic Nerve Glioma

The biologic behavior of lesions grouped histologically as gliomas (Figs. 91–1 through 91–3) varies sufficiently

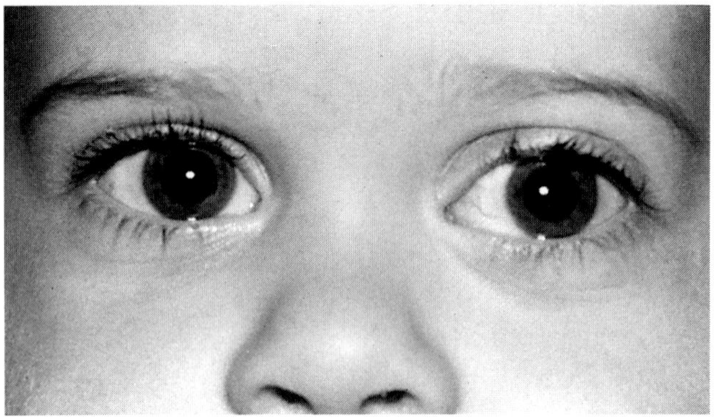

Figure 91 – 1. A 3-year-old child presented with left axial proptosis produced by an optic nerve glioma.

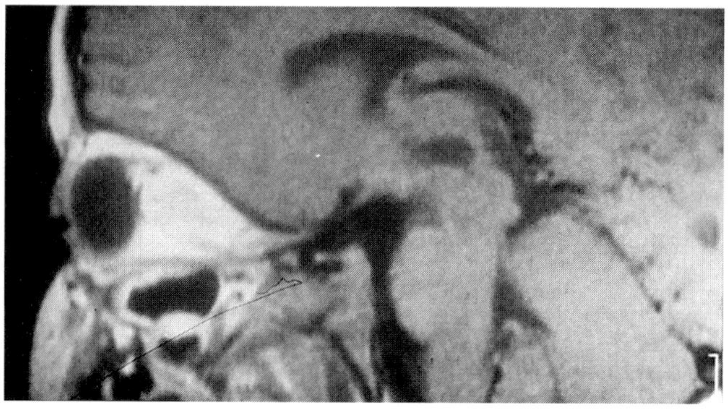

Figure 91 – 3. Optic nerve glioma. On magnetic resonance scan sagittal section, enlargement of the optic nerve within the optic canal identifies potential intracranial extension.

that predictions regarding the growth potential of a given tumor or conclusions of a retrospective analysis are imprecise. All attempts at identifying clinical, radiographic, or histologic markers that consistently predict behavior or outcome have failed. Most gliomas are solitary lesions. The tumor may be located solely within the orbit, bridge the orbitocranial space, or reside within the intracranial space alone. Modern imaging permits this classification, which is the keystone to management of these cases.

Retrospective studies provide conflicting data. Alvord and Lofton compiled the data of 623 previously reported cases of optic nerve or chiasmal glioma and applied a mathematical model to derive more statistically significant results. They found that although the behavior of the tumors varied overall there was a general trend toward declining growth rate over time. This result suggests classification of the tumors as low-grade pilocytic astrocytomas. The majority of tumors are diagnosed within the first 2 decades of life. Increasing age at the time of diagnosis correlates with worse long-term prognosis. Those younger than age 20 years at the time of diagnosis had a 20-year survival rate of 65%, while the group diagnosed when older than 50 years had a 10-year mortality rate of 80%. Mortality rates were higher among patients with chiasmal involvement at the time of diagnosis and higher still when the hypothalamus or ventricle was involved.

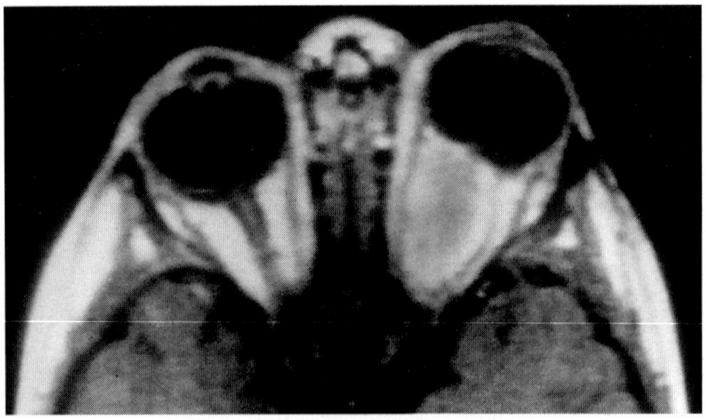

Figure 91 – 2. Optic nerve glioma. Magnetic resonance scan shows fusiform enlargement of the right optic nerve. There is no calcification. A normal optic nerve is not apparent within the enlarged nerve sheath.

In this study, 25% of tumors had invaded the chiasm at the time of surgical excision. Although this figure may represent cases that involved the chiasm early in the course, it also includes cases from the pre-CT era when data from plain film radiographs and tomograms came late in the course of the disease. Earlier diagnosis with MRI and the ability to closely monitor the growth of the tumor may change the statistics.

Recurrences developed in 5% of cases in which a "complete" intraorbital resection was performed. We would routinely advocate a combined intracranial and intraorbital approach to excision of the involved optic nerve from the globe to the chiasm to minimize such recurrences.

In 15% to 50% of cases associated with neurofibromatosis, multifocal disease is found. Bilateral optic nerve glioma is nearly uniformly associated with neurofibromatosis. Investigators differ regarding prognosis in the multifocal cases. Although most have no long-term increase in mortality there is an increase in the rate of distant sarcomas or glioblastoma multiforme, unrelated to the treatment rendered.

Clinical Presentation. The clinical signs and symptoms depend on the size and location of the tumor. Intraorbital gliomas produce axial proptosis and visual loss. The vision loss varies and is often severe and out of proportion to the proptosis. In children, the vision loss may be manifest as amblyopia or strabismus. Profound proptosis may limit ocular rotations and produce corneal decompensation and spontaneous prolapse of the globe. Papilledema is generally present, although long-standing disease may produce optic disc pallor.

Tumors predominantly within the intracanalicular segment of the optic nerve, the chiasm, or optic radiations may be difficult to detect in the pediatric population. In the absence of proptosis, loss of vision is the sole clinical barometer. Similarly, tumors involving the optic radiations will not produce proptosis; rather, typical visual field defects will be present.

The increased risk of optic nerve gliomas in patients with neurofibromatosis mandates screening neuro-ophthalmic examinations and radiologic investigation when indicated by the clinical findings.

Radiographic Findings. The standard diagnostic imaging modality for optic gliomas is CT. Images should be rendered in the axial and coronal planes with and without contrast medium enhancement. Optic nerve gliomas produce fusiform enlargement of the optic nerve. The optic nerve is not identified within the tumor, and calcification is rarely present. The nerve and sheath are often kinked at nearly 90 degrees in the anterior third of the orbit. Invasion of the optic canal, chiasm, or optic radiations is best imaged by MRI. Enlargement of the optic canal may be seen with parasagittal views. Optic gliomas are hypointense or isointense on T1-weighted images and hyperintense on T2-weighted images.

Treatment. Treatment is guided by the location of the tumor and visual potential. Bilateral optic nerve or chiasmal involvement precludes surgical treatment. We generally monitor these cases closely. Those tumors that appear static are not treated. Measurements of optic nerve function, proptosis, corneal decompensation, and optic disc edema are made every 3 months. Deterioration of the clinical picture or radiographic evidence of disease progression necessitates treatment. Obstructive hydrocephalus requires shunting, and chiasmal involvement may produce pituitary insufficiency that may require treatment. Trials are being conducted to determine the efficacy of radiation therapy and chemotherapy in such cases.

Surgery is reserved for unilateral cases that radiographically invade the optic canal but spare the chiasm or when proptosis produces uncontrollable corneal decompensation or gross disfigurement. We prefer a transcranial approach and resection of the optic nerve from the globe to the chiasm to ensure complete extirpation of the tumor. If tumor is evident at the proximal end of the resected specimen at the time of histopathologic inspection, we do not attempt to resect the residual tumor within the chiasm, because surgical damage to the contralateral visual pathway may result. Additionally, there is no assurance that further resection into the chiasm will identify a tumor-free margin. The prognosis is unclear in individual cases. Each patient is monitored closely, and if progression is noted, consideration is given to radiation therapy or chemotherapy.

Meningioma

Orbital meningiomas involve either the optic nerve or the sphenoid bone and are discussed separately.

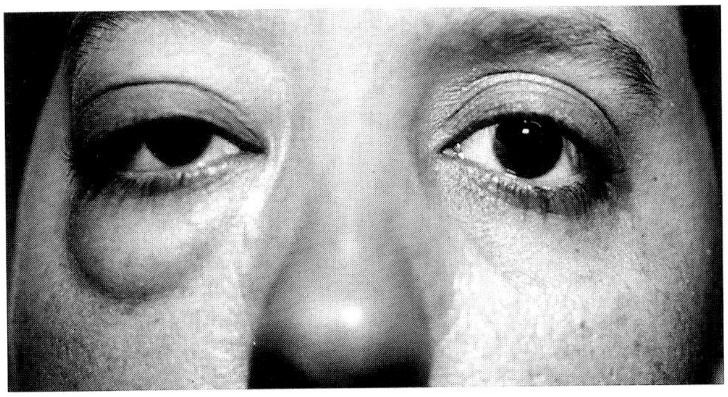

Figure 91-4. A 34-year-old woman had slowly progressive, right axial proptosis and sudden vision loss due to an optic nerve meningioma. Marked papilledema was present, and no cilioretinal artery was identified.

Optic Nerve Meningioma

Meningiomas of the optic nerve (Figs. 91-4 through 91-10) generally affect women in their third or fourth decade. Early in the course of the disease, visual loss may be mild and apparent only with threshold perimetry. More profound visual loss evolves over decades. Although the occasional patient seeks attention for proptosis, it is generally a late finding. The slow evolution of signs and symptoms argues for a conservative approach to management.

Radiographic Findings. CT identifies two morphologic tumor types. The en plaque variety appears as a focal exophytic tumor that may be present at any point along the course of the intraorbital segment of the optic nerve. The tumor enhances with intravenous contrast dye. The morphologic MRI findings are much the same as those of CT. The tumor is intense on both T1- and T2-weighted sequences and is hyperintense with gadolinium enhancement.

The second more common variety produces a fusiform enlargement of the optic nerve. On CT the tumor is denser than the normal nerve and is identified by the

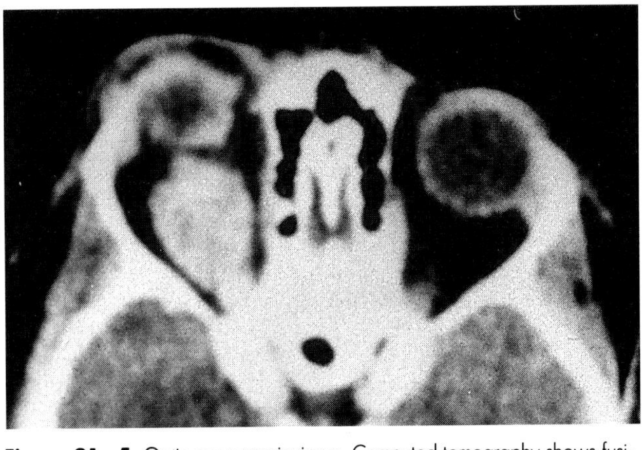

Figure 91-5. Optic nerve meningioma. Computed tomography shows fusiform enlargement of the right optic nerve with calcifications.

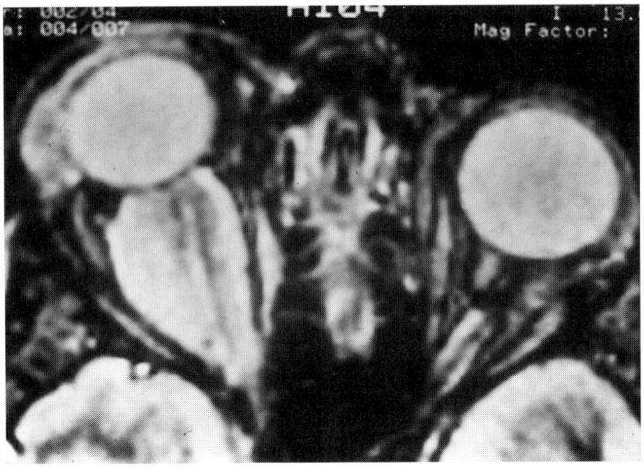

Figure 91–6. Optic nerve meningioma. On magnetic resonance scan, the centrally located optic nerve is identified within the enlarged nerve sheath.

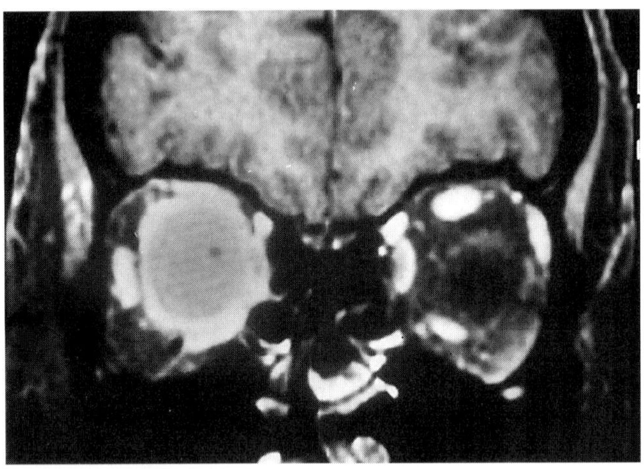

Figure 91–7. Optic nerve meningioma. Viewed in this magnetic resonance scan coronal projection, the centrally located optic nerve within the expanded sheath is clearly identified.

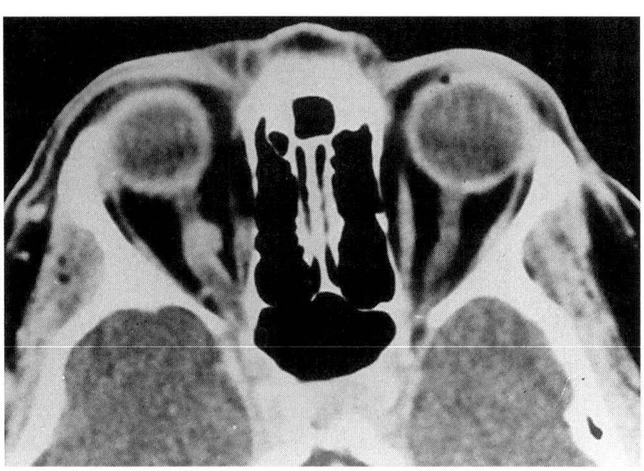

Figure 91–8. En plaque optic nerve meningioma. A radiodense focal enlargement of the optic nerve is apparent in the middle third of the right optic nerve on this computed tomographic scan.

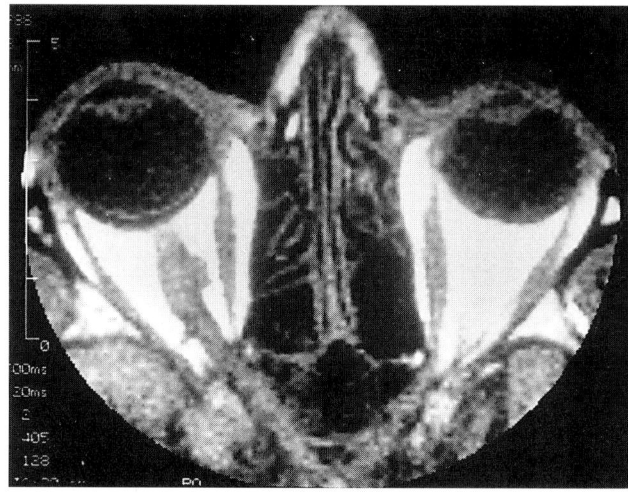

Figure 91–9. En plaque optic nerve meningioma. The tumor is clearly delineated from the normal optic nerve by magnetic resonance scan.

classic "railroad track" sign produced by calcification within the tumor. This sign is not, however, uniformly identified. With MRI the tumor is hyperintense on T2 weighting and with a contrast medium enhancement. Generally, the normal centrally located optic nerve is identified within circumferentially expanded tumor mass. This is most helpful in distinguishing a meningioma from a glioma. MRI provides the earliest evidence of optic canal invasion by tumor.

Management. Treatment is dictated by the degree of visual acuity loss, development of proptosis, and evidence of intracranial extension. Although there have been isolated reports of surgical removal of en plaque optic nerve tumors with preservation or improvement in

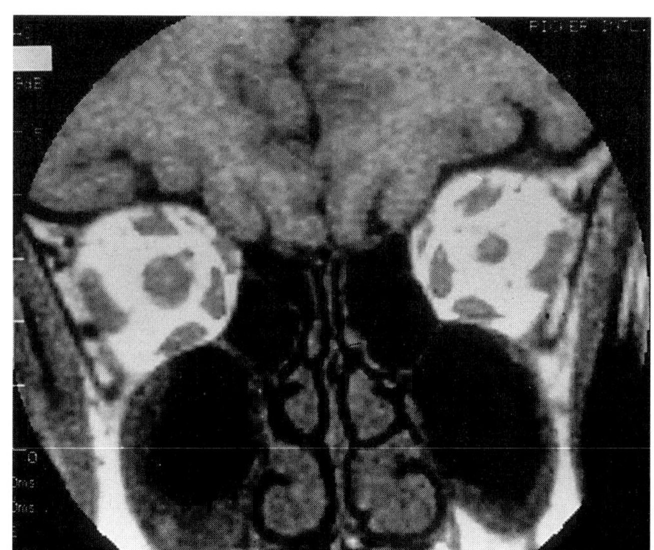

Figure 91–10. En plaque optic nerve meningioma. In coronal magnetic resonance projection the lesion is circumferential to the right optic nerve in the middle third of the orbit.

vision, complete loss of vision is most common. Decompression of the nerve sheath has been advocated. We avoid this approach because it has been associated with massive orbital extension requiring exenteration. We avoid surgery except to prevent intracranial extension. Invasion of the optic canal is identified by MRI and associated with rapid vision loss. Resection is approached through a cranio-orbitotomy to permit complete removal of the tumor and prevent intracranial spread. If intracranial extension occurs, treatment is more complicated and less successful. We favor the same surgical approach if resection is performed to treat profound proptosis.

As an alternative, some have applied radiation therapy to halt the progression of visual loss. We reserve this modality for cases in which vision has deteriorated to 20/80 or less. In such cases we have seen preservation of useful vision in cases treated with 4000 cGy to the tumor. In cases in which the vision is better than 20/80, the risk of radiation therapy–induced damage to the optic nerve and retina is not warranted. Observation is in order and surgical resection indicated in those few cases in which the tumor grows into the optic canal.

Sphenoid Wing Meningioma

Meningiomas of the sphenoid wing (Figs. 91–11 through 91–14) produce clinical disease as mass-occupying lesions. Straddling the sphenoid wing they produce proptosis and orbital congestion. If large or apically located, there may be associated compressive optic neuropathy. This is best detected and monitored using automated threshold visual field testing. Fullness of the temporalis fossa is common when the tumor bulk is large. The tumor may involve the intracranial dura and produce pain, but pain is not a common feature. Intracranial extension may be associated with cranial neuropathy and ultimate compromise of the brain-stem function.

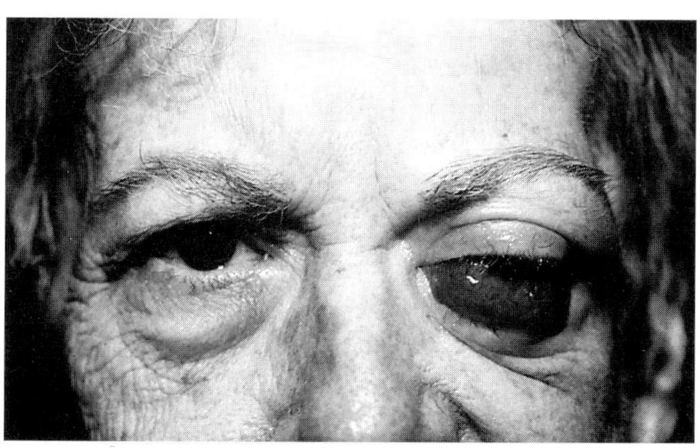

Figure 91–11. This 78-year-old woman presented with left proptosis, marked chemosis, restriction of motility, compressive optic neuropathy, and fullness of the temporalis fossa.

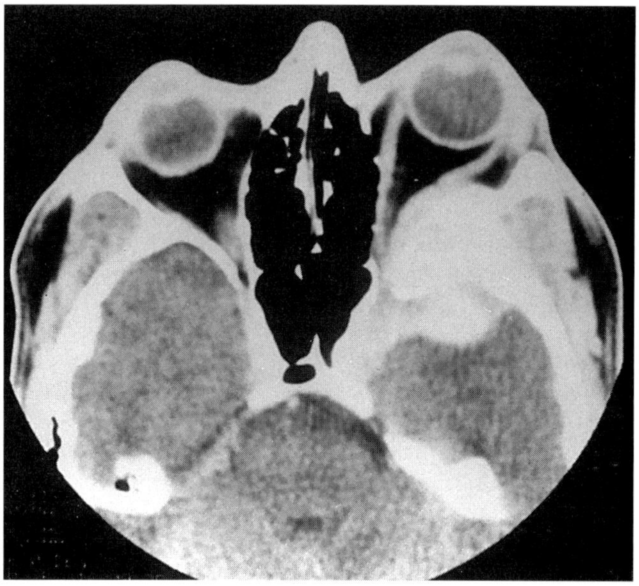

Figure 91–12. Sphenoid wing meningioma. Marked hyperostosis of the left sphenoid wing produced mass effect in the adjacent orbit. Associated soft tissue component to the tumor is apparent within the associated dura and temporalis fossa.

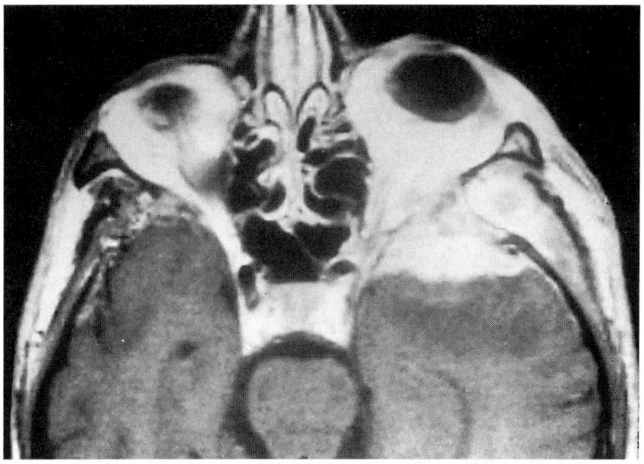

Figure 91–13. Sphenoid wing meningioma. Use of gadolinium-enhanced magnetic resonance scan clearly defines the soft tissue extent of the tumor, layering along the dura and temporalis fossa.

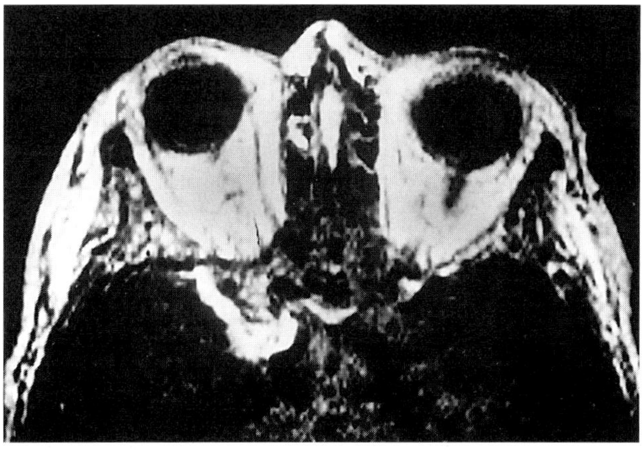

Figure 91–14. Cavernous sinus meningioma. Enlargement with gadolinium-enhanced magnetic resonance scan of the right cavernous sinus.

Radiographic Findings. CT reveals hyperostosis of the involved bone. A soft tissue component may be present in association with the bony lesion and appear hyperintense after the administration of contrast dye.

MRI with gadolinium enhancement is the optimal examination for detecting the extent of the tumor, which may be difficult to define using CT alone. MRI is especially useful in the detection of tumor growth along the dura, where it will produce a hyperintense signal with gadolinium as compared with uninvolved tissue.

Treatment. Meningiomas of the sphenoid wing are nonencapsulated and invasive, making complete surgical resection very difficult. Relief of signs and symptoms can, however, be achieved by gross total resection. The tumors produce symptoms by invading the superior ophthalmic fissure, optic foramen, or cavernous sinus. Surgical resection should be considered in cases of compressive optic neuropathy, disfiguring proptosis, corneal decompensation, or disabling diplopia. Although these tumors are generally slow growing, we have seen one case of sphenoid wing meningioma that behaved aggressively. Four gross total resections of the tumor were performed over 3 years. In each case, histopathologic findings were benign. The patient ultimately died of brain stem involvement.

Resection should be approached in a combined fashion to the orbital and intracranial segments of the tumor. Where possible, the tumor should be dissected from the periorbita. The periorbita should be preserved even when gross tumor remains because it may provide a barrier to orbital invasion. The surgically created defects in the sphenoid wing should not be reconstructed. Postoperative pulsatile proptosis generally resolves spontaneously, and the defect provides space into which inevitable tumor regrowth may occur. When both the lateral wall and roof of the orbit are resected, repair of the anterosuperior orbital defect with either autologous bone or a titanium mesh is advisable. Invasion of the cavernous sinus is problematic. Removal of tumor from the cavernous sinus is indicated for cranial nerve decompression or when gross total excision is attainable.

Postoperative radiation therapy is controversial, but reports of slowed tumor regrowth after radiation therapy are encouraging and the modality should be considered in selected cases. An evolving technology, radiosurgery may prove of particular value when residual, surgically unresectable tumor is potentially symptomatic. Clinical trials of RU 486 suggest that hormonal treatment may slow tumor growth and be an effective adjunct.

Neurofibroma

Neurofibromas (Figs. 91–15 through 91–17) are grouped into three classes: (1) isolated, (2) diffuse, and (3) plexiform. Each will be discussed separately. Although all may be manifestations of neurofibromatosis, only the plexiform variety is uniformly associated with the syndrome. The diffuse and isolated forms are associated with neurofibromatosis in only 10% of cases. In all classes the histology features proliferation of schwannian and endoneural elements.

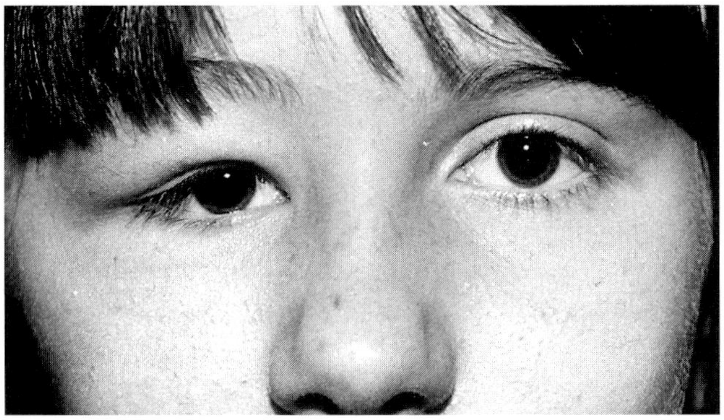

Figure 91–15. Sixteen-year-old with a plexiform neurofibroma of the right orbit. Fullness and an S-shape of the right upper lid results from extension of the tumor through the orbital septum. The bony orbit is expanded and the globe is depressed by the superiorly based mass.

Neurofibromatosis

Neurofibromatosis is an autosomally inherited trait with highly variable and incomplete penetrance affecting approximately 1 in 3000 births. Diagnostic criteria include six or more café-au-lait spots of greater than 15 mm in diameter, axillary freckling, cutaneous neurofibromas, and a family history of neurofibromatosis. Peripheral neurofibromatosis features the appearance of café-au-lait spots in the first year of life, followed by neurofibromas in adolescence. Visceral neurofibromas and skeletal abnormalities, most notably absence of the sphenoid wing, may be identified. Growth and mental disorders are possible. The disease may be associated with pheochromocytomas or neurilemomas, and there is a 10% rate of malignant degeneration of neurofibromas in

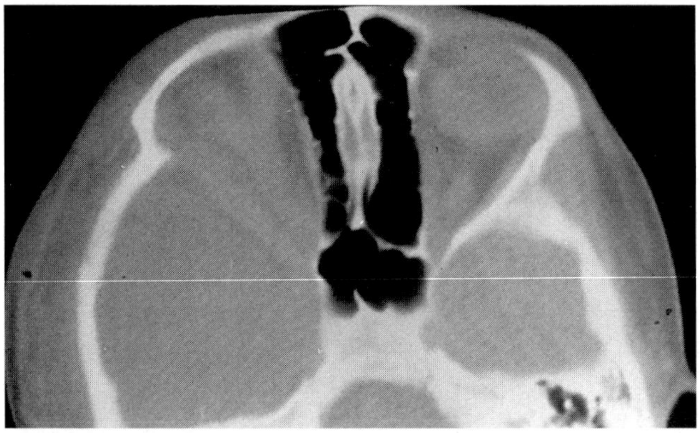

Figure 91–16. Neurofibroma. Computed tomographic scan shows agenesis of the sphenoid wing in the right orbit.

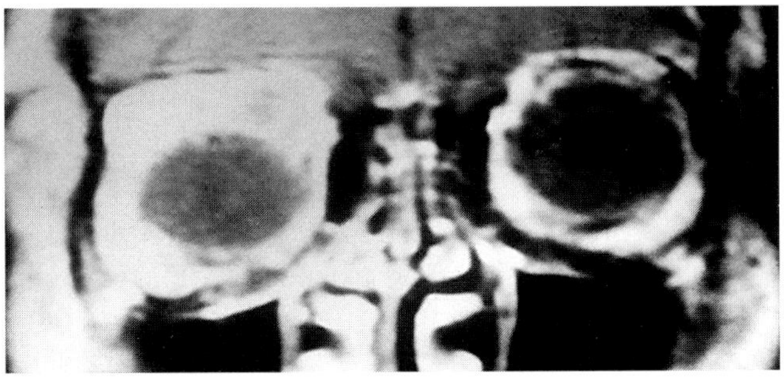

Figure 91 – 17. Neurofibroma. On magnetic resonance scan, a high-signal soft tissue mass exists superiorly and laterally in the right orbit.

the setting of neurofibromatosis. Central neurofibromatosis is associated with astrocytomas, meningiomas, schwannomas, and ependymomas, with few peripheral manifestations. The orbital findings of neurofibromatosis include gliomas and meningiomas of the optic nerve, orbital neurofibromas and schwannomas, and dysgenesis of the sphenoid wing. Lisch nodules (iris hamartomas) are present in 90% of patients with neurofibromatosis. Also seen are choroidal hamartomas, café-au-lait spots and neurofibromas of the eyelids, prominent corneal nerves, and glaucoma, which may produce buphthalmos.

Plexiform Neurofibromas. Plexiform neurofibromas are the most common form of the disease. They may affect any nerve, although there is a predilection for sensory nerves. Proliferation produces a "bag of worms" within the soft tissue. Management is complicated by the lack of encapsulation and the substantial vascularity. Malignant degeneration is rare.

A moderately enhancing soft tissue density without clearly defined borders is identified on CT. Involvement of the extraocular muscles, intraconal sensory or motor nerves, or cavernous sinus produces nodular enlargement of these structures. Absence of the sphenoid wing is the most typical bony orbital deformity, but long-standing soft tissue volume expansion may produce enlargement of the bony orbit when compared with the contralateral orbit. On MRI most lesions are hypointense on T1 weighting and hyperintense on T2 weighting and have the same gross features as seen on CT.

Lack of encapsulation and profound vascularity complicates management. Surgical excision is generally incomplete, bloody, and subject to significant postoperative edema, which is slow to resolve. The goals of excision are to provide modest cosmetic improvement with minimal risk to normal tissues. This requires multiple operative procedures over the life of the patient with decreasingly satisfactory results. Use of the CO_2 laser minimizes intraoperative bleeding.

Isolated Neurofibromas. Isolated neurofibromas are rarely identified in the orbit. Generally affecting sensory nerves, they enlarge slowly, producing mass-occupying effects not generally appreciated until the middle age. These may include proptosis, strabismus, and optic neuropathy. Although markedly adherent to the involved nerve, they do not possess the substantial vascularity that exists in the plexiform variety.

CT reveals a homogeneous and well-circumscribed soft tissue density that has uniform contrast medium enhancement. MRI demonstrates lesions hypointense to isointense on T1-weighted images and hyperintense on T2-weighted images.

Treatment of these lesions is dictated by the severity of the mass effect that is produced. Resection is considered for lesions producing compressive optic neuropathy or disfigurement. The surgical approach is dictated by the location of the mass. Less vascular than the plexiform variety, solitary neurofibromas pose fewer surgical complications. Efforts should be made to identify the function of the involved nerve both before surgery and intraoperatively. Sensory nerve function loss is of lesser consequence than motor loss. In the latter case, attempts should be made to preserve the function of the nerve by careful dissection of the tumor from the nerve with the assistance of the operating microscope.

Diffuse Neurofibromas. Diffuse neurofibromatosis is a rare form, generally affecting the skin and sparing the orbit. Involvement of the orbit produces diffuse infiltration of the soft tissues. Radiologically it has much the same features as the plexiform variety. Surgical resection is subtotal and complicated by significant vascularity and lack of encapsulation. Resection should be avoided and, if necessary, limited in extent.

Schwannoma

Schwannomas (Figs. 91 – 18 and 91 – 19) are benign proliferations of the Schwann cell envelope of peripheral

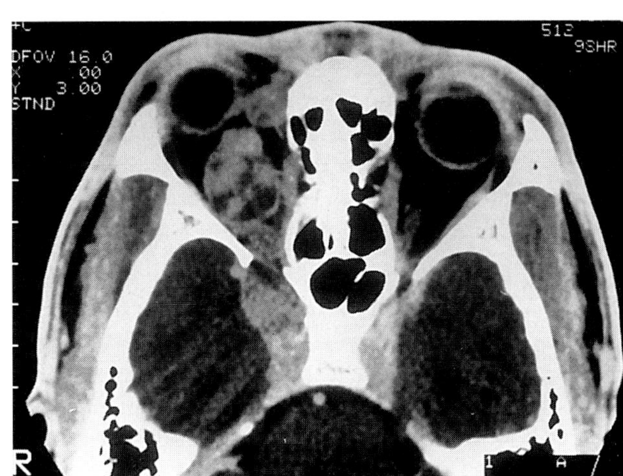

Figure 91 – 18. Schwannoma. Multilobulated soft tissue tumor extending from the intraconal space of the right orbit to the cavernous sinus where it produces widening of the sinus. Mild enhancement of the tumor is produced with contrast medium injection on this computed tomographic scan.

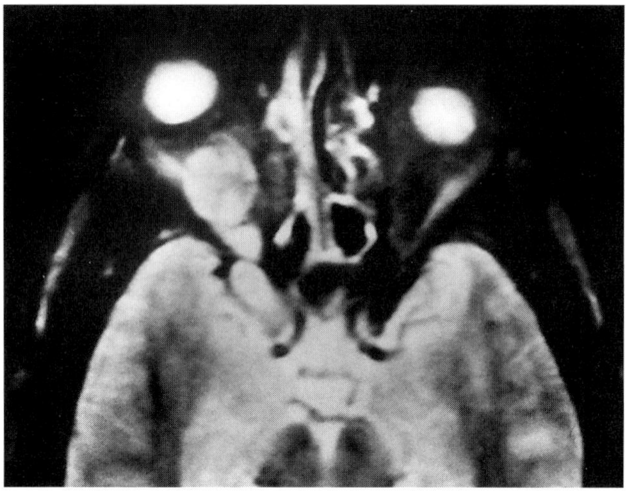

Figure 91–19. Schwannoma of the right orbit shown by magnetic resonance scan.

nerves. Within the orbit they may affect any of the sensory or motor nerves. They become clinically apparent in the fourth to fifth decades, producing slowly progressive painless proptosis. They do not affect nerve function until late in their course. Optic neuropathy is an inconsistent feature that depends on the critical size and location of the tumor producing secondary compression of the optic nerve. Small, apically located tumors may produce profound visual symptoms before there is evidence of proptosis, while a more anteriorly located mass will feature proptosis before optic neuropathy is documented. Mass effect of the tumor may also produce choroidal folds. Rare are malignant schwannomas that appear to be degenerations of more benign histologic forms. Growth in these cases is explosive.

Radiographic Features. CT scan reveals a homogeneous well-circumscribed soft tissue density that may be either intraconal or extraconal. It displaces surrounding structures, and long-standing lesions may produce remodeling or frank erosion of surrounding bone. Contrast dye may produce a small degree of enhancement.

MRI features a discrete, homogeneous, soft tissue density that is hypointense on T1-weighted images and hyperintense on T2-weighted images. There is little enhancement with the use of gadolinium.

Treatment. Treatment is primary excision when mass effect (e.g., optic neuropathy, proptosis) is significant or if the pattern of tumor growth accelerates, suggesting malignant degeneration. The route for orbitotomy is determined by the site of the tumor. The mass may be removed whole if small or in a fragmented fashion if larger. In such cases we find a CO_2 laser coupled to an operating neurosurgical microscope to aid the dissection and removal of the mass. Small volumes of residual tumor generally do not recur and are best left to preserve the surrounding normal structures. If histopathologic inspection reveals a malignant schwannoma, then exenteration is recommended.

Melanoma

Melanocytes are derived developmentally from the neural crest and are therefore grouped with the foregoing tumors. Primary orbital melanomas are extremely rare. More commonly, melanomas occur within the orbit as the result of extension through the sclera from a primary ocular tumor or as a metastatic lesion from an unknown or unsuspected primary cutaneous source. Tumors become clinically apparent by producing painless, progressive proptosis without substantial impairment of ocular motility or optic nerve function.

Radiographic Findings. Imaging with either CT or MRI identifies a soft tissue, contrast-enhancing mass that is most often located within the intraconal space. The tumors are usually homogeneous, although spontaneous hemorrhage, heralded clinically by rapid evolution of proptosis, is most easily identified by MRI, which can distinguish new and old clotted blood. There are no radiologic features that are pathognomonic of this lesion.

Treatment. Primary orbital melanomas are exceedingly rare, and most often identified after orbitotomy and histopathologic inspection. Orbital melanomas are usually pigmented and may be friable. The intraoperative identification and diagnosis are made more difficult if the lesion is amelanotic. Cure is not assured even if a gross total removal of the mass is achieved. Long-term outcome is poor regardless of the treatment, but current recommendations favor exenteration. Chemotherapy and orbital radiation therapy appear to be of no benefit.

SUGGESTED READING

Alper MG: Management of primary optic nerve sheath meningiomas: Current status—therapy in controversy. J Clin Neuro Ophthalmol 1:101, 1981.

Alvord EC, Lofton S: Gliomas of optic nerve or chiasm. J Neurosurg 68:85–98, 1988.

Borit A, Richardson EP Jr: The biological and clinical behaviour of pilocytic astrocytomas of the optic pathways. Brain 105:161, 1982.

Brand WN, Hoover SV: Optic glioma in children: Review of 16 cases given megavoltage radiation therapy. Childs Brain 5:459, 1979.

Coppetto JR, Jaffe R, Gillies CG: Primary orbital melanoma. Arch Ophthalmol 96:2255, 1978.

Daniels DL, Williams AL, Syvertsen A, et al: CT recognition of optic nerve sheath meningioma: Abnormal sheath visualization. AJNR 3:181, 1982.

Danoff BF, Kramer S, Thompson N: The radiotherapeutic management of optic nerve gliomas in children. Int J Radiat Oncol Biol Phys 6:45, 1980.

Desai R, Bruce J: Meningiomas of the cranial base. J Neuroradiol 20:255, 1994.

Glaser JS, Hoyt WF, Corbett J: Visual morbidity with chiasmal glioma. Arch Ophthalmol 85:3, 1971.

Gurland JE, Tenner M, Hornblass A, et al: Orbital neurofibromatosis. Arch Ophthalmol 94:1723, 1976.

Haik BG, et al: Magnetic resonance imaging in the evaluation of optic nerve gliomas. Ophthalmology 94:709, 1987.

Hart M Jr, Burde RM, Klingele TG, et al: Bilateral optic nerve sheath meningiomas. Arch Ophthalmol 98:149, 1980.
Holman RE, Grimson BS, Drayer BP, et al: Magnetic resonance imaging of optic gliomas. Am J Ophthalmol 100:596, 1985.
Holt JF: Neurofibromatosis in children. AJR 130:615, 1978.
Horwich A, Bloom HJG: Optic gliomas: Radiation therapy and prognosis. Int J Radiat Oncol Biol Phys 11:1067, 1985.
Hoyt WF, Baghdassarian SA: Natural history and rationale for conservative management. Br J Ophthalmol 53:793, 1969.
Hoyt WF, Meshal LG, Lessel S, et al: Malignant optic glioma of adulthood. Brain 96:121-132, 1973.
Jackson IT, Laws ER, Martin RD: The surgical management of orbital neurofibromatosis. Plast Reconstr Surg 71:751, 1983.
Jakobiec FA, Depot MJ, Kennerdell JS, et al: Combined clinical and computed tomographic diagnosis of orbital glioma and meningioma. Ophthalmology 91:137, 1984.
Jakobiec FA, Ellsworth R, Tannenbaum M: Primary orbital melanoma. Am J Ophthalmol 78:24, 1974.
Jakobiec FA, Jones IS: Neurogenic tumors. *In* Jones IS, Jakobiec FA (eds): Diseases of the Orbit. Philadelphia, Harper & Row, 1979, p 371.
Jones IS, Desjardins L: Management of orbital neurofibromatosis and lymphangiomas. *In* Jakobiec FA (ed): Ocular and Adnexal Tumors. Birmingham, AL, Aesculapius, 1978, p 375.
Kennerdell JS, Dekker A, Johnson BL, et al: Fine-needle aspiration biopsy: Its use in orbital tumors. Arch Ophthalmol 97:1315-1317, 1979.
Kennerdell JS, Maroon JC: Intracanalicular meningioma with chronic optic disc edema. Ann Ophthalmol 7:507, 1975.
Krohel GB, Rosenberg MD, Wright JE Jr et al: Localized orbital neurofibromas. Am J Ophthalmol 100:458, 1985.
MacMichael IM, Cullen JF: Primary intraorbital meningiomas. Br J Ophthalmol 53:169, 1969.
Mark LE, Kennerdell JS, Maroon JC, et al: Microsurgical removal of a primary intra-orbital meningioma. Am J Ophthalmol 86:704, 1978.
Mehra KS, Khanna S, Dube B: Primary meningioma of the intraorbital optic nerve. Ann Ophthalmol 11:758, 1979.
Reed D, Robertson WD, Rootman J, et al: Plexiform neurofibromatosis of the orbit: CT evaluation. AJNR 7:259, 1986.
Rush JA, Younge BR, Campbell RJ, et al: Long-term follow-up of 85 histopathologically verified cases. Ophthalmology 89:1213, 1982.
Sibony PA, Krauss HR, Kennerdell JS, et al: Optic nerve sheath meningiomas. Ophthalmology 91:11, 1984.
Smith JL, Vuksanovic MM, Yates BM, et al: Radiation therapy for primary optic nerve meningiomas. J Clin Neuro Ophthalmol 1:85, 1981.
Spoor TC, Kennerdell JS, Martinez AJ, Zorub D: Malignant gliomas of the optic nerve pathways. Am J Ophthalmol 89:284, 1980.
Tenny RT, Laws ER Jr, Younge BR, et al: The neurosurgical management of optic glioma: Result in 104 patients J Neurosurg 57:452, 1982.
White HR: Survival in malignant schwannoma: An 18-year study. Cancer 27:720, 1971.
Wright JE: Primary optic nerve meningiomas: Clinical presentation and management. Trans Am Acad Ophthalmol Otolaryngol 83:617, 1977.
Wright JE, McNab AA, McDonald WI: Optic nerve glioma and the management of optic nerve tumors in the young. Br J Ophthalmol 73:967-974, 1989.

CHAPTER 92

Mesenchymal and Fibro-osseous Tumors

Michael Clarke

MYOGENIC ORBITAL TUMORS

Skeletal Muscle Origin

Rhabdomyosarcoma

Epidemiology. Rhabdomyosarcoma is the most common soft tissue sarcoma of childhood and is also the most common primary malignant tumor of the orbit in childhood.[1] Up to 5% of childhood malignancies are rhabdomyosarcomas,[2] but the tumor is rare in adults older than age 45.[3] The overall incidence of rhabdomyosarcoma is 4 per 1 million per year.[4] Forty-four percent of rhabdomyosarcomas occur in the head and neck, and 25% to 50% of these originate in the orbit.[1] Seventy percent of rhabdomyosarcomas occur in the first decade. There is a bimodal age distribution, with a higher prevalence in children younger than 3 years old or older than 6 years old.[5] Congenital rhabdomyosarcoma has been reported.[6] There is a male to female predominance of 3:2, which increases to 5:3 when the tumor is in the orbit.[7] Knowles and Jakobiec[8] have suggested that rhabdomyosarcoma may be more common in Caucasians.

Presentation. There are two common modes of presentation of orbital rhabdomyosarcoma. The first is the acute onset of painless, rapidly progressive proptosis. The other common mode of presentation is with swelling and ptosis of the upper lid caused by a palpable mass.[9, 10] The mass is commonly in the upper inner quadrant of the orbit and may cause displacement of the globe and diplopia. Vision is usually preserved in the early stages. There are no distinguishing features on palpation that identify the tumor. Jones and colleagues,[10] in an analysis of 62 cases, found that in 50% the mass was predominantly retrobulbar, in 25% it was above the globe, and in 12% it was below the globe. The remainder were temporal or nasal.

Differential Diagnosis. Trauma may be suspected, and there is often a history of minor trauma before the onset of symptoms, but this is not considered to be an etiologic factor. Other differential diagnoses include inflammatory orbital lesions and other rapidly progressive orbital tumors. Children with orbital cellulitis are usually febrile and systemically unwell, and the swollen tissues are hot and painful, in contrast to children with rhabdomyosarcoma. The distinction from other rapidly progressive tumors may be more difficult and underlines the requirement for pediatric consultation at an early stage. Secondary deposits of leukemia and neuroblastoma may masquerade as rhabdomyosarcoma. It is usually possible to identify infantile hemangioma and dermoids on the basis of clinical examination.

Investigation. Investigation of suspected orbital rhabdomyosarcoma is required for tumor identification and staging. Computed tomography (CT) is preferred to magnetic resonance imaging (MRI) for orbital rhabdomyosarcoma, because CT better demonstrates orbital bone invasion, which is a poor prognostic sign. Arteriography is not usually indicated, but it should be performed if there is significant expansion of the lesion in response to a Valsalva maneuver. Biopsy is necessary to confirm the diagnosis and should be performed by an experienced orbital surgeon. The size of the lesion on CT is often deceptive, since the tumor is frequently surrounded by edema. Frozen section may be helpful but is usually not necessary. Biopsy is primarily for histologic confirmation of the diagnosis, but as much of the tumor as possible should be removed without damaging orbital structures. Staging investigations include CT of the chest, bone marrow examination, examination of the cerebrospinal fluid, liver function tests, and other tests as indicated.

Histopathology. Rhabdomyosarcoma develops from undifferentiated orbital mesenchyme rather than differentiated striated muscle. Four histologic patterns are described[11]: embryonal, botryoid, alveolar, and adult pleomorphic. However, there is considerable overlap between categories, with different patterns being present in one lesion, except in the case of embryonal rhabdomyosarcoma. Some tumors are so poorly differentiated that they are difficult to identify as rhabdomyosarcoma.

The presence of cross-striations in tumor cells is pathognomonic, but the vast majority of rhabdomyoblasts do not demonstrate this. Cross-striations are seen in 50% to 60% of embryonal and 30% of alveolar rhabdomyosarcomas. In the absence of cross-striations, staining for glyocogen and immunostaining for desmin are helpful and immunostaining for myoglobin is diagnostic of rhabdomyosarcoma. Genetic studies to identify chromosomal translocations may also be helpful in both diagnosis and prognosis.

Embryonal rhabdomyosarcoma makes up two thirds of cases and is usually seen in children younger than 10 years of age. Embryonal tumors mainly occur in the head and neck. The cellularity of the tumor may be loose (myxoid) or compact and varies in different regions of the same tumor. There is a range of microscopic appearances, with more differentiated tumors showing a larger proportion of rhabdomyoblasts and resembling fetal muscle tissue. Relatively undifferentiated embryonal tumors consist of small, round cells with indistinct cytoplasm and darkly staining nuclei, showing high levels of mitotic activity. Rhabdomyoblasts may be difficult to identify and rarely show cross-striations. More differentiated forms show multiple round or oval rhabdomyoblasts with eosinophilic cytoplasm and fibrillary material arranged around the nuclei. Intracellular glycogen is a pronounced feature of well-differentiated rhabdomyoblasts, and "spider web" cells from which intracellular glycogen has been washed out may be seen. With increasing differentiation, fusiform rhabdomyoblasts become apparent, with well-marked cross-striations.

Botryoid rhabdomyosarcoma refers to an embryonal tumor adjacent to mucous membrane. Such tumors show rapid, unrestricted growth in polypoid grape-like fashion. This growth pattern may rarely occur in the orbit if tumor prolapses through conjunctiva. Microscopically, cells are sparse and there is an abundance of mucoid stroma.

Alveolar rhabdomyosarcoma was described in 1956. When compared with embryonal tumors, rhabdomyosarcomas affect an older age group (10–25 years) and the tumors are poorly differentiated. The typical histologic pattern permits diagnosis even in the absence of rhabdomyoblasts. This type of rhabdomyosarcoma carries a relatively poor prognosis. Light microscopy shows ill-defined aggregates of poorly differentiated cells showing loss of cellular cohesion, leading to the "alveolar" appearance. These "alveoli" are surrounded by fibrous septa to which relatively well preserved cells adhere. Fusiform rhabdomyoblasts with cross-striations may very rarely be found in this area. "Spider web" cells are scarce. Cells in the center of the "alveoli" are often necrotic, and in some tumors it may be difficult to identify any cells at all. At the periphery of many alveolar tumors, more solidly packed cells are seen, and these probably represent the initial stages of growth. Multinucleate giant cells are common in alveolar rhabdomyosarcoma and help differentiation from embryonal tumors. The giant cells are probably formed by fusion with rhabdomyoblasts, but cross-striations are not seen.

Adult pleomorphic rhabdomyosarcoma is seen in less than 1% of tumors. Patients are usually older than age 45. These tumors are usually seen in the peripheral skeleton rather than in the orbit. Distinction from other pleomorphic sarcomas is difficult histologically, and immunostaining characteristics are very helpful in making the diagnosis. Tadpole-shaped rhabdomyoblasts are seen with granular cytoplasm, but cross-striations are very rare. Stains for myoglobin, desmin, and glycogen may assist in the differential diagnosis.

Differential Diagnosis. Rhabdomyosarcomas need to be differentiated from poorly differentiated round or spindle cell sarcomas, including Ewing's tumor, neuroblastoma, malignant melanoma, granulocytic sarcomas, and malignant lymphoma. Small cell carcinoma must also be considered in patients older than 40 years of age. Again, immunostaining can often resolve this problem, as can electron microscopy.

Genetics. Familial cases of rhabdomyosarcoma have been documented,[12] and the tumor has been seen in some families with the Li-Fraumeni syndrome, who are genetically predisposed to some malignancies.[13] A number of chromosomal abnormalities have been demonstrated in tumor cells from patients with rhabdomyosarcoma,[14–17] and these may be a frequent event during tumor development. The translocation t(2;13) (q35;q14) may be specific for rhabdomyosarcoma[15] and can be helpful diagnostically.[14]

Treatment. Prior to 1960, most patients with orbital rhabdomyosarcoma died. In the 1960s, aggressive surgical excision was the treatment of choice.[10] Chemotherapy for rhabdomyosarcoma was first suggested by Wilbur in 1974.[18] Survival rates have improved since the introduction of a multidisciplinary approach to management. The publications of the Intergroup Rhabdomyosarcoma Study have greatly increased the understanding of this condition.[19–26]

Surgical excision is now conservative and is followed by multiagent chemotherapy with or without radiation. The choice of therapy depends on the results of staging investigations.

The Intergroup Rhabdomyosarcoma Study distinguishes four stages:

I: Local disease, resection complete
II: Regional positive and negative lymph nodes, grossly resected but microscopic residual
III: Incomplete resection with gross residual disease
IV: Distant metastases

Treatment of stage I and II tumors consists of biopsy, followed by chemotherapy. It is not necessary to attempt total removal of the tumor at biopsy; however, as much of the tumor mass as possible should be removed, while leaving orbital structures intact. Stage III and IV lesions receive radiation therapy in addition. The current regimen of chemotherapy consists of vincristine and dactinomycin, together with cyclophosphamide when indicated. Other agents such as ifosphamide and etoposide are also used in some centers.

Courses of drugs are given every 3 weeks, and reassessment is made after four courses. Chemotherapy is usually continued for 6 months and, in the case of alveolar rhabdomyosarcoma, for 12 months. The dose of radiation for gross residual disease is 4500 to 5500 cGy over 6 weeks. This dose is sufficient to induce a variety of ocular side effects, including dry eye and cataract.

Lymphatic spread is unusual in orbital rhabdomyosarcoma. Spread through bone to the paranasal sinuses, and to the anterior and middle cranial fossae, may occur and is a poor prognostic sign.[9] Hematogenous spread most commonly occurs to the lung and bone marrow. Nonorbital, head and neck rhabdomyosarcoma is often referred to as parameningeal rhabdomyosarcoma because of the predisposition of these lesions to invade intracranially, leading to a poorer prognosis.

Prognosis. Before the use of combined surgery and chemotherapy, survival rates of 35% were reported, irrespective of age.[7, 10, 11] The prognosis has improved dramatically in recent years. There is now a 95% 5-year survival rate following therapy for orbital rhabdomyosarcoma.[27] The few fatalities that do occur are usually due to contiguous spread into the central nervous system. Five-year survival of 65% is the rule for lesions elsewhere in the body. Alveolar lesions carry the worst prognosis. Orbital lesions have a relatively good prognosis because of early presentation and the absence of orbital lymphatics.

Rhabdomyoma

The term *rhabdomyoma* was used synonymously with rhabdomyosarcoma in the older literature. True rhabdomyoma, a benign tumor of striated muscle, is rare in the orbit. Knowles and Jakobiec[28] reported a well-documented case in an 8-year-old boy. The tumor was initially misdiagnosed as rhabdomyosarcoma. Fetal rhabdomyoma is a clinically benign but cytologically immature variant seen in children younger than 3 years of age.[29] It has not been reported in the orbit.

Smooth Muscle Tumors

Tumors of smooth muscle origin are rare in the orbit and probably arise from neural crest, and are therefore classified as mesectodermal tumors.[30] The cells of origin are likely to be blood vessel associated. Distinction from striated muscle tumor is made histologically by the presence of intracellular nonstriated longitudinal cytoplasmic filaments, with intense cytoplasmic eosinophilia.[31] The diagnosis is difficult and may be confused with nerve sheath and vascular tumors.

Leiomyoma

The few reported cases of orbital leiomyoma have shown slowly progressive proptosis.[32–34] Patients tend to be younger than those with leiomyosarcoma. The tumor is encapsulated and lobulated. Local recurrence occurs if excision is incomplete, but metastatic spread does not occur. Treatment is surgical. Radiation therapy is ineffective and may induce sarcoma.[31]

Leiomyosarcoma

Leiomyosarcoma may arise as a primary orbital lesion,[35] spread into the orbit from the paranasal sinuses,[36] or metastasize to the orbit from a distant primary site.[37] Occurrence of leiomyosarcoma as a second tumor after orbital irradiation for retinoblastoma is well documented.[38, 39] Leiomyosarcoma is a highly malignant lesion, and most reported patients have died of distant metastases occurring after exenteration.

ADIPOSE TUMORS

Lipoma

True lipomas of the orbit are rare, and a pathology report stating "normal orbital fat" usually indicates failure to correctly identify the lesion to be biopsied. There are occasional reports of slowly enlarging orbital lesions composed of mature, nonencapsulated adipose tissue. Brown and coworkers[40] have described such a lesion as a lipomatous hamartoma and speculate that it may represent the evolution of a tumor of immature adipose tissue—lipoblastomatosis.

Variants of lipoma have been described in the orbit. One case of angiolipoma has been described, a tumor more commonly seen on the forearm and trunk.[41] Two cases of spindle cell lipoma have been described in the orbit.[42, 43] In these lesions, usually found on the shoulders and neck of men, mature adipose tissue is replaced by collagen forming spindle cells. One lesion was removed intact, and the other was debulked.

Liposarcoma

Common soft tissue tumors in the thigh and retroperitoneum, liposarcomas are rare in the head and neck.[1, 44] Jakobiec and colleagues[44a] reported five patients aged between 22 and 57 years. In all, diplopia and proptosis had been present for many months and visual acuity was preserved. The lesions were of irregular radiodensity on CT, which gave rise to the impression that they were cystic. However, ultrasonography showed them to be solid. There was a surrounding pseudocapsule consisting of compressed orbital tissues. The extraocular muscles were bowed and displaced by the tumor, and this was helpful in distinguishing liposarcoma from Graves' disease. There are often no specific features on CT to suggest malignancy.[45] In one of the cases in the series of Jakobiec and colleagues[44a] and in one of the cases reported by Lane and associates,[46] the patient had undergone orbital decompression for presumed dysthyroid orbitopathy. The appearance on light microscopy varied, with some tumors showing a myxoid stroma. There were characteristic "signet ring" lipoblasts at the tumor margin. Mitoses were absent, and all of Jakobiec and colleagues' patients were alive and free of distant metastases at followup of between 9 months and 4 years. Other clinicians have reported a fatal outcome.[47] Treatment consisted of local excision, followed by radiation or exenteration for recurrent disease. Lane and associates[46] concluded that radiation therapy and chemotherapy were ineffective. They suggested radical excision as a lifesaving procedure in young patients and a more conservative surgical approach in the elderly.

FIBROUS TISSUE TUMORS AND PROLIFERATIONS

Fibroma

True orbital fibromas and fibrosarcomas are rare.[48-50] Desmoid tumor, a nonmalignant, locally invasive, well-differentiated proliferation of musculoaponeurotic fibrous tissue, has rarely been reported in the orbit.[51, 52] Juvenile ossifying fibroma occurs in the orbit, predominantly on the orbital plate of the frontal bone and the ethmoid. The lesions can reach a large size. Margo and coworkers[53] described characteristic histology in juvenile ossifying fibroma of the orbit, consisting of "psammoma-like" ossicles in a spindle cell stroma. Treatment is by local excision. Recurrence occurs if this is incomplete. Rarely these lesions have been reported to arise from the maxillary sinus.[54] The differential diagnosis includes fibrous dysplasia, orbital inflammatory lesions with fibrosis, and bony tumors. Epibulbar fibroma, possibly arising from Tenon's capsule, has also been reported,[55] but reports of orbital fibroma are otherwise rare in the recent literature.

Fibromatosis

The term *fibromatosis* encompasses those proliferative lesions of fibroblast origin that invade locally but do not metastasize.[56] Some of these lesions have been referred to as myofibromatosis.[57, 58] Solitary, multicentric and generalized forms are seen. Treatment consists of wide local excision.

Fibrosarcoma

Fibrosarcoma of the orbit is a rare cause of proptosis in infants. Tumor cells are immature fibroblasts arranged in a herringbone pattern. The differential diagnosis includes rhabdomyosarcoma and fibrous histiocytoma. Of the five cases reported by Weiner and Hidyat,[59] two had local recurrence, but none developed distant metastases. Fibrosarcoma of the orbit can develop after radiation therapy for retinoblastoma.[60]

Nodular Fasciitis

Nodular fasciitis is a benign lesion that usually presents as a rapidly growing, solitary mass on the upper trunk of a young adult. More rarely it may affect the head and neck, and the lids and conjunctiva may be involved.[61] Occasionally the deeper orbit may be affected.[62] Treatment consists of surgical removal.

REFERENCES

1. Enzinger F, Weiss S: Soft Tissue Tumors. St. Louis, CV Mosby, 1988.
2. Miser J, Pizzo P: Soft tissue sarcomas in childhood. Pediatr Clin North Am 32:779–800, 1985.
3. Nakhleh R, Swanson P, Dehner L: Juvenile (embryonal and alveolar) rhabdomyosarcoma of the head and neck in adults: A clinical, pathologic and immunohistochemical study of 12 cases. Cancer 67:1019–1024, 1991.
4. Grufferman S, Wang H, Delong E, et al: Environmental factors in the aetiology of rhabdomyosarcoma in childhood. J NCI 68:107–113, 1982.
5. Knowles D, Jakobiec F, Potter G, Jones I: Ophthalmic striated muscle neoplasms. Surv Ophthalmol 21:219–261, 1976.
6. Himmel S, Siegel H: Congenital embryonal rhabdomyosarcoma in a newborn. Arch Ophthalmol 77:662–665, 1967.
7. Ashton N, Morgan G: Embryonal sarcoma and embryonal rhabdomyosarcoma of the orbit. J Clin Pathol 18:699–714, 1965.
8. Knowles D, Jakobiec F, Potter G, Jones I: The diagnosis and treatment of rhabdomyosarcoma of the orbit. *In* Jakobiec FA (ed): Ocular and Adnexal Tumors. Birmingham, AL, Aesculapius, 1978.
9. Abramson DH, Ellsworth RM, Tretter P, et al: The treatment of orbital rhabdomyosarcoma with irradiation and chemotherapy. Ophthalmology 86:1330–1335, 1979.
10. Jones I, Reese A, Kraut J: Orbital rhabdomyosarcoma: An analysis of 62 cases. Am J Ophthalmol 61:721–736, 1966.
11. Horner R, Enterline H: Rhabdomyosarcoma: A clinicopathological study of 39 cases. Cancer 11:181–184, 1958.
12. Howard G, Casten V: Rhabdomyosarcoma of the orbit in brothers. Arch Ophthalmol 70:319–322, 1963.
13. Malkin D, Li F, Strong L, et al: Germ line p53 mutations in a familial syndrome of breast cancer, sarcomas, and other neoplasms. Science 250:1233–1238, 1990.
14. Brichard B, Ninane J, Gosseye S, et al: A disseminated alveolar rhabdomyosarcoma in a nine year old boy disclosed by chromosomal translocation. Pediatr Hematol Oncol 8:215–219, 1991.
15. Douglas E, Valentine M, Etcubanas E, et al: A specific chromosomal abnormality in rhabdomyosarcoma. Cytogenet Cell Genet 45:148–155, 1987.
16. Magnani I, Faustinella F, Nanni P, et al: Karyotypic characterization of a new human embryonal rhabdomyosarcoma cell line. Cancer Genet Cytogenet 54:83–89, 1991.
17. Voullaire L, Petrovic V, Sheffield L, Campbell P: Two forms of ring 13 in a child with rhabdomyosarcoma. Am J Med Genet 39:285–287, 1991.
18. Wilbur J: Combination chemotherapy for embryonal rhabdomyosarcoma. Cancer Chemother Rep 58:281–284, 1974.
19. Tefft M, Lindberg R, Gehan E, and Intergroup Rhabdomyosarcoma Study Committee: Radiation of rhabdomyosarcoma in children combined with systemic chemotherapy: Local control in

patients enrolled into the Intergroup Rhabdomyosarcoma Study (IRS). NCI Monogr 56:75, 1981.
20. Palmer N, Sachs N, Foulkes M: Histopathology and prognosis in rhabdomyosarcoma (IRS-I). ASCO Abstracts C660:170, 1982.
21. Suton W, Lindberg R, Gehan E, et al: Report from Intergroup Rhabdomyosarcoma Study: Three-year relapse-free survival rates in childhood rhabdomyosarcoma of the head and neck. Cancer 49:2217, 1982.
22. Palmer N, Foulkes M: Histopathology and prognosis in the second Intergroup Rhabdomyosarcoma Study (IRS-II). ASCO Abstracts C897:229, 1983.
23. Maurer H, Foulkes M, Gehan E: Intergroup Rhabdomyosarcoma Study (IRS) II: A preliminary report. Proc Am Soc Clin Oncol 2:70, 1983
24. Maurer H, Beltangady M, Gehan E, et al: The Intergroup Rhabdomyosarcoma Study I: A final report. Cancer 61:209–220, 1988.
25. Maurer H, Gehan E, Crist W: Intergroup Rhabdomyosarcoma Study III: A preliminary report of the overall outcome. Proc Am Soc Clin Oncol 8:296, 1989.
26. Crist W, Garnsey L, Beltangady M, et al: Prognosis in children with rhabdomyosarcoma: A report of the Intergroup Rhabdomyosarcoma Studies I and II. Clin Oncol 8:443–452, 1990.
27. Wharam M, Beltangady M, Hays D, et al: Localized orbital rhabdomyosarcoma. Ophthalmology 94:251–254, 1987.
28. Knowles D II, Jakobiec F: Rhabdomyoma of the orbit. Am J Ophthalmol 80:1011–1018, 1975.
29. Dehner L, Enzinger F, Font R: Fetal rhabdomyoma: An analysis of nine cases. Cancer 30:160, 1972.
30. Jakobiec F, Tannenbaum M: Embryological perspectives on the fine structure of orbital tumors. Int Ophthalmol Clin 15:85–110, 1975.
31. Jakobiec F, Howard G, Rosen M, Wolff M: Leiomyoma and leiomyosarcoma of the orbit. Am J Ophthalmol 80:1028–1042, 1975.
32. Jakobiec F, Jones I, Tannenbaum M: Leiomyoma: An unusual tumor of the orbit. Br J Ophthalmol 57:825–831, 1973.
33. Vigstrup J, Glenthoj A: Leiomyoma of the orbit. Acta Ophthalmol 60:992–997, 1982.
34. Sanborn G, Valenzuela R, Green W: Leiomyoma of the orbit. Am J Ophthalmol 87:371–375, 1979.
35. Meekins B, Dutton J, Proia A: Primary orbital leiomyosarcoma: A case report and review of the literature. Arch Ophthalmol 106:82–86, 1988.
36. Jakobiec F, Mitchell J, Chauhan P, Iwamoto T: Mesectodermal leiomyosarcoma of the antrum and orbit. Am J Ophthalmol 85:51–57, 1978.
37. Kaltreider S, Destro M, Lemke B: Leiomyosarcoma of the orbit: A case report and review of the literature. Ophthalmic Plast Reconstr Surg 3:35–41, 1987.
38. Font R, Jurco S. III, Brechner R: Postradiation leiomyosarcoma of the orbit complicating bilateral retinoblastoma. Arch Ophthalmol 101:1557–1561, 1983.
39. Folberg R, Cleasby G, Flanagan J, et al: Orbital leiomyosarcoma after radiation therapy for bilateral retinoblastoma. Arch Ophthalmol 101:1562–1565, 1983.
40. Brown H, Kersten R, Kulwin D: Lipomatous hamartoma of the orbit. Arch Ophthalmol 109:240–243, 1991.
41. Feinfeld R, Hesse R, Scharfenberg J: Orbital angiolipoma. Arch Ophthalmol 106:1093–1095, 1988.
42. Johnson B, Linn JJ: Spindle cell lipoma of the orbit. Arch Ophthalmol 97:133–134, 1979.
43. Bartley G, Yeatts R, Garrity J, et al: Spindle cell lipoma of the orbit. Am J Ophthalmol 100:605–609, 1985.
44. Naeser P, Mostrom U: Liposarcoma of the orbit: A clinicopathological case report. Br J Ophthalmol 66:190–193, 1982.
44a. Jakobiec FA, Rini F, Char D, et al: Primary liposarcoma of the orbit: Problems in the diagnosis and management of five cases. Ophthalmology 96:180–191, 1989.
45. McNab A, Moseley I: Primary orbital liposarcoma: Clinical and computed tomographic features. Br J Ophthalmol 74:437–439, 1990.
46. Lane C, Wright J, Garner A: Primary myxoid liposarcoma of the orbit. Br J Ophthalmol 72:912–917, 1988
47. Mortada A: Rare primary orbital sarcomas. Am J Ophthalmol 68:919–927, 1969.
48. Reese A: Tumors of the Eye. Hagerstown, MD, Harper & Row, 1976.
49. Rootman J: Diseases of the Orbit. Philadelphia, JB Lippincott, 1988.
50. Mortada A: Fibroma of the orbit. Br J Ophthalmol 55:350–352, 1971.
51. Schutz J, Rabkin M, Schutz S: Fibromatous tumor (desmoid type) of the orbit. Arch Ophthalmol 97:703–704, 1979.
52. Craig R, Studd D: Extra-abdominal desmoid of the face involving the orbit. Br J Surg 65:131–134, 1978.
53. Margo C, Ragsdale B, Perman K, et al: Psammomatoid (juvenile) ossifying fibroma of the orbit. Ophthalmology 150–159, 1985.
54. Shields J, Peyster R, Handler S, et al: Massive juvenile ossifying fibroma of maxillary sinus with orbital involvement. Br J Ophthalmol 69:392–395, 1985.
55. Herschorn B, Jakobiec F, Hornblass A, et al: Epibulbar subconjunctival fibroma: A tumor possibly arising from Tenon's capsule. Ophthalmology 90:1490–1494, 1983.
56. Campbell R, Garrity J: Juvenile fibromatosis of the orbit: A case report with review of the literature. Br J Ophthalmol 75:313–316, 1991.
57. Nasr A, Blodi F, Lindahl S, Jinkins J: Congenital multicentric myofibromatosis with orbital involvement. Am J Ophthalmol 102:779–787, 1986.
58. Waeltermann J, Huntrakoon M, Beatty EJ, Cibis G: Congenital fibromatosis (myofibromatosis) of the orbit: A rare cause of proptosis at birth. Ann Ophthalmol 20:394–396, 1988.
59. Weiner J, Hidyat A: Juvenille fibrosarcoma of the orbit and eyelid: A study of five cases. Arch Ophthalmol 101:253–259, 1983.
60. Soloway H: Radiation induced neoplasms following curative therapy for retinoblastoma. Cancer 19:1984–1988, 1966.
61. Font R, Zimmerman L: Nodular fasciitis of the eye and adnexa. Arch Ophthalmol 75:475–481, 1966.
62. Perry R, Ramani P, McAllister V, et al: Nodular fasciitis causing unilateral proptosis. Br J Ophthalmol 59:404–408, 1975.

CHAPTER 93

Lacrimal Gland Neoplasia

Geoffrey E. Rose

Lacrimal gland tumors constitute a small, but significant, proportion of orbital disease[1-4] and present particular difficulty in their clinical diagnosis and management. Inflammation, sarcoidosis, and other non-neoplastic conditions of the lacrimal gland are more common than such tumors but may have a similar clinical presentation; neoplasia should, therefore, enter the differential diagnosis for most lacrimal gland disorders.

Secondary tumors within the lacrimal gland may arise from a systemic disease, such as metastasis from distant primary tumors[5] or as a multifocal systemic lymphoma,[6] or may result from direct invasion of the gland by primary tumors arising in other orbital tissues. Primary tumors of the gland, benign or malignant, are more common than such secondary tumors.

The benign primary tumor of the lacrimal gland is almost exclusively pleomorphic adenoma (benign mixed tumor), in which proliferating ductular elements occur within a diffuse stroma; the stroma comprises spindle-shaped cells in a myxoid or hyaline ground, and cartilage-like areas, with or without calcification, may occur rarely. Various components of this benign tumor are thought to be derived from glandular ectoderm and myoepithelial cells.[7, 8] The slowly expanding, very hard tumor attenuates and compresses surrounding lacrimal tissue, and this normal tissue forms a "pseudocapsule" around the adenoma and it is recognized that small extensions of the tumor lie outside the main bulk of the tumor and within this pseudocapsule.[9]

Malignant tumors form up to half of the primary epithelial neoplasms of the lacrimal gland,[1-4, 9-12] with the several forms of adenoid cystic carcinoma being the most common variants[13] and mucoepidermoid or squamous carcinomas or adenocarcinomas occurring infrequently. Carcinomas, particularly poorly differentiated adenocarcinomas,[13] can arise within a preexisting pleomorphic adenoma and are termed *malignant mixed tumors*; such malignant transformation may be limited to within the original benign tumor or may extend beyond the parental pleomorphic adenoma.

EPIDEMIOLOGY, CLINICAL PRESENTATION, AND RADIOLOGIC FEATURES

Pleomorphic adenomas are rare and present, with a male predominance, from childhood, although their peak incidence is in middle age.[1, 4, 11] Malignant mixed tumors occur in a similar age range to pleomorphic adenomas, but without an overall sex bias. Adenoid cystic carcinomas are the predominant primary epithelial malignancy of the lacrimal gland.[1-3, 9-12] They occur in either sex with a peak incidence around the fourth decade but may rarely present in childhood. Adenocarcinomas are much rarer, have a male predominance, and present in an older age group than the more common adenoid cystic carcinoma. Mucoepidermoid or squamous carcinomas are extremely rare.

Tumors in the body of the lacrimal gland may present as a palpable lump and cause proptosis or displacement of the globe inferomedially[3, 4]; such displacement may be symptomatic as binocular diplopia or facial asymmetry, the latter often being noted by friends (Fig. 93-1). Diplopia may be intermittent, with limitation of eye movements occurring at extremes of gaze or with larger tumors. Distortion of the globe by a firm tumor mass (Fig. 93-2) may cause a symptomatic alteration of visual acuity. Painful tumors tend to present earlier since smaller tumors and objective signs may be limited to a subtle change in the upper lid profile and skin crease (Fig. 93-3) or a palpable mass in the lacrimal gland fossa. Lacrimal gland tumors almost never cause ocular irritation, although episodic epiphora occurs with some pleomorphic adenomas.[4] Tumor extension to the superior orbital fissure (Fig. 93-4) may cause secondary congestion of the episcleral veins (Fig. 93-5) or may cause ptosis, diplopia, or sensory loss owing to involvement of cranial nerves passing through the fissure (Fig. 93-6).

Palpebral lobe tumors are less common than those in the body of the gland.[4, 15, 16] Because of the anterior location, these tumors typically present with a short history of a palpable mass in the upper eyelid or an alteration of lid contour; examination generally reveals a mobile hard

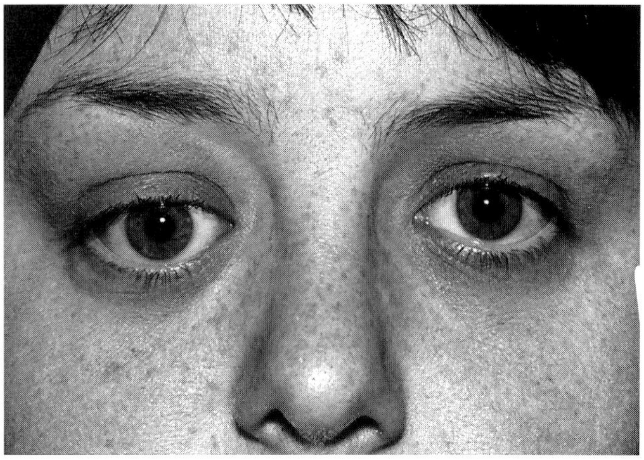

Figure 93 – 1. Facial asymmetry due to pleomorphic adenoma of the right lacrimal gland; the asymmetry was first noted by relatives.

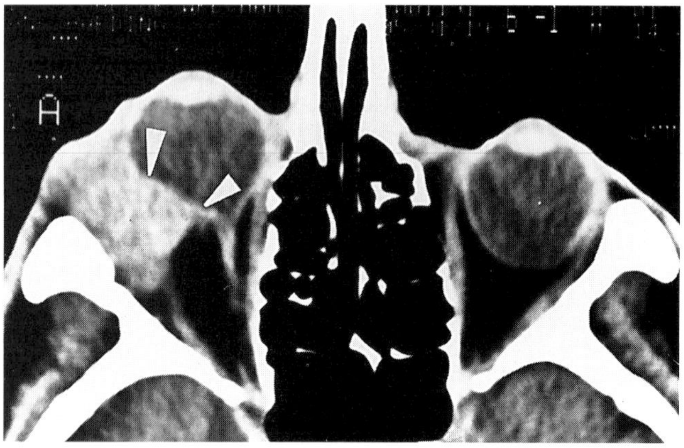

Figure 93 – 2. Marked flattening of the contour of the right globe due to a pleomorphic adenoma *(arrowheads)*.

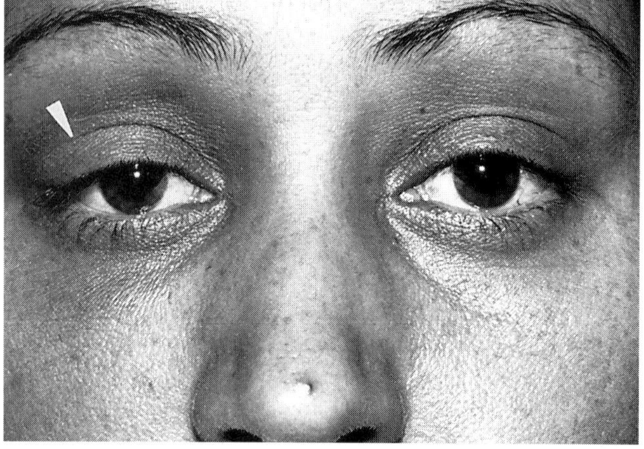

Figure 93 – 3. Alteration or effacement of the upper eyelid skin crease *(arrowhead)* may, as in this patient with right-sided disease, be the first sign of a lacrimal gland tumor.

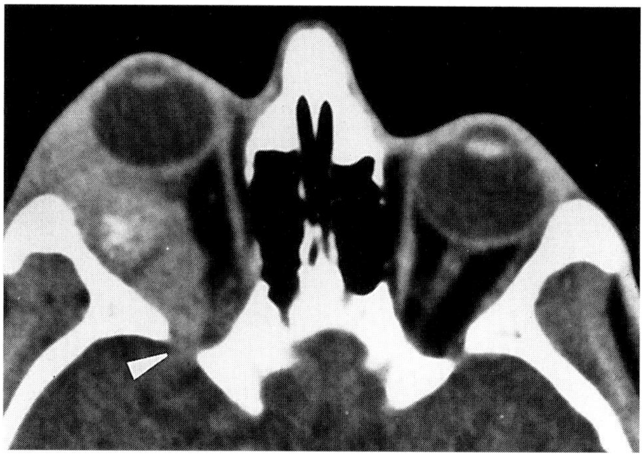

Figure 93 – 4. Adenoid cystic carcinoma of the lacrimal gland extends backward along the lateral wall of the right orbit and through the superior orbital fissure *(arrowhead)*.

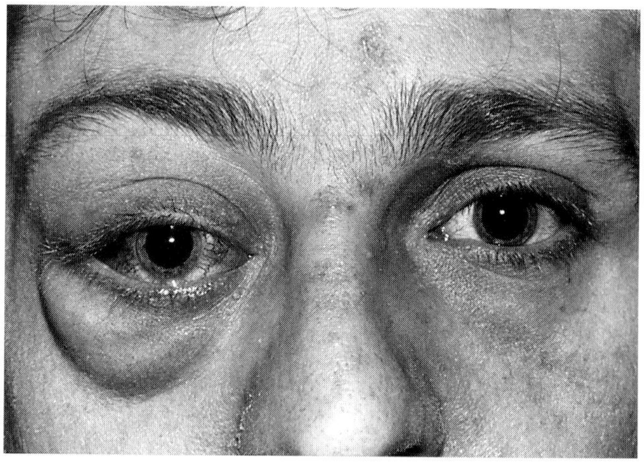

Figure 93 – 5. Congestion of right orbital veins due to adenoid cystic carcinoma invading the superior orbital fissure (same patient as in Fig. 93 – 4).

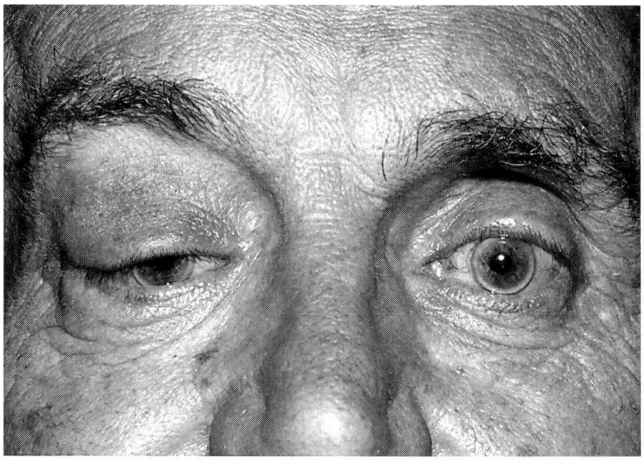

Figure 93 – 6. Partial neurogenic ptosis due to an adenocarcinoma of the right lacrimal gland extending to the superior orbital fissure.

mass in the lateral aspect of the upper lid or a prominence of the palpebral lobe in the upper conjunctival fornix.

Orbital pain is rare with lacrimal lymphoma and occurs in only a minority of pleomorphic adenomas.[4] In contrast, persistent pain is common with primary lacrimal carcinomas[3] or tumors metastatic to the gland; this stresses the importance of malignancy entering the differential diagnosis for all painful lacrimal disorders, such as acute or chronic dacryoadenitis or reactive lymphoid hyperplasia. Persistent pain is an important determinant in the practical management of lacrimal gland tumors[3, 4, 17, 18] and is considered later.

The features of a lacrimal mass on high-resolution computed tomographic (CT) scans, particularly configuration, are valuable in the differentiation of lacrimal gland disorders.[19] Palpebral lobe tumors lie anteriorly to the orbit and may be shown on high-resolution CT scans (Fig. 93–7). Tumors in the body (orbital lobe) tend to be larger and compress (see Fig. 93–2) and displace (Fig. 93–8) the globe. Expansion of the lacrimal fossa may occur with these firm, slowly growing tumors (see Fig. 93–8) and may also be evident on plain radiographs (Fig. 93–9). Rapidly growing or softer tumors, such as carcinomas or lymphomas, tend to be less well defined and mold to, rather than indent, the contour of the globe (Fig. 93–10). Carcinomas frequently extend along the lateral orbital wall toward the superior orbital fissure, displacing the lateral rectus medially (see Fig. 93–4).

Most tumors show some variation of density on CT scan, with moderate enhancement after intravenous contrast medium. Calcification occurs in about a third of lacrimal gland carcinomas,[3] relatively rarely with pleomorphic adenoma[4] or metastases, and extremely rarely with lymphomas; calcification in carcinomas tends to be present as diffuse flecks (Fig. 93–11), whereas that with pleomorphic adenomas may be more discrete (Fig. 93–12).

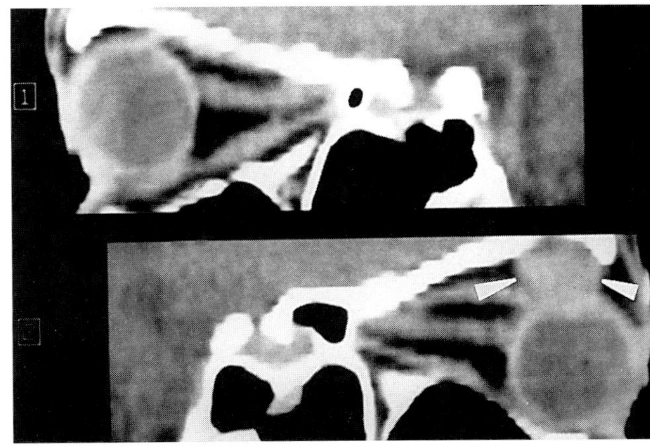

Figure 93–8. Sagittal computed tomographic scans of both orbits show a right-sided pleomorphic adenoma *(arrowheads)* displacing the globe downward.

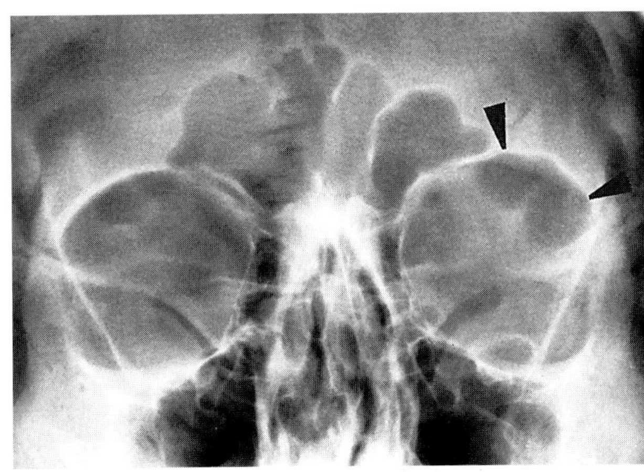

Figure 93–9. Clearly defined enlargement of the left lacrimal gland fossa *(arrowheads)* on plain radiograph, caused by a long-standing pleomorphic adenoma.

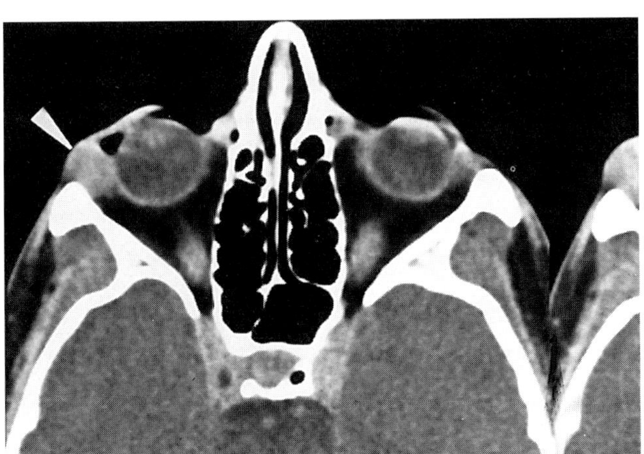

Figure 93–7. Pleomorphic adenoma in the palpebral lobe of the right lacrimal gland *(arrowhead)*.

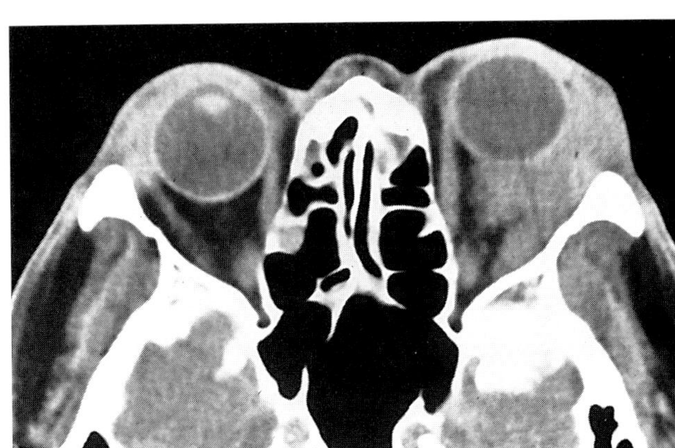

Figure 93–10. Lymphoma of both lacrimal glands, showing the characteristic "molding" to the contour of the globes.

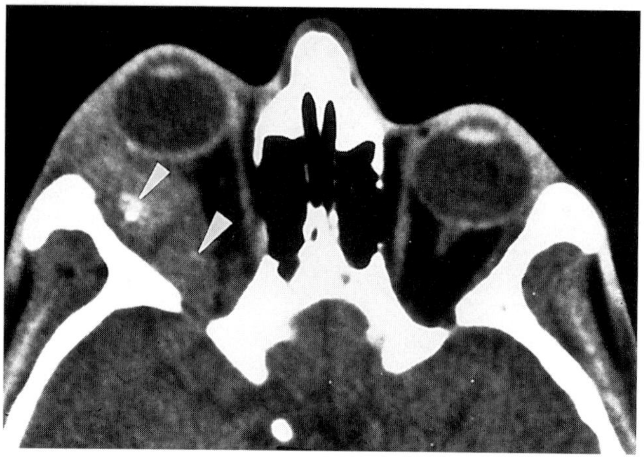

Figure 93–11. Soft tissue calcification *(arrowheads)* in an adenoid cystic carcinoma (same patient as in Figs. 93–4 and 93–5).

NATURAL HISTORY

The natural course for lacrimal gland tumors can be estimated from typical clinical histories and from radiologic or historical evidence. The value of an accurate clinical history in the management of all lacrimal gland disorders has been proposed by Wright and colleagues[17] and confirmed by subsequent studies.[4, 18]

Pleomorphic adenomas progress very slowly and are probably asymptomatic for many years; symptoms in such patients are often present for at least 1 year before seeking medical attention.[1, 2, 4, 17, 18] Malignant transformation of a pleomorphic adenoma is evidenced by an acceleration of symptoms that were previously only slowly progressive.[20] It has been estimated that up to 20% of pleomorphic adenomas may undergo malignant transformation by 30 years after inadequate surgical excision or biopsy.[11]

In contrast to orbital lobe tumors, pleomorphic adenomas arising in the palpebral lobe are generally detected and treated early in their natural history.

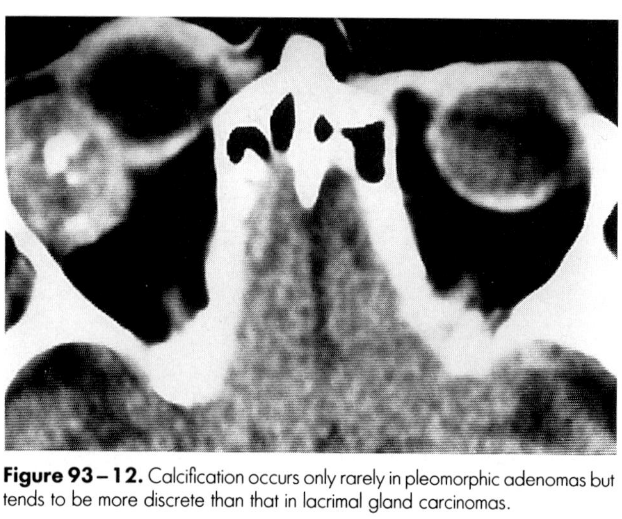

Figure 93–12. Calcification occurs only rarely in pleomorphic adenomas but tends to be more discrete than that in lacrimal gland carcinomas.

Primary malignant lacrimal gland tumors tend to infiltrate neighboring orbital tissues and breach the orbital periosteum. Once through periosteum, these tumors typically invade bone and spread into the temporalis fossa, cranial diploe, or intracranial cavity. Many carcinomas also extend posteriorly within the orbit and pass through the superior orbital fissure (see Fig. 93–4); this probably reflects the propensity for adenoid cystic carcinoma to extend beyond the main tumor bulk by perineural spread.[21] Malignant tumors show various rates of growth: adenocarcinomas appear to progress rapidly[3] whereas well-differentiated mucoepidermoid carcinomas may progress relatively slowly.[21] The growth of adenoid cystic carcinomas can vary from an aggressive to a chronic, but relentlessly progressive, local disease. Despite variations in the growth rate for primary malignancies, most tend to have a short history and show, relative to their short history, a large tumor on CT scan; this is in contrast to pleomorphic adenomas, which tend to show a smaller mass with respect to the length of history.[4]

Lacrimal gland lymphoma will, in some cases, be part of a systemic disease, possibly active for years before presentation. Progression of lymphomas can be very variable, although tumors within the lacrimal gland tend to follow a relatively indolent course and have a reasonable prognosis.[6]

Metastatic secondary tumors will tend to follow the course of the parent tumors, but most such tumors are fast growing and associated with a poor prognosis.

PRINCIPLES AND PROBLEMS OF MANAGEMENT

Management of lacrimal gland disease presents the surgeon with diagnostic difficulty and several opposing requirements.

The extent of a malignant tumor is often underestimated by clinical or radiologic signs, and many tumors thought to be localized are found, at surgery, to have breached the orbital periosteum. Moreover, the extension of pleomorphic adenomas into a "pseudocapsule" of compressed tissues[9] and the perineural spread of adenoid cystic carcinomas[21] also means that many primary lacrimal tumors extend beyond the main bulk of tumor. These factors dictate that the curative resection of benign or malignant lacrimal tumors must include an adequate buffer of surrounding normal tissues—in some cases orbital exenteration or more extensive en bloc cranio-orbital resection.

The rapid progression of primary lacrimal gland malignancies necessitates early biopsy to differentiate this diagnosis from other, medically treatable, disorders, such as inflammations or lymphomas; this is particularly so when pain is present. Biopsy, with definitive (paraffin) sectioning rather than frozen section, is also mandatory before considering any extensive or disfiguring surgery for eradication of malignancy. Biopsy of pleomorphic adenomas is, however, strictly contraindicated: if biopsy is done before excision, the 5-year recurrence rate is estimated to be 32%, compared with 3% if tissue is not sampled; many of these recurrences undergo malignant transformation.[11] Pleomorphic adenomas should be identified preoperatively and biopsy avoided.[4, 17]

Adequate access for the intact resection or pleomorphic adenomas of the body of the gland is provided only by a lateral orbitotomy. When dealing with malignant disease, however, it is preferable to maintain an intact orbital periosteum. Lateral orbitotomy, with its breach of periosteum and craniofacial bone, might be providing a route for the extraorbital dissemination of malignant cells and, in turn, prejudice the cure of lacrimal gland malignancies.

DIFFERENTIAL DIAGNOSIS

In 1979, Wright and colleagues, having recognized the need for preoperative differentiation of pleomorphic adenoma from primary malignancy, proposed a clinical algorithm for the management of suspected lacrimal gland malignancy; this was based on the duration of symptoms (an indirect indication of the rate of tumor growth) and the presence of pain.[17] Painless lesions with symptoms for more than a year were typically pleomorphic adenomas, whereas carcinomas tended to have shorter histories with persistent pain; review of a larger clinical series has confirmed the practical value of the algorithm,[4] although high-resolution CT scanning is of particular value in refining the preoperative clinical diagnosis (Table 93–1).[4, 19]

TABLE 93–1

Management Plan for Masses Within the Orbital Lobe of the Lacrimal Gland

Characteristic	Score −1	Score +1
Clinical		
Duration of acute symptoms	< 10 months	> 10 months
Persistent pain	Present	Absent
Sensory loss	Present	Absent
*Radiologic**		
Well-defined round or oval mass	Absent	Present
Molding of mass to globe or along the lateral orbital wall	Present	Absent
Tumor calcification	Present	Absent
Invasion of bone	Present	Absent
Duration of symptoms in relation to the tumor size	Large tumor; brief symptoms	Small tumor; extended symptoms

*Features on high-resolution computed tomography studies.

Total Score: −8 to +2; probably carcinoma (for incisional biopsy)
−6 to +2; probably malignant mixed tumor (for incisional or excisional biopsy)
+3 to +8; probably pleomorphic adenoma (for excision *without* prior biopsy)

From Rose GE, Wright JE: Pleomorphic adenoma of the lacrimal gland. Br J Ophthalmol 76:395–400, 1992.

When symptoms have been present for more than 10 to 12 months, especially in the absence of pain, the differential diagnosis is principally that of pleomorphic adenoma, lymphoma, sarcoidosis, chronic mild dacryoadenitis, and other non-neoplastic conditions. On high-resolution CT scans, pleomorphic adenomas typically have a round or oval configuration, tend to flatten the globe and often expand, not invade, the bone of the lacrimal gland fossa (see Figs. 93–2, 93–8, and 93–9); such a tumor should be excised intact through a lateral orbitotomy. An elongated enlargement of the gland, with molding to the globe (see Fig. 93–10), is suggestive of lymphoma, chronic dacryoadenitis, or sarcoidosis, with these diagnoses being particularly likely if changes are bilateral; in such cases a transseptal biopsy should clarify the diagnosis.

A diagnosis of malignant transformation within a pleomorphic adenoma (malignant mixed tumor) should be considered when long-term symptoms (>10–12 months) give way to a dramatic acceleration in apparent tumor growth or a recent onset of pain.[14, 20] A well-circumscribed tumor on CT scan should be treated like a pleomorphic adenoma, with intact excision; where radiologic evidence, such as bone invasion, suggests extraorbital extension, a biopsy should be performed before definitive treatment.

Acute onset of a painful, swollen, and tender lacrimal gland is likely to be inflammatory, either idiopathic or of bacterial or (presumed) viral etiology; most episodes resolve rapidly with appropriate systemic antibiotics. Lacrimal gland swelling that persists for more than a few weeks should be investigated with orbital CT scans and transseptal biopsy, since acute inflammatory episodes may be related to an underlying carcinoma.[17]

A patient with a 1- to 12-month history of a lacrimal gland mass, especially when painful, should be examined as a matter of urgency. A diffuse mass molding to the globe and extending along or invading the lateral orbital wall (see Figs. 93–4, 93–10, and 93–11) suggests a differential diagnosis between primary or secondary neoplasia, lymphoma, subacute dacryoadenitis or sarcoidosis, and other non-neoplastic conditions; in such cases a transseptal biopsy is mandatory. A well-defined mass with smooth expansion of the lacrimal fossa and flattening of the globe (see Figs. 93–2, 93–8, and 93–9) is probably of long standing and has become symptomatic only recently; the likelihood of pleomorphic adenoma in such cases would favor exploration through a lateral orbitotomy.

When continued doubt exists, the lacrimal gland may be approached through an incision in the lateral part of the brow. If inspection and palpation suggests a pleomorphic adenoma (generally smooth, pale gray, and very hard) or a mass localized to the gland, the skin incision can be extended laterally and lateral orbitotomy performed. However, if the gland is replaced by a friable tissue or if there is evidence of a breach of the periosteum, then the gland should be sampled and the brow incision closed.

Henderson and Neault suggest another approach, whereby all lacrimal gland tumors are approached through a lateral orbitotomy and resected en bloc with a portion of the lateral orbital wall; the technique may be modified for intraoperative histopathology by frozen section.[22] The failure to preserve an intact orbital periosteum in the presence of malignancy might, however, jeopardize a subsequent cure for such tumors.

Fine-needle aspiration biopsy can be available for orbital diagnosis,[23] and its advocates suggest that tumor seeding is unlikely along a fine needle track. In the case of pleomorphic adenomas, however, followup studies from such biopsy techniques have not been sufficiently long to justify this claim; recurrence of pleomorphic adenomas is very slow and occurs over several decades after biopsy.[11]

TREATMENT AND PROGNOSIS

Secondary tumors presenting as lacrimal gland masses, although rare,[5] should be treated according to the parent tumor. However, being within the cranial vascular territory, such metastasis is a likely sentinel for intracranial or other widespread disease and will generally carry a poor prognosis.

Systemic lymphoma is present in about 24% of patients at the time of presentation with orbital lymphoma and develops later in another 9%.[6] Investigations for systemic disease should be performed and patients reviewed for the onset of systemic disease (or recurrence of orbital disease) for many years after first presentation. A rapid resolution of clinical signs may follow the use of local external beam radiation therapy for orbital disease, but, in some cases, systemic chemotherapy may be required for widespread disease. Atrophy of normal lacrimal gland tissue leads, in a minority of cases, to reduced tear secretion and keratoconjunctivitis sicca.

Pleomorphic adenomas should be excised intact, with a cuff of normal tissues. Small adenomas within the palpebral lobe are readily resected through a transcutaneous anterior orbitotomy (with division of the lateral horn of the levator aponeurosis) or through the upper conjunctival fornix.[4, 15, 16] Orbital lobe adenomas should be approached through a lateral orbitotomy[24] and the tumor mobilized on an island of intact periosteum; the tumor should not be handled with forceps (but rather with malleable retractors) and at all times a "buffer" of normal tissues should be maintained around the tumor.[4] When spillage of cells occurs during surgery, or when the orbital periosteum appears completely attenuated by the tumor, the breach should be treated by strict surgical isolation and lavage of the operative field after tumor removal. The intraoperative use of a tissue adhesive to seal breaches of the tumor "pseudocapsule" may also be considered.

Subtotal dacryoadenectomy for orbital lobe tumors decreases the incidence of dry eyes and secondary corneal disease.[4] This technique, developed by Wright, preserves a functional palpebral lobe by transection of tissues between the two lobes. The effect of this modification on the long-term outcome for such tumors remains to be established.

The generally accepted treatment for a recently biopsied pleomorphic adenoma is tumor excision through lateral orbitotomy and resection of the whole biopsy track; long-term results from such therapy are, however, limited. Recurrence of a biopsied pleomorphic adenoma often involves several orbital tissues, and tumor clearance may necessitate extensive resection or exenteration.[4, 11, 12, 21]

The primary carcinomas of the lacrimal gland, particularly adenoid cystic carcinoma (the most common variant), present great difficulty in their management and in the assessment of clinical outcome.

Mucoepidermoid and squamous differentiation may coexist in carcinomas of the lacrimal gland, and these tumors are extremely rare. Consensus suggests treatment should be by wide surgical resection, and marked squamous differentiation would appear to be associated with a worse prognosis.[21]

Primary adenocarcinomas of the lacrimal gland, albeit rare, progress rapidly to involve other tissues of the orbit, temporalis fossa, and cranium. Curative local resection or exenteration for such tumors is hardly ever possible, and the response to high-dose radiation therapy tends to be transient (Fig. 93–13), with most patients surviving less than 3 years after diagnosis.[3]

The prognosis for adenoid cystic carcinomas of the lacrimal gland is, in contrast to adenocarcinomas, variable. Comparison of treatments of adenoid cystic carcinoma is complicated by both the late and the slowly progressive nature of tumor recurrence; these two characteristics give little value to absolute survival times as a measure of prognosis, with many patients suffering a tumor recurrence for many years before death. Recurrences of adenoid cystic carcinoma are typically localized and may be related to perineural spread of neoplastic cells beyond the main bulk of tumor.[21] Such recurrences often progress slowly and relentlessly by intraorbital and intracranial spread (Fig. 93–14) or by widespread metastasis (Fig. 93–15). Late recurrence of tumor (in some cases more than 10 years after initial treatment[3]) limits the value of series with shorter follow-up intervals and

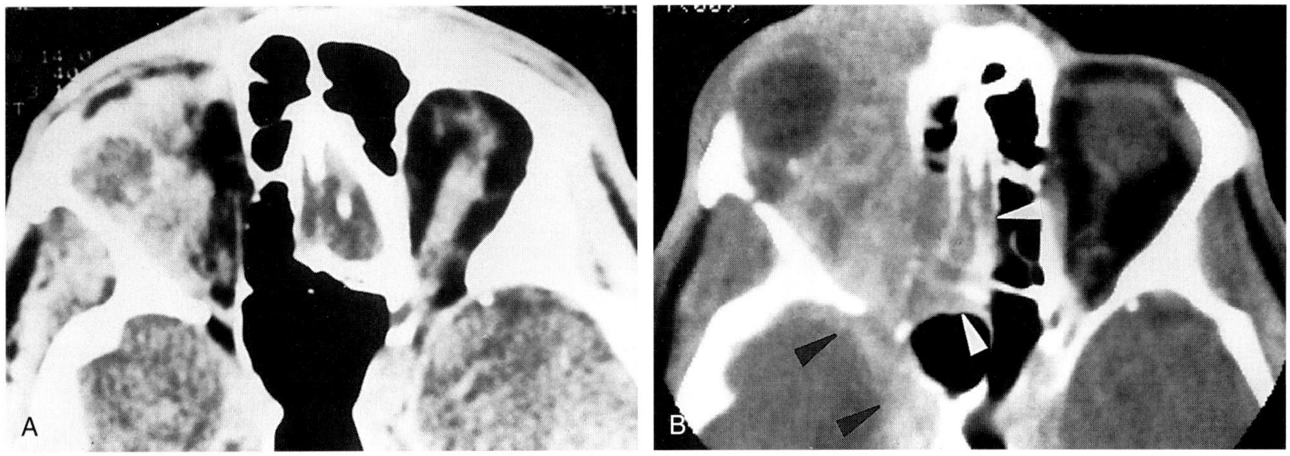

Figure 93–13. Cavitation due to necrosis within an adenocarcinoma of the right lacrimal gland at presentation *(A)*. By a year after radiation therapy *(B)* the tumor has spread intracranially *(black arrowheads)* and into the ethmoidal sinuses and nose *(white arrowheads)*.

makes assessment of therapeutic outcome extremely difficult; indeed, Henderson has questioned whether this particular tumor can ever be considered cured.[25]

Various treatments for adenoid cystic carcinomas have been advocated, although most are based on small series with short followup intervals[26–29]; as such, these are of interest, but provide poor estimates of disease-free survival.

Adenoid cystic carcinomas localized (clinically and radiologically) to the orbit may be considered for curative surgical resection, although some will be found to be extraorbital at the time of surgery. Cranio-orbital resection is generally required to achieve an adequate clear margin around the tumor. Although actuarial analysis has failed to demonstrate an alteration in the disease-free survival with cranio-orbital resection, this form of treatment was used in a considerably higher proportion of those patients surviving more than 10 years after therapy in the series of Wright and associates.[3] Over 20 years' followup might show cranio-orbital resection to be warranted in the very small group of patients with solely orbital disease; if tumor is demonstrated preoperatively to be extraorbital, exposure of the diploe during cranio-orbital resection might serve only to accelerate local recurrence by tumor seeding into the cranium.

Radiation therapy might slow the growth or delay the recurrence of adenoid cystic carcinomas, although there is no definitive evidence to support this[3, 30]; with this treatment, median disease-free survival is about 3 years[3] and overall median survival is about 10 years.[29] It is doubtful whether the maximum tolerated dose from external sources (50–70 Gy) is adequate for a cure of these tumors.[3] Debulking of adenoid cystic carcinomas before radiation therapy delays significantly the onset of tumor recurrence and slightly prolongs survival, as compared with the use of external source radiation therapy alone[3]; interpretation of this observation is difficult, however, because of clinical selection of patients for different treatments. There has been interest in the use of implanted sources of radiation (brachytherapy) for high-

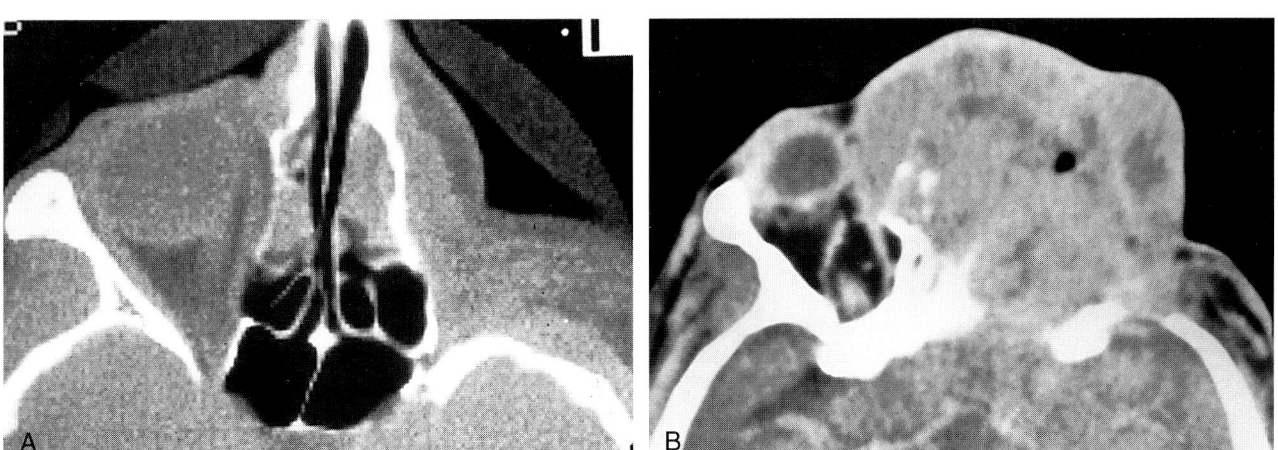

Figure 93–14. Left cranio-orbital resection for adenoid cystic carcinoma *(A)* and extensive local recurrence of tumor 10 years later *(B)*. The patient is still alive, with active disease, at 17 years after the primary surgery.

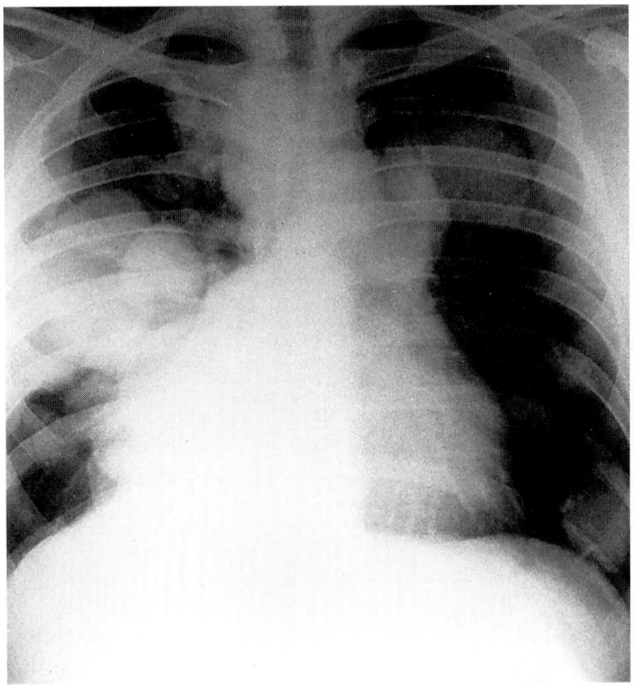

Figure 93 – 15. Widespread pulmonary metastases from adenoid cystic carcinoma, detected 12 years after treatment of the primary lacrimal gland tumor. The patient (same as in Fig. 93 – 14) has survived 17 years since the first treatment and 5 years since the detection of pulmonary metastases.

dose irradiation of these tumors, but long-term results for such treatment modalities are unknown.

No widely recognized chemotherapeutic regimen is available for the treatment of extensive localized or disseminated adenoid cystic carcinoma.

At present the most influential determinant of disease-free survival outcome after treatment of adenoid cystic carcinoma is the histologic morphology of the tumor: tumors of the "basaloid" variant have a much worse prognosis,[3, 13] and tumors of the "cribriform" variant carry a better prognosis.[30]

REFERENCES

1. Henderson JW, Farrow GM: Orbital Tumors, 2nd ed. New York, BC Decker, 1980, pp 394–424.
2. Rootman JA: Diseases of the Orbit: A Multidisciplinary Approach. Philadelphia, JB Lippincott, 1988, pp 384–405.
3. Wright JE, Rose GE, Garner A: Primary malignant neoplasms of the lacrimal gland. Br J Ophthalmol 76:401–407, 1992.
4. Rose GE, Wright JE: Pleomorphic adenoma of the lacrimal gland. Br J Ophthalmol 76:395–400, 1992.
5. Goldberg RA, Rootman J, Cline RA: Tumors metastatic to the orbit: A changing picture. Surv Ophthalmol 35:1–24, 1990.
6. Knowles DM, Jakobiec FA, McNally L, Burke JS: Lymphoid hyperplasia and malignant lymphoma occurring in the ocular adnexa (orbit, conjunctiva and eyelids): A prospective multiparametric analysis of 108 cases during 1977 to 1987. Hum Pathol 21:959–973, 1990.
7. Dardick I, van Hostrand AWP, Phillips MJ: Histogenesis of salivary gland pleomorphic adenoma (mixed tumor) with an evaluation of the role of the myoepithelial cell. Hum Pathol 13:62–75, 1982.
8. Grossniklaus HE, Abbuhl MF, McLean IW: Immunohistologic properties of benign and malignant mixed tumor of the lacrimal gland. Am J Ophthalmol 110:540–549, 1990.
9. Zimmerman LE, Sanders TE, Ackerman LV: Epithelial tumors of the lacrimal gland: Prognostic significance of histologic types. Int Ophthalmol Clin 2:337–367, 1962.
10. Ashton N: Epithelial tumours of the lacrimal gland. Mod Probl Ophthalmol 4:306–338, 1975.
11. Font RL, Gamel JW: Epithelial tumours of the lacrimal gland: An analysis of 265 cases. *In* Jakobiec FA (ed): Ocular and Adnexal Tumors. Birmingham, AL, Aesculapius, 1978, pp 787–805.
12. Ni C, Cheng SC, Dryja TP, Cheng TY: Lacrimal gland tumors: A clinicopathological analysis of 160 cases. Int Ophthalmol Clin 22:99–120, 1982.
13. Gamel JW, Font RL: Adenoid cystic carcinoma of the lacrimal gland: The clinical significance of a basaloid histologic pattern. Hum Pathol 13:219–225, 1982.
14. Perzin KH, Jakobiec FA, Livolsi VA, Desjardins L: Lacrimal gland malignant mixed tumors (carcinomas arising in benign mixed tumors): A clinicopathologic study. Cancer 45:593–606, 1980.
15. Auran J, Jakobiec FA, Krebs W: Benign mixed tumor of the palpebral lobe of the lacrimal gland: Clinical diagnosis and appropriate surgical management. Ophthalmology 95:90–99, 1988.
16. Parks SL, Glover AT: Benign mixed tumours arising in the palpebral lobe of the lacrimal gland. Ophthalmology 97:526–530, 1990.
17. Wright JE, Stewart WB, Krohel GB: Clinical presentation and management of lacrimal gland tumours. Br J Ophthalmol 63:600–606, 1979.
18. Wright JE: Factors affecting the survival of patients with lacrimal gland tumours. Can J Ophthalmol 17:3–9, 1982.
19. Jakobiec FA, Yeo JH, Trokel SL, et al: Combined clinical and computed tomographic diagnosis of primary lacrimal fossa lesions. Am J Ophthalmol 94:785–807, 1982.
20. Font RL, Patipa M, Rosenbaum PS, et al: Correlation of computed tomographic and histopathologic features in malignant transformation of benign mixed tumor of lacrimal gland. Surv Ophthalmol 34:449–452, 1990.
21. Jakobiec FA: Tumors of the lacrimal gland and lacrimal sac. *In* Anderson RL, et al (eds): Symposium on Diseases of the Lids, Lacrimal Apparatus and Orbit. Transactions of the New Orleans Academy of Ophthalmology. St. Louis, CV Mosby, 1982, pp 190–202.
22. Henderson JW, Neault RW: En bloc removal of intrinsic neoplasms of the lacrimal gland. Am J Ophthalmol 82:905–909, 1976.
23. Midena E, Segato T, Piermarocchi S, Boccato P: Fine needle aspiration biopsy in ophthalmology. Surv Ophthalmol 29:410–422, 1985.
24. Wright JE: Orbitotomy. *In* Heilman K, Paton D (eds): Atlas of Ophthalmic Surgery. Stuttgart, Georg Thieme, 1985.
25. Henderson JW: Adenoid cystic carcinoma of the lacrimal gland, is there a cure? Trans Am Ophthalmol Soc 85:312–319, 1987.
26. Byers RM, Berkeley RG, Luna M, Jesse RH: Combined therapeutic approach to malignant lacrimal gland tumors. Am J Ophthalmol 79:53–55, 1975.
27. Janecka I, Housepian E, Trokel S, et al: Surgical management of malignant tumors of the lacrimal gland. Am J Surg 148:539–541, 1984.
28. Cheeseman AD, Quiney RE, Wright JE: Craniofacial resection for orbital tumours. Ann R Coll Surg Engl 71:333–337, 1989.
29. Brada M, Henk JM: Radiotherapy for lacrimal gland tumours. Radiother Oncol 9:175–183, 1987.
30. Lee DL, Campbell RJ, Waller RR, Ilstrup DL: A clinico-pathologic study of adenoid cystic carcinoma of the lacrimal gland. Ophthalmology 92:128–134, 1985.

C H A P T E R 9 4

Metastatic Tumors

Jan W. Kronish

Two to 12% of all orbital neoplasms are metastatic tumors to the orbit.[1,2] The clinical manifestations are diverse because of the variation in the intrinsic aggressiveness and histologic type of the primary source. Although most tumors metastatic to the orbit present in patients with known systemic disease, some will represent the initial sign of an unsuspected primary cancer. Due to advances in local treatment and systemic control of disease, the recognition of a metastatic lesion to the orbit has become increasingly important as it relates to patient survival and quality of life.

The biologic process of cancer metastasis is a cascade of linked sequential steps involving numerous tumor–host interactions. Primary tumor proliferation initiates the sequence with invasion of tumor cells in preexisting host blood vessels and defective tumor vessels formed by tumor angiogenesis. Tumor cells may also enter the regional lymphatic channels and nodes and are eventually released into the venous system, leading to systemic dissemination. Circulating tumor cells can adhere to the endothelial surface of the arterioles in the target organ where a metastatic lesion will develop. Following a complex response between the tumor cells and arteriolar cellular elements, the tumor cells eventually invade the basement membrane and, with the aid of angiogenesis, proliferate in an extravascular location. Throughout this metastatic cascade, host defenses, such as natural killer cells and macrophages, must be overcome to allow the growth of such tumor colonies.[3] Future advances in our understanding of tumor cell biology and molecular genetics will play a key role in the strategy to control and treat malignancies.

Metastasis to the orbit occurs less frequently than to the eye. Ferry and Font[4] reported only 28 (12.3%) cases of tumors isolated to the orbit in 227 patients with intraocular and ocular adnexal metastases. Freedman and Folk[5] found a similar trend with 42% of 112 patients with eye and orbital metastases having involvement of the orbit alone. The prevalence of metastatic disease to the orbit in patients with known systemic malignant disease has been estimated to be 1% to 2%.[6,7] An increase in the number of reported cases of orbital metastatic disease has been recorded over the past few decades and is attributed to improved therapy and prolonged survival of cancer patients.[1]

CLINICAL FEATURES

The majority of patients with metastatic orbital tumors present after the primary tumor has been diagnosed. The time interval between detection of the primary malignancy and ophthalmologic presentation averages 31 months, although it is largely dependent on the tumor of origin. In the literature review by Goldberg and associates,[1] 42% of patients presented with an orbital metastasis before the detection of a primary tumor. Such cases of occult primary tumors were most commonly identified in patients with carcinomas of the lung, kidneys, gastrointestinal tract, and thyroid.

Metastatic tumors to the orbit in infants and children are typically undifferentiated sarcomas, with neuroblastoma being the most common type. Postembryonal carcinomas are the predominant source of metastases in adults (Table 94–1). The most common primary site, according to most published series, is breast carcinoma in women. Lung cancer is the second most frequent source, followed by prostatic carcinoma in men. Melanoma, kidney, carcinoid, gastrointestinal, and thyroid malignancies are the remaining common primary sites.[1,4,5,8–10] Unknown primary tumors represented 14% of cases in the combined series of orbital metastases of Rootman and colleagues.[2]

Although some authors have reported a higher frequency of metastatic tumors to the left orbit,[11–13] Goldberg and coworkers[1] found no statistically significant predilection for either side from a review of combined case reports. Seven percent of cases have been reported to be bilateral.[1,10] The lateral and superior quadrants of the orbit are the most common locations. Certain tumors have a propensity for specific components of the orbit, such as prostate carcinoma that tends to metastasize to bone. Melanoma has a strong preference for the extraocular muscles, and breast carcinoma most often spreads to the orbital soft tissues.[1,14]

The presenting clinical manifestations are largely de-

TABLE 94-1

Prevalence Of Orbital Metastatoc Primary Sites

Tumor Type	Percentage
Breast	42.0
Lung	11.0
Unknown	11.0
Prostate	8.3
Melanoma	5.2
Gastrointestinal	4.4
Renal	3.2
Squamous cell	2.0
Other	12.9

Modified from Goldberg RA, Rootman J, Cline RA: Tumors metastatic to the orbit: A changing picture. Surv Ophthalmol 35:1-24, 1990.

pendent on the histologic type of tumor and an orbital location. Proptosis, diplopia, and pain are the most common symptoms of orbital metastatic disease.[1, 8-10] In a comprehensive literature review, proptosis was the most common initial sign (64% of patients), followed by motility disturbance (58%), palpable mass (27%), blepharoptosis (21%), decreased vision (22%), nonaxial displacement of the globe (18%), and chemosis (15%). Enophthalmos was seen in 10% of the cases and is a distinctive feature of scirrhous carcinomas such as from the breast and stomach. The temporal course of disease is largely determined by the primary source. For example, metastases of lung cancer and melanoma tend to behave aggressively with a rapid course of onset, as opposed to breast and thyroid carcinomas that progress subacutely because of slow tumor growth.[1]

The evaluation of a patient with orbital disease must begin with a thorough clinical history. A remote history of a preexistent tumor is often missed when assessing patients with an orbital metastasis. The ophthalmologic findings in a patient with orbital metastatic disease typically conform to one of four patterns of presentation including an infiltrative syndrome, orbital mass effect, inflammatory disease, or functional disorder.[15] Radiographic imaging studies of the orbit are of primary importance and can be diagnostic. Metastatic tumors have characteristic features on standardized echography, including irregular shape, moderate to highly reflective, irregular internal structure, little sound attenuation, and lack of vasculature.[16] Orbital computed tomography (CT) has the advantage over magnetic resonance imaging (MRI) in its ability to demonstrate bony destruction or hyperostosis secondary to metastatic disease.[17] MRI, however, is an ideal method to image tumor infiltration of bone marrow and may show characteristic signal properties to help differentiate metastatic lesions from other orbital diseases.[17, 18] Fine-needle aspiration or open biopsy may be necessary to ascertain the diagnosis and provide the basis for a treatment plan.

The pathologic features of metastatic orbital tumors vary considerably. Special techniques such as histochemical stains, immunohistochemical studies, and electron microscopy are often necessary to determine the tumor source.[1, 2] Special histologic stains such as alcian blue, mucicarmine, and periodic acid-Schiff may help to differentiate the origin of the primary tumor by characterizing the composition of cytoplasmic organelles. For example, adenocarcinomas were found in 15 of 28 metastatic orbital tumors in Font and Ferry's[10] series in which mucicarmine-positive and alcian blue-positive material was identified. Immunohistochemical markers are not only useful for pathologic diagnosis but also may have implications with regard to treatment, such as the higher response rate of breast tumors to hormone therapy when estrogen and progesterone receptors are present. A specified amount of fresh tissue and proper handling of the orbital biopsy specimen is necessary to process the tissue for these specialized tests and should, therefore, be discussed with the pathologist in advance.

A complete workup for systemic disease is mandatory in patients who present with a suspected orbital metastasis. A careful physical examination and appropriate radiologic studies and laboratory tests should be obtained by an oncologist. A nonspecific test that may be helpful in identifying metastatic disease is the carcinoembryonic antigen (CEA). The CEA may be elevated in patients with carcinoma of the breast, lung, prostate, and gastrointestinal tract, and the degree of elevation may be proportional to the extent of disease.[1, 19] Laboratory tests that are more specific for certain carcinomas include prostate-specific antigen and prostate acid phosphatase associated with prostate tumors; human chorionic gonadotropin, which may be produced by seminomas; and 5-hydroxyindoleacetic acid detected in the urine of patients with carcinoid tumors. Once a general evaluation is completed, the stage of disease is determined and used to guide a treatment protocol.

Orbital metastatic disease is rarely curable and, therefore, treatment goals are usually palliative. Radiation therapy, hormonal therapy, and chemotherapy are the available modes of treatment. Localized radiation therapy to the orbit is utilized most frequently and is indicated in patients with acute ophthalmologic complications such as visual dysfunction and pain. A tumor dose of 30 to 40 Gy delivered in divided doses over a 2- to 3-week period has been demonstrated to be effective in 72% to 89% of cases.[20, 21] With proper shielding of the globe, ocular complications may be avoided and long-term effects such as retinopathy, cataract, and optic neuropathy are rarely encountered, owing to relatively short-term patient survival. Hormone therapy is efficacious in the treatment of prostate and breast carcinoma orbital metastases, especially when the tumors are well differentiated with hormone receptors present on the cell surfaces. Chemotherapy provides adjunctive treatment for the palliation of orbital metastases in addition to management of concurrent generalized metastatic disease.

METASTATIC ORBITAL TUMORS

Breast Carcinoma

Carcinoma of the breast is the most common malignancy and the second leading cause of cancer death in women in North America. Endocrinologic factors, such as the age of menarche and menopause, environment, and genetics are believed to play a role in the etiology of breast cancer. Infiltrating ductal adenocarcinoma represents the most common histologic type and is usually poorly differentiated. The development of this malignancy in men is rare and accounts for 1% of such cases. Breast carcinoma may metastasize to any organ in the body, although the lungs, pleura, bones, and liver are the most frequently involved sites.[22]

Primary breast cancer is the most common site of origin for metastasis to the eye and orbit. Intraocular involvement is more frequently encountered than orbital disease.[4] Ten patients presented with tumors in the orbit in Bullock and Yanes' series[19] of 30 cases of metastatic breast cancer to the eye and ocular adnexa. In a combined series of orbital metastases, Goldberg and coworkers[1] reported a prevalence of 42% for breast cancer, which represented the largest group of primary tumors. Patients with orbital metastases usually present in the fifth or sixth decade of life, and the majority have a known primary tumor. The mean interval between the diagnosis of breast cancer and onset of orbital signs or symptoms is 4.5 to 6.5 years, although there are numerous case reports of prolonged latency, including one case of 27 years.[1, 19, 23] The orbital metastasis may be the presenting symptom of disease in up to one third of patients.[1, 24]

The most common features of orbital involvement include blepharoptosis, extraocular motility restriction, pain, and displacement of the globe. Exophthalmos may result from the mass effect of tumor. Alternatively, infiltration and fibroblastic contraction of scirrhous adenocarcinoma of the breast in the orbit causes enophthalmos, blepharoptosis, and limitation of ocular motility (Fig. 94–1).[1, 9, 19, 25] Enophthalmos was found in 54% of cases of metastatic breast carcinoma in the series by Goldberg and Rootman.[15] Less frequently, breast carcinoma may manifest a "pseudoinflammation"[25] or may metastasize to the extraocular muscles.[14] Orbital computed tomography typically reveals a soft tissue mass with irregular borders infiltrating adjacent structures including bony erosion. Characteristic features of breast metastases on MRI include hypointensity to orbital fat on T1-weighted images, hyperintensity on T2-weighted images, and contrast enhancement with gadolinium-DTPA.[18] Serum CEA levels may be helpful in differentiating metastatic breast carcinoma from other orbital tumors, as advocated by Bullock and Yanes,[19] and are elevated above 3 ng/mL in 55% of patients with metastases.[26]

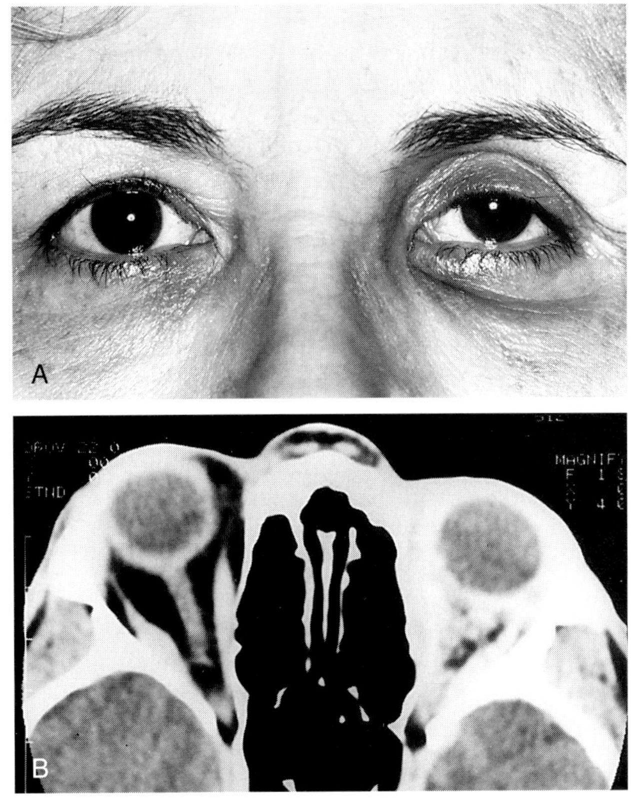

Figure 94–1. *A*, A 58-year-old woman presented with enophthalmos and ptosis caused by metastatic scirrhous carcinoma of the breast in the left orbit. *B*, Axial computed tomographic scan demonstrates an infiltrative mass in the intraconal space of the left orbit with posterior retraction of the globe.

Orbital biopsy of a tumor suspected to be metastatic breast carcinoma is indicated not only to obtain a definitive pathologic diagnosis but also to provide nonfixative treated tissue for analysis of estrogen and progesterone receptors. The presence of such hormone receptors indicates a higher response rate to endocrine therapies. Pathologically, infiltrating ductal carcinoma tumor cells have oval nuclei and may form columns or strands that surround lumina. Different patterns may be seen, including papillary, mucinous, histiocytoid, and anaplastic. Intracytoplasmic vacuoles containing mucicarmine-positive material, Alcian blue haloes, and PAS-positive central target cells are histochemical features associated with breast carcinoma; however, their presence or absence may not differentiate these tumors from other sources of adenocarcinoma. Electron microscopy may reveal intracytoplasmic lumina and mucinous vacuoles.[2, 27]

Metastatic breast carcinoma is incurable, and no therapeutic protocol has been shown to significantly prolong survival. Therefore, treatment goals are palliative and should be directed toward management of the patient's symptoms. For example, patients with acute orbital signs and visual compromise should initially receive radiation therapy to the orbit in conjunction with systemic therapy. Radiation doses of 35 to 40 Gy are effective in local tumor control.[21] The number of sites of disease, location of metastases, menstrual status, and time interval between the initial diagnosis of breast cancer and findings of metastatic disease have prognostic implications and influence treatment choices.

Metastatic breast cancer is highly responsive to hormonal therapy, particularly in patients whose tumors have both estrogen and progesterone receptors. In premenopausal women, tamoxifen is the initial treatment of choice, followed by oophorectomy, progestins, and finally aminoglutethimide. Tamoxifen is also the first line of treatment in postmenopausal patients, with secondary endocrine therapies including progestins, aminoglutethimide, and estrogens. Adrenalectomy and hypophysectomy are also effective but have been replaced by the less toxic forms of medical treatment. Symptomatic patients who are not candidates for or do not respond to endocrine therapy should receive chemotherapy. Combination regimens provide a greater response rate than single-agent therapy and consist mainly of alkaloid and anthracycline agents. Cyclophosphamide, methotrexate, 5-fluorouracil, and prednisone are commonly employed in combination, whereas doxorubicin is the most effective agent used as a single drug.[26]

Lung Carcinoma

Lung cancer is the leading cause of cancer death in men and women 35 years of age or older. Most cases are seen between the ages of 35 and 75 years, with a peak incidence in the fifth and sixth decades.[9, 28] Smoking is a widely recognized risk factor in the development of lung carcinoma, as are other environmental carcinogens such as asbestos and radon particles. Unlike breast carcinoma, which tends to have a prolonged time interval from the onset of primary tumor to the first appearance of metastasis, lung cancer has a more fulminant course. In fact, 70% of patients have regional lymph node or distant metastases at the time of initial diagnosis.[28] Orbital metastases usually present a few months before or after the primary tumor is identified. The orbital tumor in 6 of 10 patients in Henderson and Farrow's series[9] and 7 of 9 cases in Goldberg and associates' review[1] represented the initial sign of lung cancer in patients with an occult primary tumor. The prognosis of patients with metastatic carcinoma of the lung is poor, with a median survival time of 6 months after ophthalmic presentation.[5]

Carcinoma of the lung is the second most common metastatic tumor to the orbit[1, 5, 9] Eleven percent of tumors in Goldberg and associates' review were metastatic from the lung,[1] and 23% of the 43 patients in Henderson and Farrow's series[9] had metastatic disease that arose from the lung. Lung cancer metastasizes much more frequently to the choroid than the orbit.[4, 5] The tumor may present with a mass effect or may infiltrate the orbital soft tissues and usually progresses at a rapid rate.[2, 9] Pain, ophthalmoplegia, chemosis, visual disturbance, palpable mass, and proptosis are typical presenting symptoms and signs.[9] CT scan characteristics include a well-demarcated mass that may have focal areas of necrosis and calcification.[2] The four major histologic types of lung cancer are squamous cell (or epidermoid) carcinoma, small cell (or oat cell) carcinoma, adenocarcinoma, and large cell carcinoma. Although epidermoid carcinoma and adenocarcinoma occur with the greatest frequency,[28] undifferentiated small cell carcinoma is the most common form that metastasizes to the orbit.[2]

Local irradiation and systemic corticosteroids may be used for palliation of symptoms caused by orbital metastases.[9, 28] Doses of 30 to 40 Gy over a 2- to 4-week period are administered, usually starting with 3- to 4-Gy fractions. Combination chemotherapy with such agents as cyclophosphamide, doxorubicin, vincristine, and etoposide has an overall response rate of 90% and prolongs survival in patients with small cell lung cancer. On the other hand, patients with non–small cell lung cancer have a low response rate to chemotherapy with no effect on survival.[28]

Prostate Carcinoma

Carcinoma of the prostate is a common malignancy in men that typically develops in late adulthood. Five-year survival rates are approximately 60%, and prognosis is dependent on tumor differentiation and the stage of disease at the time of detection. Adenocarcinoma is the most frequent histologic type, and poorly differentiated tumors are more likely to metastasize. The majority of tumors are detected at advanced stages of disease with local invasion, lymph node involvement, and distant metastases. The most common sites of metastasis are the axial skeleton and proximate long bones, and most are osteoblastic. Assessment of serum levels of prostate-specific antigen is a sensitive method to monitor response and recurrence of tumor after therapy.[22]

Prostate carcinoma is the third most frequent site of origin for metastasis to the orbit.[1, 29] In a review of the literature by Goldberg and coworkers[1] that included 42 cases, approximately half of the patients presented after the primary tumor had been detected and median survival was less than 12 months after the onset of ophthalmic presentation. The most common site of involvement is the orbital bones, characterized as osteoblastic or osteolytic, with an associated mass effect. The tumor may be localized in the orbital soft tissues, resulting in ocular dysfunction on the basis of infiltration, tumor expansion, or cicatrization.[1, 2] Presenting symptoms and signs include proptosis, diplopia, pain, eyelid swelling, ptosis, and decreased vision (Fig. 94–2).[29]

Computed tomographic features of osteoblastic lesions of the bony orbit include hyperostotic bone with irregular, spiculated borders invading the adjacent soft tissues. Osteolytic metastatic lesions are associated with

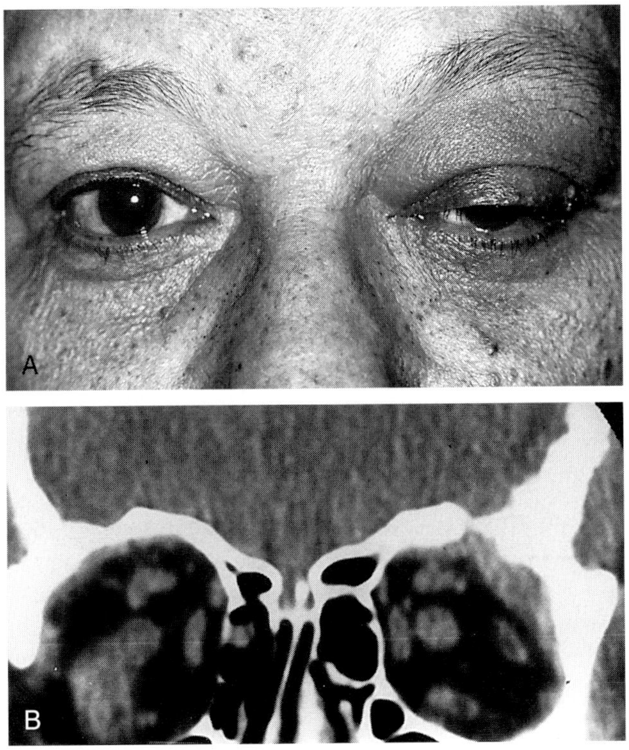

Figure 94–2. *A*, A 67-year-old man presented with left upper eyelid ptosis and proptosis associated with pain of 4 months' duration. *B*, Axial computed tomographic scan shows an irregular osteoblastic lesion of the left superolateral orbit with medial displacement of the orbital soft tissues.

bony destruction and infiltration of orbital structures. Standardized echography is typically characterized by a mass with irregular margins and a V-shaped echogram.[29] Fine-needle aspiration biopsy or direct open biopsy may be necessary in selected cases. The detection of prostate-specific antigen and prostate acid phosphatase with immunohistochemical techniques on biopsy specimens provide accurate pathologic confirmation of the tissue of origin.[2, 30]

Therapeutic options include radiation therapy, hormonal therapy, and chemotherapy. Local irradiation is an effective treatment for palliation of symptoms and is the modality of choice for orbital metastases.[20, 29] Reduction of the androgenic stimulation of prostatic carcinoma by hormonal manipulation is effective in pain control and prolongs remission. Orchiectomy eliminates the source of most of the circulating testosterone and provides long-lasting reduction in androgens. Suppression of the pituitary gonadotropic release can be achieved with estrogens, progestational agents, and luteinizing hormone-releasing hormone (LHRH) agonists. LHRH agonists may cause an initial testosterone surge within the first 2 weeks of therapy that could lead to sudden tumor growth; therefore, these agents are contraindicated in lesions that could compress the spinal cord or optic nerve. Other hormonal modulating agents include inhibitors of androgen synthesis, such as aminoglutethimide and ketoconazole, and progestational antiandrogens, including cyproterone acetate and flutamide.[22, 29] Individual and combination cytotoxic chemotherapy is reserved for hormone-refractory patients, although the antitumor effects are minimal.[22]

Neuroblastoma

Neuroblastoma is the most common tumor of infancy and comprises 8% of malignancies in children younger than 15 years of age. This malignant neoplasm of undifferentiated embryonic neural crest cells may arise from any site along the sympathetic nervous system, including the adrenal gland (40%), paraspinal ganglion (25%), thorax (15%), and pelvic region (5%). Chromosomal abnormalities and oncogenes are believed to play a role in its pathogenesis. In children younger than 1 year old, the disease tends to be localized in the thorax[31] and has an 85% to 90% three-year survival rate.[2, 31] On the other hand, 75% of older children have metastatic disease at the time of diagnosis, which most commonly involves the lymph nodes, bone marrow, bone, liver, and subcutaneous tissue and is associated with a high mortality rate.[31]

Neuroblastoma is the second most frequent orbital tumor encountered in juveniles occurring after rhabdomyosarcoma. Most orbital metastases originate from the abdomen[2, 32] and present a few months after diagnosis of the primary tumor. Approximately 50% of patients have bilateral orbital disease.[32] Proptosis typically progresses rapidly, owing to sphenoid bone involvement and invasion of the orbital soft tissues. Palpebral ecchymosis is a common finding resulting from hemorrhagic necrosis of tumor that outgrows its blood supply.[2, 31] Orbital CT scan features may include bone destruction and a soft tissue mass that contains lucent areas due to necrosis.[2] Other ocular manifestations include heterochromia and ptosis in patients with cervical tumors and opsoclonus in cases with or without orbital or central nervous system metastases.[33]

Laboratory studies are often useful in the diagnosis of neuroblastoma. Urinary excretion of vanillylmandelic acid (VMA) and homovanillic acid (HVA), 3-methoxy-4-hydroxyphenylethyleneglycol (HMPG), and cystathionine may be increased. Neuron-specific enolase levels are elevated in most patients with neuroblastoma. Histopathologically, the tumor consists of nests of small, round cells with hyperchromatic nuclei separated by fibrovascular stroma. Necrosis, calcification, hemorrhage, and mitotic figures are common. Homer-Wright rosettes with central neurofibrils may be seen. Electron microscopy findings include dense core neurosecretory granules in the peripheral cytoplasm, neurotubules, and axons. Immunohistochemical techniques are applied to help differentiate neuroblastoma from other small round cell tumors such as Ewing's sarcoma, lymphoma, and rhabdomyosarcoma.[2, 31]

Chemotherapy is the primary therapeutic modality for metastatic disease. The most effective agents used in various combinations are cyclophosphamide, doxorubicin, cisplatin, epipodophyllotoxins, vincristine, dacarbazine, and melphalan. Radiation therapy may be indicated in patients who have an incomplete response to chemotherapy or for palliation of bone pain or orbital lesions.[31]

Gastrointestinal Carcinoma

Cancer of gastrointestinal tract is the second leading cause of cancer deaths in the United States. Carcinoma of the stomach, ileum, colon, and rectum is slightly more common in men with a peak incidence in the sixth decade. In spite of the high frequency of these tumors, fewer than 12 cases of orbital metastases have been reported in large series.[1, 2, 9] The majority of patients have regional or distant metastatic spread at the time of diagnosis. Goldberg and coworkers[1] found a similar trend in which 7 of 10 patients with gastrointestinal metastases to the orbit had an occult primary tumor. The tumor may spread to the orbital bones or soft tissues and present with symptoms related to infiltration or mass effect. Pain is commonly encountered in patients with mucin-producing cancers. Unique features of gastrointestinal carcinomas in the orbit include enophthalmos associated with scirrhous carcinoma of the stomach, hyperostosis of the bony orbit, and a high incidence of bilaterality.[2, 9]

The majority of tumors are adenocarcinomas, and the well-differentiated metastases, histologically, may be composed of mucus-producing signet ring cells. Poorly differentiated lesions are more likely to arise from the stomach[9] and portend a worse prognosis. Chemotherapy and irradiation are the major forms of treatment for metastatic gastrointestinal carcinomas. Stomach carcinoma has a response rate of up to 35% to single-agent or combination chemotherapy with 5-fluorouracil, mitomycin C, doxorubicin, and semustine (methyl-CCNU). Colorectal carcinoma is usually treated with 5-fluorouracil. Radiation therapy of orbital lesions may be effective for palliation,[2, 34] but survival is typically less than 6 months after ophthalmic presentation.[1]

Melanoma

More than 90% of malignant melanomas arise in the skin, while the remainder may originate in the eye, meninges, respiratory tract, and gallbladder. The incidence of cutaneous melanoma has been rising over the past 50 years and is predicted to develop in 1 in 90 individuals by the year 2000. The malignancy predominantly affects Caucasians with risk factors that include fair skin, a familial background of melanoma, and previous history of a primary melanoma.[35] The most common sites of metastases are the skin and subcutaneous tissues, lung, pleura, liver, brain, bone, and gastrointestinal tract.

Most cases of metastatic melanoma to the orbit are from the skin; however, a few cases of choroidal melanoma spreading to the contralateral orbit have been reported. Orbital metastases are usually associated with widespread dissemination occurring late in the course of disease.[1, 8, 36] The unique propensity of melanoma to involve the extraocular muscles was demonstrated in the literature review by Goldberg and coworkers,[1] who found 41% of patients had tumors localized to the rectus muscles. Presenting symptoms and signs include diplopia with limited extraocular movement, proptosis, pain, blepharoptosis, and decreased vision.[36] Histologically, metastatic melanoma is composed of epitheloid cells that may be pigmented or amelanotic infiltrating the orbital tissues. Histochemical stains and electron microscopy may be useful in the identification of melanin or premelanosomes.[2] Mean survival after ophthalmic presentation is approximately 6 months.[1, 36] Dacarbazine is the most active chemotherapeutic agent used for metastatic melanoma,[36] and its action may be complemented with the antiestrogen drug tamoxifen.[37] Immunologic agents, such as interferon, the interleukins, and monoclonal antibodies, have shown some efficacy in controlling disseminated disease.[35] Radiation therapy and corticosteroids are usually palliative in patients with orbital pain, inflammation, or progressive proptosis.[2, 36]

Renal Cell Carcinoma

Renal cell carcinoma comprises 3% of adult cancers, occurs in men twice as commonly as women, and has a peak incidence in the sixth decade. The tumor often remains clinically occult until the disease is relatively advanced. Metastases are present in 30% of patients at the time of diagnosis and most frequently affect the lungs, bone, and soft tissues.[38, 39] Ferry and Font,[4] in their review of metastatic renal cell carcinoma to the eye and orbit, found 8 of 9 patients presented with ophthalmologic symptoms before detection of the primary tumor. On the other hand, orbital metastasis have been reported to present as long as 15 years after excision of the primary tumor.[38] Orbital metastases present as a distinct mass in the soft tissues and, due to their rich vascularity, may cause pulsating exophthalmos.[9, 38]

Histologically, renal cell carcinoma consists of nests of large granular or clear cells that contain glycogen or lipid surrounded by a vascular stroma. Radical nephrectomy is performed in selected patients with metastatic disease to decrease tumor burden or to alleviate symptoms such as pain and hemorrhage. Conventional chemotherapy for renal cell carcinoma involves vinblastine with or without other agents, but response rates are generally low. Biologic agents, including lymphokine-activated cells, interleukin-2, interferon, and monoclonal antibodies, appear promising in their antitumor effects. Palliative radiation therapy is the treatment of choice for orbital metastases.[39]

Other Metastatic Tumors

In children, solid tumor metastases other than neuroblastoma are rare and include Ewing's sarcoma and Wilms' tumor. Less common orbital metastases in adults may arise from the thyroid, pancreas, liver, uterus, adrenal glands, bladder, and testes.[1, 9] Thyroid carcinomas may be aggressive tumors with increased vascularity causing pulsatile proptosis.[2, 9] Carcinoid tumors, which arise from neuroendocrine cells in the gastrointestinal mucosa, rarely metastasize to the orbit. Metastatic carcinoid tumors are the rare exception to the usual treatment approach to orbital metastases in that total surgical excision may improve survival and relieve symptoms.[1, 40]

REFERENCES

1. Goldberg RA, Rootman J, Cline RA: Tumors metastatic to the orbit: A changing picture. Surv Ophthalmol 35:1–24, 1990.
2. Rootman J, Ragaz J, Cline R, Lapointe JS: Orbital metastasis. *In* Rootman J (ed): Diseases of the Orbit. Philadelphia, JB Lippincott, 1988, pp 405–427.
3. Liotta LA, Stetler-Stevenson WG: Principles of molecular cell biology of cancer: Cancer metastasis. *In* Devita VT, Hellman S, Rosenberg SA (eds): Cancer: Principles and Practice of Oncology. Philadelphia, JB Lippincott, 1989, pp 98–115.
4. Ferry AP, Font RL: Carcinoma metastatic to the eye and orbit: I. A clinicopathologic study of 227 cases. Arch Ophthalmol 92:276–286, 1974.
5. Freedman KI, Folk JC: Metastatic tumors to the eye and orbit: Patient survival and clinical characteristics. Arch Ophthalmol 105:1215–1219, 1987.
6. Bloch RS, Garner S: The incidence of ocular metastatic carcinoma. Arch Ophthalmol 85:673–675, 1971.
7. Albert DM, Rubenstein RA, Scheie HG: Tumor metastasis to the eye: I. Incidence in 213 patients with generalized malignancy. Am J Ophthalmol 63:723–726, 1967.
8. Shields CL, Shields JA, Peggs M: Tumors metastatic to the orbit. Ophthalmic Plast Reconstr Surg 4:73–80, 1988.
9. Henderson JW, Farrow GM: Orbital Tumors, 2nd ed. New York, Thieme-Stratton, 1980, pp 451–471.
10. Font RL, Ferry AP: Carcinoma metastatic to the eye and orbit: III. A clinicopathologic study of 28 cases metastatic to the orbit. Cancer 38:1326–1335, 1976.
11. Hart WM. Metastatic carcinoma to the eye and orbit. Int Ophthalmol Clin 2:465–482, 1962.
12. Castro PA, Albert DM, Wang WJ, Ni C. Tumors metastatic to the eye and adnexa. Int Ophthalmol Clin 22:189–223, 1982.
13. Silva D: Orbital tumors. Am J Ophthalmol 65:318–339, 1968.
14. Capone A Jr, Slamovits TL: Discrete metastasis of solid tumors to extraocular muscles. Arch Ophthalmol 108:237–243, 1990.
15. Goldberg RA, Rootman J: Clinical characteristics of metastatic orbital tumors. Ophthalmology 97:620–624, 1990.
16. Byrne SF, Green RL: Orbital echography. *In* Tasman W, Jaeger EA (eds): Duane's Clinical Ophthalmology, vol 2. Philadelphia, JB Lippincott, 1992, chap 26, pp 1–66.
17. Dortzbach RK, Kronish JW, Gentry LR: Magnetic resonance imaging of the orbit: II. Clinical applications. Ophthalmic Plast Reconstr Surg 5:160–170, 1989.
18. Kronish JW, Dortzbach RK: Magnetic resonance imaging of the orbit. *In* Tasman W, Jaeger EA (eds): Duane's Clinical Ophthalmology, vol 2. Philadelphia, JB Lippincott, 1992, chap 25, pp 1–25.
19. Bullock JD, Yanes B: Ophthalmic manifestations of metastatic breast cancer. Ophthalmology 87:961–973, 1980.
20. Glassburn JR, Klionsky M, Brady LW: Radiation therapy for metastatic disease involving the orbit. Am J Clin Oncol 7:145–148, 1984.
21. Huh SH, Nisce LZ, Simpson LD, Chu FCH: Value of radiation therapy in the treatment of orbital metastasis. Am J Roentgenol Radium Ther Nucl Med 120:589–594, 1974.
22. Perez CA, Fair WR, Ihde DC: Carcinoma of the prostate. *In* Devita VT, Hellman S, Rosenberg SA (eds): Cancer: Principles and Practice of Oncology. Philadelphia, JB Lippincott, 1989, pp 1023–1058.
23. Henderson JW, Farrow GM: Orbital Tumors, 2nd ed. New York, Thieme-Stratton, 1980, pp 451–471.
24. Glazer LC, Harris GJ, Simons KB: Orbital metastasis as the presenting sign of adenocarcinoma of the breast. Ophthalmic Plast Reconstr Surg 7:252–255, 1991.
25. Mottow-Lippa L, Jakobiec FA, Iwamoto T: Pseudoinflammatory metastatic breast carcinoma of the orbit and lids. Ophthalmology 88:575–580, 1981.
26. Henderson IC, Harris RJ, Kine DW, Hellman S: Cancer of the breast. *In* Devita VT, Hellman S, Rosenberg SA (eds): Cancer: Principles and Practice of Oncology. Philadelphia, JB Lippincott, 1989, pp 1197–1268.
27. Jakobiec FA, Austin P, Iwamoto T, et al: Primary infiltrating signet ring carcinoma of the eyelids. Ophthalmology 90:291–299, 1983.
28. Minna JD, Pass H, Glatstein E, Ihde DC. Cancer of the lung. *In* Devita VT, Hellman S, Rosenberg SA (eds): Cancer: Principles and Practice of Oncology. Philadelphia, JB Lippincott, 1989, pp 591–705.
29. Boldt HC, Nerad JA: Orbital metastases from prostate carcinoma. Arch Ophthalmol 106:1403–1408, 1988.
30. Reifler DM, Kini SR, Liu D, Littleton RH: Orbital metastasis from prostatic carcinoma. Arch Ophthalmol 102:292–295, 1984.
31. Pizzo PA, Horowitz ME, Poplack DG, et al: Solid tumors of childhood. *In* Devita VT, Hellman S, Rosenberg SA (eds): Cancer: Principles and Practice of Oncology. Philadelphia, JB Lippincott, 1989, pp 1612–1670.
32. Albert DM, Rubenstein RA, Scheie HG: Tumor metastasis to the eye: II. Clinical study in infants and children. Am J Ophthalmol 63:727–732, 1967.
33. Feman SS, Apt L: Eye findings associated with pediatric malignancy. J Pediatr Ophthalmol 9:224–231, 1972.
34. MacDonald JS, Steele G, Gunderson LL: Cancer of the stomach. *In* Devita VT, Hellman S, Rosenberg SA (eds): Cancer: Principles and Practice of Oncology. Philadelphia, JB Lippincott, 1989, pp 765–799.
35. Balch CM, Houghton A, Peters L: Cutaneous melanoma. *In* Devita VT, Hellman S, Rosenberg SA (eds): Cancer: Principles and Practice of Oncology. Philadelphia, JB Lippincott, 1989, pp 1499–1542.
36. Orcutt JC, Char DH: Melanoma metastatic to the orbit. Ophthalmology 95:1033–1037, 1988.
37. Cocconi G, Bella M, Calabresi F, et al: Treatment of metastatic malignant melanoma with dacarbazine plus tamoxifen. N Engl J Med 327:516–523, 1992.
38. Kindermann WR, Shields JA, Eiferman RA, et al: Metastatic renal cell carcinoma to the eye and adnexae. Ophthalmology 88:1347–1350, 1981.
39. Linehan WM, Shipley WU, Ongo DL: Cancer of the kidney and ureter. *In* Devita VT, Hellman S, Rosenberg SA (eds): Cancer: Principles and Practice of Oncology. Philadelphia, JB Lippincott, 1989, pp 979–1007.
40. Shetlar DJ, Font RL, Ordonez N, et al: A clinicopathologic study of three carcinoid tumors metastatic to the orbit. Ophthalmology 97:257–264, 1990.

CHAPTER 95

Ophthalmic Manifestations of Mucoceles

Barrett G. Haik and Ronald G. Amedee

Mucoceles are benign, expansile masses that arise within paranasal sinuses and are locally destructive. It is theorized that mucoceles arise after obstruction of the normal drainage pathways of the paranasal sinuses. The sequestered respiratory epithelium continues to produce mucus within the closed cavity, resulting in a fluid-filled cyst. The increasing fluid pressure within the sinus cavity will cause the sinus walls to slowly expand in the directions of least resistance. The etiology of mucoceles is, however, debated since not all sinuses with mechanically obstructed ostia develop mucoceles or not all mucoceles are found in sinuses with obstructed ostia. An infected mucocele is referred to as a *mucopyocele.*

The initial obstruction of the sinus ostia or nasofrontal duct most commonly occurs after accidental or surgical trauma involving the frontal or ethmoidal sinuses (e.g., facial fracture repair, sinus surgery, or neurosurgical procedures), chronic inflammation (e.g., allergic or infectious), benign tumors (e.g., osteomas, polyps, or congenital goblet cell cysts), or sinus neoplasms.[1] Mucoceles rarely occur in children with predisposing systemic conditions. Examples of these include cystic fibrosis[2, 3] in which mucous hyperviscosity may result in inspissated material blocking drainage channels, ciliary dyskinesis with mucous stagnation, and osteopetrosis, in which abnormal bone remodeling occurs and the bony foramina are compressed or obliterated (Fig. 95–1). The incidence of orbital mucoceles is difficult to determine since these patients are managed by physicians of various subspecialties, including ophthalmology, otolaryngology, and neurosurgery. In a large series of patients, mucoceles accounted for 4% to 8.5% of expanding orbital lesions.[4, 5] The frontal and ethmoidal sinuses are by far the most common sites for mucocele formation (>90%). Additionally, their anatomic proximity commonly results in frontoethmoidal mucoceles, which simultaneously involve both of these sinus cavities. Although maxillary and sphenoidal sinus mucoceles are extremely rare lesions, they are important entities because they may result in significant ophthalmic sequelae such as diplopia, nasolacrimal duct obstruction, and visual loss from optic nerve compression. To fully discuss the ophthalmic manifestations of mucoceles and their therapy, a brief review of pertinent sinus anatomy, pathophysiology, physical examination, and diagnostic imaging is presented.

THE PARANASAL SINUSES

There are eight paranasal sinuses, four on the left and four on the right side of the nose. These accessory sinuses are the ethmoidal sinuses (anterior and posterior), the maxillary sinuses, the sphenoidal sinuses, and the frontal sinuses. Under normal physiologic conditions each sinus is filled with air and communicates with the nasal cavity through an ostium. They are lined with a respiratory type of mucous membrane that is continuous with that of the nasal cavity.

The sinuses are divided clinically into two groups, anterior and posterior, depending on location in reference to the line of attachment of the middle turbinate. The anterior group consists of the frontal, maxillary, and anterior ethmoidal sinuses, all of which drain anterior to the middle meatus of the nose near the infundibulum. The posterior group includes the sphenoidal and posterior ethmoidal cells, which drain above the attachment of the middle turbinate.

The ethmoidal sinuses appear during the third or fourth fetal month as evaginations of the lateral nasal wall in the region of the middle meatus (anterior ethmoidal sinuses) and the superior meatus (posterior ethomoidal sinuses). They are present along the medial orbit and along the maxillary sinuses, the only sinus cavities large enough to be of clinical significance at birth. Because of this earlier development, they may occupy positions in which they bulge into the later-developing frontal and sphenoidal sinuses. The ethmoidal cells, which collectively form the ethmoidal sinuses, vary from 3 to 18. The anterior group of ethmoidal cells drain into the infundibulum of the middle meatus, and the posterior group drains into the superior meatus. The two groups vary

This work was supported in part by an unrestricted grant from The St. Giles Foundation, New York, New York.

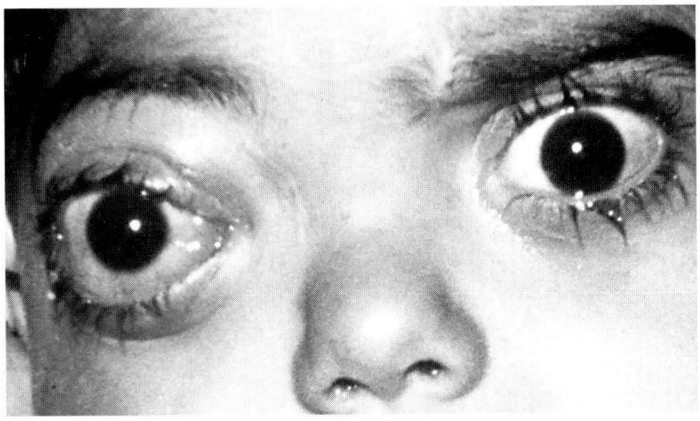

Figure 95–1. Infant with right ethmoidal mucocele secondary to abnormal bony architecture associated with osteopetrosis.

considerably in size, but generally the anterior ethmoidal cells are smaller and more numerous than the posterior cells.

The maxillary sinuses are the first of the paranasal sinuses to begin development in the human fetus at about day 65 of gestation. The maxillary sinuses enlarge from birth until the last permanent teeth have erupted around age 16 to 18. These sinuses occupy the body of the maxilla and in the adult represent the largest of the paranasal sinuses. The maxillary sinuses drain through one or more openings into the middle meatus of the nasal cavity through the hiatus semilunaris. This main sinus ostium generally drains into the posterior third of the hiatus.

The sphenoidal sinuses originate during the third fetal month as paired evaginations of the mucosa in the superior portion of the nasal cavity near the sphenoethmoidal recess. Pneumatization of the sphenoidal sinuses begins at approximately 3 years of age. The carotid artery and cranial nerves III, IV, VI, and V_1 are found lateral to the sphenoidal sinuses. The two sinuses vary much in size and are rarely symmetric. The bony septum between them is usually deviated to one side. Each sinus opens by an ostium in the superior portion of its anterior wall and drains into the sphenoethmoidal recess of the nasal cavity.

The frontal sinuses begin development during the fourth month of gestation as upward extensions of the anterior portion of the nasal capsule in the region of the frontal recess. They generally begin to pneumatize after the second year of life and complete this process usually in the late teens. They are absent in 5% of the population and are unilateral in about 15%. These sinuses drain beneath the anterior portion of the middle concha either into the ethmoidal infundibulum or into the frontal recess.

PATHOPHYSIOLOGY

The epithelium of the sinus mucosa is composed of ciliated pseudostratified columnar cells with interspersed basal cells and goblet-type mucus-secreting cells in a ratio of one goblet cell to approximately five ciliated cells. The purpose of this mucosa is to provide an uncontaminated supply of mucus to the nasal mucosa.[6] No proven function has been determined for the paranasal sinuses, but several theories have been entertained. These include increased olfaction, lightening of the skull, voicer resonation, and aiding in the humidification of inspired air. Some believe they are useless products of human evolution.[7]

Messerklinger studied the clearance of sinus mucous extensively using endoscopy in patients.[8] He noted that wherever two nasal mucosal layers came into direct contact, localized disruption of clearance of mucus occurred, resulting in retention of secretions in the area of contact with increasing potential for infection even in the presence of a normal draining sinus ostium. These areas of direct mucosal contact were consistently located at the anatomic level of the narrow mucosa-lined channels of the middle meatus and anterior ethmoidal sinuses. The importance of this anatomic level in the ultimate pathogenesis of frontal and maxillary sinusitis resulted in it being named the osteomeatal complex.[9] Mucosal disease at the level of the maxillary and frontal sinuses (which was previously considered irreversible) will usually undergo resolution when normal aeration and clearance of mucus are restored and osteomeatal complex disease is eradicated.[8]

Histopathology

The mucocele wall consists of thinned bone, mucosal lining, and thickened mucus. Chronic inflammation of the subepithelial connective tissue is common. The mucosal lining may display pseudostratified ciliated epithelium, goblet cells, flattened cuboidal epithelium, or squamous metaplasia. The viscous mucus filling the sinus is typically creamy white or tan but may vary in color if infection or intracavitary hemorrhage is present.

DIAGNOSTIC IMAGING

Ultrasonography, conventional radiography, computed tomography (CT), and magnetic resonance imaging (MRI) evaluations are valuable ancillary diagnostic techniques for the evaluation of mucoceles involving the orbit. In addition to detecting a mucocele and outlining its morphology, diagnostic tests may also depict associated conditions, such as evidence of an old fracture, osteoma, sinus tumor, polyps, or coexisting disease in other sinuses.

Ultrasonography

Ultrasonography serves to complement the other established diagnostic modalities by adding helpful infor-

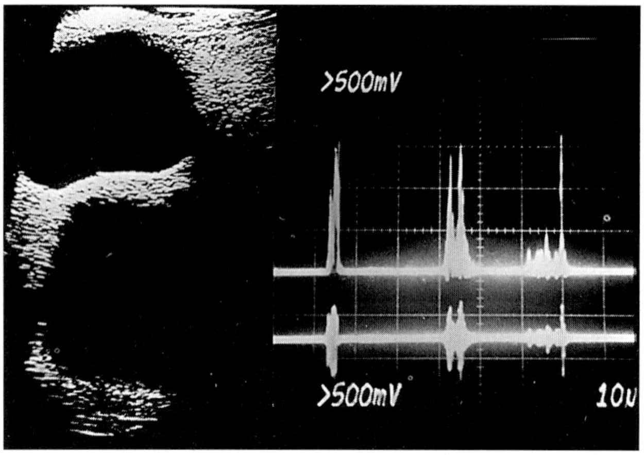

Figure 95–2. B-scan immersion ultrasonogram demonstrating a large spherical, acoustically hollow mass compressing the posterior globe. A-scan ultrasonogram demonstrates good sound transmission and minimal internal reflectivity.

mation that enables fast and reliable diagnosis, particularly in dealing with anterior ethmoidal, maxillary, and frontal sinus disease. Ultrasonographic evaluation is most valuable in detecting and delineating frontal or ethmoidal mucoceles. The tumor appears as a large spherical or oval mass located in the superior nasal orbit. The distinct and highly reflective anterior border indents the anterior orbital fat and may locally compress or flatten the globe. Typically, the mass is acoustically hollow and its interior appears as a solid black cavity (Fig. 95–2). Very little sound is absorbed by the viscous fluid within the cyst, and the sound waves easily penetrate the tumor. Therefore, the highly reflective posterior borders of the mass are well outlined.[10, 11] Although more easily seen on radiographic evaluation, ultrasonographic detection of a bony defect is possible. On A-scan evaluation the tumor cavity is anechoic, but it may occasionally demonstrate low internal reflectivity secondary to debris or hemorrhage within the tumor cavity.

Conventional Radiography

Conventional radiography (plain sinus films) usually includes a series of four different views (Waters, Caldwell, lateral, and submentovertex). These views are usually obtained with the patient in the upright position because the level of fluid in the sinus becomes more obvious in this position. The normal air-containing sinuses appear as radiographically dark, but pathologic conditions may alter this by opacifying the sinuses or by destroying bone.

Computed Tomography

The use of CT in the clinical evaluation of anatomic and pathologic conditions involving the paranasal sinuses is paramount. The axial projection is the most important scan and is usually obtained on a plane parallel to the infraorbital meatal line using 5-mm sections. A direct coronal view is often difficult to obtain, owing to dental fillings, but 60- to 80-degree sections are useful. Reconstruction of images with excellent resolution usually allows less radiation exposure to the patient. CT offers both soft tissue and bony detail not only of the paranasal sinuses but also of the anatomic structures that intimately surround them, including the orbits and brain.

Magnetic Resonance Imaging

On spin-echo MRI, mucoceles are depicted as well as circumscribed spherical or oval masses arising within the affected sinus cavity. The cyst contents are homogeneous and typically isointense or moderately hyperintense on T1-weighted studies and markedly hyperintense on T2-weighted studies (Fig. 95–3).[12] The cyst contents may be markedly hyperintense on T1-weighted studies if hemorrhage, infection, or inflammatory debris is present. The cyst contents do not enhance after gadolinium-DTPA contrast medium administration, but the mucosal lining

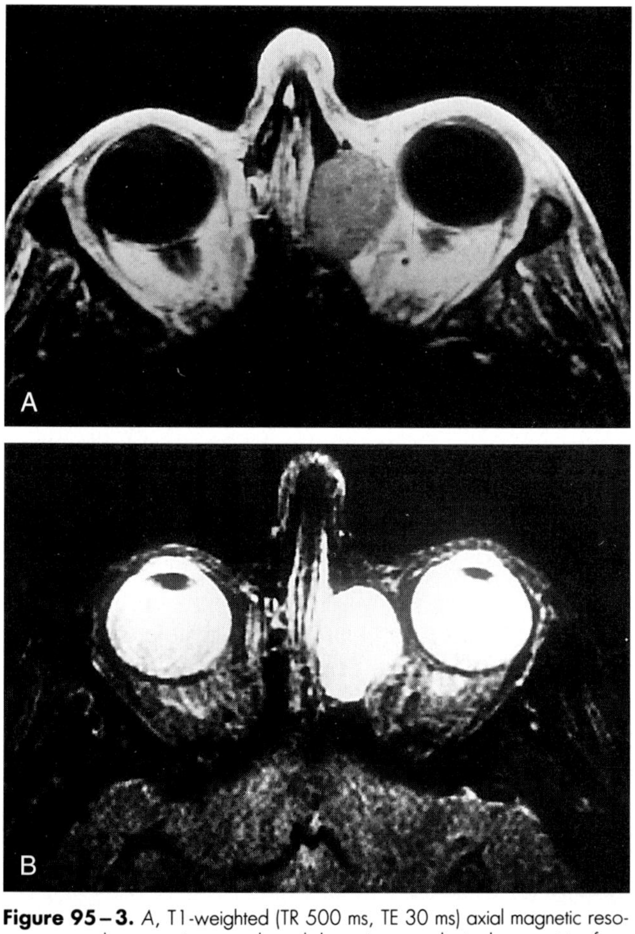

Figure 95–3. *A*, T1-weighted (TR 500 ms, TE 30 ms) axial magnetic resonance scan demonstrating a moderately hyperintense spherical mass arising from the ethmoidal sinus and displacing the left glove laterally, *B*, Axial T2-weighted study (TR 2000 ms, TE 90 ms) shows markedly hyperintense cyst contents.

may enhance. Associated soft tissue abnormalities, such as polyps, may affect the clinical picture. MRI is particularly valuable in posterior ethmoidal or sphenoidal mucoceles for the delineation of the optic chiasm and suprasellar structures and for determining the status of the carotid vasculature. MRI is less valuable for evaluating the status of surrounding bone, since orbital bone will be depicted as a signal void. Absence of a signal void surrounding the orbital cyst is indicative of bony destruction.

FRONTAL SINUS MUCOCELES

The patient with a frontal sinus mucocele may present with headache, lid swelling, proptosis, diplopia, or decreased vision. The disease process develops slowly and often in patients with a history of sinus disease. The headache is most commonly frontal and may display diurnal variation. A nontender mass is usually palpable underneath the superior nasal orbital rim. The mass may be firm, reflecting the presence of remodeled bone, crepitant due to shifting plaques of thin bone bordering the mass, or "doughy" when the bone is totally destroyed and the cystic mass is palpated directly.[5]

Erosion of the anterior wall of the frontal sinus results in a tender fluctuant mass beneath the periosteum of the frontal bone known as Pott's puffy tumor.[13, 14] A subcutaneous abscess, a fistula, and/or may develop if the mass erodes through the anterior wall. Erosion of the posterior bony wall of the frontal sinus may result in a progressive series of complications beginning with epidural abscess, subdural empyema, meningitis, and brain abscess.

The upper eyelid may be edematous and ptotic, particularly medially. The globe is characteristically displaced inferiorly and laterally (Fig. 95–4). Both globe displacement and periocular swelling may vary during upper respiratory tract infections. Extraocular motility may be affected and diplopia noted particularly in extremes of gaze. Limited elevation and adduction are most common. Globe indentation may result in refractive changes and choroidal striae.[5, 14]

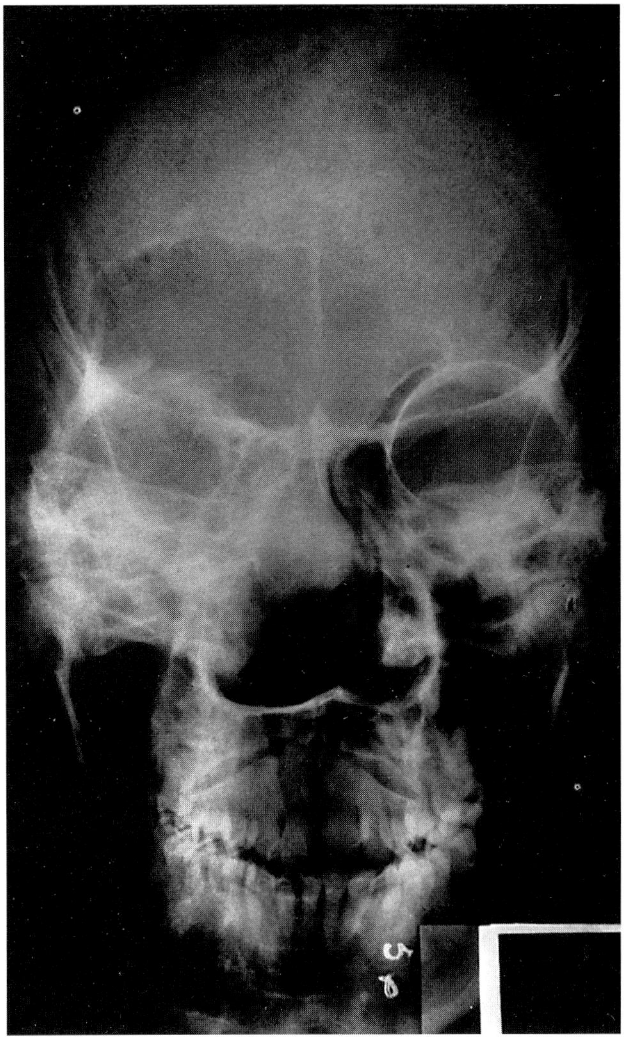

Figure 95–5. Plain radiograph of a patient with a frontal mucocele displaying an expanded sinus with loss of scalloping and increased radiolucency due to extensive bony reabsorption.

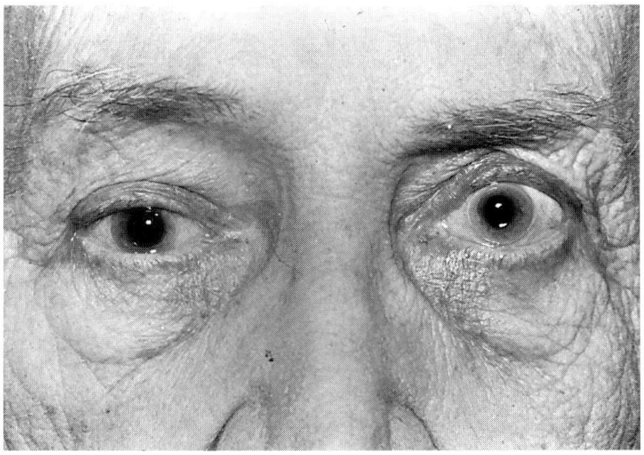

Figure 95–4. Patient with frontal sinus mucocele resulting in ptosis and inferior temporal displacement of the right globe.

Radiographic Findings

The frontal sinus is expanded with loss of scalloping and downward displacement of the supraorbital ridge (Fig. 95–5). The sinus is usually opaque but may appear radiolucent because of extensive bony destruction. Margins are round and thickened or may show evidence of destruction. On computed tomography, the expanding sinus mass is homogeneous and similar in density to brain. The radiodensity of the mass does not increase after contrast medium injection, but the rim of the mass may enhance. Careful examination of the posterior wall of the frontal sinus using CT with bone windows is advisable to detect osteolysis (Fig. 95–6).

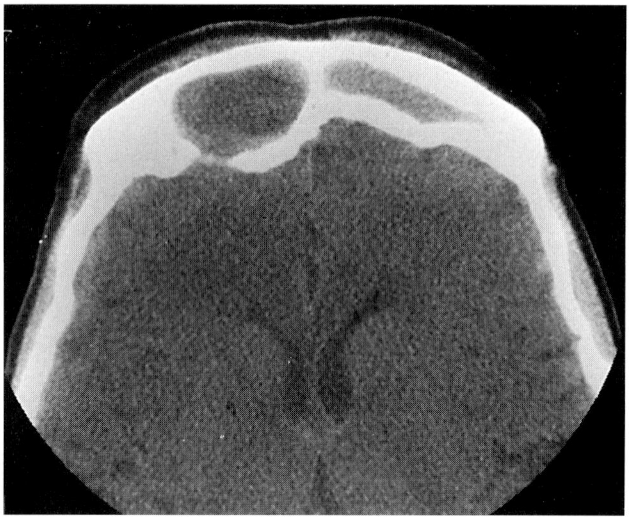

Figure 95–6. Axial computed tomographic scan demonstrating right frontal mucocele with osteolysis of the posterior wall of the frontal sinus.

Treatment

The osteoplastic frontal sinus operation is extremely useful in the removal of mucoceles. When there is adequate hair, a coronal incision at or slightly into the hairline is used. If balding is a concern, an incision just superior to the eyebrow is used. Reliable entrance into the sinus depends on the creation of a frontal sinus template prepared from a Caldwell plain film that is sterilized before surgery. The procedure is carried out under general anesthesia, and the patient's face and abdomen are prepped and draped. Lidocaine 1% with epinephrine is used before making the incision. The flap tissues are elevated in a plane between the frontalis muscle and the frontal periosteum. The template is placed over the periosteum of the frontal bone, and the periosteum is incised 0.5 cm from the anterior sinus wall. A beveled bone cut is made in the outer table of the sinus with either a small straight chisel or an oscillating bone saw. Next, the anterior wall of the sinus is carefully elevated with a chisel. The frontal wall hinges on the periosteum inferiorly after fracturing of the sinus floor is completed. Cultures are routinely taken, and all evidence of disease is removed. The sinus mucosa is carefully resected, and the interior of the sinus is then polished with a diamond bur. Adipose tissue removed from the left lower quadrant of the abdomen is subsequently used to pack the sinus and occlude the nasofrontal ducts. The osteoplastic flap is replaced, and the periosteum is sutured with Vicryl or Dexon. The skin is closed in a routine manner, and stainless steel staples are usually used for closure of the coronal incision. A pressure dressing is applied for 24 to 48 hours, and postoperative antibiotics are administered.

ETHMOIDAL MUCOCELES

Ethmoidal mucoceles most commonly arise in the anterior air cells. The lamina papyracea offers little resistance to this expanding mass, and the globe is displaced anteriorly and laterally. A mass may be seen and palpated in the medial canthal region. Epiphora may result from compression of the lacrimal sac or nasolacrimal duct. Diplopia is common, as are adduction defects. Pain is a rare finding and usually associated with secondary infection. Occasionally sterile mucus will leak through the wall of ethmoidal mucoceles, resulting in a swollen, painful orbit mimicking orbital cellulitis (Fig. 95–7). This inflammation is nonresponsive to antibiotics but responds rapidly to systemic corticosteroid therapy.

Radiographic Findings

Ethmoidal mucoceles are often difficult to diagnose on plain radiography. Nonspecific findings include loss of sinus translucence, destruction of ethmoidal septa, lateral expansion of the medial orbital wall, and expansion into the frontal sinus. CT (Fig. 95–8) and MRI will usually easily define the nature and extent of the mass.

Treatment

Ethmoidal mucoceles may be removed using an external approach. General anesthesia is preferred for external ethmoidectomy and mucocele removal. The skin is marked for a curvilinear incision (Lynch) extending from the inferior medial eyebrow along the lateral nasal wall between the dorsum of the nose and medial canthus. If encountered, the angular vessels are ligated or retracted. The supraorbital nerve may at times be identified

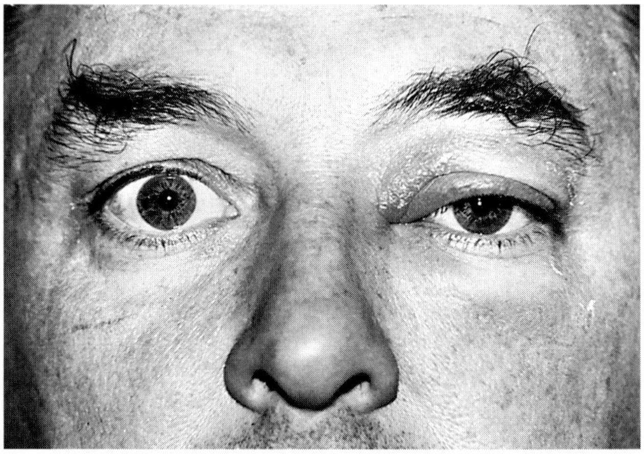

Figure 95–7. A patient with an ethmoidal mucocele and sterile orbital inflammation due to leakage of cyst contents.

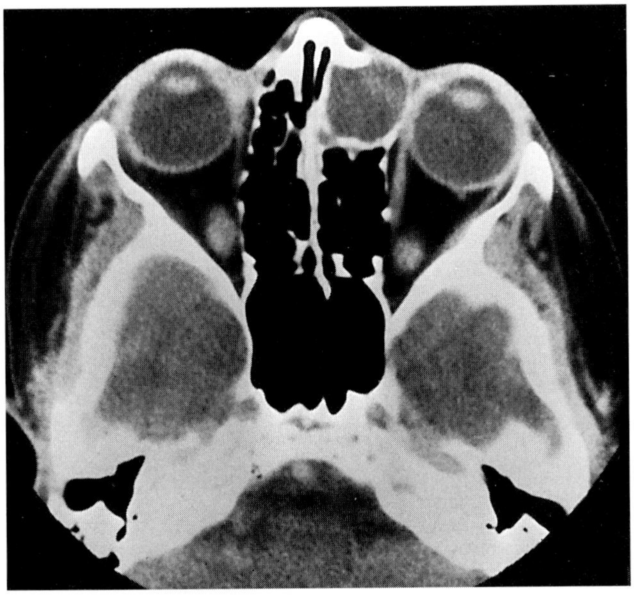

Figure 95–8. Axial computed tomographic scan through mid orbit demonstrating left anterior ethmoidal mucocele expanding the medial orbital wall and displacing the globe laterally.

and retracted laterally. The incision is carried down to the periosteum with sharp and blunt dissection or electrocautery. Periosteum is next incised and elevated. Resistance is encountered at the trochlea, which is detached from the trochlear fossa of the orbital plate of the frontal bone. The bulging mass is usually easily seen at this point. Although the anterior ethmoidal artery in adults is normally approximately 20 mm posterior to the posterior lacrimal crest in the frontoethmoidal suture, the tumor mass commonly distorts these anatomical relationships. The posterior ethmoidal artery is normally 10 mm posterior to the anterior ethmoidal vessels, and the optic foramen is located an additional 10 mm posteriorly. However, as noted earlier, the mucocele may distort or destroy these anatomic landmarks. Once the periosteum is adequately retracted, laterally exposing the orbital portion of the mass, the cyst wall is then palpated to detect an area of thin or absent bone. A large syringe (10 to 20 mL) with a 16-gauge needle is passed gently through the wall and cyst contents are aspirated. This decompresses the cyst, thus minimizing spillage of mucus into the surrounding tissues when the wall is opened. This also provides an uncontaminated specimen for Gram stain, cytology, and microbiologic studies. The cyst wall is then opened widely, and the remainder of the cavity is evacuated with suction. Abnormal bone extending into the orbit, and the remaining lamina papyracea are removed with rongeurs. The mucosa is removed and submitted for histopathologic evaluation. Ethmoidal air cells adjacent to the mucocele are removed as well as the medial and inferior wall of the mucocele. An instrument placed intranasally should be easily seen through the surgical site. Recurrence rates are lowest when all mucosa has been removed and unobstructed drainage has been established. The periosteum, subcutaneous tissue, and skin are each closed in separate layers. With reapproximation of the periosteum, the trochlea will reattach without significant sequelae in nearly all patients.

With the advent of functional endoscopic sinus surgery, these lesions also are commonly removed transnasally. The principle of this technique is to provide for a limited resection of inflammatory tissues or anatomic defects that interfere with the normal clearance of sinus mucous, resulting in localized persistent inflammation. This technique involves limited surgical resection rather than wide exenteration. It avoids external incisions and is cosmetically acceptable. Accurate diagnosis and an understanding of the pathogenesis of sinus disease and anatomy are essential to successful surgical outcome.

Local or general anesthesia may be used. Telescopic or microscopic approaches have both been described.[15, 16] Lidocaine 1% with epinephrine is injected in specific sites of the lateral nasal wall. A sickle knife is then used to expose the ethmoidal infundibulum, which is then subluxed and removed with forceps. This maneuver allows access to the anterior ethmoidal area. The extent of surgical resection from this point is variable and based on preoperative radiographic evaluation. A complete ethmoidectomy, sphenoidotomy, and middle meatal antrostomy (to access the maxillary sinus) may be performed. This technique is therefore useful in the drainage of ethmoidal, frontal, sphenoidal, and maxillary sinus mucoceles. Simply stated, persistent disease (including mucocele) in one of the paranasal sinuses is most likely caused by undiagnosed, untreated, anterior ethmoidal disease. Relief of obstruction at the level of the anterior ethmoidal sinuses allows the other contiguous sinuses to drain and the mucosa to return to normal.

SPHENOIDAL MUCOCELES

Mucoceles of the sphenoidal and posterior ethmoidal paranasal sinuses are extremely rare but clinically important lesions. The peak incidence for development is between the ages of 40 and 60 years. These tumors cause a myriad of signs and symptoms due to the proximity of the sphenoidal sinus to many vital structures. They frequently affect the nerves and vessels passing through the optic foramen and superior orbital fissure. The protean manifestations of this disorder may result in a delayed diagnosis. Patients will typically present with a headache, visual impairment, strabismus, or proptosis.

Headache is a common nonspecific symptom.[17, 18] The pain may be retrobulbar, periorbital, frontotemporal, or occasionally occipital. The headache may be bilateral and slowly progressive over long periods of time. The pain is often more intense in the supine position. A positional change in the intensity and character of the headache may be related to stretching of the dura in the region of the planum sphenoidale or the anterior cranial fossa. Additionally, irritation of the gasserian ganglion or the first two branches of the trigeminal nerve could account for such pain.

Visual impairment occurs when the mucocele expands, compresses the chiasm or optic nerves, or compromises the vasculature of the optic nerve or retina.[19, 20] Optic disc edema is occasionally observed; however, the most typical ophthalmoscopic finding is slowly progressive optic atrophy. The combination of orbital pain and decreased vision has led to the inaccurate diagnosis of optic neuritis in some patients. Visual field defects may be unilateral, bilateral, and include bitemporal hemianopsia, and central scotomas. Complete blindness in one eye and a temporal field cut in the opposite eye have been noted.[21] Several patients developed sudden blindness after compromise of the optic nerve or retinal vasculature.[22, 23] Diplopia and strabismus occur secondary to third (pupil involvement variable), fourth, or sixth nerve palsies. These nerves or their nutrient vessels may be compressed as the mass encroaches on the cavernous sinus or superior orbital fissure. A complete orbital apex syndrome can occur. Unilateral or bilateral proptosis or lateral ocular displacement often occurs. Pulsating exophthalmos[24] occurs occasionally when cerebrospinal fluid pulsations are transmitted through the mucocele to the orbit. Other signs and symptoms include dysfunction of the first and second branches of the fifth cranial nerve, pituitary dysfunction, nasal obstruction, anosmia, and rhinorrhea. The differential diagnosis includes a slowly expanding lesion in the sphenoidal region, including pituitary tumors, carotid aneurysms, craniopharyngioma, and sinus neoplasms. Before the development of CT, most sphenoidal mucoceles were diagnosed at craniotomy or sphenoidectomy.

Radiographic Findings

The sphenoidal sinus will be opacified and expanded. The affected sinus may be radiolucent since bone loss cancels out the increased density related to mucus accumulation.[12] The tumor may be seen eroding and remodeling the surrounding bone, as well as compressing adjacent structures. The tumor margins are distinct, and no adjacent structures are infiltrated. The orbital bone has a smooth outline, and the wall displays rarefaction. The sella turcica may be destroyed, as well as the clinoid processes. The lamina papyracea may be displaced laterally, and the interseptum destroyed. The carotid artery will often be displaced laterally, and the anterior cerebral arteries will be elevated.[25]

On computed tomography, an isodense (to brain) or hyperdense nonenhancing mass occupies and expands the sphenoidal sinus. On MRI a smooth, oval, nonenhancing cyst is depicted (Fig. 95–9). The mucocele wall

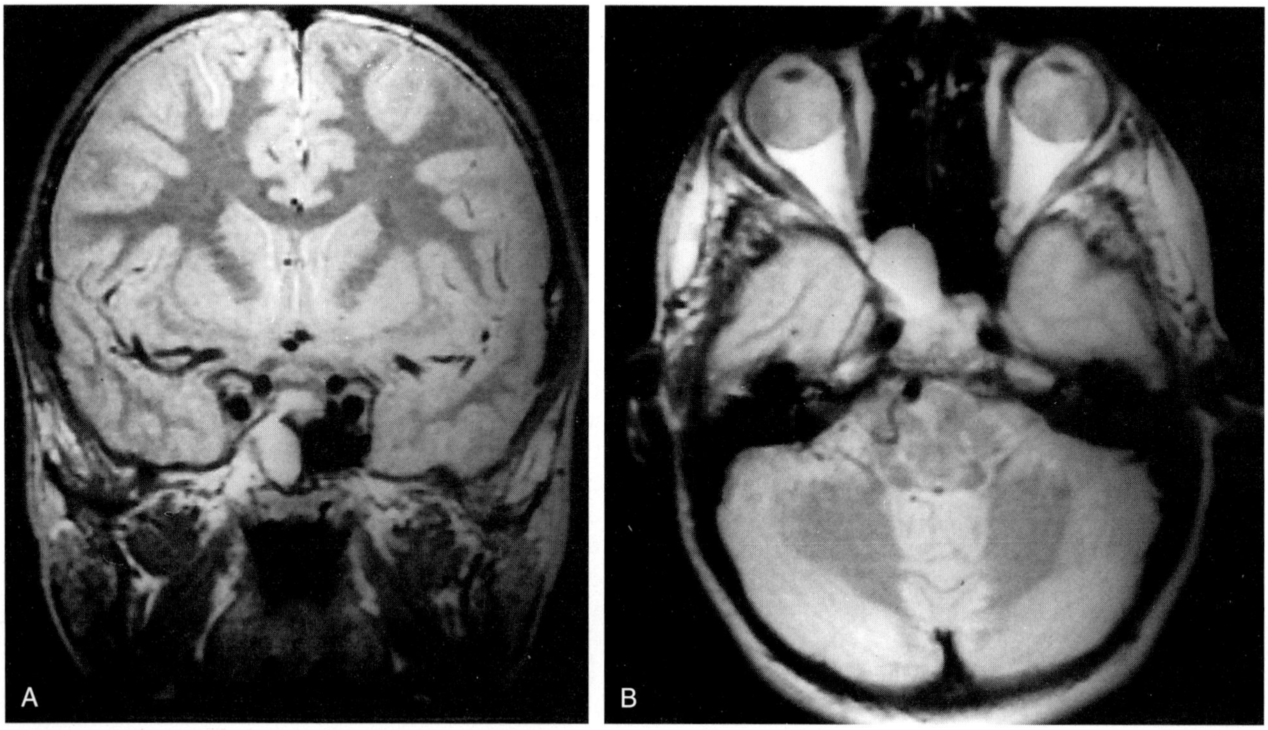

Figure 95–9. *A*, Axial proton density (TR 3000 ms, TE 18 ms) magnetic resonance (MR) scan reveals a sphenoidal mucocele compressing the right optic nerve. *B*, Coronal proton density (TR 3000 ms, TE 18 ms) MR scan reveals a sphenoidal mucocele compressing the right optic nerve.

often enhances after contrast medium administration. The mass may erode the base of the cranium at the level of the sella turcica, extend through the cribriform plate into the anterior cranial fossa, and invade the sphenoid with some involvement in the middle cranial fossa. Erosion of the lamina papyracea may also be present.

Treatment

Drainage of sphenoidal sinus mucoceles may be performed after a complete functional endoscopic ethmoidectomy with sphenoidectomy as previously described. When the bulge of the sphenoidal sinus is evident in the inferomedial aspect of the most posterior ethmoidal sinus, it is opened under direct vision. When the bulge is not evident, the natural ostium may be identified medial to the middle turbinate and the sinus opened from this area. Excessive removal of mucosa is to be avoided since natural dehiscences in the bony wall are common and iatrogenic injuries may occur (e.g., internal carotid artery laceration).

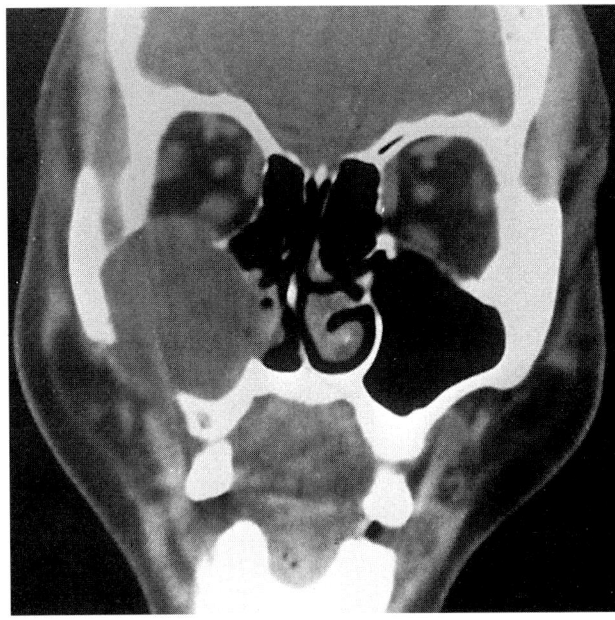

Figure 95–10. Coronal computed tomogram of a patient with a right maxillary sinus mucocele.

MAXILLARY SINUS MUCOCELES

Maxillary sinus mucoceles are rare lesions that demonstrate slow, but unremitting growth.[26] Mucoceles in the sinus are usually small and asymptomatic. They are typically seen on plain films of the sinus and are sometimes referred to as mucous retension cysts. As with all expanding lesions within the maxillary antrum, presenting symptoms may be orbital, nasal, dental, or facial, depending on the direction of mucocele growth.[26] Frequently, patients have a history of previous maxillary sinus surgery. This high incidence is associated with postoperative compartmentalization of the maxillary antrum.

Ophthalmic manifestations of maxillary mucoceles include globe displacement, diplopia, lid abnormalities, epiphora, palpable masses, and infraorbital hypesthesia. Globes may be proptotic and displaced superiorly or enophthalmic and displaced inferiorly. This nontraumatic acquired enophthalmos results from erosion of the orbital floor with herniation of orbital contents and is associated with a superior sulcus deformity.[27, 28] Vertical diplopia is a common symptom. Lid abnormalities include ptosis, pseudoptosis, and lower lid malpositions. Epiphora may occur after compression of the nasolacrimal duct or lacrimal sac. Nonophthalmic manifestations include nasal obstruction, maxillary pain, facial swelling, and loose teeth. Infraorbital hypesthesia may occur when the mass compresses the infraorbital nerve.

Radiographic Findings

Radiographically, the maxillary sinus is enlarged and opacified. Bony erosion, thickening, and remodeling may be depicted. On CT, the enlarged sinus is filled with a homogeneous material isodense with brain tissue (Fig. 95–10). The cystic tumor mass does not enhance, but the mucosal lining may. The orbital floor is typically thinned, destroyed, or remodeled, and the lesion may extend to the nasal cavity, ethmoidal sinus, and pterygopalatine fossa.[27] Reactive bony thickening from reactive osteoblastic activity has been documented in one patient with inferior bowing of the orbital floor.[27] It is speculated that downward pressure of the orbital tissues, aided by gravity, must have exceeded upward pressure from the mucocele.[27]

Treatment

Maxillary sinus mucoceles usually do not require treatment. They are seen as asymptomatic opacifications on plain films of the sinus. The Caldwell-Luc antrostomy is the traditional approach for removal of these mucoceles. This involves an incision in the respective upper gingivobuccal sulcus with fenestration of the anterior bony wall using a gouge or osteotome. The opening is enlarged, and the diseased sinus contents are removed. An opening in the inferior meatus of the nose is usually performed, the sinus packed, and the incision closed. The packing is removed on the first or second postoperative day.

Acknowledgment

The authors gratefully acknowledge the assistance of Grace Shin, MD, in the preparation of this manuscript.

REFERENCES

1. Weaver DT, Bartley GM: Malignant neoplasia of the paranasal sinuses associated with mucocele. Ophthalmology 98:342–346, 1991.
2. Stool S, Kertesz E, Sibinga M, Frayer W: Exophthalmos due to pyocele to the sinus in children with cystic fibrosis. Trans Am Acad Ophthalmol 70:811–816, 1966.
3. Levine MR, Kim Y, Witt W: Frontal sinus mucopyocele in cystic fibrosis. Ophthalmic Plast Reconstr Surg 4:221–225, 1988.
4. Reese AB: Expanding lesions of the orbit (Bowman lecture). Trans Ophthalmol Soc UK 91:85–104, 1971.
5. Henderson JW: Orbital Tumors, 2nd ed. New York, BC Decker, pp 96–105, 1980.
6. Herzon FS: Nasal ciliary structural pathology. Laryngoscope 93:63–67, 1983.
7. Amedee RG: Anatomy, physiology, and evaluation of the paranasal sinuses. *In* Ballinger JJ (ed): Diseases of the Nose, Throat, Ear, Head and Neck. Malvern, PA, Lea & Febiger, 1991, pp 168–183.
8. Messerklinger W: On the drainage of the normal frontal sinus of man. Acta Otolaryngol 63:176–179, 1967.
9. Naumann H: Pathologische Anatomie der chronischen Rhinitis und Sinusitus: *In* Proceedings of the VII International Congress of Otorhinolaryngology. Amsterdam, Excerpta Medica, 1965.
10. Coleman DJ, Lizzi FL, Jack RL: Ultrasonography of the Eye and Orbit. Philadelphia, Lea & Febiger, 1977.
11. Byrne SF, Green RL: Ultrasound of the Eye and Orbit, St. Louis, Mosby-Year Book, 1992.
12. Eisele DW, Crane RD, Yarington CT: Magnetic resonance imaging of the sphenoethmoid mucoceles. Ear Nose Throat J 67:713–725, 1988.
13. Abrahamson IA, Baluyot ST, Tew JM, Scioville G: Frontal sinus mucocele. Ann Ophthalmol 11:173–178, 1979.
14. Mauriello JA, Flanagan JC (eds): Management of Orbital and Ocular Adnexal Tumors and Inflammations. New York, Field & Wood, 1990, pp 91–94.
15. Amedee RG, Mann W, Gisbach J: Microscopic endonasal surgery of the paranasal sinuses and the parasellar region. Arch Otolaryngol Head Neck Surg 115:1103–1106, 1989.
16. Amedee RG, Mann W, Gisbach J: Microscopic endonasal surgery: Clinical update for treatment of chronic sinusitus with polyps. Am J Rhinol 4:203–205, 1990.
17. Alper MG: Mucoceles of the sphenoid sinus neuro-ophthalmologic manifestations. Trans Am Ophthalmol Soc 74:53–81, 1977.
18. Bregeat P: Ophthalmic manifestations of sphenoidal mucoceles. Ann Ophthalmol 9:259–266, 1977.
19. Blum ME, Larson A: Mucocele of the sphenoid sinus with sudden blindness. Laryngoscope 83:2042–2049, 1973.
20. Larson CH, Adkins WY, Osguthorpe JD: Post-traumatic frontal and frontoethmoid mucoceles causing reversible visual loss. Otolaryngol Head Neck Surg 91:691–694, 1983.
21. Nugent GR, Sprinkle P, Bloor BM: Sphenoid sinus mucoceles. J Neurosurg 32:443–451, 1970.
22. Heitzman ER, Markarian B: Unilateral proptosis with loss of vision. NY State J Med 73:1671–1675, 1973.
23. Wurster CF, Levine TM, Sisson GA: Mucocele of the sphenoid sinus causing sudden onset of blindness. Otolaryngol Head Neck Surg 94:257–259, 1986.
24. O'Shea HV: Pulsating exophthalmous due to sphenoidal sinus mucocele. Lancet 1:1253, 1932.
25. Chen HJ, Kao LY, Lui CC: Mucocele of the sphenoid sinus with the apex orbitae syndrome. Surg Neurol 25:101–104, 1986.
26. Sharp JF: Non-axial proptosis without diplopia secondary to maxillary pyomucocele. J Royal Soc Med 82:507–508, 1989.
27. Traustason OI, Feldon SE: Cause of enophthalmos secondary to maxillary sinus mucocele. Am J Ophthalmol 95:838–840, 1983.
28. Cline RA, Rootman J: Enophthalmos: A clinical review. Ophthalmology 91:229–237, 1984.

C H A P T E R 9 6

Radiation Therapy in Orbital Disease

Steven J. Rubin

One of my professors once said, "Radiotherapy is like operating without a knife."[1] Instead of that cutting utensil used in surgery radiation therapists use physics. Therefore, to understand radiation therapy one must understand some basic physics.

The radiograph in Figure 96–1 is a simulation film taken on a machine built like a treatment machine with a diagnostic x-ray head instead of a treatment head. The film in Figure 96–2 is a port film taken with therapeutic x-rays (6-MeV photons) by a treatment machine. The diagnostic film clearly shows bone and metal; the port film gives a fuzzier image. At diagnostic energies most photons are absorbed by the photoelectric effect. The likelihood of an interaction with the photoelectric effect is proportional to Z^3, where Z is the atomic number. Therefore, far more interactions occur with bone (calcium; $Z = 20$) than with tissue (water is a good approximation for tissue; $Z_{ave} = 3.3$), making the bone look sharper on the diagnostic film. At therapeutic energies, most of the interactions occur by means of the Compton effect, which deposits energy in a Z-independent manner. Instead, this effect is only dependent on the electron density of the material, or roughly the physical density. Therefore, lung tumors sometimes show up better on therapy films than on diagnostic ones; and tungsten is a better marker for therapy films than lead because of its high electron density.

These effects are energy dependent (Table 96–1). At diagnostic energies, the photoelectric effect predominates; at about 1 MeV*(cobalt-60 = 1.1 MeV), the Compton effect occurs; and at energies greater than 10 MeV another process starts to be common, pair production, which is proportional to Z^2. At 24 MeV, the highest energy that is generally used in routine clinical practice, pair production is about 50% of all interactions. In the old days, pre-megavoltage or before cobalt-60, orthovoltage was used in which the photoelectric effect predominated. Therefore, bone (i.e., the orbit) got a much higher dose, resulting in more complications.

Photons produce electrons through the photoelectric or Compton effect or pair production. These electrons produce ion radicals, which in turn produce free radicals, which damage DNA.[2] Then when a cell divides, it dies. Thus radiation is sometimes said to cause a reproductive or mitotic death. As the energy of the incident photon increases, so does the energy or the range of the secondary electron. Therefore, at the skin, because there is no contribution of electrons from the air, there is a lower dose (Fig. 96–3). The higher the energy, the deeper the depth of maximal energy deposition (D_{max}) (Table 96–2). So, in the old days, patients had very bad skin reactions. The skin was the dose-limiting organ.

If we give a human a lethal total-body dose of radiation, for example, 400 cGy, the amount of energy deposited would be equivalent to drinking a sip of hot coffee.[2] Why does this amount of radiation kill? The energy is quantized or absorbed in packets. These energy packets are large enough in the case of ionizing radiation to produce high-energy electrons or to break chemical bonds. The coffee delivers energy through heat, which consists of very small quanta, only enough to vibrate such bonds.

How is dose measured? The first attempt to measure dose was the skin erythema dose, literally the dose it took to turn human skin red. This is a biologic dosimeter, where the old-timers used to stick their hands in the beam.[3] The roentgen (R) is a unit of exposure that is proportional to the number of ionizations in air. The roentgen was used because devices existed that could measure it. The rad (radiation absorbed dose) is a better unit, representing the amount of energy deposited by ionizing radiation per gram of tissue. For most practical purposes, there are 0.962 rad/R.[4] This number actually varies with energy and tissue type. The gray (Gy) is the SI unit where 1 Gy = 100 rad or 1 cGy (centigray) = 1 rad.

RADIOBIOLOGY

All radiobiology is a post hoc attempt to explain an empiric fact: fractionation. This is giving the treatment over

*MeV is an abbreviation for million electron volts, a unit of energy, which is used in radiation therapy because it is practical and because this is how high-energy physicists talk. An eV is the energy an electron has when accelerated across a potential of 1 volt. In diagnostic machines this has a direct physical meaning: this is the actual voltage between two plates over which electrons are accelerated.

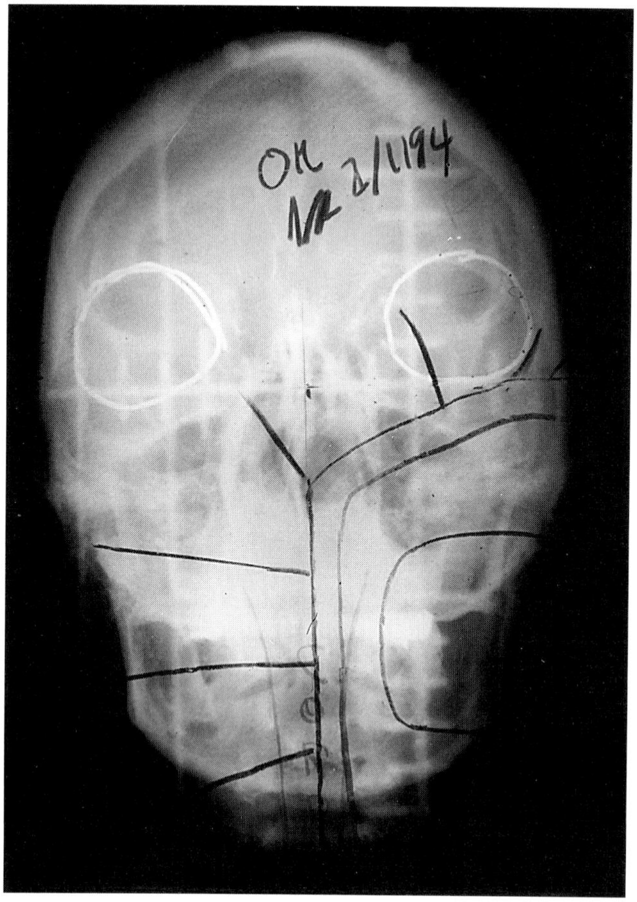

Figure 96–1. A simulation radiograph taken with diagnostic-energy x-rays.

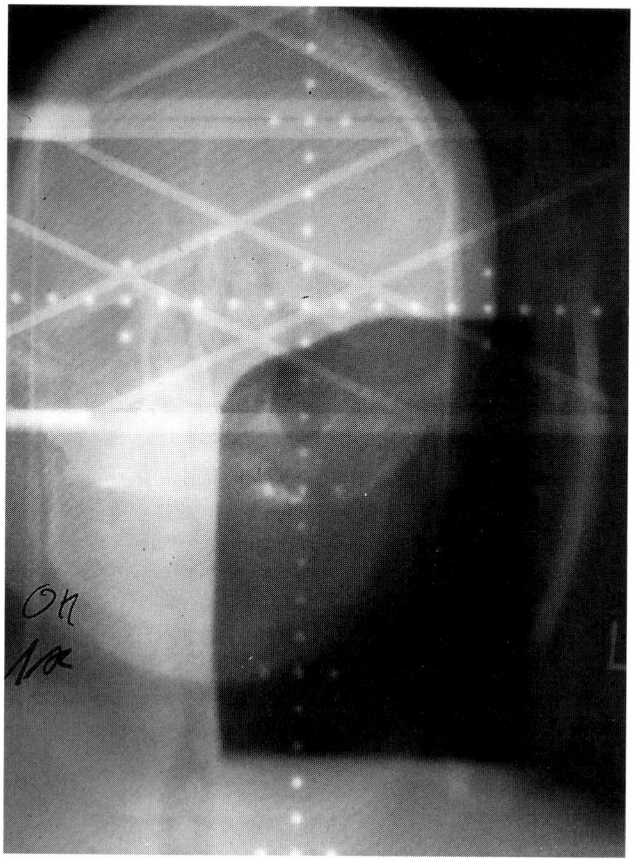

Figure 96–2. A port radiograph taken with 6-MeV x-rays of the same patient as in Figure 96–1.

many divided doses rather than in one large dose; it gives better local control and lower complication rates. The French, in particular Coutard[5] and Baclesse,[6] invented fractionation for several reasons, some practical and others scientific. Since there was no skin sparing, fractionation reduced the severity of their patients' skin reactions; thus the smaller the fraction size, the slower the treatment, the less the acute side effects. An experiment by Regaud and Ferroux[7] showed that they could lower the normal tissue effects on the skin while improving the sterilization rates by fractionating when irradiating rams' testicles. (This experiment assumes that spermatogonia are like cancer cells.) Therefore, the French school uses relatively small fractions, roughly 200 cGy/d. Around the same time in Manchester, England, Paterson[8] believed shorter treatment times were important to prevent tumor regrowth. Therefore, he recommended larger fractions (300–400 cGy/d). Today, most centers in the British Commonwealth still tend to use larger fraction sizes. Radiotherapy in the United States is in the French school thanks to Coutard's arrival in the 1930s.

Long-term complication rates are exquisitely sensitive to fraction size. In 1976, Harris and Levene[9] reported that no optic complications occurred in the treatment of pituitary adenomas with a fraction size less than 250 cGy/d and an 18% complication rate with larger fraction sizes. Parsons and colleagues[10] report that when 6000 to 7000 cGy is given to the optic nerves, there is an 8% incidence of complications with fraction sizes less than or equal to 195 cGy and a 40% incidence with greater fraction sizes. In the treatment of Hodgkin's disease, at the

TABLE 96–1

Relative Importance of Photoelectric (τ), Comptom (σ), and Pair Production (Π) Processes in Water

Photon Energy (MeV)	Relative Number of Interactions (%)		
	τ	σ	Π
0.01	95	5	0
0.026	50	50	0
0.060	7	93	0
0.150	0	100	0
4.00	0	94	6
10.00	0	77	23
24.00	0	50	50
100.00	0	16	84

From Khan FM: The Physics of Radiation Therapy, 2nd ed. Baltimore, Williams & Wilkins, 1994.

Data from Johns HE, Cunningham JR: The Physics of Radiology, 3rd ed. Springfield, IL, Charles C Thomas, 1969.

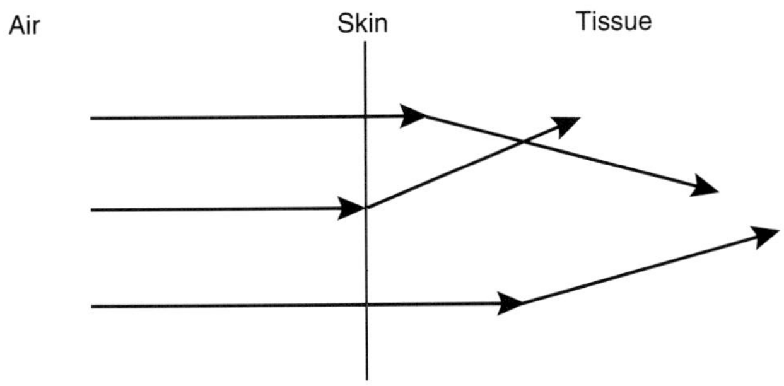

Figure 96–3. A representation of skin sparing with megavoltage irradiation. High-energy photons interact with tissue, producing high-energy electrons. The higher the energy of the secondary electron, the longer is its range. Because virtually no electrons are produced by interacting with the air, the dose near the skin is lowered.

TABLE 96–2

Table of D_{max} Versus the Energy of the Incident Photon Beam

Energy	D_{max}
Orthovoltage	Surface
Cobalt-60	0.6 cm
6 MV	1.5 cm
10 MV	2.5 cm
24 MV	4.5 cm

D_{max}, depth where the maximal dose deposition occurs.

University of California, San Francisco, researchers reported an incidence of pericarditis of 3.2%, treating at 200 cGy/d, while at Stanford University a 6.6% incidence at 250 cGy/d was reported.[11]

Tumor control probably is dependent on fraction aize as well. Eichorn[12] performed a human experiment on fractionation in patients with lung cancer. All patients were operated on or autopsy was performed. The best tumor control rate was with the most standard fractionation (250 cGy/d).

Radiobiology can be thought of as having four Rs: radiosensitivity, reoxygenation, repopulation, and redistribution.[13] Radiosensitivity is the laboratory measure of cell line survival when irradiated (Fig. 96–4) and has very little to do with how a tumor responds clinically. Sarcomas are quite radiosensitive in the laboratory[14] but are not radioresponsive (i.e., they do not shrink). Most of their cells are not clonogenic (tumor) cells but are stromal cells. Sarcomas, however, are radiocurable.[15] Head and neck cancer cell lines are relatively radioresistant in the laboratory, are clinically radioresponsive, and are radiocurable.[13] Small cell carcinomas of the lung are radiosensitive and radioresponsive but are not radiocurable.

Cells lines are 2.8 times more sensitive to radiation with oxygen than without.[16] The centers of large tumors are hypoxic (Fig. 96–5) and thus may be radioresistant. In clinical practice the first fraction would kill off the well-oxygenated cells. By the next day some of the previously hypoxic cells would become well oxygenated and thus radiosensitive. Clinical trials in which patients were randomly assigned to be treated with and without hyperbaric oxygen, however, showed an improvement in local tumor control in head and neck and cervical cancers when hyperbaric oxygen was used.[17, 18] For practical reasons, these trials were hypofractionated, using only a few large fractions, thus limiting the potential benefit of reoxygenation.

Repopulation simply means that the longer it takes to treat a tumor, the longer it has to grow. Withers and colleagues[19] suggest that accelerated repopulation occurs after fractionated radiation therapy is discontinued. In the 1960s and 1970s patients were commonly treated with a "split course," receiving a 2-week break in the middle of their treatment, thus lowering their acute reactions. The long-term outcome of these patients is definitely worse than patients treated in a continuous manner.[20] Mendenhall and associates[21] showed that smaller fraction sizes (<225 cGy/d) in the treatment of the glottic

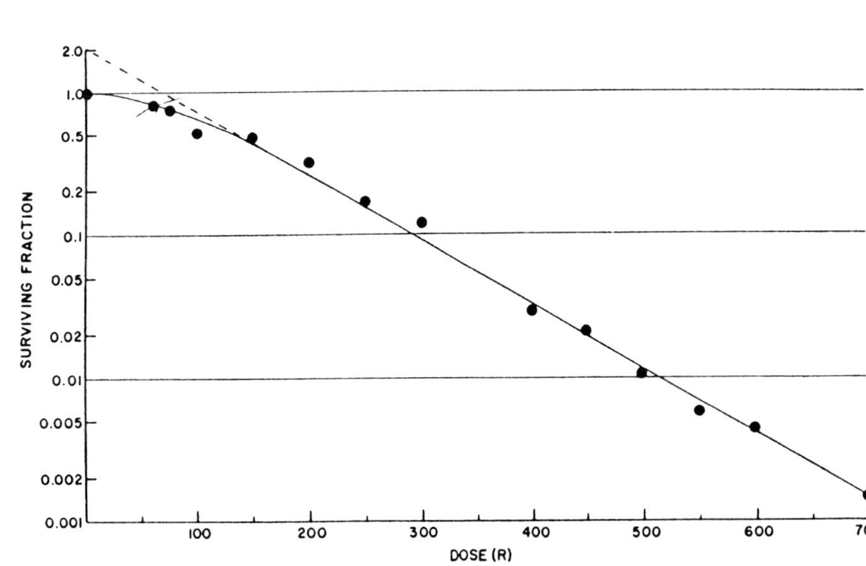

Figure 96–4. Survival curve for HeLa cells in culture exposed to x-rays. Characteristically, this cell line has a small initial shoulder. (Reproduced from The Journal of Experimental Medicine, 1956, 103, pp 653–656 by copyright permission of The Rockefeller University Press.)

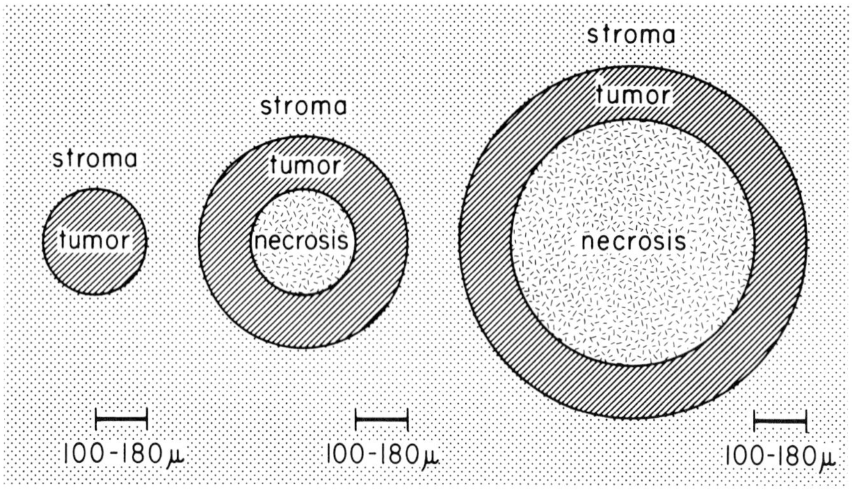

Figure 96–5. The conclusions reached by Thomlinson and Gray[16a] from a study of histologic sections of human bronchial carcinoma. No necrosis was seen in small tumor cords with a radius smaller than about 160 μm. No tumor cord with a radius exceeding 2100 μm was without a necrotic center. As the diameter of the necrotic area increased, the thickness of the sheath of viable tumor cells remained essentially constant at 100 to 180 μm. (From Hall EJ [ed]: Radiobiology for the Radiologist, 4th ed. Philadelphia, JB Lippincott, 1994.)

larynx led to lower cure rates. They believe that this is secondary to longer treatment times. Therefore, I try to give my patients as few treatment breaks as possible.

Figure 96–6 represents the four categories of cells in a tumor. The proliferating cells are most sensitive to radiation in late G_2 and M stages and most resistant in S.[22] Most tumor cells (90–98%), however, are not even in the cell cycle. They are quiescent or in G_0. These cells are thought to be radioresistant because they have time to repair damage. If the treatment is fractionated, the cells in the cell cycle, the sensitive ones, are killed; then the cells in G_0 are recruited into the cycle and thus become sensitive. This type of redistribution was Eichorn's explanation for his results.

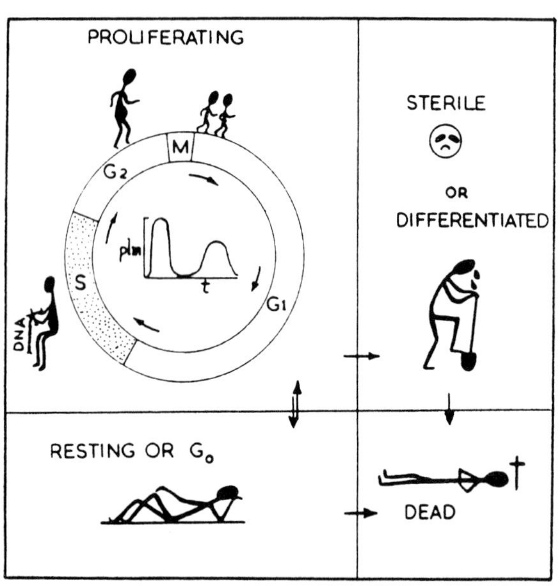

Figure 96–6. The neoplastic component of a tumor compromises four categories of cells: proliferating, resting, differentiated, and dead. (From Steel GG [ed]: Basic Clinical Radiobiology for Radiation Oncologists. London, England, Edward Arnold, 1993. Reproduced by permission of Edward Arnold [Publishers] Limited.)

PRACTICAL APPLICATIONS

If small fractions equal small complications, then why not use smaller fractions while treating to a higher dose? This is, in fact, being done. Hyperfractionation gives small fractions (110–120 cGy) twice a day to avoid prolonged treatment times to a higher total dose (7400–8000 cGy) than is standard.[23] The European Organization for Research on Treatment of Cancer showed such a treatment schema to be superior to standard treatment in oropharyngeal cancers excluding the base of tongue.[24] To avoid accelerated repopulation, investigators at M. D. Anderson Hospital in Houston treat patients in a manner called accelerated fractionation.[25] The patients are treated at 180 cGy/d once a day for the first 3 weeks and for the last 3 weeks at 180 cGy in the morning and 150 cGy in the afternoon to standard total doses (7000 cGy). This shortens overall treatment time. Most authors believe that in any multiple fraction per day schema the interval between doses should be kept to at least 6 hours.[26, 27] Another technique that, in effect, gives infinitely small fractions is brachytherapy or implants.

A RAD IS NOT A RAD

It really does matter how the treatment is given and prescribed. Figure 96–7 represents treatment with a single field of 6-MeV photons prescribed to 10.0 cm. Note that there is a "hot spot" of 300+ cGy. Thus if a patient were treated in such a manner some of the normal tissue would not get the prescribed fractions size of 200 cGy but rather 300 cGy. If that "hot spot" was over a critical structure (e.g., the spinal cord), a complication could result. This problem could be avoided by using a higher energy beam (a 240+ cGy "hot spot") (Fig. 96–8) or treating with opposed fields (a 210+ cGy "hot spot") (Fig. 96–9). Consider the following situation: someone has a

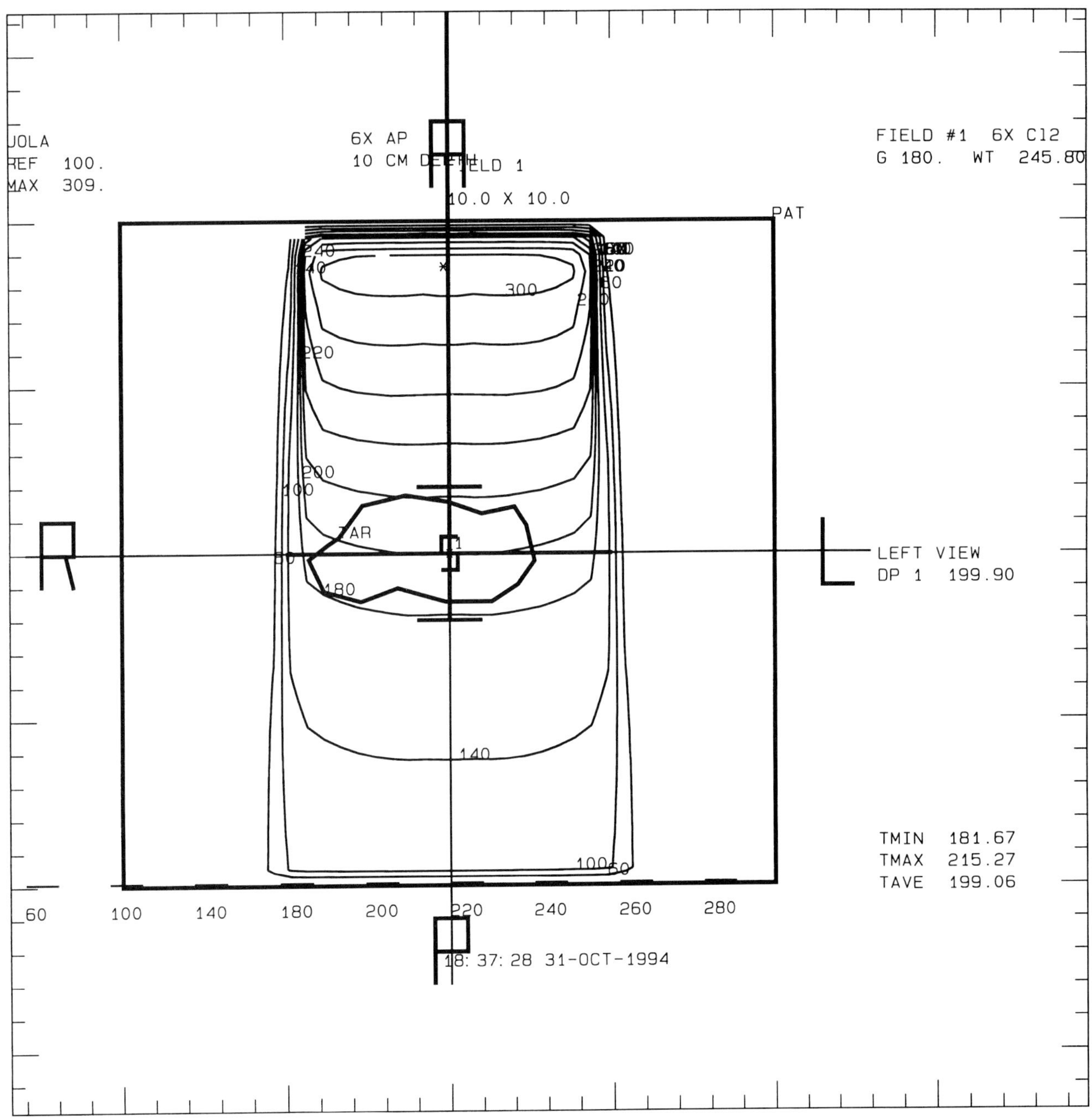

Figure 96–7. Depth dose profile of a 10 × 10-cm 6-MeV photon field prescribed to deliver 200 cGy at 10-cm depth in tissue. The numbers on the curves are in centigrays. The TAR represents a hypothetical target or tumor. Note the "hot spot" of greater than 300 cGy for a given dose of 200 cGy. The maximal dose delivered to this volume is 309 cGy, which occurs when the * is seen.

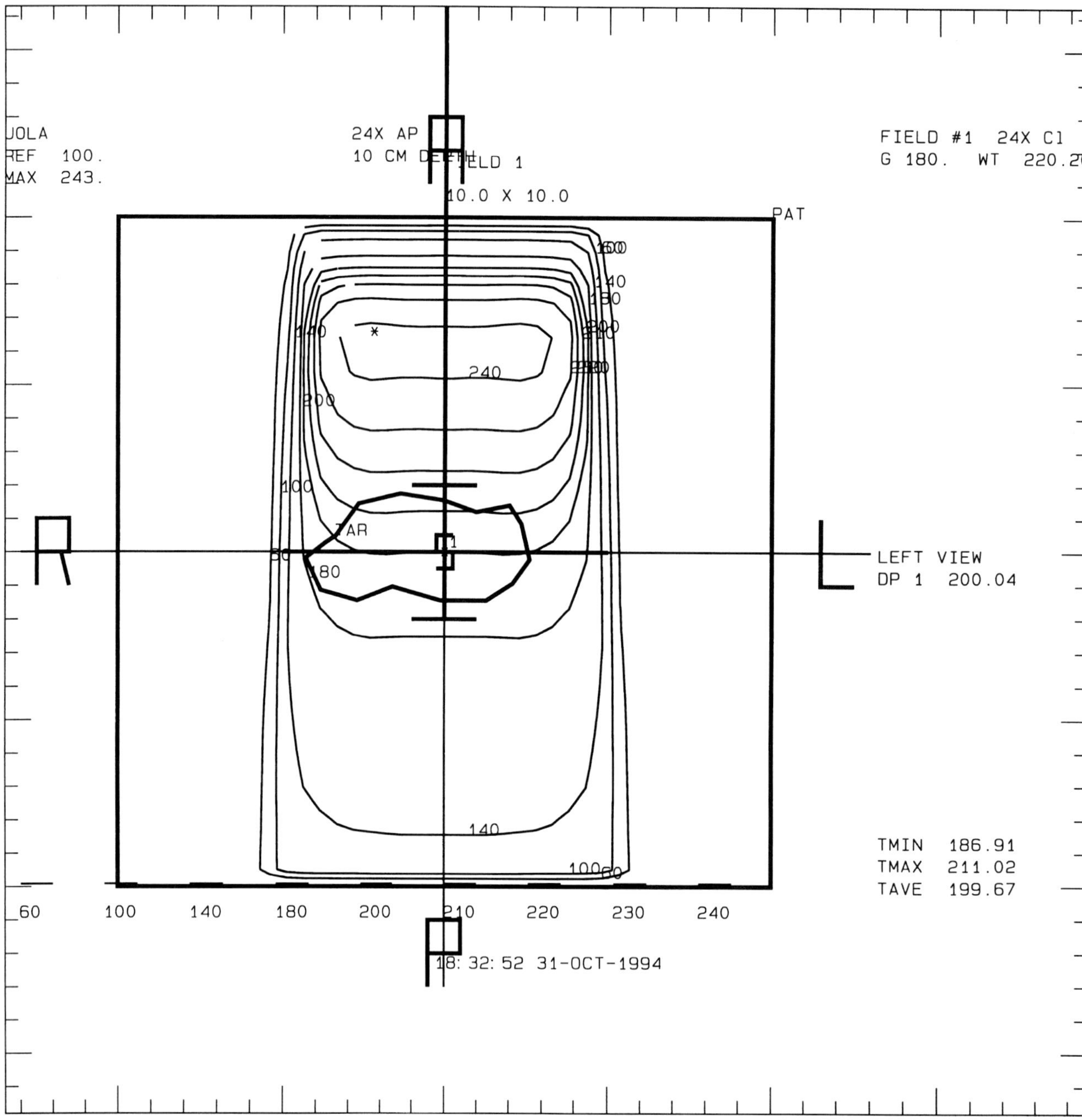

Figure 96–8. Depth dose profile of a 10 × 10-cm 24-MeV photon field prescribed at 10-cm depth in tissue. Note that the "hot spot" here has been reduced to 240 cGy by using the higher energy.

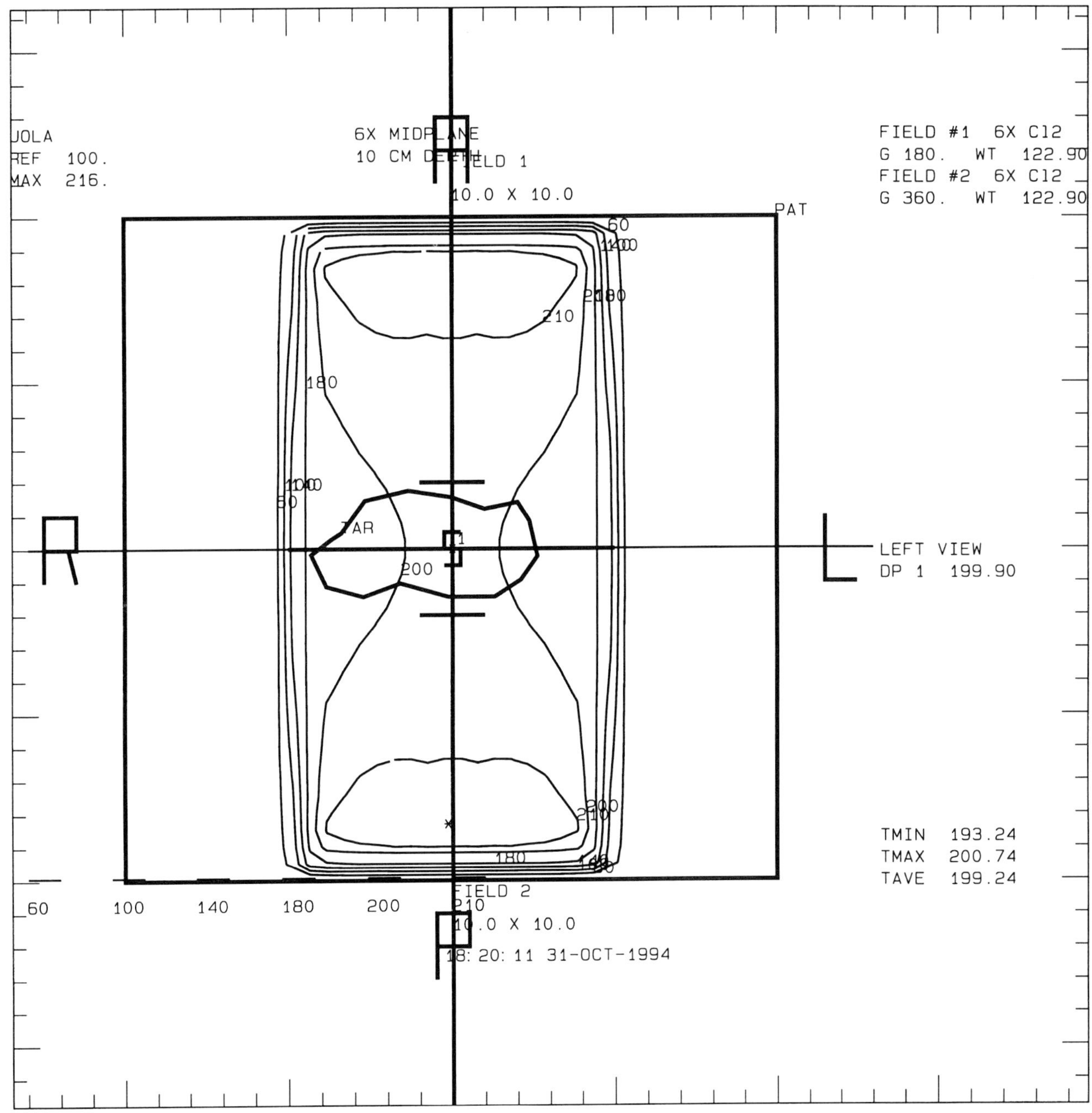

Figure 96–9. Depth dose profile of two opposed (AP/PA) 10 × 10-cm 6-MeV fields, each of which is prescribed to deliver 100 cGy at 10-cm depth in tissue. (This "patient" is 20 cm thick.) This delivers a planned dose to the midplane of 200 cGy. Note the "hot spot" has been reduced to 210 cGy.

TABLE 96-3

Incidence of Side Effects of Radiation Therapy for Eyelid Carcinoma Among 1166 Patients*

Side Effect†	Incidence (%)
Skin atrophy	64
Ectropion	36‡
Entropion	6
Epiphora	27‡
Keratinization	21
Keratitis	5
Cataract	11
Perforated globe	3

*Treated at Princess Margaret Hospital, Toronto, Canada.

†Moderate skin changes and epilation are considered equivalent to a surgical scar and are not listed as complications.

‡Often present before treatment.

From Perez CA, Brady LA (eds): Principles and Practice of Radiation Oncology. Philadelphia, JB Lippincott, 1992.

very busy clinic and plans on using opposed fields but for efficiency's sake treats only one field a day. This is poor form because the whole tumor is not treated each day. In addition, although a very high total dose is not given to a "hot spot," the daily fraction size to the "hot spot" on alternate days is quite high. The conclusion, therefore, is to treat a target volume in as homogeneously a manner as possible.

CLINICAL APPLICATIONS

Radiation therapy is efficacious for the treatment of a variety of benign and malignant conditions. Postoperative irradiation of pterygia using a strontium-90 applicator lowers the local recurrence rate from as high as 67%[28] to less than 20%.[29] Fractionation for this varies considerably.[29] I usually give applications of 1000 cGy once a week for 3 weeks. Giving 2000 cGy in 10 fractions of external-beam radiation therapy improves symptoms in 75% of patients with Graves' ophthalmopathy.[29] One radomized trial demonstrated superior efficacy for radiation therapy over corticosteroids.[30] Simulation, customized blocking, and careful patient immobilization are required to avoid giving a significant dose to either lens, the most radiosensitive organ in the entire body.

Treatment of orbital malignancies falls into two categories: metastatic and nonmetastatic. The most common malignancy to metastasize to the orbit is breast cancer. If the orbital metastasis is the only site of disease or the patient has a long disease-free interval, a dose greater than the standard palliative dose of 3000 cGy in 300-cGy fractions may be indicated in smaller fractions.[31]

Of the nonmetastatic cancers the most common are basal and squamous cell carcinomas of the eyelid. Fitzpatrick and colleagues[32] reviewed their experience in 1166 tumors treated at the Princess Margaret Hospital. This showed a 5% recurrence rate for basal cell carcinomas and 6.7% rate for squamous cell carcinomas. The incidence of side effects is shown in Table 96-3. The technique used is shown in Figure 96-10. Low-energy photons are used along with a lead eye shield to lower the dose to the lens. Electrons can be used as well. Only meticulous attention to detail, including a computed tomographic scan before treatment planning to accurately determine tumor extent[33] makes a good outcome possible. Although controversial, some authors believe radiation therapy gives a better cosmetic result than surgery.[34] In the era of managed care this argument may become moot since radiation therapy is less expensive than surgery.

Lymphomatous diseases of the orbit consist of pseudolymphoma and lymphoma, which are pathologically difficult to differentiate. Pseudolymphoma is generally recommended to receive 2000 to 2500 cGy in standard

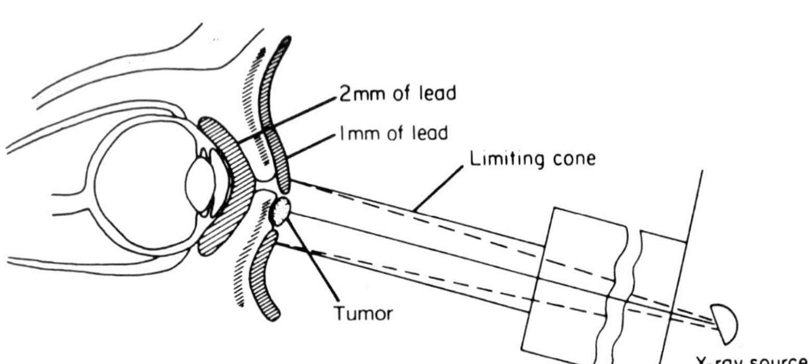

kV	HVL mm	SSD cm	% Transmission
100	0.7 Al	20	< 0.3
250	1.1 Cu	50	3.0

Figure 96-10. The most common way to treat eyelid tumors by radiation therapy. The radiovulnerable anterior segment of the eye gets less than 0.3% of the prescribed dose at 100 kV and only 3% at 250 kV. (From Perez CA, Brady LA [eds]: Principles and Practice of Radiation Oncology. Philadelphia, JB Lippincott, 1992.)

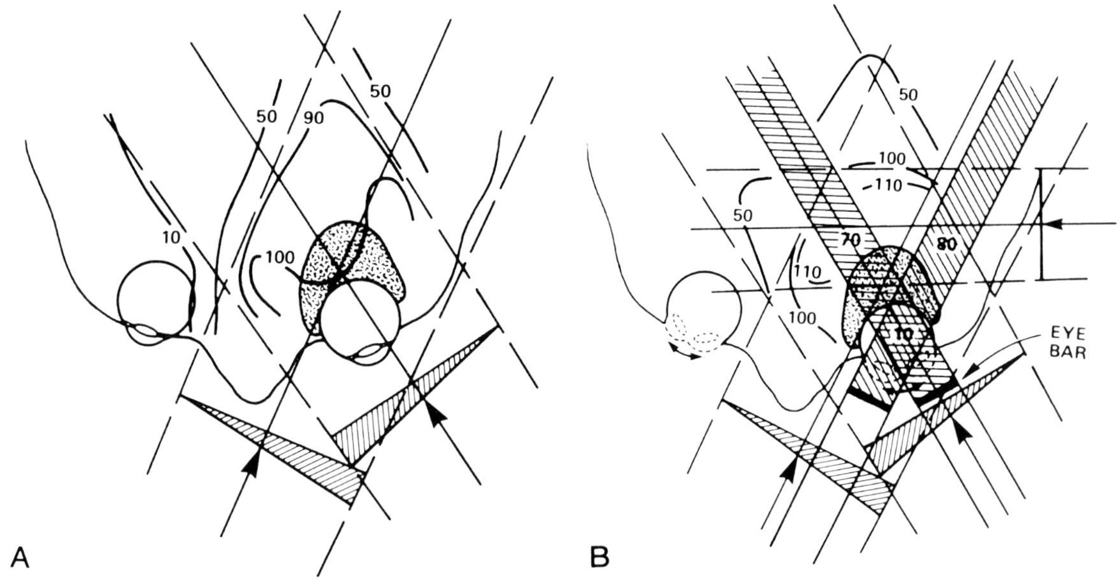

Figure 96–11. *A*, Isodose distribution using the isocentric technique for a unilateral treatment volume (*stippled area*). Numbers indicate percentages of the absorbed dose at the isocenter. Two wedged oblique fields are used to optimize the 90% isodose contour to the treatment volume. *B*, At the level of the lens, an eye bar is inserted in both oblique fields, with the patient looking at the eye bar for each oblique treatment field. (Reprinted from The International Journal of Radiation Oncology, Biology, Physics, vol. 1, Austin-Seymour MM, Donaldson SS, Egbert PR, et al: Radiotherapy of lymphoid diseases of the orbit, pp. 371–379, Copyright 1985, with kind permission. From Elsevier Science Ltd, The Boulevard, Langford Lane, Kidlington OX5 1GB, UK.)

fraction sizes (180–200 cGy). Roughly one third of these cases eventually convert to malignant lymphoma. For localized lymphoma of the orbit, 3500 to 4000 cGy is generally recommended.[35] Techniques for treatment of such lesions are shown in Figures 96–11 and 96–12.

Rhabdomyosarcoma of the orbit is generally seen in children and has an excellent prognosis with combined

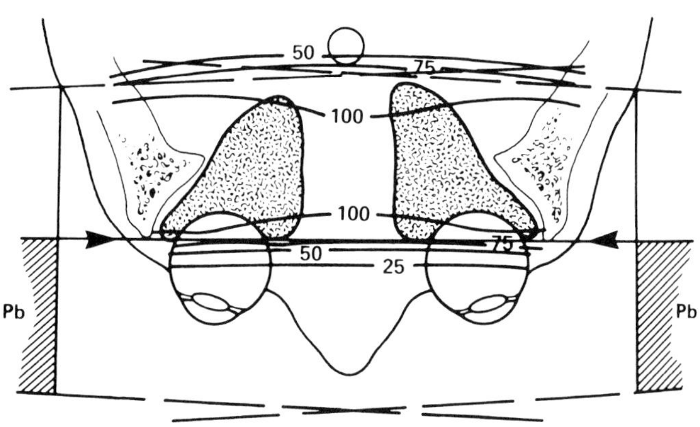

Figure 96–12. Isodose distribution for the split-beam technique on an outline through the orbit demonstrating the central axis of the treatment beam at the anterior border of the effective treatment area, here located at the anterior border of the lateral orbital rim. (Reprinted from The International Journal of Radiation Oncology, Biology, Physics, vol. 1, Austin-Seymour MM, Donaldson SS, Egbert PR, et al: Radiotherapy of lymphoid diseases of the orbit, pp. 371–379, Copyright 1985, with kind permission. From Elsevier Science Ltd, The Boulevard, Langford Lane, Kidlington OX5 1GB, UK.)

radiation therapy and chemotherapy; 4500 to 5000 cGy can control approximately 90% of these tumors.[36]

COMPLICATIONS

Permanent epilation of the eyelashes occurs with 2300 to 2800 cGy in 2 weeks with a 100-kV beam.[37] If the complete lacrimal apparatus is irradiated to 3200 to 4800 cGy in standard fractions, about one fourth of the patients will develop a dry eye so severe that enucleation will be required.[38] A severe dry eye in all patients results from treatment with 5400 cGy. Fifteen percent of patients treated to 6000 cGy developed severe corneal ulcerations during a 2-year followup period.[39] Radiation-induced cataracts generally occur in the posterior pole. The best study in the literature regarding this phenomenon is that of Merriam and Focht (Fig. 96–13).[40] A retinal dose in excess of 5000 cGy carries with it a significant risk of damage.[38] The key is to try to avoid irradiating the macula to such doses. When irradiating tumors of the paranasal sinuses, patients at one time were told to look away from the beam so as to reduce the risk of cataracts. This brought the macula right into the field. Today it is generally not recommended.[41] As noted earlier, fraction size is the strongest predictor of optic nerve damage (Fig. 96–14).

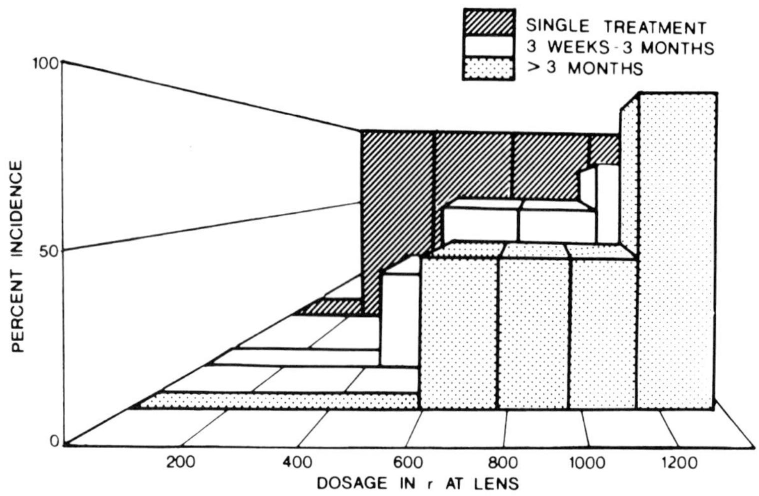

Figure 96–13. This composite histogram demonstrates that the incidence of cataract production is related to both total dosage and fractionation. Delivery of 600 cGy over 3 months (*dotted bars*) produced cataract in approximately 50% of the patients. Delivery of 600 cGy in a single treatment (*hatched bars*) produced cataract in 100% of the patients. (From Merriam GR, Focht E: A clinical study of radiation cataracts and the relationship to dose. Am J Roentgenol Radiat Ther 77:759, 1957.)

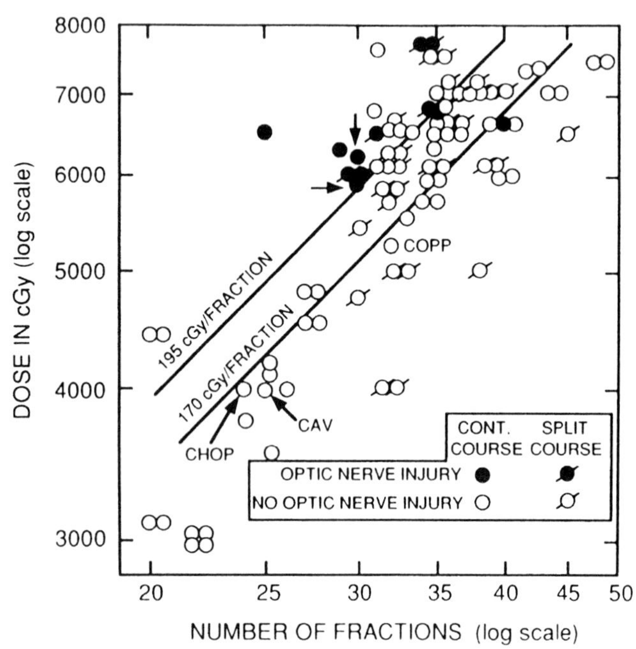

Figure 96–14. Dose versus number of fractions for optic nerve injury secondary to irradiation. Included are data on 92 optic nerves in 55 patients after continuous or split-course irradiation (cobalt-60 or 2 MV) of a variety of head and neck tumors at the University of Florida (October 1964 through March 1979). All patients had 3 to 14 years of followup; patients who died within 3 years without developing optic nerve injury are excluded. Eyes that lost sight due to severe retinal injury are also excluded. The mean followup was 6.35 years, and median 6.5 years, for the 80 optic nerves that showed no clinical evidence of injury after irradiation. Eight of 12 injuries were detected by 3 years. Reference lines for treatments administered at 170 cGy per fraction and 195 cGy per fraction have been added for convenience of interpreting the data; these lines are not isoeffect lines. Two optic nerves (*arrows*) received an additional small dose from a radium implant (approximately 200 cGy to the optic nerves) after external irradiation. Three patients who received concomitant chemotherapy are so designated. (Reprinted from The International Journal at Radiation Oncology, Biology, Physics, vol. 9, Parsons JT, Fitzgerald CR, Hood CI, et al: The effects of irradiation on the eye and optic nerve, pp. 609–622, Copyright 1983, with kind permission from Elsevier Science Ltd, The Boulevard, Langford Lane, Kidlington OX5, 1GB, UK.)

REFERENCES

1. Weichselbaum RR: Personal communication, 1985.
2. Hall EJ: The physics and chemistry of radiation absorption. *In* Hall EJ: Radiobiology for the Radiologist. Philadelphia, JB Lippincott, 1994.
3. Cohen L: Personal communication, 1987.
4. Khan FM: The Physics of Radiation Therapy. Baltimore, Williams & Wilkins, 1994, pp 135–137.
5. Coutard H: Roentgen therapy of epitheliomas of the tonsillar region, hypopharynx, and larynx from 1920 to 1926. AJR 28:313, 1932.
6. Baclesse F: Carcinoma of the larynx. Br J Radiol 3:1, 1949.
7. Regaud C, Ferroux R: Discordance des effects de rayons X, d'une part dans le testicule, par le peau, d'autre part dans le fractionment de la dose. Comp Rend Soc Biol 97:431, 1927.
8. Paterson R: The Treatment of Malignant Disease by Radium and X-rays. Baltimore, Williams & Wilkins, 1949.
9. Harris JR, Levene MB: Visual complications following irradiation for pituitary adenomas and craniopharyngiomas. Radiology 120:167, 1976.
10. Parsons JT, Fitzgerald CR, Hood CI, et al: The effects of irradiation on the eye and optic nerve. Int J Radiat Oncol Biol Phys 9:619, 1983.
11. Stewart R, Fajardo LF: Dose response in human and experimental radiation-induced heart disease. Radiology 99:403, 1971.
12. Eichorn HJ: Different fractionation schemes tested by histological examination of autopsy specimens from lung cancer patients. Br J Radiol 54:132, 1981.
13. Withers HR: The four R's of radiotherapy. Adv Radiat Biol 5:241, 1975.
14. Weichselbaum RR, Beckett MA, Vijayakumar S, et al: Radiobiological characterization of head and neck and sarcoma cells derived from patients prior to radiotherapy. Int J Radiat Oncol Biol Phys 19:313, 1990.
15. Tepper JE, Suit HD: Radiation therapy of soft tissue sarcomas. Cancer 55:2273, 1985.
16. Horseman MR, Overgaard J: The oxygen effect. *In* Steel GG (ed): Basic Clinical Radiobiology. London, Edward Arnold, 1993.

16a. Thomlinson RH, Gray LH: The histological structure of some human lung cancers and possible implications for radiotherapy. Br J Cancer 9:539, 1955.

17. Watson ER, Halnan KE, Dische S, et al: Hyperbaric oxygen and radiotherapy: A medical research council trial in carcinoma of the cervix. Br J Radiol 51:879, 1978.

18. Henk JM, Smith CW: Radiotherapy and hyperbaric oxygen in head and neck cancer. Lancet 2:104, 1977.
19. Withers HR, Taylor JMF, Maciejewski B: The hazard of accelerated tumor clonogen repopulation during radiotherapy. Acta Oncol 27:131, 1988.
20. Parsons JT, Bova FJ, Million RR: A re-evaluation of the University of Florida split-course technique for squamous carcinoma of the head and neck. Int J Radiat Oncol Biol Phys 6:10645, 1980.
21. Mendenhall WM, Parsons JT, Million RR, et al: T1-T2 squamous cell carcinoma of the glottic larynx treated with radiation therapy: Relationship of dose-fractionation factors to local control and complications. Int J Radiat Biol Phys 15:1271, 1988.
22. Sinclair WK, Morton RA: X-ray sensitivity during the cell generation cycle of cultured Chinese hamster cells. Radiat Res 29:4500, 1966.
23. Parsons JT: Hyperfractionation. *In* Million RR, Cassisi NJ (eds): Management of Head and Neck Cancer: A Multidisciplinary Approach. Philadelphia, JB Lippincott, 1994.
24. Horiot JL, Le Fur R, N'Guyen T, et al: Hyperfractionation versus conventional fractionation in oropharyngeal carcinoma: Final analysis of a randomized trial of the EORTC cooperative group of radiotherapy. Radiother Oncol 25:231, 1992.
25. Knee R, Fields RS, Peters LJ: Concomitant boost radiotherapy for advanced squamous cell carcinoma of the head and neck. Radiother Oncol 4:1, 1985.
26. Parsons JT: Time-dose-volume relations in radiation therapy. *In* Million RR, Cassisi NJ (eds.): Management of Head and Neck Cancer: A Multidisciplinary Approach. Philadelphia, JB Lippincott, 1994.
27. Withers HR: Biologic basis of radiation therapy. *In* Perez CA, Brady LW (eds): Principles and Practice of Radiation Oncology. Philadelphia, JB Lippincott, 1992.
28. de Keizer RJ, Swart-van-den-Berg M, Baartse WJ: Results of pterygium excision with Sr-90 irradiation, lamellar keratoplasty and conjunctival flaps (abstract). Doc Ophthalmol 67:33, 1987.
29. Order SE, Donaldson SS: Radiation Therapy of Benign Disease. Berlin, Springer-Verlag, 1990.
30. Prummel MF, Mourits MP, Bland L, et al: Randomized double-blind trial of prednisone versus radiotherapy in Graves' ophthalmopathy. Lancet 342:949, 1993.
31. Kagan AR: Radiation therapy in palliative cancer management. *In* Perez CA, Brady LW (eds): Principles and Practice of Radiation Oncology. Philadelphia, JB Lippincott, 1992.
32. Fitzpatrick PJ, Thompson GA, Easterbrook WM, et al: Basal and squamous cell carcinomas of the eyelids and their treatment by radiotherapy. Int J Radiat Oncol Phys 10:449, 1984.
33. Sloan MJ, Brady LW, Binnick SA, Fitzpatrick PJ: Skin. *In* Perez CA, Brady LW (eds): Principles and Practice of Radiation Oncology. Philadelphia, JB Lippincott, 1992.
34. Petrovich Z, Parker R, Luxton G, et al: Carcinoma of the lip and selected sites of the head and neck: A clinical study of 896 patients. Radiother Oncol 8:11, 1987.
35. Markoe AM, Brady LW, Karlsson UL, et al: *In* Perez CA, Brady LW (eds): Principles and Practice of Radiation Oncology. Philadelphia, JB Lippincott, 1992.
36. Wharam M, Beltangady M, Hays D, et al: Localized orbital rhabdomyosarcoma: An interim report of the Intergroup Rhabdomyosarcoma Committee. Ophthalmology 94:251, 1987.
37. Moss WT: The orbit. *In* Radiation Oncology: Rationale, Technique, Results. St. Louis, CV Mosby, 1989.
38. Parsons JT, Fitzgerald CR, Hood CI, et al: The effects of irradiation on the eye and the optic nerve. Int J Radiat Oncol Biol Phys 9:611, 1983.
39. Chan RC, Shukovsky LJ: Effects of irradiation on the eye. Radiology 120:673, 1976.
40. Merriam GR, Focht EF: A clinical study of radiation cataracts and the relationship to dose. Am J Roentgenol Radiat Ther 77:609, 1983.
41. Parsons JT: The effect of radiation on normal tissues of the head and neck. *In* Million RR, Cassisi NJ (eds): Management of Head and Neck Cancer: A Multidisciplinary Approach. Philadelphia, JB Lippincott, 1994.

CHAPTER 97

Enucleation and Evisceration

William R. Nunery and William P. Chen

Enucleation is the removal of the eye from the orbit while preserving all other orbital tissue. Evisceration is the removal of the contents of the eye (i.e., uvea, retina, lens, vitreous, and aqueous) while leaving the sclera and extraocular muscles intact. In this chapter we discuss indications, techniques, and considerations in enucleation and evisceration surgery.

ENUCLEATION

Indications

Indications for enucleation include (1) a painful eye with no useful vision; (2) an intraocular tumor, suspected to be malignant; (3) ocular trauma, to avoid sympathetic ophthalmia in the second eye; (4) phthisis with degeneration, to prevent increased risk of malignancy or to avoid use of a poorly fitting cover shell; (5) congenital anophthalmia or severe microphthalmia, with poor development of the bony orbit; (6) endophthalmitis unresponsive to antibiotics; and (7) improvement of cosmesis in a blind eye.

Evisceration is also considered for these last two indications. It is contraindicated in cases of suspected intraocular malignancy and may not relieve the pain associated with a blind eye since ciliary nerves remain intact after evisceration. Evisceration also may not prevent sympathetic ophthalmia following trauma and is technically difficult or impossible in cases of phthisis bulbae with degenerating globes. In addition, evisceration has a higher risk of implant extrusion and exposure when compared with enucleation.[1]

Sympathetic ophthalmia occurs in 1 in 20,000 to 25,000 cases of corneal or scleral rupture with uveal prolapse.[2] Sympathetic ophthalmia is a delayed hypersensitivity immune response that occurs from 2 weeks to 50 years after corneoscleral perforation. Therefore, if a traumatized eye is beyond the hope of recovery of functional vision, enucleation should be performed within 10 to 14 days after trauma to reduce the risk of sympathetic ophthalmia.

Enucleation is the procedure of choice in many cases of intraocular tumor, especially tumors considered to be malignant. Evisceration should not be performed in any case of suspected intraocular malignancy. In cases of a blind eye with opaque media, ultrasonography or computed tomography must be done preoperatively before considering evisceration. In cases of phthisis with opaque media, the eye should be followed with ultrasonography on a yearly basis to rule out occult malignancy.

Retinoblastoma in childhood may also be treated with enucleation or radiation therapy. Enucleation is often chosen in the more involved eye of bilateral cases, while irradiation is often recommended for the less involved eye. Since retinoblastoma may be present in the suprachoroidal space of the optic nerve head, the objectives during enucleation are to perform surgery with minimal manipulation and to obtain a long section of optic nerve for histologic evaluation. A lateral canthotomy may be performed to facilitate the enucleation and placement of the implant. Clamps across the optic nerve are avoided to lessen the amount of artifact compression of the optic nerve specimen. After the globe is removed, the section of the optic nerve is measured and submitted separately. The distal edge of the optic nerve should be examined

Portions of this chapter are adapted from an earlier work by the authors, first published in Chen WP: Enucleation, evisceration, and exenteration. *In* McCord CD, Tanenbaum M, Nunery WR (eds): Oculoplastic Surgery, 3rd ed. New York, Raven Press, 1995, pp 581–608.

with interoperative frozen sections to determine if tumor is present and if further surgical resection is required.

Shields and Shields[3] have advocated the use of an 8-mm trephine to create a scleral window adjacent to the main lesion on the enucleated specimen and curette out fresh tissue for DNA analysis while the remainder of the globe is preserved in formalin for axial sectioning and permanent pathologic examination.

Evisceration is a shorter and less complex procedure compared with enucleation and is easier to perform using local anesthesia. Some surgeons believe evisceration may result in better prosthetic motility when compared with enucleation, but this may depend on the enucleation technique and the placement of extraocular muscles during enucleation. Evisceration is preferred for patients who are not good surgical risks for general anesthesia or who have bleeding dyscrasias. Evisceration, traditionally, has been considered preferable in cases of endophthalmitis to avoid spreading of infection along the optic nerve sheath. Scant evidence exists, however, that risk of meningitis increases after enucleation in those cases. We routinely employ enucleation in cases of endophthalmitis.

The use of a cosmetic cover shell may be an alternative to enucleation or evisceration to improve the cosmesis of a blind and degenerating eye. Careful followup, however, must be done to avoid development of intraocular malignancy in these cases. Also, continuing degeneration of the phthisical eye may prevent satisfactory fitting of the cover shell and lead to socket inflammation and discharge. In some patients with painful degenerating eyes cover shells are not well tolerated.

After enucleation or evisceration, a volume implant is usually placed in the orbit (in the case of enucleation) or in the scleral shell (after evisceration). Spherical implants may be made of silicone, acrylic, or hydroxyapatite. Dermal fat grafts are also sometimes used as volume replacement. Spherical implants such as the Iowa, Allen, or Universal implants have been used by some surgeons to improve prosthetic motility.

Inert spherical implants of silicone or acrylic have been used for nearly 100 years. Efficacy is well proven, but spherical implants have been criticized for implant migration, high rate of extrusion, and poor prosthetic motility. We believe these failings of the sphere implant are related more to older Frost-Lang enucleation techniques than to the implants themselves. Specifically, imbrication of extraocular muscles over the anterior surface of the spherical implant promotes superotemporal migration of the implant and decreases prosthetic motility. Purse-stringing of Tenon's fascia and conjunctiva promotes easy extrusion of the implant. We suture extraocular muscles to the implant in the normal anatomic locations and also suture extraocular muscles to the fornices to increase implant stability and prosthetic motility. Tenon's fascia and conjunctiva are closed separately, in multiple layers. With this technique, extrusion rates of spherical implants are less than 1% and motility is good.[1]

Asymmetric implants have anterior surface projections that push the prosthesis through overlying conjunctiva. Muscles are usually sutured to the asymmetric implants to initiate movement. Motility with these implants is good, but pressure between the implant and prosthesis may lead to erosion, pain, and eventual extrusion. Later designs of Universal implants have smaller and more spherical projections to reduce the incidence of painful extrusion.

Dermal fat grafts avoid extrusion and have fair motility, but have an increased incidence of secondary absorption and eyelid retraction.[4] Secondary spherical implants behind dermal fat grafts are often necessary to avoid volume deficit in the anophthalmic socket. Dermal fat grafts do increase the conjunctival surface area by reepithelialization of dermal surface by the conjunctival mucosa. This may be helpful in cases of inadequate fornices or multiple implant extrusions.

Hydroxyapatite is a naturally occurring substance found in coral. A lattice-like structure similar to bone matrix is present in hydroxyapatite, and this may lead to vascularization and incorporation of the hydroxyapatite as living tissue after implantation. After successful vascularization of the hydroxyapatite implant, a secondary hole may be surgically drilled to allow placement of a peg that couples the implant to the prosthesis. This may result in superior prosthetic motility.

Hydroxyapatite, however, is associated with an increased risk of inflammation,[5] tissue breakdown, and infection, as well as higher cost compared with silicone sphere implants. We recommend hydroxyapatite for young adult patients who prefer superior motility and who can tolerate a higher risk of exposure as well as a higher cost. We avoid hydroxyapatite in children undergoing socket expansion, in patients with sockets with poor vascularization, in patients who have diabetes, or in patients who desire the lowest risk and cost and are willing to sacrifice some prosthetic motility.

Regardless of the implant chosen, implants are often wrapped to allow fixation of extraocular muscles and to decrease the risk of extrusion or migration. Wrapping the implant may be done with autogenous fascia, autogenous sclera, or preserved sclera or fascia. Preserved sclera or preserved fascia is an easy substance for wrapping the implant, but autogenous tissue has the advantage of being free of exogenous viral contamination. A sheet of fascia approximately 2 inches square is adequate to cover a 20-mm sphere. The fascia lata is sutured like a wrap around the sphere, using nonabsorbable suture. The recti muscles are then sutured to the fascia lata in the normal anatomic locations. Eye bank sclera or preserved fascia may be used for wrapping alloplastic implants. There is a substantial cost involved in obtaining these preserved tissues, and current screening for human immunodeficiency virus (HIV) is not fail-safe. Freeze-dried bank tissues that have been hyper-radiated with gamma rays may have less risk for HIV transmission than glycerin-preserved sclera.

Autogenous sclera from the enucleated eye may be used after enucleation in some selected cases. The cornea is removed from the enucleated globe, and the contents of the globe are completely eviscerated and inverted for thorough cleansing of uveal tissue. The remaining scleral shell may then be used to wrap the implant. The implant is placed in the anophthalmic socket with the excised corneal button window facing posteriorly. Autogenous fascia lata or temporalis fascia may also be used, but this necessitates a second surgical site.

Preoperative Counseling

Perhaps one of the most important settings in which the patient needs the physician's reassurance, explanations, and psychological support is before and after enucleation. The patient should be aware that enucleation involves complete removal of the diseased or deformed eye, that there will not be a globe inside the orbit after surgery, and that an ocular prosthesis will be fitted approximately 2 months after the surgery. The indications, whether pain, poor visual prognosis, the risk of sympathetic ophthalmia, or the presence of an intraocular tumor, need to be clearly explained. The patient and his or her family must understand the final, permanent nature of the enucleation procedure and the permanent loss of that eye.

The patient should be informed of the choices between enucleation versus evisceration, the availability of various synthetic orbital implants or hydroxyapatite implants, the advantages and disadvantages or autogenous versus preserved tissue, and the risk of communicable diseases such as syphilis, hepatitis, and HIV infection with preserved (donor) tissue use. The patient should be aware that to maximize the prosthetic motility after a hydroxyapatite implant in primary enucleation or evisceration there is a need for a second-stage procedure to be performed (i.e., secondary drill hole formation for the placement of a peg).

Psychological Impact of Enucleation

After enucleation, patients undergo a predictable grief reaction. All patients are affected to varying degrees and in a variety of ways. The common elements of this loss or grief reaction include (1) denial, (2) depression or anger, and (3) acceptance and rehabilitation. The goal of the ophthalmologist is to facilitate the passage of these three phases and assist in the acceptance and rehabilitation phase.

It is common for patients losing one eye to initially experience a denial reaction. During this phase, patients often seem to handle the situation well. They may remain upbeat and cheerful, and often the physician may be impressed with the patient's strength and coping mechanisms. This phase, however, is not permanent and eventually will give way to the second phase of depression and anger in virtually every patient.

When patients begin to experience the effect of depression over the loss of one eye, they may experience diminished self-esteem, diminished self-image, and a loss of eye contact communication skills. This may lead to a feeling of hopelessness and helplessness. In severe cases, patients may become suicidal. Although the suicidal extreme is uncommon, the surgeon should be alert to signs of sleep and appetite disorders or suicidal ideation. Under these circumstances, suitable psychiatric referral may be life saving. Lesser degrees of depression may be adequately addressed by the surgeon's empathy and counseling that the reaction is expected and will be temporary. Encouragement to move on to the acceptance and rehabilitation phase is often an important part in diminishing the severity and length of the depression stage.

Some patients may experience anger rather than depression. The anger may be directed toward the person responsible for the loss of the eye or may be transferred inappropriately to the physician caring for the patient. The physician must listen empathetically without internalizing or reacting to the patient's expression of anger and realize that this is simply an alternative expression of the depression cycle that is common to virtually every patient. Returning the patient's anger is counterproductive and unprofessional.

The final phase of the loss-grief reaction is the acceptance phase in which the patient realizes that he or she is able to lead a full life and is not restricted in any normal activities. With very few exceptions, the monocular patient may participate in a full range of home, professional, athletic, and industrial activities. The few exceptions refer to the loss of depth perception. This eliminates the patient considering a career as an airline pilot or operating heavy machinery in which depth perception is essential for industrial safety. Although many monocular patients do drive cars, they should begin this process slowly and carefully, since the loss of binocular depth perception may present a hazard to themselves or others until they are adequately adjusted to the monocular condition.

We believe that the patient should be encouraged to resume normal work duties early after surgery and avoid use of an eye patch. Encouraging the patient to feel positive about the appearance of a new prosthesis is an important motivating factor in the rehabilitation of the anophthalmic patient.

Eye Protection

After enucleation, we recommend safety glasses for both normal daily wear and in industrial wear. For normal or street activities, 2-mm polycarbonate lenses with sturdy frames are probably adequate. For athletic, industrial, and workshop activities, we recommend 3-mm polycarbonate lenses with wraparound frames for both frontal and side protection. We do not recommend wearing a contact lens, especially the extended-wear type, in the remaining eye. We prefer instead to avoid the small but present risk of corneal infection, and we also prefer the use of spectacle lenses for mechanical protection.

Surgical Anatomy

It is important to remember the following points:

1. The medial rectus inserts 5.3 mm from the limbus. The inferior rectus inserts 6.8 mm from the limbus. The lateral rectus inserts 6.9 mm from the limbus. The superior rectus inserts 7.9 mm from the limbus.
2. The average horizontal diameter of the cornea is 11.75 mm. The average vertical diameter of the cornea is 10.6 mm.
3. The medial rectus insertion is separated from the lateral rectus insertion by an arc distance of approximately 24 mm. Similarly, the vertical recti muscles are 25 mm apart. The extraocular muscles retain their optimal physiologic contractile function when they are placed at an ideal length, close to its normal physiologic length-tension relationship.
4. The intraorbital segment of the optic nerve is 25 mm long.
5. The inferior oblique muscle inserts to a point of the sclera overlying the macula and is 8 mm inferior to the inferior border of the lateral rectus insertion on the globe.
6. The inferior oblique and the inferior rectus are enclosed by fascial connective layers that are continuous with the inferior capsulopalpebral fascia and form Lockwood's ligament.
7. The capsulopalpebral fascia (rudimentary equivalent to the levator aponeurosis and levator muscle) shares its origin with the inferior rectus through the inferior palpebral head and splits into fascial insertions into the apex of the inferior fornix, the lower margin of the inferior tarsus, and subdermally over the lower lid skin. Medially, the capsulopalpebral fascia connects the ligamentous attachments of the medial canthal ligaments (anterior and posterior lacrimal crests) and laterally the lateral canthal ligaments (lateral canthal tubercle).
8. Traction on any of the extraocular muscles, levator muscle, or optic nerve can result in the oculocardiac reflex, a sudden slowing of the heart rate. Clamping of the optic nerve alone, without traction, has also been reported to cause bradycardia.[6]
9. The volume of an average size globe is 7.0 ml. The volume of a 16-mm spherical implant is 2.15 ml. The volume of an 18-mm sphere is 3.05 ml. The volume of a 20-mm sphere is 4.19 ml. The volume of a 22-mm sphere is 5.58 ml. A 20-mm sphere, wrapped with sclera or fascia, when added to the volume of an average-sized prosthesis, approximately replaces the volume of an average-sized eye.

Presurgical Setup

Removal of the wrong eye is one of the greatest disasters that can occur to the ophthalmic surgeon and patient. Every ophthalmologist and surgeon must be aware of this possibility, no matter how remote.

Preoperatively, the ophthalmic surgeon may mark the forehead or trim the lashes on the appropriate side. These methods, however, are not fail safe. In the operating room, the surgeon must compulsively review the chart, including the operative permit and examination notes. The surgeon may prefer to personally apply the prep and drape to the patient. Traquair[7] has suggested the use of local anesthesia as a means of preventing the removal of the wrong eye. It must never happen that a surgeon hurries into the operating room where the patient is already under general anesthesia and begin an operation without suitable review of the situation.

Once a sterile operative field is set up, the surgeon must again verify that the correct eye is about to undergo enucleation. In situations of enucleation after severe trauma, the correct eye is often externally deformed. In cases in which the external appearance of both eyes is normal, the surgeon must compulsively reexamine the fundus. Intraoperative direct ophthalmoscopy is necessary to confirm that the surgical field has been set up correctly.

Surgical Steps

Although enucleation may be performed adequately with local and retrobulbar anesthesia, we favor the use of general anesthesia because it lessens the psychological impact of the procedure.

In addition to general anesthesia, a retrobulbar injection is given of lidocaine (Xylocaine) 2%, bupivacaine (Marcaine) 0.5%, with epinephrine 1 : 100,000 and hyaluronidase (Wydase). The epinephrine improves hemostasis, and the local anesthetic blocks the potential reflex cardiac arrythmias associated with extraocular muscle and optic nerve manipulations. The addition of bupivacaine to the mixture prolongs the duration of postoperative pain relief.

For situations in which regional anesthesia is preferred instead of general anesthesia (e.g., a medically unstable patient), the surgeon may elect to give a retrobulbar injection of local anesthetic, supplemented by a frontal nerve block for the upper lid and a mid-inferior fornix block for the lower eyelid (branches of the infraorbital nerve).

Enucleation with Myoconjunctival Attachments

A self-retaining eyelid speculum is applied. The conjunctiva is dissected from the limbus in a 360-degree periotomy fashion using a pair of sharp Wescott scissors. The underlying Tenon layer is undermined in all quadrants to the equator. Each of the four recti commencing with the medial rectus is hooked, identified, secured on a double-armed 6-0 Dexon suture, and detached from the globe. During this maneuver, care should be taken not to sever the intermuscular septum and the sheath along each rectus muscle as one normally would perform in strabismus repair. It is, however, necessary to dissect in a plane between the sclera and overlying orbital tissues in the quadrants between the four recti muscles to facilitate the isolation of the oblique muscles and the subsequent enucleation. The superior oblique tendon is hooked, is detached from the globe, and may be attached to the superior rectus suture. The inferior oblique muscle is hooked and isolated on a 6-0 Dexon suture and saved for attachment to the inferior border of the lateral rectus close to its insertional end (Fig. 97–1*A*).

At this point, the four recti and two oblique muscles have been isolated with double-armed 6-0 Dexon, while the globe remains attached to the orbital apex by the optic nerve. To facilitate access to the optic nerve, 4-0 silk sutures are applied over the muscle stumps of the medial and lateral recti for use as traction sutures (see Fig. 97–1*B*). The eyelid speculum should be removed at this point in the procedure to facilitate forward traction on the globe. With gentle traction on the two sutures, the globe is pulled forward, and then the medial traction suture is pulled slightly more to rotate the globe laterally. The optic nerve is made more accessible from the medial direction; the maneuver prolapses the globe in a forward position and separates itself from the posterior half of the extraocular muscle cone, thereby avoiding inadvertent transection of any of the five muscles that have been tagged.

From a medial direction, a gently curved hemostat is used to clamp the optic nerve, usually several millimeters behind the globe. Since the optic nerve is still encased with orbital tissue behind the posterior Tenon layer, the hemostat is ideally introduced closed and the tips used to strum the optic nerve. When the optic nerve is identified, the two ends of the clamp are opened and applied over the optic nerve. How posterior the clamp is placed will influence the size of the opening in the posterior Tenon layer after transection of the optic nerve. With the hemostat in place, a pair of slender, curved Metzenbaum scissors is then used to transect the optic nerve between the globe and the hemostat, again, approaching from a medial direction. Alternately, one may elect to use a tonsil snare with a no.18 gauge wire loop, looping it around and behind the globe but in front of the clamp.

Before submission for pathologic study, the surgeon should carefully examine the enucleated globe. Should there be any evidence of extrascleral extension of tumor, or involvement of the optic nerve with tumor, one should consider further excision of the adjacent orbital tissues or additional optic nerve. Havre[8] described the technique of obtaining a longer section of the optic nerve with the enucleation specimen. Whether it is a snare or a scissors, the surgical instrument may be used to walk along the optic nerve posteriorly to obtain up to 10 mm or more of optic nerve. In patients with retinoblastoma, an intraoperative frozen section analysis of the distal optic nerve can be used to verify clear margins of resection.[9]

The clamped optic nerve and its central retinal vessels are lightly cauterized with a unipolar cautery, effectively eliminating the major source of hemorrhage in enucleation. The clamp is removed, and an open gap in the posterior Tenon layer is seen (see Fig. 97–1*C*).

For an average-sized adult orbit, we favor the use of a 20-mm spherical orbital implant. The selected implant size can, of course, vary, and the implant may also be wrapped in autogenous fascia or donor sclera. We prefer wrapping a 20-mm sphere with autogenous fascia lata to avoid possible viral contamination associated with preserved donor tissue.

With the spherical implant in place, the four recti muscles, with the inferior oblique attached to the lateral rectus and the superior oblique attached to the superior rectus, are gently pulled forward by the double-armed 6-0 Dexon sutures and secured to the implant in their appropriate anatomic locations (see Fig. 97–1*D*). The needles on the sutures are left intact. The anterior Tenon layer and subjacent orbital tissues at the level of the anterior one third of the implant are closed from opposite oblique quadrants (superotemporal to inferonasal, superonasal to inferotemporal) using interrupted, nonabsorbable sutures (see Fig. 97–1*E*).

As the tissues are brought together, adjacent quadrants are similarly closed with interrupted sutures. Each of the four rectus muscle sutures is then passed through overlying conjunctiva. The superior and inferior recti are each placed approximately 12 mm from the horizontal edges of the conjunctival wound in their respective fornix. The medial and lateral recti are attached myoconjunctivally to the medial and lateral fornices about an inch (25 mm) apart (see Fig. 97–1*F*). Thus, the four recti are hooked to the subconjunctival plane of each fornix, approximating the normal physiologic position. By now, the conjunctiva should be without wound tension and may be easily closed with a continuous 6-0 absorbable suture.

Coston[10] was the first to describe suturing extraocular muscle to the fornix. Chen[11] described the interrelationship of forniceal movement and prosthetic motility (see Fig. 97–1*G*), and together with McCord outlined the technique of enucleation with myoconjunctival attachment. Nunery and Hetzler[12] presented their enucleation technique using the above principle with the addition of ear cartilage graft.

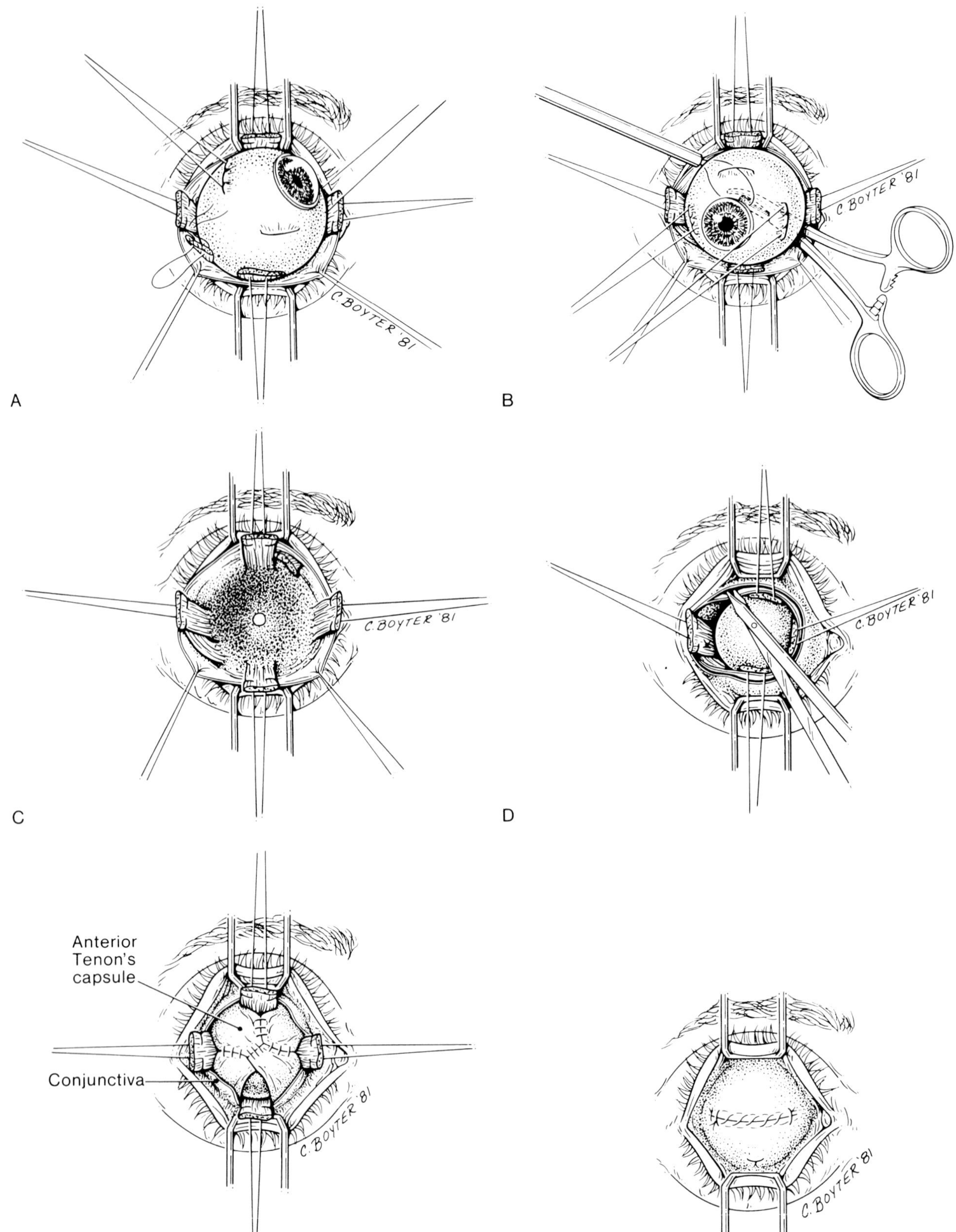

Figure 97 – 1. Steps in enucleation with myoconjunctival attachment. *A*, Each of the four recti is isolated with 6-0 Dexon suture. The superior oblique tendon is sutured to the superior rectus muscle. The inferior oblique is sutured to the inferior border of the lateral rectus; 4-0 silk traction sutures are in place over the medial and lateral rectus stump. *B*, The globe is rotated laterally while a curved clamp is introduced from the medial direction. Either a curved scissors or an enucleation snare may be used to transect the optic nerve. *C*, The central retinal vessels are cauterized before the clamp is released. The orbit is examined for hemostasis. *D*, A spherical implant is placed in the orbit without closure of the posterior Tenon layer. *E*, With the recti muscles tunneling forward, the anterior Tenon layers are closed from opposite oblique quadrants with interrupted sutures. (Some surgeons prefer suturing the recti muscles to the sphere implant before the anterior Tenon closure.) *F*, Myoconjunctival attachment. Each of the four recti is attached subconjunctivally to its respective fornix, spacing them about an inch apart vertically and horizontally. The conjunctiva is then closed horizontally with a 6-0 absorbable suture.

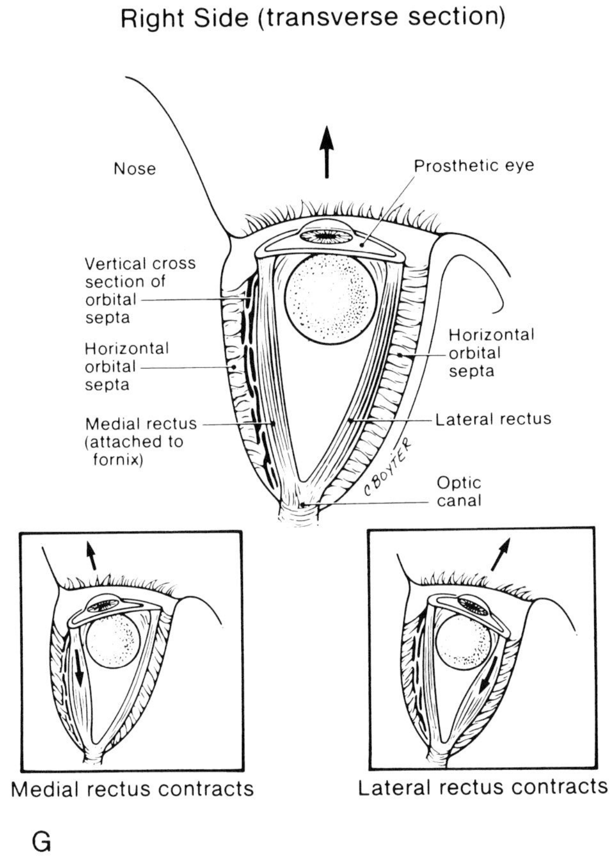

Figure 97-1 *Continued.* G, A cross-sectional view of the right orbit containing a spherical implant with myoconjunctival attachment. Movement of the fornices as a result of contraction of the recti is transmitted to the prosthetic eye. (From Chen WP: Enucleation, evisceration, and exenteration. *In* McCord CD, Tanenbaum M, Nunery WR [eds]: Oculoplastic Surgery, 3rd ed. New York, Raven Press, 1995, pp 586-588.)

Figure 97-2 shows socket motility after enucleation with myoconjunctival attachment. Optical antibiotic ointment (bacitracin or bacitracin-polymixin) is applied to the fornices. A soft silicone conformer with holes is fashioned to the proper size and placed to maintain the fornices. The lid margins should appose each other. In some patients, an intermarginal tarsorrhaphy suture is maintained for 5 to 7 days postoperatively. A light pressure bandage consisting of a piece of Telfa dressing and two eyepatches are applied. There is seldom any need to apply a heavy bandage since uncontrolled orbital hemorrhage with this technique is rare.

Postoperative Care

The patient is seen on the fifth day, and the dressing is removed. The lids should retain the conformer well. The patient is gently introduced to the new appearance of his or her socket, which has a clear or acrylic conformer in the palpebral fissure. Instructions are given on daily cleaning and on the instillation of optical antibiotic ointment to the socket. The patient is encouraged to allow the socket to remain uncovered and while at home. A shield may be worn for social occasions. Although there is variation in the time interval before prosthetic fitting, it is generally necessary to wait at least 6 to 8 weeks for the wound to heal.

Enucleation with Hydroxyapatite Implant

The porous coralline structures of hydroxyapatite contain 500-μm diameter pores that are similar to the haversian systems of cancellous bone. The placement of a sclera-wrapped, windowed hydroxyapatite implant instead of an inert solid sphere allows fibrovascular ingrowth into the implant. This buried, vascularized hydroxyapatite implant can then be secondarily drilled and fitted with a peg. The drill hole becomes lined with host fibrovascular tissue, and the inserted peg can be directly coupled to the ocular prosthesis. This enhances prosthesis motility.

At the time of surgery, the enucleated socket is presized with sterile trial spheres. A sterile 18- or 20-mm hydroxyapatite implant is presoaked in dilute gentamicin solution. It is wrapped with a shell of donor sclera or autogenous fascia lata and oriented with the hexagonal rosettes of the coralline exoskeleton aligned axially to the anteroposterior direction of the orbit, with the area of the optic nerve of the sclera oriented anteriorly in the orbit. The sclera or fascia effectively adds 1 to 1.5 mm to the overall diameter of the implant. Four rectangular windows are made through the sclera, measuring 2 to 3 $\times$ 4 to 6 mm each, preferably 6 to 7 mm from the center of the anteriorly oriented optic nerve head. The posteriorly oriented corneal window serves as the fifth window for vascular ingrowth. At each of the five windows, a 1-mm hole is drilled to the core center to further promote early fibrovascular ingrowth. These drill holes can be made with a hand-held 20-gauge needle. The sclera-wrapped implant is inserted into the orbit. Each of the four recti is sutured to the anterior scleral lip of the corresponding rectangular window. The anterior Tenon layer is closed with interrupted 4-0 Vicryl, while the conjunctiva may be closed with 5-0 plain in a continuous fashion.

Ferrone[13] and Dutton[14] using technetium-99m DP bone scans have shown that vascularization can occur as early as 10 weeks. Shields and colleagues[15-17] reported magnetic resonance imaging evidence of vascular ingrowth as early as 4 weeks. A minimal period of 6 months is recommended for complete fibrovascular ingrowth. During this period, a preliminary fitting of ocular prosthesis is performed.

After an adequate time period, a second-stage procedure can be performed in which a drill hole 10 mm long $\times$ 3 mm in diameter is made through the conjunctiva and the scleral shell and into the anterior portion of the vascularized hydroxyapatite implant. A threaded receptacle is

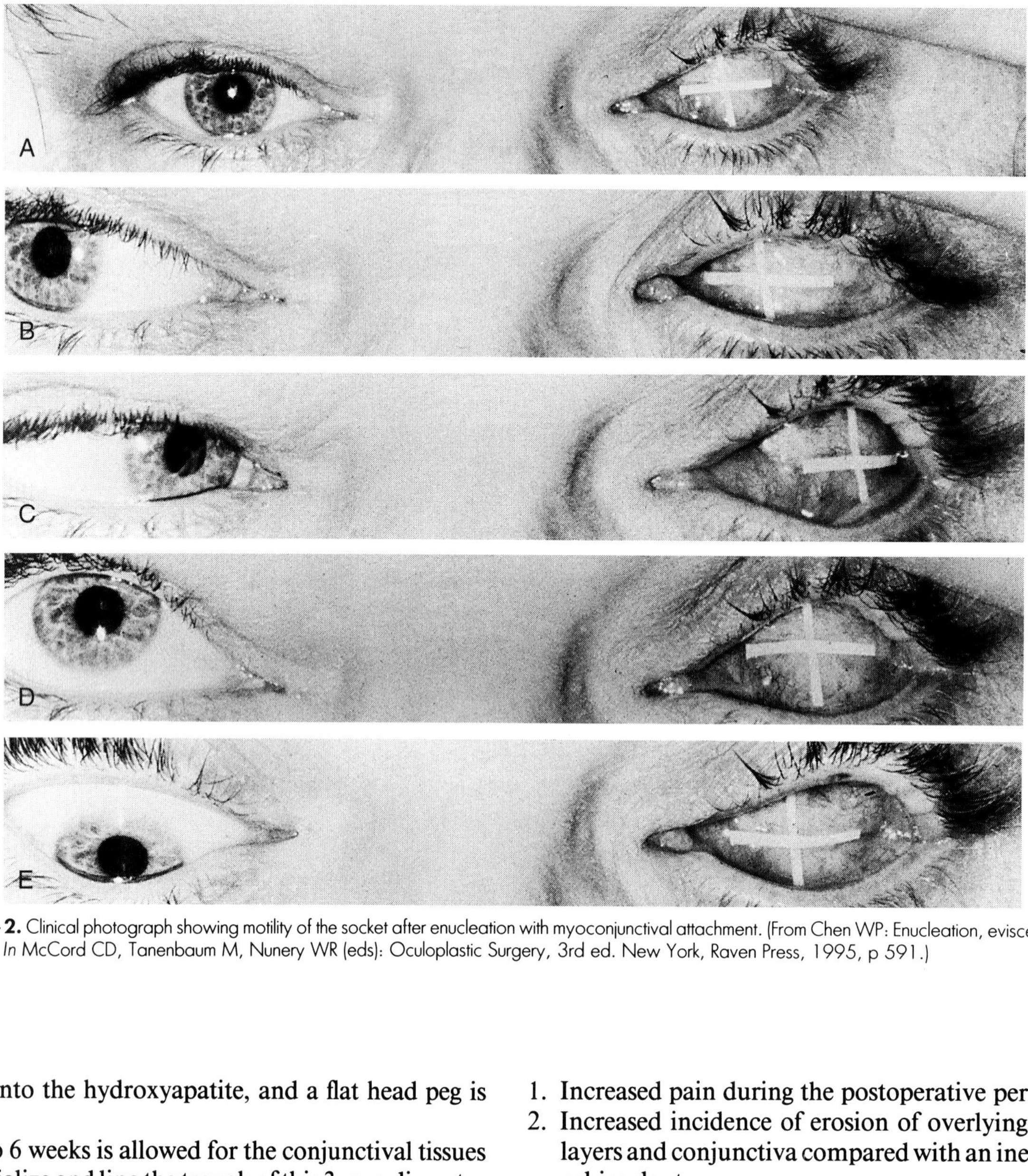

Figure 97 – 2. Clinical photograph showing motility of the socket after enucleation with myoconjunctival attachment. (From Chen WP: Enucleation, evisceration, and exenteration. *In* McCord CD, Tanenbaum M, Nunery WR (eds): Oculoplastic Surgery, 3rd ed. New York, Raven Press, 1995, p 591.)

screwed into the hydroxyapatite, and a flat head peg is inserted.

Four to 6 weeks is allowed for the conjunctival tissues to epithelialize and line the trough of this 3-mm diameter pit. When this is complete, a peg with a round hemispheric head is then placed in the hole in place of the flat head peg or sleeve. A final prosthesis is made with a posterior concavity in its center to fit over the round head peg sitting over the implant.

Contraindications to hydroxyapatite use include deficient muscle movement, orbital malignancy with potential for recurrence that may be masked by the vascularized presence of hydroxyapatite implant, and orbital infection. In general, sockets with a compromised vascular supply or known impaired healing should not have hydroxyapatite implants. These implants may also fail to vascularize well in elderly patients.

Several authors[18-21] have reported complications of hydroxyapatite implantation. These complications include higher incidence of exposure, infection, and reoperation when compared with silicone implants. Other disadvantages of hydroxyapatite include the following:

1. Increased pain during the postoperative period
2. Increased incidence of erosion of overlying Tenon's layers and conjunctiva compared with an inert spherical implant
3. Increased cost, including the price of the hydroxyapatite implant, of the donor sclera for wrapping the implant, and of postoperative bone scan or magnetic resonance image, and the cost of a second procedure if drilling of a peg hole is chosen
4. A variable waiting period for vascular ingrowth, up to 6 to 12 months
5. Need for preliminary fitting of ocular shell before final prosthetic fitting

Whether the increased cost and complication rate are justified by the improved ocular motility remains to be determined. We recommend hydroxyapatite in young adult patients with healthy sockets who are willing to bear the higher risk and cost for the possibility of improved motility. We do not recommend using hydroxyapatite in elderly patients or in patients with compromised sockets or other contraindications.

Congenital Anophthalmia and Severe Microphthalmia

Congenital anophthalmia or severe microphthalmia may lead to orbit bony hypoplasia if not encouraged to grow by early enucleation and replacement of adequate volume. Cepala and coworkers[22] have demonstrated that orbital bony growth in kittens is related to the amount of volume replaced, while Heinz and associates[23] demonstrated the slope of orbit bony growth and eventual volume obtainable decreases with elapsed time and age of kittens. We, therefore, recommend volume replacement as early as possible in patients with congenital anophthalmia or severe microphthalmia.

We develop eyelids and fornices in these cases with progressively enlarging conformers during the first 6 months of life. We then proceed with volume implantation through a lateral orbitotomy approach. The implant is placed through the lateral orbital wall and into the posterior Tenon fascia. The implant is left in the muscle cone posteriorly in the orbit. This minimizes the risk of extrusion through a conjunctival incision. We place 18-mm implants if possible, but we may initially place a 14- to 16-mm implant in very small infants. We then progressively enlarge the implant to a size of 19 or 20 mm in one or two subsequent procedures before the age of 3 to 4 years. In this manner, orbital volume can be encouraged while lids and fornices are developing. This will greatly reduce the risk of facial asymmetry secondary to hypoplastic orbital bony growth.

EVISCERATION

Evisceration removes the contents of an eye while leaving the scleral shell and muscle attachments intact. The cornea may or may not be removed. The scleral shell is usually filled with a spherical implant and sutured closed. Evisceration is especially helpful in situations in which there is a shortage of conjunctiva, since enucleation may cause further shortening of the conjunctival fornices.

Evisceration is a simpler procedure than enucleation and provides good prosthetic motility. Evisceration may have a higher postoperative incidence of sympathetic ophthalmia compared with enucleation, particularly after scleral laceration with uveal prolapse. Also, evisceration may not always relieve preoperative ocular pain since sensory ciliary nerves remain.

Presurgical Setup

The same degree of diligence and compulsion, as described in the section on enucleation, must be exercised by the surgeon to make sure that the correct eye is being eviscerated.

Surgical Steps

Evisceration can be performed under regional anesthesia. A mixture of 2% lidocaine, 0.5% bupivacaine, with 1:100,000 dilution epinephrine and hyaluronidase is given in a retrobulbar injection into the muscle cone. The upper and lower lids are anesthetized with a frontal nerve block and infiltration along the infraorbital nerve over the inferior orbital rim.

The cornea may be left in place or excised. For a well-vascularized cornea, a 360-degree conjunctival periotomy is initiated and undermining carried out in the sub-Tenon fascia plane to the equator. An incision through the limbus is started using a sharp blade followed by extension to each side with corneoscleral scissors.

The wound is extended to over 10 clock hours, leaving the cornea attached at the 5 and 7 o'clock positions. An alternative scleral incision can be made through the pars plana. With one forceps grasping the cornea, a cyclodialysis spatula is introduced to completely separate the iris root and ciliary body from the sclera. A small or medium-sized evisceration spoon can be used to scoop the intraocular contents from the sclera. Besides the spoon, the sharp edge of a Freer elevator with a suction instrument can be used to remove uveal tissues. Cotton-tipped applicators moistened with absolute alcohol (100% ethanol) may be used to denature any residue uveal pigment. The scleral shell is then rinsed thoroughly with saline solution. Relaxing cuts may be made through the sclera to facilitate exposure. A frequent source of vascular bleeding are the four exit sites of emissary veins and the optic nerve head. They should be very gently cauterized to control the oozing of blood.

It is often difficult to place a sphere of greater than 16 mm unless expansion sclerotomies are performed in a radial fashion through the internal surface of the scleral shell.[24] This can be performed using a needle-tipped cautery on cutting mode, making one to two splits per oblique scleral quadrant. An 18- to 20-mm sphere can then be placed in the expanded scleral shell. The limbal corneal wound is closed using interrupted transparent 6-0 nylon sutures. The cornea epithelium is meticulously scraped off. The anterior Tenon layer is then pulled over the cornea and closed using 5-0 Vicryl sutures in an interrupted fashion, followed by conjunctival closure with a running 6-0 plain suture. A conformer and light bandage are applied.

The use of a hydroxyapatite implant at the time of evisceration requires that the posterior part of the sclera be excised to provide a large window for fibrovascular growth. An 18- to 20-mm hydroxyapatite implant that has been predrilled with 10 to 20 holes using an 18-gauge needle is inserted into the scleral pocket. An excessively large implant will result in less socket depth for the ocularist to make a deep anterior chamber in the prosthesis. The use of a hydroxyapatite implant with evisceration is associated with a greater degree of postoperative pain than silicone spheres.

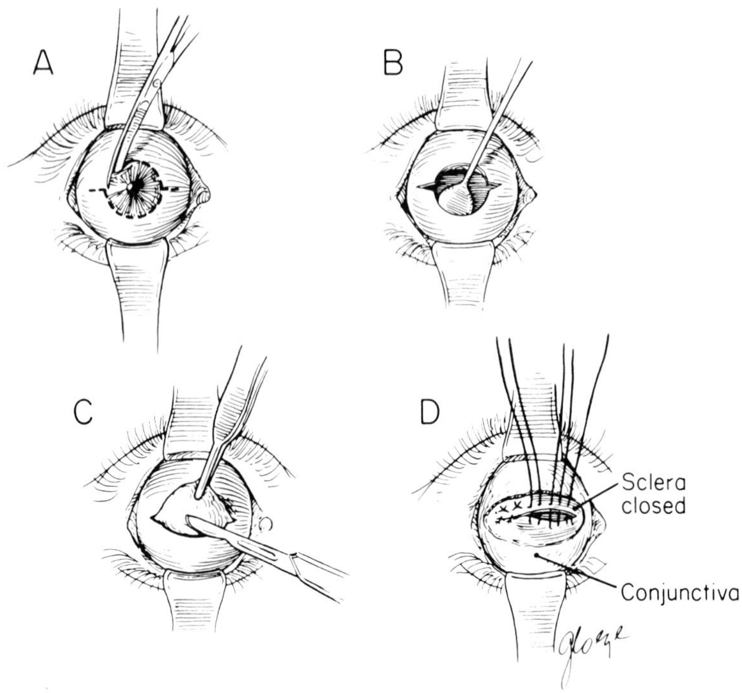

Figure 97 – 3. Basic steps in evisceration. *A*, After a periotomy is made and the conjunctiva is reflected, the cornea is excised. *B*, The evisceration spoon is used to separate and remove the ocular contents from the sclera. *C*, The posterior sclera is pulled forward through the wound and curetted to remove all uvea. *D*, The interior scleral wound edge is brought under the superior scleral wound edge, and the superior edge is then imbricated over the inferior sclera. (From Chen WP: Enucleation, evisceration, and exenteration. *In* McCord CD, Tanenbaum M, Nunery WR [eds]: Oculoplastic Surgery, 3rd ed. New York, Raven Press, 1995, p 595.)

Evisceration with removal of the cornea is indicated for those patients who may still have corneal sensation or corneal pain or when there is a chance of corneal thinning, such as connective tissue disorders or rheumatoid arthritis.

After a 360-degree conjunctival peritomy and undermining of the sub-Tenon fascial plane to the equator, the steps may proceed as in the previously discussed method. Relaxing scleral cuts are made at the 3 and 9 o'clock meridians, extending up to 12 mm in length. The corneal button, still attached to the limbus by a stalk, is helpful for grasping with a forceps while eviscerating the intraocular contents (Fig. 97 – 3). The cornea button is then excised. Relaxing radial sclerotomies are helpful[24] to allow for placement of a larger sphere (e.g., 18 mm). The scleral edges are overlapped and secured with double-armed, nonabsorbable sutures in a mattress fashion.

Trimming at each side of the scleral wound is usually necessary to avoid redundant dog-ears. The free edge of the sclera is then secured to the underlying sclera with a separate row of interrupted sutures, forming a secure closure. The Tenon layer is closed with interrupted 5-0 absorbable suture and the conjunctiva with running 6-0 absorbable suture. A conformer and light bandage are applied.

SUMMARY

Enucleation and evisceration are performed for a variety of indications. Meticulous technique and placement of extraocular muscles will decrease incidence of extrusion and improve prosthetic motility. Early enucleation and volume expansion in microphthalmic children will encourage orbital bony growth. The role of hydroxyapatite in improving prosthetic motility is not yet well determined, although it holds promise. Emotional support for the enucleation patient is important in the long-term rehabilitation of the patient. Eye protection of the remaining eye is an important aspect in preservation of vision.

REFERENCES

1. Nunery WR, Cepela MA, Heinz GW, et al: Extrusion rate of silicone spherical anophthalmic socket implants. Ophthalmic Plast Reconstr Surg 9:90 – 95, 1993.
2. Duke-Elder S: System of Ophthalmology. Vol IX, Diseases of the Uveal Tract. St. Louis, CV Mosby, 1966, pp 558 – 593.
3. Shields JA, Shields CL: Intraocular Tumors: A Test and Atlas. Philadelphia, WB Saunders, 1992.
4. Nunery WR, Hetzler KJ: Dermal fat graft as a primary enucleation technique. Ophthalmology 92:1256 – 1261, 1985.
5. Nunery WR, Heinz GW, Bonnin JM, et al: Exposure rate of hydroxyapatite spheres in the anophthalmic socket: Histopathic correlation and comparison with silicone sphere implants. Ophthalmic Plast Reconstr Surg 9:96 – 104, 1993.
6. Munden PM, Carter KD, Nerad JA: The oculocardiac reflex during enucleation. Am J Ophthalmol 111:378 – 379, 1991.
7. Traquair HM: Local anaesthesia in enucleation of the eyeball. Ophthalmic Rev 35:75 – 89, 1916.
8. Havre DC: Obtaining long sections of the optic nerve at enucleation: A new surgical technique based on the anatomy of the posterior fascia bulbi. Am J Ophthalmol 60:272 – 277, 1965.
9. Karcioglu ZA, Halk BG, Gordon RA: Frozen section of the optic nerve in retinoblastoma surgery. Ophthalmology 95:674 – 676, 1988.
10. Coston TO: The spherical implant. Trans Am Acad Ophthalmol Otolaryngol 74:1284 – 1286, 1970.
11. Chen WP: Enucleation with myoconjunctival attachment: Biome-

chanics of socket and prosthetic motility. Thesis for Fellowship Candidacy to American Society of Ophthalmic Plastic and Reconstructive Surgery, Atlanta, GA, 1981.
12. Nunery WR, Hetzler, KJ: Improved prosthetic motility following enucleation. Ophthalmology 90(9):1110–1115, 1983.
13. Ferrone PJ, Dutton JJ: Rate of vascularization of coralline hydroxyapatite ocular implants. Ophthalmology 99:375–379, 1992.
14. Dutton JJ: Coralline hydroxyapatite as an ocular implant. Ophthalmology 98:370–377, 1991.
15. DePotter P, Shields CL, Shields JA, et al: Role of magnetic resonance imaging in the evaluation of the hydroxyapatite orbital implant. Ophthalmology 99:824–830, 1992.
16. Shields CL, Shields JA, Eagle RC, DePotter P: Histopathologic evidence of fibrovascular ingrowth four weeks after placement of the hydroxyapatite orbital implant. Am J Ophthalmol 111:363–366, 1991.
17. Shields CL, Shields JA, DePotter P: Hydroxyapatite orbital implant after enucleation. Arch Ophthalmol 110:333–338, 1992.
18. Buettner H, Bartley GB: Tissue breakdown and exposure associated with orbital hydroxyapatite implants. Am J Ophthalmol 113:669–673, 1992.
19. Goldberg RA, Holds BH, Ebrahimpour J: Exposed hydroxyapatite orbital implants, reports of six cases. Ophthalmology 99:832–836, 1992.
20. Perry A: Presented at the First International Symposium on Hydroxyapatite Implant, La Jolla, California, January 1993.
21. Nunery WR, Heinz GW, Bonnin JM, et al. Exposure rate of hydroxyapatite spheres in the anophthalmic socket: Histopathologic correlation and comparison with silicone sphere implants. Ophthalmic Plast Reconstr Surg 9:96–104, 1993.
22. Cepala M, Nunery W, Martin R: Stimulation of orbital growth by the use of expandable implants in anophthalmic cat orbits. Ophthalmic Plast Reconstr Surg 8:157–169, 1992.
23. Heinz GW, Nunery WR, Martin RT: Stimulation of orbital growth in the anophthalmic cat orbit. (submitted for publication)
24. Stephenson CM: Evisceration of the eye with expansion sclerotomies. Ophthalmic Plast Reconstr Surg 3:249–251, 1987.

CHAPTER 98

Indications for Orbital Surgery

Ted H. Wojno

Orbital surgery is among the most complex and challenging of procedures undertaken by ophthalmologists. Because of the large number of orbital disorders, indications for surgery are, of necessity, relative. The final decision to intervene is based on the individual circumstances of each case and on the health of the patient.

BIOPSY

Numerous neoplastic and inflammatory conditions affect the orbit. The diagnosis is often obvious, as in the case of a typical intraconal cavernous hemangioma. Frequently, however, the physician is faced with an infiltrative process or unknown space-occupying lesion for which there are little or no diagnostic clues from the history, physical examination, imaging, or systemic evaluation. It is important to establish the benign or malignant nature of such problems to determine prognosis and direct any potential therapy. Biopsy with appropriate histopathologic study dictates whether further, more aggressive surgery is indicated or if the patient will be treated by irradiation, chemotherapy, or observation. Before biopsy the surgeon should consider consultation with the pathologist to determine the amount of tissue needed, appropriate handling of the specimen, media into which the specimen will be placed, and the transportation of the specimen to the laboratory. Frozen sections are often necessary to determine whether the surgeon has located the sought-after pathology. This is especially important with infiltrative lesions that do not cause a distinct, grossly identifiable tumefaction but are only microscopically visible.

EXCISION

In the case of many benign neoplasms the diagnosis is often obvious before intervention and the surgeon may decide to seek a complete removal. Well-localized, noninfiltrative lesions, such as cavernous hemangioma, leiomyomas, and neurilemomas, are relatively easy to excise with minimal morbidity. Removal may be indicated if the tumor is causing visual loss through optic nerve compression or involvement of the vascular supply to the globe. Proptosis and globe displacement may result in exposure with corneal decompensation or unacceptable cosmetic appearance. Diplopia may occur from impairment of the extraocular muscles or motor nerves.

The level of patient anxiety is an important factor to consider. There are patients who on finding that they have an orbital neoplasm, albeit a benign one causing only minimal functional problems, will suffer emotional stress until the tumor is removed. Others, in spite of advancing functional problems, will delay surgical intervention because of fear of the surgical procedure. The surgeon should counsel both types of patients so that each one is comfortable with the decision to operate and can accept any complications that may result.

Pain is not a common feature of most slowly growing orbital neoplasms. Some patients do complain of nonspecific headaches or ocular discomfort and relate this to the neoplasm. I am reluctant to tell any patient that pain will be relieved by removal of such tumors. To the extent that a tumor causes proptosis and exposure, however, excision will often make a patient more comfortable.

Many benign orbital neoplasms grow very slowly and occasionally cease growing all together. Visual loss and other functional problems may permanently stabilize. Observation may therefore be a viable option in some patients.

For all the neoplasms that cannot be completely resected, such as an extensive sphenoid wing meningioma, partial excision may be indicated because of proptosis and discomfort. Partial excision is indicated in malignant neoplasms of the orbit for the same reason.

DRAINAGE

Orbital abscess and hemorrhage may accumulate in the orbit and compromise vision and motility. Drainage, usually performed by a frontal orbitotomy, is indicated for treatment of these problems and to prevent spread of infection to the surrounding tissues.

EXENTERATION

Exenteration is the removal of all orbital contents down to and including the periosteum. The eyelids may be included in the resection, as in the case of sebaceous cell carcinoma, or may be left behind, as in certain deep orbital neoplasms or in the case of extrascleral extension of an intraocular neoplasm. Exenteration is usually done to provide a cure for malignancy or to palliate a malignant or benign neoplasm that has resulted in disfiguring proptosis with visual loss or pain. If the neoplasm involves the orbital walls, bone may also need to be removed.

TRAUMA AND RECONSTRUCTION

Orbital fractures are often handled in a multidisciplinary fashion, depending on the severity of the fracture, concomitant injuries, and local custom. The ability to work harmoniously with other specialists who treat facial trauma will make the experience more enjoyable for the surgeons involved and improve the overall care of the patient.

Reconstruction of congenital orbital defects usually falls in the domain of the craniofacial surgeon. The ophthalmologist will often play a role in management of associated ocular problems.

FOREIGN BODIES

In general, organic material such as wood is poorly tolerated in the orbit and provokes an intense inflammatory reaction with abscess formation. Removal of such foreign bodies is mandatory, followed by appropriate cultures and antibiotics. By contrast, glass, stone, and plastic are often well tolerated but do occasionally work their way to the surface of the eyelids and extrude. Metallic fragments such as bullets and BBs are usually not problematic and only rarely become infected. Many patients request removal of metallic orbital foreign bodies, but if they cause no problems the risk of surgical removal generally outweighs any potential complications of leaving them in tissue.

DECOMPRESSION

The term *decompression* is applied to three distinctly different surgical procedures of the orbit.

Nerve Sheath Decompression (Fenestration)

Pseudotumor cerebri threatening vision and nonresponsive to weight loss, diuretics, and corticosteroids is an indication for optic nerve sheath decompression. Such patients may also be treated by lumboperitoneal shunt.

Optic Canal Decompression

Indirect trauma to the optic nerve may result in contusion, concussion, edema, or infarction of the nerve with visual loss. Decompression of the optic canal may relieve pressure on the nerve and improve the visual prognosis. The surgery may be performed through a transorbital-ethmoidal approach, an intracranial approach, or a transantral approach. Despite numerous papers on this subject, optic canal decompression for traumatic optic neuropathy remains controversial. Therapy with high doses of corticosteroids is an alternative.

Orbital Decompression

Orbital decompression is indicated in Graves' eye disease with compressive optic neuropathy, severe orbital congestion, or severe proptosis leading to exposure and cosmetic disfigurement. Radiation therapy and corticosteroids are alternative and sometimes adjunctive treatment approaches.

CHAPTER 99

Operative Principles and Instrumentation

Ted H. Wojno

There are three basic principles of orbital surgery: good exposure, careful dissection, and meticulous hemostasis. Instrumentation for orbital surgery is designed to help the surgeon abide by these principles.

EXPOSURE

Adequate exposure of orbital tissue is of paramount importance. Without it, complications are more likely and the surgery will be more difficult. In general, orbital lesions are deeper and less accessible than they appear on radiologic scans. The surgeon should therefore carefully plan and expose the area involved. After draping, care must be taken not to inadvertently put pressure on the opposite globe. It is often helpful to drape the other eye into the field as a reminder of its presence. If the globe on the operative side is to be exposed for any length of time, a moistened corneal protector will decrease the need for frequent irrigation.

Proper exposure is achieved through good lighting, magnification, wide bone removal, and retraction. A variety of instruments are available to accomplish this.

1. *Lighting.* For surgery on superficial orbital lesions the overhead room lights are often adequate. For surgery on deeper lesions, however, a headlight is helpful and with some adjustments can be worn in addition to loupes. Alternatively, a headlight may be directly attached to some models of loupes.
2. *Magnification.* There are numerous brands of loupes available, and the surgeon should choose one based on comfort, magnification, and depth and width of field. In general, loupes with higher magnification have less depth of field and smaller areas of view. The degree of magnification is based on personal preference but somewhere between two and three times normal is most common. The operating microscope can be used for procedures requiring higher magnification but can be awkward if the surgeon is working in a wide field or if the depth must be frequently changed.
3. *Bone removal.* Bone removal is accomplished with combinations of saws, drills, and rongeurs. In general, it is easier to drill wire holes before making saw cuts for bone that will be replaced at the end of the procedure. Saw blades may be oscillating, reciprocating, or sagittal, with oscillating being the most commonly used in orbital surgery. Insertion of malleable retractors inside the orbital walls protects the soft tissue from inadvertent injury by the saw blade or drill. After saw cuts are completed, bone flaps can be removed with a small bone-holding clamp. A variety of rongeurs, from small to large, are used to remove additional bone. Bone is usually wired back at the end of the surgical procedure but can also be secured with nonabsorbable 2-0 polypropylene or nylon, thus avoiding interference with subsequent radiologic scans. Bone may also be secured with titanium miniplates or Vitallium microplates that do not interfere with magnetic resonance imaging.
4. *Retraction.* Skin and muscle edges may be retracted with 4-0 silk traction sutures at the wound edges or with a variety of self-retaining retractors. Self-retaining retractors are quickly placed, while silk traction sutures allow for more precise adjustment of the wound edges. A sophisticated system of self-retaining orbital retractors was developed by Kennerdell and Maroon.[1] Although expensive and somewhat time consuming to assemble, it gives the surgeon precisely adjustable instrumentation adaptable to both medial and lateral orbitotomy.

The surgeon encounters orbital fat after opening the septum or periorbita. The fat causes difficulty in orbital dissection because of its tendency to billow into the operative field, obstructing the view of deeper structures. It is helpful to place a neurosurgical patty (Codman and Shurtleff, Randolph, MA) against the fat and then a malleable retractor over the patty. The rough, absorptive surface holds the fat more securely than the smooth malleable surface. Malleable retractors, used for the temporalis muscle and orbital soft tissue, are either bare metal or plastic-coated and come in varying widths. Smaller, more delicate malleable orbital retractors are also available (Wright Retractors, John Weiss & Son, London, England).

DISSECTION

Instruments chosen for orbital dissection are as varied as the number of surgeons doing orbital surgery. Most dissections are accomplished with relatively simple equipment, however. Fine-toothed (0.3 and 0.5 mm) Castroviejo-type forceps are used for grasping. Cottle and Joseph elevators are useful for adherent periorbita at the orbital rim, while a Freer elevator works well on the loosely attached periosteum deeper in the orbit. A Tenzel elevator (Storz, St. Louis, MO) combines both a Freer and Cottle at opposite ends. A small nerve hook is useful for delicately mobilizing nerves and blood vessels deep within the orbit.

Blunt and sharp Wescott scissors are useful for fine cutting within the orbit. A bayonet-style modification of Wescott scissors is useful to avoid impaired visualization when working in a small field (Storz, St. Louis, MO).

Cotton-tipped applicators are beautifully suited for orbital dissection. Their small size, soft tips, and somewhat adhesive surfaces make them ideal for manipulating fat and the surface of tumors.

HEMOSTASIS

Uncontrolled bleeding can lead to disastrous complications in orbital surgery. Knowledge of the location of major vessels helps the surgeon to dissect in as bloodless a plane as possible and to cauterize such vessels before they are inadvertently cut. Fat should be retracted gently since all orbital tissues are interconnected. Excessive traction can tear small vessels deep within the orbit and be tremendously difficult to locate. The surgeon should never close the incision until certain that adequate hemostasis was obtained since bleeding will most certainly continue. If the patient bucks or strains excessively on awakening, bleeding may suddenly restart. To avoid this, the anesthesiologist may be able to extubate the patient while the patient is still relatively deeply anesthetized. Postoperatively, the head of the bed is elevated to decrease venous pressure in the operative site and appropriate medication is used to avoid coughing, sneezing, and a Valsalva maneuver.

A Bovie-type unipolar cautery is useful to both cut and coagulate in areas such as the temporalis fossa and for major perforating blood vessels such as the ethmoidal arteries. A needle point gives finer control than the larger spatula-style tip. A red rubber catheter may be cut and fashioned as a guard to avoid inadvertent coagulation of surrounding tissue. A suction Bovie tip, although a bit more difficult to use, has distinct advantages (Valleylab, Boulder, CO). Lighted suctions are also available (Vital-Vue, San Diego, CA).

Bipolar cautery is usually used within the orbit and whenever the surgeon desires only minimal lateral destruction of tissue. A variety of styles are available.

The carbon dioxide (CO_2) and yttrium-aluminum-garnet (YAG) contact laser are occasionally useful adjuncts in orbital surgery, especially when dealing with vascular lesions such as lymphangiomas. The CO_2 laser will coagulate vessels up to 1.0 mm in diameter and can also be used for tissue evaporation. The contact YAG laser provides a distinct advantage of tactile feedback and also cuts and provides hemostasis on vessels 1.0 mm in diameter or larger, depending on the tip chosen.

Vascular clips are sometimes useful for large perforating vessels in the orbital walls or for control of bleeding for vascular neoplasms such as orbital varices. Small, bony perforating vessels or bleeding from the cut edge of bone is usually well controlled by the application of bone wax.

Persistent capillary ooze can be controlled by providing a surface on which a clot may form. Topical agents for this purpose are made from gelatin (Gelfoam, Upjohn, Kalamazoo, MI), collagen (Avitene, Alcon, Humacao, Puerto Rico; Instat, Johnson & Johnson, New Brunswick, NJ), or cellulose (Surgicel, Johnson & Johnson, New Brunswick, NJ). All of these agents are absorbed from the site of implantation in several days to a few weeks.

If there is any possibility that blood may accumulate in the retrobulbar space, the surgeon should leave a suction drain in place for at least overnight. A variety of drains are available, or the surgeon may make one from a butterfly needle by cutting off the Luer-Lok tip and cutting multiple holes in the plastic tubing.

REFERENCE

1. Kennerdell JS, Maroon, JC: Microsurgical approach to intraorbital tumors. Arch Ophthalmol 94:1333–1336, 1976.

CHAPTER 100

Surgical Approaches to the Orbit*

Giulio Bonavolontà

Although the history of orbital surgery is quite ancient, the first publication of interest is a reference to Bartish, in 1583, which describes for the first time the exenteration of the orbit.[1] The modern history of orbital surgery must be dated to the invention of computed tomography. Only after the advent of the computed tomographic scan has it been possible to have preoperative knowledge of the shape, dimensions, structural details, and relations and secondary changes due to an orbital lesion. This has been an enormous development and has substantially enlarged the operative indications. Modern orbital surgery revolves around four basic areas of orbital pathology: (1) orbital tumors, (2) trauma, (3) Graves' orbitopathy, and (4) congenital and acquired malformations.

The surgical approaches to the orbit are much less diverse than the variations in orbital pathology, and I shall explain some principles guiding the selection of a surgical route of attack for the variety of problems that an orbital surgeon confronts.

GENERAL PRINCIPLES

Orbital surgery has many aspects that are significantly different from other ophthalmic surgical techniques. The surgical approach of the orbital surgeon is much closer to the approach of a neurosurgeon than to that of an ophthalmologist. Surgical maneuvers alternate between relatively gross techniques and fine or microscopic ones. The orbital surgeon must be able to navigate in deep tissue planes; must be able to recognize veins, arteries, and nerves; and must be able to prevent and control significant bleeding. He or she must also have familiarity with surgical bone techniques, because some orbital procedures require demolition and reconstruction of the orbital walls. It is also important that the anesthesiology team be acquainted with this type of surgery.

SURGICAL INSTRUMENTATION

To the normal ophthalmic armamentarium the orbital surgeon must add instruments specifically for orbital work. Required are suction catheters, malleable retractors (Fig. 100–1), neurosurgical dissectors, an oscillating saw for bone removal, and bipolar forceps. A fiberoptic headlight and operating loupes are necessary. Many orbital surgeons use an operating microscope for the more delicate phases of surgery. A neurosurgical microscope is frequently more suitable than an ophthalmic microscope, but the ophthalmic microscope will be adequate if necessary. I have used carbon dioxide and Nd-YAG lasers, but others have not found their use necessary.

Bone wax should be available in the operating suite to stop bleeding from the orbital walls, and neurosurgical cottonoids are used for absorption of blood and to protect vital structures during retraction. A cryoextractor is useful in the case of encapsulated tumors to facilitate extraction while diminishing the risk of capsular rupture.

SURGICAL APPROACH TO THE ORBIT

The orbit is an osseous cavity of pyramidal shape consisting of four walls and containing the globe and its adnexae. The orbit is adjacent to the brain superiorly and posteriorly, the sphenoidal and ethmoidal sinuses medially, the maxillary antrum inferiorly, and the temporal fossa laterally.

The term *orbitotomy*, from the Greek, "to cut into the orbit," has been inappropriately used for all of the surgical approaches to the orbit. Its use should ideally be reserved for the approaches to the orbit that involve opening of one or more of the osseous walls of the orbit.

The orbit can be approached from five routes: superior, lateral, inferior, medial, or anterior. Each route presents characteristic advantages and disadvantages. It is up to the skills and experience of the surgeon to choose a route that minimizes the disadvantages and maximizes the advantages of the route taken and is appropriate to the pathologic process in question.

*Original manuscript translated by Dr. Jeffrey Schiller.

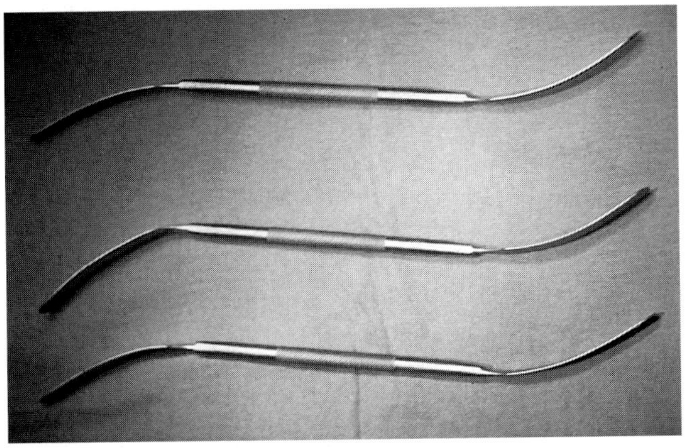

Figure 100–1. Malleable nonreflective retractors of different sizes, designed by the author for orbital surgery.

In the following sections the surgical approaches to the most frequently seen diseases of the orbit are discussed: (1) treatment of orbital tumors, (2) treatment of orbital trauma, (3) reconstruction of the anophthalmic socket, and (4) surgery related to diseases of the paranasal sinuses. Before establishing the general rules that dictate one approach over another in a particular case, it is appropriate to give some short accounts of the anatomic structures encountered depending on the route selected.

ANATOMIC PLANES AND SURGICAL EXPOSURE OF DIFFERENT ROUTES

Within the orbit, the structures encountered depend on the route of surgical exposure taken (Table 100–1).

TABLE 100–1

Anatomic Planes and Structures Encountered During Surgical Exposure

Superior orbitotomy (neurosurgical route)
Scalp
Galea
Pericranium
Skull
Brain
Orbital roof
Lateral orbitotomy
Skin and subcutaneous tissues
Temporal muscle
Zygomatic arch and lateral orbital wall
Medial approach
Nasal mucosa
Medial wall
Inferior approach (transantral)
Buccal sulcus mucosa
Maxilla
Mucosa of maxillary sinus
Orbital floor
Transcutaneous anterior approach
Skin and subcutaneous tissues
Orbicularis
Orbital septum
Orbital periosteum
Transconjunctival anterior approach
Direct or subperiosteal approach

From the superior approach, medially one encounters the body of the superior oblique, centrally the body of the levator, below it the body of the superior rectus, and, anteriorly, the trochlea. In the superomedial quadrant are the supraorbital nerves and vessels. Through the lateral approach, as in the superoanterior aspect, is the lacrimal gland; and posterior to this is the lacrimal nerve and vessels with the lateral rectus muscle below. In the inferior approach, the lacrimal excretory system is seen medially, with the inferior oblique muscle, the inferior rectus muscle, and the infraorbital neurovascular bundle. Finally, from the medial approach, the medial rectus muscle and the anterior and posterior ethmoidal arteries are encountered (Fig. 100–2).

How should we select the best route of approach to the orbit? The approach should satisfy the following requirements:

1. It should involve the least surgical trauma to the orbital structures and to the patient.
2. It should provide good surgical exposure of the pathologic process.
3. It should be the simplest and most direct approach.
4. It should give the best possible cosmetic result.

Sometimes all these requirements cannot be met, and the emphasis must be placed on obtaining the best surgical exposure with the least surgical trauma.

SURGICAL APPROACH BASED ON PATHOLOGIC PROCESS

Neoplasms

In oncologic surgery, the surgical approach is selected with regard to the (1) shape and consistency of the lesion, (2) location, (3) nature and progression of the lesion, and (4) age of the patient.

Shape and Consistency of the Lesion. Examples include

1. Circumscribed lesion with hard consistency: osteomas (Fig. 100–3).
2. Circumscribed lesion with "duroelastic" consistency: cavernous hemangiomas, mixed tumors of the lacrimal gland, schwannomas (Fig. 100–4).
3. Circumscribed lesion with fluid contents: dermoid cysts (Fig. 100–5).
   Strategy. The surgical approach in these cases should allow the resection of the lesion in toto without rupture of the capsule where present. In cystic lesions with fluid contents, it is often preferable to aspirate the fluid from the lesion to facilitate its resection in toto if there is a restricted surgical space.
4. Poorly demarcated lesions with firm consistency: adenoid cystic carcinoma (Fig. 100–6).

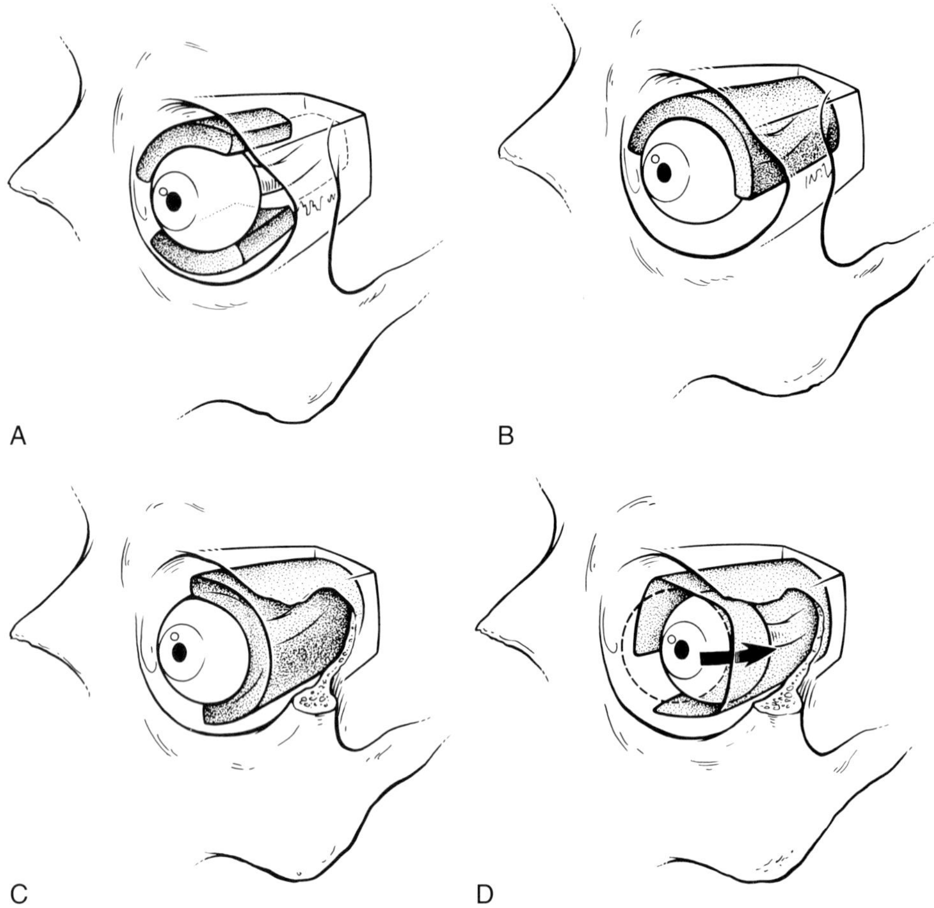

Figure 100–2. Scheme of surgical exposure obtained by various orbitotomies. *A*, Anterior orbitotomy: approxidative surgical field of exposure for superior and inferior-anterior orbitotomy (60 degrees superior, 60 degrees inferior). *B*, Coronal orbitotomy: approxidative surgical field of exposure (200 degrees). *C*, Osteoplastic lateral orbitotomy: approxidative surgical field of exposure (180 degrees). *D*, Coronal orbitotomy: the surgical field of exposure is improved opening the lateral wall (200 degrees).

5. Poorly demarcated lesions with soft consistency: lymphatic lesions, lymphomas (Fig. 100–7).
   Strategy. These lesions can only be partially resected; success of the treatment depends on other modalities, including radiation therapy and chemotherapy.

Location. Examples include

1. Anterior lesions. Normally an osteotomy is not necessary, and the lesion can be reached through an anterior transcutaneous or transconjunctival route.

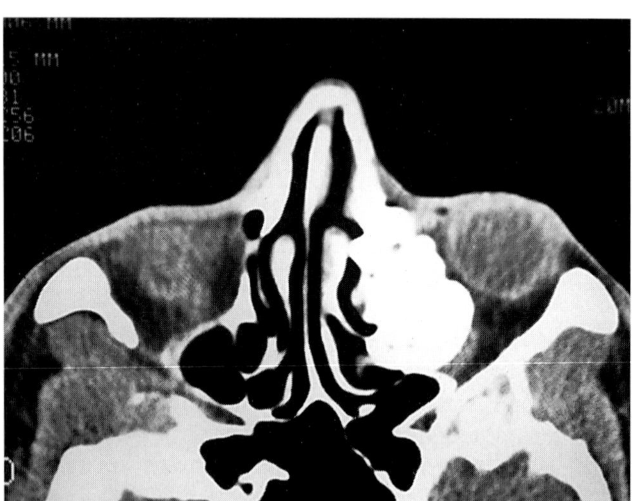

Figure 100–3. Computed tomographic scan of osteoma of ethmoidal sinus without orbital invasion.

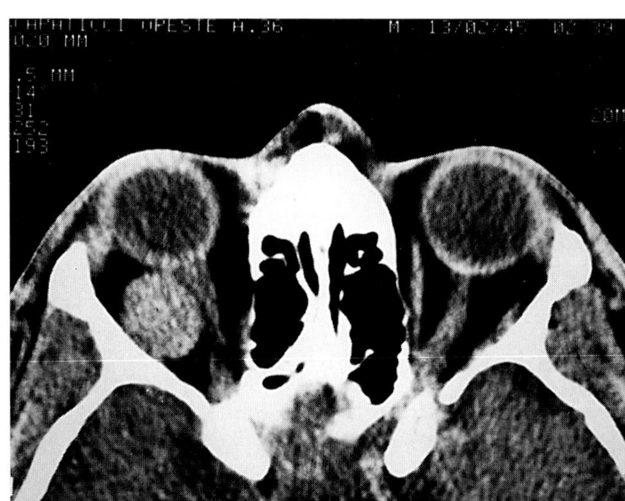

Figure 100–4. Computed tomographic scan of cavernous hemangioma (dimensions: 1.7 × 1.5 cm), lateral to optic nerve.

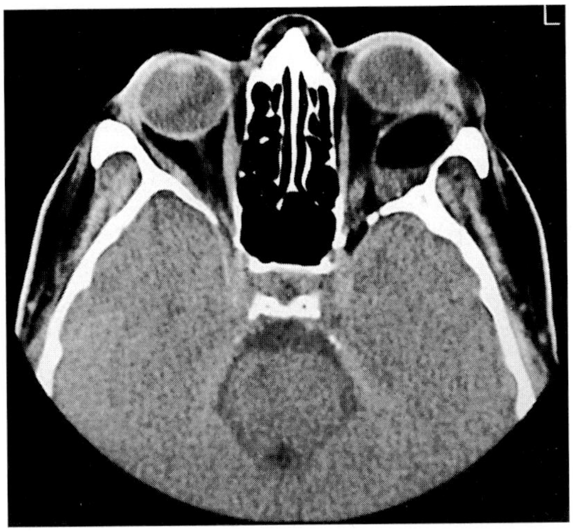

Figure 100–5. Computed tomographic scan of dermoid cyst lateral to the optic nerve. Note air–fluid level and deformation of the orbital wall.

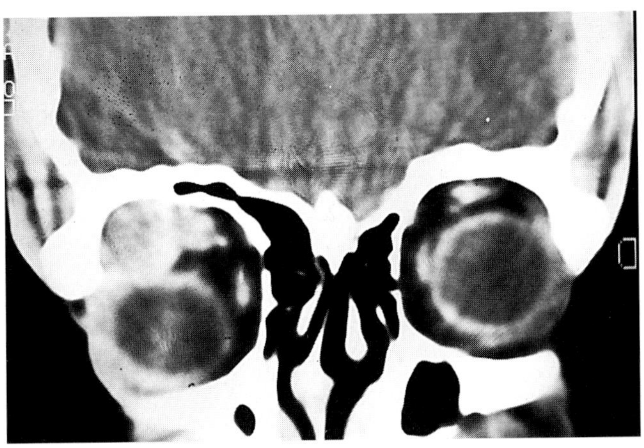

Figure 100–6. Computed tomographic scan of adenoid cystic carcinoma of the lacrimal gland. Note the indistinct margins and erosion of the bone of the orbital roof.

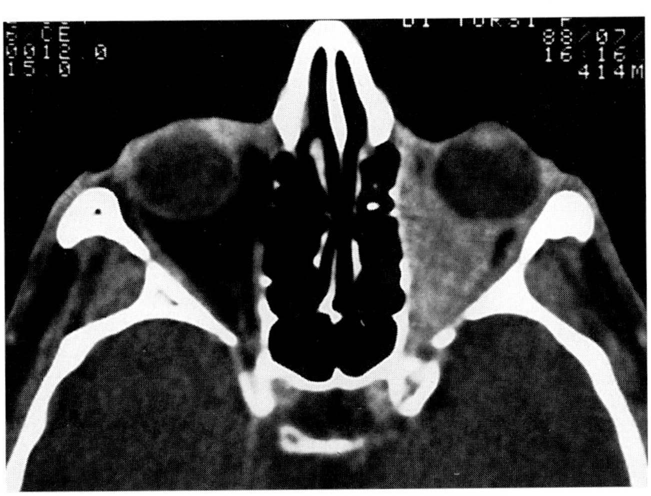

Figure 100–7. Computed tomographic scan of orbital lymphoma. Note the consistency and the poorly defined margins of the lesion.

Strategy. Extraperiosteal lesions are approached through an extraperiosteal route, while intraconal lesions are reached through a transseptal route; and it is often sufficient to biopsy diffuse lesions through the transconjunctival route.

2. Posterior lesions. An osteotomy is almost always necessary.
   Strategy. Lesions superior, lateral, and inferior to the optic nerve can be easily treated through a lateral orbitotomy. Lesions medial to the optic nerve often require a superomedial approach, either a transcutaneous extraperiosteal route or through a coronal incision associated with a prior lateral orbitotomy to allow more space in the superonasal sector.
3. Lesions not confined to the orbit.
   Strategy. A combined approach is used depending on the individual case.

Nature and Progression of the Lesion. Examples include

1. Benign lesions. These generally require a wide incision, since they usually require medical attention when they have grown large enough to cause problems.
   Strategy. In these circumstances, surgery represents the only chance of cure; the surgical approach should allow safe and total resection with the smallest chance of iatrogenic damage.
2. Malignant lesions. Modern oncology has demonstrated that malignant neoplasms are rarely cured simply by resection and are generally considered as systemic diseases. In some cases, the surgery can exacerbate the situation, rendering the tumor more aggressive and favoring dissemination of the neoplastic cells.
   Strategy. The surgical game plan varies depending on whether the tumor is sensitive to irradiation or chemotherapy; if so, a limited surgical approach is prudent in consultation with the consulting oncologist. In certain cases in which medical therapy is of limited value, radical surgery is unfortunately necessary.

Age. Osteotomy techniques should not be used in the very young patient to avoid inciting developmental abnormalities. Fortunately, even the posterior orbit can be reached in young individuals owing to the reduced dimensions of the orbit.

Strategy. An anterior transseptal orbitotomy that is extraperiosteal and transconjunctival is done. Greater exposure to the orbit can be obtained by coronal incision in complicated cases.

Anophthalmic Socket

The topic of the anophthalmic socket is more thoroughly covered in other parts of this volume. Here, several general principles are presented.

The primary goal in the treatment of the anophthalmic socket is to correct socket contraction, allowing retention of the prosthesis.

In the great majority of cases of recurrent prolapse of the prosthesis, the cause is shrinkage or contraction of the fornices. This is most frequently due to conjunctival loss or contraction alone, and this is treated elsewhere. The most severe cases of socket incompetence are due to disease processes involving the entire orbit, including orbital infections, irradiated orbits, and congenital anophthalmia. In these cases, orbital surgery proper is necessary.

The surgery is directed toward reconstituting a deep vascularized bed over which one can reconstruct an anterior socket capable of retaining the prosthesis. The techniques that I use involve transfer of temporalis or frontalis muscle tissue into the orbit.[4] These techniques almost always require a bicoronal approach. This allows a wide exposure of all of the orbital walls, combined with exposure of the frontalis and temporalis muscles, which are transposed into the orbital cavity.

Trauma

In the approach to orbital trauma, we distinguish three occurrences that require diverse surgical approaches: (1) orbital foreign body, (2) orbital hematoma, and (3) orbital fracture.

Orbital Foreign Body. The best approach in the case of a retained orbital foreign body is to follow the trajectory of the foreign body, beginning by enlarging the entry wound. Some have proposed the possibility of an endoscopic approach, but I have used the traditional surgical approach, respecting anatomic planes. This approach is less risky and allows the removal of the foreign body by an "open sky" technique. Of course, small, well-tolerated foreign bodies can often be observed and not removed.

Orbital Hemorrhage. Any collection of blood is potentially dangerous, whether by compressive effect on the optic nerve or by toxic effect produced by hemosiderin. It usually should be evacuated. The surgical approach is the transcutaneous transseptal route in the quadrant of the hematoma. A drain should be left in place for 48 hours.

Orbital Fracture. Orbital fractures are treated in detail in another part of this volume. I would stress here that although a classic blow-out fracture can be approached by an anterior transcutaneous or transconjunctival extraperiosteal approach, complex orbital fractures often require wider surgical exposure. Often the best approach to these fractures is a bicoronal approach, which allows visualization of the entire bony orbit.

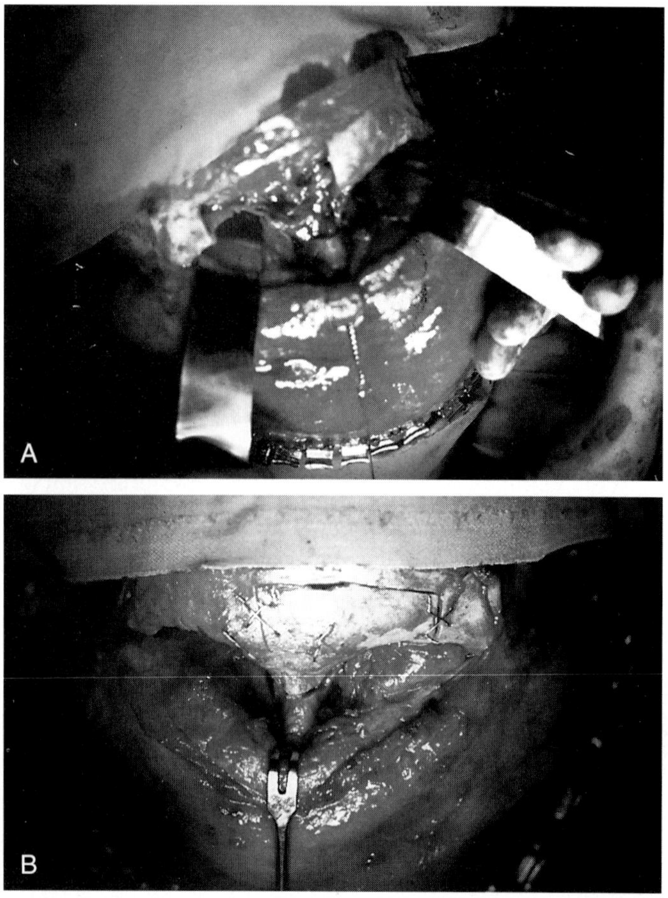

Figure 100–8. View of frontal sinus and orbital cavity through bicoronal incision with removal of orbital rim. *B*, Repositioning of the bony orbital rim at the end of the procedure in *A*.

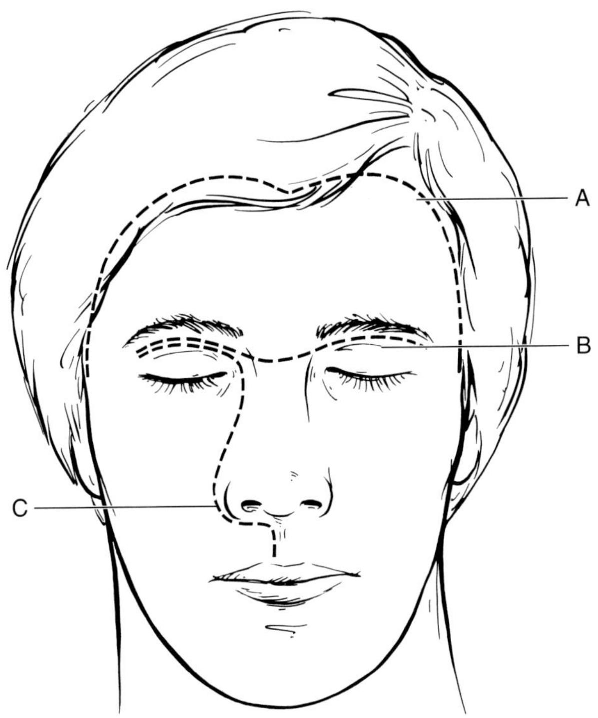

Figure 100–9. The most common surgical approaches to the paranasal sinuses. *A*, Coronal approach to the frontal sinus. *B*, Subciliary approach to the frontal and ethmoidal sinuses. *C*, Enlarged paralateral-nasal incision for exposure of frontal, ethmoidal, and maxillary sinuses.

Associated Sinus Surgery

Although disease of the paranasal sinuses per se is not part of the field of the orbital surgeon, there are cases in which the invasion of the orbit by pathologic processes or lesions originating in the orbit will involve the orbital surgeon. The most common of these cases are mucoceles of the frontal and ethmoidal sinuses, osteomas of the frontoethmoidal region, and malignancies originating in the maxillary and ethmoidal sinuses. The routes of approach must provide exposure of the orbital region invaded as well as the adjacent sinus (Fig. 100–8). The most common approaches used are shown in Figure 100–9.[6]

REFERENCES

1. Henderson JW: Orbital Tumors. Philadelphia, WB Saunders, 1973.
2. Ambrose JAE, Lloyd GAS, Wright JE: A preliminary evaluation of fine matrix computerized axial tomography (EMI scan) in the diagnosis of orbital space-occupying lesions. Br J Radiol 47:747–751, 1974.
3. Frezzotti R: Patologia Clinical e Terapia delle Malattie Dell'orbital. Siena, Soi, 1985.
4. Rougier J, Tessier P, et al: Chirurgie Plastique Orbito-palpebrale. Paris, Masson, 1971.
5. Bosniak S: Complex Socket Deformities. New York, McGraw-Hill, 1992.
6. Thawley SE, Pauje WR, et al: Comprehensive Management of Head and Neck Tumors. Philadelphia, WB Saunders, 1987.

CHAPTER 101

Optic Nerve Sheath Decompression

Marc S. Cohen

The primary purpose of this chapter is to provide a practical, step-by-step approach to the technique of optic nerve sheath decompression.

Optic nerve sheath decompression is a surgical procedure in which the intraorbital meningeal sheath of the optic nerve is fenestrated to allow drainage of cerebrospinal fluid. The operation is widely accepted as the procedure of choice for the treatment of visual loss due to chronic papilledema. Additionally, optic nerve sheath decompression has been proposed as a treatment of other vision-threatening disorders.

Pseudotumor cerebri is a relatively common disorder that results in idiopathic elevation of the intracranial pressure. This results in headaches and chronic papilledema. Although pseudotumor cerebri has been termed *benign intracranial hypertension*, 50% of patients have some visual complaints and 25% develop serious visual loss.[1-4] Severe visual loss in pseudotumor cerebri is the result of an optic neuropathy that is secondary to prolonged, elevated intracranial pressure that is transmitted along the nerve sheath. In patients with visual loss, medical management generally consists of weight loss and high doses of carbonic anhydrase inhibitors. Corticosteroids and diuretics have also been used.

When there is progressive visual loss despite medical therapy, surgery is indicated. Until the mid 1980s the surgical procedure of choice for progressive visual loss in pseudotumor cerebri was placement of a lumboperitoneal shunt. It is now widely accepted that, as compared with lumboperitoneal shunt, optic nerve sheath decompression is more effective and offers less morbidity in the treatment of vision-threatening papilledema.[5-7]

The mechanism of action of optic nerve sheath decompression is still debated. It has been proposed that optic nerve sheath decompression results in scarring in the subarachnoid space that blocks the transmission of increased pressure to the optic nerve head.[8, 9] Many authors believe that optic nerve sheath decompression is a filtering procedure that simply lowers the pressure around the optic nerve.[10, 11] Seiff and Shah[12] have suggested that fenestration reduces pressure on the optic nerve in accordance with Bernoulli's equation of fluid dynamics. Sergott and coworkers[13] have proposed that optic nerve sheath decompression improves optic nerve function by reducing optic nerve ischemia.

Other possible indications for optic nerve sheath decompression include treatment of progressive nonarteritic ischemic optic neuropathy,[14-16] traumatic optic nerve sheath hemorrhage,[13] acute retinal necrosis syndrome,[13] and chronic papilledema secondary to a nonresectable central nervous system mass.[13] These indications remain controversial, and the reader is referred to the growing body of literature regarding this topic.

SURGICAL TECHNIQUE

Two approaches have been employed to perform optic nerve sheath decompression. The optic nerve can be approached by a medial orbitotomy or a lateral orbitotomy. If the lateral approach is taken, a Krönlein-Berke lateral orbitotomy is performed. This technique offers the advantage of more complete exposure of the optic nerve. It has the disadvantage of requiring the removal of bone that is not necessary in the medial approach. In this chapter the medial approach is emphasized because, with the technique described, the procedure can be performed easily with adequate exposure. Because bone is not removed, the medial approach offers less morbidity and a shorter postoperative recovery. The medial approach was popularized by Galbraith and Sullivan.[17] The technique described was modified by Sergott.[18]

1. The surgery is performed with the patient under general anesthesia. A protective shield is placed over the unoperated eye. In other orbital procedures local injection with epinephrine is often employed to aid in hemostasis. Epinephrine should *not* be used in this procedure because it may dilate the pupil and hinder intraoperative assessment of optic nerve function.
2. After the patient is prepped and draped, a lateral canthotomy is performed. It is not necessary to disinsert the lateral canthal tendon from the orbital rim. A 270-degree peritomy is performed 4 mm posterior to the limbus. The lateral 90 degrees of the conjunctiva is not incised. The intramuscular septal attach-

ments between the medial rectus and the superior and inferior rectus are then severed.

3. Traction sutures of 4-0 silk are passed under the superior and inferior rectus muscle and tied. The medial rectus is held with a self-retaining muscle hook and cleared of its connective tissue attachments. The medial rectus is then attached to a double-armed 6.0 polyglactin (Vicryl) suture in standard manner for strabismus surgery. The medial rectus is then disinserted from the globe with Aebli scissors. The operating microscope is then brought into place.
4. A 6-0 Vicryl traction suture is then placed deep to the muscle stump of the medial rectus. This suture is placed as an intrascleral running suture. Approximately eight bites are made. It is important that the entire length of the muscle stump be included because this will be necessary to help orient the globe during the subsequent steps.
5. The surgical assistant then retracts the globe. Proper retraction of the globe is the key to success in performing a medial approach optic nerve sheath decompression. The three traction sutures are used to retract the globe. The assistant must first slightly prolapse the globe and then retract it laterally. While this is being done it is essential that the globe retain its proper orientation. Any induced cyclotortion will make finding the optic nerve difficult. If cyclotortion occurs, the assistant must place differential traction on the holding sutures to orient the globe. The important points of this step are to continue to prolapse the globe while retracting it laterally and maintain orientation of the globe.
6. The surgeon then places a Fisher malleable retractor medially with moderate pressure against the medial wall of the orbit. A surgical space is then created between the medial orbital wall and medial rectus, medially, and the globe, laterally (Fig. 101–1). The operating microscope is then focused posteriorly. There will be a reflection of Tenon's capsule that will be seen as a transparent membrane just anterior to orbital fat. This should be carefully incised. At this point the assistant holds the medial retractor, remembering to maintain an upward, lateral traction on the traction sutures in the other hand. The surgeon then employs two cotton-tipped applicators to sweep the orbital fat away from the optic nerve. The long posterior ciliary nerve has an intrascleral course that runs directly toward the optic nerve. This nerve can be easily identified as a slightly bluish ridge on the medial aspect of the globe. By following the long posterior ciliary nerve posteriorly, the optic nerve is easily found. The cotton-tipped applicators are then placed directly superiorly and inferiorly to the optic nerve (Fig. 101–2).
7. At this point it is important to observe the pupil. Because the operating microscope shines light in the operated eye while the contralateral eye is covered, optic nerve function can be accessed by pupillary size. If the optic nerve becomes ischemic and its function is compromised, the pupil will dilate by the same mechanism that occurs when a patient has a relative afferent pupillary defect. If at any point the pupil dilates, the traction sutures are relaxed and the retractor is removed from the orbit for several minutes. All patients undergoing this procedure have compromised optic nerve function and are susceptible to the ischemia that occurs by retracting the globe. Even if pupillary dilation does not occur, the eye should be placed in the resting position every few

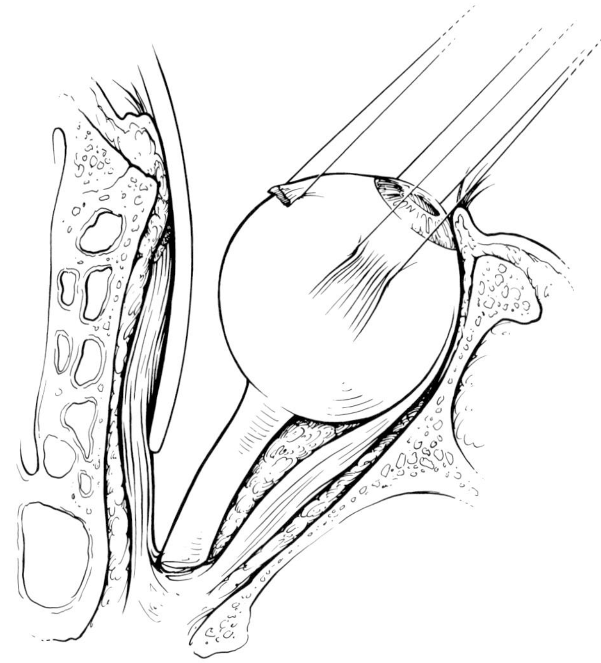

Figure 101–1. The intraconal space is entered between the medial orbital wall and the medial rectus medially, and the globe laterally.

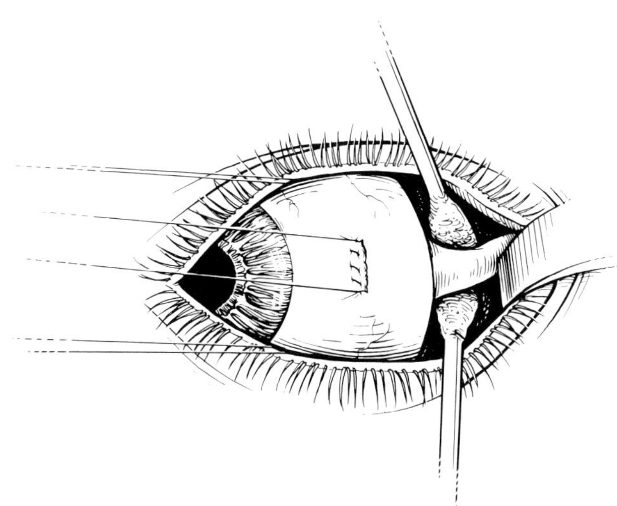

Figure 101–2. Cotton-tipped applicators are used to sweep the orbital fat from the nerve.

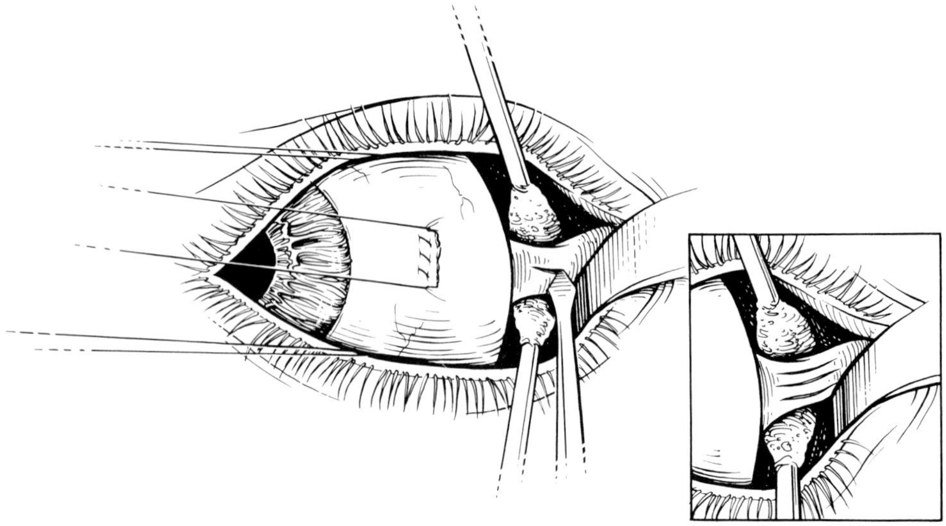

Figure 101–3. The optic nerve sheath is incised with a long-handled tympanic membrane blade 2 mm posterior to the globe. The incision is made in a lengthwise direction for about 4 mm.

minutes. Pupillary dilation can also occur secondary to compromised function of the long posterior ciliary nerves. This generally results in a segmental dilation of the pupil.

8. Fenestration can now be performed. An avascular portion of the meningeal sheath is identified on the medial aspect of the globe. The incision is initiated with a long-handled tympanic membrane blade (Fig. 101–3). The incision is made lengthwise starting 2 mm posterior to the globe. A gush of cerebrospinal fluid is encountered as the subarachnoid space is entered. The incision is extended posteriorly for 4 mm. This can be accomplished with the tympanic membrane blade or a trans-sphenoidal scissors. The incision is never extended beyond 8 mm posterior to the globe because the central retinal artery, as it enters the nerve, must be avoided. A small Stevens tenotomy hook is then placed in the opening, and subarachnoidal adhesions are lysed. There is often a second gush of loculated fluid as this is performed. Three or four similar cuts are made on the medial half of the nerve sheath (Fig. 101–4). The surgeon is assured that each cut is full thickness by the fact that the tenotomy hook can be passed from one opening to the other through the subarachnoid space (Fig. 101–5). The procedure described employs multiple slits. Some surgeons prefer to make rectangular windows in the sheath. Both techniques seem equally effective.
9. The globe is returned to the resting position for several minutes. The orbit is then inspected again for any orbital bleeding. All three holding sutures are removed, and the medial rectus is reattached to the muscle stump with the preplaced Vicryl sutures. Retraction of the globe tends to pull the medial rectus muscle stump anteriorly. It is suggested that the medial rectus be attached 5.5 mm posterior to the limbus.
10. The conjunctiva is carefully closed with 6-0 gut suture in a running fashion. Every third pass is locked. Careful closure is important because there is now an open communication between the subarachnoid space and the subconjunctival space. In fact, a bleb is often seen postoperatively.

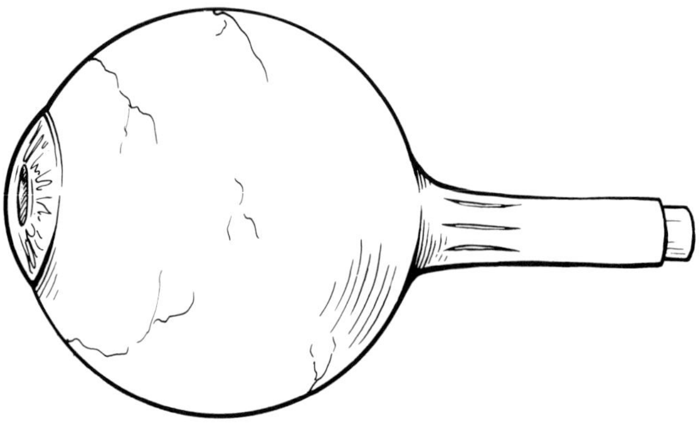

Figure 101–4. Three incisions are made on the medial half of the optic nerve sheath.

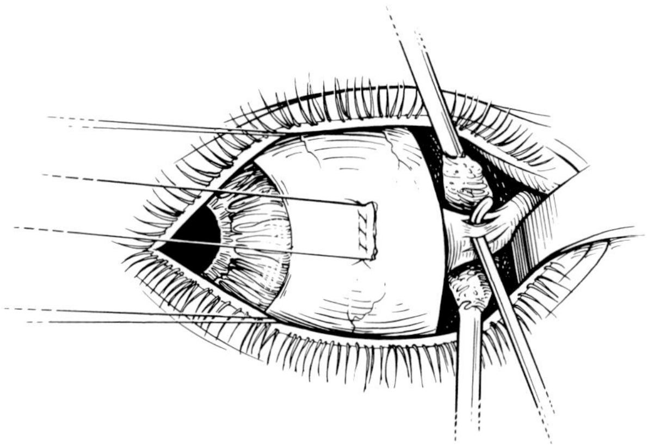

Figure 101 – 5. A Fisher tenotomy hook is placed through each of the cuts, and any subarachnoid adhesions are lysed. If the hook can be passed from one opening to another, the surgeon is assured that full-thickness dural incisions have been made.

11. Subconjuctival injections are *not* given because they could enter the subarachnoid space. Antibiotic ointment is placed in the eye, and the eye is patched.

POSTOPERATIVE CARE

The patient is examined several hours after surgery and then daily for 3 days. The patch is removed on postoperative day 1. Vigorous ocular lubrication is used for the first week after surgery. Carbonic anhydrase inhibitors are discontinued after surgery.

COMPLICATIONS

By far the most common complication of medial approach optic nerve sheath decompression is a transient adduction deficit. This is most likely due to trauma to the medial rectus or its innervation. This is self-limited in most patients, and resolution occurs within 3 months. Rarely, patients may require prisms or even strabismus surgery if diplopia persists. It is important to reattach the medial rectus to its proper position during surgery.

The most severe complication of optic nerve sheath decompression is permanent visual loss after surgery. There have been reported cases of visual loss due to central retinal artery occlusions and direct trauma to the optic nerve. The combined incidence of visual loss from this procedure is about 2%.[13]

In a small percentage of patients a corneal dell can form after surgery. Rarely, a dell can develop into a corneal ulcer. This is best avoided by adequate lubrication after surgery.

Occasionally, a repeat optic nerve sheath decompression is indicated. The procedure is identical to that previously described. However, the orbital dissection is more difficult because of the intraorbital septa and fat.

In conclusion, optic nerve sheath decompression is the procedure of choice for the treatment of vision-threatening papilledema that is unresponsive to medical therapy. Reports have indicated that optic nerve sheath decompression may result in visual improvement in patients with the progressive form of nonarteritic ischemic optic neuropathy and other disorders that have been poorly responsive to other therapeutic modalities. Optic nerve sheath decompression is gaining wider acceptance. It is hoped that the many controversies regarding this procedure will be resolved and its indications clearly elucidated.

REFERENCES

1. Corbett JJ, Savino PJ, Thompson HS, et al: Visual loss in pseudotumor cerebri: Follow-up of 57 patients from five to 57 years and a profile of 24 patients with permanent severe visual loss. Arch Neurol 39:461 – 474, 1982.
2. Wall M, Hart WM, Burde RM: Visual field defects in idiopathic intracranial hypertension (pseudotumor cerebri). Am J Ophthalmol 96:654 – 668, 1983.
3. Orcutt JC, Page NGR, Sander MD: Factors affecting visual loss in benign intracranial hypertension. Ophthalmology 91:1303 – 1312, 1984.
4. Lessell S, Rosman NP: Permanent visual impairment in childhood pseudotumor cerebri. Arch Neurol 43:801 – 804, 1986.
5. Brourman ND, Spoor TC, Ramochi JM: Optic nerve sheath decompression for pseudotumor cerebri. Arch Ophthalmol 106: 1378 – 1383, 1988.
6. Sergott RC, Savino PJ, Bosley TM: Modified optic nerve sheath decompression provides long-term visual improvement for pseudotumor cerebri. Arch Ophthalmol 106:1384 – 1390, 1988.
7. Corbett JJ, Nerad JA, Tse DT, Anderson RL: Results of optic nerve sheath fenestration for pseudotumor cerebri. Arch Ophthalmol 106:1391 – 1397, 1988.
8. Davidson SI: A surgical approach to plerocephalic disc oedema. Trans Ophthalmol Soc UK 89:669 – 690, 1969.
9. Davidson SI: The relief of papilledema. *In* Cant JS (ed): The Optic Nerve. London, Henry Kimpton, 1972, pp 174 – 179.
10. Keltner JL, Albert DM, Lubow M, et al: Optic nerve decompression: A clinical pathologic study. Arch Ophthalmol 95:97 – 104, 1977.
11. Hupp SL, Glaser JS, Frazier-Byrne S: Optic nerve sheath decompression: Review of 17 cases. Arch Ophthalmol 105:386 – 389, 1987.
12. Seiff SR, Shah L: A model for the mechanism of optic nerve sheath fenestration. Arch Ophthalmol 108:1326 – 1329, 1990.
13. Sergott RC, Savino PJ, Bosley TM: Optic nerve sheath decompression: A clinical review and proposed pathophysiologic mechanism. Aust NZ J Ophthalmol 18:365 – 373, 1990.
14. Sergott RC, Cohen MS, Bosley TM, Savino PJ: Optic nerve decompression may improve the progressive form of nonarteritic ischemic optic neuropathy. Arch Ophthalmol 107:1743 – 1754, 1989.
15. Kelman SE, Elman MJ: Optic nerve sheath decompression for nonarteritic ischemic optic neuropathy improves multiple visual function measurements. Arch Ophthalmol 109:667 – 671, 1991.
16. Spoor TC, Wilkinson MJ, Ramocki JM: Optic nerve sheath decompression for the treatment of progressive nonarteritic ischemic optic neuropathy. Am J Ophthalmol 111:724 – 728, 1991.
17. Galbraith JEK, Sullivan JH: Decompression of the perioptic meninges for relief of papilledema. Am J Ophthalmol 76:687 – 692, 1973.
18. Sergott RC: Diagnosis and management of vision-threatening papilledema. Semin Neurol 6:176 – 184, 1986.

CHAPTER 102

Anterior, Medial, Lateral, and Combined Surgical Approaches to Orbital Tumor Resection*

Giulio Bonavolontà

In Chapter 100 the various indications for the different surgical approaches to orbital pathology were discussed. In this chapter the steps of the most commonly employed surgical techniques for management of orbital neoplasms are presented. The anterior, medial, lateral, and combined approaches are considered. All approaches except the transconjunctival involve a skin incision. Various approaches have been advocated by different authors, but here the discussion is limited to the description of those approaches that we prefer and that we believe provide the best surgical exposure while allowing the best aesthetic result (Fig. 102–1).

ANTERIOR APPROACH

There are three types of anterior approaches: transconjunctival, transseptal, and extraperiosteal.

Transconjunctival Approach

The indications for the transconjunctival approach include transconjunctival biopsy, orbital lymphoma, lipodermoids, and optic nerve biopsy (Fig. 102–2).

The conjunctiva is incised through the fornix at the quadrant of interest. Traction sutures are passed through the insertions of the rectus muscles bordering the involved quadrant, which allows greater exposure of the area while preventing inadvertent trauma to these rectus muscles. Sometimes for greater exposure a lateral canthotomy is required. To gain access to the retrobulbar intraconal space it is necessary to disinsert a horizontal rectus muscle—the medial for the optic nerve and the lateral for exposure of the lateral intraconal space.

The scleral stump of the resected rectus muscle is imbricated with a silk traction suture for rotation of the globe, which allows access to the deeper orbital space. Dissection is accomplished by delicate blunt dissection in anatomic planes. Use of a headlight or operating microscope helps to identify vital orbital structures and prevent their inadvertent damage. Closure includes reattachment of the disinserted rectus muscle and closure of the conjunctiva with a fine absorbable suture. Postoperative bandages and care are similar to that after surgery of the globe. No drain is necessary.

Anterior Transseptal Approach

The indications for the anterior transseptal approach are excisional biopsy of malignant tumors, rhabdomyosarcoma, and orbital lymphoma (Fig. 102–3).[2]

The skin incision is over the preseptal orbicularis fibers, following the skin creases to make it as acceptable aesthetically as possible. The orbicularis is divided horizontally, and the dissection is carried to the orbital septum. Traction sutures through the skin and orbicularis facilitate exposure and hemostasis. The septum is opened with blunt scissors centrally. This will expose the orbital fat. Use of a malleable retractor allows dissection through the fat and exposure of the tumor. It is often necessary to use a muscle hook to retract the levator or tendon of the superior oblique in the superior orbit, and the inferior oblique in the inferior orbit, to allow better exposure and to prevent trauma to these structures. After performing the resection, biopsy, or drainage procedure, a suction drain is placed and the orbicularis and skin are closed in layers, avoiding incorporation of the septum in the closure. The orbicularis is closed with an absorbable suture, and the skin is closed with 6-0 silk or nylon. A light pressure dressing is placed. Postoperative treatment is similar to after eyelid surgery, with the exception of the drain, which is removed after 48 hours.

Anterior Extraperiosteal Approach

The indications for the anterior extraperiosteal approach are an orbital dermoid or a well-defined anterior orbital mass (Fig. 102–4).[3]

The anterior extraperiosteal approach is executed using a skin incision parallel to the rim in the quadrant of

*Original manuscript translated by Dr. Jeffrey Schiller.

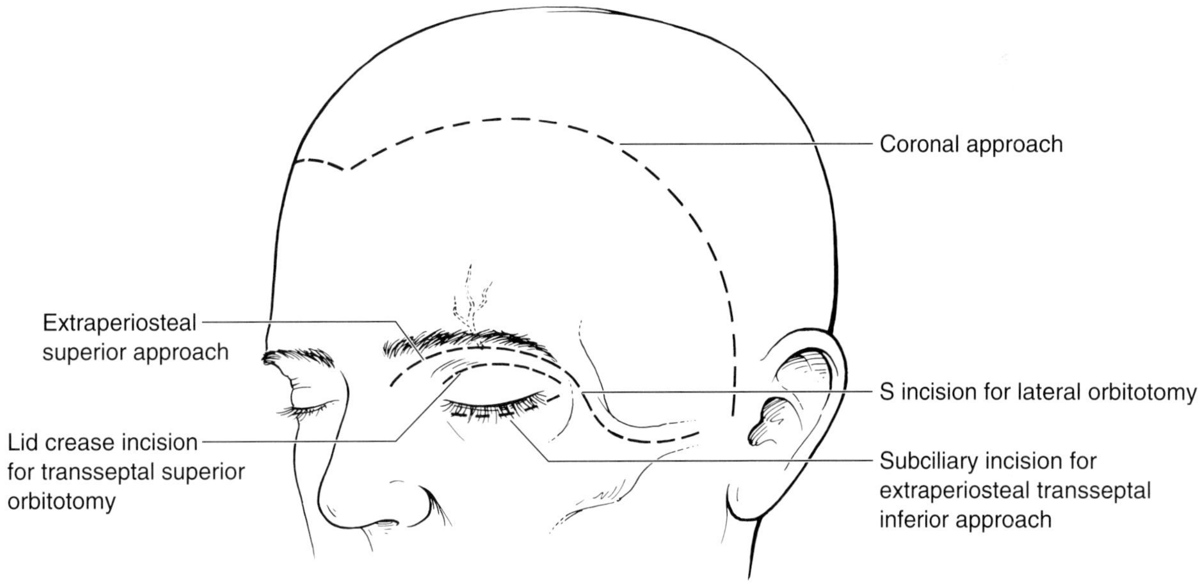

Figure 102–1. The most utilized skin incisions in orbital surgery.

interest. The most common is the superomedial incision just inferior to the brow. Infiltration with anesthetic and epinephrine facilitates hemostasis, as in the transseptal approach, even if the patient is under general anesthesia. The skin incision is carried down to the periosteum in one movement. Once the periosteum is encountered, it is incised, taking care to preserve the supraorbital nerve and vascular bundle. The dissection is then carried out in the subperiosteal plane with periosteal elevators. In this procedure, the virtual subperiosteal space is developed and is easily penetrated. There are only a few attachments between the bone and periosteum of which one must be aware. In the medial sector these are the anterior and posterior ethmoidal arteries, and in the lateral orbit is Hertel's canal, which transmits a branch of the medial meningeal artery into the orbit. Once the area overlying the tumor has been reached, the periosteum is opened longitudinally, between the bodies of the levator and the superior oblique superonasally and between the levator and lateral rectus superolaterally. Careful dissection prevents damage to the trochlea and tendon of the superior oblique medially and the lacrimal gland and its vasculature laterally. Neurosurgical cottonoids can be used in conjunction with malleable retractors to retract and protect these delicate structures. After resection of the tumor, a suction drain is inserted. The periorbita in the orbit need not be sutured, but the periosteum at the orbital rim is closed with 4-0 catgut or other absorbable suture. The orbicularis and skin are closed in the traditional manner, depending on the preference of the surgeon, with 5-0 nylon, silk, or Prolene. A pressure dressing is placed that allows inspection of the globe, and it is left in place for 48 hours. The drain is removed at 48 hours, and antibiotics are given for 72 hours. We prefer to use corticosteroids postoperatively in patients undergoing anterior orbitotomy.

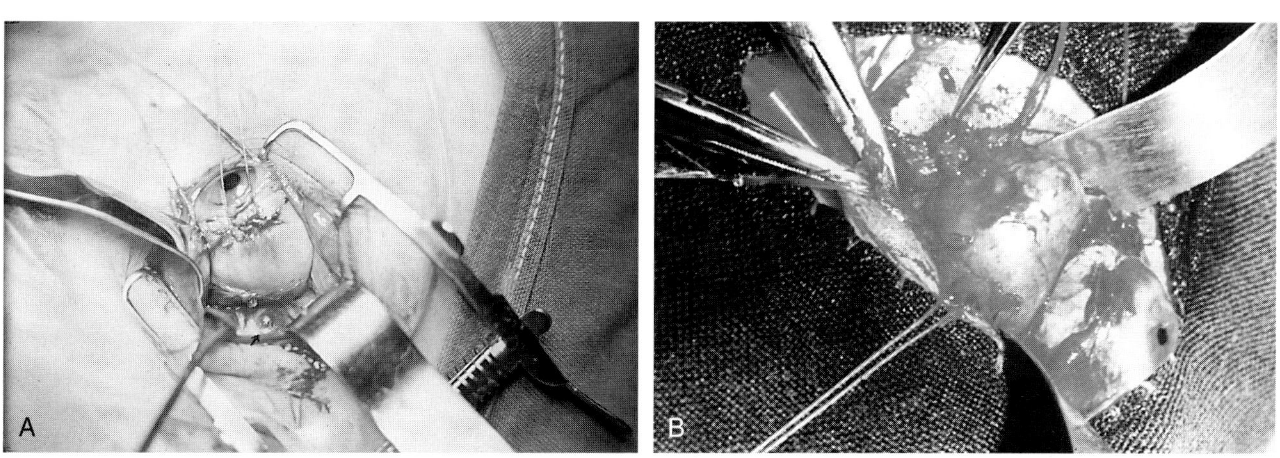

Figure 102–2. *A*, Exposure of an arachnoid cyst of the optic nerve using a transconjunctival approach. *B*, A large schwannoma resected through a transconjunctival approach. Disinsertion of the lateral rectus and lateral cantholysis improves the surgical exposure.

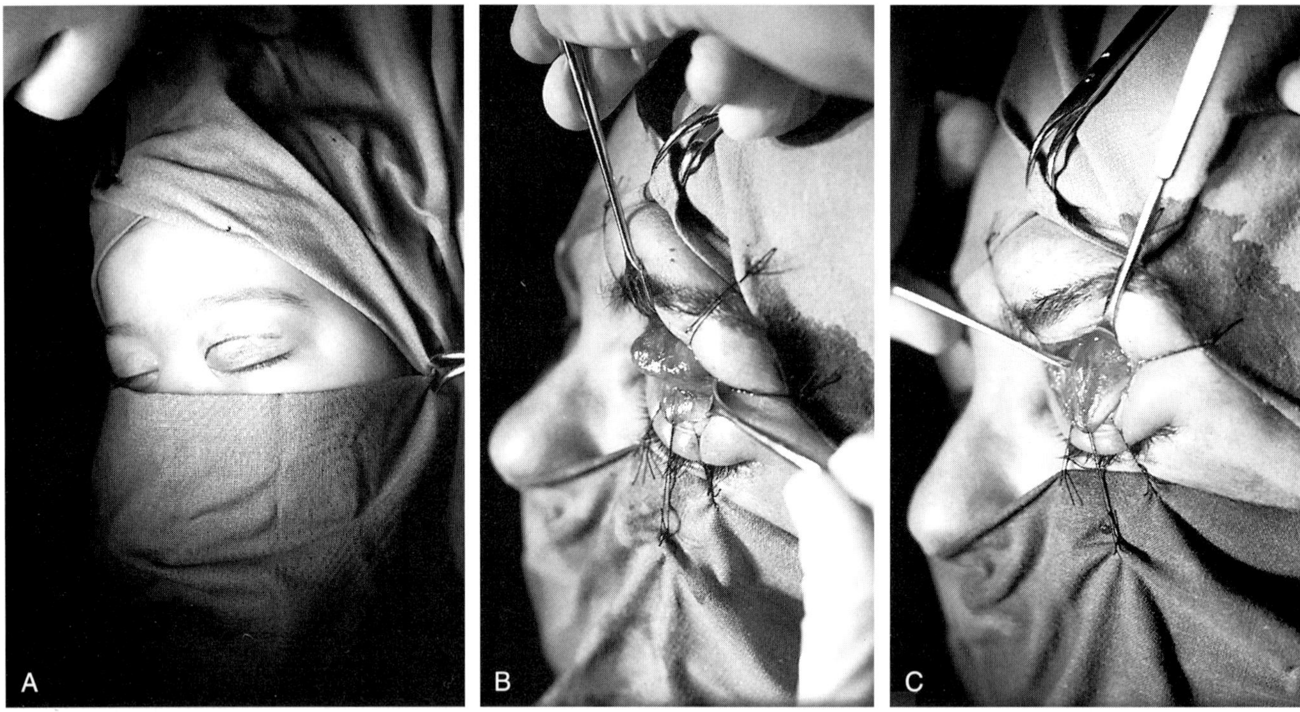

Figure 102–3. *A*, Design for the surgical incision in a transseptal approach. *B*, A retroseptal angiomatous mass exposed with the transseptal approach. *C*, The levator aponeurosis is preserved after dissection of the mass.

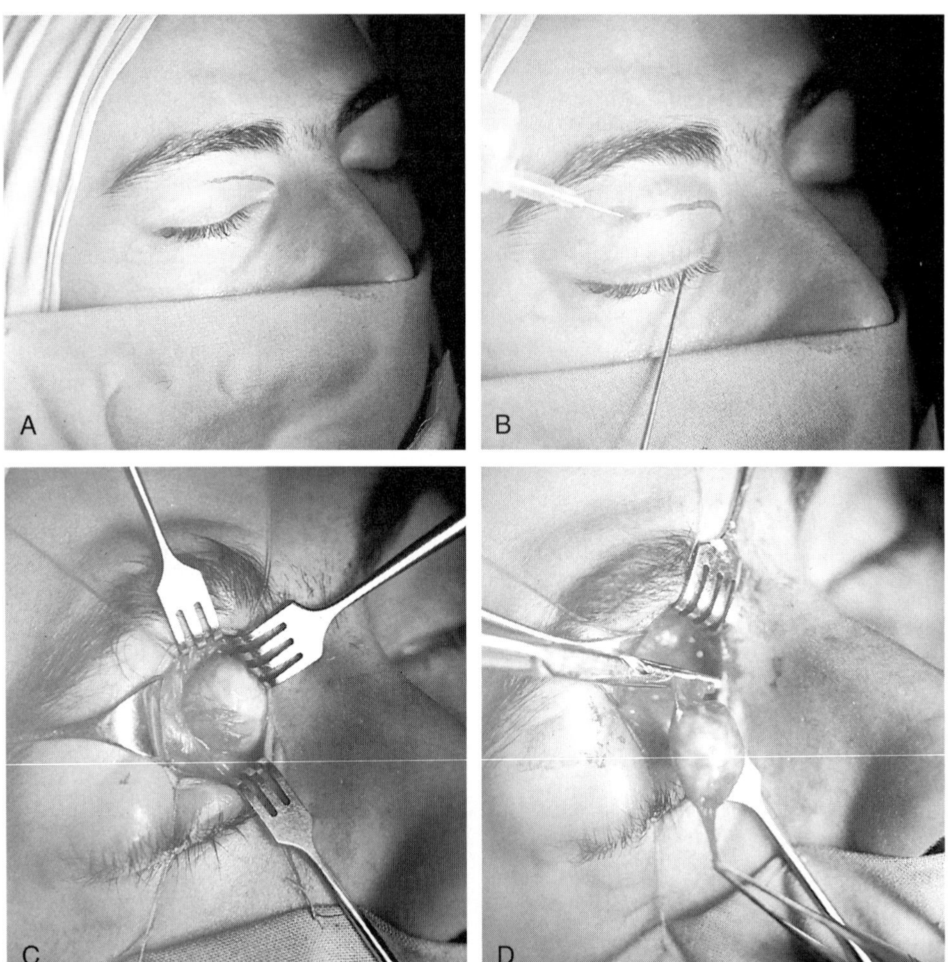

Figure 102–4. *A*, The design for skin incisions for the extraperiosteal superior and medial approach. *B*, Local infiltration with anesthetic and epinephrine. *C*, Direct exposure of an extraperiosteal dermoid cyst after dissection of the orbicularis. *D*, Complete resection of the cyst.

LATERAL ORBITOTOMY

The indications for lateral obitotomy are lacrimal gland tumors and encapsulated tumors in the deep orbit.

Although many cutaneous incisions have been proposed for the lateral orbitotomy, we prefer the classic curvilinear S-shaped incision, beginning above the brow and descending inferolaterally along the lateral orbital rim to the zygoma and then laterally across the zygomatic arch to the hairline (Fig. 102–5). The dissection is carried through the subcutaneous tissues and the orbicularis to the level of the periosteum and the fascia of the temporalis muscle. Bleeding is controlled during this phase by retraction sutures through the skin, which also provide exposure of the surgical field (see Fig. 102–5*B*). Remaining bleeding vessels are cauterized. The periosteum is incised 2 mm outside the orbital rim parallel to the bony margin. The periosteum is elevated off of the rim including the temporalis muscle, exposing the temporal fossa, and inside the rim, exposing the extraperiosteal space of the lateral quadrant. Once the lateral wall of the orbit is completely exposed, one can proceed with the osteotomy. Before making the cuts one should inspect the lateral orbital rim where it joins the zygoma. In a small percentage of patients it is perforated by a superficial branch of the zygomaticotemporal vessels; these vessels should be cauterized and cut before the osteotomy. The osteotomy is performed with an oscillating saw, making two cuts parallel to the zygomatic arch, one above the frontozygomatic suture and one just above the horizontal ramus of the zygoma (see Fig. 102–5*C*). A third incision is made vertically in the temporalis fossa, and this is connected with the two previous incisions. While making these osteotomies, two malleable retractors are used to retract and protect both the orbital contents and the temporalis muscle. Once the osteotomy is completed, the fragment of bone is preserved in warm saline until it is repositioned at the end of the procedure. The bony opening is enlarged posteriorly using rongeurs. The lateral wall is nibbled away until the hard bone is reached, signifying the junction of the orbital rim with the wall of the middle cranial fossa. Bleeding is controlled with bone wax. At this point one has an excellent view of the superotemperal portions of the periorbita. The periorbita is then incised with one vertical and one horizontal incision to form a T (see Fig. 102–5*D*). Once the periorbita is open, orbital fat will spontaneously prolapse. To enter the intraconal space, it is necessary to identify the lateral rectus muscle, which is placed on a traction suture and retracted inferiorly or superiorly depending on which sector one plans to explore. The dissection is carried out with caution, with the use of blunt neurosurgical or orbital dissectors, a headlight, and operating loupes. Only rarely is the operating microscope necessary to distinguish the fine structures at the orbital apex. After carefully dissecting the tumor from the neighboring vital structures, it can be extracted either with a standard forceps (see Figs. 102–5*E* and 102–5*F*) or using a standard retinal cryoprobe. The cryoprobe facilitates traction on the tumor without the risk of capsular rupture and consequent diffusion of neoplastic cells.

After the resection, the bed is inspected for bleeding sites before closure of the periorbita. The periorbita is not closed too tightly, to allow any postoperative blood to escape. An aspirating drain further assists in the evacuation of any blood. The bony fragment is drilled and repositioned in place (see Fig. 102–5*G*). It has traditionally been fixated with stainless steel sutures. However, if magnetic resonance imaging is contemplated, use of a nonmetallic suture is suggested. The periosteum is closed over the orbital rim and zygomatic arch, which will bring into anatomic position the temporalis muscle and the lateral canthal ligament. A drain is placed in the temporal fossa and exits through a stab incision in the cheek. The skin and subcutaneous layers are closed in two layers using a running suture of 3-0 Prolene through the dermis and 6-0 interrupted nylon through the skin. A compressive dressing is applied. The skin sutures are removed in 5 days and the running Prolene suture is removed in 10 days. There is generally a significant amount of postoperative edema, which peaks in 48 hours, and there may be transient dysfunction of the extraocular muscles. We prefer to prescribe a corticosteroid and antibiotic postoperatively.

The procedure described represents a standard lateral orbitotomy; however, in selected cases to obtain the best possible cosmetic result, we sometimes use a bicoronal scalp incision, which results in a scar entirely concealed beneath the hair and which also allows a greater surgical exposure.[5] The surgical details of this technique are described elsewhere.

MEDIAL APPROACH

The medial approach is utilized for localized orbital masses medial to the optic nerve (Fig. 102–6).[5]

Deep lesions located medial to the optic nerve are the least accessible to an ophthalmologic approach. The approaches inappropriately called medial orbitotomy described in the surgical literature are in effect modifications of the anterior approach. The approach that we use in these circumstances is a compromise between the superomedial subperiosteal approach and the neurosurgical transfrontal approach; it gives a better exposure than the former and with less danger than the latter. With the goal of gaining more exposure to the medial orbit, we use a coronal incision and a 360-degree incision through the orbital periosteum at its bony insertion. The orbital contents, thus freed from their bony attachments, can be subluxated laterally through a lateral wall osteotomy of the temporal fossa, thus giving a wide exposure to the medial sector of the orbit.

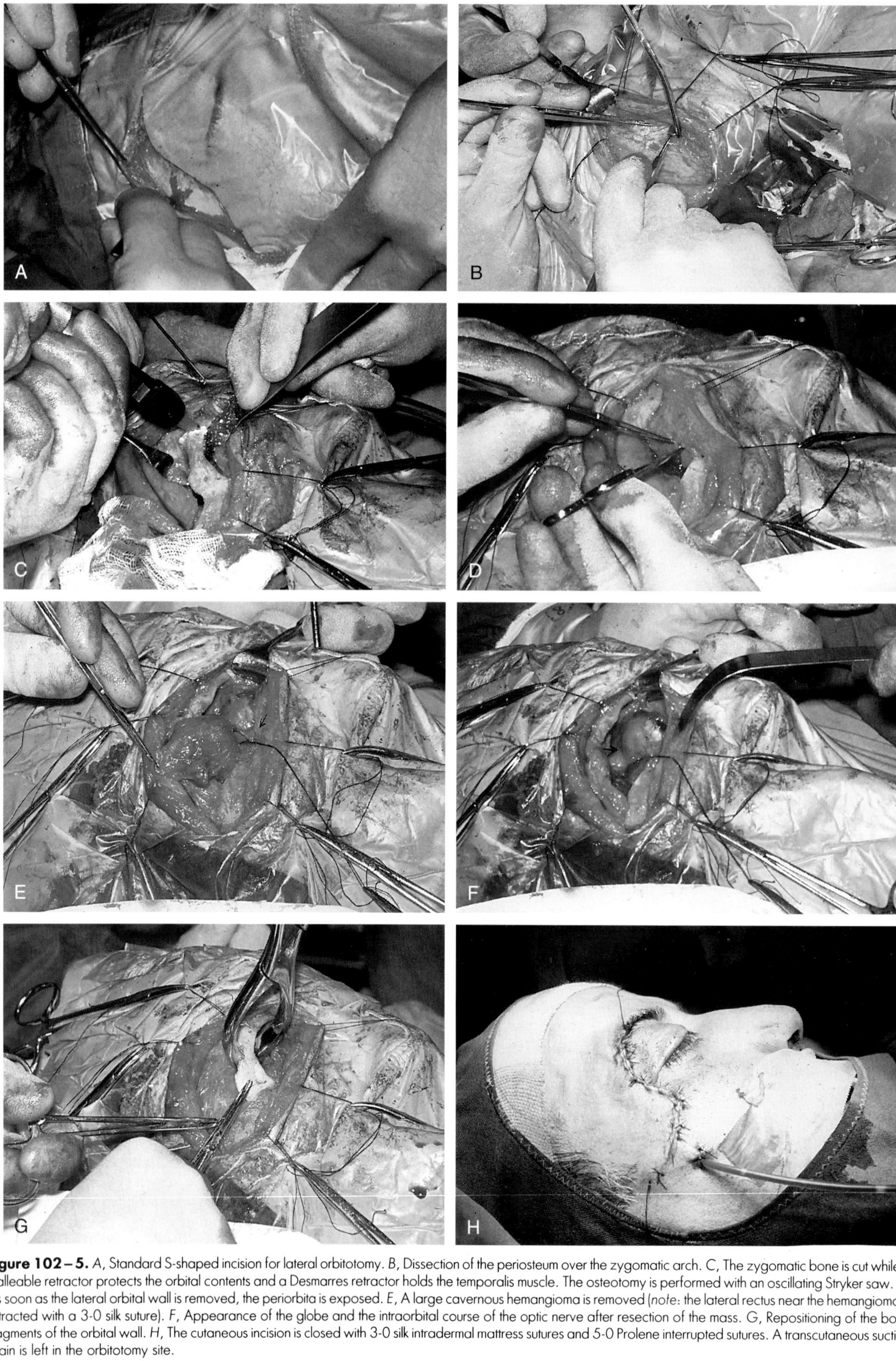

Figure 102–5. *A*, Standard S-shaped incision for lateral orbitotomy. *B*, Dissection of the periosteum over the zygomatic arch. C, The zygomatic bone is cut while a malleable retractor protects the orbital contents and a Desmarres retractor holds the temporalis muscle. The osteotomy is performed with an oscillating Stryker saw. *D*, As soon as the lateral orbital wall is removed, the periorbita is exposed. *E*, A large cavernous hemangioma is removed (*note*: the lateral rectus near the hemangioma is retracted with a 3-0 silk suture). *F*, Appearance of the globe and the intraorbital course of the optic nerve after resection of the mass. *G*, Repositioning of the bone fragments of the orbital wall. *H*, The cutaneous incision is closed with 3-0 silk intradermal mattress sutures and 5-0 Prolene interrupted sutures. A transcutaneous suction drain is left in the orbitotomy site.

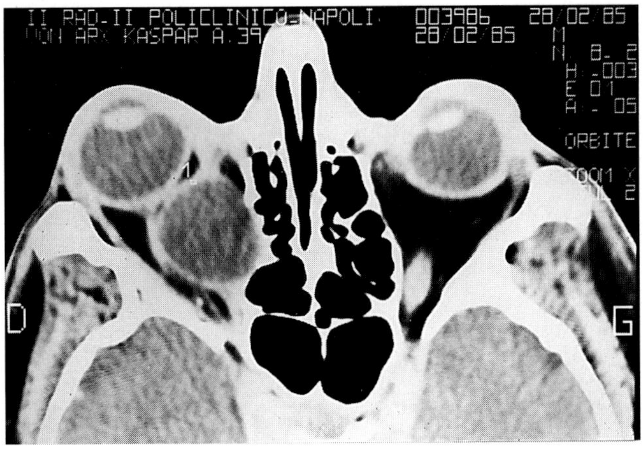

Figure 102–6. Computed tomographic scan of a cystic lesion medial to the optic nerve in the deep orbit. This is the typical situation for the use of a modified medial orbitotomy.

The line of the incision parallels the coronal suture from one tragus to the other, with a lazy V at the center to allow accurate repositioning of the coronal flap at the end of the procedure (Fig. 102–7*A*). Saline solution is injected beneath the scalp to facilitate the dissection off the skull (see Fig. 102–7*B*). The incision is carried through the skin and subcutaneous layers and galea to the periosteum centrally and down to the temporalis fascial plane laterally. The superficial temporal arterial branches that lie superior and anterior to the ear should be identified and ligated before cutting them. Once the incision has been completed, the dissection is carried out in the surgical space of Meckel, which is the plane between the galea and the periosteum of the skull. The dissection in the temporal region is kept deep, at the level of the temporalis fascia, to avoid damage to the branches of the facial nerve, which travel in the subdermal level (see Fig. 102–7*C*). At the temporal region the dissection exposes the fat pad that is situated between a split in the temporalis fascia immediately above the zygomatic arch. The arrival of the dissection to the depth of the fat pad assures the surgeon that the dissection is deep enough. The dissection is much easier in the central region because the scalp separates easily from the underlying skull (see Fig. 102–7*D*). The dissection stops 1 cm above the orbital rim. At this point the periosteum is incised parallel to the superior orbital rim (see Fig. 102–7*E*). The dissection then continues subperiosteally to the superior orbital rim. At this point the emergence of the supraorbital nerve and artery can be seen. The supraorbital neurovascular bundle emerges either from a canal through the bone or a notch at the rim. If it emerges through a canal, a mallet and osteotome are used to open the canal and free the bundle so that it can be mobilized inferiorly. This allows access to the superior orbit through the subperiosteal space. The periosteum is stripped along the lateral and superior orbital walls. The dissection is continued to the lateral aspect of the lateral wall where the temporalis muscle is separated from the lateral aspect of the zygoma (see Fig. 102–7*F*). A lateral wall osteotomy is performed, similar to the standard lateral orbitotomy (see Fig. 102–7*G*). This allows a wide access to the lateral and superior orbit. With the use of a periosteal elevator, the dissection is continued along the orbital floor, in a medial direction, until the nasolacrimal canal is reached. At this point, the entire orbital contents are freed of any attachments to the bone along the orbital walls and rim. To complete the mobilization of the orbital contents, the deep medial dissection should free the bony insertion of the trochlea and the anterior and posterior ethmoidal arteries must be cauterized and cut. At this point it is possible to mobilize the entire orbital contents laterally through the lateral orbitotomy (see Fig. 102–7*H*). The surgical exposure thus obtained is about 2 cm wider than the standard superomedial orbitotomy. This also reduces traction and pressure on the optic nerve by providing a preventive orbital decompression laterally.

The periorbita is incised vertically between the body of the superior oblique and the levator, which allows access to the intraconal space (see Fig. 102–7*I*). The tumor can now be resected with the aid of the cryoprobe (see Fig. 102–7*J*). After the resection, the lateral bone is refixated, and the temporal muscle is reinserted on the periosteum of the lateral orbital wall (see Fig. 102–7*K*), and the scalp is closed with interrupted sutures of 3-0 nylon. Suction drains are inserted bilaterally, concluding the operation (see Fig. 102–7*L*).

COMBINED PROCEDURES*

Combined procedures are those surgical techniques that use a combination of two different approaches to provide improved exposure.[6] Two combined procedures frequently used in orbital surgery are the combined transcutaneous and transconjunctival technique and the combined transfrontal neurosurgical and lateral orbital approach.

Combined Lateral and Inferior Orbitotomy

A lateral orbitotomy can be combined with an inferior fornix-based flap. This technique may be useful in the excision of large inferiorly located lesions. It consists of a Berke orbitotomy and the extension of the incision laterally. The transconjunctival incision in the inferior fornix is combined with a lateral canthotomy and inferior cantholysis to allow wide exposure of the floor and medial and lateral walls of the orbit (Fig. 102–8).

*This section was translated by Maurizio Sentella.

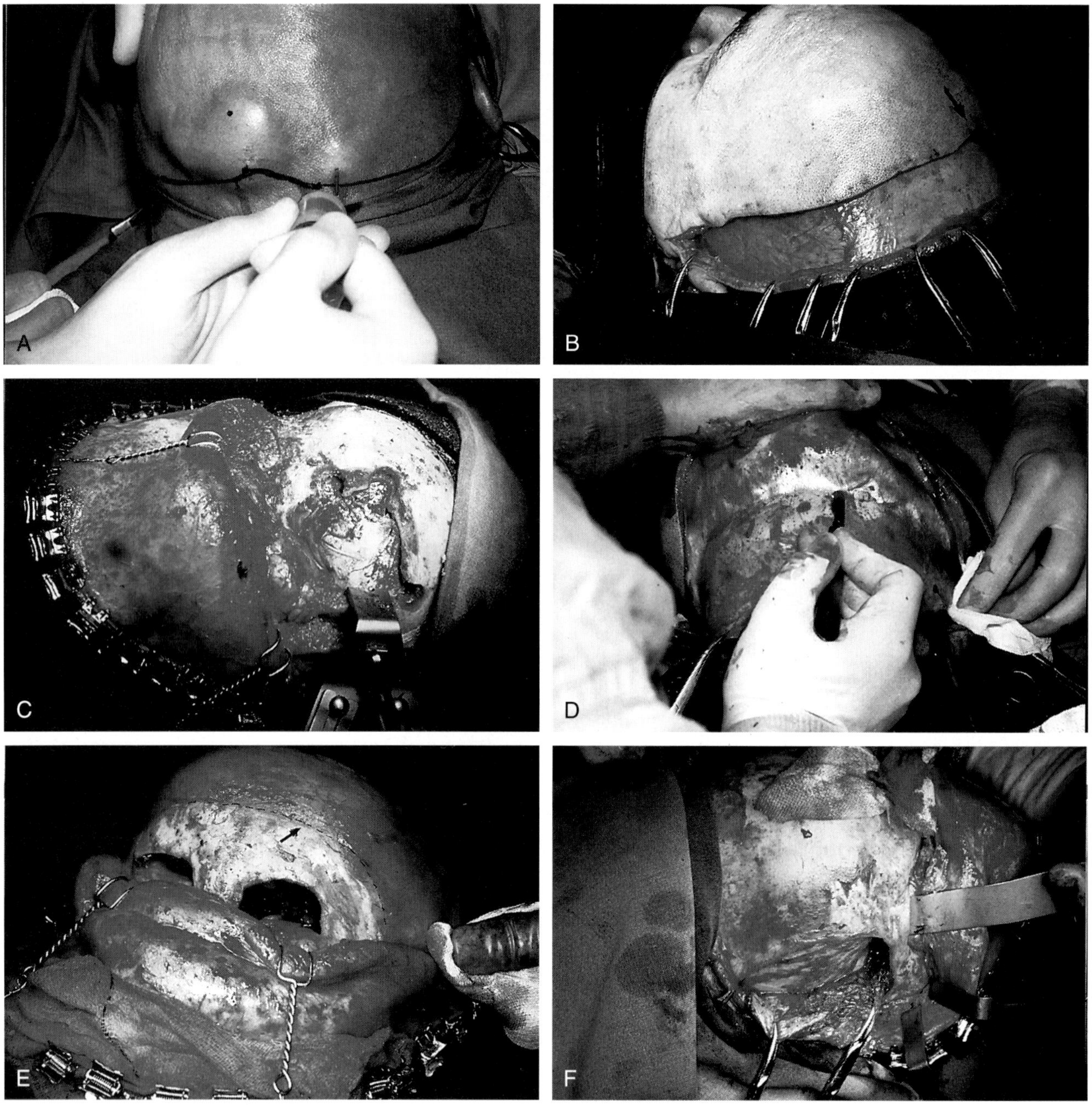

Figure 102–7. *A*, A "lazy V" incision and subcutaneous infiltration. *B*, A deep incision is made into the periosteum (the *arrow* indicates V-shaped coronal flap). *C*, Dissection to the level of the temporalis muscle (*note*: the fat pad above the levator aponeurosis is exposed). *D*, Separation of the periosteum 2 cm above the orbital rim. *E*, Exposure of the orbital rim (*dashed line*) (note: limited between the subperiosteal dissection and the extraperiosteal dissection). *F*, Exposure of the temporal fossa after resection of the temporalis muscle and then exposure of the lateral orbital wall.

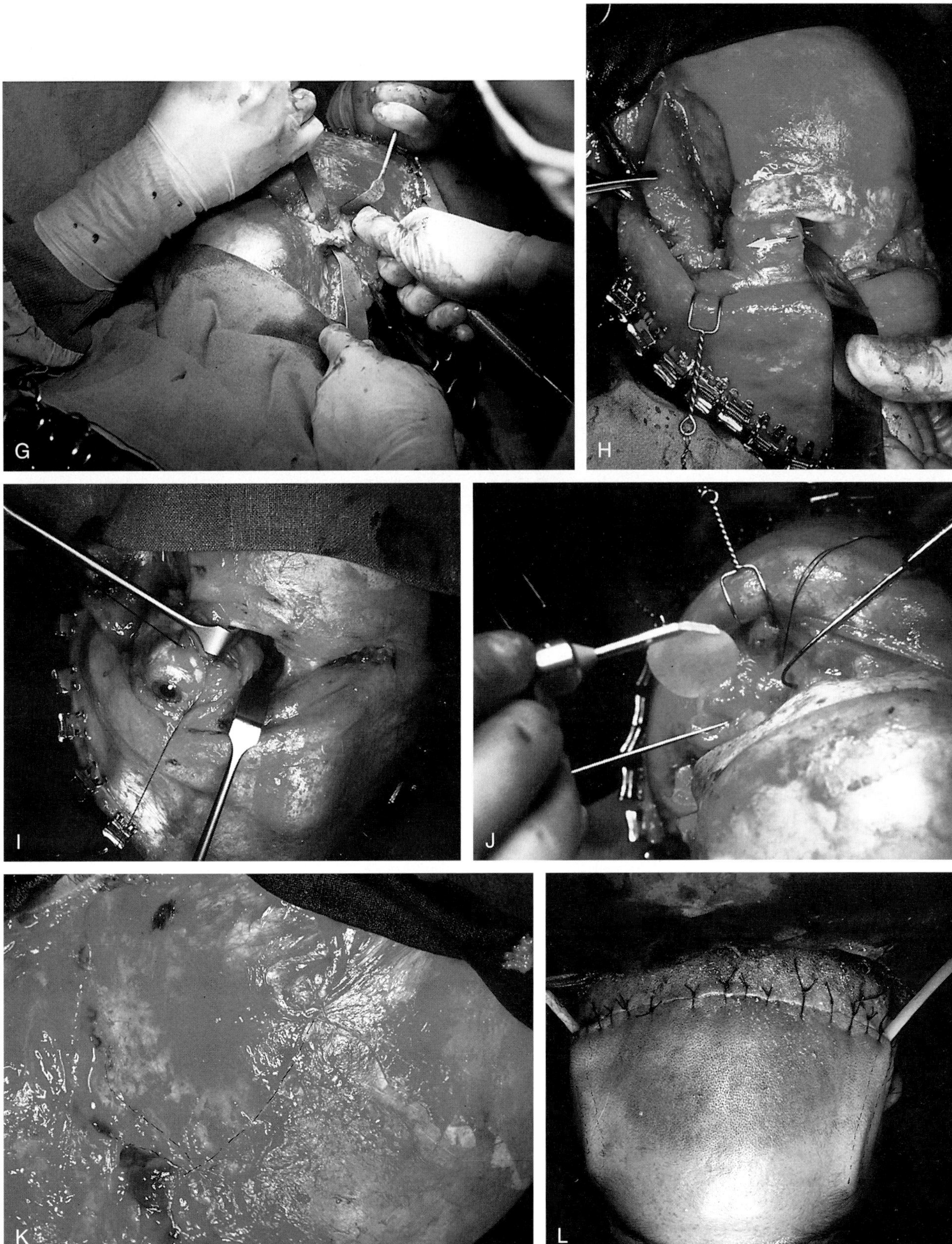

Figure 102–7 *Continued.* *G*, Osteotomy of the lateral orbital wall. *H*, Lateral displacement (*arrow*) of the temporal fossa with the orbital contents. *I*, After opening the orbital fascia, the globe is free to move laterally in the temporal fossa, providing ample exposure of the nasal segment of the orbit. *J*, Dissection and resection of a large echinococcus cyst removed with a cryoprobe. *K*, Appearance after repositioning the orbital rim and the temporalis muscle and resuturing the surgical site (the *dashed line* shows the suture site). *L*, Cutaneous sutures and bilateral drains.

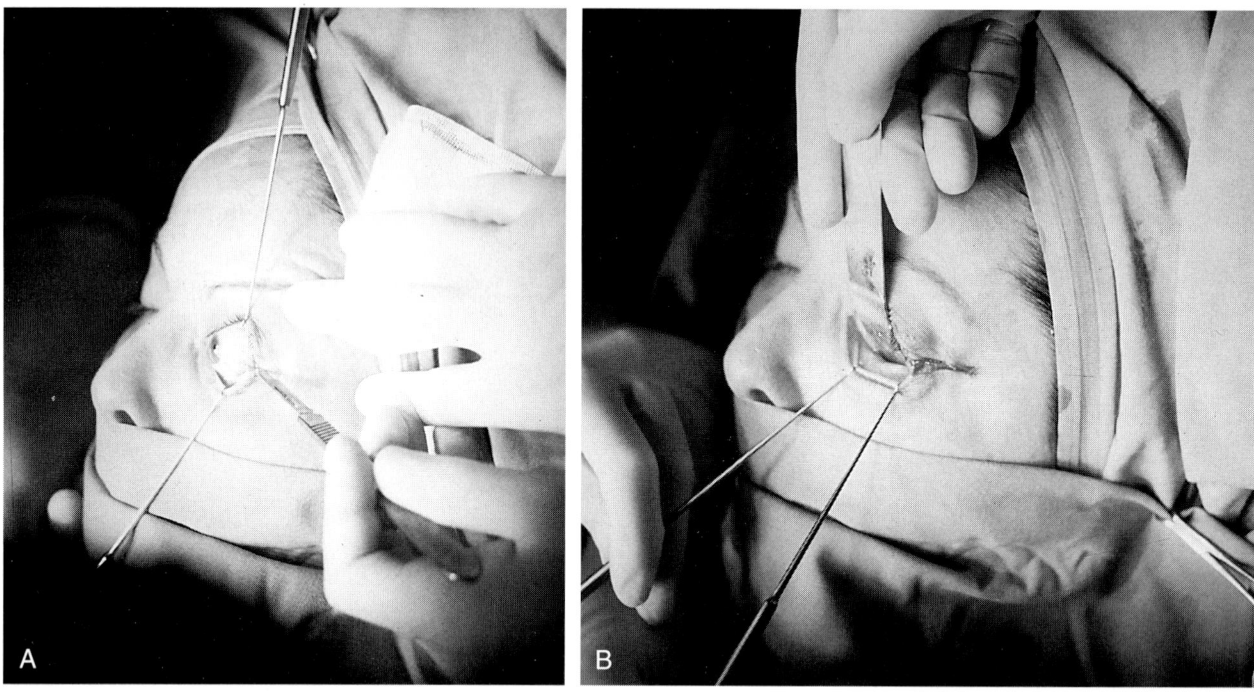

Figure 102–8. *A*, Lateral cantholyses. *B*, Exposure of the orbital floor after a transconjunctival incision in the inferior fornix.

Combined Superior and Lateral Orbitotomy

This technique allows the en bloc resection of the superior and lateral walls of the orbit.

The panoramic orbitotomy (Fig. 102–9) is the preferred method for accessing the orbital apex. This procedure allows the resection of the superior and lateral orbital walls with adequate exposure of the adjacent intracranial structures. In short, this approach consists of a coronal incision and removal of a segment of frontal bone. This is followed by the dissection of the temporal fossa and of the periorbita. Osteotomies can be made on the orbital roof near the zygomaticotemporal suture that will allow en bloc resection of the superior and lateral orbital walls. This approach is particularly indicated with apical orbital tumors or combined orbital and intracranial lesions, such as tumors of the optic nerve or sphenoid wing.

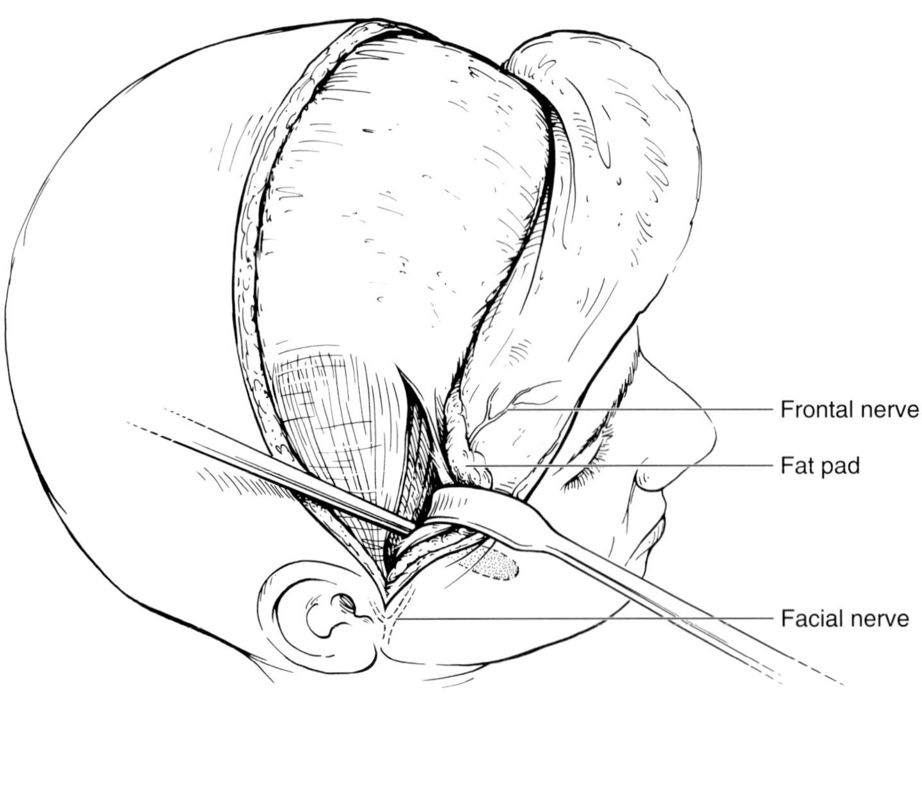

Figure 102–9. Complete exposure of the cranial fossa and orbits through a panoramic orbitotomy.

REFERENCES

1. Knap A: Un cas de carcinome de la gaine externe du nerf optique, extirpe en conservant l'oeil. Arch Augenheilked Ohrenhilkunde 2:209, 1875.
2. Rollet: Arch Ophthalmol 27:273, 1907.
3. Benedict WL: Surgical treatment of tumors and cysts of the orbit. Am J Ophthalmol 32:763–773, 1949.
4. Krohel GB, Stewart WB, et al: Orbital Disease: A Practical Approach. New York, Grune & Stratton, 1981, pp 102–111.
5. Buonavolonta G: Acta XXIV, International Congress of Ophthalmology 2:1036, 1982.
6. Rootman J: Disease of the Orbit. Philadelphia, JB Lippincott, 1988, pp 597–598.

CHAPTER 103

Orbital Exenteration

Peter S. Levin

Orbital exenteration is the removal of the eye and entire orbital contents, including the eyelids, ocular muscles, and orbital fat. Because of the radical nature of this procedure and the relatively poor reconstructive alternatives, orbital exenteration is usually only performed after other therapies have failed or are deemed inappropriate.

INDICATIONS

Orbital exenteration is generally performed to cure presumed life-threatening neoplasms or infections or to treat severe orbital pain or deformity.[1] Since exenteration is severely disfiguring, it is performed only if there is a reasonable expectation that disease or deformity will be eliminated. Consultation with medical or radiation oncologists, otolaryngologists, or hospital-based tumor boards may help to evaluate the patient for metastatic disease and educate the patient on treatment options.

The most frequent reason for performing exenteration is to treat presumed life-threatening neoplasia. The histopathologic processes leading to orbital exenteration in six large series are shown in Table 103–1.[1–6] Predominant in frequency are the epithelial malignancies, particularly squamous cell, basal cell, and sebaceous carcinoma.

The sites of the primary malignancy accounting for orbital exenteration are by no means limited to the orbit and may include the eyelid skin, facial skin, and paranasal sinuses (Table 103–2). The high incidence of eyelid and facial skin lesions leading to exenteration lends support to current concepts in management of periocular cutaneous neoplasms that recommend early and definitive treatment.[7, 8]

Primary paranasal sinus tumors may involve the orbit in as many as 60% of cases at the time of detection.[9, 10] Interestingly, in three of our reported 18 cases of exenteration for presumed orbitosinus disease,[1] no intraorbital tumor was found. This attests to the difficulty in determining the spread of sinus disease into the orbit and to the tendency of surgeons to pursue aggressive extirpation of tissue in the pursuit of tumor-free margins. It is hoped that current orbitosinus examination and imaging techniques can be trusted to exclude orbital involvement with neoplasia and allow preservation of the orbit without diminishing the chances for cure.[11, 12]

Current trends in orbital and ocular oncology have diminished the indications for orbital exenteration in many specific disease entities. In the management of conjunctival squamous cell carcinoma[13] and melanoma,[14] recent trends favor local resection of involved tissue without exenteration, as long as the tumor remains superficial. Exenteration is generally only proposed after failure of previous nonsurgical therapies for rhabdomyosarcoma.[15] Although the issue remains controversial, orbital exenteration does not appear to improve the poor prognosis of patients with intraocular melanoma with extrascleral extension.[16–18]

In our review of orbital exenteration at Duke (1969–1988),[1] exenterations were performed for what later histopathologic examination showed to be one case of a benign lymphoepithelial lesion (Mikulicz's syndrome), two cases of intraepithelial carcinoma of the conjunctiva, and one case of benign mixed tumor of the lacrimal gland. This experience reinforces the importance of establishing certain histopathologic diagnoses by conclusive biopsy before exenteration.

Orbital exenteration is performed to treat life-threatening infection, usually of fungal origin in a diabetic or immunocompromised host. Fungi multiply in the paranasal sinuses and invade the orbit by contiguous spread. Although orbital exenteration may be indicated along with débridement of the sinus cavities, some cases can be successfully managed without orbital exenteration.[19, 20]

Exenteration has been used to treat benign processes such as severe orbital contracture with pain and inability to wear a prosthesis,[21] disfiguring (but not life threatening) proptosis from orbital tumors such as meningioma and lymphangioma,[1] severe unremitting orbital inflammatory processes,[6] and neurofibromatosis with orbital deformity and visual loss.[22]

This chapter was supported in part by a grant from Research to Prevent Blindness, Inc., New York, New York.

TABLE 103-1

A Comparison of Orbital Exenteration at Six Institutions*

	Wilmer Institute 1927–1953 (N = 48)	Univeristy of California at San Francisco 1940–1971 (N = 48)	University of Kansas 1951–1964 (N = 31)	Mayo Clinic 1967–1986 (N = 102)	University of Naples 1976–1986 (N = 39)	Duke University 1969–1988 (N = 99)
Squamous cell carcinoma	4	6	3	33	7	32
Skin	3	2	1	NA	6	12
Sinus	1	0	2	NA	1	13
Conjunctiva	0	3	0	NA	0	6
Tear sac	0	1	0	NA	0	1
Basal cell carcinoma	11	14	11	21	9	8
Sebaceous carcinoma	0	1	0	6	0	6
Other epithelial tumors	6	8	5	9	10	15
Malignant melanoma	12	8	7	16	8	18
Conjunctiva	3	5	NA	NA	1	10
Sinus	0	0	NA	NA	0	3
Choroid	9	2	NA	8	7	1
Other	0	1	NA	NA	0	4
Rhabdomyosarcoma	2	5	2	2	2	2
Infectious	1	0	0	1	0	6
Other	12	6	3	14	3	12

*At Wilmer, University of California at San Francisco, and University of Naples only, exenterations performed by ophthalmology departments were surveyed; at University of Kansas, Mayo Clinic, and Duke University, all exenterations were reported, regardless of the department performing the operation.
NA, no data available.
From Levin PS, Dutton JJ: A 20-year series of orbital exenteration. Am J Ophthalmol 112:496–501, 1991.

TECHNIQUE

Orbital exenteration is surgical excision of the entire orbital contents including the periorbita. However, this procedure must be tailored to the specific disease entity. Anteriorly invasive processes, such as cutaneous or conjunctival tumors, can sometimes be successfully treated by removal of the conjunctiva, globe, and anterior orbital structures without excision of the mid and posterior orbital tissues. Primary orbital disease with bony involvement, such as some lacrimal gland tumors and diseases arising in contiguous cavities (e.g., the paranasal sinuses or the skull base), may require removal of the orbit, adjacent bone, sinuses, and soft tissues.

With the patient under general anesthesia, the eyelids are sewn closed and sutures are left long to allow mobilization of the specimen. The bony orbital margin is marked, and infiltrative anesthetic is injected to aid with hemostasis (Fig. 103–1). The scalpel or cutting cautery is used to incise skin, orbicularis, and periosteum down to the bony orbital margin (Fig. 103–2). The procedure may be slightly modified by saving the skin and muscle of the eyelid if they are normal, but there is no advantage to preserving the eyelashes and eyelid margin. If the skin and muscle are involved with tumor, then clear margins

TABLE 103-2

Orbital Exenteration for Presumed Life-Threatening Malignancy: Duke University 1969–1988

Site of Neoplasm	No. of Cases (N = 89)
Eyelid skin	20
Paranasal sinuses	18
Conjunctiva	18
Orbit excluding lacrimal gland	14
Skin excluding eyelid	13
Lacrimal gland	4
Ocular	1
Unknown	1

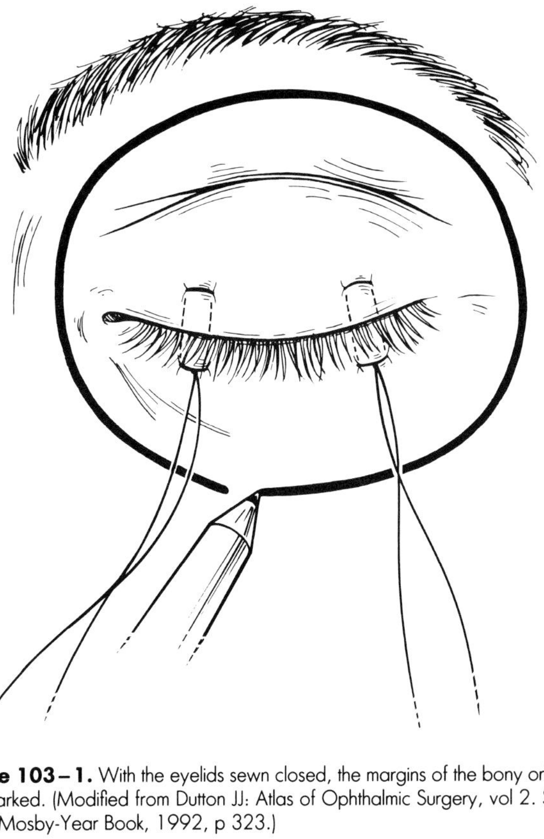

Figure 103–1. With the eyelids sewn closed, the margins of the bony orbit are marked. (Modified from Dutton JJ: Atlas of Ophthalmic Surgery, vol 2. St. Louis, Mosby-Year Book, 1992, p 323.)

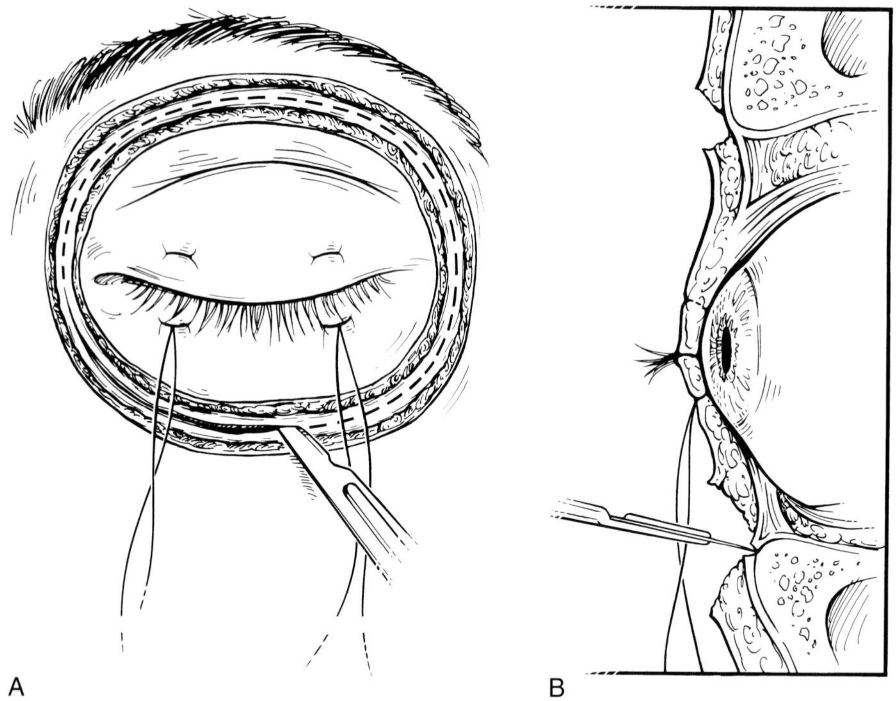

Figure 103–2. Skin, muscle, and periosteum are incised, exposing the bone of the orbital margin. (Modified from Dutton JJ: Atlas of Ophthalmic Surgery, vol 2. St. Louis, Mosby-Year Book, 1992, p 323.)

can be obtained using frozen section techniques. A periosteal elevator separates the periorbita from the bony orbit along the entire circumference of the cavity (Fig. 103–3). At the inferior and superior orbital fissures, trochlea, lateral orbital tubercle, and the origin of the inferior oblique muscle, the periorbita is closely fixed to bone but can be freed with careful dissection. Special care is taken in the superior orbit, since violation of the superior bony orbit may predispose to cerebrospinal fluid leak,[23] and at the thin lamina papyracea of the medial orbit, since penetration may result in a fistulous tract with the ethmoidal sinus. The nasolacrimal duct should be cut as it enters the bony nasolacrimal canal. The canal can be followed surgically into the nose, if tumor has involved the lacrimal drainage system.[24]

An enucleation scissors or wire snare[25] is used to divide the specimen from the orbital apex (Fig. 103–4). The specimen is removed, and the orbital cavity is packed with gauze to achieve hemostasis. After 5 to 10 minutes, the packs are removed and any bleeding vessels are cau-

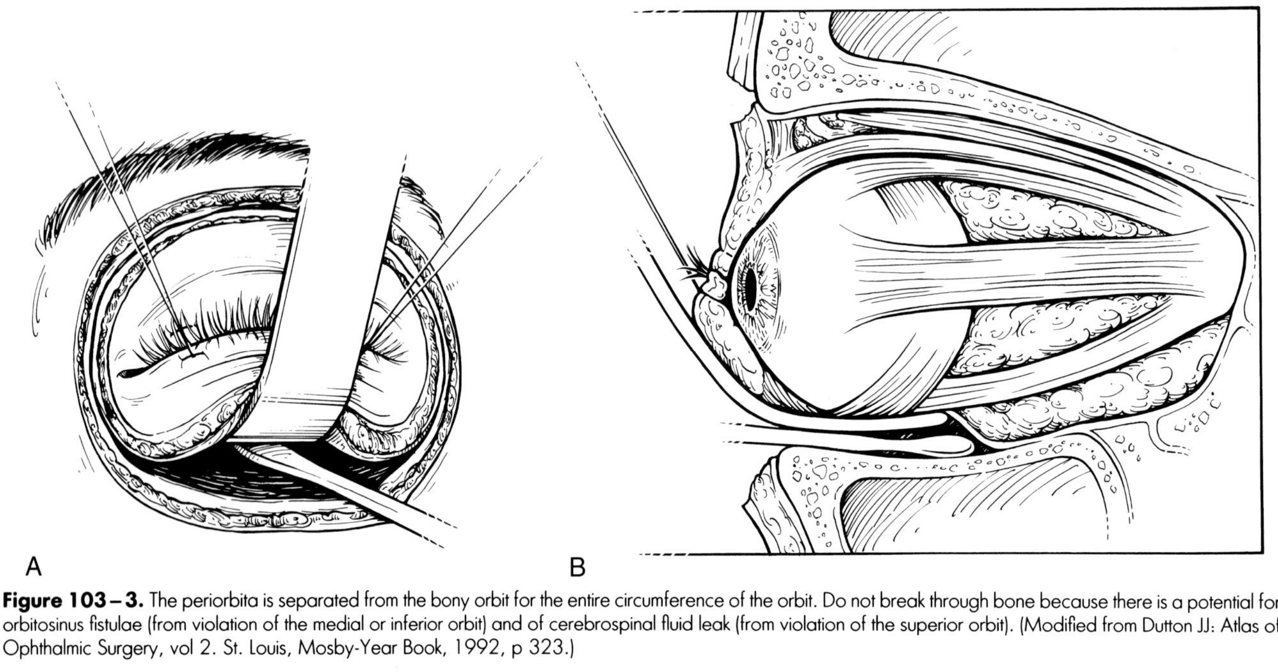

Figure 103–3. The periorbita is separated from the bony orbit for the entire circumference of the orbit. Do not break through bone because there is a potential for orbitosinus fistulae (from violation of the medial or inferior orbit) and of cerebrospinal fluid leak (from violation of the superior orbit). (Modified from Dutton JJ: Atlas of Ophthalmic Surgery, vol 2. St. Louis, Mosby-Year Book, 1992, p 323.)

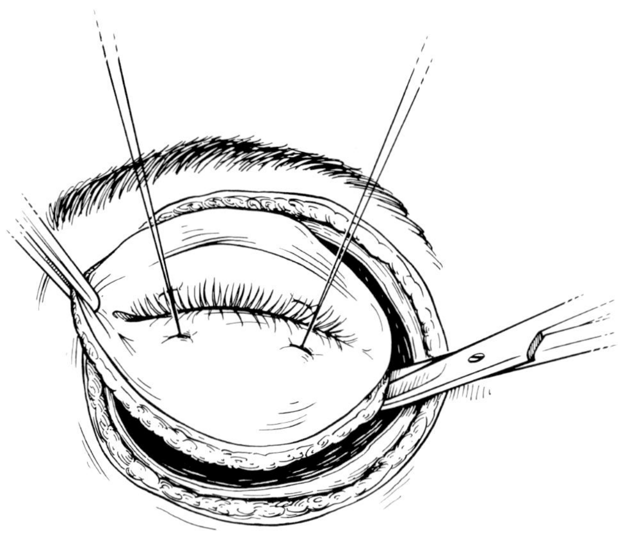

Figure 103–4. The specimen is cut at the orbital apex and delivered. The orbital cavity is packed with gauze. (Modified from Dutton JJ: Atlas of Ophthalmic Surgery, vol 2. St. Louis, Mosby-Year Book, 1992, p 323.)

terized (Fig. 103–5). The most apical tissue, which is difficult to remove, can be excised with the scalpel or scissors. Cautery is only used conservatively since it will prevent histopathologic examination of apical tissues and has been implicated in cerebrospinal fluid leaks after exenteration. Once hemostasis is obtained the surgeon

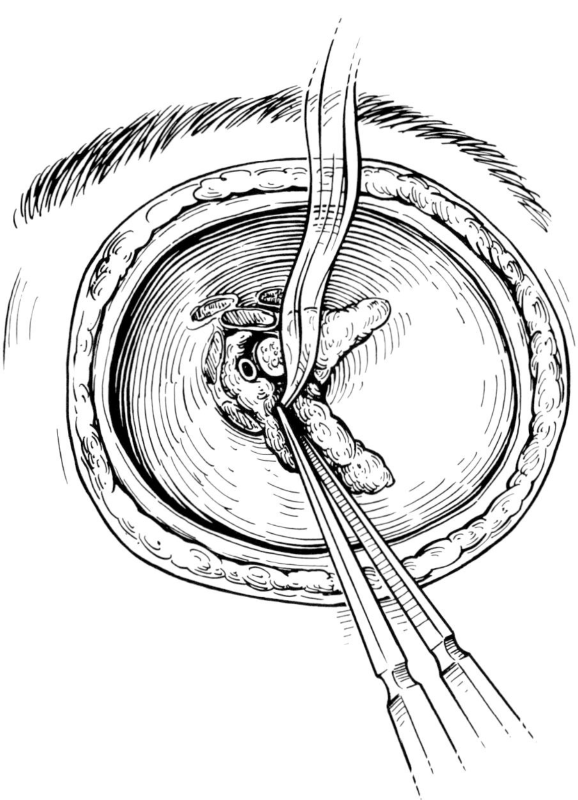

Figure 103–5. After the orbital packing is removed, conservative electrocautery may be needed to obtain hemostasis. (Modified from Dutton JJ: Atlas of Ophthalmic Surgery, vol 2. St. Louis, Mosby-Year Book, 1992, p 323.)

turns to the reconstructive options discussed in the next section.

Complications of orbital exenteration include bleeding from the ophthalmic artery and its branches, fistulas between the sinuses and orbit, and cerebrospinal fluid leaks.[23] Most fistulas result from inadvertent penetration of the lamina papyracea during surgery, causing chronic hygiene problems, malodorous discharge, difficulty in blowing the nose, or change in voice.[26] The exact cause of cerebrospinal fluid leaks is uncertain, but leaks from the superior orbital roof have been reported, possibly due to iatrogenic defects in the bone or the application of monopolar cautery.[6, 23]

RECONSTRUCTIVE AND PROSTHETIC OPTIONS

Surgery must incorporate a reconstructive plan that achieves several goals.[27] First, in cases of malignancy, a solution must be sought that allows for detection of recurrent disease. Second, when contiguous structures are violated, the boundaries between the orbit and adjacent cavities such as the brain, sinuses, and nasopharynx need to be re-established. Third, the optimal aesthetic result must be pursued, remembering that most patients wish to camouflage their surgical defect by using patches or oculofacial prostheses. With these goals in mind, the physician depends on local, regional, and distant surgical solutions as well as skilled prosthetic solutions to the problems of the exenterated orbit.[27, 28]

After removal of the surgical specimen, the orbit may be left to heal by granulation. The empty socket is packed with sponges coated with an antibiotic-lubricant for several days while the patient is maintained on systemic antibiotics. After the dressing is removed, the cavity is cleaned daily with soap or hydrogen peroxide. In about 3 months the apex of the orbital cavity is filled by granulation tissues and is covered by squamous epithelium. A simple eye patch or an oculofacial prosthesis can be placed over the orbit. This simple and effective technique is particularly well suited to the critically ill patient since operative time is minimized. A disadvantage is the occasional contraction of adjacent tissues, most visibly the eyebrow.[29]

Another local solution to the problems of the exenterated socket is to place a split-thickness skin graft.[30] A dermatome is applied to the anterior thigh, and a 0.015-inch thick skin graft is harvested. The donor site is covered with topical ointment or an occlusive membranous dressing. The graft is carefully spread over several pieces of lubricated gauze and then draped into the orbital cavity. At the orbital margin, the graft is sewn to the patient's skin with chromic sutures. The orbit is packed with lubricated gauze, and systemic antibiotics are initiated. One to 2 weeks later, the packing is removed and the socket has largely epithelialized. Split-thickness grafts provide for speedier healing than does healing by granulation. Like sockets that heal by granulation, the cavity may be covered by a patch or prosthesis, and recurrent disease may be detected by inspection.

Many other techniques have been described that depend on the local vascularity of the exenteration cavity to ensure healing. Dermal grafts have been substituted for split-thickness skin grafts as an orbital lining.[31] In cases in which the eyelid skin has been preserved, the eyelids may be sewn together over the empty orbital cavity[32] or over a methyl methacrylate implant.[33] Regional flaps and distant flaps or composite grafts may be used at the time of initial exenteration or after a disease-free interval has passed. These procedures bring tissue into the orbit to partially or completely fill the orbital cavity. When contiguous cavities have been violated, these techniques can also separate the orbit from adjacent structures. As the orbital cavity is shallowed, however, the ability to detect recurrent disease by physical examination is compromised. This is unimportant after exenteration for infection or deformity but very important in following patients with malignant processes. Although shallowing the orbital cavity often has great aesthetic advantages, oculofacial prostheses cannot be fitted over an extremely shallow orbital cavity.

Many regional and distant solutions to the problems of the exenterated socket have been described.[27] Such solutions may involve rotation of the temporalis muscle[34-37] or forehead tissues[38, 39] into the orbit, use of a temporoparietal fascia flat[27, 40, 41] or a long pectoralis muscle flap,[42] or anastomosis of a free composite graft such as

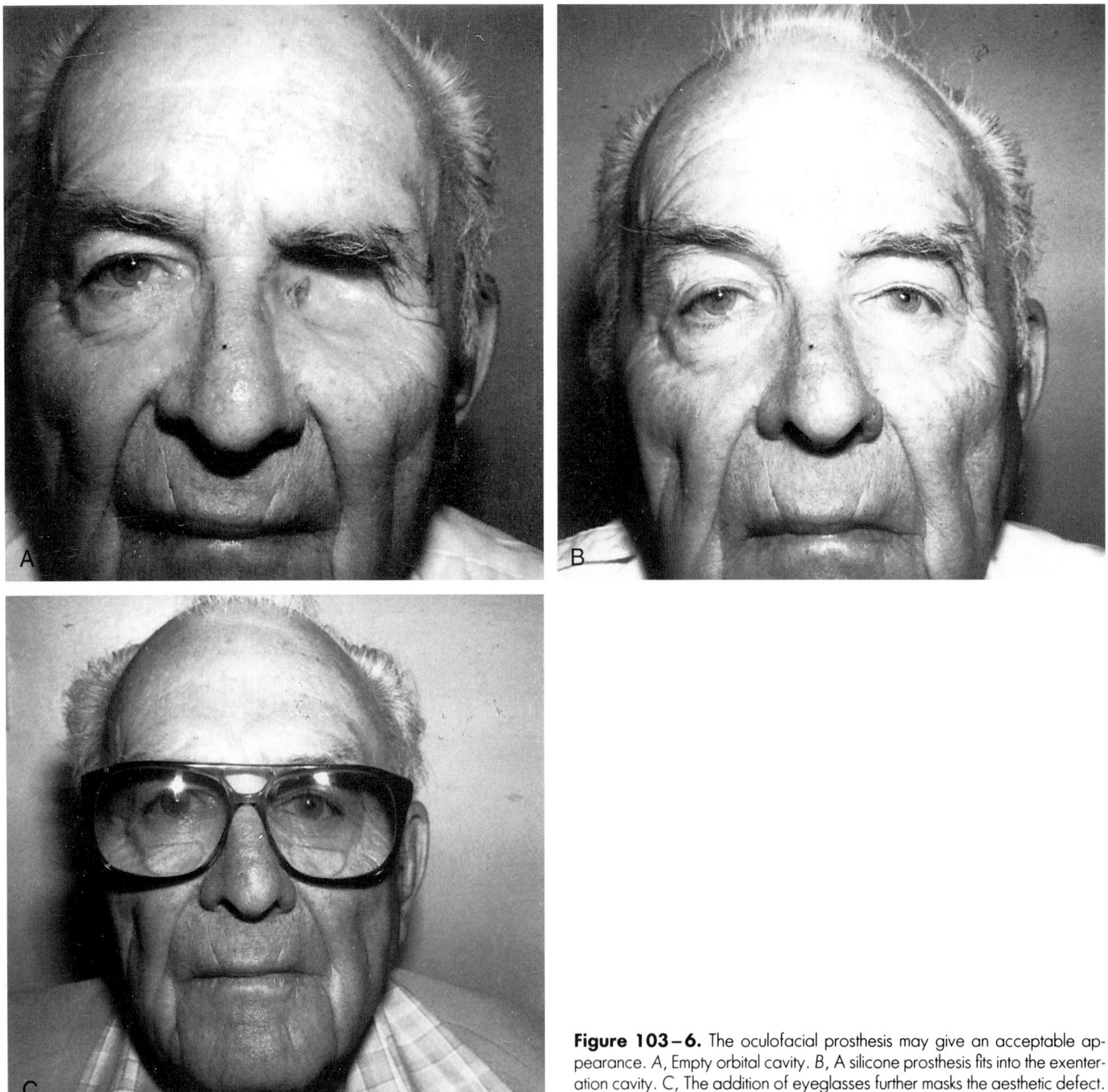

Figure 103–6. The oculofacial prosthesis may give an acceptable appearance. *A*, Empty orbital cavity. *B*, A silicone prosthesis fits into the exenteration cavity. *C*, The addition of eyeglasses further masks the aesthetic defect. (*A* to *C* courtesy of Steven Young, BCO.)

that from the latissimus dorsi.[43] Selection of the optimal procedure is highly individual and depends on the specific surgical defect and the needs of the patient.

Prostheses

Wearing a simple occlusive patch is an inexpensive and simple measure that many patients choose. The patch can fit over the empty cavity and covers the defect. The result is a rugged image that many patients, particularly men, find acceptable. Since patients are often concerned that the patch may become dislodged and expose their deformity, surgical sponges, towels, or custom-made silicone moulages may be placed beneath the patch.

Contemporary oculofacial prostheses consist of a standard methacrylate ocular prosthesis mimicking the eye coupled to a silicone mold that fills the orbital defect and matches the opposite side. The appearance of these prostheses can be outstanding, particularly when viewed head-on (Fig. 103–6). Spectacles with concave lenses may be incorporated to help mask the defect. However, even the best prostheses are imperfect. Neither the prosthetic eyelids nor the eye moves. Even when the colored silicone is made to match the color of adjacent skin, exposure to sun and wind may bring out stark contrast between the prosthesis and neighboring skin. Prostheses have the potential to become dislodged, which can be a constant worry to some patients.

Borrowing from dental technology, prostheses can now be integrated to the orbital and facial skeleton by linking the prosthesis to titanium screws incorporated into the bony orbit.[44, 45] The great advantage of this technique is in preventing migration and displacement of the prosthesis. It is too early to know if this technology will gain widespread acceptance.

CONCLUSION

Orbital exenteration remains the treatment of last resort for patients with severe orbital problems. Before performing orbital exenteration, the physician and patient must consider alternatives to exenteration, the extent to which orbital and adjacent tissues should be excised, and the means by which the empty orbital cavity will be covered or masked.

REFERENCES

1. Levin PS, Dutton JJ: A 20-year series of orbital exenteration. Am J Ophthalmol 112:496–501, 1991.
2. Naquin HA: Exenteration of the orbit. Arch Ophthalmol 51:850, 1954.
3. Rathbun JE, Beard C, Quickert MH: Evaluation of 48 cases or orbital exenteration. Am J Ophthalmol 72:191, 1971.
4. Simons JN, Robinson DW, Masters FW: Malignant tumors of the orbit and periorbital structures treated by exenteration. Plast Reconstr Surg 37:100, 1966.
5. Bartley GB, Garrity JA, Waller RR, et al: Orbital exenteration at the Mayo Clinic: 1967–1986. Ophthalmology 96:468, 1989.
6. de Conciliis C, Bonavolontà G: Incidence and treatment of dural exposure and CSF leak during orbital exenteration. Ophthalmic Plast Reconstr Surg 3:61, 1987.
7. Doxanas MT, Green WR, Iliff CE: Factors in the successful surgical management of basal cell carcinoma of the eyelids. Am J Ophthalmol 91:726, 1981.
8. Mohs FE: Micrographic surgery for the microscopically controlled excision of eyelid cancers. Arch Ophthalmol 103:901, 1986.
9. Johnson LN, Krohel GB, Yeon EB, Parnes SM: Sinus tumors invading the orbit. Ophthalmology 91:209, 1984.
10. Conley J, Baker DC: Management of the eye socket in cancer of the paranasal sinuses. Arch Otolaryngol 105:702, 1979.
11. Perry C, Levine PA, Williamson BR, Cantrell RW: Preservation of the eye in paranasal sinus cancer surgery. Arch Otolaryngol Head Neck Surg 114:632–634, 1988.
12. Graamans K, Slootweg PJ: Orbital exenteration in surgery of malignant neoplasms of the paranasal sinuses: The value of preoperative computer tomography. Arch Otolaryngol Head Neck Surg 115:977–980, 1989.
13. Iliff WJ, Marback R, Green WR: Invasive squamous cell carcinoma of the conjunctiva. Arch Ophthalmol 93:119, 1975.
14. Jakobiec FA, Brownstein S, Albert W, et al: The role of cryotherapy in the management of conjunctival melanoma. Ophthalmology 89:502, 1982.
15. Wharam M, Beltangady M, Hays D, et al: Localized orbital rhabdomyosarcoma. Ophthalmology 94:251, 1987.
16. Kersten RC, Tse DT, Anderson RL, Blodi FC: The role of orbital exenteration in choroidal melanoma with extrascleral extension. Ophthalmology 92:436, 1985.
17. Pach JM, Robertson DM, Taney BS, et al: Prognostic factors in choroidal and ciliary body melanomas with extrascleral extension. Am J Ophthalmol 101:325, 1986.
18. Rini FJ, Jakobiec FA, Hornblass A, et al: The treatment of advanced choroidal melanoma with massive orbital extension. Am J Ophthalmol 103:634–640, 1987.
19. Gamba JL, Woodruff WW, Djang WT, Yeates AE: Craniofacial mucormycosis: Assessment with CT. Radiology 160:207, 1986.
20. Kohn R, Hepler R: Management of limited rhino-orbital mucormycosis without exenteration. Ophthalmology 92:1440, 1985.
21. Small RG, LaFuente H: Exenteration of the orbit in selected cases of severe orbital contracture. Ophthalmology 90:236–238, 1983.
22. Jackson IT, Laws ER Jr, Martin RD: The surgical management of orbital neurofibromatosis. Plast Reconstr Surg 71:751–758, 1983.
23. Wulc AE, Adams JL, Dryden RM: Cerebrospinal fluid leakage complicating orbital exenteration. Arch Ophthalmol 107:827–830, 1989.
24. Levin PS, Dutton JJ: Orbital exenteration. *In* Stewart WB (ed): Ophthalmic Plastic and Reconstructive Surgery. San Francisco, CA, American Academy of Ophthalmology, in press.
25. Buus DR, Tse DT: The use of the enucleation snare for orbital exenteration. Arch Ophthalmol 108:636–637, 1990.
26. Tse DT, Bumsted RM: A two-layer closure of sino-orbital fistula. Ophthalmology 86:1673–1678, 1989.
27. Levin PS, Ellis DS, Stewart WB, Toth BA: Orbital exenteration: The reconstructive ladder. Ophthalmic Plast Reconstr Surg 7:84, 1991.
28. Jackson IT: Reconstruction of the orbit after exenteration. *In* Stark RB (ed): Plastic Surgery of the Head and Neck, vol 1. New York, Churchill Livingstone, 1987, pp 439–452.
29. Putterman AM: Orbital exenteration with spontaneous granulation. Arch Ophthalmol 103:139–140, 1986.
30. McLaren LR: Primary skin grafting after exenteration of the orbit. Br J Plast Surg 11:57–61, 1959.
31. Mauriello JA, Han KH, Wolfe R: Use of autogenous split-thickness dermal grafts for reconstruction of the lining of the exenterated orbit. Am J Ophthalmol 100:465–467, 1985.
32. Shields JA, Shields CL, Suvarnami C, et al: Orbital exenteration with eyelid sparing: Indications, technique, and results. Ophthalmic Surg 22:292–297, 1991.
33. Gass JDM: Technique of orbital exenteration utilizing methyl methacrylate implant. Arch Ophthalmol 82:789–791, 1969.

34. Holmes AD, Marshall KA: Uses of the temporalis muscle flap in blanking out the orbits. Plast Reconstr Surg 63:336, 1979.
35. Naquin HA: Orbital reconstruction: Utilizing temporalis muscle. Am J Ophthalmol 41:519, 1956.
36. Shagets FW, Panje WR, Shore JW: Use of temporalis muscle flaps in complicated defects of the head and face. Arch Otolaryngol Head Neck Surg 112:60–65, 1986.
37. Reese AB, Jones IS: Exenteration of the orbit and repair by transplantation of the temporalis muscle. Am J Ophthalmol 51:217–227, 1961.
38. Sevel D: Exenteration of the orbit using a frontal periosteal flap. Head Neck Surg 4:154–160, 1981.
39. Dortzbach RK, Hawes MJ: Midline forehead flap in reconstructive procedures of the eyelids and exenterated socket. Ophthalmic Surg 12:257–268, 1981.
40. Brent B, Upton J, Acland RD, et al: Experience with the temporoparietal fascial flap. Plast Reconstr Surg 76:177, 1985.
41. Jackson IT Adham MN, Marsh WR: Use of the galeal frontalis myofascial flap in craniofacial surgery. Plast Reconstr Surg 77:905–910, 1986.
42. Ariyan S: The pectoralis major for single-stage reconstruction of the difficult wounds of the orbit and pharyngoesophagus. Plast Reconstr Surg 72:468–477, 1983.
43. Donahue PJ, Liston SL, Falconer DP, Manlove JC. Reconstruction of orbital exenteration cavities. The use of the latissimus dorsi myocutaneous free flap. Arch Ophthalmol 107:1681, 1989.
44. Nerad JA, Carter KD, LaVelle WE, et al: The osseointegration technique for the rehabilitation of the exenterated orbit. Arch Ophthalmol 109:1032, 1991.
45. Jackson IT, Tolman DE, Desjardins RP, Brånemark P-I: A new method for fixation of external prostheses. Plast Reconstr Surg 77:668–672, 1986.

CHAPTER 104

Harvesting and Use of Biological Tissue Grafts

Craig D. Friedman, Fred S. Bodker, and Robert A. Weiss

HARVESTING OF AUTOGENOUS BONE GRAFTS

Progress in orbital reconstructive techniques has been based on the use of bone grafts for the success of complex osseus reconstructions. Historically, a spectrum of donor sites has been employed. Basic scientific research on bone healing and repair has improved the understanding of how autogenous bone grafts heal.[1] The use of grafts from different embryologic sites of membranous bone versus endochondral bone has been delineated by several investigators and summarized by Habal and Reddi.[2] The application of autogenous bone grafts to orbital reconstruction has evolved from the use of these grafts to correct severe orbitofacial deformities of congenital and traumatic origin.[3, 4] Significant emphasis has been placed on techniques of harvesting autogenous bone grafts. The most common donor sites are iliac crest, costal rib, and calvarial bone. Although other donor sites can be utilized (i.e., tibia and ulna), reconstructive surgeons most frequently choose iliac and cranial bone for orbital reconstruction. Additionally, the use of vascularized bone transfers utilizing microvascular techniques can be another source of bone graft materials; however, this is infrequently chosen for most orbital reconstructions because of the success of free autologous bone grafts. The focus in the remainder of this discussion is on specific harvesting techniques and associated potential complications. For additional techniques for harvesting and use of tissue grafts, please refer to Chapter 106.

Harvesting of Iliac Bone Grafts

As stated by Wolfe,[5] the iliac crest has served as the "workhorse" donor site for craniomaxillofacial reconstructive surgery. The ability to obtain grafts that are easily shaped and contoured make it ideal for orbital floor and roof defects and augmentations. Of paramount consideration in any donor harvest is to minimize complications and deformity. Careful attention to technique will allow for safe and effective harvesting.

The patient is placed supine with supportive elevation to the undersurface of the hip-iliac area. The incision should be placed to avoid crossing over the crest itself and, depending on patient gender and clothing style, be just inferior or superior to the iliac crest and posterior to the iliac spine. The incision need not be longer than 4 cm. Dissection should proceed to the crest surface. Care is taken to preserve muscular attachments, thus avoiding most serious postoperative sequelae. It is preferable to obtain corticocancellous grafts from the medial surface of the ilium. Maintaining the crest itself is important and avoids donor site deformity. Exposure and access can be achieved by splitting the medial and lateral crest lips or by creating a trap door of the crest with a free osteotome. Then periosteal elevation is performed to expose the surface from which the graft is harvested. With the use of either surgical saws or osteotomes corticocancellous grafts are obtained of the desired shape and size for the reconstruction (Figs. 104-1 and 104-2). Once the necessary amount of grafting material is harvested, closure of the wound follows with repositioning of the previously split medial and lateral portions of the crest. With proper technique this can usually be accomplished with resorbable suture material and then closure of the skin and subcutaneous tissues. Suction drains are reserved for those instances in which large amounts of bone are harvested.

Kurz and colleagues[6] in a review of the literature, reported the following complications after iliac crest bone graft harvest: persistent postoperative pain, nerve injury (particularly affecting the lateral femoral cutaneous and the ilioinguinal nerves), arterial injury (especially of the superior gluteal artery), cosmetic deformity, hemorrhage (including postoperative hematomas), and infection. More unusual and devastating complications include peritoneal perforation with potential intraperitoneal contents with associated ileus. Although rare, bladder and ureteral injuries are also possible and have been reported.

Harvesting of Costal Rib Grafts

Rib grafts have been relegated to a secondary role for most orbital and facial applications. Their main application is for osteochondral grafts and pure cartilage grafts.

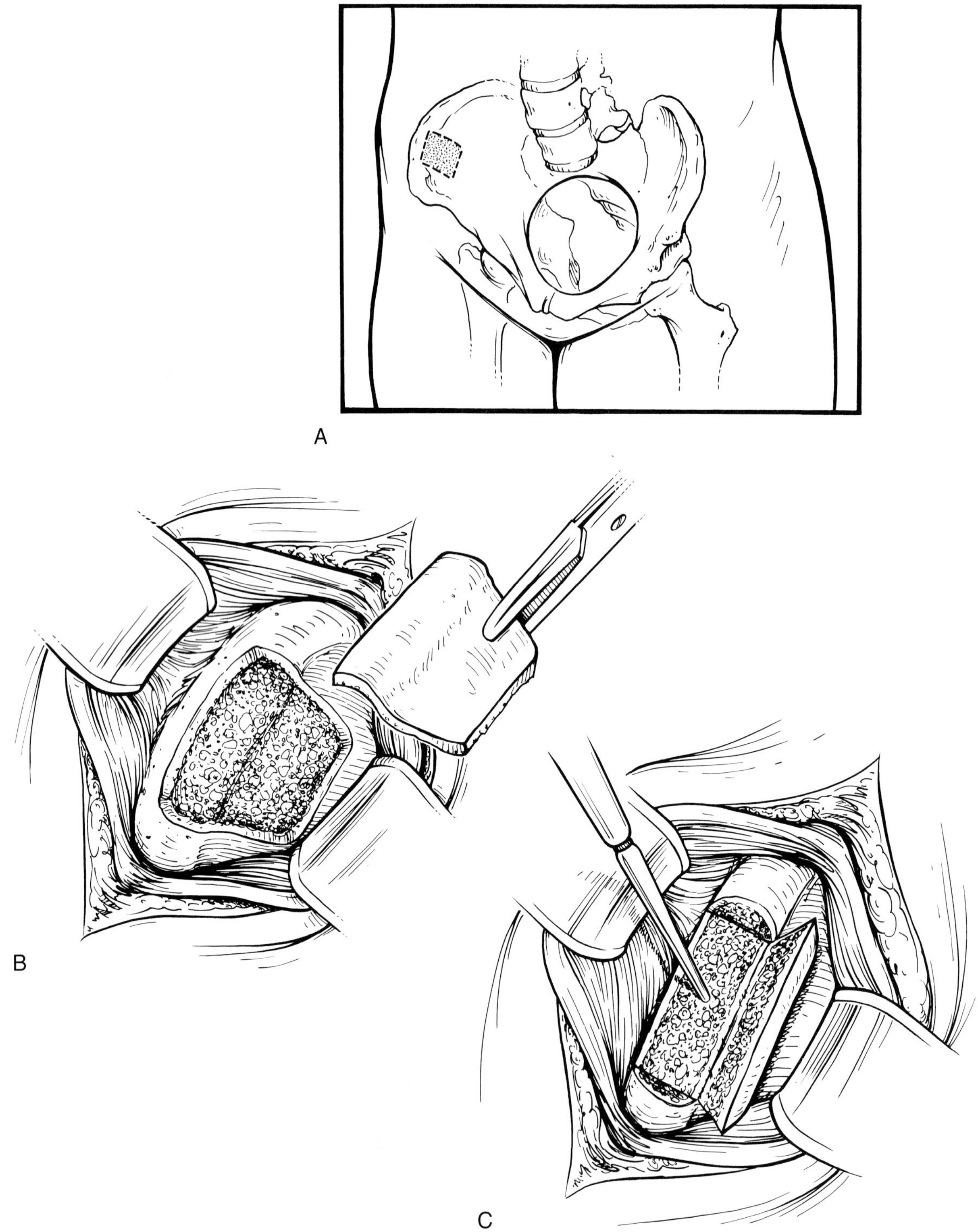

Figure 104–1. *A*, Iliac crest approach. *B* and *C*, Use of an osteotomy to preserve the crest.

For osseous reconstruction they have been replaced by cranial bone grafts in most procedures. The technique of harvest utilizes an incision that begins at the costochondral junction in the inframammary crease extending for approximately 5 cm. Dissection is taken down to the periosteum, and the elevation and stripping of the muscular attachments with long periosteal or Doyen elevators circumferentially is performed, avoiding pleura. The costochondral junction is disarticulated, and the rib is sectioned laterally (Fig. 104–3). The most obvious and significant complication is that of pneumothorax. Pneumothorax is usually managed by drainage of intrathoracic air and closure of the pleura; if significant, chest tube drainage is indicated.

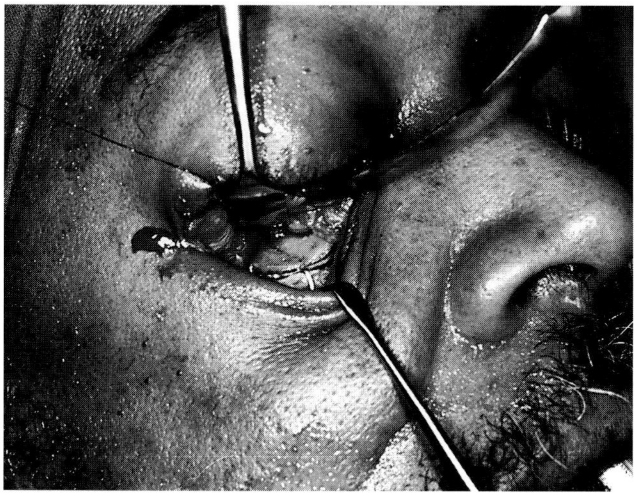

Figure 104–2. Corticocancellous block of Iliac crest bone graft in orbital floor defect.

Harvesting of Cranial Bone Grafts

Cranial bone grafts have become the donor site of choice for complex orbitocranial reconstructions. Although many historical precedents existed, it was Tessier who promoted the use of the skull as donor site for orbitocranial surgery. Subsequently, numerous reports and investigations of cranial bone grafts have been performed. The primary advantages of this site are minimal donor site morbidity and easy access with a concealed scar in most cases. Morphogenetically, cranial bone is the same as the osseous components of the orbit and thus a more appropriate reconstructive instrument. The major limitation of cranial bone grafts is the poor malleability and limited ability to contour the graft in three dimensions; yet with careful planning this is often easily overcome.

Because the significant complications of cranial bone

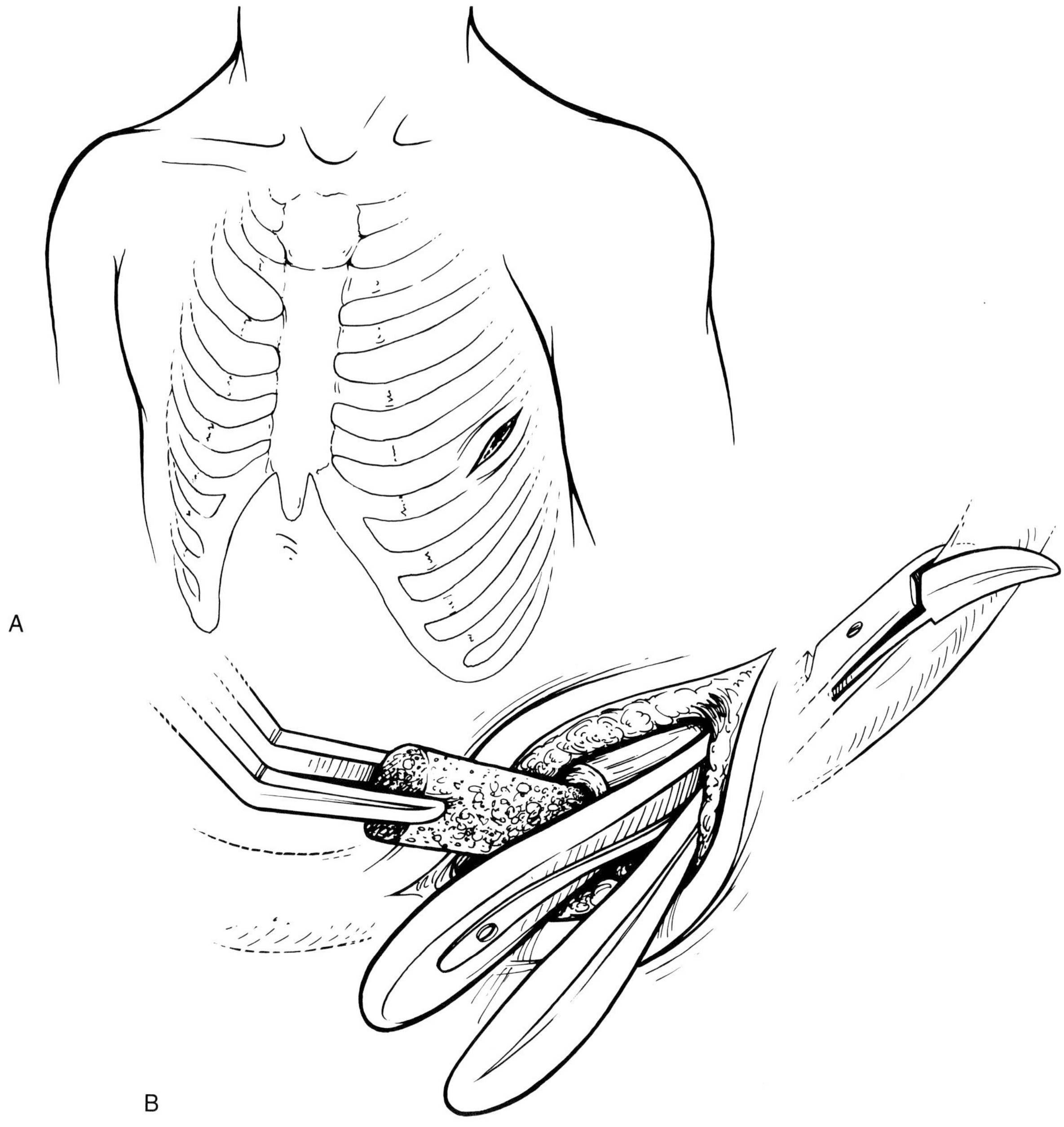

Figure 104–3. *A* and *B*, Rib graft harvest technique and sectioning.

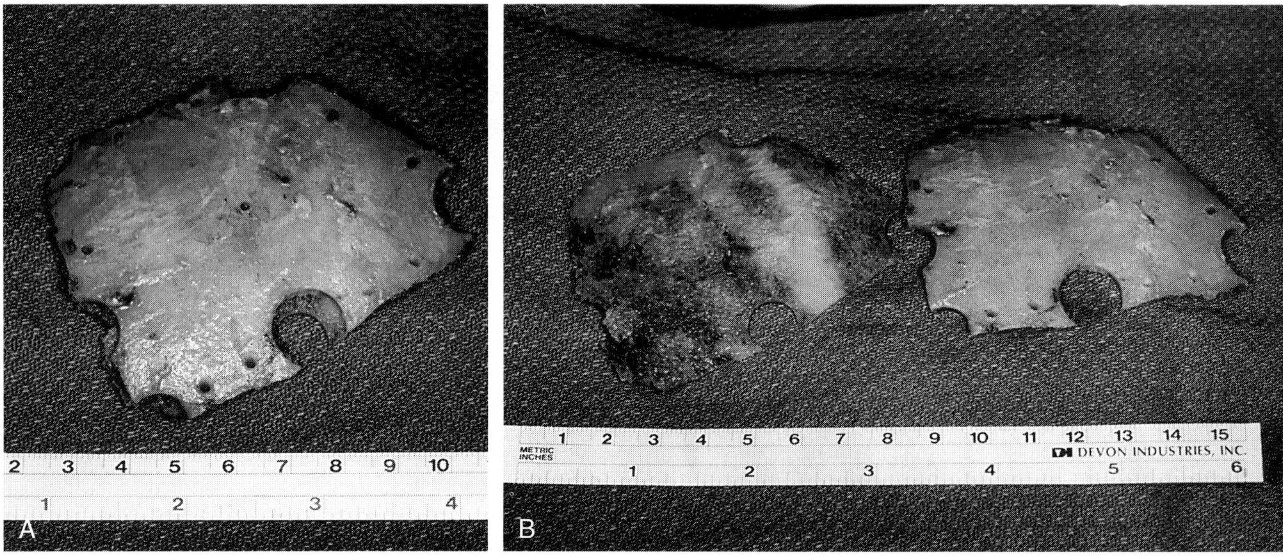

Figure 104–4. *A*, Craniotomy bone flap. *B*, After splitting of the bone flap with surgical saws and osteotomes. Large inner table graft is available.

harvesting are intracranial it is prudent to have neurosurgical collaboration available if injury is suspected. Essentially two approaches are utilized. First is formal craniotomy and harvesting of the split bone flap for major reconstruction (Fig. 104–4). Second, outer table grafts can be obtained directly. The parietal skull over the nondominant hemisphere is the preferred site since it is usually the thickest portion of the skull with a developed diploic space. It is important to review imaging studies before surgery in cases in which poorly developed diploic spaces may mandate a limited craniotomy.

Outer table grafts from the parietal skull are approached from a coronal scalp incision starting from the root of the auricular helix and extending the dissection superior and posterior (Fig. 104–5). The graft is then outlined with a perforating drill bit or surgical saw blade through the cortical surface to the diploic space. The trough that is created is deepened in the diploic space, allowing for the use of thin curved and straight osteotomes or, if the surgeon prefers, an oscillating saw. Once the grafts are obtained, the perimeter of the donor site can be contoured so as to minimize the palpable and sometimes visible skull defect.

This defect is usually minimal and well tolerated, the site can be reconstructed, and our current recommendations are for the use of well-tolerated alloplasts of hydroxyapatite or the newly developed hydroxyapatite cement,[7] which allows for effective reconstruction of such defects (Fig. 104–6). Intracerebral hematoma and superior sagittal sinus laceration as complications of cranial bone graft harvest have been reported.[8, 9] If there is any concern about intracranial entry and bleeding, then the wound exposure needs to be wider, including formal craniotomy.

MUCOUS MEMBRANE GRAFT HARVESTING

Nasal Septal Mucosa and Cartilage

Uses for nasal septal mucosa and cartilage grafting include major eyelid reconstruction and severe symblepharon with cicatricial entropion. Both lid-sharing procedures and free grafts may be considered surgical options. Its indication is generally believed to be for the posterior lamella of the upper eyelid since it is too thick for use in the lower eyelid. Scleral tissue is more elastic and lacks rigidity to substitute for the tarsal plate. Similarly, fascia is also less stiff than tarsus. Auricular cartilage provides excellent support, but it is must stiffer than tarsus and causes an unnaturally firm eyelid. Composite tarsal-conjunctival grafts such as nasal septum chondromucosa have the advantage of replacing both layers of posterior lamella with better host site incorporation and less keratopathy from contraction and shrinkage than the above options.

Both sides of the nasal septum should be inspected for maximal exposure. If the convex side is preferable due to severe deviation of exposure, one should proceed from that side. One should not worry that the curvature of the graft will be inverted because later trimming of the cartilage from the concave side will cause contraction of the remaining layer of perichondrium and subsequent curling in the opposite direction.

Anesthesia and vasoconstriction should be achieved by applying cocaine and phenylephrine hydrochloride to the mucosa using cotton-tipped applicators. Additional vasoconstriction and expansion of the musosa may be secured by injection of lidocaine hydrochloride (1%) with epinephrine (1 : 100,000) and hyaluronidase.[10] Alterna-

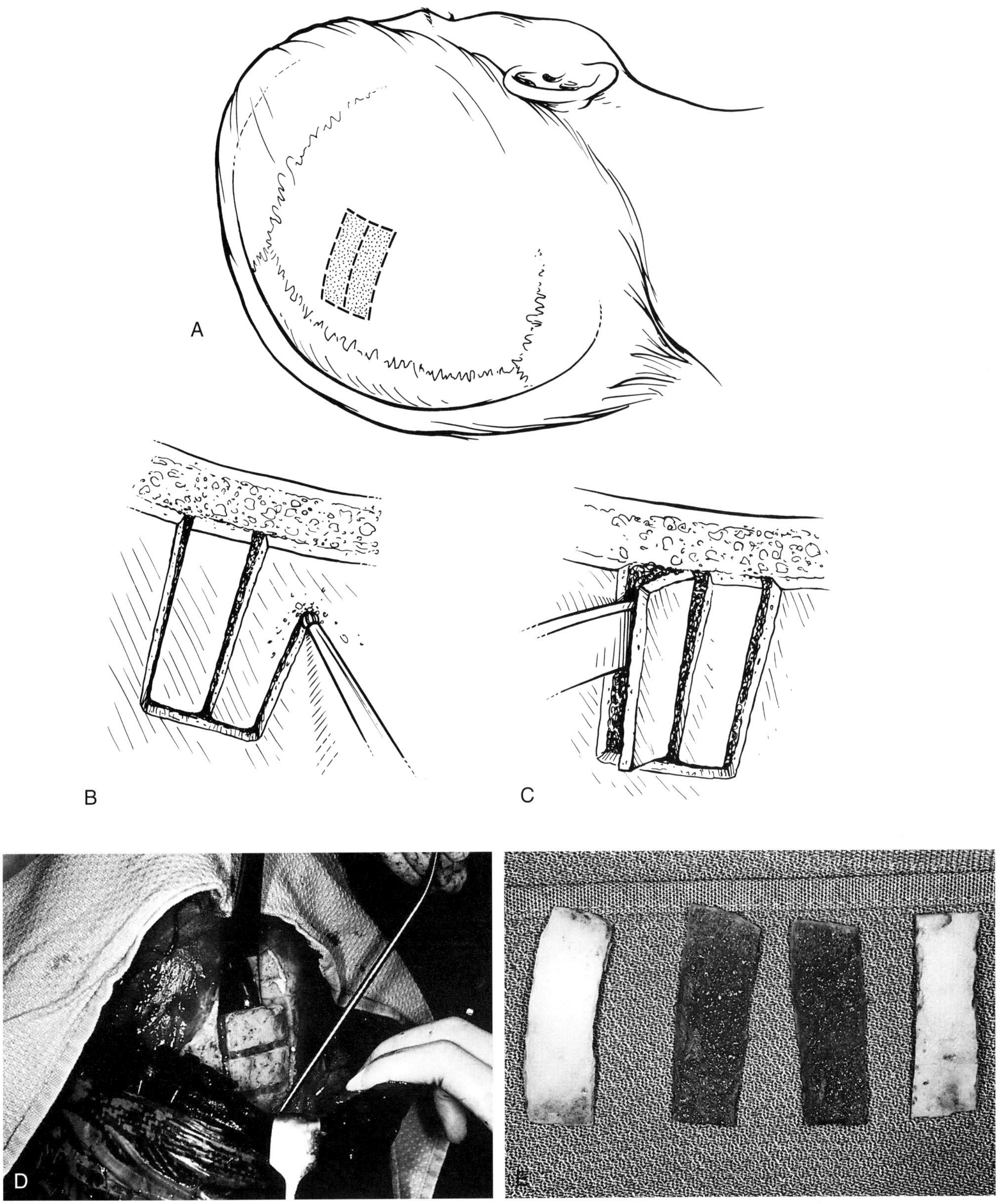

Figure 104–5. *A* to *C*, Cranial bone graft technique. Note the position of the donor site in the parietal skull, creation of trough in the bone down to the diploic space, and use of an osteotome to separate the outer table graft. *D*, Intraoperative view of cranial bone graft harvest using an osteotome. *E*, Examples of harvested cranial bone grafts.

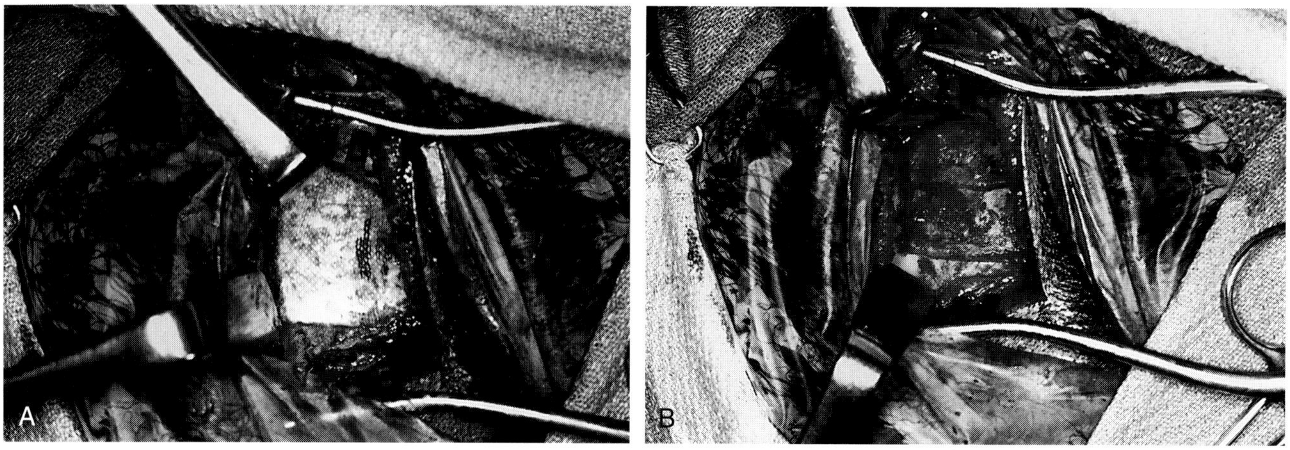

Figure 104–6. *A* and *B*, Use of hydroxyapatite cement in cranial defect reconstruction.

tively, one can pack the donor site with gauze soaked in cocaine[11] or insert cotton-tipped applicators soaked in cocaine into the floor of the nose, between the inferior and middle turbinates, and toward the roof of the nose[12] before the submucosal injection of lidocaine, epinephrine, and hyaluronidase. While performing the submucosal injection, one should be careful not to disinsert the mucosa and perichondrium from the underlying cartilage on the donor side. Conversely, infiltration beneath the mucosa and perichondrium on the opposite side will facilitate the harvest without perforating both mucosal layers.

A nasal speculum should be inserted into the nostril with the blades oriented horizontally to provide adequate exposure. A no. 15 Bard-Parker blade should be used to make the incision vertically through the mucosa, perichondrium, and cartilage approximately 1 cm from the anterior border of the cartilaginous septum. This location should allow sufficient cartilaginous support for the nasal tip in the form of a strut. The blade should be advanced slowly from the top of the cartilaginous septum down to the maxillary bone. After the vertical incision is completed, the nasal speculum should be rotated 90 degrees to increase exposure of the vestibule. Dissection of the cartilage from the perichondrial sling is achieved using a periosteal elevator. This instrument is best utilized by making short sweeps from inferior to superior since the firmest adherence between the perichondrial sling and cartilaginous septum occurs superiorly.

Horizontal incisions both inferiorly and superiorly are made with angled nasal scissors. The graft should be grasped with long-handled Adson forceps with caution not to separate the individual layers. At the posterior edge of the graft, the horizontal cuts should be angled toward each other to facilitate removal without tearing. The final detachment requires the use of a scalpel blade. A composite graft of 25 × 50 mm can be obtained in this manner and should be adequate for most reconstructive purposes. On removal, the graft should be soaked in an antibiotic solution. Any attached bone (ethmoid and vomer) must be excised before placement adjacent to the globe.

The nasal cavity must be inspected for active bleeding after the harvest. Despite the preoperative use of vasoconstrictors, a combined suction-cautery instrument should be employed to establish hemostasis. Any anterior perforation of the contralateral mucosa should be firmly sutured; if located posteriorly, the defect will not cause significant disability. Both nasal cavities should be packed tightly with petrolatum gauze containing an antibiotic ointment to ensure equal pressure on both sides. The gauze pack may be removed on postoperative day 1 or 2; this procedure may be followed by slight epistaxis for 5 to 10 minutes. Forceful blowing of the nose is prohibited for the following week.[10]

The cartilage of the composite graft is typically thicker than that required for eyelid reconstruction (in severe cicatricial entropion from Stevens-Johnson syndrome or trachoma, the full nasal cartilage thickness will prevent recurrence of entropion).[10] A medium-sized scalpel blade is frequently used to thin it to 1.5 mm. This process will also serve to curl the cartilage side toward the mucosal side in the configuration required in the eyelid. A 1- to 2-mm edge of cartilage should be cut from the periphery, leaving a border of mucosal fringe. This border should be 2 to 3 mm wide on the side that will become the lid margin, such that the mucosa can extend anteriorly over the cartilage toward the cutaneous tissue.[12]

Once the graft is trimmed to appropriate size, it may be secured with 7-0 chromic catgut sutures in a running fashion, except at the corners, where it should be tied in an interrupted fashion. Burying the knots will reduce the amount of keratopathy. The placement of a conformer, symblepharon ring, or rubber bolster over the graft in the early postoperative period improves healing by maintaining tissue apposition and pressure.

Hard Palate Mucosa Grafts

Indications for use of hard palate mucosa grafts have included postblepharoplasty lower eye lid retraction, cicatricial entropion, trichiasis, eyelid retraction secondary to thyroid eye disease, and lagophthalmos after surgery for paralytic ptosis. It is a composite material and is believed to be more flexible than ear or nasal cartilage.[13] It is also plentiful enough to supply graft tissue for all four eyelids if necessary.

Anesthetic block is achieved by submucosal injection of lidocaine (2%) with epinephrine (1 : 100,000) and hyaluronidase (1 mL/50 mL). Much of the palatine mucosa and submucosa is tightly adherent to the underlying periosteum, making infiltration of anesthesia challenging. Directing the needle toward the loose connective tissue near the incisive and greater palatine foramina regions enables the surgeon to infiltrate up to 0.5 mL of anesthetic without difficulty. In addition, one will improve hemostasis since most palatal vessels enter through the foramina with the nerves. The mucosa should be ballooned from the underlying mucoperiosteum.

The greater palatine foramen is located 3 to 4 mm anterior to the border of the hard and soft palates at the distal half of the last molar. The needle must be introduced tangentially at the distal half of the second to last molar, rather than vertically into the foramen, owing to the shape and size of the oral cavity. The site of entrance should be made at the apex of the barrel-shaped mucosal arch between the roof of the mouth and the alveolar process. The needle is directed superiorly, laterally, and posteriorly.

The nasopalatine nerve and vessels enter the oral cavity just posterior to the central incisors. The incisive papilla in this region is extremely pain sensitive; thus the needle should puncture lateral to them. The needle is directed superiorly, medially, and posteriorly. A properly placed block will achieve bilateral anterior palatal anesthesia since the two nasopalatine nerves are located near the midline.

The harvest of hard palate mucosa is performed as described. The hard palate is dried with gauze pads. The estimated size of the graft is marked onto the mucosa with a marking pen between the median raphe and the alveolar process. A no. 15 Bard-Parker blade is then used to incise the marked area. The edge of the graft is then lifted using 0.12 Castroviejo forceps while dissection in the submucosal plane is performed with a Wescott scissors or a no. 15 Beaver blade[13] or iris scissors.[14] The junction between hard and soft palate should be avoided cautiously because of the location of the palatine artery. Aggressive suction should be employed to control any bleeding that might drip into the patient's throat. The wound should be covered with a Telfa pad with an overlying moist 2 × 2-inch gauze pad. Digital pressure may be applied through the gauze pad for excessive bleeding; cautery is not usually needed. Alternatively, collagen periodontal tape[13] or oxidized regenerated cellulose[15] may be used to cover the wound. The fatty portion of the submucosa and any adherent mucus glands are trimmed from the graft. The tissue is then wrapped in a saline-moistened gauze pad and rinsed in solution of neomycin and bacitracin.

As the eyelid is prepared for grafting, the harvested tissue is cut to appropriate proportions. An infratarsal incision should separate tarsus from conjunctiva and lower eyelid retractors extending from the punctum to the lateral canthus. Wescott scissors are used to dissect the newly created space. The graft is then placed between the inferior border of the tarsus and the superior edge of recessed conjunctiva and retractors. The graft is secured to conjunctiva with closely placed, running 6-0 double-armed chromic gut suture. Both superior and inferior needles are passed full thickness through the lid and tied on the skin surface. The lid is positioned with three Frost-type sutures. A corticosteroid-antibiotic combination ointment is applied to the eye, and a pressure dressing is placed over the eye for the ensuing week. Patients should understand that the pressure patch immobilizes the eyelid to allow adequate healing. One week after surgery the patch and the Frost-type sutures are removed.

Hard palate mucosa has a variable amount of keratinized epithelium that can cause irritation and discharge. Over time, metaplasia to nonkeratinized epithelium has been found to occur, resulting in rare complaints at the 6-month followup visit.[14]

REFERENCES

1. Manson PN: Bone grafts: Clinical review of factors affecting survival. *In* Proceedings of the Portland Bone Symposium, Portland, Oregon. 1993, pp 356–380.
2. Habal M, Reddi AH: Bone Grafts & Bone Substitutes. Philadelphia, WB Saunders, 1992.
3. Tessier P: Autogenous bone grafts taken from the calvarium for facial and cranial applications. Clin Plast Surg 9:531–538, 1982.
4. Jackson IT: Classification and treatment of orbitozygomatic and orbitoethmoid fractures: The place of bone grafting and plate fixation. Clin Plast Surg 16:77–91, 1989.
5. Wolfe SA: Autogenous bone grafts versus alloplastic materials. *In* Plastic Surgery of the Facial Skeleton. Boston, Little, Brown & Co, 1989, p 30.
6. Kurz LT, Garfin SR, Booth RE: Harvesting autogenous iliac bone grafts: A review of complications and technique. Spine 14:1324–1331, 1989.
7. Costantino PD, Friedman CD, Jones K, Chow LC, Sisson GA: Experimental hydroxyapatite cement cranioplasty. Plast Reconstr Surg 90:174–185, 1992.
8. Young VL, Shuster RH, Harris LW: Intracerebral hematoma complicating split calvarial bone graft harvesting. Plast Reconstr Surg 86:763–765, 1990.
9. Cannella DM, Hopkins LN: Superior sagittal sinus laceration complicating an autogenous calvarial bone graft harvest: Report of a case. J Oral Maxillofac Surg 48:741–743, 1990.
10. Callahan MA, Callahan A: Ophthalmic Plastic and Orbital Surgery. Birmingham, AL, Aesculapius, 1979, pp 23–25, 90–92.
11. Kohn R: Textbook of Ophthalmic Plastic and Reconstructive Surgery. Philadelphia, Lea & Febiger, 1988, pp 52–53.
12. Mustardé JC: Repair and Reconstruction in the Orbital Region: A Practical Guide. Edinburgh, Churchill Livingstone, 1988, pp 378–381.
13. Cohen MS, Shorr N: Eyelid reconstruction with hard palate mucosa grafts. Ophthalmic Plast Reconstr Surg 8:183–195, 1992.
14. Kersten RC, Kulwin DR, Levartovsky S, Tiradellis H, Tse DT: Management of lower-lid retraction with hard palate mucosa grafting. Arch Ophthalmol 108:1339–1343, 1990.
15. Bartley GB, Kay PP: Posterior lamellar eyelid reconstruction with a hard palate mucosal graft. Am J Ophthalmol 107:609–612, 1989.

Orbital Trauma

CHAPTER 105

Orbital Fractures

Sara A. Kaltreider

The seven bones that constitute the bony orbit may be disrupted by blunt or sharp trauma. The soft tissues and ocular structures may be injured by the trauma itself or entrapped and damaged by bony fragments. Edema and hemorrhage may be followed by fibrosis and loss of function. Distortion of tissues and loss of function may become permanent if repair, when indicated, is not implemented in a timely fashion.

The incidence of ocular injuries among patients with orbital fractures is around 10%. Most of those injuries are associated with supraorbital and complex fractures (80%), and fewer are associated with trimalar and orbital floor fractures or trimalar fractures alone (20%).[1] Ocular injuries range in severity from traumatic iritis to globe rupture and optic nerve avulsion.

Facial fractures resulting from sports injuries or assault are low-velocity injuries, whereas motor vehicle accidents result in high-velocity injuries. The latter are much more destructive and more often associated with life-threatening injuries. Forces causing fractures may be categorized according to impact delivered or impact tolerance of the affected bones. These forces are many times greater than the force of gravity.[2] The glabellar area, nasal bridge, and malar eminence have the lower resistance to impact compared with the supraorbital region and the lower maxilla.[2–4] Injuries associated with high-velocity facial injuries include central nervous system injuries, skull or basilar skull fractures, airway obstructive injuries, chest injuries with contusion, pneumothorax or hemothorax, and intra-abdominal injuries. These serious injuries are two to three times more common in high-velocity trauma than in low-velocity trauma. Airway and ventilatory support and injuries to the thorax, intra-abdominal structures, and central nervous system take precedence over trauma to the eye and orbit. Specialized care of the ocular and orbital problems should be initiated as quickly and efficiently as possible after the life-threatening conditions have been stabilized.

The many types of orbital fractures may occur alone or in various combinations. The most common types of orbital fractures are blow-out fractures of the orbital floor, with or without medial wall fractures, and malar fractures. Other fractures include LeFort II and III fractures, nasoethmoid fractures, frontobasal fractures (including supraorbital, glabellar, and isolated superior orbital rim fractures), orbital roof blow-in or blow-out fractures, orbital apex fractures with or without optic canal fractures, and localized fractures produced by sharp objects thrust into the orbit.

EVALUATION OF ORBITAL FRACTURES

Assessment of orbital fractures should begin with a thorough examination and documentation of vision and pupillary findings and a complete ocular evaluation to rule out rupture or laceration of the eye and intraocular foreign bodies. Adnexal examination is essential, documenting findings such as edema, ecchymosis, crepitus, entry wounds, and avulsion of tissue. Globe position, intercanthal distance, medial and lateral canthal position, lid position, and integrity of the lacrimal excretory apparatus should be noted in a systematic fashion. Extraocular motility should be determined as accurately as possible. This aspect of the examination may be limited by the patient's ability to cooperate, which in turn is dependent on age, mental status, and pain tolerance. Forced duction testing is important and may be done preoperatively if the patient can tolerate it and if globe rupture has been ruled out with certainty. Forced duction testing should be repeated intraoperatively before repair of the orbital fracture and again after the repair and placement of orbital implants. The finding of restricted forced ductions not only is synonymous with muscle entrapment in the fracture site, but also may be a consequence of edema, hemorrhage, or entrapment of fat and fibrous septa in the fracture site.

Skull radiography or computed tomography (CT) may be indicated not only for orbital fractures but also for evaluation of the eye, optic nerve, and possible intraocular or orbital foreign bodies. The role of routine radiography is mainly one of screening for fractures and radiopaque foreign bodies. When the examination of the eye and orbit is unremarkable, the vitreoretinal examination reveals no evidence of foreign bodies, and no entry wounds are seen, but the history suggests the possibility of an occult foreign body (hammering metal on metal, working with or near power equipment generating high-velocity missiles), then a plain radiograph may be a helpful screening tool. A routine radiograph should not be relied on for proof or disproof of small metallic foreign bodies or nonmetallic foreign bodies that may easily escape detection on plain radiographs. CT provides more accurate and complete information regarding ocular and orbital foreign body identification and localization and the extent of soft tissue and bony injuries.

CT is an exceptionally valuable modality for imaging the relationship of the soft tissues to the fracture sites; defining the secondary effects of trauma, such as retrobulbar hemorrhage, optic nerve sheath hemorrhage, and subperiosteal fluid collections; and confirming complications of trauma such as cellulitis, abscess, and retained foreign body.[5-7] Radiographic studies should be coordinated with other subspecialty consultants as indicated to include all injured anatomy in the scan. If trauma to the intracranial space is suspected, then the study should be extended posteriorly and superiorly to look for intracranial hemorrhage, contusion, pneumocephalus, foreign bodies, and bone fragments in the cerebral cortex.

High-resolution multiplanar CT scanning gives the clinician a three-dimensional concept of fractures and soft tissue disruption. Scanning in at least two planes is extremely helpful for assessing the full extent of the injury and planning the surgical approach for the best intraoperative exposure. Several constraints may preclude an optimum study such as patient obtundation, combativeness, hemodynamic instability limiting the patient's time in the scanner, and cervical fractures preventing extension of the neck. When direct multiplanar imaging is not possible or practical, reconstructed views using thin sections may provide helpful information.

Three-dimensional computer reconstructions of the orbital bony anatomy are a useful adjunct before reconstruction of the traumatized orbit.[8] These images elucidate areas of bony depression and volume loss and assist the surgeon in planning late repairs and reconstruction. Three-dimensional CT reconstruction of a patient with trimalar, orbital floor, and glabellar fractures is seen in Figure 105–1. The volume deficits in these areas are obvious. Many views in one or two planes are necessary to convey the information shown on just one three-dimensional view. Very thin (1.5 mm) sections are required for a meaningful reconstruction.[8]

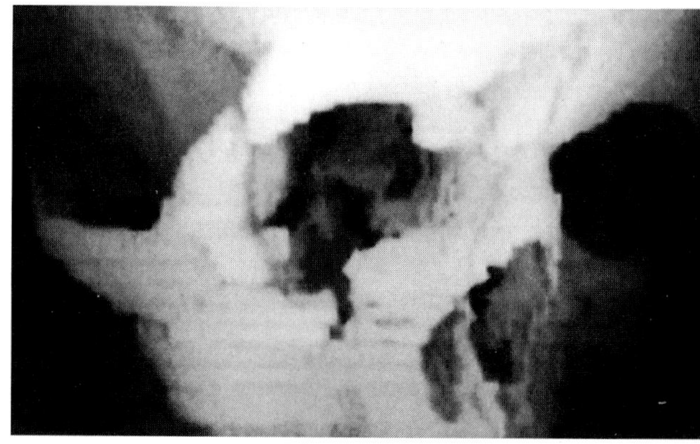

Figure 105–1. In this three-dimensional computed tomographic reconstruction, note the comminuted malar fracture with fragments of the zygoma rotated and displaced downward, the depressed orbital floor fracture, the depressed glabellar fracture, and the medial wall fracture. (From Kaltreider SA, Dortzbach RK: Orbital trauma. *In* Stephenson C [ed]: Ophthalmic Plastic, Reconstructive, and Orbital Surgery. Stoneham, MA, Butterworth-Heinemann, in press.)

The presence of ferromagnetic foreign bodies and the inability of magnetic resonance imaging (MRI) to image cortical bone are contraindications to its use in evaluating the acutely traumatized orbit, particularly when fractures or metallic foreign bodies are possibilities.[9, 10] Vitreoretinal damage during an MRI has been reported in a sheet metal worker with an unsuspected intraocular foreign body.[11] Other contraindications include the presence of a pacemaker, metallic implants, and clips.[9] Makeup and tattooing have been reported to cause artifacts interfering with the resolution of the MRI.[12] Patient movement and claustrophobia may also preclude an accurate study. Although not appropriate in the setting of acute trauma, MRI may have a role in characterizing fluid collections in the orbit and subperiosteal space. Fresh hemorrhage is isointense compared to white matter and later becomes hypointense because of conversion of methemoglobin to hemosiderin.[13] The MRI may prove useful in detecting nonmetallic foreign bodies and may be complementary to CT in imaging post-traumatic structural abnormalities.[13]

PRINCIPLES OF FIXATION

Surgical treatment of fractures with internal fixation with wires was first proposed in the late 1700s.[14] Over 100 years later Hansmann performed bone plate fixation of a fracture.[15] The concept of improved stability and healing of bone with absolute immobilization and compression of the fracture ends prompted the development of compression plate fixation for fractures of the extremities.[16]

Advances in materials and technology led to the development of smaller rigid (noncompression) plates adaptable to midface fractures. Microfixation systems with tiny plates and screws for very thin bone are available.[17, 18]

Collective experience indicates that several conditions are prerequisite to optimal fracture healing. Absolute immobility, adequate blood supply to bone fragments, and contact of fracture ends allows healing with functional use of the injured area.[19] Rigid fixation maximizes these conditions and minimizes extensive callus formation and instability of the bone fragments, thereby eliminating malunion and secondary deformities.

The use of miniplate fixation requires a stock of system-specific instruments, plates, and screws. In addition, the surgeon must be familiar with the use of these devices.[20] When applying miniplates to the maxilla, one must avoid the dental roots. Distraction of the bone may occur if the plate is not in the proper configuration for the bone where it is placed.[20] The plate and screws may be palpable through the soft, thin tissues of the eyelids.

The advantages of miniplate fixation over conventional wiring outweigh the disadvantages for many types of facial fractures. Miniplate fixation allows greater stability and ease of fixation in comminuted fractures. Rotation of the zygoma by the forces of the masseter muscle is eliminated with the use of rigid fixation.[20] Whereas traditional three-point fixation with wires is necessary for reasonable stability of tripod fractures, two-plate, and even one-plate, fixation provides greater stability of the zygoma.

Differences in bone thickness may dictate the applicability of miniplates for facial fractures. The nasal bones are among the thinnest, 1.0 to 1.5 mm. The thickness of the anterior wall of the maxillary sinus is variable and may be 1.0 mm in some areas.[19] The zygoma, frontal, and maxillary bones in the area of the orbital rim are much thicker. Although the orbital rim areas can accommodate the plates and screws, isolated orbital rim fractures may be wired into place successfully. Unlike tripod fractures, in which the force of the masseter muscle may rotate the bone, the fragments of bone in an isolated rim fracture are not subjected to the displacing forces of muscle.

Materials must have biocompatibility and resistance to corrosion. Titanium is optimal because of its stability in air and tissues, a result of its conversion to titanium oxide that resists corrosion.[19] Another advantage is the ability to obtain CT and MRI scans without artifact despite the presence of this material. Miniplates are available in multiple configurations and lengths that may be used for orbital and midface fractures. The screws are 2 mm in diameter and 5 to 15 mm in length.[19]

FRACTURES OF THE ORBITAL FLOOR

The orbital floor blow-out fracture is the most common of the orbital fractures. Although this type of fracture was documented as early as 1844 by MacKenzie, it was designated "blow-out fracture" in 1956 by Converse and Smith.[21, 22] Blunt trauma to the orbital soft tissues causes downward displacement and fracturing of the thin orbital floor. Buckling forces transmitted from the orbital rim to the orbital floor is another mechanism explaining the occurrence of a blow-out fracture.[23] The soft tissues recoil more slowly than the bone, and, therefore, the soft tissues may become entrapped in the fracture.[24] Cadaver and other experimental models have shown that several mechanisms are valid.[24, 25]

Lid edema, ecchymosis, vertical diplopia, enophthalmos or exophthalmos, and infraorbital nerve hypesthesia are the usual presenting symptoms and signs. Diplopia may be present in primary gaze, upward gaze, and downward gaze. Tethering of the muscle in the fracture site or hemorrhage and edema may produce diplopia in both downward and upward gaze.[22, 26] Eighteen percent of motility defects may be produced by extraocular muscle or cranial nerve palsy rather than mechanical restriction of the muscle and periorbita.[26]

Expansion of the orbital volume by inferior displacement of the floor and orbital contents into the maxillary sinus may produce enophthalmos. Fat atrophy may contribute to late enophthalmos. Exophthalmos rather than enophthalmos may occur acutely in the presence of orbital edema and hemorrhage.

Blow-in fractures of the orbital floor may result from blunt trauma with the primary force directed at the maxillary rim and inferior orbital rim.[27, 28] Unlike blow-out fractures, the fragmented bones are displaced upward into the orbit because of the forces from the maxillary sinus below. These patients may present with exophthalmos rather than enophthalmos and may be more likely to experience visual dysfunction and extraocular muscle or cranial nerve palsies. Increased intraorbital hydraulic pressure does not play a role in blow-in fractures.[27]

In all patients with orbital fractures, the initial evaluation should begin with visual acuity and pupillary testing, followed by slit lamp examination, intraocular pressure, and dilated fundus examination. Generally, when the orbital floor gives way, the globe does not rupture, but this possibility should not be overlooked. Globe position and the adnexa should then be examined.

Extraocular motility should be documented in degrees or prism diopters of tropia. This initial examination will provide the basis for subsequent therapeutic decisions and therefore should be documented as carefully and accurately as possible. Red glass testing is extremely helpful in mapping areas of diplopia. The patient may find recognition and quantitation of the diplopia easier with this test and may also be more aware of improvements that may occur over the next few days.

Early forced duction tests may not add much information to the management decisions because restriction may be a result of edema or hemorrhage within the muscle sheath rather than entrapment of tissue. Forced duction testing is very useful in patients under general anesthesia before repair of the fracture and intraoperatively to ensure release of entrapped tissues and proper placement of the floor implant.

Management

The indications for repair of a blow-out fracture are unresolving extraocular muscle dysfunction and diplopia, 2 mm or more of enophthalmos, and a large fracture according to CT scan.[29] Persistent infraorbital nerve dysfunction is a less compelling indication. Compromise of vision produced by bone fragments (as in blow-in fractures) and compartment syndromes are encountered occasionally and are also indications for intervention. Rarely is the eye displaced into the maxillary sinus, but this occurrence should be treated immediately to ensure the best visual outcome.[30]

The CT scan provides useful guidelines in predicting those patients who will require surgical repair. Patients at high risk for developing enophthalmos and persistent diplopia may be identified by coronal CT scan.[31] Muscles that are surrounded by fat density and are not adjacent to any bone densities are unlikely to be restricted, and these patients are unlikely to experience continued diplopia. Patients whose muscles are contiguous with bone on one side but surrounded on other sides by orbital fat are also not likely to develop clinically bothersome diplopia. Conservative management is appropriate in these cases. Muscles that are contiguous with bone density on both the nasal and temporal sides are entrapped, and surgical repair is necessary to eliminate the diplopia.[31] The patient whose CT scan is seen in Figure 105–2 illustrates this situation. No spontaneous improvement in diplopia occurred, and the patient underwent repair within 2 weeks of injury. The amount of orbital expansion and soft tissue herniation seen on CT is predictive of later enophthalmos.[32] Those patients with large fractures and

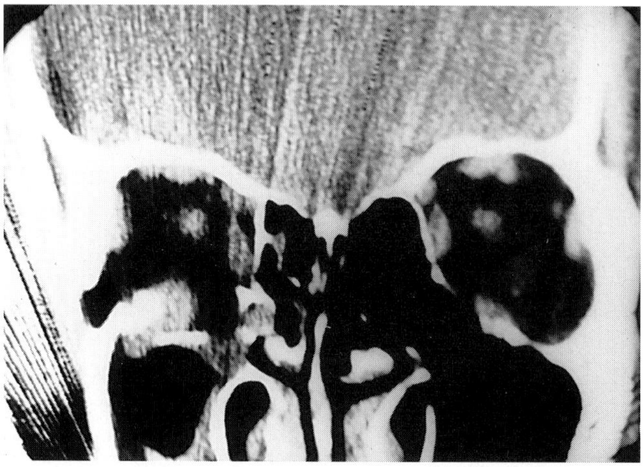

Figure 105–2. In this blowout fracture, the inferior rectus muscle is entrapped and contiguous with bone laterally and medially. Resolution of diplopia in this situation is unlikely, and early repair is indicated.

marked herniation of orbital tissues should have repair of their fractures.

Nonsurgical or late management has been advocated in the past because many patients clinically improve with respect to diplopia and infraorbital nerve dysfunction.[33, 34] Several methods to disguise the enophthalmos have been recommended. Late corrective surgery such as an orbital floor implant, Müller's muscle–conjunctival resection, or excision of skin and orbital fat on the opposite side may improve symmetry.[34] Extraocular muscle surgery on the uninvolved eye has been recommended for bothersome diplopia.[34]

Early repair is technically easier and yields a better clinical result with respect to diplopia and enophthalmos.[29, 35] Ample evidence exists suggesting that the longer one waits to repair the fracture, the more difficult repair becomes as fibrosis intervenes. Therefore, it becomes imperative to identify early those patients who will need surgery. The timing of blow-out fracture repair is dependent on the findings on serial examinations and the CT scan. When repair is imminent, then surgery within 2 weeks of injury is preferable. The patient in Figure 105–3 had no improvement in diplopia over a 12-day period and therefore underwent early repair on the 15th day after injury. Recovery was complete. If serial examinations indicate continued improvement over a 2-week period and diplopia is becoming less bothersome, then surgery may be delayed. Repair after 8 weeks is likely to be much more difficult and produce less predictable results.

The use of corticosteroid treatment to accelerate the resolution of post-traumatic edema of the injured periorbital and inferior rectus has been proposed to facilitate differentiation between those patients who will need surgery and those who will not.[32] In a randomized prospective double-blind study, patients receiving 1 mg/kg prednisone daily for 10 days, with doses tapered over 4 days, experienced more rapid clearing of their edema, allowing early determination of those patients who will require surgery because of persistent motility defects and significant enopththalmos. Pretreatment with corticosteroids may decrease the morbidity and enhance the surgical outcome.[32] Further studies will be necessary to determine whether corticosteroid treatment improves the long-term outcome, and whether prediction of those patients who ultimately require surgery is just as accurate by CT criteria and serial clinical examinations, without corticosteroid treatment.

The objective information obtained by clinical examination and CT should be combined with more subjective information regarding the patient's overall condition, livelihood, aspirations, and daily activities to reach the final decision regarding surgical intervention. For example, the surgeon may be less inclined to repair a blow-out fracture in a debilitated individual with minimal residual diplopia and more inclined to repair one in an aspiring young athlete with even less diplopia. If occupation or

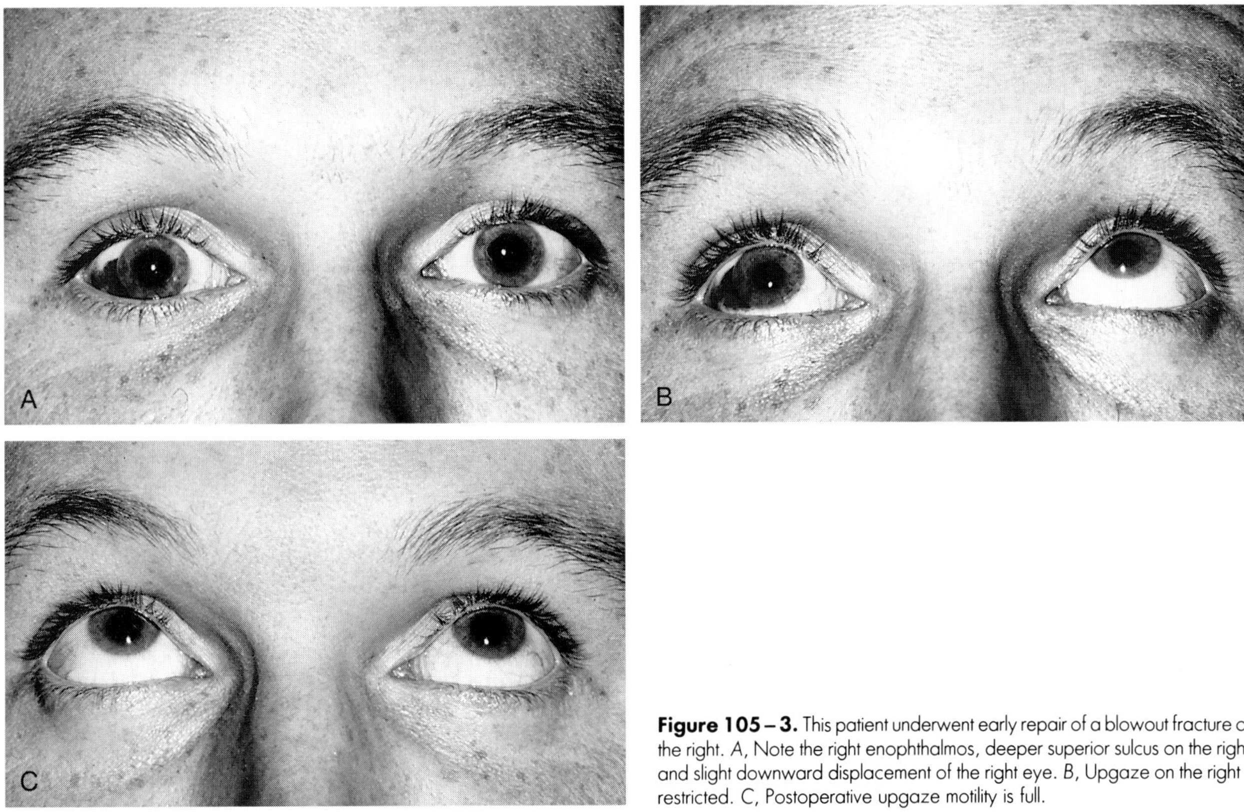

Figure 105–3. This patient underwent early repair of a blowout fracture on the right. *A*, Note the right enophthalmos, deeper superior sulcus on the right, and slight downward displacement of the right eye. *B*, Upgaze on the right is restricted. *C*, Postoperative upgaze motility is full.

recreation involves consistent use of upward gaze (e.g., postal workers, airline pilots, and basketball players) then a patient with any amount of bothersome diplopia should have the fracture repaired.

The surgical approaches to the floor of the orbit include a subciliary incision, inferior fornix incision, lower eyelid crease incision, and orbital rim incision. The latter two approaches leave the patient with pronounced lid edema for a greater period of time postoperatively compared with the first two approaches. The subciliary skin incision may produce a noticeable scar, although this is much less noticeable than the lid crease incision. This approach allows intraoperative protection of the globe and cornea by the lower lid, which may be elevated with lid margin traction sutures. The traction sutures may be left in place for several days to prevent postoperative lid retraction. The greatest advantage of the inferior fornix incision is the elimination of the skin incision (except for a small canthotomy incision) and potential scarring. A canthotomy and lower cantholysis may be performed before the conjunctival incision.[36] Through this approach one transects the lower lid retractors. Closure of the conjunctiva and retractors at the end of the procedure will prevent possible problems later with lid malpositions. Prolonged conjunctival chemosis may occur following this approach to the orbital floor.

After the orbital rim is exposed, the periosteum is incised and elevated from the orbital rim and the floor of the orbit. The fracture is generally recognized very quickly as a depression of the periorbita into a defect in the floor, usually medially. Cautious dissection will avoid damage to the entrapped tissue. The infraorbital nerve should be identified as soon as possible to avoid inadvertent damage. Removal of some of the bone fragments may be required to safely reposition the orbital tissue above the orbital floor (Fig. 105–4). The maxillary sinus

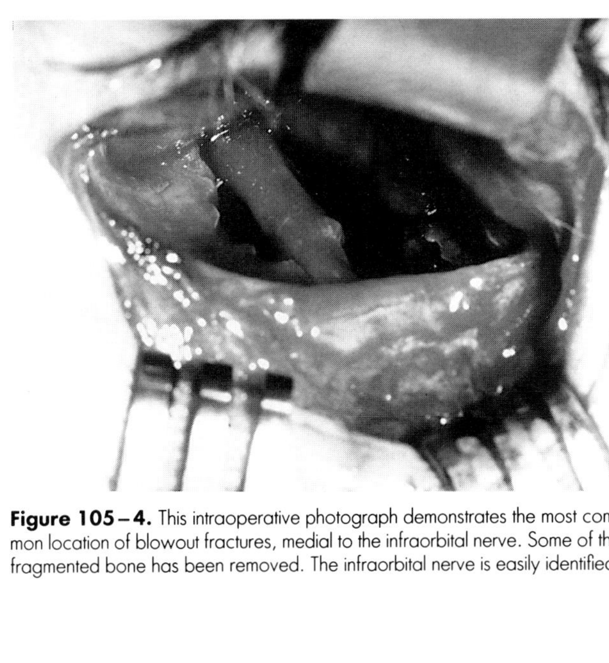

Figure 105–4. This intraoperative photograph demonstrates the most common location of blowout fractures, medial to the infraorbital nerve. Some of the fragmented bone has been removed. The infraorbital nerve is easily identified.

mucosa becomes adherent to the periorbita very soon after injury, and this should be removed from the orbital tissue as it is elevated into the socket. Sequestration of secreting mucosal tissue in the orbit may lead to formation of a cyst around the orbital floor implant.[37]

A variety of materials have been used to cover orbital floor bone defects and prevent the periorbita from sagging down into the maxillary sinus. Supramid and Silastic are readily available and, if cautiously sized and shaped for the defect, are unlikely to extrude or migrate. If late removal of the implant is necessary, the alloplastic materials are easily removed. Bone may be used, but requires a second surgical site to harvest and creates more discomfort for the patient.

After placement of the orbital floor implant, forced duction testing should be done again. The periosteum is closed securely over the anterior orbital rim. It is seldom necessary to directly suture the implanted material over the defect since the periosteum will hold it in position. The orbital septum should not be tethered in the closure if a subciliary or lid crease incision has been used. If the septum is caught up in the closure, lid retraction may result.

Immediate postoperative care should include bed rest with elevation of the head of the bed, medication for pain and nausea, ice compresses, and systemic antibiotics if the patient has a previous history of sinusitis. Dressings are not necessary; but if they are used, they should be removed the following day or sooner if acute pain develops. Traction sutures used in the lower lid margin may be kept in place for several days and may help to prevent lower lid retraction. Duration of the hospitalization may vary, depending on the patient. One night may be sufficient to observe the patient for immediate postoperative complications and provide pain relief. However, if painful ecchymosis of the lids and decreased vision occur, then intervention for postoperative hemorrhage and a longer stay in the hospital may be necessary.

Orbital cellulitis may occur after orbital fractures into the adjacent paranasal sinuses, with or without a previous history of sinusitis.[38] Systemic antibiotic treatment should be considered in patients with blow-out fractures, particularly those with a history of sinusitis.

Postoperatively, the patient should be advised to avoid nose blowing, lifting, bending, and straining for at least 2 weeks. Activities should be limited for an even longer period of time, particularly if the patient's livelihood involves lifting heavy objects. The patient should be instructed to return to the ophthalmologist immediately if pain, tense ecchymosis or edema of the lids, or decreased vision occurs.

Complications

Complications of blow-out fractures may arise from the trauma or from the surgical repair. Optic nerve injury and blindness may result from direct force of the trauma, shearing force on the vessels of the optic nerve sheath, or pterygomaxillary force (as in blow-in fractures).[39] Compartment syndromes including hemorrhage in the retrobulbar space or subperiosteal space may compromise vision early or late. The patient in Figure 105–5 underwent blow-out fracture repair 5 years before her presentation with acute painful proptosis, lid ecchymosis, and diffuse decrease in extraocular motility caused by a subperiosteal hematoma. She was admitted for intravenous antibiotic therapy and close followup of the visual acuity. No surgical intervention was pursued because of 20/20 visual acuity and rapid improvement of the proptosis and motility.

Loss of vision after surgery indicates intraoperative compression of the nerve by the implant or surgical instruments. Exploration and removal of the implant should be considered. Painful loss of vision associated with tense ecchymosis of the lids and decreased motility

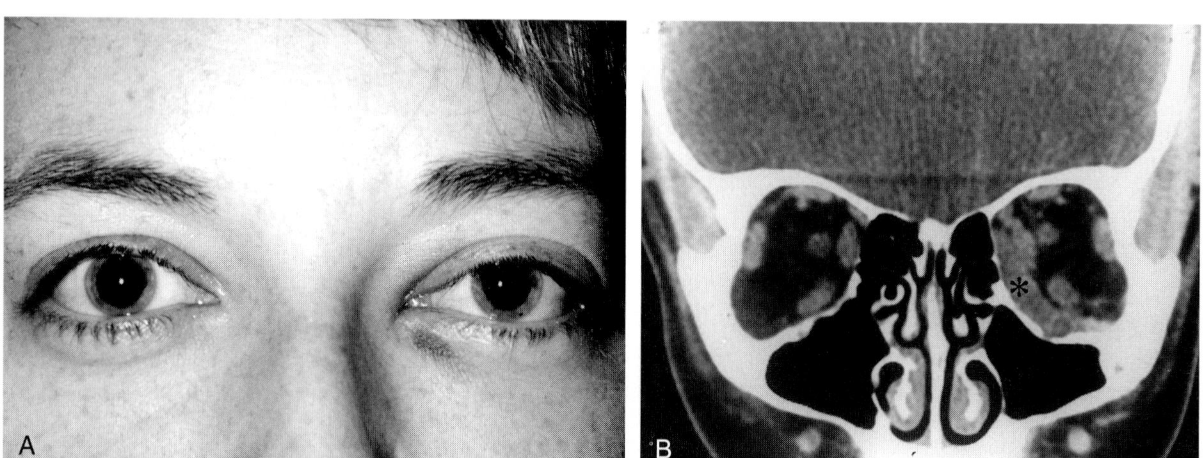

Figure 105–5. *A*, Left proptosis, lid ecchymosis, and edema are evident in this patient with a superiosteal hematoma. *B*, Computed tomographic scan showing a superiosteal fluid collection *(asterisk)* with lateral and upward displacement of the medial rectus and inferior rectus muscles. (From Kaltreider SA, Dortzbach RK: Orbital trauma. In Stephenson C [ed]: Ophthalmic Plastic, Reconstructive, and Orbital Surgery. Stoneham, MA, Butterworth-Heinemann, in press.)

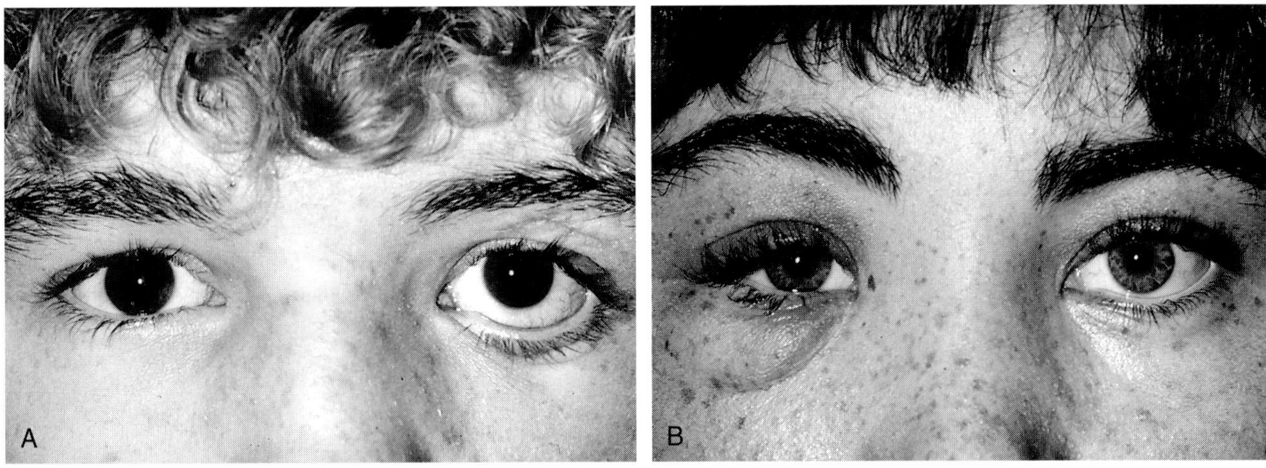

Figure 105–6. *A*, Lid retraction usually follows inadvertent capturing of the orbital septum when closing the periosteum over the implant or when closing the skin. Surgical repair is necessary except with very small amounts of retraction, which may repond to massage. *B*, This patient was referred for edema and ptosis 1 month following blowout fracture repair. During the next 6 months, the edema and ptosis gradually resolved spontaneously.

is characteristic of hemorrhage. Immediate exploration is indicated. Postoperative visual loss may be prevented by avoiding excessive pressure on the eye and optic nerve intraoperatively, intermittent tonometry readings intraoperatively, using the minimum-sized implant needed to cover the defect, keeping the implant under the periosteum, and notching the posterior margin of the implant.[40, 41] Caution should be exercised when using antral packing since this may also exert pressure on the optic nerve. Dressings, if used at all, should be removed early to monitor the pupils, vision, and fundus examination.

Certain complications are inherent in the surgical approach selected by the surgeon or may result from inadvertent capturing of the septum while closing the incision. Lid retraction complicated by lagophthalmos and exposure keratopathy may be seen with the subciliary approach. The patient in Figure 105–6*A* was referred for lid retraction after blow-out fracture repair. This complication is easily prevented by avoiding pulling the septum downward into the closure of the periosteum and by placing the lid on traction sutures for several days postoperatively. Prolonged lid edema and scarring may result from a lid crease or orbital rim incision. The patient in Figure 105–6*B* experienced prolonged edema of the lower lid and ptosis secondary to edema after repair of her blowout fracture through an incision directly over the orbital rim. This type of approach to the orbital floor is the least desirable. An inferior fornix incision avoids an obvious incision and subsequent potential for scarring. Inferior chemosis may be seen after this approach but resolves in time.

Persistent diplopia may be a result of inadequate release of entrapped tissue or paresis of the inferior rectus muscle (Fig. 105–7). Residual entrapment with dense scar tissue formation occurs when the initial surgical dissection is not carried posteriorly enough to free all of the entrapped tissue. Damage to the muscles or nerves may also occur as a result of the trauma or the corrective surgery. Hypertropia may occur after blowout fracture repair (Fig. 105–8). CT, forced ductions, and forced generations will help to clarify the cause of the residual strabismus. Therapeutic options include reexploration if the diplopia and motility defects are severe and restrictive, prisms if the diplopia is minimal, or extraocular muscle surgery to eliminate the diplopia in primary gaze. Recession of the ipsilateral superior rectus and inferior rectus muscles eliminates bothersome diplopia and expands the field of single binocular vision.[42]

Despite repair, enophthalmos may persist because of fat atrophy. Late enophthalmos related to fat atrophy may be partially corrected by building up the floor of the orbit with an implant. Alloplastic materials, fascia, bone, and dense hydroxyapatite have been used for this purpose.[43] If a maximal size implant is present, and a larger implant is likely to elevate the globe above the level of the contralateral eye, then another alternative is removal of the fat from the opposite upper lid to create a deeper superior sulcus similar to the injured side.[35]

Slowly developing enophthalmos after a blow-out fracture is also a presenting sign of a maxillary sinus mucocele, as seen in the patient in Figure 105–9.[38] Sequestered mucosal epithelium, compartmentalization of the maxillary sinus by bone fragments, or an obstructed sinus ostium are the etiologic mechanisms. The orbital floor becomes remodeled and descends, expanding the volume of the orbit. A CT scan should be obtained before correction of the enophthalmos to investigate this possibility. Surgery is directed at elevating the orbital contents with an implant, extirpating the maxillary sinus mucocele, and providing adequate drainage for the sinus.

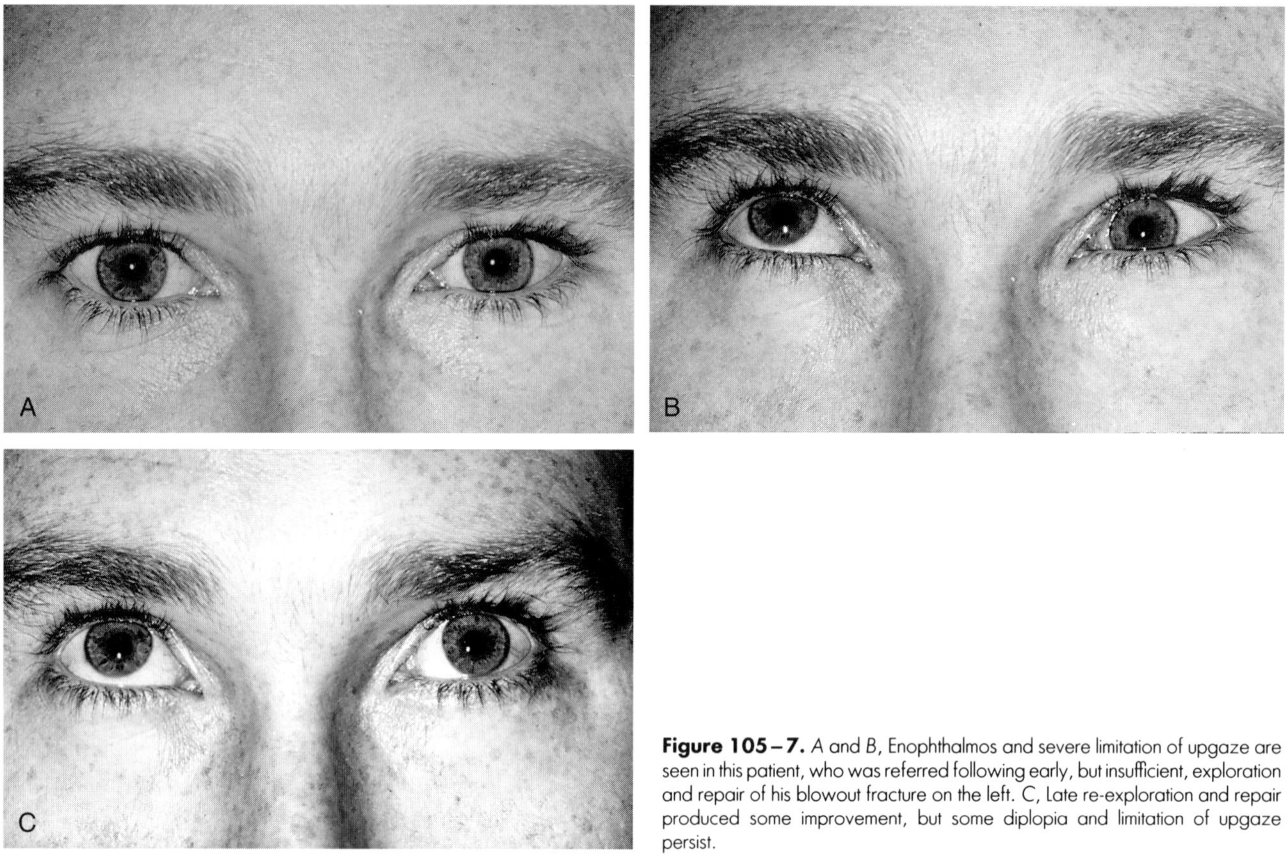

Figure 105–7. *A* and *B*, Enophthalmos and severe limitation of upgaze are seen in this patient, who was referred following early, but insufficient, exploration and repair of his blowout fracture on the left. *C*, Late re-exploration and repair produced some improvement, but some diplopia and limitation of upgaze persist.

MEDIAL ORBITAL WALL FRACTURES

Medial orbital fractures sometimes occur alone, but more often they accompany orbital floor fractures or nasoethmoidal fractures. Medial wall blow-out fractures occur in 20% or more of those patients who have orbital floor blow-out fractures.[44–46] Medial wall fractures resulting from crushing injuries to the nasal bridge may be more accurately classified as blow-in rather than blow-out fractures. The blunt force over the nasal bridge expands the ethmoidal sinus air cells, pushing the medial wall of the orbit laterally.

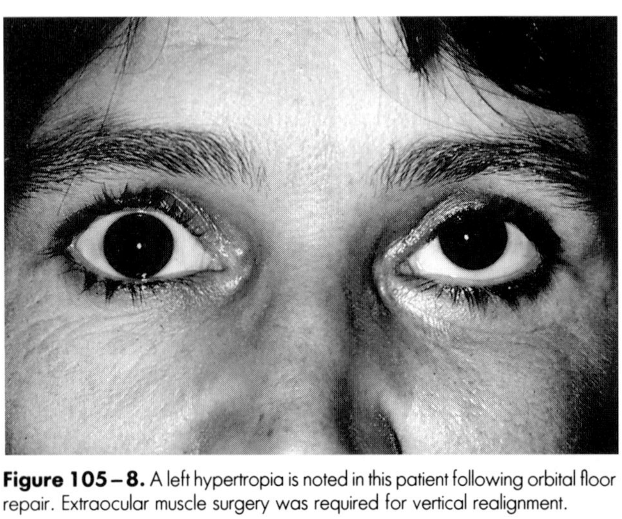

Figure 105–8. A left hypertropia is noted in this patient following orbital floor repair. Extraocular muscle surgery was required for vertical realignment.

These patients typically present with restriction of abduction and retraction of the globe and with limitation of adduction.[47] Periorbital edema, ecchymosis, orbital or lid emphysema, epistaxis, and enophthalmos may be seen on examination. Concomitant medial canthal tendon dehiscence and cerebrospinal fluid rhinorrhea may also occur.

Repair of medial wall fractures may be approached from a subciliary or an inferior fornix incision if the patient also has an orbital floor fracture. After releasing the entrapped orbital tissue, the implant is placed, avoiding pressure on the lacrimal apparatus anteriorly and the optic nerve posteriorly. Better visualization is provided by a medial canthal approach, as described in detail by Leone.[47] The lacrimal sac may be easily identified, and the anterior and posterior ethmoidal vessels may be cauterized and transected. A thin silicon implant is placed over the defect and sutured to the periorbita. Although an implant was not used in two patients in this series, placement of an implant is recommended. Just as in blow-out fractures of the orbital floor, forced duction testing is an important maneuver preoperatively and intraoperatively to ensure release of the entrapped orbital tissue.

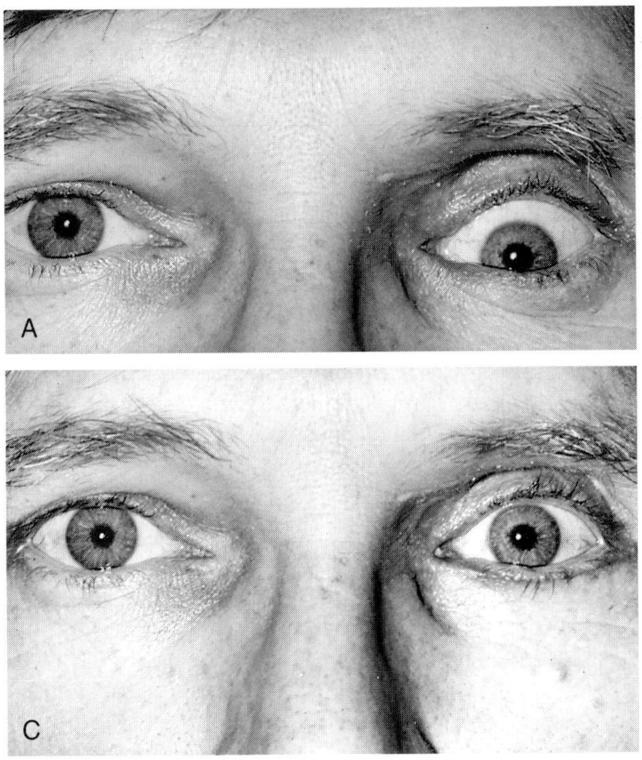

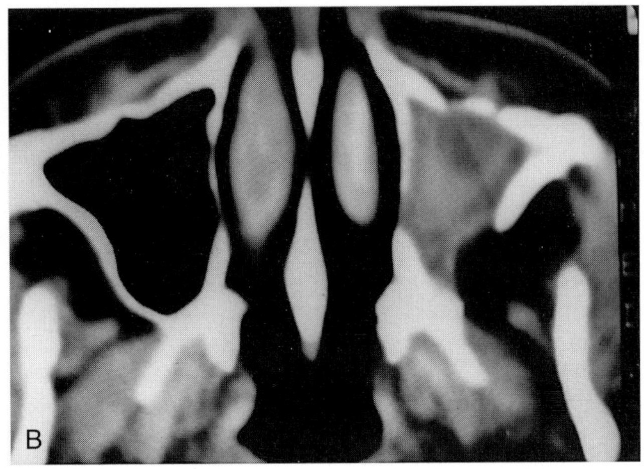

Figure 105–9. *A*, Eight months following blowout fracture that was not repaired, this patient presented with gradually progressive enophthalmos, downward displacement of the left eye, diplopia in extreme upgaze, and chronic irritation and foreign body sensation of the left eye. *B*, Computed tomographic scan showed opacification of the left maxillary sinus. *C*, Following exploration and repair of the orbital floor, and Caldwell-Luc exploration and nasal antrostomy to drain the maxillary sinus, the patient has 2 mm of residual enophthalmos and minimal diplopia in extreme upgaze. (From Kaltreider SA, Dortzbach RK: Destructive cysts of the maxillarly sinus affecting the orbit. Arch Ophthalmol 105:1398–1402, 1988. Copyright 1988, American Medical Association.)

ZYGOMATIC FRACTURES

The tripod fracture is one of the most common orbital fractures and, by nature of its location and the anatomy of the orbit, always involves the orbital floor. Most tripod fractures are a result of assault or automobile accidents.[48, 49] Sports, falls, and industrial accidents are responsible for a smaller number of tripod fractures. LeFort II and III fractures may also be present in these patients.[48]

Ocular and optic nerve injuries may be associated with tripod fractures and should be addressed first in examination of the patient. Orbital hemorrhage, edema, or displaced bone fragments may impinge on the optic nerve in the orbital apex, causing traumatic optic neuropathy. Blindness may result from the injury itself or from manipulation of the bone during repairs.[50–52]

Clinical findings may include flattening of the cheek, downward displacement of the lateral canthal tendon and globe, enophthalmos, superior sulcus deformity, and lower lid retraction. The patient may experience diplopia, trismus, infraorbital nerve hypesthesia, and epistaxis. These findings may be more pronounced in those patients with marked displacement of the malar bone.

Although the tripod fracture often may be adequately visualized on Water's and submentovertex radiographs, the CT scan best delineates the fracture and the relationship of the soft tissues to the fracture sites. The tripod fracture generally involves the zygomatic arch, the zygomaticofrontal suture, the lower zygomatic buttress, and the orbital floor along the infraorbital foramen.[19] Axial views to picture the apex and medial wall of the orbit and coronal views to evaluate the roof, medial wall, and floor are helpful.

Treatment

Stabilization of the displaced malar bone by a combination of wiring and miniplate fixation is indicated in those patients with a displaced or unstable zygoma. Three-point wire fixation may be adequate, but miniplate fixation (with one or two plates) has the advantage of greater stability and fewer late complications.[19, 53] One- or two-point fixation with wire does not resist the powerful rotational forces exerted by the masseter muscle. Those patients whose fractures are repaired with wire sutures more frequently have asymmetry and infraorbital nerve dysfunction and more often require orbital floor exploration.[19]

Prein and coworkers[19] recommend an incision in the lateral superciliary area to expose the zygomaticofrontal suture. A plate is then placed in this location, carefully shaping the plate to the proper contour to avoid displacement of the bone on tightening of the screws. If the stability of the zygoma is still in question, then an infraciliary incision is made, the inferior orbital rim and orbital floor are explored, and a second plate is placed along the inferior orbital rim.[19] Antral balloons and packing have been used in the repair of tripod fractures, but they may be associated with impingement on the optic nerve, overcorrection, and exophthalmos.[48, 49] Jackson[54] emphasizes three-point fixation, with the third point located along the zygomaticomaxillary buttress. He recommends the use of wires along the inferior and lateral orbital rims and a miniplate on the buttress.

Conventional approaches to repair are skin incisions near the fracture sites; however, safer access and better visualization of the orbital contents and fractures can be provided by a lateral canthotomy and inferior fornix approach.[54, 55] This excellent orbital exposure allows direct visualization as bone fragments are manipulated into position, provides access for medial wall and floor fracture repair, permits decompressing of the apex or removal of apical bone fragments, and avoids further trauma to the orbital apex, which might be induced by poor surgical exposure.[55, 56] Ideally, repair should be done within 1 week to minimize late complications and avoid the technical difficulties arising from fibrous proliferation along the fracture lines.[48]

Complications

Late sequelae of zygomatic fractures are facial asymmetry due to insufficient reduction of the fracture, diplopia, infraorbital nerve anesthesia, enophthalmos and downward displacement of the globe, and restricted jaw opening.[48, 51] Overcorrection with upward displacement of the globe is also a possibility. Delayed treatment is associated with more complications.[48] Edema, masseter force, wire fixation, antral packing alone, severe comminution of the bone, and scar tissue contracture are factors predisposing to the above complications.[51] The patient shown in Figure 105–10 demonstrates residual deformity after repair of a comminuted zygomatic fracture. Wire sutures were used at the zygomaticofrontal junction and at the site of another fracture line along the lower lateral orbital rim. Miniplate fixation was used to stabilize the orbital rim and the malar arch. Additional late reconstruction with bone grafts was planned 6 months after the primary repairs.

Several approaches to late reconstruction may be used.[53] The post-traumatic deformities may be disguised with alloplastic materials or bone grafts. The use of osteotomies along the fracture sites with mobilization, reduction, and fixation is another alternative. A combination of these approaches may also be effective. Perino and associates[53] recommend alloplastic materials or bone grafts in those patients who have minimal displacement and no loss of function. Osteotomy yields superior results in those patients with functional deficits such as depression of the lateral canthus, infraorbital nerve entrapment, and restricted mandibular excursion. Bone grafts along the rim or arch and orbital floor implants or grafts may be needed to restore normal contour and eliminate some of the enophthalmos.

Fibrous proliferation present in 3 to 5 weeks makes mobilization of the bone fragments extremely difficult.[53] Within 3 months the callus may be curetted and the bone mobilized; however, after this time period, osteotomes, chisels, and rotary devices are necessary.[53] Maximum exposure with minimal risk to the facial nerve branches is provided by a temporal flap approach. An infraciliary or inferior fornix incision may be added to expose the orbital floor.

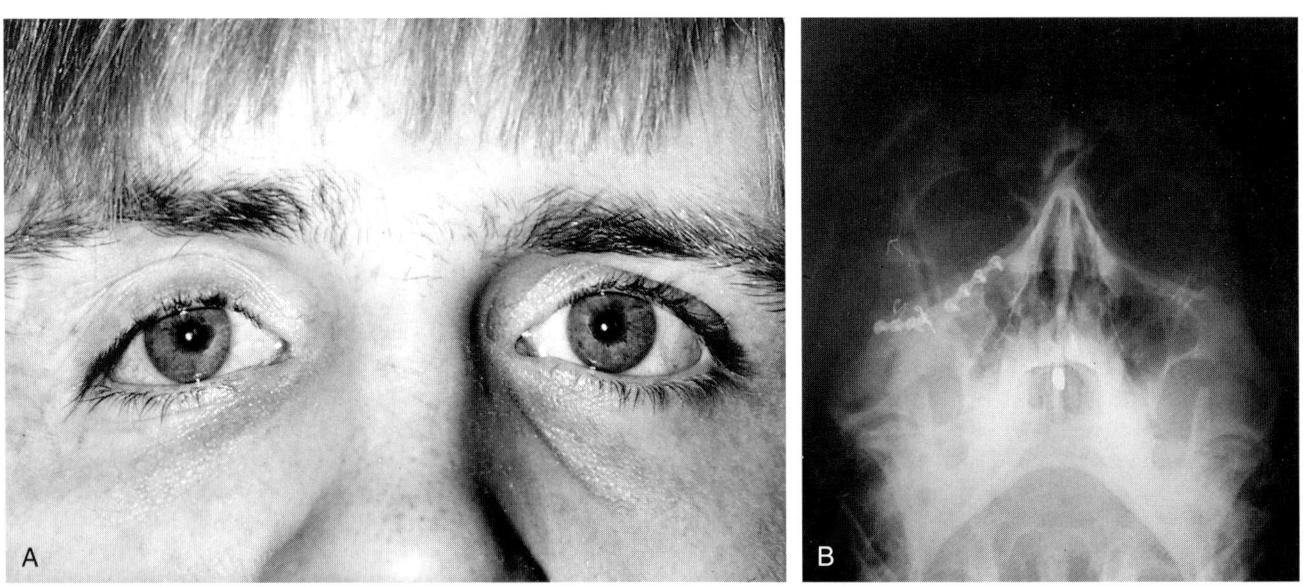

Figure 105–10. *A*, One month after repair of a comminuted zygomatic fracture, this patient has residual flattening of the malar area, downward displacement of the lateral canthal angle, and enophthalmos. *B*, A Water's view shows the wire sutures and miniplates used for repair of this comminuted fracture. (From Kaltreider SA, Dortzbach RK: Orbital trauma. In Stephenson C [ed]: Ophthalmic Plastic, Reconstructive, and Orbital Surgery. Stoneham, MA, Butterworth-Heinemann, in press.)

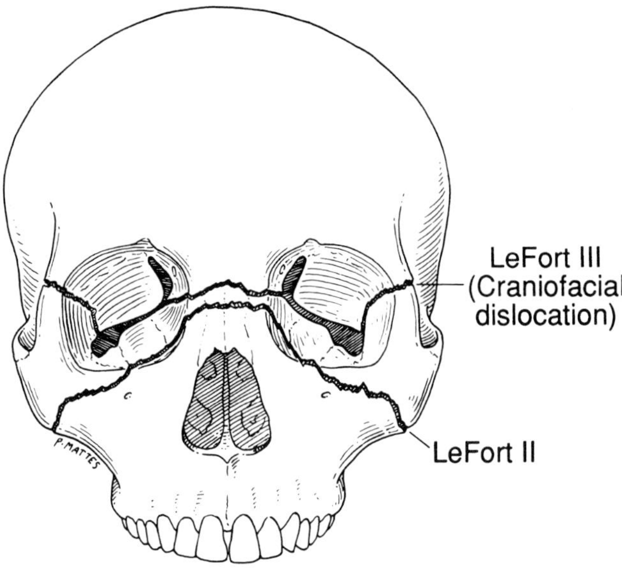

Figure 105–11. LeFort II and III fractures directly involve the orbital bones. Both may be associated with traumatic telecanthus. LeFort II fractures may involve the lacrimal excretory apparatus. LeFort III fractures may produce an elongated midface, with downward displacement of the lid and canthal structures. These fractures may occur together or in combination with other types of fractures. (From Kaltreider SA, Dortzbach RK: Orbital trauma. *In* Stephenson C [ed]: Ophthalmic Plastic, Reconstructive, and Orbital Surgery. Stoneham, MA, Butterworth-Heinemann, in press.)

LeFORT FRACTURES

LeFort described and classified midface fractures in 1900.[57] These fractures result from severe crushing blows to the midface, most occurring in the setting of motor vehicle accidents. Although LeFort I fractures may be associated with LeFort II or III fractures or other craniofacial fractures, this type of fracture does not directly involve the orbit. LeFort II and III fractures directly involve the orbital bones (Fig. 105–11). LeFort II fractures may disrupt the medial canthal tendon, whereas LeFort III fractures (craniofacial disjunction) produce an elongated midface. Both may interfere with the lacrimal excretory system. Ocular adnexal examination should include evaluation of the medial canthal tendon, the lateral canthal tendon, and the lacrimal excretory system.

Treatment

Exploration and fixation may be undertaken through a combination of skin incisions and a Caldwell-Luc approach. A transconjunctival incision may be added for floor exploration and repair if indicated. A coronal incision is particularly advantageous for extensive facial fractures and especially LeFort III fractures.[58, 59] Miniplate fixation provides the greatest stability and functional use of the jaw, often eliminating the need for intermaxillary fixation as discussed in the section on rigid fixation.

NASO-ORBITAL FRACTURES

Nasoethmoidal fractures often occur in combination with other facial fractures. Orbital floor and rim fractures, frontal and glabellar fractures, orbital roof fractures, LeFort fractures, and orbital apex fractures may be seen in these patients. The ethmoidal plates and nasal or vomer bone fragments may be thrusted posteriorly by the trauma, piercing through the region of the crista galli and penetrating into the cerebral tissue.

A high incidence of visual loss is associated with nasoethmoidal fractures. Globe perforation and optic nerve injury occur in 30%, and central nervous system injury occurs in 51%.[60] The patient in Figure 105–12 sustained crushing midface injuries that included naso-orbital, ethmoidal, and LeFort III fractures and avulsion of the left optic nerve. He underwent open reduction with wiring and extensive miniplate fixation using Luhr miniplates. Automobile accidents are a common cause of crushing midface injuries associated with visual loss.

Stabilization of the airway and evaluation of life-threatening and neurosurgical injuries are the first priority. Frontal and skull base fractures should be sought. As with all other types of orbital trauma, a thorough ocular examination is mandatory to exclude disruption of the globe and intraocular complications and to thoroughly document the preoperative status of the anterior and posterior visual pathways. Multispecialty involvement in the care of the patient is essential.

Adnexal examination typically reveals traumatic telecanthus and saddle deformity of the nose.[61] Rounding of the medial canthal angle and widening of the intercanthal distance occurs when the medial canthal tendon is dehisced along with bony fragments and pulled in a lateral direction with contraction of the orbicularis oculi. The lacrimal excretory apparatus may be disrupted by bone fragments or by the shearing forces of the injury. This may occur at the level of the canaliculi, common canaliculus, sac, or nasolacrimal duct. Lid edema, ecchymosis, and crepitus may be observed.

Cerebrospinal fluid leak occurs in approximately 20% of all patients with midface trauma and in 42% of patients with nasoethmoidal fractures.[60, 62] Frontal sinus fractures with dural lacerations may cause the leak. A cerebrospinal fluid leak may be detected on examination as a clear watery discharge or may be perceived by the patient as a salty-tasting fluid in the nasopharynx.[62] Cerebrospinal fluid may also collect in the interseptal or subperiosteal spaces of the orbit, forming a fluctuant mass.

A thin-section, axial CT scan of the orbits will provide a detailed picture of the extent of the fractures and the relationship of the bone fragments to the soft tissues of the orbit. One should systematically look for intraocular and intraorbital air, optic nerve or globe disruption, hemorrhage in the various orbital compartments, associated orbital roof or apex fractures, and intracranial air, bone fragments, or hemorrhage.

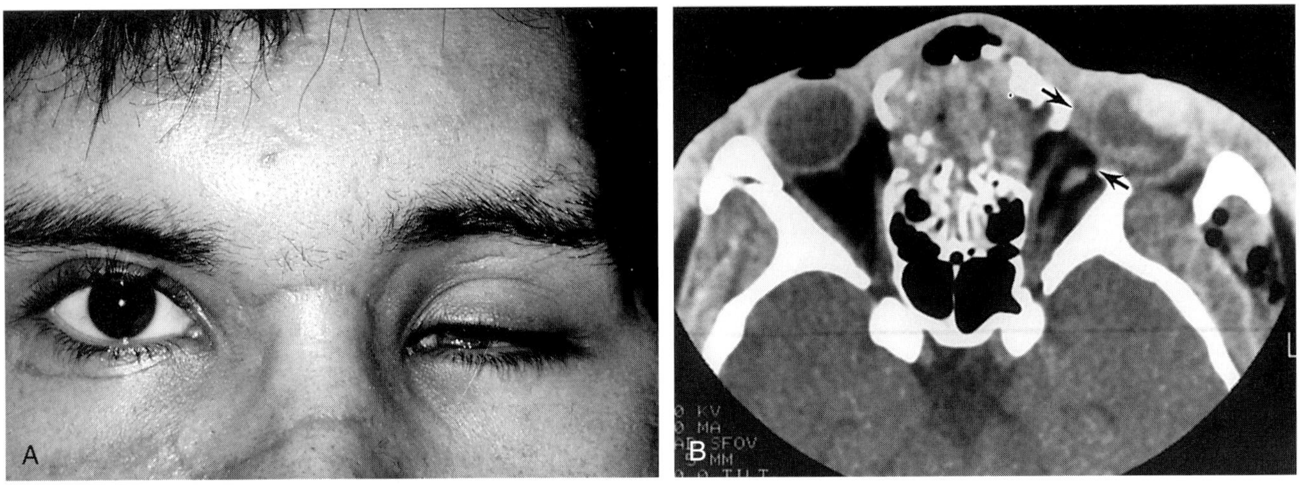

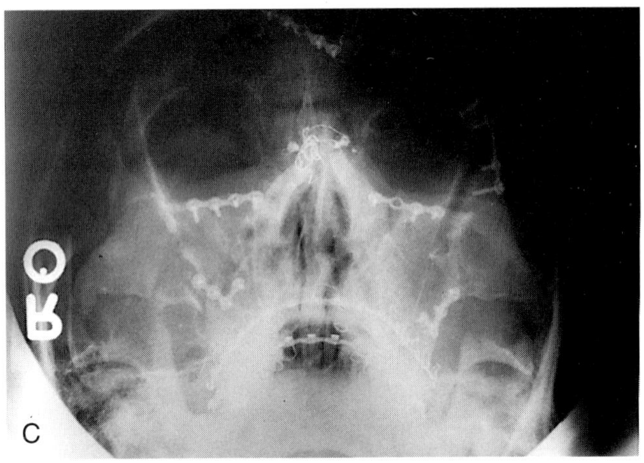

Figure 105–12. *A*, This patient sustained a crushing midface injury in an automobile accident several months before this photograph was taken. The enophthalmic left eye has no light perception. *B*, Computed tomographic scan shows the forces of the bone fragments *(arrows)* that snapped the optic nerve from the globe. The eye was pushed laterally by the medial orbital rim (frontal process of the maxillary bone), and the nerve was restricted in its lateral movement by the tip of the sphenoid wing. The optic nerve was totally avulsed from the eye. *C*, Wiring of the nasal bones, miniplate fixation, and intermaxillary fixation were techniques used for repairs. (From Kaltreider SA, Dortzbach RK: Orbital trauma. *In* Stephenson C [ed]: Ophthalmic Plastic, Reconstructive, and Orbital Surgery. Stoneham, MA, Butterworth-Heinemann, in press.)

Treatment

After stabilization of the patient, neurosurgical evaluation, and examination of the eyes, appropriate exploration and repairs of the nasal and adnexal abnormalities may proceed. Investigation of the lacrimal excretory system should be performed. Lacrimal probing and irrigation with methylene blue or fluorescein will aid in defining abnormalities. Absence of reflux may not be indicative of an intact system since the irrigating fluid may be diverted through a tear in the sac, conducting fluid into the surrounding wound or orbit. The surgeon may want to ensure patency of the nasolacrimal system at the conclusion of the reconstructive procedures by repeating the probing and irrigation to rule out kinking of the canaliculi, sac, or duct or mechanical obstruction by wires or sutures.

Transnasal wiring for bilateral medial canthal tendon dehiscence or ipsilateral or transnasal wiring for unilateral dehiscence may be necessary. The wiring may be executed through an existing wound, through a dacryocystorhinostomy incision, or with an H-shaped incision over the bridge of the nose, depending on the extent of the fractures and the need for exposure for other aspects of the reconstruction.[61] When multidisciplinary surgical intervention is required for extensive fractures or neurosurgical exploration, a coronal incision may be advantageous.[58–60]

Medial canthal tendon wiring is achieved by drilling holes in stable bone unilaterally or transnasally through osteotomies, passing the wire through the bone with a Veirs needle or awl, and then passing the wire through the tendon.[61] The medial canthal tendon should be drawn medially and posteriorly, well behind the anterior lacrimal crest, to avoid pulling the lid margins away from the anterior surface of the globe.

FRONTOBASAL FRACTURES

Fractures in the supraorbital and glabellar region are relatively less common than the fractures already discussed but have serious consequences if the fractures extend through the inner table of the frontal bone to involve the central nervous system. Interference of the frontal sinus duct may also cause major long-term complications. Most of these fractures result from high-velocity impact to the frontal area, as in automobile accidents. They may be associated with other facial fractures, especially nasal, zygomatic, and maxillary fractures.[63] Isolated fractures of the superior orbital rim and glabellar area not involving the inner table of bone or the frontal sinus duct are a subset of frontobasal fractures that are less worrisome with respect to serious complications.

Clinical examination reveals lid edema and ecchymosis, tenderness and crepitus over the frontal area, decrease in frontalis action, diplopia, and cerebrospinal fluid rhinorrhea. Routine skull radiographs may disclose the fractures; however, CT is a far superior diagnostic imaging technique to determine the presence of intracranial air and visualize the inner table of the frontal bone. Thin-section axial CT views with bone window settings are optimal for evaluating this type of fracture.[64]

Treatment

The management of frontobasal fractures depends on the involvement of the cerebral wall of the frontal sinus and the status of the dural and cerebral tissues. The anterior wall of the frontal sinus may be reconstructed using miniplate fixation. Large defects may require onlay of cranial bone grafts. Stents for maintaining patency of the frontal ostium may be necessary if extensive damage to the mucous membrane of the sinus and the inner wall of the sinus exists.[19] Intervention may therefore require interdisciplinary collaboration between the neurosurgeon and the otolaryngologist.

Exploration and repair of depressed fragments of bone should be undertaken after stablilization of the patient. Small nondisplaced fractures without involvement of the inner table of bone may be observed. Grossly displaced fragments of bone along the orbital rim may be repositioned and fixed in place if they do not remain in the desired anatomic position.[63] The superior orbital rim area may be approached through an existing laceration, infrabrow incision, suprabrow incision, forehead incision within a relaxed skin tension line, or upper lid crease incision. The patient whose CT scan is seen in Figure 105–13 was struck with a bat over the right superior orbital rim. This isolated rim fracture was repaired through a lid crease incision rather than reopening the brow wound that had been sutured before referral.

Neurosurgical evaluation is indicated in the event of intracranial involvement. Neurosurgical exploration and reconstruction of the frontal area may be indicated, and, if so, exposure of the affected orbital bones is excellent through a bicoronal flap approach.[65] Bone fragments are then gently maneuvered into position with periosteal elevators and wired or fixed with miniplates if the periosteum itself does not support the bone fragments in a normal anatomic location.[63] Secondary reconstruction may be necessary using onlay split rib grafts or alloplastic implants to restore normal contour to visibly depressed areas, although primary repair using the existing bone fragments may be preferable.[65] Intravenous antibiotics such as penicillin or a cephalosporin are an important safeguard against infectious complications.

Complications

Complications of frontobasal fractures arise from infections and obstruction of the nasofrontal duct. Meningitis and brain abscess may arise from the entry of organisms through the fracture site. Sinusitis, osteomyelitis, mucocele, and osteomyelitis may occur when the drainage of the sinus is compromised.[64] The nasofrontal duct is located above the nasofrontal suture and empties into the middle meatus or adjacent to the ethmoid infundibulum. Fractures medial to the supraorbital notch, and those involving the anterior table and nasoethmoid bones, are more likely to cause obstruction of the duct and long-term complications.[64] Intersinus septectomy with stenting or sinus obliteration may be necessary to prevent or treat complications.

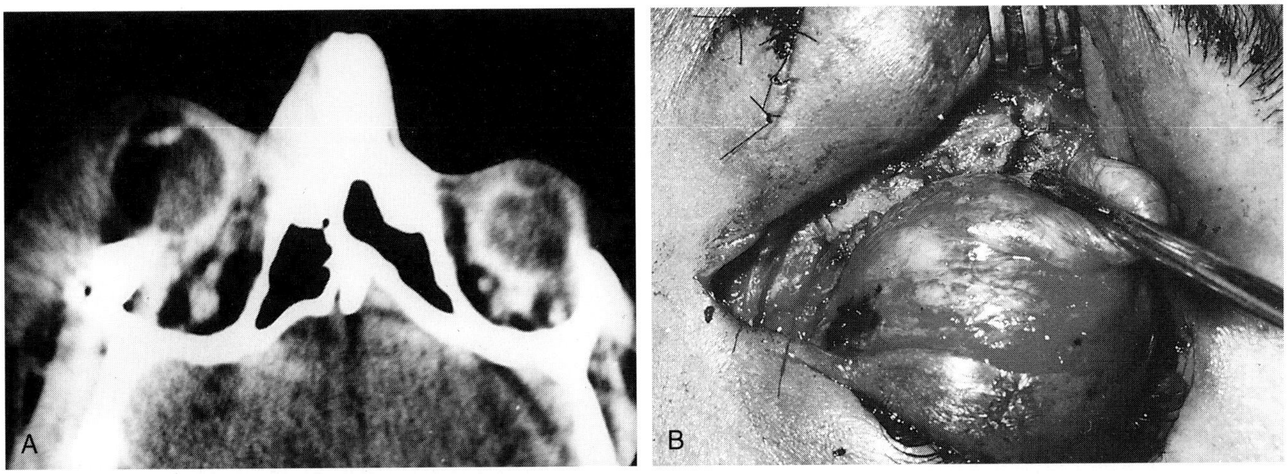

Figure 105–13. *A*, A superolateral orbital rim fracture with the displaced fragment abutting the posterior globe is seen in this computed tomographic scan. *B*, Intraoperative view of the two orbital rim fragments wired into place.

A cerebrospinal fluid leak may also complicate frontobasal fractures and is of concern because of the potential for ascending infection. Close neurosurgical followup, antibiotic therapy, and surgical intervention for persistent leak are indicated.[65]

ORBITAL ROOF FRACTURES

Orbital roof fractures are found in 5% of patients with facial fractures and are usually a result of severe crush injuries from falls, motor vehicle accidents, and blows to the facial area with heavy objects.[66] Fractures of this type may be produced by a blow-out mechanism, by extension of fractures of the superior orbital rim, or by direct injury from penetrating objects.[66, 67] Anterior fractures of the orbital roof may extend into the frontal sinus alone, into the cranial cavity, or both.

These fractures may be associated with nasal or ethmoidal fractures. Fragments of bone may telescope into the intracranial fossa. Posterior fractures of the roof with or without other orbital apex fractures may result in optic nerve injury. The patient in Figure 105–14 sustained a right orbital roof fracture in an automobile accident. On initial examination, the visual acuity was 20/20 without a visual field defect or afferent pupillary defect. Lid edema, ecchymosis, proptosis, and third cranial nerve palsy were also noted. Over the next 2 days the vision decreased to 20/200 and a superior altitudinal defect developed. Intravenous high-dose corticosteroids were begun, and surgery was planned to remove bone fragments impinging on the optic nerve at the apex of the orbit. After intracranial exploration and removal of displaced bone fragments, the vision recovered to 20/20 and the third cranial nerve palsy and visual field defect resolved.

Childhood orbital roof fractures may be isolated and associated with relatively minor trauma, such as a fall or birth trauma.[68] Fractures in this age group may also be associated with extensive craniofacial fractures. Softer bone and lack of frontal sinus pneumatization may make infants and children more susceptible to this type of fracture.[68] On the other hand, forces of the fracture may be more readily transmitted to the apex of the orbit in adults, thereby making optic nerve damage more likely in older patients.[68]

In children, the classic picture is one of an evolving lid hematoma after frontal injury. In all age groups, the spectrum of ocular and orbital findings includes visual loss, levator dysfunction, lid or orbital hematoma or crepitus, and extraocular motility defects. Neurologic

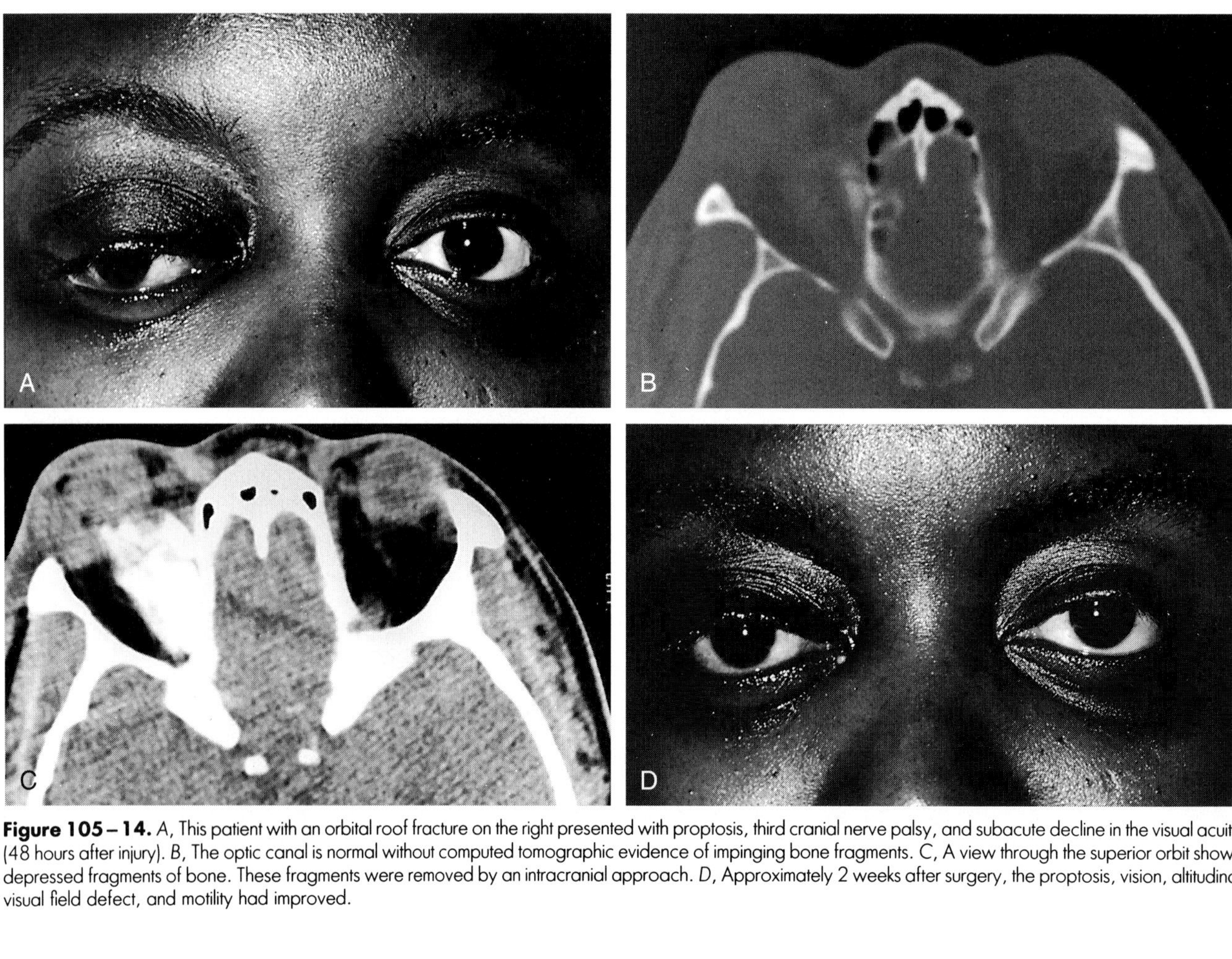

Figure 105–14. *A*, This patient with an orbital roof fracture on the right presented with proptosis, third cranial nerve palsy, and subacute decline in the visual acuity (48 hours after injury). *B*, The optic canal is normal without computed tomographic evidence of impinging bone fragments. *C*, A view through the superior orbit shows depressed fragments of bone. These fragments were removed by an intracranial approach. *D*, Approximately 2 weeks after surgery, the proptosis, vision, altitudinal visual field defect, and motility had improved.

manifestations such as headache, cerebrospinal fluid leak, meningismus, and stupor or loss of consciousness may be present. Intracranial hemorrhage, pneumocephalus, and cerebral contusion or laceration by bone fragments may be evident on CT. Orbital and neurologic sequelae may include traumatic optic neuropathy, ptosis, superior rectus or superior oblique dysfunction, trigeminal first- or second-division sensory deficits, persistent orbital structural deformities and enophthalmos, anosmia, meningitis, brain abscess, frontal sinus mucocele, encephalocele, encephalomalacia, and persistent cerebrospinal fluid leak.[68, 69]

Evaluation of patients suspected of having orbital roof fractures should include a thorough neurologic examination and ocular and orbital evaluation after potentially life-threatening issues have been addressed. CT scan, particularly coronal CT imaging, is most helpful in defining the extent of the fractures, presence of displaced bone spicules, entrapment of orbital tissues in the fracture site, and intracranial involvement.

Treatment

Treatment of orbital roof fractures with no displacement of bone and no evidence of intracranial complications may be conservative; however, the incidence of meningitis and brain abscess is a major risk, particularly if cerebrospinal fluid rhinorrhea and intracranial air are present.[66] The latter two findings establish the existence of a communication between the nasopharynx or sinuses and the cranial vault.

Selection of the surgical approach is based on the extent of cerebral involvement and dural tears. If dural tears and intracranial damage are not evident, then an anterosuperior orbitotomy approach may be used to expose and release entrapped orbital tissue and remove displaced bone fragments.[66] Persistent or large cerebrospinal fluid leaks, cerebral injuries, or presence of retained intracranial foreign bodies mandate an intracranial approach by the neurosurgeon or a collaborative approach by both the neurosurgeon and the ophthalmologist.[66]

Intravenous antibiotics are an absolute necessity since many patients go on to develop brain abscess or meningitis, particularly those with foreign-body injuries and those with intracranial air, indicating a communication with the paranasal sinuses. Delayed complications may arise many weeks later and, therefore, close extended followup by both the ophthalmologist and neurosurgeon is important.

ORBITAL APEX FRACTURES

Orbital apex fractures may be associated with cranial vault, skull base, facial, or other orbital fractures. Motor vehicle accidents, beatings, falls, and other types of crushing injuries are capable of producing apex fractures. The sphenoid bone is the portal through which all important neurovasular structures enter the orbit. The clinical impact of the apex fracture is a direct reflection of this anatomy. Sensory, motor, and vascular input to the extraocular muscles, lacrimal gland, and globe enter through the superior orbital fissure flanked by the greater and lesser wings of the sphenoid bone. The optic nerve, vascular supply to the optic nerve and retina, and sympathetic input enter through the optic canal in the sphenoid body.

Different syndromes may result from fractures in the apex.[70] Ophthalmoplegia, ptosis, and sensory deficits may arise from trauma involving the superior orbital fissure. Blindness secondary to direct or indirect injury to the optic nerve or its blood supply may result from trauma to the optic canal area. Visual loss from traumatic optic neuropathy even in the absence of orbital apex or optic canal fractures has been well documented in the literature before and after the advent of CT.[69, 71–74] Conversely, fractures across the apex of the orbit are not necessarily associated with loss of vision and may produce variable degrees of ophthalmoplegia. In a review of 17 patients with orbital apex fractures, Unger noted that most of these patients had other craniofacial fractures.[70] Twenty of 23 fractures were comminuted, 1 was linear, and 2 were avulsion fractures with an intact optic foramen. Six patients had a superior orbital fissure syndrome, and three had optic neuropathy.

Manfredi reviewed 379 consecutive patients with facial fractures and found that 21 (6%) had visual loss secondary to facial trauma.[56] In 12 of these patients, a CT scan had been performed. Seven had ocular rupture, vitreous hemorrhage, or retinal detachment explaining the visual loss. The remaining 5 had a fracture through the optic canal seen on CT scan. One other patient had frontal trauma with blindness, but no fracture evident on CT scan. In 5 of 6 of these patients with optic nerve injury, the impact was at the level of the orbital roof, and in the other patient the primary impact was at the level of the orbital floor. The latter patient also had frontal sinus fractures, indicating impact at the level of the roof as well as the floor. Significant CT findings associated with optic nerve injury were fractures of the lesser wing of the sphenoid or hemorrhage into the optic nerve sheath. Another important observation was an association between sphenoethmoidal sinus hemorrhage and optic canal fracture (31%).[56]

Diagnosis of orbital apex fractures is best accomplished by high-resolution, thin-section CT. Multiplanar views are helpful in determining the three-dimensional anatomy of the injury, detecting displaced bone fragments, and revealing possible areas of impingement on the optic nerve. Sections should extend well above the orbit to detect fractures involving the orbital roof, intracranial bone fragments, foreign bodies, hemorrhage, or

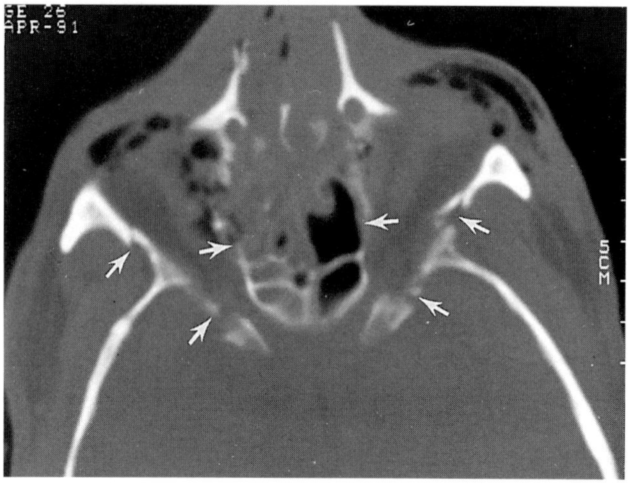

Figure 105–15. Computed tomographic scan of a patient who was in a multiple vehicle accident and sustained a crushing injury to the midface. Notice the air in the orbit and the lids and the opacities in the ethmoid and sphenoid sinuses. The fractures of the greater wings of the sphenoids, the orbital apices adjacent to the superior orbital fissures, and the ethmoids are marked by the arrows from the lateral to the medial direction respectively. The optic canals appear intact. This patient had no evidence of traumatic optic neuropathy on either side. (From Kaltreider SA, Dortzbach RK: Orbital trauma. *In* Stephenson C [ed]: Ophthalmic Plastic, Reconstructive and Orbital Surgery. Stoneham, MA, Butterworth-Heinemann, in press.)

air. Likewise, CT sections should also extend through the paranasal sinuses to detect other midface fractures. The patient whose CT scan is seen in Figure 105–15 was an unrestrained passenger in a motor vehicle accident. Crushing forces to the midface produced orbital apex and LeFort II and III fractures. Visual acuity was 20/30 on both sides without afferent pupillary defects. Open reduction and internal fixation of the LeFort fractures was performed along with intermaxillary fixation.

Treatment

Management of orbital apex fractures in essence amounts to treatment of the resulting syndromes or the intracranial complications. The ophthalmologist must therefore consider the indications for intervention for direct or indirect optic nerve trauma, superior orbital fissure syndrome, or orbital apex syndrome. Intervention for neurosurgical complications supercedes ocular or orbital considerations but may provide an opportunity to explore the optic nerve in its canal by a superior approach. Indications for surgical intervention in cases of traumatic visual loss are discussed in another chapter. Potential deterioration of vision or injury to the optic nerve during surgical fixation of facial fractures must be remembered when treating facial fractures with or without associated orbital apex fractures.[40, 50–52]

PANFACIAL FRACTURES

Panfacial fractures involve bony elements of the upper, middle, and lower face. Thus, the combination of nasoethmoidal, zygomatic or LeFort, and mandibular fractures constitutes panfacial fracture. High-energy impact injuries such as those sustained in automobile accidents are largely responsible for these fractures. The individual components of panfacial fractures have been discussed, however, a brief discussion of the approach to the patient with multiple fractures might be helpful. Guidelines to prioritizing the repairs are based on the three-dimensional anatomy of the facial bones and the vertical and horizontal facial buttresses.[75]

The nasomaxillary, zygomaticomaxillary, and pterygomaxillary vertical buttresses must be normally aligned to preserve the height of the face. The horizontal and anteroposterior dimensions are preserved by properly aligning the supraorbital rims and glabella, the infraorbital rims, the zygomatic arches, and the horizontal or basal segments of the mandible.[75] Attention to the above relationships will maintain the width, height, and projection of the facial features.

The mandibular and maxillary arches must be aligned perfectly to establish normal occlusion.[75] Once the occlusion has been addressed, the vertical mandibular rami are repaired. The upper facial reconstruction may require neurosurgical intervention and attention to the naso-orbital complex to establish normal width. The intercanthal distance may require overcorrection to achieve a normal anatomy and appearance. Exploration of the orbit and the zygomatic complex is performed next. Finally, reduction of the midface fractures with attention to the major anterior buttresses is done. Assessment for primary bone grafting using split-rib grafts for the orbit and nose and calvarial grafts for the LeFort fractures may be done.[75]

In summary, one often encounters patients requiring reconstruction of multiple facial fractures. Unless intracranial intervention is required initially, then the preferred sequence for fixation is (1) the occlusion and lower face, (2) the upper face and orbits, and (3) the midface. An interdisciplinary team is often essential for optimal outcome. The diagnostic capabilities of multiplanar high-resolution CT and advances in biotechnology often allow reconstruction to a normal or nearly normal functional anatomy.

REFERENCES

1. Petro J, Tooze FM, Bales CR, et al: Ocular injuries associated with periorbital fractures. J Trauma 19:730, 1979.
2. Hoehn RJ: Facial injuries. Surg Clin North Am 53:1479, 1973.
3. Luce EA, Tubb TD, Moore AM: Review of 1,000 major facial fractures and associated injuries. Plast Reconstr Surg 63:26, 1979.
4. Swearingen JJ: Tolerance of the Human Face to Crash Impact.

Oklahoma City, Office of Aviation Medicine, Federal Aviation Agency, Civil Aeromedical Research Institute, 1965.

5. Grove AS: Computed tomography in the management of orbital trauma. Ophthalmology 89:433, 1982.
6. Grove AS, Tadmor R, New PFJ, et al: Orbital fracture evaluation by coronal CT. Am J Ophthalmol 85:679, 1978.
7. Lindahl S: Computed tomography of intraorbital foreign bodies. Acta Radiol 28:235, 1987.
8. Koornneef L, Zonneveld FW: The role of direct multiplanar high resolution CT in the assessment and management of orbital trauma. Radiol Clin North Am 25:753, 1987.
9. Bilaniuk LT, Atlas SW, Zimmerman RA: Magnetic resonance imaging of the orbit. Radiol Clin North Am 25:509, 1987.
10. Lagouros PA, Langer BG, Peyman GA: Magnetic resonance imaging and intraocular foreign bodies. Arch Ophthalmol 105:551, 1987.
11. Kelley WM, Paglen PG, Pearson JA, et al: Ferromagnetism of intraocular foreign body causes unilateral blindness after MR study. AJNR 7:243, 1986.
12. Wright PM, Swietek PA, Simmons ML: Eye artifacts from mascara in MRI. Am J Neuroradiol 6:652, 1985.
13. Wilson WB, Dreisbach JN, Lattin DE, et al: Magnetic resonance imaging of nonmetallic orbital foreign bodies. Am J Ophthalmol 105:612, 1988.
14. Tucker MR, Terry BC, White RP, Van Sickels JE (eds): Rigid Fixation for Maxillofacial Surgery. Philadelphia, JB Lippincott, 1991.
15. Hansmann H: Eine neue Methode zur Fixierung der Fragmente bei complicierten Frakturen. Verh Dtsch Ges Chir 15:134, 1886.
16. Key JA: Positive pressure in arthrodesis for tuberculosis of the knee joint. South Med J 25:909, 1932.
17. Luhr HG: Zur stabilen Osteosynthese bei Unterkieferfrakturen. Dtsch Zahnarztl Z 23:754, 1968.
18. Luhr HG: A micro-system for cranio-maxillofacial skeletal fixation. J Craniomaxillofac Surg 16:312, 1988.
19. Prein J, Schilli W, Hammer B, et al: Rigid fixation of facial fractures. Fonseca RJ, Walker RV (eds): *In* Oral and Maxillofacial Trauma, vol 2. Philadelphia, WB Saunders, 1991, p 1172.
20. Marsh JL: The use of the Wurtzberg system to facilitate fixation in facial osteotomies. Clin Plast Surg 16:49, 1989.
21. MacKenzie W: Traite Pratique des Maladies des Yeux. Laugier S, Richelot G (trans). Paris: B Dusillon, 1884, p vii.
22. Converse JM, Smith B: Enophthalmos and diplopia in fractures of the orbital floor. Br J Plast Surg 9:265, 1956.
23. Smith B, Regan WF: Blowout fracture of the orbit. Am J Ophthalmol 44:733, 1957.
24. Fujino T, Sato TB: Mechanisms, tolerance limit curve and theoretical analysis in blow-out fractures of two and three dimensional orbital wall models. *In* Proceedings of the Third International Symposium on Orbital Disorders, Amsterdam, 1967.
25. Jones DEP, Evans JNG: "Blow-out" fracture of the orbit: An investigation into the anatomic basis. J Laryngol Otol 81:1109, 1967.
26. Wojno T: The incidence of extraocular muscle and cranial nerve palsy in orbital floor blow-out fractures. Ophthalmology 94:682, 1987.
27. Raflo GT: Blow-in and blow-out fractures of the orbit: clinical correlations and proposed mechanisms. Ophthalmic Surg 15:114, 1984.
28. Dingman RO, Natvig P: Surgery of Facial Fractures. Philadelphia, WB Saunders, 1964.
29. Hawes MJ, Dortzbach RK: Surgery on orbital floor fractures: Influence of time of repair and fracture size. Ophthalmology 90: 1056, 1983.
30. Berkowitz RA, Putterman AM, Patel DB: Prolapse of the globe into the maxillary sinus after orbital floor fracture. Am J Ophthalmol 91:253, 1981.
31. Gilbard SM, Mafee MF, Lagouros PA, et al: Orbital blow-out fractures: The prognostic significance of computed tomography. Ophthalmology 92:1523, 1985.
32. Millman AL, Della Rocca RC, Spector S, et al: Steroids and orbital blow-out fractures: A new systematic concept in medical management and surgical decision-making. Adv Ophthalmic Plast Reconstr Surg 6:291, 1987.
33. Putterman AM, Stevens T, Urist MJ: Nonsurgical management of blow-out fractures of the orbital floor. Am J Ophthalmol 77:232, 1974.
34. Putterman AM: Late management of blow-out fractures of the orbital floor. Trans Am Acad Ophthalmol Otolaryngol 83:650, 1977.
35. Dortzbach RK: Orbital floor fractures. Ophthalmic Plast Reconstr Surg 1:149, 1985.
36. McCord CD, Moses JL: Exposure of the inferior orbit with fornix incision and lateral canthotomy. Ophthalmic Surg 10:53, 1989.
37. Kaltreider SA, Dortzbach RK: Destructive cysts of the maxillary sinus affecting the orbit. Arch Ophthalmol 105:1398, 1988.
38. Goldfarb MS, Hoffman DS, Rosenberg S: Orbital cellulitis and orbital fractures. Ann Ophthalmol 19:97, 1987.
39. Cullen GCR, Luce CM, Shannon GM: Blindness following blow-out orbital fractures. Ophthalmic Surg 8:60, 1977.
40. Nicholson DH, Guzak SV: Visual loss complicating repair of orbital floor fractures. Arch Ophthalmol 86:369, 1971.
41. Browning CW: Materials in orbital repair. Am J Ophthalmol 63:955, 1967.
42. Kushner BJ: Paresis and restriction of the inferior rectus muscle after orbital floor fracture. Am J Ophthalmol 94:81, 1982.
43. Zide MF: Late posttraumatic enophthalmos corrected by dense hydroxyapatite blocks. J Oral Maxillofac Surg 44:804, 1986.
44. Converse JM, Smith B: Naso-orbital fractures. Trans Am Acad Ophthalmol Otolaryngol 67:622, 1963.
45. Prasad SS: Blow-out fracture of the medial wall of the orbit. Mod Probl Ophthalmol 14:493, 1975.
46. Thering HR, Bogart JN: Blowout fracture of the medial orbital wall with entrapment of the medial rectus muscle. Plast Reconstr Surg 63:848, 1979.
47. Leone CR, Lloyd WC, Rylander G: Surgical repair of medial wall fractures. Am J Ophthalmol 97:349, 1984.
48. Souyris F, Klersy F, Jammet P, et al: Malar bone fractures and their sequelae. J Craniomaxillofac Surg 17:64, 1989.
49. Ellis E, El-Attar A, Moos KF: An analysis of 2,067 cases of zygomatico-orbital fractures. J Oral Maxillofac Surg 43:417, 1985.
50. Gordon S, MacRae H: Monocular blindness as a complication of the treatment of a malar fracture. Plast Reconstr Surg 6:228, 1950.
51. Miller GR: Blindness developing a few days after a midfacial fracture: Case report. Plast Reconstr Surg 42:384, 1968.
52. Kaplan LJ: Unilateral disk edema following tripod fracture repair necessitating optic nerve decompression. Plast Reconstr Surg 70:375, 1982.
53. Perino KE, Zide MF, Kinnebrew MC: Late treatment of malunited malar fractures. J Oral Maxillofac Surg 42:20, 1984.
54. Jackson IT: Classification and treatment of orbitozygomatic and orbitoethmoid fractures: The place of bone grafting and plate fixation. Clin Plast Surg 16:77, 1989.
55. Nunery WR: Lateral canthal approach to repair of trimalar fractures of the zygoma. Ophthalmic Plast Reconstr Surg 1:175, 1985.
56. Manfredi SJ, Raji MR, Sprinkle PM, et al: Computerized tomographic scan findings in facial fractures associated with blindness. Plast Reconstr Surg 68:479, 1981.
57. LeFort R: Fractures de la Machoire Superieure. Paris, Congress of Internal Medicine, 1900, p 275.
58. Shaw RC, Parsons RW: Exposure through a coronal incision for initial treatment of facial fractures. Plast Reconstr Surg 56:254, 1975.
59. Tessier P: Total osteotomy of the middle third of the face for faciostenosis or for sequelae of LeFort III fractures. Plast Reconstr Surg 48:533, 1971.
60. Cruse W, Blevins PK, Luce EA: Naso-ethmoid-orbital Fractures. J Trauma 20:551, 1980.
61. Beyer CK, Fabian RL, Smith B: Naso-orbital fractures, complications, and treatment. Ophthalmology 89:456, 1982.
62. Lewin W: Cerebrospinal fluid rhinorrhea in closed head injuries. Br J Surg 42:1, 1954.
63. Schultz RC: Supraorbital and glabellar fractures. Plast Reconstr Surg 45:227, 1970.
64. Stanley RB: Fractures of the frontal sinus. Clin Plast Surg 16:115, 1989.
65. Nadell J, Kline DG: Primary reconstruction of depressed frontal

skull fractures including those involving the sinus, orbit, and cribriform plate. J Neurosurg 41:200, 1974.
66. McLachlan DL, Flanagan JC, Shannon GM: Complications of orbital roof fractures. Ophthalmology 89:1274, 1982.
67. Curtin HD, Wolfe P, Schramm V: Orbital roof blow-out fractures. Am J Radiol 139:969, 1982.
68. Greenwald MJ, Boston D, Pensler JM, et al: Orbital roof fractures in childhood. Ophthalmology 96:491, 1989.
69. Anderson RL, Panje WR, Gross CE: Optic nerve blindness following blunt forehead trauma. Ophthalmology 89:445, 1982.
70. Unger JM: Orbital apex fractures: The contribution of computed tomography. Radiology 150:713, 1984.
71. Kline LB, Morawetz RB, Swaid SN: Indirect injury of the optic nerve. Neurosurgery 14:756, 1984.
72. Lessell S: Indirect optic nerve trauma. Arch Ophthalmol 107:382, 1989.
73. Chadwick J, Mann WN: The Medical Works of Hippocrates. Oxford, England, Blackwell, 1950.
74. Pringle JH: Atrophy of the optic nerve following diffused violence to the skull. Br Med J 2:1156, 1922.
75. Markowitz BL, Manson PN: Panfacial fractures: Organization of treatment. Clin Plast Surg 16:105, 1989.

SECTION

VIII

Anophthalmic Socket

SECTION EDITORS

Robert A. Weiss
Stephen Bosniak

CHAPTER 106

Evaluation and Management of the Anophthalmic Socket

Michael E. Migliori

Managing the complications associated with the anophthalmic socket presents a variety of complex challenges to the ophthalmic plastic surgeon. A functionally and cosmetically acceptable anophthalmic socket must have all of the following components;

1. An orbital implant of sufficient volume centered within the orbit
2. Eyelids with a normal appearance and sufficient tone to support a prosthesis
3. Fornices of sufficient depth to hold a prosthesis
4. A socket lined by conjunctiva or mucous membrane
5. A comfortable ocular prosthesis that is similar in appearance to the normal eye

It is essential that these components be established and maintained to avoid chronic irritation, difficulty in retaining a prosthesis, and an unsatisfactory appearance.

The defects observed in the congenital anophthalmic or microphthalmic socket are usually secondary to developmental abnormalities. The complications that develop in acquired anophthalmos are usually due to involutional, cicatricial, or iatrogenic alterations.

CONGENITAL ANOPHTHALMOS

True congenital anophthalmos is rare. In most cases there is some vestigial ocular tissue present. Mild cases of microphthalmos, in which a small eye may be the only defect, can be treated with a cosmetic scleral shell, in the same way a scleral shell would be used to cover a phthisical eye (Fig. 106–1). In more severe cases, the bony orbit is underdeveloped and other deformities are often present. There may be decreased horizontal and vertical dimensions of the palpebral fissure, shallow fornices, hypoplastic lids, ptosis, and poor levator function. Without treatment, these patients may develop a 25% decrease in the size of the orbital entrance and up to 60% reduction in orbital volume.[1]

The initial treatment is progressive socket expansion, which should begin in the first few weeks of life. A microphthalmic eye should not be removed unless pathologic examination of the tissue is necessary. Progressively larger conformers are placed in the socket in an attempt to expand the conjunctiva and the socket. A Gunderson flap can be used if the cornea does not tolerate the conformer. Lateral canthotomies may be necessary to enable the insertion of large prostheses, even though repeated canthotomies may cause disruption of the canthal tendons and make subsequent eyelid reconstruction difficult.

Dumbbell expanders transmit pressure to the posterior orbit by the application of pressure on the external aspect of the conformer with tape or a headband. This technique does not always generate deep fornices and adequate socket expansion. It should be considered a temporary measure until the child becomes a candidate for definitive socket expansion surgery.

Ultimately, expansion of the bony orbital cavity is necessary to allow retention of a cosmetically acceptable prosthesis. Osteotomies are made in the orbital rim, and the cavity is expanded in all directions.[2] The fornices are deepened with mucosal grafts several months later. Reconstruction of the hypoplastic lids and canthus is performed last.

ACQUIRED ANOPHTHALMOS

Proper management of deformities of the acquired anophthalmic socket requires a thorough understanding of the alterations in the complex relationships among orbital structures after surgical removal of the eye. The complications most likely to develop are enophthalmos, superior sulcus depression, upper lid ptosis, and lower lid laxity and malposition. This group of complications has been termed the *anophthalmic orbit syndrome*.[3] Migration or extrusion of the orbital implant may also occur. Contraction of the socket and the resulting inability to retain a prosthesis is perhaps the most difficult condition to treat.

Before any surgical correction, the patient should be referred to an ocularist to determine whether revision of the prosthesis can affect an adequate improvement. Small to moderate amounts of enophthalmos can be corrected with a custom impression molded prosthesis (Fig.

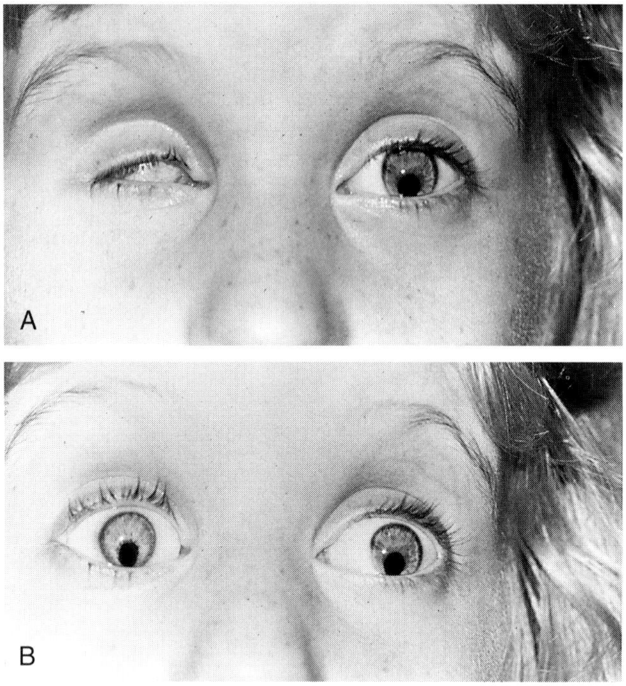

Figure 106–1. *A*, Microphthalmic right eye and iris coloboma in the left eye. *B*, Same patient with a custom-molded prosthesis. (*A* and *B* courtesy of Raymond C. Jahrling, BCO.)

106–2). Extending the prosthesis into the superior fornix reduces the superior sulcus depression. A horizontal cutback on the superior projection of the prosthesis reduces mild to moderate upper lid ptosis (Fig. 106–3).[4] Cutting back the inferior aspect of the prosthesis reduces the downward displacement of the lower lid (Fig. 106–4). It is important to remember that enlarging the prosthesis may cause further sagging of the lower lid if there is significant lower lid laxity. The resulting inferior displacement of the prosthesis will deepen the superior sulcus and worsen upper lid ptosis. Also, large prostheses do not move as well as smaller ones.

All patients with unilateral anophthalmos must be instructed to wear polycarbonate safety glasses to protect the remaining eye. Optics can also be used to camouflage asymmetry. If the anophthalmic palpebral fissure is larger than the normal fissure, a minus lens will make the larger fissure appear smaller (Fig. 106–5). Conversely, if the anophthalmic side is smaller, a plus lens will magnify the image of the smaller eye. Prisms can be used to project the image of the dystopic orbit in line with the normal eye.[5] An additional benefit of cosmetic optics is that it may induce reluctant patients to wear their glasses.

The Lax Socket

Enucleation of an eye alters the structural and functional relationships of the orbital soft tissue: extraocular muscles (including the levator muscle), Tenon's capsule, orbital fat, connective tissue septa, and vasculature. The "anophthalmic orbit syndrome" described by Nolan and coworkers[3] consists of enophthalmos, superior sulcus depression, upper lid ptosis, and lower lid ptosis. The pathophysiology of these complications is not completely understood. Soll[6] noted that thermography studies performed on anophthalmic patients showed colder readings on the anophthalmic side when compared with the normal side. He concluded that atrophy of orbital fat is most likely due to the decreased circulatory and metabolic requirements of the anophthalmic socket.

Kronish and associates[7, 8] studied the pathophysiology of the anophthalmic socket both in terms of orbital blood flow and analysis of orbital fat in a cynomolgus monkey model. They found no difference in the vasculature or capillary blood flow in the anophthalmic socket compared with the normal orbit and no change in adipocytes. They did find a statistically significant increased weight of the fat and connective tissue compartments in the anophthalmic orbit. The increase in mass was attributed to an increase in fibrous tissue and scar proliferation in the operated socket. Kaltreider and colleagues[9] found that myofibroblasts are present in anophthalmic sockets. They postulated that contraction of orbital scar tissue would decrease orbital volume without fat atrophy.

Mechanical alterations in the complex orbital muscular and connective tissue network also cause displace-

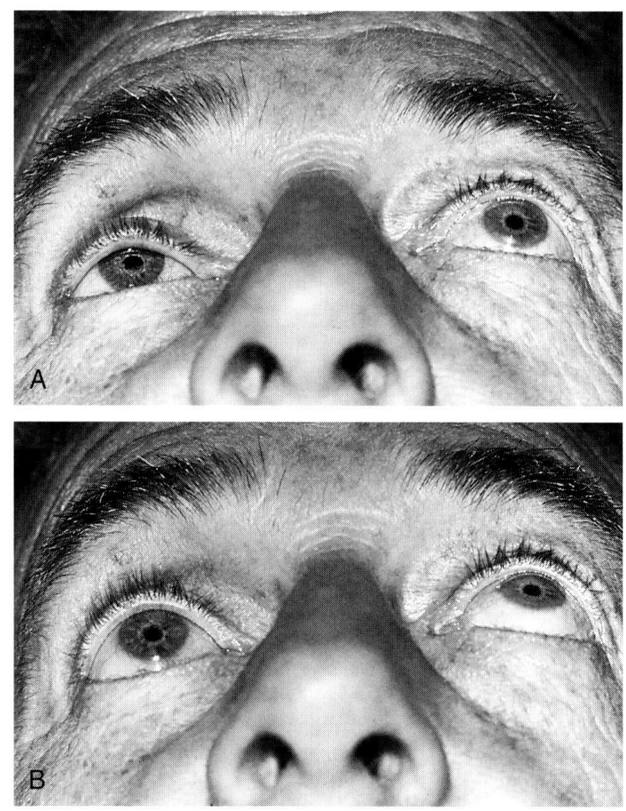

Figure 106–2. *A*, Enophthalmic appearance with a stock prosthesis. *B*, Reduction of enophthalmos with a custom-molded prosthesis. (*A* and *B* courtesy of Raymond C. Jahrling, BCO.)

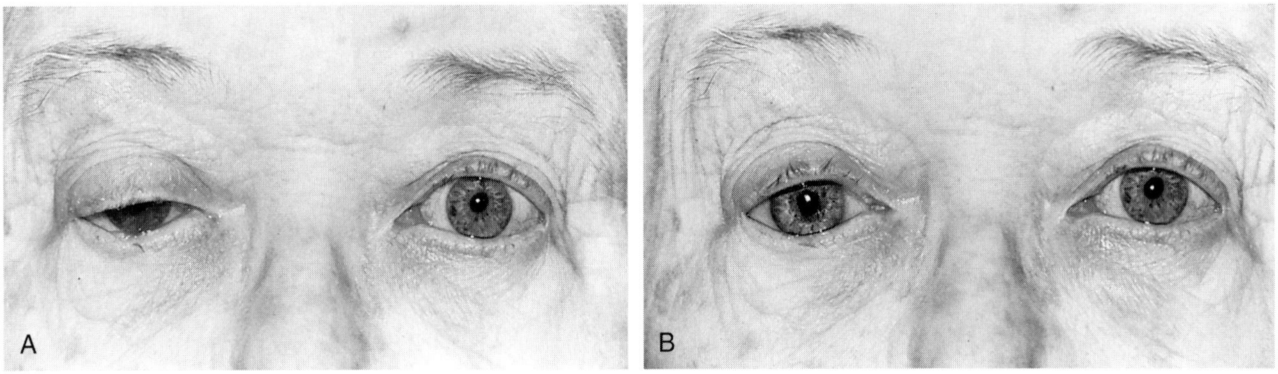

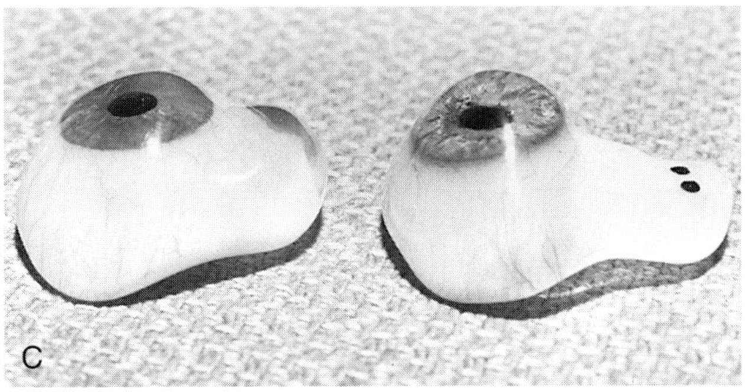

Figure 106–3. *A*, Right upper lid ptosis. *B*, Correction of ptosis with a modified custom-molded prosthesis. C, Old *(left)* prosthesis and new *(right)* prosthesis with superior extension and modified anterior curvature. (*A* to C courtesy of Raymond C. Jahrling, BCO.)

ment of the orbital contents. Since enucleation is often preceded by trauma, there may be associated orbital fractures that increase the dimensions of the bony orbit and further accentuate a volume deficit.

Surgical correction of deformities in the anophthalmic orbit should be performed in a logical, sequential manner. Orbital volume should be augmented first. Increasing the volume of the orbital soft tissue advances the prosthesis anteriorly, reducing superior sulcus depression and perhaps relieving upper lid ptosis. Lower lid lax-

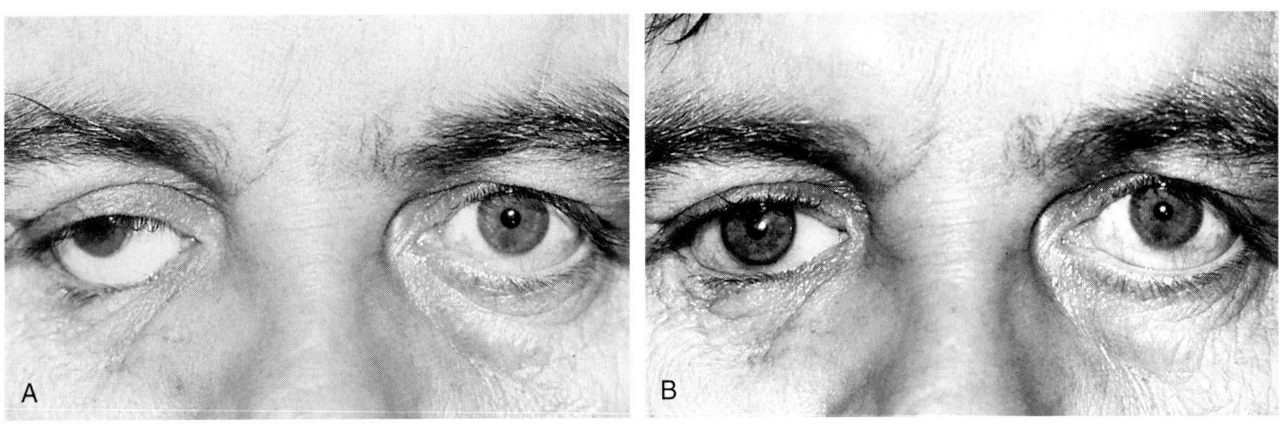

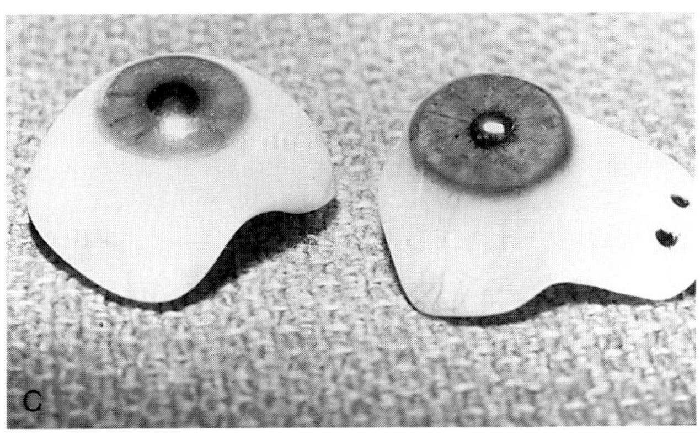

Figure 106–4. *A*, Right upper lid ptosis and loss of inferior fornix due to stock prosthesis. *B*, Improved ptosis and lower lid position with a modified custom-molded prosthesis. C, Old stock prosthesis *(left)* and modified prosthesis *(right)* with superior extension and reduced inferior curvature. (*A* to C courtesy of Raymond C. Jahrling, BCO.)

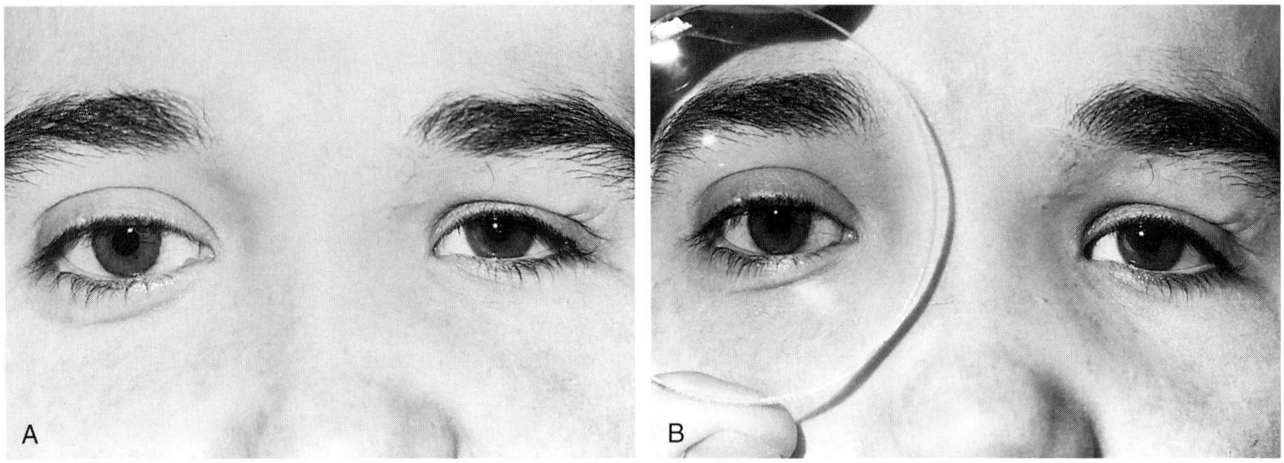

Figure 106–5. *A*, Large anophthalmic palpebral fissure. *B*, −4.00-Diopter lens reduces image of larger fissure. (*A* and *B*, courtesy of Raymond C. Jahrling, BCO.)

ity should be corrected next, either at the same time as volume augmentation or as the second procedure. The lower lid can then support the prosthesis, thereby eliminating its inferior displacement. If ptosis or superior sulcus deformity persists after these corrections have been made, and they cannot be corrected with a new prosthesis, surgical repair of the sulcus deformity is next, followed by repair of any residual ptosis.

Enophthalmos

The human eye has a volume of 7 to 8 mL. After enucleation, an additional 3 to 4 mL of orbital volume may be lost due to either atrophy of orbital tissue, predominantly orbital fat,[10] or contraction of orbital connective tissue.[7, 8] This may result in a total deficit of 10 to 12 mL.

A deep superior sulcus will accentuate the enophthalmic appearance. Reduction of the apparent enophthalmos and improvement of the superior sulcus deformity is accomplished by either increasing the volume of the orbital contents, specifically increasing the size of the orbital implant, or by reducing the dimensions of the orbital cavity with subperiosteal implants to displace the orbital tissue anteriorly.

Migration of the orbital implant may also contribute to an anophthalmic appearance. If the implant migrates inferiorly, it will obliterate the inferior fornix. The inferior edge of the prosthesis is pushed up and forward, and the superior aspect of the prosthesis is tipped back away from the superior fornix. This further deepens the superior sulcus (Fig. 106–6).

When enophthalmos occurs because there is no implant in the socket, a secondary implant should be inserted. An alloplastic spherical implant made of silicone, Proplast, high-density porous polyethylene, or hydroxyapatite should be wrapped in donor sclera, donor fascia, or autogenous fascia and sutured behind Tenon's capsule to minimize the chance of migration (Fig. 106–7).[11–13] Some degree of conjunctival shrinkage can be expected if there has been no implant in the socket, making it necessary to use a smaller spherical implant than would be placed initially, and leaving a significant volume deficiency.

A dermis–fat graft is a better alternative as a secondary implant. This technique was first described by Smith and Petrelli[14] and offers several distinct advantages. First, more volume can be replaced than with a spherical implant. Second, there has never been a reported case of migration or extrusion of a dermis–fat graft; and since it is the patient's own tissue, there is no risk of allergic reaction or rejection. Third, in cases of mild contraction of the socket, a dermis–fat graft will increase the amount of available conjunctiva and deepen the fornices. The conjunctiva is incised horizontally in the palpebral fissure

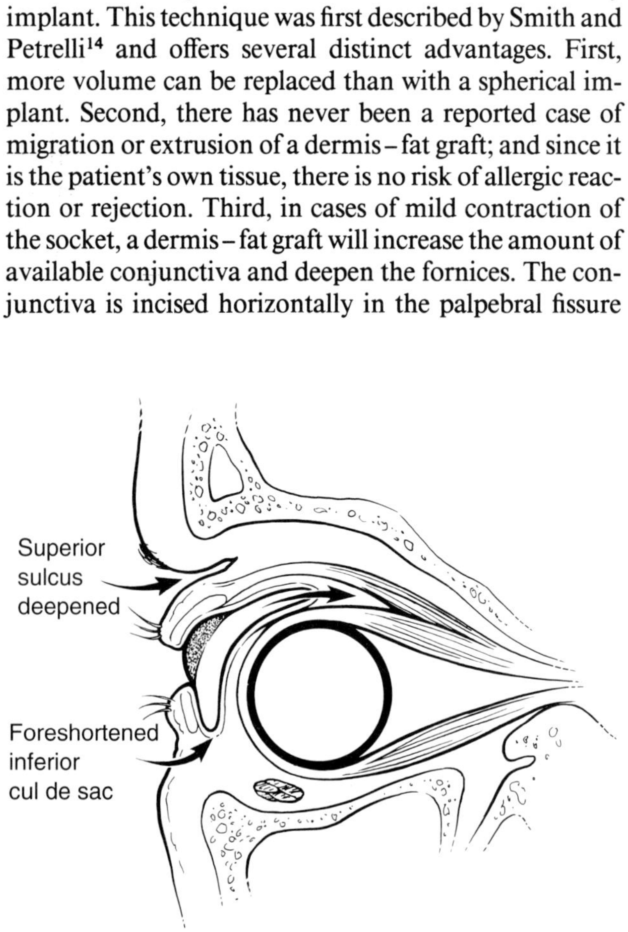

Figure 106–6. Inferiorly migrated orbital implant causes shortening of inferior fornix, rotation of prosthesis and deepening of superior sulcus. (Modified and published courtesy of *Ophthalmology* [1984; 91: 494–6] for Figure 1 from Neuhaus et al's article "Enucleation with Implantation of a Proplast Sphere.")

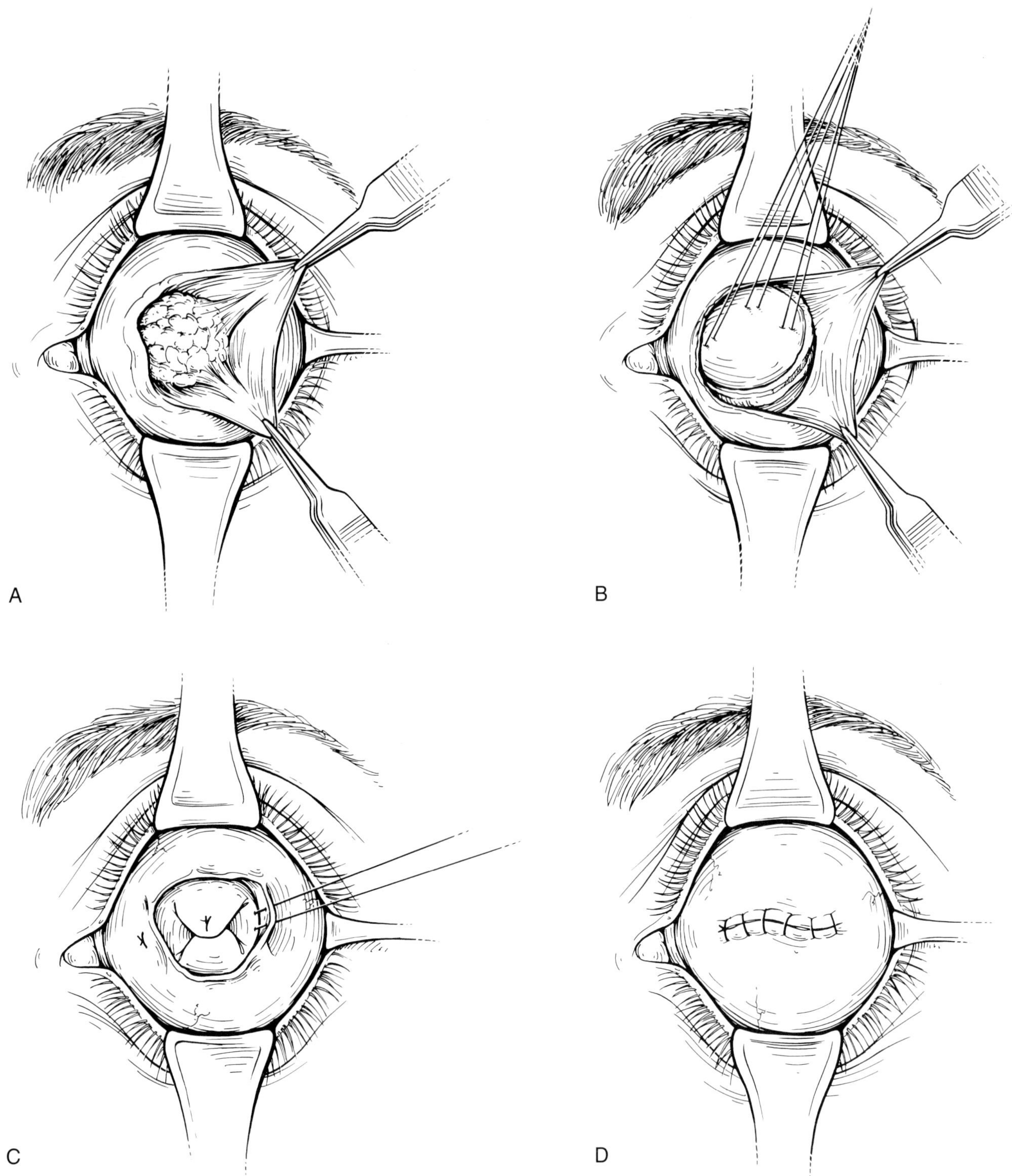

Figure 106–7. Surgical technique for implantation of secondary implant. *A*, Posterior Tenon's capsule opened. *B*, Wrapped implant with fixation sutures placed in muscle cone posterior to Tenon's capsule. *C*, Posterior Tenon's capsule closed over implant. Fixation sutures passed through posterior and anterior Tenon's capsule and conjunctiva. *D*, Conjunctiva closed. (Modified and published courtesy of *Ophthalmology* [1982; 89: 407–23] for Figures 9 and 16 from Soll's article "The Anophthalmic Socket.")

and then allowed to retract. The graft is placed in the center of the socket and the conjunctiva is sutured to the edge of the dermis, not closed over it as it would be over a spherical implant. The area of the conjunctiva is thereby increased by the area of the dermis. This deepens the fornices and relieves some of the contraction. The prosthesis can then be thinner and lighter since it will not have to replace as much orbital volume. Thinner prostheses are usually more comfortable, move better, and are more easily supported by the lower lid.

If the graft is being placed as a secondary implant after extrusion or migration of an orbital implant, the conjunctival incision is made horizontally through the center of the socket in the palpebral fissure and is extended to within several millimeters of the medial and lateral canthal angles. If there is an implant, it is removed, and the capsule surrounding the implant cavity is entirely excised. Every attempt is made to locate the rectus muscles because the anterior ciliary arteries within them become the major source of blood supply to the graft.[15, 16] The rectus muscles should only be sutured to the dermis in opposing pairs, or the graft will rotate toward the unopposed muscle.

The dermis–fat graft is taken from the buttock or lateral hip area. A 25-mm diameter circle is drawn over the donor site. The epidermis within the circle is removed with an air-driven dermabrader. The circle of dermis is then incised with a no.15 Bard-Parker blade. A 25-mm long cylinder of fat with the dermis attached is excised. The cylinder is flared out so that the diameter of the base of the graft is slightly larger than the diameter of the dermis cap. The graft is then placed fat side down into the recipient site. The superior rectus muscle is sutured to the superior edge of the dermis. The medial rectus muscle is sutured to the medial edge, and the inferior rectus muscle is sutured to the inferior edge. Excess fat is trimmed from the base of the graft, and then the graft is tucked into the socket with the scalpel handle. The lateral rectus muscle is sutured to the temporal edge and the conjunctiva is sutured to the edge of the dermis with interrupted 5-0 absorbable sutures. If no muscles can be isolated, the conjunctiva is simply sutured to the edge of the dermis after excess fat is trimmed. A symblepharon ring is placed in the socket to maintain the fornices.

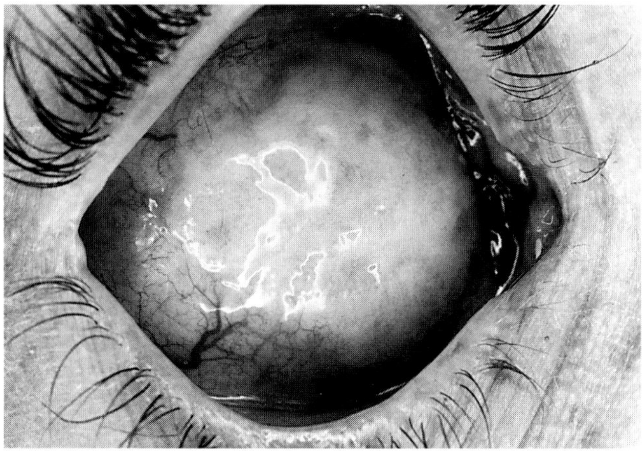

Figure 106–8. Domed dermis–fat graft with deep fornices.

The domed dermis–fat graft creates deeper fornices than a standard flat-surfaced dermis–fat graft and allows better contact between the prosthesis and the dermis as the graft moves (Fig. 106–8). Four 3-mm equilateral base-out triangles of dermis are excised from the periphery of the graft. The triangles are taken from the 1:30, 4:30, 7:30, and 10:30 positions. The resulting wedge-shaped defects are closed with interrupted 5-0 absorbable sutures. This creates a domed shape to the surface of the dermis once the graft is sutured into place (Fig. 106–9). A

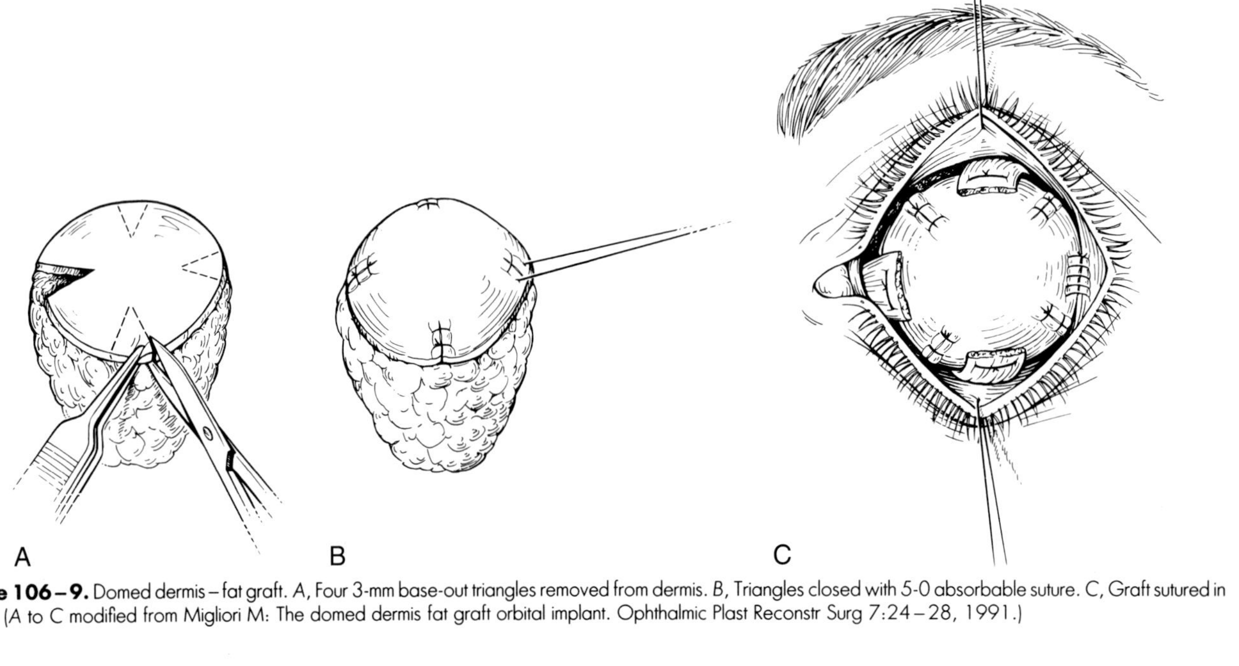

Figure 106–9. Domed dermis–fat graft. *A*, Four 3-mm base-out triangles removed from dermis. *B*, Triangles closed with 5-0 absorbable suture. C, Graft sutured in place. (*A* to *C* modified from Migliori M: The domed dermis fat graft orbital implant. Ophthalmic Plast Reconstr Surg 7:24–28, 1991.)

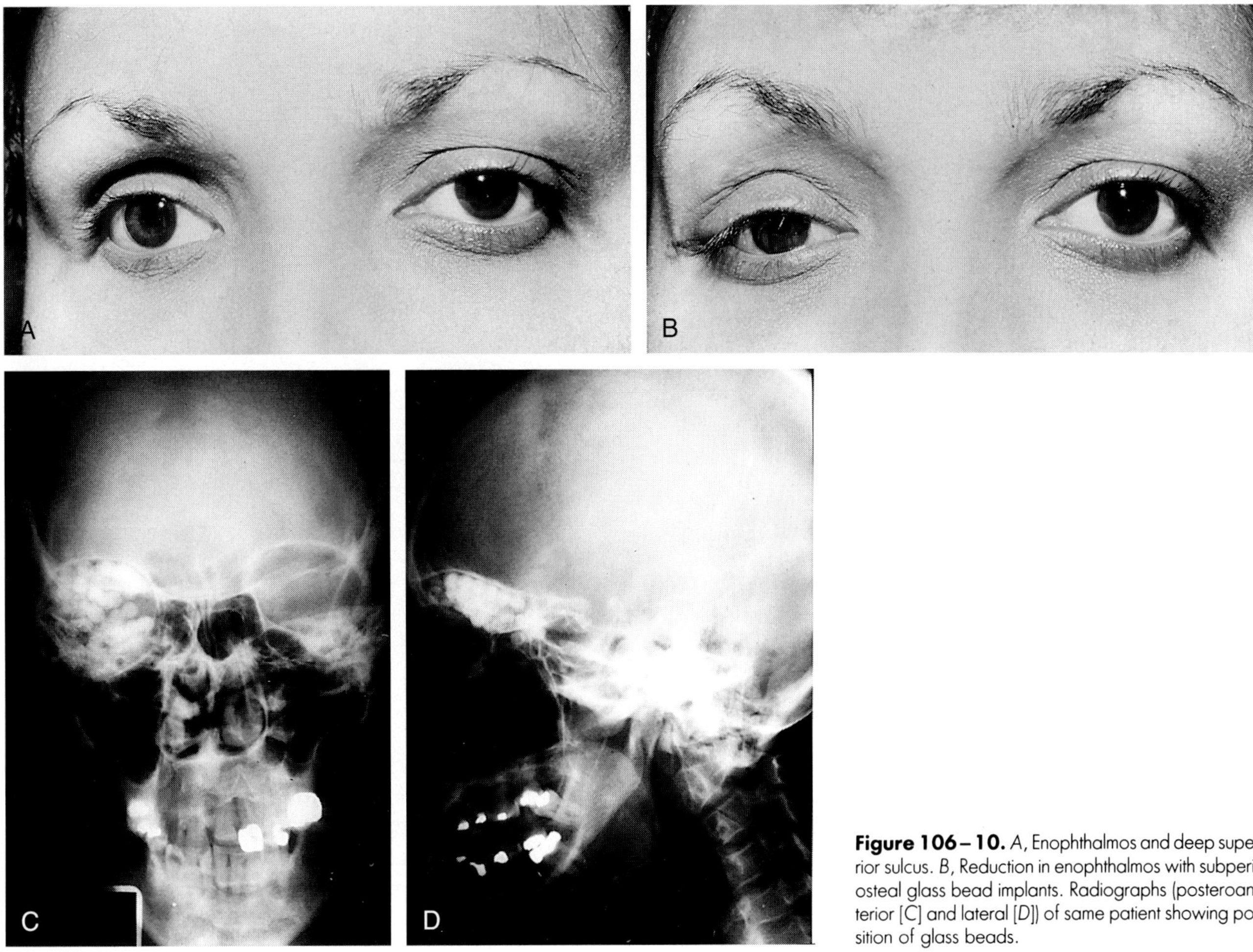

Figure 106–10. *A*, Enophthalmos and deep superior sulcus. *B*, Reduction in enophthalmos with subperiosteal glass bead implants. Radiographs (posteroanterior [*C*] and lateral [*D*]) of same patient showing position of glass beads.

prosthesis molded for a domed dermis–fat graft is thinner centrally and lighter than a prosthesis fabricated for a socket with a standard dermis–fat graft or spherical implant. Motility of the prosthesis is generally better.[17]

If the orbital implant is in a satisfactory position, or if there is a dermis–fat graft present but enophthalmos is still a problem, subperiosteal implants are used to reduce the dimensions of the orbital cavity and displace the orbital contents anteriorly and superiorly (Fig. 106–10). There have been many techniques reported. Glass[18,19] or silicone[20] bead implants, carved silicone implants, molded methyl methacrylate implants,[21] and RTV silicone have all been described. Glass beads are no longer recommended because they have been shown to migrate into the sinuses, alimentary tract, and cranial cavity.[22,23]

RTV silicone has been very effective in reducing enophthalmos and the associated deep superior sulcus (Fig. 106–11). A small incision is made at the lateral canthus, and the periorbita is incised. A pocket is created along the orbital floor posteriorly, and the RTV silicone is mixed with its catalyst and injected into the subperiosteal space. The amount of silicone injected can be titrated with the prosthesis in place to precisely replace orbital volume.[10,24–26]

A carved silicone block, a prefabricated orbital floor implant, or preserved cartilage[27] can be placed beneath the periorbita through a subciliary or fornix incision as is normally used for repair of an orbital floor fracture. The implant should be taller posteriorly to push the orbital contents superiorly and anteriorly. The implant should also not extend as far forward as the inferior orbital rim to avoid compromising the inferior fornix.

Sulcus Deformity

There are several possible mechanisms for superior sulcus depression, including contraction and malposition of the superior rectus and levator muscles,[28] inferior migration of the orbital implant,[21] levator disinsertion, and inferior displacement of the prosthesis from loss of lower eyelid support.[10,29]

The diameter of a spherical orbital implant is smaller than the diameter of the normal eye, and therefore it cannot support the superior orbital structures. This downward displacement of the prosthesis and orbital tissues causes the deep superior sulcus deformity. Enlargement of the superior projection of the prosthesis improves the superior sulcus deformity if there is minimal lower lid

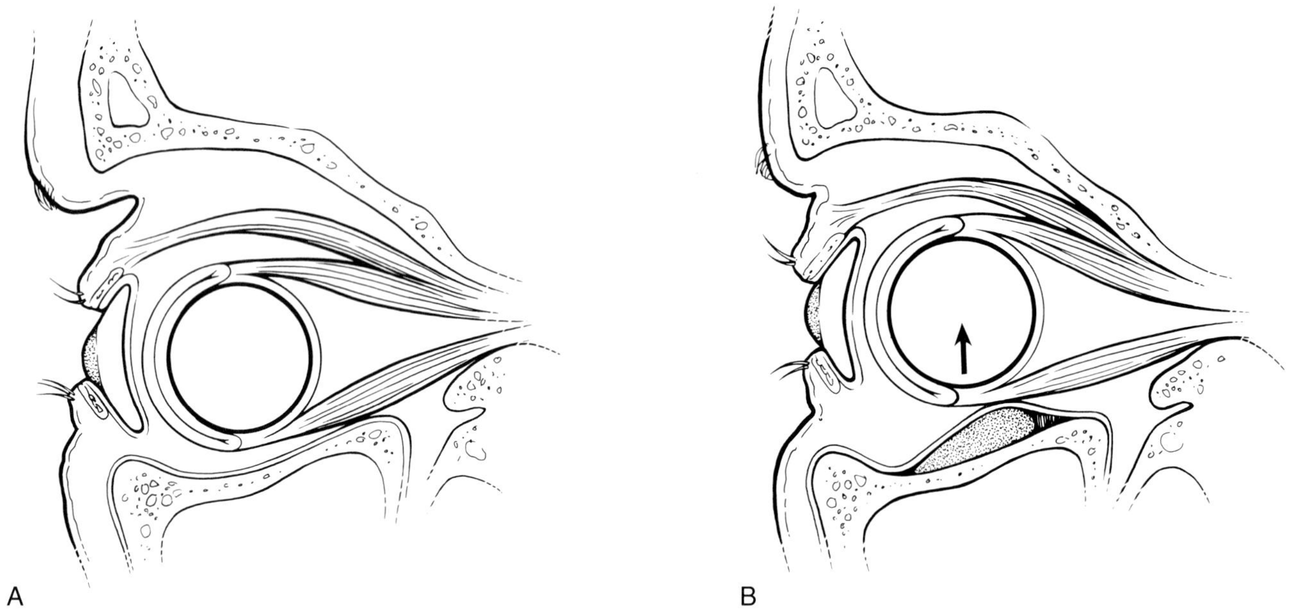

Figure 106–11. *A*, Enophthalmos, deep superior sulcus and inferior displacement of orbital contents. *B*, Subperiosteal implant elevating the orbital contents, reducing enophthalmos and superior sulcus depression. (Modified from McCord C, Tannenbaum M: The Anophthalmic Socket: Evaluation and Management of Surgical Problems. *In* Oculoplastic Surgery. New York, Raven Press, 1987, p 427.)

laxity. A larger prosthesis is heavier and puts more pressure on the lower lid, eventually causing more pronounced sagging of the lower lid and inferior displacement of the prosthesis. Resuspending the lower lid, either with a lateral tarsal tightening procedure or a fascia lata sling, gives more support to a heavy prosthesis and maintains it in proper position to fill the superior sulcus. Replacing a spherical implant with a dermis–fat graft will reduce the superior sulcus depression by adding volume to the orbit, giving more support to the superior orbital structures (Fig. 106–12).

Grafts can be used to augment the volume deficit in the upper lid. Strips of autogenous fascia, auricular cartilage, pearl fat grafts,[30] or donor sclera[31] can be implanted in the preaponeurotic space to fill the superior fornix. The strips of tissue are stacked to the appropriate thickness to fill the sulcus deformity, and the ends are sutured together. Five-millimeter horizontal incisions are made in two places in the upper lid, each one just above the medial and lateral lid crease. A hemostat is passed through the lateral incision, posterior to the orbital septum in the preaponeurotic space, and exits through the medial incision. This stack of material is then grasped with the hemostat and tunneled through the space. The skin incisions are sutured closed (Fig. 106–13).

A dermis–fat graft will also satisfactorily fill the sulcus depression. An elliptical graft is taken from the lateral hip or buttock and implanted in the superior sulcus. The incision is made in the upper lid crease, and the preaponeurotic space is opened. The de-epithelialized graft is placed into this space so that the dermis is facing anteriorly and the fat sits posteriorly. The 6-0 absorbable su-

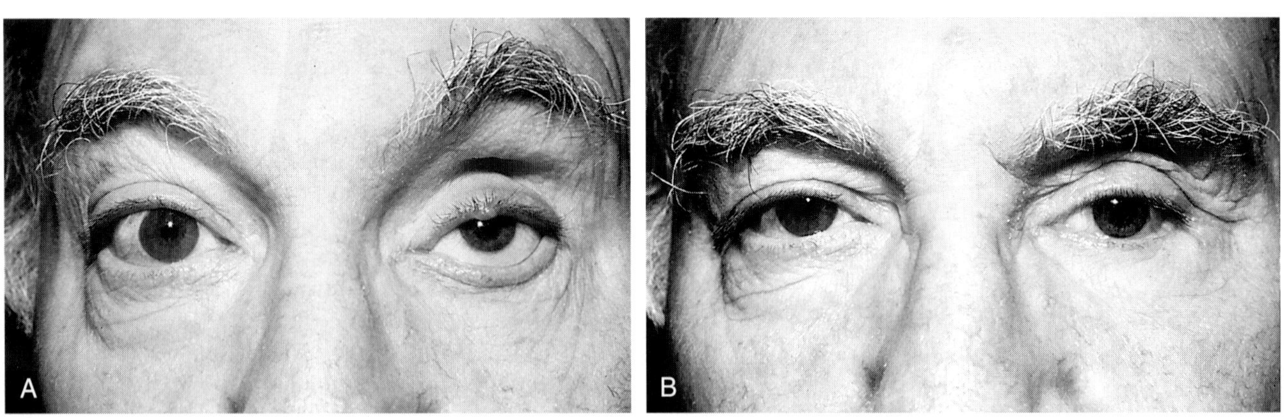

Figure 106–12. *A*, Enophthalmic appearance of the left eye due to volume deficit. *B*, Elimination of enophthalmos by replacing a spherical implant with dermis–fat graft.

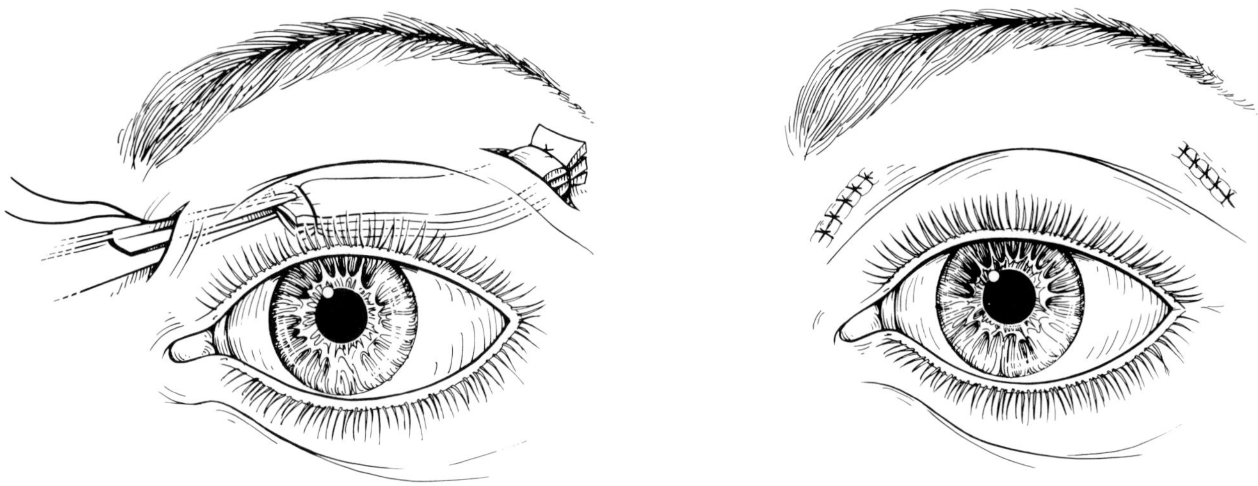

A B

Figure 106–13. Technique for augmenting a deep superior sulcus with fascia or cartilage. *A*, Fascia tunneled under orbicularis. *B*, Incisions closed. (Modified from Oberfeld S, Levine M: Diagnosis and treatment of complications of enucleation and orbital implant surgery. Adv Ophthalmic Plast Reconstr Surg 8:107–111, 1990.)

tures passed through the superior edge of the dermis are passed through orbicularis and skin so that the inferior edge of the dermis sits at the level of the lid crease (Fig. 106–14).[32] Alternatively, the incision can be made through conjunctiva, Müller's muscle, and levator aponeurosis in the superior fornix and the graft placed with the fat in the preaponeurotic space and the dermis facing the fornix. The conjunctiva is sutured to the edges of the dermis (Fig. 106–15).[33]

Lower Lid Malposition

The normal eye is supported by the extraocular muscles, Tenon's fascia, and the intraorbital fascial network. The lids do not provide support for the globe. The orbital implant in an anophthalmic socket is predominantly supported by the lower lid, as is the prosthesis. The constant stress of these elements on the lower lid commonly leads to lower lid laxity. Vistnes and associates[29] reported this complication in 40% of patients in his series.

The average prosthesis weighs 20g.[34] The constant pressure of the prosthesis on the lower lid eventually stretches the canthal tendons. There also may be a dehiscence of the canthal tendons from previous trauma or chronic orbital inflammation and edema. Facial palsy may contribute to lower lid laxity.

As the lower lid becomes more lax, the prosthesis loses its support and drops down. The superior aspect of the prosthesis may also tip forward. Disinsertion of the inferior retractors causes flattening of the inferior fornix and the subsequent inability to retain a prosthesis.

Lower lid laxity is corrected by reinforcing the canthal tendons. A lateral tarsal strip procedure horizontally tightens the lower lid (Fig. 106–16). A lateral canthotomy is completed, and then the inferior crus of the lateral canthal tendon is severed. With the prosthesis in place, the lower lid is pulled temporally under moderate tension. A mark is made at the point where the lower lid margin overlaps the edge of the upper lid. The tarsus lateral to this mark is cleared of skin, orbicularis muscle, and conjunctiva. This tarsal strip is then sutured to the periosteum at the lateral orbital tubercle (Fig. 106–17).[35, 36]

Alternatively, a fascia lata sling can elevate and support a sagging lower lid without shortening the lid. The strip of fascia lata acts like a hammock to support the prosthesis.[3, 10, 29] Small horizontal incisions are made over the medial and lateral canthal tendons, and centrally 2 mm below the lashes. A strip of fascia lata is tunneled under the orbicularis muscle and each end is wrapped around the canthal tendon. If there is significant canthal tendon laxity, the fascia should either be sutured to the periosteum or passed through holes drilled into the orbital rim (Fig. 106–18).

Involutional ectropion of the lower lid occurs because of horizontal laxity. In some cases, the lower lid retractors may be detached. The lid can neither support the prosthesis nor maintain it in the socket. Horizontally shortening the lid with a lateral tarsal strip procedure repairs this type of ectropion. A pentagonal resection should not be used to tighten the lower lid in the anophthalmic socket because it does not correct the basic defect, which is canthal tendon laxity. Also, a pentagonal resection removes conjunctiva from the inferior fornix, which may cause the formation of vertical bands of scar tissue in the inferior fornix that will shorten the fornix and limit motility of the prosthesis.

Trauma, surgery, or radiation causes a vertical shortage of the anterior lamella of the lid, which results in cicatricial ectropion. A full-thickness skin graft combined

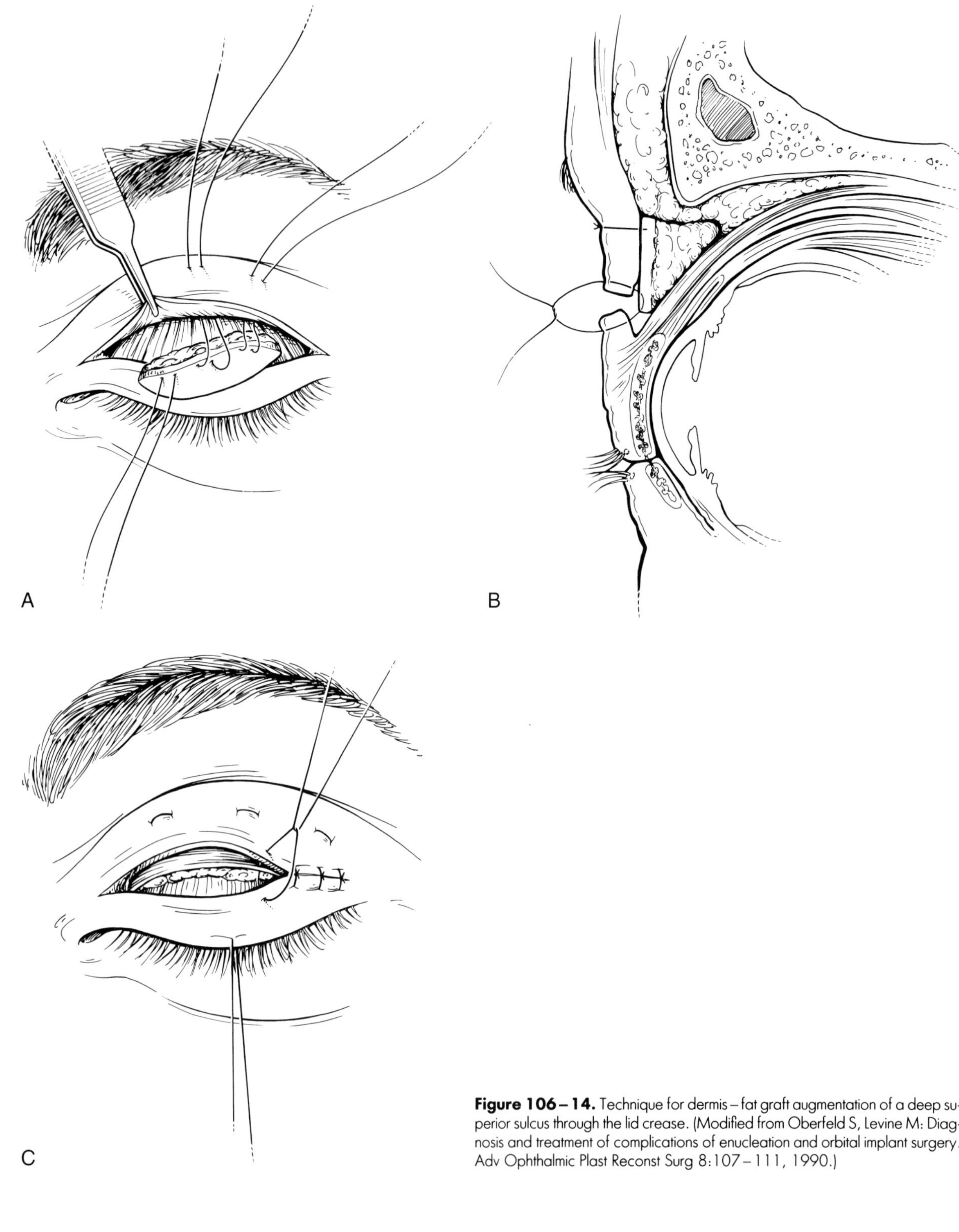

Figure 106–14. Technique for dermis–fat graft augmentation of a deep superior sulcus through the lid crease. (Modified from Oberfeld S, Levine M: Diagnosis and treatment of complications of enucleation and orbital implant surgery. Adv Ophthalmic Plast Reconst Surg 8:107–111, 1990.)

with a horizontal shortening procedure is usually necessary to repair this type of ectropion.

Involutional entropion is caused by horizontal laxity of the lower lid combined with detachment of the lower lid retractors. Enophthalmos worsens an entropion. Horizontally shortening the lid and reattaching the lower lid retractors to the inferior tarsal border corrects this type of entropion. Entropion repair should be done after enophthalmos is corrected.

Cicatricial entropion is usually secondary to chronic inflammation in the socket, whether from chronic conjunctivitis, a poorly fitting prosthesis, prior trauma, or multiple surgical procedures. Mild cases of cicatricial entropion can generally be repaired with a standard trans-

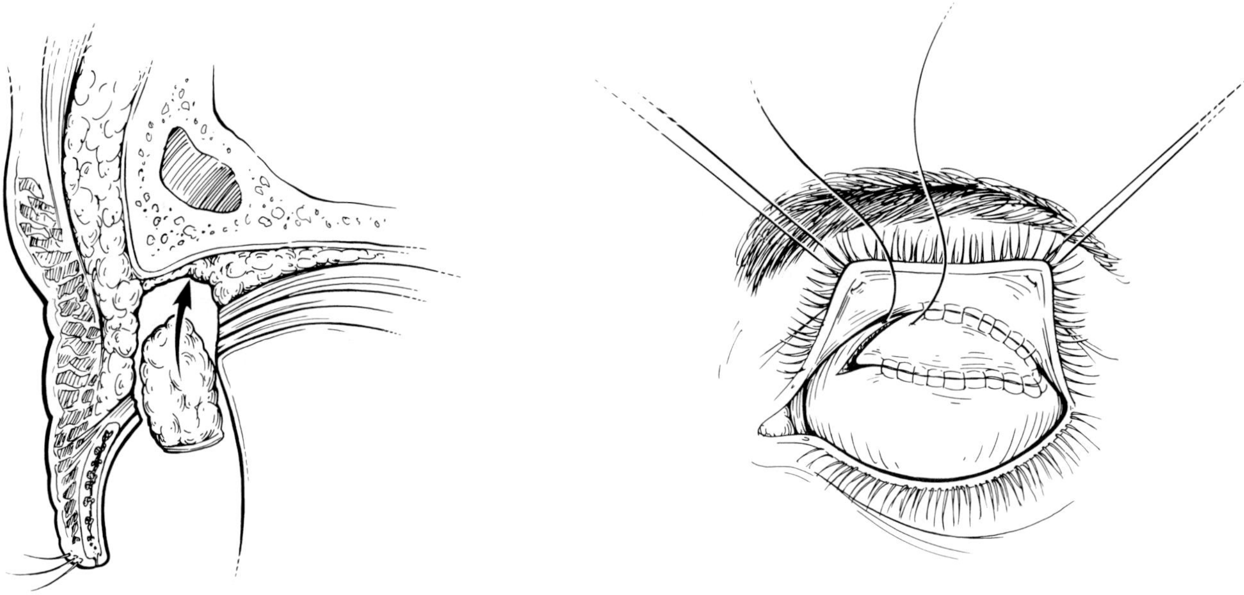

A B

Figure 106–15. Technique for dermis–fat graft augmentation of a deep superior sulcus through the superior fornix. *A*, Dermis–fat graft sutured into superior sulcus. *B*, Dermis sutured to conjunctiva. (Modified from Oberfeld S, Levine M: Diagnosis and treatment of complications of enucleation and orbital implant surgery. Adv Ophthalmic Plast Reconstr Surg 8:107–111, 1990.)

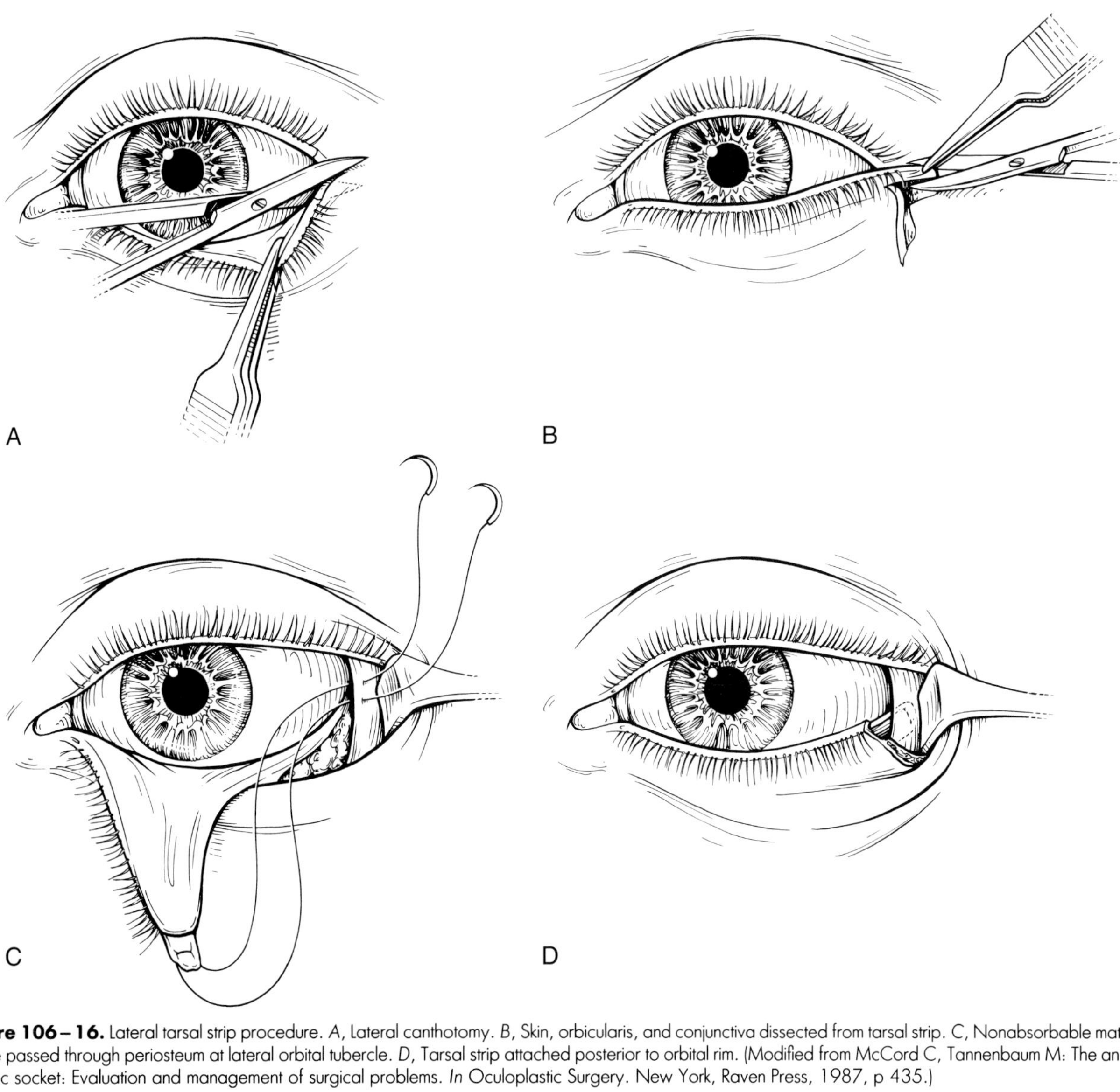

Figure 106–16. Lateral tarsal strip procedure. *A*, Lateral canthotomy. *B*, Skin, orbicularis, and conjunctiva dissected from tarsal strip. C, Nonabsorbable mattress suture passed through periosteum at lateral orbital tubercle. *D*, Tarsal strip attached posterior to orbital rim. (Modified from McCord C, Tannenbaum M: The anophthalmic socket: Evaluation and management of surgical problems. *In* Oculoplastic Surgery. New York, Raven Press, 1987, p 435.)

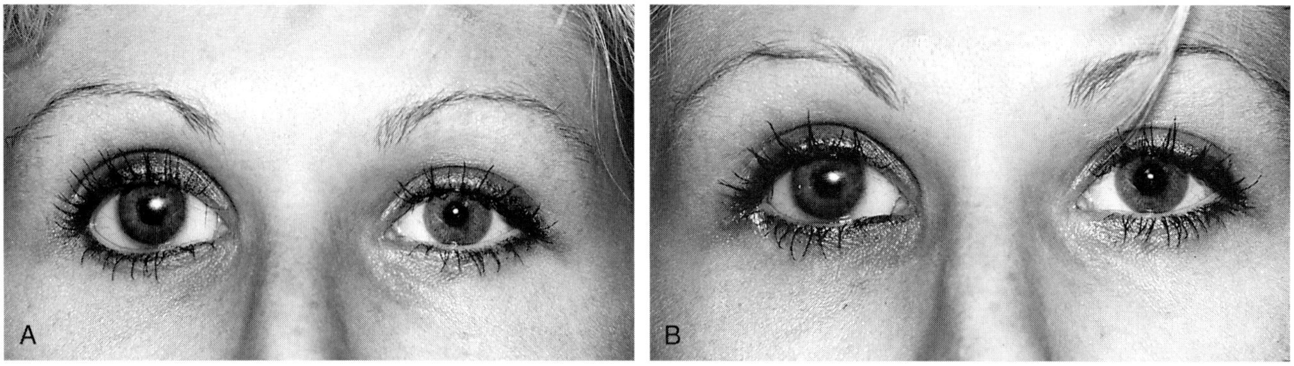

Figure 106–17. *A*, Sagging of temporal right lower lid due to lid laxity. *B*, Improvement of lower lid position after lateral tarsal strip procedure.

verse blepharotomy.[37] The skin and orbicularis are incised parallel to and 4 mm from the anterior lid margin. The lid is then everted and a parallel incision is made through conjunctiva and tarsus 4 mm from the posterior lid margin. The transverse blepharotomy is completed with scissors. Two incisions are made to ensure that the heights of the anterior and posterior aspects of the lid margin flap are the same. A chalazion clamp or transmarginal rotation clamp is used to stabilize the lid. Double-armed 4-0 silk mattress sutures are passed through conjunctiva and tarsus of the proximal segment, exiting between tarsus and orbicularis. Both arms of the suture are then passed into the marginal segment, entering between tarsus and orbicularis. The degree of marginal rotation is determined by suture placement. If the sutures exit anterior to the cilia, rotation is minimal; when they exit near the meibomian gland orifices, maximum rotation is achieved. The sutures are tied over cotton pled-

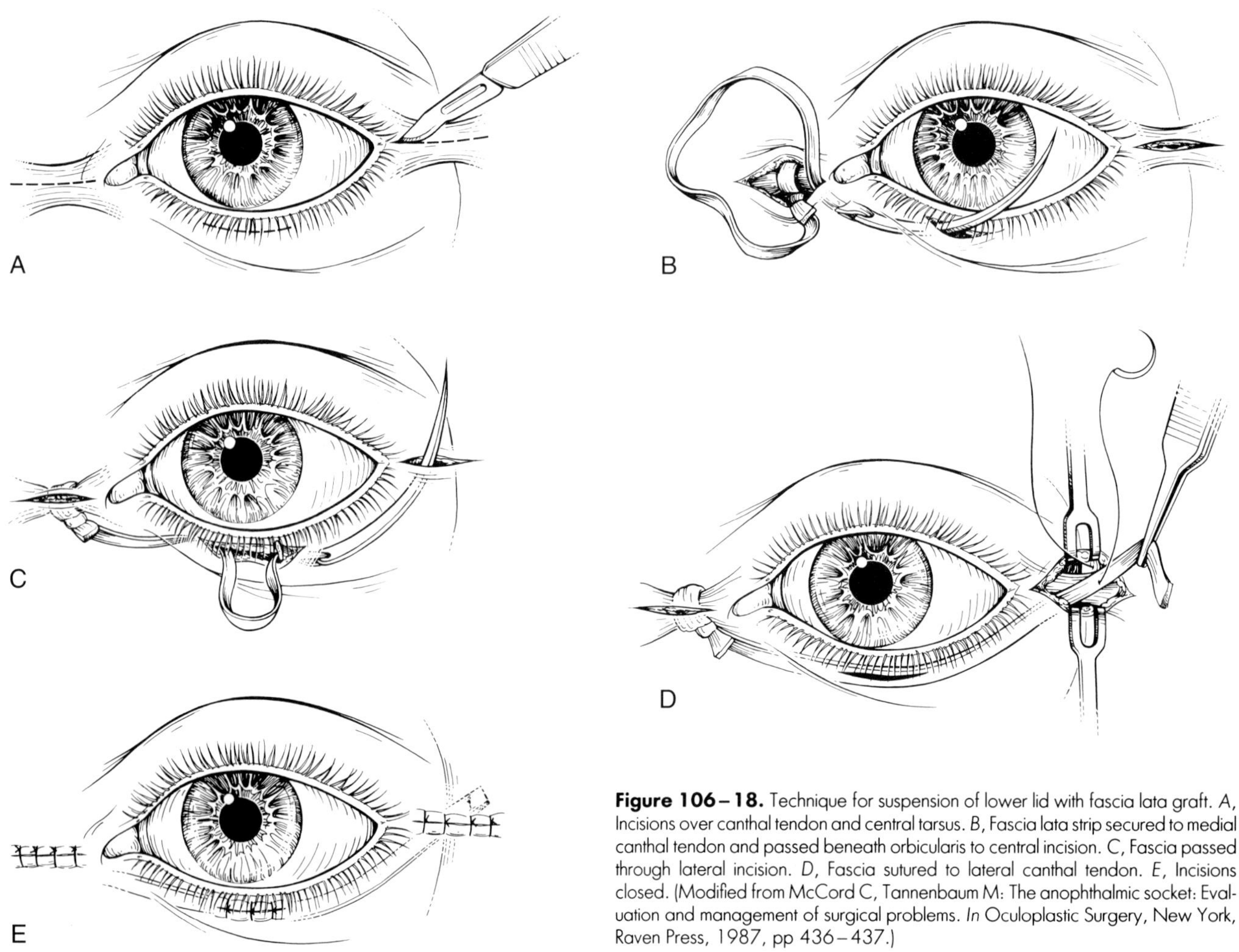

Figure 106–18. Technique for suspension of lower lid with fascia lata graft. *A*, Incisions over canthal tendon and central tarsus. *B*, Fascia lata strip secured to medial canthal tendon and passed beneath orbicularis to central incision. *C*, Fascia passed through lateral incision. *D*, Fascia sutured to lateral canthal tendon. *E*, Incisions closed. (Modified from McCord C, Tannenbaum M: The anophthalmic socket: Evaluation and management of surgical problems. *In* Oculoplastic Surgery, New York, Raven Press, 1987, pp 436–437.)

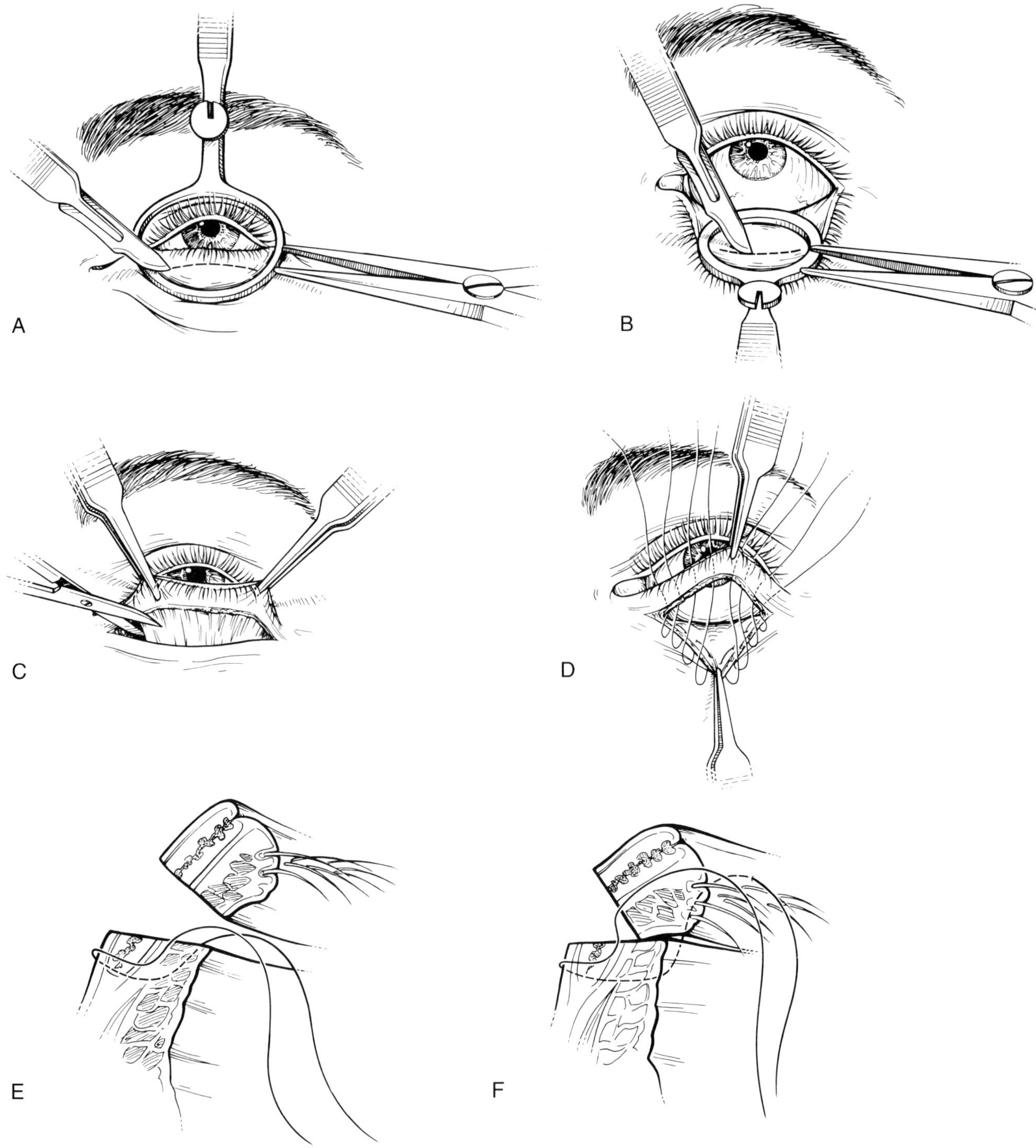

Figure 106–19. Technique for marginal rotation. Degree of marginal rotation is determined by suture placement. *A*, Clamp applied to eyelid and incision made through skin and orbicularis. *B*, Parallel incision made through conjunctiva and tarsus. *C*, Full-thickness blepharotomy completed with scissors. *D*, Rotational sutures placed before tying. *E* and *F*, Detail of rotational suture placement. (Modified from Millman AL, Katzen LB, Putterman AM: Cicatricial entropion: An analysis of its treatment with transverse blepharotomy and marginal rotation. Ophthalmic Surg 20:575–579, 1989.)

gets. The skin is closed with a running 6-0 nylon or silk suture (Fig. 106–19). This procedure works equally well on upper or lower lids (Fig. 106–20).

In severe cases of cicatricial entropion, a graft is needed to lengthen the posterior lamella of the lid. Fascia, ear cartilage, hard palate mucosa,[38] and polytetrafluoroethylene grafts[39] have all been used successfully. A transverse incision is made in the upper lid through conjunctiva and tarsus 4 mm above the posterior lid margin. The upper lid retractors are recessed and a spacer graft is placed in

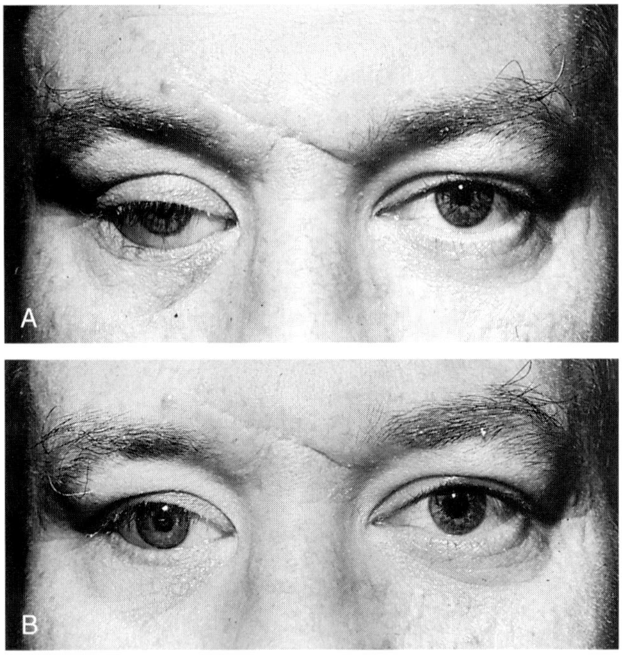

Figure 106–20. *A*, Right upper lid ptosis and lower lid cicatricial entropion. *B*, Same patient after levator advancement and marginal rotation of lower lid.

the defect. In the lower lids, the incision is made at the inferior tarsal border, the retractors are recessed, and the spacer is placed in the defect.

Ptosis

Before surgical correction of an upper lid ptosis in the anophthalmic patient, it is necessary to determine if a true ptosis exists. A poorly fitting or inferiorly displaced prosthesis will cause a pseudoptosis.

The patient should be referred to the ocularist before surgical repair of the ptosis is recommended. If there is a pseudoptosis or a mild to moderate true ptosis, revising the prosthesis may be sufficient to elevate the lid to a satisfactory level, but consequently it may add pressure to the lower lid, contributing to laxity and loss of support. Any lower lid laxity should be corrected if the prosthesis cannot be supported by the lower lid.

To determine if the lower lid laxity is contributing to the ptosis, the prosthesis can be digitally elevated from below. If this eliminates the ptosis, then horizontally shortening the lower lid should improve the upper lid position. Usually this will also reduce the superior sulcus depression. Any other socket abnormalities should be corrected, and if there is residual ptosis after all of these steps have been taken, then surgery is recommended.

The levator muscle originates at the orbital apex and courses anteriorly to pass through Whitnall's ligament near the equator of the globe. At Whitnall's ligament, the aponeurosis shifts to a vertical direction. A spherical orbital implant, which has a smaller diameter than a normal eye, may not adequately support the levator complex. Once the eye is removed, the levator muscle may sag and lose its vertical orientation. This functionally lengthens the levator muscle, causing the upper lid to drop.[40] Soll[41] has shown in Yucatan miniature swine that, despite placement of a spherical implant, the levator muscle separates from the orbital roof.

Dehiscence or disinsertion of the levator aponeurosis may also be responsible for the upper lid ptosis. This may occur as a result of the trauma that was responsible for the enucleation or possibly during the course of the enucleation. Preexisting acquired or congenital ptosis may also be a factor. Oculomotor nerve injury may occur as a direct result of the initial trauma or rarely during enucleation surgery. A mechanical ptosis may be caused by a superiorly displaced migrated orbital implant or after surgery to correct socket contraction or reduce the superior sulcus depression.

Fasanella-Servat and conjunctival-Müller's muscle resection operations are effective and relatively simple procedures[42, 43] that produce consistent results in the lax socket (Fig. 106–21). They should be avoided when socket contraction is present. Both procedures entail resection of conjunctiva, which may worsen some cases of contraction. If there is significant socket contraction, or if the lid does not elevate to a satisfactory level after applying phenylephrine drops, either an external levator aponeurosis advancement or external levator resection is the procedure of choice.

When levator function is poor or absent, as is often seen with a contracted socket, a frontalis suspension

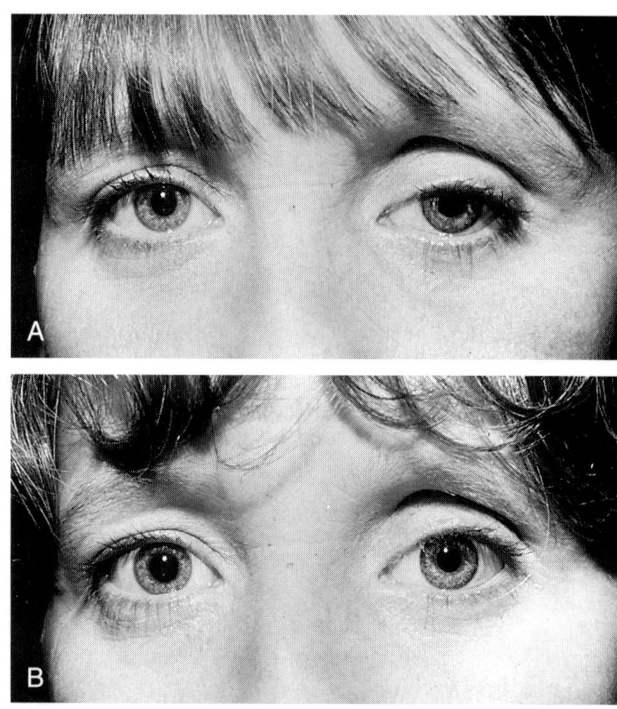

Figure 106–21. *A*, Left upper lid ptosis. *B*, Correction of ptosis by Müller's muscle resection.

using autogenous fascia lata or a silicone rod is effective to repair the ptosis.

Implant Complications

Migrated Implant

As many as 65% of implants placed within Tenon's capsule migrate out of position.[41] Orbital implants can migrate out of the muscle cone, most commonly superotemporally or inferiorly, especially if the rectus muscles are imbricated over the implant at the time of enucleation.[44] If the implant moves into the superior fornix, the prosthesis will be displaced inferiorly and tipped downward. If the implant migrates into the inferior fornix, it will obliterate the fornix and interfere with the ability to retain the prosthesis. An inferiorly migrated implant may also cause superior sulcus depression and pseudoptosis.

An implant may extrude early in the postoperative period when there is poor wound closure due to conjunctival shortage, poor surgical technique, or if the implant is too large. A socket infection may cause a dehiscence of the wound.

Late extrusion may be caused by erosion of the conjunctiva, infection, or a poorly fitting prosthesis. Mesh implants have a high extrusion rate, presumable because the sharp edges of the mesh create excessive friction on the orbital soft tissue as the prosthesis moves over the implant. Late extrusion is usually associated with fistula formation and cicatricial scarring of the conjunctiva and fornices.[45] The shortage of conjunctiva may make placement of an adequate size spherical implant impossible.

A migrated implant should be removed and replaced by either a spherical implant wrapped in sclera, fascia, or polytetrafluoroethylene, or by a dermis–fat graft (Fig. 106–22). The wrapped sphere is sutured to Tenon's capsule to reduce the chance of a repeated migration or extrusion.[11–13, 46] A dermis–fat graft is the better alternative in this situation.[14, 15, 17, 33] The principal advantage is that more orbital volume can be replaced with a dermis–fat graft than with an alloplastic implant, even when there is mild to moderate socket contraction. There have not been any reported cases of a dermis–fat graft migration or extruding. A dermis–fat graft can be used in moderately contracted sockets, but if the vascular supply of the orbit is severely compromised as in traumatized sockets, the graft may contract or become necrotic.[47]

Exposed or Extruded Implant

If a dehiscence or extrusion is due to a socket infection, the socket should be packed and systemic antibiotics should be administered until the infection is cleared. A

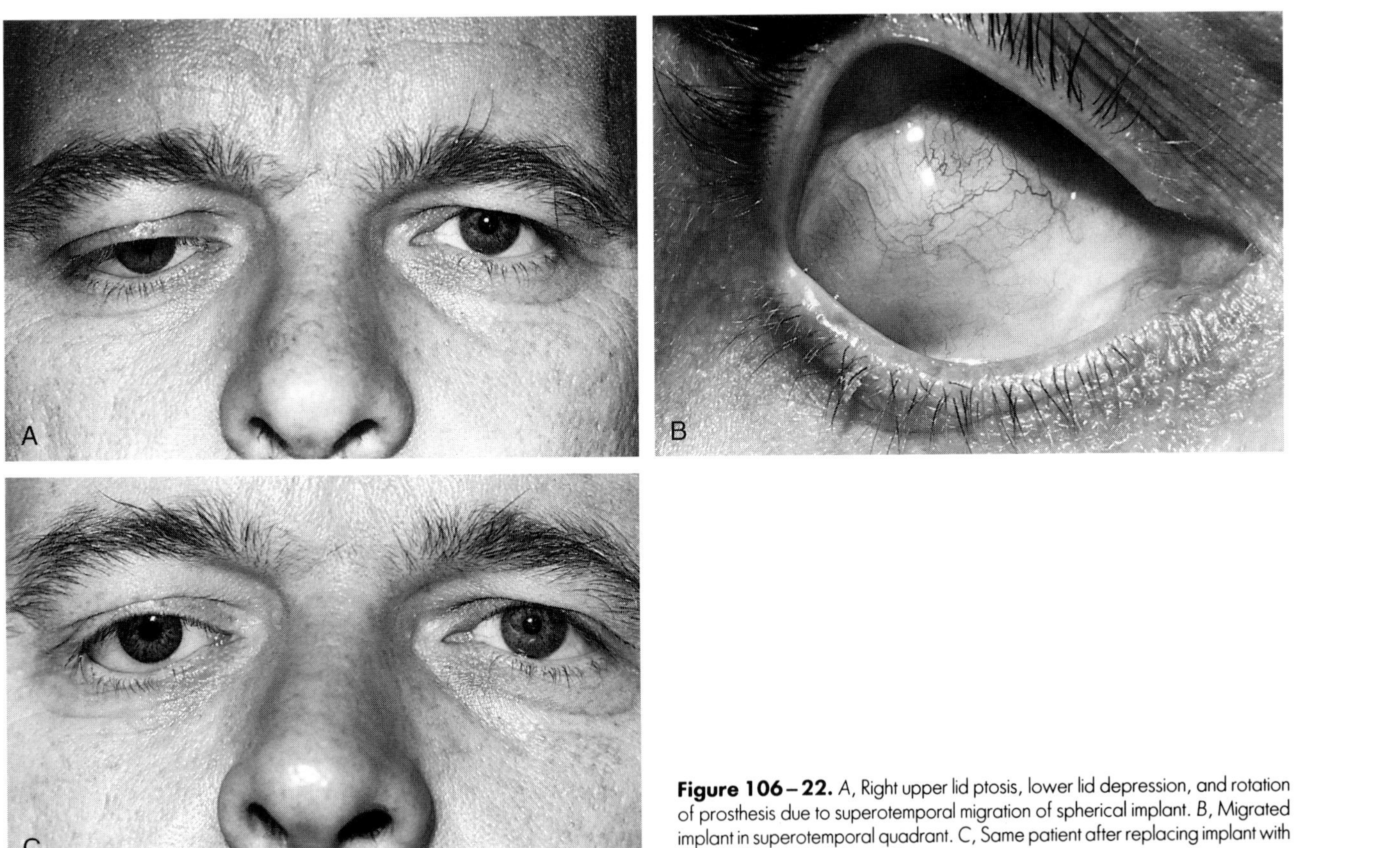

Figure 106–22. *A*, Right upper lid ptosis, lower lid depression, and rotation of prosthesis due to superotemporal migration of spherical implant. *B*, Migrated implant in superotemporal quadrant. *C*, Same patient after replacing implant with dermis–fat graft and levator aponeurosis advancement.

secondary implant can be placed after resolution of the infection.

If a small dehiscence in the conjunctiva exposes the implant, the defect can be repaired with a scleral[48] or autogenous fascia[34] patch graft if the dehiscence is noted in 3 to 4 postoperative days and there is no evidence of infection. The scleral or fascial graft is cut several millimeters larger than the dehiscence. Several 6-0 double-armed absorbable sutures are passed from the posterior to the anterior surface around the periphery of the graft. The graft is then tucked under the conjunctiva, covering the exposed implant. The sutures are passed through the conjunctiva in the fornices and tied externally. The conjunctiva is then imbricated over the graft (Fig. 106–23).

If the defect is larger than 3 or 4 mm, or if it has been present longer than 3 or 4 days, the implant should be removed and the surrounding capsule excised. If conjunctival epithelium has grown into the implant cavity, it forms an epithelial-lined pouch around the implant, leading to the formation of orbital cysts. Both factors may increase the change of implant extrusion.[45] A secondary spherical implant wrapped in sclera or fascia, or preferably a dermis–fat graft, should be implanted. It is often necessary to place a smaller spherical implant than

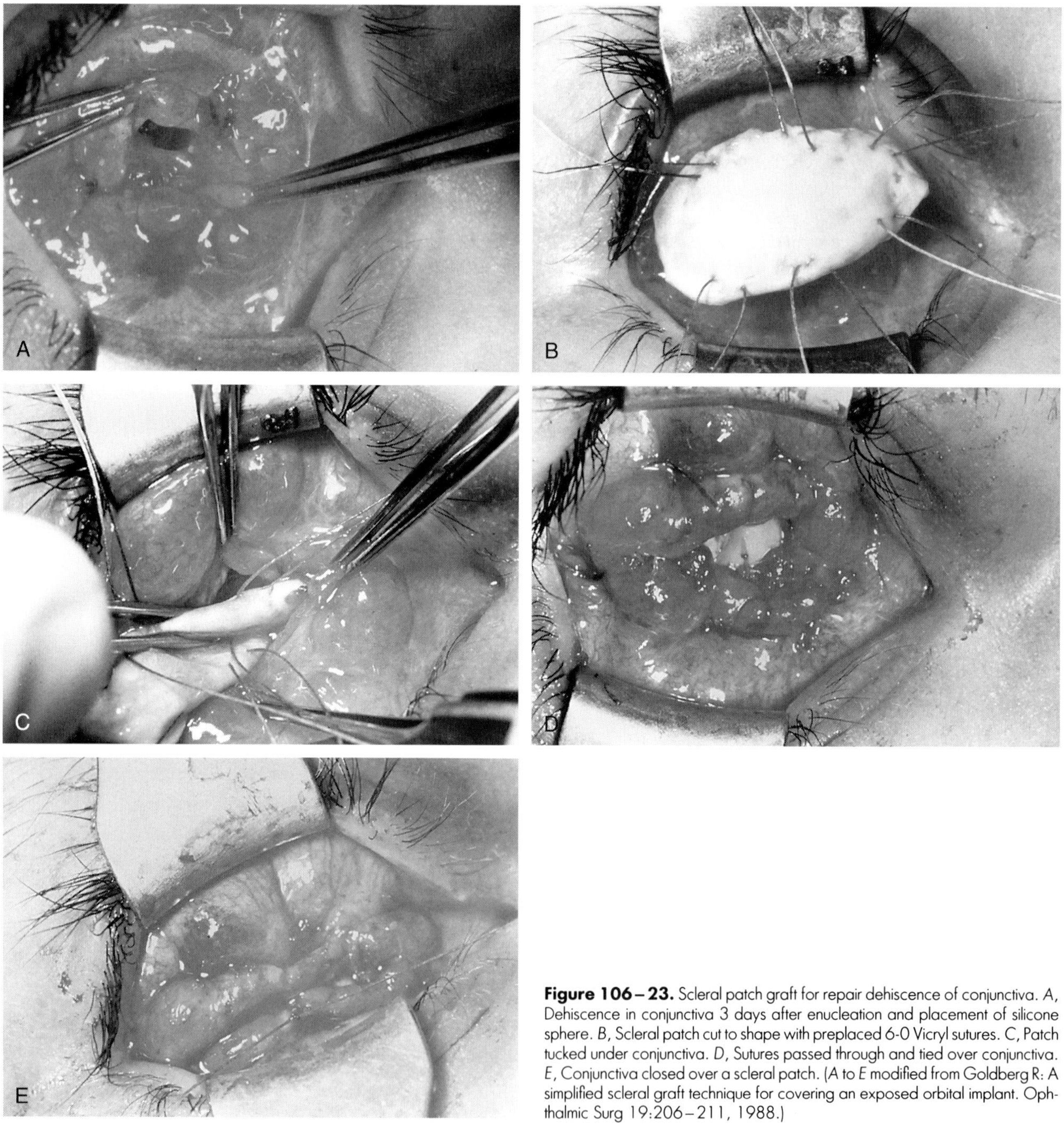

Figure 106–23. Scleral patch graft for repair dehiscence of conjunctiva. *A*, Dehiscence in conjunctiva 3 days after enucleation and placement of silicone sphere. *B*, Scleral patch cut to shape with preplaced 6-0 Vicryl sutures. *C*, Patch tucked under conjunctiva. *D*, Sutures passed through and tied over conjunctiva. *E*, Conjunctiva closed over a scleral patch. (*A* to *E* modified from Goldberg R: A simplified scleral graft technique for covering an exposed orbital implant. Ophthalmic Surg 19:206–211, 1988.)

the one that extruded because of the associated contraction of the conjunctiva and orbit. This may further amplify the orbital volume deficit. Soll[49] reported using an inflatable evisceration sphere inserted through a lateral brow incision to avoid incision conjunctiva and Tenon's capsule. A hydroxyapatite implant permits fibrovascular ingrowth, so the implant should not extrude or migrate. There is still a limit to the size of the hydroxyapatite implant that can be placed into the socket without stressing the conjunctival incision. The prosthesis must make up the additional lost volume. The implant peg may provide additional support to the prosthesis, reducing the stress on the lower lid. A dermis–fat graft more effectively reduces the orbital volume deficit and allows for a thinner, lighter prosthesis.

Motility of the prosthesis with a secondary hydroxyapatite implant or dermis–fat graft is generally better than the motility with a standard spherical secondary implant.

Orbital Deformity

Cosmetic and functional reconstruction of the anophthalmic socket can be complicated by disruption of the bony orbit. Unrepaired fractures of the orbital floor or medial wall will accentuate the enophthalmos. Displaced orbital rim fractures may aggravate socket laxity and contribute to difficulty retaining a prosthesis. Loss of the orbital skeleton from trauma or surgery creates a cosmetically objectionable appearance.

Reestablishing the normal dimensions of the orbit after trauma is important to minimize post-traumatic deformities. If enophthalmos is due to an unrepaired orbital blow-out fracture, then subperiosteal implants of carved silicone, preserved cartilage, high-density porous polyethylene, or Vitallium or titanium mesh may be necessary to reduce the dimensions of the orbital cavity.

Orbital rim deformities should be repaired either by advancing the depressed rims or with onlay bone grafts,[27] preserved cartilage, or alloplastic material such as Proplast,[50] high-density porous polyethylene, or silicone.[51]

Socket Contraction

Contraction of the ocular socket is commonly seen after extrusion of an orbital implant, in the presence of chronic conjunctivitis, and in severely traumatized sockets. Iatrogenic causes of socket contraction include multiple surgical procedures and radiation.

Enucleation in childhood may result in retarded orbital growth and facial asymmetry.[52] Orbital radiation given at a young age to treat retinoblastoma or rhabdomyosarcoma may cause progressive contraction of orbital soft tissue and bony abnormalities. These irradiated sockets are also predisposed to develop secondary malignancies, especially osteogenic sarcoma. They should be examined yearly, and radiographic studies or biopsies should be performed if there is a suspected malignancy.

The contraction may be localized to the fornices or may involve the entire socket. Treatment is aimed at reestablishing the fornices as well as maintaining sufficient volume to permit wearing of a comfortable and cosmetically acceptable prosthesis.

In mild cases of socket contraction there may be only mild cicatricial entropion of the lids. More severe contraction involves the fornices. The inferior fornix is most frequently affected. Treatment consists of excising subconjunctival scar tissue and replacing scarred mucous membrane.

If the contraction is limited to either fornix, the scar tissue is excised. A full-thickness mucous membrane graft from the lip or cheek can be placed in the fornix and held in place with retinal implant sponges sutured through the inferior fornix to the orbital rim (Fig. 106–24). Full-thickness grafts are preferred because split-thickness grafts shrink.

Severely contracted sockets require more extensive repair. The goal is to achieve deep fornices while replacing scarred mucous membrane. Procedures that deepen the cul-de-sac by suturing the conformer to the orbital rim do not always create adequate fornices. The deep ocular socket reconstruction described by Putterman and Scott usually provides satisfactory deepening of the fornices (Fig. 106–25).[53, 54] The conjunctiva is incised horizontally in the center of the socket and then undermined anteriorly to the tarsus. Subconjunctival bands of scar tissue are excised from the fornices. The conformer is wrapped with full-thickness buccal mucous membrane with the mucosal side toward the conformer and the raw surface facing outward. The mucous membrane–covered conformer is then placed within the socket. The posterior extensions of the oversized conformer push the mucous membrane deep into the superior and inferior orbit. The conformer is sutured to the orbital rim and left in place for 6 months (Fig. 106–26).

A socket that has contracted after multiple surgical procedures or radiation presents a more difficult challenge. If the mucous membrane graft shrinks, the socket should then be lined with a split-thickness skin graft. Skin grafts will survive better than mucous membrane will in a poorly vascularized socket, but they frequently become a hygiene problem because of the chronic discharge from sockets lined with keratinized epithelium. A vascularized free flap[55] or a temporalis muscle flap will add volume and a vascular bed to these relatively avascular sockets, improving the chances for a successful mucous membrane graft.

Severely contracted sockets that have failed reconstructive surgery may achieve the best cosmetic result from a limited exenteration and fitting of a facial prosthesis.[56]

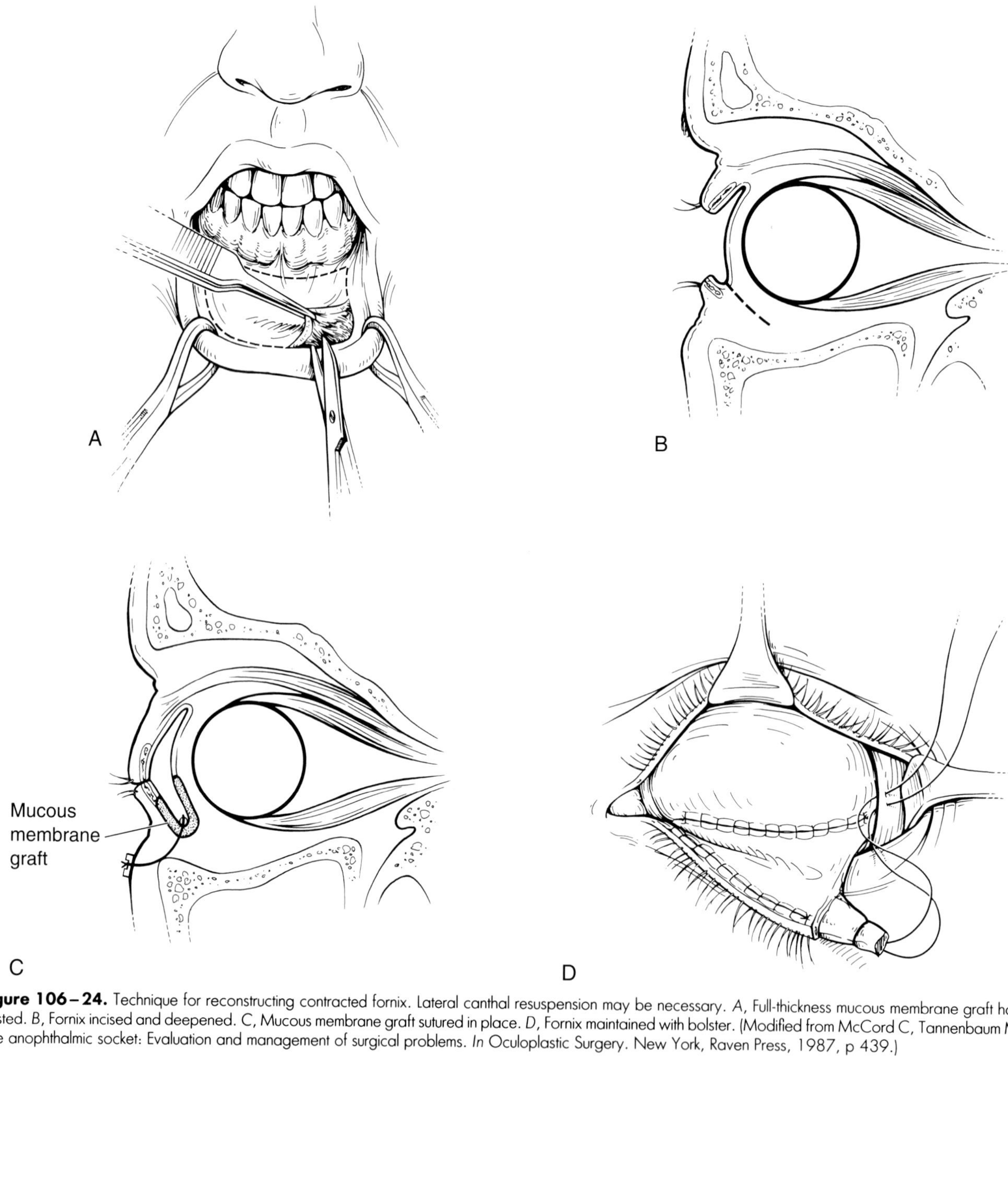

Figure 106–24. Technique for reconstructing contracted fornix. Lateral canthal resuspension may be necessary. *A*, Full-thickness mucous membrane graft harvested. *B*, Fornix incised and deepened. C, Mucous membrane graft sutured in place. *D*, Fornix maintained with bolster. (Modified from McCord C, Tannenbaum M: The anophthalmic socket: Evaluation and management of surgical problems. *In* Oculoplastic Surgery. New York, Raven Press, 1987, p 439.)

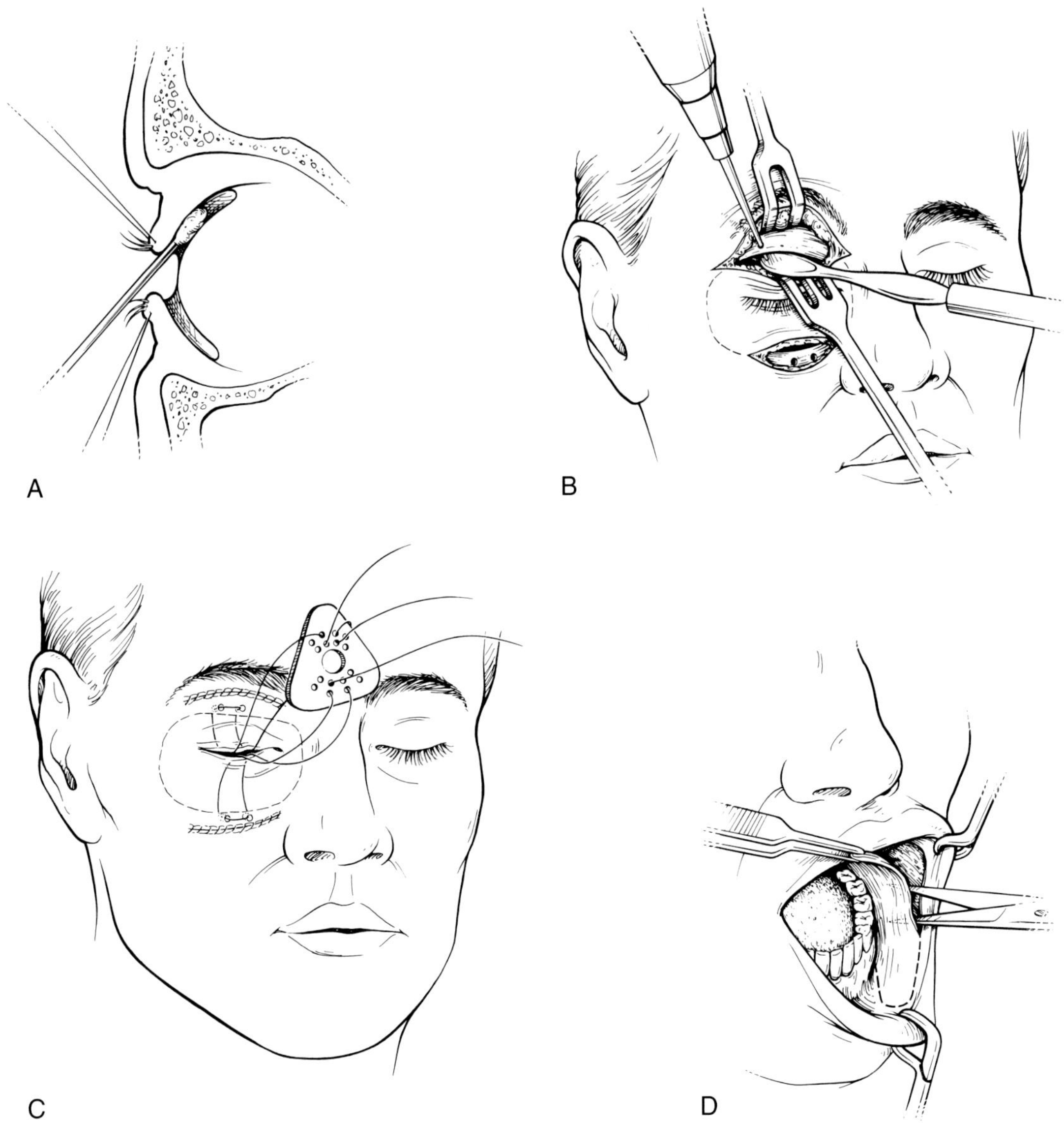

Figure 106–25. Technique for deep ocular socket reconstruction. *A*, Fornices incised and deepened. *B*, Anchor holes drilled through superior and inferior orbital rims. *C*, Sutures passed through C-shaped conformer. *D*, Full-thickness mucous membrane graft harvested.

Illustration continued on following page

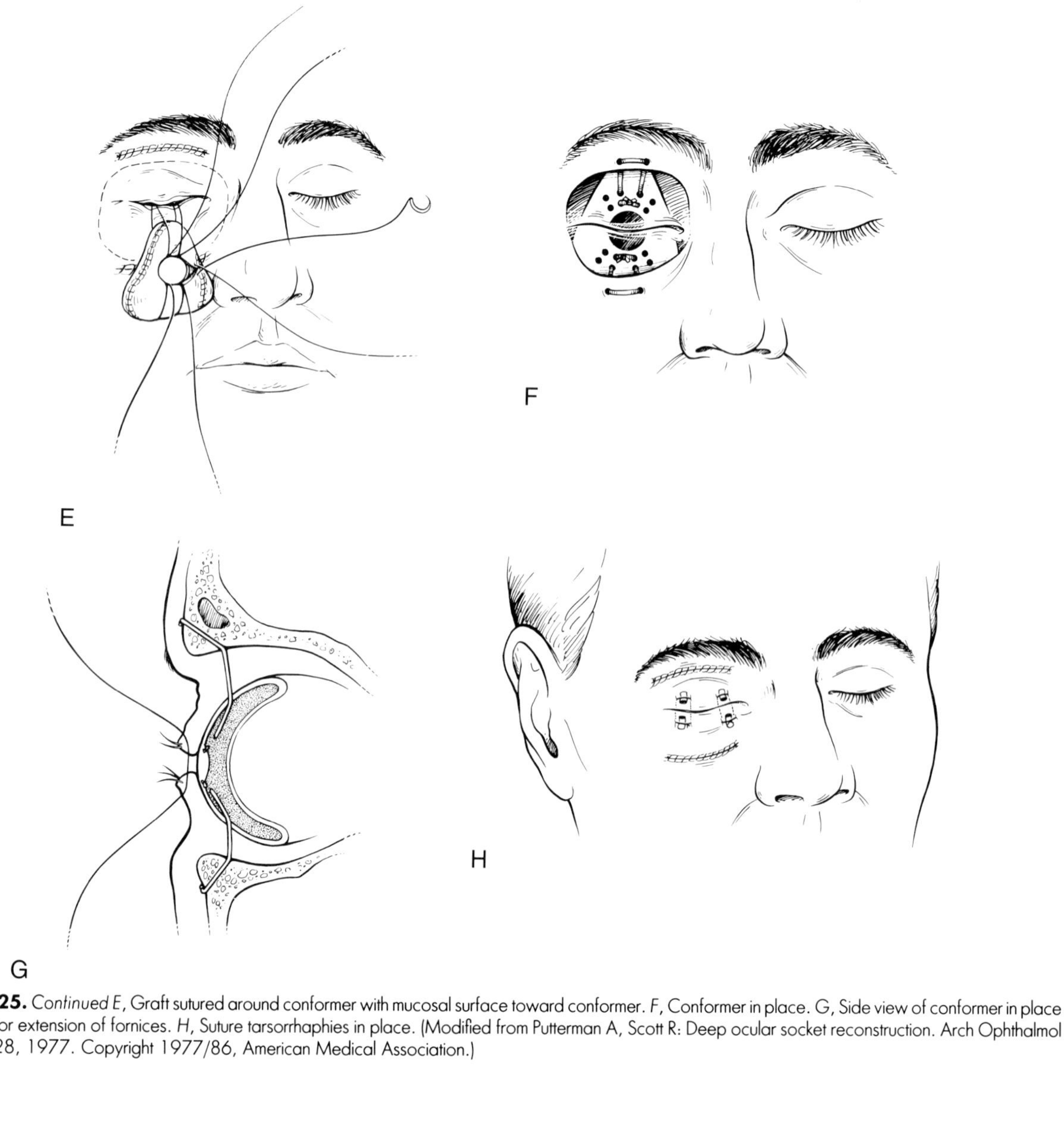

Figure 106–25. *Continued E*, Graft sutured around conformer with mucosal surface toward conformer. *F*, Conformer in place. *G*, Side view of conformer in place showing posterior extension of fornices. *H*, Suture tarsorrhaphies in place. (Modified from Putterman A, Scott R: Deep ocular socket reconstruction. Arch Ophthalmol 95:1221–1228, 1977. Copyright 1977/86, American Medical Association.)

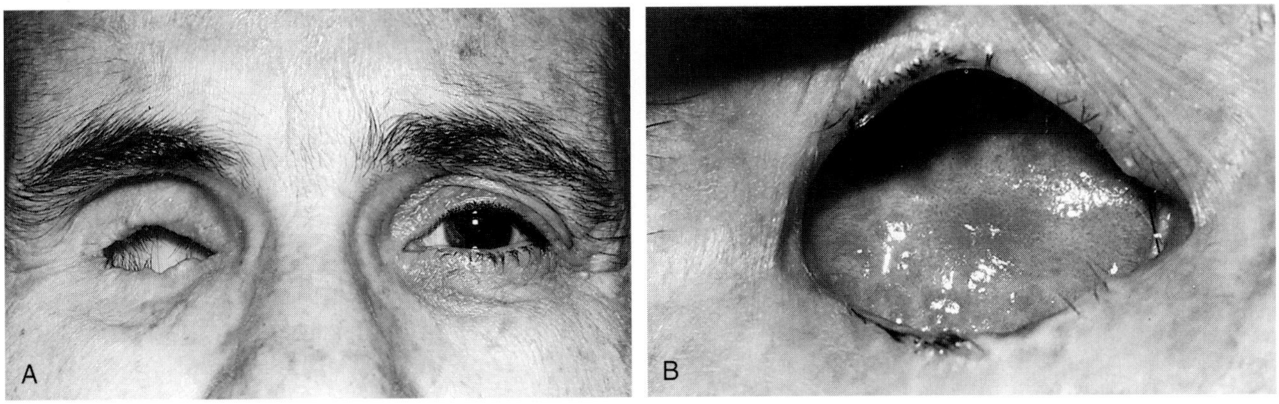

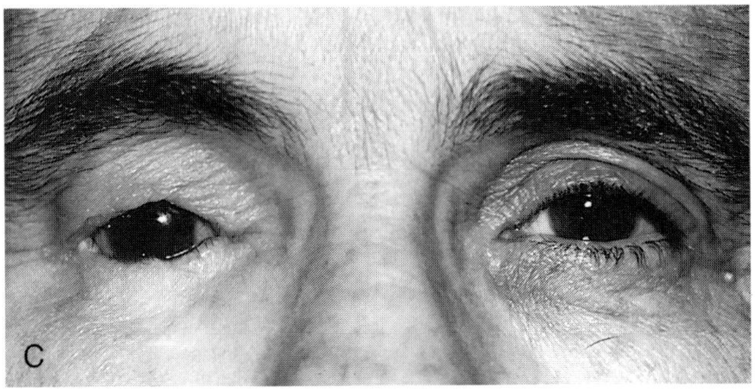

Figure 106–26. *A*, Contraction of socket, in which patient is unable to insert prosthesis. The patient has had multiple surgical procedures, including a full-thickness skin graft to line the socket. *B*, Appearance of socket after removal of skin and replacement with full-thickness buccal mucous membrane graft. *C*, Patient is able to wear cosmetically acceptable prosthesis.

REFERENCES

1. Silverstone PJ, Beyer-Machule CK, Schaefer DP, Della Rocca RC: Treatment of anophthalmos and socket reconstruction. *In* Della Rocca RC, Nesi FA, Lisman RD (eds): Ophthalmic Plastic and Reconstructive Surgery. St. Louis, CV Mosby, 1987, pp 1329–1359.
2. Marchac D, Cophignon J, Achard E, Dufourmentel C: Orbital expansion for anophthalmia and micro-orbitism. Plast Reconstr Surg 59:486–491, 1977.
3. Nolan WB, Vistnes LM: Correction of lower eyelid ptosis in the anophthalmic orbit: A long-term follow-up. Plast Reconstr Surg 72:289–292, 1983.
4. Jahrling RC: Prosthetics for upper lid deformities. Int Ophthalmol Clin 10:813–822, 1970.
5. Allen L: Cosmetic optics. Int Ophthalmol Clin 10:783–787, 1970.
6. Soll DB: The anophthalmic socket. Ophthalmology 89:407–423, 1982.
7. Kronish JW, Gonnering RS, Dortzbach RK, et al: The pathophysiology of the anophthalmic socket: Analysis of orbital blood flow. Ophthalmic Plast Reconstr Surg 6:77–87, 1990.
8. Kronish JW, Gonnering RS, Dortzbach RK, et al: The pathophysiology of the anophthalmic socket: II. Analysis of orbital fat. Ophthalmic Plast Reconstr Surg 6:88–95, 1990.
9. Kaltreider SA, Wallow IHL, Gonnering RC, Dortzbach RK: The anatomy and histology of the anophthalmic socket: Is the myofibroblast present? Ophthalmic Plast Reconstr Surg 3:207–230, 1987.
10. Paris GL, Spohn WG: Correction of enophthalmos in the anophthalmic orbit. Ophthalmology 87:1301–1308, 1980.
11. Soll DB: The use of sclera in surgical management of extruding implants. Ophthalmology 85:863–868, 1978.
12. Frueh BR, Felker GV: Baseball implant: A method of secondary insertion of an intraorbital implant. Arch Ophthalmol 94:428–430, 1976.
13. Stewart WB, Gratiot JB, Soll DB: Surgical management of orbital implant extrusion by implant placement posterior to Tenon's fascia. Ophthalmic Surg 13:807–811, 1982.
14. Smith B, Petrelli R: Dermis–fat graft as a movable implant within the muscle cone. Am J Ophthalmol 85:62–66, 1978.
15. Guberina C, Hornblass A, Meltzer MA, et al: Autogenous dermis–fat orbital implantation. Arch Ophthalmol 101:1586–1590, 1983.
16. Guberina C, Hornblass A, Smith B: Pitfalls of autogenous lipodermal implantation to the orbit. Ophthalmic Plast Reconstr Surg 3:65–70, 1987.
17. Migliori ME, Putterman AM: The domed dermis–fat graft orbital implant. Ophthalmic Plast Reconstr Surg 7:23–30, 1991.
18. Smith B, Obear M, Leone CR Jr: The correction of enophthalmos associated with anophthalmos by glass bead implantation. Am J Ophthalmol 64:1088–1093, 1967.
19. Taiara C, Smith B: Correction of enophthalmos and deep supratarsal sulcus by posterior subperiosteal glass bead implantation. Br J Ophthalmol 57:741–746, 1973.
20. White RH, Shannon GM, Yassin J: A modification of the correction of enophthalmos. Arch Ophthalmol 87:652–654, 1972.
21. Spivey BE, Allen L, Stewart WB: Surgical correction of superior sulcus deformity occurring after enucleation. Am J Ophthalmol 82:365–370, 1976.
22. Walter WL: Complications associated with the orbital bead implant operation. Ophthalmic Surg 8:68–75, 1977.
23. Helms HA, Zeiger HE. Callahan A: Complications following enucleation and implantation of multiple glass spheres in the orbit. Ophthalmic Plast Reconstr Surg 3:87–89, 1987.
24. Vistnes LM, Paris GL: Uses of RTV silicone in orbital reconstruction. Am J Ophthalmol 83:577–581, 1977.
25. Neuhaus RW, Shorr N: The use of room temperature vulcanizing silicone in anophthalmic enophthalmos. Am J Ophthalmol 94:408–411, 1982.
26. Sergott TJ, Vistnes LM: Correction of enophthalmos and superior sulcus depression in the anophthalmic orbit: A long-term follow-up. Plast Reconstr Surg 79:331–338, 1987.
27. Linberg JV, Anderson RL, Edwards JJ, et al: Preserved irradiated homologous cartilage for orbital reconstruction. Ophthalmic Surg 11:457–462, 1980.
28. Spaeth PG: Superior sulcus deformity and ptosis: Surgical correction. Int Ophthalmol Clin 10:791–797, 1970.
29. Vistnes LM, Iverson RE, Laub DR: The anophthalmic orbit: Surgical correction of lower eyelid ptosis. Plast Reconstr Surg 52:346–351, 1973.
30. Shorr N, Christenbury JD, Goldberg RA: Free autogenous "pearl fat" grafts to the eyelids. Ophthalmic Plast Reconstr Surg 4:37–40, 1988.
31. Smith B, Lisman RD: Use of sclera and liquid collagen in the camouflage of superior sulcus deformities. Ophthalmology 90:230–235, 1983.

32. Van Gemert JV, Leone CR Jr: Correction of a deep superior sulcus with dermis–fat implantation. Arch Ophthalmol 104:604–607, 1986.
33. Smith B, Bosnia S, Nesi F, Lisman R: Dermis–fat orbital implantation: 118 cases. Ophthalmic Surg 14:941–943, 1983.
34. Oberfeld S, Levine M: Diagnosis and treatment of complications of enucleation and orbital implant surgery. *In* Bosniak SL (ed): The Anophthalmic Socket. New York, Pergamon Press, 1990, pp 107–117.
35. Anderson RL: The tarsal strip. Trans New Orleans Acad Ophthalmol 30:352–363, 1982.
36. Nowinski T, Anderson RL: Advances in eyelid malpositions. Ophthalmic Plast Reconstr Surg 1:145–148, 1985.
37. Millman AL, Katzen LB, Putterman AM: Cicatricial entropion: An analysis of its treatment with transverse blepharotomy and marginal rotation. Ophthalmic Surg 20:575–579, 1989.
38. Bartley GB, Kay PP: Posterior lamellar eyelid reconstruction with a hard palate mucosal graft. Am J Ophthalmol 107:609–612, 1989.
39. Karesh JW, Fabrega MA, Rodrigues MM, Glaros DS: Polytetrafluoroethylene as an interpositional graft material for the correction of lower eyelid retraction. Ophthalmology 96:419–423, 1989.
40. Vistnes LM: Mechanism of upper lid ptosis in the anophthalmic orbit. Plast Reconstr Surg 58:539–545, 1976.
41. Soll DB: Evolution and current concepts in the surgical treatment of the anophthalmic orbit. Ophthalmic Plast Reconstr Surg 2:163–171, 1986.
42. Beard C (ed): Ptosis, 3rd ed. St. Louis, CV Mosby, 1981, pp 84–143.
43. Karesh JW, Putterman AM, Fett DR: Conjunctiva–Müller's muscle excision to correct anophthalmic ptosis. Ophthalmology 93:1068–1071, 1986.
44. Allen L: The argument against imbricating the rectus muscles over spherical orbital implants after enucleation. Ophthalmology 90:1116–1120, 1983.
45. Dryden R, Leibsohn J: Postenucleation orbital implant extrusion. Arch Ophthalmol 96:2064–2065, 1978.
46. Karesh JW: Polytetrafluoroethylene as a graft material in ophthalmic plastic and reconstructive surgery: An experimental and clinical study. Ophthalmic Plast Reconstr Surg 3:179–185, 1987.
47. Shore JW, McCord CD, Bergin DJ, et al: Management of complications following dermis–fat grafting for anophthalmic socket reconstruction. Ophthalmology 92:1342–1350, 1985.
48. Goldberg MF: A simplified scleral graft technique for covering an exposed orbital implant. Ophthalmic Surg 19:206–211, 1988.
49. Soll DB: Insertion of secondary intraorbital implants. Arch Ophthalmol 89:214–216, 1973.
50. Bello VM, Levine MR: Superior sulcus deformity. Arch Ophthalmol 98:2215–2216, 1980.
51. Callahan MA, Thomas R: Complex socket deformity: The team approach to physical and psychologic patient rehabilitation. Ophthalmology 86:1636–1639, 1979.
52. Osborne D, Hadden OB, Deeming LW: Orbital growth after childhood enucleation. Am J Ophthalmol 77:756–759, 1974.
53. Putterman AM, Scott R: Deep ocular socket reconstruction. Arch Ophthalmol 95:1221–1228, 1977.
54. Putterman AM, Karesh JW: A surgical technique for the successful and stable reconstruction of the totally contracted ocular socket. Ophthalmic Surg 19:193–201, 1988.
55. Tahara S, Susuki T: Eye socket reconstruction with free radial forearm flap. Ann Plast Surg 23:112–116, 1989.
56. Small RG, LaFuente H: Exenteration of the orbit in selected cases of severe orbital contracture. Ophthalmology 90:236–238, 1983.

CHAPTER 107

The Perfect Socket: The Ocularist's View

Walter J. Johnson

Obviously, the overall condition of the enucleated socket affects the chances for superior cosmesis. The ocularist's goal is to complement the ophthalmologist's surgical procedure by fabricating an ocular prosthesis that matches the patient's remaining eye and surrounding orbital symmetry. Ocularists who have been working for many years become adept at forecasting the cosmetic result before the prosthesis is fabricated. The severity of the patient's injury or trauma, the surgical technique, the depth of orbital volume lost, and the head structure surrounding the enucleated socket are just a few of the many significant details that will suggest the probability of prosthetic result. The better those situations are, the greater chance of a good prosthetic result. What is the possibility of creating a "perfect socket"? History tells us that perfection and enucleation are opposites. For how can we obtain perfection, when we are creating an imperfection? The surgeon, however, is trying to leave the enucleated socket as close to the original structures as possible. When this result is at its best, it leads to better prosthetic results.

In Tillman's excellent book *An Eye for an Eye,* he discusses the opinions of many experts in ophthalmology and ocularistry regarding eye loss, enucleation, and the anophthalmic socket. Demonstrating that good surgical results help lead to acceptable prosthetic cosmesis, Tillman, in 1973, listed the various conditions that ocularists are faced with according to difficulty in attaining superior cosmesis[1]:

1. Any evisceration
2. Microphthalmic or phthisical eye
3. Enucleation — Iowa or Allen implant
4. Full globe — blind eye
5. Enucleation — sphere implant
6. Full globe — esotropic or exotropic
7. Enucleation — no implant
8. Exophthalmos
9. Contracted sockets, anophthalmos
10. Orbital exenteration

NONSURGICAL MONOCULAR CONDITIONS

Most ocularists would agree that when fitting the thin ocular prosthesis or scleral cosmetic shell, nonsurgical methods, when possible, lead to the most consistently good results. If the monocular patient has a blind, slightly distorted eye that need not be removed, is well centered, and is slightly atrophied with decreased corneal sensitivity, then fitting the scleral cosmetic shell can produce excellent cosmesis and is quite comfortable (Fig. 107–1).

Many persons are not aware of the comfort that patients with scleral shells enjoy today. When a well-made scleral shell is fit properly over a blind globe with slight sensitivity, the patient will have few of the common problems that the ocular prosthetic patient may be faced with. Most of my patients with scleral shells who have healthy blind eyes experience few discomforts. In fact, 95% of all my patients wear their scleral shells at least 16 hours a day, and 50% of those wear their scleral shells 24 hours per day with more consistent comfort than any other prosthetic patients. This was true as far back as 1973, when Tillman stated that "the state of the art has advanced so that today a patient can not only wear a scleral shell comfortably, but it is not unusual to hear of 24-hour wearing schedules."[2]

There are some situations in which removing the blind unsightly eye is an advantage to the patient, from both a cosmetic and a comfort standpoint. Those situations would include (1) eyes that are too sensitive, resulting in inconsistent wearing schedules; (2) eyes that are severely esotropic or exotropic, creating tilts in the eyelids and awkward motility of the shell; (3) eyes that are larger than the remaining sighted globe, obviously appearing even larger once the scleral shell is in place; and (4) eyes that have exaggerated irregularities, leading to discomfort and poor cosmesis. But, if the disfigured, blind eye can be left in place, not causing the patient either pain or discomfort, and a scleral shell can be properly fitted over the eye with cosmetic success, then the first choice of therapy

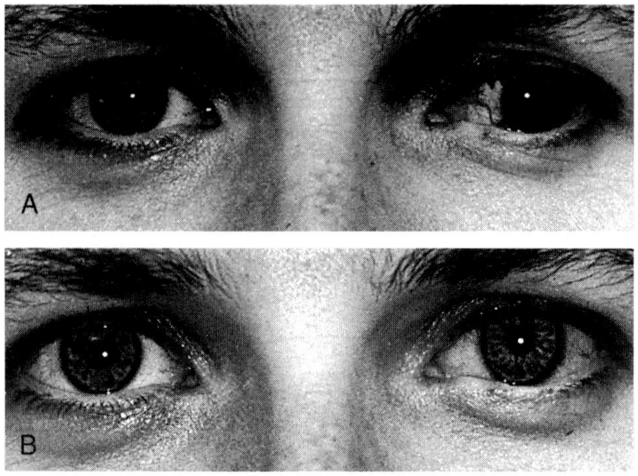

Figure 107–1. *A*, Patient with blind disfigured left eye. *B*, The same patient with a scleral cosmetic shell.

would be nonsurgical. This is not a new concept. Allen[3] made this observation years ago:

> My first choice is nonsurgical. In our concentration upon and absorption in the controversy over enucleation vs. evisceration, we must not overlook the fact that many persons with injured and unsightly eyes do not require either partial or complete eye removal. If retained eyes have reduced corneal and ciliary body sensitivity, they can be fitted with flush-fitting cosmetic contact shells. These are my first choice because there is very little distortion of the eyelids and orbital tissues, offering the best chance for excellent cosmesis, including fine motility, when fitted from an impression of the globe.

SURGICAL CONDITIONS: ANOPHTHALMIC SOCKET

Even though many ocularists would agree that the ideal scleral shell candidate is their most successful type of prosthetic patient, this is not the situation that the majority of us see most often. Most of the time we are dealing with eye removal, either enucleation or evisceration. How do we achieve the best socket results in those two procedures? How do we make the enucleated socket closely resemble the structures of the ideal scleral shell candidate?

Excellent socket results are more common today than in the past. Improved surgical techniques and the ophthalmologists' awareness that this patient will have to live the rest of his or her life with this deformity have resulted in more time and detail spent during the enucleation and evisceration procedures.

Since enucleation is not an easy procedure in which one consistently achieves good results, patience, immaculate efforts, and a full understanding of the techniques are essentials. The first enucleation procedure that I had the privilege to observe demonstrated the importance of time, effort, and technique. I doubt the entire operation lasted 30 minutes, and although I was a relatively inexperienced ocularist at the time, I was quite sure that the levator had been cut. Unfortunately, when I saw this patient about 5 weeks later, my observation had been correct. Obviously, with any surgical procedures, there are certain risk factors. On the other hand, I doubt that anyone can perform a successful enucleation in less than 30 minutes.

For many years, both oculoplastic surgeons and experienced ophthalmologists have stressed the importance of good initial surgical techniques. As Young[4] pointed out in *Today's Ocularist* in 1977:

> An enucleation is a very important procedure. A simple removal of the globe without meticulous forethought generates most of the subsequent problems when it comes to fitting the prosthesis. Enucleation is not a menial task. It is the first step toward an acceptable appearance for the rest of the patient's life.

Both oculoplastic surgeons and ocularists are well aware that there are dozens of factors that contribute to the ideal anophthalmic situation. Many of these factors are beyond our control. Certainly traumatic accidents resulting in eye removal and multiple facial deformities may limit restoration of the patient's original looks. Although good surgical technique is extremely important in all situations, with many accident casualties the end result will never be close to pretraumatic conditions.

So what are the conditions that help lead to the perfect socket situation?

1. When pre-enucleation or evisceration trauma is nonexistent or minimal (Fig. 107–2):
   a. Noncomplicated diseased eye
   b. Nontraumatic
   c. Usually not related to cancer
2. When the surgical procedure leaves a patient with few complications (Fig. 107–3):
   a. No superior sulcus defect, lid ptosis, enophthalmos, entropion, or ectropion
   b. Presence of a well-placed implant
   c. Adequate fornices
   d. Usually a primary procedure

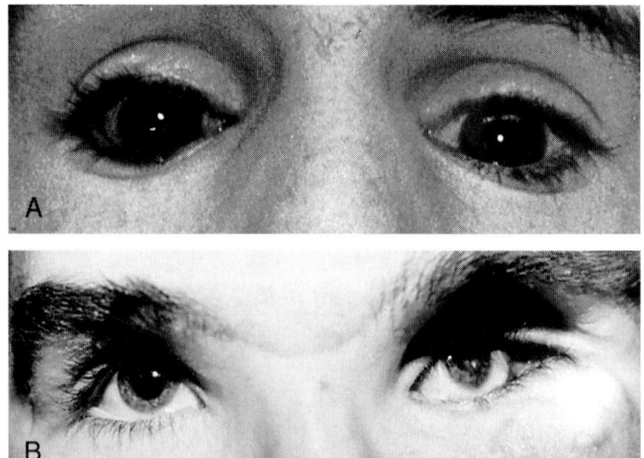

Figure 107–2. *A*, Patient with retinoblastoma after irradiation with enucleation of right eye. *B*, Patient after trauma from vehicular accident resulted in phthisical left eye.

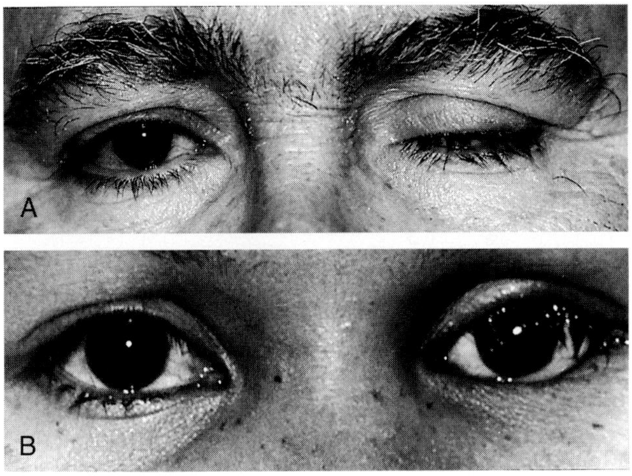

Figure 107–3. *A*, Severe blepharoptosis and anophthalmic left socket. *B*, Contraction of left eye socket.

Of course it is very rare when no defects are found after enucleation, for perfection is not easily achieved when removing part of the human body structure. According to Bayliss and associates,[5] "The anophthalmic socket is a uniquely complex system of structural and functional elements in which a change in any single element profoundly affects the other elements."

3. When the patient is fortunate enough to have the ideal head structure and symmetry that aids the surgeon and ocularist in achievement of a good cosmetic prosthetic result (Fig. 107–4):
   a. Strong and high cheekbones
   b. Low to mid-low brow
   c. Deep-set eyes

The patient with what we will call ideal anophthalmic head structure has an advantage over the patient with lower cheekbones, higher brows, and prominent eyes. This is due to the head structure somewhat camouflaging the facial defect. Ideal head structure will sometimes negate the lack of motility of the implant or a poor eye socket. On the other hand, low cheekbones and removal of a large eye almost always result in the appearance of a dropped eye socket, even when the surgical procedure is excellent.

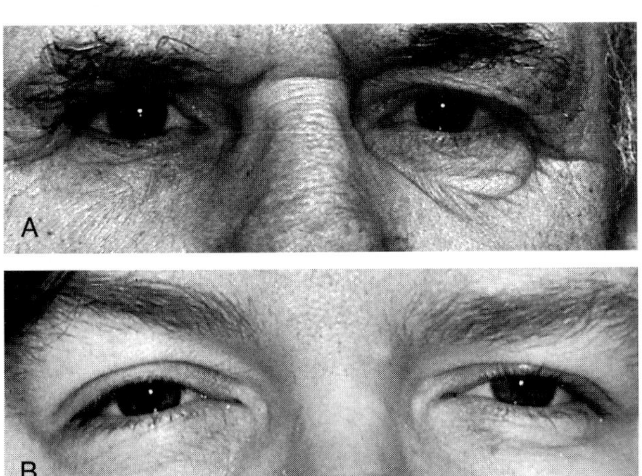

Figure 107–4. *A*, Deep-set eyes and prosthetic right eye. *B*, Low brow with prosthesis in left socket.

The graphs in Figure 107–5 illustrate the ideal surgically implanted sphere and a patient with good and with poor head structure for maintaining the symmetry surrounding the anophthalmic socket. Figure 107–5*A* illustrates that the closer the postenucleated structures match the pre-enucleated condition, the more desirable is the anophthalmic socket result. Figures 107–5*B* and 107–5*C* attempt to show how head structure affects the overall symmetry and settling of the postenucleated areas.

One thing is clear through everything ever written in regard to accomplishing a superior anophthalmic situation: preservation of as much of the preexisting conditions before either enucleation or evisceration is essential in achieving the perfect socket.

ENUCLEATION VERSUS EVISCERATION

If the procedure of choice is between enucleation and evisceration, the consensus would be to eviscerate, leaving the anatomic structures for the most part intact. With the exception of scleral shells over blind eyes and a few other new techniques, eviscerations lead to the best prosthetic cosmetic results. According to Ruedemann,[6] "Those who have had a reasonably long experience with this procedure know that it is eminently favorable to the patient; it provides superior cosmesis to any enucleation procedure as well as a functional orbit." Soll[7] stated that "Irrespective of the surgical technique or modifications used in both enucleation and evisceration surgery, certain changes occur in all anophthalmic sockets. These changes are somewhat less in the post-evisceration state because there is less disturbance of the extraocular anatomic structures."

From the ocularist viewpoint, Allen[3] can argue the benefits of the choice of evisceration.

> My second choice is evisceration with retained cornea and 18-mm spherical methyl methacrylate resin implant. It is my first choice as far as surgical mechanics are involved. This is because anatomy of the orbit and eyelids is practically unaffected. Cosmetic shell prostheses for these eye sockets should be fitted from impressions. Patient comfort and cosmesis, including motility, are nearly perfect in most cases.
>
> Evisceration with excised cornea and 16-mm spherical methyl methacrylate resin implant is my third choice. The supraorbital fold tends to be a little higher, exposing slightly more expanse of the upper lid than in the preceding evisceration.

As Allen describes, excessive secretion is not as much a concern in eviscerations as in enucleations. Any anophthalmic patient will relate that discharge on a regular basis is his or her first concern. In addition, as many ocu-

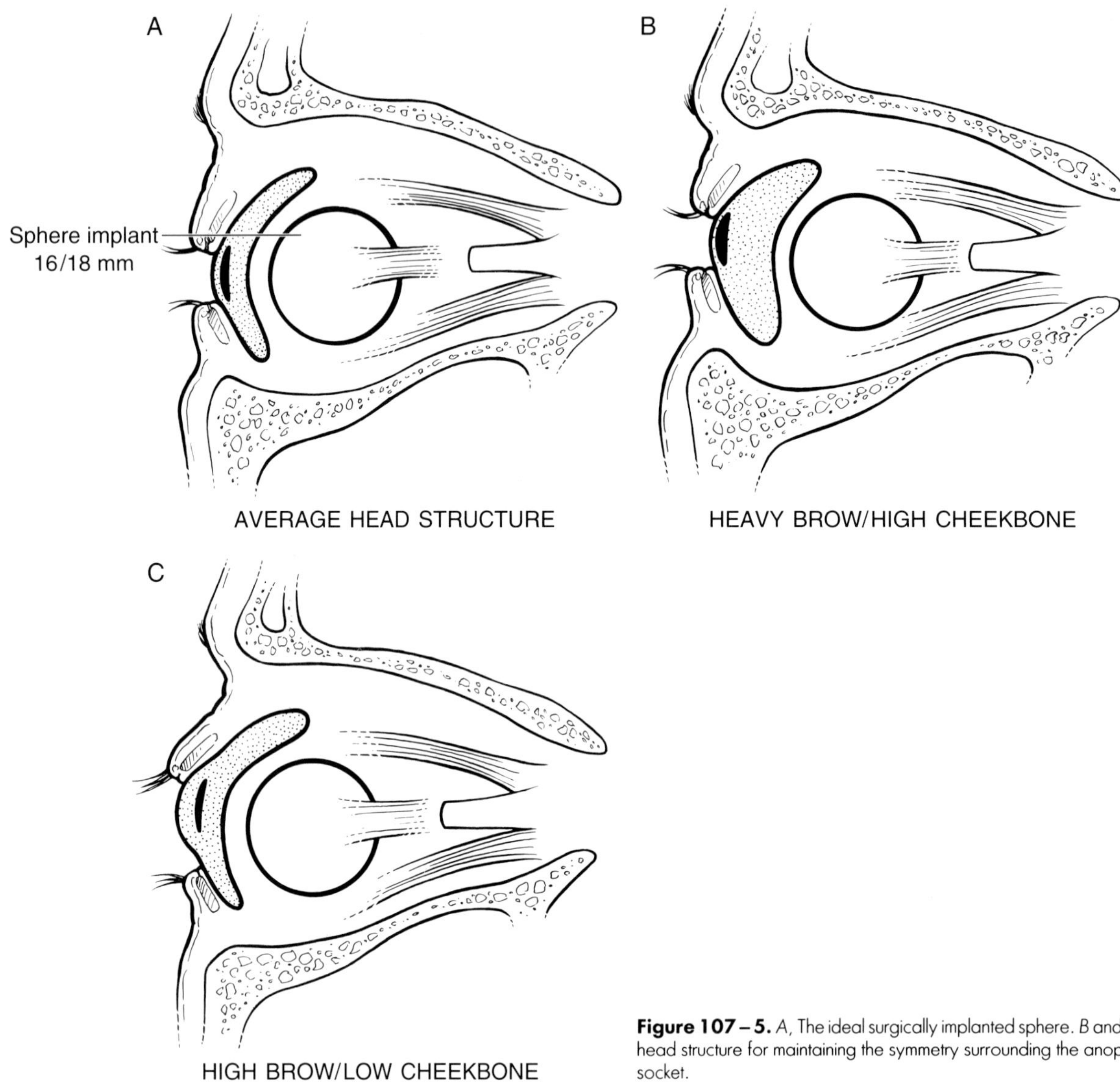

Figure 107–5. *A*, The ideal surgically implanted sphere. *B* and *C*, Poor head structure for maintaining the symmetry surrounding the anophthalmic socket.

larists are aware, most patients are adamant regarding preservation of their eye, if at all possible. Evisceration gives some prosthetic patients the comfort that the entire eye was not removed. According to Ruedemann,[6] "There is a strong psychological advantage to performing an evisceration instead of an enucleation: the patient may be aware that the globe is nonfunctional; this is not unpleasant. It may also be painful and unsightly, but the patient does not want to face removal of the globe."

EVALUATION OF IDEAL ANOPHTHALMIC SITUATIONS

So, let's analyze the situations that lead to the perfect socket. What comes first? What do we have control of? What is the responsibility of the surgeon or the ocularist?

Head Structure

We are born with the head structure we will live with the rest of our lives. Some head structures are conducive to the possibility of losing an eye. It is fortunate to have deeper-set eyes, a low brow, and high cheekbones when faced with the loss of an eye (Fig. 107–6).

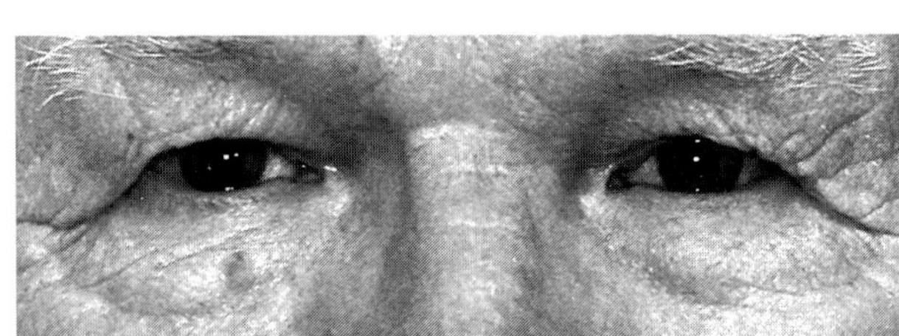

Figure 107–6. Patient with a good head structure for orbital reconstruction.

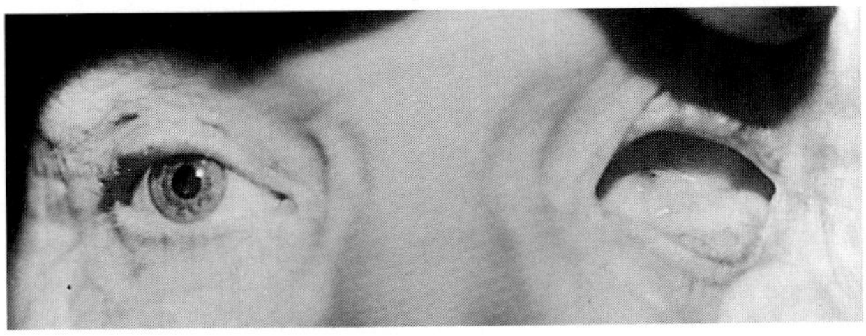

Figure 107–7. Well-healed socket.

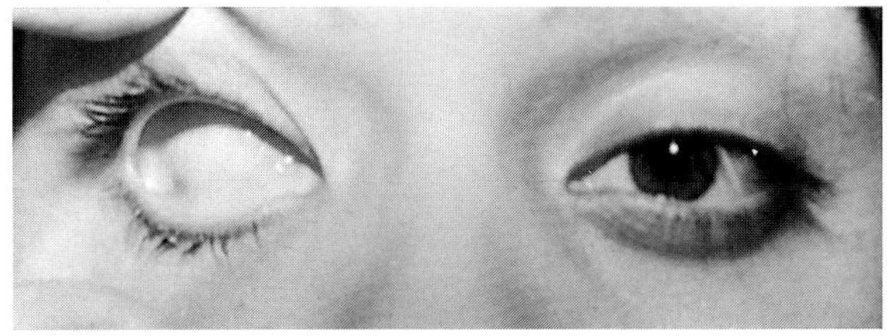

Figure 107–9. Centrally located implant.

Condition of Socket

The condition of the socket depends entirely on how the patient lost the eye and on the surgical result. Obviously, if the patient has an eye removed due to disease or a relatively minor accident causing little damage to the orbital area, the greater is the chance of the surgical result being excellent. The least damage done before evisceration or enucleation gives the surgeon a positive situation. The better the socket looks, the better the prosthetic result should be (Fig. 107–7).

Eyelid Symmetry

Eyelid symmetry can differ even before surgery. The more symmetric the eyelids before and after surgery leads to a superior balance between the prosthesis and the companion eye (Fig. 107–8).

Implant Location

The implant location is one of the most important areas in the final cosmetic success for the anophthalmic patient. If the implant (1) is the right size (with the sphere, somewhere between 16 and 20 mm should be used in almost all cases); (2) is totally balanced within the socket, leaving the same space superiorly, inferiorly, medially, and laterally; and (3) leaves just enough room for the thickness of the prosthesis (ideally between 2 and 4 mm thickness, which allows for adequate depth for the artwork in the prosthesis), then the situation is optimal. This goal is more difficult than one can imagine. Critical judgments must be made by the surgeon, and it is no doubt a very tedious endeavor (Fig. 107–9).

Volume Loss in Socket

The volume loss reflects, for the most part, the correct choice in the size and type of implant. It is more extensive after extreme accidents (Fig. 107–10).

Motility of Implant

Eviscerations generally lead to superior motility, but I have seen enucleations that could compare to the best in scleral shell results for cosmetic excellence. In the past few years, much has been done regarding the motility of ocular implants. The hydroxyapatite and porous acrylic implants are two types of porous implants. Both allow the ingrowth of tissue into the implant, thus increasing motility and decreasing both migration and extrusion, and both have had great success. Thy hydroxyapatite implant has been accepted worldwide and may be the most popular implant. In the past, the well-placed plastic sphere and Iowa implant provided the best in enucleation results. These implants are still widely used and will continue to be used, owing to their past success. I have seen the best results in sphere and hydroxyapatite implants wrapped in fascia. These fascia-wrapped implants may provide a cleaner socket for the patient, good motility, and excellent volume replacement (Fig. 107–11).

POSTSURGICAL CONSIDERATIONS

A well-placed, proper-sized plastic conformer will always help the socket heal properly, because of the comfort it provides the patient. Anyone who wears a prosthesis knows how uncomfortable it is for the inside of the

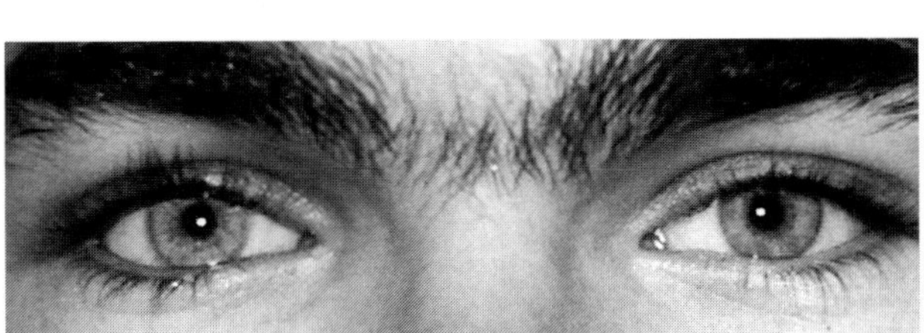

Figure 107–8. Good symmetry of eyelids with prosthesis in right socket.

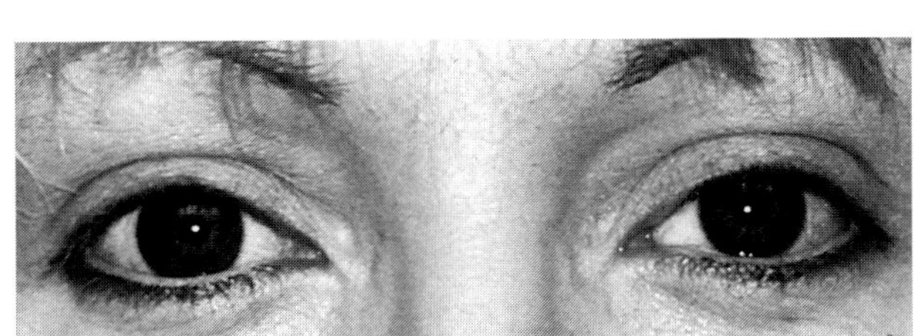

Figure 107–10. Very little volume loss after enucleation with prosthesis in left socket.

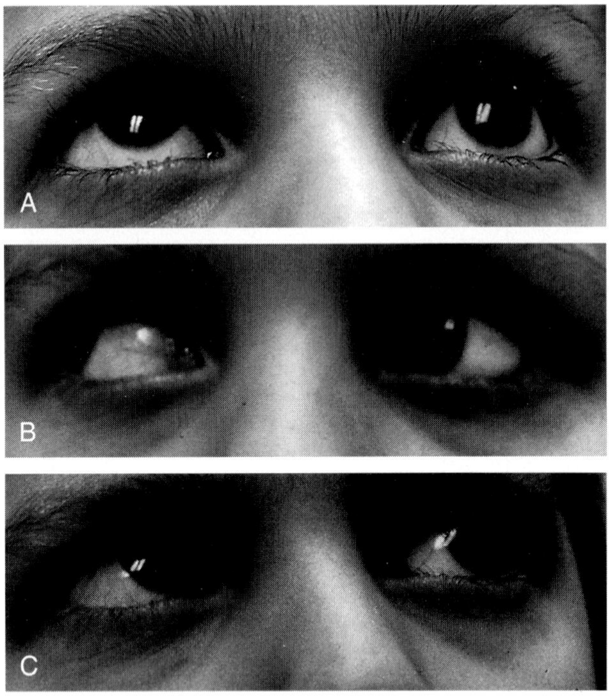

Figure 107–11. A to C, Good motility with prosthesis in left socket.

eyelids to touch the socket. The conformer gets the patient used to having something in the socket, thus preparing him or her for the prosthesis. Use of silicone-type conformers should be avoided because they irritate most sockets, which can interfere with initial prosthetic fitting.

Most patients are ready for prosthetic fitting at 4 to 6 weeks after enucleation. I believe it is safer and smarter to wait the entire 6 weeks. This extra 2 weeks always seems to eliminate discomfort in the fitting procedure for the patient and generally leads to a more accurate impression of the socket.

It is always helpful for the ocularist to know what type and size of implant has been placed in the patient's socket. Good communication between the surgeon and the ocularist always benefits the anophthalmic patient.

NEW MOTILITY IMPLANTS

Over the past 50 years there have been hundreds of different types of motility implants composed of a variety of materials. The sphere, whether it be glass, plastic, or silicone, has without a doubt been the most commonly used, owing in a large part to the fact that when a sphere migrates, it is still possible to fit. Many quasi-integrated implants, such as the Allen or more popular Iowa implant, have led to excellent results. However, if these implants migrate in the socket, fitting the prosthesis successfully is extremely difficult.

During the late 1940s and early 1950s, many integrated implants (an implant that eventually connects directly to the ocular prosthesis) were introduced. Although the motility of these implants proved excellent, the majority of these implants led to necrosis, infection, and exposure and ultimately were removed. This outcome led to the almost complete disappearance of the integrated implant for over 25 years.

A new version of the integrated implant, the hydroxyapatite implant, is becoming the implant of choice for many oculoplastic surgeons. Developed by Perry in 1983, the success of this innovation in motility implants has been monumental. The hydroxyapatite ocular implant was approved by the Food and Drug Administration in 1989 after 6 years of thorough research. The implant was able to be directly attached to the artificial eye by drilling a hole into the implant through the tissues that cover it. Originally, after the drilling procedure, either a flat or ball peg was inserted directly into the hole with the prosthesis being attached to the peg. This method proved very successful for a few years until it was observed that over time the ingrowth of tissue into the drilled hole would eventually push the peg out. This discovery led to the innovation of the threaded sleeve peg, which is widely used today. It will be years before we know how successful this threaded sleeve peg has been.

Since the motility aspect is so important to the anophthalmic patient, the motility peg after drilling is the major selling point of the implant. Unfortunately this supercedes some of the other qualities that this implant offers. Because the material, hydroxyapatite, is porous, it allows the ingrowth of tissue directly into the implant. This negates both migration and extrusion, two of the least desirable problems for the anophthalmic patient, ocularist, and surgeon.

This tissue ingrowth is also very responsible for excellent prosthetic motility. I believe that when this implant is wrapped in the patient's own fascia, it provides possibly the most consistent prosthetic result that I have ever seen. Whether the drilling procedure stands the test of time remains to be seen. However, regardless of the drilling and peg placement, the implant on its own is quite successful.

At the present time, there are many other implants being worked on that would increase motility, stability, and comfort for the anophthalmic patient. Perry's fine discovery has opened the door to research in finding the best for ocular prosthetic patients (Fig. 107–12).

CONCLUSION

Certainly, every ocularist and oculoplastic surgeon would prefer all their patients to leave the office with the best of prosthetic and surgical results. Unfortunately, sometimes this is not a reality. Innovations and improvements in both related fields have resulted in the overall advancement in cosmesis and comfort for the anophthalmic patient. In the future, this will unquestionably continue to improve. However, we are still dealing with a

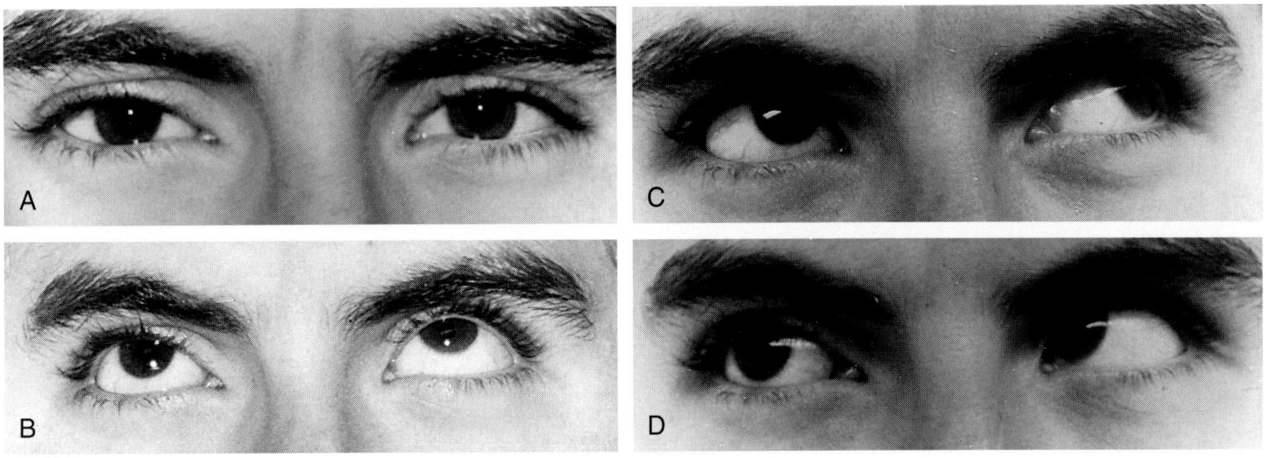

Figure 107–12. *A* to *D*, Patient with hydroxyapatite implant in right socket. Patient shows great prosthetic motility superiorly, medially, and laterally.

physical loss, and so far no one has found a way to replace an eye with anything that compares to the original.

> One thing we should all recognize is once an enucleation is performed, a deformity is present. This is quite an important concept. It is virtually impossible to take out an individual's eye and make him or her perfectly normal. Probably the most important part of this entire concept is that the ophthalmologist should let the patient know that from the beginning so that his expectations are realistic.[8]

REFERENCES

1. Tillman WT: Cosmetic anomalies following enucleation. Today's Ocularist, 4th ed, 1974, p 9.
2. Tillman WT: Various cosmetic complications. *In* Guibor, Gougelmann (eds): Problems and Treatment of Enucleation, Evisceration, and Exposure. Symposia Specialists, 1974, p 165.
3. Allen L: Prosthesis fitting, cosmesis and motility criteria. *In* Guibor, Gougelmann (eds): Problems and Treatment of Enucleation, Evisceration, and Exposure. Symposia Specialists, 1974, p 138.
4. Young C: Lack of motility in ocular prosthetics. Today's Ocularist, 7th ed, 1977, pp 10–11.
5. Bayliss H, Shorr N, Tanenbaum M, McCord CD Jr: The anophthalmic socket: Evaluation and management of surgical problems: *In* McCord CD, Tanenbaum M (eds): Oculoplastic Surgery, 2nd ed. New York, Raven Press, 1987, p 425.
6. Ruedemann AD Jr: Evisceration and sympathetic ophthalmia. *In* Guibor, Gougelmann (eds): Problems and Treatment of Enucleation, Evisceration, and Exposure. Symposia Specialists, 1974, p 97.
7. Soll DB: The anophthalmic socket. Ophthalmology 89:410, 1982.
8. Soll DB: Complications of enucleation surgery. Today's Ocularist, 7th ed, 1977, p 7.

CHAPTER 108

Orbital Prostheses

Gregory G. Gion

Patients who have undergone an orbital exenteration have few options from which to choose in dealing with their defect cavity. Although it is likely that some patients will choose to ignore the cavity and make no attempts to distract attention from it or conceal it, most exenteration patients will opt for some means of appearing less conspicuous. This would include the employment of either some type of eye patch or an orbital prosthesis.

The options in terms of eye patches are the homemade gauze and tape patch, the prepackaged flesh tone ophthalmic patches, and the traditional leather or fabric patch intended for extended use. In general, the patch offers an inexpensive and immediate means of covering the defect cavity. In some instances the wearer of the traditional patch may even take a certain satisfaction in sporting the patch as a well-integrated wardrobe accessory.

Many patients, however, do not feel comfortable wearing an eye patch. Any type of patch identifies the wearer as someone who has sustained an eye injury or loss. The wearer is then constantly reminded of the exenteration by the extra attention paid to the patch in the form of curious looks or inquiries from strangers. Exenteration patients often feel that people react to their loss or the patch covering it, rather than to them as an individual. The orbital prosthesis, then, is the final attempt to normalize the appearance.

FUNCTIONS OF THE ORBITAL PROSTHESIS

The orbital prosthesis functions primarily as an aesthetic device. It is a simulation of human anatomy, using prosthetic materials to create the illusion of a perfectly normal healthy eye and surrounding tissue. Fabrication of orbital prostheses that are aesthetic is a challenge. Since conversation with others is initiated with eye contact, slight discrepancies in position of the eye, lid contour, and color of the prosthesis are immediately noticed by even the most casual observer. Anteroposterior, mediolateral and inferosuperior positioning of the ocular component should mimic the exact position of the normal eye if a successful prosthesis is to be fabricated (Figs. 108–1 and 108–2). Ideally, the skin texture and pigmentation of the companion orbit are mimicked in the prosthesis to such a degree of accuracy and naturalism that the casual observer, even at a distance of perhaps 1 meter, believes the prosthesis to be a normal eye. The desired result of wearing such a prosthesis is the wearer will be able to interact more naturally, unencumbered by the obligation to explain his or her exenteration. In some cases it may not be possible to duplicate the appearance and contour of the remaining normal eye and adjacent structures. In orbital defects in particular an unaesthetic prosthesis could create more psychological trauma than no prosthesis at all.

While covering and, in some cases, filling the exenteration cavity, the prosthesis can also perform other functions. By virtue of the fit and seal of the prosthesis, the exenteration cavity is effectively protected from any harsh agents the wearer may come in contact with. Windblown debris is kept out of the cavity, as are large amounts of water encountered during swimming or bathing. This is particularly helpful when the exenteration presents a communication with the nasal cavity. When this occurs, the prosthesis may also be designed to obturate the opening. The purpose of this would be to prevent mucus from entering the exenteration cavity. Mucus that enters the cavity tends to accumulate and form crusts if it is not removed regularly by the patient. This crusting is not only detrimental to the hygiene of the cavity but can also hinder the proper positioning of the prosthesis within the cavity.

Individuals who have undergone a hemimaxillectomy along with the orbital exenteration are also likely to experience problems associated with a connection between the exenteration cavity and the oral cavity. However, the solutions to these problems are the responsibility of the dental specialists, specifically the maxillofacial prosthodontist. Only after the prosthodontist has fit the patient with a definitive obturator prosthesis to restore eating, speaking, and breathing function should the prosthetist begin designing the orbital prosthesis. The orbital prosthesis can then be designed to mechanically attach to the dental obturator via the absent orbital floor. This con-

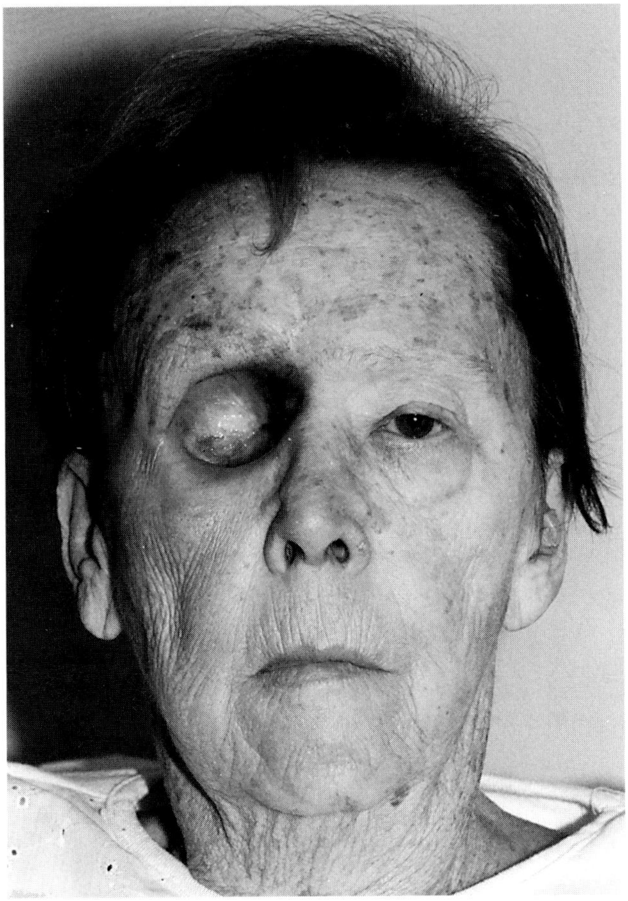

Figure 108 – 1. Exenteration of right orbit.

nection retains and stabilizes both the orbital and dental prosthesis to some degree and thereby increases the patient's overall confidence in his or her restoration.

BASIC SURGICAL CONSIDERATIONS

The success of an orbital prosthesis can be enhanced by careful presurgical planning and communication involving the patient, the surgeon, and the facial prosthetist. In this regard it is important for the facial prosthetist to be aware of what is involved with an orbital exenteration.

Exenteration is the removal of the entire contents of the orbit including the extraocular muscles.[1] The eyelid may or may not be involved with the disease process. If the eyelids are involved with the disease process, they must be removed during the surgical procedure. If the eyelids are not involved, the surgeon can (1) leave the eyelids intact (partial exenteration), (2) preserve and split the eyelids using the eyelid skin to cover the surgical defect, or (3) remove the eyelids totally. Removing the eyelids totally is the treatment of choice when the internal portion of the orbital defect is large. When the internal orbital defect is large, preserving the eyelids will leave a relatively small external opening, which can lead to infection, drainage problems, and prosthetic difficulties. In this situation it is difficult, if not impossible, for the facial prosthetist to construct a prosthesis that resides behind the eyelids. The defect is best treated by an external prosthesis lying totally outside the eyelids. The converse situation is encountered when the orbital defect is shallow, owing to the use of a muscle flap to fill the defect. The shallowness of the defect forces the facial prosthetist to fabricate a thin prosthesis, which loses its natural appearance because of lack of depth in the final prosthesis.

During an orbital exenteration, the surgeon should round any sharp bony edges on the lateral and superior bony wall of the orbit. The sharp edges can be painful when a prosthetic restoration is placed against them. Adequate contouring of these walls is also necessary to allow for proper positioning of the prosthesis superiorly. When the inferior bony margin of the orbit is removed, it should be re-created using fascia lata, muscle slings, or other means to prevent the margin from sagging postoperatively.

In most circumstances the orbital defect should be covered with a split-thickness skin graft, which provides for a firm, dry defect that allows for impression making, prosthetic support, visualization of the defect for recurrent disease, and the retention of the prosthesis by anatomic undercuts. On some occasions the orbital defect can be allowed to heal by second intention; however, careful presurgical planning and communication by the patient, surgeon, and facial prosthetist is necessary to ensure that there is enough space to allow for proper positioning of the prosthesis to obtain a good cosmetic appearance.

PROSTHETIC MATERIALS

A number of different materials are used today for the fabrication of orbital prostheses. Perhaps, the most widely used material is medical-grade silicone elastomer. Although other materials may possess some desirable properties, the silicone elastomer seems to demonstrate an optimum combination of several desirable properties for creating a successful prosthesis. Important properties include translucency for simulating tissue depth and pigmentation, adequate elongation and tear strength for durability, flexibility for comfort and compliance with facial mobility, and biocompatibility.

Polymethyl methacrylate acrylic, otherwise known as denture plastic, is also used for orbital prostheses. The hardness of the material makes for a very durable prosthesis. However, the margins of the prosthesis must be designed rather thick and blunt to avoid a knife edge that could cut the patient. Often, the prosthetist employing this material will permanently attach the prosthesis to the patient's eyeglasses, thereby avoiding the need for adhesive for retention. This, of course, greatly simplifies the management of the prosthesis since the patient need

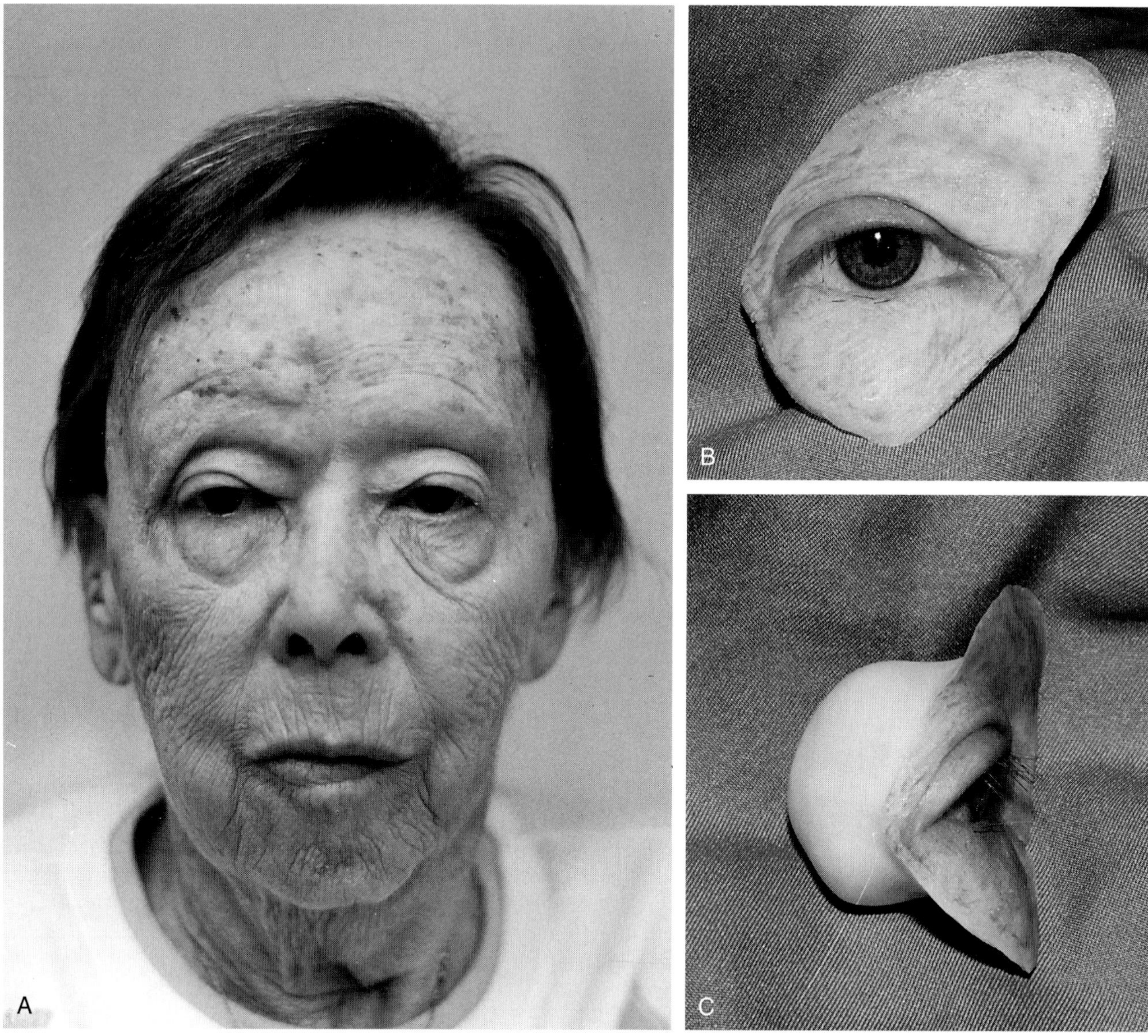

Figure 108–2. *A*, Orbital prosthesis in place. Anterior (*B*) and lateral (*C*) views of the prosthesis.

only put on the eyeglasses to quickly and correctly position the orbital prosthesis. The major disadvantage is that the margins, being rigid, thick edged, and not adhered to the skin, often allows gaps to form, particularly in areas where there is tissue mobility. Gaping margins of any prosthesis tend to be a major cause for concern for the patient trying to gain confidence in the effectiveness of the prosthesis. The other disadvantage to this arrangement is that the patient must always wear the eyeglasses to wear the prosthesis and may not remove the eyeglasses without also removing the orbital prosthesis. Although polymethyl methacrylate acrylic is not the ideal material in which to fabricate the entire orbital prosthesis, its density, rigidity, and alterability make it ideal for fabricating the more functional components of larger, more complex composite orbital prostheses.

Another material used in conjunction with the silicone elastomer is polyurethane sheet material. The clear polyurethane sheeting, 0.002 to 0.008 inches in thickness, is vacuum formed and chemically bonded to the posterior surface of the orbital prosthesis. The polyurethane is essentially a lining or backing of the prosthesis that serves several purposes. The thinness and transparency of the material produces an almost imperceptible prosthesis margin, while the very high tear strength produces a durable margin that is more resistant to damage commonly caused by adhesive removal. Also, the polyurethane seems to hold the adhesives more strongly than the silicone, adding to the patient's confidence in the security of the attachment. Finally, the polyurethane acts as an effective barrier to the glandular secretions produced by the underlying tissue.

Other properties of the polyurethane backing, however, lessen its desirability for use in the fabrication of the orbital prostheses. The polyurethane material yellows more rapidly than does the silicone. Therefore, the margin areas where the polyurethane is in view become prematurely conspicuous by their darker, yellow tone. The rate of yellowing may be difficult to predict, however. Exposure to sunlight and cigarette smoke seem to be factors largely responsible for accelerating this discoloration. Therefore, the prosthetist should consider these factors along with the patient's manual dexterity and attitude toward caring for the prosthesis before deciding on whether to integrate the polyurethane backing.

The polyurethane is also very technique sensitive. The need for vacuum forming limits the application to small to medium-sized defects and those that are relatively shallow without undercut areas. Delamination of the polyurethane is also a problem. Subsequent attempts to reattach or repair the polyurethane backing are often tedious and ineffective. Just as polymethyl methacrylate and polyurethane are valuable as adjunct prosthetic materials, the silicone family has grown to include several other useful forms. The medical-grade silicone foams, dispersions, gels, and encapsulants all possess some useful properties.

The low-density silicone foam may be used to produce a relatively lightweight bulb prosthesis that fills the exenteration cavity, engaging undercuts, thus retaining the orbital prosthesis. However, the foam can still be quite firm and irritating to a thinly grafted cavity. Also, the foam bulb, acting like a sponge, is susceptible to infiltration of dirt and body fluids if not positively sealed in an envelope of silicone.

Silicone dispersions are sometimes employed to produce thin-walled, bulb, or balloon prostheses. Again, this type of design is utilized to take advantage of cavity undercuts for anatomic retention. The dispersions are low viscosity silicone and solvent mixtures that enhance the technical ease of producing a thin flexible silicone bulb or balloon of uniform thickness.

Silicone gels used in conjunction with a coating or encapsulating silicone layer are available to produce a more flesh-like softness for the prosthesis. Although a prosthesis that is softer to the touch is more desirable, the real advantage lies in the ability of the softer prosthesis to move more freely and naturally with the underlying mobile tissue. Ideally, this would allow the design of an orbital prosthesis that would reflect to some degree the changing expression of the wearer such as in smiling. When the patient smiles with this type of orbital prosthesis in place, the muscle movement beneath the prosthesis may actually cause the inferior and lateral portions of the prosthesis to crease or fold momentarily. This slight movement or animation in the orbital prosthesis may add an extra level of naturalism.

The drawbacks to the encapsulated gel prosthesis for the orbit include technique sensitivity, biocompatibility considerations, and durability.

For the most part, the materials mentioned here and others such as polydimethyl siloxane, polyvinyl chloride, and other forms of polyurethane all have been employed as prosthetic materials because they demonstrated reasonable durability, a life-like appearance when pigmented, or both qualities. As long as the orbital prosthesis remains an external removable device to be managed daily by the patient, the search for the ideal prosthetic material or combination of materials will continue.

TREATMENT PLAN

Before the design of the orbital prosthesis is begun, the exenteration cavity, whether lined with skin graft or allowed to granulate, should be fully healed and free of edema. If the prosthesis was to be designed and fit based on an impression taken prematurely of a transitional exenteration cavity, the likelihood of gaping, poor retention, and patient dissatisfaction would increase. For this reason, it is advantageous to have the patient wait several weeks or even months before beginning the prosthesis. The patient's surgeon is helpful in monitoring the progress of the exenteration cavity and the periorbital contours that are particularly important to margin adaptation. Once the cavity appears to be well stabilized, the design of the orbital prosthesis may begin. Because this section is aimed at providing basic information about fabricating standard orbital prostheses, the interested reader is referred to other sources for additional techniques and information.[2–20]

The length of time required to make the orbital prosthesis depends on the size and complexity of the anticipated prosthesis. The small simple prosthesis might require three sessions while the larger or more complex design might require five or more patient visits for design and fitting. The prosthetist usually tries to schedule the patient sessions with enough time in between to allow his or her laboratory work to be performed unhurried and uncompromised. The patient traveling a great distance for the orbital prosthesis is often scheduled for an entire week stay, during which time the prosthetist can focus his or her attention almost exclusively to that patient. This allows the patient to receive the prosthesis in a reasonable amount of time while enjoying a brief retreat from other concerns.

The first of the patient's visits to the prosthetist's office is primarily for consultation. The prosthetist will assess the exenteration cavity to make certain it can safely and comfortably support a prosthesis. The prosthetist will also note how the prosthesis will be retained—with or without adhesive. At this point, the prosthetist can give the patient an accurate picture of what to expect out of his or her orbital prosthesis. Photographs of patients wearing

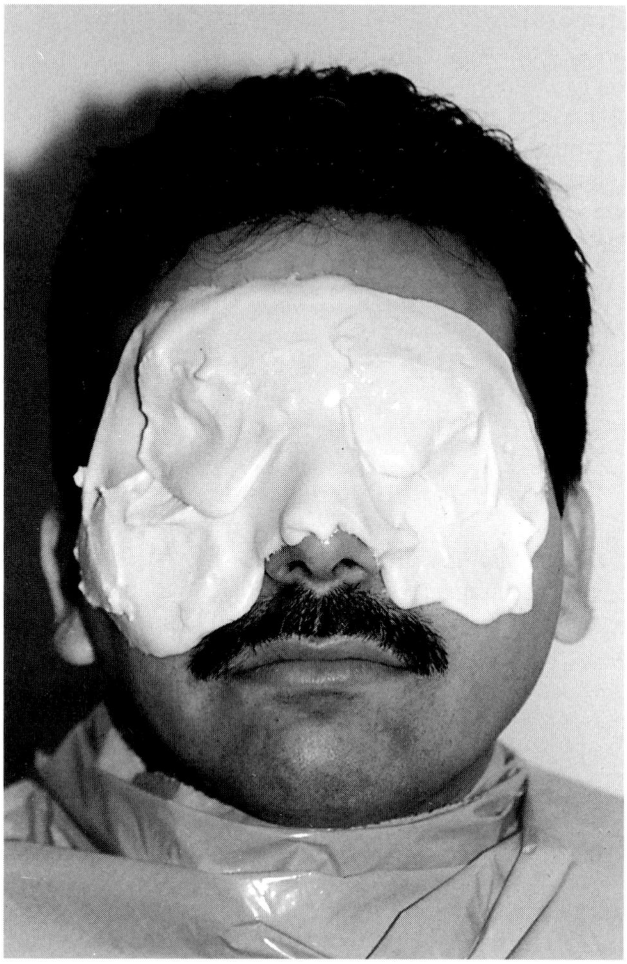

Figure 108–3. Facial impression using alginate, an irreversible hydrocolloid.

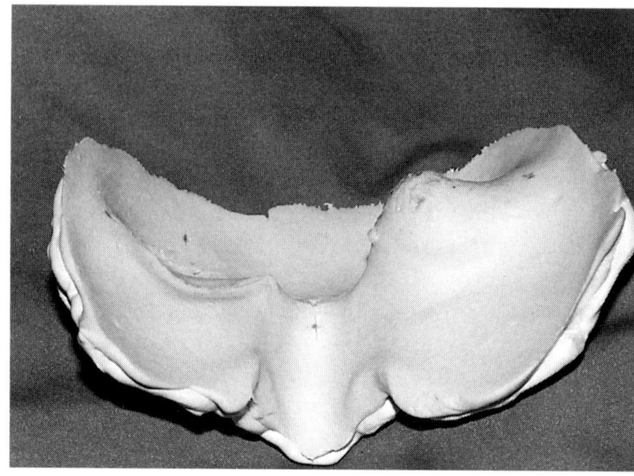

Figure 108–4. Inverted alginate impression showing transferred orientation marks.

similarly designed prostheses or actual orbital prostheses may be shown to the patient and family to demonstrate the nature of the restoration, the effectiveness of the restoration, and also the inherent compromises and limitations associated with the restoration.

If the patient presents a well-healed cavity and is anxious to begin, the facial impression may be taken at the time of the consultation. The impression procedure causes no discomfort to the patient. The creamy alginate impression material is injected or spatulated into and around the exenteration cavity. Also, the impression material may be spread over the forehead, the closed companion eye, across the nasal bridge, and well down onto the mid face (Fig. 108–3). Backed with a layer of fast-setting plaster for support, the impression is carefully removed, producing a very accurate negative relief of the patient's cavity and adjacent facial contour (Fig. 108–4). Onto this negative impression is poured a denser and stronger plaster or dental stone, producing an accurate, positive working cast of the patient's exenteration cavity and surrounding facial contour (Fig. 108–5).

The patient's skin coloration is also observed and noted. Silicone color swatches representing base skin tones, vascularity, mottling, and so on are selected and photographed next to the patient's face to help guide the prosthetist during later steps involving color and characterization. The frontal photographs of the patient will also be helpful to refer to in the laboratory during the preliminary sculpting. The acrylic ocular component is also chosen from a selection and modified or custom fabricated to match the patient's iris size and color, sclera, and so on (Fig. 108–6).

From measurements and photographs taken of the patient at the time of the impression, the preliminary sculpting may be accomplished in the laboratory (Fig. 108–7). The patient returns to the office so that the ocular placement within the wax model and the accuracy of

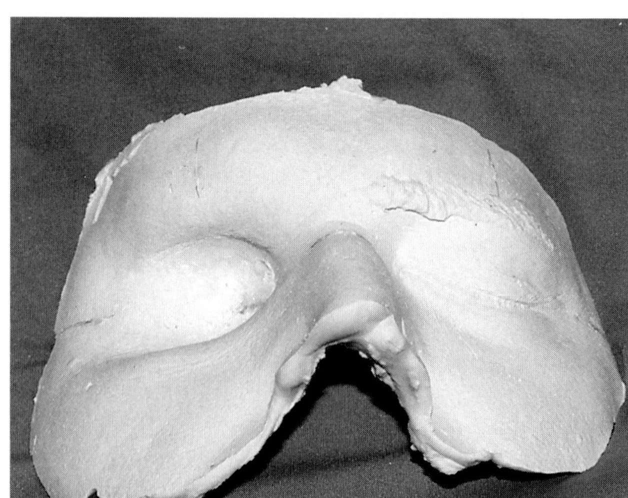

Figure 108–5. Plaster cast produced from the alginate impression. The orientation marks have been transferred from the impression and redefined.

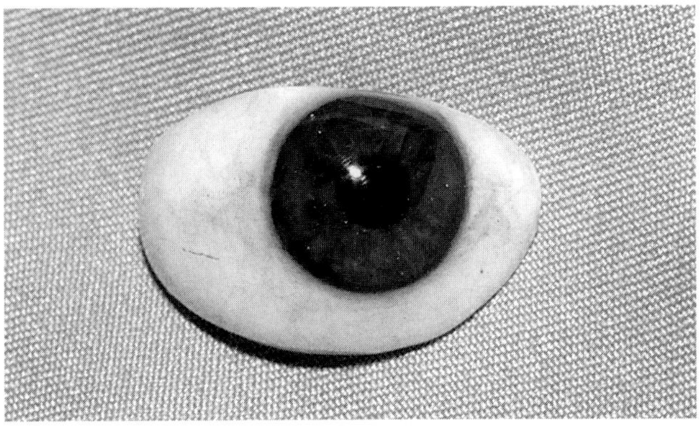

Figure 108–6. Ocular component of the orbital prosthesis.

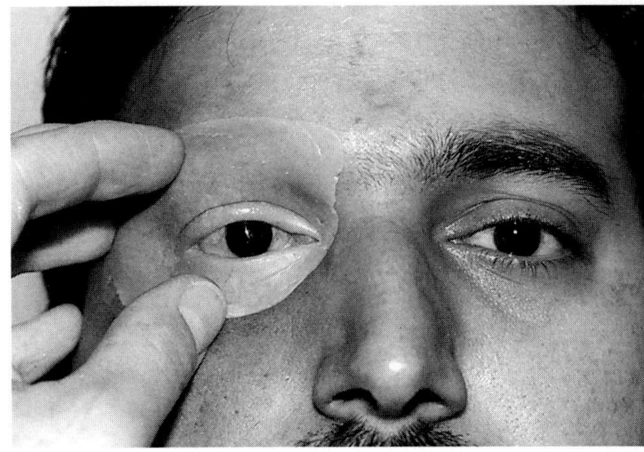

Figure 108–8. Wax model is repeatedly positioned on the patient during the sculpting session to adjust the ocular position and sculpt the eyelid anatomy.

the impression may be checked and to model for the facial prosthetist as he or she sculpts the anatomic detail in the wax model to achieve bilateral symmetry with the remaining open eye (Fig. 108–8). A second or even third sculpting or design session may be scheduled to avoid an unusually lengthy and possibly hurried single session.

A discussion should also take place during the final sculpting session concerning the use of eyeglasses. Any monocular person should always wear eyeglasses, prescription or not, to protect the vision of the remaining eye. In addition, carefully selected frames and lenses can do much to enhance the overall aesthetics of the restoration. In general, frames should be chosen that cover the margins of the prosthesis when viewed from the front. This helps to obscure any margins that are difficult to blend or camouflage. New lenses should be of the same prescription, both left and right. This ensures that the sighted eye and prosthetic eye will appear the same regardless of the magnification or other optical effect caused by the prescription. The patient may also be encouraged to experiment with lightly tinted lenses to suit his or her complexion. Attractive frames and graded tint lenses can effectively detract from the lack of animation in the prosthetic eye. This discussion as the sculpting is finalized allows the patient to anticipate the size of the eventual prosthesis and the type of eyeglasses he or she will want to consider.

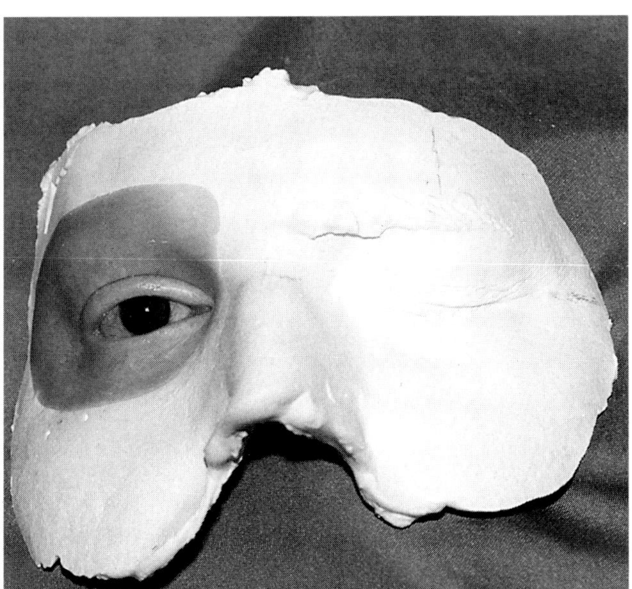

Figure 108–7. Flesh-toned wax mixture is sculpted on the plaster cast in preparation for the patient-sculpting session.

When the patient returns, the prosthesis, having been fabricated in the interim, is positioned in the exenteration cavity. The fit is checked, and the final external coloration is completed (Fig. 108–9).

Once the external coloration is cured sufficiently for purpose of handling, human hair fashion eyelashes are anchored into the prosthesis, matching the color and thickness of the patient's lashes as closely as possible (Fig. 108–10*A*). Eyebrows can also be incorporated into the prosthesis by embedding some of the patient's own hair into a thin layer of clear silicone (see Fig. 108–10*B*). This makes for a more durable eyebrow since the hair is protected from the frictional effort of adhesive removal.

The finished orbital prosthesis (Figs. 108–11 through 108–13) is delivered to the patient along with thorough instructions for its proper management and care. The patient is encouraged to practice positioning the prosthesis without adhesive at first. This allows multiple attempts at proper positioning and increases the patient's skill and confidence before the adhesive is used.

The patient is also assured that although deterioration of the prosthesis is inevitable, repairs and retinting of the prosthesis are possible. In the event of loss or irreparable damage of the prosthesis or if the prosthesis is simply worn out, a fresh replacement can be fabricated from the existing mold, usually at a significantly lower cost.

At the outset of the treatment plan it should be re-

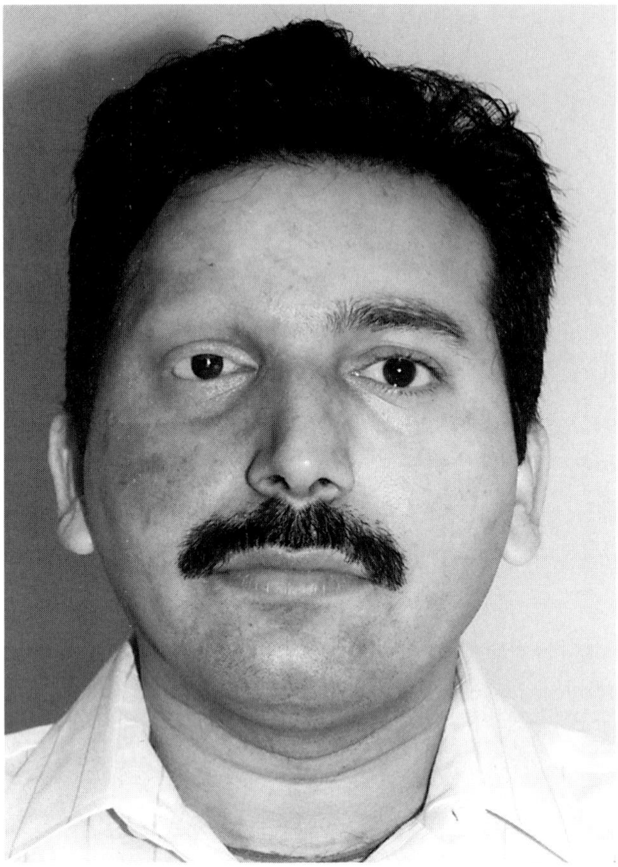

Figure 108–9. Extrinsic coloration complete except for the entire inferior margin. The dark-red irradiated tissue of the patient's right cheek does not allow aesthetic margin color blending at this time.

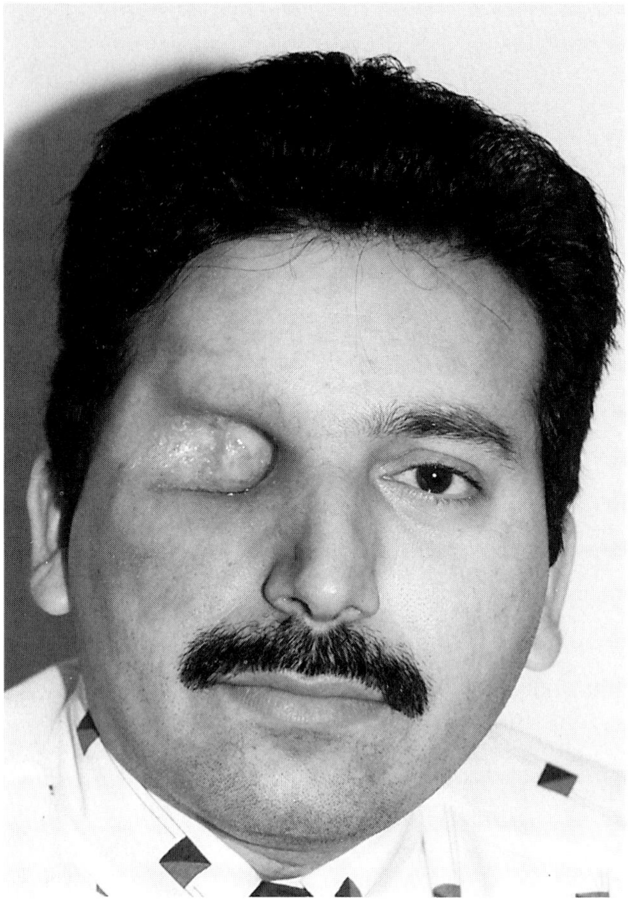

Figure 108–11. Patient without orbital prosthesis.

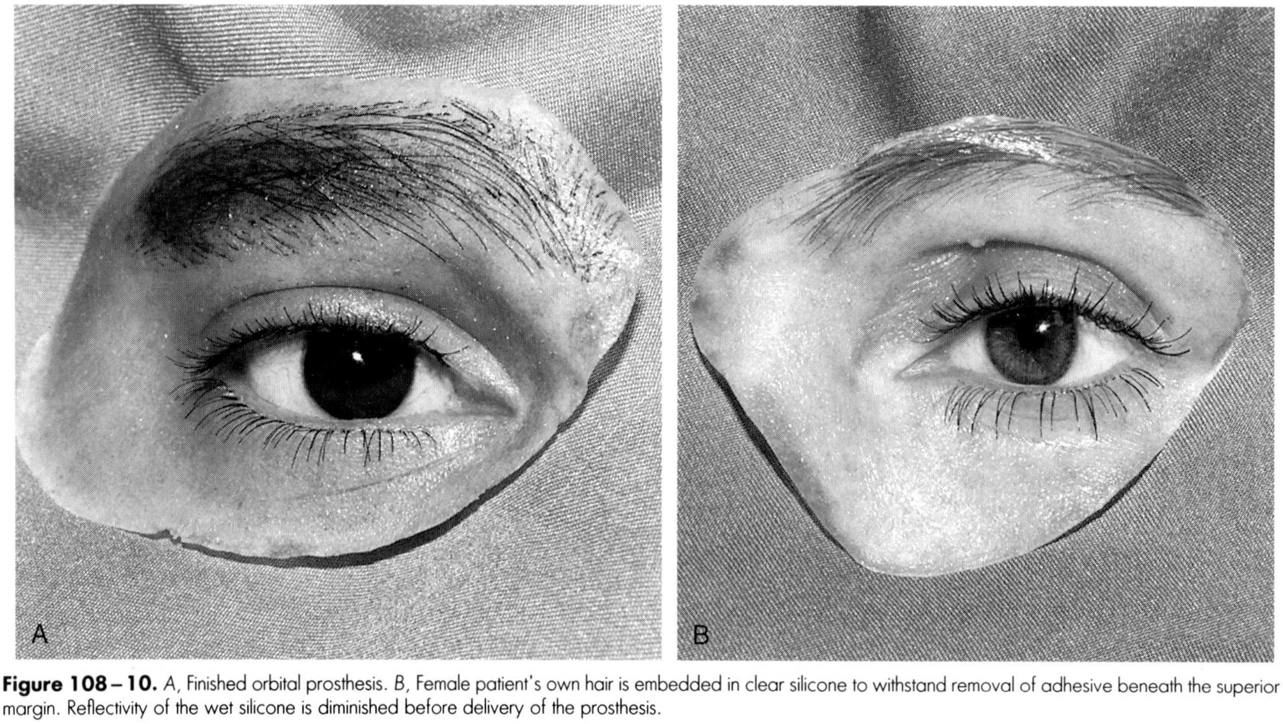

Figure 108–10. *A*, Finished orbital prosthesis. *B*, Female patient's own hair is embedded in clear silicone to withstand removal of adhesive beneath the superior margin. Reflectivity of the wet silicone is diminished before delivery of the prosthesis.

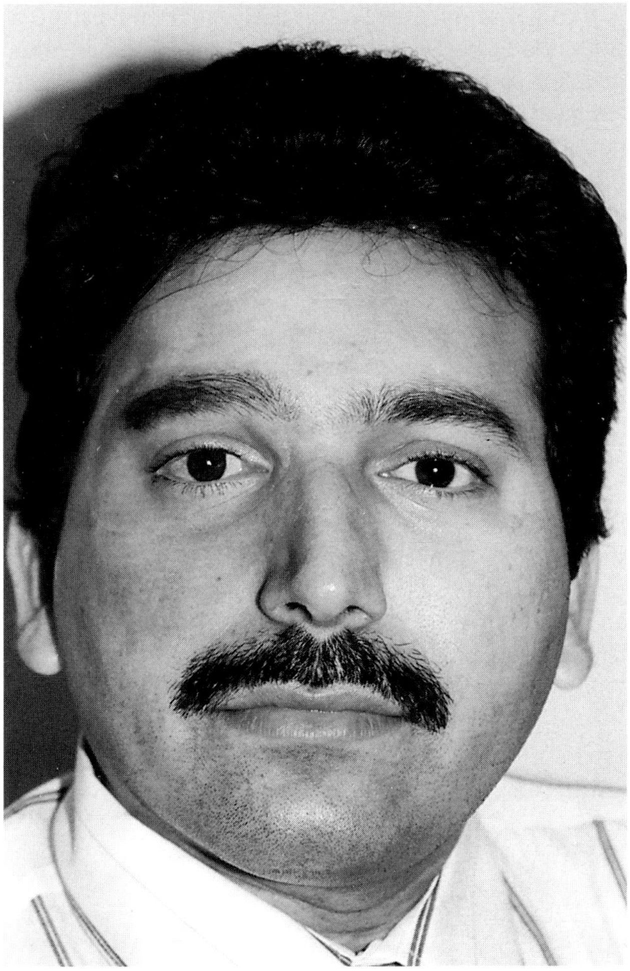

Figure 108 – 12. Same patient as in Figure 108 – 11 with orbital prosthesis in position. Note untinted prosthesis margins due to color-compromised irradiated tissue.

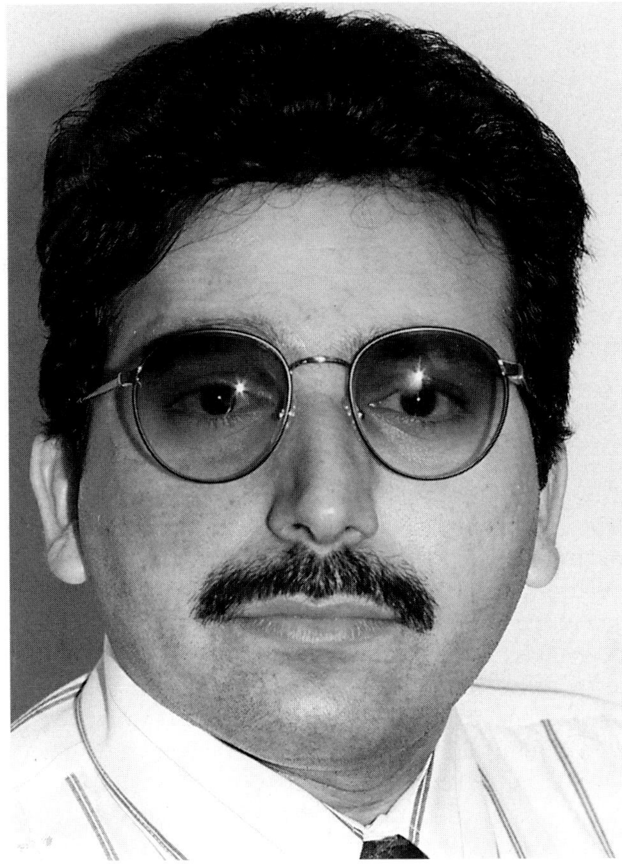

Figure 108 – 13. Same patient as in Figures 108 – 11 and 108 – 12. Use of graded tint lenses and personally selected frames of eyeglasses helps enhance the overall aesthetic result of the restoration.

membered that the primary purpose of making an orbital prosthesis is to camouflage the patient's exenteration by restoring normal external anatomy. Only with painstaking attention to detail will a very life-like and convincing prosthesis result. This should be remembered because any prosthesis that does not achieve accurate coloration, bilateral symmetry, and close margin adaptation will fail to fulfill its purpose. A conspicuous prosthesis may actually become a greater burden than the eye patch.

SURGICAL NUANCES FOR OPTIMUM RESULTS

If the patient has had a complete exenteration, the surgeon can do a great service to the patient by creating a defect cavity that allows for the design of an anatomically retained prosthesis. The advantage to such a prosthesis system is that no adhesive is necessary to retain the prosthesis. As a result, the patient is spared the difficulties that are common in managing medical adhesives. These include messiness of applying adhesive, the deterioration of the prosthesis from adhesive removal, the difficulty of positioning the sticky prosthesis, and the time and energy spent working with the prosthesis and adhesive. Also, the adhesive retained prosthesis must be designed to cover greater surface area beyond the defect for adhesive contact. This, and the need for thicker margins to prevent tearing, compromise the aesthetics of the prosthetic result. Conversely, the anatomically retained prosthesis may be designed to cover only the cavity and deficient contour while featuring feather-edged margins for nearly imperceptible transitions from prosthesis to skin. Beyond the practical and aesthetic advantages, the anatomic retention instills greater confidence in the patient who does not have to be worried about adhesive failure and the embarrassment of untimely loosening or loss of the prosthesis.

The ideal exenteration cavity features a continuous split-thickness skin graft lining the entire cavity (Fig. 108 – 14). The skin graft maintains cavity depth and recessed areas or undercuts. These undercut areas behind the bony rim of the orbit should be of such a depth that seating the prosthesis is easy for the patient yet a positive engagement takes place superiorly, laterally, and inferi-

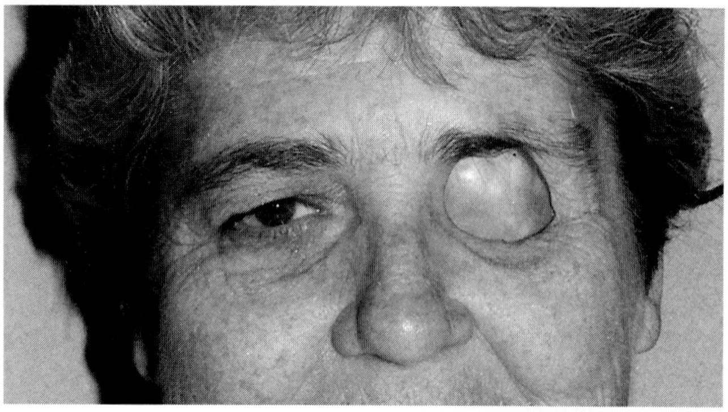

Figure 108–14. Orbital exenteration cavity well-prepared to support an anatomically retained orbital prosthesis.

orly (Fig. 108–15). In my experience the superior and lateral undercuts are often more than adequate for good retention while the infraorbital rim is sometimes inadequate and allows the prosthesis to slip outward, causing a gap at the inferior prosthesis margin. This situation can be avoided by surgical augmentation of the inadequate infraorbital rim area. By using fascia lata, muscle slings, or other means, an infraorbital rim or lip should be created behind which the prosthesis can be designed to engage for secure retention. The presence of an undercut inferiorly is particularly important since facial muscle movement caused by smiling could, along with gravity, help to dislodge the prosthesis.

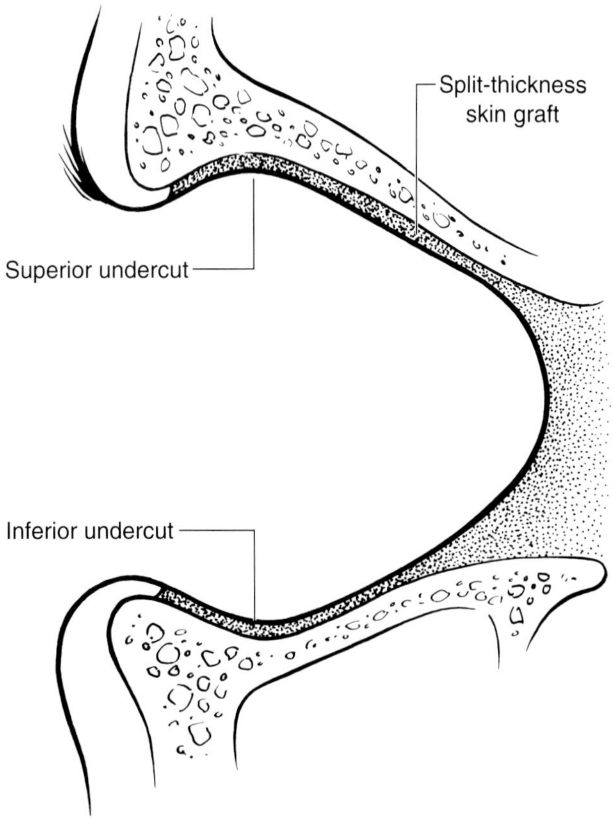

Figure 108–15. Sagittal section through the orbit demonstrating superior and inferior undercuts.

Another problematic area relative to orbital exenterations is the preservation of a normal eyebrow. Care must be taken to prevent the eyebrow from being pulled into the defect during healing and scar contracture. The presence of eyebrow hair beneath the superior margin of the prosthesis can interfere with the use of skin adhesives and will tend to lift the prosthesis away from the skin. Consequently, the patient's eyebrow must be kept shaven and an artificial eyebrow incorporated into the orbital prosthesis. Although acceptable results are possible under these circumstances, the presence of a normal eyebrow is a great aid in achieving an aesthetic-appearing orbital prosthesis. In this case, the superior margin of the prosthesis is neatly hidden beneath the inferior margin of the eyebrow (Figs. 108–16 and 108–17).

In summary, the surgeon can greatly enhance the patient's success in managing the orbital prosthesis by considering the eventual morphology of the exenteration cavity. Lining the cavity with split-thickness skin graft and preserving or creating cavity undercuts superiorly, laterally, and inferiorly will allow for the design of an anatomically retained prosthesis. Preserving a normal eye-

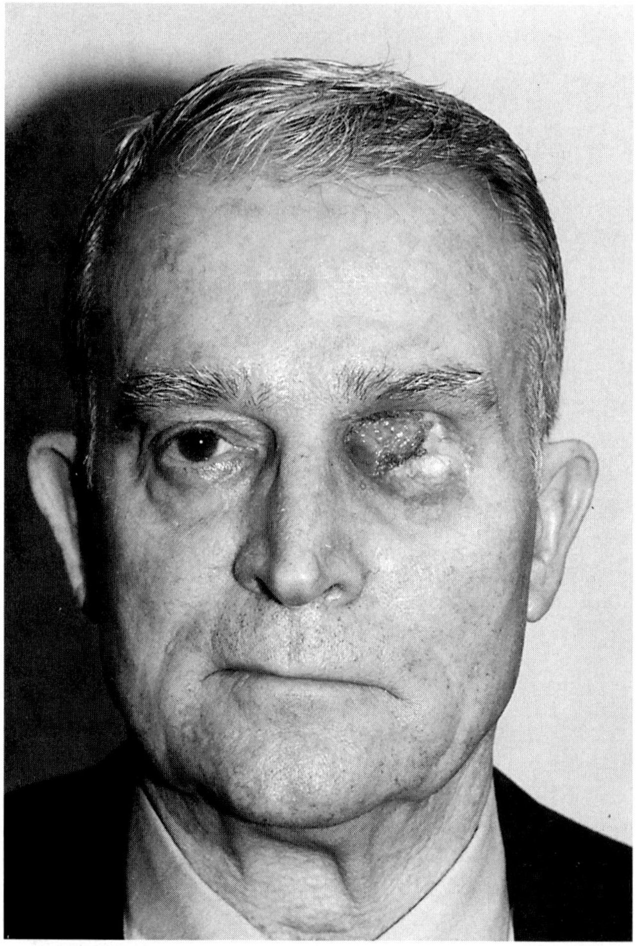

Figure 108–16. Preservation of normal eyebrow position after exenteration of left orbit.

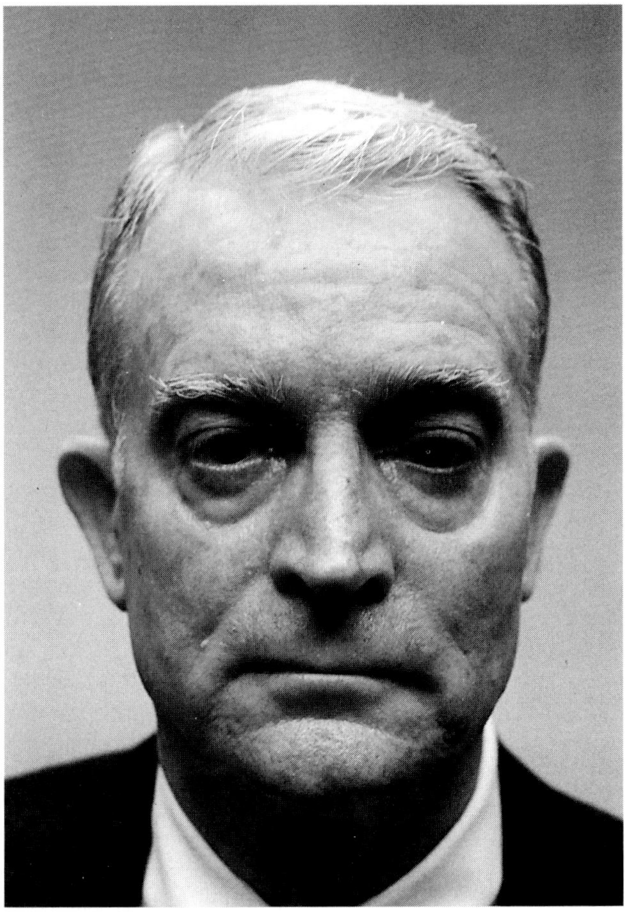

Figure 108–17. Same patient as in Figure 108–16. Prominence of supraorbital rim and eyebrow help to camouflage the superior margin of the prosthesis.

brow will keep to a minimum the overall dimension of the orbital prosthesis and further enhance the aesthetics of the restoration.

DESIGN OF THE ANATOMICALLY RETAINED PROSTHESIS

For the exenteration cavity featuring adequate undercuts, a bulb-style orbital prosthesis may be created. Although it is also possible to design the back of the prosthesis to extend only deep enough into the cavity to engage the undercuts behind the orbit rim, this approach puts a greater force over a relatively small area. As a result, pressure points can occur, causing the patient discomfort. This approach also requires significantly more time to design the mold.

The bulb-style prosthesis (Fig. 108–18) on the other hand covers nearly all of the surface area within the exenteration cavity. The greater area of surface contact creates an additional measure of retention through surface tension between the silicone and tissue in addition to creating a more intimate and stable fit. The greater area of contact also allows the walls of the bulb portion of the prosthesis to be thin (1–2 mm) so that trauma to the delicate tissues is avoided while secure retention is achieved. This is particularly important in areas of the cavity where a thin graft overlies prominent bone such as the infraorbital rim. Here, the prosthesis should be very thin (≤ 1 mm) so it will not exert too much pressure that could cause pressure breakdown of the tissue.

The bulb-style prosthesis may be created by several methods. The bulb may contain a center portion of low-density silicone foam or even one of a variety of low-durometer silicone gels. Of course, either the foam or gel should be contained and sealed with an envelope of silicone elastomer, silicone dispersion, or other compatible material. This is because the foam acts like a sponge to retain water, dirt, body fluids, and so on and also has poor durability. The gels typically possess poor tensile strength and, therefore, also lack durability. The bulb portion of the prosthesis is often made hollow to greatly reduce weight, provide suppleness, promote hygiene, and produce good retention. One way to achieve the hollow bulb is by casting. In this approach, an internal mold piece is created within the mold cavity to displace the silicone and produce the void or hollow space. However, this internal mold piece that creates the void must be pulled through an opening of sufficient diameter in the posterior of the prosthesis (Fig. 108–19). This opening unfortunately reduces the integrity and thus retentiveness of the bulb.

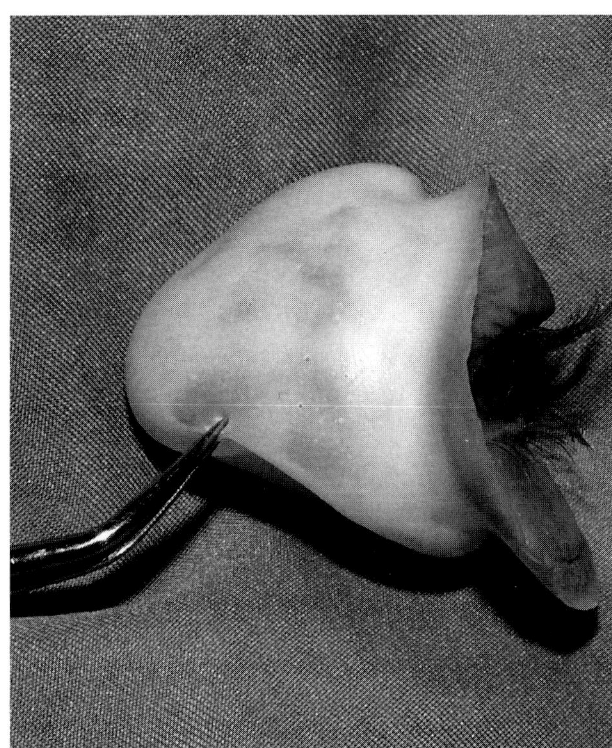

Figure 108–18. Thin-walled hollow-bulb orbital prosthesis, medial view.

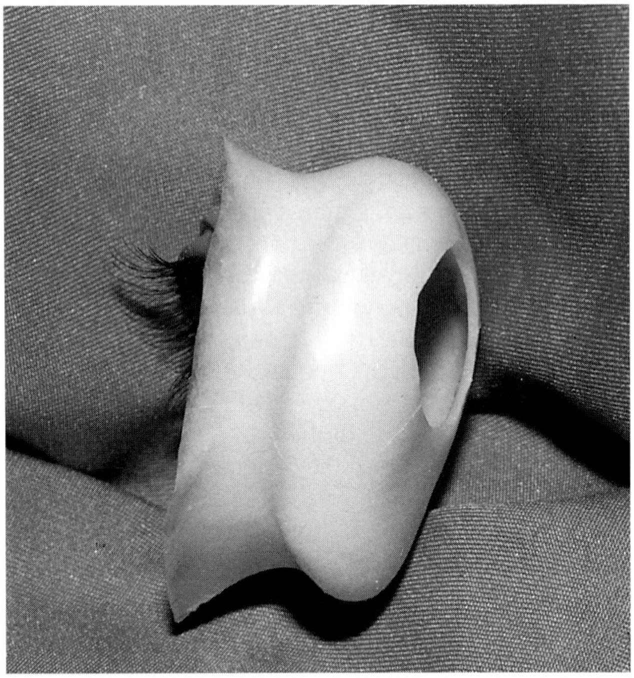

Figure 108–19. Hollow-bulb prosthesis with a hole for evacuation of the internal mold piece, postero-medial view.

The bulb prosthesis may also be made hollow by slush molding, dipping, or simply brush coating the mold pieces with a thin layer of silicone. In the last case, a fast-setting silicone elastomer is ideal because the thickness of the different areas of the prosthesis may be controlled by the application of the silicone. The silicone is brushed very thin into areas of the mold that correspond to the patient's sensitive areas, such as the infraorbital rim. The recesses behind the orbital rim may be given slightly more thickness, perhaps 1 to 2 mm, for slightly more retention, while the mold piece that creates the anterior or cosmetic surface of the prosthesis is heavily coated to perhaps 3 to 4 mm so that the necessary opacity is achieved.

The air-filled hollow bulb prosthesis should be vented in some fashion to allow air pressure within the bulb and the environment to remain equal. A 5-mm diameter hole cut through the silicone behind the ocular component allows restricted venting to that the bulb maintains a cushioned fullness while pressure will not be allowed to build. The hidden location of this vent also prevents excessive amounts of water from collecting in the bulb from regular washing of the prosthesis. However, the patient is still able to remove the ocular component and flush the bulb as needed to maintain hygiene (Fig. 108–20).

In summary, the anatomically retained hollow bulb prosthesis offers many advantages to the patient. This type of prosthesis is designed with feather-thin margins that cover only deficiencies in contour and blend inconspicuously with the patient's skin. Its lightweight construction and inherent suppleness allow for comfort. The elimination of adhesive for retention increases durability and enhances the patient's attitude toward the prosthesis and its care (Figs. 108–21 through 108–23).

CHALLENGES TO THE PROSTHETIST

To some extent there is an inverse relationship between the size of the defect and the success of the orbital restoration. In many cases, the smaller the defect is, the greater the difficulty the prosthetist encounters in offering a successful and manageable prosthesis. This is primarily due to the lack of space available for ocular placement and the delicateness of the small wafer-like prosthesis. This prosthesis may consist only of the ocular component and upper and lower eyelids and eyelashes. The difficulty arises as the patient applies the liquid medical adhesive to the back of the prosthesis and attempts to position the prosthesis without disturbing the adhesive layer or crushing the delicate artificial eyelashes. However, it is sometimes surprising to see how well many of these patients surmount the awkwardness of this task and manage the prosthesis successfully. This type of prosthesis is typically hidden very effectively behind the frames of the patient's eyeglasses.

Smaller and more challenging to the prosthetist and patient is the case of the enucleated patient with eyelids, but without a viable socket. In this case, the ocular com-

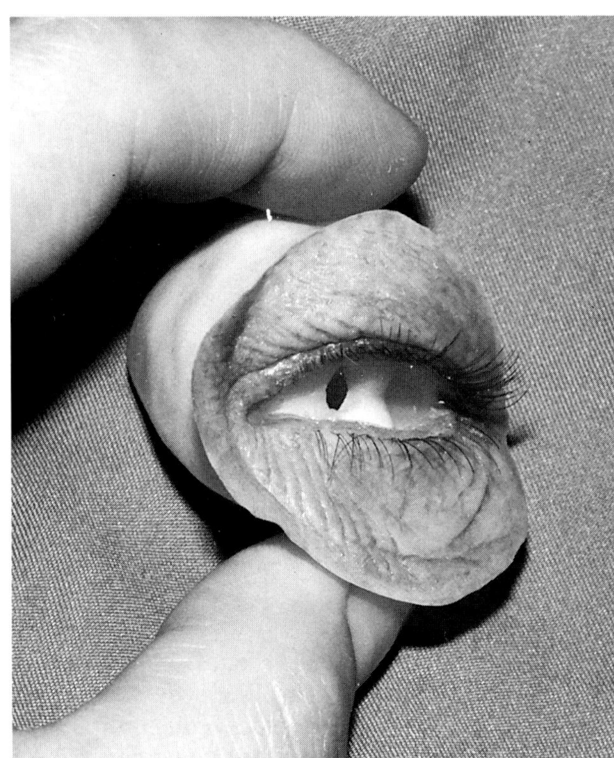

Figure 108–20. Hollow-bulb prosthesis with ocular component removed to show vent/valve hole also used for flushing.

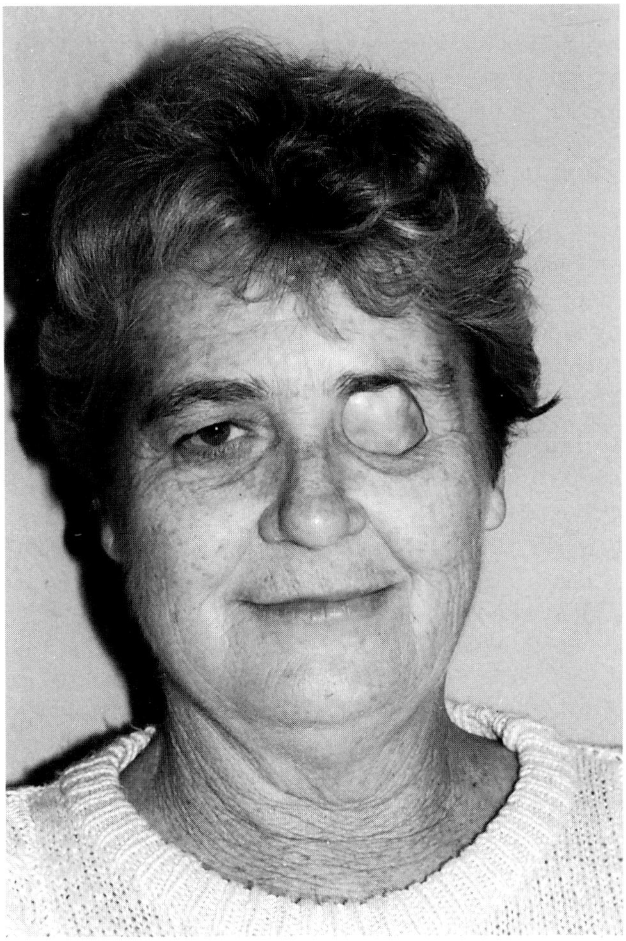

Figure 108–21. Patient without orbital prosthesis.

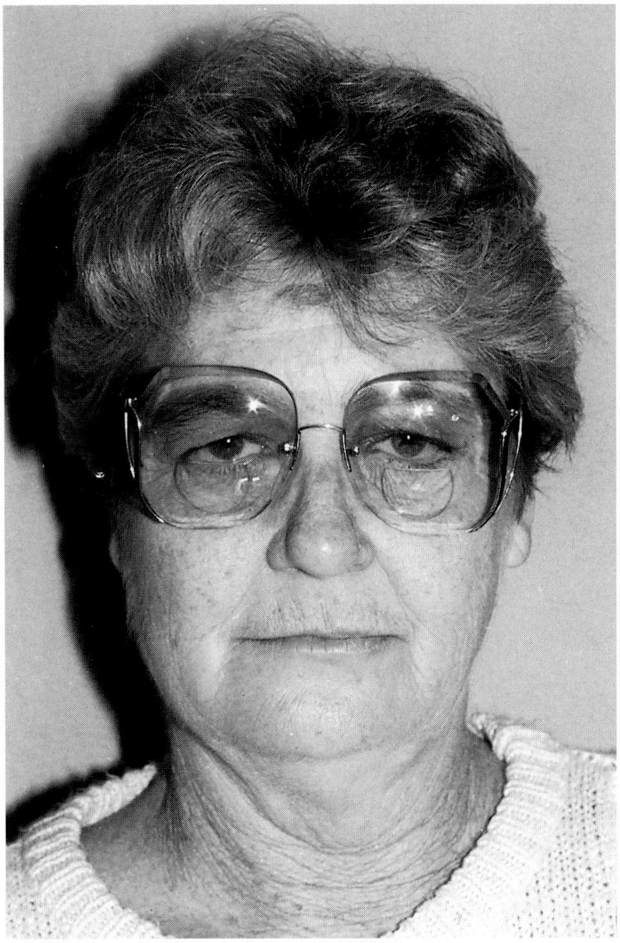

Figure 108–22. Same patient as in Figure 108–21 with orbital prosthesis in position. Eyeglasses with lightly graded tint lenses and attractive frames complete the cosmetic result. No adhesive is used.

ponent is shaved to sliver-like thinness and positioned on the eyelids to achieve the necessary depth, if possible. More than likely, the eyelids will not allow the ocular component to be positioned deep enough to be symmetric with the companion eye. Therefore, the aesthetic result is compromised by the remaining eyelid tissue. In addition to this, the socket may produce discharge that would accelerate the failure of the adhesive bond and lead to retention problems. To compound the situation, movement of the eyelids during blinking further contributes to the loosening of the prosthesis. Therefore, if the surgeon is definitely not going to attempt to reconstruct the socket to accept an ocular prosthesis, then he or she should consider the removal of the eyelid tissue in the interest of ensuring success with the orbital prosthesis.

At the other end of the spectrum in terms of prosthesis size is that which results from orbital exenteration with hemimaxillectomy. While the large cavity requires significantly more time to restore, the resulting large prosthesis is often more easily handled by the patient because there is more room to grasp the prosthesis without touching the adhesive-coated surfaces. In fact, this type of prosthesis often requires only small amounts of adhesive, if any at all, because secure retention can be achieved anatomically by engagement of cavity undercuts (Fig. 108–

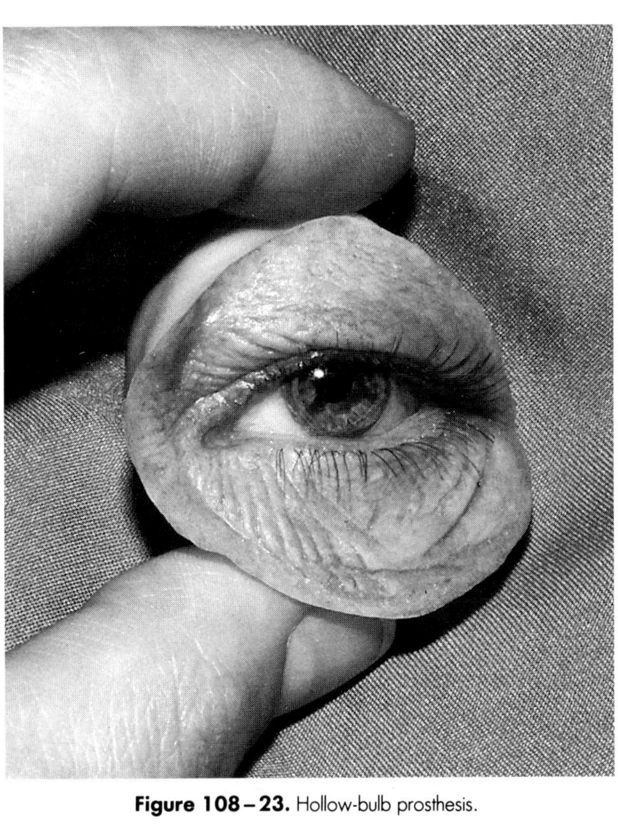

Figure 108–23. Hollow-bulb prosthesis.

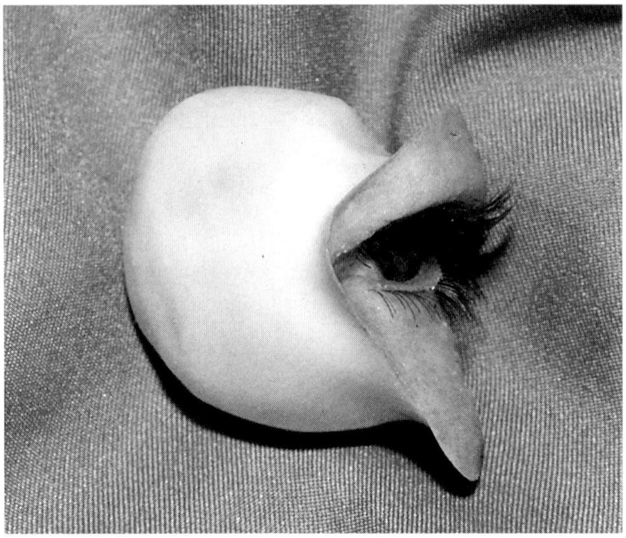

Figure 108–24. Medial view of an orbital prosthesis formed to fit into and engage exenteration cavity undercuts.

24), magnetically by the use of acrylic extensions that attach to the superior surface of the intraoral obturator prosthesis (Fig. 108–25), or by a combination of the two systems (Figs. 108–26 and 108–27).

The greatest detractor from the success of this large prosthesis is the inferior margin of the prosthesis, which typically falls inferior to the frames of the eyeglasses. This margin is somewhat more conspicuous because it is not hidden by the eyeglasses and lies on the flat, mobile, soft tissue of the midface. The prosthetist may decide to end this margin more superior so that it lies behind the frames of the eyeglasses. However, this strategy is often a compromise, leaving the midfacial defect unrestored. The prosthodontist may attempt to restore the midfacial deficiency with the anterior buildup of the obturator prosthesis. However, there are limits to the size and shape of the appliance that the patient can insert into the mouth and tolerate.

SUMMARY

The orbital prosthesis can be a valuable option for the patient who has undergone orbital exenteration. The orbital prosthesis is primarily an aesthetic device to restore the patient's normal appearance. Secondary to this, the prosthesis serves a rehabilitative purpose in restoring or upholding the patient's self-image during the period of physical and psychological adjustment after exenteration. The orbital prosthesis in many cases also encloses

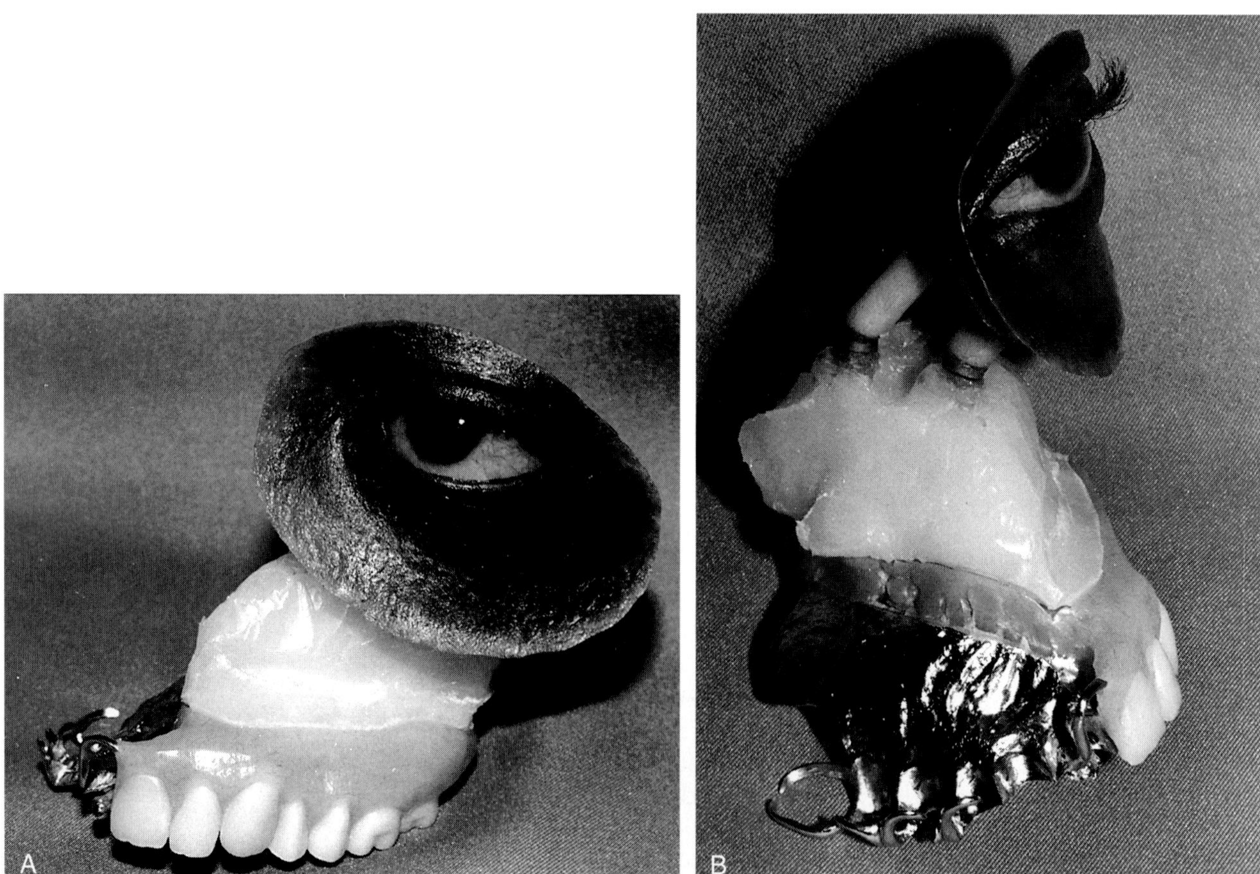

Figure 108–25. *A*, Anterior view of orbital prosthesis attached magnetically to an obturator (hemimaxillectomy) prosthesis. *B*, Medial view. Acrylic extensions with magnets (three) attach to mating magnets embedded in obturator.

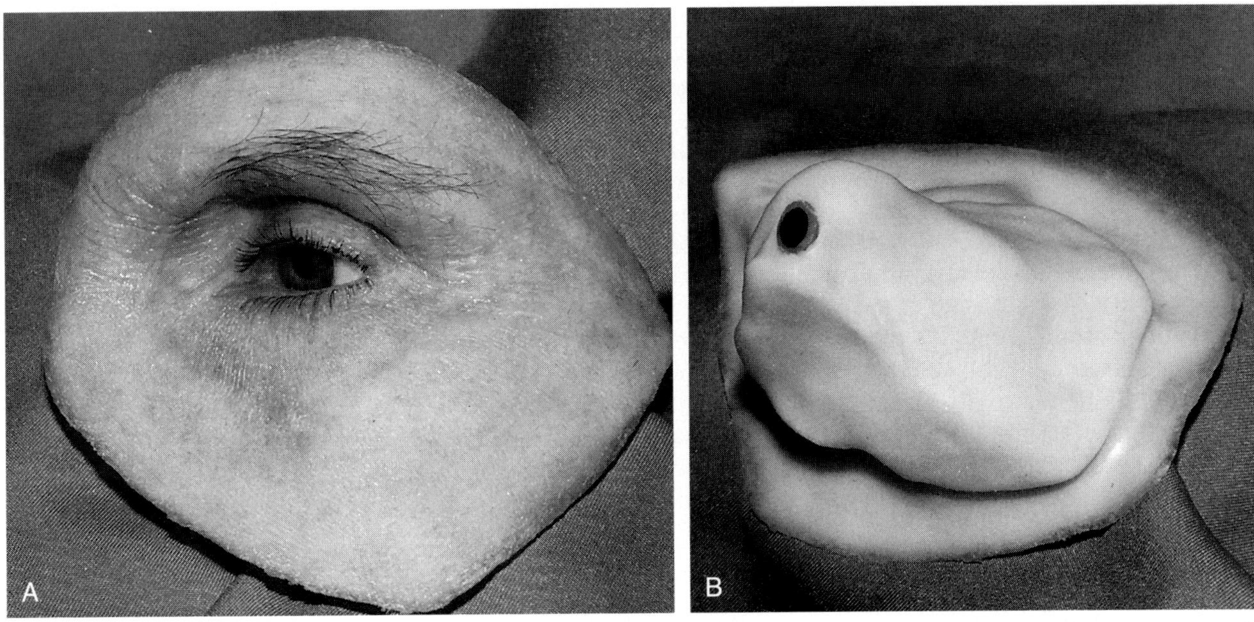

Figure 108–26. *A*, Large orbital prosthesis. *B*, Large orbital prosthesis with hollow bulb to engage cavity undercuts and one strong neodymium magnet to attach to the dental obturator prosthesis, posterior view.

and protects delicate tissues that have been left exposed by the ablative surgery.

To improve the art and science of facial prosthetics, many attempts have been made to develop the optimum combination of prosthetic materials and methods to retain the prosthesis. While prosthetists routinely choose among the medical-grade silicone elastomers, many other materials have been developed or borrowed from other biomedical applications to accommodate the particular dynamics of varying postoperative defect cavities. In terms of methods used to retain the orbital prosthesis, those that reduce the dependence on medical adhesive have gained almost universal support. Although adhesive is effective in holding the prosthesis margins close to the skin for excellent cosmetic results, its extended use is often detrimental to the prosthesis. Regular removal of the adhesive from the margins can contribute to the deterioration of the prosthesis if considerable care is not exercised by the patient. The unpredictability of patient compliance with adhesive management along with the

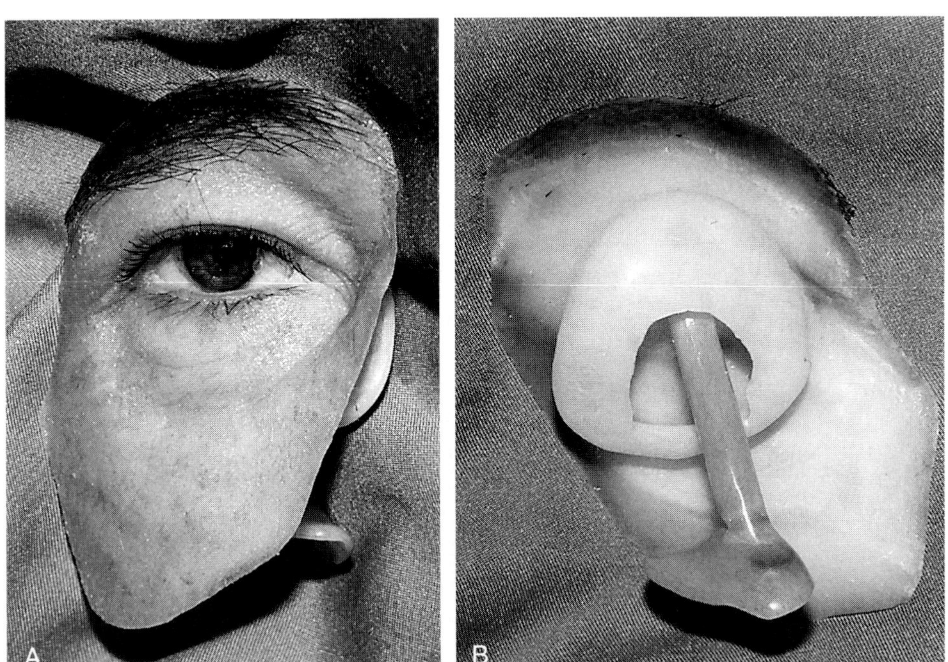

Figure 108–27. *A*, Large orbital prosthesis. *B*, Large orbital prosthesis with hollow bulb and acrylic extension for dual (anatomic and magnetic) retention, posterior view.

susceptibility of adhesive failure due to perspiration, facial movement, and so on are reasons the facial prosthetist utilizes anatomic or mechanical retention whenever possible.

The surgeon should be aware of nuances that he or she can create within the exenteration cavity that in turn create the possibility for the prosthetist to design an aesthetically successful anatomically retained orbital prosthesis. The preservation of the position of the eyebrow is very important to the aesthetics of the restoration. Augmenting the infraorbital rim, if necessary to ensure the presence of superior, lateral, and inferior anatomic undercuts, and lining the cavity with split-thickness skin graft create the ideal exenteration cavity to accept an anatomically retained orbital prosthesis. The orbital prosthesis that attaches by magnets or other devices to the dental obturator of the hemimaxillectomy patient is an example of the mechanically retained prosthesis.

The value placed on prosthetic restoration of the orbit is apparent in view of recent contributions from the field of implantology. The Brånemark implant system[21-24] and the Bud implant system [25, 26] both feature titanium oxide endosseous implants installed in the lateral and superior orbital rim. The transcutaneous components called abutments penetrate the skin, forming a biologic seal, and support small magnets or a bar splint to which the orbital prosthesis is finally designed to attach (Fig. 108–28). These implant systems almost completely remove the parameters of durability and manageability that compromise aesthetics in the design of the adhesive-retained orbital prosthesis.

Despite the method of retention used, the orbital pros-

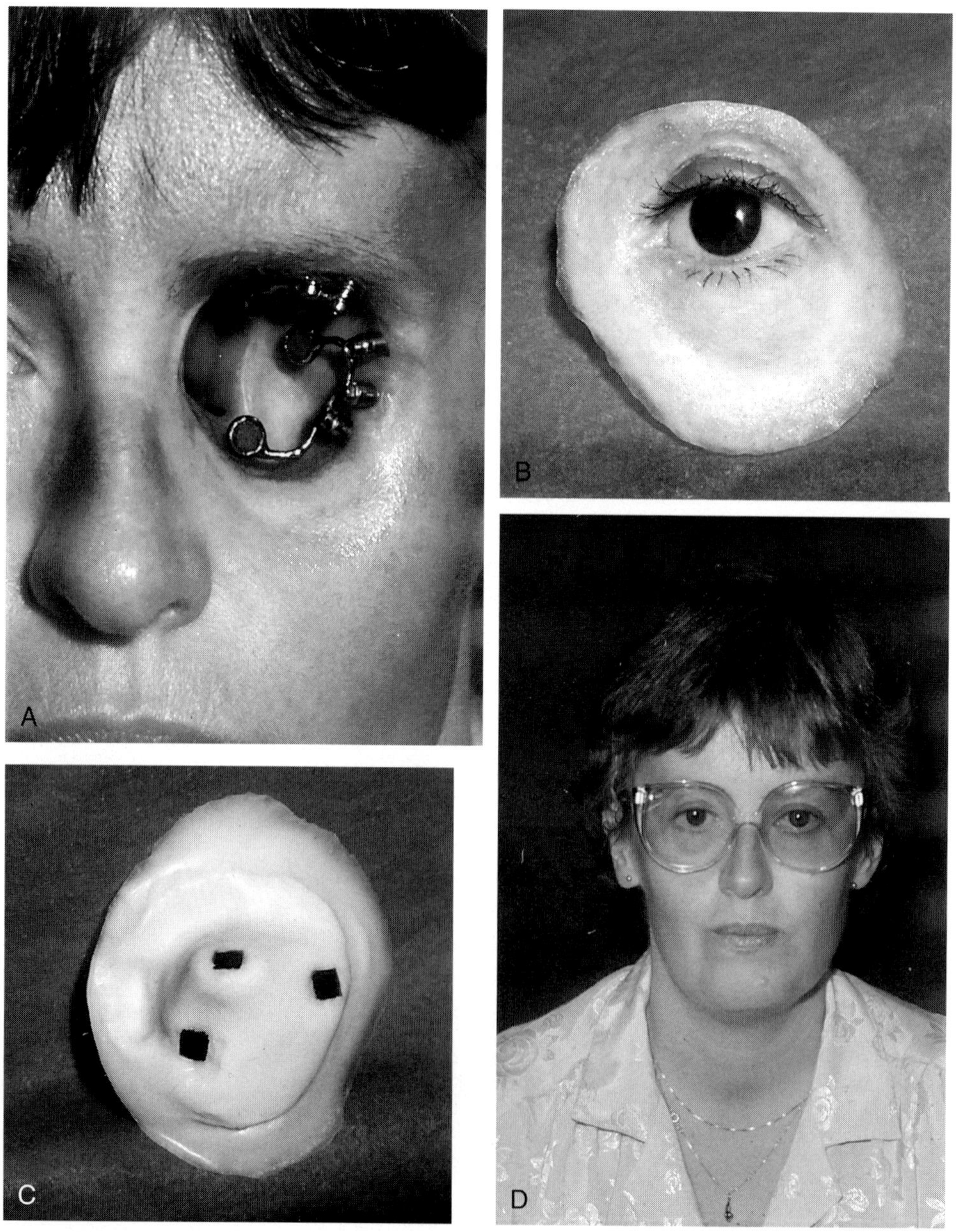

Figure 108–28. *A,* Osseointegrated implants anchor transcutaneous abutments and a magnet-loaded bar splint for adhesive-free retention of the orbital prosthesis. *B,* Implant-retained orbital prosthesis. Note the thin translucent margins. *C,* Same implant-retained orbital prosthesis as in *B*, posterior view. Magnets embedded in the silicone mate with those embedded in the acrylic of the bar splint. *D,* Brånemark implant-retained prosthesis in place.

thesis remains as a valuable alternative for the patient who has undergone orbital exenteration. Ideally, communication will take place before the exenteration between the surgeon and the individual responsible for creating the orbital prosthesis. This individual, whether titled facial prosthetist, medical artist, prosthodontist, medical sculptor, head and neck prosthetist, or anaplastologist, should be trained and devoted to the art and science of providing quality prostheses. Through this collaborative effort an optimal exenteration cavity and orbital prosthesis will result, enhancing the patient's rehabilitation both in body and spirit.

REFERENCES

1. Parr G, Goldman BM, Rahn AO: Surgical considerations in the prosthetic treatment of ocular and orbital defects. J Prosthet Dent 49:379–385, 1983.
2. Brown KE: Fabrication of orbital prostheses. J Prosthet Dent 22:592–607, 1969.
3. Rahn AO, Boucher LJ: Maxillofacial Prosthetics. Philadelphia, WB Saunders, 1970.
4. Chalian VA, Drane JB, Standish SM: Maxillofacial Prosthetics. Baltimore, Williams & Wilkins, 1971.
5. Joneja OP, Madan SK, Mehra MD, Dogra RN: Orbital prostheses. J Prosthet Dent 36:306–311, 1976
6. Oral K, Zini I, Aramany MA: Construction of orbital prostheses using the silicone pattern technique. J Prosthet Dent 40:430–433, 1978.
7. Beumer J, Curtis TA, Firtell DN: Maxillofacial Rehabilitation: Prosthodontic and Surgical Considerations. St Louis, CV Mosby, 1979.
8. Levy M, Shortz RH, Blumenfeld I, Lepley JB: A flexible moulage for the fabrication of an orbital prosthesis. J Prosthet Dent 43:436–438, 1980.
9. Parr G, Goldman BM, Rahn AO: Maxillofacial prosthetic principles in the surgical planning for facial defects. J Prosthet Dent 46:323–329, 1981.
10. Kent K, Schaaf NG: Use of a previously completed prosthesis in the construction of a new orbital prosthesis. J Prosthet Dent 48:313–318, 1982.
11. Taicher S, Bergen SF, Rosen A, Levy M, Lepley JB: Hollow polydimethylsiloxane prostheses using anatomic undercuts. J Prosthet Dent 48:444–447, 1982.
12. Barron JB, Rubenstein JE, Archibald D, Manor RE: Two-piece orbital prosthesis. J Prosthet Dent 49:386–388, 1983.
13. Wolfaardt JF, Hacqueboard A, Els JM: A mold technique for construction of orbital prostheses. J Prosthet Dent 50:224–226, 1983.
14. Eaton LD, Dryden RM, Popp JC, Harner D: Functional anatomical reconstruction in an oculofacial prosthesis. Ophthalmology 91:984–986, 1984.
15. Stanley RB, Beumer J: Orbital rehabilitation: Surgical and prosthetic. Otolaryngol Clin North Am 21: 189–198, 1988.
16. Couillard P, Schaaf NG: Fabrication of the ocular portion of an orbital prosthesis. J Prosthet Dent 35:478–481, 1976.
17. McArthur DR: Aids for positioning prosthetic eyes in orbital prostheses. J Prosthet Dent 37:320–326, 1977.
18. Jooste CH: A method for orienting the ocular portion of an orbital prosthesis. J Prosthet Dent 51:381–382, 1984.
19. Nusinov NS, McCartney JW, Mitchel DL: The orbital shell: An aid in positioning the ocular component and verifying margin contours for oculofacial prostheses. J Prosthet Dent 61:337–339, 1989.
20. McKinstry RE: Fundamentals of Facial Prosthetics. Arlington, VA, ABI Professional Publications, 1994.
21. Parel SM, Brånemark PI, Tjellstrom A, Gion GG: Osseointegration in maxillofacial prosthetics: II. Extraoral applications. J Prosthet Dent 55:600–606, 1986.
22. Parel SM, Holt RG, Brånemark PI, Tjellstrom A: Osseointegration and facial prosthetics. Int J Oral Maxillofac Implants 1:27–29, 1986.
23. Parel SM, Tjellstrom A: The United States and Swedish experience with osseointegration and facial prostheses. Int J Oral Maxillofac Implants 6:75–79, 1991.
24. Holt RG, Parel SM, Brånemark PI: Osseointegrated titanium implants. Facial Plast Surg 3(2):113–124, 1986.
25. Schaaf NG, Meenagham MA, Duthie RE: Advantages of endosseous implants for retaining facial prostheses. Transactions of the Academy of Dental Materials, vol 5. University of Louisville, 1992, pp 65–76.
26. Bielat KL, Meenaghan MA, Worth JE, Schaaf NG: SEM of extraoral osseointegrated implants. J Dent Res 69:290, 1990.

CHAPTER 109

Osseointegration for the Exenterated Orbit

Jeffrey A. Nerad

After orbital exenteration the patient is left with a severe facial defect. Reconstruction using standard plastic surgical procedures cannot provide a satisfactory result. Facial rehabilitation may be undertaken with a silicone prosthesis, but problems exist with retention and alignment of these prosthetic devices. The prosthesis may be attached to spectacle frames, but then the eyeglasses may not be removed in public. Adhesives or double-sided tape may be used to secure the prosthesis in place, but this may cause skin reaction, prosthetic discoloration, poor edge adhesion, and loss of retention. Because many of the patients undergoing exenteration are older, problems with inaccurate alignment occur. Fear of misalignment or of losing the prosthesis in public often causes these patients to lose confidence in their appearance. Many patients stop wearing the prosthesis. Bone-anchored orbital implants, placed by means of the osseointegration procedure, provide patients who have undergone exenteration with an excellent means of retention and accurate alignment of their orbital prostheses.[1] The technique of osseointegration is also being applied in the rehabilitation of maxillofacial defects resulting from trauma or tumor.[2-4]

THE OSSEOINTEGRATION TECHNIQUE

The osseointegration procedure[4-6] is performed in two stages. The stage I procedure consists of implanting three or four titanium fixtures into the bony orbital rim. The fixtures are covered with skin and subcutaneous tissues while osseointegration occurs. Stage II is undertaken 4 months later. The skin over the fixtures is opened, and an abutment is screwed into the fixture. The abutment protrudes from the skin. After healing takes place a prosthesis is made that attaches directly to the abutments or to a framework connected to the abutments (Fig. 109-1).

Stage I: Implant Installation

Stage I (Fig. 109-2) is performed with the use of local anesthesia in most cases.[1] A skin incision is marked along the superior and lateral orbital rim. Local anesthesia consisting of 2% lidocaine and 0.75% bupivacaine is injected subcutaneously in the area of the proposed incision (Fig. 109-3). The surgical field is prepped and draped in the usual manner. A skin incision is made, and a periosteal flap is formed (Fig. 109-4). Three or four implant sites are chosen, with two or three sites above and one or two sites below the frontozygomatic suture.

Drilling is accomplished with a sharp, disposable cutting drill. A slow drilling speed (1200 to 1500 rpm) and abundant irrigation are mandatory to prevent thermal injury to the bone since viable bone is required to accomplish osseointegration. The first drilling is performed with a cutting bur (Fig. 109-5). A small drill hole is made to assess the quality and depth of the bone. If the bone appears strong and thick enough to permit a larger hole, a 3- or 4-mm sleeve is fitted over the bur and the hole is completed. If the bone is too thin, the site is abandoned and a new site is chosen. After this preliminary drilling a spiral drill with a countersink is used to make a hole of the final width and direction. The spiral drill (Fig. 109-6*A*) is used at the same slow speed with similar precautions with regard to irrigation. As the drill reaches the final depth, the countersink on the drill engages the rim and a flat area is cut that will seat the flange of the implant against the bone (see Fig. 109-6*B*).

The spiral drill is exchanged for a titanium threading tap (Fig. 109-7). The threading is performed at only 8 to 15 rpm to allow precise cutting of the bone. Again, irrigation is used to cool the bone during threading. A titanium screw-shaped implant of the corresponding length of the threaded hole (3 or 4 mm) is selected. The implant is screwed into the threads of the bone using a fixture mount on the drill (Fig. 109-8). Only bone touches the implant threads to avoid surface contamination with talc or other debris. The implant turns at 8 to 15 rpm until small shavings of bone from the flat area of countersink appear in the small holes in the flange of the implant. The fixture is then tightened by hand using a small ratchet. Extreme care is taken not to overtighten the implant and strip the threads in the bone. A coverscrew is threaded into the internal threads of the implant (Fig. 109-9). These internal threads will be used later to attach the

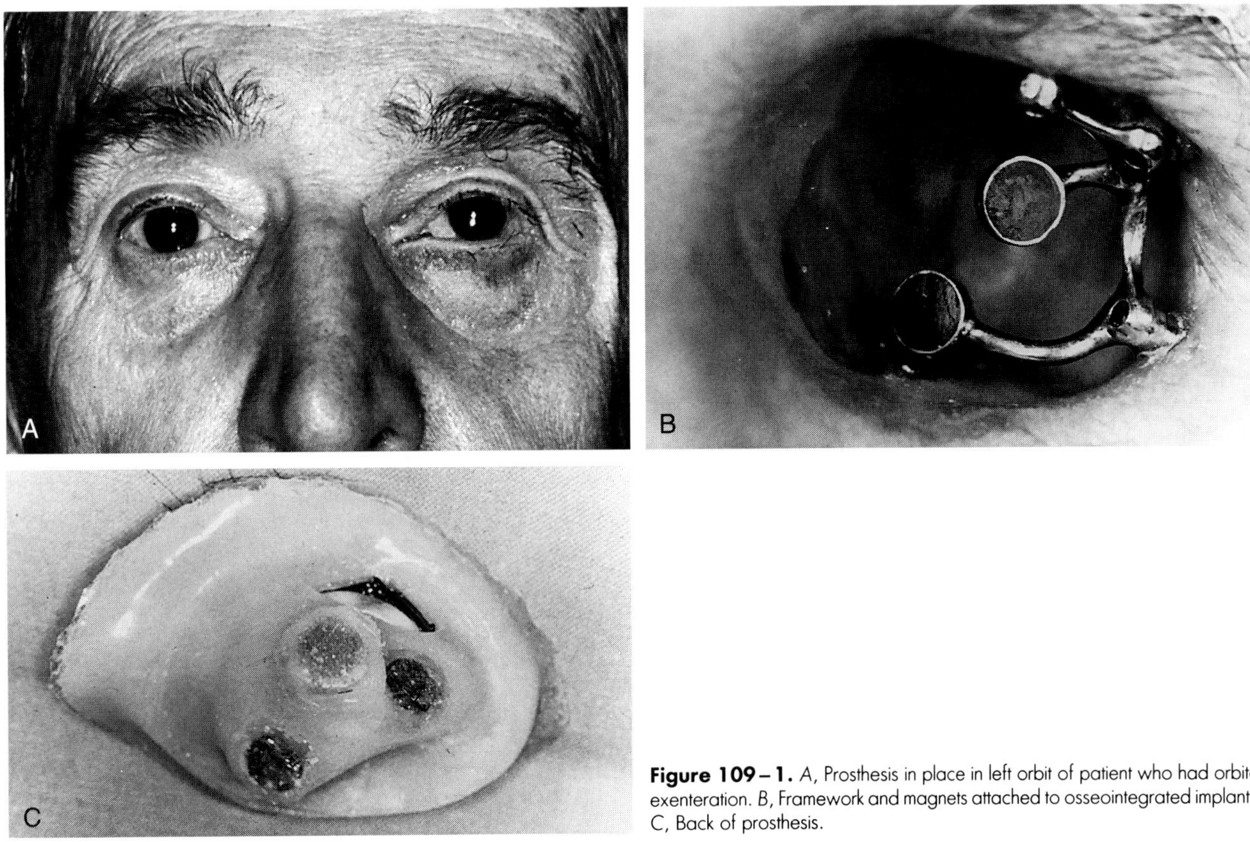

Figure 109–1. *A*, Prosthesis in place in left orbit of patient who had orbital exenteration. *B*, Framework and magnets attached to osseointegrated implants. *C*, Back of prosthesis.

skin-penetrating abutments. After placement of three or four fixtures the periosteal flap is closed with interrupted 5-0 Vicryl sutures (Fig. 109–10). The skin is closed with either 7-0 Vicryl or 7-0 nylon interrupted sutures. Topical antibiotic ointment is applied, and the wounds are dressed with a pressure bandage for 1 week. These steps complete the stage I procedure.

Stage II: Abutment Installation

Stage II is undertaken not less than 3 months later. The goal of the stage II procedure is to connect a titanium cylinder, known as an abutment, to the implant that has become integrated with the bone (Fig. 109–11). This procedure involves thinning of the subcutaneous tissues and penetration of the skin with the abutment. Again the procedure is performed on an outpatient basis using local anesthesia.

After satisfactory anesthesia, prepping, and draping, the previously placed implants are identified using a sharp probe. In some cases intraoperative photographs of stage I are consulted to help locate the implants, which may not be palpable under the skin. Preoperative skull radiographs (Fig. 109–12) may be helpful if photographs are not available. A skin incision is made at the side of the implant. If the implants are close together, a single continuous incision may be used rather than an incision over each fixture. Any soft tissue or bony overgrowth is freed from the surface of the implant. Any loose fixture has not undergone osseointegration and should be removed. A plane of dissection superficial to the periosteum is made surrounding the fixture for 5 to 7 mm. The skin overlying and surrounding the implant is thinned such that there is no subcutaneous tissue between the periosteum and the dermis of the skin (Fig. 109–13). This thinning is essential to prevent movement of the skin around the implant, thereby interfering with eventual integration of the soft tissue to the abutment. Any skin containing eyebrow hairs should be removed and replaced with a skin graft of non–hair-bearing skin. The thinned skin flap is laid over the implants, and a trephine is used to cut a hole in the skin overlying the implant. Alternatively, a suitable hole may be fashioned using a scalpel or scissors. A 3- or 4-mm abutment is placed through the hole in the skin and screwed into the implant (Fig. 109–14). The procedure is repeated for each of the implants. The skin is sutured with interrupted 7-0 Vicryl sutures (Fig. 109–15).

A plastic healing cap is screwed into the top of the abutment. Gauze coated with antibiotic ointment is wrapped around the abutments to compress and immobilize the skin (Fig. 109–16). The dressing is changed after 1 week and replaced with a similar one for an additional week. Four weeks after this procedure fitting of the prosthesis is started.

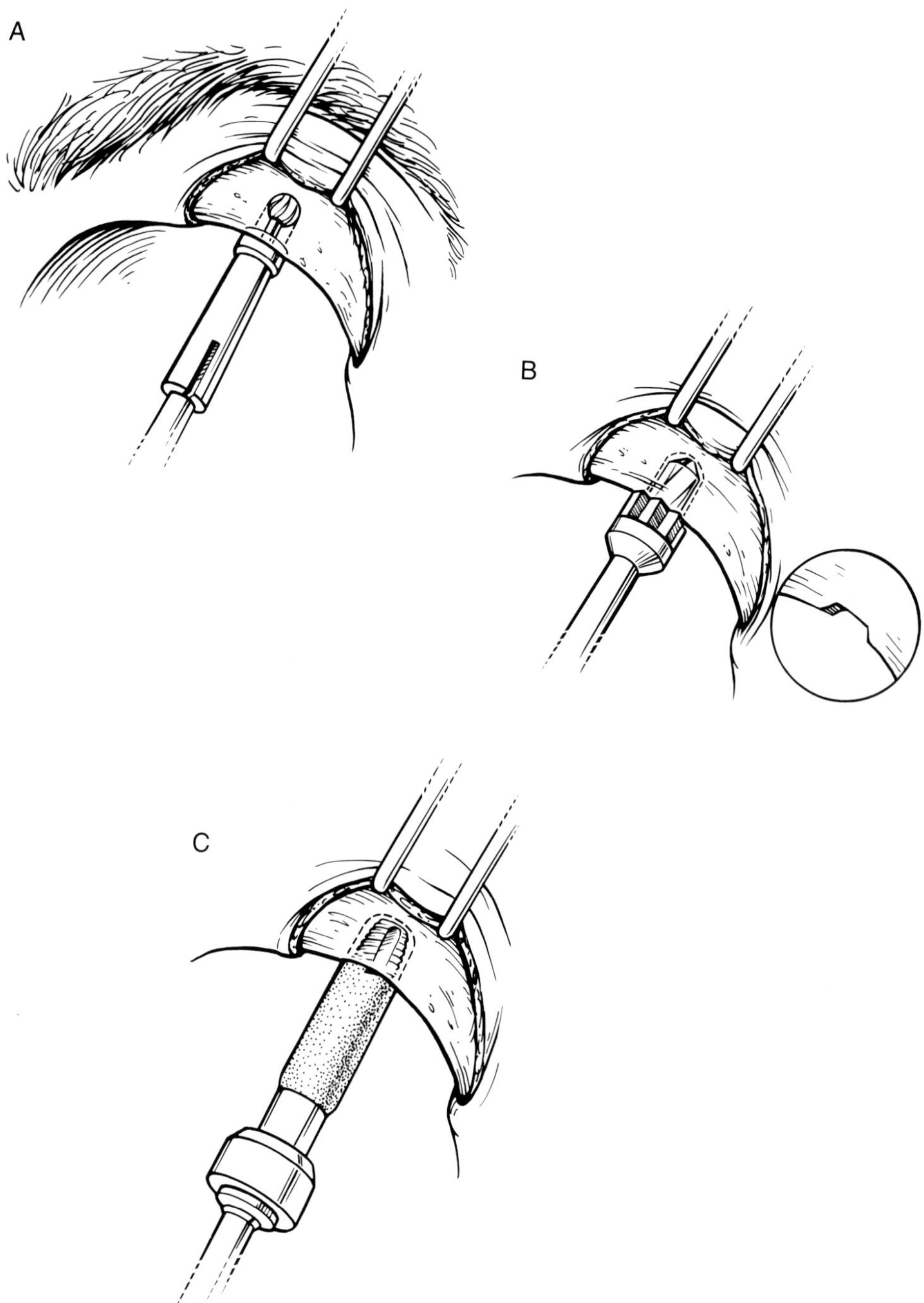

Figure 109–2. Schematic diagram summarizing implant installation (stage I).

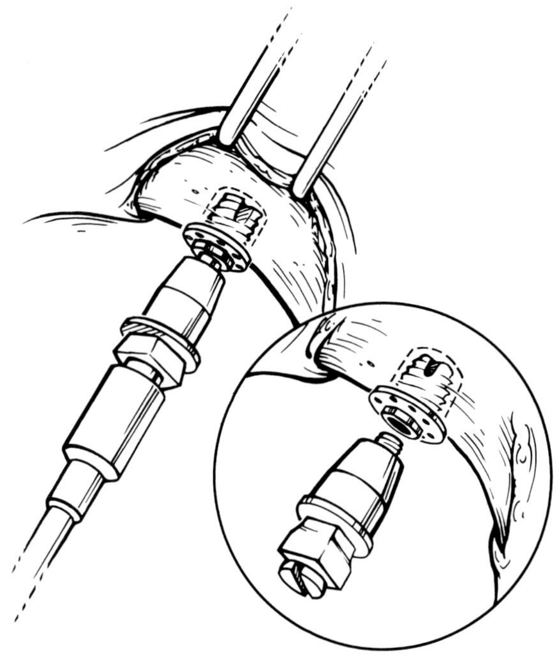

D

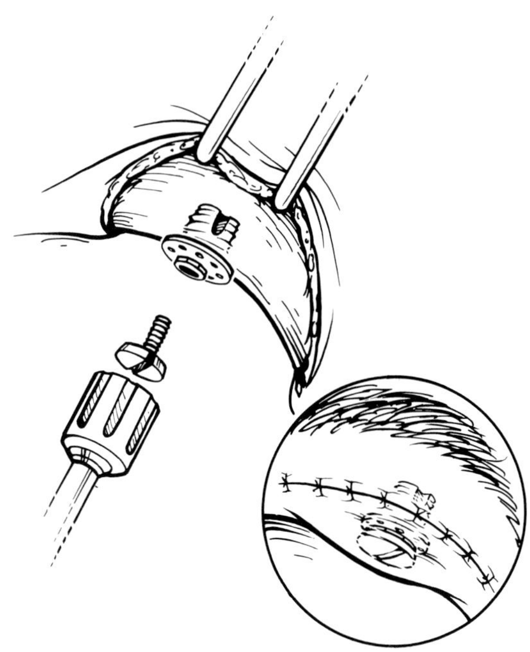

E

Figure 109–2 *Continued*

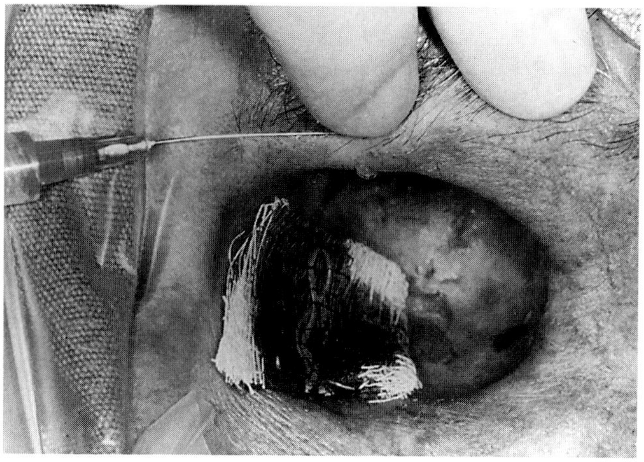

Figure 109–3. Subcutaneous tissues infiltrated with local anesthetic containing epinephrine.

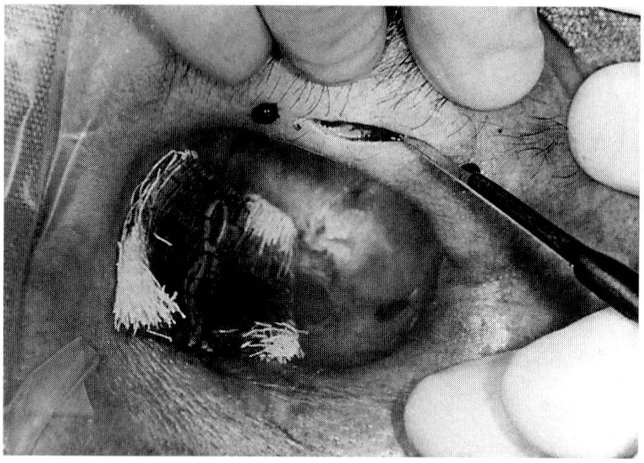

Figure 109–4. Skin incision prior to periosteal flap elevation.

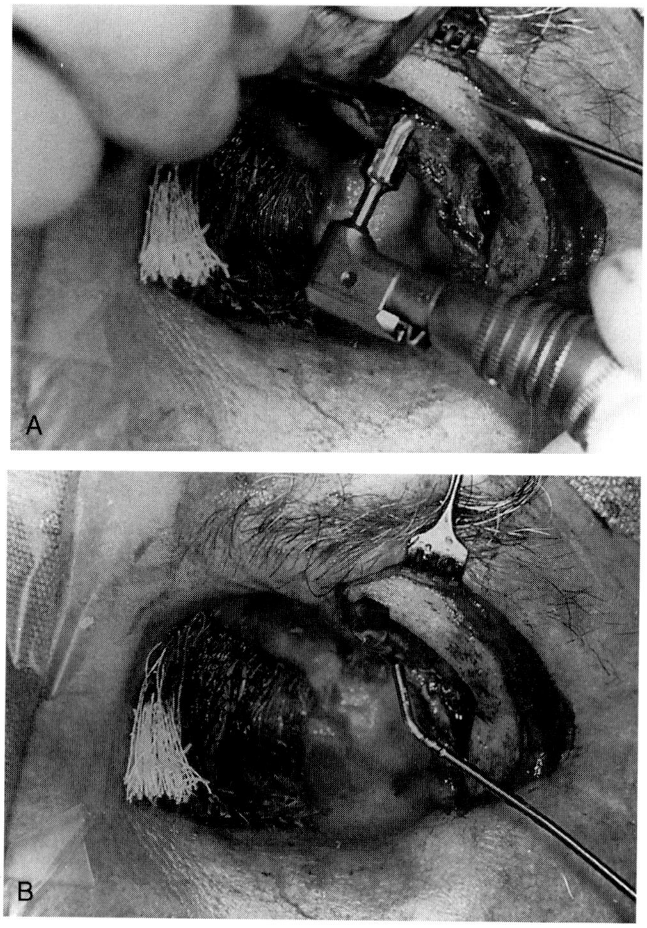

Figure 109–6. *A*, Spiral drill used at slow speed to cut implant site. *B*, Flat area on bony rim cut by countersink on spiral drill to seat flange of implant against bone.

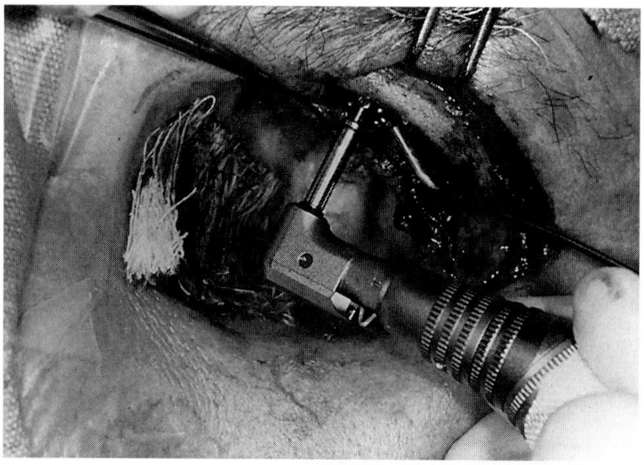

Figure 109–5. Preliminary drilling with cutting bur.

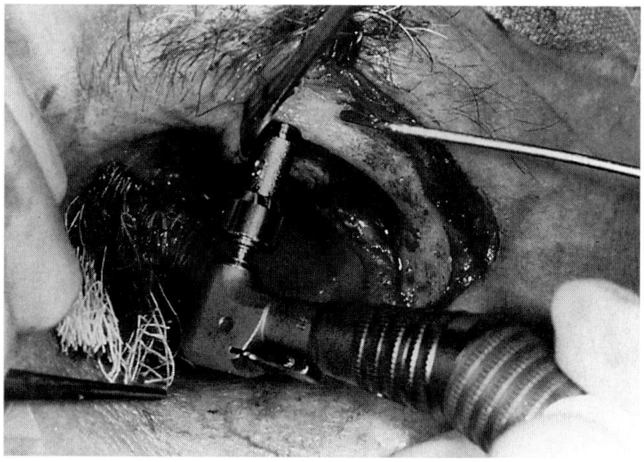

Figure 109–7. Threading tap cutting threads into bone at 8 to 15 rpm.

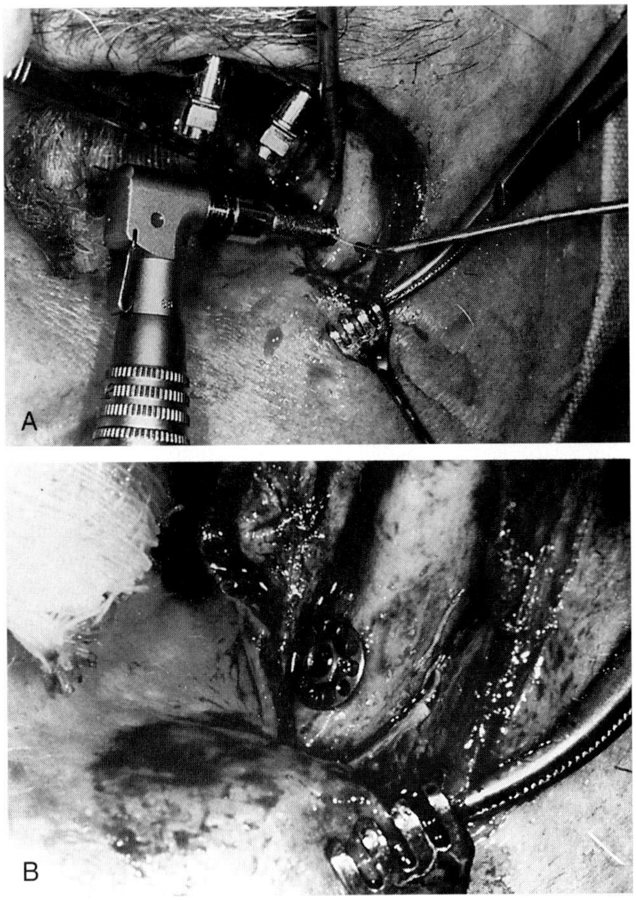

Figure 109–8. *A*, Fixture mount screwing implant into bony rim. *B*, Implant in place.

FACIAL PROSTHESIS

Once the skin has healed, a cast of the socket is made.[7] The technique is similar to the procedures described for the fitting of osseointegrated dental implants.[8] The cast is a negative impression of the socket including the exact position of the abutment cylinders. This cast is used to

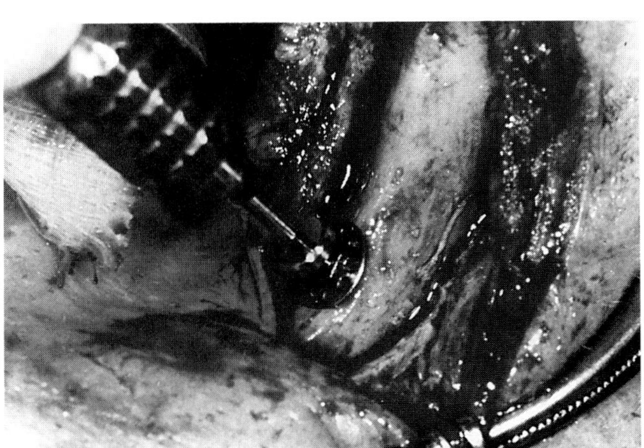

Figure 109–9. Coverscrew threaded into internal threads of the implant.

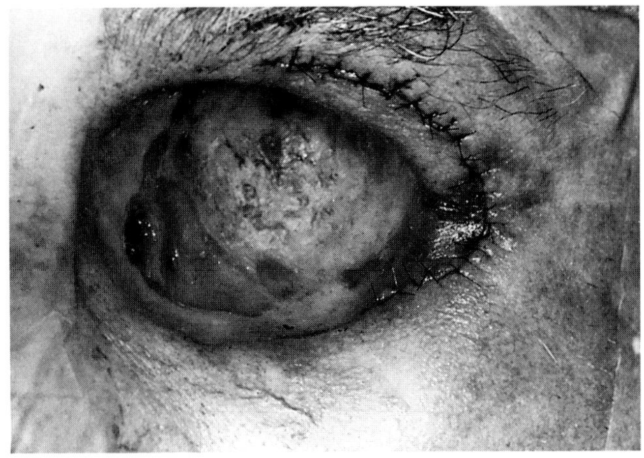

Figure 109–10. Closure of the wound.

create a metal bridge that will fit precisely with the abutments. Either small clips or magnets are attached to this framework. In some cases magnets may be attached directly to the abutment (Fig. 109–17). A silicone orbital prosthesis is made. Magnets of opposite polarity to those on the bridge are cast into the back of the prosthesis. To place the prosthesis into position the patient brings the prosthesis up to the socket and the magnetic forces pull the prosthesis into position and hold it in precise alignment. Retention is excellent. No additional means of support are necessary.[7, 8]

BIOLOGY OF OSSEOINTEGRATION

The success of the osseointegration procedure depends on the physical properties of the materials used as well as on the meticulous technique described. The search for suitable materials started in the 1950s as interest developed in finding a suitable implant material and technique to permanently anchor dentures to the edentulous jaw. A variety of metallic implants ranging from stainless steel to tantalum were tried.[9] All met the same fate, that is, fibrous encapsulation and eventual extrusion. It was assumed that permanent implantation was not possible without connective tissue intervening between the implant and the surrounding bone.[10] In 1969, during in vivo microscopic studies of bone marrow, Brånemark found that screw-shaped titanium optical chambers implanted into the bone could not be easily removed. These titanium implants were anchored to bone without fibrous encapsulation such that high stress loads could be tolerated.[11] This technique of implantation was refined, enabling a stable direct implant anchorage into living bone tissue, and was termed *osseointegration*.[9] Long-term studies showed that the intraosseous anchorage was stable and caused no undesirable effects on the soft tissues.

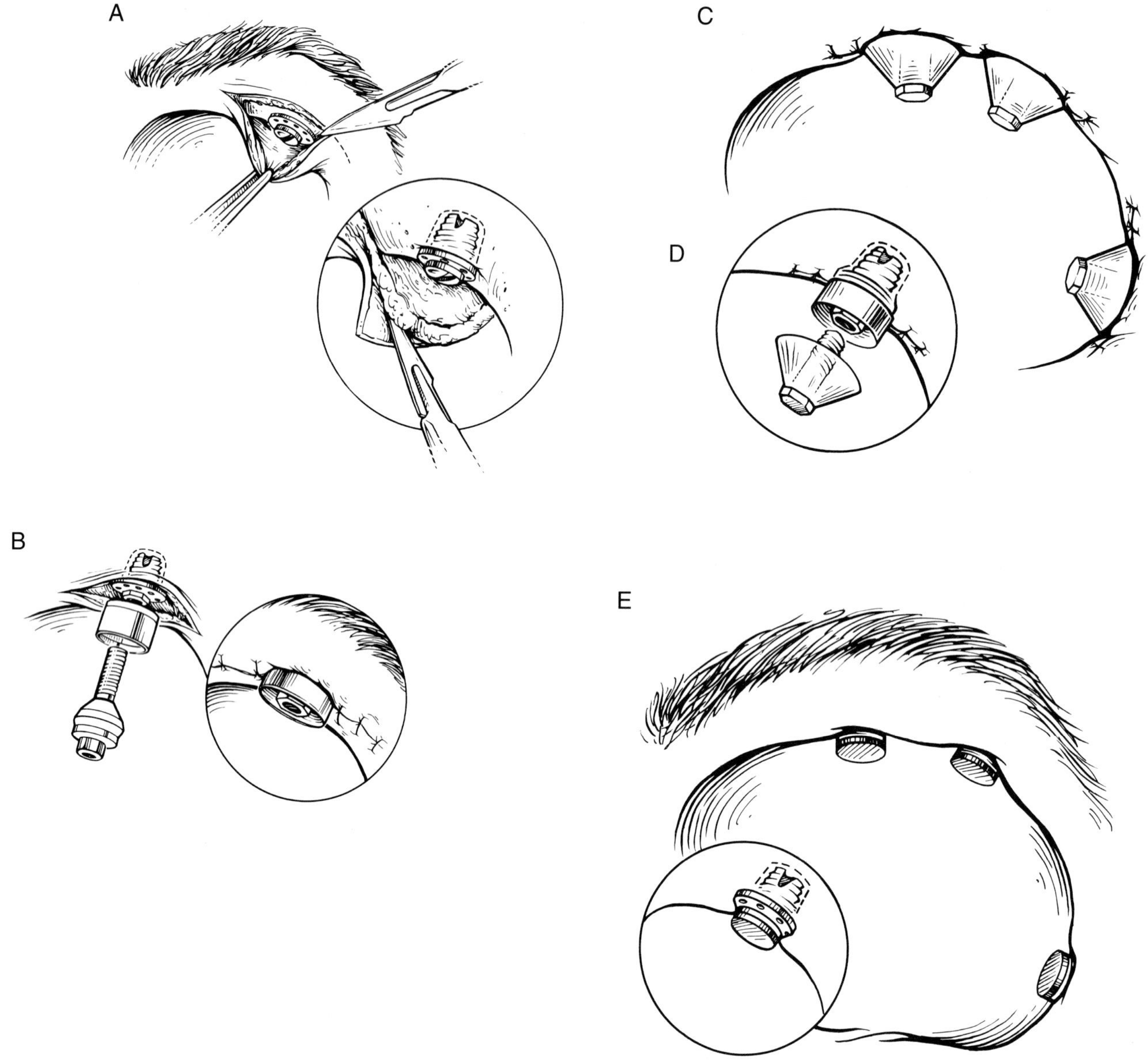

Figure 109–11. Schematic diagram summarizing abutment installation (stage II).

Further experimental work by Brånemark[12] showed that similar direct integration of a titanium implant into vertebral bone of dogs could be achieved even if the implant was allowed to penetrate the skin. The first osseointegrated implants used in humans were in 1965 when edentulous patients were treated. Unlike dental implants anchored in fibrous tissue bone, anchored oral implants gave long-lasting results.[1] Adell and associates,[11, 13, 14] in three studies, reported on implants in the upper and lower jaw after 10, 15, and 20 years. The success rate after 10 years was better than 80% for implants in the upper jaw and better than 90% for those in the lower jaw.[1] As of May 1988, more than 100,000 implants of the Brånemark Nobelpharma type had been used all over the world.[1]

Before the work of Brånemark it was thought that direct contact between living bone and implant would be possible only if the implant was a nonmetallic porous mineral, a ceramic. Experimental work with ceramic implants did prevent connective fibrous tissue encapsulation, but ceramic implants showed poor mechanical characteristics and fractured when loaded at the implant site. The strength of the osseointegration bond is the result of interaction between the bone and a thin oxide layer of the titanium. Except under rare conditions the surface of titanium becomes instantaneously coated with an oxide layer when exposed to air. The oxide layer is built up of a combination of TiO, TiO_2, TiO_3, and Ti_3O_4. This stable oxide coating of about 10 nm prevents a direct contact between bone and metal, acting as a porous ce-

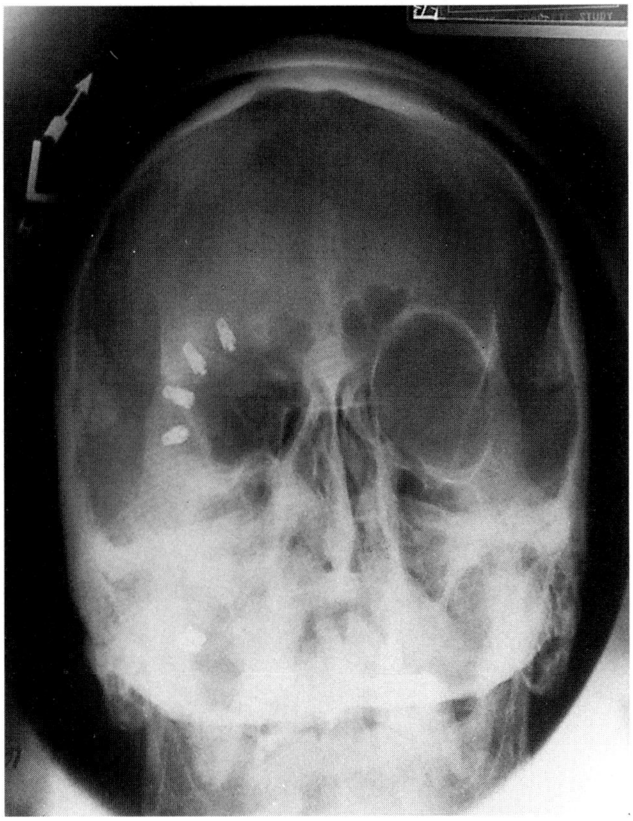

Figure 109–12. Plain skull radiograph showing the site of integrated implants.

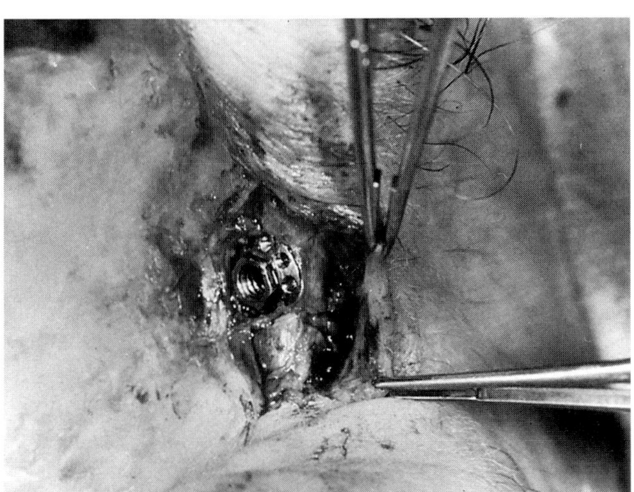

Figure 109–13. Exposure of implant and thinning of subcutaneous tissue.

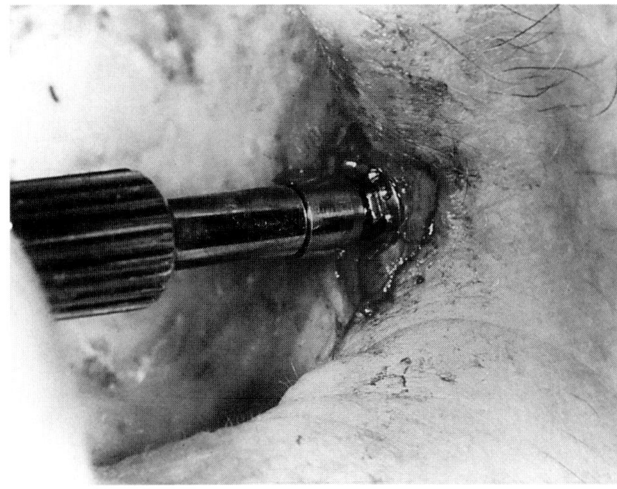

Figure 109–14. Screwing abutment into implant.

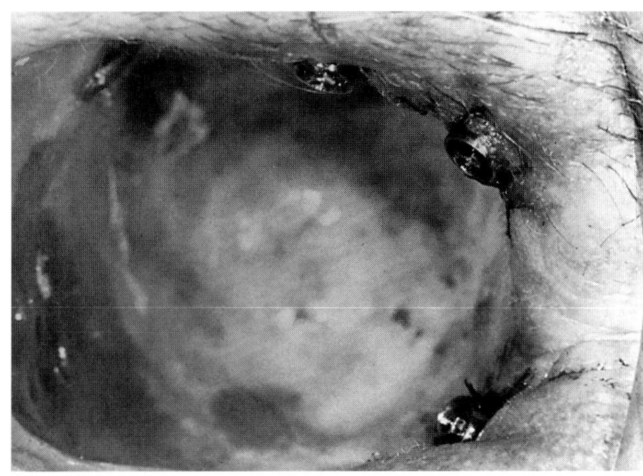

Figure 109–15. Skin closure around exposed abutments.

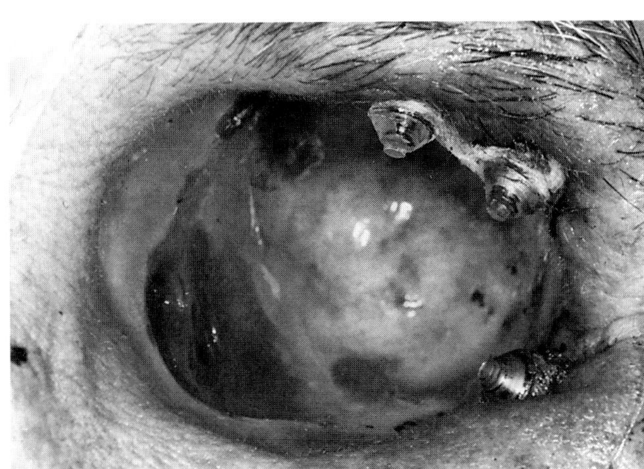

Figure 109–16. Gauze coated with antibiotic ointment compressing and immobilizing skin surrounding abutments.

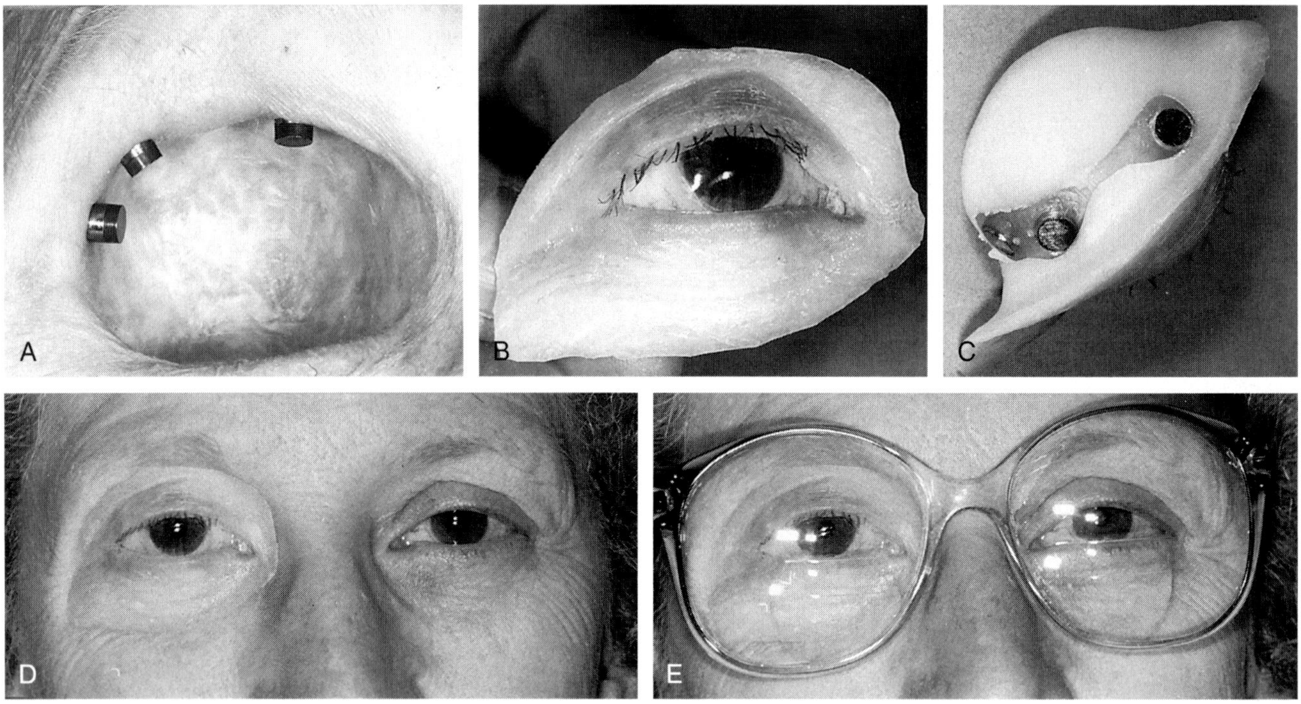

Figure 109–17. *A*, Magnets attached directly to abutments. *B*, Front of prosthesis. *C*, Back of prosthesis showing reverse polarity magnets. *D*, Patient wearing prosthesis. *E*, Patient wearing prosthesis (eyeglasses help hide the edge of the prosthesis).

ramic layer. Consequently, the exact composition of the oxide layer appears to be important in terms of the osseointegration process.[9]

A great deal of research has been done on the composition of the bone–implant interface. Radiographic and histologic analyses[15] of the anchoring tissue in dogs revealed incorporation of the titanium implants into the jaw bone. There was no evidence of any intermediary connective tissue layer between the implant and the bone. There were also no histologic signs of inflammation in the bone bordering the implant. Even when the anchoring elements were exposed to unlimited masticatory forces, the tissues retained their integrity and vitality. In 1981, Brånemark and Albrektsson[15] studied the interface zone between bone and the implant using radiograph, scanning electron microscopy, transmission electron microscopy, and light microscopy.[9] There were no signs of a connective tissue layer between the bone and the implant. The implants showed no signs of corrosion. The bone covering the implants was of a dense lamellar type, forming well-organized concentric lamellae. The close relationship between the bone and the implant was thought to be responsible for the mechanical stability. The collagenous fibers of the bone were tightly adhered to the titanium surface. Transmission electron microscopic analysis showed a direct bone to implant interface contact, suggesting the possibility of direct chemical bonding between bone and titanium.[9]

Brånemark and colleagues[11] first noted that titanium implanted subcutaneously did not cause inflammation or infection even at the site where the implant projected through the skin. In a study of 12 human volunteer subjects, Brånemark and Albrektsson,[14] in 1982, studied the possibilities for skin penetration of the implant without subsequent infection. They showed that a biologic seal around the titanium implant was possible, preventing descending infection. The critical factor seemed to be immobilization of the epithelial tissue around the implant. Where skin mobility was permitted, all implants had to be removed due to infection. In volunteers in whom all relative movement between the implant and the skin was eliminated there were no extrusions or soft tissue reactions. Thus, it appears that the immobility of the skin achieved by thinning the soft tissues at the time of the stage II osseointegration is important.

Albrektsson and associates[9] also studied the soft tissue–implant interface. The soft tissues were closely adhered to the titanium implant, thereby forming a biologic seal, preventing microorganism infiltration along the implant. There were no white blood cells nor any other types of inflammatory cells infiltrating the border of the soft tissues. No breakdown products from the implants could be found in the soft tissues.

The effects of irradiation on the success of osseointegration have been studied. Jacobsson and coworkers[16] studied nine patients, aged 4 to 72 years, who had radiation therapy before the osseointegration procedure. The patients received from 25.0 to 72.8 Gy. A total of 35 implants were placed. After an average follow-up time of 25 months, 29 of the 35 implants remained in stable position. Five fixtures (14.3%) were removed because of nonintegration or insufficient integration. Additionally 3 implants were available from postmortem specimens, all of which were clinically stable. Light microscopy of the loose implants showed a fibrous capsule around the implant. In contrast, when the clinically stable implants were examined the implant was in direct contact with the bone. Jacobsson and coworkers[16] concluded that osseointegration was possible in irradiated patients, but when it was compared with other studies, bone healing was delayed. The number of patients available was too small to try to establish a relationship between failure of osseointegration and the irradiation dosage or the time span between the radiation and the implantation procedure. They suggested that at least 1 year pass between the time of radiation and implantation. Currently, when osseointegration is used in radiated bone, hyperbaric oxygen treatments are recommended before and after the procedure.

EXTRAORAL APPLICATION

Encouraged by good results in the oral cavity, Tjellström and associates operated on the first three patients for bone-anchored hearing aids in 1977.[1] Since that time the use of bone-anchored implants has become a routine clinical practice in Sweden. Tjellström and associates[17] reported the first osseointegrated auricular prosthesis. Tjellström and coworkers,[10] in 1983, showed a very favorable 1- to 5-year outcome in patients with bone-anchored auricular prostheses and hearing aids. A success rate of over 95% in the temporal bone has been reported.[2] Tjellström and colleagues[17] concluded that titanium fixtures can be permanently integrated into the human temporal bone and can penetrate the skin without soft tissue infection or inflammation. In the oral surgery literature, Parel and coworkers[3, 4] reported excellent success with facial prosthetics using osseointegration in the combined experience in Gothenberg, Sweden, and San Antonio, Texas. My colleagues and I[18] have reported success in the rehabilitation of the exenterated socket.

SUMMARY

The goal of osseointegration is to achieve a direct contact between living bone and implant in an attempt to allow a permanent anchor for a prosthesis. Several key features of the osseointegration process are stressed. The implant material, titanium, is extremely corrosion resistant and is able to withstand stress.[9] The implant design and finish contribute to the initial mechanical stability while osseointegration occurs.[9] The bone should be healthy, not infected, and thick enough to support the fixture. A gentle surgical technique should be employed to keep bone and soft tissue damage to a minimum. Thermal damage[1] is avoided using sharp tools, a slow drilling speed, adequate cooling, and little, or no, cautery. Surface contaminants should not be introduced onto the surface of the titanium oxide. This is accomplished by handling the implants with only titanium instruments. There must be no pressure on the implants until osseointegration occurs. A period of 3 to 4 months should pass before stage II is undertaken. In irradiated bone a period of 1 year should pass before stage II is started. Hyperbaric oxygen treatments should be considered. The skin surrounding the abutments should be immobilized for at least 2 weeks such that a bond can form at the skin–abutment interface.

The technique of osseointegration in the orbit appears to offer patients an excellent means of wearing an orbital prosthesis. The prosthesis is easy to attach and remove. Retention is excellent, even during sporting activities. Inspection of the socket can be easily accomplished. Older patients have no problems with alignment. The exenteration patient is able to function in society without fear of looking abnormal or having the prosthesis fall out. This technique is worthy of consideration for all patients who have undergone orbital exenteration.

REFERENCES

1. Tjellström A: Osseointegrated systems and their applications in the head and neck. Adv Otolaryngol Head Neck Surg 3:39–70, 1989.
2. Hallén O, Magnusson S, Jacobsson M (eds): Bone-anchored implants in the head and neck region. Presented at the State-of-the-Art Conference, Göteborg, Sweden, September 1988.
3. Parel SM, Holt R, Brånemark PI, Tjellström A: Osseointegration and facial prosthetics. Int J Oral Maxillofac Implant 1:27–29, 1986.
4. Parel SM, Brånemark PI, Tjellström A, Gion G: Osseointegration in maxillofacial prosthetics: II. Extraoral applications. J Prosthet Dent 55:600–606, 1986.
5. Tjellström A, Lindström J, Hallén O, et al: Osseointegrated titanium implants in the temporal bone, a clinical study on bone-anchored hearing aids. Am J Otol 2:304–310, 1981.
6. Albrektsson T, Brånemark PI, Jacobsson M, Tjellström A: Present clinical applications of osseointegrated percutaneous implants. Plast Reconstr Surg 79:721–731, 1987.
7. Seals RR, Cortes AL, Parel SM: Fabrication of facial prostheses by applying the osseointegration concept for retention. J Prosthet Dent 61:712–716, 1989.
8. Lundqvist S, Carlsson GE: Maxillary fixed prostheses on osseointegrated dental implants. J Prosthet Dent 50:262–270, 1983.
9. Albrektsson T, Brånemark PI, Hansson HI, Lindström J: Osseointegrated titanium implants, requirements for ensuring a long-lasting, direct bone-to-implant anchorage in man. Acta Orthop Scand 52:155–170, 1981.
10. Tjellström A, Rosenhall U, Lindström J, et al: Five-year experience with skin-penetrating bone-anchored implants in the temporal bone. Acta Otolaryngol 95:568–575, 1983.
11. Brånemark PI, Breine U, Adell R, et al: Intraosseous anchorage of dental prostheses: I. Experimental studies. Scand J Plast Reconstr Surg 3:81–100, 1969.
12. Brånemark PI: Osseointegration and its experimental background. J Prosthet Dent 50:399–410, 1983.
13. Brånemark PI, Adell R, Albrektsson T, et al: Osseointegrated titanium implants in the rehabilitation of the edentulous patient. *In* Lee AJC, Albrektsson T, Brånemark PI (eds): Clinical Applications of Biomaterials. New York, John Wiley & Sons, 1982, pp 133–141.

14. Brånemark PI, Albrektsson T: Titanium implants permanently penetrating human skin. Scand J Plast Reconstr Surg 16:17–21, 1982.
15. Brånemark PI, Hansson BO, Adell R, et al: Osseointegrated Implants in the Treatment of the Edentulous Jaw, Experience from a 10-year Period. Stockholm, Sweden, Almquist & Wiksell International, 1977, pp 7–132.
16. Jacobsson M, Tjellström A, Albrektsson T, et al: Integration of titanium implants in irradiated bone: Histologic and clinical study. Ann Otol Rhinol Laryngol 97:337–340, 1988.
17. Tjellström A, Lindström J, Nylén O, et al: The bone-anchored auricular episthesis. Laryngoscope 91:811–815, 1981.
18. Nerad JA, Carter KD, LaVelle WE, et al: The osseointegration technique for the rehabilitation of the exenterated orbit. Arch Ophthalmol 109:1032–1038, 1991.

SECTION

IX

Craniofacial Deformities

SECTION EDITOR

Robert A. Weiss

CHAPTER 110

Craniofacial Congenital Anomalies: The Subcranial Approach

Joram Raveh, Kurt Laedrach, and Thierry Vuillemin

The conventional surgical approaches and procedures for the correction of the fronto-orbital anomalies are well known and extensively described in the literature. These can be summarized as follows:

1. Total resection of the midline including the cribriform plate and the median part of the nasal buttress as well as the septum[1-6]
2. Partial preservation of the midline skull base structures[7-13]
3. Paramedian resection, leaving the skeletal midline undamaged[14-23]

Common to these procedures is that the osteotomies of the skull base, roof of orbits, and optic nerve decompression are performed by the intracranial, transfrontal approach, which requires adequate retraction of the frontal lobes and adjacent dura.

The major disadvantages related to these procedures alluded to are the often resulting brain edema, damage to the olfactory filaments along with resulting anosmia, and the relatively high rate of morbidity and protracted hospitalization. Furnas and coworkers[19] and Jackson[20] described the exposure of the anterior skull base through the frontal sinus walls so as to accomplish the paramedian resection. The authors emphasize the limited visualization and exposure, as well as the risk of a via falsa, representing major disadvantages directly related to this procedure. Others accentuate that simple paramedian resection is often insufficient for optimal reduction of the interorbital distance.[15] Indeed, the classic rhinosurgical transethmoidal approach is inadequate for such a procedure. To avoid the previously mentioned disadvantages, we developed the subcranial procedure to provide a broad exposure of the ethmoidal-orbital roofs and lateral orbital walls as well as the entire frontal region and skull base, thus permitting an optimal approach for the osteotomies and bone resection. This procedure enables radical reduction of the interorbital distance with simultaneous optic nerve decompression.[24, 25] This method has already been used extensively in traumatic cases exposed to severe high-velocity force impact resulting in nasoethmoidal, frontobasal, and midface fractures.[25, 26]

In contrast to conventional procedures, exposure and osteotomy of the frontoethmoidal and orbital skull base planes, as well as orbital advancement, are performed by the subcranial approach. Thus, the transfrontal intracranial procedure, implying adequate frontal lobe retraction for exposure of the anterior skull base planes, can be avoided. This is particularly apparent in cases of hypertelorism without indication of anterior advancement in which osteotomy and resection of the paramedian frontonasal and ethmoidal roof have to be performed without further displacements along the calvaria. The word "subcranial" as such should not be understood as a terminologic controversy to the intracranial procedure. Visualizing the dura after the osteotomy, of course, implies penetration into the intracranial spaces, but the exposure and osteotomy are performed underneath the skull base planes, by definition, subcranially. Thus, the subcranial exposure is not a problem concerning simple semantics but represents a different technique.

A further major advantage rendered by this method is the optic nerve decompression. The subcranial approach facilitates the resection of the medial optic nerve canal wall, thus enabling the expansion of the same toward the subcranial cavity created after radical resection of the ethmoidal compartment. The further advantages of this extracranial decompression in comparison to the neurosurgical approach are highlighted later in this chapter.

SURGICAL PROCEDURES

Osteotomy and resection are conventionally performed after craniotomy by the transfrontal intracranial approach, along with retraction of the frontal lobes. In contrast to this approach, the subcranial exposure enables resection of the ethmoidal compartment, paramedian osteotomy, and resection of the frontoethmoidal roof and nasal segments, as well as the osteotomy of the orbital roofs and lateral walls (Figs. 110–1 and 110–2) by the external route. Thus, although the dura is visualized after osteotomy and resection of the bone segments, the whole procedure is not performed by the transfrontal intracranial access but by the subcranial exposure. Thus, no frontal lobe retraction is necessary. As in most cases,

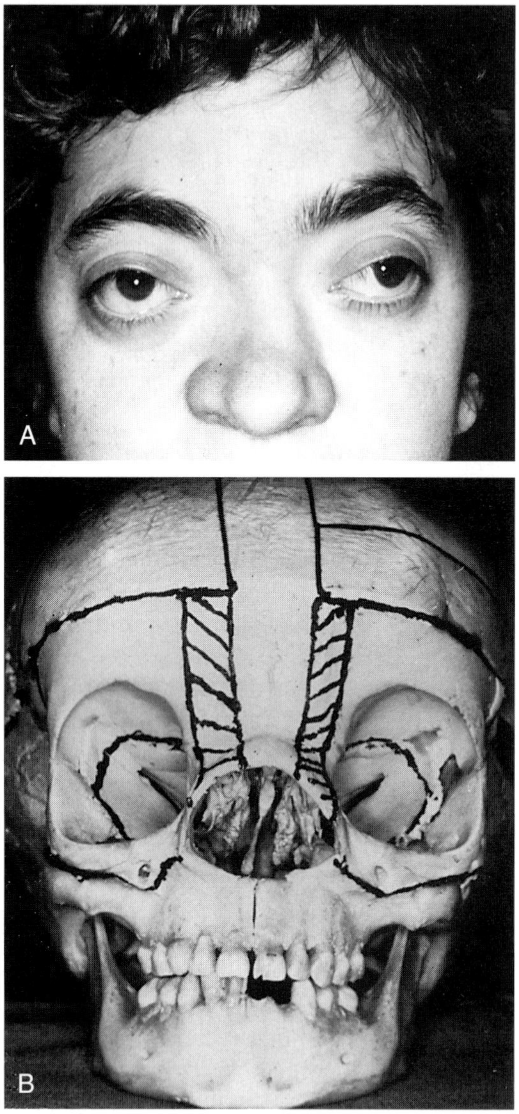

Figure 110–1. *A,* Patient with Apert's syndrome. Complex osteotomies of the frontal, orbital nasal, and maxillary regions are necessary to correct deformities. *B,* The current methods as shown include either total midline or paramedian resection, including craniotomy and transfrontal approach.

the ethmoidal compartment and not the cribriform plate is enlarged,[25, 27] and there is no indication to expose or resect the cribriform plate. We always prefer to spare this area, which includes the olfactory filaments as well as the nasal midline structures, so as to guarantee normal physiologic function.

Total resection of the ethmoidal compartment, including exposure of the sphenoid and ligature of the ethmoidal and further vessels, enables significant reduction in blood loss. Additionally, through this access the osteotomy and the resection of the ethmoidal roofs are performed.

The optic nerve decompression is then undertaken (Fig. 110–3). The extracranial optic nerve decompression by the transethmoidal,[28–33] transantral,[34] as well as the transorbital[35, 36] approach has already been described. Yet this access was restrictively and sporadically utilized in trauma limited to only selected cases in regard to the limited exposure and visualization of the area restricted to the paramedian skull base planes. These studies mainly include optic nerve decompression for other reasons than trauma or anomaly cases. In contrast to this the exposure and resection of the medial optic nerve canal wall facilitated by the subcranial approach can optimally be performed routinely in all the cases (see Fig. 110–3). The subcranial compartment created after radical removal of the ethmoidal cells enables optimal visualization of the medial canal wall. Apart from that and compared with the intracranial procedure, the decompression at this site is most efficient. The nerve can expand underneath the subcranial plane medially toward the compartment created after resection of the ethmoidal cells. This is crucial after orbital advancement, so as to avoid optic nerve compression. Because the nerve can expand medially and the subcranial drainage is guaranteed by a Portex tube externalized to the nasal lumen, postoperative development of pressure as a result of hematoma or edema along the orbital cone and nerve canal with consequent Apex syndrome and optic nerve damage can be avoided.

Correct preoperative studies, as well as the performance of radiographs, computed tomography, and three-dimensional scans (Fig. 110–4), are necessary for optimal planning. In particular, aberrative configuration of the midline skull base structures and optic nerve canal can be detected.

A further advantage after the fronto-orbital osteotomy is the correct symmetric advancement enabled by the subcranially exposed skull base planes: the centripetal symmetric compression of the canthal ligaments and orbitozygomatic complex. As shown in Figure 110–5, this procedure was developed for our trauma cases as well as for our teleorbitism cases. The thread, once passed through the canthal ligaments and the medial orbital–lateral nasal wall segment, is guided underneath the exposed anterior skull base and perpendicular lamella into the contralateral frontal sinus lumen and through two bur holes applied to the anterior segment of the frontal sinus wall. Tightening of the thread and performance of the procedure on both sides results in compression of the canthal ligaments as well as of the nasal bone fragments. The canthal ligaments are thus compressed not only toward the midline but also down and inward, achieving an optimal relation in regard to the vertical, horizontal, and sagittal levels. In the absence of, or with insufficient bone support at, the medial aspect of the orbit, a bone graft should be applied to which the canthal ligament must be attached; otherwise, postoperative lateral distraction and displacement of the ligament is usually inevitable.

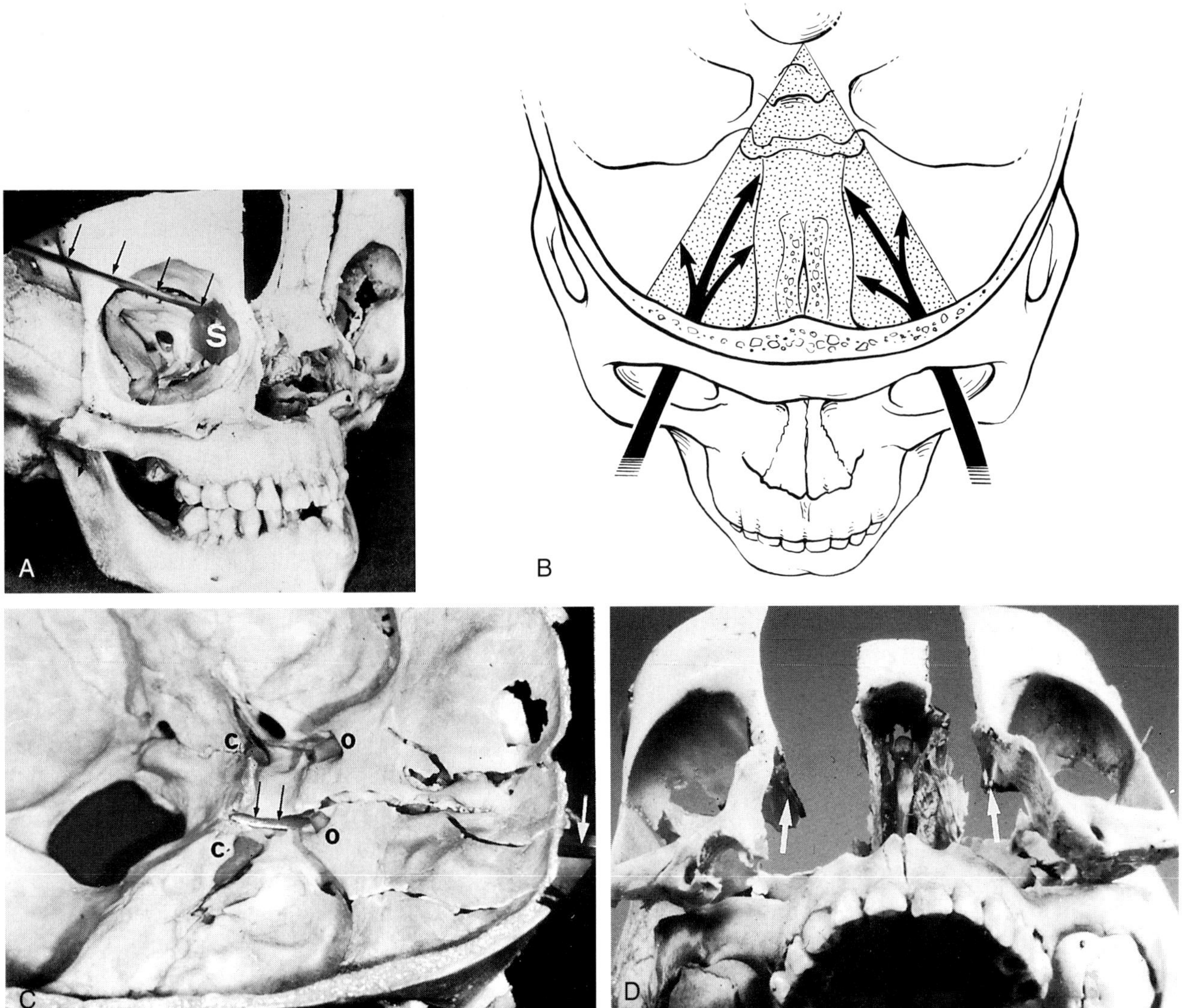

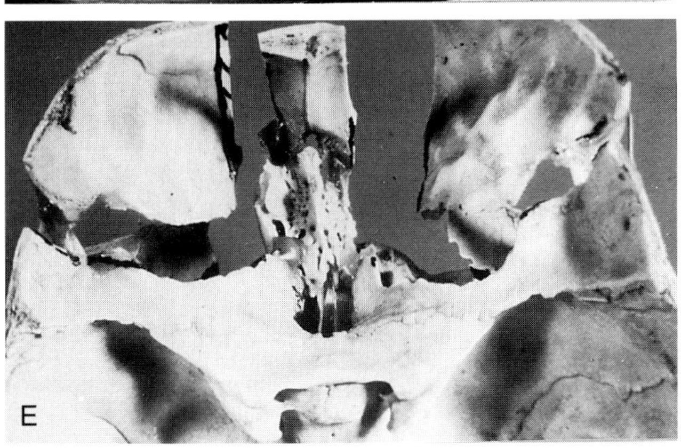

Figure 110–2. Principles of the subcranial approach. *A*, Before resection after radical ethmoidectomy, all skull base, orbital, ethmoidal roof, and sphenoidal planes are exposed by the subcranial approach (S). The *arrows* indicate a sonde. *B*, The *arrows* indicate the extent of the subcranial exposure. C, Intracranial view illustrating the optimal visualization of the dura, the optic nerve (O), the carotid artery (C), and the ethmoidal vessels rendered by the subcranial access. The *arrows* indicate a sonde. *D*, Schematic illustration of the paramedian bone segment resections sparing the nasal and skull base midline structures and optic nerve decompression (*arrows*) performed by the subcranial access. *E*, Intracranial schematic illustration of the skull base planes after osteotomy and resection by the subcranial approach obviating the transfrontal procedure and frontal lobe retraction.

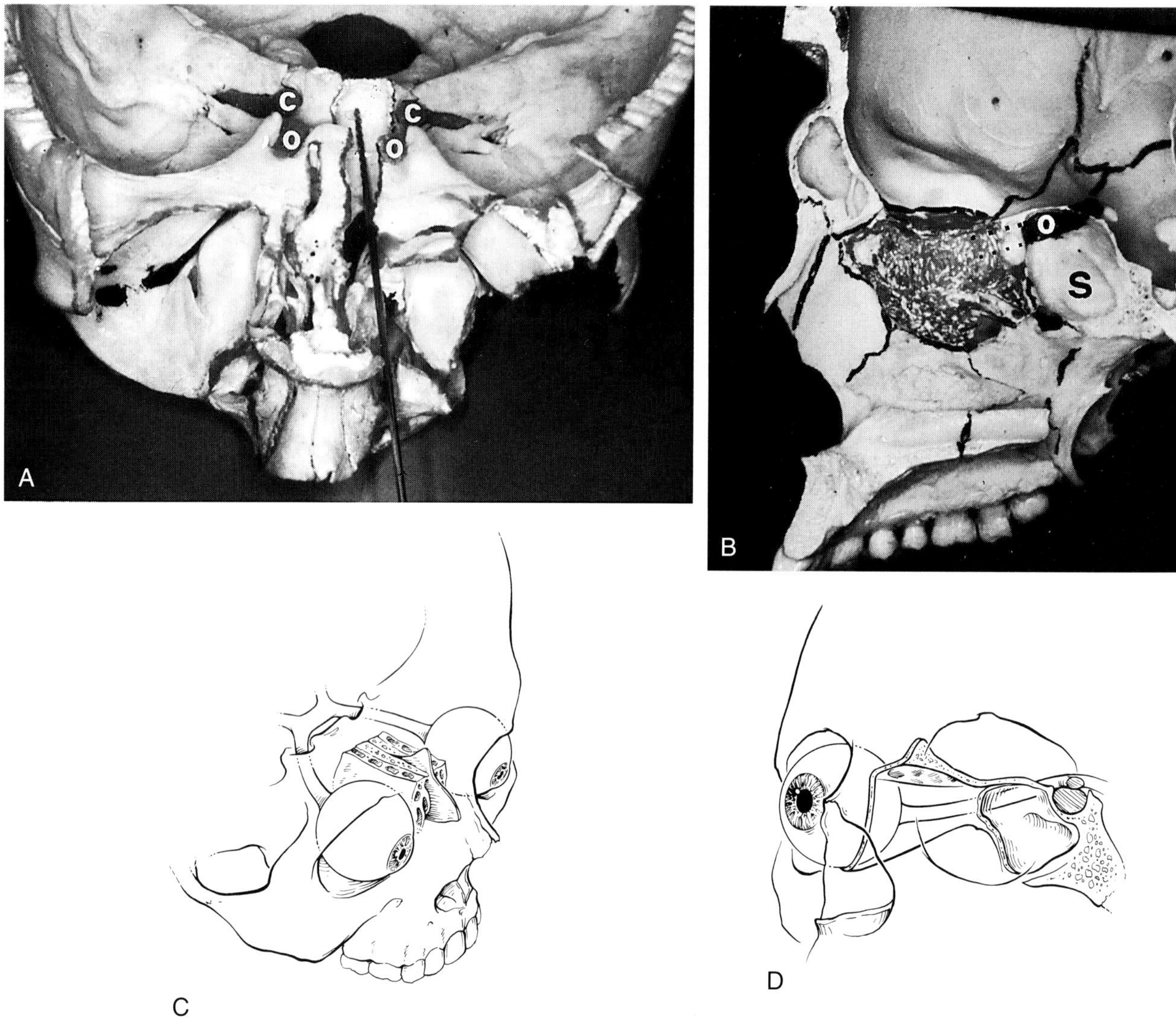

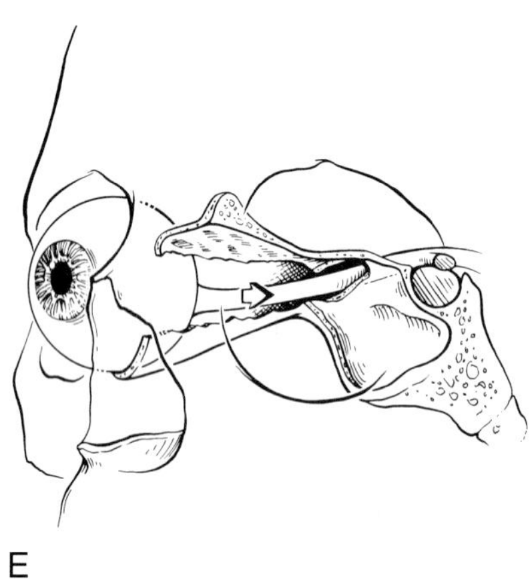

Figure 110–3. Schematic illustration of the optic nerve decompression by the subcranial approach. *A*, The subcranial exposure includes the sphenoid (located where the sonde is pointing). O, optic nerve; C, carotid artery (note its adjacency to the sphenoid). *B*, The *dotted lines* indicate the projection of the medial optic nerve canal wall to be resected. O, optic nerve; S, sphenoid. *C*, Lateral view depicting the anatomic relation of the canal to the skull base and lateral ethmoidosphenoidal walls. *D*, Medial view of the orbital and ethmoidosphenoidal walls along the nerve canal. *E*, Borders of medial orbital and canal wall resection enabling expansion of the nerve toward the created subcranial compartment as well as drainage of apical orbital cone.

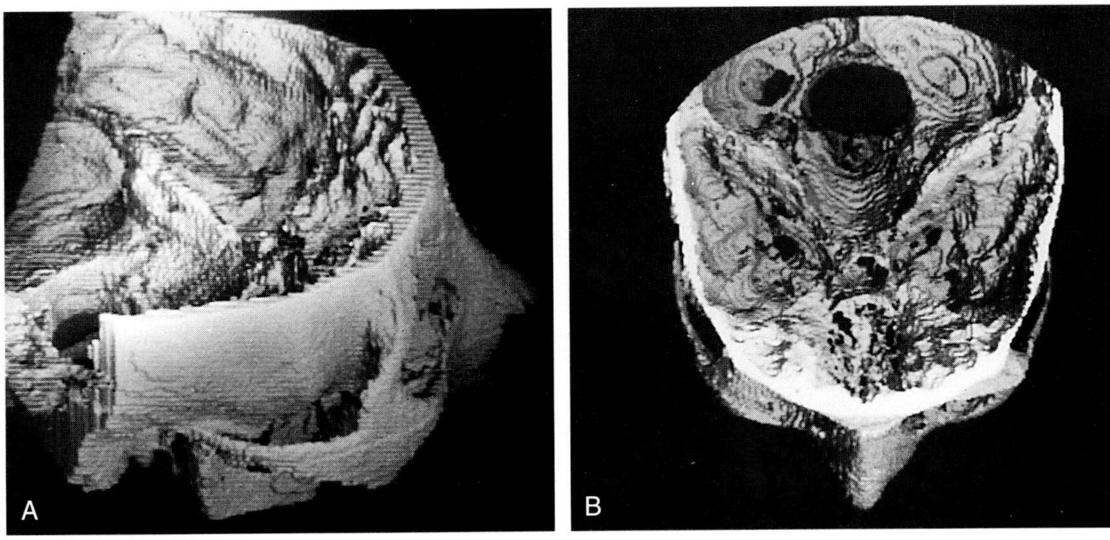

Figure 110–4. *A* and *B*, Before surgery a three-dimensional computed tomographic scan is recommended for relevant information concerning the skull base configuration.

The same procedure can be extended to the orbitozygomatic complex for compression toward the midline (see Fig. 110–5*C* and *D*). The thread is then guided through bur holes applied to the zygomatic prominence underneath the orbital floor and skull base to the contralateral side, resulting in optimal symmetric reduction of the interorbital distance. This compression, in concert with miniplate osteosynthesis of the supraorbital-frontal area, contributes significantly to the symmetric three-dimensionally correct advancement of the orbital frame complex.

Particularly apparent are the advantages in hypertelorism cases in which only limited calvarial or frontal bone segmentation and advancement has to be performed. As indicated in Figure 110–6*A*, the enlarged interorbital distance and marked broad nasal buttress are evident. Before the paramedian osteotomy and resection of the nasofrontal segments, exposure of the entire subcranial basal area including the orbital-ethmoidal and the both-sided optic nerve decompression is accomplished (see Fig. 110–6*B* through *D*).

After paramedian resection of the anterior frontal sinus wall and ethmoidal roof, the exposed posterior wall of the frontal sinus is osteotomized and resected. The bur holes, applied at the frontotemporal junction (see Fig. 110–6*B* through *D*), are connected by an osteotomy line toward the resection borders are the posterior frontal sinus wall, visualized by a further bur hole at the anterior wall. A further osteotomy along the orbital lateral wall and floor toward the zygomatic-maxillary arch, as well as along the orbital roof, is then accomplished.

The intraoperative view after both-sided orbitozygomatic mobilization is shown in Figure 110–6*C* and *D* depicting the osteotomy borders along the orbital roofs and visible dura at these locations. Reduction of hypertelorism and medial advancement of the orbitae included 3.8 cm (see Fig. 110–6*E*). A craniotomy for the transfrontal approach or frontal lobe retraction is unnecessary in these cases. The blood loss during surgery as measured by the anesthetist was, in this case, reduced to only 1.260 L, also being representative for the other cases. It is of utmost importance that the globes are symmetrically positioned toward the midline as well as in all the other planes. Optimal alignment and isolation of the dura and the skull base planes is indicated with fascia lata. The alignment of the subcranial planes, including the orbital roofs, sphenoid, and paramedian skull base area provides a watertight isolation toward the subcranial and paranasal spaces. This is crucial for the reduction of postoperative cerebrospinal fluid leaks or meningitis. The drainage of the subcranial compartment and frontal sinuses is provided by an inserted Portex tube, externalized into the nasal cavity, and this again is most advantageous in regard to the reduction of complications such as immediate postoperative development of an Apex syndrome, sinus dysfunction, mucus retention, empyema, or ascending infection and meningitis later on.

The fixation of the fronto-orbital segments is achieved by miniplate osteosynthesis; thus optimal retention of the mobilized segments is achieved. Only after definitive advancement and fixation are the skull base planes and dura aligned with fascia lata layers adapted with the help of fibrin glue by the subcranial access. The resulting gaps along the orbital walls and floor after orbital advancement are bridged by lyophilized cartilage layers or bone grafts harvested from the external calvarial table.

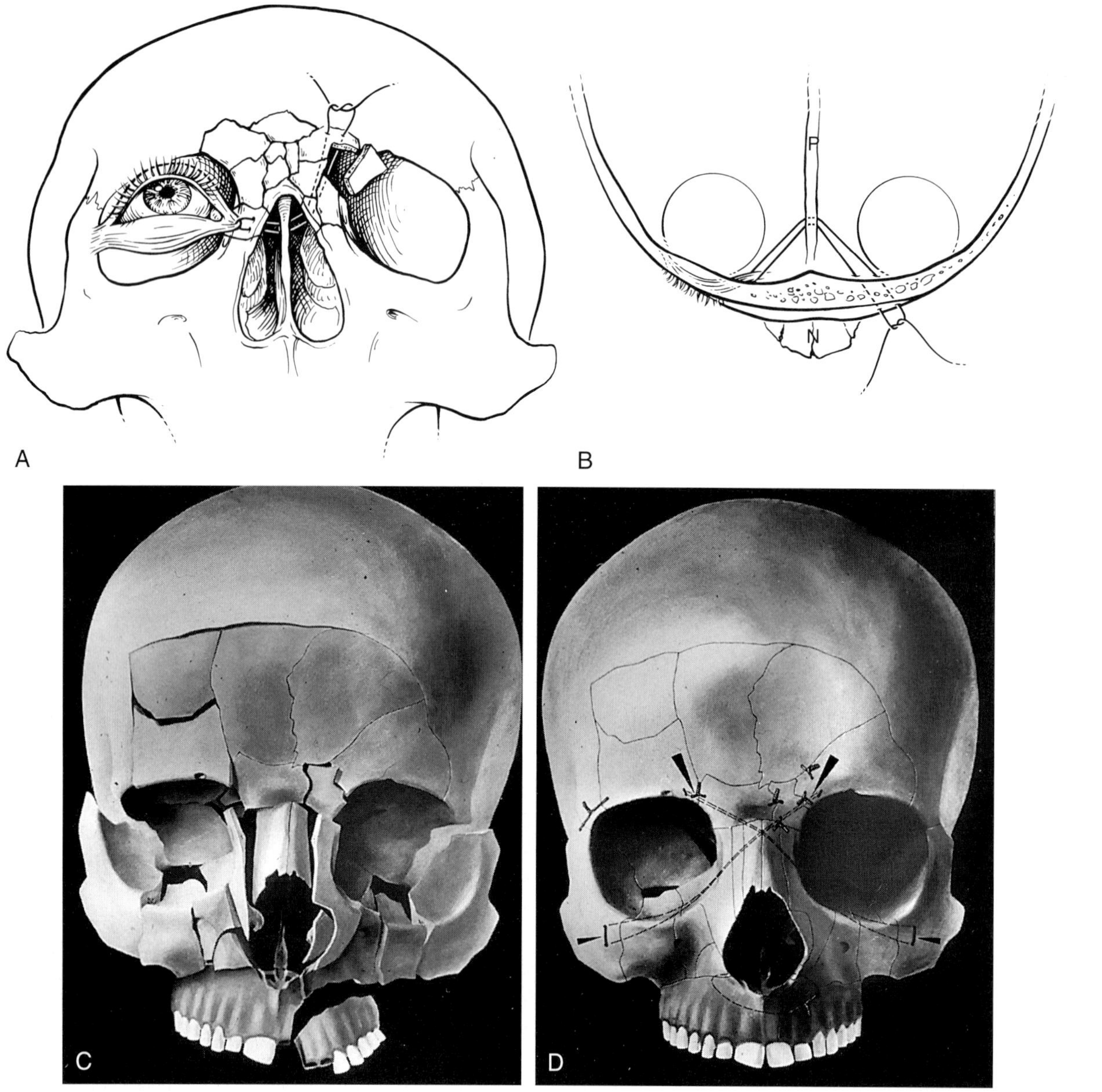

Figure 110–5. Schematic illustration of the cross-sided centripetal canthal ligament and naso-orbital compression method. *A*, Schematic illustration of multiple naso-frontal fragments and disattached canthal ligaments common to high-velocity trauma cases, which represent a far more complicated configuration compared with simple osteotomies. The canthal ligament and lateral nasal wall fragment are fixed by a thread guided underneath the exposed anterior skull base into the frontal sinus to be fixed to the anterior wall. This both-sided procedure enables the compression of the medial orbital and nasal wall fragment towards the midline in the correct vertical, horizontal, and sagittal levels. For further details see text. *B*, Transfrontal projection of the technique. N, nasal buttress; P, lamina perpendicularis. *C* and *D*, Same procedure as in *A* and *B*, extended to the zygomatic complex. The thread fixed to the zygomatic prominence is guided underneath the orbital floor, thus compressing the entire osteotomized orbitozygomatic complex (see text for details). This method is applied in trauma as well as anomaly cases.

Figure 110–6. Hypertelorism (Woakes' syndrome). *A*, Intraoperative view depicting the broad nasal buttress (N) and orbital distance. Note bicoronal flap and subcranial exposure (S). *B*, Intraoperative view depicting the performed segment osteotomy of the frontonaso-orbital segments performed by the subcranial approach with preliminary ethmoidal roof resection and optic nerve decompression. No craniotomy is performed. C, Schematic illustration of the orbital advancement. The *arrows* indicate the direction of the advancement. *D*, Situation after removal of the paramedian segments, sparing the midline structures. The *arrowheads* indicate the bur holes used to guide the osteotomy. D, exposed dura; O, osteotomized and mobile orbitae. The *arrows* indicate the orbital roof resection borders. The osteotomy of the caudal part of the zygoma and orbital floor is performed by the intraoral and transconjunctival approach. Both-sided optic nerve decompression was performed as discussed. *E*, Miniplate osteosynthesis and fixation of the fronto-orbital segments reducing the intercanthal distance. The borders of the bur holes (*arrows*) indicate the degree of advancement toward the midline. *F* and *G*, Preoperative and postoperative views, respectively, of the same patient.

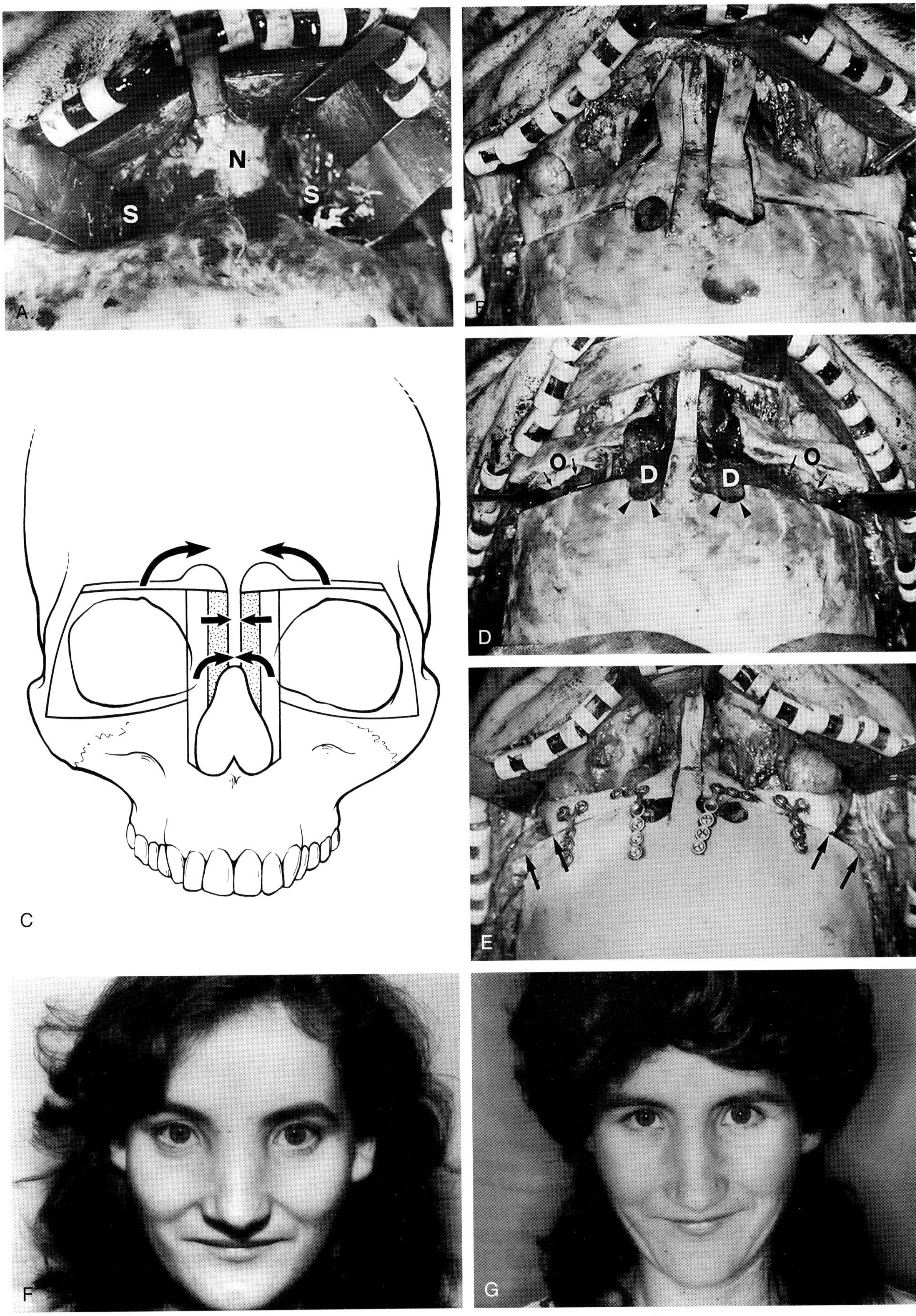
N
S
S
A
B
O
O
D
D
D
C
E
F
G

The postoperative care in the intensive care unit in such cases can usually be reduced to 24 hours, and the entire hospitalization period is 5 to 6 days if no packing of the skull base was necessary. If packing was necessary, the detamponade is performed on the 10th and 11th days, and the patient can then be dismissed on the 11th day. The expenditure and risks of this type of surgery can be reduced to the level of a routine surgical procedure if the subcranial approach is used.

This is also apparent in the case illustrated in Figure 110–7. The asymmetry and laterocaudal displacement of the orbitozygomatic complex on the right side made a medial and upward mobilization necessary. The subcranial exposure including the right-sided skull base planes facilitates this surgical procedure, obviating any transfrontal approach (see Fig. 110–7*C*). In this case splitting of the orbital complex in two segments was indicated in regard to the incongruency and asymmetry of the infraorbital and supraorbital sections: moving the zygomatico-orbital complex in one unit would have fulfilled neither the aesthetic nor the functional requirements. After completion of the osteotomy along the orbital walls and zygoma, the frontosupraorbital and part of the medial and lateral orbital walls were temporarily removed as one segment. After the resection, this segment was replaced in an upward and medial position and slightly advanced at the lateral aspect, including part of the orbital roof. Only then the distal segment of the orbit, including part of the lateral and medial walls, infraorbital rim, orbital floor, and zygomatic prominence, was moved so as to meet the upper segment. This procedure enabled us to move the periorbital tissue and the globe medially and upward, particularly accentuated along the lateral aspect of the globe. The watertight alignment with fascia lata of the dura and skull base and optic nerve canal decompression and drainage were performed as alluded to. Since no packing was indicated, the patient was dismissed after 6 days without the need of any care in an intensive care unit. The postoperative view is shown in Figure 110–7*F*.

In cases such as Apert's and Crouzon's syndromes, not only reduction of the hypertelorism but also correction of the exophthalmus by fronto-orbital and midface advancement (Figs. 110–8 through 110–10) and osteotomy of the frontal and calvarial regions is indicated. Obviously, craniotomy has to be performed, yet the osteotomies of the fronto-orbital segments, as well as the paramedian osteotomy and optic nerve decompression, are performed by the subcranial approach as alluded to.

In this case, after the osteotomies of the frontonaso-orbital sections, the midface osteotomized by a LeFort III procedure is advanced and the correct occlusion was set and retained temporarily by intermaxillary fixation. Then the calvarial and fronto-orbital segments are advanced and moved medially. After the fixation of the midface with miniplates the intermaxillary function is removed. The medial optic nerve canal walls are removed by the subcranial approach and the drainage externalized to the nasal lumen. Bone grafts and lyophilized cartilage layers were applied to bridge the resulting defects. Particular attention should be paid to the bridging of defects and adequate compensation along the orbital cone so as to avoid divergence and asymmetry of the globes. Figures 110–8 through 110–10 show a comparison of various views of a patient undergoing this procedure. In such cases, a limited 24-hour stay in an intensive care unit is advised and dismissal is scheduled after 11 days.

In deformities limited to the frontonasal region, as shown in Figures 110–11 and 110–12, the subcranial approach facilitates the surgical management, reducing the complication rate as alluded to. This patient was accordingly dismissed from the intensive care unit after 24 hours, with dismissal from the hospital after 9 days.

RESULTS

There were 52 anomaly cases that were managed by the subcranial approach. Another 124 cases with fronto-orbital asymmetry and hypertelorism were due to trauma and insufficient reduction or during childhood, resulting in asymmetric growth.

As indicated in Tables 110–1 through 110–3, the results reveal a significant reduction of the complication rate. The followup included a minimum of 1 and a maximum of 5 years in the anomaly cases and up to 8 years in the remaining cases.

In one of the anomaly cases, Apert's syndrome, postoperative development of an Apex syndrome on one side, was manifested 2 days postoperatively. This was due to insufficient orbital periosteal incisions and drainage and resulted in partial optic nerve atrophy. In none of the remaining cases was pressure development along the orbital cone and decompressed optic nerve observed. Meningitis occurred in one patient and subsided after antibiotic therapy. The further postoperative course was uneventful. The low rate of sinus dysfunction and mucocele and the fact that in none of the cases was anosmia related to surgery observed should particularly be pointed out.

The intensive care period was reduced to 1 to 2 days. The patients with orbital advancement were dismissed from the hospital after 5 to 7 days, and those who had additional frontal advancement after 11 to 12 days.

DISCUSSION

The term *subcranial exposure* only means that the extended frontobasal exposure is performed so as to enable

(*Text continued on page 1177*)

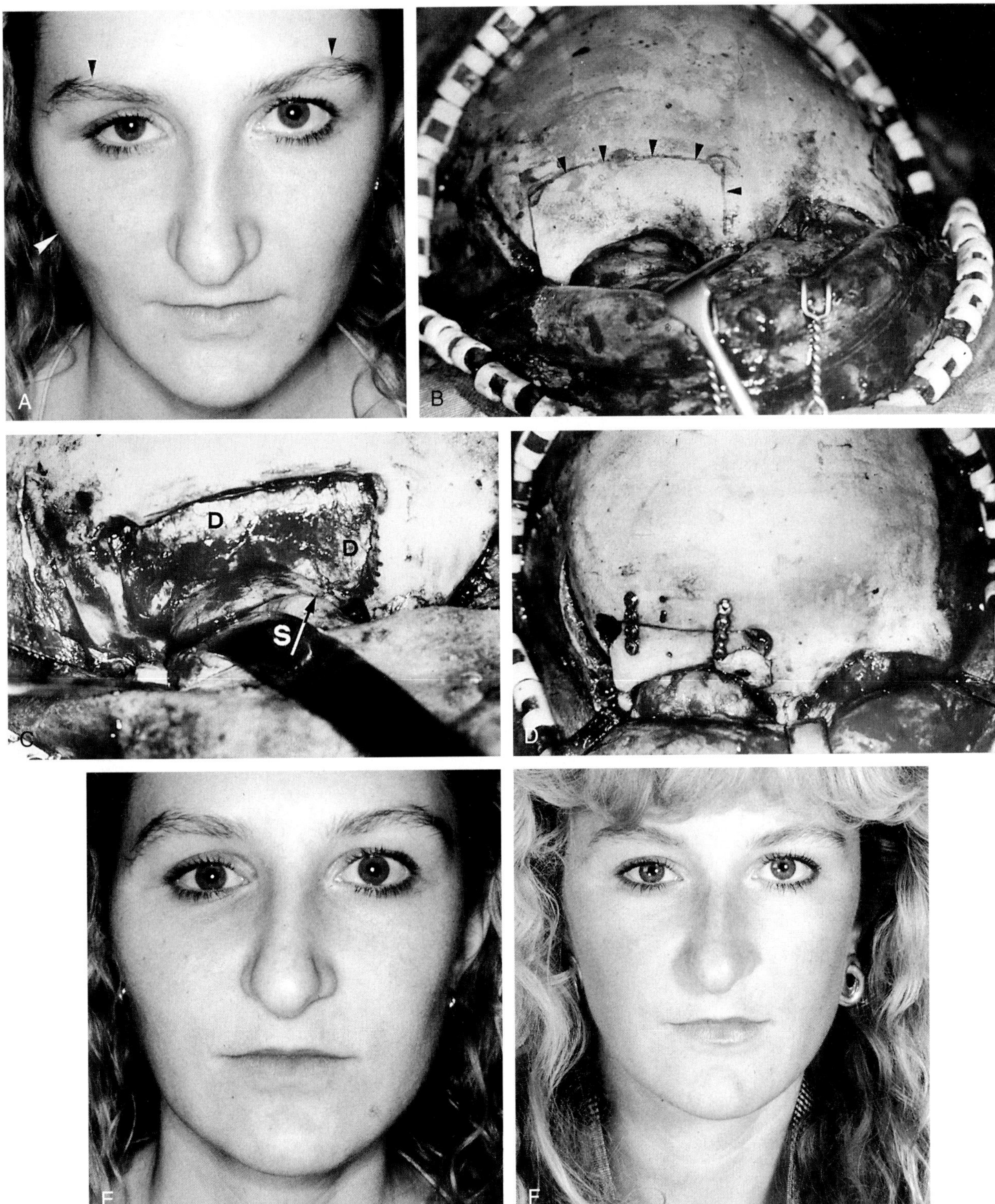

Figure 110–7. A, Asymmetry of the right fronto-orbital and zygomatic complex (*arrowheads*). B, Subcranial exposure and osteotomy (*arrowheads*) as referred to without any craniotomy-transfrontal procedure. C, Temporary removal of the upper half of the orbit revealing the dura (D). Optic nerve decompression and exposure of the skull base up to the sphenoid were performed by the subcranial access (S) (*arrow*). D, After the osteotomy of the superfluous bone, the orbital segments were fixed in the correct new location. E and F, Preoperative and postoperative views, respectively, in the same patient.

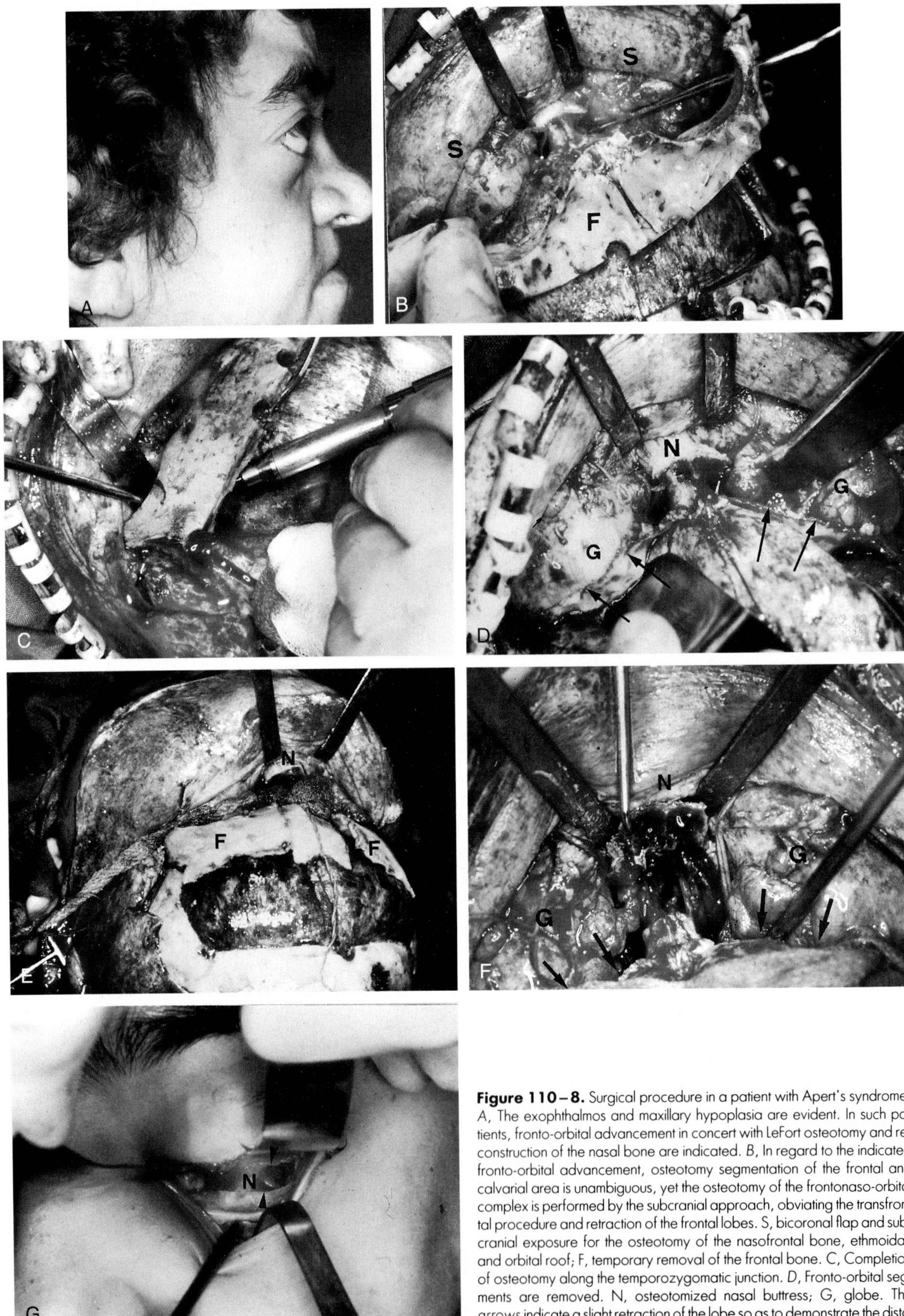

Figure 110–8. Surgical procedure in a patient with Apert's syndrome. *A*, The exophthalmos and maxillary hypoplasia are evident. In such patients, fronto-orbital advancement in concert with LeFort osteotomy and reconstruction of the nasal bone are indicated. *B*, In regard to the indicated fronto-orbital advancement, osteotomy segmentation of the frontal and calvarial area is unambiguous, yet the osteotomy of the frontonaso-orbital complex is performed by the subcranial approach, obviating the transfrontal procedure and retraction of the frontal lobes. S, bicoronal flap and subcranial exposure for the osteotomy of the nasofrontal bone, ethmoidal, and orbital roof; F, temporary removal of the frontal bone. C, Completion of osteotomy along the temporozygomatic junction. *D*, Fronto-orbital segments are removed. N, osteotomized nasal buttress; G, globe. The *arrows* indicate a slight retraction of the lobe so as to demonstrate the distal resection border of the orbital roof performed by the subcranial approach. *E*, Patient after midface advancement. N, advanced nasal buttress; F, osteotomized fronto-orbital segments. *F*, The same patient as in *E* after temporary removal of the segments with fully mobilized midface and nasal buttress. G, globes. Osteotomized distal orbital roof borders. The *arrows* indicate the subcranial access. G, Transconjunctival approach for the orbital floor osteotomy. The *arrowhead* indicates the resulting defect after anterior midface advancement to alignment with lyophilized cartilage (see text). N, intact infraorbital nerve.

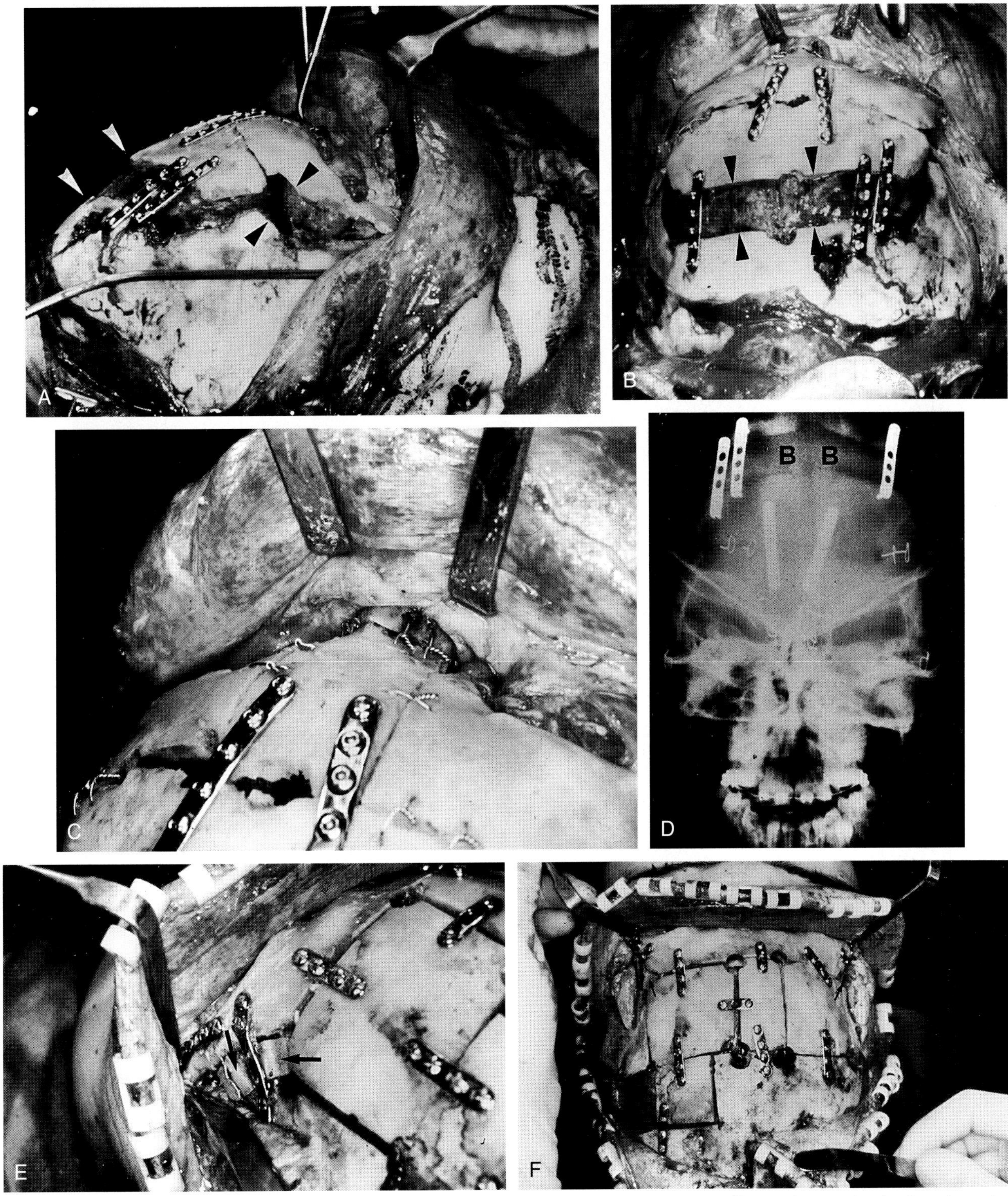

Figure 110–9. *A* and *B*, The same patient as in Figure 110–8*A* after fronto-orbital and midface advancement and fixation. The *arrowheads* indicate the resulting gap, demonstrating the degree of advancement to be bridged by bone grafts and lyophilized cartilage. C, Combined miniplate and wire ligature osteosynthesis of the frontonaso-orbital segments. *D*, Postoperative radiograph showing costal bone grafts. *E* and *F*, Midface, fronto-orbital and calvarial segment advancement, as well as external table bone grafting (*arrows*).

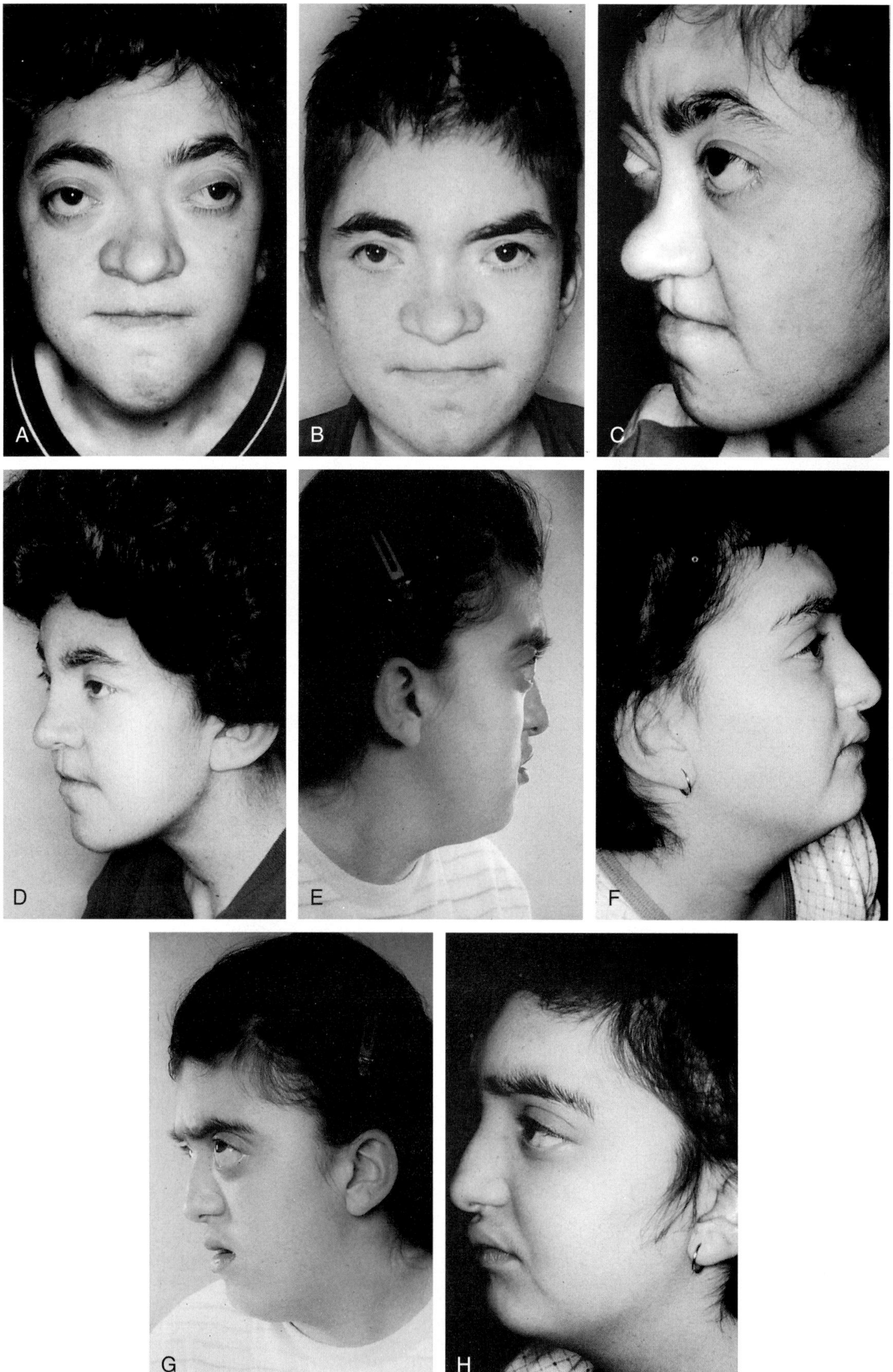

Figure 110–10. *A* to *D*, Preoperative and postoperative frontal and lateral views of the patient shown in Figure 110–8*A* to *F* illustrating the degree of midface advancement, reduction of the intercanthal distance. and correction of the exophthalmus. *E* to *H*, Preoperative and postoperative frontal and lateral views of the patient shown in Figure 110–9*E* and *F* with corrected exophthalmus and advanced midface.

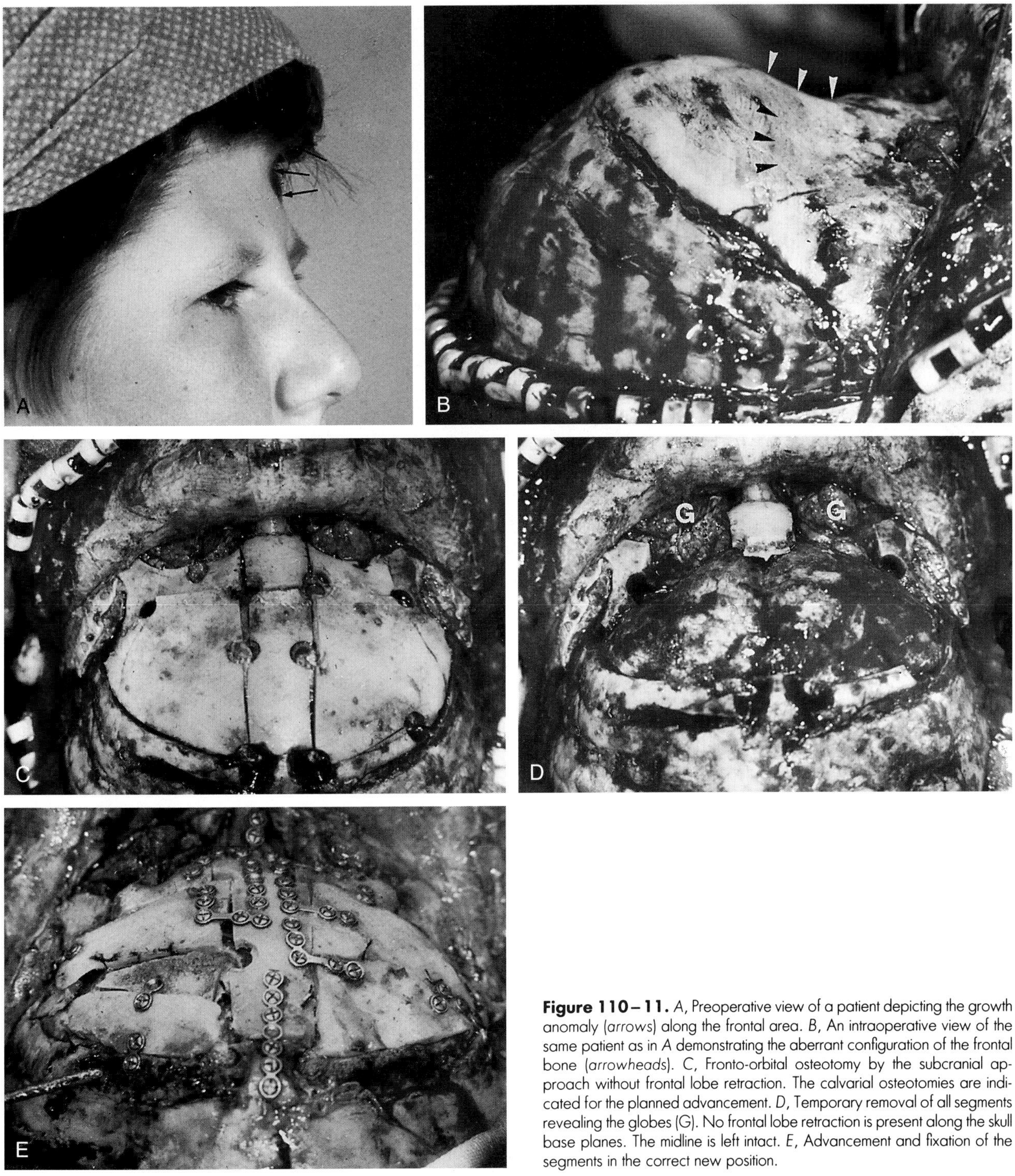

Figure 110–11. *A*, Preoperative view of a patient depicting the growth anomaly (*arrows*) along the frontal area. *B*, An intraoperative view of the same patient as in *A* demonstrating the aberrant configuration of the frontal bone (*arrowheads*). *C*, Fronto-orbital osteotomy by the subcranial approach without frontal lobe retraction. The calvarial osteotomies are indicated for the planned advancement. *D*, Temporary removal of all segments revealing the globes (G). No frontal lobe retraction is present along the skull base planes. The midline is left intact. *E*, Advancement and fixation of the segments in the correct new position.

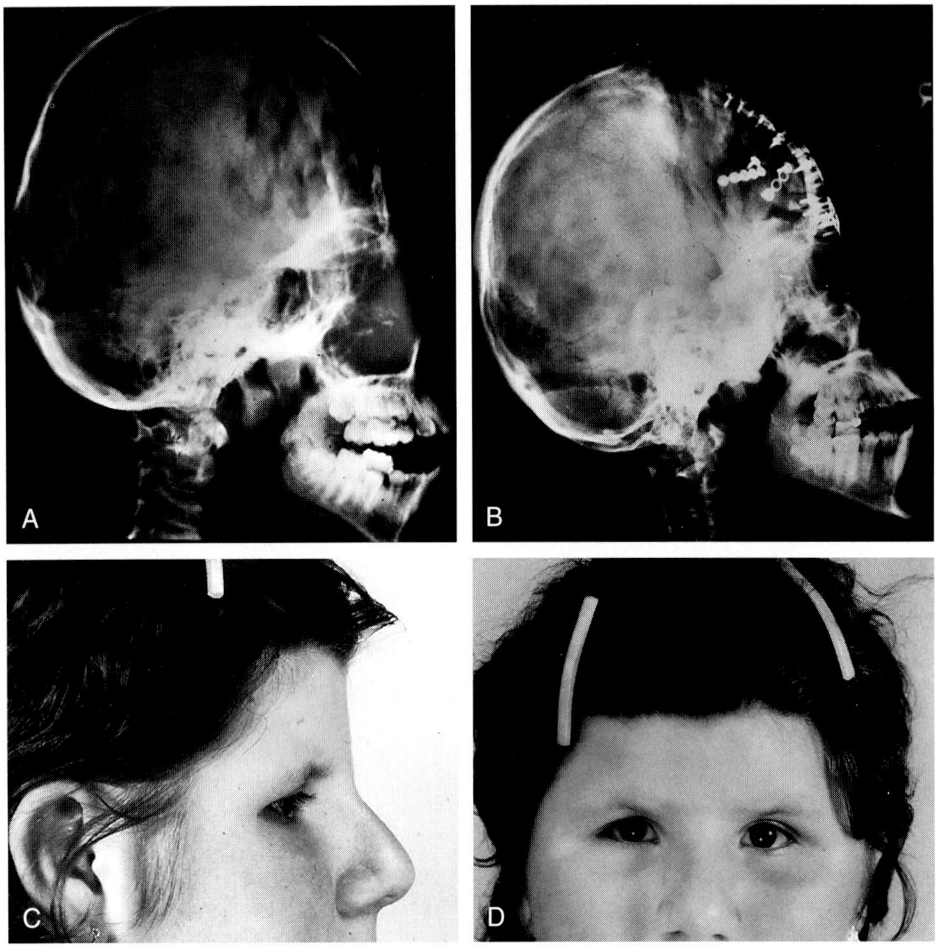

Figure 110–12. *A* and *B*, The same patient as in Figure 110–11 shown in preoperative and postoperative radiographs demonstrating the degree of advancement. *C* and *D*, A postoperative view of the patient with correct relation of the frontosupraorbital region.

TABLE 110–1

Complications After Surgical Fronto-orbital Management

Anomalies	No. of Cases	Cerebrospinal Fluid Leaks (%)	Meningitis	Mortality
Plagiocephaly, Apert's and Crouzon's syndromes	52	1.9	1.9	0
Fronto-orbital asymmetry, hypertelorism	124	2.5	0	0

TABLE 110–2

Ophthalmologic Complications After Surgical Fronto-orbital Management

Anomalies	No. of Cases	Apex Syndrome, Optic Nerve Damage (%)	Double Vision (%)	Strabismus (%)
Plagiocephaly, Apert's and Crouzon's syndromes	52	0.9	1.9	3.8
Fronto-orbital asymmetry, hypertolerism	124	0	2.4	3.2

TABLE 110–3

Complications After Surgical Fronto-orbital Management

Anomalies	No. of Cases	Sinus Dysfunction, Mucocele (%)	Insufficient Reduction of Canthal Ligament (%)	Facial Nerve Damage (%)
Plagiocephaly, Apert's and Crouzon's syndromes	52	0	5.7	0
Fronto-orbital asymmetry, hypertelorism	124	4.0	4.8	0

the osteotomy and management of the frontal region and orbitoethmoidal and sphenoidal planes, obviating the transcranial approach. This, of course, does not exclude that the dura along the frontoethmoidal and orbital roofs is not exposed; yet the brain–frontal lobe retraction is thus reduced to an absolute minimum. The major advantages are as follows:

1. Craniotomy and the transfrontal-intracranial procedure along with frontal lobe retraction for the osteotomy of the skull base planes and orbital advancement can be avoided. Even in those cases in which the osteotomy of frontal and calvarial segments has to be performed, the procedure remains the same
2. Optimal exposure for the efficient decompression of the optic nerve
3. Drainage of the subcranial compartment, apical orbital cone, avoiding postoperative development of an Apex syndrome
4. Establishment of efficient drainage of the sinuses
5. Correct placement of the canthal ligaments by the centripetal compression method
6. Watertight alignment of the dura and the subcranial compartment

The subcranial access to the frontal and skull base planes enabled reduction of the morbidity rate significantly. The reduction of postoperative cerebrospinal fluid leaks, meningitis, and optic nerve damage due to development of pressure along the orbital apex should particularly be emphasized. This access has proved to be most advantageous in all cases in which the skull base and orbital roof have to be exposed.

REFERENCES

1. Derome PJ, Tessier P: Craniofacial reconstruction in patients with craniofacial malformations: The neurosurgical approach. Clin Neurosurg 24:642, 1977.
2. Lejoyeux E, Tulsane JF, Tessier PL: Maxillary growth following total septal resection in correction of orbital hypertelorism. *In* Marsh JL (ed): Long-Term Results in Craniofacial Surgery. Burlington, Ontario, BC Decker, 1986, p 27.
3. Maillard GF, Montandon D, Goin JL: Die Kraniofaziale Chirurgie, vol. 1. Hexagon "Roche." Basel, Switzerland, Roche, 1986.
4. Murray JE, Swanson LT, Strand RD, Hricko GM: Reconstructive surgery for major craniofacial deformities. Surg Clin North Am 56:495, 1976.
5. Tessier P, Guiot G, Rougerie J: Ostéotomies cranio-naso-orbito-faciales: Hypertélorisme. Ann Chir Plast 12:103, 1967.
6. Van der Meulen JCH, Vaandrager JM: Surgery related to the correction of hypertelorism. Plast Reconstr Surg 71:6–19, 1983.
7. Anderl H, Mühlbauer W, Twerdy K, et al: Craniofaciale Chirurgie. Klin Monatsbl Augenheilkd 181:331, 1986.
8. Atkinson L, Emmet A, Pabari M: Craniofacial surgery. Med J Aust 1:541, 1979.
9. David D, Poswillo D, Simpson D: The craniosynostoses: Causes, natural history and management. *In* David D (ed): Die Craniosynostosen. Berlin, Springer, 1982.
10. Freihofer HP: Results of osteotomies of the facial skeleton in adolescence. J Maxillofac Surg 5:276, 1977.
11. Goldin H, Hockley A, Wake M, Beasley J: Craniofacial surgery. Br J Hosp Med 35:368, 1986.
12. Obwegeser HL, Farmand M: Hypertelorism associated with other facial anomalies. *In* Caronni EP (ed): Craniofacial Surgery. Boston, Little, Brown & Co, 1985, p 166.
13. Ortiz-Monaterio F, Fuente-del-Campo A: Nasal correction in hyperteleorbitism. Scand J Plast Reconstr Surg 15:277, 1981.
14. Benedetti A, Curioni C, Rubini L: Combined maxillofacial and neurological surgery for the correction of teleorbitism. J Neurosurg Sci 23:47, 1979.
15. Caronni EP: Early correction of some orbital anomalies. *In* Caronni EP (ed): Craniofacial Surgery. Boston, Little, Brown & Co, 1985, p 163.
16. Converse JM, Ransohoff J, Mathews E, et al: Ocular hypertelorism and pseudohypertelorism. Plast Reconstr Surg 45:1, 1970.
17. Converse JM, McCarthy JG: Orbital hypertelorism. Scand J Plast Reconstr Surg 15:265, 1981.
18. Epstein FJ, Wood-Smith D, Converse JM, et al: Radical one-stage correction of craniofacial anomalies. J Neurosurg 42:522, 1975.
19. Furnas DW, DeFeo DR, Kusske JA: Glabellar osteotomy and orbital craniotomies with microscopic control for correction of hypertelorism: A preliminary report of microcraniofacial surgery in two patients. Plast Reconstr Surg 70:51, 1982.
20. Jackson IT: The wide world of craniofacial surgery. J Oral Maxillofac Surg 41:103, 1983.
21. Matthews D: Craniofacial surgery: Indications, assessment and complications. Br J Plast Surg 32:96, 1979.
22. Munro IR: Craniofacial surgical techniques for aesthetic results in congenital and acute traumatic deformities. Clin Plast Surg 8:303, 1981.
23. Pruzansky S: Craniofacial surgery: The experiment on nature's experiment: Review of three patients operated by Paul Tessier. Eur J Orthod 4:151, 1982.
24. Raveh J, Kaiser G: Die kraniofaziale Chirurgie: Vorteile der Transethmoidalen radikalen Ethmoidresektion. Ther Umsch 43:844, 1986.
25. Raveh J, Vuillemin T: The surgical one-stage management of combined cranio-maxillofacial and frontobasal fractures: Advantage of the subcranial approach in 374 cases. J Craniomaxillofac Surg 16:160, 1988.
26. Raveh J, Redli M, Markwalder T. Operative management of 194 cases of combined maxillofacial-frontobasal fractures: Principles and modification. J Oral Maxillofac Surg 42:555, 1984.
27. Gruss JS: Fronto-naso-orbital trauma. Clin Plast Surg 9:577, 1982.
28. Escher F: Ein Beitrag zur Versorgung frontobasaler Hirnverletzungen. ORL J Otolaryngol Relat Spec 6:326, 1944.
29. Escher F: Die frontobasalen Schädelverletzungen. Schweiz Med Wochenschr 90:1481, 1960.
30. Escher F: Clinical classification and treatment of the frontobasal fractures. *In* Nobel Symposium, Stockholm, 1968, Vol 10, Disorders of the Skull Base Region. Stockholm, Almqvist and Wiksell International, 1969, p 343.
31. Fukado Y: Diagnosis and surgical correction of optic canal fracture after head injury. Ophthalmologica (Suppl) 00:307, 1969.
32. Fukado Y: Results in 400 cases of surgical decompression of the optic nerve. *In* Proceedings of the Second International Symposium in Orbital Disorders, vol 14. 1973, p 474.
33. Fukado Y, Nagai M: A five-year review of ocular injuries. Acta Soc Ophthalmol Jpn 22:70, 1971.
34. Kennerdell JS, Ambaugh GA, Myers EN: Transantral ethmoidal decompression of optic nerve fractures. Arch Ophthalmol 94:1040, 1976.
35. Habal MB, Maniscalco JE, Rhoton AL: Microsurgical anatomy of the optic canal: Observations on the anatomical relations and exposure of the optic nerve. Surg Forum 25:542, 1976.
36. Habal MB: Clinical observations on the isolated optic nerve injury. Ann Plast Surg 6:603, 1978.

CHAPTER 111

Diagnostic and Presurgical Evaluation of Congenital Craniofacial Anomalies

Jay M. Pensler

Diagnosis of a congenital craniofacial abnormality is predicated on an understanding of normal physiology. Normal craniofacial growth is a differential developmental process. A delicate and continuous balance is achieved between resorption of old bone and deposition of new bone. The initial growth of the craniofacial region is spurred to a large extent by the push of the underlying brain. The normal brain grows at an astounding rate during the first several years of life. During the first year of life 60% of the adult volume is achieved. Furthermore, by 3 years of age 80% of the adult volume is attained.

Virchow,[1] in 1859, observed that growth occurs in the cranial vault at right angles to the sutures. He postulated that cranial deformities could be explained by growth inhibition at right angles to a fused suture with compensatory overexpansion of the cranium at the patent (noninvolved) suture sites. Abnormal growth that occurs in response to fusion of a cranial vault suture involves both the bone and soft tissue components of the face.[2–5]

Since virtually any portion of the craniofacial complex may be involved by an acquired or congenital process, the team assembled to evaluate these patients should contain appropriate expertise to ensure experienced evaluation of each patient's problems. The multidisciplinary team should include an anesthesiologist, audiologist, geneticist, neurologist, neuroradiologist, neurosurgeon, ophthalmologist, orthodontist, otolaryngologist, pediatrician, plastic surgeon, speech pathologist, and social worker.

After initial evaluation of the patient by appropriate members of the team the specific findings are reviewed and a detailed treatment plan that should encompass treatment through skeletal maturity of the patient is formulated. This initial plan is communicated to the parents and patient (depending on the individual's age). The initial plan may be revised in future years depending on the outcome of specific surgical interventions or growth and development of the individual. In fact, the long-term treatment plan should be viewed as a dynamic process that is critically reevaluated after each clinical visit.

SPECIFIC BONY ABNORMALITIES

Sagittal Synostosis

Premature closure of the sagittal suture results in elongation of the anteroposterior diameter of the skull and narrowing of the width or biparietal diameter of the skull. As Virchow predicted, growth appears to be inhibited at right angles to the sagittal suture and compensatory growth occurs parallel to the suture.[1]

The result of premature fusion of the sagittal sutures is termed *scaphocephaly* or *dolichocephaly*. In contrast to other types of simple craniosynostoses, sagittal synostosis initially results in minor secondary changes to the anterior portion of the cranium and orbits.

The diagnosis should be made on the basis of clinical examination of an elongated and narrowed cranium (Fig. 111–1). The diagnosis is then confirmed using skull radiographs or computed tomographic (CT) scan. The CT scan, in addition to identifying closure of the sagittal suture, may be required to identify the underlying pathology of the ventricles or brain when suspected preoperatively. Surgery is performed at 6 to 12 weeks of age. The frontal bossing that is present initially resolves over 4 to 8 weeks postoperatively. Isolated fusion of the sagittal suture results in minimal early changes of the frontal bone and orbits. The changes observed in the neonatal period tend to resolve postoperatively in the overwhelming majority of patients. Patients with scaphocephaly require only an extensive median strip craniectomy with lateral extensions if surgery is performed at several months of age. We have not found it necessary to require an extensive preoperative ophthalmologic examination if normal vision, extraocular movement, and ocular position are noted.

If the initial diagnosis of premature fusion of the sagittal suture is delayed until after 1 year of age, the cranial base has become fixed and, consequently, the frontal bossing has become more severe and the decreased width of the skull is more noticeable (see Fig. 111–1). The delayed diagnosis alters the treatment from an operation in

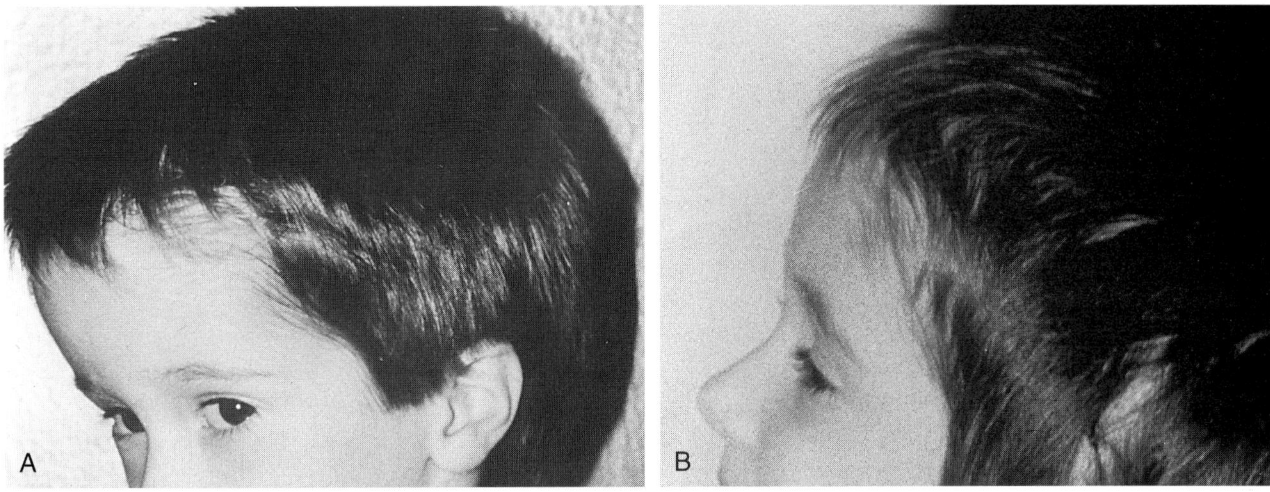

Figure 111 – 1. *A*, Five-year-old boy with isolated fusion of the sagittal suture. Note the elongated and narrowed appearance of cranium. *B*, Postoperative result after 1 year.

which a strip craniectomy may be performed into one in which the majority of the cranium must be removed and reshaped. It should be noted that in cases of delayed diagnosis of sagittal synostosis the orbits still retain a normal appearance and position. The surgery is confined to the cranium above the supraorbital bar (Fig. 111 – 2).

Unilateral Coronal Synostosis

Premature closure of the coronal suture unilaterally frequently occurs in utero. The premature fusion results in an asymmetric configuration of the calvaria termed *plagiocephaly*, which is derived from the Greek *plagios* (oblique) and *kefali* (head). The deformity is detectable in the neonate and worsens progressively throughout infancy and childhood if untreated.

A constellation of bony and soft tissue abnormalities may be noted in patients with plagiocephaly secondary to premature unilateral coronal synostosis.[2, 3] Skeletal malformations consist of underdevelopment and flattening of the forehead on the side of the premature synostosis along with elevation and posterolateral angling of the ipsilateral supraorbital rim. This elevation of the ipsilateral supraorbital rim and sphenoid may easily be appreciated on plain radiographs. The resultant characteristic appearance has been termed a *devil's eye* (Fig. 111 – 3). The sagittal suture is deviated toward the synostosed side as are the nasoethmoid junction, the root of the nose, the posterior cranial fossa, and the foramen magnum. The parietal bone is flattened on the involved side. The orbit is elevated along with the lesser wing of the sphenoid on the involved side. The posterior fossa on the side of the synostosis is deepened, and the petrus ridge is depressed. Associated findings may include depression of the temporomandibular fossa, shortening of the anterior cranial fossa, enlargement of the middle cranial fossa, and thinning of the parietal bone. Soft tissue changes in patients with premature fusion of the coronal suture include protrusion of the anthelix and helical rim on the side of the synostosis, elevation of the ipsilateral brow, and medial canthal dystopia (see Fig. 111 – 3).[2–62]

We have noted that the majority of patients with premature unilateral coronal synostosis exhibit preoperative abnormal ocular findings. These have ranged from visual abnormalities, such as amblyopia or nystagmus to problems with refraction and strabismus. Strabismus is the most common presentation of extraocular muscle dysfunction preoperatively in patients with plagiocephaly. Since 1985 we have noted strabismus in 66% of patients seen with this disorder. The superior oblique on the side of premature fusion may exhibit a paresis in up to half of the patients with strabismus.

Because patients with premature fusion of the unilateral coronal suture exhibit a staggering percentage of ophthalmologic complications it becomes paramount to distinguish this type of plagiocephaly from a commonly observed variant, deformational plagiocephaly, in which there is no synostosis of the coronal suture. Patients with deformational plagiocephaly may exhibit a large number of skeletal and soft tissue deformities similar to those found in patients with premature unilateral coronal synostosis, such as muscular torticollis, unequal ear size, flattening of the forehead, and epicanthal folds. Early distinction of the type of plagiocephaly is important since the treatment of these two entities is quite different.[2, 3, 46, 52, 56, 57] We have identified several clinical features that enable one to easily delineate between patients with premature synostosis of the coronal suture and

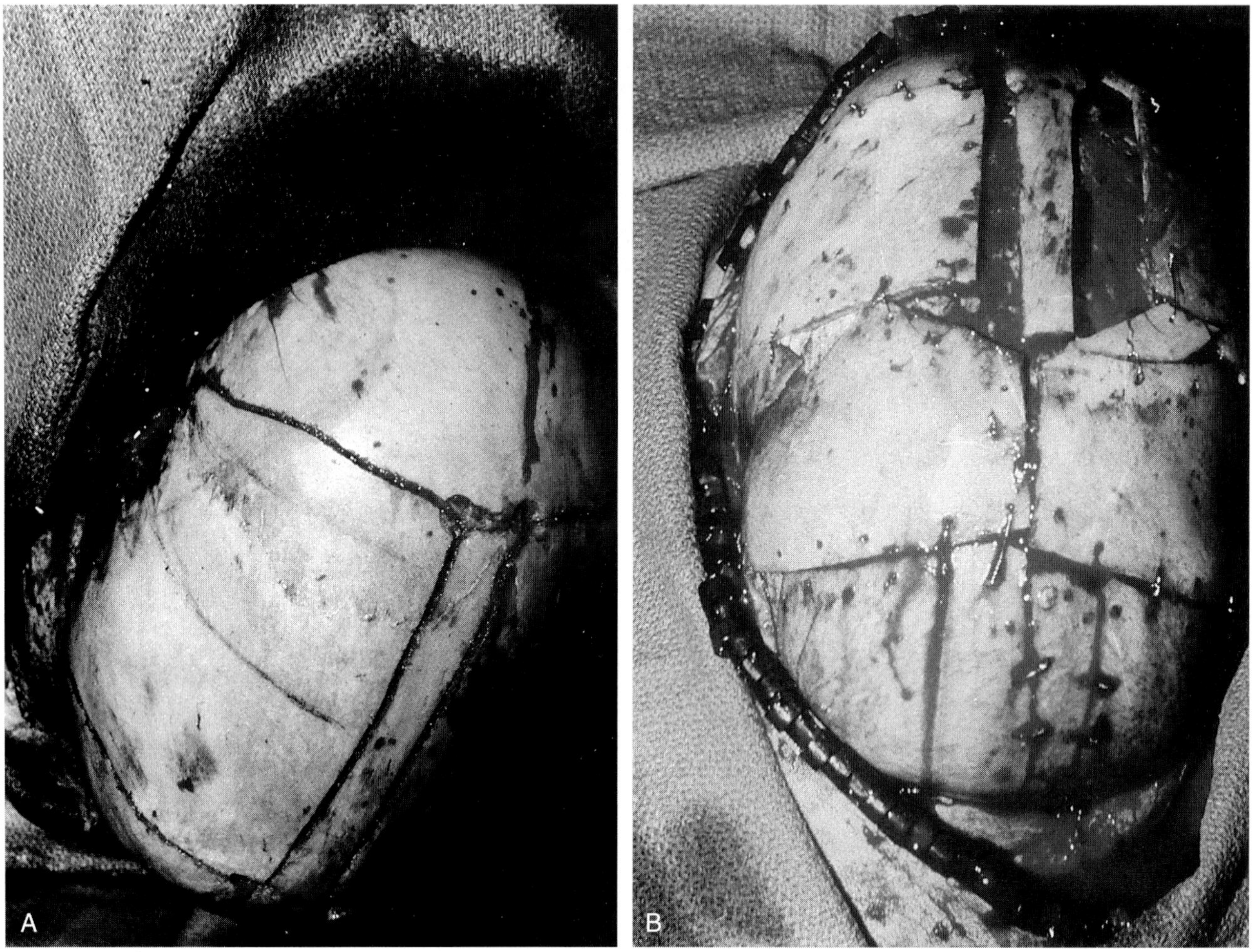

Figure 111–2. *A*, Postoperative view of the patient shown in Figure 111–1 after surgical repositioning of the bony cranium. *B*, Note increased width and decreased length of the cranium after manipulation.

those with a patent suture and cranial deformation (deformational plagiocephaly). Patients with unilateral coronal synostosis exhibit flattening of the ipsilateral supraorbital rim but projection of the ipsilateral infraorbital rim anterior to the coronal plane of the ipsilateral supraorbital rim and the contralateral maxilla. This was distinctly different from what we observed in a group of sex- and age-matched patients with the deformational variant of plagiocephaly who exhibited frontal bone and infraorbital rim flattening on the side of the deformation.[2] The key to diagnosis of this entity therefore rests with the position of the ipsilateral infraorbital rim. In patients with premature synostosis of the coronal suture it is displaced anteriorly on the involved side, and in patients with the deformational variant of plagiocephaly the rim is displaced posteriorly on the involved side.

Patients with premature fusion of the coronal suture undergo surgical release of the suture and advancement of the frontal bone and supraorbital bar. In addition, these patients have the orbital roof and parietal region reshaped and repositioned. The bony surgery optimally occurs between 5 and 7 months of age. Patients with deformational plagiocephaly usually do not require surgery of the frontal bone or bony orbit. These patients are treated with repositioning the patient, keeping weight off the retrodisplaced region. One method that is very effective is to use shock blocks on one side of the individual's crib.

Brachycephaly

Patients with premature bilateral coronal synostosis develop brachycephaly. Half of the children with brachycephaly do not have synostosis of another type of suture.[31–34] Plain skull radiographs may demonstrate absence of the coronal suture; however, the anteroposterior view will invariably demonstrate the bilateral harlequin eye deformity.[34, 40, 43, 45] The patients exhibit retrusion of the supraorbital rims, a shortened anterior cranial fossa,

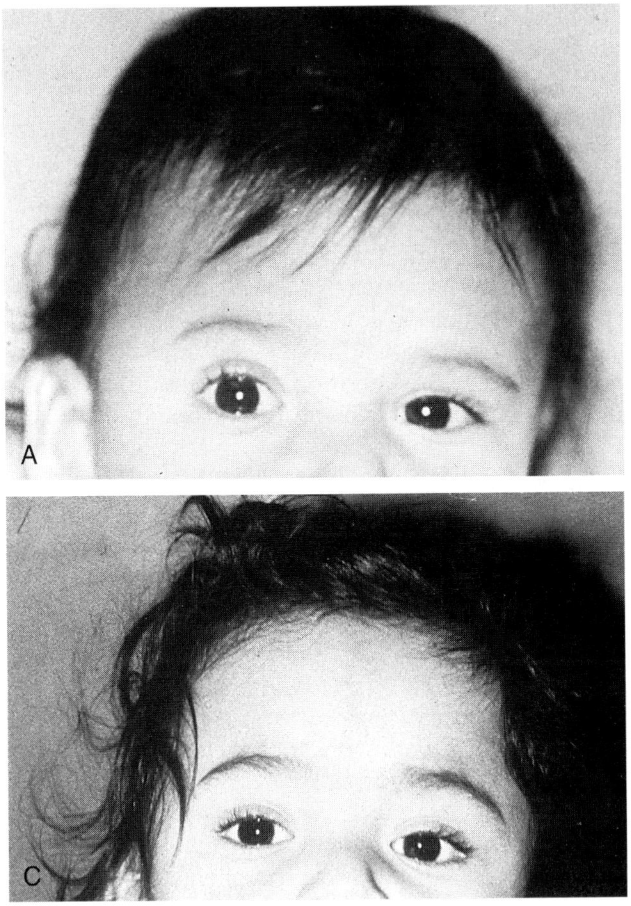

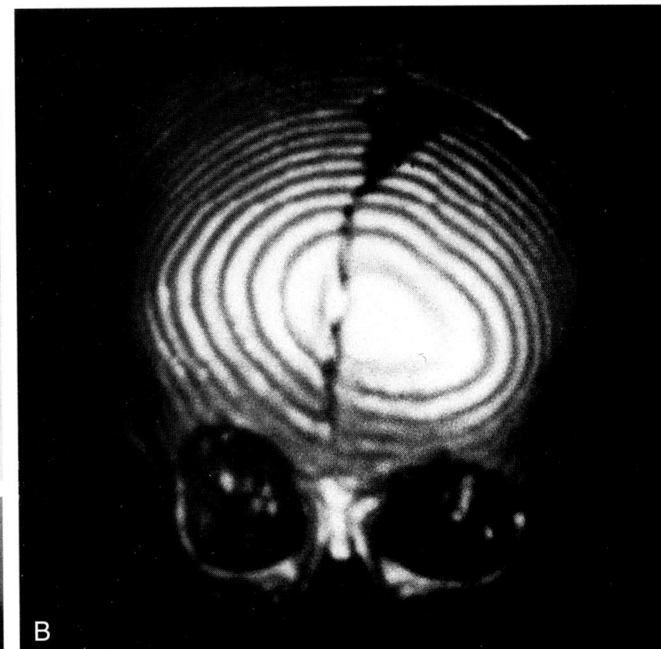

Figure 111–3. *A*, Six-month-old infant with premature fusion of the right coronal suture. Note the flattened right forehead and the elevation of the right supraorbital rim. *B*, A three-dimensional computed tomographic scan that illustrates the right "devil's eye deformity." Note the retrusion of the right supraorbital rim and frontal bone. *C*, Postoperative result at 18 months.

anterior bossing, and varying degrees of exorbitism (Fig. 111–4). Brachycephaly may be associated with other craniofacial anomalies, such as Apert's syndrome (in which case there is acrosyndactyly), or with a complete complex syndactyly of the hands and feet, or it may be an isolated finding. There is also severe retrusion of the middle third of the face exaggerating the tendency toward exorbitism (Fig. 111–5). In the most severe cases the lids may retract posteriorly to the globes. If retraction of the lids occurs, the lids may be manually repositioned anteriorly.

The immediate concern on evaluation of a patient with brachycephaly is corneal ulceration that may result from exposure. Ophthalmologic assessment should include identification of the presence of corneal ulceration and appropriate lubrication before skeletal repositioning.

Patients with Crouzon's or Apert's syndrome who present with brachycephaly also have retrusion of the midface and accompanying exorbitism due to the shallow orbits (Fig. 111–6). Divergent strabismus and a mild hypertelorism are often associated with these syndromes. The maxillary arch may be constricted, and the upper airway is often impeded by the reduced size of the dental arch and retropositioning of the maxilla. We prefer to defer any surgical correction involving the extraocular musculature until after the frontal bone and supraorbital region have been advanced, which is performed at 6 to 8 months of age. The maxilla is surgically repositioned, usually when the patient reaches mixed dentition (age 6 to 7 years). We prefer to intervene to correct the extraocular muscle pathology in the time window between the two bony procedures. Because the frontal orbital advancement relieves a portion of the exorbitism by expanding the superior half of the orbital volume the patients should be reexamined for possible corneal ulceration after frontal orbital advancement. If severe exorbitism is present, this may be reduced by either earlier frontal orbital advancement or midface advancement. The risk associated with earlier surgery for frontal bone or maxillary advancement is the possible requirement for repetition of the operation.

Trigonocephaly

The metopic suture is normally open until age 2. It then gradually becomes obliterated over the next several years. In approximately 10% of the population the metopic suture may remain patent throughout life. Prema-

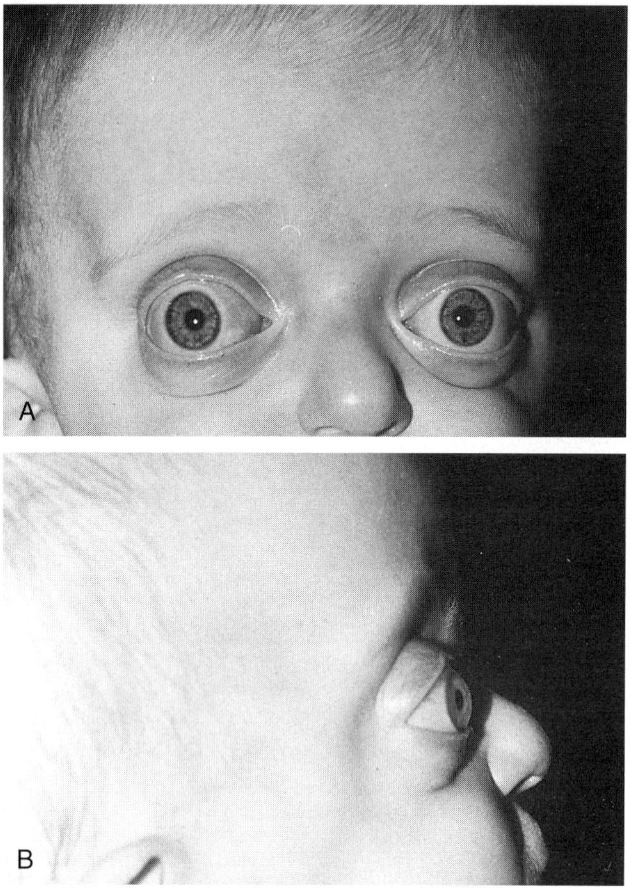

Figure 111–4. *A* and *B*, Patient with isolated bilateral fusion of the coronal sutures. Note the extreme exorbitism.

ture closure of the metopic suture results in trigonocephaly, in which there is a keel-shaped deformity of the frontal bone (Fig. 111–7). The patients exhibit varying degrees of hypotelorism and may often exhibit strabismus. CT scan demonstrates ethmoidal sinuses that are hypoplastic and an intact crista galli. The medial walls of the orbit tend to be thickened, which results in the orbits being highest medially, often slanting as they proceed inferiorly and laterally.[34]

Orbital hypotelorism may also be seen in holoprosencephaly. Holoprosencephaly may be associated with a midline cleft of the lip, palate, or both. If any of the variants of holoprosencephaly are suspected, a CT scan should be performed to identify the anatomy of the brain.

Although patients with premature metopic synostosis exhibit orbital hypertelorism preoperatively, this improves markedly postoperatively after repositioning the frontal bone and supraorbital ridge at 6 months of age. Extraocular muscle imbalances that are present in over half of the children are reevaluated after the bony correction of the deformity. Since 40% of my patients have exhibited a discernible change in muscle balance postoperatively I believe that any effort to improve the muscular balance should be deferred until after the bony repositioning is complete. The repositioning of the frontal bone and supraorbital rim is usually performed at 5 to 7 months of age.

Lambdoidal Synostosis

Lambdoidal synostosis may also result in plagiocephaly. There is flattening of the skull posteriorly, but this may result in bulging anteriorly. This may give the clinician the false impression of premature closure of the coronal suture, but the position of the infraorbital rim on the retruded side should delineate the etiology. A CT scan should be performed. Patients with lambdoidal synostosis have not been found to have a significantly increased incidence of ocular abnormalities.

Multiple Suture Synostosis

A combination of the sutures may be closed at birth. This results in a cloverleaf skull also termed *Kleeblatt-Schaedel.* These patients with multiple synostosis exhibit an unforgettable deformation of the cranial vault (Fig. 111–8). Any number of the sutures may be involved, and the deformity may present as an isolated problem or in association with a syndrome (i.e., Apert's, Crouzon's, or Carpenter's syndrome). Hydrocephalus is often associated with this deformity, and, as with the other types of multiple cranial synostoses, its presence should be evaluated through a preoperative CT scan. These patients are at risk for development of significantly increased intracranial pressure and may exhibit papilledema, decreased vision, or both on initial examination. Problems with extraocular muscles are common in these patients since a majority (70%) will exhibit some extraocular imbalance before the first surgical correction of the bony abnormality, which typically occurs at 6 weeks of age to release the constriction resulting from closure of the sagittal suture. A second operation to address the frontal bone deformation characteristically occurs at 6 months of age. Any correction of extraocular muscle imbalance should be deferred until completion of the fronto-orbital repositioning since, as noted in previous types of craniosynostosis, the preoperative extraocular imbalance may exhibit improvement or deterioration of the muscle balance postoperatively.

Preoperative Evaluation in Patients with Craniofacial Deformities

Preoperative evaluation should begin with a detailed history since it is important to establish any genetic connection between members of the family who have been similarly affected. Physical examination should include observation and palpation of the entire cranium and

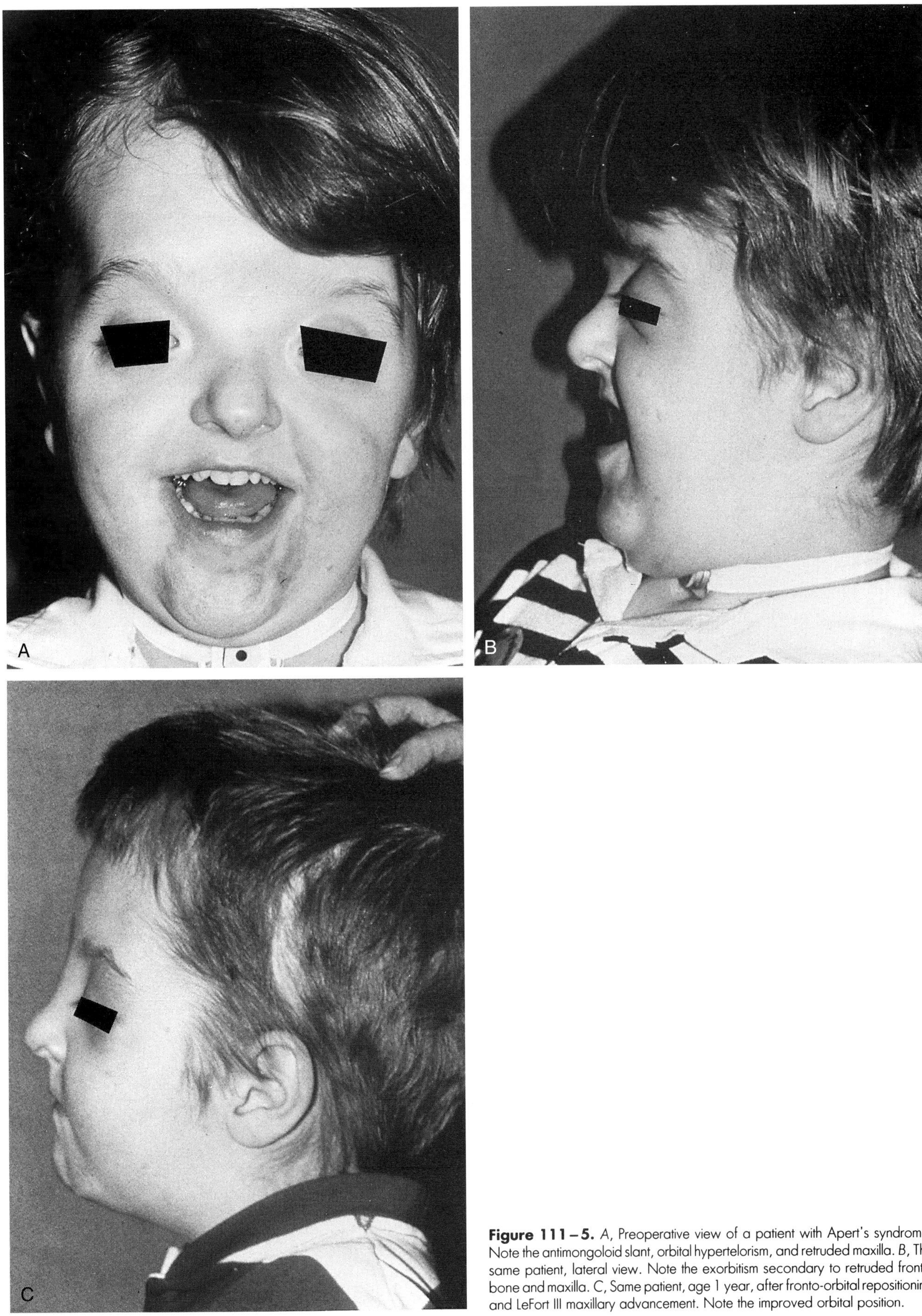

Figure 111–5. *A*, Preoperative view of a patient with Apert's syndrome. Note the antimongoloid slant, orbital hypertelorism, and retruded maxilla. *B*, The same patient, lateral view. Note the exorbitism secondary to retruded frontal bone and maxilla. C, Same patient, age 1 year, after fronto-orbital repositioning and LeFort III maxillary advancement. Note the improved orbital position.

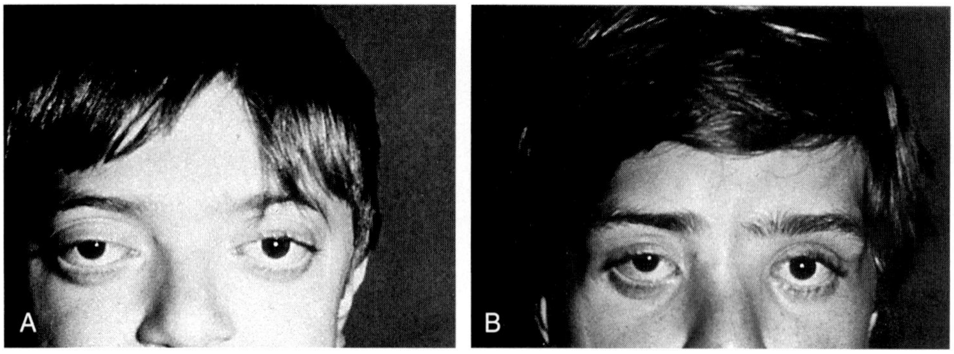

Figure 111–6. *A* and *B*, Patient with Crouzon's syndrome. Note the exorbitism and strabismus before repositioning of the frontal bone and maxilla and improved orbital position (*A*) subsequent to LeFort III and frontal bone repositioning.

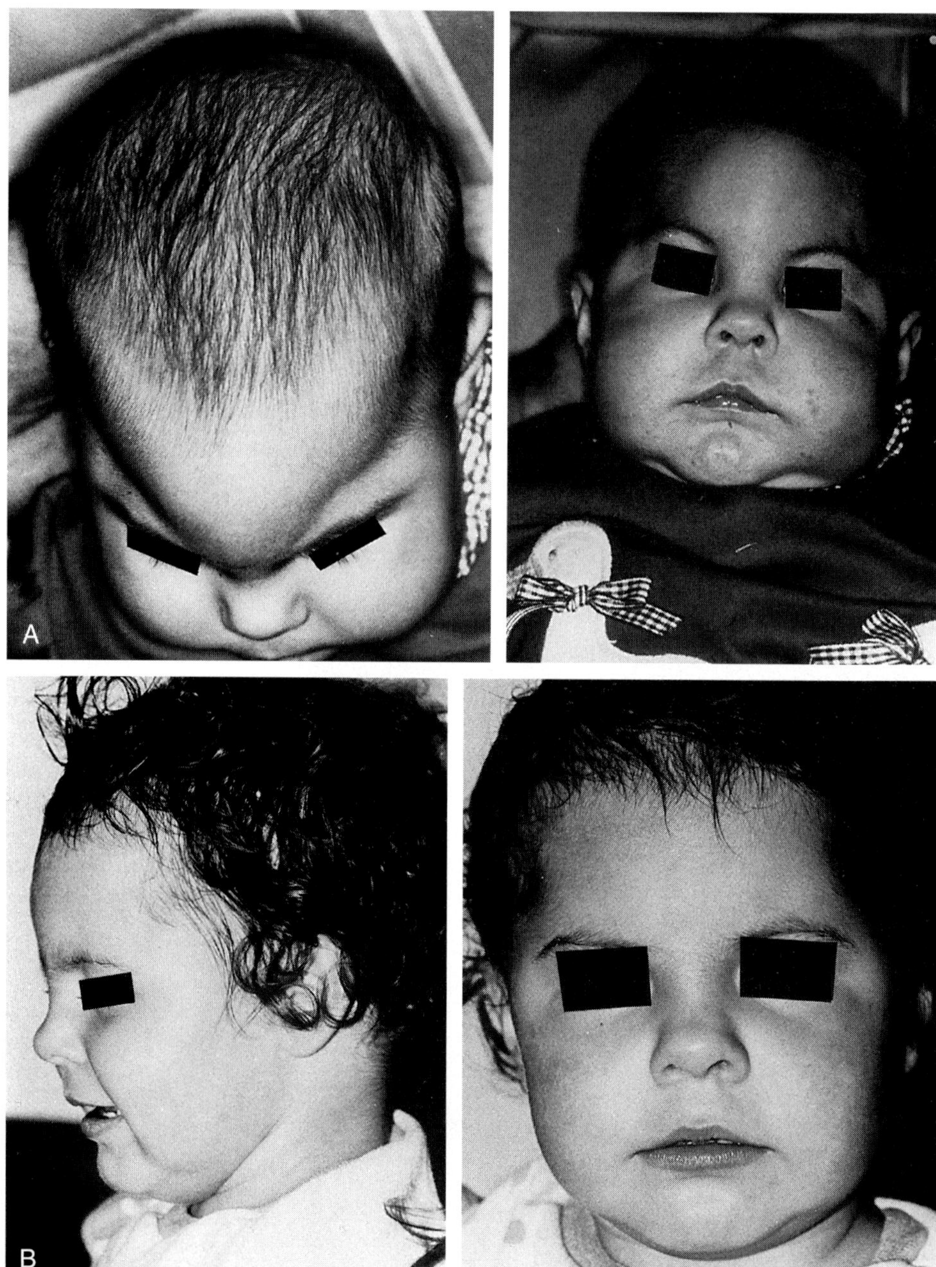

Figure 111–7. *A*, Two views of a patient with premature closure of the metopic suture at 6 months of age. Note the hypotelorism and deformation of the frontal bone. *B*, Lateral and frontal views show result at 4 years after supraorbital repositioning and frontal bone development.

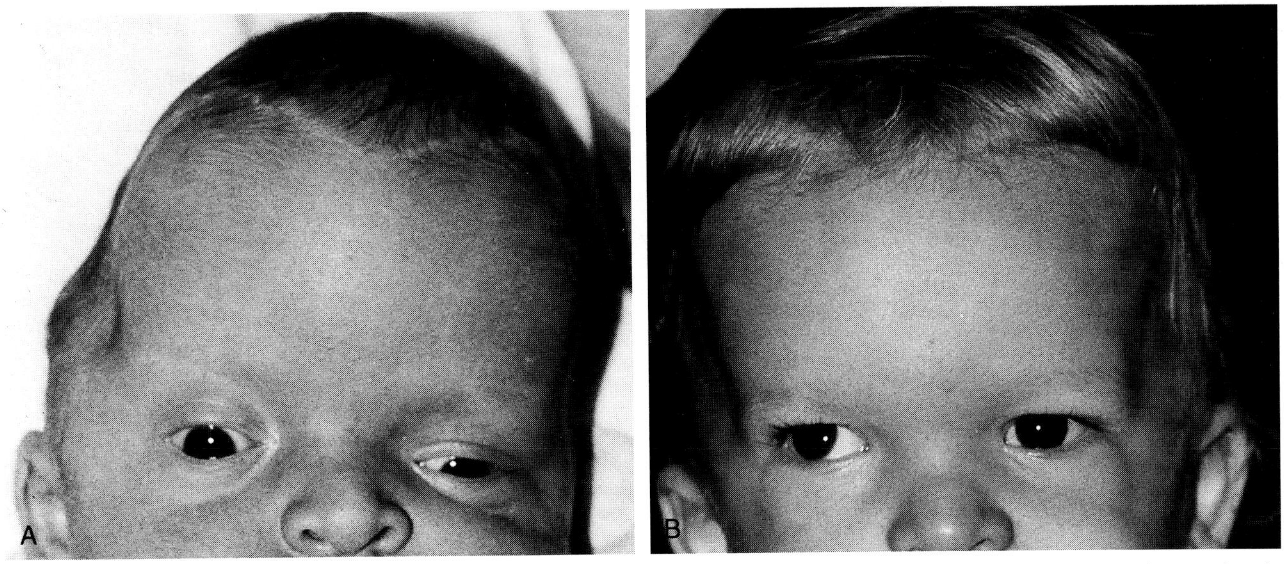

Figure 111-8. *A*, Patient with premature closure of multiple cranial vault suture. *B*, The same patient after cranial vault repositioning. Note the strabismus in the right eye.

face. All abnormalities, regardless of their relative importance, should be noted. A detailed ophthalmologic examination is routinely performed. This should include examination of visual acuity and ocular motility, evaluation of pupil size, and slit lamp and dilated funduscopic examination. Since elevated intracranial pressure or hydrocephalus has been reported in as many as 13% of patients with multiple cranial stenoses, radiologic examination should be performed before any surgical intervention in this group. I routinely obtain a CT scan in all cases except those of simple isolated sagittal synostosis. CT scan is performed preoperatively to assess the status of the brain and to define the bony anatomy. Newer three-dimensional re-formations have enabled one to more clearly visualize the sutures and assess their patency. Both axial and coronal views should be obtained on CT scans for optimal definition of orbital anatomy and position.

Determination of the severity of enophthalmos or exorbitism should be performed in all patients routinely and the preoperative plan adjusted to compensate for any abnormalities that are present. The position of the medial and lateral canthal tendons should be ascertained, and the long-term treatment plan should be designed to incorporate repositioning of these tendons as needed.

The definitive treatment plan should represent an attempt to encompass all of the individual's problems—medical, psychological, and social—and it should be well defined but adjusted on an ongoing basis. The order of treatment of the respective problems should be organized so that previous treatments will not be affected in a deleterious manner. Teams treating patients with craniofacial disorders must remember that the overwhelming majority of these patients exhibit ocular abnormalities. Surgical manipulation of the bony components of the orbit will effect changes in the extraocular balance in approximately 25% of patients. Therefore, bony manipulation of the craniofacial skeleton will, in general, precede correction of extraocular muscle imbalances. Above all, the final result should represent the coordinated input of appropriate members of the treatment team.

REFERENCES

1. Virchow R: Knochenwachstrum und Schaedelformen mit besonderer Rucksicht auf Cretinismus. Virchow's Arch (Pathol Anat) 13:323, 1859.
2. Loomis MG, Radkowski MA, Pensler JM: Maxillary deformation in unilateral coronal synostosis. J Craniofacial Surg 1:73-76, 1990.
3. Bruneteau RJ, Mulliken JB: Frontal plagiocephaly: Synostotic, compensational, or deformational. Plast Reconstr Surg 89:21-31, 1992.
4. Aase J: Structural defects as a consequence of late intrauterine constraint: Craniotabes, loose skin, and asymmetric ear size. Semin Perinatol 7:270-273, 1983.
5. Clarren SK: Plagiocephaly and torticollis: Etiology, history and helmet treatment. J Pediatr 98:92-95, 1981.
6. Clarren SK, Smith DW, Hanson JW: Helmet treatment for plagiocephaly and congenital muscular torticollis. J Pediatr 94:43-46, 1979.
7. Connor J, Conner A, Connor R, et al: Genetic aspects of early childhood scoliosis. Am J Med Genet 27:419-421, 1987.
8. David DJ, Poswillo D, Simpson D (eds): The Craniosynostoses: Causes, Natural History and Management. New York, Springer-Verlag, 1982.
9. Dunn PM: Congenital sternomastoid torticollis: An intrauterine postural deformity. Arch Dis Child 49:824-825, 1974.
10. Graham J: Alterations in head shape as a consequence of fetal head constraint. Semin Perinatol 7:257-269, 1983.
11. Jones M: Unilateral epicanthal fold: Diagnostic significance. J Pediatr 108:702-704, 1986.
12. Kreiborg S: Craniofacial growth in plagiocephaly and Crouzon's syndrome. Scand J Plast Reconstr Surg 15:187-197, 1981.
13. Kreiborg S, Pruzansky S: Craniofacial growth in premature craniofacial synostosis. Scand J Plast Reconstr Surg 15:171-186, 1981.
14. Marchac D: Radical forehead remodeling for craniostenosis. Plast Reconstr Surg 61:823-835, 1978.
15. Marsh JL, Vannier MW: Comprehensive Care for Craniofacial Deformities. St. Louis, CV Mosby, 1985, p 135.

16. Editorial: Plagiocephaly and torticollis in young infants. Lancet 2:789–790, 1986.
17. Poole M, Briggs M, Rayne J, Cheng H: Craniofacial surgery. Br Med J 290:693–696, 1985.
18. Renier D, Sainte-Rose C, Marchac D, Hirsch JF: Intracranial pressure in craniostenosis. J Neurosurg 57:370–377, 1982.
19. Robb R, Boger W: Vertical strabismus associated with plagiocephaly. J Pediatr Ophthalmol Strabismus 20:58–62, 1983.
20. Stratoudakis A, Gaines C: Treatment of plagiocephaly in infancy. South Med J 80:1097–1104, 1987.
21. Tulasne JF, Tessier P: Analysis and late treatment of plagiocephaly. Scand J Plast Reconstr Surg 15:257–263, 1981.
22. Bertelsen TI: The premature synostosis of the cranial sutures. Acta Ophthalmol (Suppl) 51:1, 1958.
23. DuBoulay EPG, O'Connell JEA: The x-ray characteristics of particular diseases of the skull and brain. *In* Cochrane Shanks S, Kerley P (eds): A Text-book of X-Ray Diagnosis. London, Lewis, 1969, p 143.
24. Danby PM: Plagiocephaly in some 10-year-old children. Arch Dis Child 37:500, 1962.
25. Watson GH: Relation between side of plagiocephaly, dislocation of hip, scoliosis, bat ears and sternomastoid tumors. Arch Dis Child 46:203, 1971.
26. Rout PGJ, Price C: Plagiocephaly. Br J Oral Surg 16:163, 1978–1979.
27. Vulliamy DG: Problems of the newborn: Less urgent problems and minor abnormalities. Br Med J 4:547, 1971.
28. Bhatia KK, Nanda S, Bhatian B, Nanda S: Persistent plagiocephaly with congenital dislocation of hip. Ind Pediatr 25:800, 1988.
29. Marsh JL, Vannier MW: Three-dimensional surface imaging from CT scans for the study of craniofacial dysmorphology. J Craniofac Genet Dev Biol 9:61, 1989.
30. Shillito J, Matson DD: Craniosynostosis: A review of 519 surgical patients. Pediatrics 41:829, 1968.
31. Tessier P: Relationship of craniostenosis to craniofacial dysostoses, and to faciostenoses: A study with therapeutic implications. Plast Reconstr Surg 48:224, 1971.
32. Hunter AGW, Rudd NL: Craniosynostosis: II. Coronal synostosis, its familial characteristics and associated clinical findings in 109 patients lacking bilateral polysyndactyly or syndactyly. Teratology 15:301, 1977.
33. Laitinen L: Craniosynostosis: Premature fusion of the cranial sutures. Ann Pediatr Fenn 2 (Suppl 6):1, 1956.
34. Fernbach SK, Naidich TP: Radiological evaluation of craniosynostosis. *In* Cohen MM Jr (ed): Craniosynostosis: Diagnosis, Evaluation, and Management. New York, Raven Press, 1986, pp 191–214.
35. Oakes JW: Craniosynostosis. *In* Serafin D, Georgiade NG (eds): Pediatric Plastic Surgery. St. Louis, CV Mosby, 1984, pp 404–439.
36. Chasler CN: Atlas of Roentgen Anatomy of the Newborn and Infant Skull. St. Louis, Warren H. Green, 1972, pp 68–71.
37. Venes JL: Surgery of craniosynostosis. *In* Bosma JE (ed): Symposium on Development of the Basicranium (DHEW publication NIH 76-989). Bethesda, MD, National Institutes of Health, 1976, pp 443–454.
38. Nathan MH, Newman A: The skewed nasal septum: A pathognomonic sign of premature unilateral coronal suture stenosis. Br J Radiol 43:139, 1970.
39. Griscom NT: Craniosynostosis. *In* Kaufman HJ (ed): Skull, Spine, and Contents. Part II: Progress in Pediatric Radiology, vol 6. Basel, Karger, 1978, pp 3–38.
40. Carmel PW, Luken MG III, Ascherl GF Jr: Craniosynostosis: Computed tomographic evaluation of skull base and calvarial deformities and associated intracranial changes. Neurosurgery 9:366, 1981.
41. Furaya Y, Edwards MSB, Alpers CE, et al: Computerized tomography of cranial sutures: I. Comparison of suture anatomy in children and adults. J Neurosurg 61:53, 1984.
42. Furuya Y, Edwards MSB, Alpers CE, et al: Computerized tomography of cranial sutures: II. Abnormalities of sutures and skull deformities in craniosynostosis. J Neurosurg 61:59, 1984.
43. Marsh JL, Gado MH, Vannier MW, Stevens WG: Osseous anatomy of unilateral coronal synostosis. Cleft Palate J 23:87, 1986.
44. Gates GF, Dore EK: Detection of craniosynostosis by bone scanning. Radiology 115:665, 1975.
45. Tait MV, Gilday DL, Ash JM, et al: Craniosynostosis: Correlation of bone scans, radiographs and surgical findings. Radiology 133:615, 1979.
46. Kawamoto HK: Torticollis versus plagiocephaly. *In* Marchac D (ed): Craniofacial Surgery: First International Congress of the International Society for Cranio-Maxillo-Facial Surgery. New York, Springer-Verlag, 1987, pp 105–109.
47. Delaire J: Malformations faciales et asymetrie de labase du crane. Rev Stomatol 66:379, 1965.
48. Kreiborg S, Bjork A: Craniofacial asymmetry in a dry skull with plagiocephaly. Eur J Orthod 3:195, 1981.
49. Jones KL: Smith's Recognizable Patterns of Human Malformations, 4th ed. Philadelphia, WB Saunders, 1988, pp 2–4.
50. Graham JM Jr, Badura RJ, Smith DW: Coronal craniosynostosis: Fetal head constraint as one possible cause. J Pediatr 65:995, 1980.
51. Graham JM Jr: Smith's Recognizable Patterns of Human Deformation, 4th ed. Philadelphia, WB Saunders, 1988, pp 50–52, 64.
52. Higginbottom MC, Jones KL, James HE: Intrauterine constraint and craniosynostosis. Neurosurgery 6:39, 1980.
53. Koskinen-Moffett LK, Moffett BC Jr, Graham JM Jr: Cranial Synostosis and Intrauterine Compression: A Development Study of Human Sutures—Factors and Mechanisms Influencing Bone Growth. New York, Alan R. Liss, 1982, pp 365–378.
54. Sullivan PK, Melsen B, Mulliken JB: Calvarial sutural abnormalities: Metopic synostosis and coronal deformation: An anatomic, three-dimensional radiographic, and pathologic study. Plast Reconstr Surg 86:1072, 1990.
55. Wynne-Daves R: Infantile idiopathic scoliosis: Causative factors, particularly in the first six months of life. J Bone Joint Surg [Br] 578:138, 1975.
56. Dunn PM: Congenital postural deformities. Br Med Bull 32:71, 1976.
57. Miller ME, Dunn PM, Smith DW: Uterine malformation and fetal deformation. J Pediatr 94:387, 1979.
58. Frexes-Keusch CF, Mulliken JB, Kaplan LC: Craniofacial anomalies in twins. Plast Reconstr Surg 87:16, 1991.
59. Johnstone RN, Kellar RJ: A Textbook of Midwifery, 16th ed. London, Black, 1955.
60. Record RG, Edwards JH: Environmental influences related to the aetiology of congenital dislocation of the hip. Br J Prev Soc Med 12:8, 1958.
61. Brooks B: Pathologic changes in muscle as a result of disturbances of circulation. Arch Surg 5:188, 1922.
62. Robb RM, Boger WP: Vertical strabismus associated with plagiocephaly. J Pediatr Ophthalmol Strabismus 20:58, 1983.

CHAPTER 112

Orbital Deformities: Anterior Cranial Base Approach

Jeffrey C. Posnick

HISTORICAL PERSPECTIVE

An anterior cranial base approach to the orbits has evolved gradually. A review of the historical landmarks in its evolution is important for understanding what we have yet to accomplish.

The numerous combined soft tissue and hard tissue facial injuries that resulted from the trench warfare of World War I required urgent treatment and later secondary reconstruction. Two physicians in particular, Kazanjian[1] and Gillies,[2] stand out for their work during this period. During World War I, between the wars, and again during World War II, these men laid the foundation of what we know now as craniomaxillofacial surgery.

After World War II, Sir Harold Gillies applied the knowledge he had gained from treating wartime facial injuries to the treatment of craniofacial malformations of the previously neglected patients now seeking his help. In 1950, he reported an encouraging experience involving an elective LeFort III osteotomy to advance the midface for Crouzon's syndrome.[3] His early enthusiasm later turned to discouragement when the patient's facial skeleton relapsed to its preoperative position.

In 1967, Tessier described a new cranial base approach to the orbits and midface for the management of Crouzon's and Apert's syndromes.[4] His landmark presentation and publications were the beginning of modern craniofacial surgery.[5–7] To overcome Gillies' earlier problems, Tessier developed a new basic approach that involved a bifrontal craniotomy for retraction of the brain, giving exposure to the anterior cranial base so that safe orbital and midface osteotomies could be carried out. He worked with a neurosurgeon through a coronal (skin) incision, designed new locations for osteotomies, interposed autogenous bone grafts, and applied an external fixation device to help maintain stability of the bone until healing had occurred.

Rougerie and coworkers applied this concept of simultaneous cranial vault suture release and forehead reshaping to infants in 1972.[8] Later, in 1976, Hoffman and Mohr[9] advanced the concept of a cranial base suture release and of cranial vault and orbital reshaping for unilateral coronal synostosis in infancy (lateral canthal advancement procedure). In 1977, Whitaker and associates[10] proposed a more formal cranial vault and orbital reshaping for unilateral coronal synostosis. In 1979, Marchac and Renier published their experience with this cranial base approach for simultaneous suture release and cranial vault and orbital reshaping (floating forehead technique) to manage either unilateral or bilateral coronal synostosis in infancy.[11] The common denominator was an anterior cranial base approach to the orbits.

One of the spinoffs of Tessier's craniofacial–cranial base approach to facial deformity has been the development of surgical approaches to tumors involving the orbits and cranial base. Ablative surgeons gained familiarity with the coronal (skin) incision and the concept of exposure craniotomies for access to the anterior cranial base for tumor removal while reconstructive surgeons used this approach to assist with orbital and midfacial osteotomies. The idea of completing orbital osteotomies, to gain exposure and facilitate anterior skull base tumor resection, was a natural progression of thinking. Derome and colleagues[12–14] pioneered this facial osteotomy approach for cranial base tumor exposure and management. Jackson and associates[15–17] and others[18–30] have refined this approach for cranial base tumor exposure and removal in adults and children.

A coordinated interdisciplinary approach to the management of pediatric congenital, traumatic, and neoplastic anterior cranial base and orbital problems is essential. The pediatric neurosurgeon, craniofacial/plastic surgeon, pediatric neuro-ophthalmologist, pediatric anesthesiologist, and skilled nursing staff work together to complete effective urgent and elective cranial base and orbital procedures.

REFINEMENTS IN PEDIATRIC CRANIOFACIAL SURGERY

In 1968, Hans Luhr, proposed that small metal bone plates could be constructed and used for mandibular fracture fixation.[31] Despite his early enthusiasm, these concepts of internal fixation for the craniofacial skeleton were not put into practice until the mid 1980s.[32, 33] We realize that this form of fixation increases the ease of three-dimensional shaping of the osteotomies and bone graft units, increases the ability of the placed osteotomy units to withstand the natural deforming forces (i.e., scar tissue, congenitally inadequate soft tissue drape, muscles of mastication, postural molding, trauma, and wound contracture), and encourages primary bone healing.[34-37] In addition, the incidence of infection and late skeletal relapse may be diminished,[38, 39] and there should be less overall bone graft resorption.[40] The development and current use of a micro bone plate and screw internal fixation system further facilitates this form of internal fixation when osteotomies and bone graft reconstruction are required in immature and non-weight-bearing facial bones (i.e., cranial vault, orbits, zygomas, and nasal bones).[41, 42]

The widespread use of autogenous cranial bone grafts that has virtually eliminated the rib and hip grafts when bone replacement or augmentation is required in cranio-orbitozygomatic procedures represents another of Tessier's contributions to craniofacial surgery.[43] Zins and Whitaker[44] and Kusiak and associates,[45] working with both New Zealand rabbits and rhesus monkeys, placed membranous and endochondral autogenous onlay bone grafts in a subperiosteal pocket but without any form of fixation. They demonstrated less resorption of the membranous than the endochondral bone grafts. Phillips and Rahn studied onlay autogenous bone grafts in mature sheep from a slightly different perspective.[40] They examined the differences between membranous and endochondral onlay autogenous bone graft and considered fixation technique an additional variable. They concluded that the stable fixation of grafts (lag-screw technique) results in less graft resorption. The nonfixed membranous grafts resorb less than the nonfixed endochondral grafts, but the difference in graft resorption patterns was much less when a stable form of fixation (lag-screw technique) was used.

Effective craniofacial reconstruction demands both subjective (qualitative) and objective (quantitative) assessment. Various methods have been used in the past to indirectly analyze the skeletal morphology, patterns of growth and development, and normative standards of the craniofacial skeleton. Computed tomography (CT) has now been established as an important modality in the diagnosis, surgical planning, and longitudinal study of craniofacial deformities.[46-53]

The normal range of CT measurement values and growth patterns for the cranial vault and orbital and zygomatic regions have been developed.[48] The knowledge of these differential craniofacial growth patterns and normal measurement values helps make an accurate diagnosis, perform reconstructive surgery more precisely, and follow patients more effectively.[50-53] With the combination of two- and three-dimensional CT scans of the craniofacial skeleton, we can now gain qualitative impressions[46] as well as make quantitative assessments.[50-54]

The use of microvascular free tissue transfers was initially limited to older children, adolescents, and adults. More recently, elective free tissue transfers have been carried out in 6-month to 1-year-old infants and young children with reliable success.[27-29, 55, 56] When indicated, free tissue transfers can be designed to limit morbidity by closing dead space, providing vascularized tissue to line mucosal surfaces or provide skin cover over exposed osteotomy units or bone grafts. Vascularized bone grafts can be especially useful in the reconstruction of pediatric mandibular tumor defects to limit morbidity and to improve functional and aesthetic rehabilitation.[55]

EXPOSURE OSTEOTOMIES AND CRANIOTOMIES FOR ACCESS TO TUMORS OF THE ANTERIOR CRANIAL BASE AND ORBITS

Tessier introduced the concept of exposure craniotomies to provide access to the orbital and midfacial bones through the anterior cranial base for reconstruction of craniofacial malformations in adults.[4] During the following 25 years, this concept has been applied to persons of all ages and to reconstruction of a variety of congenital and traumatic deformities and secondary defects after tumor ablation.

Derome and coworkers' concept of exposure orbital osteotomies combined with craniotomies to provide access to the anterior cranial base and posterior orbits for safe tumor resection was a unique concept.[12] Facial osteotomies for exposure to anterior cranial base and posterior orbital tumors are now frequently completed through the anterior orbits, nasal bones, maxilla, zygomas, and mandible.[14-20, 22, 23, 25, 26, 30, 35] Exposure facial osteotomies are also used for the management of craniofacial malformations (i.e., encephaloceles and intracranial nasal dermoids) and for the repair of traumatic defects (i.e., orbital roof blow-in fractures and traumatic encephaloceles with dural leaks).[34, 36, 57]

INDICATIONS

Traumatic Upper Orbital Deformities

Principles of Management of Acute Pediatric Traumatic Cranio-orbital Injuries and Secondary Deformities

Pediatric craniofacial trauma with anterior cranial base and upper orbital involvement is best managed at a pediatric trauma referral center.[36, 57-59] Initial evaluation by the pediatric craniofacial team should include neurosurgical evaluation, neuroradiologic studies (i.e., high-resolution CT scanning, angiography, and magnetic resonance imaging as indicated), neuro-ophthalmologic assessment, and craniofacial/plastic surgical evaluation.

There are frequent patterns of craniofacial fractures with anterior cranial base–orbital involvement that will require a combined neurosurgical and craniofacial/plastic surgeon approach.[58, 59] They include unilateral forehead and upper orbital fractures with orbital roof blow-in, naso-orbitoethmoid fractures with associated brain and dural injury, frontal bone and anterior cranial base fractures, cerebrospinal fluid leak, and meningitis with secondary forehead defects. When these injuries are recognized early they are best repaired primarily or as a delayed primary repair. There is very little justification for a neurosurgical brain and dural repair followed weeks or months later by craniofacial/plastic surgical reconstruction. All aspects of the craniofacial repair should be discussed in advance by the surgeons and anesthetist, including type of airway management, preparation and draping of the patient, location of scalp incision, location of expected craniotomies and osteotomies, perioperative medications (i.e., antibiotics, corticosteroids, and anticonvulsants), and postoperative management. A further consideration is the effect of the injury and the surgical intervention on further growth of the craniofacial skeleton. The late correction of secondary deformities requires a similar approach for evaluation and reconstruction, but the reconstructive results may be more modest owing to previous scar tissue and malunion.

Unilateral Forehead and Upper Orbital Fractures with Orbital Roof "Blow-in." The 10-year-old boy shown in Figure 112–1 was downhill skiing when he ran into a stationary metal post and sustained trauma to the right fronto-orbital region.[36] He suffered right frontal bone–cranial base–supraorbital ridge displaced fractures with an orbital roof and upper medial orbital wall blow-in fracture resulting in right eye proptosis with limited upward gaze. After neurosurgical, craniofacial/plastic surgical, neuro-ophthalmologic, and CT scan evaluation he underwent a combined single-staged intracranial-cranial base approach. Through a coronal incision, a right frontal craniotomy was completed. The dural tears were repaired with a patch of temporalis fascia. Autogenous cranial bone was harvested from the right parietal region, contoured to reconstruct a new orbital roof and superior medial orbital wall, and fixed with titanium microplates and screws. The supraorbital ridge fracture and right frontal craniotomy and fractures were reduced and fixed with microplates and screws. He had a full and early recovery.

Naso-orbitoethmoid Fracture with Associated Brain and Dural Injury. The 8-year-old girl shown in Figure 112–2 was involved in a motor vehicle accident, having been an unbelted back seat passenger.[60] Clinical and CT scan evaluation confirmed displaced and comminuted naso-orbitoethmoid fractures with brain contusion, dural tears, and cerebrospinal fluid leakage through the nose.

One day after injury she underwent a combined neurosurgical and craniofacial/plastic surgical procedure. A coronal (skin) incision was made, a frontal craniotomy was completed, and after anterior cranial base exposure all dural tears were repaired and a patch graft was placed. Through this cranial base approach the comminuted nasal and upper orbital fractures were reduced and fixed with multiple titanium microplates and screws. The frontal bone fractures and craniotomy units were also reduced and fixed with microplates and screws. The patient's recovery was uneventful.

Frontal Bone and Anterior Cranial Base Fracture, Cerebrospinal Fluid Leak with Resulting Meningitis, and Secondary Forehead and Orbital Defects. A 16-year-old girl was in a motor vehicle accident and sustained fronto-orbital and cranial base fractures, brain concussion, dural tear, and cerebrospinal fluid leak (Fig. 112–3).[37] She was initially treated with conservative débridement, dural repair, and repositioning of her frontal and orbital fragments without the use of bone stabilization techniques. She suffered an ongoing cerebrospinal fluid leak with resulting meningitis and frontal bone loss due to infection.

As a secondary procedure, a combined intracranial-cranial base approach was used to gain exposure of the anterior cranial base. This exposure provided access for repair of the traumatic encephalocele and dural tears. The orbital roof, supraorbital ridge, and forehead defects were then reconstructed using autogenous cranial bone grafts and stable (miniplate and microplate and screw) fixation. The cerebrospinal fluid leak has remained closed, and the initially achieved orbital and forehead contour has remained.

Congenital Orbital Anomalies

Craniofacial Malformations with Anterior Cranial Base–Orbital Involvement

There are a number of craniofacial malformations with anterior cranial base–orbital involvement.[4–8, 34, 61–64] The most frequent are the craniofacial dysostosis syndromes, including Crouzon's syndrome, Apert's syndrome, Pfeiffer's syndrome, Saethre-Chotzen syndrome, and Kleeblattschädel's anomaly. The craniofacial dysostosis syndromes present as varied forms of cranial vault, cranial base, and midface suture synostosis. Other frequent craniofacial malformations with anterior cranial base–orbital involvement include frontonasal dysplasia (with or without craniosynostosis), microphthalmia, encephalocele, dermoids, and Klippel-Feil anomaly.

Principles of Management of Anterior Cranial Base–Orbital Craniofacial Malformations

An initial craniofacial team assessment is essential to evaluate brain, eye, auditory, and airway function very early in life. As the infant grows through childhood and

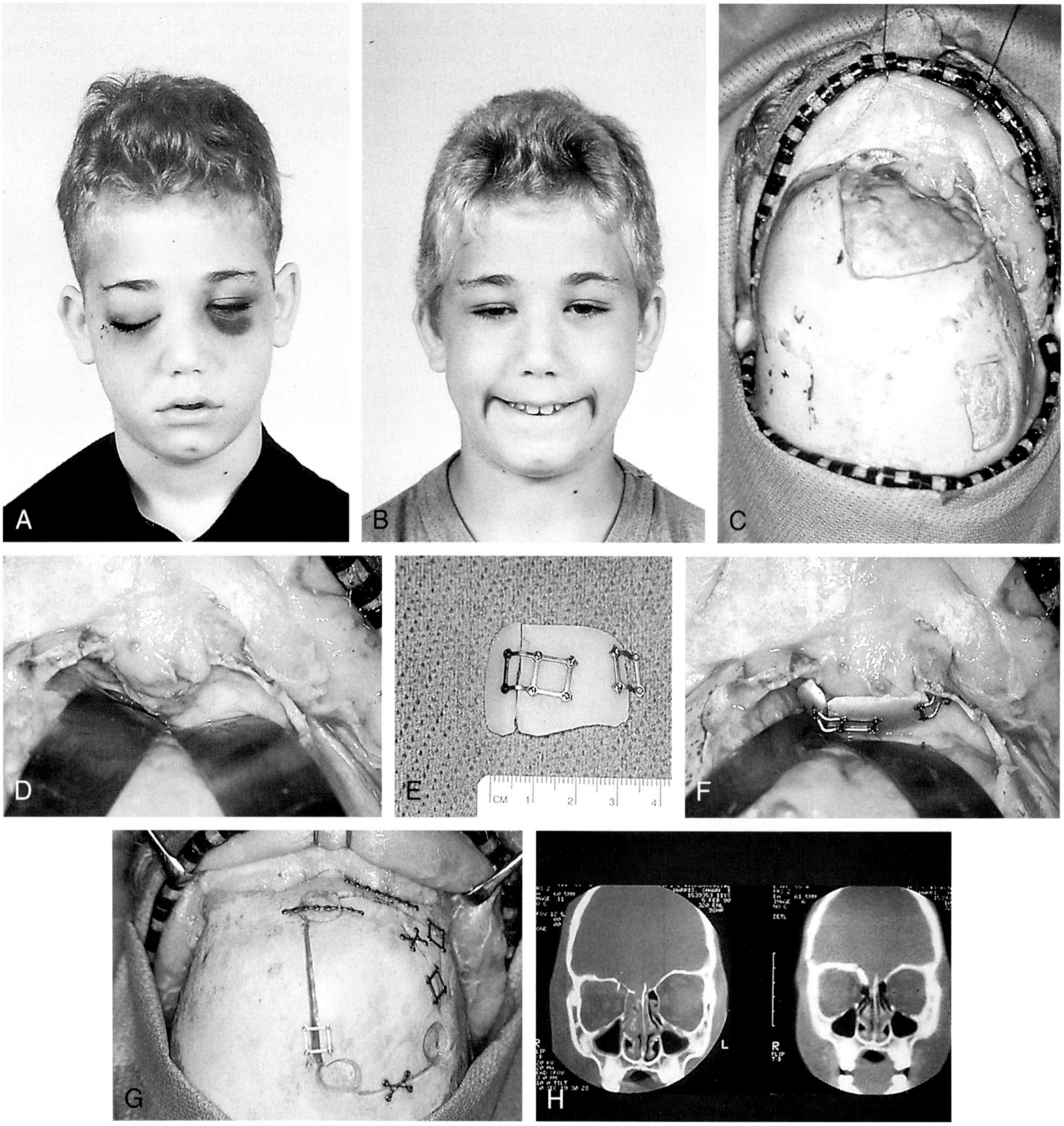

Figure 112–1. A 10-year-old boy who was in an accident sustained a unilateral forehead and upper orbital fracture with orbital roof "blow-in" combined with brain and dural injury. *A*, Preoperative frontal view of the patient 5 days after injury and 1 day before reconstruction. *B*, Postoperative view of the patient 6 months after reconstruction. C, Coronal incision and right frontal craniotomy have been completed, and cranial bone graft harvested from right parietal region for orbital reconstruction. *D*, Close-up view with exposure of orbital roof defect after dural lacerations have been repaired and brain retracted. *E*, Cranial bone grafts from right parietal region have been contoured and fixed with microplates and screws for orbital roof reconstruction. *F*, Orbital roof graft in position and fixed to the cranial base. *G*, Supraorbital ridge and frontal bone fractures reduced and craniotomy segments replaced and fixed with microplates and screws. *H*, Coronal computed tomographic scans demonstrating right orbital roof before (*left*) and after (*right*) reconstruction. (*A* to *H* from Posnick JC: The role of plate and screw fixation in the treatment of paediatric facial fractures. *In* Gruss JS, Manson PM, Yaremchuk MJ [eds]: Rigid Fixation of the Craniofacial Skeleton. Stoneham, MA, Butterworth-Heinemann, 1992, pp 396–419.)

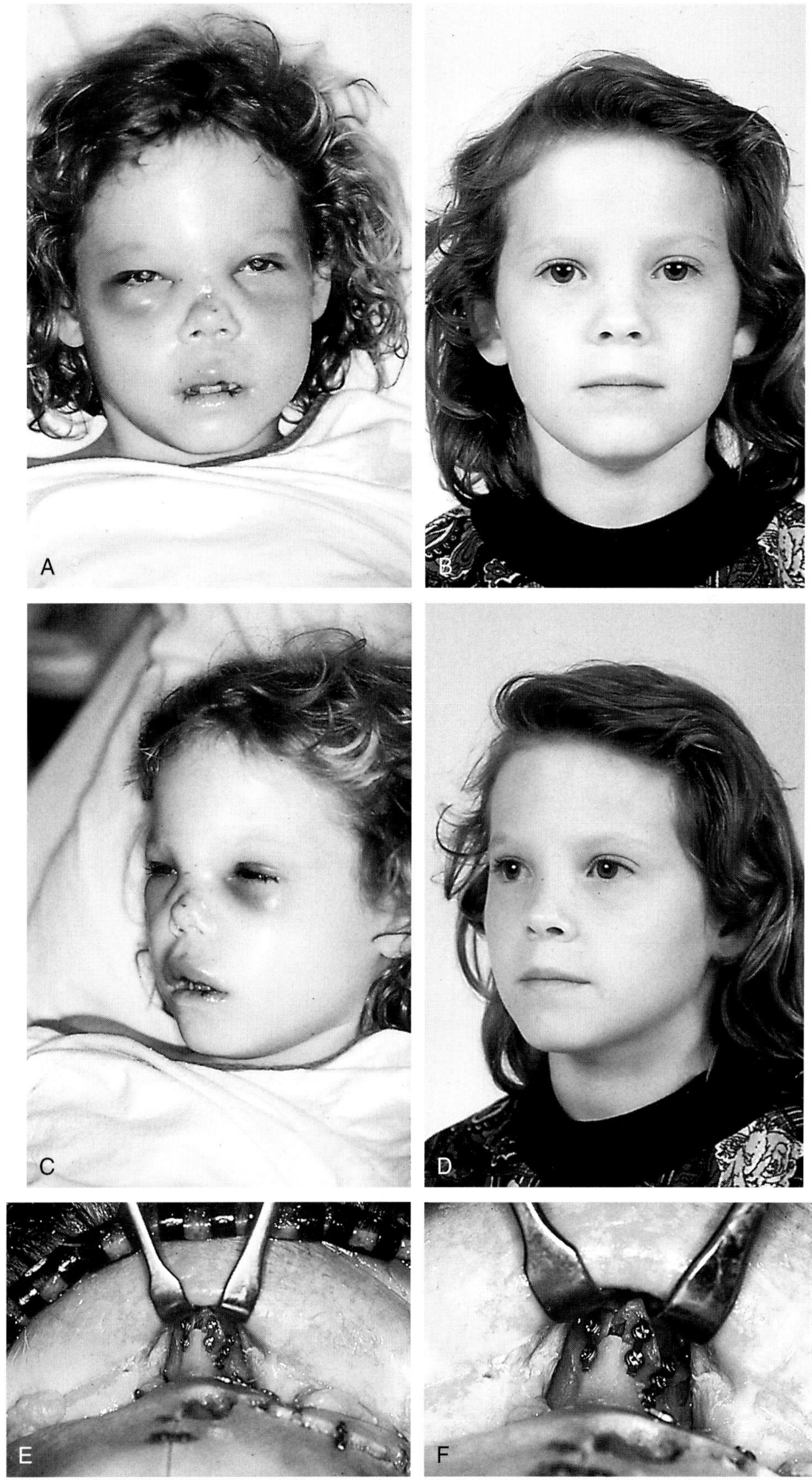

Figure 112–2. An 8-year-old girl who was in a motor vehicle accident sustained naso-orbitoethmoid fractures with associated brain and dural injury with cerebrospinal fluid leak. She required a combined neurosurgical and craniofacial/plastic surgical procedure. *A*, Frontal view before reconstruction. *B*, Frontal view 1 year after reconstruction. *C*, Oblique view before reconstruction. *D*, Oblique view 1 year after reconstruction. *E*, Intraoperative view of reconstructed naso-orbital frontal fractures. *F*, Close-up view of reduced, comminuted naso-orbital frontal fractures fixed with titanium microplates and screws. (*A* to *F* from Posnick JC: Pediatric cranial base surgery. Prob Plast Reconstr Surg 3:107, 1994.)

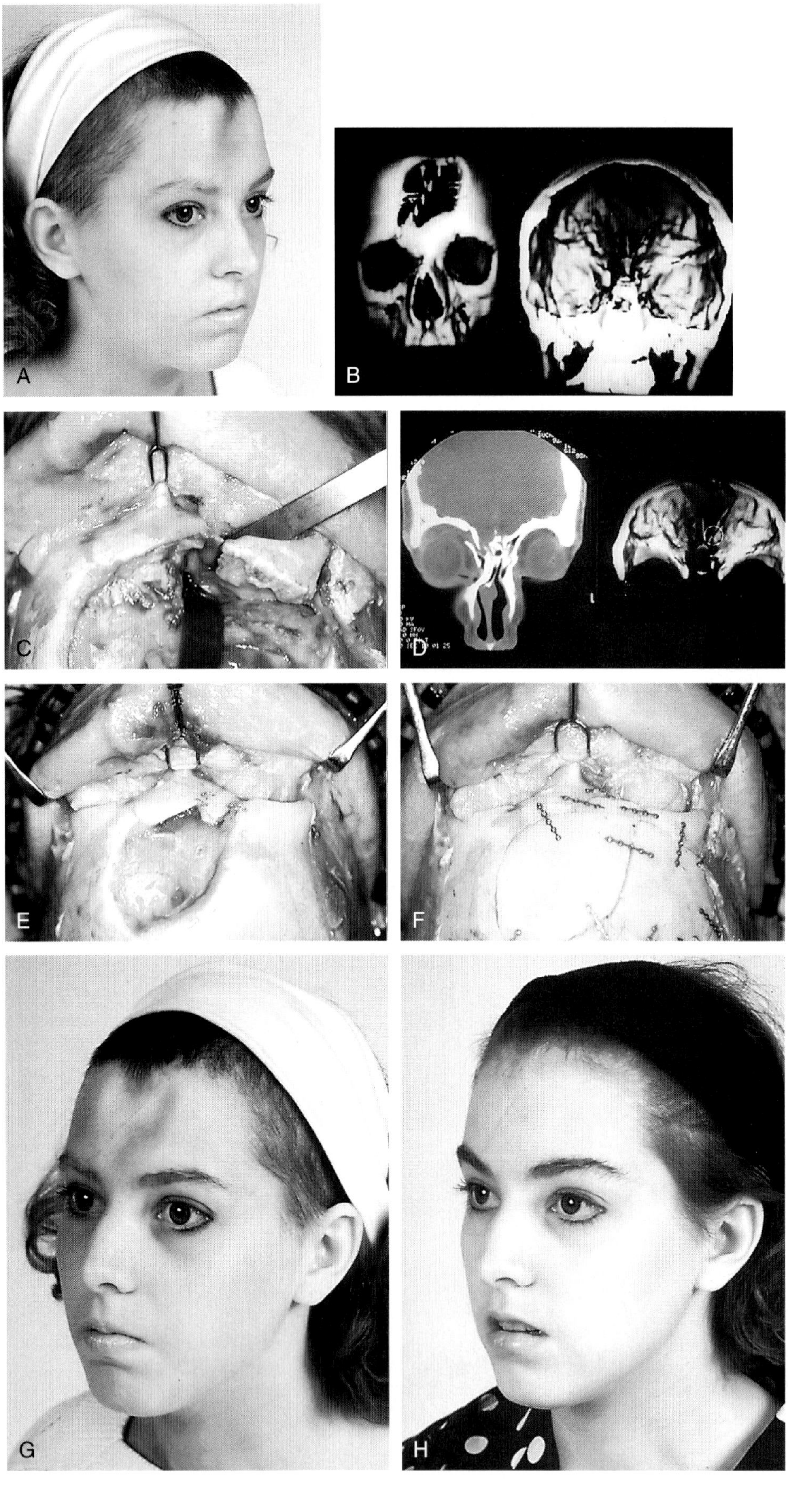

Figure 112–3. A 16-year-old girl who was in a motor vehicle accident sustained fronto-orbital fractures and cerebrospinal fluid leak with resulting meningitis and required bone flap débridement. She arrived with a fronto-orbital defect requiring secondary reconstruction. *A*, Oblique facial view revealing frontal defect. *B*, Three-dimensional craniofacial computed tomographic (CT) scans indicating extent of frontal and cranial bone defects. *C*, Intraoperative view, after coronal incision, soft tissue dissection extended craniotomy and repair of traumatic encephalocele. *D*, Two- and three-dimensional CT view of orbital and cranial base defects. *E*, Intraoperative view of fronto-orbital region before reconstruction. *F*, Intraoperative view of reconstruction with microplate-fixed cranial grafts. *G*, Oblique facial view before reconstruction. *H*, Oblique facial view 1 year after reconstruction. (*A* to *H* from Posnick JC, Goldstein JA, Armstrong D, Rutka JT: Reconstruction of skull defects in children and adolescents using fixed cranial bone grafts: Long-term results. Neurosurgery 91:1241–1244, 1933.)

into adolescence reassessment at intervals is critical to monitor progress and consider time intervals for surgical intervention.

Selection of the right time and extent of reconstruction will vary according to syndrome type, severity of deformity, and functional and psychosocial concerns. As an example, my general approach to the staging of reconstruction for the craniofacial dysostosis syndromes includes cranio-orbital and cranial base decompression and reshaping in infancy; further cranial vault, anterior cranial base, and upper orbital decompression and reconstruction in childhood to manage signs and symptoms of increased intracranial pressure secondary to inadequate anterior intracranial volume; total midface osteotomies with reshaping and advancement generally carried out through an intracranial anterior cranial base approach later in childhood; and routine jaw surgery combined with orthodontic (i.e., LeFort III, monobloc or facial bipartition osteotomies) treatment to resolve jaw discrepancies and malocclusion (i.e., LeFort I, sagittal splits of the mandible and genioplasty).[57–59]

The staged reconstruction of craniofrontonasal dysplasia generally includes (1) cranio-orbital and cranial base reconstruction in infancy to release fused sutures and initially reshape the forehead and upper orbits; (2) correction of orbital and upper midface hypertelorism through a cranial base approach later in childhood (facial bipartition osteotomies); (3) augmentation of the dorsum of the nose in adolescence; and (4) frequently jaw surgery (i.e., LeFort I, sagittal splits of the mandible and genioplasty) combined with orthodontic treatment at the time of skeletal maturity to normalize jaw relations and occlusion.

The craniofacial malformations that require osteotomies of the orbits and upper midface are generally approached with the exposure provided to the anterior cranial base by the coronal (skin) incision and bifrontal craniotomy with retraction of the frontal and temporal lobes of the brain. Bone grafting is generally required and completed with autogenous calvarial grafts; osteotomy and bone graft fixation are achieved with a combination of microplates and miniplates and screws. The airway is managed without the need for tracheostomy.

Anterior Plagiocephaly (Unilateral Coronal Synostosis). The 8-month-old infant described in Figure 112–4 had craniofacial asymmetry at birth.[63] The left ipsilateral forehead was flat and retruded. On the same side the supraorbital ridge and lateral orbital rim was displaced posteriorly. The root of the nose was constricted to the left side. The left infraorbital rim and anterior zygoma also displayed a degree of flatness. The right (contralateral) side of the forehead bulged forward with inferior and anterior displacement of the orbital roof and supraorbital ridge. The tip of the nose was shifted to the side away from the flat forehead.

A CT scan of the craniofacial skeleton was completed, revealing a left coronal suture fusion. The left sphenoid wing was elevated superiorly (harlequin shaped), and the anterior cranial base was short in the anterior posterior dimension on the left side.[26]

At operation, a coronal incision was carried out with soft tissue dissection and exposure for a bifrontal craniotomy and then retraction of the frontal and temporal lobes of the brain. The three-quarter orbital osteotomies were completed across the orbital roof, lateral orbital wall, and orbital floor into the inferior orbital fissure and down to the mid-infraorbital rim region. The symmetrically reshaped orbital osteotomy units were then reinset between the ocular globes and the brain. The previously removed anterior cranial vault bone was sectioned and units used to reconstruct a new forehead. Stabilization was with direct transosseous wires (or microplates and screws) as needed.

Apert's Syndrome with Total Cranial Vault and Midface Dysplasia. The 5-year-old girl shown in Figure 112–5 was born with Apert's syndrome.[61] She underwent suture release and forehead and upper orbital reshaping at 6 months of age. She presented with a retruded and wide anterior cranial base (residual brachycephaly). The forehead was flat at the supraorbital ridge level with bitemporal constrictions and bulged superiorly. The orbits were shallow, with eye proptosis and a moderate degree of orbital hypertelorism. The midface lacked a normal convexity when viewed from above. The total midface was horizontally and vertically deficient, with a marked anterior open bite and Angle Class III malocclusion.

A craniofacial CT scan was completed and confirmed evidence of fingerprinting along the inner table of the cranial vault and anterior cranial base. The CT scan confirmed that the anterior cranial base was short, with bitemporal constrictions and a recessed supraorbital ridge. The superior forehead bulged anteriorly. The orbits were shallow, and moderate orbital hypertelorism was present. The midface was deficient, and the nasal air passages were diminished.

At operation, the dysplastic cranial vault bone was removed through a coronal (skin) incision. With the frontal and temporal lobes of the brain retracted, exposure was gained to the cranial base for completion of facial bipartition osteotomies (orbits and midface). With the midface, orbits, and cranial vault reshaped, stabilization was with autogenous cranial bone and titanium miniplate and screw fixation. The patient has maintained good function and facial aesthetics. Routine orthognathic surgery and orthodontic treatment are planned for the teenage years.

Midline Craniofacial Cleft with Orbital and Upper Facial Hypertelorism. The child described in Figure 112–6, who was born with a Tessier 0 and 14 midline craniofa-

(Text continued on page 1199)

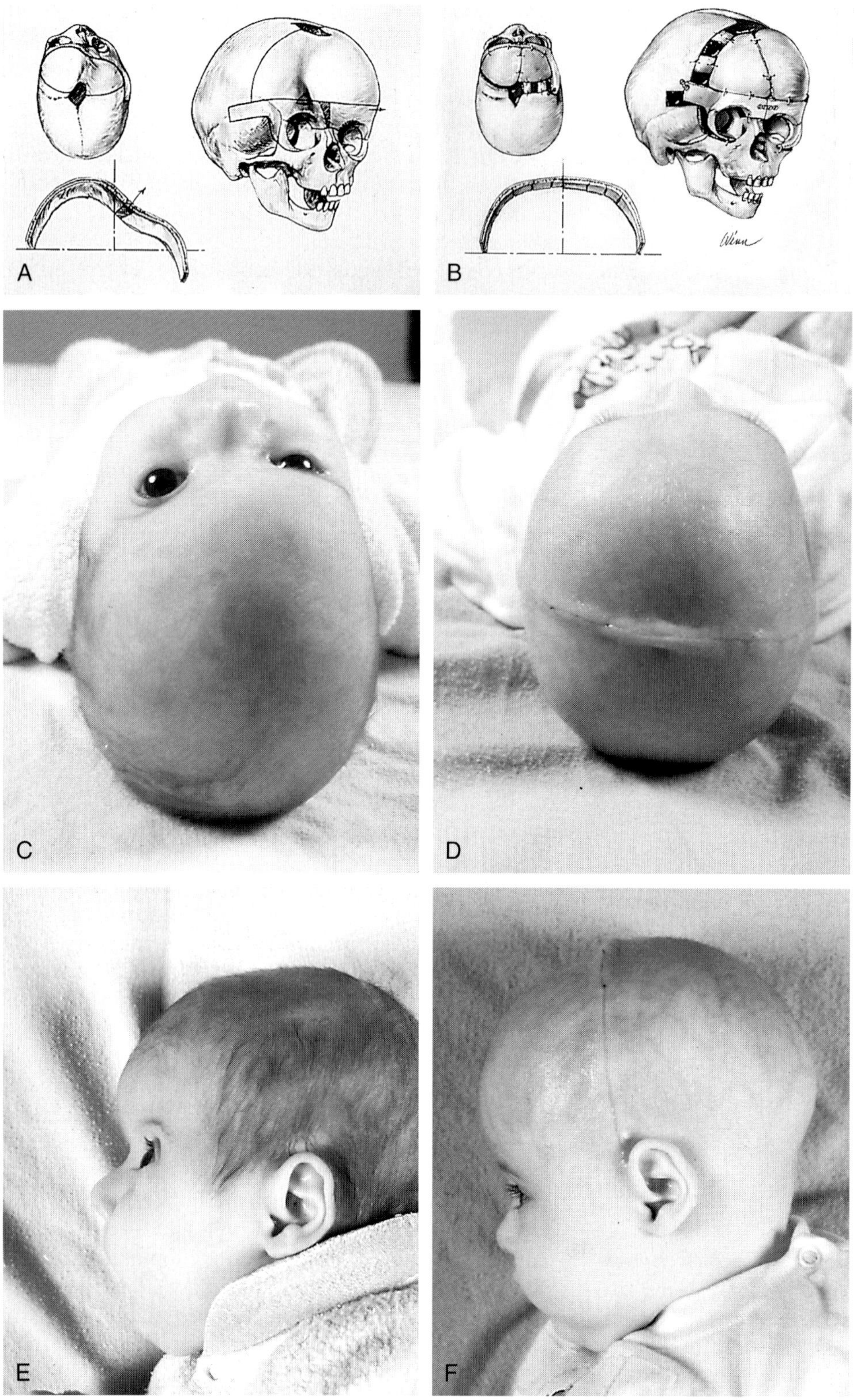

Figure 112–4. An 8-month-old infant with unrepaired unilateral coronal synostosis required suture release and anterior cranial vault and three-quarter orbital osteotomies with reshaping and advancement. *A*, Craniofacial morphology resulting from unilateral coronal synostosis. Proposed osteotomies are outlined. *B*, Craniofacial morphology after cranial vault and three-quarter orbital osteotomies with reshaping, advancement, and fixation. *C*, Preoperative bird's-eye view. *D*, Bird's-eye view early after reconstruction. *E*, Preoperative profile view. *F*, Profile view early after reconstruction.

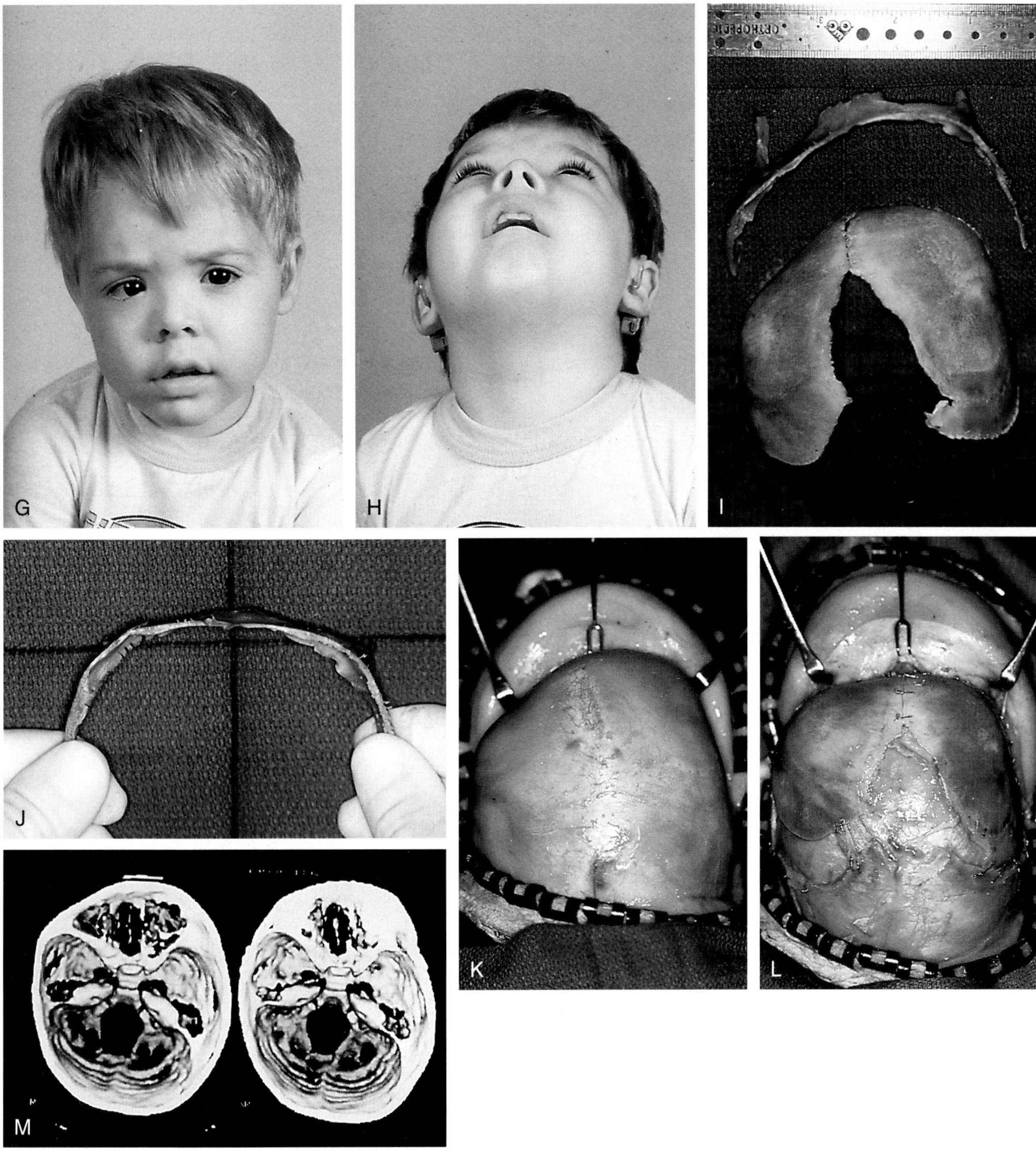

Figure 112–4 *Continued.* G, Frontal view at 3 years of age. *H*, Worm's-eye view at 3 years of age. *I*, View of misshapen orbital unit and anterior cranial vault bone before reinsertion. *J*, Same view of orbital unit after reshaping before reinsertion. *K*, Craniofacial skeleton from above in unilateral coronal synostosis before and after (*L*) reconstruction. *M*, Three-dimensional computed tomographic scan re-formations of cranial base before (left) and after (right) reconstruction. (*A* to *M* from Posnick JC: Craniosynostosis: Surgical management in infancy. *In* Bell WH [ed]: Orthognathic and Reconstructive Surgery, vol 3. Philadelphia, WB Saunders, 1992, pp 1888–1931.)

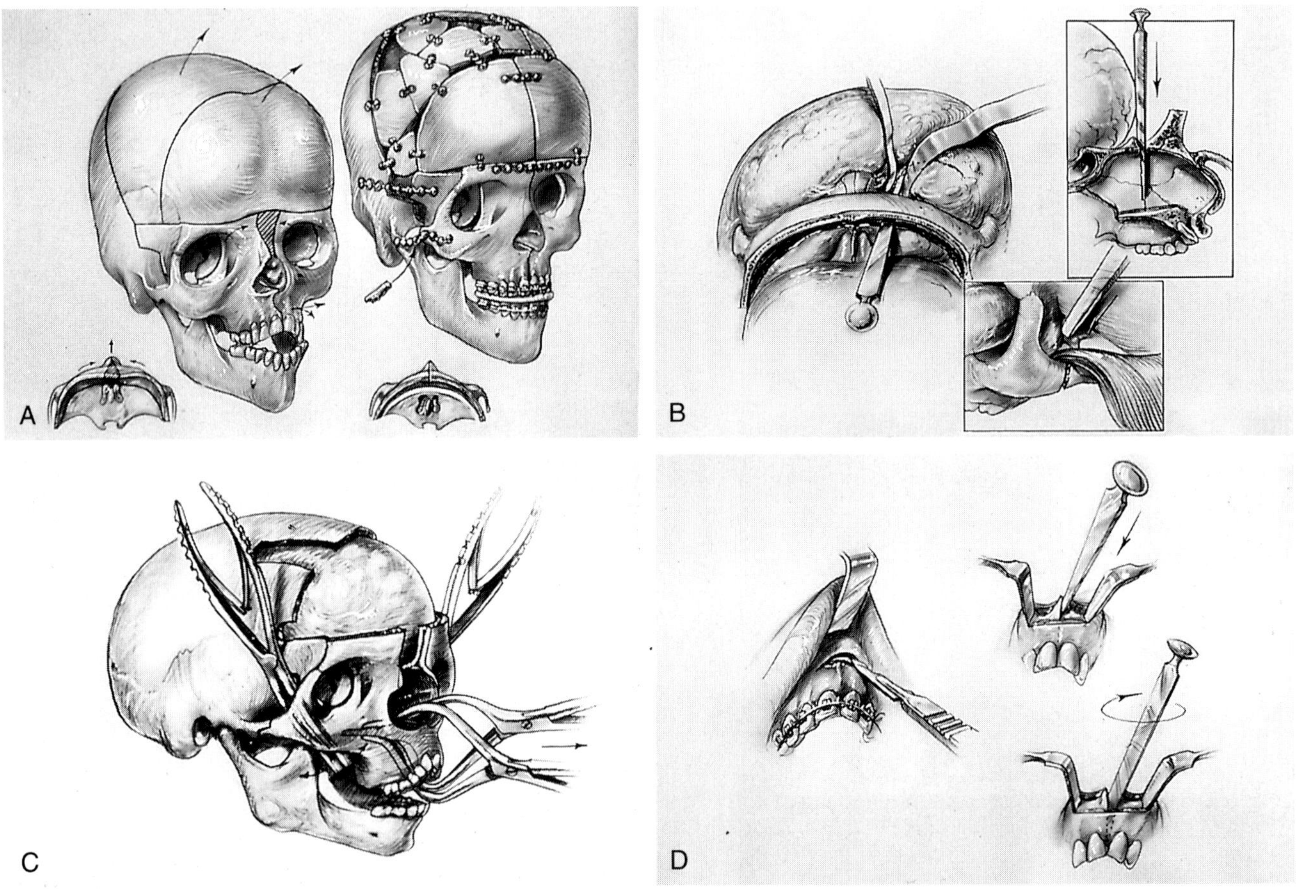

Figure 112–5. A 5-year-old girl with Apert's syndrome underwent suture release and forehead reshaping at 6 months of age. She presented for cranial vault and facial bipartition osteotomies with reshaping and anterior repositioning. *A*, Preoperative craniofacial morphology with planned and completed osteotomies and reshaping. Stabilization is with cranial bone grafts and miniplate fixation. *B*, Osteotomies requiring completion with a chisel. Osteotomy of medial orbital wall is completed posterior to the medial canthi and nasolacrimal apparatus; with the chisel placement through the anterior cranial base, osteotomy is completed through anterior cranial base down through the bony septum of the nose; osteotomy through the exposure provided by the coronal incision and infratemporal fossa to the pterygomaxillary suture, which is then separated. *C*, After completing the facial bipartition osteotomies, Tessier disimpaction forceps are placed through the nose and mouth with pterygomaxillary spreader forceps placed through coronal incision and infratemporal fossa to pterygomaxillary suture regions for disimpaction of midface. *D*, Intraoral buccal vestibular incision, dissection down to anterior nasal spine region with osteotomy down the midline of the hard palate as part of facial bipartition osteotomies. *E*, Preoperative frontal view. *F*, Postoperative frontal view at 2 years after reconstruction. *G*, Preoperative lateral view. *H*, Postoperative lateral view at 2 years after reconstruction. *I*, Intraoperative lateral view of cranial vault, orbits, and zygomatic arch through coronal incision after osteotomies. Stabilization with cranial bone grafts and miniplate fixation. *J*, Preoperative (*left*) and postoperative (*right*) axial-sliced computed tomographic scans through midorbits, demonstrating improvement in orbital hypertelorism and orbital depth with diminished eyeball proptosis. (*A* to *J* from Posnick JC: Craniofacial dysostosis: Staging of reconstruction and management of the midface deformity. Neurosurg Clin North Am 2:683–702, 1991.)

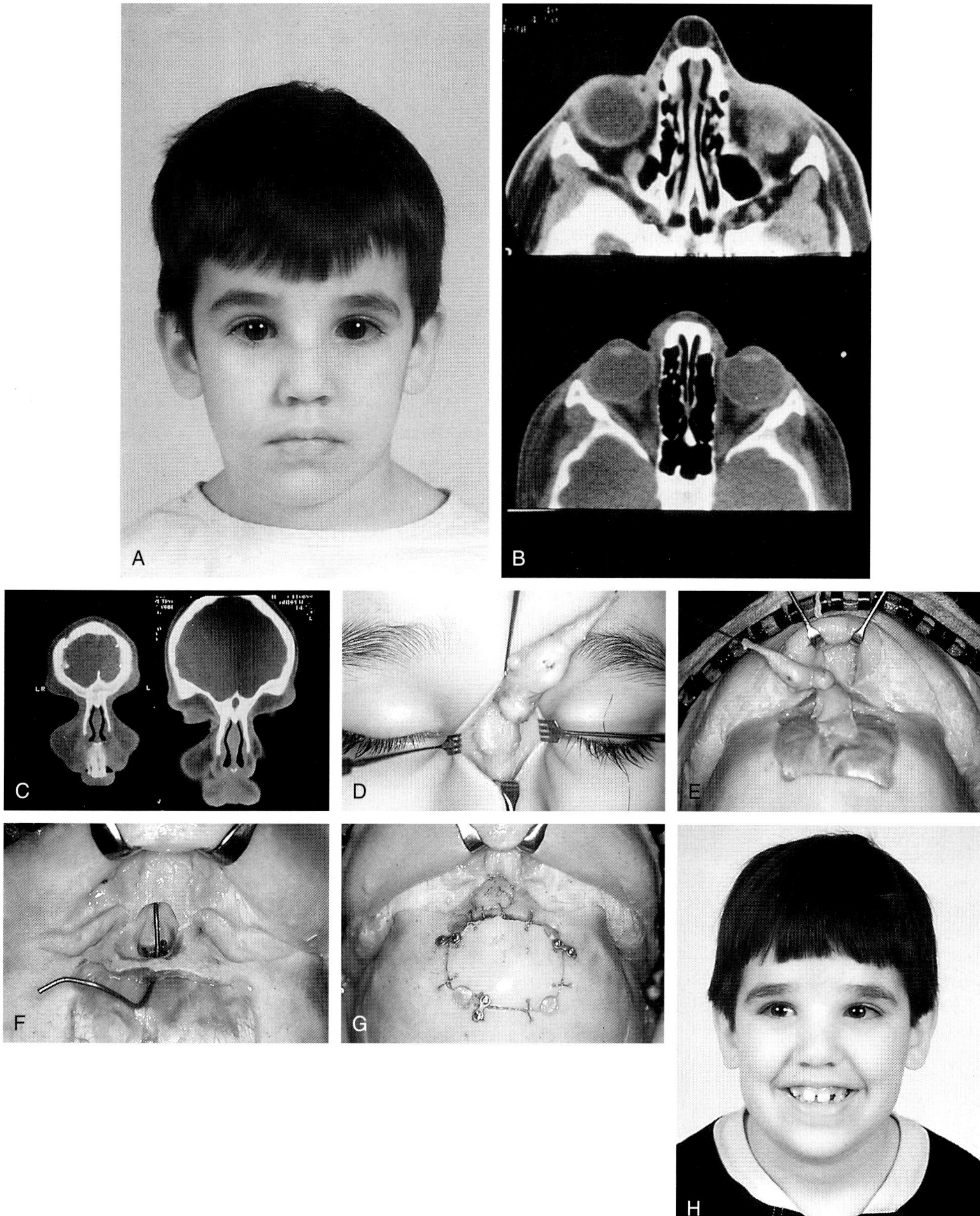

Figure 112–7. A 3½-year-old boy born with a cystic mass over the dorsum of the nose. *A*, Preoperative frontal view demonstrating mass over dorsum of nose. Axial (*B*) and coronal (*C*) computed tomographic scans demonstrating cyst overlying dorsal aspect of nasal bones and separation of the cristi galli. *D*, Intraoperative view, through a direct vertical nasal incision. The multiple cystic mass is being dissected for excision. *E*, Intraoperative view, through a coronal incision and after a frontal craniotomy; the dermoid nasal sinus cyst tract is followed toward the dura. *F*, With the mass excised, an intraosseous dead space remains in the glabella region of the frontal bones. *G*, The intraosseous dead space is closed with autogenous cranial bone shavings. The frontal bone was initially fixed with direct wires, but replaced bone tended to collapse. Miniplates were therefore used to secure the bone in the anatomically correct position. *H*, Frontal view 3 years after the excision. There is no evidence of recurrence. (*A* to *H* from Posnick JC, Bertolluzi P, Armstrong D: Intracranial nasal dermoid sinus cysts: Computed tomography scan findings and surgical results. Plast Reconstr Surg 93:750, 1994.)

cial cleft, underwent repair of the soft tissue midline cleft of the lip, nasal skin, and palate during infancy. She presented with total upper midface hypertelorism including the cranial base, orbits, and nasal, zygomatic, and upper maxillary bones.[34] At operation, the exposure gained to the anterior cranial base allowed effective facial-bipartition osteotomies for repositioning of the two halves of her face medially to correct her facial hypertelorism, bringing her left and right nasal bones and orbits back into the midline. The palatal arch width was corrected, and excess midline nasal skin was excised. Stabilization of the osteotomies was accomplished with autogenous cranial bone grafts and multiple titanium miniplates and screws. She recovered well and has maintained good facial aesthetics. Further augmentation of the dorsum of the nose is planned for the teenage years.

Congenital Midline Nasal Dermoid with Intracranial Extension. The 3½-year-old boy in Figure 112–7 presented with a history of a cystic mass over the dorsum of the nose present since birth.[65] A craniofacial CT scan was completed in the axial and coronal planes. The scans demonstrated a cyst overlying the dorsal aspect of the nasal bones and separation of the crista galli.

A combined single-staged intracranial-extracranial approach was used to excise the lesion. A direct vertical nasal incision was combined with a coronal (skin) incision to allow adequate soft tissue exposure and dissection. A frontal craniotomy allowed adequate exposure to follow the congenital cyst tract up to its dural extension without rupture. Immediate reconstruction was carried out with autogenous cranial bone and stable fixation techniques. There has been no evidence of cyst recurrence or facial growth distortions.

Congenital Frontonasalethmoidal Encephalocele. The 8-year-old girl shown in Figure 112–8 was referred from the Philippines with an unrepaired congenital frontonasalethmoidal encephalocele.[60] Although she started first grade on schedule, she was not allowed to continue because her appearance upset the other children.

She arrived for evaluation and possible treatment. Clinical and CT scan examination confirmed the large encephalocele extending from the right frontal lobe of the brain through a large defect in the anterior cranial base. There was splaying of the ethmoidal sinus air cells and displacement of the orbits and nasal bones (left greater than right). The encephalocele bulged anteriorly through a large defect in the nasal bones.

At operation, a combined single-staged intracranial-extracranial approach was used to excise and plicate the encephalocele. A direct vertical nasal incision was combined with a coronal incision to allow adequate soft tissue exposure and dissection. The bifrontal craniotomy combined with segmental orbital osteotomies allowed adequate exposure for effective removal and plication of the encephalocele without disruption of the structures in the pituitary region. Dismantling and then reconstructing the orbits and nasal and frontal bones required autogenous cranial bone grafting, and titanium miniplate and microplate and screw internal fixation allowed for satisfactory immediate reconstruction. The patient's recovery was uneventful; she returned to the Philippines where she lives with her family and attends public school. Ideally, further nasal reconstruction should be performed to shorten the nose.

Pediatric Tumors and Neoplasms

Principles of Management of Anterior Cranial Base–Orbital Tumors and Neoplasms of Childhood

Tumors of the head and neck are rare in children.[66–70] In contrast to adults, in whom most head and neck tumors are primarily squamous cell carcinomas or salivary gland neoplasms, head and neck tumors in children represent a heterogeneous group of conditions. Only 2% to 3% of all pediatric tumors are located in this region and range from neoplasms (both malignant and benign) to hamartomas and congenital growths.[67] I prefer to divide pediatric head and neck tumors into two main categories: (1) congenital growths and benign tumors and (2) malignant tumors.[35]

Congenital growths and benign tumors often require immediate treatment at whatever age they present because of progressive deformation and immediate functional concerns affecting the brain, eyes, breathing, swallowing, speaking, hearing, and chewing, as well as for psychosocial reasons.[30, 35, 55, 56, 71] Anterior cranial base–orbital involvement is a frequent finding in fibrous dysplasia, neurofibroma, and meningioma.

Patients with congenital growths and benign tumors should be evaluated in a similar fashion as described for craniofacial malformations.[34] Patients with tumors that may be malignant should be assessed by an interdisciplinary team consisting of a pediatric medical oncologist, radiation therapist, and oncologic-reconstructive surgeon. In this way, maximum control of both local and systemic disease can be achieved if a malignancy is diagnosed.

Most malignant tumors of the head and neck that arise in infancy and childhood appear as a solid mass and grow very rapidly.[67] Malignant tumors of lymphoid tissue account for a high percentage of head and neck tumors in children. Treatment often involves biopsy followed by chemotherapy; major surgery is usually not needed. Rhabdomyosarcomas account for almost one third of malignancies of the head and neck in children.[72] The interdisciplinary treatment of this type of tumor generally involves adjuvant chemotherapy to manage micrometastatic disease.[72–77] The local disease is frequently treated with surgical resection and immediate reconstruction using craniofacial techniques.[27–29, 35, 56, 70]

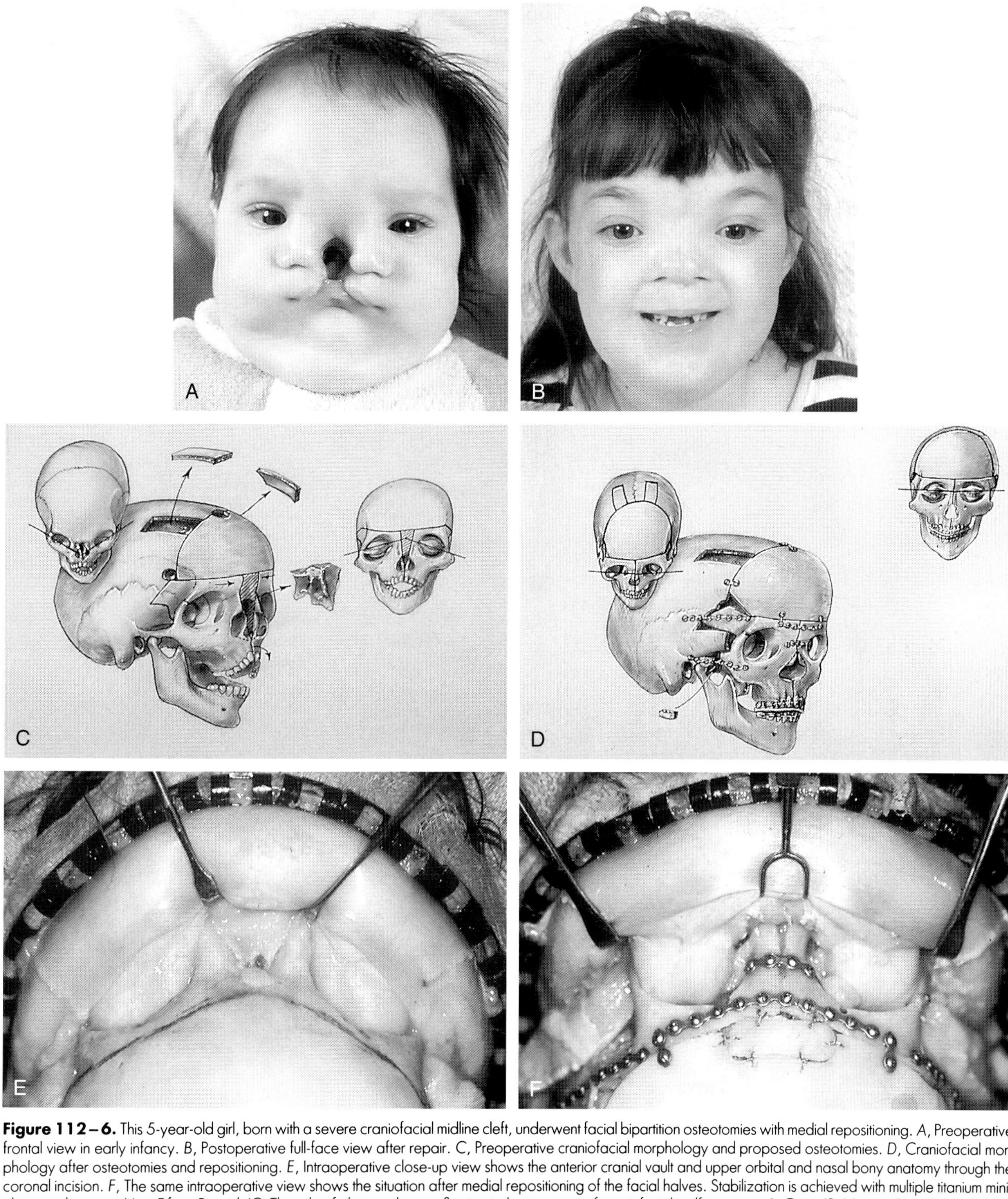

Figure 112–6. This 5-year-old girl, born with a severe craniofacial midline cleft, underwent facial bipartition osteotomies with medial repositioning. *A*, Preoperative frontal view in early infancy. *B*, Postoperative full-face view after repair. C, Preoperative craniofacial morphology and proposed osteotomies. *D*, Craniofacial morphology after osteotomies and repositioning. *E*, Intraoperative close-up view shows the anterior cranial vault and upper orbital and nasal bony anatomy through the coronal incision. *F*, The same intraoperative view shows the situation after medial repositioning of the facial halves. Stabilization is achieved with multiple titanium miniplates and screws. (*A* to *F* from Posnick JC: The role of plate and screw fixation in the treatment of craniofacial malformations. *In* Gruss JS, Manson PM, Yaremchuk MJ [eds]: Rigid Fixation of the Craniomaxillofacial Skeleton. Stoneham, MA, Butterworth-Heinemann, 1992, pp 512–526.)

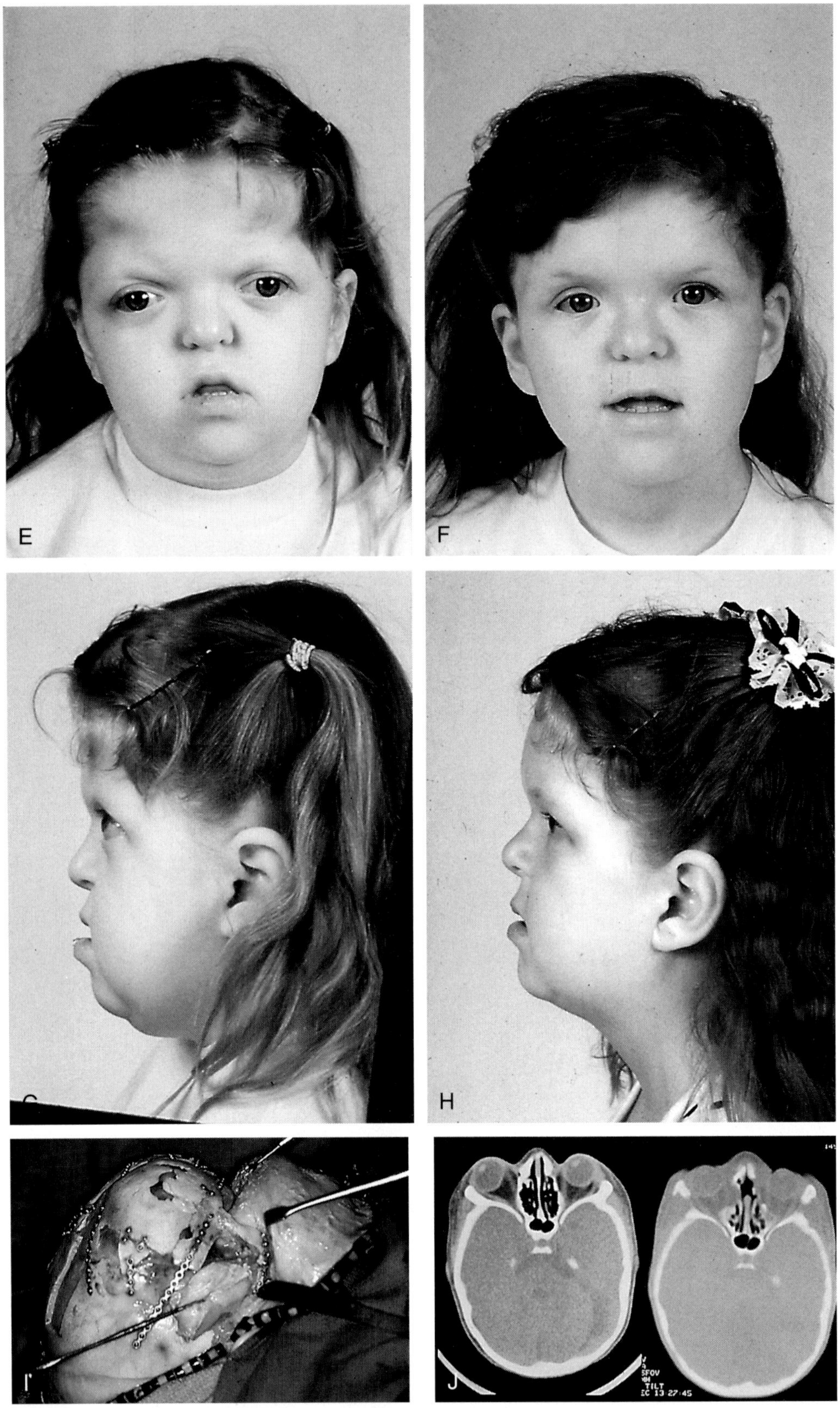

Figure 112–5 *Continued.*

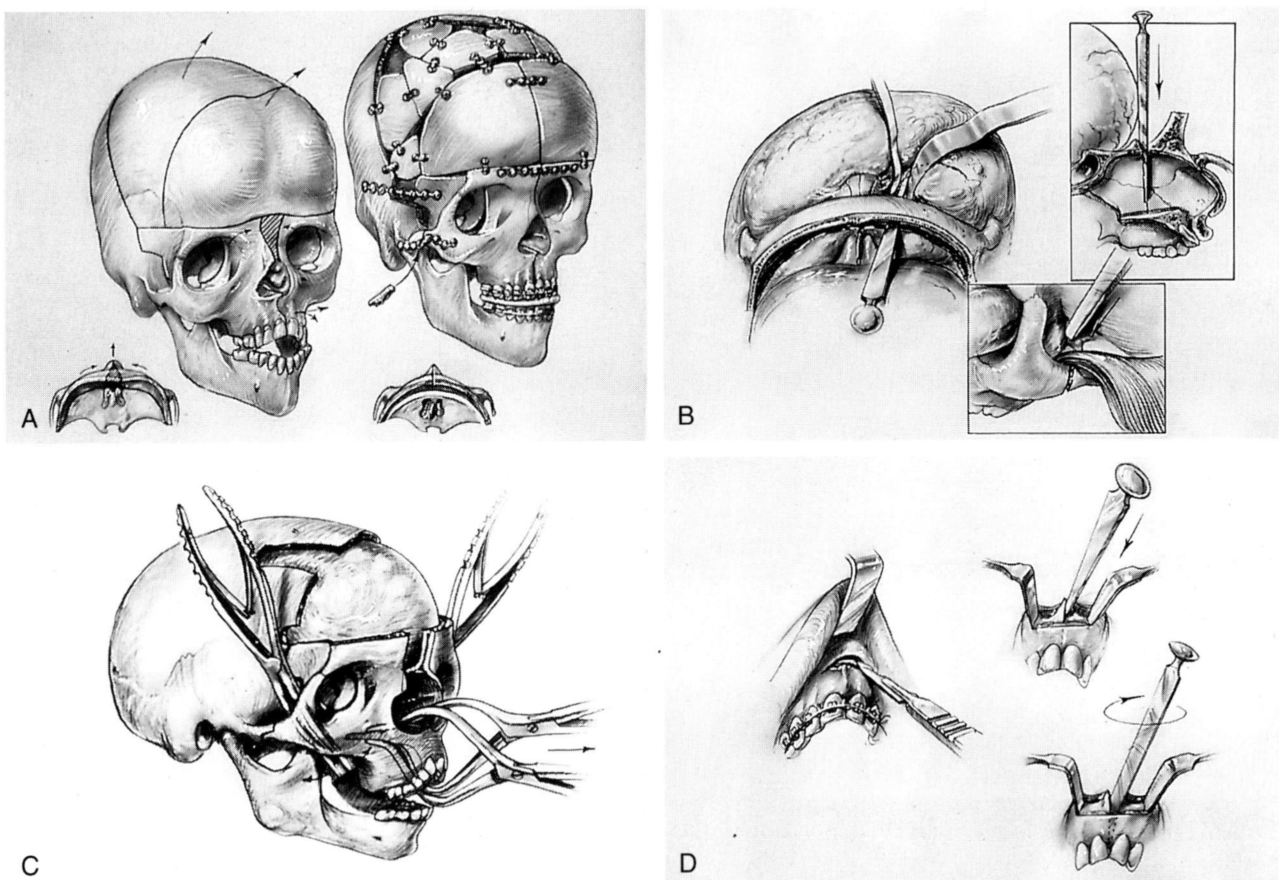

Figure 112–5. A 5-year-old girl with Apert's syndrome underwent suture release and forehead reshaping at 6 months of age. She presented for cranial vault and facial bipartition osteotomies with reshaping and anterior repositioning. *A*, Preoperative craniofacial morphology with planned and completed osteotomies and reshaping. Stabilization is with cranial bone grafts and miniplate fixation. *B*, Osteotomies requiring completion with a chisel. Osteotomy of medial orbital wall is completed posterior to the medial canthi and nasolacrimal apparatus; with the chisel placement through the anterior cranial base, osteotomy is completed through anterior cranial base down through the bony septum of the nose; osteotomy through the exposure provided by the coronal incision and infratemporal fossa to the pterygomaxillary suture, which is then separated. *C*, After completing the facial bipartition osteotomies, Tessier disimpaction forceps are placed through the nose and mouth with pterygomaxillary spreader forceps placed through coronal incision and infratemporal fossa to pterygomaxillary suture regions for disimpaction of midface. *D*, Intraoral buccal vestibular incision, dissection down to anterior nasal spine region with osteotomy down the midline of the hard palate as part of facial bipartition osteotomies. *E*, Preoperative frontal view. *F*, Postoperative frontal view at 2 years after reconstruction. *G*, Preoperative lateral view. *H*, Postoperative lateral view at 2 years after reconstruction. *I*, Intraoperative lateral view of cranial vault, orbits, and zygomatic arch through coronal incision after osteotomies. Stabilization with cranial bone grafts and miniplate fixation. *J*, Preoperative (*left*) and postoperative (*right*) axial-sliced computed tomographic scans through midorbits, demonstrating improvement in orbital hypertelorism and orbital depth with diminished eyeball proptosis. (*A* to *J* from Posnick JC: Craniofacial dysostosis: Staging of reconstruction and management of the midface deformity. Neurosurg Clin North Am 2:683–702, 1991.)

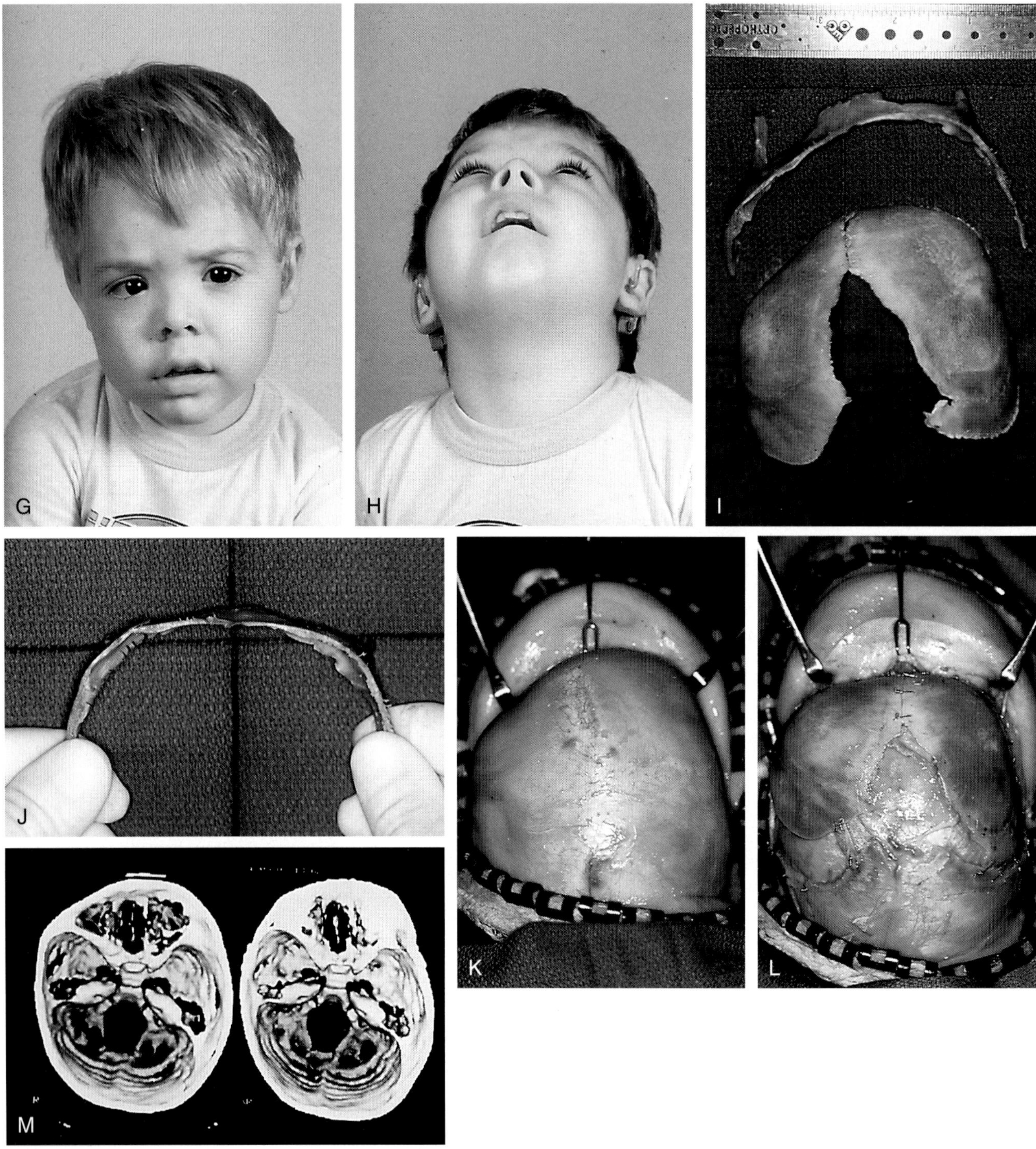

Figure 112–4 *Continued. G*, Frontal view at 3 years of age. *H*, Worm's-eye view at 3 years of age. *I*, View of misshapen orbital unit and anterior cranial vault bone before reinsertion. *J*, Same view of orbital unit after reshaping before reinsertion. *K*, Craniofacial skeleton from above in unilateral coronal synostosis before and after (*L*) reconstruction. *M*, Three-dimensional computed tomographic scan re-formations of cranial base before (left) and after (right) reconstruction. (*A* to *M* from Posnick JC: Craniosynostosis: Surgical management in infancy. *In* Bell WH [ed]: Orthognathic and Reconstructive Surgery, vol 3. Philadelphia, WB Saunders, 1992, pp 1888–1931.)

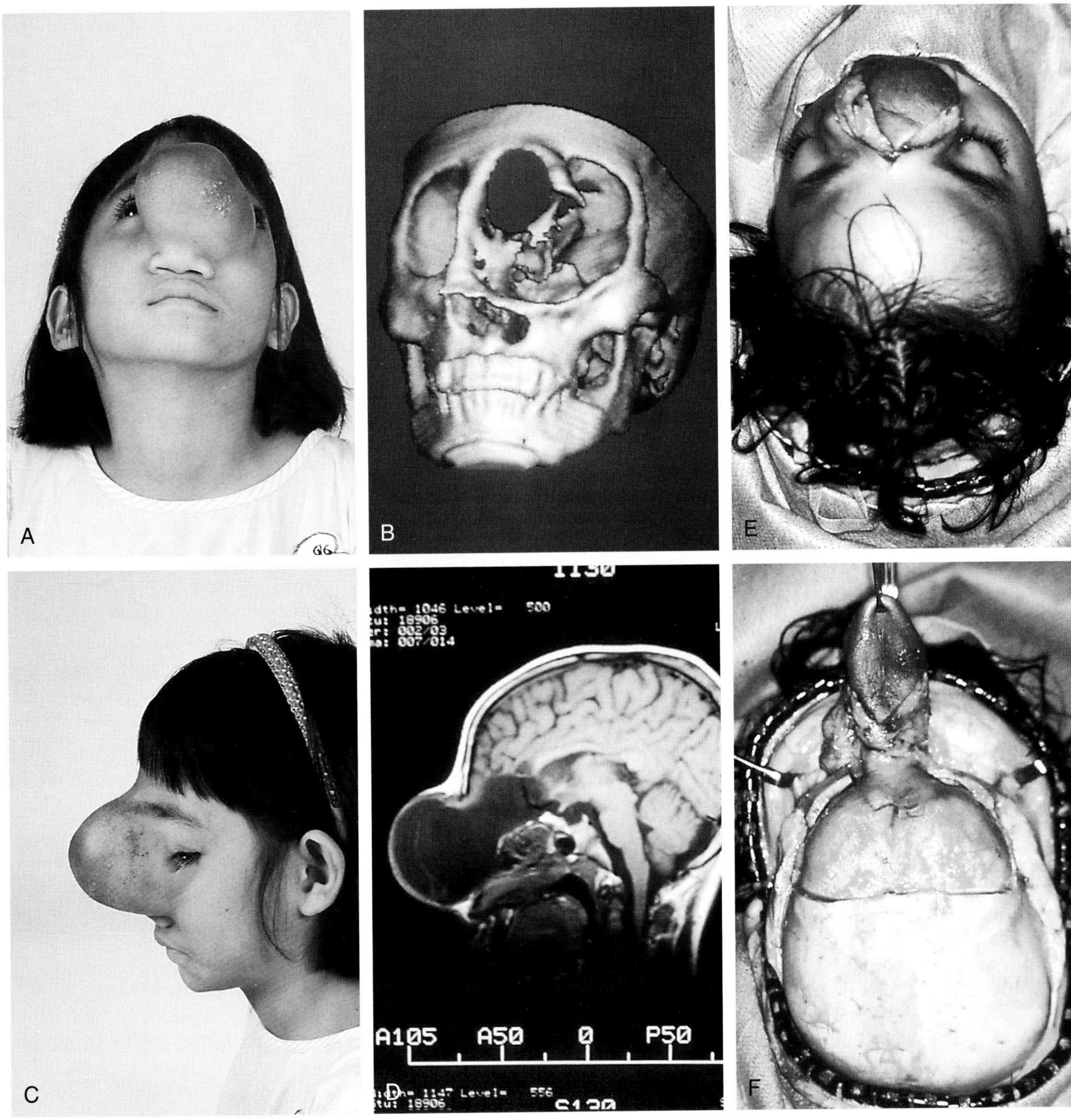

Figure 112–8. An 8-year-old girl was referred from the Philippines with a previously unrepaired congenital frontonasoethmoidal encephalocele. *A*, Bird's-eye view before repair and reconstruction. *B*, Preoperative computed tomographic scan view demonstrating the size and location of the encephalocele and the extent of the bony deformation. C, Lateral view before repair and reconstruction. *D*, Lateral midsagittal sliced magnetic resonance image demonstrating the extent of encephalocele. *E*, Intraoperative view, through a direct nasal skin excision; the encephalocele is being dissected. *F*, Intraoperative view, through a coronal incision, after bifrontal craniotomies and removal of the mid-supraorbital ridge; the encephalocele is followed to the cranial base.

Illustration continued on following page

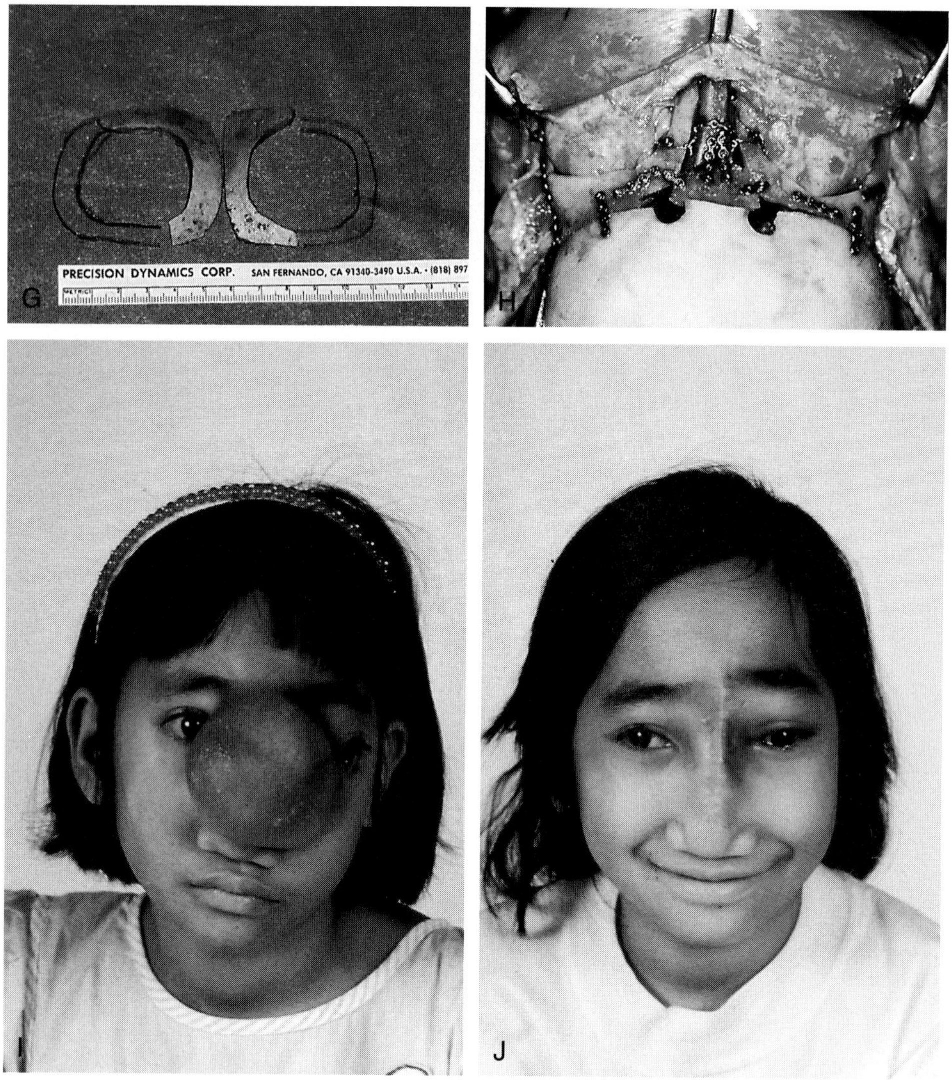

Figure 112–8 *Continued.* G, New medial orbital rims are constructed from autogenous cranial bone grafts. *H*, Intraoperative view, through a coronal incision, after skeletal reconstruction. Fixation is with titanium miniplates and microplates and screws. *I*, Frontal view before repair and reconstruction. *J*, Frontal view 2 months later. (*A* to *J* from Posnick JC: Pediatric cranial base surgery. Plast Reconstr Surg 3:107, 1994.)

Fibrous Dysplasia of Anterior Skull Base and Orbits Presenting as Blindness. The 3-year-old boy in Figure 112–9 presented to the emergency department with progressive visual loss and a degree of proptosis of the left eye.[30] At the time of presentation, he had central, steady, and maintained fixation of the right eye but had difficulty locating objects placed before his left eye, which showed axial proptosis of 3 mm. Both optic nerves were severely atropic on funduscopy, particularly in the left proptotic eye. The boy was judged to have only light perception in the left eye and a mild to moderate loss of vision in the right eye.

A large, partially cystic and bony mass was centered in the region of the body of the sphenoid bones. It extended laterally along the greater and lesser wings of the sphenoid bones, inferiorly as far as the clivus, and anteriorly into the ethmoids and the medial walls of the orbits. The left optic nerve in particular was depressed inferiorly and laterally. The clinical and radiographic findings were consistent with the diagnosis of fibrous dysplasia.[15, 25, 26]

At operation, a bifrontal craniotomy was completed through a coronal (skin) incision. Bilateral upper orbital osteotomies were completed, and the orbital units were removed to adequately expose the cranial base for direct tumor removal, minimizing the need for excessive traction on the frontal lobes or optic nerves. The entire procedure was carried out extradurally. The resultant defect included both orbital roofs, medial orbital walls, and anterior cranial base.

Autogenous cranial bone was selected from the posterior cranial vault to reconstruct the orbital roof defects. The grafts were shaped to reconstruct the resected segments and then secured with microplates and screws. All dural rents were repaired, and the orbital units and frontal bones were replaced and secured with microplates and screws. The child's recovery was uneventful without further visual deterioration.

Extensive Malignant Melanoma of the Uvea Extending to the Cranial Base. A female infant (Fig. 112–10) was born with a large left-sided facial mass involving the

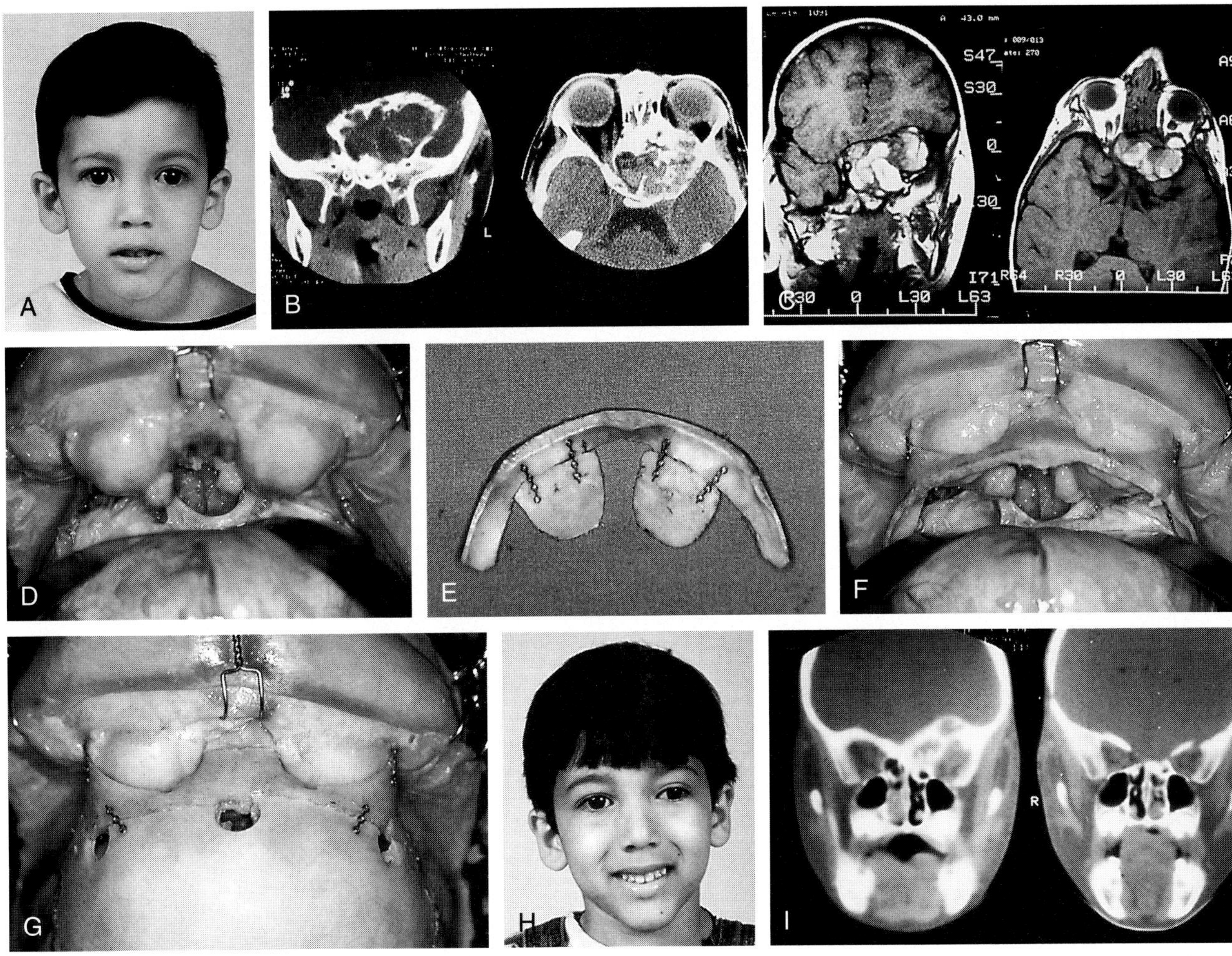

Figure 112–9. A 3-year-old boy with progressive visual loss and a degree of proptosis of the left eye resulting from fibrous dysplasia originating at the anterior skull base and orbits. *A*, The patient is shown in frontal view. *B*, Coronal and axial computed tomographic (CT) scan slices through the cranial base and orbits, demonstrating extent of abnormal fibro-osseous process of bone resulting in optic nerve compression. C, Coronal and axial magnetic resonance scans demonstrating mass of anterior skull base and orbits. *D*, With completion of access frontal and upper orbital osteotomies and decompression of the surrounding contents of both superior orbital fissures, optic nerves and dura, the optic chiasm is visualized. *E*, The orbital roofs are reconstructed with cranial grafts and fixed in place with microplates and screws to the orbital unit before being reinset. *F*, Orbital osteotomy unit reinset and then fixed with microplate and screws. *G*, Frontal bones reinset and fixed in place with microplates and screws. *H*, Full-face view 1½ years after surgery. *I*, Coronal-sliced CT scan close to optic foramen before (*left*) and after (*right*) tumor resection. Reconstructed orbital roofs can be seen. (*A* to *I* from Posnick JC, Wells MC, Drake JM, et al: Childhood fibrous dysplasia presenting as blindness: A skull base approach for resection and immediate reconstruction. Pediatr Neurosurg 19:260–266, 1993; reprinted by permission of S. Karger AG, Basel.)

orbit, forehead, and cheek.[29] A CT scan and magnetic resonance image of the infant's face showed a lobulated mass filling the orbit and the temporal, infratemporal, and pterygopalatine fossa; destruction of the maxilla; and distortion of the nasal bones and left nasal passage. The globe was completely filled with tumor, and there was erosion of the skull base. The results of a metastatic workup were negative. A biopsy was performed, and a malignant melanoma was confirmed.

Resection and satisfactory reconstruction was not considered possible. The patient underwent two courses of chemotherapy and, concomitantly, low-dose radiation therapy of 1000 rads using a tangential field to spare the brain. However, the size of the tumor remained unaffected.

The patient was referred to me for assessment. Surgical resection with immediate reconstruction was judged technically possible. At 4 months of age, the patient underwent total resection of the tumor. The excision included en bloc resection of the soft tissue of the forehead, cheek, preauricular area, lateral portion of the nose, adnexal area, and cutaneous portion of the upper lip; enucleation of the eyeball; resection of the total zygoma, glenoid fossa, lateral orbital wall, and orbital floor; a partial maxillectomy; and resection of the soft tissue of the pterygomaxillary space, temporal and infratemporal space, and nasopharynx on the left side. The mandible, although degloved for tumor resection, was preserved. The cranial base was dissected free of tumor from the facial side without the need for formal craniotomy.

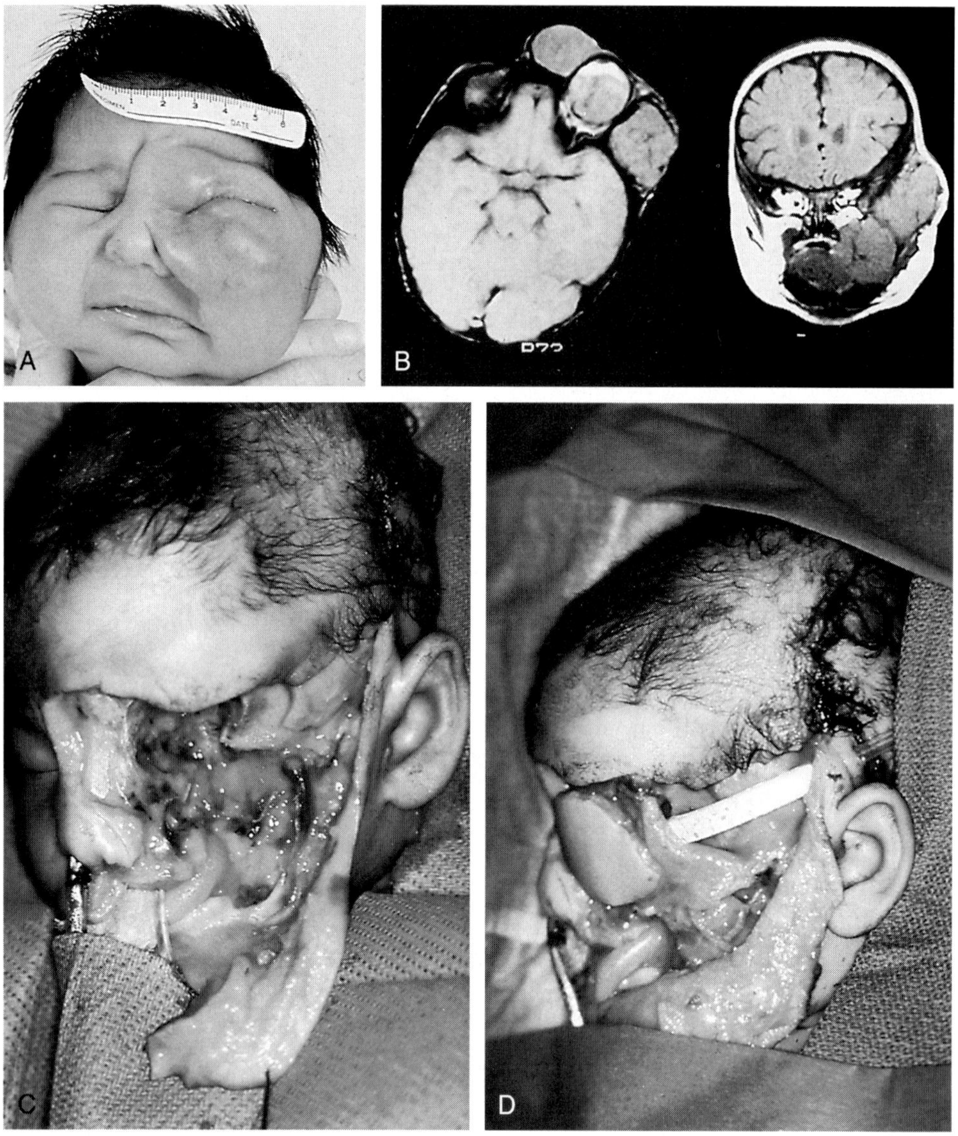

Figure 112–10. Extensive malignant melanoma of the uvea in a child. *A*, Full-face frontal view shortly after birth. *B*, Axial-sliced computed tomographic scan and coronal-sliced magnetic resonance scan of craniofacial region demonstrating the extent of the congenital tumor. *C*, Intraoperative view after tumor resection before soft tissue reconstruction. *D*, Intraoperative view showing the serratus anterior–latissimus dorsi free tissue transfer in place before the wound was closed.

A combined free serratus anterior–latissimus dorsi myocutaneous flap was transferred to the resection defect and tailored for satisfactory reconstruction. The vascular pedicle of the flap was anastomosed to the superficial temporal vessels. There has been no evidence of tumor recurrence. This patient's breathing, swallowing, speech, and chewing are all in the normal range 3 years later.

Cranio-orbital Neurofibromatosis. The child shown in Figure 112–11 was born with von Recklinghausen's disease with extensive plexiform neurofibromatosis involving the left cranio-orbital region. He underwent initial resection and reconstruction through an intracranial approach at 3 years of age.[60] There was significant regrowth of the residual tumor, and he was referred to me when he was 11 years of age. Clinical and CT scan examination confirmed the presence of extensive left facial neurofibroma extending from the cavernous sinus, through the widened superior orbital fissure, the cone of the globe, and the upper eyelid tissue into the dermis of the skin. There was marked proptosis of the left eye with intermittent globe herniation.

At 11 years of age, he underwent a combined neurosurgical and craniofacial/plastic surgical anterior cranial base–orbital approach to debulk his tumor and improve his eye position. A craniotomy was completed of the left frontal and temporal bone through a coronal incision.

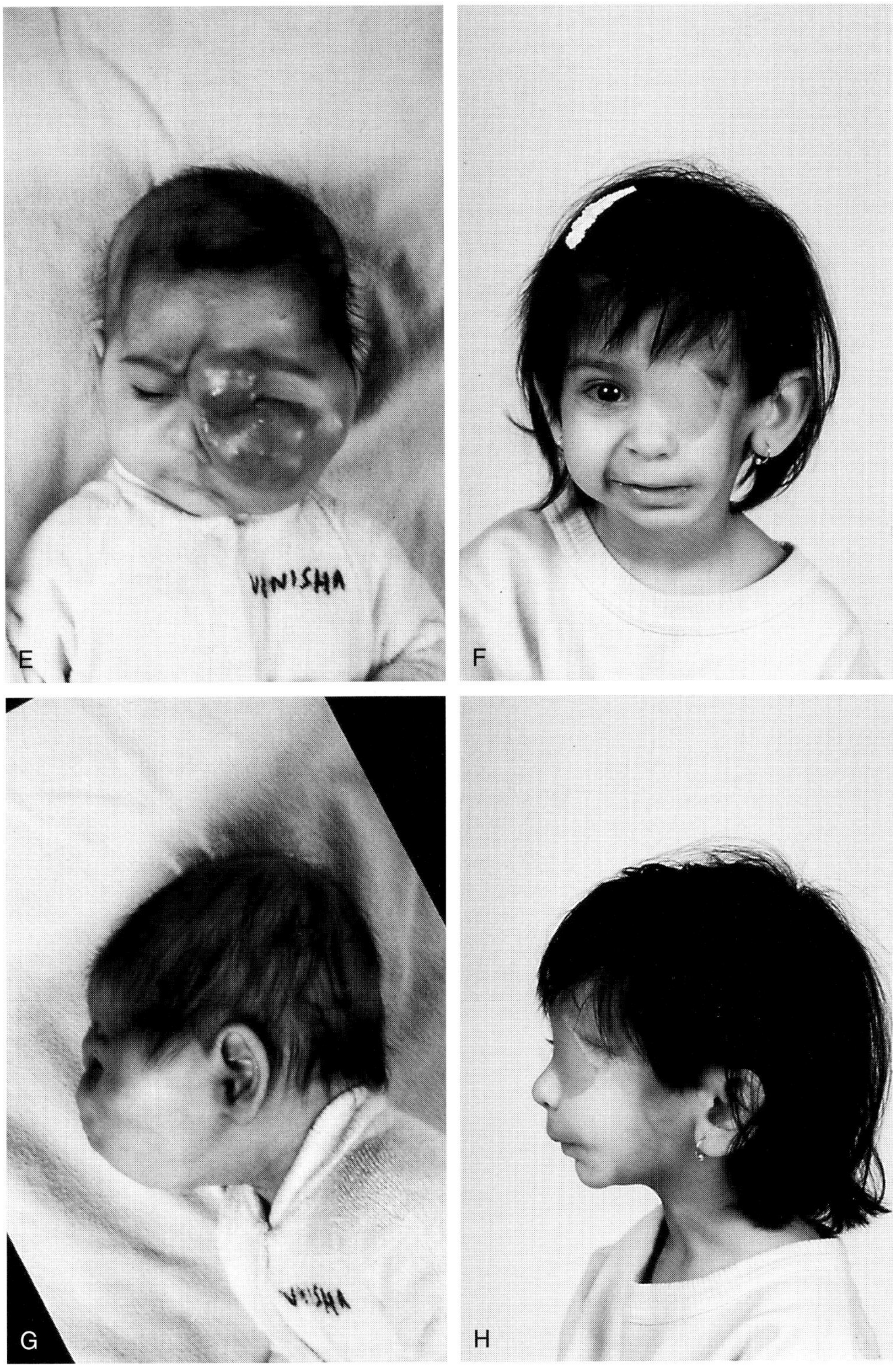

Figure 112–10. *Continued E*, Full-face frontal view at 4 months of age, after a course of chemotherapy and radiation therapy before surgical resection that included immediate reconstruction. *F*, Full-face frontal view, 2 years following tumor resection and reconstruction. *G*, Full-face lateral view at 4 months of age. *H*, Full-face lateral view, 2 years following tumor resection and reconstruction. (*A* to *H* from Posnick JC, Chen P, Zuker R, et al: Extensive malignant melanoma of the uvea in childhood: Resection and immediate reconstruction with microsurgical and craniofacial techniques; reprinted with permission from Ann Plastic Surg 31:265–270, 1993.)

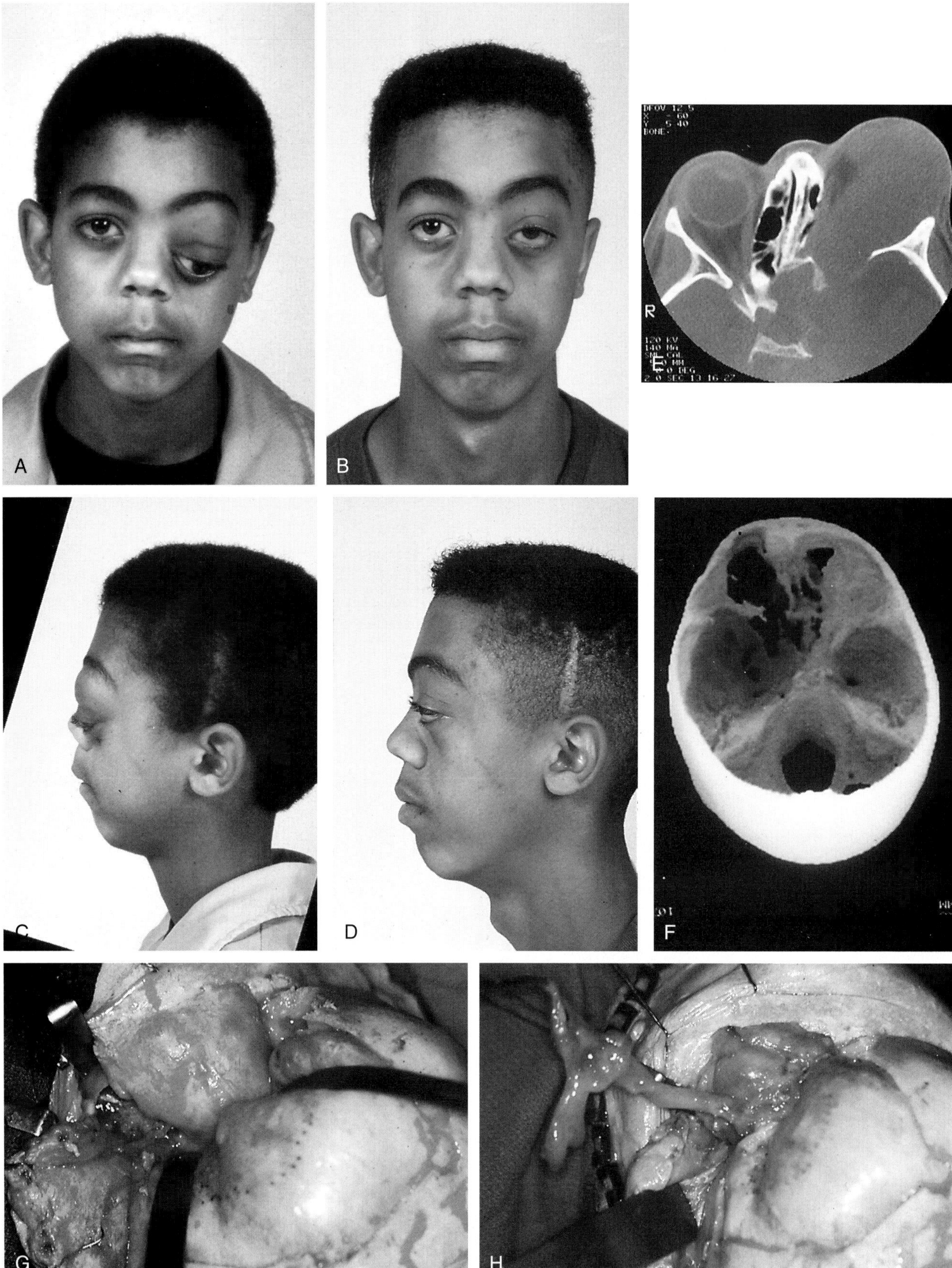

Figure 112–11. An 11-year-old boy born with von Recklinghausen's disease with extensive neurofibromatosis involving the left cranio-orbital region. *A*, Frontal view before tumor rebulking and reconstruction. *B*, Frontal view 4 years later. *C*, Lateral view before tumor debulking and reconstruction. *D*, Lateral view 4 years later. *E*, Axial-sliced computed tomographic scans demonstrating extensive cranio-orbital neurofibromatosis and bony deformation before surgery. *F*, Three-dimensional reconstruction of cranial bone demonstrating a large defect in the anterior cranial fossa. *G*, Intraoperative view after coronal incision and cranial vault and orbital osteotomies with exposure of tumor excision. *H*, Intraconal removal of plexiform neurofibromatosis. (*A* to *H* from Posnick JC: Pediatric cranial base surgery. Prob Plast Reconstr Surg 3:107, 1994.)

After the orbit and zygoma were dismantled, the neurofibroma was debulked from the cavernous sinus intradurally, the globe intraconally, and within the upper eyelid. The orbit, zygoma, and temporal and frontal bones having been dismantled were then reconstructed. The patient's recovery was uneventful. His vision is intact, and he participates in all routine and sports-related activities.

CONCLUSIONS

Surgery of the anterior cranial base and orbits in children has become a routine component of the practice of neurosurgeons, craniofacial/plastic surgeons, neuro-ophthalmologists, and head and neck otolaryngologists. Selective craniotomies and facial osteotomies can improve exposure to the anterior cranial base and orbits for tumor removal. Once the anterior cranial base–orbital work is completed, the access craniotomies and osteotomies are replaced with minimal morbidity. In other clinical situations, craniotomies are completed to retract the frontal and temporal lobes of the brain to minimize morbidity and allow for effective osteotomies of the orbits and midface through the anterior cranial base. This approach offers the opportunity to solve difficult congenital, post-traumatic, and postneoplastic orbital and midface problems.

A coordinated interdisciplinary approach to the management of these pediatric congenital, traumatic, and neoplastic anterior cranial base–orbital problems is essential. When this approach is combined with recent technical advances (including the use of pedicle flaps, microvascular free tissue transfers, microneural repairs, tissue-expansion techniques, autogenous cranial bone grafts, and the use of refined plate and screw internal fixation for osteotomy and bone graft stabilization), the craniofacial team is able to achieve satisfactory results in most patients.

REFERENCES

1. Converse JM, Kazanjian VH: Surgical Treatment of Facial Injuries, 2nd ed. Baltimore, Williams & Wilkins, 1982.
2. Gillies H, Millard DR Jr: The Principles and Art of Plastic Surgery. Boston, Little, Brown & Co, 1957.
3. Gillies H, Harrison SH: Operative correction by osteotomy of recessed malar maxillary compound in case of oxycephaly. Br J Plast Surg 3:123–127, 1950.
4. Tessier P: Osteotomies totales de la face: Syndrome de Crouzon, syndrome d'Apert: Oxycephalies, scaphocephalies, turricephalies. Ann Chir Plast 12:273, 1967.
5. Tessier P: Relationship of craniosynostoses to craniofacial dysostoses and to faciostenoses: A study with therapeutic implications. Plast Reconstr Surg 48:224, 1971.
6. Tessier P: Total osteotomy of the middle third of the face for faciostenosis or for sequelae of LeFort III fractures. Plast Reconstr Surg 48:533, 1971.
7. Tessier P: The definitive plastic surgery treatment of the severe facial deformities of craniofacial dysostosis: Crouzon's and Apert's diseases. Plast Reconstr Surg 48:419, 1971.
8. Rougerie J, Derome P, Anquez L: Craniostenoses et dysmorphies cranio-faciales: Principes d'une nouvelle technique de traitement et ses resultats. Neurochirurgie 18:429–440, 1972.
9. Hoffman HJ, Mohr G: Lateral canthal advancement of the supraorbital margin: A new corrective technique in the treatment of coronal synostosis. J Neurosurg 45:376, 1976.
10. Whitaker LA, Schut L, Kerr LP: Early surgery for isolated craniofacial dysostosis. Plast Reconstr Surg 60:575, 1977.
11. Marchac D, Renier D: "Le front flottant": Traitement précoce des faciocraniostenoses. Ann Chir Plast 24:121, 1979.
12. Derome PJ, et al: Les tumeurs sphenoethmoidales: Possibilités d'exerese et de réparation chirurgicales. Neurochirurgie 18 (suppl I), 1972.
13. Derome PJ: The transbasal approach to tumors invading the base of the skull. *In* Schmidek MH, Sweet WH (eds): Current Technics in Operative Neurosurgery. New York, Grune & Stratton, 1977, pp 223–245.
14. Derome PJ, Visot A: Osseous lesions of anterior and middle base. *In* Sekhar LN, Janecka IP (eds): Surgery of Cranial Base Tumors. New York, Raven Press, 1993.
15. Jackson IT, Hide TAH, Gomuwka PK, et al: Treatment of cranio-orbital fibrous dysplasia. J Maxillofac Surg 10:138, 1982.
16. Jackson IT, Laws ER Jr, Martin RD: A craniofacial approach to advanced recurrent cancer of the central face. Head Neck Surg 5:474–488, 1983.
17. Jackson IT, Marsh WR: Anterior cranial fossa tumors. Ann Plast Surg 11:479–489, 1983.
18. Alperin KM, Levine HL, Wood BG, Tucker HM: Approach to and reconstruction for lesions of the posterior third of the tonque via midline labiomandibular glossotomy. Head Neck Surg 6:744, 1984.
19. Tessier P, Rougier J, Hervouet F, et al (eds): Plastic Surgery of the Orbits and Eyelid. New York, Masson, 1977.
20. Ray BS, McLean JM: Combined intracranial and orbital operation for retinoblastoma. Arch Ophthalmol 30:437, 1943.
21. Sisson GA, Bytell DE, Becker SP, Ruge D: Carcinoma of the paranasal sinuses and craniofacial resection. J Laryngol Otol 90:59, 1976.
22. Shah JP, Galicich JH: Craniofacial resection for malignant tumours of the ethmoid and anterior skull base. Arch Otolaryngol 103:514, 1977.
23. Schram VL Jr, Myers EN, Maroon JC: Anterior skull base surgery for benign and malignant disease. Laryngoscope 89:1077, 1979.
24. Attia EL, Bentley KC, Head T, Mudder D: A new external approach to the pterygomaxillary fossa and parapharyngeal space. Head Neck Surg 6:884, 1984.
25. Moore AT, Buncic JR, Munro IR: Fibrous dysplasia of the orbit in childhood: Clinical features and management. Ophthalmology 92:12–20, 1985.
26. Chen Y-R, Noordoff MS: Treatment of craniomaxillofacial fibrous dysplasia: How early and how extensive? Plast Reconstr Surg 86:835–842, 1990.
27. Posnick JC, Polley JW, Zuker RM, Chan H: Chemotherapy and surgical resection combined with immediate reconstruction in a one-year-old child with rhabdomyosarcoma of the maxilla. Plast Reconstr Surg 89:320–325, 1992.
28. Zuker RM, Posnick JC: The role of microsurgery in pediatric craniofacial reconstruction. Clin Plast Surg 4:833, 1992.
29. Posnick JC, Chen P, Zuker R, et al: Extensive malignant melanoma of the uvea in childhood: Resection and immediate reconstruction with microsurgical and craniofacial techniques. Ann Plast Surg 3:265–270, 1993.
30. Posnick JC, Wells MC, Drake JM, et al: Childhood fibrous dysplasia presenting as blindness: A skull base approach for resection and immediate reconstruction. Pediatr Neurosurg 19:260–266, 1993.
31. Luhr HG: Zur stabilen Osteosynthese bei Unterkiefer-frakturen. Dtsch Zahnaerztl Z 23:754, 1968.
32. Horster W: Experience with functionally stable palate osteosynthesis after forward displacement of the upper jaw. J Oral Surg 8:176, 1980.
33. Drommer P, Luhr HG: The stabilization of osteotomized maxillary segments with Luhr mini-plates in secondary cleft surgery. J Oral Surg 9:166, 1981.
34. Posnick JC: The role of plate and screw fixation in the treatment of craniofacial malformations. *In* Gruss JS, Manson PM, Yaremchuk MJ (eds): Rigid Fixation of the Craniomaxillofacial Skeleton. Stoneham, MA, Butterworth, 1992, pp 512–526.

35. Posnick JC: The role of plate and screw fixation in the management of pediatric head and neck tumors. *In* Gruss JS, Manson PM, Yaremchuck MJ (eds): Rigid Fixation of the Craniomaxillofacial Skeleton. Stoneham, MA, Butterworth, 1992, pp 656–670.
36. Posnick JC: The role of plate and screw fixation in the treatment of pediatric facial fractures. *In* Gruss JS, Manson PM, Yaremchuk MJ (eds): Rigid Fixation of the Craniomaxillofacial Skeleton. Stoneham, MA, Butterworth, 1992, pp 396–419.
37. Posnick JC, Goldstein JA, Armstrong D, Rutka JR: Reconstruction of skull defects in children and adolescents using fixed cranial bone grafts: Long-term results. Neurosurgery 32:785–791, 1993.
38. Posnick JC, Ewing MP: The role of plate and screw fixation in the treatment of cleft lip and palate jaw deformities. *In* Gruss JS, Manson PM, Yaremchuk MJ (eds): Rigid Fixation of the Craniomaxillofacial Skeleton. Stoneham, MA, Butterworth, 1992, pp 466–485.
39. Posnick JC, Ewing M: Skeletal stability after LeFort I maxillary advancement in patients with unilateral cleft lip and palate. Plast Reconstr Surg 80:706–710, 1989.
40. Phillips JH, Rahn BA: Fixation effects on membranous and endochondral onlay bone-graft resorption. Plast Reconstr Surg 82:872, 1988.
41. Luhr HG: A micro-system for craniomaxillofacial skeletal fixation: Preliminary report. J Craniomaxillofac Surg 16:312–314, 1988.
42. Manson P: Commentary on the long-term effects of rigid fixation on the growing craniomaxillofacial skeleton. J Craniofac Surg 2:69–70, 1991.
43. Tessier P: Autogenous bone grafts taken from the calvarium or facial and cranial applications. Clin Plast Surg 9:531, 1982.
44. Zins JE, Whitaker LA: Membranous versus endochondral bone: Implications for craniofacial reconstruction. Plast Reconstr Surg 72:778, 1983.
45. Kusiak JF, Zins JE, Whitaker LA: The early revascularization of membranous bone. Plast Reconstr Surg 76:510, 1985.
46. Marsh JL, Vannier MW: The "third" dimension in craniofacial surgery. Plast Reconstr Surg 71:759, 1983.
47. Waitzman AA, Posnick JC, Armstrong DC, Pron G: Craniofacial skeletal measurements based on computed tomography: I. Accuracy and reproducibility. Cleft Palate Craniofac J 29:112–117, 1992.
48. Waitzman AA, Posnick JC, Armstrong DC, Pron G: Craniofacial skeletal measurements based on computed tomography: II. Normal value and growth trends. Cleft Palate Craniofac J 29:118–128, 1992.
49. Carr M, Posnick JC, Pron G, Armstrong DC: Cranio-orbito-zygomatic measurements from standard CT scans in unoperated Crouzon and Apert infants: Comparison with normal controls. Cleft Palate Craniofac J 29:129–136, 1992.
50. Posnick JC, Goldstein JA, Waitzman A: Surgical correction of the Treacher Collins malar deficiency with quantitative CT scan analysis of long-term results. Plast Reconstr Surg 92:12–22, 1993.
51. Posnick JC, Lin KY, Chen P, Armstrong D: Sagittal synostosis: Quantitative assessment of presenting deformity and surgical results based on CT scans. Plast Reconstr Surg 92:1015–1024, 1993.
52. Posnick JC, Lin KY, Ghawar BJ, Armstrong D: Crouzon syndrome: Quantitative assessment of presenting deformity and surgical results based on CT scans. Plast Reconstr Surg 92:1027–1037, 1993.
53. Posnick JC, Lin KY, Chen P, Armstrong D: Metopic synostosis: Quantitative assessment of presenting deformity and surgical results based on CT scans. Plast Reconstr Surg 93:16–24, 1994.
54. Murovic JA, Posnick JC, Drake JM, et al: Hydrocephalus in Apert syndrome: A retrospective review. Pediatr Neurosurg 19:151–155, 1993.
55. Posnick JC, Cleland HJ, Zuker RM, Mock D: Recurrent giant cell lesion of the nasomaxillary region in a child: Excision and immediate reconstruction with a free rectus abdominus muscle transfer. J Oral Maxillofac Surg 50:1009–1015, 1992.
56. Posnick JC, Wells MD, Zuker RM: Use of free fibula flap in the immediate reconstruction of paediatric mandibular tumours. J Oral Maxillofac Surg 51:189–196, 1993.
57. Posnick JC: Diagnosis and management of pediatric craniomaxillofacial fractures. *In* Peterson LJ, Indresano AT (eds): Principles of Oral and Maxillofacial Surgery, vol I, part V. Philadelphia, JB Lippincott, 1992, pp 623–640.
58. Posnick JC, Wells M, Pron GE: Pediatric facial fractures: Evolving patterns of treatment. J Oral Maxillofac Surg 51:836–844, 1993.
59. Posnick JC: Pediatric orbital trauma. Oral Maxillofac Surg Clin North Am 5:495–506, 1993.
60. Posnick JC: Pediatric cranial base surgery. Prob Plast Reconstr Surg 3:107–129, 1993.
61. Posnick JC: Craniofacial dysostosis: Staging of reconstruction and management of the midface deformity. Neurosurg Clin North Am 2:683–702, 1991.
62. Posnick JC: Craniofacial dysostosis: Management of the midface deformity. *In* Bell WH (ed): Orthognathic and Reconstructive Surgery, vol III. Philadelphia, WB Saunders, 1992, pp 1888–1931.
63. Posnick JC: Craniosynostosis: Surgical management in infancy. *In* Bell WH (ed): Orthognathic and Reconstructive Surgery, vol III. Philadelphia, WB Saunders, 1992, pp 1838–1887.
64. Cohen MM Jr: Craniosynostosis: Diagnosis, Evaluation and Management. New York, Raven Press, 1986.
65. Posnick JC, Bortolluzi P, Armstrong D, Drake JM: Intracranial nasal dermoid sinus cysts: Computed tomography scan findings and surgical results. Plast Reconstr Surg 93:745–755, 1994.
66. Gaisford JC: Tumors of the head and neck in children. *In* Gaisford JC (ed): Symposium on Cancer of the Head and Neck. St. Louis, CV Mosby, pp 162–172, 1969.
67. Green DM (ed): Diagnosis and Management of Malignant Solid Tumors in Infants and Children. Boston, Martinus Nijhoff, 1985, pp 1–13.
68. Rapids AD, Economidis J, Goumas PD, et al: Tumors of the head and neck in children: A clinico-pathological analysis of 1,007 cases. J Craniomaxillofac Surg 16:279–286, 1988.
69. Pizzo PA, Poplack DG (eds): Principles and Practice of Pediatric Oncology, vol 5. Philadelphia, JB Lippincott, 1989, p 778.
70. Posnick JC, Louie G, Zuker RM, Weitzman S: Ewing's sarcoma: Primary involvement of the zygoma undergoing resection and immediate reconstruction. Plast Reconstr Surg 89:956–961, 1992.
71. Posnick JC, Al-Qattan MM, Zuker RM: Large vascular malformation of the face undergoing resection with facial nerve preservation in infancy. Ann Plast Surg 30:67–70, 1993.
72. Albores-Saavedra J, Martin RG, Smith JL Jr: Rhabdomyosarcoma: A study of 35 cases. Ann Surg 157:186, 1963.
73. Flamant F, Hill C: The improvement in survival associated with combined chemotherapy in childhood rhabdomyosarcoma: A historical comparison of 345 patients in the same center. Cancer 53:2417, 1984.
74. Heyn RM, Holland R, Newton WA Jr, et al: The role of combined chemotherapy in the treatment of rhabdomyosarcoma in children. Cancer 34:2128, 1974.
75. Sagerman RH, Tretter P, Ellsworth RM: The treatment of orbital rhabdomyosarcoma of children with primary radiation therapy. AJR 114:31, 1972.
76. Abramsom DH, Ellsworth RM, Tretter P, et al: The treatment of orbital rhabdomyosarcoma with irradiation and chemotherapy. Ophthalmology 86:1330, 1979.
77. Batsakis JG: Tumors of the Head and Neck: Clinical and Pathological Considerations, 2nd ed. Baltimore, Williams & Wilkins, 1979, pp 269–279, 291–311.

Index

Note: Page numbers in *italics* refer to illustrations; page numbers followed by t refer to tables.

Abducens nerve, anatomy of, 845
Abducens nerve palsy, eyelid retraction associated with, 74, *75*
  in diabetic patient, 139
Abscess, subperiosteal, diagnostic and therapeutic features of, 941t–942t
    MRI scan of, 889–890, *890*
  with preseptal cellulitis, 310, *310*
Absorbable suture(s), 284, 284t
Acantholysis, in pemphigus, 103
Acanthosis nigricans, *23,* 23–24
  differential diagnosis of, 24
  disorders associated with, 23t
  drug-induced, 23
  in diabetic patient, 140
  malignant, 23–24
ACE (angiotensin-converting enzyme), in sarcoidosis, 108
Acetylcysteine, to reduce ulceration, after chemical injury, 225
ACLE (acute cutaneous lupus erythematosus), 4. See also *Lupus erythematosus (LE).*
  diagnosis of, 6
  ocular complications of, 4–5, 5t
  revised criteria for, 4t
  treatment of, 6–7
Acne rosacea, 38, *38*
Acoustic neuroma, 474
Acquired immunodeficiency syndrome (AIDS), 525–533
  conjunctival Kaposi's sarcoma in, 236, 242, *243*
  eyelid manifestation(s) of, 526–529
    herpes zoster ophthalmicus in, 526
    infection as, 526
    Kaposi's sarcoma as, 526–528, *527*
    molluscum contagiosum in, 526, *526*
    non-Hodgkin's lymphoma as, 528
    sebaceous cell carcinoma as, 528–529
    verruca vulgaris in, 526
  management of, 525
  ocular manifestation(s) of, 532–533
    cytomegalovirus retinitis as, 533
    Kaposi's sarcoma as, 532
  orbital manifestation(s) of, 529–532
    aspergillosis as, 529, *530*
    eosinophilic granuloma as, 532
    infection as, 529
    inflammatory diseases as, 529–530
    non-Hodgkin's lymphoma as, 530–532, *531*
    Pneumocystis carinii infection and, 529
    tumors as, 532, *532*
Acquired immunodeficiency syndrome (AIDS) *(Continued)*
  seborrheic dermatitis in, *37,* 38
  transmission of, 525
  virus causing, 525
Acrochordon (skin tag), of eyelid, 324, *324*
Acromegaly, 142–143
Acrospiroma, eccrine, of eyelid, 334
Actinic keratoses, chemical peels for, 663
Actinomycosis, involving eyelids, 314
Acuity, visual. See *Visual acuity.*
Acupuncture, 695
  auricular, equipment for, 719
    for blepharospasm, 718–720, 719t
    mapping studies in, 718
    point localization in, 718–719, *719*
    preparation for, 718
    technique of, 719, *720*
Acute cutaneous lupus erythematosus (ACLE), 4. See also *Lupus erythematosus (LE).*
  diagnosis of, 6
  ocular complications of, 4–5, 5t
  revised criteria for, 4t
  treatment of, 6–7
Acute disseminated epidermal necrosis (ADEN), 35, 106
Addison's disease, 141
ADEN (acute disseminated epidermal necrosis), 35, 106
Adenoacanthoma (adenoid squamous carcinoma), of eyelid, 350
Adenocarcinoma, metastatic, to eyelid, *54*
  of lacrimal glands, 999, *1000*
    treatment of, 1004
Adenoid cystic carcinoma, of lacrimal glands, 68–69, *69,* 303, *304*
    metastasis from, 1004, *1006*
    prognosis for, 1004–1005, *1005*
    radiologic features of, 1001, *1001–1002*
    treatment of, 1005
  of orbit, 68–69, *69*
Adenoid squamous carcinoma (adenoacanthoma), of eyelid, 350
Adenoma, pleomorphic, of eyelid, 334, *334*
  of lacrimal glands, epidemiology of, 999, 1001
    malignant transformation of, 1002, 1003
    natural history of, 1002
    presentation of, *1000,* 1001
    radiologic features of, 1001, *1001–1002*
    treatment of, 1004
Adenoma *(Continued)*
  sebaceous, in tuberous sclerosis, 27
    of eyelid, 337, *337*
Adie's pupil, 877
Adipose tumor(s), of orbit, 996–997
Adult pleomorphic rhabdomyosarcoma, 995
Aesthetician, role of, before and after surgery, 576–577
Aesthetics, definition of, 573
  in plastic and reconstructive surgery, 573–575
    patient benefits of, 574–575
    physician benefits of, 573–574
  medical, certification courses in, 574t
African American(s), exophthalmometry in, 699t
  oculoplastic surgery in, considerations for, 715–717, *716–717,* 717t
Age, osteotomy and, 1053
Age distribution, of orbital lesions, 854t–856t, *857–858,* 858t
AIDS. See *Acquired immunodeficiency syndrome (AIDS).*
Alfentanil, as anesthetic agent, 296
Alginate impression, used in design and making of prosthesis, 1138, *1138*
Alkali burns, 222–230. See also *Chemical injury(ies).*
Alkylating agents, pharmacology of, 97
Allergic granulomatous angiitis, 113
Allergic reaction(s), to anesthesia, 297
Allergy, causing tearing, 751
  pseudonasolacrimal duct obstruction secondary to, 751–752
"Alligator" tears, 735
Alloplasty, and spontaneous epithelialization, in conjunctival mucous membrane replacement, 171–172, *171–172*
Alopecia, brow, electropigmentation for, 676
Alopecia areata, *44,* 44–45
Alopecia mucinosa, 44, *44*
Alopecia totalis, 44
Alopecia universalis, 44, *44*
Alpha-hydroxy acids, for wrinkles, 563–564, *564*
  used in chemical peels, 666t, 666–667
Alveolar rhabdomyosarcoma, 995
Amebiasis, involving eyelids, 317
Amphotericin B, for phycomycosis, 138
Ampicillin, for sinus infections, 939
Amyloid A, 18, 238
Amyloid AA, 944

Amyloid fibrils, cause and structure of, 944–945
Amyloid L, 18, 238
Amyloidosis, *17,* 17–19, 944–947
  classification of, 18t, 945
  conjunctival, *65,* 65–66, 238–240
    classification of, 238, 239t
    primary localized, 238–239, 239t
      amyloid in, 239, *239–240*
      management of, 239–240
    ptosis due to, 240
    secondary localized, 239t, 240
  differential diagnosis of, 19
  eyelid as site of, *65,* 65–66
  localized forms of, 238, 239t
  myeloma-associated, 18
  ocular presentation of, 945–946, *945–946*
  pathology of, 946–947, *947*
  secondary systemic form of, 238, 239t
  systemic manifestations of, 945
Anaphylactic response (hypersensitivity type I), 96
Anesthesia, "balanced," 297
  for blepharoplasty, 706
  for enucleation, 1038
  for harvesting of tissue grafts, 1080, 1083
  for oculoplastic surgery, 294–299
    commonly used agents in, 296–297
    in pediatric patients, 298–299
    intraoperative problems in, 298
    local or monitored approach to, advantages and disadvantages of, 297–298
    management of concurrent medications with, 295–296
    monitoring during, 298
    preoperative evaluations and screening tests in, 294–295
  for tarsal polishing with mucous membrane grafting, 203
  for transantral approach to orbital decompression, 974
  for transorbital antroethmoidal orbital decompression, 969
  general, agents for, 297
  monitored care during, 296–297
  regional, advantages of, 297
    for eyelid surgery, 278–279, 442, 550
    for lower eyelid blepharoplasty, 619–620, 627
    for male blepharoplasty, 636
    for pterygia removal, 212
    for upper eyelid blepharoplasty, 589–599, *599*
      variations in, 606–607
Anesthetic agents, allergy to, 297
  anxiolytics as, 296
  barbiturates as, 297
  for general anesthesia, 297
  narcotics as, 296–297
  use of, monitored care during, 296–297
Angiitis, allergic granulomatous, 113
  orbital, 966
Angioedema, 40, *40*
Angiolymphoid hyperplasia, with eosinophilia, 949–950, *949–950*
  of eyelid, 332
Angiotensin-converting enzyme (ACE), in sarcoidosis, 108
Angular vein, anatomy of, 275, *276*
Animal bite(s), eyelid injury caused by, 453, 455
Anisocoria, in Horner's syndrome, 78
Ankyloblepharon, congenital, 409
Annulus of Zinn, anatomy of, 847, *847,* 848
Anophthalmic orbit syndrome, 1105. See also *Anophthalmos, acquired.*
Anophthalmic socket, 1127–1133
  complications associated with, evaluation and management of, 1105–1125
  enucleation vs. evisceration procedures and, 1129–1130
  ideal, condition of socket in, 1131, *1131*
    evaluation of, 1130–1131
    eye symmetry in, 1131, *1131*
    head structure in, 1130, *1130*
    implant location in, 1131, *1131*
    implant mobility in, 1131, *1132*
    surgical conditions leading to, 1128–1129, *1128–1130*
    volume loss in, 1131, *1131*
  lax, 1106–1108
  new mobility implants for, 1132, *1133*
  nonsurgical monocular conditions of, 1127–1128, *1128*
  postsurgical considerations for, 1131–1132
  severe contracture in, repair of, 1121, *1122–1125*
    split-thickness skin grafts for, 167–168
  surgical approach to, 1053–1054
Anophthalmos, 905
  acquired, 1105–1125, *1106–1108.* See also *Enucleation.*
    enophthalmos in, 1108–1111, *1108–1112*
    implant complication(s) following, 1119–1121
      exposure or extrusion as, 1119–1121, *1120*
      migration as, 1119, *1119*
    lax socket in, 1106–1108
    lower lid malposition in, 1113–1114, *1115–1118,* 1116–1118
    orbital deformity after, 1121
    ptosis in, *1118,* 1118–1119
    socket contraction after, 1121, *1122–1125*
    sulcus deformity in, 1111–1113, *1112–115*
  congenital, 1105, *1106*
    volume replacement in, 1043
Anterior chamber, paracentesis of, following chemical injury, 223–224
Anthrax, causing necrotic eschars of eyelid, 313
Antibiotics, for orbital cellulitis, 148
  for preseptal cellulitis, in children, 310
  for sinus infections, 939
Antibody(ies), 95
  monoclonal, 96
Antibody-dependent cell-mediated cytotoxicity, 95
Anticholinergics, for essential blepharospasm and Meige's syndrome, 507
Anticonvulsants, chronic patient use of, anesthetic considerations with, 295
  for hemifacial spasm, 511
Antigen(s), epidermolysis bullosa acquisita, 105
  factor VIII–related, in Kaposi's sarcoma, 242
  histocompatibility, 96
Antihypertensives, chronic patient use of, anesthetic considerations with, 295
Antimetabolites, pharmacology of, 97
Anti-Ro/SSA, in subacute cutaneous lupus erythematosus, 5–6
Antrostomy, Caldwell-Luc, 974
Anxiolytics, as anesthetic agents, 296
Aorta, irradiated, used in upper eyelid reconstruction, 365
Apert's syndrome, brachycephaly associated with, 1181, *1183*
  subcranial approach to, 1170, *1172–1173*
    results of, 1176t
  with cranial vault and midface dysplasia, anterior cranial base approach to, 1193, *1196–1197*
Apocrine sweat gland(s), 273, *273,* 324
  benign adnexal lesions originating in, 334–335, *334–335*
Aqueous humor, accumulation of inflammatory products in, glaucoma resulting from, 222–223
Aqueous layer, and precorneal tear film, 736
Argon laser, postoperative use of, for pterygia, 219
Arion sling, in surgical management of facial paralysis, 478–479, *479*
Arlt's line, 203
Arterial arcades, tarsal, *275*
Arteriovenous malformation(s), of eyelid, 331
Arteritis, temporal, 112
Artery(ies). See also specific artery, e.g., *Ophthalmic artery.*
  of ocular region, 273–274, *274–275*
Arthropod venom, disruption of neuromuscular transmission by, 83
Ascorbate, to reduce corneal ulceration, after chemical injury, 229
Asian patient(s), anatomic differences among, 696t, 696–700, 697t, 698t, 699t, 700t
  blepharoplasty in, 702–713. See also *Blepharoplasty, in Asian patients.*
  Chinese view of medicine and, *692–694,* 692–695, 693t
  cultural background of, 691–692
  eyelid tumor(s) in, 721–727
    basal cell carcinoma as, 723, *723*
    lid reconstruction with donor sclera for, 724–727, *725–727*
    sebaceous gland carcinoma as, 721–722, *727*
    squamous cell carcinoma as, 721, *727*
    statistics on, 723–724
Aspergillosis, orbital, diagnostic and therapeutic features of, 941t–942t
  in AIDS patients, 529, *530*
Aspirin, chronic patient use of, anesthetic considerations with, 296
Asteroid bodies, 65
Astrocytoma, juvenile pilocytic, imaging of, 899–900, *899–900*
Atenolol, for thyrotoxicosis, 125, 128
Atopic dermatitis, 41–42, *42*
  treatment of, 42
Atrial fibrillation, evaluation of, prior to oculoplastic surgery, 294–295
Atypia, definition of, 179
Auricular cartilage, used in upper eyelid reconstruction, 364, *364*
Auricular prosthesis, osseointegrated, 1159
Auspitz's sign, in psoriasis vulgaris, 39
Autograft(s). See also *Graft(s).*
  bone, harvesting of, 1077–1080, *1078–1082*
  conjunctival, for management of pterygia, 214–215, *216–217,* 217
    complications of, 217
    graft harvesting in, 215, *216*
    for repopulation of corneal epithelium,

Autograft(s) *(Continued)*
indications for, 249–250
surgical technique of, 250, *250*
Autoimmune syndrome(s), cicatricial pemphigoid associated with, 199
polyglandular, 141
Autologen, 670–675
clinical results with, 673–674, *673–674*
clinical use of, 672–673
collagen dispersion in, 671
collagen fibers in, 672, *672–673*
injection implant site and, histopathologic changes at, 674–675, *674–675*
preparation of, 671
tissue source for, 671–672, 672t
Avitene, for hemostasis in wound repair, 283
Avulsion, in pterygia removal, 211
Azathioprine, for cicatricial pemphigoid, 199
pharmacology of, 97
Azelaic acid, used in chemical peels, 666

B cell(s), 94–95
Bacillus anthracis infection, 313
Bacterial infection(s), causing nasolacrimal duct obstruction, 797–799, 798t, *799*
of eyelid, 313–315
of orbit, in AIDS patients, 529
Baker's phenol solution, used in chemical peels, 667–668
Balloon cell nevus, of eyelid, 338
Barbiturates, as anesthetic agents, 297
Bare-sclera technique (BST), concept of, 212
of pterygia removal, 212–214, *213*
administration of beta radiation after, 217–218
Bartonellosis, of eyelid, 314
Basal cell carcinoma, of eyelid, 300
clinical presentation of, 342–343
histologic features of, 343, *344*
in African American patients, 716, *717*
in Asian patients, 723, *723*
morphea pattern of, 344, *345*
nodular pattern of, 343, *344*
orbital invasion of, 300, *301*
superficial spreading (multicentric) pattern of, 344–345, *345*
ulcerative pattern of, 344, *344*
Basal cell nevus syndrome, of eyelid, 67, *68*
Basilar hyperplasia, definition of, 179
Basophil(s), 95
Bell's palsy, 470, 473
in diabetic patient, 139
ptosis following, 91, *91*
Benign reactive lymphoid hyperplasia, involving orbit, 61–62
Benzodiazepines, for essential blepharospasm and Meige's syndrome, 507
for hemifacial spasm, 511
Béraud valve, 742, *743*
Beta radiation, as adjunct to surgery for pterygia, 217–218
Beta-adrenergic antagonists, for thyroid storm, 130
for thyrotoxicosis, 125, 128
Bianchi valve, 742, *743*
Biologic agents, for metastatic renal cell carcinoma, 1012
Biopsy, diagnostic, of neurogenic tumors of orbit, 984
excisional, for conjunctival lymphoid tumors, 236, *236*
for idiopathic orbital inflammation, 955
Biopsy *(Continued)*
indications for, 1046
of eyelid, for suspected sebaceous gland carcinoma, 193
Birbeck granules, 64
Bite(s), eyelid injury caused by, 452–453, *454*, 455
spider, eyelid necrosis due to, 313
Blastomycosis, of eyelid, 318
Blend modality, used in eyebrow contouring, 593
vs. other techniques, 593–594
Blending, of skin color tone, in micropigmentation, 536
Blepharoconjunctivitis, chronic, sebaceous gland carcinoma masquerading as, 346
sebaceous carcinoma presenting as, 301, *303*
Blepharophimosis syndrome, 411, *411*
Blepharopigmentation, 535, 536–537, *537–538*. See also *Electropigmentation; Micropigmentation.*
Blepharoplasty, complication(s) of, 643–650
brow displacement as, 649, *649*
diplopia as, 644
double crease as, 648, *648*
eyelash loss or misdirection as, 649
incomplete or excessive fat removal as, 646–647, *647*
infection as, 648
lacrimal disorders as, 648–649
lagophthalmos as, 646, *646*
lid necrosis as, 650
lower lid malposition as, 644–645, *645–646*
medial canthal folds as, 649
meibomianitis as, 649
oculocardiac reflex as, 650
prominent pigmentation as, 648
ptosis as, 644, *644*
refractive changes as, 649
round eye deformity as, 646, *646*
scarring as, 648
sensory nerve damage as, 649–650
skin asymmetry as, 648
suture tracts as, 649
visual loss as, 643–644
wound dehiscence as, 648
cosmetic, 543–550
anesthesia for, 550
documentation and patient instructions for, *549*, 549–550
fat excision in, 638, *639–642*, 640–642. See also *Fat excision.*
patient examination prior to, 545–549
baseline tear function in, 549
blepharochalasis in, 548
brow contour in, *546*, 546–547
brow position in, 546, *546*
crow's feet in, 548, *549*
glabellar wrinkles in, 547, *547*
Graves' disease in, 548, *548*
ptosis in, 547
redundant upper and lower lid skin in, 547, *547*
scleral in, 548, *548*
seventh nerve function in, 548–549
surgical modalities used in, *544*
in African American patients, 715–716, *716*
in Asian patients, 702–713
anesthesia for, 706
determination and marking of lid crease in, 706, *706*
Blepharoplasty *(Continued)*
incision techniques in, 706–708, *707–708*
complications of, 709
postoperative care following, 708–709
preoperative evaluation in, 705–706
procedures in, 706–713
suture technique(s) in, 709–713
buried mattress, 710–711, *710–711*
combined buried sutures and small incisions as, 712, *713*
complications of, 712–713
continuous suturing as, 711–712, *712*
postoperative care following, 712
lower eyelid, 617–624
anesthetic injection for, 619–620
draping of patient for, 619
evaluation for, 617–619, *618*
postoperative care in, 624, *624*
repair of lid laxity in, 622–624, *623–624*
skin flap approach to, 620, *620*
skin-muscle flap approach to, 620–622, *621–622*
transconjunctival approach to, 626–631
complications of, 630
inspection of anatomy in, 626, *627*
local anesthesia for, 627
postoperative care in, 629–630
preoperative evaluation and considerations in, 626–627
surgical technique of, 627–629, *628–629*
male, 632–637
anatomic differences in, 633, *633–634*
anesthesia for, 636
lower eyelid correction in, 636–637, *637*
preoperative evaluation in, 633–635
psychosocial issues in, 632
surgical technique in, 635–637, *636*
variations in, 637, *637*
upper eyelid, 596–614
concurrent ptosis repair with, 602–603, *603*
variations of, 609
crease formation and skin closure in, 603, *603–604*
variations of, 609–610
excision and incision of orbital septum in, 600, *600*
variations of, 607–608
excision of fat in, 601, *601*
variations of, 608–609
excision of skin and muscle in, 599–600, *599–600*
variations of, 607
functional indications for, 596–597
historical landmarks in, 597t
local anesthetic infiltration for, 598–599, *599*
variations in, 606–607
postoperative care in, 603–604
variations of, 611
preoperative considerations in, 597, 597t
preparation and draping of patient for, 598
variations in, 605
repair of prolapsed lacrimal gland in, 601–602, *602*
variations of, 609
results of, 611–612, *612–614*
skin closure in, variations of, 610–611
skin marking for, 598, *598–599*
variations in, 605–606
surgical steps in, 597t

Blepharoplasty *(Continued)*
surgical techniques in, 597t, 597–604
variations of, 604–611
Blepharoptosis, in Graves' ophthalmopathy, 515, *515*
Blepharosis, moniliform, 20
Blepharospasm, 89
atypical, 90
auricular acupuncture for, 718–720, 719t, *719–720*
essential, 89, *89*
clinical features of, 504, 506, *506*
diagnostic features of, 505t
management of, 507–510
botulinum A toxin injection in, 507–508, *508*, 509t
future directions in, 509–510
general eye care in, 507
pharmacotherapy in, 507
surgery in, 508–509, *509*
pathogenesis of, 506
management of, 90
Blindness, after blepharoplasty, 643–644
Blood cyst(s), drainage of, 925
Blood supply, to conjunctiva, 161
to facial nerve, *468*, 469
to lacrimal gland, 734, 849
to orbit, 843–844, *843–844*
Blue nevus, of eyelid, 338–339
Bochdalek valve, 742, *743*
Bone(s), craniofacial, abnormality of, 1178–1182, *1179–1185*. See also specific anomaly, e.g., *Brachycephaly.*
male vs. female, 633, *633*
Paget's disease of, causing nasolacrimal duct obstruction, 813
Bone graft(s), autogenous, harvesting of, 1077–1080, *1078–1082*
Bone removal, in orbital surgery, 1048
in transorbital antroethmoidal decompression, *971*, 971–972
Bone wax, for hemostasis in wound repair, 283–284
Bone-anchored hearing aids, 1159
Borrelia burgdorferi, 473
Botryoid rhabdomyosarcoma, 995
Botulinum A toxin, injection of, for essential blepharospasm and Meige's syndrome, 507–508, *508*, 509t
for hemifacial spasm, *508*, 509t, 511
Botulism, cranial nerve paresis in, 152
ptosis from, 83, *84*
Bournville's disease, 26–27, 27t
Brachycephaly, 1180–1181, *1182*
associated with Apert's and Crouzon's syndromes, 1181, *1183–1184*
Bradycardia, during oculoplastic surgery, 298
Breast carcinoma, metastatic orbital disease from, *1009*, 1009–1010
Brightness desaturation, in optic nerve dysfunction, 874–875
Brittle hair (trichothiodystrophy), in ichthyosis, 46
Brow ptosis. See *Ptosis, brow.*
Brown tumor (osteoclastoma), in hyperparathyroidism, 133–134, *134–135*
Browpexy procedure, translid, 587, *587–588*
Brueghel's syndrome, 504
BST (bare-sclera technique), concept of, 212
of pterygia removal, 212–214, *213*
administration of beta radiation after, 217–218
Buccal mucous membrane graft(s), for cicatricial entropion and trichiasis, 203–206
anesthesia and, 203
complications of, 205
harvesting of lower lip membrane in, 204–205, *205*
results of, 205, *206*
surgical methods of, 203–205, *204–206*
for pterygia, 217
"Buff-peel," for wrinkled skin, 565, *565*
Bulbar conjunctiva, 159. See also *Conjunctiva.*
Bulla(e), 29
Bullous disease(s), 98–106. See also specific disease for details.
cicatricial pemphigoid as, 98–100
epidermolysis bullosa as, 103–105
erythema multiforme as, 100–102
pemphigus as, 102–103
toxic epidermal necrolysis as, 105–106
Bullous pemphigoid, vs. cicatricial pemphigoid, 198–199
Bundle of energy theory, *582*, 592
Burkitt's lymphoma, Epstein-Barr virus associated with, 530, 959
Burn(s), alkali, 222–230. See also *Chemical injury(ies).*
facial, micropigmentation for, 535. See also *Micropigmentation.*
thermal, 222

Café-au-lait spots, in neurofibromatosis, 25
Calcification, orbital, dystrophic, differential diagnosis of, 887t
metastatic, differential diagnosis of, 887t
Calcifying epithelioma, Malherbe's, of eyelid, 336, *336*
Calcinosis cutis, in childhood dermatomyositis, 7
Calcium metabolism, regulation of, 132
Caldwell-Luc antrostomy, 974
Caliper(s), used in ophthalmic plastic surgery, *290*
Calymmatobacterium granulomatis infection, 314
Camera, for medical photography, 551–554
automatic film advance in, 551
film in, 554
flash-cord receptacle on, 551
focusing screens of, 552, *552*
lens of, 552–554, *553*
shutter and shutter speed of, 551
Camouflage make-up, 657–661, *658–659*
application principles in, 659–660
choice of, 657, 659t
color principles in, application of, 658, *660*
colors in, choice of, 657–658, *659*
cosmetics used in, 569–571
"faking faults" in, 661
good lighting for, 659
highlighting and contouring in, 660–661
in neutralization of skin discoloration, 658
referral of patient for, 657
use of, 657
in facial rejuvenation, 570–571
Canaliculitis, 153
diagnosis of, 826, *828*
treatment of, 827–829
Canaliculodacryocystorhinostomy, for canalicular stenosis, 830–831
Canaliculus(i), 739–740, *739–741*
agenesis of, 782
Canaliculus(i) *(Continued)*
anatomy of, 821
congenital malformations of, 740, *740*, 821–822, *822*
treatment of, *822*, 822–823
elastic properties of, 745
lower eyelid defects involving, 406
physiology of, 821
stenosis of, 829–831
epiphora due to, 751, *752*
trauma to, 824–825
repair of, 825–826, *826–828*
tumors of, 823–824, *824*
upper eyelid lacerations of, repair of, 359–361, *362*
Candidal infection(s), of eyelid, 318
Cantalano stents, for nasolacrimal duct obstruction, 780
Canthal folds, medial, after blepharoplasty, 649
Canthal ligament(s), medial, 265, *267*
Canthal obliquity, in Graves' ophthalmopathy, surgical techniques for, 521
Canthal tendon, injuries to, repair of, 361–363, *363*
medial, anatomy of, 744
fixation/reconstruction of, 388–390
cantilevered miniplates in, 389–390, *390*
creation of new tendon in, 388, *389*
Nelson screw in, 389, *390*
suturing in, 388–389, *390*
transnasal wiring with dacryocystorhinostomy in, 388, *389*
reconstruction of, in surgical management of facial paralysis, 480, *480–481*
Cantholysis, inferior, in transorbital antroethmoidal orbital decompression, 970, *970*
lateral, in lower eyelid reconstruction, 400, *401*
Canthoplasty, lateral, for paralytic ectropion, 432, *433–435*
Canthotomy, lateral, in transorbital antroethmoidal orbital decompression, 970, *970*
Canthus, injury to, sequence of repair following, 458, *459*
lateral, migration of, as complication of medial reconstruction, 398
rounding of, after blepharoplasty, 646, *646*
medial, laxity of, plication for, 426–427, *426–427*
reconstruction of, 387–398
complications of, 398
composite graft in, 391
direct closure in, 388
glabellar flap in, 391, 393, *395*
goals in, 387
insertion of pretarsal muscles in, 387, *388*
island forehead flap in, 393, *396*
lacrimal involvement in, 396, 398
midline forehead flap in, 393, *396*
Mustardé flap in, 390–391, *392*
myocutaneous flap in, 390, *391*
pedicle flap in, 391, *395*
skin grafts in, 393, 396, *397*
sliding tarsoconjunctival flap in, 391, *394*
spontaneous granulation in, 387
tendon fixation in, 388–390, *388–390*
Tenzel flap in, 391, *393*

Cantilevered miniplates, in fixation/
reconstruction of canthal tendon, 389–390, *390*
Capillary hemangioma. See *Hemangioma, capillary.*
Capnography, monitoring of, during anesthesia, 298
Carbon dioxide, solid, used in chemical peels, 666
Carbon dioxide laser, fat removal by, 638, 640
treatment of lymphangioma with, 926
ultrapulse, used in blepharoplasty, *544*
Carcinoembryonic antigen (CEA), in diagnosis of metastatic disease, 1008
Carcinoid tumor(s), metastatic, to orbit, 57, *58*
Carcinoma, adenoid cystic, of lacrimal glands. See *Adenoid cystic carcinoma, of lacrimal glands.*
of orbit, 68–69, *69*
adenoid squamous, of eyelid, 350
basal cell. See *Basal cell carcinoma.*
breast, metastatic orbital disease from, *1009,* 1009–1010
gastrointestinal, metastatic orbital disease from, 1012
lung, metastatic orbital disease from, 1010
mucoepidermoid, of lacrimal glands, 68, *69,* 999
of orbit, 68, *69*
of sebaceous glands. See *Sebaceous gland carcinoma.*
prostate, metastatic orbital disease from, 1010–1011, *1011*
renal cell, metastatic orbital disease from, 1012
squamous cell. See *Squamous cell carcinoma.*
thyroid, metastatic, to rectus muscle, *55*
Carotenemia, in diabetic patient, 141
Carotid artery, to eyelids, 273–274, *274–275*
Carotid cavernous fistula, CT scan of, 897, *898*
Cartilage, auricular, used in upper eyelid reconstruction, 364, *364*
Cartilage graft(s), harvesting of, 1080, 1082
in surgical management of facial paralysis, 481–482, *481–482*
Cartilage-mucosal compound graft(s), 176
Caruncle, of conjunctiva, 159
Castanares' classification, of baggy eyelid deformity, 597, 597t
Cataract surgery, for cicatricial pemphigoid, 201
Cat-scratch disease, 149
Caucasian(s), exophthalmometry in, 699t
orbits in, 696, 696t
Cautery, thermal, for hemostasis in wound repair, 282–283
Cavernous hemangioma. See *Hemangioma, cavernous.*
Cavernous lymphangioma (cystic hygroma), of eyelid, 331
Cavernous sinus thrombosis, diagnostic and therapeutic features of, 941t–942t
CCLE (chronic cutaneous lupus erythematosus), 4. See also *Lupus erythematosus (LE).*
common form of, 6
CEA (carcinoembryonic antigen), in diagnosis of metastatic disease, 1008
Ceftriaxone, for sinus infections, 939
Cell(s). See also named cell.
of immune system, 94–95
Cellulitis, eyelid, 313
orbital, 146–148, *147,* 889
bacteriology of, 146–147
complications of, 148
diagnostic and therapeutic features of, 941t–942t
medical management of, 148
radiographic diagnosis of, 147–148, *148*
role of paranasal sinus disease in, 935–940, 941t–942t
signs and symptoms of, 147t
postseptal, 146, *147*
preseptal, 144, *147,* 310–312, 889
CT scan of, *148*
diagnostic and therapeutic features of, 941t–942t
in children and neonates, 310
post-traumatic, 311
treatment of, 311–312
with abscess formation, 310, *310*
Centigray (cGy), 1023
Central core myopathy, ptosis in, 84, *85*
Centronuclear (myotubular) myopathy, ptosis in, 84
Cerebellar artery, anteroinferior, 468, *468*
Cerebellopontine angle, *468,* 468–469
Cervicofacial nerve, anatomy of, 277, *277*
Cestode infection(s), of eyelid, 317–318
cGy (centigray), 1023
Chagas' disease, of eyelid, 316–317
periorbital edema in, 152
Chalazion, development of, 308
marginal, 308
recurrent, sebaceous gland carcinoma masquerading as, 346
sebaceous carcinoma presenting as, 190, 301, *303*
surgical removal of, 168, 309
treatment of, 308–309
Chancroid, of eyelid, 314
Chemical agents, topically applied, for hemostasis in wound repair, 283–284
Chemical injury(ies), 222–230
aqueous component of tear film after, reduced, 226
classification of, 223, *224*
emergency care for, 223–225
epidemiology of, 222–223
clinical history in, 222–223
natural repair in, 223
intermediate care for, 225
nature of, 222
perilimbal epithelial loss after, influence of, 226–227, *227*
prognosis of, 223
reevaluation of conjunctiva and tear frame after, 226
treatment of, epidermal growth factor in, 229–230
fibronectin in, 229
orthomolecular approaches to, 229
visual rehabilitation after, 227–228, *228*
Chemical peel(s), 662–669
agents used in, 665–668, 666t, *667–668*
application technique for, 665, *665*
complications of, 668t, 668–669
consent for, 664t
depths of, 662, 663t
evaluation of patient for, 664, 664t, 665t
for wrinkles, 564
indications for, 662–664, 663t
skin preparation for, 664–665
Chemosis, 160
Chemotherapy, causing secondary acquired nasolacrimal duct obstruction, 804
for lymphoid tumors, 961–962
for metastatic breast carcinoma, 1010
for metastatic gastrointestinal carcinoma, 1012
for metastatic lung carcinoma, 1010
for metastatic melanoma, 1012
for non-Hodgkin's lymphoma, 531
for orbital metastatic disease, 1008
for orbital metastatic tumors, 57
for rhabdomyosarcoma, 995–996
Chest radiography, for sarcoidosis, 108
prior to oculoplastic surgery, 294
Chiasmal syndrome, anterior, 883, *884*
Chickenpox, 152
Child(ren), myasthenia gravis in, acquired, 80–81
Prostigmin test for, 82, *82*
oculoplastic surgery in, anesthesia for, 298–299
orbital deformities in, anterior cranial base approach to, access to tumors in, 1188
indications for, 1188–1207
surgical refinement for, 1187–1188. See also *Craniofacial surgery, pediatric.*
orbital rhabdomyosarcoma in. See *Rhabdomyosarcoma, orbital.*
preseptal cellulitis in, 310
Chinese, epicanthal folds in, prevalence of, 699, 700t, 705t
exophthalmometry measurements in, 698, 698t
eyelid dimensions of, 698–700, 699t, 700t
lacrimal fossa in, 696–698, 697t, 698t
optic nerve foramen in, 696–697
orbits in, 696, 696t, 697t, 698t
male vs. female, 696, 696t
tarsus and fat pad in, 699, 700t
Chinese culture, and medicine, *692–694,* 692–695, 693t
Chinese diet, in balance of yin and yang, 695
Chlamydia trachomatis, 154
lymphogranuloma venereum caused by, 315
trachoma caused by, 314
Chloroma (granulocytic sarcoma), orbital, 61, *61*
Chocolate cyst, 926, *926*
Chondrodysplasia punctata syndrome(s), 46
Chondroid syringoma, of eyelid, 334, *334*
Choristoma, of eyelid, *327,* 327–328
phakomatous, 328, *328*
Choroidal detachment, imaging of, 906–907, *906–907*
Choroidal folds, presence of, in orbital disease, 881, *881*
Choroidal hemangioma, imaging of, 910–911, *910–911*
Chromic gut suture, 284, 284t
Chronic cutaneous lupus erythematosus (CCLE), 4. See also *Lupus erythematosus (LE).*
common form of, 6
Chronic progressive external ophthalmoplegia (CPEO), 86–88
neurologic deficits associated with, 88
pigmentary retinopathy in, 87–88, *88*
ptosis in, 87, *87*
ragged-red fibers in, 86
Churg-Strauss syndrome, 11
criteria for classification of, 11t
ocular abnormalities of, 10t

Cicatricial ectropion, as cause of tearing, 765, 767–768, *767–769*
Cicatricial entropion. See *Entropion, cicatricial.*
Cicatricial pemphigoid, *31,* 31–32
associated with secondary acquired nasolacrimal duct obstruction, 801, 802, *803*
clinical stages of, 99
cutaneous manifestations of, 196
differential diagnosis of, 100, 198t, 198–199
disorders associated with, 199
drug-induced, *197,* 197t, 197–197
epidemiology of, 98
general aspects of, 196–199
histopathology of, 99, 198
immunopathology of, 198
nonocular mucous membrane manifestations of, 196
ocular manifestations of, 98, 196–197
staging of, 196–197, *197,* 197t
pathogenesis of, 99–100
systemic manifestations of, 98–99
treatment of, 32, 100, 199–201
medical, 199–200
surgical, *200,* 200–201
Ciliary ganglion, 846, *847*
CIN (conjunctival intraepithelial neoplasia), 231–232
recurrence rates for, 232
Cirrhosis, hepatic, eyelid retraction associated with, 75, *76*
Citrate, to reduce corneal ulceration, after chemical injury, 229
Clamp(s), used in ophthalmic plastic surgery, *290*
Clamp-cut-cauterize technique, of fat removal, 638, *639*
Clavulanate, for sinus infections, 939
Clear cell hidradenoma, of eyelid, 334
Cleft, craniofacial, with orbital and facial hypertelorism, anterior cranial base approach to, 1193, *1198,* 1199
Clindamycin, for sinus infections, 939
Clonazepam, for essential blepharospasm and Meige's syndrome, 507
Clostridial myonecrosis (gas gangrene), of eyelid, 312
Clostridium botulinum, 83, 152
Clostridium tetani, 83, 152
Closure, direct, of eyelid defect, 366
Coats' disease, CT scan of, 908, *910*
Cocaine test, for Horner's syndrome, 79, *79*
Coccidioidomycosis, of eyelid, 318–319
Collagen, autologous dermal, for wrinkles, 670–675. See also *Autologen.*
Zyderm, for wrinkles, *566,* 566–567, 670
Collagen fibers, in Autologen, 672, *672–673*
Collagen vascular disease(s), 3–12. See also specific disease for detail.
Churg-Strauss syndrome as, 10t, 11, 11t
dermatomyositis as, 7, 7t
lupus erythematosus as, 3–7, *4,* 4t, 5t
lymphomatoid granulomatosis as, 10t, 11–12
scleroderma as, 7–9, *8,* 8t
Wegener's granulomatosis as, 9–11, 10t
Collier's sign, in dorsal mesencephalic syndrome, 72, *73*
Coloboma, congenital, 407–409, *408*
creation of, 408–409
definition of, 407
in Goldenhar's syndrome, 407–408
management of, 409
imaging of, 905
Color(s), correct, for camouflage, 657–658, *659*
Color adjustment, in micropigmentation, 536
Color desaturation, in optic nerve dysfunction, 874
Color film, photographic, 554
Color matching, in micropigmentation, 536
of prosthesis, 1138, 1139, *1140*
Color mixing procedure, in micropigmentation, 538–541, *540*
Color perception, altered (dyschromatopsia), 860
Combined nevus, of eyelid, 339
Comedones, nodular elastosis with, of eyelid, 327, *327*
Complement system, 95–96
Complexion-associated melanosis, clinical features of, 180–181, *180–181*
Composite graft(s), used in medial canthal reconstruction, 391
used in upper eyelid reconstruction, 382, *383*
Compound nevus, of eyelid, 337, *337*
Compton effect, 1023, *1025*
Computed tomography (CT), diagnostic, for tearing, 760
of capillary hemangioma, 893, *893*
of carotid cavernous fistula, 897, *898*
of cavernous hemangioma, 894, *894*
of cellulitis, 147–148, *148*
of choroidal detachment, 906–907, *906–907*
of Coats' disease, 908, *910*
of dermoid cyst, 886–888, *888*
of hemangiopericytoma, 895–896, *896*
of idiopathic orbital inflammation, 954, *954*
of lacrimal gland lesions, 903, *904*
of lacrimal gland tumors, 1001, *1001–1002*
of lymphoid tumor, 957, *957*
of lymphoma, *892,* 892–983
of mucoceles, in paranasal sinuses, 1016
of neurofibroma, *990*
of neurogenic tumors, 984
of optic nerve glioma, *899,* 899–900
of optic nerve meningioma, *987,* 987–988
of optic nerve sheath meningioma, 897, *898*
of orbit, 885–886
of pseudotumor, *890,* 890–891
of retinoblastoma, *907,* 907–908
of rhabdomyosarcoma, 902, *903*
of schwannoma, *991,* 992
of subperiosteal phlegmon, *889,* 889–890
of thyroid orbitopathy, 891, *892*
of uveal malignant melanoma, 909, *910*
of varices, 896, *897*
Computer-controlled cooling-heating mask, used in blepharoplasty, *544*
Congenital anomaly(ies), craniofacial. See *Craniofacial congenital anomaly(ies).*
of eyelids, 407–411. See also specific anomaly, e.g., *Coloboma, congenital.*
Congenital dacryocystocele, *781,* 781–782
Congenital erythropoietic porphyria, 29
Congenital ichthyosiform erythroderma, 45, *45*
Congenital nevus, of eyelid, 338, *339*
Conjunctiva, 159–161
alkali burns to, 222–230. See also *Chemical injury(ies).*
amyloidosis of, 65–66, 238–240. See also *Amyloidosis, conjunctival.*
anatomy of, 178, *179*
macroscopic, 159–160
Conjunctiva *(Continued)*
microscopic, *160,* 160–161
blood supply to, 161
bulbar, triangular tumor of. See *Pterygium(ia).*
embryology of, 159
epithelium of, 160, *160*
loss of, 170, *171.* See also *Conjunctival mucous membrane(s), replacement of.*
glandular structure of, 160–161
lacerations of, 168–169
lymphatic supply to, 161
neoplasms of. See *Conjunctival neoplasm(s).*
nerve supply to, 161
physiology of, 161
prolapse of, management of, 253–254
reevaluation of, after chemical injury, 226
sarcoidosis of, 65, *65*
scarring of, in cicatricial pemphigoid, 98
stroma of, 160
thermal burns to, 222
tissue of, handling of, 161
xeroderma pigmentosum of, 66–67, *67*
Conjunctival autograft(s), for management of pterygia, 5, *214–215,* 216–217
complications of, 217
graft harvesting in, 215, *216*
for repopulation of corneal epithelium, indications for, 249–250
surgical technique of, 250, *250*
Conjunctival flap(s), 163–165
complete, 164–165, *166*
disadvantages of, 165
for management of pterygia, 214, *215*
Gundersen-type, 248, *249*
partial, 163–164, *164–165*
transpositional, 163, *164*
types of, 163
Conjunctival graft(s), 165–168
free, 165–167
mucous membrane, full-thickness, 167
split-thickness, 167
skin, split-thickness, 167–168
Conjunctival intraepithelial neoplasia (CIN), 231–232
recurrence rates for, 232
Conjunctival mucous membrane(s), replacement of, 170–176
alloplastic grafting and spontaneous epithelization in, 171–172, *171–172*
cartilage-mucosal compound grafts in, 176
free tarsoconjunctival grafts in, 175, *175–176*
oral mucous membrane grafts in, 172–175, *173–174*
spontaneous granulation in, 170–171
transplantation in, 172
Conjunctival neoplasm(s), 231–237
complexion-associated melanosis as, clinical features of, 180–181, *180–181*
intraepithelial, 231–232
recurrence rates for, 232
Kaposi's sarcoma as, 236–237, 242, *243,* 532
lymphoid tumors as. See *Lymphoid tumor(s), of conjunctiva.*
malignant melanoma as, 233–235, *234*
clinical features of, 183, *183*
treatment of, 187t, 187–188, *188,* 188t
nevi as, clinical features of, 181–182, *181–182*

Conjunctival neoplasm(s) *(Continued)*
differential diagnosis of, 181, *182*
histopathological classification of, 181
treatment of, 185
pigmented, 178–189
classification of, 179–180, 180t
clinical evaluation of, 183t, 183–185
examination in, *184,* 184–185
history in, 183–184, *184*
clinical features of, 180–183
management of, *185–186,* 185–188
terminology used for, 178–179
primary acquired melanosis as, clinical features of, 182, *182–183*
treatment of, 185–187, *186*
squamous cell carcinoma as, 231–232, *232–233*
squamous papilloma as, 68, *69,* 251, *252*
treatment of, 251–252
Conjunctival surgery, 163–169
flaps in, 163–165, *164–166*
for superior limbic keratoconjunctivitis, indications for, 248–249
technique in, 249
grafts in, 165–168
miscellaneous techniques in, 168–169
Conjunctival-retractor excision, for involutional ectropion, 425, *425*
Conjunctivitis, ligneous, 20
Connective tissue, orbital, 840–842, *842*
Connective tissue disease(s). See *Collagen vascular disease(s);* specific disease.
Contact dermatitis, *42,* 42–43
treatment of, 43
Contact yttrium-aluminum-garnet (YAG) laser, fat removal by, *641,* 641–642
Contouring, as cosmetic technique, used in facial rejuvenation, 570
Contrast sensitivity testing, for optic nerve dysfunction, 874, *875*
Cooling-heating mask, computer-controlled, used in blepharoplasty, *544*
Cornea, alkali burns to, 222–230. See also *Chemical injury(ies).*
thermal burns to, 222
Corneal disease, conjunctival procedure(s) for, 248–250
autografting as, 249–250
Gundersen flap as, 248, *249*
resection as, 248–249
Corneal epithelium, repopulation of, conjunctival autograft for, indication for, 249–250
surgical technique of, 250, *250*
Corneal transplantation, after chemical injury, 228, *228*
Corneal ulcer(s), prevention of, after chemical injury, 225, 229
Corneoscleral graft(s), lamellar, in management of pterygia, 214, *214*
Coronal flap, for brow ptosis, 585–586, *586*
Coronal synostosis, unilateral, 1179–1180, *1181*
Corrugator supraciliaris muscle, 262, *263,* 264
contraction of, 262
Cortical tubers, in tuberous sclerosis, 27
Corticosteroids, chronic patient use of, anesthetic considerations with, 295
for capillary hemangioma, 919–920
for lymphoid tumors, 961
for orbital floor fractures, 1088
pharmacology of, 97
topical, for pterygia, 211, 219
Corynebacterium diphtheriae infection, 313
Cosmeceutical(s), alpha-hydroxy acids as, 563–564
tretinoin as, 562–563
Cosmetic(s), camouflage. See *Camouflage make-up.*
Cosmetic blepharoplasty. See *Blepharoplasty, cosmetic.*
Costal rib graft(s), harvesting of, 1077–1078, *1079*
Cowpox, involving eyelids, 316
CPEO. See *Chronic progressive external ophthalmoplegia (CPEO).*
Cranial arteritis, 112
Cranial base–orbital tumor(s), pediatric, anterior cranial base approach to, 1199, 1202–1204, *1203–1206*
Cranial bone graft(s), harvesting of, 1079–1080, *1080–1082*
Cranial nerve(s). See also specific nerve, e.g., *Facial nerve.*
assessment of, in orbital disease, 877–878, *878–879*
function of, testing, 470–471
Cranial nerve palsy(ies), in diabetic patient, 138t, 138–139
infectious diseases causing, 152
Cranial suture(s), premature closure of, 1178–1182, *1179–1185*
Craniocervical dyskinesia(s), 504. See also specific disorder, e.g., *Blepharospasm, essential.*
Craniofacial cleft, with orbital and facial hypertelorism, anterior cranial base approach to, 1193, *1198,* 1199
Craniofacial congenital anomaly(ies), 1163–1207
anterior cranial base approach to, 1187–1207. See also *Craniofacial surgery, pediatric.*
historical perspective on, 1187
indications for, 1189–1207
refinements in, 1187–1188
brachycephaly as, 1180–1181, *1182–1184*
diagnosis of, 1178
evaluation of, 1178–1185
lambdoidal synostosis as, 1182
multiple suture synostosis as, 1182, *1185*
preoperative evaluation of, 1182, 1184
sagittal synostosis as, 1178–1179, *1179–1180*
subcranial approach to, 1163–1177
advantages of, 1163
results of, 1170, 1176t
surgical procedures in, 1163–1164, *1164–1169,* 1170, *1171–1176*
trigonocephaly as, 1181–1182, *1184*
unilateral coronal synostosis as, 1179–1180, *1181*
Craniofacial surgery, pediatric, anterior cranial base approach to, access to tumors in, 1188
for congenital orbital anomalies, 1189, 1193, *1194–1198,* 1199, *1200–1202*
for traumatic upper orbital deformities, 1188–1189, *1190–1192*
for tumors and neoplasms, 1199, 1202–1204, *1203–1206,* 1207
indications for, 1188–1207
refinements in, 1187–1188
Cranio-orbital neurofibromatosis, anterior cranial base approach to, 1204, *1206,* 1207
Cranio-orbital trauma, pediatric, anterior cranial base approach to, 1188–1189, *1190–1192*
Craniotomy, modified, for transcranial approach to tumors, 985
CREST syndrome, 9
Cretinism, 14
"Crocodile" tears, 735
Crouzon's syndrome, brachycephaly associated with, 1181, *1184*
subcranial approach to, results of, 1176t
Crow's feet, chemical peels for, 662
Cruveilhier valve, 742, *743*
Cryoablation, for districhiasis and trichiasis, 201
Cryotherapy, care following, 188t
complications of, 187t
excision with, for conjunctival malignant melanoma, 235
for conjunctival squamous cell carcinoma, 232
for hyperpigmented facial lesions, 568
for Kaposi's sarcoma, 528
for pagetoid spread of sebaceous gland carcinoma, 348
for pigmented conjunctival neoplasms, *185–186,* 185–188
for sebaceous gland carcinoma, 193–194, *194*
Cryptophthalmos, 407, *408*
Crypts of Henle, 160, *273*
CT. See *Computed tomography (CT).*
Curette(s), used in ophthalmic plastic surgery, *290*
Current, in electrolysis, density of, 590
polar effects of, 589
radio-frequency, heating effects of, 592
Customized suborbital implant, 490–491, *491,* 495–498, *496–499*
Cutaneous. See also *Skin* entries.
Cutaneous horn, of eyelid, 326, *326*
Cutler-Beard flap, used in upper eyelid reconstruction, technique of, 374–375, *375–378*
Cyclophosphamide, for cicatricial pemphigoid, 199
pharmacology of, 97
Cyclosporine, pharmacology of, 97–98
Cylindroma (turban tumor), of eyelid, 334–335, *335*
Cyproheptadine, for essential blepharospasm and Meige's syndrome, 507
Cyst(s), blood, drainage of, 925
chocolate, 926, *926*
dermoid, nasal, with intracranial extension, anterior cranial base approach to, 1199, *1200*
of eyelid, *327,* 327–328
of orbit, 886–888, *888–889*
epidermal inclusion, of eyelid, 326–327, *327*
epidermoid, of orbit, 886–888, *888*
horn, 325
hydatid, 151
Moll's, 334, *334*
nodular elastosis with, of eyelid, 327, *327*
pseudohorn, 325
L-Cysteine, to reduce ulceration, after chemical injury, 225
Cystic hygroma (cavernous lymphangioma), of eyelid, 331
Cysticercosis, 151
Cytomegalovirus retinitis, in AIDS patients, 533

Cytotoxic response (hypersensitivity type II), 96
Cytotoxicity, antibody-dependent cell-mediated, 95

Dacron suture, 284
Dacryoadenitis, 965
associated with infection, 153, *153*
clinical manifestations of, 964–966
diagnostic evaluation of, 954
Dacryocystitis, chronic, in primary acquired nasolacrimal duct obstruction, 785, *785*
Dacryocystocele, congenital, *781,* 781–782
Dacryocystography, in evaluation of tearing, 759, *759–760*
Dacryocystorhinostomy, for canalicular stenosis, 830–831
for nasolacrimal duct obstruction, 781
for primary acquired nasolacrimal duct obstruction, *786–792,* 786–794
endonasal, 792–794, *793–795*
history in, 786–787
incisions in, 788, *789*
Kerrison rongeur for bone removal in, 789–790, *790*
lacrimal sac flaps in, 790–792, *791–792*
nasal packing for, 787, *788*
sedation for, 787
transnasal wiring with, in fixation/reconstruction of canthal tendon, 388, *389*
Dacryolith(s), causing nasolacrimal duct obstruction, 812
Dapsone, for cicatricial pemphigoid, 199
Darier's disease (keratosis follicularis), 21
Darier's sign, in mastocytoma, 43
Daylight, for photography, 554
Daylight film, photographic, 554
DDAVP (desmopressin), for hemostasis in wound repair, 283
de Hertoghe's sign, in atopic dermatitis, 42
Decompression, optic nerve sheath, 1056–1059
complications of, 1059
indications for, 1047
mechanism of action of, 1056
postoperative care following, 1059
technique of, 1056–1059, *1057–1059*
orbital, for Graves' disease, 967–982. See also *Graves' disease, orbital decompression for.*
indications for, 1047
Dehiscence(s), wound, after blepharoplasty, 648
Zuckerkandl's, 935
Delayed reaction (hypersensitivity type IV), 96
Dendritic cell(s), of eyelid, 323
Dengue fever, involving eyelids, 316
Dennie-Morgan fold, in atopic dermatitis, 42
Dermabrasion, for wrinkles, 565, *565*
Dermal fillers, autologous, for wrinkles, 670. See also *Autologen.*
Dermatitis, atopic, 41–42, *42*
treatment of, 42
contact, *42,* 42–43
treatment of, 43
seborrheic, *37,* 37–38
Dermatochalasis, in Graves' ophthalmopathy, 515–516, *516*
Dermatofibroma, of eyelid, 333
Dermatomyositis, 7
diagnostic criteria for, 7t
Dermatoses, 37–46. See also specific type.
Dermis. See also *Skin.*
of eyelid, 324
benign lesions of, 328–333. See also under *Eyelid tumor(s).*
Dermoid cyst, nasal, with intracranial extension, anterior cranial base approach to, 1199, *1200*
of eyelid, *327,* 327–328
of orbit, 886–888, *888–889*
Dermolipoma(s), 255–257, *256*
complications of, 255–256
treatment of, 256–257
excision of, 256
Desmopressin (DDAVP), for hemostasis in wound repair, 283
"Devil's eye," 1179
Dexamethasone, for thyroid storm, 130
Diabetes mellitus, complication(s) of, 137–141, 138t
acanthosis nigricans as, 140
carotenemia as, 141
eruptive xanthomas as, 140–141
granuloma annulare as, 140
hemochromatosis as, 141
idiopathic optic disc edema as, 138–139
malignant external otitis as, 138
necrobiosis lipoidica diabeticorum as, 139–140
phycomycosis as, 137–138
rhinoscleroma as, 138
vitiligo as, 140
Diathermy, lipolytic, fat removal by, 640–641, *640–641*
Diazepam, as anesthetic agent, 296
DIDMOAD (Wolfram) syndrome, in diabetic patient, 138t, 139
Diet, Chinese, in balance of yin and yang, 695
Diffuse cutaneous leishmaniasis, of eyelid, 150, *150*
Digoxin, chronic patient use of, anesthetic considerations with, 295
Diphtheria, involving eyelids, 313
Diplopia, after blepharoplasty, 644
persistent, as complication of orbital floor fractures, 1091, *1092*
Discoid lupus erythematosus (DLE), 3. See also *Lupus erythematosus (LE).*
characteristic features of, 6
Dissection, in orbital surgery, 1049
Disseminated neonatal hemangioma, 920t, 920–921, *920–921*
Distichiasis, congenital, 409, *409*
in cicatricial pemphigoid, correction of, 201
Diuretics, chronic patient use of, anesthetic considerations with, 295–296
DLE (discoid lupus erythematosus), 3. See also *Lupus erythematosus (LE).*
characteristic features of, 6
Documentation, for medicolegal considerations with eyelid trauma, 457
Dog bite(s), eyelid injury caused by, 453, *454*
Dolichocephaly, 1178
Doll's eye maneuver, 72
Donor sclera, for eyelid reconstruction, 364
in Asian patients, 724–727
histology of homograft and, 726, *726–727*
immunopathology of homograft and, 726–727
results with, 727, *727*
surgical technique and, 725, *725*
Dorsal mesencephalic syndrome, eyelid retraction in, 72–73, *73*
Dorsonasal artery, anatomy of, 274, *275*
Down syndrome, epicanthal folds associated with, 411
Doxycycline, for trachoma, 155
Drainage, indications for, 1046
of blood cysts, 925
of orbital abscess, 939–940
Dressing(s), eyelid, 384
Drug(s). See also specific drug or drug group.
associated with cicatricial pemphigoid, *197,* 197–198
chronic patient use of, anesthetic considerations with, 295
disruption of neuromuscular transmission by, 83–84
for hemostasis in wound repair, 283
Dry eye, treatment of, after chemical injury, 226
Dye disappearance test, in tearing, 753–754, *754*
Dyschromatopsia, 860
Dysplastic nevus syndrome, 67–68, *68*

Ear cartilage, used in upper eyelid reconstruction, 364, *364*
Eaton-Lambert syndrome, 83
EBV (Epstein-Barr virus), associated with Burkitt's lymphoma, 530
Ecchymosis, due to blepharoplasty, 709
Eccrine sweat gland(s), *273,* 323–324
benign adnexal lesions originating in, 333–334, *333–334*
Ecthyma gangrenosum, of eyelid, 312–313
Ectropion, 422–437
after blepharoplasty, 644–645, *645–646*
as complication of medial canthal reconstruction, 398
cicatricial, as cause of tearing, 765, 767–768, *767–769*
congenital, 410, *410*
infection causing, 308t
involutional, 422–429
as cause of tearing, 762–765, *763–764, 766–767*
etiology of, 422, *423–424*
medical treatment of, 424
preoperative evaluation of, 422–424, *424*
surgical treatment of, 424–429, 763–765
conjunctival-retractor excision in, 425, *425*
horizontal full-thickness eyelid shortening in, 427, *428,* 764–765
inferior punctoplasty in, 424–425, *425*
lateral tarsal strip procedure in, 427, 429, *429–430,* 765, *766–767*
medial plication for canthal laxity in, 425–427, *426–427*
posterior lamellar shortening procedure in, 763–764, *764*
Smith lazy-T procedure in, 425, *426*
paralytic, 429–437
as cause of tearing, 768–770, *769*
etiology of, 429
medical management of, 430
pathology of, 429, *430*
preoperative evaluation of, 429–430
surgical management of, 430–437
eyelid sling procedure in, 432, 434, *435*
indications for, 430
lateral canthoplasty in, 432, *433–435*
tarsorrhaphy in, 430–432, *431–432*
temporalis transfer in, 434, 436–437, *436–437*

Edema, due to blepharoplasty, 709
eyelid, in Graves' ophthalmopathy, 515–516, *516*
optic disc, in diabetic patient, 138t, 138–139
periorbital, diseases and organisms associated with, 308t
infectious causes of, 151–152
postoperative, manual lymphatic drainage for, 653–654
preseptal, in sinus disease, 938–939
Edinger-Westphal nucleus, preganglionic fibers from, 846
EDTA (ethylenediaminetetra-acetic acid), to reduce ulceration, after chemical injury, 225
Electrocardiography, prior to oculoplastic surgery, 294, 295
Electrocautery, for hemostasis in wound repair, 283
Electrology, and eyebrow contouring, 589–595
Electrolysis, 589–591
and current density, 590
and polar effects of current, 589
chemical and physiologic effects of, 590
galvanic, advantages of, 590–591
disadvantages of, 591
multiple-needle, 590
single-needle, 589
principle of time and intensity in, 590
removal of metal jewelry before, 589–590
vs. other epilating techniques, 593–594
Electronic flash, for photography, 555
Electropigmentation, 676–681. See also *Micropigmentation.*
and pigment removal, 681
complications of, 681
contraindications to, 677t
indications for, 676, 677t
patient evaluation for, 676, *677*
tattoo pigments used in, 677, 681
technique of, 676–677, *678–681*
Elephantiasis neuromatosa, 25
ELISA (enzyme-linked immunosorbent assay), 97
Ellman Surgitron radiosurgical unit, used in removal of hyperpigmented facial lesions, 568, *568*
used in treatment of telangiectasia, 569
Embolus, cerebral, ptosis caused by, 75–76, *77*
Embryonal rhabdomyosarcoma, 995
Encephalocele, frontonasalethmoidal, anterior cranial base approach to, 1199, *1201–1202*
Endocrine disease. See also specific disease.
non-thyroid-related, ocular manifestations of, tarsal polishing with, 137–143
Endophthalmitis, sclerosing, imaging of, 908–909
Endoscope(s), used for endonasal dacryocystorhinostomy, 793, *793*
Endoscopic sinus surgery kit, *292*
Endoscopy, in evaluation of tearing, 760
Endothelial hyperplasia, intravascular papillary, of eyelid, 332
Enophthalmos, 1108–1111, *1108–1112*
as complication of orbital floor fracture, 1091, *1092–1093*
associated with orbital disease, 881
Entamoeba histolytica infection, 317
Entropion, 413–421
cicatricial, 414, *415*
as cause of tearing, 771
Entropion *(Continued)*
buccal mucous membrane grafting for, 203–206
anesthesia in, 203
complications of, 205
results of, 205, *206*
surgical methods of, 203–205, *204–206*
correction of, *200,* 200–201
surgical approach to, 417–421, *418*
technique in, 418–419, *419–420,* 421
congenital, 409, *410,* 413
in Graves' ophthalmopathy, 515, *516*
surgical techniques for, 521
involutional, 414–415
as cause of tearing, 770–771, *772–773*
surgical approach to, 415–416, *416–417*
spastic, 414
as cause of tearing, 771, *773*
Enucleation, 1035–1043. See also *Anophthalmos, acquired.*
care following, 1041
eye protection following, 1037–1038
hydroxyapatite implant and, 1041–1042. See also *Prosthesis.*
contraindications to, 1042
indications for, 1035–1037
lax socket following, 1106–1108
preoperative counseling for, 1037
presurgical set-up for, 1038
psychological impact of, 1037
surgical anatomy for, 1038
surgical steps in, 1038
vs. evisceration, 1129–1130
with myoconjunctival attachments, 1039, *1040–1042,* 1041
Enucleation and evisceration kit, *290*
Enzyme-linked immunosorbent assay (ELISA), 97
Eosinophil(s), 95
Eosinophilia, angiolymphoid hyperplasia with, 949–950, *949–950*
of eyelid, 332
Eosinophilic granuloma, of orbit, 62, *63*
in AIDS patients, 532
Ephelides (freckles), in neurofibromatosis, 25
of eyelid, 339, *339*
Epiblepharon, as cause of tearing, 775, *775*
congenital, 409–140
Epiblepharon fold(s), 261
Epicanthal fold(s), 261, 704–705
congenital, 410–411
prevalence of, 699, 700t, 705t
Epidermal growth factor (EGF), wound healing with, after chemical injury, 229–230
Epidermal inclusion cyst, of eyelid, 326–327, *327*
Epidermal necrolysis, toxic. See *Toxic epidermal necrolysis (Lyell's syndrome).*
Epidermal nevus, linear, of eyelid, 327
Epidermis. See also *Skin.*
of eyelid, 323
benign lesions of, 324–328. See also under *Eyelid tumor(s).*
Epidermoid cyst, of orbit, 886–888, *888*
Epidermolysis bullosa, 29–31, 103–105
classification of, 103
epidemiology of, 104
immunohistopathology of, 104–105
ocular manifestations of, 30t, 104
subgroups and types of, 30–31
systemic manifestations of, 104
treatment of, 31, 105
types of, 30
Epidermolysis bullosa acquisita antigen, 105
Epilation, permanent, of eyelashes, radiation therapy and, 1031
Epinephrine, for hemostasis in wound repair, 283
Epiphora, 729–730, 749, 751, *752.* See also *Tearing.*
age of onset of, 730
causes of, 751–752
definition of, 729
Episcleritis, in AIDS patients, 529
Epithelial eyelid tumor(s), malignant, 342–350. See also *Eyelid tumor(s), malignant.*
Epithelialization, in wound repair, 281, 282t
spontaneous, alloplastic grafting and, in conjunctival mucous membrane replacement, 171–172, *171–172*
Epithelioid (spindle) nevus, of eyelid, 338
Epithelioma, Malherbe's calcifying, of eyelid, 336, *336*
Epithelium, conjunctival, 160, *160*
loss of, 170, *171*
corneal, repopulation of, conjunctival autograft for, 249–250, *250*
perilimbal, loss of, after chemical injury, 226–227, *227*
Epstein-Barr virus (EBV), associated with Burkitt's lymphoma, 530
Erdheim-Chester disease, of orbit, 64, *64*
xanthogranulomas of, 948
Eruptive xanthoma, in diabetic patient, 140–141
Erythema multiforme, *34–35,* 34–37
causes of, 36t
differential diagnosis of, 36–37
epidemiology of, 100
immunohistopathology of, 101
major (Stevens-Johnson syndrome), *34,* 34–35, 100
minor, 34, 100
ocular manifestations of, 100–101
pathogenesis of, 101–102
systemic manifestations of, 101
toxic epidermal necrolysis form of, 34, 35, *35*
drugs causing, 35, 36t
treatment of, 37, 102
Erythema nodosum, in sarcoidosis, 16
Erythroderma, congenital ichthyosiform, 45, *45*
exfoliative, 41
Erythromycin, for trachoma, 155
Erythropoietic porphyria, congenital, 29
Erythropoietic protoporphyria, 29
Ethmoidal sinus(es), anatomy of, 1014–1015
mucoceles in, *1018,* 1018–1019
radiographic findings in, 1018, *1019*
treatment of, 1018–1019
Ethylenediaminetetra-acetic acid (EDTA), to reduce ulceration, after chemical injury, 225
Euthyroid Graves' disease, 121
Euthyroid hyperthyroxinemia, 129
causes of, 129t
Evisceration, enucleation and, kit for, *290*
presurgical set-up for, 1043
surgical steps in, 1043–1044, *1044*
vs. enucleation, 1129–1130
Excimer laser, postoperative use of, for pterygia, 219
Excision, conjunctival-retractor, for involutional ectropion, 425, *425*
for rhabdomyosarcoma, 995
indications for, 1046
of capillary hemangioma, 918–919
of cavernous hemangioma, 928–929

Excision *(Continued)*
of conjunctival lymphoid tumors, 236, *236*
of hemangiopericytoma, 931–932, *932*
of lymphangioma, 925
of sebaceous gland carcinoma, 348
of skin, in ptosis surgery, 450–451
with cryotherapy, for conjunctival malignant melanoma, 235
for conjunctival squamous cell carcinoma, 232
Exenteration, for conjunctival malignant melanoma, 235
indications for, 1047
orbital, indications for, 1070, 1071t
reconstructive and prosthetic options in, 1073–1075, *1074*
technique of, 1071–1073, *1071–1073*
osseointegration following, 1150–1159. See also *Osseointegration, for exenterated orbit.*
Exfoliative erythroderma, 41
Exophthalmometry, in Caucasian and African American adults, 699t
in Chinese and Taiwanese adults, 698, 698t
Exophthalmos, systemic diseases associated with, 13t
Exposure, adequate, in orbital surgery, 1048
Extraocular muscles, anatomy of, 841
enlarged, causes of, 886t
Extremity(ies), manual lymphatic drainage of, pressure bandages with, 655
Eye(s), "devil's," 1179
dry, treatment of, after chemical injury, 226
enucleation of, 1035–1043. See also *Enucleation.*
ocular protection following, 1037–1938
evisceration of. See *Evisceration.*
wet, 726–730. See also *Epiphora.*
Eyebrow(s), 262, *263–265,* 264. See also *Hair; Hair follicles.*
contouring of, 594–595, *594–595*
technique(s) used in, 589–595
blend modality as, 593
comparison of, 593–594
electrolysis as, 589–591
regulatory agencies and, 591–593
short-wave or thermolysis method as, 591
displacement of, after blepharoplasty, 649, *649*
elevation of, endoscopic approach to, 550
for ptosis, 585, *585.* See also *Ptosis, brow.*
male vs. female, 633, *634*
reconstruction of, electropigmentation in, 676
micropigmentation in, 537–538, *539–540,* 685–688, *686–688*
Eyelash(es), 273. See also *Hair; Hair follicles.*
epilation of, permanent, radiation therapy and, 1031
loss or misdirection of, after blepharoplasty, 649
misdirected. See *Trichiasis.*
pigmentary treatment of, 536–537, *537–538,* 676
sebaceous glands of, 323. See also *Sebaceous gland(s).*
Eyelid(s), 261–279
acquired immunodeficiency syndrome affecting, 526–529. See also *Acquired immunodeficiency syndrome (AIDS), eyelid manifestation(s) of.*
amyloidosis of, 65–66
anatomy of, 261, *262,* 413, *414*

Eyelid(s) *(Continued)*
ancillary techniques involving, in management of facial paralysis, 482
and precorneal tear film, 738
apraxia of, *89,* 90
arterial supply to, 273–274, *274–275*
basal cell carcinoma of. See *Basal cell carcinoma, of eyelid.*
basal cell nevus syndrome of, 67, *68*
chalazion of. See *Chalazion.*
chancroid of, 314
changes of, in orbital disease, 865–868, *867–868*
congenital anomaly(ies) of, 407–411. See also specific anomaly, e.g., *Ectropion.*
ankyloblepharon as, 409
blepharophimosis syndrome as, 411, *411*
coloboma as, 407–409, *408*
cryptophthalmos as, 407, *408*
distichiasis, 409, *409*
ectropion as, 410, *410*
entropion as, 409, *410*
epiblepharon as, 409–410
epicanthal folds as, 410–411
lid retraction as, 411, *411*
crease in. See *Eyelid crease(s).*
dimensions of, in Chinese adults, 698–700, 699t, 700t
disorders of, 72–91. See also specific disorder, e.g., *Ptosis.*
injury to. See *Eyelid trauma.*
innervation of, 275, 277–278, *277–278*
lower, blepharoplasty for, 617–624. See also *Blepharoplasty, lower eyelid.*
bony support of, 485, *486–487*
defects in, closure of, 400, *401*
involving canaliculus, 406
lacerations of, 455–456, *455–457*
malposition of, after blepharoplasty, 644–645, *645–646*
correction of, 1113–1114, *1115–1118,* 1116–1118
muscles retracting, anatomy of, 269–272, *270–272*
reconstruction of, 400–406. See also *Eyelid reconstruction, lower.*
retraction of, 438–446. See also *Eyelid retraction, lower.*
transconjunctival approach to, complications of, 630
lymphatic drainage of, 275, *276*
margins of. See *Eyelid margin.*
mycosis fungoides of, 62
necrosis of, after blepharoplasty, 650
nodular eruptions of, infectious causes of, 149–150, *150*
pseudoptosis of, *88–91,* 89–91
retraction of, 72–75. See also *Eyelid retraction.*
sebaceous glands of, benign lesions originating in, 336–337, *337*
carcinoma of, 190–194, 301–303. See also *Sebaceous gland carcinoma.*
inflammation of, 307–310, *309*
causes of, 308t
shortening of, after chemical injury, 226
horizontal full-thickness, for involutional ectropion, 427, *428*
skin folds (laugh lines) around, 261–262, *263*
skin of, 262
histology of, 323–324
symmetry of, anophthalmic socket and, 1131, *1131*
tumors of. See *Eyelid tumor(s).*

Eyelid(s) *(Continued)*
ulcerative lesion of, causes of, 308t
upper, blepharoplasty for, 596–614. See also *Blepharoplasty, upper eyelid.*
components of, 356
double, 703–704, *704,* 705t
prevalence of, 705t
horizontal section through, *266*
lacerations of, repair of, 359–361, *362*
protractors of, anatomy of, 264–265, 267–269, *267–269*
reconstruction of, 356–384. See also *Eyelid reconstruction, upper.*
single, 703, *704*
venous supply to, 274–275, *276*
vertical, and suborbital augmentation, 498–499, *499–502,* 501
xeroderma pigmentosum of, 66–67
Eyelid crease(s), 261, *262–263*
double, after blepharoplasty, 648, *648*
formation of, in upper eyelid blepharoplasty, 603, *603–604*
variations of, 609–610
high, surgery for, 450
male vs. female, 633
upper, determination and marking of, 706, *706*
Eyelid deformity, baggy, Castanares' classification of, 597, 597t
Eyelid dressings, 384
Eyelid edema, in Graves' ophthalmopathy, 515–516, *516*
Eyelid lag, definition of, 514
in Graves' ophthalmopathy, 514
in orbital disease, 866–867
Eyelid laxity, as complication of medial canthal reconstruction, 398
in involutional ectropion, 762–763, *763,* 764
pinch test for, 762, *763*
repair of, 622–624, *623–624*
Eyelid margin, 272–273, *273*
contour of, abnormal, 450
injury to, evaluation of, *455,* 455–456
sequence of repair following, 458, 460, *460*
inward rotation of. See *Entropion.*
outward rotation of. See *Ectropion.*
pigmentary treatment of, 536–537, *537–538*
reapproximation of, following injury, 357–358, *359–360*
Eyelid necrosis, *312,* 312–313
causes of, 308t, 312
Eyelid reconstruction, donor sclera for, in Asian patients, 724–727, *725–727*
results with, 727, *727*
lower, 400–406
closure of defects in, 400, *401*
Hughes flap for, 402–404, *403–404*
severing of, 404, *405*
lateral cantholysis in, 400, *401*
Mustardé flap for, 404–405, *405*
Tenzel rotation flap for, 400–402, *401–402*
Trepier flap (rotated myocutaneous) for, 403, *403–404*
upper, 356–384
dressings used in, 384
objectives of, 356
technique(s) used in, 363–384
auricular cartilage for, 364, *364*
autogenous tarsus for, 363–364
composite grafting as, 382, *383*

Eyelid reconstruction *(Continued)*
Cutler-Beard flap as, 374–375, *375–378*
direct closure as, 366
donor sclera for, 364
hard palate mucosa for, 364–365
irradiated tarsal plates and aorta for, 365
lateral transpositional skin flap as, 371, *372*
median forehead flap as, 371, *373*
myocutaneous flap as, 369, *369–370*
nasochondral tissue for, *356,* 365
nasojugal myocutaneous flap as, 373–374, *374*
oral mucosa for, 365
pedicle flap from lower lid to upper lid as, 382–383, *383*
semicircular flap as, 366, *367*
skin grafting as, 366–367, *368,* 369
sliding tarsal flap as, 380, 382, *382*
split-level full-thickness grafts as, 384, *384*
tarsal rotational flap as, 375–378, *379–380*
tarsal substitutes for, 363
tarsoconjunctival flap as, 378–380, *381*
traumatic injury requiring, 356–363, *357*
canalicular lacerations as, 359–361, *362*
canthal tendon injury as, 361–363, *363*
extensive, 358–359, *360–361*
lid margin reapproximation and, 357–358, *359–360*
with no tissue loss, 357, *358*
with tissue loss, 357
Eyelid retraction, 72–75
as complication of orbital floor fractures, 1091, *1091*
congenital, 411, *411*
in Graves' disease, 514–523. See also *Graves' disease, eyelid retraction in.*
lower, 438–446
anterior lamellar defects in, 438
surgical repair of, 439–440, *440*
causes of, 438
functional and cosmetic complaints associated with, 438–439
middle and posterior lamellar defects in, 438
surgical repair of, 440–446
greater palatine nerve block in, 442
hard palate graft in, 441–442, *442*
harvesting of, 442–444, *443–444*
nasopalatine nerve block in, 442
technique of, 444–446, *444–446*
myopathic, 74–75, *76*
neuromuscular, 74, *76*
neuropathic, nuclear and infranuclear lesions causing, 73–74, *74–76*
supranuclear lesions causing, 72–73, *73*
pseudoptosis and, 89–91
upper, in orbital disease, 867, *867*
Eyelid retractor(s), lower, with spacers, 440
used in ophthalmic plastic surgery, *290*
Eyelid sling procedures, for paralytic ectropion, 432, 434, *435*
Eyelid sulcus, *262*
Eyelid surgery, anesthesia for, 278–279
cosmetic. See *Blepharoplasty.*
hemostasis in, 282–284
pharmacologic agents for, 283
Eyelid surgery *(Continued)*
pressure tamponade for, 282
thermal cautery and electrocautery for, 282–283
topically applied chemical agents for, 283–284
lower, greater palatine nerve block for, 442
hard palate graft for, 441–442, *442*
harvesting of, 442–444, *443–444*
nasopalatine nerve block for, 442
technique of, 439–440, 444–446, *444–446*
ophthalmic plastic instruments used in, 289, *290–292*
suture material used in, 284, 284t
suture needles used in, 284–285, *285*
suturing techniques used in, 285–286, *285–289,* 288
wound healing following, primary, 281, 282t
secondary, 281–282
Eyelid trauma, 452–463
bites causing, 452–453, *454,* 455
blunt, 452
evaluation of, 452–457, *454*
mechanism of injury in, 452
patient evaluation in, 453, 455–457
extramarginal injuries and, 456, *456–457*
formulation of treatment plans and, 456–457
marginal injuries and, *455,* 455–456
medicolegal considerations and, 457
systemic considerations and, 453, 455
sharp, 452
treatment of, 457–463
surgical, 457–461
care following, 461
secondary procedures in, 461–463
sequence of repair in, 458, *459–462,* 460–461
wound decontamination in, 457–458, *458*
upper, canalicular lacerations in, 359–361, *362*
canthal tendon injuries in, 361–363, *363*
penetrating injuries in, 357–359
lid margin reapproximation and, 357–358, *359–360*
with no tissue loss, 357, *358*
with tissue loss, 357
reconstruction for, 356–363
techniques used in, 363–384. See also *Eyelid reconstruction, upper, technique(s) used in.*
Eyelid tumor(s), benign, 323–340
classification of, 342, 343t
diagnosis and management of, 324
of dermis, 328–333
angiolymphoid hyperplasia with eosinophilia as, 332
arteriovenous malformation as, 331
capillary hemangioma (strawberry nevus) as, 330, *330*
cavernous hemangioma as, 330
dermatofibroma as, 333
glomus tumor as, 332
granular cell tumor as, 329
intravascular papillary endothelial hyperplasia as, 332
juvenile xanthogranuloma as, 64, 333
leiomyoma as, 329
lymphangioma as, 331, *331*
neurilemoma (schwannoma) as, 328–329
Eyelid tumor(s) *(Continued)*
neurofibroma as, 328, *329*
neuroma as, 329
nevus flammeus (port wine stain) as, *329,* 329–330
pyogenic granuloma as, 331, *331*
varix as, 330–331
xanthelasma as, 332, *332*
xanthoma as, 332
of epidermis, 324–328
acrochordon (skin tag) as, 324, *324*
cutaneous horn lesion as, 326, *326*
dermoid cyst as, *327,* 327–328
inclusion cyst as, 326–327, *327*
inverted follicular keratosis as, 326, *326*
keratoacanthoma as, 325–326, *326*
linear nevus as, 327
milia as, *324,* 324–325
nodular elastosis with cysts and comedones as, 327, *327*
oncocytoma as, 328
phakomatous choristoma as, 328, *328*
seborrheic keratosis as, 325, *325*
pigmented, 337–339
blue nevus as, 338–339
congenital nevus as, 338, *339*
freckles as, 339, *339*
lentigo simplex as, 339
nevocellular nevi as, 337–338, *337–338*
Ota's nevus as, 339
solar lentigo as, 339, *340*
in Asian patients, 721–727
basal cell carcinoma as, 723, *723*
lid reconstruction with donor sclera for, 724–727, *725–727*
sebaceous gland carcinoma as, 721–722, *722*
squamous cell carcinoma as, 721, *722*
statistics on, 723–724
malignant, 300–306, 342–350
basal cell carcinoma as, 300, 342–345, *343–345*
in African American patients, 716, *717*
in Asian patients, 723, *723*
classification of, 342, 343t
metastatic, *54,* 56
sebaceous gland carcinoma as. See *Sebaceous gland carcinoma.*
squamous cell carcinoma as, 300–301, *302,* 349–350, *349–350*
in Asian patients, 721, *722*
low-grade, 325
types of, 343t
painless, diseases and organisms associated with, 308t
Eyelid twitch response, in myasthenic patients, 80
Eyeliner reconstruction, with micropigmentation, 536–537, *536–537*

Face, "ideal," artist's rendition of, 560, *561*
skin tension lines in, 285, *285*
Face-lift (rhytidectomy), 565
Facial anomaly(ies), anomalies of nasolacrimal drainage system with, 783
Facial expression, muscles of, 262, *263,* 264
Facial movement, disorders of. See also specific disorder, e.g., *Hemifacial spasm.*
overview of, 504
Facial myokymia, 510
diagnostic features of, 505t

Facial nerve, aberrant regeneration of, 91, *91*
anatomy of, 275, 277, *277*
blood supply to, *468*, 469
disorders of, 473–474
injury to, 473–474
lesions of, 474
diagnosis of, 471t–472t
motor branches of, 469, *469*
motor nucleus of, 465–466, *467*
supranuclear pathways of, 465, *466*
Facial paralysis, 465–482
diagnostic considerations in, 473t
examination of, 470–471, 471t–472t
history of, 470
medical management of, 474–475, *475*
pontine, diagnosis of, 465–466, *467*
surgical management of, 475–482
ancillary eyelid techniques in, 482
Arion sling in, 478–479, *479*
fascial strip in, 480–481
gold weight in, 475–476, *476–477*
lateral canthal tendon reconstruction in, 480, *480–481*
palpebral spring in, 476–478, *477–478*
retractor recession with ear cartilage graft in, 481–482, *481–482*
transposition of temporalis muscle to lids in, 479–480, *480*
unilateral brow ptosis and, 482
symptoms of, 470
Facial rejuvenation, 560–571
cosmetic technique(s) used in, 569–571
camouflage, 570
fashion, 570–571
for pigmentary problems, 567–568, *568*
for telangiectasia, 569, *569*
for wrinkled skin, 562–567
alpha-hydroxy acids used in, 563–564, *564*
chemical peels used in, 564
dermabrasion used in, 565, *565*
Fibrel used in, 567, *567*
filler substances used in, 565–567
tretinoin used in, *562*, 562–563
Zyderm collagen used in, *566*, 566–567
harmful effects of ultraviolet light and, prevention of, 561–562
Facial spasm(s), diagnostic features of, 505t
Facial synkinesis, diagnostic features of, 505t
Facial tic, diagnostic features of, 505t
Facial vein, anatomy of, 275, *276*
Factor VIII–related antigen, in Kaposi's sarcoma, 242
Familial periodic paralysis, ptosis in, 85–86, *86*
Fasanella-Servat procedure, 448
Fascia, orbital, anatomy of, 841–842, *842*
Fascial strip, in surgical management of facial paralysis, 480–481
Fasciitis, necrotizing, of eyelid, 312
nodular, of orbit, 997
Fashion cosmetics, used in facial rejuvenation, 570–571
Fat excision, in cosmetic blepharoplasty, technique(s) of, 638–642
carbon dioxide laser as, 638, 640
clamp, cut, and cauterize as, 638, *639*
contact yttrium-aluminum-garnet laser as, *641*, 641–642
fat repositioning as, 641
lipocauterization as, 638, *639*
lipolytic diathermy as, 640–641, *640–641*
monopolar dissection as, 638
radio-frequency lipocontouring as, 642, *642*
Fat excision *(Continued)*
in transconjunctival lower blepharoplasty, inadequate, 630
in upper eyelid blepharoplasty, 601, *601*
variations of, 608–609
incomplete or excessive, 646–647, *647*
Fat pad, orbital, 269, *269*
anatomy of, 842, *842*
pseudoherniation of, evaluation of, 635
removal of. See *Fat excision.*
repositioning of, 640–641, *640–641*
sub-brow, surgical management of, 586–587, *586–588*
tarsus and, in Chinese adults, 699, 700t
Fat transplantation, autologous, for wrinkles, 565
Favre-Racouchot syndrome, 327, *327*
Fc receptors, 95
Fenestration, indications for, 1047
Fentanyl, as anesthetic agent, 296
Fibrel, for wrinkles, 567, *567*, 670
Fibroblastic phase, of wound repair, 281, 282t
Fibroma, orbital, 997
Fibromatosis, orbital, 997
Fibronectin, wound healing with, after chemical injury, 229
Fibrosarcoma, orbital, 997
Fibrous tissue, benign eyelid tumors derived from, 333
Fibrous tissue tumor(s), of orbit, 997
Filamentary keratitis, associated with dry eye, 226
Filler substance(s), for wrinkles, 565–567
Fibrel as, 567, *567*
Zyderm as, *566*, 566–567
Film, photographic, automatic advance of, 551
color, 554
speed of, 554
radiographic, 1023, *1024*
Fissure, orbital. See *Orbital fissure.*
Fistula, carotid cavernous, CT scan of, 897, *898*
lacrimal sac, 782–783, *783*
naso-orbital, as complication of medial canthal reconstruction, 398
Fitzpatrick classification, of photodamage, 662, 663t
Flap(s), conjunctival. See *Conjunctival flap(s).*
coronal, for brow ptosis, 585–586, *586*
skin, used in lower eyelid blepharoplasty, 620, *620*
skin-muscle, used in lower eyelid blepharoplasty, 620–622, *621–622*
used in lower eyelid reconstruction, Hughes, 402–404, *403–404*
severing of, 404, *405*
Mustardé, 404–405, *405*
Tenzel rotation, 400–402, *401–402*
Trepier (rotated myocutaneous), 403, *403–404*
used in medial canthal reconstruction, 390–391, 393
composite, 391
glabellar, 391, 393, *395*
island forehead, 393, *396*
midline forehead, 393, *396*
Mustardé, 390–392, *392*
myocutaneous, 390, *391*
pedicle, 391, *395*
tarsoconjunctival, 391, *394*
Tenzel, 391, *393*
used in upper eyelid reconstruction, Cutler-Beard, 374–375, *375–378*
forehead, 371, *373*
Flap(s) *(Continued)*
lateral transpositional, 371, *372*
myocutaneous, 369, *369–370*
nasojugal, 373–374, *374*
pedicle, from lower lid to upper lid, 382–383, *383*
semicircular, 366, *367*
sliding tarsal, 380, 382, *382*
tarsal rotational, 375–378, *379–380*
tarsoconjunctival, 378–380, *381*
sliding, 380, 382, *382*
Flash-cord receptacle, of camera, 551
Flower tear trough implant, 488, *489*, 492–493, *492–495*, 495
Focusing screen, of camera, 552, *552*
Fogo selvagem, 33
Follicles, hair. See *Hair follicles.*
Follicular keratosis, inverted, of eyelid, 326, *326*
Foltz valve, 742, *743*
Forceps, used in ophthalmic plastic surgery, *290*
Forehead flap, used in medial canthal reconstruction, island, 393, *396*
midline, 393, *396*
used in upper eyelid reconstruction, technique of, 371, *373*
Forehead fracture, unilateral, orbital fracture and, anterior cranial base approach to, 1188–1189, *1190*
Foreign body(ies), causing secondary acquired nasolacrimal duct obstruction, 812
removal of, 1047
surgical approach in, 1054
Fornical conjunctiva, 159. See also *Conjunctiva.*
Foster's classification, of cicatricial pemphigoid, 197, 197t
Four-wall orbital decompression, for Graves' disease, combined transorbital-neurosurgical, 980. See also *Graves' disease, orbital decompression for.*
Fracture(s), orbital. See *Orbital fracture(s).*
Francisella tularensis, 149
tularemia caused by, 313
Freckles (ephelides), in neurofibromatosis, 25
of eyelid, 339, *339*
Free thyroxine index (FTI), in thyrotoxicosis, 124
Fresh tissue technique, for removal of skin cancer, 352
advantages of, 354–355
steps in, 352–354, *353–355*
Frontal nerve, anatomy of, 277, *278*
Frontal sinus(es), anatomy of, 1015
mucoceles in, *1017*, 1017–1018
radiographic findings in, 1017, *1017–1018*
treatment of, 1018
Frontalis muscle, *263*, 264, *266*
contraction of, 262
Frontobasal fracture(s), 1096–1098
complications of, 1097–1098
treatment of, 1097, *1097*
Frontonasalethmoidal encephalocele, anterior cranial base approach to, 1199, *1201–1202*
Fronto-orbital asymmetry, subcranial approach to, results of, 1176t
Fronto-orbital fracture, cerebrospinal fluid leak with, anterior cranial base approach to, 1189, *1192*
Fronto-orbital osteotomy, subcranial approach to, 1163–1164, *1165–1167*
Frost-type sutures, in eyelid surgery, 439, *440*

FTI (free thyroxine index), in thyrotoxicosis, 124
Fuchs, islets of, 208
Fungal infection(s), of eyelid, 318–319

Gangrene, gas, of eyelid, 312
progressive synergistic, of eyelid, 312
Gas gangrene (clostridial myonecrosis), of eyelid, 312
Gastrointestinal carcinoma, metastatic orbital disease from, 1012
Gelfoam, for hemostasis in wound repair, 283
Giant cell arteritis, 112
Glabellar flap, used in medial canthal reconstruction, 391, 393, *395*
Glanders, involving eyelids, 313
Glaucoma, development of, following alkali burn, 222–223
in cicatricial pemphigoid, 98
Glioma, midbrain, ptosis caused by, 76
optic canal, 881–882, *882*
optic nerve, 985–987, *986*
clinical presentation of, 986–987
imaging of, 899–900, *899–900*
radiographic findings in, 987
treatment of, 987
Globe, anatomy of, 846–847, *847*, 904
examination of, evidence of orbital disease in, 868–870, *869–870*
malignant melanoma of, 909, *910–911*
metastasis of, *911*, 911–912
neuroradiologic imaging of, 904–912
techniques in, 904–905
ocular pathology of, 905–909
position and movement of, in orbital disease, 861–862, *863–865*
prominent, 486–487, *488–489*
cause of, 487–488
Glogau's classification, of photodamage, 662, 663t
Glomus tumor, of eyelid, 332
Glucocorticoids, for thyroid storm, 130
for thyrotoxicosis, 128
Gold weight, in surgical management of facial paralysis, 475–476, *476–477*
Goldberg lateral orbital rim implant, 488, *489*
Goldenhar's syndrome, 255
congenital colobomas in, 407–408
Goldmann perimetry, kinetic, 860
Gottron's papules, in dermatomyositis, 7
Gradenigo's syndrome, 473
Graft(s). See also *Autograft(s); Homograft(s).*
alloplastic, and spontaneous epithelialization, in conjunctival mucous membrane replacement, 171–172, *171–172*
bone, harvesting of, 1077–1080, *1078–1082*
buccal mucous membrane. See *Buccal mucous membrane graft(s).*
cartilage, harvesting of, 1080, 1082
in surgical management of facial paralysis, 481–482, *481–482*
cartilage-mucosal compound, 176
composite, used in medial canthal reconstruction, 391
used in upper eyelid reconstruction, 382, *383*
conjunctival. See *Conjunctival graft(s).*
hard palate, harvesting of, 442–444, *443–444*, 1082–1083
harvesting of, 1077–1083
for eyelid surgery, 440
lamellar corneoscleral, in management of pterygia, 214, *214*

Graft(s) *(Continued)*
nasal septal mucosa, harvesting of, 1080, 1082
oral mucosal. See *Oral mucosal graft(s).*
skin, used in medial canthal reconstruction, 393, 396, *397*
used in upper eyelid reconstruction, 366–367, *368*, 369
split-level full-thickness, used in upper eyelid reconstruction, 384, *384*
tarsoconjunctival, free, 175, *175–176*
Granular cell tumor, of eyelid, 329
Granulation, spontaneous, in conjunctival mucous membrane replacement, 170–171
of medial canthal area, 387
Granulocyte(s), 95
Granulocytic sarcoma, involving orbit, 61, *61*
Granuloma, eosinophilic, of orbit, 62, *63*
in AIDS patients, 532
in sarcoidosis, 107
lethal midline, 114
midline idiopathic, of orbit, 66, *66*
pyogenic, of eyelid, 331, *331*
Granuloma annulare, 43, *43*
in diabetic patient, 140
Granuloma faciale, 43
Granuloma inguinale, involving eyelids, 314
Granulomatosis, lymphomatoid, 10t, 11–12, 113–114
Wegener's. See *Wegener's granulomatosis.*
Granulomatous angiitis, allergic, 113
Graves' disease, *12*, 12–14
canthal obliquity in, surgical techniques for, 521
euthyroid, 121
eyelid retraction in, clinical features of, 514–516, *515–516*
historical background to, 516–518
lower, surgical techniques for, 520–521, *520–521*
surgical techniques for, 518–521
complications of, 521–523, *522–523*
upper, surgical techniques for, 518–520, *519–520*
lower eyelid entropion in, surgical techniques for, 521
orbital decompression for, 967–982
four-wall, combined transorbital-neurosurgical, 980
in patients with compressive optic neuropathy, *973*, 973–974
indications for, 968
overview to surgery in, *968*, 968–969
preoperative evaluation in, 967–968
three-wall, transorbital approach to, 976–980, *976–980*
tissue compliance impacting on, 969
transantral approach to, 974–976, *974–976*
transorbital antroethmoidal, 969–973, *970–973*
orbital expansion for, complications of, 981–982
craniofacial approach to, 980–981
postoperative management in, 981
Graves' ophthalmopathy, 13–14
Gray (Gy), defined, 1023
Ground substance, of wound repair, 281
Gundersen conjunctival flap(s), contraindications to, 248
indications for, 248
postoperative management of, 248, *249*
surgical technique of, 248, *249*
Gundersen flap, 164–165
Günther's disease, 29

Guttate, in scleroderma, 8
Gy (gray), defined, 1023

Haemophilus ducreyi, chancroid caused by, 314
Hair. See also *Eyebrow(s); Eyelash(es).*
direction of, in adult, 264, *265*
in infant, 264, *264*
permanent removal of, 589–594
blend modality in, 593
comparison of techniques in, 593–594
electrolysis in, 589–591
regulatory agencies and, 591–593
short-wave or thermolysis method in, 591
Hair follicles, 268, 324
benign adnexal lesions originating in, 335–336, *335–336*
Hand-Schüller-Christian disease, 62
Hansen's disease (leprosy), 153–154
involving eyelids, 313
Hard palate, anatomy of, 441, *442*
mucosa of, used in upper eyelid reconstruction, 364–365
Hard palate graft(s), harvesting of, 442–444, *443–444*, 1082–1083
Hard palate surgery, 441–442
Harlequin fetus, 45, *45*
Harvesting, of auricular cartilage, technique in, 364, *364*
of autogenous bone grafts, 1077–1080, *1078–1082*
of hard palate graft(s), 442–444, *443–444*, 1082–1083
of mucous membrane grafts, 173, *173*, 1080, 1082–1083
of nasochondral tissue, technique in, 365, *365*
Hasner valve, 742, *743*
Hasner's membrane, 777
rupture of, 778, 780
Hasner's valve, 777
Hauschka technique, of lymphatic drainage, 654–655
Head structure, anophthalmic socket and, 1130, *1130*
Hearing aids, bone-anchored, 1159
Heerford's syndrome, 16, 901
Heliotrope, 7
Helminthic infection(s), of eyelid, 317–318
Hemangioendothelioma, benign, imaging of, 893, *893–894*
malignant, 929
Hemangioma, capillary, of eyelid, 330, *330*
of orbit, 913–920
clinical course of, 913–916, *915–916*
complications of, 917, *918*
corticosteroids for, 919–920
diagnostic testing for, 916–917, *916–917*
histopathology of, 913, *914–915*
imaging of, 893, *893–894*
radiation therapy for, 919
surgical excision of, 918–919
treatment of, 917–920
indications for, 917–918
cavernous, of eyelid, 330
of orbit, 926–929
clinical course of, 927–928
diagnostic testing for, 928, *928–929*
histopathology of, 926–927, *927*
imaging of, 894, *894–895*
treatment of, 928–929
choroidal, imaging of, 910–911, *910–911*
disseminated neonatal, 920–921

Hemangioma *(Continued)*
clinical course of, 921, *921*
histopathology of, 920, *920*
ocular and ophthalmic manifestations of, 920t
treatment of, 921
eruptive (pyogenic granuloma), of eyelid, 331, *331*
retinal, 910–911
Hemangiopericytoma, 929–932
clinical course of, 930, *931*
diagnostic testing for, 930–931, *931*
histopathology of, 930, *930–931*
orbital, imaging of, 895–896, *896*
treatment of, 931–932, *932*
Hematoma, as complication of medial canthal reconstruction, 398
Hemiexophthalmos, 488
Hemifacial spasm, 90, *90*, 510–512
botulinum A toxin injection for, *508*, 509t, 511
clinical features of, 510, *510*
diagnostic features of, 505t
drug therapy for, 511
etiology of, 510–511, *511*
management of, 90
surgical therapy for, 511–512
Hemochromatosis, in diabetic patient, 141
Hemorrhage, as complication of orbital decompression surgery, 981–982
retrobulbar, causing blindness, 643
surgical approach to, 1054
Hemostasis, in orbital surgery, 1049
in wound repair, 282–284
pharmacologic agents for, 283
pressure tamponade for, 282
thermal cautery and electrocautery for, 282–283
topically applied chemical agents for, 283–284
Hemostats, used in ophthalmic plastic surgery, *290*
Hepatic cirrhosis, eyelid retraction associated with, 75, *76*
Hepatoblastoma, metastatic, to orbit, *56*
Hereditary hemorrhagic telangiectasia (Osler-Weber-Rendu disease), 9
Hering's law of equal innervation, 878
eyelid retraction secondary to, 74, *76*
Herpes simplex infection, of eyelid, 315, *315*
treatment of, 315
Herpes zoster infection, 152
of eyelid, 315
treatment of, 315–316
Herpes zoster ophthalmicus, of eyelid, in AIDS patients, 526
Hidradenoma, clear cell, of eyelid, 334
Hidrocystoma, apocrine (Moll's cyst), of eyelid, 334, *334*
Highlighting, as cosmetic technique, used in facial rejuvenation, 570
Highlighting and contouring, with camouflage make-up, 660–661
Histiocytes, benign eyelid tumors derived from, *332*, 332–333
Histiocytic disorder(s), involving orbit, 62, *63*, 64
Histiocytosis, Langerhans' cell, 62
sinus, associated with secondary acquired nasolacrimal duct obstruction, 801
Histiocytosis X. See *Eosinophilic granuloma.*
Histocompatibility leukocyte antigen (HLA), 96
HIV (human immunodeficiency virus), 525
infection by. See *Acquired immunodeficiency syndrome (AIDS).*
HLA (histocompatibility leukocyte antigen), 96
HMB-45 marker, for malignant melanoma, 57
Hollow bulb prosthesis, 1143–1144, *1143–1145*. See also *Prosthesis.*
Homograft(s). See also *Graft(s).*
scleral, for eyelid reconstruction, 724–727
results with, 727, *727*
histology of, 726, *726–727*
immunopathology of, 726–727
Hordeolum (stye), 307, *309*
treatment of, 307–308
Hormonal therapy, for orbital metastatic disease, 57, 1008
Horn cyst, 325
Horner's muscle, *850*, 744850
Horner's syndrome, 77–79
anisocoria in, 78
cocaine test for, 79, *79*
evaluation of, 78–79
Paredrine test for, 79
postganglionic, orbital disease causing, 877
ptosis in, 77–78, *78*
Hrytl valve, 742, *743*
Hudson-Stähli line, 208
Hughes flap, in lower eyelid reconstruction, 402–404, *403–404*
severing of, 404, *405*
Human immunodeficiency virus (HIV), 525
infection by. See *Acquired immunodeficiency syndrome (AIDS).*
Huschke valve, 742, *743*
Hutchinson's freckle (lentigo maligna), definition of, 179
of eyelid, 339
Hyalinosis cutis et mucosae, 20–21
Hyaloid detachment, posterior, MRI of, 905, *905*
Hydatid cyst, 151
Hydralazine lupus, 5, 5t. See also *Lupus erythematosus (LE).*
Hydrocystoma, eccrine, of eyelid, 334
Hydroxyapatite implant. See also *Prosthesis.*
enucleation with, 1036, 1041–1042
complications of, 1042
contraindications to, 1042
Hygroma, cystic (cavernous lymphangioma), of eyelid, 331
Hypercalcemia, causes of, 133t
evaluation of, parathyroid hormone in, 132–133
hyperparathyroidism causing, 132
severe, definition of, 135
treatment of, 135–136
Hyperparathyroidism, 132–136
clinical manifestations of, 133–135, *134–135*
diagnostic considerations in, 132–133, 133t
management of, 135–136, 136t
Hyperpigmentation, periorbital, chemical peels for, 663
Hyperplasia, angiolymphoid, with eosinophilia, of eyelid, 332
intravascular papillary endothelial, of eyelid, 332
sebaceous gland, of eyelid, 336–337
Hypersensitivity reaction(s), types of, 96
Hypertelorism, subcranial approach to, results of, 1176t
Hyperthyroidism, 12–14
in pregnancy, 129–130
thyrotoxicosis vs., 123
Hyperthyroxinemia, euthyroid, 129
causes of, 129t
Hypertropia, as complication of orbital floor fractures, 1091, *1092*
Hypothalamic-pituitary-thyroid axis, physiologic regulation of, 122–123, *123*
Hypothyroidism, associated with myxedema, 14, *14*
due to ^{131}iodine therapy, 128
Hypotonia, lower lid, evaluation of, prior to male blepharoplasty, 635

"Ice pack" test, for myasthenia gravis, 82
Ichthyosis, *45*, 45–46
treatment of, 46
Ichthyosis vulgaris, 45
Idiopathic midline destructive disease, of orbit, 66, *66*
Idiopathic optic disc edema, in diabetic patient, 138t, 138–139
Idiopathic orbital inflammation, 952–956
acute form of, 952–953, *953*
biopsy of, 955
CT scans of, 954, *954*
diagnosis of, 953–954
histopathology of, 954–955, *955*
historical perspective on, 952
imaging of, 890–891, *890–891*
immunopathogenesis of, 955
subacute, 953
treatment of, 955–956
Idiopathic orbital pseudotumor, 965
IgA (immunoglobulin A), 95
IgD (immunoglobulin D), 95
IgE (immunoglobulin E), 95
IgG (immunoglobulin G), 95
IgM (immunoglobulin M), 95
Iliac bone graft(s), harvesting of, 1077, *1078–1079*
Immune complex reaction (hypersensitivity type III), 96
Immune disease, ocular manifestation(s) of, 94–114
allergic granulomatous angiitis and, 113
cicatricial pemphigoid and, 98–100
epidermolysis bullosa and, 103–105
erythema multiforme and, 100–102
lethal midline granuloma and, 114
lymphomatoid granulomatosis and, 113–114
pemphigus and, 102–103
polyarteritis nodosa and, 111–112
polymorphic reticulosis and, 113–114
sarcoidosis and, 106–108
temporal arteritis and, 112
toxic epidermal necrolysis and, 105–106
Wegener's granulomatosis and, 109–111
Immune reaction(s), classic, 96
Immune system, 94–98
cells of, 94–95
histocompatibility antigens of, 95
hypersensitivity reactions of, 95
monoclonal antibodies of, 95
Immunity, cell-mediated, 94, 96
Immunoglobulin(s), classes of, 95
Immunosuppressive therapy, for cicatricial pemphigoid, 199
complications of, 199–200
goal of, 200
Imperforate punctal membrane, 782, *782*
Implant(s). See *Prosthesis.*

Impression(s), alginate, used in design and making of prosthesis, 1138, *1138*
Incision(s), for blepharoplasty, 707–708, *707–708*
  for brow ptosis, 579, *579,* 581, *581–583,* 583
  for orbital surgery, 1060, *1061*
Infection(s). See also specific infection.
  after blepharoplasty, 648
  causing nasolacrimal duct obstruction, 797–799, 798t, *798–800*
  of eyelid, 313–319
    bacterial, 313–315
    fungal, 318–319
    in AIDS patients, 526
    parasitic, 317–318
    viral, 315–316, *315–316*
  of orbit, 146–155, 888–891
    causing edema, 151–152
    causing nodular eruptions, *140,* 149–150
    cellulitis due to, 146–148, 147t, *147–148*
    Chlamydia trachomatis causing, 154t, 154–155, *155*
    dacryoadenitis associated with, 153, *153*
    herpes zoster virus causing, 152
    in AIDS patient(s), 529
    in diabetic patient, 137–138, 138t
    miscellaneous, 150–151, *151*
    Mycobacterium leprae causing, 153–154
    Mycobacterium tuberculosis causing, 152–153
    syphilis and, 153
Infiltrative myopathy, 88
Inflammation, of eyelid, 307–310, *309*
    causes of, 308t
  of orbit, idiopathic. See *Idiopathic orbital inflammation.*
    in AIDS patients, 529–530
Inflammatory cause(s), of secondary acquired nasolacrimal duct obstruction, 799, 801t, 801–804, *802–804*
Inflammatory myopathy, 88
Inflammatory phase, of wound repair, 281, 282t
Infranuclear factor(s), tearing due to, 750
Infranuclear lesion(s), eyelid retraction caused by, 73–74, *74–76*
  ptosis caused by, 77, *78*
Injury. See *Trauma.*
Inorganic pigment, 541. See also *Pigment(s).*
Insulin, chronic patient use of, anesthetic considerations with, 295
Intensity, principle of, in electrolysis, 590
Interferon(s), for Kaposi's sarcoma, 528
Interrupted suture(s), deep, 286, *287*
  simple, 286, *286*
Intracranial hypertension, benign, optic nerve decompression for, 1056–1059, *1057–1059*
Intradermal nevus, of eyelid, 337–338, *338*
Intravascular papillary endothelial hyperplasia, of eyelid, 332
Iodide, oral (Lugol's solution), for thyroid storm, 130
    for thyrotoxicosis, 128
^{131}Iodine therapy, for thyrotoxicosis, 128
  side effects of, 128
Irrigation, immediate, following chemical injury, 223
Islets of Fuchs, 208

Jaw winking phenomenon, Marcus Gunn, 73, *74*
Jessner's solution, used in chemical peels, 666, 666t
Jewelry, metal, removal of, before electrolysis, 589–590
Jones I test, in tearing, 754–755
Jones II test, in tearing, 755
Jones' muscle, 744
Junctional nevus, of eyelid, 337
Juvenile melanoma, of eyelid, 338
Juvenile pilocytic astrocytoma, imaging of, 899–900, *899–900*
Juvenile xanthogranuloma, of eyelid, 64, 333
  of orbit, 64

K (killer) cell(s), 95
Kaposi's sarcoma, of conjunctiva, in AIDS patients, 236–237, 242, *243,* 532
  of eyelid, in AIDS patients, 526–528, *527*
Kearns-Sayre syndrome, 87
  in diabetic patient, 138t, 139
  pigmentary retinopathy in, 87–88, *88*
Keloid(s), in African American patient, 715–716, *716*
  pigmentary management of, 535–536
  vs. hypertrophic scarring, 717t
Keratinocyte(s), of eyelid, 323
Keratoacanthoma, of eyelid, 325–326, *326*
Keratoconjunctivitis, superior limbic, conjunctival resection for, indications for, 248–249
    surgical technique of, 249
Keratosis, actinic, chemical peels for, 663
  of eyelid, inverted follicular, 326, *326*
    seborrheic, 325, *325*
Keratosis follicularis (Darier's disease), 21
KID syndrome, 46
Kiem test, for sarcoidosis, 108
Killer (K) cell(s), 95
Kimura's disease (angiolymphoid hyperplasia with eosinophilia), 949–950, *949–950*
  of eyelid, 332
Kissing nevus, of eyelid, 337, *337*
Klebsiella rhinoscleromatis, 138
  rhinoscleroma caused by, 314
Kleeblatt-Schaedel's anomaly, 1182
Koenen's tumors, in tuberous sclerosis, 27
Krause gland(s), 161, *273,* 732, *732, 737*
Krause (Béraud) valve, 742, *743*
Krönlein-Berke orbitotomy, technique of, 1056–1059, *1057–1059*
Kuhnt-Szymanowski procedure, Smith modification of, for involutional ectropion, 427, *428*
Kveim test, for sarcoidosis, 65

Laceration(s), conjunctival, 168–169
  lower eyelid, evaluation of, 455–456, *455–457*
  upper eyelid, repair of, 359–361, *362*
Lacrimal artery, anatomy of, 274, *274–275*
Lacrimal diaphragm, 744
Lacrimal ductule(s), destruction of, treatment for, 255
Lacrimal fossa, 731
  in Chinese skulls, 696–698, 697t, 698t
Lacrimal gland(s), 273, *273,* 731–736
  adenoid cystic carcinoma of, 68–69, *69,* 303, *304*
Lacrimal gland(s) *(Continued)*
  anatomy of, 731–732, *732–733*
  blood supply to, 849
  direct stimulation of, tearing and, 750–751
  disorders of, after blepharoplasty, 648–649
  embryology of, 731
  histology of, 732–734, *734*
  innervation of, 734–736, *735*
  lesions of, imaging of, 902–904, *904*
  mucoepidermoid carcinoma of, 68, *69*
  prolapse of, in Graves' ophthalmopathy, 515–516, *516*
    repair of, in upper eyelid blepharoplasty, 601–602, *602*
      variations of, 609
  pseudocapsule of, 732
  secretion of, 735–736
  tumor(s) of, 999–1006
    benign, 999
    differential diagnosis of, 1003t, 1003–1004
    epidemiology of, 999, 1001
    malignant, 999
    natural history of, 1002
    presentation of, 1001
    prognosis for, 1006
    radiologic features of, *1000–1002,* 1001
    secondary, 999
    treatment of, 1004–1006, *1005–1006*
      principles and problems in, 1002–1003
  vascular supply to, 734
Lacrimal nerve, 849
  anatomy of, 277, *278*
Lacrimal nucleus, stimulation of, tearing due to, 750
Lacrimal probes, for nasolacrimal duct obstruction, 778, *779*
  for ophthalmic plastic surgery, *290*
Lacrimal pump, disorders of, epiphora due to, 751
  integrity of, affecting tearing, 762
Lacrimal pump mechanism, composition of, 267
Lacrimal sac, 740–741, *742*
  anatomy of, 268, *268,* 850
  fistula of, 782–783, *783*
  tumors of, 304–305, *305*
Lacrimal surgery, for altered tear production, 201
Lacrimal system, 731–746
  anatomy of, 784, *785*
  congenital abnormalities of, 777–783. See also specific anomaly, e.g., *Nasolacrimal duct obstruction, congenital.*
  excretory, 738–746, *739*
    anatomy of, 849–850, *850*
    canaliculi of, 739–740, *739–741*
    embryology of, *738,* 738–739
    lacrimal sac in, 740–741, *742*
    nasolacrimal duct in, 741–745, *743–746*
    pump system in, 744–745, *746*
    puncta of, 739
  glands in, 731–738
    anatomy of, 731–72, *732–733*
    embryology of, 731
    histology of, 732–734, *734*
    innervation of, 734–736, *735*
    vascular supply to, 734
  injury to, sequence of repair following, 458
  involvement of, in medial canthal reconstruction, 396, 398
  secretory, anatomy of, 849

Lacrimation. See also *Tearing.*
afferent and efferent pathways of, 734, *735*
causes of, 750–751
Lagophthalmos, after blepharoplasty, 646, *646*
in Graves' ophthalmopathy, 514
Lambdoidal synostosis, 1182
Lamellar corneoscleral graft(s), in management of pterygia, 214, *214*
Langerhans' cell histiocytosis, 62
Large cell lymphoma, 959
Laser(s), carbon dioxide, fat removal by, 638, 640
treatment of lymphangioma with, 926
ultrapulse, used in blepharoplasty, *544*
in treatment of endonasal dacryocystorhinostomy, 794
in treatment of hyperpigmented facial lesions, 568
in treatment of telangiectasia, 569
postoperative use of, for pterygia, 219
YAG, fat removal by, *641,* 641–642
treatment of lymphangiomas with, 926
Laugh line (skin folds), around eyelids, 261–262, *263*
LE. See *Lupus erythematosus (LE).*
LeFort fracture(s), 1095, *1095*
Leiomyoma, of eyelid, 329
of orbit, 996
Leiomyosarcoma, metastatic, to orbit, *58*
of orbit, 996
Leishmaniasis, diffuse cutaneous, of eyelid, 150, *150*
involving eyelids, 316
Lens, of camera, 552–554, *553*
Lentigines, chemical peels for, 663–664
Lentigo maligna (Hutchinson's freckle), definition of, 179
of eyelid, 339
Lentigo maligna melanoma, 179
of eyelid, 339
Lentigo senilis, of eyelid, 339, *340*
Lentigo simplex, of eyelid, 339
Leprosy (Hansen's disease), 153–154
involving eyelids, 313
Lethal midline granuloma, 114
Leukemia, involving orbit, 60
Leukocoria, 907
Levator aponeurosis, applied anatomy of, 448
Levator palpebrae superioris muscle, anatomy of, 270–271, 849
superior view of, *272*
Lichen planus, 40–41
treatment of, 41
Lichen simplex chronicus, 41
Lid(s). See *Eyelid(s).*
Lidocaine (Xylocaine), for aponeurotic surgery, 448
for lower eyelid blepharoplasty, 619, 627
for male blepharoplasty, 636
for transantral approach to orbital decompression, 974
for transorbital antroethmoidal orbital decompression, 969
for upper eyelid blepharoplasty, 599
recommended maximal dosage of, 298
Lighting, for orbital surgery, 1048
for photography, 554–555, *556–559,* 557–559
proper set-up of, *556*
sources of, 554–555
Ligneous conjunctivitis, 20
Limbal tumor(s), 69–70
Lipocauterization, in fat removal, 638, *639*
Lipocontouring, radio-frequency, in fat removal, 642, *642*
Lipodermoid(s). See *Dermolipoma(s).*
Lipoid proteinosis, 20–21
differential diagnosis of, 21
Lipolytic diathermy, fat removal by, 640–641, *640–641*
Lipoma, orbital, 996
Liposarcoma, orbital, 996–997
Lisch nodules, in neurofibromatosis, 25
Lithium, for thyroid storm, 130
for thyrotoxicosis, 128
Loa loa infection, of eyelid, 317
Local anesthesia. See *Anesthesia, regional.*
Lockwood's ligament, anatomy of, 841–842, *842*
Löfgren's syndrome, 16
Lorazepam, for essential blepharospasm and Meige's syndrome, 507
Lubricants, topical, for facial paralysis, 474
Lugol's solution, for thyroid storm, 130
for thyrotoxicosis, 128
Lung carcinoma, metastatic orbital disease from, 1010
Lupus erythematosus (LE), 3–7, *4*
acute cutaneous, 4
chronic cutaneous, 4
common form of, 6
clinical manifestations of, 3–4
discoid, 3
characteristic features of, 6
drug-related, 5, 5t
mucocutaneous lesions of, classification of, 4t
subacute cutaneous, 3
serologic marker for, 5–6
systemic manifestations of, 5
systemic, 3
diagnosis of, 6
ocular complications of, 4–5, 5t
revised criteria for, 4t
treatment of, 6–7
Lupus miliaris disseminatus faciei, 38, *38*
treatment of, 39
Lupus panniculitis, 6
Lupus profundus, 6
Lutzner's cells, 62
Lyell's syndrome. See *Toxic epidermal necrolysis (Lyell's syndrome).*
Lyme disease, 473
Lymphadenopathy, sinus histiocytosis with, of orbit, 62, *62*
Lymphangioma, 921–926
clinical course of, 923–924, *923–924*
diagnostic testing for, 924–925, *924–926*
histopathology of, *922,* 922–923
of eyelid, 331, *331*
orbital, imaging of, 894–895, *895*
treatment of, 925–926, *926*
Lymphangion, 652, *652*
Lymphatic drainage, manual, 651–656
contraindications to, 655t
features of, 655
Hauschka technique of, 654–655
indications for, 655, 655t
mechanical methods of, 655
of extremities, pressure bandages with, 655
Vodder technique of, 654
of conjunctiva, 161
of eyelid, 275, *276*
Lymphatic flow, pulse-wave nature of, 653, *653*
Lymphatic fluid, 651
forward propulsion of, *652,* 652–653
osmotic pressure of, 654
protein concentration of, 654
Lymphatic system, anatomy and physiology of, 651, *652*
Lymphatic vessels, 651–652, *652–653*
pharmacology of, 655
pumping action of, 652
Lymphoblastic lymphoma, 959
Lymphocyte(s), subpopulations of, 94–95
Lymphocytic lymphoma, small cell, 959
Lymphogranuloma venereum, involving eyelids, 315
Lymphoid cells, gene rearrangement unique to, 960
Lymphoid granulomatosis, ocular abnormalities of, 10t
Lymphoid hyperplasia, benign reactive, involving orbit, 61–62
Lymphoid tumor(s), of conjunctiva, 58–59, 235–236, *235–236,* 244–246, 956–957
classification of, 244
clinical features of, 244, *245*
demographics and, 245
histology of, 244
histopathologic analysis of, 244
immunophenotypic analysis of, 244–245
molecular genetic analysis of, 245
patient evaluation for, 245–246
prognosis for, 245
treatment of, 246
of orbit, 58–60, *59,* 303–304, 956–962
benign, 958
classification of, 956
clinical course of, 960
clinical presentation of, 956–957, *956–957*
differential diagnosis of, 960–961
historical perspective on, 952
laboratory evaluation of, 957–960, *958*
malignant, 958–959
treatment of, 961–962
Lymphoma, 58–60, *59,* 303–304
Burkitt's, Epstein-Barr virus associated with, 530, 959
imaging of, 892–983, *893*
large cell, 959
lymphoblastic, 959
mantle cell, 959
non-Hodgkin's. See *Non-Hodgkin's lymphoma.*
of lacrimal glands, natural history of, 1002
radiologic features of, 1001, *1001*
treatment of, 1004
small cell lymphocytic, 959
Lymphomatoid granulomatosis, 11–12, 113–114
Lymphoproliferative disease(s), of orbit, in AIDS patients, 530–532, *531*

MacCallan classification, of trachoma, 314–315
Macrophage(s), 94
Macrophthalmia, 905
"Madame Butterfly" procedure, for ectropion, 645
Magnetic resonance imaging (MRI), of capillary hemangioma, 893, *894*
of cavernous hemangioma, 894, *895*
of choroidal hemangioma, 910, *911*
of dermoid cyst, 886–888, *889*
of epidermoid cyst, 886–888, *888*
of hemangiopericytoma, 895–896, *896*
of lacrimal gland lesions, 904, *904*
of lymphangioma, 894–895, *895*
of lymphoid tumor, 957

Magnetic resonance imaging (MRI) *(Continued)*
of lymphoma, 892-983, *893*
of mucoceles, in paranasal sinuses, *1016*, 1016-1017
of neurofibroma, *991*
of neurogenic tumors, 984
of optic nerve glioma, 900, *900*, *986*, 987
of optic nerve meningioma, 988, *988*
of optic nerve sarcoidosis, 900-901, *902*
of optic nerve sheath meningioma, 899, *899*
of optic neuritis, 900, *900*
of orbit, 885-886
of persistent hyperplastic primary vitreous, 908, *909*
of posterior hyaloid detachment, 905, *905*
of pseudotumor, 890-891, *891*
of retinal detachment, 905-906, *906*
of retinoblastoma, 907-908, *908*
of rhabdomyosarcoma, 902, *903*
of schwannoma, 992, *992*
of sphenoid wing meningioma, *989*, 990
of subperiosteal abscess, 889-890, *890*
of uveal malignant melanoma, 909, *910-911*
of uveal metastatic disease, *911*, 911-912
Magnification, in orbital surgery, 1048
Maier's sinus, 740, *742*, 850
Make-up, camouflage. See *Camouflage make-up.*
Malar fold, *262-263*, 484
Malar hypoplasia, evaluation of, prior to male blepharoplasty, 635
Malherbe's calcifying epithelioma (pilomatricoma), of eyelid, 336, *336*
Malignancy. See also specific neoplasm.
acanthosis nigricans associated with, 23-24
dermatomyositis associated with, 7
life-threatening, orbital exenteration for, 1070, 1071t
Malignant external otitis, in diabetic patient, 138
Malignant hemangioendothelioma, 929
Malignant melanoma, metastatic orbital disease from, 1012
of conjunctiva, 233-235, *234*
clinical features of, 183, *183*
primary acquired melanosis associated with, 233, 234
treatment of, 187-188, *188*
care following, 188t
complications of, 187t
of lacrimal sac, 305
of orbit, 57-58, *58*, 992
imaging of, 909, *910-911*
of uvea, anterior cranial base approach to, 1202-1204, *1204-1205*
Mantle cell lymphoma, 959
Manual lymphatic drainage, 651-656
contraindications to, 655t
features of, 655
Hauschka technique of, 654-655
indications for, 655, 655t
mechanical methods of, 655
of extremities, pressure bandages with, 655
Vodder technique of, 654
Manz gland(s), 160, *273*, 736, 737, *737*
Marcus Gunn jaw winking phenomenon, 73, *74*
Marcus Gunn pupil, 876
reverse, 876, *877*
Marcus Gunn swinging light test, 860-861
Mask, computer-controlled cooling-heating, used in blepharoplasty, *544*
Masquerade syndrome, in sebaceous gland carcinoma, 190
Massage techniques, of lymphatic drainage, 651-656. See also *Manual lymphatic drainage.*
Mast cell(s), 95
Mastocytoma, 43
Mastocytosis, 43
Mattress suture(s), buried, 710-711, *710-711*
combined with small incisions, 712, *713*
horizontal, 288, *288*
half-buried, 288, *289*
vertical, 288, *289*
Maturation phase, of wound repair, 281, 282t
Maxillary nerve, anatomy of, 278
Maxillary sinus(es), anatomy of, 1015
mucoceles in, 1021, *1021*
as complication of orbital floor fracture, 1091, *1093*
Maxillary vein, anatomy of, 275
McReynolds operation, for pterygia removal, 211
Mechanical cause(s), of nasolacrimal duct obstruction, 812t, 812-813, *812-813*
Mechanobullous disease(s), 29-31, 30t
Medical device, migrated or retained, causing nasolacrimal duct obstruction, 812, *812*
Medical photography, 551-559
camera feature(s) for, 551-554
automatic film advance as, 551
film as, 554
flash-cord receptacle as, 551
focusing screens as, 552, *552*
lens as, 552-554, *553*
shutter and shutter speed as, 551
lighting for, 554-555, *556-559*, 557-559
daylight as, 554
electronic flash or strobe as, 555
proper set-up and, *556*
tungsten bulbs as, 555
Medical tattooing. See *Micropigmentation.*
Medicine, Chinese view of, *692-694*, 692-695, 693t
Meibomian gland(s), 273, *273*, 736, *737*
carcinoma arising in, 190. See also *Sebaceous gland carcinoma.*
hyperplasia of, 336-337
inflammation of, 307, *309*
Meibomitis, acute, 307
after blepharoplasty, 649
chronic, 307, *309*
Meige's syndrome, 89-90, 504, 506
diagnostic features of, 505t
management of, 90, 507-510
botulinum A toxin injection in, 507-508, *508*, 509t
future directions in, 509-510
general eye care in, 507
pharmacotherapy in, 507
surgery in, 508-509, *509*
unconventional therapies in, 507
Melanocytosis, oculodermal, of eyelid, 339
Melanoma, choroidal, 182, *182*
juvenile, of eyelid, 338
malignant. See *Malignant melanoma.*
nodular, 179
superficial spreading, 179
Melanosis, complexion-associated, clinical features of, 180-181, *180-181*
definition of, 178-179
primary acquired. See *Primary acquired melanosis (PAM).*
Melasma, chemical peels for, 662-663
Melkersson-Rosenthal syndrome, 15-16
differential diagnosis of, 16
MEN I (Wermer's syndrome), 22, 142
MEN II (Sipple's syndrome), 22, 142
MEN III (multiple endocrine neoplasia III), 21-23, 22t, 142
Meningioma, optic nerve, 882, *883*, 987-989
management of, 988-989
radiographic findings in, 987-988, *987-988*
optic nerve sheath, imaging of, 897, *898-899*, 899
sphenoid wing, 989-990
radiographic findings in, *989*, 990
treatment of, 990
Metabolic disease(s). See *Systemic and metabolic disease(s).*
Metabolism, calcium, regulation of, 132
Metal jewelry, removal of, before electrolysis, 589-590
Metastatic disease, causing nasolacrimal duct obstruction, 804, *805-810*, 806-807
from adenoid cystic carcinoma, of lacrimal glands, 1004, *1006*
of eyelid, *54*, 56
of orbit, 53-56, *54-57*, 1007-1013. See also *Orbital tumor(s), metastatic.*
prevalence of, 53
of uvea, *911*, 911-912
progressive palsy and, 474
Methimazole, for thyroid storm, 130
for thyrotoxicosis, 125
Methohexital, as anesthetic agent, 297
for aponeurotic surgery, 448
Methotrexate, pharmacology of, 97
Methyl methacrylate rings, insertion of, following chemical injury, 225
Metoprolol, for thyrotoxicosis, 125, 128
Microabscess, Pautrier's, 62
Microdissection, monopolar, fat removal by, 638
Microphthalmia, 905
severe, volume replacement in, 1043
Micropigmentation, 535-541. See also *Electropigmentation.*
aesthetic goals of, 683, 684t
consultation and preoperative teaching concerning, 683, 685
equipment for, 683
eyebrow reconstruction with, 537-538, *539-540*
technique of, 685-688, *686-688*
eyeliner reconstruction with, 536-537, *537-538*
technique of, 685, *686*
facial, 535-538
color adjusting in, 536
color matching in, 536
shading and blending in, 536, *536-537*
history of, 535
pigment color matching procedure in, 538-541, *540*
pigments for, 682-683
inorganic and organic, 541
selection of, 538
skin testing prior to, guidelines for, 541
techniques of, 685
Midazolam, as anesthetic agent, 296
Midbrain, glioma of, ptosis caused by, 76
Midbrain ptosis, *77*
Mikulicz's cells, in rhinoscleroma, 138
Mikulicz's syndrome, 107
Milia, of eyelid, *324*, 324-325
Miliary sarcoid, 16
Millard-Gubler syndrome, 470

Mini-driver, used in ophthalmic plastic surgery, *291*
Miniplates, cantilevered, in fixation/reconstruction of canthal tendon, 389–390, *390*
Miosis, ipsilateral, and unilateral ptosis. See *Horner's syndrome.*
Mitomycin C, as adjunct to surgery for pterygia, 218–219
Mixed eccrine tumor, of eyelid, 334, *334*
Mobility prosthesis, new, 1132, *1133*
Mohs' surgery, for periorbital malignancy, 352–355
  advantages of, 354–355
  drawbacks to, 352
  fresh tissue technique in, 352–354, *353–355*
Moisture bubble, for facial nerve palsy, 474, *475*
Moisture chamber glasses, for facial nerve palsy, 475, *475*
Moll's cyst (apocrine hidrocystoma), of eyelid, 334, *334*
Moll's gland(s), 273, *273*, 324, 737, *737*
Molluscum contagiosum, involving eyelids, 316, *316*
  in AIDS patients, 526, *526*
Mondino and Brown classification, of cicatricial pemphigoid, 196–197, 197t
Monoamine oxidase inhibitors, chronic patient use of, anesthetic considerations with, 296
Monoclonal antibody(ies), 96
Monocular condition(s), nonsurgical, for anophthalmic socket, 1127–1128, *1128*
Mononucleosis, periorbital edema in, 151
Monopolar microdissection, fat removal by, 638
Morning glory anomaly, 905
Moxibustion, 695
MRI. See *Magnetic resonance imaging (MRI).*
Mucin, 160
  reduced production of, after chemical injury, 226
Mucin layer, and precorneal tear film, 737
Mucocele(s), causing secondary acquired nasolacrimal duct obstruction, 813, *813*
  in paranasal sinuses, 1014–1021, *1015*
    as complication of orbital floor fracture, 1091, *1093*
    diagnostic imaging of, 1014–1017, *1016*, 1017–1018, *1017–1021*, 1020–1021
    histopathology of, 1014
    pathophysiology of, 1014
    treatment of, 1018–1019, 1021
Mucoepidermoid carcinoma, of lacrimal glands, 68, *69*, 999
Mucopyocele, 1014
Mucormycosis (phycomycosis), diagnostic and therapeutic features of, 941t–942t
  in diabetic patient, 137–138, 138t
    treatment of, 138
  rhinocerebral, 150–151, *151*
Mucosa, used in upper eyelid reconstruction, hard palate, 364–365
  oral, 365
Mucosal graft(s), oral. See *Oral mucosal graft(s).*
Mucous glands, conjunctival, 160–161
Mucous membrane(s), conjunctival, replacement of. See *Conjunctival mucous membrane(s), replacement of.*
  nonocular, involvement of, in cicatricial pemphigoid, 196
Mucous membrane graft(s), harvesting of, 1080, 1082–1083
Mular lesions, of eyelid, 314
Mulberry lesion, in squamous cell carcinoma of conjunctiva, *232*
Müller's muscle, anatomy of, 272, *273*
  in aponeurotic surgery, 448
Multicore disease, ptosis in, 84
Multiple endocrine neoplasia I (Wermer's syndrome), 22, 142
Multiple endocrine neoplasia II (Sipple's syndrome), 22, 142
Multiple endocrine neoplasia III (MEN III), 21–23, 22t, 142
Multiple mucosal neuroma syndrome, 21–23
  differential diagnosis of, 22–23
  ocular manifestations of, 22, 22t
  treatment of, 23
Multiple myeloma, of orbit, 62, *63*
Multiple suture synostosis, 1182, *1185*
Multiple-needle galvanic electrolysis, 590. See also *Electrolysis.*
Muscle(s). See also specific muscle, e.g., *Orbicularis oculi muscle.*
  excision of, in upper eyelid blepharoplasty, 599–600, *599–600*
    variations in, 607
  extraocular, enlarged, causes of, 886t
  of facial expression, 262, *263*, 264
Muscle of Riolan, 268
Muscle retraction, in orbital surgery, 1048
Muscular dystrophy, 84
Mustardé flap, in lower eyelid reconstruction, 404–405, *405*
  in medial canthal reconstruction, 390–391, *392*
Myasthenia gravis, 79–83
  acquired, in children, 80–81
  autoimmune disorders associated with, 83
  clinical findings in, 79–80
  eyelid retraction in, 74, *76*
  "ice pack" test for, 82
  ophthalmoparesis of, 80
  Prostigmin test for, in children, 82, *82*
  ptosis in, 80, *80–81*
  sleep test for, 82, *82*
  Tensilon test for, *80*, 81
    advantages and disadvantages of, 81–82
Myasthenic syndrome(s), 83
Mycobacterial infection(s), of eyelid, 313–314
Mycobacterium leprae, 153
  Hansen's disease caused by, 313
Mycosis cells, 62
Mycosis fungoides, of eyelid, 62
Myeloma, multiple, of orbit, 62, *63*
Myocutaneous flap, nasojugal, used in upper eyelid reconstruction, technique of, 373–374, *374*
  rotated, used in lower eyelid reconstruction, 403, *403–404*
  used in medial canthal reconstruction, 390, *391*
  used in upper eyelid reconstruction, 369, *369–370*
Myokymia, facial, 510
  diagnostic features of, 505t
Myonecrosis, of eyelid, clostridial, 312
  streptococcal, 312
Myopathy(ies), structural, ptosis caused by, 84, *85*
Myositis, ocular, in AIDS patients, 529
  orbital, 965–966
Myotonia, ptosis in, 85–86, *85–86*
Myotonic dystrophy, facial nerve disorders and, 474
  ptosis in, 85, *85–86*
Myxedema, 14, *14*

Narcotics, as anesthetic agents, 296
  reversal of, 296–297
Nasal dermoid, with intracranial extension, anterior cranial base approach to, 1199, *1200*
Nasal septal mucosa graft(s), harvesting of, 1080, 1082
Nasal telangiectasia, treatment of, 569, *569*
Nasochondral tissue, used in upper eyelid reconstruction, 365, *365*
Nasociliary nerve, anatomy of, 277, *278*
Nasoethmoidal fracture(s), 1095–1096
  treatment of, 1096
Nasojugal fold, *262–263*, 484
Nasojugal myocutaneous flap, used in upper eyelid reconstruction, technique of, 373–374, *374*
Nasolabial fold, *263*
Nasolacrimal duct, 741–745, *743–746*, 850
  congenital malformations of, 742–743, *743*
  stenosis of, epiphora due to, 751
  valves of, 742, *743*
Nasolacrimal duct obstruction, congenital, 777–778, *779*, 780
    probing of, 778, *779*
      failed, 780–781
    variant of, 780–781, *782*
  primary acquired, 784–796
    cause of, 784–785
    clinical presentation of, *785*, 785–786
    dacryocystorhinostomy for, *786–792*, 786–794
      endonasal, 792–794, *793–795*
      history in, 786–787
      incisions in, 788, *789*
      nasal packing for, 787, *788*
      procedure in, 787–792, *788–792*
      sedation for, 787
  secondary acquired, 797–813
    infectious causes of, 797–799, 798t, *798–800*
    inflammatory causes of, 799, 801t, 801–804, *802–804*
    mechanical causes of, 812t, 812–813, *812–813*
    neoplastic causes of, 804, 805t, *805–810*, 806–807
    traumatic causes of, 809–811, 810t, *810–812*
Nasolacrimal excretory system, dimensions of, 268, *268*
Nasolacrimal sac, narrowing of, epiphora due to, 751
Naso-orbital fistula, as complication of medial canthal reconstruction, 398
Naso-orbital fracture(s), 1095–1096
  treatment of, 1096
Naso-orbitoethmoid fracture, with associated brain and dural injury, anterior cranial base approach to, 1189, *1191*
Nasopalatine nerve block, 442
Natural killer (NK) cell(s), 95
Necrobiosis lipoidica diabeticorum, in diabetic patient, 139–140
Necrobiotic xanthogranuloma, 19–20
Necrosis, eyelid, *312*, 312–313
  causes of, 308t, 312

Necrotizing fasciitis, of eyelid, 312
Needle(s), suture, 284–285, *285*
Needle holder(s), used in ophthalmic plastic surgery, *290*
Nelson stainless steel screw, in fixation/reconstruction of canthal tendon, 389, *390*
Nemaline myopathy, ptosis in, 84
Nematode infection(s), of eyelid, 317
Neodymium:yttrium-aluminum-garnet (Nd:YAG) laser(s), used in removal of hyperpigmented facial lesions, 568
Neonate(s), disseminated hemangioma in, 920t, 920–921, *920–921*
  preseptal cellulitis in, 310
Neoplasm(s). See *Tumor(s)*; specific neoplasm.
Nerve(s). See also specific nerve, e.g., *Facial nerve.*
  conjunctival, 161
  lacrimal, 734
  of ocular region, 275, 277–278, *277–278*
Nerve block(s), for eyelid surgery, 442
Nerve tissue, benign eyelid tumors derived from, 328–329, *329*
Neurilemoma (schwannoma), of eyelid, 328–329
  of orbit, 991–992, *991–992*
Neuritis, optic, MRI scan in, 900, *900*
Neuroblastoma, metastatic orbital disease from, 1011–1012
Neurodermatitis circumscripta (lichen simplex chronicus), 41
Neurofibroma, of eyelid, 328, *329*
  of orbit, 990, *990–991*
    diffuse, 991
    isolated, 991
    plexiform, 991
Neurofibromatosis, *24*, 24–26, 990–991
  cranio-orbital, anterior cranial base approach to, 1204, *1206*, 1207
  diagnostic criteria for, 24t
  ocular features of, 25–26, 26t
  types of, 25
Neurogenic tumor(s), of orbit, 983–992. See also *Orbital tumor(s), neurogenic.*
Neuroma, acoustic, 474
  of eyelid, 329
Neuromuscular toxin(s), ptosis caused by, 83–84, *84*
Neuropathy, optic, transorbital decompression for, *973*, 973–974
Neuroradiologic imaging. See also specific imaging technique, e.g., *Computed tomography (CT).*
  of globe, 904–912
  of orbit, 885–904
Neutrophil(s), 95
Nevocellular nevus, of eyelid, 337–338, *337–338*
  variants of, 338
Nevoxanthoendothelioma (juvenile xanthogranuloma), of eyelid, 64, 333
Nevus(i), definition of, 179
  of conjunctiva, clinical features of, *181*, 181–182
    differential diagnosis of, 181, *182*
    histopathological classification of, 181
    treatment of, 185
  of eyelid, blue, 338–339
    combined, 339
    compound, 337
    congenital, 338, *339*
    intradermal, 337–338, *338*
    junctional, 337
    kissing, 337, *337*
Nevus(i) *(Continued)*
    linear epidermal, 327
    nevocellular, 337–338, *337–338*
      variants of, 338
    Ota's, *181*, 339
    strawberry, 330, *330*. See also *Hemangioma, capillary.*
Nevus flammeus (port wine stain), of eyelid, *329*, 329–330
Nevus ichthyosiformis, 20–21
Newton's groove, in surgical management of pterygia, 214
Nicotinic acid, chronic patient use of, anesthetic considerations with, 296
Nikolsky's sign, 29
  in pemphigus, 34, 102
  in toxic epidermal necrolysis, 35, 105
Nodular elastosis, with cysts and comedones, of eyelid, 327, *327*
Nodular fasciitis, of orbit, 997
Nodular melanoma, 179
Nonabsorbable suture(s), 284
Non-Hodgkin's lymphoma, of eyelid, in AIDS patients, 528
  of orbit, 60
    in AIDS patients, 530–532, *531*
Nonsteroidal anti-inflammatory drugs (NSAIDs), chronic patient use of, anesthetic considerations with, 296
Nose, evaluation of, tearing and, 755, *757–758*, *758*
NSAIDs (nonsteroidal anti-inflammatory drugs), chronic patient use of, anesthetic considerations with, 296
Nuclear lesion(s), eyelid retraction caused by, 73–74, *74–76*
  ptosis caused by, 77, *77*
Null cell(s), 95
Nylon suture, 284

Oblique muscle(s), inferior, 849
  superior, 848
Ocular adnexa. See also specific part, e.g., *Eyelid(s).*
  benign lesion(s) of, apocrine sweat gland origin of, 334–335, *334–335*
    eccrine sweat gland origin of, 333–334, *333–334*
    hair follicle origin of, 335–336, *335–336*
    sebaceous gland origin of, 336–337, *337*
  collagen vascular disease(s) affecting, 3–12
    Churg-Strauss syndrome as, 10t, 11, 11t
    dermatomyositis as, 7, 7t
    lupus erythematosus as, 3–7, *4*, 4t, 5t
    lymphomatoid granulomatosis as, 10t, 11–12
    scleroderma as, 7–9, *8*, 8t
    Wegener's granulomatosis as, 9–11, 10t
  dermatosis(es)/hypersensitivity disorder(s) affecting, 37–46
    alopecia areata as, 44–45
    alopecia mucinosa as, 44, *44*
    angioedema as, 40, *40*
    atopic dermatitis as, 41–42, *42*
    contact dermatitis as, *42*, 42–43
    exfoliative erythroderma as, 41
    granuloma annulare as, 43, *43*
    granuloma faciale as, 43
    ichthyosis as, *45*, 45–46
    lichen planus as, 40–41
    lichen simplex chronicus as, 41
    mastocytoma and mastocytosis as, 43
    pityriasis rubra pilaris as, 39
Ocular adnexa *(Continued)*
    psoriasis as, 39–40, *39–40*
    rosacea as, *38*, 38–39
    seborrheic dermatitis as, *37*, 37–38
    ulerythema ophryogenes as, 43–44
    urticaria as, 40
  systemic and metabolic disease(s) affecting, 12–29
    acanthosis nigricans as, *23*, 23t, 23–24
    amyloidosis as, *17*, 17–19, 18t
    congenital erythropoietic porphyria as, 29
    Darier's disease as, 21
    erythropoietic protoporphyria as, 29
    hyperthyroidism as, *12*, 12–14, 13t
    ligneous conjunctivitis as, 20
    lipoid proteinosis as, 20–21
    Melkersson-Rosenthal syndrome as, 15–16
    multiple mucosal neuroma syndrome as, 21–23, 22t
    myxedema as, 14, *14*
    necrobiotic xanthogranuloma as, 19–20
    neurofibromatosis as, *24*, 24t, 24–26, 26t
    sarcoidosis as, *16*, 16–17, 17t
    scleredema as, 15
    scleromyxedema as, *14*, 14–15
    tuberous sclerosis as, 26–28, 27t
    variegate porphyria as, 28
  vesicobullous disease(s) affecting, 29–37
    cicatricial pemphigoid as, *31*, 31–32
    epidermolysis bullosa as, 29–31, 30t
    erythema multiforme as, *34–35*, 34–37, 36t
    pemphigus as, 33–34
Oculocardiac reflex, after blepharoplasty, 650
Oculodermal melanocytosis (Ota's nevus), of eyelid, 339
Oculofacial prosthesis, following orbital exenteration, *1074*, 1075
Oculoglandular syndrome of Parinaud, 149
Oculomotility disorder(s), in orbital disease, 877–878, *878–879*, 880
Oculomotor nerve, anatomy of, 277, 844–845
Oculomotor nerve palsy, in diabetic patient, 139
  ptosis caused by, 77, *78*
Oculopharyngeal dystrophy, 86
Oculoplastic surgery. See also specific procedure, e.g., *Blepharoplasty.*
  aesthetician in, patient benefits of, 574–575
    physician benefits of, 573–574
  anesthesia for, 294–299
    commonly used agents in, 296–297
    in pediatric patients, 298–299
    intraoperative problems in, 298
    local or monitored care approach to, 297–298
    management of concurrent medications with, 295–296
    monitoring during, 298
    preoperative evaluation and screening tests in, 294–295
  in African American patient, considerations for, 715–717, *716–717*, 717t
  in Asian patient, cultural background and anatomic considerations for, 691–700
  medical photography for, 551–559. See also *Medical photography.*
  role of aesthetician in, before and after surgery, 576–577

Oil layer, and precorneal tear film, 737–738
Onchocerca volvulus infection, of eyelid, 317
Onchocercomata, of eyelid, 317
Oncocytoma, of eyelid, 328
Ophthalmia, sympathetic, enucleation for, 1035
Ophthalmic artery, anatomy of, 274, *275*, 843, *843*
Ophthalmic nerve, anatomy of, 277, *278*
Ophthalmic plastic instrument(s), 288, *290–292*
Ophthalmic vein(s), anatomy of, 275, *276*, 844, *844*
Ophthalmoparesis, of myasthenia gravis, 80
Ophthalmopathy, Graves,' 13–14
  thyroid-associated, 121–122
    clinical features of, 122
    management of, 122
Ophthalmoplegia, painful, 892
Ophthalmoscopy, in orbital disease, 875, *875*
Optic canal, decompression of, indications for, 1047
  glioma of, 881–882, *882*
  orbital disease invasion via, 881–882, *882–883*
Optic disc(s), edema of, in diabetic patient, 138t, 138–139
Optic nerve, anatomy of, 844
  function of, index of, 860
    status of, orbital disease and, 874–876, *875–876*
  glioma of. See *Optic nerve glioma.*
  meningioma of. See *Optic nerve meningioma.*
  nontumoral enlargement of, 900
  sarcoidosis of, MRI scan of, 900–901, *902*
Optic nerve decompression, subcranial approach to, 1164, *1166*
Optic nerve foramen, in Chinese skulls, 696–697
    measurement of, 697t
Optic nerve glioma, 985–987, *986*
  clinical presentation of, 986–987
  imaging of, 899–900, *899–900*
  radiographic findings in, 987
  treatment of, 987
Optic nerve meningioma, 882, *883*, 987–989
  management of, 988–989
  radiographic findings in, 987–988, *987–988*
Optic nerve sheath, meningioma of, imaging of, 897, *898–899*, 899
Optic nerve sheath decompression, 1056–1059
  care following, 1059
  complications of, 1059
  indications for, 1047
  mechanism of action of, 1056
  technique of, 1056–1059, *1057–1059*
Optic neuritis, MRI scan in, 900, *900*
Optic neuropathy, compressive, transorbital decompression for, *973*, 973–974
Oral mucosa, used in upper eyelid reconstruction, 365
Oral mucosal graft(s), in conjunctival mucous membrane replacement, 172–175, *173–174*
    complications of, 174–175
    harvesting and storage of, 173, *173*
  technique of, 173–174, *174*
Orbicularis oculi muscle, 261, *263*
  contraction of, 262
  shortening of, laugh lines caused by, 261, *263*
  superficial relations of, 264–265, *266*
Orbit. See also *Orbital* entries.
  acquired immunodeficiency syndrome affecting, 529–532. See also *Acquired immunodeficiency syndrome (AIDS), orbital manifestation(s) of.*
  adenoid cystic carcinoma of, 68–69, *69*
  amyloidosis affecting, *65*, 65–66
  anatomy of, 146, *147*, 837–849
  anterior structures of, parasagittal section of, 270, *271*
  basal cell carcinoma of, 300, *301*
  basal cell nevus syndrome affecting, 67, *68*
  benign reactive lymphoid hyperplasia of, 61–62
  blood supply to, 843–844, *843–844*
  cellulitis of. See *Cellulitis, orbital.*
  compartments of, 885, 886t, 887t
  connective tissues of, 840–842, *842*
  deformity(ies) of, after acquired anophthalmos, management of, 1121
    anterior cranial base approach to, 1187–1207
      historical perspective on, 1187
      in children, surgical refinement for, 1187–1188. See also *Craniofacial surgery, pediatric.*
        access to tumors in, 1188
        indications for, 1188–1207
  dysplastic nevus syndrome affecting, 67–68, *68*
  embryology of, 850–851, *851*
  exenteration of, 1070–1077. See also *Exenteration, orbital.*
  fibrous dysplasia of, presenting as blindness, anterior cranial base approach to, 1202, *1203*
  idiopathic inflammation of. See *Idiopathic orbital inflammation.*
  infections of, 146–155, 888–891. See also *Infection(s), of orbit.*
  leukemia involving, 60
  mucoepidermoid carcinoma of, 68, *69*
  mycosis fungoides of, 62
  neoplastic and related condition(s) affecting, 53–70
    diagnosis of, 53–57, *54–57*
    Erdheim-Chester disease as, 64, *64*
    histiocytic disorders as, 62, *63*, 64
    idiopathic midline destructive disease as, 66, *66*
    laboratory tests for, 57
    treatment of, 57
  neuroradiologic imaging of, 885–904
    anatomic and developmental considerations on, 885, *886*
  of Caucasian adult, 696, 696t
  of Chinese adult, male vs. female, 696, 696t
    relationship between lacrimal fossa and ethmoidal cells in, 697t
    relationship between lacrimal fossa and middle turbinate in, 698t
  osteology of, 837–840, *838–840*
    shape and dimensions in, 837, *838*
  paraneoplastic syndromes affecting, 58
  pathology of, epidemiology of, 853, 854t–856t, 856, *857–858*, 858t, 859
  prosthesis for. See *Prosthesis.*
  pseudorheumatoid nodules of, 67
  pseudotumor of. See *Pseudotumor(s), orbital.*
  sarcoidosis of, 64–65, *64–65*
  sinus histiocytosis with lymphadenopathy affecting, 62, *62*
  soft tissue of, *842–845*, 842–849, *847–848*
  squamous cell carcinoma of, 300–301, *302*
Orbit *(Continued)*
  vascular conditions of, imaging of, 893–897, *893–898*
  xeroderma pigmentosum affecting, 66–67, *67*
Orbital and lacrimal kit, *291*
Orbital apex, anatomy of, 839–840, *840*
  fractures of, 1099–1100, *1100*
    treatment of, 1100
Orbital apex inflammatory syndrome, 965
Orbital apex syndrome, 148
Orbital calcification, dystrophic, differential diagnosis of, 887t
  metastatic, differential diagnosis of, 887t
Orbital cyst, 886–888. See also *Dermoid cyst; Epidermoid cyst.*
Orbital decompression, for Graves' disease, 967–982. See also *Graves' disease, orbital decompression for.*
Orbital disease, 860–873
  clinical signs of, 860
  evidence of, within globe, 868–870, *869–870*
  extent of, 862–863, 865, *866*
  eyelid changes in, 865–868, *867–868*
  globe position and movement in, 861–862, *863–865*
  neuro-ophthalmic conditions in, 874–884
    clinical method(s) of assessment of, 874–880
      motility disorders as, 877–878, *878–879*
      pupillary function as, 876–877, *877*
      status of optic nerve function as, 874–876, *875–876*
      trigeminal function as, *879*, 879–880
    localization of disease process(es) in, 880–883
      choroidal folds and, 881, *881*
      enophthalmos and, 881
      oculomotility disturbances and, 880
      perturbation of acuity and visual field and, 880
      proptosis and, 880–881
      pupillary disturbances and, 880
  periorbital function changes in, 868
  periorbital injury and, 871, *873*
  pupillary reflex changes in, 868
  radiation therapy in, 1023–1032
  systemic signs of, 870–871, *871–872*
Orbital expansion, craniofacial approach to, 980–981
Orbital fascia, anatomy of, 841–842, *842*
Orbital fat pad, 269, *269*
  anatomy of, 842, *842*
  pseudoherniation of, evaluation of, 635
  removal of. See *Fat excision.*
Orbital fissure, inferior, neuroradiologic imaging of, 885
  superior, neuroradiologic imaging of, 885
    orbital disease invasion via, 882–883, *884*
Orbital floor, fractures of, 1087–1091
    blow-out, 1087
    complications of, 1090–1091, *1090–1093*
    management of, *1088–1089*, 1088–1090
Orbital fracture(s), 1085–1100
  evaluation of, 1085–1086, *1086*
  fixation of, principles in, 1086–1087
  incidence of, 1085
  management of, 1047
  site of, 1087–1100. See also specific site, e.g., *Orbital floor, fractures of.*

Orbital fracture(s) *(Continued)*
surgical approach to, 1054
unilateral forehead fracture and, anterior cranial base approach to, 1188–1189, *1190*
Orbital lesion(s), age distribution of, *857–858,* 858t
clinicopathologic classification of, 854t–856t
extraconal, 887t
intraconal, 886t
pathology of, epidemiology of, 853, 856, 859
subperiosteal, 887t
Orbital margins, anatomy of, 837, *838*
Orbital nerve(s), anatomy of, 844–846, *845*
paresis involving, 152
Orbital rim, sulcus of, sculpturing and recontouring of, 707, *707*
Orbital roof, fractures of, *1098,* 1098–1099
treatment of, 1099
Orbital septum, anatomy of, 268–269, *269*
excision and incision of, in upper eyelid blepharoplasty, 600, *600*
variations of, 607–608
Orbital surgery. See also specific procedure, e.g., *Orbitotomy.*
anatomic planes and exposure of different routes during, 1051, 1051t, *1052*
approach(es) to, 1050–1051
anophthalmic socket and, 1053–1054
associated with paranasal sinus disease, 1055, *1055*
based on pathologic process, 1051–1055
neoplasms and, 1051–1053, *1052–1053*
trauma and, 1054
dissection in, 1049
exposure in, 1048
general principles in, 1050
hemostasis in, 1049
incisions utilized in, 1060, *1061*
indications for, 1046–1047
instrumentation for, 1050, *1051*
operative principles in, 1048–1049
Orbital tumor(s). See also specific tumor.
adipose, 996–997
carcinoid, 57, *58*
fibrous, 997
in AIDS patients, 532, *532*
lymphoid, 58–60, 303–304, 956–962
malignant, 300–306
surgical approach to, 1053
metastatic, 1007–1013
clinical features of, 1007–1008, 1008t
from breast carcinoma, *1009,* 1009–1010
from gastrointestinal carcinoma, 1012
from lung carcinoma, 1010
from melanoma, 1012
from neuroblastoma, 1011–1012
from prostate carcinoma, 1010–1011, *1011*
from renal cell carcinoma, 1012
pathologic features of, 1008
primary sites of, 1008t
tests for, 1008
treatment of, 1008
myogenic, 994–996
neurogenic, 983–992
biopsy of, 984
clinical examination of, 983–984
general approach to, 983–984
noninvasive imaging of, 984
transcranial approach to, 984–985
preparation for, 984
Orbital tumor(s) *(Continued)*
technique of, 984–985
treatment of, 984
pediatric, anterior cranial base approach to, 1199, 1202–1204, *1203–1206*
resection of, 1060–1068
anterior approach to, 1060–1061, *1061–1062*
combined procedures in, 1065, *1067–1068,* 1068
lateral approach to, 1063, *1064*
medial approach to, 1063, 1065, *1065–1067*
secondary, 68
surgical approach to, 1051–1053, *1052–1053*
vascular, 913–932
Orbital varices, CT scan of, 896, *897*
Orbital wall(s), anatomy of, 837–839, *838–839*
medial, fractures of, 1092
Orbitocheek fold, *485*
Orbitoethmoidal osteotomy, transcranial approach to tumors via, 985
Orbitopathy, thyroid, CT scan of, 891, *892*
Orbitotomy, 1051
anterior extraperiosteal approach to, 1060–1061, *1062*
anterior transseptal approach to, 1060, *1062*
combined lateral and inferior, 1065, *1067–1068*
combined superior and lateral, 1068, *1068*
Krönlein-Berke, technique of, 1056–1059, *1057–1059*
lateral approach to, 1063, *1064*
medial approach to, 1063, *1065–1067*
transconjunctival approach to, 1060, *1061*
Orchiectomy, for metastatic prostate carcinoma, 1011
Orf, involving eyelids, 316
Organic pigment, 541. See also *Pigment(s).*
Oriental sore, 150
Orphenadrine, for essential blepharospasm and Meige's syndrome, 507
Osler-Weber-Rendu disease (hereditary hemorrhagic telangiectasia), 9
Osmotic pressure, of lymphatic fluid, 654
Osseointegration, biology of, 1155–1156, 1158–1159
effects of irradiation on, 1158–1159
for exenterated orbit, 1150–1159
abutment installation in, 1151, *1156–1157*
implant installation in, 1150–1151, *1152–1155*
technique of, 1150–1151, *1151*
placement of bone-anchored implants by, 1159
Osteoclastoma (brown tumor), in hyperparathyroidism, 133–134, *134–135*
Osteotomy, age and, 1053
fronto-orbital, subcranial approach to, 1163–1164, *1165–1167*
orbitoethmoidal, transcranial approach to tumors via, 985
Ota's nevus, of eyelid, 339
Otitis, malignant external, 138
Otitis media, acute, 473
Oxycel, for hemostasis in wound repair, 283
Oxymetazoline, for hemostasis in wound repair, 283
P component, of amyloid fibrils, 944
Pagetoid spread, definition of, 179
of sebaceous gland carcinoma, 190, *191,* 347, *347*
management of, 348
Paget's disease of bone, causing nasolacrimal duct obstruction, 813
Palate, hard. See *Hard palate* entries.
Palatine nerve block, 442
Palpebral conjunctiva, 159. See also *Conjunctiva.*
Palpebral spring, in surgical management of facial paralysis, 476–478, *477–478*
Palsy(ies). See also *Paralysis.*
abducens nerve, eyelid retraction associated with, 74, *75*
in diabetic patient, 139
Bell's, 470, 473
in diabetic patient, 139
ptosis following, 91, *91*
cranial nerve, in diabetic patient, 138t, 138–139
oculomotor nerve, in diabetic patient, 139
ptosis caused by, 77, *78*
progressive, metastatic lesions in, 474
PAM. See *Primary acquired melanosis (PAM).*
PANDO. See *Nasolacrimal duct obstruction, primary acquired.*
Panfacial fracture(s), 1100
Papillary endothelial hyperplasia, intravascular, of eyelid, 332
Papilloma, of eyelid, 324, *324*
squamous, of conjunctiva, 68, *69,* 251, *252*
treatment of, 251–252
of orbit, 68, *69*
Papillomavirus, warts caused by, eyelid presentation of, 316
Papular sarcoid, 16
Paracentesis, of anterior chamber, following chemical injury, 223–224
Paracoccidioidomycosis, of eyelid, 318
Paralysis, 469, *469.* See also *Palsy(ies).*
facial, 465–482. See also *Facial paralysis.*
familial periodic, ptosis in, 85–86, *86*
partial, involving orbital nerves, 152
Paranasal sinus(es). See also *Sinus* entries.
anatomy of, 935, *936–938,* 937, 1014–1015
disease of, approach to orbital surgery associated with, 1055, *1055*
role of, in orbital cellulitis, 935–943
mucoceles in, 1014–1021, *1015*
diagnostic imaging of, 1014–1017, *1016*
histopathology of, 1014
pathophysiology of, 1014
Parasitic infection(s), of eyelid, 317–318
Parathyroid hormone (PTH), calcium regulation by, 132
Paredrine test, for Horner's syndrome, 79
Parinaud's syndrome, 149
Patch test, for micropigmentation, 541
Patient, evaluation of, for chemical peels, 664, 664t, 665t
for electropigmentation, 676, *678*
pediatric. See *Child(ren).*
preparation and draping of, for lower eyelid blepharoplasty, 619
for upper eyelid blepharoplasty, 598
variations in, 605
Pautrier's microabscess, 62
Pediatric patient. See *Child(ren).*
Pedicle flap, upper eyelid, used in medial canthal reconstruction, 391, *395*
used in upper eyelid reconstruction, from lower lid to upper lid, 382–383, *383*

Pemphigoid, cicatricial. See *Cicatricial pemphigoid.*
Pemphigus, 33–34
  differential diagnosis of, 103
  epidemiology of, 102
  immunohistopathology of, 103
  ocular manifestations of, 102
  pathogenesis of, 103
  systemic manifestations of, 102–103
  treatment of, 34, 103
  variants of, 33
Pemphigus vulgaris, vs. cicatricial pemphigoid, 198
Penetrating trauma. See also *Trauma.*
  to upper eyelid, 357–358
    extensive, 358–359, *360–361*
    lid margin reapproximation following, 357–358, *359–360*
    with no tissue loss, 357, *358*
    with tissue loss, 357
Perilimbal epithelial loss, after chemical injury, 226–227, *227*
Periorbita, anatomy of, 840–841
  changes in function of, in orbital disease, 868
  vascularization of, 841
    anatomy of, 841
Periorbital edema, diseases and organisms associated with, 308t
  infectious causes of, 151–152
Periorbital hyperpigmentation, chemical peels for, 663
Periorbital malignancy, Mohs' surgery for, 352–355
    advantages of, 354–355
    drawbacks to, 352
    fresh tissue technique in, 352–354, *353–355*
Persistent hyperplastic primary vitreous, imaging of, 908, *909*
Phakoma, in tuberous sclerosis, 27
Pharmacologic testing, for myasthenia gravis, *80,* 81–82, *82*
Pharmacology, of therapeutic agents, 97–98
Phenol solution, Baker's, used in chemical peels, 667–668
Phenylephrine, for hemostasis in wound repair, 283
Pheochromocytoma(s), 141–142
Phlegmon, subperiosteal, CT scan of, *889,* 889–890
Photodamage, chemical peels for, 662, 663t
Photoelectric effect, 1023, *1025*
Photographs, for medicolegal considerations with eyelid trauma, 457
Photography. See *Medical photography.*
Phycomycosis. See *Mucormycosis (phycomycosis).*
Pigment(s), changes in, management of, 535–541. See also *Micropigmentation.*
    resulting from facial trauma, 535–536
  for micropigmentation, 682–683
  inorganic, 541
  organic, 541
  removal of, 681
  selection of, for micropigmentation, 538
  tattoo, used in electropigmentation, 677, 681
Pigmentary retinopathy, in Kearns-Sayre syndrome, 87–88, *88*
Pigmentation, prominent, after blepharoplasty, 648
Pigmented lesion(s). See also specific lesion, e.g., *Nevus(i).*
  of aging skin, treatment for, 567–568, *568*
Pigmented lesion(s) *(Continued)*
  of conjunctiva, 179–189, 183t, *184–186*
  of eyelid, benign, 337–339, *337–340*
Pilocytic astrocytoma, juvenile, imaging of, 899–900, *899–900*
Pilomatricoma (Malherbe's calcifying epithelioma), of eyelid, 336, *336*
Pinch test, for lid laxity, 762, *763*
Pinta, involving eyelids, 314
Pityriasis rubra pilaris, 39
Plagiocephaly, 1179
  subcranial approach to, results with, 1176t
Plague, involving eyelids, 314
Plain gut suture, 284, 284t
Plasma cell tumor(s), of orbit, 62, *63*
Plastic instrument(s), ophthalmic, 288, *290–292*
Plastic wrap, creation of moist chamber with, following chemical injury, 225
Plastic wrap occlusive dressing, for facial nerve palsy, 474, *475*
Pleomorphic adenoma, of eyelid, 334, *334*
  of lacrimal glands, 999–1004
Pleomorphic rhabdomyosarcoma, in adults, 995
Plica semilunaris, of conjunctiva, 159. See also *Conjunctiva.*
Plication, medial, for canthal laxity, in involutional ectropion, 426–427, *426–427*
PMNs (polymorphonuclear neutrophil leukocytes), role of, in injured eye repair, 223
Pneumatic drill, used in ophthalmic plastic surgery, *291*
Pneumocystis carinii infection, of orbit, in AIDS patients, 529
Poliomyelitis, cranial nerve paresis in, 152
Polyarteritis nodosa, differential diagnosis of, 112
  epidemiology of, 111
  laboratory findings in, 111–112
  ocular manifestations of, 111
  pathogenesis of, 112
  systemic manifestations of, 111
  treatment of, 112
Polyclonal antibody(ies), 96
Polydioxanone suture, 284, 284t
Polyendocrine disease, acromegaly as, 142–143
  Addison's disease as, 141
  MEN syndromes as, 142
  pheochromocytoma as, 141–142
  polyglandular autoimmune syndromes as, 141
  polyostotic fibrous dysplasia as, 143
Polyglactin suture, 284, 284t
Polyglandular autoimmune syndrome(s), 141
Polymethyl methacrylate acrylic, for prosthesis, 1135–1136
Polymorphic reticulosis, 114
Polymorphonuclear neutrophil leukocytes (PMNs), role of, in injured eye repair, 223
Polyostotic fibrous dysplasia, 143
Polypropylene suture, 284
Polytetrafluoroethylene (polytef) graft, and spontaneous epithelialization, in conjunctival mucous membrane replacement, 171–172, *171–172*
Polyurethane sheet, for prosthesis, 1136–1137
Pons, cross section of, *467*
Porphyria, 28–29
  congenital erythropoietic, 29
  variegate, 28–29
Porphyria cutanea tarda, 27–28
Port wine stain (nevus flammeus), of eyelid, *329,* 329–330
Potassium abnormality(ies), evaluation of, prior to oculoplastic surgery, 294
Pott's puffy tumor, 1017, *1017*
Prednisone, for capillary hemangioma, 919
  for idiopathic orbital inflammation, 955–956
  for orbital floor fractures, 1088
  in preoperative treatment of malignant melanoma, 187
  with dapsone, for cicatricial pemphigoid, 199
Pregnancy, hyperthyroidism in, 129–130
Premature ventricular contraction, evaluation of, prior to oculoplastic surgery, 295
Preseptal cellulitis, 310–312
  CT scan of, *148*
  in children and neonates, 310
  post-traumatic, 311
  treatment of, 311–312
  with abscess formation, 310, *310*
Preseptal muscles, anatomy of, 744
Pressure bandages, with manual lymphatic drainage of extremities, 655
Pressure tamponade, for hemostasis in wound repair, 282
Pretarsal muscles, anatomy of, 744
  insertion of, in medial canthal area, 387, *388*
Primary acquired melanosis (PAM), of conjunctiva, classification of, 79–180, 180t
    clinical features of, 182, *182–183*
    malignant melanoma arising from, 233
    treatment of, 185–187, *186*
    types of, 234
Probing, in evaluation of tearing, 755, *756–757*
Procerus muscle, 262, *263,* 264
Progressive synergistic gangrene, of eyelid, 312
Prolapse, conjunctival, management of, 253–254
  lacrimal gland, repair of, in upper eyelid blepharoplasty, 601–602, *602*
      variations of, 609
Propofol, as anesthetic agent, 297
Propranolol, for thyroid storm, 130
  for thyrotoxicosis, 125, 128
Proptosis, in orbital disease, 880–881
Propulsion, forward, of lymphatic fluid, *652,* 652–653
Propylthiouracil (PTU), for hyperthyroidism, 129–130
  for thyrotoxicosis, 125
Prostate carcinoma, metastatic orbital disease from, 1010–1011, *1011*
Prosthesis, 1134–1149
  after enucleation, 1036–1037
    hydroxyapatite, 1036, 1041–1042
      complications of, 1042
      contraindications to, 1042
  anatomically retained, design of, 1143–1144, *1143–1145*
  auricular, osseointegrated, 1159
  bulb-style, 1143–1144, *1143–1145*
  challenges regarding, 1144–1146, *1146–1148*
  design, making, and fitting of, treatment plan in, 1137–1139, *1138–1141,* 1141
  for acquired anophthalmos, complications of, *1119–1120,* 1119–1121
  functions of, 1134–1135, *1135–1136*

Prosthesis *(Continued)*
  installation of, for exenterated orbit, 1150–1151, *1152–1155*
  location of, in anophthalmic socket, 1131, *1131*
  magnet attachments to, 1155, *1158*
  material(s) for, 1135–1137
    polymethyl methacrylate acrylic as, 1135–1136
    polyurethane sheet as, 1136–1137
    silicone elastomer as, 1135
    silicone foam as, 1137
    silicone gels as, 1137
  mobility, new, 1132, *1133*
  mobility of, in anophthalmic socket, 1131, *1131*
  ocular component of, 1138, *1139*
  oculofacial, following orbital exenteration, *1074,* 1075
  optimal results with, surgical nuances for, 1141–1143, *1142–1143*
  suborbital rim, 488, 490–498
    complications associated with, 501–503
    customized, 490–491, *491,* 495–498, *496–499*
    Flower tear trough, 488, *489,* 492–493, *492–495,* 495
    Goldberg lateral, 488, *489*
    malposition of, 503
    prefabricated, 488, *489–491,* 490
  surgical considerations for, 1135
Prosthetist, challenges for, 1144–1146, *1146–1148*
Prostigmin test, for myasthenia gravis, in children, 82, *82*
Protein, concentration of, in lymphatic fluid, 654
Proteinosis, lipoid, 20–21
Protoporphyria, erythropoietic, 29
Pseudocapsule, of lacrimal gland, 732
Pseudo-Graefe's sign, 74, *75*
Pseudoherniation, of orbital fat pad, evaluation of, 635
Pseudohorn cyst, 325
Pseudomelanocytic lesion, *184*
Pseudomonas aeruginosa, 138
Pseudomonas mallei, glanders caused by, 313
Pseudo-ocular pemphigoid syndrome, 203
Pseudoporphyria, 28
Pseudopterygium, vs. true pterygium, 209
Pseudoptosis, and eyelid retraction, 89–91
  associated with vertical strabismus, *88,* 89
Pseudorheumatoid nodule(s), of orbit, 67
Pseudotumor(s), idiopathic inflammatory, associated with nasolacrimal duct obstruction, 801–802
  orbital, classification of, 890
    imaging of, 890–891, *890–891*
    in AIDS patients, 530
Pseudotumor cerebri, optic nerve decompression for, 1056–1059, *1057–1059*
Psoriasis vulgaris, 39–40, *39–40*
  treatment of, 40
Psychosocial issues, in male blepharoplasty, 632
Pterygium(ia), 208–220
  adjunctive therapy for, 217–219
    argon laser in, 219
    beta radiation in, 217–218
    corticosteroids in, 219
    excimer laser in, 219
    mitomycin C in, 218–219
    thiotepa in, 218
  aggressive, 210
  anatomy of, 208
  differential diagnosis of, 209–210
Pterygium(ia) *(Continued)*
  general considerations concerning, 219–220
  histopathology of, 208–209
  inactive, 210
  nonsurgical management of, 210–211
  pathogenesis of, 209
  prognosis for, 210
  recurrent, 209, 210
  surgical management of, anesthesia in, 212
    bare-sclera technique in, 212–214, *213*
    buccal mucous membrane graft in, 217
    conjunctival autograft in, 214–215, *216–217,* 217
    conjunctival flaps in, 214, *215*
    current, 211–217
    historical, 211
    indications for, 210
    lamellar grafts in, 214, *214*
    preoperative evaluation in, 211
    treatment alternatives in, 211
  vs. pseudopterygium, 209
Pterygoid plexus, venous drainage into, 275, *276*
PTH (parathyroid hormone), calcium regulation by, 132
Ptosis, 75–88
  after blepharoplasty, 644, *644*
  after dermolipoma excision, treatment of, 256
  aponeurotic, 447–451
    evaluation of, 447
    residual, 450
      correction of, 450–451
    surgery for, applied anatomy used in, 448
      choice of, 448
      complications of, 449
      contour abnormality in, 450
      overcorrection in, 449–450
      skin excision in, 450–451
      undercorrection in, 450
  as complication of conjunctival amyloidosis, 240
  brow, 578–588
    asymmetric, 578–579
    in facial paralysis, surgical management of, 482
    presenting complaints in, 578
    surgical management of, 579–581, *579–588,* 583–587
      coronal flaps in, 585–586, *586*
      incisions in, 579, *579,* 581, *581–583,* 583
      prominent sub-brow fat pad and, 586–587, *586–588*
  correction of, *1118,* 1118–1119
  following Bell's palsy, 91, *91*
  myopathic, 84–88
    in chronic progressive external ophthalmoplegia, 86–88, *87–88*
    in inflammatory and infiltrative myopathies, 88
    in muscular dystrophy, 84
    in myotonia and myotonic disorders, 85–86, *85–86*
    in structural myopathies, 84, *85*
  neuromuscular, 79–84
    in myasthenia gravis, 79–83, *80–82*
    in myasthenic syndromes, 83
    toxins causing, 83–84, *84*
  neuropathic, 75–77
    infranuclear lesions causing, 77, *78*
    nuclear lesions causing, 77, *77*
    supranuclear lesions causing, 75–77, *76–77*
    sympathetic lesions causing, 77–79, *78–79*
Ptosis *(Continued)*
  repair of, concurrent with upper eyelid blepharoplasty, 602–603, *603*
    variations of, 609
PTU (propylthiouracil), for hyperthyroidism, 129–130
  for thyrotoxicosis, 125
Pulmonary function test(s), for sarcoidosis, 108
Pulse oximetry, monitoring of, during anesthesia, 298
Pulse-wave flow, of lymph, 653, *653*
Pumping action, of lymphatic vessels, 652
Punctoplasty, inferior, for involutional ectropion, 424–425, *425*
Punctum(a), 739
  anatomy of, 268, *268,* 821
  atresia of, 782, *782*
  congenital abnormalities of, 740, *740,* 821–822, *822*
    treatment of, 822–823
  imperforate membrane of, 782, *782*
  physiology of, 821
  stenosis of, 829, *829*
  supernumerary, *741*
  trauma to, 824–825
  tumors of, 823–824, *824*
Pupil(s), Adie's, 877
  Marcus Gunn, 876
    reverse, 876, *877*
Pupillary function, in orbital disease, assessment of, 876–877, *877*
  disturbances of, 880
Pupillary reflex, changes in, with orbital disease, 868
Pyogenic granuloma, of eyelid, 331, *331*
Pyruvic acid, used in chemical peels, 667

Quartz iodine lamp, for photography, 555

R (roentgen), defined, 1023
Rabies, cranial nerve paresis in, 152
  prophylaxis for, 458
Rad (radiation absorbed dose), 1026, *1027–1029,* 1030
Radiation, beta, as adjunct to surgery for pterygia, 217–218
  ultraviolet, exposure to, pterygia due to, 209
Radiation absorbed dose (rad), 1026, *1027–1029,* 1030
Radiation therapy, 1023–1032
  causing nasolacrimal duct obstruction, 803–804
  clinical applications of, *1030,* 1030t, 1030–1031
  complications of, 1031, *1032*
  diagnostic energies in, 1023, 1024t
  film in, 1023, *1024*
  for capillary hemangioma, 919
  for conjunctival lymphoid tumors, 246
  for idiopathic orbital inflammation, 956
  for Kaposi's sarcoma, 242, 528
  for lacrimal gland tumors, 1005–1006
  for lymphangioma, 925
  for lymphoid tumors, 961
  for metastatic breast carcinoma, 1009–1010
  for metastatic gastrointestinal carcinoma, 1012
  for metastatic lung carcinoma, 1010
  for metastatic melanoma, 1012

Radiation therapy *(Continued)*
for metastatic prostate carcinoma, 1011
for non-Hodgkin's lymphoma, 531
for orbital metastatic disease, 57, 1008–1012
for rhabdomyosarcoma, 303, 996
for sebaceous gland carcinoma, 302–303, 348
measurement of dose in, 1023
photoelectric or Compton effect in, 1023, *1025*
practical applications of, 1026
prior to osseointegration, effects of, 1158–1159
rad in, 1026, *1027–1029,* 1030
side effects of, incidence of, 1030t
Radioactive iodine therapy, for thyrotoxicosis, 128
Radiobiology, 1023–1026. See also *Radiation therapy.*
long-term complication rates in, 1024–1025
radiosensitivity in, 1025, *1025*
redistribution in, 1026
reoxygenation in, 1025, *1026*
repopulation in, 1025–1026
Radio-frequency current, heating effects of, 592
Radio-frequency lipocontouring, in fat removal, 642, *642*
Radio-frequency surgical unit, used in blepharoplasty, *544*
Radiography, chest, for sarcoidosis, 108
prior to oculoplastic surgery, 294
of mucoceles, in paranasal sinuses, 1016
Radiosensitivity, in radiobiology, 1025, *1025*
Radiosurgical unit, Ellman Surgitron, used in removal of hyperpigmented facial lesions, 568, *568*
used in treatment of telangiectasia, 569
Ramsay Hunt syndrome, 470, 473
RAPD (relative afferent pupillary defect), 860–861
Rappaport classification, of non-Hodgkin's lymphoma, 60
Reconstructive plan, in orbital exenteration, 1073–1075, *1974*
goals of, 1073
Rectus muscle(s), horizontal, 847
inferior, 848
capsulopalpebral head of, 269–270, *270*
medial, 848
metastasis of thyroid carcinoma to, *55*
superior, 841, 848
Redistribution, in radiobiology, 1026
Reflex, oculocardiac, after blepharoplasty, 650
pupillary, changes in, with orbital disease, 868
Reflex tearing, 750
Refraction, changes in, after blepharoplasty, 649
Refsum's disease, 46
Regional anesthesia. See *Anesthesia, regional.*
Regulatory agency(ies), 591–593
Rehabilitation, visual, after chemical injury, 227–228, *228*
Rejuvenation, facial, 560–571. See also *Facial rejuvenation.*
Relative afferent pupillary defect (RAPD), 860–861
Renal cell carcinoma, metastatic orbital disease from, 1012
Reoxygenation, in radiobiology, 1025, *1026*
Repopulation, in radiobiology, 1025–1026
Reptile venom, disruption of neuromuscular transmission by, 83
Reticulosis, polymorphic, 114
Retinal detachment, MRI of, 905–906, *906*
Retinal hemangioma, 910–911
Retinitis, cytomegalovirus, in AIDS patients, 533
Retinoblastoma, enucleation for, 1035–1036
imaging of, 907–908, *907–908*
Retinopathy, pigmentary, in Kearns-Sayre syndrome, 87–88, *88*
Retraction, skin and muscle, in orbital surgery, 1048
Retrobulbar hemorrhage, causing blindness, 643
Rhabdomyoma, orbital, 996
Rhabdomyosarcoma, alveolar, 995
botryoid, 995
embryonal, 995
orbital, 303, *303,* 994–996
differential diagnosis of, 994, 995
epidemiology of, 994
histopathology of, 994–995
imaging of, 901–902, *903*
presentation of, 994
prognosis of, 996
treatment of, 995–996
pleomorphic, in adults, 995
Rhinocerebral mucormycosis, 150–151, *151*
Rhinoscleroma, in diabetic patient, 138
of eyelid, 314
Rhinosporidiosis, of eyelid, 319
Rhinosporidium seeberi, rhinosporidiosis caused by, 319
Rhytidectomy (face-lift), 565
Rhytides. See *Wrinkles (rhytides).*
Rib graft(s), costal, harvesting of, 1077–1078, *1079*
Rickettsial disease, involving eyelids, 313
Riley-Day syndrome, 736
"River blindness," caused by *Onchocerca volvulus,* 317
Rod myopathy, ptosis in, 84
Roentgen (R), defined, 1023
Romaña's sign, 152
in Chagas' disease, 316
Rosacea, *38,* 38–39
treatment of, 39
Rose bengal testing, of tearing, 759
Rosenmüller valve, 744
Round eye deformity, after blepharoplasty, 646, *646*
Ruby laser(s), used in removal of hyperpigmented facial lesions, 568
Running suture(s), percutaneous, 286, *286*
subcuticular, 288, *288*
Russell body(ies), in rhinoscleroma, 138

Sagittal synostosis, 1178–1179, *1179–1180*
SALDO. See *Nasolacrimal duct obstruction, secondary acquired.*
"Salmon patches," in conjunctival lymphoid tumors, 235, *235*
Sarcoid, 106
miliary (papular), 16
Sarcoidosis, 106–108
associated with secondary acquired nasolacrimal duct obstruction, 801, *803*
diagnosis of, 108
differential diagnosis of, 108
epidemiology of, 106–107
Sarcoidosis *(Continued)*
erythema nodosum in, 16
immunohistopathology of, 107–108
ocular manifestations of, 16–17, 17t, 107
of conjunctiva, 65, *65*
of optic nerve, MRI scan of, 900–901, *902*
of orbit, *64,* 64–65
systemic manifestations of, 107
treatment of, 17, 108
Sarcoma, granulocytic, involving orbit, 61, *61*
Kaposi's, of conjunctiva, in AIDS patients, 236–237, 242, *243,* 532
of eyelid, in AIDS patients, 526–528, *527*
Sawdust, exposure to, pterygia due to, 209
Scaphocephaly, 1178
Scar(s), facial, electropigmentation for, 676. See also *Electropigmentation.*
micropigmentation for, 535. See also *Micropigmentation.*
hypertrophic, vs. keloids, 717t
prominent, after blepharoplasty, 648
Schaumann's bodies, 65
Schirmer's test, of tearing, 758–759
without anesthesia, 470
Schistosomiasis, of eyelid, 318
Schwannoma (neurilemoma), of eyelid, 328–329
of orbit, 991–992
radiographic findings in, *991–992,* 992
treatment of, 992
Scintillography, lacrimal, in evaluation of tearing, 759–760
Scissors, used in ophthalmic plastic surgery, *290*
SCLE (subacute cutaneous lupus erythematosus), 3. See also *Lupus erythematosus (LE).*
serologic marker for, 5–6
systemic manifestations of, 5
Sclera, donor. See *Donor sclera.*
Scleredema, 15
Scleroderma, 7–9
facial linear, *8,* 8–9
ocular manifestations of, 8t
localized, 8
systemic, 9
treatment of, 9
Scleromyxedema, *14,* 14–15
differential diagnosis of, 15
treatment of, 15
Sclerosis, systemic, 9
tuberous, 26–27
diagnostic criteria for, 27t
ocular manifestations of, 27t
Scratch test, for micropigmentation, 541
Sebaceous gland(s), of eyelid. See also specific gland, e.g., *Zeis gland(s).*
benign lesions originating in, 336–337, *337*
carcinoma of. See *Sebaceous gland carcinoma.*
inflammation of, 307–310, *309*
Sebaceous gland carcinoma, 190–194, 345–348
clinical features of, 190–192, *191–192*
clinicopathologic features of, 346, *346*
diagnosis of, 347–348
excision with cryotherapy for, 302, 348
histopathologic features of, 346–347, *347*
in AIDS patients, 528–529
in Asian patients, 721–722, *722*
management of, 193–194, *194,* 348
metastasis of, 194
mortality rates in, 301

Sebaceous gland carcinoma *(Continued)*
multicentric, 347
pagetoid involvement of epithelium in, 190, *191*, 347, *347*
management of, 348
pathology of, 192–193, *192–193*
prognosis of, 193, 348
radiation therapy for, 302–303, 348
Sebaceous gland hyperplasia, of eyelid, 336–337
Seborrheic dermatitis, *37*, 37–38
Seborrheic keratosis, of eyelid, 325, *325*
Secondary tumor(s), from ocular lesions, 68
Sedation, "startle reaction" following, 298
Seizure(s), ptosis caused by, 75, *76*
Semicircular flap, used in upper eyelid reconstruction, 366, *367*
Senear-Usher syndrome, 33
Sensory nerve, damage to, after blepharoplasty, 649–650
Septum, orbital. See *Orbital septum.*
Shading, of color distortion, in micropigmentation, 536, *536–537*
Shadowing, as cosmetic technique, used in facial rejuvenation, 570
Shagreen patches, in tuberous sclerosis, 27
Short-wave modality, for epilation, 591
cautions associated with, 592–593
point effect in, 593
vs. other techniques, 593–594
Shutter, of camera, 551
Silicone droplets, for wrinkles, 566
Silicone elastomer, for prosthesis, 1135
Silicone foam, for prosthesis, 1137
Silicone gels, for prosthesis, 1137
Silicone intubation, for canalicular stenosis, 830
for nasolacrimal duct obstruction, 780–781
Silk suture, 284
Single-needle galvanic electrolysis, 589. See also *Electrolysis.*
Sinus(es), Maier, 740, *742*, 750
maxillary. See *Maxillary sinus(es).*
paranasal. See *Paranasal sinus(es).*
sphenoidal. See *Sphenoidal sinus(es).*
Sinus histiocytosis, with lymphadenopathy, of orbit, 62, *62*
Sinus infection(s), bacterial, 937–940, *938*
fungal, complications of, 940
orbital extension of, 937–943
preseptal edema associated with, 938–939
surgical exploration and drainage for, 939–940
Sinus surgery kit, endoscopic, *292*
Sinus thrombosis, cavernous, diagnostic and therapeutic features of, 941t–942t
Sinusitis, causing orbital cellulitis, 889
Sipple's syndrome (multiple endocrine neoplasia II), 22, 142
Sjögren-Larsson syndrome, 46
Sjögren's syndrome, 736
Skeletal muscle tumor(s), of orbit, 994–996
Skin, aging of, factors contributing to, 560
pigmentary problems in, treatment of, 567–568, *568*
asymmetry of, after blepharoplasty, 648
disorders of, in diabetic patient, 138t, 139–141
excision of, in ptosis surgery, 450–451
in upper eyelid blepharoplasty, 589–599, 599–600, *599–600*
variations in, 607
facial, rejuvenation of, 560–571. See also *Facial rejuvenation.*
Skin *(Continued)*
inflammation of. See *Dermatitis.*
involvement of, in cicatricial pemphigoid, 196
of eyelid, 262
histology of, 323–324
wrinkled. See *Wrinkles (rhytides).*
Skin cancer, removal of, Mohs' fresh tissue technique in, 352
advantages of, 354–355
steps in, 352–354, *353–355*
Skin closure, in upper eyelid blepharoplasty, 603, *603–604*
variations of, 609–610, 610–611
Skin discoloration, neutralization of, application of color principles in, 658, *660*
Skin flap(s), used in lower eyelid blepharoplasty, 620, *620*
Skin folds (laugh lines), around eyelids, 261–262, *263*
Skin graft(s), for eyelid surgery, harvesting of, 439
for medial canthal reconstruction, 393, 396, *397*
for upper eyelid reconstruction, 366–367, *368*, 369
Skin marking, for upper eyelid blepharoplasty, 598, *598–599*
variations in, 605–606
Skin retraction, in orbital surgery, 1048
Skin staples, 284
Skin tag (acrochordon), of eyelid, 324, *324*
Skin tension lines, in face, 285, *285*
Skin testing, for anesthetic allergies, 297
for micropigmentation, guidelines in, 541
Skin wrinkling, in transconjunctival lower blepharoplasty, 630
Skin-muscle flap(s), used in lower eyelid blepharoplasty, 620–622, *621–622*
Skull base, fibrous dysplasia of, presenting as blindness, anterior cranial base approach to, 1202, *1203*
SLE. See *Systemic lupus erythematosus (SLE).*
Sleep test, for myasthenia gravis, 82, *82*
Sliding tarsal flap, used in upper eyelid reconstruction, technique of, 380, 382, *382*
Small cell lymphocytic lymphoma, 959
Smallpox, involving eyelids, 316
Smith lazy-T procedure, for involutional ectropion, 426, *426*
Smooth muscle, benign eyelid tumors derived from, 329
Smooth muscle tumor(s), of orbit, 996
Soemmering's ligament, 732
Soft contact lens, corneal reepithelialization with, following chemical injury, 225
Soft tissue, orbital, *842–845*, 842–849, *847–848*
Solar lentigo, of eyelid, 339, *340*
Sore, oriental, 150
Spasm(s), eyelid. See *Blepharospasm.*
facial, diagnostic features of, 505t
hemifacial. See *Hemifacial spasm.*
Sphenoid wing meningioma, 989–990
radiographic findings in, *989*, 990
treatment of, 990
Sphenoidal sinus(es), anatomy of, 1015
mucoceles in, 1019–1021
radiographic findings in, *1020*, 1020–1021
treatment of, 1021
Spider bite(s), eyelid necrosis due to, 313
Spindle (epithelioid) nevus, of eyelid, 338
Spiradenoma, eccrine, of eyelid, 333–334
Spiral of Tillaux, *847*, 847–848
Spirochetal infection(s), of eyelid, 314
Split-level full-thickness graft, used in upper eyelid reconstruction, technique of, 384, *384*
Sporotrichosis, of eyelid, 150, *150*, 319
Squamous cell carcinoma, of conjunctiva, 231–232, *232–233*
recurrence rates for, 232
treatment of, 232, *233*
of eyelid, 300, 349–350
clinical presentation of, 349, *349*
histologic features of, 349–350, *350*
in Asian patients, 721, *722*
low-grade, 325
management of, 350
metastatic potential of, 350
orbital invasion by, 300–301, *302*
radiotherapy as etiologic factor in, 349
variation of, 350
of lacrimal sac, 305, *305*
Squamous papilloma, of conjunctiva, 68, *69*, 251, *252*
treatment of, 251–252
of orbit, 68
Stainless steel screw, Nelson's, in fixation/reconstruction of canthal tendon, 389, *390*
Stainless steel wire suture, 284
"Startle reaction," following sedation, 298
Stenosis. See under anatomy, e.g., *Canaliculus(i), stenosis of.*
Steroids, topical, after chemical injury, 225
Stevens-Johnson syndrome, *34*, 34–35, 100
and ocular pemphigoid, 203
definition of, 35
differential diagnosis of, 36
treatment of, 37
vs. cicatricial pemphigoid, 198
vs. toxic epidermal necrolysis, 35
Stocker's line, in corneal epithelium, 208
Strabismus, after dermolipoma excision, treatment of, 256
vertical, pseudoptosis associated with, *88*, 89
Strawberry nevus. See also *Hemangioma, capillary.*
of eyelid, 330, *330*
Streptococcal myonecrosis, of eyelid, 312
Strobe lighting, for photography, 555
Stroma, conjunctival, 160
Strontium 90, as source of beta radiation, 217
ST-T segment, changes in, evaluation of, prior to oculoplastic surgery, 295
Stye (hordeolum), 307, *309*
Subacute cutaneous lupus erythematosus (SCLE), 3. See also *Lupus erythematosus (LE).*
serologic marker for, 5–6
systemic manifestations of, 5
Subcutaneous suture(s), buried, 286, *287*
Suborbital region, anatomy of, 484–485, *485–487*
augmentation of, 484–503
implants in, 484, 488, 490–498
complications associated with, 501–503
custom, 490–491, *491*, 495–498, *496–499*
Flower tear trough, 488, *489*, 492–493, *492–495*, 495
Goldberg lateral, 488, *489*
malposition of, 503

Suborbital region *(Continued)*
prefabricated, 488, *489–491,* 490
vertical eyelid and, 498–499, *499–502,* 501
deficiency of, inadequate projection in, 487–488
prominent globe in, 486–487, *488–489*
tear trough deformity in, *486,* 487, *489*
Substantia propria, of conjunctiva, 160, *160,* 178
Sulbactam, for sinus infections, 939
Sulcus, deformity of, 1111–1113, *1112–1115*
Summerskill's sign, *76*
Sunscreen(s), use of, 561–562
Supranuclear lesion(s), eyelid retraction caused by, 72–73, *73*
ptosis caused by, 75–77, *76–77*
Supraorbital artery, anatomy of, 843
Supratarsal fixation technique, of eyelid crease creation, 708, *708*
Surgery, role of aesthetician before and after, 576–577
Surgicel, for hemostasis in wound repair, 283
Suture(s), buried mattress, 710–711, *710–711*
combined with small incisions, 712, *713*
continuous, 711–712, *712*
cranial, premature closure of, 1178–1182, *1179–1185*
Frost-type, in eyelid surgery, 439, *440*
horizontal mattress, 288, *288*
half-buried, 288, *289*
in fixation/reconstruction of canthal tendon, 388–389, *390*
interrupted, deep, 286, *287*
simple, 286, *286*
running percutaneous, 286, *286*
running subcuticular, 288, *288*
subcutaneous, buried, 286, *287*
used in blepharoplasty, 709–713, *710–713*
used in brow ptosis, 580, *580*
vertical mattress, 288, *289*
Suture material, absorbable, 284, 284t
nonabsorbable, 284
Suture needle(s), 284–285, *285*
Suture tracts, after blepharoplasty, 649
Sweat gland(s), apocrine, 273, *273,* 324
benign adnexal lesions originating in, 334–335, *334–335*
eccrine, *273,* 323–324
benign adnexal lesions originating in, 333–334, *333–334*
Symblepharon, conjunctival, treatment of, 226
Sympathetic innervation, to orbit, 846
Sympathetic lesion(s), ptosis caused by, 77–79, *78–79*
Synkinesis, facial, diagnostic features of, 505t
physiologic, 74, *74*
Synostosis(es), lambdoidal, 1182
multiple suture, 1182, *1185*
sagittal, 1178–1179, *1179–1180*
unilateral coronal, 1179–1180, *1181*
anterior cranial base approach to, 1193, *1194–1195*
Synthes mini- and microplating kit, *292*
Syphilis, 153
involving eyelids, 314
Syringocystadenoma papilliferum, of eyelid, 335
Syringoma, of eyelid, 333, *333*
chondroid, 334, *334*
Systemic and metabolic disease(s), 12–29. See also specific disease for detail.
Systemic and metabolic disease(s) *(Continued)*
acanthosis nigricans as, *23,* 23t, 23–24
amyloidosis as, *17,* 17–19, 18t
congenital erythropoietic porphyria as, 29
Darier's disease as, 21
erythropoietic protoporphyria as, 29
hyperthyroidism as, *12,* 12–14, 13t
ligneous conjunctivitis as, 20
lipoid proteinosis as, 20–21
Melkersson-Rosenthal syndrome as, 15–16
multiple mucosal neuroma syndrome as, 21–23, 22t
myxedema as, 14, *14*
necrobiotic xanthogranuloma as, 19–20
neurofibromatosis as, *24,* 24t, 24–26, 26t
porphyria cutanea tarda as, 27–28
sarcoidosis as, *16,* 16–17, 17t
scleredema as, 15
scleromyxedema as, *14,* 14–15
tuberous sclerosis as, 26–27, 27t
variegate porphyria as, 28
Systemic lupus erythematosus (SLE), 3. See also *Lupus erythematosus (LE).*
diagnosis of, 6
ocular complications of, 4–5, 5t
revised criteria for, 4t
treatment of, 6–7

T cell(s), 94–95
T_3 (triiodothyronine), in thyrotoxicosis, 124
T_4 (thyroxine), in thyrotoxicosis, 124
Taenia solium, 151
Taillefer valve, 742, *743*
Taiwanese, epicanthal folds in, prevalence of, 705t
exophthalmometry in, 698, 698t
Takayasu's arteritis, 112
Tamoxifen, for metastatic breast carcinoma, *1009,* 1009–1010
Tamponade, pressure, for hemostasis in wound repair, 282
Taoist view, of medicine, 692–693, *692–693*
Tarsal arterial arcades, *275*
Tarsal flap, rotational, in upper eyelid reconstruction, 375–378, *379–380*
sliding, in upper eyelid reconstruction, 381–382, *382*
Tarsal strip procedure, lateral, for involutional ectropion, 427, 429, *429–430*
Tarsal substitutes, used in upper eyelid reconstruction, 363
Tarsoconjunctival flap, in upper eyelid reconstruction, 378–380, *381*
sliding, in medial canthal reconstruction, 391, *394*
in upper eyelid reconstruction, 380, 382, *382*
Tarsoconjunctival graft(s), free, 175, *175–176*
Tarsoconjunctival polishing, with mucous membrane grafting, for cicatricial entropion and trichiasis, 203–205, *204–206*
Tarsorrhaphy, for paralytic ectropion, 430–432, *431–432*
Tarsus, and submuscular fat pad, in Chinese adults, 699, 700t
used in upper eyelid reconstruction, autogenous, 363–364
irradiated, 365
Tattoo machine, 676, *678*
Tattoo pigments, used in electropigmentation, 677, 681
Tattooing, medical. See *Micropigmentation.*
Tear(s), "alligator" or "crocodile," 735
artificial, in management of pterygia, 211
drainage of, 762
Tear break-up time, 759
Tear film, abnormalities in, pterygia due to, 209
precorneal, *736–737,* 736–738
aqueous layer of, 736
eyelids and, 738
mucin layer of, 737
oil layer of, 737–738
quantity and quality of, after chemical injury, 226
Tear frame, reevaluation of, after chemical injury, 226
Tear production, altered, lacrimal surgery for, 201
Tear trough, 484, *485*
deformity of, *486,* 487, *489*
Tear trough implant, Flower, 488, *489,* 492–493, *492–495,* 495
Tearing, anatomic location responsible for, 749–750
cause(s) of, 750–751
eyelid, cicatricial ectropion as, 765, 767–768, *767–769*
cicatricial entropion as, 771
epiblepharon as, 775, *775*
involutional ectropion as, 762–765, *763–764, 766–767*
involutional entropion as, 770–771, *772–773*
paralytic ectropion as, 768–770, *769*
spastic entropion as, 771, *773*
trichiasis as, 771, *774,* 774–775
evaluation of, 748–760
from blocked outflow. See *Epiphora.*
history of, 748–752, *749*
physical examination of patient with, 752–760, *753*
computed tomography in, 760
dacryocystography in, 759, *759–760*
dye disappearance test in, 753–754, *754*
endoscopy in, 760
Jones I test in, 754–755
Jones II test in, 755
lacrimal scintillography in, 759–760
nasal evaluation in, 755, 757–758, *758*
probing in, 755, *756–757*
rose bengal testing in, 759
Schirmer testing in, 758–759
tear break-up time in, 759
ultrasonography in, 760
reflex, 750
Teflon-coated Dacron suture, 284
Telangiectasia, treatment of, 569, *569*
Temporal arteritis, 112
Temporal nerve, anatomy of, 277, *277*
Temporalis muscle transfer, for paralytic ectropion, 434, 436–437, *436–437*
in surgical management of facial paralysis, 479–480, *480*
TEN. See *Toxic epidermal necrolysis (Lyell's syndrome).*
Tendon(s). See also named tendon, e.g., *Canthal tendon.*
creation of, in fixation/reconstruction of canthal tendon, 388, *389*
Tensilon test, for myasthenia gravis, *80,* 81–82

Tenzel flap, in lower eyelid reconstruction, 400–402, *401–402*
in medial canthal reconstruction, 391, *393*
Tetanus, 83
cranial nerve paresis in, 152
Tetracycline, for hordeolum, 308
for rosacea, 39
for trachoma, 155
Therapeutic agent(s), pharmacology of, 97–98
Thermal cautery, for hemostasis in wound repair, 282–283
Thermal injury, 222. See also *Chemical injury(ies).*
Thermolysis method, of epilation, 591
Thiopental, as anesthetic agent, 297
Thiotepa, as adjunct to surgery for pterygia, 218
Thiourea drug(s), for thyroid storm, 130
for thyrotoxicosis, 125
Three-wall orbital decompression, for Graves' disease. See also *Graves' disease, orbital decompression for.*
transorbital approach to, 976–980, *976–980*
Thrombin, for hemostasis in wound repair, 283
Thrombophlebitis, orbital, 966
Thrombosis, cavernous sinus, diagnostic and therapeutic features of, 941t–942t
Thyroid carcinoma, metastatic, to rectus muscle, *55*
Thyroid drugs, chronic patient use of, anesthetic considerations with, 296
Thyroid dysfunction, ocular manifestations of, 13
Thyroid orbitopathy, CT scan of, 891, *892*
Thyroid storm, management of, 129–130
Thyroid-associated ophthalmopathy, 121–122
clinical features of, 122
management of, 122
Thyroidectomy, subtotal, for thyrotoxicosis, 128–129
Thyroid-stimulating hormone (TSH), in thyrotoxicosis, 124
Thyrotoxicosis, 121–130
"apathetic," 124
biochemical diagnosis of, 124–125
causes of, 125t
clinical manifestations of, 123–124
during pregnancy, management of, 129–130
etiology of, characteristic test results in, 126t–127t
determination of, 125
management of, 125, 128–129
drug therapy in, 125, 128
radioactive iodine therapy in, 128
subtotal thyroidectomy in, 128–129
signs and symptoms associated with, 123t
thyroid storm and, management of, 129–130
vs. hyperthyroidism, 123
Thyroxine (T_4), in thyrotoxicosis, 124
Tic, facial, diagnostic features of, 505t
Ticarcillin, for sinus infections, 939
Tillaux, spiral of, *847,* 847–848
Time, principle of, in electrolysis, 590
Tissue, conjunctival, handling of, 161
Tissue flap(s). See *Flap(s).*
Tissue graft(s). See also *Graft(s).*
harvesting of, 1077–1083
Tolosa-Hunt syndrome, 882, 892, 965
Torre's syndrome, 337, *337*
Touton giant cell, 64
Toxic epidermal necrolysis (Lyell's syndrome), 34, 35, *35*
differential diagnosis of, 36–37, 106
drug-induced, 35, 36t
epidemiology of, 105
immunohistopathology of, 105–106
ocular manifestations of, 105
pathogenesis of, 106
systemic manifestations of, 105
treatment of, 37, 106
vs. Stevens-Johnson syndrome, 35
Toxin(s), neuromuscular, ptosis caused by, 83–84, *84*
Toxocariasis, ocular, imaging of, 908–909
Trachoma, bacteriology of, 154
clinical presentation of, 155, *155*
diagnosis of, 155
epidemiology of, 154
eyelid retraction caused by, 315
MacCallan classification of, 314–315
pathogenesis of, 154–155
staging system for, 154t
treatment of, 155
Transnasal wiring, with dacryocystorhinostomy, in fixation/reconstruction of canthal tendon, 388, *389*
Transplantation, corneal, after chemical injury, 228, *228*
fat, autologous, for wrinkles, 565
in conjunctival mucous membrane replacement, 172
Transpositional skin flap, in upper eyelid reconstruction, 371, *372*
Trauma. See also specific anatomic site, e.g., *Eyelid trauma.*
causing nasolacrimal duct obstruction, 809–811, 810t, *810–812*
chemical, 222–230. See also *Chemical injury(ies).*
facial nerve, 473–474
orbital, surgical approach to, 1054
Trepier flap, in lower eyelid reconstruction, 403, *403–404*
Treponema carateum, pinta caused by, 314
Treponema pallidum, syphilis caused by, 314
Treponema pertenue, yaws caused by, 314
Tretinoin, for wrinkles, *562,* 562–563
used in chemical peels, 665–666
Triamcinolone, for capillary hemangioma, 919
Trichiasis, as cause of tearing, 771, *774, 774–775*
cicatricial, buccal mucous membrane grafting for, 203–206
anesthesia in, 203
complications of, 205
results of, 205, *206*
surgical methods of, 203–205, *204–206*
correction of, 201
infection causing, 308t
Trichilemmoma, of eyelid, 336
Trichinella spiralis, causing periorbital edema, 151
Trichloroacetic acid, used in chemical peels, 667, *667–668*
Trichoepithelioma, of eyelid, *335,* 335–336
Trichofolliculoma, of eyelid, 336
Trichothiodystrophy (brittle hair), in ichthyosis, 46
Trigeminal nerve, anatomy of, 277–278, *278, 845,* 845–846
function of, assessment of, in orbital disease, *879,* 879–880
Trigonocephaly, 1181–1182, *1184*
Trihexyphenidyl, for essential blepharospasm and Meige's syndrome, 507
Triiodothyronine (T_3), in thyrotoxicosis, 124
Trochlea, *848,* 848–849
Trochlear nerve, anatomy of, 845
Trypanosoma cruzi, 152
Chagas' disease caused by, 316
TSH (thyroid-stimulating hormone), in thyrotoxicosis, 124
Tuberculosis, 152–153
eyelid involvement due to, 313
Tuberous sclerosis, 26–27
diagnostic criteria for, 27t
ocular manifestations of, 27t
Tularemia, 149
involving eyelids, 313–314
Tumor(s). See also specific tumor.
causing nasolacrimal duct obstruction, 804, 805t, *805–810,* 806–807
conjunctival. See *Conjunctival neoplasm(s).*
eyelid, benign, 323–340
malignant, 300–306, 342–350
facial nerve, 474
lacrimal gland, 999–1006
orbital. See *Orbital tumor(s).*
pediatric, anterior cranial base approach to, 1199, 1202–1204, *1203–1206*
prognosis of, markers in, 53
Tungsten light, for photography, 555
Tungsten-balanced film, photographic, 554
Turban tumor (cylindroma), of eyelid, 334–335, *335*

Ulcer(s), corneal, prevention of, after chemical injury, 225, 229
eyelid, causes of, 308t
Ulerythema ophryogenes, 43–44
Ultrapulse carbon dioxide laser, used in blepharoplasty, *544*
Ultrasonography, diagnostic, for tearing, 760
of mucoceles, in paranasal sinuses, 1015–1016, *1016*
of neurogenic tumors of orbit, 984
Ultraviolet light, harmful effects of, prevention of, 561–562
Ultraviolet radiation, exposure to, pterygia due to, 209
Unilateral coronal synostosis, 1179–1180, *1181*
anterior cranial base approach to, 1193, *1194–1195*
Urbach-Wiethe disease, 20–21
differential diagnosis of, 21
Urticaria, 40
Urticaria pigmentosa, 43
Uvea, malignant melanoma of, anterior cranial base approach to, 1202–1204, *1204–1205*
metastatic disease of, *911,* 911–912
Uveoparotid fever (Heerfordt's syndrome), 16, 901

Varicella zoster. See *Herpes zoster infection.*
Variegate porphyria, 28–29
Varix (varices), of eyelid, 330–331
of orbit, CT scan of, 896, *897*
Vascular tissue, benign eyelid tumors derived from, *329–331,* 329–332
Vascular tumors, of orbit, 913–932. See also specific tumor, e.g., *Hemangioma.*